KT-549-115

0807586

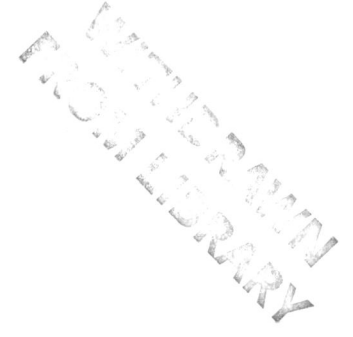

BRITISH MEDICAL ASSOCIATION

Nathan and Oski's Hematology and Oncology of Infancy and Childhood

NATHAN AND OSKI'S HEMATOLOGY AND ONCOLOGY OF INFANCY AND CHILDHOOD

Stuart H. Orkin, MD
David G. Nathan Professor of Pediatrics
Harvard Medical School
Chair, Department of Pediatric Oncology
Dana-Farber Cancer Institute
Boston Children's Hospital
Investigator, Howard Hughes Medical Institute
Boston, Massachusetts

David E. Fisher, MD, PhD
Chief, Department of Dermatology
Director, Cutaneous Biology Research Center
Massachusetts General Hospital
Director, Melanoma Program
Massachusetts General Hospital Cancer Center
Boston, Massachusetts

David Ginsburg, MD
James V. Neel Distinguished University Professor
Departments of Internal Medicine, Pediatrics and Communicable Diseases, and Human Genetics
Investigator, Howard Hughes Medical Institute
University of Michigan Medical School
Ann Arbor, Michigan

A. Thomas Look, MD
Professor of Pediatrics
Harvard Medical School
Vice Chair for Research
Department of Pediatric Oncology
Dana-Farber Cancer Institute
Boston Children's Hospital
Boston, Massachusetts

Samuel E. Lux, MD
Robert A. Stranahan Professor of Pediatrics
Harvard Medical School
Chief Emeritus, Hematology/Oncology
Boston Children's Hospital
Boston, Massachusetts

David G. Nathan, MD
President Emeritus
Dana-Farber Cancer Institute
Physician-in-Chief Emeritus
Boston Children's Hospital
Stranahan Distinguished Professor of Pediatrics and Professor of Medicine
Harvard Medical School
Boston, Massachusetts

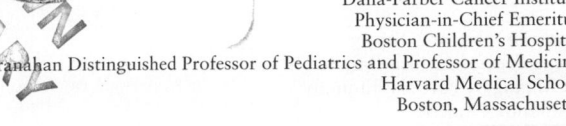

ELSEVIER
SAUNDERS

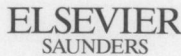

ELSEVIER
SAUNDERS

1600 John F. Kennedy Blvd.
Ste 1800
Philadelphia, PA 19103-2899

NATHAN AND OSKI'S HEMATOLOGY AND ONCOLOGY OF   ISBN: 978-1-4557-5414-4
INFANCY AND CHILDHOOD, ED 8
Copyright © 2015, 2009, 2003, 1998, 1993, 1987, 1981, 1974 by Saunders, an imprint of Elsevier Inc.

No part of this publication may be reproduced or transmitted in any form or by any means, electronic or mechanical, including photocopying, recording, or any information storage and retrieval system, without permission in writing from the publisher. Details on how to seek permission, further information about the Publisher's permissions policies and our arrangements with organizations such as the Copyright Clearance Center and the Copyright Licensing Agency, can be found at our website: www.elsevier.com/permissions.

This book and the individual contributions contained in it are protected under copyright by the Publisher (other than as may be noted herein).

Notices

Knowledge and best practice in this field are constantly changing. As new research and experience broaden our understanding, changes in research methods, professional practices, or medical treatment may become necessary.

Practitioners and researchers must always rely on their own experience and knowledge in evaluating and using any information, methods, compounds, or experiments described herein. In using such information or methods they should be mindful of their own safety and the safety of others, including parties for whom they have a professional responsibility.

With respect to any drug or pharmaceutical products identified, readers are advised to check the most current information provided (i) on procedures featured or (ii) by the manufacturer of each product to be administered, to verify the recommended dose or formula, the method and duration of administration, and contraindications. It is the responsibility of practitioners, relying on their own experience and knowledge of their patients, to make diagnoses, to determine dosages and the best treatment for each individual patient, and to take all appropriate safety precautions.

To the fullest extent of the law, neither the Publisher nor the authors, contributors, or editors, assume any liability for any injury and/or damage to persons or property as a matter of products liability, negligence or otherwise, or from any use or operation of any methods, products, instructions, or ideas contained in the material herein.

Library of Congress Cataloging-in-Publication Data

Nathan and Oski's hematology and oncology of infancy and childhood / [edited by] Stuart H. Orkin, David E. Fisher, A. Thomas Look, Samuel E. Lux, IV, David Ginsburg, David G. Nathan.—Eighth edition.
    p. ; cm.
    Hematology and oncology of infancy and childhood
    Preceded by: Nathan and Oski's hematology of infancy and childhood / edited by Stuart H. Orkin ... [et al.]. 7th ed. c2009; and, Oncology of infancy and childhood / [edited by] Stuart H. Orkin ... [et al.]. 1st ed. c2009.
    Includes bibliographical references and index.
    ISBN 978-1-4557-5414-4 (hardcover : alk. paper)
    I. Orkin, Stuart H., editor.   II. Title: Hematology and oncology of infancy and childhood.
    [DNLM: 1. Hematologic Diseases. 2. Neoplasms. 3. Child. 4. Infant. WS 300]
    RC281.C4
    618.92′994—dc23
                                                                    2014033436

Senior Content Strategist: Suzanne Toppy
Content Development Specialist: Lisa Barnes
Publishing Services Manager: Patricia Tannian
Project Manager: Amanda Mincher
Art and Design: Amy Buxton

Printed in Canada

Last digit is the print number: 9 8 7 6 5 4 3 2 1

Working together
to grow libraries in
developing countries

www.elsevier.com • www.bookaid.org

Sarah Alexander, MD
Assistant Professor, University of Toronto, Clinical Director of Hematology/Oncology, Hospital for Sick Children, Toronto, Canada
Pediatric Lymphoma

James Amatruda, MD, PhD
Associate Professor of Pediatrics, Molecular Biology and Internal Medicine, UT Southwestern Medical Center, Dallas, Texas
Pediatric Germ Cell Tumors

Megan E. Anderson, MD
Attending, Department of Orthopedic Surgery, Children's Hospital Boston; Attending, Department of Orthopedic Surgery, Beth Israel Deaconess Medical Center; Instructor, Department of Orthopedic Surgery, Harvard Medical School, Boston, Massachusetts
Pediatric Surgical Oncology

Pedram Argani, MD
Director of Immunohistochemistry Laboratory, Johns Hopkins Hospital, Baltimore, Maryland
Pediatric Renal Tumors

Scott A. Armstrong, MD, PhD
Leukemia Center, Human Oncology and Pathogenesis Program and Department of Pediatrics, Memorial Sloan Kettering Cancer Center, New York, New York
Infant Leukemias

Pratiti Bandopadhayay, MD, PhD
Pediatric Medical Neuro-Oncology, Department of Pediatric Oncology, Dana-Farber/Boston Children's Cancer and Blood Disorders Center, Boston, Massachusetts
Tumors of the Brain and Spinal Cord

Raymond Barfield, MD, PhD
Associate Professor of Pediatrics and Christian Philosophy, Director, Pediatric Quality of Life and Palliative Care Program, Director, Theology, Medicine, and Culture, Duke University, Durham, North Carolina
Ethical Considerations in Pediatric Oncology Clinical Trials

Frederic G. Barr, MD, PhD
Senior Investigator and Deputy Chief, Laboratory of Pathology, National Cancer Institute, Bethesda, Maryland
Rhabdomyosarcoma

Kenneth A. Bauer, MD
Professor of Medicine, Harvard Medical School; Chief, Hematology Section, Medical Service, VA Boston Healthcare System, Jamaica Plain, Massachusetts; Director, Thrombosis Clinical Research, Department of Medicine, Beth Israel Deaconess Medical Center, Boston, Massachusetts
Rare Hereditary Coagulation Factor Abnormalities
Inherited Disorders of Thrombosis and Fibrinolysis

Susanne H.C. Baumeister, MD
Instructor of Pediatrics, Harvard Medical School; Attending Physician, Pediatric Hematology and Oncology, Dana-Farber Cancer Institute, Boston Children's Hospital, Boston, Massachusetts
Immunotherapy of Cancer

Charles B. Berde, MD, PhD
Chief, Division of Pain Medicine, Department of Anesthesiology, Perioperative and Pain Medicine, Boston Children's Hospital; Professor of Anesthesia and Pediatrics, Harvard Medical School, Boston, Massachusetts
Symptom Management in Children with Cancer

Guillaume Bergthold, MD, PhD
Service de Pédiatrie III, Pédiatrie Onco-Hématologie, Progression Tumorale et Microenvironnement, Approches Translationnelles et Épidémiologie, Université de Strasbourg, Strasbourg, France
Tumors of the Brain and Spinal Cord

Jason N. Berman, MD
Associate Professor, Pediatrics, Microbiology and Immunology, and Pathology, Dalhousie University, IWK Health Centre, Halifax, Nova Scotia, Canada
Pediatric Myeloid Leukemia, Myelodysplasia, and Myeloproliferative Disease

Monica Bessler, MD, PhD
Professor of Pediatrics, The Children's Hospital of Philadelphia; Professor, Department of Medicine, University of Pennsylvania School of Medicine, Philadelphia, Pennsylvania
Inherited Bone Marrow Failure Syndromes

Smita Bhatia, MD, MPH
Chair, Population Sciences, City of Hope Medical Center, Duarte, California
Epidemiology of Leukemia in Childhood

Amy Louise Billett, MD
Director of Safety and Quality, Dana-Farber/Boston
  Children's Cancer and Blood Disorders Center;
  Associate Professor of Pediatrics, Harvard Medical
  School, Boston, Massachusetts
Symptom Management in Children with Cancer

Deborah Billmire, MD
Professor of Surgery, Indiana University School of
  Medicine, Indianapolis, Indiana
Pediatric Germ Cell Tumors

Michael Bishop, MD, MS
Staff Physician, Department of Oncology, St. Jude
  Children's Research Hospital, Memphis, Tennessee
Rare Tumors of Childhood

Francisco A. Bonilla, MD, PhD
Director, Clinical Immunology Program, Division of
  Immunology, Boston Children's Hospital; Associate
  Professor of Pediatrics, Harvard Medical School,
  Boston, Massachusetts
Primary Immunodeficiency Diseases

Niels Borregaard, MD, DMedSci
Professor of Hematology, National University Hospital;
  Professor of Hematology, Faculty of Health Sciences,
  University of Copenhagen, Copenhagen, Denmark
Phagocyte System and Disorders of Granulopoiesis and
Granulocyte Function

Brian Branchford, MD
Instructor of Pediatrics, Hematology/Oncology/Bone
  Marrow Transplant, University of Colorado School
  of Medicine, Children's Hospital Colorado, Aurora,
  Colorado
Approach to the Child with a Suspected Bleeding Disorder

†Patricia A. Branowicki, MS, RN, NEA-BC, FAAN
Associate Chief Nurse, Medicine Patient Services,
  Boston Children's Hospital; Associate Chief Nurse,
  Pediatric Oncology, Dana-Farber Cancer Institute,
  Boston Children's Hospital, Boston, Massachusetts
Nursing Care of Patients with Childhood Cancer

Carlo Brugnara, MD
Professor of Pathology, Harvard Medical School;
  Director of the Hematology Laboratory, Department
  of Laboratory Medicine, Boston Children's Hospital,
  Boston, Massachusetts
Diagnostic Approach to the Anemic Patient
Appendices: Reference Values in Infancy and Childhood

Kathleen Brummel-Ziedins, PhD
Associate Professor of Biochemistry, University of
  Vermont, Burlington, Vermont
Blood Coagulation

T. Andrew Burrow, MD
Assistant Professor of Clinical Pediatrics, University of
  Cincinnati Department of Pediatrics, Cincinnati
  Children's Hospital, Cincinnati, Ohio
Lysosomal Storage Diseases

Alan B. Cantor, MD, PhD
Assistant Professor of Pediatrics, Division of Pediatric
  Hematology and Oncology, Dana-Farber Cancer
  Institute, Boston Children's Hospital, Harvard
  Medical School, Boston, Massachusetts
Hemostasis in the Newborn and Infant

Ralph Carmel, MD
Department Medicine, New York University Medical
  Center, New York, New York
Megaloblastic Anemia

Susan N. Chi, MD
Clinical Director, Pediatric Neuro-Oncology,
  Department of Pediatric Oncology, Dana-Farber/
  Boston Children's Cancer and Blood Disorders
  Center, Boston, Massachusetts
Tumors of the Brain and Spinal Cord

Stella T. Chou, MD
Assistant Professor of Pediatrics, Division of
  Hematology, The Children's Hospital of Philadelphia,
  Philadelphia, Pennsylvania
Autoimmune Hemolytic Anemia

Susanne B. Conley, MSN, RN, CPON
Clinical Nurse Specialist, Dana-Farber Cancer Institute,
  Boston Children's Hospital, Boston, Massachusetts
Nursing Care of Patients with Childhood Cancer

George Q. Daley, MD, PhD
Samuel E. Lux, IV, MD, Professor of Hematology and
  Oncology, Boston Children's Hospital; Director, Stem
  Cell Transplantation Program, Dana-Farber Cancer
  Institute, Boston Children's Hospital, Boston,
  Massachusettes
Anatomy and Physiology of Hematopoiesis

Ian J. Davis, MD, PhD
Associate Professor of Pediatrics and Genetics, Member,
  Lineberger Comprehensive Cancer Center, University
  of North Carolina at Chapel Hill, Chapel Hill, North
  Carolina
Nonrhabdomyosarcoma Soft Tissue Sarcomas and Other Soft
Tissue Tumors

Barbara A. Degar, MD
Senior Physician of Pediatric Oncology, Dana-Farber
  Cancer Institute, Boston Children's Hospital;
  Assistant Professor, Department of Pediatrics,
  Harvard Medical School, Boston, Massachusetts
Histiocytoses

†Deceased.

Claire F. Dickson
Menzies Research Institute Tasmania, University of Tasmania, Hobart, Tasmania, Australia
Normal and Abnormal Hemoglobins

Lisa Diller, MD
Professor of Pediatrics, Harvard Medical School; Chief Medical Officer, Dana-Farber/Boston Children's Cancer and Blood Disorders Center, Boston, Massachusetts
Childhood Cancer Survivorship

Mary C. Dinauer, MD, PhD
Fred M. Saigh Distinguished Chair of Pediatric Research, Department of Pediatrics, Department of Pathology and Immunology, Washington University School of Medicine, St. Louis, Missouri
Phagocyte System and Disorders of Granulopoiesis and Granulocyte Function

Barthelemy Diouf, PhD, PharmD
Staff Scientist of Pharmaceutical Sciences, St. Jude Children's Research Hospital, Memphis, Tennessee
Cancer Chemotherapy for Pediatric Patients

Jorge Di Paola, MD
Associate Professor of Pediatrics and Human Genetics, Hematology/Oncology/Bone Marrow Transplant, University of Colorado School of Medicine, Children's Hospital Colorado, Aurora, Colorado
Approach to the Child with a Suspected Bleeding Disorder
Hemophilia and von Willebrand Disease

Jeffrey S. Dome, MD, PhD
Chief of Hematology and Oncology, Children's National Medical Center, Washington, District of Columbia
Pediatric Renal Tumors

Elissa Downs, MD, MPH
Pediatric Gastroenterology Fellow, Department of Pediatric Gastroenterology, Hepatology, and Nutrition, University of Minnesota, Minneapolis, Minnesota
Neonatal Jaundice and Disorders of Bilirubin Metabolism

Glenn Dranoff, MD
Professor of Medicine, Department of Medical Oncology, Dana-Farber Cancer Institute, Boston Children's Hospital, and Harvard Medical School, Boston, Massachusetts
Immunotherapy of Cancer

Steven G. DuBois, MD, MS
Associate Professor, Department of Pediatrics, University of California, San Francisco School of Medicine; Attending Physician, Department of Pediatrics, University of California, San Francisco, Benioff Children's Hospital, San Francisco, California
Ewing Sarcoma

Christine N. Duncan, MD, MSc
Assistant Professor of Pediatric Hematology and Oncology, Dana-Farber Cancer Institute, Boston Children's Hospital, Boston, Massachusetts
Principles of Bone Marrow and Stem Cell Transplantation

Janet Duncan, PNP
Program Founder and Director of Comfort Care Research and Program Development, Mattel Children's Hospital; Adjunct Assistant Professor of Pediatrics, University of California Los Angeles, Los Angeles, California
Palliative Care in Pediatric Oncology

Michael Dyer, MD
Investigator, HHMI, Member, Department of Developmental Neurobiology, Head, Division of Developmental Biology, St. Jude Children's Research Hospital, Memphis, Tennessee
Retinoblastoma

Alaa El-Haddad, MD
Professor of Pediatric Hematology/Oncology, Dean, National Cancer Institute, Cairo University; Director of Pediatric Bone Marrow Transplant, Children's Cancer Hospital, Cairo, Egypt
Principles of Bone Marrow and Stem Cell Transplantation

Elana Evan, PhD
Program Founder and Director of Comfort Care Research and Program Development, Mattel Children's Hospital; Adjunct Assistant Professor of Pediatrics, University of California Los Angeles, Los Angeles, California
Palliative Care in Pediatric Oncology

William E. Evans, PharmD
Director and CEO of St. Jude Children's Research Hospital; Professor of Pediatrics and Clinical Pharmacy, University of Tennessee, Colleges of Medicine and Pharmacy; Member (Professor) of Pharmaceutical Sciences, St. Jude Children's Research Hospital, Memphis, Tennessee
Cancer Chemotherapy for Pediatric Patients

Carolyn A. Felix, MD
Professor of Pediatrics, University of Pennsylvania School of Medicine; Attending Physician, Division of Oncology, Joshua Kahan Endowed Chair in Pediatric Leukemia Research, The Children's Hospital of Philadelphia, Philadelphia, Pennsylvania
Cytogenetic and Molecular Pathology of Pediatric Cancer

Adolfo A. Ferrando, MD, PhD
Associate Professor of Pediatrics, Associate Professor of Pathology and Cell Biology, Associate Profrressor, Institute for Cancer Genetics, Columbia University Medical Center, New York, New York
Pediatric Lymphoma

Brian T. Fisher, DO, MPH, MSCE
Assistant Professor of Pediatrics, Division of Infectious
  Diseases, Perelman School of Medicine at the
  University of Pennsylvania, Philadelphia,
  Pennsylvania
Infectious Disease in the Pediatric Cancer Patient

David E. Fisher, MD, PhD
Chief, Department of Dermatology, Director, Cutaneous
  Biology Research Center, Massachusetts General
  Hospital; Director, Melanoma Program,
  Massachusetts General Hospital Cancer Center,
  Boston, Massachusetts
Nonrhabdomyosarcoma Soft Tissue Sarcomas and Other Soft
Tissue Tumors

Mark D. Fleming, MD
S. Burt Wolbach Professor and Chairman, Department
  of Pathology, Boston Children's Hospital, Boston,
  Massachusetts
Disorders of Iron and Copper Metabolism, the Sideroblastic
Anemias, and Lead Toxicity
Histiocytoses

Jonathan A. Fletcher, MD
Pathologist, Brigham and Women's Hospital; Associate
  Professor of Pathology and Pediatrics, Harvard
  Medical School, Boston, Massachusetts
Cytogenetic and Molecular Pathology of Pediatric Cancer

Veronica Flood, MD
Associate Professor of Pediatric Hematology and
  Oncology, Medical College of Wisconsin, Milwaukee,
  Wisconsin
Hemophilia and von Willebrand Disease

A. Lindsay Frazier, MD, ScM
Institute Physician of Pediatric Hematology and
  Oncology, Dana-Farber Cancer Institute, Boston
  Children's Hospital; Associate Professor of Pediatrics,
  Harvard Medical School; Associate Professor of
  Epidemiology, Harvard School of Public Health,
  Boston, Massachusetts
Pediatric Germ Cell Tumors

Patrick G. Gallagher, MD
Professor of Pediatrics, Pathology, and Genetics, Yale
  University School of Medicine, New Haven,
  Connecticuit
The Neonatal Erythrocyte and Its Disorders

Glenn Gardener, MB, BS
Director, Center for Maternal Fetal Medicine, Mater
  Mothers' Hospital, Brisbane, Australia
Immune Hemolytic Disease

Mark C. Gebhardt, MD
Surgeon-in-Chief, Department of Orthopaedic Surgery,
  Beth Israel Deaconess Medical Center; Orthopedic
  Surgeon, Department of Orthopedics, Children's
  Hospital; Frederick W. and Jane M. Ilfeld Professor
  of Orthopedic Surgery, Department of Orthopedic
  Surgery, Harvard Medical School, Boston,
  Massachusetts
Pediatric Surgical Oncology

David A. Gell, PhD
Menzies Research Institute Tasmania, University of
  Tasmania, Hobart, Tasmania, Australia
Normal and Abnormal Hemoglobins

Rani E. George, MD, PhD, MRCP
Associate Professor of Pediatrics, Harvard Medical
  School; Department of Pediatric Hematology and
  Oncology, Dana Farber Cancer Institute, Boston
  Children's Hospital, Boston, Massachusetts
Neuroblastoma

Joan Cox Gill, MD
Professor of Pediatrics and Medicine, Medical College
  of Wisconsin; Senior Investigator, Medical Sciences
  Institute, BloodCenter of Wisconsin, Milwaukee,
  Wisconsin
Hemophilia and von Willebrand Disease

John M. Goldberg, MD
Assistant Professor of Clinical Pediatrics, Director,
  Pediatric Oncology Early Phase Clinical Trials
  Program, UM Sylvester Comprehensive Cancer
  Center, Division of Pediatric Hematology and
  Oncology, Miami, Florida
Rare Tumors of Childhood

Neil Goldenberg, MD, PhD
Director of Research, Chief Research Officer, All
  Children's Hospital–Johns Hopkins Medicine, St.
  Petersburg, Florida
Acquired Disorders of Hemostasis

Liliana C. Goumnerova, MD, FRCSC, FAANS
Director for Pediatric Neurosurgical Oncology, Boston
  Children's Hospital/Dana Farber Cancer Institute;
  Associate Professor of Neurosurgery, Harvard
  Medical School, Boston, Massachusetts
Tumors of the Brain and Spinal Cord

Glenn R. Gourley, MD
Professor of Pediatrics, Research Director, Pediatric
  Gastroenterology, University of Minnesota,
  Minneapolis, Minnesota
Neonatal Jaundice and Disorders of Bilirubin Metabolism

Gregory A. Grabowski, MD
Human Genetics, Cincinnati Children's Research
  Foundation, Cincinnati, Ohio
Lysosomal Storage Diseases

Rachael F. Grace, MD, MMSc
Assistant Professor of Pediatrics, Harvard Medical School; Director, Hematology Clinic, Boston Children's Hospital, Dana-Farber Cancer Institute, Boston Children's Hospital, Boston, Massachusetts
Hematologic Manifestations of Systemic Diseases

Eric Gratias, MD, FAAP
Associate Professor of Pediatric Hematology and Oncology, Children's Hospital at Erlanger; Associate Professor of Pediatrics, University of Tennessee College of Medicine Chattanooga, Chattanooga, Tennessee
Oncologic Emergencies

Mel Greaves, PhD
Professor of Molecular Pathology, Institute of Cancer Research, London, United Kingdom
Origins and Evolution of Pediatric Cancers

Adam L. Green, MD
Instructor of Pediatrics, University of Colorado Denver; Attending Physician, Center for Cancer and Blood Disorders, Children's Hospital Colorado, Denver, Colorado
Tumors of the Brain and Spinal Cord

Holcombe E. Grier, MD
Professor, Department of Pediatrics, Harvard Medical School, Dana-Farber/Boston Children's Cancer and Blood Disorders Center, Boston, Massachusetts
Ewing Sarcoma

Alejandro Gutierrez, MD
Assistant Professor of Pediatrics, Division of Hematology and Oncology, Dana-Farber Cancer Institute, Boston Children's Hospital, and Harvard Medical School, Boston, Massachusetts
Acute Lymphoblastic Leukemia

W. Nicholas Haining, BM, BCh
Assistant Professor of Pediatrics, Department of Pediatric Oncology, Dana-Farber Cancer Institute, Boston Children's Hospital, and Harvard Medical School, Boston, Massachusetts
Principles of Bone Marrow and Stem Cell Transplantation

Katherine Amberson Hajjar, MD
Brine Family Professor and Chair, Cell and Developmental Biology, Professor of Pediatrics, Professor of Medicine, Weill Cornell Medical College, New York, New York
Molecular Basis of Fibrinolysis

Matthew M. Heeney, MD
Associate Chief of Hematology, Division of Hematology and Oncology, Boston Children's Hospital; Assistant Professor of Pediatrics, Harvard Medical School, Boston, Massachusetts
Sickle Cell Disease

Kathleen E. Houlahan, MSN, MHA, RN, NE-BC
Director, Nursing/Patient Care Services, Pediatric Oncology, Dana-Farber Cancer Institute, Boston Children's Hospital, Boston, Massachusetts
Nursing Care of Patients with Childhood Cancer

Hiroto Inaba, MD, PhD
Associate Member (Associate Professor) of Oncology, St. Jude Children's Research Hospital; Associate Professor of Pediatrics, University of Tennessee Health Science Center, Memphis, Tennessee
Cancer Chemotherapy for Pediatric Patients

Katherine Janeway, MD, MMSc
Assistant Professor of Pediatrics, Harvard Medical School; Senior Physician of Pediatric Oncology, Dana-Farber/Boston Children's Cancer and Blood Disorders Center, Boston, Massachusetts
Osteosarcoma

Lisa B. Kenney, MD, MPH
Assistant Professor of Pediatrics, Harvard Medical School; Senior Physician, Dana-Farber/Boston Children's Cancer and Blood Disorders Center, Boston, Massachusetts
Childhood Cancer Survivorship

Alex Kentsis, MD, PhD
Department of Pediatrics, Molecular Pharmacology and Chemistry Program, Memorial Sloan-Kettering Cancer Center, Sloan-Kettering Institute, New York, New York
Genetics and Epigenetics of Childhood Cancers

Mark W. Kieran, MD, PhD
Director of Pediatric Medical Neuro-Oncology, Department of Pediatric Oncology, Dana-Farber/Boston Children's Cancer and Blood Disorders Center, Boston, Massachusetts
Tumors of the Brain and Spinal Cord

Nancy E. Kline, PhD, RN, CPNP, FAAN
Director, Nursing Research, Department of Medicine Patient Services, Boston Children's Hospital, Boston, Massachusetts
Nursing Care of Patients with Childhood Cancer

Rachel Kobos, MD
Department of Pediatrics, Memorial Sloan Kettering Cancer Center, New York, New York
Infant Leukemias

Eric Kodish, MD
Director, Center for Ethics, Humanities, and Spiritual Care, FJ O'Neill Professor and Chair, Department of Bioethics, Cleveland Clinic, Cleveland, Ohio
Ethical Considerations in Pediatric Oncology Clinical Trials

Andrew Y. Koh, MD
Assistant Professor, Director of Pediatric Hematopoietic
Stem Cell Transplantation, Pediatrics, University of
Texas Southwestern Medical Center, Dallas, Texas
Infectious Disease in the Pediatric Cancer Patient

James P. Kushner, MD
M.M.Wintrobe Distinguished Professor of Medicine
Emeritus, Department of Internal Medicine, Division
of Hematology, University of Utah School of
Medicine, Salt Lake City, Utah
Porphyrias

Dominic P. Kwiatkowski, FRCP
Group Head/PI and Consultant Physician, Wellcome
Trust Center for Human Genetics, University of
Oxford, Oxford, United Kingdom
Hematologic Manifestations of Systemic Diseases in Children of
the Developing World

Michele P. Lambert, MD, MTR
Assistant Professor of Pediatrics, Perelman School of
Medicine, University of Pennsylvania; Attending
Physician, Division of Hematology, The Children's
Hospital of Philadelphia, Philadelphia, Pennsylvania
Inherited Platelet Disorders

Leslie E. Lehmann, MD
Assistant Professor of Pediatric Hematology and
Oncology, Dana-Farber/Boston Children's Cancer and
Blood Disorder Center, Boston, Massachusetts
Principles of Bone Marrow and Stem Cell Transplantation

Nancy D. Leslie, MD
Professor of Pediatrics, Division of Human Genetics,
Cincinnati Children's Hospital Medical Center,
Cincinnati, Ohio
Lysosomal Storage Diseases

Stephen L. Lessnick, MD, PhD
Director, Center for Children's Cancer Research, Jon
and Karen Huntsman Presidential Professor in
Cancer Research, Huntsman Cancer Institute;
Professor of Pediatrics, Division of Pediatric
Hematology and Oncology, University of Utah, Salt
Lake City, Utah
Ewing Sarcoma

Keith L. Ligon, MD, PhD
Department of Pathology, Dana-Farber Cancer Institute,
Boston Children's Hospital; Department of Pathology,
Division of Neuropathology, Brigham and Women's
Hospital, Boston, Massachusetts
Tumors of the Brain and Spinal Cord

Helen G. Liley, MB, ChB
Senior Staff Specialist, Newborn Services, Mater
Mothers' Hospital, South Brisbane, Queensland;
Associate Professor, Pediatrics and Child Health,
School of Medicine, The University of Queensland,
Brisbane, Queensland
Neonatal Immune Hemolytic Disease

Corinne M. Linardic, MD, PhD
Associate Professor of Pediatrics, Division of
Hematology and Oncology, Associate Professor of
Pharmacology and Cancer Biology, Duke University
School of Medicine, Durham, North Carolina
Rhabdomyosarcoma

Robert B. Lindell, MD
Division of General Pediatrics, Children's Hospital of
Philadelphia, Philadelphia, Pennsylvania
Genetic Predisposition to Cancer

Daniel C. Link, MD
Alan and Edith Wolff Professor, Department of
Medicine, Washington University, St. Louis, Missouri
Inherited Bone Marrow Failure Syndromes

Cori Liptak, PhD
Senior Psychologist, Director of Pediatric
Neurooncology Survivorship Behavioral Health
Programs, Dana-Farber/Boston Children's Center for
Cancer and Blood-Related Disorders; Instructor,
Department of Psychiatry, Harvard Medical School,
Boston, Massachusetts
Psychosocial Care of the Child and Family

A. Thomas Look, MD
Professor of Pediatrics, Harvard Medical School; Vice
Chair for Research, Department of Pediatric
Oncology, Dana-Farber Cancer Institute, Boston
Children's Hospital, Boston, Massachusetts
Pediatric Myeloid Leukemia, Myelodysplasia, and Myeloproliferative
Disease

Enrico Lopriore, MD, PhD
Pediatrician-Neonatologist, Leiden University Medical
Center, The Hague, Netherlands
Immune Hemolytic Disease

Samuel E. Lux, MD
Robert A. Stranahan Professor of Pediatrics, Harvard
Medical School; Chief Emeritus, Hematology/
Oncology, Boston Children's Hospital, Boston,
Massachusetts
Red Cell Membrane
Disorders of the Red Cell Membrane

Lucio Luzzatto, MD
Istituto Toscano Tumori and Department of
Haematology, University of Florence, Florence, Italy
Glucose-6-Phosphate Dehydrogenase Deficiency

Shannon M. MacDonald, MD
Radiation Oncology, Massachusetts General Hospital,
Harvard Medical School, Boston, Massachusetts
Pediatric Radiation Oncology

Jennifer W. Mack, MD, MPH
Assistant Professor of Pediatrics, Department of
Pediatric Hematology and Oncology, Dana-Farber
Cancer Institute, Boston Children's Hospital;
Assistant Professor of Pediatrics, Harvard Medical
School, Boston, Massachusetts
Palliative Care in Pediatric Oncology

Peter E. Manley, MD
Director, Pediatric Neuro-Oncology Outcomes Clinic,
Dana-Farber Boston Children's Cancer and Blood
Disorders Center; Instructor in Pediatrics, Harvard
Medical School, Boston, Massachusetts
Tumors of the Brain and Spinal Cord

Kenneth G. Mann, PhD
Professor Emeritus of Biochemistry and Medicine,
College of Medicine, University of Vermont,
Burlington, Vermont; Chairman, Haematologic
Technologies Incorporated, Essex Junction, Vermont
Blood Coagulation

Karen Jean Marcus, MD
Pediatric Radiation Oncology, Dana-Farber/Boston
Children's Cancer and Blood Disorders Center;
Associate Professor of Radiation Oncology, Harvard
Medical School, Boston, Massachusetts
Pediatric Radiation Oncology
Tumors of the Brain and Spinal Cord

Philip J. Mason, PhD
Professor of Pediatrics, Children's Hospital of
Philadelphia, Philadelphia, Pennsylvania
Inherited Bone Marrow Failure Syndromes

William C. Mentzer, Jr., MD
Professor Emeritus of Pediatrics, University of
California, San Francisco, San Francisco, California
Pyruvate Kinase Deficiency and Disorders of Glycolysis

Robert R. Montgomery, MD
Senior Investigator, Blood Research Institute,
BloodCenter of Wisconsin; Professor of Pediatric
Hematology and Pediatrics, Medical College of
Wisconsin, Milwaukee, Wisconsin
Hemophilia and von Willebrand Disease

Andres E. Morales La Madrid, MD
Neuro-Oncology Unit, Department of Pediatric
Hematology and Oncology, St. Joan de Déu
Children's Hospital, Barcelona, Spain
Tumors of the Brain and Spinal Cord

Elizabeth A. Mullen, MD
Attending Physician of Pediatric Oncology, Dana-Farber
Cancer Institute, Boston Children's Hospital;
Associate Professor of Pediatrics, Harvard Medical
School, Boston, Massachusetts
Pediatric Renal Tumors
Oncologic Emergencies

David G. Nathan, MD
President Emeritus, Dana-Farber Cancer Institute;
Physician-in-Chief Emeritus, Boston Children's
Hospital; Stranahan Distinguished Professor of
Pediatrics and Professor of Medicine, Harvard
Medical School, Boston, Massachusetts
Diagnostic Approach to the Anemic Patient
Thalassemias

Peter E. Newburger, MD
Ali and John Pierce Professor of Pediatric Hematology
and Oncology, Department of Pediatrics, University
of Massachusetts Medical School, Worcester,
Massachusetts
Phagocyte System and Disorders of Granulopoiesis and
Granulocyte Function

Debra K. Newman, PhD
Investigator, Blood Research Institute, BloodCenter of
Wisconsin, Milwaukee, Wisconsin
Platelets and the Vessel Wall

Peter J. Newman, PhD
Vice President for Research, BloodCenter of Wisconsin;
Professor, Departments of Pharmacology and Cellular
Biology, Medical College of Wisconsin, Milwaukee,
Wisconsin
Platelets and the Vessel Wall

Kim E. Nichols, MD
Chief, Division of Hereditary Cancer Predisposition, St.
Jude Children's Research Hospital, Division of
Oncology, Memphis, Tennessee
Genetic Predisposition to Cancer

Luigi D. Notarangelo, MD
Professor of Pediatrics and Pathology, Department of
Medicine, Division of Immunology, Children's
Hospital Boston, Harvard Medical School, Boston,
Massachusetts
Primary Immunodeficiency Diseases

John S. Olson, PhD
Ralph and Dorothy Looney Professor, Department of
Biochemistry and Cell Biology, Rice University,
Houston, Texas
Normal and Abnormal Hemoglobins

Stuart H. Orkin, MD
David G. Nathan Professor of Pediatrics, Harvard
Medical School; Chair, Department of Pediatric
Oncology, Dana-Farber Cancer Institute, Boston
Children's Hospital; Investigator, Howard Hughes
Medical Institute, Boston, Massachusetts
Thalassemias

†Frank A. Oski, MD
Distinguished Service Professor, Johns Hopkins
University School of Medicine, Baltimore, Maryland
Diagnostic Approach to the Anemic Patient

†Deceased.

Maureen J. O'Sullivan, MD, MBBCh
Professor of Histopathology, University of Dublin,
  Trinity College; Consultant Pediatric Pathologist,
  Department of Pathology, Our Lady's Children's
  Hospital, Crumlin; Principal Investigator of Cancer
  Genetics, The National Children's Research Centre,
  Crumlin, Dublin, Ireland
Cytogenetic and Molecular Pathology of Pediatric Cancer

Sung-Yun Pai, MD
Assistant Professor of Pediatrics, Department of
  Medicine, Boston Children's Hospital; Department of
  Pediatric Oncology, Dana-Farber Cancer Institute,
  Boston Children's Hospital, Boston, Massachusetts
Immune Response

Alberto S. Pappo, MD
Director, Solid Tumor Division, St. Jude Children's
  Research Hospital, Memphis, Tennessee
Rare Tumors of Childhood

Charles J. Parker, MD
Professor of Medicine, Division of Hematology and
  Hematologic Malignancies, University of Utah School
  of Medicine, Salt Lake City, Utah
Paroxysmal Nocturnal Hemoglobinuria

Antonio R. Perez-Atayde, MD
Director of Special Techniques and Diagnostic Surgical
  Pathology, Boston Children's Hospital; Associate
  Professor of Pathology, Harvard Medical School,
  Boston, Massachusetts
Nonrhabdomyosarcoma Soft Tissue Sarcomas and Other Soft
Tissue Tumors

John D. Phillips, PhD
Associate Professor of Medicine, University of Utah
  School of Medicine, Salt Lake City, Utah
Porphyrias

Steven Pipe, MD
Professor of Pediatrics and Pathology, University of
  Michigan, Ann Arbor, Michigan
Acquired Disorders of Hemostasis

Vincenzo Poggi, MD
Chief of Oncology, AORN Santobono-Pausilipon,
  Naples, Italy
Glucose-6-Phosphate Dehydrogenase Deficiency

Mortimer Poncz, MD
Division Chief of Hematology, Department of
  Pediatrics, Children's Hospital of Philadelphia,
  Perelman School of Medicine, University of
  Pennsylvania, Philadelphia, Pennsylvania
Inherited Platelet Disorders

Sanjay P. Prabhu, MBBS, FRCR
Assistant Professor of Radiology, Harvard Medical
  School; Director, Advanced Image Analysis Lab,
  Boston Children's Hospital, Boston, Massachusetts
Tumors of the Brain and Spinal Cord
Imaging in the Evaluation and Management of Childhood Cancer

Carlos E. Prada, MD
Assistant Professor of Human Genetics, Assistant
  Director, Biochemical Genetics Laboratory, Human
  Genetics, Cincinnati Children's Hospital Medical
  Center, Cincinnati, Ohio; Director, Centro de
  Medicina Genómica y Metabolismo, Fundación
  Cardiovascular de Colombia, Bucaramanga,
  Santander, Colombia
Lysosomal Storage Diseases

Christopher J. Recklitis, PhD, MPH
Director of Research and Support Services, Perini
  Family Survivors' Center, Dana-Farber Cancer
  Institute, Boston Children's Hospital; Assistant
  Professor, Department of Pediatrics, Harvard Medical
  School, Boston, Massachusetts
Psychosocial Care of the Child and Family

Ellis L. Reinherz, MD
Dana-Farber Cancer Institute, Boston Children's
  Hospital, Harvard Medical School, Boston,
  Massachusetts
Immune Response

Charles W.M. Roberts, MD, PhD
Associate Professor of Pediatric Oncology, Dana-Farber
  Cancer Institute, Boston Children's Hospital;
  Associate Professor of Pediatric Oncology, Harvard
  Medical School, Boston, Massachusetts
Genetics and Epigenetics of Childhood Cancers

David J. Roberts, MB ChB, D Phil
Consultant Hematologist, National Health Service
  Blood and Transplant, John Radcliffe Hospital;
  Professor of Haematology, Nuffield Department of
  Clinical Laboratory Sciences, University of Oxford,
  Oxford, England
Hematologic Manifestations of Systemic Diseases in Children of
the Developing World

Leslie L. Robison, PhD
Chair, Epidemiology and Cancer Control, St. Jude
  Children's Research Hospital, Memphis, Tennessee
Epidemiology of Leukemia in Childhood

Nathan J. Robison, MD
Assistant Professor of Pediatrics, University of Southern
  California Keck School of Medicine, Division of
  Hematology/Oncology and BMT, Children's Hospital
  Los Angeles, Los Angeles, California
Tumors of the Brain and Spinal Cord

Carlos Rodriguez-Galindo, MD
Director, Solid Tumor Program, Dana-Farber Cancer Institute and Boston Children's Cancer and Blood Disorders Center, Harvard Medical School, Boston, Massachusetts
Retinoblastoma
Histiocytoses

Barrett J. Rollins, MD, PhD
Linde Family Professor of Medicine, Department of Medical Oncology, Dana-Farber Cancer Institute, Boston Children's Hospital; Linde Family Professor of Medicine, Department of Medicine, Brigham & Women's Hospital; Linde Family Professor of Medicine, Department of Medicine, Harvard Medical School, Boston, Massachusetts
Histiocytoses

David S. Rosenblatt, MD, CM
Professor, Departments of Human Genetics, Medicine, and Biology, McGill University; Director, Division of Medical Genetics, McGill University Health Centre, Montreal, Quebec, Canada
Megaloblastic Anemia

Philip M. Rosoff, MD, MA
Professor of Pediatrics and Medicine, Duke University Medical Center, Durham, North Carolina
Ethical Considerations in Pediatric Oncology Clinical Trials

Vijay G. Sankaran, MD, PhD
Assistant Professor of Pediatrics, Division of Hematology and Oncology, Dana-Farber Cancer Institute, Boston Children's Hospital, Harvard Medical School, Boston, Massachusetts
Thalassemias

Nadine P. Sauer, MD, MPH
Pediatric Hematology Oncology, Lafayette Family Cancer Center, Brewer, Maine
Tumors of the Brain and Spinal Cord

Joshua D. Schiffman, MD
Associate Professor of Pediatrics and Oncological Sciences, Division of Pediatric Hematology and Oncology, University of Utah School of Medicine, Salt Lake City, Utah
Genetic Predisposition to Cancer

Alan D. Schreiber, MD
Professor of Medicine, University of Pennsylvania Perelman School of Medicine, Philadelphia, Pennsylvania
Autoimmune Hemolytic Anemia

Rosalind A. Segal, MD, PhD
Professor of Neurobiology, Dana-Farber Cancer Institute, Boston Children's Hospital, Boston, Massachusetts
Tumors of the Brain and Spinal Cord

William R. Sellers, MD
Vice President and Global Head of Oncology Research, The Novartis Institute for BioMedical Research, Cambridge, Massachusetts
Targeted Therapies in Oncology

Raja Shaikh, MD
Interventional Radiologist, Department of Radiology, Boston Children's Hospital, Boston, Massachusetts
Imaging in the Evaluation and Management of Childhood Cancer

Robert C. Shamberger, MD
Chief of Surgery, Boston Children's Hospital; Robert E. Gross Professor of Surgery, Harvard Medical School, Boston, Massachusetts
Pediatric Surgical Oncology

Anish V. Sharda, MB, BS
Instructor in Medicine, Beth Israel Deaconess Medical Center, Harvard Medical School, Boston, Massachusetts
Rare Hereditary Coagulation Factor Abnormalities

Akiko Shimamura, MD, PhD
Associate Member of the Clinical Research Division, Fred Hutchinson Cancer Research Center; Associate Professor, Department of Pediatrics, University of Washington; Hematology and Oncology, Seattle Children's Hospital, Seattle, Washington
Acquired Aplastic Anemia and Pure Red Cell Aplasia

Neerav Shukla, MD
Department of Pediatrics, Memorial Sloan Kettering Cancer Center, New York, New York
Infant Leukemias

Suzanne Shusterman, MD
Assistant Professor of Pediatrics, Harvard Medical School; Department of Pediatric Hematology and Oncology, Dana Farber Cancer Institute, Boston Children's Hospital, Boston, Massachusetts
Neuroblastoma

Colin A. Sieff, MBBC, FRCPath
Associate Professor of Pediatrics, Division of Pediatric Hematology and Oncology, Dana-Farber/Boston Children's Cancer and Blood Disorders Center; Senior Associate in Medicine, Division of Hematology, Boston Children's Hospital, Boston, Massachusettes
Anatomy and Physiology of Hematopoiesis

Lewis B. Silverman, MD
Director, Pediatric Hematologic Malignancy Service, Dana-Farber Cancer Institute, Boston Children's Hospital; Associate Professor of Pediatrics, Harvard Medical School, Boston, Massachusetts
Acute Lymphoblastic Leukemia

Steven R. Sloan, MD, PhD
Blood Bank Medical Director, Laboratory Medicine,
Director, Pediatric Transfusion Medicine, Joint
Program in Transfusion Medicine, Boston Children's
Hospital; Assistant Professor of Pathology, Harvard
Medical School, Boston, Massachusetts
Transfusion Medicine

Vivianne Smits-Wintjens, MD, PhD
Pediatrician-Neonatologist, Leiden University Medical
Center, The Hague, Netherlands
Immune Hemolytic Disease

Kimberly Stegmaier, MD
Associate Professor of Pediatrics, Harvard Medical
School; Co-Director of the Pediatric Hematologic
Malignancy Program, Dana-Farber Cancer Institute,
Boston Children's Hospital, Boston, Massachusetts
Targeted Therapies in Oncology

Lillian Sung, MD, PhD
Associate Professor, Division of Hematology and
Oncology, The Hospital for Sick Children, Toronto,
Ontario, Canada
Infectious Disease in the Pediatric Cancer Patient

Christopher S. Thom, PhD
Perelman School of Medicine, University of
Pennsylvania, Philadelphia, Pennslyvania
Normal and Abnormal Hemoglobins

Gail E. Tomlinson, MD, PhD
Professor and Division Director, Pediatric Hematology
and Oncology, Greehey Children's Cancer Research
Institute, University of Texas Health Science Center
at San Antonio, San Antonio, Texas
Hepatoblastoma and Other Liver Tumors in Children

Cameron C. Trenor, III, MD
Staff Physician, Department of Hematology and
Oncology, Boston Children's Hospital; Instructor in
Pediatrics, Harvard Medical School, Boston,
Massachusetts
Inherited Disorders of Thrombosis and Fibrinolysis

Christina K. Ullrich, MD, MPH
Assistant Professor of Pediatrics, Harvard Medical
School; Physician, Pediatric Oncology and Pediatric
Palliative Care, Dana-Farber Cancer Institute, Boston
Children's Hospital, Boston, Massachusetts
Symptom Management in Children with Cancer

Samuel L. Volchenboum, MD, PhD, MS
Assistant Professor, Department of Pediatrics, Director,
Center for Research Informatics, University of
Chicago, Chicago, Illinois
Informatics

Stephan D. Voss, MD, PhD
Division Chief, Oncologic Imaging, Director of Nuclear
Medicine and Molecular Imaging, Associate Professor
of Radiology, Harvard Medical School, Boston,
Massachusetts
Imaging in the Evaluation and Management of Childhood Cancer

Lynda Vrooman, MD, MMSc
Instructor in Pediatrics, Harvard Medical School;
Attending Physician, Dana-Farber/Boston Children's
Cancer and Blood Disorders Center, Boston,
Massachusetts
Childhood Cancer Survivorship

Russell E. Ware, MD, PhD
Professor, Department of Pediatrics, University of
Cincinnati College of Medicine; Director, Division of
Hematology, Co-Executive Director, Cancer and
Blood Diseases Institute; Associate Director, Global
Health Center, Cincinnati Children's Hospital
Medical Center, Cincinnati, Ohio
Paroxysmal Nocturnal Hemoglobinuria
Sickle Cell Disease

David Watkins, PhD
Research Associate of Human Genetics, McGill
University, Montreal, Quebec, Canada
Megaloblastic Anemia

David J. Weatherall, MD, FRCP, FRS
Weatherall Institute of Molecular Medicine, University
of Oxford, Oxford, United Kingdom
Hematologic Manifestations of Systemic Diseases in Children of
the Developing World

Mitchell J. Weiss, MD, PhD
Professor of Pediatrics, The Children's Hospital of
Philadelphia; Professor of Pediatrics, The University
of Pennsylvania, Philadelphia, Pennsylvania;
Department of Hematology, St. Jude Children's
Research Hospital, Memphis, Tennessee
Normal and Abnormal Hemoglobins

Christopher B. Weldon, MD, PhD
Assistant in Surgery, Department of Pediatric Surgery,
Boston Children's Hospital; Assistant Professor of
Surgery, Harvard Medical School, Boston,
Massachusetts
Pediatric Surgical Oncology

David A. Williams, MD
Chief of Hematology and Oncology, Boston Children's
Hospital; Leland Fikes Professor of Pediatrics,
Harvard Medical School, Boston, Massachusetts
Acquired Aplastic Anemia and Pure Red Cell Aplasia

David B. Wilson, MD, PhD
Associate Professor of Pediatrics, Washington
   University, St. Louis, Missouri
   Inherited Bone Marrow Failure Syndromes
   Acquired Platelet Defects

Matthew W. Wilson, MD
Professor of Ophthalmology, University of Tennessee
   Health Sciences Center, St. Jude Children's Research
   Hospital, Memphis, Tennessee
   Retinoblastoma

Joanne Wolfe, MD, MPH
Division Chief, Pediatric Palliative Care, Departments
   of Psychosocial Oncology and Palliative Care and
   Medicine, Dana-Farber Cancer Institute, Boston
   Children's Hospital; Associate Professor of Pediatrics,
   Harvard Medical School, Boston, Massachusetts
   Palliative Care in Pediatric Oncology

Richard B. Womer, MD
Senior Physician, Department of Pediatrics, Division of
   Oncology, The Children's Hospital of Philadelphia;
   Professor of Pediatrics, Perelman School of Medicine,
   University of Pennyslvania, Philadelphia,
   Pennsylvania
   Rhabdomyosarcoma

Kristin Zelley, MS, LCGC
Department of Oncology, Children's Hospital of
   Philadelphia, Philadelphia, Pennsylvania
   Genetic Predisposition to Cancer

Lonnie M. Zeltzer, MD
Director, Children's Pain and Comfort Care Program,
   Distinguished Professor of Pediatrics, Anesthesiology,
   Psychiatry, and Biobehavioral Sciences, David Geffen
   School of Medicine at UCLA, Las Angeles, California
   Psychosocial Care of the Child and Family

Leonard I. Zon, MD
Grousbeck Professor of Pediatrics, Department of
   Medicine—Hematology and Oncology, HHMI/
   Boston Chilldren's Hospital, Boston, Massachusettes
   Anatomy and Physiology of Hematopoiesis

On behalf of the editors, I welcome you to the eighth edition of *Nathan and Oski's Hematology of Infancy and Childhood*, which has been renamed *Nathan and Oski's Hematology and Oncology of Infancy and Childhood* to reflect the new format begun with the last edition. The classic *Nathan and Oski* text continues to evolve in concert with development in the field of pediatric hematology and oncology. Four decades ago David Nathan and Frank Oski had the vision of creating a resource for students, practitioners, and clinical and basic investigators in which pathophysiology relating to diseases of children would inform clinical care and research in the present and for the future. They hoped to stimulate bench-to-bedside and bedside-to-bench activities in order to understand and treat pediatric patients with hematologic disorders and cancer. The first six editions were decidedly hematology-centric. They concentrated on normal blood cells and their abnormalities, hemostasis, and immune disorders. Except for relatively brief discussion of childhood leukemias, the emphasis was on what might be classified as non-malignant hematology. In recognition of the enormous growth of interest, new knowledge, and treatment possibilities in pediatric oncology, we expanded the scope of the seventh edition with extensive coverage of cancer therapeutics, solid tumors, and oncologic supportive care. In some respects the seventh edition was an experiment. We intentionally separated hematology and oncology into two volumes, thereby allowing readers to consider and purchase either *Hematology of Infancy and Childhood* or *Oncology of Infancy and Childhood*. To accomplish the task of creating an oncology volume de novo, we invited our colleagues Tom Look and David Fisher to join as editors.

By branding the eighth edition with a unified title, the editors have declared the experiment of the seventh edition a success. We believe the expanded scope of the textbook has been well received by readers and more accurately reflects the state of the entire field of pediatric hematology and oncology. The rather artificial distinction between hematology and oncology pained us as editors. Where would we now place leukemia if restricted to one or the other volume? Don't the bone marrow failure syndromes that often evolve to frank malignancy constitute an important bridge between the two areas? As many trainees and practitioners in pediatric hematology and oncology devote a majority of their time to oncology, the need to bring a unified package forward was clear.

We hope that the current form of *Hematology and Oncology of Infancy and Childhood* captures the enormous progress in our understanding and management of non-malignant and malignant conditions in pediatrics. The last two decades have been revolutionary in terms of discovery. The impact of molecular biology, human genetics, immunology, and chemistry on pediatric hematology and oncology, as on all medicine, has been extraordinary. It is now commonplace to anticipate that the entire genome of every child with cancer or a blood disorder will be determined going forward based on the expectation that a full genetic profile will lead to personalized and more effective treatment. To encompass areas of broad relevance that were not covered previously, we have added new chapters. Mel Greaves, a distinguished leader in childhood leukemia, has graced our text with his views on the origin and evolution of cancer, indeed retracing some of Darwin's logic for us. Because informatics has become a critical component of all genomic efforts, we solicited a new chapter on informatics that has been written by Sam Volchenboum. Given the increasing excitement and relevance of epigenetics to childhood cancer, we asked two experts in this area, Charles Roberts and Alex Kentsis, to provide a new contribution on this topic. As always, we hope that readers will provide frank and constructive feedback on this edition. To do justice to the entire field of pediatric hematology and oncology may be a near impossible task. The editors have given their best efforts on behalf of the cause. The readers are our judges.

The eighth edition has truly been a team effort. I cannot thank the other editors enough for their dedication to this project. We are most grateful to the authors of each chapter for their contributions. The editorial staff at Elsevier kept us on course, even when it seemed that we would not make our deadlines. We appreciate everything they have done and more.

It is an honor to be in the field of pediatric hematology and oncology.

Stuart H. Orkin, MD

CONTENTS

Volume II

A

A2: annexin 2
AA: arachidonic acid
AABB: American Association of Blood Banks
AAE: acquired angioedema
AAIR: age-adjusted incidence rate
AAP: American Academy of Pediatrics
AAV: adeno-associated virus
ABC: ATP-binding cassette transporter superfamily
ABCB7: ATP-binding cassette subfamily B member 7, mitochondrial
ABL: Abelson kinase, Abelson gene product
ABO: ABO(H) blood group system
ABP: actin-binding protein
ABP-1: actin-binding protein-1
ACO1: aconitase 1
ACS: acute chest syndrome
ACE: angiotensin-converting enzyme
ACIP: Advisory Committee on Immunization Practices
ACTH: adrenocorticotropic hormone, adrenocorticotropin
AD: anauxetic dysplasia; autosomal dominant
ADA: adenosine deaminase
ADAD: ADA deficiency
ADC: apparent diffusion coefficient
ADCC: antibody-dependent cellular cytotoxicity; antibody-dependent cell-mediated cytotoxicity
AdoCbl: adenosylcobalamin, 5′-deoxyadenosylcobalamin
AdoHcy: *S*-adenosylhomocysteine
AdoMct: *S*-adenosylmethionine
ADP: adenosine diphosphate; ALA-D deficiency porphyria; antibody-dependent phagocytosis
ADPase: adenosine diphosphatase
AE1: anion exchange protein 1 (band 3 protein of the red cell membrane)
AFP: α-fetoprotein
AGLT: acidified glycerol lysis test
AGM: aorta-gonad-mesonephros
aGVHD: acute graft-versus-host disease
AH50: alternative pathway complement hemolysis 50%
AHA: acute hemolytic anemia
AHG: antihuman globulin
AHSP: α-hemoglobin–stabilizing protein
aHUS: atypical hemolytic uremic syndrome
AICAR: amino-4-imidazolecarboxamide ribonucleotide
AICD: activation-induced cell death
AICDA: activation-induced cytidine deaminase (gene)
AID: activation-induced cytidine deaminase, activation-induced deaminase
AIDS: acquired immunodeficiency virus
AIHA: autoimmune hemolytic anemia
AIN: autoimmune neutropenia
AIP: acute intermittent porphyria

AIRE: autoimmune regulator
AIS: arterial ischemic stroke
AK: adenylate kinase
AK2: adenylate kinase 2
ALA: δ-aminolevulinic acid
ALA-D: δ-aminolevulinic acid dehydratase
ALA-S: δ-aminolevulinic acid synthase
ALCL: anaplastic large-cell lymphoma
ALD: adrenoleukodystrophy
ALDH: aldehyde dehydrogenase
ALG: antilymphocyte globulin
ALK: anaplastic lymphoma kinase
ALL: acute lymphoblastic leukemia; acute lymphocytic leukemia; acute myeloblastic leukemia; acute myeloid leukemia
ALM: activation loop mutations
ALPS: autoimmune lymphoproliferative syndrome
AMKL: acute megakaryoblastic leukemia
AML: acute myelogenous leukemia; acute myeloid leukemia
AMT: amegakaryocytic thrombocytopenia
ANC: absolute neutrophil count
ANCA: antineutrophil cytoplasmic antibody
α₂-AP: $α_2$-antiplasmin
AP3B1: adaptor protein 3 complex β3A subunit
APA: antiphospholipid antibody
APC: activated protein C, adenomatous polyposis coli, antigen-presenting cell
APCC: activated prothrombin complex concentrate
APECED: autoimmune polyendocrinopathy–candidiasis–ectodermal dystrophy
APHON: Association of Pediatric Hematology/Oncology Nurses
APL: acute promyelocytic leukemia
APLA: antiphospholipid antibody
APOL1: apolipoprotein L1
APRCA: acquired pure red cell aplasia
APRIL: α-proliferation–inducing ligand
APS-1: autoimmune polyglandular syndrome type 1
APTT: activated partial thromboplastin time
AQP1: aquaporin-1
AR: autosomal recessive; androgen receptor
Ara-CMP: arabinosylcytosine 5′ monophosphate
ARC: Australia Research Council
ARF: alternate reading frame
ARSB: arylsulfatase B
ARTUS: amegakaryocytic thrombocytopenia with radio-ulnar synostosis
ASA: arylsulfatase A
ASBMT: American Society for Blood and Marrow Transplantation
ASCO: American Society of Clinical Oncology
ASCT: autologous stem cell transplant
ASH: American Society of Hematology

ASL: arterial spin labeling
ASM: acid sphingomyelinase; aggressive systemic mastocytosis
AST: aspartate aminotransferase
AT: antithrombin; ataxia-telangiectasia
ATG: antithymocyte globulin
ATLS: acute tumor lysis syndrome
ATM: ataxia-telangiectasia mutated
ATOX1: antioxidant 1 copper chaperone
ATP: adenosine triphosphate
ATPase: adenosine triphosphatase
ATP7A: ATPase, Cu^{2+} transporting, alpha polypeptide
ATRA: all-*trans*-retinoic-acid
ATRUS: amegakaryocytic thrombocytopenia with radio-ulnar synostosis
AUC: area under the plasma concentration vs. time curve
AVN: avascular necrosis
AVWS: acquired von Willebrand syndrome
AZT: zidovudine

B

β-LCR: β-locus control region
BACT: BCNU (carmustine)/Ara-C (cytarabine)/cyclophosphamide/6-thioguanine
BACH1: BTB and CNC homology 1
BAEP: brainstem auditory evoked potential
BAER: brainstem auditory evoked responses
BAF: BRG1-associated factor
BAFF: B-cell–activating factor
BAFFR: BAFF receptor
BAL: bronchoalveolar lavage
BAL: British anti-Lewisite
B-ALL: B-cell acute lymphoblastic leukemia; B-precursor ALL
BCAM: basal cell adhesion molecule
BCG: bacille Calmette-Guérin
BCL10: B-cell lymphoma 10
BCNU: carmustine
BCR: B-cell receptor; breakpoint cluster region
BDNF: brain-derived neutrotrophic factor
BEAM: BCNU (carmustine)/etoposide/Ara-C (cytarabine)/melphalan
BET: bromodomain and extraterminal
BFU-E: burst-forming unit–erythrocyte
BFU-Meg: burst-forming unit–megakaryocyte
bHLH: basic helix-loop-helix
BiPAP: bilevel positive airway pressure
BIRC4: baculoviral IAP repeat-containing 4
BiTEs: bispecific T-cell engagers
BLM: Bloom syndrome, RecQ helicase-like
BLNK: B-cell linker protein
BM: bone marrow
BMD: bone mineral density
BMF: bone marrow failure
BMI: body mass index
BMP: bone morphogenetic protein
BMT: bone marrow transplantation
BMT-MA: bone marrow transplantation–associated microangiopathy

BPGM: 2,3-bisphosphoglycerate mutase
BPI: bactericidal/permeability-increasing protein
BRB: blood-retinal barrier; blood-eye barrier
BRCA1: breast cancer 1, early onset
BrdU: bromodeoxyuridine
BrOb: bronchiolitis obliterans
BRM: biologic response modifier
BSAP: B-cell–specific activator protein
BSP: bromsulfophthalein
BSS: Bernard-Soulier syndrome
BT: bleeding time
Btk: Bruton tyrosine kinase
BU: Bethesda units, busulfan
BUGT: bilirubin UDP-glucuronyltransferase
BWS: Beckwith-Wiedemann syndrome
bZIP: basic region–leucine zipper domain

C

C282Y: cysteine 282 to tyrosine
C: constant
CAD: cold agglutinin disease
CADP: collagen/adenosine diphosphate
CAFC: cobblestone area–forming cell
CAIV: carbonic anhydrase IV
CALGB: Cancer and Leukemia Group B
CaM: calmodulin
CAM: complementary and alternative medicine
cAMP: cyclic adenosine monophosphate
CAMT: congenital amegakaryocytic thrombocytopenia
CaNaEDTA: calcium disodium-ethylenediaminetetraacetic acid
CAR: Central African Republic; chimeric antigen receptor
CARD: caspase recruitment domain family member
CASP: caspase
CAT: calibrated automated thrombography
CB: cord blood
CBB: cord blood bank
C4bBP: C4b-binding protein
CBF: core-binding factor
CBP: cyclophosphamide/BCNU (carmustine)/cisplatin
CBV: cyclophosphamide/BCNU (carmustine)/VP-16 (etoposide)
CCG: Children's Cancer Study Group
CCI: corrected count increment
CCSK: clear cell sarcoma of the kidney
CCyR: complete cytogenetic response
CD: cluster of differentiation
CD3D, CD3E, CD3G, CD3Z, CD3: δ, ε, γ, chains, respectively
CD40L: CD40 ligand
CDA: congenital dyserythropoietic anemia
CDA: cytidine deaminase
CDC: complement-dependent cytotoxicity
Cdc42: cell division control protein 42
CDK: cyclin-dependent kinase
CDP: CCAAT displacement protein; cytidine diphosphate
CDR3: complementarity-determining region 3
C/EBP: CCAAT/enhancer-binding protein α
CEP: congenital erythropoietic porphyria

CEPI: collagen/epinephrine
CESD: cholesteryl ester storage disease
CFC: colony-forming cell
CFC-Eo: eosinophil colony-forming cell
CFU-C: colony-forming unit in culture
CFU-E: colony-forming unit–erythrocyte
CFU-Eo: colony-forming unit–eosinophil
CFU-GEMM: colony-forming unit–multipotent (granulocyte, erythrocyte, macrophage, megakaryocyte)
CFU-GM: colony-forming unit–granulocyte-macrophage
CFU-Meg: colony-forming unit–megakaryocyte
CFU-S: colony-forming unit–spleen
CGD: chronic granulomatous disease
CGH: comparative genomic hybridization
cGMP: current good manufacturing practice; cyclic guanosine monophosphate
CGP: circulatory granulocyte pool
cGVHD: chronic graft-versus-disease
CH: calponin homology domain
CHBA: congenital Heinz body hemolytic anemia
CHF: congestive heart failure
CH50: classical pathway complement hemolysis 50%
CHH: cartilage-hair hypoplasia
CHO: Chinese hamster ovary
CHL: classic Hodgkin lymphoma
CHOP: cyclophosphamide, hydroxydaunorubicin, oncovin, and predsinone or prednisolone
CHR: complete hematologic response
CHr: cellular hemoglobin of the reticulocyte
CHS: Chédiak-Higashi syndrome
CIBMTR: Center for International Blood and Marrow Transplant Research
CIK: cytokine-induced killer cell
CIITA: class II *trans*-activator
C1-INH: C1 esterase inhibitor
CI: confidence interval
CIS: cytokine-inducible SH2-containing protein
Cl⁻: chloride anion
CLABSI: central line–associated bloodstream infection
CLC: Charcot-Leyden crystal
ClC: chloride channel (may be followed by -7 or other number)
CLIA: Clinical Laboratory Improvement Amendment
CLL: chronic lymphocytic leukemia
CLN-1: neuronal ceroid lipofuscinosis type 1
CLP: common lymphoid progenitor
CMC: chronic mucocutaneous candidiasis
CML: chronic myelocytic leukemia; chronic myelogenous leukemia
CMN: cellular congenital mesoblastic nephroma
cMOAT: canalicular multispecific organic anion transporter
CMP: common myeloid progenitor; cytidine monophosphate
CMV: cytomegalovirus
CN: Crigler-Najjar syndrome, type I (CNI) or type II (CNII); cyanide; cystic nephroma
CNB: core needle biopsy
CNCbl: cyanocobalamin
CNS: central nervous system

CNSHA: congenital nonspherocytic hemolytic anemia
CNTF: ciliary neurotrophic factor
CNV: copy number variation
CO: carbon monoxide
CO_2: carbon dioxide
CoA: coenzyme A
COG: Children's Oncology Group
COJEC: cisplatin, vincristine, carboplatin, etoposide, and cyclophosphamide
COL1A1: collagen, type I, α1
COPA: cancer outlier profile analysis
COX-1: cyclooxygenase-1
COX-2: cyclooxygenase-2
CP: connecting peptides
CPAP: continuous positive airway pressure
CPD: citrate-phosphate-dextrose
CPDA-1: citrate-phosphate-dextrose-adenosine
CPDN: cystic, partially differentiated nephroblastoma
CPO: coproporphyrinogen oxidase
CPP: choroid plexus papillomas
CR: complete remission
CR1: complement receptor 1
CRAC: calcium release–activated calcium
CREG: cross-reactive group
CRF: chronic renal failure
CRHR1: corticotropin-releasing hormone receptor 1
CRIg: complement receptor of the immunoglobulin superfamily
CRISPR: clustered regularly interspaced short palindromic repeats
CRLF2: cytokine receptor-like factor 2
CRM: cross-reacting material
CRP: cross-reactive protein; C-reactive protein
CRT: catheter-related thrombosis
CRX: cone-rod homeobox
CSA: congenital sideroblastic anemia
CSF: cerebrospinal fluid; colony-stimulating factor
c-SMAC: central supramolecular activation cluster
CSR: class switch recombination
CSC: cancer stem cells
CSSCD: Cooperative Study of Sickle Cell Disease
CSVT: cerebral sinovenous thrombosis
CT: closure time; computed tomography
CTCL: cutaneous T-cell leukemia
CIITA: MHC class II transactivator
CT-1: cardiotropin-1
CTD: C-terminal domain
CTL: cytotoxic T lymphocyte
CTLA-4: cytotoxic T-lymphocyte antigen 4
CTP: cytidine triphosphate
CTR1: copper transporter 1
Cu-ATPase: adenosine triphosphatase transmembrane copper transporter
CVID: common variable immunodeficiency
CVL: central venous line
CVS: chorionic villus sampling
CXCR4: CXC chemokine receptor 4
CXR: chest radiography
CY: cyclophosphamide
CYP: cytochrome P

D

D: diversity
DA: diffuse anaplasia
DAF: decay accelerating factor
DAG: diacylglycerol
DAMP: damage-associated molecular pattern
DAP: DNAx activating protein (au query; set OK?)
DAT: direct antibody test, direct antiglobulin test
dATP: deoxyadenosine triphosphatase
DBA: Diamond-Blackfan anemia
DC: dyskeratosis congenita
DCC: delayed cord clamping
DCE: downstream core element
DCK: deoxycytidine kinase
DCLRE1C: DNA cross-link repair enzyme 1C
DCRLRE1C: DNA cross-link repair enzyme 1C
DCT1: divalent cation transporter 1
DDAVP: 1-deamino-8-D-arginine vasopressin
DEB: diepoxybutane
deoxy-Hb: deoxygenated hemoglobin
DFMO: a-difluoromethylornithine
DFS: dermatofibrosarcoma; disease-free survival
DGS: DiGeorge syndrome
dGTP: deoxyguanosine triphosphatase
DHAP: dihydroxyacetone phosphate
DHF: dengue hemorrhagic fever; 7,8-dihydrofolate
DHFR: dihydrofolate reductase
DHR 123: dihydroxyrhodamine 123
DIC: disseminated intravascular coagulation
DIDMOAD: diabetes insipidus, diabetes mellitus, optic atrophy, and deafness
DIDS: 4,4′-diisothiocyanostilbene-2,2′-disulfonate (anion channel inhibitor)
DIIHA: drug-induced immune hemolytic anemia
DJS: Dubin-Johnson syndrome
DLI: donor lymphocyte infusion
DLBCL: diffuse large B-cell lymphoma
DLT: dose-limiting toxicity
DMS: demarcation membrane system
DMSO: dimethyl sulfoxide
DMT1: divalent metal transporter 1
DNA: deoxyribonucleic acid
DNA-PKcs: DNA-dependent protein kinase catalytic subunit
DNET: dysembryoplastic neuroepithelial tumors
DNM3TA: DNA methyltransferase 3A
DNM3TB: DNA methyl transferase 3B
DNTs: double-negative T cells
DOCK8: dedicator of cytokinesis 8
DLI: donor lymphocyte infusion
DOPA: 3,4-dihydroxyphenylalanine
DOT1L: Histone-*lysine*-N-methyltransferase, H3 *lysine*-79–specific
DP: double-positive
2,3-DPG: 2,3-diphosphoglycerate
DPT: diphtheria and tetanus toxoids and pertussis
DRESS: drug rash with eosinophilia and systemic symptoms (syndrome)
dRTA: distal renal tubular acidosis
DRVVT: dilute Russell viper venom time
DS: Down syndrome

DS-AMKL: Down syndrome–acute megakaryoblastic leukemia
DSRCT: desmoplastic small round blue cell tumors
DSS: dengue shock syndrome
DS-TMD: Down syndrome–transient myeloproliferative disorder
DTB: ditaurobilirubin
DTI: Diffusion tensor imaging
dTMP: thymidylate (deoxythymidine monophosphate)
DTS: dense tubular system
DVI: partial D category VI phenotype
DVT: deep venous thrombosis
DWI: diffusion-weighted imaging

E

EA: early antigen
EBA140: *Plasmodium falciparum* erythrocyte binding antigen 140
EBMT: European Group for Blood and Marrow Transplantation
EBP: elastin-binding protein
EBRT: external beam radiation therapy
EBV: Epstein-Barr virus
EC: Enzyme Commission
ECLT: euglobulin clot lysis time
ECMO: extracorporeal membrane oxygenation
EDA-ID: anhidrotic ectodermal dysplasia with immunodeficiency
EDAS: encephaloduroarteriosynangiosis
EDAMS: encephaloduroarteriomyosynangiosis
EDS: Ehlers-Danlos syndrome
EDTA: ethylenediaminetetraacetic acid
EFS: event-free survival
EGA: estimated gestational age
EGF: epidermal growth factor
EGFR: epidermal growth factor receptor
EHEC: enterohemorrhagic *Escherichia coli*
EKLF: erythroid Krüppel-like factor
ELISA: enzyme-linked immunoabsorbent assay
EM: extramedullary
eNOS: endothelial nitric oxide synthase
ENU: *N*-ethyl-*N*-nitrosourea
EPCR: endothelial cell protein C receptor
EPEC: enteropathogenic *Escherichia coli*
EPO: erythropoietin
EpoR: erythropoietin receptor
EPP: erythropoietic protoporphyria
EPR: electron paramagnetic resonance
ER: endoplasmic reticulum; estrogen receptor
ERGIC-53: endoplasmic reticulum–Golgi intermediate compartment, 53 kilodalton protein
ERT: enzyme replacement therapy
ES: embryonic stem
ESC: embryonic stem cell
ESL-1: E-selectin ligand-1
ESRD: end-stage renal disease
ET: essential thrombocythemia
ETANTRs: embryonal tumors with abundant neuropile and true rosettes
EV: epidermodysplasia verruciformis

EVER: epidermodysplasia verruciformis
EZH2: enhancer of zeste 2

F

FA: Fanconi anemia; focal anaplasia
FAAP: Fanconi anemia–associated protein
FAB: French-American-British (staging)
Fab: antigen-binding fragment
FACS: fluorescence-activated cell sorting
FACT: Foundation for the Accreditation of Cell Therapy
FAD: flavin adenine dinucleotide
FADD: Fas-associated via death domain
FAH: fumarylacetoacetate hydrolase
FAICAR: formamido-4-imidazolecarboxamide ribonucleotide
FAK: focal adhesion kinase
FASLG: FAS ligand
FBN: fibronectin
FBXL5: F-box and leucine-rich repeat protein 5
FCP: F-cell production (locus)
FcR: Fc receptor
FcγR: IgG Fc receptor
FDA: Food and Drug Administration
FDC: follicular dendritic cell
FDG-PET: fluorine 18–labeled deoxyglucose positron emission tomography
FDP: familial platelet deficiency; fibrin(ogen) degradation product; fructose 6-diphosphate
FECH: ferrochelatase
FEIBA: factor eight inhibitor–bypassing activity
FEP: free erythrocyte protoporphyrin
Fe-SIH: ferric salicylaldehyde-isonicotinyl-hydrazone
FFP: fresh-frozen plasma
FGAR: formylglycinamide ribonucleotide
FGF: fibroblast growth factor
fH: factor H
FHL: familial hemophagocytic lymphohistiocytosis
fI: factor I
FIGlu: formiminoglutamic acid
FISH: fluorescence in situ hybridization
FKBP: FK-binding proteins
FL: ligand for the Flks/Flt3 receptor
FLAER: fluorescent aerolysin
FLAIR: fluid-attenuated inversion recovery
FLIP: FLICE-like inhibitory protein
FLT3: fms-related tyrosine kinase 3
FMH: fetomaternal hemorrhage
FN: fever and neutropenia
FNA: fine needle aspiration
FOG-1: friend of GATA-1
FOX: forkhead box transcription factor
FPA: fibrinopeptide A
FPB: fibrinopeptide A
F-PCT: familial porphyria cutanea tarda
FPN1: ferroportin 1
FRAP: fluorescence recovery after photobleaching
FSGS: focal sclerosing glomerulosclerosis
FTCD: formiminotransferase-cyclodeaminase
5-FU: 5-fluorouracil
FUO: fever of unknown origin

G

γc: cytokine receptor common gamma chain
G6PD: glucose-6-phosphate dehydrogenase
GABA: γ-aminobutyric acid
GAG: glycosaminoglycan
β-gal: β-d-galactosidase
GalNAc-T: N-acetylgalactosaminyltransferase
GALNS: N-acetylgalactosamine-6-sulfatase
GAP: GTPase-activating protein
GAR: glycinamide ribonucleotide
GAS: IFN-γ–activated sequence
GAT: granulocyte agglutination test
GBS: Guillain-Barré syndrome
GC: germinal center; glucocorticoids
GCase: acid β-glucosidase; glucocerebrosidase (i.e, the Gaucher disease enzyme)
G-CSF: granulocyte colony-stimulating factor
G-CSFR: granulocyte colony-stimulating factor receptor
GDF: growth and differentiation factor
GDF15: growth differentiation factor 15
GDP: guanosine diphosphate
GEMMs: genetically engineered mouse models
GFR: glomerular filtration rate
GH: growth hormone
GI: gastrointestinal
GIF: gastric intrinsic factor
GIFT: granulocyte immunofluorescence test
GIST: gastrointestinal stromal tumors
GITMO: Gruppo Italiano Trapianti di Midollo Osseo
GlcNAc: N-acetylglucosamine
GLRX5: glutaredoxin 5
Glu-Plg: glutamic acid plasminogen
GluR1: glutamate receptor type 1
GM2A: GM2 activator protein
GM-CSF: granulocyte-macrophage colony-stimulating factor
GMP: granulocyte-monocyte precursor, guanosine monophosphate; granulocytic-monocytic–restricted progenitors
GMTZ: gemtuzumab ozogamicin
GNPT: UDP-N-acetylglucosamine:lysosomal-enzyme N-acetylglucosamine-1-phosphotransferase
GnRH: gonadotropin-releasing hormone
GP: glycoprotein
GPA: glycophorin A
GPB: glycophorin B
GPC: glycophorin C
GPCR: G protein–coupled receptor
GPD: glycophorin D
G3PD: glyceraldehyde-3-phosphate dehydrogenase
G6PD: glucose-6-phosphate dehydrogenase
GPE: glycophorin E
GPI: glucose phosphate isomerase, glycosylphosphatidylinositol
GPIb: glycoprotein Ib
GPS: gray platelet syndrome
GRF: guanine nucleotide–releasing factor
GRO: growth regulated oncogene
GS: Gilbert syndrome; Griscelli syndrome
GS2: Griscelli syndrome type 2

GSCbl: glutathionylcobalamin
GSH: reduced glutathione, γ-secretase inhibitor
GSK3: glycogen synthase kinase 3
GSL: glycosphingolipid
GSSG: oxidized glutathione
GSHPX: glutathione peroxidase
GST: glutathione-S-transferase
GT: Glanzmann thrombasthenia
GTP: guanosine triphosphate; guanosine nucleotide phosphate
GTPase: guanosine triphosphatase
GV: gemcitabine and vinorelbine
GVHD: graft-versus-host disease
GVL: graft versus leukemia

H

H3K27: lysine 27 of histone 3
H3K79: lysine 79 of histone 3
H63D: histidine 63 to aspartic acid
H⁺: hydrogen cation
HAART: highly active antiretroviral therapy
HABA: 2(4′-hydroxyazobenzene) benzoic acid
HAE: hereditary angioedema
HAMP: hepcidin antimicrobial peptide
Hb: hemoglobin
HB: Heinz body
HbA: adult hemoglobin
HbF: fetal hemoglobin
HBV: hepatitis B virus
HC: homocysteine; haptocorrin (also called transcobalamin I or R binder)
4-HC: 4-hydroperoxycyclophosphamide
HCP: hereditary coproporphyria, hematopoietic cell phosphatase
HCV: hepatitis C virus
HD: Hodgkin disease; homodimerization
HDAC: Histone deacetylase
HDL: high-density lipoprotein
HDN: hemolytic disease of the fetus and newborn; hemorrhagic disease of the newborn
HDW: hemoglobin distribution width
HE: hereditary elliptocytosis
HELLP: hemolytic anemia, elevated liver enzymes, low platelet count
HEMPAS: hereditary erythroblastic multinuclearity with a positive acidified serum lysis test
HEP: hepatoerythropoietic porphyria
HES: Hairy and Enhancer of Split, hypereosinophilic syndrome
HETE: 15(S)-hydroxyeicosatetraenoic acid
Hex-A: hexosaminidase A
Hex-B: hexosaminidase B
HFE: HLA-linked human hemochromatosis protein
HGF: hematopoietic growth factor; hepatocyte growth factor
HGFR: hematopoietic growth factor receptor
HHS: Hoyeraal-Hreidarsson syndrome
HHV-6: human herpesvirus 6
HHV-8: human herpesvirus 8
HiB: *Haemophilus influenzae* type B
HIDA: hepatobiliary iminodiacetic acid

HIES: hyperimmunoglobulin E syndrome (hyper-IgE syndrome)
HIF: hypoxia-inducible factor
HIF-1: hypoxia-inducible factor 1
HIM: hyper-IgM syndrome
HIT: heparin-induced thrombocytopenia
HITTS: HIT with thrombosis syndrome
HIV: human immunodeficiency virus
HJV: hemojuvelin
HK: hexokinase
HLA: human leukocyte antigen
HLH: hemophagocytic lymphohistiocytosis
HMB: hydroxymethylbilane
HMGB1: high–molecular group box 1 protein
HMP: hexose monophosphate
HMPV: human metapneumovirus
HMS: hyperreactive malarial splenomegaly
HMWK: high-molecular-weight kininogen
HNE: hydroxynonenal
hnRNA: heterogeneous nuclear RNA
HO: heme oxygenase
HOCl: hypchlorous acid
H₂O₂: hydrogen peroxide
H₂OCbl: aquocobalamin
holo-HC: holohaptocorrin
holo-TC: holotranscobalamin
HOX: homeobox transcription factor
HPA-1a: human platelet antigen 1a
HPC: hematopoietic progenitor cell
HPCHA: high-phosphatidylcholine hemolytic anemia
HPFH: hereditary persistence of fetal hemoglobin
HPLC: high-performance liquid chromatography; high-pressure liquid chromatography
HPP: hereditary pyropoikilocytosis
HPP-CFCs: high–proliferative potential colony-forming cells
HPRT: hypoxanthine phosphoribosyltransferase
HPS: Hermansky-Pudlak syndrome
HPV: human papillomavirus
HR: homologous recombination
HRE: hypoxia response element
HRI: heme-regulated inhibitor kinase
HRM: heme regulatory motif
HRQoL: Health-related quality of life
HS: hereditary spherocytosis; hypersensitivity site
HSC: hematopoietic stem cell
HSCT: hematopoietic stem cell transplantation
HSP: heat shock protein; Henoch-Schönlein purpura
HSt: hereditary stomatocytosis
HSV: herpes simplex virus
5-HT: 5′-hydroxytryptamine (serotonin)
HTLV: human T-cell leukemia/lymphoma virus; human T-cell lymphotropic virus
HUS: hemolytic uremic syndrome
HUSOFT: Hydroxyurea Safety and Organ Toxicity
HUVEC: human umbilical vein endothelial cell

I

IAP: integrin-associated protein or CD47
IAS: ischemic arterial stroke
IBMFS: inherited bone marrow failure syndrome

IBMTR: International Bone Marrow Transplant Registry

ICAM: intercellular adhesion molecule

ICE: ifosfamide, carboplatin, and etoposide

ICD-9: International Classification of Diseases, 9th revision

ICF: immunodeficiency-centromeric instability facial anomalies

ICG: indocyanine green

ICH: intracranial hemorrhage

ICN: intracellular domain of Notch

ICOS: inducible costimulator; inducible T-cell costimulator

ICOSL: inducible costimulator ligand

IDO: indolamine 2,3-dioxygenase

IDS: iduronate 2-sulfatase

IDUA: α-l-iduronidase

IE: ineffective erythropoiesis

IEF: isoelectric focusing

IF: intrinsic factor

IFAR: International Fanconi Anemia Registry

IFI: invasive fungal infection

IFN: interferon

IFN-α: interferon-α

IFN-γ: interferon-γ

IFNGR: interferon γ receptor

IFRT: involved-field radiotherapy

IFS: infantile sarcoma

IgA: immunoglobulin A

IGAD: IgA deficiency

IGF-1: insulin-like growth factor 1

IGFBP: insulin-like growth factor binding protein

IgE: immunoglobulin E

IgG: immunoglobulin G

IgM: immunoglobulin M

IGGSD: IgG subclass deficiency

IHC: immunohistochemistry

IκB: inhibitor of NF-κB

IKBA: inhibitor of NF x-B α chain

IKK: IκB kinase

IL: interleukin

IL-1RA: IL-1 receptor antagonist

IL-2: interleukin-2 (also IL-1, IL-3, IL-4, etc.)

IL2RG: interleukin-2 receptor gamma (IL-2R γ)

IL-6R: interleukin-6 receptor

IL-"X"R: IL-"X" receptor

ILNR: intralobar nephrogenic rests

IMP: inosine 5′-monophosphate; intramembrane particle

IMRT: intensity-modulated radiation therapy

IMT: inflammatory myofibroblastic tumor

iNKT: invariant natural killer T cell

iNOS: inducible nitric oxide synthase

INPC: International Neuroblastoma Pathology Classification

INR: international normalized ratio

INRG: International Neuroblastoma Risk Group

INSS: International Neuroblastoma Staging System

IRS: Intergroup Rhabdomyosarcoma Study

IP₁: isoprostenoid

IP₃: inositol 1,4,5-triphosphate

IPEX: immune dysregulation, polyendocrinopathy, enteropathy, X-linked (syndrome)

IPH: idiopathic pulmonary hemosiderosis

IPT: intraperitoneal fetal transfusion

IRAG: IP₃ receptor–associated cGMP

IRAK-4: interleukin-1 receptor–associated kinase 4

IRE: iron response element, iron responsive element

IREG1: iron-regulated transporter

IRF: interferon regulatory factor

IRIDA: iron-refractory iron deficiency anemia

IRP: IRE-binding protein, iron regulatory protein

IRSS: International Retinoblastoma Staging System

ISBT: International Society for Blood Transfusion

ISC: irreversibly sickled cell

ISH: in situ hybridization

ISHAGE: International Society for Hematotherapy and Graft Engineering

ISI: International Sensitivity Index

ISM: indolent systemic mastocystosis

ISP: intermediate single positive

ISRE: interferon-stimulated response element

IST: immunosuppressive therapy

ISTH: International Society on Thrombosis and Hemostasis

ITAM: immunoreceptor tyrosine–based activation motif, immunoreceptor tyrosine activation motif

ITCH: itchy E3 ubiquitin protein ligase

ITD: internal tandem duplication

ITIM: immunoreceptor tyrosine–based inhibitory motif, immunoreceptor tyrosine activation motif

ITP: immune thrombocytopenia purpura

ITK: IL-2 inducible tyrosine kinase

iTreg: inducible Treg

IVIG: intravenous immune serum globulin, intravenous immunoglobulin

IVS: intervening sequence (intron)

IVT: intravascular transfusion

J

J: joining

JAK: Janus kinase

JAK-STAT: Janus kinase–signal transducer and activator of transcription

JAM-1: junctional adhesion molecule 1

JCML: juvenile chronic myelomonocytic leukemia

JIA: juvenile idiopathic arthritis

JME: juxtamembrane expansion

JMML: juvenile myelomonocytic leukemia

K

kb: kilobase

KCC: K⁺-Cl⁻ cotransporter

K_d: dissociation constant

KD: Kostmann's disease, kyphomelic dysplasia

KEYY: lysine–glutamic acid–tyrosine-tyrosine

KIF1B: kinesin family member 1B

KIR: killer cell immunoglobulin-like receptor

KL: Klotho (gene)

K_m: Michaelis constant

KRAS: v-Ki-ras2 Kirsten rat sarcoma viral oncogene homolog

KTLS: c-Kit⁺, Thy-1ˡᵒ, Lin⁻, Sca-1⁺ cell

KLF4: Krüppel-like factor 4
KLH: keyhole limpet hemocyanic
KSS: Kearns-Sayre syndrome

L

LA: lupus anticoagulant
LAD I: leukocyte adhesion deficiency type I
LAD II: leukocyte adhesion deficiency type II
LAD III: leukocyte adhesion deficiency type III
LAL: lysosomal acid lipase
LAMP-3: lysosome-associated membrane protein 3
LASD: lysosomal autophagy system disease
LAP: localized aggressive periodontitis; leukocyte alkaline phosphatase
LAT: linker for activation of T cells
LCAT: lecithin-cholesterol acyltransferase
Lck: lymphocyte-specific protein tyrosine kinase
LCL: large cell lymphoma
LCR: locus control region
LDH: lactate dehydrogenase
LDHL: lymphocyte-depleted Hodgkin lymphoma
LD-RIPA: low-dose ristocetin-induced platelet aggregation
LDL: low-density lipoprotein
LEF-1: lymphoid enhancer–binding factor 1
LELY: low-expression allele Lyon
LEPRA: low-expression allele Prague
LFA-3: lymphocyte function antigen 3
LFS: Li-Fraumeni syndrome
LGL: large granular lymphocyte leukemia
LHRF: luteinizing hormone–releasing factor
LIC: leukemia-initiating cells
LIF: leukemia inhibitory factor
LIFR: leukemia inhibitory factor receptor
LIG4: DNA ligase IV
LIR: leukocyte immunoglobulin-like receptor
LJP: localized juvenile periodontitis
LL: lymphoblastic lymphoma
LMIC: low- and middle-income countries
LMO2: LIM domain only 2 (rhombotin-like 1)
LMWH: low-molecular-weight heparin
LMWK: low-molecular-weight kininogen
LNR: Lin12-NOTCH repeats
LOH: loss of heterozygosity
LPS: lipopolysaccharide
LRHL: lymphocyte-rich Hodgkin lymphoma
LRP: lipoprotein receptor–related protein
LRRC8: leucine-rich repeat–containing 8
LSD: lysosomal storage disease
LSP1: lymphocyte-specific protein 1
LT: leukotriene
LTB$_4$: leukotriene B$_4$
LTC-IC: long-term culture–initiating cell
LTR: long terminal repeat
LTR-HSCs: long-term–reconstituting hematopoietic stem cells
LW: Landsteiner-Weiner glycoprotein
Lyso-PC: lysophosphatidylcholine
Lys-Plg: lysine plasminogen
LYST: lysosomal trafficking regulator

M

mAbs: monoclonal antibodies
MAGE: melanoma antigen-encoding gene
MAGT1: magnesium transporter protein 1
MAGUK: membrane-associated guanylate kinase
MAIT: mucosa-associated invariant T
MALT1: mucosa-associated lymphoid tissue lymphoma translocation gene 1
MAP: mitogen-activated protein
MAPK: mitogen-activated protein kinase
MARCKS: myristoylated alanine-rich C kinase substrate
MAS: macrophage activation syndrome
MASP: MBL-associated serine protease
MASCC: Multinational Association of Supportive Care in Cancer
Mb: myoglobin
MBD: membrane-binding domain
MBL: mannose-binding lectin
MBP: major basic protein
MCH: mean corpuscular hemoglobin
MCHL: mixed-cellularity Hodgkin lymphoma
MCHC: mean corpuscular hemoglobin concentration
MCL: mast cell leukemia
MCM4: mini-chromosome maintenance-deficient 4
MCP: membrane cofactor protein
MCP-1: monocyte chemotactic protein 1
M-CSF: macrophage colony-stimulating factor
MCV: mean cell volume; mean corpuscular volume
MCV4: meningococcal conjugate vaccine
MCyR: major cytogenetic response
MDCK: Madin-Darby canine kidney (cells)
MDM2: murine double minute 2
MDS: myelodysplastic syndrome
MDWH: metaphyseal dysplasia without hypotrichosis
MeCbl: methylcobalamin
MEK: MAPK kinase
MELAS: mitochondrial myopathy, encephalopathy, lactic acidosis, and strokelike episodes
MEN1: multiple endocrine neoplasia type I
MEP: megakaryocyte, erythroid, and basophil (lineage); megakaryocyte/erythroid precursor
met-Hb: methemoglobin
5-methyl-THF: 5-methyltetrahydrofolate
α$_2$-MG: α$_2$-macroglobulin
MGF: myelomonocytic growth factor
MGP: marginating granulocyte pool
MGSA: melanoma growth stimulatory activity
mHA: minor histocompatibility antigen
MHA: May-Hegglin anomaly
MHC: major histocompatibility complex
MIBG: metaiodobenzylguanidine
micro-PET: micro–positron emission tomography
MIDAS: metal ion–dependent adhesion site
MIM: Mendelian Inheritance in Man
MIP-1α: macrophage inflammatory protein 1α
miR: micro–ribonucleic acid
MIS: minimally invasive surgery
MKI: mitosis-karyorrhexis index
MLASA: mitochondrial myopathy with lactic acidosis and sideroblastic anemia

MLD: metachromatic leukodystrophy
MLL: mixed-lineage leukemia
mM: millimolar
MMA: methylmalonic acid
MMC: mitomycin C
MMF: mycophenolate mofetil
MMP: matrix metalloproteinase
MMP-25: membrane type matrix metalloproteinase 25; the membrane-associated metalloproteinase leukolysin
MoAb: monoclonal antibody
M6P: mannose 6-phosphate
MPD: myeloproliferative disease
MPCF: multiparameter flow cytometry
MPGM: monophosphoglycerate mutase
Mpl: ligand for the myeloproliferative ligand receptor
MPO: myeloperoxidase
MMR: major molecular response
MRP: multidrug resistance-associated protein
MPS: Montreal platelet syndrome, mucopolysaccharidosis
MPS I: mucopolysaccharidosis I
MPS I H: Hurler disease
MPS III: Sanfilippo disease
MPS III A: Sanfilippo disease III A
MPS III B: Sanfilippo disease III B
MPS VI: Maroteaux-Lamy disease
MPS VII: Sly syndrome
MPSV4: meningococcal polysaccharide vaccine
MPV: mean platelet volume
M_r: molecular weight
MRA: magnetic resonance angiography
MRI: magnetic resonance imaging
MRC: Medical Research Council
MRE11A: meiotic recombination 11 homolog A
mRNA: messenger RNA
mRNP: messenger ribonucleoprotein
MRP2: multidrug resistance–associated protein 2 (a.k.a. ABCC2, cMOAT)
MRT: malignant rhabdoid tumor
ms: millisecond
MSC: multipotent mesenchymal stem cells
MSCV: murine stem cell virus
MSH: Multicenter Study of Hydroxyurea
MSH6: MutS homologue 6
MSMD: mendelian susceptibility to mycobacterial diseases
MSP1: *Plasmodium falciparum* merozoite surface protein 1
MST: metanephric stromal tumor
MTD: maximum tolerated dose
mtDNA: mitochondrial DNA
mTEC: medullary thymic epithelial cell
MTHFD1: methylenetetrahydrofolate dehydrogenase (NADP+ dependent) 1
MTHFR: methylenetetrahydrofolate reductase (methylene-THF reductase)
mTOR: mammalian target of rapamycin
MTTP: microsomal triglyceride transfer protein
MTP1: metal tolerance protein 1
Munc: mammalian homolog of *Caenorhabditis elegans* unc

MVB: multivesicular body
MWC: Monod, Wyman, and Changeaux model
MYD88: myeloid differentiation primary response gene (88)
MYHIIA: myosin heavy chain IIA
MYO5A: myosin 5 Va

N

NAA: *N*-acetylaspartate
NACHRI: National Association of Children's Hospitals and Related Institutions
NAD: nicotinamide adenine dinucleotide
NAD 47/89: neutrophil actin dysfunction with 47- and 89-kD protein abnormalities
NADH: reduced nicotinamide adenine dinucleotide
NADP: nicotinamide adenine dinucleotide phosphate
NADPH: reduced nicotinamide adenine dinucleotide phosphate
NAFLD: nonalcoholic fatty liver disease
NAIT: neonatal alloimmune thrombocytopénia
NANT: the New Approaches to Neuroblastoma Therapy consortium
NAP: neutrophil-activating protein
NAP-2: neutrophil-activating protein 2
NAT: nucleic acid testing
NATP: neonatal alloimmune thrombocytopenic purpura
NB-DGJ: *N*-butyldeoxygalactonojirimycin
NBS: Nijmegen breakage syndrome
NBT: nitroblue tetrazolium
NCI: National Cancer Institute
NCV: nerve conduction velocity
NDPase: nucleoside diphosphatase
NE: neutrophil elastase
NEMO: NF-κB essential modulator
NET: neutrophil extracellular trap
NF-1: neurofibromatosis type 1
NF-AT: nuclear factor of activated T cells
NF-κB: nuclear factor κB
NGAL: neutrophil gelatinase–associated lipocalin
NGF: nerve growth factor
NH: neonatal hemochromatosis
NHANES: National Health and Nutrition Examination Survey
NHEJ: nonhomologous end joining
NHL: non-Hodgkin's lymphoma
NHLBI: National Heart, Lung, and Blood Institute
NICU: neonatal intensive care unit
NIH: National Institutes of Health
NIK: NF-κB–inducing kinase
NK: natural killer (cell)
NKT: natural killer T cell
NLR: NOD-like receptor
NLPHL: nodular lymphocyte–predominant Hodgkin lymphoma
nm: nanometer
NMDP: National Marrow Donor Program
NMR: nuclear magnetic resonance
NNJ: neonatal jaundice
NO: nitric oxide
NOD: nonobese diabetic

NOS: nitric oxide synthase
NOX: NAD(P)H oxidase
NPA: Niemann-Pick disease type A
NPB: Niemann-Pick disease type B
NPC: Niemann-Pick disease type C
NR: nephrogenic rest
Nramp2: natural resistance-associated macrophage protein 2
NRAS: neuroblastoma RAS viral (v-ras) oncogene homolog
Nrf-1: nuclear regulatory factor 1
NRTI: nucleoside reverse transcriptase inhibitors
ns: nanosecond
NS: Noonan syndrome
NSAID: nonsteroidal anti-inflammatory drug
NSE: nonspecific esterases
NSCLC: non–small cell lung cancer
NSHL: nodular sclerosis Hodgkin lymphoma
NTBI: non–transferrin-bound iron
NTD: neural tube defect
nTreg: natural Treg
NuMA: nuclear mitotic apparatus (protein)
NWTSG: National Wilms Tumor Study Group

O

O$_2$: oxygen
OATP: organic acid–transporting polypeptide
OCA: oral contraceptive agent
OCS: open canalicular system
OCT1: organic cation transporter-1
ODC1: ornithine decarboxylase–1
OF: osmotic fragility
OGT: orogastric tube
OHCbl: hydroxycobalamin
OLTX: orthotopic liver transplant
OMIM: Online Mendelian Inheritance in Man
OMS: opsoclonus-myoclonus syndrome
OPG: Optic pathway gliomas
OPSI: overwhelming postsplenectomy infection
OR: odds ratio
OS: Omenn syndrome; overall survival
OSA: osteosarcoma
OSM: oncostatin M
OSMR: oncostatin M receptor
oxy-Hb: oxygenated hemoglobin

P

PA: phosphatidic acid
PAF: platelet-activating factor
PAFc: polymerase-associated factor complex
PAGE: polyacrylamide gel electrophoresis
PAI-1: plasminogen activator inhibitor 1
PAIgG: platelet-associated IgG
PALS: periarterial (or periarteriolar) lymphoid sheath
PAMP: pathogen-associated molecular pattern
PANDAS: pediatric autoimmune neuropsychiatric disorders associated with streptococcal infections
PAR: protease-activated receptor
PAS: periodic acid–Schiff

PBG: porphobilinogen
PBG-D: porphobilinogen deaminase
PBREM: phenobarbital-responsive enhancer module
PBSC: peripheral blood stem cell
PC: phosphatidylcholine
PCBP1: poly C–binding protein 1
PCC: prothrombin complex concentrate
PCFT: proton-coupled folate transporter
PCH: paroxysmal cold hemoglobinuria
PCP: *Pneumocystis carinii* pneumonia
PCR: polymerase chain reaction
PCT: porphyria cutanea tarda
PCV: polycythemia vera
PCV7: 7-valent pneumococcal polysaccharide vaccine
PCV23: 23-valent pneumococcal polysaccharide vaccine
PD-1: programmed death 1
PDB: Protein Data Bank
PDGF: platelet-derived growth factor
PDGFB: platelet-derived owth factor β
PE: phosphatidylethanolamine; pulmonary embolism
PEBP2: polyomavirus enhancer–binding protein 2
PECAM-1: platelet–endothelial cell adhesion molecule 1
PEG: polyethylene glycol
PEG-ADA: polyethylene glycol conjugated ADA
PEG-MGDF: pegylated megakaryocyte growth and development factor
PEMR: progressive epilepsy with mental retardation
PET: partial exchange transfusion
PF4: platelet factor 4
PFA-100: Platelet Functional Analyzer 100
PFK: phosphofructokinase
PFS: progression-free survival
PFT: pulmonary function test
PGC-1a: peroxisomal proliferator–activated cofactor 1α
PGD: preimplantation genetic diagnosis
6-PGD: 6-phosphogluconate dehydrogenase
PGI$_2$: prostaglandin I$_2$ (prostacyclin)
PGK: phosphoglycerate kinase
PH: Pleckstrin homology
PHA: phytohemagglutinin
PHS: polycythemia hyperviscosity syndrome
PHT: primary hypertension; pulmonary hypertension
P$_i$: inorganic phosphate
PI: phosphatidylinositol
PIDD: primary immunodeficiency disease
PIG-A: phosphatidylinositol glycan class A (gene: *PIGA*)
PI3: phosphoinositide 3′
PI3K: phosphatidylinositol 3′-kinase
PIK3R2: phosphoinositide-3-kinase, regulatory subunit 2 (beta)
PIP: phosphatidylinositol 4-phosphate
PIP$_2$: phosphatidylinositol 4,5-bisphosphate
PIP$_3$: phosphatidylinositol 3,4,5-triphosphate
PIT: plasma iron turnover
PIVKA: protein induced by vitamin K antagonists
PK: pyruvate kinase
PKA: protein kinase A
PKB: protein kinase B
PKC: protein kinase C
PKG: protein kinase G
PKR: protein kinase regulated by RNA

PLC: phospholipase C
PLCγ: phospholipase Cγ
PLCγ2: phospholipase Cγ2
PLDN: pallidin
PLK1: polo-like kinase–1
PLNR: perilobar nephrogenic rests
PLP: pyridoxal 5-phosphate
PLTP: phospholipid transfer protein
PM: primary myelofibrosis
PMA: phorbol myristate acetate
PMBCL: Primary mediastinal (thymic) large B-cell lymphoma
PMD: AU QUERIED
PML: progressive multifocal leukoencephalopathy
PMN: polymorphonuclear neutrophil
PMPS: Pearson marrow-pancreas syndrome
PMS2: postmeiotic segregation 2
PN: parenteral nutrition
P-5′-N: pyrimidine-5′-nucleotidase
PN2/APP: protease nexin-2/amyloid β-protein precursor
PNET: primary neuroectodermal tumor
PNH: paroxysmal nocturnal hemoglobinuria
POD: PML oncogenic domains
POG: Pediatric Oncology Group
PNP: purine nucleoside phosphorylase
PNPD: purine nucleoside phosphorylase deficiency
PO$_2$: partial pressure of oxygen
PPCA: protective protein cathepsin A
PPO: protoporphyrinogen oxidase
PPP: platelet-poor plasma
PPTID: pineal parenchymal tumor of intermediate differentiation
PPTP: Pediatric Preclinical Testing Program
PR: partial remission
pRBCs: packed red blood cells
PRC2: Polycomb repressive complex 2
PRCA: pure red cell aplasia
PRCC: papillary renal cell carcinoma
PRES: Posterior reversible leukoencephalopathy
PRETEXT: pretreatment imaging-defined staging protocol
PRF1: perforin
PRKDC: protein kinase, DNA-activated, catalytic polypeptide
PROWESS: Protein C Worldwide Evaluation in Severe Sepsis (trial)
PRP: platelet-rich plasma
PRPP: 5-phosphoribosylpyrophosphate
PRR: pattern recognition receptor
PS: Pearson's marrow-pancreas syndrome; phosphatidyl-serine
PSA: prostate-specific antigen
PSD95: postsynaptic density protein of 95 kD
PSGL-1: P-selectin glycoprotein ligand-1
p-SMAC: peripheral central supramolecular activation cluster
PT: prothrombin time
PTB: phosphotyrosine binding
PTD: partial tandem duplication
P-TEFB: positive transcription elongation factor b
PTH: parathyroid hormone

PTK: phosphotyrosine kinase
PTLD: posttransplant lymphoproliferative disease
PTP: posttransfusion purpura
PTS: postthrombotic syndrome
PTT: partial thromboplastin time
PUS1: pseudouridylate synthase 1
PV: polycythemia vera
PXA: Pleomorphic xanthroastrocytomas

Q

QoL: quality of life

R

RA: refractory anemia
RAB27A: member *RAS* oncogene family 27A
RAD: recombinase-activating gene
RAEB: refractory anemia with an excess of blasts
RAEBIT (RAEB-T): RAEB in transformation
RAG: recombination-activating gene
RAG1 and *RAG2*: recombinase activating gene 1 and 2
RANK: receptor activator of nuclear factor κB
RANTES: regulated on activation, normal T-cell expressed and secreted
RAR: retinoic acid receptor
RARS: refractory anemia with ringed sideroblasts
RBC: red blood cell
RCC: renal cell carcinoma
RCT: randomized control trial
RDA: recommended dietary allowance
REAL: Revised European-American Classification of Lymphoid Neoplasms
RECIST: Response Evaluation Criteria in Solid Tumors
REM: rapid eye movement
RES: reticuloendothelial system
RDS: respiratory distress syndrome
RDW: red cell distribution width, red cell volume distribution width
RFC: reduced folate carrier
RFLP: restriction fragment length polymorphism
rFVIIa: recombinant activated factor VII
RFX5: regulatory factor X, 5
RFXANK: regulatory factor X-associated ankyrin-containing protein
RFXAP: regulatory factor X-associated protein
RGD: arginine, glycine, aspartic acid
Rh: rhesus
RhAG: Rh-associated glycoprotein
rhG-CSF: recombinant human granulocyte colony-stimulating factor
RhoH: Ras homology family member H
r-HuEPO: rhEPO, rHuEPO, recombinant human erythropoietin
RIG: retinoic acid–inducible gene
RIAM: Rap1$_{GTP}$-interacting adaptor molecule
RIS: reduction of immunosuppression
RLR: RIG-1–like receptor
RMC: renal medullary carcinoma
RMRP: RNase mitochondrial RNA processing

RNA: ribonucleic acid

rNAPc2: recombinant nematode anticoagulant protein c2

RNP: ribonucleoprotein

ROHHAD: rapid-onset obesity with hypothalamic dysfunction, hypoventilation, and autonomic dysregulation

ROS: reactive oxygen species

RPA: replication protein A

RPE: retinal pigment epithelium

RPL: ribosomal protein of the large ribosomal subunit

RPS: ribosomal protein of the small ribosomal subunit

RPS19: ribosomal protein S19

RR: rate ratio; response rate

rRNA: ribosomal RNA

RS: Rotor syndrome

RSC: reversibly sickled cell

RSP-2: ring surface protein 2

RSV: respiratory syncytial virus

RT: reverse transcriptase

RTA: renal tubular acidosis

RTK: receptor tyrosine kinase; rhabdoid tumor of the kidney

rVIIa: recombinant factor VIIa

RVT: renal vein thrombosis

RVV: Russell viper venom

S

SAA: severe aplastic anemia

SABD: spectrin-actin binding domain

SADNI: specific antibody deficiency with normal immunoglobulins

SAHA: suberoylanilide hydroxamic acid

SAGE: serial analysis of gene expression

SAO: Southeast Asian ovalocytosis

SAP: SLAM-associated protein

SARS: severe acute respiratory syndrome

SBB: Sudan black B

SBDS: Shwachman-Bodian-Diamond syndrome

SCA: sickle cell anemia

Sca-1: stem cell antigen 1

SCI: silent cerebral infarct

SCID: severe combined immunodeficiency disease

SCD: sickle cell disease

SCDSC: subacute combined degeneration of the spinal cord

SCF: stem cell factor

SCFR: stem cell factor receptor

scFv: single-chain variable fragments

SCID: severe combined immunodeficiency

SCN: severe congenital neutropenia

SCNIR: Severe Chronic Neutropenia International Registry

SCT: sacrococcygeal teratomas; stem cell transplantation

SD: standard deviation

SDF-1: stromal cell–derived factor 1

SDS: Shwachman-Diamond syndrome; sodium dodecyl sulfate

SDS-PAGE: sodium dodecyl sulfate–polyacrylamide gel electrophoresis

SEER: Surveillance Epidemiology and End Results

SEGA: subendymal giant cell astrocytoma

SERCA: sarcoplasmic/endoplasmic reticulum Ca^{2+}-ATPase

SF3B1: splicing factor 3B subunit 1

SGD: specific (secondary) granule deficiency

SH2: src homology domain 2

SHD: sex hormone–binding domain

SH2D1A: SH2-containing protein 1A, Src homology 2 domain–containing protein

Shh: Sonic hedgehog

SHIP1: SH2 domain–containing inositol 5′-phosphatase 1

sHLH: secondary hemophagocytic lymphohistiocytosis

SHML: sinus histiocytosis with massive lymphadenopathy

SHP-2: SH2 domain–containing protein tyrosine phosphatase-2

SIFD: sideroblastic anemia, immunodeficiency, fever, and developmental delay

SIGAD: selective IgA deficiency

sIgM: surface IgM

SIOP: International Society of Paediatric Oncology

SIR: standardized incidence ratio

SIV: simian immunodeficiency virus

S-JIA: systemic onset juvenile idiopathic arthritis

SLAM: signaling lymphocyte activation molecule

SLC4A: solute carrier family 4A

SLC11A2: solute carrier family 11, member 2

SLC19A2: solute carrier family 19 (thiamine transporter), member 2

SLC25A37: solute carrier family 25 (mitochondrial iron transporter), member 37

SLC40A1: solute carrier family 40 member 1

SLE: systemic lupus erythematosus

SL-IC: severe combined immunodeficiency (SC)-ID mouse leukemia–initiating cell

SLP3: stomatin-like protein 3

SLP76: SH2 domain–containing leukocyte protein of 76 kD

SM: sphingomyelin; systemic mastocytosis

SMAC: supramolecular activation cluster

SMARCAL1: SWI/SNF related, matrix associated, actin dependent regulator of chromatin, subfamily a-like 1

SMC3 and SMC1A: structural maintenance of chromosomes 3 and 1A

SMD: spondylometaphyseal dysplasia

SMMHC: smooth muscle myosin heavy chain

SMN: second malignant neoplasms

Smo: Smoothened receptor

SMRT: silencing mediator of retinoid and thyroid receptors

SNARE: soluble N-ethylmaleimide–sensitive attachment protein receptor

snoRNA: small nucleolar RNA

SNP: single nucleotide polymorphism

SOCbl: sulfitocobalamin

SOCS: suppressor of cytokine signaling

SOD2: superoxide dismutase 2

SOS: sinusoidal obstruction syndrome; son of sevenless (protein)

SOT: solid organ transplantation

S-PCT: sporadic porphyria cutanea tarda

SP: single-positive

SP110: SP110 nuclear body protein
SPD: storage pool deficiency
sPLA2: secretory phospholipase A_2
SQUID: superconducting quantum interference device
SRC: SCID-reconstituting cell
SREBP: sterol regulatory element-binding proteins
SRT: substrate reduction therapy
SSCP: single-strand conformation polymorphism
SSP: stage-selector protein
STAG: stromal antigen 2
STAT: signal transducer and activator of transcription
STEAP3: six-transmembrane epithelial antigen of prostate 3
sTfR: serum transferrin receptor
STIM1: stromal interacting molecule 1
STOP: Stroke Prevention Trial in Sickle Cell Anemia
STR-HSC: short-term–reconstituting hematopoietic stem cell
Stx: Shiga-like toxin
STX11: syntaxin 11
STXBP2: syntaxin binding protein 2
SUMF1: sulfatase-modifying factor
SVC: superior vena cava
SWI/SNF: switch/sucrose nonfermentable
SWiTCH: Stroke With Transfusions Changing to Hydroxyurea study

T

TACI: transmembrane activator and calcium modulator and cyclophilin ligand interactor
TACL: Therapeutic Advances in Childhood Leukemia and Lymphoma consortium
TAFI: thrombin-activatable fibrinolysis inhibitor
TALEN: transcription activator-like effector nucleases
T-ALL: T-cell acute lymphoblastic leukemia
T antigen: Thomsen-Friedenreich cryptoantigen
TAM: transient abnormal myelopoiesis
TAMs: tumor-associated macrophages
TAMV: time-averaged maximum velocity
TAP1 or TAP2: transporter associated with antigen processing 1 or 2
TAPS: Alternatives Preoperatively in SCD
TAPA1: target of antiproliferative antibody 1
TAR: thrombocytopenia–absent radius (syndrome)
TAT: thrombin-antithrombin complex
TBI: total-body irradiation
TBK1: TANK-binding kinase 1
TBP: TATA-binding protein
TBX1: T-box 1
TcB: transcutaneous bilirubin
TCD: transcranial Doppler
TCDD: 2,3,7,8-tetrachlorodibenzo-*p*-dioxin
TCN2: transcobalamin II
TCR: T-cell antigen receptor, T-cell receptor
TCT: thrombin clotting time
TD: thymus dependent (antigen)
TdT: terminal deoxyribonucleotidyl transferase
TE: thromboembolism
TEC: transient erythroblastopenia of childhood
TEG: thromboelastography

TEMRA: T effector memory cell CD45RA+
TERT: telomerase reverse transcriptase
TF: tissue factor
TFEB: transcription factor EB
TFH: follicular helper T cell
TFPI: tissue factor pathway inhibitor
TFR2: transferrin receptor 2
TGA: thrombin generation assay
TGN: thioguanine nucleotides
TGF-β: transforming growth factor β
TGTP: 6-thioguanosine 5-triphosphate
TH: tyrosine hydroxylase
tHcy: plasma total homocysteine
THF: 5,6,7,8-tetrahydrofolate
THI: transient hypogammaglobulinemia of infancy
TI: thymus independent (antigen)
TIA: transient ischemic attack
TIBC: total iron-binding capacity
TIC: tumor-initiating cell
TICAM1: TIR domain-containing adapter molecule 1
TIMP: tissue inhibitor of matrix metalloproteinase-2
TIPS: intrahepatic portosystemic shunting
TKI: tyrosine kinase inhibitor
TL: transient leukemia
TLR: Toll-like receptor
TLR2: Toll-like receptor 2
TLS: translesion synthesis
TLT-1: TREM cells–like transcript-1
TM: tropomyosin
TMC: transmembrane channel-like
TMD: transient myeloproliferative disorder
TM8: transmembrane domain 8
TMD: transient myeloproliferative disorder
TMod: tropomodulin
TMP-SMX: trimethoprim-sulfamethoxazole
TMPRSS6: transmembrane protease, serine 6
7-TMR: seven-transmembrane–spanning receptor
7-TMS: seven-transmembrane–spanning domain
TNF: tumor necrosis factor
TNF-α: tumor necrosis factor-α
TNFRSF: TNF receptor superfamily
TNFSF: TNF superfamily
TNM: tumor-nodes-metastasis
TOF: time-of-flight (imaging)
TORCH: toxoplasmosis, rubella, cytomegalovirus, and herpesvirus infections
tPA: tissue plasminogen activator
TPE: therapeutic plasma exchange
TPH: transplacental hemorrhage
TPI: triose phosphate isomerase
TPMT: thiopurine methyltransferase
TPN: total parenteral nutrition
TPO: thrombopoietin
TPOR: thrombopoietin receptor
TPR: tetratricopeptide repeat
TQM: total quality management
TRAF: TNF receptor–associated factor
TRAF3: TNF receptor-associated factor 3
TRAIL: tumor necrosis factor–related apoptosis-inducing ligand
TRALI: transfusion-related acute lung injury

TRAP: Trial to Reduce Alloimmunization to Platelets
TREC: T-cell receptor excision circle, T-cell receptor gene excision circle
Treg: T-regulatory
TREM, TREM-1, TREM-2: triggering receptor expressed on myeloid cells (1, 2, etc)
TfR: transferrin receptor
TRIF: Toll-interleukin-1 receptor domain-containing adapter protein inducing interferon β
TRJV: tricuspid regurgitant jet velocity
TRK: tropomyosin receptor kinase
TRM: treatment-related mortality
TRMA: thiamine-responsive megaloblastic anemia
tRNA: transfer RNA
TSB: total serum bilirubin
TSH: thyroid-stimulating hormone
TSLC: tumor suppressor in lung cancer–1
TSLP: thymic stromal thymopoietin
TT: thrombin time
TTP: thrombotic thrombocytopenic purpura
TTT: transpupillary thermotherapy
TTTS: twin-twin transfusion syndrome
TVTG: topotecan, vinorelbine, thiotepa, dexamethasone, and gemcitabine
TWSG1: twisted gastrulation 1
TXA$_2$: thromboxane A$_2$
TYK2: tyrosine kinase 2
TYMS: thymidylate synthetase

U

UBIL: unconjugated bilirubin
UCB: umbilical cord blood
UDP: uridine diphosphate
UDPG: uridine diphosphate glucose
UDPGA: uridine diphosphate glucuronic acid
UDPGT1: Uridine diphosphogluconosyl transferase 1
UDPNAG: uridine diphosphate N-acetylglucosamine
UGT1A1: UDP glucuronosyltransferase 1A1 gene
UKCCG: United Kingdom Children's Cancer Group
ULVWF: unusually large multimers of VWF
UMP: uridine monophosphate
UNC: unc homolog (C. elegans)
UNG: uracil nucleoside glycosylase
UNOS: United Network of Organ Sharing
uPA: urokinase plasminogen activator
uPAR: uPA receptor
UPR: unfolded protein response
URD: unrelated donor
URO-D: uroporphyrinogen decarboxylase
URO3-S: uroporphyrinogen III synthase
UTI: urinary tract infection
UTP: uridine triphosphate
UTR: untranslated regions
UV: ultraviolet

V

V: variable
VACTERL: vertebral abnormalities, anal atresia, cardiac abnormalities, tracheoesophageal fistula, and/or esoph-ageal atresia, renal agenesis and dysplasia, and limb defects
VAMP-1, -2: vesicle-associate membrane protein 1, 2, etc
VASP: vasodilator-stimulated phosphoprotein
VATER: vertebral defects, imperforate anus, tracheo-esophageal fistula, renal defects and radial dysplasia
VCA: viral capsid antigen
VCAM-1: vascular cell adhesion molecule 1
Vd: volume of distribution
VDJ: variable, diversity, joining
VDRL: Venereal Disease Research Laboratory
VEGF: vascular endothelial growth factor
VHL: von Hippel-Lindau (protein)
VK: vitamin K
VK1: phylloquinone
VK2: menaquinone
VKDB: vitamin K–dependent bleeding
VKDP: vitamin K–dependent protein
VKOR: vitamin K 2,3-epoxide reductase
VLA-4: very late antigen 4
VLBW: very low birth weight
VLDL: very-low-density lipoproteins
VOD: veno-occlusive disease
VODI: veno-occlusive disease with immunodeficiency
VP: variegate porphyria
VP-16: etoposide
VTE: venous thromboembolism
V/Q: ventilation-perfusion
VWD: von Willebrand disease
VWF: von Willebrand factor
VWF:Ag: von Willebrand factor antigen
VWF:CB: collagen-binding assay for von Willebrand factor
VWFpp: von Willebrand factor propeptide
VWF:RCo: VWF activity by ristocetin cofactor assay
VZV: varicella-zoster virus

W

WAGR: Wilms tumor, Aniridia, Genitourinary abnor-malities, and Retardation
WAS: Wiskott-Aldrich syndrome
WASP: Wiskott-Aldrich syndrome protein
WBC: white blood cell
WBRT: whole-brain radiotherapy
WHIM: warts, hypogammaglobulinemia, infections, myelokathexis (syndrome)
WIP: WASP-interacting protein
WIPF1: WAS/WASL interacting protein family, member 1
WNDP: Wilson disease protein
WNV: West Nile virus
WRK: Woodward's reagent K
WSXWS: Trp-Ser-Xaa-Trp-Ser

X

X-CGD: X-linked chronic granulomatous disease
XHIM: X-linked immunodeficiency with normal or ele-vated IgM
XIAP: X-linked inhibitor of apoptosis

XLA: X-linked agammaglobulinemia
XLF: XRCC4-like factor
XLP1, XLP2: X-linked lymphoproliferative syndrome type 1 and 2
XLPD: X-linked lymphoproliferative disease
XLSA: X-linked sideroblastic anemia
XLSA/A: X-linked sideroblastic anemia with ataxia
XLT: X-linked thrombocytopenia
XPD: xeroderma pigmentosum disease
XRT: x-ray therapy; pulmonary radiation therapy
XSCID: X-linked severe combined immunodeficiency

Y

YARS2: tyrosyl-tRNA synthetase 2, mitochondrial
YTRF: tyrosine-threonine-arginine-phenylalanine (sequence)

Z

ZAP-70: TCRζ–associated protein of 70 kD
ZBTB24: zinc-finger and bric-a-brac, tramtrack, broad complex-domain-containing 24
ZIP: zinc transporter
ZFN: zinc-finger nucleases
ZPI: protein Z–dependent protease inhibitor
ZPP: zinc protoporphyrin

BIOLOGY OF CANCER

CHAPTER 39

Origins and Evolution of Pediatric Cancers

Mel Greaves

CHAPTER OUTLINE

PEDIATRIC VERSUS ADULT CANCERS

CHILDHOOD ACUTE LYMPHOBLASTIC LEUKEMIA AS A MODEL OF CLONAL EVOLUTION

EVOLUTIONARY PENETRANCE OF DISEASE

EVOLUTIONARY DYNAMICS AND CLINICAL OUTCOME

"Nothing in biology makes sense except in the light of evolution" was Dobzhansky's bold but persuasive claim, and nothing is as natural in biology as natural selection. It has been occurring for approximately 3 billion years whenever heritable traits vary in replicating populations, affecting the survival and reproductive fitness of molecules, unicellular or multicellular organisms, each in the face of environmental selective pressures.

When complex multicellular organisms evolved some 600 million years ago,[1] the potential for individual cells to be selectable, or to clone, was suppressed or rendered subservient to the fitness of the entire individual.[1] Two classic exceptions to this rule exist, however: the immune system and cancer. In the former, lymphoid cells genetically diversify their immunoglobulin heavy chain in B cells or T-cell receptor in T cells antigen recognition gene segments by recombinase-mediated rearrangement[2] to produce more than 10^{11} potentially selectable variants, collectively covering the recognition of essentially any infectious antigenic epitope. This naturally selected or adaptive system is under tight network control, although collapse of regulation can result in autoimmune disease or lymphoid cell cancers.

All pediatric and adult cancers are nonphysiologic, nonbeneficial clonal evolutions that follow the same rules of engagement as speciation in ecosystems (Fig. 39-1).[3] They are, in essence, breaking a 600-million-year-old covenant. It has been known for some time that cancer is a paradigmatic Darwinian, adaptive system.[4] The implications for cancer risk, progression of disease, prognosis, drug resistance, and clinical response have only more recently been appreciated.[3,5,6] Genomics has contributed significantly to this sharpness of focus,[7] just as it has reinforced the underlying principles of evolutionary phylogeny and natural selection of species and variants.[8,9] As in speciation, what emerges in cancer in terms of

functionally important mutations (the so-called *drivers*) or subclones is the consequence of selective pressures exercised via the tissue habitat or ecosystem (Fig. 39-2), with outcome being heavily modulated both by variation in inherited susceptibility and by chance. Inherited susceptibility is a marked feature of pediatric cancers, both in terms of familial syndromes and in sporadic cases with little or no family history, as revealed by genomewide association studies.[10-13] The element of chance applies in both cancer and evolution in general because mutations arise throughout the genome in a stochastic manner and independently of the functions encoded by particular genes.[14] For mutations to have a functional impact in cancer requires that they occur in a manner that alters protein function (and consequently cell fitness) and in the appropriate context with respect to cell type and the presence (or absence) of other mutations with which they may be epistatic or interactive. The vast majority of mutations are neutral passengers of no consequence. The mutations we see recurrently are the result of natural or therapeutic selection.

As clones evolve over time (within a few years for most pediatric cancers compared with decades for adult carcinomas) they also move in space or throughout tissue ecosystems, both within the primary site and to secondary sites.[15,16] This characteristic has important implications for biopsy-based sampling, because anything other than the complete tumor will be a biased selection of subclones.[3] This phenomenon has been well documented for adult cancers, and we assume that the same phenomenon must apply to most if not all pediatric solid tumors.

In evolutionary or Darwinian selection, it is the phenotype that is the focus of selectability—for example, a predator with sharp teeth, a thermoresistant bacteria, or a drug-resistant bacterium or cell. In addition, stable phenotypes are initiated and sustained by genotypic

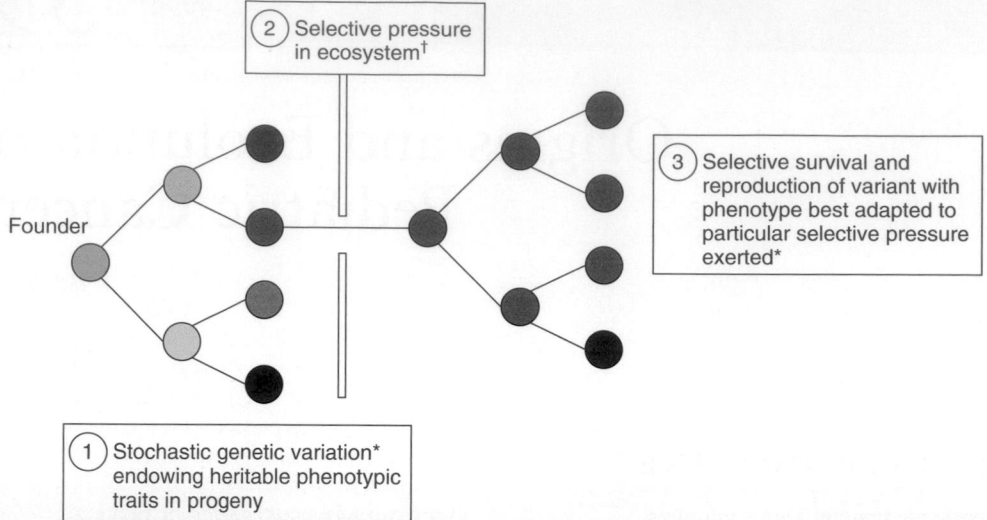

Figure 39-1 Principles of evolution by natural selection. *Different colored circles* represent genetic variants. If selection is stringent, there may be a selective sweep (winner takes all), as shown in the figure, with one or a few individuals surviving. A selective sweep may occur in key junctures in the evolution of cancer—for example, with in situ carcinoma to invasive cancer transition in adults, with metastases (which are usually monoclonal), and with the emergence of drug-resistant mutants in postchemotherapy relapse or recurrence. However, note that winners can become losers if the selective conditions change; as George Williams noted, "Evolution has no eyes to the future." *Must be present in germ cells for sexually reproducing multicellular organism selection, or, in cancer, in self-renewing stem cells.[22] †A wide variety of selective pressures exist in a diverse ecosystem, including interspecies competition for limited resources (food or mates), predation, and climatic factors.

alterations that are either mutational or epigenetic. However, any evolutionary system must have a "unit of selection," which is defined classically as any unit that replicates and in which a stable phenotype is linked to survival and/or reproductive success.[17] For bacteria and protists, this unit is the single cell. For multicellular organisms, it is the entire individual.[1] For cancer it will be somatic cells but probably not every cancer cell. The key attribute of any unit of selection is extensive replicative potential plus expression of the selectable phenotype. Extensive replication capacity, or self-renewal, is the key and exclusive feature of cancer stem cells.[18] The numbers of stem cells vary greatly in individual cancers and are generally increased in frequency with progression of

disease and clinical malignancy.[19] In addition, the stem cell state may not be entirely stable, and under some circumstances (microenvironmental or mutational), non–stem cell progenitors can acquire or reacquire stem cell status.[20,21] Despite these variables, it is likely that cancer stem cells are the units of selection that drive and sustain the evolution of cancer clones and are the repositories of drug resistance.[22]

PEDIATRIC VERSUS ADULT CANCERS

All cancers are consequences of stable variation in somatic cells that facilitate clonal escape.[23] However, fundamental differences exist between pediatric and adult cancers

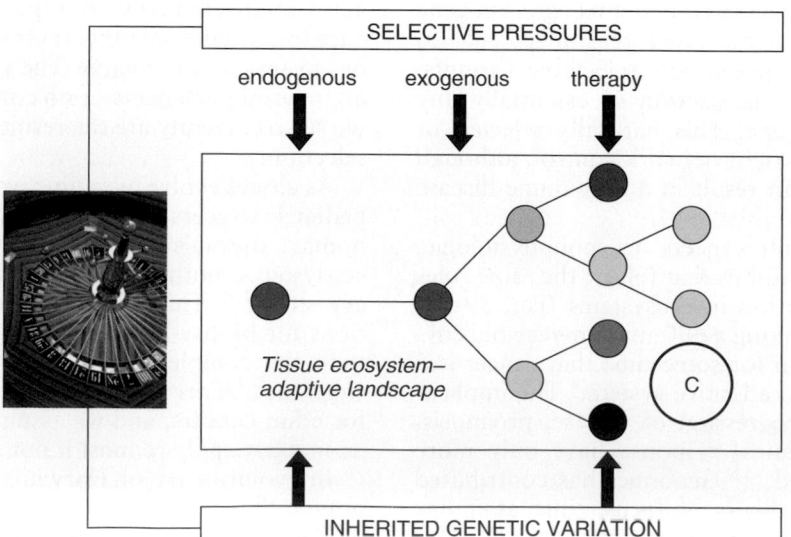

Figure 39-2 Determinants of clonal selection in cancer. The *roulette wheel* represents chance. *Different colored* circles represent genetically distinct cancer cells. C, Cancer.

TABLE 39-1   Differences Between Pediatric and Adult Cancers

Variable	Pediatric	Adult
Predominant lineage origins	Transient/developmental tissue progenitors in embryo and fetus Fetal blood	Epithelia Adult blood
Time frame of natural history	Months to 15 yr	2-3 decades
Number of "driver" mutations required	2 (?)	5-8 (?)
Genetic instability	Rare	Common
Major risk factors	Endogenous proliferative stress (?)	Genotoxic exposures, persistent proliferative stress (hormonal), or infection
Cumulative risk	~1 in 800 (0-15 yr)	~1 in 3 (16-90 yr)
Age-associated incidence distribution	Defined, age-linked peak incidence in infancy or childhood	Increases as power of age*

*Some exceptions are testicular cancer and Hodgkin lymphoma in young adults and choriocarcinoma.

(Table 39-1). The most striking of these differences is the context of tissue or cell type involved, which in turn can be rationalized in terms of underlying risk factors. Most adult cancers are the consequences of protracted environmental or lifestyle exposures to epithelia.[24] In contrast, most pediatric cancers can best be viewed as developmental accidents arising during very restricted windows of tissue morphogenesis in the embryo or fetus when particular stem or progenitor cells are proliferating.[25-27] This view is supported by the finding that many of the inherited gene variants that contribute to the risk of pediatric cancer[11,13] and many of the somatic mutations that are restricted to the cancer cells themselves[28] are encoded by genes that are critical for the normal developmental biology and differentiation of the cells involved. Very few pediatric cancers are attributable to any known in utero external exposure (i.e., via the pregnant mother), despite an epidemiologic quest to find them lasting decades. This is not to say that pediatric cancers are not subject to variable risk factors. Aside from inherited variation in susceptibility, the numbers of cells at risk and proliferative stress may play a part. Higher birth weight is consistently associated with excess risk of pediatric cancer[29] and may operate by simply increasing the number of proliferating "target" cells at risk. Patterns or timing of infection (especially in affluent, "hygienic" societies) may promote or trigger the clinical development of childhood B-cell precursor acute lymphoblastic leukemia (ALL).[30] This mechanism is likely to operate via proliferative stress on preleukemic clones that are generated in utero (rather than via specific viral transformation).[30] Similarly, the striking peak of incidence of long bone osteosarcoma in adolescents might reflect the clinical emergence of a cancer initiated long before (prenatally) but promoted by the proliferative stress of the long bone growth spurt associated with puberty.[31]

A few types of cancer occur in both children and ageing adults, with acute leukemias and gliomas being clear examples. However, it is interesting that the genetics or mutational spectrum of these cancers,[32] and probably their etiology, is very different according to age. Two nonexclusive "seed or soil" interpretations of this distinction have been proposed. One interpretation is that the mutations are different because the microenvironments and selective pressures are different, resulting in different mutant genes providing clonal advantage. A second interpretation is that the mutations are cell context–sensitive and that the cell type of origin is different and developmentally constrained. Evidence for the latter interpretation came from mouse modeling of the impact of GATA1 mutations, which revealed that the cellular targets that, with this mutation, lead to acute megakaryocytic leukemia in infants with Down syndrome, are developmentally restricted to the yolk sac and fetal liver.[33]

The tissue distribution, composite phenotypes (or cell type), and gene expression profiles of pediatric cancers provide a strong indication of the possible lineage and cell type or origin,[34-38] and this indication is endorsed by animal models (Table 39-2).[39-41] Subtypes of some cancers, such as medulloblastoma, may have distinct developmental origins.[42] No unambiguous way exists to identify precisely when and where any childhood cancer is initiated by somatic mutations. Most mutations are assumed to originate prenatally either in the embryo or the developing fetus, possibly when the cell lineage stem or progenitor cell "targets" are under maximum risk from proliferation.[43]

CHILDHOOD ALL AS A MODEL OF CLONAL EVOLUTION

Childhood leukemias lend themselves to interrogation of their natural history more than any other pediatric cancer type. This situation occurs because, although it is initiated in tissue sites such as fetal liver, bone marrow, or thymus, the clone disseminates very readily into the accessible blood, including in the early stages of clinical covert natural history, such as at the birth of the child. Figure 39-3 illustrates a minimal two-stage model proposed for the development of the common form of B-cell precursor ALL in children.[30,44] The challenge was to backtrack clonal history from the point of diagnosis when the genetic features of the clone were definable. For this task, chromosome translocation–generated chimeric gene fusion sequences are the ideal markers for clonal tracking, as illustrated in Figure 39-4 for the most frequent of such fusion genes, ETV6-RUNX1 (formerly TEL-AML1).[45,46] Three tactics have been successfully adopted for backtracking clonal history in ALL (Fig. 39-5),[44,47] and collectively they have provided persuasive evidence for the in utero origin of disease and the two-step model that has been proposed. Formal proof of a prenatal origin of other

TABLE 39-2 Developmental, Lineage Origins of Pediatric Cancers

1. Central nervous system	Gliomas	Glial precursor (different brain regions)
	Ependymoma	Radial glial cells
	Medulloblastoma*	
	(i)	Cerebellum (granule neuron precursor cells)
	(ii)	Dorsal brain stem
2. Neuroblastoma		Embryonic neural crest cells
3. Rhabdomyosarcoma		Muscle stem/progenitor cells (Satellite cells?)
4. Hepatoblastoma		Embryonic liver precursor cells (?)
5. Osteosarcoma		Bone progenitor cells
6. Retinoblastoma		Embryonal retinoblasts
7. Ewing sarcoma		Mesenchymal stem cells (?)
8. Wilms tumor		Embryonic urogenital ridge (mesenchymal) progenitor/stem cells
9. Acute leukemias		Fetal, hematopoietic stem/progenitor cells
	(i) Childhood ALL	B (or T) progenitor cells (fetal liver or bone marrow)
	(ii) Infant ALL	Fetal B/monocytic progenitor?
	(iii) AML	Myeloid restricted stem/progenitor cells
	(iv) Down syndrome AMKL	Fetal liver megakaryocytic erythroid progenitors

ALL, Acute lymphoblastic leukemia; *AMKL*, acute megakaryoblastic leukemia; *AML*, acute myelogenous leukemia.
*More distinctive subtypes in terms of cellular and anatomic origin probably exist than are listed here.

pediatric cancers is not available, although the very young age of many patients at diagnosis and the embryonal phenotypes of some make a prenatal origin very likely.[43] The oldest age at diagnosis of ALL to date with backtracking evidence for an in utero origin is 14 years.[48] However, it is possible that some leukemias and other tumors in older children and even young adults are initiated prenatally with a protracted clinically silent latent period—for example, osteosarcoma in teenagers and testicular cancer in adults in their twenties and thirties.[37] This scenario has yet to be formally assessed, however.

Monozygotic twins with concordant or discordant clinical ALL have been especially informative in defining the sequence of prenatal and later secondary but essential genetic hits (Fig. 39-6, *A* and *B*).[47,49,50,51] These data strongly suggest that fusion genes (or hyperdiploidy) are common initiating, prenatal genetic events in childhood

ALL. This suggestion is supported by modeling experiments with murine and human blood cells, which indicate that *ETV6-RUNX1* can initiate a preleukemic phenotype but that additional genetic changes are required for progression of disease and overt clinical ALL.[52,53] When coupled with in-depth second-generation, whole-genome sequencing, it becomes possible to define the genetic landscape of ALL as assembled via the two independent prenatal and postnatal steps (Fig. 39-7).

This explanation still leaves unclear how the "set" of secondary abnormalities (copy number alterations and single nucleotide variants) are accrued; that is, are they sequentially acquired, and if so, does this acquisition occur in any preferential order or as some type of bolus? This question has been resolved by single-cell genetic analysis and inferred clonal phylogeny (Fig. 39-8).[54,55] The striking—although, from an evolutionary perspective, not

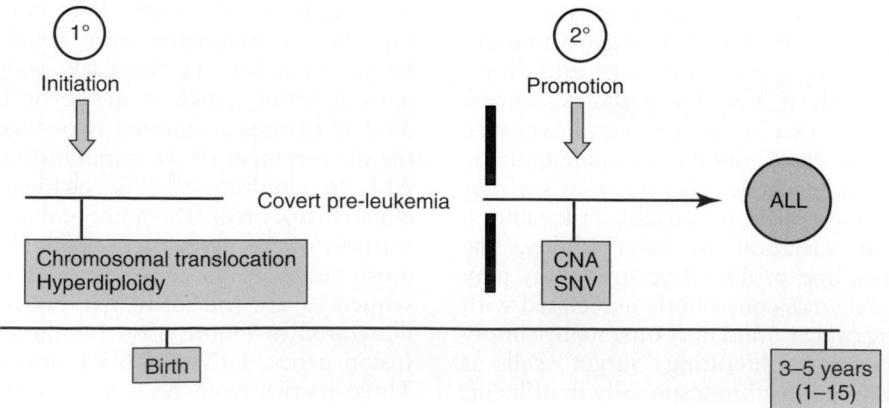

Figure 39-3 A two-step model for childhood acute lymphoblastic leukemia (ALL). *CNA,* Copy number (gene/locus/chromosome) alteration (i.e., gain or loss from diploid normal), identified by single nucleotide polymorphism arrays; *SNV,* single nucleotide variant (or mutation), identified by exome sequencing; *3-5 years,* peak age incidence of diagnosis; *1-15 years,* age range of diagnoses in B-cell precursor ALL (hyperdiploid or *ETV6-RUNX1*⁺). (*Modified from Greaves M: Infection, immune responses and the aetiology of childhood leukaemia. Nat Rev Cancer 6:193–203, 2006.*)

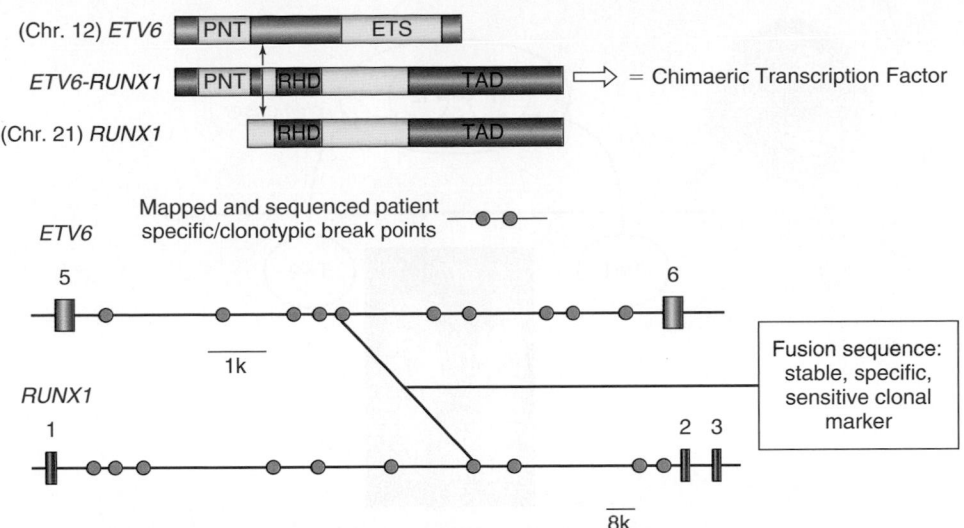

Figure 39-4 The t(12;21) *ETV6-RUNX1* gene fusion in acute lymphoblastic leukemia. *Circles* represent individual, patient-specific (clonotypic) break points determined by long-range polymerase chain reaction amplification of genomic deoxyribonucleic acid, sequencing, and mapping. The diagram is for the purpose of illustration. Actual sequencing mapping data is provided in references 80 and 81. *Chr,* Chromosome; *ETS,* Ets domain (DNA binding); *PNT,* pointed domain (dimerisation); *RHD,* runt homology domain (DNA binding and interaction with CBFb); *TAD,* transactivation domain.

surprising—result is the branching clonal architecture, which is now seen as a hallmark feature of cancer,[3,7] just as it is seen as a hallmark feature of biological speciation and evolution in general (Fig. 39-9). Relapse can originate from within either major or minor subclones that are present at diagnosis[54,56] and can involve positive selection of prior, very rare subclones with mutations that render these cells resistant to particular drug therapies.[57] An implication of these data is that a patient with ALL (and other pediatric cancers) has multiple subclones with malignant potential. This implication in turn implies that

distinct subclones should be generated and sustained by genetically distinct (and diverse) self-renewing stem cells. This situation has been shown to be the case for ALL by comparing single-cell genetics and clonal phylogenies of diagnostic samples with those generated by serial transplantation in NOD/SCID-IL2Rγ[-/-] (NSG) mice.[54] Stem cells are the "units of selection" in the evolutionary development of cancer,[22] and as such their genetic diversity and plasticity of phenotype (including quiescence option) is a key or even possibly the key parameter in clinical outcome.

- Monozygotic (monochorionic) twins with concordant ALL
    comparative genomics

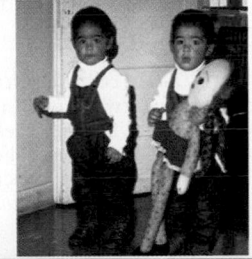

- Archived neonatal blood spots (Guthrie cards) of patients with ALL
    clonotypic fusion gene sequences

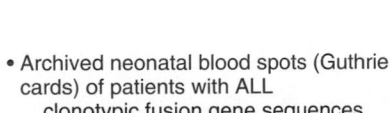

- Frozen cord bloods
  - patients with ALL (rare)
  - unselected cohort
    fusion gene[+] preleukemic clones

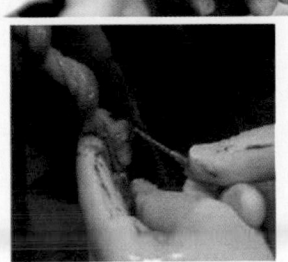

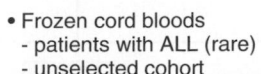

Figure 39-5 Three strategies for backtracking the prenatal origins of childhood leukemia. *ALL,* Acute lymphoblastic leukemia. (*Reviewed in references* 44 *and* 47. *The photograph of the twins is used with the permission of the parents.*)

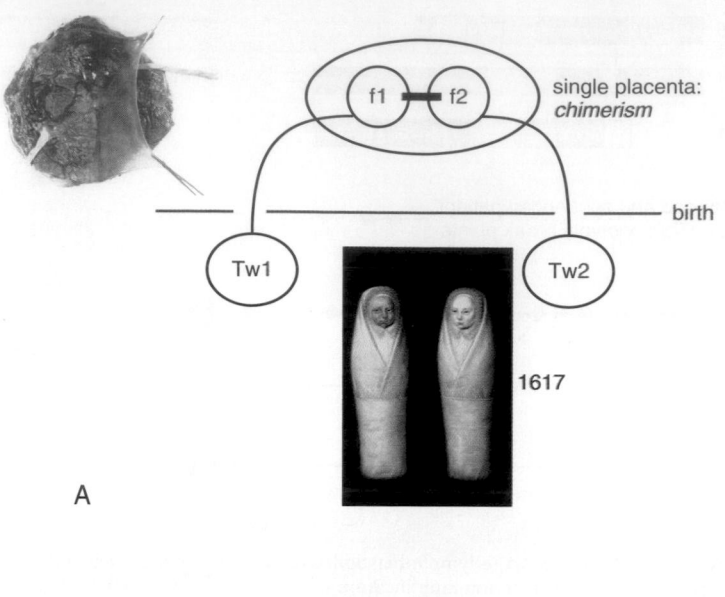

A

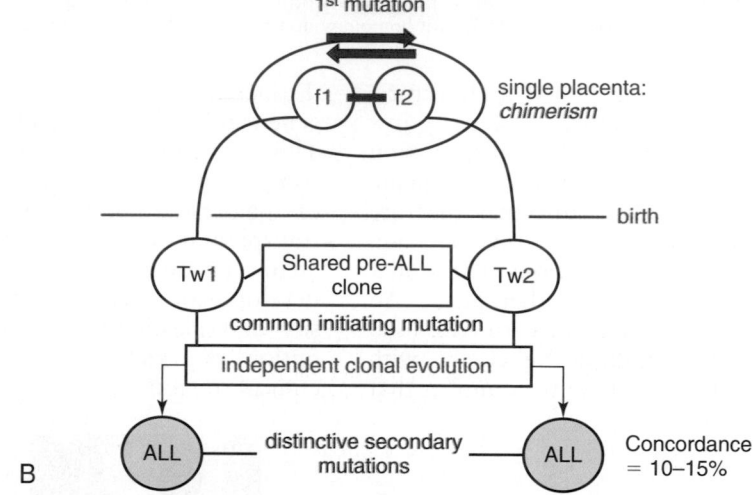

B

Figure 39-6 Leukemia in identical twins. **A,** Blood cell chimerism in monozygotic, monochorionic twins. The photograph of the twins is from a 1617 painting of Dutch twins who likely had twin-twin transfusion syndrome (the twin on the right is anemic and the one on the left is polycythemic, which is a common morbidity of twinning). The upper left photograph is of a single (monochorionic) placenta. Two cords are visible at 2 and 7 o'clock. **B,** Concordance of leukemia and divergent clonal evolution in monozygotic, monochorionic twins. *ALL,* Acute lymphoblastic leukemia; *f1, f2,* two fetuses with shared blood circulation (via vascular anastomoses); *Tw1, Tw2,* two twins after birth. *(A, Photograph of painting of twins from Berger HM, de Waard F, Molenaar Y: A case of twin-to-twin transfusion in 1617. Lancet 356:847–848, 2000.)*

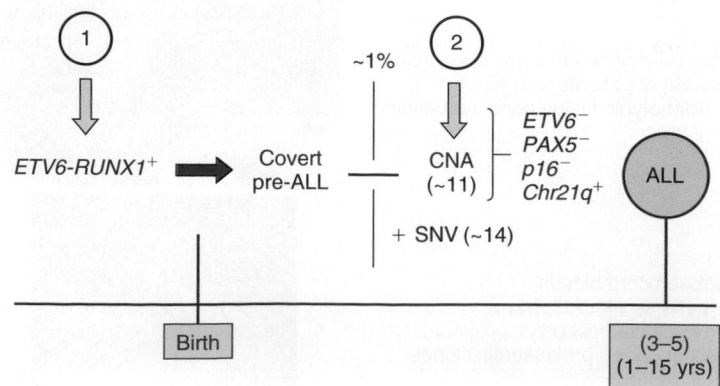

Figure 39-7 Sequential evolution in B cell precursor acute lymphoblastic leukemia (ALL). *Chr21q+,* Extra copy of most of long arm of chromosome 21; *CNA,* copy number alterations (~7): average number per patient sample; *ETV6⁻, PAX5⁻,* one copy/heterozygous loss of *ETV6; p16⁻,* loss of one copy of *p16/CDKN2A; SNV,* single nucleotide variants, nonsynonymous (~7): average number per patient sample; *3-5 years,* peak age incidence of diagnosis; *1-15 years,* age range of diagnosis of *ETV6-RUNX1⁺* ALL; *~1%,* probability of transition between covert preleukemia and overt, clinically silent diagnosed ALL. *(From Mori H, Colman SM, Xiao Z, et al: Chromosome translocations and covert leukemic clones are generated during normal fetal development. Proc Natl Acad Sci U S A 99:8242–8247, 2002.)*

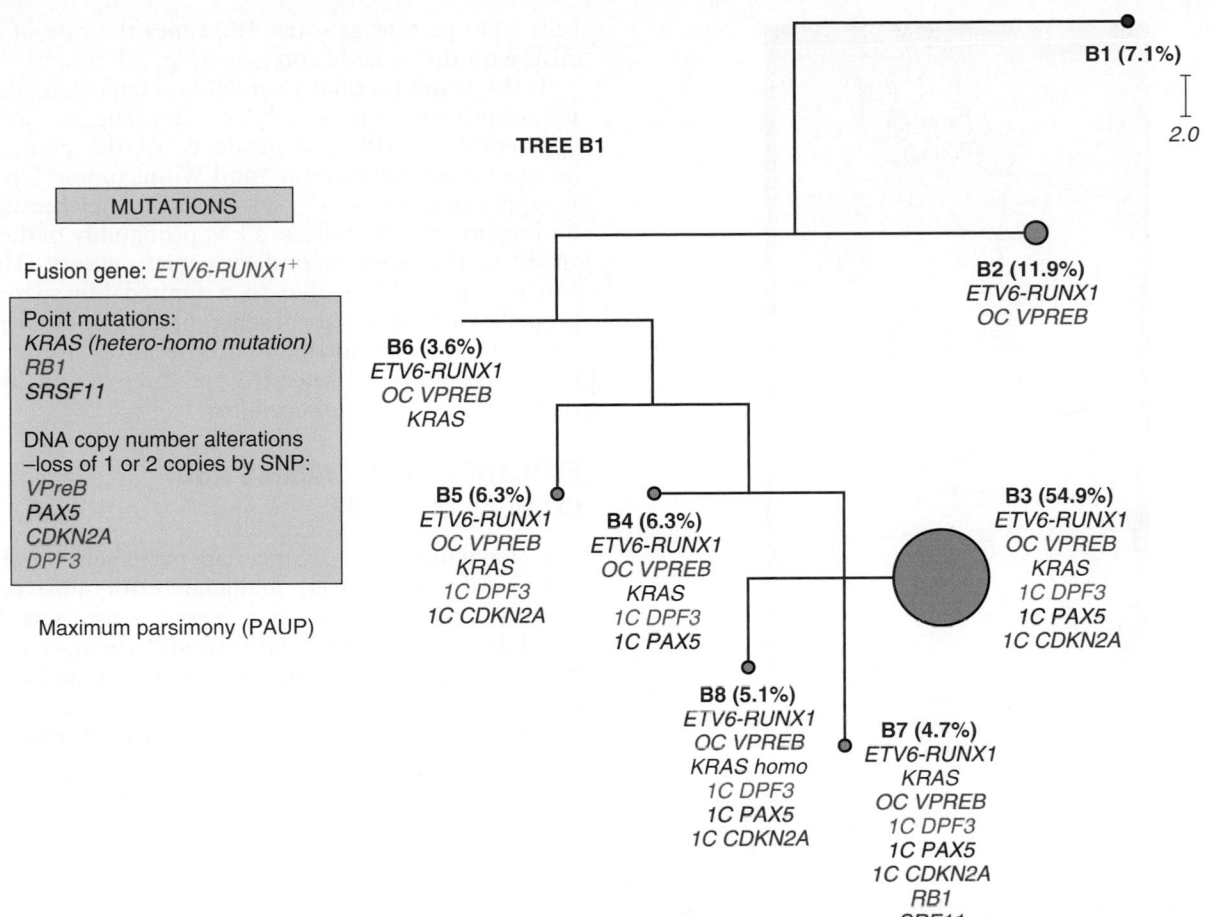

Figure 39-8 Inferred clonal architecture and phylogenetic tree in acute lymphoblastic leukemia (ALL). B1, Normal cells; B2-7, ALL subclones with individual genotypes listed alongside with the percentage representation in the entire population. B3 at 54.0% is the dominant subclone. Mutations listed were determined by whole exome sequencing (depth 100×). Deoxyribonucleic acid copy number alterations were determined by single nucleotide polymorphism array.[55] Single cells were flow sorted and genotyped by multiplex quantitative polymerase chain reaction using the Fluidigm BioMark microfluidic platform (Fluidigm, South San Francisco, Calif.). Maximum parsimony (PAUP) was the method used for assembling the phylogenic tree and the software that was used. *(From Potter N, Ermini L, Papaemmanuil E, et al: Single cell mutational profiling and clonal phylogeny in cancer.* Genome Res *23:2115–2125, 2013.)*

Another marked feature of ALL clonal architecture and its genetic variegation is the finding that the same gene is frequently altered, or mutated, independently in distinct subclones (or phylogenetic branches) of ALL in individual patients.[54,58] Reiterated gene mutation is seen in some other leukemias and solid tumors[16] and presumably reflects strong selection for particular gene alterations that have an impact on cell fitness. Additionally, however, some mutations may not be entirely stochastic or random. Bioinformatic scrutiny of *ETV6-RUNX1*–positive ALL genomes have revealed that half or more of all recurrent copy number alterations, mostly deletions, have lymphoid recombinase, *RAG1/RAG2* recognition motif heptamer nonamer sequences close to the break points.[59] Recombination-activating genes are expressed constitutively in normal B- and T-cell precursors as part of the physiologic program of immunoglobulin heavy chain and T-cell receptor gene rearrangement.[60] These enzymes continue to be expressed in ALL, where they may saturate their physiologic targets and mutate other substrates.

EVOLUTIONARY PENETRANCE OF DISEASE

Pediatric cancers are rare in human and animal species. Were they not, their highly deleterious impact on reproductive fitness (prior to the advent of successful therapy) would have led, by natural selection, to more potent suppressive mechanisms. The evolution of complex multicellular organisms required the elaboration of suppressor gene functions[31,61] to ensure cohesion and integration of diverse cell functions. That this mechanism so clearly fails in ageing adult humans is, we assume, a reflection of the weak impact of natural selection postreproductively and the chronic exposure patterns associated with human societies that can overwhelm suppression.[14]

It might then be assumed that the 1 in 800 risk of childhood cancer is a compound of the various components of risk (Fig. 39-2). However, it is well recognized that the evolutionary progression of adult cancers is both sluggish and inefficient because substantially more covert, early or premalignant lesions (e.g., carcinomas in situ) exist than ever emerge as a clinical malignancy.[62] This situation

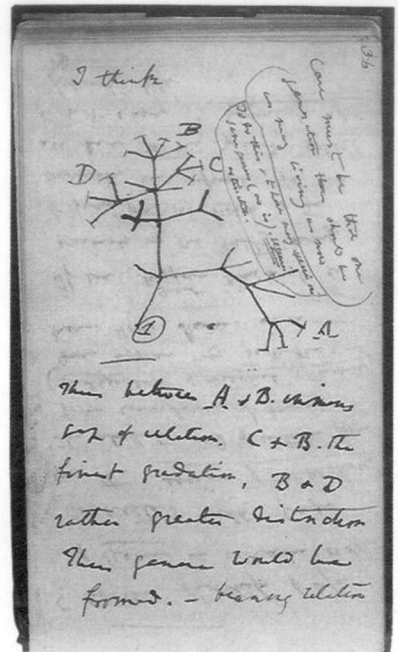

Figure 39-9 Branching phylogeny in speciation as depicted by Charles Darwin in his 1837 notebook. Founder individual 1 gives rise via a branching architecture to descendents A, B, C, and D.

raises an interesting question with regard to pediatric cancer: how often is the disease initiated prenatally but then stalls or regresses and fails to evolve to overt cancer? Presumably more frequently than 1 in 800 instances? An answer to this question has been determined for ALL using a tactic available for bloodborne premalignant cells. Careful molecular screening of a large series (approximately 600) of unrelated cord blood samples revealed that expanded clones of *ETV6-RUNX1*–positive B lineage

cells were present at some 100 times the rate of clinical ALL with the same fusion gene (Fig. 39-10).[63]

Is this result peculiar to childhood leukemia? Probably not. Autopsy histopathologic data suggest a similar approximately 100-fold incidence of the premalignant lesions for neuroblastoma[64] and Wilms tumor[65] (resulting in approximately a 1% incidence in newborns). This finding presumably reflects a low probability of the acquisition of necessary secondary genetic events. This low penetrance could be due to a limited life span of the premalignant clone, an absence of the required promotional impact of postnatal proliferative stress, altered microenvironmental selective pressures, or an influence of inherent genetic susceptibility.

EVOLUTIONARY DYNAMICS AND CLINICAL OUTCOME

The clonal dynamics of cancer are extremely variable, but the time frame to overt malignancy for most pediatric cancers is measured in a few years versus a few decades in adults. As in ecologic speciation,[66] the pace of evolution is not constant or steady; periods of stasis or slow, parallel clonal evolution and codominance (or even regression) are occasionally punctuated by major selective sweeps where, in cancer, one subclone emerges to dominance. Genetic analysis of both adult[67] and pediatric cancers[68] suggests that these key transition times in clonal evolution occur when in situ tumors become diffuse, with metastases and posttherapeutic recurrence or relapse. These changes reflect the imposition of stringent selective pressures.

In contrast with the common adult carcinomas, a striking feature of pediatric cancers is the low mutational burden.[69] Most pediatric cancers have around 10 nonsynonymous exomic nucleotide alterations compared with

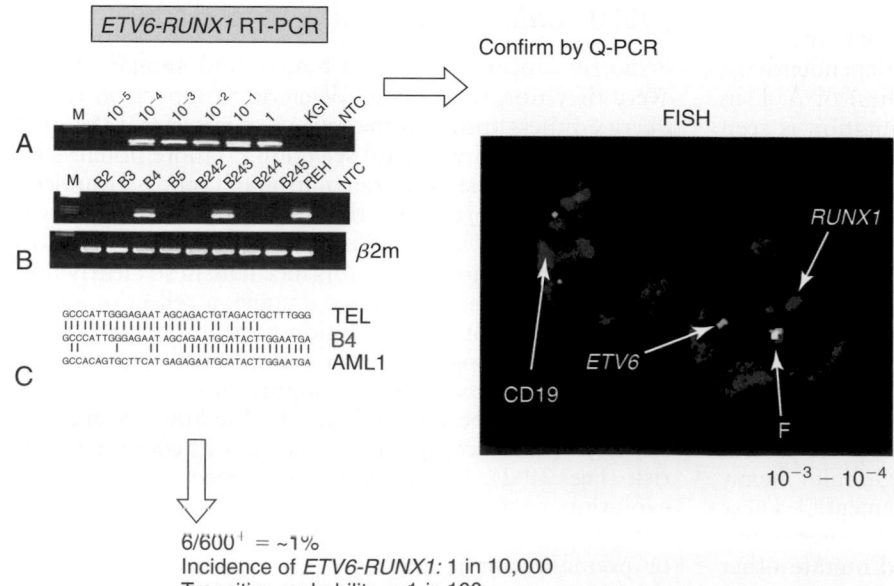

Figure 39-10 Determining the transition probability for acute lymphoblastic leukemia (ALL). Multicolor fluorescence in situ hybridization of interphase nuclei (of cord blood cells). The cell on the left has two normal signals of *RUNX1* *(red)* and *ETV6* *(green)* and is normal. The cell on the right has fused *(yellow)* *ETV6-RUNX1* signal, plus loss of one *ETV6* *(green)* signal with one normal *RUNX1* *(red)* signal and one remnant *RUNX1* *(small red)* signal resulting from translocation. 10^{-3}-10^{-4}: Frequency of positive cells within the CD19+ *(blue)* population. Reverse transcription polymerase chain reaction *(RT-PCR)* for *ETV6-RUNX1* (ribonucleic acid). **A,** Dilution series using positive cell line (REH) versus negative cell line (KG1) and no template control (NTC). **B,** Results with eight cord blood samples. B4 and B243 give positive results. **C,** Sequencing of amplicons from sample B4 showing a bona fide, in frame *ETV6-RUNX1* sequence. *(Data from Mori H, Colman SM, Xiao Z, et al: Chromosome translocations and covert leukemic clones are generated during normal fetal development.* Proc Natl Acad Sci U S A 99:8242–8247, 2002.)

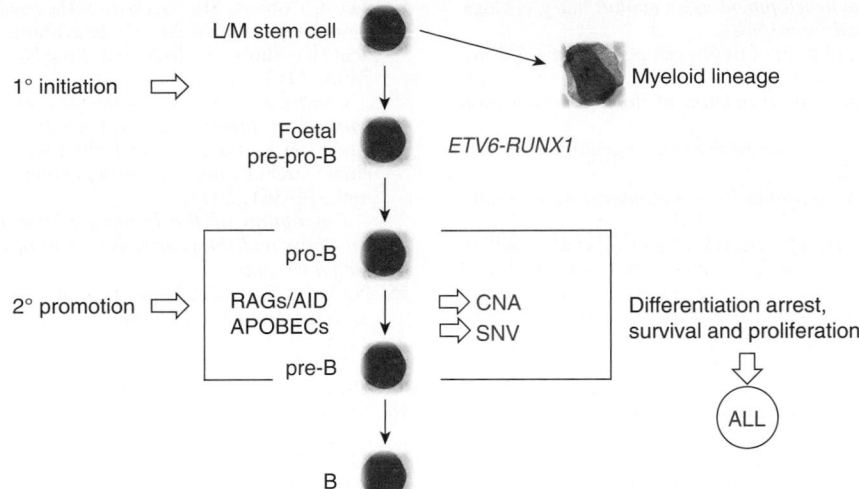

Figure 39-11 Developmental model for childhood B-cell precursor acute lymphoblastic leukemia (ALL). Lymphomyeloid (L/M) stem/progenitor cells. The model shows preleukemic ALL clones initiated (by gene fusion or hyperdiploidy) in the fetal, early pre-pro-B stage. An overt ALL clone with secondary genetic changes (copy number alterations [CNA]/single nucleotide variants [SNV]) becomes trapped in differentiation arrest. Off-target RAG1/RAG2 recombinase activity (R) generates reiterated and highly recurrent CNA. APOBEC enzymes induce SNV.[59]

50 to 70 for many adult cancers and several thousand for the adult cancers associated with known genotoxic exposures (e.g., lung cancer and melanoma).[69] Part of this distinction can be attributed to the frequent presence of genetic instability in many adult cancers, which itself is a possible adaptive cellular response to genotoxic exposure.[70] However, it is also possible that within the architectural constraints of a structured epithelium, more restraints on cancerous growth must be abrogated by mutations. The minimal number of mutations necessary for the evolution of malignant pediatric cancer is difficult to determine, but it could be as few as two or even one for rare pediatric cancers in which the initiating genetic lesion is a major chromatin modifier with pleiotropic impact on multiple pathways, such as *MLL-AF4* fusion in infant ALL[71] and *SMARCB1* in rhabdoid cancer.[72] Two mutations might be sufficient for most pediatric cancers if these mutations effectively uncoupled proliferation from differentiation and if, in the developmental context, this uncoupling caused relatively rapid onset of a diagnosable disease, leading to relatively early detection of these cancers in their evolutionary trajectory.

These considerations may be relevant to the success in treatment of pediatric cancer. Prior to the advent of combination chemotherapy, all cases of childhood ALL were universally fatal within around 12 months.[73] The current long-term remission and possible cure rate for *ETV6-RUNX1+* ALL is close to 100%.[74] Other rarer subtypes of ALL are considerably more intransigent.[75] What is it about the evolutionary biology of the major, or common, subtypes of pediatric ALL that render them curable with use of relatively generic cytotoxics? In adult cancers, evidence indicates that the extent of clonal, genetic diversity is a strong predictor of progression of disease[76] or eventual clinical outcome.[77] One interpretation of this situation is that genetic diversity is fueled by genetic instability and high diversity, which substantially increases the likelihood of acquisition of drug-resistant mutations. Minimal

genetic diversity arising at the time of "early" diagnosis may therefore be critical to the curability of *ETV6-RUNX1+* ALL. However, other factors probably also contribute, including an origin from a progenitor (B) population that is intrinsically very sensitive to deoxyribonucleic acid (DNA) damage and apoptosis.[78] The same dynamic may apply to embryonic progenitors that give rise to other pediatric cancers that are intrinsically sensitive to radiation and chemotherapy.[25] In addition to mutation rate or load, the particular mutations selected may also be crucial. Adult cancers with genetic instability have a very high frequency of *TP53* mutations or deletions,[79] which may reflect an adaptive cellular response to DNA damage; the downside is resistance to chemotherapy. *TP53* mutations are rarer in pediatric cancer and absent from *ETV6-RUNX1+* ALL.[59] Also missing from curable *ETV6-RUNX1+* ALL are kinase mutations[59] that are a hallmark feature of high-risk childhood ALL.[75] Although deletions of the cell cycle inhibitor *CDKN2A* (*p16*) are very common in all ALL (and other pediatric cancers), the lack of proliferative "driver" oncogene mutations (i.e., activated kinases) is striking. This finding supports the notion that the common variants of childhood ALL and possibly several other types of pediatric cancer, including Wilms and germ cell tumors, are in effect minimally modified, albeit expanded, clones in differentiation arrest and that this status renders them chemosensitive (Fig. 39-11).

References available online at ExpertConsult.

KEY REFERENCES

1. Buss LW: *The evolution of individuality*, Princeton, 1987, Princeton University Press.
   Broad review of how evolutionary selection has operated over the past 2 billion years at the hierarchical levels of molecules, individual cells, and multicellular organisms.
3. Greaves M, Maley CC: Clonal evolution in cancer. *Nature* 481:306–313, 2012.

Review of cancer clone development as an evolutionary, ecological process and its clinical importance.

4. Nowell PC: The clonal evolution of tumor cell populations. *Science* 194:23–28, 1976.
   Seminal paper describing cancer in terms of clonal diversification and selection.

7. Yates LR, Campbell PJ: Evolution of the cancer genome. *Nat Rev Genet* 13:795–806, 2012.
   Interpretation of cancer genomes from a dynamic, evolutionary viewpoint.

13. Papaemmanuil E, Hosking FJ, Vijayakrishnan J, et al: Loci on 7p12.2, 10q21.2 and 14q11.2 are associated with risk of childhood acute lymphoblastic leukemia. *Nat Genet* 41:1006–1010, 2009.
    Identification of major inherited risk alleles for childhood acute lymphoblastic leukemia via a genome-wide association study.

15. Sottoriva A, Spiteri I, Piccirillo SGM, et al: Intratumor heterogeneity in human glioblastoma reflects cancer evolutionary dynamics. *Proc Natl Acad Sci U S A* 110:4009–4014, 2013.
    Description of temporal-spatial segregation and evolution of genetically distinct subclones in glioblastoma.

25. Maris JM, Denny CT: Focus on embryonal malignancies. *Cancer Cell* 2:447–450, 2002.
    Review of evidence linking subtypes of pediatric cancers to developmental abnormalities in embryogenesis.

28. Mullighan CG, Goorha S, Radtke I, et al: Genome-wide analysis of genetic alterations in acute lymphoblastic leukaemia. *Nature* 446:758–764, 2007.
    First genome-wide description of copy number alterations in childhood acute lymphoblastic leukemia.

30. Greaves M: Infection, immune responses and the aetiology of childhood leukaemia. *Nat Rev Cancer* 6:193–203, 2006.
    Review of the evidence implicating abnormal immune responses to common infections in the etiology of childhood leukemia.

32. Armstrong SA, Look AT: Molecular genetics of acute lymphoblastic leukemia. *J Clin Oncol* 23:6306–6315, 2005.
    Review of chromosome translocations in different subtypes of acute lymphoblastic leukemia at different ages.

33. Li Z, Godinho FJ, Klusmann JH, et al: Developmental stage-selective effect of somatically mutated leukemogenic transcription factor GATA1. *Nat Genet* 37:613–619, 2005.
    Experimental evidence that some mutations have selective value at particular stages of development. Fetal liver in this case.

39. Chesler L, Weiss WA: Genetically engineered murine models—contribution to our understanding of the genetics, molecular pathology and therapeutic targeting of neuroblastoma. *Semin Cancer Biol* 21:245–255, 2011.
    Review of the establishment of mouse models of neuroblastoma and their potential clinical value.

41. Johnson RA, Wright KD, Poppleton H, et al: Cross-species genomics matches driver mutations and cell compartments to model ependymoma. *Nature* 466:632–636, 2010.
    Comparison of transcriptomes of subtypes of clinical ependymomas with those of murine neural stem cells from different regions of the brain suggest possible cells of origin.

42. Gibson P, Tong Y, Robinson G, et al: Subtypes of medulloblastoma have distinct developmental origins. *Nature* 468:1095–1099, 2010.
    Genetically distinct subtypes of clinical medulloblastoma have different anatomical localizations in the brain and can be mimicked in murine models driven by the same mutations.

43. Visvader JE: Cells of origin in cancer. *Nature* 469:314–322, 2011.
    Review of the evidence used to deduce the possible target cell of origin in different cancers.

44. Greaves MF, Wiemels J: Origins of chromosome translocations in childhood leukaemia. *Nature Rev Cancer* 3:639–649, 2003.
    Review of the evidence that most childhood leukemias originate in utero.

47. Greaves MF, Maia AT, Wiemels JL, et al: Leukemia in twins: lessons in natural history. *Blood* 102:2321–2333, 2003.
    Review of the evidence that concordance of leukemia in monozygotic twins arises in one twin followed by spread to the co-twin via intraplacental anastomoses.

50. Ma Y, Dobbins SE, Sherborne AL, et al: Developmental timing of mutations revealed by whole-genome sequencing of twins with acute lymphoblastic leukemia. *Proc Natl Acad Sci U S A* 110:7429–7433, 2013.
    Comparative whole genome sequencing of acute lymphoblastic leukemia in identical twins. Reveals early initiating genetic events.

54. Anderson K, Lutz C, van Delft FW, et al: Genetic variegation of clonal architecture and propagating cells in leukaemia. *Nature* 469:356–361, 2011.
    Description of the branching clonal architecture of leukemia subclones and the genetic variation of leukemic stem cells in individual patients.

55. Potter N, Ermini L, Papaemmanuil E, et al: Single cell mutational profiling and clonal phylogeny in cancer. *Genome Res* 23:2115–2125, 2013.
    Proof of principle paper illustrates single cell genetics and clonal phylogenies in leukemia using Q-PCR microfluidics.

56. Mullighan CG, Phillips LA, Su X, et al: Genomic analysis of the clonal origins of relapsed acute lymphoblastic leukemia. *Science* 322:1377–1380, 2008.
    Genetic analysis backtracking relapses to subclones in the primary, diagnostic material.

57. Meyer JA, Wang J, Hogan LE, et al: Relapse-specific mutations in NT5C2 in childhood acute lymphoblastic leukemia. *Nat Genet* 45:290–294, 2013.
    Genetic, sequencing study reporting that relapse clones are selected via mutations in target for drugs being used.

59. Papaemmanuil E, Rapado Martinez I, Li Y, et al: RAG mediated recombination is the predominant driver of oncogenic rearrangement in ETV6-RUNX1 acute lymphoblastic leukemia. *Nat Genet* 46:116–125, 2014.
    Genomic analysis of mutational signatures in childhood leukemia revealing likely mechanisms of mutations involved.

63. Mori H, Colman SM, Xiao Z, et al: Chromosome translocations and covert leukemic clones are generated during normal fetal development. *Proc Natl Acad Sci U S A* 99:8242–8247, 2002.
    Discovery of putative pre-leukemic clones in normal newborns, suggesting relatively high frequency initiation of childhood acute lymphoblastic leukemia.

68. Wu X, Northcott PA, Dubuc A, et al: Clonal selection drives genetic divergence of metastatic medulloblastoma. *Nature* 482:529–533, 2012.
    Genetic analysis of both clinical medulloblastoma and equivalent murine models show that metastatic cells have an altered mutational spectrum but are derived from a minor subclone in the primary tumor.

69. Vogelstein B, Papadopoulos N, Velculescu VE, et al: Cancer genome landscapes. *Science* 339:1546–1558, 2013.
    Comprehensive review of mutational spectra in different types of cancer.

72. Lee RS, Stewart C, Carter SL, et al: A remarkably simple genome underlies highly malignant pediatric rhabdoid cancers. *J Clin Invest* 122:2983–2988, 2012.
    Evidence indicating that in rhabdoid cancer a single mutation, in an epigenetic modifier (SMARCB1), may be sufficient to produce a malignant clone.

74. Bhojwani D, Pei D, Sandlund JT, et al: ETV6-RUNX1-positive childhood acute lymphoblastic leukemia: improved outcome with contemporary therapy. *Leukemia* 26:265–270, 2012.
    Striking clinical evidence that optimal therapy of a major subtype of childhood acute lymphoblastic leukemia can now deliver almost 100% cure rates.

75. Roberts KG, Morin RD, Zhang J, et al: Genetic alterations activating kinase and cytokine receptor signaling in high-risk acute lymphoblastic leukemia. *Cancer Cell* 22:153–166, 2012.
    Presents data indicating that high risk childhood acute lymphoblastic leukemias are driven by mutation activating kinases similar to BCR-ABL1-positive ALL.

CHAPTER 40

Epidemiology of Leukemia in Childhood

Smita Bhatia and Leslie L. Robison

CHAPTER OUTLINE

Leukemias of childhood are a highly heterogeneous group of diseases. In reviewing the descriptive and analytic epidemiology of these malignancies, we have, when possible, emphasized specific subgroups as defined by morphologic, cytogenetic, or molecular features. In selected instances, evidence indicates that specific subgroups of leukemia may have distinct causes and that molecular abnormalities associated with particular subgroups may be linked with specific causal mechanisms. In assessing risk factors, studies of the childhood leukemias present several methodologic advantages compared with those addressing adult leukemias. For example, because the interval between exposure to putative risk factors and the onset of leukemia is shorter, recall of exposures is likely to be more accurate and intervening factors are less likely to be of importance than are those associated with adult leukemias. These characteristics of childhood leukemia better lend themselves to an approach that includes both population studies and molecular epidemiologic techniques, permitting the design of studies to assess interactions between genes and the environment. However, in striking contrast to the impressive advances in the treatment and biology of childhood leukemia, remarkably little has been achieved regarding our understanding of the cause of leukemia, the most common form of childhood malignancy.

DESCRIPTIVE EPIDEMIOLOGY

Leukemias are the most common cancers affecting children, accounting for 32% of all occurrences of cancer among children younger than 15 years and 27% of occurrences of cancer among children younger than 20 years.[1] Each year in the United States, leukemia is diagnosed in approximately 3540 children who are younger than 20 years. Of these occurrences, acute lymphoblastic leukemia (ALL) accounts for 73%, acute myeloid leukemia (AML) accounts for approximately 18%, and chronic myeloid leukemia (CML) is rarely seen, accounting for less than 4%.

International Patterns

A wide variation exists in the incidence of childhood leukemia by geographic location. The highest annual incidence rates are reported in Costa Rica, Ecuador, Hong Kong, Denmark, and Singapore (57.9 to 51.0 per million population), whereas some of the lowest rates are found in Zimbabwe, India, Israel, and Algeria (23.1 to 26.0 per million).[1] The annual incidence of childhood leukemia for many regions, including North America, Australia, Northern and Western Europe, China, Japan, the Philippines, and Singapore, ranges between 35 and 50 per million (Table 40-1). When evaluating geographic variation in disease incidence, concerns always exist regarding the quality and completeness of reporting. Ecologic studies of childhood leukemia incidence according to annual per-capita gross national income demonstrates substantial variation within low-income countries and a much narrower range in middle- and high-income countries.[2] In addition, a significant correlation exists between the incidence of childhood leukemia and population mortality rates for children younger than 5 years in low- and middle-income countries. Some of the lowest reported childhood leukemia rates are within countries with high mortality rates for children younger than 5 years, suggesting that children with undiagnosed leukemia may die in some low-income countries as a result of anemia or fever that is attributed to infectious disease.

Age-Specific Incidence and Sex Ratio

The incidence rate for all leukemias is highest among children younger than 5 years and decreases with age.[3] The age-adjusted incidence for boys exceeds that for girls, with a sex ratio typically between 1.1:1 and 1.4:1.[1]

TABLE 40-1 Incidence of all Childhood Leukemias, ALL, and AML in Selected International Sites

Country	ANNUAL INCIDENCE RATE (PER MILLION POPULATION)*		
	Leukemia	ALL	AML
Costa Rica	57.9	46.3	8.9
Ecuador	56.3	39.6	9.1
Hong Kong	53.9	40.6	3.9
Denmark	53.0	42.8	8.4
Singapore	51.0	39.5	6.9
Canada	50.8	41.0	6.3
Finland	49.9	41.9	5.4
Australia	49.9	39.9	8.0
Italy	49.1	37.9	7.9
Sweden	48.7	40.1	6.7
Norway	48.6	38.3	8.0
Philippines	48.1	25.2	8.6
United States (white)	46.9	38.0	6.0
Germany	46.6	39.0	6.7
Uruguay	44.0	29.3	7.4
Colombia	42.8	31.5	6.4
United Kingdom	40.8	32.8	6.3
France	40.5	31.7	6.1
China	40.3	17.4	6.7
Netherlands	40.1	30.9	5.8
Japan	38.5	22.6	7.2
Korea	38.1	20.2	8.7
Cuba	37.7	25.4	5.7
Czech Republic	37.1	28.4	5.1
India (Delhi)	36.0	23.1	6.1
Peru	35.9	25.4	6.9
Brazil	33.7	21.9	5.3
Thailand	29.8	19.8	5.8
United States (black)	29.4	20.8	6.2
Algeria	26.0	14.3	5.7
Israel	25.7	18.6	5.3
India (Bombay)	25.4	16.0	4.8
Zimbabwe	23.1	11.6	11.0

Data from Parkin DM, Kramárová PE, Draper GJ, et al, editors: International incidence of childhood cancer, vol II (IARC Scientific Publications No. 144). Lyon, France, 1998, International Agency for Research on Cancer.
ALL, Acute lymphocytic leukemia; AML, acute myeloid leukemia.
*Children 0 to 14 years of age.

Acute Lymphoblastic Leukemia

In developed countries, the age-incidence curve for ALL is characterized by a peak between the ages of 1 and 4 years (Fig. 40-1).[4] Thus a sharp peak in ALL incidence is seen among 2- to 3-year-olds (>100 per million), which decreases to a rate of 20 per million for 8- to 10-year-olds. The incidence of ALL among 2- to 3-year-olds is approximately fourfold greater than that for infants and is nearly tenfold greater than that for 19-year-olds. Although this age distribution is well recognized and attributable to common ALL (cALL),[5] it has not always been present. It was first observed in England and Wales in the 1920s,[6] among American whites in the 1940s,[6] among African Americans[7] and in Japan in the 1960s,[8,9] and among Jews and non-Jews in Israel in the 1970s.[10] In Kuwait, where the incidence was low during the 1970s, the age peak has recently been observed, whereas in the African series, in which the incidence is also low, the peak has not yet been reported.[11]

An exaggerated peak incidence among 2- to 3-year-olds, with a very low incidence of ALL in older children, was observed in certain areas of England and Wales and in the rural north of Scotland and coincided with a high socioeconomic status. These observations have led to a hypothesis that an elevated risk of ALL is influenced by community characteristics such as isolation, high socioeconomic status, and population mixing,[12] which in turn are related to immunologic isolation in infancy and influence patterns of exposure to common infectious agents in the early years of life before the appearance of leukemia.[13] These hypotheses are discussed in detail later. The ratio of incidence rates of ALL for boys and girls ranges between 1.1:1 and 1.3:1.[11]

Acute Myeloid Leukemia

Among children, the incidence rates for AML are highest in infancy and are fairly uniform in older children (see Fig. 40-1).[4] In the United States, during 1986 to 1995, the incidence in the 0- to 4-year-old age group was 10.3 per million, and in the 5- to 9-year-old and 10- to 14-year-old groups it was 5.0 per million and 6.2 per million, respectively. Comparable rates have been reported elsewhere in Europe and in England. The male-to-female ratio is close to unity for AML.[1]

Chronic Myeloid Leukemia

The incidence rates of CML in one of the largest series, originating from the United Kingdom, were 1.2 per million for infants and 1.6, 0.5, and 0.7 for children aged 1 to 4 years, 5 to 9 years, and 10 to 14 years, respectively,[14] which are comparable to rates observed in the United States for these age ranges.[4] The rate for CML increases during the 15- to 19-year age interval. The male-to-female sex ratio is 1.6:1.[1]

Myelodysplastic Syndrome and Other Myeloproliferative Diseases

The International Classification of Childhood Cancer[15] includes a classification for myelodysplastic syndrome (MDS) and other myeloproliferative diseases. In the 0- to 19-year age group, rates for MDS are very similar to those for CML; however, in contrast, the incidence of MDS is highest among infants and drops essentially to 0 by age 8 years.[4] The incidence is almost twice as high among males.

Ethnic Origin

In the United States, substantial variation is seen in the incidence rates of ALL by ethnicity. The highest rates are reported among Hispanics, Filipinos, and Chinese, and the lowest rates are reported among African Americans.[4] The incidence rates among whites are moderate to high by international standards, whereas those for American Indians are somewhat lower.

On the other hand, two studies have investigated the incidence of childhood cancer by ethnicity in England, but results were negative. The lack of variation in the incidence of ALL among ethnic groups in England, in conjunction with the markedly lower incidence of ALL in the Indian subcontinent and Africa than in England, suggests that the incidence of ALL depends to some extent on environmental factors in association with geographic location. The contrast between the ethnic variations in incidence could be a reflection of the socioeconomic differences by ethnicity (or the lack thereof) in the two countries.[14] A recent report from the Malaysia-Singapore Leukemia Study Group describes differences in prognostically important chromosomal abnormalities among an unselected multiethnic Asian population.[16] Ethnic groups differed significantly with regard to the proportion of patients with ALL who had T-cell ALL (the incidence is higher in Chinese and Indians), ETV6-RUNX1 (with a lower incidence in Chinese persons), and BCR-ABL (with a lower incidence in Indian persons). Beyond ethnic differences in the occurrence of childhood ALL, it has been well documented that race/ethnicity is associated with prognosis.[17] The black-to-white ratio of the incidence of AML in the United States is 0.85. The rates are highest among Hispanics.[1,18] This higher rate of AML contributed to the higher incidence of acute promyelocytic leukemia seen among Hispanics than among non-Hispanics, thus raising the question of genetic predisposition to acute promyelocytic leukemia or exposure to distinct environmental factors.[19] As with ALL, race/ethnicity also has prognostic importance.[20]

Socioeconomic Status

Socioeconomic factors have been proposed as an explanation for the age peak in childhood leukemia.[21] Thus it has been hypothesized that with economic development, poorer communities move from a situation in which leukemia is rare (T-cell ALL is the predominant type of ALL) through an intermediate stage in which cALL begins to appear to a state of high socioeconomic status that is associated with a high incidence of ALL and cALL. Numerous descriptive studies have investigated the relationship between leukemia and socioeconomic status.[22-28] In the vast majority of these studies, the area of residence of the patients (or those who died) was used as a measure of socioeconomic status. Other measures used included household income and years of schooling. In most of

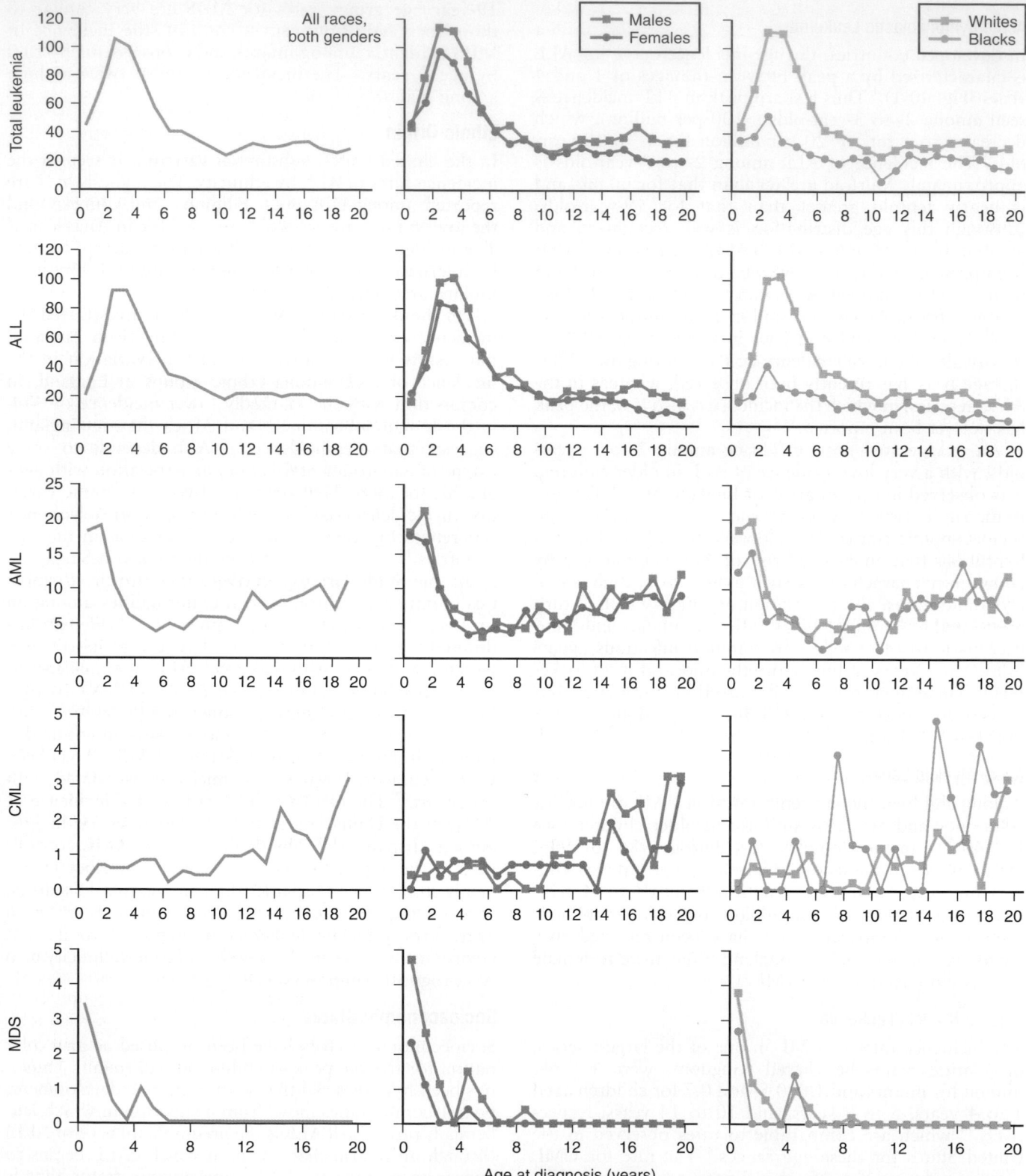

Figure 40-1 Incidence of leukemia (per million children) by age at diagnosis. *ALL,* Acute lymphoblastic leukemia; *AML,* acute myeloid leukemia; *CML,* chronic myeloid leukemia; *MDS,* myelodysplastic syndrome.

these studies, a weak positive association between leukemia and high socioeconomic status was observed, with a few exceptions.[24,27,29-31] In contrast, several investigators have examined the relationship between AML and socioeconomic status and have failed to show an association.[23]

Time Trends

Several investigators have examined temporal trends for leukemia, but the findings are difficult to interpret,[32-37] primarily because of the varying periods covered and different methods of analysis used. Some investigators analyzed the 0- to 14-year-old age group as a whole, whereas others examined trends in specific age groups. Some investigators reported trends for each sex, whereas others combined the two sexes in their analyses. In some analyses all leukemias were grouped together, whereas others conducted their analyses by the leukemia subtype. In addition, diagnostic improvements have led to more accurate and precise classification of leukemias over time, which could contribute to the observed temporal trends in incidence.

In the studies reporting an increase in the incidence of ALL, the increase is fairly modest and is confined to the 0- to 4-year-old age group. Moreover, in some reports, the increase in incidence of ALL appeared to be accompanied by a decrease in the incidence of AML or other leukemias, which could reflect diagnostic shifts and more accurate and precise classification.[38-40] A temporal increase in the incidence of childhood ALL has been reported in England[41] and is attributed to an increase in the precursor B-cell subtype.[42] Between 1974 and 2000, the average annual increase in childhood ALL was 0.7% overall but 1.4% for cALL. Similarly, analyses of childhood ALL time trends in Italy demonstrated increases, some of which were related to maternal time variables that included maternal age and maternal birth cohort, which were considered to be consistent with an infectious cause.[43,44] On the other hand, in another study, Linet and associates[45] report no substantial change in the incidence of childhood leukemia diagnosed in the United States between 1975 and 1995. The Czech national registries reported a 1.5-fold increase in childhood ALL incidence between the ages of 1 to 4 years during the period of substantial socioeconomic transition in the European postcommunist countries.[46]

Clustering of Leukemia in Space and Time

Spatial clustering of childhood leukemia has been observed to varying degrees in England,[47,48] France,[49] and Greece[50] but not in the United States.[51-55] Where spacial clustering was identified, it was strongest for leukemias diagnosed in younger children. Although spatial clustering was confined to sparsely populated areas in England, such clustering was found only in urban areas in Greece. Birch and colleagues[56] addressed the issue of space-time clustering by using the Manchester Children's Tumor Registry. All methods showed highly significant evidence of space-time clustering on the basis of place of birth and time of diagnosis of childhood leukemia. The authors concluded that the results were consistent with an infection hypothesis (discussed later). Furthermore, the investigators found an excess of instances in males versus females in space-time pairs, thus suggesting gender-specific susceptibility to infections. More recently they have reported statistically significant cross-clustering among childhood leukemia and central nervous system (CNS) tumors and between ALL and astrocytoma, suggesting possible common causes, possibly of an infectious nature.[57] The correlation between childhood leukemias and CNS tumors is of interest, given the recently reported correlation in international rates for these two pediatric cancers.[58]

Historically, clusters of childhood leukemia have been observed in which the number of cases reported exceed those expected within a given time and geographic location. Investigation of these clusters has typically not identified any causal agent. A recent leukemia cluster in the United States gained substantial public and scientific attention because of the marked excess observed within a small population.[59] Comprehensive investigation including biologic samples from persons within the population that were analyzed for chemicals, viral markers, and genetic polymorphisms, in conjunction with air, water, soil, and dust sampling, failed to identify any leukemia risk factor.[60]

GENETIC FACTORS AND FAMILIAL AGGREGATION

Certain genetic syndromes are associated with an increased susceptibility to leukemia.[61] These syndromes include Down syndrome,[62] neurofibromatosis type 1,[63] and chromosome breakage syndromes, such as ataxia telangiectasia,[64] Bloom syndrome,[65] Shwachman syndrome,[66,67] Fanconi anemia, and Langerhans cell histiocytosis.[68] Shaw and associates[69] reported an association between Klinefelter syndrome and childhood leukemia on the basis of an observation of two children with ALL who had a 47XXY karyotype. However, Hasle and colleagues[70] subsequently reported no increase in the incidence of childhood leukemia in a cohort of 696 men with Klinefelter syndrome. In a recent study of malformation syndromes among children with cancer, an association was reported between Bardet-Biedl syndrome and ALL.[71]

Although specific associations have been described mainly as case reports, data on the proportion of instances of leukemia that are known to have a genetic etiology or are associated with specific genetic syndromes are limited. In a study from England, 2.6% of children with leukemia were reported to have a recognized genetic condition, and this percentage was almost entirely accounted for by Down syndrome (2.3% of all leukemias).[72] This proportion is similar to that found in studies from the United States and Nordic countries.[73-75]

Population-based studies using record-linkage approaches have documented that approximately 97% of cancers occurring among children with Down syndrome are leukemia.[76] Persons with Down syndrome have an estimated 56-fold increase in leukemia between the ages of 0 to 4 years, which declines to tenfold for leukemia risk between the ages of 5 to 29 years. More recently, interest has been increasing in the identification of environmental factors that may contribute to the development of leukemia among patients with Down syndrome.[77] Case-control investigations comparing persons with Down syndrome who have leukemia with persons with Down syndrome who do not have leukemia have found that reduced risk of leukemia is associated with maternal vitamin supplementation in the periconceptional period and reported history of infection in the first 2 years of life.[78,79]

Concordance of Childhood Leukemia in Twins

Assessment of concordance for childhood leukemia in twins may provide etiologic clues. If childhood leukemia were to have a predominantly genetic cause, monozygotic twins would be expected to be concordant for leukemia more often than dizygotic twins because of their genetic similarity. If childhood leukemia were caused by an abnormal intrauterine environment, it would be expected that if one member of a dizygotic twin pair were affected, the other twin would be affected more often than a nontwin sibling because of the shared environment. Recently, in a study of leukemia in a pooled series from the United States, Canada, and England, only three concordant pairs (1.5%) were found among 197 pairs in which one or both twins had leukemia, with the concordance rate for monozygotic twins reported to be 3.9% (95% confidence interval [CI], 0.8 to 11.1).[80] Although the concordance rate in twins of like sex (probably monozygotic twins) is higher than the zero concordance rate reported for twins of unlike sex (dizygotic twins), the concordance rate in twins of like sex is quite variable.[80,81] These findings suggest that inherited genetic factors most likely play a relatively small part in the cause of childhood leukemia.

The occurrence of concordant leukemic pairs has been hypothesized to be due to parallel expansions of clones descended from a single, ancestral cell transformed in utero, with a malignant clone arising in one monozygotic twin and entering the circulation of the co-twin through anatomizing placental vessels. This mechanism would account for the early and similar age of onset of leukemia and the similar cytogenetic findings.[82,83] Support for this hypothesis is provided by the recent observation of shared clonal but nonconstitutional mixed lineage leukemia gene (MLL) rearrangements in the leukemic cells of three pairs of monozygotic twins concordant for infant acute leukemia.[84] The rearrangements were not observed in nonleukemic cells of the twins and were not present in the maternal or paternal blood of two of the three twins.

Leukemia and Cancer in the Families of Children with Leukemia

In studies of leukemias of all types combined, no excess of cancer was observed among siblings, parents, or offspring.[85-91] In studies focusing on acute leukemia, an excess of acute leukemia was observed among siblings, in whom the expected rates were extremely low.[92-94] Limitations of these studies include the inclusion of distant relatives, in whom verification of cancer becomes problematic, incomplete follow up, and, finally, the inclusion of families with a history of consanguinity.

Cancer in Offspring of Patients Treated for Childhood Leukemia

Few studies have reported the rate of occurrence of cancer in the offspring of patients treated for childhood leukemia. Only recently have enough patients survived that the number of their offspring permitted estimates of their risk of developing malignant neoplasms. After performing a review of the literature, Hawkins and associates[89] estimated that the proportion of heritable cases among survivors is unlikely to exceed 5%, assuming that the age of onset of all heritable cases is 15 years of age or younger and that the diseases had a penetrance of 70% or more. Chromosomal instability was examined in 20 apparently healthy children of survivors of childhood malignancy. Compared with control subjects, no increases in spontaneous or bleomycin-induced aberrations were found in these "index children." The results suggest that the offspring of subjects who previously received chemotherapy, radiotherapy, or both for childhood malignancy probably have no increased risk of latent chromosomal instability.[95]

Other Conditions in Relatives of Patients with Leukemia

Savitz and Ananth[96] reported an excess of major birth defects among the siblings of patients with ALL (relative risk [RR], 3.2; 95% CI, 1.3 to 7.7; adjusted for age at diagnosis, sex, and year of diagnosis). Mann and colleagues[97] reported an excess of congenital defects among parents, uncles, aunts, and other distant relatives of patients with ALL compared with community control subjects. Buckley and associates[98] reported an excess of a number of conditions in siblings, parents, and grandparents of index patients with various types of ALL. These conditions included musculoskeletal disorders among relatives of patients with the common cell type; gastrointestinal, hematologic, and musculoskeletal disorders and allergies for those with the pre–B-cell type; an excess of gastrointestinal disorders for those with the T-cell type; and an excess of congenital heart and lung disease for those with the null cell type. The offspring of adult survivors of childhood ALL were not found to have an increased risk of occurrence of congenital anomalies compared with the offspring of sibling control subjects.[98] Similarly, Kenney and colleagues[99] reported no excess of congenital anomalies among the offspring of adult survivors of childhood cancer compared with the offspring of sibling control subjects.

Human Leukocyte Antigen–DR and Susceptibility to Childhood ALL

Both genetic and environmental factors could possibly play an interactive role in the development of childhood ALL. Because of the demonstration of the influence of major histocompatibility complex on mouse leukemia, a human leukocyte antigen (HLA) association has been considered as a possible genetic risk factor. Dorak and associates[100] demonstrated a moderate association with the most common allele in the HLA-DR53 group, HLA-DRB1*04, which was stronger in males. In addition, homozygosity for HLA-DRB4*01, encoding the HLA-DR53 specificity, was increased among patients. Confounding these associations was a male-specific increase in homozygosity for HLADRB4*01. The cross-reactivity between HLA-DR53 and H-2Ek, extensive mimicry of the immunodominant epitope of HLA-DR53 by several carcinogenic viruses, and the extra amount of deoxyribonucleic acid (DNA) in the vicinity of the *HLA-DRB4* gene provide arguments for the case that HLA-DRB4*01 may be one of the genetic risk factors for childhood ALL. Comparison of DQA1 and DQB1 alleles in 60 children with ALL and 78 newborn infants (control subjects) revealed that male but not female patients had a higher rate of occurrence of DQA1 *0101/*0104 and DQB1 *0501 than did appropriate control subjects.[101] The authors concluded that this finding represented a male-associated susceptibility haplotype in ALL, supporting an infectious cause. Additional investigations from the United Kingdom have suggested that cALL in children may be associated with HLA-DPB1 through a mechanism that involves the presentation of specific antigenic peptides, possibly derived from infectious agents, which leads to activation of helper T cells that mediate proliferative stress on preleukemic cells.[102]

Susceptibility to Childhood ALL: Genetic Polymorphisms

In the search for gene-environment interactions in the cause of childhood leukemia, investigations have focused on the genetic variability in xenobiotic metabolism, DNA repair pathways, and cell-cycle checkpoint functions that might interact with environmental factors to influence leukemia risk. Although much of the research in this area has been limited by small sample size, data suggest a potential role for polymorphisms in genes encoding cytochrome P450, glutathione S-transferase, reduced nicotinamide adenine dinucleotide phosphate quinone oxidoreductase, methylenetetrahydrofolate reductase (MTHFR), cycle-cycle inhibitors, and DNA-repair polymorphisms.[103-111]

In general, few reports have addressed the potential role of these polymorphic genes in childhood leukemia, and in many instances they provide contradictory findings. This situation is particularly true with regard to studies of GSTM1 and GSTT1 and CYP-P450 enzymes.[112,113] Low folate intake or alterations in folate metabolism as a result of polymorphisms in the enzyme MTHFR have been associated with neural tube defects and some cancers. Polymorphic variants of MTHFR lead to enhanced thymidine pools and better quality DNA synthesis that could afford some protection from the development of leukemias, particularly those with translocations. Wiemels and colleagues[103] and Smith and colleagues[111] reported an association of MTHFR polymorphisms in infant leukemias with *MLL* gene rearrangements and childhood leukemia with either *ETV6-RUNX1* fusions or hyperdiploid karyotypes. These studies provide evidence that molecularly defined subgroups of childhood leukemias may have different causes and also suggest a role for folate in the development of childhood leukemia. In a case-control study, MTHFR genotypes TT677/AA1298 and CC677/CCC1298 were

associated with a reduced risk of childhood ALL.[114] Moreover, the findings of these studies suggested a gene-environment interaction based on timing of implementation of folic acid supplementation in the Canadian population. To date, no direct gene-environment associations have been established convincingly. When considering the potential importance of the prenatal origin of childhood leukemia, it becomes important to consider the genotypic profile of the mother with respect to metabolizing enzymes. Investigation of maternally mediated genetic effects through reduced nicotinamide adenine dinucleotide phosphate quinone oxidoreductase did not affect risk for childhood ALL.[115]

PRENATAL ORIGIN OF CHILDHOOD ALL

As mentioned earlier, molecular studies on several pairs of identical twins, aged between 2 months and 14 years at diagnosis, first provided strong evidence that concordant ALL arises in monozygotic twins after mutation and clonal expansion of one cell in one fetus in utero.[84,116,117,118,119] Because the disease in the twins is not clinically or biologically different from that in singletons, Gale and associates[119] hypothesized that some of the singletons are likely to have a prenatal initiation of their leukemia. They further hypothesized that an additional event or exposure postnatally results in the clinically overt leukemia at a variable time after birth. To test these hypotheses, they used the neonatal blood spots or Guthrie cards[119] to identify the presence of clonotypic or patient-specific leukemia fusion-gene sequences *(ETV6-RUNX1)*.[120] The association between the t(12;21) and the deletion of the nontranslocated allele of *TEL* is among the most frequent abnormalities observed in B-lineage ALLs.[121] Neonatal blood samples are routinely used to screen for inherited metabolic disorders. By reverse-transcriptase polymerase chain reaction screening of blood or bone marrow, the investigators identified *ETV6-RUNX1* fusion in 12 children and a pair of identical twins, aged 2 to 5 years, with newly diagnosed ALL. They identified *ETV6-RUNX1* fusion sequences in blood spots from the identical twins and in six of the nine studied ETV6-RUNX1–positive patients. Gale and colleagues concluded that childhood ALL is often initiated by a chromosome translocation event in utero. This important observation has been more extensively investigated and characterized.[122,123] Screening of neonatal cord/blood samples has revealed a putative leukemia clone with the *ETV6-RUNX1* fusion gene in 1% of newborn babies,[124] which represents a frequency 100 times greater than the prevalence of ALL defined by this fusion gene later in childhood. In children with cALL who have a *ETV6-RUNX1* fusion gene, deletion of the unrearranged or normal *TEL* allele is a common secondary occurrence. The causal events that lead to the initial *ETV6-RUNX1* fusion in utero and any postnatal secondary mutations are not known.[125] Some epidemiologic data provide support for the idea that an abnormal immunologic response under particular social conditions could account for certain critical postnatal events.[13,126] Further epidemiologic studies need to focus on in utero exposures that could result in the initial *ETV6-RUNX1* fusion and postnatal exposures or events that could explain the secondary mutations.

INFECTION

Considerable interest and research has focused on the potential role of infection in the cause of childhood ALL through a mechanism of stimulation of an inappropriate immune response or via a direct transformation.[127] This avenue of research, proposed and spearheaded by British researchers, reflects two different but conceptually related hypothesized mechanisms.

The Kinlen Hypothesis: Residence in Areas with High Population Mixing

In 1988 Kinlen[128] hypothesized that the high incidence of leukemia in children in the vicinity of the Sellafield and Dounreay nuclear reprocessing plants in England could be due to a rare response to some unidentified mild and subclinical infection, the transmission of which is facilitated by contacts between large numbers of people. An influx of people of diverse origin into a previously isolated area would particularly facilitate transmission. Thus a high incidence of leukemia in childhood would be expected in isolated areas into which a significant influx of people had occurred. The hypothesis was first tested in an area in Scotland. Glenrothes New Town was identified a priori as an area where, after a period of relative isolation, a sudden burst of in-migration occurred in 1964 because of the opening of the Forth Road bridge.[128] A significant number of persons younger than 25 years who died of leukemia were identified during the period from 1951 to 1967. The incidence of leukemia was not excessive in the period from 1968 to 1985, when the community became much less isolated. The hypothesis has been tested in a number of other situations in England, France, and other parts of Europe and Hong Kong.* A 3.6-fold increase in childhood leukemia was observed in the wartime cohort compared with national Scottish rates in Orkney and Shetland (England's northernmost islands) during World War II, when the local people were outnumbered by servicemen stationed there. The rates normalized to the national rates in the postwar period.[141] A recent analysis of the U.S. Surveillance Epidemiology and End Results data also provided confirmatory evidence for the population mixing hypothesis, with findings that changes in rural county population sizes from 1980 to 1989 were associated with increased incidence rates for childhood ALL.[142]

Infections during the Index Pregnancy

An alternative model for the cause of childhood ALL places the critical infectious event during pregnancy rather than early childhood. In this model, the etiologic agent causing the primary infection in the mother is transmitted to the fetus, and as a consequence of this in utero infection, the child is at increased risk for the development of ALL before the age of 5 years. The characteristics that the causative infectious agent should possess include:

*References 6, 12, 25, 49, 129-134, **135**, 136-140.

(1) the ability to induce genomic instability, (2) specific effects on B lymphocytes and not on T lymphocytes, (3) higher rates of infection in regions with lower socioeconomic status, (4) limited general oncogenic potential, (5) minimal symptoms associated with the primary infection, and (6) the ability to cross the placenta and infect the fetus but not result in severe fetal abnormalities. A virus that meets several of these criteria is the JC virus, a member of the polyomavirus family.[143]

The possibility that maternal infection during pregnancy could potentially be leukemogenic is supported by the observation that leukemia in cats is caused by a feline virus transmitted from the mother to the fetus.[144] Three cohort studies of maternal infection during pregnancy and subsequent childhood cancer revealed an excess of cancer in these children compared with the age- and sex-matched general population.[145-147] In case-control studies, no association between maternal infection with influenza or varicella and subsequent childhood cancer was seen.[98,148-153] With regard to maternal infection in general, a twofold excess of childhood cancer has been reported. However, the studies are small or the reported prevalence of exposure is low and may be attributed to recall bias. Neonatal blood spots have been used to identify evidence of selected in utero viral infections.[154,155] Investigation of cytomegalovirus and human parvovirus B19 infection failed to identify DNA in the small groups of childhood ALL cases compared with healthy control subjects. First-trimester serum samples from mothers of children diagnosed with ALL derived from large maternal cohorts in Finland and Iceland have been tested for antibodies to *Chlamydia trachomatis, Helicobacter pylori,* and *Mycoplasma pneumonae.*[156] Comparison of ALL cases to control subjects identified an increased risk associated with *M. pneumoniae* immunoglobulin M and, in Iceland, *H. pylori* immunoglobulin G. Within the same maternal cohort, evidence was found for activation of maternal Epstein-Barr virus infection in both childhood ALL and non-AML cases.[157]

Smith and colleagues[158] sought to assess the relationship of childhood ALL with hygiene conditions, an aspect of socioeconomic development affecting rates of exposure to infectious agents. The data suggested that improved public hygiene conditions measured by decreased prevalence of hepatitis A virus infection (an agent with a fecal-oral route of transmission) were associated with high childhood ALL incidence rates. The model presented in this study supports the plausibility of the hypothesis that decreased childhood exposure to a leukemia-inducing agent associated with hygiene conditions leads to higher rates of ALL in children by increasing the incidence of in utero transmission caused by primary infection during pregnancy (or by increasing the number of persons infected in early infancy because of a lack of protective antibodies).

Antibiotic Use and Immunizations during the Index Pregnancy

No association between antibiotic use during pregnancy and leukemia has been identified.[148,150,152,159-161] No consistent association has been reported between vaccination during pregnancy and leukemia. Salonen and Saxen[162] found a positive association between leukemia and maternal polio vaccination during pregnancy. Similarly, Gilman and associates[160] reported a positive association between total childhood deaths and vaccination during pregnancy that was largely accounted for by neoplasms of the reticuloendothelial system. However, results of a population-based study in the Netherlands showed no association between vaccination during pregnancy and ALL.[150]

Association of Childhood Leukemia with Factors Related to the Immune System

It has been proposed that some instances of pediatric ALL arise as a rare response to a common childhood infection and that the leukemia-inducing potential of the agent is related to the timing of infection, with a greater leukemogenic effect for later infections compared with those occurring during infancy.[163] In this context, factors related to the child's immune system are of special interest. Several investigators have sought to identify factors such as birth order and breastfeeding that can potentially be used as markers of infections or confer protection against infection before the diagnosis of leukemia.[164]

Breastfeeding

Breastfeeding is well known to have a protective effect against infection in infants.[165] Data regarding the association between breastfeeding and subsequent childhood leukemia are important because of the proposed hypothesis about the etiologic role of infections, taking into consideration the fact that breastfeeding protects against infections. This association was examined in several studies with mixed results. Whereas some researchers failed to show any association between breastfeeding and childhood leukemia,[152,166-172] other researchers do show that a protective effect is offered by breastfeeding.[173] A report of a large North American case-control study revealed that breastfeeding was associated with a reduced risk of childhood acute leukemia.[173] The inverse association was stronger with a longer duration of breastfeeding for patients with ALL and AML. A recent meta-analysis suggested that breastfeeding of any duration was associated with a 9% lower risk of ALL, but little evidence was found of an association for risk of childhood AML.[174]

Immunizations

Previous studies suggested that vaccinations during infancy may reduce the risk of subsequent childhood leukemia. No consistent association between leukemia and immunization has been identified, although two recent studies suggested that early immunization against *Haemophilus influenzae* type b may reduce the incidence of childhood leukemia.[175,176] Auvinen and associates[176] compared the vaccination histories of 439 children in whom ALL was diagnosed and 439 community control subjects matched to patients with regard to age, race, and telephone exchange. No association was demonstrated between most infant vaccinations such as oral poliovirus, diphtheria-pertussis-tetanus, and measles-mumps-rubella. However, Infants receiving the conjugate *H. influenzae* type b vaccine had a reduced risk for subsequent childhood ALL. Confirmatory studies are needed.

Sibship Size

Sibship size might be an indirect indicator of exposure to common childhood infections. However, although no consistent association between ALL and sibship size has been identified,[177] authors of a study from Canada reported that when all variables defining family structure are included in a model, having older siblings at the time of diagnosis was a risk factor among children in whom ALL was diagnosed before 4 years of age, whereas having older siblings in the first year of life was a protective factor among children in whom ALL was diagnosed at 4 years or later.[171] More recently, analysis of the Swedish Family-Cancer Database demonstrated that having three or more older siblings is associated with a significantly reduced risk of childhood AML and ALL.[178]

Early Child Care and Preschool Experiences

Day care of the index child and of siblings has been used as a proxy measure of exposure to infections. The findings of case-control studies have been inconsistent regarding association between attendance at day care centers and risk of leukemia.[177,179-185] A recent study conducted by the United Kingdom Childhood Cancer Study (UKCCS) investigators was specifically designed to test the early infection hypothesis, including the role of day care. These investigators found that increasing levels of social activity were associated with reductions in the risk of ALL in a dose-response manner.[185]

Infection and Related Exposures during the Lifetime of the Index Child

Studies of an association between childhood cancer and postnatal infection of the index child are problematic because of the difficulty in assessing whether the episodes of infectious disease were a possible cause of the childhood cancer or represented a prediagnostic sign of the disease. Some investigators have attempted to overcome this concern by restricting attention to infection during the first year or first 6 months of life or by considering infections reported only during a specified period before diagnosis in patients and during a reference time in control subjects. Specifically, investigators explored the role of parvovirus B19 with its hematotropic effects and the potential to precipitate varying forms of cytopenia in patients before or after the diagnosis of ALL,[186] but they failed to find an association between parvovirus B19 and childhood ALL. Other epidemiologic studies have provided inconsistent findings for an association between leukemia and recorded or reported infections in early life.[98,149,153,167,186-191] In the UKCCS investigation, which utilized general practitioner records for visits during the first year of life, it was found that children with ALL who were diagnosed between the ages of 2 to 5 years had significantly more clinically diagnosed infectious episodes in infancy.[191] Another case-control study from the UKCCS group explored the relationship between childhood leukemia, infant infection, and three markers of infection exposure: birth order, infant day care attendance, and area-based deprivation. The study findings indicated that immune dysregulation among children who are diagnosed with ALL is detectable from an early age.[192] Moreover, recent epidemiologic data indicate that the risk of cALL is increased by higher socioeconomic status, isolation, and other community characteristics suggestive of abnormal patterns of infection during infancy,[13] and population-based incidence patterns have identified small peaks in the incidence of childhood ALL that coincide with years immediately following influenza epidemics.[42]

Chloramphenicol

Chloramphenicol can cause bone marrow suppression and could potentially play an etiologic role in childhood leukemia. Shu and colleagues[193] reported a positive association with the use of chloramphenicol from a study conducted in Shanghai. The risk of leukemia associated with chloramphenicol use increased with an increasing total number of reported days of use. The association was stronger for AML than for ALL. A major limitation of the study was the long interval between diagnosis (1974 to 1986) and interview (1985 to 1986) for the patients, whereas the control subjects were recruited in the 2-year period of 1985 to 1986.

Index Child's Contact with Animals

Although considerable interest has been generated in a possible role of feline leukemia virus because of similarities between human and feline ALL in clinical findings, laboratory data, and response to treatment,[194] evidence is lacking for a biologic association.[195]

Bovine leukemia virus has also been studied for a possible role in the cause of human leukemia. A case-control study of 131 children with leukemia and 136 regional population control subjects was conducted to investigate this association. However, none of the DNA samples from patients or control subjects hybridized with a bovine leukemia virus DNA probe, providing strong evidence that genomic integration of bovine leukemia virus is not a factor in childhood ALL.[196]

Buckley and associates[98] reported a positive association with exposure of the mother, father, and index child to farm animals, compared with control subjects who had other types of cancer or community control subjects. However, no overall association with cat ownership was identified. A recent large case-control study failed to show any association between pet ownership and childhood acute leukemia.[197]

Leukemia and Bacillus Calmette-Guérin Vaccination

Laboratory evidence that tubercle bacilli of the Calmette-Guérin strain (BCG) can prevent or suppress challenge from leukemia or tumor grafts in laboratory animals[199] led investigators to explore whether BCG vaccination might reduce the incidence of cancer in humans and of leukemia in particular. However, no consistent association between BCG vaccination and the subsequent risk of leukemia was found.[198-201]

Seasonal Variations in the Onset of Childhood Leukemia

Seasonal variations in onset of disease could provide supportive evidence of an infectious cause. Westerbeek and colleagues[202] demonstrated significant seasonal variation in the date of the first symptom of childhood ALL, with peaks occurring in November. However, a larger study of 15,835 patients with childhood leukemia failed to reveal any evidence of seasonality in either month of birth or month of diagnosis overall or in any subgroups by age, sex, histologic analysis, or immunophenotype.[203] However, this study did find a statistically significant February peak in month of birth for patients born before 1960 and an August peak in month of diagnosis for patients in whom leukemia was diagnosed before 1962. Although these findings may be due to chance, they are also consistent with changes over time in the seasonality of exposure or immunologic response to a relevant infection. Changes in the seasonal variation in the fatality rate of a preleukemic illness, such as pneumonia, could be another explanation. Ross and associates[204] examined data from the Children's Cancer Group and the Pediatric Oncology Group for seasonal variation patterns. A statistically significant seasonal variation for ALL was found, with a peak in the summer. Biologic mechanisms underlying these seasonal patterns are probably multifactorial and need to be investigated.

ENVIRONMENTAL EXPOSURES

Although a large body of literature describes the associations between a variety of environmental exposures and childhood leukemia, insufficient evidence exists for a causal relationship in most exposure studies, with the exception of those for ionizing radiation. Retrospective studies are limited because of the reliance placed upon parental self-report of the exposure in the context of a case-control study design, which can be hampered by recall bias. In addition, the nonspecific nature of the exposure being assessed makes it difficult to explore causal mechanisms involved with the associations. Moreover, a majority of the exposure assessment has focused on paternal exposures, with little emphasis placed on maternal exposures. To more clearly evaluate the importance of these exposures in future investigations, improvement is needed in the following areas: (1) importance given to maternal exposures; (2) sophisticated exposure techniques used; (3) attention paid to the mechanism, timing, and route of exposure; and (4) the provision of evidence that the exposure is actually transferred to the child's environment.

Radiation Exposure

In utero exposure to radiation has been reported to be associated with a small yet statistically significant increased risk of development of childhood leukemia in numerous case-control studies.[†] Reported estimated risks generally ranged from 1.1 to 2.0, with most of the risk ratios being equal to or lower than 1.6. It is reasonable to expect that in utero levels of exposure to radiation would have declined substantially over time given the knowledge of health-related risks associated with radiation exposure and the reduced level of radiation required for diagnostic procedures. Studies from Sweden, England,

---

[†]References 166, 205-208, **209**, 210-213.

and the United States have demonstrated higher risk estimates among children born in earlier eras (e.g., the 1930s to 1950s) compared with more recent periods.[213-216] Nonetheless, the potential role of in utero exposure to radiation in childhood leukemia has remained controversial. Much of the debate has focused on the lack of an observed association among offspring of mothers who were exposed while pregnant at the time of the Hiroshima and Nagasaki atomic bombs[217,218] coupled with concerns regarding the lack of good exposure assessment and the potential for recall bias in case-control studies of the topic. Results from a large case-control study in North America did not identify an overall increased risk associated with in utero pelvimetric diagnostic x-rays or associations within subgroups defined by immunophenotype.[219] It is likely that the reduced rate and dose of exposure in North America has resulted in an inability to detect the small risk that may exist.

In contrast to the in utero data, postnatal exposure to radiation has not been consistently associated with the risk of childhood leukemia.[166,206,212] Regardless, even if leukemia risk is increased, the potential number of instances of leukemia that currently might be attributed to in utero or postnatal exposure to radiation would probably be very small when one considers the modest magnitude of risk and the limited level of exposure. Results of a case-controlled study of 302 cases of infant leukemia suggested that paternal low-level radiation exposure before conception is associated with an increased risk of infant leukemia, although the nature of this association needs to be further evaluated.[220]

A number of investigations of environmental exposures of children to sources of radiation from nuclear detonations and power plants were conducted to determine the potential impact on leukemia risk. In studies of children who survived the atomic bombs of Hiroshima and Nagasaki, an increased occurrence of leukemia 5 to 15 years later was seen.[221] Leukemia risk was positively correlated with the dose of radiation among the atomic bomb survivors. Reports relating to follow-up of nuclear accidents at Three Mile Island and early reports from Chernobyl did not provide strong evidence of an increased risk of childhood leukemia. Analyses that included residents in the area surrounding the Three Mile Island facility did not reveal an increase in the ratio of observed to expected incidence of leukemia.[222] Similarly, investigation of specific regions of the former Soviet Union did not reveal increased rates of childhood leukemia within the first 5 years after the Chernobyl accident.[223] Because of the widespread fallout from Chernobyl, a series of investigations were undertaken in affected countries, including Sweden,[224] Finland,[225] England,[226] Scotland,[227] Germany,[228] and Greece.[229] With the exception of higher rates in Scotland and an observed excess of infant leukemia (i.e., in children younger than 1 year) in Greece,[230] results were generally negative for an observed increase after the accident. The most recent investigation of the acute and long-term risks for childhood leukemia resulting from radiation exposure (a median estimated dose of <10 mGy) after the Chernobyl power station accident identified a significant increase in leukemia risk with increasing

radiation dose to the bone marrow.[231] However, the potential overestimate of childhood leukemia risk within one region raised serious concerns about conclusions that could be drawn with regard to the level of risk resulting from the Chernobyl accident.

During the 1950s, testing of nuclear weapons took place in Nevada, with nuclear fallout affecting regions of Nevada and Utah. Studies were carried out in Utah to determine the potential impact on childhood leukemia, using geographic region–specific radiation dose estimates to the bone marrow. No significant trend between estimated dose and risk of leukemia mortality was found.[232] However, the risk of death from leukemia was found to be higher in those exposed at the highest dose level (6 to 30 mGy) compared with those in the lowest dose group (0 to 2.9 mGy).

During the past several decades, the potential impact of nuclear facilities, either nuclear energy plants or nuclear reprocessing plants, has generated considerable interest with regard to cancer risk among surrounding residents. Studies addressing childhood leukemia have been conducted in England,[233,234] France,[235,236] the United States,[237,238] Germany,[239] and Canada.[240] In aggregate, these investigations have not provided strong evidence of an increased occurrence of childhood leukemia, although several have reported increases in incidence and mortality.

Although the biologic plausibility of indoor radon exposure and the cause of childhood leukemia are speculative[241] and debatable,[242] studies have been conducted to address the topic. Although ecologic investigations have provided some evidence for a correlation,[241-243] case-control studies incorporating measurement of indoor radon levels have not found higher levels within homes of children with ALL[244] or AML.[245]

Parental Occupational Exposures

Occupational exposure of parents and its association with childhood leukemia have been the subject of several investigations.[246-249] Occupations and exposures of fathers were investigated more often than were those of the mother. Detailed assessment with use of a job exposure matrix to classify occupational exposures identified an increased risk for childhood AML in association with maternal exposure to 1,1,1-tricholorethane, toluene, mineral spirits, alkanes, and mononuclear aromatic hydrocarbons, although dose-response associations were not present.[249] Exposure in the home was not associated with increased risk. Investigation within the UKCCS identified small but statistically significant increased risks among children with ALL whose fathers reported their occupation to involve motor vehicle driving and were exposed to exhaust fumes and/or inhaled particulate hydrocarbons.[248] The studies have several limitations related to the quality of exposure assessment, small numbers of exposed children, multiple comparisons, and possible bias toward the reporting of positive results. Although some evidence exists for an association between childhood leukemia and paternal exposure to solvents, paint, and employment in motor vehicle–related occupations, clearly established associations between parental occupation and childhood leukemia are lacking.

Exposure to Chemicals and Dust

Pesticides

The association between pesticides—including insecticides, fungicides, and herbicides—and childhood leukemia has generated considerable interest, primarily because of the observed higher incidence of leukemia in rural areas and because of the biologic activity of these chemicals. Leiss and Savitz[250] reported a positive association between the use of pest strips and childhood leukemia. The insecticide used in pest strips was dichlorvos, an organophosphate that has been associated with adult-onset leukemia in men.[251] Authors of another study reported an association between the use of pesticides in gardens and farms and childhood leukemia,[252] but no association of leukemia with reported home pest extermination was found in this study. A positive association between maternal exposure during pregnancy and lactation and paternal exposure to household pesticides and garden pesticides or herbicides during the time the mother was pregnant was reported by Lowengart and associates.[253] A recent study provides further evidence for an association between an increased risk of leukemia and rural residence and use of household pesticides.[254] Authors of several other studies report an association between pesticide exposure and childhood leukemia.[255,256]

In a multicenter study of 404 patients who had ALL and individually matched community control subjects, Buckley and associates[98] reported a positive association between ALL and both paternal exposure (RR, 2.8; $P < .001$) and exposure of the index child (RR, 5.0; $P < .001$) to insecticides. The strongest associations for both paternal exposure and exposure of the index child were apparent for T-cell and common cell ALL.

In another case-control study consisting of 204 patients with AML and matched community control subjects, Buckley and associates[257] reported a positive association with maternal occupational exposure to pesticides before, during, and after pregnancy and paternal occupational exposure during the same period. In addition, an independent association of maternal exposure to household fly sprays, pesticides, and garden and agricultural sprays and treatment of the house by insect exterminators in the month before the last menstrual cycle and during the index pregnancy was found, along with direct exposure of the index child to household and garden insecticides. These associations were independent of parental occupational exposure.

Thus, although a large body of literature exists regarding the association between pesticide exposure and childhood leukemia,[255,256] the studies are limited by the nonspecific nature of the exposure, the reliance of these studies on parental self-report, and the lack of sufficient evidence for a causal relationship. Moreover, use of pesticides may be an indicator of rural isolation, and thus there is a possible confounding effect because of the patterns of exposure to infection that may be associated with population mixing.

Agent Orange. Wen and colleagues[258] reported a small increase in the risk of the diagnosis of AML before the age 2 years among offspring of veterans who had served in Cambodia or Vietnam.[258] The etiologic importance of these observations remains to be determined. Exposure to Agent Orange was evaluated in this study, but no association was identified. Other studies also concluded that exposure to the herbicides in Agent Orange was not associated with an increased risk of childhood leukemia among the children born to veterans who reported the exposure.[259]

Hydrocarbons and Solvents

Parental exposure to hydrocarbons at work has been investigated as a potential risk factor for childhood leukemia, with no consistent association between paternal or maternal occupational exposure to hydrocarbons and leukemia (all types and specifically ALL).[260-264] Similarly, no association between paternal exposure to benzene and leukemia has been found.[253,257,262-265] Maternal occupational exposure has been less well studied, but in two of the three studies, a positive association with maternal occupational exposure to hydrocarbons was found that is compatible with the observation that benzene is associated with AML in adults.[162,193,257] Two studies indicated that maternal exposures to hydrocarbons during the preconception period, during pregnancy, and during the postnatal period were related to an increased risk of ALL.[266] A positive association between ALL and paternal exposure to hydrocarbons during the preconception period was also found.

No clear association with residential proximity to industrial sources of hydrocarbons has been observed,[267,268] although authors of one study reported an increased risk of childhood leukemia, and AML in particular, associated with living near petrol stations and/or repair garages.[264] An increased risk of childhood leukemia associated with paternal occupational exposure to chlorinated solvents was reported by several investigators.[253,257,263] The risk has been assessed for exposure during the periods of 1 year before pregnancy, during pregnancy, and after delivery.[257] Several investigators reported a positive association with postnatal exposure of the index child to solvents.[98,153] No consistent association with maternal exposure to solvents is apparent.[269] A recent study revealed a significant association between substantial participation by household members in some common household activities involving organic solvents and childhood leukemia,[270] but further substantiation of these findings is necessary.

Metal Dusts and Fumes

A positive association between the total reported duration of paternal occupational exposure to lead and AML has been reported by Buckley and associates.[257] In the same study, these investigators reported an association between maternal occupational exposure to "metal dusts and fumes." Similar findings were reported by Shu and colleagues[193]; in their study in Shanghai, maternal occupational exposure to lead was associated with an increased risk of acute leukemia. A positive association between maternal exposure to molten metal and ALL (null cell and T cell) and a positive association between paternal exposure to metals and T-cell ALL have been reported.[98] However, ecologic studies have failed to show an association between leukemia and proximity to industrial facilities with an increased exposure to metal or metal fumes.[271,272]

Wood Dust

An association between maternal occupational exposure to wood dust before conception of the index child and childhood leukemia and non-Hodgkin lymphoma has been reported. A few women were exposed during or after pregnancy.[263] Significantly elevated RRs have been reported for paternal occupational exposure to wood dust before conception, during the periconceptional and gestational periods, and postnatally.[246] The association of exposure to wood dust and leukemia was studied by Buckley and associates.[98,257] They found that the risk was elevated compared with that for other cancers and also compared with that for community control subjects.

Traffic

Occupational exposure to elevated concentrations of benzene is a known cause of leukemia in adults. Concentrations of benzene from motor vehicle exhaust fumes could be elevated along highly trafficked streets. The hypothesis that exposure to traffic-related air pollution increases the risk of development of childhood cancer was examined by several investigators.[273-275] Results indicate that an association might exist between residence on a busy street and childhood leukemia. However, these results need to be viewed with caution, because most of the results are based on ecologic studies, with an imperfect assessment of individual exposure.

Electromagnetic and Radiofrequency Field Exposure

An initial report in 1979 suggested an association between childhood leukemia and residential proximity to sources of electric and magnetic fields, as assessed by wiring configurations.[276] Subsequently, a large number of investigations have been conducted to further evaluate the hypothesis that exposure to extremely low-level electric and magnetic fields may influence the risk of childhood leukemia and other pediatric malignancies.[‡] These studies, although they provide some consistent findings, are difficult to interpret given the inconsistencies observed in associations between inferred exposure (i.e., wire configuration) compared with measured fields.

Moreover, many of these studies are limited by small sample size and the inability to adequately consider potential confounding factors within the analysis. Three of the more recently reported investigations from the United States,[287] Canada,[288] England,[289,290] and Japan[291] provide rather convincing evidence that electric and magnetic field exposure is not associated with a significantly increased risk of childhood ALL. Nonetheless, results of meta-analyses[292,293] have been interpreted to suggest that risk may be increased at the highest exposure levels (i.e., >0.4 µT). However, it is important to note that even if an increased risk does exist at this highest exposure level,

‡References 228, 277, 278, **279-286, 287-289**.

the proportion of the population exposed is extremely small and thus the attributable risk would be negligible. Beyond investigation of risk for leukemia, reports have been made of possible associations between electric and magnetic field exposure and prognosis.[294,295]

Although not as extensively studied as electric and magnetic fields, radiofrequency exposure has been suggested as a possible cancer-related risk factor.[296] A recent report investigating radiofrequency exposure in 1928 patients with childhood leukemia observed a twofold risk associated with living within 2 km of an amplitude modulation radio transmitter, which was statistically significant in a dose-dependent fashion for childhood ALL.[297]

LIFESTYLE

Maternal Diet and Vitamin Supplement Use during Pregnancy

Diet and use of vitamin supplements have been shown to be associated with the risk of several cancers among adults. In pediatric malignancies, research has focused primarily on use of vitamin supplements during pregnancy, with little attention given to diet.[159,298] Investigation of maternal diet during pregnancy of children with ALL between the ages of 1 to 5 years found that ALL risk was statistically significantly lower with increased consumption of fruits, vegetables, and fish/seafood, with a significantly higher risk related to increased maternal intake of sugar/syrups and meat products, but these findings will require confirmation in other populations.[299]

Among the available studies of childhood leukemia and maternal consumption of vitamin supplements during pregnancy, no association was found,[159,162,298] with the exception of one study reporting a decrease in risk of ALL among mothers who took iron supplements during the index pregnancy.[300]

Nearly 80% of infants with leukemia have a specific genetic abnormality in their leukemic blast cells involving the MLL gene on chromosome band 11q23.[301] Abnormalities involving 11q23 have also been reported in persons with secondary AML after exposure to topoisomerase inhibitors. Therefore Ross and colleagues[301] hypothesized that infant leukemias involving 11q23 may result from exposure to naturally occurring topoisomerase inhibitors. These agents include caffeine and a variety of fruit and vegetables. A subset of mothers of infants with leukemia diagnosed at 1 year of age or less and control children selected by random digit dialing included in three multicenter case-control studies of childhood leukemia in the United States[257,298] was reapproached to obtain additional information on maternal diet during the index pregnancy.[302] On the basis of data from a food-frequency questionnaire assessing consumption of 26 food items during the index pregnancy, no association was found between total estimated dietary intake of topoisomerase II inhibitors and leukemia of all types combined or ALL. However, a statistically significant positive association for AML was noted with increasing consumption of dietary topoisomerase II inhibitors. A study conducted in 2000 identified bioflavonoids, which are natural substances in food and in dietary supplements that cause site-specific DNA cleavage in the *MLL* breakpoint cluster region in vivo.[303] These results suggest that maternal ingestion of bioflavonoids may induce MLL breaks and potentially induce translocations in utero, leading to infant leukemia. In utero exposures and their association with infant acute leukemia were assessed by Alexander and associates.[304] Use of cigarettes and alcohol, the ingestion of certain herbal medicines and drugs classified as "DNA damaging," and exposure to pesticides were associated with an increased risk of leukemias associated with alterations in *MLL*.

Postnatal Diet of the Index Child and Use of Vitamin Supplements

The role of diet of the index child in the development of childhood leukemia has not been the subject of intensive investigation. Results of investigations exploring the association between the intake of certain food items thought to be precursors or inhibitors of N-nitroso compounds have been controversial. Some investigators report a positive association with hot dogs,[253] whereas others have failed to show any association with consumption of hot dogs or other cured meats.[298] No associations have been reported with postnatal use of vitamins by the index child[98] or consumption of fish, dried milk, fruit juice, or canned foods.[207]

Tobacco Smoking by Parents

Parental smoking and its association with childhood leukemia has been the focus of several investigations. However, issues such as publication bias (with a greater likelihood of positive associations being published) limit the quality of the data. In summary, the literature shows no consistent association between childhood leukemia and parental exposure to tobacco.

Furthermore, no consistent association between maternal smoking during pregnancy and leukemia[305-308] or between paternal smoking and all types of leukemia combined or AML has been found. In most studies, the period of exposure considered has been up to the birth of the index child. Although a positive association between paternal smoking and ALL has been reported by several investigators,[309-312] other investigators have failed to show any association.[305-308,313,314] The largest investigation of maternal smoking and risk of childhood leukemia, which was conducted in Sweden, included more than 1.4 million children born between 1983 and 1997.[315] In this study it was found that maternal smoking was associated with a lower risk of ALL but a higher risk of AML, particularly among heavy smokers. Sandler and associates[316] evaluated the cancer risk from cumulative household exposure to cigarette smoke in a case-control study. Cancer risk was greater for persons who were exposed during both childhood and adulthood than for persons who were exposed during only one period. Some evidence indicates that the effect of parental smoking could be modified to some extent by variant alleles in the *CYP1A1* gene.[306]

An earlier study reported an association between AML (type M1 or M5) and reported use of mind-altering drugs (primarily marijuana) by the mother in the year before or during the index pregnancy.[159] However, a subsequent investigation by the same investigators that was designed to test the hypothesis of maternal marijuana exposure failed to reproduce the association.[317] Thus, overall, maternal smoking during pregnancy or the exposure of infants to cigarette smoke shortly after birth is unlikely to contribute substantially to the risk of childhood leukemia. Moreover, it seems unlikely that passive smoke inhalation during childhood strongly affects the risk of development of childhood leukemia. However, the demonstration of genotoxic effects on the fetus of exposure to metabolites of tobacco smoke should lead to strong recommendations aimed at fully protecting fetuses, newborns, and infants from tobacco smoke.

Alcohol

The majority of studies pertain solely to alcohol consumption by the mother and only to consumption during the pregnancy leading to the birth of the index child. No consistent associations have been found between maternal alcohol consumption before or during the index pregnancy and leukemia of all types combined or ALL.[149,161,193,310] A recent report indicates that maternal alcohol consumption before (adds ratio [OR], 1.37; 95% CI, 0.99-1.9) or during pregnancy (OR, 1.39; 95% CI, 1.01-1.93) may contribute to an increased risk of childhood leukemia.[318] However, some evidence from a number of studies shows an association between maternal alcohol consumption and AML, primarily among persons in whom leukemia is diagnosed early in life. Severson and colleagues[305] reported an increased risk of AML among children in whom leukemia was diagnosed at or before 2 years of age and whose mothers reported consuming alcohol during their pregnancies; the association was particularly pronounced among patients with monocytic and myelomonocytic leukemia. However, the authors advised cautious interpretation of the data because of the small number of subjects included in the subgroup analysis. A positive association between alcohol consumption and AML has also been reported by others.[161,310] The risk appears to be increased for alcohol consumption during each of the three trimesters of pregnancy and for each type of beverage. A dose-response relationship is also suggested.[305,310] No association between paternal alcohol consumption and childhood leukemia has been found.[193,305,310]

MATERNAL REPRODUCTIVE HISTORY

Maternal Age and Birth Order

Accumulation of chromosomal aberrations and mutations during the maturation of germ cells are mechanisms hypothesized for the association between increasing maternal age and cancer in offspring. Most studies have failed to show an association between leukemia and maternal age.[193,319-322] However, a report from 1999 using the Swedish Family-Cancer Database revealed a maternal age effect for childhood leukemia (of about 50% greater in persons older than 35 years).[323]

Most studies based on index cases do not show a positive association with first birth. However, one of the largest of these studies revealed a decreasing trend with increasing birth order for children in whom ALL was diagnosed between the ages of 0 and 4 years.[322] This study also showed a positive association between AML and birth order, adjusted for age, sex, calendar period, and maternal age at the birth of the child. This association was also reported from a combined analysis of data for children who had AML that was diagnosed before 1 year of age in the United States.[319]

Prior Fetal Loss

The association between childhood leukemia and prior fetal loss has been examined by many investigators, with the reported RRs ranging from 0.3 to 1.8.[153,319,320] Data from a Children's Cancer Group case-control study were analyzed to test the hypothesis that this association depended on the number of previous fetal losses and age at leukemia diagnosis. Overall, a modestly increased risk of leukemia was found to be associated with a history of fetal loss. Stratification by age at diagnosis of leukemia showed that this association was significant only for patients in whom ALL and AML was diagnosed before 4 years of age and was most significant in patients in whom leukemia was diagnosed before 2 years of age.[324] Ross and associates[319] also reported a positive association between infantile AML and prior fetal loss. These reports suggested that childhood acute leukemia occurring at younger ages may be associated with an underlying genetic abnormality or chronic environmental exposure, which can be either lethal to the developing fetus or mutagenic and result in the development of acute leukemia.[319]

Oral Contraceptives

McKinney and associates[152] reported no association between leukemia and an interval of less than 3 months between when a woman stopped taking oral contraceptives and conception. Van Steensel-Moll and colleagues[150] reported no association between childhood leukemia and any use of oral contraceptives.

Maternal Illness and Use of Medications during the Index Pregnancy

Ever since the use of diethylstilbestrol to treat women during pregnancy was causally linked with clear-cell adenocarcinoma of the vagina and cervix, several investigators have explored a possible association between use of medications during pregnancy and childhood cancer.

Van Steensel-Moll and colleagues[150] reported a significant positive association with "threatened miscarriage" and "drugs to maintain pregnancy." Another study reported a positive association with hormonal treatment for infertility in the preconceptual period and reported infertility investigations.[148] However, in 1991 Kobayashi and associates[325] from Japan showed that no instance of maternal ovulation induction was recorded for the mothers of 2301 children with leukemia. The Northern California Childhood Leukemia Study investigators observed a significantly increased risk of ALL among mothers reporting influenza/pneumonia during the index pregnancy.[300] Lastly, in the Children's Oncology Group study of 1840 childhood ALL cases, it was reported that significant associations existed with parental use of amphetamines or diet pills and mind-altering drugs before and during the index pregnancy.[326]

Ultrasound Examinations

No association has been found between routine ultrasound exposure in pregnancy and childhood leukemia.[219,327-329]

Anesthesia during Labor

No consistent association has been found between childhood leukemia and cesarean section, which is an indication for anesthesia during labor.[148,190,321] McKinney and associates[152] found a positive association between leukemia and use of narcotic and opioid analgesics, mainly dextropropoxyphene hydrochloride, and between leukemia and the use of barbiturates in labor, but other investigators failed to show any association.[148]

MEDICAL HISTORY OF THE INDEX CHILD

Wen and colleagues[330] investigated the association between childhood ALL and allergic disorders (e.g., asthma, hay fever, food or drug allergies, eczema, and hives) using a case-control study design. The results of this study were in agreement with those of most previous studies of adult cancer, suggesting that allergic disorders may be associated with reduced risk of childhood ALL.

Congenital Anomalies

The presence of cancer and congenital anomalies in the same child may sometimes be explained by an underlying genetic abnormality. A study of these associations might provide clues to the identification of genes that are important to the cause of childhood leukemia. The increased risk of leukemia associated with congenital anomalies appears to be accounted for largely by Down syndrome.[331] Children with Down syndrome have a thirtyfold increased risk of developing childhood leukemia, with the proportion of leukemia attributable to Down syndrome by age 14 years estimated to be 2.7%.[332] To evaluate the risk of leukemia associated with congenital anomalies, a series of matched case-control studies was carried out by the Children's Cancer Group.[333] A total of 2117 children in whom ALL was diagnosed and 605 children in whom AML was diagnosed were compared with matched regional population control subjects. Data on congenital anomalies in the index child were collected by telephone interview with the biologic mother. More congenital anomalies were reported in index case patients who had ALL than in control subjects and included statistically significant increases in multiple birthmarks, Down syndrome, congenital heart defects, and gastrointestinal anomalies. Similarly, birth defects were reported more often among index case patients with AML than among control subjects and included a significant increase in multiple birthmarks, Down syndrome, mental retardation, and congenital heart defects. Exclusion of patients with Down syndrome from the analysis did not change the statistically significant excess of gastrointestinal anomalies in patients with ALL or the excess of birthmarks in patients with AML. However, the majority of the observed associations with congenital anomalies occurred in children with Down syndrome.

In a study of 20,029 children with cancer in England between 1971 and 1986, the occurrence of congenital anomalies was significantly lower in children with leukemia or lymphoma (2.6%) than in children with solid cancers (4.4%).[334] This finding is compatible with the hypothesis that mutations leading to the development of leukemias and lymphomas occur at a much later stage in development in the cells committed to hematopoiesis.

Birth Weight and Length at Birth

Birth weight might serve as an indirect indicator of the intrauterine stresses to the fetus and therefore has been studied by numerous investigators for its association with leukemia.[§] The accumulating literature on high birth weight and risk of childhood ALL, particularly at younger ages, is becoming increasingly convincing as demonstrated in a meta-analysis.[340] High levels of insulin-like growth factor–1, which might both produce a larger baby and contribute to leukemogenesis, has been postulated as an explanation for this association.[341] No consistent association has been reported between length of child at birth and leukemia.[152,321]

Vitamin K

Several studies have explored the association between vitamin K administered in the neonatal period and leukemia, with inconsistent results.[148,342-347] The initial studies by Golding and associates[342,343] from England showed an association between intramuscularly (but not orally) administered vitamin K and childhood leukemia. The biologic basis for the association between vitamin K and childhood leukemia was the observation that concentrations of vitamin K in the infants 12 to 24 hours after injection have been shown to increase sister chromatid exchanges in human placental lymphocytes in vitro and sheep fetal lymphocytes in vitro.[348] However, in vivo studies in human neonates did not substantiate this observation.[349] Moreover, the positive association between leukemia of all types and vitamin K reported by Golding and associates has not been confirmed by analytic studies in England,[346] Germany,[345] Denmark,[350] Sweden[344] and the United States.[351] Parker and associates[352] reported a positive association between parenterally administered vitamin K and childhood ALL diagnosed between the ages of 1 and 6 years, although no association was seen in a cohort-based study. The authors stated that a definite conclusion regarding the relationship between vitamin K and childhood leukemia has not yet been reached. Thus the relationship between vitamin K and childhood leukemia is tenuous at best and the attributable risk is extremely small, with some as yet unidentifiable biologic predisposition placing the patients at increased risk of the development of childhood leukemia.[353]

FUTURE DIRECTIONS

The occurrence of cancer during childhood remains one of the leading causes of childhood mortality, even with the marked improvements in the treatment and cure of pediatric malignancies during the past three to four decades. Although the volume of epidemiologic research addressing the cause of childhood cancer is considerable, relatively little has been achieved regarding our understanding of the cause of childhood leukemia, which would have direct impact on potential future prevention strategies. The absence of progress is not the result of a lack of research in populations around the world directed toward investigation of environmental and genetic factors. This body of research includes large case-control epidemiologic studies including thousands of pediatric leukemia cases, with many incorporating state-of-the-art clinical and biological characterization of cases along with environmental sampling designed to enhance exposure assessment. Future research in this, the most common malignancy of childhood, will probably need to focus on patients with a common primary genetic lesion, such as those with BRC-ABL, MML-AF4, or ETV6-RUNX1 fusion, or hyperdiploidy. By investigating within such well-defined groups, the potential exists to identify common environmental and genetic factors that result in the specific genetic lesion.

References available online at ExpertConsult.

KEY REFERENCES

12. Kinlen LJ, Petridou E: Childhood leukemia and rural population movements: Greece, Italy, and other countries. *Cancer Causes Control* 6:445–450, 1995.

    The infection hypothesis was tested by examining the impact of major rural-urban migration on mortality from childhood leukemia in the 1950s and 1960s—an era that preceded the decline in mortality brought about by effective chemotherapy. Greece and Italy, the two countries with the most striking levels of rural migration, also had the highest mortality rates from childhood leukemia, suggesting that marked rural population mixing in Greece and Italy may have contributed to their high mortality rates from childhood leukemia in the 1950s and 1960s.

13. Greaves MF, Alexander FE: An infectious etiology for common acute lymphoblastic leukemia in childhood? *Leukemia* 7:349–360, 1993.

    Epidemiologic data, reviewed in this article, indicate that risk of B-cell precursor, a form of ALL (cALL), is increased among persons with higher socioeconomic status, isolation, and other characteristics suggestive of abnormal patterns of infection during infancy. The authors conclude that these data may be compatible with the concept that cALL may be a rare response to common infection(s).

17. Bhatia S, Sather HN, Heerema NA, et al: Racial and ethnic differences in survival of children with acute lymphoblastic leukemia. *Blood* 100:1957–1964, 2002.

    African-American and Hispanic children with ALL who were treated with Children's Cancer Group protocols had worse outcomes and Asian children had better outcomes when compared with non-Hispanic white children. The poorer outcomes among black children were most apparent among patients with standard-risk features, whereas poorer outcomes in Hispanic children were most evident among patients with high-risk features. Asian children had better outcomes than all racial and ethnic groups among high-risk patients, particularly in the recent era.

61. Shannon K: Genetic predispositions and childhood cancer. *Environ Health Perspect* 106(Suppl 3):801–806, 1998.

    The role of genetic susceptibility in childhood cancer is discussed, with a particular emphasis on problems with ascertaining inherited cancer risk and the role of tumor-suppressor gene mutations in cancer predispositions. The association between

---

§References 98, 319, 322, 324, 335, **336**-339.

neurofibromatosis type 1 and childhood leukemia is used to illustrate issues related to identifying and analyzing at-risk persons.

62. Zipursky A, Poon A, Doyle J: Leukemia in Down syndrome: a review. *Pediatr Hematol Oncol* 9:139–149, 1992.

    The authors use observations from their own experience, reports in the literature, and data accumulated in the Canadian Down Syndrome Leukemia Registry to describe the epidemiologic and clinical characteristics of leukemia in children with Down syndrome.

71. Merks JH, Caron HN, Hennekam RC: High incidence of malformation syndromes in a series of 1,073 children with cancer. *Am J Med Genet A* 134A:132–143, 2005.

    The authors describe the prevalence and nature of malformation syndromes associated with childhood cancer in 1073 children with cancer. They observe that the prevalence of patients with a proven or suspected syndrome is high, suggesting a possible association.

72. Narod SA, Stiller C, Lenoir GM: An estimate of the heritable fraction of childhood cancer. *Br J Cancer* 63:993–999, 1991.

    The authors reviewed the records of the 16,564 cases of childhood cancer diagnosed from 1971 to 1983 that were reported to the National Registry of Childhood Tumours in Great Britain to estimate the proportion that results from inherited mutations. The total genetic fraction was estimated to be 4.2%.

80. Buckley JD, Buckley CM, Breslow NE, et al: Concordance for childhood cancer in twins. *Med Pediatr Oncol* 26:223–229, 1996.

    The authors of this study determined the concordance rates for childhood cancer in twins to clarify the importance of constitutional predisposition. The monozygotic casewise concordance rate was 5%. The results suggest that a strong constitutional genetic component for childhood cancers other than retinoblastoma does not exist.

84. Ford AM, Ridge SA, Cabrera ME, et al: In utero rearrangements in the trithorax-related oncogene in infant leukaemias. *Nature* 363:358–360, 1993.

    This report describes three pairs of infant twins with concordant leukemia who each share unique but nonconstitutive HRX rearrangements in their leukemic cells, demonstrating that the leukemogenic event originates in utero and provides support for intraplacental "metastasis" for leukemia concordance in twins.

102. Taylor GM, Dearden S, Ravetto P, et al: Genetic susceptibility to childhood common acute lymphoblastic leukaemia is associated with polymorphic peptide-binding pocket profiles in HLA-DPB1*0201. *Hum Mol Genet* 11:1585–1597, 2002.

    *This study demonstrates an association between childhood cALL and an allele at the HLA-DPB1 locus, DPB1*0201, pointing to a mechanism of cALL susceptibility that involves the presentation of specific antigenic peptides, possibly derived from infectious agents, by DPbeta1*0201–related allotypic proteins and leading to the activation of helper T cells, mediating proliferative stress on preleukemic cells.*

103. Wiemels JL, Smith RN, Taylor GM, et al: Methylenetetrahydrofolate reductase (MTHFR) polymorphisms and risk of molecularly defined subtypes of childhood acute leukemia. *Proc Natl Acad Sci U S A* 98:4004–4009, 2001.

    This study examines the role for alterations in folate metabolism as a result of polymorphisms in the enzyme methylenetetrahydrofolate reductase (MTHFR) in the risk of three subgroups of pediatric leukemias: infant leukemias with MLL rearrangements and childhood lymphoblastic leukemias with either ETV6-RUNX1 fusions or hyperdiploid karyotypes. Carriers of C677T demonstrated protection from leukemias with MLL translocations. A1298C homozygotes and C677T homozygotes offer protection from hyperdiploid leukemia, providing preliminary evidence for a role of folate in the development of childhood leukemia.

117. Ford AM, Bennett CA, Price CM, et al: Fetal origins of the TEL-AML1 fusion gene in identical twins with leukemia. *Proc Natl Acad Sci U S A* 95:4584–4588, 1998.

    The ETV6-RUNX1 genomic sequence has been characterized in a pair of monozygotic twins with common ALL diagnosed at ages 3 years, 6 months and 4 years, 10 months. The twin leukemic DNA shared the same ETV6-RUNX1 fusion sequence, suggesting a single cell origin of the TEL-AML fusion in one fetus in utero,

probably as a leukemia-initiating mutation, followed by intraplacental metastasis of clonal progeny to the other twin.

118. Wiemels JL, Ford AM, Van Wering ER, et al: Protracted and variable latency of acute lymphoblastic leukemia after TEL-AML1 gene fusion in utero. *Blood* 94:1057–1062, 1999.

    This study describes the natural history of disease in a pair of identical twins with concordant ALL separated temporally by 9 years. The genomic fusion sequence was identical in the two leukemias, indicative of a single cell origin in one fetus, in utero. These data suggest that consequent to a prenatal initiation of a leukemic clone, most probably by TEL-AML fusion, the latency of ALL can be protracted.

119. Gale KB, Ford AM, Repp R, et al: Backtracking leukemia to birth: identification of clonotypic gene fusion sequences in neonatal blood spots. *Proc Natl Acad Sci U S A* 94:13950–13954, 1997.

120. Maia AT, van der Velden VH, Harrison CJ, et al: Prenatal origin of hyperdiploid acute lymphoblastic leukemia in identical twins. *Leukemia* 17:2202–2206, 2003.

121. Raynaud S, Cave H, Baens M, et al: The 12;21 translocation involving TEL and deletion of the other TEL allele: two frequently associated alterations found in childhood acute lymphoblastic leukemia. *Blood* 87:2891–2899, 1996.

122. Hong D, Gupta R, Ancliff P, et al: Initiating and cancer-propagating cells in TEL-AML1-associated childhood leukemia. *Science* 319:336–339, 2008.

    This study explores the clonal evolution of ETV6-RUNX1 ALL. A cell compartment in leukemic children that can propagate leukemia when transplanted in mice is identified. The study suggests that ETV6-RUNX1 functions as a first-hit mutation by endowing preleukemic cells with altered self-renewal and survival properties.

125. Greaves MF, Wiemels J: Origins of chromosome translocations in childhood leukemia. *Nat Rev Cancer* 3:639–649, 2003.

    This commentary describes the etiopathogenesis of leukemia by describing the timing of the occurrence of chromosome translocations and discussing the role of these genetic changes as necessary but not usually sufficient to cause leukemia.

126. Kinlen LJ: Epidemiologic evidence for an infective basis in childhood leukemia. *Br J Cancer* 71:1–5, 1995.

    This review provides a broad overview for the infectious etiology for childhood ALL.

135. Kinlen LJ, O'Brien F, Clarke K, et al: Rural population mixing and childhood leukemia: effects of the North Sea oil industry in Scotland, including the area near Dounreay nuclear site. *BMJ* 306:743–748, 1993.

    This study demonstrates a significant excess of leukemia and non-Hodgkin lymphoma in 1979-1983 in the group of rural home areas with the largest proportion of oil workers, following closely after large increases in the workforce, supporting the infection hypothesis that population mixing can increase the incidence of childhood leukemia in rural areas.

209. Murray R, Heckel P, Hempelmann LH: Leukemia in children exposed to ionizing radiation. *N Engl J Med* 261:585–589, 1959.

    This article provides evidence for the observed increased risk of leukemia among children with a prior history of exposure to ionizing radiation reported by Stewart, Webb, and Hewitt. These findings are placed in the context of studies describing the experience of the Japanese inhabitants in Hiroshima and Nagasaki at the time of nuclear explosions, patients who have ankylosing spondylitis, children treated in infancy for enlargement of the thymus gland, and American radiologists.

230. Petridou E, Trichopoulos D, Dessypris N, et al: Infant leukaemia after in utero exposure to radiation from Chernobyl. *Nature* 382:352–353, 1996.

    Infants exposed in utero to ionizing radiation from the Chernobyl accident had 2.6 times the incidence of leukemia compared with unexposed children; those born to mothers residing in regions with high radioactive fallout were at higher risk of developing infant leukemia. No significant difference in leukemia incidence was found among children aged 12 to 47 months. Preconception irradiation had no impact on leukemia risk.

279. Savitz DA, Wachtel H, Barnes FA, et al: Case-control study of childhood cancer and exposure to 60-Hz magnetic fields. *Am J Epidemiol* 128:21–38, 1988.

This study was one of the first to examine the impact of extremely low frequency magnetic fields (e.g., proximity to electric power distribution lines) on the risk of childhood cancer. Exposure was characterized through in-home electric and magnetic field measurements under low and high power use conditions and wire configuration codes, a surrogate measure of long-term magnetic field levels. Measured magnetic fields under low power use (and not under high power use) conditions had a modest association with cancer incidence. Wire codes associated with higher magnetic fields were more common among case than control homes.

287. Linet MS, Hatch EE, Kleinerman RA, et al: Residential exposure to magnetic fields and acute lymphoblastic leukemia in children. *N Engl J Med* 337:1–7, 1997.

This study investigated the impact of measuring a single home and then imputing information from another home among subjects who lived in two homes in a subset of an investigation of residential exposure to magnetic fields and risk of childhood leukemia. All methods with measurements from one of the homes in conjunction with imputation of measurements for the second home led to attenuation of risk estimates. These results provided little evidence to support a risk of electric and magnetic field and cautioned against attempting to estimate lifetime magnetic field exposure from imputed values derived from current residences to fill in gaps caused by unmeasured residences previously lived in.

302. Ross JA, Potter JD, Reaman GH, et al: Maternal exposure to potential inhibitors of DNA topoisomerase II and infant leukemia (United States): a report from the Children's Cancer Group. *Cancer Causes Control* 7:581–590, 1996.

This study tested the hypothesis that de novo infant leukemias (with MLL gene rearrangements commonly associated with topoisomerase II inhibitors) may occur as a result of maternal exposure to agents in diet and medications that inhibit DNA topoisomerase II. No significant trends for ALL were found with increasing maternal consumption. However, a statistically significant positive association was found between AML and increasing consumption of foods containing DNA topoisomerase II inhibitors.

315. Mucci LA, Granath F, Cnattingius S: Maternal smoking and childhood leukemia and lymphoma risk among 1,440,542 Swedish children. *Cancer Epidemiol Biomarkers Prev* 13:1528–1533, 2004.

In this investigation, population-based registries in Sweden were used to examine maternal smoking during pregnancy and childhood risk of leukemia. Maternal smoking was associated with a lower risk of ALL but a higher risk of AML.

322. Westergaard T, Andersen PK, Pedersen JB, et al: Birth characteristics, sibling patterns, and acute leukemia risk in childhood: a population-based cohort study. *J Natl Cancer Inst* 89:939–947, 1997.

In this population-based record linkage study, a direct association between birth weight and childhood leukemia was observed. In addition, a weak inverse association between birth order and ALL risk was observed among children younger than 5 years.

336. McLaughlin CC, Baptiste MS, Schymura MJ, et al: Birth weight, maternal weight and childhood leukaemia. *Br J Cancer* 94:1738–1744, 2006.

This case-cohort study reports increased risk of ALL associated with birth weight of 3500 g or more, as well as evidence of effect modification with birth weight and maternal prepregnancy weight. High birth weight was associated with ALL only when the mother was not overweight, and heavier maternal weight was associated with ALL only when the infant did not have a high birth weight. Increased pregnancy-related weight gain was associated with ALL.

CHAPTER 41

Informatics

Samuel L. Volchenboum

CHAPTER OUTLINE

The first genome to be sequenced came at a cost of $100 million. Only 13 years later, the price for sequencing an entire genome is nearing $1000 (Fig. 41-1). Rapid increases in the speed and complexity of genomic sequencing technologies, coupled with dramatically decreasing costs, have created an overwhelming array of platforms, methods, and informatics analysis algorithms. In many publications the authors assume the reader is facile with the platform used in the study described, yet most clinicians and researchers have a limited or narrow knowledge of the wide range of methods capable of describing the genomic or proteomic content of a biologic sample. This chapter focuses on describing the basic framework with which to understand most of the common platforms in use today.

Genomic platforms can be classified in many ways, and one can consider the starting material (e.g., deoxyribonucleic acid [DNA], ribonucleic acid [RNA], proteins, and small molecules) or the questions being asked (e.g., copy number, mutations, loss of heterozygosity [LOH], transcript expression, and methylation). The classification scheme shown in Table 41-1[1,2] classifies each platform according to the underlying structure, and the remainder of this chapter is organized in this fashion.

DNA-BASED METHODS

Most of the time the goal of studying DNA is to learn about the genes encoded, including mutations, rearrangements, and changes in copy number. Low-resolution methods prevailed for years as the standard way of understanding copy number variations and rearrangements (e.g., karyotyping and fluorescent in situ hybridization [FISH]), and low-throughput techniques were required to evaluate point mutations and pathogenic sequences (e.g., capillary sequencing, pyrosequencing, polymerase chain reaction [PCR], and microbial arrays). The emergence of high-throughput, high-resolution techniques has revolutionized the study of the genome.

Comparative Genomic Hybridization

Until the development of comparative genomic hybridization (CGH), chromosomal or subchromosomal gains and losses were discovered though Giemsa banding ("karyotyping") or FISH. Although similar in resolution to these techniques (5 to 10 megabases[3]), CGH can be used in an unbiased and agnostic way to detect unbalanced chromosomal abnormalities by competitive FISH using different fluorophores for two different isolates of DNA (e.g., test and control).[4-6] The technique was also

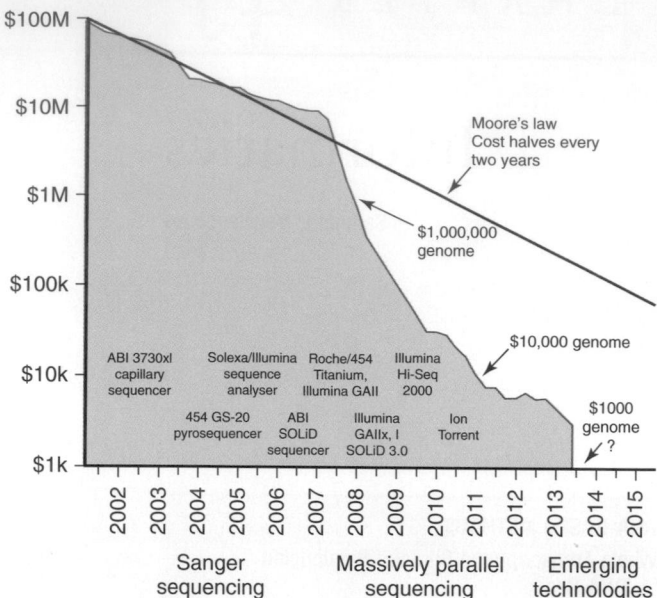

Figure 41-1 The decreasing cost of genome sequencing. Note that the price has been falling faster than Moore's law would predict. *(Modified from MacConaill LE: Existing and emerging technologies for tumor genomic profiling. J Clin Oncol 31:1815–1824, and Mardis ER: Next-generation DNA sequencing methods. Annu Rev Genomics Hum Genet 9:387–402, 2008.)*

novel because it did not require cells to be undergoing active cellular division.[7] With the popularization of DNA microarrays, a higher resolution technique was developed: array CGH (aCGH).[8-10] As is common to all microarray techniques, probes (oligonucleotides) are deposited onto a solid support (glass slide), with the resolution dependent on the size of the probes and the genomic distance separating them.[11] DNA from a test sample and control are extracted, labeled with different fluorescent dyes, and applied to the probes (Fig. 41-2). Complementary strands will bind and can be visualized with use of a digital imaging system to quantify the relative amounts of each target bound. The ratio of test to control for each DNA region can then be used to determine copy number variation throughout the genome. Compared with prior methods, aCGH can detect copy number changes at any locus, as long as it is represented in the array. The technique has been productively applied to the study of thousands of diseases and complex traits, and despite the emergence of newer high-resolution methods, aCGH continues to be a significant platform for the study of copy numbers.

Genotyping

Genotyping is simply determining the genetic variation in an individual. Many methods may be used to perform genotyping with varying degrees of throughput. Restriction fragment length polymorphism analysis was productively applied to describe human leukocyte antigen polymorphisms, followed by PCR-based methods using membranes or bead-bound sequence specific oligonucleotide probes and sequence-specific priming (reviewed in references 12 and 13).[12,13] For the specific application of identifying a point mutation or allelic variant, genotyping via PCR followed by restriction digestion is a simple approach that has been applied to many diseases and conditions, including fatty acid binding protein mutations in insulin resistance[14,15] and identification of polymorphisms in thiopurine methyltransferase in leukemia[16] and methylenetetrahydrofolate reductase in childhood acute leukemia.[16]

Capillary (Sanger) Sequencing

Sanger sequencing, which was first developed in 1977, has been routinely used for more than 25 years for genomic studies.[17,18] In the classic method (Fig. 41-3), chain-terminating nucleotides are incorporated by DNA polymerase during DNA replication with a synthesized primer specific to the region of interest. Compared with normal deoxynucleoside triphosphates, terminating dideoxynucleoside triphosphates lack a 3′-hydroxyl group, and DNA polymerase is unable to create the phosphodiester bond between two nucleotides, thus halting transcription. Four DNA replication samples are prepared, each with a different radiolabeled or fluorescently tagged dideoxynucleoside triphosphate, and the resulting DNA products are separated by electrophoresis and visualized by autoradiography or ultraviolet light. Current instruments use dye terminators instead of fluorescent labels, resulting in faster and more accurate readings.[19,20] The relatively high cost for reagents and the nonautomated nature of traditional Sanger sequencing have been largely obviated by the development of microfluidic technology.[21-24] All of the steps for Sanger sequencing are carried out on a small chip using nanoliter volumes. This "lab-on-a-chip" or "sequencing-on-a-chip" technique increases speed and accuracy while decreasing costs. Despite limited resolving power for the first 25 to 50 bases and read lengths fewer than 1000 bases, Sanger sequencing is still being used for smaller scale projects or when a long contiguous read is desired.

Pyrosequencing

In pyrosequencing, liberated pyrophosphates from nucleotide incorporation are detected and the DNA sequence is determined by light emitted upon nucleotide incorporation.[25-28] Because only one nucleotide at a time is presented to the DNA template and DNA polymerase, the base responsible for the emitted light is the one incorporated into the growing strand. The pyrophosphate release during the reaction is converted to adenosine triphosphate, fueling a luciferase-based fluorescent reaction. Although the reads are shorter (300 to 500 base pair [bp]), multiple reactions can be detected simultaneously, thereby increasing throughput.

DNA Microarrays

A microarray is simply a small piece of DNA (the "probe") that is attached to a solid support, which is usually a glass, plastic, or silicon chip (e.g., an Affymetrix [Santa Clara, CA] genome chip, gene array, or DNA chip) or polystyrene beads (Illumina, San Diego, CA). The process of "printing" the array refers to the deposition of the DNA onto the solid support, either through "spotting"

TABLE 41-1 Types of "-omics" Data

Underlying Structure	"-omics"	Alterations in Disease	Technologies
DNA	Genome	Point mutations	Capillary (Sanger) sequencing Pyrosequencing Genotyping Targeted-sequencing/WES RNA-seq
		Copy number gains or losses	FISH Array CGH SNP array Targeted-sequencing/WES WGS
		Rearrangements/fusion genes	Karyotyping FISH WGS RNA-seq
		Pathogenic sequences	PCR Microbial arrays WGS RNA-seq
	Epigenome	DNA methylation Histone modifications	Bisulfite sequencing Methyl-specific PCR ChIP-seq
mRNA	Transcriptome	Altered transcript expression Altered allele-specific expression Differential alternative splicing	Microarrays RNA-seq
microRNA	Epigenome	Altered transcriptional control	Microarrays
Proteins	Proteome	Mutated or deleted proteins Altered posttranslational modification Increased or decreased regulation	Microarrays Mass spectrometry
Small molecules	Metabolome	Modulations in small molecules	Mass spectrometry NMR spectroscopy

Modified from Chadeau-Hyam M, Campanella G, Jombart T, et al: Deciphering the complex: methodological overview of statistical models to derive OMICS-based biomarkers. Environ Mol Mutagen 54:542–557, 2013, and MacConaill LE: Existing and emerging technologies for tumor genomic profiling. J Clin Oncol 31:1815–1824, 2013.

CGH, Comparative genomic hybridization; ChIP-seq, chromatin immunoprecipitation followed by massively parallel sequencing; DNA, deoxyribonucleic acid; FISH, fluorescent in situ hybridization; mRNA, messenger ribonucleic acid; NMR, nuclear magnetic resonance; PCR, polymerase chain reaction; RNA, ribonucleic acid; RNA-seq, ribonucleic acid sequencing (transcriptome sequencing); SNP, single nucleotide polymorphism; WES, whole exome sequencing; WGS, whole genome sequencing.

(complementary DNA [cDNA] microarray[29]) or by synthesizing the oligonucleotides directly onto the array surface.[30-32] For a spotted array, the probes are produced beforehand, either through the production of a cDNA library, by PCR, or by the generation of oligonucleotides that are then "spotted" directly onto the support surface, often by a robot.[33,34,35]

Single Nucleotide Polymorphism Arrays

A single nucleotide polymorphism (SNP) is any sequence variation in the genome for which both alleles occur at a relatively high frequency. The vast majority do not appear to confer functional consequences.[36] Although they are located most often in noncoding regions, SNPs can occur

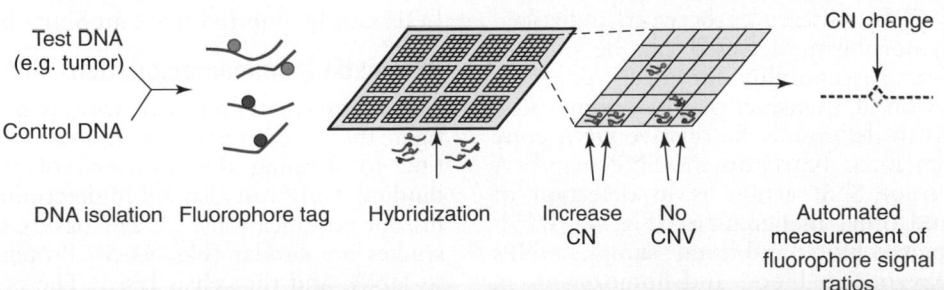

Figure 41-2 Array comparative genomic hybridization workflow. Deoxyribonucleic acid (DNA) is isolated from patient/tumor and control, differentially labeled with fluorophores, hybridized to oligonucleotides on a solid support, and analyzed for differences in ratios of fluorescence. CN, Copy number; CNV, copy number variation.

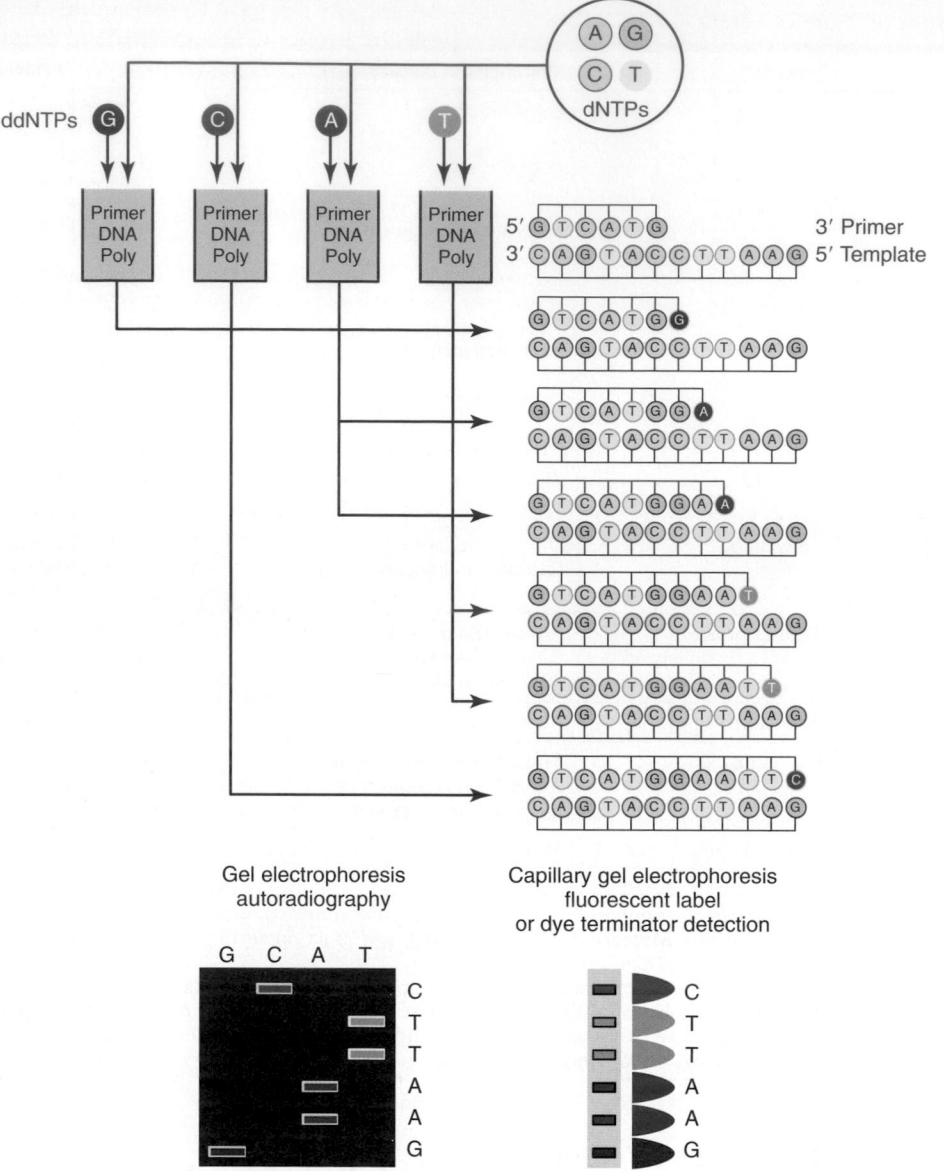

Figure 41-3 Capillary (Sanger) sequencing. The dideoxynucleoside triphosphates *(ddNTPs; black)* terminate the elongation reaction by deoxyribonucleic acid *(DNA)* polymerase. Results are visualized by autoradiography or fluorescence detection. *dNTPs,* Deoxynucleoside triphosphates.

anywhere throughout the genome. More than 50 million SNPs have been cataloged in the SNP database.[37] High-density SNP arrays can be used for genetic linkage studies to map disease loci and complex traits.[38,39] Because SNP arrays can detect slight differences between individual genomes, the polymorphisms detected can be used to characterize disease susceptibility or drug effectiveness.[40,41] A comparison of intensities of DNA-bound SNP probes can be used to determine the relative DNA copy number for a given locus based on the SNP map.[42] A specific application of SNP arrays is in detection of LOH in tumors and other malignancies (Fig. 41-4).[43-46] When examining paired blood and tumor samples, SNPs detected as heterozygous in blood and homozygous in tumor (LOH) may be part of a region where a normal copy of a tumor suppressor gene was lost. A special case of LOH called uniparental disomy is a copy-neutral gene

conversion.[47-49] Instead of a deletion leading to the loss of the normal allele, a nondisjunction event results in LOH without a change in copy number. Although undetectable by FISH or karyotyping, this important type of LOH can be inferred from an SNP virtual karyotype.

Chromatin Immunoprecipitation, ChIP-Chip, ChIP-Seq

Chromatin immunoprecipitation (ChIP) is used to investigate the interaction between proteins and DNA. In addition to defining the locations of transcription factor binding, ChIP can also aid in determining the location of histone modifications.[50-52] The basic concepts for all ChIP studies are similar (Fig. 41-5). Proteins are cross-linked to DNA, and the cell is lysed. The protein-bound DNA is sheared, and immunoprecipitation is used to "pull down" the protein-bound DNA regions of interest.[53] The DNA is then isolated and purified, and different

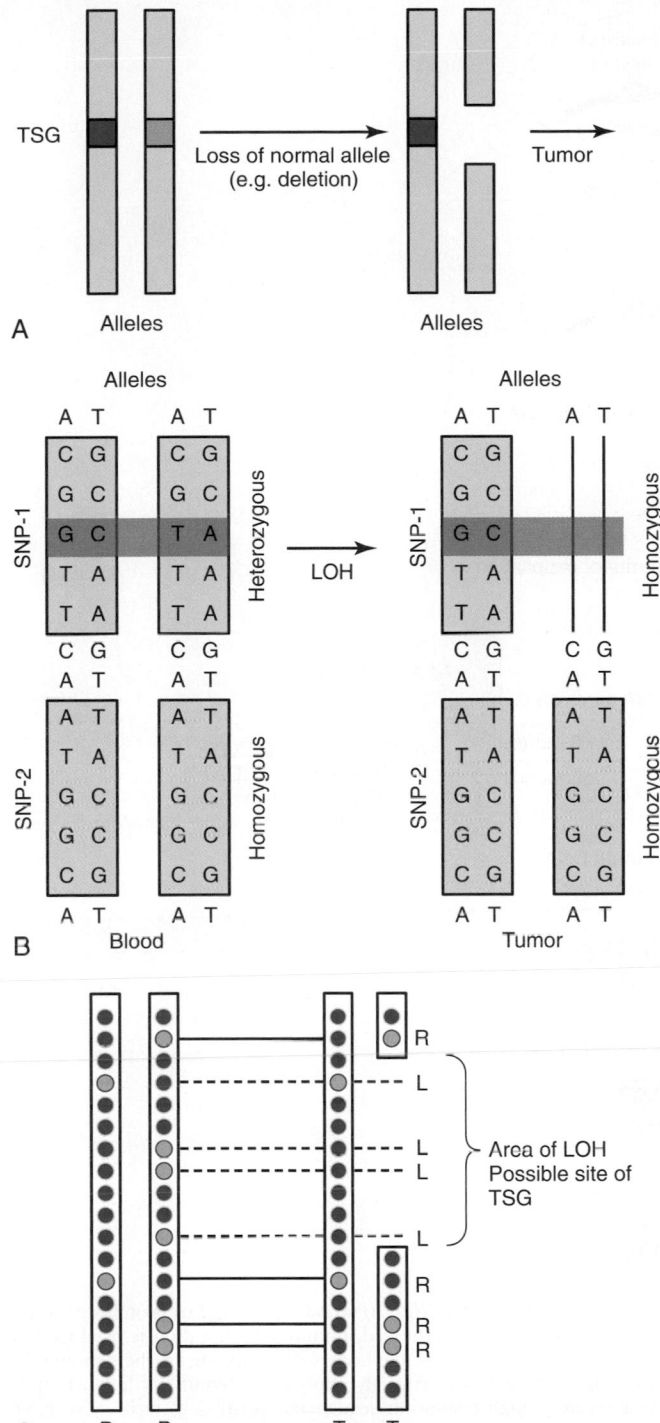

Figure 41-4 Using single nucleotide polymorphism *(SNP)* array technology to detect loss of heterozygosity (LOH) with detection of a possible tumor suppressor gene *(TSG)*. **A,** Part of a chromosome with a mutated *(black)* and normal *(gray)* copy of a TSG. Loss of the normal TSG leads to tumor formation, because the remaining TSG is not functional. **B,** Region of chromosome from blood and tumor showing two SNPs. The subject is homozygous for SNP-2 in the blood but heterozygous for SNP-1. In the tumor sample from the same patient, SNP-1 is detected as homozygous, because one of the alleles has been lost. This "loss of heterozygosity" can be a marker for chromosomal deletion. **C,** An expanded view of both alleles showing many SNPs. In the tumor, several of the heterozygous SNPs have been lost, indicating the site of a possible TSG. Homozygous SNPs are noninformative, because the loss of an allele will not be detected.

techniques are used to determine the sequence and region of DNA bound by the protein. In standard ChIP, low-resolution, traditional sequencing methods[54] or PCR are used, followed by genome mapping. ChIP has been productively applied to study histone binding,[55,56] histone acetylation,[57] and cell differentiation in myeloid leukemia cells.[58] To increase the coverage and depth of DNA binding site discovery, the analysis of protein-bound DNA was extended to DNA microarrays ("ChIP-chip" or "ChIP-on-chip").[59-61] This technique has been applied to describe histone binding patterns,[62,63] identify therapeutic targets in persons with acute myelogenous leukemia,[64] and describe and map transcriptional networks and histone modifications in leukemia.[65,66] With the development and popularization of next-generation sequencing (NGS) techniques, the products of ChIP can be subjected to high-resolution sequencing ("ChIP-seq"). This technique has been used to describe a genome-wide map of chromatin binding in stem cells,[67] delineate histone phosphorylation,[68] identify transcription factor binding sites,[69] demonstrate the requirement of histone ligase in mixed-lineage leukemia–rearranged leukemia,[70] describe transcriptional networks,[65] and provide overall maps of chromatin binding and histone modifications in leukemia.[66]

Genome-Wide Association Studies

The purpose of a genome-wide association study (GWAS) is typically to compare two groups (e.g., cases/control) to find common genetic variants associated with either group.[71-73] As a by-product of sequencing the human genome, the discovery of large numbers of SNP variants facilitated an unbiased interrogation of the genome. Useful SNPs must be selectively neutral and have relatively high frequencies (generally >0.05). More than 1 million SNPs were collected for the HapMap project, capturing most of the genomic variation in a select number of human populations.[74] GWA studies are only dependent on linkage disequilibrium between the genotyped SNP and the nongenotyped causal variants, with the strength of the association depending on their allele frequencies (Fig. 41-6). Hundreds of loci have been discovered for many complex diseases and traits such as Crohn disease,[75] ulcerative colitis,[76] and short stature.[77] Metabolic traits, autoimmune diseases, cancer, and many complex traits have been studied extensively and with large sample sizes by GWA studies.[77a] Data from a GWA study are typically visualized with use of a Manhattan plot (Fig. 41-7).[78] Much of the statistical analysis of GWA study data focuses on determining the significance threshold given the sample size and the large number of features (multiple testing).[79]

Exome Sequencing/Targeted Sequencing

Although GWA studies have identified many loci contributing to diseases and complex traits, most findings account for only a small proportion of the heritability.[80,81] Many mendelian disorders have been attributed to underlying genetic changes through linkage analysis and resequencing. Nevertheless, the causative mutations for more than half of the ~6000 known mendelian disorders remain

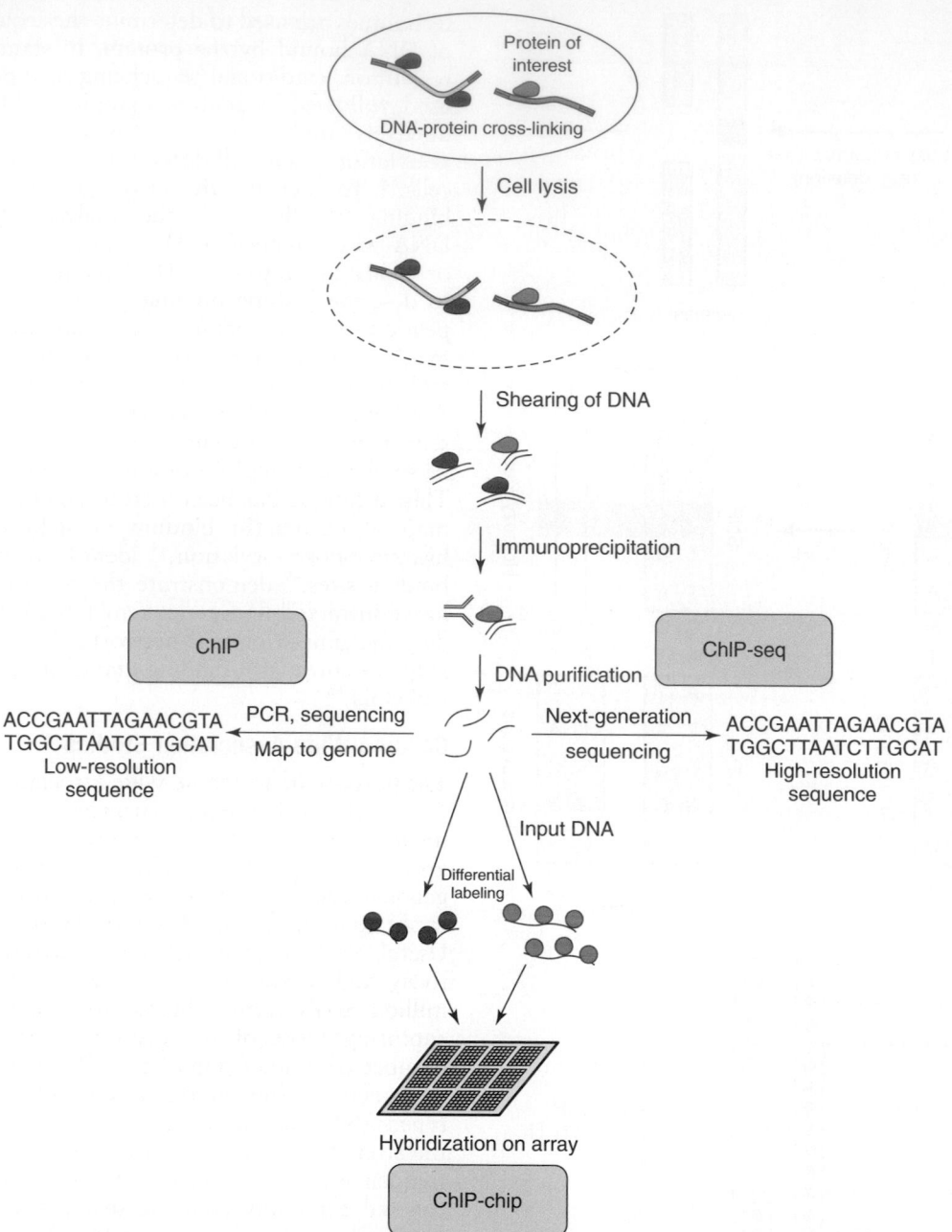

Figure 41-5 Chromatin immunoprecipitation *(ChIP)* is used to determine the deoxyribonucleic acid *(DNA)* sequences bound to proteins of interest. In traditional ChIP *(left)*, proteins are cross-linked to DNA, the cells are lysed, and the DNA is sheared. Immunoprecipitation is used to pull down the protein-DNA complexes. Purified DNA is then subjected to sequencing through traditional methods with mapping to the genome. In ChIP-chip (ChIP-on-chip), the DNA is not sequenced but is instead labeled and applied to a DNA array. By applying differentially labeled input DNA, the regions to which the proteins were bound can be ascertained. Most recently, high-resolution sequencing (ChIP-seq) techniques have emerged in which the isolated and purified DNA is subjected to high-resolution next-generation sequencing. *PCR,* Polymerase chain reaction.

unknown, mostly because of the paucity of cases and low penetrance.[82-84] Therefore an abundance of low-penetrant common variants are now described that reportedly contribute to the inheritance of common diseases (Fig. 41-8).[85] Highly penetrant but rare mutations that contribute to diseases with mendelian inheritance are being identified through NGS high-throughput methods that parallelize the sequencing process, producing millions of concurrent sequences.[86-89,90-92] To better focus on these potential causes of disease, target enrichment strategies

were developed to facilitate a focused sequencing to determine the coding variation in the entire genome (Fig. 41-9).[93,94] The exome represents the 1% of the genome (30 megabases) that is translated into proteins.[95] Although the untranslated regions are part of the exon, exome sequencing studies usually do not include these regions. The general workflow for whole exome sequencing (WES) involves DNA extraction, fragmentation, exome segment isolation, and sequencing (Fig. 41-10).[96] For many diseases for which conventional approaches have failed,

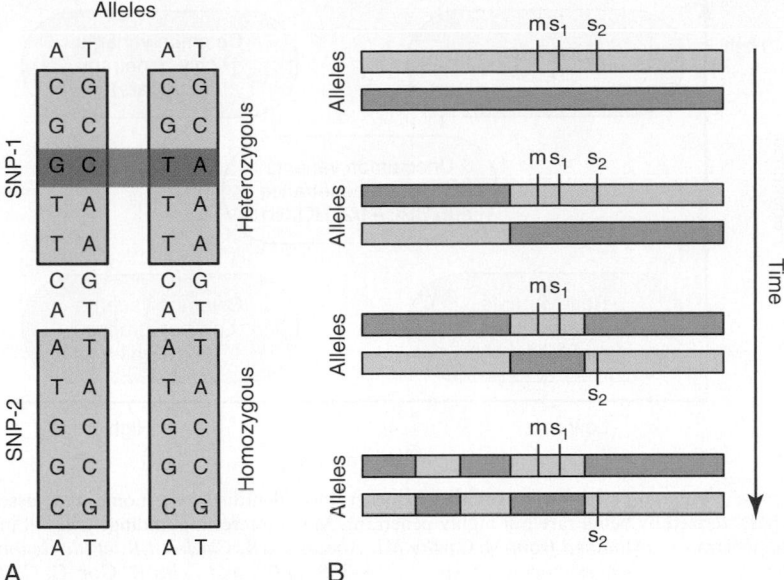

Figure 41-6 **A**, Two single nucleotide polymorphisms *(SNPs)* are shown, both on the same chromosome. This individual is heterozygous for SNP-1 and homozygous for SNP-2. **B**, A gene mutation is shown, along with two SNPs. The first SNP is closely associated with the mutation, whereas the second is in strong linage disequilibrium. Note how during recombination, the haplotype block containing the mutation and SNP-1 remains intact, whereas SNP-2 does not remain associated. By comparing large numbers of SNPs in persons with a disease to persons without a disease, one can infer the location of mutations associated with the condition.

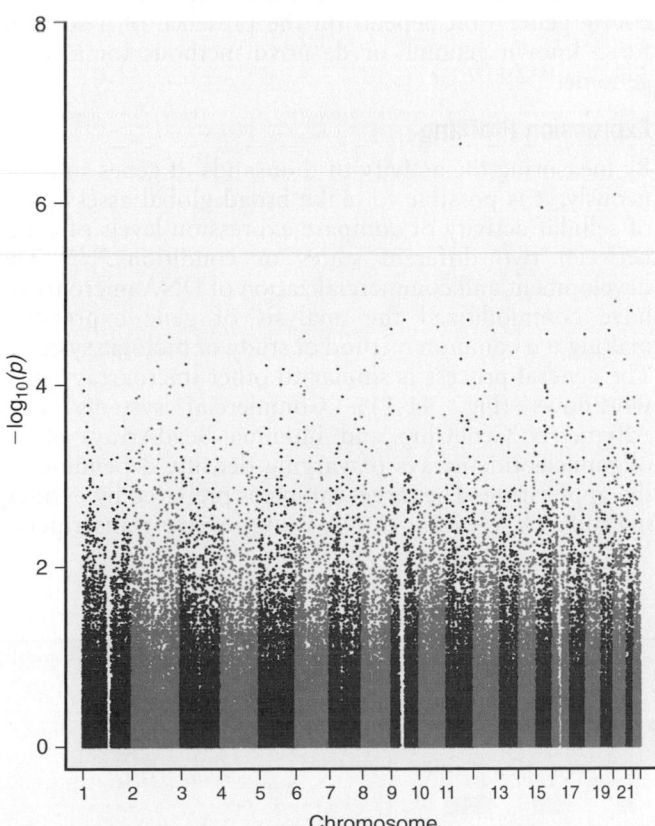

Figure 41-7 A typical Manhattan plot showing the significance of genetic variants (single nucleotide polymorphisms) along each chromosome. The highest ones are most likely to be statistically significant.

exome sequencing has led to candidate gene identification.[97,98,99,100] Targeted exome sequencing has also provided evidence for alternative transcriptional start sites in colorectal carcinoma,[101] RET gene fusion in lung cancer in nonsmokers,[102] and stage-specific alternative splicing in neuroblastoma.[103] Of course, identifying the disease-related genes among all of the sequencing errors and non–disease-causing polymorphisms remains a considerable challenge. The application of exome sequencing typically results in identification of more than 20,000 single nucleotide variants, and although most are known polymorphisms, other details are necessary, such as the pedigree, mode of inheritance, and sample size. The informatics techniques for identifying causal and alternatively spliced variants are well established.[97,104-106] Although the costs of whole genome sequencing (WGS) are decreasing, WES remains a mainstay for identifying causal variants of genetic diseases.

Whole Genome Sequencing

NGS methodologies can be applied to determine the entire sequence of an organism's genome. A current role for WGS and WES is to study whether common complex diseases are driven by rare variants ("rare variant hypothesis")[107-109] or by many common variants with small effects on risk ("common disease–common variant").[110-112] Methods for WGS are similar to exome and whole transcriptome sequencing (Fig. 41-10). Isolated and fragmented DNA is subjected to repetitive and overlapping sequencing to achieve the most robust coverage. Although the cost of WGS remains relatively high, identification of rare disease-causing variants is often achieved by family studies in which sequencing efforts are focused on individuals at the extremes of the trait's

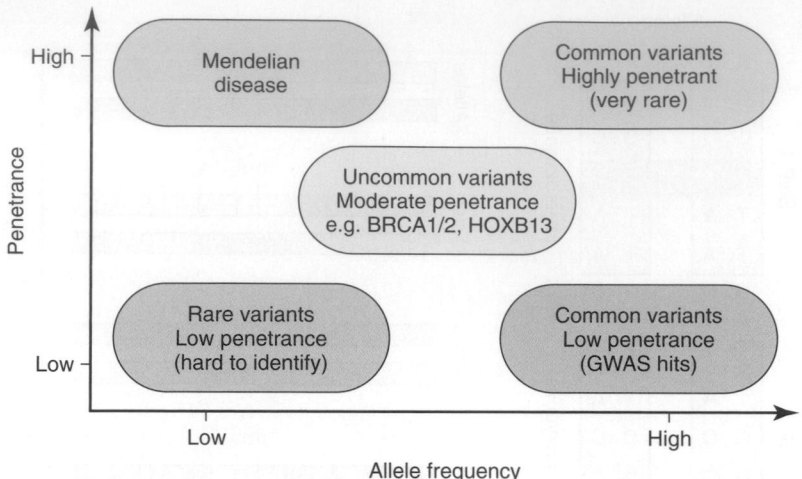

Figure 41-8 Genetic architecture showing common variants with low penetrance identified by genome-wide association studies (GWAS). Conversely, mendelian diseases are characterized by being rare but highly penetrant. Many interesting findings will fall in the middle range with modest variant frequency with moderate penetrance. *(Modified from McCarthy MI, Abecasis GR, Cardon LR, et al: Genome-wide association studies for complex traits: consensus, uncertainty and challenges. Nat Rev Genet 9:356–369, 2008, and Eeles R, Goh C, Castro E, et al: The genetic epidemiology of prostate cancer and its clinical implications. Nat Rev Urol 11:18–31, 2014.)*

distribution or by studying the most distant coaffected subjects.[109] As might be expected, considerable informatics challenges exist for determining significant rare variants.[113]

RNA-BASED METHODS

Whole Transcriptome Shotgun Sequencing (RNA-Seq)

Although hybridization-based (e.g., microarray) studies target the millions of common alleles (SNPs) in the genome, such libraries are limited in their ability to detect rare variants that cause disease. NGS methodologies facilitate the unbiased sequencing of all RNA transcripts in a cell (RNA-seq[114,115]; Fig. 41-9), providing a means to study gene fusions,[116] mutations, alternative splicing,[117-119] and modulation in gene expression levels.[120-124] Subpopulations of RNA such as microRNA (miRNA), transfer RNA, and ribosomes can be characterized as well.[125-129] Sequencing of the transcriptome has been applied to many malignancies, including prostate cancer,[130] mesothelioma,[131] squamous cell lung cancer,[132] Fanconi anemia,[133] and breast cancer.[134] The general

workflow for transcriptome sequencing is similar to WGS and WES, except that isolated RNA must first be converted into a cDNA library (Fig. 41-10). Once sequencing data have been collected, alignment and contig generation depend on the presence of a scaffold for a known genome or de novo methods for a novel genome.[114,135-137]

Expression Profiling

By measuring the activity of thousands of genes simultaneously, it is possible to make broad global assessments of cellular activity or compare expression levels of genes between two different states or conditions.[35,138] The development and commercialization of DNA microarrays have commoditized the analysis of gene expression, making it a common method of study of biologic systems. The general process is similar to other microarray-based workflows (Fig. 41-11). Commercial systems (e.g., Affymetrix GeneChip and Illumina BeadArray) utilize oligonucleotide arrays of varying density, depending on the application. The target sample is prepared by extracting miRNA, creating cDNA using reverse transcriptase,

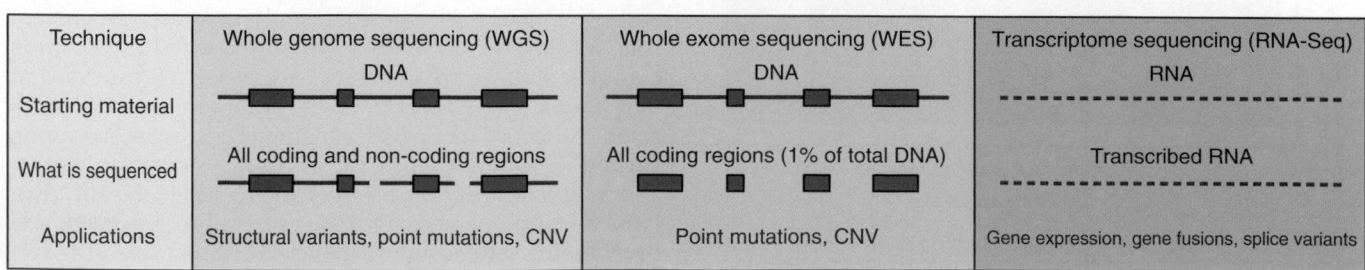

Figure 41-9 Strategies for next-generation sequencing *(NGS)*. Whole genome sequencing determines the deoxyribonucleic acid *(DNA)* sequence for all DNA, both introns and exons, whereas whole exome sequencing only describes the coding portions. In transcriptomics, the transcribed ribonucleic acid *(RNA)* is sequenced, leading to information about gene expression, gene fusions, and splice variants. *CNV,* Copy number variation. *(Modified from Simon R, Roychowdhury S: Implementing personalized cancer genomics in clinical trials. Nat Rev Drug Discov 12:358–369, 2013.)*

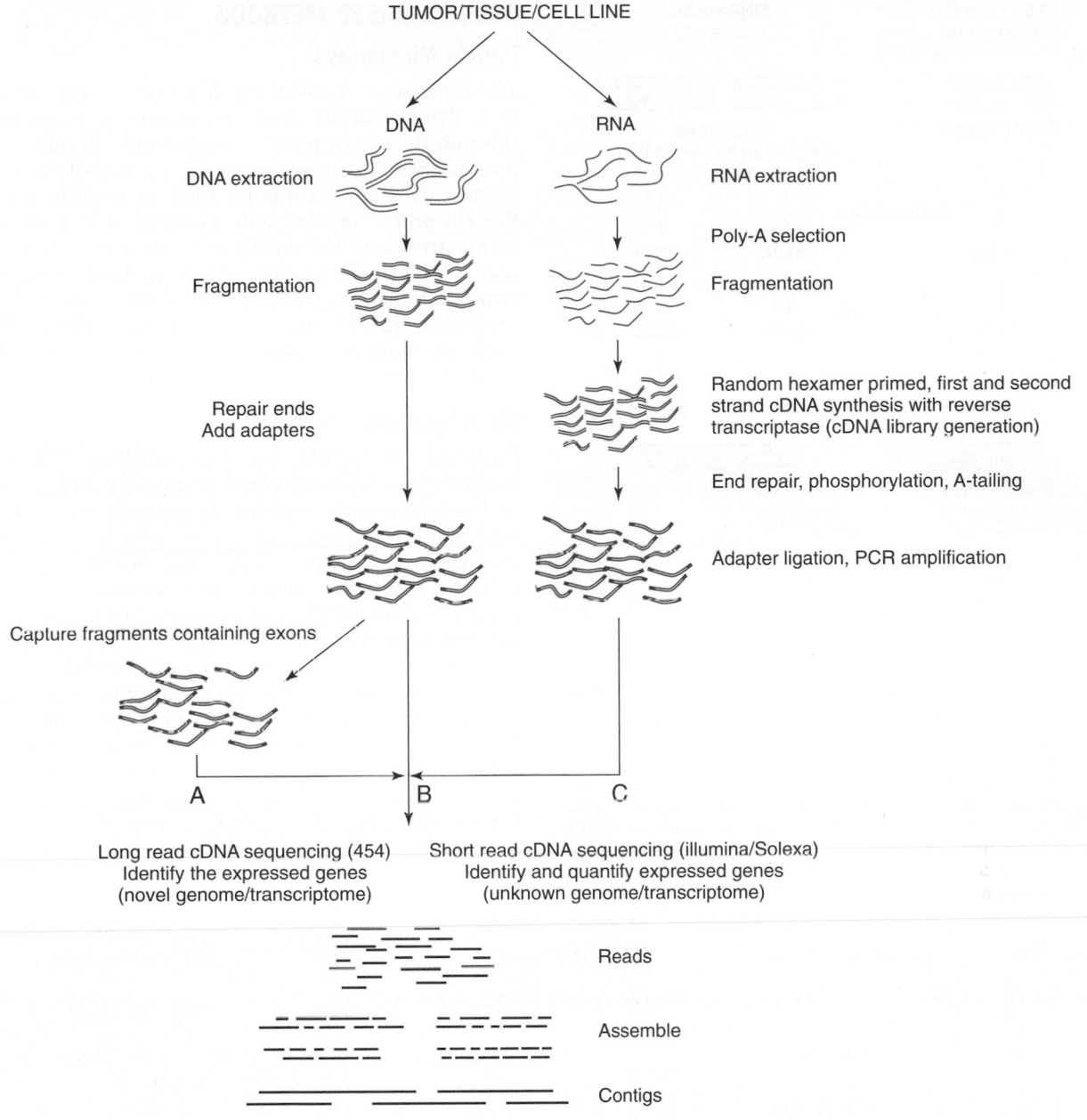

Figure 41-10 Workflow for whole exome sequencing *(A)*, whole genome sequencing *(B)*, and ribonucleic acid *(RNA)*-seq/whole transcriptome sequencing *(C)*. DNA, Deoxyribonucleic acid; *cDNA*, complementary DNA; *PCR*, polymerase chain reaction. *(Partially modified from Bras J, Guerreiro R, Hardy J: Use of next-generation sequencing and other whole-genome strategies to dissect neurological disease.* Nat Rev Neurosci 13:453–464, 2012.)

and then labeling the DNA. Even though each chip characterizes a single sample, the high reproducibility of the system facilitates comparison of expression levels between more than one condition. To compare two conditions directly, they are first differentially labeled (e.g., green and red), combined, and then applied to a cDNA array with subsequent measurement of the intensity ratios.[139] Three applications for gene expression profiling are: (1) class comparison, (2) class prediction, and (3) class discovery.[138] For class comparison, the objective is to understand which genes are differentially expressed between

two known disease subtypes or conditions (Fig. 41-12).[140] The goal of class prediction is to define a classifier that can facilitate class membership for a sample based on its gene expression profile.[141-143,144-146] Class discovery is useful when trying to define clinically relevant molecular subtypes.[140,146-150] MiRNA functions as a regulator of gene expression both during and after transcription.[151] The expression of miRNA can be monitored with use of microarrays, as described earlier.[152,153] Such methods were used to show a novel miRNA profile for chronic lymphocytic leukemia.[154-156]

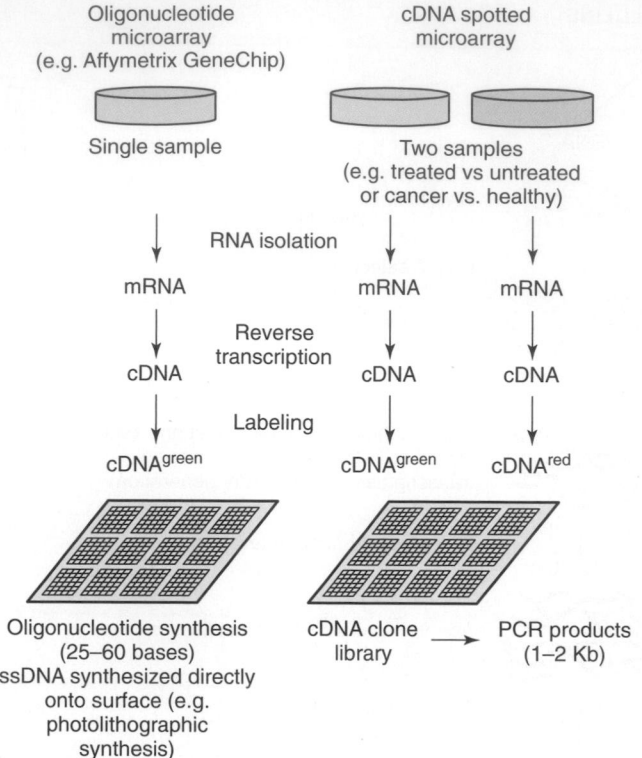

Figure 41-11 Oligonucleotide arrays *(left)* require synthesis of the deoxyribonucleic acid *(DNA)* sequence directly onto the solid support, whereas complementary DNA *(cDNA)* spotted arrays *(right)* are produced by the deposition of DNA onto the slide. Because of the high reproducibility of the oligonucleotide arrays, comparisons between chip analyses can be performed to determine differential levels of gene expression. To compare two conditions using cDNA microarrays, a single experiment using two different color fluorophores is required. *mRNA,* Messenger ribonucleic acid; *PCR,* polymerase chain reaction; *ssDNA,* single-stranded DNA.

PROTEIN-BASED METHODS

Protein Microarrays

The large-scale monitoring of protein expression, function determination, and interaction can be assessed through the use of protein microarrays. Similar to DNA microarrays in concept, proteins are immobilized on the surface of a solid support, such as a glass slide.[157,158] Protein probes labeled with fluorescent dye are applied to the array and the interactions are monitored by laser scanning. Protein microarrays have been used to construct interactome maps,[159] monitor protein levels in patients with chronic graft-versus-host disease,[160] and facilitate biomarker identification for cancer and other diseases.[161-164]

Mass Spectrometry

Proteomic analysis by mass spectrometry (MS) remains the mainstay of comprehensive protein analysis in cells and other complex systems. In general, most MS-based studies follow a paradigm of protein isolation, enzymatic digestion, separation, MS, and informatic analysis (Fig. 41-13).[165] For quantitative studies,[166] cells can be grown in differential isotopic media (with stable isotope labeling by amino acids in culture) or labeled during or after enzymatic digestion (oxygen-18 [18O],[167] isobaric tag for relative and absolute quantitation [iTRAQ][168]) so that amounts of nonlabeled (light) and labeled (heavy) peptides can be compared. Traditional proteomic approaches involving data-dependent acquisition are based on selecting the top most abundant precursor ions for fragmentation. As a result, protein identifications are disproportionate, with the abundant proteins in a sample

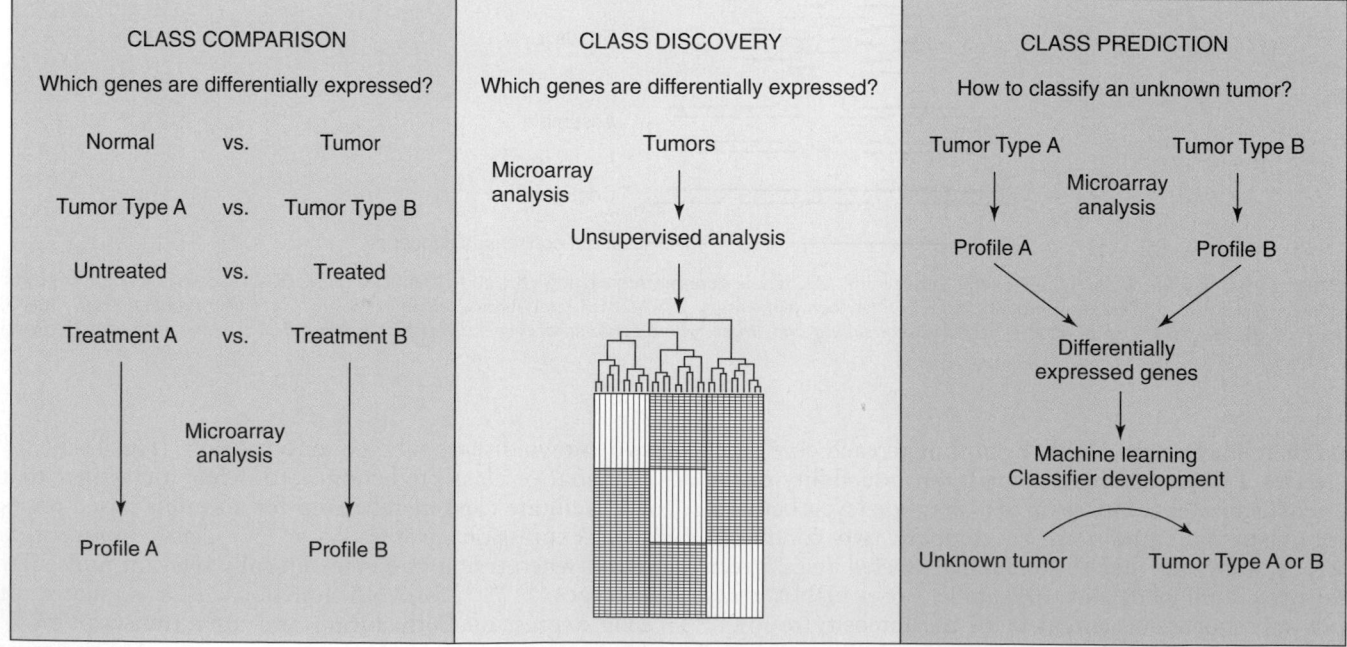

Figure 41-12 Applications for gene profiling include class comparison *(left)* in which two different conditions or tumors are compared to determine which genes are differentially expressed. Class discovery *(middle)* does not require prior knowledge about the tumor types but instead looks for subgroups of differentially expressed genes. Class prediction *(right)* results in the discovery of a gene classifier that can predict the class of an unknown sample.

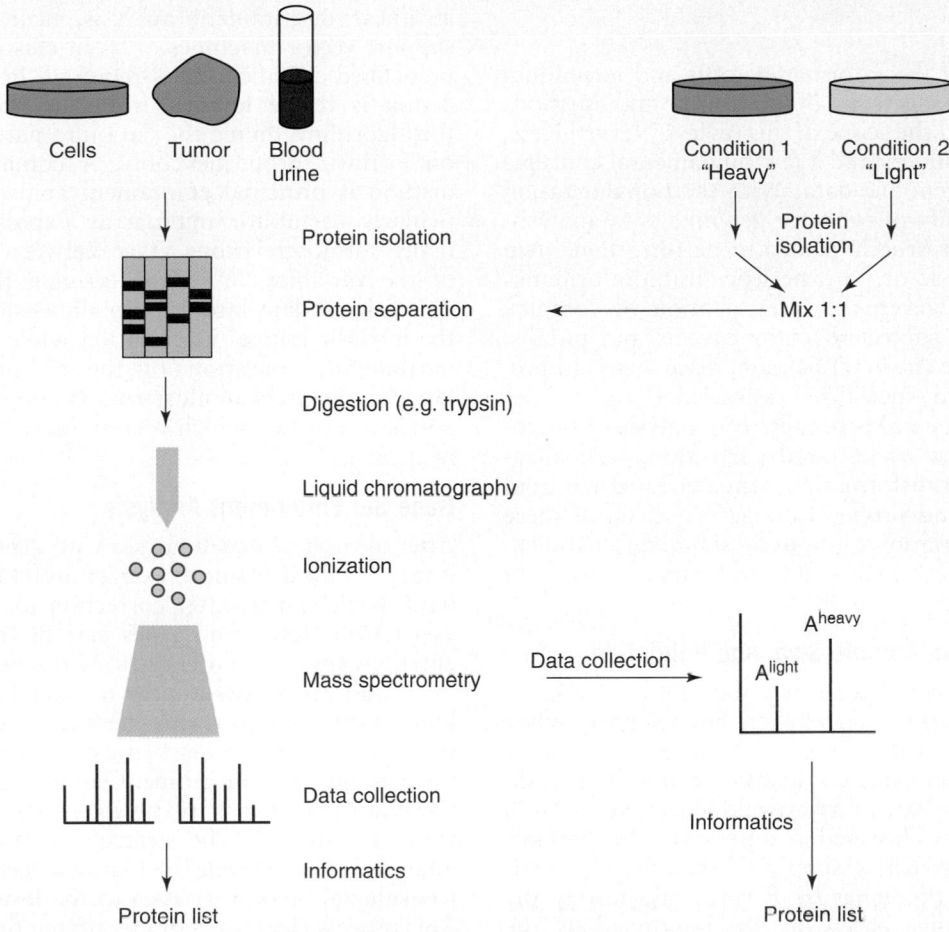

Figure 41-13 The standard workflow for mass spectrometry–based proteomics *(left)* includes isolation of proteins from a complex sample followed by separation, usually by gel electrophoresis. The proteins are then subjected to trypsin digestion and then separated by liquid chromatography prior to ionization and injection onto the mass spectrometer. All data are collected and then analyzed offline to match spectra to peptides and to create the most parsimonious protein list. A quantitative proteomics experiment *(right)* often involves growing cells in a "light" (normal) and "heavy" isotope-labeled media. The proteins are then mixed in equal amounts and subjected to a similar workflow. Peptides from each condition can be identified by the characteristic mass shift, and their relative peak heights correspond to quantitative differences.

getting more coverage and low-abundance (and often more interesting) proteins being missed entirely. The downside of narrow dynamic range is evident in MS analysis of complex samples such as human serum, wherein the most abundant proteins account for more than 85% to 90% of total protein content,[169,170] whereas the more informative proteins remain in the low molecular weight serum proteome.[171-173] To circumvent these issues, researchers typically incorporate the use of labeled cell lines, enrichment strategies, fractionation techniques, and protein depletion methods (e.g., Agilent [Santa Clara, Calif.] Multiple Affinity Removal System column) into experimental protocols.[171,174] On the analysis front, inclusion lists and single/multiple reaction monitoring assays for targeted proteomics are used and have been shown to be sensitive[175,176] even in the context of biomarker validation in human plasma.[177,178] However, these methods still have a fundamental flaw in that the candidates for inclusion are chosen without regard for the overlap between the proteins of interest and the dominant background. Thus, in the context of analyzing important cancer protein markers, the complexity of the

human proteome makes it difficult for the MS platform to characterize a few select proteins effectively. Informatics challenges present a second major obstacle to the effective use of proteomics in a clinical setting. Providing researchers and clinicians with access to powerful computing resources and data management tools that are capable of rapidly processing the hundreds of samples in large-scale clinical settings remains a challenge. Existing proteomics pipelines such as the Trans-Proteomic Pipeline,[179] OpenMS,[180] and ProteoWizard[181,182] run on workstations but do not work effectively at these scales. On-demand cloud computing services, such as that operated by Amazon Web Services, provide an intriguing alternative,[183] and cloud-based options for data processing are available.[184-186] Galaxy-P (https://usegalaxyp.org/), developed at the University of Minnesota, is a framework for performing computation-intensive proteomic data processing on their computer cluster. Inspired by the public Galaxy server[187,188] that is used for genomics at the University of Pennsylvania, Galaxy-P offers key proteomics software applications on a freely available platform.

INFORMATICS

A full summary of the informatics tools and techniques across the broad spectrum of platforms and methods discussed is beyond the scope of this review. Nevertheless, it is important to understand a few fundamental concepts when evaluating genomic data. With the popularization and wide availability of tools for genomic data analysis, it is common for research groups to perform their own analysis despite little or no experience in bioinformatics and statistics. However, the interpretation of complex and dense data is subject to many caveats and pitfalls. The algorithms for class comparison, discovery, and prediction all require specialized knowledge for proper application. The general procedure for analysis of microarray data includes background correction, normalization, logarithmic transformation, batch effect correction, outlier removal, and probe filtering.[189-193] Each of these steps has many variations, and understanding the indications and caveats for each is an important part of data analysis.

False-Positive Rate, Sample Size, and Validation

With a large number of features, the number of false-positive results becomes significant. For instance, when testing 20,000 genes for differential expression, even if none is truly significant (i.e., no true-positives), a traditional false-positive rate of 5% would indicate that 1000 genes will be falsely classified as differentially expressed. One possible approach is simply to increase the stringency by ranking the genes by P value and testing the value for significance based on 5% multiplied by the rank of the P value divided by the number of features, thus limiting the false-discovery rate to less than 5%. A simpler method is the Bonferroni correction, in which the P value is divided by the number of tests.[194] The most important factors influencing the P value are the absolute proportion of true-positive differentially expressed genes, the distribution of the differences, the variability in expression, and the sample size.[195] Of course, overly aggressive methods for controlling for the false-discovery rate will raise the false-negative rate. Increasing the sample size can help alleviate this problem.[195,196] It is critical that differentially expressed genes be validated, either in another experiment using a different sample set or by using an alternative method such as reverse transcriptase–PCR.[196]

Clustering and Classification

Classification is the process of predicting membership in predetermined groups and requires training data with known class assignments for each point.[197] For example, with a set of gene expression data on patients with leukemia of known risk group status, one could use classification techniques to predict which features (genes) could be used to classify an unknown patient. Classification is a form of supervised learning and requires knowledge of not only the feature values (gene expression) but also the class of each sample. Supervised learning methods are usually neighbor based, such as k-nearest neighbors, or based on discriminating hyperplanes, such as linear discriminant analysis, neural networks, and support vector machines.[198,199] In clustering analysis, no predefined classification is required. Instead, the classification is to be learned from the data only, because the algorithms divide the data into natural groups based on intrinsic properties only. A common unsupervised method is principal component analysis, which is particularly useful for microarray expression data where many intracorrelations exist between a large number of the variables.[200,201] Transforming the original high-dimensional data into a lower dimensional space retains the intrinsic critical information while still facilitating a meaningful separation of the samples into relevant groups. Hierarchical clustering is another form of unsupervised analysis, which is commonly visualized through heat maps.[197]

Gene Set Enrichment Analysis

After using statistical analyses with gene expression data, it may still be difficult to extract useful meaning from the data. For instance, after correction for multiple hypotheses testing, few or no genes may be found to be differentially expressed. Alternatively, the list of differentially expressed genes may appear to have no underlying biologic theme. Additionally, the overall effect of pathway interactions may be masked as a result of the measurement of one gene at a time. One way to compensate for these shortcomings is to apply gene set enrichment analysis to the data.[202] The strategy in gene set enrichment analysis is to use predefined knowledge of gene pathways to evaluate microarray data at the level of the gene set. This process is a means of identifying functionally related groups of genes.[203]

CONCLUSIONS

It remains challenging to keep pace with the rapid advancements in systems biology technology. The development and widespread adoption of NGS technologies have resulted in torrents of data. The informatics challenges are considerable and include issues of storage, access, and analysis. These problems will only continue to grow because the rate of data accumulation is likely to increase. As more institutions adopt genomic testing platforms, informaticists, geneticists, pathologists, and other clinicians will need to work together to apply these tools appropriately.[204] With the concurrent popularization and widespread availability of genomics analysis tools, it is increasingly important to retain expertise in the acquisition and analysis of high-density genomic data. Many successful research institutions have established bioinformatics core service teams that serve as collaborators throughout the experimental process, from planning to data collection to analysis and interpretation. Bioinformatics experts are most likely to have access to the most current and advanced tools and will understand the subtleties and nuances inherent to complex data analysis and interpretation. For the nonexpert, it is most important to understand the context in which the technology or platform is being used. As old methods are supplanted by new ones, the most well-informed scientist, researcher, or clinician will recognize the progression and adoption of newer technologies and appreciate any positive and negative implications. We have never experienced a more exciting time in medicine. In the next 10 years, enormous growth will occur in our knowledge about complex biological processes, resulting in new methods of disease prevention and therapy.

References available online at ExpertConsult.

KEY REFERENCES

2. MacConaill LE: Existing and emerging technologies for tumor genomic profiling. *J Clin Oncol* 31:1815–1824, 2013.

   An excellent overview of the range of technologies being applied to tumor genomic profiling.

18. Sanger F, Coulson AR: A rapid method for determining sequences in DNA by primed synthesis with DNA polymerase. *J Mol Biol* 94:441–448, 1975.

   Sanger's original article describing DNA sequencing—remarkably only 40 years old.

34. Yershov G, Barsky V, Belgovskiy A, et al: DNA analysis and diagnostics on oligonucleotide microchips. *Proc Natl Acad Sci U S A* 93:4913–4918, 1996.

   One of the original microarray DNA analysis descriptions.

36. Venter JC, Adams MD, Myers EW, et al: The sequence of the human genome. *Science* 291:1304–1351, 2001.

   A landmark publication of the first human genome sequence.

52. Bernstein BE, Meissner A, Lander ES: The mammalian epigenome. *Cell* 128:669–681, 2007.

   A comprehensive survey of epigenomics.

73. Manolio TA: Genomewide association studies and assessment of the risk of disease. *N Engl J Med* 363:166–176, 2010.

   An important review of genome-wide association studies and implications for clinical research.

74. International HapMap Consortium: A haplotype map of the human genome. *Nature* 437:1299–1320, 2005.

   A landmark article including the description of the human genome haplotype map.

85. McCarthy MI, Abecasis GR, Cardon LR, et al: Genome-wide association studies for complex traits: consensus, uncertainty and challenges. *Nat Rev Genet* 9:356–369, 2008.

   An older review of genome-wide association studies that is interesting in its context at the edge of the NGS revolution.

90. Shendure J, Ji H: Next-generation DNA sequencing. *Nat Biotechnol* 26:1135–1145, 2008.

   Evolution and development of NGS.

93. Simon R, Roychowdhury S: Implementing personalized cancer genomics in clinical trials. *Nat Rev Drug Discov* 12:358–369, 2013.

   The authors discuss the challenges of integrating cancer genomics into clinical practice.

97. Bamshad MJ, Ng SB, Bigham AW, et al: Exome sequencing as a tool for Mendelian disease gene discovery. *Nat Rev Genet* 12:745–755, 2011.

   A good introduction to exome sequencing and how it is used to study complex traits.

99. Yang Y, Muzny DM, Reid JG, et al: Clinical whole-exome sequencing for the diagnosis of mendelian disorders. *N Engl J Med* 369:1502–1511, 2013.

   Demonstrates how whole exome sequencing will revolutionize the diagnosis of genetic disorders for which no known cause has been found.

110. Plomin R, Haworth CMA, Davis OSP: Common disorders are quantitative traits. *Nat Rev Genet* 10:872–878, 2009.

   An interesting discussion of the theory that common disorders are due to the complex interplay of the small effects of many common genes.

114. Wang Z, Gerstein M, Snyder M: RNA-Seq: a revolutionary tool for transcriptomics. *Nat Rev Genet* 10:57–63, 2009.

   A review of RNA-seq, its development, and its use.

139. Shalon D, Smith SJ, Brown PO: A DNA microarray system for analyzing complex DNA samples using two-color fluorescent probe hybridization. *Genome Res* 6:639–645, 1996.

   One of the first large-scale demonstrations of two-channel detection in DNA microarrays.

144. Shipp MA, Ross KN, Tamayo P, et al: Diffuse large B-cell lymphoma outcome prediction by gene-expression profiling and supervised machine learning. *Nat Med* 8:68–74, 2002.

   A very important article illustrating the importance of supervised clustering algorithms and the need for classifier validation.

150. Armstrong SA, Staunton JE, Silverman LB, et al: MLL translocations specify a distinct gene expression profile that distinguishes a unique leukemia. *Nat Genet* 30:41–47, 2002.

   A landmark article describing the discovery of a novel form of childhood leukemia, as determined through gene expression profiling and clustering analysis.

151. Yates LA, Norbury CJ, Gilbert RJC: The long and short of microRNA. *Cell* 153:516–519, 2013.

   An in-depth primer on microRNA.

171. Mayne J, Starr AE, Ning Z, et al: Fine tuning of proteomic technologies to improve biological findings: advancements in 2011-2013. *Anal Chem* 86:176–195, 2014.

   An excellent current review of a broad range of proteomics topics.

187. Hillman-Jackson J, Clements D, Blankenberg D, et al: Using Galaxy to perform large-scale interactive data analyses. *Curr Protoc Bioinformatics* Chapter 10:Unit10.5, 2012.

   Galaxy has emerged as a key tool for genomics and proteomics work, as outlined in this review.

189. Cordero F, Botta M, Calogero RA: Microarray data analysis and mining approaches. *Brief Funct Genomic Proteomic* 6(4):265–281, 2007.

   This article covers in an accessible way many of the issues inherent to microarray data analysis.

202. Subramanian A, Tamayo P, Mootha VK, et al: Gene set enrichment analysis: a knowledge-based approach for interpreting genome-wide expression profiles. *Proc Natl Acad Sci U S A* 102(43):15545–15550, 2005.

   This article introduces gene set enrichment analysis, and it remains a good review of the theory and practice.

CHAPTER 42

Genetic Predisposition to Cancer

Kristin Zelley, Robert B. Lindell, Joshua D. Schiffman, and Kim E. Nichols

CHAPTER OUTLINE

It is currently estimated that 1% to 10% of children with cancer develop the disease due to an underlying genetic predisposition.[1-4] Over the last 3 decades, there has been an explosion in knowledge regarding the heritable causes of cancer, including the discovery of many genes that when mutated in the germline significantly increase the risk for tumor formation in children. This knowledge has allowed for a better understanding of the mechanisms leading to tumor formation and provided insights into the development of novel cancer therapies targeting defective genetic pathways. Through presymptomatic genetic testing, it is also now possible to identify children who are at increased risk for tumor formation and to initiate surveillance protocols with the intent to improve overall outcomes through the detection of early-stage tumors that are more readily cured with less invasive and/or toxic therapies. In this chapter, we review the principles of cancer predisposition, steps involved in the recognition and testing of children for heritable cancer syndromes, and concepts underlying tumor surveillance. We also describe the clinical and genetic features typifying specific syndromes and review current recommendations regarding management. As there are too many conditions to discuss in this chapter, we focus on several syndromes that are associated primarily with the development of solid tumors. For a review of additional childhood cancer syndromes, including those that increase the risk for hematologic malignant tumors, we refer the reader to several excellent recent reviews.[5-8]

PRINCIPLES OF CANCER PREDISPOSITION

Seminal insights into cancer predisposition were gained in 1971 when Alfred Knudson developed the *two-hit hypothesis* to explain the epidemiology of retinoblastoma (RB), the most common pediatric eye tumor.[9] Children with RB show two patterns of tumor formation, including: (1) early-onset disease characterized by bilateral eye involvement and autosomal dominant inheritance; or (2) later-onset disease typified by unilateral eye involvement with no family history of RB. According to the two-hit hypothesis, children with bilateral RB are at increased risk for tumor formation because they carry an altered copy of a growth regulatory gene within the cells of the body; this constitutional (germline) mutation is known as the first hit. Knudson proposed that if the second gene copy underwent an inactivating mutation within a developing retinal cell (i.e., the second hit), that cell would then become susceptible to tumor formation. Because every cell in a child with heritable RB carries the first hit, children with this form are likely to develop more than one tumor (multifocal and/or bilateral RB) at a very young age. In contrast, for those with nonheritable RB, both hits would need to occur within a single retinal cell. As these mutational events are exceedingly rare, it is expected that the process would take longer and be less likely to occur. Thus, children with nonheritable RB would be older at presentation and only develop unilateral tumors.

In 1986, Stephen Friend confirmed Knudson's prediction by demonstrating that patients with bilateral RB harbor inactivating germline mutations in the RB susceptibility gene *RB1*, the first tumor suppressor gene to be identified.[10] Since this initial observation, many additional tumor suppressor genes have been cloned, and it is now clear that inactivating tumor suppressor gene mutations account for the majority of heritable cancers in humans. Other genetic mechanisms that contribute to heritable cancers include the presence of constitutional activating or "gain-of-function" mutations involving one copy of a growth-promoting oncogene, inactivating mutations in one or both alleles of an X-linked or autosomal recessive gene, and larger structural chromosomal abnormalities such as translocations, deletions, and duplications that disrupt or enhance the expression of a tumor suppressor gene or oncogene, respectively.

IDENTIFICATION OF A CHILD WITH A CONDITION PREDISPOSING TO CANCER

Pediatric oncologists play an important role in recognizing hereditary cancer syndromes in children and their families. Toward this end, there are several possible clues that point to the existence of a condition that predisposes a child to cancer, including: (1) a positive family history of cancer; (2) the diagnosis of specific tumor types in the child; (3) tumors that involve paired organs; and (4) the presence of associated physical or syndromic features. Pediatric oncologists should consider each of these factors when evaluating a patient and refer the child to a geneticist or genetic counselor when there is a suspicion of an underlying cancer predisposition.

Features of Family History Suggestive of a Heritable Predisposition to Cancer

Features of the family history that are suggestive of a genetic predisposition to cancer include the presence in the child or his or her close relatives of one or more cancers presenting at a younger than expected age, involving both of paired organs (e.g., eyes, kidneys, or adrenal glands) or exhibiting multifocality (more than one discrete tumor within an organ). Other suspicious features include the existence of multiple individuals on the same side of the family (maternal or paternal lineage) with the same type of cancer or cancers known to cluster together in certain syndromes (e.g., the clustering of soft tissue and bone sarcomas, early-onset breast cancer, brain tumors,

adrenocortical cancers, and leukemia in Li-Fraumeni syndrome [LFS]).

Pediatricians and pediatric oncologists should take a careful family history and generate a pedigree as a routine part of each patient's initial clinic visit. Ideally, the pedigree should include information about the child being seen (the proband), as well as his or her first-degree relatives (parents and siblings), second-degree relatives (aunts, uncles, and grandparents), and third-degree relatives (first cousins). For any individuals who have developed a cancer, its type, site of origin, stage (laterality, focality), and the age at which it was diagnosed should be determined. It is important to note whether individuals have had more than one cancer, and if so, to distinguish whether multiple cancers represent recurrence of the initial tumor or development of a second primary malignant tumor. Finally, it is important to gather information about the ethnic background of the family, as some genetic syndromes manifest more commonly in individuals from specific geographic regions (as is the case with hereditary breast and ovarian cancer, which is more common in Ashkenazi Jewish individuals with ancestors from Eastern Europe). Information about the biologic relationship between parents can provide insights into the mode of inheritance. For example, if parents are closely related or both come from a similar geographic region, there is a greater chance for consanguinity and the presence of an autosomal recessive condition.

The importance of collecting a family history cannot be underestimated; however, this procedure can have its limitations. Some hereditary syndromes exhibit incomplete penetrance where not everyone with the inherited mutation will develop a cancer. Variable expressivity can be a complicating factor, with affected individuals manifesting in different ways within a given family. One must recognize that family histories evolve over time. A child may have an affected parent; however, this parent might be young or not yet have developed a cancer or other features typical of the condition. In some cases, affected family members may die of other causes before they develop a cancer. Finally, the family history may be unrevealing when there is a de novo germline mutation in an affected child, the presence of autosomal recessive or X-linked recessive conditions (where carriers are clinically unaffected), nonpaternity, or situations in which a child is adopted and there is little knowledge of the biologic parents' family history. Due to these factors, it may be difficult to ascertain from a pedigree whether a specific syndrome is present. Nonetheless, the family history remains an important tool in recognizing conditions predisposing a child to cancer, and one should be obtained, regularly updated, and reviewed for the presence of a possible predisposition.

Tumor Features Suggestive of a Heritable Predisposition to Cancer

In addition to whether the tumor is unilateral or bilateral, unifocal or multifocal, specific tumor types should raise the suspicion of a syndrome predisposing to cancer, even in the absence of a positive family cancer history (Table 42-1). RB is an excellent example as there is a hereditable

TABLE 42-1 Pediatric Tumor Types and Underlying Syndromes Predisposing to Cancer

Tumor Type	Predisposition Syndrome	Gene(s)
Adrenocortical carcinoma*	Li-Fraumeni syndrome (LFS)	TP53
Astrocytoma	LFS	TP53
	Tuberous sclerosis	TSC1, TSC2
Atypical teratoid or rhabdoid tumor*	Rhabdoid tumor syndrome	SMARCB1/INI1
Basal cell carcinoma	Nevoid basal cell carcinoma syndrome (NBCCS)	PTCH1
Choroid plexus carcinoma*	LFS	TP53
Cystic nephroma* Bilateral or multifocal	Pleuropulmonary blastoma (PPB) family tumor and dysplasia syndrome/DICER1 syndrome	DICER1
Endolymphatic sac tumors	von Hippel–Lindau syndrome (VHL)	VHL
Fibroma	Familial ademonatous polyposis (FAP)	APC
Gardner fibroma (desmoid fibroma)		
Cardiac fibroma	NBCCS	PTCH1
Hemangioblastoma	VHL	VHL
Glioblastoma	LFS	TP53
	Constitutional mismatch repair–deficiency syndrome (CMMR-D)	MLH1, MSH2, MSH6, PMS2
Hepatoblastoma	Beckwith-Wiedemann syndrome (BWS)	11p15, CDKN1C
	FAP	APC
Leukemia		
Pre-B acute lymphoblastic (low-hypodiploid)* leukemia	PAX5-associated familial leukemia	PAX5
	LFS	TP53
Other types†	CMMR-D	MLH1, MSH2, MSH6, PMS2
	Neurofibromatosis type 1 (NF1)	NF1
Lipoma	PTEN hamartoma tumor syndrome (PHTS)	PTEN
Malignant peripheral nerve sheath tumor	NF1	NF1
Medulloblastoma	FAP	APC
	NBCCS	PTCH1
Neuroblastoma* Bilateral or multifocal	Hereditary neuroblastoma	ALK
		PHOX2B
Optic pathway glioma	NF1	NF1
Ovarian sex-cord stromal tumors	PPB family tumor and dysplasia syndrome/DICER1 syndrome	DICER1
	Peutz-Jeghers syndrome (PJS)	STK11/LKB1
Papillary cystadenoma of epididymis or broad ligament	VHL	VHL
Paraganglioma (PGL)/ pheochromocytoma (PCC)*	Hereditary PGL/PCC syndrome	SDHA, SDHB, SDHC, SDHD, SDHAF2, MAX, TMEM127
	Multiple endocrine neoplasia type 2 (MEN2)	RET
	NF1	NF1
	VHL	VHL
Pineoblastoma	Hereditary retinoblastoma (RB)	RB1
PPB*	PPB family tumor and dysplasia syndrome/DICER1 syndrome	DICER1
Retinoblastoma*	Hereditary RB	RB1
Sarcoma		
Liposarcoma	LFS	TP53
Rhabdomyosarcoma	LFS	TP53
	PPB family tumor and dysplasia syndrome/DICER1 syndrome	DICER1
	Costello syndrome	HRAS

TABLE 42-1 Pediatric Tumor Types and Underlying Syndromes Predisposing to Cancer (Continued)

Tumor Type	Predisposition Syndrome	Gene(s)
Osteosarcoma	Hereditary RB	*RB1*
	LFS	*TP53*
Schwannoma		
Acoustic neuroma*	Neurofibromatosis type 2 (NF2)	*NF2*
Schwanommatosis	Rhabdoid tumor syndrome	*SMARCB1/INI1*
Thyroid		
Medullary*	MEN2	*RET*
Nonmedullary	PHTS	*PTEN*
Wilms tumor	BWS	11p15, *CDKN1C*
Bilateral or multifocal*	*WT1*-related syndromes	*WT1*
Or with associated GU defects in males (hypospadias, undescended testicles)		

Seif AE: *Pediatric leukemia predisposition syndromes: clues to understanding leukemogenesis.* Cancer Genet 204(5):227-244, 2011; and Stieglitz E, Loh ML: *Genetic predispositions to childhood leukemia.* Ther Adv Hematol 4(4):270-290, 2013.

*Tumor types that warrant genetic testing even if there is no other personal or family history of cancer (where noted, only if tumor is bilateral or multifocal).

†Several other leukemia predisposition syndromes exist that are not discussed here.

component in 40% of patients.[11,12] Additional tumor types associated with a high likelihood of an underlying genetic predisposition include: (1) Wilms tumor (WT), where features such as bilaterality, early age of onset, and genitourinary anomalies in boys indicate a higher likelihood of a germline *WT1* mutation[13,14]; (2) pheochromocytoma (PCC) and paraganglioma (PGL), where more than 70% carry a germline mutation in *SDHB* or other associated PCC/PGL genes[15,16]; (3) atypical teratoid/rhabdoid tumor, where 35% carry a mutation in the *INI1/SMARCB1* gene[17]; (4) pleuropulmonary blastoma (PPB), where more than 70% of cases in one study carried a germline *DICER1* mutation[18]; (5) hepatoblastoma (HB), where up to 10% carry a mutation in the *APC* gene that is causative of familial adenomatous polyposis (FAP)[19]; (6) medullary thyroid cancer (MTC), where 20% to 25% carry a mutation in the *RET* protooncogene[20]; (7) medulloblastoma, where onset at an age younger than 5 years and desmoplastic histology are indicative of possible nevoid basal cell carcinoma syndrome (NBCCS, Gorlin syndrome)[21,22], where patients harbor germline mutations of *PTCH1*; and (8) adrenocortical carcinoma (ACC), choroid plexus carcinoma (CPC), and rhabdomyosarcoma presenting under the age of 3 years, where 50% to 80%, 35% to 100%, and 20% of children, respectively, carry germline mutations in the *TP53* gene.[23-27] The diagnosis of an adult-onset tumor in a child should also raise suspicion for a predisposing condition. For example, the presence of colorectal cancer could indicate a constitutional mismatch repair–deficiency (CMMR-D).[28-30]

Other Clinical Features Suggestive of a Heritable Predisposition to Cancer

Specific clinical features can provide clues to the diagnosis of an underlying cancer predisposition. These features include physical findings, cognitive or developmental disabilities, and the presence of benign tumors (Table 42-2). Primary physicians and pediatric oncologists should be alert to the presence of these manifestations in their patients. If suspicion of a hereditary cancer syndrome is raised, the child should be referred to a geneticist or genetic counselor, as well as appropriate specialist(s) for evaluation, genetic testing, and management.

Dermatologic Findings

Benign or malignant skin findings are a common feature of several cancer predisposition syndromes, and evaluation by a dermatologist may be helpful in characterizing these findings and facilitating the diagnosis. Café-au-lait macules and axillary and inguinal freckling are a well-known example and are crucial in establishing a clinical diagnosis of neurofibromatosis type 1 (NF1)[15,31] (Fig. 42-1). Café-au-lait macules are often the earliest clinical manifestation of NF1, as they are present in 99% of affected children by 1 year of age.[32] Café-au-lait macules are also a cardinal feature of CMMR-D.[33,34] Skin pigmentation differences may also provide a clue to the diagnosis of PTEN hamartoma tumor syndrome (PHTS). For example, boys with PHTS may exhibit pigmented macules of the glans penis, which should raise the suspicion of the diagnosis, especially if features such as macrocephaly, developmental delay, or autism are present. Other skin findings are also found in PHTS, including trichilemmomas and papillomatous papules; however, these may not be diagnosed until later in life.[35] Individuals with Peutz-Jeghers syndrome (PJS) commonly exhibit mucocutaneous pigmentation resembling "freckling" around the mouth, eyes, or nostrils, or on the buccal mucosa or perianal area. Skin cancers in children may also indicate the presence of a syndrome predisposing to cancer. NBCCS predisposes individuals to basal cell carcinomas, which generally appear in the late teens or early adult years, but can occasionally develop in young children. Benign skin findings such as palmar and plantar pits and facial milia may be present in individuals with NBCCS.[36]

TABLE 42-2   Clinical Manifestations of Syndromes Predisposing to Cancer

Manifestation	Predisposition Syndrome	Gene(s)
Cutaneous		
Café-au-lait macules	Neurofibromatosis type 1 (NF1)	*NF1*
	Constitutional mismatch repair–deficiency syndrome (CMMR-D)	*MLH1, MSH2, MSH6, PMS2*
Axillary or inguinal freckling	NF1	*NF1*
Penile freckling	PTEN hamartoma tumor syndrome (PHTS)	*PTEN*
Mucosal pigmentation	Peutz-Jeghers syndrome (PJS)	*STK11*
Plantar or palmar pits	Nevoid basal cell carcinoma syndrome (NBCCS)	*PTCH1*
Pilomatrixomas	Familial adenomatous polyposis (FAP)	*APC*
Dental anomalies		
Extra or missing teeth	FAP	*APC*
Jaw osteomas	FAP	*APC*
Jaw keratocysts	NBCCS	*PTCH1*
Ear anomalies		
Earlobe creases or pits	Beckwith-Wiedemann syndrome (BWS)	11p15 abnormalities, *CDKN1C*
Eye abnormalities		
Aniridia	Wilms tumor (WT), aniridia, genitourinary malformations, retardation syndrome (WAGR)	*WT1*
Cataracts	Neurofibromatosis type 2 (NF2)	*PTCH1*
	NBCCS	*NF1*
Lisch nodules	NF1	*NF2*
Congenital hypertrophy of retinal pigmented epithelium (CHRPE)	FAP	*APC*
Strabismus or leukocoria	Hereditary retinoblastoma (RB)	*RB1*
Genitourinary anomalies	*WT1*-related WT syndromes	*WT1*
Hypospadias, undescended testes, undermasculinized male external genitals, streak gonads		
Kidney abnormalities	*WT1*-related WT syndromes	*WT1*
Horseshoe kidney		
Nephroblastomatosis		
Overgrowth		
Macrosomia	BWS	11p15 abnormalities, *CDKN1C*
	Simpson Golabi Behmel syndrome	*GPC3, CXORF5*
	NBCCS	*PTCH1*
Macrocephaly	PHTS	*PTEN*
Macroglossia	BWS	11p15 abnormalities, *CDKN1C*
Hemihypertrophy	BWS	11p15 abnormalities, *CDKN1C*
Marfanoid habitus	Multiple endocrine neoplasia type 2B	*RET*
Neurologic issues		
Ataxia	Ataxia-telangiectasia	*ATM*
Autism-spectrum disorders	PHTS	*PTEN*
Cognitive delays	WAGR	*WT1*
	NF1	*NF1*
	NF2	*NF2*
Seizures	NF1	*NF1*
	NF2	*NF2*

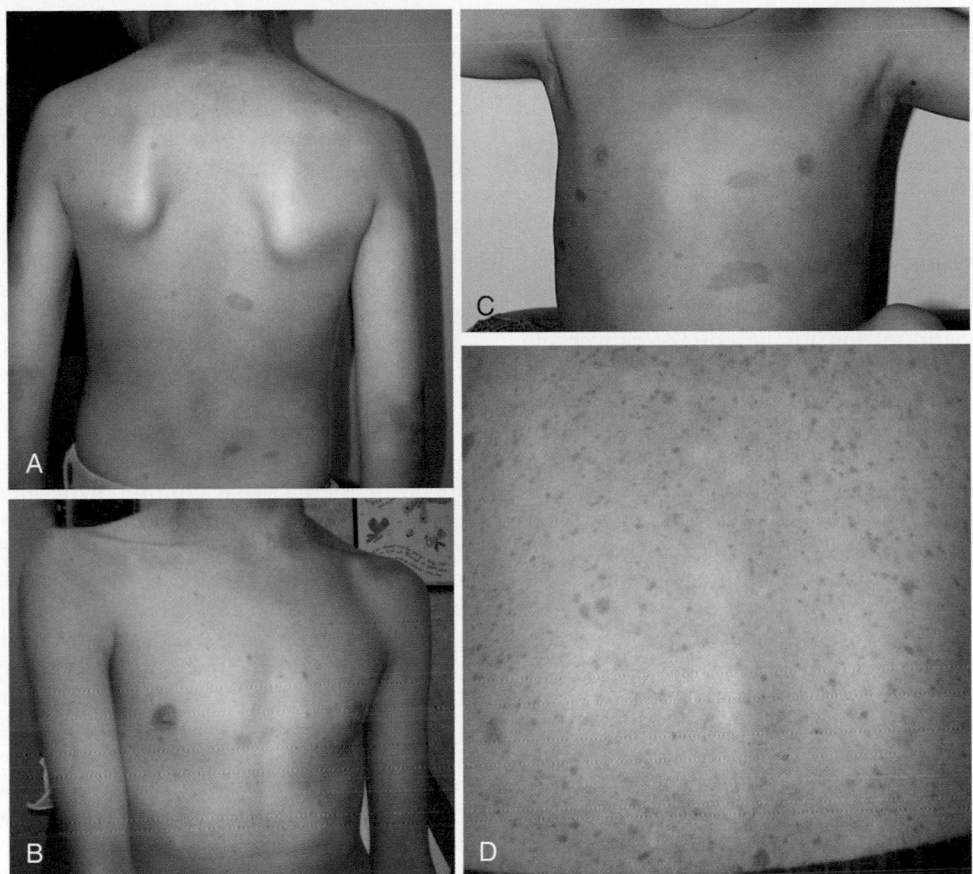

Figure 42-1 Café-au-lait spots in neurofibromatosis type 1 (NF1). (**A** to **D**). Photographs depicting the appearance of typical café-au-lait spots, as seen in NF1. Café-au-lait spots exhibit distinct edges and are slightly darker than the surrounding skin. Café-au-lait spots can increase in size, number, and darkness throughout childhood. Multiple café-au-lait spots alone are not a definitive indication for NF1; they must be present with other established criteria in order to make the diagnosis. In (C), there is also evidence of bilateral axillary freckling.

Developmental or Cognitive Abnormalities

Developmental or cognitive disabilities, including delays in achieving motor milestones, intellectual disabilities, and autism-spectrum disorders are commonly seen in cancer predisposition syndromes, including PHTS; WT, aniridia, genitourinary malformations, and retardation (WAGR) syndrome; tuberous sclerosis; 13q deletion syndrome (which predisposes to RB); and NF1. Seizures may also be a feature, where they are often seen in NF1 and tuberous sclerosis, and may indicate the presence of an underlying tumor. Any child with cancer who has a history of developmental or intellectual disabilities, autism-spectrum disorders, seizures, and/or other neurologic features should be considered a candidate for referral for a possible cancer genetics evaluation.

Overgrowth

Generalized or focal overgrowth of specific parts of the body can be a feature of a condition predisposing to cancer, such as Beckwith-Wiedemann syndrome (BWS), PHTS, and Simpson Golabi Behmel syndrome. In BWS overgrowth may manifest with generalized macrosomia at birth, and some patients may also exhibit macroglossia and/or asymmetric overgrowth of one side of the body

(hemihypertrophy). Hemihypertrophy may involve the extremities or external physical features (face, labia, buttocks), as well as internal organs (where, for example, one kidney may be larger than the other). Macrosomia is also a feature of Simpson Golabi Behmel syndrome and Proteus syndrome (PS), while macrocephaly can be a manifestation of PHTS and NBCCS.

Specific Congenital Anomalies

In some cases, the presence of specific congenital anomalies can serve as an early indicator of a condition predisposing to cancer. For example, an omphalocele or umbilical hernia, especially in a child with macrosomia, macroglossia, ear pits or creases, or neonatal hypoglycemia, can point to the diagnosis of BWS. Another good example is WAGR syndrome, where affected children have aniridia, often in combination with genitourinary abnormalities such as hypospadias or cryptorchidism.

Other Physical Features

Other physical manifestations may also suggest an underlying hereditary cancer syndrome. Examples include individuals with multiple endocrine neoplasia type 2B (MEN2B), who often present with mucosal neuromas of the lips and tongue, ganglioneuromas, and marfanoid habitus, and those with FAP, who may present with dental abnormalities (missing or extra teeth), epidermal cysts or pilomatrixomas, Gardner fibromas (also known as desmoid tumors), osteomas (usually involving the jaws), and congenital hypertrophy of the retinal pigmented epithelium. Generally these manifestations present prior to the development of colon polyps.

Incidental Identification of a Child with a Condition Predisposing to Cancer

Until recently, genetic testing for hereditary cancer syndromes was only offered when an individual presented with a specific cancer type, physical or developmental features consistent with a known syndrome predisposing to cancer, or a suggestive family history. Due to the increasing use of genome-wide approaches to establish a genetic diagnosis, including single-nucleotide polymorphism arrays, multigene panels, and whole-exome sequencing, the "incidental" discovery of a gene mutation that predisposes to cancer is becoming more and more common. This information can lead to the unintended diagnosis of a predisposing syndrome prior to its clinical manifestation in the child and/or his or her family. Toward this end, several recent studies of genome-wide microarrays have reported the identification of copy number variations involving genes predisposing to cancer in individuals presenting with a noncancer phenotype.[37-39] In these studies, the frequency of incidental findings involving genes predisposing to cancer was estimated to be between 0.18% and 0.60%.[40-42]

The testing of tumor samples for somatic genetic mutations is also being pursued with the intent of facilitating "personalized" cancer care by identifying and therapeutically targeting mutated genetic pathways in tumors. When evaluating tumors, it is often necessary to compare tumor-derived sequences to those obtained using normal tissue from the same individual. As a result, it is possible to identify incidental constitutional mutations that are indicative of an underlying cancer predisposition or other nononcologic condition.[43,44] In one recent study, most patients undergoing tumor genetic testing expressed interest in receiving incidental germline genetic test results, as most thought this information would be valuable to family members. However, some perceived it to be an additional burden on top of their cancer diagnosis.[45] Many laboratories have specific policies regarding the sequencing of normal tissue and return of incidental results. Therefore, prior to ordering tumor testing, pediatric oncologists should be familiar with the performing laboratory's policy, discuss the possibility of obtaining incidental genetic findings with the patient and his or her parents, and determine whether or not they would like to receive these results as part of the informed-consent process.

Genetic Testing for a Heritable Predisposition to Cancer
Complexities of Childhood Cancer Genetic Testing

Genetic testing for cancer predisposition is a complex process that should be explored with the patient and

family, preferably by a genetic counselor or trained genetics professional, prior to performing the testing. Counseling should include information about the natural history of the condition under consideration, methods of testing and its possible outcomes, as well as the potential risks, benefits, and limitations of testing. Patients may have concerns about privacy, confidentiality, insurance coverage, and genetic discrimination, all of which must be addressed. For the oncologist, it is important to recognize that genetic test results have implications not only for the individual being tested but also for his or her family members. This factor necessitates counseling of the whole family and discussion of how the results will be communicated between various members. When the individual under consideration is a minor (defined here as a person <18 years), the importance of these issues is further magnified by the fact that children generally do not have the capacity to fully understand the risks, benefits, and limitations of genetic testing. Therefore, they are not able to make their own informed decisions about whether or not to be tested. Instead, this decision falls to the child's parent(s) or guardian(s), and strips the child of the opportunity to make an autonomous decision about genetic testing later in life. Testing in childhood and disclosure of results to parents, guardians, and/or other family members may violate the child's privacy, confidentiality, and right not to know.[46,47,48] Many also fear that performing genetic testing on a child may have adverse psychological consequences, such as depression, anxiety, fear of the future, altered self-image, limited horizons (i.e., impact on thoughts about future education and career choices), and altered family relationships.[49] However, others have argued for the possible benefits of genetic testing in childhood, such as relief if test results are negative, providing certainty about genetic risk, and allowing the child to integrate genetic information into the self-concept at a younger age, when it is less disruptive to the sense of self. Until recently, the concerns about testing children have more or less superseded the possible benefits of such testing.

Despite much debate, available evidence suggests that the negative consequences of cancer genetic testing may be fewer and less severe than anticipated. Studies of the psychosocial consequences of genetic testing in adults have generally shown minimal or no negative consequences and suggested that emotional outcomes may be more dependent on factors such as pretest emotional state and social support than on the actual genetic test result itself.[50,51] Several studies report that adults undergoing genetic testing for LFS consider obtaining certainty about cancer risk a psychological benefit of testing, even if adults are found to be affected.[51,52] Data on the outcomes of presymptomatic cancer genetic testing of children are more limited. Much of the data comes from testing for FAP, where affected individuals are prone to develop multiple gastrointestinal polyps, which if left untreated invariably lead to early-onset colorectal cancer. In FAP, polyps generally begin to form during adolescence. Consequently, it is recommended that children begin surveillance with colonoscopy around the age of 10 to 12 years. Based on these factors, it is deemed appropriate to offer

FAP genetic testing to minors. Published reports describing the psychosocial consequences of pediatric FAP genetic testing reveal that children by and large do not experience significant distress related to this testing.[53,54,55] One report describing the psychological outcomes of genetic testing of minors for LFS did not note any significant negative outcomes after up to 12 years of follow-up.[56] However, in this study, the participation rate in testing for minors was low, with only 4 of 26 parents who were offered testing for their children actually following through with the test. Therefore, it remains to be determined whether and how genetic testing for these or other conditions predisposing to cancer impacts the well-being of children and their families.

Guidelines for Testing Children for a Heritable Predisposition to Cancer

The controversies surrounding genetic testing of children have prompted several groups to issue guidelines and recommendations. Most recommendations indicate that the primary justification for presymptomatic (i.e., predictive) genetic testing is medical benefit for the child. Therefore, testing should be offered to minors only if the condition is known to manifest in childhood and there are effective preventive or therapeutic interventions available. Conversely, if cancer risk is not increased in childhood or if there are not effective surveillance or intervention measures, it is recommended that testing be delayed until adulthood, when a child can then independently decide whether or not to pursue the testing. Families must be counseled about the benefits, risks, and limitations of genetic testing in order to give informed consent for genetic testing on behalf of their child. As with other medical interventions, it is the role of the health care provider to advocate for the best interests of the child when discussing the option of genetic testing. If possible, minors should be encouraged to participate in decision making about genetic testing; however, the capacity of children to understand genetic information is variable and depends upon their age, maturity, education, and cognitive abilities. Disclosure of results to tested minors is also encouraged once the minor reaches the legal age of majority, or possibly sooner if it is felt that the minor is capable of understanding and coping with the results.[49,56-61,62]

Management of Children with a Heritable Predisposition to Cancer

The identification of a presymptomatic child with a heritable predisposition to cancer has the potential to improve survival and minimize morbidity by allowing prospective monitoring for tumor formation and often life-saving prophylactic surgeries or other preventive measures. This information can also benefit children who already have cancer, as it can influence choice of the most appropriate or least toxic cancer-directed therapy. For example, one should avoid the use of radiation therapy in children with hereditary RB or LFS, as these children are at increased risk of developing secondary irradiation induced malignant disease due to their constitutional genetic mutations. Similarly, in a child with a WT predisposition syndrome,

it is recommended that a renal tumor be removed using nephron-sparing surgery and not total nephrectomy. Because the remaining kidney tissue remains at risk for tumor formation and could thus become the target of future surgical procedures, it is deemed advisable to leave as much healthy kidney in place as possible. Below, we review some of the salient principles of tumor surveillance and cancer risk reduction for children with heritable predisposition to cancer.

Principles of Tumor Surveillance

Cancer surveillance guidelines exist or are being developed for several conditions predisposing to childhood cancer. The primary goal of surveillance is to detect cancers at the earliest and most curable stage. For this reason, cancer surveillance protocols are best suited for solid tumors, where survival is often linked to the size and extent of spread of the tumor at diagnosis. Tumors identified in individuals undergoing regular monitoring may be smaller. As a result, surveillance allows for less invasive surgical procedures and can also reduce or eliminate the need for additional chemotherapy and/or irradiation. However, surveillance can also be complicated by the possibility of false-positive results, which often lead to worry about cancer, excess rates of follow-up imaging and/or biopsy, and possibly increased costs of care.

Several factors must be taken into account in the development and implementation of a cancer surveillance protocol. First, there must be a benefit for early cancer detection in an individual undergoing monitoring (i.e., there should be an effective treatment available and preferably also demonstration that early detection improves outcome). Second, the age-specific tumor risks for syndromes predisposing to cancer must be known and deemed high enough to warrant surveillance (generally, a tumor incidence of ≥5% is considered sufficiently high to initiate monitoring). This information helps to identify candidates for surveillance, when it should be initiated, and how long it should be continued. The surveillance method(s) and interval between specific tests must also be carefully considered in light of the specific tumor risks and growth rate associated with a given syndrome. Ideally, surveillance methods should be readily available, safe, and have high sensitivity and specificity. Whenever possible, screening tools that involve no or minimal irradiation should be used, as patients with hereditary cancer syndromes may be at increased risk to develop irradiation-induced cancers (as is the case for hereditary RB, LFS, ataxia telangiectasia, and other genetic syndromes associated with defects in DNA repair).

Cancer Prevention Strategies

For some syndromes, early identification of at-risk children allows for the elimination or dramatic reduction of cancer risk through prophylactic surgery. MEN2 and FAP are excellent examples, where removal of the at-risk organ may be considered early in a patient's lifetime to prevent the development of thyroid or colorectal cancer, respectively. In MEN2, there is a nearly 100% lifetime risk for MTC, an aggressive type of thyroid cancer with a high metastatic potential. As a result, it is recommended that individuals with MEN2 undergo prophylactic thyroidectomy, a procedure that has greatly reduced the likelihood of developing MTC.[63] It should be noted that while all individuals with MEN2 are at increased risk for MTC, there are significant genotype-phenotype correlations that predict the age of thyroid cancer onset, and this information can dictate the appropriate timing for prophylactic removal of the thyroid.[20] In FAP, individuals have a similarly high risk of early-onset colon cancer that nears 100% if colonic polyps are not removed. To prevent colon cancer, affected individuals should undergo colectomy when polyps become too numerous to clinically follow or remove, generally in the late teens to early 20s. Studies of the efficacy of colectomy reveal a significant reduction in colon cancer risk.[6] Due to the morbidities associated with colectomy, alternatives to surgery are being sought. Nonsteroidal antiinflammatory medications such as sulindac and Cox-2 inhibitors reduce polyp formation in adults with FAP[64-66]; however, these medications are currently under examination for use in children with the condition.[67]

SPECIFIC SYNDROMES PREDISPOSING TO CANCER

There currently exist more than 30 genetic conditions that predispose to cancer in which children are at risk for tumor formation (several examples are summarized in Table 42-3). Each of these conditions is typified by distinct clinical and genetic manifestations. For some of these conditions, recommendations regarding genetic testing, surveillance, and management are well established. However, for others these issues are only recently emerging. Here we focus on some of these conditions, including the clinical and molecular features and current recommendations regarding management.

Hereditary Retinoblastoma

Incidence

Hereditary RB is an example of a classic syndrome predisposing to cancer and the first for which the underlying genetic mechanism was recognized. RB is a malignant tumor of the embryonic neural retina that has an

TABLE 42-3   Clinical and Genetic Features of Selected Childhood Syndromes Predisposing to Cancer

Syndrome	Gene(s)	Inheritance	Cancers or Tumors	Other Features
Beckwith-Wiedemann syndrome	Chromosome 11p15, CDKN1C	Imprinting defects Autosomal dominant (AD)	Hepatoblastoma (HB) Wilms tumor (WT) Others (rare): Adrenocortical cancer Neuroblastoma Pheochromocytoma (PCC) Rhabdomyosarcoma Rhabdoid tumor Gonadoblastoma	Macrosomia Macroglossia Omphalocele Umbilical hernia Hypoglycemia Hemihypertrophy Ear pits or creases
Constitutional mismatch repair–deficiency syndrome	MLH1 MSH2 MSH6 PMS2	Autosomal recessive (AR)	Gastrointestinal polyps (adenomas) Colon cancer Brain cancer Leukemia or lymphoma Endometrial cancer	Café-au-lait spots Axillary or inguinal freckling Lisch nodules
DICER1 syndrome	DICER1	AD	Pleuropulmonary blastoma Cystic nephroma Sertoli–Leydig cell tumor Thyroid goiter WT Rhabdomyosarcoma Colon polyps (hamartomas)	Pulmonary cysts
Familial adenomatous polyposis	APC	AD	Gastrointestinal polyps Colorectal cancer Small bowel cancer Papillary thyroid cancer HB Medulloblastoma Soft tissue tumors Gardner fibroma Desmoid tumor Osteomas	Epidermoid cysts Pilomatrixomas Supernumerary or missing teeth Congenital hypertrophy of retinal pigmented epithelium (CHRPE)
Hereditary paraganglioma (PGL)-PCC syndrome	SDHA/B/C/D/AF2 MAX TMEM127	AD	PCC PGL Papillary thyroid cancer Renal cancer Gastrointestinal stromal tumor (GIST)	

TABLE 42-3   Clinical and Genetic Features of Selected Childhood Syndromes Predisposing to Cancer (Continued)

Syndrome	Gene(s)	Inheritance	Cancers or Tumors	Other Features
Hereditary neuroblastoma	ALK PHOX2B	AD	Neuroblastoma	Hirschsprung disease (PHOX2B) Congenital central hypoventilation (PHOX2B)
Hereditary retinoblastoma	RB1	AD	Retinoblastoma Pineoblastoma Soft tissue or bone sarcoma Melanoma	Multiple congenital anomalies (13q syndrome)
Juvenile polyposis syndrome	BMPR1A SMAD4	AD	Colon cancer Gastric cancer Pancreatic cancer Gastrointestinal polyps Juvenile type	Arteriovenous malformations (SMAD4)
Li-Fraumeni syndrome	TP53	AD	Adrenocortical carcinoma Choroid plexus carcinoma Bone or soft tissue sarcoma Breast cancer Brain cancer Leukemia Colon cancer Many other cancers	None
Multiple endocrine neoplasia type 1	MEN1	AD	Parathyroid adenoma Gastrinoma-insulinoma Anterior pituitary adenoma Carcinoid tumor Angiofibroma Collagenoma Lipoma	None
Multiple endocrine neoplasia type 2	RET	AD	Medullary thyroid cancer PCC Parathyroid adenoma (MEN2A) Mucosal neuroma (MEN2B) Ganglioneuroma (MEN2B)	Hyperparathyroid (due to parathyroid adenomas) (MEN2A) Marfanoid habitus (MEN2B) Mucosal neuromas (MEN2B)
Neurofibromatosis type 1	NF1	AD	Neurofibromas Optic pathway gliomas Astrocytomas Schwannomas Juvenile myelomonocytic leukemia Acute myeloid leukemia PCCs	Café-au-lait macules Axillary or inguinal freckling Lisch nodules Tibial bowing Macrocephaly Developmental delay, intellectual disability, or autism
Neurofibromatosis type 2	NF2	AD	Vestibular schwannomas Meningiomas Astrocytomas Schwannomas Gliomas Neurofibromas	Posterior subcapsular lenticular opacities Hearing loss Peripheral neuropathy Seizures
Nevoid basal cell carcinoma syndrome (Gorlin syndrome)	PTCH1	AD	Basal cell carcinoma Medulloblastoma Cardiac and ovarian fibromas	Macrocephaly Palmar or plantar pits Jaw keratocysts Bifid ribs Calcificiation of falx Developmental delay, intellectual disability, autism

Continued on following page

TABLE 42-3   Clinical and Genetic Features of Selected Childhood Syndromes Predisposing to Cancer (Continued)

Syndrome	Gene(s)	Inheritance	Cancers or Tumors	Other Features
Peutz-Jeghers syndrome	STK11/LKB1	AD	Gastrointestinal polyps (Peutz-Jeghers type) Colon cancer Gastric cancer Breast cancer Lung cancer Pancreatic cancer Ovarian cancer Cervical cancer	Mucocutaneous hyperpigmentation
PTEN hamartoma tumor syndrome	PTEN	AD	Breast cancer Thyroid cancer (nonmedullary) Endometrial cancer Renal cancer Lipomas Thyroid nodules or goiter Gastrointestinal polyps (hamartomas)	Macrocephaly Arteriovascular malformations Trichilemmomas Papillomatous papules Developmental delay, intellectual disability, or autism
Rhabdoid tumor syndrome	SMARCB1/INI1	AD	Atypical teratoid/rhabdoid tumors (CNS) Malignant rhabdoid tumors (renal or extrarenal) Schwannomatosis	None
Tuberous sclerosis	TSC1 TSC2	AD	Astrocytoma Cortical tuber Subependymal nodules Cardiac rhabdomyoma Angiomyolipomas Renal cell carcinoma (RCC) Colon polyps (hamartomas)	Facial angiofibroma Hypopigmented macules (ash leaf macules) Ungual fibromas Shagreen patch Confetti skin lesions Dental pits Gingival fibromas Developmental delay, intellectual disability, or autism Seizures or infantile spasms

Von–Hippel Lindau syndrome	VHL	AD	Hemangioblastoma (retinal or cerebellar)
			RCC
			Pancreatic neuroendocrine tumors
			PCCs
			Endolymphatic sac tumors
			Papillary cystadenomas
			  Epididymis (males)
			  Broad ligament (females)
				Renal cysts
				Pancreatic cysts

WT1-related syndromes	WT1	AD	WT Gonadoblastoma	Aniridia (WAGR syndrome) Genitourinary abnormalities Developmental delay, intellectual disability, or autism

WAGR, Wilms tumor, aniridia, genital anomalies, and retardation.

incidence of two to five cases per million children per year and accounts for 3% to 4% of all pediatric cancers.[4] Nonhereditary RB accounts for 60% of cases and is associated with development of unilateral eye tumors at a median age of 22 months.[68,69] The remaining 40% of patients have hereditary RB, which involves both eyes in more than 80% of cases and presents at a median age of 11 months.[68,69] Heritable RB is highly penetrant, with more than 90% of patients developing RB and 0.5% to 15% also developing intracranial tumors of the pineal gland.[70,71] Over the course of their lives, survivors of hereditary RB remain at increased risk to develop second malignant neoplasms, including bone and soft tissue sarcomas, which commonly occur in previously irradiated sites, as well as melanomas and cancer of the lungs, gastrointestinal tract, and bladder.[72]

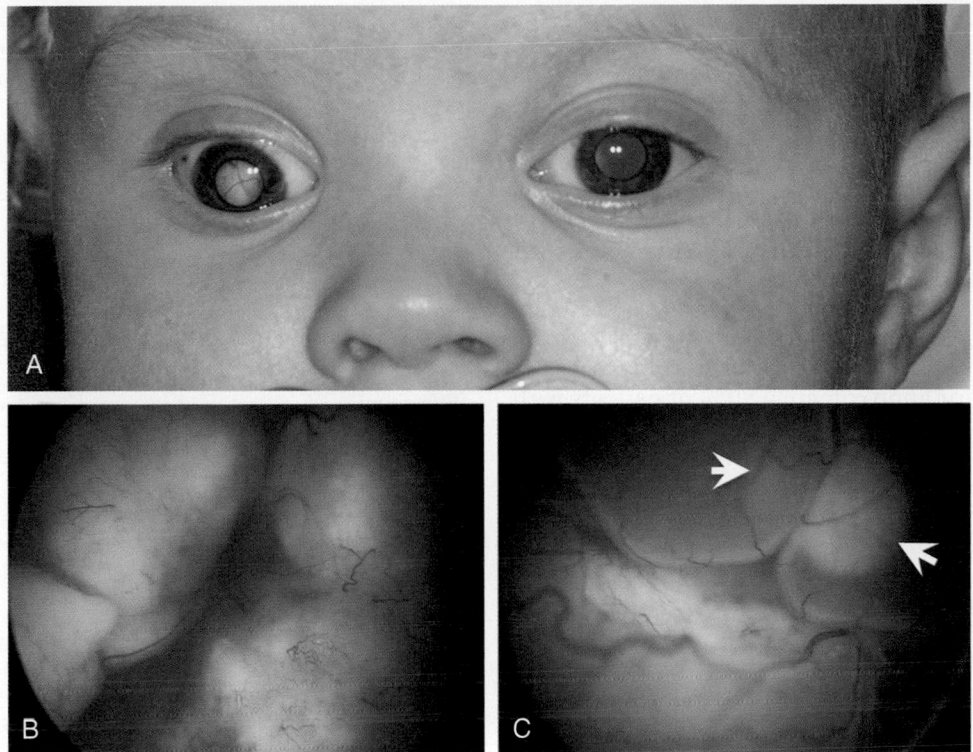

Figure 42-2 A child with hereditary retinoblastoma (RB) with bilateral eye involvement. **A,** The face of an infant with bilateral RB demonstrating bilateral leukocoria, one of the most common presentations for this eye tumor. **B** and **C,** Retinal photographs of this child's ocular tumors, which appear as large white masses. In **B,** the right eye has an advanced-stage (group E) tumor. In **C,** the left eye has a large (group D) tumor with evidence for subretinal seeding (*arrows*).

Genetics

RB is caused by mutations in *RB1*, which resides at chromosomal locus 13q14.[10] *RB1* encodes the RB protein (pRB), a potent tumor suppressor that regulates cell growth by inhibiting the function of the E2F family of transcription factors and preventing inappropriate S-phase entry. pRB also regulates cellular glucose tolerance, mitogenesis, glutathione synthesis, and the expression of genes involved in carbon metabolism.[73] When both RB1 alleles are mutated within a developing retinal cell, pRB expression and/or function are diminished, cell division proceeds in a dysregulated manner, and, ultimately, RB tumors form.

In patients with nonhereditary RB, both RB1 gene copies are mutated within a single postzygotic retinal cell. In contrast, patients with hereditary RB harbor one mutated RB1 allele within the germline. This mutation is inherited from a similarly affected parent in 10% to 20% of cases.[69] In the remaining cases, the RB1 mutation arises de novo within one of the parent's gametes[74] or a cell of the developing embryo. Mutation of the remaining RB1 allele occurs somatically. Genetic testing for germline RB1 gene mutations can identify mutations in more than 90% of individuals with hereditary disease.[75,76] While most patients can be identified clinically due to the presence of multifocal or bilateral eye tumors and/or a positive family history, 10% to 15% of patients have single eye tumors and no family history of RB. These latter factors make them indistinguishable from those with the sporadic form of disease. The identification of RB1 mutations in unilateral patients enables appropriate primary eye tumor treatment as well as initiation of surveillance for involvement of the pineal gland and later second cancers. Identification of a germline RB1 mutation in any child with RB also allows for presymptomatic testing of other family members, including siblings who may not yet have developed RB but carry a mutated RB1 gene copy, as well as children of RB survivors.

Tumor Risks and Surveillance

Individuals harboring germline RB1 mutations are at greatly increased risk to develop bilateral RB tumors, generally during the first 5 years of life (Fig. 42-2). During this time period patients are also at increased risk to develop tumors involving the pineal gland (so-called trilateral RB). Later in life, individuals with hereditary RB can develop second malignant neoplasms. While the risk for these cancers is greatest in those treated with external-beam radiation therapy, nonirradiated long-term survivors of hereditary RB have an approximately 10% to 15% risk of developing one or more second malignant neoplasms[77]

The early detection of eye tumors has been shown to significantly increase ocular retention and preserve vision.[78] Therefore, it is recommended that children at risk for RB be examined by fundoscopy beginning 1 to 2 weeks after birth and then every 2 weeks until the age of 3 months.[78] Subsequently, examinations should be performed under general anesthesia until the age of 4 to 5 years.[79] The frequency of examination depends upon the age of the patient, with examinations recommended every 2 months during the first year of life and then gradually spaced to every 6 months during the fourth to fifth years of life.[79] A study by Abramson and colleagues[80] showed that patients with a positive family history who received ophthalmologic examinations from birth had an overall survival rate of 93.2% and an ocular retention rate of 67.7%. This is in contrast to patients who did not receive screening, whose survival rate measured 87.4% and ocular retention rate only 38.2%. In addition to increased ocular retention, early screening and close follow-up results in a long-term visual acuity measuring between 20/20 and 20/40 for approximately 90% of patients with hereditary disease.[78] To screen for pineal tumors, it is recommended that children undergo magnetic resonance imaging (MRI) examination of the brain every 6 months until the age of 5 years.[71] Screening in this manner successfully identifies tumors when they are smaller and has been reported to increase the 5-year survival rate from 0% to 27%.[71] While the basis for ocular and pineal gland surveillance is well established, it remains unclear whether monitoring for second malignant neoplasms is of benefit. As a result, monitoring for these tumors is not yet recommended and remains the subject of investigation.

Li-Fraumeni Syndrome

Incidence

LFS is a highly penetrant cancer syndrome first described in 1969 in four families with soft tissue sarcoma and early-onset breast cancer.[81] Since this initial observation, more than 500 families have been reported with complete or partial LFS phenotypes, and it is possible that many more families exist that have not yet been identified. In 1990, it was determined that germline TP53 mutations were responsible for most cases of LFS.[82] The TP53 mutation carrier rate has been reported to be about 1 in 5000 births,[23] although the true incidence and prevalence of germline TP53 mutations are unknown. TP53 germline mutations are more common in southern Brazil, due to a founder mutation with a high population prevalence of nearly 0.3%.[83-85,86]

Genetics

TP53 encodes p53, which is often referred to as the "guardian of the genome" because it is a critical transcription factor that mediates cellular stress responses and initiates DNA repair, cell-cycle arrest, senescence, and apoptosis. TP53 somatic alterations have been detected in nearly every type of human cancer, and patients with LFS who harbor a mutated copy of this important cancer-preventing gene are much closer to the threshold of developing cancer in any of their body tissues. Although there are no strong genotype-phenotype correlations, early tumor onset has been reported to be more common in those with nonsense, frameshift, or splice site mutations.[87] Modifiers of tumor risk have included increased burden of copy number variants,[88] shorter telomeres,[89] a single-nucleotide polymorphism at codon 72 (R72) of TP53,[90,91] and a single-nucleotide

polymorphism (rs2279744) affecting the p53 inhibitor MDM2.[91] As more LFS families are studied, these associations and the genotype-phenotype correlations will be more clearly elucidated.

Over the years, several classification systems have been developed to help identify possible LFS families and determine those to whom TP53 genetic testing should be offered (Table 42-4). Currently, TP53 mutations are

TABLE 42-4 Clinical Classification Schemes for Li-Fraumeni Syndrome

Classification Criteria	Description
Classic Li-Fraumeni syndrome (LFS)	Proband with sarcoma diagnosed before 45 years of age and First-degree relative with cancer diagnosed before 45 years of age and First- or second-degree relative on same side of family with cancer diagnosed before 45 years of age or sarcoma at any age
Chompret classification	Proband with LFS spectrum cancer diagnosed before 36 years of age and At least one first- or second-degree relative on same side of family with cancer (other than breast cancer if proband has breast cancer) diagnosed before 56 years of age or A relative with multiple primary cancers at any age
	A proband with cancer with a relative with cancer or multiple primaries, two of which are sarcoma, brain tumor, breast cancer, and/or adrenocortical carcinoma, with the initial cancer occurring before 46 years of age, regardless of family history
	A proband with adrenocortical carcinoma or choroid plexus carcinoma at any age, regardless of family history
Birch classification	Proband with any childhood cancer or sarcoma, brain tumor, or adrenocortical carcinoma diagnosed before 45 years of age and First- or second-degree relative with typical LFS cancer (sarcoma, breast cancer, brain tumor, leukemia, or adrenocortical carcinoma) diagnosed at any age and First- or second-degree relative on same side of family with any cancer diagnosed before 60 years of age
Eeles classification	Two first- or second-degree relatives with LFS-related malignant disease (sarcoma, breast cancer, brain tumor, leukemia, adrenocortical carcinoma, melanoma, prostate cancer, or pancreatic cancer) at any age

identified in 70% or more of patients who meet the strict diagnostic criteria for LFS. The mutation detection rate drops to 20% in families classified as "Li-Fraumeni–like," who exhibit some but not all of the features associated with LFS (such as very early onset or multiple primaries).[92] Even without an identified *TP53* mutation, cancer-prone families with an LFS pedigree are considered to be at high risk for an inherited cancer syndrome, and it is recommended that members of these families be monitored carefully for early cancer development using modalities currently in place for those with genetically verified LFS.

Tumor Risks and Surveillance

Patients with classic LFS are at risk for nearly every type of cancer, and the lifetime cancer risk is extraordinarily high, with a 68% risk in men and 93% risk in women.[93] Patients with LFS most commonly present with breast cancer (nearly 30% of patients), soft tissue sarcomas (<20%), brain tumors (<14%), osteosarcomas (12% to 14%), and ACCs (6.5% to 10%).[23,85,87,93] In children, the tumors most strongly associated with LFS include ACC, CPC, rhabdomyosarcoma presenting before 3 years of age, and osteosarcoma presenting before 5 years of age.[23,27,87] Recently, *TP53* germline mutations have been described in nearly half of patients with hypodiploid pre-B acute lymphoblastic leukemia,[94] most notably those children whose leukemia cells are considered "low hypodiploid" and contain a median of 32 to 39 chromosomes. A germline *TP53* mutation was also described in an additional kindred with familial transmission of acute lymphoblastic leukemia.[95] Nearly half of cancers in LFS present before 30 years of age.[93] The phenomenon of genetic anticipation has been observed in LFS, with a decrease in age and increase in cancer onset in successive generations.[96] Subsequent tumors also are an issue in LFS, with more than an 80-fold relative risk for a second malignant neoplasm in patients with their first cancer under the age of 20, a 10-fold relative risk if diagnosed between 20 and 44 years, and a 1.5-fold relative risk if diagnosed at over 45 years.[97]

The recommendations for cancer surveillance in patients with LFS are emerging, although no formal guidelines for affected children are in place at this time. For *TP53* mutation carriers, a healthy lifestyle with avoidance of ionizing radiation and DNA-damaging agents is encouraged. Annual dermatology visits are recommended, along with avoidance of unprotected sun exposure. Annual physical examinations are also recommended, with careful attention to the thyroid and abdomen for masses and a neurologic examination for indication of brain tumors. For adults, colonoscopy is recommended beginning at age 25 years; if there is a family history of colorectal cancer, the patient can consider screening at an age 5 to 10 years younger than the earliest age at which colorectal cancer has been diagnosed in other family members. For women, annual mammograms and breast MRI are recommended beginning at age 25 years, with these procedures alternated so that the breasts are screened every 6 months. The cost versus benefit of mammography in this high-risk population is still being explored, and these recommendations may change in the future.[98]

Currently, studies are ongoing to determine whether newer radiologic approaches, alone or in combination with other screening measures, are effective in detecting tumors in patients with LFS. One study of rapid whole-body MRI combined with other imaging and laboratory measures has reported increased survival rates in patients with LFS,[99] and this now can be considered an option for surveillance (Fig. 42-3). Additional measures being offered include abdominal ultrasound (to screen for ACC or other intraabdominal tumors), assessments of complete blood count (to detect leukemia), and measurements of adrenal hormones (to screen for ACC). Although it has not yet been definitively proven that surveillance is beneficial, many practitioners will test for *TP53* mutations in order to begin a tumor surveillance program in children who are determined to be at increased cancer risk. Cancers identified in LFS patients can be treated according to standard protocols, although the avoidance of agents that might damage DNA (e.g., exposure to ionizing radiation) is recommended due to the increased risk for second malignant tumors in this population.

WT1-Related Wilms Tumor Predisposition Syndromes

Incidence

Wilms tumor (WT, also known as nephroblastoma) is the most common renal tumor of childhood, accounting for 8% of all pediatric cancers[100] and 95% of pediatric renal cancers.[101] As many as 10% of WTs develop in the setting of a hereditary predisposition, where it is estimated that up to 5% of tumors are caused by germline mutations in the *WT1* tumor suppressor gene.[102] As with other predisposition syndromes, children with germline *WT1* mutations are more likely to present with bilateral kidney involvement[103] and at a younger-than-expected age.[100] Patients may also exhibit a variety of nononcologic clinical manifestations.[13]

Genetics

The *WT1* gene, located at chromosomal locus 11p13, encodes a zinc finger transcription factor that regulates mesenchymal to epithelial transition in embryonic renal and genitourinary development[104] and thus functions as a tumor suppressor gene.[105] The *WT1* gene consists of 10 exons, which encode an N-terminal proline and glutamine-rich transactivation domain, and a C-terminal zinc-finger domain involved in DNA binding.[106,107] Loss of heterozygosity at 11p13 in WT samples suggests a key role as a tumor suppressor,[108] and numerous constitutional mutations in *WT1* have been described in association with familial WT.[100] In cases of *WT1*-associated WT, a second mutation in either CTNNB1 or *IGF2* is often also required for oncogenesis.[101]

Tumor Risks and Surveillance

Patients harboring a germline *WT1* mutation develop WT in the context of several distinct clinical syndromes (Table 42-5), including WT, aniridia, genital anomalies, and retardation (WAGR), Denys-Drash syndrome (DDS),

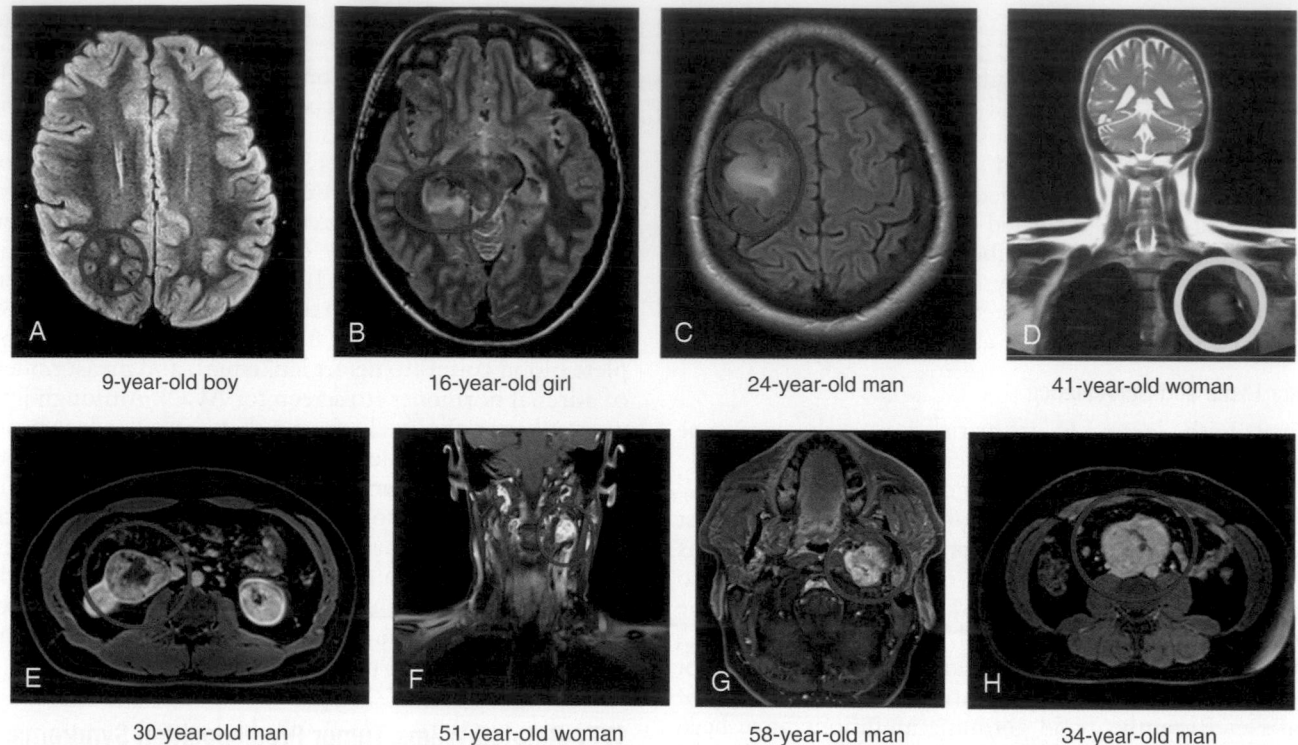

9-year-old boy   16-year-old girl   24-year-old man   41-year-old woman

30-year-old man   51-year-old woman   58-year-old man   34-year-old man

Figure 42-3 Tumors identified by magnetic resonance imaging (MRI)-based surveillance of asymptomatic TP53 and SDHB mutation carriers. A to D, Examples of lesions in *TP53* mutation–positive patients with Li-Fraumeni syndrome. A, Unknown lesion, followed regularly on brain MRI. B, Diffuse astrocytoma (World Health Organization [WHO] grade II), resected. C, Diffuse fibrillary astrocytoma (WHO grade II), resected. D, Lung adenocarcinoma, resected. E to H, Examples of lesions found in patients with hereditary paraganglioma/pheochromocytoma (PCC), who carried mutations in *SDHB*. E, Renal cell carcinoma, removed by nephrectomy. F, Carotid body tumor, resected. G, Carotid body tumor, resected. H, PCC in the organ of Zuckerkandl, resected.

and Frasier syndrome (FS). In a large study of WT patients, only 20% with a germline *WT1* mutation did not have associated congenital abnormalities.[103]

Wilms Tumor, Aniridia, Genital Anomalies, Retardation Syndrome

WAGR syndrome is caused by a contiguous gene deletion at 11p13, which leads to the loss of a single copy of *WT1* as well as neighboring genes, including *PAX6*, a transcription factor critical for development of the eye and other neural organs. Haploinsufficiency for WT1 is believed to result in genitourinary abnormalities, which are most notable in males and include hypospadias and undescended testes,[101] as well as an almost 50% risk of developing WT.[109] Haploinsufficiency for PAX6 contributes to the development of complete or partial aniridia. The etiology of the cognitive delay in WAGR syndrome has not been elucidated, though it is likely that haploinsufficiency for genes adjacent to *WT1* are responsible for this finding.

TABLE 42-5 Clinical and Genetic Features of *WT1*-Related Syndromes Predisposing to Wilms Tumor

Syndrome	Genetic Alteration	Molecular Pathogenesis	Wilms Tumor Risk	Clinical Phenotype
Familial Wilms tumor (WT)	*WT1* mutation or deletion	Altered *WT1* function	Variable risk of WT	Nonsyndromic, hypospadias or undescended testes in males
WAGR syndrome	*WT1* deletion	*WT1* haploinsufficiency	~50% risk of developing WT	Aniridia, genital abnormalities, developmental delays, possibility for streak gonads in girls
Denys-Drash syndrome	*WT1* missense mutation	Dominant negative mutation	>90% risk of WT	Development of diffuse mesangial sclerosis, undermasculinized genitalia in 46 XY males
Frasier syndrome	*WT1* splice site mutation	Altered ratio of *WT1* splice forms	5% to 10% risk of WT	Development of focal segmental glomerulosclerosis, gonadoblastoma, undermasculinized genitalia in 46 XY males

Denys-Drash Syndrome

DDS is characterized by the development of WT, renal diffuse mesangial sclerosis, and undermasculinized external genitalia in 46 XY males. It is caused by missense mutations affecting exon 8 or 9 of *WT1*,[103] which lead to the generation of a WT1 protein with impaired DNA-binding capacity. These WT1 mutants function in a dominant negative fashion, and as a result patients with DDS exhibit a very high incidence (>90%) of WT.[13] Furthermore, approximately 74% of patients develop end-stage renal disease within 20 years of diagnosis.[110] While the molecular pathogenesis of the diffuse mesangial sclerosis remains unclear, murine studies have implicated *WT1* in the regulation of podocyte formation,[111] suggesting a central role for *WT1* in lifelong renal homeostasis. Genitourinary abnormalities of varying severity are common in males with DDS, and there is also an increased risk for gonadoblastoma. In contrast, most females with DDS have normal genitourinary development and no risk for gonadal tumors.[112]

Frasier Syndrome

FS is typified by the development of renal focal segmental glomerulosclerosis, gonadoblastoma, and undermasculinized external genitalia in 46 XY males. FS is caused by point mutations in the WT1 intron 9 donor splice site.[113] Normally, distinct messenger RNA (mRNA) isoforms are produced by WT1 as the result of alternative splicing. The intron 9 alternative splice donor site mutation seen in FS leads to loss of three amino acids (KTS, or lysine, threonine, and serine), thus disrupting the normal ratio of WT1 isoforms critical for proper gonadal and renal development. The altered ratio of WT1 isoforms is associated with decreased expression of *SRY* and *SOX9*, which both encode transcription factors required for normal testicular development.[114] Interestingly, most patients with FS do not develop WT; however, a few cases have been reported,[115] with overall estimates for WT of 5% to 10%.[116] Most males with FS, however, have severe genitourinary abnormalities, resulting in a high risk for gonadoblastoma.[112]

The management of children with WT1-associated WT predisposition syndromes involves genetic testing, tumor surveillance, and organ-sparing therapies. It is recommended that children presenting with WT, genitourinary abnormalities, and/or early-onset renal failure be tested for germline *WT1* mutations.[103] Testing should also be considered for patients with bilateral WT without associated abnormalities, although the yield of testing in this instance is lower.[103] Generally, it is not recommended that children with unilateral WT and no associated abnormalities be tested, as the prevalence of *WT1* mutations in these patients is only 1.4%.[100] All children with aniridia should be screened by fluorescence in situ hybridization studies or single-nucleotide polymorphism array, as up to one third of patients will exhibit loss of one copy of *WT1*[117] and thus be at increased risk for WT formation.

As the treatment strategies for WT have become more successful, screening programs are unlikely to affect these outcomes. However, the goal of screening is to promote earlier detection and, thus, easier surgical management, less intensive chemotherapy, and possible avoidance of radiotherapy. Ninety-eight percent of children with *WT1*-associated WT are diagnosed with their tumors by 7 years of age.[118] As a result, it is generally recommended that patients with germline *WT1* mutations undergo kidney surveillance with renal ultrasound examinations every 3 months through the first 7 years of life.[116] Given the increased risk for multifocal and bilateral disease, it is recommended that for those who do develop WT, nephron-sparing surgery be used whenever possible. Newer areas of investigation focus on the use of neoadjuvant chemotherapy to eradicate renal tumors and thereby avoid the use of surgery. Patients with a germline *WT1* mutation are particularly at risk for this end-stage renal disease. Therefore patients should undergo lifelong monitoring of blood pressure and renal function, with early treatment of hypertension and avoidance of nephrotoxic medications.[110]

Hereditary Paraganglioma/ Pheochromocytoma Syndrome

Incidence

PGLs and PCCs are neuroendocrine tumors that generally involve the parasympathetic and sympathetic chains or adrenal glands. PGLs are rare in the general population, occurring at an estimated incidence of 1:30,000 to 1:1 million.[119-121] However, in the presence of an underlying predisposing condition, the tumor rate can be extraordinarily high.[122,123] Toward this end, a recent study demonstrated that 30% and 81% of children with nonmetastatic and metastatic PGLs/PCCs, respectively, carried germline mutations in genes encoding subunits of the succinate dehydrogenase (SDH) complex.[124] In addition to *SDH* genes, germline mutations in *NF1*, *VHL*, *RET*, *TMEM127*, and *MAX* also predispose to PGL/PCC. Therefore, the true incidence of germline mutations in children with these tumors may be even higher than currently estimated.[125]

Genetics

Hereditary PGL/PCC is caused by germline mutations in the *SDHA*, *SDHB*, *SDHC*, *SDHD*, and *SDHAF2* genes (collectively *SDHx*), which encode components of *SDH*, a mitochondrial enzyme complex responsible for converting succinate to fumarate as part of the tricarboxylic acid cycle.[126] *SDHA*, *SDHB*, *SDHC*, and *SDHD* encode for proteins that make up SDH, while *SDHAF2* encodes for SDH assembly factor 2, a protein needed to assemble the SDH proteins into a fully functioning complex.[16] Mutations in the *SDHx* genes lead to a faulty tricarboxylic acid cycle with increased levels of succinate and subsequent increases in hypoxia-inducible factor (HIF) signaling and histone deregulation. It was recently reported that *SDHx* mutations are associated with a hypermethylator phenotype, which may also contribute to tumorigenesis.[127,128] PGLs are usually benign tumors, but when caused by an *SDHx* mutation, particularly *SDHB*, they exhibit an aggressive metastatic phenotype. The biology behind this clinical difference is not yet known. Hereditary PGL/PCC is inherited in an autosomal dominant fashion; however, *SDHD* and *SDHAF2* are maternally imprinted, with only the children of fathers, not mothers, developing tumors. Nevertheless, mothers can still pass along *SDHD* and *SDHAF2* mutations to their children, who will not develop PGL/PCC but remain at 50% risk to transmit the disease to future generations.

Tumor Risks and Surveillance

The SDHx-related tumor spectrum is broad and includes PGL (*SDHA, SDHB, SDHC, SDHD, SDHAF2*), PCC (*SDHA, SDHB, SDHC, SDHD*), gastrointestinal stromal tumors (GISTs) (*SDHA, SDHB, SDHC, SDHD*), papillary thyroid cancer (*SDHB, SDHD*), renal cell carcinoma (RCC) and oncocytoma (*SDHB, SDHC*), neuroblastoma (*SDHD*), and, most recently, pituitary adenoma (*SDHA*).[93,126,129,130] Patients who develop PGLs as well as GISTs have a condition known as Carney-Stratakis syndrome.[131] In rare instances, PGLs, GISTs, and pulmonary chondromas occur together, in which case they are referred to as the Carney triad. Traditionally, tumors occurring in the context of Carney triad have not been associated with underlying SDHx mutations.[131,132]

Hereditary PGL/PCC has no defining clinical criteria other than a possible family history of *SDHx*-related tumors. Therefore, any child diagnosed with a PGL, PCC, or GIST should undergo genetic testing due to the strong association between these tumors and underlying *SDHx* mutations. Immunohistochemical staining of tumor tissue for *SDHB* protein expression can identify patients at risk for underlying germline *SDHx* mutations.[133,134] Specifically, absent *SDHB* staining indicates that the SDH protein complex is not intact, and this finding may be caused by a mutation in any of the *SDH*-related genes. Clinical laboratories have started to offer *SDHB* immunohistochemical staining to facilitate genetic diagnosis of hereditary PGL/PCC, although the sensitivity and specificity of this test needs to be determined.

Due to the aggressive nature of *SDH*-related tumors, early identification of small tumors in asymptomatic patients may reduce morbidity and mortality. No consensus screening guidelines exist for tumor surveillance, but many clinicians will perform annual physical examinations, blood pressure checks (to detect hypertension due to increased secretion of catecholamines), and blood work for serum metabolites (fractionated catecholamines, including epinephrine, norepinephrine, dopamine; fractionated free metanephrines, including metanephrine and normetanephrine; and chromogranin A).[135,136] Regular imaging can also identify PGL/PCC, and this is especially important for those with non–catecholamine-secreting tumors.[137-140] Common imaging approaches include computed tomography, ^{18}F-fluorodeoxyglucose positron-emission tomography, and [^{123}I]-metaiodobenzylguanidine scintigraphy. Some centers are beginning to use rapid-sequence whole-body MRI, with or without dedicated neck MRI, as a screening measure for individuals with germline *SDHx* mutations (see Fig. 42-3). Recently, the University of Utah published findings showing that this approach has a sensitivity of 88% and specificity of 95%

for detecting new tumors compared with isolated biochemical testing, which exhibited a sensitivity of 38% and specificity of 95%.[141] As *SDHx* mutations are increasingly recognized and studied, we will learn more about the genetic, epigenetic, and metabolic alterations linked to cancer and discover novel approaches to tumor prevention and treatment.

Neurofibromatosis Type 1
Incidence

Neurofibromatosis type 1 (NF1) is considered one of the most common inherited cancer predisposition syndromes, affecting 1 in 3000 children.[142,143] NF1 is caused by germline heterozygous inactivating mutations in the *NF1* gene, which is located on chromosome 17 and encodes the protein neurofibromin.[142-144] In addition to cancer, patients with NF1 are at increased risk to develop benign tumors such as neurofibromas and Lisch nodules (iris hamartomas), as well as nononcologic manifestations, including café-au-lait macules and intertriginous freckles (see Fig. 42-1), bone deformities (long bone pseudarthrosis, skeletal dysplasias, scoliosis, osteoporosis), vascular abnormalities, short stature, and neurocognitive delay.[145-148]

Genetics

The *NF1* gene encodes a cytoplasmic protein, neurofibromin, which is mainly expressed in neurons, Schwann cells, oligodendrocytes, and leukocytes. Neurofibromin functions as a tumor suppressor by restricting cell proliferation through its effects on the RAS signaling pathway. Interestingly, there is wide variation in the phenotypic presentation of NF1, even among family members with the identical *NF1* mutation. Szudek and associates[149] examined familial aggregation of NF1 phenotypes in 904 affected individuals from 373 families with NF1 and concluded that unlinked modifying genes are likely to contribute to the distinct presentations.[149] Most recently, Sabbagh and colleagues[150] evaluated phenotypic correlations between affected relatives in 750 patients with NF1 in 275 multiplex families; they also concluded that genetic modifiers unlinked to the *NF1* locus contribute to the variable phenotypic severity observed in NF1. Thus, similar to other hereditary cancer disorders, loss of *NF1* serves as the first hit but the presence of other modifying genes and/or accumulation of tissue-specific second hits may ultimately dictate the phenotype.

Tumor Risks and Surveillance

The tumors that develop in children with NF1 include malignant peripheral nerve sheath tumors (MPNSTs) and astrocytomas (including optic gliomas [OPGs]), and, less commonly, rhabdomyosarcomas and neuroblastomas. Adults with NF1 remain at increased risk for MPNSTs and gliomas, as well as GISTs, somatostatinomas, and PCCs.[151] Half of patients with NF1 develop plexiform neurofibromas, the majority of which grow slowly but can cause significant disfigurement and pain. A small proportion transform to MPNST, which can be aggressive and resistant to therapy.[152-154] OPGs occur in up to 25% of patients and may lead to blindness if left untreated.

OPGs usually present before 6 years of age, although they may not become problematic until later in life as they encroach along the optic pathway.[156-159]

The diagnosis of NF1 is often clinical and based on a patient having at least two or more of the following criteria: (1) six or more café-au-lait macules measuring more than 5 mm in greatest diameter in prepubertal individuals and more than 15 mm in postpubertal individuals; (2) two or more neurofibromas of any type or one plexiform neurofibroma; (3) freckling in the axillary or inguinal regions; (4) an OPG; (5) two or more Lisch nodules (iris hamartomas); (6) osseous lesions such as sphenoid dysplasia or tibial pseudarthrosis; or (7) a first-degree relative (parent, sibling, offspring) with NF1 as defined by the above criteria. The clinical features of NF1 increase with age. Therefore, many children meet the criteria for diagnosis by 8 years.[32,156] Young children who manifest only with café-au-lait macules should be followed closely for development of other manifestations and considered to have NF1 unless proven otherwise.[160]

Surveillance for early cancers remains controversial in NF1.[58,145,161-163] Upon diagnosis, patients should undergo a thorough physical examination with a complete ophthalmologic evaluation (to assess for compromised vision, which could indicate an underlying OPG) and developmental assessment. Currently, some institutions order baseline and annual head MRIs to screen for OPGs. Other institutions order MRIs only if patients are symptomatic or if visual or central nervous system abnormalities are detected. Avoidance of radiation therapy is encouraged in patients with NF1 as this treatment may be associated with a higher risk for developing subsequent MPNSTs.[153,164]

Von Hippel–Lindau Syndrome

Incidence

Von Hippel–Lindau syndrome (VHL) is an autosomal dominant disorder caused by mutation of the *VHL* gene, which resides at chromosomal locus 3p25.5. VHL is a rare disease, with a prevalence of 1:36,000 live births and an estimated de novo mutation rate of 1% to 3%.[165,166] VHL is primarily considered to be a genitourinary cancer syndrome because of its strong association with RCC, but as discussed below, several different tumor types are associated with germline VHL mutations.

Genetics

VHL encodes a protein with diverse functions, including activity as an ubiquitin ligase as well as a tumor suppressor involved in transcriptional regulation, posttranscriptional gene expression, apoptosis, and extracellular matrix formation.[166,167] The VHL protein functions as part of a complex that targets other proteins for degradation, including HIF1α-.[168] The fact that it participates in the same pathway that is affected by *SDHx* mutations could explain the clinical similarities between VHL and hereditary PGL/PCC; both are characterized by the development of PGL, PCC, and RCC. It is also proposed that VHL's involvement in HIF1α signaling might explain the tendency of patients to form highly vascularized tumors such as hemangioblastomas.[166]

Tumor Risks and Surveillance

VHL is associated with an increased risk of developing benign as well as malignant tumors, including retinal angiomas; central nervous system hemangioblastomas; clear cell RCC; pancreatic islet cell tumors; endolymphatic sac tumors of the inner ear; renal, pancreatic, and epididymal cysts; PGLs; and PCCs. Of these tumors, RCC is one of the most common and develops in nearly 70% of VHL patients by the age of 60 years. Although RCC is common, it is rarely the first tumor to present.[169] In fact, over a third of patients initially present with cerebellar hemangioblastomas decades prior to RCC.[170] Unfortunately, most VHL patients succumb to RCC, the leading cause of mortality in this disorder.[165,169] Somatic *VHL* mutations are found in inherited and sporadic RCC, and are thus recurring drivers of RCC formation.[171]

Any patient who presents with a VHL-related tumor becomes a candidate for *VHL* genetic testing. Asymptomatic children born to a parent with VHL should be tested within the first year of life, given the 50% risk for inheriting the syndrome and the importance of early intervention. *VHL* germline mutations are typically identified in close to 100% of affected individuals, making the genetic test a very reliable one.[172] VHL is typified by strong genotype-phenotype correlations, which can guide the approach to genetic testing and/or screening.[167,173] For example, the VHL "type 1" phenotype lacks PCCs and is associated with *VHL* deletions, insertions, and truncations. The VHL "type 2" phenotype presents with PCCs and is associated with *VHL* missense mutations. "Type 2A" lacks RCC and pancreatic cysts and is associated with specific missense alterations, including the pathogenic *VHL* Y98H, Y112H, and V116F variants. "Type 2B" patients develop RCC and pancreatic cysts, and harbor R167Q and R167W variants. Finally, VHL "type 2C" is associated with PCC only, and is associated with the V155L, R238W, and L188V variants of *VHL*.

Although no evidence-based guidelines exist, many clinicians follow a similar protocol for tumor surveillance. In affected individuals, ophthalmologic examinations should be initiated by 5 years of age or earlier to examine for retinal angiomas. In those at risk for PGL or PCC, plasma catecholamines and metanephrines should be measured annually, along with regular blood pressure monitoring and abdominal ultrasound examinations starting before the age of 10 years. Rapid whole-body MRI may be useful as a means of locating various tumors; however, this approach has not yet been systematically evaluated in VHL. Audiology assessments are suggested to occur every 2 to 3 years starting at age 5 to assess for the presence of endolymphatic sac tumors. In those with hearing loss, tinnitus, or vertigo, hearing evaluation and/or MRI scans should be completed annually. MRI of the brain and spine is recommended to commence around midadolescence to assess for the presence of central nervous system hemangioblastomas, and close neurologic examinations starting at birth and continuing throughout life are also recommended. Collectively, these approaches have proven to be effective in VHL, where they have greatly decreased morbidity and increased life expectancy for affected children and adults.[174]

Beckwith-Wiedemann Syndrome and Isolated Hemihyperplasia

Incidence

BWS is an overgrowth syndrome characterized by macrosomia, neonatal hypoglycemia, abdominal wall defects (omphalocoele, umbilical hernia), hemihyperplasia, macroglossia, ear anomalies, and increased risk for tumor formation.[175] BWS is estimated to affect 1 in 13,700 live births, with 85% of cases being sporadic and 15% familial.[175] Approximately 7.5% to 10% of BWS patients develop malignancy, most commonly hepatoblastoma (HB) or WT.[175,176] ACC, neuroblastoma, and rhabdomyosarcoma are also rarely encountered.[3,33,63] Atypical teratoid/rhabdoid tumor and PCC have been identified in single case reports but may be coincidental findings.[177-179] Isolated hemihyperplasia (IHH) is defined by asymmetric overgrowth of one or more body parts in the absence of the other clinical findings associated with BWS. IHH may represent part of the clinical spectrum of BWS as, in many cases, it has a similar genetic etiology and profile of cancer predisposition.[180]

Genetics

Multiple genetic and epigenetic abnormalities are observed in patients with BWS or IHH, all of which affect chromosomal locus 11p15.5. Among the genes included this region are *IGF2*, which encodes insulin-like growth factor 2, and *CDKN1C*, which encodes cyclin-dependent kinase inhibitor 1C. These and surrounding genes are "imprinted," or differentially methylated, depending on whether the gene copy is inherited from the mother or the father. As a result, only the maternal or paternal copy is expressed at any given time. The epigenetic aberrations in BWS/IHH lead to hypomethylation, and thus overexpression, of *IGF2*, as well as hypermethylation and, thus, reduced expression of *CDKN1C*.[175,181] The overexpression of growth-promoting genes and inhibition of growth-controlling genes may contribute to the overgrowth and tumor predisposition that occur in BWS/IHH.

Fifty-five percent to 65% of BWS patients have a defect at one of two imprinting control centers that determine methylation of the genes in the region. Paternal uniparental disomy at chromosome 11p15.5, in which a child has two copies of the chromosome or chromosomal region from the father and none from the mother, is the genetic abnormality identified in 20% to 25% of patients with BWS.[175,182] About 5% of patients with sporadic BWS harbor germline mutations in *CDKN1C*, a tumor suppressor gene encoding a cell cycle inhibitor, whereas approximately 40% of familial cases display this defect.[175,182] In total, about 75% to 80% of patients with clinical BWS have identifiable constitutional genetic abnormalities. The remaining patients may harbor mutations in novel genes, or be genetic mosaics for alterations in known genes linked to BWS. In mosaicism, the genetic or epigenetic alteration occurs during embryogenesis, with the result that only a subpopulation of cells displays the genetic abnormality. When mosaicism is present, the disease-associated genetic abnormality may be difficult to detect if only a small percentage of cells is affected, or if it is isolated to tissues that are not as easily sampled as the blood.

Tumor Risks and Surveillance

Cancer screening recommendations for patients with BWS or IHH are aimed primarily at detecting HB and WT. Although the incidence of neuroblastoma is higher in patients with BWS than in the general population, it is not considered high enough to warrant screening. Screening should be used for all patients with a clinical diagnosis of BWS or IHH, even if no underlying molecular abnormality is identified. Screening for HB begins when the diagnosis of BWS is made or suspected. It is recommended that patients undergo abdominal ultrasound examinations every 3 months, as well as serial evaluations of serum alpha-fetoprotein (AFP), as AFP is typically increased in patients with HB and thus serves as a very sensitive tumor marker. Although the timing of when to obtain AFP levels remains a subject of debate, it is generally recommended that levels be measured at a minimum of every 3 months.[183] AFP levels tend to be higher in patients with BWS, even in the absence of HB. In addition, levels tend to decrease more slowly over time.[183] Therefore, if the initial AFP level is elevated but there is no abnormality on ultrasound or other imaging, the test may be repeated in 4 to 6 weeks. If the levels are falling, they may be rechecked every 4 to 6 weeks until they return to normal. If the initial elevation is accompanied by a radiologic abnormality, if it fails to fall, or if it exponentially increases, the patient should be referred to an oncologist for further evaluation. Screening for HB can be discontinued at age 4 years as the majority of these tumors develop before this time.

Screening for WT consists of serial ultrasound examinations every 3 months from the time of diagnosis until the age of 8 years. In the first 4 years, the abdominal ultrasound performed to screen for HB is also used to evaluate for renal masses.[184] After age 4 years, imaging may be limited to renal ultrasound, which is faster and less expensive than abdominal ultrasound and does not require that the child fast for the examination. For HB and WT screening, ultrasound is favored over MRI or computed tomography as it is widely available, is noninvasive, leads to no radiation exposure, only rarely requires sedation, and is generally faster and less expensive.

There is increasing evidence to suggest that within the spectrum of BWS and/or IHH, distinct molecular abnormalities confer different risks for tumor development. For example, paternal uniparental disomy and abnormalities at the imprinting control center 1 have the highest risk of tumor development, whereas mutations of *CDKN1C* may not increase a child's risk for malignancy.[62,182,185,186] However, these genetic findings have not yet been used to direct decisions in most screening programs. It is likely, however, that future screening programs will be more precisely designed to take into account the particular risks related to the underlying genetic abnormality.

Data pointing to the benefits of screening in BWS are sparse but encouraging. Choyke and associates[187] report that patients with BWS or IHH who did not undergo screening had an increased rate of high-stage WT (stage III or IV) compared with patients who underwent screening. A report from the National Wilms Tumor Study Group examining 4669 children between 1980 and 1995 found that 1.1% of children with WT had BWS.[188] Interestingly, the children with BWS were diagnosed at younger ages (mean 28 months) than children without BWS (mean 44 months) and with lower-stage WT (71.7% of BWS patients with stage I or II tumors vs. 55% of non-BWS patients). Furthermore, none of the BWS patients presented with metastatic disease, compared with 12% of the non-BWS children. It is not possible to discern how much these differences were affected by screening. Nonetheless, it remains feasible that some of them were due to the positive effects of the monitoring for tumors in this population. Few studies exist evaluating the efficacy of screening for HB, although case reports document presymptomatic detection of tumors in some BWS patients.[189]

Rhabdoid Tumor Predisposition Syndrome

Incidence

Rhabdoid tumors are rare, highly aggressive malignant growths that generally present in infancy or early childhood[190] and are most commonly found in the kidney or central nervous system.[191] The annual incidence of rhabdoid tumors in children under 15 years of age in the United States is 0.19 per million for renal tumors, 0.89 per million for central nervous system tumors, and 0.32 per million for tumors involving other sites (SEER data, 2011). The characteristic somatic genetic abnormality and the primary initiating event includes mutation of the INI1/SMARCB1 gene located on chromosome 22q11.2.[192]

Genetics

SMARCB1 is part of a chromatin-remodeling complex involved in regulating gene expression, including genes involved in cell cycle control, DNA repair, and differentiation.[193] Both alleles must be inactivated in order for a tumor to arise, consistent with its function as a tumor suppressor gene. Approximately 35% of rhabdoid tumor patients have germline INI1/SMARCB1 alterations.[194] While the majority of germline mutations are de novo, families with rhabdoid tumor predisposition have been reported in which multiple siblings have been affected. In rare cases, a parent is an unaffected carrier, and can have multiple children with rhabdoid tumor before the condition comes to the attention of a clinical geneticist. Additionally, there have been reports of families in which some members were diagnosed with schwannomatosis, a disorder in which an individual develops two or more benign tumors of the nerve sheath, commonly referred to as schwannomas, while others developed rhabdoid tumors.[194] Most cases of familial schwannomatosis are associated with germline INI1/SMARCB1 mutations.[10,27,195,196] The penetrance and expressivity of INI1/SMARCB1 abnormalities are under investigation, and may vary with the specific genetic mutation.[194]

Tumor Risks and Surveillance

The major tumor risk in rhabdoid tumor predisposition syndrome (RTPS) is for the development of renal or extrarenal rhabdoid tumors, which generally have a very aggressive phenotype. In National Wilms Tumor Study Group trials, patients with stage I or II renal rhabdoid tumors had an overall survival rate of 42% at 4 years; those with stage III, IV, or V disease fared less well, with a survival rate of about 16% when evaluated as a group.[190] For those with central nervous system disease, the prognosis is comparably dismal, with a registry review identifying a median overall survival time of 16.75 months.[197] Event-free survival appears to be better in patients with gross total resection compared with those who had subtotal resections of their central nervous system tumors.[197] Thus, if central nervous system tumors were detected earlier, they might be more easily resected and the outcome might be improved. Individuals with RTPS have also been reported to develop multiple schwannomas and meningiomas later in life.[194]

Currently, there are no standard recommendations for surveillance in patients with RTPS. Experts in the field have suggested that patients have thorough physical and neurologic examinations as well as head ultrasound imaging studies monthly during the first year of life to detect the presence of central nervous system tumors. It is also suggested that patients undergo abdominal ultrasound imaging every 1 to 3 months to assess for the presence of renal lesions. After age 4 years, the risk of developing a rhabdoid tumor rapidly declines, and at this point one could consider periodic screening using whole-body MRI. Although there are as yet no studies to confirm the benefit of screening patients with germline INI1/SMARCB1 mutations, the aggressive natural history of the disease, apparently high penetrance, and well-defined age of onset for central nervous system rhabdoid tumors suggest that screening could prove beneficial. Given the potential survival benefit of surgically resectable disease, it is reasonable to postulate that early detection might improve overall survival rates.

DICER1-Related Tumor Predisposition Syndrome

Incidence

PPB is a rare cancer of embryonal lung tissue, which presents in infancy or early childhood. The first known case was reported in 1945, and the term PPB was proposed in 1988 to describe a range of rare pulmonary and pleural tumors made up primarily of fetal tissues.[198] Over 50 cases have been described, with a median age of 34 months at diagnosis.[199] Hereditary PPB has been observed in a small number of families worldwide, and in 2009 germline DICER1 mutations were identified as the cause of hereditary PPB.[200] Since this discovery, germline mutations in DICER1 have been implicated in up to 60% to 70% of PPB cases. Furthermore, careful review of DICER1-mutation–positive individuals and families reveals that there are many additional tumors associated with germline DICER1 mutations, including cystic nephroma, ovarian Sertoli-Leydig cell tumor, embryonal rhabdomyosarcoma, intraocular medulloepithelioma, and supratentorial primitive neuroectodermal tumor.[201]

Genetics

The *DICER1* gene, located at 14q32.13, encodes a cytoplasmic endoribonuclease, which cleaves precursor molecules into microRNAs (miRNAs) that subsequently modulate cellular mRNA expression.[201] Impaired miRNA processing decreases the posttranslational regulation of mRNAs, and germline *DICER1* mutations have recently been shown to promote tumorigenesis via this mechanism.[202] Interestingly, all individuals with familial PPB show haploinsufficiency at 14q32.13 due to germline mutations affecting a single *DICER1* allele.[201] Studies of zebrafish[203] and mice[204] suggest that *DICER1* haploinsufficiency with retention of a single wild-type allele is sufficient for cancers to develop. Perturbations in miRNA concentrations have been implicated in studies of many human cancers, including lung, breast, ovarian, and skin cancers, with diverse and unclear associations between defects in miRNA processing and tumor phenotype depending on the tissue and mutation studied.[205] Consistent with this observation, several recent studies have implicated somatic mutations in *DICER1* in a variety of adult solid tumors.[206,207] Further translational studies will be necessary to explain the exact cause of miRNA-mediated oncogenesis, but it seems likely that miRNA dysregulation represents a new and important pathway in tumor formation.

Tumor Risks and Surveillance

DICER1 syndrome should be considered and clinical gene testing pursued in patients who present with PPB, cystic nephroma, ovarian Sertoli-Leydig cell tumors, embryonal rhabdomyosarcoma, intraocular medulloepithelioma, supratentorial primitive neuroectodermal tumor, or multinodular goiter. In a large retrospective cohort, 11 of 14 (79%) PPB cases, 2 of 3 (67%) cystic nephromas, and 3 of 6 (50%) cases of ovarian Sertoli-Leydig cell tumor were associated with germline *DICER1* mutations.[18] *DICER1* mutations are inherited in an autosomal dominant manner with variable expressivity and incomplete penetrance.[18] A negative family history does not exclude the diagnosis, especially in patients with typical tumors due to de novo germline *DICER1* mutations.

Since *DICER1* syndrome has been only recently described, the understanding of its phenotype and associated tumor risks is evolving. As a result, there are not yet consensus guidelines for surveillance among individuals harboring *DICER1* mutations. In cross-sectional studies, many individuals harboring a *DICER1* mutation do not develop cancer.[18] Given the rare and varied nature of malignant disease associated with *DICER1* germline mutations, individual practitioners will need to account for penetrance, age of tumor onset, clinical impact of early diagnosis, and risk of false-positive screening tests when weighing the risks and benefits of surveillance. Once PPB develops, complete surgical resection (often combined with adjuvant chemotherapy) is indicated and can lead to cure.[199] The overall 5-year survival rate in a cohort of 50 PPB patients was 45%,[13] although there was significant biologic variability within the cohort. A recent European review of 65 cases of PPB reveals that stage, grade, and degree of resection were highly correlated with survival,[208] suggesting that screening and early detection may indeed improve patient outcomes. Patients with *DICER1* mutations warrant close follow-up, and patients and their physicians should remain vigilant for changes in respiratory function, alterations in menses, and development of goiter, as each of these manifestations can herald the development of malignancy in this high-risk patient population.

Constitutional Mismatch Repair–Deficiency Syndrome

Incidence

CMMR-D (also known as CoLoN [Colon tumors and/or Leukemia/Lymphoma and/or Neurofibromatosis features],[210] childhood cancer syndrome,[211] and Lynch III syndrome[212]) is a recently described predisposition syndrome associated with the development of several different types of cancer, and sometimes multiple cancers, in children.[213] CMMR-D is caused by homozygous or compound heterozygous germline mutations in the genes that function in DNA mismatch repair (MMR), including *MLH1*, *MSH2*, *MSH6*, and *PMS2*. Individuals who carry a heterozygous mutation in one of these genes have a condition known as hereditary nonpolyposis colon cancer, or Lynch syndrome [LS]), which predisposes to many cancer types, including early-onset colorectal cancer, endometrial cancer, and ovarian cancer, with an average age of onset of cancer in the 40s or 50s. CMMR-D was first described in two consanguineous LS families in which the children were noted to have features of NF1 and early-onset hematologic and gastrointestinal malignancies.[214,215] To date, about 100 cases have been reported[216,217]; however, the exact incidence of CMMR-D is not known. In addition to cancer, children with CMMR-D develop café-au-lait macules, axillary and/or inguinal freckling, and Lisch nodules. Due to its similarity to NF1, children may be misdiagnosed as having neurofibromatosis.

Genetics

The normal role of the MMR proteins is to identify and repair small errors, such as base pair mismatches and small insertions and deletions, which occur during DNA replication. Additionally, the DNA MMR system has a role in apoptosis in response to DNA damage. Defective MMR leads to the accumulation of additional mutations, which eventually lead to tumor development. MMR-deficient tumors are often characterized by instability in microsatellites, short repeated sequences of DNA that are highly susceptible to errors during DNA replication. In LS, the second copy of an affected MMR gene is lost during tumor development. Therefore, LS-associated tumors are MMR-deficient and high in microsatellite instability (MSI).

Some genotype-phenotype correlations have been reported in CMMR-D. Individuals with biallelic mutations in *MLH1* or *MSH2* are more frequently diagnosed at younger ages and with hematologic malignant disease compared with individuals who carry mutations affecting *MSH6* or *PMS2*. In contrast, brain and other LS-associated tumors are more common in individuals with *MSH6* or *PMS2* mutations compared with *MLH1* or *MSH2*.[213] There is some evidence that individuals with more severe mutations (deletions or truncating mutations resulting in no functional protein) exhibit a more severe phenotype, with hematologic and brain cancers developing in the first decade of life, compared with individuals with less damaging mutations. These latter individuals are more likely to develop hematologic, brain, and gastrointestinal malignant disease in the second to fourth decades of life.[212,213]

Establishing a molecular diagnosis of CMMR-D is similar to making the diagnosis of LS, which can be accomplished in a stepwise manner beginning with testing for MSI and/or loss of expression of an MMR protein, followed by mutational analysis of the appropriate MMR genes. Because patients with CMMR-D have constitutional MMR deficiency, MSI and lack of MMR protein expression should theoretically be detectable in tumor as well as normal tissue. Interestingly, immunohistochemical staining of tumor was recently shown to be 100% sensitive and specific in diagnosing MMR deficiency, whereas MSI was neither sensitive nor specific and thus did not help in making the diagnosis.[209] If one or more of the familial MMR mutations are already known, it may be possible to proceed directly to genetic testing in the individual in question. It is important to note that diagnostic and genetic testing for this disorder is challenging, and it should be coordinated by professionals with experience in the diagnosis of LS and/or CMMR-D.[212,213,218]

Tumor Risks and Surveillance

The cancers most commonly associated with CMMR-D include hematologic malignant tumors, brain tumors, and LS-associated cancers (most notably, very early-onset gastrointestinal cancer).[209] Less common cancers include neuroblastoma and rhabdomyosarcoma.[212,213,217] In recent reviews, LS-associated cancers (mostly gastrointestinal) accounted for 32% to 37% of all cancers, brain tumors for 32% to 48%, and hematologic cancers for 15% to 24%; 5% to 7% were other types of cancer.[209,213] Multiple primary tumors have been reported in 20% to 40% of patients.[216,217] Age of onset varies by tumor type, with hematologic malignant tumors presenting in early childhood (mean age of onset, 5.5 years), brain tumors presenting in slightly older children (mean age of onset, 8 years), and LS-associated tumors in adolescence and young adulthood (mean age of onset, 15 to 16 years for gastrointestinal and genitourinary tract cancers and 24 years for endometrial cancer). LS-associated tumors may present as a second or third malignancy in patients who survive their initial cancer diagnosis.[213] In one study, gastrointestinal polyps or cancers were the first manifestation of CMMR-D in up to one third of patients.[217]

CMMR-D should be considered for young children who present with hematologic malignant disease, brain tumors, and/or LS-related cancers, in conjunction with: (1) café-au-lait macules and/or other signs of NF1 and/or hypopigmented skin lesions; (2) consanguineous parents; (3) a family history of LS-related cancers; (4) a second malignant tumor; and (5) siblings with childhood cancer. The lack of a family history of LS-related cancers should not rule out the possibility of CMMR-D, as some families could carry less penetrant mutations and thus not meet clinical criteria for a diagnosis of LS.[212,216,219] Because CMMR-D shares clinical features with NF-1, FAP, and LFS, it is important to keep this diagnosis in mind when evaluating children who present with one or more of these features.[213,216,217,220]

Development of a surveillance protocol has been challenging in CMMR-D because of the variety of associated cancers and the possibility of multiple primary cancers. There are currently no standard cancer screening guidelines, although some groups have suggested protocols including surveillance for colon and other gastrointestinal, hematologic, endometrial and ovarian, and other cancers.[217,221] Recently, it was reported that a surveillance protocol including semiannual brain MRI, annual gastrointestinal endoscopy, and blood work every 4 months successfully identified 39 asymptomatic tumors in a cohort of 23 children with CMMR-D, including 2 malignant gliomas, 2 gastrointestinal carcinomas, and 6 cases of polyposis.[209] There are currently very few data regarding the optimal treatment of cancers in patients with CMMR-D. However, clinicians should be aware of the possibility of increased toxicity and reduced efficacy of chemotherapy, as well as increased risk of second primary malignant tumors.[219,222]

CONCLUSIONS, CHALLENGES, AND LOOKING TO THE FUTURE

Since the isolation of *RB1* as the first gene predisposing to cancer, we have experienced tremendous advances in cancer genetics, including sequencing of the human genome and elucidation of DNA, RNA, and the epigenetic landscape of several different cancers. These new data have led to a profound increase in our knowledge of genes that predispose to cancer and the heritable basis of cancer. The characterization of these genes has highlighted critical roles for the encoded proteins in processes ranging from cell cycle control, DNA repair, apoptosis, signaling, miRNA processing, and metabolism. Because many of these predisposing genes are also mutated on a somatic level in a wide array of sporadic cancers, the study of rare cancer syndromes— many of which affect children—has provided invaluable insights into the processes underlying tumor formation.

Along with these advances have come many challenges. For example, we continue to know little about the psychosocial, developmental, and behavioral issues related to the genetic testing of children or adults for heritable predisposition to cancer. We do not yet understand which factors influence the pursuit and uptake of genetic testing by families, whether patients truly understand genetic test results and their implications, how individuals choose to communicate results within their immediate and/or extended families, and how genetic information influences the health-promoting and risk-taking behaviors of children and other family members. For many conditions predisposing to cancer, it is impossible to know when and what types of cancer will occur. This uncertainty makes it difficult to establish effective surveillance protocols. Assessment of the costs and benefits of these protocols is further compounded by the rarity of specific syndromes.

These challenges are only likely to exponentially increase as genetic technologies evolve and are increasingly applied to the clinical setting. Although these technologies will further our knowledge of the pathogenic mutations linked to cancer, they will also reveal many less-damaging variants. In many cases, it may not be readily evident whether these variants influence the expression or function of an encoded protein. Therefore, it will be difficult to know how to react to these results. Will these variants influence disease susceptibility, response to treatment, and/or therapy-associated toxicities? How do these variants cooperate with one another or with environmental factors during the process of tumor formation? As more information is gained and functional assays are developed, variants may eventually be reclassified as benign polymorphisms or disease-causing mutations. Who will be responsible for reanalyzing these data, reporting the updated results, and explaining their implications to clinicians and patients? Finally, how will we translate the increasing body of genetic information to the clinical setting to predict cancer risk, direct tumor screening, and prevent tumors from occurring? Although it is expected that genetic discoveries will enable development of new and more effective therapies or preventive measures, unfortunately we are yet to realize these benefits for the majority of human cancers. Ultimately, the challenge lies in establishing national and international collaborations, where information on these rare, yet informative, syndromes predisposing to cancer can be gathered, integrated, and analyzed to address these important and as yet unanswered questions.

ACKNOWLEDGEMENTS

This work was funded in part by the Grundy Vision of Life Fund at The Children's Hospital of Philadelphia. We thank Dr. Carol Shields for providing the retinoblastoma images shown in Figure 42-2.

References available online at ExpertConsult.

KEY REFERENCES

9. Knudson AG, Jr: Mutation and cancer: statistical study of retinoblastoma. *Proc Natl Acad Sci U S A* 68(4):820–823, 1971.
   This is the original article by Knudson in which he puts forth the two-hit" hypothesis underlying the development of hereditary RB.
18. Slade I, Bacchelli C, Davies H, et al: DICER1 syndrome: clarifying the diagnosis, clinical features and management implications of a pleiotropic tumour predisposition syndrome. *J Med Genet* 48(4):273–278, 2011.
   Researchers screened more than 800 blood samples from children with a broad range of solid tumors and more than 750 cancer cell lines to determine the impact of somatic DICER1 mutations. DICER1 mutation was associated with a variety of solid tumors, but in families with DICER1 syndrome, most mutation carriers did not develop malignant disease. The authors also give recommendations for DICER1 mutation testing in at-risk families.
34. Wimmer K, Kratz CP: Constitutional mismatch repair–deficiency syndrome. *Haematologica* 95(5):699–701, 2010.
   Describes the phenotypic spectrum, including tumor and non-tumor features, of CMMR-D syndrome. Genotype-phenotype correlations, diagnostic testing, and treatment and surveillance strategies for CMMR-D are also reviewed.
35. Pilarski R: Cowden syndrome: a critical review of the clinical literature. *J Genet Couns* 18(1):13–27, 2009.
   An overview of Cowden syndrome, including a review of tumor and nontumor features, genetics and genetic testing, and medical management.
36. Gabree M, Seidel M: Genetic testing by cancer site: skin. *Cancer J* 18(4):372–380, 2012.
   An overview of hereditary cancer syndromes with associated skin cancer risks and/or benign skin findings. Reviews clinical features, genetic testing, and medical management for each syndrome.
44. Lolkema MP, Gadellaa–van Hooijdonk CG, Bredenoord AL, et al: Ethical, legal, and counseling challenges surrounding the return of genetic results in oncology. *J Clin Oncol* 31(15):1842–1848, 2013.
   Discusses the promises and challenges of next-generation sequencing in oncology. Specifically, the authors point out the possibility of incidental findings from tumor sequencing and the potential ethical, legal, and counseling challenges involved in disclosure of the results to patients.
45. Miller FA, Hayeems RZ, Bytautas JP, et al: Testing personalized medicine: patient and physician expectations of next-generation genomic sequencing in late-stage cancer care. *Eur J Hum Genet* 22:391–395, 2014.
   A qualitative interview study examining patient and physician perceptions and expectations of next-generation tumor sequencing. Patients with late-stage cancers who were participating in a pilot feasibility study of targeted-tumor DNA sequencing and their physicians were interviewed about patients' motivations for participating in the tumor-sequencing study, interpretation of tumor genetic test results, and the possibility of incidental information about inherited cancer risk.
47. Borry P, Stultiens L, Nys H, et al: Presymptomatic and predictive genetic testing in minors: a systematic review of guidelines and position papers. *Clin Genet* 70(5):374–381, 2006.
   This article provides a review of guidelines and position statements on presymptomatic and predictive genetic testing of children. Reviews special issues to be considered in the testing of children and focuses on particular areas of discussion and disagreement among various guidelines.
54. Michie S, Bobrow M, Marteau TM: Predictive genetic testing in children and adults: a study of emotional impact. *J Med Genet* 38(8):519–526, 2001.
   A study examining the psychological impact of positive genetic test results on adults and children. Psychological responses, including anxiety and depression, were measured in adults and children undergoing genetic testing for FAP. Compares the reactions of children and adults to test results and reviews possible factors affecting psychological outcomes.
61. Riley BD, Culver JO, Skrzynia C, et al: Essential elements of genetic cancer risk assessment, counseling, and testing: updated recommendations of the National Society of Genetic Counselors. *J Genet Couns* 21(2):151–161, 2012.
   Recommendations of the National Society of Genetic Counselors regarding all elements of cancer genetic risk assessment. Reviews the impact of identifying patients at increased risk of developing cancer on cancer surveillance and treatment; cancer risk assessment tools such as family history and cancer risk assessment software programs; when genetic testing should be offered; and elements of informed consent, disclosure of genetic test results, and psychosocial assessment.
81. Li FP, Fraumeni JF, Jr: Rhabdomyosarcoma in children: epidemiologic study and identification of a familial cancer syndrome. *J Natl Cancer Inst* 43(6):1365–1373, 1969.
   This is the original article describing the original cluster of familial cancers that eventually became known as LFS, named after the two coauthors. This article is of historical interest and helps the reader to understand the initial description of an important hereditary cancer syndrome.

82. Malkin D, Li FP, Strong LC, et al: Germ line p53 mutations in a familial syndrome of breast cancer, sarcomas, and other neoplasms. *Science* 250(4985):1233–1238, 1990.

This article offers the first association between LFS and the TP53 gene. It helps the reader to learn how genes linked to hereditary cancer syndromes are discovered and described.

85. Mai PL, Malkin D, Garber JE, et al: Li-Fraumeni syndrome: report of a clinical research workshop and creation of a research consortium. *Cancer Genet* 205(10):479–487, 2012.

This article describes the creation of a clinical research workshop dedicated to LFS hosted by the National Institutes of Health and a subsequent research consortium. The article highlights the topics discussed at the workshop and the research objectives of the consortium. It can serve as a model for other types of hereditary cancer syndromes.

88. Shlien A, Tabori U, Marshall CR, et al: Excessive genomic DNA copy number variation in the Li-Fraumeni cancer predisposition syndrome. *Proc Natl Acad Sci U S A* 105(32):11264–11269, 2008.

This article offers a nice example of further molecular characterization of germline DNA in patients with LFS and the identification of copy number variants as genomic modifiers of disease risk. The authors found that excessive copy number variants correlated with patients with LFS and increased risk for cancer presentation.

99. Villani A, Tabori U, Schiffman J, et al: Biochemical and imaging surveillance in germline TP53 mutation carriers with Li-Fraumeni syndrome: a prospective observational study. *Lancet Oncol* 12(6):559–567, 2011.

This landmark article offers the first definitive example of the benefits of intensive early tumor screening in patients with LFS. The authors demonstrate that whole-body MRI and targeted laboratory work in patients with LFS resulted in 100% survival at 3 years for patients found to have tumors through screening versus 20% survival in patients without screening.

101. Royer-Pokora B: Genetics of pediatric renal tumors. *Pediatr Nephrol* 28(1):13–23, 2013.

Focusing on both sporadic and familial WT, this extensive review article summarizes the epidemiology, histology, genetics, and epigenetics of WT and discusses current literature on WT cancer predisposition syndromes. Other types of pediatric renal tumors are also covered in less depth.

105. Pelletier J, Bruening W, Li FP, et al: WT1 mutations contribute to abnormal genital system development and hereditary Wilms' tumour. *Nature* 353(6343):431–434, 1991.

This describes the original mapping of WT1 to 11p13 and provides early evidence of the two-hit model of tumorigenesis associated with tumor suppressor genes. These findings also were instrumental in defining the role of WT1 in WAGR syndrome and the pathways involved in normal urogenital development.

123. Pasini B, Stratakis CA: SDH mutations in tumorigenesis and inherited endocrine tumours: lesson from the phaeochromocytoma-paraganglioma syndromes. *J Intern Med* 266(1):19–42, 2009.

This review summarizes the association between SDH mutations and tumorigenesis, as well as the different types of SDH mutations, and the association of PGLs with several different tumor subtypes, and biologic hypotheses to explain genotype-phenotype correlations. It is a very thorough description and an excellent article for readers interested in learning about the clinical spectrum of SDH mutations.

125. Schiffman JD: No child left behind in SDHB testing for paragangliomas and pheochromocytomas. *J Clin Oncol* 29(31):4070–4072, 2011.

Reviews the significant hereditary component of PCCs and PGLs, particularly when they are diagnosed in childhood. Discusses the importance of identifying children with these conditions to allow for appropriate surveillance and medical management of both patients and their at-risk family members.

126. Rutter J, Winge DR, Schiffman JD: Succinate dehydrogenase: assembly, regulation and role in human disease. *Mitochondrion* 10(4):393–401, 2010.

This review describes the spectrum of SDH mutations, with an emphasis on the biochemistry responsible for the observed clinical phenotypes.

141. Jasperson KW, Kohlmann W, Gammon A, et al: Role of rapid sequence whole-body MRI screening in SDH-associated hereditary paraganglioma families. *Fam Cancer* 2013. [Epub ahead of print].

This study is the first to demonstrate that as in LFS, whole-body MRI is a useful modality for identifying tumors in patients with underlying germline SDH mutations.

156. Friedman JM, Birch PH: Type 1 neurofibromatosis: a descriptive analysis of the disorder in 1,728 patients. *Am J Med Genet* 70(2):138–143, 1997.

This report describes the National Neurofibromatosis Foundation International Database, which is a multicenter collaborative system for collecting information about patients with NF1. It is a nice example of the power and potential of what a multiinstitutional collaboration can do to advance the research field in hereditary cancer syndromes.

173. Chen F, Kishida T, Yao M, et al: Germline mutations in the von Hippel–Lindau disease tumor suppressor gene: correlations with phenotype. *Hum Mutat* 5(1):66–75, 1995.

This important study helps to explain the genotype-phenotype correlation in patients with VHL mutations. As emphasized by the authors, this information is useful for presymptomatic diagnosis through targeted screening in patients with VHL mutations who are at risk for specific phenotypic presentations.

201. Foulkes WD, Bahubeshi A, Hamel N, et al: Extending the phenotypes associated with DICER1 mutations. *Hum Mutat* 32(12):1381–1384, 2011.

In this recent study, researchers review the variety of malignant diseases associated with DICER1 syndrome in earlier literature. They additionally suggest a new association between DICER1 and several malignant diseases and congenital abnormalities based on careful review of seven new families with DICER1 mutation.

209. Bakry D, Aronson M, Durno C, et al: Genetic and clinical determinants of constitutional mismatch repair deficiency syndrome: report from the constitutional mismatch repair deficiency consortium. *Eur J Cancer* 50:987–996, 2014.

This is a comprehensive description of a cohort of 23 children with CMMR-D, including their clinical presentations, tumor spectrum, genetic data, and results of tumor surveillance.

CHAPTER 43

Genetics and Epigenetics of Childhood Cancers

Alex Kentsis and Charles W.M. Roberts

CHAPTER OUTLINE

The first scientific reports of childhood cancers such as Virchow glioma (neuroblastoma), Wilms tumor (nephroblastoma), and Ewing sarcoma provided a classification system based on organ involvement but shed little light on the natural causes of these diseases. Subsequent study of cancer cells and animal tumors, and in particular Boveri's analysis of cell mitoses and Rous' study of oncogenic viruses, revealed that cancer is at least in part a disease of genes and their aberrations.[1,2]

With the advent of molecular biology, we learned that animal oncogenic viruses contain mutant versions of cellular genes, termed *oncogenes*, as well as gene products that negatively regulate endogenous tumor suppressor genes.[3] Expressed in normal cells, these tumorigenic viral genes can cause unrestrained proliferation and, ultimately, immortalization and malignant transformation, leading to the concept that human cancer is caused by the dysregulation of endogenous protooncogenes and tumor suppressor genes.[4-6]

In particular, the idea of endogenous tumor suppressor gene inactivation in human cancers is strongly supported by (1) the analysis of the age dependence of retinoblastoma incidence and (2) the finding that in children who inherit one mutant allele, bilateral tumors develop at an earlier age than in persons who have tumors that develop as a result of spontaneous biallelic inactivation.[6] Although this "two-hit" model provides a powerful explanation of the incidence of retinoblastomas, similar analyses of other human cancers led to the conclusion that at least six different genetic mutations are needed to explain the apparent age-dependent incidence of some human tumors.[7,8] Indeed, a large majority of human cancers contain many gene mutations in a complex clonal architecture, as revealed by recent analysis of tumor genomes by next-generation sequencing. Some tumors, however—particularly those in children—can have surprisingly low mutation rates. Finally, even cancers with extremely low numbers of gene mutations contain mutations outside of genes that could contribute to tumorigenesis. Consequently, the extent to which alterations in noncoding genetic elements and epigenetic changes have the potential to cooperate with or substitute for genetic mutations has become an active area of investigation.

In addition to the polygenic nature of human cancers, many features of tumor cells are not directly explained by the mutation of cancer-causing genes but instead involve complex cell and tissue biologic systems. These "hallmarks of cancer," which include limitless cell replication, self-sufficiency in growth signaling, circumvention of cell death, immune system evasion, and the ability to metastasize, provide an expedient phenomenologic model to understand cancer cell behavior.[9,10]

Recently, contributions from changes in the chemical modifications of deoxyribonucleic acid (DNA) and chromatin have been increasingly implicated in cancer pathogenesis. These changes are often referred to as "epigenetic" because they may have the potential to result in somatically heritable changes in gene expression and phenotype that do not result directly from changes in DNA composition. Normal development provides a vivid illustration of the power of epigenetic changes, because virtually every cell in the body contains mostly identical coding DNA sequences and yet cells display markedly different behaviors and fates. For example, mature neurons have a distinct differentiated appearance and never divide, whereas hematopoietic stem cells divide throughout a person's lifetime. Further, these cellular fates remain stable over years of somatic cell division. Given the role of epigenetic regulation in the control of cell fate, perhaps it is not surprising that epigenetic perturbations may also contribute to oncogenesis. Although they are conceptually distinct, genetic and epigenetic dysregulation can be closely associated in cancer cells, while genetic mutations of epigenetic regulators are increasingly recognized, particularly in childhood tumors.

Whereas somatic cancer mutations are relatively easy to identify by comparing the sequence of DNA between tumor and nontumor cells, epigenetic causes of cancer are much more difficult to discern because the normal epigenetic state varies with cell type, which makes defining aberrant features a challenge. With respect to DNA methylation, it has become evident that cancer genomes overall tend to be hypomethylated compared with normal tissues and that they have focal areas of hypermethylation in the promoters of specific genes associated with silencing of gene expression. Similarly, the recent discovery of mutations in genes that regulate chromatin structure suggests that aberrant chromatin modifications may contribute to tumorigenesis via epigenetic dysregulation rather than through the induction of additional genetic mutations, although in most cases this conjecture has yet to be proven.

Arguably, our ability to decipher the biologic basis of human cancer will depend on understanding the relationship between molecular aberrations and dysregulated properties of cancer cells. Awareness of the importance of this problem is increasing in the field of pediatric oncology, leading to the recognition that although some childhood tumors can have a remarkably low number of recurrently mutated genes, others can contain thousands of DNA substitutions and complex chromosomal rearrangements. Pediatric cancers may be conceptually distinct from those that occur in adults, because in the absence of a syndromic predisposition, children otherwise have relatively low rates of somatic genetic alterations and toxin exposures due to aging. Thus childhood cancers may involve unique mechanisms of tumorigenesis.

In this chapter we review the mechanisms of molecular pathogenesis of childhood cancers. Our goal is not to provide a comprehensive encyclopedia (electronic publishing and online databases* now enable ready access to this information) but to develop a systematic classification of the molecular lesions responsible for childhood tumors, with a focus on biologic mechanisms and functional principles. Instead of organizing this chapter on the basis of cancer types, which are covered individually in other chapters of this volume, we have attempted to develop a functional framework that we hope will provide helpful insights into the relationship between molecular aberrations and behaviors of cancer cells *sui generis*. Such an approach should inform the development of improved clinical therapies, particularly if cancer treatment is to become more precise through the use of rationally targeted agents.

FUNCTIONAL GENETICS OF CHILDHOOD CANCER PREDISPOSITION SYNDROMES

The study of childhood cancer predisposition syndromes is an important source of information about the genetic basis of human cancers. Indeed, the retinoblastoma 1 *(RB1)* gene, which is mutated in familial retinoblastomas, was the first human tumor suppressor gene identified.[6,11,12] What follows is an overview of known genes mutated in childhood cancer predisposition syndromes based on the major cell biologic pathways thought to be perturbed by the inherited gene mutations.

DYSREGULATION OF CELL DIVISION AND GROWTH

A large number of childhood cancer predisposition syndromes involve mutations of genes that regulate cell growth and division. One of the first to be described, the *RB1* gene, is mutated in children who are predisposed to the development of retinoblastoma, pinealoblastoma, and osteosarcoma. The *RB1* gene is part of the G1 cell cycle checkpoint, where its product directly binds and regulates the activity of the E2F family of transcription factors and the DREAM chromatin remodeling complex in response to stress.[13] Cancer-causing deletions and nonsense mutations of *RB1* can cause entry into the cell cycle by otherwise quiescent cells and mitigation of senescence that limits cellular life span.[14] Whereas loss of *RB1* in cellular and mouse models causes defects in mitotic chromosome segregation that lead to aneuploidy,[15,16] most human retinoblastomas are largely diploid,[17] suggesting that the canonic chromosome segregation effects of *RB1* inactivation in human retinoblasts are functionally compensated. Human retinoblastomas invariably exhibit biallelic inactivation of *RB1*, but otherwise often have a comparatively low mutation rate. One study found that *RB1* was the only known cancer gene mutated in these tumors.[17] However, additional subclonal DNA mutations were observed, with some mutations located outside of coding regions, which may cooperate with *RB1* loss to drive retinoblastoma formation. In addition, epigenetic alterations have also been implicated in cooperating with *RB1* mutation.[17]

The adenomatous polyposis coli *(APC)* gene, which is mutated in children with familial adenomatous polyposis who are predisposed to hepatoblastoma and colon carcinoma, also controls the G1 cell cycle checkpoint.[18] APC serves as a ubiquitin ligase that regulates the protein stability of β-catenin, which controls transcription of cyclins, including cyclin D, which in turn associates with

*At the time of this writing, the following publicly accessible databases of cancer-associated mutations and structural aberrations are available: http://target.cancer.gov; http://pediatriccancergenomeproject.org; http://www.sanger.ac.uk/genetics/CGP; and http://cansar.icr.ac.uk.

cyclin-dependent kinase (CDK)4/6 to negatively regulate *RB1* activity.[19] Disease-associated dominant mutations of *APC* tend to occur in distinct regions of the gene, leading to the generation of truncated protein products, consistent with the requirement of residual or neomorphic activity of the mutant proteins.[20] Because *APC* regulates the stability of many proteins—and because, in addition to the cell cycle progression, β-catenin also regulates cell adhesion and differentiation—the mechanism of tumorigenesis induced by *APC* mutations is thought to be pleiotropic.

In addition to mutations of genes whose products regulate cell division, cancer-causing mutations also directly dysregulate mitogenic signaling and cell growth. The most common cancer predisposition syndrome, neurofibromatosis, is predominantly caused by autosomal-dominant inheritance of inactivating mutations of the neurofibromin 1 *(NF1)* gene, with the less frequent form caused by mutations of neurofibromin 2 *(NF2)* or *merlin*. Children with mutations of *NF1* are predisposed to the development of benign and malignant tumors, including gliomas, peripheral nerve sheath tumors, pheochromocytomas, and leukemias.[21] NF1 is a large protein that is not completely understood but is known to regulate the activity of rat sarcoma (Ras).[22,23] In turn, *NF1* mutant tumors exhibit increased Ras guanosine triphosphate hydrolase activity, which stimulates the mitogen-activated protein and AKT kinase cascades that, among other effects, result in the transcription of genes involved in cell growth and stimulation of protein synthesis.[24-26] Although most patients with germline *NF1* mutations experience the development of neurofibromas, which harbor biallelic inactivation of the gene, only a minority of these tumors evolve to become malignant. This finding indicates that disease-associated *NF1* mutations have limited transforming ability, and that additional lesions are required for carcinogenesis.

The complex relationship between cancer-causing gene mutations and their effects on tumorigenesis is also evident from mutations of *ras* genes themselves. Genes related to *ras*, including Kirsten rat sarcoma *(KRAS)*, neuroblastoma rat sarcoma *(NRAS)*, and Harvey rat sarcoma *(HRAS)*, are some of the first human protooncogenes identified, based on the involvement of the corresponding viral oncogenes in the pathogenesis of rat sarcomas.[27] However, whereas *NF1* mutations stimulate Ras activity and cause neurofibromatosis, patients with inherited mutations of the *ras* genes instead experience the development of cardiofaciocutaneous, Noonan, LEOPARD, and Costello syndromes. Inherited mutations of the *ras* genes are missense activating mutations, analogous to the oncogenic viral *ras* mutations, yet the spectrum of tumor phenotypes in these patients is distinct. In addition to gliomas these phenotypes also include leukemias, neuroblastomas, and rhabdomyosarcomas.[28,29] These differences between *NF1*- and *ras*-mutant cancer predisposition syndromes are not simply due to differences in tissue expression of the two genes, because both appear to be expressed in neuronal, mesenchymal, and hematopoietic tissues. Rather, they may reflect the developmental consequences of Ras activation as a result of the inactivation

of an endogenous negative regulator as opposed to direct mutational activation of an oncogenic signaling pathway, a property that may inform the development of strategies to target these lesions therapeutically.

DNA REPAIR AND GENOME INSTABILITY

The prevention of de novo cancer-causing mutations ultimately depends on efficient DNA repair and maintenance of genome stability. Indeed, several cancer predisposition syndromes involve defective DNA repair. For example, inherited mutations of the tumor protein 53 (*TP53*) tumor suppressor gene cause most cases of Li-Fraumeni syndrome, which is associated with the predisposition to sarcomas, leukemias, and breast carcinomas.[30] The genotype-phenotype relationship of *TP53* cancer-causing mutations is complex, with some mutations having apparent loss-of-function, dominant-negative, or gain-of-function properties in experimental models.[31-34] p53 regulates the expression of genes involved in cell division, apoptosis, and DNA repair, and its mutation in cells leads to chromosomal instability.[35,36] This process is mediated partly by direct effects of p53 on the transcription and translation of target genes, as well as via feedback interaction with its ubiquitin ligase murine double minute 2 (MDM2), which also has oncogenic effects independent of its negative regulation of p53.[37] As a result, the dysregulation of cellular DNA damage and stress response by *TP53* mutations is profoundly tumorigenic, contributing to the somatic pathogenesis of most human cancers. The p53-MDM2 feedback regulation also complicates therapeutic targeting, because inhibition of MDM2 aimed at restoring p53 tumor suppression may in effect enhance the deleterious activity of gain-of-function p53 mutant proteins.[38]

Defective DNA damage response is also a hallmark of Fanconi anemia (FA), a cancer predisposition syndrome characterized by bone marrow failure and development of myelodysplasia, leukemia, and carcinomas.[39,40] Although mutations of more than 15 different genes can cause FA, most of the known FA-mutant gene products physically interact with the components of a conserved DNA damage response mechanism, breast cancer 1 (BRCA1), ataxia telangiectasia mutated (ATM), Nijmegen breakage syndrome 1 (NBS1), and radiation-sensitive 51 (RAD51), and are required for the repair of chromosome defects that occur during homologous recombination.[39] FA pathway–deficient cells are hypersensitive to DNA-damaging agents, and over time they accumulate deleterious gene mutations (usually segmental deletions).[41]

Several other chromosome-breakage syndromes with cancer predisposition involve defects in closely related biochemical pathways of DNA repair of homologous recombination errors, such as ataxia telangiectasia (due to mutations of *ATM*), Nijmegen breakage syndrome (due to mutations of *NBS1*), and Bloom syndrome (due to mutations of *BLM*). Genes involved in nucleotide excision or transcription-coupled DNA repair can also be mutated and cause the cancer predisposition syndromes xeroderma pigmentosum and Cockayne syndrome, usually due to accumulation of ultraviolet radiation–induced mutations (typically nucleotide substitutions).[42]

ABERRANT GENE EXPRESSION

Another hallmark of cancer cells is expression of genes in inappropriate developmental states, often driven by mutations of gene products that regulate gene expression. For example, patients with inherited mutations of the Wilms tumor 1 (WT1) gene experience development of the Denys-Drash syndrome (due to loss-of-function missense mutations) or the Wilms tumor, aniridia, genitourinary anomalies, and mental retardation (WAGR) syndrome (due to gene deletions), both with predisposition to the development of bilateral Wilms tumors.[43] In spite of years of study, the function of the WT1 protein is incompletely understood. WT1 is a key regulator of mesenchymal cell development, including kidney mesenchyme, in part through its functions as a transcriptional repressor.[44] However, WT1 also interacts with messenger RNA (mRNA) and splicing factors, consistent with possible posttranscriptional functions in regulation of gene expression.[45] In addition, although recessive mutations of WT1 appear consistent with its tumor suppressive functions in Wilms tumorigenesis, in other developmental and tissue contexts, particularly myeloid leukemias, WT1 can enhance cell survival and proliferation and as a result can act as an oncogene or haploinsufficient tumor suppressor gene.[46] Such tissue-dependent phenotypes are characteristic of cancer-associated genes that affect gene expression and cell fate determination, insofar as the functional consequences of mutations depend on the spectrum of expressed genes themselves and differentiation state in general.

Tumorigenesis due to aberrant regulation of gene expression can also occur posttranscriptionally, as in the case of inherited mutations of the DICER1 gene, which predispose to the development of pleuropulmonary blastoma, cystic nephroma, and rhabdomyosarcoma.[47] DICER1 is a ribonuclease that is required for the generation of endogenous microRNAs (miRNAs), which negatively regulate gene expression by inducing degradation and translational blockade of specific mRNAs.[48] Cancer-associated mutations affect conserved, enzymatically required residues in DICER1 and cause defective miRNA processing, leading to increased expression of target genes.[49] The reason inherited DICER1 mutations predispose specifically to the development of pleuropulmonary blastoma, cystic nephroma, and rhabdomyosarcoma is not understood, but it is reasonable to hypothesize that this predisposition is due to the specific requirements for miRNA-mediated gene expression in these tissues or expression of specific target protooncogenes.

SOMATICALLY ACQUIRED GENE MUTATIONS AND CANCER GENOMICS

Many cancer-causing gene mutations that are inherited as part of familial cancer predisposition syndromes can also be acquired somatically in tumor cells. These mutations include most of the genes described in the preceding sections, but with notable differences in pathogenic mechanisms.

First, in many instances of somatic mutations of tumor suppressor genes, only one of the alleles is mutated, leaving the other wild-type allele intact and expressed.[50] Such haploinsufficient mutations, as opposed to the classic "two-hit" tumor suppressor gene mutations, are thought to exert their effects through reduced tumor suppressive activities as part of tumor initiation. In addition, the functional contributions of the wild-type allele may be required for tumor maintenance in some cases. This distinction may be crucial for the development of therapeutic strategies to target haploinsufficient tumor suppressors, because restoration of tumor suppressor gene functions may be not be useful in tumors in which residual wild-type activity is required for tumor maintenance.[51]

Second, the tumor spectrum and phenotype, and therefore the exact mechanism of tumorigenesis, are often different for the same mutation when it is developed somatically as opposed to inherited in the germline. For example, inherited mutations of WT1 cause Denys-Drash syndrome and predisposition to Wilms tumors but never leukemias, whereas somatic mutations of WT1 occur in 10% of cases of acute myeloid and T-cell acute lymphoblastic leukemias (ALLs).[52] This difference may be due to the differences in gene expression and differentiation state of cells that are transformed by these tumorigenic mutations. The same principle is likely responsible for the nonequivalence of many other somatically acquired tumor mutations that have counterparts that occur as part of inherited developmental syndromes, such as the loss-of-function mutations of BCL6 corepressor (BCOR) that occur somatically in medulloblastomas and myeloid leukemias but cause oculofaciocardiodental syndrome without cancer predisposition when inherited in the germline.[53-55]

Finally, recent whole-genome surveys have revealed that recurrence rates of somatically acquired gene mutations may be rare when considered individually but can involve coherent biologic pathways that are mutated frequently as a functional group. This functional co-occurrence is often suggested by the mutual exclusivity of the individual mutations. We review the mechanisms of tumorigenesis by these mutations, as organized below by shared biochemical activities or biologic pathways.

GENOMIC REARRANGEMENTS AND CHROMOTHRIPSIS

Structural genomic rearrangements and copy number changes are particularly prevalent in adult cancers, both at the level of whole chromosomes and chromosomal segments, particularly in advanced or histologically anaplastic diseases, but they are generally somewhat less prominent in pediatric cancers. The mechanisms of their generation and tumorigenic sequelae at least in part appear to be related to the dysfunction of DNA repair and maintenance of genome stability. In particular, whole chromosome aneuploidy, often as a result of chromosomal instability due to defects in mitosis such as centrosome amplification or failure of spindle assembly, is a prevalent feature of anaplastic tumors.[56] In some cases, such as acute myeloid leukemias, mutations of the components of the mitotic cohesin complex, including stromal antigen 2 (STAG2), structural maintenance of chromosomes 3 and 1A (SMC3 and SMC1A), and radiation-sensitive 21 (RAD21), may lead to chromatin cohesion defects and aneuploidy.[57] However, identification of such cohesin complex mutations in karyotypically normal acute myeloid leukemia (AML) raises the possibility that their tumorigenic effects rely on nonmitotic functions of the cohesin complex components.[58]

In model systems, aneuploid cells appear to have increased rates of mutation and susceptibility to DNA damage.[59,60] Noncancerous aneuploid human cells tend to be nonviable, with the exception of cells with trisomies of chromosomes 13, 18, and 21 and certain ring chromosomes.[61] However, somatically acquired chromosomal aneuploidy is far more prevalent in tumors than in constitutional syndromes, suggesting that additional molecular changes that enable tumor cells to tolerate aneuploidy must exist. Indeed, tumors with characteristic aneuploidies often have specific additional mutations—for example, overexpression and mutational activation of cytokine receptor-like factor 2 (CRLF2) signaling in B-cell ALL (B-ALL) with trisomy of chromosome 21.[62-64] Defining the molecular basis of these interactions may reveal potential opportunities to therapeutically target mechanisms that permit tolerance of aneuploidy in cancer cells.[65]

One of the best-studied genomic aberrations in cancer cells is recurrent chromosomal translocations. These chromosomal rearrangements generally lead either to the aberrant expression of protooncogenes as a result of juxtaposition of regulatory transcriptional elements or to the generation of chimeric fusion gene products that have gain-of-function tumorigenic effects.[66] Chromosomal translocations are frequently observed in hematopoietic cancer cells, where they lead to increased survival, growth, and malignant transformation, such as MYC-overexpressing t(8;14) translocation in Burkitt lymphomas and t(9;22) translocation generating the BCR-ABL1 fusion proteins in B-ALL and chronic myeloid leukemia. In lymphoid cells, these translocations are generated at least in part by aberrant V(D)J recombination and activation-induced deaminase activities that occur at the immunoglobulin and T-cell receptor loci undergoing somatic hypermutation. In addition, recombination of endogenous repetitive elements and DNA topoisomerase II failures also appear to cause chromosomal translocations, such as those generating mixed-lineage leukemia (MLL) fusion proteins.[67,68]

The chimeric fusion proteins generated by these translocations have been found to disrupt cell differentiation and specification, along with enhanced cell survival and growth.[69] For example, the TEL-AML1 fusion protein leads to abnormal self-renewal of hematopoietic stem cells, making them susceptible to additional mutations and ultimate transformation to B-ALL.[70,71] The EWS-FLI1 fusion protein in Ewing sarcoma disrupts specification of mesenchymal progenitors, blocking cell differentiation.[72-74]

By virtue of being tumor-specific, fusion gene products generated by chromosomal translocations represent attractive targets for rational therapy. Indeed, introduction of all-*trans*-retinoic acid and arsenic trioxide to induce the degradation of the chimeric PML-RARA fusion protein caused by the t(15;17) chromosomal translocation in the majority of cases of acute promyelocytic leukemia has revolutionized the treatment of this disease by eliminating the need for chemotherapy.[75]

In addition to the gains and losses of whole chromosomes and their segments, cancer cells can exhibit other distinct and complex types of genomic rearrangements. In particular, some tumors such as neuroblastomas and gliomas, for example, have been found to contain short episomal DNA fragments, termed *double minutes,* that lack centromeres and telomeres.[76,77] In neuroblastomas, these double minutes contain multiple copies of the *MYCN* protooncogene, leading to its high-copy amplification and overexpression. The mechanisms generating these episomal DNA fragments are not well defined but may involve recombination or transposition events involving endogenous *Alu, LINE,* and *MER* elements, or microhomology-based aberrant nonhomologous end-joining reactions.[77]

Recently a highly complex form of genomic rearrangements, termed *chromothripsis,* has been described in a variety of tumors, including neuroblastomas, medulloblastomas, and osteosarcomas.[78-80] This phenomenon is defined by extensive intrachromosomal rearrangements, often numbering in the thousands, of a single chromosome.[81] It has been proposed to be caused by aberrant DNA replication and microhomology-based nonhomologous end-joining repair, as well as by damage of chromosomes trapped in micronuclei as a result of mitotic errors.[80,82,83] The mechanisms of the generation of these complex rearrangements and their functional consequences remain to be defined but promise to reveal important insights into the mechanisms of human tumorigenesis, given their marked prevalence in distinct tumor types.

DNA METHYLATION, CHROMATIN, AND THE EPIGENETICS OF CHILDHOOD CANCER

Structural abnormalities in the genomes of cancer cells seem essential for tumorigenesis, but increasingly, the contribution of aberrant epigenetic regulation to the development of human cancers in general and pediatric cancers in particular is also becoming recognized. Methylation of cytosines in DNA can cause profound changes in transcription, and methylation of CpG islands in the promoters of genes can lead to transcriptional silencing.[84,85] In addition, nuclear DNA is tightly bound to histones as part of chromatin, and sequence-specific posttranslational modification of histones, including acetylation, methylation, and ubiquitination, have all been shown to modulate DNA accessibility and transcription.[86,87] Consequently, the transcription of individual genes depends both on the degree of DNA compaction and accessibility, as well as on the individual chemical modifications of histones surrounding specific genes.

DNA METHYLATION

Methylation of cytosines in DNA is a key regulator of mammalian cell development, and changes in DNA methylation have long been known to be associated with human cancer. For example, loss of normal DNA methylcytosine imprinting patterns on chromosome 11 causes Beckwith-Wiedemann syndrome, a developmental disorder that predisposes to the formation of hepatoblastomas and Wilms tumors.[88] Indeed, abnormal patterns of cytosine methylation are frequently observed in tumor cells, and recently mutations of enzymes that control DNA methylation have been found in AML and myelodysplastic syndromes.

The de novo DNA methyltransferase 3A (DNMT3A) is recurrently mutated in a large fraction of cases of AML.[89,90] The mutations tend to be missense and heterozygous, involving an evolutionarily conserved DNA-binding interface of DNMT3A, consistent with a possible gain-of-function effect that presumably alters locus-specific DNA methylation. Loss-of-function deletions and nonsense mutations of methylcytosine dioxygenase 2 (TET2) are also observed in AML and myelodysplastic syndromes.[91-93] TET2 functions by hydroxylating methylcytosine, and these mutations are thought to lead to the loss of DNA hydroxymethylcytosine, although whether this is carcinogenic in itself or transforms cells indirectly via its effects on histone modifications and DNA demethylation remains to be determined.[94,95] Consistent with this notion, the CpG island methylator phenotype, which is a key factor in the tumorigenesis of adult colorectal carcinomas, is yet to be definitively established in tumors with defects in DNA methylation.[96]

CHROMATIN-MODIFYING ENZYMES

Whereas perturbation of nuclear appearance in cancer cells was long ago realized to represent a change in chromatin structure, the molecular underpinnings of this phenomenon have begun to be elucidated only recently. Perhaps the strongest evidence implicating perturbation of chromatin structure in carcinogenesis is the finding that chromatin-remodeling complexes are mutated at a high frequency in a wide variety of cancers. Some of these include genes that encode proteins that contribute to the methylation and acetylation of histone lysines. Others include those that encode subunits of complexes that mobilize histones and remodel chromatin structure. Numerous other modifications of histones also occur, such as arginylation, succinylation, and glycosylation, but their significance is only beginning to be assessed.

One of the earliest genes involved in chromatin modification that was identified as being mutated in pediatric cancers is the MLLT1 gene, which contains the SET lysine N-methyltransferase domain that is characteristically lost as a result of chromosomal translocations that generate chimeric MLL fusion proteins in infant and topoisomerase inhibitor–induced leukemias.[97,98] Wild-type MLL and mutant MLL fusion proteins physically interact with a large supramolecular complex involved in regulation of gene expression by chromatin modification.[99] MLL fusion–induced leukemias are characterized by unique patterns of gene expression associated with a distinct spectrum of chromatin modifications, particularly those involving methylation of lysine 79 of histone 3 (H3K79), which in turn is associated with high levels of gene expression.[100] Notably, these activities require the preferential recruitment of the DOT1L lysine methyltransferase by the MLL fusion proteins compared with wild-type MLL, and DOT1L activity is required for leukemogenesis in preclinical models, potentially offering a therapeutic strategy.[101,102] Aberrant methylation of H3K79 at target genes of the MLL fusion protein therefore likely contributes to MLLT1 translocation-induced leukemogenesis.

Whereas increased target gene H3K79 methylation by aberrant recruitment of a lysine methyltransferase represents a gain-of-function of tumorigenic methyltranferase activity, loss-of-function mutations of lysine methyltransferases have also been observed in tumors. In particular, loss-of-function frameshift and nonsense mutations of the suppressor of zeste 12 homologue (SUZ12), embryonic ectoderm development (EED), and enhancer of zeste homologue 2 (EZH2) genes are frequently found in T-cell ALL (T-ALL).[103,104] Similar mutations have also been observed in cases of myelodysplastic syndromes.[105,106] These gene products are physical components of the Polycomb repressive complex (PRC) 2, which methylates lysine 27 of histone 3 (H3K27), a modification associated with silencing of target gene expression.[107] It is important to note that whereas EZH2 undergoes loss-of-function mutations in T-ALL, gain-of-function missense mutations of EZH2, which are associated with neomorphic enzymatic activity of the mutant protein, are observed in cases of diffuse large B-cell lymphoma.[108] The complexity of the tumorigenic mechanism of these mutations is further emphasized by the recent finding of loss-of-function mutations of the H3K27 demethylase UTX, which, when mutated, ought to potentiate H3K27 methylation in some cases of B-ALL.[109] The importance of regulation of H3K27 modifications was recently further highlighted by the finding that H3K27 itself is frequently mutated in pediatric diffuse pontine gliomas, in which lysine to methionine mutations occur in histone 3.3 or 3.1[110,111] and result in inhibition of PRC2.[112] Collectively, these findings indicate that the developmental and epigenetic state of the cell likely makes key contributions to tumorigenesis by the mutant chromatin-modifying enzymes by providing specific substrates for their altered enzymatic activities.

The recognized role of chromatin modifiers has continued to expand via cancer genome sequencing efforts and has led to identification of the switch/sucrose nonfermentable (SWI/SNF) chromatin remodeling complex as the most frequently mutated chromatin regulatory complex. Genes that encode subunits of this complex are mutant in 20% of all human cancers.[113] This 12-to 15-protein complex serves important roles in transcriptional regulation by utilizing adenosine triphosphate hydrolysis to modulate chromatin structure at the promoters and enhancers of its target genes. Identification of biallelic inactivating mutations of *SNF5/INI1/SMARCB1*, a core SWI/SNF subunit, in nearly all cases of malignant rhabdoid tumors represented the first identified link between an adenosine triphosphate–dependent chromatin remodeler and cancer.[114,115] Heterozygous *SMARCB1* mutation was also identified as the basis of a familial cancer predisposition syndrome.[114] Other SWI/SNF subunits have also recently been found to be recurrently mutated in pediatric malignancies, including *ARID1A* in Burkitt lymphoma, *ARID1A* and *ARID1B* in neuroblastoma, and *ARID1A* and *SMARCA4* in medulloblastoma. Although these findings broadly implicate the SWI/SNF complex in tumor suppression, the mechanisms by which these mutations drive cancer formation remain unclear.

The complex serves roles in transcriptional regulation by modulating the chromatin landscape at promoters and enhancers of its target genes; in addition, the complex has also been implicated in DNA repair.[116-121] However, recent sequencing of rhabdoid tumor genomes indicates that these cancers contain a remarkably simple protein coding genome, with mutations of *SMARCB1* essentially the sole recurrent genetic mutation; in some cases it is sole coding sequence mutation identified.[122-124] These findings have been interpreted as suggesting that oncogenesis caused by the mutation of the SWI/SNF complex occurs not via induction of genomic instability but rather via epigenetic dysfunction.[125] Perhaps providing mechanistic insight, mutation of *SMARCB1* was reported to result in unbalanced epigenetic antagonism between the SWI/SNF and PRC2 complexes, generating a unique dependence upon EZH2.[126] Preclinical small molecule inhibition of EZH2 has been reported to be effective against rhabdoid tumors in preclinical models but has yet to be tested in humans.[127]

Cancer genome sequencing has also identified other chromatin remodelers mutated in cancer. For instance, alpha-thalassemia mental retardation syndrome, X-linked *(ATRX)* and death-domain associated protein *(DAXX)*, which encode subunits of a chromatin-remodeling complex required for replication-independent deposition of histone H3.3, were identified in glioblastoma and were present in 100% of tumors that also contained G34R or G34V mutations in H3.3 itself, raising the possibility of mutations with coordinate effects upon chromatin structure.[110] Mutations in *ATRX* also occur in older patients with neuroblastoma.[78] Collectively, chromatin modifiers have emerged as a major new class of tumor suppressors.

SPLICING FACTORS

In addition to mutations affecting factors that regulate chromatin, recent studies have also identified recurrent mutations of genes encoding components of the spliceosome, including mutations of the *U2AF35*, *ZRSR2*, *SRSF2*, and *SF3B1* genes in myelodysplastic syndromes, AML, and juvenile myclomonocytic leukemia.[128,129] The mutations tend to be missense and mutually exclusive, and they cluster in distinct conserved parts of the genes, suggesting gain-of-function phenotypes. All of these genes encode components of the spliceosome that are involved in splicing of pre-mRNAs, suggesting that their tumorigenic mechanism may involve dysfunctional control of gene expression arising from aberrant mRNA splicing. Indeed, mutated splicing factor gene products participate in the 3′ splice site selection during pre-mRNA processing, inducing abnormal splicing in reporter assays.[128] However, SF3B1 can also interact with components of the Polycomb complex involved in regulation of chromatin structure and gene transcription, raising the possibility that its mutation and tumorigenesis may involve mechanisms other than splicing.[130] Because transcription and splicing are often coregulated in normal cells and mutations of splicing factor genes often co-occur with mutations affecting regulators of gene expression in tumor cells, a definition of their tumorigenic mechanisms and phenotypic consequences may require a comprehensive analysis of the potential interactions of the co-occurring mutations.

METABOLIC ENZYMES

Another unanticipated finding from the analysis of tumor genomes has been the discovery of mutations in metabolic enzymes. Initially observed in gliomas, missense mutations of the isocitrate dehydrogenase 1 and 2 *(IDH1* and *IDH2)* genes that encode isocitrate dehydrogenase enzymes, which are components of the mitochondrial citric acid cycle, have also been found in a large fraction of AMLs.[131,132] The majority of mutations involve conserved arginine residues in the enzymatic active sites, which aberrantly generate 2-hydroxyglutarate that accumulates to high concentrations in tumor cells, tissues, and even circulating blood.[133,134] Because 2-oxoglutarate, the normal metabolite of *IDH1* and *IDH2*, is an essential cofactor of many cellular enzymes, the effects of oncogenic *IDH1* and *IDH2* mutations and excess production of 2-hydroxyglutarate may be pleiotropic.[135] Indeed, *IDH1* and *IDH2* mutations can lead to the inhibition of enzymatic activity of *TET2* that hydroxylates 5-methylcytosine in DNA, as well as associated changes in DNA methylation and gene expression in leukemia cells.[136] Mutations of IDH and production of 2-hydroxyglutarate have also been found to inhibit H3K9 demethylase KDM4C in glioma cells.[137] In addition, in glioma cells, generation of 2-hydroxyglutarate by mutant IDH enzymes also inhibits EGLN prolyl hydroxylases, leading to diminished hypoxia-inducible factor levels and enhanced cell growth.[138]

The stereospecific nature of the effects of 2-hydroxyglutarate—wherein the (R)- but not the (S)-enantiomer appears to be oncogenic yet both metabolites can inhibit 2-oxoglutarate–dependent cellular enzymes—may lead to the definition of specific mechanisms and their ultimate therapeutic blockade.[139] Mutations of other metabolic enzymes, such as succinate dehydrogenase and fumarate hydratase, can also be tumorigenic, causing gastrointestinal stromal tumors, paragangliomas, and renal cell carcinomas,[140] which suggests that aberrant metabolic properties of cancer cells may be not only adaptive but in and of themselves tumorigenic.

CONCLUSIONS AND FUTURE OUTLOOK

The study of the genetic basis of pediatric cancers has revealed important principles of human carcinogenesis that help explain the diverse traits of cancer cells. In particular, the study of human cancer predisposition syndromes, many of which clinically present in childhood, has established the prevalence of mutations of tumor suppressor genes and oncogenes that cause the dysregulation of cell growth, DNA repair, and gene expression in human cancers. These studies have also established the essential contributions of the cellular state on the effects of tumorigenic mutations, with the same mutations having distinct functional consequences and phenotypic effects that depend on the cancer cell of origin. Likewise, the increasing recognition of epigenetic alterations in human cancers may reveal fundamental developmental pathways that are required for normal and cancerous cell growth. Finally, because tumorigenesis is inherently a multistep process, the accumulation of genetic lesions that ultimately lead to symptomatic disease is nonrandom, establishing discrete combinations of molecular lesions that functionally cooperate to transform cells. As a result, the clonal structure of tumors is organized hierarchically, and its future study will reveal important principles of biologic cell function and dysfunction. This notion is further bolstered by the frequent observation of somatically acquired gene mutations that are rare when considered individually but involve coherent biologic pathways that are mutated frequently as a functional group. Consequently, future studies of the biologic basis of human cancer that are faithful and therapeutically relevant may necessitate the generation of compendia of molecular lesions and cancer models based on such ontogenies.

References available online at ExpertConsult.

KEY REFERENCES

8. Armitage P, Doll R: The age distribution of cancer and a multistage theory of carcinogenesis. *Br J Cancer* 8:1–12, 1954.
   A seminal model of age-dependent cancer incidence informing the underlying mechanisms of tumorigenesis.
10. Hanahan D, Weinberg RA: Hallmarks of cancer: the next generation. *Cell* 144:646–674, 2011.
    A comprehensive analysis of cancer cell phenotypes.
26. Karnoub AE, Weinberg RA: Ras oncogenes: split personalities. *Nat Rev Mol Cell Biol* 9:517–531, 2008.
    A detailed review of the contributions of Ras to carcinogenic cell signaling.
46. Huff V: Wilms' tumours: about tumour suppressor genes, an oncogene and a chameleon gene. *Nat Rev Cancer* 11:111–121, 2011.
    A comprehensive review of mixed oncogenic and tumor suppressive functions of WT1.
51. Berger AH, Knudson AG, Pandolfi PP: A continuum model for tumour suppression. *Nature* 476:163–169, 2011.
    A revised concept of tumor suppressor genes incorporating haploinsufficiency.
55. Pugh TJ, Weeraratne SD, Archer TC, et al: Medulloblastoma exome sequencing uncovers subtype-specific somatic mutations. *Nature* 488:106–110, 2012.
    A report of the genomic survey of medulloblastomas.
58. Cancer Genome Atlas Research Network: Genomic and epigenomic landscapes of adult de novo acute myeloid leukemia. *N Engl J Med* 368:2059–2074, 2013.
    A report of the genomic survey of acute myeloid leukemias.
65. Gordon DJ, Resio B, Pellman D: Causes and consequences of aneuploidy in cancer. *Nat Rev Genet* 13:189–203, 2012.
    A review of the mechanisms and effects of chromosomal aneuploidy in cancer cells.
66. Rabbitts TH: Chromosomal translocations in human cancer. *Nature* 372:143–149, 1994.
    An essential description of the causes and consequences of carcinogenic chromosomal translocations.
78. Molenaar JJ, Koster J, Zwijnenburg DA, et al: Sequencing of neuroblastoma identifies chromothripsis and defects in neuritogenesis genes. *Nature* 483:589–593, 2012.
    A report of the genomic survey of neuroblastomas.
87. Cantone I, Fisher AG: Epigenetic programming and reprogramming during development. *Nat Struct Mol Biol* 20:282–289, 2013.
    An excellent overview of the factors and processes of normal epigenetic development.
107. Hock H: A complex Polycomb issue: the two faces of EZH2 in cancer. *Genes Dev* 26:751–755, 2012.
    Analysis of the mechanisms of methyltransferase effects of mutations of EZH2.
112. Lewis PW, Muller MM, Koletsky MS, et al: Inhibition of PRC2 activity by a gain-of-function H3 mutation found in pediatric glioblastoma. *Science* 340:857–861, 2013.
    The mechanism of tumorigenic histone mutations in glioblastoma.
126. Wilson BG, Wang X, Shen X, et al: Epigenetic antagonism between polycomb and SWI/SNF complexes during oncogenic transformation. *Cancer Cell* 18:316–328, 2010.
    A study demonstrating blockade of Snf5 chromatin remodeling factor mutant tumors by inhibition of Polycomb repressive complex 2.
139. Losman JA, Kaelin WG, Jr: What a difference a hydroxyl makes: mutant IDH, (R)-2-hydroxyglutarate, and cancer. *Genes Dev* 27:836–852, 2013.
    Tumorigenic mechanisms of oncometabolite 2-hydroxyglutarate.

CHAPTER 44

Targeted Therapies in Oncology

Kimberly Stegmaier and William R. Sellers

CHAPTER OUTLINE

With the discovery of nitrogen mustard as an anticancer agent in the 1940s, medicinal and hence systemic cancer therapy became a reality. The identification and application of cytotoxic agents dominated the next 60 years of cancer treatment. The success of imatinib for *BCR-ABL* rearranged chronic myelogenous leukemia (CML), the dramatic responses seen in patients with *BRAF*-mutated melanoma and *ALK* rearranged non–small cell lung cancer to targeted inhibitors, and the unparalleled ability to systematically characterize cancer genomes have catapulted the community into a new era of targeted cancer therapy. Nonetheless, there is much to learn from the 60-year experience in empiric-based therapy that should be directly applicable to the development of molecularly targeted therapy. Cytotoxic chemotherapy, although often regarded as largely unsuccessful, has led to substantial cure rates in a number of well-defined malignancies, particularly pediatric. In this chapter we will discuss the fundamental concepts, advantages, and disadvantages of cytotoxic cancer therapy and their relevance to targeted drug therapy for malignancy. We will define targeted therapy, its advantages and disadvantages, discuss the credentialing of targets, and provide a system for categorizing classes of targets and classes of therapies. We will then focus on particular lessons learned in the early development and testing of new targeted therapies for adult malignancies, with examples from each of the target classes. Our intent is to highlight illustrative examples rather than to provide an exhaustive list of all targeted therapies in development. We will conclude with a discussion of the challenges facing us in the development of targeted therapies for children and highlight emerging pediatric cancer-based targets.

TRADITIONAL CHEMOTHERAPY

Conventional Chemotherapy: Not Entirely Nonspecific

Although conventional chemotherapy agents are often seen as nonspecific cytotoxic drugs, over the years more information has come to light about their mechanisms of action in killing tumor cells. In general, these agents were designed to interfere with molecular pathways required for nucleotide synthesis, DNA replication, and the mechanics of cell division. Thus these agents have significant but often predictable, or at least stereotypical, morbidity related to target-mediated suppression of hematopoiesis or of the cell-division process required for homeostasis of other organ systems. These agents are discussed in greater detail in Chapter 45.

Lessons Learned from Cytotoxic Chemotherapy

The use of cytotoxic chemotherapy agents is an imperfect science at best, but researchers have learned many lessons over the years about the medicinal treatment of cancer,

Box 44-1   Lessons Learned from Cytotoxic Chemotherapy

1. Combination therapy is required for cure.
2. Appropriate dose intensity is required for improved outcome.
3. Toxicity is acceptable when therapy is curative.
4. Establish curative regimens, and then attempt to reduce toxicity.

lessons to strongly consider in the development of targeted therapy (Box 44-1).

Combination Therapy Is Required for Cure

The goals of combination therapy are numerous. First, because it is difficult to predict which single agent will be most effective against an individual patient's tumor, the use of multiple drugs increases the potential for an initial complete response. Second, combination therapy is likely critical for preventing the development of therapeutic resistance. Third, drug combinations may have additive or synergistic interactions, increasing the total activity of the drugs and potentially enabling lower dosing and reduced toxicity. One example is the successful dose reduction of cytotoxic chemotherapy with the addition of all-*trans*-retinoic acid (ATRA) for the treatment of patients with acute promyelocytic leukemia (APL).[1,2] With few exceptions, curative systemic therapy has required the combination of highly active agents rather than combinations of active and inactive agents.

The need for multiagent therapy was first appreciated in the treatment of acute lymphoblastic leukemia (ALL). At best, 60% of patients are estimated to achieve complete remission with single-agent chemotherapy. Despite continued use, almost all patients will relapse within 6 to 9 months with single-agent therapy. However, complete remission rates exceed 95% in patients treated with combination chemotherapy, and cure rates today for children with ALL exceed 80% with multiagent treatment regimens.[3,4] Similarly, patients with APL had very poor remission and cure rates until the discovery of ATRA differentiation therapy for this disease. ATRA achieved a high complete remission rate in use as a single agent, but virtually all patients ultimately relapsed.[5,6] It was not until the combination of cytotoxic chemotherapy with ATRA and the recent combination of ATRA with arsenic trioxide that these patients obtained the best long-term survival rates of any acute myeloblastic leukemia (AML) subtype.[1,7]

Appropriate Dose Intensity Is Required for Improved Outcome

A guiding principle in the delivery of cytotoxic chemotherapeutic agents is the concept of the maximum tolerated dose (MTD): the simple idea that more is better. Drugs are delivered at the maximum dose possible, a dose greater than which unacceptable toxicity is encountered. Here, without a clear cellular biomarker of cytotoxic activity, it is not possible to relate the maximum molecular effect to maximum achievable efficacy. Thus cytotoxic drugs are first evaluated in phase I studies with the primary study goal of establishing the MTD. Subsequent phase II and III trials are then based on this dosing

schedule. MTD assumes that some toxicity is acceptable and, in fact, expected in the pursuit of cure. The most extreme example of this concept has been the use of autologous stem cell transplantation to deliver what otherwise would be lethal doses of chemotherapy. In this case the MTD is surpassed by replacing the dose-limiting factor, the hematopoietic system, with stem cells harvested from the patient before delivery of the conditioning chemotherapy. While clearly a brute force approach, the MTD paradigm also established an important corollary: significant side effects can be tolerated when therapy is administered with curative intent (discussed later).

Many retrospective studies of chemotherapy dose intensity and outcome support this premise, particularly in the pediatric setting. In high-stage neuroblastoma the addition of dose intensification with stem cell transplantation has improved the outcome for patients with metastatic disease.[8-11] In pediatric ALL several studies suggest that dose intensification is important for long-term outcome, including one randomized study comparing standard versus dose-reduced methotrexate with mercaptopurine.[12-15] Moreover, in Ewing sarcoma chemotherapy intensification through interval compression in a randomized trial was also associated with an improved outcome in patients with localized disease.[16] However, fewer prospective studies than retrospective studies have been performed to address the issue of dose intensity and outcome for pediatric tumors. Significantly, while these studies begin to emerge, some previous assumptions about MTD have come into question. For example, retrospective studies support the notion that doxorubicin or methotrexate dose intensity is important for outcome in patients with localized high-grade osteosarcoma.[17,18] However, prospective studies involving large patient numbers have called into question the role of further dose intensification for this disease.[19,20] Furthermore, randomized trials for malignancies such as breast cancer have demonstrated that massively increasing dose with stem cell transplantion does not always improve long-term survival.[21,22] Well-controlled prospective trials are critical to address the issue of dose intensification, even for cytotoxic agents.

Toxicity Is Acceptable When Therapy Is Curative

The oncology community has accepted toxicity as inherent in the mission of cure. With the implementation of dose-intensive regimens, however, comes additional toxicity. Because of the relatively nonspecific nature of traditional chemotherapy, morbidity from these treatment regimens is significant. Acute toxicity takes the form of infection, transfusion dependence, renal injury, and hepatic injury. There are also potential long-term consequences such as cardiac injury, infertility, chronic renal insufficiency, hearing loss, skeletal injury, and secondary malignancies.[23] Ongoing efforts are focused on decreasing these short- and long-term side effects. For example, to minimize acute toxicity, chemotherapy dosing is usually individualized on the basis of body surface area (mg/m^2). For some cytotoxic agents, such as methotrexate and busulfan, drug levels can be monitored to minimize toxicity. Dose intensity can also be achieved with regional tumor delivery, growth factor support, or rescue with stem cells. Furthermore, better supportive care, such as infection prophylaxis, has enabled tolerance of prolonged immunosuppression. To decrease long-term morbidity, "safe" maximum cumulative doses are being established, such as maximum cumulative doxorubicin to minimize late cardiac effects. Although toxicity can be tolerated, it is essential that the level of toxicity be commensurate with the level of benefit. Marginally effective therapeutic regimens that result in substantial toxicity should not become accepted standards.

Establish Curative Regimens and Attempt To Reduce Toxicity

Treatment strategies for most of the pediatric malignancies, including ALL and the solid tumors, have used disease stratification to decrease dose in treatment regimens. A dose-intensive regimen is initially used to establish efficacy. Then, patients with a good prognosis are treated with less intensive regimens, with the goal of comparable disease-free outcomes but decreased treatment-related morbidity. This is particularly important for pediatric disease, in which the long-term toxicity of treatment is experienced over a lifetime. Historically, these stratifications were based on factors such as age, stage, and histology, but now they include molecular genetic markers, such as *MYCN* amplification in neuroblastoma, and *MLL* rearrangement in pediatric ALL. For example, the National Wilms' Tumor Study evaluated a half-dose chemotherapy regimen for infants with low-risk disease in an attempt to decrease the incidence of toxic deaths without compromising long-term survival. These infants had acceptable toxicity with no toxic deaths, and long-term survival was not compromised.[24] A similar approach has been taken with infants and young children with low-stage neuroblastoma,[25,26] and therapy for children with ALL has been dose-reduced based on rapid clearance of minimal residual disease.[27]

While our understanding of the molecular basis of malignancy improves, so will our ability to develop fine-grained prognostic categories and patient-tailored treatment regimens, perhaps even for traditional chemotherapy agents. While we implement targeted therapy, it is expected that disease stratification and patient selection will be based on molecular genetic findings related to the credentialed target. In the clinical development of targeted therapies, we must continue to consider these key concepts: combination therapy, appropriate dose intensification, tolerance of toxicity for substantial efficacy and cure, and treatment adjustment within established favorable prognostic groups.

Shortcomings of Cytotoxic Chemotherapy

Although clinicians have made great progress with the cytotoxic armamentarium, further strides in the treatment of cancer are limited with this approach alone. Several shortcomings of this approach are intimately related to the lack of specific target knowledge (Box 44-2).

1. Toxicity is significant.
2. Optimization of anticancer effect versus side effects is difficult.

> **Box 44-2 Shortcomings of Cytotoxic Chemotherapy**
>
> 1. Toxicity is significant.
> 2. Optimization of anticancer effect versus side effects is difficult.
> 3. Mechanistic understanding of nonresponding and resistant disease is lacking.
> 4. Predictors of patient response to a specific drug are poor.
> 5. Cytotoxics have explored a narrow range of cellular and molecular mechanisms.

3. Mechanistic understanding of nonresponding and resistant disease is lacking.
4. Predictors of patient response to a specific drug are poor.
5. To date cytotoxics have explored a narrow range of cellular and molecular mechanisms.

One major shortcoming to cytotoxic therapy is morbidity. Because these agents are relatively nonspecific, there is significant toxicity to normal host cells. Patients can expect to experience short- and long-term morbidity from these drugs and even incur the risk of therapy-related fatality. Furthermore, because the most relevant targets of these drugs are poorly understood, it is difficult to optimize the anticancer effect versus the toxicity, and it is difficult to separate on-target from off-target toxicities. Often, there is no relationship between the administered dose (pharmacokinetics) or the MTD and inhibition of the putative target (pharmacodynamics). Developing a strong correlation between the pharmacokinetics of a drug and its pharmacodynamic effect is obviously impossible when the target of a drug is unknown. Similarly, in the absence of target knowledge, our understanding of resistant or refractory disease is poor at best, and it is very difficult to predict responders a priori. This has necessitated long clinical development programs with large trials to identify responsive subpopulations of patients and then follow-up trials to more thoroughly investigate response in this patient subset. Targeted therapy has the potential to address these shortcomings, to enable more rational tumor-specific therapy with less morbidity risk, and to explore previously unexploited cancer-related molecular mechanisms. With the sequencing of the human genome, the development of high-throughput genomic technologies, and an ever-increasing understanding of the molecular pathogenesis of cancer, this promise is likely to be realized.

INTRODUCTION TO TARGETED THERAPY

What Is Targeted Therapy?

Although we have made great strides with the cytotoxic armamentarium, further strides in the treatment of cancer are limited with this approach alone. We still fail to cure many patients with this approach, and several shortcomings of this approach are closely related to the lack of specific target knowledge (see Box 44-2). Targeted therapy, defined as a therapeutic procedure whose preclinical development focused on modulation of a single molecular target (typically inhibition but occasionally activation of the molecular entity), has the potential to address these shortcomings. Targeted therapy relies on the concept of cancer cell dependence—that is, the malignant cell or tumor as a whole depends for its survival or proliferation on the particular gene product or pathway. The discovery of targeted therapy differs significantly from that of cytotoxics. Historically, cytotoxic therapy discovery relied on simple, phenotypic cell death assays in which small-molecule libraries were screened in vitro against a panel of cancer cell lines. Because cytotoxic compounds are believed to cause nonspecific cell death, effective compounds should, in principle, have efficacy for all cancer types. In practice, however, this has not proved to be the case. Thus although phenotypic screens may be of significant value in identifying molecules with complex mechanisms of action, the direct prediction of clinical efficacy from limited in vitro testing remains problematic. This is in sharp contrast to the concept of targeted therapy.

There are three critical elements to the implementation of targeted therapy. First, on the basis of available data, a hypothesis is generated suggesting a causal or pathogenic link between a specific protein or gene (the potential drug target) and cancer. Experiments are then performed and data generated to test the validity of this hypothesis. Is this candidate target relevant to oncogenesis or the maintenance of the malignant phenotype? Second, there must be a valid therapeutic approach to interfering with the target activity through small molecules, antibodies, or protein- or cell-based biologics. Third, the clinician must estimate the likely impact of target manipulation in a relevant clinical application. For example, a targeted therapeutic may have limited clinical application if the disease state is already readily cured. The process of evaluating potential targets that emerge is target "validation."

Advantages of Targeted Therapy

Targeted therapy offers several potential advantages over nonspecific cytotoxic treatments (Box 44-3).
1. Improved patient selection is enabled.
2. Drug efficacy and target inhibition are linked, enabling rational dosing.
3. Side effects are more predictable.
4. Understanding of target and pathway increases options for the subsequent development of therapeutics with improved efficacy.

Box 44-3   Advantages of Targeted Therapy

1. Improved patient selection is enabled.
2. Drug efficacy and target inhibition are linked, enabling rational dosing.
3. Side effects are more predictable.
4. Understanding of target and pathway increase options for the subsequent development of therapeutics with improved efficacy.
5. The mechanisms of resistance may, in some cases, be more readily discovered and interdicted with second-generation therapeutics or specific combinations.
6. Rational pathway-based combination regimens can be tested.

---

5. The mechanisms of resistance may, in some cases, be more readily discovered and interdicted with second-generation therapeutics or specific combinations.
6. Rational pathway-based combination regimens can be tested.

By way of example, hormonal therapy has become standard of care for patients with estrogen receptor (ER)–positive breast cancer. In this case there is a lineage-dependent target in the malignant cell, the ER, and antiestrogen agents, such as tamoxifen, have been developed to inhibit competitive binding of estrogen to the ER. Numerous studies exploring estrogen antagonist therapy with tamoxifen for patients with ER-positive versus ER-negative disease demonstrate benefit only in the ER-positive patients.[28-31] In conjunction with diagnostic tools to identify hormonal receptor status, patients are now rationally chosen for therapy, thus eliminating exposure to drug toxicity for patients not likely to respond.

A second advantage of targeted therapy is the strong link between the target inhibition and efficacy. The dosing goal is achievement of complete target inhibition, not MTD. Thus there is no need to suffer undue toxicity in the achievement of an MTD. In fact, studies have shown that tamoxifen treatment responses do not correlate with serum levels and that doses greater than 20 mg daily do not increase efficacy compared with that of this dose.[32] A related third advantage of targeted therapy is that the side effects can generally be anticipated and serve as a marker for on-target inhibition. For example, the side effects of tamoxifen are predominantly related to the antiestrogen effects of this drug: vaginal dryness, hot flashes, and irregular menses. Because this drug also has proestrogen effects, thromboses and endometrial cancer can be seen.

A fourth advantage of targeted therapy is that understanding the target and the pathway increases the possibilities for therapeutic design. In the case of modifying ER signaling, there are several methods to accomplish this other than direct ER antagonism. One method is to decrease ovarian production of estrogen with luteinizing hormone–releasing factor agonists, which induce a medical ovarian ablation. A second method of interfering with ER signaling is to decrease estrogen production through the inhibition of aromatase activity. Aromatase is the final enzyme in estrogen synthesis converting the androgens androstenedione and testosterone to the estrogens estrone and estradiol. Aromatase inhibitors work by decreasing this conversion and thus decreasing circulating estrogens. Aromatase inhibitors have improved efficacy over tamoxifen and have the advantage of fewer side effects in terms of hot flashes, endometrial disease, and ischemic cerebrovascular effects.[33,34] Because of the clear dependence of some breast cancers on ER and detailed knowledge regarding estrogen biosynthesis and signaling, multiple agents could be developed to inhibit this pathway.

The fifth advantage of targeted therapeutics is the ability to more readily understand the molecular mechanisms associated with resistance. The success of targeted inhibition of BCR-ABL in CML and of epidermal growth factor receptor (EGFR) in lung cancer was rapidly followed by the specific elucidation of direct resistance mutations in the target leading to decreased activity of the relevant small-molecule inhibitors, imatinib and erlotinib or gefitinib, respectively.[35,36] In the case of CML, new agents were developed in short order to treat resistance in patients by more efficient inhibition of the mutant BCR-ABL proteins.[37]

The final advantage of targeted therapies may be the ability to generate rational and novel combination regimens. Currently, the vast majority of combination strategies derive from combining a novel agent with components of existing standards of care without regard to mechanism. This strategy is largely based on clinical expedience, existing clinical efficacy (for the standard of care) and tolerability. The difficulty of empirically discovering new synergistic combinations stems from the large number of permutations required to test all possible combinations against multiple in vitro and in vivo models or multiple cancer types. Targeted therapeutics are often related to one another in the context of a pathway. This allows testing of specific pathway-related hypotheses. For example, combinations might target upstream and downstream components of the same pathway to defeat feedback mechanisms, target components of parallel pathways to defeat pathway redundancy, or target distinct antiproliferative and prosurvival pathways.

Classes of Targets

Much of current cancer therapy development focuses on specific changes that alter the malignant cell, setting it apart from its normal counterpart and creating distinct molecular or pathway dependence for cell survival and replication. These may be genetic mutations, gene rearrangements, epigenetic modifications such as altered patterns of methylation or acetylation, lineage legacies, or other metabolic liabilities. Genes whose expression and activation have been increased, resulting in a cancer-dependent state, are prime targets for therapy development. On the basis of cancer dependencies, cancer targets can be categorized in four classes: genetic, lineage, host, and synthetic lethal or empiric (Box 44-4).[38] Although some targets may cross over from one class to another, this classification may be useful in the design of clinical trials and elucidation of the parallel biomarker strategy.

Genetics Track

The genetics track relies on the idea that a cancer develops from a finite number of genetic alterations, that these alterations give the malignant cell a selective advantage, and that these genetic changes are selected for during malignant cell replication. Hence the malignant cell becomes dependent on a set of these changes for continued survival, a process sometimes referred to as *oncogene*

Box 44-4   Classes of Targets
1. Genetics track
2. Lineage track
3. Host track
4. Synthetic lethal or empiric track

---

addiction.[39,40] This cancer cell dependence or addiction should provide a window for drug specificity for the malignant cell compared with normal cells. Targeted therapeutics taking advantage of genetic abnormalities should, in theory, be more injurious to the malignant cell than to the normal cellular counterpart. Advances in cytogenetic studies, high-throughput gene sequencing, detection of copy number alteration, whole genome expression profiling, and proteomic approaches have revolutionized candidate genetic target discovery. Now, tens of thousands of genes in hundreds of tumor samples can be analyzed simultaneously. These candidate targets must then be carefully credentialed for their suitability as a drug target. Is there cancer cell dependence on the genetic abnormality, and can the target be pharmacologically manipulated? Imatinib is one of a number of examples of clinically validated targeted therapeutics exploiting a genetic dependence, in this case the dependence of CML on the activity of the Abelson kinase (ABL). The very existence of the cancer-dependent state is dramatically illustrated by the emergence of resistance mechanisms that largely appear to restore Abelson activity (see further discussion later in this chapter).

Lineage Track

Cancer cells often maintain developmental features of the lineage from which they were derived. This is well supported with gene expression studies that report tumor cells more closely resembling the normal lineage counterpart than tumors of a different cell type. The notion that lineage or "legacy" features of a tumor cell may be exploited with targeted therapy is known as *lineage addiction.*[41] One of the earliest examples of the success of this approach has been the antagonism of ER and its signaling pathway in patients with ER-positive breast cancer. Similarly, the vast majority of patients with prostate cancer derive significant benefit from antagonism of the androgen receptor (AR). In both ER-positive breast cancer and in prostate cancer (virtually all forms of which express AR), the emergence of hormone-refractory disease largely appears to rely on mechanisms that restore steroid receptor signaling.[42] Thus as in the case of imatinib resistance, the dependent state is illustrated by these resistance mechanisms. In many cases lineage dependence may also derive from the normal hierarchy of differentiation beginning with the stem cell.

Host Track

The importance of tumor cell environment to the development and maintenance of the malignant state has become increasingly recognized and represents another potential inroad to targeted therapy. It is possible that tumors, by evolving in a particular environmental context, may become dependent on certain growth factors or neighboring cells for survival in that niche. Preclinical evidence suggests that many tumors require de novo blood vessel development for their growth and maintenance. The identification of these angiogenesis factors has enabled the development of modifiers of the angiogenesis process, leading to the successful clinical application of bevacizumab, an anti–vascular endothelial growth factor

(VEGF) antibody, in patients with colorectal cancer and the approval of kinase insert dependent receptor inhibitors (sunitinib and sorafenib) in renal cell carcinoma (see further discussion later in this chapter). The interaction of tumors with the bone microenvironment has also been targeted using inhibitors of osteoclastogenesis. Here, multiple bisphosphonate agents are approved for the prevention of cancer-related fractures.[43]

Synthetic Lethal or Empiric Track

A number of highly efficacious anticancer agents do not conveniently map to the first three categories. Admittedly, we can say that the understanding of the mechanisms of efficacy of such agents remains opaque. Nonetheless, it is quite likely that such agents, including many of the cytotoxic agents described previously, take advantage of aspects of cancer cell biology that remain unknown but may be broadly termed as *synthetic lethal interactions*. Synthetic lethal genetic interactions are defined as mutations that are lethal in combination but that do not produce a lethal phenotype as a single event. In a similar way, gain-of-fitness alterations in a malignant cell, which give the cell a survival advantage, can sensitize the cell to other stresses that have no consequence in a normal state but may be lethal with the malignancy promoting alteration. Thus cancer-promoting mutations give the malignant cell a survival advantage, but they may also incur a distinct liability that can be exploited therapeutically. Rather than two synthetic lethal genetic events, the clinician can also apply such synthetic lethal concepts to a preceding cancer-related molecular alteration followed by the application of a therapeutic. For example, a striking synthetic lethal relationship was discovered between loss of BRCA1 or BRCA2 function and inhibition of the poly(ADP-ribose) polymerase I enzyme (PARP). Here, loss of PARP1 was found to induce double-strand DNA breaks that required the recruitment of the RAD51 homologous recombination repair complex to the site of these breaks for effective repair. Because it was known that BRCA1 and 2 were required for RAD51 recruitment to such complexes, it was hypothesized that loss of BRCA1 or BRCA2 would create sensitivity to PARP inhibition. This was demonstrated both with siRNA and small-molecule inhibitors of PARP.[44] Moreover, clinical activity of PARP inhibitors has now been seen in patients with *BRCA1* and *BRCA2* mutations with ovarian or breast cancer.[45-48]

Credentialing Targets

By the strictest of measures, a drug target is not validated until a selective inhibitor of the target of interest has proven clinical activity *and* when resistance emerges through specific alterations in the direct target. Although very few cancer targets have achieved this degree of validation, we can envision preclinical experimental methods that will allow the researcher to credential a target for further drug discovery efforts. In this effort, the goals are to build data sets that either prove or disprove certain target-based hypotheses and to use such data sets to prioritize target selection for future drug discovery efforts.

Box 44-5   Credentialing Targets

Target epidemiology: study of a target in human cancers
  Target expression
  Genetic alteration
  • Gain-of-function
    • Translocation
    • Activating point mutations
    • Copy number gain
  • Loss-of-function
    • Translocation
    • Inactivating point mutations
    • Deletion
      a. Homozygous
      b. Heterozygous
      c. Loss of heterozygosity
  Protein Epidemiology
Functional validation: study of a target in a model system of tumor
  biology
  Gain-of-function: address sufficiency of target
  Loss-of-function: address necessity of target

We can consider three key questions regarding the relevance of any given target to anticancer therapy:

1. Is the activity of the target required for the development and maintenance of the cancer-dependent state?
2. Is it possible to identify a strategy for developing a therapeutic for the target of interest?
3. Is there a clinical application for the eventual therapeutic?

In the subsequent sections we will focus on the approaches relevant to addressing the role of a given target in cancer dependence. In this specific regard there are two general sources of information: the study of a target in human cancers (target epidemiology) and the functional study of a target in model systems of tumor biology (functional validation) (Box 44-5).

Target Epidemiology

Preclinical models of cancer are limited in both number and in their qualitative relationship to human cancers. Comprehensive collection of human tumor specimens could, in theory, be used to study a given target in a large array of samples broadly covering tissue distribution and stage distribution (primary versus metastatic sites). In practice, however, there are limited sets of comprehensive tumor collections, and generally the largest tumor-type specific collections are limited to fixed, paraffin-embedded specimens. The availability of tissue samples paired with robust clinical data remains limited. Furthermore, the vast majority of human cancer collections come from surgical resection samples, which do not necessarily reflect the disease state in which a therapeutic will be initially tested. Despite these limitations, molecular epidemiology studies in tissue samples, enabled by tissue microarrays, single nucleotide polymorphism (SNP) arrays, expression microarrays, reverse protein arrays, and next-generation sequencing technologies remain critical to building a case for the cancer relevance of a given target.

Target Expression. The desire to discover genes "selectively" expressed in cancer led first to the development of differential expression methods, including the subtractive hybridization cDNA libraries, differential display, and serial analysis of gene expression (SAGE) as examples.[49,50] Following the elucidation of the human genome sequence and the development of DNA-based microarrays, comparative expression profiling largely replaced difference methods, and more recently, RNA sequencing has become a commonly used tool. In all cases the basic premise has been to identify genes overexpressed in cancer with the assumption that overexpression will equate with increased sensitivity to target inhibition and hence serve to improve the therapeutic index. This basic idea, however, must be challenged and carefully considered for each target, for the simple reason that resistance to therapeutics can likewise be engendered through overexpression. Indeed, on the basis of standard biochemical principles, increased target expression should necessitate a higher drug concentration to achieve target inhibition. This is clearly the case in the amplification of dihydrofolate reductase (DHFR) in generating resistance to methotrexate.[51] Likewise, data suggest that increased expression of AR can lead to resistance to AR blockade.[42] Thus caution is required before proceeding with target selection based solely on expression data in the absence of a demonstrated causal or functional link to the maintenance of a cancer state.

Genetic Alterations. As illustrated by the success of ATRA, trastuzumab, and imatinib, direct genetic alteration leading to gene activation of a given drug target remains perhaps the best evidence for the causal role of a given gene in carcinogenesis. Genetic alterations that are highly frequent in a given tumor type and are present in the majority of cells are a strong indicator of causality. In the era of large-scale resequencing projects, it is critical that one distinguishes "driver" mutations (causal mutations) from so-called passenger mutations.[52] In addition, driver mutations that arise late in the course of disease, are present in only a minor fraction of the tumors, or are present in only a fraction of tumor cells in a given single tumor must be given less weight. These findings would suggest a reduced likelihood of this lesion possessing a strong causal link to the initiation of the disease state, although they may pose an eventual mechanism of drug resistance. The types of genetic alterations (e.g., point mutations, focal amplifications, broad amplifications, and translocations) are also distinguished with respect to the extent to which they can be used to establish causality or to infer dependence.

Gain-of-Function Genetic Alterations. Gain-of-function genetic alterations include translocations, activating point mutations, and increases in gene copy number. Translocations were among the first discovered genetic alterations initially described using chromosome spreads. Approaches to the discovery of chromosomal rearrangements include exon microarrays, which can potentially detect imbalanced or amplified translocations, cancer outlier profile analysis (COPA), paired-end resequencing of BAC clones from a genomic library (giving a structural map of a cancer genome),[53] and newer methods of single-molecule sequencing (discussed later). Translocations are highly informative with respect to causality because they typically alter only two genes, and because background or random translocation events are relatively rare, with chromothripsis (massive DNA rearrangements affecting one or a few chromosomes that occur as a result of one catastrophic event) as a notable exception.[54]

Amplifications are now routinely detected by methods of DNA copy number analyses: comparative genomic hybridization (CGH) array, high-density SNP arrays, and whole exome or whole genome sequencing. There are two general types of increases in gene copy: focal amplifications and broad copy number increases covering an entire chromosome or chromosome arm. With sufficient sample numbers it is possible to discern one to several genes contained within a focal amplicon. Typically, the minimal region of amplification is a guide. However, methods for detecting copy number alterations (e.g., genomic identification of significant targets in cancer [GISTIC]) also use the amplitude of amplification as an important parameter.[55] Although it is not definitive proof, amplification lends evidence to a causal relationship between a given gene within an amplicon and a cancer state. In some amplicons, multiple genes remain strong candidates for oncogenes targeted by the amplification. One notable example is the 11q13 amplification with genes including *Cyclin D1*, *FGF3*, and *FGF4*.[56]

Larger-scale chromosomal alterations leading to trisomy or gain of an entire chromosome arm are frequent yet are far more difficult to study. As such, identifying single genes (or drug targets) within such broad regions remains a challenge. In this case the number of genes implicated in such large-scale alterations is so large that almost no importance can be ascribed to the cancer relevance of a gene contained within such broad chromosomal-level alterations. Outlier analysis may begin to allow the elucidation of multigene targeting by such broad regions and is illustrated by the analysis of trisomy 7 in glioma revealing a dependence on cMET and its ligand HGF, both located on chromosome 7.[57]

Subtle nucleic acid level alterations, including point mutations and small insertions and deletions, are an important mechanism for the activation of oncogenes. Point mutations leading to the constitutive guanosine triphosphate (GTP)–bound and hence activated form of N-RAS and K-RAS,[58] as well as genetic events leading to activation of the BRAF kinase in melanoma, thyroid cancer, colorectal cancer,[59] pediatric pilocytic astrocytoma,[60-62] and Langerhans cell histiocytosis[63] are exemplars of this mechanism. Large-scale sequencing projects that unveiled new mutations activating oncogenes such as *EGFR*[36] and *PIK3CA*[64] have led to national and international cancer genome sequencing projects. From these studies it has become apparent that the detection of passenger mutations, constituting the background rate of mutation, can pose a significant challenge. These passenger mutations must be separated from the more prevalent and recurrent driver mutations.[52] Such passenger mutations may be exceedingly high in certain types of tumors, particularly those bearing mutations in mismatch repair genes. Indeed, in one case inactivating mutations in the mismatch repair gene *MSH6* were discovered in glioma tumors recurring after treatment with temozolomide. Here the sequencing of *MSH6* was triggered by the very high rate of observed passenger mutations in treated versus untreated tumors.[65,66] These data suggest that cautious interpretation of low-frequency events is warranted when considering mutation analysis from larger-scale modalities. A framework for context-specific mutation analysis has been provided by a systematic study of mutation data across many cancer types in The Cancer Genome Atlas (TCGA) project and others, and these studies are revealing remarkably simple genomes in many pediatric cancers (Fig. 44-1).[67]

Loss-of-Function Genetic Alterations. Loss-of-function alterations do not typically directly indicate or point to a specific gene as a candidate drug target. However, such alterations may predict sensitivity to agents acting against protein targets contained within downstream or parallel pathways. For example, clinical trials are under way testing inhibitors of mammalian target of rapamycin (mTOR) function against sporadic tumors or hereditable cancer predisposition syndromes resulting from loss of the tumor suppressors PTEN and TSC1 or TSC2. In both cases loss-of-function mutations in these tumor-suppressor genes are thought to lead to constitutive activation and hence constitutive dependence on mTOR (discussed later in this chapter).

Similarly, in the hedgehog pathway, a key development pathway regulating cell patterning, deletions or muta-tions in the gene encoding the Patched receptor (PTCH) are associated with hereditary and sporadic basal cell carcinomas and sporadic medulloblastoma.[68-70] Loss of PTCH, a receptor for the ligands in the hedgehog family, leads to constitutive activation of the atypical G protein–coupled receptor (GPCR)–like protein Smoothened (Smo).[71] Cyclopamine, a naturally derived inhibitor of Smo, and other, newer small-molecule inhibitors, have had significant activity in preclinical models lacking *PTCH* gene function[72] and in clinical trials.[73,74] These examples illustrate that identification of loss-of-function mutations can reveal downstream target molecules in critical cancer pathways.

Translocations are typically thought of as gain-of-function genetic events in that they act dominantly. However, they can functionally inactivate endogenous genes through the creation of dominant-negative protein fusions. For example, the PML-RARα fusion protein is believed to act, at least in part, as a dominant-negative inhibitor of endogenous RARα function.[75] This type of molecular action can be difficult to elucidate in functional experiments. Nonetheless, it is worth remembering this possibility when evaluating proteins or genes as drug targets when they are involved in new or existing translocations.

Chromosomal-level alterations leading to loss-of-function events include homozygous deletions, heterozygous deletions, and loss of heterozygosity. Homozygous deletions are typically highly focal in their nature. When the boundaries are defined with large sample sets, in

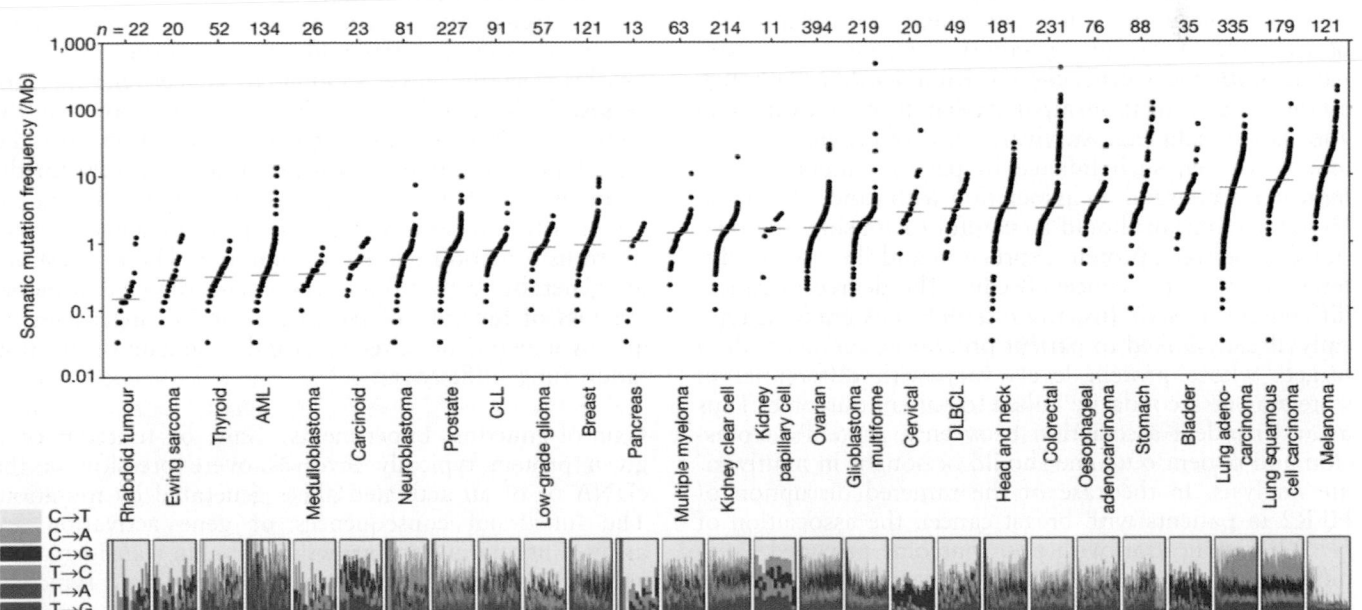

Figure 44-1 Somatic mutation frequencies observed in exomes from 3083 tumor-normal pairs. Each *dot* corresponds to a tumor-normal pair, with vertical position indicating the total frequency of somatic mutations in the exome. Tumor types are ordered by their median somatic mutation frequency, with the lowest frequencies *(left)* found in pediatric tumors and hematologic malignancies, and the highest *(right)* in tumors induced by carcinogens such as tobacco smoke and ultraviolet light. Mutation frequencies vary more than 1000-fold between lowest and highest across different cancers and also within several tumor types. The *bottom panel* shows the relative proportions of the six different possible base-pair substitutions, as indicated in the label on the left. *AML,* Acute myeloblastic leukemia; *CLL,* chronic lymphocytic leukemia; *DLBCL,* diffuse large B-cell lymphoma. *(Modified from Lawrence, et al: Mutational heterogeneity in cancer and the search for new cancer-associated genes.* Nature *499:214–218, 2013.)*

many cases, only a few genes are found in the overlapping region. For example, in the case of focal deletions on 9p, the typical minimal deleted regions in tumors such as melanoma contain only CDKN2A and CDKN2B.[76] Heterozygous deletions are typically larger and usually involve entire chromosomes or chromosome arms. As in the case of amplifications, such large-scale broad genetic alterations make it difficult to ascertain the cancer relevance of any single gene contained within a larger region. Loss of heterozygosity (LOH) can occur as an event associated with heterozygous deletion leaving only one parental chromosome behind, which is thus homozygous. LOH can also occur when duplication of the remaining parental chromosome creates a situation known as *uniparental disomy*. This is significant because it may indicate preservation of a mutated allele, leading to two mutant alleles of a given gene. In the case of the tumor suppressor gene *p53*, copy-neutral LOH is common.

Inactivating point mutations are a common means of gene inactivation. In this case stop codons are the most efficient mechanism for disrupting gene function. As a result, tumor suppressor gene mutations often are enriched for stop or truncating mutations. This creates certain technical and cost difficulties in sequencing genes for inactivating mutations because it is necessary to sequence all coding exons, consider sequencing of the regulatory elements governing splicing, and consider the detection of promoter mutations. As a result of these difficulties, precise clinical analysis of tumor suppressor gene mutations remains challenging even with the application of next-generation sequencing technologies.

Protein Molecular Epidemiology by Immunohistochemistry. It is important to understand the relationship between the expression or activity of a gene product and patient outcome or other clinicopathologic data. Although establishing a relationship between protein expression and clinical data (e.g., survival) does not provide a causal link to cancer, such linkage to patient outcome likely indicates a nonrandom association with cancer behavior. Here the clinician should be careful to consider the relationship between protein expression and the state of differentiation of the cancer. Because the degree of cancer differentiation state (usually referred to as *grade*) is typically already linked to patient prognosis, candidate drug targets whose protein levels vary with differentiation state may be secondarily linked to patient outcome. Thus an independent association between a protein's expression and patient outcome should be sought in multivariate analysis. In the case of the targeted disruption of HER2 in patients with breast cancer, the association of *HER2* amplification with poor outcome provided a significant motivation for the development of trastuzumab, an anti-HER2 monoclonal antibody.[77]

The ability to perform larger-scale epidemiology analyses typically relies on archived tissue for which longer-term clinical follow-up is available. This largely dictates that target epidemiology be carried out in paraffin-embedded, fixed tissue. Here RNA and DNA can be examined by in situ hybridization (ISH), fluorescence in situ hybridization (FISH), or next-generation sequencing

approaches. Historically, the most common method for interrogating human tissue samples is protein-based immunohistochemistry (IHC). These studies have been made higher throughput by the advent of tissue microarrays. Such arrays align hundreds of tumor samples on a single slide, facilitating the experimental procedures. IHC is primarily limited by the quality of the antibody reagents that are used and the care with which such reagents are subject to rigorous validation. Too often, poorly described or unvalidated antibodies are used in IHC studies after a quality assessment based solely on the observed staining pattern in tissue sections. In all cases where IHC is used, the controls should include experimental, fixed cell blocks derived from negative control cells or tissues known to lack the antigen of interest and positive control cells or tissue known to harbor the antigen of interest. These controls can typically be obtained from blocks created from cell lines where the negative controls can be generated by using short hairpin RNA (shRNA). With the development of protocols for next-generation sequencing from paraffin-embedded tissues, the use of such approaches has become more commonplace for the interrogation of archived primary patient tissues.[78,79]

Functional Studies to Address Cancer Dependence

Ideally, the functional relevance of a putative cancer target should be elucidated before embarking on the lengthy process of drug discovery. The concept is simple: It is preferable to "fail" or invalidate a putative target in preclinical studies than to fail later in the clinic. Although there are multiple reasons for the failure of a given therapeutic in clinical development, ideally failure should be avoided because the drug is made against an irrelevant target. Hence one should develop a robust understanding of the science surrounding a given drug target and tie this scientific understanding to cancer-relevant processes. It is useful to consider two questions in the context of designing experiments for functional validation. First, is the putative cancer target *necessary* for the maintenance of a cancer-related phenotype? Second, is the putative cancer target *sufficient* for inducing a cancer or transformation-related phenotype? These questions are generally answered by experiments directed at inducing loss of function of the target (addressing necessity) and by experiments directed at inducing gain of function (addressing sufficiency).

Gain-of-Function Experiments. Gain of function of a given protein typically involves overexpression of the cDNA or of an activated allele generated by mutation. The functional consequences of gene activation are assayed first in in vitro growth assays, in transformation assays, and in cotransformation experiments. Typically, gain of function in transformation assays would be assessed in murine embryonic fibroblasts, in immortalized NIH3T3 cells, Ba/F3 cells, or in Rat1a fibroblasts. In addition, the ability to transform human primary epithelial cells has been made possible through the use of telomerase and has provided a set of assays that can be used to measure the ability of a given gene to induce transformation in human cells.[80]

Short-term validation experiments using in vivo systems have become more attractive with the advent of tissue reconstitution murine models, enabling rapid genetic manipulation. Examples of this approach include the use of murine hematopoietic cells or murine fetal hepatoblast cells. In each case retroviruses directing the expression of the relevant candidate oncogene can be introduced into the respective primary cells that are then re-introduced into host animals. As an example, mutations in *JAK2* discovered in myeloproliferative syndromes recapitulate the disease entity when re-introduced in retroviral vectors into the hematopoietic reconstitution system.[81-83] Similarly, the use of hepatoblasts has been useful in demonstrating that certain gene activation events can induce hepatocellular carcinoma.[84,85] These systems provide some of the speed and flexibility of in vitro systems but maintain the more authentic relationship between stroma and the generated tumor cells.

Fully genetically engineered models, including transgenic mice, can be useful in studying gene activation in the specific tissue of origin depending on the extent to which promoter regulation can be used to direct gene expression to the indicated cell. Knock-in animals have also been generated in which mutant *RAS* alleles are re-introduced into the endogenous murine *RAS* gene locus.[86] Such animals have been used to demonstrate sufficiency of *K-RAS* for the induction of lung adenocarcinomas,[86] carcinomas of the pancreas[87] and myeloproliferative disease.[88] These engineered models also provide a stable resource for testing candidate drug compounds in highly defined mechanistically driven models.

Loss-of-Function Experiments. For many years there were no feasible methods for readily inducing loss-of-function alterations in mammalian systems. Consequently, the elaboration of a cell-penetrant small-molecule inhibitor or tool compound was one of the only ways to achieve the desired inhibitory effect. The development of robust small interfering RNA (siRNA) methods, taking advantage of the endogenous siRNA processing systems, now allows for transient, stable, or regulated knockdown of nearly any mammalian gene product.[89,90] Genome-editing technologies, such as transcription activator-like effector nucleases (TALEN) and the CRISPR (clustered regularly interspaced short palindromic repeats)/Cas system have also been developed to enable targeted gene-disruption events.[91,92] These powerful new tools are complemented by existing methods for loss-of-function experiments, including the use of inhibitory antibodies for extracellular targets, soluble protein traps for extracellular ligands and receptors, dominant-negative proteins expressed from cDNAs, murine germline knockouts, and inducible knockouts. Generally, loss-of-function experiments would be attempted first in human cancer cell line models. Increasingly, cell line models are being characterized in greater genetic detail, enabling more rational selection of models for functional inactivation experiments by either small molecules or genetic perturbations.[93,94,95] Additionally, shRNAs have been merged with the bone marrow transplantation and the hepatoblast tissue reconstitution models described previously (Fig. 44-2).[96] Finally, regulated germline shRNAs can now be engineered in the mouse as a rapid method for generating tissue-specific and temporally regulated gene knockdowns.[97]

Genetic Studies in Lower Organisms

The topic of genetic studies in lower organisms is too broad for a complete discussion in this chapter. However, it is worth noting the utility of defining genetic dependence in the context of highly conserved pathways that are shared between mammals, flies *(Drosophila melanogaster)* and worms *(Caenorhabditis elegans)*. In some cases lower organisms have a reduced set of homologues for any given pathway member, and thus the necessity of a single gene can be tested directly. Although establishing the relationship between a gene and a cancer phenotype in these organisms is not usually possible, the genetic dependence or epistatic relationships elucidated in such model systems have proved highly informative in humans. A notable example is the discovery of the relationship between loss-of-function mutations in the tuberous sclerosis genes and activation of the mTOR and S6K (ribosomal S6 kinase) pathway (discussed later).

Target Credentialing Summary

The credentialing of drug targets ultimately must be conceived as a set of hypotheses to be tested experimentally. In each case these hypotheses must be built around the relevant biology. It is important to distinguish targets with cell-autonomous effects versus those in which the interaction between cancer cell and host factors is critical. In the case of drug targets that are encoded by bona fide human oncogenes with definitive genetic alterations, one can have a high degree of confidence in the likely therapeutic effect of inhibitory molecules. Unfortunately, this group is the minority of the drug targets for consideration. Thus the intent of credentialing is to enable a rational stratification of potential drug targets and a rational application of resources to specific drug discovery efforts.

Classes of Targeted Therapies

Targeted therapies can be divided into two main classes: drugs (small molecules, natural products, antisense, and siRNA) and biologics (antibody, protein/peptide, and cell-based) (Box 44-6). Biologics, as defined by the U.S. Food and Drug Administration (FDA), include a wide range of products such as vaccines, blood and blood components, somatic cells, gene therapy, tissues, and recombinant therapeutic proteins. They can be composed of sugars, proteins, or nucleic acids or complex combinations of these substances, or they may be living entities such as cells and tissues. Biologics are isolated from a variety of natural sources—human, animal, or microorganism—and may be produced by biotechnology methods. From a practical point of view, drugs entering the market require the filing of a New Drug Application (NDA), whereas biologics require the filing of a Biologic License Application (BLA).

Drugs

Small molecules are defined as carbon-containing compounds that usually have a molecular weight of less than

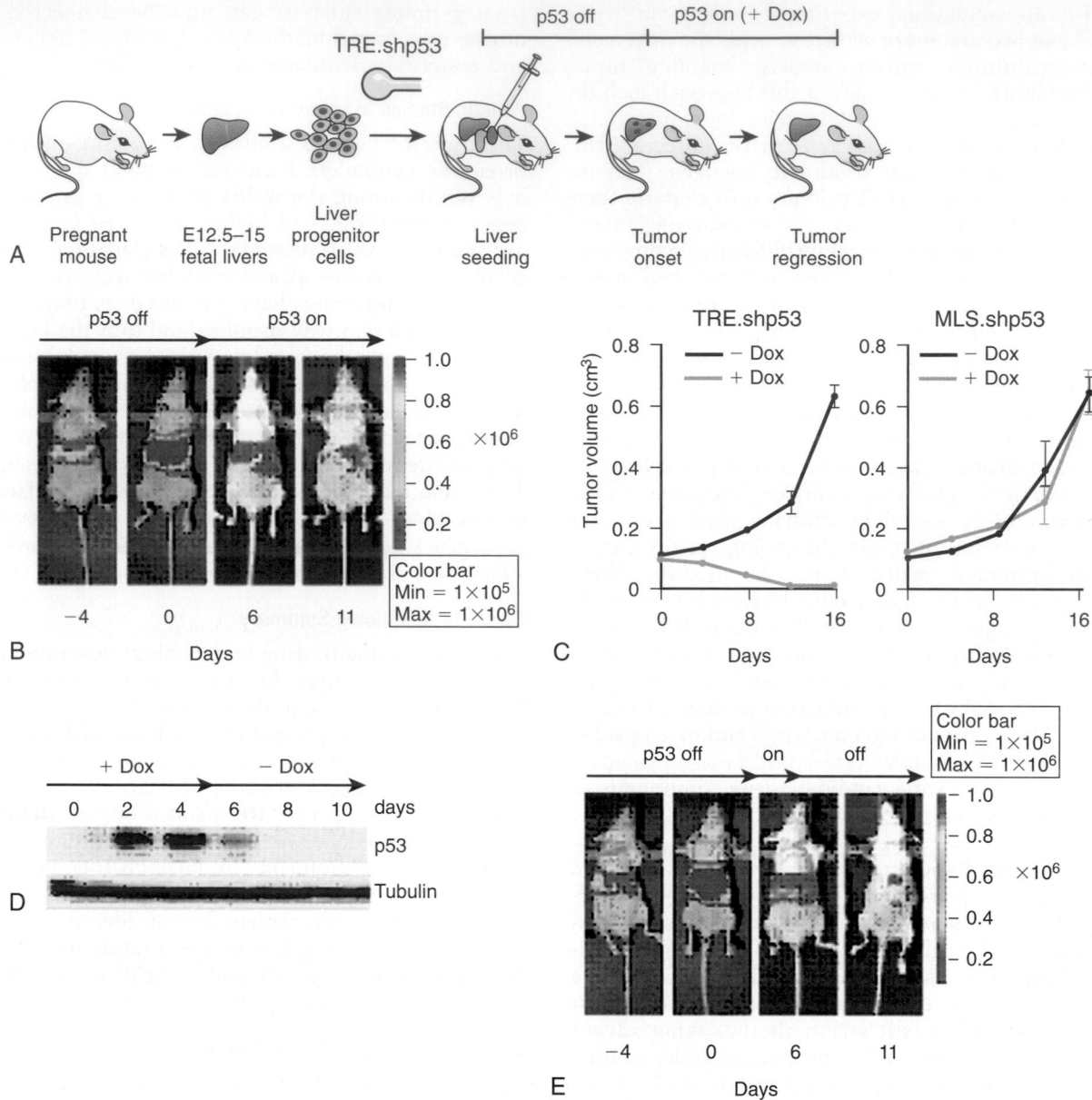

Figure 44-2 Reactivation of p53 results in liver tumor regression. **A,** Embryonic liver progenitor cells were transduced with a tetracycline-regulatable p53 shRNA (TRE.shp53), tTA, and H-rasV12. After onset of liver tumors, p53 expression could be restored by doxycycline (Dox) treatment. **B,** Reactivation of p53 leads to rapid tumor regression. Tumor-bearing mice were treated with Dox starting at day 0 and imaged at the indicated time points ($n = 9$). **C,** Subcutaneous tumors derived from ras-transformed liver progenitor cells with tet-off shRNA (TRE.shp53) or a nonregulatable shRNA (MLS.shp53) were grown in nude mice. Values represent mean s.d. ($n = 4$). **D,** p53 reactivation is reversed by Dox withdrawal. Protein lysates from liver progenitor cells pulse-treated with Dox for 4 days were immunoblotted for p53. **E,** Representative mice ($n = 6$) as in **B** were pulse-treated with Dox for 4 days and imaged at the indicated time. *(Modified from Xue, et al: Senescence and tumour clearance is triggered by p53 restoration in murine liver carcinomas.* Nature *445:656–60, 2007.)*

2000 g/mol. These small organic compounds have the advantage of purity, high permeability into target cells, ease of manufacturing, and stability, and they remain the primary class amenable to oral delivery. However, disadvantages include insufficient selectivity resulting in off-target toxicity, challenges with poor bioavailability, and challenges with metabolism of the molecule. Over the last decade synthetic methods have been developed for producing a diversity of chemical structures, either by using directed medicinal chemistry approaches or by using com-

binatorial chemistry, the synthesis of numerous organic compounds by combining variations of each of the building blocks that make up the compounds.[98] Similarly, there has been the elaboration of a diverse set of methods for identifying the initial small-molecule hits against a desired target. High-throughput screening involves the in vitro assay of target activity against chemical libraries. In silico screening can be used to dock millions of compounds into known or modeled three-dimensional structures of a given target. Fragment-based screening uses either

Box 44-6 **Classes of Therapies**

DRUGS
  Small molecules
  Natural products
  Antisense oligonucleotides
  RNA interference
BIOLOGICALS
  Antibody
  Protein
    Whole protein
    Peptides
    Soluble receptors
CELLULAR

radiographic or nuclear magnetic resonance–based structural approaches to identify very-low-molecular-weight fragments that can interrogate the binding surface of a new target.[99] Finally, target-specific cell-based screens can be used to identify cell-penetrant small molecules perturbing a target-specific reporter or phenotype.

Natural products have been important in drug development and have played a dominant role in cancer therapy.[100] Approximately three fourths of the current anticancer drugs are natural products or derived from natural products.[101] The chemical diversity of natural products complements that of synthetic libraries. As a result of a long evolutionary process, natural products tend to be sterically complex with greater diversity of ring systems compared with synthetic and combinatorial libraries.

Natural products are classified according to shared scaffolding elements and can be divided into several structural classes, such as terpenes, alkaloids, polyketides, and nonribosomal peptides. The building blocks for the natural products are most often monomeric components of primary metabolic pathways that are then shunted into secondary metabolic pathways. Plants and soil microbes are traditional sources of natural products with new sources, such as fungi and marine life (e.g., sponges and algae), under active exploration.[102]

Drug development with natural products may have specific advantages to that of synthetic molecules. The complexity of natural products may lead to greater specificity. In addition, unanticipated activities may be discovered that would be difficult to engineer into a small molecule. For example, rapamycin (derived from a soil fungus from Easter Island [Rapa Nui]), creates a novel protein-drug-protein interaction between the protein FKBP12, rapamycin, and the mTOR kinase, resulting in an exquisitely selective inhibition of mTOR.[103,104] However, although the natural products have been developed into very successful drugs, there are several disadvantages to these libraries. First, natural product extracts are generally impure, and hence identifying the active compound can be difficult. Second, the synthesis of these compounds in production level quantities for medicinal purposes can be challenging. Third, subsequent optimization of the lead natural product can be difficult in the absence of a complete in vitro synthesis of the relevant natural product. New high-throughput strategies are under development to tackle roadblocks to the use of natural products for medicinal purposes.

Antisense oligonucleotides are single strands of short deoxynucleotide sequences (18-21 oligomers) that bind to target mRNA sequence by Watson-Crick hybridization and induce transcript destruction. They interact with the target transcript with sequence specificity and inhibit production of the target protein by several potential mechanisms. First, they activate endogenous nucleases, such as RNAse H, which then cleave the RNA strand of an RNA-DNA heteroduplex. A second potential mechanism of antisense activity is a noncatalytic effect with steric inhibition of the translational machinery with induction of translational arrest and inhibition of protein synthesis. A third mechanism is interference with normal RNA splicing, resulting in the inhibition of specific splice variants. Antisense therapeutics held the promise of pharmacologically inhibiting targets that had been intractable with small molecule approaches. In theory, virtually any gene can be targeted with antisense approaches with an expectation of high target selectivity. However, the development of antisense therapy has faced many challenges, including poor solubility, limited intracellular uptake, and rapid degradation. To overcome these issues, subsequent antisense therapy focused on chemical modification of the backbone to which the nucleoside bases are attached.

Despite these efforts, the utility of antisense therapy for cancer has been disappointing. However, there have been some clinical responses seen in trials. Oblimersen (Genasense), a phosphorothioate antisense therapy targeting BCL-2, has shown some activity in patients with heavily pretreated chronic lymphocytic leukemia (CLL).[105] Furthermore, recent data from a randomized phase III trial for patients with relapsed or refractory CLL comparing fludarabine plus cyclophosphamide with or without oblimersen demonstrated an increase in complete response and nodular partial response in patients in the oblimersen arm, particularly for those patients with fludarabine-sensitive disease.[106,107]

RNA interference (RNAi) is a more recent approach to nucleic acid–based therapy. Similar to antisense therapy, RNAi may have therapeutic application, particularly for targets that have been considered intractable by traditional drug discovery approaches. RNAi is a double-stranded RNA (dsRNA)–induced mechanism of gene silencing naturally occurring in plants and animals. Over the last few years, it has become possible to target virtually any gene in the genome for knockdown with small, dsRNA gene-silencing by using siRNAs or expressed shRNAs. The RNAi pathway is hypothesized to have evolved early in eukaryotes as a protection against viral and genetic pathogens. Double-stranded RNA viruses and genetic elements are subject to RNAi-dependent gene silencing as a means of cell-based immunity. Furthermore, endogenously expressed shRNAs may regulate gene expression during development through the RNAi pathway.[89,90] If exploited as a potential cancer therapy, RNAi has the potential advantages of (1) relative specificity for a particular gene target, (2) efficiency with the potential to achieve more than 90% knockdown, and

(3) widespread applicability with the potential of targeting any gene in the human genome. Unlike antisense oligonucleotides, RNAi takes advantage of a naturally occurring cellular mechanism for gene silencing.

As in the case of oligonucleotides, there are impasses to the development of RNAi-based therapies, including the difficulty of delivering large nucleic acid molecules to intracellular targets in humans. Unmodified siRNAs have a short half-life in human plasma and are rapidly excreted by the kidneys. Furthermore, to have activity the siRNA or shRNA must reach the cytoplasm of the targeted cell, and naked siRNAs are not efficiently taken up by mammalian cells unaided. One method of delivering shRNA that is commonly used in the laboratory to develop stable knockdown is the use of viral vectors. However, with viral vector delivery, there remains significant concern regarding insertional mutagenesis, carcinogenesis, direct cellular toxicity and short-lived on-target effects.[108-111] Other nonviral methods of delivery are actively under exploration. One possibility is to chemically modify the siRNA to increase its stability with modifications such as locked nucleic acid (LNA) residues[112,113] or phosphorothioates.[114] A second approach to increase the stability of the siRNA is to package it in liposomes[115] or other nanoparticles such as the cationic polymer polyethylenimine[116] or to use cholesterol modifications.[117] These packaging systems can also be modified to contain tissue-specific homing signals, such as the attachment of specific antibodies. Despite the problems with delivery and stability of RNAi, novel therapeutics using RNAi have entered clinical trials for multiple diseases.[118-120]

Biologicals

Antibody therapy with monoclonal antibodies (Mabs) is an increasingly important mode of targeted therapy for cancer. Early attempts at antibody-based therapy with murine Mabs were limited by immunogenicity, short half-life in humans, and poor ability to activate human immune effector mechanisms. With the evolution of recombinant DNA technology, it is now routine to create humanized Mabs. Recombinant antibodies with human crystallizable fragments (Fc) regions are much less immunogenic in humans than murine Mabs and can facilitate activation of immune effector mechanisms. Thus recombinant Mabs may have a dual mechanism of anticancer activity secondary to the specificity of epitope targeting with the antigen-binding fragment (Fab) and the recruitment of immune effectors with the Fc region. As a direct effect of the Mab variable domain binding to the target, they can have antagonist effects on receptor-ligand interactions and receptor-receptor interactions or agonistic effects on the target's biological activity. Second, if engineered to be of the immunoglobulin G1 (IgG1) subclass and to contain an Fc region, they induce immune effector function against I the target cell after their interactions with complement or with receptors for the Fc region, such as FcγR, a class of surface glycoproteins expressed predominantly on white blood cells. The Fc region interactions with FcγR can induce antibody-dependent cell-mediated cytotoxicity (ADCC), phagocytosis, endo-

Box 44-7   **Advantages and Disadvantages of Antibody-Based Therapy**

ADVANTAGES
1. High-degree of specificity results in reduced off-target effects.
2. Pharmacokinetic properties are similar across different antibodies.
3. Spectrum of targets amenable to antibody-based therapy differs from that of small molecules.

DISADVANTAGES
1. Intravenous administration is necessary.
2. Preclinical in vivo studies are difficult to perform.
3. Neutralizing antibodies can develop.
4. Antibodies cannot access intracellular antigens.
5. Volume of distribution is limited by large molecular weight of antibody.
6. The cost of production is higher.

cytosis of immune complexes followed by antigen presentation, and release of inflammatory mediators.[121] Antibodies can be linked to chemical moieties with additional antitumor activity, such as in gemtuzumab ozogamicin, where an antibody to CD33 was conjugated to the antitumor antibiotic calicheamicin.

Bispecific antibodies: Whereas MAbs that are clinically effective usually recruit immune cells expressing an Fc receptor, T cells are notably FcR negative. To engage T cells in the antitumor response, bispecific antibodies (bsAbs) can be deployed. These are artificially designed molecules that bind simultaneously to two different antigens, one on the tumor cell, the other one on an immune cell, such as T cells, cross-linking tumor cells and T cells. For example, blinatumomab, a bsAb that directs T cells to CD19-expressing tumor cells, such as B-ALL and non-Hodgkin lymphoma (NHL) cells, has been demonstrated to have compelling activity in clinical trials, including complete responses.[122-124]

Antibody-based therapy has several advantages to small molecule–based therapy (Box 44-7). First, there is a high degree of specificity for the target of interest, resulting in reduced off-target effects. Second, pharmacokinetic properties are very similar from one antibody product to another, with the half-life of an infused antibody generally lasting 2 weeks. Unlike the case of small molecules, there is a consistent path for metabolism, thus eliminating a highly variable aspect of low-molecular-weight drug development. Third, the spectrum of targets amenable to antibody-based therapeutics is largely distinct from small molecules and includes large extracellular domains and secreted ligands that are otherwise "undruggable."

On the other hand, there are several disadvantages of antibody-based therapy compared with small-molecule therapy. Currently antibody-based therapies are generally delivered intravenously. A second disadvantage is that preclinical in vivo studies can be difficult to conduct.[125] The researcher must address whether the antibody in development will recognize the appropriate antigen in the animal model being tested. In some cases only primates conserve the relevant human epitope, limiting the selection of species available for toxicology studies. Efficacy studies, in particular against stromal or host factors, may require generation of a "murine equivalent" antibody, although equivalence is difficult to quantitate. The robust evaluation of host effector function elicited by an antibody and the role of this function in antitumor activity is also difficult to assess in the typical human tumor xenotransplant study in rodents. A third challenge with antibody-based therapy is that the patient can develop neutralizing antibodies to the therapy. This was particularly problematic with murine-based antibody therapy. Fourth, antibodies cannot easily gain access to intracellular antigens. Fifth, the volume of distribution of antibodies is limited by the large molecular weight, and tumor penetration is therefore a concern, at least theoretically. Finally, antibody-based treatment is generally more costly to produce compared with small-molecule therapy.

Cellular Adoptive Therapy

Most recently, cell-based biological products have also seen dramatic clinical responses. The transfer of autologous T cells modified to express chimeric antigen receptors (CARs) specific for the B-cell antigen CD19 has shown antitumor activity in low-grade B-cell malignancies and in refractory adult and pediatric B-cell ALL.[126,127] These exciting advances are discussed in more detail in Chapter 46.

Targeted Therapy: Lessons Learned from Adult Oncology

With rare exceptions, most drugs are first tested in adults before evaluation in children. This has been true for targeted agents as well. In the following section several examples of successful targeted therapies for the treatment of adult patients with cancer are briefly discussed, with an emphasis on particular lessons learned in the development and testing of these early agents.

Genetics Examples of Targeted Therapy

Treatment of Acute Promyelocytic Leukemia with All-Trans-Retinoic Acid. The successful treatment of patients with M3-AML (acute promyelocytic leukemia, or APL) with ATRA is one of the earliest examples of targeted therapy in the genetic class. This therapeutic discovery was serendipitous. The observation that myeloid blasts differentiate in response to retinoic acid derivatives preceded the discovery of the involvement of the retinoic acid receptor in the pathogenesis of APL.[128,129] ATRA treatment is one example of how discovery of a compound inducing a phenotypic alteration can lead to greater understanding of the mechanisms underlying the state change. By morphologic examination APL is characterized by a predominance of malignant hypergranular cells blocked at the promyelocyte stage of differentiation. At the molecular level a reciprocal translocation involving the *retinoic acid receptor α (RARα)* gene on chromosome 17q21 is invariably present. This translocation most commonly fuses *RARα* to the *PML* gene on chromosome 15q22. RARα is a hormone-dependent, DNA-binding, nuclear receptor transcription factor that can act as a transcriptional activator or inhibitor.[75,130,131] In the presence of physiologic amounts of retinoic acid, it

normally functions as a transcriptional activator. Abnormal RARα fusion proteins function as transcriptional repressors, enhancing interactions with the corepressor complex.[132,133] Pharmacologic doses of ATRA appear to overcome the PML-RARα–induced transcriptional repression by dissociating the corepressors from PML-RARα and restoring normal ATRA-mediated myeloid differentiation.[134] Furthermore, the PML-RARα protein undergoes proteolytic cleavage in APL cells after ATRA treatment.[135] ATRA treatment increases the fraction of differentiated cells with functional characteristics of neutrophils, induces a mature membrane phenotype, inhibits leukemia cell proliferation, and ultimately induces apoptosis. Historically, APL was among the most fatal subtypes of AML. However, with the addition of ATRA to APL therapy regimens, the overall 2-year survival rate is more than 75%. APL now has the highest cure rate of the AML subtypes.[1,5,136]

The success of ATRA in the treatment of PML-RARα rearranged AML illustrates several important issues regarding targeted therapy. First, specific somatic rearrangements, such as PML-RARα, can be exploited with targeted therapy, and the specific underlying genetic event predicts response, not the phenotype. For example, other RARα rearrangements, such as PLZF- RARα, are associated with an APL phenotype. However, the PLZF-RARα fusion protein is associated with nuclear corepressor interactions that are resistant to ATRA therapy. Patients with the *PLZF-RARα* rearrangement are resistant to ATRA therapy.[137] A second important concept that emerges from the success of ATRA is that differentiation therapy is feasible for some malignancies. In general, terminally differentiated cells lose the capacity to divide and ultimately undergo apoptosis. This is indeed the case for APL cells treated with ATRA, which raises the possibility that such approaches may be more broadly applicable. A third important lesson from this example is that modulation of transcription factors is therapeutically feasible. Rearrangements involving transcription factors are a common event in the acute leukemias and in the pediatric solid tumors. Although well-characterized contributors to the malignant state, these transcription factor abnormalities have been considered "undruggable" or pharmacologically intractable because there is no obvious approach to inhibiting their function. However, ATRA therapy for the genetic lesion PML-RARα lends credence to the idea that these lesions can be targeted and that their modulation can have therapeutic efficacy. Finally, this example reinforces the importance of combination therapy not only for cytotoxic agents but also for targeted therapy. Although the majority of patients with APL in early trials achieved a complete remission with ATRA as a single agent, it was only in combination with conventional chemotherapy or arsenic trioxide that long-term cure rates were achieved.[6,136,138,7]

Imatinib in Chronic Myelogenous Leukemia. The development of imatinib for the treatment of CML stands out as the first example of a designed small-molecule inhibitor developed for the purpose of targeting an activated oncogene. Moreover, its dramatic single-agent activity in its initial phase I and II trials, along with the rapid path to registration, has provided the impetus for attempting to identify highly responsive patient populations during preclinical and early clinical development. In 1960 Nowell and Hungerford first detected the presence of the then-named *Philadelphia chromosome* in nearly all patients with CML.[139] This aberrant chromosome, resulting from the fusion of chromosomes 9 and 22, was subsequently shown to encode a fusion protein linking a gene of unknown function (*BCR*, or *breakpoint cluster region*) to the product of the *Abelson* gene—the cellular homologue of an oncoprotein activated by the Abelson leukemia virus. The discovery that the *Abelson* gene product (ABL) could function as a protein tyrosine kinase and that the normal autoregulatory domain of ABL was replaced with coding sequences from BCR led to the idea that constitutive activation of ABL kinase activity was likely a causal genetic event in CML.[140-142] In animal models production of BCR-ABL was sufficient to induce both acute and chronic leukemia.[143] These data, along with the presence of a catalytic domain, made BCR-ABL kinase an attractive drug target. Based on these elements, a drug-discovery program was launched, culminating in the discovery and clinical testing of imatinib (Gleevec), a small molecule inhibitor of BCR-ABL.

In the initial phase I trial by Druker and colleagues, 83 patients with interferon-refractory CML were enrolled and treated with doses of imatinib ranging from 25 to 1000 mg per day. No MTD was reached, and nausea, myalgias, edema, and diarrhea were the most frequent side effects. Remarkably, at a dose of 140 mg or higher, all patients had a hematologic response. At doses of 300 mg per day or greater, 53 of 54 patients had complete hematologic responses, 17 had major cytogenetic responses, and 7 had complete cytogenetic remissions.[144] Numerous subsequent trials demonstrated remarkable activity in CML and CML in accelerated phase, lymphoid or myeloid blast crisis or with Ph+ ALL in adults, including complete molecular responses.[144-148]

On the basis of these data, imatinib became the gold standard for first-line therapy of CML. Nonetheless, resistance to imatinib does occur. In vitro experiments conducted by using randomly mutagenized *ABL* cDNA libraries inserted into sensitive CML cells revealed that a defined spectrum of mutations in the *ABL* gene itself could preserve kinase activity but could disrupt binding to imatinib.[149] More important, sequencing of the *ABL* kinase domain in patients relapsing on imatinib revealed a similar spectrum of mutations in patient samples.[150,151] When these mutations were isolated and placed into ABL kinase constructs and re-inserted into sensitive CML cells in vitro, these mutant ABL constructs also rescued lethality induced by imatinib inhibition. These data, although initially concerning because of the potential for long-term control of the CML disease state, definitively demonstrated in humans the absolute requirement for ABL kinase activity in CML and closed the loop on the notion of a fully validated drug target. Moreover, the identification of such mutants provided the impetus for testing second-generation inhibitors that might overcome these resistance alleles. Here, two separate approaches were

considered. First, although imatinib is a fairly selective inhibitor, it is not a particularly potent inhibitor. Because many mutations shifted the IC_{50} of the kinase activity, it remained possible that a more potent inhibitor might be able to overcome or prevent the emergence of these resistance alleles. Nilotinib is a second-generation inhibitor designed to target BCR-ABL and preserve the interaction with the inhibited form of the ABL kinase, the type II binding mode.[152] Nilotinib is more potent in biochemical and cellular assays of ABL activity and in phase I and phase II trials had significant activity in imatinib-resistant CML.[153] Nilotinib was later demonstrated to be superior to imatinib in patients with newly diagnosed chronic phase CML.[154] Dasatinib, initially developed as a src kinase inhibitor, binds to the "active" form of its kinase targets. Src kinases are highly related to ABL kinase activity, and in vitro testing showed that dasatinib had activity against imatinib-resistance alleles.[155] In phase I and II trials dasatanib has shown significant activity in imatinib-resistant patients.[156] Both dasatinib and nilotinib have gained FDA approval in imatinib-resistant patients with CML and in CML-accelerated phase and blast crisis. Ultimately, both drugs were approved for upfront therapy of patients with CML.[157]

Unfortunately, both nilotinib and dasatinib lack activity against a common but difficult to target *ABL* mutation, the T315I or "gatekeeper" mutation. This mutation creates a steric problem in the adenosine triphosphate–binding domain. This particular kinase domain conformation creates challenges in the drug design process. Notably, it has been difficult to make potent *and* selective inhibitors of this conformation inhibition. Recently, a drug with activity against the T315I mutation, ponatinib, was granted accelerated approval by the FDA for the treatment of adult patients with chronic, accelerated, or blast-phase CML that is resistant or intolerant to prior tyrosine kinase inhibitor therapy or BCR-ABL–positive ALL that is resistant or intolerant to prior tyrosine kinase inhibitor therapy (Fig. 44-3).[158] However, the safety of this drug was later called into question secondary to concerns about drug-related arterial thrombotic events.[159,160]

Imatinib and Other Malignancies. Imatinib, in addition to inhibiting ABL kinase activity, also inhibits c-KIT and platelet-derived growth factor receptor (PDGFR). In preclinical cell line models of gastrointestinal stromal tumors (GIST), a tumor defined by frequent mutations in the *c-KIT* gene, efficacy of imatinib both in vitro and in murine xenograft models was demonstrated.[161] Based on these early preclinical findings, a patient with inoperable, recurrent, and treatment-refractory *c-KIT*-mutated GIST was treated with imatinib. After 4 weeks of therapy, the fludeoxyglucose-positron emission tomography scan showed a complete resolution of tracer uptake compared with the pretreatment scan, and over the ensuing 8 months the patient had a progressive diminution in the tumor volume.[162] Multiple subsequent studies demonstrated response to tyrosine kinase inhibitors in GIST,[163-166] and in 2008 the FDA granted accelerated approved for imatinib in the adjuvant setting for completely resected primary GISTs 3 cm and larger.

Imatinib   Nilotinib

Dasatinib   Ponatinib

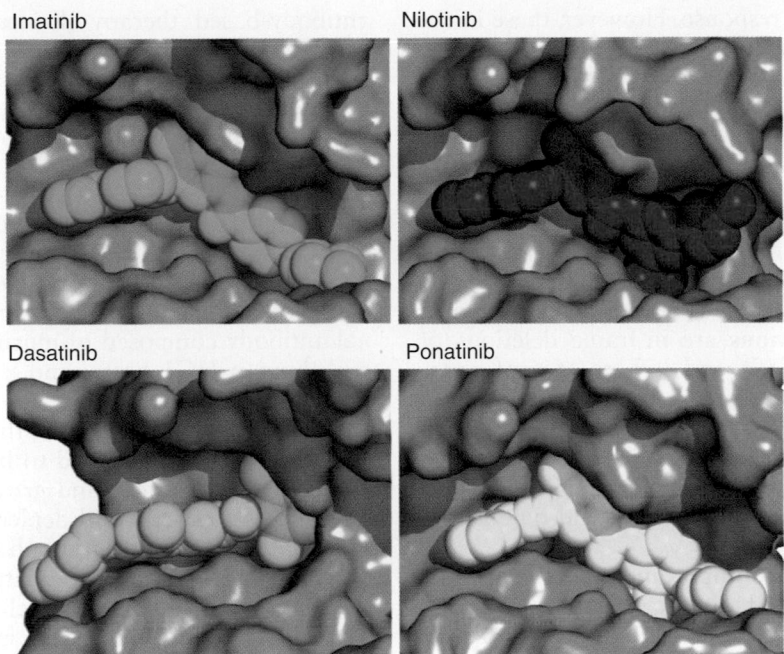

Figure 44-3 Abl inhibitors. Shown are representative structural images of the indicated small molecule inhibitors *(colored)* bound to the ABL kinase domain *(gray)*. Imatinib, nilotinib, and ponatinib are type II inhibitors and contain molecular components that occupy the hydrophobic pocket that is exposed when the kinase is in an "inactive" conformation. Dasatinib is a type I inhibitor and does not have extended interactions with the hydrophobic pocket and instead binds to the "active" conformation of the kinase. *(Courtesy Sandra Jacobson, Novartis Institutes for BioMedical Research, Emeryville, Calif.)*

The activity of imatinib against PDGFR or KIT has enabled clinical development in other diseases characterized as harboring specific genetic alterations activating these receptors. In the case of dermatofibrosarcoma (DFS) the majority of patient lesions harbor translocations between chromosomes 17 and 22 fusing the *PDGFB* ligand gene downstream of the *Col1a* promoter.[167] This leads to constitutive ligand production and receptor activation and sensitivity to imatinib in in vitro models, transplantable primary tumors from patients, and in patients treated with the drug.[168-170] In hypereosinophilic syndrome (HES) Schaller and Burkland report that empiric imatinib treatment of a patient with HES induced a complete and rapid remission of the disease.[171] Similarly, other studies revealed patients with HES responding to imatinib.[172] Gleich and colleagues reported the empiric treatment of five HES patients, four of whom had a prompt and sustained response to imatinib with a resolution of the eosinophilia.[173] The basis for these dramatic observations was uncovered in 2003, when Cools and coworkers reported the discovery of an intrachromosomal deletion that placed *PDGFRA* downstream of the promoter of the *FIP1L1* gene, resulting in constitutive upregulation of the receptor.[174]

The remarkable finding in the examples of the FDA-approval of imatinib for CML, GIST, dermatofibrosarcoma, and HES is that in each case a specific genetic event leads to constitutive activation of a molecular target of imatinib, and in each case a high degree of efficacy is achieved. Moreover, we have learned that efficacy is identified rapidly in selected patient populations, with dramatic responses even in phase I. We have learned that

MTD does not necessarily set the appropriate effective dose, and, indeed, MTD end points were not reached in a number of the early phase I trials.

Dramatic Responses in Select Genotypes. With the success of imatinib for the treatment of patients with CML, a high bar was set for subsequent small-molecule kinase inhibitors. The possibilities that this targeted approach held for the poorly treated adult epithelial malignancies generated great excitement. The EGFR pathway is believed to be important in the development, maintenance, and proliferation of many malignancies, and EGFR is frequently overexpressed in epithelial solid tumors. For these reasons EGFR was an attractive target for small-molecule inhibition. Gefitinib (Iressa) and erlotinib (Tarceva), both orally administered tyrosine kinase inhibitors, were developed to bind competitively at the adenosine triphosphate pocket of EGFR, inhibiting autophosphorylation, and suppressing downstream EGFR signaling. Surprisingly, these EGFR inhibitors have been largely ineffective in the treatment of solid tumors with one exception: the treatment of a subset of patients with non–small cell lung cancer (NSCLC).[175-179]

After these initial clinical studies, numerous reports characterized the clinical predictors of tumor response (as opposed to survival) in patients. It soon became apparent that these patients frequently shared similar demographic features: a nonsmoking history, a well-differentiated adenocarcinoma histology, female sex, and Asian origin, although the underlying genetic reason for these response differences was not known.[178-180] One hypothesis was that expression levels of EGFR correlated with these clinical characteristics and hence response. However, these initial clinical trials failed to identify a correlation between receptor expression and clinical outcome.

Later, in 2004, two research groups independently identified a correlation between mutations in the tyrosine kinase domain of the EGFR and patient responders.[36,181] These *EGFR* mutations enhance ligand-dependent EGFR activation and sensitivity to gefitinib/erlotinib and are more common in nonsmokers, women, Asians, and patients with adenocarcinoma. Approximately 90% of these mutations occur in a few amino acids. Between 45% and 50% of mutations are in-frame deletions of exon 19 (codons 746 to 750), and 35% to 45% of mutations are missense mutation leucine to arginine at codon 858 (L858R) in exon 21.[182-185] Several studies have also reported that patients with EGFR mutant tumors have a longer survival when treated with EGFR small- molecule inhibitors compared with patients with wild-type EGFR tumors.[184,186-188]

This work highlights the importance of developing a molecular understanding of disease and response. The molecular characterization of EGFR abnormalities in NSCLC and their relationship to response to tyrosine kinase inhibitors have been illuminating for the clinical application of targeted therapy. More recently, the dramatic responses seen to B-RAF inhibition in patients with V600E *B-RAF*-mutant melanoma and to ALK inhibition in patients with *EML4-ALK* rearranged lung cancer underscores the critical role of matching tumor genotype with targeted drug therapy (Fig. 44-4).[189,190-192,193]

Lineage-Dependence Examples of Targeted Therapy

Several successful targeted cancer therapies capitalize on the lineage dependence of the tumor as exemplified by antibody-based therapy directed against cancers with hematologic lineage markers such as rituximab (Rituxan). As discussed in the subsequent sections, these therapies have the advantage of target specificity, with predictability of side effects based on the expression pattern of the lineage marker.

Rituximab Therapy for Non-Hodgkin Lymphoma. Rituximab (Rituxan) in 1997 became the first monoclonal antibody approved by the FDA for the treatment of malignancy (NHL). It is a chimeric, anti-CD20 monoclonal antibody composed of murine variable regions fused with human IgG1 heavy and κ light chains. CD20 is a transmembrane protein expressed on normal and malignant mature B lymphocytes[194] thought to be important in calcium transportation and to be involved in B-cell activation, differentiation, and growth regulation.[195] Rituximab binds to CD20 and depletes CD20-positive B cells in the circulation and in lymph nodes.

The first trials evaluating rituximab were in patients with indolent lymphoma, which has no curative therapy. The pivotal multicenter trial in patients with relapsed low-grade or follicular lymphoma demonstrated an overall response rate of 50% and a complete remission rate of 6%. These results were comparable with the best single-agent cytotoxic therapy for relapsed follicular lymphoma.[196] Rituximab has also been evaluated in combination with cytotoxic chemotherapy for patients with indolent B-cell lymphomas. One of the earliest studies, published in 1999, evaluated 40 patients with low-grade or follicular lymphoma treated with six cycles of CHOP (cyclophosphamide, hydroxydaunorubicin, oncovin, and prednisone or prednisolone) and rituximab (R-CHOP). The initial report suggested an additive benefit of

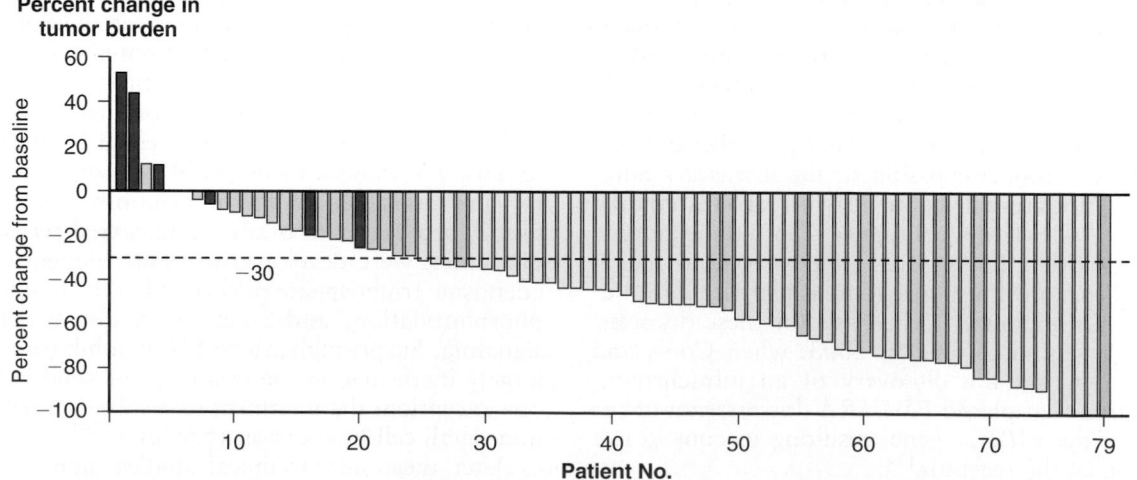

Figure 44-4 Response to ALK inhibition in patients with ALK-positive non–small cell lung cancer. Shown is the best response of patients with *ALK*-positive tumors who were treated with crizotinib, compared with pretreatment baseline. Numbers along the *x* axis indicate arbitrarily assigned patient numbers from 1 to 79. The *bars* indicate the percentage of change in tumor burden from baseline. *Black bars* indicate disease progression, *blue* stable disease, *yellow* partial response, and *orange* complete response. Four patients had complete resolution of their target lesions but were classified as having had a partial response on the basis of stability in nontarget lesions. Eight patients had tumor shrinkage of more than 30% but were classified as having stable disease either because confirmatory scans were not available by the data-cutoff point or early restaging was performed at 6 weeks after crizotinib initiation. The *dashed line* indicates a tumor reduction of 30% from baseline, the minimal percentage of decrease that constitutes a partial response, according to Response Evaluation Criteria in Solid Tumors. *(Modified from Kwak, et al: Anaplastic lymphoma kinase inhibition in non-small-cell lung cancer. N Engl J Med 363:1693–703, 2010.)*

rituximab with no additional toxicity when these two therapies are used in combination.[197] The overall response rate was 95%, and the complete response rate was 55% in the intent-to-treat group. One of the larger clinical trials of 428 patients with previously untreated, advanced-stage follicular lymphoma assigned to CHOP or R-CHOP demonstrated an overall response rate of 90% with CHOP and 96% with R-CHOP and estimated survival rate at 2 years of 90% and 95%, respectively.[198]

The combination of rituximab with cytotoxic chemotherapy has also been evaluated for aggressive NHL. In a randomized phase III study comparing CHOP with R-CHOP in elderly patients with diffuse large B-cell lymphoma, the rate of complete response was higher in the group receiving R-CHOP (76% versus 63%, $P = 0.005$). Furthermore, at 2 years both event-free and overall survival rates were higher in the R-CHOP arm, with no significant additional toxicity.[199] A randomized study of CHOP-like chemotherapy alone or in combination with rituximab in adult patients ages 18 to 60 years with good-prognosis diffuse large B-cell lymphoma demonstrated a 3-year event-free survival rate of 59% with chemotherapy alone versus 79% with the addition of rituximab and at 6 years of 56% and 74%, respectively.[200,201]

Thus R-CHOP is now considered the standard of care for the first-line treatment of CD20-positive diffuse large B-cell lymphoma and for CD20-positive follicular B-cell NHL in combination with chemotherapy. Rituximab is also indicated for the treatment of patients with relapsed or refractory CD20-positive low-grade or follicular NHL.

Host Track Example of Targeted Therapy

Bevacizumab and Colorectal Cancer. Angiogenesis plays an important role in tumor formation. Continued tumor growth is dependent on new blood vessels for the supply of oxygen and critical nutrients. Moreover, certain somatic and germline alterations, including those disrupting the function of the *von Hipple-Landau (VHL)* tumor-suppressor gene, appear to act largely by triggering dysregulated hypoxic and angiogenic responses.[202-205] Over the last several years, numerous angiogenic growth factors have been characterized, including vascular endothelial growth factor (VEGF). VEGF is a member of a large family of dimeric glycoproteins acting as growth factors. It is essential for the normal development of blood vessels and is a growth factor for vascular endothelium.[206,207] VEGF binds to the transmembrane tyrosine kinase receptors VEGFR1, VEGFR2, and VEGFR3. In the malignant state VEGF secreted by the tumor or surrounding stroma leads to endothelial cell proliferation and migration. Because VEGF and its receptors play a critical role in tumor formation, progression, and maintenance, VEGF or VEGFR inhibition became a focus of targeted antiangiogenesis therapy.[208] Several approaches are in development, but the two with the most success thus far are (1) neutralizing antibodies that inhibit the binding of VEGF to its receptors and (2) small-molecule tyrosine kinase inhibitors that block downstream signaling from the VEGFR.

Bevacizumab (Avastin) is a recombinant, humanized monoclonal antibody that binds to VEGF-A, preventing its interaction with the VEGF receptors. It is believed that bevacizumab affects tumor vasculature by several mechanisms: (1) inducing regression of tumor vasculature, (2) normalizing the tumor vasculature, (3) inhibiting new blood vessel formation, and (4) preventing recruitment of progenitor cells from the marrow. It may also improve chemotherapy delivery by altering tumor vasculature and decreasing interstitial pressure.[209] Bevacizumab has been approved by the FDA for first- (2004) and second- (2006) line treatment of patients with metastatic colorectal cancer and the treatment of nonsquamous metastatic lung cancer, although it extends survival by less than 6 months.[210-214]

As with most of the targeted therapies, many of the side effects of bevacizumab were predictable. Some of the reported side effects include hypertension, proteinuria, arterial thromboembolic events, bleeding, poor wound healing, gastrointestinal perforation, and reversible posterior leukoencephalopathy syndrome (RPLS). Most of these side effects are predictable from the known activity of VEGF. For example, VEGF is a homeostatic factor for regulating blood pressure. Blocking of VEGF or VEGFR leads to increased vascular tension and thus problems with hypertension and RPLS. It is interesting to note that the side effects of VEGF inhibition are similar to the signs of preeclampsia and eclampsia (hypertension, proteinuria, and mental status changes), a disease in which soluble VEGFR-1, which antagonizes VEGF functions, has been implicated.[215,216]

Other VEGFR pathway inhibitor development has focused on inhibition of the kinase activity of the VEGF receptor. In December of 2005 the FDA approved the drug sorafenib (Nexavar), a small-molecule VEGFR inhibitor, for the treatment of patients with advanced renal cell carcinoma, and in January of 2006 the FDA approved the multitargeted inhibitor (including VEGFR and KIT) sunitinib (Sutent) for the treatment of patients with both advanced renal cell carcinoma and for patients with GIST who are intolerant of, or who have had disease progression with, imatinib treatment.

The "success" of bevacizumab for colorectal cancer is a humbling one for drug development. In reality, there is a long way to go when the successful drug extends overall survival by less than 6 months. In pediatric cancer care this would hardly be deemed a victory. However, many lessons have been learned from this experience. One is that antiangiogenesis-directed therapy can play a role in some disease treatments. A second is the continued importance of combination therapy, even for targeted therapy. Bevacizumab alone had very little activity. It was in combination with standard cytotoxic agents that a clinical benefit was demonstrated. Third, careful evaluation of targeted therapy benefits and toxicities may provide new insight into human disease.

Empiric or Synthetic Lethal

As described previously, classical chemotherapy is likely to exploit cancer-dependent states that are not fully understood. For example, microtubule inhibitors, such as the taxanes, specifically interact with protein components of microtubules and are efficacious in a number of cancers, although there is no current scientific rationale for their selective efficacy. A number of emerging targeted therapeutics target highly selective protein targets involved in diverse basic cellular processes and were elaborated according to specific synthetic lethal hypotheses.

Histone Deacetylase Inhibitors. Histone deacetylase (HDAC) inhibitors are an example of an empirically acting targeted agent. Transcriptional repression and transcriptional activation, at least in part, reflect the balance of histone modification of chromatin structures surrounding gene regulatory regions. Histone acetylation is of particular importance. In many cases transcriptional activators recruit histone acetylase activity to gene regulatory regions, whereas transcriptional repression complexes typically recruit HDAC to the same regions. In keeping with the notion that repression might underlie the function of oncogenic transcription factor translocations, HDAC enzymes are recruited to the critical promoters by various translocation partners, including RARα and ETO. These data provide a compelling rationale for the development and testing of HDAC inhibitors. In keeping with the underlying concept of synthetic lethality, it is possible to hypothesize an enhanced dependence on, or constitutive requirement for, HDAC enzymes by the aforementioned repressive oncogenes. Although the original therapeutic concept evolved from a link between leukemogenesis and transcriptional repression, a large array of proteins are now known to be modulated through acetylation at the hands of 11 related HDACs.[217] This will invariably create difficulty in elucidating the underlying therapeutic mechanisms linked to the anticancer activity now observed in the clinic with relatively broad-acting HDAC inhibitors.

An array of HDAC inhibitors targeting the major classes of HDAC enzymes are now in the clinic. The majority of these inhibitors have a core hydroxamate structure that sits deep in the enzymatic pocket, making contacts with a key coordinated zinc atom in the enzyme. The most advanced of these compounds, vorinostat (suberoylanilide hydroxamic acid [SAHA]), was approved for the treatment of cutaneous T-cell lymphoma (CTCL).[218] In initial phase I studies testing vorinostat, diarrhea, anorexia, dehydration, and fatigue were found to be the limiting side effects. Thrombocytopenia was also frequent.[219] Based on early evidence of efficacy in patients with CTCL, a phase II trial of vorinostat was conducted exploring three dose levels.[218] Eight of 33 patients achieved a partial response. A phase IIB multicenter trial was subsequently conducted. In this trial of 74 patients who had all progressed or relapsed on at least two prior treatment regimens, 30% achieved an objective response and 77% of patients had some measure of disease improvement. One patient achieved a complete response.[220] These data provided the basis for the FDA approval of vorinostat for CTCL in 2006.

Romidepsin (depsipeptide, FR901228, FK228), a natural product bicyclic depsipeptide originally isolated from a broth culture of *Chromobacterium violaceum,* was discovered to have potent transcriptional activation properties and to be a potent inhibitor of HDAC enzymatic activity.[221] In the early clinical experiences with romidepsin, in addition to the observed toxicities with HDAC inhibitors discussed previously, cardiac abnormalities were also reported.[222,223] In a phase I trial conducted in pediatric patients taking romidepsin, the dose-limiting toxicities were T-wave inversions and transient sick sinus syndrome, which were asymptomatic.[224] In phase II trials romidepsin was tested in patients with neuroendocrine tumors and in patients with metastatic renal cell carcinoma. The neuroendocrine study was terminated because of serious cardiac adverse events, including ventricular arrythmias and prolonged QTc.[225] In the renal cancer trial, prolonged QTc interval (two), grade 3 atrial fibrillation and tachycardia (one), and sudden death (one) were observed.[226] There was insufficient antitumor activity to warrant further development in these indications. A phase II trial of romidepsin in patients with CTCL reported an overall response rate of 38%.[227] In 2009 the FDA approved romidepsin for CTCL in patients who have received at least one prior systemic therapy. Similarly, panobinostat (LBH589), a synthetic hydroxamic acid–based small-molecule inhibitor that was specifically designed as part of a drug-discovery effort directed at producing a pan-HDAC inhibitor, has been demonstrated to have activity in patients with CTCL but also to have the potential liability of cardiac toxicity.[228]

It is clear from the summation of these emerging data that HDAC inhibition results in significant activity in CTCL, although the reason for this empiric observation remains obscure. HDAC inhibitors are now being tested more widely in other solid tumor and hematologic malignancies. The key to these studies will be the elucidation of effective yet well-tolerated dosing regimens.

NEW AND EMERGING OPPORTUNITIES IN PEDIATRIC CANCER

Targeted therapies have been introduced into the pediatric cancer therapeutic arsenal.[229] Thus far, nearly all of these agents have already been tested in the adult community. Several have had success in the pediatric setting where the potential target is shared by the phenotypically identical adult and pediatric tumor, such as ATRA for children with APL,[230,231] imatinib for BCR-ABL–rearranged CML[232] and ALL,[233] and rituximab for lymphoma.[234,235] There are many targets—those shared by both adult and pediatric malignancies and targets specific to pediatric cancers—not yet thoroughly explored with targeted approaches. In the following sections we will discuss these new and emerging targets and the special considerations in bringing targeted therapy to the pediatric setting (Box 44-8).

Special Considerations in Targeted Therapy Development for Children
Majority of Children with Cancer Are Cured

There are numerous special considerations in the development of targeted therapy for pediatric cancer. In contrast to adults with cancer, the majority of children with cancer will be cured of the malignancy, making the selection of pediatric patients for testing of new targeted

Box 44-8   Special Considerations in Pediatric Targeted Therapy Development

1. Most children with cancer are cured.
2. Pediatric cancer is rare.
   a. Market incentive is reduced.
   b. Clinical trial design and accrual are difficult.
   c. Limited number of agents can be reasonably tested
3. Toxicity may be specific to developmental stage.
4. Ethical considerations are more difficult.
   a. Informed consent for experimental therapy must be obtained.
   b. Informed consent for participation in biological study must be obtained.

therapies more challenging and raising the required level of activity necessary for "success." For example, in de novo pediatric pre–B-cell ALL, with cure rates greater than 80%, it is difficult to introduce a new targeted agent for fear of detracting from an already excellent cure rate by diluting curative agents. Although there are many interesting new targets emerging, such as *PAX5* and other genes important in B-cell developmental pathways,[236] it would be difficult to justify the inclusion of upfront novel targeted therapy in patients with this excellent outcome. Thus it is likely in the relapsed setting, or in de novo disease with poor outcome, that novel targeted therapies will undergo initial testing. If efficacy and safety are demonstrated, researchers may then consider incorporation into upfront clinical trials.

Pediatric Cancer Is Rare

A total of 1,660,290 new diagnoses of cancer and 580,350 cancer deaths are projected to occur in the United States in 2013.[237] In contrast, it is estimated that only 14,023 children in the United States younger than age 20 years were diagnosed with cancer in 2009, and 1964 died of cancer in 2009.[238] Hence pediatric cancers are quite rare compared with adult malignancies, and there is a reduced market incentive for pediatric-specific targeted drug development by the pharmaceutical industry. Furthermore, researchers have been understandably hesitant to test new drugs in children. For these reasons, there are virtually no drugs that have been developed specifically for pediatric malignancies. Even when a common target has been identified in adult and pediatric cancer, it may be years before a drug reaches a pediatric trial. Because pediatric cancers are rare, even with a drug in hand to test, clinical trials are difficult. A rare disease incidence means slow accrual of patients and necessitates large cooperative groups to power the trial with appropriate patient numbers. The limited number of patients also precludes testing of all possible new agents. New methods are needed to more rationally choose novel targeted agents for testing in children.

One national attempt to prioritize the selection of new agents for testing in children with cancer was the development of the Pediatric Preclinical Testing Program (PPTP) by the National Cancer Institute. This group is prospectively testing new agents against a panel of xenografts and genetic models of pediatric cancer, such as neuroblastoma, rhabdomyosarcoma, osteosarcoma, and ALL. The PPTP builds on earlier work demonstrating the ability of preclinical testing of new agents in rhabdomyosarcoma and neuroblastoma xenografts to predict in vivo activity in children with these malignancies.[239,240] The development of new genetically engineered models of pediatric cancer should also facilitate preclinical evaluation of targeted therapies and better prioritization of new agents for clinical trial, particularly for diseases such as Ewing sarcoma, for which no such model yet exists.

Developmental Considerations in Targeted Therapy for Children

Children may tolerate targeted therapies differently from adults secondary to age-specific differences in physiology that result in altered pharmacokinetics or to drug interference with critical developmental pathways. In normal development, vascularization of cartilage is prominent during embryogenesis and during periods of growth when neoangiogenesis occurs at growth plates.[241,242] Inhibition of VEGF signaling has been reported in animal models to result in thickening of the epiphyseal growth plates secondary to an expansion of the hypertrophic chondrocyte zone.[243,244] These findings have been attributed to a delayed vascular invasion of the epiphyseal growth plate with a subsequent reduced rate of chondrocyte apoptosis. Inhibition of VEGF signaling has also been reported to impair trabecular bone formation, induce dental dysplasia, and cause ovarian atrophy.[245] Although the animal data are concerning, the actual long-term effects of this class of drug on human children is unknown.

Ethical Considerations in Targeted Therapy for Children

The testing of drugs in children raises issues universal to cytotoxic and targeted therapies, as well as challenges more specific to targeted treatments. Adults can make informed decisions about the risk and potential benefit of experimental therapies and biological studies and actively participate in treatment decisions. Particularly for young children, however, true informed consent from the patients for experimental therapies cannot be obtained. Here it is the parent or legal guardian making decisions about participation in a trial. In light of this potential conflict of interest, special regulations have been instituted to afford additional protection to children. These include the Code of Federal Regulations, Part 46; Protection of Human Subjects, Subpart D; and the related FDA regulation, Part 50, Protection of Human Subjects, Subpart D. These regulations outline allowable research in children based on the risk to the child, potential benefit to the child or other children, and alternative therapies. In the testing of targeted therapies, pharmacodynamic studies with sampling of tumor tissue before and after therapy initiation become more critical. For obvious reasons these studies can be difficult to perform with the current regulations, particularly for solid tumors or brain tumors. In general, tissue collection in children for the purpose of biological studies must be considered no greater than a minor increase in minimal risk. Innovative methods are needed to evaluate pharmacodynamic response, such as new imaging technologies, and better methods are needed to assess surrogate tissues.

Emerging Genetic Targets in Pediatric Cancer

Significant progress has been made in our understanding of the pediatric leukemias and solid tumors. As such, numerous potential genetic targets have emerged over the past 10 years. In light of the excellent cure rates for some pediatric malignancies, it might be difficult to incorporate target-directed therapies associated with good outcome genetic lesions, such as *TEL-AML1* in pediatric ALL. In these early stages of targeted therapy for pediatric malignancies, the focus will likely be on lesions associated with poor outcome. In the following section we will discuss some of these genetic lesions with potential for therapeutic targeting.

FLT3 and the Acute Leukemias

Although much progress has been made in the treatment of childhood leukemias, patients with AML with mutations in the Fms-like tyrosine kinase 3 *(FLT3)* gene remain a high-risk group. FLT3 is a class III receptor tyrosine kinase that plays a critical role in normal hematopoiesis and shares structural homology with PDGFR, c-KIT, and CSF1R. Upon the binding of FLT3 ligand, wild-type receptors dimerize and become activated by phosphorylation, leading to activation of downstream signal transduction pathways. Mutations in *FLT3* can be identified in blasts from 30% of adult patients with AML with constitutive activation of the kinase resulting from internal tandem duplications (ITD) in the juxtamembrane domain or point mutations in the activation loop.[246] The *FLT3* ITD is present in 15% and *FLT3* point mutations in 7% of pediatric AML, and children with FLT3 ITD have a particularly poor prognosis.[247,248]

FLT3 has also been implicated as a target in pediatric patients with *MLL*-rearranged ALL. Gene-expression profiling studies comparing *MLL*-rearranged ALL with all other ALL and AML have demonstrated a unique expression profile for *MLL*-rearranged leukemia. *FLT3* is the gene most frequently overexpressed in *MLL*-rearranged leukemia compared with the other acute leukemias.[249,250] An initial study reported mutations in *FLT3* in approximately 15% of samples of *MLL*-rearranged ALL. All of these were point mutations in the activation loop, including mutations not previously reported in patients with AML (deletion of isoleucine 836). These mutations lead to constitutive activation of the kinase and increased sensitivity to small-molecule inhibitors of FLT3. Furthermore, *MLL*-rearranged lymphoblasts with high levels of wild-type FLT3 were sensitive to the FLT3 inhibitor PKC412.[251] Subsequent studies have reported an incidence of *FLT3* mutations in infant MLL samples ranging from 3% to 18%. These studies also confirmed increased expression of FLT3 in *MLL*-rearranged infant ALL compared with both infant and noninfant patients with germline *MLL*. Even in the absence of documented mutation, a high level of FLT3 expression was associated with FLT3 ligand independence and with increased sensitivity to the FLT3 inhibitor PKC412.[252,253] In addition to its role as a target in *MLL*-rearranged ALL, FLT3 is a potential target in children with T-cell ALL (T-ALL), particularly with early precursor T-ALL, and in children with hyperdiploid ALL, wherein *FLT3* mutations have been reported.[253-257]

Several FLT3 inhibitors have been tested in clinical trials for adults with AML.[258-263] Most of the early trials testing these compounds have had some transient responders with decreased peripheral blood or marrow blasts, and the compounds have generally been well tolerated. However, very few patients enter a complete remission, and the majority of patients eventually progress. The high rate of initial response failure, as well as the development of progressive disease despite an initial clinical response, has tempered enthusiasm for FLT3 inhibitors in AML.[264] There are several possible explanations for the lack of dramatic clinical responses, including issues related to pharmacology and the failure to achieve sustained, complete inhibition of FLT3.[265,266] Another explanation is the acquisition of resistance mutations in *FLT3* itself. Indeed, the newer drug quizartinib (AC220), with greater potency and sustained inhibition of FLT3, has had promising initial results in clinical trials.[267] Moreover, point mutations within the kinase domain of *FLT3*-ITD, conferring quizartinib resistance, were recently reported.[268] This finding is similar to the emergence of *BCR-ABL*–resistance mutations in patients with CML treated with imatinib. Significantly, this study provided gold-standard validation that FLT3-ITD is an oncogenic driver of AML.

The clinical study of FLT3 inhibitors in children with leukemia is ongoing. A phase I trial testing the multikinase inhibitor sorafenib, with activity against FLT3, in children with refractory solid tumors and leukemia, was reported by the Children's Oncology Group (COG).[269] This trial established a recommended phase II dose of sorafenib for children with leukemias. Rash, diarrhea, and liver enzyme elevation were the most common sorafenib-related toxicities. Two patients with AML with the FLT3-ITD achieved less than 5% bone marrow blasts with 4 or 5 cycles of sorafenib. A second phase I trial evaluated the effects of sorafenib in combination with clofarabine and cytarabine in children with relapsed or refractory leukemia.[270] On day 8 of this trial, 10 of 12 patients demonstrated a decrease in blast percentage after sorafenib alone. After combination chemotherapy, six patients (three of these with FLT3-ITD) achieved a complete remission, two with FLT3-ITD had a complete remission with incomplete count recovery, and one patient with FLT3 wild-type had a partial remission. This trial also demonstrated downregulation of AKT, RPS6, and 4E-BP1 phosphorylation in leukemic blasts. Finally, there was another report of three patients with relapsed FLT3-ITD AML who achieved a sustained remission with sorafenib in combination with other cytotoxic chemotherapy.[271] Based on these encouraging initial results, there are now multiple ongoing trials to test the efficacy of FLT3 inhibitors in pediatric patients with leukemia.

JAK Mutations in Pediatric Leukemia

With the marked success of imatinib in the treatment of *BCR-ABL*-rearranged ALL in children (Fig. 44-5), there has been interest in the identification of other kinase abnormalities in childhood cancers, including leukemia.[233] Recurrent mutations in Janus kinases (JAKs) have

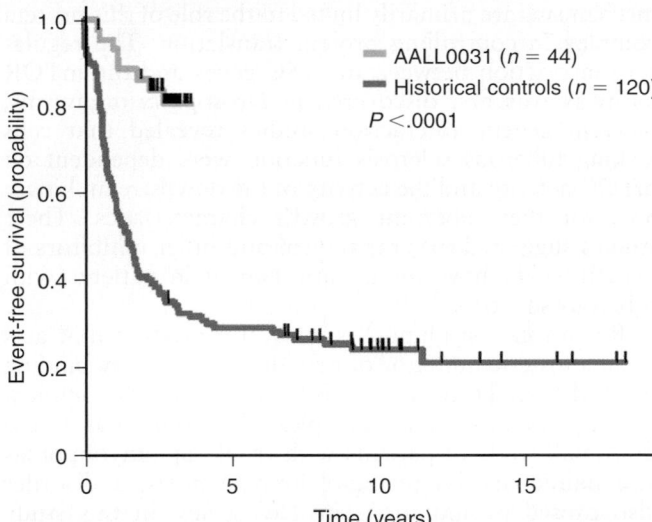

Figure 44-5 Early event-free survival in patients with Philadelphia chromosome–positive acute lymphoblastic leukemia treated with imatinib. Treated patients in cohort 5 (*n* = 44) were compared with patients previously treated on Pediatric Oncology Group protocols AL inC 14, 15, and 16 from January 1986 through November 1999 (*n* = 120). *(Modified from Schultz, et al: Improved early event-free survival with imatinib in Philadelphia chromosome-positive acute lymphoblastic leukemia: a children's oncology group study.* J Clin Oncol 27:5175-5181, 2009.)

emerged as immediately targetable in a subset of pediatric patients with leukemia. JAKs phosphorylate substrates, including STAT proteins, on ligand binding to a type I cytokine receptor, leading to altered transcription of growth-enhancing and anti-apoptotic genes. Interest in targeting JAK2 was sparked by the finding of recurrent *JAK2* mutations (most frequently involving valine 617) in patients with myeloproliferative disorders.[81-83,272] Subsequently, activating mutations in *JAK2* and *JAK3* were reported in patients with AML and Down syndrome–associated acute megakaryoblastic leukemia[273,274] and in 18% to 28% of patients with Down syndrome–associated ALL.[275-278] In the case of Down syndrome–associated ALL, the mutations affect a highly conserved arginine residue (R683) in the pseudokinase domain of JAK2 and have been demonstrated to induce JAK/STAT activation and promote growth factor independence in BaF3 cells and response to JAK inhibitors.

In a subgroup of pediatric patients with poor-outcome ALL, a gene expression signature similar to that observed in patients with *BCR-ABL*–rearranged ALL was identified by genome-wide expression profiling in patients lacking the *BCR-ABL* rearrangement.[279] It was hypothesized that these *BCR-ABL*–negative cases might harbor other kinase abnormalities. Indeed, recurrent mutations in *JAK1*, *JAK2*, and *JAK3* were identified in approximately 11% of patients with high-risk B-precursor ALL (B-ALL), with mutations in *JAK2* being the most common.[280,281] As was seen in Down syndrome, the mutations in *JAK2* frequently involved the R683 residue. Mutations in *JAK2* are also frequently associated with overexpression of CRLF2 (cytokine receptor–like factor 2), a type I cytokine receptor subunit also referred to as

thymic stromal lymphopoietic receptor.[282,283] Overexpression of CRLF2 has been linked to genomic rearrangement of *CRLF2* by way of a translocation of the immunoglobulin heavy chain (*IGH*) gene and by way of an interstitial deletion centromeric of *CRLF2* that results in a P2RY8-CRLF2 fusion.

There has been some controversy regarding the prognostic significance of *CRLF2* overexpression/genomic lesions and *JAK* mutations. In a study of 1061 pediatric patients with B-precursor ALL (both high risk and standard risk) treated on COG trials, it was found that only 50% of patients with high CRLF2 expression had *CRLF2* genomic lesions; the reason for high CRLF2 in the other 50% remains unclear. All *CRLF2* genomic lesions and nearly all *JAK* mutations were observed in samples with high CRLF2 expression. In this study high CRLF2 expression was associated with a very poor outcome in the high-risk patients with ALL but not in the standard-risk patients.[284] Thus targeting of JAKs, particularly JAK2, is of interest given its association with CRLF2 overexpression and poor outcome and the preclinical data supporting activity of JAK inhibitors in *JAK*-mutated ALL.[285] Clinical trials testing JAK inhibitors in pediatric patients are now ongoing.

ALK in Anaplastic Large Cell Lymphoma and Neuroblastoma

The discovery of the recurrent translocation t(2;5) (p23;q35) in anaplastic large cell lymphoma led to the cloning of *ALK*, a novel tyrosine kinase, as the key oncogene dysregulated by the gene fusion. Subsequently, *ALK* was found to be the transforming partner fused to the *EML4* promoter in approximately 4% of patients with adenocarcinoma of the lung[189] and to be activated by point mutations in neuroblastoma[286] and in inflammatory myoblastic tumors.[287,288] These data, in particular the findings in lung adenocarcinoma, triggered attempts to exploit this genetic information for therapeutic gain. Cells driven by the EML4-ALK fusion were shown to be sensitive to ALK inhibition in the original work describing the fusion event,[189] and it was known that crizotinib, originally developed as a MNNG HOS transforming gene (MET) inhibitor, was also a potent ALK inhibitor. Indeed, crizotinib showed significant preclinical efficacy in models of anaplastic lymphoma.[289] These data led to the rapid clinical testing of crizotinib in patients with lung adenocarcinoma tumors bearing ALK fusions. In the phase I testing of crizotinib, there was an overall response rate of 57%, including one complete response, and an additional 33% of patients achieved disease stabilization.[190] These data led to a randomized phase III trial comparing crizotinib with chemotherapy in patients with tumors harboring *ALK* translocations. In this trial the response rate to crizotinib was 65% compared with 20% in the chemotherapy arm (*P* >.001) and progression-free survival was 7.7 months in the crizotinib-treated patients compared with 3 months in the chemotherapy group.[290] Crizotinib received FDA market approval for the treatment of ALK-positive lung adenocarcinoma in August of 2011.

Crizotinib has recently been tested in pediatric patients with solid tumors enriched for those with ALK alterations.[291] The investigators enrolled 79 patients with a diversity of tumor types in children with an average age of 10.1 years. Crizotinib was well tolerated in children. Efficacy was marked in patients with tumor types known to harbor genetic alterations in *ALK*. In nine patients with anaplastic lymphoma, there were eight responders, including seven who responded completely and one whose disease remained stable. In addition, three of seven patients with inflammatory myofibroblastic tumors also responded to crizotinib, and the remainder all had stable disease. One patient (out of 11) with neuroblastoma also had a response. In summary, crizotinib is a promising agent in pediatric patients with these diseases.

In adenocarcinoma of the lung, treatment with crizotinib, although achieving marked efficacy, is eventually associated with the development of therapeutic resistance. In some cases this is accompanied by point mutations in the kinase domain creating specific resistance to the binding of the drug. Significantly, the most common de novo mutation in *ALK* observed in children with neuroblastoma is the *ALK* F1174L, a mutation reported to engender crizotinib resistance. Novel ALK inhibitors are now entering clinical trials in the hopes of both overcoming resistance and improving on the upfront therapy of tumors bearing genetic alterations in *ALK*. NVP-LDK378 is a selective ALK inhibitor that is more potent than crizotinib and has activity against some of the resistance mutations seen with crizotinib.[292] In a phase I trial of NVP-LDK378 in adults, both crizotinib-naïve and crizotinib-refractory patients were enrolled on ascending doses. Among 88 patients receiving doses greater than 400 mg daily, the overall response rate was 70% with a response rate of 73% in the crizotinib-refractory setting. NVP-LDK378 was well tolerated in this trial. On the basis of these data, the FDA granted Breakthrough designation to LDK387 in March 2013. Early clinical data for AP26113, a second-generation ALK inhibitor that also inhibits EGFR, have been reported. Here, among 18 evaluable ALK-positive patients there were 10 responses. In the 12 patients previously treated with an ALK inhibitor, eight patients responded (67%).[293] Finally, the ALK inhibitor CH5424802 showed a remarkable 93.5% response rate in Japanese patients with ALK-positive lung cancer not previously treated with crizotinib.[294] The evolution of this field has been rapid and promises to bring highly active ALK inhibitors to pediatric patients with *ALK*-mutant cancers, including anaplastic lymphoma, neuroblastoma, and inflammatory myoblastic tumors.

Mammalian Target of Rapamycin in Tuberous Sclerosis

Tuberous sclerosis is a rare disorder characterized by skin and mucosal manifestations, including angiofibromas and subungual fibromas and by central nervous system manifestations, including cortical tubers and a high incidence of seizures. Two notable tumors in this disorder are renal angiomyolipomas and subependymal giant cell astrocytoma (SEGA). Tuberous sclerosis arises from inactivating germline mutations in the tumor-suppressor genes *TSC1* or *TSC2*. The protein products of these genes, known as hamartin and tuberin, are negative regulators of the kinase known as mTOR, a critical regulator of cell growth and cell size. These cellular control mechanisms are primarily linked to the role of this protein complex in controlling protein translation. The regulatory interaction between the TSC genes and the mTOR pathway was first discovered in *Drosophila* organisms, wherein genetic interaction studies revealed that cells lacking tuberous sclerosis function were dependent on mTOR activity and the activity of the downstream kinase S6K for their aberrant growth characteristics. These studies suggested that rapamycin and other inhibitors of mTOR might have therapeutic benefit in patients with tuberous sclerosis.[295,296]

Rapamycin (sirolimus) is a natural product that acts as an allosteric inhibitor of mTOR. It does so by binding to FKBP12 and recruiting FKBP12 to the mTOR complex, creating an inactivated complex. Sirolimus was tested in a small study of patients with renal angiomyolipomas and pulmonary lymphangioleiomyomatosis, a disorder also caused by mutations in *TSC* genes. In this study five patients with renal angiomyolipomas had a tumor response over a 24-month period.[297] Everolimus is a derivative of rapamycin that has improved oral availability and demonstrated efficacy and market approval in a number of adult malignancies, including renal cell carcinoma, neuroendocrine tumors, and breast cancer. Everolimus has been tested in patients with tuberous sclerosis who have either angiomyolipomas or SEGA tumors. In a phase III randomized trial 35% of patients with SEGA (EXIST-1) responded to everolimus compared with 0% in the placebo control arm. Significantly, no patients in the treated arm progressed during the trial.[298] Similarly, in a phase III trial (EXIST-2) patients with angiomyolipoma had a response rate of 42% in the everolimus-treated arm compared with 0% in the placebo control arm.[299] On the basis of these data, everolimus was approved for use in these indications.

In earlier uncontrolled studies there was evidence of a reduction in seizure frequency that appeared independent of the effect on SEGA tumor volume reduction. This raised the possibility that ongoing dysregulation of mTOR signaling in the central nervous system could contribute directly to seizure frequency. To further understand these findings, a phase II study examining seizure frequency was conducted. Here, everolimus reduced the seizure frequency by 50% or more in 12 of 20 patients, and in total 17 of the 20 patients experienced seizure reduction with an overall median decrease of 73% ($P < .001$).[300] Together these data support the notion that everolimus is a highly effective agent in the treatment of SEGA and angiomyolipomas in children with tuberous sclerosis disease. In addition, everolimus might be effective in seizure control, although additional randomized data will be required.

RAS Pathway Activation and Inhibition in Childhood Cancers

Genetic alterations leading to activation of the RAS-MAPK pathway are frequent in pediatric cancers and precancer syndromes. Germline mutations in RAS pathway components, including *NF1*, *KRAS*, *NRAS*, *SHP2* (*PTPN11*), *MEK2*, *SHOC2*, and *CBL*, result in a set of related disorders known collectively as "RASopathies." These disorders include neurofibromatosis, Noonan syndrome,

LEOPARD syndrome, Costello syndrome, cardiofaciocutaneous syndrome, and Legius syndrome.[301] Moreover, somatic activating mutations in *KRAS* and *NRAS* are also common in a diversity of pediatric tumors. Juvenile myelomonocytic leukemia (JMML), in both syndromic and nonsyndromic forms, appears to be a disease wherein RAS is activated in nearly all settings. In this disorder loss-of-function mutations in *NF1*, gain-of-function mutations in *SHP2*, and activating mutations in *RAS* genes all lead to constitutive RAS pathway activation.[302] In B-ALL, mutations in *NRAS* and *KRAS* are among the most common mutations found.[281,303] Similarly, *NRAS*, *KRAS*, *BRAF*, *SHP2*, and *NF1* are, in aggregate, frequently mutated in pediatric T-ALL.[257] In pediatric AML activating mutations in *NRAS* are seen in 10% of patients.[304]

Outside of the hematologic malignancies, recent discoveries highlight the role of alterations in BRAF, a key immediate downstream mediator of RAS signaling. In pilocytic astrocytoma duplications of the *BRAF* locus occurred in 28 of 53 patients (53%).[62] This genomic rearrangement results in a *KIAA1549-BRAF* fusion gene and constitutive activation of BRAF. Another surprising discovery was the finding of the oncogenic mutation *BRAFV600E*, most commonly seen in melanoma, in 57% of patients with Langerhans cell histiocytosis[63] and 50% of patients with the related disorder Erdheim-Chester disease.[305] In aggregate, both germline and somatic genetic alterations in RAS pathway components frequently occur in pediatric cancers, and these observations strongly support the rationale for testing RAS pathway inhibitors in these pediatric indications.

Emerging data from the targeted treatment of adult patients with melanoma suggest that we divide the therapeutic approach to the RAS pathway into two distinct categories: *BRAF* mutant tumors and those tumors with direct *RAS* mutation or with upstream genetic events (e.g., *NF1*) that lead to RAS activation. BRAF inhibitors have had dramatic efficacy in patients with melanoma bearing the V600E *BRAF* mutation.[306,307] These data have led to the market approval of vemurafenib and dabrafenib. In the NRAS or KRAS setting, however, BRAF inhibitors are not effective. In addition, the current generation of BRAF inhibitors all share the property of *activating* rather than inhibiting other RAF family members (CRAF or ARAF), especially in the setting of *KRAS* mutation. Hence although in the setting of *BRAF* mutation these drugs indeed turn off pathway signaling and lead to tumor regression, in settings of the wild-type RAS pathway or in the setting of *KRAS* mutation the drugs lead to pathway activation. Indeed, this so-called paradoxical activation results in a plethora of vemurafenib-mediated dermatologic side effects, including the induction of keratoacanthomas. In addition, at least one patient was found to have a *KRAS* mutant leukemia while on therapy for metastatic melanoma. Withdrawal of the vemurafenib led to partial regression of the leukemia,[308] suggesting that the drug was inducing tumor growth. These findings imply that the use of BRAF inhibitors is likely to be restricted to indications in which *BRAF* itself is mutated.

Studies attempting to elucidate the mechanisms of resistance to BRAF inhibition, both preclinical and clinical, have identified a number of alterations leading to therapeutic resistance primarily linked to activation of downstream signaling by MEK or ERK. These observations have led to combination clinical trials in which MEK inhibition has been combined with BRAF inhibition. Although many such trials are under way, the most advanced is the trial of dabrafenib and the MEK inhibitor trametinib. A phase II randomized study comparing this combination with dabrafenib alone found that median progression-free survival rate was increased from 5.8 months to 9.4 months. In addition, the response rate increased from 54% to 76%. Notably, the incidence of skin manifestations caused by "paradoxical activation" was significantly reduced, and hence the combination was well-tolerated.[309] These data suggest that the BRAF/MEK inhibitor combination will become a standard of care for *BRAF*-mutant melanoma.

Do these findings apply to pediatric patients? At the time of this review, phase I trials of dabrafenib and vemurafenib were ongoing in pediatric patients. Although results in pilocytic astrocytoma were not yet reported, Haroche and coworkers reported treating three patients with Erdheim-Chester disease with vemurafenib. For all three patients, treatment led to substantial and rapid clinical improvement, with tumor responses confirmed by imaging studies.[310] These exciting results support the notion that BRAF inhibition will find significant clinical utility in these disorders.

Therapeutic intervention in tumors driven by RAS or upstream activation event has proved more challenging. It has not been possible to develop direct inhibitors of RAS. Therefore current efforts are focused on interrupting the outputs of oncogenic RAS, including downstream effectors in the MAP kinase pathway, such as MEK, or downstream effectors in the PI3K pathway, such as PI3K or mTOR. In adult *NRAS*-mutant melanoma there is evidence for activity of MEK inhibitors, notably MEK162 which had a 20% response rate among *NRAS*-mutant patients in a phase II trial in melanoma.[311] In pediatric patients MEK inhibitor phase I trials are under way primarily in glioma, but on the basis of preclinical data there is also strong support for the clinical testing of MEK inhibitors in JMML.[312] As mentioned previously, mutations in the *NF1* gene result in activation of RAS. To date, most therapeutic interventions have focused on inhibiting mTOR downstream of RAS in patients with type 1 neurofibromatosis. Although clinical trials are progressing, no results have been reported. As in the case of *BRAF*-mutant tumors, it is likely that combination therapy will be required. In this case there is a rationale for testing the combinations of mTOR or PI3K pathway inhibitors and MEK inhibitors in pediatric disorders resulting from RAS activation.

Notch1 in T-ALL

With intensive chemotherapy the majority of children with T-ALL will be cured. However, ALL is still a leading cause of death from cancer in children, and intensive chemotherapy is not without toxicity. One important

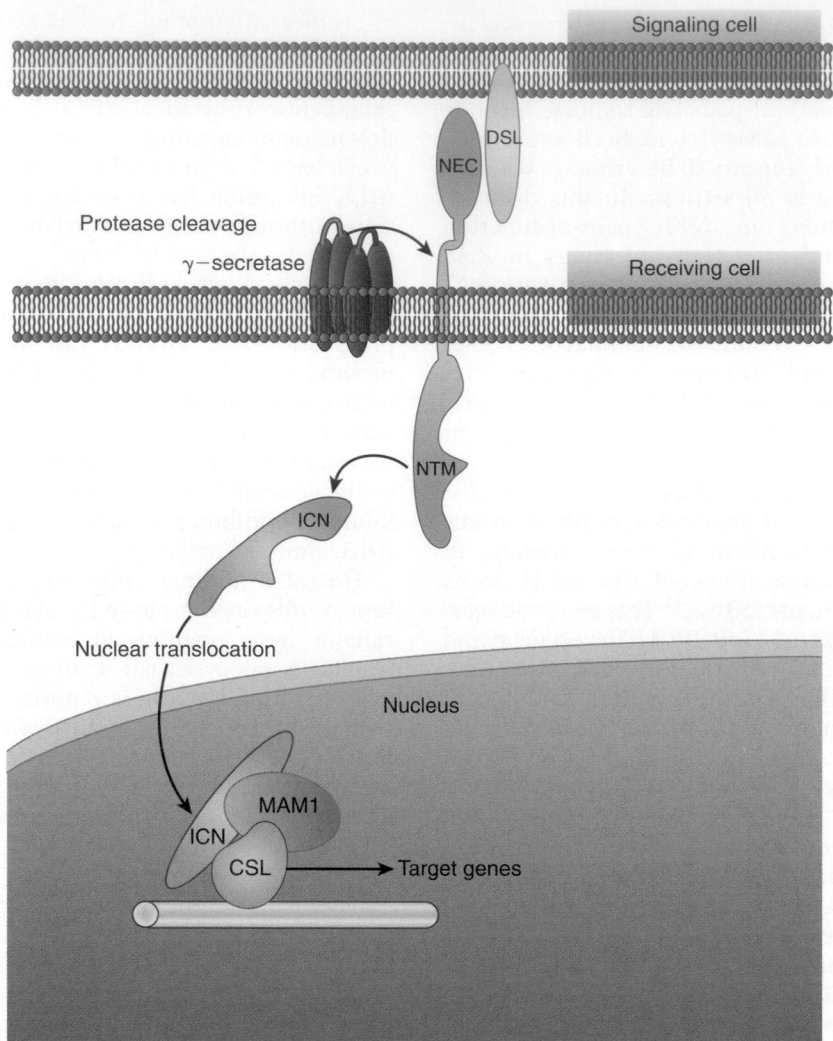

Figure 44-6 Notch1 signaling. Notch is activated by the binding of the ligands of the Delta-Serrate-Lag2 (DSL) family, which trigger a series of proteolytic cleavages. Notch receptors are cleaved by ADAM metalloproteases producing two noncovalently associated subunits, NEC and NTM. Next, cleavage by γ-secretase releases the intracellular domain of Notch (ICN), which translocates to the nucleus and forms a transcriptional activation complex with CSL and Mastermind-like (MAM1) cofactors. *CSL,* CBF1, Suppressor of Hairless, Lag-1; *NEC,* notch extracellular subunit; *NTM,* notch transmembrane subunit.

target in T-ALL is Notch1. *NOTCH1* encodes a transmembrane receptor required for T-cell differentiation and for the assembly of pre–T-cell receptor complexes in immature thymocytes (Fig. 44-6). Notch is activated by the binding of ligands of the Delta-Serrate-Lag2 (DSL) family that triggers a series of proteolytic cleavages, with the last step catalyzed by the γ-secretase complex, releasing the intracellular domain of Notch (ICN) into the cytoplasm, for subsequent translocation to the nucleus. Once in the nucleus, Notch acts as a transcriptional activator complexed with the DNA-binding protein CSL (CBF1, Suppressor of Hairless, Lag-1) and the transcriptional co-activators of the Mastermind-like family (MAML1).[313,314]

The oncogenic role of *NOTCH1* was first identified through its involvement in a rare (7;9) translocation in T-ALL.[315] Later, mutations in *NOTCH1* were discovered in 50% to 60% of T-ALL samples,[316,317] and

NOTCH1 mutations have also been reported in numerous murine models of T-ALL.[318-320] Enforced Notch signaling also induces T-ALL in mice.[321] In humans these mutations are activating mutations that involve the heterodimerization domain or the PEST domain of *NOTCH1* (or both), leading to constitutive activation or increased stability of the protein. Inhibition of γ-secretase is one possible approach to inhibiting Notch signaling. Initially, γ-secretase inhibitors (GSIs) were developed because of their potential therapeutic role in Alzheimer disease in cleaving amyloid precursor protein.[322] However, they were tested in Notch-dependent cancers in an attempt to block the production of the processed, nuclear form of Notch.[323] Many human T-ALL cell lines with Notch mutation showed a G0/G1 cell-cycle arrest in response to a GSI.[316] A Notch pathway inhibitor clinical trial with the GSI MK-0752 was opened in 2005 for patients with refractory T-ALL.[324] The drug was tolerated in a limited number of patients at doses below 300 mg/m². However, further dose escalation by continuous infusion was discontinued secondary to diarrhea. This gastrointestinal toxicity is thought to result from blockade of Notch1 and Notch2 in the gut, leading to intestinal secretory metaplasia, an increased number of goblet cells, and arrested proliferation in the crypts of the small intestine.[325] Because of the limited antileukemic activity in this trial and the severe gastrointestinal toxicity, studies were conducted to identify combination therapies with gamma secretase inhibitors (GSIs). One promising combination identified is GSI with glucocorticoids (GCs). This combination has been demonstrated to alleviate the gut toxicity by induction of cyclin D2 (CCND2), a cyclin associated with cell-cycle progression, and by the downregulation of Krüppel-like factor 4 (KLF4), a negative regulator of the cell cycle that is required for goblet cell differentiation.[326] It also potentiates the antileukemia effect of either drug given alone.[327,328] Alteration in the schedule of GSI delivery has also been evaluated, and a 3 day on, 4 day off dosing schedule was better tolerated.[329] Other approaches to Notch inhibition are being explored, including antibody-based targeting of the Notch1 receptor,[330,331] targeting of Notch ligands,[332] direct inhibition of the Notch1 complex,[333] and selective targeting of the maturation of the mutant receptor.[334]

Although the genetic and functional data to support targeting Notch1 in hematologic malignancy are compelling, and multiple approaches to targeting Notch may be feasible, there are still numerous challenges that lie ahead. One difficulty is the on-target side effects of inhibiting Notch, as discussed previously. Another concerning toxicity, reported in a recent trial performed in patients with Alzheimer disease, is the development of secondary malignancies because Notch pathway loss-of-function mutations have been reported in squamous cell carcinomas of the head and neck,[335,336] skin, and lung.[337] Here the hope is that intermittent dosing of the Notch inhibitor will mitigate this risk of secondary malignancy. A second concern in targeting Notch1 has been the largely cytostatic effect of Notch1 inhibition with GSIs and antibody-based therapy in preclinical testing. As in the case of cytotoxic therapy for cancer, targeted therapies will likely need to be used in combination with other drugs to achieve maximal clinical efficacy. In addition to the combination of GSI with GCs discussed previously, several studies support the combination of Notch1 inhibitors with inhibitors of the PI3K-AKT-mTOR pathway for T-ALL.[338,339] Notch pathway inhibitors have yet to be brought to pediatric testing.

Sonic Hedgehog Signaling and Medulloblastoma

Medulloblastoma is the most common malignant pediatric brain tumor. The sonic hedgehog signaling pathway, implicated in the pathogenesis of this disease, is a potential pathway for targeted therapy. Aberrant sonic hedgehog signaling was first implicated in the pathogenesis of medulloblastoma with the discovery of germline mutations in the sonic hedgehog (Shh) receptor gene *PTCH1* in patients with Gorlin syndrome (basal cell nevus syndrome) who have an underlying predisposition to develop

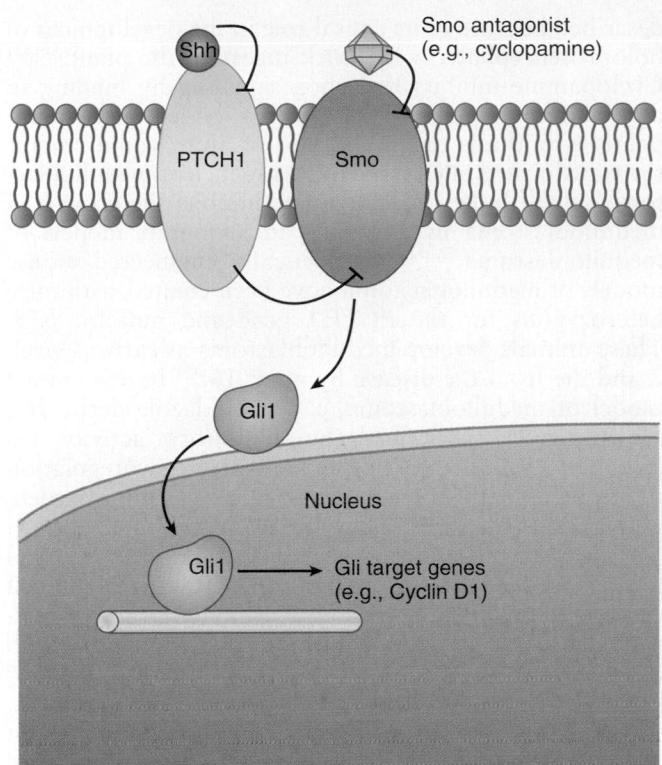

Figure 44-7 Hedgehog signaling. Patched (Ptch1) is a transmembrane receptor for the ligand sonic hedgehog (Shh). In the absence of Shh, Ptch1 inhibits Smo, a transmembrane protein with homology to G protein–coupled receptors. Upon Shh binding to Smo, this repression is relieved and signal is transduced through Smo to the nucleus, upregulating Gli1 transcription factors, which turn on a host of other transcriptional targets, including cyclin D1. *(Courtesy of Curtis Glavin and William Sellers.)*

medulloblastoma.[68,69] Heterozygous loss of *PTCH1* occurs in approximately 10% of sporadic medulloblastoma. Mutations in the downstream members of the hedgehog pathway, *Smo*, and *suppressor of fused (SUFU)*, have also been reported.[340-345] Furthermore, the hedgehog pathway is activated in approximately 30% of human medulloblastoma based on gene expression studies.[346]

PTCH1 is a transmembrane receptor for the ligand Shh (Fig. 44-7). In the absence of Shh, PTCH1 inhibits Smo, a transmembrane protein with homology to G-protein–coupled receptors. Upon Shh (ligand) binding to PTCH1, the repression is relieved and signal is transduced through Smo to the nucleus. This activity upregulates the Gli1 transcription factors, which in turn induces a set of transcriptional targets, including cyclin D1, PTCH1, and Gli1 themselves. SUFU appears to have a role in the repression of hedgehog signaling by interacting with GLI proteins in the cytoplasm and the nucleus.[347-349] The hedgehog pathway is critical for the development of the cerebellum and regulates the proliferation of granule neuron precursor cells in the cerebellum. Medulloblastoma is thought to originate from these immature granule cells.[343]

The goal of identifying inhibitors of the pathway began with the identification of cyclopamine, a plant-derived alkaloid from *Veratrum calcifornicum* initially described because of its causal role in the development of holoprosencephaly in livestock ingesting the plant.[350,351] Cyclopamine inhibits hedgehog signaling by binding to and inhibiting Smo, and this observation led to the therapeutic hypothesis that inhibition of Smo would reverse the transformed phenotype of Ptch-deficient medulloblastoma cells.[72] Indeed, cyclopamine inhibits the growth of medulloblastoma in vitro and in xenograft models of medulloblastoma.[72,352,353] Genetically engineered mouse models of medulloblastoma have been created with mice heterozygous for the PCTH1 gene and null for p53. These animals develop medulloblastoma as early as week 2 and die from the disease by week 16.[354] In this animal model of medulloblastoma, a benzimidazole derivative, Hh-Antag691, with hedgehog-inhibitory activity via binding to Smo, led to a dose-dependent downregulation of hedgehog pathway members, decreased tumor burden, and increased disease-free survival rates in treated mice.[355]

These data led to the development and early clinical testing of Smo inhibitors in patients with basal cell carcinoma and medulloblastoma. Among the Smo inhibitors that have been in clinical testing are vismodegib (GDC-0449), sonidegib (NVP-LDE225), BMS-833923, PF04449913, LY2940680, saridegib (IPI-962) and TAK-441. Clinical trials of the latter two molecules have been discontinued. Vismodegib is the first Smo inhibitor and is currently approved in basal cell carcinoma on the basis of the tumor response rates in metastatic and locally advanced basal cell carcinoma (30% and 43%, respectively).[356,357] In the first report of its activity in medulloblastoma, a heavily pretreated patient with medulloblastoma had short-term tumor regression followed by progression at 3 months.[74] Analysis of this patient's tumor revealed an acquired point mutation in the Smo receptor likely mediating therapeutic resistance.[358] These data in aggregate suggested that medulloblastomas bearing a mutationally activated hedgehog pathway would be responsive to Smo inhibitors while also pointing out the potential problems of emergent resistance. Phase I testing of vismodegib led to a recommended phase II dose from this trial of 150 mg by mouth based on a maximal plasma exposure and pharmacodynamics reponse.[359] The activity of vismodegib in medulloblastoma is being evaluated in an ongoing phase II trial. Early results from the first 32 patients with refractory or relapsed medulloblastoma treated daily with 150 mg of vismodegib have been presented in preliminary form. Among 20 patients with sonic hedgehog–positive tumors, there were three with sustained response compared with no response among the patients with either no evidence of Shh activity or indeterminate tumors, and six patients remained on trial for longer than 6 months.[360]

Sonidegib (NVP-LDE225) is a potent Smo inhibitor with reasonable blood-brain barrier penetration as a feature of the molecule.[292] In phase I testing sonidegib was escalated from 100 to 3000 mg daily and also tried at 400 and 750 mg twice daily. Sonidegib was tolerated with doses as high as 800 mg daily. The MTD was defined by exposure-related creatine kinase elevations thought to be related to target-mediated effects on muscle. Gli1 mRNA, a marker of hedgehog pathway activity, was

reduced by as much as 95% and 99% in skin and tumor biopsies. Preliminary evidence of activity was noted with one partial remission and one metabolic partial remission in medulloblastoma and one complete remission and four partial remissions in advanced basal cell carcinoma. Based on these data a phase II trial is being conducted in pediatric and adult patients with medulloblastoma in which post hoc evaluation of hedgehog activity is being conducted by using a five-gene hedgehog pathway mRNA signature. Preliminary results have been presented from 37 patients with medulloblastoma treated with sonidegib. In this cohort six patients responded (two complete remissions and four partial remissions) to sonidegib, and all responders were predicted to have hedgehog pathway–activated tumors. Of the remaining 31 patients, 29 were predicted to have hedgehog-inactive tumors and two were predictive to be hedgehog active. These latter two patients had stable disease. Based on the high concordance between the five-gene signature and patient response, this signature is now being used for patient selection to a randomized phase III trial comparing sonidegib with temozolamide in refractory or relapsed adult and pediatric medulloblastoma.[361] Taken together the aforementioned clinical data for vismodegib and sonidegib strongly support the notion that such inhibitors have significant clinical activity in hedgehog-activated medulloblastoma.

The hedgehog pathway is also thought to play a role in the maintenance of cancer stem cells. In particular, the preclinical data suggests that leukemia stem cells may be particularly dependent on hedgehog-pathway signaling.[362-364] To test this hypothesis the Smo inhibitor PF-0449913 has been tested clinically and found to have preliminary evidence of efficacy in AML; a complete remission with incomplete blood count recovery was noted in one patient, and five patients with AML had 50% or greater reduction in bone marrow blast counts. In addition, a major cytogenetic response with loss of the T315I mutation was observed in one patient with CML. These data suggest the Smo inhibitors may also find a role outside of tumor types driven by genetic mutations in the hedgehog pathway.

Transcription Factors and Pediatric Cancer

Abnormalities of transcription factors are a common genetic theme in the development of pediatric solid tumors, as well as leukemia. Often, the transcription factor is involved in a translocation rendering a new protein with aberrant transcriptional activity. Some examples of common transcription factor rearrangements are as follows: Ewing sarcoma (EWS-FLI, EWS-ERG), alveolar rhabdomyosarcoma (PAX3-FKHR, PAX7-FKHR), infantile fibrosarcoma (TEL-NTRK3), ALL (TEL-AML1, MLL rearrangements, E2A-PBX), and AML (PML-RARα, AML1-ETO, CBFβ-MYH11, MLL rearrangements). A second mechanism of transcription factor aberrancy is upregulation by amplification, such as amplification of MYCN in neuroblastoma and medulloblastoma. The high frequency of these abnormalities and the tumor cell specificity make these genetic lesions attractive targets. However, transcription factors have been considered "undruggable." Unlike enzymatic targets, such as kinases, transcription factors are not easily amenable to high-throughput screening assays. With the exception of the treatment of *PML-RARα*–rearranged APL, no current therapy directly targets these transcription factor abnormalities. Alternative approaches to small molecule discovery are needed. Technologies, such as RNAi, may facilitate therapeutic targeting of oncogenic transcription factors as better delivery methods are developed. Furthermore, these evolving technologies have enabled new methods for drug screening.

One approach to address the challenges to transcription-factor targeting exploits gene expression signatures. With this method gene expression signatures, defined by using genome-wide expression profiling, are used to identify different biological states. Then a small molecule library is screened with a low-cost, higher-throughput assay to identify compounds that induce the change in gene expression signature from "state A" to "state B." The gene expression signature definition, amplification, and detection are generic. Furthermore, a priori knowledge of a target is not needed. The gene expression signature serves as a surrogate for the biological state in question. The method is thus well suited for discovery of modulators of oncogenic transcription factors in which the mutant transcription factor's transforming mechanism is not known. One method developed, gene expression–based high-throughput screening (GE-HTS), used Affymetrix microarrays to define expression signatures of the two biological states of interest. From these high-complexity arrays, as many as 100 genes are selected as marker genes for each state. These signature genes are then amplified and detected with a high-throughput assay.[365,366] This approach was successfully used in a proof-of-concept experiment to identify inducers of AML differentiation. It was then extended to the modulation of transcription factors in an effort to identify small-molecule modulators of EWS-FLI in Ewing sarcoma, AML1-ETO in AML, and Notch1 in T-ALL.[334,367,368] GE-HTS provides an avenue for identifying tool compounds for the study of these genetic lesions and for identifying therapeutic leads. In fact, there are industry-based efforts incorporating gene expression fingerprints for drug discovery.

A second signature-based approach to address this problem uses a reference collection of gene expression profiles from cells treated with bioactive small molecules. This approach was initially demonstrated to be feasible in yeast with a pivotal study confirming that gene expression data could be used to functionally annotate small molecules and genes.[369] A pilot study next demonstrated the feasibility of this approach in human cell lines with the expression profiling of 164 distinct small molecule perturbagens, including many FDA-approved drugs and known bioactive compounds. Here the goal was to create an in silico tool (the Connectivity Map, or C-Map) for discovering the relationships among diseases, physiologic processes, and small molecule interventions.[370,371] One example pertinent to pediatric leukemia identified rapamycin as a small molecule candidate to reverse dexamethasone resistance in ALL.[372] In this example the C-Map was screened for molecules whose profile overlapped with a gene expression signature of GC sensitivity

or resistance in ALL cells. The screen indicated that the mTOR inhibitor rapamycin profile matched the signature of GC sensitivity. Rapamycin was confirmed to sensitize ALL to GC-induced apoptosis, suggesting that the combination of rapamycin and GCs has potential utility in lymphoid malignancies. A clinical trial testing this hypothesis for pediatric patients with relapsed ALL is ongoing.

One approach to target the interface between proteins involved in transcriptional regulation uses peptides. One example is the use of specific peptide interference with BCL6 (B-cell lymphoma 6) transcriptional mechanisms in B-cell lymphoma.[373] Regulatory elements of the *BCL6* gene are frequently mutated in human diffuse large B-cell lymphoma, leading to sustained expression of BCL6.[374,375] This is thought to enhance B-cell survival, proliferation, and block differentiation. BCL6 possesses an N-terminal BTB/POZ (Bric-a-brac, Tramtrack, Broad complex/Poxvirus zinc finger) domain, and the BTB domain recruits the corepressors SMRT (silencing mediator of retinoid and thyroid receptors), NCoR (nuclear receptor corepressor) and BCoR (BCL6 corepressor).[376] The interface through which BCL6 recruits corepressor proteins was characterized with x-ray crystallography, and based on this structure a peptide inhibitor blocking the interaction of these proteins was designed.[377] This peptide disrupted BCL6-mediated repression and reactivated the expression of BCL6 target genes. Furthermore, in B-cell lymphoma cells positive for BCL6, the peptide caused apoptosis and cell cycle arrest. With improved methods of delivering peptides to cells, peptide therapy has become more feasible. One method fuses the peptide with protein transduction domains, which mediate receptor-independent cell penetration by binding the peptide to lipid rafts and triggering macropinocytosis.[378]

A second potential peptide-based approach to achieving this goal might use a reported stapled peptide technology. This approach has been applied to the activation of apoptosis by using a hydrocarbon-stapled BH3 peptide.[379,380] In contrast to the use of helical peptides to interfere with protein-protein interactions, which has been limited because of the loss of secondary structure in solution, susceptibility to degradation, and poor penetration of intact cells, the hydrocarbon-stapled peptides proved to be helical, protease-resistant, and cell-permeable molecules that bound with increased affinity to target pockets. Hydrocarbon stapling of native peptides may provide a useful strategy for experimental and therapeutic modulation of protein-protein interactions, especially in disrupting transcription factor homodimers and heterodimers requiring extended helical interaction surfaces, as is the case for the MYC family.

Finally, multiple recent studies have used high-throughput in vitro screening of cancer cell lines to define genetic-, lineage-, and gene expression–based predictors of drug response. These studies focused primarily on adult cancers and involved the testing of a limited number of small molecules. Nevertheless, two of the most remarkable insights to emerge from those studies (discussed in greater detail later) were the discovery of marked sensitivity of Ewing sarcoma cell lines with EWS-ETS rearrangements to PARP inhibitors and the marked sensitivity of

MYCN-amplified neuroblastoma cell lines to BET bromodomain inhibitors.[381] These discoveries illustrate the potential power of comprehensive, pediatric cancer–focused screening to identify either compounds that directly interfere with aberrant transcription factors or synthetic lethal relationships in the presence of a transcription factor abnormality. Moreover, the potential of small molecule inhibitors of epigenetic regulators to alter aberrant transcriptional programs is revealed in the preclinical efficacy of BET bromodomain inhibitors in *MYCN*-amplified neuroblastoma tumors.

Emerging Lineage-Dependent Targets in Pediatric Cancer

Anti-GD2 and Neuroblastoma

Cure rates for children with high-stage neuroblastoma have improved with dose intensity of chemotherapy. However, even with double autologous stem cell transplantation, most children with stage 4 disease will relapse. For long-term survivors, therapy-related morbidity is high. Alternative approaches to cytotoxic therapy are clearly needed. One approach to targeted therapy for this disease has exploited the high-density expression of the neuronal lineage marker disialoganglioside, GD2, on neuroblastoma cells.[382] Several anti-GD2 monoclonal antibodies have been developed and tested in clinical trials.

One of the first was a murine IgG3 monoclonal antibody 3F8 directed at GD2. According to reports, 3F8 mediates neuroblastoma cell death by human complement activation and by activation of lymphocytes, monocytes, and neutrophils.[383-385] Initial studies testing 3F8 showed evidence of activity, particularly in children with minimal disease at the time of immunotherapy initiation.[386] Subsequent studies evaluated whether the addition of granulocyte-macrophage colony-stimulating factor (GM-CSF) to 3F8 would increase response by increasing the number of granulocytes and by priming effector cells for greater cytotoxicity. There were 45 patients with high-stage disease not in remission enrolled in the study.[387] Of the 15 patients with refractory bone marrow disease, 80% had a complete remission in bone marrow. Eleven patients were treated for recurrent neuroblastoma that was refractory to salvage therapy. Five of ten with marrow disease had complete remission in the marrow, but the one patient with soft tissue disease progressed. Additionally, the 15 patients treated for progressive disease did quite poorly, with all continuing to progress. The combination of GM-CSF and 3F8 was well tolerated, with the principal side effects of pain and rash. The authors concluded that the combination of 3F8 and GM-CSF was well tolerated and shows promise for treatment of minimal residual neuroblastoma in the bone marrow.

Another anti-GD2 antibody, 14.G2a, a murine monoclonal IgG2a antibody, has been tested in a clinical trial.[388,389] In an attempt to improve this antibody, a chimeric human/murine anti-GD2 monoclonal antibody (ch14.18) was developed and tested in phase I clinical trials, with some encouraging results.[390,391] This construct uses the 14.G2a variable region's heavy and light chains

and human constant region genes for IgG1 heavy chain and kappa light chain. However, a large retrospective study of 334 assessable children older than 1 year of age (166 received ch14.18 consolidation treatment, 99 received 12-month low-dose maintenance chemotherapy, and 69 received no additional treatment) failed to demonstrate an advantage to ch14.18 in event-free survival or overall survival with multivariate analysis.[392] Similarly, an analysis of infants younger than 1 year of age failed to show a difference in outcome with ch14.18 consolidation therapy.[393]

Ch14.18 was also tested in combination with GM-CSF in a phase I study with manageable toxicities, including pain, urticaria, and emesis.[394] Testing was performed with humanized ch14.18 linked to IL-2 (hu14.18-IL2) with the hypothesis that IL-2 would augment activation of preexisting antigen specific T cells, enhancing destruction of tumor cells and activation of natural killer cells. A phase I trial demonstrated manageable side effects: hypotension, allergic reaction, fever, pain, marrow suppression, and blurred vision. Three patients out of 27 experienced some antitumor activity, with decreased tumor burden in the bone marrow.[395]

A landmark phase III trial evaluated ch14.18 administered in combination with interleukin-2 (IL-2) and GM-CSF and isotretinoin versus isotretinoin alone for patients after stem cell transplantation with a total of 226 eligible patients randomly assigned to each treatment group.[396] With a median duration of follow-up of 2.1 years, this immunotherapy was superior to standard therapy with event-free survival of $66 \pm 5\%$ versus $46 \pm 5\%$ and overall survival of $86 \pm 4\%$ versus $75 \pm- 5\%$, and the trial was stopped early owing to efficacy based on event-free survival. This study reported that 52% of patients experienced grade 3, 4, or 5 pain; 23% capillary leak syndrome; and 25% hypersensitivity reactions, expected side effects attributable to antibody binding to GD2 on normal nerves, cytokine-mediated leak, and hypersensitivity to either antibody or cytokines, respectively. Immunotherapy was also more effective in patients with minimal, rather than high, levels of residual disease. Patients who had biopsy-proven persistent disease before entering the study were nonrandomly assigned to immunotherapy, and event-free survival for these patients was only $36\% \pm 10\%$ at 2 years. Nevertheless, this study suggests the more routine use of lineage-directed immunotherapy for patients with neuroblastoma with minimal residual disease after stem cell transplantation.

Emerging Synthetic Lethal or Empiric Track: Targets in Pediatric Cancer

Insulin-like Growth Factor Receptor Signaling and Pediatric Solid Tumors

More than 10 years ago, the insulin-like growth factor-1 receptor (IGF-1R) signaling pathway was implicated in Ewing sarcoma. It has also been implicated in other pediatric and adult tumors.[397] With the evolution of small molecule inhibitors of receptor tyrosine kinases and the development of antibody-based therapy, therapeutic inhibition of this pathway has become a reality. IGF-1R is a heterodimeric tyrosine kinase receptor. IGF-1 and IGF-2, and to a lesser extent insulin, bind to IGF-1R, leading to receptor activation, autophosphorylation, and phosphorylation of downstream targets. The receptor is important for development, cell growth, transformation, and the prevention of apoptosis.

One early study demonstrated that IGF-1 mRNA was expressed in 90% of Ewing tumor samples positive for the EWS-FLI translocation. Furthermore, this work demonstrated that blockade of the IGF-1R with a monoclonal antibody inhibited serum free growth in a Ewing cell line.[398] Next, it was demonstrated that IGF-1R is essential for EWS-FLI transformation of fibroblasts and that expression of the EWS-FLI fusion may alter the IGF-1R signaling pathway.[399] In addition, the expression of insulin-like growth factor binding protein (IGFBP-3) is strongly induced with siRNA against EWS-FLI, and EWS-FLI can bind the IGFBP-3 promoter and repress its activity, suggesting that dysregulation of IGFBP-3 contributes to the development of Ewing sarcoma.[400,401] With the advent of inhibitors of IGF-1R, it was next demonstrated that small molecule inhibitors of IGF-1R, such as NVP-AEW541, a pyrrolopyrimidine derivative with selectivity for IGF-1R versus insulin receptor, had activity in vitro and in vivo models of Ewing sarcoma.[402,403] Furthermore, a dominant negative mutant IGF-1R inhibited tumorigenesis and induced apoptosis in Ewing sarcoma cells.[404]

In addition to Ewing sarcoma, IGF-1R has been implicated in numerous other pediatric solid tumors. One study reported inhibition of proliferation in several pediatric cancer–related cell lines (neuroblastoma, rhabdomyosarcoma, and osteosarcoma) with an antagonistic, monoclonal antibody (EM164) directed against IGF-1R.[405] Other evidence implicating IGF-related signaling in rhabdomyosarcoma, particularly for alveolar, includes upregulation of IGF-2 in cell lines, cooperation of IGF-2, and PAX3-FKHR, and inhibition of rhabdomyosarcoma growth with overexpression of IGFBP-6, an inhibitor of IGF-2.[406-408] In osteosarcoma, expression of IGF-1R has been reported in both canine and human cells.[409] In neuroblastoma the small molecule inhibitor NVP-AEW541 has had in vitro and in vivo activity,[410] and data suggest that IGF-1R expression may regulate metastases to bone.[411]

Initial phase I trials testing monoclonal antibodies against IGF-1R demonstrated tolerability of this approach in patients with sarcoma, with excitement generated about responses seen specifically in patients with Ewing sarcoma.[412-414] However, this initial excitement was tempered in subsequent follow-up trials wherein moderate activity has been observed. A phase I/II study of figitumumab, a fully human IgG2 monoclonal antibody against the IGF-1R, enrolled 106 evaluable patients with Ewing sarcoma in the phase II component of the trial.[415] Of these, 15 had a partial response (overall response rate = 14.2%) and 25 had stable disease. However, the median duration of response was only 4.7 months, and median overall survival was only 8.9 months. Another phase II study testing R1507, the fully human IgG1 monoclonal antibody against the IGF-1R, enrolled 115 patients with Ewing sarcoma.[416] For all patients the overall response rate was 10% with a 29-week median duration of response and a median overall survival of 7.6 months. This study identified patients with bone primaries as more likely to respond to antibody therapy compared with patients with extraskeletal sites. A third phase II study tested the fully human monoclonal antibody antagonist of IGF-1R, ganitumab, in patients with Ewing sarcoma and desmoplastic small round blue cell tumors (DSRCT).[417] In this trial, of the 35 evaluable patients, only two had an objective response for an overall response rate of 6%, although 49% of patients had stable disease.

Although the data suggest modest activity of anti–IGF-1R antibody therapy in a subset of patients with Ewing sarcoma, and possibly DSRCT, biomarkers of sensitivity have yet to be identified. The IGF1R gene is not commonly mutated in Ewing sarcoma, and although some studies have correlated IGF-1 serum levels with a longer median overall survival, neither serum IGF-1 nor tumor IGF-1R have been demonstrated to be associated with response to IGF-1R antibody therapy.[415,417-419] Identification of biomarkers of response and mechanisms of rapid resistance to IGF-1R therapy are critical next steps in determining the role of IGF-1R–directed therapy for patients with Ewing sarcoma. Moreover, the identification of highly efficacious combination therapies with IGF-1R antibodies is another active avenue of pursuit.[420]

Poly(ADP-ribose) Polymerase Inhibitors in Ewing Sarcoma

In an effort to uncover new biomarkers of drug sensitivity and resistance, several groups have screened large collections of genetically annotated cancer cell lines against hundreds of drugs.[93,94] Although well-known connections between genotype and chemosensitivity have been validated (e.g., BCR-ABL–positive cell lines are sensitive to multiple ABL inhibitors), new tumor vulnerabilities are emerging. For example, in a study conducted by Garnett and colleagues, 639 human cancer cell lines were screened with 130 drugs under clinical preclinical testing. Ewing sarcoma cell lines expressing EWS-FLI fusions were identified as highly sensitive to multiple structurally distinct PARP inhibitors, undergoing apoptosis in vitro.[94] Tumors harboring either BRCA1 or BRCA2 mutations have been demonstrated to have increased sensitivity to PARP inhibitors owing to defects in homologous recombination and reliance on alternative pathways to repair DNA damage that are targeted by these inhibitors. Ewing sarcoma tumors, however, have not been demonstrated to have genomic events involving BRCA1 or BRCA2. Rather, these investigators confirmed that the presence of the EWS-FLI fusion engenders sensitivity to PARP inhibitors by demonstrating that mouse mesenchymal cells transformed with EWS-FLI were more sensitive to the PARP inhibitor olaparib than when they were transformed with FUS-CHOP. Expression of EWS-FLI in NIH3T3 cells also conferred greater sensitivity to this compound class compared with a control.

Although the precise mechanism of Ewing sarcoma cell line sensitivity to PARP inhibitors is still under consideration, a study by Brenner and colleagues suggests that EWS-FLI or EWS-ERG fusions themselves promote DNA damage.[421] In this study the authors report that Ewing sarcoma cell lines have DNA double-strand breaks induced by the expression of the EWS-ETS fusion and that treatment with PARP inhibitors potentiates this DNA damage. Moreover, they found that EWS-FLI enhances the expression of PARP in a positive feedback loop, and a synergistic response was seen when PARP inhibitors were combined with the DNA-damaging agent temozolomide in preclinical models of Ewing sarcoma. These initial preclinical observations were rapidly translated to phase I/II trials for patients with Ewing sarcoma, with results of these trials still pending.

BRD4 in Pediatric Cancers

Another example of the power of high-throughput in vitro screening of cancer cell lines to define genetic, lineage, and gene expression–based predictors of drug response is provided by the identification of the sensitivity of MYCN-amplified neuroblastoma cells to BET bromodomain inhibitors.[381] The BET family is composed of BRD2, BRD3, BRD4, and BRDT. All are defined by two N-terminal bromodomains sharing high levels of sequence conservation. BET family members are epigenetic "readers," which recognize covalent modifications of histone proteins or DNA.[422] One important modification associated with open chromatin, and thus transcriptional activation, is the ε-N-acetylation of lysine residues on histone tails.[423] Context-specific molecular recognition of acetyl-lysine residues is mediated by 61 diverse bromodomains, comprising 46 human proteins.[424]

The BET family member BRD4 has been reported to be a critical mediator of cell cycle progression and transcriptional elongation, functioning to recruit the positive transcription elongation factor b (P-TEFb).[425-427] BRD4 has been identified as a component of a recurrent t(15;19) chromosomal translocation in NUT midline carcinoma (NMC), resulting in the expression of the twin N-terminal bromodomains of BRD4 as an in-frame chimera with the NUT protein.[428] Functional studies in patient-derived NMC cell lines have validated the essential role of the BRD4-NUT oncoprotein in maintaining a proliferation advantage and differentiation block.[429]

Recently, multiple BET bromodomain small molecule inhibitors have been developed that displace BET bromodomains from chromatin by competitively binding to the acetyl-lysine recognition pocket. Not only have these molecules had remarkable preclinical activity in NMC, but they have also been shown to modulate the transcriptional function of MYC in several diseases, including AML, T-ALL, and multiple myeloma.[430-434] BET proteins bind to acetylated histone lysines and modulate transcription by recruiting transcriptional activators; MYC-regulated transcription is associated with increases in histone lysine acetylation. Unexpectedly, however, it was discovered that MYC itself is transcriptionally regulated by BET bromodomains.[431,432,434] In multiple myeloma cells JQ1 treatment leads to depletion of the MYC oncoprotein and downregulation of the coordinated MYC transcriptional program, leading to cell cycle arrest and senescence. This was associated with significant therapeutic responses in orthotopic xenograft studies as well as

genetically engineered mouse models of multiple myeloma. Moreover, in AML, JQ1 treatment inhibited MYC transcription and promoted AML differentiation and response in a mouse model of MLL-rearranged leukemia,[432] and in ALL, BET inhibition targeted IL7R with prolonged survival in mice xenografted with primary human CRLF2-rearranged B-ALL treated with JQ1.[435]

An unbiased screen of a collection of 673 genetically characterized cancer cell lines was conducted to understand response and resistance to BET inhibition and to find new opportunities for therapeutic development. Neuroblastoma was identified as one of the most JQ1-sensitive diseases and MYCN amplification as the most predictive marker of sensitivity.[381] Subsequent studies revealed a strong correlation between MYCN amplification and sensitivity to bromodomain inhibition. Bromodomain-mediated inhibition of MYCN impaired growth and induced apoptosis in neuroblastoma and suppressed the MYCN pattern of gene expression. BRD4 knockdown phenocopied these effects, establishing BET bromodomains as transcriptional regulators of MYCN. BET inhibition conferred a significant survival advantage in three in vivo neuroblastoma models, including a primary human orthotopic xenograft and a MYCN GEMM, and this efficacy correlated with blockade of both MYCN and of MYCN target genes, providing a strong rationale for developing BET bromodomain inhibitors in patients with neuroblastoma. The preclinical evaluation of BET bromodomain inhibitors in other MYCN-driven malignancies, such as medulloblastoma, is ongoing.

BET bromodomain inhibitors have entered the clinic, with trials now ongoing in adult diseases. Indeed, investigators reported the safety of chronic administration of the BET inhibitor RVX-208 from a clinical trial to treat atherosclerosis.[436] Future trials are under development for pediatric malignancies.

EZH2 in Pediatric Cancer

Whereas some targets have emerged from high-throughput screening efforts, other pediatric cancer vulnerabilities have been uncovered through the detailed study of genetic models of specific diseases. One recent example is the discovery of epigenetic antagonism between the polycomb family member EZH2 and SWI/SNF complexes in malignant rhabdoid tumors. Polycomb group proteins contribute to epigenetic-driven gene silencing during development, and increasing evidence supports a critical role for this protein class in oncogenesis. EZH2 is the core catalytic protein in the polycomb repressor complex 2 (PRC2) and catalyzes the trimethylation of histone 3 lysine 27 (H3K27), leading to the repression of hundreds of genes in embryonic stem cells.[437] EZH2 forms a complex with other PRC2 components, including the cofactors SUZ12 and EED and the protein Jarid2, which recruit PRC2 to promoters. EZH2 has been implicated in numerous malignancies. It is highly expressed in many tumors, including those of the breast, prostate, colon, and pancreas, as well as lymphomas and sarcomas.[438] In 2010 the discovery was made of recurrent Tyr 641 mutations in the catalytic SET domain of EZH2 in diffuse large

B-cell lymphomas and in follicular lymphomas, which increase H3K27me3 in an interaction with the remaining wild-type *EZH2* allele.[439-441] More recently, a tumor-suppressor function of EZH2 in some malignancies has been described. Homozygous deletions or inactivating mutations have been reported in approximately 6% of myelodysplastic syndrome and in certain subsets of myeloproliferative disease.[442-445] Moreover, loss of *EZH2* is reported to cause aggressive T-ALL in mice, and loss-of-function mutations in multiple members of the PRC2 complex, including *EZH2*, *SUZ12*, and *EED*, have been reported in adult and early precursor T-ALL.[257,446,447]

Recent studies support the role for EZH2 dependency in malignant rhabdoid tumor. The first line of evidence that SWI/SNF complexes oppose epigenetic silencing by polycomb group proteins was supported by genetic studies in *Drosophila* species in which defects in body segment identity induced by mutations in polycomb proteins were suppressed by mutations in the SWI/SNF complex.[448] It was later discovered that polycomb proteins can oppose the enzymatic activity of the SWI/SNF complex.[449,450] Malignant rhabdoid tumors, a highly aggressive pediatric malignancy, arise from the biallelic inactivation of *SNF5*, a SWI/SNF complex member.[451,452] It was reported that EZH2 expression and H3K27me3 levels at lineage-specific target genes are upregulated in these SNF5-deficient tumors, with SNF5 directly repressing EZH2 expression.[453] Reduction of EZH2 levels in primary cells lacking SNF5 expression led to downregulation of stem cell signatures. Moreover, it was determined that EZH2 is required for the development and growth of tumor cells with biallelic inactivation of *SNF5*. Although these studies were performed with genetic manipulation, it has only recently become possible to selectively inhibit the enzymatic activity of EZH2 with a small molecule inhibitor with the development of EZH2 inhibitors by multiple pharmaceutical companies.

Small molecule inhibitors of EZH2 were initially described and reported in *EZH2*-mutated lymphoma, in which as many as 22% of germinal center diffuse large B-cell lymphoma and follicular lymphomas harbor mutations in the Y641, located in the catalytic SET domain of *EZH2*. GSK126, a selective S-adenosyl-methionine competitive small molecule inhibitor of EZH2 methyltransferase activity, was reported to decrease global H3K27me3 levels, activate the expression of genes suppressed by PRC2, and inhibit *EZH2*-mutated lymphoma in vitro and in xenograft mouse models of the disease.[454] Similarly, the compound EPZ005687 was reported to reduce H3K27 methylation in lymphoma cells, resulting in apoptosis of lymphoma cells with heterozygous mutations in Y671 or A677, but with little effect on lymphoma cells with wild-type EZH2.[455] A second-generation EZH2 inhibitor, EPZ-6438, with improved potency and pharmacokinetics from EPZ005687, was developed and tested in malignant rhaboid tumor.[456] This compound had remarkable activity, with treatment leading to a dose-dependent regression of malignant rhabdoid tumors in mouse models of disease, a decrease in intratumoral levels of H3K27me3, and even prevention of regrowth after treatment was discontinued. This study demonstrated the dependency of rhabdoid tumors on not only the EZH2 protein but specifically the enzymatic activity of this molecule.

EZH2 has been implicated in other pediatric malignancies. For example, in Ewing sarcoma EWS-FLI has been reported to directly upregulate the expression of EZH2.[457,458] In this study EZH2 was reported to regulate the expression of genes related to stemness and to genes involved in neuroectodermal and endothelial differentiation. Furthermore, in this study the downregulation of EZH2 by shRNA suppressed oncogenic transformation in Ewing sarcoma cells by inhibiting in vitro clonogenicity. Whether Ewing cells depend on the enzymatic activity of EZH2 or another function of the EZH2 protein (as has been implicated in prostate cancer)[459] has yet to be determined. Finally, a potential role for EZH2 has been implicated in neuroblastoma. Here, EZH2 has been found to be physically associated with MYCN in a complex and shRNA directed against EZH2 to alter growth of neuroblastoma cells.[460,461] However, as in Ewing sarcoma, the therapeutic role of EZH2 inhibition in neuroblastoma has not been fully explored. As in the examples discussed previously for other epigenetic modifying drugs, EZH2 inhibitors are now entering clinical trials for adults with cancer.

DOT1L in Mixed-Lineage Leukemia-Rearranged Leukemia

As discussed before, epigenetic modifiers have come to the forefront as therapeutic targets in multiple pediatric cancers. Mixed-lineage leukemia (MLL)-rearranged leukemia represents another illustrative example of a defined genetic subtype of childhood leukemia in which multiple epigenetic vulnerabilities have been identified.[462,463] There are two primary genetic aberrations of *MLL* in leukemia. The most common event is a balanced translocation; more than 70 different fusion partners with *MLL* have been described. A second class of aberration of the *MLL* gene creates a repeat within the N-terminal of MLL resulting in an internal partial tandem duplication (PTD). As noted above, BRD4 has emerged as one potential target in this genetic subtype of leukemia. Another potential target is the H3K79 methyltransferase DOT1L (Fig. 44-8). Whereas MLL-fusion proteins have lost the histone H3K4 methyltransferase activity of wild-type MLL, many of these fusion proteins have been shown to copurify with protein complexes normally involved in transcriptional elongation and activation, such as polymerase-associated factor complex (PAFc), P-TEFb, and DOT1L.[464] It has thus been hypothesized that MLL-fusion proteins promote leukemia through enhanced elongation or activation of leukemia-promoting genes.

The association of MLL fusions with DOT1L precipitated the study of H3K79 methylation levels in *MLL*-rearranged leukemia. Numerous studies demonstrate enhanced H3K79 methylation associated with genes overexpressed in *MLL*-rearranged leukemia cells.[465-467] As in the studies of EZH2 and malignant rhaboid tumor, a therapeutic effect of targeting DOT1L in the context of certain MLL fusions has been demonstrated with both genetic and chemical approaches. In one study abnormal H3K79me2 profiles were identified on MLL-AF9 fusion

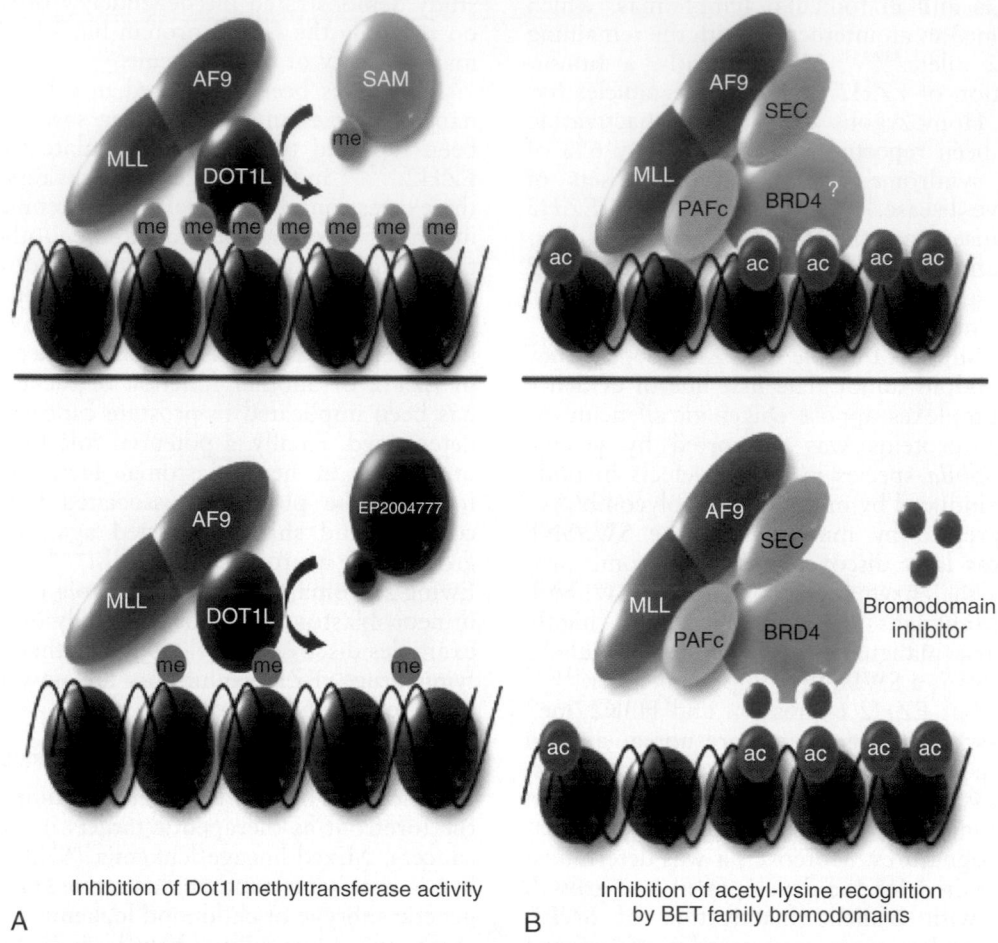

Inhibition of Dot1l methyltransferase activity

A

Inhibition of acetyl-lysine recognition
by BET family bromodomains

B

Figure 44-8 Pharmacologic targeting of chromatin regulator pathways in mixed-lineage leukemia (MLL)-rearranged leukemias. **A,** Depiction of the association of DOT1L with the AF9 component of the MLL-AF9 fusion. DOT1L methylates histone 3 at lysine residue 79 by using S-(5′-adenosyl)-1-methionine (SAM) as a donor. The use of a SAM mimetic (e.g., EPZ004777), as shown in the lower panel, can potently inhibit DOT1L activity and target oncogenic H3K79 hypermethylation. **B,** MLL fusions recruit polymerase-associated factor complex (PAFc) through the N-terminal portion of MLL. A number of nuclear fusion partners, such as AF9 and ENL, are members of the super elongation complex (SEC), which includes positive transcription elongation factor b (P-TEFB). Both PAFc and P-TEFb have been implicated in MLL-fusion positive leukemias. The BET family member BRD4 was shown to co-purify with several components of the PAFc and SEC. Small molecule inhibitors of BRD4, which inhibit its recognition of acetyl lysine, impair the targeting of the PAFc and SEC components to chromatin, leading to altered gene expression. BRD4 inhibitors might therefore inhibit MLL-mediated leukemogenesis. *(Modified from Deshpande, et al: Chromatin modifications as therapeutic targets in MLL-rearranged leukemia.* Trends Immunol 33:563–570, 2012.)

target loci in leukemic stem cells and inactivation of Dot1l led to the downregulation of MLL-AF9 target genes.[468] Moreover, in this study, by using an experimentally derived mouse model of MLL-AF9 leukemia, it was determined that Dot1l is required in vivo for both leukemic transformation and maintenance. Similar findings were observed in an independent study by using a tamoxifen-inducible Cre-mediated loss-of-function mouse model in which it was demonstrated that Dot1l is required for the initiation and maintenance of MLL-AF9–induced leukemogenesis in vitro and in vivo.[469] The critical relevance of the enzymatic activity of DOT1L in *MLL*-rearranged leukemia was determined with the testing of EPZ004777, a selective small molecule inhibitor of DOT1L. Treatment of MLL cells with the compound inhibited H3K79 methylation, blocked expression of leukemogenic genes, resulted in the selective killing of

MLL-rearranged leukemia cells, and led to a modest extension of survival in a mouse MLL-leukemia xenograft model.[470] Subsequently, it was demonstrated that other MLL fusions, including MLL-AF6, MLL-AF10, and CALM-AF10, require the H3K79 methyltransferase activity of DOT1L.[471,472] As in the case of BET bromodomain and EZH2 inhibitors, DOT1L inhibitors are just beginning to enter clinical trials.

CONCLUSIONS

Tremendous progress has been made in the treatment of pediatric cancer over the last century. The empiric combination of cytotoxic agents has proved curative for many patients, but at the expense of toxicity. Over the last decade, heralded by the success of targeting BCR-ABL in CML, we have entered a new era of drug discovery with an emphasis on target-based treatment with the promise of improved cure rates and decreased toxicity. New and developing high-throughput genomic and proteomic technologies are dramatically altering the landscape of research, enabling the identification and credentialing of new targets with a speed previously unfathomable. In this chapter we have provided a framework for classifying and credentialing new targets. We have highlighted examples of successful targeted approaches from the treatment of adults with cancer and have discussed emerging targets for pediatric cancer. Although it is an exciting time in cancer therapy, there are many sobering challenges that lie ahead in the development of targeted therapy, particularly for pediatric cancer. Continued advancement will require innovative approaches to intractable targets (e.g., transcription factors), rational approaches to combination therapy, and collaborative efforts between industry and academic centers to identify new pediatric targets along with target-specific drugs. For maximal progress in the treatment of children with cancer, we will need to collectively solve the issues that confront the clinical development of novel therapeutics. Trials that allow for biopsies, genetic profiling of tumors, and "window" treatment periods may be necessary to bring targeted therapies into the pediatric realm.

References available online at ExpertConsult.

KEY REFERENCES

36. Paez JG, Janne PA, Lee JC, et al: EGFR mutations in lung cancer: correlation with clinical response to gefitinib therapy. *Science* 304:1497–1500, 2004.
    This article documents one of the earliest examples of dramatic responses to targeted therapies seen in select genotypes.
38. Benson JD, Chen YN, Cornell-Kennon SA, et al: Validating cancer drug targets. *Nature* 441:451–456, 2006.
    This review article provides a summary of approaches used to validate cancer drug targets.
67. Lawrence MS, Stojanov P, Polak P, et al: Mutational heterogeneity in cancer and the search for new cancer-associated genes. *Nature* 499:214–218, 2013.
    This manuscript describes the problem of mutational heterogeneity across cancers, revealing the marked simplicity of many pediatric cancer genomes, and provides a computational solution for accounting for this heterogeneity in the search for new cancer-associated genes.
74. Rudin CM, Hann CL, Laterra J, et al: Treatment of medulloblastoma with hedgehog pathway inhibitor GDC-0449. *N Engl J Med* 361:1173–1178, 2009.
    Among the first studies to document the activity of hedgehog pathway inhibitors in treating patients with medulloblastoma with activation of this pathway.
93. Barretina J, Caponigro G, Stransky N, et al: The Cancer Cell Line Encyclopedia enables predictive modelling of anticancer drug sensitivity. *Nature* 483:603–607, 2012.
94. Garnett MJ, Edelman EJ, Heidorn SJ, et al: Systematic identification of genomic markers of drug sensitivity in cancer cells. *Nature* 483:570–575, 2012.
    Two articles describing the power of systemative screening of genetically characterized cancer cell lines to uncover new gentoype-chemosensitivity relationships.
96. Xue W, Zender L, Miething C, et al: Senescence and tumour clearance is triggered by p53 restoration in murine liver carcinomas. *Nature* 445:656–660, 2007.
    Article demonstrating that p53 loss is required for the maintenance of some aggressive malignancies.
126. Grupp SA, Kalos M, Barrett D, et al: Chimeric antigen receptor–modified T cells for acute lymphoid leukemia. *N Engl J Med* 368:1509–1518, 2013.
    Article demonstrating striking early response data to chimeric antigen receptor–modified T cells for patients with relapsed/refractory ALL.
136. Warrell RP, Jr, Frankel SR, Miller WH, Jr, et al: Differentiation therapy of acute promyelocytic leukemia with tretinoin (all-trans-retinoic acid). *N Engl J Med* 324:1385–1393, 1991.
    Among the first articles to describe the clinical success of differentiation therapy targeting the PML-RARα fusion in patients with APL.
144. Druker BJ, Talpaz M, Resta DJ, et al: Efficacy and safety of a specific inhibitor of the BCR-ABL tyrosine kinase in chronic myeloid leukemia. *N Engl J Med* 344:1031–1037, 2001.
    A pivotal study demonstrating the safety and clinical activity of imatinib in patients with CML.
149. Azam M, Latek RR, Daley GQ: Mechanisms of autoinhibition and STI-571/imatinib resistance revealed by mutagenesis of BCR-ABL. *Cell* 112:831–843, 2003.
    A critical study demonstrating that resistance mutations to targeted therapies can be predicted and modeled in the preclinical setting.
163. Demetri GD, von Mehren M, Blanke CD, et al: Efficacy and safety of imatinib mesylate in advanced gastrointestinal stromal tumors. *N Engl J Med* 347:472–480, 2002.
    A pivotal clinical trial documenting that the unintended targets of some targeted therapies can be leveraged in new indications, in this case, the application of the KIT inhibitory activity of imatinib in the treatment of patients with c-KIT–mutated GIST.
174. Cools J, DeAngelo DJ, Gotlib J, et al: A tyrosine kinase created by fusion of the PDGFRA and FIP1L1 genes as a therapeutic target of imatinib in idiopathic hypereosinophilic syndrome. *N Engl J Med* 348:1201–1214, 2003.
    A study demonstrating that unusual responders to targeted therapies can be studied to uncover the mechanistic reason behind their response.
181. Lynch TJ, Bell DW, Sordella R, et al: Activating mutations in the epidermal growth factor receptor underlying responsiveness of non–small cell lung cancer to gefitinib. *N Engl J Med* 350:2129–2139, 2004.
    This article documents one of the earliest examples of dramatic responses to targeted therapies seen in select genotypes.
190. Kwak EL, Bang YJ, Camidge DR, et al: Anaplastic lymphoma kinase inhibition in non–small cell lung cancer. *N Engl J Med* 363:1693–1703, 2010.
    One of the initial trials demonstrating dramatic responses in patients with ALK-positive NSCLC to ALK inhibition with crizotinib.
192. Sosman JA, Kim KB, Schuchter L, et al: Survival in BRAF V600-mutant advanced melanoma treated with vemurafenib. *N Engl J Med* 366:707–714, 2012.
    Pivotal trial demonstrating a survival advantage in patients with BRAF-mutant melanoma treated with the BRAF inhibitor vemurafenib.
199. Coiffier B, Lepage E, Briere J, et al: CHOP chemotherapy plus rituximab compared with CHOP alone in elderly patients with diffuse large-B-cell lymphoma. *N Engl J Med* 346:235–242, 2002.
    Landmark trial for antibody-based lineage-targeted therapy demonstrating efficacy of rituximab in elderly patients with diffuse large-B-cell lymphoma.
229. Janeway KA, Place AE, Kieran MW, et al: Future of clinical genomics in pediatric oncology. *J Clin Oncol* 31:1893–1903, 2013.
    Review article that features currently druggable targets and their small molecule modulators relevant to pediatric malignancies.
233. Schultz KR, Bowman WP, Aledo A, et al: Improved early event-free survival with imatinib in Philadelphia chromosome-positive acute lymphoblastic leukemia: a children's oncology group study. *J Clin Oncol* 27:5175–5181, 2009.
    Study demonstrating the efficacy of imatinib in BCR-ABL–positive ALL.

268. Smith CC, Wang Q, Chin CS, et al: Validation of ITD mutations in FLT3 as a therapeutic target in human acute myeloid leukaemia. *Nature* 485:260–263, 2012.

Landmark study validating FLT3 as a therapeutic target in AML, a much debated topic, by demonstrating resistance mutations in FLT3 in patients who develop clinical resistance while receiving a FLT3 inhibitor.

297. Bissler JJ, McCormack FX, Young LR, et al: Sirolimus for angiomyolipoma in tuberous sclerosis complex or lymphangioleiomyomatosis. *N Engl J Med* 358:140–151, 2008.

This report demonstrated the efficacy of the inhibition of mTOR as an approach to inhibit tumor progression in patients with TSC1 or TSC2 loss-of-function mutations.

316. Weng AP, Ferrando AA, Lee W, et al: Activating mutations of NOTCH1 in human T cell acute lymphoblastic leukemia. *Science* 306:269–271, 2004.

First article to report frequent activating mutations in NOTCH1 in T-ALL and dependency of these T-ALLs on NOTCH1.

381. Puissant A, Frumm SM, Alexe G, et al: Targeting MYCN in neuroblastoma by BET bromodomain inhibition. *Cancer Discov* 3:308–323, 2013.

This study, which demonstrates the power of cell line screening to match genotype with drug sensitivity, identifies MYCN amplification as a predictor of response to BET inhibitors.

396. Yu AL, Gilman AL, Ozkaynak MF, et al: Anti-GD2 antibody with GM-CSF, interleukin-2, and isotretinoin for neuroblastoma. *N Engl J Med* 363:1324–1334, 2010.

Landmark phase III trial demonstrating efficacy of lineage-directed anti-GD2 therapy coupled with immune modulation in neuroblastoma.

416. Pappo AS, Patel SR, Crowley J, et al: R1507, a monoclonal antibody to the insulin-like growth factor 1 receptor, in patients with recurrent or refractory Ewing sarcoma family of tumors: results of a phase II Sarcoma Alliance for Research through Collaboration study. *J Clin Oncol* 29:4541–4547, 2011.

One representative trial of the modest activity of anti–IGF-1R antibody therapy for patients with Ewing sarcoma.

430. Filippakopoulos P, Qi J, Picaud S, et al: Selective inhibition of BET bromodomains. *Nature* 471:235–239, 2010.

Report describing the first protypical BET bromodomain inhibitor and its application to cancer therapy.

453. Wilson BG, Wang X, Shen X, et al: Epigenetic antagonism between polycomb and SWI/SNF complexes during oncogenic transformation. *Cancer Cell* 18:316–328, 2010.

Manuscript demonstrating the dependency of rhaboid tumors on EZH2 for oncogenic transformation.

454. McCabe MT, Ott HM, Ganji G, et al: EZH2 inhibition as a therapeutic strategy for lymphoma with EZH2-activating mutations. *Nature* 492:108–112, 2012.

One of the first papers describing the development and testing of an EZH2 inhibitor in EZH2 mutated lymphoma.

470. Daigle SR, Olhava EJ, Therkelsen CA, et al: Selective killing of mixed lineage leukemia cells by a potent small-molecule DOT1L inhibitor. *Cancer Cell* 20:53–65, 2011.

Article demonstrating dependency of MLL-rearranged leukemia on the enzymatic activity of DOT1L.

CHAPTER 45

Cytogenetic and Molecular Pathology of Pediatric Cancer

Maureen J. O'Sullivan, Carolyn A. Felix, and Jonathan A. Fletcher

CHAPTER OUTLINE

Cytogenetic and molecular analyses have provided pivotal biologic and clinical insights into pediatric neoplasia. It is increasingly evident that genetic assays of various types can provide essential diagnostic or prognostic information about pediatric solid tumors and hematologic malignancies (Tables 45-1 to 45-3). In this chapter we offer an overview of the methods in use for the analysis of cytogenetic and molecular aberrations (Table 45-4) in pediatric cancers together with their relative attributes, discuss the causes of these genetic aberrations, and summarize their diagnostic and predictive relevance in clinical practice.

CYTOGENETIC AND MOLECULAR METHODOLOGIES

The pathognomonic genetic aberrations in pediatric cancer can be evaluated by various methods. Because each of these methods has a different profile of substrate requirements, sensitivity, and specificity (see Table 45-4), the optimal approach must be tailored individually in regard to both the nature and quantity of material available and to the precise information being sought.

Karyotyping

The traditional karyotype provides a low-resolution snapshot of the entire genome. Cells are cultured, arrested in metaphase, and then subjected to staining of the chromosomes to produce characteristic banding patterns,[1-4] which are described using standardized nomenclature (Box 45-1). Probably the major advantage of karyotypic analysis is the provision of a global overview of the chromosomal composition of a cultured cellular population without any requirement for preknowledge, especially enabling the identification of completely novel aberrations (Fig. 45-1). However, karyotyping has distinct limitations, including the requirement for fresh material in sufficient amounts and slow turnaround because of time required for tumor cell growth.

Need for Sufficient Viable Tumor Cells

Solid tumors may comprise substantial nonviable or hypocellular regions containing few neoplastic cells. Such regions may be extensively necrotic because the tumor cells have died, having outstripped their blood supply.

Text continued on p. 1345

TABLE 45-1   Typical Genetic Aberrations in Soft Tissue and Bone Tumors

Histologic Findings	Cytogenetic Events	Molecular Events	Frequency (%)	Clinical Relevance
Alveolar soft part sarcoma	t(X;17)(p11;q25)	ASPSCR1 (ASPL)-TFE3 fusion	>90	
Aneurysmal bone cyst (extraosseous)	16q22 and 17p13 rearrangements	USP6 fusion genes	>50	
Angiomatoid fibrous histiocytoma	t(12;16)(q13;p11)	FUS-ATF1 fusion EWSR1 (EWS)-GREB1 fusion	10 80	
Chondromyxoid fibroma	Deletion of 6q		>75	

Chondrosarcoma
  Skeletal
  Extraskeletal myxoid
	Complex*
	t(9;22)(q22;q12)
	t(9;17)(q22;q11)
	t(9;15)(q22;q21)
		EWS-NR4A3 fusion
		TAF15-NR4A3 fusion
		TCF12-NR4A3 fusion
			>75
			>75
			<10
			<10	

Clear cell sarcoma—melanoma of soft parts	t(12;22)(q13;q12)	EWS-ATF1 fusion	>	
Dermatofibrosarcoma protuberans	Ring form of chromosomes 17 and 22 t(17;22)(q21;q13)	COL1A1-PDGFB fusion COL1A1-PDGFB fusion	>75 10	PDGFRB therapeutic inhibition PDGFRB therapeutic inhibition
Desmoplastic small round cell tumor	t(11;22)(p13;q12)	EWS-WT1 fusion	>75	
Endometrial stromal tumor	t(7;17)(p15;q21)	JAZF1-SUZ12	30	
Ewing sarcoma	t(11;22)(q24;q12) t(21;22)(q12;q12) t(2;22)(q33;q12) t(7;22)(p22;q12) t(17;22)(q12;q12) t(16;21)(p11;q12) t(2;16)(q33;p11) inv(22)(q12q12)	EWS-FLI1 fusion EWS-ERG fusion EWS-FEV fusion EWS-ETV1 fusion EWS-ETV4 fusion FUS-ERG fusion FUS-FEV fusion EWS-PATZ1 (ZSG) fusion	>80 5-10 <5 <5 <5 <5 <5 <5	
Fibromatosis (desmoid)	Trisomies 8 and 20 Deletion of 5q	APC inactivation CTNNB1 mutation	30 10 70	Association with germline APC mutation and familial adenomatous polyposis
Fibromyxoid sarcoma, low-grade	t(7;16)(q33;p11)	FUS-CREB3L2 (BBF2H7) fusion	50	
Fibrosarcoma, infantile	t(12;15)(p13;q26) Trisomies 8, 11, 17, and 20	ETV6 (TEL)-NTRK3 fusion	>75 >75	NTRK3 therapeutic inhibition
Gastrointestinal stromal tumor	Monosomies 14 and 22 Deletion of 1p	KIT or PDGFRA mutation	>75 >25 >90	KIT-PDGFRA therapeutic inhibition

Giant cell tumor
  Bone
  Tenosynovial
	Telomeric associations
	Trisomies 5 and 7
	t(1;2)(p13;q35)
		CSF1-COL6A3 fusion	>50
			>25
			25
				CSF1R therapeutic inhibition

Hibernoma	11q13 rearrangement		>50	

TABLE 45-1   Typical Genetic Aberrations in Soft Tissue and Bone Tumors (Continued)

Histologic Findings	Cytogenetic Events	Molecular Events	Frequency (%)	Clinical Relevance
Inflammatory myofibroblastic tumor	2p23 rearrangement	*ALK* fusion genes	50	ALK therapeutic inhibition
Leiomyoma				
Uterine	t(12;14)(q15;q24) or deletion of 7q	*LHFP (HMGIC)* rearrangement	40	
Extrauterine	Deletion of 1p		?	
Leiomyosarcoma	Deletion of 1p		>50	
Lipoblastoma	8q12 rearrangement or polysomy 8	*PLAG1* oncogenes	>80	
Lipoma				
Typical	12q15 rearrangement	*HMGIC* rearrangement	60	
Spindle cell or pleomorphic	Deletion of 13q or 16q		>75	
Chondroid	t(11;16)(q13;p12-13)		?	
Liposarcoma				
Well-differentiated	Ring form of chromosome 12		>75	
Myxoid, round cell	t(12;16)(q13;p11)	*FUS-DDIT3 (CHOP)* fusion	>75	Trabectedin therapeutic response
	t(12;22)(q13;q12)	*EWS-CHOP* fusion	<5	
Pleomorphic	Complex*		90	
Malignant fibrous histiocytoma				
Myxoid	Ring form of chromosome 12		?	
High-grade	Complex*		>90	
Myxofibrosarcoma	(see "Malignant fibrous histiocytoma")			
Malignant peripheral nerve sheath tumor	(see "Schwannoma")			
Mesothelioma	Deletion of 1p	*?BCL10* inactivation	>50	
	Deletion of 9p	*p15*, *p16*, and *p19* inactivation	>75	
	Deletion of 22q	*NF2* inactivation	>50	
	Deletions of 3p and 6q		>50	
Neuroblastoma				
Good prognosis	Hyperdiploid, no 1p deletion		40	
Poor prognosis	1p deletion		40	
	Double-minute chromosomes	*MYCN* amplification	>25	
Oligodendroglioma	Deletion of 1p and 19q			Therapeutic response to CDDP
Osteochondroma	Deletion of 8q	*EXT1* inactivation	>25	
Osteosarcoma				
Low-grade	Ring chromosomes		>50	
High-grade	Complex*	*RB1* and *TP53* inactivation	>80	
Pericytoma	t(7;12)(p22;q13-15)	*GLI-ACTB* fusion	?	
Pigmented villonodular synovitis	(see "Giant cell tumor: Tenosynovial")			
Primitive neuroectodermal tumor	(see "Ewing sarcoma")			
Rhabdoid tumor	Deletion of 22q	*SMARCB1 (INI1)* inactivation	>90	

Continued on following page

TABLE 45-1   Typical Genetic Aberrations in Soft Tissue and Bone Tumors (Continued)

Histologic Findings	Cytogenetic Events	Molecular Events	Frequency (%)	Clinical Relevance
Rhabdomyosarcoma				
Alveolar	t(2;13)(q35;q14)	*PAX3-FOXO1* fusion	60	Prognosis
	t(1;13)(p36;q14), double minutes	*PAX7-FOXO1* fusion	10-20	Prognosis
Embryonal	Trisomies 2q, 8 and 20		>75	
		Loss of heterozygosity at 11p15	>75	
Schwannoma				
Benign	Deletion of 22q	*NF2* inactivation	>80	
Malignant, low-grade	None			
Malignant, high-grade	Complex*		>90	
Synovial sarcoma				
Monophasic	t(X;18)(p11;q11)	*SS18 (SYT)-SSX1* or *SYT-SSX2* fusion	>90	Prognosis
Biphasic	t(X;18)(p11;q11)	*SYT-SSX1* fusion	>90	
Wilms tumor	Deletion 11p13	*WT1* inactivation		Association with syndromic Wilms tumor
	1p deletion			Adverse prognosis in low-stage FH
	16q deletion			Adverse prognosis in low-stage FH
	1q gain			Increased relapse risk

CDDP, cis-Diamminedichloroplatinum; *FH*, favorable histology; *PDGFRA*, platelet-derived growth factor receptor alpha; *PDGFRB*, platelet-derived growth factor receptor beta.
*Indicates presence of complicated numeric and structural chromosomal aberrations.

TABLE 45-2   Typical Genetic Aberrations in Pediatric Lymphomas

Histologic Findings	Cytogenetic Events	Molecular Events	Frequency (%)
Hodgkin, classic	Complex*	Clonal Ig rearrangements	95
		Clonal *IGH* translocations	17
		Clonal *IGK* translocations	1
		Clonal *IGL* translocations	3
		Clonal TCR rearrangements	1-2
Hodgkin, nodular lymphocyte predominance	t(3;14)(q27;q32)	*BCL6* rearrangement	50
Burkitt	t(8;14)(q24;q32)	*IGH-MYC* rearrangement	80
	t(2;8)(p11;q24)	*IGK-MYC* rearrangement	5
	t(8;22)(q24;q11)	*IGL-MYC* rearrangement	15
Lymphoblastic (see Table 45-4) ALL			
Anaplastic large cell	t(2;5)(p23;q35)	*NpM1 (NPM)-ALK* fusion	80
	Various inversions and translocations	*ALK* fusions with *TPM3, ATIC, CLTC* and others	10-20
Diffuse large B-cell	Complex*		
Subcutaneous panniculitic T-cell		Clonal T-cell receptor rearrangements	
Hepatosplenic T-cell	Isochromosome 7q; trisomy 8	Clonal T-cell receptor rearrangements	>75

*Indicates presence of complicated numeric and structural chromosomal aberrations.

TABLE 45-3 Typical Genetic Aberrations in Pediatric Leukemias and Myeloproliferative Disorders

Histologic Findings	Cytogenetic Events	Molecular Events	Frequency	Clinical Relevance
Early T-cell precursor ALL	*MEF2C* rearrangements (e.g., *MEF2C-PITX2*) or related rearrangements (*NKX2-5/BCL11B, SPI1(PU.1)/BCL11B, ETV6/NCOA2*) *RUNX1-AFF3* rearrangement	AML-like aberrations: Cytokine receptor and RAS signaling mutations (*NRAS, KRAS, NF1, FLT3, IL7R, JAK3, JAK1, SH2B, BRAF;* 67%) Inactivating hematopoietic transcription factor mutations (*GATA3, ETV6, RUNX1, IKZF1;* 58%) Inactivating histone modifier mutations (*EZH2, EED, SUZ12, SETD2; EP300;* 48%) Novel and other mutations (*WT-1, DNM2, ECT2L, RELN*)	Accounts for 5-16% pediatric T-ALL	Associated with poor prognosis, early T-cell differentiation arrest (CD1a−, CD8−, CD5weak, stem-cell or myeloid marker+, biallelic *TRG* deletions absent)
T-cell ALL	t(1;14)(p34;q11)	*SCL(TAL1)*-TCR alpha-delta locus fusions *or SIL-SCL* rearrangements	30% T-cell ALL	
	t(1;3)(p34;p21)	*SCL-TCTA* fusion	Rare	
	Chromosome band 11p13 translocations	*LMO2*-TCR loci fusions	10%-20% T-cell ALL	
	Chromosome band 11p15, 19p13.2, or 10q24 translocations	*LMO1, LYL1, TLX1 (HOX11)*-TCR loci fusions	?	
	t(7;9)(q34;q34)	*TRB (TCRB)-NOTCH1* fusion, activating *NOTCH1* mutations	<1% T-cell ALL	Gamma secretase inhibitor sensitivity
	t(6;7)(q23;q34)	*TCRB-MYB (CMYB)* fusion		Associated with young age
		Activating *NOTCH1* mutations	50% T-cell ALL	
		PTEN gene mutation	8% T-cell ALL	Associated with disease progression
	t(10;14)(q24;q11)	*HOX11(TLX1)* overexpression, *HOX11(TLX1)-TCRD* fusion		Favorable prognosis
	Chromosome band 9p21 deletion	*CDKN2A (p16^{INK4A}-p14^{ARF})* deletion; variable *CDKN2B (p15^{INK4B})* deletion		Associated with relapse, poor prognosis
Cortical T-cell ALL	*NKX2-1* or *NKX2-2* rearrangement *TLX1* rearrangement *MYB* rearrangement			CD1+ immunophenotype, associated with favorable prognosis
T-cell ALL, precursor B-cell ALL	Translocations, inversions involving chromosome bands 14q32, 14q11, 7q34, 7p14	Hybrid antigen receptor gene rearrangements	?	
	Chromosome band 9p21 deletion	*CDKN2A (p16^{INK4A})/p14^{ARF})* deletion/ variable *CDKN2B (p15^{INK4B})* deletion	60% T-cell ALL, 20% childhood precursor B-cell ALL	

Continued on following page

TABLE 45-3   Typical Genetic Aberrations in Pediatric Leukemias and Myeloproliferative Disorders (Continued)

Histologic Findings	Cytogenetic Events	Molecular Events	Frequency	Clinical Relevance
Precursor B-cell ALL	Chromosome band 11q23 translocations	*MLL (KMT2A)* gene rearrangements	80% of infant ALL	Poor prognosis especially in ALL and therapy-related cases, associated with FAB M4, FAB M5, other AML morphologies, leukemia cutis, extramedullary involvement, and topoisomerase II (TOP2) poison exposure
	Hyperdiploidy		30% precursor B-cell ALL	Favorable prognosis if >50 chromosomes and specific trisomies
	Hypodiploidy		6%-8% precursor B-cell ALL	Unfavorable prognosis if <44 chromosomes, −7, dicentric chromosome
	t(12;21)(p13;q21) (cryptic; detectable by FISH only)	*TEL-AML1* fusion	25% of "common" ALL	Favorable prognosis
	t(9;22)(q34;q11)	*BCR-ABL1* fusion	5% precursor B-cell ALL	Poor prognosis, associated with older age, imatinib mesylate sensitivity
	t(1;19)(q23;p13.3)	*E2A-PBX1* fusion	~4% Precursor B-cell ALL; 25% cIg+ cases; <1% cIg− cases	Poor prognosis in cIg+ cases
	t(17;19)(q22;p13.3)	*E2A-HLF* fusion	1% precursor B-cell ALL	Coagulopathy, poor prognosis
	t(5;14)(q31;q32)	*IGH-IL3* fusion	<1% precursor B-cell ALL	Peripheral eosinophilia
	t(6;14)(p22.3;q32)	*IGH-ID4* fusion	?	Favorable prognosis
	t(1;19)(q23;p13.3)	*MEF2D-DAZAP1* fusion	?	
		FLT3 point mutation	5% childhood precursor B-cell ALL, 16% infant ALL, ~21%-28% high hyperdiploid ALL, 18% *MLL*-rearranged ALL	Poor prognosis, increased FLT3-ITD allelic ratio associated with AML relapse, sensitivity to FLT3 tyrosine kinase inhibition
		*FLT3*ITD	2% precursor B-cell ALL	Poor prognosis, increased FLT3-ITD allelic ratio associated with AML relapse, sensitivity to FLT3 tyrosine kinase inhibition
		IKZF1 mutations	10%-15% of precursor B-cell ALL	Poor prognosis
	iAMP21	Accompanying *IKZF1*, *CDKN2A/B*, *PAX5*, *ETV6*, and *RB1* alterations	~2% of B-cell precursor ALL in older children	Poor outcome with standard regimens
Precursor B-cell ALL,	Chromosome band 9p21 deletion	*CDKN2A (p16^{INK4A}-p14^{ARF}* deletion; variable *CDKN2B (p15^{INK4B})* deletion		Associated with relapse, poor prognosis
Precursor B-cell ALL "Ph-like ALL"	Cryptic rearrangements *EBF1-PDGFRB*, *BCR-JAK2*, *STRN3-JAK2*, *PAX5-JAK2*, *NUP214-ABL1*, *ETV6-ABL1*, *RANBP2-ABL1*, *RCSD1-ABL1*, *IGH-EPOR* *SH2B3* deletion	May also have *IL7R* mutation. Accompanying *IKZF1* deletions (40%) Accompanying *JAK* mutations	10% of precursor B-cell ALL, ~15% of cases of high-risk precursor B-cell ALL	Poor prognosis, preclinically responsive to TKI and JAK inhibition

TABLE 45-3 Typical Genetic Aberrations in Pediatric Leukemias and Myeloproliferative Disorders (Continued)

Histologic Findings	Cytogenetic Events	Molecular Events	Frequency	Clinical Relevance
Precursor B-cell ALL and precursor B-cell ALL in DS	CRLF2 rearrangements (Xp22.3/Yp11.3) with IGH (14q32) CRLF2 interstitial deletion (P2RY8-CRLF2 rearrangement)	CFLF2 lesion may be F232C point mutation Accompanying JAK1 or JAK2 mutations in 50% Accompanying IKZF1 mutation/deletion Accompanying IL7R	Ph-like ALL, 15% of high-risk precursor B-cell ALL, 60% Down syndrome ALL, in non-DS high-risk ALL	Associated with poor prognosis high relapse rate, high MRD, associated with Hispanic ethnicity; preclinically responsive to signal transduction inhibitors (JAK, PI3K/mTOR)
B-cell ALL	t(8;14)(q24;q32) t(2;8)(p12;q24) t(8;22)(q24;q11)	IGH-MYC fusion IGK-MYC fusion IGL-MYC fusion	Rare Rare Rare	Poor prognosis
AML	t(8;21)(q22;q22)	AML1-ETO fusion	~12% pediatric AML	Associated with FAB M2 morphology, granulocytic sarcoma presentation, favorable prognosis
	Chromosome band 11q23 translocations	MLL gene rearrangements	80% myelomonocytic-monoblastic AML in infants and young children; ~7%-18% pediatric AML	Poor prognosis especially in ALL and therapy-related cases, associated with FAB M4, FAB M5, other AML morphologies, leukemia cutis, extramedullary involvement, TOP2 poison exposure
	inv(16)(p13q22) or t(16;16)(p13;q22)	CBF-MYH11 fusion	~7% pediatric AML	Associated with abnormal eosinophils (adults), FAB M2 or M4 AML without eosinophilia (pediatrics), favorable prognosis
	t(8;16)(p11;p13)	MOZ-CBP fusion	Rare	Unfavorable prognosis, erythrophagocytosis, coagulopathy, associated with leukemia cutis and spontaneous remission in neonates
	t(6;9)(p23;q34)	DEK-NUP214 (CAN) fusion	Rare	Unfavorable prognosis
	May be associated with t(8;21) or inv(16)	KIT mutation	37% CBF AML	Sensitivity to imatinib, sensitivity to FLT3 tyrosine kinase inhibition
		NPM mutation	~7%-8% pediatric AML	Favorable prognosis in absence of FLT3 ITD
		FLT3 point mutation	7%-9% pediatric AML	Poor prognosis, increased FLT3-ITD allelic ratio associated with AML relapse, sensitivity to FLT3 tyrosine kinase inhibition
		FLT3-ITD	~12%-15% pediatric AML	Poor prognosis, increased FLT3-ITD allelic ratio associated with AML relapse, sensitivity to FLT3 tyrosine kinase inhibition
APL	t(11;17)(q23;q21)	PLZF-RARA fusion FLT3-ITD	Rare ~30% pediatric APL	Insensitive to ATRA
Therapy-related APL	t(15;17)(q22;q21)	PML-RARA fusion		Favorable prognosis, ATRA sensitivity, arsenic trioxide sensitivity
Therapy-related MDS/AML, de novo MDS/AML	Monosomy 7/del(7q)		~40% pediatric MDS, 49% RC, 4%-5% pediatric AML	Alkylating agent exposure, associated with disease progression, poor prognosis, can be familial
De novo or therapy-related AML, ALL, MDS	Chromosome band 11p15 translocations	NUP98 gene rearrangements	?	

Continued on following page

TABLE 45-3   Typical Genetic Aberrations in Pediatric Leukemias and Myeloproliferative Disorders (Continued)

Histologic Findings	Cytogenetic Events	Molecular Events	Frequency	Clinical Relevance
Therapy-related MDS/ AML	Monosomy 5, del(5q)			Alkylating agent exposure
	May be associated with segmental jumping translocations	TP53 mutation	? (more common in therapy-related than de novo MDS, AML)	Alkylating agent exposure, associated with AML in Li-Fraumeni syndrome
Therapy related ALL and AML after exposure to TOP2 poisons	Chromosome band 11q23 translocations	MLL gene rearrangements		Poor prognosis especially in ALL and therapy-related cases, associated with FAB M4, FAB M5, other AML morphologies, leukemia cutis, extramedullary involvement, TOP2 poison exposure
5q− syndrome, refractory anemia	del(5q)	RPS14 deletion	?—not described in children	Lenalidomide sensitivity
JMML, AML, MDS, precursor B-cell ALL		PTPN11 mutation	30%-35% of JMML, 4% of AML, 18% of FAB M5 AML	Associated with Noonan syndrome
JMML	May be associated with monosomy 7	NF1 mutation	~30% of JMML, ~50% of JMML in constitutional NF1 syndrome	Associated with constitutional NF1 syndrome
JMML, AML, MDS	May be associated with monosomy 7 in JMML/MDS or with t(8;21) or inv(16) in AML	KRAS or NRAS mutation	20%-30% JMML, ~20%-30% pediatric AML, 30% monosomy 7 MDS	
CMML	t(5;12)(q33;p13)	TEL-PDGFRB fusion	Rare	Associated with eosinophilia, progression to AML
TAM, AMKL	May be associated with +8 if progression to AMKL	GATA1 mutations		Associated with Down syndrome
Non–Down syndrome AMKL	t(1;22)(p13;q13)	OTT-MAL fusion	Rare	Found in neonates
Refractory cytopenia (RC)	Trisomy 8		9% of RC	

ALL, Acute lymphocytic leukemia; AMKL, acute megakaryoblastic leukemia; AML, acute myeloid leukemia; APL, acute promyelocytic leukemia; CBF, core-binding factor; CMML, chronic myelomonocytic leukemia; FAB, French-American-British classification; FISH, fluorescence in situ hybridization; ITD, internal tandem duplication; JMML, juvenile myelomonocytic leukemia; MDS, myelodysplastic syndrome; MRD, minimal residual disease; NF1, neurofibromatosis type 1; TAM, transient abnormal myelopoiesis.

TABLE 45-4   Complementary Nature of Cytogenetic and Molecular Assays

Assay Consideration	METHOD				
	Karyotyping	FISH	CGH	SNP	PCR Sequencing
Cost of assay	High	Low	High	High	Low
What types of tumor material can be used?	Fresh	Any	Fresh, frozen*	Fresh, frozen*	Any
Does assay detect translocations?	Yes	Yes	No	No	Yes
Does assay detect point mutations?	No	No	No	No	Yes
Does assay detect deletions?	Yes	Yes	Yes	Yes	Yes, if qPCR
Does assay detect amplifications?	Yes	Yes	Yes	Yes	Yes, if qPCR
Does assay detect low-frequency mutations?	No	Yes; 1 in 100	No	No	Yes; 1 in 10,000
Does assay permit genome-wide evaluation?	Yes	No	Yes	Yes	No

CGH, Comparative genomic hybridization; FISH, fluorescence in situ hybridization; PCR, polymerase chain reaction; qPCR, quantitative PCR; SNP, single-nucleotide polymorphism analysis.
*Can be performed using DNA extracted from paraffin materials, but with some loss of resolution.

Box 45-1   Cytogenetic Abbreviations and Definitions

cDNA: complementary DNA
cen: centromere
CGH: comparative genomic hybridization
CISH: chromogenic in situ hybridization
del: deletion
dmin; double minute chromosome (extrachromosomal amplicon)
FISH: fluorescence in situ hybridization
hsr: homogeneously staining region (intrachromosomal amplicon)
ins: insertion within chromosome
inv: inversion of chromosome segment
ISH: in situ hybridization
mar: marker chromosome (aberrant chromosome whose origin cannot be ascertained)
p: chromosome short arm
q: chromosome long arm
r: ring chromosome
SKY: spectral karyotyping
t: translocation
tel: telomere

Other regions of a tumor mass may be composed largely of blood (hemorrhage) or scar tissue (fibrosis). Therefore in the case of solid tumor karyotyping, it is crucial that the pathologist select a maximally viable region for analysis.

Unpredictable Tumor Cell Growth in Culture

Even when tumor tissue has been selected from an optimal region, the unpredictable growth of neoplastic cells in culture remains a major consideration. Benign tumors often contain only few mitotic cells and so one generally has to wait several days before such specimens proliferate actively in culture. In the meantime, the culture may become overgrown by nonneoplastic cells, such as fibroblasts. Perhaps surprisingly, even highly malignant solid tumors may grow poorly in tissue culture, despite the fact that they grew well in the patient. Such tumor cultures may occasionally be stimulated by the use of specialized culture media or growth factors,[5] but it is impractical in most clinical cytogenetic laboratories to troubleshoot tissue cultures to optimize the growth of each tumor type. Therefore in practice it may be challenging to culture and

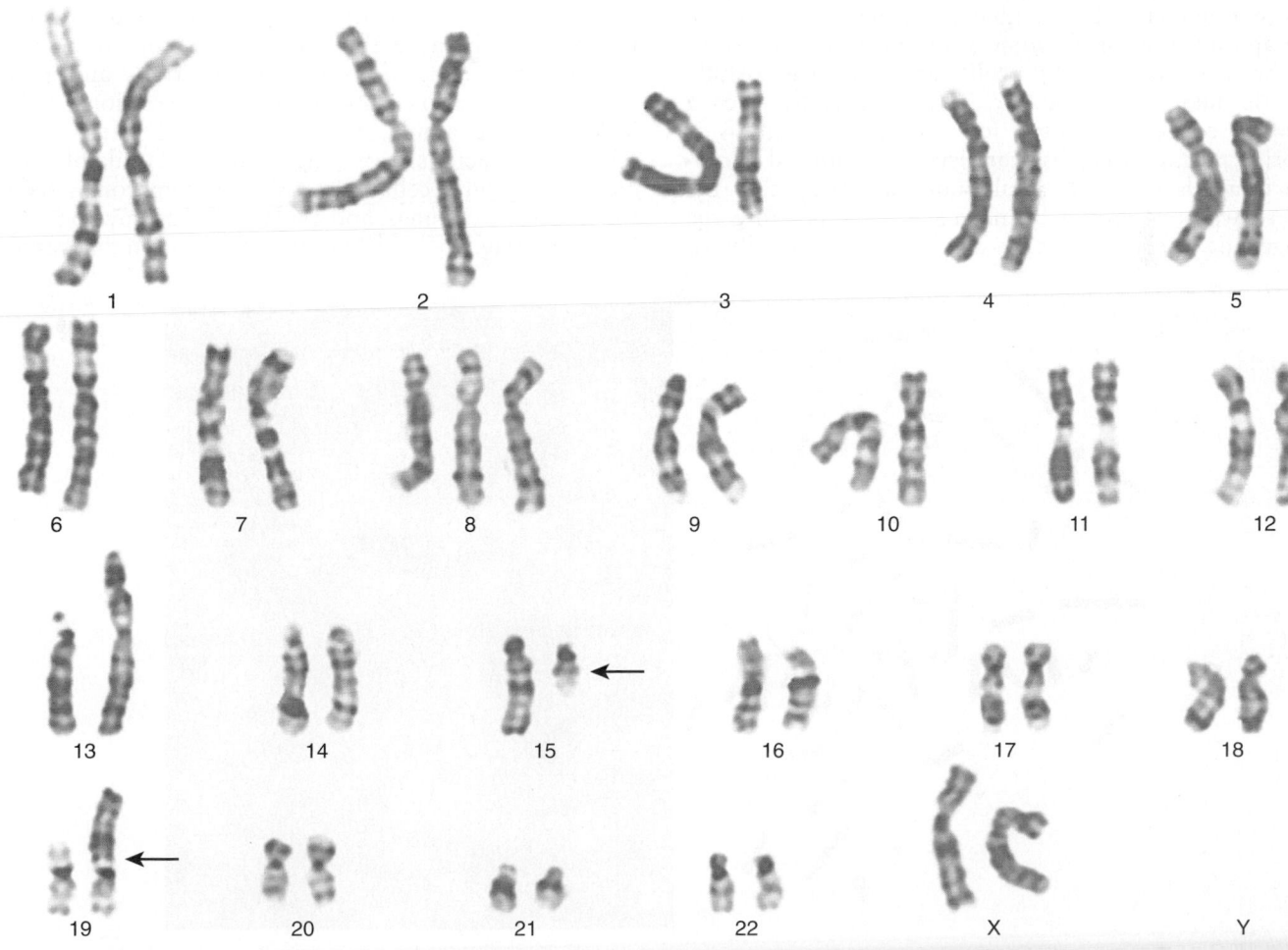

Figure 45-1 Giemsa-banded karyotype of highly lethal NUT midline carcinoma, demonstrating balanced t(15;19) with *arrows* indicating the translocation breakpoints. Other cytogenetic findings, including chromosome 3 and 13 rearrangements and trisomy 8, are secondary aberrations.

karyotype certain types of pediatric tumors in the clinical laboratory. In the case of bone marrow cytogenetics, it is well known that posttherapeutic specimens can be difficult to analyze, being hypocellular and containing cells—reactive and/or neoplastic—that have been temporarily growth-arrested by therapy and therefore fail to give rise to metaphases in culture.

Nonrepresentative Cell Culture

It is also important to recognize that only a subpopulation of cells within a given sample might be capable of growing under a particular set of culture conditions. Therefore one cannot necessarily assume that a clonally abnormal karyotype is representative of the overall neoplastic process. For example, in a given tumor, the final karyotype might be representative of the components of the tumor that were more or less clinically aggressive, depending on which component was best suited for growth under the particular culture conditions used at that time.

Culture Overgrowth by Nonneoplastic Cells

All tumor samples contain mixtures of neoplastic and nonneoplastic cells. The nonneoplastic elements may include hematopoietic cells, fibroblasts, normal epithelial cells, endothelial cells, or glial cells, depending on the type and location of the tumor. Any of these reactive or support cell types might proliferate more successfully than the neoplastic cells in culture. Invariably, when a pediatric cancer submitted for cytogenetic analysis is reported to have a normal karyotype, the normal karyotype is a false-negative result, only signifying that the culture was overgrown by normal cells. Therefore the cytogenetic analysis must always be timed carefully, so

that metaphases are analyzed at a point at which the neoplastic population is actively dividing. This technical challenge can, in the case of solid tumors, be met if the cytogeneticist develops familiarity with the distinctive morphologies of the various neoplastic and reactive cell types and then inspects the tissue cultures daily to determine when the neoplastic cells have the proliferative advantage.[5]

Complex Karyotype

Beyond the initial challenges incurred at the culture stage, various additional considerations influence the success of cytogenetic evaluation in different types of pediatric cancer. For example, conventional karyotyping can be challenging in many high-grade solid tumors, in which the karyotypes are often complex compared with those seen in leukemias and lymphomas. A single metaphase cell from such cancers can contain dozens of clonal and nonclonal chromosomal aberrations, making it impractical to characterize the exact mechanisms of rearrangement responsible for each chromosomal aberration or to estimate the relative significance of any of these abnormalities.

Technical Limitations in Detecting Aberrations

There are certain aberrations that cannot be detected by karyotyping, because the resolution is too low. These include smaller deletions or amplifications and point mutations, but also cryptic or masked aberrations, which include, for example, the chromosomal translocation t(12;15) characteristic of congenital or infantile fibrosarcoma, congenital cellular mesoblastic nephroma, secretory breast carcinomas, and a subset of acute myelogenous leukemias (Fig. 45-2).[6,7] Another translocation that cannot

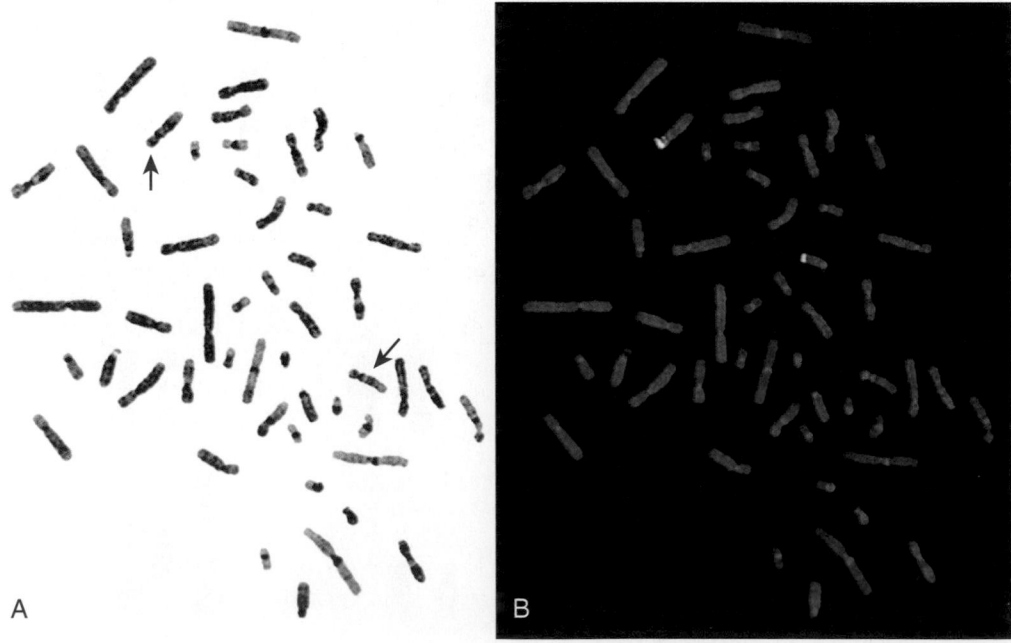

Figure 45-2 **A**, Giemsa banding studies in infantile fibrosarcoma do not reveal the characteristic, but cytogenetically cryptic t(12;15), associated with *TEL-NTRK3* oncogenic fusion. *Black arrows* indicate the normal *(top)* and rearranged *(middle)* copies of chromosome 12, as demonstrated by *TEL* break-apart fluorescence in situ hybridization (FISH). **B**, The FISH studies reveal yellow probe fusion signal on the normal chromosome 12, whereas the t(12;15) results in split red and green FISH signals on rearranged chromosomes 12 and 15, respectively.

be resolved by conventional karyotype analysis is the t(12;21), which is the most common translocation in pediatric leukemia. It is found in a large fraction of common acute lymphoblastic leukemia (ALL) in children and fuses the *ETV6 (TEL)* and *RUNX1 (AML1)* genes.

In essence, then, the major advantage of karyotypic evaluation of solid tumors is the breadth of the data provided. Notable challenges include the successful culture of representative tumor cells, particularly because this is essentially a one-shot approach, with no opportunity to return to the specimen, because the window of opportunity for culture is confined to the short period of viability of fresh cells after biopsy. Even when culture is successful, meaningful interpretation of the findings on karyotype may represent a further challenge, depending on the number and nature of the aberrations.

Although solid tumors are less readily accessible for biopsy compared with hematologic neoplasms, minimally invasive sampling by a percutaneous approach is becoming more common. Needle biopsy is often performed under ultrasound or computed tomographic (CT) guidance and can involve fine-needle aspiration or needle core biopsy of the tumor. Solid tumor samples obtained by these methods can be karyotyped successfully,[8-11] but the small amount of starting material is a constraint in that fewer cultures can be established. Because the successful cytogenetic evaluation of tumors in standard practice is limited by these factors, alternative, more robust methods are needed for the successful routine demonstration of genetic aberrations. Traditionally, these have included fluorescence in situ hybridization (FISH) and polymerase chain reaction (PCR) techniques, which have the distinct advantage of applicability to fixed material and therefore also to large cohorts of archival cases. Both FISH and molecular analyses can be straightforward also in fine-needle specimens.[12,13]

Molecular Cytogenetics

Recombinant DNA Technologies

Southern Blot Analysis. In pediatric solid tumors, leukemias, and lymphomas, recombinant DNA technologies, including Southern blot analyses of candidate genes relevant to particular disease states, can overcome limitations of conventional karyotype analysis for the detection of chromosomal aberrations (Fig. 45-3). Although no longer used extensively in most clinical diagnostic laboratories, Southern blotting has served an important role in gene discovery. That is, genomic Southern blot analyses, coupled with PCR-based molecular cloning and gene sequencing strategies, have identified unknown partner genes fused to various known genes in chromosomal translocations. For example, the demonstration of immunoglobulin *(IG)* and T-cell receptor *(TCR)* loci rearrangements in leukemias and lymphomas, as evidenced by altered size of restriction enzyme fragments on genomic Southern blot analyses, has been essential in highlighting crucial regions that could be studied by molecular cloning strategies and that characterize the genomic translocation breakpoint junction sequences that define these tumors (Fig. 45-4). The molecular

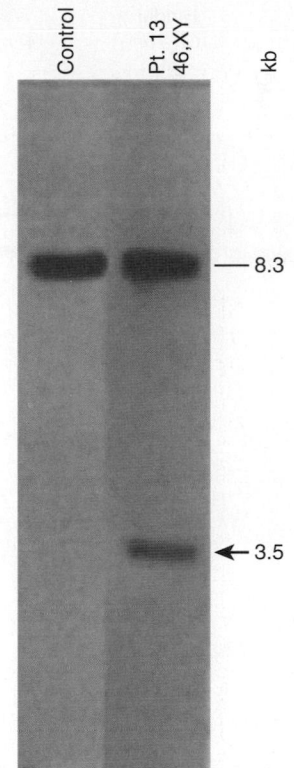

Figure 45-3 Detection of cryptic *MLL* bcr rearrangement by Southern blot analysis in treatment-associated acute myelogenous leukemia (AML). The karyotype was normal, but the French-American-British (FAB) M4 morphology and clinical history of dactinomycin exposure informed further analysis of *MLL*. The *dash* indicates the germline pattern, and the *arrow* shows a rearrangement, which panhandle polymerase chain reaction molecular cloning revealed to be an *MLL* internal tandem duplication. *(Modified from Megonigal MD, Rappaport EF, Jones DH, et al: Panhandle PCR strategy to amplify* MLL *genomic breakpoints in treatment-related leukemias. Proc Natl Acad Sci U S A 94:11583–11588, 1997.)*

principles that provide the basis for current clinical molecular cytogenetic diagnostic strategies (e.g., FISH) in pediatric leukemias and solid tumors are not substantially different from the recombinant DNA concepts used in Southern blotting. Some seminal examples of gene rearrangements characterized originally by Southern blotting and now detected routinely by FISH include *MYC* gene rearrangements, involving the *IGH* or *IGL* chain loci in Burkitt lymphoma,[14] and *MLL (KMT2A)* rearrangements, of which the first characterized type was associated with t(4;11), resulting in *MLL-AFF1 (AF4)* fusion.[15]

Another application of Southern blot analysis has been in discerning gene copy number variation. One example is *MLL* gene amplification (see Fig. 45-4), involving an interlocus DNA rearrangement known as segmental jumping translocation in which the unrearranged *MLL* DNA segment is amplified and translocated to various regions of the genome.[16]

Fluorescence and Chromogenic in Situ Hybridization. Whereas conventional cytogenetic analyses are performed using staining techniques that highlight chromosomal banding patterns (1;2), the various molecular cytogenetic

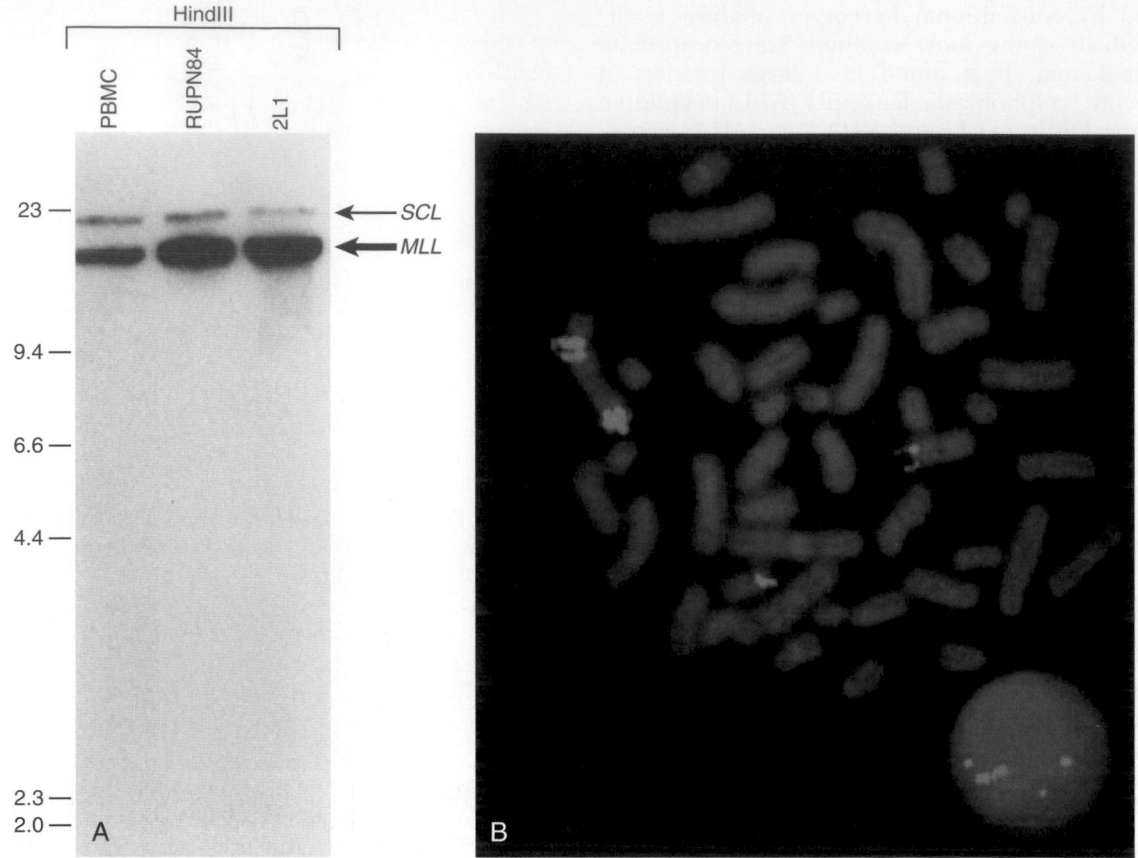

Figure 45-4 A, Southern blot analysis indicating *MLL* gene amplification in treatment-related acute myelogenous leukemia (AML). Southern blot analysis of *HindIII*-digested genomic DNA from French-American-British M4 AML cells (RUPN84) of a patient whose AML karyotype showed no evidence of chromosome band 11q23 rearrangement that would suggest *MLL* gene rearrangement and a cell line established from the same AML (2L1). Cohybridization with a *MLL* bcr-region probe and a loading control *SCL* probe demonstrates unrearranged but amplified *MLL* with signal intensity of 4.3 : 1 in the AML compared with normal peripheral blood mononuclear cell (PBMC) control DNA. **B,** Fluorescence in situ hybridization confirms *MLL* genomic amplification in RUPN84. *(Modified from Felix CA, Megonigal MD, Chervinsky DS, et al: Association of germline p53 mutation with* MLL *segmental jumping translocation in treatment-related leukemia.* Blood *91:4451–4456, 1998.)*

methods interrogate chromosomal regions of interest by using nucleic acid probes.[17,18] Most molecular cytogenetic methods use some variant of in situ hybridization (ISH), in which DNA probes are hybridized and evaluated in the cellular context. These probes are usually cosmids, containing an approximately 40-kb sequence of interest or bacterial artificial chromosomes, containing hundreds to a few thousand kilobases of sequence. ISH assays can be performed with fluorescence or enzymatic detection, referred to as FISH and CISH (chromogenic in situ hybridization), respectively (Figs. 45-5 and 45-6).[18]

Flexibility of in Situ Hybridization: Substrate Options. FISH and CISH analyses are performed routinely in cytogenetic preparations (metaphase spreads) and in paraffin sections and other archival pathologic preparations. Substantial advantages of using paraffin sections include the following: (1) the abundance of source material for each case permits retrospective and repeat analyses; and (2) the well-preserved cell morphology can guide evaluation of the chromosomal events in the relevant cell populations. However, a drawback in the use of paraffin sections is that the nuclei are generally incomplete, having been sliced through during preparation of the sections by

microtomy.[19] This limitation can be addressed by performing the ISH assays with nuclei disaggregated from thick (50- to 60-μμ) paraffin sections[20] or from thin cores of the paraffin block.[21]

Resolution. Most ISH studies have a resolution of one to several megabases on metaphase spreads. Notwithstanding the aforementioned problems of interphase FISH on fixed material, the technique offers the advantage of higher resolution, given the less compact arrangement of DNA in interphase nuclei. Higher-resolution FISH techniques have been developed in which the DNA is essentially stretched out over a slide, as in direct visual hybridization (DIRVISH), resulting in a resolution of between 700 and 5 kb,[22] or fiber FISH, in which the resolution is between 500 kb and just a few kilobases.[23]

Highly Combinatorial Modifications of FISH. Various molecular cytogenetic methods have expanded the capabilities of FISH, enabling evaluation of the entire genome or karyotype. Examples include comparative genomic hybridization (CGH)[24,25] and spectral karyotyping (SKY).[26] CGH is performed by extracting total genomic DNA from a tumor of interest and from a nonneoplastic control cell population. These DNAs are differentially

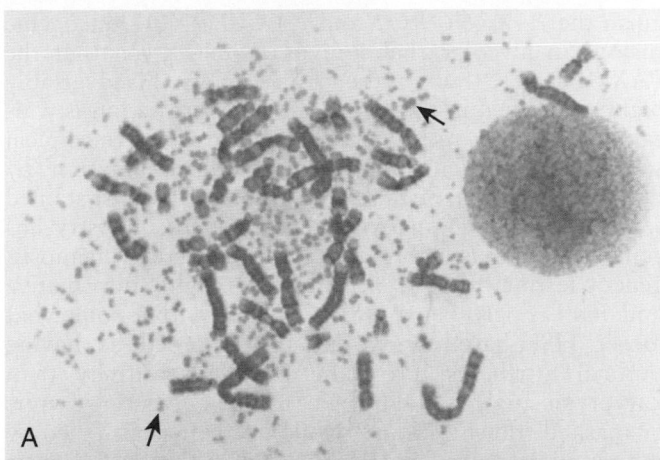

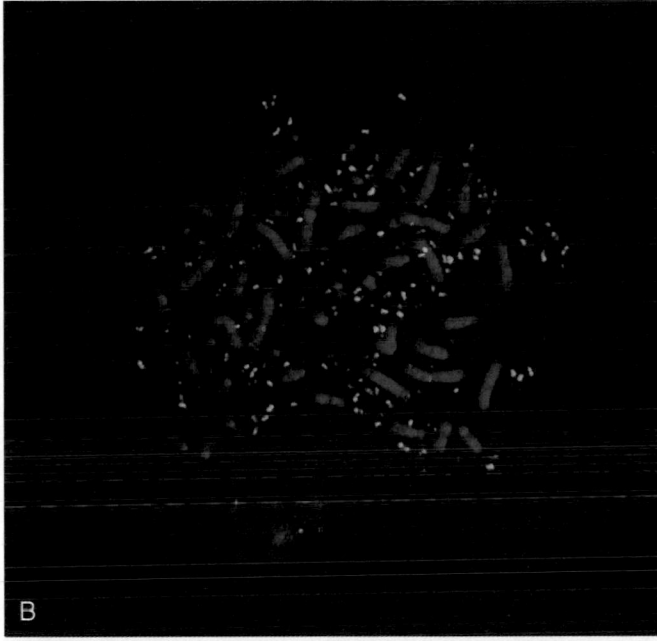

the in vivo situation, although diluted by the admixture of support stromal DNA. In addition, the array CGH methods (discussed later) can detect very small deletions, which would be overlooked by traditional cytogenetic banding assays and might even be missed by FISH. However, CGH does not detect the balanced chromosomal rearrangements, particularly the translocations that are the genetic hallmarks of many pediatric cancers. Furthermore, while detecting chromosomal amplifications and deletions reliably, the technique does not provide a functional assay in terms of expression level changes.

Genome-wide molecular cytogenetics can be performed using spectral karyotyping or M-FISH, in which entire panels of DNA probes are simultaneously hybridized against tumor metaphase cells.[26] Whereas conventional FISH techniques involve hybridization of one or two fluorescence-tagged probes, the spectral karyotyping and M-FISH methods use probes for each chromosome or chromosome arm (24 or more probes). Each probe is then detected combinatorially, using different ratios of fluorescence markers, such as fluorescein and rhodamine. By varying the ratio of fluorescence tags, each chromosome can be visualized with a unique color (Fig. 45-7). Thus spectral karyotyping enables a comprehensive ISH screen of the entire tumor cell karyotype. Spectral karyotyping and M-FISH are powerful research tools in tumor cytogenetics and have been useful in identifying rearrangements that are cryptic by conventional cytogenetic banding methods or that are highly complex.[27,28] However, these techniques have generally been supplanted by array CGH and SNP profiling methods (see later).

Routine Applications of FISH. Most ISH studies performed in clinical laboratories are focused on investigating deletions, rearrangements, or amplifications of particular gene loci or chromosomes. The probes used for

Figure 45-5 A, Giemsa-stained neuroblastoma metaphase cell (and with nucleus from a different cell on right) showing hundreds of variably sized double-minute chromosomes, as indicated by *arrows.* **B,** *MYCN* fluorescence in situ hybridization (FISH) evaluation of neuroblastoma metaphase cell, showing numerous extrachromosomal double minutes containing *MYNC (green)* whereas the reference chromosome 2 pericentromeric FISH probe *(red)* shows two copies.

labeled (e.g., tumor DNA with fluorescein and control DNA with rhodamine) and in the earliest applications were cohybridized against normal metaphase cells (metaphase CGH), although these methods have been rapidly supplanted by higher-resolution assays in which the sample DNAs are hybridized against arrayed clones (array CGH) or interrogated for presence of informative single nucleotide polymorphisms (SNPs) as an indicator of copy number and heterozygosity across the genome (discussed later).

An advantage of CGH, compared with conventional karyotyping, is that the tumor DNA can be isolated from frozen or even paraffin specimens, without any need for cell culture, thereby avoiding the selection pressures imposed by culture and instead capturing an overview of

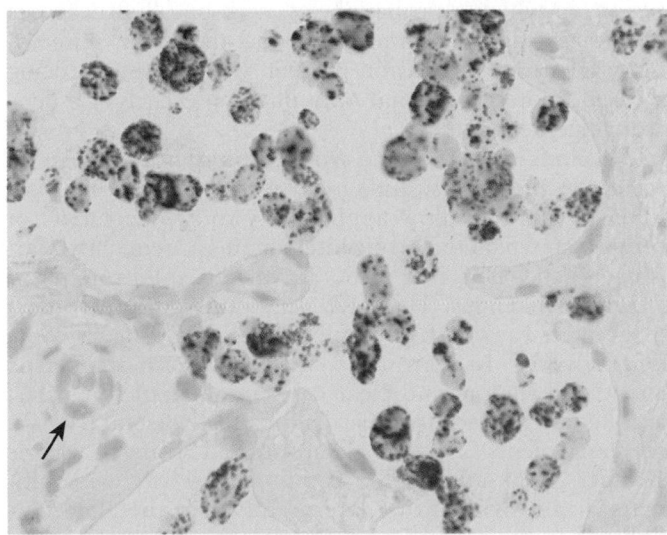

Figure 45-6 *MYCN* chromogenic in situ hybridization in a neuroblastoma paraffin section. Peroxidase-DAB detection *(brown)* of *MYCN* fluorescence in situ hybridization probe demonstrates high-level *MYCN* amplification in neuroblastoma cells but not in fibrovascular nonneoplastic cells *(arrow).*

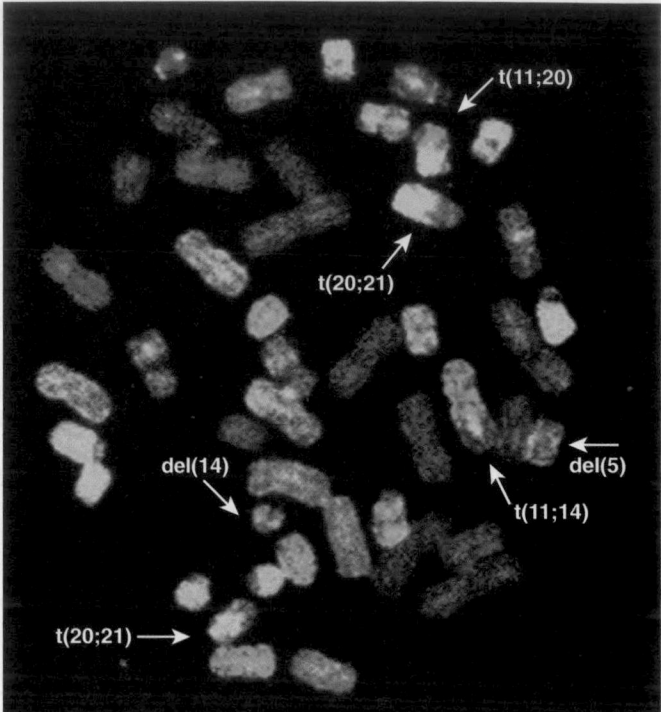

Figure 45-7 Metaphase spectral karyotype in treatment-associated acute myelogenous leukemia, showing typical 5q deletion, among other clonal aberrations. *(Courtesy Hesed, National Institutes of Health, Bethesda, Md.)*

FISH analysis of chromosomal translocations (and other balanced cytogenetic rearrangements) generally fall into two categories. First, there are those that hybridize to a region spanning a breakpoint on one involved chromosome, producing a split signal in the presence of chromosomal rearrangement (see Fig. 45-2), Second, there are probes designed to come together in the presence of a fusion, in which a probe labeled with one fluorochrome hybridizes to one partner gene and the other, differentially labeled, to its fusion partner, with these producing a fused fluorescent signal only in the presence of a gene rearrangement.

Maximizing Data Yield from Individual FISH Probes for Rearrangements. Judicious selection of break-apart FISH probes can allow applicability to a wide variety of tumors, in which the probe interrogates a frequently rearranged gene such as *EWSR1* in various solid tumors or *MLL* in leukemias. The *EWS* gene undergoes rearrangement with various ETS family genes in Ewing sarcoma and *EWSR1* is rearranged in pediatric desmoplastic round cell tumors and clear cell sarcomas of soft parts, among others. Each of these diagnostically useful *EWSR1* rearrangements can be demonstrated using a single *EWSR1* break-apart FISH probe (Fig. 45-8), with ultimate diagnosis requiring interpretation of the molecular findings in the context of the histology.

Additional gross genetic aberrations routinely accompanying chromosomal translocation may be exploited to refine interpretation of FISH-based analysis in certain contexts. For example, *FOXO1* gene FISH can distin-

guish the *PAX7-FOXO1* and *PAX3-FOXO1* oncogenic fusions in alveolar rhabdomyosarcoma, given that the *PAX7-FOXO1* (but not the *PAX3-FOXO1*) is invariably highly amplified in these tumors. This distinction is warranted because of its prognostic significance. In the typical scenario, in which routine pathologic evaluation by light microscopy of hematoxylin and eosin (H&E)-stained sections with accompanying immunohistochemistry has generated a reasonably narrow differential diagnosis, genetic testing by this type of assay is highly informative and increasingly being used. Generally, this somewhat looser FISH-based assay may be regarded as having optimal attributes, providing greater sensitivity than karyotypic analysis and being capable of detecting cryptic or masked translocations[29] while not being burdened by the restrictive specificity of PCR-based assays, a feature that is especially advantageous for detection of variant translocations.

FISH in the Analysis of Gains and Losses. Although quantitative assessment of gene amplifications and deletions can be obtained by quantitative PCR (qPCR) or FISH, in practice such assays are more often conducted in clinical laboratories by FISH-based methods. In the example of *MYCN* amplification in neuroblastoma, FISH detection is performed routinely (see Figs. 45-5 and 45-6). Assessment of *MYCN* amplification may alternatively be done by semiquantitative PCR, using a standard PCR assay with normal (unamplified) and known amplified controls and multiplexing the reaction to include a housekeeping gene along with the gene of interest. However, such assessments can be confounded by intratumoral

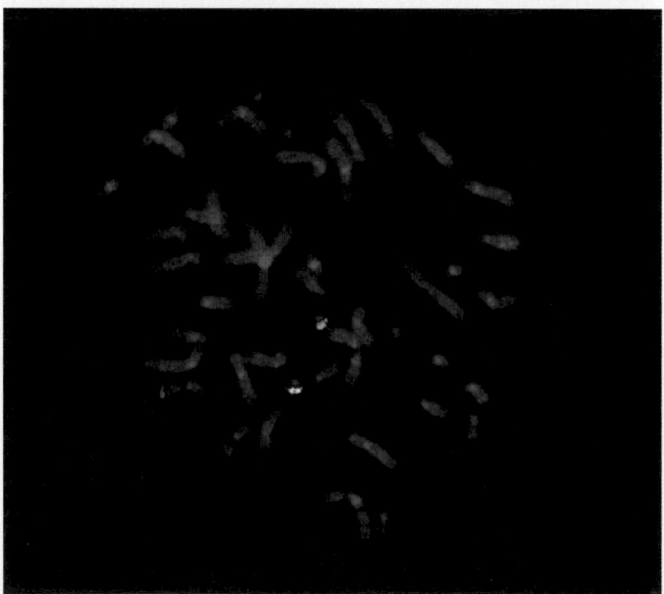

Figure 45-8 *EWS* break-apart fluorescence in situ hybridization probe, hybridized to Ewing sarcoma metaphase cell, in which probe components centromeric and telomeric to *EWSR1* are detected with fluorescein isothiocyanate *(green)* and rhodamine *(red)*, respectively. *EWSR1* rearrangement is indicated by the breaking apart of the normal yellow *(green-red fusion)* signal into the red and green components, which localize to different chromosomes as a result of translocation.

heterogeneity. In neuroblastoma, this heterogeneity may encompass substantial variations in cellular composition and maturation, and thus careful selection of tumor tissue for analysis is essential. The analysis of poorly selected tissue for *MYCN* evaluation (e.g., submission of schwannian stroma) will otherwise yield a false-negative result.[30] Moreover, contributions of different components of the neuroblastic tumor in the final DNA isolate can dilute out regional (neuroblast-specific) *MYCN* amplification, again yielding false-negative results. In this context, there is a distinct advantage to the FISH assays for *MYCN* amplification, because such methods permit correlation with cytology or morphology for the detection of regional heterogeneity of *MYCN* amplification, particularly when performed in tissue sections or multifocal touch imprints.

Detection of deletions by FISH is a more complex matter and particularly challenging when using fixed tissue, in which the assay is for an absence of signal and one is dealing with interphase nuclei, by definition incomplete (sliced through by microtomy), with an admixture of normal stromal cells further confounding the picture. Where cytogenetically abnormal metaphase spreads are available, these problems are largely circumvented, but there are other potentially more suitable technical strategies that might be used, including PCR-based assays—again with the caveat of normal cell admixture—to establish loss of heterozygosity (LOH). The immunohistochemical stain may provide a ready assay for such detection, as in the case of the *SMARCB1* gene on chromosome 22q, commonly deleted in malignant rhabdoid tumors (Fig. 45-9), and atypical teratoid rhabdoid tumors.[31]

Polymerase Chain Reaction–Based Molecular Assays

General Applications of PCR-Based Methods

Since the initial description of the basic PCR assay,[32] critical modifications of the technique have led to massive expansion of the applicability of this technology. The initial methodology involved the use of a DNA template from which a sequence of interest could selectively be amplified. This methodology provides the basis for testing for LOH, which relies on the natural allelic heterogeneity of repeat sequences in the vicinity of a gene of interest.[33] Where a genomic region is deleted, the concomitant loss of an adjacent allelic repeat sequence results in PCR amplification of only one version of the repeat sequence, thus producing hemizygosity (seeming homozygosity) at that locus.

Reverse-Transcriptase PCR Assay. When a particular question revolves around the presence of a specific transcript, the starting material is RNA, which is subjected to reverse-transcriptase PCR (RT-PCR), a highly sensitive technique.[34] The principle is that total RNA extracted from fresh, flash-frozen, or fixed material is reverse-transcribed into first-strand complementary DNA (cDNA). This provides the template[34,35] for testing for the presence of fusion oncogene transcripts using primers complementary to the involved partner genes flanking the fusion point in the chimeric transcript and which cannot therefore generate a product from unrearranged normal transcript. The technique is extraordinarily sensitive, able to detect as few as 1 in 10,000 cells bearing a fusion transcript.[36] The presence of just a small neoplastic component within a tissue sample for genetic testing is therefore sufficient for detection. Thus this PCR-based technology is useful for the detection of minimal residual disease[35] and well suited for the surveillance of hematologic malignancy, in which serial peripheral blood or bone marrow specimens are obtained for routine follow-up of patients. However, this same sensitivity of PCR-based methods carries with it the risk for false-positive results, from cross-contamination of minute amounts of fusion gene templates within assays or detection of very-low-level biologically insignificant fusion transcripts within specimens. Although moot in the context of demonstrating uniquely tumor-associated aberrations (e.g., fusion products), ideally DNAse I treatment of the RNA substrate should be performed to eliminate the possibility of inadvertent genomic amplification during RT-PCR.

Specificity of RT-PCR Reaction. Breakpoint variability within the genes involved in translocation-generated fusion oncogenes has prognostic implications in some cases. This is reported for Ewing sarcoma and synovial

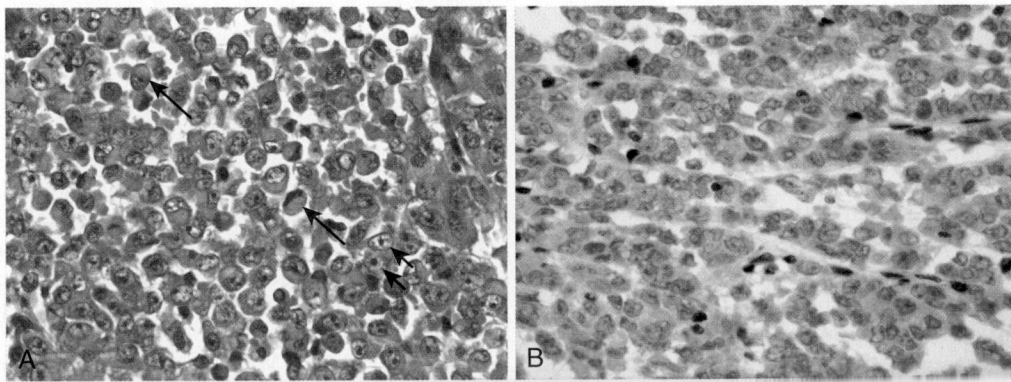

Figure 45-9 **A,** Rhabdoid tumor showing loosely cohesive cells, many containing intracytoplasmic inclusions *(arrows)*. Nuclei are vesicular and contain prominent nucleoli *(short arrows)* (H&E stain). **B,** INI1 immunohistochemistry, showing entirely negative reaction in the neoplastic cells, reflecting loss of 22q, and with only the endothelial and occasional admixed inflammatory cells staining positively.

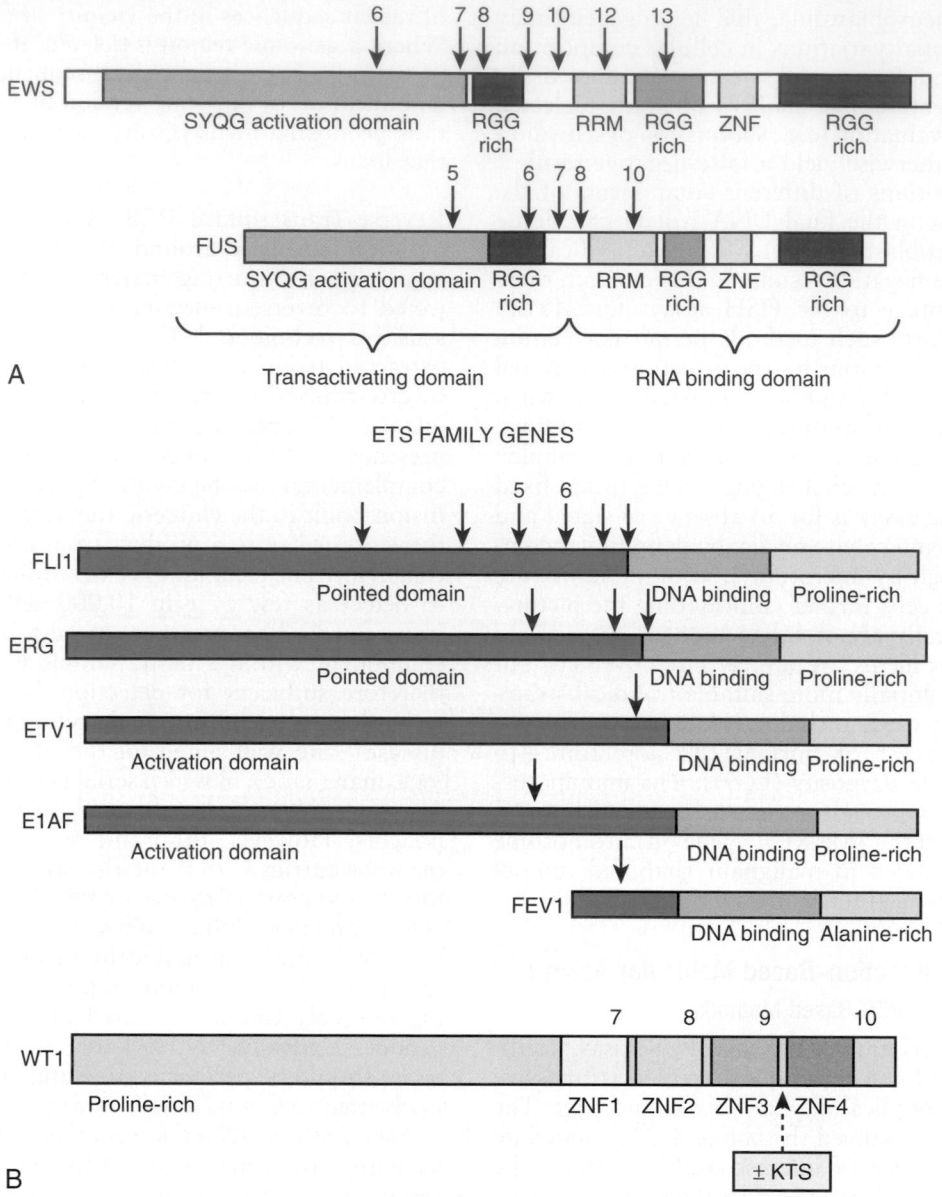

Figure 45-10 A, *EWS* and *FUS* genes encode an N-terminal transcriptional activation domain, RGG-rich regions, RNA recognition motif, and a zinc finger. *Arrows* indicate various breakpoints reported in *EWS* or *FUS* oncogenes. **B** *(top)*, Domains encoded by the various ETS-family genes fused with *EWS* or *FUS* in Ewing sarcoma. *Arrows* indicate various breakpoints that have been reported in fusion rearrangements. The most common oncogenic rearrangements in Ewing sarcoma involve the fusion of the *EWS* exon 7 to *FLI1* exon 6 (type 1 transcript) or exon 5 (type 2 transcript). **B** *(bottom)*, Domains encoded by the *WT1* gene, which is fused with *EWS* in desmoplastic small round cell tumor. Two WT1 isoforms are produced by an alternative spicing event (±KTS) between zinc fingers 3 and 4.

sarcoma, in which a favorable prognosis is associated with a type I fusion of *EWS* exon 7 to *FLI1* exon 6 compared with all other combinatorial variations in Ewing sarcoma (Fig. 45-10).[37-39] *SYT-SSX2* fusion in synovial sarcoma is similarly reportedly associated with better patient outcome.[40,41] Assays may be designed to address breakpoint variability through choice of primers, selectively amplifying only one variant product, or by choosing consensus primers that will amplify several transcripts[12,17] and then sequencing the product to establish the precise nature of the transcript. An indication of transcript type might already have been obtained from

gel electrophoresis demonstrating the product size (Fig. 45-11; see Fig. 45-10). PCR-based assays are best suited to the detection of such fine genetic detail, which cannot be detected by karyotypic analysis and only by specifically designed FISH assays. Currently, distinction among variant transcripts generally remains of academic interest because it provides no basis for therapeutic stratification.

In the case of *MLL* translocations, not only can one of more than 50 different partner genes be fused to *MLL* but it has also been suggested that the various partner genes of *MLL* affect the prognosis.[44] In this case, PCR

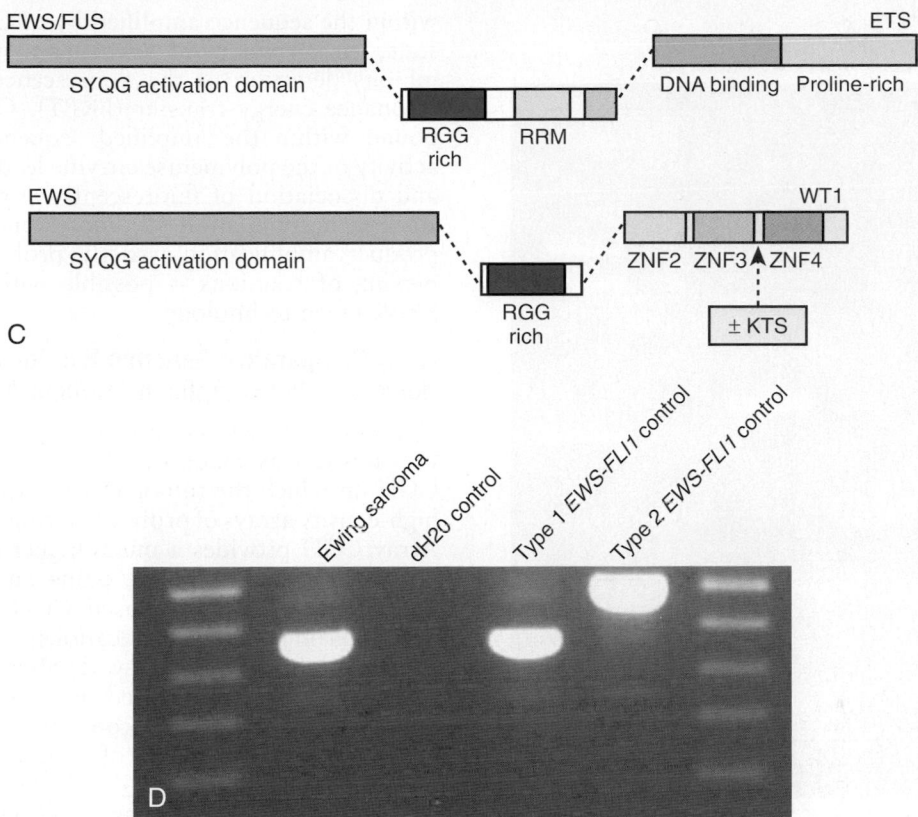

Figure 45-10, cont'd C *(top)*, Domains encoded by oncogenic fusions between *EWS* or *FUS* with an ETS family member in Ewing sarcoma. *Dotted lines* indicate regions that are variably included, depending on the breakpoint locations. C *(bottom)*, Domains encoded by the *EWS-WT1* fusion oncogene in desmoplastic small round cell tumor. *Dotted lines* indicate encoded sequences that are variably included, depending on the breakpoint locations (RGG-rich region) and alternative splicing events (KTS). **D,** Reverse-transcriptase polymerase chain reaction demonstration of type 1 *EWS-FLI1* transcript in Ewing sarcoma (lane 1). Positive controls for types 1 and 2 transcripts are in lanes 3 and 4, respectively.

with gene-specific primers has been one approach to identify fusion transcripts involving some of the more common partner genes of *MLL*, and primer combinations for different *MLL* transcripts can be combined in a multiplex PCR reaction. This is most feasible in ALL, where the *MLL* partner genes are less heterogeneous than in acute myeloid leukemia (AML). Alternatively, approaches such as cDNA panhandle PCR can detect the fusion transcript produced by the 5'-*MLL* partner gene 3' rearrangement using primer sequences derived from MLL. This is accomplished by the generation of a stem loop template in which a known *MLL* sequence has been attached to the unknown partner sequence by reverse transcribing the first-strand cDNA from total RNA using a 5'-*MLL*-random hexamer adapter-3' primer for the primer extension.[45]

Additionally, genomic panhandle PCR approaches[46-48] and long distance inverse PCR approaches[49,50] are alternatives for characterizing translocations in which the sequence of only one of the involved genes is known. And increasingly, intron-capture methods, coupled with sequencing, are used in high-throughput sequencing screens to identify oncogene fusion partners.

One clinical scenario that requires the ability to detect a broad range of chromosomal translocations, including unknown or rare fusion variants, is in surveillance screening for evidence of a preleukemic state in chemotherapy-exposed patients, before these patients manifest frank secondary leukemia.[51] Advances in sensitive molecular PCR-based screening methods and molecular cytogenetic screening methods such as FISH will better enable the prospective detection of chromosomal translocations, which is crucial in such applications.

Quantitative PCR Assay. Simultaneous PCR of a constitutively expressed housekeeping gene provides an internal control. A standard positive control may be used as a comparator across a series of cases to rank these in a semiquantitative approach.[52] Use of qPCR methods can provide precise information about the actual copy number of oncogene transcripts (gene expression level) by qRT-PCR or gene copy number when genomic DNA is used as template material. qPCR has advantages of increased reliability and reproducibility over conventional PCR. Because it provides data accrued during the entire cycle, rather than just end-point analysis, as in standard PCR, it will discriminate between different assays quantitatively rather than based on product size differences. Additionally, the graphic readout of accumulating fluorescence generated within each tube or well during the reaction is instantaneous (real time) and therefore no delaying additional step for product analysis is

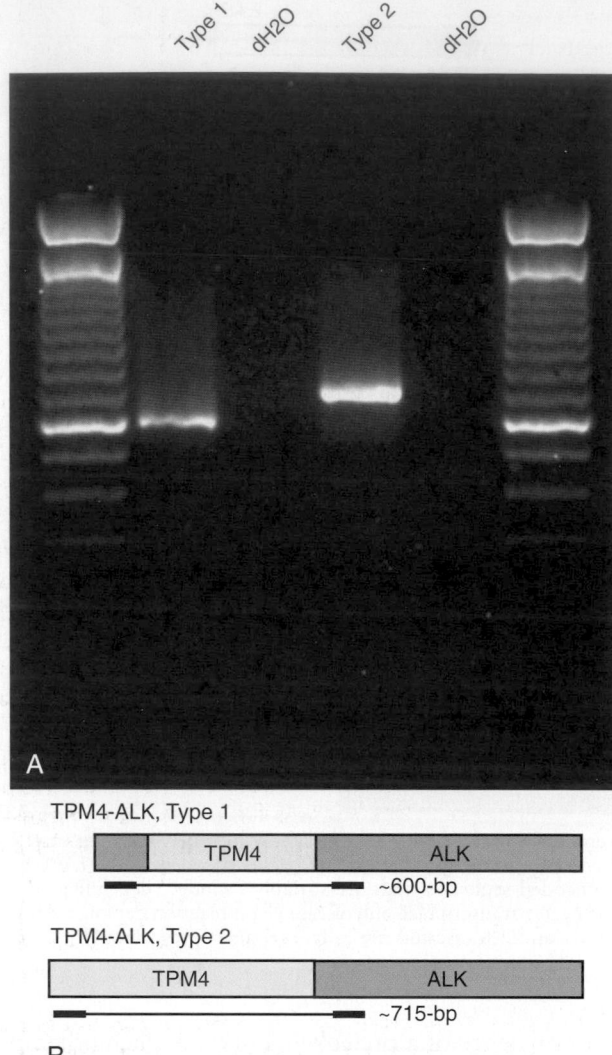

TPM4-ALK, Type 1

	TPM4	ALK	

~600-bp

TPM4-ALK, Type 2

TPM4	ALK

~715-bp

B

Figure 45-11 Reverse-transcriptase polymerase chain reaction (RT-PCR) demonstration of various *TPM4-ALK* fusion oncogene transcripts in inflammatory myofibroblastic tumors, as distinguished by gel electrophoresis of PCR products generated with the same primers (**A**), with primer hybridization sites as indicated (**B**).

required. In conventional PCR, the amplification products must typically be evaluated by gel electrophoresis. Therefore the assay turnaround time is minimized in qPCR, so that a complete analysis can be performed in only a few hours. qPCR is more sensitive, with an ability to detect twofold changes in expression level as opposed to a tenfold cutoff for standard PCR assays. If desired, the products can still be subjected to gel electrophoresis (e.g., to evaluate product size). Various forms of qPCR are available, including (1) an SYBR green-based method, detecting double-stranded DNA product accumulation by binding to the minor groove of double-stranded DNA nonspecifically and thus being more readily subject to false positivity because of contamination or detection of primer-dimer; and (2) TaqMan methodology, based on highly specific primer-probe combinations. In TaqMan qPCR, a probe labeled with a fluorescent dye at one end (5′) and a quencher at the other (3′) is designed to bind

within the sequence amplified by qPCR. In the unbound state, the proximity of quencher to the fluorescent dye inhibits detection of the fluorescence through Foerster resonance energy transfer (FRET). Once the probe has bound within the amplified sequence, 5′ exonuclease activity of the polymerase enzyme leads to probe cleavage and dissociation of fluorescent dye and quencher, with ensuing accumulation of fluorescence proportional to product amplification (strictly probe cleavage). Multiplexing of reactions is possible with TaqMan but not SYBR green technology.

Array Comparative Genomic Hybridization and Single Nucleotide Polymorphism Profiling Assays

Conventional metaphase CGH, which was summarized previously, was made obsolete by the advent of array CGH, in which the tumor DNA is hybridized instead to high-density arrays of probes covering the entire genome.[53] Array CGH provides a much higher-resolution genome-wide definition of genetic gains and losses. However, conventional and array-based CGH do not detect balanced chromosome translocations, a hallmark of many pediatric cancers. Genome-wide SNP assays (Fig. 45-12), like array CGH, are used increasingly as a higher-resolution alternative to conventional karyotyping for genome-wide assessments of gene copy number alterations, and, unlike array CGH, the SNP methods have the advantage of demonstrating LOH, even in situations in which gene copy number is normal (copy number neutral LOH). However, SNP profiling generally provides less quantitative assessment of copy number gains compared with array CGH.

Next-Generation Sequencing and Other Techniques

In light of the ever-increasing number of gene fusions identified in pediatric sarcomas and hematologic neoplasms, the need for more efficient, multiplexed methods for their detection is becoming more pressing. Increasingly, molecular diagnostic laboratories are implementing variations of next-generation sequencing toward these ends. Whereas few laboratories now employ comprehensive genome sequencing (exome, whole genome, or whole transcriptome) in routine diagnostics, more targeted high-throughput sequencing panels have become commonplace. Typically, these panels focus on gene perturbations with known prognostic, predictive, or diagnostic relevance in cancer, detecting hundreds of clinically relevant mutations in a single panel. Although the translation of these new approaches based on next-generation sequencing into routine diagnostic assays is moving quickly,[54] there remain challenges to routine implementation for diagnosis, including the need for relatively large amounts of high-quality nucleic acids. In addition to next-generation sequencing, there are various other novel and promising methods for detecting the ever-expanding variety of diagnostically relevant gene rearrangements in cancer. These include the NanoString nCounter system, which detects individual messenger RNA (mRNA) molecules without PCR amplification in a quantitative and highly multiplexed fashion[55] and antibody detection of translocations assays.[56]

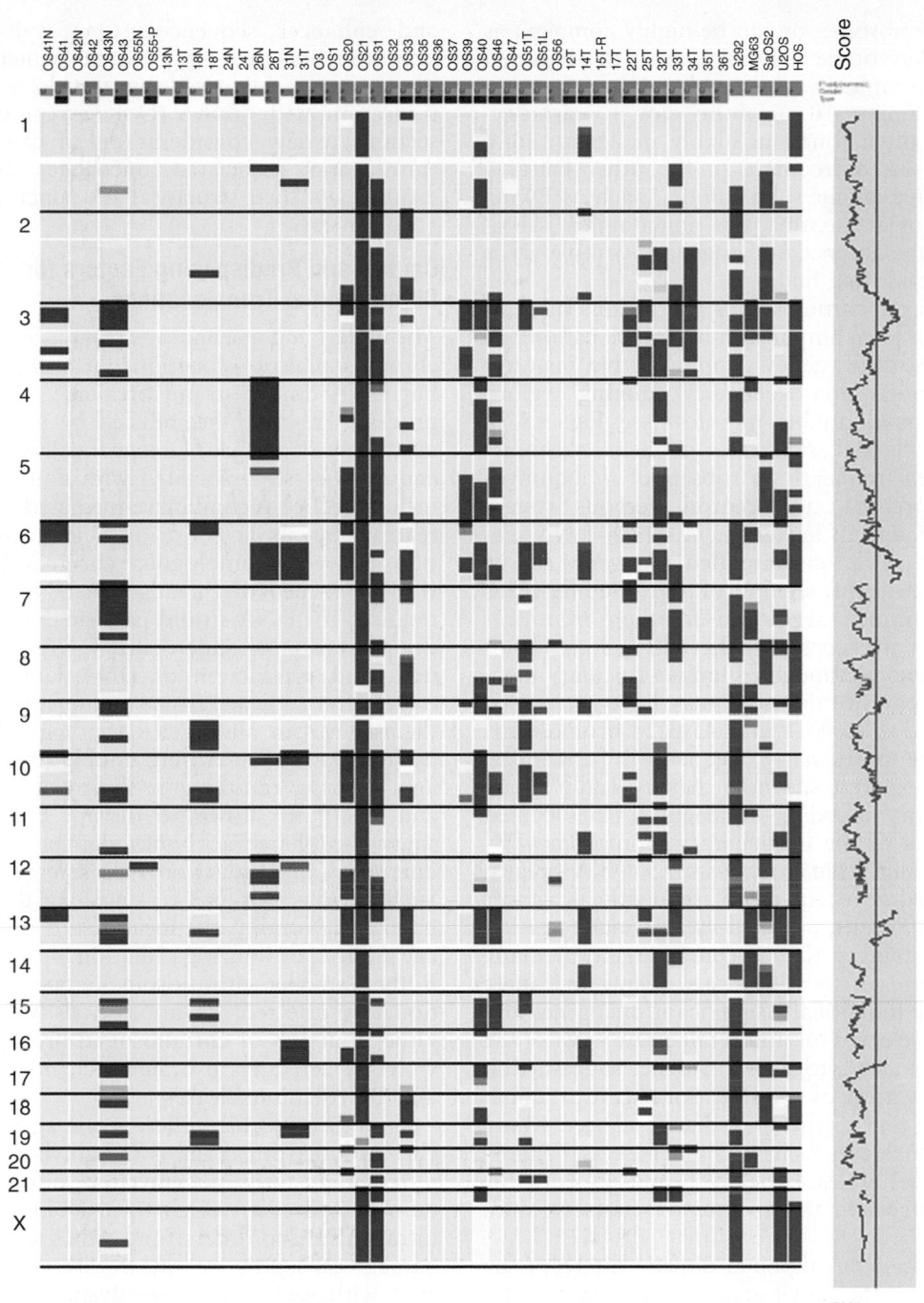

Figure 45-12 Genome-wide single-nucleotide polymorphism (SNP) analysis of osteosarcomas, with each column showing data from an individual case and the rows showing SNP data for each chromosome. Most osteosarcomas have numerous regions of SNP loss of heterozygosity, which are indicated in *blue*, whereas admixed regions of retained heterozygosity are in *yellow*.

It might be surmised that the optimal setup of a tumor genetics laboratory in the pediatric context would strive to culture cells from all newly diagnosed tumors. It would largely rely on FISH-based assays to screen for rearrangements or amplifications of commonly involved genes such as *EWSR1, FOXO1, MYCN, MLL,* and *ALK* but retain expertise in PCR for detection of gene rearrangements and minimal residual disease and array-based or sequenc-ing screens for more comprehensive evaluations of action-able mutations across the broad spectrum of pediatric hematologic neoplasms and solid tumors.

GENOMIC MECHANISMS IN PEDIATRIC TUMORS

The cytogenetic aberrations in pediatric tumors can be extremely simple, involving loss or rearrangement of only a single chromosome, or can be highly complex, as manifested by a karyotype showing dozens of abnormal chromosomes. Complexly abnormal pediatric cancer karyotypes, containing 10 or more clonal rearrangements, are most often found in highly malignant solid tumors, such as osteosarcoma. On the other hand, a subset of highly malignant solid tumors, such as Ewing sarcoma and synovial sarcoma, has noncomplex karyotypes. Therefore the absence of cytogenetic complexity is not, in itself, a reassuring finding.

Clinically relevant chromosomal aberrations in pediatric tumors result in amplification, translocation, or deletion of various target genes. Amplifications, manifest as intrachromosomal homogeneously staining regions or extrachromosomal double minutes (see Fig. 45-5), are of greatest clinical relevance in neuroblastoma. They are also seen frequently in subsets of rhabdomyosarcoma, osteosarcoma, and central nervous system (CNS) tumors[57,58] and in leukemia, in which DNA segments encompassing various amplified oncogenes can be translocated to different regions of the genome. This phenomenon is termed *segmental jumping translocation*.[16,59] Deletions are generally believed to target tumor suppressor gene loci. Although of limited ancillary diagnostic value, detection of deletions may have prognostic implications (see Tables 45-1 and 45-3). Chromosomal translocations are particularly frequent in leukemias, lymphomas, and sarcomas, where they typically create fusions of regulatory or coding sequences in genes located at the breakpoints of the participant chromosomes.[60,61] Translocations result from double-strand DNA breaks, which are believed to occur more frequently in cancer cells than in normal cells, presumably as a manifestation of the genetic instability that is characteristic of many cancers. Most random translocations arising in cancer cells do not create functionally significant oncogenes and are therefore not selected for and retained by most of the cells in that cancer. The cytogenetic evidence suggests that at most a limited variety of translocations serve an oncogenic role in any given type of pediatric cancer. Many such recurring translocations have clinical use as diagnostic biomarkers (see Tables 45-1, 45-2, and 45-3) or for identifying tumor-specific therapeutic targets (see Tables 45-1 and 45-3).

Some translocation breakpoints directly interrupt the coding sequences of the target genes, leading to the creation of a fusion oncogene. Other breakpoints are outside of the gene coding sequences but nonetheless alter transcriptional regulation of the target gene. In the case of coding sequence fusions, important functional domains from the two component genes are generally brought together by the chromosomal rearrangement. For example, fusion kinase oncogenes often result from apposition of the kinase gene catalytic domain with a translocation partner's protein-protein association domain (oligomerization domain). Such fusions lead to constitutive activation of the kinase. In other translocations, the intact coding sequence of a particular gene, usually one expressed at weak to undetectable levels in the nonneoplastic progenitor cell, is overexpressed by translocational juxtaposition to highly active promoter and enhancer sequences. One well-known example occurs in Burkitt lymphomas, in which *MYC* oncogene expression is increased by translocation into various transcriptionally active *IG* gene regions. The following sections review considerations of causative factors for translocation-associated oncogenes and provide key examples of their structural and functional roles in pediatric cancers.

Causes and Predisposing Factors for Chromosomal Translocations

The underlying mechanisms responsible for the genesis of chromosomal translocations are still poorly understood, but DNA double-strand breakage is a key step in this process. This may be induced by intracellular (endogenous) or extracellular (exogenous) agents. Some endogenous processes associated with double-strand breakage include V(D)J recombinase-mediated intrachromosomal rearrangements at *IG* or *TCR* loci, meiotic recombination between homologous chromatids, topoisomerase II (TOP2)–mediated changes in DNA topology that are required for DNA strand passage during mitosis and for the relaxation of supercoiled DNA for RNA transcription, and production of DNA-damaging agents (e.g., oxygen free radicals) from spontaneous hydrolysis, which themselves can alter DNA topology. Among the many exogenous insults causing double-stranded DNA breakage, ionizing radiation is the most extensively studied and has been shown to disrupt hydrogen bonds and sugar-phosphate backbones, damage purine and pyrimidine bases, and induce cross-links between DNA strands. Such damage can lead to single- or double-strand DNA breakage. Notably, the locations of chromosomal breakage induced by ionizing radiation are not entirely random. Rather, smaller chromosomes appear to be disproportionately affected, as are regions rich in GC repeats. Other inducers of chromosomal breakage include ultraviolet A–activated psoralens, chemotherapeutic agents, and DNA endonucleases.

One class of chemotherapeutic agents that can induce chromosomal breakage is the alkylating agents, such as nitrogen mustards, mitomycin C, nitrosoureas, and platinum compounds, which form DNA adducts and cause intrastrand and interstrand DNA cross-linkage. DNA damage caused by treatment with these agents is associated with secondary myelodysplastic syndrome (MDS) and secondary leukemias, whose salient molecular cytogenetic features include complex numerical and structural abnormalities that often involve loss of chromosome 5, 5q, 7, or 7q. Noteworthy also is that germline and somatic mutations in the TP53 tumor suppressor protein, which is critical for DNA damage recognition, are frequent in secondary leukemias with chromosome 5q abnormalities and a complex karyotype, suggesting that genomic instability caused by loss of TP53 predisposes to this treatment complication.[16,62] The second class of chemotherapeutic agents that can induce chromosomal breakage are the TOP2 poisons, which target the nuclear enzyme topoisomerase II (e.g., the epipodophyllotoxins etoposide and teniposide; the anthracyclines doxorubicin, daunorubicin, and idarubicin; the anthracenedione mitoxantrone; and the combined topoisomerase I/topoisomerase II poison dactinomycin).[63]

Studies on genomic instability mechanisms in the yeast *Saccharomyces cerevisiae* have implicated defects in double-strand DNA breakage repair as causative factors in chromosomal translocations.[64] These repair defects can involve homologous recombination repair or nonhomologous end joining. Homologous recombination repair necessitates guidance of the DNA repair mechanism by two homologous sister chromatids and is therefore more active in the G2 and S phases of the cell cycle. Nonhomologous end joining is intrinsically mutagenic and does not require extensive homology (usually <10 base pairs [bp]) between the two sequences that are joined. Nonhomologous end joining does not require the presence of guiding sister chromatids and is therefore most active during the G1 phase of the cell cycle. Malfunction of these DNA repair systems is responsible for the chromosomal instability in some cancer and premature aging syndromes such as Bloom syndrome, an autosomal recessive disorder caused by inactivating mutations of the *BLM* gene. *BLM* encodes a nuclear protein related to the RecQ family of helicases, which are DNA-unwinding proteins involved in homologous recombination. Bloom syndrome patients show increased rates of chromosomal breakage and exhibit sister chromatid exchanges in the form of quadriradials, which are four-armed structures composed of two chromosomes intersecting at regions of chromatin homology. Bloom syndrome patients develop various benign and malignant tumors, generally occurring at an earlier age than in the normal population.

Other chromosomal instability syndromes result from defects in RecQ helicase proteins. For example, both Werner and Rothmund-Thompson syndromes are autosomal recessive disorders with germline mutations of *RECQL2 (WRN2)* and *RECQL4 (WRN4)*, respectively. Affected individuals develop various tumors, with osteosarcomas being particularly characteristic of patients with the Rothmund-Thompson syndrome. Ataxia-telangiectasia is an autosomal recessive disorder conferring exquisite sensitivity to ionizing radiation.[65] Ataxia-telangiectasia generally results from mutations in the *ATM* gene, which encodes a protein kinase that participates in surveillance for double-strand DNA breakage. Lymphocytes from ataxia-telangiectasia patients show increased levels of chromosomal rearrangement.

Nijmegen breakage syndrome shares several features with ataxia-telangiectasia but is caused by mutations of the *NBN (NBS1)* gene. The NBN (NBS1) protein participates in a complex with apparent roles in homologous recombination repair and nonhomologous end joining. Patients with ataxia-telangiectasia and Nijmegen breakage syndromes are particularly susceptible to the development of leukemias and lymphomas.

Fanconi anemia is a heterogeneous group of autosomal recessive disorders with predisposition to cancer, particularly leukemias and squamous cell carcinomas. At least eight distinct genes involved in DNA double-strand breakage repair have been implicated in the genesis of Fanconi anemia.[66] The chromosomes of patients with Fanconi anemia exhibit increased sensitivity to DNA cross-linking agents, such as diepoxybutane, and this feature can be useful in diagnosis of the disease. Fanconi anemia DNA repair defects can also result from germline mutations of the *BRCA2* gene.

The Li-Fraumeni syndrome is a familial cancer predisposition syndrome that manifests as early onset of a constellation of tumors (rhabdomyosarcoma, breast carcinoma, osteogenic sarcoma, astrocytic brain tumors, adrenal cortical carcinoma, acute myelogenous leukemia) caused by germline mutation in the TP53 tumor suppressor protein.[67]

Certain DNA sequences may be targeted for chromosomal rearrangements. For example, certain sequences within the *MLL* transcription factor gene might comprise TOP2 DNA-binding sites that promote leukemia-associated rearrangements, and this has been studied in detail.[68] Notably, *MLL* is typically rearranged in secondary leukemias after exposure to topoisomerase II poisons, including epipodophyllotoxins, and in leukemia in infants in whom maternal-fetal exposures to dietary or environmental topoisomerase II poisons have been implicated.[63] Even though there is not a clear consensus TOP2 DNA-binding sequence in *MLL* and the preferred sites of enzyme recognition are modified by specific chemotherapeutic agents, it has been shown that *MLL* translocation breakpoints occur near functional sites of chemotherapy-enhanced TOP2 cleavage in in vitro assays.[63] TOP2 is an essential cellular enzyme that relaxes supercoiled DNA by transiently cleaving and religating both strands of the double helix. TOP2 catalyzes the sequential reactions of double-strand DNA cleavage, DNA strand passage, and DNA strand rejoining (religation). The DNA cleavage reaction occurs when each subunit of the TOP2 enzyme homodimer covalently attaches to and introduces staggered nicks in the DNA, with the nicked DNA remaining tethered to the enzyme subunits, forming a fleeting TOP2/DNA intermediate called the cleavage complex. Particular anticancer drugs such as etoposide alter the cleavage-religation equilibrium by decreasing the rate of religation, which damages the DNA by increasing cleavage complexes. Chemotherapeutic agents that interact with TOP2 in this manner are termed *topoisomerase II poisons* because the enzyme is converted to a cellular toxin that promotes strand breakage. Although sometimes called TOP2 inhibitors when used clinically, these agents are distinct in their activity from catalytic inhibitors of this enzyme. The association of various chemotherapeutic TOP2 poisons used for anticancer treatment with secondary leukemias characterized by balanced chromosomal translocations has suggested that TOP2 has a role in other balanced translocations, such as t(8;21), t(15;17), and inv(16) in addition to those involving *MLL*.

Other examples of recombination-promoting sequences are the heptamer-nonamer sequences adjacent to translocation breakpoints in many B-cell lymphomas. These sequences serve as sites of V(D)J recombination and are, therefore, recombination signals in the B-cell context. Similarly, the sites of V(D)J recombination also promote translocations of *TCR* genes with heterologous gene loci in T-cell ALL and T-cell lymphomas.

Physical proximity of genes in interphase nuclei has also been implicated in their incorporation into fusion genes. For example, radiation-induced thyroid carcinomas frequently exhibit rearrangements of the protein tyrosine kinase gene *RET* on chromosome 10q11, which is most often fused with the *H4* locus, telomeric (band 10q21) to *RET* on the same chromosome arm.[69,70] *RET* and *H4* are physically juxtaposed in 35% of normal human thyroid cells, providing a hypothesis as to why these two particular genes are disproportionately likely to be fused after radiation-induced double-strand DNA breakage.[71] Indeed, the three-dimensional topography of the genome explains why certain rearrangements, particularly between neighboring regions on a given chromosome, are commonplace both in cancer and nonneoplastic cells.[72] Accordingly, whole transcriptome evaluations in various cancers have revealed hundreds of apparent intrachromosomal rearrangements in a given tumor, many of which involve closely neighboring genome regions and most of which are unlikely to create functionally important oncogenes. The constraints of genome organization and nuclear proximity likely determine that certain genes are the favored partners in cancer-associated rearrangements, even in situations in which other members of the same gene family would appear to be equally suitable, biologically, in the oncogenic roles. As one example, *MYC*, rather than its biologically similar family member, *MYCN*, is rearranged with an *IG* locus in Burkitt lymphoma; however, *MYCN* if moved to the *MYC* genomic locus effectively undergoes oncogenic rearrangement with *IGH*.[73]

One intriguing aspect of cancer chromosomal translocations is that they are sometimes amplified, providing additional copies of the associated fusion oncogenes. After their formation, the translocation breakpoint regions can be amplified as tandem repeats within the original chromosome or can be amplified as extrachromosomal structures, such as double-minute chromosomes. One example of intrachromosomal amplification occurs with the typically low-level amplification of *PDGFB* fusion genes in the spindle cell sarcoma dermatofibrosarcoma protuberans (Fig. 45-13, *A*).[74,75] An example of extrachromosomal amplification is found in a subset of alveolar rhabdomyosarcomas, in which double-minute chromosomes contain numerous copies of the *PAX7-FOXO1* fusion oncogene (see Fig. 45-13, *B*).[76] In either of these situations, the amplification event suggests that multiple copies of the fusion oncogenes are required to accomplish cellular transformation.

The *EWSR1* gene is rearranged in a striking number of pediatric sarcomas including Ewing sarcoma and desmoplastic small round cell tumor. There are, however, striking racial discrepancies with respect to Ewing sarcoma incidence, such that children of European ancestry are affected with a higher frequency than African-American, Asian, or Native American children. A recent study has shown, however, that the incidence of EWSR1-rearranged sarcoma is not uniformly higher in European descendants, because desmoplastic small round cell tumor (DSRCT), for example, occurs with higher frequency in African-American children.[77]

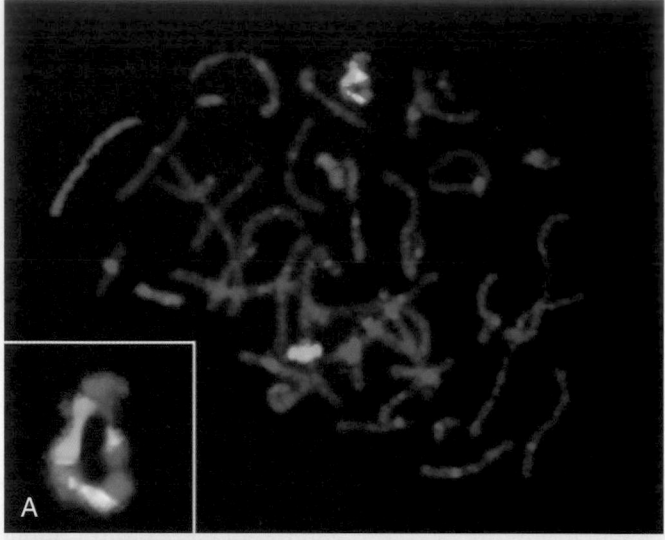

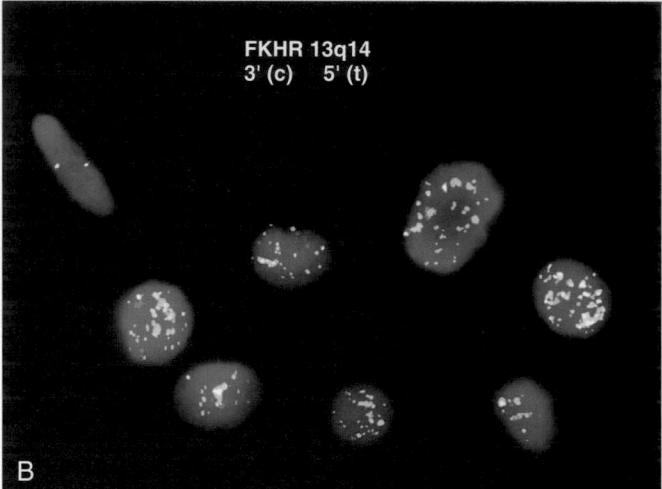

Figure 45-13 **A**, Fluorescence in situ hybridization (FISH), with whole chromosome "painting" probes to chromosomes 17 *(pink)* and 22 *(green)*, demonstrates alternating segments of chromosomes 17 and 22 in a dermatofibrosarcoma protuberans ring chromosome *(magnified in inset)*, resulting in threefold amplification of the characteristic *COL1A1-PDGFB* fusion oncogene. **B**, FISH demonstration of highly amplified and rearranged *FOXO1* gene *(green)* in an alveolar rhabdomyosarcoma with *PAX7-FOXO1* oncogenic fusion. Break-apart probe components 5′ and 3′ to the *FOXO1* gene are *red* and *green*, respectively. Normal fibroblast nucleus at upper left contains two normal fusion probe signals.

BIOLOGIC CONSEQUENCES OF CHROMOSOMAL TRANSLOCATION

Chromosomal Rearrangements Involving Transcription Factor Genes

Transcription factors are a heterogeneous group of DNA-binding proteins, most of which have domains involved in DNA binding, protein dimerization (for interaction with homologous proteins), and gene transactivation (for activation of gene transcription) or transcriptional repression. There are several classes of transcription factors, primarily relating to the structure of their DNA-binding domains. Some of the major categories include homeodomain proteins, zinc finger proteins, leucine zipper proteins, forkhead proteins, and helix-loop-helix proteins. Transcription factor genes are disrupted by many chromosomal translocations, resulting in their aberrant expression and function. Often, these transcription factor genes control lineage-specific developmental pathways and their abnormal activation can induce ectopic or asynchronous expression of corresponding lineage-specific antigenic markers, which then become a defining aspect of the transformed phenotype.

Many chromosomal translocations involving transcription factors have been described in leukemias and lymphomas. Chromosomal translocations in leukemias often interfere with the normal differentiation program of myeloid and lymphoid lineages,[78] although the presence of a chromosomal translocation per se does not prevent subclone evolution via further lineage-associated differentiation (e.g., progression from IGH gene rearrangement only to IGH plus IGL-chain rearrangement in precursor B-cell ALL). In acute leukemias, the targets for various chromosomal translocations are genes encoding hematopoiesis-related transcription factors, including AML1 (also known as RUNX1) and CBFB (see Fig. 45-12).

AML1 is a DNA-binding protein with significant homology to the Drosophila melanogaster developmental protein Runt. AML1 binds to the DNA enhancer sequence TGTGGT; the DNA-binding capabilities of AML1 are enhanced through interactions with the non–DNA-binding protein subunit of CBF (core-binding factor) called CBFB, thereby regulating expression of several genes involved in hematopoiesis. One of the most common chromosomal translocations observed in AMLs (approximately 12% of cases) is the t(8;21)(q22;q22), which fuses AML1 on chromosome 21q to RUNX1T1 (ETO) on chromosome 8.[79] ETO encodes a nuclear phosphoprotein expressed in the nervous system and in CD34+ hematopoietic progenitor cells. ETO is a transforming protein that normally participates in a multiprotein complex involved in chromatin remodeling and transcriptional repression. The fusion protein AML1-ETO retains the Runt domain of AML1 and almost the entire sequence of ETO.[80] It appears that the ETO domains incorporated into the fusion oncoprotein can dominantly repress transcription of certain genes, the expression of which is normally activated by AML1. As an example, the tumor suppressor protein p14^{ARF} normally is transcriptionally activated by AML1, but p14^{ARF} is transcriptionally repressed by AML1-ETO.[81,82] AML1 is also involved in several other chromosomal translocations in leukemias and myeloproliferative disorders, including AML1-MDS1 in myelodysplastic (preleukemic) syndromes, AML1-EVI1 in chronic myelogenous leukemia in blast crisis, and TEL (ETV6)-AML1 in pre-B ALL. All these fusion genes retain the AML1 Runt domain.[83]

Another example of a fusion gene affecting the normal function of the AML1-CBFB DNA-binding transcription factor protein complex is CBFB-SMMHC, which results from rearrangement of chromosome 16 in the French-American-British (FAB) M4Eo subtype of AML.[84] CBFB-SMMHC can result from translocation or pericentric inversion of chromosome 16, thereby fusing sequences from the 5' end of CBFB to the 3' end of SMMHC. The resultant fusion oncoprotein contains the AML1-binding heterodimerization domain of CBFB juxtaposed to the coiled-coil domains of the MYH11 (SMMHC) protein. The fusion protein CBFB-SMMHC binds to the AML1 Runt domain more effectively than the normal CBFB and has a dominant negative effect on the AML1-CBFB complex.[85]

MLL is a transcription factor protein in which the amino and carboxyl aspects contribute transcriptional repression and activation activities, respectively. MLL undergoes posttranslational processing so that the transcriptional repression and activation regions are separated by cleavage, but they then reassociate with one another in a large multiprotein chromatin remodeling complex. MLL maintains but does not initiate expression of its target genes via histone methyltransferase activity, which is provided by a SET domain within the MLL carboxyl terminus.[86] A wide range of MLL fusion oncoproteins resulting from translocations of the MLL gene at chromosome band 11q23 contain the amino terminus of the MLL transcription factor and the carboxyl terminus of partner proteins that are themselves involved in transcriptional regulation. However, there is substantial diversity in MLL partner protein function and not all MLL partner proteins are transcription factors.[86]

Chimeric (fusion) transcription factor oncogenes are also featured in many soft tissue tumors. A much-studied example is the EWS-FLI1 fusion oncogene resulting from the t(11;22)(q24;q12) translocation[87] in Ewing sarcoma. This translocation fuses EWS 5' sequences to FLI1 3' sequences. EWS encodes a ubiquitously expressed protein involved in DNA transcription, and FLI1 is a member of a large family of DNA transcription factors that contain the highly conserved ETS domain. The EWS-FLI1 fusion oncogene structure varies, depending on which EWS and FLI1 exons are retained in the chimeric gene (see Fig. 45-10). EWS can be fused with other ETS family members to provide the oncogenic impulse in Ewing sarcoma, and, alternatively, FUS (an EWS family member) can instead be fused with ETS family members in Ewing sarcomas. EWSR1-ETS fusion proteins are necessary but insufficient for cellular transformation,[88,89] a process for which IGF1R is vital.[90] Some progress has been made in recent years in understanding the oncogenic mode of action of the EWSR1-ETS fusion protein, with a rather complex and multifaceted picture emerging whereby gene targets may be direct or indirect and include transcriptional regulators such as EZH2,[89,91] NROB1,[92] and NKX2.2,[93] as well as genes involved in signal transduction or genes involved in cell cycle control. EWS-FLI1 can directly bind promoters of target genes and modulate gene expression[94,95] by upregulating (e.g., IGF1, CCND1, hTERT[96]) or repressing targets (e.g., cyclin-dependent kinase inhibitors and IGFBP3, the latter potentially allowing increased IGF1 signaling). Reduced target expression may result from decreased transcription through EWS-FLI1 reducing Pol II at the target gene promoter or through posttranscriptional reduction of transcript half-life.[97] Any additional posttranscriptional role, for example, of microRNAs putatively targeted by the fusion oncogene remains to be elucidated fully,[98] and there is emerging evidence that posttranslational protein modification is a further important function of *EWS-ETS* fusions. The direct binding of EWSR1-ETS to the *EZH2* promoter specifically with upregulation of EZH2 is interesting in relation to the ongoing debate regarding the cell of origin of Ewing sarcoma. EZH2 is a subunit of the Polycomb repressor complex, PRC2, and its expression holds cells through reversible epigenetic means, in an undifferentiated state of "stemness."[99]

Similarly, *EWS* or *FUS* is fused with other genes (not belonging to the ETS family) in various Ewinglike and frankly non-Ewing mesenchymal small round blue cell neoplasms, always resulting in fusion oncoproteins with EWS or FUS at the amino-terminal end of the fusion protein. DSRCT, a clearly defined tumor that is considered absolutely distinct from Ewing sarcoma, is an exceptionally malignant cancer composed of nests of small round tumor cells sharply delineated by a reactive fibroblastic proliferation. It is cytogenetically characterized by t(11;22)(p13;q12), which fuses *EWS* to the *WT1* gene.[100] The EWS-WT1 fusion oncoprotein retains the EWS transactivation domain and the WT1 DNA-binding domain. *WT1*, located on chromosome 11p13 encodes a zinc finger transcription factor with crucial roles in genitourinary tract development. Germline *WT1* mutations cause Wilms tumor syndromes, including Denys-Drash and WAGR (Wilms-Aniridia-Genitourinary abnormalities and mental Retardation) syndromes. Further examples of fusion genes involving *EWSR1* or *FUS* and non-ETS genes include isolated cases or small cohorts of small round blue cell tumors, which to a variable degree share histologic features with Ewing sarcoma. The partner genes may again be transcription factors, as seen with POU5F1 or NFATc2,[101,102] or in the case of SMARCA5,[103] a chromatin remodeler, whereas single reports each of a small round blue cell tumor with EWS-SP3[104] and of EWS-ZSG[105] represent fusions of EWS with zinc finger proteins. The latter case particularly has more similarity with

DSRCT, insofar as it failed to react with CD99, a classic marker of Ewing sarcoma, but did express desmin. Indeed with respect to both these cases, fusion with a zinc finger gene resonates with the situation in DSRCT. The rarity of such cases precludes major comment on their likely biologic relationship with Ewing sarcoma versus DSRCT.

A recently described undifferentiated small round cell tumor is characterized by recurrent chromosomal translocations t(4;19)(q35;q13.1) or t(10;19)(q35;q26) fusing the high mobility group box [HMG] transcription factor *CIC* with one or other of the *DUX4* double homeobox transcription factor genes located within macrosatellite repeats on 4q and 10q[106]; thus these tumors are known as CIC-DUX4 tumors. An isolated report documenting t(18;19)(q23;q13.2) in a soft tissue tumor resembling Ewing sarcoma most likely represents a variant also involving *CIC*.[107]

Tumors of epithelial differentiation (carcinomas) often have complex karyotypes, which can obfuscate recurrent translocations. However, translocations involving transcriptional regulatory genes have been identified in several pediatric carcinomas, including follicular thyroid carcinomas, renal cell carcinomas, and NUT midline carcinoma.[108,109,110] Follicular thyroid carcinomas can feature *PAX8-PPARγ* fusion transcription factor genes resulting from t(2;3)(q13;p15)[108] (Fig. 45-14), whereas in the highly lethal NUT midline carcinomas, the translocation t(15;19)(q13;p13) (Fig. 45-15) results in oncogenic fusion of the bromodomain transcriptional regulator *BRD4* with a novel testis-restricted gene, *NUT*.[110] Although exhibiting epithelial immunophenotypic features, NUT midline carcinomas typically have a primitive round cell morphology (see Fig. 45-15).

Chromosomal Rearrangements Involving Protein Tyrosine Kinase Genes

Chromosomal translocations in various neoplasms produce protein tyrosine kinase fusion genes, and such

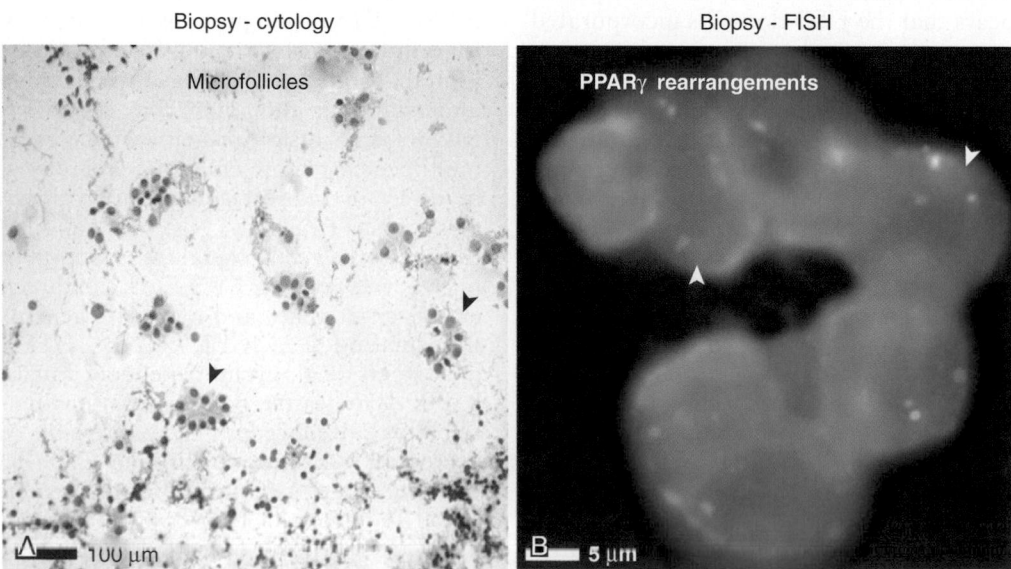

Figure 45-14 **A,** Cytology and **B,** fluorescence in situ hybridization (FISH) of follicular thyroid carcinoma, demonstrating rearrangement of the *PPARγ* gene, using break-apart probe, in microfollicle cells. *(Courtesy Dr. Todd Kroll.)*

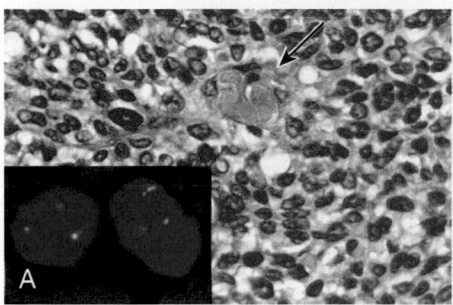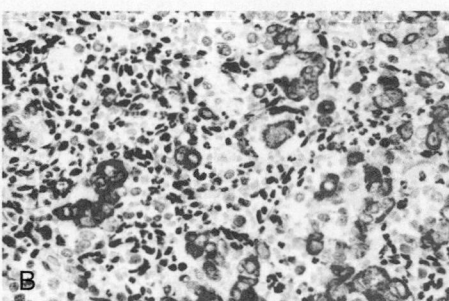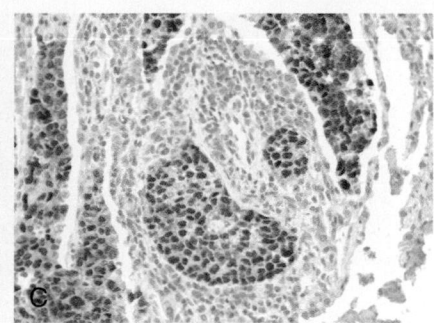

Figure 45-15 **A,** NUT midline carcinoma (sinonasal primary) composed of undifferentiated rounded cells with focal keratinization *(arrow)*. *Inset,* *BRD4* break-apart fluorescence in situ hybridization reveals rearrangement. Immunohistochemical study demonstrates reactivity for pan-keratin **(B),** indicating epithelial differentiation (alkaline phosphatase red). The NUT protein **(C)** (peroxidase DAB) is expressed in tumor cells but not in admixed histiocytes and lymphocytes.

oncogenes are of considerable clinical importance. Protein tyrosine kinases comprise a large family of proteins, which are primarily involved in signal transduction. All tyrosine kinase proteins contain a highly conserved kinase (catalytic) domain, which mediates the phosphorylation of tyrosine residues in protein substrates. Phosphorylated tyrosines serve to stabilize various protein-protein interactions and to enhance kinase activity in those substrates with intrinsic kinase function. Tyrosine kinase fusion oncoproteins resulting from chromosomal translocations in cancer have a consistent structure. The carboxyl-terminal end of these fusion oncoproteins typically contains the entire kinase domain from the tyrosine kinase protein, whereas the amino-terminal end contains an oligomerization domain from the other fusion partner. The oligomerization domain facilitates spontaneous interactions between kinase fusion oncoproteins, and the complexed oncoproteins can then phosphorylate each other, resulting in further upregulation of kinase activity.

The Philadelphia (Ph) chromosome is the cytogenetic hallmark of chronic myelogenous leukemia (CML) and was the first diagnostic translocation identified in a human cancer, also providing the best known example of a fusion tyrosine kinase oncogene.[111] The Ph chromosome results from chromosomal translocation between chromosomes 9 and 22, in which the *BCR* gene on chromosome 22 is fused with the *ABL1 (ABL)* kinase gene on chromosome 9. This translocation is found in most CMLs, 25% of ALLs in adults, 5% of ALLs in children and, less often, in AML. *ABL* encodes a 145-kD nonreceptor protein tyrosine kinase that shuttles between the nucleus and cytoplasm and is involved in various cellular processes, such as cell cycle regulation and apoptosis. *BCR* encodes a 160-kD protein with dimerization, serine-threonine kinase, Rho-GEF (guanine nucleotide exchange factor), and Rac-guanosine triphosphatase (GTPase) domains. The BCR-ABL fusion oncoprotein is expressed as three structural variants, depending on the location of the breakpoint in the *BCR* gene. The BCR-ABL fusion transcript types segregate with specific neoplasms so that the 190-, 210-, and 230-kD BCR-ABL proteins are typically expressed in ALL, CML, and chronic neutrophilic leukemia, respectively. In AML, BCR-ABL fusion oncoproteins can be the P210 or P190 form.[112] The BCR-ABL

fusion oncoproteins feature constitutive activation of the ABL kinase domain, resulting in autophosphorylation and tyrosine phosphorylation of various substrates. The phosphotyrosine residues serve as binding sites for various signaling proteins, resulting in activation of signaling pathways, such as Ras/MAPK (implicated in cell proliferation) and PI3K/AKT (implicated in cell survival).

Translocation-associated fusion kinase oncogenes are also found in various soft tissue tumors, including congenital fibrosarcoma, a pediatric spindle cell neoplasm with an excellent prognosis. Cytogenetically, congenital fibrosarcoma is characterized by the balanced translocation t(12;15)(p13;q25), which fuses the 5′ end of the transcription factor gene *TEL* to the 3′ end of the *NTRK3* protein tyrosine kinase gene (see Fig. 45-2).[113] The TEL-NTRK3 fusion oncoprotein retains the TEL helix-loop-helix dimerization domain and the NTRK3 kinase domain. *TEL* is also rearranged with other genes, including protein tyrosine kinase genes in various leukemias. The *TEL-NTRK3* fusion gene is seen in pediatric renal tumors known as congenital cellular mesoblastic nephromas, which are histologically similar to congenital fibrosarcoma (Fig. 45-16).[7] This finding suggests that congenital fibrosarcoma and cellular mesoblastic nephroma belong to the same spectrum of tumors. TEL-NTRK3 is also found occasionally in AML[6] and is one of a few fusion oncogenes known to play transforming roles not only in soft tissue and hematopoietic neoplasms[114] but also in epithelial neoplasia (secretory breast carcinoma).

Inflammatory myofibroblastic tumor (IMT) is an unusual entity that arises predominantly in the abdominal cavity/peritoneum of young patients. Similar to congenital fibrosarcoma, IMT is usually associated with an excellent prognosis and metastases are rare. However, a subset of patients with IMT do develop disseminated disease and it is notable that many IMTs have chromosomal translocations that create activated fusion forms of the *ALK* receptor tyrosine kinase gene detectable by immunohistochemical means (Fig. 45-17).[114] *ALK* oncogenic fusion genes were initially described as a consequence of the chromosomal translocation t(2;5)(p23;q35), which occurs in a subset of anaplastic large cell lymphomas (ALCLs).[115] At least nine *ALK* fusion genes have now been described in IMT and ALCL; in all of them,

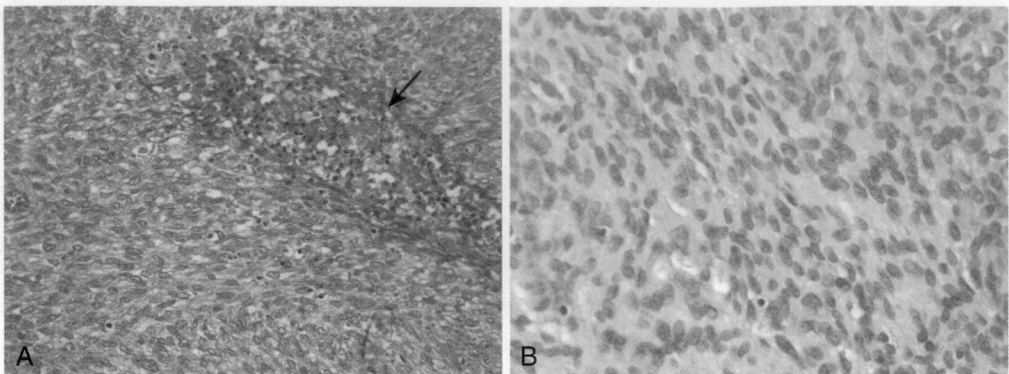

Figure 45-16 **A,** Congenital mesoblastic nephroma and **B,** infantile fibrosarcoma are histologically indistinguishable tumors composed of mitotically active plump spindle cells, with varying extent of fascicular arrangement and showing islands of spontaneous necrosis as a characteristic feature *(arrow).*

the resultant fusion oncoproteins contain the ALK kinase domain fused to an oligomerization domain of another protein. Two of the *ALK* fusion genes, *TPM3-ALK* and *CLTC-ALK*, have been found in IMT and ALCL, indicating that an identical oncogenic mechanism can contribute to these different tumors.[114,116] Most recently, *ALK* kinase domain mutations and gene amplification have been demonstrated in hereditary and sporadic neuroblastoma.[117,118,119] Other receptor tyrosine kinase translocations in pediatric cancer include those in papillary thyroid cancers, which can target the *RET* or *NTRK1* genes.[120,121] In these fusion oncoproteins, the RET or NTRK1 kinase domains are activated by fusion with various oligomerization-inducing domains.

A further mechanism of protein tyrosine kinase activation by chromosomal translocation is seen in dermatofibrosarcoma protuberans (DFSP).[122] DFSP is a subcutaneous plump spindle cell sarcoma that exhibits high local recurrence rates but rarely metastasizes. Cytogenetically, this tumor is characterized by the chromosomal translocation t(17;22)(q21;q13), often amplified within a circular or ring chromosome (see Fig. 45-13A). The t(17;22) creates a *COL1A1-PDGFB* fusion gene, in which the entire *PDGFB* coding sequence is placed under the transcriptional control of the highly active *COL1A1* promoter in

an event referred to as promoter swapping. This mechanism results in *PDGFB* overexpression, with resultant autocrine activation of the PDGFB receptor.[122] The same genetic event underlies the development of giant cell fibroblastoma, which is a pediatric tumor believed to be closely related to DFSP.[74,123]

Chromosomal Rearrangements Associated with Transcriptional Upregulation of Nonfusion Oncogenes

Many pediatric lymphomas feature juxtaposition of intact protooncogenes to transcriptionally active loci (e.g., the *IG* locus in B-cell lymphomas or the *TCR* locus in T-cell lymphomas). V(D)J recombination and class switch recombination, which normally occur within the *IG* or *TCR* loci in lymphocytes, have been implicated in the genesis of these nonfusion genes.[124] V(D)J recombination and class switch recombination mechanisms are exemplified by the nonfusion genes targeting *MYC*, a regulator of cell growth and survival, in many Burkitt lymphomas. V(D)J recombination facilitates the chromosomal translocation t(8;14)(q24;q32) in endemic Burkitt lymphomas found in patients from equatorial Africa. This translocation juxtaposes *MYC* to the intronic *IG* heavy chain gene enhancer, leading to MYC overexpression. In contrast, most nonendemic Burkitt

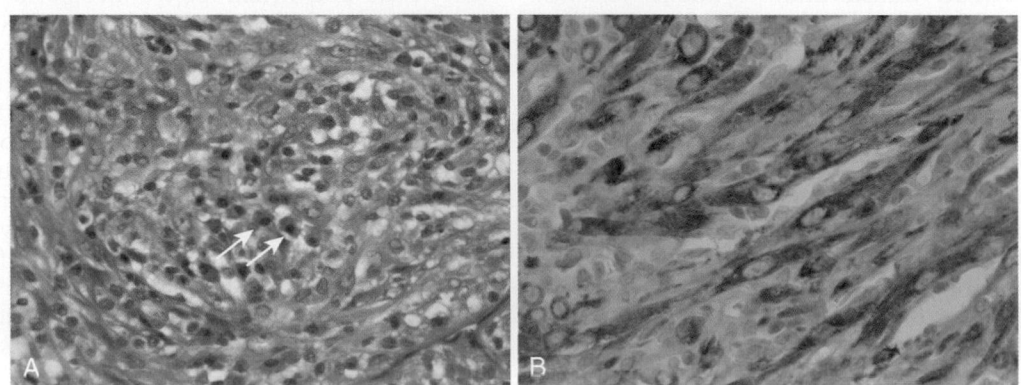

Figure 45-17 **A,** Inflammatory myofibroblastic tumor composed of plump neoplastic spindle cells with a reactive infiltrate featuring abundant plasma cells *(arrows).* **B,** Immunohistochemistry in a case with *TPM4-ALK* fusion, showing diffuse cytoplasmic staining with nuclear sparing in spindle cell (myofibroblastic) component and absence of immunoreactivity in the inflammatory cell infiltrate.

lymphomas have translocation breakpoints downstream elsewhere in the *IG* heavy chain gene locus, juxtaposing *MYC* to other enhancers. Alternatively, *MYC* overexpression can result from juxtaposition to the *IG* κ or λ light chain genes resulting from t(2;8) or t(8;22).

Like Burkitt lymphomas, follicular cell lymphomas of B-cell origin also feature rearrangements of *IG* loci, but with *BCL2* or *BCL6*, rather than *MYC*, typically overexpressed by translocation into the region of an *IG* gene promoter. *BCL2* alterations, conferring well-described antiapoptotic effects, often result from *IG* heavy chain V(D)J recombination, with a breakpoint in exon 3 of *BCL2* becoming fused to the 5′ end of J_H or D-J_H heavy chain segments. These mechanisms result in *BCL2* transcriptional upregulation, mediated by the *IG* heavy chain gene enhancer. Although deregulated BCL2 expression provides a survival advantage in such lymphomas, additional gene mutations are needed for full neoplastic transformation.[125] However, in the pediatric population, follicular lymphomas are uncommon and the vast majority of cases feature elevated BCL6 expression. Cases with t(14;18) fusing the *IGH* chain locus with the BCL2 gene comprise only a small subset of the cases, which is in contrast to adults, but increased BCL2 expression is associated with advanced disease and a poor prognosis in pediatric lymphoma.[126]

TCR locus rearrangements are demonstrable in many T-cell leukemias and lymphomas, resulting in transcriptional upregulation of various translocated genes, similar to the mechanisms involving *IG* gene regions in various B-cell malignancies. The T-cell leukemia and lymphoma cytogenetic rearrangements dysregulate expression of transcription factor genes, such as *MYC, HOX11, TLX3 (HOX11L2), TAL-SCL, LYL1, LMO1*, and *LMO2*, by placing these genes under the control of highly active *cis*-acting transcriptional regulatory *TCR* elements, although dysregulation of these T-cell oncogenes can also occur in the absence of cytogenetic *TCR* rearrangements.[127,128]

Translocations resulting in nonfusion oncogenes can be found in pediatric solid tumors; one example is the *PDGFB* fusion gene in DFSP (see earlier). Other examples include translocations of chromosome 8, targeting the *PLAG1* gene, a zinc finger transcription factor, in salivary gland pleomorphic adenoma and the primitive adipose tumor lipoblastoma. In both tumor types, the chromosomal breakpoints occur in the 5′ noncoding regions of the involved genes, resulting in promoter swapping, in which the transcriptionally inactive *PLAG1* promoter is replaced by the highly active promoter of the translocation partner gene, leading to *PLAG1* overexpression.[129-131]

BIOLOGIC BASIS FOR SPECIFICITY OF BALANCED CHROMOSOMAL REARRANGEMENTS: DIAGNOSTIC RELEVANCE

Recurrent chromosomal rearrangements involving specific breakpoint regions are increasingly being used as diagnostic markers in various pediatric cancers. Translocations are the most extensively studied of these rearrangements, but other mechanisms include chromosomal insertions, inversions, and interstitial deletions. Although diagnostic rearrangements, such as those involving chromosome 22 in Ewing sarcoma, have become useful biomarkers, it is unclear whether most such characteristic rearrangements are initiating tumorigenic events or later events responsible for tumor progression. However, their oncogenic nature is generally convincing in that they can transform cells, as can be demonstrated by expressing the oncogenes in nonneoplastic cells in vitro or in mice. Although *EWS* and its family member *TLS-FUS* are frequently rearranged in chromosomal translocation in sarcomas, the partner gene varies and appears occasionally to dictate the tumor phenotype (see Table 45-1). For example, *EWS-WT1* transcripts are found in DSRCT but not Ewing sarcoma, whereas *EWS-ATF1* fusion occurs in soft tissue clear cell sarcoma but not other sarcomas. It has not yet been clearly established whether it is the partner gene that determines lineage in these tumors or whether only certain cells, already lineage committed, might tolerate the presence of these oncogenic transcripts.

Translocations of the *MLL* gene at chromosome band 11q23 are examples of leukemia-associated chromosomal translocations that create potent fusion oncoproteins. *MLL* translocations are believed to be the events that initiate these leukemias.[132] Analogous to *EWS* variant rearrangements in pediatric solid tumors, particular *MLL* partner genes are more likely to occur in ALL than in AML, even though there is some overlap, and leukemias with *MLL* translocations can also exhibit dual lineage or actually switch lineage.[133]

There is substantial evidence that single genetic aberrations are insufficient to produce cancer. Rather, tumor development requires many gene mutations, perturbing different aspects of the cell biology (including apoptosis, proliferation, differentiation, and adhesion), which collectively results in the neoplastic phenotype. Even with *MLL* translocations in which there is a short latency from the in utero occurrence of the translocation to manifestation of disease, which is often in the young infant (<3 months old) or even in the neonate or the fetus,[134] there are characteristic secondary alterations in addition to the translocations.[135]

Some of the same characteristic genetic alterations, including chromosomal translocations, observed in human cancers have been detected at very low levels (e.g., 1 in 10,000 cells) in nonneoplastic cell populations.[136,137] The rare cells containing these alterations are individually at low risk for progression to malignancy, presumably because it is unlikely that they will acquire the other mutations required to result in clinically evident cancer. However, this likely is more pertinent to solid tumors, in which a greater number of events generally is believed to be required for full oncogenesis than in leukemias. Similarly, it is likely that various diagnostic genetic alterations can be detected at very low levels in cancer types in which they are not characteristically encountered and where they likely are not serving an important transforming role for the vast majority of cells in that cancer. Therefore when using genetic alterations as diagnostic markers, it is important to have some sense that the alteration is found in most cells in the cancer, rather than being a rare and perhaps trivial event. It is similarly crucial to correlate the genetic findings with the histology, thereby confirming that the molecular diagnosis is credible.

The recurring and relatively specific association of chromosomal translocations with one or a few types of cancer has enabled the development of assays in which the translocations serve as ancillary diagnostic markers. There is a biologic basis to such tumor specificity because the neoplastic phenotype is essentially a symbiotic interaction between cell environment and translocation product, and certain genetic alterations, particularly those resulting from translocations, appear oncogenic in only a limited number of cancer cell environments.[138] Support for this concept is provided by B-cell lymphomas, in which diagnostic translocations often juxtapose oncogenes to the *IG* loci. The *IG* gene promoters are extremely active in the B-cell context, and ectopic placement of oncogenes near these promoters results in striking overexpression of the oncogenes, provided that the chromosomal rearrangement occurs in the B-cell context. By contrast, this same chromosomal rearrangement would presumably be irrelevant in other cell types, in which the *IG* genes are transcriptionally silent. Translocations that occur in B-cell lymphoma have not been found in other varieties of human cancer. Another factor accounting for tumor specificity is the restriction of transforming properties of translocation-associated oncoproteins to certain cell lineages. Fusion oncoproteins always require interactions with other cellular proteins that facilitate and support the effect of that oncoprotein. Therefore cell lineages lacking the relevant interacting proteins will not be transformed by a given fusion oncoprotein. These concepts are underscored by the observation that the BCR-ABL fusion oncoprotein, which is highly transforming in hematopoietic progenitor cells, fails to transform fibroblast cell lines.[139]

In pediatric tumors, genetic aberrations useful for testing as ancillary diagnostic findings are especially frequent in sarcomas, leukemias, and lymphomas. Interestingly, in contrast to adult tumors, diagnostic alterations are also found in many pediatric carcinomas, including papillary and follicular thyroid carcinomas, renal cell carcinomas, and lethal midline carcinoma. Although cytogenetic and molecular profiles are diagnostic in some pediatric cancers, there are many others that lack specific genetic or cytogenetic aberrations or have extremely complex karyotypes in which the specific aberrations, if present at all, are difficult to identify.

CYTOGENETIC AND MOLECULAR PATHOLOGY: MAJOR TUMOR TYPES

Cytogenetic and molecular analyses have provided extraordinary insights into the biology and pathogenesis of pediatric cancer and, in some cases, these insights have then formed the basis for more accurate assessment of diagnosis and prognosis. However, neither cytogenetic nor molecular methods are required routinely in the clinical setting. In some pediatric solid tumors, there is not yet a basis for genetic testing because recurrent genetic aberrations are unknown. In others, particularly those that are benign clinically, the histopathology diagnosis and prognosis are generally straightforward and genetic adjuncts are therefore irrelevant. Some pediatric solid tumors, such as high-grade osteosarcoma, have extremely complex karyotypes, so that to date, there is little clinical advantage in genetic analysis, given the formidable task of describing the many genetic aberrations in a given tumor and the questionable prognostic relevance of the individual genetic perturbations. Widespread application of genetic assays in such tumors awaits the identification of key genetic predictors, which might then be determined in tumor interphase cells by molecular cytogenetic assays.

The following sections will highlight applications of cytogenetic and molecular assays in subsets of pediatric tumors, in which the technical challenges of genetic assays are manageable, and in which genetic findings are acknowledged to provide important diagnostic or prognostic information.

Mesenchymal Neoplasms: Soft Tissue and Bone Tumors

Ewing Sarcoma

Ewing sarcomas are highly aggressive tumors, characteristically occurring in bone and soft tissue, but also, less commonly, in viscera, and in which the neoplastic cells are generally of the small, round, blue cell type. Ewing sarcoma and peripheral primitive neuroectodermal tumor (pPNET), although historically considered distinct entities, share molecular and morphologic features and are now regarded as essentially the same entity (herein referred to simply as Ewing sarcoma). Ewing sarcomas typically contain chromosomal translocations involving the Ewing sarcoma gene (*EWS* or *EWSR1*), which is located on the long arm of chromosome 22. These translocations involve a number of partner genes (see Table 45-1), with the most common translocation being t(11;22)(q24;q12), resulting in oncogenic fusion of 3′ sequences of the *FLI1* gene on chromosome 11 with 5′ sequences of *EWS*.[140-144] *FLI1* belongs to the winged helix-loop-helix transcription factor family that share a conserved 85-amino acid ETS domain that is present in all EWS-ETS fusions. The oncogenic *EWSR1-FLI1* fusion gene encodes an activated version of transcription factor in which the DNA binding domain of *FLI1* is fused to the more potent *trans*-activating domain (TAD) of *EWSR1*, replacing the TAD of *FLI1*. In variant translocations, *EWS* is fused with alternative ETS transcription factor family members (see Fig. 45-10 and Table 45-1)[145-149] and, rarely, the *EWS*-related gene, *FUS*, can also be fused with an alternative ETS family member in Ewing sarcomas (Fig. 45-18; see Table 45-1).[150] The *EWS* family and ETS family gene translocations are apparently essential for oncogenesis, being found in almost all Ewing sarcomas.

These translocations are readily detected by conventional cytogenetic methods, even using needle biopsy material, because Ewing sarcoma cells grow well in tissue culture.[9] The translocations can also be detected by FISH,

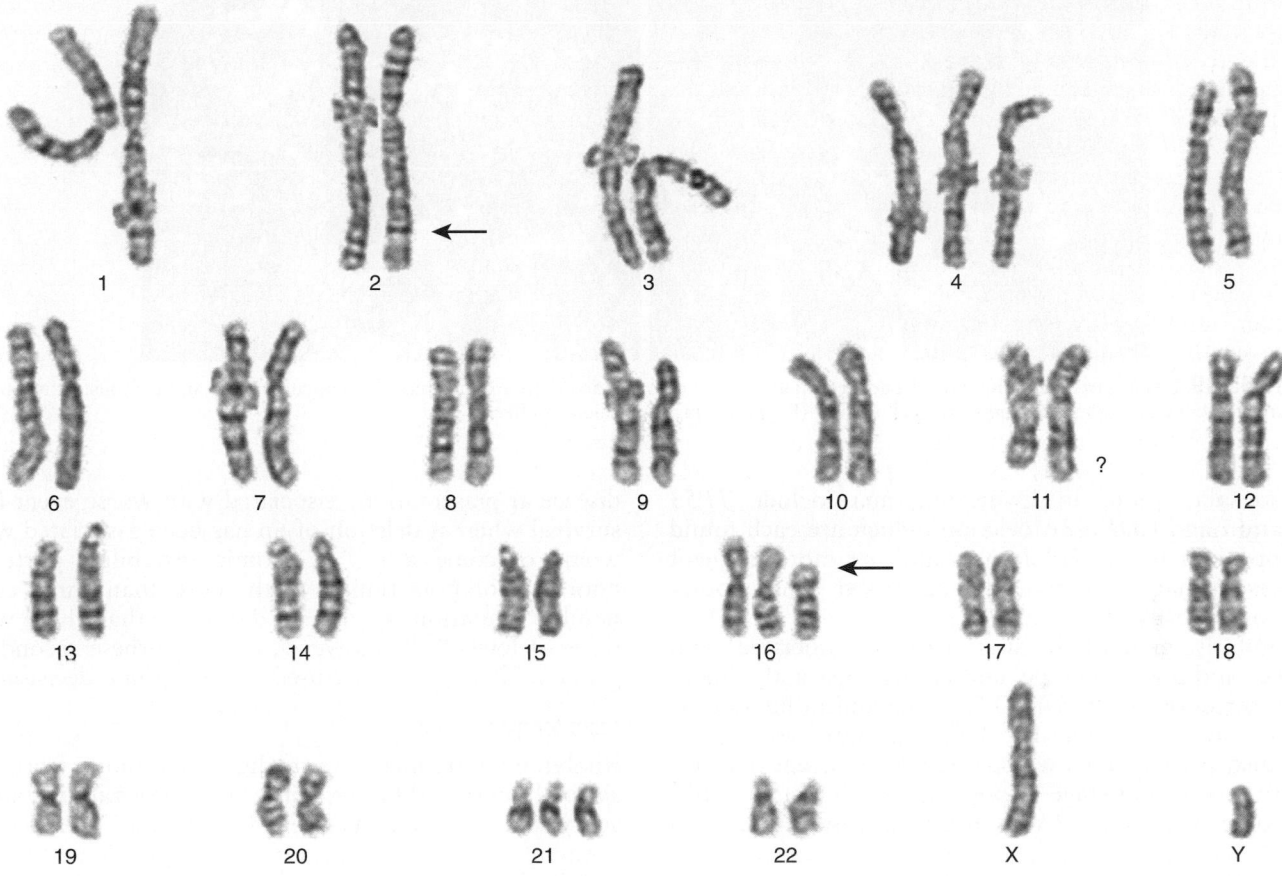

Figure 45-18 Ewing sarcoma with t(2;16)(q35;p11), resulting in oncogenic fusion of the *FEV1* and *FUS* genes (*arrows* indicate translocation breakpoints).

typically using dual-color probes flanking the *EWSR1* locus (see Fig. 45-8).[151] Although this does not identify the partner gene fused to *EWSR1,* that information is generally unnecessary for diagnostic purposes. Another method for detecting these translocations is RT-PCR.[152] Advantages of PCR include superior sensitivity, identification of the *EWS* fusion partner gene, and identification of the breakpoint locations within the genes. The most common fusion is between *EWS* exon 7 and *FLI1* exon 6, known as type I fusion, whereas type II fusion involves fusion of *EWSR1* exon 7 with *FLI1* exon 5, and many further variants have been described (see Fig. 45-10). Although several studies have indicated that *EWSR1-FLI1* breakpoint locations might be prognostic in Ewing sarcoma,[37,39,153] with tumors bearing the type I transcript doing better than all others, more recent studies do not confirm this, and such information is not used routinely to guide therapeutic decisions.

Although histomorphologic and immunohistochemical features are often sufficient to establish the diagnosis of Ewing sarcoma, genetic corroboration of the diagnosis is highly reassuring in distinguishing Ewing sarcoma from other small round blue cell tumors, particularly in situations in which tumor arises at an unusual site, or outside the typical age range, in the context of smaller biopsies, or if tumor cell preservation is compromised and/or

immunohistochemistry is suboptimal. Although the cells are essentially undifferentiated, and superficially similar or identical to those in many other small round cell tumors, there are nonetheless characteristic findings, such as subtle cytologic features and crisp cytoplasmic membrane–associated expression of the CD99 (O13-HBA71, pseudoautosomal gene-encoded membrane glycoprotein [Fig. 45-19], or specifically for *Erg*-rearranged Ewing sarcoma, anti-Erg monoclonal antibody[154]) that aid the diagnosis.

Thus the combined traditional histologic evaluation of H&E-stained sections, together with immunohistochemical profiling, enables distinction of Ewing sarcoma from, for example, a reasonable mimic in alveolar rhabdomyosarcoma by the demonstration of CD99 expression in Ewing sarcoma versus expression of myogenic markers such as myogenin, MyoD1, and desmin in rhabdomyosarcoma (Fig. 45-20). The characteristic oncogene fusions in Ewing sarcoma *(EWS-FLI1)* and alveolar rhabdomyosarcoma *(PAX-FOXO1)* might contribute to the distinct cell differentiation profiles that separate these two round cell tumors immunophenotypically and morphologically. Evidence to this effect has been obtained from in vitro studies in which *EWS-ETS* oncogenes can induce neuroectodermal differentiation,[155] whereas *PAX-FOXO1* induces a myogenic program.[156,157] Secondary

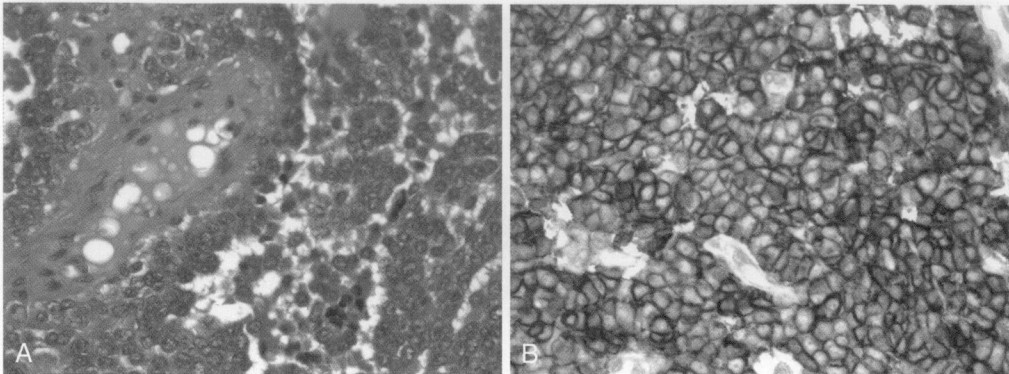

Figure 45-19 Ewing sarcoma composed of undifferentiated round cells (**A**) arranged around thick fibrovascular cores and demonstrating strong and crisp CD99 expression confined to the cell surface (**B**), producing a mosaic-like effect.

genetic aberrations in Ewing sarcoma include *TP53* mutation and *CDKN2A* deletion, which are each found in approximately 25% of cases and are more frequent in cases that are clinically aggressive and poorly chemoresponsive.[158]

Similarly, gain of 1q was strongly associated with relapse and poor outcome, and this is apparently due to overexpression of *DTL (CDT2)*, a ubiquitin ligase gene located on chromosome 1q.[159,160] Independent loss of 16q was also predictive of worse overall and event-free survival regardless of stage at presentation.[159] In that study, gain of chromosome 12 was, at least in cases of localized

disease at presentation, associated with worse event-free survival whereas deletion of 6p has been associated with worse outcome also.[161] Genomic instability portends poorly insofar as tumors with more than three copy number alterations reportedly did worse than those with three of fewer.[162,163] However, currently these secondary genomic findings are not used in therapeutic decisions.

Rhabdomyosarcoma

Rhabdomyosarcomas are malignant tumors featuring skeletal muscle differentiation, with several histologic subtypes (see Fig. 45-20). The major varieties in

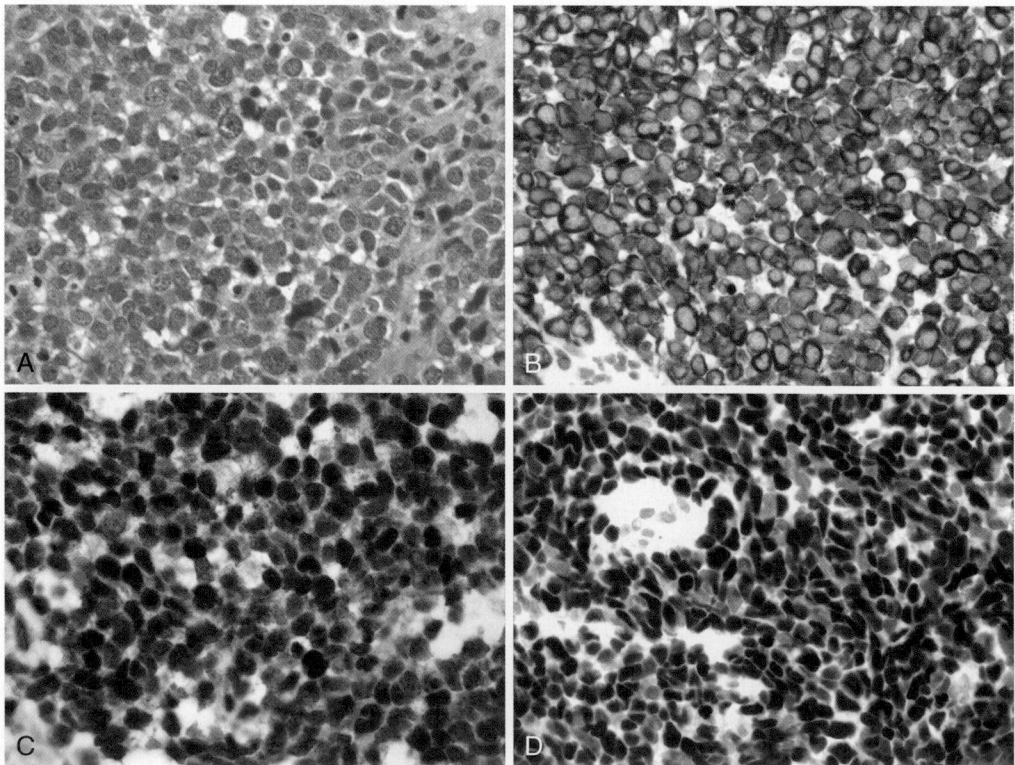

Figure 45-20 Solid variant of alveolar rhabdomyosarcoma composed of undifferentiated, moderately pleomorphic round cells histologically (**A**), but with convincing evidence of myogenic differentiation, as demonstrated by strong and diffuse cytoplasmic expression of desmin (**B**) and nuclear reactivity for MyoD1 (**C**) and myogenin (**D**). Of note, the percentage of nuclei reacting for both myogenin and MyoD1 is very high, as is typical of the alveolar variant of rhabdomyosarcoma.

childhood are the embryonal and alveolar subtypes and, although there are classic morphologies of alveolar and embryonal rhabdomyosarcoma, the distinction is not always clear-cut, because a solid variant alveolar rhabdomyosarcoma exists and composite cases also occur. Therefore especially with decreasing biopsy size, traditional morphologic distinction between embryonal and alveolar subtypes of rhabdomyosarcoma is not always a reliable means of subclassifying the tumors but is nonetheless essential for appropriate therapeutic stratification of patients with these two biologically different tumors. Alveolar rhabdomyosarcoma exhibits a higher proportional nuclear reactivity for both myogenin and MyoD1 than embryonal rhabdomyosarcoma,[164] but even this feature may be unconvincing in small biopsies and thus be of little value in firmly establishing the diagnosis. The biologically distinct nature of embryonal and alveolar subtypes is confirmed by genetic studies, which show translocations targeting the chromosome 13 *FOXO1A* (forkhead transcription factor) gene in most alveolar rhabdomyosarcomas, and nontranslocation cytogenetic alterations, including 11p deletion, trisomy 8, and trisomy 20, in embryonal rhabdomyosarcomas. In 70% to 80% of alveolar rhabdomyosarcomas there is fusion of the *FOXO1* gene with the *PAX3* gene on chromosome 2,[165-167] and approximately 10% have fusions of *FOXO1* with the *PAX7* gene on chromosome 1.[168] The *PAX7-FOXO1* fusion is often highly amplified in the form of double-minute chromosomes (see Fig. 45-13B), whereas the *PAX3-FOXO1* fusions are not usually amplified. This difference appears to reflect the lower intrinsic expression of *PAX7-FOXO1*, relative to that of *PAX3-FOXO1*, with genomic amplification therefore required to provide a comparable and sufficient level of oncogenic transcript.[169] The *FOXO1*, *PAX3*, and *PAX7* genes encode transcription factors, and the *PAX3-FOXO1* and *PAX7-FOXO1* fusion oncogenes encode activated forms of those transcription factors[170,171] that function to induce myogenic differentiation programs.[156,157,172] Notably, alveolar rhabdomyosarcomas with *PAX7-FOXO1* rearrangements were reported in one study to have better prognoses than those with *PAX3-FOXO1* when comparing patients presenting with metastatic disease.[173] Furthermore, an argument has been made for movement

toward designation of rhabdomyosarcomas based on translocation status rather than on morphology; and in that vein, cases of morphologic alveolar rhabdomyosarcoma have been termed *fusion-positive* versus *fusion-negative*. The observation that gene expression profiles of fusion-negative alveolar rhabdomyosarcomas are indistinguishable from those of embryonal rhabdomyosarcomas[174-177] might lend considerable support to such subclassification. Whether molecular categorization however translates well to clinical prognosis and treatment stratification remains unresolved,[176,178,179] and a combined morphomolecular diagnosis is currently considered best practice.[180]

A proportion of cases of rhabdomyosarcoma lacking the canonical *PAX-FOXO1* fusions show t(2;2)(p23;q35) or t(2;8)(q35;q13) in which *PAX3* is fused with either *NCOA1* or *NCOA2*, which are nuclear receptor transcriptional coactivators,[181] whereas isolated individual cases of rhabdomyosarcoma were reported to show t(2;6)(p23;p21.1),[182] t(4;22)(q35;q12) fusing *EWSR1* with *DUX4*,[183] and a complex t(8;13;9)(p11.2;q14;q32) apparently resulting in amplification of *FGFR1-FOXO1* fusion.[184]

Synovial Sarcoma

Synovial sarcomas may be monophasic (Fig. 45-21), in which the tumor is predominantly composed of spindle cells, or biphasic, in which the tumor contains both spindle cell and epithelioid elements, with the latter exhibiting more convincing epithelial immunophenotypic characteristics or, uncommonly, poorly differentiated, with a primitive round cell morphology reminiscent of Ewing sarcoma. Apart from the epithelial markers epithelial membrane antigen (EMA) and cytokeratins, transducer-like enhancer protein 1 (TLE1) also has been validated from gene expression profiles as a reliable marker for synovial sarcoma.[185-187] Synovial sarcomas feature translocation of chromosomes X and 18, t(X;18)(p11;q11).[188,189] t(X;18) is found in more than 90% of synovial sarcomas but not generally in histologic mimics such as hemangiopericytoma, mesothelioma, leiomyosarcoma, or malignant peripheral nerve sheath tumor. The molecular underpinnings of t(X;18) are complex in that the oncogene on chromosome 18 (*SYT* or *SS18*) can be

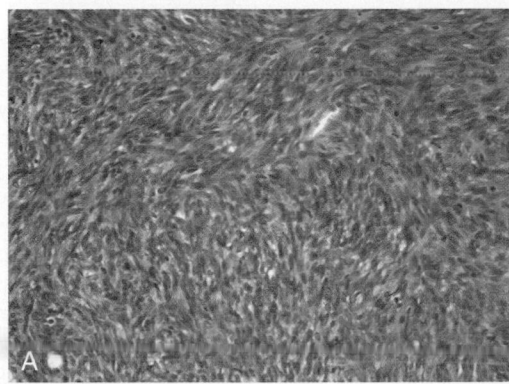 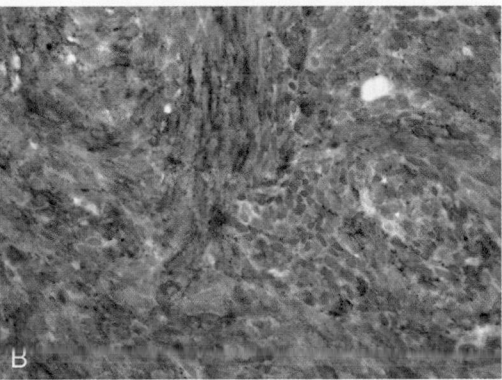

Figure 45-21 **A,** Monophasic synovial sarcoma, with interdigitating fascicular arrangement of fusiform spindle cells. **B,** Weak, patchy immunohistochemical staining for epithelial membrane antigen (EMA) in the spindle cells.

fused with one of several almost identical genes (generally *SSX1* or *SSX2* and, rarely, *SSX4*) on chromosome X.[190,191] *SSX1* and *SSX2* are adjacent genes and, given their close proximity, it is impossible to distinguish *SS18-SSX1* and *SS18-SSX2* translocations using conventional chromosomal banding methods. However, the alternative *SSX* fusions can be demonstrated by FISH or RT-PCR using specific probes or primers, respectively.[192,193] One study has suggested that synovial sarcomas with the *SS18-SSX1* fusion are typically biphasic, whereas those with *SS18-SSX2* can be biphasic or monophasic and have better metastasis-free survival compared with those bearing *SS18-SSX1* fusions.[194] This morphologic-genotypic correlate is substantiated by studies of SS18-SSX1 and SS18-SSX2 interactions with SNAIL and SLUG, both transcriptional repressors of E-cadherin, which mediates mesenchymal to epithelial transition.[195]

The SS18-SYT fusion protein is both necessary and sufficient for cellular transformation.[196] SS18 and SSX contribute, respectively, transcriptional coactivator and repressor domains to the SS18-SSX fusion proteins, and, despite the lack of any DNA binding domain, exert an effect on gene transcriptional dysregulation apparently through association with chromatin remodeling proteins Trithorax (TRX) and the Polycomb repressor complex (PRC2).[197-200] Mass spectrometry has revealed that SS18-SSX fusion proteins bind TLE1 and ATF2 to form a complex necessary for tumor cell survival. ATF2 is the DNA binding partner of SS18-SSX, and the epigenetic repression of ATF2 is dependent on TLE1, the recruitment of which can be abrogated by HDAC inhibitors, which have already shown considerable promise in preclinical trials.[201] In addition, SS18-SSX competes physically with wild-type SS18, forming an altered complex lacking SMARCB1. This altered complex transactivates *SOX2*, which is a diagnostic marker that is universally overexpressed in synovial sarcoma and essential for synovial sarcoma proliferation.[202]

Adipose Tumors

Most subtypes of adipose tumors, whether benign or malignant, contain distinctive genetic aberrations (see Table 45-1). Useful diagnostic markers include 8q rearrangement in lipoblastoma, 12q rearrangement in lipoma, ring chromosomes in well-differentiated and dedifferentiated liposarcoma, and t(12;16) in myxoid or round cell liposarcoma.

Lipoblastomas are pediatric adipose tumors containing variable numbers of primitive cells (lipoblasts) and generally bearing translocations of the chromosome 8 long arm at bands 8q11-12, resulting in rearrangement of the *PLAG1* zinc finger oncogene.[130] Reports of individual cases each of lipoblastoma[203] and lipoma[204] bearing translocations involving 8q21.1 region in each case as well as with a t(9;12)(p22;q14) in a pediatric intramuscular lipoma[205] add to the variability in observations in these benign fatty neoplasms. Hibernomas, which contain adipose cells with a brown fat phenotype, generally have rearrangements of the chromosome 11 long arm,[206] although the gene target of that translocation has not been identified.

Another diagnostically useful aberration is the translocation of chromosomes 12 and 16 found in myxoid liposarcomas.[207-209] This translocation is also found in round cell liposarcomas and is retained in myxoid liposarcomas that acquire round cell features and thereby undergo transition to higher histologic grade.[210,211] t(12;16) results in fusion of the *DDIT3 (CHOP)* transcription factor gene on chromosome 12 to the *TLS* gene on chromosome 16,[212,213] and the resultant fusion oncoprotein is an activated transcription factor. t(12;16) has not been found in other subtypes of liposarcoma or in other types of myxoid soft tissue tumors.[214,215] It appears to be relevant therapeutically, in that patients with myxoid or round cell liposarcoma show impressive responses to trabectedin chemotherapy.[216] However, liposarcoma is rare in childhood and virtually unheard of in the first decade of life.

Clear Cell Sarcoma: Malignant Melanoma of Soft Parts

Clear cell sarcomas of the soft tissues resemble cutaneous melanomas histologically, and therefore have been referred to as melanoma of soft parts. Immunohistochemically, the tumors are consistently positive for S-100 protein, usually at least focally for HMB45, microphthalmia transcription factor (MITF), and Melan A.[217] Despite their histologic and immunohistochemical overlaps, clear cell sarcoma and true melanoma are different clinically. Whereas most melanomas are of cutaneous origin, clear cell sarcomas generally present as isolated masses in deep soft tissues, without apparent origin from, or involvement of, skin. Less commonly they arise in the gastrointestinal tract. Most clear cell sarcomas contain a chromosomal translocation, t(12;22)(q13;q12), while those arising in the gastrointestinal tract will more commonly bear the variant t(2;22)(q34;q12).[218] The latter has, however, also been described in a minor subset of soft tissue–based clear cell sarcoma.[154,219] These translocations have never been reported in cutaneous melanoma and therefore serve as a reliable markers in distinguishing these two tumor types (Fig. 45-22). t(12;22) fuses the *ATF1* gene on chromosome 12 with the *EWS* gene on chromosome 22.[219,220] *ATF1* encodes a transcription factor, and the biologic implications of the translocation are probably similar to those in Ewing sarcoma translocations (see earlier). t(2;22) fuses the *CREB1* gene on chromosome 2, a *CREB* gene family member closely related to *ATF1*, with the *EWSR1* gene.

Desmoplastic Small Round Cell Tumor

DRSCTs are aggressive and chemotherapy-resistant neoplasms that arise most commonly from the peritoneum or intraabdominal soft tissues, particularly in adolescent males.[221] They are composed of undifferentiated malignant small round cells in a striking desmoplastic reaction, ensnaring sharply demarcated islands of tumor cells (Fig. 45-23).[222] Almost all cases express an *EWSR1-WT1* fusion oncogene[222,223] resulting from translocation between the chromosome 11 short arm and chromosome 22 long arm.[110,223] The EWS-WT1 oncoproteins are expressed as several isoforms (see Fig. 45-10), each of which is composed of the EWSR1 amino-terminal

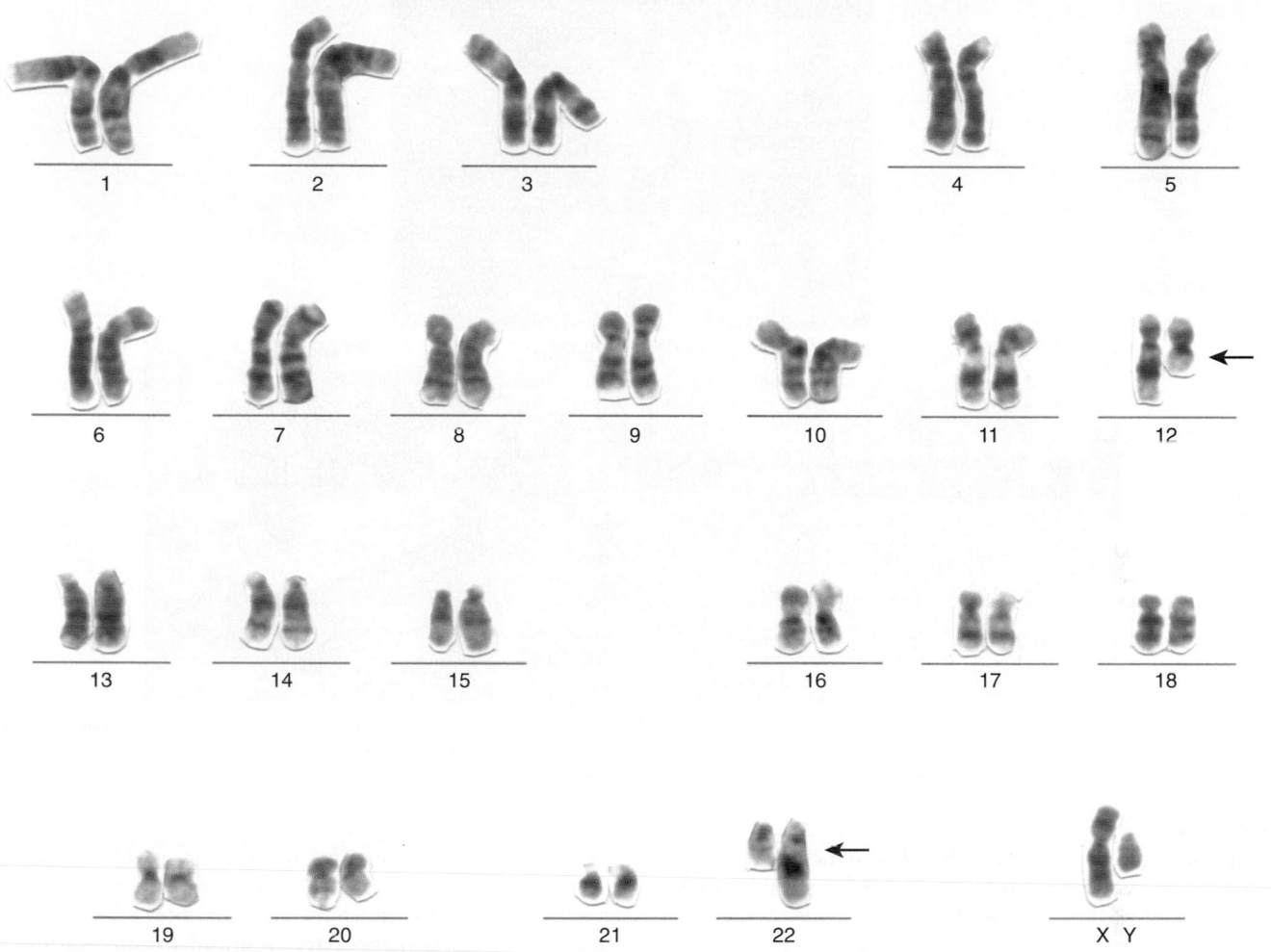

Figure 45-22 Clear cell sarcoma karyotype showing balanced translocation, t(12;22), as the only cytogenetic aberration. *Arrows* indicate translocation breakpoints.

transactivation region fused to the last three of four zinc fingers at the WT1 carboxyl-terminal end.[226,227] These oncoproteins result from fusion of *EWSR1* exon 7, 8, or 9 to *WT1* exon 8. The *EWSR1-WT1* fusion typically results in expression of the carboxyl-terminal but not amino-terminal aspect of WT1 in DSRCT, which may be detected by immunohistochemistry using appropriate antibodies (see Fig. 45-23). Quantitatively minor secondary transcripts lacking exon 6 of *EWSR1* and/or exon 9 of *WT1* are also expressed, although the functional relevance of these transcripts is unknown.[226] However, it is worth noting that the usual immunostaining pattern was not observed in an isolated reported case with atypical transcript that lacked *WT1* exons 9 and 10.[228] The EWSR1-WT1 oncoprotein retains an alternative splicing site (±KTS) between the third and fourth WT1 zinc fingers (see Fig. 45-10). The KTS– isoform regulates genes that are believed to have important biologic roles in DSRCTs, including platelet-derived growth factor-α (PDGFA) and insulin-like growth factor receptor I, whereas the KTS+ isoform regulates a different set of genes.[229] Notably,

only the KTS– isoform has shown transforming activity when evaluated in vitro.[230] PDGFA is known to activate potent receptor (platelet-derived growth factor receptor [PDGFR])-mediated mitogenic signaling pathways in fibroblasts,[231] and EWSR1-WT1 might therefore induce desmoplastic proliferation via PDGFA transcriptional upregulation.[227]

Dermatofibrosarcoma Protuberans

DFSP is a low-grade spindle cell tumor, which can occasionally progress to a more aggressive fibrosarcomatous phase. Most DFSPs contain ring chromosomes composed of sequences from chromosomes 17 and 22 (see Fig. 45-13A).[232,233] The ring chromosomes contain multiple copies of a fusion gene, *COL1A1-PDGFB*, in which *COL1A1* (a collagen gene) is contributed from chromosome 17 and *PDGFB* (platelet-derived growth factor-β gene) from chromosome 22.[75,122] Alternatively, DFSP, particularly in pediatric patients, occasionally has t(17;22) translocations, resulting in a single copy of the *COL1A1-PDGFB* fusion gene.[234] The *COL1A1-PDGFB* oncogene

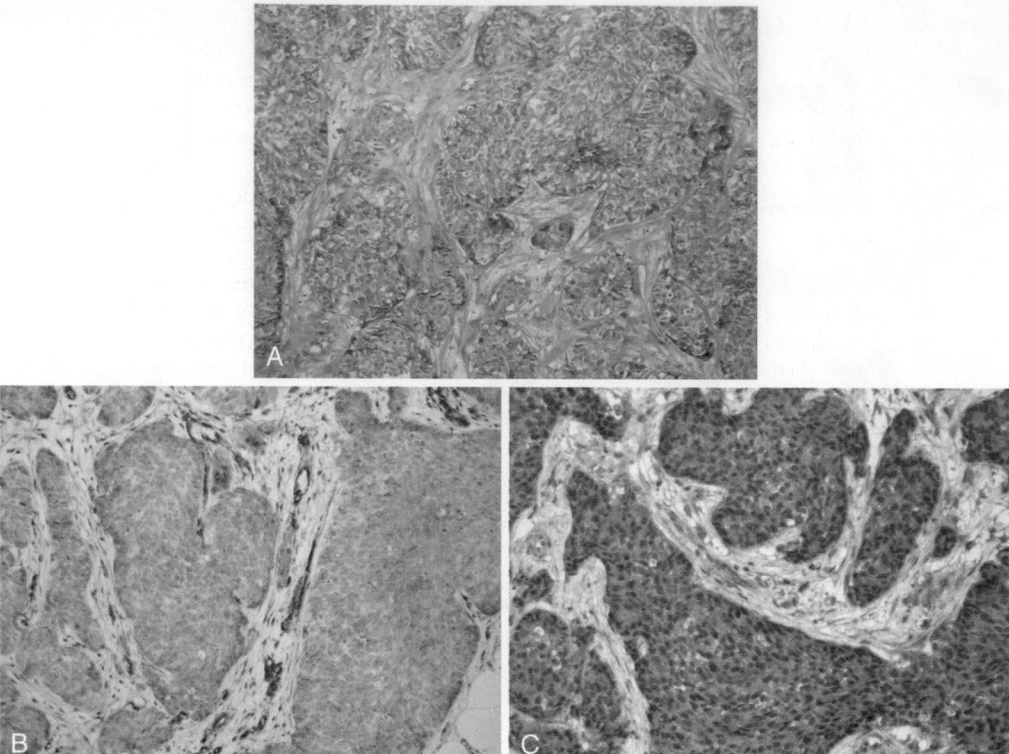

Figure 45-23 **A**, Desmoplastic small round cell tumor with sharply demarcated islands of blue tumor cells separated by pink densely fibrotic "desmoplastic" stroma. Immunoreactivities with antibodies to N-terminal (**B**) and C-terminal (**C**) regions of WT1 are negative and strongly positive, respectively, in the tumor cells, in keeping with EWS-WT1 fusion oncoprotein expression.

results in overexpression of PDGFB, which is a growth factor that activates platelet-derived growth factor receptor-β (PDGFRB) and PDGFRA. This cytogenetic observation has suggested that patients with inoperable DFSP might benefit from treatment with PDGFR inhibitors such as imatinib, and this hypothesis has been confirmed by impressive clinical responses to PDGFRB therapeutic inhibition with imatinib.[235,236,237,238] *COL1A1-PDGFB* oncogenic fusion is also seen in giant cell fibroblastoma (GCF), a pediatric neoplasm closely related to DFSP.[123,239] Studies of GCF and composite GCF/DFSP cases have shown the presence of a single translocation t(17;22) and the resultant *COL1A1-PDGFB* fusion, in the GCF component, with acquisition of additional copies of the oncogene being associated with progression to DFSP.[74]

Desmoid Tumors

Desmoid tumors, also known as deep fibromatoses, contain various genetic aberrations, including the *APC* (adenomatous polyposis coli) gene or *CTNNB1* mutations,[240,241] and trisomies for chromosomes 8 or 20.[242] Cytogenetic deletions of the chromosome 5 long arm are seen in occasional desmoids, resulting in loss of the *APC* tumor suppressor gene.[243,244] However, the most common mutations, particularly in nonfamilial desmoid tumors, are activating *CTNNB1* mutations, which are found in at least 50% of cases.[240,241] Both *APC* inactivating and β-catenin activating mutations result in stabilization and resultant overexpression, of the β-catenin protein with roles in cell proliferation, motility, and differentiation. This overexpression of β-catenin can be detected immunohistochemically in a nuclear distribution.[245] In a retrospective analysis of primary desmoid tumor, the precise β-catenin mutation type was strongly predictive of recurrence, with S45F being associated in multivariate analysis with decreased time to recurrence and overall percentage recurrence.[246] The cytogenetic aberrations in most desmoid tumors, particularly the trisomies 8 and 20, are mechanisms of progression and are acquired subsequent to the *APC* or *CTNNB1* mutations. Interestingly, an as yet unexplained association of desmoidal fibromatosis in patients with gastrointestinal stromal tumor (GIST) has been reported.[247]

Infantile Fibrosarcoma

Infantile (also congenital/infantile) fibrosarcomas characteristically present within the first year of life. These are tumors composed of plump fibroblast-like cells (see Fig. 45-16), which often show high mitotic activity, and feature trisomies of chromosomes 8, 11, 17, and 20.[248] This same group of trisomies occur in the histologically identical pediatric renal tumor, congenital cellular mesoblastic nephroma (see Fig. 45-18).[249] Most infantile fibrosarcomas and congenital cellular mesoblastic nephromas also contain a diagnostic chromosomal translocation, t(12;15)(p13;q26), which is cryptic when studied by traditional cytogenetic banding methods (see Fig. 45-2).[7,113,250] A complex three-way t(12;15;19) translocation has also been reported in infantile fibrosarcoma.[251] t(12;15) (p13;q26) results in fusion of the *TEL* gene on chromosome 12 to the *NTRK3* receptor tyrosine kinase gene on chromosome 15, producing constitutive tyrosine kinase activation. Although challenging to detect by banding methods, the t(12;15) translocation is demonstrated readily by FISH with a dual-color break-apart TEL probe (see Fig. 45-2) or RT-PCR assay.[7,113,250]

Inflammatory Myofibroblastic Tumor

Inflammatory myofibroblastic tumors, belonging to the group of inflammatory pseudotumors, are relatively rare tumors occurring primarily in children and young adults. They are composed of myofibroblastic cells admixed with an infiltrate of lymphocytes and plasma cells (see Fig. 45-17). The inflammatory component of these tumors is nonneoplastic and therefore lacks cytogenetic aberrations, whereas the myofibroblastic cells often contain clonal chromosomal aberrations[252-254] involving rearrangement and oncogenic activation of the *ALK* receptor tyrosine kinase gene at chromosome band 2p23.[114] The *ALK* oncogenes cause constitutive activation of the ALK kinase by enhanced oligomerization resulting from fusion of the ALK kinase domain to the oligomerization domain of the partner gene.[114] *ALK* oncogenic activation is associated with strong, immunohistochemically detectable ALK expression in the inflammatory myofibroblastic tumor spindle cells in about 50% of cases (see Fig. 45-17).[114] The ALK immunohistochemical staining pattern reflects the fusion type, insofar as fusion of ALK with most of the various partners (TPM3, TPM4, CARS, CLTC, SEC31A (SEC31L1),[255] PPFIBP1,[256] ALO17) produces cytoplasmic staining, whereas ALK-RANBP2 fusion produces nuclear membrane–associated reactivity.[257,258] These immunohistochemical findings can distinguish inflammatory myofibroblastic tumor from its histologic mimics, but, given the considerable rate of nonimmunoreactivity, demonstration of *ALK* rearrangement is especially helpful in confirming the diagnosis. An aggressive form of IMT characterized by round cell or epithelioid morphology is described that typically arises intraabdominally in male patients and shows in virtually all cases ALK immunoreactivity in a nuclear, or less commonly, cytoplasmic and perinuclear distribution.[259]

ALK-rearranged inflammatory myofibroblastic tumors are effectively treated with ALK inhibitor crizotinib; however, the emergence of secondary resistance can limit efficacy.[260,261]

Gastrointestinal Stromal Tumor

Most adult GISTs contain activating mutations of the *KIT* or *PDGFRA* oncogenes[262-264] or rarely *BRAF.*[265] These mutations have been targeted with considerable success using the KIT and PDGFRA inhibitor imatinib (Gleevec)[266,267] and second-line tyrosine kinase inhibitors in the context of resistant disease.[268] In addition, germline (inherited) *KIT* mutations are responsible for rare syndromes of familial, multifocal GISTs.[269] However, because most pediatric GISTs do not contain *KIT* or *PDGFRA* mutations they have been termed *wild-type GISTs,* and these predominate as gastric tumors in prepubescent girls.[270-272] In keeping with this, children with metastatic GISTs show only very limited benefit from the KIT-PDGFRA kinase inhibitor therapies. Moreover, pediatric GISTs lack the typical sequential cytogenetic deletions that seem to drive genetic and clinical progression in adult GISTs.[273] Largely through an appreciation of the occurrence of GIST as a component of Carney-Stratakis syndrome/dyad, which is the dominantly inherited predisposition to paraganglioma and GIST,[274,275] underpinned by germline inactivation of subunits B, C or D of succinate dehydrogenase (SDH), it has become evident that deficiency in cellular respiration in fact appears to provide the pathologic basis to all pediatric/wild-type GISTs, despite the low incidence of SDH mutation in such tumors.[276] Germline *SDHA* mutations have been described in isolated cases of paraganglioma and adult wild-type GIST.[277,278] Inactivation of any of the four subunits A, B, C, or D of SDH leads to enzyme complex destabilization and inactivation. Immunohistochemical staining for the B subunit of succinate dehydrogenase (SDHB) provides a surrogate marker for SDH function and is characteristically negative in all pediatric/wild-type GISTs. On this basis, a proposal has been made that GISTs no longer be classed as "mutant" and "wild-type" based on receptor tyrosine kinase mutation but rather be designated type 1 and type 2 as SDHB-positive and SDHB-negative, respectively.[279] Although a strong association with neurofibromatosis type 1 (NF1) exists, in this particular context GISTs usually arise only in adulthood.[280]

Malignant Peripheral Nerve Sheath Tumors

Benign peripheral nerve sheath tumors and malignant peripheral nerve sheath tumors (MPNSTs) are frequent complications in patients with hereditary neurofibromatosis syndromes. These syndromes are the most common tumor predisposition syndromes, affecting 1 in 3500 individuals worldwide. Neurofibromas and malignant peripheral nerve sheath tumors are common in those NF1, whereas benign schwannomas are common in neurofibromatosis type 2 (NF2, central neurofibromatosis). Characterization of the neurofibromatosis syndrome genes has shed substantial light on the pathogenesis of peripheral nerve sheath tumors. The *NF1* and *NF2* genes are located on chromosomes 17 and 22, respectively, and both these genes encode tumor suppressor proteins that normally constrain cellular proliferation.[281-286] NF1 protein tumor suppressor mechanisms involve regulation of RAS GTPase activity,[282,283] with *NF1* gene deletion therefore resulting in constitutive RAS activation, suggesting that therapeutics targeting RAS (or downstream signaling intermediates such as RAF and MEK-MAPK) might be useful for clinical management of MPNSTs and other NF1-associated cancers.[287] MPNSTs often have *NF1* gene deletions, which can be demonstrated by FISH assay. The *NF1* gene aberrations are accompanied by a generally complex karyotype, suggesting that genetic instability plays a prominent role in the development of MPNSTs. Notably, *NF1* gene deletions can be shown in only the Schwann cell component of neurofibromas.[288] This observation supports the view that neurofibromas are clonal Schwann cell neoplasms, whereas the other admixed cell lineages—including fibroblasts, mast cells, and perineural cells—are reactive.

Recent studies demonstrated that the evolution of benign peripheral nerve sheath tumors to MPNST is accompanied predominantly by *loss* of expression of a large number of genes, including, in a vast majority of cases, inactivation of TP53[289] with associated downregulation of the pro-apoptotic miR-34a. MiR-10b, which specifically targets NF1, is upregulated in NF1-associated MPNSTs.[290] Homozygous loss of CDKN2A is also associated with malignant transformation,[291,292] whereas high-resolution copy number profiling has shown, among others, recurrent gains of *PDGFRA, MET, HGF, TP73, EGFR, TERT, MYC,* and *IGF1R* and losses of *NF1, p16^{INK4A}/CDKN2A, RB1,* and *TP53,*[293,294] providing potential basis for novel therapeutic agents[294,295] in this therapeutically challenging sarcoma.

Neuroblastoma

Most neuroblastomas have distinctive cytogenetic features that correlate with their clinical behavior. Favorable prognosis neuroblastomas, which respond well to chemotherapy and can even undergo spontaneous regression, generally feature near-triploid karyotypes without 1p deletion or *MYCN* amplification.[296] Unfavorable prognosis neuroblastomas (Fig. 45-24), by contrast, feature near-diploid or near-tetraploid karyotypes, often accompanied by 1p deletion, 17q amplification, and/or *MYCN* amplification,[297] whereas deletions of 3p and 11q are reportedly predictive of metastasis.[298] In essence, gains of whole chromosomes are more typical of low- or intermediate-risk neuroblastoma whereas segmental chromosomal aberrations are more commonly seen in high-risk cases. *MYCN* amplification, typically manifested as double-minute chromosomes (see Figs. 45-5 and 45-6), is arguably the most ominous of the adverse genetic markers. *MYCN*-amplified neuroblastomas are rarely curable,

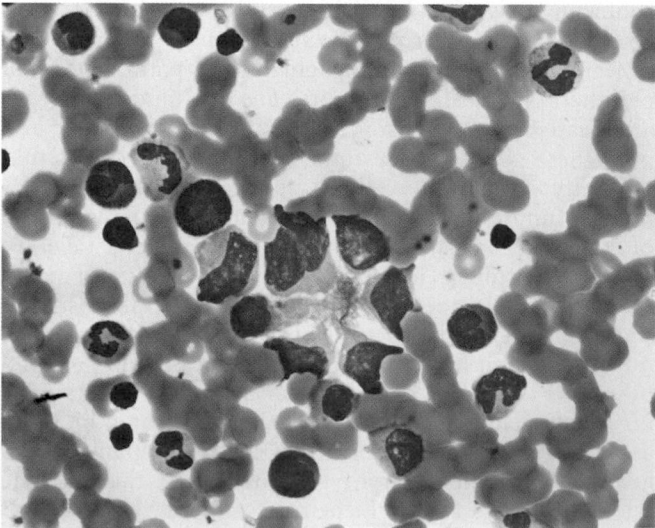

Figure 45-24 Bone marrow involvement by disseminated neuroblastoma, showing a classic rosette of tumor cells, with bluish cytoplasm and neuropil. (*Courtesy Marybeth Helfrich, Children's Hospital of Philadelphia.*)

although complete remission can be achieved through intensive myeloablative chemotherapy. Therefore genetic parameters can be useful adjuncts for determining appropriate intensity of therapy, particularly for those children whose prognoses are not clear based on clinical parameters alone.[297] Cytogenetic analysis of neuroblastoma has been difficult, however, because the tumor cells from most favorable prognosis neuroblastomas fail to divide in culture.[297] *MYCN* amplification and chromosome 1p or 11q deletion and 17q gain can be demonstrated in interphase cells by FISH or CISH (see Fig. 45-6), obviating the need for tumor cell culture.[299,300] It remains unclear whether one or more conventional tumor suppressor genes are targeted by the 1p deletions found in most poor-prognosis neuroblastomas. However, several microRNAs in the critical 1p deletion region function to maintain neuroblastoma survival and activate *MYCN* transcription.[301,302] *ALK* kinase domain mutations and gene amplifications have been demonstrated in hereditary neuroblastoma that may otherwise be underscored by *PHOX2B* germline mutation.[117-119,303,304] About 15% of sporadic neuroblastomas also show aberrations of ALK,[117-119,305] suggesting that ALK inhibitors might be useful therapeutically in neuroblastoma. SNP variations at 6p22.3,[306] 2q35 (the *BARD1* gene),[307] and copy number aberration at 1q21 (the *NBPF23* gene)[308] are associated with increased risk for development of neuroblastoma but without further elucidation of the likely mechanisms involved biologically.

Rhabdoid Tumor

Malignant rhabdoid tumors generally have dismal outcomes, particularly those presenting in infancy, and most cases, whether arising in soft tissues, kidney, or CNS (where they are known as atypical teratoid/rhabdoid tumors), have deletions of the chromosome 22 long arm, targeting the *SMARCB1 (INI1)* tumor suppressor gene. Biallelic *SMARCB1* mutation is present in the vast majority of rhabdoid tumors, with frequent truncating mutations occurring. In a small number of cases, instead of *SMARCB1,* the *SMARCA4 (BRG1)* gene is inactivated.[309] *SMARCB1* encodes a member of the SWI/SNF protein complex involved in chromatin remodeling.[310,311] Chromosome 22 deletion is often the only detectable cytogenetic aberration, suggesting that *SMARCB1* inactivation is an early oncogenic event in these remarkably aggressive tumors,[312,313] which are classically diploid and genomically stable.[314,315] Indeed, sequencing studies have revealed a remarkably simple tumor genome otherwise with virtually no oncogenic mutations identifed.[315,317] Additional evidence of an essential tumorigenic role includes the finding of germline *INI1* mutations in some individuals with rhabdoid tumors[311,318,319] and the development of rhabdoid tumor models in mice with inactivating *SMARCB1* mutations.[320] Notably, germline *SMARCB1* mutations are not restricted to rhabdoid tumors but have been implicated also in familial schwannomatosis[321] and in nonrhabdoid CNS tumors, including medulloblastoma.[318] and multiple meningiomas[322] SMARCB1 inhibits cyclin D1 expression by recruiting a histone deacetylase 1 complex to the *CCND1* (cyclin D1) promoter, resulting in G1 cell cycle arrest.[323] The relevance of cyclin D1 in *SMARCB1*-mediated tumorigenesis is underscored by the observation that rhabdoid tumors develop in SMARCB1+/– mice expressing cyclin D1 whereas SMARCB1+/– mice with cyclin D1 deficiency (cyclin D1–/–) do not develop rhabdoid tumors.[324] These observations suggest that drugs targeting cyclin D1 might be relevant for rhabdoid tumors,[325] and clinical trials testing this are planned.

Recent work has unraveled an epigenetic antagonism between SMARCB1 and Polycombs of the PRC2 complex.[326] The Polycomb proteins are transcriptional repressors that modulate chromatin structure to silence gene expression, and they are key regulators of cell fate transitions. Their function frequently becomes deregulated in cancer.[327] The Polycombs have been shown to be required for the repression of differentiation genes in stem cells[328,329] so that this repression of differentiation might be facilitated by loss of the PRC2 antagonist SMARCB1.

Rhabdoid tumors are characteristically composed of cells with vesicular nuclei and prominent nucleoli, with the nucleus often being pushed to an eccentric location within the cell by a dense intracytoplasmic inclusion (see Fig. 45-9), which, as seen by electron microscopy, consists of a tightly arranged whorl of intermediate filaments. These filaments stain nonspecifically for various markers, giving the tumor a polyphenotypic appearance. Absence of SMARCB1 expression in the tumor cells but not the normal stromal support nuclei, as is readily demonstrable by immunohistochemistry, is useful for diagnosing rhabdoid tumor (see Fig. 45-9).[31,330]

Alveolar Soft Part Sarcoma

Alveolar soft part sarcoma is a rare tumor, occurring mostly in adolescents and young adults, with a predilection for involvement of soft tissues in the head and neck region. However, other soft tissue and even hollow viscera may be involved. Characterized by a distinctive morphology, with nested or alveolar-like growth, the tumor cells are epithelioid, with abundant clear to eosinophilic cytoplasm, sharply defined cellular borders, and diastase-resistant, periodic acid–Schiff (PAS)-positive intracytoplasmic crystals (Fig. 45-25), which on electron microscopic examination are rhomboidal. Alveolar soft part sarcoma generally exhibits indolent behavior but nonetheless has

a high risk for late metastases and indeed represents the sarcoma most likely to metastasize to the CNS.[331] There are no histologic features to predict clinical behavior. The classic cytogenetic feature of ASPS is t(X;17)(p11;q25), producing fusion of the *ASPSCR1* and *TFE3* genes.[332] This same translocation is seen in a subset of pediatric renal cell carcinomas, with the distinct difference that the *ASPS*-related translocation is *un*balanced and involves gain of Xp telomeric to *TFE3* and loss of 17q sequence telomeric to q25[333] while the renal carcinoma–associated translocation is balanced. The ASPSCR1-TFE3 fusion protein induces strong expression of MET tyrosine kinase in tumor cells.[334] Antibody raised to the carboxyl terminus of TFE3 produces strong nuclear reactivity in *ASPSCR1-TFE3* fusion-positive tumors.[335]

Nonmesenchymal Solid Tumors

Renal Tumors

Most pediatric renal tumors contain characteristic cytogenetic aberrations. Deletion of 11p is a well-known aberration in Wilms tumor, but several other aberrations, including extra copies of chromosome 12, are more frequent and have apparent prognostic relevance, as does LOH of 1p and 16q.[336,337] Another pediatric renal tumor with consistent cytogenetic aberrations is congenital cellular mesoblastic nephroma, in which various chromosomal trisomies and oncogenic fusion of the TEL and NTRK3 proteins are observed reliably.[7,250] More recently, it has emerged that translocation-associated carcinomas make up a majority of pediatric renal carcinomas.[338,339] In addition, neuroblastoma patients are at hugely increased risk (329-fold)[340] of developing oncocytoid renal carcinoma[341]; however, pediatric renal carcinoma may also follow certain sarcomas.[342,343]

Pediatric Renal Cell Carcinomas with Xp11 or 6p21 Translocations. Pediatric renal cell carcinomas are uncommon and they generally have a papillary morphology, accompanied by translocations involving chromosomes X or 6.[344] By comparison, adult papillary renal cancers typically have a distinctive profile of chromosomal trisomies, although a rare few contain the same translocations seen in pediatric renal cancers. The

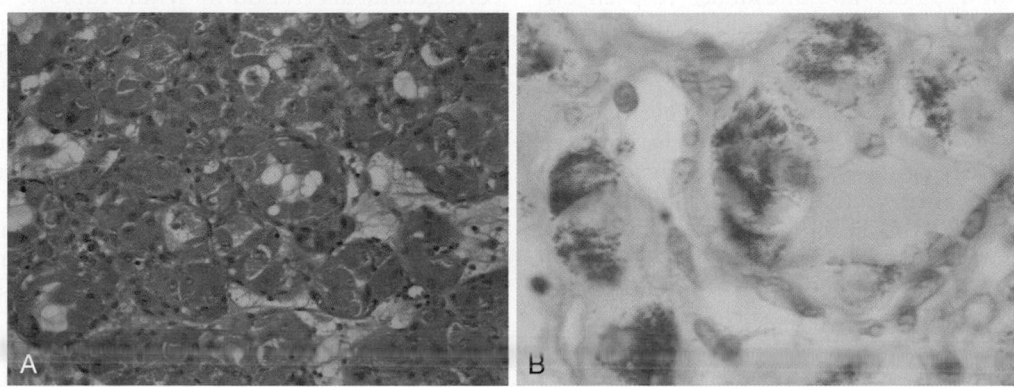

Figure 45-25 Characteristic histologic features of alveolar soft part sarcoma include an alveolar-like arrangement of cells with abundant deeply eosinophilic cytoplasm (**A**) and diastase-resistant, periodic acid–Schiff-positive intracytoplasmic crystals (**B**).

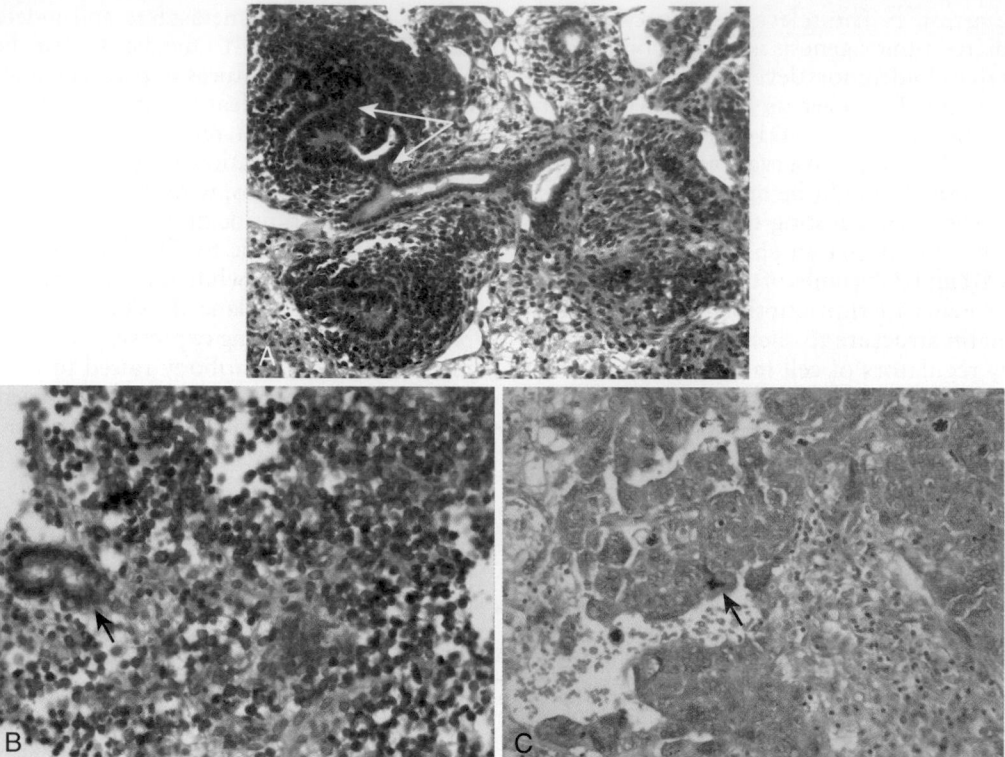

Figure 45-26 **A,** Wilms tumor with triphasic histology. The tumor recapitulates nephrogenesis with condensation of mesenchyme at tips of tubular branch-points. Here, the blastema is condensed around a focus of tubular differentiation *(arrows)*. **B,** High-power image showing undifferentiated blastema, which in the absence of obvious tubular differentiation *(arrow)* might be difficult to distinguish from other undifferentiated small round cell tumors. **C,** Anaplastic Wilms tumor with bizarre mitoses and massively enlarged hyperchromatic nuclei *(arrow)*.

unifying theme for the pediatric carcinoma translocations is that they target various members of the MiT family of transcription factors. These include t(X;1)(p11;q21), resulting in fusion of *PRCC* (at chromosome band 1q21) and the MiT family member *TFE3* (at chromosome band Xp11). There are variants of this translocation, including t(X;17)(p11;q25), in which *TFE3* is fused with the *ASPSCR1* gene at chromosome band 17q25.[345] Also involving an MiT family member is t(6;11)(p21;q13), which fuses *TFEB* (at chromosome band 6p21) with the *Alpha* gene (at chromosome band 11q13).[346] The *TFEB*-rearranged tumors more consistently express melanocytic markers HMB45 and Melan A than do *TFE3*-translocated cases.[347] TFE3 and TFEB immunostains, respectively, show specific reactivity in a nuclear distribution in the correspondingly rearranged cases but may rarely be negative in the presence of molecular proof of a translocation, and a robust FISH assay has also been developed to confirm rearrangement of *TFEB*.[347] Intriguingly, however, whereas ASPS cases with ASPSCR1-TFE3 fusion were found to uniformly express cathepsin K, a target of MiTF, and the majority of PRCC-TFE3 rearranged carcinomas did similarly, the ASPSCR1-TFE3 fusion-positive carcinomas were all negative for cathepsin K,[348] a feature that might be exploited in certain diagnostic settings.

Wilms Tumor. Wilms tumors are the most common type of renal cancer in children. They typically contain primitive blastemal cells that differentiate into tubular epithe-lial, glomerular, and/or mesenchymal populations. The classic triphasic Wilms tumor contains an admixture of blastemal, epithelial, and mesenchymal components (Fig. 45-26), and all three cell types may contain the same clonal chromosomal aberrations.[349] Various genetic alterations are found in subsets of Wilms tumors, including trisomies 6, 8, 12, and 18, and deletions of 11p13 (see later). Deletions of 11p15, 1p, and 16q bode ill in patients with low-stage favorable histology tumors and 1q gains are associated with relapse. These can all readily be tested on interphase nuclei by FISH assay (see Table 45-1).[337,350-352]

Deletion 11p13 is the most extensively characterized cytogenetic aberration in Wilms tumors. This aberration became the focus of many studies after reports that individuals with the WAGR syndrome (**W**ilms, **A**niridia, **G**enitourinary abnormalities, and mental **R**etardation) often had constitutional deletions at chromosome band 11p13, harboring the Wilms tumor suppressor gene *(WT1)*.[244,245] WAGR phenotype, however, results from deletions of several genes, with the *WT1* gene deletion responsible for predisposition to Wilms tumors and with deletion of a neighboring gene, *PAX6*, responsible for aniridia.[246] Although most or all WAGR-associated Wilms tumors have complete inactivation of *WT1*, such inactivation is found in fewer than 20% of sporadic Wilms tumors, and here again it appears to function as a tumor suppressor gene, the homozygous deletion of which is essential for Wilms tumorigenesis.[353] Familial Wilms tumor predisposition is rare and primarily linked to loci on 17q or 19q and only uncommonly to *WT1*.[354,355] Approximately 7% to 30% of Wilms tumors have deletion of the *WTX* gene, which notably is the first putative tumor suppressor gene identified on chromosome X.[247-249] *WTX* loss, invariably a somatic event in Wilms tumor, results from truncating mutations or more commonly from deletion of the corresponding region on the single copy of chromosome X in males, although there is controversy as to whether the deletion in females invariably involves the active copy of chromosome X.[250,251] Interestingly, although germline mutation of WTX is associated with osteopathia striata congenita with cranial sclerosis, these patients have no increased risk for developing Wilms tumor.[356] The WTX protein promotes β-catenin ubiquitination and degradation,[254] and it is therefore expected that *WTX* gene deletions in Wilms tumors would hyperactivate WNT–β-catenin signaling pathways. This is in keeping with the finding of virtually mutual exclusivity of β-catenin mutations (found in about 15% Wilms tumors) and *WTX* mutations.[255-258] On the other hand, CTNNB1 (protein)-stabilizing mutations largely overlap with inactivating mutations of *WT1*[357,358] but occur later in oncogenesis. The suggestion has been made that WTX inactivation, although frequent in Wilms tumor, is a late event and of unclear clinical significance.[359]

Loss of heterozygosity (LOH) or loss of imprinting (LOI) of 11p15 is seen in approximately 70% of Wilms tumors and leads to upregulation of IGF2,[359-361] which occurs through biallelic expression of IGF2 owing to germline mutation of imprinting in Beckwith-Wiedemann syndrome.[362,363]

Nephrogenic rests—persistent islands of uncompleted organogenesis believed to represent precursor lesions— are found in surrounding kidney in approximately 30% of sporadic Wilms tumors and almost all bilateral or multifocal Wilms tumors.[364,365] These may take the form of intralobar or perilobar nephrogenic rests (ILNR and PLNR, respectively), each being associated with particular histologic phenotype[364,366] and genetic mutations, such that PLNRs are more commonly blastema rich, associated with overgrowth syndromes and show aberrations in the 11p15 imprinted region, whereas ILNRs typically are rich in stroma, including skeletal muscle or adipose elements, are associated with Denys-Drash and WAGR syndromes, and have *WT1* or β-catenin mutations.[367,368]

Various cytogenetic findings are associated with anaplastic histology in Wilms tumor. Complex karyotypes with chromosome counts in the triploid to tetraploid range are generally found in tumors with diffuse or focal anaplasia.[259] Similarly, Wilms tumors with *TP53* tumor suppressor gene mutations generally show anaplasia (see Fig. 45-26),[260] a finding linked more with therapy resistance than to a more biologically aggressive phenotype per se.

Clear Cell Sarcoma of the Kidney. Also formerly known as bone-metastasizing renal tumor, clear cell sarcoma of the kidney lacks any specific immunomarker and may show very variable histological features, making diagnosis a potential challenge. This tumor has a propensity to occur in boys younger than age 5 years.[369,370] Until recently, virtually nothing was known about the biology of this tumor of unfavorable histology, apart from individual case reports of a t(10;17)(q22;p13) recently characterized to show a fusion of the gene encoding the 14-3-3 ε family member of ubiquitously expressed modulators of phosphoserine-containing proteins (YWHAE) with *NUTM2* genes on 10q22, which encode proteins that are related to the NUT protein (see later).[371] This transcript was found to be expressed in 12% of clear cell sarcomas of the kidney and is similar to the translocation underpinning high-grade endometrial stromal sarcoma.[372] Although the full functional consequences of this translocation remain to be elucidated, upregulation of CCND1 is a feature in high-grade endometrial stromal sarcoma bearing YWHAE-FAM rearrangements.[372]

Mesoblastic Nephroma. Mesoblastic nephromas are the most common renal tumors diagnosed in infancy and may rarely also be encountered in older children. Histologically, mesoblastic nephroma falls into two categories: those tumors composed of bland, benign-appearing spindle cells interdigitating with the surrounding tissues, essentially recapitulating the morphology of fibromatosis, are known as classic mesoblastic nephroma,[261] whereas those with greater cellularity, sometimes in a fascicular arrangement, that are well delineated with a pushing border and composed of cells with plump nuclei, less cytoplasm, more mitoses, blood lakes, and often zonal necrosis, are known as cellular mesoblastic nephroma (Fig. 45-27; see Fig. 45-16).[262] Trisomy 11 is a consistent cytogenetic aberration in mesoblastic nephromas but is found only in the cellular group.[187,263] Approximately 70% of cellular mesoblastic nephromas contain trisomy 11, often accompanied by trisomies for chromosomes 8 and 17.[187] By contrast, clonal chromosomal aberrations have not been identified in classic mesoblastic nephroma. These findings suggest that trisomy 11, with or without other clonal chromosomal aberrations, is associated with

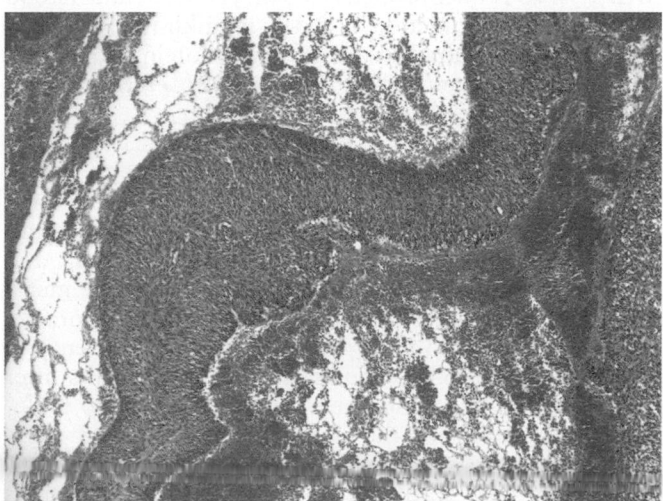

Figure 45-27 Cellular congenital mesoblastic nephroma with prominent blood lakes.

progression from classic to cellular histology in mesoblastic nephroma.[187] Mesoblastic nephromas with trisomy 11 generally also contain a balanced translocation t(12;15) (p13;q26), resulting in oncogenic fusion of the *TEL* and *NTRK3* genes. The t(12;15)(p13;q26) is cryptic by cytogenetic evaluation using chromosomal banding but is readily demonstrable by FISH or RT-PCR (see Fig. 45-2). These cytogenetic associations have been useful diagnostically, because Wilms tumors (the entity most likely confused with mesoblastic nephroma on small biopsy when blastema only has been sampled) rarely have trisomy 11 and have not been found to bear t(12;15).[241,242]

NUT Midline Carcinomas

Based on initial case reports, NUT midline carcinoma was considered a malignancy of children and adolescents arising in midline structures, especially upper aerodigestive tract and thymus.[110,373,374] Midline origin below the diaphragm is now well recognized, and the entity may also present in adulthood.[375,376] With the exception of an isolated atypical case,[377] all reported patients have died of disease or treatment complications within months of diagnosis. The histologic appearance is variable, typically including undifferentiated cells but often accompanied by immunohistochemical evidence of epithelial differentiation and, in some cases, with histologically convincing squamous differentiation (see Fig. 45-15). This entity was initially defined by the midline location, undifferentiated carcinoma–like histology, highly lethal course, and characteristic cytogenetic feature of t(15;19) (see Fig. 45-1). The t(15;19) results in oncogenic fusion of the *BRD4* (bromodomain-containing) and *NUT* genes on chromosomes 19 and 15, respectively, encoding a BRD4-NUT fusion oncoprotein. A subset of NUT midline carcinomas features similar oncogenic mechanisms in which *NUT* is fused with *BRD3*, or with yet unidentified translocation partners.[375] Diagnosis can be confirmed by karyotypic demonstration of t(15;19), molecular cytogenetic demonstration of *NUT* gene rearrangement, or RT-PCR demonstration of *BRD4-NUT* or *BRD3-NUT* fusion oncogenes.[375,376,378] The oncogenic function of BRD3-4-NUT oncoproteins is not yet well understood and the normal function of NUT is unknown. Interestingly, however, the NUT fusion oncoproteins do appear to block squamous differentiation in epithelial cell precursors.[378]

Thyroid Carcinomas

Thyroid malignancies include medullary carcinoma, which may be sporadic, or familial in the setting of multiple endocrine neoplasia type IIA (MEN-IIA) and MEN-IIB with germline *RET* tyrosine kinase gene mutations. Papillary thyroid carcinomas may also be sporadic, but are encountered with greatly increased frequency in individuals exposed to radiation, including adults after external-beam irradiation and children exposed to radioactive fallout, as from the Chernobyl disaster. Regardless of the patient's age or exposure to radiation, papillary carcinomas can feature chromosomal rearrangements resulting in oncogenic *RET* fusions.[70,379] *BRAF* mutations, on the other hand, although found in many adult papillary thyroid carcinomas, are uncommon in childhood thyroid carcinomas.[380,381] Follicular thyroid carcinomas are uncommon but are associated with a diagnostic translocation t(2;3), resulting in oncogenic fusion of the *PAX8* and *PPARγ* genes (see Fig. 45-14).[108]

Blastomas

The central tumorigenic role of RB1 inactivation in retinoblastoma has served as a paradigm for tumor suppressor genes in oncology, but little is known of the other genetic mechanisms responsible for tumor progression in this disease. Recently, specificity of the cone-rod homeobox-containing gene *(CRX)* as an immunohistochemical marker for metastatic retinoblastoma versus other extracranial small round blue cell tumors was described.[383] Similarly, the molecular underpinnings of hepatoblastoma, pancreatoblastoma, and pleuropulmonary blastoma are only poorly understood. Trisomies of chromosomes 2 and 8 are found in many hepatoblastomas and pleuropulmonary blastomas,[384,385] but the genes targeted by these trisomies have not been identified. The identification in patients with familial pleuropulmonary blastoma of germline inactivating mutations of *DICER1*, an RNAse endonuclease essential in the processing of microRNAs,[386,387] has led to the recognition of a "DICER1 syndrome," predisposing patients to a wide variety of tumors, notably pleuropulmonary blastoma, cystic nephroma, and ovarian Sertoli-Leydig tumors.[388] The risk for tumors, however, is low, because most mutation carriers do not develop tumors. In contrast to the classic tumor suppressor model, monoallelic loss of DICER1 predisposes to tumor development through haploinsufficiency whereas loss of the second allele is inhibitory.[389,390]

Central Nervous System Tumors

Although heritable syndromes, including neurofibromatosis 1 and 2, von Hippel-Lindau syndrome, tuberous sclerosis, Li-Fraumeni syndrome, Gorlin syndrome, and Turcot syndrome account for a minor proportion of childhood CNS tumors, they have provided considerable pathogenetic insights including the important roles of Wnt, SHH, and TP53 pathways in medulloblastoma, for example.[391] Medulloblastomas are now, on a molecular basis, categorized into four groups based on alterations of SHH and Wnt pathways.[392-396] Dysregulation of Notch and HGF/MET pathways are also important in medulloblastoma. It has long been known that isochromosome 17 i(17)q was a common aberration in medulloblastoma and correlates with poor clinical outcome.[397,398] Further, cytogenetic aberrations also occur in medulloblastoma and many of these can be established by FISH assay, which has been used to generate a molecular stratification system from worst to best, including *MYC/MYCN* amplification, 6q gain, 17q gain, 6q/17q balance, and 6q loss.[397] Catastrophic DNA rearrangements were reported in pediatric medulloblastoma in the context of TP53-associated chromothripsis.[399] Meanwhile, high-resolution SNP arrays have identified recurrent copy number alterations indicative of epigenetic modification contributing to tumorigenesis[400] and evidence is emerging of a role for microRNA dysregulation also contributing.[400,401] Recently, somatic copy number aberration analysis has shown novel potentially targetable alterations in medulloblastoma including transforming growth factor β (TGF-β) and nuclear factor κB (NF-κB) signaling pathways.[402] In supratentorial PNET, deletion of *CDKN2A* was associated with metastatic progression[403] and amplification of *KIT* and *PDGFRA* have been described in some cases also,[404] potentially providing therapeutic targets. Recently, considerable further progress has been made in understanding supratentorial PNET (also known as CNS PNET).[405] Copy number and gene expression analyses detected three molecular subgroups of sPNET: primitive neural, oligoneural, and mesenchymal lineage based on differential expression of cell lineage markers Lin28 and OLIG2 with distinct survival and metastatic characteristics. These markers can be evaluated by immunohistochemistry.

Many genetic alterations have been identified in ependymoma without further pointers as to candidate genes until recent studies,[406-409] which have helped generate three subsets of ependymoma. Until very recently little if anything was known about the biology of diffuse pontine gliomas, because these are rarely sampled. Oligo array CGH conducted on archival postmortem cases has now provided initial insights into this tumor.[410] Response predictors identified in oligodendroglioma include amplification of *EGFR* (epidermal growth factor receptor) at 7p12 and homozygous deletion of *CDKN2A* at 9p21, which correlate with poor response to chemotherapy and reduced survival.[411] *EGFR* amplification in high-grade gliomas and amplification of *PDGFRA* in 15% malignant pediatric gliomas similarly call for investigation of its role as a molecular therapeutic target in that tumor.[412,413] More than half of pilocytic astrocytomas bear tandem duplications, translocations, or activating mutations of *BRAF*, which are associated with improved prognosis.[414-417]

Germ Cell Tumors

Many germ cell tumors contain a diagnostic cytogenetic marker, isochromosome 12p, often found in the context of a moderately complex karyotype, among other clonal chromosomal aberrations (Fig. 45-28).[418] Isochromosome 12p results from duplication of the chromosome 12 short arm on either side of the centromere and is uncommon in carcinomas and sarcomas.[419] Therefore demonstration of isochromosome 12p, particularly in any poorly differentiated cancer, should provoke strong suspicion of a germ cell origin.

Hematologic Neoplasms

Hodgkin Lymphoma

Hodgkin disease (HD), first described by Thomas Hodgkin in 1832, remained a poorly understood disease for over a century and a half, largely because of the sparse nature of neoplastic cells (typically <1%) within the tumor mass, even raising occasional doubt as to

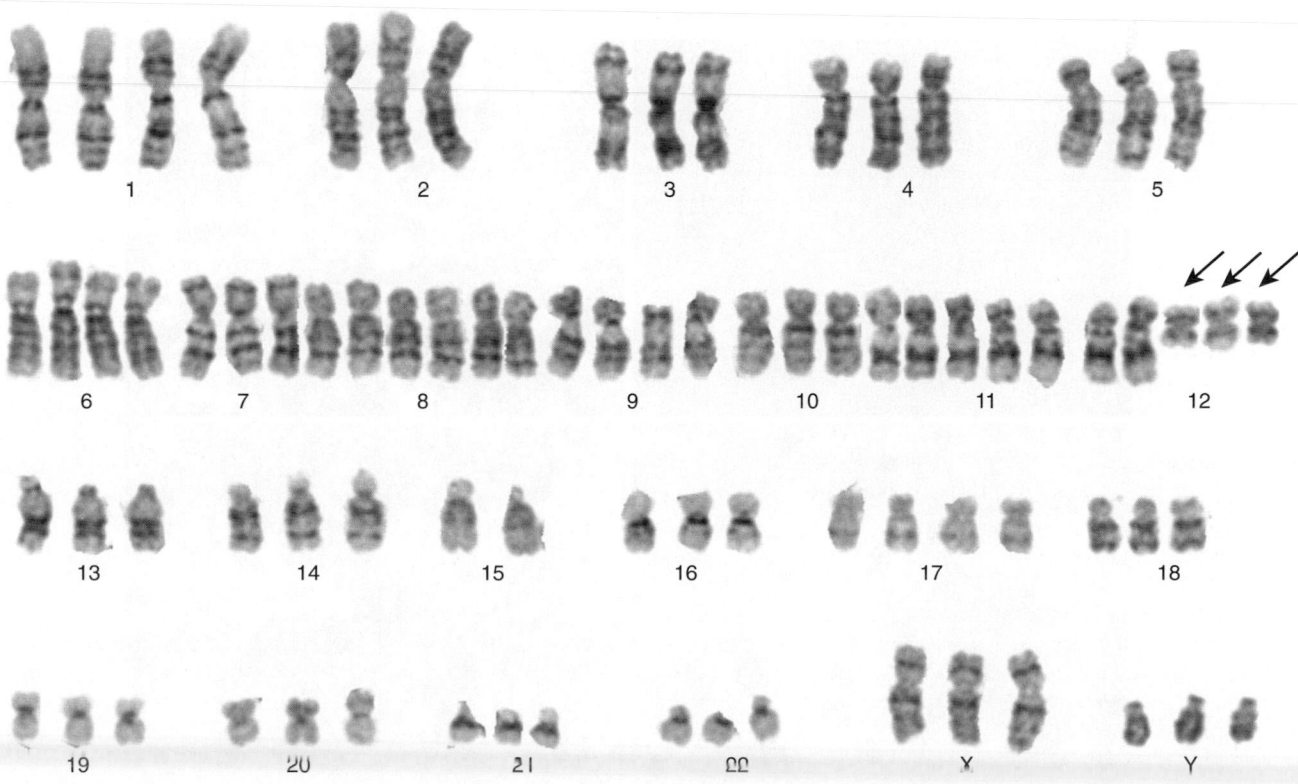

Figure 45-28 Malignant germ cell tumor karyotype showing three copies of the pathognomonic isochromosome 12p *(arrows)*.

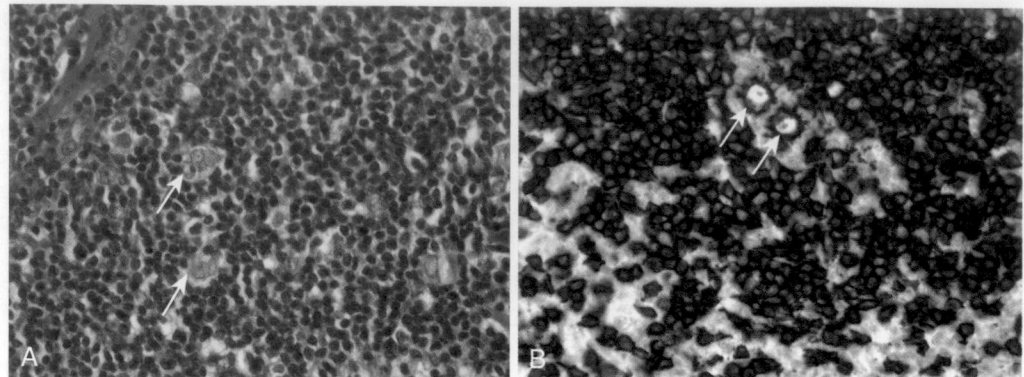

Figure 45-29 Nodular lymphocyte-predominance Hodgkin lymphoma featuring lymphocyte and histiocyte popcorn neoplastic cells (**A,** *arrows*) among small reactive lymphocytic infiltrate, and with immunohistochemical reactivity for the CD20 pan-B marker in both reactive and neoplastic cells (**B,** *arrows*).

the neoplastic nature of the entity. This sparseness of malignant cells, combined with their poor proliferative index, confounded attempts to investigate the molecular basis of HD. Karyotypic evaluations have been challenging, but nonetheless yielded early insights into the nature of HD. The capacity to grow Hodgkin cells continuously in vitro and the fact that injection of these cells into athymic nude mice produced tumors supported a neoplastic nature,[420] as did the aneuploid karyotypes demonstrated in Hodgkin lymphoma (HL) cell cultures.[421]

Light microscopic examination has permitted morphologic assignment of HL into classic and nodular lymphocyte-predominance subtypes,[422-424] a categorization recognized by the World Health Organization

(WHO); this provided an attempt at cell of origin classification. The nodular lymphocyte-predominant subtype features a lymphocyte and histiocyte (L&H) neoplastic cell population, also known as popcorn cells (Fig. 45-29), with B-cell immunophenotype—expressing CD45, CD20, and BCL6 but lacking CD15 and CD30—whereas classic Hodgkin-Reed-Sternberg (H-RS) cells show only equivocal expression of the pan–B-cell marker CD20 and lack CD45 reactivity but express CD15 and CD30 in a membrane and Golgi staining pattern (Fig. 45-30).[425,426] Classic HL is subclassified into nodular sclerosis, mixed cellularity, lymphocyte-depleted, and lymphocyte-rich variants, depending on the composition of the background nonneoplastic elements in the tumor. The lack of any obvious

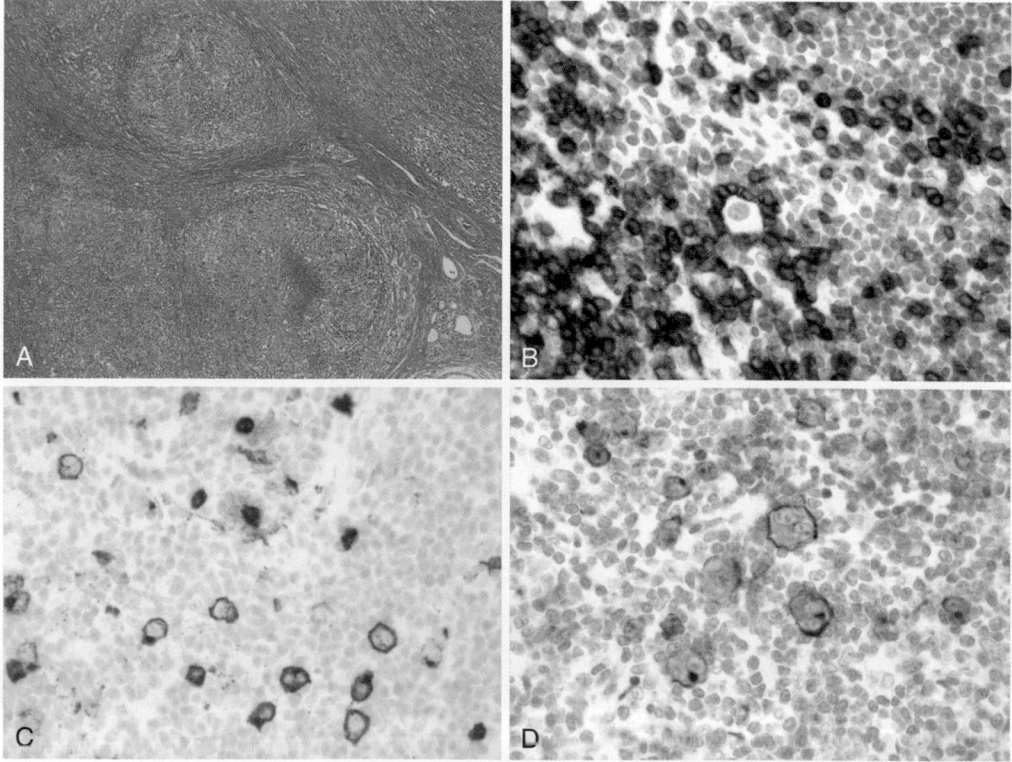

Figure 45-30 Nodular sclerosis Hodgkin lymphoma showing prominent fibrotic bands (**A**) and rimming of characteristic Reed-Sternberg cells by CD57+ lymphocytes (**B**). The Reed-Sternberg elements show cell membrane and Golgi expression of CD15 (**C**) and CD30 (**D**).

physiologic counterpart, together with its otherwise non-committal immunophenotype, initiated a search to reveal the true nature of the H-RS cell, and molecular studies have assisted substantially in these efforts (see later).

Substantial insights into HL pathogenesis have come from single-cell studies showing that L&H and the vast majority of H-RS cells are B cells and clonal in nature.[427] These neoplastic H-RS cells seem to be of germinal center B-cell derivation,[428] with 96% featuring clonal *IG* rearrangements but lacking *IG* gene transcripts because of defects in *IG* gene regulatory elements. These findings apply in both Epstein-Barr virus (EBV)-associated and EBV-unassociated HL.[429] L&H cells express BCL6, in keeping with a germinal center differentiation stage, whereas H-RS cells express CD138 (syndecan), more in keeping with a postgerminal center differentiation stage.[430] Single-cell studies of H-RS cells have shown clonal *IG* gene rearrangements supporting a B-cell phenotype in 95% of cases. Even the 15% of HL with H-RS cells expressing T-cell markers generally contain clonal *IG* gene rearrangements and, overall, only 1% to 2% of classic HL cases have clonal *TCR* gene rearrangements.[431-434] Thus T-cell marker expression is generally considered aberrant in H-RS cells.

Both classic and nodular lymphocyte-predominance HL (NLPHL) are characterized by chromosomal instability, which is manifest by extremely complex cytogenetic aberrations in the neoplastic cells.[435] Molecular cytogenetic studies typically demonstrate chromosomal aberrations in the hyperdiploid range.[436]

Nodular Lymphocyte-Predominance Hodgkin Lymphoma. The observation that NLPHL corresponds to germinal center stage B-cell differentiation is in keeping with the finding of recurrent *IGH-BCL6* fusions, resulting from t(3;14)(q27;q32).[437] HL karyotyping evaluations have not revealed IGH region 14q32 rearrangements in NLPHL; these aberrations are undoubtedly being masked by the overall complexity of the HL karyotypes, with the recurring t(3;14) being cytogenetically cryptic.[438] However, molecular cytogenetic studies have demonstrated *BCL6* rearrangements in almost 50% of NLPHL.[437,439-441] CGH analyses in NLPHL have underscored the genomic complexity of these tumors, with frequent copy number gains involving chromosomes 1, 2q, 3, 4q, 5q, 6, 8q, 11q, 12q, and X and copy number losses for chromosome 17.[442] The copy number gains involving 2q, 4q, 5q, 6, and 11q are otherwise uncommon in hematologic neoplasia, and therefore might signify genomic aberrations of unique importance in the pathogenesis of NLPHL.

Classic Hodgkin Lymphoma. In classic HL, gains of 2p and 9p are identified in 30% to 50% of cases and 12q aberrations are also noted.[443] FISH studies have confirmed that the aberrations involve the locus of the *JAK2* gene at 9p23-24[444] and *MDM2* at 12q14-15.[445,446] The 2p copy number gains, which involve the *REL* gene (encoding one of the five subunits of NF-κB), might contribute to constitutive NF-κB activation, which is a hallmark of HL.[447]

Evaluations of *IG* gene aberrations in classic HL have demonstrated *IGH*, *IGL*, and *IGK* rearrangements in 17%, 3%, and 1% of cases, respectively.[448] These rearrangements juxtaposed the *IG* loci with genes at 2p16 *(REL)*, 3q27 *(BCL6)*, 8q24 *(MYC)*, 14q24, 16p13.1, 17q12, and 19q13.2 *(BCL3-RELB)*. *IGH-BCL6* fusions were found in 4 of 70 cases, although a previous study had not shown such events in 40 cases of nodular sclerosis and mixed cellularity classic HL.[441] t(14;18), resulting in the typical *IGH-BCL2* fusion, has been reported in one case of follicular lymphoma evolving into Hodgkin lymphoma.[449]

Non-Hodgkin Lymphoma

Non-Hodgkin lymphomas (NHLs) account for 7% to 10% of all pediatric malignancies. Cytogenetic and molecular genetic aberrations have been studied extensively in adult NHL, but there have been few comparable studies in pediatric NHL, with the exception of well-characterized *MYC* gene rearrangements in Burkitt lymphomas. Most pediatric NHLs belong to one of four overall categories: Burkitt (40%), lymphoblastic (30%), large B-cell (20%), and anaplastic large cell (10%). Cytogenetic hallmarks include *MYC* rearrangements in Burkitt lymphomas, 14q11 rearrangements in T-cell lymphoblastic leukemia and lymphomas, and *ALK* rearrangements in anaplastic large cell lymphomas.[450] The proposed WHO classification of lymphoid neoplasms incorporates the Revised European American Lymphoma (REAL) classification, which takes into account morphologic, immunophenotype, genetic, and clinical features. Notably, there can be marked differences in molecular mechanisms and clinical response when comparing pediatric with adult forms of the same NHL subtype. For example, adult large B-cell lymphomas are heterogeneous entities, many of which have a phenotype suggesting follicular center cell origin and containing *IGH* region translocations that upregulate the *BCL2* or *BCL6* genes. Pediatric large B-cell lymphomas, by contrast, generally have gene expression and immunophenotypic features of germinal center cell origin and lack *IGH-BCL2* rearrangements but have a better prognosis than adult cases.[451] Lymphoblastic lymphomas are on a biologic continuum with ALL, and the biology of this subtype is discussed in the later section on ALL.

Burkitt Lymphoma. The cytogenetic underpinnings of Burkitt lymphoma were first reported in 1972, when Manolov and Manolova described aberrations of the chromosome 14 long arm[452]; these were later shown to represent t(8;14)(q24;q32), resulting in rearrangement of the *IGH* gene with the chromosome 8q *MYC* oncogene region.[14,453] *IGH-MYC* rearrangements are found in approximately 80% of Burkitt lymphomas, irrespective of whether the tumors are EBV positive or EBV negative and whether they are sporadic or arise in an endemic region.[454] However, *IGH-MYC* rearrangement can be found rarely in diffuse large cell lymphomas, so this cytogenetic aberration is not diagnostic of Burkitt lymphoma. Alternative cytogenetic mechanisms dysregulate *MYC* transcription by juxtaposing *MYC* with the κ or λ *IG*

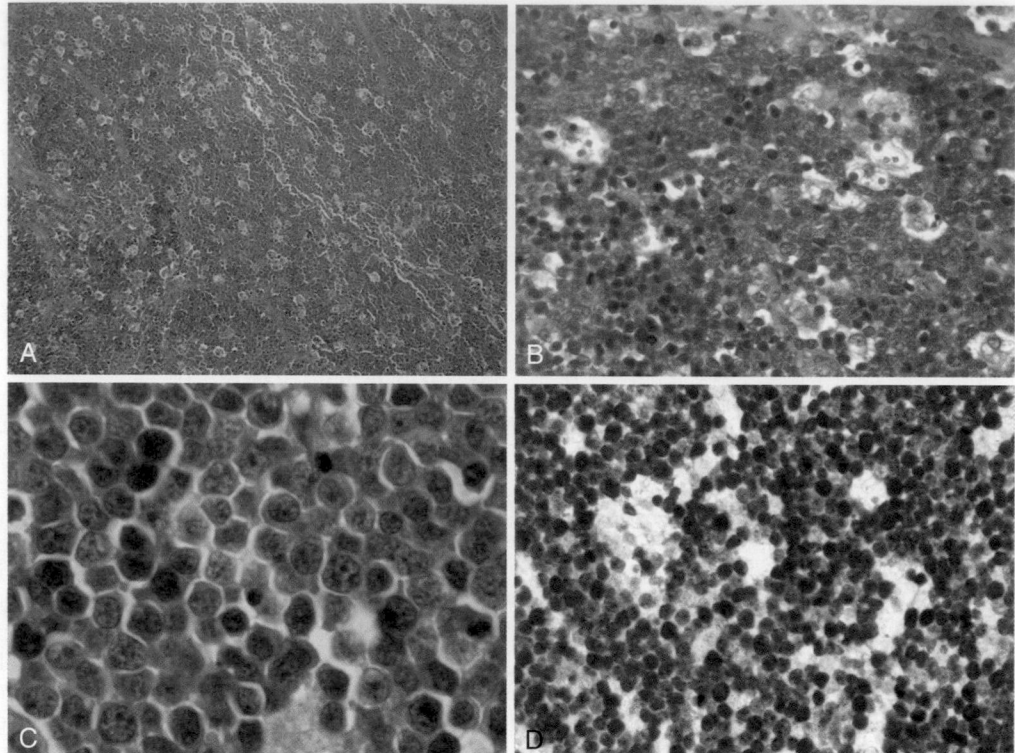

Figure 45-31 Burkitt lymphoma low-power (**A**) and intermediate-power (**B**) views show starry sky appearance resulting from engulfment of cellular apoptotic debris by interspersed macrophages; higher-power view shows typical squaring off of cells from one another (**C**). The Ki-67 proliferation marker is expressed strongly by almost 100% of the lymphoma cells (**D**).

gene loci.[455] The κ and λ *IG* rearrangements result from t(2;8) and t(8;22), which are found in 5% and 15% of Burkitt lymphomas, respectively.

Burkitt lymphoma has a characteristic cytomorphologic appearance in which the cells are squared off from each other. A starry sky appearance results from engulfment of cellular apoptotic debris by interspersed macrophages, whereas the actual neoplastic cells have relatively uniform intermediate-sized nuclei and exhibit at least a 99% proliferative index, as demonstrated by immunostaining for Ki-67 (Fig. 45-31). *MYC* region genomic breakpoints vary between the endemic and sporadic types of Burkitt lymphoma. The breakpoints in endemic Burkitt lymphomas can be as much as 300 kb upstream or downstream of the *MYC* coding sequences, whereas those in sporadic Burkitt lymphomas typically involve the first exon or first intron of *MYC*.[455] Despite this considerable variability in genomic breakpoint location, all the rearrangements serve the purpose of dysregulating *MYC* expression and can be detected by a simple dual-color *MYC* break-apart FISH assay, in which the probe components are more than 300 kb upstream and downstream of *MYC*, thereby flanking most *MYC* region translocation breakpoints (Fig. 45-32). Secondary cytogenetic aberrations occur in conjunction with *MYC* translocations in some Burkitt lymphomas. Several of these, particularly 1q duplication and 13q deletion, may be associated with worse prognosis, although the numbers of patients studied have been few.[456]

Follicular Lymphoma. Follicular lymphoma is uncommon in childhood. When diagnosed, it more commonly affects boys and presents as localized disease in lymph nodes or tonsils. Such cases generally lack *BCL2* rearrangement and BCL2 expression.[457]

Diffuse Large B-Cell Lymphoma. Diffuse large B-cell lymphomas may be categorized into germinal center, activated B-cell–like, or primary mediastinal types. In children, diffuse large B-cell lymphomas are frequently of the germinal center type and associated with an overall better prognosis than for adults. Despite the germinal center phenotype, however, diffuse large B-cell lymphomas in children generally lack t(14;18), which is seen in a proportion of adult cases of this subtype.[451]

Anaplastic Large Cell Lymphoma. ALCLs are predominantly mature T-cell disorders with excellent prognosis in the pediatric population.[458] ALCL is a diagnostic pitfall for the pathologist, although the morphology is uniquely different from all other hematopoietic malignancies. The cells often appear relatively cohesive and have abundant cytoplasm, so they may mimic an epithelial neoplasm more so than suggesting a lymphoid one; ALCLs, furthermore, classically express epithelial membrane antigen (Fig. 45-33). The cells typically react for CD30 and often also express the anaplastic ALK receptor tyrosine kinase protein (see Fig. 45-33), which is constitutively activated by oncogenic fusions to various partners containing

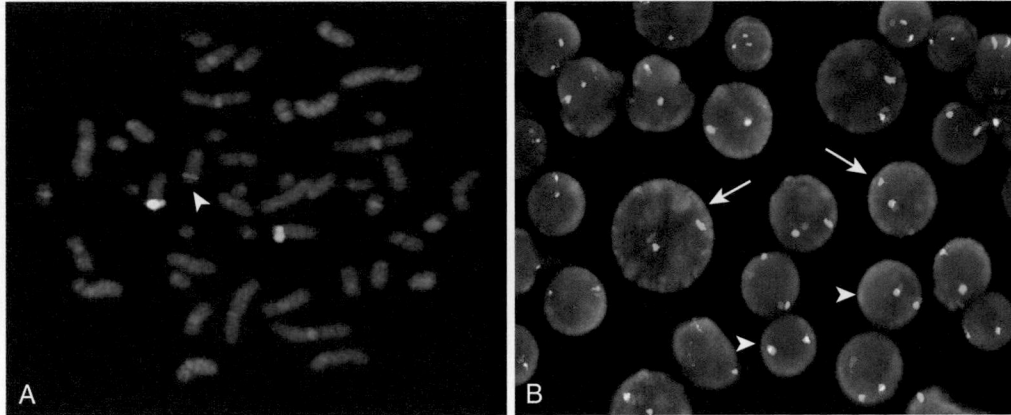

Figure 45-32 Burkitt lymphoma fluorescence in situ hybridization (FISH) using *MYC* break-apart probe in metaphase cell (**A**) and interphase cells (**B**) from malignant pleural effusion in a 5-year-old child. The metaphase cell shows a t(8;14), indicative of *IGH-MYC* fusion, in which the centromeric *(red)* and telomeric *(green)* FISH probe components localize to chromosomes 8 *(arrowhead)* and 14, respectively. The interphase cells include *MYC*-rearranged Burkitt lymphoma *(arrows)* and reactive nonneoplastic lymphocytes *(arrowheads)*.

dimerization domains. The most common of these fusions, found in 80% of ALCLs, results from t(2;5) fusing the 3′ end of the *ALK* gene to the 5′ end of *NPM*,[459] and serving as a useful diagnostic marker of ALCL. Less common *ALK* fusions involve *ATIC, TFG, CLTC, TPM3, TPM4,* and *MSN*.[116,460-462] ALCL occurs in a cutaneous form, which is usually ALK-negative, whereas nodal and extranodal systemic forms express ALK in about 95% of pediatric cases. ALK encodes a receptor tyrosine kinase that is normally expressed in neural cells of the intestine,

testis, and brain but not in nonneoplastic lymphoid cells. A smaller number of pediatric ALCLs are B-cell disorders, and these cases often feature oncogenic fusions of the *ALK* and clathrin genes.[458] The pattern of ALK immunostaining in association with *ALK-NPM1 (NPM)* fusion resulting from t(2;5) is one of nuclear and cytoplasmic staining, with distinctive nucleolar accentuation (see Fig. 45-33). Similarly, other ALK oncoproteins are associated with distinctive immunostaining patterns, including the granular cytoplasmic staining with clathrin-*ALK*

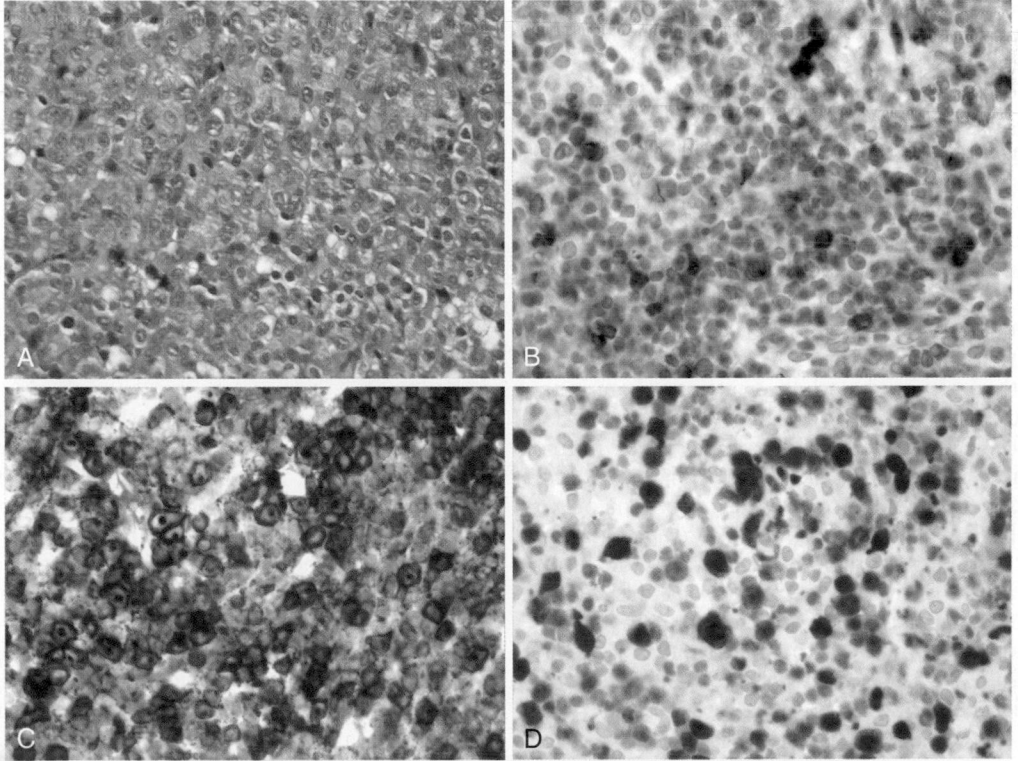

Figure 45-33 In anaplastic large cell lymphoma, histologic features include cohesive cells with abundant cytoplasm, imparting an epithelioid appearance (**A**). Immunohistochemical features include patchy expression of epithelial membrane antigen (**B**), strong membrane and Golgi reactivity for CD30 (**C**), and anaplastic lymphoma kinase immunostain (**D**), which in this t(2;5)-positive case shows reactivity in both nuclear and cytoplasmic compartments.

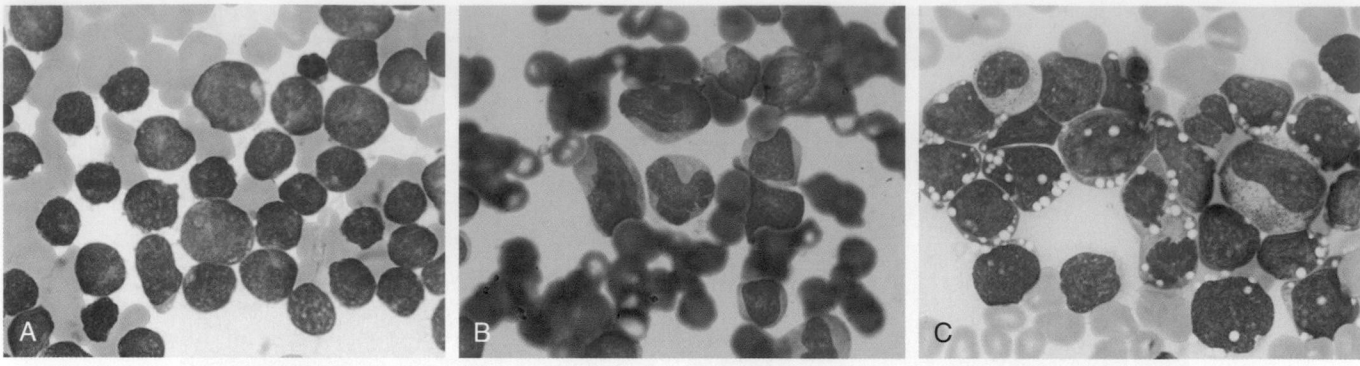

Figure 45-34 Acute lymphoblastic leukemia historical French-American-British subtypes. **A,** L1, with smaller, more uniform cells and a high nuclear-to-cytoplasmic ratio. **B,** L2, with somewhat larger cells, and a more varied nuclear-to-cytoplasmic ratio. **C,** L3 (Burkitt), with larger cells and numerous vacuoles. *(Courtesy Marybeth Helfrich, Children's Hospital of Philadelphia.)*

rearrangement, diffuse cytoplasmic staining in the case of *TFG-ALK* and *ATIC-ALK* rearrangements, diffuse membranous and cytoplasmic staining with *TPM3-ALK*, and nuclear membrane staining with *RANBP2-ALK* rearrangement. However, *ALK* staining is not specific for ALCL. As noted earlier (see "Mesenchymal Neoplasms: Soft Tissue and Bone Tumors"), *ALK* oncoprotein expression is also characteristic of inflammatory myofibroblastic tumors. In the hematopoietic group of neoplasms, *ALK* reactivity as an indicator of clathrin-*ALK* fusion oncoproteins also has been described for large B-cell neoplasms.[463]

Subcutaneous Panniculitic T-Cell Lymphoma. This lymphoma subtype produces firm nodular infiltrates of skin, which occasionally progress to ulceration. These infiltrates are generally confined to subcutaneous fat, with sparing of the overlying dermis and epidermis. Other helpful histologic features include evidence of cellular atypia and characteristic rimming of adipocytes by the neoplastic cells. In the presence of such histologic features, demonstration of *TCR* gene rearrangement confirms the diagnosis.

Hepatosplenic T-Cell Lymphoma. This is an extranodal lymphoma of γδ T-cells. Clinical presentation is generally that of hepatosplenomegaly without accompanying lymphadenopathy, although other anatomic locations, typically also extranodal, may be involved. The histologic findings on a diagnostic liver biopsy may mimic those of hepatitis. The neoplastic infiltrate is sinusoidal in distribution, sparing the portal tracts. Expansion of the sinusoids by a monotonous lymphoid population should prompt consideration of this diagnosis. Demonstration of *TCRγ* gene rearrangement is confirmatory, and another helpful genetic feature, seen in many cases, is the cytogenetic finding of isochromosome 7q,[464,465] often accompanied by trisomy 8.[466] Development of hemophagocytic syndrome may ensue and heralds poor outcome.

Acute Lymphoblastic Leukemia

ALL, the most common childhood cancer, comprises a heterogeneous spectrum of diseases characterized by clonal proliferations of lymphoid precursor cells at varying stages of development but traditionally assigned to one of three FAB subtypes (Fig. 45-34). Classic teaching has been that the ALL cell of origin is a committed lymphoid progenitor, with the particular stage of lymphoid differentiation during which the transforming event occurs being highly variable. However, although controversial, studies have suggested that leukemic transformation in ALL may occur in a more primitive stem cell.[467] Irrespective of whether the nonneoplastic cell that is targeted for transformation is a committed lymphoid cell, the major demonstrable immunophenotypic ALL subsets are B- or, less often, T-cell precursors. About 85% of cases are B-cell precursor ALL, whereas 10% to 15% are T-cell precursors. Expression of the CD10 B-cell differentiation antigen characterizes common ALL, which is the most frequent form of childhood ALL (Fig. 45-35). By contrast, the vast majority of cases of ALL in infants (defined as <1 year old) are negative for CD10 cell surface antigen expression. Burkitt leukemias, with their characteristic phenotype of mature B-cell surface IG expression, account for only approximately 0.5% of cases of childhood ALL.[2] Heterogeneous primary molecular genetic aberrations cause leukemic transformation and are associated with distinctive biologic properties and clinical features in the different major subtypes of childhood ALL.

Intralocus *IG* and *TCR* Gene Rearrangements. Historically, the patterns of *IG* and *TCR* gene rearrangements in pediatric ALL have provided insights into the ordered hierarchy of rearrangements of *IG* and *TCR* genes in lymphoid maturation.[468,469] The diversity of rearrangements of variable (V), diversity (D), and joining (J) segments generated within these loci in the human immune response affords a signature of unique markers of lineage, clonality, and maturation stage in each ALL. This is particularly true because *TCR* gene rearrangements can be identified even in precursor B-cell ALL and, conversely, *IG* gene rearrangements can occur in T-cell ALL. Furthermore, *IG* and *TCR* gene rearrangements are not static but can evolve after leukemic transformation via subclone progression (e.g., from D-J to complete V[D]J assembly or from *IGH* to *IGK* light-chain gene

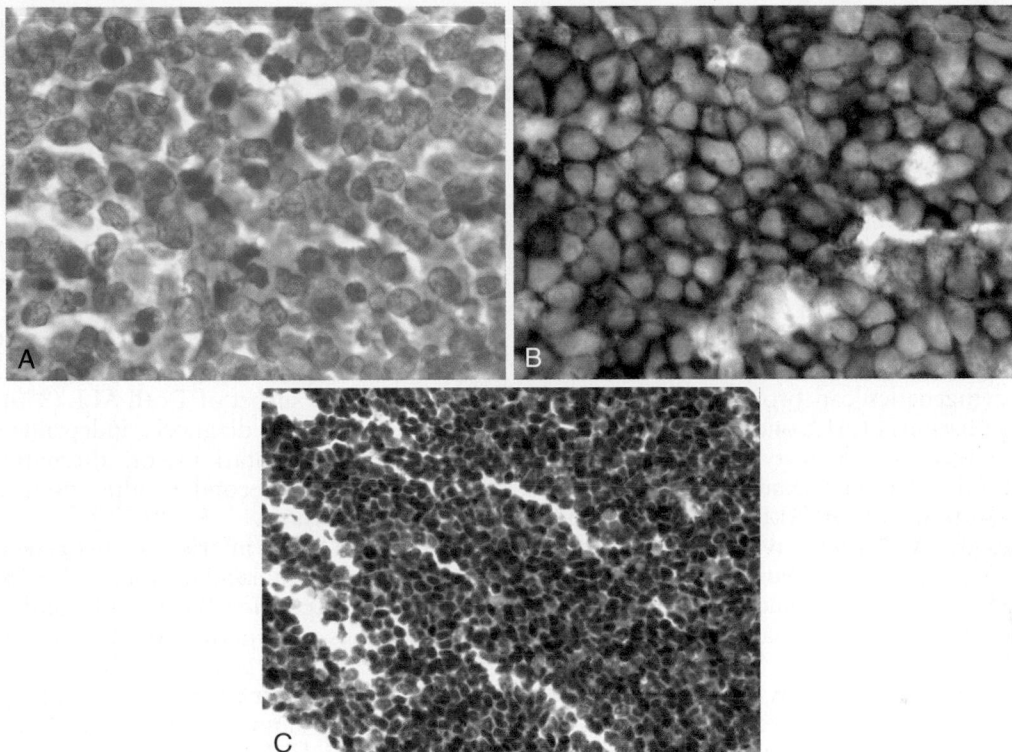

Figure 45-35 A, Lymph node infiltration by pre–B-cell acute lymphoblastic leukemia lacking any appreciable cytoplasm and with slightly irregular nuclear contours. The nuclear chromatin is finely dispersed. This case shows typical strong immunohistochemical staining for CD10 (common ALL antigen) **(B)** and nuclear TdT expression **(C).**

rearrangement).[470] However, because of the related nature of the ALL subclones in any given patient, *IG* and *TCR* gene rearrangements can serve as sensitive markers for detecting minimal residual disease and predicting relapse.[471,472] Comparable sensitivity in detecting minimal residual disease can also be achieved by multiparameter flow cytometric analysis of various antigens, expression of which is restricted to leukemic cells.[473]

One study has suggested that about 25% of cases of B-cell precursor ALL undergo transformation at the pro–B- to pre–B-cell stage, characterized by cytoplasmic μ expression and assembly of the pre–B-cell receptor complex. The pre–B-cell differentiation stage is a critical cell survival checkpoint because most normal B cells cannot form intact immunoglobulin and instead undergo apoptosis.[474] The subset of ALL transitioning from pro-B to pre-B cells exhibits steroid sensitivity.[474]

Interlocus *IG* and *TCR* Gene Rearrangements and Translocations. Not only do *IG* and *TCR* genes undergo intralocus rearrangements, but their aberrant recombination also causes interlocus chromosomal translocations and inversions. These chromosomal rearrangements can create hybrid antigen receptor genes when two different antigen receptor loci recombine with each other. A small fraction of pediatric ALLs of B- or T-cell lineage harbor those hybrid antigen receptor gene rearrangements.[475] Alternatively, chromosomal rearrangements can juxtapose transformation-inducing non-*IG*/non-*TCR* genes with the regulatory enhancer and promoter elements of

IG or *TCR* genes as a second type of interlocus rearrangement. V(D)J recombination errors of this type,[476] causing transcriptional upregulation of the juxtaposed non-*IG*/non-*TCR* genes, occur in subsets of pediatric ALL, especially in T-cell ALL.

SIL-SCL rearrangements and *SCL* translocations disrupting *TCR* genes are present in approximately 30% of cases of T-cell ALL overall. The *SCL (TAL1)* gene at chromosome band 1p34, which encodes a basic helix-loop-helix (bHLH) transcription factor, was first discovered at the t(1;14)(p34;q11) breakpoint junction involving the *TCR*αδ locus in a stem cell leukemia.[477] Other T-cell ALL cases harbor a different type of *SCL* rearrangement, in which illegitimate V(D)J recombinase activity at recombinase-like signal sequences in *SCL* and *SIL* (SCL-interrupting locus) creates an interstitial deletion on chromosome 1p. The *SIL-SCL* rearrangement causes aberrant regulation of *SCL* expression by the *SIL* promoter.[478,479] The t(1;3)(p34;p21) translocation, fusing *SCL* and the nonantigen receptor gene *TCTA*, is mediated by a similar mechanism of illegitimate V(D)J recombinase activity.[480]

In other recurrent translocations in T-cell ALL, various oncogenic transcription factor genes such as *LMO1*, *LMO2*, *LYL1*, and *HOX11 (TLX1)* are fused to different *TCR* loci, leading to unscheduled expression of the relevant transcription factor protein.[78] *LMO2* translocations occur in 10% to 20% of T-cell ALLs. Microarray experiments have shown that oncogenic transcription factor genes can be overexpressed in T-cell ALL subsets at distinct maturation stages and are prognostic markers, even when conventional karyotyping studies do not reveal such translocations.[481] For example, dual-color FISH analysis and a ligation-mediated PCR assay have revealed cryptic translocations of the *HOX11 (TLX1)* gene with the *TCRD* locus in most T-cell ALLs in which there was high *HOX11* expression.[482] This finding is particularly intriguing because high-level *HOX11* expression in T-cell ALL correlates with a favorable prognosis.[482] In addition, the CD34–, CD1a+, CD4/CD8 double-positive cortical immunophenotype has suggested that the immature β pre-αβ stage of maturation arrest is associated with high *HOX11* expression.[482] These results have demonstrated that molecular cytogenetics can provide more sensitive and consistent evaluations of ALL oncogenic mechanisms compared with conventional karyotyping.

The most recently identified example of a recurrent *TCR* gene translocation in T-cell ALL is t(6;7)(q23;q34), which juxtaposes the *MYB* gene at chromosome band 6q23 with the *TRB* locus.[483] Although the subtelomeric locations of *TRB* and *MYB* precluded recognition of this rearrangement by conventional karyotyping, the rearrangement is readily detectable with methods such as FISH, Southern blotting, or PCR assay.[483] Molecular cloning has revealed a heptamer-like sequence adjacent to the translocation breakpoint in the *MYB* gene, consistent with illegitimate V(D)J recombinase activity as the mechanism of this translocation. In this translocation, placement of *MYB* in close proximity with the *TRB* enhancer regulatory element results in aberrant expression of the translocated *MYB* allele and a gene expression signature consistent with upregulation of various proliferation and mitosis genes.[483] t(6;7) is of clinical interest because the median age of the patients is only 2.2 years old,[483] which is unusual because T-cell ALL is otherwise infrequent in young children. This translocation exemplifies the importance of cooperating mutations in pediatric ALL pathogenesis, because many cases of T-cell ALL with t(6;7) also contain *NOTCH1* mutations and *CDNK2A (p16^ARF)* deletions.[483] Dysregulated *MYB* expression in T-cell ALL of the very young can also result from gene duplications, as demonstrated by molecular and fiber FISH analyses of *MYB* gene copy number.[483] *MYB* is expressed at high levels in the thymus, and it has been suggested that *MYB* deregulation results from sustained rather than ectopic expression[483]; in that sense, it differs from several other transcription factor oncogenes disrupted in T-cell ALL.

Another T-cell ALL translocation, t(7;9)(q34;q34.3), fuses *TCRB* to the gene encoding the NOTCH1 transmembrane receptor protein, which regulates T-cell maturation.[484] This is an extremely uncommon translocation, occurring in less than 1% of cases of T-cell ALL; however, it was more recently shown that at least 50% of T-cell ALL cases have activating intragenic *NOTCH1* mutations, including cases with other major translocations.[485] Activating *NOTCH1* mutations affecting the extracellular heterodimerization domain result in ligand-independent activation, whereas those affecting the intracellular PEST (proline [P], glutamic acid [E], serine [S], and threonine [T]) domain cause increased stability of the protein. The

mutant NOTCH1 protein is a potential therapeutic target of gamma secretase inhibitors, which can block NOTCH1-mediated signaling in T-cell ALL.[485] Inhibition of NOTCH1 signaling by gamma secretase inhibitors is associated with upregulation of the phosphatase and tensin homologue (PTEN) tumor suppressor protein.[486] Although a phase I/II clinical trial of γ secretase inhibition did not show efficacy in T-cell ALL, the observed drug resistance could be attributed in part to *PTEN* gene deletion. PTEN inhibits the PI3K/AKT pathway, and loss of PTEN function is associated with AKT activation and a switch in oncogene addiction from the NOTCH1 to the AKT signaling pathway. *PTEN* mutational analyses have indicated that a subset of T-cell ALL (8%) harbors mutations of this gene at diagnosis, independently or together with *NOTCH1* mutations, or, alternatively, the *PTEN* mutations can be secondary alterations associated with disease progression.

Analogous to the interlocus *TCR* gene rearrangements in T-cell ALL, molecular approaches have also been revealing in precursor B-cell ALL, and recurrent novel translocations that juxtapose *IG* genes with oncogenic transcription factor genes have been identified and characterized. One recent example is the t(6;14)(p22.3;q32.22) that fuses the joining region of the *IGH* gene with the gene encoding *ID4*.[487] The translocation causes overexpression of the ID4 bHLH transcription factor and is associated with a CD19+, CD10+, HLADR+, TdT+ common precursor B-cell immunophenotype, low-risk clinical features, and favorable prognosis.[487] This translocation is often accompanied by deletion of the chromosome 9p genes *CDKNA* and *PAX5*, suggesting cooperativity of these alterations in the pathogenesis of this disease.[487] Another example of *IGH* gene rearrangement is seen with t(5;14), which occurs in less than 1% of cases of precursor B-cell ALL. t(5;14) places the *IL3* gene under transcriptional regulatory control of the *IGH* locus, resulting in the hallmark clinical feature of peripheral eosinophilia associated with this translocation.[78]

In the rare entity of Burkitt leukemia, expression of *MYC* is altered by translocation into the *IGH* or, less often, the *IGK* or *IGL* light chain locus, but oncogenic transformation at a more mature B-cell developmental stage is reflected by IgM expression on the leukemia cell surface.

Another area of interest has been in the application of molecular approaches to determine the temporal origins of ALL-specific *IG*, *TCR*, or transcription factor gene rearrangements. Studies of ALL in monozygous twins and studies of ALL molecular cytogenetic aberrations in neonatal Guthrie blood spots have been useful in indicating whether various ALL subtypes arise before or after birth. In the case of T-cell ALL there is recent evidence that the disease is not initiated in utero or that the clonal aberration in most cases is present below the detection sensitivity of PCR at the time of birth.[488] However, these findings are in contrast to PCR-based findings on *TCR* gene rearrangements in two other studies, which were consistent with a prenatal origin of T-cell ALL.[489,490] In one of three cases of T-cell ALL with *NOTCH1* mutation, the *NOTCH1* mutation was detectable in neonatal

Guthrie blood spot DNA, whereas the *SIL-SCL* rearrangement in the same case occurred later as a postnatal event.[491] Thus ALL-specific *IG* and *TCR* gene rearrangements and/or leukemia-associated transcription factor alterations in at least some T-cell ALLs are in utero events, even though the latency to clinically evident disease can be protracted. Most subtypes of precursor B-cell ALL also initiate in utero (see later).

Chromosomal Translocations Not Involving *IG* or *TCR* Genes

TEL-AML1 *Translocations*. Several of the major recurrent chromosomal translocations in pediatric ALL do not involve *IG, TCR,* or other genes with obvious V(D)J recombination signal sequences. The most frequent chromosomal translocation in all pediatric cancers[492] is t(12;21), which is present in 25% of cases of CD10+ B-cell lineage common ALL. This translocation is cryptic by conventional Giemsa-banded karyotyping and must be detected by FISH or molecular analyses. The leukemogenic fusion of the *TEL (ETV6)* gene from chromosome band 12p13 to the *RUNX1 (AML1)* gene from chromosome band 21q21 is associated with recruitment of complexes containing histone deacetylases to AML1 target genes, causing aberrant transcriptional repression.[493] There is evidence that t(12;21) occurs as an in utero event[493,494] in cells that are at a stem or B-cell progenitor developmental stage, before *IG* and *TCR* gene rearrangement. Rearrangement of the immune receptor loci occurs after the initiating *TEL-AML1* translocation.[495] *TEL-AML1* translocations occur in cord blood specimens of healthy neonates at 100 times the incidence of *TEL-AML1* translocations in leukemia, indicating that progression to overt ALL is rare in *TEL-AML1*–positive cells. Similarly, the low concordance (5% to 10%) of *TEL-AML1* leukemia in monozygous twins has suggested that postnatal mutations are required for transformation of *TEL-AML1*–positive progenitor cells into frank ALL.[496] These additional mutations often include loss of the normal *TEL* allele.[492] The *TEL-AML1* translocation is associated with a favorable outcome.[492]

TCF3 (E2A) *Gene Translocations*. t(1;19) occurs in approximately 5% of cases of pediatric ALL, fusing the *E2A* gene on chromosome band 19p13.3 to the *PBX1* gene on chromosome band 1q23. This translocation is most often found in cIg+ (pre-B) rather than cIg– B-cell precursor ALL (25% vs. <1% of cases).[497] t(1;19)(q23;p13.3) is associated with a poor prognosis in the cIg+ (pre-B) cases. *E2A* is a critical B-cell developmental gene that encodes an IG enhancer binding protein. The *E2A* gene encodes three different bHLH transcription factors via alternative splicing of the *E2A* transcript. The *PBX1* gene product is a homeobox transcription factor, and t(1;19) results in the production of a fusion oncoprotein from the der(19) chromosome, in which the DNA-binding domain of PBX1 replaces the carboxyl DNA-binding bHLH domain of *E2A*. t(1;19)(q23;p13.3) is detectable in neonatal Guthrie cards in only about 10% of cases, suggesting a postnatal origin, and is different in that sense from the other major subtypes of pediatric ALL.[496,498] Split-signal FISH using different color probes

for the *E2A* and *PBX1* genes is a useful tool for the definitive identification of this translocation,[499] which is otherwise indistinguishable karyotypically from a different translocation sharing breakpoints in the same chromosome bands. The alternate form of t(1;19)(q23;p13.3) in ALL does not disrupt the *TCF3 (E2A)* and *PBX1* genes but rather fuses the *DAZAP1* RNA-binding protein gene on chromosome band 19p13.3 to the *MEF2D* DNA-binding protein gene on chromosome band 1q23.[500]

A rare t(17;19) *E2A* variant occurs in 1% of cases of childhood B-cell precursor ALL, which creates a E2A-HLF (hepatic leukemia factor) fusion gene. t(17;19) is associated with coagulation abnormalities and has a poor prognosis.[497]

BCR-ABL1 *Translocations*. About 5% of cases of B-cell precursor ALL harbor t(9;22)(q34;q11), fusing *BCR* with the *ABL1* tyrosine kinase gene. This translocation is associated with the clinically high-risk features of older age and high white blood cell count and an especially grim prognosis.[78] However, emerging data have indicated that the molecularly targeted ABL kinase inhibitor imatinib mesylate has clinical activity against BCR-ABL+ ALL in the pediatric population as well as in adults.[501]

MLL (KMT2A) *Translocations*. Leukemia is the second most common malignancy during infancy. The infant cases comprise 2.5% to 5% of ALLs and 6% to 14% of AMLs in the pediatric population overall. The annual incidence of infant ALL and AML is 19 and 10/million, respectively.[133,502] Infant leukemia is a special subtype of pediatric leukemia characterized by chromosomal translocations that generate fusion oncoproteins, and 75% to 80% of cases of infant ALL and myelomonocytic-monoblastic AMLs feature balanced chromosomal translocations of the *MLL* gene at chromosome band 11q23.[503] Cases of ALL with *MLL* translocations often coexpress myeloid-associated surface antigens, especially CD15. Additionally, *MLL* translocations can be associated with true bilineal acute leukemias, in which there are separate lymphoid and myeloid cell populations (Fig. 45-36), and acute leukemias with *MLL* translocations can undergo lineage switch. *MLL* translocations are also found in secondary leukemias in patients treated with chemotherapeutic TOP2 poisons.[63] The *MLL* gene encodes a large complex oncoprotein that regulates transcription[15,504-507] and has regional amino acid similarity to that of *Drosophila* Trithorax (TRX).[132,505,506] Whereas TRX is involved in the maintenance of expression of homeotic gene complexes during embryonic development,[508] of relevance to leukemia, MLL maintains *HOX* gene expression during hematopoiesis.[509] *MLL* translocations in various types of pediatric leukemia disrupt an 8.3-kb breakpoint cluster region and fuse the 5' portion of *MLL* with one of more than 80 different partner genes, generating diverse leukemogenic fusion oncoproteins containing the amino-terminus of MLL and the carboxyl-terminus of the partner protein.[49,68,86,510]

The native MLL protein has complex transcriptional regulatory functions. MLL undergoes proteolytic cleavage into amino- and carboxyl-segments that reassociate with one another in a multiprotein complex,[511-513]

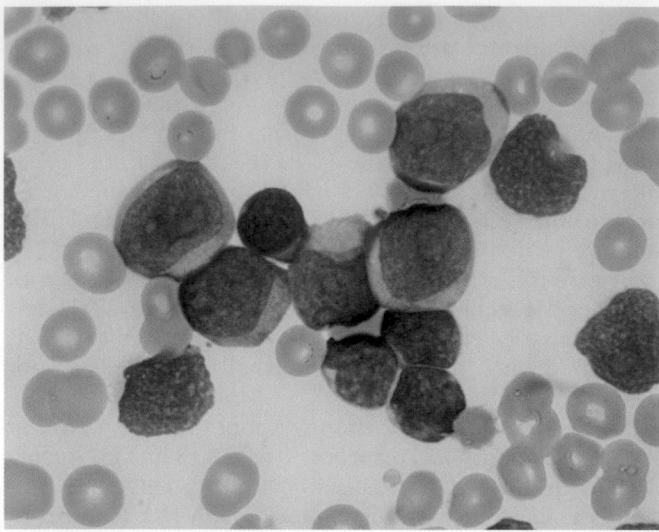

Figure 45-36 Infant bilineal acute leukemia with *MLL* translocation showing lymphoid and myeloid blast cell populations. *(Courtesy Marybeth Helfrich, Children's Hospital of Philadelphia.)*

regulating *HOX* gene expression and epigenetic modifications of nucleosomes and histones.[514] The MLL chimeric oncoproteins resulting from the various *MLL* partner gene rearrangements lack the MLL proteolytic cleavage site and affect leukemogenic transformation through transcriptional dysregulation of MLL target genes.[515] Although many *MLL* partner genes themselves encode important proteins in transcriptional regulation or cell signaling pathways,[132,515] it is unclear how the partner gene disruption contributes to leukemogenesis mediated by *MLL* translocations.

Of the approximately 75% of infant ALL cases with *MLL* translocations, 70% and 13% of cases, respectively, involve the *AF4* (chromosome band 4q21) or *MLLT1 (ENL)* (chromosome band 19p13) transcription factor partner genes.[516] In AML, the partner genes of *MLL* are much more heterogeneous, including not only genes that encode nuclear transcription factors and transcriptional regulatory proteins but also cytoplasmic proteins and proteins in various cellular organelles.[49]

MLL translocations in infant leukemias exemplify another principle in the molecular cytogenetics of pediatric leukemias, namely, the association of host risk factors and gene-environment interactions with specific aberrations. The *MLL* translocation in infant leukemia is an in utero event, the origin of which has been established by the detection of identical nonconstitutional *MLL* rearrangements in leukemias of monozygous twins,[517,518] as well as the detection of *MLL* translocations in neonatal Guthrie blood spot DNA in nontwin cases.[519] Maternal-fetal exposure from consumption of food containing TOP2–interacting substances during pregnancy has been implicated as a risk factor in *MLL*-rearranged infant AML.[520] Moreover, an inactivating polymorphism in the gene encoding reduced nicotinamide adenine dinucleotide phosphate (NADPH) quinone oxidoreductase 1 (NQO1) increases the risk for all *MLL*-rearranged infant acute leukemias, especially cases with t(4;11) fusing *MLL* to

AF4, which are primarily ALL.[521,522] The inactivating NQO1 polymorphism is a plausible host predisposition factor because the *p*-benzoquinone detoxified by NQO1 is a TOP2 poison[523] and four-base 5′ overhangs from TOP2 cleavage lend readily to DNA damage resolution by nonhomologous end joining (NHEJ) repair, features of which usually are evident at *MLL* translocation breakpoint junctions.[47,524] Infant leukemia risk is also modulated by a genetic polymorphism in the methylene tetrahydrofolate reductase *(MTHFR)* gene; it has been suggested that the resultant increased thymidine synthesis, which enhances DNA repair, protects against *MLL* translocations.[525]

Infant ALLs with *MLL* translocations are composed of CD10– early B progenitor cells, but they may have monocytic features and they typically express the myeloid-associated CD15 cell surface antigen.[133] Clinically, *MLL* translocations are important because of their unfavorable prognosis.[516] The *MLL* translocation in infant ALL is associated with a high leukemia burden manifest as marked hyperleukocytosis, massive hepatosplenomegaly, and meningeal involvement.[133] Neonatal leukemia (leukemia in the first month of life) has an annual incidence of 4.7/million live births[526] and comprises an important fraction of leukemia in infants. The clinical manifestations of neonatal leukemia include stillbirth, signs of leukemia at birth, or hematologic abnormalities preceding the leukemia diagnosis within a few weeks.[134] Clinical hallmarks include hepatosplenomegaly, hydrops, and polyhydramnios detected antenatally, and the archetypal marked hyperleukocytosis, hepatosplenomegaly, leukemia cutis, and CNS involvement detected after birth.[134] *MLL* translocations in infant and neonatal leukemia have significant adverse effects on response to treatment, especially in cases of early B-cell lineage ALL.[44,134,516,527] The substantial adverse impact of *MLL* translocations on prognosis places infant ALL at the extreme of pediatric ALL in which outcome is the poorest.[44,134,516,527] However, in AML, in which outcome is less favorable overall than in ALL, *MLL* translocations are not independent prognostic factors. Overexpression of *FLT3* mRNA is a common secondary alteration in infant ALL with *MLL* translocations.[528] In these cases, the *FLT3* gene may be mutated or upregulated and the FLT3 protein is highly expressed.[135,529,530]

There is limited copy number variation[531] and few additional mutations have been detected, (e.g., in *NRAS, KRAS, FLT3,* and *IKZF1*[532-534]) in *MLL*-R infant ALL beyond the translocations. In contrast, altered methylation, especially hypermethylation, is a very characteristic epigenetic aberration of *MLL*-rearranged(R) ALL and the altered methylation within different subsets of *MLL*-R ALL is similar.[535]

In a microarray analysis of an infant ALL cohort (n = 97) from the COG P9407 trial representing the largest group of infants to be studied in this manner, the most significant determinant of gene expression was infant age at diagnosis.[536] Remarkably, there was a very distinct change in the gene expression pattern at approximately 90 days of age, which also corresponds with the cutoff for worst outcome. Interestingly, whereas the gene expression signature of older infants was that of a more differentiated B-cell lineage precursor, in infants younger than 90 days of age, interleukin-related genes, heat-shock proteins, and human leukocyte antigen genes linked through IL13 and IL1A were more prominent, suggesting different pathways in leukemogenesis. In addition, outcome predictors beyond age and *MLL* rearrangement status were discovered that were highly predictive of event-free survival.

Molecular Aberrations in Subsets of Precursor B-Cell ALL Identified by Integration of Gene Expression Profiling, Analysis of Copy Number Alterations, and Genomic Sequencing. The subtypes of precursor B-cell ALL that are distinguishable by distinctive cytogenetic aberrations also are able to be distinguished by their gene expression profiles. Conversely, application of integrated genomic approaches including gene expression profiling, analysis of copy number alterations, and, later, next-generation sequencing has led to the identification of clusters of precursor B-cell ALL otherwise classified as "high-risk" by conventional definition (age, white blood cells, cytogenetics) encompassing subsets with well-recognized molecular cytogenetic aberrations, such as *KMT2A* gene rearrangements and t(1;19), but also subsets lacking molecular cytogenetic markers and subsets with particularly favorable or poor outcome. For example, a cluster with 94% 4-year relapse-free survival defined by high *AGAP1, CCNJ, CHST2/7, CLEC12A/B,* and *PTPRM* expression and intragenic *ERG* deletions was identified as well as a cluster with 9.4% 4-year relapse-free survival with high *BMPR1B, CRLF2, GPR110, GPR171, IGJ, LDB3,* and *MUC4* expression and *EBF1, NUP160-PTPRJ, IL3RA-CSF2RA, SLX4IP, ADD3, IKAROS/IKZF1,* and *VPREB1* deletions.[537] The genomic basis for the differences in gene expression were subsequently elucidated and continue to be elucidated by next-generation sequencing initiatives.

Through the application of sophisticated bioinformatics algorithms, the patterns of gene expression not only have been correlated with molecular cytogenetic subtypes, but they also have been used to develop classifiers that are predictive of minimal residual disease at the end of induction and the risk for relapse within cases characterized by the presence of, for example, *JAK* mutations, kinase signatures, *IKAROS/IKZF1* deletions, or t(1;19). Whereas high expression of *RGS2, NFKBIB, NR4A3, DDX21,* and *BTG3* was associated with 87% relapse-free survival, high expression of genes including *BMPR1B, CTGF (CCN2), TTYH2, IGJ, PON2, CD73, CDC42EP3, TSPAN7,* and *SEMA6A* was associated with relapse-free survival of only 29%.[538] Additionally a 21-gene classifier in the diagnostic marrow was discerned that was able to predict the minimal residual disease burden at the end of induction.[538] Such gene expression signatures underscore the heterogeneity in gene expression within ALL in general and high-risk ALL in particular, and they are significant because they are possibly expected to have prospective therapeutic utility in the near future.

IKZF1 Deletions in B-Cell Precursor ALL. Deletion of the *IKZF1* tumor suppressor gene is present in 10% to 15% of B-cell precursor ALL. Findings from a large international study of 1128 cases of childhood B-cell precursor ALL have suggested that *IKZF1* gene deletion, as detected by approaches including PCR assay, array CGH, and Sanger sequencing, is an independent poor prognostic feature.[539]

"BCR-ABL1–like" B-Cell Precursor ALL. *IKZF1* deletions are also a frequent finding marking approximately 40% of cases of "BCR-ABL1-like" B-cell precursor ALL,[539] a molecular subtype of high-risk precursor B-cell ALL without *BCR-ABL1* rearrangement but with a "BCR-ABL1–like" gene expression signature.[540] The "BCR-ABL1–like" gene expression signature is estimated to be present in approximately 10% of cases of B-cell precursor ALL and approximately 15% of cases of high-risk precursor B-cell ALL and has been associated with a poor prognosis.[539-541] By mRNA-seq analysis, the "BCR-ABL1–like" cases were found to be characterized by cryptic chromosomal rearrangements such as *EBF1-PDGFRB, BCR-JAK2, STRN3-JAK2, PAX5-JAK2, NUP214-ABL1, ETV6-ABL1, RANBP2-ABL1,* and *RCSD1-ABL1; IGH-EPOR* fusions; *IL7R* mutations; or *SH2B3* deletion.[541] *JAK1, JAK2,* and *JAK3* mutations also have been linked to the "BCR-ABL1–like" gene expression signature.[542] Of therapeutic interest, consistent with the ABL1 and/or JAK/STAT signaling activation in these cases, in preclinical experiments the "BCR-ABL1–like" leukemias are sensitive to tyrosine kinase inhibitors (e.g., imatinib, dasatinib) as well as to the JAK2 inhibitor roxolitinib.[541]

CRLF2 Aberrations in Precursor B-Cell ALL. The "BCR-ABL1–like" precursor B-cell ALLs also encompass cases with *CRLF2* aberrations.[540,541] This subset of high-risk precursor B-cell ALL has surfaced through cytogenetic and FISH analyses, as well as advanced genomics studies, including microarray analysis, analysis of copy number alterations, and next-generation sequencing, and is characterized by rearrangement or mutation of the chromosome pseudoautosomal region 1 Xp22.3/Yp11.3 gene *CRLF2* (cytokine receptor-like factor 2), which encodes the TSLP (thymic stromal lymphopoietin) receptor.[543,544] *CRLF2* rearrangements are present in approximately 60% of ALL occurring in patients with Down syndrome.[545] *CRLF2* aberrations also account for approximately 8% and 15%, respectively, of pediatric precursor B-cell ALL and high-risk precursor B-cell ALL.[546-548] The *CRLF2* gene can be disrupted by rearrangements with the *IGH* locus at chromosome band 14q32, by *CRLF2* interstitial deletion resulting in *P2RY8-CRLF2* rearrangement or, alternatively, by F232C point mutation.[543,547,549] The *CRLF2* aberrations are frequently associated with *JAK1/JAK2* mutations, *IKZF1* mutations, and, less often, *IL7R* mutations. Clinically, the *CRLF2* aberrations are important because they have been correlated with a poor prognosis.[543,547] Within high-risk ALL, the poor outcome has been further linked to high minimal residual disease burden and high *CRLF2* expression.[547] They also have been linked to Hispanic/Latino ethnicity.[550] In contrast, in a recent large international study of Down syndrome ALL[545] and a number of smaller studies of Down syndrome ALL,[544] the *CRLF2* aberrations did not affect prognosis. The *CRLF2* aberrations may have further significance for therapeutic targeting because they result in sensitivity to JAK and PI3K/AKT/mTOR (mammalian target of rapamycin) signaling inhibition in preclinical models.[551,552]

iAMP21 (Intrachromosomal Amplification of Chromosome 21) in Precursor B-Cell ALL. iAMP21 is a cytogenetic abnormality that occurs in approximately 2% of B-cell precursor ALL in older children, which has a known association with inferior outcome in standard treatment protocols and for which the molecular basis has been poorly understood. In a recent analysis of leukemia cells from 94 patients with this abnormality, the common region of amplification was narrowed to a 5.1-Mb region of chromosome 21 that encompasses *RUNX1*, miR-802, and genes in the Down syndrome critical region.[553] Genomic abnormalities affecting *IKZF1*, *CDKN2A/CDKN2B*, *PAX5*, *ETV6*, and *RB1* also were frequently detected in these cases in addition to iAMP21.[553] Interestingly, a very detailed analysis of the heterogeneous leukemic subclones that were present and their relationships to the iAMP21 suggests that iAMP21 and not these other abnormalities was the initiating alteration and that other aberrations such as *P2RY8-CRLF2* were secondary alterations to iAMP and were acquired later in the subclones.[553] However, the specific chromosome 21 gene within the 5.1-Mb regions that is most relevant to leukemogenesis remains to be determined.

Hereditary Susceptibility to B-Cell Precursor ALL. Until recent genome-wide association studies, few heritable factors influencing B-cell precursor ALL susceptibility had been identified by candidate gene approaches (e.g., *ABCB1*; *MTHFR*; *GSTM1*, *GSTT1*; SNPs in *CDKN2A*, *CDKN2B*, *CDKN1A*, *CDKN1B* promoters; *CYP1A1*). However, a number of genetic variants modulating disease susceptibility with predilection to influence the development of particular subsets of this disease have recently been discovered. One genome-wide association study conducted on a large number of cases and controls implicated variants in three different genes as risk loci.[554] The cases studied were predominantly B-cell precursor (824 B-cell ALL, 83 T-cell ALL). The most significant variant was rs4132601 in the *IKZF1* transcription factor gene, which encodes a master regulator of lymphoid development. The rs7089424 polymorphism in the gene encoding ARID5B (AT-rich interactive domain 5B), a member of the AT-rich interaction domain family of transcription factors involved on B-cell development, was a particularly strong risk variant. A variant (rs2239633) in the gene *CEBPE*, encoding CCAAT/enhancer binding protein, epsilon, was also associated with increased risk.[554] Interestingly, the *ARID5B* variant is particularly selective for hyperdiploid ALL,[554] an association validated by a second study.[555] The latter study determined that 18 different SNPs varied in allele frequencies between cases and controls and also found that an OR2C3 variant is particularly linked to *ETV6-RUNX1* leukemia.[555] Most recently, two different polymorphisms (rs3824662 and rs3781093) in the hematopoietic transcription factor *GATA3* gene were found to significantly increase the risk for "BCR ABL1–like" disease both relative to nonleukemia controls and relative to non–"BCR-ABL1–like" leukemia cases.[556]

Molecular Alterations in Early T-Cell Precursor Leukemia. Early T-cell precursor (ETP) ALL is a recently recognized form of T-cell ALL characterized by a CD1a–, CD8–, CD5^weak, CD34+ stem cell and CD33 and/or CD13 myeloid marker+ immunophenotype and absence of biallelic *TCRG* deletions consistent with a differentiation arrest at an immature T-cell developmental stage.[557] Whole-genome sequencing in 12 pediatric cases has shown that ETP leukemia is characterized by AML-like aberrations.[558] These include cytokine receptor and *RAS* signaling mutations affecting *NRAS*, *KRAS*, *NF1*, *FLT3*, *IL7R*, *JAK3*, *JAK1*, *SH2B3*, or *BRAF* in 67% of cases; inactivating mutations in hematopoietic transcription factor genes (*GATA3*, *ETV6*, *RUNX1*, *IKZF1*) in 58% of cases; and inactivating mutations in genes encoding histone modifying factors (*EZH2*, *EED*, *SUZ12*, *SETD2*, *EP300*) in 48% of cases, as well as other novel types of mutations not otherwise seen in T-cell ALL (e.g., *WT1*, *DNM2*, *ECT2L*, *RELN*).[558] Interestingly, adult ETP ALL has been shown by whole-exome sequencing to manifest mutations in *ETV6*, *NOTCH1*, *JAK1*, and *NF1*; frequent recurrent novel mutations involving *FAT1* (25%), *FAT3* (20%), and *DNM2* (35%); as well as other mutations in the *MLL2*, *BMI1*, and *DNMT3A* genes encoding epigenetic regulators and at least a single mutation in *DNMT3A*, *FLT3*, or *NOTCH1* in 60% of cases.[559] Moreover, based on gene expression profiling and cluster analysis of pediatric T-cell ALL, ETP ALL comprises a unique cluster and it has been suggested that the driving aberration in ETP leukemia involves upregulation of expression of the *MEFC2* transcription factor gene on chromosome 5q14, which is a member of the MADS-box family of transcription factors, as a consequence either of novel *MEFC2* gene rearrangements (e.g., *MEF2C-PITX2*) or of rearrangements of related factors, examples of which include *NKX2-5/BCL11B*, *SPI1(PU.1)/BCL11B*, and *ETV6/NCOA2* translocations.[560] The NKX2-5 regulatory protein directly binds the *MEF2C* promoter.[560] The PU.1 transcription factor controls *MEF2C* expression during lymphoid development.[560] NCOA2 is also a *MEF2C* coregulator. The ETP leukemias highly express *HHEX*, *LYL1*, and *LMO2*, which are MEF2C-regulated targets.[560] Interestingly, *MEF2C* has been implicated as a target gene of HOXA9 and is also highly expressed in *MLL*-rearranged AML. Yet another case was characterized by a variant reciprocal *RUNX1-AFF3* translocation with upregulated *MEF2C* expression by an unknown mechanism. ETP leukemia is clinically important because of its poor outcome.

Alterations Associated with T-Cell ALL with Cortical Arrest and a Proliferative Gene Expression Profile. The same study that identified *MEFC2* and related aberrations in ETP leukemia also has identified a novel proliferative cluster of T-cell ALL characterized by a CD1+ immunophenotype consistent with a cortical arrest, expression of cell cycle genes, and ectopic *NKX2-1* or *NKX2-2* expression, also resulting from a number of novel *NKX2-1* and *NKX2-2* gene rearrangements or *TLX1* rearrangements.[560] These include *NKX2-1* inversions to the *TCRA* or *IGH* genes, a translocation with

TCRB [t(7;14)(q34;q13)] and a *TCRD/NKX2-2* gene rearrangement. In one case, array-CGH suggested *NKX2-1* amplification due to duplication or insertion into another chromosome. The subset of cases in the proliferative cluster marked not by *NKX2-1* or *NKX2-2* rearrangement but by *TLX1* gene rearrangements are also characterized by *NKX2-1* expression. Less often there are *MYB* gene translocations in the proliferative cluster of T-ALL. This subset of leukemia is clinically important because of its more favorable prognosis.[560]

Other Clinically Important Genomic Aberrations in Acute Lymphoblastic Leukemia

FLT3 *Mutations.* Aberrations of the FMS-like tyrosine kinase 3 (FLT3) receptor tyrosine kinase protein are crucial oncogenic events that contribute to cellular proliferation and survival and arrested differentiation in a subset of ALL.[561,562] *FLT3* mutations have been proposed to function as secondary oncogenic events in ALL, in which there is already a proliferation-inducing primary oncogenic mutation involving another gene.[532] *FLT3* molecular aberration types include in-frame deletions and internal tandem duplications (ITDs) in the juxtamembrane region and point mutations in the activation loop of the kinase domain.[135,532,563] All of these are associated with FLT3 protein overexpression and constitutive activation of FLT3 signaling pathways through STAT5, MAP kinase, and AKT.[532,564] *FLT3*-ITD mutations are found in approximately 2% of childhood ALL,[565] and *FLT3* point mutations are found in approximately 5% and 16% of childhood B-cell lineage ALL and infant ALL, respectively.[532,565] *FLT3* mutations have a predilection for particular molecular/cytogenetic ALL subtypes, being found in 21% to 28% of cases of high hyperdiploid ALL[135,530,532] and in 18% of ALL with *MLL* gene translocations, which consequently also express high levels of constitutively active FLT3 protein.[529,530] Overexpression of the wild-type FLT3 protein is another mechanism of FLT3 activation in leukemias with *MLL* translocations,[135] and microarray analyses have demonstrated increased *FLT3* mRNA expression as a distinguishing feature of ALL cases with *MLL* translocations.[528,566] Alternatively, the expression of FLT3 ligand by leukemia cells can cause autocrine activation of FLT3 signaling by increasing constitutive FLT3 phosphorylation.[135,530,567] *FLT3* mutations are clinically important in infant ALL because they are associated with a poor prognosis.[532]

Alterations in BCL2 *Expression.* In addition to classic oncogenes and tumor suppressor genes, genes that control cell death and survival decisions are clinically important, not only in pediatric ALL but in all types of pediatric cancer because they have an impact on chemosensitivity and resistance. The intrinsic (mitochondrial) cell death pathway is regulated by the formation of homotypic and heterotypic dimers involving BCL2 and many other BCL2 family protein members with opposing pro-apoptotic or anti-apoptotic actions that collectively determine the apoptosis threshold.[568-572] Almost all cases of pediatric ALL express detectable BCL2 protein.[573] BCL2 mRNA and protein are particularly abundant in infant and pediatric leukemias with t(4;11) or other *MLL* translocations

compared with ALL and AML cases without *MLL* translocations,[574] but *BCL2* expression is not exclusively a feature of *MLL* disease.[573,575,576]

CDKN2 *Tumor Suppressor Gene Deletions.* Chromosome band 9p21 is a site of recurring deletions in pediatric ALL. The critical deleted region at chromosome band 9p21 contains the *CDKN2A* gene, which encodes two different tumor suppressor proteins p16^{INK4A} and p14^{ARF}. The adjacent gene *CDKN2B* encodes p15^{INK4b} and is often codeleted with the *CDKN2A* gene.[577] p16^{INK4A} and p15^{INK4b} inhibit the cyclin D–dependent kinases CDK4 and CDK6.[578] Deletions of the *CDKN2B* and *CDKN2A* tumor suppressor genes at the *CDKN2* loci are present in 60% and 20% of cases, respectively, of T-cell and B-cell precursor ALL, and the p15 promoter is inactivated by hypermethylation in additional cases. *CDKN2* alterations have been implicated in relapse and poor response to treatment,[577-582] and homozygous loss of p16^{INK4A} is more frequent in pediatric ALL at relapse than at diagnosis, indicating that this aberration portends disease progression.[583] Notably, hemizygous *CDKN2A* deletion may be constitutional and confer susceptibility to leukemia and other forms of cancer.[584]

SMAD3 *Alterations.* Loss of *SMAD3* expression is important in the pathogenesis of pediatric T-cell ALL.[585] TGF-β is a cytokine family composed of three isoforms that have a role in tumor suppression. The *SMAD3* component protein in the TGF-β signaling pathway was discovered to be absent or barely detectable in each of 10 cases of T-cell ALL, but sequencing of the corresponding *MADH3* gene from the leukemia cells of affected patients did not reveal mutations and the mechanism of loss of *SMAD3* expression is unknown. Nonetheless, the loss of *SMAD3* impairs the growth-suppressive effects of TGF-β on T cells. *SMAD3* loss is apparently restricted to T-cell ALL and is not observed in precursor B-cell ALL or AML.[585] Deletions resulting in haploinsufficiency of the cyclin-dependent kinase inhibitor *CDKN1B (p27^{Kip1})* at chromosome band 12p12 are also recurring abnormalities in T-cell ALL,[586] and *SMAD3* loss has been demonstrated to cooperate *CDKN1B* loss in a murine leukemogenesis model.[585]

Numerical Chromosomal Abnormalities. The largest cytogenetic subset of childhood precursor B-cell ALL (approximately 30%) is characterized by a hyperdiploid karyotype, which results when nondisjunction of chromosomes causes chromosomal gains. Hyperdiploidy can be of prenatal origin, as evidenced by its presence in cord blood and neonatal Guthrie blood spots, suggesting that hyperdiploidy itself may be the initiating event in this form of ALL.[587,588] High hyperdiploid ALL (>50 chromosomes) has a favorable prognosis, especially when there are specific chromosomal trisomies, such as +4, +10, +18[589] or +10, and +17.[78,590] About 25% of cases of high hyperdiploid ALL have *FLT3* mutations, whereas other cases exhibit overexpression of the FLT3 protein through autocrine activation.[135,530]

In contrast, hypodiploidy occurs in only 6% to 8% of childhood ALL, is frequently associated with chromosomal translocations, and is a poor prognostic factor.[590,591] In one study, the adverse prognosis was especially pronounced in cases with near-haploid karyotypes containing 24 to 28 chromosomes.[590] In a more recent study there was no difference in outcome when 24 to 29, 33 to 39, or 40 to 43 chromosomes were present.[592] Nonetheless, hypodiploidy with less than 44 chromosomes is generally regarded as a marker of poor prognosis. Patients with ALL containing 44 or 45 chromosomes have a better outcome unless there is monosomy 7 or a dicentric chromosome.[592]

Importantly, the major pediatric ALL leukemia subtypes recognizable at the cytogenetic and molecular levels can now be distinguished based on their unique gene expression profiles. These broad gene expression profile differences provide new insights into ALL biology and predictive markers and might be useful in identifying novel, molecularly targeted treatments.[593]

MicroRNA Aberrations. A burgeoning class of abnormalities in cancer cells involves changes in gene expression mediated by the aberrant activity of microRNAs, which affect the translation of coding mRNAs into their respective proteins.[594,595] MicroRNAs, which are short noncoding RNAs, originate via the excision of 19 to 25 nucleotide (nt) segments after formation of a hairpin pre-microRNA loop from a larger primary pri-microRNA transcript. The base pairing interactions of microRNAs with protein coding mRNAs[595] result in microRNA-mediated translational repression. Using microRNA profiling arrays, it recently has been possible to discern unique microRNA signatures and microRNA mutations in particular leukemia subtypes.[596] For example, ALL and AML can be distinguished by differential expression of microRNAs. The microRNAs miR-128a and miR-128b are overexpressed, and the microRNAs let-7b and miR-223 are underexpressed in ALL compared with AML.[597] MicroRNAs can regulate oncoprotein expression, as shown by mir-203 regulation of BCR-ABL, as relevant in CML and BCR-ABL+ ALL.[598] It has also been suggested that microRNA signatures have prognostic relevance in leukemias in adults.[599,600] Therefore the further characterization of microRNA mechanisms has important implications for the development of new antileukemia targeted therapeutics.

Aberrant DNA Methylation Patterns in B- and T-Lineage ALL. In addition to the granularity with which recurring structural aberrations and mutations have been characterized with new developments and applications of next-generation sequencing and other genomics methods, genome-wide analysis of cytosine methylation profiles has demonstrated an overarching signature of methylation across all subtypes of B-cell lineage ALL relative to normal B cells regardless of genetic subset, but also that the different ALL genetic subtypes, whether of B- or T-cell lineage, are characterized by distinct methylation patterns.[535] The common methylation signature in B-cell lineage ALL affects cell signaling genes *(TIE1, MOS, CAMLG, GPRC5C),* cell cycle regulatory genes *(MCTS1, DGKG),* RNA metabolism genes *(PABPN1, PABPC5),* transcription factor and transcriptional regulatory genes *(PROP1, TAF3, H2AFY2, ELF5, ZBTB16, CNOT1, TADA2A),* and HOX genes *(HOXA5, HOXA6).*

Interestingly, however, different and robust ALL clusters defined by hypomethylation and hypermethylation signatures were associated with the different genetic subtypes. At one extreme, high hyperdiploid B-ALL was the most hypomethylated, B-ALL characterized by ERG alterations was more balanced in regard to hypermethylated versus hypomethylated loci, and *CRLF2*-rearranged cases exhibited few differentially methylated regions. Moreover, the subtype-specific methylation signatures also were well correlated with gene expression patterns and there was differential methylation of genes associated with T-cell versus B-cell differentiation that were lineage dependent.[535]

However, the molecular complexity of ALL extends beyond the primary aberration, acquisition of secondary alterations, and epigenetic signatures. In a study of the molecular complexity of subclone evolution that occurs within *ETV6-RUNX1* ALL, Anderson and associates used multiplex FISH to determine in unprecedented detail the relationships of cells within leukemia subclones to one another to understand their "clonal architecture."[601] The results suggested a tremendous amount of genetic variegation that includes continued diversification in propagating cells relative to ancestral cells in the development of subclones.[601] This genetic diversification has substantial implications for the understanding of the results of genome-wide analyses that are now more commonly being undertaken.[601]

Acute Myeloid Leukemia

Pediatric AMLs exhibit heterogeneous but characteristic clinical and biologic features, which reflect underlying molecular and cytogenetic abnormalities. Many of the characteristic AML cytogenetic aberrations are similar to those in adult AML, although the relative frequencies of the aberrations differ between pediatric and adult AML. The major FAB morphologic subtypes of AML (Fig. 45-37) are, in general, associated with typical balanced chromosomal translocations.[602] The WHO has reclassified AML based on molecular and cytogenetic aberrations, which underlie unique biologic subgroups, have clinical importance, and form the basis for assignment to appropriate treatment regimens.[603] The current WHO classification system incorporates genetic, immunophenotypic, clinical, and biologic features for diagnosis of the myeloid neoplasms.[603]

Major molecular cytogenetic aberrations in AML recognized in the WHO classification system are the following: AML with t(8;21)(q22;q22), *(AML1-ETO);* AML with abnormal bone marrow eosinophils and inv(16)(p13q22) or t(16;16)(p13;q22), *(CBFB-MYH11);* acute promyelocytic leukemia (APL) with t(15;17)(q22;q21), *(PML-RARA),* and variants; and AML with 11q23 *(MLL)* abnormalities. It has been estimated that the t(8;21), t(15;17), inv(16), and *MLL* translocations are present in 12%, 7%, 12%, and 7% of cases of pediatric AML, respectively.[602,604] However, these frequencies are inexact, with another study using standard cytogenetic analyses finding *MLL* translocations in approximately 18% of cases.[605] Furthermore, other characteristic recurrent molecular cytogenetic aberrations are observed.

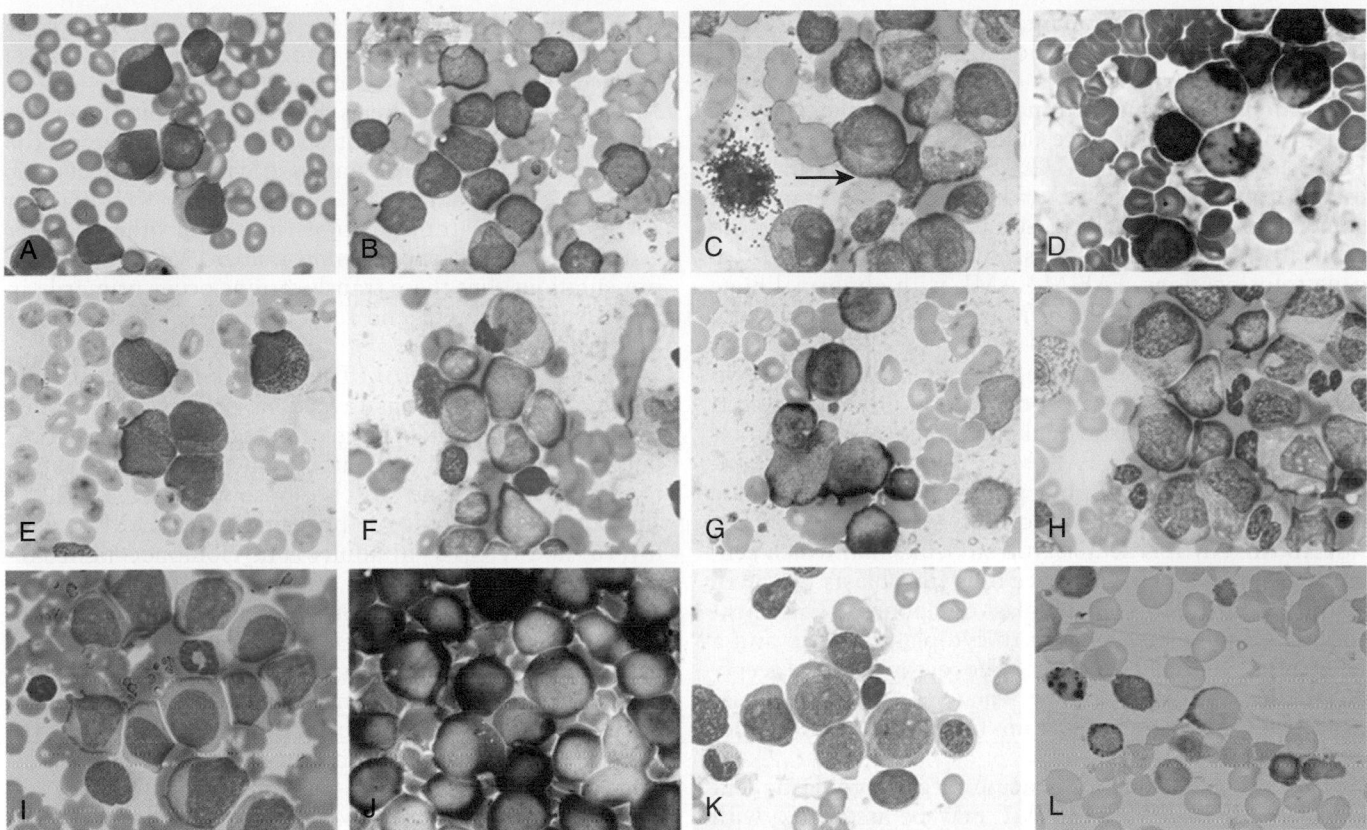

Figure 45-37 Major acute myeloid leukemia subtypes. M0 (**A**) and M1 (**B**) have minimal differentiation. **C**, M2 shows greater myeloid differentiation and may feature Auer rods *(arrow)* along with strong myeloperoxidase staining (**D**). **E**, M3 promyelocytic leukemia with typical coarse cytoplasmic granules. **F**, M4 myelomonocytic leukemia with staining for chloroacetate esterase *(blue)* in the myeloblasts, and nonspecific esterase *(brownish red)* in the monoblasts (**G**). **H**, M4eo with pronounced eosinophilic features. **I**, M5 monoblastic leukemia with staining for nonspecific esterase (**J**). **K**, M6 erythroleukemia with staining for periodic acid–Schiff (**L**). *(Courtesy Marybeth Helfrich, Children's Hospital of Philadelphia.)*

Although morphology no longer serves as the diagnostic gold standard for AML, the observation of a dyshesive, monotonous, immature cell population should trigger and guide further investigations by histochemical, immunophenotypic (including flow cytometric), and molecular cytogenetic methods. AML may exhibit morphologic features of any of the various hematopoietic progenitors or even of several simultaneously. The cytologic features, cytochemical staining pattern, and immunotype all assist in the subclassification of AML morphology by the FAB system, which recognizes the eight different subcategories (see Fig. 45-37) described here.

In FAB M0 AML there are more than 30% blasts with no or minimal features of myeloid differentiation. FAB M0 AML nuclei are generally large, with remarkably fine nuclear chromatin, prominent nucleoli, and high nuclear-to-cytoplasmic ratio.[606] The cytoplasm may exhibit focal granularity, and Sudan black reactivity is typical. Myeloperoxidase expression is inapparent by light microscopy but can be demonstrated by electron microscopy.

In FAB M1 AML, like in FAB M0, there are more than 30% blasts with minimal differentiation but, unlike in FAB M0, myeloperoxidase expression is readily demonstrable and accompanies Sudan black and chloracetate esterase positivity.

The diagnosis of FAB M2 AML is based on the observation of myeloblasts with some maturation, generally requiring more than 30% total blasts, with more than 10% of the blasts showing granulocytic differentiation. FAB M2 AML blasts also exhibit myeloperoxidase and chloracetate esterase staining. FAB M2 morphology is typical in AML with t(8;21).[607] Although the typical morphology of AML with inv(16)(p13;q22) is FAB M4eo, in one series a substantial fraction of pediatric AML with inv(16)(p13;q22) showed FAB M2 morphology.[608]

The classic FAB M3 APL has coarse cytoplasmic granules, the nuclear chromatin is less fine than in myeloblasts, and the nucleus often is eccentric. FAB M3v is an APL microgranular variant in which the cytoplasmic granules are finer than in classic FAB M3 APL, and the nuclei may have irregular contours, appearing reniform or folded. The genetic underpinnings, typically associated with t(15;17), are similar to FAB M3, but FAB M3v APL does not carry the risk for massive hemorrhage during chemotherapy induction that is associated with classic FAB M3 APL.

FAB M4 AML is acute myelomonocytic leukemia, which is composed of myeloblasts, monoblasts, and promonocytes. The monoblast has a substantially lower nuclear-to-cytoplasmic ratio than the myeloblast or promyelocyte; its nucleoli are more prominent and its cytoplasm is more abundant, with fine granularity and occasional vacuolation. Although the promonocyte has similar features, it shows a different cytoplasmic hue. Both monoblasts and promonocytes, whether in FAB M4 or FAB M5 AML, are nonspecific esterase positive. FAB M4 and FAB M5 AMLs also express chloracetate esterase, myeloperoxidase, and α-naphthol acetate, and some stain with PAS. FAB M4 and FAB M5 AMLs are typically, although not exclusively, associated with *MLL* gene translocations. FAB M4 AML with abnormal bone marrow eosinophils (FAB M4eo) is associated with inv(16)(p13;q22).

FAB M5 acute monocytic leukemias encompass two subcategories; one subcategory with no differentiation is FAB M5a (monoblastic leukemia), whereas the other with differentiation is FAB M5b. Monoblasts predominate in FAB M5a AML, but promonocytes predominate in the FAB M5b morphologic subtype.

FAB M6 AML is acute erythroid leukemia, which generally exhibits a predominance of erythroblasts but often also has a substantial myeloblast component. The erythroblast shows a high nuclear-to-cytoplasmic ratio and a condensed rounded nucleus. The cytoplasm is deeply basophilic and may contain vacuoles. FAB M6 cases express glycophorin and stain for PAS but not other cytochemical markers.

The FAB M7 category is acute megakaryoblastic leukemia (AMKL). FAB M7 AML may be associated with prominent marrow fibrosis, making aspiration difficult. The cells are pleomorphic (see Fig. 45-39) and the megakaryocytic nature may not be obvious by morphology alone. FAB M7 AMKL cells may express α-naphthol acetate. Expression of glycoprotein Ia, IIb, or IIIa or factor VIII can aid in the diagnosis of FAB M7 AMKL. As described in more detail later, AML in Down syndrome is AMKL; however, the t(1;22) is found in some non–Down syndrome cases.[609]

Major Chromosomal Translocations

t(8;21). The archetypal chromosomal translocation in FAB M2 AML is the t(8;21), which fuses the 5′ terminus of the *AML1 (RUNX1, CBFA2)* gene at chromosome band 21q22, with almost the entire *ETO* gene from chromosome band 8q22.[79] In one series, 82% of pediatric AML with this translocation had FAB M2 morphology.[607] These morphologic-cytogenetic correlates, although compelling, are imperfect. Therefore some classifications have taken account of cytogenetic abnormalities, thereby highlighting crucial biologic pathways and, in some cases, therapeutic targets.[603] The t(8;21) also is strongly associated with extramedullary granulocytic sarcoma presentations.[607,610] Leukemias with this translocation, which disrupt the *AML1* gene encoding the DNA-binding subunit of core binding factor, comprise one of the two subtypes of core binding factor leukemias. The AML1 fusion oncoprotein binds the non–DNA-binding subunit of core binding factor, CBFB, as does native AML1, but the fusion oncoprotein interacts with nuclear corepressors that inhibit AML1-mediated transcriptional activation through the deregulation of histone deacetylation.[79] The t(8;21) has been associated with a favorable prognosis in studies conducted by the Pediatric Oncology Group[611] and the Children's Cancer Group.[612] The t(8;21) has been associated with a mixed outcome in the experience of St. Jude Children's Research Hospital, but the treatment regimens did not specify repetitive high-dose cytarabine as did other regimens in which the t(8;21) was associated with a favorable prognosis.[607,612,613] Variant *AML1 (CBFA2)* translocations involving other partner genes have heterogeneous morphologic MDS and AML presentations, but these translocations occur primarily in adult leukemias and tend to be treatment related rather than to occur de novo.[614]

inv(16) and t(16;16). The second subtype of core binding factor AML has inversions or, less often, translocations fusing the *CBFB* gene encoding the non–DNA-binding subunit of CBF at chromosome band 16p13 to the *MYH11* gene at chromosome band 16q22.[615] The classic morphologic presentation of AMLs with inv(16) and t(16;16) in adults is myelomonocytic leukemia with eosinophilia (FAB M4eo)[616] but many pediatric cases present as FAB M2 or M4 AML, without eosinophilia.[608,617] RT-PCR analysis and FISH are particularly useful and important for the detection of this rearrangement.[618-621] Additionally, the leukemic blast cells may coexpress the CD2 T-cell surface antigen.[622] The inv(16) is leukemogenic via a mechanism of dominant transcriptional repression of AML1-regulated genes, so that the pathways involved and the biologic consequences are similar to those resulting from the t(8;21).[79] The outcome associated with this aberration is also favorable in several pediatric series, similar to the t(8;21).[623] In one large study of adults and children, the outcomes were comparable in patients undergoing allotransplantation and receiving high-dose or low-dose cytarabine, and the outcome was better in the younger patients.[624] Pediatric studies have found that current regimens incorporating intensive high-dose cytarabine into postremission treatment are associated with event-free survival rates of approximately 70% or higher.[605,612]

t(15;17). The t(15;17) fusing the *PML* and *RARA* genes at chromosome bands 15q22 and 17q21, respectively, is associated with FAB M3 APL.[625,626] The t(15;17) and variant translocations associated with APL disrupt the function of the retinoic acid receptor α (RARα), also called the RARA protein, which is a ligand-dependent transcription factor important in myeloid differentiation. The RARα protein forms a heterodimer with another ligand-dependent protein, retinoic X receptor protein (RXR). The natural ligand of RARα is all-*trans*-retinoic acid (ATRA), whereas RXR is responsive to ATRA or 9-*cis*-retinoic acid.[625] In the presence of ligand, the heterodimeric complex interacts with transcriptional co-activators to induce myeloid differentiation. In contrast, the molecular pathogenesis of APL involves the aberrant recruitment of transcriptional co-repressors and the histone deacetylase complex to RARα target genes. Notably, the first molecularly targeted agent ever to be implemented for antileukemia treatment was ATRA. Variant translocations fuse *RARA* with partner genes other than *PML*, including *NPM*, *NUMA1 (NuMA)*, *STAT5b*, *PRKAR1A*, and *ZBTB16 (PLZF)*.[625,627-630] The

PRKAR1A-RARA fusion was first identified by *RARA* FISH analysis in an ATRA-sensitive adult with APL who had normal cytogenetics by conventional karyotype analysis.[630] *PRKAR1A* encodes the regulatory subunit type 1α of cyclic adenosine monophosphate–dependent protein kinase,[630] and the karyotypically cryptic nature of the translocation highlights the importance of molecular cytogenetic testing. APLs with *PLZF-RARA* translocation are insensitive to ATRA, whereas those with the other *RARA* fusion types are ATRA responsive.[625]

Mixed-Lineage Leukemia (MLL) *Gene Translocations.* In contrast to ALL, in which *MLL* partner genes are limited and *AF4* is the most common, the partner genes are much more diverse in AML.[631] Nonetheless, *MLL* partner genes in ALL and AML, and in de novo and treatment-related leukemias, are at least partially overlapping. Many MLL partner proteins have structural motifs of nuclear transcription factors,[15,132,506] transcriptional regulatory proteins,[632] or other nuclear proteins.[633-635] Others are cytoplasmic proteins or cell membrane proteins.[132,518,636-642] *MLL* also undergoes self-fusion in a type of rearrangement termed *partial tandem duplication;* therefore in AML, MLL itself is an MLL partner protein.[45,643,644] As in ALL, cDNA panhandle PCR analysis has been applied to detect novel and rare partner genes of *MLL* and covert *MLL* rearrangements in AML.[645-647] There is no obvious functional relationship between the many partner genes of *MLL* but some are members of the same gene families.[518,638-640,648,649] It has been suggested that the nuclear partner proteins mediate transcriptional activation[132,649,650] and that cytoplasmic partner proteins cause forced MLL dimerization or oligomerization.[651] Several MLL partner proteins also interact with one another.[652] Fusion proteins from the der(11) chromosome, which retain the AT hook, SNL, and MT domains of MLL but replace the MLL PHD, transactivation, and SET domains with the carboxyl partner protein, transform hematopoietic progenitors and cause leukemia in mice.[653,654] In murine models, MLL fusion proteins constitutively activate *Hoxa9*, and *Hoxa9* activation is essential for leukemogenesis with some MLL fusion proteins (e.g., MLL-ENL).[515] However, altered *Hox* expression is not essential for leukemogenesis with other MLL fusion proteins, including MLL-AF9 and MLL-GAS7.[654,655]

As described earlier, balanced *MLL* gene translocations are the primary molecular aberrations underlying most cases of acute leukemia in infants.[503] AML is more common than ALL in neonates, unlike during the rest of infancy and childhood.[134,656] It has been estimated that *MLL* translocations are present in half of all ALLs and AMLs diagnosed during the neonatal period.[134] *MLL* translocations also comprise 5% to 10% of acquired chromosomal rearrangements in childhood AML.[657] The particular partner gene fused to *MLL* affects cell lineage and differentiation features, which are reflected in the immunophenotype. *MLL* translocations in AML are often associated with myelomonocytic and monoblastic features.[133] Leukemias with *MLL* translocations can also present as treatment-associated myelodysplastic syndrome or AML[658,659]; this is particularly characteristic of cases with t(11;16) fusing *MLL* with *CBP* (CREB binding protein).[632,660-662] Unlike in

ALL, the presence of an *MLL* translocation is not an independent prognostic factor in pediatric AML with current treatment. However, in some series, the *MLL-MLLT3 (AF9)* fusion resulting from t(9;11) has been associated with a more favorable outcome than other *MLL* translocations[617] (e.g., *MLL-MLLT10 [ALF10]*).[663]

Certain clinical and laboratory features are associated with the archetypal neonatal FAB M4 and FAB M5 leukemias with *MLL* translocations. These features include cutaneous nodules (leukemia cutis), petechiae, and ecchymoses, in addition to the hematologic abnormalities (hyperleukocytosis, anemia, thrombocytopenia) and CNS involvement.[134,656,664] Curiously, congenital *MLL*-rearranged AML may be present predominantly in the skin and not in the marrow (aleukemic leukemia cutis) and, on occasion, can undergo spontaneous remission.[664,665] In these situations, molecular analysis of bone marrow and skin biopsy material is warranted because of the propensity for progressive disease when a clonal *MLL* rearrangement is identified.[664,665]

As discussed earlier for infant ALL, the *MLL* translocations in many infant AMLs are in utero events.[518] In some cases, however, an in utero origin cannot be demonstrated, possibly because the clonotypic sequences of the translocations are present below the detection limit of the PCR assay.[666] The occasional stillbirth presentations[134] and the presentation of monoblastic AML with an *MLL-ELL* rearrangement as a granulocytic sarcoma diagnosed by prenatal ultrasonography[667] further substantiate that *MLL* translocations arise in utero in infant AML. However, latency to leukemia underscores that additional secondary alterations are important, and perhaps required, for the development of leukemia with an *MLL* translocation.[132]

t(8;16). The chromosome 16 rearrangement in t(8;16) (p11;p13) is in the same band (16p13) disrupted by inversions and translocations of the *MYH11* gene in M4Eo AML.[615,668,669] However, the 16p13.3 breakpoints in t(8;16) target a different gene, encoding the transcriptional coactivator CREB binding protein (CBP; CREBBP) at chromosome band 16p13.3, which is fused with the *MOZ (MYST3)* gene on chromosome 8.[670] The CBP protein contains RARA and CREB binding domains, a bromodomain, and E1A and transcription factor IIB (TFIIB) binding regions, whereas MOZ contains zinc finger motifs and a MYST acetyltransferase domain.[670-674] The *CBP-MOZ* fusion transcript encoded by the der(16) chromosome is not in-frame, whereas the *MOZ-CBP* transcript is believed to have transforming properties and clinical relevance.[670,675,676] MOZ-CBP tumorigenic mechanisms have been proposed to involve inhibition of AML1-mediated transcriptional activation.[677] The *MOZ-CBP* rearrangement is associated with a gene expression signature that includes *HOXA9*, *MEIS1*, and *FLT3* overexpression, similar to the gene expression profiles in AML with *MLL* translocations.[678] Notably, *CBP* is also an occasional fusion partner of *MLL* in MDS.[632,660-662] *CBP* oncogenic aberrations can be constitutional, as evidenced by the germline *CBP* point mutations, microdeletions, and translocations that underlie the Rubinstein-Taybi syndrome.[679-681]

The t(8;16) is associated with a prognostically unfavorable subset of FAB M4 and FAB M5 AMLs, other features of which include erythrophagocytosis and coagulopathy.[682,683] Therefore recognition of this AML subset is clinically important and can be accomplished by molecular cytogenetic detection of the rearrangement. Although a rare translocation, accounting for only approximately 2% of pediatric AML,[684] most AMLs with this translocation have occurred in infants and children.[670,683] The t(8;16) in neonatal AML, like translocations in several other AML subtypes, can be associated with leukemia cutis and spontaneous remission.[685,686]

A variant t(10;16) translocation fuses the *KAT6B (MORF)* gene at chromosome band 10q22 to *CBP* and was discovered in a case of childhood FAB M5a AML.[687] The MORF protein contains zinc fingers, nuclear localization signals, and a histone acetyltransfersase domain[687] and, similar to MOZ, contributes to chromatin remodeling.[674] Additional variant translocations result in fusion of *MOZ* with the *NCOA2 (TIF2)* or *EP300 (p300)* genes[688-690]; p300 is related structurally to CBP, and the MOZ-TIF2 oncoprotein recruits CBP. Therefore CBP-mediated oncogenic transcriptional regulatory functions appear crucial in the several translocation variants that compose this AML molecular cytogenetic subset.

t(6;9). The t(6;9) (p23;q34) translocation is a rare recurrent translocation in AML, primarily seen in adults, the clinical and molecular features of which include myelodysplasia, basophilia, a CD34– immunophenotype and *FLT3* mutations.[691-693] AML with t(6;9) in children and adolescents has had a poor prognosis.[684,695-696] The translocation occurs in various morphologic AML subtypes, including FAB M1, M2, and M4, and fuses the 5' end of the *DEK* gene (chromosome 6) to the 3' end of the *NUP214 (CAN)* gene (chromosome 9), creating a *DEK-CAN* oncogene.[697-699] The *DEK* gene product is a multimeric chromatin protein, regulated by CK2 kinase, which modifies DNA topology by the introduction of supercoils into closed circular DNA.[700,701] The *CAN* gene at chromosome band 9q34 (also called *CAIN*, because of its chromosomal proximity to *ABL*), encodes the nucleoporin protein NUP214 of the nuclear pore complex. DEK-CAN oncogenic roles in leukemogenesis involve a myeloid lineage-specific increase in protein translation, which occurs in conjunction with increased eIF4E translation initiation factor phosphorylation.[702] Leukemias with the *DEK-CAN* fusion may have oncogenic mechanisms in common with other AML subtypes, as is suggested by the observation that nucleoporin-specific FG repeats in the fusion oncoprotein can induce transcriptional activation by recruitment of the transcriptional coactivators CBP and p300. Reverse-transcriptase and real-time PCR methods have been helpful for AML monitoring in patients with this rearrangement, because the persistence of the fusion transcript identifies patients at risk for relapse.[703-705] A translocation variant resulting in the *SET-CAN* oncogenic fusion gene has been observed in AML of the FAB M0 subtype.[697]

NUP98 Translocations. The *NUP98* gene at chromosome band 11p15 encodes a nucleoporin protein that serves as a structural component of nuclear pore complex.

The NUP98 protein is located on the nucleoplasmic side of the nuclear pore and provides a docking site for the export of mRNA between the nucleus and cytoplasm.[706,707] Various chromosomal translocations produce *NUP98* oncogenic fusions and, depending on exactly which partner gene is fused with *NUP98*, these translocations can be associated with de novo or treatment-related AML, ALL, or MDS.[706-726] Many of the *NUP98* partner genes encode homeobox transcription factors, but some of the partner genes, including *TOP1* and *TOP2B*, have more diverse functions.[708,717,723] Several *NUP98* fusions, such as those involving *NSD1*, *HOXD13*, and *PSIP1 (LEDGF)*, are found in infant and pediatric de novo AML.[718,724,725] t(7;11)(p15;p15), which fuses *NUP98* with *HOXA9*, and t(10;11)(q23;p15), which fuses *NUP98* with *HHEX,* have been shown to shift the cellular distribution of NUP98 away from the nuclear pore complex and into intranuclear aggregation bodies.[711,719] Because of the substantial variety of *NUP98* partner genes, it is most feasible to detect these rearrangements using a general *NUP98* break-apart FISH strategy.[723,727] cDNA panhandle PCR assay has also been applied as a gene discovery tool to identify new partner genes in leukemias with *NUP98* translocations.[728]

Therapy-Related Acute Myeloid Leukemias and Myelodysplastic Syndromes

Therapy-related AMLs and MDS comprise a separate WHO AML subgroup[603] relevant to pediatrics; two major categories have been recognized. Therapy-related leukemias are of increasing concern in children, in whom survivorship—as a percentage of patients diagnosed with cancer—is greater than in the adult cancer population.[729] Therapy-related leukemia or MDS is also well-recognized as a long-term complication after autologous hematopoietic stem cell transplantation.[730-732] The two major categories of chemotherapies associated with leukemia and MDS are alkylating agents and TOP2 poisons. The forms of leukemia associated with these agents have distinctive molecular cytogenetic features, which can also be found in subsets of leukemia arising de novo.

All alkylating agents engender some risk for leukemia as a treatment complication, but the risk is variable, depending on the particular agent(s), cumulative dose, patient age, and superimposed effects of radiation therapy.[733-736] The latency period is variable, ranging from 2 to 12 years after exposure, but the peak incidence occurs at approximately 6 years.[737] The archetypal cytogenetic features in alkylating agent–related leukemias are complete or partial deletions of chromosomes 5 and 7 and complex, unbalanced, numeric and structural cytogenetic abnormalities.[738] The chromosome 7 aberrations are the most common cytogenetic events in leukemias after alkylating agent treatment.[739,740] Most cases with chromosome 7q deletions exhibit allelic loss of the chromosomal segment between bands 7q22 and 7q31 but, despite identification of various candidate genes in this genomic region, the exact tumor suppressor gene(s) have not been convincingly identified.[741-745] In treatment-associated MDS and AML lacking chromosome 5 aberrations, the monosomy 7 or del(7q) may be acquired by subclone evolution and accompanied by other key mutational aberrations, including t(3;21), *RAS* mutation, and CDKN2B promoter hypermethylation.[740]

Monosomy 5 and del(5q) are the next most common aberrations in alkylating agent–related MDS and AML. FISH analyses have revealed that the chromosome 5q abnormalities frequently are covert unbalanced translocations.[740] The chromosome 5q abnormalities arise as primary aberrations and not by subclone evolution, and additional aberrations in therapy-related MDS and AML with monosomy 5 or del(5q) can include monosomy 7 or del(7q), *TP53* mutations, and gene duplications, such as *MLL* segmental jumping translocations.[16,740,746] The critical genes targeted by 5q deletion have been difficult to pinpoint because of variable involvement of a large genomic region that encompasses chromosome bands 5q13 to 5q33.[739,747-753] Two recently implicated chromosome 5q31 candidate genes are *CTNNA1* encoding the α-catenin protein[754] and the *EGR1* gene,[755] although there have been several others.[739,747-753] Epigenetic dysregulation may also contribute to the pathogenesis, with transcriptional silencing in the retained nondeleted *CTNNA1* allele resulting from promoter methylation and histone deacetylation.[754]

A tumor suppressor gene, *RPS14*, has been identified as the target of 5q– in the syndrome of refractory anemia, in which there is preservation of megakaryopoiesis and myelopoiesis,[756] but the role of *RPS14* in therapy-related MDS and AML remains to be determined. This gene encodes a ribosomal protein required for processing of 18S pre-rRNA.[756] The strategy of screening normal human CD34+ cells with short hairpin RNAs (shRNAs) against various genes in the minimal 5q– deletion region has revealed that *RPS14* silencing causes erythroid maturation block and increased apoptosis in differentiating erythroid cells, similar to the increased apoptosis observed in MDS.[756] Furthermore, lentiviral RPS14 expression restored erythroid differentiation in bone marrow cells from patients with 5q– refractory anemia syndrome.[756] These insights underscore the role of ribosomal genes in anemia, given that other ribosomal genes, *RPS19* and *RPS24,* contribute to Diamond-Blackfan anemia.

Most AMLs developing after autologous hematopoietic stem cell transplantation have complex numeric and structural karyotypic aberrations, including losses of chromosomes 5 and 7; these are also features of AML arising after exposure to alkylating agents.[732,757-759] The secondary AMLs can occur early after transplantation, and the cytogenetic aberrations in these treatment-associated leukemias are often demonstrable in pretransplantation specimens, suggesting that the genotoxic damage results from the prior therapy.[757,760] On the other hand, such cytogenetic aberrations are not demonstrable in the peripheral blood stem cell autografts.[761]

Therapy-related leukemias can be caused by exposure to various chemotherapeutic TOP2 poisons, including epipodophyllotoxins and anthracyclines, the anthracenedione mitoxantrone, and the TOP1/TOP2 interacting agent dactinomycin.[63] Balanced translocations, often involving the *MLL* gene,[562] are the most typical molecular alterations in leukemias related to TOP2 poisons.

The typical latency is 2 to 2½ years after chemotherapy exposure,[658,762] although more protracted latencies of up to 10 years have been described.[645,763] A particularly high risk has been reported in association with high cumulative doses of etoposide and anthracyclines,[764] but other studies have not found a correlation between etoposide cumulative dose and secondary leukemia risk.[765] Intermittent weekly or twice-weekly etoposide dose schedules, and semicontinuous schedules, have also been associated with increased risk for secondary AML.[764,765] The *MLL* translocations in therapy-related AML (as is the case in de novo AML) are often associated with myelomonocytic and monoblastic morphology.[766,767] Other translocations in therapy-related MDS and AML include t(8;21) and its variants,[614,768-777] t(15;17),[778] inv(16) and t(16;16),[762,779-782] t(8;16),[783,784] t(9;22),[783] and various translocations involving the *NUP98* gene at chromosome band 11p15.[708,709,711,785-788]

Treatment-related MDS/AML can present as bizarre and highly abnormal morphology in some cases (Fig. 45-38) but, in others, can be insidious and challenging to diagnose, particularly in patients actively receiving treatment, in whom the hematologic features of cytopenia and monocytosis can be indistinguishable from ordinary side effects of chemotherapy and recovery of the marrow. Additionally, some patients with treatment-related MDS and AML, particularly in the early stages, have no obvious peripheral blood cell abnormalities at all.[51,637] Therefore one front-line pediatric neuroblastoma treatment protocol has specified routine bone marrow surveillance every 3 to 6 months, not only for neuroblastoma relapse but also for leukemia-associated aberrations.[51] In addition to the insidious nature of the clinical presentations, the spectrum of known molecular cytogenetic abnormalities associated with therapy-related MDS and AML is constantly increasing and is already very large, creating the yet-unmet need for broad molecular cytogenetic screening

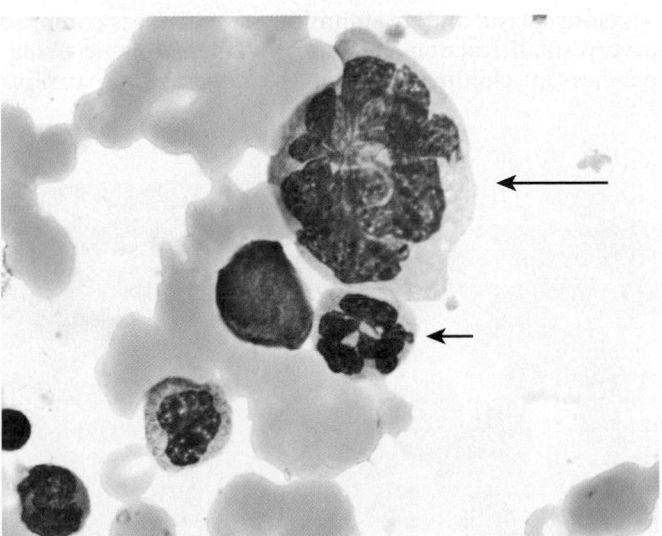

Figure 45-38 Therapy-related MDS showing hypersegmented granulocyte *(short arrow)* below an extremely dysplastic hypersegmented neutrophil *(arrow). (Courtesy Marybeth Helfrich, Children's Hospital of Philadelphia.)*

methods with which to monitor high-risk patients. For example, even though there are few data on patients observed in this manner, it seems that most of the protean *MLL* translocations emerging during treatment, which involve many different partner genes, are harbingers of MDS or AML.[51,637,789] An *MLL-FRYL* translocation that was traced prospectively by molecular cytogenetic testing (FISH, panhandle PCR assay) caused clonal replacement of the bone marrow without affecting differentiation, only after a long latency culminated in clear-cut therapy-related MDS.[51] However, clinical progression is apparently not inevitable because, in one patient, the morphologically normal clone harboring an *MLL-ARHGEF17* translocation gradually regressed and neither leukemia nor MDS ensued.[790]

Additional challenges for molecular characterization result from the variable locations of *MLL* translocation breakpoints, which can be within or outside a breakpoint hot spot region.[45,47,51,63,121,134,139,155,463,465-470,632,647,791,792] Secondary myeloid disorders are particularly challenging to diagnose in patients previously diagnosed with AML, for example, the *MOZ* oncogenic rearrangement resulting from a novel t(2;8)(p23;p11.2) translocation in treatment-related MDS after AML in a pediatric patient.[793]

Clinically, the molecular cytogenetic features of the therapy-related leukemias are important prognostic factors. Most cases, except those with favorable translocations—t(8;21), inv(16), t(15;17)—are resistant to current treatment strategies, but intensive regimens, including hematopoietic stem cell transplantation, have been more successful. Prognosis is affected further by the reduced tolerance to additional intensive antileukemia therapy after primary cancer treatment.[794] Nonetheless, just as in the de novo leukemias, additional targeted therapy options are emerging from an understanding of the molecular cytogenetic aberrations in these challenging disorders.

Myelodysplasia and Myeloproliferative Diseases

Myelodysplasia and myeloproliferative diseases comprise a very small fraction (<10%) of all hematologic malignancies in children. Incomplete coverage of various unique features of pediatric MDS and myeloproliferative diseases in the current WHO classification system has led to the development of diagnostic guidelines for MDS and myeloproliferative categories applicable specifically to children.[795] To fulfill minimal diagnostic criteria for MDS, at least two of the following four features are required: (1) sustained unexplained cytopenia; (2) bi-lineage morphologic myelodysplasia; (3) acquired clonal hematopoietic cell cytogenetic abnormality; and (4) 5% or more blasts in the marrow.[795] In contrast to AML, which is defined by a bone marrow blast threshold of 20% and aberrant differentiation, and to MDS, myeloproliferative disorders are characterized by expansion of one or more hematopoietic lineages but retained differentiation.[795,796] Three major categories of MDS and myeloproliferative diseases are applicable to children: (1) a group of myelodysplastic-myeloproliferative disorders comprising primarily juvenile myelomonocytic leukemia (JMML); (2) myeloid leukemia of Down syndrome; and (3) MDS.[795]

Juvenile Myelomonocytic Leukemia. The constellation of hepatosplenomegaly, lymphadenopathy, pallor, and rash, especially in children younger than 3 years old, comprises the clinical features of JMML, the diagnostic criteria for which include peripheral monocytosis, absence of the *BCR-ABL* rearrangement, less than 20% blasts in the bone marrow, and at least two of the following: increased fetal hemoglobin, circulating myeloid precursors (Fig. 45-39), a white blood cell count more than 10 × 10⁹/L, presence of a clonal cytogenetic abnormality, and in vitro hypersensitivity of myeloid precursors to granulocyte-macrophage colony-stimulating factor (GM-CSF).[796] Children with neurofibromatosis type 1 (NF1) or Noonan syndrome are predisposed to JMML. Notably, several of the key molecular abnormalities contributing to JMML pathogenesis result in RAS signaling pathway hyperactivation.

Many hematopoietic growth factors transduce signals from the cell surface to the nucleus through RAS family proteins, which regulate cellular proliferation and differentiation by cycling between active guanosine triphosphate (GTP)-bound and inactive guanosine diphosphate

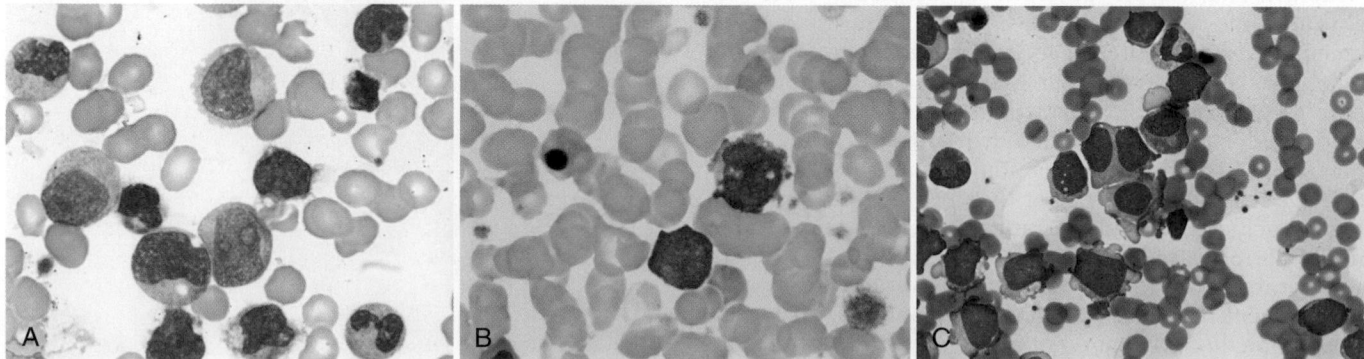

Figure 45-39 A, Juvenile myelomonocytic leukemia peripheral blood showing leukocytosis, monocytosis, myeloid left shift, and myelodysplasia. B, Down syndrome transient abnormal myelopoiesis (TAM). This peripheral blood specimen shows a megakaryoblast, nucleated red blood cell, and giant platelet. C, Acute megakaryoblastic leukemia (FAB M7) featuring pleomorphic blasts and cytoplasmic blebbing. *(Courtesy Marybeth Helfrich, Children's Hospital of Philadelphia.)*

(GDP)-bound states.[797,798] Somatic mutations in *RAS* oncogenes are one mechanism of RAS pathway activation and are found in 20% to 30% of JMMLs,[798,799] often involving *KRAS* or *NRAS* at codons 12, 13, or 61. Some cases of *RAS*-mutant JMML undergo spontaneous regression,[800] whereas *NRAS*-mutant JMML can progress with loss of the remaining normal *NRAS* allele.[801] Monosomy 7 is also found in some cases of JMML with *RAS* oncogene mutations.[802]

The *NF1* tumor suppressor gene product, neurofibromin, is a GTPase activating protein that accelerates GTP hydrolysis on RAS proteins.[803] Germline mutations in the *NF1* gene, often with accompanying loss of the normal *NF1* allele, result in elevated levels of GTP-bound RAS. Thus germline *NF1* mutations comprise an alternative mechanism for hyperactivating the RAS signaling pathway, predisposing to JMML.[803,804] LOH at the *NF1* locus is observed in approximately 50% of JMML arising in patients with NF1.[803] In NF1 kindreds, JMML is seen particularly in boys with maternal transmission of the mutant *NF1* allele.[805] Additional mutations in the *NF1* gene, with or without LOH, occur in sporadic JMML that is not associated with the NF1 syndrome.[806] In some of these cases, the *NF1* mutations are germline, with JMML being the presenting feature of the NF1 syndrome. Overall, it is estimated that *NF1* mutations are present in approximately 30% of all JMMLs.[806] Monosomy 7 occurs in addition to *NF1* mutation in some JMMLs.[803] However, *NF1* and *RAS* mutations in JMMLs are mutually exclusive.[806]

Noonan syndrome is an autosomal dominant disorder associated with germline mutations in the *PTPN11 (SHP2)* gene in approximately 50% of cases and is characterized by JMML, facial dysmorphology, short stature, and cardiac defects.[807] The *PTPN11* gene product, SHP2 phosphatase, regulates RAS-MAPK pathway signaling but is inactive in its baseline state.[808,809] *PTPN11* mutations in Noonan syndrome result in SHP2 activation and, consequently, hyperactivation of RAS-MAPK signaling.[808] In pediatric patients without Noonan syndrome, *PTPN11* somatic mutations can be found in sporadic cases of JMML, MDS, AML (particularly the FAB M5 subtype), and B-cell lineage ALL.[810-814] Somatically acquired *PTPN11* mutations are present in 30% to 35% of de novo JMML.[811,814] Generally, the types of *PTPN11* mutations occurring as somatic events in nonsyndromic cases are more strongly activating than the germline *PTPN11* mutations in patients with Noonan syndrome.[796,815] The fact that *PTPN11* mutations are less strongly activating in patients with Noonan syndrome might explain why syndromic JMML is associated with less severe hematologic abnormalities and can resolve spontaneously.[796,811] Thus dysregulation of the RAS signaling pathway by *RAS*, *NF1*, or *PTPN11* mutations is instrumental to the aberrant cell growth and differentiation in JMML, and these three mechanisms of RAS dysregulation are usually mutually exclusive.[814]

The myeloproliferative disorder known as monosomy 7 syndrome has clinical overlap with JMML and is characterized by myelodysplasia, thrombocytopenia, anemia, and hepatosplenomegaly.[816] However, this disorder is not included in the more recent classification system for pediatric myelodysplastic and myeloproliferative diseases.[795]

Chronic Myelomonocytic Leukemia. Chronic myelomonocytic leukemia (CMML) is a clonal bone marrow stem cell disorder characterized by monocytosis, myelodysplasia, and absence of *BCR-ABL* fusion.[41,603] t(5;12)(q33;p13), which generates the *TEL-PDGFRB* fusion product, is a recurring but rare rearrangement in CMML.[603] The case in which the fusion transcript was first described occurred in an adolescent patient.[817] t(5;12) is associated with eosinophilia and progression to AML on acquisition of additional cytogenetic changes.[817] However, only secondary and not de novo CMML is included as a diagnostic category in the pediatric adaptation of the WHO classification of myelodysplastic and myeloproliferative diseases.[795]

Transient Abnormal Myelopoiesis and Acute Megakaryoblastic Leukemia of Down Syndrome. Ten to 20 percent of neonates with Down syndrome are affected with transient abnormal myelopoiesis (TAM), and 20% to 30% of TAM will progress to AMKL by 4 years of age (see Fig. 45-39).[818-820] Several laboratories have identified truncating *GATA1* point mutations as in utero mutational oncogenic events that initiate both TAM and AMKL.[818,821] GATA1 is a hematopoietic transcription factor that, via interactions with the FOG1 cofactor and GATA2, regulates erythroid and megakaryocyte maturation.[818] However, whereas the *GATA1* mutation is sufficient for TAM, postnatal secondary changes such as *TP53* mutation and/or trisomy 8 are required for subsequent clonal expansion, a prerequisite for disease progression to AMKL.[822] In many cases of TAM, however, there is no disease progression because the clone with *GATA1* mutation is ultimately extinguished in the absence of requisite secondary alterations.[818] The TAM and AMKL in Down syndrome have distinct gene expression profiles.[819]

Several chromosome 21 genes, including *CBS* (cystathionine beta-synthase), at band 21q22 may contribute to the unique forms of leukemogenesis in Down syndrome.[823] The *CBS* gene is overexpressed, above and beyond the levels predicted based on the trisomy 21 increased gene dosage. This upregulation seems to result from mechanisms involving transcriptional upregulation through the *CBS* promoter.[823] Consequences of *CBS* overexpression include reduced levels of plasma homocysteine, methionine, *S*-adenosylmethionine and *S*-adenosylhomocysteine, resulting in altered CpG methylation and consequent dysregulation of gene expression. Other effects include perturbed folate metabolism and genetic instability (increased DNA mutations), which may predispose to accumulation of the secondary genetic mutations in AMKL.[823] Another consequence of *CBS* overexpression is increased cytarabine sensitivity,[823] which contributes to increased treatment-related toxicities and to the more favorable outcome associated with myeloid leukemia of Down syndrome.[824]

t(1;22)(p13;q13), which fuses *RBM15 (OTT)* and *MLK1 (MAL)*, is associated with non–Down syndrome

AMKL, another distinct form of AMKL peculiar to neonates.[134,503,825]

Myelodysplastic Syndrome. The three MDS morphologic subtypes of greatest relevance in pediatrics are refractory cytopenia, refractory anemia with excess blasts (RAEB), and RAEB in transformation (RAEB-T).[796] Monosomy 7 or del(7q) occurs in approximately 40% of cases and is the most commonly acquired cytogenetic aberration in pediatric MDS.[826] In cases of refractory cytopenia, monosomy 7 is associated with disease progression and poor outcome.[795,827] Similarly, monosomy 7, with or without other cytogenetic abnormalities, is a frequent finding in RAEB-T.[826] Despite the generally poor prognosis of −7/del(7q) in MDS, spontaneous and durable hematologic remissions have been described in some children diagnosed with MDS characterized by this cytogenetic feature.[828] Rarely, MDS with monosomy 7 is familial and observed in siblings.[805,829] In one study of refractory anemia of childhood, which is a form of refractory cytopenia, cytogenetic analyses have demonstrated monosomy 7 in 49% of cases, whereas trisomy 8 was the next most common abnormality, found in 9% of cases.[827] The 5q− syndrome associated with an indolent refractory anemia but with preservation of megakaryopoiesis and myelopoiesis[756] has not been described in children.[795] FISH analysis with chromosome-specific probes in combination with immunophenotyping has enabled characterization of the cell lineages affected by the clonal aberrations in MDS[830] as well as evaluation of the lineages affected by MDS clonal expansion.[831] MDS secondary to prior therapy has been discussed earlier. As is true for adults,[734] pediatric patients with MDS secondary to cytotoxic therapies (see earlier) often have chromosome 5 and 7 abnormalities.[832] Constitutional disorders associated with congenital bone marrow failure syndromes and acquired aplastic anemia are included in the differential diagnosis of MDS in children.[795]

Other Clinically Important Genomic Aberrations in Myeloid Disorders

It has been proposed that in addition to the major chromosomal aberrations that underlie the various AML morphologic subtypes, cooperating mutations affecting proliferation and differentiation are essential in AML pathogenesis[503] and may affect prognosis and treatment. The balanced chromosomal translocations that disrupt major hematopoietic transcription factor genes are generally regarded as the primary molecular alterations in the associated AML morphologic subsets. Translocations that disrupt major hematopoietic transcription factor genes generally alter differentiation,[503] whereas additional aberrations, including kinase or RAS-RAF pathway gene mutations, often contribute to hyperproliferative behavior.

FLT3 Alterations. Although less common than in adult AML, FLT3 mutations are nonetheless found in a considerable minority of pediatric AML cases, with juxta membrane region ITD and activation loop point mutations identified in 12% to 15% and 7% to 9% of pediatric

cases, respectively.[565,833,834] Indeed, FLT3 mutations might represent the most frequently occurring molecular abnormalities in AML. FLT3 mutations are common in pediatric AML with MLL translocations; 23% of MLL-rearranged AML in one large series harbored either FLT3-ITD or kinase domain mutations.[565] Also, FLT3 mutations are particularly common in AMLs with normal karyotypes, in which they are demonstrable in up to 60% of cases.[565] Another subset of AML features autocrine FLT3 activation caused by the expression of FLT3 ligand, resulting in constitutive FLT3 phosphorylation and signaling.[834] FLT3-ITD mutations in pediatric AML are associated with poor outcomes, similar to those in adult cases.[834-836] An increased FLT3-ITD allelic ratio is associated with relapse, and molecular diagnostic tests have been developed to detect FLT3 mutations and quantify the FLT3-ITD allelic ratio.[837,838] FLT3-ITD mutations occur in approximately 30% of childhood APL.[837] FLT3-ITD mutations, although common in de novo AML, are infrequent in treatment-related cases, as reported in an adult series.[839]

KIT Mutations. Mutations in the KIT receptor tyrosine kinase gene are also common in pediatric AML and occur most often in cases with t(8;21) or inv(16), which disrupt DNA or non–DNA-binding subunits of CBF.[840] The KIT mutations are associated with constitutive, ligand-independent activation of the KIT protein. One recent study has estimated that 37% of all AML in children with either t(8;21) or inv(16) harbor KIT mutations. KIT mutations do not affect prognosis but are nonetheless significant because preclinical studies have indicated that AML with KIT mutations are sensitive to imatinib mesylate and FLT3 inhibition.[840]

RAS Mutations. It has long been recognized that the RAS oncogene family members can be activated by mutations in myeloid neoplasms,[841] although these mutations do not usually have prognostic relevance.[840] Mutations of NRAS or KRAS codons 12, 13, or 16 have been described in approximately 20% of pediatric AMLs with MLL translocation[842] and in approximately 30% of pediatric AMLs with t(8;21) or inv(16).[840] RAS mutations are also found in about one third of MDS with monosomy 7.[843] In secondary AML, RAS mutations are less common than in de novo disease[844,845] but are seen more often in alkylating agent–related cases, especially cases with monosomy 7, than in AML arising after exposure to TOP2 poisons. Additional evidence of RAS pathway oncogenic roles is seen in the germline RAF1 mutations in adult therapy-related AML.[846] RAF1 is activated by RAS binding and participates in RAS signaling.

PTPN11 Mutations. The RAS/RAF/MEK/ERK signaling pathway can also be activated by mutations in the SHP2 phosphatase gene, PTPN11. Although somatic PTPN11 mutations are uncommon, and occur in only approximately 4% of childhood AMLs overall, PTPN11 mutations have a predilection for the FAB M5 morphologic subtype, in which they are found in approximately 18% of cases.[813]

PI3K/AKT/mTOR Pathway Aberrations. The PI3K/AKT/mTOR pathway is a signaling pathway that promotes cell proliferation and survival in leukemia. In adults, constitutive AKT activation, leading to downstream mTOR activation, contributes to the progression of MDS to AML.[847,848]

PTEN is a tumor suppressor protein that inhibits the PI3K/AKT/mTOR signaling pathway. Although *PTEN* gene mutations and LOH are uncommon in AML, aberrant *PTEN* mRNA splicing has been demonstrated, primarily in adult AML.[849] Constitutive PTEN phosphorylation, which results in PTEN inactivation, may contribute to AML,[850,851] whereas reduced PTEN expression may be important in MDS progression.[847] These oncogenic mechanisms may impede normal PTEN functions, which include not only attenuation of PI3K survival signaling but also promotion of hematopoietic stem cell quiescence and preservation of the self-renewal capacity of the hematopoietic stem cell compartment.[852]

TP53 Mutations. TP53 is a crucial cell cycle regulatory tumor suppressor protein that senses and responds to DNA damage by regulation of the G1-S cell cycle checkpoint. *TP53* mutations are features of alkylating agent–related leukemias in adults and children.[16,746,845,853] In contrast to *RAS* mutations, *TP53* mutations are more common in therapy-related than de novo cases.[845] Segmental jumping translocations are chromosomal abnormalities in which multiple copies of various oncogenes are dispersed extrachromosomally and throughout the genome.[16] Gene amplification accompanies loss of wild-type TP53 after exposure to genotoxic agents, and *TP53* mutations and *MLL* segmental jumping translocations are strongly associated, with both occurring after alkylating agent treatment.[746] The *TP53* mutations may be of germline origin.[16,854] Similarly, *TP53* gene mutations are associated with *AML1* gene amplification or duplication in MDS and AML after alkylating agent treatment.[855] *TP53* mutations occur in de novo AML in patients affected with the Li-Fraumeni syndrome.[67,856]

NPM1 (Nucleophosmin) Mutations. The *NPM1* gene encodes a nucleolar shuttle protein with multiple functions in protein trafficking, preribosomal assembly, and ARF-TP53 pathway regulation.[857,858] t(5;17), a variant translocation in APL, involves fusion of the *NPM1* gene to *RARA*,[628] and *NPM1* is fused to *ALK* in a subset of anaplastic large cell lymphomas.[859] Identification of *NPM1* point mutations in adult AML without karyotypic abnormalities has led to the recent analysis and discovery of *NPM1* mutations in childhood AML. The mutations cause loss of nucleolar localization with accumulation of nucleophosmin in the cytoplasm. Leukemic cells with *NPM1* mutations have a particular gene expression signature of *HOXB2*, *HOXB3*, *HOXB6*, and *HOXD4* upregulation.[860] In contrast to adult AML, in which *NPM1* mutations are present in 25% to 35% of cases, and even in up to 60% of cases with a normal karyotype, the frequency of *NPM1* mutations in pediatric AML is only 7% to 8%. Similar to adult AML, however, *NPM1* mutations are concentrated in patients with normal cytogenetics and, in the absence of *FLT3*-ITD mutations, *NPM1* mutations are associated with an especially good prognosis.[857,858] *NPM1* mutations in AML are more common in older than younger children and in girls than boys.[857] In addition, *NPM1* mutations are significant because they may facilitate risk stratification and allow for minimal residual disease detection in cases in which no other molecular cytogenetic markers are available.[858]

Monosomy 7 and del(7q). Monosomy 7 or del(7q) occurs with or without other cytogenetic aberrations in only 4% to 5% of pediatric AMLs but in 40% of pediatric MDSs.[826] Because of the infrequency of these aberrations, an international retrospective study was conducted to characterize −7 and del(7q) in pediatric AML and MDS. del(7q) is more common than −7 in AML cases with favorable cytogenetic features, such as t(8;21), inv(16), t(15;17), or t(9;11), whereas −7 is more common in cases with inv(3), t(9;22), i(17q), or +21. Further subgroup analysis, which was enabled by the size of the study, has demonstrated that −7 is associated with inferior survival compared with del(7q) and that survival is worse in the del(7q) subgroup without other favorable cytogenetic features compared with the del(7q) group having other favorable cytogenetic features.[826]

IDH1 and IDH2 Mutations. A novel type of mutations in AML affects the isocitrate dehydrogenase 1 *(IDH1)* and isocitrate dehydrogenase 2 *(IDH2)* genes, which encode the metabolic enzymes responsible for conversion of isocitrate to α-ketoglutarate.[861] These mutations result in the production of an aberrant oncometabolite 2-hydroxyglutarate. They are associated with a global pattern of DNA hypermethylation because of the dependence of *TET2* on α-ketoglutarate and the resultant impaired oxidation of 5mC by the TET2 enzyme.[862] Somatic *IDH1* and *IDH2* mutations characterize 15% to 23% of cases of adult AML, and they occur in AML cases in which there are few other molecular cytogenetic abnormalities.[861,863] A genomic classifier in adult AML has suggested that the co-occurrence of *IDH1* or *IDH2* mutation with *NPM* mutation in absence of the *FLT3*-ITD predicts a favorable prognosis.[863] However, in pediatric AML, *IDH1* and *IDH2* mutations appear to be much less common. In studies conducted by the Children's Oncology Group, there were no *IDH1* mutations[864] and *IDH2* mutations were detected in 2.2% of cases, in which accompanying t(8;21), MLL translocation, or *NPM* mutation was detected.[865] In another study, two *IDH1* and one *IDH2* mutations were detected in 206 cases of pediatric AML. Interestingly, both *IDH1* mutations occurred in cases with MLL–partial tandem duplication of FAB M0 morphology.[866]

TET2 Mutations. The TET2 DNA methylase enzyme catalyzes the oxidation of 5mC to 5-hydroxymethylcytosine (5hmC) in a reaction that is dependent on α-ketoglutarate.[862] Circos maps have suggested that *IDH1* or *IDH2* mutations and *TET2* mutations in adult AML are mutually exclusive.[862] Both *IDH1* and *IDH2* mutations as well as *TET2* mutations are associated with impaired hematopoietic differentiation programs.[862] *TET2* mutations have been reported in 6% of pediatric AML, a frequency more similar to that in adult AML.[863,865] In a second pediatric study, their frequency was only 1.7% and they were found with *FLT3*-TKD, *FLT3*-ITD plus *CEBPα*, and *KRAS* plus *WT1* mutations.[866] *TET2* mutations in adult AML are most often associated with an intermediate prognosis.[862] The results of the latter pediatric study, which also examined the mutation frequency in *ASXL1* (1.1%) and *DNMT3* (0), altogether indicate that the occurrence of mutations in genes whose products regulate DNA methylation and histone modification is less in pediatric AML than in AML in adults, but also that, when present, there are more accompanying molecular cytogenetic aberrations in the pediatric cases.[866]

MicroRNA Abnormalities

Levels of a particular microRNA, miR-223, are low in AML with the t(8;21) translocation.[597] The underlying mechanism was shown to involve epigenetic transcriptional silencing of miR-223 by the AML1-ETO fusion oncoprotein through the recruitment of several chromatin-remodeling enzymes, including DNA methyltransferases and HDAC1 to the pre–miR-223 gene.[867] The ages of the patients studied were not specified (they were presumably adults), but t(8;21) is a feature of AML in adult and pediatric patients.

CONCLUSION

It is now possible to characterize and understand the cytogenetic and molecular pathobiology of the many forms of pediatric cancer in unprecedented detail using a panoply of approaches starting with decades-old conventional cytogenetic analysis of larger chromosomal aberrations that have withstood the test of time, advanced genomic methods reliant on the many derivatives of recombinant DNA technologies that followed later on and, now, next-generation sequencing of the whole transcriptome, genome, and epigenome, not only globally but within single cells. The ascertainment of cancer gene alterations and the cytogenetic and molecular subclassification of the many pediatric cancers outlined in this chapter is significant because the disruption of particular oncogenic pathways has prognostic and therapeutic relevance and is leading to the discovery of therapeutic targets that provide opportunities for new directed treatments.

References available online at ExpertConsult.

KEY REFERENCES

54. Lipson D, Capelletti M, Yelensky R, et al: Identification of new *ALK* and *RET* gene fusions from colorectal and lung cancer biopsies. *Nat Med* 18:382–384, 2012.
    This study demonstrates identification of novel, therapeutically relevant kinase fusion genes through targeted gene sequencing in standard paraffin-embedded pathology materials.
91. Richter GH, Plehm S, Fasan A, et al: *EZH2* is a mediator of EWS/FLI1 driven tumor growth and metastatic blocking endothelial and neuro-ectodermal differentiation. *Proc Natl Acad Sci U S A* 106:5324–5329, 2009.

This study shows that EWSR1-FLI1 oncogenic programs involve EZH2-mediated gene silencing, which are in turn dependent on histone deacetylase (HDAC) activity.
97. France KA, Anderson JL, Park A, et al: Oncogenic fusion protein EWS/FLI1 down-regulates gene expression by both transcriptional and posttranscriptional mechanisms. *J Biol Chem* 286:22750–22757, 2011.
    This study demonstrates that EWSR1-FLI1 regulates target gene expression by modulating both transcript synthesis and degradation.
106. Italiano A, Sung YS, Zhang L, et al: High prevalence of *CIC* fusion with double-homeobox *(DUX4)* transcription factors in *EWSR1*-negative undifferentiated small blue round cell sarcomas. *Genes Chromosomes Cancer* 51:207–218, 2012.
    Whereas previous studies demonstrated that a subset of small round cell sarcomas had CIC-DUX4 oncogenic fusions resulting from a t(4;19) translocation, this report shows that a similar fusion can result from a t(4;10) translocation, given that another copy of the DUX4 gene is located at 10q26. CIC-DUX4 fusions are found in many Ewing-like tumors that lack ETS-family gene rearrangements, suggesting that a subgroup of primitive round cell sarcomas characterized by CIC rearrangements are distinct from the Ewing sarcoma family of tumors.
114. Lawrence B, Perez-Atayde A, Hibbard MK, et al: *TPM3-ALK* and *TPM4-ALK* oncogenes in inflammatory myofibroblastic tumors. *Am J Pathol* 157:377–384, 2000.
    A subset of inflammatory myofibroblastic tumors, particularly those diagnosed in younger individuals, were found to have chromosomal rearrangements resulting in constitutive activation of the ALK receptor tyrosine kinase.
117. George RE, Sanda T, Hanna M, et al: Activating mutations in ALK provide a therapeutic target in neuroblastoma. *Nature* 455:975–978, 2008.
    This study demonstrates that gain of function ALK receptor tyrosine kinase mutations are a novel therapeutic target in a subset of neuroblastoma.
118. Janoueix-Lerosey I, Lequin D, Brugieres L, et al: Somatic and germline activating mutations of the ALK kinase receptor in neuroblastoma. *Nature* 455:967–970, 2008.
    This study demonstrates that gain of function ALK receptor tyrosine kinase mutations in neuroblastoma can result from either germline or somatic events.
135. Armstrong SA, Kung AL, Mabon ME, et al: Inhibition of *FLT3* in *MLL*: validation of a therapeutic target identified by gene expression based classification. *Cancer Cell* 3:173–183, 2003.
    This study suggested that the high level FLT3 expression that is characteristic of MLL-rearranged ALL and occurs as a consequence of either overexpression of the wild-type protein or mutations also provides a therapeutic opportunity for FLT3 signaling inhibition.
201. Su L, Sampaio AV, Jones KB, et al: Deconstruction of the SS18-SSX fusion oncoprotein complex: insights into disease etiology and therapeutics. *Cancer Cell* 21:333–347, 2012.
    This study characterizes proteins complexing with the SS18-SSX fusion oncoprotein in synovial sarcoma. SS18-SSX was shown to serve as a bridge between activating transcription factor 2 (ATF2) and transducin-like enhancer of split 1 (TLE1), resulting in repression of ATF2 target genes. These findings implicate ATF2 transcriptional dysregulation in the etiology of synovial sarcoma.
202. Kadoch C, Crabtree GR: Reversible disruption of mSWI/SNF (BAF) complexes by the SS18-SSX oncogenic fusion in synovial sarcoma. *Cell* 153:71–85, 2013.
    This study demonstrates that the SS18-SSX fusion protein competes for assembly with wild-type SS18, forming an altered transcriptional regulatory complex lacking the tumor suppressor BAF47 (hSNF5). This altered complex transcriptionally activates Sox2, which is uniformly expressed in synovial sarcoma and is essential for proliferation.
237. McArthur GA, Demetri GD, van Oosterom A, et al: Molecular and clinical analysis of locally advanced dermatofibrosarcoma protuberans treated with imatinib. Imatinib Target Exploration Consortium Study B2225. *J Clin Oncol* 23:866–873, 2005.

Oncogenically upregulated PDGFRB kinases were shown to be a clinically effective therapeutic target of the tyrosine kinase inhibitor imatinib.

250. Knezevich SR, Garnett MJ, Pysher TJ, et al: *ETV6-NTRK3* gene fusions and trisomy 11 establish a histogenetic link between mesoblastic nephroma and congenital fibrosarcoma. *Cancer Res* 58:5046–5048, 1998.

This paper demonstrates shared genetic mechanisms in mesoblastic nephroma and congenital fibrosarcoma, providing an explanation for the histologic overlap in these two neoplasms of infancy.

276. Janeway KA, Kim SY, Lodish M, et al: Defects in succinate dehydrogenase in gastrointestinal stromal tumors lacking *KIT* and *PDGFRA* mutations. *Proc Natl Acad Sci U S A* 108:314–318, 2011.

Most pediatric GISTs were shown to have loss-of-function mutations that destroy succinate dehydrogenase activity. These GISTs lack the KIT *and* PDGFRA *mutations found in most adult GISTs.*

326. Wilson BG, Wang X, Shen X, et al: Epigenetic antagonism between polycomb and SWI/SNF complexes during oncogenic transformation. *Cancer Cell* 18:316–328, 2010.

This paper sheds light on the mechanisms by which the rhabdoid tumor suppressor gene SNF5 (SMARCB1) results in dysregulated cell growth. In these studies, SNF5 loss was shown to induce expression of the Polycomb gene EZH2 (which might serve as a therapeutic target).

330. Sigauke E, Rakheja D, Maddox DL, et al: Absence of expression of SMARCB1/INI1 in malignant rhabdoid tumors of the central nervous system, kidneys and soft tissue: an immunohistochemical study with implications for diagnosis. *Mod Pathol* 19:717–725, 2006.

This study demonstrates that immunohistochemistry can be an efficient tool for demonstrating diagnostically relevant genetic loss-of-function events in cancer cells. Here, the authors use immunohistochemistry to confirm that SMARCB1 is silenced in rhabdoid tumors arising in various primary locations.

396. Northcott PA, Shih DJ, Peacock J, et al: Subgroup-specific structural variation across 1,000 medulloblastoma genomes. *Nature* 488:49–56, 2012.

Somatic copy number aberrations were characterized in 1,087 medulloblastomas. These studies showed that highly localized genomic copy number alterations and rearrangements were associated with specific medulloblastoma subtypes. As one example, the most frequent focal copy number gain, a tandem duplication of SNCAIP, was restricted to medulloblastoma group 4a. Potentially targetable aberrations were identified, including recurrent events targeting TGF-β signalling in group 3, and NF-κB signaling in group 4.

399. Rausch T, Jones DT, Zapatka M, et al: Genome sequencing of pediatric medulloblastoma links catastrophic DNA rearrangements with *TP53* mutations. *Cell* 148:59–71, 2012.

This study demonstrates massive chromosomal rearrangements (i.e. chromothripsis) in a medulloblastoma associated with germline TP53 mutation. The authors further show that TP53 inactivation is associated with chromothripsis in many types of cancer, providing a genetic basis for understanding particularly aggressive subtypes of cancer.

485. Weng AP, Ferrando AA, Lee W, et al: Activating mutations of *NOTCH1* in human T cell acute lymphoblastic leukemia. *Science* 306:269–271, 2004.

This work demonstrated the significance of activating intragenic NOTCH1 mutations in 50% of T-cell ALL, including cases with other major translocations, and pointed to the mutant NOTCH1 protein as a potential therapeutic target of gamma secretase inhibitors.

517. Ford AM, Ridge SA, Cabrera ME, et al: In utero rearrangements in the Trithorax-related oncogene in infant leukaemias. *Nature* 363:358–360, 1993.

Through the detection of identical nonconstitutional MLL gene rearrangements in leukemias of monozygous twins, this study was the first of its kind to establish that the MLL translocation in infant leukemia is an in utero event.

535. Figueroa ME, Chen SC, Andersson AK, et al: Integrated genetic and epigenetic analysis of childhood acute lymphoblastic leukemia. *J Clin Invest* 123:3099–3111, 2013.

This study coupled a genome-wide analysis of cytosine methylation profiles with gene expression profiling and discerned an overarching signature of methylation across all subtypes of B-cell lineage ALL, as well as distinct methylation patterns within different leukemia subtypes.

536. Kang H, Wilson CS, Harvey RC, et al: Gene expression profiles predictive of outcome and age in infant acute lymphoblastic leukemia: a Children's Oncology Group study. *Blood* 119:1872–1881, 2012.

This study from the COG P9407 trial, which represents the largest existing gene expression profiling analysis of infant ALL to date, determined distinct gene expression patterns in ALL of infants younger than 90 days of age at diagnosis indicative of different pathways to leukemogenesis compared with older infants and also discerned gene expression markers that are predictive of EFS in infant ALL beyond age and MLL rearrangement status.

541. Roberts KG, Morin RD, Zhang J, et al: Genetic alterations activating kinase and cytokine receptor signaling in high risk acute lymphoblastic leukemia. *Cancer Cell* 22:153–166, 2012.

This work defined the spectrum of cryptic chromosomal rearrangements and mutations associated with the "BCR-ABL1-like" gene expression signature, a poor prognostic feature within high-risk B-cell precursor ALL. Because these abnormalities result in activated kinase signaling, it also tested and validated that this subtype of leukemia is sensitive to tyrosine kinase and JAK2 inhibition.

560. Homminga I, Pieters R, Langerak AW, et al: Integrated transcript and genome analyses reveal *NKX2-1* and *MEF2C* as potential oncogenes in T-cell acute lymphoblastic leukemia. *Cancer Cell* 19:484–497, 2011.

This study combined gene expression profiling and advanced genomic approaches in order to unravel the molecular aberrations underlying ETP ALL as well as those underlying a cluster of T-cell ALL with an immunophentype indicative of cortical arrest as two different recently recognized subsets of T-cell ALL. Whereas novel rearrangements of the MADS-box transcription factor MEFC2 or rearrangements of related factors were found to underlie the former, the cortical subset was defined by NKX2-1, NKX2-2, TLX1, or, less often, MYB gene rearrangements.

601. Anderson K, Lutz C, van Delft FW, et al: Genetic variegation of clonal architecture and propagating cells in leukaemia. *Nature* 469:356–361, 2011.

This work utilizes a highly novel application of multiplex FISH analysis to determine in unprecedented detail the relationships of cells within ETV6/RUNX1 leukemia subclones to one another in order to understand their "clonal architecture," and the results unravel tremendous genetic variegation and continued diversification in propagating cells relative to ancestral cells in subclone evolution.

803. Shannon KM, O'Connell P, Martin GA, et al: Loss of the normal NF1 allele from the bone marrow of children with type 1 neurofibromatosis and malignant myeloid disorders. *N Engl J Med* 330:597–601, 1994.

This study comprises the original description of germline transmission of the mutant NF1 allele and loss of heterozygosity due to deletion of the wild-type allele as a means to dysregulation of RAS signaling in the myeloid malignancies occurring in children with type 1 neurofibromatosis and implicates NF1 as a critical tumor suppressor locus in this leukemia predisposition syndrome.

810. Tartaglia M, Niemeyer CM, Fragale A, et al: Somatic mutations in *PTPN11* in juvenile myelomonocytic leukemia, myelodysplastic syndromes and acute myeloid leukemia. *Nat Genet* 34:148–150, 2003.

This study points to dysregulation of the RAS signaling pathway via somatic mutations in the PTPN11 gene in sporadic myeloid malignancies and establishes the importance of these mutations in the myeloid malignancies beyond the germline PTPN11 mutations occurring in JMML associated with Noonan syndrome.

PEDIATRIC CANCER THERAPEUTICS

CHAPTER 46

Cancer Chemotherapy for Pediatric Patients

Hiroto Inaba, Barthelemy Diouf, and William E. Evans

CHAPTER OUTLINE

In the past two decades we have seen substantial advances in the number of available chemotherapeutic agents to treat a variety of neoplastic diseases, as well as in the discovery and development of new anticancer drugs, while our understanding of the biology and genetics of cancer continues to grow.[1,2,3,4] The tools at our disposal now include classes of molecules with highly distinct structures and innovative mechanisms of action and an impressive array of new techniques and novel uses for existing agents. In this chapter we will review the principles of chemotherapy in children, discuss the factors that influence individual responses to chemotherapy, and describe how pharmacokinetic, pharmacodynamic, and/or pharmacogenetic principles are used when conducting clinical trials that provide therapy tailored to individual patients.

CHEMOTHERAPEUTIC AGENTS

Chemotherapeutic agents used to treat pediatric cancer are generally similar to those used with adults, including conventional cytotoxic drugs and molecularly targeted agents. The former class can be subdivided into two large groups based on the dependence of their mechanism of action on the cell cycle. Cell cycle–nonspecific agents, which include alkylating agents, platinum agents, and most antitumor antibiotics, kill both quiescent and cycling tumor cells. Cell cycle–specific agents include antimetabolites and agents that interact with tubulin and topoisomerases. Conventional cytotoxic agents can target both malignant and normal cells and often cause adverse effects. During the past decade, the development of molecularly targeted chemotherapy has been revolutionized by a greater understanding of the biologic and genetic features of malignant disease.[2-4] Table 46-1 provides an overview of the drugs used to treat childhood cancers and their key pharmacologic features.

CLINICAL APPLICATION OF CHEMOTHERAPY

Chemotherapy has four major roles in the management of cancer: (1) primary cytoreduction therapy, (2) adjuvant therapy, (3) neoadjuvant therapy, and (4) site-directed therapy. Primary cytoreduction therapy is used when no superior alternative treatment is available (such as surgery and radiation therapy). Hematologic malignancies and some solid tumors of childhood are significantly chemosensitive and can be cured by serial courses of chemotherapy (e.g., induction, consolidation, and continuation therapy for acute lymphoblastic leukemia [ALL]). The chemosensitive malignancies also include acute myeloid leukemia (AML), lymphomas (both non-Hodgkin and Hodgkin), germ cell tumors, Wilms tumor, and embryonal rhabdomyosarcoma. Chemotherapy can also be used as an adjuvant therapy, wherein systemic treatment is applied to enhance local tumor control and to eradicate occult disseminated disease after surgery and/or radiation therapy. Occult residual disease at original sites and micrometastases are frequently present even after

Text continued on p. 1414

TABLE 46-1   Key Features of Drugs Used in Pediatric Oncology

Drug (Trade Name; Chemical Class)	Mechanism of Action	Antitumor Activity	Route of Administration	Primary Pathway of Elimination	Enzymes and Transporters	Principal Adverse Effects
Alkylating Agents						
Mechlorethamine (Mustargen; nitrogen mustard, mustine, HN2)	Alkylation; DNA cross-linking	Hodgkin lymphoma (MOPP)	IV injection	Hydrolysis; liver	N-demethylation (CYP)	A, M, N&V, Mu, HU, Derm, V, Phleb, G, SM
Melphalan (Alkeran; mechlorethamine analogue)	Alkylation; DNA cross-linking	HDCT	IV injection or infusion; oral	Hydrolysis; renal	GSTP1, LAT1, ABCB1	A, M, N&V, D, Mu, Derm, Vas, Phleb, SIADH, G, SM
Chlorambucil (Leukeran; mechlorethamine analogue)	Alkylation; DNA cross-linking	Hodgkin lymphoma (ChlVPP)	Oral	Hydrolysis	GSTP1, ABCC2	A, M, N&V, HU, P, S, G, SM
Cyclophosphamide (Cytoxan; mechlorethamine analogue)	Alkylation (prodrug); DNA cross-linking	Leukemias, lymphomas, neuroblastoma, sarcoma	IV infusion; oral	Hydrolysis; liver	CYP2B6, CYP2C9, CYP3A4, CYP3A5, GSTA1, GSTP1, ALDH1A1, ALDH3A1	A, M, N&V, Cy, SIADH, C, P, G, SM
Ifosfamide (Ifex; mechlorethamine analogue)	Alkylation (prodrug); DNA cross-linking	Sarcomas, germ cell	IV infusion	Hydrolysis; liver	CYP2A6, CYP2B6, CYP3A4, CYP2C19, OCT2	A, M, N&V, Met, Cy, SIADH, NT, C, P, R, G, SM
Bendamustine (Treanda)	Alkylation; DNA cross-linking; blocks purine synthesis	Hodgkin lymphoma, lymphoma, leukemia	IV infusion	Liver	CYP1A2	M, N&V, H, P, PE, NT
Thiotepa (Thioplex; aziridine)	Alkylation; DNA cross-linking	HDCT	IV injection or infusion; intrathecal, intravesical	Liver	NA	A, M, N&V, HU, Derm, Cy, G, SM
Busulfan (Myleran; alkyl alkane sulfonate)	Alkylation; DNA cross-linking	HDCT	IV infusion; oral	Conjugation with glutathione; liver	CYP3A4, GSTA1, GSTP1	A, M, N&V, Mu, Derm, HU, AI, NT, VOD, P, S, G, SM
Carmustine (BiCNU; BCNU, nitrosourea)	Alkylation; DNA cross-linking; carbamoylation	Brain tumors, Hodgkin lymphoma, lymphoma	IV infusion; wafer implant (glioblastoma)	Chemical hydrolysis; liver	CYP	M, N&V, Phleb, S (wafer), C, H, P, R, G, SM

TABLE 46-1   Key Features of Drugs Used in Pediatric Oncology (Continued)

Drug (Trade Name; Chemical Class)	Mechanism of Action	Antitumor Activity	Route of Administration	Primary Pathway of Elimination	Enzymes and Transporters	Principal Adverse Effects
Lomustine (CeeNU; CCNU, nitrosourea)	Alkylation; DNA cross-linking; carbamoylation	Brain tumors, Hodgkin lymphoma, lymphoma	Oral	Chemical hydrolysis; liver	CYP2D6	M, N&V, NT, C, H, P, R, G, SM
Dacarbazine (DTIC, DTIC-Dome; imidazole-carboxamide)	Methylation inhibition (prodrug)	Hodgkin lymphoma, neuroblastoma, sarcomas	IV infusion	Chemical hydrolysis; liver, renal	N-demethylation (CYP); CYP1A2, CYP2E1	M, N&V, Flu, H
Procarbazine (Mutulane; imidazole-carboxamide)	Methylation inhibition (prodrug)	Brain tumors; Hodgkin lymphoma (ChlVPP)	Oral	Chemical hydrolysis; liver, renal	CYP, MAO	M, N&V, Mu, Flu, NT, Derm, G, SM
Temozolomide (Temodar; imidazole-carboxamide)	Methylation inhibition (prodrug)	Brain tumors	Oral	Chemical hydrolysis	CYP (minor)	M, N&V, NT, PE, H
Antimetabolites						
Cytarabine (Cytosar; Ara-C, cytosine arabinoside; cytidine analogue)	Incorporated into DNA; inhibits DNA polymerase; terminates DNA chain elongation	Leukemias	IV injection or infusion; intrathecal; SC	Activated to triphosphate; deamination	Cytidine deaminase, CNT1, ENT1, ENT2, ABCC4, ABCC11	M, N&V, Mu, GI, HU, Derm, HFS, PE, Conj, NT, H, PE
Azacytidine (Vidaza; cytidine analogue)	Hypomethylation of DNA (low dose)	MDS, AML	SC	Activated to triphosphate; chemical degradation; deamination	Cytidine deaminase	M, N&V, F, Mu, D, Inj, Derm
Decitabine (Dacogen; cytidine analogue)	Hypomethylation of DNA (low dose)	MDS, AML	IV infusion	Activated to triphosphate; chemical degradation; deamination	Cytidine deaminase	M, N&V, F, Mu, D, Derm
Gemcitabine (Gemzar; cytidine analogue)	Incorporated into DNA; inhibits DNA polymerase; terminates DNA chain elongation; inhibits ribonucleotide reductase (prodrug)	Solid tumors, lymphoma	IV infusion	Activated to triphosphate; deamination	Cytidine deaminase, CNT1, ENT1	M, N&V, Mu, D, F, Flu, Derm, NT, PE, H, R
Cladribine (Leustatin; adenosine analogue)	Incorporated into DNA; inhibits DNA polymerase; terminates DNA chain elongation; inhibits ribonucleotide reductase (prodrug)	Leukemias	IV infusion	Activated to triphosphate; renal; liver	Oxidative cleavage, oxidation, conjugation, CNT1, CNT2, CNT3, ENT1, ABCG2	M, N&V, D, Derm, NT

Continued on following page

TABLE 46-1   Key Features of Drugs Used in Pediatric Oncology (Continued)

Drug (Trade Name; Chemical Class)	Mechanism of Action	Antitumor Activity	Route of Administration	Primary Pathway of Elimination	Enzymes and Transporters	Principal Adverse Effects
Clofarabine (Clolar; adenosine analogue)	Incorporated into DNA; inhibits DNA polymerase; terminates DNA chain elongation; inhibits ribonucleotide reductase (prodrug)	Leukemias	IV infusion	Activated to triphosphate; extrahepatic	NA	M, N&V, D, C, H, R
Fludarabine (Fludara; adenosine analogue)	Incorporated into DNA; inhibits DNA polymerase; terminates DNA chain elongation; inhibits ribonucleotide reductase (prodrug)	AML, CML, indolent lymphomas	IV infusion	Activated to triphosphate; renal	NA	M, HA, Derm, fever, H, NT, TLS
Nelarabine (Arranon)	Incorporated into DNA; inhibits DNA synthesis	ALL	IV infusion	Activated to ara-guanine triphosphate; liver, renal	Adenosine deaminase	M, N&V, NT, P, PE
6-Mercaptopurine (Purinethol; hypoxanthine analogue)	Incorporated into DNA, RNA; blocks purine synthesis (prodrug)	ALL	Oral	Liver, renal (high dose)	TPMT, HGPRT, ENT2, OAT2, OAT3, ABCC4	M, H, Mu, N&V, HU, crystalluria, GI
6-Thioguanine (guanine analogue)	Incorporated into DNA, RNA; blocks purine synthesis (prodrug)	ALL, AML	Oral	Liver	TPMT, HGPRT, CNT3, ENT2, OAT3, ABCC5	M, H, Mu, N&V, HU, crystalluria
Hydroxyurea (Hydrea, Droxia)	Interferes with synthesis of DNA synthesis; inhibits ribonucleoside diphosphate reductase	ALL, AML	Oral	Liver, renal	OATP1B3, UT-A, UT-B1	M, H, Mu, N&V
5-Fluorouracil (fluoropyrimidine)	Incorporated into RNA, DNA; inhibits thymidine synthase (prodrug of 5′-DFUR)	Carcinomas, hepatic tumors	IV injection or infusion	Liver	DPD, GSTP1, hNT1, OAT2,	M, Mu, N&V, HFS, D, Derm, NT, C
Capecitabine (Xeloda; fluoropyrimidine)	Incorporated into RNA, DNA; inhibits thymidine synthase (prodrug of 5′-DFUR)	Colorectal cancer (in development)	Oral	Urine	CES2, CES1A1, cytidine deaminase, thymidine phosphorylase, DPD, CNT1, ABCA1	M, Mu, N&V, HFS, D, Derm, NT, C

TABLE 46-1 Key Features of Drugs Used in Pediatric Oncology (Continued)

Drug (Trade Name; Chemical Class)	Mechanism of Action	Antitumor Activity	Route of Administration	Primary Pathway of Elimination	Enzymes and Transporters	Principal Adverse Effects
Methotrexate (Trexall; antifolate)	Interferes with folate metabolism	Leukemias, lymphomas, osteosarcoma	Oral; IM; SC; IV injection; intrathecal	Renal	FPGS, GGH, OAT1, OAT2, OAT3, OAT4, OATP1A2, OATP1B1, OATP1B3, OATP4C1, RFC, PCFT, ABCB1, ABCC1, ABCC2, ABCC3, ABCC4, ABCG2	M, Mu, Derm, H, R, NT
Pemetrexed (Alimta; antifolate)	Interferes with folate metabolism	Various (in development)	IV infusion	Renal	NA	M, fatigue, Mu, HFS, Derm
Antitumor Antibiotics						
Bleomycin (Blenoxane)	Free radical–mediated DNA strand breaks	Lymphomas, germ cell tumor	IV injection; IM, SC	Renal	OCT6	P, Derm, fever, Mu, A, HSR, N&V
Dactinomycin (Cosmegen)	DNA cross-linking	Solid tumors	IV injection	Renal, liver	NA	M, Mu, N&V, D, A, H, V
Mitomycin C (Neulasta)	DNA cross-linking	Carcinomas	IV injection or infusion; intravesical	Liver	ABCB1	M, N&V, Mu, HU, anemia, VOD
Daunorubicin (Daunomycin; anthracycline)	DNA strand breaks (topo II)	ALL, AML, lymphomas	IV injection or infusion	Renal, liver	OCTN1, ABCB1, aldoketoreductase	M, Mu, N&V, D, A, C, V
Doxorubicin (Adriamycin; anthracycline)	DNA strand breaks (topo II)	ALL, AML, lymphomas, solid tumors	IV infusion	Liver	CYP2D6, CYP3A4, GSTP1, OCT6, OCTN1, ABCB1, ABCB5, ABCG2, aldoketoreductase	M, Mu, N&V, A, D, C, V
Epirubicin (Ellence; anthracycline)	DNA strand breaks (topo II)	Solid tumors, leukemia (in development)	IV infusion	Renal, liver	ABCB1, ABCC1, ABCG2, aldoketoreductase	M, Mu, N&V, A, C, V
Idarubicin (Idamycin; anthracycline)	DNA strand breaks (topo II)	ALL, AML, lymphomas	IV injection or infusion; oral	Renal, liver	ABCB1, aldoketoreductase	M, Mu, N&V, D, A, C, V
Mitoxantrone (Novantrone; anthracenedione)	DNA strand breaks (topo II)	ALL, AML, lymphomas	IV infusion; IP	Renal, liver	OCTN1, ABCB1, ABCG2	M, Mu, N&V, A, urine, veins and nail discoloration
Asparaginases						
l-Asparaginase (Elspar, Kidrolase; native asparaginase from *Escherichia coli*)	Depletion of plasma asparagine	ALL, lymphomas	IV infusion (>30 min), IM	Nonrenal	NA	HSR, thrombosis, GI, glucose intolerance, coagulopathy, hyperglycemia, H
Crisantaspase (Erwinase; Erwinia l-asparaginase, native asparaginase from *Erwinia chrysanthemi*)	Depletion of plasma asparagine	ALL, lymphomas	IV infusion (>30 min), IM	Nonrenal	NA	HSR, thrombosis, GI, glucose intolerance, coagulopathy, hyperglycemia, H

Continued on following page

TABLE 46-1   Key Features of Drugs Used in Pediatric Oncology (Continued)

Drug (Trade Name; Chemical Class)	Mechanism of Action	Antitumor Activity	Route of Administration	Primary Pathway of Elimination	Enzymes and Transporters	Principal Adverse Effects
Pegasparaginase (Oncaspar; PEG-asparaginase, from *E. coli*)	Depletion of plasma asparagine	ALL, lymphomas	IV infusion (1-2 hours)	Nonrenal	NA	HSR, thrombosis, GI, glucose intolerance, coagulopathy, hyperglycemia, H
Corticosteroids						
Dexamethasone (Decadron)	Receptor-mediated lympholysis	Leukemias, lymphomas	Oral, IV injection; IM	Liver	CYP3A4, ABCB1	Muscle weakness, osteoporosis, Derm, hypertension, N&V, headache
Prednisolone (Orapred OTD, Pediapred)	Receptor-mediated lympholysis	Leukemias, lymphomas	Oral; IV injection	Renal, liver	CYP3A4, sulfation, glucuronidation	Muscle weakness, osteoporosis, Derm, hypertension, N&V, headache
Prednisone (Deltasone)	Receptor-mediated lympholysis (prodrug)	Leukemias, lymphomas	Oral	Renal, liver	CYP3A4, sulfation, glucuronidation	Muscle weakness, osteoporosis, Derm, hypertension, N&V, headache
Platinum Compounds						
Carboplatin (Paraplatin)	Platination; DNA cross-linking	Brain tumors, neuroblastoma, sarcomas	IV infusion	Renal	CTR1, ATP7A	M, N&V, NT, EA, HSR
Cisplatin (Platinol)	Platination; DNA cross-linking	Testicular, brain tumors, osteosarcoma, neuroblastoma	IV infusion	Renal	GSTP1, OCT1, OCT2, CTR1, ABCC2, ABCC4, ATP7B, MATE1	N&V, R, NT, M, EA, O, HSR
Oxaliplatin (Eloxatin)	Platination; DNA cross-linking	Colorectal cancer, lymphoma (in development)	IV infusion	Renal	GSTP1, OCT1, OCT2, OCT3, OCTN1, OCTN2, MATE1, MATE2-K	NT, N&V, D, M, R, HSR
Retinoids						
All-*trans*-retinoic acid (ATRA; Vesanoid; tretinoin; retinol derivative)	Differentiation agent	Acute promyelocytic leukemia	Oral	Liver	CYP2C8, CYP2A6, CYP2B6, CYP2C9	Retinoic acid syndrome, pseudotumor cerebri, cheilitis
13-*cis*-retinoic acid (Accutane; retinol derivative)	Differentiation agent	Neuroblastoma	Oral	Liver	CYP2B6, CYP2C8, CYP2C9, CYP3A4/5, CYP2A6, CYP2D6	Cheilitis, conjunctivitis, dry mouth, xerosis, pruritus, headache

TABLE 46-1   Key Features of Drugs Used in Pediatric Oncology (Continued)

Drug (Trade Name; Chemical Class)	Mechanism of Action	Antitumor Activity	Route of Administration	Primary Pathway of Elimination	Enzymes and Transporters	Principal Adverse Effects
Topoisomerase-Interactive Agents						
Etoposide (VePesid; VP-16)	DNA strand breaks (topo II)	ALL, AML, lymphomas, neuroblastoma, sarcomas, brain tumors	IV infusion	Renal, liver	CYP3A4, CYP3A5, CYP1A2, CYP2E1, UGT1A1, OCTN2, OATP1B1, ABCB1, ABCC1, ABCC2	M, N&V, hypotension, HSR, SM
Teniposide (Vumon; VM-26)	DNA strand breaks (topo II)	ALL	IV infusion; oral	Liver	CYP3A4, ABCB1	M, N&V, HSR, hypotension, SM
Irinotecan (Camptosar; CPT-11; camptothecin analogue)	DNA strand breaks (topo I; prodrug of SN-38)	Rhabdomyosarcoma, solid tumors	IV infusion	Renal, liver	CYP3A4, CYP3A5, CYP2B6, CES2, UGT1A1, OATP1B1, ABCB1, ABCC2, ABCC4, ABCG2,	M, D, N&V, A, H
Topotecan (Hycamptin; camptothecin analogue)	DNA strand breaks (topo I)	Neuroblastoma; rhabdomyosarcoma	IV infusion	Renal	OAT3, ABCB1, ABCC4, ABCG2	M, Mu, D, N&V, A, Derm, H
Tubulin-Interactive Agents						
Docetaxel (Taxotere; taxanes)	Microtubule depolarization inhibitor	Solid tumors	IV infusion	Liver	CYP3A4/5, CYP2C8, OAT2, OATP1B3, ABCB1, ABCC2, ABCC10	M, HSR, A, NT, Derm, Mu
Paclitaxel (Taxol; Abraxane; taxane)	Microtubule depolarization inhibitor	Solid tumors	IV infusion	Liver	CYP2C8, CYP2C9, CYP3A4/5, OAT2, OATP1B1, OATP1B3, ABCB1, ABCC2, ABCC10	M, HSR, A, NT, M, C
Vinblastine (Velban; Vinca alkaloid)	Microtubule polarization inhibitor	Histiocytosis, Hodgkin lymphoma, testicular cancer	IV push or infusion	Liver	CYP3A4, CYP2D6, ABCB1, ABCC1, ABCC2, ABCC10, ABCG2	M, A, Mu, NT, V
Vincristine (Oncovin; Vinca alkaloid)	Microtubule polarization inhibitor	ALL, lymphomas, solid tumors	IV injection	Liver	CYP3A5, CYP3A4, ABCB1, ABCC1, ABCC2, ABCC10	NT, A, SIADH hypotension, V
Vinorelbine (Navelbine; Vinca alkaloid)	Microtubule polarization inhibitor	Solid tumor, Hodgkin lymphoma (in development)	IV injection of infusion	Liver	CYP3A4, CYP2D6	M, NT, A, V
Tyrosine Kinase Inhibitors						
Imatinib (Gleevec; STI-571, benzamide analogue)	Abl inhibitor	Ph+ CML, ALL	Oral	Liver	CYP3A4, CYP3A5, CYP2D6, CYP2C9, CYP2C19, OATP1A2, OATP1B3, OCT1, ABCB1, ABCC1, ABCC4, ABCG2	N&V, F, D, H, M

Continued on following page

TABLE 46-1   Key Features of Drugs Used in Pediatric Oncology (Continued)

Drug (Trade Name; Chemical Class)	Mechanism of Action	Antitumor Activity	Route of Administration	Primary Pathway of Elimination	Enzymes and Transporters	Principal Adverse Effects
Dasatinib (Sprycel; carboxamide analogue)	Src-Abl inhibitor	Ph+ CML, ALL	Oral	Liver	CYP3A4, FMO3, OATP1B3, ABCB1, ABCC4, ABCG2	M, D, N&V, Derm, fatigue, P, headache
Nilotinib (Tasigna)	Abl inhibitor	Ph+ CML, ALL	Oral	Liver	CYP3A4, OATP1B1, OATP1B3, ABCB1, ABCG2	M, N&V, D, C, Derm, MS, P
Ponatinib (Iclusig)	Src-Abl inhibitor	Ph+ CML, ALL (in development)	Oral	Liver	CYP3A4, CYP2C8, CYP2D6, CYP3A5	M, N&V, D, C, Derm, H, GI, MS
Sunitinib (Sutent; carboxamide analogue)	VEGFR, PDGFR inhibitor	In development	Oral	Liver	CYP3A4, CYP1A2, OATP1B1, ABCB1, ABCG2	M, D, Derm, anorexia, hypertension, fatigue, headache
Sorafenib (Nexavar; carboxamide analogue)	Raf and FLT3 inhibitor	In development	Oral	Liver	CYP3A4, UGT1A9, OATP1B1, OATP1B3, ABCB1, ABCG2	M, D, Derm, anorexia, hypertension, fatigue, headache
Erlotinib (Tarceva; OSI-774, quinazolinamine analogue)	EGFR inhibitor	Solid tumors (in development)	Oral	Liver	CYP3A4/5, CYP1A2, ABCG2	Derm, D, anorexia, fatigue, N&V, dyspnea, fatigue
Gefitinib (Iressa; ZD1839, anilinoquinazoline analogue)	EGFR inhibitor	Solid tumors (in development)	Oral	Liver	CYP3A4/5, CYP2D6, OATP1B3, ABCB1, ABCG2	D, Derm, N&V
Crizotinib (Xalkori)	ALK inhibitor	ALCL, non–small cell lung cancer, neuroblastoma (in development)	Oral	Liver, Renal	CYP3A4/5, OATP1B1, OATP1B3, ABCB1	Ocular, N&V, Edema, H, NT
Pazopanib (Votrient)	Vascular endothelial growth factor inhibitor	Solid tumors (in development)	Oral	Liver	CYP3A4, CYP1A2, CYP2C8, OATP1B1, OATP1B3, ABCB1, ABCG2	D, N&V, M, H, C, MS, P
Vemurafenib (Zelboraf)	BRAF inhibitor	Melanoma	Oral	Liver	CYP3A4, OATP1B3, ABCB1	Derm, N&V, MS, PE
Proteasome Inhibitors						
Bortezomib (Velcade)	Proteasome inhibitor	Leukemia, lymphoma (in development)	IV injection, SC	Liver	CYP2C19, CYP3A4, CYP1A2	M, N&V, NT, D, P
Histone Deacetylase Inhibitors						
Vorinostat (Zolinza)	Histone deacetylase inhibitor	Leukemia, lymphoma (in development)	Oral	Liver, Renal	NA	D, N&V, PE, A, M, NT, R

TABLE 46-1 Key Features of Drugs Used in Pediatric Oncology (Continued)

Drug (Trade Name; Chemical Class)	Mechanism of Action	Antitumor Activity	Route of Administration	Primary Pathway of Elimination	Enzymes and Transporters	Principal Adverse Effects
Other Molecular Targeting Agents						
Arsenic trioxide (Trisenox)	Degrades PML-RARA and induces apoptosis	Acute promyelocytic leukemia, MDS	IV infusion	Hydrolysis	NA	C, NT, Derm, N&V, D, M, H, P
Everolimus (Afinitor)	mTOR kinase inhibitor	Solid tumor, leukemia, subependymal giant cell astrocytoma (in development)	Oral	Liver	CYP3A4, ABCB1	N&V, D, HR, P, PE, Derm, M, Mu
Temsirolimus (Torisel)	mTOR kinase inhibitor	Solid tumor, leukemia (in development)	IV infusion	Liver	CYP3A4, ABCB1	N&V, D, HR, P, PE, Derm, M, Mu
Ruxolitinib (Jakavi)	Janus kinase inhibitor	In development	Oral	Liver	CYP3A4	M, D, N&V, H, P, PE
Vismodegib (Erivedge)	Hedgehog inhibitor	In development	Oral	Liver	CYP2C9, CYP3A4, ABCB1	M, A, MS
Antibodies						
Rituximab (Rituxan)	CD20 antibody	Leukemia, lymphoma	IV infusion	NA	NA	M, N&V, F, PE, NT
Gemtuzumab ozogamicin	CD33 antibody, DNA double-strand break	AML	IV infusion	NA	NA	M, H, C, F, N&V, R
Brentuximab vedotin (Adcetris)	CD30 antibody, disrupt microtubule network	Hodgkin lymphoma, ALCL	IV infusion	Liver	CYP3A4	NT, F, PE, Derm, N&V, D, M, P
Alemtuzumab (Campath)	CD52 antibody	Leukemia, lymphoma, HSCT	IV infusion, SC	NA	NA	F, M, MS, C
Bevacizumab (Avastin)	Vascular endothelial growth factor antibody	Solid tumors (in development)	IV infusion	NA	NA	M, C, D, D, N&V, MS, P, R
Biological Response Modulator						
Aldesleukin (Proleukin)	Interleukin-2	Melanoma, leukemia, cell therapy	IV infusion, SC	Renal	NA	D, F, Flu, C, PE, Derm, N&V, M, R, P

A, Alopecia; *ABC*, adenosine triphosphate–binding cassette transporter; *AI*, adrenal insufficiency; *ALCL*, anaplastic large cell lymphoma; *ALDH*, aldehyde dehydrogenase; *ALK*, anaplastic lymphoma kinase; *ALL*, acute lymphoblastic leukemia; *AML*, acute myeloid leukemia; *ANC*, absolute neutrophil count; *AS*, addisonian syndrome; *BRAF*, v-raf murine sarcoma viral oncogene homolog B; *C*, cardiac toxicity; *CES*, carboxylesterase; *ChlVPP*, chlorambucil, vinblastine, procarbazine, and prednisolone; *CML*, chronic myelogenous leukemia; *CNT*, concentrative nucleoside transporter; *Conj*, conjunctivitis; *CTR*, copper transporter; *Cy*, cystitis; *CYP*, cytochrome P-450 enzyme; *D*, diarrhea; *Derm*, dermatologic toxicity (skin rash and/or nail changes); *5′-DFUR*, 5′-deoxy-5-fluorouridine; *DNA*, deoxyribonucleic acid; *DPD*, dihydropyrimidine dehydrogenase; *EA*, electrolyte abnormalities; *EGFR*, epidermal growth factor receptor; *ENT*, equilibrative nucleoside transporter; *F*, fever; *FLT3*, fms-related tyrosine kinase 3; *Flu*, flu-like syndrome; *FMO3*, flavin-containing monooxygenase 3; *G*, gonadal toxicity; *GGH*, γ-glutamyl hydrolase; *GI*, gastrointestinal (ulcers, pancreatitis); *GST*, glutathione-S-transferase; *H*, hepatic; *HA*, hemolytic syndrome; *HDCT*, high-dose chemotherapy; *HFS*, hand-foot syndrome; *hNT1*, human nucleoside transporter 1; *HSR*, hypersensitivity reactions; *HU*, hyperuricemia; *IM*, intramuscular injection; *Inj*, injection site reaction or irritation; *IP*, intraperitoneal injection; *IV*, intravenous; *LAT*, L-type amino acid transporter; *M*, myelosuppression; *MAO*, monoamine oxidase; *MATE*, multidrug and toxin extrusion transporter; *MDS*, myelodysplastic syndrome; *Met*, metabolic acidosis; *MOPP*, mechlorethamine, vincristine, prednisone, and procarbazine; *MS*, muscular skeletal; *mTOR*, mammalian target of rapamycin; *Mu*, mucositis; *NA*, information not available; *N&V*, nausea and vomiting; *NT*, neurotoxicity; *O*, ototoxicity; *OAT*, organic anion transporter; *OATP*, organic anion-transporting polypeptide; *OCT*, organic cation transporter; *P*, pulmonary toxicity; *PCFT*, proton-coupled folate transporter; *PDGFR*, platelet-derived growth factor receptor; *PE*, peripheral edema; *Ph+*, Philadelphia chromosome–positive; *Phleb*, phlebitis; *Plt*, platelets; *PML-RARA*, promyelocytic leukemia-retinoic acid receptor, alpha; *R*, renal toxicity; *RFC*, reduced folate carrier, *RNA*, ribonucleic acid; *S*, seizures; *SC*, subcutaneous injection; *SIADH*, syndrome of inappropriate antidiuretic hormone; *SM*, secondary malignancy; *TLS*, tumor lysis syndrome; *UGT*, uridine diphosphate glucuronosyltransferase; *UT*, urea transporter; *V*, vesicant; *Vas*, vasculitis; *VEGFR*, vascular endothelial growth factor receptor; *VOD*, veno-occlusive disease.

macroscopic resolution of local disease. Before the routine use of adjuvant chemotherapy, 60% to 95% of children with localized solid tumors experienced relapse at primary or metastatic sites after receiving local control therapy alone. Thus the goal of adjuvant chemotherapy is to reduce the risk of local and systemic recurrence by eradicating microscopic residual disease or micrometastases in lungs, bone, bone marrow, lymph nodes, or other sites. The efficacy of adjuvant chemotherapy for Wilms tumor, Ewing sarcoma, rhabdomyosarcoma, osteosarcoma, and brain tumors (e.g., medulloblastoma) is well established. Neoadjuvant therapy may be used to reduce the size of primary and metastatic tumors, allow definitive surgical resection, and eradicate possible micrometastases when localized cancers cannot otherwise be optimally managed. This approach is often used with childhood solid tumors, including osteosarcomas, neuroblastomas, hepatoblastomas, and Wilms tumors. Examples of site-directed therapy include instillation of chemotherapy agents into sanctuary sites, such as intrathecal chemotherapy for leukemia and site-directed perfusion therapy (e.g., injection of agents into the feeding artery of tumors such as sarcomas in the extremities, liver tumors, and retinoblastoma).

CHEMOTHERAPY IN CHILDREN

The current strategy is to administer chemotherapeutic agents at the maximum tolerated dose—that is, the dose just below that which causes unacceptable toxicity. This approach is based on a series of prospective and retrospective analyses showing that the greater the dose intensity (i.e., the dose delivered over a standard time interval), the better the outcome.[5,6] However, the narrow therapeutic index (i.e., the ratio of the theoretical minimum effective dose to the maximum tolerated dose) of most anticancer drugs demands a rigorous effort to optimize these regimens (Fig. 46-1). Effective systemic treatment requires judicious application of cytotoxic drugs that differ only slightly in their toxicity to normal cells and their therapeutic lethality to malignant cells. Pediatric oncologists and pharmacologists have studied multiple approaches in search of the best way to exploit this narrow therapeutic margin, including the use of drug combinations with different dose-limiting toxicities, the rescue or reconstitution of normal tissues (e.g., administration of leucovorin after methotrexate and use of bone marrow transplantation after high-dose chemotherapy), and the use of biologic modifiers to counteract specific mechanisms of resistance.

The therapeutic approaches used in adults cannot be directly transferred to growing children because certain agents have an extremely narrow therapeutic range in pediatric patients, and in most cases little or no information is available about the intrinsic sensitivity of a tumor to a particular agent and the tolerability of a given dose. Physiologic differences between children and adults, such as body composition, hepatic metabolism, and renal function, may affect the pharmacokinetics of a drug (i.e., drug disposition involving its absorption, distribution, metabolism, and excretion and the plasma concentration–time profile of the drug in the body) and thus the

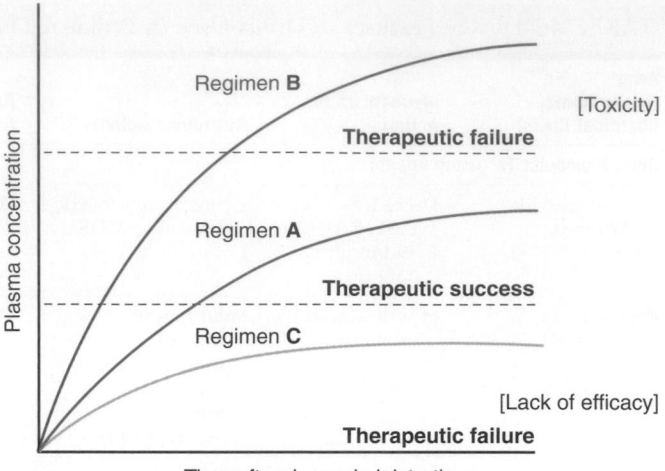

Figure 46-1 Narrow therapeutic index for chemotherapy administration. When a drug is given at a fixed dose and at fixed time intervals, it accumulates within the body until a plateau is reached. With regimen A, therapeutic success is achieved after a period of time. With regimen B, the therapeutic plasma concentration is achieved more quickly, but the plasma concentration ultimately becomes too high and causes toxicity. Regimen C does not reach therapeutic plasma concentration.

pharmacodynamics of a drug (i.e., drug action; the quantitative study of the effects of a drug, including efficacy and toxicity).[7,8] Children may also be more susceptible than adults to the toxicity of agents even when the pharmacokinetics are similar, as in the case of all-*trans*-retinoic acid for pseudotumor cerebri.[9] Further, pharmacokinetic studies have shown substantial interpatient variability in drug disposition and systemic drug exposure in children; these findings may underlie the observed variability in toxicity and response. The pharmacokinetics and pharmacodynamics of a drug, and thus its anticancer effects, are also influenced by physiologic factors that differ in children and adults, by drug-drug interactions, and by genetic influences (pharmacogenomics). Although pediatric cancer is rare compared with adult cancer, optimizing treatment in a patient group with a higher cure rate and a longer expected survival becomes critical to minimize the incidence of preventable acute and late complications in children while maintaining efficacy.

PHARMACOKINETIC CHANGES DURING CHILDHOOD

Pharmacokinetic parameters include half-life ($T_{1/2}$), area under the plasma concentration versus time curve (AUC), bioavailability, volume of distribution (Vd), steady state concentration, and clearance (Table 46-2). Body composition and organ function at the extremes of age can affect drug disposition and effect.[10,11] Changes as a child develops and matures may alter absorption, distribution, metabolism, and excretion of chemotherapeutic agents (Fig. 46-2).

The importance of understanding the influence of age on the pharmacokinetics and pharmacodynamics of

TABLE 46-2   Pharmacokinetic Parameters

Parameter	Units	Definition
Half-life ($T_{1/2}$)	Time (h)	The time necessary to halve the plasma concentration. Useful for determination of frequency of drug administration to obtain the desired plasma concentration. The half-life of a particular drug is usually independent of the dose administered. However, it may change according to the saturation of a mechanism (e.g., elimination, catabolism, or binding to plasma proteins).
Area under the curve (AUC)	Concentration × time ($\mu M \times h$)	Calculated as f ([C] × Dt); [C] is measured concentration and Dt is the interval of time between two measurements. The integral of the plasma concentration versus an interval of definite time. It represents an important quantitative measure of total systemic drug exposure. Also, it is required for the calculation of other pharmacokinetic parameters such as clearance and bioavailability.
Bioavailability (F)	Fraction (%)	The percentage of the administered drug concentration that is achieved in the central compartment. Generally measured by comparing the AUCs obtained after intravenous administration with those obtained after oral administration. For example, the AUC obtained after intravenous administration usually corresponds to bioavailability (i.e., 100%). After oral administration, the AUC corresponds at best to an identical bioavailability; it is generally lower.
Volume of distribution (Vd)	Volume (L)	The fictitious volume in which the drug would have been distributed by supposing that its concentration is homogeneous (i.e., the average tissue concentration is identical to that of plasma). Expressed as Vd = dose/C0 (initial concentration). For example, after intravenous injection of 100 mg of a drug whose initial concentration, C0, in plasma is 10 mg/L, the volume of distribution is 10 L. For a given drug, the knowledge of its desired concentration in blood and of its volume of distribution allows evaluation of the dose to administer.
Steady state concentration (Css)	Concentration (μM)	The state of equilibrium obtained at the end of a certain number of administrations. To obtain an increase in the plasma concentration with repeated administrations, it is necessary that a residual concentration persists at the time of the following administration. At the steady state, if the dose and the frequency of administration remain constant, the concentration obtained will also be constant. The steady state is usually obtained at the end of approximately five half-lives.
Clearance (Cl)	Volume/Time (mL/min)	Defined as the theoretic volume from which drug is completely removed per unit time. Plasma clearance is the apparent volume of plasma from which drug is cleared per unit of time. Total clearance is the fraction of the volume of distribution, Vd, which is completely cleared per unit of time. The total clearance depends on the constant of elimination and thus on $T_{1/2}$ and on Vd, which is considered to be sum of metabolic and spontaneous chemical degradation, as well as biliary/fecal and renal elimination.

individual anticancer agents has increased steadily with advances in the treatment of infant and childhood malignancies. Although the influence of age has been formally evaluated for a limited number of cytotoxic drugs, further efforts to improve the individualization of drug therapy on the basis of maturation and development are necessary to enhance the odds of therapeutic success.

Absorption

Medications are typically administered via the gastrointestinal tract (mainly orally), intravenously (IV), intramuscularly, and via the skin (subcutaneous or transdermal). Orally administered agents must surmount multiple barriers to reach the systemic circulation (Figs. 46-2 and 46-3). Gastric pH, gastrointestinal motility, transporter-mediated uptake and efflux, and metabolism before a drug enters the systemic circulation play important roles in the absorption of many drugs. Although chemotherapy is rarely administered intramuscularly or transdermally, the lack of muscle and fatty tissue in newborns and infants and their thin skin would cause erratic absorption and increase the risk of toxicity.

Gastric pH is neutral during the first few weeks of life and does not approximate adult values until the age of 2 years, which may affect the bioavailability of compounds.[7,8] Higher pH delays the absorption of weak acids and increases the absorption of weak bases. Methotrexate absorption, for example, is significantly reduced by coadministration with milk, which may further increase gastric pH.[12] The solubility of tyrosine kinase inhibitors (e.g., dasatinib and nilotinib) is also dependent on pH.[13] Further, pH-dependent drug degradation in the stomach affects the quantity of intact drug that reaches the small intestine. Absorption of lipophilic drugs requires their micellar solubility, which is dependent on biliary acids, whose secretion in turn is affected by food intake. Bile acid secretion is low at birth and increases to the adult level at approximately 6 months.

Gastric emptying time varies with gestational age and is typically longer in premature infants and neonates than in older children.[14] Low gastrointestinal motility persists until 6 to 8 months of age and may cause delayed absorption or increased absorption because of greater contact time. In addition, drugs may be administered in altered

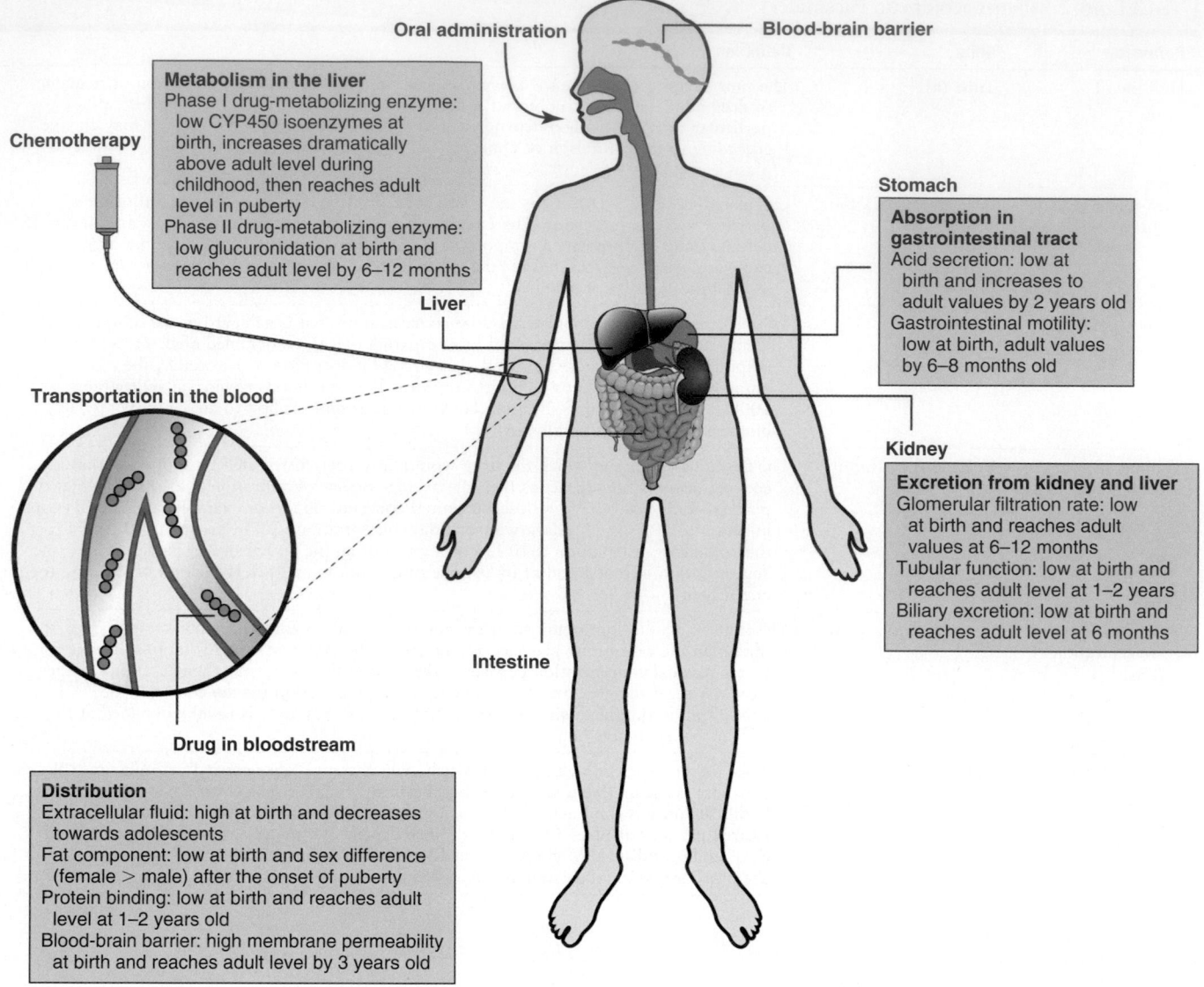

Figure 46-2 Pharmacokinetic changes during childhood development. Changes in body composition and organ function during childhood development can affect drug disposition and effects by altering absorption, distribution, metabolism, and excretion of chemotherapeutic agents. *CYP450*, Cytochrome P450.

forms to small children. For example, tablets may be crushed and added to food or slurries/suspensions and sometimes may be given via nasogastric tube, which may alter their rate and extent of absorption.

Transporter proteins are involved in drug uptake and movement across the intestinal epithelium (Fig. 46-3). Intestinal epithelial cells contain several uptake transporters, including one or more members of the organic anion-transporting polypeptide (OATP) family, peptide transporter (PEPT)–1 (PEPT1; solute carrier [SLC]–15A1 [SLC15A1]), ileal apical sodium/bile acid cotransporter (SLC10A2), and monocarboxylic acid transporter 1 (SLC16A1) in their apical (luminal) membranes (Fig. 46-4, *A*). Adenosine triphosphate–binding cassette (ABC) transporters such as ABCB1 (P glycoprotein, multidrug resistance protein [MDR]-1), ABCC1 (multidrug resistance-associated protein [MRP]–1), ABCC2 (MRP2), and

ABCG2 (breast cancer resistance protein [BCRP]) are located on the apical membranes of intestinal epithelial cells, where they secrete substrates back into the intestinal lumen, thereby limiting intestinal absorption and decreasing bioavailability.[15,16] The basolateral membranes of intestinal epithelial cells contain organic cation transporter–1 (OCT1; SLC22A1), heteromeric organic solute transporter α-β, and ABCC3 (MRP3). Some drugs are eliminated by hepatocytes into the bile before they are metabolized (Figs. 46-3 and 46-4, *B*). Phase I (e.g., cytochrome P [CYP]–450) and phase II (e.g., glutathione *S*-transferase) drug-metabolizing enzymes in the gastrointestinal tract can metabolize drugs before they enter the systemic circulation (see Fig. 46-3). Although the data are limited, some studies have shown that developmental changes in at least some of these enzyme activities and transporter proteins can affect drug absorption.[17-19]

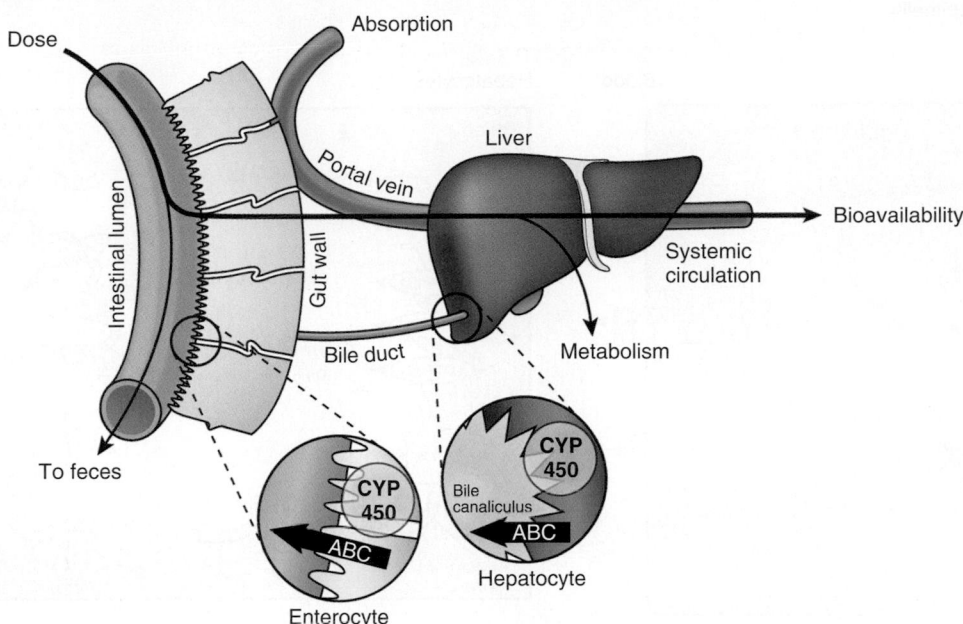

Figure 46-3 Absorption of orally administered medications and their bioavailability and metabolism. The role of active transport toward the gut lumen and bile by adenosine triphosphate–binding cassette *(ABC)* transporters expressed in the intestinal epithelium and liver, respectively, after oral administration of chemotherapeutic agents. Cytochrome P450 *(CYP450)* isoenzymes can metabolize drugs before they reach systemic circulation.

Volume of Distribution

The volume of distribution (Vd) of a systemically absorbed drug is the extent to which the drug penetrates extravascular tissues (see Fig. 46-2 and Table 46-2). Vd is affected by body composition (water and fat) and plasma proteins. Changes in body composition between birth and adolescence can alter pharmacokinetic parameters. The proportions of body water compartments, particularly extracellular fluid volume, change dramatically between birth and adulthood; extracellular fluid volume represents 50% of body weight in premature infants, 35% in infants 4 to 6 months old, and 20% in adolescents and adults.[20] Thus polar drugs, which are distributed primarily in body water, will have a larger volume of distribution in infants than in older children and adults. The net result of an isolated increase in Vd is a lower peak concentration and prolonged terminal half-life, assuming that drug clearance remains unchanged.

Newborns have less skeletal muscle mass and subcutaneous fat than do older infants. Fat components gradually increase after birth, but they differ in boys and girls after the onset of puberty. During adolescence, boys actually lose body fat (reaching a mean of 12% of body weight), whereas girls gain body fat (reaching a mean of 25% of body weight). Therefore gender-related differences in Vd and clearance of lipophilic drugs may be more prominent during adolescence than in preadolescent children or older adults.

Drug distribution may also be affected by plasma proteins. Theoretically, drug displacement from blood components by lower protein binding increases the apparent distribution volume. Although the resulting increase in the free drug fraction may make the drug more available to its target, it also enhances metabolic and renal elimination. Protein binding may be reduced because of persistence of fetal albumin or by low plasma protein content, particularly albumin, α1-acid glycoprotein, and gamma globulin.[21,22] Although the protein binding of acidic drugs may reach adult levels between 1 and 2 years of age, adult gamma-globulin levels are not reached until age 7 to 12 years.

One unique aspect of infancy is the immaturity of specific organs. For example, the myelin content of the brain is lower in newborns. Because of incomplete maturation of the blood-brain barrier (which reaches adult level by age 3 years), membrane permeability is greater in the infant brain, and the brain-to-plasma ratio of some drugs has been shown to vary with age.[23,24]

Hepatic Metabolism

The liver plays an important role in drug metabolism (see Fig. 46-2). Drug-metabolizing enzymes are divided into two classes: phase I (oxidation, reduction, hydrolysis, or demethylation) and phase II (conjugation or coupling of endogenous molecules, including glucuronide, sulfate, acetate, amino acid, methyl, and glutathione moieties, to the parent drug or a phase I metabolite; Table 46-3). Immature organ systems in infants and young children can alter the disposition of many classes of drugs, including antibiotics, anticonvulsants, and antineoplastic agents.[7,8,10] Phase I enzymes (e.g., CYP450 microsomal enzymes) are highly expressed in the liver. They can diminish the pharmacologic activity of a drug but can also convert a prodrug to its biologically active form (e.g., cyclophosphamide and codeine). CYP3A4 is the phase I

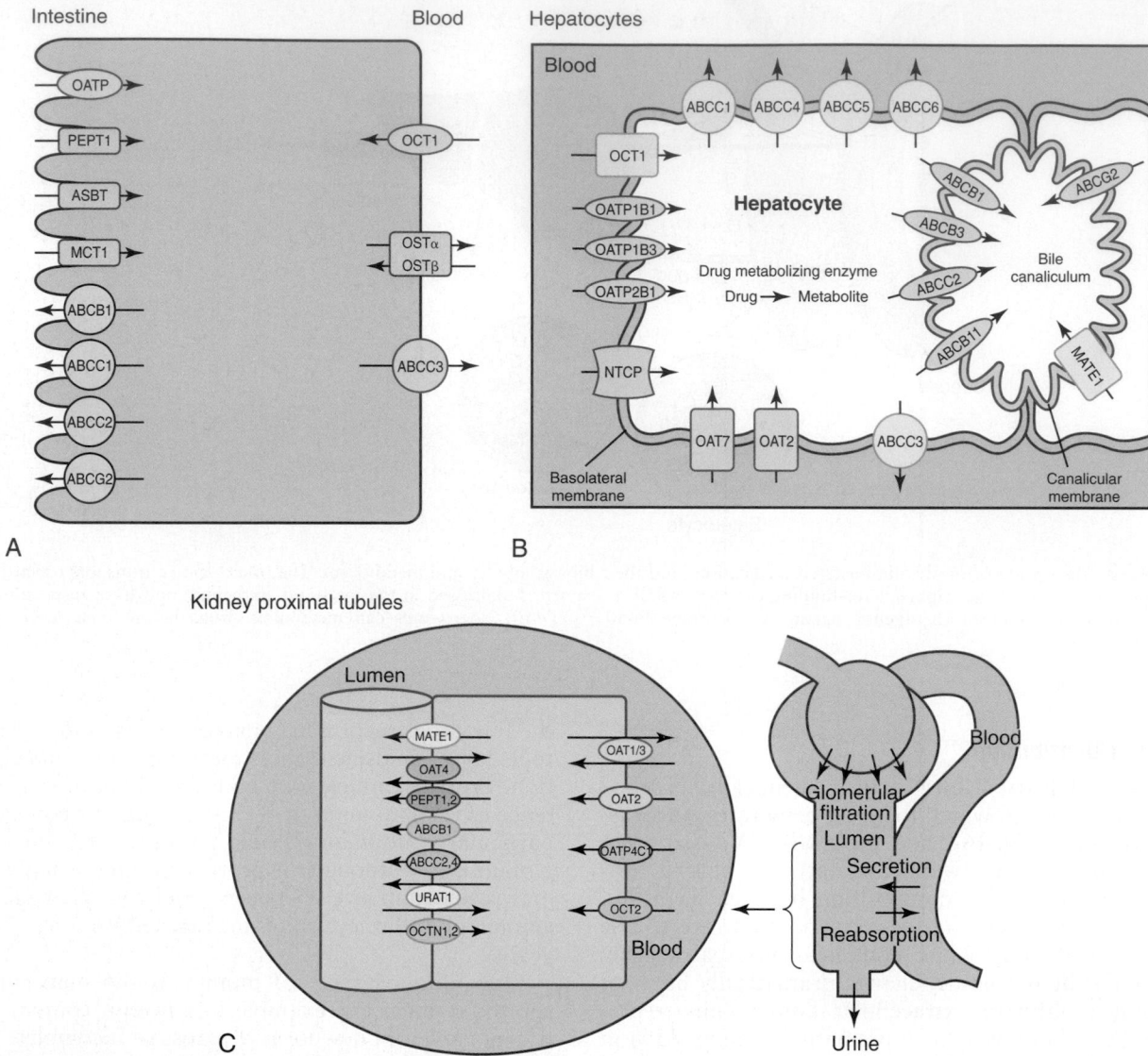

Figure 46-4 Common mechanisms involved in anticancer drug uptake and elimination through the gastrointestinal tract (**A**), liver (**B**), and kidney (**C**). *ABC,* Adenosine triphosphate–binding cassette transporter; *ASBT,* ileal apical sodium/bile acid cotransporter; *MATE,* multidrug and toxic extrusion transporter; *MCT,* monocarboxylic acid transporter; *NTCP,* (Na⁺)-taurocholate cotransporting polypeptide; *OAT,* organic anion transporter; *OATP,* organic anion-transporting polypeptide; *OCT,* organic cation transporter; *OCTN,* novel organic cation transporter; *OST,* organic solute transporter; *PEPT,* peptide transporter; *URAT,* urate transporter.

enzyme involved in the metabolism of the largest number of drugs, followed in approximate order by CYP2D6, CYP2C8/9/19, CYP1A2, CYP2B6, CYP2A6, and CYP2E1.[7] CYP3A7 is highly expressed in the fetus and then decreases rapidly after birth.[25] The metabolic activity of other CYP450 enzymes (e.g., CYP3A4, CYP2D6, and CYP2C9) is low in neonates but increases dramatically between age 2 weeks and 3 years. Clearance rates by CYP450 enzymes rise from 20% of that in adults to two to six times that in adults between infancy and adolescence, and then they decline gradually to adult values during puberty.[26] Low hydrolysis rates have been reported for drugs such as procaine in premature infants and neonates, but normal activity is measurable by 12 months. Phase II glucuronidation is almost exclusively a

detoxification mechanism that inactivates a compound and facilitates its excretion by enhancing its hydrophilicity and its recognition by biliary canicular efflux proteins. The activity glucuronidation enzyme rises to 30% of adult activity by 3 months of age and then reaches adult levels between 6 and 12 months of age.[27] Esterase activity, which is important for the metabolisms of agents such as irinotecan, gradually increases during the first year of life.[28]

Renal and Hepatic Excretion

The kidney is predominantly responsible for excretion of drugs and their metabolites (see Fig. 46-2). The immature kidney has a low glomerular filtration rate (GFR). In full-term infants, the GFR is 40 mL/min/1.73 m² and varies

TABLE 46-3 Drug Metabolizing Enzymes

Enzymes	Reactions
Phase I Enzymes	
Cytochrome P450s	C and O oxidation, dealkylation, others
Flavin-containing monooxygenases	N, S, and P oxidation
Epoxide hydrolases	Hydrolysis of epoxides
Phase II Enzymes	
UDP-glucuronosyltransferases	Addition of glucuronic acid
Glutathione-S-transferases	Addition of glutathione
Sulfotransferases	Addition of sulfate
N-acetyltransferases	Addition of acetyl group
Methyltransferases	Addition of methyl group
Other Enzymes	
Alcohol dehydrogenases	Reduction of alcohols
Aldehyde dehydrogenases	Reduction of aldehydes
NADPH-quinone oxidoreductase	Reduction of quinones

C, Carbon; N, nitrogen; NADPH, nicotinamide adenine dinucleotide phosphate; O, oxygen; P, phosphorus; S, sulfur; UDP, uridine diphosphate.

substantially among individuals.[29,30] The GFR gradually increases, reaching adult values between age 6 and 12 months. Tubular function and passive resorption may also be significantly lower in the neonate. Because tubular resorption matures more slowly than does glomerular filtration, toddlers may have remarkably high clearance rates for compounds that undergo tubular resorption in older children.

GFR, as assessed by technetium-99m diethylenetriamine pentaacetic acid filtration, was related to body surface area (BSA) in children 2 months to 17 years of age, but GFR was not related to age when normalized to BSA.[29] Premature and term infants require dose adjustments based on GFR measurement or estimation for drugs eliminated primarily by glomerular filtration, such as carboplatin. Formulas are available for estimation of creatinine clearance in infants and older children on the basis of serum creatinine and height[30,31] or on another endogenous surrogate marker of GFR, such as cystatin C.[32]

Many drugs are excreted in bile as the parent compound or as a metabolite. Biliary excretion favors compounds that have a molecular weight greater than 300 and contain both polar and lipophilic groups. Conjugation, particularly with glucuronate, increases biliary excretion. After the bile empties into the intestine, a fraction of the drug may be reabsorbed and eventually return to the liver (enterohepatic cycling). The remainder is excreted into the feces. Biliary excretion is low at birth and reaches adult levels at approximately 6 months of age.

Many SLC family transporters and ABC family transporters have been identified; these transporters mainly facilitate cellular drug uptake and elimination in kidney and liver (see Fig. 46-4, B and C).[33] The apical (luminal) membranes of renal proximal tubules contain organic anion transporter (OAT)–4 (OAT4, SLC22A11), urate transporter–1 (SCL22A12), PEPT1 (SLC15A1) and PEPT2 (SLC15A2), ABCC2 and ABCC4 (MRP4), multidrug and toxin extrusion (MATE) protein–1 (MATE1, SLC47A1), ABCB1, organic cation/ergothioneine transporter (OCTN1; SLC22A4), and organic cation/carnitine transporter (OCTN2; SLC22A5). The basolateral membranes of the proximal tubules contain the uptake transporters OATP4C1 (SLCO4C1); OCT2; and OAT1, OAT2 (SLC22A7), and OAT3 (SLC22A8).

Uptake transporters in the hepatocyte basolateral (sinusoidal) membrane include the sodium/taurocholate cotransporting peptide (SLC10A1), three members of the OATP family (OATP1B1 [SLCO1B1], OATP1B3 [SLCO1B3], and OATP2B1 [SLCO2B1]), OAT2 and OAT7 (SLC22A9), and OCT1. Efflux pumps in the hepatocyte basolateral membrane include ABCC1 (MRP1), ABCC3, ABCC4, ABCC5 (MRP5), and ABCC6 (MRP6). Apical (canalicular) efflux pumps of the hepatocyte comprise ABCB1, ABCC2, ABCB3 (transporter associated with antigen processing 2 [TAP2]), ABCB11 (bile salt export pump [BSEP] or sister of P-glycoprotein [SPGP]), ABCG2, and MATE1.

ABCB1 activity in lymphocytes peaks at birth, decreases between ages 0 and 6 months, and stabilizes at the adult level between the ages of 6 months and 2 years.[34] Developmental changes in the functions of other transporters have not been fully defined, but many are under investigation.

Influence of Underlying Disease on Metabolism

Pathophysiologic changes associated with specific pediatric malignancies may alter drug disposition. For example, the clearance of antipyrine and lorazepam was observed to increase between diagnosis and the end of remission induction therapy in children with ALL.[35] The clearance of unbound teniposide is lower in children with relapsed ALL than during first remission.[36] Because leukemic infiltration of the liver is common at the time of diagnosis of ALL, drugs metabolized by the liver may have reduced clearance, as has been documented in preclinical models.[37]

In mouse models, certain tumors elicited an acute-phase response that coincided with downregulation of human hepatic CYP3A4 and of the mouse orthologue Cyp3a11.[38] The reduction of murine hepatic Cyp3a gene expression in tumor-bearing mice resulted in decreased Cyp3a protein expression and consequently a significant reduction of Cyp3a-mediated metabolism of midazolam. These findings support the possibility that tumor-derived inflammation may alter the pharmacokinetic and pharmacodynamic properties of CYP3A4 substrates, leading to reduced drug metabolism in humans.

Unique Drug Effects in Pediatric Patients

Experience has shown that children often tolerate the conventional toxicities of chemotherapy better than adults, and that children (with the exception of neonates) experience very low regimen-related mortality. This finding may be partly explained by relatively low drug exposure caused by higher drug clearance rather than by altered pharmacodynamics. Lower exposure may explain briefer periods of neutropenia, less mucositis, and rare hepatic veno-occlusive disease. Children's greater ability to tolerate intensive therapy may partly explain why children with ALL have a higher cure rate compared with adults.[39,40]

However, the immature organ systems of the very young may be more susceptible to certain aspects of toxicity, including late cardiomyopathy, neuron developmental disorders, delayed puberty, growth plate arrest, and infertility. Children appear to be more sensitive to the cardiotoxic effects of anthracyclines (e.g., doxorubicin, daunorubicin, idarubicin, and mitoxantrone).[41,42] Follow-up studies have shown that months or years after intrathecal therapy for central nervous system (CNS) leukemia, with or without cranial irradiation, children treated for ALL may experience a chronic demyelinating encephalopathy and/or cognitive late effects.[43,44] Further, the latent effects of chemotherapy on fertility appear to vary with the developmental stage of the patient at the time of treatment. Treatment of leukemia and lymphoma in prepubertal boys, for example, does not appear to produce sustained testicular damage unless large cumulative doses of alkylating agents (e.g., cyclophosphamide >6 g/m^2) are used.[45] Treatment during puberty is more likely to permanently damage the germinal epithelium, although sexual maturation may proceed on a normal schedule.[46] Most prepubertal girls treated for leukemia with antimetabolites achieve menarche and progress through puberty.[47] Ovarian failure is associated mainly with alkylating agents and gonadal radiotherapy and is directly related to cumulative dose and age at exposure.[48] Nearly 30% of survivors treated with alkylating agents and abdominal-pelvic irradiation experienced nonsurgical primary ovarian failure (defined as cessation of menses before age 40 years).[49] Procarbazine exposure at any age, cyclophosphamide exposure from age 13 to 20 years, and ovarian radiation doses greater than 10 Gy were independent risk factors for acute ovarian failure (defined as loss of ovarian function within 5 years after diagnosis).[50] Most girls treated for brain tumors with procarbazine and/or nitrosourea and with neuraxis radiation showed evidence of ovarian hormonal failure.[51]

DRUG INTERACTIONS

Combination Chemotherapy

The vast majority of pharmacologic studies of anticancer agents have modeled the effects of a single drug. However, as a consequence of somatic mutations and/or selection of genetically resistant clones, tumor cytotoxicity tends to diminish over subsequent courses of single-agent treatment. Therefore cancer chemotherapy is most frequently given as a combination of drugs that individually have shown activity against the specific cancer to be treated but that have different pharmacologic mechanisms of action. The selection of agents that exert maximal anticancer effects and minimal adverse effects requires a clear understanding of the biochemical, molecular, and pharmacokinetic mechanisms of action and of individual and overlapping toxicities of the agents. The treatment for ALL provides an example of excellence.[3] Most of the drugs used were developed before 1970. However, their dosage and schedule of administration have been optimized on the basis of leukemic-cell biologic features, response to therapy (e.g., minimal residual disease), and patient pharmacodynamic and pharmacogenomic findings. The 5-year survival rate for pediatric ALL has been approximately 90% in recent trials.[52]

Optimal combination chemotherapy theoretically should meet the following criteria:

- Drugs that show single-agent activity should be selected. Because of primary resistance, rates of complete response to a single agent rarely exceed 20%.
- Drugs with different mechanisms of action should be combined. The various classes of anticancer agents have different cellular targets. The use of multiple agents with different mechanisms of action enables independent killing of cells by each agent. Cells resistant to one agent may be sensitive to another drug or drugs in the regimen. Known patterns of cross-resistance must be taken into consideration.
- Drugs with different mechanisms of resistance should be combined. Resistance to many agents may be the result of mutations selected by those agents. However, a single mutational change can also cause resistance to multiple drugs. The number of known mechanisms of resistance is continuously increasing and is partly drug dependent. Because drug-resistant mutants may be present at the time of clinical diagnosis, the earliest possible use of non–cross-resistant drugs is recommended to avoid the selection of double mutants. Adequate cytotoxic doses of drugs must be administered as frequently as possible to achieve maximal killing of sensitive and moderately resistant cells.
- If possible, drugs with different dose-limiting toxicities should be combined, because it is more likely that drugs with nonoverlapping toxicities can be used at the full dosage, optimizing their potential effectiveness.

As noted, multidrug therapy can give rise to clinically important drug-drug interactions, which typically occur when the pharmacokinetic behavior of one drug is altered by the other (Fig. 46-5 and Table 46-1). These interactions are important in the design of drug combinations, because diminished therapeutic efficacy or increased toxicity of one or more of the administered agents can occur. Combinations of drugs may also show pharmacodynamic interactions that cannot be explained by altered pharmacokinetic profiles. Some of these interactions are at the cellular level or are related to the cell cycle. Interactions can be classified as synergistic (i.e., the effect of the combination is greater than the sum of the individual effects), additive (the effect of two drugs is the sum of the effects of each), or antagonistic (the effect of two drugs is less than the sum of their individual effects). Provided that the drugs used are active against a particular disease,

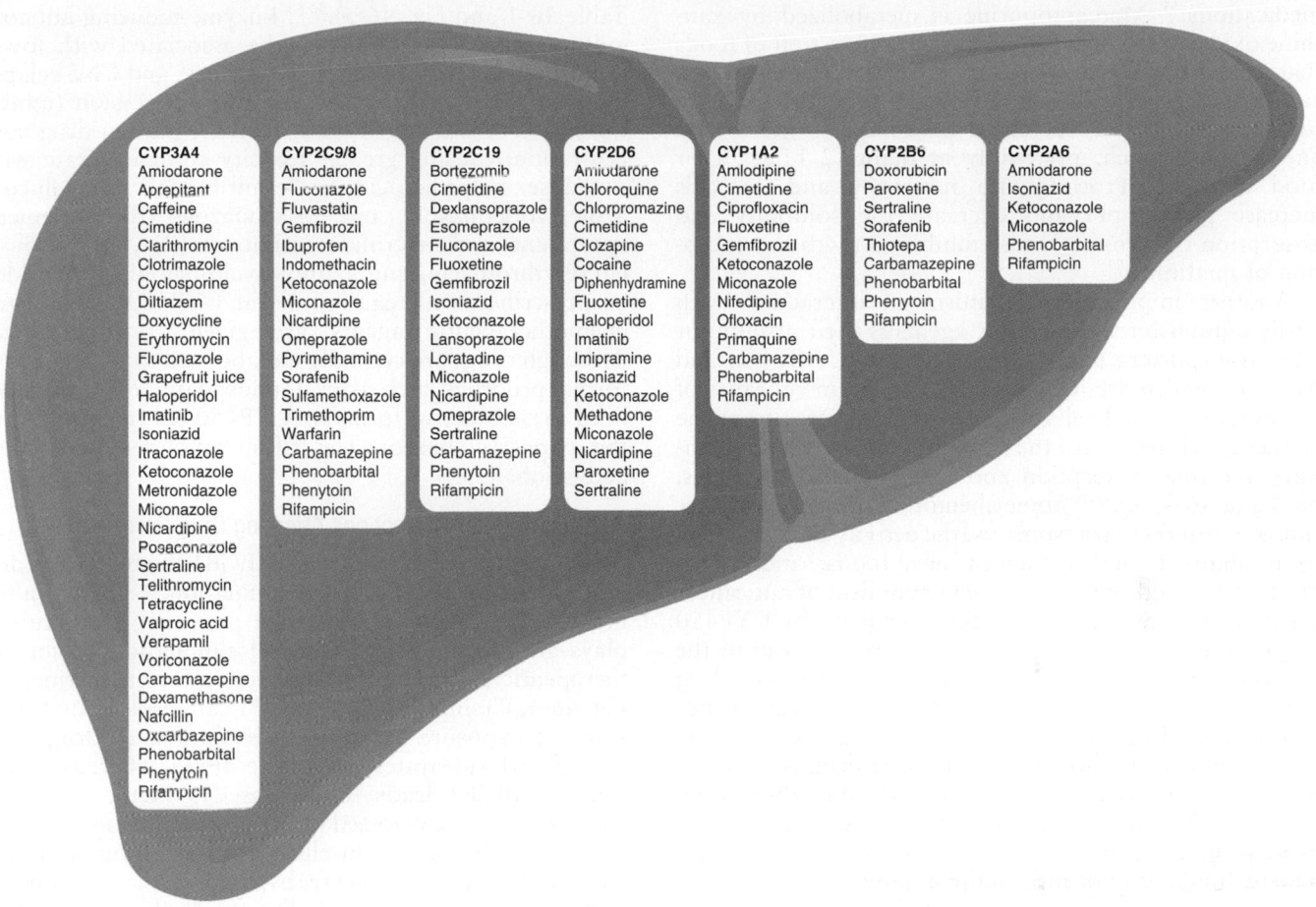

Figure 46-5 The main cytochrome P450 isoenzyme–inducing and P450 isoenzyme–inhibiting agents used in pediatric oncology. Drugs listed in *red* are inhibitors and those listed in *green* are inducers of the cytochrome P450 enzyme system.

knowledge of cellular kinetics can be used to consider the use of non–cell cycle phase-specific agents (e.g., alkylating agents, platinum agents, and anthracyclines), first to reduce tumor bulk and second to recruit slowly dividing cells into active deoxyribonucleic acid (DNA) synthesis. After the latter is achieved, treatment can be continued with cell-cycle phase-specific agents (e.g., methotrexate or fluoropyrimidines), which affect cells mainly during DNA synthesis. Similarly, repeated courses of S-phase–specific drugs, such as cytarabine and methotrexate, are most effective if administered during the rapid rebound recovery of DNA synthesis that follows suppression of DNA synthesis in the previous course.[53] If pharmacokinetic and pharmacodynamic interactions exist, the drug doses and sequence of administration that allow safe administration of combination chemotherapy are typically defined during early clinical trials (i.e., phase I and phase II studies).

Coadministration of Non-Anticancer Drugs

Many prescription and over-the-counter medications are used during chemotherapy to improve quality of life or to treat other diseases, but they may interact with anticancer agents, thus altering their pharmacokinetic char-

acteristics, clinical effectiveness, and/or toxicities.[54,55,56] More than 100,000 deaths per year in the United States alone are attributed to drug-drug interactions, placing these interactions between the fourth and sixth leading cause of death.[57] Clearly, all aspects of pharmacokinetics (i.e., absorption, distribution, metabolism, and excretion) may be affected when a drug is given in combination with another drug. The generally narrow therapeutic index of cytotoxic chemotherapy means that drug-drug interactions would predispose some persons to excessive toxicity or inadequate efficacy.

Pharmacokinetic Interactions Affecting Drug Absorption

Because many chemotherapeutic agents are given via an IV line, factors that affect absorption have little effect on their pharmacokinetics. However, absorption plays a crucial role in the bioavailability of orally administered drugs; absorption is contingent on adequate intestinal uptake and circumvention of intestinal and subsequent hepatic metabolism of the drug (see Figs. 46-2 and 46-3).[13,58,59] Food intake can delay gastric emptying, raise intestinal pH, increase hepatic blood flow, and slow gastrointestinal transit, which may significantly affect the pharmacokinetic profile of orally administered medications.[55] Mercaptopurine is metabolized by xanthine oxidase into inactive metabolites. Ingestion of foods that contain xanthine oxidase, such as dairy products, can reduce the effectiveness of mercaptopurine.[58] Therefore patients are instructed to take mercaptopurine on an empty stomach, preferably at night (2 hours after food intake).[56] Proton-pump inhibitors and antacids increase gastric pH and decrease the solubility and absorption of tyrosine kinase inhibitors (with the exception of imatinib).[60]

Another important mechanism of interaction with orally administered anticancer agents is their affinity for ABC transporters (e.g., ABCB1, ABCC1, ABCC2, and ABCG2), which are located on the apical membranes of intestinal epithelial cells and secrete substrates from the epithelial cell back into the intestinal lumen, thereby limiting intestinal absorption and bioavailability (see Figs. 46-3 and 46-4, A).[15,16] Some chemotherapeutic agents are substrates of these transporters, the activity of which may be inhibited by other medications, foods, and herbal products. In addition, extensive metabolism of anticancer drugs in the gut wall and/or the liver (e.g., by CYP450 enzymes) during the first pass can keep them out of the systemic circulation and is another potential drug-drug interaction mechanism (see Fig. 46-3). An ideal chemotherapeutic drug would have an adequate absolute bioavailability, as shown by little drug-drug interaction or interpatient/intrapatient variability in absorption. However, the most commonly used oral agents, including mercaptopurine, methotrexate, etoposide, and cyclophosphamide, do not meet these criteria.

Pharmacokinetic Interactions Affecting Drug Distribution

Chemotherapeutic agents can bind to several blood components, including albumin, lipoproteins, immunoglobulins, and α1-acid glycoprotein, and the increased free-drug fraction caused via displacement by another drug may make the displaced drug more available to the target and enhance metabolism and elimination.[55] Highly protein-bound drugs, such as warfarin, may interact with protein-bound cytotoxic drugs such as etoposide and paclitaxel. The hematologic toxicity of etoposide is more closely related to systemic exposure to the unbound drug than to the total drug.[61] However, the therapeutic implications of displacement of many anticancer drugs from their protein-bound state are as yet undefined.

Pharmacokinetic Interactions Affecting Drug Metabolism

Most important drug-drug interactions involve altered liver metabolism—for example, altered expression or functionality of CYP450 isoenzymes, such as CYP3A4, 2C9/8, 2D6, and 2C19 isoforms, which oxidize anticancer drugs to more polar and usually inactive metabolites (see Table 46-1).[62] Induction of CYP450 activity, which increases a drug's metabolic rate, may reduce plasma drug concentration and thus reduce the therapeutic effect. For example, anticonvulsant drugs (such as phenytoin, phenobarbital, and carbamazepine) induce drug-metabolizing CYP450 enzymes and thereby increase the clearance of various anticancer agents (e.g., anthracyclines, epipodophyllotoxins, and vinca alkaloids) in children (see

Table 46-1 and Fig. 46-5).[56,63] Enzyme-inducing anticonvulsants have been shown to be associated with lower event-free survival, hematologic relapse, and CNS relapse in persons with ALL.[63] Conversely, suppression (inhibition) of CYP450 activity may increase plasma drug concentration, causing greater toxicity commensurate with overdose. Valproic acid, azole antifungals (e.g., fluconazole, voriconazole, and posaconazole), the antiemetic aprepitant, and macrolide antibiotics (e.g., clarithromycin, erythromycin, and azithromycin) should be avoided or prescribed with caution when CYP450-metabolized chemotherapeutic agents are given concomitantly.[56] Although drugs are typically metabolized to their inactive forms, prodrugs such as cyclophosphamide are metabolized to their active forms by CYP450 enzymes and have the opposite consequences of metabolic inhibition or activation.

Pharmacokinetic Interactions Affecting Drug Excretion

ABC transporters such as ABCB1, ABCC1/2, and ABCG2 are involved in drug elimination.[33] ABCB1 in the brush-border membrane of the proximal renal tubule plays an important role in renal elimination of chemotherapeutic agents by active secretion into the urine (see Fig. 46-4, C). Inhibition of ABCB1 can result in increased systemic exposure and tissue distribution of drugs that are ABCB1 substrates (see Table 46-1), whereas induction of ABCB1 leads to decreased systemic exposure. ABCB1 is also expressed in canalicular membranes of the liver; it has a role in elimination of drugs into bile, from which they can be reabsorbed in the intestine or eliminated in the feces (see Fig. 46-4, B). Excretion of irinotecan and its metabolites is mediated by several ABC transporters (e.g., ABCB1 and ABCG2).[64] Substrates and/or inhibitors of these transporters (e.g., cyclosporine and gefitinib) may interfere with renal and/or biliary excretion of irinotecan and its metabolite, SN-38, and increase the plasma concentration and toxicity. Organic anion transporters (e.g., OAT1, OAT3, and OAT4) are highly expressed on the renal proximal tubules and are involved in the renal elimination of methotrexate.[65] Nonsteroidal antiinflammatory drugs (e.g., salicylate, ibuprofen, and indomethacin), probenecid, and penicillin can inhibit these OATs and delay renal excretion of methotrexate, leading to severe and even life-threatening drug interactions, including bone-marrow suppression and acute renal failure.[66,67]

Coadministration of Complementary and Alternative Medicine

In recent years, interest in complementary and alternative medicine (CAM) has grown rapidly in the industrialized world.[68,69] No compelling clinical trial data support the use of CAM in children with cancer, and the potential interaction of CAM agents with conventional, possibly curative, treatment may be harmful. Families are more likely to use CAM for their child if a parent uses CAM, if the child has a poor prognosis, or if the parents are older and better educated.[68,69] Surveys within the past decade have estimated that CAM is used in 31% to 84% of pediatric oncology cases, and in many cases the treating clinician is unaware of the patient's use of CAM.[68,69] In addition to nonherbal therapies (e.g., hypnosis, guided imaginary, massage, and acupuncture), many children use herbal treatments, such as St. John's wort (*Hypericum perforatum*), garlic, and ginseng (*Panax ginseng*), in combination with allopathic therapies.[68,69] The risk of herb-drug interactions is a growing concern, and the need is increasing to understand possible adverse interactions. This concern is of particular relevance to pediatric oncology, because CAM use is more common in this group than in the general population.

During the past decade, a wealth of in vitro and in vivo evidence has shown that many herbal preparations interact extensively with drug-metabolizing enzymes and drug transporters. A number of clinically important interactions are now recognized, although causal relationships have not consistently been established and confirmatory studies in children are lacking. Most of the observed interactions suggest that the herbs inhibit or induce several isoforms of the CYP family, and concurrent use of some herbs with chemotherapy is likely to have serious clinical and toxicologic implications. An additional consideration for cancer chemotherapy is that herb-mediated induction or inhibition of phase I and II metabolic enzymes and ABC/SLC transporters may alter response. Therefore rigorous testing is urgently required to identify the pharmacokinetic interactions of anticancer drugs with widely used herbs. Drug-drug interaction potential has been investigated for only a limited number of herbs. For example, St. John's wort, melatonin, and whey protein are CYP450 inducers, and curcumin, goldenseal *(Hydrastis canadensis)*, and grapefruit juice *(Citrus paradise)* are strong inhibitors.[68,69] Milk thistle *(Silybum marianum)*, *Echinacea (Echinacea purpurea)*, saw palmetto, *Ginkgo biloba*, valerian, and green tea have showed no significant interactions. Because of the widespread use of herbal medicines in the United States, physicians should include it in their routine drug histories and review potential hazards with individual patients. Detailed information can be obtained from the following websites[68,69]:

- National Center for Complementary and Alternative Medicine, National Institutes of Health: *http://nccam.nih.gov*
- Office of Cancer Complementary and Alternative Medicine, National Cancer Institute, National Institutes of Health: *http://cam.cancer.gov/*
- PDQ Cancer Information Summaries: Complementary and Alternative Medicine, National Cancer Institute, National Institutes of Health: *http://www.cancer.gov/cancertopics/pdq/cam*
- Integrative Therapies Program for Children with Cancer, Columbia University Medical Center: *http://integrativetherapies.columbia.edu/*
- About Herbs, Botanicals and Other Products, Memorial Sloan Kettering Cancer Center: *http://www.mskcc.org/mskcc/html/11570.cfm*
- Complementary/Integrative Medicine, MD Anderson Cancer Center: *http://www.mdanderson.org/departments/cimer/*
- Natural Standard: *http://www.naturalstandard.com/*

PHARMACOGENETICS AND PHARMACOGENOMICS OF CHEMOTHERAPEUTIC AGENTS IN CHILDREN

Pharmacogenetics/pharmacogenomics investigates the influence of human genomic variation in drug response. Inherited (germline) or acquired (somatic) variation in genes encoding drug-metabolizing enzymes, drug receptors, drug transporters, and drug targets have all been shown to influence anticancer drug response in humans and they may also influence drug toxicity.[70]

A single nucleotide polymorphism (SNP) is defined as a single base change in a DNA sequence.[71] Unless it occurs in at least 1% of the population, it is considered a variant or a mutation. Accumulation of mutations during evolution, in concert with random selection, has made SNPs the most common form (about 90%) of genetic variation in the human genome.

The advent of pharmacogenomics was characterized by the passage from a candidate gene approach to a genome-wide approach. This advance was initially made possible by the international HapMap project, which included 270 samples from three geographic areas of genetic descent—African descent (Yoruban population); European descent (Center d'Étude du Polymorphisme Humain population), and Asian descent (Japanese and Han Chinese population)—and more than 2 million publicly available SNPs.[72] Subsequently, the "1000 Genomes Project" has provided the most detailed catalogue of human genetic variation. The recent development of next-generation sequencing technologies has allowed better coverage of all genetic variants.[73]

Advances in treatment have greatly improved the survival rates of children with cancer. However, the efficacy of therapy, as well as its short- and long-term adverse effects, can vary among patients, even when their chemotherapeutic or radiologic treatment is identical. Thus it is very important to identify inherited (germline) genomic variations that can alter the absorption, distribution, metabolism, and/or excretion of chemotherapeutic agents, thereby altering their effects and toxicities (Table 46-4).

Thiopurines

Thiopurines frequently used for the treatment of childhood ALL are 6-mercaptopurine and 6-thioguanine (see Table 46-1). As prodrugs, they require conversion to thioguanine nucleotides (TGNs) via the purine-salvage pathway, and 6-thioguanosine 5'-triphosphate (TGTP) and deoxy-TGTP are then incorporated into ribonucleic acid (RNA) or DNA, respectively (Fig. 46-6). The active DNA mismatch repair system identifies these base-pair mismatches and induces cell cycle arrest and apoptosis.[74,75] An alternative protein complex that includes high mobility group box 1 and 2 proteins, heat shock cognate protein 70 (HSC70), protein disulfide isomerase (ERp60), and glyceraldehyde 3-phosphate dehydrogenase trigger apoptosis when it detects changes in DNA structure caused by incorporation of nonnatural nucleosides.[76] Thiopurines are inactivated by methylation catalyzed by thiopurine methyltransferase (TPMT). The relation between *TPMT* polymorphisms and thiopurine efficacy and toxicity provides a well-established example of the

TABLE 46-4   Pharmacogenomics of Chemotherapeutic Agents Used for Pediatric Cancer

Agent	Genes Involved	Effects
Thiopurines	TPMT*3A (460 G>A and 719 A>G), TPMT*3C (719 A>G), and TPMT*2 (238G>C)	Higher incidence of hematopoietic cell toxicities, secondary malignancies in ALL
6-mercaptopurine	PACSIN2 (rs2413739, T allele)	Lower TPMT activity and higher incidence of severe gastrointestinal toxicity in ALL
6-thioguanine	ITPA (rs41320251, C>A)	Higher methylmercaptopurine nucleotides and higher incidence of febrile neutropenia when mercaptopurine dose was adjusted with TPMT genotype in ALL
Methotrexate	SLC19A1 (G80A, AA or AG vs. GG)	Worse EFS and higher gastrointestinal toxicities in ALL
	SLC19A1 AA80 and positive GSTM1	Higher incidence of hepatotoxicity in ALL
	DHFR (G308A, AA or AG vs. GG) and DHFR *1b haplotype	Worse EFS in ALL
	TYMS (3/3 vs. 2/3 or 2/2)	Increased risk of hematologic relapse in ALL
	MTHFR (C677T, TT vs. CC)	Increased risk of relapse in ALL
	MTHFR (T677A1298 haplotype)	Lower EFS in ALL, especially in the presence of TYMS (3/3)
	MTHFD1 (A1958 variant, AA or GA vs. GG)	Lower EFS in ALL, especially in the presence of TYMS (3/3)
	SLCO1B1 (rs11045879 [T allele], rs4149081 [G allele], and rs4149056 [TT])	Higher methotrexate clearance and higher incidence of gastrointestinal toxicity in ALL
Glucocorticoids Prednisone Prednisolone Dexamethasone	NR3C1 (-627 AA vs. AG or GG, intron 2+646 CG or GG vs. CC, and 9b TT vs. CC or TC)	Worse EFS in ALL
	NR3C1 (1088 AG vs. AA)	Increased risk of hematologic relapse in ALL patients with GSTM1 null genotype
	GSTT1 (*0/0 vs. *A/A)	Better early response to prednisone in ALL
	GSTP1 (codon105 Val/Val or Val/Ile vs. Ile/Ile, codon 114 Ala/Ala vs. Ala/Val or Val/Val)	Increased central nervous system relapse in ALL
	GSTM1 (null vs. normal)	Severe infection in ALL
	SNPs in CNTNAP2, LEPR, CRHR1, NTAN1, SLC12A3, ALPL, BGLAP, and APOB	Association with hypertension during remission-induction therapy in ALL
	ACP1 (rs 12714403 AA or AG vs. GG)	Higher incidence of symptomatic osteonecrosis in ALL
	TYMS (2/2 vs 3/3 or 2/3) and VDR (rs2228570, CC vs. TT or CT)	Higher incidence of osteonecrosis in ALL
	PAI-1 (rs6092, AA or GA vs. GG)	Higher incidence of osteonecrosis in ALL
Asparaginase Escherichia coli asparaginase	ATF5 T1562C (TT or CT vs. CC)	Inferior EFS when treated with Escherichia coli asparaginase in ALL
PEG-asparaginase	SNPs in ADSL, DARS, ASS1, DARS2, NARS2, ADSSL1	Association with in vitro asparaginase sensitivity in ALL
Erwinia asparaginase	GRIA1 (rs4958381, A allele vs. G allele)	Higher incidence of asparaginase hypersensitivity in ALL
Vincristine	VDR intron 8 (AA or AG vs. GG), CYP3A5*3 (AA or AG vs. GG)	Increased peripheral neuropathy in ALL
	PMP22 duplication (Charcot-Marie-Tooth disease)	Increased peripheral neuropathy in ALL
Anthracycline Daunorubicin	CBR3 V244M (GG vs. GA or AA)	Increased cardiomyopathy, especially with anthracycline dose at 1-250 mg/m^2
Doxorubicin	SLC28A3 (rs7853758, L461L)	Decreased risk of cardiotoxicity
Mitoxantrone	ABCC1 (rs3743527TT, combination of rs3743527TT-rs246221TC/TT)	Increased cardiotoxicity in ALL
Idarubicin	CAT (rs10836235; c.66 + 78C > T, CC vs. TC)	Increased cardiotoxicity in ALL
Cytarabine	SLC29A1 haplotype with −1345C>G, −1050G>A, or −706G>C	Associated with high hENT1 expression
	DCK −360G allele (GG or CG vs. CC)	Increased risk of mucositis after low-dose cytarabine in ALL
	CDA A79C (CC vs. AA or AC)	Higher postinduction treatment-related mortality in AML
	CDA G208A (GA or AA vs. GG)	Lower activity of CDA and increased sensitivity to cytarabine in ALL, AML, and NHL

TABLE 46-4   Pharmacogenomics of Chemotherapeutic Agents Used for Pediatric Cancer (Continued)

Agent	Genes Involved	Effects
Etoposide	*ABCB1* exon 26 (3435C>T, CC or CT or TT)	Higher clearance in patients with ALL who have prednisone pretreatment
	CYP3A5*3 (AA vs. AG or GG) and *GSTP1* (313 A>G, AA vs. AG or GG)	Lower clearance in black patients with ALL who have prednisone pretreatment
	VDR intron 8 (GG vs. AG) and *VDR* Fok 1 (CC vs. CT or TT)	Higher clearance in black patients with ALL who do not have prednisone pretreatment
	UGT1A1 (7/7 vs. 6/7 or 6/6)	Lower clearance in black patients with ALL who do not have prednisone pretreatment
	SNPs in *AGPAT2*, *IL1B*, and *WNT5B*	Higher etoposide catechol AUC in black and white patients with ALL
	SNPs in *UVRAG*, *SEMA5A*, *SLC7A6*, and *PRMT7*	Association with etoposide cytotoxicity
		Association with etoposide cytotoxicity
	MDM2 309T>G	Decreased sensitivity to etoposide
Cyclophosphamide	*CYP2B6*4* (AG or GG vs. AA), recipient	Higher incidence of oral mucositis in patients with leukemia who received MSD HSCT
	CYP2B6*2 (CT or TT vs. CC), recipient	Higher incidence of hemorrhagic cystitis in patients with leukemia who received MSD HSCT
	CYP2B6*6 (GG vs. GT or TT), donor	Higher incidence of SOS in patients with leukemia who received MSD HSCT
	CYP2B6 rs3211371, R487C (Arginine), recipient	Reduced toxicity <100 days after allogeneic HSCT
	SOD2 rs4880, V16A (Valine), recipient	Higher overall toxicity after allogeneic HSCT
Platinum compounds Cisplatin Carboplatin Oxaliplatin	*ERCC2* Lys751Gln G allele (TG or GG vs. TT)	Poor tumor response and shorter EFS in patients with osteosarcoma treated with cisplatin
	GSTM3 (*B allele vs. *A allele)	Protective effect for cisplatin-induced ototoxicity in solid tumor and CNS malignancies
	GSTP1 (^{105}Val/^{105}Val vs. ^{105}Ile/^{105}Ile or ^{105}Ile/^{105}Val)	Protective effects in long-term cisplatin-induced hearing impairment in testicular cancer
	GSTM1 and *GSTT1* polymorphisms (≥1 null type vs. non-null type)	More cognitive impairment after therapy in children with medulloblastoma
	TPMT (rs12201199, A allele) and *COMT* (rs9332377, A allele)	Increased cisplatin-induced hearing loss in patients with solid tumor and CNS malignancies
	Megalin (rs2075252, AG or AA vs. GG)	Increased cisplatin-induced hearing loss in patients with solid tumor and CNS malignancies
Irinotecan	*UGT1A1*28* (7/7 vs. 6/7 or 6/6)	No association with severe toxicity when treated with low dose and protracted schedule

ALL, Acute lymphoblastic leukemia; *AML,* acute myeloid leukemia; *AUC,* area under the plasma concentration versus time curve; *CDA,* cytidine deaminase; *CNS,* central nervous system; *EFS,* event-free survival; *hENT1,* human equilibrative nucleoside transporter; *HSCT,* hematopoietic stem cell transplantation; *MSD,* matched sibling donor; *NHL,* non-Hodgkin lymphoma; *SNP,* single nucleotide polymorphism; *SOS,* sinusoidal obstruction syndrome; *TPMT,* thiopurine methyltransferase.

potential clinical importance of pharmacogenomics (Fig. 46-7 and Table 46-4).[77-79] SNPs in the *TPMT* gene are associated with different inherited levels of TPMT enzyme activity.[80-83] One in approximately 400 white persons has profound TPMT deficiency resulting from inheritance of two nonfunctional variants of *TPMT*, 6% to 11% have intermediate activity by having heterozygous variants of *TPMT*, and 89% to 94% have normal activity (homozygous wild-type *TPMT*).[74,84,85] Ethnic differences exist in the frequency of occurrence of these variant alleles and thus in the frequency of TPMT deficiency. To date more than 20 *TPMT* variants have been identified, but three variants—*TPMT*3A* (460 G>A and 719 A>G), *TPMT*3C* (719 A>G), and *TPMT*2* (238 G>C)— account for more than 90% of inactivating alleles.[86,87]

The specific activity of TPMT determines the efficacy of thiopurine treatment and serves as an indirect indicator of hematologic toxicity.[88] At conventional thiopurine doses, patients with inherited TPMT deficiency accumu-

late excess intracellular concentrations of thioguanine nucleotides (TGN) especially in hematopoietic cells, predisposing them to moderate to severe hematologic toxicity depending on their deficiency status (i.e., heterozygous vs. homozygous).[77,89] In addition, several studies have found a relationship between low TPMT activity and secondary neoplasms, especially at high doses (e.g., mercaptopurine, 75 mg/m^2/day).[90,91] Patients with homozygous and heterozygous TPMT deficiency can be treated safely with appropriate adjustment of the thiopurine dosage.[92,93]

Because some patients with wild-type *TPMT* experience toxicities during mercaptopurine treatment, a genome-wide association study was performed to identify additional genetic determinants of thiopurine toxicity (see Table 46-4). In an analysis of a panel of human HapMap cell lines followed by validation in patients with ALL, the protein kinase C and casein kinase substrate in neurons–2 *(PACSIN2)* gene was among the top genes

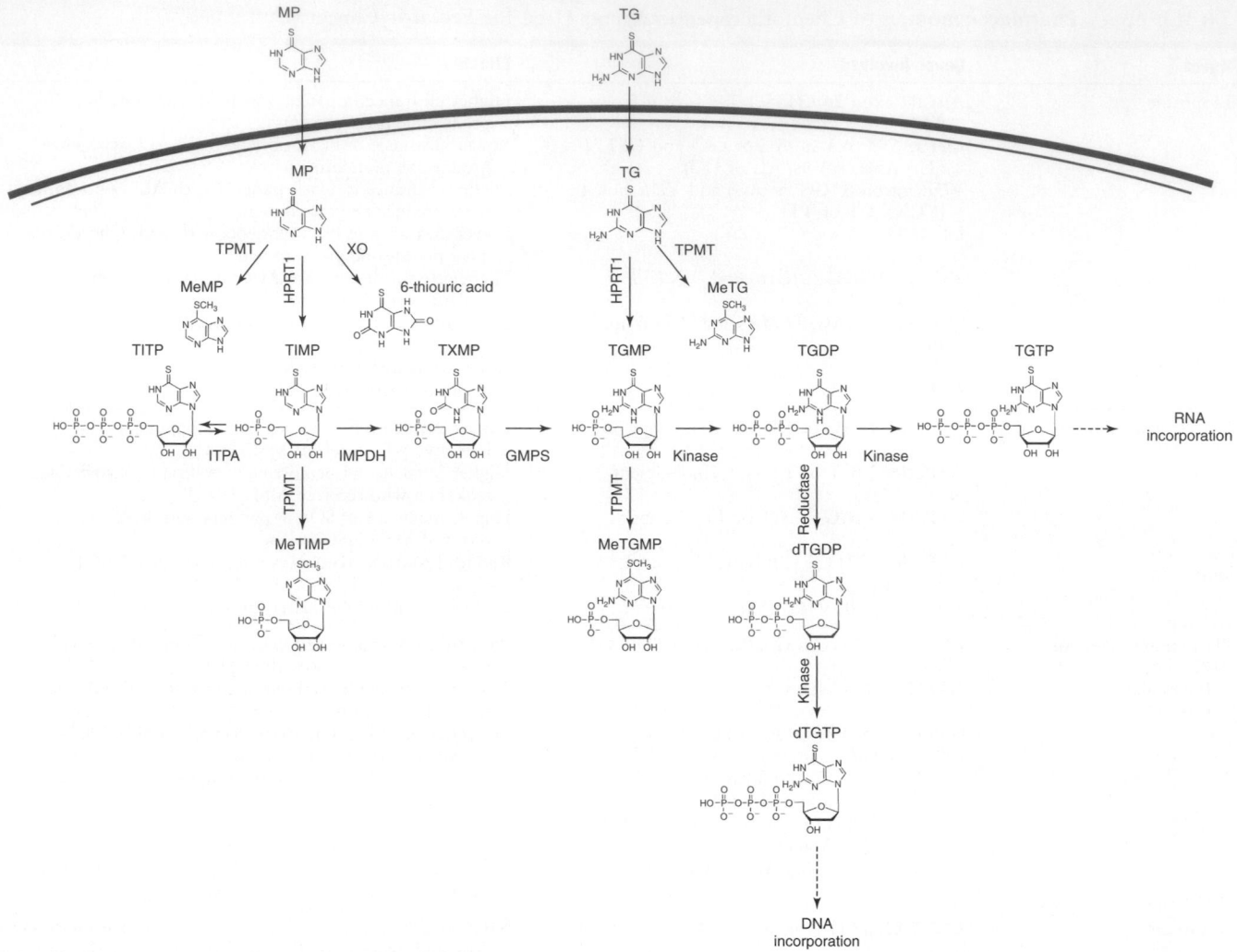

Figure 46-6 Metabolic pathways of 6-mercaptopurine and 6-thioguanine. 6-Mercaptopurine *(MP)* and 6-thioguanine *(TG)* are prodrugs that require conversion to thioguanine nucleotides (TGNs) via the purine-salvage pathway. The TGNs are incorporated into deoxyribonucleic acid *(DNA)* or ribonucleic acid *(RNA)*. Thiopurines are inactivated by thiopurine methyltransferase *(TPMT)* through catalytic methylation and by xanthine oxidase *(XO)*. Inosine triphosphate pyrophosphatase *(ITPA)* catalyzes the hydrolysis of thioinosine triphosphate *(TITP)* to 6-thioinosine 5′-monophosphate *(TIMP)*. *dTGDP,* Deoxy-6-thioguanosine 5′-diphosphate; *dTGTP,* deoxy-6-thioguanosine 5′-triphosphate; *GMPS,* guanosine monophosphate synthetase; *HPRT1,* hypoxanthine phosphoribosyltransferase 1; *IMPDH,* inosine-5′-monophosphate dehydrogenase; *Me,* S-methyl; *TGDP,* 6-thioguanosine 5′-diphosphate; *TGMP,* 6-thioguanosine 5′-monophosphate; *TGTP,* 6-thioguanosine 5′-triphosphate; *TXMP,* 6-thioxanthosine 5′-monophosphate.

identified, and the T allele of the *PACSIN2* SNP rs2413739 was significantly associated with lower TPMT activity and a higher incidence of severe gastrointestinal toxicity during consolidation therapy for ALL.[94] PACSIN2, also called syndapin II, has a role in various biologic processes, including endocytosis, cell-cycle control, and autophagy. PACSIN2 may influence TPMT activity by influencing *TPMT* messenger RNA levels and/or TPMT protein degradation. Furthermore an SNP (rs41320251, C>A) in the inosine triphosphate pyrophosphatase *(ITPA)* gene was associated with significantly higher accumulation of methylmercaptopurine nucleotides and a higher incidence of febrile neutropenia during ALL therapy in patients whose mercaptopurine doses had been individualized to the *TPMT* genotype.[95] These findings illustrate that even when treatment has been adjusted for the

strongest genetic determinant of drug response, additional genetic variants may emerge as determinants of a drug's effects.

Methotrexate

Methotrexate is a folate analogue commonly used in the treatment of certain pediatric malignancies, including ALL and osteosarcoma (Fig. 46-8 and Table 46-1).[96] Cellular uptake is mediated mainly by the reduced folate carrier RFC1 (also known as SLC19A1).[97-99] In cells, cytosolic folylpolyglutamyl synthase converts methotrexate to methotrexate polyglutamates (MTXPGs) by adding as many as five glutamate residues. Methotrexate and MTXPG inhibit dihydrofolate reductase (DHFR), the enzyme responsible for conversion of dihydrofolate to its active form, tetrahydrofolate. In addition, MTXPG

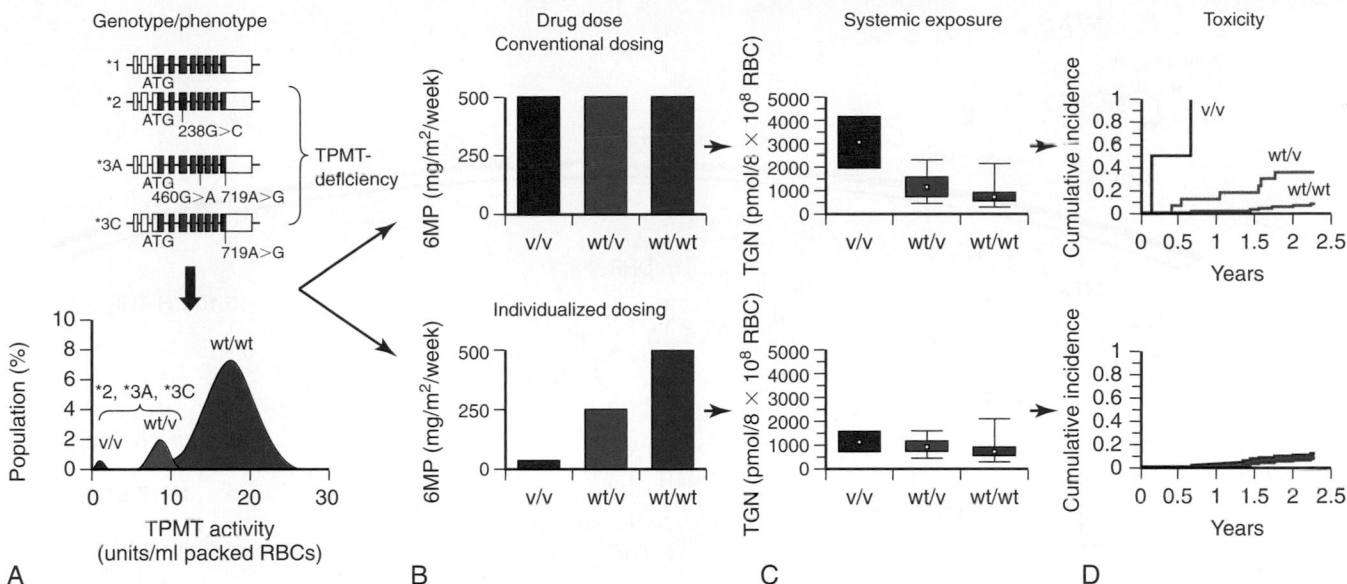

Figure 46-7 Polymorphisms in thiopurine methyltransferase and their effects on the pharmacogenetics of mercaptopurine toxicity. Wild-type thiopurine methyltransferase (*TPMT*1*) and the three predominant *TPMT* variant alleles (*TPMT*2*, *TPMT*3A*, and *TPMT*3C*) are shown (**A**). These changes cause autosomal codominant inheritance of TPMT activity in humans. The wild-type *(wt/wt)* enzyme is most active, homozygous variants *(v/v)* are least active, and the heterozygous wild-type/variant enzyme *(wt/v)* has intermediate activity. When mercaptopurine (MP) treatment is given to a cohort of patients, dosing can be conventional or individualized according the patient's genotype (**B**). When conventional doses of mercaptopurine are given, TPMT-deficient patients *(v/v)* have a systemic exposure to active thioguanine nucleotides *(TGN)* 10 times that of wild-type patients *(wt/wt)*, and heterozygous patients have TGN concentrations about two times that of wild-type patients (**C**). The higher concentrations of TGN cause a significantly higher frequency of hematopoietic toxicity (**D**). When doses specifically adjusted to the genotype are given in an individualized therapeutic regimen, similar cellular TGN concentrations are achieved in all patients, and all three TPMT phenotypes can be treated without acute toxicity. *RBC*, Red blood cell. *(Modified from Cheok MH, Evans WE: Acute lymphoblastic leukaemia: a model for the pharmacogenomics of cancer therapy.* Nat Rev Cancer *6:117–129, 2006.)*

inhibits thymidylate synthetase (TYMS), thereby blocking purine and thymidine synthesis, as well as DNA and RNA synthesis. MTXPG is not readily effluxed from cells, making its formation advantageous for anticancer effects of methotrexate. Other enzymes such as 5,10-methylenetetrahydrofolate reductase (MTHFR) and methylenetetrahydrofolate dehydrogenase–1 (MTHFD1) are also key elements in folate metabolism and in methotrexate effects.[100,101] MTHFR catalyzes the reduction of 5,10-methylenetetrahydrofolate to 5-methyltetrahydrofolate, a cosubstrate of homocysteine remethylation to methionine, and MTHFD1 catalyzes interconversion of 1-carbon derivatives of tetrahydrofolate, which are substrates for methionine, thymidylate, and de novo purine synthesis. MTXPG can be degraded via cleavage by lysosomal γ-glutamyl hydrolase. Several transporters (e.g., ABCG2, ABCC2, OATP1B1 [SLCO1B1], OAT1, OAT3, and OAT4) also participate in methotrexate clearance.

Interpatient variability in the efficacy and toxicity of methotrexate treatment is associated with genetic variations in methotrexate metabolic pathways (see Table 46-4). The G80A polymorphism of *SLC19A1* replaces Arg with His at position 27 of the major methotrexate transporter RFC1 (encoded by *SLC19A1*). ALL patients with the A80 variant had lower event-free survival estimates than did those with the GG genotype.[102,103] However, this association has not been widely replicated, and patients homozygous for A80 had higher plasma levels of methotrexate than the other genotype groups; the mechanism by which this SNP might confer a worse prognosis is not clear.[103] In other studies, the G80A *SLC19A1* genotype was associated with a substantially higher incidence of gastrointestinal toxicity,[104] and patients with AA80 and positive *GSTM1* (glutathione S-transferase mu–1) had a higher incidence of hepatotoxicity.[105] Patients with Down syndrome experience greater methotrexate toxicity, requiring dose reduction and early leucovorin rescue.[106] This toxicity may partly reflect enhanced intracellular uptake of methotrexate, because *SLC19A1* is located on chromosome 21 and thus three copies are present in all cells of persons with Down syndrome, although other mechanisms, such as enhanced methotrexate polyglutamination and reduced folate depletion, may also be involved.

Altered levels of DHFR expression have been found in patients with relapsed ALL and in ALL cells with a methotrexate-resistant phenotype.[107,108] Genetic variations in both a major promoter and a noncoding minor transcript region of *DHFR* have been identified.[109] Patients with ALL who had an A allele of the G308A polymorphism and the *1b haplotype of *DHFR* had a significantly poorer outcome because of increased DHFR expression.

The promoter region of the *TYMS* gene exhibits a genetic polymorphism, having either two or three 28-base-pair tandem repeat sequences.[110] *TYMS* (3/3) was associated with greater TYMS expression and a

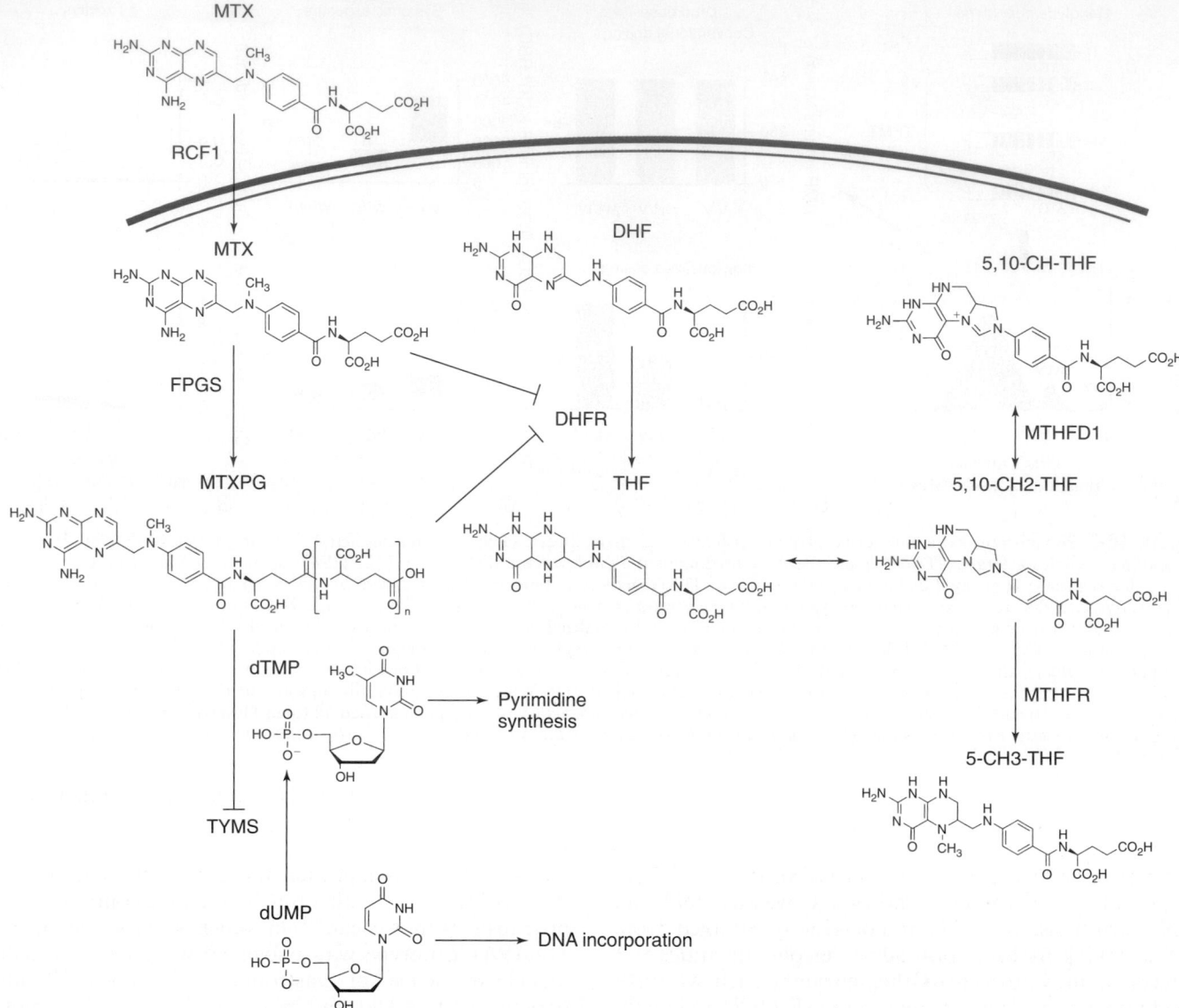

Figure 46-8 Metabolic pathways of methotrexate. Cellular uptake is mediated mainly by reduced folate carrier–1 *(RFC1)*. Within cells, cytosolic folylpolyglutamyl synthase *(FPGS)* converts methotrexate to methotrexate polyglutamates *(MTXPGs)* by adding glutamate residues. Methotrexate *(MTX)* and MTXPGs inhibit dihydrofolate reductase *(DHFR)*, the enzyme responsible for conversion of dihydrofolate *(DHF)*, to its active form, tetrahydrofolate *(THF)*. In addition, MTXPGs inhibit thymidylate synthetase *(TYMS)*, thereby blocking purine and thymidine synthesis, as well as deoxyribonucleic acid *(DNA)* and ribonucleic acid synthesis. 5,10-methylenetetrahydrofolate reductase *(MTHFR)* and methylenetetrahydrofolate dehydrogenase 1 *(MTHFD1)* are also key elements in folate metabolism and in methotrexate effects. *5,10-CH-THF,* 5,10-methenyltetrahydrofolate; *5,10-CH2-THF,* 5,10-methylenetetrahydrofolate; *5-CH3-THF,* 5-methyltetrahydrofolate; *dTMP,* deoxythymidine monophosphate; *dUMP,* deoxyuridine monophosphate.

greater risk of hematologic relapse of ALL than was observed in children with a 2/2 or 2/3 genotype, possibly implicating resistance to methotrexate, which targets this enzyme.[111,112]

Polymorphisms in the *MTHFR* gene, such as C677T and A1298C, which result in reduced enzymatic activity, have been implicated in the response to methotrexate treatment.[113-115] The *MTHFR* C677T polymorphism is a common genetic variant, and enzyme activity is reduced by 70% in patients with the homozygous TT polymorphism, conferring a greater risk of relapse in children with ALL.[116,117] Patients with either the *MTHFR* T677A1298 haplotype or the *MTHFD1* A1958 variant

also had a lower rate of event-free survival, which became more evident in the presence of *TYMS* (3/3).[100]

A genome-wide analysis has identified common inherited variations in *SLCO1B1*, encoding OATP1B1, as important determinants of methotrexate pharmacokinetics and clinical effects.[118] Two SNPs, rs11045879 and rs4149081, were in linkage disequilibrium with each other and with the functional polymorphism T521C (rs4149056). These SNPs were associated with methotrexate clearance and gastrointestinal toxicity. The association of *SLCO1B1* SNP rs4149056 with methotrexate clearance was further validated in five different treatment regimens.[119] Of note, rare genetic variants of the

SLCO1B1 gene have been shown to have a greater impact on methotrexate clearance than common variants and to contribute to the inherited basis of methotrexate clearance and toxicity.[120]

Glucocorticoids

Glucocorticoids (prednisone or prednisolone and dexamethasone) are important components of ALL treatment (see Table 46-1). Glucocorticoids diffuse into the cell and bind to the glucocorticoid receptor, leading to its translocation into the nucleus.[121-123] In the nucleus, the glucocorticoid receptor transactivates or transrepresses glucocorticoid-responsive genes,[124] leading to inhibition of cytokine production, alteration of oncogene expression, cell-cycle arrest, and apoptosis.[125] Glucocorticoids can be metabolized by CYP450 enzymes (mainly CYP3A4) and glutathione-S-transferases (GSTs) and are transported by ABCB1.[126-129]

Sensitivity to glucocorticoid therapy is variable among patients, both in efficacy and the prevalence and severity of adverse effects. Numerous polymorphic sites in the glucocorticoid receptor gene (*NR3C1*) are described as being associated with prognosis (see Table 46-4).[130] Polymorphisms −627A/G, intron 2 +646C/G, and 9bT/C of *NR3C1* have each been associated with event-free survival in childhood ALL.[131] The *NR3C1* AG genotype (1088A>G) showed a greater association with hematologic relapse than did the *NR3C1* AA genotype among children with the *GSTM1*-null genotype.[111] Association between polymorphisms of the phase II enzyme GST and prognosis has also been reported. A deletion polymorphism in glutathione-S-transferase theta–1 *(GSTT1)* modulates the early response to glucocorticoids in childhood ALL; patients with *GSTT1*0/0* had a better early response to prednisone than did patients with *GSTT1*A/A*.[132] Polymorphisms in glutathione-S-transferase pi–1 *(GSTP1)* codon 105 (Ile/Val) and codon 114 (Ala/Val) were associated predominantly with CNS relapse.[133]

The acute and late adverse effects associated with glucocorticoids include hypertension, infection, and osteonecrosis. Among 203 candidate polymorphisms, those in eight genes (*CNTNAP2* [contactin-associated protein-like–2], *LEPR* [leptin receptor], *CRHR1* [corticotropin releasing hormone receptor–1], *NTAN1* [N-terminal asparagine amidase], *SLC12A3*, *ALPL* [alkaline phosphatase, liver/bone/kidney], *BGLAP* [bone gamma-carboxyglutamate (gla) protein], and *APOB* [apolipoprotein B]) were associated with hypertension during remission-induction therapy (prednisone, 40 mg/m²/day for 28 days) for childhood ALL.[134] In another candidate gene study that included *NR3C1*, *ABCB1*, *GSTM1*, *GSTP1*, *GSTT1*, and interleukin 10 *(IL10)* genes, the *GSTM1*-null genotype was associated with severe infections.[135] Glucocorticoid-induced osteonecrosis causes severe pain, limited range of motion of joints, and eventual joint destruction and mechanical failure because of compromised bone vascularization, demineralization, and trabecular thinning.[136] Clinically, older age, greater treatment intensity, lower serum albumin levels, higher cholesterol, and low dexamethasone clearance rates were important prognostic factors for osteonecrosis.[137,138,139,140,141,142] Polymorphisms (AA/AG) in acid phosphatase–1, soluble *(ACP1;* e.g., rs12714403), which regulates lipid levels and osteoblast differentiation, were associated with a greater risk of osteonecrosis and with lower albumin and higher cholesterol concentrations compared with those in patients with the GG genotype.[141] In addition, variants in *TYMS* (enhancer 2-repeat allele), vitamin D (1,25-dihydroxyvitamin D3) receptor *(VDR)* Fok I (rs2228570), and plasminogen activator inhibitor–1 *(PAI1;* rs6092) have been found to be associated with a higher incidence of osteonecrosis.[137,143]

Asparaginase

Asparaginase catalyzes the hydrolysis of asparagine to aspartic acid and ammonia (see Table 46-1). ALL cells have a low level of asparagine synthetase (ASNS) and are therefore dependent on external sources of asparagine.[144,145] Depletion of circulating endogenous asparagine by asparaginase therapy selectively kills leukemic cells by decreasing their protein synthesis. Three different formulations of asparaginase are available: native asparaginase derived from *Escherichia coli* (*E. coli* asparaginase); a pegylated form of the native *E. coli* asparaginase (polyethylene glycol [PEG] asparaginase); and asparaginase isolated from *Erwinia chrysanthemi* (*Erwinia* asparaginase).[146,147] The different asparaginase preparations have different pharmacokinetic properties, and thus the dosing schedule of each preparation is adjusted based on the half-life of the preparation; serum asparaginase concentrations at or above 0.1 international units/mL are believed to deplete asparagine levels to below the limit of detection.[148]

Asparaginase resistance appears to be caused by various mechanisms, and ASNS plays a variable functional role (see Table 46-4).[149-152] An analysis of 14 polymorphisms in the regulatory and coding regions of *ASNS*, activating transcription factor–5 *(ATF5)*, and argininosuccinate synthase–1 *(ASS1)* genes showed that *ATF5* T1562C was associated with lower event-free survival rates in patients with ALL who were treated with *E. coli* native asparaginase.[153] T1562 was associated with greater *ATF5* promoter activity, which may increase ASNS expression and lead to worse outcome. In a genome-wide study seeking to identify determinants of asparaginase sensitivity in lymphoblastoid HapMap cell lines and patient-derived ALL cells, the aspartate metabolic pathway was the most overrepresented.[154] SNPs primarily involved in this pathway included those in adenylosuccinate lyase *(ADSL)*, aspartyl-tRNA synthetase *(DARS)*, *ASS1*, *DARS2*, asparaginyl-tRNA synthetase–2 *(NARS2)*, and adenylosuccinate synthase-like–1 *(ADSSL1)*.

Asparaginase may be associated with adverse effects, including hypersensitivity, pancreatitis, hyperglycemia, and thrombosis.[155-158] Asparaginase hypersensitivity can lead to antibody formation, which is more commonly observed with native *E. coli* asparaginase than with PEG asparaginase.[159,160] Antibody formation was related to low systemic exposure to asparaginase and even to higher systemic clearance of dexamethasone.[161,162] A genome-wide association approach identified variations in the glutamate receptor, ionotropic, AMPA1 (GRIA1) gene, especially SNP rs4958381, as being associated with the risk of hypersensitivity to asparaginase among children with ALL.[163]

Vincristine

Vincristine is a natural alkaloid isolated from *Catharanthus roseus* (the Madagascar periwinkle) and is widely used in the treatment of both hematologic and solid malignancies (see Table 46-1).[164] Vincristine interferes with microtubule formation and mitotic spindle dynamics by interacting specifically with β-tubulin, causing mitotic arrest and cell death.[165] Vincristine is metabolized by CYP3A4 and CYP3A5 in the liver, mainly forming a secondary amine, M1 metabolite.[166-168] Vincristine appears to be exported from cells by ABCB1, ABCC1, ABCC2, and ABCC10.[169-173]

Vincristine is associated with a dose-limiting peripheral neurotoxicity, and several factors may influence its incidence and severity (Table 46-4). For example, underlying neuropathy (e.g., Charcot-Marie-Tooth disease [especially with duplication of peripheral myelin protein–22 (PMP22)] and Guillain-Barré syndrome) or myopathy (e.g., muscular dystrophy) and malnutrition have been reported to be associated with greater vincristine neuropathy.[165] The mechanism of vincristine-induced peripheral neuropathy has not been fully elucidated. *CYP3A5* is highly polymorphic, with variants including *CYP3A5*3*, *CYP3A5*6*, and *CYP3A5*7*.[168,174,175] The association of genetic polymorphisms with vincristine-induced neurotoxicity appears to be inconsistent and may be influenced by the treatment context (e.g., disease and concomitant therapy). VDR regulates CYP3A4, CYP3A5, and ABCB1.[176] Variants in *VDR* intron 8 (AA or AG) and *CYP3A5*3* (AA or AG) were associated with a higher incidence of peripheral neurotoxicity during continuation therapy in children with ALL,[104] and children with ALL who express a functional CYP3A5 experienced less vincristine-induced peripheral neuropathy.[177] In another study, however, patients with the *CYP3A4*1B* and *CYP3A5*3* variant genotypes had a decreased risk of peripheral neuropathy that was statistically significant in a univariate analysis but not in a multivariate analysis.[178] Expression of the efflux transporters ABCB1 and ABCC1 in cancer cells has been reported to be associated with reduced accumulation of, and in vitro resistance to, vincristine.[179] However, a retrospective analysis of children with ALL showed no association between the *ABCB1* SNPs C3435T and G2677T and vincristine pharmacokinetics or toxicity.[180] Thus additional studies are needed to identify genomic variations associated with vincristine neurotoxicity and/or cancer cell resistance.

Anthracyclines

The anthracyclines (e.g., daunorubicin, doxorubicin, mitoxantrone, and idarubicin) are antibiotic chemotherapeutic agents used for both hematologic and solid malignancies (Table 46-1).[181,182] The antitumor activity of anthracyclines is attributed to their ability to intercalate between base pairs of DNA and inhibit the topoisomerase II enzyme, preventing the relaxing of supercoiled DNA

and thus blocking transcription and replication.[183-185] Daunorubicin differs from doxorubicin by the substitution of a hydroxyl group for a hydrogen atom in the acetyl radical.[186] Although anthracyclines are considered to enter the cell via passive diffusion, transport proteins are also involved.[187,188] Within cells, the anthracyclines are substrates for the ABC efflux transporters. The mechanism of resistance to anthracyclines can involve increased efflux via ABCB1, ABCC1, and/or ABCG2.[189-191] To overcome this resistance, functional modulation of the ABC drug transporters has been investigated, mainly in adults.[192,193]

The cumulative dose of anthracyclines is limited by their selective toxicity to cardiomyocytes, which are vulnerable to free radical damage due to low activity of antioxidant enzymes. Free oxygen radicals cause DNA damage and mitochondrial dysfunction.[194] Daunorubicin and doxorubicin are metabolized to the more cardiotoxic hydroxyl derivatives, daunorubicinol and doxorubicinol, respectively, by the myocardial cytosolic carbonyl reductases (CBRs) and aldo-keto reductases. In humans, two monomeric CBRs (CBR1 and CBR3) are encoded by genes located on chromosome 21.[195,196] The *CBR3* V244M polymorphism showed a trend toward association with the risk of congestive heart failure (see Table 46-4).[197] Although the risk of cardiomyopathy generally increases with cumulative doses of anthracycline greater than 250 mg/m², a homozygous G allele in *CBR3* V244M increases the risk of cardiomyopathy even at low to moderate cumulative doses (1 to 250 mg/m²), suggesting that no safe dosage exists for patients with this SNP (Fig. 46-9).[198] In a study of 2977 SNPs in 220 key drug biotransformation genes, it was found that the synonymous coding variant rs7853758 (L461L) within the *SLC28A3* gene had a significantly protective effect

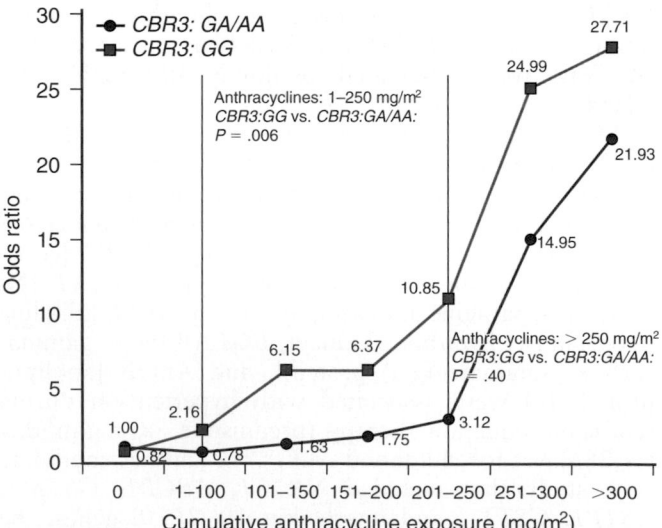

Figure 46-9 Dose-response relationship between cumulative anthracycline exposure and risk of cardiomyopathy, stratified by patients' carbonyl reductase–3 (*CBR3*) genotype (*CBR3*:GG or *CBR3*:GA/AA). Patients with the *CBR3*:GA/AA genotype who were not exposed to anthracyclines served as the reference group. Magnitude of risk is expressed as odds ratio. (*From Blanco JG, Sun CL, Landier W, et al: Anthracycline-related cardiomyopathy after childhood cancer: role of polymorphisms in carbonyl reductase genes—a report from the Children's Oncology Group.* J Clin Oncol 30:1415–1421, 2012.)

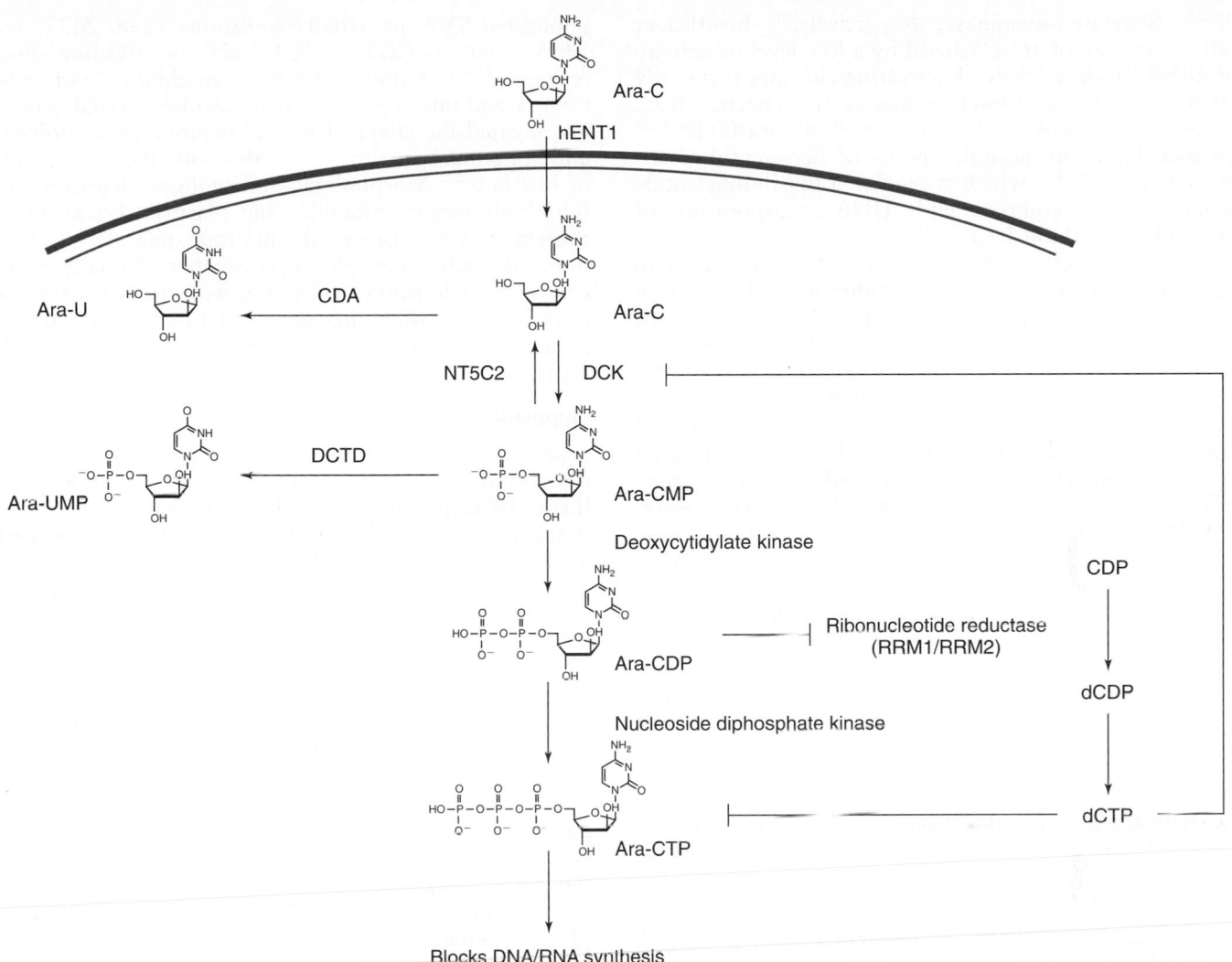

Figure 46-10 Metabolic pathways of cytarabine. Cytarabine *(Ara-C)* is transported through the cell membrane by the human equilibrative nucleoside transporter *(hENT1)*. It is first phosphorylated by deoxycytidine kinase *(DCK)* to form arabinosylcytosine 5′-monophosphate *(ara-CMP)*, which is then phosphorylated by deoxycytidylate kinase to arabinosylcytosine 5′-diphosphate *(ara-CDP)* and converted by nucleoside diphosphate kinase to the active arabinosylcytosine 5′-triphosphate *(ara-CTP)*. Ara-CMP can be dephosphorylated back to ara-C by 5′-nucleotidase *(NT5C2)*. Both ara-C and ara-CMP can be converted to inactive forms (uracil arabinoside *[ara-U]* and uracil arabinoside monophosphate *[ara-UMP]*) by cytidine deaminase *(CDA)* and deoxycytidylate deaminase *(DCTD)*, respectively. Larger intracellular pools of deoxycytidine triphosphate *(dCTP)*, which is regulated by ribonucleotide reductase, can compete with deoxyribonucleic acid *(DNA)* incorporation of ara-CTP and inhibit DCK activity. *CDP,* Cytidine diphosphate; *dCDP,* deoxycytidine diphosphate; *RNA,* ribonucleic acid; *RRM,* ribonucleotide reductase M.

against anthracycline-induced cardiotoxicity.[199] Risk and protective variants in other genes included *SLC28A1* and several ABC transporters (*ABCB1*, *ABCB4*, and *ABCC1*). Combination of these multiple variants into a single prediction model that included clinical risk factors was able to identify patients at high risk of anthracycline cardiotoxicity. Other studies found cardiotoxicity to be associated with the *ABCC1* rs3743527TT genotype and the rs3743527TT-rs246221TC/TT genotype combination[200] and with CC homozygosity at rs10836235 of the catalase gene (*CAT* c.66 + 78C > T) in childhood ALL.[201]

Cytarabine

Cytarabine (cytosine arabinoside, ara-C, 1-β-arabinofuranosylcytosine), is one of the most effective chemotherapeutic agents for treatment of AML and ALL (see Table

46-1). Ara-C is a deoxynucleoside analogue and is transported through the cell membrane by the human equilibrative nucleoside transporter (hENT1/SLC29A1) (Fig. 46-10). Within the cell, ara-C undergoes a series of phosphorylations. It is first phosphorylated by deoxycytidine kinase (DCK) to form arabinosylcytosine 5′-monophosphate (ara-CMP), which is then phosphorylated by pyrimidine kinases to the active 5′-triphosphate derivative, arabinosylcytosine 5′-triphosphate (ara-CTP).[202-204] Ara-CTP is incorporated into DNA and causes chain termination, blocking DNA and RNA synthesis.[205,206] Ara-CMP can be dephosphorylated back to ara-C by 5′-nucleotidase (NT5C2). Both ara-C and ara-CMP can be converted into inactive forms (uracil arabinoside [ara-U] and uracil arabinoside monophosphate [ara-UMP]) by cytidine deaminase (CDA) and deoxycytidylate deaminase, respectively.[207] Insufficient cellular uptake of ara-C caused by a low level or activity of hENT1 reduce levels of activating enzymes (primarily DCK), and increased levels of inactivating enzymes (e.g., NT5C2 and CDA) reduce the level of ara-CTP.[208,209] Further, larger intracellular pools of deoxycytidine triphosphate (dCTP), which is regulated by ribonucleotide reductase, can compete with DNA incorporation of ara-CTP and inhibit DCK activity.

The expression of hENT1 appeared to be related to the cytarabine sensitivity of childhood AML cells in vitro,[210] and haplotypes including −1345C>G, −1050G>A, and −706G>C of the SLC29A1 promoter region were related to higher hENT1 expression, which may alter ara-C chemosensitivity (see Table 46-4).[211]

DCK activity and expression vary widely in normal and malignant cells but may be related to ara-C sensitivity and patient survival.[212] Polymorphisms in the DCK gene differ between races; SNPs in the 5′ regulatory region (−201C>T and −360C>G) are common in the Chinese population and less common in Caucasians.[213] Adult Chinese patients with AML who have the −360CG/−201CT and −360GG/−201TT compound genotype had higher levels of DCK mRNA and a greater response to chemotherapy than patients with the −360CC/−201CC compound genotype.[214] The DCK −360G allele was found to increase the risk of mucositis after exposure to low-dose cytarabine in Asian children with ALL.[215]

Analysis of functional SNPs in human CDA led to the identification of three polymorphisms (A79C, G208A, and T435C) in the coding region. Analysis of the impact of the CDA A79C genotype on therapy outcomes in children with AML showed that postinduction treatment-related mortality was significantly greater in patients with the CC genotype, which is associated with low CDA activity.[216] The G208A polymorphism results in an alanine to threonine substitution (A70T) within the conserved catalytic domain, and the 208A genotype was associated with lower CDA activity and greater sensitivity to ara-C in pediatric leukemia cells.[217] Another polymorphism in the CDA promoter, SNP C-451T, reduces the expression level and enzymatic activity of CDA.[218] CDA SNP C-451T was found to be a significant, independent predictor of survival in adult AML, in which the TT genotype predicted higher risk.

Imatinib Mesylate

Imatinib mesylate (Gleevec) or 4-[(4-methyl-1-piperazinyl)methyl]-N-[4-methyl-3-[[4-(3-pyridinyl)-2-pyrimidinyl]amino]-phenyl] benzamide methanesulfonate is a breakpoint cluster region-Abelson (BCR-ABL) tyrosine kinase inhibitor commonly used for the treatment of chronic myeloid leukemia and Philadelphia chromosome–positive ALL (see Table 46-1).[219-222] Imatinib is metabolized to the active metabolite N-desmethyl-imatinib by CYP3A4; CYP3A5 and other CYP enzymes (e.g., CYP2D6, CYP2C9, and CYP2C19) play minor roles.[223] Imatinib is a substrate of the ABC transporters ABCB1 and ABCG2. It is bound to plasma proteins, predominantly albumin and α1-acid glycoprotein.[224] Pharmacogenetic studies of imatinib, conducted mainly in adults,

implicated SNPs in ABCB1 (positions 1236, 2677, and 3435) and ABCG2 (rs2231142) as affecting drug response.[225-228] Authors of a study in children with solid tumors and adults with gastrointestinal stromal tumors investigated the effect of several demographic, biologic, and pharmacogenetic covariates on the disposition of imatinib.[229] Morphologic and biologic characteristics (i.e., body weight, albumin, and plasma α1-acid glycoprotein levels) influenced imatinib pharmacokinetics more strongly than pharmacogenetics. Somatic DNA changes or selection of subclones with preexisting mutations in the tyrosine kinases targeted by imatinib are the predominant genetic mechanisms underlying imatinib resistance.[230]

Etoposide

Etoposide (VP-16), 4′-demethylepipodophyllotoxin-9-(4,6-O-ethylidene)-β-D-glucopyranoside, is a semisynthetic derivative of podophyllotoxin that inhibits DNA topoisomerase II and is used for the treatment of several malignancies, including AML and solid tumors (see Table 46-1).[231] Etoposide is metabolized to a catechol etoposide through an O-demethylation reaction catalyzed mainly by CYP3A4 and CYP3A5 and to a minor degree by CYP1A2 and CYP2E1.[232,233] CYP3A4 and CYP3A5 expression is regulated in part by the VDR.[176] Etoposide catechol metabolite binds covalently to DNA and cellular proteins and displays intrinsic cytotoxic properties.[234] Etoposide metabolites can be conjugated to glutathione by GSTs and can be glucuronidated by the uridine diphosphate–glucuronosyltransferase 1A1 (UGT1A1) gene.[235] Etoposide and its metabolites are substrates for the efflux transporters ABCB1, ABCC1, and ABCC2 and for the influx transporter OCTN2.[236,237] In addition, the pharmacokinetics of etoposide in children are reported to be influenced by other factors, including body weight and excessive urinary carnitine loss.[237,238]

Genetic variants that contribute to etoposide metabolism and etoposide-induced cytotoxicity have been identified (see Table 46-4). A study in children with ALL showed that the pharmacokinetics of etoposide and its catechol metabolite are related to polymorphisms in CYP3A5, ABCB1, GSTP1, UGT1A1, and VDR in a manner influenced by race and by prednisone use.[239] Etoposide clearance rates were significantly higher in patients who had recently received prednisone, which can modulate expressions of CYP3A and ABCB1. The ABCB1 exon 26 (3435C>T) CC genotype was associated with higher etoposide clearance for patients on day 29 of remission-induction therapy, after 28 days of prednisone treatment, and the CYP3A5*3 AA and GSTP1 (313 A>G) AA genotypes predicted lower clearance in black patients. At week 54 of continuation treatment without preceding prednisone treatment, the VDR intron 8 GG and VDR Fok 1 CC genotypes predicted higher etoposide clearance, and UGT1A1 7/7 predicted lower clearance, in black patients. The UGT1A1 7/7 genotype predicted higher etoposide catechol AUC in both black and white patients.

A genome-wide study using the HapMap human lymphoblastoid cell lines identified 63 genetic variants that contribute to interindividual variation in etoposide cytotoxicity.[240] These variants included genes previously reported to be associated with carcinogenesis and sensitivity to etoposide (e.g., 1-acylglycerol-3-phosphate O-acyltransferase–2 [AGPAT2], interleukin-1 beta [IL1B], and wingless-type MMTV integration site family, member 5B [WNT5B]) and genes not yet known to be associated with sensitivity to etoposide. The influence of heritable genetic variation on etoposide cytotoxicity was confirmed by the identification of additional genomic regions and SNPs in UVRAG (UV radiation resistance–associated), SEMA5A (sema domain, seven thrombospondin repeats [type 1 and type 1-like], transmembrane domain [TM] and short cytoplasmic domain, [semaphorin] 5A), SLC7A6, and PRMT7 (protein arginine methyltransferase–7), which may also be associated with adverse effects, including myelosuppression, therapy-related leukemia, and neurotoxicity.[241] Cell lines homozygous for the MDM2 (murine double minute 2) SNP309 T to G change in the promoter region showed a lower response to etoposide that was attributable, at least in part, to the lower expression of topoisomerase II.[242]

Cyclophosphamide

Cyclophosphamide is an alkylating agent widely used in the treatment of childhood cancers, including leukemia, lymphoma, neuroblastoma, rhabdomyosarcoma, and brain tumor (Table 46-1). Cyclophosphamide is a prodrug first metabolized into 4-hydroxycyclophosphamide (4-OHCP) in the liver, which is mediated by CYP2B6, CYP2C9, and CYP3A4.[243,244] 4-OHCP exists in equilibrium with the aldophosphamide, which spontaneously degrades to the active DNA-alkylating agent phosphoramide mustard and to acrolein. Cyclophosphamide and 4-OHCP can be transformed to the inactive metabolites dechloroethylcyclophosphamide and 4-keto-cyclophosphamide, respectively, by CYP3A4 and CYP3A5.[243,245] Cyclophosphamide metabolites are detoxified by aldehyde dehydrogenase (ALDH) enzymes (ALDH1A1 and ALDH3A1) and the glutathione-S-transferase enzyme system (GSTP1 and glutathione-S-transferase alpha–1 [GSTA1]).[246]

The adverse effects of cyclophosphamide include cardiotoxicity, nephrotoxicity, and hemorrhagic cystitis, but these effects vary among patients (see Table 46-4). In children and adults with leukemia who received human leukocyte antigen–identical sibling-donor hematopoietic stem cell transplants, recipient CYP2B6*4 (AG or GG), recipient CYP2B6*2 (CT or TT), and donor CYP2B6*6 (GG) were associated with oral mucositis, hemorrhagic cystitis, and hepatic sinusoidal obstruction syndrome, respectively.[247] Another study showed that CYP2B6 rs3211371 R487C, which inhibits the activation of cyclophosphamide, was significantly associated with reduced toxicity less than 100 days after transplantation.[248] Superoxide dismutase–2 (SOD2) is a mitochondrial enzyme that converts endogenous toxic superoxides to hydrogen peroxide, and the valine variant has lower enzymatic activity. In SOD2 rs1000 V16A polymorphism, the valine allele was associated with significantly greater overall toxicity.

In adult women with breast cancer who were treated with cyclophosphamide, women with at least 1 GSTP1 (rs1695) variant G allele had a lower risk of neutropenia and leukopenia than those with the AA genotype,[249] and women with GSTA1*B/*B, which has reduced enzyme activity, had a higher survival rate than those with GSTA1*A/*A and GSTA1*A/*B.[250]

Platinum Compounds

Platinum-based drugs (cisplatin, carboplatin, and oxaliplatin) are widely used for the treatment of childhood solid tumors, including osteosarcoma, neuroblastoma, and hepatoblastoma (see Table 46-1).[251] Cisplatin (cis-diamminedichloroplatinum[II]) was first approved by the Food and Drug Administration in 1978, followed by carboplatin (cis-diammine[cyclobutane-1,1-dicarboxylate-O,O′] platinum[II]) in 1989 and oxaliplatin ([1R,2R]-cyclohexane-1,2-diamine[ethanedioato-O,O′] platinum[II]) in 2002. Although passive diffusion through the cellular lipid bilayer was hypothesized,[252-254] recent studies have shown the significant role of a variety of ion pumps and transporters.[255,256] The copper transporter protein copper transporter–1 (SLC31A1), which is involved in copper homeostasis, appears to be a major influx transporter of the platinum compounds.[257,258] ABCC2, ABCC4, copper-transporting P-type adenosine triphosphatases (ATP7B), MATE1, OCT1, and OCT2 are suggested to have a role in the cellular accumulation of platinum compounds.[259-263] GST catalyzes the conjugation of cisplatin with glutathione, which leads to its inactivation and excretion. Within cells, the platinum compounds are aquated and are then more reactive with the drug's cellular targets.[264-267] They bind to DNA and induce lesions that are recognized by multiple repair pathways, mainly the nucleotide excision repair system.[268-272] However, the mismatch repair system is also implicated in the recognition and repair of these lesions.[273,274] When the lesions cannot be repaired, apoptosis is induced through different signaling cascades.[275,276]

Previous studies using the lymphoblastoid cell lines have identified genetic variants associated with cisplatin-induced cytotoxicity (see Table 46-4).[277,278] ERCC2 (excision repair cross-complementation group–2) is one of the genes involved in the nucleotide excision repair pathway; common variations in the ERCC2 Lys751Gln G allele (TG or GG) were associated with poorer tumor response and shorter event-free survival than the TT allele in pediatric and young adult patients with osteosarcoma who were treated with cisplatin, suggesting that polymorphic variants in DNA repair genes could be useful predictors of response.[279]

Platinum compounds can cause adverse effects (e.g., ototoxicity and nephrotoxicity) in children, and cisplatin, carboplatin, and oxaliplatin have different toxicity profiles.[280] Cisplatin-induced hearing loss is usually bilateral and irreversible, affecting 41% to 61% of children treated, and several candidate genes may be associated with ototoxicity.[281] The GSTM3*B allele was found to provide a protective effect against cisplatin-induced ototoxicity, compared with the GSTM3*A allele.[282] GST genes were also associated with cisplatin-induced long-term hearing impairment in testicular cancer survivors; the genotype [105]Val/[105]Val-GSTP1 appeared to be protective in comparison with [105]Ile/[105]Ile- or [105]Ile/[105]Val-GSTP1.[283] The role of GST genes in other cisplatin-induced toxicities was confirmed by the discovery that GSTM1 and GSTT1 polymorphisms may affect cognitive impairment in children after treatment for medulloblastoma; patients with at least one null genotype were at greater risk than those without a null genotype.[284] Authors of another genotyping study of 1949 SNPs in 220 drug-metabolism genes in children identified genetic variants in TPMT (rs12201199, A allele) and catechol-O-methyltransferase (COMT; rs9332377, A allele) that were associated with cisplatin-induced hearing loss.[285] TPMT and COMT are methyltransferases dependent on the S-adenosylmethionine methyl donor substrate in the methionine pathway. The authors of this study proposed that higher levels of this substrate could provide a putative mechanism for cisplatin ototoxicity mediated by reduced TPMT and COMT activity. They suggested that decreased TPMT enzyme activity may also reduce the inactivation of cisplatin-purine compounds, thereby increasing cisplatin cross-linking efficiency and cisplatin toxicity, but no mechanistic data were provided. Megalin is a member of the low-density lipoprotein receptor family and is highly expressed in marginal cells of the stria vascularis of the inner ear, which accumulate high levels of platinum DNA adducts. The nonsynonymous SNP rs2075252 in megalin was found to be associated with cisplatin-induced ototoxicity.[286]

Irinotecan

Irinotecan, known as 7-ethyl-10-[4-(1-piperidino)-1-piperidino] carbonyloxycamptothecin or CPT-11, is a semisynthetic analogue of the natural alkaloid camptothecin (Fig. 46-11 and Table 46-1). It is a prodrug converted to its active metabolite, 7-ethyl-10-hydroxycamptothecin (SN-38), by carboxylesterases in the liver and gastrointestinal tract.[287,288] SN-38 is a potent topoisomerase I inhibitor and has shown promising activity against pediatric solid tumors alone or in combination with other chemotherapeutic agents.[289-291] Irinotecan is inactivated after oxidation by CYP3A4 to 7-ethyl-10-[4-N-(5-aminopentanoic acid)-1-piperidino] carbonyloxycamptothecin and 7-ethyl-10-(4-amino-1-piperidino) carbonyloxycamptothecin.[292,293] The majority of irinotecan and its metabolites are excreted in bile; bile excretion is enhanced by the formation of SN-38 glucuronide (SN-38G), catalyzed primarily by UGT1A1.[294]

The UGT1A1*28 polymorphism reflects a change in the number of TA repeats in the TATA box of the UGT1A1 promoter from the wild-type 6 repeats to the variant 7 repeats (Table 46-4).[295] Approximately 7% to 19% of the white population is homozygous (7/7) for the variant allele, as seen in Gilbert syndrome, which leads to reduced enzyme expression. Several studies in adults found that patients with the UGT1A1*28 7/7 genotype had lower SN-38G/SN-38 AUC ratios and greater toxicity after treatment with a high dosage of irinotecan (e.g., 350 mg/m², once a month) than did those with the 6/6 or 6/7 genotype.[296,297] Children with the UGT1A1*28 7/7 genotype who received low-dose irinotecan (15 to

75 mg/m²) on a protracted schedule (5 days weekly for 2 consecutive weeks) tended to have higher SN-38 AUC values and lower SN-38G/SN-38 AUC ratios.[298] However, severe toxicity was not increased in these patients, suggesting that UGT1A1 genotyping is not a useful predictor of severe toxicity for patients treated with this irinotecan dosage and schedule.

Temozolomide

Temozolomide is one of the imidazotetrazinone derivatives discovered in the 1980s and is used to treat CNS malignancies (see Table 46-1).[299] Temozolomide is a prodrug that undergoes spontaneous conversion to the reactive metabolite 5-(3-methyltriazen-1-yl-) imidazole-4-carboxamide (MTIC) under physiologic conditions.[300,301] MTIC is degraded to the methyldiazonium cation, which transfers its methyl group to DNA and to the final degradation product, 4-amino-5-imidazole carboxamide. The most common methylation site in DNA is the N^7 position of guanine, followed by the N^3 position of adenine and the O^6 position of guanine.[300,302] N^7-methylguanine and N^3-methyladenine, which constitute nearly 90% of the total methylation events, are efficiently repaired by the base excision repair pathway and have low cytotoxicity potential. O^6-methylguanine represents only 5% to 10% of methylation events, but these adducts trigger the DNA mismatch repair pathway and are highly cytotoxic. O^6-methylguanine methyltransferase (MGMT) is a cellular DNA repair protein that rapidly reverses alkylation (including methylation) at the O^6 position of guanine, thereby neutralizing cytotoxic effects.[303] MGMT can be silenced by abnormal methylation of CpG islands in its promoter region, which prevents DNA damage repair.[304,305] In several studies, adult patients with glioblastoma who had a methylated MGMT promoter had longer survival after temozolomide treatment than did patients without methylation.[306-308] Thus the methylation status of the MGMT gene promoter may provide a marker of temozolomide sensitivity. Results in the pediatric population are inconsistent, and more studies in larger cohorts are needed.[115,117,309]

Pharmacogenetics, Pharmacogenomics, and the Future

Many studies are underway to relate interindividual variability in pharmacokinetics to drug efficacy and toxicity and their implications for improving the therapeutic index of anticancer agents in children. Evaluation of the whole genome in a large series of patients will deepen our understanding of how pharmacogenetics and pharmacogenomics can be used to improve patient outcomes. This knowledge can be used to develop individualized therapy for patients. However, thus far the clinical application of pharmacogenomics research findings has been slow. The cost of genotyping will diminish over time and with advances in genomic technology, but the consistent interpretation of results and their efficient communication to the clinician are essential. Key components to successful clinical implementation of pharmacogenomics will include not only clinician understanding of pharmacogenomic test results but also availability of clinical prescription guidelines based on the test results,

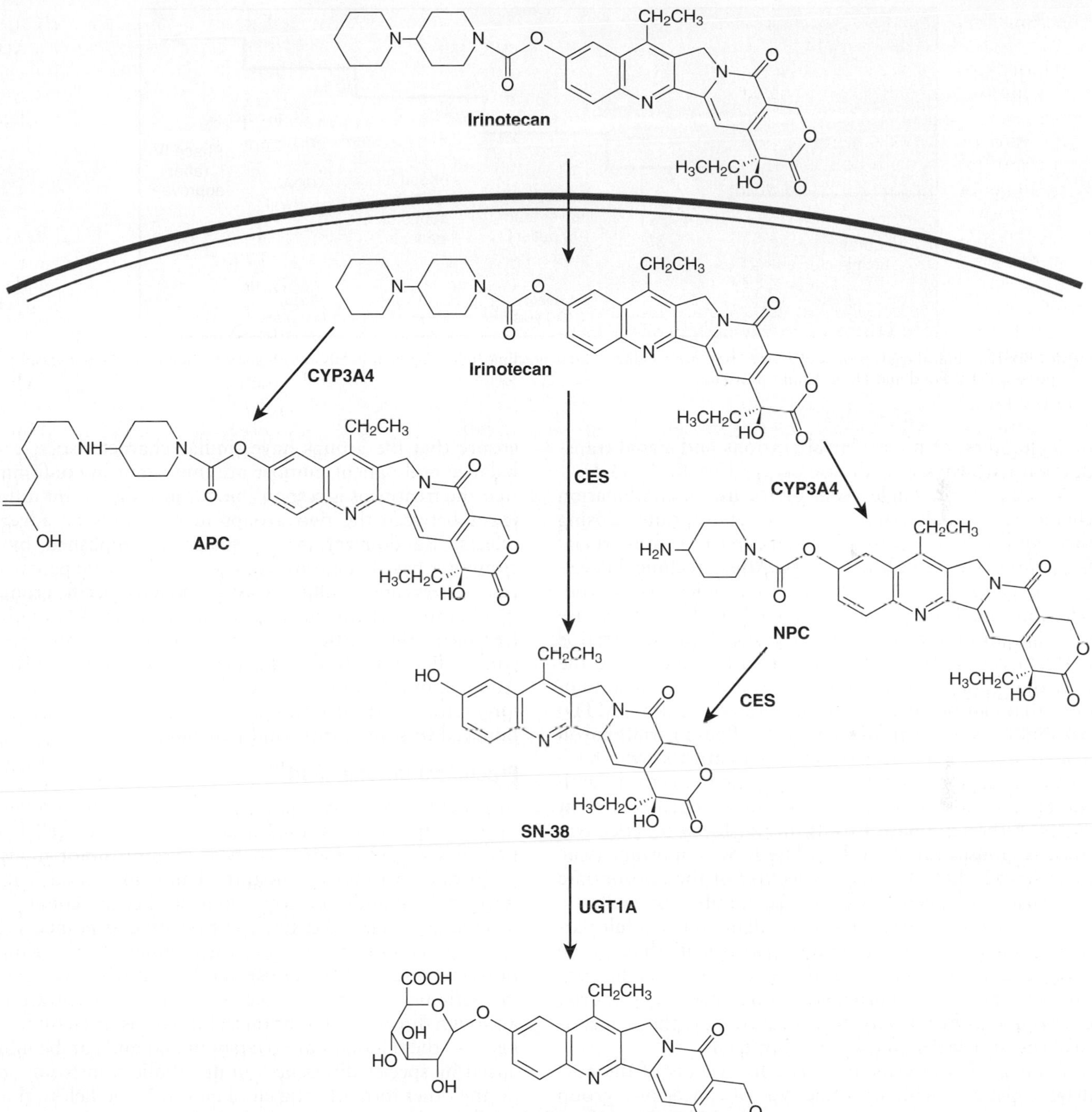

Figure 46-11 Metabolic pathways of irinotecan. Irinotecan is a prodrug converted to its active metabolite, 7-ethyl-10-hydroxycamptothecin (SN-38), by carboxylesterases *(CES)* in the liver and gastrointestinal tract. Irinotecan is inactivated after oxidation by CYP3A4 to 7-ethyl-10-94-N-[5-aminopentanoic acid]-1-piperidino) carbonyloxycamptothecin *(APC)* and 7-ethyl-10-(4-amino-1-piperidino) carbonyloxycamptothecin *(NPC)*. The majority of irinotecan and its metabolites are excreted in bile; bile excretion is enhanced by the formation of SN-38 glucuronide *(SN-38G)*, catalyzed primarily by uridine diphosphate *(UDP)*–glucuronosyltransferase 1A1 *(UGT1A1)*.

knowledge/evidence-based decision support systems, and appropriate sharing of this sensitive information with patients. Pharmacogenomics data cannot substitute for close clinical monitoring of patients, but they can be used to improve outcomes through informed treatment planning and anticipation of toxicities.

NEW DRUG DEVELOPMENT

The era of molecular targeted therapy arrived with the approval of the *BCR-ABL1* inhibitor imatinib for treatment of chronic myeloid leukemia.[219] Numbers of new agents have been tested in clinical trials along with further

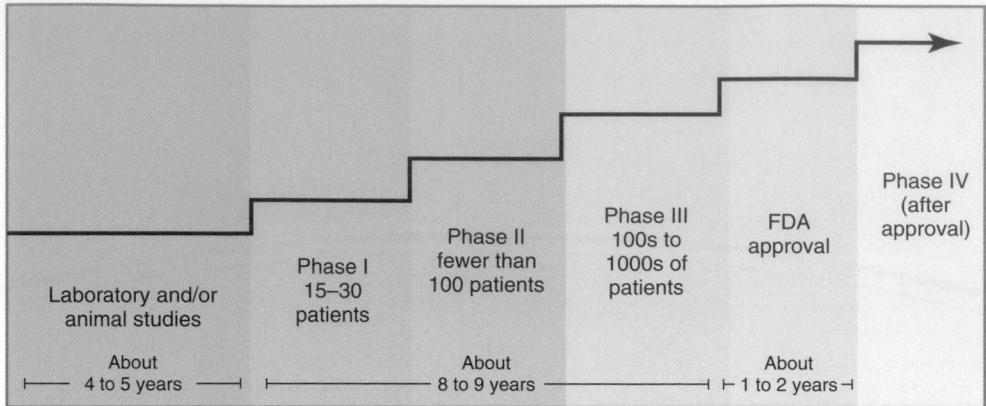

Figure 46-12 Clinical trials process. Clinical trials are conducted after preclinical development in laboratory and/or animal studies and encompass four phases. *FDA,* Food and Drug Administration.

understanding of molecular alterations and signal transduction pathways in pediatric cancer (see Table 46-1).

Whether for a single agent or for use in combination chemotherapy, determination of appropriate dosing through preclinical evaluation and clinical trials is crucial for appropriate use of new drugs. After preclinical development in cellular or animal models, clinical trials progress through four phases (Fig. 46-12).[310,311] The entire process can take more than 10 years. A phase I trial is performed to evaluate the safety of a new agent and the tolerable dosage. The study determines the maximum dose that can be given (maximum tolerated dose, MTD) without causing harmful side effects. Phase I trials enroll a small number of patients (15 to 30 patients) who have advanced cancers that cannot be treated effectively with standard regimens or for which no standard treatment exists. Although phase I trials do not focus on effectiveness, responses are recorded. The most important issue in pediatric phase I trials is selection of the appropriate investigational agent, because the number of pediatric participants is remarkably smaller than that of adult participants and therefore the number of agents that can be investigated is limited. Also, the new agent must be continuously available to progress through the stages of drug development, but it may be withdrawn by pharmaceutical firms if it lacks efficacy in adult trials.

A phase II trial evaluates the effectiveness of the new drug in patients with a specific type of cancer or a group of related cancers, typically by using the MTD determined in the phase I trial. Safety is also monitored. These studies usually enroll fewer than 100 patients but may include as many as 300, depending on the breadth of cancer diagnoses evaluated. The patients who participate in phase II trials may or may not have been treated previously with standard therapy for their type of cancer. Although efficacy in a specific population is the main question of phase II studies, these studies are almost never designed to compare the efficacy of an intervention with that of standard therapy. This comparison is done in phase III trials, which usually enroll large groups of patients (100 to several thousand). Participants are randomly assigned to groups that are typically stratified according to patient characteristics such as age, sex, and extent of disease to ensure that the groups have similar characteristics. This balance and patient number are important in confirming that the treatment is responsible for any significant differences between the two groups in responses or adverse effects. Randomization is usually accomplished by a computer-based algorithm, and trial participants or researchers cannot influence assignment to specific groups. Neither the participants nor their doctors may know what treatment the participants are receiving (double-blind study). Phase IV trials take place after Food and Drug Administration approval to evaluate the effectiveness and long-term safety of drugs in larger populations (several hundred to several thousand patients).

Preclinical Development

In general, preclinical data come from cytotoxic effects in vitro in various animal and human cancer cell lines and in vivo antitumor activity in mouse tumor models or in human tumors xenografted into immunodeficient mice.[312,313] In addition, toxicology studies are conducted in various species to determine toxicity end points, such as the lethal dose for 10% of the animals. These evaluations in vitro and in mouse models clearly have value in defining the target plasma drug concentrations, although direct extrapolation to humans is often difficult, because these models are oversimplified and can be influenced by species differences in metabolic transformation or any other form of drug elimination. Nonetheless, these studies may guide the choice of starting dosage and schedules of administration for phase I clinical trials. For example, if drug cytotoxic activity is shown to be S-phase–specific, prolonged exposure may be required, suggesting the use of a prolonged IV infusion if the agent has a relatively short terminal half-life. Preclinical data can also be valuable in defining the therapeutic window. Theoretically, it is possible to define a two-dimensional plasma concentration-versus-time window, the lower limit of which is the plasma concentration at which antitumor activity begins and whose upper limit is the plasma concentration at which unacceptable toxicity begins (see Fig. 46-1).[314] This approach is used to define the plasma concentration parameters for therapeutic drug monitoring and is widely used for cancer drugs and for numerous noncancer drugs, including antibiotics and antiretroviral agents.[315] In the United States, the Pediatric Preclinical Testing Program of the National Cancer Institute evaluates the therapeutic potential of new agents against molecular characteristics of pediatric cancers identified by the work of the St. Jude Children's Research Hospital and Washington University Pediatric Cancer Genome Project and others.[316]

Choice of Starting Dose for Clinical Studies

Historically, the starting dose of anticancer agents for early clinical trials has been selected empirically on the basis of toxicologic studies in rodents (mice and rats) and dogs; 10% of the murine lethal dose for 10% of the animals is often selected as the starting dose for safety studies in patients, because intolerable toxicity is unlikely at this dose.[312,313,317] Theoretical considerations and an extensive review of preclinical toxicologic studies support the appropriateness and safety of using toxicologic models based on mouse and rat data for anticancer drug development.[318,319] Importantly, however, much higher plasma concentrations can generally be achieved in animals than in humans, and this difference is not always explained by a difference in drug clearance. Therefore, in extrapolating the results of efficacy studies in tumor-bearing animals to clinical use, it is important to remember that these tumors have been exposed to drug levels that in most cases cannot be achieved in patients. This factor is particularly relevant when the relationship between plasma levels and antitumor effects is poorly understood.

Drug development for pediatric cancer has had to evolve while survival rates have improved, making fewer patients eligible for investigational drug studies.[311,313] Agents developed for use in adults may readily be investigated for potential pediatric use. However, new agents targeted to specific molecular abnormalities in adult cancers may have little value in treating pediatric cancers, which typically do not have the same underlying molecular abnormalities.

In a retrospective comparison of phase I studies performed between 1999 and 2004, the pediatric MTD was strongly correlated with the adult MTD. Adult data, such as MTD, pharmacokinetics, toxicity profile, and efficacy findings, are available for many candidate agents. Dose-finding pediatric phase I studies often start at approximately 80% of the adult MTD,[313] even though the MTD in children is often higher when adjusted to BSA. Pediatric formulations (e.g., liquid formulation or crushed form of tablets) are often necessary for younger children who cannot swallow capsules or tablets. However, pharmaceutical companies have little financial incentive to invest in the development of pediatric formulations, which have a very small market. It should also be recognized that the "starting dosage" is typically a dosage that has been tolerated by essentially everyone and thus will be lower than the MTD for patients with rapid drug clearance, and perhaps intolerable for a small subset of patient with very slow drug clearance (possibly because of an inherited defect in drug metabolism, as exemplified by TPMT and mercaptopurine, in which 1 in ~400 children can tolerate only 10% of the standard dosage).

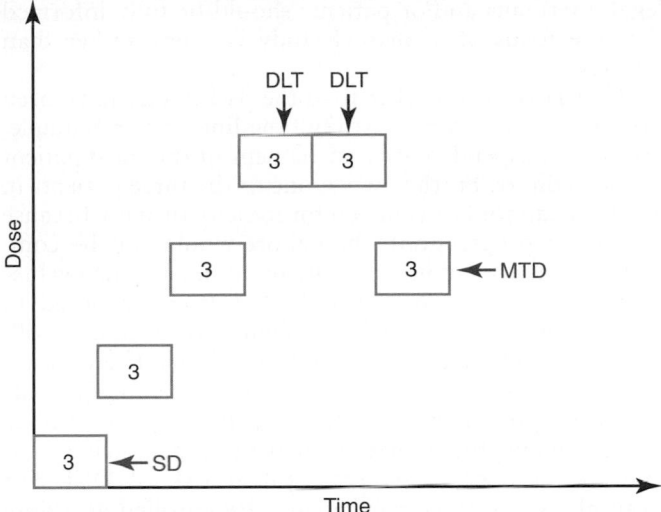

Figure 46-13 Graphic depiction of dose escalation methods using the traditional 3+3 design in phase I cancer clinical trials. Each box represents a cohort consisting of the indicated number of patients treated at a given dose level. After three patients have undergone treatment without experiencing dose-limiting toxicity *(DLT)*, the dose is escalated for the next set of three patients. *MTD,* Maximum tolerated dose; *SD,* starting dose.

Dose Escalation Schemes

Most phase I oncology trials use rule-based designs, which include the traditional 3+3 design or its variations.[312] This model implements any prior assumptions of the dose-toxicity curve. Doses are escalated or de-escalated by using the "up-and-down" methods created by Dixon and Mood in 1948.[320] In the 3+3 model, a minimum of three participants are evaluated at each dose level (Fig. 46-13). If none of the three experiences a dose-limiting toxicity (DLT), an additional three participants are enrolled at the next higher dose level. If one of the three experiences a DLT, an additional three participants are evaluated at the same dose level. Dose escalation continues in this manner until at least two participants in a cohort of three or six experience DLT (i.e., >33% of participants have a DLT at this dose level). Because the MTD is exceeded at this level, an additional three participants (as high as a total of six) are treated at the next lower dose level, which is defined as the MTD if no more than one of six participants (0% to 17%) experience DLT.

Dose escalation is usually based on the modified Fibonacci sequence, in which steps escalate in decreasing increments (e.g., 100%, 67%, 50%, 40%, and 30% to 35% of preceding doses). Because good correlation between adult and pediatric MTDs has been shown, little value exists in testing more than four dose levels or testing dose levels greater than 1.6 times the adult MTD.[321] Limiting pediatric phase I trials to a maximum of four dose levels increasing in 30% increments (e.g., 0.7, 1.0, 1.3, and 1.6 times the adult MTD) would significantly shorten the time required for study completion and can expect therapeutic activity, although it is not the major purpose. Historically, children participating in phase I studies have been treated with therapeutic intent, although legal guardians and/or patients should be fully informed that the focus of a phase I study is safety rather than efficacy.[322]

Alternative rules other than the 3+3 design have been proposed to shorten the study time line.[312] For example, accrual is suspended after enrollment of the third patient in each cohort. Further, when one of the three patients in a cohort cannot be evaluated for toxicity (usually because of disease progression), the cohort would not be completed until one additional patient completes the evaluation. The "rolling 6" design[323] has been proposed to shorten the time frame by allowing concurrent enrollment of two to six patients at a dose level. The decision about the dose level at which to enroll upcoming patients is based on the number of the patients currently enrolled and evaluable, the number of patients experiencing DLT, and the number of patients still at risk of DLT. For example, when three participants are enrolled at a dose level, if toxicity data are available for all three and no DLTs have been observed, the fourth participant is enrolled at the next higher dose level. If toxicity data are not yet available for all three participants but no DLT has been observed, or if one patient has experienced DLT, the new participant is enrolled at the same dose level. If two or more of the three participants have experienced DLT, the dose level is de-escalated. This process is repeated for the fifth and sixth participants. Accrual is suspended only when a cohort of six is filled. A discrete-event simulation study showed that the rolling 6 model significantly shortened the duration of pediatric phase I trials without increasing the risk of toxicity; this strategy has been incorporated into pediatric phase I studies.[324]

Parameter Estimates

The pharmacokinetic parameters of the investigational agent, including peak concentration, drug clearance, half-life, Vd, AUC, and metabolic profile, should be defined at different dose levels to be used clinically.[312,313] Because the effect of a therapeutic agent in the body is generally a function of its concentration at the (molecular) site of action, a description of the spatial-temporal behavior of the drug in the body is helpful, if not essential, for understanding and predicting normal tissue toxicity and optimizing tumor response.[312,313] Measures of drug exposure (e.g., AUC) are clearly more informative than the absolute dose. Ideally, drug exposure should be measured at the molecular locus of action or at least at the tissue or tumor level, but with the exception of leukemia, drug concentrations are usually measured only in plasma, which is the only readily accessible surrogate. The detection of metabolites and definition of their pharmacokinetic behavior and pharmacologic activity are also extremely important, particularly in the case of agents that require metabolic activation, such as cyclophosphamide and irinotecan.

Data from early clinical studies can be used to define the therapeutic window of the agent and design more rational schedules of administration and combination therapies; it may also provide clues about potential cumulative toxicity or organ-specific toxicity. The measured parameters can be compared with the observed clinical outcome, particularly in terms of toxicity, to help define pharmacokinetic-pharmacodynamic relationships that may be of use in further clinical testing of the agent. In addition, dose-effect relationships, at least in terms of toxicity, can best be assessed at this early stage of clinical development, when a wide range of doses is being administered to patients.

After a dose is selected, the same dose is usually maintained throughout treatment unless serious toxicity occurs, in which case the dose is empirically decreased during subsequent treatment courses. In contrast, the dose of chemotherapy is rarely increased in the absence of toxicity, despite the possibility of undertreatment. Although wide interpatient variability has been demonstrated in all aspects of anticancer drug pharmacokinetics, several studies have observed reasonably predictive relationships between a measure of drug exposure and toxicity or antitumor efficacy in pediatric patients (Table 46-5). These findings would add to the argument to

TABLE 46-5   Pharmacokinetic-Pharmacodynamic Relationships of Chemotherapeutic Agents

Drug	Toxicity/Efficacy (Disease)	Pharmacokinetic Parameter
Busulfan	Hepatotoxicity	AUC
Carboplatin	Thrombocytopenia	AUC
Cisplatin	Nephrotoxicity	C_{max} (unbound drug)
	Neurotoxicity	C_{max} (unbound drug)
Cyclophosphamide	Cardiotoxicity	AUC
Docetaxel	Neutropenia	AUC
Doxorubicin	AML	$C_{3\ hr}$
	Leukocytopenia	AUC
	Thrombocytopenia	Doxorubicinol AUC
5-Fluorouracil	Mucositis	AUC $>30\ \mu g \times h/mL$
	Leukocytopenia	AUC and C_{ss}
Irinotecan	Neutropenia	AUC
	Diarrhea	Biliary index
6-Mercaptopurine	ALL	AUC; RBC 6-TGN levels
Methotrexate	Mucositis, myelosuppression	$C_{48\ hr} >0.9\ \mu M$
Paclitaxel	Neutropenia	Time above $0.05\ \mu M$
Teniposide	Lymphoma, leukemia	C_{ss} and CL
Topotecan	Myelosuppression	Lactone AUC
Vinblastine	Neutropenia	C_{ss}
Vincristine	Neurotoxicity	AUC

ALL, Acute lymphoblastic leukemia; *AML,* acute myeloid leukemia; *AUC,* area under the plasma concentration vs. time curve; C_{3-hrs}, plasma concentration 3 h after intravenous bolus administration; $C_{48\ hr}$, plasma concentration at 18 h; C_{max}, peak plasma concentration; C_{ss}, plasma concentration at steady state; *CL,* total plasma clearance; *RBC,* red blood cell; *6-TGN,* 6-thioguanine nucleotide (intracellular active metabolite of 6-mercaptopurine).

increase the dose in cases of limited toxicity, although this question remains unresolved.

Various mathematical models have been used to analyze the relation between drug concentration in biologic fluids (e.g., plasma) and the pharmacologic effects of anticancer agents. One such model is the modified Hill equation or the E_{max} model—that is, the drug concentration producing the maximum effect. The Hill equation reflects the sigmoidal relationship of pharmacologic response to AUC, steady state exposure, and threshold concentration, respectively; the response is usually measured as hematologic toxicity, expressed as a percentage. A number of commonly used anticancer drugs, including carboplatin, doxorubicin, etoposide, teniposide, mercaptopurine, 5-fluorouracil, paclitaxel, and vinblastine, have demonstrated this type of relationship.[325] When nonhematologic toxicities are dose limiting, they can be more difficult to model because of the subjective nature of grading them, in contrast to hematologic toxicity, which is a more quantitative continuous variable. However, efforts to model these adverse effects have yielded useful correlations between nephrotoxicity and cisplatin AUC and between gastrointestinal toxicity and glucuronidation rates of the irinotecan metabolite, SN-38.[326]

Clinical trials in childhood ALL that revealed a relation between drug clearance or drug exposure (AUC or steady state plasma concentration) and treatment efficacy (event-free survival) also have been conducted[327,328]; therefore treatment outcome may be improved by randomized clinical trials that adjust doses on the basis of drug clearance.[5]

STRATEGIES TO IMPROVE THE THERAPEUTIC INDEX

Dosage Based on Body Surface Area

The traditional method of individualizing anticancer drug dosage in children is by using body surface area (BSA) (Table 46-6).[329,330] BSA has become the standard variable for determining the dose of anticancer agents in pediatric patients for several reasons. First, an established correlation exists between BSA and some relevant individual patient characteristics, such as GFR, blood volume, and basal metabolic rate.[331] Second, the starting dose of agents in phase I studies is based on data derived from animal models, in which the drug dose is calculated on the basis of weight (mg/kg) or BSA (mg/m²). Third, in the 1950s, when attempts were first made to define a more accurate method for administration of cytotoxic drugs to children, several studies suggested that BSA be used in dose calculation. In 1958, Pinkel[332] reported a retrospective analysis that used a BSA-based formula for adults and children and Meeh's formula for animals to determine the pediatric and adult doses of five cytotoxic drugs (mercaptopurine, methotrexate, mechlorethamine, triethylene thiophosphoramide, and actinomycin). When the conventional doses were calculated according to unit surface area, similar values were obtained for all agents tested in children and adults except for mercaptopurine; therefore, the author recommended that doses of cytotoxic agents be normalized by using BSA.

TABLE 46-6 Strategies to Improve Therapeutic Index of Anticancer Drugs in Children

Dose Adjustment Method	Example
Based on Patient Characteristics	
Body surface area*	All drugs
Based on Pharmacokinetic-Pharmacodynamic Principles	
Therapeutic drug monitoring	Methotrexate, 5-fluorouracil, busulfan, etoposide, cisplatin
Feedback-controlled dosing	Methotrexate
Circadian rhythm–based dosing	6-Mercaptopurine, busulfan, carboplatin, docetaxel, 5-fluorouracil, oxaliplatin
Biomodulation	
Pharmacokinetic modulation	CYP3A4 inhibitor (erythromycin, quinidine, ketoconazole, cyclosporin A) ABCB1 inhibitor (cyclosporin A)
Pharmacodynamic modulation	Leucovorin for methotrexate and 5-fluorouracil Amifostine for cisplatin Dexrazoxane for anthracycline Cefixime for irinotecan
Drug scheduling	Etoposide, methotrexate, dexamethasone
Drug administration sequence	Methotrexate–5-fluorouracil Lestaurtinib–chemotherapeutic agents in acute lymphoblastic leukemia Deoxyadenosine analogues (fludarabine, cladribine, clofarabine)–cytarabine
Based on Pharmacogenetic Principles	
Pharmacogenetics-based dosing	6-Mercaptopurine (*TPMT*)

ABC, Adenosine triphosphate–binding cassette transporter; *CYP*, cytochrome P-450 enzyme; *TPMT*, thiopurine methyltransferase.
*Weight (mg/kg) is used in children who weigh less than 10 kg.

BSA is commonly estimated by using a formula derived primarily to determine basal metabolism from weight and height alone; more recently, the original formula has been confirmed as surprisingly accurate, considering the small sample size used in deriving it.[330] The formulas by Mosteller

$$BSA = \sqrt{\frac{W \times H}{3600}} = 0.016667 \times W^{0.5} \times H^{0.5}$$

and Du Bois

$$(BSA = 4.688 \cdot W^{(0.8168 - 0.0154 \cdot \log W)})$$

are most commonly used.[333] Because of the difficulty of measuring height in infants and their physiologic differences from older children (e.g., a higher proportion of body water and a lower proportion of body fat, immature enzyme systems, and lower renal clearance rates), the majority of pediatric protocols apply a 10-kg cutoff for surface area–based dosing.[333] Below this weight, the dosing of chemotherapeutic drugs is specified on a mg/kg basis, usually based on the assumptions that an individual with BSA of 1-m² weighs 30 kg and that there is a linear relationship between weight and BSA. This method may result in significantly lower calculated doses for children whose body weight is less than 10 kg. This lower dose may avert excessive toxicity in infants and younger children, who have immature hepatic and renal function. However, some patients may receive subtherapeutic dosing, and a significant step-up in dosage can occur as children cross the 10 kg boundary by moving from mg/kg to mg/m² dosing during their treatment.

The usefulness of normalizing anticancer drug dose to BSA in adults has recently been questioned, because BSA does not vary as widely in adults as in children and is not related to the clearance of most anticancer drugs in adults.[334] BSA is considered more important for drug dose calculation in pediatric patients, whose BSA values vary over a greater range.[335]

Pathophysiologic Status

Most pharmacologic studies of anticancer agents have shown important interindividual and intraindividual variability in pharmacokinetic behavior. In some cases, this variation is caused by cancer-induced changes in physiologic status or dysfunction of specific organs involved in drug elimination (Table 46-7). For example, if urinary excretion is an important elimination route for a given drug, any decrement in renal function could decrease drug clearance and result in drug accumulation and toxicity. It would therefore be logical to reduce the drug dose relative to the degree of impaired renal function to maintain plasma concentration within a targeted therapeutic window, as has been well documented for bleomycin, carboplatin, cisplatin, cyclophosphamide, etoposide, methotrexate, and topotecan.[336] The best known example of this a priori dose adjustment of an anticancer agent is carboplatin, which is excreted renally, almost entirely by glomerular filtration. Various strategies have been developed to estimate carboplatin dose on the basis of renal function of patients, either by using creatinine clearance[337] or radioisotopically measured GFR.[338] Use of these methods has

substantially reduced pharmacokinetic variability, such that carboplatin is one of the few drugs routinely administered to achieve a targeted exposure rather than on a mg/m² or mg/kg basis.

Although a decline in renal clearance of drugs can be predicted when glomerular filtration is impaired, it is less easy to predict the effect of impaired liver function on drug clearance. The main problem is that hepatic enzymes are typically poor indicators of metabolizing activity or anticancer drug pharmacokinetics. A proposed alternative dynamic measure of liver function is based on the sum of serum bilirubin, alkaline phosphatase, and either alanine aminotransferase or aspartate aminotransferase values (each scored according to the World Health Organization grading system) to provide a hepatic dysfunction score.[339] Guidelines based on carefully conducted pharmacokinetic studies in patients with normal and impaired hepatic function have been proposed for adjustment of the doses of several agents, including anthracyclines (doxorubicin and daunorubicin), etoposide, and vinca alkaloids (vinblastine and vincristine), for patients with liver dysfunction.[340]

The binding of drugs to plasma proteins, particularly when drugs are highly bound, may also have significant clinical implications for therapeutic outcome.[341] Although protein binding is a major determinant of drug action, it is clearly only one of a myriad of factors that influence drug disposition. The extent of protein binding is a function of drug and protein concentrations, the affinity constants for the drug-protein interaction, and the number of protein-binding sites per class of binding site. Because only unbound (or free) drug in plasma is available for diffusion from the vascular compartment to the tumor interstitium, the therapeutic response will be related to free drug concentration rather than total drug concentration. Several clinical factors, including liver and renal disease, can significantly decrease the extent of plasma binding and may increase free drug concentration and the risk of unexpected toxicity, despite unaltered total (free plus bound forms) plasma drug concentration. High systemic exposure to asparaginase induces hypoalbuminemia and is associated with lower apparent clearance of dexamethasone in patients with ALL.[342] Hepatic synthesis of proteins involved in dexamethasone clearance, rather than decreased plasma protein binding, is thought to be implicated in such cases. Third-space fluid collection, such as pleural effusion and ascites, alters the pharmacokinetics of chemotherapeutic agents (e.g., methotrexate), and dose modification and strict monitoring are required.

Adjustment of the dosage a posteriori on the basis of a patient's tolerance is also widely practiced, although it may result in dose reduction, which can compromise dose intensity and lead to treatment failure. Clearly, the seriousness of the first adverse effect is the major determinant of whether it can be used as an end point. Examples of this type of dose adjustment are the platelet nadir-directed individualized approach to carboplatin dosage[343] and leukopenia targeted dosing of methotrexate and mercaptopurine in children with ALL.[344] However, this approach can be untenable when, as often occurs, treatment

TABLE 46-7   Characteristics That Affect the Pharmacokinetics of Chemotherapeutic Agents in Children

Parameter	Anticancer Drug
Renal function	Bleomycin, carboplatin, cisplatin, cyclophosphamide, etoposide, methotrexate, topotecan
Hepatic function	Anthracyclines, vinblastine, vincristine
Serum albumin	Etoposide, dexamethasone
Third spaces	Methotrexate

consists of multiple anticancer agents with overlapping toxicities (especially hematologic toxicity).

Dose Adaptation Using Pharmacokinetic-Pharmacodynamic-Pharmacogenetic Principles

Therapeutic Drug Monitoring

Prolonged infusion schedules offer a very convenient setting for anticancer drug dose adaptation in individual patients. When steady state concentration is achieved, it is possible to modify the infusion rate for the remainder of the treatment course if a relationship is known between this steady state concentration and a desired pharmacodynamic end point (see Table 46-6). This method has been successfully used to adapt the dose during continuous infusions of methotrexate, 5-fluorouracil, busulfan, and etoposide, and for repeated oral administration of etoposide or repeated IV administration of cisplatin.[340] Methotrexate plasma concentration is routinely monitored after administration of high-dose methotrexate to identify patients at high risk of toxicity and to adjust leucovorin rescue and hydration in patients with delayed excretion. In some cases, ongoing methotrexate infusion can be slowed or discontinued if the concentration is considered to be critically high. Such monitoring has significantly reduced the incidence of serious toxicity (including toxic death) and has in fact improved outcome by eliminating unacceptably low systemic exposure.[5]

Feedback-Controlled Dosing

It remains to be seen how information about variability can eventually be used to devise an optimal dosage regimen of a drug for the treatment of a given disease in an individual patient. Obviously, the desired objective would be most efficiently achieved if the individual's dosage requirements could be calculated before the drug is administered. Although this ideal cannot be completely met in clinical practice, some success may be achieved by adopting feedback-controlled dosing, as in the case of methotrexate (see Table 46-6).[5,345] In adaptive dosage with feedback control, population-based predictive models are initially used but allow the possibility of dosage alteration based on feedback revision. In this approach, patients are first treated with the standard dose, and then during treatment pharmacokinetic information is estimated by a limited-sampling strategy, and compared with that predicted from the population model with which dosage was initiated. More patient-specific pharmacokinetic parameters are calculated on the basis of this comparison, and dosage is adjusted accordingly to maintain the target exposure that produces the desired pharmacodynamic effect for subsequent courses. It has been proposed that, despite its mathematical complexity, this approach may be the only way to achieve the desired precise exposure of an anticancer agent. The use of population pharmacokinetic models is increasingly studied in adults in an attempt to accommodate as much pharmacokinetic variability as possible in terms of measurable characteristics, and mathematical equations based on BSA, gender, and protein levels are provided, for example, to predict drug clearance with an acceptable degree of precision.

Circadian Rhythm–Based Dosing

Administration at certain times of the day may improve the therapeutic index of several anticancer drugs (see Table 46-6).[346,347] For example, significant improvement in survival has been demonstrated for children with ALL who received 6-mercaptopurine in the evening compared with the morning.[348] Chronotherapy schedules based on this concept showed improved tolerability in several clinical trials using other anticancer drugs, including busulfan, carboplatin, docetaxel, 5-fluorouracil, and oxaliplatin.[349-351]

Although the precise mechanisms are still unknown, such findings have led to the assumption that tolerability rhythms are coupled with the rest-activity cycle in patients with cancer. For example, one of the major limiting factors for 6-mercaptopurine is bone marrow toxicity. Normal bone-marrow cells are thought to have their nadir of DNA synthesis activity at night.[352] Thus administration of 6-mercaptopurine in the evening could provide normal cells an advantage over leukemic cells, which have minimal and variable diurnal changes in DNA synthesis. It remains unclear whether the potential benefits will justify the major inconvenience of drug administration in the middle of the night.

Pharmacogenetics-Based Dosing

The *TPMT* genetic polymorphism probably best illustrates the potential impact of pharmacogenetics on pediatric oncology (Figs. 46-6 and 46-7; see also Table 46-6).[87] TPMT plays an important role in inactivation of thiopurines (6-mercaptopurine, 6-thioguanine, and azathioprine) by catalyzing the transfer of the methyl group from S-adenosyl methionine to the sulfur atoms of thiopurines. TPMT-deficient patients accumulate excessive concentrations of thioguanine nucleotides after conventional doses of thiopurines, leading to severe and potentially fatal hematologic toxicity.[353,354] Heterozygous patients have an intermediate risk of toxicity and typically require only a modest dose reduction (as much as 50%), whereas patients who have inherited two nonfunctional alleles require treatment with only 5% to 10% of the standard dose to avoid toxicity without compromising efficacy.[92,355,356] Pretreatment knowledge of a patient's TPMT status is now used for dose optimization to reduce the likelihood of toxicity.[356] *TPMT* genotyping (e.g., use of restriction fragment length polymorphism or high-throughput DNA arrays such as the Affymetrix DMET chip [Affymetrix, Santa Clara, Calif.]) is highly efficient in identifying patients at risk of thiopurine-related toxicity. TPMT enzymatic activity in erythrocytes can also be directly measured by radiochemical assay, but heterologous red blood cell transfusions within the past ~30 to 60 days can cause spurious results.

Mercaptopurine, thioguanine, and their metabolites (e.g., thioguanine nucleotides) can be quantified by reverse-phase high-performance liquid chromatography assay.[357] A significant inverse relationship between TGN and TPMT activity in erythrocytes has been observed in several studies, and acute hematologic toxicity (e.g., neutropenia) has been clearly related to erythrocyte TGN concentration; unacceptable toxicity is reported when doses of 50 to 75 mg/m^2 per day are given to children with *TPMT* deficiency.[353,358] When thiopurines are administered according to genotype, comparable cellular thioguanine nucleotide concentrations are achieved; therefore all patients, regardless of *TPMT* phenotypes, can be treated without adverse effects and without compromising efficacy. It is unclear whether adjustment of thiopurine doses on the basis of TGN levels improves treatment efficacy, but TGN measurement is helpful for detecting noncompliance and explaining hematopoietic toxicity.[358,359]

Intentional Biomodulation

Pharmacokinetic Alterations. Intestinal metabolic systems and drug efflux pumps located in the intestinal mucosa are another limitation of the bioavailability of orally administered drugs.[360] Several enzymes located in enterocytes, such as CYP3A4, are involved in the presystemic metabolism of many cytotoxic agents, including cyclophosphamide and etoposide, thereby limiting the oral absorption of these drugs.[361] The bioavailability of these drugs might be substantially enhanced by pharmacologic modulation of enteric CYP3A4 activity (see Table 46-6). Several investigators confirmed that coadministration of specific inhibitors of CYP3A4 activity, such as erythromycin, quinidine, ketoconazole, and cyclosporin A, increase the oral bioavailability of various anticancer agents such as etoposide while also diminishing variability in absorption.[362] Similarly, ABCB1, which is abundantly present in the gastrointestinal tract, has been shown to limit intestinal absorption of numerous (anticancer) agents.[363] Combined inhibition of intestinal ABCB1 and CYP3A4 by cyclosporin A was shown to substantially increase systemic exposure to oral paclitaxel in adult patients with cancer,[364] suggesting that simultaneous modulation of transporter and enzyme could be considered when anticancer agents that have poor bioavailability are given orally.

Pharmacodynamic Alterations. The coadministration of specific agents with anticancer drugs to increase the therapeutic index has made a substantial impact in certain diseases (see Table 46-6). One of the most widely used biomodulating agents is leucovorin, a reduced folate used in combination with both methotrexate and 5-fluorouracil. This agent has been shown to decrease methotrexate-induced toxicity in various normal tissues and to enhance 5-fluorouracil–mediated cytotoxicity to tumor cells by inhibition of thymidylate synthase, thereby allowing escalation of the anticancer drug dose without affecting its disposition profile.[365] Other examples of agents that interfere with anticancer drug pharmacodynamics to reduce toxicity include (1) the use of amifostine to reduce cisplatin-associated myelosuppression, nephrotoxicity, and neurotoxicity,[366] (2) dexrazoxane to decrease anthracycline-induced cardiotoxicity,[367] and (3) coadministration of cefixime to ameliorate irinotecan-induced diarrhea.[290] Pharmacodynamic biomodulation with ABCB1-blocking agents has also been extensively studied in adults in an attempt to improve the therapeutic index of anticancer agents.[368] This multidrug-resistant drug-efflux

transporter encoded by the *ABCB1* gene is abundant in various types of human cancer. Studies performed during the past several years have shown that intrinsic and acquired expression of ABCB1 may play a role in clinical drug resistance in specific hematologic malignancies. Consequently, in clinical trials performed worldwide, ABCB1 blockers such as verapamil and cyclosporin A have been administered with anticancer drugs with the intent of attenuating carrier-mediated tumor-cell drug resistance. Unfortunately, decreased systemic clearance of the anticancer drugs became a serious problem in these trials and necessitated substantial dose reductions, thereby precluding the potential benefits of increased antitumor activity.[368] In most cases, pharmacokinetic interference appears to be the result of competition for enzymes (mainly CYP3A4) involved in drug metabolism.[369]

Although this modulation can be beneficial in pediatric cancer treatment, prospective pharmacokinetic and pharmacodynamic studies must be conducted to determine at which level (i.e., kinetics or dynamics) the interaction takes place and whether biomodulation ultimately improves the therapeutic index of anticancer agents.

Drug Scheduling and Sequence of Administration

The antitumor activity of certain chemotherapeutic agents is highly schedule dependent (see Table 46-6). For these drugs, the antitumor response or toxicity profile of a dose fractionated over several days can differ from those of the same dose given over a shorter period. For example, markedly greater efficacy in adult patients with small-cell lung cancer was documented when an identical total dose of etoposide was administered on a 5-day divided-dose schedule rather than as a 24-hour infusion.[370] Pharmacokinetic analysis showed that both schedules produced very similar overall systemic drug exposure (as measured by AUC) but that the divided-dose schedule produced twice the duration of exposure to an etoposide plasma concentration >1μg/mL. This observation was consistent with preclinical data, and the authors speculated that the duration of exposure to this threshold concentration was important in achieving clinical efficacy. This finding has led to the use of prolonged oral administration of etoposide to treat pediatric leukemia and solid tumors.[371,372] Similar schedule dependency has been demonstrated for a number of other anticancer agents. In children with ALL, 24-hour infusion of high-dose methotrexate (1 g/m^2) produced significantly greater accumulation of MTXPG$_{1-7}$ in leukemia cells than did 4-hour infusion.[373] The 24-hour infusion increased the duration of methotrexate exposure greater than 1 μmol/L by a factor of 2.5, producing greater inhibition of de novo purine synthesis in bone-marrow ALL cells and greater reduction of circulating leukemia cells. Furthermore, alternate-week (10 mg/m^2 per day on days 0 to 6 and 14 to 20) rather than continuous (10 mg/m^2 per day on days 0 to 20) administration of dexamethasone in childhood ALL significantly reduced osteonecrosis despite delivering a higher cumulative dose.[142]

Combinations of anticancer drugs can also exhibit schedule-dependent toxicity or antitumor activity,

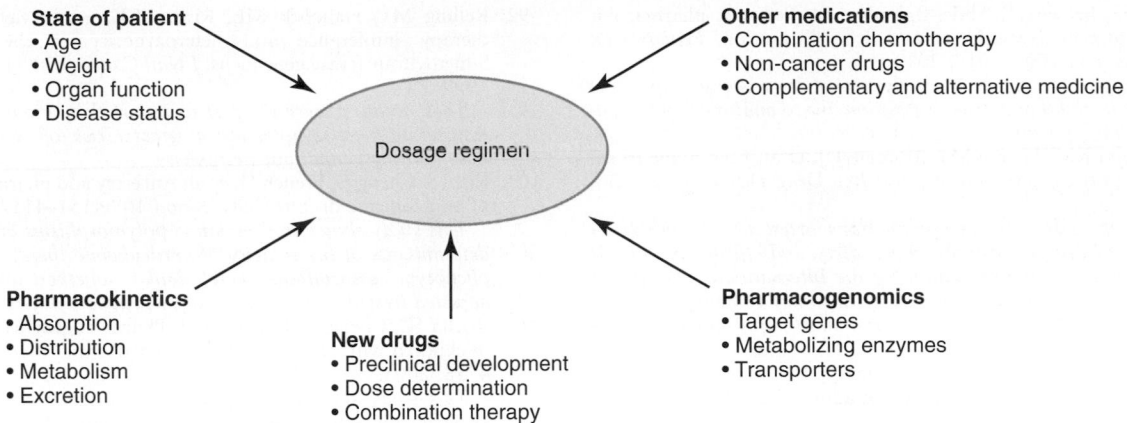

Figure 46-14 Determinants of the dosage regimen for an anticancer drug.

reflecting either pharmacokinetic or pharmacodynamic modulation. For example, the sequence of administration of 5-fluorouracil and methotrexate seems to determine the tumor cytotoxicity of this combination. In vitro, if methotrexate precedes 5-fluorouracil by at least 1 hour, synergistic results are obtained,[374] which may be due to increased activation of 5-fluorouracil to its nucleotide form. The opposite sequence of administration leads to drug antagonism due to blockage of the thymidylate synthase pathway by 5-fluorouracil. This blockage preserves the intracellular folates in their active tetrahydrofolate form, which diminishes the inhibition of dihydrofolate reductase by methotrexate. Similarly, a sequence-dependent interaction was observed in the treatment of *MLL*–rearranged ALL cells with the fms-related tyrosine kinase–3 (FLT3) inhibitor lestaurtinib and six chemotherapeutic agents (dexamethasone, vincristine, L-asparaginase, daunorubicin, cytarabine, and etoposide).[375] When chemotherapy was given before lestaurtinib, the combination was markedly synergistic, whereas the opposite sequence was antagonistic. This sequence dependence was caused by cell cycle suppression via FLT3 inhibition. Deoxyadenosine analogues such as fludarabine, cladribine, and clofarabine have been used in patients with leukemia.[376-378] They inhibit ribonucleotide reductase and decrease de novo synthesis of deoxynucleotide, lessening the feedback inhibition of deoxycytidine kinase. When combined with cytarabine in patients with AML, deoxyadenosine analogues are given first to increase the intracellular ara-CTP accumulation in leukemia cells.

In vitro and in vivo studies and phase I and II trials of combination chemotherapy typically reveal relevant pharmacokinetic and pharmacodynamic interactions and define drug doses and sequences of administration that can be safely administered.

CONCLUSION AND PERSPECTIVES

Substantial progress has been made in the optimization of cancer chemotherapy in recent years with the contribu-

tions of pharmacokinetics, pharmacodynamics, and pharmacogenetics and our increasing knowledge about physiologic changes associated with growth and development, the role of disease status, and drug-drug interactions (Fig. 46-14). Pharmacogenomics studies now include the application of next-generation sequencing technologies to cover all genetic variants,[284,285] and the inherited nature of differences in drug disposition and pharmacodynamic effects is being elucidated to provide a stronger scientific basis for optimization of drug therapy on the basis of an individual patient's genome.[30,286] The development of technologies such as cancer genome analysis, high-throughput drug screening, and combinatorial chemistry is likely to exponentially increase the number of drug targets and candidate compounds, and a deeper understanding of each compound's pharmacologic properties is expected to emerge during the exploratory stages of drug development.[287] In addition, the enormous quantity of patient-oriented information will require the use of models and computer simulation to guide clinical decisions for individualized therapy (i.e., systems biology).[288,289] In the next several years we should see the growth of targeted anticancer chemotherapy designed to exploit genetic abnormalities in individual tumors, with the reduction of toxicity and the enhancement of efficacy through judicious analysis of constitutional and genomic factors that modulate the pharmacokinetics (e.g., absorption, distribution, metabolism, and excretion) and pharmacodynamics (e.g., sensitivity and resistance) of chemotherapeutic agents.

References available online at ExpertConsult.

KEY REFERENCES

2. Horton TM, Berg SL: Educational paper. The development of new therapies for pediatric oncology. *Eur J Pediatr* 170:555–559, 2011.
   This article provides an overview of molecular agents at different stages of drug development: agents that have been approved for use in children, have been approved for use in adults, have shown promise in early clinical trials, or are supported by strong preclinical data.

7. Funk RS, Brown JT, Abdel-Rahman SM: Pediatric pharmacokinetics: human development and drug disposition. *Pediatr Clin North Am* 59:1001–1016, 2012.

   To support rational drug use, this report describes age-dependent changes in childhood drug disposition due to anatomic and physiologic development.

33. Giacomini KM, Huang SM, Tweedie DJ, et al: Membrane transporters in drug development. *Nat Rev Drug Discov* 9:215–236, 2010.

   This report describes membrane transporters as the major determinants of drug pharmacokinetic, safety, and efficacy profiles. It also provides recommendations of the International Transporter Consortium, including decision trees intended to help guide clinical studies on the currently recognized most important drug transporter interactions.

40. Schafer ES, Hunger SP: Optimal therapy for acute lymphoblastic leukemia in adolescents and young adults. *Nat Rev Clin Oncol* 8:417–424, 2011.

   This review explores the reasons and potential solutions for the disparate survival rates of adolescents and young adults versus younger children.

52. Inaba H, Greaves M, Mullighan CG: Acute lymphoblastic leukaemia. *Lancet* 381:1943–1955, 2013.

   This article comprehensively describes the epidemiology, pathobiology, and management of the most common pediatric cancer, acute lymphoblastic leukemia.

55. Scripture CD, Figg WD: Drug interactions in cancer therapy. *Nat Rev Cancer* 6:546–558, 2006.

   This article outlines the types of drug-drug interactions that occur in oncology and their underlying mechanisms.

56. Haidar C, Jeha S: Drug interactions in childhood cancer. *Lancet Oncol* 12:92–99, 2011.

   This report discusses the most common interactions between chemotherapeutic and supportive-care pediatric oncology drugs. It also reviews interactions of chemotherapy drugs with food and herbal supplements and provides recommendations for preventing adverse and potentially fatal interactions in children with cancer.

68. Sencer SF, Kelly KM: Complementary and alternative therapies in pediatric oncology. *Pediatr Clin North Am* 54:1043–1060, xiii, 2007.

   This article provides an overview of the use of complementary and alternative medicine in children with cancer.

72. International HapMap Consortium: The International HapMap Project. *Nature* 426:789–796, 2003.

   This study determined for the first time the genotypes and frequencies of 1 million or more sequence variants, and the degree of association between them, in deoxyribonucleic acid samples from populations of African, Asian, and European ancestry, allowing the discovery of sequence variants.

73. 1000 Genomes Project Consortium, et al: A map of human genome variation from population-scale sequencing. *Nature* 467:1061–1073, 2010.

   This study describes the location, allele frequency, and local haplotype structure of approximately 15 million single nucleotide polymorphisms, 1 million short insertions and deletions, and 20,000 structural variants.

79. Stanulla M, Schaeffeler E, Flohr T, et al: Thiopurine methyltransferase (TPMT) genotype and early treatment response to mercaptopurine in childhood acute lymphoblastic leukemia. *JAMA* 293:1485–1489, 2005.

   This study demonstrates the importance of the thiopurine methyltransferase genotype and its association with the early response to treatment of acute lymphoblastic leukemia.

80. Krynetski EY, Schuetz JD, Galpin AJ, et al: A single point mutation leading to loss of catalytic activity in human thiopurine S-methyltransferase. *Proc Natl Acad Sci U S A* 92:949–953, 1995.

   This report describes the cloning and characterization of the first human thiopurine methyltransferase variant allele.

89. Cheok MH, Evans WE: Acute lymphoblastic leukaemia: a model for the pharmacogenomics of cancer therapy. *Nature Rev Cancer* 6:117–129, 2006.

   This article reviews the pharmacogenomics of acute lymphoblastic leukemia and its translation to new chemotherapeutic approaches as a model for treatment optimization.

92. Relling MV, Hancock ML, Rivera GK, et al: Mercaptopurine therapy intolerance and heterozygosity at the thiopurine S-methyltransferase gene locus. *J Natl Cancer Inst* 91:2001–2008, 1999.

   These authors were the first to report that thiopurine methyltransferase heterozygotes are at greater risk of mercaptopurine dose-limiting hematopoietic toxicity.

104. Kishi S, Cheng C, French D, et al: Ancestry and pharmacogenetics of antileukemic drug toxicity. *Blood* 109:4151–4157, 2007.

   This study shows that germline polymorphisms are significant determinants of the toxicity of antileukemic therapy. Genotype-phenotype associations were similar whether analyses were adjusted by self-reported race or by genetic markers of ancestry.

111. Rocha JC, Cheng C, Liu W, et al: Pharmacogenetics of outcome in children with acute lymphoblastic leukemia. *Blood* 105:4752–4758, 2005.

   This study showed that polymorphisms interact to influence antileukemic outcome and represent determinants of response that can be used to optimize therapy.

120. Ramsey LB, Bruun GH, Yang W, et al: Rare versus common variants in pharmacogenetics: SLCO1B1 variation and methotrexate disposition. *Genome Res* 22:1–8, 2012.

   References 118, 119, and 120 are studies that identified variants associated with methotrexate pharmacokinetics at a genome-wide level.

125. Inaba H, Pui C-H: Glucocorticoid use in acute lymphoblastic leukaemia. *Lancet Oncol* 11:1096–1106, 2010.

   This article reviews glucocorticoid treatment for acute lymphoblastic leukemia.

141. Kawedia JD, Kaste SC, Pei D, et al: Pharmacokinetic, pharmacodynamic, and pharmacogenetic determinants of osteonecrosis in children with acute lymphoblastic leukemia. *Blood* 117:2340–2347, 2011.

   This study identified not only pharmacogenetic but also pharmacokinetic and pharmacodynamic determinants of osteonecrosis in children with acute lymphoblastic leukemia.

142. Mattano LA, Jr, Devidas M, Nachman JB, et al: Effect of alternate-week versus continuous dexamethasone scheduling on the risk of osteonecrosis in paediatric patients with acute lymphoblastic leukaemia: results from the CCG-1961 randomised cohort trial. *Lancet Oncol* 13:906–915, 2012.

   This report describes the clinical characteristics of osteonecrosis and shows that its incidence is influenced by the administration schedule of dexamethasone.

146. Pieters R, Hunger SP, Boos J, et al: L-asparaginase treatment in acute lymphoblastic leukemia: a focus on Erwinia asparaginase. *Cancer* 117:238–249, 2011.

   This article provides an overview of asparaginase in the treatment of acute lymphoblastic leukemia.

162. Kawedia JD, Liu C, Pei D, et al: Dexamethasone exposure and asparaginase antibodies affect relapse risk in acute lymphoblastic leukemia. *Blood* 119:1658–1664, 2012.

   This report describes the influence of antiasparaginase antibodies on acute lymphoblastic leukemia therapy, showing that patients with antibodies have higher systemic dexamethasone clearance rates. Lower exposure to both drugs was associated with greater risk of relapse.

199. Visscher H, Ross CJ, Rassekh SR, et al: Pharmacogenomic prediction of anthracycline-induced cardiotoxicity in children. *J Clin Oncol* 30:1422–1428, 2012.

   References 198 and 199 report the identification of genetic variants associated with anthracycline cardiotoxicity in children with cancer.

212. Lamba JK: Genetic factors influencing cytarabine therapy. *Pharmacogenomics* 10:1657–1674, 2009.

   This article summarizes the metabolism of cytarabine and the pharmacogenomics of cytarabine therapy.

219. Druker BJ, Talpaz M, Resta DJ, et al: Efficacy and safety of a specific inhibitor of the BCR-ABL tyrosine kinase in chronic myeloid leukemia. *N Engl J Med* 344:1031–1037, 2001.

   This study was the first to show significant activity of imatinib against chronic myeloid leukemia.

222. Biondi A, Schrappe M, De Lorenzo P, et al: Imatinib after induction for treatment of children and adolescents with Philadelphia-chromosome-positive acute lymphoblastic leukaemia (EsPhALL):

a randomised, open-label, intergroup study. *Lancet Oncol* 13:936–945, 2012.

The authors of references 221 and 222 assessed the safety and efficacy of imatinib for pediatric patients with Philadelphia-chromosome–positive acute lymphoblastic leukemia.

311. Balis FM, Fox E, Widemann BC, et al: Clinical drug development for childhood cancers. *Clin Pharmacol Ther* 85:127–129, 2009.

This article describes current issues in clinical drug development for childhood cancers.

312. Le Tourneau C, Lee JJ, Siu LL: Dose escalation methods in phase I cancer clinical trials. *J Natl Cancer Inst* 101:708–720, 2009.

The authors of this article review dose escalation methods for phase I trials, including the rule-based and model-based methods developed to evaluate new anticancer agents.

316. Downing JR, Wilson RK, Zhang J, et al: The Pediatric Cancer Genome Project. *Nat Genet* 44:619–622, 2012.

This perspective article describes the rationale for the Pediatric Cancer Genome Project, presents some of its early results, and discusses the major lessons learned and how they will affect the application of genomic sequencing in the clinic.

356. Relling MV, Gardner EE, Sandborn WJ, et al: Clinical Pharmacogenetics Implementation Consortium guidelines for thiopurine methyltransferase genotype and thiopurine dosing: 2013 update. *Clin Pharmacol Ther* 93:324–325, 2013.

In references 77 and 356, dosing recommendations are provided for azathioprine, mercaptopurine, and thioguanine based on the thiopurine methyltransferase genotype.

CHAPTER 47

Immunotherapy of Cancer

Susanne H.C. Baumeister and Glenn Dranoff

CHAPTER OUTLINE

The role of the immune system in controlling cancer was subject to debate for decades, reflecting the limited understanding of the immune system at the time and the complexity of tumor immunology. However, over time a wealth of evidence from murine and human studies[1-3] has demonstrated that the immune system can control cancer. Numerous animal models have demonstrated the ability of T cells to reject tumors, revealed the importance of cytokines for antitumor immunity, and showed the susceptibility of immunodeficient mice to tumor formation. Compelling evidence of tumor immunosurveillance in humans is provided by reports of rare spontaneous tumor regressions in persons with melanoma and renal cell carcinoma,[4] particularly after infection,[5] paraneoplastic

diseases (which are autoimmune neurologic manifestations of an antitumor response), and the higher incidence of melanoma in patients undergoing chronic pharmacologic immunosuppression after organ transplantation.[6] Pediatric patients with immunodeficiencies are at risk for lymphoma, and posttransplant lymphoproliferative disease (PTLD) is a well-known entity in iatrogenically immunosuppressed patients. The immune system can prevent virus-induced malignancies, eliminate tumor cells via recognition of tumor antigens that distinguish them from "self," and promptly terminate inflammation to avoid tumorigenesis. However, when the latter process is in disarray, such as in chronic inflammatory conditions and autoimmunity, the immune system is implicated in tumorigenesis. The control of tumor growth by the immune system also applies selection pressure, which may ultimately promote tumor progression. In this process, termed "cancer immunoediting,"[7] cancer cells develop immune escape mechanisms and establish a tumor microenvironment that interferes with antigen presentation, T-cell activation, and differentiation, thereby leading to a gradual loss of control by T cells (Fig. 47-1).[8] An expanding body of preclinical and clinical experiences has established that the immune system can be manipulated in increasingly sophisticated ways to prevent, control, or aid in the control of established cancers.

Careful selection of the appropriate target antigen(s) and consideration of preexisting immunologic memory are key features in the pursuit of successful immunotherapy. Antigens that are unique to the tumor and absent on healthy tissues often require priming of the immune system but possess the advantage that the induced antitumor response is unlikely to have autoimmune adverse effects. In the case of antigens that are present or overexpressed on tumor cells but are also detectable in some healthy tissues, depletion of T-cell clones with high avidity to the antigen may have polarized existing memory T cells toward tolerance. In this scenario, effective

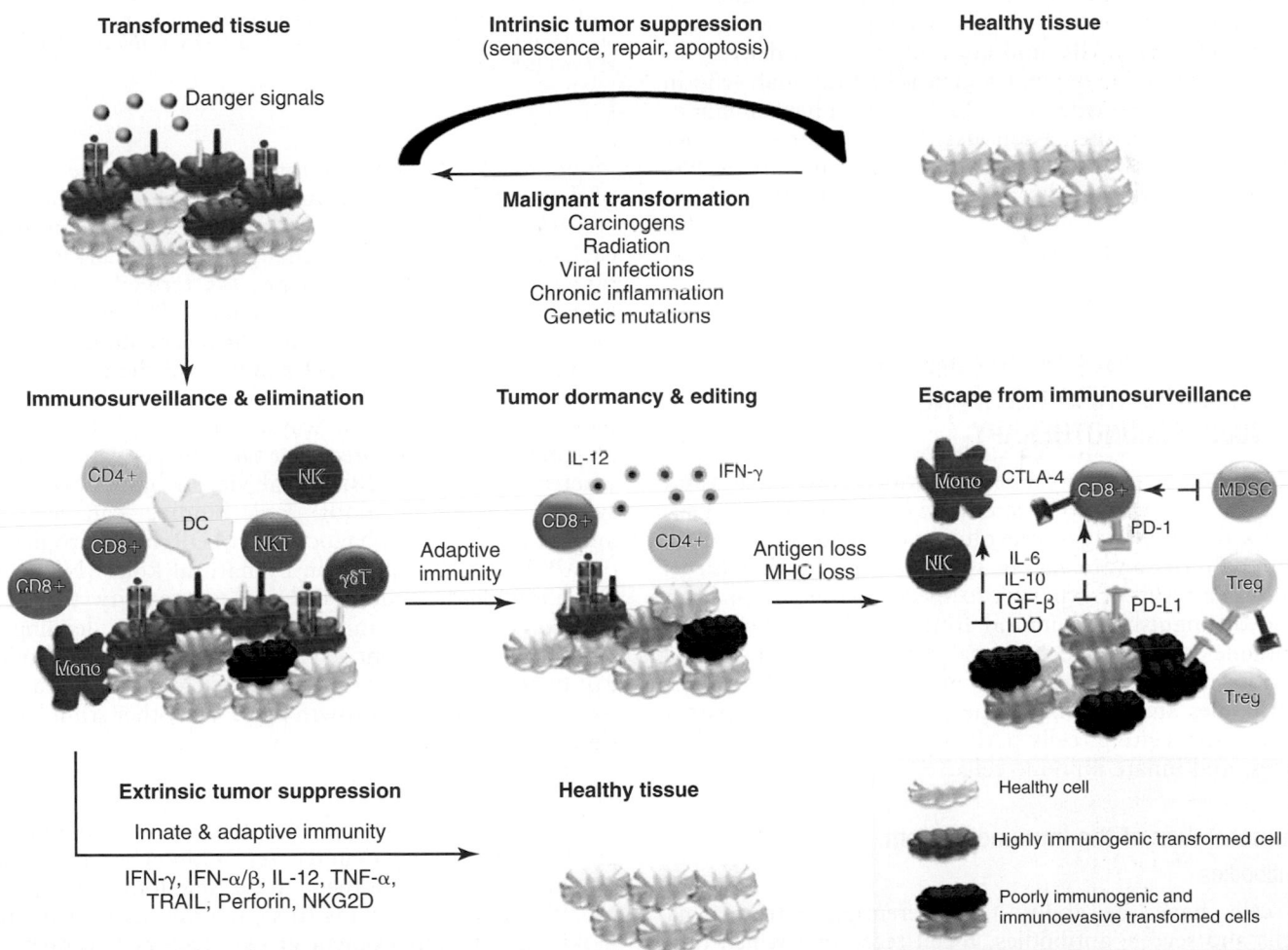

Figure 47-1 The concept of cancer immunoediting. Malignant transformation can be triggered by multiple insults, including inherited or acquired genetic mutations, exposure to radiation, carcinogens, infections, and chronic inflammation. Intrinsic tumor suppression mechanisms such as deoxyribonucleic acid repair, apoptosis, and senescence are in place to eliminate transformed cells. The extrinsic tumor suppressor mechanism of cancer immunoediting involves both the innate and adaptive arms of immunity and contributes to the control of a developing tumor by recognition of danger signals from immunogenic malignant cells (such as expression of tumor antigens and stress ligands specific for receptors on innate immune cells). If complete elimination of transformed cells is achieved, the person remains free of cancer. However, if rare tumor cell variants or poorly immunogenic cells survive elimination, they may enter a phase of equilibrium during which adaptive immune mechanisms control tumor outgrowth but do not achieve complete elimination. The immune selection pressure may lead to editing of tumor immunogenicity and emergence of tumor escape mechanisms. These mechanisms include (1) loss of antigen or stress ligand expression and major histocompatibility complex–I downregulation to escape recognition by adaptive immunity, (2) desensitization to immune effector mechanisms, and (3) induction of an immunosuppressive tumor microenvironment. If tumor outgrowth is no longer blocked by immune mechanisms, tumor cells emerge to cause clinically apparent disease. *DC*, Dendritic cell; *IDO*, indolamine 2,3 dioxygenase; *IFN*, interferon; *IL*, interleukin; *MDSC*, myeloid-derived supressor cell; *NK*, natural killer cell; *NKT*, natural killer T cell; *PD-1*, programmed cell death–1; *PD-L1*, programmed cell death–1 ligand; *TGF-β*, transforming growth factor β; *TNF-α*, tumor necrosis factor-α; *TRAIL*, TNF-related apoptosis-inducing ligand; *Treg*, regulatory T cell. *(Modified from Schreiber RD, Old LJ, Smyth MJ: Cancer immunoediting: integrating immunity's roles in cancer suppression and promotion.* Science *331:1565–1570, 2011.)*

immunotherapy has to break tolerance and is more likely to induce undesired autoimmunity. The clinical use of immunotherapeutic modalities such as monoclonal antibodies (mABs), vaccines against oncogenic viruses, cytokines, and hematopoietic stem cell transplantation (HSCT) has been the standard of care in the prevention, treatment, and supportive care of cancer for many years. More recently, an exciting renaissance in cancer immunotherapy occurred as a result of the success of proof-of-concept clinical trials for a variety of novel immune-modulating strategies. As will be discussed further, these strategies include cellular therapies such as chimeric antigen receptor (CAR) T-cells (CARTs) and the first Food and Drug Administration (FDA)–approved cancer vaccine (sipuleucel-T); blockade of regulatory pathways with anti–cytotoxic T-lymphocyte antigen 4 (anti-CTLA-4) mABs; and antibody-targeted delivery of drugs via immunoconjugates such as brentuximab vedotin and trastuzumab emtansine. Many early-phase immunotherapy trials are being conducted for adult malignancies first and will be discussed when they are applicable. While promising results and toxicity data emerge from adult trials, the benefits of immunotherapy will also increasingly become available to pediatric patients with cancer.

KEY COMPONENTS OF THE IMMUNE SYSTEM AND THEIR RELEVANCE IN CANCER IMMUNOTHERAPY

The immune response can be divided into innate and adaptive immunity to differentiate between an early, generalized response against evolutionarily conserved molecular patterns and a highly specific response that forms fully as a result of exposure to specific antigens. One can also distinguishe a humoral from a cellular arm of the immune system. The humoral arm consists of soluble factors that are secreted by immune cells and includes antibodies and cytokines. The cellular arm encompasses antigen-presenting cells (APCs), phagocytes, lymphocytes, and innate immune cells.

Humoral Arm of the Immune System
Antibodies

B cells have the ability to differentiate into plasma cells and secrete antibodies. B-cell receptors, which represent surface-expressed antibodies against a vast variety of potential antigens, are created by somatic V(D)J-recombination. Subsequent antigen exposure leads to clonal expansion of B cells with the cognate B-cell receptor and facilitates large-scale antibody production. Antibodies consist of two heavy chains (γ, δ, α, μ, or ε) and two light chains (λ or κ). The composition of the heavy chains determines the immunoglobulin (Ig) subclass, which can be IgM, IgG, IgA, IgE, or IgD. These immunoglobulin subclasses have different binding valencies and functions; for example, IgM is produced early in the immune response followed by a class switch to IgG, whereas IgA is predominantly involved in mucosal

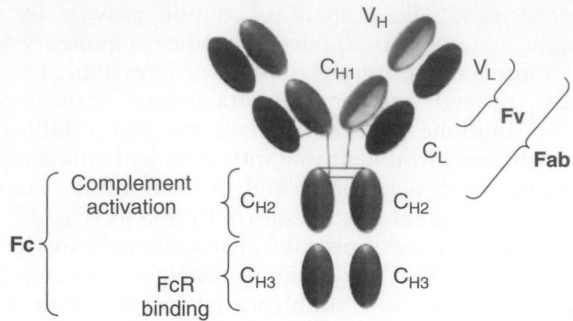

Figure 47-2 Structure of an antibody molecule. Antigen-binding fragment *(Fab)* and crystallizable fragment *(Fc)* regions are distinguished on the basis of proteolytic cleavage by papain. Functionally, the variable region *(Fv)* represents the antibody binding site, whereas the Fc region mediates complement activation and binding to Fc receptors *(FcRs)*. Structurally, one further differentiates heavy chains *(blue;* γ, δ, α, μ, or ε) from light chains *(red;* λ or κ).

immunity. Antibodies function by binding to the antigen of their specificity via the antigen-binding fragment (Fab; consisting of one constant and one variable domain from each of the heavy and light chains), thereby marking their target for destruction in a process termed "opsonization." Cellular destruction is mediated by the crystallizable fragment (Fc) component, which is composed of two heavy chains (Fig. 47-2). Depending on the effector cell and type of Fc receptor (FcR), the immune response can be modulated in multiple ways. Activating FcRs contain a cytoplasmic immunoreceptor tyrosine activation motif, whereas inhibitory FcRs signal via an immunoreceptor tyrosine inhibition motif. FcR binding can lead to antibody-dependent phagocytosis (ADP) by macrophages or APCs or cell destruction by natural killer (NK) cells via antibody-dependent cellular cytotoxicity (ADCC). The Fc component can also fix complement, leading to complement-dependent cytotoxicity (CDC). Antibodies can further kill tumor cells by direct induction of apoptosis and blockade of growth factors or other stimulatory signals (Fig. 47-3).

Cytokines

Cytokines are soluble proteins that are predominantly produced by leukocytes and carry out intercellular signaling function. Based on their varied functions, they can be classified into interleukins (ILs), interferons (IFNs), chemokines, and hematopoietic growth factors. Several cytokines have been used in cancer immunotherapy either as a single agent or to enhance the effect of other therapeutic agents. Growth factors such as granulocyte-colony stimulating factor (G-CSF) also play an important role in facilitating the neutrophil recovery necessary for compressed chemotherapy regimens, which have led to improved survival for children with multiple types of pediatric solid tumors. Lastly, analysis of the cytokine response triggered by immune therapies is informative in elucidating the mechanism of action and associated toxicities and can guide lifesaving therapeutic interventions, as demonstrated by the successful use of an IL-6 receptor (IL-6R) antagonist in the treatment of cytokine

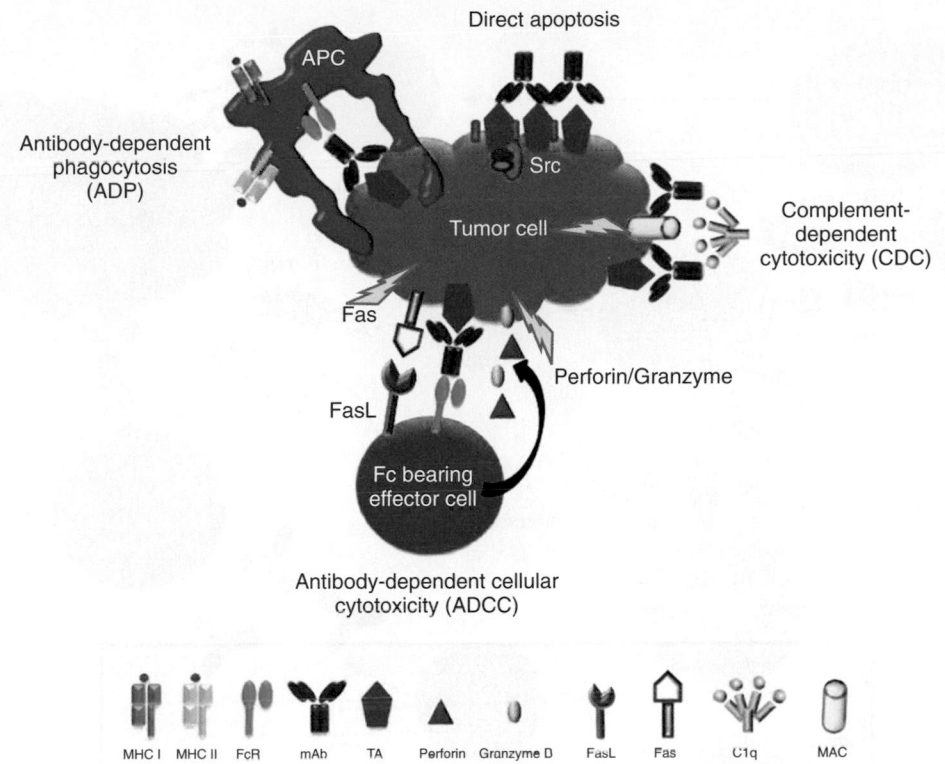

Figure 47-3 Antibody-mediated mechanisms of tumor cell destruction. Antibody-dependent phagocytosis *(ADP)*: Via the antibody-dependent phagocytosis pathway, antibodies entice crystallizable fragment receptor *(FcR)*–bearing phagocytes to take up tumor cells, process a variety of different tumor antigens, and present them in major histocompatibility complex *(MHC)*–restricted fashion to cluster of differentiation (CD)4+ and CD8+ cells. This process can lead to the vaccinal effect of monoclonal antibody *(mAb)* therapy. Antibody-dependent cellular toxicity *(ADCC)*: FcR-bearing effector cells such as natural killer cells can mediate antibody-dependent cellular cytotoxicity via perforin/granzyme B or induce apoptosis via Fas ligand *(FASL)*/Fas after recognition of the crystallizable fragment *(Fc)* portion of the bound antibody. Complement-dependent cytotoxicity *(CDC)*: The C1q protein of the complement system binds to antigen:antibody complexes on the tumor cell surface and causes activation of the complement cascade, resulting in formation of the membrane attack complex *(MAC)* and tumor cell lysis. Direct apoptosis: Cross-linking of antibody molecules and tumor antigens *(TAs)* in the lipid raft can activate signaling pathways involving Src kinases that mediate direct apoptosis. *APC,* Antigen-presenting cell.

release syndrome associated with cluster of differentiation (CD)19-CAR therapy.

Cellular Arm of the Immune System

T Cells

T cells are a major component of the adaptive immune system (Fig. 47-4). They are derived from bone marrow, but in contrast to B cells, they travel to the thymus to undergo V(D)J-recombination of their T-cell receptors (TCRs), editing, and maturation. Somatic recombination of the α- and β-chains of the TCR results in the incredibly diverse T-cell repertoire from which clonal expansion can occur upon encounter of a specific antigen. To prevent autoimmunity, TCRs specific for "self" undergo negative selection in the thymus but also are subject to regulatory mechanisms in the periphery. Generation of an adaptive antitumor response begins with capture of tumor antigens by dendritic cells (DCs) in the peripheral tissues. DCs then travel to the draining lymph nodes, where they interact with T cells. Successful activation of a T-cell response (T-cell priming) requires presentation of the antigen on major histocompatibility complex class I

(MHC-I) or class II (MHC-II) molecules for TCR-mediated recognition (signal 1), as well as a costimulatory signal (signal 2). Classically, the costimulatory signal is delivered to CD28 on T cells via the B7 family (CD80 and CD86) on APCs, but many other costimulatory molecules have been identified. The absence of costimulation leads to anergy. T cells may also receive inhibitory signals via CTLA-4, programmed death 1 (PD-1), and various other receptors, which play a physiologic role in terminating an immune response. The tumor microenvironment exploits some of these mechanisms to escape immune surveillance by MHC downregulation, as well as expression of inhibitory ligands such as PD-1 ligand (PD-L1). The discovery and characterization of other modulatory signaling pathways is ongoing and will continue to be a platform for therapeutic intervention.

T cells express CD3 and are divided in CD8+ cytotoxic T lymphocytes (CTLs) and CD4+ helper T cells. DCs can process and present antigens via MHC I and MHC-II pathways. CD8+ CTLs are generally activated via MHC-I. This pathway predominantly processes antigens derived from the cell itself (such as viral antigens), but it can also

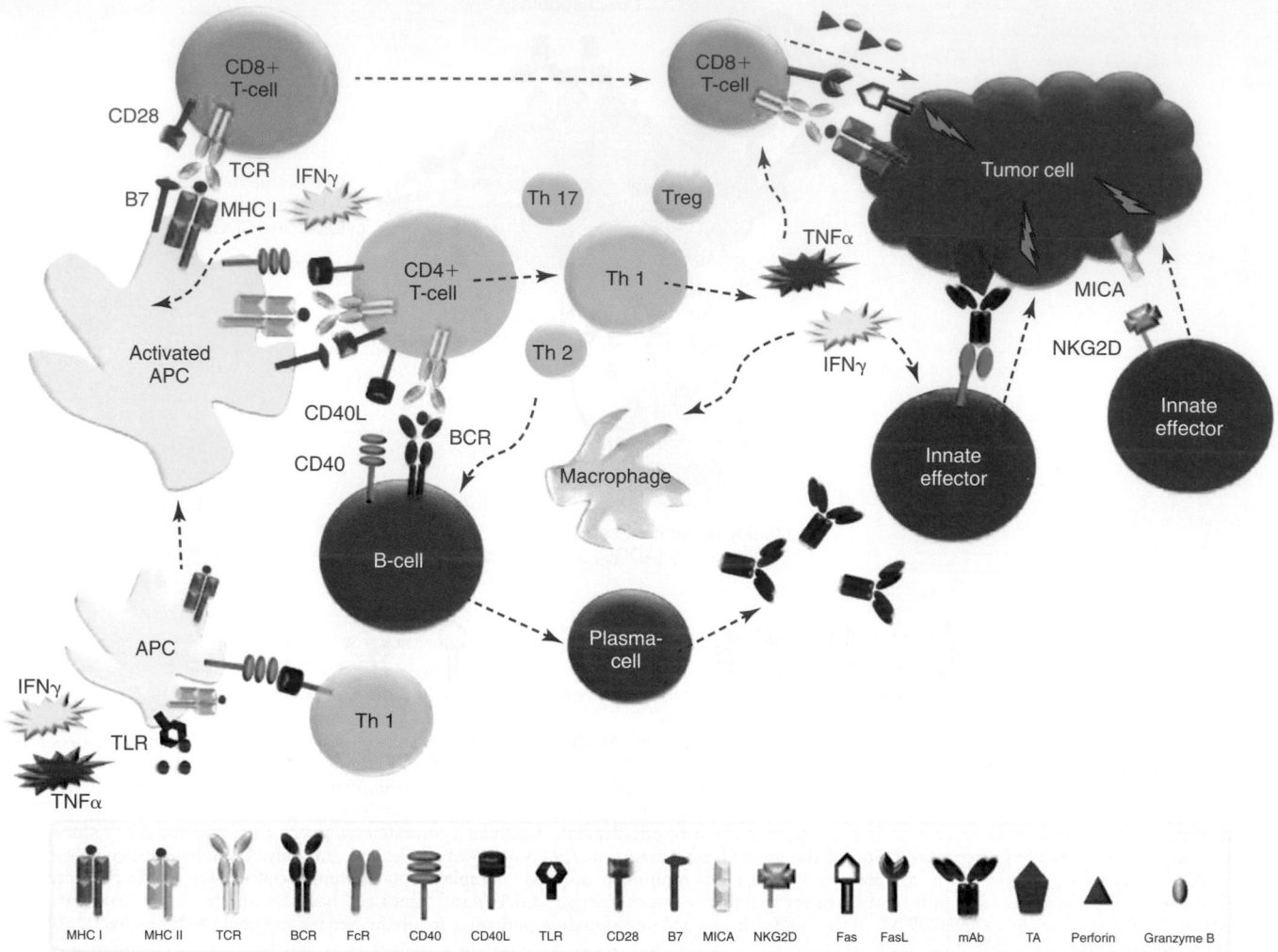

Figure 47-4 Antitumor effects of the immune system. Innate effector cells (such as natural killer cells) are regulated by a system of activating and inhibitory receptors and often recognize major histocompatibility complex *(MHC)*-I or MHC-I–related molecules that are upregulated by cells under the stress of malignant transformation. They are capable of rapid killing of tumor cells or mediation of apoptosis upon recognition of such ligands. They also mediate antibody-dependent cellular toxicity via interaction of their crystallizable fragment receptor *(FcR)* with the Fc portion of antibodies directed against tumor antigens *(TAs)*. Initiation of the adaptive immune response to tumors relies on TA uptake by an antigen-presenting cell (APC) in the context of appropriate maturation signals such as Toll-like receptor *(TLR)* signaling, cluster of differentiation (CD)40/CD40L interaction with CD4+ T cells, and cytokines. In its activated state the APC presents TAs on MHC molecules and provides the necessary costimulatory signals (e.g., CD80/CD86, also referred to as B7) to activate a T-cell response in lymph nodes. Via the MHC-I pathway, APCs prime CD8+ cytotoxic T lymphocytes (CTLs), which then clonally expand, recognize the TA on tumor cells via their cognate T-cell receptor *(TCR)*, and mediate tumor cell lysis. APCs present antigens to CD4+ helper cells via MHC-II molecules. CD4+ T cells do not directly partake in tumor cell destruction but provide help to other immune cells. They are polarized toward functionally distinct subtypes. T helper *(Th)*1 cells mediate tumor immunity through production of cytokines such as interferon *(IFN)*-γ and tumor necrosis factor *(TNF)*-α, which enhance macrophage and CTL functions, and provision of CD40L signals that enhance APC maturation. Th2 cells are crucial for the induction of B-cell responses and antibody production against TAs. Regulatory T cells *(Tregs)* are immunosuppressive, and their presence in the tumor microenvironment dampens a vigorous antitumor immune response. *BCR,* B-cell receptor; *FasL,* Fas ligand; *mAb,* monoclonal antibody; *MICA,* MHC class I–related chain A.

present antigens taken up by the cell through a mechanism referred to as cross-presentation. MHC-I is present on all nucleated cells, and upon recognition of the MHC-restricted cognate antigen on a tumor cell, primed CD8+ CTLs mediate tumor cell death by virtue of releasing perforin/granzyme B or by inducing apoptosis through interactions of death receptors such as Fas/Fas ligand. MHC-II expression is limited to APCs such as DCs, macrophages, and B cells, which process phagocytosed antigens and activate CD4+ T cells via the MHC-II pathway.

CD4+ T cells do not generally directly mediate tumor cell lysis, but they critically support and influence the immune response by producing cytokines and providing "help" to CD8+ T cells and B cells via CD40 signaling. Depending on the polarization of their cytokine profile and function, CD4+ helper T cells are divided into Th1, Th2, Th17, and follicular helper T-cell subtypes and regulatory T cells (Tregs). Th1 responses are characterized by proinflammatory cytokines such as IFN-γ and tumor necrosis factor (TNF)-α, which enhance macrophage and CTL function and promote secretion of immunostimulatory cytokines, such as IL-12 by APCs. Th2 responses are essential for antibody production and class switching of B cells, are involved in allergic responses, and produce an array of cytokines such as IL-4, IL-9, IL-10, and IL-13 that contribute to eosinophil and mast cell activation. The Th17 subset was only described relatively recently. Although it is involved in the pathogenesis of autoimmune and inflammatory diseases, it may also play an important role in tumor immunity.[9] Lastly, Tregs express CD25 and the forkhead box (FOX)P3 transcription factor in addition to CD4+. They serve to inhibit immune activation, induce self-tolerance under physiologic conditions, and notably expand in response to IL-2. Treg blockade or elimination is an important factor in facilitating an effective antitumor immune response, and therapeutic expansion of Tregs may play a role in controlling graft-versus-host disease (GVHD).

γδ T Cells

γδ T cells represent a small subgroup of circulating T cells that function at the interface of innate and adaptive immunity. Their TCR also undergoes somatic recombination and editing but consists of a γδ heterodimer. This subset may recognize specific antigenic determinants via the TCR or by a TCR independent pathway similar to that of NK cells.

Natural Killer T Cells

Natural killer T cells (NKTs) are a unique subset of T cells with a highly restricted TCR repertoire, allowing recognition of certain glycolipid antigens, such as GD2, in conjunction with the nonclassical MHC-I molecule CD1d. They contribute to antitumor immunity as an early source of cytokine production, resulting in activation of other effector cells. Higher numbers of tumor-infiltrating NKTs have been associated with improved long-term disease-free survival (DFS) in children with stage IV neuroblastoma.[10] NKTs are thought to inhibit tumor growth by targeting tumor-associated macrophages (TAMs) that have been shown to have clinical significance in neuroblastoma,[11] Hodgkin lymphoma (HL),[12] and other malignancies. NKTs are attracted by the chemokine (C-C motif) ligand 2 (CCL2). *MYCN*, the hallmark of aggressive neuroblastoma, mediates CCL2 repression and therefore reduces NKT infiltration.[13] Via another escape mechanism, TAMs in the neuroblastoma microenvironment produce a different chemokine, CCL20, in response to hypoxia, thereby attracting NKTs into hypoxic traps. IL-15 was shown to protect NKTs from the inhibitory effects of hypoxia and enhances antimetastatic activity of NKTs.[14]

NK Cells

NK cells play a key role in the innate immune response, in an early defense against infection or malignant transformation. NK cells can be phenotypically distinguished from other peripheral blood mononuclear cells because they are CD56+ and lack B-cell (CD19), T-cell (CD3), and monocytic (CD14) markers. Subsets of NK cells also express the FcRs CD16 and CD11b that mediate ADCC

and participate in CDC. Contrary to T and B cells, NK-cell receptors do not undergo somatic recombination and do not require recognition of a cognate antigen to mediate cytotoxicity. Traditionally it has been thought that they do not develop immunologic memory, although this paradigm may be changing.[15] Their function is tightly regulated by a complex system of activating and inhibitory receptors, which often recognize MHC-I or MHC-I–related molecules. These interactions provide the basis for the therapeutic exploitation of NK-cell alloreactivity. The key regulators of NK cells are activating and inhibitory killer cell immunoglobulin-like receptors (KIRs), which activate natural cytotoxicity receptors including NKp30, NKp46, and NKp44 and the activation receptor NKG2D. NK cells are capable of rapid killing via degranulation and release of toxic granules, primarily through a perforin and granzyme B–dependent pathway. They can also mediate apoptosis by utilizing Fas ligand or TNF-related apoptosis-inducing ligand (TRAIL) and execute ADCC via their FcRIII (CD16) receptor. NK cells further secrete chemokines such as CCL2 through CCL5, XCL1, and CXCL8. Their clinical significance in pediatrics is underscored by the susceptibility of infants born with NK-cell deficiencies to fulminant viral infections and the NK-cell defects underlying primary hemophagocytic lymphohistiocytosis. NK cells facilitate stem cell engraftment, fight infection, and control cancer, yet they do not cause GVHD. These characteristics make them attractive therapeutic candidates for adoptive NK-cell therapies.

Dendritic Cells

Dendritic cells (DCs) represent a small subset of peripheral blood mononuclear cells (1% to 2%). They are mobile sentinels that collect antigen from peripheral tissues and carry it to the secondary lymphoid organs to activate T cells. DCs are termed "professional APCs" based on their ability to process and present antigenic peptides on MHC-I or MHC-II molecules. In steady state, they reside in the periphery in an immature state and play an important role in maintaining tolerance by taking up self-antigens. Successful T-cell activation requires DC activation. Upon activation, DCs upregulate MHC molecules, costimulatory molecules (which provide the second signal for T-cell activation), and chemokine receptors (which enhance homing to lymphoid organs) and secrete inflammatory cytokines such as IL-12.[16] DC activation can occur in response to a variety of signals, such as the receipt of exogenous and endogenous danger signals via Toll-like receptors (TLRs), which recognize evolutionarily conserved molecular patterns from products of damaged or dying cells and from pathogens.[17] DCs are also matured by proinflammatory cytokines secreted by other cells (e.g., innate effectors) or by CD40 ligation. In addition, DCs are important in launching humoral immunity, partly because of their capacity to directly activate B cells.[18]

Myeloid DCs and plasmacytoid DCs are the two main subsets among various other DCs. They express high levels of human leukocyte antigen (HLA)-DR (MHC-II), but they differ in their expression of CD11c (myeloid DCs), CD123 (plasmacytoid DCs), and TLRs, among other markers. DCs are critical regulators of adaptive T- and B-cell responses and are central to the development of successful tumor vaccines. Because of their low abundance in the peripheral blood, sufficient numbers of DCs can be generated in vitro either by expansion of isolated DCs or by generation from monocytes using cytokine cocktails. DCs further play a role in the pathogenesis of GVHD and are required for full graft-versus-leukemia (GVL) effects, and thus their therapeutic manipulation is of relevance in HSCT.

Neutrophils

Neutrophils are crucial to the rapid destruction of pathogens, particularly bacterial, fungal, and certain parasitic organisms, as evidenced by the high risk of sepsis during periods of neutropenia in the oncology population. However, neutrophils also contribute to antitumor activities of the immune system. Through their FcRs, they can be involved in ADCC-mediated tumor destruction. In addition, neutrophil activation at sites of the tumor via administration of cytokines such as GM-CSF can play a role in tumor cell degradation and enhance antigen presentation.[19]

Monocytes/Macrophages

Monocytes are myeloid-derived phagocytic cells that differentiate into resident macrophages upon recruitment into tissues. Macrophages are able to ingest apoptotic cells and opsonized cells via their FcRs. Aside from their role in clearing cellular debris, they are able to present antigenic peptides of the digested cells in an immunogenic way. Activated macrophages prominently secrete cytokines such as IL-12, which may be critical in activating local immune responses by NK cells and T cells. Macrophages were originally classified into M1 (proinflammatory) and M2 (antiinflammatory) macrophages according to their polarization status. Although this classification remains conceptually helpful, it is now clear that tissue macrophages display a high degree of functional and phenotypic plasticity in response to changing microenvironmental stimuli and that M1 and M2 polarization represent extremes of a continuum of activation states. Increasing evidence indicates that TAMs are implicated in protumor effects and can play a role in tumor initiation, progression, and distant metastasis.[20,21] Limited evidence suggests that myeloid-derived suppressor cells develop from a common myeloid progenitor without a monocytic intermediate and have predefined immunosuppressive properties, whereas monocytes lack suppressive activity in steady state and acquire this function in response to certain stimuli. In persons with cancer, the majority of studies support an association between high TAM density and poor clinical outcome, as has been demonstrated in several malignancies, including neuroblastoma.[11,12] However, TAM function in tumor immunity appears to be dynamic and heterogeneous depending on the tumor type, tumor progression, location within the tumor, and perhaps most importantly, polarization of the TAM. In this regard, increased density of M2-like TAMs is a marker of poor prognosis, whereas the presence of M1-like subsets is advantageous. Based on these findings, subpopulations of TAMs are now being explored as new therapeutic targets.[20]

TARGET ANTIGENS IN CANCER IMMUNOTHERAPY

Tumor antigens (TAs) are molecules that enable the recognition of tumors by components of the immune system. A wide array of target antigens have been identified and may be classified into various subgroups according to their origins. Tumor-specific antigens are epitopes that are found exclusively on malignant cells. This group includes proteins arising from mutated oncogenes, clonally rearranged immunoglobulin genes, and oncoviral gene products. Tumor-associated antigens are expressed on some healthy and malignant tissues alike. Tumor-associated antigens may arise from overexpressed normal proteins, oncofetal proteins, lineage-restricted markers, histocompatibility molecules, and proteins that are normally expressed in immune-privileged sites.

Antigens Arising from Genetic Alterations

A number of malignancies are associated with specific genetic mutations or translocations, resulting in the synthesis of novel proteins that are foreign to the host's immune system, thereby offering the potential of immune recognition while sparing healthy tissues. Commonly they are drivers of or contribute to tumorigenesis, as is the case for oncogenes or mutated tumor suppressor genes, but they may also arise from mutations not directly involved in the neoplastic process. A variety of malignancies express gene products derived from mutated tumor suppressor genes, such as *p53* or *ras*. Examples of antigens derived from mutated oncogenes include the EWS-FLI fusion protein resulting from the t(11:22) translocation characteristic of Ewing sarcoma and the p210 and p190 products of the bcr/abl translocation in chronic myelogenous leukemia (CML) and Philadelphia chromosome–positive acute lymphoblastic leukemia (ALL), respectively.

Oncoviral Proteins

Viral infections play a causal role in several malignancies and give rise to immunogenic viral proteins that can be recognized and eliminated by the immune system. This process is underscored by the fact that immunosuppressed persons, particularly those with impairment of T-cell immunity, have a higher propensity to develop Epstein-Barr virus (EBV)–associated lymphomas and human papillomavirus (HPV)–associated skin and cervical cancers. Examples of oncoviral proteins are the expression of the EBV antigens EBNA-1, EBNA-3, LMP-1, and LMP-2 in PTLD and some lymphomas and the papillomavirus E6 and E7 proteins in cervical carcinomas.

Clonally Rearranged Immunoglobulin Genes

Surface immunoglobulin is a marker of B-cell maturity and is present in mature B-cell non-Hodgkin lymphomas (NHLs) and multiple myeloma. Because surface immunoglobulin expression results from separate somatic recombination events in each B cell, all malignant cells in a monoclonal B-cell malignancy express the clonally unique immunoglobulin variable region, or idiotype. Immunoglobulins are proteins and can therefore be immunogenic and lead to the development of idiotype vaccines. Another approach to targeting this group of TAs includes the generation of anti-idiotype mABs in mice, which in turn are immunogenic and amplify the immune response upon administration to the patient as a type of vaccine.

Altered Glycolipid and Glycoprotein Antigens

Most human tumors express higher levels or abnormal forms of surface glycoproteins and glycolipids, which serve as targets for immunotherapy. Some aspects of the malignant phenotype of tumors, including tissue invasion and metastatic behavior, may reflect altered cell surface properties as a result of the abnormal glycolipid and glycoprotein synthesis. Most of these epitopes are not exclusively expressed on tumors but are present at higher levels on cancer cells compared with healthy tissues. Examples of such glycolipids are GD2, which is expressed in neuroblastoma and some osteosarcomas, as well as GM2, GD2, and GD3 in melanomas. These molecules are actively being explored in vaccination strategies, and mABs against the carbohydrate groups or peptide cores of such molecules have been generated and clinically used with success.

Oncofetal Antigens

Oncofetal antigens are proteins that are expressed at high levels in cancer cells and during normal fetal development, but not in adult tissues. Alpha-fetoprotein expression in hepatoblastomas and germ cell tumors and carcinoembryonic antigen in colorectal cancer are examples of aberrant expression of fetal antigens. Although they are largely utilized as biomarkers, they are also being explored as targets of CART therapy.

Products of Genes That Are Selectively Expressed in Immune-Privileged Sites

An interesting group of antigens are the so-called "cancer-testes antigens." These nonmutated proteins arise from germline-associated genes that are preferentially expressed in immune-privileged sites such as the testes and placenta. These antigens include NY-ESO, MAGE, BAGE, and RAGE and are expressed in melanomas and many carcinomas. They are promising targets given their relatively tumor-specific distribution and have been explored in the context of tumor vaccination.

Histocompatibility Antigens

Histocompatibility antigens are of importance in the allogeneic HSCT setting. Because HLAs are widely expressed in normal tissues and are immunologic targets for T-cell responses, donor selection intends to maximize major histocompatibility matches between the donor and recipient to minimize GVHD. However, minor histocompatibility antigens (mHAs) may generate a GVL response both in matched sibling and in unrelated donor (URD) transplantation. mHAs may have tissue restricted expression, such as HA-1 and HA-2, which are expressed only on hematopoietic cells. Such mHAs are particularly

appealing immunologic targets because the induced immunologic response will not cause GVHD in nonexpressing tissues.

Molecules That Activate Recognition of the Innate Immune System

Cells of the innate immune system do not require presentation of antigens via MHC molecules but instead have the ability to respond to MHC-I–related ligands, which tissues may express inducibly in association with cell stress, infection, or malignant transformation, thus allowing for a system in which the body alerts the immune system by creating internal danger signals. Such molecules may not be recognized by endogenous T and B cells but can induce potent responses by innate effector cells. The advantage of such danger signals is that they are absent or expressed at very low levels in steady state. In healthy humans, MICA and MICB, which are ligands for the NKG2D receptor on NK cells and CD8+ T cells, are expressed only by intestinal epithelial cells at low levels, likely as a consequence of stimulation by the local bacterial flora. However, these molecules are significantly upregulated in a variety of tumor types[22] and are thus promising targets.

Normal Proteins Overexpressed in Tumor Tissue

Increased gene transcription or amplification of normal genes in tumor cells may result in aberrantly high expression of proteins. Examples include MYCN amplification in high-risk neuroblastoma, overexpression of human epidermal growth factor receptor 2 (Her2/neu) in a subset of breast and ovarian cancers, as well as some sarcomas, and gp100 and MART in melanomas. Because these proteins are also found at lower levels in some healthy tissues, immune tolerance to such antigens may have developed and needs to be overcome by effective immunotherapy.

Lineage-Specific Tumor Antigens

Many tumors express differentiation antigens that are not restricted to the malignant cell but rather to their lineage of origin. Examples include CD19 and CD22 in pre–B-cell ALL (pre–B-ALL), CD33 in acute myeloid leukemia (AML), and prostate-specific antigen (PSA) in prostate cancer. Similar to overexpressed proteins, the utility of these antigens as targets for tumor immunotherapy is highly dependent on the expression pattern on healthy tissues. As such, the B-cell aplasia accompanying CD19-targeted therapies may be transient and can be managed with exogenous administration of immunoglobulin. Similarly, targeting of PSA may be associated with immune destruction of normal prostate cells, yet this destruction is pathophysiologically tolerable. In contrast, lineage-specific antigen expression on vital organs would be prohibitive to this approach.

TUMOR VACCINES

One of medicine's great successes was the introduction of vaccines for the prevention of infectious diseases.

Vaccines that provide protection against oncogenic viruses effectively prevent certain cancers as well. Based on Center for Disease Control and Prevention estimates, approximately 26,000 new cervical cancers each year are attributable to HPV.[23] Therefore the quadrivalent HPV vaccine, which was implemented in 2007 and is recommended for female and male adolescents, has tremendous potential to prevent cervical cancer.[24,25,26] Another example is the prevention of hepatocellular carcinoma by way of hepatitis B virus vaccination.[27] The generation of therapeutic cancer vaccines is much more challenging, given that such vaccines must overcome preestablished tumor tolerance. However, the discovery that patients can harbor CD8+ and CD4+ T cells specific for antigens expressed in their tumors[28] gave rise to the idea that therapeutic cancer vaccines could activate and amplify this preexisting reaction and possibly induce new immune responses. Adjuvants such as keyhole limpet hemocyanin (KLH) or Montanide are important components of cancer vaccines because they act to enhance the immunogenicity of the antigen, activate DCs, and help overcome preexisting tolerance.

Dendritic-Cell Vaccines

Because of the central role of DCs in the orchestration of adaptive immune responses, DCs have been a special focus of tumor vaccination strategies. Immature DCs take up antigen and rely on appropriate maturation signals to effectively prime T cells, whereas antigen presentation by immature DCs leads to immune tolerance. It is essential to consider the complexity of DC biology in the context of DC vaccine design.[29] Delivery of the TA to DCs and provision of maturation signals can be provided ex vivo or in vivo. Because of the low frequency of DCs in the peripheral blood, approaches have been developed to generate inflammatory DCs from monocytes under culture conditions with cytokine combinations such as GM-CSF and IL-4[30] and then pulse them with the desired antigen ex vivo. Such vaccines have been clinically tested for more than a decade,[31] and it has been concluded that they are safe and can induce expansion of circulating tumor-specific CD4+ and CD8+ T cells, with objective and potentially long-lasting responses in some patients.[32,33] Sipuleucel-T, a vaccine based on enriched blood APCs that are briefly cultured with a fusion protein of prostatic acid phosphatase and GM-CSF, was the first tumor vaccine to be approved by the FDA after it demonstrated a prolonged median survival of patients with metastatic prostate cancer in a randomized phase I trial.[34] In pediatrics, the experience has been limited to a few early nonrandomized trials. Administration of tumor lysate/ KLH pulsed autologous DCs to children with relapsed solid tumors was well tolerated and demonstrated induction of specific T-cell responses. Significant regression of metastatic sites was observed in one patient, with several other patients having sustained stable disease.[35] In a related approach, patients with metastatic or relapsed sarcomas or neuroblastomas are receiving Treg-depleted autologous lymphocytes in combination with tumor lysate/KLH pulsed DCs ± IL-7 (trial NCT00923351). An initial study demonstrated that consolidative immu-

notherapy consisting of adoptive T-cell transfer with peptide-pulsed DCs can improve survival compared with historic control subjects when given in a minimal residual disease (MRD) setting of high-risk solid tumors.[36] An ongoing trial of decitabine followed by vaccination with autologous DCs pulsed with overlapping peptides derived from full-length MAGE-A1, MAGE-A3, and NY-ESO-1 antigens may hold promise in the induction of remission of relapsed neuroblastoma[37] or sarcoma (trial NCT01241162).

DCs can also be targeted in vivo by fusing the selected antigen to an antibody directed against a DC surface receptor. This technique has been shown to elicit potent antigen-specific CD4+ and CD8+ T-cell responses.[38] The choice of a DC receptor that is targeted is an important consideration because distinct DC subsets induce different types of T-cell polarization, which determine in part the elicited immune response.[39] The engagement of DC receptors by such targeting antibodies also provides activation signals, which are crucial to avoid the induction of T-cell anergy. In fact, it is now accepted that the adjuvant components of vaccines (even non–DC-based vaccines) primarily act by triggering DC maturation.

The delivery of antigens and adjuvants into the same intracellular DC compartment has been shown to be crucial.[40] Nanovaccines are a promising preclinical technology to achieve synchronized delivery of antigen and adjuvant cargo to DCs. Nanoscale complexes such as polymer-based or lipid-based nanoparticles provide protection against unwanted antigen degradation or systemic immune activation by soluble adjuvants. Upon injection into the skin, nanovaccines are transported to the lymph nodes by cell-based drainage or free interstitial lymphatic flow (depending on particle size), where they are internalized by lymph node resident DCs and generally directed to the MHC-II pathway.[41] Another bioengineering-based approach is now entering clinical trials and involves implantation of absorbable polymer scaffolds, pulsed with tumor lysate and adjuvants, to facilitate DC-based T-cell priming in situ.[42]

Peptide-Based Vaccines

The immunogenicity of peptide epitopes depends on their associations with specific polymorphic variants of MHC molecules, such that a given peptide might only elicit a response in persons with a certain HLA allele. Studies with HLA-restricted peptides thus must be carried out in patients with unique HLA alleles. Given that the population of pediatric patients is small a priori, the exploration of peptide vaccines has been much more feasible in adults who have common malignancies. Largely as a result of a poor understanding of the mechanisms of immunization and the role of DCs, in many early trials patients were unsuccessfully treated with short peptide-based vaccines in the absence of effective adjuvants.[43] Short peptides have pharmacokinetic properties that make them susceptible to rapid clearance in the absence of an adjuvant that can effectively trigger DC maturation and may promote tolerance rather than immunity. A notable exception is the administration of a short-peptide vaccine derived from gp100 in conjunction with

IL-2, which augmented tumor responses and prolonged progression-free survival (PFS) compared with IL-2 alone in persons with advanced melanoma.[44] Longer peptides (~20-mer) require further processing by DCs but have the potential to prime against a greater variety of antigens and capture CD8+ and CD4+ lymphocyte responses more efficiently compared with peptides (10- to 12-mer) that fit the MHC-I antigen-binding groove unedited. A long-peptide vaccine against HPV-16 oncoproteins administered in incomplete Freund adjuvant to patients with vulvar intraepithelial neoplasia proved to have good efficacy, including complete responses in a phase II trial.[45] These favorable results may be based on the selection of viral gene products for vaccination that are more readily recognized as foreign. In contrast, a long-peptide vaccine derived from p53 (a tumor suppressor protein mutated in many cancers), which was delivered in the emulsion-adjuvant Montanide, induced no tumor regressions in patients with advanced ovarian cancer, emphasizing preexisting tolerance and the need to optimize these formulations.[46]

Full-length protein vaccines harbor a wider profile of epitopes, and a diverse set of targets—including two cancer testes antigens, MAGE-A3 and NY-ESO-1—have been explored.[47,48] Phase I and II trials have been conducted with adjuvant-mixed, recombinant MAGE-A3 vaccines in melanoma and non–small cell lung cancer, demonstrating potent antitumor B- and T-cell responses, tumor-specific cell persistence for years after vaccination, and encouraging clinical effects.[49,50] "MAGRIT"—an ongoing large, randomized phase III trial accruing more than 2500 HLA-A2–positive patients with non–small cell lung cancer—is exploring a recombinant MAGE-A3 fusion protein in combination with an adjuvant consisting of a saponin/lipid-A emulsion and TLR4 and TLR9 agonists.[51]

Whole-Cell Vaccines

Whole-cell vaccines contain the broadest range of TAs, including mutated proteins. A meta-analysis of 173 immunotherapy trials involving a variety of solid tumors revealed that patients vaccinated with whole-cell vaccines had low objective response rates that were nonetheless significantly higher than those of patients treated with molecularly defined antigen vaccines.[52] GVAX, a vaccine strategy in which autologous or allogeneic whole tumor cells are engineered to secrete GM-CSF (to activate APCs at the site of vaccination) and are irradiated prior to injection, reached the furthest in clinical development. Phase I trials of GVAX were conducted in adults who had a variety of malignancies.[53] These early-stage trials were not powered to assess clinical endpoints, yet they consistently demonstrated immune cell infiltration at the sites of vaccination, as well as extensive tumor necrosis mediated by dense infiltrates of intratumoral CD4+ and CD8+ lymphocytes and plasma cells. Although some patients had promising results after receiving GVAX in preceding trials, a phase III trial in persons with prostate cancer that used allogeneic tumor cell lines did not demonstrate clinical efficacy.[54] This results indicate that this strategy may be most effective when autologous tumor cells are used

or when it is combined with other immune-modulating therapies. Administration of anti-CTLA4-mAb to patients previously immunized with GVAX evoked objective responses of metastatic melanoma with minimal toxicities.[55] Furthermore, administration of GVAX early after allogeneic HSCT for adult AML or myelodysplastic syndrome was shown to be safe and immunogenic,[56] with encouraging responses that have led to further exploration in a randomized phase II study (trial NCT01773395). In a similar approach, a pediatric phase I trial with IL-2-transduced autologous neuroblastoma cells in 10 patients resulted in the generation of antitumor antibodies and increased antitumor cytotoxic activity, which correlated well with clinical responses. This study observed one complete response, one partial response, and three patients with stable disease, of whom one patient entered complete remission (CR) after oral etoposide therapy.[57] In a subsequent study of 21 patients treated with an allogeneic neuroblastoma vaccine engineered to secrete lymphotactin and IL-2, two complete responses and one partial response were induced.[58]

Idiotype Vaccines

The clonal immunoglobulin idiotype, which is displayed on the surface of most malignant B cells, is a patient- and tumor-specific antigen that can be used for therapeutic vaccination. An idiotype vaccine conjugated with KLH and administered with GM-CSF indicated prolonged PFS in one phase III trial, whereas several other trials failed to demonstrate a therapeutic benefit.[59]

DNA Vaccines

Deoxyribonucleic acid (DNA) vaccines consist of viral vectors that encode TAs and are based on the idea that strong immune responses against the viral vaccine components enhance the reactivity to the TA. A phase II trial, PROSTVAC, utilized a recombinant vaccinia virus that encoded PSA along with costimulatory and adhesion molecules with the intention of rendering infected cells into surrogate APCs, followed by administration of a similarly configured fowlpox vector in a prime-boost strategy. For additional immune stimulation, GM-CSF was administered with the vectors. This trial demonstrated a median overall survival (OS) benefit of 25.1 months in the treatment group versus 16.6 in the control group[60] and prompted initiation of a phase III trial.

CYTOKINES

Interferons

IFNs are a class of cytokines that were initially investigated for their ability to interfere with viral infections, and they play an important role in the propagation of an immune response. Clinically meaningful activity of IFN-α has been shown against CML,[61] although its clinical use in CML has largely been abandoned with the advent of tyrosine kinase inhibitors. IFN-α remains a very relevant agent in the adjuvant therapy of high-risk operable melanoma, and high-dose IFN-α has demonstrated a consistent and significant improvement in DFS and OS.[62]

Interleukin-2

IL-2 plays a crucial role in T-cell growth and proliferation. It is primarily produced by CD4+ T cells after antigen stimulation, and to a lesser extent by CD8+ cells, NKT cells, activated DCs, and mast cells. IL-2 transcription is mediated by multiple transcription factors, including the nuclear factor of activated T cells (NF-AT) family proteins, AP-1 and NF-κB. The immunosuppressive drugs cyclosporine and tacrolimus act by blocking NF-AT translocation to the nucleus. The IL-2 receptor (IL-2R) is composed of an α, β, and γ chain. The IL-2R β chain is shared with IL-15, and the common γ chain receptor (γcR) is shared with six other cytokines. The crucial role of IL-2 in T-cell growth is evidenced by the severe combined immunodeficiency phenotype of patients with γcR defects. IL-2 preferentially promotes differentiation of Th1 and Th2 cells while inhibiting Th17 and follicular helper T-cell development, yet it can promote Th17 expansion once polarization has occurred. Importantly, IL-2 also drives the development of Tregs, which promote tolerance, and is essential for activation-induced cell death, an important regulator of T-cell homeostasis. Besides its potent effect on T cells, IL-2 induces proliferation and cytolytic activity of NK cells and promotes B-cell proliferation and antibody production.[63]

Clinical administration of IL-2 in an effort to activate immune cells has been in use for many years, with FDA approval in 1992 for metastatic renal cell carcinoma and in 1998 for metastatic melanoma.[64] In a small subset of 5% to 10% of patients with these malignancies, IL-2 treatment has resulted in long-term CRs, and the addition of adoptive therapy approaches have improved cure rates for metastatic melanoma to a range of 20% to 40%.[65] A limitation of IL-2 is its toxicity, including the propensity for severe capillary leak syndrome.

In pediatrics, a randomized children's oncology group trial of 289 children with AML in CR1 who received either no further therapy or two short courses of IL-2 after intensive chemotherapy did not show improvement in DFS or OS.[66] However, IL-2 administration plays a role in the treatment of high-risk neuroblastoma, where it is used in conjunction with anti-GD2 mAb therapy, GM-CSF, and isotretinoin, an approach that has led to significant improvements in outcome.[67] The rationale underlying coadministration of IL-2 is the promotion of ADCC via FcRs of IL-2–activated NK cells and macrophages, which demonstrated an enhanced antitumor effect in murine models compared with IL-2 or mAb alone.[68]

As the effects of IL-2 on Tregs have become more clearly delineated, exogenous administration of IL-2 and therapeutic interventions that may prompt high levels of endogenous IL-2 production are being considered carefully. In fact, the tolerance-inducing aspect of IL-2 administration is now being explored for the treatment of GVHD. It has been shown that daily low-dose IL-2 can be safely administered in patients who have chronic GVHD, leading to a preferential and sustained Treg expansion in vivo and ameliorating chronic GVHD symptoms in a substantial portion of patients.[69,70]

Furthermore, IL-2 remains an invaluable tool for the in vitro expansion and preparation of adoptive T-cell therapeutics.

Interleukin-7

IL-7 is produced by nonhematopoietic stromal cells and in small amounts by DCs but is not produced by T cells, B cells, or NK cells. It signals through the IL-7 receptor (IL-7R), a heterodimer consisting of IL-7Rα and the γcR, and mediates antiapoptotic and costimulatory proliferative signals through activation of phosphatidylinositol 3-kinase (P13K) and Janus kinase (JAK) signal transducers and activators of transcription (STAT), as well as antiapoptotic pathways such as B-cell lymphoma–2 (B-CL2). IL-7 is required for normal human T-cell development as demonstrated by the absence of T cells in patients with severe combined immunodeficiency as a result of mutations in the IL-7Rα or γcR, and it may play a role in normal B-cell development. Further, IL-7–mediated signaling in DCs has been implicated as a regulator of peripheral CD4+ T-cell homeostasis. Contrary to typical activation cytokines that do not act on resting T cells, IL-7 primarily affects naive T cells, which then downregulate IL-7R upon T-cell activation. An exception to this rule occurs during primary immune responses when IL-7R expression is maintained on a small subset of T cells destined to enter the central memory pool. Whereas IL-7 is continuously available in secondary lymphoid organs, plasma IL-7 is a limited resource and increases in lymphopenic states as a result of decreased use, thereby enhancing T-cell proliferation.[71] In preclinical models, IL-7 therapy augments antigen-specific T-cell responses after vaccination and adoptive cell therapy.[72,73] It also facilitates immune reconstitution in lymphopenic settings, largely via thymus-independent homeostatic expansion of peripheral T-cell populations,[74,75] and has been implicated in antagonizing inhibitory networks.[76]

In light of the preclinical promise, several clinical trials are using recombinant human IL-7 (rhIL-7) to treat patients with malignancies, chronic viral infections, and idiopathic CD4+ lymphopenia, as well as after HSCT. In the first adult human trial of patients with refractory malignancies, rhIL-7 was well tolerated apart from mild toxicities. After an initial decline in the numbers of circulating lymphocytes, IL-7 showed consistent biologic activity with substantial increases of CD8+ and CD4+ cells in the peripheral blood, as well as in spleen and lymph nodes, whereas proliferation rates of Tregs inversely correlated with IL-7 treatment. Notably, rhIL-7 preferentially induced the nonclonal proliferation of naive T cells, resulting in broadening of the TCR repertoire diversity without increasing thymopoiesis. However, in this subset of highly refractory patients, no significant antitumor effects were observed.[77] The first trial that used rhIL-7 after allogeneic HSCT was performed in recipients of T-cell–depleted grafts, given that IL-7 had boosted alloreactive T cells and GVHD in murine models.[78] IL-7 was well tolerated, with only one case of acute GVHD of the skin. In contrast to other clinical scenarios, IL-7 in the posttransplant setting preferentially expanded effector memory T cells rather than naive T cells but increased

TCR diversity and functional viral-specific T cells.[79] Further studies are needed to determine whether these effects translate clinically into reduced morbidity and mortality and protection from infection. In pediatric sarcomas, IL-7 therapy is currently being explored in the context of DC vaccination (trial NCT00923351).

Interleukin-15

IL-15 was discovered in 1994 and has pleiotropic immune-enhancing properties. It is thought to be critical for the stimulation and differentiation of NK cells, NKTs, and memory CD8+ T cells. It also promotes proliferation and differentiation of CD4+ T cells, nonmemory CD8+ T cells, and B cells; it further enhances cytolytic activity of CD8+ T cells and induces DC maturation and immunoglobulin synthesis by B cells. Although IL-15 messenger ribonucleic acid (mRNA) is expressed by a large number of tissues, the detection of IL-15 protein is largely limited to DCs and monocytes/macrophages. Free soluble IL-15 is limited, indicating tight regulation of this proinflammatory cytokine. The composition of the heterotrimeric IL-15 receptor (IL-15R) and the main signaling mechanism of IL-15 via presentation in trans are unique. IL-15 shares the β chain (IL-2Rβ/IL-15Rβ) and γcR chain with the IL-2R and signals through these domains via the JAK1/JAK3/STAT5 signaling pathway. Contrary to IL-2 signaling, where the IL-2Rα domain assembles with the IL-2Rβ and γc subunits on the recipient cell, the IL-15Rα domain is located on APCs, binds IL-15 with high affinity, and then presents IL-15Rα–bound IL-15 to the IL-15Rβ/γcR heterodimer on NK or T cells in trans. IL-15 is also thought to have minor signaling pathways that involve direct binding to the IL-15Rβ/γcR as well as binding to IL-15Rα on the target cell and presentation in cis to the IL-15Rβ/γcR on the same target cell.[80] Unlike IL-2, IL-15 does not stimulate immunosuppressive Tregs and has an antiapoptotic effect on T cells. Preclinical and clinical data suggest a dual role for IL-15. Through the link between inflammation and cancer, it has been suggested that IL-15 plays a proleukemic role in hematologic malignancies. In adults with pre–B-ALL, IL-15 expression was associated with an inferior 5-year relapse-free survival (RFS), as well as mediastinal and lymph node involvement.[81] In children without central nervous system involvement at diagnosis, high IL-15 expression levels were associated with a higher risk of central nervous system relapse.[82] A phase I clinical trial blocking IL-15 presentation in trans for patients with T-cell large granular leukemia was well tolerated but showed no responses.[83] On the other hand, evidence for a protective role of IL-15 through enhanced tumor immunosurveillance is provided with the antitumor effects of IL-15 in several preclinical tumor models.[84,85] Ongoing phase I trials for adults with advanced melanoma are investigating the administration of rhIL-15, either alone or after transfer of tumor-infiltrating lymphocytes (TILs; trials NCT01021059 and NCT01369888). IL-15 is also used for ex vivo preparation of cellular immunotherapies such as in a pediatric trial of haploidentical HSCT and IL-15–stimulated NK cells for refractory solid tumors (trial NCT01337544).

ANTIBODY-BASED IMMUNOTHERAPY

The specific recognition of surface antigens on pathogens or tumor cells was first conceptualized by Paul Ehrlich more than a century ago. In contrast to cellular immunotherapy, which often requires costly and individualized preparation, antibody-based immunotherapy is feasible for off-the-shelf use and thus is more cost effective. Antibody-based therapy may rely on recognition of TAs or interfere with tumor cell growth by disrupting negative regulatory and survival pathways as well as ligand receptor–dependent cell growth. Unconjugated antibodies predominantly function by recruiting other immune effector cells and initiating pathways such as ADCC, CDC, ADP, and direct apoptosis. Via the ADP pathway, antibodies entice APCs to take up not only the targeted antigen but also a variety of tumor contents that are processed to induce T-cell responses in MHC-restricted fashion.[86] This effect is termed the "vaccinal effect" of antibody therapy because it promotes not only immediate tumor cell death, but also vaccinelike antitumor effects with ensuing humoral and cellular immunologic memory. Clinically this effect has been shown to be relevant in solid tumors and lymphomas.[87] Although conventional antibodies activate innate effector mechanisms, they do not trigger T-cell immunity directly. The development of bispecific antibodies represents a promising approach to recruit and activate T cells directly at the site of the tumor cell by providing specificity not only to the TA but also to CD3 (Fig. 47-5).

Unconjugated Antibodies

Rituximab, a genetically engineered chimeric mouse antihuman CD20 mAb, was the first mAb to be approved by the FDA for the treatment of cancer in 1997. The murine Fab domain of rituximab binds CD20 on mature B-cell malignancies and healthy B cells, and the humanized Fc domain mediates effector functions. The mechanism of cytotoxicity is primarily via ADCC and CDC, although rituximab has also been shown to sensitize resistant lymphoma cells to chemotherapy and Fas ligand–induced apoptosis,[88] which led to its synergistic use with chemotherapy regimens in clinical practice. It may also have a vaccinal effect, leading to T-cell priming and lasting antilymphoma immunity. Rituximab is now a well-established component of therapeutic regimens for adult CD20+ NHL[89,90] and chronic lymphocytic leukemia (CLL) in the United States and Europe.[91] CD20 is expressed by almost all cases of pediatric B-cell NHL,[92] yet clinical experience with rituximab in pediatric lymphomas is still limited and in evolution. Pediatric randomized controlled trials of antibody therapy for B-cell lymphoma have not been published, but a limited number of phase I and II studies suggest a low incidence of adverse effects and encouraging response rates.[93] In a study of 38 children with stage III/IV B-cell NHL who were treated with a combination of FAB/LMB96 chemotherapy and rituximab, the 3-year event-free survival (EFS) and OS was 95%.[94] As rituximab is studied further in the pediatric population, it may improve outcomes

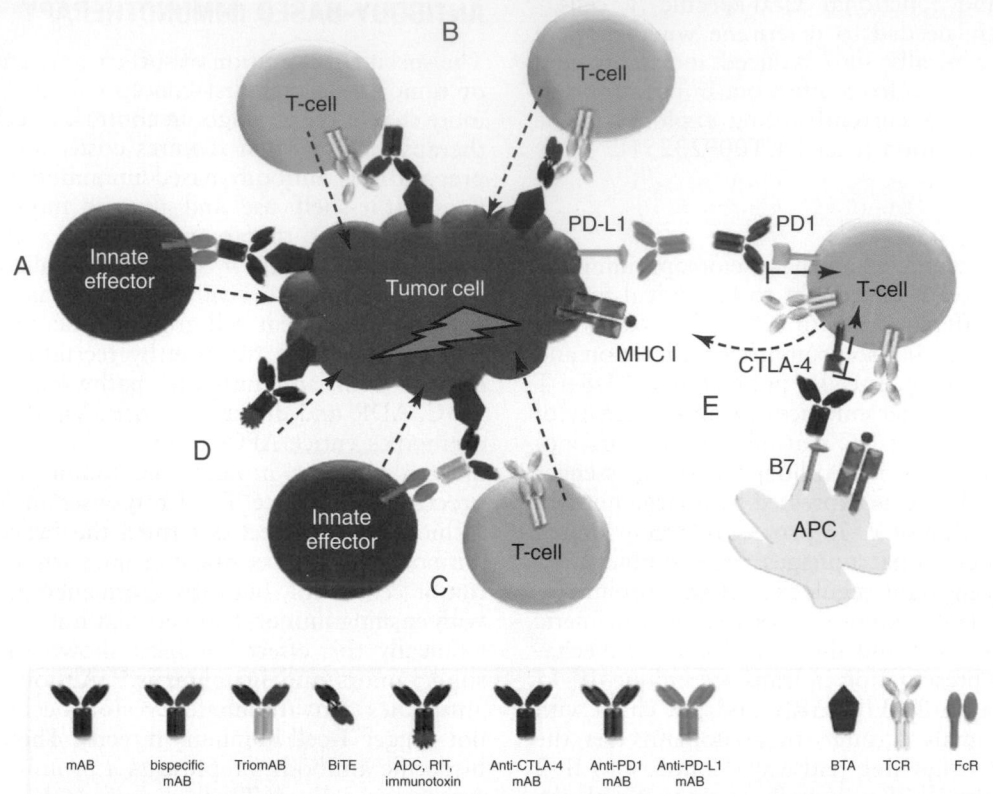

Figure 47-5 Mechanisms of antibody-based immunotherapy approaches. Various iterations of monoclonal antibodies *(mABs)* have been developed for the treatment of cancer. **A,** Unconjugated mABs bind to their target and engage effector cells (see Fig. 47-4). **B,** Bispecific mABs and bispecific T-cell engagers *(BiTEs)* are engineered to bind to the tumor antigen *(TA)* and engage cluster of differentiation (CD)3 on cytotoxic T lymphocytes (CTLs), thereby activating CTLs against tumor cells, independent of their T-cell receptor *(TCR)* specificity. **C,** Triomab antibodies *(TriomABs)* bind to TA and CD3 but also recruit natural killer cells and macrophages via their crystallizable fragment receptor *(FcR)*. **D,** Immunoconjugates deliver cytotoxic agents directly to the target cell. **E,** Antagonistic mABs to cytotoxic T-lymphocyte antigen 4 *(CTLA-4)*, programmed death–1 *(PD-1)*, programmed death–1 ligand *(PD-L1)*, or programmed death–2 ligand block ligand-receptor interactions that otherwise deliver inhibitory signals to the T cell and unleash their antitumor potential. *ADC,* Antibody drug conjugate; *APC,* antigen-presenting cell; *MHC,* major histocompatibility complex; *RIT,* radioimmunotherapy. *(Modified from Baumeister SH, Dranoff G: Principles of targeted immunotherapy. Translational cancer research: molecular therapeutics. In Kurzrock R, editor:* Targeted therapy in cancer, *Wiley Publications, Hoboken, N.J., in press.)*

both for newly diagnosed patients and patients who have had a relapse or have refractory disease, and facilitate chemotherapy regimens with reduced toxicity. Rituximab further finds application in the treatment of PTLD, either as a single agent or in combination with low-dose chemotherapy.[95] Isolated reports also indicate its utility in the treatment of pediatric paraneoplastic syndromes.[96] It should be emphasized that rituximab temporarily depletes healthy B cells, and thus patients may require immunoglobulin replacement.

Specific to the treatment of pediatric high-risk neuroblastoma is a highly effective unconjugated mAb against the disialoganglioside GD2. When immunotherapy (consisting of ch14.18 anti-GD2 mAb in conjunction with IL-2 and GM-CSF) was administered with isotretinoin after standard intensive multimodal therapy in a phase III trial, 2-year EFS increased dramatically to 66% versus 46% and OS increased to 86% versus 75%.[67]

Also noteworthy is trastuzumab, an antibody against HER2, which is approved by the FDA for the treatment of HER2-overexpressing breast cancer and gastric adenocarcinoma.

Bispecific Antibodies

Staerz and colleagues[97] first introduced the concept of bispecific antibodies to engage CTLs for cancer cell lysis. Such antibodies have dual specificity for both CD3 and the TA of interest, thereby bringing CTLs in close proximity to the tumor cell and facilitating the killing of tumor cells, regardless of the T-cell's TCR specificity. Increasingly sophisticated constructs have been developed with time. Bispecific T-cell engagers (BiTEs) can be distinguished from other bispecific constructs by their high potency at picomolar range and support of serial lysis at low effector-to-target ratios. BiTEs against multiple different target antigens including CD19, GD2, epithelial cell adhesion molecule (EpCAM), Her2/neu, epidermal growth factor receptor (EGFR), carcinoembryonic antigen (CEA), CD33, ephrin type A receptor 2 (EphA2), and melanoma-associated chondroitin sulfate proteoglycan (MCSP) have been constructed. Conventional EGFR antibodies such as cetuximab can mediate an ADCC effect via FcRs but appear to act predominantly by blocking EGFR, based on analyses showing that patients with downstream mutations in *KRAS* and *BRAF* genes do not have an overall survival advantage.[98] EGFR-BiTE antibodies, however, can activate T cells via CD3 when engaging a tumor cell and have been shown to lyse even KRAS-mutated colorectal cancer cell lines.[99] EpCAM is frequently expressed on human adenocarcinomas and some squamous cell carcinomas, but also on cancer stem cells.[100,101] MT110,[102] an EpCAM BiTE, is being tested in a phase I trial for lung, gastrointestinal (GI), breast, ovarian, and prostate cancers (trial NCT00635596). Blinatumomab, a CD19 BiTE that targets B-cell malignancies, first demonstrated efficacy in persons with advanced NHL[103] and has shown promising phase II results as a single agent in adult patients with ALL who have persistence or recurrence of MRD, leading to a 80% response rate with elimination of MRD[104] and a 61% hematologic RFS at a median follow-up of 33 months.[105] Of note, some but not all of the patients who experienced a relapse had CD19-negative relapses. As expected, blinatumomab treatment resulted in B-cell depletion, but interestingly, it also resulted in a transient decline followed by a significant expansion of T cells bearing the early activation marker CD69.[106] CD4+ T cells expanded more profoundly than did CD8+ T cells, but Treg numbers generally remained low. A single-arm phase II multicenter international trial is currently evaluating blinatumomab in pediatric and adolescent patients with relapsed or refractory ALL (trial NCT01471782). In the first reported pediatric experience of compassionate blinatumomab use in patients with refractory ALL who had experienced multiple relapses after HSCT, all three patients were able to reach MRD-negative CRs, although only one patient who was able to undergo subsequent HSCT had a lasting remission.[107] From a practical standpoint, blinatumomab is administered as a continuous 24-hour infusion for 4 weeks per 6-week cycle via a portable mini pump. The most prominent adverse effects of blinatumomab include lymphopenia, pyrexia, hypogammaglobulinemia, and hypokalemia, but reversible neurologic toxicities such as seizures and ataxia have been reported. Other BiTEs such as a CD33/CD3 BiTE for AML[108] and BiTEs engaging NK cells via CD16[109] are still in preclinical development.

In yet another iteration, Triomab antibodies are specific for the TA and engage T cells via CD3, but they also recruit NK cells and macrophages via their FcR. Catumaxomab, a Triomab antibody against EpCAM, was approved in Europe in 2009 for the treatment of malignant ascites in a variety of EpCAM+ abdominal tumors, following its success in a phase II/III clinical trial.[110] Other Triomab antibodies are in phase I/II adult clinical trials, such as a CD20 Triomab antibody in the therapy of B-cell lymphoma in conjunction with donor lymphocyte infusion (DLI) after allogeneic HSCT (trial NCT01138579) and ertumaxomab, a Triomab antibody against HER2/neu+ advanced solid tumors (trial NCT01569412). An anti-GD2 Triomab antibody has thus far been tested in animal models of neuroblastoma.[111]

Immunoconjugates

Various immunoconjugates have emerged from the idea that mABs against TAs could be exploited to deliver cytotoxic agents directly to the tumor cell site and minimize systemic adverse effects. In this approach, mABs are linked to radionuclides (radioimmunotherapies), drugs (antibody-drug conjugates, or ADCs), toxins (immunotoxins), enzymes (antibody-directed enzyme prodrug therapy), and cytokines (immunocytokines) to boost the cytotoxic mAb effects on target cells. Two radioimmunotherapies targeting CD20 have been approved by the FDA for adults. Yttrium-90 ibritumomab tiuxetan, approved in 2002, is used in the therapy of follicular NHL or relapsed/refractory low-grade NHL. Iodine-131 tositumomab was approved by the FDA in 2003 and is now indicated in the treatment of CD20+ relapsed or refractory follicular or transformed NHL.[112,113]

A very promising recent ADC, brentuximab vedotin, carries the antimitotic drug monomethyl auristatin E and targets CD30, leading to tumor cell apoptosis. It has shown remarkable efficacy in adults with relapsed or refractory HL or anaplastic large-cell lymphoma (ALCL).[114-116] These results led to accelerated FDA approval for brentuximab in 2011 for the treatment of HL and ALCL; it was the first new drug to be approved for HL in more than 30 years. Brentuximab has also been used successfully prior to allogeneic HSCT, as well as for relapse after allogeneic HSCT.[117,118] Its efficacy in other CD30+ adult malignancies is being tested in the phase II trials NCT01461538 and NCT01421667, and several clinical trials are being conducted to evaluate its safety and efficacy in conjunction with combination chemotherapy as a frontline agent (e.g., trial NCT01060904). In the pediatric population, brentuximab is currently being explored in a phase I/II trial for relapsed or refractory ALCL and HL (trial NCT01492088), but successful single-agent remission induction in a pediatric patient with ALCL who has experienced multiple relapses has been reported.[119] The Children's Oncology Group is planning to evaluate inclusion of brentuximab in the upfront therapy of newly diagnosed patients with classic HL across all risk strata in an effort to improve initial response and minimize radiotherapy, as well as to evaluate administration of brentuximab in conjunction with gemcitabine for relapsed/refractory HL.[120] Cooperative groups are also pursuing evaluation of brentuximab vedotin in combination with standard chemotherapy in children with ALCL.[121] Based on CD30 expression in patients with GVHD,[122] brentuximab is also being investigated as an agent to treat and prevent GVHD (trials NCT01596218 and NCT 01700751).

Trastuzumab emtansine most recently gained FDA approval in 2013 for the treatment of Her2+ metastatic breast cancer. This ADC combines the Her2-targeting antitumor properties of the mAb trastuzumab with the cytotoxicity of the microtubule inhibitory agent DM1, a derivative of maytansine. In a randomized international phase III trial it showed significantly prolonged PFS with less toxicity compared with a standard chemotherapeutic regimen[123] and further compared favorably to trastuzumab and docetaxel in a phase II trial of patients with metastatic breast cancer who had progressed after receiving Her2-targeted therapy with trastuzumab.[124] This drug has not been evaluated in children but may hold promise, given reports of Her2 expression in subgroups of patients with osteosarcoma,[125] Ewing family tumors,[126] neuroblastic tumors, and some Wilms tumors.

Gemtuzumab ozogamicin (GO) is a humanized anti-CD33 mAb conjugated with the anthracycline calicheamicin. It targets CD33, which is expressed in more than 80% of patients with AML. In phase II results of adults older than 60 years who had their first relapse, GO as a single agent was associated with a 30% overall response rate,[127] leading to accelerated FDA approval in 2000. Other randomized phase II trials comparing GO with induction chemotherapy and chemotherapy alone confirmed these results.[128,129] However, a large phase III study evaluating the effects of GO in combination with chemotherapy versus standard induction therapy in adults younger than 60 years with newly diagnosed AML failed to show superiority of the GO arm with respect to overall efficacy, RFS, and OS and demonstrated increased induction mortality in the GO arm.[130] Based on results from this study and concerns about high frequencies of hematologic and liver toxicity, approval for GO was voluntarily withdrawn in 2010. Since then, resurrection of GO has been widely discussed, citing the exceptionally low induction mortality of 1% in the control arm of the aforementioned study and typical induction mortality of 5% in the GO arm, as well as a lower dose of daunorubicin in the GO arm, complicating direct comparison of both groups.[131] Several other large randomized trials in adults with newly diagnosed AML have shown no difference in remission rates but a significantly higher EFS and OS in patients receiving GO in conjunction with chemotherapy, with particular benefit for younger adults who have favorable cytogenetics.[132,133] Furthermore, trials using lower dose GO either at single or fractionated dosing no longer showed an increase in hepatotoxicity or veno-occlusive disease.[133] In pediatric patients, an increased incidence of veno-occlusive disease was also limited to high-dose GO, and a phase I study of GO in combination with busulfan and cyclophosphamide conditioning for 12 children with CD33+ AML showed no GO-associated dose-limiting toxicities.[134] CD33 expression in childhood AML is heterogeneous, but high CD33 expression is associated with adverse disease characteristics such as fms-related tyrosine kinase 3 internal tandem duplication (FLT3-ITD) and independently predicts poor outcome.[135] Initial phase I and compassionate use data suggested efficacy of GO monotherapy in some patients,[136,137] and subsequent studies established that combination of GO with chemotherapy was well tolerated in the pediatric population.[138,139] In a study that administered chemotherapy in combination with GO to patients with poor end-induction MRD responses, 27 of 29 patients had a reduction in MRD and 13 of 29 patients became MRD negative, including 4 of 8 patients who had MRD levels greater than 25%.[140] However, no published pediatric trials have compared GO with chemotherapy versus chemotherapy alone in a randomized fashion.

Inotuzumab ozogamicin is a calicheamicin-linked mAb directed against CD22, a marker that is highly expressed in ALL. It has been evaluated in a phase II trial for relapsed or refractory adult ALL with promising responses and in a phase I/II trial for adults with relapsed NHL, where it showed high response rates and PFS in combination with rituximab.[141] It is currently undergoing further evaluation in several adult trials. No pediatric clinical trials have been conducted thus far, although preclinical studies suggest sensitivity of pediatric B-ALL blasts to inotuzumab ozogamicin in vitro.[142]

Within the group of immunotoxins, BL22 is an antibody that is bound to a modified Pseudomonas exotoxin and directed against CD22. A phase I trial of BL22 in pediatric patients with relapsed or refractory CD22+ ALL or NHL had an acceptable safety profile but did not show any responses, leading to an ongoing phase I trial of a second-generation antibody, CAT-8015, with improved binding affinity and in vitro cytotoxicity (trial NCT00659425). BL22 has shown promise in phase II trials for the treatment of hairy cell leukemia in adults,[143] and CAT-8015 is also being investigated in a phase I trial. Neutralizing antibody responses to BL22 have been documented in some patients and present an obstacle to retreatment.

Antibodies in the Modulation of Regulatory Pathways

During a physiologic T-cell response, the balance between costimulatory and inhibitory signals (so-called immune checkpoints) is critical to allow for efficient T-cell activation while limiting the duration and amplitude of T-cell responses, thereby protecting against chronic inflammation and autoimmunity.[144] CTLA-4 and PD-1 are examples of inhibitory receptors that are upregulated by T cells during the course of an immune response and inhibit T cells upon binding to their respective ligands. In the process of immunoediting, tumor cells or nontransformed cells in the tumor microenvironment express inhibitory ligands to escape immune surveillance.[145] However, given that many of these immune checkpoints are mediated by ligand-receptor interactions, they lend themselves to therapeutic blockade with mABs. In contrast to TA-specific mABs, such mABs do not target the tumor but rather target lymphocyte receptors or their ligands to unleash intrinsic antitumor activity.

CTLA-4 was the first inhibitory receptor to be clinically targeted. CTLA-4 is upregulated on activated T cells, where it dampens T-cell activation upon engagement with the B7 (CD80/CD86) receptors on DCs. Although expressed by CD8+ T cells, its major impact is the inhibition of CD4+ helper T cells and enhancement of the activity of Tregs, which express CTLA-4 constitutively.[146] Although the exact mechanism by which CTLA-4 enhances Treg function is not known, numerous studies have documented that the ratio of effector T cells to Tregs in the tumor microenvironment plays a crucial role in the control of tumors and correlates with outcome.[147,148] After demonstration of significant tumor regressions by single-agent anti-CTLA-4 mAb in conjunction with GVAX by Leach et al.[149] and van Elsas et al.,[150] two fully humanized anti-CTLA-4 mABs, ipilimumab and tremelimumab, entered phase I clinical trials in 2000. These mABs demonstrated ~10% objective response rates in patients with refractory metastatic melanoma who received either GVAX[151] or gp100 peptide vaccines.[152] The initial phase III trial with tremelimumab plus dacarbazine compared with dacarbazine alone did not show benefit at the dose used,[153] but a later trial comparing ipilimumab plus dacarbazine versus dacarbazine plus placebo showed improved outcomes with ipilimumab.[154] After a phase III trial with ipilimumab alone or combined with a gp100 peptide vaccine versus gp100 alone, which demonstrated a survival benefit in both ipilimumab groups, ipilimumab was approved in 2011 by the FDA for use in persons with advanced melanoma.[155] Up to 30% of patients may experience severe immune-related adverse effects (the most common being colitis) with ipilimumab, which modestly correlate with response. Steroids and TNF blockade have been used in clinical management; some adverse effects such as hypophysitis may be long lasting or irreversible, although they are readily managed with hormone replacement therapy. Trials in several adult malignancies are assessing Ipilimumab alone or in combination regimens such as with chemotherapy (trials NCT01331525 and NCT01473940), in combination with GM-CSF (trial NCT 01530984), or with androgen ablation in persons with prostate cancer (trial NCT 01377389). The necessity for rigorous evaluation of novel combination regimens is highlighted by significant hepatotoxicity observed during concurrent administration of ipilimumab and the BRAF inhibitor vemurafenib.[156] In the pediatric population, a first phase I trial is underway to evaluate ipilimumab in the treatment of refractory solid tumors and lymphoma (trial NCT01445379).

The PD-1/PD-L1 axis has been another focus of clinical investigation. PD-1 is expressed by activated T cells, B cells, and NK cells. PD-1 binding to its ligands PD-L1 or PD-L2 (expressed on DCs and in peripheral tissues) inhibits kinases that are involved in T-cell activation. Furthermore, PD-1 is expressed on Tregs, where it enhances proliferation upon PD-1 engagement with its ligand.[157] Whereas CTLA-4 regulates the immune response at the time of T-cell activation in the lymphoid organs, PD-1 primarily limits the activity of T cells in peripheral tissues. PD-1 ligands are upregulated on the tumor cell surface and on myeloid cells in the tumor microenvironment of a variety of human malignancies, where they mediate immune resistance.[145,158,159] Studies in mouse models demonstrate enhanced antitumor immunity through blockade of PD-1 or its ligands, while suggesting a favorable safety profile compared with CTLA-4 based on a comparatively mild phenotype of PD-1, PD-L1, and PD-L2 knockout mice. The first phase I trial with a single-dose fully human anti–PD-1 mAb yielded promising results, including one complete response.[160] A subsequent phase I trial evaluating sequential treatment with an anti–PD-1 mAb in adults with a variety of malignancies demonstrated quite durable objective response rates of 36% in patients with PD-L1+ tumors and a safety profile comparable with or better than that of ipilimumab.[161] Investigators of a concurrent phase I trial exploring blockade of PD-L1 rather than PD-1 reported

an objective response rate of 6% to 17% depending on the underlying malignancy but did not consider PD-L1 expression in the tumor.[162] Ongoing phase I/II trials are investigating blockade of PD-1/PD-L1 in various malignancies either alone (trial NCT01354431); with ipilimumab (trial NCT01024231); with a gp100, MART-1, and NY-ESO-1 peptide vaccine (trial NCT01176461); or in conjunction with chemotherapeutic agents (trial NCT01313416). Several other immune-checkpoint molecules are emerging as candidates for therapeutic blockade, such as lymphocyte-activation gene 3 (LAG3), 2B4, B- and T-lymphocyte attenuator (BTLA), T-cell immunoglobulin and mucin domain 3 (TIM3), A2aR, and KIR. Anti-KIR mABs aim to interfere with the interaction of inhibitory KIR receptors on NK cells and their ligands to create a missing-ligand situation and induce NK-cell–mediated tumor killing. Results from two phase I trials in adults with multiple myeloma and AML have determined safe and tolerable doses at which inhibitory KIR saturation can be achieved, and RFS in patients with AML compared favorably with that in historic control subjects.[163,164]

The stimulation of activating costimulatory pathways such as 4-1BB and inducible costimulator (ICOS) by way of therapeutic mAb administration is another strategy undergoing evaluation in early trials.[165]

ADOPTIVE CELLULAR IMMUNOTHERAPY

GVL Effect in HSCT and Donor Lymphocyte Infusions

Allogeneic HSCT is a well-established curative treatment, particularly for hematologic malignancies, and immune-mediated antileukemia effects are increasingly recognized as central to its therapeutic benefit. Myeloablative preparative chemotherapy regimens with or without total body irradiation are aimed at eradicating residual tumor cells and suppressing host immunity to prevent rejection of donor HSCs. However, patients can also be cured with reduced-intensity conditioning regimens, which facilitate engraftment but may not lead to complete eradication of leukemia cells. This outcome attests to the importance of immune recognition and eradication of residual tumor cells by donor cells in a process termed GVL, which is critical for long-term cure. Evidence of the GVL effect was provided by polymerase chain reaction–based evaluation of BCR/ABL transcripts in 92 patients with CML, of whom 80% to 83% still had detectable BCR/ABL transcripts within 6 months after transplant. Six to 24 months after transplant, 80% to 88% of patients who had received a T-cell–depleted transplant remained PCR positive compared with 26% to 30% who had received unmodified marrow.[166] Although a patient's own immune cells may have been rendered tolerant to their cancer, donor cells can recognize tumor cells through expression of TAs and mHAs. Donor and recipient are maximally matched for the HLA loci on chromosome 6 to minimize GVHD, but immune recognition of mHAs encoded by genetic polymorphisms throughout the human genome can occur.[167] Initial evidence for GVL was provided by reports that recipients of syngeneic stem cells were more likely to relapse than were HLA-matched allogeneic recipients, in whom GVHD developed.[168] Subsequently a sizable body of clinical literature established that patients experiencing GVHD were less likely to relapse, that leukemia remissions could occur in association with worsening GVHD[169] and after stopping immunosuppressive GVHD prophylaxis,[170] and that T-cell depletion of grafts was associated with higher relapse rates in persons with myeloid leukemias.[171]

Kolb and colleagues.[172] first showed that DLIs could mediate a GVL effect without additional chemotherapy or radiation, and that they induced disease remissions in patients with relapsed CML after allogeneic HSCT. The use of DLI has been less effective for patients with acute leukemias after HSCT, with CR rates ranging from 5% to 18% and 15% to 29% for ALL and AML, respectively, compared with 60% to 80% for CML.[173,174] This finding can be partially explained by higher disease burden and rate of leukemic growth, but for reasons that are not well understood, myeloid leukemias overall appear more amenable to DLI. Limited data on the efficacy of DLI are available in the pediatric population, but responses have been reported in patients with pediatric AML[175] and juvenile myelomonocytic leukemia.[176] Importantly, toxicities from DLI are not trivial and include GVHD and marrow aplasia, with a treatment-related mortality rate estimated in the 12% to 22% range.[177-179] Unfortunately, the most efficient GVL responses often arise in the setting of GVHD. Therefore efforts have focused on dissecting the immunologic mechanisms of GVL and exploiting the GVL effect while preventing GVHD. Identification of tissue-restricted expression of antigens targeted by GVL versus GVHD has been key in this endeavor. As shown in a phase I trial, adoptive transfer of T cells specific for mHAs is feasible, but restricted expression of the mHA on tumor or hematopoietic cells is crucial for a favorable toxicity profile.[180,181] Ongoing trials are exploring the infusion of donor lymphocytes specific for Wilms tumor–1 protein,[182,183] a transcription factor that is overexpressed in leukemias, as a directed DLI strategy (trials NCT00620633 and NCT00608166). Genomic approaches are likely to identify previously unknown mHAs that could be targeted.[184] Another area of interest concerns the role of alloreactive NK cells, which mediate a GVL effect and are intriguing because they do not cause GVHD.

Adoptive Therapies Exploiting NK-Cell Alloreactivity

NK cells are innate effector cells capable of rapid killing via degranulation and release of toxic granules in an early defense against malignant transformation. NK cells facilitate stem cell engraftment, fight infection, and control cancer, yet they do not cause GVHD. NK-cell alloreactivity is an important concept in haploidentical HSCT and allogeneic NK-cell therapies.[185] Human NK-cell activity is regulated by a complex system of inhibitory and activating receptors. One of the key regulators is the polymorphic KIR gene family. KIRs can be activating or inhibitory in nature and are named on the basis of their structure. This naming system distinguishes between the number of immunoglobulin-like domains

(e.g., KIR2D vs. KIR3D), as well as long and short tails (KIR2DL vs. KIR2DS), and it numbers the different receptors within the structural group in order of discovery (KIR2DL1 vs. KIR2DL2). With the exception of KIR2DL4, KIRs with long tails are generally inhibitory, whereas KIRs with short tails are activating in nature (Fig. 47-6). Three levels of KIR diversity exist: gene content, allele, and expression. A unique feature of the human KIR system is the existence of two distinctive groups of gene-content haplotypes that were identified in population studies. Group A haplotypes have a simple and constant gene content dominated by inhibitory KIRs, whereas group B haplotypes are characterized by a higher content of activating KIRs and greater gene content and variability. KIR distribution along the centromeric and telomeric motifs of the haplotype further plays a role in the ability to regulate NK-cell activity (Fig. 47-7).[186] Substantial allelic polymorphism occurs within the haplotypes, and KIR genotypic alleles are numbered analogously to HLA alleles (e.g., KIR2DL1*001 vs. KIR2DL1*002). Lastly, the expression level of each of the inherited KIR genes may vary greatly, because KIRs are clonally distributed on NK cells and individual cells express different sets of inhibitory or activating KIRs.[187] This situation illustrates why both genotyping and cell surface phenotyping are needed to accurately predict NK-cell alloreactivity between donor and recipient. Eight of the KIR family members are known to recognize MHC-I molecules, including HLA-A, HLA-B, HLA-C, and HLA-G.[188] NK cells are further regulated by a variety of other receptors, many of which recognize stress ligands that are upregulated by tissues as a signal for inflammation, infection, DNA damage, and malignant transformation (see Fig. 47-6).

An important concept of NK-cell biology is the "licensing" of NK cells. Although the exact mechanisms of licensing are yet to be fully understood, licensing provides a scientifically based concept of how NK cells maintain the balance between self-tolerance and the ability to respond to infection and malignant transformation.[189] Licensed NK cells have a matching HLA ligand for their inhibitory KIR receptor(s), which "educates" them with respect to ligand expression on healthy tissues. In steady state, ligation of the inhibitory KIR prevents them from attacking healthy tissues. However, "understanding" what normal ligand expression looks like, it renders them functional for attack in a missing ligand situation (either due to HLA class I downregulation in the tumor microenvironment or in an allogeneic setting where the recipient does not express the corresponding HLA ligand) or when tissues upregulate stress ligands that trigger activating NK-cell receptors. Unlicensed NK cells express a certain inhibitory KIR in the absence of its cognate ligand, which is possible because KIR and HLA genes are located on separate chromosomes and segregate independently. Because the ligand is lacking, unlicensed NK cells are "uneducated" and functionally are considerably less responsive in steady state.[190] However, when stress ligands are upregulated and deliver a signal to activating NK-cell receptors, unlicensed NK cells more readily mediate cytotoxicity than licensed NK cells because they do

Activating	Ligands
KIR 2DS1	HLA-C (Group C2)
KIR 2DS4	HLA-A, HLA-C
KIR 2DL4	HLA-G
CD94/NKG2C	HLA-E
KIR 3DL2	CpG
CD16 (FcR III)	IgG
NKG2D	MICA, MICB, ULBPs
NCRs	unknown, except B7-H6 (for NKp30)

Inhibitory	Ligands
KIR 2DL1	HLA-C^{Lys80} (Group C2)
KIR 2DL2/3	HLA-C^{Asn80} (Group C1)
KIR 3DL1	HLA-Bw4
CD94/NKG2A	HLA-E
KIR 3DL2	HLA-A
LIR-1	HLA-A-G
KLRG-1	Cadherins
TIGIT	PVR and PVRL2

NK Co-receptors	Ligands
DNAM-1	PVR, Nectin-2
CD96	PVR
TLR	TLRL
NKp80	AICL
CS1	CS1
NTBA	NTBA
2B4	CD48

Figure 47-6 Overview of the receptors governing natural killer-cell activity and their ligands. Natural killer *(NK)* cell surface receptors are classified based on their function as inhibitory receptors, activating receptors, or activating coreceptors. Several other receptors are involved in the regulation of NK-cell activity but are not depicted here. *AICL,* Activation-induced C-type lectin; *CD,* cluster of differentiation; *CpG,* CpG oligodeoxynucleotide; *HLA,* human leukocyte antigen; *IgG,* immunoglobulin G; *KIR,* killer cell immunoglobulin-like receptor; *KLRG-1,* killer cell lectin-like receptor subfamily G, member 1; *LIR,* inhibitory leukocyte immunoglobulin-like receptor 1; *MICA,* MHC class I–related chain A; *NCR,* natural cytotoxicity receptors; *NK,* natural killer; *NTBA,* NK-T-B antigen; *PVR,* poliovirus receptor; *TLR,* toll-like receptor; *TIGIT,* T cell immunoreceptor with Ig and ITIM domains.

not have to overcome inhibition via inhibitory KIRs (Fig. 47-8).[191]

Approximately 60% of persons have inhibitory KIRs for which they lack the cognate HLA class I ligands, and they may possess substantial numbers of unlicensed NK cells. This situation has been associated with autoimmune disease, protection from infection and cancer, and pregnancy outcome, but it may also predict the immunologic response to therapy. In an analysis of KIR-HLA immunogenetics in patients with high-risk neuroblastoma who were undergoing multimodal therapy, including autologous stem cell transplant (ASCT) and anti-GD2 mAb therapy, the presence of unlicensed NK cells was associated with significantly improved OS and reduced cumulative incidence of progression.[192] The mechanism of this benefit appeared to be due to enhanced ADCC by unlicensed NK cells during the anti-GD2 mAb therapy rather than ASCT.[193]

The importance of human NK cells in cancer surveillance was documented in an epidemiologic study by Imai and colleagues,[194] and the initial model of NK-cell alloreactivity in the HSCT setting was proposed by Valiante and Parham[195] in 1997. Ruggeri et al.[196] first reported that the KIR ligand was an important factor in determining AML relapse risk after haploidentical HSCT. These

investigators demonstrated that the probability of relapse at 5 years was 0% in 20 patients with a KIR-ligand incompatible donor, compared with 75% in 37 patients with a KIR-ligand compatible donor,[196] and later consolidated similar results in a larger cohort.[197] A plethora of clinical studies have since been conducted in the sibling donor, URD, and cord blood (CB) setting with conflicting results. As succinctly reviewed by Leung,[188] several studies showed no survival benefit or even inferior survival benefit in patients transplanted with a mismatch in the KIR/KIR-ligand system. This finding may in part be related to differences in T-cell alloreactivity and the definition and use of "KIR-mismatch" models, which varies widely in different studies.[188] The ligand-ligand mismatch model is based on the "missing-self" hypothesis, in which presence of the corresponding HLA ligand prevents NK-cell alloreactivity, whereas absence of the ligand in the HSCT recipient triggers attack by the NK cell. The receptor-ligand mismatch model takes into account that a "missing-self" ligand may go unnoticed if donor NK cells do not express the cognate KIR for this ligand and thus assesses not only the HLA-ligand repertoire in the recipient but also the donor KIR genotype and phenotype. The KIR-haplotype model is based on the presence or absence of a B-KIR haplotype in the donor. Likely as

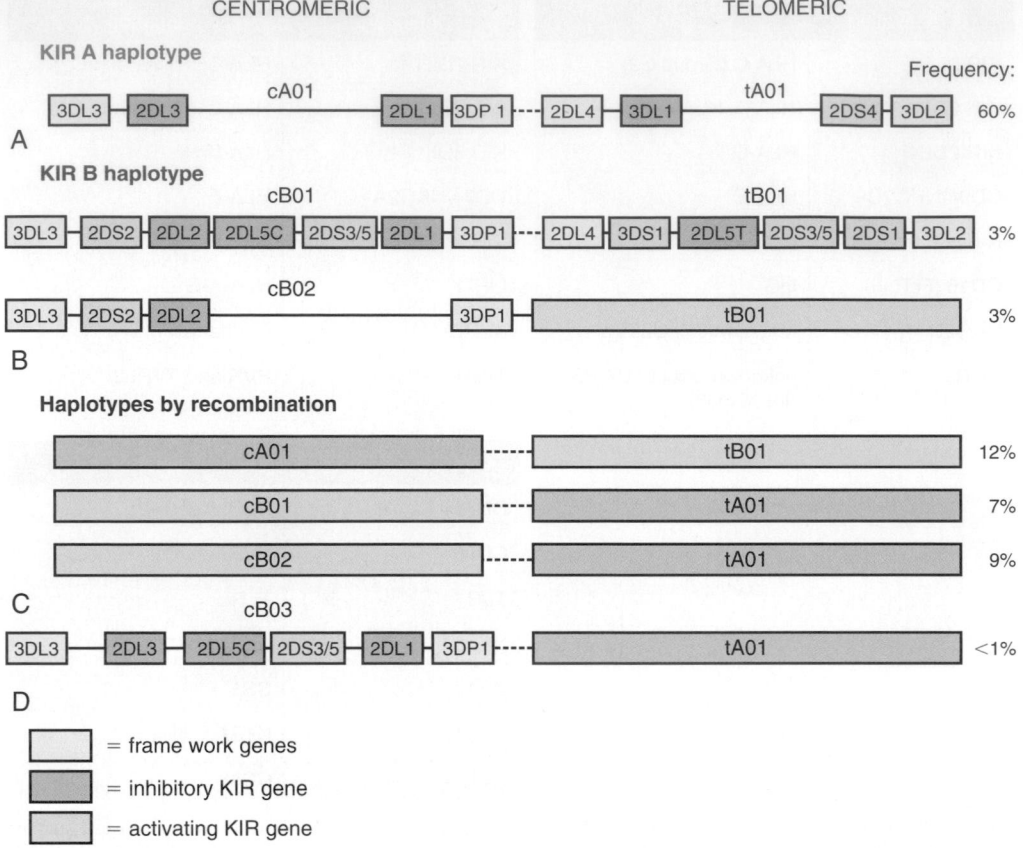

Figure 47-7 Simplified genomic map of killer cell immunoglobulin-like receptor. The human killer cell immunoglobulin-like receptor (KIR) locus maps to chromosome 19 and contains a family of highly polymorphic genes. Genetic diversity in the human KIR gene family arises from two factors: variability in KIR gene content and allelic polymorphism. Based on the combination of both, most unrelated individuals differ in KIR genotypes. A unique feature of the human KIR system is the existence of two distinctive groups of haplotypes (A and B). **A,** Approximately 60% of persons have "A" haplotype (cA01/tA01), with a simple and constant gene content, dominated by genes encoding inhibitory receptors. **B,** Group "B" haplotypes have variable and greater gene content involving genes with distinctive inhibitory receptors and a higher content of activating KIRs. The KIR haplotype model is founded on the notion that a higher number of activating KIR genes (B haplotype) in the donor increases the potential for alloreactivity and prevents relapse. **C,** Through recombination of a centromeric and telomeric cluster, various other haplotypes with "B" content have evolved, and their relative frequencies in a reference population are indicated. **D,** cB03 is an unusual B haplotype that has only been found in individuals of African descent. It contains all "A" haplotype genes but also a "B" fragment. *(Modified from Leung W: Use of NK cell activity in cure by transplant. Br J Haematol 155:14–29, 2011.)*

a result of the fact that the B haplotype carries more activating genes than does the A haplotype, it was shown that transplants from donors with the B haplotype (and specifically centromeric motifs) reduced the risk of leukemia relapse (Fig. 47-9).[198-200]

Given that ligand-ligand mismatch always equates to the presence of a major HLA class I mismatch at the antigen level, it is not surprising that such mismatch leads to significant T-cell alloreactivity and poor survival unless it is minimized by T-cell depletion (which is standard in haploidentical SCT) or in single-unit cord blood transplantation (CBT), where up to two HLA class I mismatches are acceptable and GVHD is generally lower. Presence of T cells in the graft also alters NK-cell reconstitution, leading to lower KIR expression.[201] Differences in T-cell depletion, conditioning regimens, the source and number of stem cells, the type of GVHD prophylaxis, and the clinical status of the patient population may further explain the discrepancies between different studies. Additional factors add to the complexity of the system: Activating KIRs and specifically KIR2DS1 play a substantial role in mediating alloreactivity,[202] and in adults with AML undergoing URD HSCT, those with donors who were positive for KIR2DS1 had lower rates of relapse.[203] Killing of target cells also depends on the density of KIR-independent activating receptors on NK cells and the expression of their ligands on malignant cells. Lastly, haploidentical grafts from the mother rather than the father have been shown to confer a survival advantage, whereas donor sex did not matter in haploidentical sibling HSCT.[204] Careful consideration of all factors and a more unified approach toward prospective donor selection is poised to shed light on this complicated and fascinating field. Donor selection may include consideration of the degree of receptor-ligand KIR mismatch, origin from the mother versus father, B-haplotype content, expression of specific donor-activating KIRs such as KIR2DS1, size of the alloreactive donor NK-cell pool, and in vitro cytolytic activity.

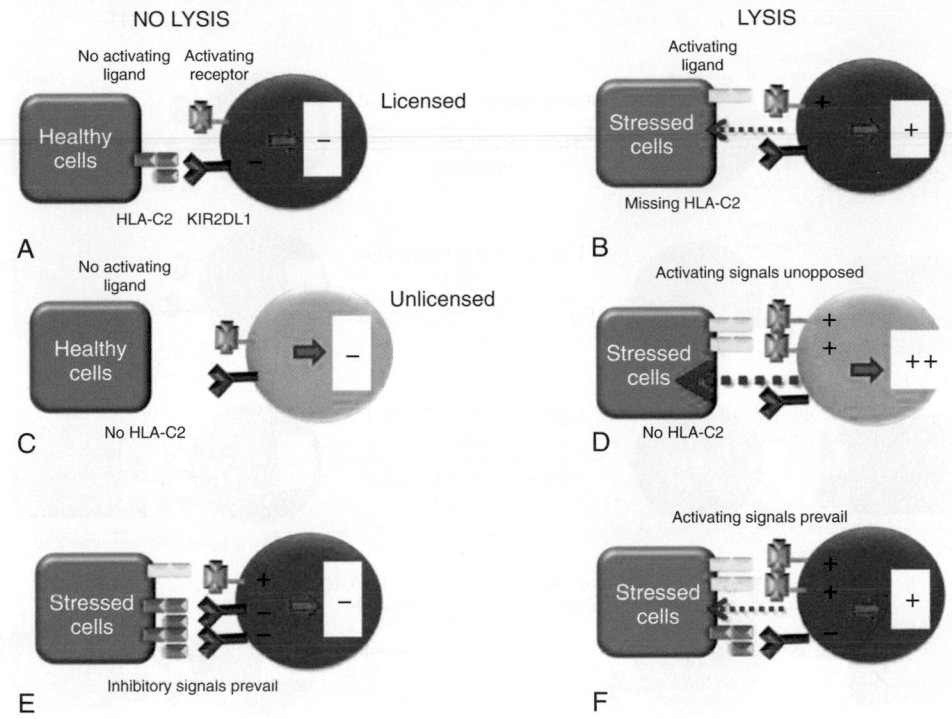

Figure 47-8 Natural killer cell reactivity is regulated by the balance of inhibitory and activating natural killer cell receptors. **A,** The presence of the appropriate ligand for an inhibitory killer cell immunoglobulin-like receptor (KIR) in an individual "licenses" the natural killer (NK) cell but delivers an inhibitory signal to the cell. **B,** If the cognate ligand is downregulated (such as in the tumor microenvironment of the same individual) or absent (in a ligand-negative allogeneic recipient), but activating ligands are expressed, NK-cell mediated killing takes place. **C,** Because of independent segregation of human leukocyte antigen (HLA; chromosome 6) and KIR (chromosome 19), an individual may lack the cognate ligand for its inhibitory receptor (autologous KIR-HLA mismatch). This scenario results in unlicensed NK cells that are hyporesponsive at baseline. **D,** However, in the presence of activating ligands, unlicensed NK cells are able to mediate killing much more readily than licensed NK cells because they do not have to overcome inhibitory signals. **E,** In contrast, licensed NK cells have to overcome inhibitory signals and will only mediate killing if activating signals prevail (**F**).

NK-cell alloreactivity is actively explored in pediatric trials by various strategies. Haploidentical HSCT involves a myeloablative or reduced-intensity conditioning regimen followed by a T-cell–depleted hematopoietic stem cell (HSC) graft from a haploidentical donor. Advantages of this approach include optimization of NK-cell alloreactive effects, immediate donor availability if no matched sibling is identified, and availability of the donor for posttransplant cellular therapies. With advances in graft manipulation and cell dose, increasingly promising results have been reported in children with malignant and benign hematologic disorders[205-208] and have led to its exploration as a treatment strategy for refractory solid tumors.[209] Novel approaches, such as use of αβ-TCR negative selection aimed at facilitating rapid engraftment and immunity by maintaining NK cells and γδ–T cells in the graft are currently being tested (trial NCT01810120). Haploidentical NK-cell transplantation as a consolidation strategy in pediatric AML (trial NCT00187096) and in relapsed or refractory neuroblastoma (trial NCT00698009) is to be distinguished by administration of a nonmyeloablative immunosuppressive regimen followed by haploidentical KIR-mismatched NK-cell infusion devoid of HSCs.[210] Yet another approach is the infusion of haploidentical KIR-mismatched NK cells without a preparative regimen after ASCT for hematologic malignancies in an effort to minimize relapse risk (trial NCT00660166).

Adoptive Therapy Using Cytokine-Induced Killer Cells

Cytokine-induced killer cells (CIKs) are ex vivo–activated cytotoxic lymphocytes characterized by a CD3+ CD56+ phenotype, acquisition of NK-cell properties, and marked upregulation of NKG2D. They can be generated from bone marrow, CB, or peripheral blood mononuclear cells by sequential addition of IFN-γ, OKT-3 (an anti-CD3 agonistic antibody), and IL-2 or IL-15.[211] Although CIKs are capable of specific MHC-restricted recognition, they can lyse a broad array of tumor targets in a non–MHC-restricted, NKG2D-dependent fashion without displaying significant alloreactive potential that could lead to GVHD.[212] Clinical experience with CIKs is still limited. Several small phase I trials demonstrated feasibility and a relatively low incidence of GVHD when donor-derived CIKs were administered to relapsed patients after allogeneic HSCT, although modest clinical benefit was limited to a few patients.[213-215] A study of CIKs in the

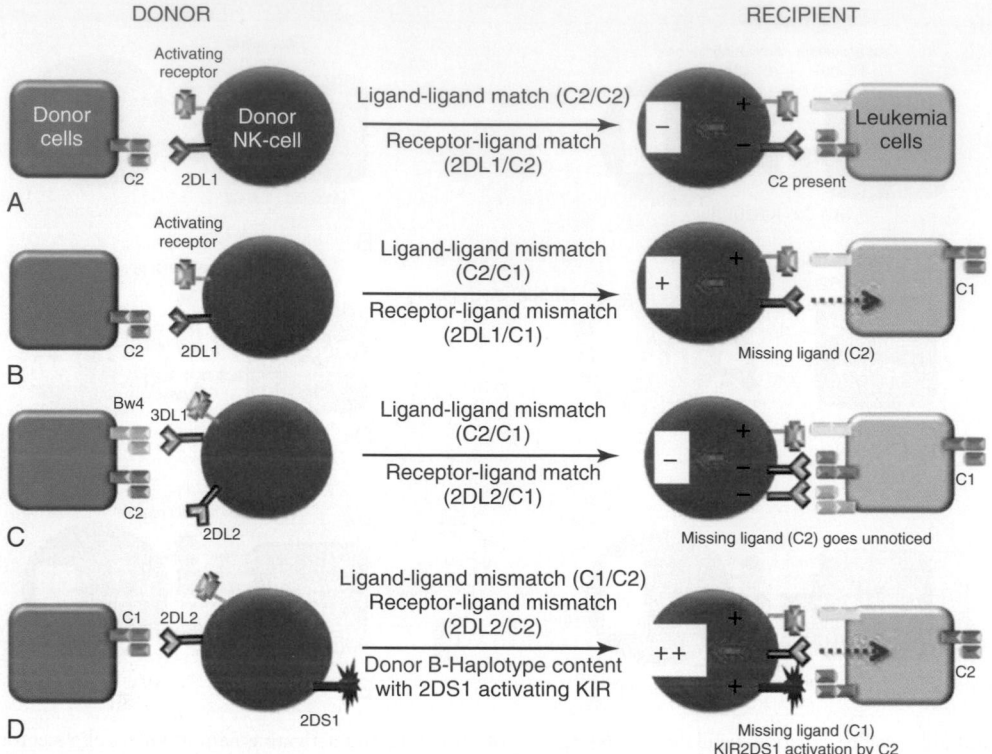

Figure 47-9 Natural killer cell alloreactivity. **A,** If donor and recipient have matching killer cell immunoglobulin-like receptor *(KIR)* ligands (C2/C2), no natural killer (NK) cell alloreactivity is expected. **B,** If the donor has a KIR ligand (C2) that is absent in the recipient (no C2; recipient has C1), lysis of recipient cells occurs, which is the basis for the ligand-ligand mismatch model. **C,** However, depending on the donor's KIR genotype and/or phenotype, the KIR for the recipient's "missing ligand" may have no or very low expression on donor NK cells. In such event, the absence of C2 in the recipient may not be noticed. This scenario forms the basis of the receptor-ligand model, which considers KIR receptors on the donor's NK cells and KIR ligands on the recipient cells, rather than respective ligands alone. **D,** Example of a scenario with optimal donor NK-cell reactivity: The donor has a strong inhibitory KIR allele (KIR2DL2) and the NK cell is licensed by recognition of KIR2DL2's cognate ligand C1 in the donor. C1 is absent in the recipient, and this missing-ligand situation is recognized by the licensed NK cell. The donor carries a B haplotype containing the strong activating KIR2DS1. KIR2DS1 may also activate the NK cell by engaging its ligand C2 on the recipient leukemia cells.

treatment of relapsed adult HL and NHL after ASCT demonstrated partial responses in select patients.[216] Pediatric patients with relapsed AML or sarcomas after haploidentical HSCT have also been reported to have received CIKs safely, but with limited efficacy in these heavily pretreated patients.[211] Novel preclinical approaches that may improve efficacy include introduction of CARs into CIKs as a mode of redirection against surface markers such as CD33 and CD123 for the treatment of AML.[217]

Adoptive T-Cell Therapy

The potential therapeutic role of lymphocytes was first revealed by studies of melanoma showing that the isolation, expansion, and adoptive transfer of TILs back into the patient[218] could result in significant clinical response rates.[219,220] Adoptive transfer of autologous TILs also showed promise in pilot clinical trials for ovarian cancer.[221,222] However, the isolation of TILs is labor intensive and technically difficult, and TILs cannot be obtained in all patients. Morgan et al.[222] developed a strategy to overcome this problem by cloning the α and β chains of a TCR recognizing the MART-1 TA from a patient with metastatic melanoma who demonstrated near-complete

regression after adoptive transfer of TILs. This strategy permitted adoptive T-cell therapy of HLA-matched patients with melanoma after their autologous T cells had been engineered to express the anti-MART1 TCR via retroviral gene transfer. With this method, select patients who sustained high levels of circulating engineered T cells achieved objective regressions of metastatic melanoma lesions.[223] However, this approach involved MHC-restricted recognition of the TA, thereby limiting availability to HLA-matched patients and remaining vulnerable to MHC downregulation in the tumor microenvironment.

CARs have since emerged as a powerful alternative tool to redirect the specificity and function of T cells and other immune cells. Gross and colleagues[224,225] pioneered the generation of TA-specific T cells by genetically modifying non–tumor-reactive T cells to express a CAR that specifically binds to TA in an MHC-unrestricted manner. CARs are hybrid receptors consisting of a single-chain variable fragment (scFv) antibody or another extracellular domain recognizing the TA of interest linked to intracellular signaling modules that mediate T-cell activation upon ligation of the CAR's extracellular domain (Fig. 47-10, *A*). Gene transfer of the CAR into T cells

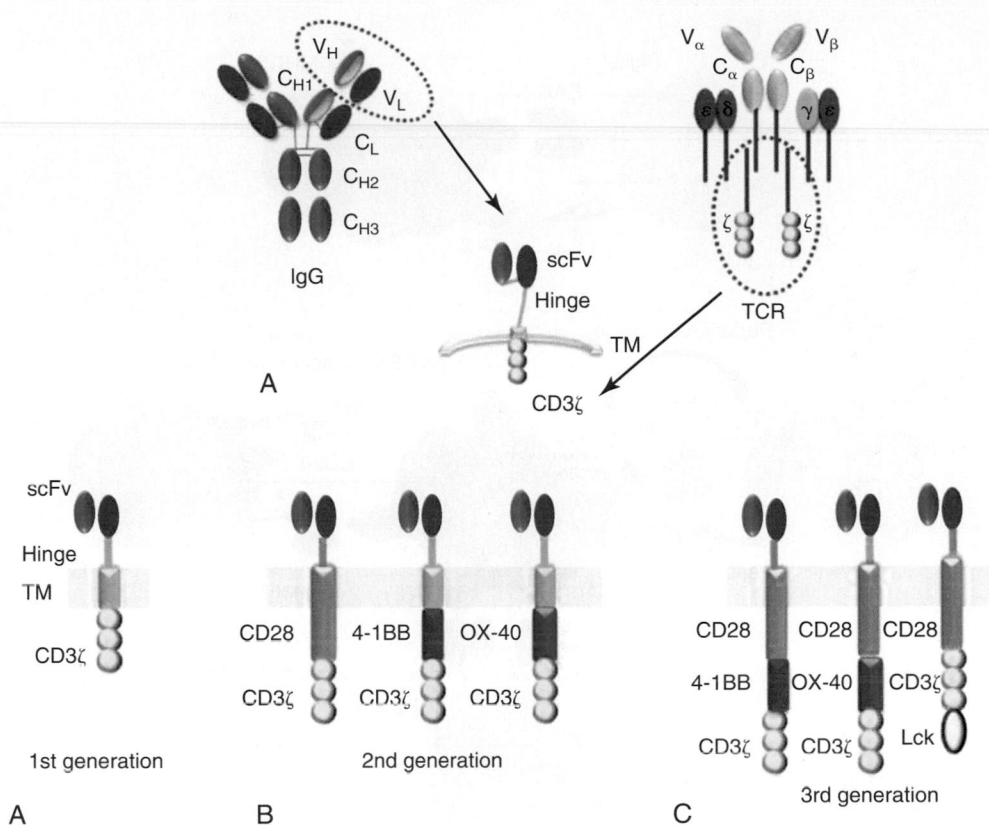

Figure 47-10 Chimeric antigen-receptor T-cells. **A,** T cells can be transduced to express chimeric antigen-receptor cells (CARs) that endow them with specificity to a particular tumor antigen (TA; signal 1), regardless of their cognate T-cell receptor *(TCR)*. Although many other iterations have been developed, the CAR commonly consists of the single-chain variable fragment *(scFv)* derived from a monoclonal antibody against a TA that is linked to an immunoreceptor tyrosine activation motif such as the CD3ζ chain. **B,** Second-generation CARs also include a costimulatory signaling domain (signal 2) in the same CAR to improve T-cell activation, expansion, and persistence. **C,** Third-generation CARs include two costimulatory signaling domains (to enhance signal 2), although it is not clear whether this is beneficial. *IgG,* Immunoglobulin G; *TM,* transmembrane region. *(Modified from Baumeister SH, Dranoff G: Principles of targeted immunotherapy. Translational cancer research: molecular therapeutics. In Kurzrock R, editor: Targeted therapy in cancer, Wiley Publications, Hoboken, N.J., in press.)*

can be achieved with use of γ-retroviral vectors, lentiviral vectors, or electroporation.[226] The transduced T cell acquires specificity for the targeted TA while retaining its endogenous TCR and can be endowed with supraphysiologic properties to carry out immediate and long-term effector functions. The ability to recognize TAs in HLA-independent fashion allows CARTs to attack tumor cells in the tumor microenvironment, where MHC downregulation is a major immune evasion mechanism. Furthermore, a single CAR construct can be used for the transduction of patient T cells regardless of HLA type and allows for large-scale production of the viral vector for clinical use. However, CARTs still have to be manufactured individually, either from a patient's autologous T cells or from matched allogeneic donor-derived T cells after HSCT. In contrast to native TCRs, which cannot recognize certain targets such as glycolipids, CARTs can be targeted to any cell surface antigen to which an mAb can be generated. Humanized scFvs have been developed from murine mABs[227] and are preferentially used to avoid CART elimination by way of an immune response against

the murine antibody fraction.[228] With emerging clinical experience and scientific insights, CAR design has become considerably more sophisticated and continues to evolve. First-generation CARs typically consist of an extracellular binding moiety such as the scFv of an mAb, linked via a hinge and transmembrane region to an intracellular immunoreceptor tyrosine activation motif such as the CD3ζ-chain or, less commonly, the FcεRIγ (see Fig. 47-10, *A*). Such CARs deliver "signal 1," resulting in modest T-cell activation, target cell lysis, IL-2 secretion, and in vivo antitumor function (Fig. 47-11, *A*). However, a costimulatory "signal 2" is required for full T-cell activation, and the lack thereof may result in T-cell anergy. To mimic physiologic T-cell activation, second-generation CARs were designed to include a costimulatory domain such as CD28, ICOS, or TNF receptor family members (e.g., 4-1BB or OX40; Fig. 47-10, *B*). Third-generation CARs include two or more costimulatory domains but may not necessarily be superior (Fig. 47-10, *C*). Costimulatory support can be provided to CARTs by different approaches. Frequently, the costimulatory

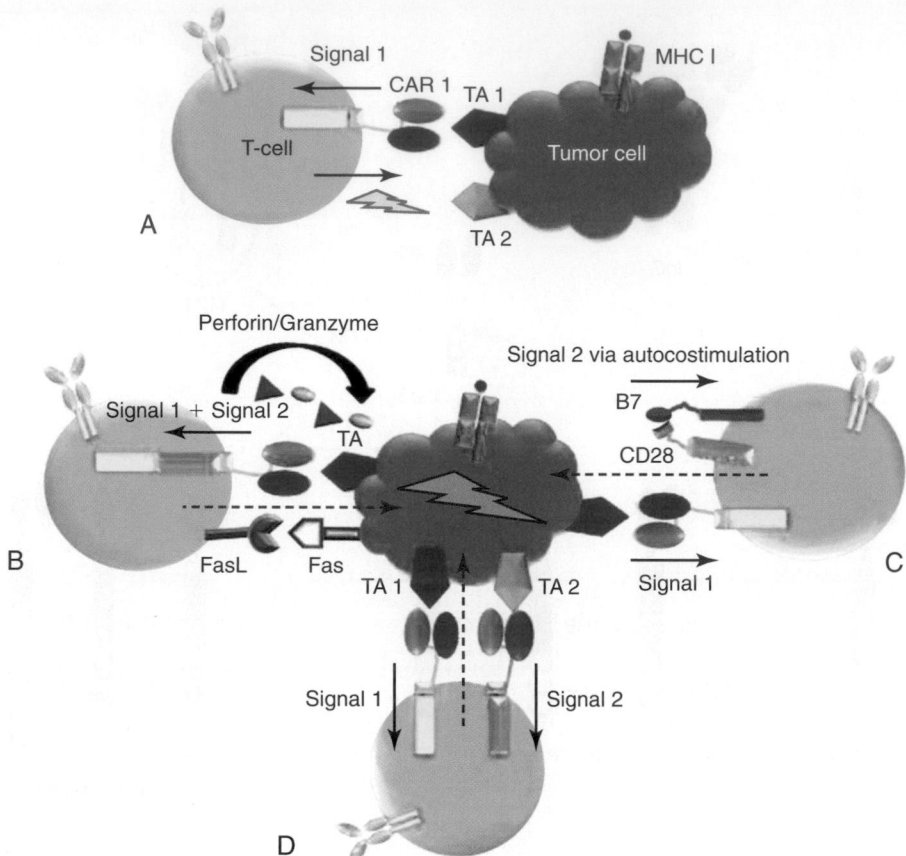

Figure 47-11 Tumor-cell elimination by chimeric antigen-receptor T cells. **A,** T cells expressing the chimeric antigen receptor (CAR) construct retain their cognate T-cell receptor but are newly endowed with specificity for the tumor antigen *(TA)*. CAR T cells can recognize the TA in major histocompatibility complex *(MHC)*–unrestricted fashion and become activated upon binding to the TA. In the absence of costimulatory signals, first-generation CARs are unable to achieve full antitumor potential and have demonstrated poor persistence in clinical phase I studies. Therefore different strategies to provide costimulatory support to CARTs were developed and significantly enhance CART-mediated killing of tumor cells and CART persistence in the patient. **B,** Costimulatory signaling domains can be embedded into the CAR construct. **C,** T cells can be engineered to express the ligand(s) for their costimulatory receptor(s) independent of the CAR, facilitating auto-costimulation. **D,** A transsignaling strategy whereby the T-cell activation signal and costimulatory signal are dissociated in two CARs with differing TA specificity not only provides a costimulatory signal but can also minimize toxicity against healthy tissues expressing one but not both of the TAs, because full CART activation is dependent on recognition of both TAs. *(Modified from Baumeister SH, Dranoff G: Principles of targeted immunotherapy. Translational cancer research: molecular therapeutics. In Kurzrock R, editor:* Targeted therapy in cancer, *Wiley Publications, Hoboken, N.J., in press.)*

domain is directly embedded into the CAR (Fig. 47-11, *B*). Alternatively, the CART can be transduced to express the ligand(s) for its costimulatory receptor(s) to enable auto-costimulation (Fig. 47-11, *C*).[229] A sophisticated strategy that also improves safety by rendering T cells specific for a tumor in the absence of a tumor-restricted antigen involves combinatorial antigen recognition and balanced, dissociated signaling; T cells are transduced both with a first-generation CAR that provides suboptimal activation upon binding of one TA and a chimeric costimulatory receptor recognizing a second TA. In this scenario, full T-cell activation is only achieved if both CARs bind to their respective antigen and tissues expressing only one of the TAs are spared from CART attack (Fig. 47-11, *D*).[230] The optimal number and configuration of costimulatory signals within a CART may vary depending on the clinical scenario and is the subject of ongoing investigation. Unifying features of second-generation CARs include enhanced cytokine production,

expression of antiapoptotic proteins in resting T cells, and proliferation in response to antigen when compared with first-generation CARs.[231-236] Compared with CARs that contain TNF receptor, CD28 costimulation leads to higher levels of IL-2 and IFN-γ secretion.[237] However, IL-2 can lead to Treg-mediated CART suppression,[238] and lower cytokine levels may be beneficial because they carry a reduced risk for cytokine release syndrome and may lead to sustained clinical activity. 4-1BB appeared superior in a xenograft model of ALL, but in a mesothelioma tumor model, CD28 and 4-1BB containing CARs were equivalent.[237,239] Stringent comparative studies to identify optimal CAR design would be prudent but are complicated by other variables such as use of different scFvs, the nature and length of extracellular spacer moieties,[100] methods of transduction, tumor models, and culture conditions.

CARs against a broad range of targets have been developed, and the identification of novel targets is ongoing. Early proof-of-principle trials were directed against carbonic-anhydrase-IX for the treatment of renal cell carcinoma,[241] folate receptor for metastatic ovarian cancer,[242] CD171 for neuroblastoma,[243] and CD20 for NHL.[244] Although these trials had a reasonable toxicity profile, T-cell persistence and efficacy were poor. Increasing evidence indicates that the degree of expansion and persistence of CARTs correlates with clinical efficacy but may also increase associated toxicity.[245,246] In an effort to improve persistence through ongoing antigenic TCR stimulation and to avoid theoretic off-target toxicity against unknown antigens via the endogenous TCR, the concept of selectively transducing EBV+ or cytomegalovirus (CMV)+ T cells has been explored. An anti-GD2-CAR trial in children with neuroblastoma utilized this approach by coinfusing EBV-specific and polyclonal anti-GD2-CARTs. Although this trial showed encouraging clinical results in several patients, CART persistence was concordant with the percentage of CD4+ T cells and central memory T cells, rather than EBV+ CARTs.[245] Consideration of the phenotypic and functional heterogeneity of the T-cell pool is key because naive T cells, effector T cells, effector memory T cells, and central memory T cells differ substantially in their readiness to deliver effector function, proliferate, and persist.[247] Depending on the therapeutic goal of achieving rapid effector function versus long-term persistence, certain T-cell subtypes may be preferentially selected for CART therapy. Furthermore, some studies identified an inverse correlation between disease burden and persistence of CARTs, suggesting that conditioning chemotherapy may be beneficial.[243,248]

Many adult and ongoing pediatric CART clinical trials have focused on CD19, which is expressed by B-cell malignancies and healthy B cells but is absent on hematopoietic stem cells, early B-precursor cells, and other tissues. Undesired on-target toxicity is thus limited to B-cell aplasia. Although transient B-cell aplasia can be supported with immunoglobulin replacement, opportunistic infections are of concern, especially if CARTs and associated B-cell aplasia might persist over the life span of a young patient. Several phase I/II clinical trials have evaluated the safety and efficacy of CD19 CARs in patients with CLL, ALL, and NHL. Although the CD19-CAR constructs used in the respective trials differ in the scFvs against CD19, the type of costimulatory domain(s) used, and lentiviral versus γ-retroviral transduction regimens, the therapeutic promise of CD19 CARTs has been demonstrated by several groups.[248,249] Brentjens et al.[250] demonstrated induction of molecular remissions with a CD19-28-ζ-CAR in five adults with MRD+ ALL. Porter et al.[246] reported on three patients with CLL who were treated with chemotherapy followed by infusion of a CD19-4-1BB-ζ-CAR, whereby two patients achieved a CR and one patient achieved a partial remission. Whereas in vivo persistence of CARTs beyond a few weeks was problematic in many of the early CART trials, this group demonstrated not only persistence of CARTs in the blood and bone marrow exceeding 6 months, but also in vivo expansion of infused CARTs by greater than three log steps. Although multiple pediatric centers are now

conducting CD19-CAR trials, Grupp et al.[251] reported first results utilizing a CD19-4-1BB-ζ-CAR construct in two pediatric patients with refractory pre–B-cell ALL who had experienced multiple relapses. Both patients achieved CRs, with one ongoing at 11 months after treatment. The second patient experienced a relapse 2 months after therapy with emergence of a CD19-negative escape variant. Similar to the adult trial, significant CART expansion and persistence occurred. Additionally, CARTs were detected in the cerebrospinal fluid. However, the remarkable therapeutic potential of CD19 CARTs is also associated with considerable toxicity. Adult and pediatric patients have been described as developing variable degrees of a febrile, potentially life-threatening cytokine-release syndrome that has been managed with Etanercept (a TNF-α blockade) and most effectively by Tocilizumab (an IL-6R blockade).[251] Transient neurologic toxicities such as mental status changes have also been observed and could be related to the presence of CD19 CARTs in the cerebrospinal fluid. In addition to CD19 CARTs, several pediatric trials are underway to evaluate CARTs directed against CD30+ lymphomas (trialsNCT01316146 and NCT01192464), Her2+ malignancies including osteosarcoma and glioblastoma multiforme (trials NCT00902044 and NCT 01109095), and GD2 in neuroblastoma (trials NCT00085930 and NCT01822652). As CARTs against new targets such as CD22+ B-precursor ALL[252] enter clinical trials, they may provide tools to prevent or treat CD19-negative escape variants. Allogeneic CART therapy after stem cell transplantation is another area of active investigation (trials NCT01087294 and NCT01475058).

From a safety perspective, one adverse event was reported for an adult with metastatic colon cancer who received a large dose of third-generation Her2-28-4-1BB-ζ-CARTs and developed an acute respiratory distress syndrome–like clinical picture followed by multiorgan failure, likely as a result of low level Her2 expression in healthy lung tissue.[253] A patient with CLL who was treated with CD19-28-ζ-CARTs after chemotherapy died within days of the T-cell infusion, but this death was ultimately attributed to an infectious cause.[254] To date, CARTs have otherwise been infused safely and with manageable and largely transient toxicity profiles. However, the relative toxicity or safety of a given target may only be evident when CARTs represent a significant amount of circulating lymphocytes, and trials with poor T-cell expansion may not be conclusive in this regard. Several strategies are being investigated to improve the safety and specificity of CARTs. These strategies include the integration of inducible suicide genes such as herpes simplex virus thymidine kinase (HSV-tk) or iCaspase-9 that can be pharmacologically activated and have been explored in the context of GVHD,[255-257] pharmacologically activated riboswitches that can regulate CAR expression and T-cell proliferation,[258] and inclusion of extracellular moieties such as human EGFR, which could allow targeted destruction via anti–human EGFR mABs.[259] Contrary to gene transfer into HSCs, transduction of differentiated T cells has not been associated with insertional mutagenesis or leukemogenesis. More than 540 patient-years of follow-up from three clinical trials evaluating a CD4-ζ-CAR for human immunodeficiency virus infection showed no evidence of persistent clonal expansion or enrichment for integration sites near genes implicated in growth control or transformation.[260]

Several interesting CAR constructs have been explored in preclinical models and hold promise for clinical application. Examples include a NKG2D-receptor-CAR targeting the natural ligands of NKG2D that are overexpressed on a multitude of tumors,[261] a CAR directed against vascular endothelial growth factor receptor 2,[262] IL-12 secreting CARTs,[263] and an anti–fluorescein isothiocyanate CAR that could be used more universally to eradicate cells marked by a fluorescein isothiocyanate–labeled antibody against various TAs.[264] Other strategies of interest include expression of chemokine receptors such as CXCR2 and CCR4 to enhance trafficking of CARTs to the site(s) of tumor[265,266] and coupling of negative T-cell regulators such as PD-1 to an activating intracellular signal, allowing the T cell to prevail over PD-L1 signals in the tumor microenvironment.[267]

CAR technology is poised to include new targets and optimize extracellular binding moieties, costimulatory domain constellations, selection of T-cell subsets, transduction regimens, safety mechanisms, and other variables. The growing body of clinical experiences should further aid in the optimal incorporation of CART therapy into existing treatment regimens and inform the prevention and management of clinical toxicities.

Allogeneic Adoptive T-Cell Therapy for the Control of Viral Infections after HSCT

Viral infections after HSCT are among the most common causes of death as a result of prolonged and profound immunosuppression of the host. This scenario is especially true after CBT or in T-cell–depleted grafts, where the graft does not contain appreciable numbers of virus-experienced T cells to confer protection. Pharmacologic therapy is available but differs in efficacy depending on the virus and may not be sufficient to eradicate infection in the absence of an intact immune system. Walter et al.[268] first established in 1995 that transfer of CMV-specific CD8+ T-cell clones derived from donor bone marrow safely and effectively boosted cellular immunity against CMV after allogeneic HSCT, whereas virus-specific CD4+ helper cells are required for persistence of the transferred CD8+ CTLs. This approach was subsequently expanded to the treatment of EBV, EBV-associated PTLD, and adenovirus and further evolved toward the generation of multivirus-specific CTLs.[269-271] However, the laborious manufacturing procedure and necessary availability of the donor with respective viral immunity presented significant challenges for a broader implementation. To overcome this barrier, third-party virus-specific CTLs were introduced.[272] Establishment of a cell bank with virus-specific lines from third-party persons possessing common HLA polymorphisms and immunity to EBV, CMV, or adenovirus permitted off-the-shelf use of these CTLs. In vitro studies predicted a high degree of alloreactivity mediated by HLA-mismatched virus-specific CTLs; however, a recent multicenter study in which 50 patients with severe, refractory viral infections after HSCT received banked third-party virus-specific CTLs reported a low incidence of de-novo GVHD in two patients with a cumulative rate of complete or partial responses of 74% in the entire group.[273]

Mesenchymal Stem Cells

Multipotent mesenchymal stem cells (MSCs) are characterized by their capacity to give rise to colony-forming–unit fibroblasts and to differentiate into tissues of mesenchymal origin in vivo and in vitro. They were first isolated from bone marrow and later from other tissues such as adipose tissue and umbilical CB. Their phenotypic definition requires expression of CD73, CD90, and CD105 in the absence of CD11b, CD14, CD34, CD45, CD19, CD79a, and HLA-DR. MSC interactions with the immune system are complex, but MSCs support hematopoiesis and co-localize with HSCs during ontogeny.[274] These characteristics generated interest in using MSCs for the prevention of graft failure and promotion of hematopoietic recovery after HSCT.[275,276] A role for MSCs in bone marrow failure syndromes has also been suggested.[277] A pediatric trial of 13 patients who received parental-derived MSC coinfusions at the time of their CBTs failed to demonstrate improved hematologic recovery or reduction in rejection, but a significantly lower risk of grade 3/4 acute GVHD was observed in the patients treated with MSC compared with historic control subjects.[278] Based on their non–HLA-restricted immunoregulatory and regenerative properties, MSCs are now being actively explored as a cellular therapy for GVHD and autoimmune/inflammatory conditions. MSCs in vivo are rare, and although they can easily be obtained by simple bone marrow aspiration, they require in vitro expansion to obtain sufficient numbers. In a multicenter phase II trial, 55 patients who had severe acute GVHD refractory to first-line steroid therapy were treated with one or more infusions of non–HLA-matched bone marrow–derived MSCs. This study reported no acute or long-term adverse effects and demonstrated 30 complete and 9 partial responses. It included 25 pediatric patients, of whom 17 achieved a complete response and four achieved a partial best response.[279] A subsequent multicenter compassionate use study evaluated a premanufactured, universal donor formulation of MSCs in 12 children who had treatment-resistant grade 3/4 acute GVHD and demonstrated an overall complete response in 58%, a partial response in 17%, and a mixed response in 25%. MSC treatment was most efficacious for GI acute GVHD, with resolution of GI symptoms in 75% of patients; however, two patients experienced recurrence of GVHD with only a partial response to retreatment.[280] Adult studies have reported a mixture of complete responses, partial responses, and nonresponses in the use of MSCs for the treatment of chronic GVHD.[281] Thus far, limited studies of MSCs in pediatric patients appear to have a very favorable toxicity profile and may offer a therapeutic option for patients with treatment-refractory GVHD.

IMMUNE RESPONSE CRITERIA

An important element of cancer immunotherapy is the accurate assessment of clinical efficacy. As has been reviewed in this chapter, immunotherapy promotes the interaction between tumor and immune cells and triggers inflammatory reactions, which often correspond with an increase in tumor size during the early phases of treatment. The Response Evaluation Criteria in Solid Tumors (RECIST) or modified World Health Organization criteria that have been used to assess chemotherapy-induced solid tumor regression may therefore not provide an adequate assessment in the context of immunotherapy. In fact, false-negative interpretation as progression could preclude the most promising immunotherapy regimens. A randomized phase III trial of ipilumimab in persons with stage IV melanoma, which showed a twofold improved OS for recipients of anti-CTLA-4 mAb, most clearly illustrated that lesions might initially increase in size, and that immunotherapy responses develop more slowly than do chemotherapy responses, reflecting the gradual buildup of a lasting immune response.[155] Clearly a need exists to develop validated biomarkers to monitor the development of an immune response after therapy and identify those that best correlate with and predict clinical efficacy.[282] Careful immune analysis will also provide further mechanistic insights and translate into improved regimens. Collaborative efforts to standardize laboratory protocols for biomarkers and to implement new immune-related response criteria are underway[283,284] and will undoubtedly benefit pediatric patients as well.

CONCLUSION AND FUTURE DIRECTIONS

Critical advances have been made in appreciating the complexity of tumor immunology and dissecting the regulatory and effector components of immunity in the tumor microenvironment and beyond. As a result, a multitude of strategies capitalizing on the immune system's ability to control cancer have emerged, both with experimental therapies and increasingly with approved clinical therapies. Ongoing preclinical discoveries and important insights from clinical trials critically inform the development of novel and optimized therapies. Although some immunotherapeutic agents have shown impressive efficacy, the overall median survival advantage may not always be overwhelming. This outcome is not surprising because phase I, II, and III studies are often performed in patients with progressive disease for whom all established therapies have failed, and the studies often use immunotherapy alone. Success in cancer therapy in general has only been achieved by using multiagent or multimodality treatments, which is likely to be the case with cancer immunotherapy as well. Immunotherapy may be most beneficial when used in upfront therapeutic regimens or in MRD states, where it can aid in the complete eradication of tumor cells and prevent relapse by establishing immunologic memory. Although lymphodepleting chemotherapeutic regimens may be important to create "space" for cellular therapies, tumor vaccines or antibody-based strategies rely on a functional immune system to carry out effector functions, and such capacity may be affected in heavily pretreated patients. Several studies suggest that the immune system has the ability to increase the efficacy of existing therapeutic modalities in cancer, and the prospect of a synergistic effect of immunotherapy is highly encouraging. Although small molecule kinase inhibitors can effectuate impressive tumor responses, these drugs are frequently limited by the emergence of drug resistance. The full effect of immunotherapy is not immediate, but once developed, it can offer a sustained response that is unparalleled by other therapeutic modalities. Tumor-specific memory T cells or persistence of infused cellular products can offer long-term control, whereas other therapies are short-lived. Upon successful initiation of antitumor immunity, the immune response can be broad and reach beyond the initially targeted antigen, thus minimizing escape mutations. The combination of targeted molecular therapy with targeted immunotherapy may thus prove to be particularly efficacious and well tolerated.[285] In pediatric oncology, effective immunotherapeutic combination regimens hold particular promise for improving survival and quality of life by sparing patients from treatment with chemotherapeutic and radiotherapeutic agents that have long-term toxicity and the propensity for secondary malignancies.

References available online at ExpertConsult.

KEY REFERENCES

7. Schreiber RD, Old LJ, Smyth MJ: Cancer immunoediting: integrating immunity's roles in cancer suppression and promotion. *Science* 331:1565–1570, 2011.
   This article provides a review of the evolution of our current understanding of tumor immunity and a discussion of the current concept of cancer immunoediting and its implications for immunotherapy.
25. Garland SM, Hernandez-Avila M, Wheeler CM, et al: Quadrivalent vaccine against human papillomavirus to prevent anogenital diseases. *N Engl J Med* 356:1928–1943, 2007.
   This randomized, placebo-controlled, phase III trial highlights the promise of preventative cancer vaccines in preventing malignant transformation caused by oncogenic viruses.
34. Kantoff PW, Higano CS, Shore ND, et al: Sipuleucel-T immunotherapy for castration-resistant prostate cancer. *N Engl J Med* 363:411–422, 2010.
   A report of the clinical trial results in prostate cancer that led to Food and Drug Administration approval of the first therapeutic cancer vaccine, Provenge, in prostate cancer.
36. Mackall CL, Rhee EH, Read EJ, et al: A pilot study of consolidative immunotherapy in patients with high-risk pediatric sarcomas. *Clin Cancer Res* 14:4850–4858, 2008.
   Results of a clinical pilot study with a dendritic cell–based tumor vaccine in pediatric patients with sarcoma, in which immunotherapy compared favorably.
45. Kenter GG, Welters MJ, Valentijn AR, et al: Vaccination against HPV-16 oncoproteins for vulvar intraepithelial neoplasia. *N Engl J Med* 361:1838–1847, 2009.
   This article demonstrates that a long-peptide vaccine of viral oncoproteins can induce clinical responses.
56. Ho VT, Vanneman M, Kim H, et al: Biologic activity of irradiated, autologous, GM-CSF-secreting leukemia cell vaccines early after allogeneic stem cell transplantation. *Proc Natl Acad Sci U S A* 106:15825–15830, 2009.
   Report of a phase I trial of the granulocyte-macrophage colony-stimulating factor–secreting whole-tumor vaccine GVAX in patients with high-risk acute myeloid leukemia and myelodysplastic

syndrome after allogeneic stem cell transplantation, which was safe and led to a number of durable complete remissions.

58. Rousseau RF, Haight AE, Hirschmann-Jax C, et al: Local and systemic effects of an allogeneic tumor cell vaccine combining transgenic human lymphotactin with interleukin-2 in patients with advanced or refractory neuroblastoma. *Blood* 101:1718–1726, 2003.

    This article describes an early approach of a pediatric whole-tumor vaccine secreting lymphotactin and interleukin-2, which led to responses in select patients with neuroblastoma.

67. Yu AL, Gilman AL, Ozkaynak MF, et al: Anti-GD2 antibody with GM-CSF, interleukin-2, and isotretinoin for neuroblastoma. *N Engl J Med* 363:1324–1334, 2010.

    This randomized phase III study established that the addition of anti-GD2 antibody-based immunotherapy to standard multimodal therapy increases event-free survival and overall survival in patients with high-risk neuroblastoma and led to a new standard of care for these patients.

70. Koreth J, Matsuoka K, Kim HT, et al: Interleukin-2 and regulatory T cells in graft-versus-host disease. *N Engl J Med* 365:2055–2066, 2011.

    The authors report that interleukin-2 can shift the ratio of conventional T cells and regulatory T cells in favor of regulatory T cells and induce clinically meaningful responses in adults with steroid-refractory chronic graft-versus-host disease.

77. Sportes C, Babb RR, Krumlauf MC, et al: Phase I study of recombinant human interleukin-7 administration in subjects with refractory malignancy. *Clin Cancer Res* 16:727–735, 2010.

    A report of the first adult trial that administered interleukin-7 to patients with refractory malignancies and achieved substantial increases in peripheral lymphocytes.

79. Perales MA, Goldberg JD, Yuan J, et al: Recombinant human interleukin-7 (CYT107) promotes T-cell recovery after allogeneic stem cell transplantation. *Blood* 120:4882–4891, 2012.

    The first report of interleukin-7 administration after T-cell–depleted allogeneic stem cell transplantation, which showed enhanced reconstitution of functional T cells, including viral-specific lymphocytes.

90. Coiffier B, Thieblemont C, Van Den Neste E, et al: Long-term outcome of patients in the LNH-98.5 trial, the first randomized study comparing rituximab-CHOP to standard CHOP chemotherapy in DLBCL patients: a study by the Groupe d'Etudes des Lymphomes de l'Adulte. *Blood* 116:2040–2045, 2010.

    This 10-year analysis confirms the benefits and tolerability of the addition of rituximab to CHOP chemotherapy in adults with diffuse large B-cell lymphoma.

93. Meinhardt A, Burkhardt B, Zimmermann M, et al: Phase II window study on rituximab in newly diagnosed pediatric mature B-cell non-Hodgkin's lymphoma and Burkitt leukemia. *J Clin Oncol* 28:3115–3121, 2010.

    This study established single-agent activity of rituximab in pediatric non-Hodgkin lymphoma.

104. Topp MS, Kufer P, Gokbuget N, et al: Targeted therapy with the T-cell-engaging antibody blinatumomab of chemotherapy-refractory minimal residual disease in B-lineage acute lymphoblastic leukemia patients results in high response rate and prolonged leukemia-free survival. *J Clin Oncol* 29:2493–2498, 2011.

    A report of encouraging clinical results in adult acute lymphoblastic leukemia with a bispecfic antibody that simultaneously engages CD19 and CD3, thereby targeting T cells to the leukemia cells.

114. Younes A, Bartlett NL, Leonard JP, et al: Brentuximab vedotin (SGN-35) for relapsed CD30-positive lymphomas. *N Engl J Med* 363:1812–1821, 2010.

    A report of the promising results with brentuximab vedotin in Hodgkin lymphoma and anaplastic large-cell lymphoma, which ultimately led to Food and Drug Administration approval of the drug in 2011.

131. Rowe JM, Lowenberg B: Gemtuzumab ozogamicin in acute myeloid leukemia: a remarkable saga about an active drug. *Blood* 121:4838–4841, 2013.

    A summary of the clinical experience with the anti-CD33 immunoconjugate gemtuzumab ozogamicin, which was approved by the Food and Drug Administration and later withdrawn, and discussion of the rationale for considering reapproval of the drug.

144. Pardoll DM: The blockade of immune checkpoints in cancer immunotherapy. *Nat Rev Cancer* 12:252–264, 2012.

    This article provides an in-depth review of various immune regulatory pathways and their therapeutic blockade.

155. Hodi FS, O'Day SJ, McDermott DF, et al: Improved survival with ipilimumab in patients with metastatic melanoma. *N Engl J Med* 363:711–723, 2010.

    A report of the phase III trial that demonstrated survival advantage conferred by the anti-CTLA-4 antibody ipilimumab and led to its approval by the Food and Drug Administration for metastatic melanoma.

161. Topalian SL, Hodi FS, Brahmer JR, et al: Safety, activity, and immune correlates of anti-PD-1 antibody in cancer. *N Engl J Med* 366:2443–2454, 2012.

    This article reports on the phase I trial experience with an anti–PD-1 antibody that induced objective responses in 36% of adults with various PD-L1+ malignancies.

162. Brahmer JR, Tykodi SS, Chow LQ, et al: Safety and activity of anti-PD-L1 antibody in patients with advanced cancer. *N Engl J Med* 366:2455–2465, 2012.

    Results of a phase I trial utilizing an anti–programmed death–1 (PD-1) ligand antibody to block the PD-1/PD-1L axis that demonstrated durable tumor regressions in 6% to 17% of patients.

168. Weiden PL, Flournoy N, Thomas ED, et al: Antileukemic effect of graft-versus-host disease in human recipients of allogeneic-marrow grafts. *N Engl J Med* 300:1068–1073, 1979.

    The first report in support of a graft-versus-leukemia effect in allogeneic hematopoietic stem cell transplantation.

188. Leung W: Use of NK cell activity in cure by transplant. *Br J Haematol* 155:14–29, 2011.

    A review of the biology of natural killer cell activity, as well as the conflicting results of clinical studies evaluating the hematopoietic stem cell transplantation outcomes associated with killer cell immunoglobulin-like receptor mismatch, depending on the model used.

197. Ruggeri L, Mancusi A, Capanni M, et al: Donor natural killer cell allorecognition of missing self in haploidentical hematopoietic transplantation for acute myeloid leukemia: challenging its predictive value. *Blood* 110:433–440, 2007.

    In an update of the results reported by the same group in 2002, this article includes a total of 112 patients with acute myeloid leukemia who underwent haploidentical hematopoietic stem cell transplantation and shows that in this cohort, donor natural killer cell alloreactivity led to lower relapse rates of patients who underwent transplantation while in complete remission and improved event-free survival in all patients.

203. Venstrom JM, Pittari G, Gooley TA, et al: HLA-C-dependent prevention of leukemia relapse by donor activating KIR2DS1. *N Engl J Med* 367:805–816, 2012.

    This article reports that the presence of the activating KIR2DS1 in the donor is associated with a lower relapse risk in adults with acute myeloid leukemia who are undergoing unrelated donor hematopoietic stem cell transplantation.

205. Leung W, Campana D, Yang J, et al: High success rate of hematopoietic cell transplantation regardless of donor source in children with very high-risk leukemia. *Blood* 118:223–230, 2011.

    Analysis of single-institution outcomes of pediatric hematopoietic stem cell transplantation in children with very high risk leukemia based on treatment era and donor source. Survival was significantly improved in recent cohorts regardless of donor source, but outcomes for haploidentical stem cell transplantation in recent cohorts were particularly encouraging.

245. Louis CU, Savoldo B, Dotti G, et al: Antitumor activity and long-term fate of chimeric antigen receptor-positive T cells in patients with neuroblastoma. *Blood* 118:6050–6056, 2011.

    This article reports on long-term results with an anti-GD2-CAR expressed in Epstein-Barr virus–specific cytotoxic T lymphocytes versus activated polyclonal T cells. Select patients with active neuroblastoma had encouraging results with this approach.

246. Porter DL, Levine BL, Kalos M, et al: Chimeric antigen receptor-modified T cells in chronic lymphoid leukemia. *N Engl J Med* 365:725–733, 2011.

    Report of clinical results in three adults with chronic lymphoid leukemia who received CD19 chimeric antigen receptor T-cell

(CART) cells. *Apart from promising clinical results, this group demonstrated significant CART expansion and persistence.*

250. Brentjens RJ, Davila ML, Riviere I, et al: CD19-targeted T cells rapidly induce molecular remissions in adults with chemotherapy-refractory acute lymphoblastic leukemia. *Sci Transl Med* 5:177ra38, 2013.

In this study, the authors successfully used CD19 chimeric antigen receptor T-cell therapy to induce molecular remissions in adults with minimal residual disease–positive acute lymphoblastic leukemia.

251. Grupp SA, Kalos M, Barrett D, et al: Chimeric antigen receptor-modified T cells for acute lymphoid leukemia. *N Engl J Med* 368:1509–1518, 2013.

The first published experience with CD19 chimeric antigen receptor T-cell therapy in two pediatric patients with relapsed, refractory acute lymphoid leukemia. Both patients experienced complete remissions, including one durable complete remission.

273. Leen AM, Bollard CM, Mendizabal AM, et al: Multicenter study of banked third party virus-specific T-cells to treat severe viral infections after hematopoietic stem cell transplantation. *Blood* 121:5113–5123, 2013.

A report on adoptive therapy with banked third-party virus-specific T cells to treat severe viral infections after hematopoietic stem cell transplantation, which shows a low rate of graft-versus-host disease and striking decreases in viral DNA and resolution of clinical symptoms.

279. Le Blanc K, Frassoni F, Ball L, et al: Mesenchymal stem cells for treatment of steroid-resistant, severe, acute graft-versus-host disease: a phase II study. *Lancet* 371:1579–1586, 2008.

This study demonstrated efficacy of mesenchymal stem cells in the treatment of steroid-resistant acute graft-versus-host disease, with 30 of 55 patients achievving complete responses and 9 showing improvement.

CHAPTER 48

Pediatric Radiation Oncology

Shannon M. MacDonald and Karen Jean Marcus

CHAPTER OUTLINE

PRINCIPLES OF RADIATION ONCOLOGY

Radiation oncology is an effective and often critical component of multidisciplinary cancer care for many childhood malignancies. The delivery of radiation for the pediatric population is highly complex because of the diversity of patients, tumor location, and biology. Additional concerns regarding the use of radiation for this patient population include a high likelihood of cure, coupled with the well-known and often lifelong complications from oncologic treatment. As survival from childhood cancer has improved, there is better recognition of the impact that long-term toxicities can have on the quality of life for patients. Practitioners have also learned a great deal over the past few decades regarding the required dose of radiation to provide cure, as well as the dose that specific healthy organs can tolerate. For each radiation plan it is now easier to deliver the desired target dose while minimizing the dose to healthy organs, allowing for disease control with decreased morbidity. Still, radiation is not without side effects and for each patient the risks and benefits must be considered to determine an acceptable treatment plan. Multimodality treatment is required for nearly all pediatric cancer patients, and physicians from different subspecialties must work closely together to determine the best management for these children. The desires of children and their parents must be taken into consideration to determine what life-long side effects are considered acceptable in order to achieve the best outcome.

THE PHYSICAL BASIS OF RADIOTHERAPY

Radiation is by no means a novel phenomenon; background radiation is ever-present. The understanding and use of radiation, however, is a relatively recent development in human history. The discoveries of x-rays in 1895 by the German physicist Wilhelm Konrad Röntgen and radioactivity in 1898 by Henri Becquerel led to the recognition of biologic effects of radiation.[1] By the early part of the twentieth century, ionizing radiation had rapidly come into use to treat malignant and benign conditions. At the 1922 International Congress of Oncology in Paris, Coutard presented the first evidence of the use of fractionated radiotherapy to cure advanced laryngeal cancer without disastrous sequelae.[2] This event marked the beginning of the field of radiation oncology.

Ionizing radiation, which includes both particulate radiation and electromagnetic waves, produces ionizations and excitations during the absorption of energy in

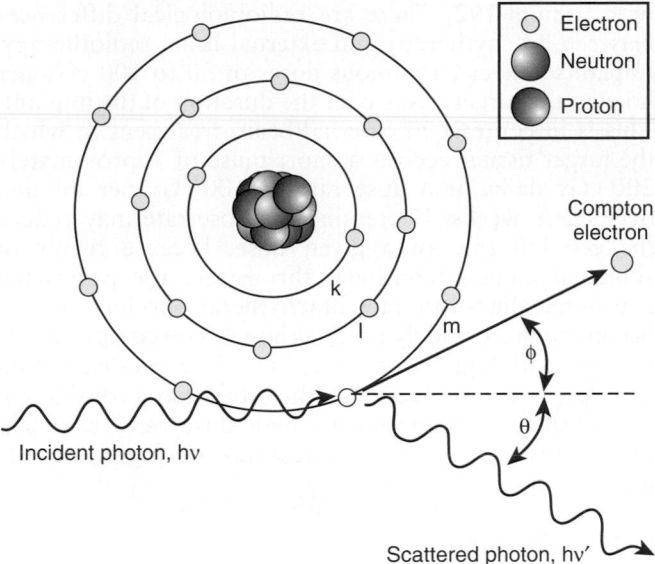

Figure 48-1 The Compton effect.

Legend:
- ○ Electron
- ● Neutron
- ● Proton

Compton electron

Incident photon, hv

Scattered photon, hv′

exposed tissue. Electromagnetic waves are part of a broad spectrum that includes radio waves, microwaves, visible light, x-rays, and gamma rays. In therapeutic radiation oncology, x-rays, gamma rays, and particulate radiation are used. Gamma rays and x-rays share similar general properties, differing in the source and energies. X-rays are produced when charged particles, generally electrons, are accelerated and bombard a high-density target. The target, most commonly tungsten, emits photons of varying energies up to the peak energy of the accelerated electrons. The energy (E) of the photons is determined using the relationship $E = hv$, where h is the constant of proportionality known as the *Planck constant*, and v is the frequency of the wave. Substituting for the frequency, the equation becomes $E = hc/\lambda$, where c is the speed of light and λ is the wavelength. In contrast, gamma rays are emitted by a source; the most commonly used source for gamma rays used in therapeutic radiation is cobalt.

Radiation may be directly ionizing or indirectly ionizing. Direct ionization results in a direct disruption of the atomic or molecular structure of tissue through which the beam of radiation passes. This disruption causes biochemical and molecular damage. Particle beams are directly ionizing. Electromagnetic waves and neutrons are indirectly ionizing; when absorbed in tissue they give up their energy by producing fast-moving charged particles. These charged particles directly damage tissue. Photons in tissue interact in several different ways, including producing the Compton effect or the photoelectric effect, coherent scattering, pair production, and photodisintegration. The dominant reaction, the Compton effect, is governed by the energy of the photons. This process, shown in Figure 48-1, involves the interaction of the photon with a loosely bound orbital electron. Part of the energy of the incident photon is transferred to the electron as kinetic energy; this Compton electron may then interact with electrons in the surrounding tissue. The remaining energy is carried away by another photon that

is less energetic than the original photon. The probability of Compton interactions is independent of the atomic number of the target tissue.

Whereas photons interact mainly with orbital electrons, protons, neutrons, and other heavy particles interact with the nuclei of atoms. Heavy particles also cause showers of lower energy and densely ionizing protons, neutrons, and other particles, depositing large amounts of energy over a very short distance. This is referred to as *linear energy transfer (LET)* and depends on the type of radiation used. Photons and electrons both have low rates of energy transfer. Heavy particles tend to deposit their energy in a track over a relatively short distance, and these particles are considered high-LET radiation.

External-beam radiation treatment systems produce ionizing radiation by radioactive decay of a nuclide, most commonly cobalt-60, or electronically through the acceleration of electrons or other charged particles such as protons. In a linear accelerator, electrons are accelerated down a waveguide by the use of alternating microwave fields. In a cobalt-60 unit the source is always on, because radioactive decay occurs continuously. The source is moved to an unshielded position to initiate a treatment. In a linear accelerator, no source is present until the unit is energized; there is an *on* switch and an *off* switch. The energy spectra are different for the two types of treatment units. Cobalt-60 units emit two monoenergetic gamma rays with each decay, producing a discrete spectrum with peaks at 1.17 and 1.33 MeV. A linear accelerator produces a continuous x-ray spectrum with a maximum energy of E_{max} (the accelerating potential) and all other photon energies down to zero. An average x-ray produces the energy of approximately one-third E_{max}. A linear accelerator can produce a treatment beam of electrons as well as photons. The accelerated electron beam exits the treatment unit under controlled conditions of scatter.

The basic components of the treatment machine include a radiation source, a collimating system to form and direct the beam, inherent shielding for protection, a light field to delineate visibly the area being treated, a control system to turn the beam on and off, a system to rotate the beam, and a support apparatus for the patient. Most treatment machines are assembled with isocentric geometry. The isocenter is a point in space at which all of the treatment machine's rotational axes intersect. Any mechanical rotation occurs around an axis that passes through the isocenter.

The linear accelerator has many degrees of geometric movement and can produce a treatment field in almost any orientation relative to the patient. Figure 48-2 shows a photon linear accelerator. The beam source is mounted on a gantry that rotates fully about the patient. The patient is on a treatment couch that can pivot with respect to the plane of gantry rotation. This degree of movement allows multiple fields to approach the target volume. In addition, the collimation assembly mounted on the gantry allows the radiation treatment field to be geometrically conformed to the target volume intersection. The delivery of proton therapy has evolved to utilize a gantry system adapted from linear accelerators and cobalt delivery systems.

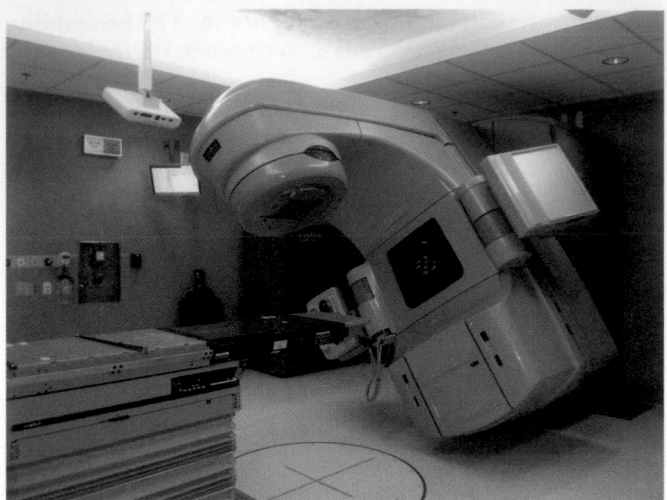

Figure 48-2 Photon linear accelerator. The patient is positioned on a couch *(black table)* that can pivot for patient positioning. The gantry can rotate fully around the patient. The radiation beam can be delivered at almost any orientation desired for treatment.

The amount of energy deposited per unit mass represents the absorbed dose of radiation. The official unit of dose is now the gray, in honor of L.H. Gray, the noted British radiobiologist who discovered the oxygen effect; it replaces the older unit, *rad.* One joule per kilogram is called a *gray (Gy)* and 1 gray equals 100 cGy. Clinical radiotherapy uses external radiation beam delivery, most often x-rays (photons) or electrons. Linear accelerators accelerate electrons to a given energy, generally 4 to 25 MeV; the electrons bombard a target, usually tungsten, resulting in the formation of an x-ray beam. The x-ray beams contain photons of varying energies up to the peak of the accelerated electrons.

In addition to external-beam radiotherapy, other radiotherapy delivery modalities are used in specific circumstances. Implanting radioactive sources directly into a tumor is known as *brachytherapy,* from the Greek *brachys,* meaning *short.* Brachytherapy can involve the placement of encapsulated sources into a body cavity (intracavitary), directly into the tumor or adjacent tissue (interstitial implants), or on the surface adjacent to the tumor (plaque therapy). Permanent implants in the form of radioactive seeds are placed under the guidance of ultrasound, computed tomography (CT), or magnetic resonance imaging (MRI). Temporary implants are performed by using hollow catheters or loading devices inserted at the time of surgery and then subsequently loaded with radioactive sources. The chief advantage of this technique is to deliver a high dose to the target tissue while sparing the nearby normal tissue. Iridium-192 and iodine-125 are the most commonly used radionuclides. Radionuclides are embedded in seeds and sealed in thin plastic strands that can be inserted into afterloading catheters. Iodine-125, with a relatively short half-life of 57 days, is often used in permanent implants. The other feature of iodine-125 that makes it appealing for use in pediatrics is the lower energy of the photons emitted, which simplify the radiation safety concerns compared

with iridium-192. There are radiobiological differences between brachytherapy and external-beam radiotherapy. Implants deliver continuous doses of 30 to 100 cGy per hour to the target tissue over the duration of the implant. This is in contrast to external-beam treatment in which the target tissue receives a short pulse of approximately 200 cGy daily, at a dose rate of 100 cGy per minute, over many weeks. Decreasing the dose rate may reduce the cell kill rate of a given dose, because repair of sublethal damage continues throughout the protracted exposure. High-dose-rate brachytherapy techniques are becoming more widely used, although late complications increase with higher dose rates.[3] For dose rates exceeding 1 Gy per hour, a reduction in the total dose is considered. In addition, fractionation of high dose rates can help to diminish the late complications of high-dose-rate delivery.

RADIOBIOLOGY

Mechanisms of Radiation Damage

The biologic effects of ionizing radiation result primarily from the formation of double-strand breaks in cellular deoxyribonucleic acid (DNA). Although most single-strand breaks in DNA caused by radiation are repaired, double-strand breaks can result in irreparable damage that leads to mitotic cell death. Photon radiation (x-rays or gamma rays) can cause damage via direct interaction with the DNA molecule or via the formation of free radicals that subsequently damage the DNA (indirect damage). Charged particles such as helium, carbon, and neon cause damage predominantly through direct interactions. High-energy neutrons interact with the nucleus of an atom, resulting in the creation of densely ionizing recoil protons, alpha particles, and nuclear fragments. LET measures the average energy deposited in tissue per unit distance traveled by a particle or photon. Conventional radiation is sparsely ionizing (low LET), whereas fast neutrons and heavy particles are more densely ionizing (high LET).[4]

Radiation causes complex cascades of molecular events that affect cell cycle checkpoints, apoptosis, DNA damage response, and DNA repair. These effects offer many potential approaches to enhancing radiation damage of tumor cells and to protecting normal tissues. These techniques are discussed in this chapter.

Clonogenic Survival Curves

A typical clonogenic survival curve is shown in Figure 48-3. The surviving fraction is plotted on a logarithmic scale, and the dose of radiation is drawn on a linear scale. The resulting cell survival curve has two distinct regions. In the initial "shoulder" portion of the curve, the fraction of cells killed increases slightly with increasing radiation doses. In the latter part of the curve, killing becomes exponential, which means that a given dose increment kills a constant fraction of cells. The slope of the exponential portion of the survival curve is called the D_0. This term is related to the inherent radiosensitivity of the cell. The smaller the D_0, the more sensitive the cells are to radiation. This is in contrast to radio responsiveness, which refers only to the rate of

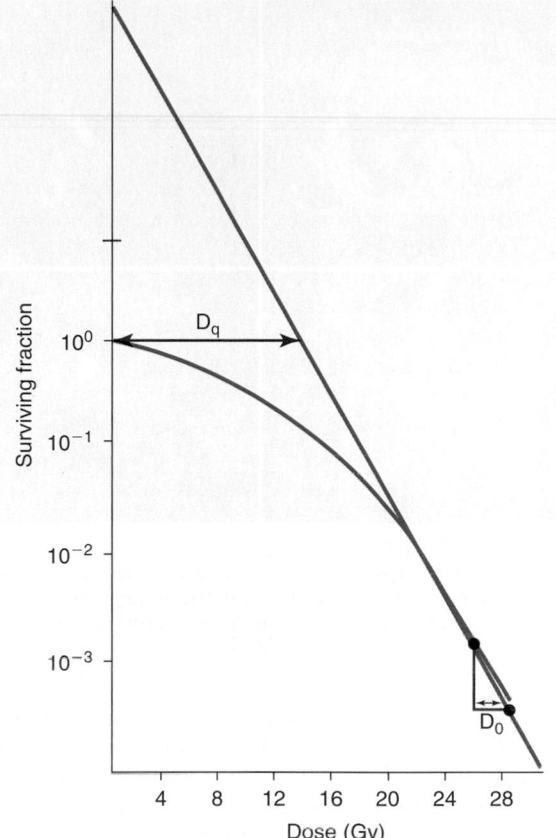

Figure 48-3 Idealized radiation cell survival curve. The fraction of surviving cells is plotted on a logarithmic scale against dose on a linear scale. The D_0 is the dose necessary to reduce the surviving fraction to 0.38 of e^{-1}. The smaller the D_0, the more sensitive the cells are to radiation. The D_q is the quasi-threshold dose and is a quantitative measure of the sublethal repair capability. *(Modified from Hall EJ: Radiobiology for the radiologist, ed 2, Hagerstown, Md., 1978, Harper Row.)*

disappearance of a tumor after irradiation and has no correlation with the innate sensitivity of the cells. The D_0 for mammalian cells in vitro generally falls between 1 and 2 Gy. The relatively narrow range of values for widely varying types of cells is striking. The initial nonexponential portion of the curve is believed to result from the capacity of most mammalian cells to repair nonlethal radiation injury. Saturation of the repair capability is thought to occur at the point where killing cells becomes exponential.[4]

Additional mathematical models have been used to characterize the cellular response to ionizing radiation. One of the most commonly used models, the linear-quadratic survival model, is routinely used to investigate how different tumor repopulation kinetics between radiation treatments influence the scheduling of radiation treatment. As various fractionation schemes have been examined clinically, including hyperfractionation, accelerated fractionation, and combined modality therapy (chemoradiation), the linear-quadratic model has been used to calculate the tolerability of specific tissues to various radiation schedules.[5] The concept of the biologically effective dose, a tool offered by the linear-quadratic

model, allows quantification of the effects of radiation schedules on tumors and on normal structures.[6] Although this model has been helpful when applying alternative fractionation schemes to patient treatment, caution must be exercised in its application, because features such as faster tumor growth rate and higher repair capacity result in greater variations in the outcome of the survival fraction. Gaps in treatment, planned or unplanned, also accentuate the differences in the survival fraction under varying growth dynamics.[7] These limitations notwithstanding, mathematical modeling of the cellular response to radiation has contributed greatly to the clinical application of radiation to combating malignancies.

The Oxygen Effect

Tissue oxygenation influences the response of tumors and normal tissues to ionizing radiation. Poorly oxygenated tissues are two to three times more resistant to radiation than are normally oxygenated tissues. Oxygen is thought to mediate indirect damage, combining with free radicals to make DNA damage irreversible. The effect of oxygenation is measured by the oxygen-enhancement ratio. This is the ratio of doses under hypoxic versus aerated conditions required to produce a given level of cell kill. As LET increases, the effect of oxygen enhancement decreases.[4]

Radiation Interactions with Chemotherapeutic Agents

A number of chemical substances may alter the radiation response of a cell.[8] The effects may be additive, such as those of most alkylating agents and antimetabolites, or they may be synergistic, such as those of the antibiotic dactinomycin.[9] Doxorubicin and dactinomycin markedly reduce the shoulder region of the radiation cell–survival curve.[9] Dactinomycin also steepens the slope of the exponential portion of the cell-survival curve and potentiates the radiation effect; thus it is thought to be a true radiation sensitizer.

Combining radiation and chemotherapy can achieve better clinical outcomes than either modality alone but can also potentiate toxicities to normal tissues. Interactions between chemotherapy and radiation can increase the risk for toxicity in normal tissues, even when the two modalities are temporally spaced. In 1959 Dr. G.J. D'Angio described an interesting yet enigmatic phenomenon termed *radiation recall*. Radiation recall describes the remembering, or reemergence, of an inflammatory reaction that occurs within the radiation field and is prompted by the administration of particular agents days to years after initial radiation exposure. In the original case described by D'Angio, dermatitis emerged within the radiation field after application of actinomycin D to the skin.[9] Although radiation recall is most commonly documented as skin reactions, other tissues and organs are also susceptible to this phenomenon, including oral and intestinal mucosa, larynx, lungs, muscles, and the central nervous system (CNS).[10] The cause of radiation recall remains poorly understood. Although timing and dosing factors clearly impact the risk and severity of the recall reaction, there is no clear radiation dose threshold.

TECHNOLOGICAL ADVANCES IN RADIATION ONCOLOGY

All technological advances in radiation oncology allow for improved dose delivery to the target or tumor and/or better avoidance of healthy tissues outside of the area at risk of disease recurrence. The field of radiation has benefited from many major developments over the past several decades in the fields of diagnostic radiation and physics, allowing for markedly improved radiation delivery to pediatric cancer patients.

The advent of three-dimensional (3D) imaging with the invention of the CT scanner in 1971 opened a new world for not only diagnostic imaging but also for radiation treatment planning.[11] The ability to define structures and tumors in 3D and to place radiation fields and beam angles with this enhanced information marked a major advancement for the field. Additional imaging developments including MRI and positron emission tomography (PET) further enhanced capabilities to define the area at risk for tumor recurrence. Most radiation centers obtain CT scans in the radiation oncology department in the desired treatment position and employ fusion software to fuse MRI and PET scans to assist in target delineation. Figures 48-4 and 48-5 show fusions used for radiation planning. By defining this region more accurately, practitioners not only improve disease control but can also decrease the volume of healthy tissue receiving unnecessary radiation. Before the use of CT, radiation oncologists used x-rays to plan fields, and beam arrangements were less well guided by anatomic detail. Because of the inability to define tumors as precisely, fields of radiation were large for fear of local recurrence. In addition, the inability to evaluate radiation plans in 3D made the details of dose

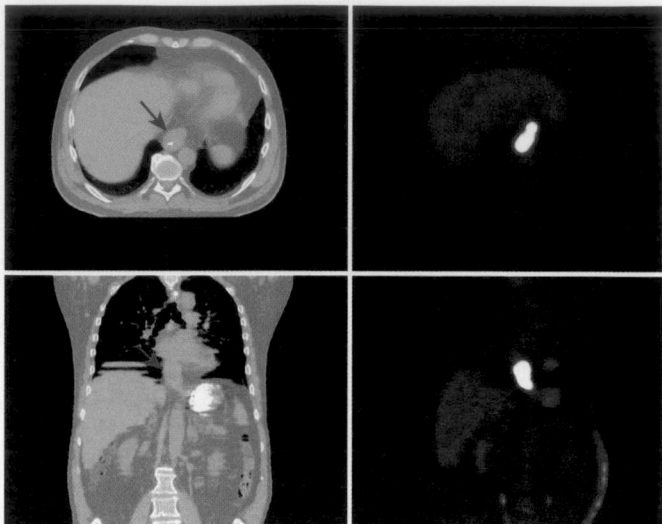

Figure 48-5 CT axial *(upper)* and coronal *(lower)* images *(left)* and PET images *(right)*. Fusion software allows for registration of PET images to planning CT so that PET avid disease *(arrow)* can be easily defined on planning CT images. Due to respiratory motion, accurate fusion can be more challenging in the chest and abdominal region.

deposition less clear. Without 3D imaging radiation oncologists would not have been capable of developing the many advanced treatment delivery techniques such as intensity modulated radiotherapy (IMRT) and stereotactic radiotherapy (SRT) that are widely available today.

Conformal radiotherapy describes treatment that delivers a high-dose volume that is shaped to conform to the target volume while minimizing the dose to critical normal tissues in the adjacent area. Because conformal radiotherapy attempts to conform the dose to the target, careful and accurate delineation of the target is critical. Patient immobilization for setup accuracy and to limit patient motion is imperative. The International Commission on Radiological Units and Measurements-50 defined target volumes that are used in treatment planning.[12] The gross tumor volume (GTV) is the volume of macroscopic tumor that is visualized on imaging studies. The clinical target volume (CTV) is the volume that should be treated to high dose, typically incorporating both the GTV and the surrounding tissues assumed to be at risk because of microscopic spread of the disease. The planning target volume (PTV) is the volume that should be treated to ensure that the CTV is appropriately covered; this takes into account systematic and random setup errors between treatments and during treatment (Fig. 48-6). The treated volume is the volume of tissue enclosed by a specific isodose line. The treated volume is greater than the PTV.

Intensity-Modulated Radiotherapy

Sophisticated planning techniques have significantly improved the ability to tailor the radiation field to the desired treatment region. IMRT is one such novel technique that allows the radiation oncologist to modulate the intensities of individual beamlets within each beam. IMRT requires highly sophisticated software that allows physicians to indicate the desired doses to tumor volumes and organs. This software then runs multiple iterations

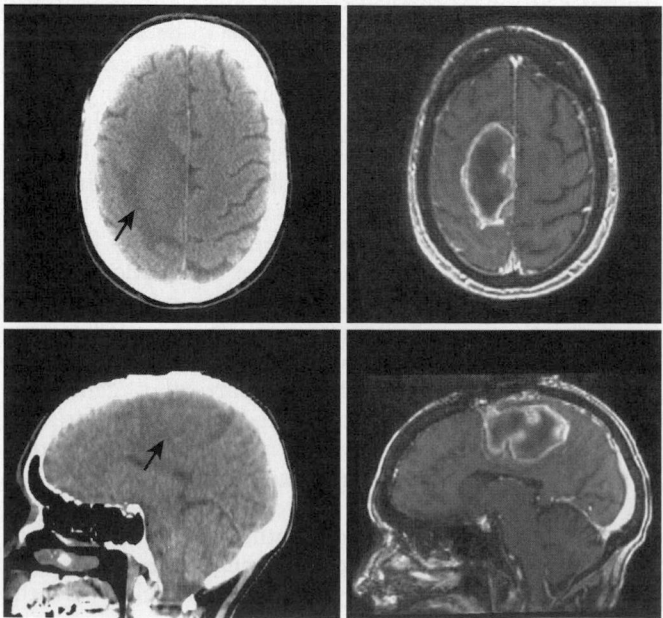

Figure 48-4 CT axial and sagittal images *(left upper and lower panels)* and MRI T1 post-gadolinium axial and sagittal images *(right)* showing brain tumor *(arrows)* that is much more easily visualized on MRI sequences. Fusion software enables more accurate delineation of tumor volumes by registering images together.

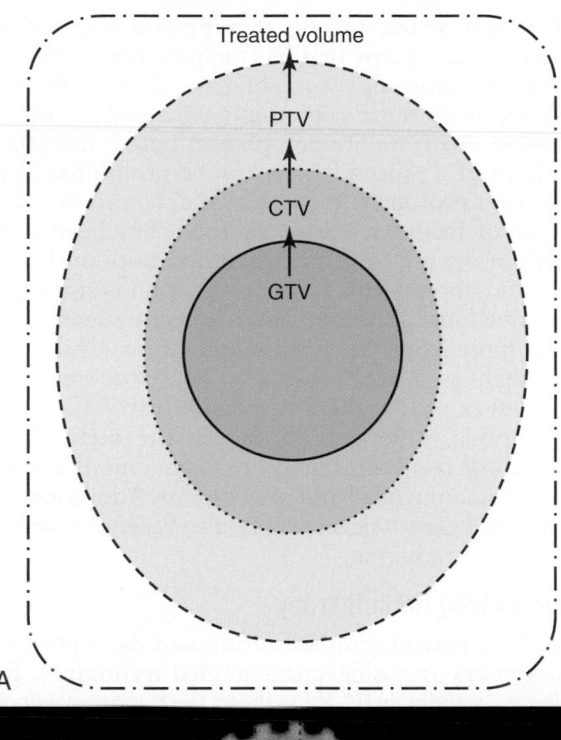

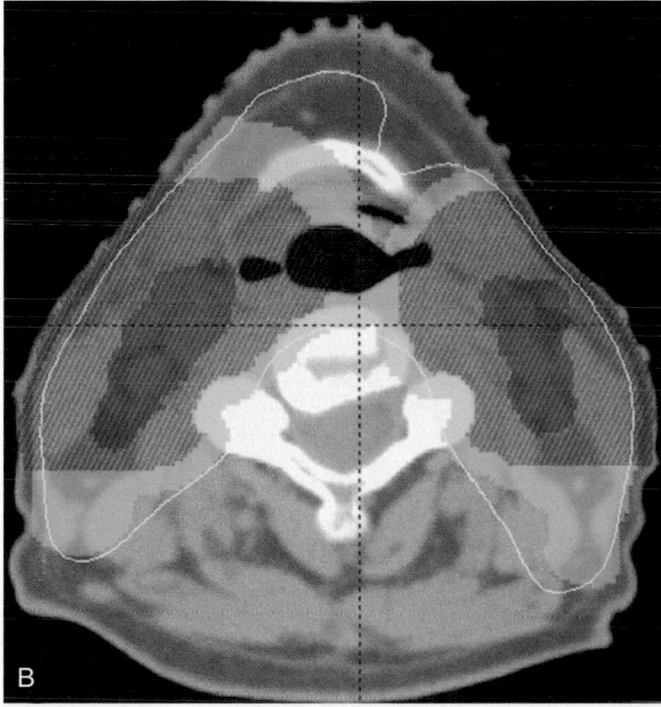

Figure 48-6 A, Target volumes for treatment planning. *CTV,* Clinical target volume; *GTV,* gross tumor volume; *PTV,* planning tumor volume. **B,** Axial CT image showing contoured target structures. Gross target volume shown in *pink*; CTV *hatched*; PTV in *green*.

of treatment plans involving numerous small fields and several beam angles. The physician either accepts the optimized plan or provides new parameters until the desired dose distribution has been met. IMRT accomplishes excellent conformity to target volumes while decreasing the high dose to nearby critical structures. Figure 48-7 demonstrates an IMRT field arrangement and plan for a young child with a localized ependymoma.

Stereotactic Radiotherapy

Stereotactic radiosurgery (SRS) is delivery of radiation to a target in a single treatment. This is generally reserved for smaller brain tumors, although stereotactic body radiosurgery has been developed in recent years. SRS is accomplished by delivering multiple small beams of radiation in order to deliver the prescription dose to the target but a much lower dose to the surrounding tissues. Precision is of paramount importance for SRS, and typically rigid frames and fiducial markers are used. Several delivery systems exist for photon-based SRS (e.g., Gamma-Knife, X-knife, Cyber-Knife). Protons can also be used to deliver SRS. Stereotactic treatments may also be delivered over several fractions; this is generally referred to as *SRT* (stereotactic radiation treatment). Figure 48-8 shows an SRS plan.

Proton-Beam Radiation

Proton-beam radiation is a form of particle radiotherapy that allows for deposition of maximum dose at a great range of depths (up to 32 cm) and complete sparing of tissues beyond the area of maximum dose deposition.[13] This is in contrast to photons that are limited in the depth at which they deliver maximum dose (less than 3 cm) and

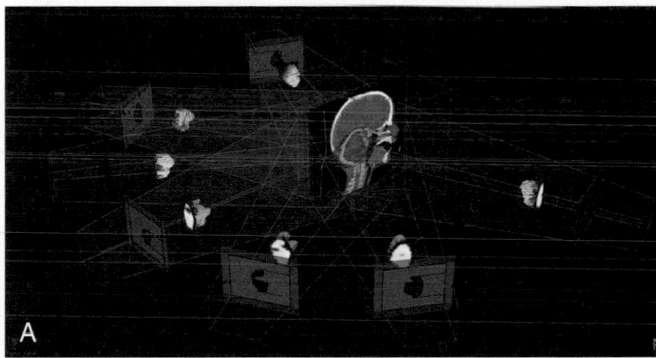

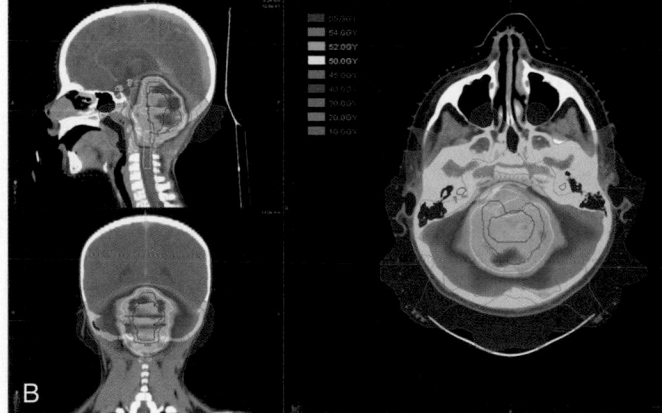

Figure 48-7 A, Multiple beam angles each deliver many small rays or beamlets of radiation that are used to conform the high dose to the target volume and minimize the high dose to avoid structures for this IMRT plan for a localized infratentorial ependymoma. **B,** Treatment plan showing dose distribution for the aforementioned beam arrangement demonstrating the high-dose region conforming very tightly to the target volume and reduced dose to critical structures such as the cochlea. This dose distribution would not be achievable with standard photon therapy.

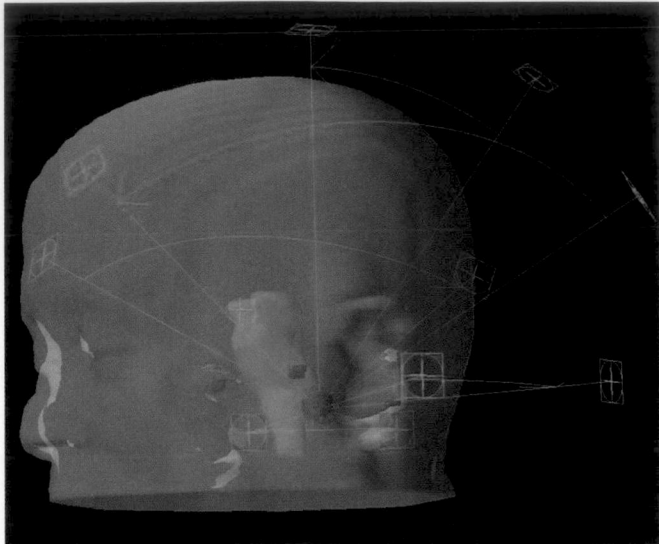

Figure 48-8 Multiple small beams of radiation deliver radiation to a small brain tumor while delivering a low dose to the surrounding healthy brain, often allowing for delivery of radiation in a single fraction.

continue to deposit the dose until passing through and exiting the body. A single proton beam delivers a small and relatively constant dose until near the end of its range, when the majority of the dose is delivered in the Bragg peak. Beyond this point, no dose is delivered.[14] Because a single Bragg peak covers only 0.5 to 1 cm, multiple Bragg peaks are required to treat a tumor.[14] CT planning is required for proton planning, because the impact of tissue inhomogeneity is greater and the density of the tissue must be taken into account by converting Hounsfield units to proton stopping power. For clinical treatment, proton beams are either combined to form a spread out Bragg peak (SOBP; 3D conformal/scattered proton treatments), or multiple proton beams are scanned across the target volume (scanning beam technique). 3D conformal radiotherapy (CRT) with protons requires patient-specific hardware to shape, or conform, the beam to the target. Lucite compensators shape the distal edge of the beam to the target volume and correct for changes in tissue density, and brass apertures or multileaf collimators shape fields to the target volume laterally. Figure 48-9 shows the delivery of 3D CRT proton treatment for a child using brass apertures and Lucite compensators. When multiple inhomogeneous scanning beam fields are used to treat a target volume, the term *intensity-modulated proton therapy (IMPT)* is used. Figure 48-10 demonstrates the use of multiple inhomogeneous beams for an IMPT plan.[15,16] Proton radiation is prescribed in gray radiobiological equivalents (Gy [RBE]) as opposed to Gy, which is used for prescribing photon radiation.[17,18] The Gy (RBE) takes into account a slightly higher average relative biologic effectiveness. Therefore the prescribed dose and biologic effects of protons are predicted to be equivalent to photons. The difference between protons and photons is the physical dose distribution. These physical properties of protons allow for a reduction in both high and low doses of radiation exposure.

In recent years, proton therapy has received much attention as a therapy that has the potential to drastically reduce late morbidity for children. Proton therapy is, however, much more capital-intensive and operationally expensive than traditional photon-based therapy. The high costs of a proton facility can be prohibitive, and for this reason proton centers are available at only a limited number of facilities. Although there has been a recent growth in the use of proton radiation both in the United States and abroad, this form of radiation is still capacity-constrained and physicians must select patients that will benefit most from this form of radiation. Children who are thought to benefit most from the tissue-sparing characteristics of proton therapy include very young children with curable tumors. Locations in the body that may benefit more from this highly conformal modality include the brain and the head and neck region. Additional malignancies and anatomic sites may also receive benefit from this form of radiation.

Image-Guided Radiotherapy

To address patient immobilization and daily positioning, some centers are using image-guided techniques. Image-guided radiotherapy (IGRT) allows the radiation oncologist

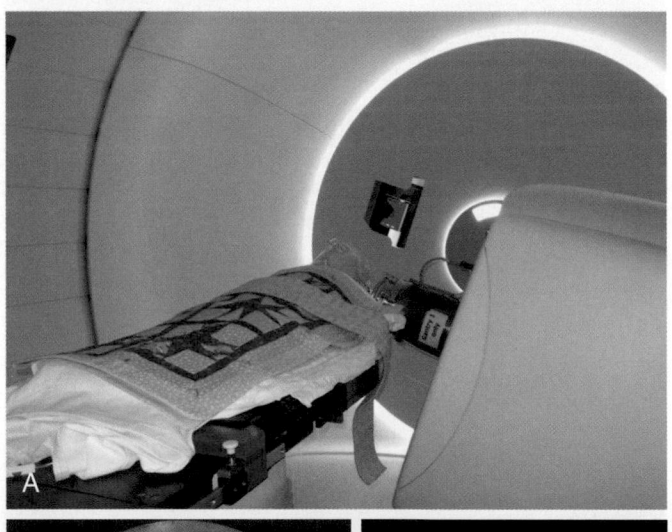

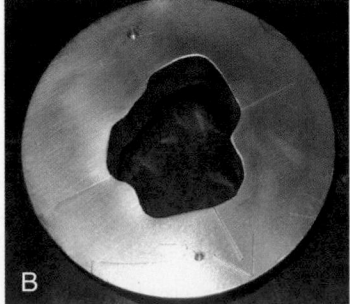

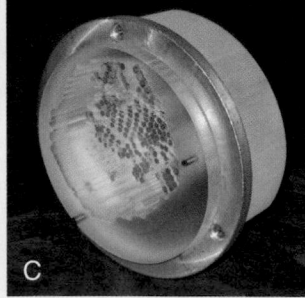

Figure 48-9 **A,** An anesthetized child receiving 3D conformal proton radiation for a brain tumor. For each field a custom brass aperture and Lucite compensator is mounted to the end of the gantry (snout). Anesthesia is required for young children to ensure that there is no movement during treatment. **B,** Brass aperture custom made to shape the field to the tumor and block healthy tissues outside of the tumor. **C,** Lucite compensator custom made to correct for tissue inhomogeneity and to shape the distal edge of the proton SOBP to the tumor.

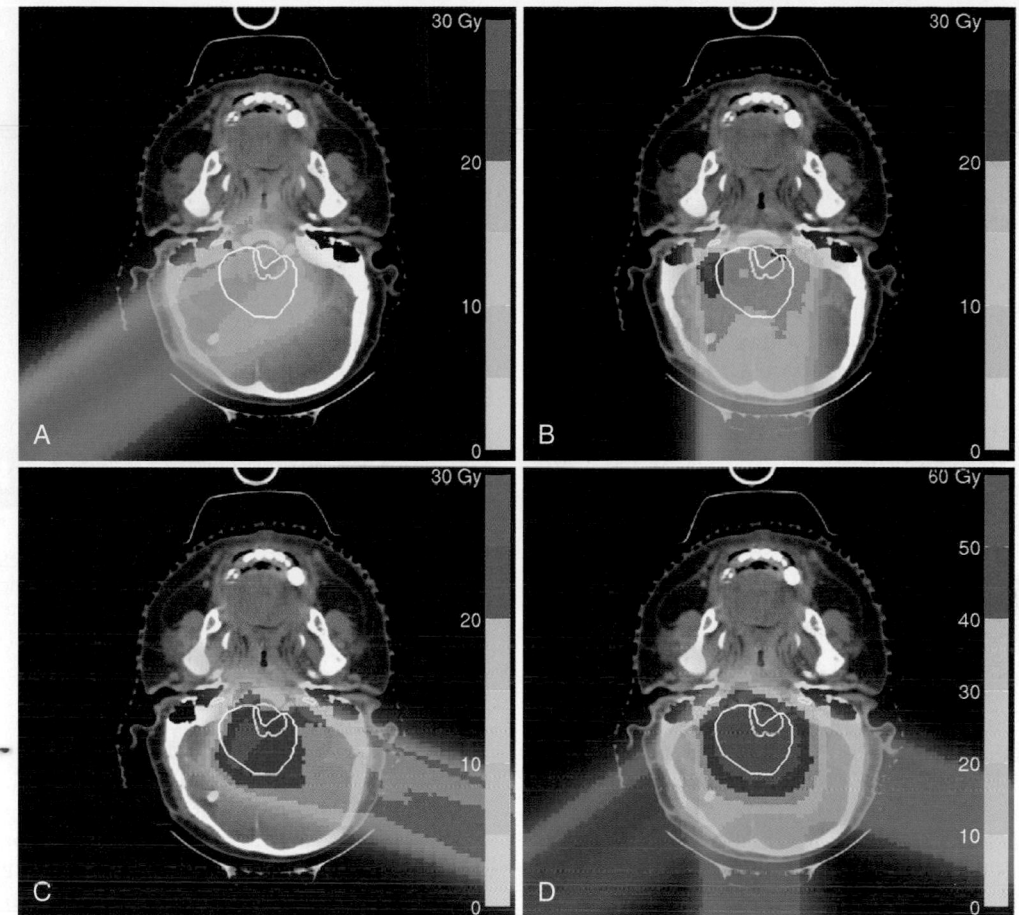

Figure 48-10 Three inhomogeneous fields composed of thousands of individual Bragg peaks are used to create a homogenous dose distribution for the composite IMPT plan. **A,** Right posterior field. **B,** Posteroanterior field. **C,** Left posterior field. **D,** Composite dose distribution of the three fields. The color scales for images **A, B,** and **C** are identical.

to confirm the tumor location every day. One technique to minimize tumor and patient movement is the use of a CT image of the patient using the "cone beam" technique that allows the generation of an image of the tumor and all surrounding normal structures using the same linear accelerator with which the patient is being treated. Appropriate adjustments can then be made daily to assure that the tumor is receiving the appropriate dose of radiation and normal tissues are receiving doses within their tolerance range. Gold seeds can be implanted into or near a tumor. The seeds can be tracked during the treatment. The technique of tracking the tumor during respiration and treating it at a particular phase of breathing is called *gated,* or *breath-synchronized radiotherapy* (BSRT) IGRT. This is also known as *four-dimensional (4D) IGRT.* (The fourth dimension is time.)

CLINICAL TREATMENT WITH RADIATION

Radiation is used for a wide variety of indications and disease sites. The decision to include radiotherapy in the management of a particular childhood malignancy, as well as the radiation dose used and volume treated is individualized for each patient and is dependent on many patient-specific and tumor-related characteristics. Primary

among these are age, biology, stage of the cancer, and tolerance of surrounding normal tissues. Radiation delivery may also depend on surgical and other adjuvant treatments. The full management of each malignancy is beyond the scope of this chapter and the reader is referred to the chapters dedicated to the specific disease sites for a full description of disease manifestations, work up, staging, and details of therapy other than radiation.

Central Nervous System Malignancies

Tumors of the CNS are the most common pediatric malignancy requiring radiotherapy. The use of radiation dose and volume is highly dependent on pathology, extent of resection, and dissemination of disease. Given the numerous critical structures in close proximity to brain tumors including the developing brain, hypothalamus, pituitary gland, visual, and auditory structures, it is highly preferable to choose a conformal modality for children who have a good prospect of long-term survival. The use of MRI to delineate target areas is crucial for this location. The use of 3D conformal planning has markedly increased capabilities for the treatment of CNS malignancies. Advanced radiation modalities including IMRT, Tomotherapy, SRS/SRT, Gamma-Knife, and proton therapy are often employed for treatment of these malignancies.

Medulloblastoma Supratentorial Primitive Neuroectodermal Tumors

Medulloblastoma, an embryonal tumor located in the cerebellum, is a common pediatric brain tumor for which radiation is an important component of curative treatment.[19] Disease extent is categorized as *standard-risk* or *high-risk,* with standard risk defined as nonmetastatic disease in children over the age of 3 with 1.5 cm^2 or less of residual disease after surgery; all others are considered to have high-risk disease. Although not included in the stratification, anaplastic histology has been shown to carry an inferior prognosis compared with classic medulloblastoma. Molecular subtypes will likely be incorporated into future stratification, which will impact radiation dose as research indicates that prognosis is contingent on molecular characteristics.[20,21] Supratentorial primitive neuroectodermal tumors (SPNETs) are embryonal tumors located in the cerebrum. The treatment for SPNETs is the same or similar to that for high-risk medulloblastoma. Patients with medulloblastoma or SPNET have a high risk of relapse in the cerebrospinal axis even if gross disease is not detected on imaging or in spinal fluid, and patients over the age of 3 years should receive craniospinal irradiation (CSI) as a component of treatment. For patients with standard-risk disease, 23.4 Gy CSI and a boost to the area of primary disease or posterior fossa to a dose of 54 Gy is recommended. Cure rates for these patients exceed 80%.[22] Outcomes are less favorable for patients with high-risk medulloblastoma and SPNET, with cure rates on the order of 60% to 70%. These patients should receive 36 Gy CSI with a boost to the primary tumor bed or posterior fossa to 54 Gy.[23-25] For medulloblastoma, the standard volume to boost is the whole posterior fossa. Although the involved field boost has become customary at some institutions, it is not yet considered to be standard of care at the time of publication, as results from the Children's Oncology Group (COG) study, *ACNS0331,* were not available.[26] This study randomized all children enrolled to whole posterior fossa radiation versus involved field radiation. This protocol also randomized standard-risk patients under the age of 8 to reduced-dose CSI (18 Gy) versus standard dose radiation (23.4 Gy). For children with high-risk medulloblastoma or SPNET, the COG protocol *ACNS0332* is evaluating the addition of daily carboplatin as a radio sensitizer concurrent with radiation and posttreatment isotretinoin.[26] Modern techniques including IMRT, Tomotherapy, and proton radiation can decrease the dose and/or volume of uninvolved tissues receiving radiation. Figure 48-11 demonstrates the ability of protons to eliminate exit dose to organs anterior to the vertebral bodies for children receiving CSI.

For children under the age of 3 years, CSI is considered to lead to unacceptable neurocognitive outcomes, and for this reason treatment of these children generally consists of chemotherapy first to delay radiotherapy, and the subsequent radiation volume is often limited to the involved field or sometimes even omitted if the child is under age 3 years at the time of radiation and did not have metastatic disease.[27,28] Outcomes are inferior, perhaps to a large extent because of the omission, deferral, or

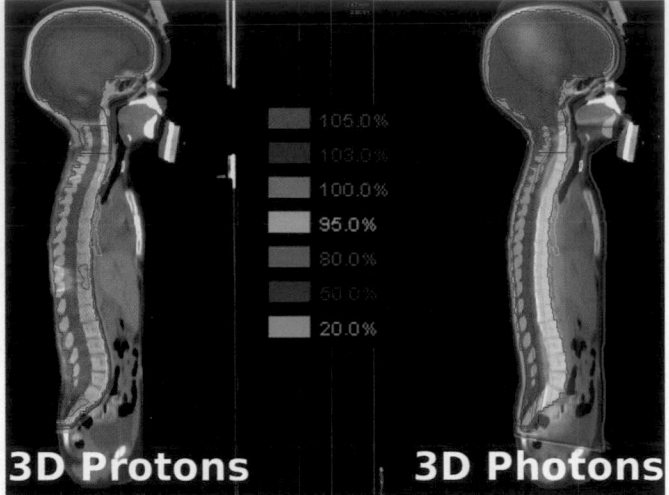

Figure 48-11 CSI delivered with protons versus photons. Protons deliver the dose to a chosen depth with no dose delivered beyond this point. This allows for sparing of all organs anterior to the vertebral bodies. Note that the entire vertebral body is treated to an even dose to prevent asymmetric growth for children who have not yet reached full height. The photon plan delivers unnecessary dose to the thyroid, heart, lung, gastrointestinal tract, and ovaries.

alteration of radiotherapy. The COG study *ACNS0334* delivers intensive chemotherapy, including high dose chemotherapy and stem-cell rescue. Radiation is optional on this trial, and when used it calls for delivery of radiation to the involved field to a dose of 50.4 to 54 Gy. Again, highly conformal techniques are recommended to achieve sparing of CNS structures from unnecessary radiation.

Low-Grade Glioma

Astrocytomas are the most common pediatric CNS tumor. Complete surgical resection can be achieved in many cases. With cure rates exceeding 90% for complete surgical resection, radiation is not required. Low-grade gliomas of the thalamus, hypothalamus, optic chiasm, tectum, or other region that is not amenable to complete resection may require radiation. Although observation may be appropriate if the child is asymptomatic, progression of the tumor will likely occur and treatment will be required at some point. Chemotherapy is also considered, although for the majority of patients this is only a temporizing measure. In general, chemotherapy is used for young patients, whereas radiation is the first choice for older patients, but there is no clear specific age to determine the appropriate treatment modality. Treatment decisions for these patients are best made in a multidisciplinary setting. Chemotherapy may allow for neurocognitive development and delay neuroendocrine or other radiation-related side effects, but there is a high risk of tumor progression that may lead to irreversible loss of function. Radiation, although more definitive, carries neurocognitive, neuroendocrine, and other risks. When radiation is used, a dose of 50.4 to 54 Gy is recommended. The treatment volume includes all gross tumor and the tumor bed as seen on MRI. Because many low-grade gliomas either do not enhance at all or have a nonenhancing component,

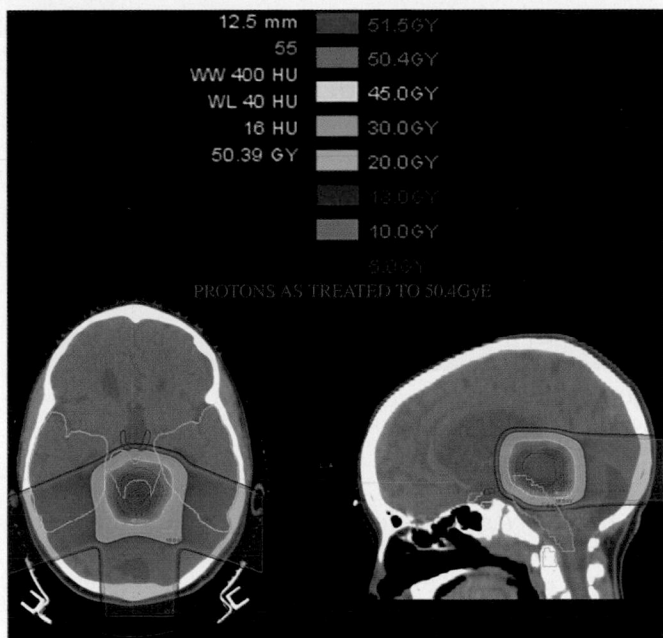

12.5 mm
55
WW 400 HU
WL 40 HU
16 HU
50.39 GY

51.5GY
50.4GY
45.0GY
30.0GY
20.0GY
15.0GY
10.0GY

PROTONS AS TREATED TO 50.4GyE

Figure 48-12 3D Conformal proton plan for a tectal glioma showing sparing of the temporal lobes and hypothalamus and pituitary gland. Protons reduce low- and high-dose radiation delivered to healthy structures of the brain.

care should be taken to include all areas of T2 abnormality that are suspicious for tumor. T2 fluid-attenuated inversion recovery (FLAIR) sequences are often useful. A margin of 5 mm to account for areas of potential microscopic disease is recommended for well-demarcated tumors. Excellent long-term outcomes have been documented after CRT.[29] Figure 48-12 shows a proton plan for a tectal glioma.

Anaplastic Astrocytoma/Glioblastoma Multiforme/Diffusely Infiltrating Pontine Glioma

Anaplastic astrocytoma and glioblastoma multiforme (GBM) carry a poor prognosis compared with other pediatric brain tumors, although long-term survival may be achieved for some patients.[30] Surgery followed by radiation with or without chemotherapy is standard. Initial treatment volumes typically include T2 FLAIR changes and enhancing tumor plus a margin for radiographically occult tumor. This volume is treated to a dose of 45 Gy. The tumor volume is then reduced to the gross tumor with a margin to deliver a total dose of 54 Gy to 59.4 Gy to this region, depending on age and adjacent critical structures.

Another highly malignant tumor is a diffusely infiltrating pontine glioma (DIPG). These tumors arise in the pons and have a classic appearance on MRI of a nonenhancing T2 bright lesion that expands the pons. Radiation is indicated for treatment of this disease, and response is typically prompt. Many patients experience a reversal of observed neurological symptoms when treated to a dose of 54 Gy. Unfortunately, response is not durable and symptoms typically recur several months after radiation. The median survival for these children is

1 year, and cure is not achievable with current available treatment.

Craniopharyngioma

Craniopharyngiomas are histologically benign tumors that can be locally destructive, causing neuroendocrine and visual disturbances. When resection is incomplete, most of these tumors recur, so radiotherapy is generally recommended. Limited surgery and radiation leads to excellent rates of control in excess of 90%. Target volume includes residual solid and cystic components and the postoperative bed with a margin of approximately 5 mm for microscopic disease. A dose of 50.4 to 54 Gy is recommended. These tumors typically have a cystic component that may change in volume during radiation, and a quick T2 MRI (Half-Fourier Acquisition Single-Shot Turbo Spin-Echo [HASTE] sequence) or CT during radiation treatment is advised so that the radiation plan can be adjusted to ensure that the cystic component remains in the treatment field with maximal sparing of uninvolved tissue. Highly conformal techniques are recommended to provide better sparing of the surrounding brain. Given neuroendocrine structures are involved by tumor, it is rarely possible to provide sparing of these structures even with the most conformal of modalities.

Ependymoma

Intracranial ependymoma represents 5% to 8% of pediatric brain tumors. The majority of these tumors arise in the fourth ventricle with fewer occurring in the supratentorial brain. Standard treatment for nondisseminated disease consists of maximal surgical resection followed by involved field radiotherapy even for children under the age of 3 years. With surgery and CRT, long-term local control rates of approximately 80% have been achieved.[31,32] Trials attempting to use chemotherapy and omit radiation have led to inferior outcomes, although chemotherapy may be recommended after a subtotal resection in attempt to allow for a second surgery and complete resection. Radiotherapy is prescribed to the tumor bed plus a margin of approximately 5 to 10 mm. Care must be taken to carefully delineate the tumor bed and areas that the tumor was in contact with before surgery as well as any areas of residual gross disease. The prescribed dose is 54 Gy to 59.4 Gy in 30 to 33 fractions to this volume. The COG protocols (*ACN0121* and *ACNS0831,* respectively) prescribe a total dose to 59.4 Gy, but *ACNS0831* requires that critical structures outside of the area of highest risk be blocked after 54 Gy.[26] Given the young age of these patients, it is important to use a very conformal technique to avoid the normal developing brain, cochlea, and neuroendocrine structures. The use of 3D CRT, IMRT, and protons has been shown to provide superior sparing of nearby critical structures while maintaining excellent outcomes.[31,32] Whereas local recurrence accounted for the majority of recurrences in historical series, recent patterns of relapse show a trend towards a more even ratio of distal and local recurrences but no absolute increase in distal recurrences; this is a reflection of the improved local control achieved as a result of advances in surgery and radiation.[31,32a]

Germ Cell Tumors

CNS germ cell tumors (GCTs) are midline CNS tumors that typically arise within the infundibulum or pineal gland but can occur elsewhere in the brain.[33] GCTs are divided into two main histologic subgroups that are highly prognostic; pure germinomas and GCTs with nongerminomatous components (NGGCTs). Pure germinoma is the most common type of GCT and typically holds the most favorable prognosis. Excellent outcomes can be achieved with radiation alone or a combination of radiation and chemotherapy. Whole-ventricle radiotherapy to a dose of 24 Gy followed by a boost to the tumor bed to total 45 Gy to 50 Gy is considered a standard treatment for pure germinoma. With the use of chemotherapy before radiotherapy, the radiation dose may be reduced, but attempts to reduce volumes to the primary tumor bed have led to an increased rate of in the ventricles. After a complete to near-complete response to chemotherapy, whole-ventricle radiation to a dose of 21 Gy followed by a dose to the tumor bed to 30 to 36 Gy is most standard. The COG protocol *ACNS1123* is investigating the use of chemotherapy followed by radiotherapy to a dose of 18 Gy to the whole ventricles, which is then followed by a boost to a total of 30 Gy for localized pure germinomas showing a good response to chemotherapy. For patients with disseminated pure germinoma, the prognosis is still excellent with radiation alone or chemotherapy followed by radiation. Doses are generally the same as stated above; however, the volume at risk for microscopic disease is the entire craniospinal axis rather than the whole ventricle. NGGCT carries a less favorable prognosis, and combined modality treatment is standard. The COG study *ACNS0122* delivered 6 cycles of induction chemotherapy (carboplatin, ifosfamide, and etoposide) followed by CSI to 36 Gy and an involved field boost to 54 Gy. Early reports suggest excellent outcomes. Reducing the volume and dose of radiation for patients who have NGGCT with localized disease and an excellent response to chemotherapy in attempt to decrease toxicity is the goal of the COG trial *ACNS1123*, which delivers the same chemotherapy as *ACNS0122* followed 30.6 Gy to the whole ventricles and 54 Gy to the tumor bed. Patients with disseminated disease still receive CSI and are not eligible for this study. A whole ventricular atlas is available on the Quality Assurance Review Center (QARC) website to help delineate this structure consistently for *ACNS1123*. Figure 48-13 shows images from this atlas.

Atypical Teratoid/Rhabdoid Tumors

Atypical teratoid/rhabdoid tumor (AT/RT) is a highly malignant, small, round, blue cell tumor that has only recently been recognized as a distinct entity since discovery of the tumor suppressor gene, *INI1*. Initial reports suggested a dismal prognosis for children with AT/RT, but studies incorporating high-dose chemotherapy have shown markedly improved outcomes compared with historical series.[34,35] Maximum surgical resection, high-dose chemotherapy with stem-cell rescue, and early radiation provide the best chance of cure.[35] Children diagnosed with AT/RT are generally very young, and children under

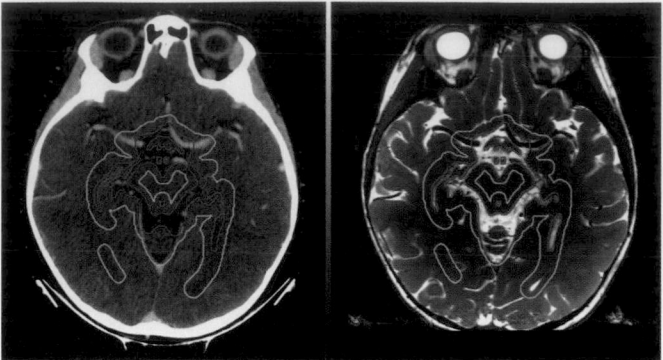

Figure 48-13 CT image *(left)* and fused T2 MRI image *(right)* showing contours for the ventricle volume. Ventricle volume is in *magenta* and PTV is in *cyan*.

the age of 3 years should receive involved field radiation to a dose of 50.4 to 54 Gy with highly conformal techniques.[36] Early radiation and CSI for children older than age 3 years seem to lead to improved outcomes and are generally recommended.[37]

Spinal Tumors

Primary spinal cord neoplasms are rare in children, accounting for approximately 5% of CNS malignancies. Most tumors are either low-grade astrocytomas or myxopapillary ependymomas. Surgical resection is the primary treatment, and radiation is reserved for situations when either complete resection is not possible or in the setting of tumor recurrence. The prescribed dose is typically 45 to 54 Gy based primarily on spinal cord tolerance, risk of relapse, and patient age.

Hematologic Malignancies

Advancements in cancer therapy have led to extraordinary improvements in outcomes for children with hematologic malignancies. Management has also greatly changed over the past few decades. Survival is excellent for children with Hodgkin disease (HD), non-Hodgkin lymphoma (NHL), and acute lymphoblastic leukemia (ALL).[38] Contemporary therapy places an emphasis on risk adaptation and avoidance of treatment-related complications while maintaining high rates of cure.[38,39] Children with hematologic malignancies are currently treated with combinations of cytotoxic chemotherapy and sometimes radiation. Advances in chemotherapy over the past several decades has allowed for a reduction in radiation dose and volume for those patients requiring it.

Hodgkin Disease

HD is a highly curable tumor with radiation alone or combined modality therapy. Contemporary treatment utilizes risk-adapted treatment with chemotherapy followed by response-based volume and dose-reduced radiotherapy. Radiotherapy alone was the first curative therapy established for HD, but the high doses used and large volumes treated with radiation led to substantial late morbidity including musculoskeletal developmental abnormalities, cardiac morbidity, and second malignancies. Many pediatric trials related to HD focus on tailoring chemotherapy and radiation to provide adequate disease control while minimizing late effects of treatment.[38,40,41] Most patients are treated with multiagent chemotherapy followed by involved field radiation to 15 to 25.5 Gy. Many studies are investigating response-adapted radiation or the omission of radiation for patients with disease showing an early favorable response to chemotherapy. Radiation volumes have been successfully reduced to the involved field, defined as a region of lymph nodes including and in close proximity to the disease as defined by diagnostic imaging. Standard involved field guidelines defining radiation field borders by anatomic landmarks are available.[42] Involved nodal radiation is being used on several trials.[43] This treatment involved contouring the areas that contained abnormal or PET-positive lymph nodes and adding a margin to these nodes to define the target for treatment. The EORTC-GELA group has established guidelines for this treatment.[43]

Leukemia

Leukemia, most often ALL, is the most common pediatric malignancy. Despite the commonality of this disease, radiation oncologists, because the development of more effective chemotherapeutic regimens, see children with leukemia less often. At present, radiation is used only in the setting of high-risk disease, refractory disease, or relapse. For patients with B-cell ALL, current guidelines indicate radiation for patients with the following high-risk features; WBC > 100,00, CNS3 disease (>5 WBC/micro-liter or blasts in the cerebrospinal fluid [CSF]), Philadelphia translocation t(9;22) ALL, T-cell phenotype, or other high-risk disease with poor response to induction chemotherapy.[44] Cranial radiation to a dose of 12 to 18 Gy is recommended. The other site for which radiation may be necessary is the testicle, but only when there is disease involvement.[45] The recommended dose for testicular radiation for leukemia is 20 to 24 Gy.

Neuroblastoma

Neuroblastoma is the most common solid non-CNS malignancy and is notable for its diverse behavior, with some cases showing spontaneous regression and others demonstrating dismal outcomes. Radiotherapy is recommended for patients with high-risk disease or sometimes for children with intermediate risk disease progressive after chemotherapy or surgery. The standard dose of radiotherapy recommended to the postchemotherapy presurgical volume is 21.6 Gy.[46,47] For children with residual disease after surgery, a total dose of 36 Gy is recommended to areas of gross disease. Radiotherapy to a dose of 21.6 Gy is also recommended to any metastatic sites that persist after induction chemotherapy. In the setting of multiple metastatic sites still metaiodobenzylguanidine (MIBG) avid after induction chemotherapy, consideration must be given to the amount of tissue to be irradiated. In this situation children are reevaluated after further chemotherapy, and an attempt is made to limit the number of metastatic sites receiving radiation to three. Urgent radiation is sometimes required for respiratory distress as a result of liver metastases in infants. If necessary, a dose of 1.5 Gy for 3 fractions is recommended. Although the radiation dose required to control neuroblastoma is low, these children are typically very young and treatment volumes may be large. Advanced radiation techniques such as IMRT, intraoperative radiation, and proton radiation should be considered.[48-50]

Wilms Tumor and other Renal Malignancies

The North American standard established by the National Wilms Tumor Study (NWTS) and COG cooperative group studies begins with up front surgery followed by radiation if indicated.[51,52] The rationale is to obtain pathology and to surgically define the extent of disease to best determine the appropriate therapy. The International Society of Paediatric Oncology (SIOP) group advises delivering chemotherapy first in attempt to decrease intraoperative tumor spillage. COG radiotherapy guidelines are based on both stage and pathology.[53] Flank radiation is recommended for patients with Stage I to III unfavorable histologies (e.g., diffuse anaplasia, focal anaplasia, clear cell sarcoma of the kidney [CCSK], and CCSK-stages II and III) and for Stage III favorable histology (FH). The standard dose is 10.8 Gy in fractions of 1.8 Gy, but higher doses are recommended for recurrent disease and stage III Diffuse Anaplasia (DA). An additional 10.8 Gy is recommended for any gross residual disease present after resection.[54] Whole abdominal radiotherapy (WART) to a dose of 10.5 Gy at 1.5 Gy per fraction is recommended for positive cytology, diffuse spillage, previous biopsy, or peritoneal seeding. COG guidelines recommend that radiotherapy commence by postoperative day 9 if feasible and no later than postoperative day 14. Whole lung irradiation (WLI) to 12 Gy is recommended for patients with anaplastic disease who have pulmonary metastases at diagnosis or children with favorable histology such as Wilms and pulmonary metastases that fail to respond to initial chemotherapy.[55] Brain, liver, and bone irradiation is indicated when metastases are present.

Rhabdomyosarcoma

Rhabdomyosarcoma (RMS) is the most common soft-tissue sarcoma of childhood and may occur in any location of the body. The COG studies stratify patients into three risk groups (low, intermediate, and high) on the basis of site, stage, histology, and group. Risk stratification is highly complex, but in general risk groups include: 1) low risk: embryonal nonmetastatic favorable sites and embryonal group 1 or 2 unfavorable sites; 2) intermediate risk: embryonal group III unfavorable sites and nonmetastatic alveolar RMS at any site; 3) high-risk: metastatic disease. See Chapter 59 for more details on prognostic factors and risk stratification of RMS.

Combined modality therapy is always used for children with RMS, and this represents another disease site that requires multidisciplinary discussion regarding best management. Radiation treatment depends on several prognostic factors and feasibility of surgery with organ preservation. Surgery is performed up front for resectable tumors and may be attempted after chemotherapy if tumors become resectable, usually with the goal of decreasing radiation dose and sometimes volume.

Contemporary treatment and the existing COG RMS trials require 3D treatment planning to allow full visualization of areas at risk and target volumes. Radiation is omitted only for patients with completely resected favorable histology disease. Thirty-six Gy is recommended for microscopic disease after surgical resection, and nodal disease is treated to a dose of 41.4 Gy. Patients with gross disease receive a dose of 50.4 Gy. Target volumes delineate prechemotherapy volume as the GTV. A margin of 1 cm around this volume to respect anatomic boundaries is recommended to encompass microscopic disease.

Osteosarcoma

Osteosarcoma is the most common primary pediatric bone tumor, but one for which radiation is less often utilized. The use of multiagent chemotherapy has led to a marked improvement in the cure of this disease. Local control is generally achieved with surgery when feasible with reasonable functional outcome. For primary tumors of the base of skull, pelvis, and spine, surgery is not possible and radiation is administered in attempt to achieve local control. Small studies indicate that high radiation doses (50 to 76 Gy) are necessary to provide a reasonable chance of durable local control.[56-60] Proton radiation or brachytherapy may be required to deliver high doses of radiation while limiting the high dose to normal surrounding structures.[56]

Ewing Sarcoma

Ewing sarcoma is the second most common pediatric sarcoma, and multimodality treatment is required. Surgery is again the preferred method of local control if feasible. Primary radiation is indicated for inoperable tumors for which surgical resection cannot be achieved or would lead to major functional impairment.[61,62] Radiotherapy is also indicated for either partially or suboptimally resected tumors. Several studies have helped define recommendations for a radiation dose in the range of 50 to 55.8 Gy to the involved area of bone with a margin for microscopic disease. Most protocols advise that definitive radiation be initiated relatively early, usually by week 12 to 14 of treatment. The initial tumor volume should be treated to a dose of approximately 45 Gy and include all areas of tumor involvement at the time of diagnosis (with adjustments for pushing tumors that have regressed with chemotherapy) and a margin for microscopic disease of approximately 1.5 cm. Gross disease at the time of treatment along with initially involved bone with a margin of approximately 1.5 cm should receive an additional dose of 10.8 Gy to total 55.8 Gy with the exception of tumors located in the vertebral body (total 45 Gy because of spinal cord tolerance).

Retinoblastoma

Retinoblastoma is a rare disease of young children who are almost all under the age of 3 years. Many patients have the hereditary form of retinoblastoma with a high propensity for bilateral disease and subsequent malignancies.[63] Treatment depends on extent of involvement,

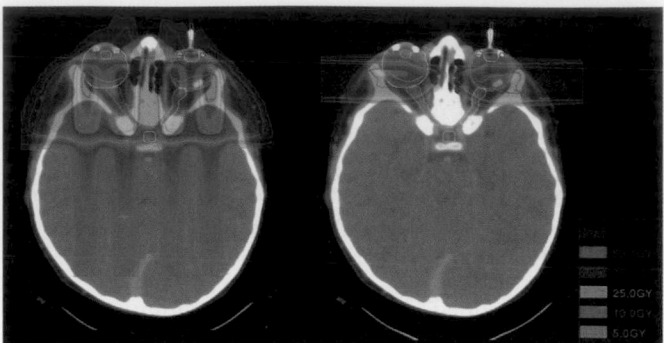

Figure 48-14 Radiation for bilateral retinoblastoma. This figure shows a radiation treatment plan with a 3D conformal photon technique from 1985 *(left)* compared with a modern proton plan from 2012 *(right)*. Protons spare tissues outside of the target volume from low and high doses of radiation. Given that these children are highly vulnerable to second malignancies, avoidance of radiation of any dose is highly desirable.

whether disease is unilateral or bilateral, hereditary status, and sometimes response to treatment and parental preference.[64] Radiation is generally recommended for disease refractory to chemotherapy and local therapies (cryotherapy and laser therapy) in an eye with useful vision, whereas enucleation is advised if it is thought that there is no meaningful visual potential. The standard dose is 45 Gy. Postoperative radiation is delivered for advanced disease after enucleation. A dose of 45 Gy to the orbit and up to the optic chiasm is necessary in cases of frank orbital disease and high-risk pathology features (transscleral extension or tumor involvement of the cut end of the optic nerve). Plaque brachytherapy may be an option for unifocal tumors that are located in the peripheral retina.[65] Radiation does provide an excellent chance at durable control of disease, but carries risks of facial hypoplasia and radiation-induced malignancies.[66] Most data for these toxicities, however, comes from old radiation series with dated techniques as far back as 1914.[67] Modern radiation treatments should maintain disease outcomes while reducing many of these risks. Figure 48-14 depicts a photon radiation plan from 1985 compared to a proton radiation plan from 2012. Given the young age of these children and the propensity of children with hereditary retinoblastoma for second malignancy, proton radiation, which provides the best sparing of involved structures from both high and low doses of radiation, may be the best radiation option for this particular group of patients.

SEQUELAE OF TREATMENT

Although the goal of therapeutic radiation is to eradicate tumors, tumors are not isolated in petri dishes but occur in the human body in the midst of normal tissues that are susceptible to damage from irradiation. This normal tissue damage occurs during the course of treatment or long after the treatment has been given. The term *acute effects* refers to reactions during or very soon after treatment; reactions occurring more than 3 months after treatment are termed *late effects*. Normal tissue tolerance to fractionated treatment is a function of the volume of the organ or tissue, the total dose, and the time course over which treatment is given. When chemotherapy is given concurrently with radiotherapy, some acute and late toxicities may be enhanced. Acute and late effects are generally restricted to tissues within the radiation field or at least to tissues that received some dose of radiotherapy. The one exception to this is the systemic fatigue, which is experienced by some patients undergoing treatment.

The most typical acute effects are those on skin, on the mucosa of the aerodigestive tract, and on bone marrow. Most acute effects require supportive care, such as topical creams for skin reactions and ongoing hydration, topical anesthetics and in severe cases, narcotics for mucositis. Abdominal irradiation can cause nausea, vomiting, and diarrhea. These toxicities are managed with antiemetics, hydration, and antidiarrheal agents if symptoms are severe. Acute toxicities can be severe and occasionally require treatment breaks. However, prolonged breaks are undesirable, because the overall treatment time is an important factor in tumor control.

The mechanisms of late complications resulting from radiotherapy, though not precisely known, are speculated to be caused by vascular endothelial damage, damage to parenchymal stem cells, or damage to DNA. The normal tissue tolerance doses for the various bodily organs have been well studied.[4] The tolerance doses for adult normal tissue are applied in children with some exceptions, as discussed later. Late effects are dependent on the total dose and fraction size.[68] The potential for late toxicity is one of the most important factors in the decisions regarding dose and volume, and it is a major concern in the treatment of children with cancer.

The late toxicities of radiotherapy are dependent upon both patient factors and treatment factors. The age of the patient, the tolerance of the normal tissue treated, and the dose of the radiotherapy delivered determine the late effects and their severity. Systems most severely affected include the musculoskeletal, endocrine, and reproductive systems, and the CNS.

In children, treatment before full development has been reached can cause abnormal or arrested development. The severity of the effect on musculoskeletal development depends on the dose of irradiation, the area treated, and the age of the patient. Doses of irradiation to the growth plate that are above 20 Gy are likely to have significant effects.[69,70] The age of the patient influences the severity of the damage. Younger children with greater growth potential are more profoundly affected. Irradiation of the pituitary gland and hypothalamus can also lead to short stature by decreasing the production of growth hormone.[71,72] Spinal irradiation in the treatment of medulloblastoma in prepubertal children causes a shortened spine or decreased sitting height.[73,74]

Neurocognitive sequelae from brain irradiation are among the most serious late effects when radiotherapy is used in children.[75,76] The age of the patient, the dose, and the volume of brain treated all influence the severity of these toxicities.[75,77,78] Irradiation of the cochlea can lead to sensory peripheral neuropathy manifested as high-frequency hearing loss.[79] Many children receive ototoxic chemotherapy such as cisplatin, which itself causes hearing loss.[80] When cochlear irradiation is combined with cisplatin, profound hearing loss or sometimes deafness can result.[80]

Germ cell survival in testes and ovaries can be impacted by radiotherapy.[81] Males treated with whole abdominal irradiation may develop gonadal dysfunction. Temporary decreases in sperm count occur in the weeks after low doses of radiotherapy (0.2 to 3 Gy). Recovery occurs in 1 to 3 years, depending on the dose and the age of the patient. Direct testicular irradiation with doses of 24 Gy as used to treat testicular relapses of ALL cause sterility and Leydig cell dysfunction.[82] Total body irradiation combined with cyclophosphamide for stem-cell transplant results in azoospermia for almost all males.[83,84]

Abdominopelvic irradiation in females damages the ovaries resulting in ovarian failure.[85] The incidence of ovarian failure depends upon the age at irradiation and the dose of radiotherapy to the ovaries.[86] When prepubertal girls were treated with WART with 20 to 30 Gy, 71% of girls did not enter puberty and 26% had premature menopause.[86a] CSI with photons can have similar results when treating prepubertal girls, depending upon the dose received by the ovaries.[87]

In addition to organ and system damage, one of the most devastating late effects of radiotherapy is the development of subsequent neoplasms. Survivors of childhood cancer have an increased risk of developing subsequent neoplasms that can be benign or malignant.[88] They can be solid tumors or myelodysplasia/acute myeloid leukemia. Treatment with radiotherapy is associated with the development of subsequent solid tumors.[88] Radiation-associated second tumors occur within the prior radiotherapy field, are of a different histology from the primary tumor, and appear after a latency period of generally at least several years. Several factors are involved in the development of second tumors, including the patient's underlying genetic predisposition, the dose of radiation, and the age and gender of the patient, as well as the specific tissue irradiated.[89] The risk of subsequent radiation-related subsequent neoplasms continues to increase with increased follow-up.[90] This is in contrast to the risk of therapy-related myelodysplasia or acute myeloid leukemia, which plateau after 10 to 15 years.

CONCLUSION

Tremendous improvements have been made in the field of pediatric radiation oncology over the past few decades. Although many children require radiation for curative treatment of their malignancy, treatment can be delivered with fewer side effects. Technological advances allow for more precise delivery of radiation and much better avoidance of healthy tissues outside of the region requiring treatment. Thanks in large part to many cooperative group studies, there is better knowledge of the dose of radiation required to control various tumors. Chemotherapy has allowed for dose reduction for many tumor sites as well as improved outcomes. Pediatric oncologists are beginning to better understand the molecular characteristics and biology of tumors. In the future, this should lead to improved risk stratification, as well as targeted agents to work synergistically with radiation and further improve outcomes for these children.

References available online at ExpertConsult.

KEY REFERENCES

4. Hall E: *Radiobiology for the radiologist*, ed 5, Philadelphia, 2000, Lippincott, Williams & Wilkins.

  This remains the leading textbook on the fundamentals of radiobiology.

5. Fowler JF, Harari PM, Leborgne F, et al: Acute radiation reactions in oral and pharyngeal mucosa: tolerable levels in altered fractionation schedules. *Radiother Oncol* 69:161–168, 2003.

  Fowler and colleagues describe the acute toxicities of altered fractionation schemes and provide the basis for current treatment approaches in a variety of malignancies.

13. MacDonald SM, DeLaney TF, Loeffler JS: Proton beam radiation therapy. *Cancer Invest* 24:199–208, 2006.

  Proton beam radiotherapy presents a major technological advance and is becoming the radiotherapy modality of choice in many curable pediatric cancer treatments.

22. Packer RJ, Gajjar A, Vezina G, et al: Phase III study of craniospinal radiation therapy followed by adjuvant chemotherapy for newly diagnosed average-risk medulloblastoma. *J Clin Oncol* 24:4202–4208, 2006.

  This phase III trial established the basis for current medulloblastoma treatment.

31. Merchant TE, Li C, Xiong X, et al: Conformal radiotherapy after surgery for paediatric ependymoma: a prospective study. *Lancet Oncol* 10:258–266, 2009.

  This reviews the management of localized ependymoma.

35. Chi SN, Zimmerman MA, Yao X, et al: Intensive multimodality treatment for children with newly diagnosed CNS atypical teratoid rhabdoid tumor. *J Clin Oncol* 27:385–389, 2009.

  The treatment of atypical teratoid rhabdoid tumors as reported by Dr. Chi showed promise.

38. Metzger ML, Weinstein HJ, Hudson MM, et al: Association between radiotherapy vs no radiotherapy based on early response to VAMP chemotherapy and survival among children with favorable-risk Hodgkin lymphoma. *JAMA* 307:2609–2616, 2012.

  Risk-adapted response-based therapy as reported here is the paradigm for pediatric Hodgkin disease.

44. Pui CH, Howard SC: Current management and challenges of malignant disease in the CNS in paediatric leukaemia. *Lancet Oncol* 9:257–268, 2008.

  This provides a thorough review of the management of CNS disease in ALL in children.

47. George RE, Li S, Medeiros-Nancarrow C, et al: High-risk neuroblastoma treated with tandem autologous peripheral-blood stem cell-supported transplantation: long-term survival update. *J Clin Oncol* 24:2891–2896, 2006.

  Dr. George reports on the pioneering approach of double autologous stem-cell transplantation for high-risk neuroblastoma.

53. Green DM: The evolution of treatment for Wilms tumor. *J Pediatr Surg* 48:14–19, 2013.

  This reviews the evolution of Wilms tumor treatment.

61. Rombi B, DeLaney TF, MacDonald SM, et al: Proton radiotherapy for pediatric Ewing's sarcoma: initial clinical outcomes. *Int J Radiat Oncol Biol Phys* 82:1142–1148, 2012.

  Proton radiotherapy for sarcomas in children shows significant benefits over photon treatment as demonstrated in this report.

67. Wong FL, Boice JD, Jr, Abramson DH, et al: Cancer incidence after retinoblastoma: radiation dose and sarcoma risk. *JAMA* 278:1262–1267, 1997.

  Secondary cancers in patients with retinoblastoma are examples of the influence of heritable defects in cancer treatment.

69. Probert JC, Parker BR, Kaplan HS: Growth retardation in children after megavoltage irradiation of the spine. *Cancer* 32:634–639, 1973.

  The effects on bone growth are a significant consequence of treatment with radiotherapy in children as discussed in this report.

78. Mulhern RK, Merchant TE, Gajjar A, et al: Late neurocognitive sequelae in survivors of brain tumours in childhood. *Lancet Oncol* 5:399–408, 2004.

  This reviews the long-term neurocognitive sequelae of children treated for brain tumors.

85. Scott JE: Pubertal development in children treated for nephroblastoma. *J Pediatr Surg* 16:122–125, 1981.

  The Childhood Cancer Survivor Study has obtained treatment details and long-term follow-up data on thousands of survivors of childhood cancer, allowing oncologists to learn the impact of treatment on quality of life and health in patients.

CHAPTER 49

Pediatric Surgical Oncology

Christopher B. Weldon, Megan E. Anderson, Mark C. Gebhardt, and Robert C. Shamberger

Successful treatment of pediatric solid tumors requires collaborative management by the disciplines of surgery, oncology, and radiotherapy. Multimodal therapy achieves the highest rate of cure in many solid tumors and often minimizes long-term morbidity. Smooth collaboration provides optimal care. The role of the surgeon varies greatly depending on the primary tumor, its site, and the presence or absence of metastatic disease. Surgeons should be involved in decisions regarding primary resection versus biopsy with neoadjuvant chemotherapy and delayed resection. The surgeon's knowledge of the risks of primary resection is critical; the method of biopsy is also very important. Inappropriate initial excisional biopsies with positive pathologic margins will require more extensive subsequent resection than if an initial incisional biopsy were performed. Similarly, inappropriate biopsies such as thoracoscopic biopsy of a chest wall Ewing sarcoma or a percutaneous or open biopsy of a Wilms tumor needlessly contaminate the thoracic and abdominal cavities, respectively, and require more intensive therapies, particularly the use of radiation therapy. A growing emphasis on minimizing the morbidity of therapy is required, because the survival for infants and children with many solid tumors is quite high. It is important,

therefore, to avoid any diagnostic or therapeutic missteps that require more intensive therapy.

Surgery is critical in the staging of pediatric solid tumors. This is well established in Wilms tumor. In a classic study by Beimann Othersen and the National Wilms Tumor Study Group (NWTSG), surgeons had a 31.3% false-negative rate in their clinical assessment of lymph-node involvement with tumor by gross inspection and a false-positive rate of 18.1%.[1] It should be stressed that in Wilms tumor the protocols of the NWTSG and the Children's Oncology Group (COG) determine the intensity of chemotherapy as well as whether or not abdominal radiotherapy is utilized. Patients with pulmonary metastases (stage IV) with local stage I or stage II tumors receive intensified chemotherapy and pulmonary radiation but no abdominal radiation.

The vital importance of adequate lymph-node biopsy has been demonstrated in several studies. An increased incidence of local relapse occurred in children enrolled in the NWTSG-4 study if no biopsy was performed of the abdominal lymph nodes, particularly in stage-I cases.[2] This finding suggests that inadequate treatment of local disease in children without lymph-node biopsy results in an increased rate of local relapse. Although lymph-node biopsy is essential in children with Wilms tumor, an extensive retroperitoneal lymph-node resection has not been demonstrated to improve local control.[3]

Lymph-node biopsy in patients with rhabdomyosarcoma is critical as well. The incidence of lymph-node involvement in rhabdomyosarcoma is determined by the primary site. Children without evidence of distant metastases have an overall 10% incidence of lymph-node involvement. It is most common in tumors arising in the prostate (41%), paratesticular (26%), and genitourinary sites (24%).[4] Lesions in the extremities have an intermediate rate of 12%, whereas the orbit (0%), truncal sites (3%), and nonorbital head and neck (7%) have the lowest rate of lymphatic dissemination. In the extremity and genitourinary sites, assessment of lymph-node involvement is essential to ensure that radiation fields are appropriately designed and sufficiently inclusive. Whether the sentinel lymph-node biopsy technique optimizes the identification of nodal spread in rhabdomyosarcoma has not been established, but it has been reported to be feasible in pediatric patients with minimal morbidity.[5] Although lymph-node biopsy is critical to identify the extent of spread, a lymph-node dissection should generally not be performed, because it may produce lymphedema that complicates radiotherapy and subsequent surgical resection of the primary tumor.

Radiographic assessment is inadequate for staging rhabdomyosarcoma as it is in Wilms tumor. In the Intergroup Rhabdomyosarcoma Study III (IRS-III), 121 boys with paratesticular rhabdomyosarcoma had a retroperitoneal lymph-node dissection to evaluate nodal status.[6] The lymph nodes were assessed to be clinically negative based on computed tomography (CT) scan in 18% of the boys, 14% of whom had positive nodes when biopsy or retroperitoneal lymph-node dissection was performed. In the boys with clinically positive lymph nodes based on the CT scans, 94% were confirmed to be positive pathologically. Retroperitoneal relapse occurred in only two of the 121 boys, one of whom had pathologically negative lymph nodes and did not receive radiotherapy. Thus CT was very accurate if lymph-node abnormalities were identified, but it was not extremely sensitive in identifying nodal involvement. In a subsequent study, Weiner and colleagues reported an increased incidence of retroperitoneal relapse in children treated during IRS-IV. The use of abdominal radiation in this study was based on thin-cut CT scans in 98% of cases as compared with children treated during the preceding IRS-III, in which 94% had retroperitoneal biopsy or lymph-node dissection. In the subsequent study, IRS-IV, a decrease in stage-2 disease (positive lymph nodes) from 35% to 17% occurred when the staging was based on radiographic findings. This resulted in a decrease in the use of abdominal radiation in this cohort. The result was a fourfold increase in retroperitoneal lymph-node relapse. Another example of how critical adequate staging is to avoid local failure.[7]

This chapter discusses some of the critical surgical issues in the treatment of infants, children, and adolescents with solid tumors. The use of anesthesia in patients with an anterior mediastinal mass, appropriate methods of biopsy, the role of neoadjuvant chemotherapy, limb salvage procedures for osseous tumors, and the management of pulmonary metastases are addressed.

ANESTHESIA IN PATIENTS WITH AN ANTERIOR MEDIASTINAL MASS

Patients presenting with an anterior mediastinal mass pose a therapeutic challenge to the anesthesiologist and the surgeon. Correct diagnosis of the tumor provides the greatest chance of cure. There are, however, a plethora of reports in the anesthesia and surgical literature of patients with an anterior mediastinal mass suffering respiratory collapse upon the induction of general anesthesia. This occurrence has led to an understandable reluctance among anesthesiologists to use general anesthesia in this setting. Respiratory symptoms are a poor index of the risk of respiratory collapse, with the clear exception of orthopnea, which suggests a high risk that respiratory collapse will occur. An initial attempt to establish the radiographic parameters that would correlate with respiratory collapse upon induction of general anesthesia involved a retrospective evaluation of 74 adults with Hodgkin disease.[8] In this study, the authors used the ratio of the transverse diameter of the mediastinal mass and the transverse diameter of the chest as the critical parameter. They found the incidence of respiratory collapse was 2.1% with a mediastinal mass less than 31% of the transverse diameter, compared with 10.5% for a mass with a ratio of 32% to 44% and 33.3% for a mass with a ratio greater than 45%. Similar results were reported by Turoff and associates.[9]

Thorne Griscom and colleagues demonstrated that CT scan can accurately determine the tracheal dimensions in children and adolescents, and he established the normative values in children.[10-12] Azizkhan first used this methodology in reviewing 50 children with anterior mediastinal masses. He found that 15 patients in his cohort had "marked" tracheal compression that was defined as a tracheal cross-sectional area less than 66% of predicted. When general anesthesia was induced in eight of these 13 patients, total airway obstruction occurred in five, all of whom had 50% or less of the predicted tracheal area. It was suggested, based on these findings, that general anesthesia should be avoided in children with less than 66% of the predicted tracheal area.

In a retrospective study at Boston Children's Hospital, 42 patients were identified who had an anterior mediastinal mass and a CT scan and underwent a surgical procedure. These patients were divided into those with tracheal area greater than 75% of expected (19 cases), those with 50% to 75% predicted area (16 cases), those with 25% to 50% (5 cases), and those with less than 25% (2 cases).[13] One clear finding of that study was that the presence or absence of respiratory symptoms did not correlate well with the degree of tracheal narrowing shown by CT scan, except for orthopnea (Fig. 49-1). General anesthesia with spontaneous ventilation was performed in four patients (with tracheal areas 33%, 73%, 76%, and 98% of predicted). General endotracheal anesthesia with paralysis was used in the remaining 32 patients, only three of whom had tracheal area of less than 50% of

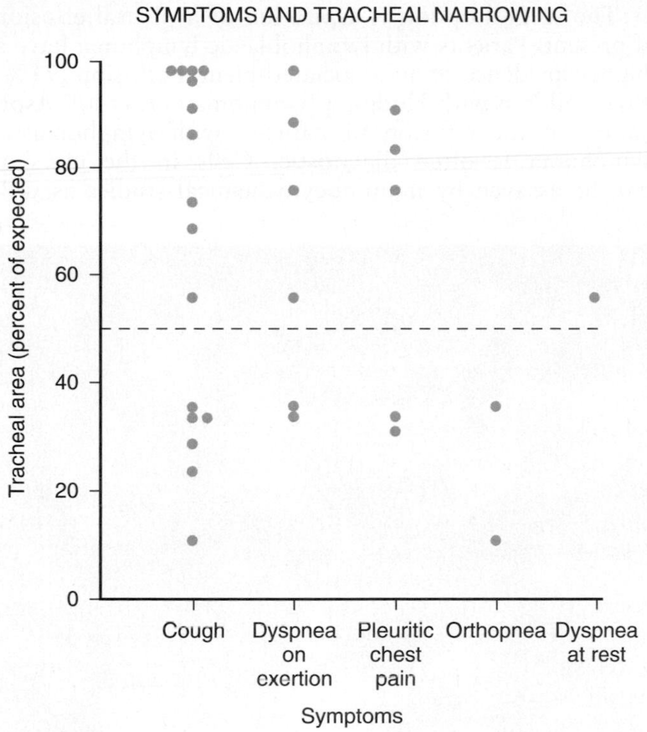

SYMPTOMS AND TRACHEAL NARROWING

Figure 49-1 Correlation of symptoms with tracheal areas is shown for a cohort of 42 children and adolescents with an anterior mediastinal mass. *(Modified from Shamberger RC, Holtzman RS, Griscom NT et al: CT quantitation of tracheal cross sectional areas as a guide to the surgical anesthetic management of children with anterior mediastinal mass. J Pediatr Surg 26:138–142, 1991.)*

predicted (30%, 26%, and 24%). One patient received preoperative radiation therapy (26%). None of these 32 patients had symptoms of orthopnea or dyspnea at rest, and only one had dyspnea on exertion. All tolerated anesthesia without difficulty, and no patients suffered respiratory or cardiovascular collapse. Adequate material for pathologic diagnosis was obtained in all cases. It was concluded in this study that general anesthesia was safe in patients with tracheal areas greater than or equal to 50% of predicted.

In a subsequent prospective study, 31 children with a mediastinal mass were evaluated with both CT scan and pulmonary function tests.[14] Although the use of pulmonary function tests had been proposed by multiple investigators as a method to assess anesthetic risk, little evaluation of this modality had been performed. Miller and Hyatt evaluated the flow volume loop curves in a series of patients with intrathoracic and extrathoracic obstruction resulting from strictures of the trachea, malignant tumors, or bilateral vocal cord paralysis.[15] The predominant distortion of the flow loops for intrathoracic obstruction was a marked reduction in the maximum expiratory flow rate. Hence in this prospective study, the peak expiratory flow rate was used as a critical factor. Patients with either a peak expiratory flow rate of less than 50% of predicted or a tracheal area of less than 50% of predicted had local anesthesia for their procedures. General endotracheal anesthesia was used only in patients with greater than 50% of predicted for both parameters.

All patients in this study did well when general anesthesia was applied (Fig. 49-2). Further analysis of this cohort revealed that patients with a tracheal area greater than 50% but a peak expiratory flow rate (PEFR) less than 50% had one of two problems: either a very low total lung capacity (38% and 55% of predicted) resulting from the massive size of the tumor or moderate to severe bronchial narrowing by qualitative estimation (four of these five patients) (Fig. 49-3).

In a subsequent study by King and coauthors, 51 children with Hodgkin lymphoma and non-Hodgkin lymphoma (NHL) were evaluated. Respiratory symptoms were present in 49% of the children in this series and were more prevalent in children with non-Hodgkin lymphoma (76%) than in those with Hodgkin lymphoma (30%). The extent of aberration in the pulmonary function test was also worse in those with non-Hodgkin lymphoma. The first-second forced expiratory volume (FEV_1) was more affected in the group with NHL (mean value of 63 +/– 27% of predicted) compared with the children with Hodgkin lymphoma (mean value of 87 +/– 16% of predicted).

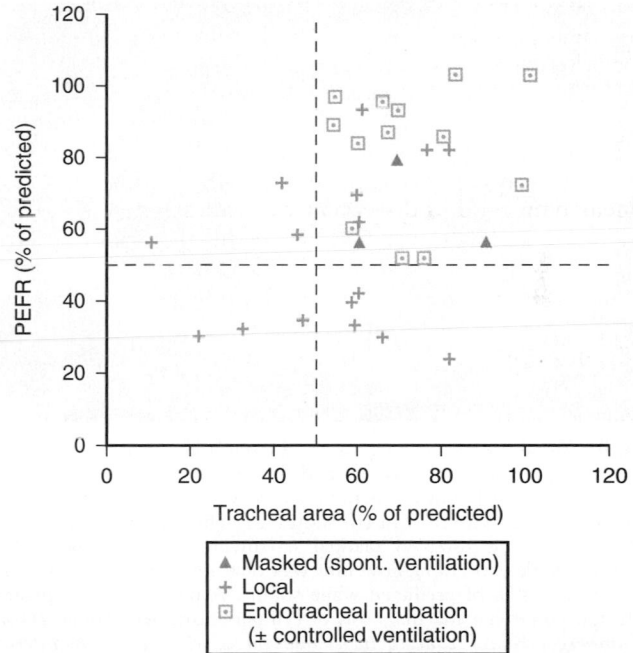

▲ Masked (spont. ventilation)
+ Local
⊡ Endotracheal intubation
(± controlled ventilation)

Figure 49-2 This figure shows the relationship between peak expiratory flow rate (PEFR) and tracheal area in a cohort of 31 children prospectively evaluated with an anterior mediastinal mass. Children with PEFR and/or tracheal area less than 50% of predicted (below or to the left of the *dotted lines*) all received local anesthetic and did well. Those children with PEFR and tracheal area greater than 50% of predicted received predominantly general anesthesia and did well *(right upper quadrant)*. The five children with tracheal areas greater than 50% of predicted but with peak PEFR less than 50% of predicted (in *lower right box*) might have been considered for general anesthesia if the tracheal area was the only parameter considered in assessing risk. Although the study could not demonstrate that these children would have had anesthetic problems, it did confirm that the parameters of greater than 50% PEFR and tracheal areas greater than 50% of predicted were safe for the administration of general anesthesia. *(Modified from Shamberger RC, Holzman RS, Griscom NT et al: Prospective evaluation of computed tomography and pulmonary function tests of children with mediastinal masses. Surgery 118:468–471, 1995.)*

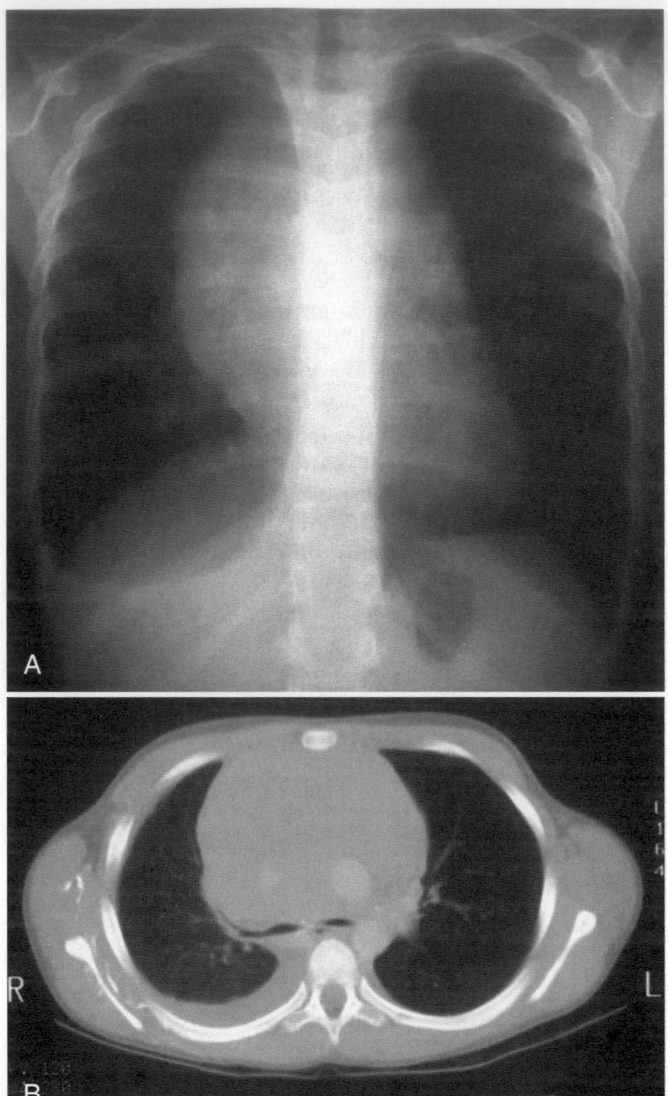

Figure 49-3 Chest imaging of an 11-year-old female who had a several-week history of a cough and dyspnea on exertion, as well as puffy eyes and orthopnea. The radiograph (**A**) reveals an anterior mediastinal mass, and a CT scan (**B**) shows a tracheal area that was 82% of predicted but revealed marked narrowing of the bronchi. The patient's peak expiratory flow rate was only 42% of predicted while sitting and 24% of predicted while supine. Aspiration of her pleural effusion confirmed the diagnosis of lymphoblastic lymphoma. *(From Shamberger RC: Preanesthetic evaluation of children with anterior mediastinal masses. Semin Pediatr Surg 8:61–68, 1999.)*

Patients with severe obstruction have one of three therapeutic options available. Patients can be treated in a preliminary fashion with either radiation therapy or steroids/chemotherapy for the most likely diagnosis based on the clinical findings (Fig. 49-4). In a series of young adults who underwent a postradiation biopsy of an anterior mediastinal mass, a histologic diagnosis could not be obtained in eight of 10 patients because of extensive necrosis.[16] In some cases, one area of tumor can be shielded for subsequent biopsy while the bulk of the tumor receives radiation. Non-Hodgkin lymphoma (NHL) is also extremely responsive to steroid therapy. Pretreatment with steroids also often obscures the histologic diagnosis.[17,18]

The second option is aspiration of a pleural effusion if present. Patients with lymphoblastic lymphoma have a higher incidence of an associated pleural effusion (71%) than children with Hodgkin lymphoma (11.4%).[19] Aspiration of the effusion in patients with lymphoblastic lymphoma is often diagnostic. Cells in the effusion can be assayed by immunocytochemical studies as well

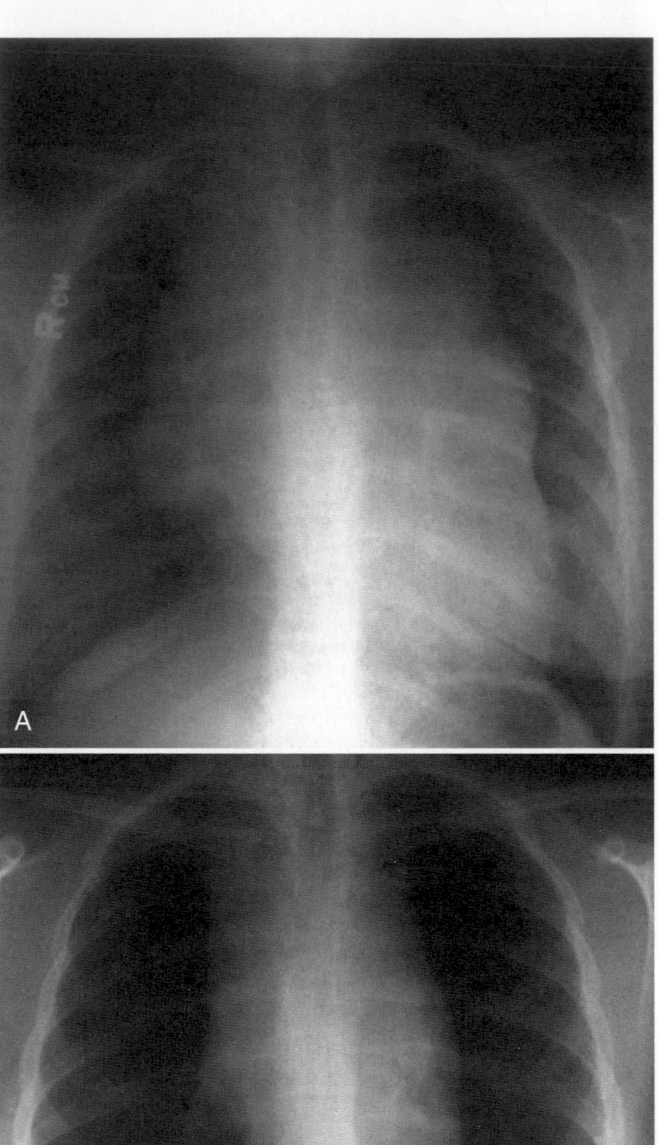

Figure 49-4 A 14-year-old girl with a nonproductive cough, retrosternal pain, 19-pound weight loss, and orthopnea. **A,** The chest radiograph showed a large anterior mediastinal mass. A biopsy was obtained in the suprasternal notch revealing lymphoblastic lymphoma. She received two courses of radiotherapy (250 cGy/per dose) over 2 days. Her chest radiograph obtained 7 days later (**B**) showed a remarkable response of the tumor to the radiation. *(From Shamberger RC: Preanesthetic evaluation of children with anterior mediastinal masses. Semin Pediatr Surg 8:61–68, 1999.)*

as by cytogenetic evaluation, immunophenotyping, and cytology.

Third, in children with significant respiratory compromise and no pleural effusion and no lymph nodes palpable outside the chest, either a percutaneous needle biopsy under radiographic guidance or an open anterior thoracotomy (Chamberlin procedure) can be performed successfully when the child is under local anesthesia. Children should be seated in a semiupright position and spontaneously ventilating to maximize their pulmonary function (Fig. 49-5). This position also decreases venous congestion if it is present. Spontaneous ventilation minimizes collapse of the trachea by the negative pressure exerted by the chest wall. It has also been shown that in children, image-guided percutaneous needle biopsy can in most instances provide a diagnosis.[20] The major challenges have been in children with Hodgkin lymphoma, where initial biopsy was able to provide a conclusive diagnosis in only 50% of the children (six of 12). An algorithm for safe management of these children and adolescents is shown in Figure 49-6.[21] Following these

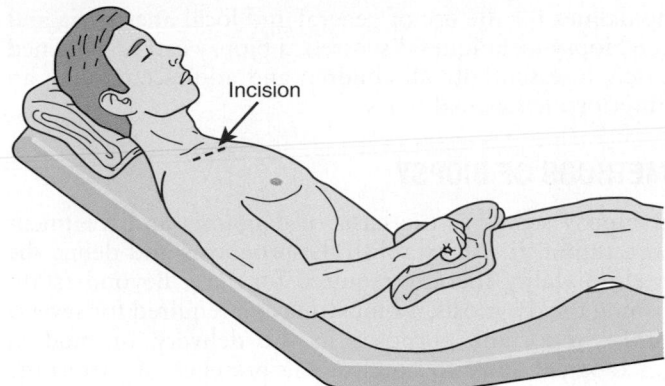

Figure 49-5 Proper position for patient with airway compromise to obtain a biopsy of an anterior mediastinal mass. The upright position optimizes pulmonary function and facilitates ventilation as well as venous drainage from potentially engorged vessels. *(From Shamberger RC: Preanesthetic evaluation of children with anterior mediastinal masses. Semin Pediatr Surg 8:61–68, 1999.)*

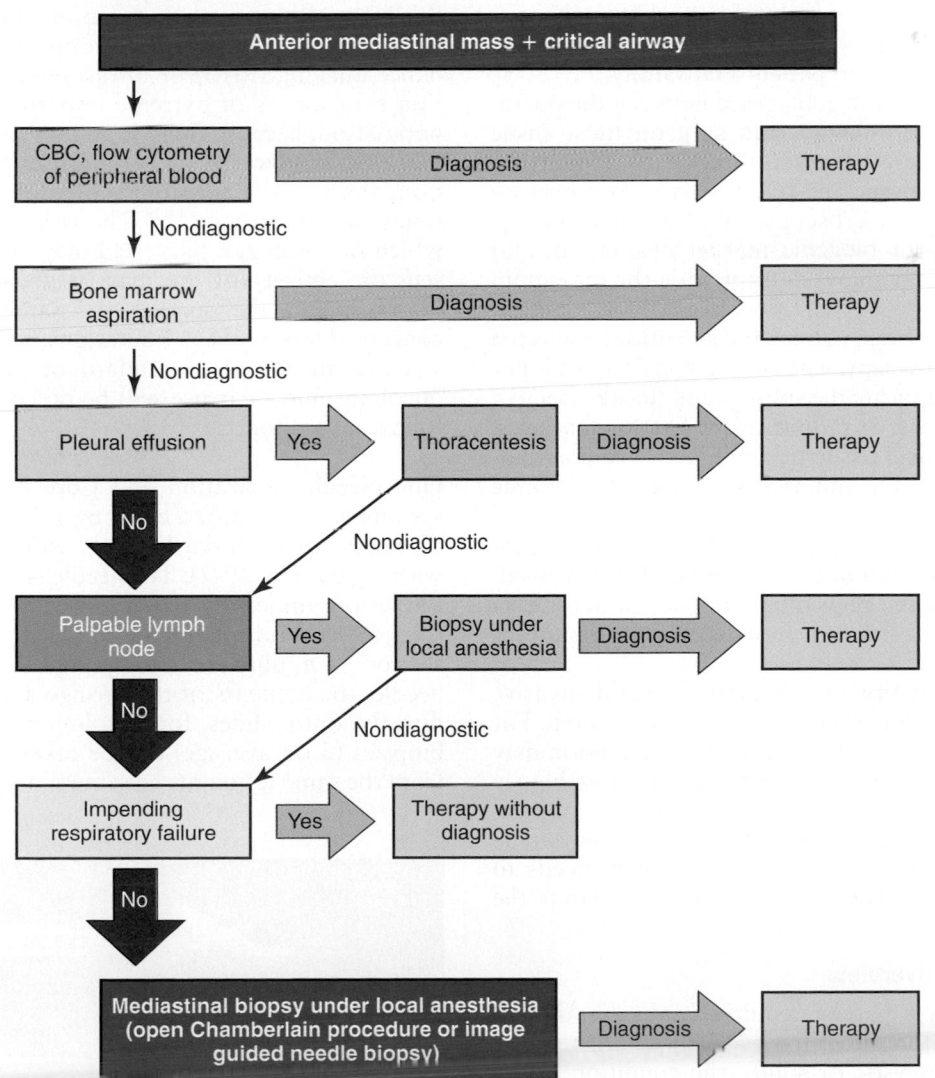

Figure 49-6 Algorithm for workup of patients with a critical airway resulting from compression by an anterior mediastinal mass. *CBC,* Complete blood count.

guidelines for the use of general and local anesthesia and the biopsy techniques discussed, a biopsy can be obtained safely in essentially all children and adolescents with an anterior mediastinal mass.

METHODS OF BIOPSY

A biopsy serves as the basis of diagnosis and treatment of a tumor. It will establish the prognosis and define the multimodality therapy required for cure. Beyond establishing the diagnosis, a biopsy may be required for several other important purposes in the delivery of modern oncological care: to confirm the presence of metastatic disease; to determine the response to treatment; and to document the presence of complications from treatment, especially suspicious lesions that may be infectious in nature and pose a significant risk to a patient with immunosuppression.

The Five Principles

Five principles must be followed when considering a biopsy. First, to minimize the psychological and physical stress for the patient and family, the need for a biopsy, how it will be performed, and the possible complications must be discussed with the patient and family.

Second, a preprocedure conference between the oncologist, pathologist, radiologist, and surgeon must ensue to determine the best biopsy technique to obtain the required amount of tissue and that the tissue is processed appropriately (light microscopy, electron microscopy, cytogenetic and other biogenic marker evaluation, and immunohistochemical analysis) to provide the maximum information.

Third, the precise biopsy route and site must be selected to facilitate future therapy. The wrong incision or biopsy site can greatly complicate the subsequent "local" therapy, whether it be resection or radiotherapy. Factors that must be considered are local tissue trauma, risk of tumor spillage or hemorrhage, and minimal violation of anatomic planes.

Fourth, the patient's general state of health, past medical history, and immune status must also be considered to fully assess the physiologic impact of anesthesia and biopsy, including risk of hemorrhagic and respiratory collapse.

Lastly, the possibility of combining several invasive procedures into one anesthetic should be considered. For example, a patient that requires a biopsy of a lesion may also need central venous access or a bone marrow biopsy and aspirate, and these procedures could all be combined. Although the grouping of procedures is not always possible, it is an option that the oncologic team needs to discuss in advance and then present a uniform plan to the patient and parents.

Method of Biopsy Overview

The type of biopsy a patient requires varies greatly and is dependent upon the site of the mass, the characteristics of the lesion itself (cystic or solid), the condition of the patient, and the diagnostic possibilities. Once the decision has been made to proceed with a biopsy, the first technical question that must be answered is the amount of tissue required and what biopsy technique will avoid increasing the stage of the patient or complicate future therapy. The fundamental separation of techniques is into small- or large-specimen biopsies.

Small-Specimen Biopsies

Small-specimen biopsies are those that are acquired through the use of hollow needles that sample an aspirate (fine needle aspiration [FNA]) or core (core needle biopsy [CNB]) of the tissue. They are often obtained with imaging assistance (ultrasound, fluoroscopy, or CT). The advantages of small-specimen biopsies are that they can often be performed with minimal or no anesthesia and are less invasive than an open procedure. Cost is also generally less for this approach, and recovery time for the patient is quicker. The disadvantages to this approach, however, are that the amount of tissue returned is quite small, which may create challenges in establishing a diagnosis or may not provide adequate tissue to complete the necessary secondary tests to adequately define the lesion. Furthermore, if imaging modalities are used to assist in this form of biopsy, then radiation exposure will occur if CT or fluoroscopy is used as opposed to magnetic resonance imaging (MRI) or ultrasound. This issue of radiation exposure is of extreme importance in the pediatric population, because there is an increased risk of developing a malignancy from radiation exposure.[22,23] In addition, there is the possibility of tumor spread in needle tracts or hemorrhage.[24-26] The risk of sampling error in which the specimen harvested may not adequately represent the entirety of the mass is always a concern with biopsies, and the smaller the sample, the larger the concern. Despite these limitations, small-specimen biopsies are an accepted standard of practice in pediatric oncology, and their use will be described in detail in the following section.

Fine Needle Aspiration and Core Needle Biopsy. FNA specimens are acquired by using a 20- to 25-gauge needle connected to a standard syringe with the plunge partially withdrawn (Fig. 49-7). The needle is inserted directly into the lesion guided by palpation or with image guidance (Fig. 49-8). Multiple passes are taken from the lesion as suction is applied to the syringe. Upon removing the needle, the contents of the syringe and needle are placed directly onto slides for cytological analysis. Multiple biopsies (3 on average) can be taken with this approach from the same lesion at the same time, and the cytological

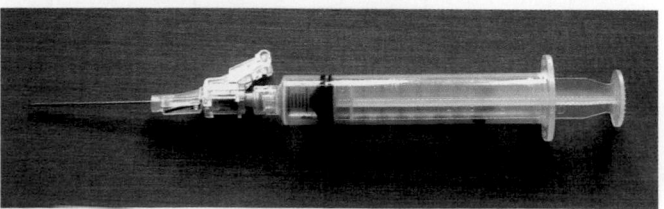

Figure 49-7 This figure shows a standard fine needle aspiration device with a 22-gauge needle attached to a 10-cc syringe that has the plunger partially withdrawn to facilitate the removal of the aspirate.

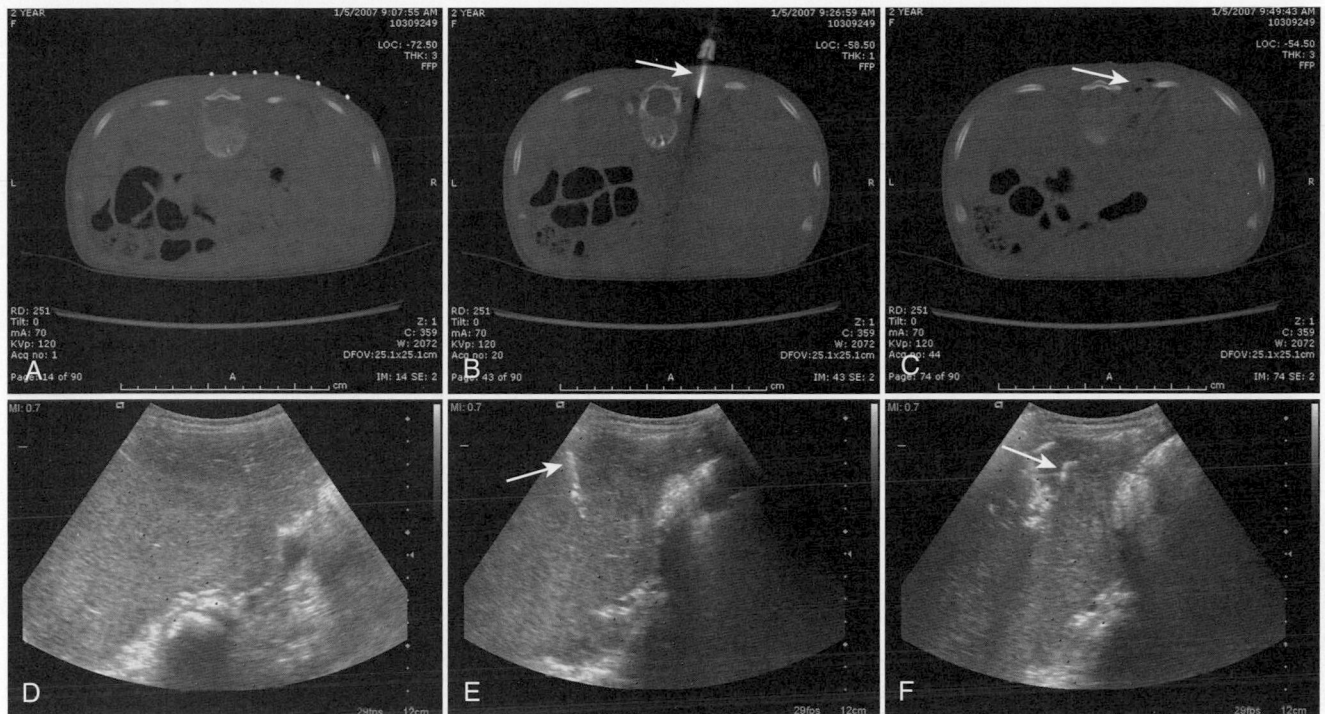

Figure 49-8 A, Prebiopsy computed tomography (CT) of a retroperitoneal mass with external grid for biopsy marking. B, The same patient with the needle in the retroperitoneal mass *(arrow)*. C, Postbiopsy CT with air in the mass and soft tissues *(arrow)* from the biopsy procedure. D, Prebiopsy ultrasound of a liver mass. E, Ultrasound-guided biopsy of a liver mass *(arrow)*. F, Postbiopsy hemorrhage in the mass is depicted *(arrow)*.

results are available for almost immediate review. However, no histologic assessment is possible using this technique, thus causing difficulty in diagnosing certain tumors with cytologic appearances that are quite similar, such as the small, round, blue cell tumors.

Histopathologic analysis is possible with a CNB. CNB specimens are retrieved using larger, hollow-bore needles (13- to 20-gauge) attached to spring-loaded devices that allow for one-step tissue harvest and extraction (Fig. 49-9). Image guidance is often used during this procedure, just as it is for the acquisition of FNA samples. The CNB device is often inserted through a coaxial sheath or cylinder that allows the operator to instill a coagulant into the tissue defects made by the CNB device to reduce the incidence of hemorrhage and tumor spillage (Fig. 49-10). Generally multiple specimens (10 or more) from different areas of the lesion are gathered with this technique to minimize sampling error and to provide more tissue for complete pathological analysis.[27-29] A representative example of the microscopic appearance of the biopsy specimens for FNA and CNB is shown in Fig. 49-11.

Imaging techniques can often distinguish areas with viable versus necrotic tissue to help identify the area best to biopsy.

The results and outcomes of small-specimen biopsies from almost any organ in the body have been reported extensively in adult patients with excellent diagnostic accuracy and minimal procedural morbidity. However, small-specimen biopsy techniques and comparison of these techniques in pediatric oncology patients, especially with abdominal lesions, have only recently gained widespread acceptance and usage.[29-35]

Hugosson and colleagues in 1999 reviewed their series of image-guided percutaneous small-specimen biopsies in children from 1992 through 1996.[31] A total of 90 biopsies (53 FNA, 37 CNB) were taken in 75 patients (mean age of 6.9 years). They compared the use of FNA with CNB (1.2 mm core specimens) under ultrasound guidance. Their cohort had many different malignant

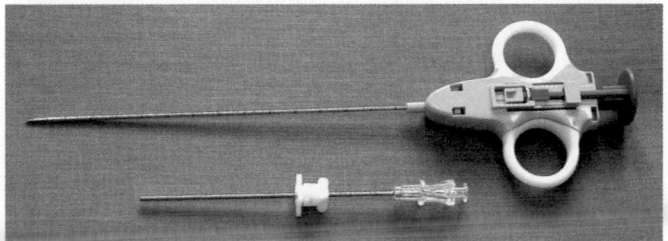

Figure 49-9 An automated 15-gauge core needle biopsy device. *(Courtesy of Easy Core Biopsy System, Boston Scientific, Natick, Mass.)*

Figure 49-10 An automated 16-gauge core needle biopsy device with a 15-gauge coaxial sheath. *(Courtesy of Coaxial Temno Evolution, Allegiance Healthcare Corporation, McGraw Park, Ill.)*

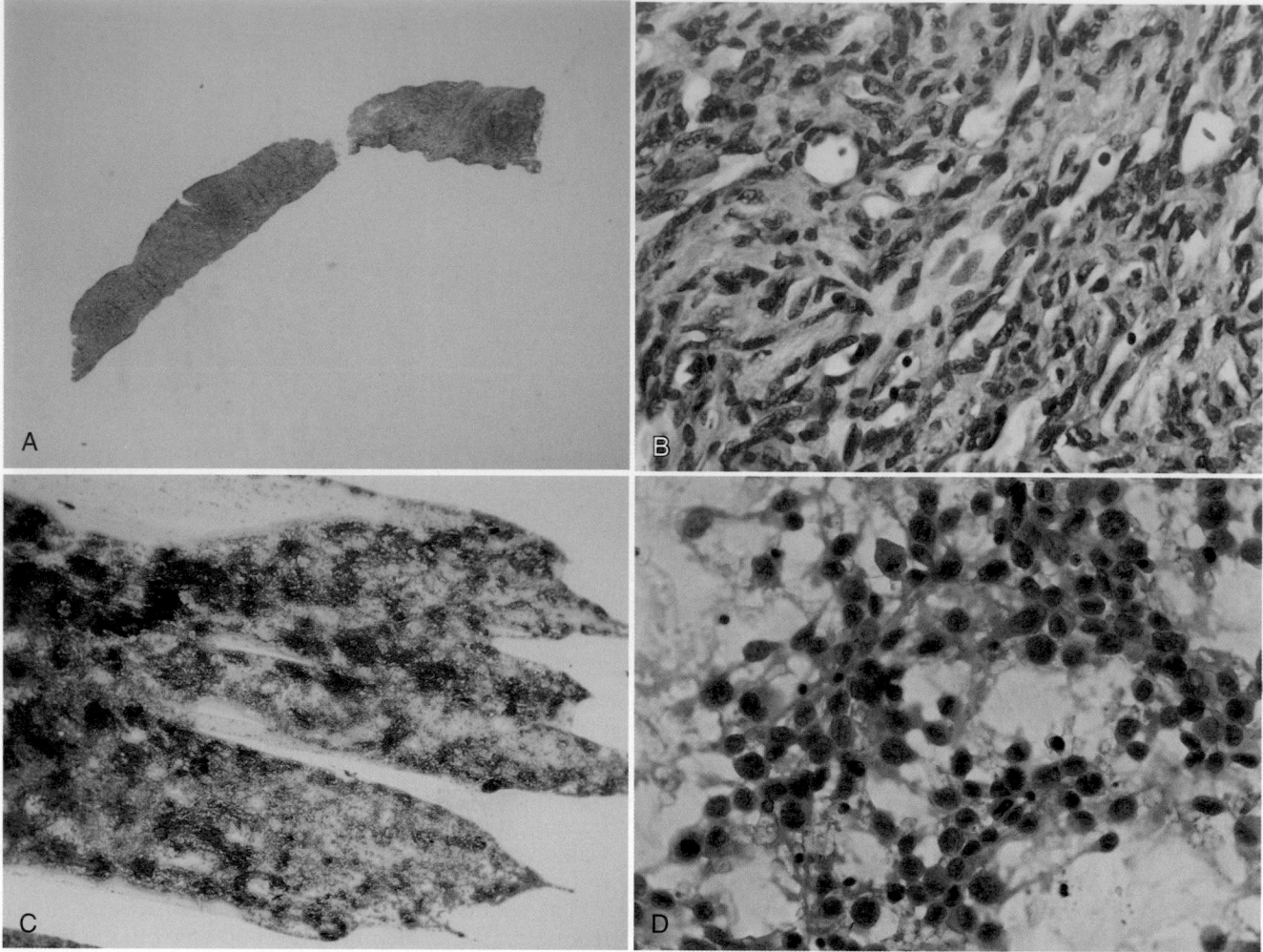

Figure 49-11 **A,** Core needle biopsy specimen from a liver mass at ×2 (angiosarcoma). **B,** CNB at ×600 with sheets of moderately pleomorphic spindled cells and lumina formation. **C,** Fine needle aspiration specimen from a submandibular lymph node at ×2 (nasopharyngeal alveolar rhabdomyosarcoma). **D,** Specimen at ×600 revealing round and elongated pleomorphic tumor cells with marked apoptosis.

processes, and they obtained biopsies from the liver, kidney, adrenal gland, spleen, pelvic masses, and enlarged abdominal lymph nodes. Their FNA diagnostic accuracy was 77% (73% for malignant lesions and 83% for benign lesions) and 95% for CNB (93% malignant lesions and 100% for benign lesions). The complication rate was 8%. They concluded that CNB is a more accurate technique with a similar complication rate to FNA. These results were echoed by Hussain and colleagues, who examined their institutional experience on image-guided percutaneous biopsies (using CNB) in children (mean age, 4 years-old).[32] Ninety-four percent of their cohort had abdominal or pelvic masses. Their reported diagnostic accuracy was 88%, and the initial diagnosis was subsequently confirmed by whole-specimen pathologic analysis. Their complication rate was approximately 8%, and they also concluded that CNB was generally successful in diagnosing tumors in children.

Sklair-Levy and colleagues published their institution's 10-year experience in small-specimen biopsies on pediatric patients.[33] They performed 69 (62 CNB) biopsies in 57 patients using image guidance. Their diagnostic

accuracy was 88.7% (55 of 62 patients). For malignant lesions, CNB had an accuracy of 98% as an isolated diagnostic technique in solid malignant tumors, although seven CNBs had to be repeated because the initial results were nondiagnostic. All seven repeated CNBs were correct on subsequent evaluation. They performed seven FNAs with a diagnostic accuracy of only 28%, and these patients then underwent surgical excision of the lesion in question. Although this accuracy rate is far lower than previously reported,[31] none of the lesions in question were abdominal or pelvic masses, and the majority of these lesions were enlarged lymph nodes. Therefore direct comparison of the utility and diagnostic accuracy of FNA in this situation is not possible. Their accuracy with primary, metastatic, or recurrent lesions was in excess of 94% for all tumor types except lymphomas, for which they were correct only 60% of the time. Interestingly, they did not have a single complication.

A more comprehensive study was published by Skoldenberg and colleagues. They examined their institution's results with 147 CNBs in 110 children (mean age 4 years) from all anatomic sites (61 abdominal and pelvic lesions of the total 110 children).[34] An overall accuracy of 89% was achieved for the CNBs performed. Twenty-four children required 37 additional biopsies for a non-diagnostic first specimen (12), a question of recurrence (22), and an insufficient quantity of tissue for all the diagnostic studies needed (3). They reported a sensitivity of 82% and a positive predictive value of 98.8%. A complication rate of 7% (10 of 141 cases) was seen, of which half were hemorrhagic in nature. Fourteen of the patients required narcotics for pain management postprocedure. A statistically significant difference in the occurrence of postprocedure pain was noted in older children. The authors strongly encourage the use of CNB in the diagnosis of pediatric malignancy, and they tout its superiority to FNA.

St. Jude's Children's Research Hospital published their experience of CNB in pediatric solid tumors over 5 years.[30] Two hundred and two CNBs were performed using image guidance and anesthesia. Ultrasound was the predominant mode of imaging assistance (124 of 202), and the biopsies were performed to evaluate both primary and metastatic sites of disease. One hundred and three primary CNBs were performed with a 96.9% sensitivity, a 100% specificity, and an accuracy of 98%. For metastatic or recurrent lesions, they measured a sensitivity of 83.1%, a specificity of 100%, and an accuracy of 87.9%. There were no false positive results. In the cohort of patients with abdominal and pelvic tumors, the sensitivity and accuracy of CNB was 100%. They had a complication rate of 13.4%, with hemorrhage being the most common. Their results and experience across all anatomic regions and pathologic lesions demonstrate that small-specimen biopsies should be considered the initial diagnostic procedure of choice. Therefore solid masses in the pediatric population should be approached where indicated with image-guided small-specimen biopsies, especially using the CNB technique.

Finally, Sebire and Roebuck[36] reported the results from a systematic literature review they conducted to determine the utility, success, and complications from image-guided CNBs. Echoing similar studies, they report that 94% of all procedures obtained adequate tissue for evaluation, and of that group an accurate diagnosis by histopathologic analysis was achieved in 94% with only a 1% complication rate.

Large-Specimen Biopsies

Large-specimen tissue biopsies involve the removal of all (excisional) or part (incisional) of a lesion using an open or minimally invasive surgery (MIS) technique. This method of biopsy should not be confused with a formal extirpative procedure, because the surgeon does not remove either part or all of the entire mass with concerns about adequate margins of resection. The goal of these procedures is to remove a piece or all of the mass in question to provide tissue for a diagnosis, not for local control of the primary site. Large-specimen biopsies are also performed in anatomic areas or on lesions where image-guided small-specimen biopsies are more difficult because of proximity to major vessels or nerves, the lesions are very vascular, or the lesions cannot be reached without damaging overlying organs and structures (i.e., retroperitoneal lymph nodes). Large-specimen biopsies may be performed sequentially with a small-specimen biopsy using the same anesthetic if there is any doubt regarding the adequacy for a histopathologic diagnosis of the FNA or CNB.

Several disadvantages of large-specimen biopsies are a longer procedural and anesthetic time, recovery time, and need for hospitalization. They can delay the initiation of adjuvant therapies and are more costly. Assuming there are no complications, the vast majority of pediatric patients who have a small-specimen biopsy performed on a solid abdominal mass do not stay more than 8 hours postprocedure, as evidenced in recent large studies.[30,32-35,37] The same cannot be said for large-specimen biopsies. Finally, operative exploration for large-specimen sampling can complicate definitive local-control therapies, especially from an operative standpoint. Violating the thoracic or peritoneal cavities induces adhesion formation that can complicate the subsequent resection.

Although significant disadvantages to large specimen biopsies exist, there are marked advantages. First, large biopsy samples are obtained, and multiple areas are sampled within the lesion, decreasing the likelihood of sampling error. Second, a detailed macroscopic evaluation of the lesion in question and all surrounding structures can be performed to search for extension or metastasis from the tumor. Third, radiation exposure is avoided for the patient and the healthcare team. Finally, hemostasis and tumor sampling is controlled and confirmed directly before closing the incision to minimize the complications of tumor spillage and hemorrhage.

In the last decade, several groups have reported success using a MIS approach for either incisional or excisional large specimen biopsies. The MIS approach relies on the same basic tenets of surgical discipline as does an open procedure, but it uses smaller incisions and advanced technology to achieve these goals. An operating telescope capable of excellent image resolution and magnification is used to display a picture on closed-circuit monitors. Dissection and biopsy is performed with long, fine instruments introduced through a percutaneously placed 2- to 12-mm canula. When operating in the peritoneal cavity, carbon dioxide gas (CO_2) is introduced by an insufflation apparatus that distends the abdominal wall to provide adequate space to assess the abdominal structures. The pressure is kept as low as possible, consistent with adequate exposure. An important point that must be discussed with the anesthesiologist is the degree of respiratory impairment that CO_2 insufflation may induce, especially in pediatric patients with extremely compliant diaphragms. If at any point the child becomes physiologically unstable, the CO_2 gas is released and the procedure is terminated. Advantages of the MIS approach are decreased postoperative pain from the small incisions, a shorter postoperative stay, improved cosmetic results, and an earlier return of bowel function.[35,30] A complication rate in the pediatric population of 4% or less has been reported in a recent large series, but this rate is clearly related to the experience of the surgeon.[38]

In 1973 Gans and Berci described their successful experiences with MIS in pediatric patients, but their procedures were not related to tumors.[39] In fact, it was not until Holcomb and colleagues' report from the Surgical Discipline Committee of the Children's Cancer Group (CCG) in 1995 that the MIS approach was formally reviewed for its efficacy in oncology.[40] In this study from 15 participating centers, 25 abdominal and 63 thoracic explorations were undertaken for the purposes of diagnosis (primary, relapsed, and metastatic lesions), staging, assessment of resectability, and the evaluation of treatment complications. All abdominal lesions (16), and 50 of 51 thoracic lesions that required biopsy were successfully diagnosed. There were no perioperative mortalities, and only seven complications—all in the thoracic cohort.

A prospective trial sponsored by the National Institutes of Health (NIH) concerning the use of MIS in pediatric oncology patients was begun by the combined Surgical Discipline Committees of the CCG and the Pediatric Oncology Group (POG) in 1996.[40] The study failed for lack of accrual, and it was closed after 2 years. A questionnaire soliciting reasons for the failure of this study documented that lack of familiarity with the MIS technique by both the surgeon and the institution, surgeon and pediatric oncologist bias against the MIS technique, and the failure to submit the necessary paperwork to local institutional review boards for study approval were statistically significant factors in the study's failure. Despite these results, MIS is gaining acceptance in pediatric oncology, especially for the diagnosis of lesions.

Spurbeck and colleagues at the St. Jude's Children's Research Hospital recently published their experience with MIS in pediatric oncology patients from 1995 through 2000.[41] One hundred and one patients underwent 113 operations (64 abdominal and 49 thoracic procedures). Abdominal biopsies were attempted in 25 patients and were successful in 23 (92%). Evaluation of resectability was determined successfully in two other cases, and seven extirpative procedures were performed. There were three complications in the abdominal group, and four MIS procedures were converted to open procedures. There were three complications reported in the abdominal cohort. The thoracoscopic procedures had similar rates of success, conversion, and complications. They reported no port-site recurrences or metastases in either the abdominal or thoracic cohorts of their study. Although a feared complication, the incidence of port-site recurrence is rare in thoracic cases (a single report by Sartorelli and colleagues).[42] However, abdominal port-site recurrence rates are higher but depend on the tumor involved.[43-46] Needless to say, these are retrospective data spanning many institutions, surgeons, tumors, and techniques. The conclusions reached by Spurbeck and colleagues attest to the safety and efficacy of MIS techniques in the successful diagnosis of pediatric tumors, but its use in the formal extirpation of tumors remains to be established.

A recent analysis by de Lijster and colleagues[47] attempted to define the role for and success of MIS techniques versus open procedures in pediatric abdominal and thoracic tumors, but they discovered that there were no randomized controlled or controlled clinical trials on this topic in the literature. Hence no formal recommendation could be made as to the effectiveness, superiority or equivalency of MIS techniques versus open procedures in childhood tumors. Obviously this topic deserves greater scrutiny and investigation through the development and completion of a rigorous controlled trial as has been done in adults.

Extremity Tumors

Biopsy of a soft-tissue or bone tumor in an extremity should be considered the first interventional procedure in limb salvage. Although the technical aspects are quite simple, the decision-making process is not. At risk are not only the patient's limb, but also overall disease control and outcome.

As noted, biopsy is truly a multidisciplinary process involving medical oncologists, surgeons, radiologists, pathologists, and radiation oncologists. Accuracy and outcome of biopsy procedures are improved when each of these specialists has a knowledge of musculoskeletal tumors and limb salvage principles. This is often best accomplished at tertiary centers with experience in the management of sarcomas.[48,49]

The first step in planning a biopsy is performing a complete work-up. Based on history and physical examination findings, suspicion is raised about a tumor. Plain radiographs are often diagnostic of a bone malignancy and are crucial. MRI is also essential for both bone and soft-tissue tumors to define the extent of the tumor itself and involvement of neighboring compartments and neurovascular structures. It should be performed before biopsy to avoid artifact signal. Ultrasound is helpful to determine whether a soft-tissue mass is cystic or solid, but MRI is the gold standard for the evaluation of a suspicious mass.

Based on the findings from the work-up, a differential diagnosis can be established through collaboration at a multidisciplinary conference. All the specialists involved should be aware of the potential of a malignancy so that proper techniques are used for the procedure itself and for handling of the tissue. The biopsy approach is selected by the surgeon based on knowledge of limb-salvage surgery. The biopsy tract should be along the planned incision for limb salvage so that the entire tract can be excised later with the resection of the tumor. This is critical, because errors in placement of the biopsy incision can contaminate neurovascular and other important structures, making limb salvage impossible or necessitating large soft-tissue flaps for coverage.[48,49] The tumor should be approached in the most direct manner and through a muscle, not in between muscles, to decrease contamination of normal tissue.

Biopsy of an extremity tumor can be performed by open or closed (CNB) techniques (Table 49-1). Open biopsy offers the advantage of a larger tissue sample so that adequate pathologic evaluation can be performed. However, the major disadvantages are a higher risk of contamination of critical structures and complications such as bleeding, infection, and pathologic fracture. It is also more expensive and requires more time. Incisional

TABLE 49-1   Comparison of Open versus Needle Biopsy

	Open	Needle
Sample size	Larger	Smaller
Accuracy	Higher or equivalent	Lower or equivalent
Morbidity	Higher	Lower
Risk of contamination	Higher	Lower
Complications	Higher	Lower

biopsy is performed by entering into the tumor itself and removing a small section of it. The pseudocapsule is repaired, and careful hemostasis is obtained to try to decrease tumor-cell spillage or creation of a hematoma. Excisional biopsy involves removing the whole tumor in one piece. This is rarely indicated for extremity tumors, because resection surgery for malignant tumors is so vastly different from that for benign tumors. Also, most musculoskeletal tumors are treated with neoadjuvant therapy before excision. This approach is used for two reasons. First, it will increase the ability to perform limb-salvage surgery. Second, it provides an in vivo assay of response to standard chemotherapy (see Neoadjuvant Therapy for Solid Tumors).

Needle biopsy on the other hand is associated with less morbidity for the patient. It carries a lower risk of complications and contamination and is often simpler to perform. However, the smaller tissue sample size is a disadvantage and decreases the accuracy rate of the diagnosis. Use of a large-bore needle to remove a core of the tumor is thus usually more advantageous than FNA, as discussed. Sampling error is another disadvantage of CNB. Image-guidance with CT (Fig. 49-12) or ultrasound improves accuracy and decreases sampling error, but it is imperative that the surgeon discuss the approach with the radiologist performing the procedure. There is a risk of local recurrence if the needle biopsy tract is not excised with the tumor, but the risk is probably less than with open biopsy.

Pathologic analysis also requires specific knowledge of musculoskeletal tumors, especially with smaller sample sizes. The specialist obtaining the biopsy should discuss the case with the pathologist. A frozen section at the time of biopsy is essential, not for definitive diagnosis, but to ensure sufficient neoplastic tissue is available to the pathologist to make a diagnosis. Proper tissue handling is also crucial for the pathologist to be able to arrive at the correct diagnosis. Hematoxylin and eosin staining as well as most immunohistochemistry can be performed on tissue placed in standard formaldehyde. However, electron microscopy, cytogenetic investigation, tissue culture, flow cytometry, and immunofluorescence all require special handling and often fresh tissue. The discovery of specific cytogenetic abnormalities in certain tumors (e.g., t[11;22] in Ewing sarcoma [EWS] and t[2;13] in alveolar rhabdomyosarcoma) has increased the ability of pathologists to make the diagnosis with small tissue samples, but they must be processed in the correct manner.

Combined discussion of the pathology completes the biopsy process. The multidisciplinary team caring for the patient can then review all of the staging studies with the known diagnosis in mind and arrive at a recommendation for treatment.

NEOADJUVANT THERAPY FOR SOLID TUMORS

Wilms Tumor

Cooperative group trials by the NWTSG in North America, the International Society of Paediatric Oncology (SIOP) in Europe, and the United Kingdom Children's Cancer Group (UKCCG) have provided a great wealth of information regarding the optimal management of Wilms tumor. A major difference in approach exists between SIOP and NWTSG. In North America, primary resection followed by chemotherapy and radiotherapy is favored. In the SIOP studies, children generally first receive either chemotherapy or radiotherapy followed by resection. This approach has been driven by a high incidence of operative tumor rupture in their early series. In SIOP 1 the use of preoperative radiation therapy (20 Gy) was randomized versus primary resection. The rate of intraoperative rupture decreased from 33% to 4% with the use of radiation.[50] Survival was not affected, and the incidence of local recurrence was not reported. The frequency of operative rupture that occurred in NWTS 1 and 2 were 22% and 12%, respectively.[51,52] In a subsequent SIOP study, preoperative therapy was randomized between abdominal radiation (20 Gy) and actinomycin D compared with those receiving vincristine and

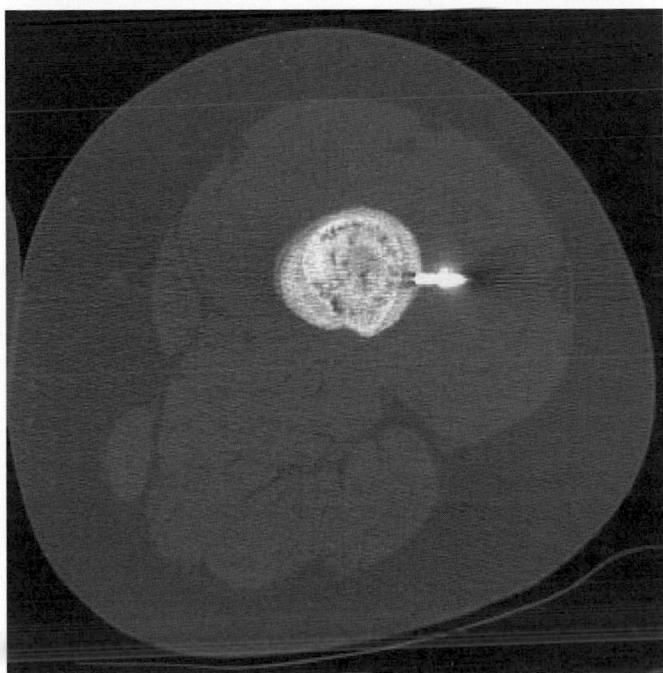

Figure 49-12 Core needle biopsy of an osteosarcoma of the femur under guidance with computed tomography.

actinomycin D. The frequency of rupture was 9% and 6%, respectively.[53]

In SIOP 6, which started in 1980, all patients received initial preoperative chemotherapy (vincristine and actinomycin D). Radiotherapy was given after resection to children with stage II N1 and stage III disease. Children with stage II N0 disease were randomized to receive either 20 Gy abdominal radiotherapy or no radiation. All children received vincristine and actinomycin D for 38 weeks. The radiotherapy randomization was halted after 123 children were randomized, 64 to radiotherapy and 59 to chemotherapy alone. Six of the 59 children who did not receive radiotherapy had local recurrences, whereas no recurrences occurred in the group who did. These findings suggest that prenephrectomy treatment altered the pathologic findings that would have led to a diagnosis of stage II N1 or stage III disease (i.e., lymph-node involvement or capsular penetration), resulting in the standard administration of local radiation. No statistical difference in survival has been seen in these children after extended follow-up observation, because those who relapsed had treatment alternatives.[54,55]

In SIOP 9, which began in 1987, preoperative therapy was randomized between 4 and 8 weeks' duration. The goal was to produce a larger proportion of stage I tumors.[56] In this study, postoperative radiotherapy for children whose disease was stage II N0 was replaced with an anthracycline (epirubicin or doxorubicin). Preoperative treatment for patients without distant metastases consisted of four weekly courses of vincristine and three 2-day courses of actinomycin D every 2 weeks versus 8 weeks of the identical therapy. There was no advantage seen from the extended therapy in terms of staging at resection (stage I, 64% versus 62%) or in intraoperative tumor rupture (1% versus 3%). Therapy after resection was based on the pathologic findings. In SIOP 9, the surgery-related complications were reported to be 8%.[57]

In both the NWTSG protocols and those of the COG, primary surgical resection is generally recommended. There are certain generally accepted situations where preoperative therapy is appropriate. These include the occurrence of Wilms tumor in a solitary kidney, bilateral renal tumors, and respiratory distress from extensive metastatic disease in the lungs. In these cases pretreatment biopsy should be obtained, and percutaneous biopsies are often used. Although needle tract seeding has been reported, this is quite rare in Wilms tumor. The aim of neoadjuvant treatment in the bilateral tumors and solitary kidney is to preserve the maximum amount of renal parenchyma and function. Current COG protocols for bilateral renal tumors have intensified the neoadjuvant therapy to include three agents (vincristine, actinomycin D, and doxorubicin) with each cycle of therapy. The duration of therapy has also been limited to avoid incremental increases in the intensity of therapy when further regression in the size of the tumor is unlikely.

The efficacy of preoperative treatment to achieve partial nephrectomy in patients with unilateral Wilms tumors has been evaluated by several centers. McLorie and associates in Toronto obtained percutaneous biopsy in 31 children with Wilms tumors. Multiagent chemo-

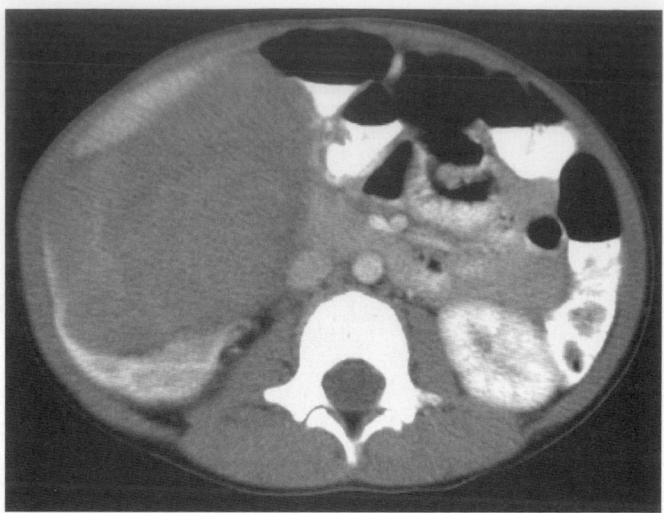

Figure 49-13 Computed tomography scan in a 4-year, 10-month-old girl who had a palpable abdominal mass. The study revealed a large tumor with a very thin renal capsule. A primary resection was performed, and the tumor was stage II with favorable histology. She went on to receive double agent therapy with vincristine and actinomycin D.

therapy was then administered for 4 to 6 weeks. Partial nephrectomy was performed in nine children (four with unilateral tumors and five with bilateral tumors).[58] Two of these children suffered an intraabdominal relapse, and only four of the 30 unilateral tumors (13.3%) were amenable to partial nephrectomy. Hence in unilateral cases not identified by prospective radiographic imaging in patients with syndromes, a partial nephrectomy is rarely possible even with preoperative therapy. Another assessment of the feasibility of partial nephrectomies was performed at St. Jude Children's Research Hospital.[59] The preoperative CT scans of 43 children with nonmetastatic unilateral Wilms tumor were reviewed. The criteria used to define those tumors suitable for partial nephrectomy were involvement by the tumor of one pole and less than one third of the kidney, a functioning kidney, no involvement of the collecting system or renal vein, and clear margins between the tumor and surrounding structures. Only two of 43 scans (4.7%) met the criteria, suggesting that a partial nephrectomy was feasible. The primary concerns regarding the administration of preoperative chemotherapy (as in the studies of Kozzi and associates and Moorman-Voestermans and co-workers) to create "resectable" small tumors is that these children may be curable by surgical resection alone without subjecting them to the toxicity of additional treatments.[60,61]

The surgical resectability of Wilms tumors has been poorly correlated with radiographic studies. In fact, extremely large tumors can be stage II lesions and be fairly safely resected (Fig. 49-13). The surgical recommendations in the NWTSG studies have been that if resection of the tumor would involve resection of adjacent organs (i.e., liver, pancreas, or spleen) because of adherence, biopsies should be obtained and subsequent chemotherapy applied before resection, because such resections are associated with an increased rate of complication (Fig. 49-14). Complications in the NWTSG-4

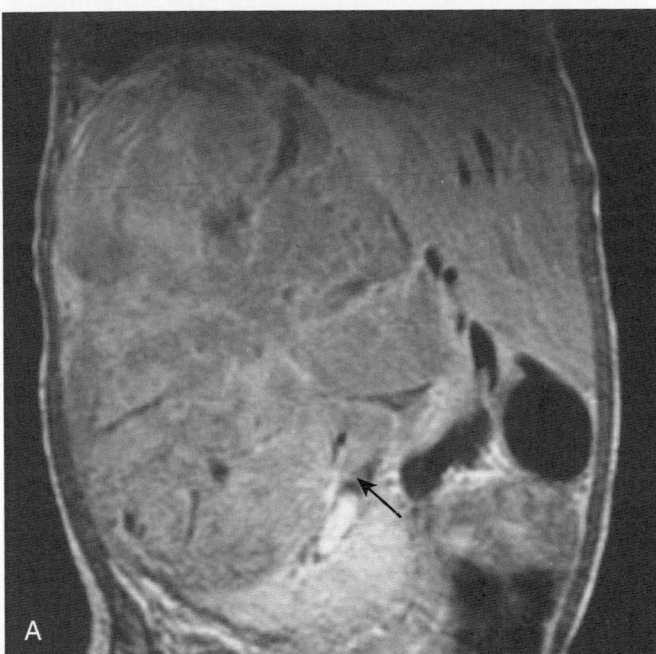

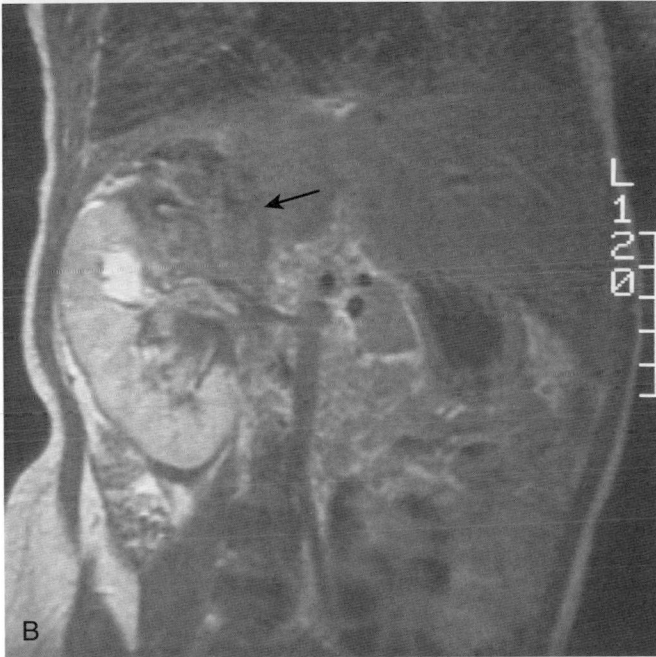

Figure 49-14 A, Magnetic resonance imaging (MRI) scan of a 2 and a half-year-old girl first seen with a massive right-sided abdominal mass *(arrow)* that appeared to arise from the kidney. Chest radiograph revealed pulmonary nodules as well as stage-IV disease. Because of the size of the primary tumor and the presence of metastatic disease, she received neoadjuvant chemotherapy after needle biopsy demonstrated a standard-risk tumor (diffuse blastemal subtype). She first received three courses of actinomycin D, vincristine, and cyclophosphamide, which achieved some shrinkage of the tumor. At attempted resection, the extensive tumor was densely adherent to the posterior aspect of the liver and the vena cava. The attempted resection was halted at that time, because it was clear that a portion of the liver would have to be resected with the nephrectomy. Repeat biopsies again demonstrated a standard histology Wilms tumor with tumor invasion into the liver. She then received more intensive therapy involving cisplatin and VP-16, as well as abdominal and thoracic radiation. **B,** MRI after additional therapy showed remarkable shrinkage of the tumor, allowing a less extensive and safer resection. A plane could be developed between the liver and kidney at this point, and hepatectomy was not required.

study have been assessed.[62] Complications occurred in 12.7% of a random sample of 534 of the 3335 patients enrolled on the study. Intestinal obstruction was the most common complication (5.1%), followed by extensive hemorrhage (1.9%), wound infection (1.9%), and vascular injury (1.5%). Factors associated with an increased incidence of complication included intravascular extension into the inferior vena cava or atrium and nephrectomy performed through a flank or paramedian incision. Tumor diameter greater than or equal to 10 cm was also associated with increased complications. In SIOP 9, complications occurred in 8% of 598 patients. These patients were pretreated with vincristine, actinomycin D, and epirubicin or doxorubicin before nephrectomy.[57] Their complications included small bowel obstruction in 3.7% and tumor rupture in 2.8%. The latter is not reported as a complication in the NWTSG reviews.

Neuroblastoma

Surgery plays a primary role in the treatment of low-stage neuroblastoma. Tumors that the surgeon deems readily resectable should generally have a primary resection for staging and to establish both the diagnosis and the biologic risk factors of the tumor. In many children with small tumors and favorable biologic factors, surgery is the only therapy required. Resection is generally accepted before administration of chemotherapy for most thoracic, pelvic, and cervical primaries and limited abdominal lesions that do not extend across the midline. This approach is used to avoid the toxicity of chemotherapy, and in many patients with low-stage favorable biology tumors, resection alone is curative. In those situations where resection would entail removal of vital organs or where there is extensive lymph-node extension, preliminary treatment with adjuvant chemotherapy, particularly in the biologically adverse tumors, would be most appropriate. In patients with favorable biologic features, even subtotal resection may be the only therapy required.[63]

Of note, however, is the report by Nuchtern and colleagues[64] documenting the results of the COG trial on expectant management in infants (younger than age 6 months) with small adrenal masses. Eighty-seven cases were enrolled, and four patients were elected for upfront surgery. Of the remaining cohort, only 16 other patients had their adrenal lesions resected, with neuroblastoma diagnosed in 10 children, low-grade adrenocortical tumors in two, adrenal hemorrhage in two, and extrapulmonary pulmonary sequestrations in two. The overall, 3-year survival rate in the entire cohort was 100%, with a neuroblastoma event-free survival (EFS) of almost 98%. These results are quite encouraging in defining a cohort of children who can be spared any treatment for small adrenal-based neuroblastomas, but the suitable application of these data to nonadrenal primary sites, larger tumors, and in older children remains to be determined.

Regrettably, the majority of infants and children have metastatic disease at diagnosis. In these cases, the diagnosis and biologic features must be established. Tissue may be obtained by either laparotomy or thoracotomy, as well as by laparoscopy and thoracoscopy. In older patients with metastatic disease where Shimada staging is not required to determine the patient's treatment, needle biopsy from either bone marrow or the primary metastatic tumor provides adequate material for both pathology and biologic grading. For patients in whom the Shimada criteria are critical to determine their therapeutic treatment, open or minimal access surgery is required to obtain adequate tissue.

In patients with extensive abdominal primary tumors, adjuvant therapy has been useful. It is well recognized by surgeons that preoperative chemotherapy decreases the vascularity and friability of the tumor and facilitates resection, particularly in developing the dissection plane between the tumor and the great vessels.[65] Lymph-node involvement surrounding the aorta, vena cava, and renal vessels is often seen in children with advanced stage abdominal adrenal or paravertebral primaries (Fig. 49-15).

Although two studies have shown no difference in the surgical complication rate between initial and postinduction resection, others have demonstrated a higher incidence of complications, including nephrectomy in the group undergoing primary resection.[66,67,68-71] Furthermore in patients with high-risk tumors who often require autologous bone-marrow transplant, preservation of the ipsilateral kidney during the resection is critical.[72] A neoadjuvant approach has contributed to decreased operative complications requiring nephrectomy.[73]

A multiinstitutional review of children treated over an 11-year interval demonstrated a 14.9% incidence of nephrectomy or renal infarction as a result of surgery for local control (52 of 349 children). There was a 25% incidence among those with initial resection (29 children) and a 9.9% incidence in the postchemotherapy resection (23 children). Children with initial resection had more than a twofold increase in their risk of nephrectomy. Hence the approach for neuroblastoma regarding primary lesions is quite different from that in Wilms tumor. The other determining factor is that the pathologic staging information is not as critical for determining local control in neuroblastoma as in Wilms tumor, and essentially all of these children with large primary lesions require adjuvant chemotherapy and radiation. Hence administration preoperatively in no way increases the chance that chemotherapy will be required and is generally recommended in most current protocols.

Of note, however, is the report from Simon and colleagues[74] reporting the results of the German cooperative trial NB97 that evaluated the role of surgery (upfront and postneoadjuvant therapy) in patients older than 18 months with stage IV disease. In this study, 278 patients were evaluated, and their data report that neither upfront surgery nor operations performed postneoadjuvant chemotherapy positively impacted EFS, local progression-free survival (LPFS), or overall survival (OS). They concluded their manuscript by calling into question the role and utility of surgery in this patient cohort secondary to the lack of compelling data supporting effective local control or survival rates. Obviously, more data are required to definitively answer these questions.

Hepatoblastoma

Surgery is the cornerstone in the treatment of hepatoblastoma, and children are rarely cured without resection. Neoadjuvant and adjuvant chemotherapy facilitates its feasibility and success. Historically, resection with complete removal of all radiographically identifiable disease cured only 25% of children; 50% of children who presented with hepatoblastoma had resectable lesions, and of those only 50% survived.[75,76] Failure was attributed to occult metastatic disease not identified radiographically,[77] and Weinblatt and colleagues[78] reported the early success of neoadjuvant chemotherapy to convert unresectable liver tumors to resectable lesions with more than 75% of the lesions becoming resectable in both series (Fig. 49-16).

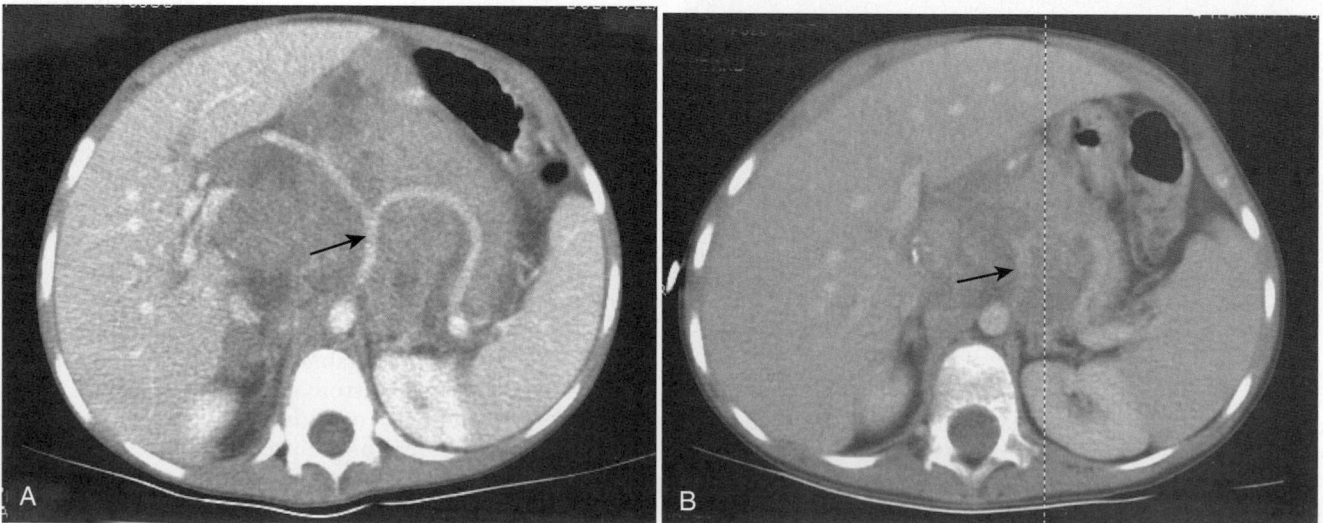

Figure 49-15 Four-year old with bone pain and palpable abdominal mass. Computed tomography (CT) showed an extensive mass arising from the adrenal gland (**A**). This scan shows extensive involvement of the lymph nodes around the aorta with the celiac axis projecting anteriorly surrounded by tumor. In this section, the splenic artery as well as the hepatic artery are demonstrated surrounded by tumor. Subsequent CT (**B**) after four courses of multiagent chemotherapy revealed marked resolution in the size of the mass, although it still surrounded the celiac axis (*arrow*).

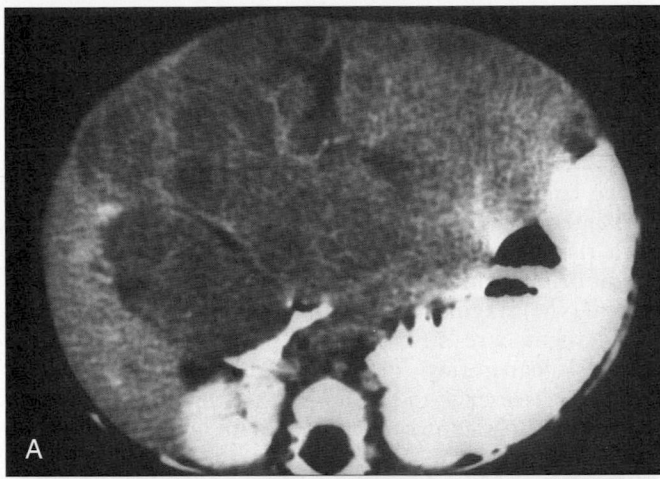

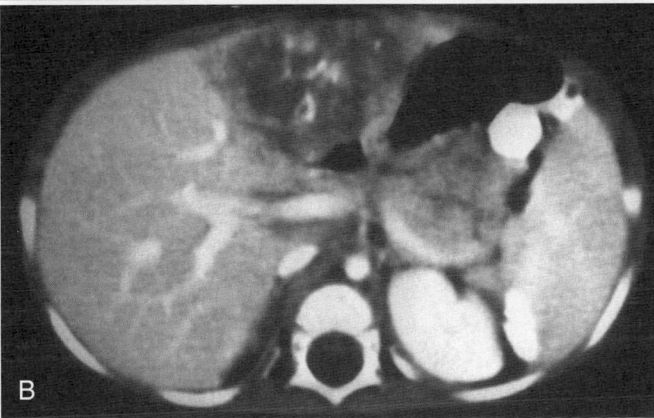

Figure 49-16 A 9-month old female with a palpable abdominal mass extending to below her umbilicus. **A**, Computed tomography (CT) scan revealed an extensive mass in her liver. **B**, CT scan after four courses of chemotherapy showed remarkable resolution of the mass that was subsequently resected by a left trisegmentectomy.

Only children with tumors with pure fetal histology do not require adjuvant therapy.[79] Subsequent reports document the utility of various chemotherapeutic regimens in hepatoblastoma to treat unresectable lesions or residual disease.[80-83,84-86] These reports establish the efficacy of doxorubicin, cisplatin, vincristine, and 5-fluorouracil alone or in various combinations. Cisplatin has been shown to be as efficacious as cisplatin with doxorubicin for standard-risk hepatoblastoma.[87] Furthermore both adjuvant and neoadjuvant regimens in combination with surgery achieved survival rates greater than 65% and tumor response rates greater than 90%. Although the regimens varied, most patients received at least two cycles before definitive surgery. The extent of tumor necrosis has also been shown to predict survival, as does negative surgical margins.[88] The critical need for resection of the primary tumor before the development of chemoresistance was demonstrated by von Schweinitz and colleagues.[84] They documented tumor regrowth as early as after the fourth course of therapy in 6 of 11 patients. Five-year survival rates for all patients with hepatoblastoma increased in just 2 decades to over 85% with the use of neoadjuvant and adjuvant chemotherapy.

Since 2000, a defined treatment protocol consisting of neoadjuvant chemotherapy and surgical resection or early orthotopic transplant evaluation for those patients with tumors that are too extensive to resect has been developed and reported by the SIOP Liver Tumor Group (SIOPEL).[89,90] This regimen was termed *PLADO,* and it consisted of a pretreatment imaging-defined staging protocol (PRETEXT), pretreatment diagnostic biopsy (core needle or incisional biopsy), neoadjuvant chemotherapy of continuous infusion cisplatin (day 1) followed by continuous infusion of doxorubicin (days 2 and 3), surgical resection after 4 to 6 cycles 12 to 20 weeks from diagnosis, and orthotopic liver transplant (OLTX) evaluation and referral for tumors confined to the liver that remained unresectable despite chemotherapy. The only tumors resected primarily were those deemed to be confined to a single section of the liver (i.e., right anterior, right posterior, left medial, left lateral; PRETEXT stage I). The overall 5-year survival rate was 75% for the entire cohort and 85% for those following the complete protocol, including neoadjuvant chemotherapy regardless of PRETEXT stage. PRETEXT stages I through IV had OS rates of 100%, 91%, 58%, and 57%, respectively, which compares favorably with survival rates achieved by Ortega and colleagues[91] through a CCG/POG cooperative trial comparing multimodality treatment protocols utilizing different chemotherapeutic regimens. Surgical mortality was 6%, and overall mortality was 24%. Twenty percent of patients had pulmonary metastases. Ninety-two percent of patients had a complete resection with this protocol, and there were 10 patients who relapsed: five with local recurrences and five with pulmonary metastases. SIOPEL's use of OLTX as primary treatment for local control was published by Otte and colleagues.[92] Those patients whose tumors involved all sectors of the liver or were intimately involved with either the hepatic or portal veins but had no evidence of metastatic disease and demonstrated some response to neoadjuvant chemotherapy were considered for a primary OLTX. Another cohort of patients who had intrahepatic recurrences of disease after resection or incomplete resections was eligible for rescue OLTX. Ten-year survival rates for the primary and rescue OLTX groups were 85% and 40%, respectively. The authors advocated, based on their results, for the following: 1) total resection of all gross disease including the retrohepatic vena cavae if needed; 2) the use of preoperative chemotherapy to control extrahepatic micrometastases and promote primary tumor regression; 3) transplantation for patients with synchronous pulmonary metastases if they had responded to neoadjuvant therapy; 4) no transplantation for those patients with evidence of metastatic disease present at surgery; 5) limiting the interval between diagnosis and OLTX to account for the rise of chemoresistance and the availability of donors (cadaveric or living); and 5) questioning the need of post-OLTX chemotherapy in the setting of a patient with immunosuppression. Although their cohort was small (12), they reviewed the world's experience with OLTX for hepatoblastoma in the same report, and the results were similar. As a corollary to this report, Austin and colleagues[93] reported on the experience of the United Network of Organ Sharing (UNOS) for 152 OLTXs performed in 135 patients in the setting of hepatoblastoma. Their actuarial 1-, 5-, and 10-year survival rates were 79%, 69%, and 66%, respectively. More than 54% of patients died of recurrent disease, and the only statistically significant predictors of favorable outcome were the preoperative condition of the patient (intensive care unit [ICU] hospitalization versus non-ICU hospitalization versus no hospitalization) and the era when the patient received the transplant (before or after December 31, 1994). These reports document not only the feasibility but also the success of OLTX as a component in the multimodality treatment of hepatoblastoma.

Rhabdomyosarcoma

Except for Wilms tumor, no other pediatric solid tumor has benefited so greatly from the combined efforts of oncologists of all disciplines in forming multimodality protocols designed to adequately diagnose, stage, and treat a lesion as has rhabdomyosarcoma. The 5-year survival rate of children with this disease was less than 25% before 1972 when the IRS study group was formed.[93,94] During the next 3 decades, this figure has increased almost threefold to 70%.[95-97] Because rhabdomyosarcoma is a tumor of mesenchymal origin, it may appear almost anywhere in the body and from almost any organ. Treatment protocols and outcomes vary greatly depending on the site and stage of the tumor. Initial pretreatment evaluations document the characteristics of the primary lesions and the regional lymph-node basins. If an extremity lesion is excised with positive margins and proves to be a rhabdomyosarcoma, it has been shown that pretreatment reexcision with generous margins (0.5 cm or greater) of uninvolved tissues and local lymph node sampling results in improved survival.[98] Debilitating resections producing loss of function are not currently warranted, except in cases with residual disease after adjuvant radiotherapy and chemotherapy. Regional and distant lymphadenopathy diagnosed clinically or radiographically must be biopsied to establish the presence or absence of tumor that will impact treatment strategies and prognosis.[99] Aggressive lymphadenectomies are not warranted, but a stepwise progression of draining lymph-node basins should be sampled to determine the lymph-node status of these contiguous basins and hence the extent of regional radiotherapy. Finally, so called "second-look" operations performed on the primary site in IRS III proved useful in the excision of residual tumor, the confirmation of the effectiveness of adjuvant therapies, and the improved prognosis of all tumors except for pelvic sites that had a pathologically confirmed complete response to therapy.[100] These principles of complete resection of the primary tumor and lymph-node biopsy determine postoperative clinical groupings that determine adjuvant treatment therapies and prognosis.

Radiotherapy is a core modality of treatment for local control, and its field is based on the size of the mass before resection. Patients receive a radiation field with at least a 2-cm margin around the primary mass. Therapy is generally begun 8 to 12 weeks after initiation of chemotherapy and continues for 5 to 6 weeks. All histopathologic subtypes except group I embryonal disease receive radiation therapy.[97] All other groups and rhabdomyosarcoma variants receive at least 4000 rads for microscopic residual disease and as much as 5000 rads for macroscopic residual disease,[97,101,102] providing a strong basis for primary resection if safely feasible.

Adjuvant chemotherapy is critical, and its use is based on a risk stratification schema that incorporates tumor site of origin, tumor histopathology, tumor-nodes-metastasis (TNM) staging, and the postoperative clinical grouping. Patients are stratified into low-, intermediate- or high-risk categories. Patients with low risk typically receive a three-drug regimen of vincristine, dactinomycin, and cyclophosphamide. Patients with intermediate risk generally receive the same three-drug regimen, but those with tumors from favorable sites and those with completely resected tumors from unfavorable sites receive dose-intensified cyclophosphamide.[102] Patients at high risk, however, should receive a two-drug regimen of ifosfamide with etoposide or doxorubicin.[103,104] Patients with metastatic disease or alveolar subtypes should also receive topotecan or irinotecan in addition to standard therapy.[105,106] Ideally, neoadjuvant chemotherapy can reduce tumor burden and convert unresectable lesions to resectable ones with decreased patient morbidity (Fig. 49-17).

Osteosarcoma, Ewing Sarcoma

The single most important factor in improved survival for patients with osteosarcoma (OSA) or Ewing sarcoma (EWS) has been the development of effective chemotherapy. Before 1970, patients with OSA had an OS of around 10%. Before the 1960s, survival was even less than 10% for patients with EWS. Ablative surgery and/or radiation were the only modalities available at that time. Local control, however, was not the issue. Patients succumbed primarily from metastatic disease that was believed to be present at diagnosis, although it could not be demonstrated radiographically. Systemic treatment was necessary to achieve improved survival and cure. Medications were identified and successfully applied in cooperative multiinstitutional trials. With modern chemotherapy protocols, OS for OSA is now 60% or better and approaches 60% for EWS.

Current protocols for OSA involve neoadjuvant chemotherapy, surgery, and then further adjuvant chemotherapy. Protocols are similar for EWS except that radiation can be used in combination with surgery or alone as local treatment. The advantages of this approach are that tumor cells in the primary tumor and in micrometastatic form are treated immediately and that histologic response to the chemotherapy can be assessed. The potential advantage of making limb salvage surgery safer is debatable, but certainly, any reduction in size of the primary tumor improves the feasibility of surgical resection (Fig. 49-18). The disadvantages are that in patients who do not respond to the usual drugs, their disease may progress, and drug resistance may develop. Because response to chemotherapy has been identified as one of the more important prognostic factors with potential

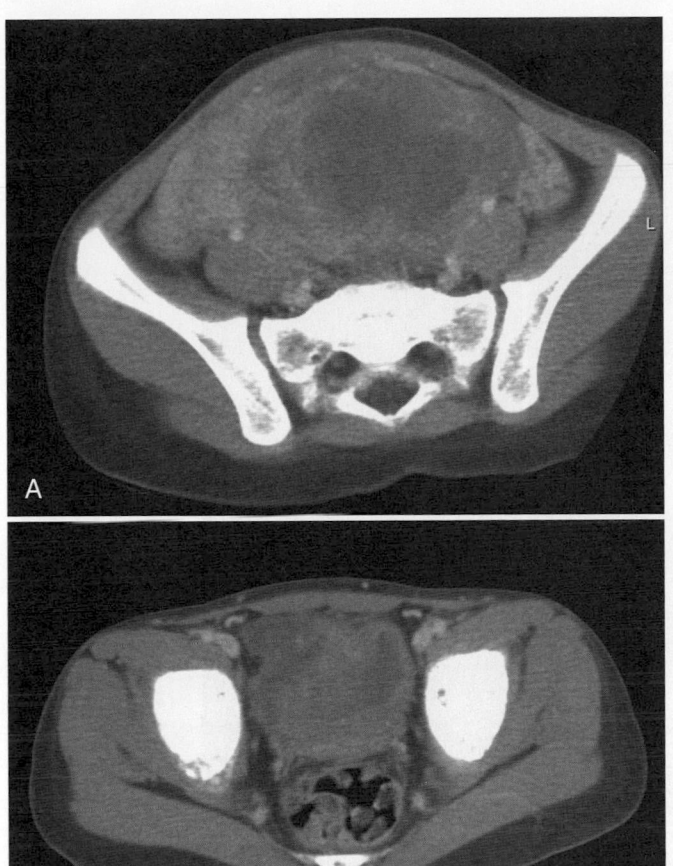

Figure 49-17 A, A 7-year-old with a large bladder rhabdomyosarcoma prechemotherapy. **B,** A significant decrease in the size of the tumor.

is not precisely known,[108-112] but at a minimum there should not be "ink on tumor." While experience with these operations grows, most surgeons now accept soft-tissue margins of 2 to 5 mm of normal soft tissue and 1 to 2 cm of marrow margin, but there is no evidence-based minimum margin that has been documented to be safe with respect to local recurrence. Neoadjuvant chemotherapy probably lessens the likelihood of a local recurrence.[113-116] Recent data would suggest that a wide margin in a patient with a good response to chemotherapy has a low likelihood of local recurrence.[117,118,119] Resections with a narrower margin (marginal or intralesional) and/or those with a poor response to chemotherapy have a higher risk of local recurrence. It is clear that a local recurrence is associated with a poor prognosis for survival.[120-123]

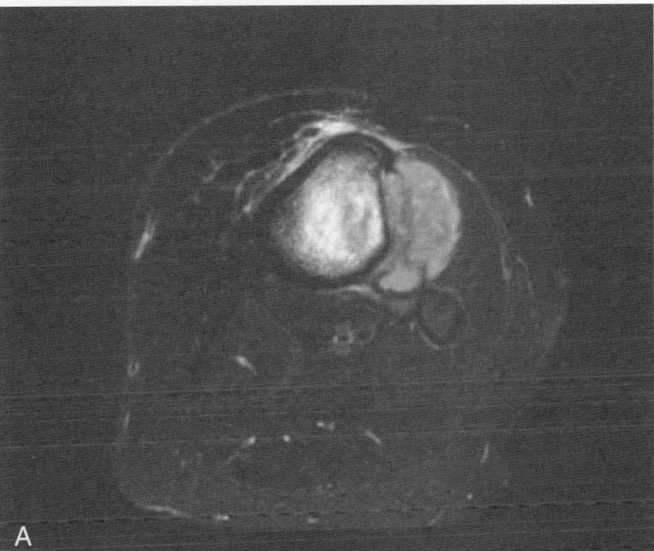

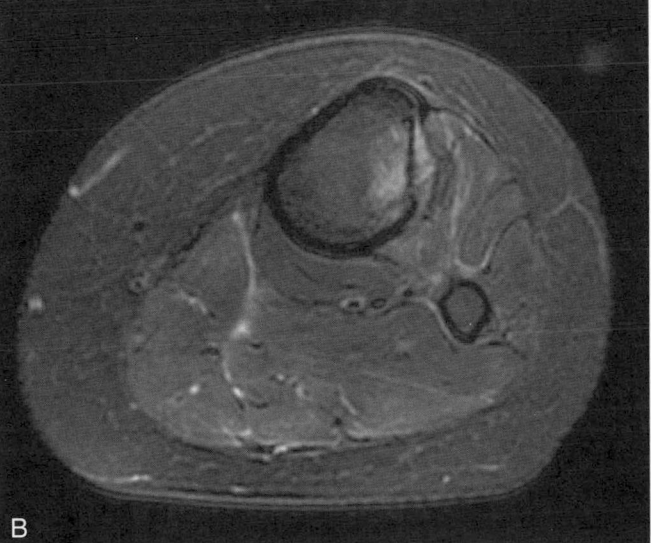

Figure 49-18 Ewing sarcoma of the proximal tibia: T2-weighted sequence with fat saturation, axial magnetic resonance imaging. **A,** At initial diagnosis; note the large anterolateral soft-tissue extension outside of the bone. **B,** After neoadjuvant chemotherapy, the soft-tissue mass has noticeably decreased in size, making surgery, especially dissection around the arterial trifurcation, less difficult.

implications for changes in therapy, this overall approach is used in the majority of trials. The reality, though, is that no new drugs or changes in therapy have been shown to improve survival to any great extent in poor responders. Efforts to improve survival for poor responders and for patients who relapse are the focus of current protocols and research.

LIMB SALVAGE PROCEDURES

Surgical Principles

The surgical treatment of bone sarcomas has evolved from the prechemotherapy era where all patients had amputations, radiation therapy, or both, to the current practice where 80% of patients or more receive a limb-salvage resection.[107] The resection can be thought of in two phases: wide resection of the tumor and involved bone and the reconstruction, for which there are multiple alternatives. A "safe" resection requires complete excision of the involved bone and soft tissues with a cuff of normal tissue surrounding the entire specimen, a so-called *wide margin*. The necessary thickness of this cuff of tissue and the length of normal marrow away from the tumor

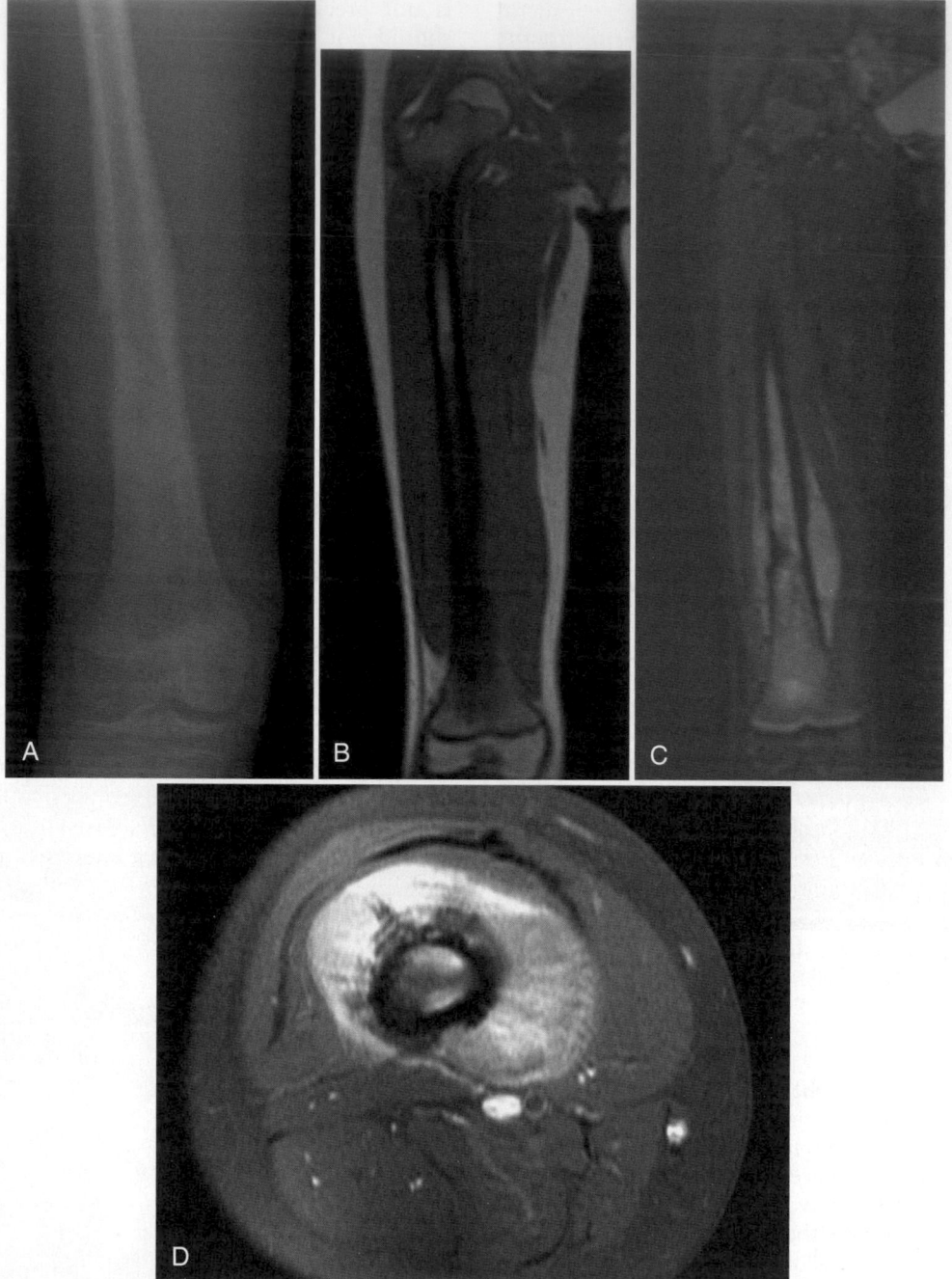

Figure 49-19 **A,** Osteosarcoma of the femur showing ill-defined bone destruction in the metaphysis and soft tissue mass. **B,** Coronal T1-weighted images show the extent of the tumor in the medullary canal. **C** and **D,** Coronal and axial images show the extent of the soft-tissue mass and the relationship to the femoral artery and vein.

The decision of resection versus amputation and the type of reconstruction requires careful evaluation of the imaging studies with a multidisciplinary team that includes an experienced musculoskeletal radiologist and a detailed discussion with the patient and family regarding the alternatives. Although most patients would prefer to save their limb if possible, it should be understood that current reconstruction options cannot restore a normal limb and most are not meant to return the patient to athletic activities. Patients with lower-extremity

primary tumors who want to continue contact and running sports are better served with an amputation or rotationplasty.

The resection requires a careful analysis of the radiograph and MRI. The entire bone should be imaged to exclude the possibility of skip metastases. MRI is the best study to assess the extent of the tumor within the bone and soft tissue (Fig. 49-19).[124-128] OSAs may cross growth plates to involve the epiphysis of the bone, but they rarely cross the articular cartilage unless there has been a fracture.[124,126] Adjacent joint involvement is rare, but if present it requires an extraarticular resection. Tumors may enter the joint by extending along the joint capsule (e.g., in the proximal humerus the metaphysis is partially intraarticular) or cruciate ligaments (knee) or ligamentum teres (hip). The major nerves and vessels must be uninvolved or resectable to achieve the required margin. Finally, there must be sufficient muscle remaining after the resection to allow soft-tissue coverage of the reconstruction and to power the limb. At times rotational flaps or free-tissue transfers may be indicated to obtain soft-tissue coverage and lessen the chance of a wound complication.[129,130] For all resection types, infection is the worst immediate complication and its incidence can be lessened with adequate soft-tissue closure.

Once the resection has been completed, the pathologist should examine the specimen grossly to ensure complete resection. The use of frozen section analysis of the marrow margins is a routine and accepted practice but is of uncertain value.[131] Bisecting the specimen with a band saw and visualizing it will reassure the surgeon that an adequate resection has been accomplished.

Types of Reconstruction in Children

Reconstruction options include the use of metallic endoprostheses, bone allografts, and rotationplasty. Some sites require no bony reconstruction. These "expendable" bones include the fibula, clavicle, rib, and iliac wing (if the acetabulum can be preserved). Most OSAs are located about the knee, hip, and shoulder and involve resection of the distal femoral, proximal tibial, proximal femoral, or proximal humeral metaphysis and epiphysis. In addition to the bony defect, a major growth center is included that in the lower extremity adds complexity to the reconstruction not encountered in adults. For patients close to skeletal maturity (10 to 12 years old in girls and 14 to 16 years in boys) this is seldom a major issue and can be addressed by reconstructing with a slightly longer implant than the length resected. Limb-length discrepancies of 2 cm or less are seldom a clinical problem and can be treated with a simple shoe lift. For tumors around the knee in younger patients, limb length must be addressed by the reconstruction chosen. The alternatives include the use of an expandable prosthesis, bone allografts, and rotationplasty. Each has advantages and disadvantages. An expandable prosthesis in theory allows "growth" of the prosthesis over time but will need to be revised to an adult prosthesis at skeletal maturity.[132-136] Some of these prostheses require several operations to achieve lengthening,[136] whereas others have nonoperative mechanisms of expansion.[132] They are expensive, complex prostheses with many potential complications. Children younger than 8 years of age have difficulty cooperating with physical therapy, so joint contractures are a problem. In addition, mechanical failure of the prosthesis, metal debris, loosening, and infection can be significant problems.[137] Bone allografts have the advantage of preserving the adjacent bone and its growth plate (i.e., the proximal tibia can be preserved after distal femoral resection) but obviously have no capacity to grow. There are also issues of finding an allograft of appropriate size and shape, but if

a suitable bone is available, length equalization can be addressed by inserting a graft 1 to 2 cm longer than the length resected and addressing limb length subsequently with standard pediatric orthopaedic techniques of contralateral epiphyseodesis. At skeletal maturity, closed femoral shortening and limb-lengthening techniques are also available. Rotationplasty addresses this issue because the prosthesis can be adjusted to the desired length while the child grows.

Bone Allografts

Bone allografts are used to reconstruct defects primarily at the distal femur, proximal tibia, proximal femur, and proximal humerus.[138-142] The obvious concern is transmission of bacterial and viral disease, but bone banks are now accredited by the American Association of Tissue Banks, and the safety record of these grafts is quite good since better testing for human immunodeficiency virus (HIV) and hepatitis became available.[143-145] The advantages in young patients are that they are intended to restore bone stock and joint structures (articular cartilage, ligaments, and joint capsule) and delay the need for metallic prostheses. In theory they restore bone stock, but experience has shown that the grafts are only partially replaced by host bone, and it is likely that most patients who receive osteoarticular grafts will require a joint arthroplasty at some point (5 to 20 years from the index procedure). Delaying artificial joints until adulthood is probably advantageous for long-term salvage of the limb; however, these secondary operations are challenging as well.[116] In a young child a major advantage of osteoarticular allografts is the avoidance of resection or placing an implant across the adjacent growth plate. These are complex operations, and they require the availability of a tissue bank and surgical expertise with the use of allografts. The procedure is associated with a significant complication rate. Infection, reported in the 0% to 20% range,[138-142] is the worst complication and usually requires removal of the graft. Nonunion of the allograft–host junction (reported to occur overall in 17%) is higher (27%) in patients receiving chemotherapy[147] but can usually be addressed by revision of the fixation and bone grafting of the osteosynthesis site. Fracture is a later complication and occurs in about 15% of patients.[138,140-142,147-149] Occasionally the fracture heals with conservative means, but more often revision to another allograft, augmentation with a vascularized fibular graft,[150] or conversion to an endoprostheses is required.[151] Postoperative management includes closed suction drains for 24 to 48 hours, preoperative and postoperative antibiotic coverage (there are no data regarding the necessary length of antibiotic coverage), venous thrombosis prophylaxis, and initial immobilization. Physical therapy to start joint motion is begun after 6 weeks, and the limbs are protected with crutches and bracing until the osteosynthesis site heals (approximately 6 to 9 months in patients getting chemotherapy).

Endoprostheses

Metallic prostheses were initially custom made to fit the expected bone resection defect. There are a number of available modular systems that allow the surgeon to

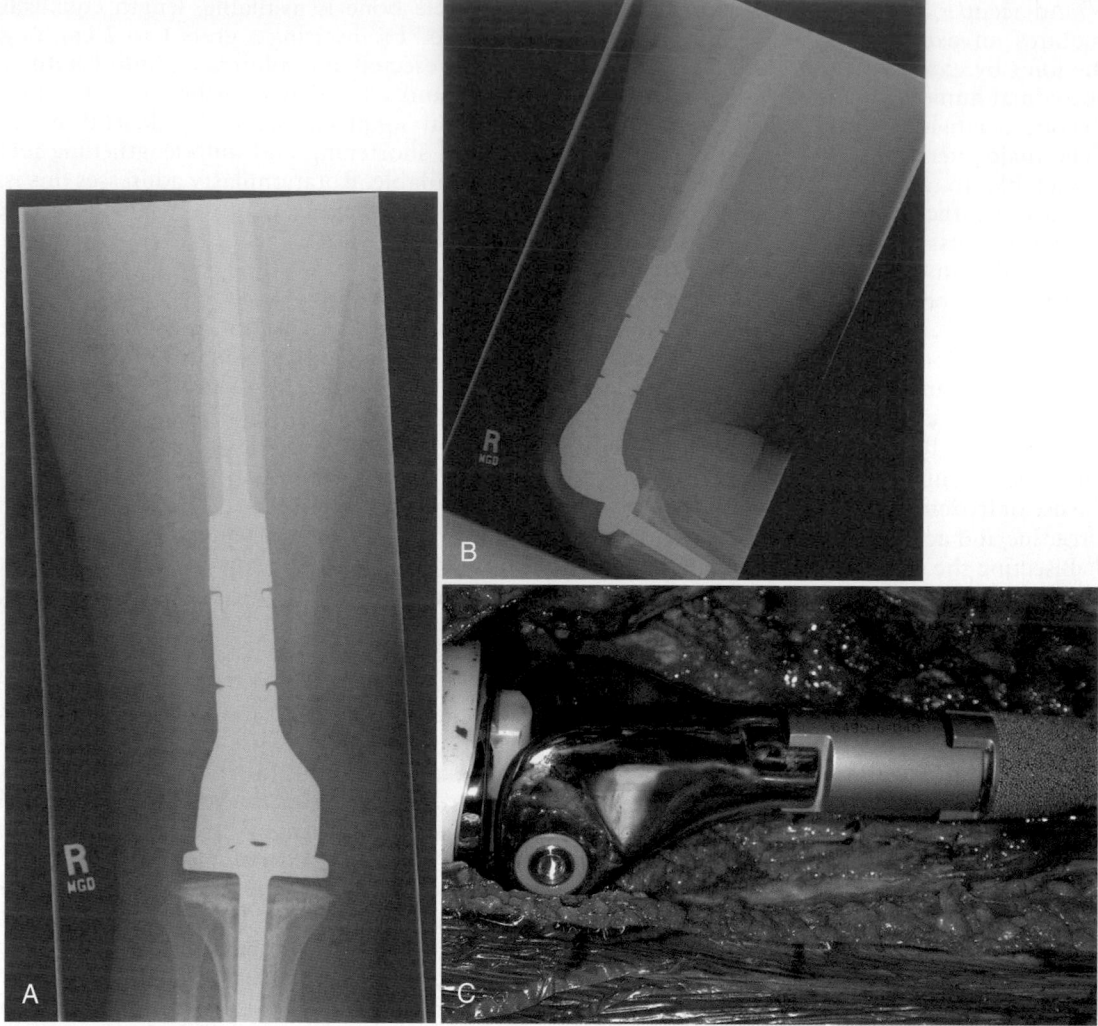

Figure 49-20 **A** and **B**, Anteroposterior and lateral views of a modular tumor prosthesis used to reconstruct after a resection for distal femoral osteosarcoma. A rotating hinge design is used, and the modular nature of the prosthesis can be appreciated. **C**, The prosthesis after insertion during the operation.

reconstruct the defect at the operating table.[152-159] In older children close to skeletal maturity, adult prostheses can be used. Most reconstructions around the knee use a rotating hinge construct that reduces the forces that are transmitted to the host-prosthesis interface, and this design is believed to increase the longevity of the implants because of delayed loosening of the stems. Modern stem designs include the option of cemented or uncemented stems, and in the femur there are curved and straight stem designs. In theory, uncemented stems offer the advantage of avoiding osteolysis and loosening, but whether bony ingrowth is reduced in patients receiving adjuvant therapies is uncertain at this time.[154,155,160,161] The main advantage to endoprostheses is that they are as stable and functional as they will ever be as soon as the wound heals, so return to function is more rapid than with allografts. Patients do not need to wait for an osteosynthesis to heal, and early weight bearing and range-of-motion exercises are permitted. The disadvantages include infection (although the reported rates are lower than with allografts), loosening or mechanical failure of the

implants, metal debris, and decreased longevity.[159,160,162-165] Because 70% to 80% of children with bone sarcomas now survive, it is unlikely that these implants will last the lifetime of the patient. Revision is possible, but multiple revisions over time may limit the options and lead to amputation. The longevity (not function) of the implants is about 60% to 80% at 5 years and 50% to 80% at 10 years for lower extremity implants depending on the specific series.* The expandable endoprostheses are more complex and likely to have a higher complication rate.[132-137,170-172]

Examples by Anatomic Site
Distal Femur and Proximal Tibia

Tumors around the knee can be reconstructed by any of these methods. A few examples will be provided. Figure 49-20 shows examples of an endoprosthesis of the distal

---

*References 136, 155, 157-163, 166-169.

femur. The implant is a modular prosthesis that is cemented into the remaining femur and proximal tibia after an intraarticular resection. Initial function of these constructs is quite good, but it is expected that loosening will occur sometime in the future. It is known from adult arthroplasty and the early experience using custom and modular prostheses that the interface between the cement and the bone will fail over time in part because of particulate debris and the biologic response to it. Design improvements such as ingrowth surfaces near the stem–implant junction that allow bony- or soft-tissue ingrowth may delay or prevent loosening.[166] Uncemented stems may also offer longevity advantages. A further concern is stress shielding. The stem takes the mechanical load from the adjacent bone, and the host responds by resorbing the cortical bone over time. The concern is that in future revisions, insufficient bone stock will remain. There are newer stem devices that load the bone to avoid stress shielding and offer the hope of more longevity. The early data from these stems is encouraging.[173] Unfortunately, there are no direct comparisons between osteoarticular allografts (Fig. 49-21) and endoprostheses at this site, but the current literature would suggest that for the distal femur, an endoprostheses is superior.[169] Some surgeons believe that in the skeletally immature, it is still advantageous to use allografts at this site for the reasons stated.

In the proximal tibia, an osteoarticular allograft offers the advantage of providing a site for attachment of the patellar tendon. This is much more difficult to achieve in an endoprostheses. As shown in Figure 49-22, an intraarticular proximal tibial resection is achieved including the host menisci (although they can be preserved depending on the extent of the tumor). The reconstruction allows repair of the cruciate ligaments, joint capsule, and patellar tendon. A gastrocnemius flap is sometimes required for soft-tissue coverage and is always required to augment soft-tissue attachment of the patellar tendon if an endoprostheses is used. Fixation is achieved with standard plates and screws used to treat fractures. Plates that span the entire length of the allograft or intramedullary fixation are desirable to lessen the fracture rate. Intramedullary rods require supplemental plate fixation to control rotation at the osteosynthesis site. Newer locking-plate designs may lessen the incidence of nonunion and fracture.[174] A variation of this construct is to combine an allograft and standard total knee prosthesis (allograft-prosthetic composite), usually a rotating hinge design for stability (Fig. 49-23). This approach allows a stable knee construct initially and a site for reattachment of the patella tendon. It has the disadvantage in a skeletally immature patient of placement of an implant across the adjacent (distal femoral) growth plate, creating a greater potential limb-length discrepancy.

A further option at the knee is an expandable prosthesis (Figs. 49-24 and 49-25). These can be used for the distal femur and proximal tibia. Many parents are now aware of these devices and are requesting them, but their long-term outcome is still uncertain. One could argue that an attempt at this is reasonable if the alternative is amputation or rotationplasty, planning to deal with complications later if the patient survives. The downside is that it restricts young children from normal activities including sports; if they pursue them, the likelihood of failure is higher.

Rotationplasty

For large tumors of the distal femur or very young patients with distal femoral sarcomas, rotationplasty is an excellent alternative to amputation.[175-177] A rotationplasty preserves the distal leg, foot, and ankle, and places it at the level of the contralateral knee (Fig. 49-26). The tibia replaces the femoral shaft, and by rotating the limb 180 degrees, the ankle and foot act like a knee, making the construct function like a below-knee amputation rather than a high-thigh amputation. A modification of this procedure can be performed for proximal tibial and proximal femoral sarcomas.[178-180] The margin achieved is wider than a standard resection, because with the exception of the sciatic nerve, no other structures need to be saved. The vessels can be dissected and coiled like the nerve at closure or resected and anastomosed after the osteosynthesis has been achieved. This procedure may be more suitable for patients with pathologic fracture because of the wider margin it achieves, but if the patient has a widely displaced fracture and a large sarcoma at diagnosis and requires spica immobilization during preoperative chemotherapy, there is a higher risk of the anastomosis failing because of venous congestion in the leg (personal observation). Rotationplasty has the advantage of avoiding phantom pain, because the sciatic nerve and its branches are preserved and growth is not an issue because the prosthesis can be adjusted as the patient grows. It usually requires a single operation with a low complication rate and allows the child to have full activities. The functional results are rewarding. The main drawback is the cosmetic appearance. Patients must be carefully selected, and it is essential that the child and parents meet a patient who has had a rotationplasty and work with an experienced therapist preoperatively so that they fully understand the operation. Many patients, parents, and surgeons refuse this option because it is distasteful, but those who accept it do extremely well functionally and emotionally. This has been documented in long-term studies.[175,181,182,183-187]

Proximal Femur

Resection of the proximal femur requires careful assessment of the hip joint (Figs. 49-27 and Fig. 49-28). If an intraarticular reconstruction can be achieved, the reconstruction options include either a metallic prosthesis or an allograft.[154,158,188,189] The likelihood that an allograft will fit perfectly into the acetabulum is low, so most allografts are used as allograft-prosthetic composites at this site. If the acetabulum requires resection, the reconstruction is much more complex. An allograft offers the theoretical advantage of a site for reattachment of the abductor muscles and lessening the abductor lurch during gait, but attaching the abductors to a metallic prosthesis or the iliotibial band has been shown to be quite successful and probably equivalent. The decision of whether to do a total hip prosthesis or a hemiarthroplasty is more difficult. Although the hemiarthroplasty is easier and

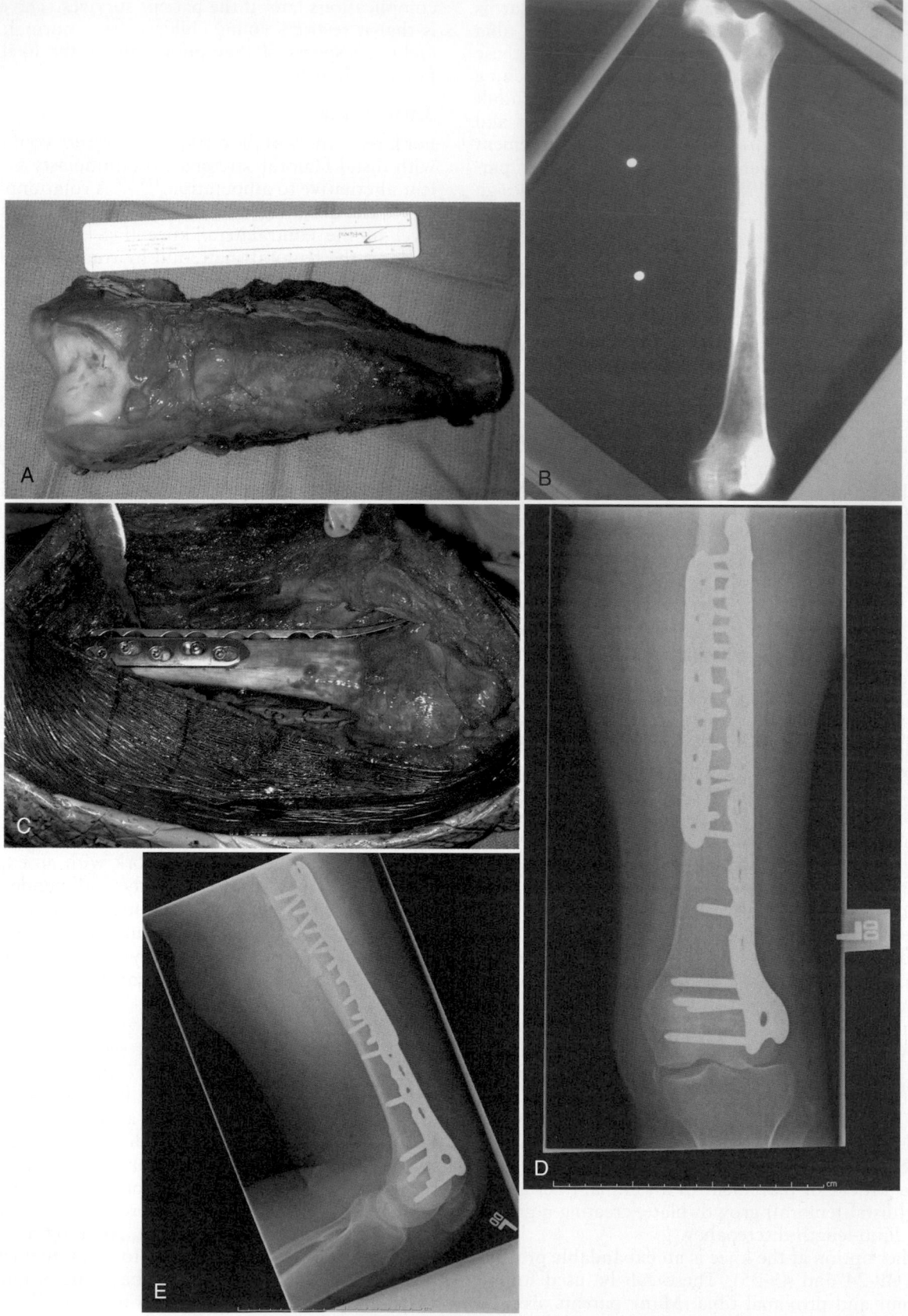

Figure 49-21 A, A resection specimen after intraarticular resection of the distal femur for osteosarcoma showing a margin of muscle surrounding the tumor. B, An osteoarticular allograft from a bone bank is thawed and then cut to fit the defect created. C, An intraoperative photograph shows the graft held in place with dynamic compression plates after ligament reconstruction. D and E, The postoperative appearance is shown on radiographs.

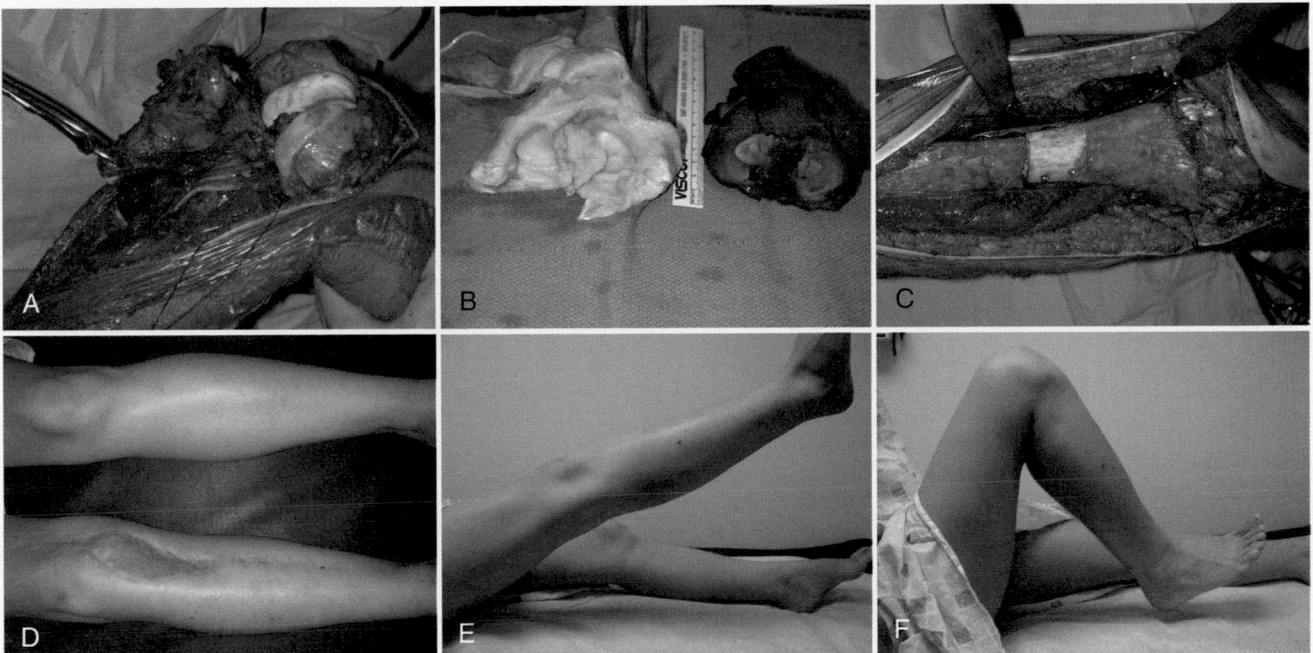

Figure 49-22 **A,** Resection of a proximal tibial osteosarcoma is shown with preservation of the tibial vessels and sacrifice of the menisci. **B,** Comparison of the resected specimen with menisci *(right)* to the allograft *(left)*. **C,** The allograft is in place after plate fixation and ligament reconstruction. The sutures in the patellar tendon are evident. **D,** The postoperative photograph shows a rotational gastrocnemius flap and skin graft. Function of a patient is demonstrated by full extension and straight leg raising (**E**) and the flexion arc (**F**).

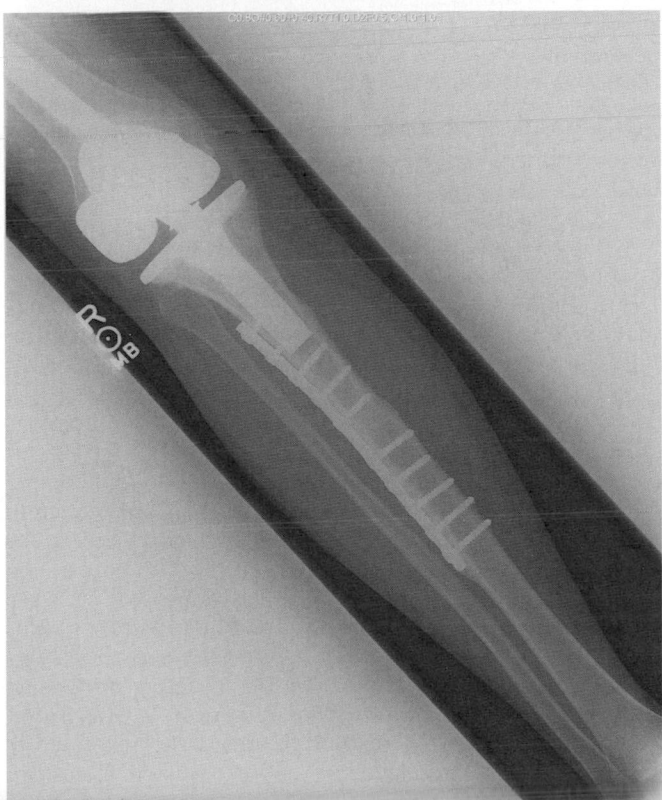

Figure 49-23 The radiographic appearance of an allograft prosthetic composite of the proximal tibia is shown.

more stable than a total hip arthroplasty, recent data in children suggest that these may subluxate as the child grows and the acetabulum develops, necessitating revision to a total-joint arthroplasty.[190]

Pelvis

In general, patients with sarcomas of the pelvis have a worse prognosis than those of the extremities.[191-196] Assessment of response to chemotherapy is critical. For EWS, the alternative of irradiation for local control is available, but for OSA surgical resection is required even if this means hemipelvectomy if the goal is cure. Resections are difficult and often require the expertise of the orthopaedic oncologist, a surgical oncologist, and at times a vascular surgeon or urologist. The site of the tumor is critical. Tumors of the iliac wing can be resected without much functional loss if the acetabulum can be preserved (Fig. 49-29). Bone grafts are sometimes used to restore the pelvic ring. Similarly tumors involving the pubic rami can be resected and require little reconstruction other than synthetic mesh to prevent herniation of the abdominal contents (Fig. 49-30). The difficult area is the acetabulum. Resection of the acetabulum or other areas of the pelvis that include the acetabulum result in complex reconstruction challenges. Often the best alternative is to leave the hip flail (Fig. 49-31). Significant shortening will occur, but function is better than an amputation even if a major nerve is sacrificed. Attempts at arthrodesis of the proximal femur to the remaining

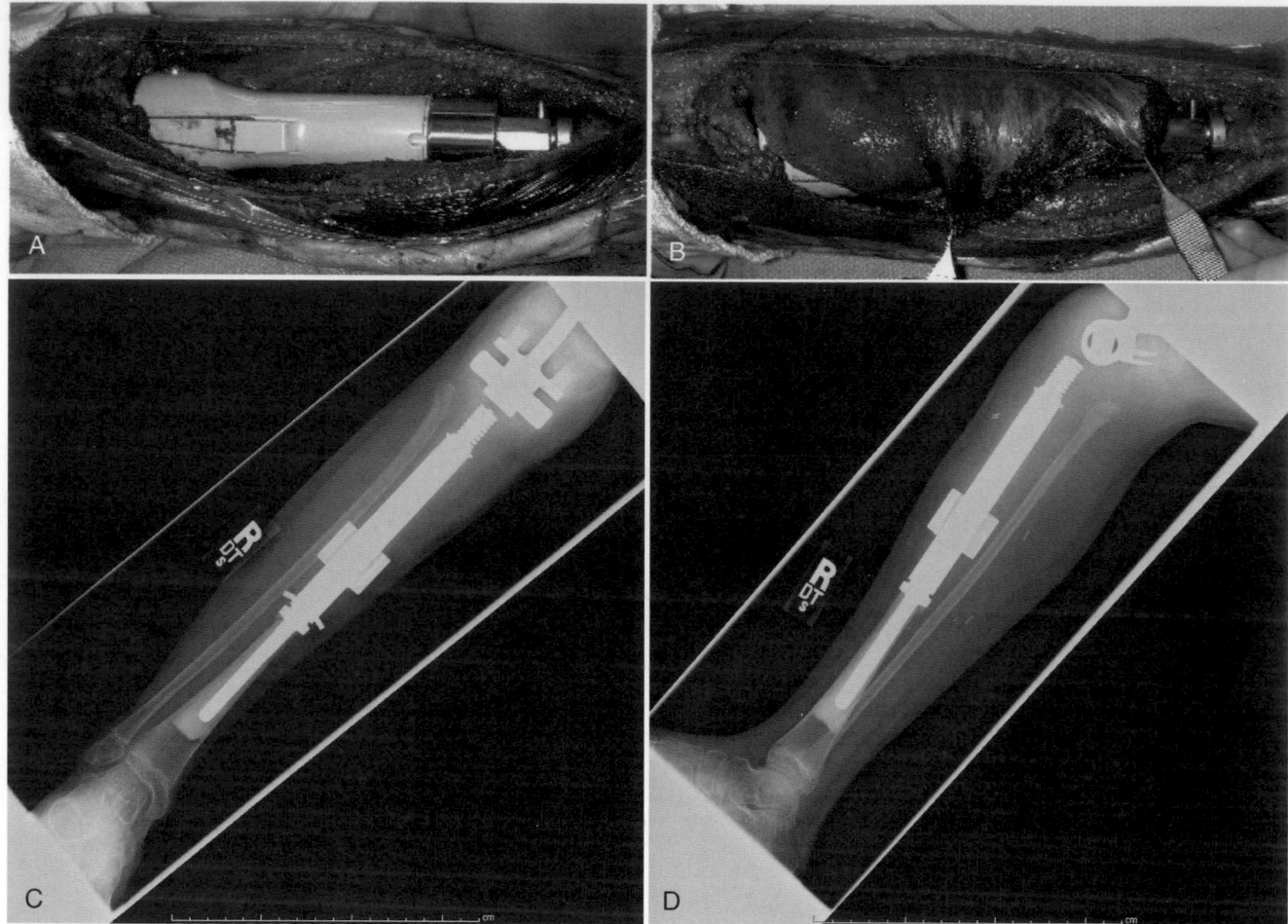

Figure 49-24 **A,** This is an example of an expandable prosthesis for the proximal tibia. The sutures for attachment of the patellar tendon are seen. **B,** The implant has been covered with a gastrocnemius and soleus flap that aid in anchoring of the patellar tendon and wound healing. This particular prosthesis allows lengthening without an operation. **C** and **D,** Anteroposterior and lateral views show the radiographic appearance of the prosthesis in place. The spring mechanism allows for the expansion after an electromagnetic field transiently melts a restraint to expansion.

pelvis can be considered but are very difficult to achieve. Allografts have been used, but are reported to have significant morbidity including a high infection rate and long-term mechanical problems such as fracture.[197-200] Custom metallic replacements have also been used,[201] but they require careful planning and have a high failure rate. All of these considerations are amplified if the adjacent sacrum requires resection as well. The multidisciplinary team and the family must have a careful discussion of the goals, resection options, reconstruction alternatives, and other treatment strategies before these pelvic resections are undertaken. Surgical expertise with the intraoperative and postoperative management of these patients is essential for success.

Proximal Humerus

All attempts should be made to avoid amputation in patients with upper extremity tumors. Unlike the lower extremity, there are no prostheses that replicate the function of the hand. Limb length in the upper extremity is usually not a major concern. A resection of the proximal humerus and scapula en bloc (Tikhoff-Linberg resection)

is preferable to a forequarter amputation and is usually possible.[202-207]

For those patients with proximal humeral sarcomas that are amenable to intraarticular resections, reconstruction can be accomplished with metallic prostheses (Fig. 49-32),[158,163,208-211] osteoarticular allografts (Fig. 49-33), or allograft-prosthetic composites.[138,212-214] Function is more a result of whether the deltoid, axillary nerve, and rotator cuff can be preserved. A flail shoulder is superior to an amputation if all these muscles must be resected. For high-grade sarcomas, the deltoid is often resected, but some active motion can be preserved if all or part of the rotator cuff can be preserved. Allografts provide sites for attachment of these motors, but metallic prostheses combined with synthetic materials around the prosthesis and synthetic suture materials can result in active motion as well. Even tumors that require resection of the radial nerve can be reconstructed and the resultant nerve deficit treated either by nerve graft or tendon transfers to restore radial nerve function in the hand. If the joint is involved, an extraarticular resection including the glenoid can be performed. The decision is between the above constructs

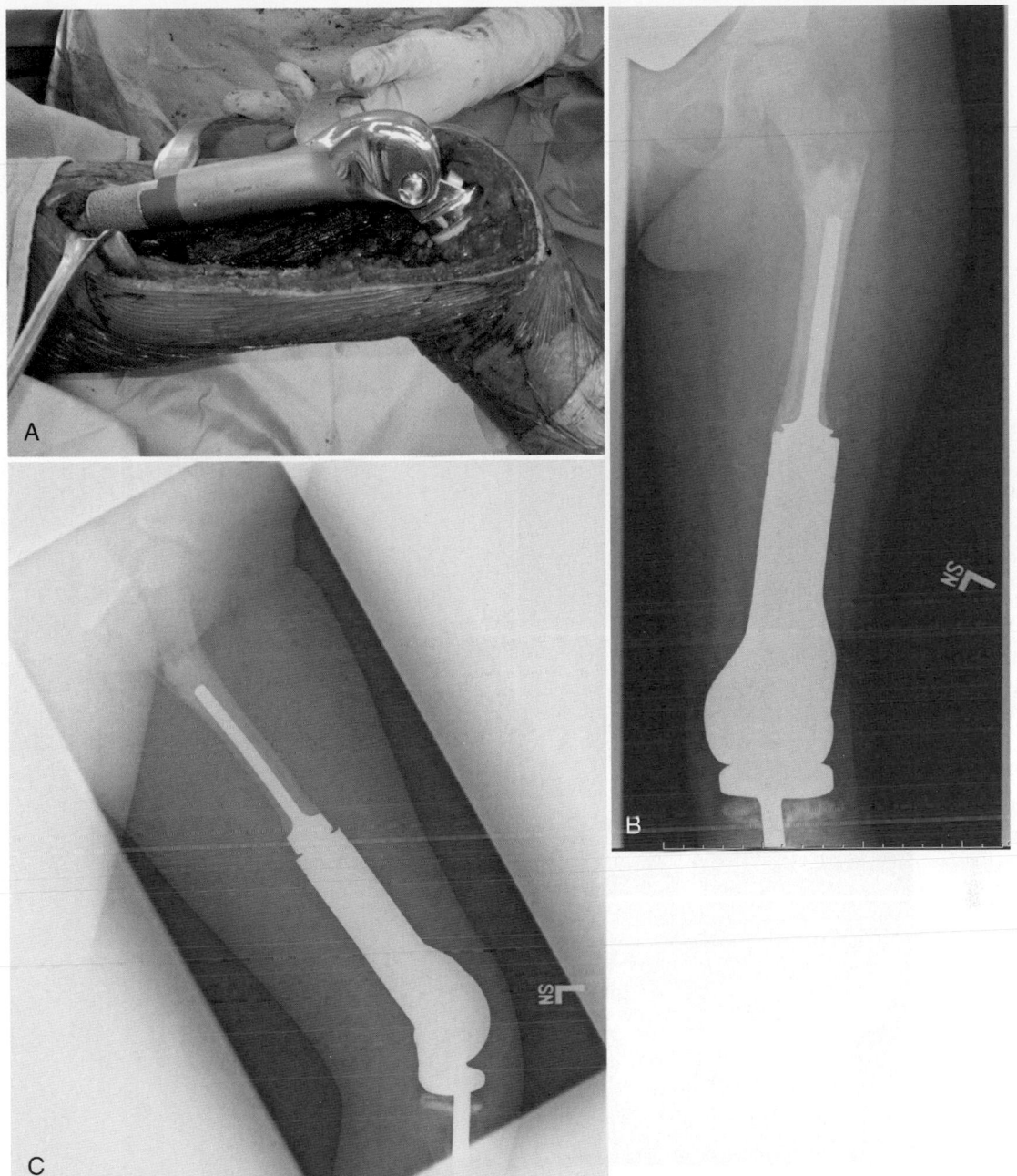

Figure 49-25 **A,** This figure shows the intraoperative appearance of another expandable prosthesis of the distal femur. This prosthesis requires an open procedure to lengthen it. **B** and **C,** The radiographic appearance of the prosthesis cemented in place. An uncemented smooth stem placed across the tibial physis allows that physis to grow.

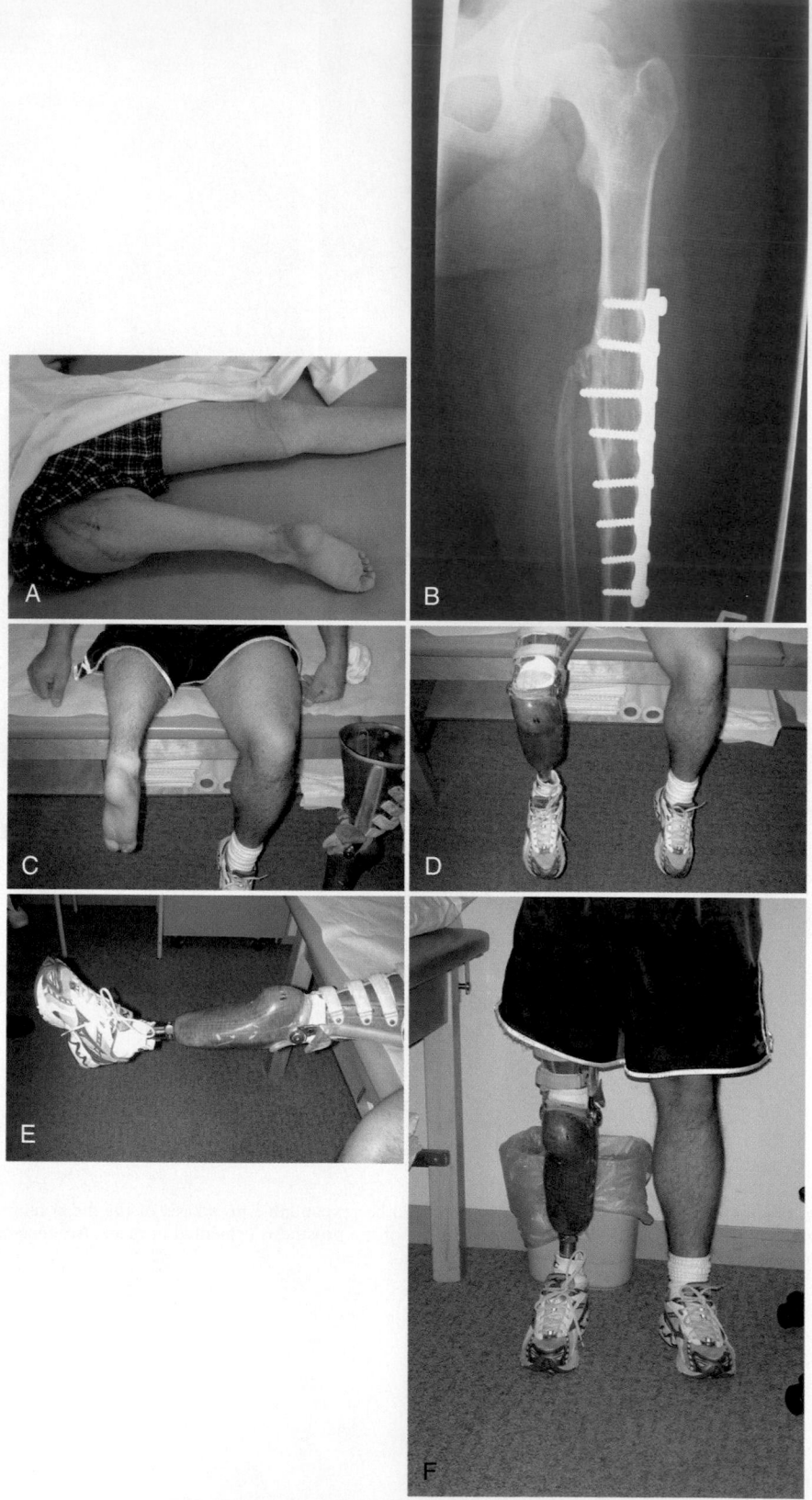

Figure 49-26 **A,** Patient with a rotationplasty for a distal femoral osteosarcoma. **B,** The radiographic appearance reveals the osteosynthesis of the tibia to the femur. **C** and **D,** These pictures show the appearance of the patient with the prosthesis off (**C**) and on (**D**). **E,** Patient has the ability to actively extend the knee against gravity. **F,** The appearance in stance.

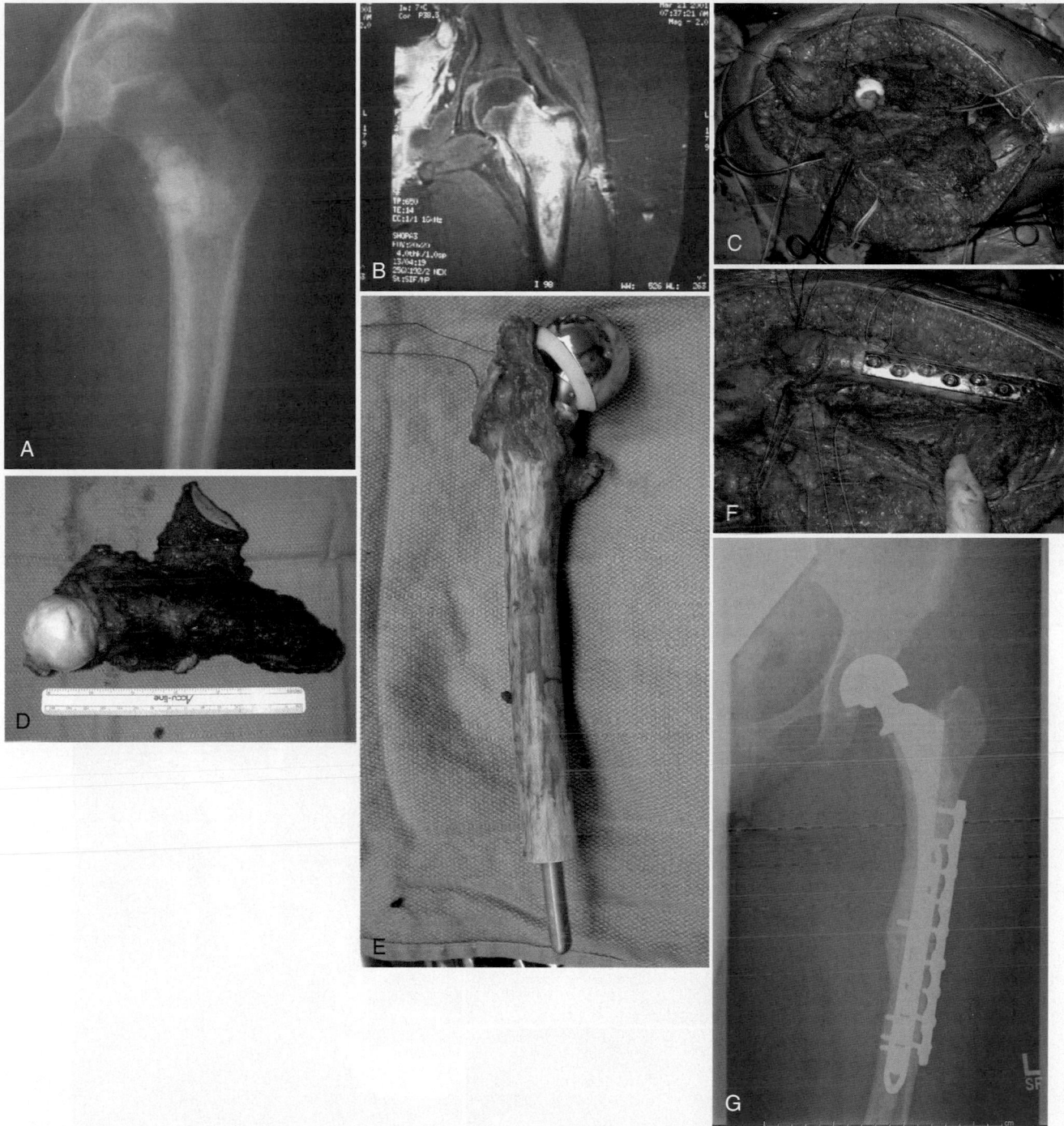

Figure 49-27 **A,** Radiograph of an osteosarcoma of the proximal femur. **B,** Magnetic resonance imaging shows that the hip joint is not involved. **C,** Intraoperative findings after resection. The acetabulum can be seen, and sutures are retracting the gluteus medius and minimus. **D,** The resected specimen is shown with the biopsy tract included. **E,** The allograft after a bipolar long-stem prosthesis has been cemented into it. **F,** Intraoperative photograph after the allograft has been fixed to the host bone. A unicortical plate is used for rotational control. The hip abductors have been sutured to the corresponding sites on the allograft. **G,** Postoperative appearance.

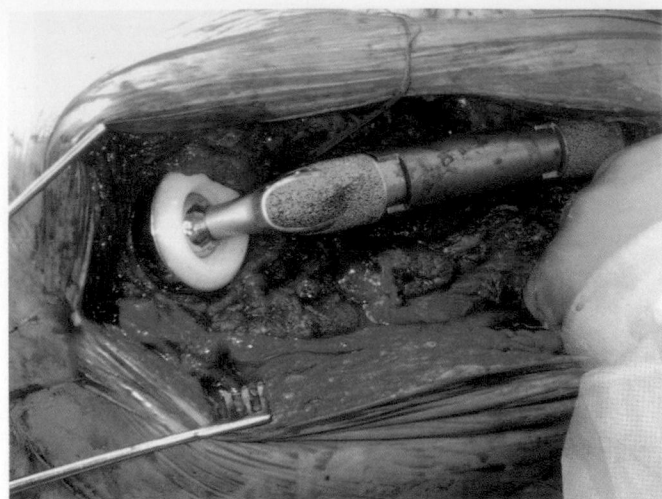

Figure 49-28 The intraoperative appearance of a modular metallic bipolar prosthesis with sites for sutures to secure the abductors. The rough surface is designed to allow tissue ingrowth with time. Distally, a similar surface allows placement of bone graft to seal the bone-cement interface and retard loosening.

and an arthrodesis using allografts with or without vascularized fibular grafts.[142,212,213,215] The latter allows for a stable shoulder, which is useful in a laborer but is difficult to achieve.

Outcomes

Although the goal of preserving a limb is laudable, and with experience the success rate of restoring functional limbs is improving, limb-sparing procedures are very complex operations. The short- and long-term complications are not trivial. It should also be remembered that young patients with amputations of the lower extremity do quite well with modern prostheses. We are only beginning to assess the quality of life and functional outcomes after these reconstructions, and the tools we have to assess these parameters are limited. The data that exists suggests that the energy cost of walking is better with a metallic prosthesis than an above-knee amputation.[216] A rotationplasty is similar to a below-knee amputation in that regard.[217] Most of the outcome studies report function using the Musculoskeletal Tumor Society rating system that has not been validated and is based on a surgeon assessment. Other outcome tools like the Short Form Health Survey 36 (SF-36) or the Toronto Extremity Salvage Score (TESS) are patient driven and not specific to sarcomas or a rare measure of disability.[218] The data

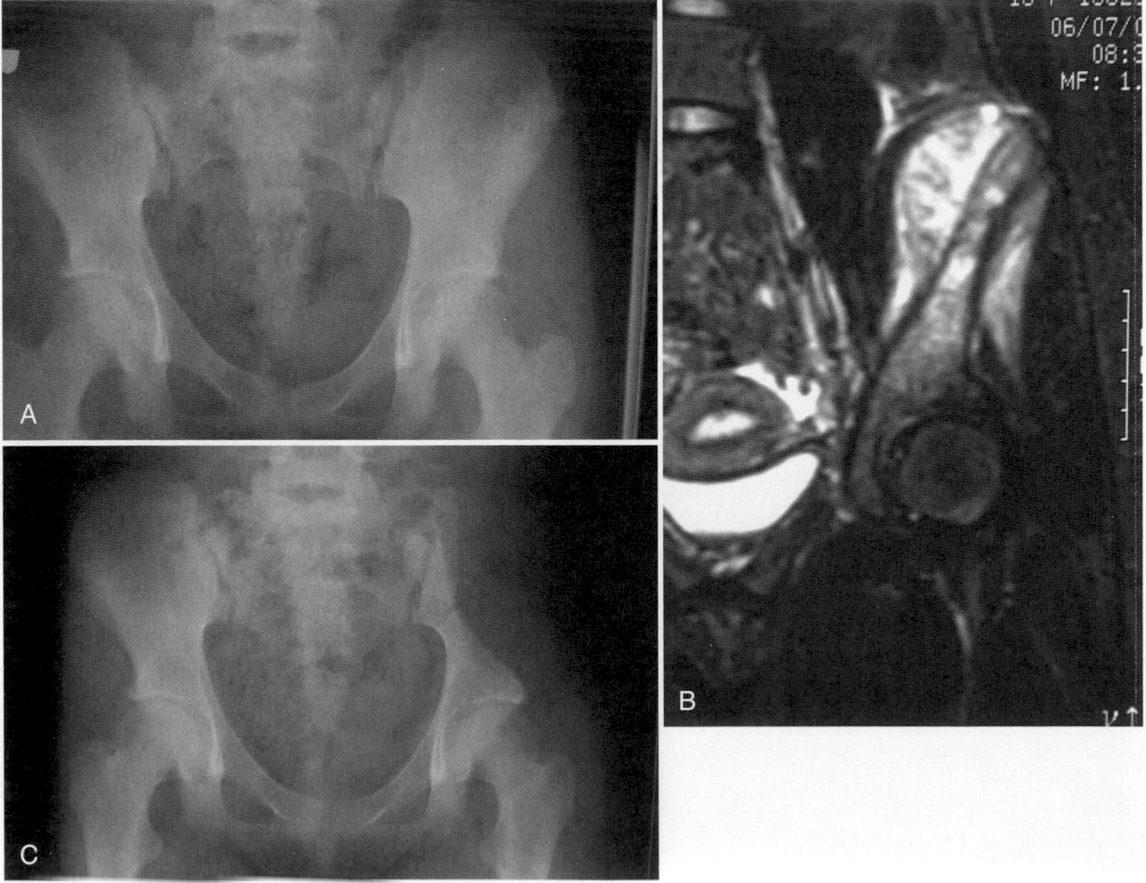

Figure 49-29 **A,** Radiograph of a Ewing sarcoma of the iliac wing. **B,** The magnetic resonance imaging reveals the extent of the soft tissue mass **C,** After chemotherapy, the soft-tissue mass was smaller, and resection was possible. The acetabulum was preserved, allowing reasonable function with a mild abductor lurch.

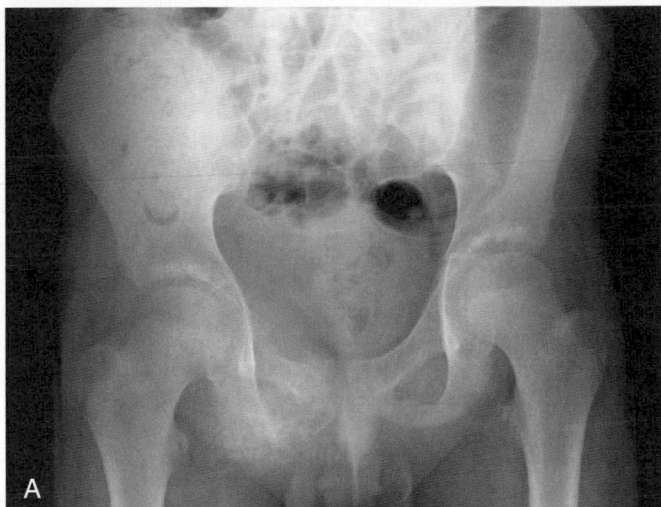

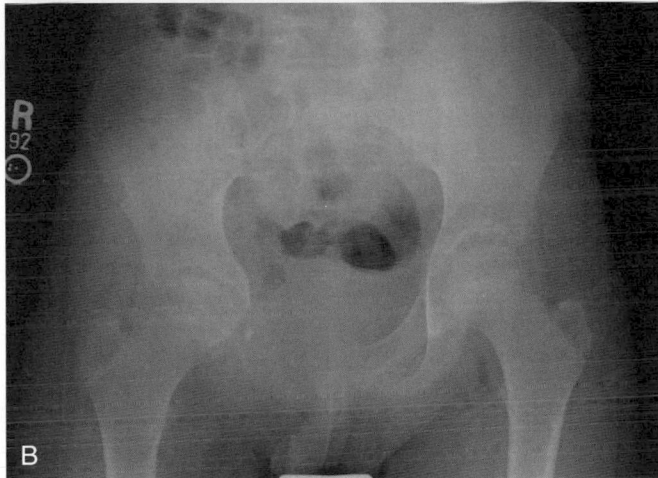

Figure 49-30 A, Preoperative radiograph of an osteosarcoma of the pubic rami. **B,** The appearance after resection showing preservation of the acetabulum is shown. Function in these situations is nearly normal, although hernia formation may be a problem.

suggest that there is little difference in outcomes and quality of life between amputees and limb-salvage patients and even less between the various types of reconstruction. However, the data are meager, and no controlled studies have been performed. This is an area for further study and development while the reconstruction options and prosthesis continue to evolve. Much progress has been made in the ability to treat pediatric bone sarcomas and to preserve limbs, but better reconstruction options are needed, including future developments in tissue engineering.

MANAGEMENT OF PULMONARY METASTASIS IN PEDIATRIC SOLID TUMORS

The value of the pediatric surgical oncologist in the locoregional control of malignant lesions in children was established well before the advent of chemotherapy or radiotherapy. However, the same cannot be said for the treatment of tumor metastases, especially in the lung. Two excellent reviews of the evolution and disease-specific

implementation of pediatric pulmonary metastasectomy have been published.[219,220] The last five decades have produced a rapid expansion in the use of pulmonary metastasectomy for pediatric cancers, but evidence-based proof of its efficacy is limited. This is the result of a general lack of tumor-specific, prospective, randomized clinical trials critically evaluating this therapeutic intervention. Reported studies are primarily from a single institution, retrospective in nature, and often span years to decades and multiple treatment protocols. The studies also generally clump multiple tumors, thereby weakening the strength of any recommendations. Despite these limitations, some general principles and lesion specific recommendations can be made.

The Four Principles

When considering the management of a suspected metastatic pulmonary lesion, four principles must be addressed for each patient. First, the primary tumor diagnosis must

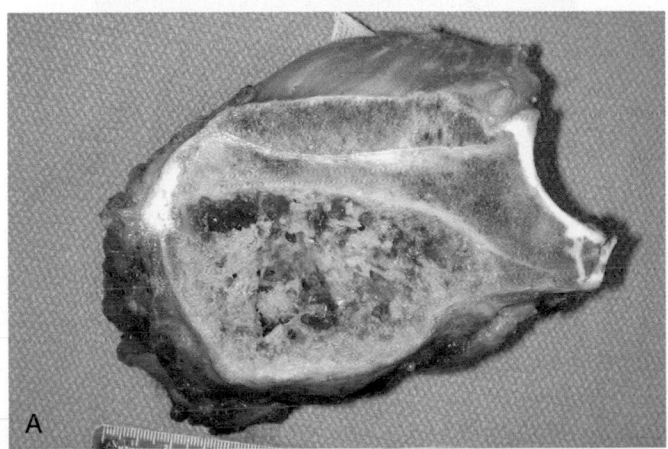

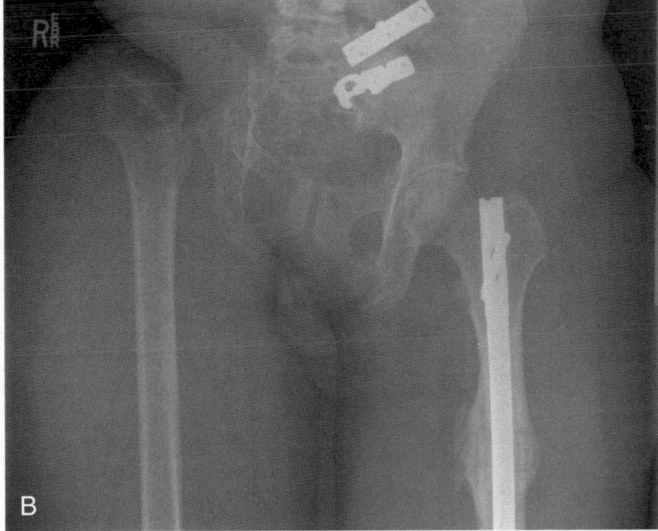

Figure 49-31 A, A specimen after resection of the iliac crest including the acetabulum for osteosarcoma (OSA). Function after these procedures is poor but better than an external hemipelvectomy. **D,** The radiograph of another patient more than 20 years after resection of her right ilium and acetabulum for OSA. She has had a closed femoral shortening on the left side to partially balance limb lengths. Despite her disabilities, she works full time and has a family.

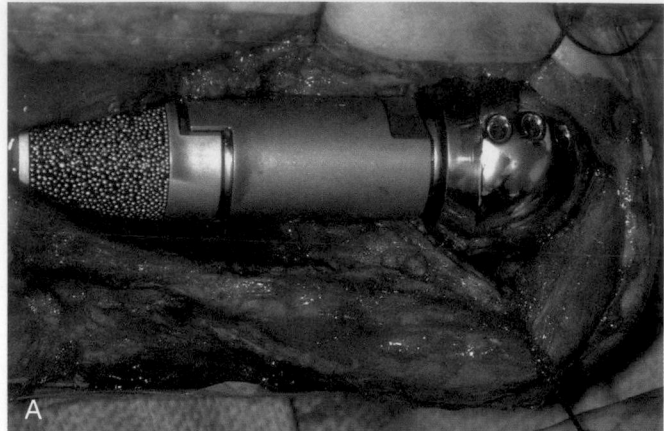

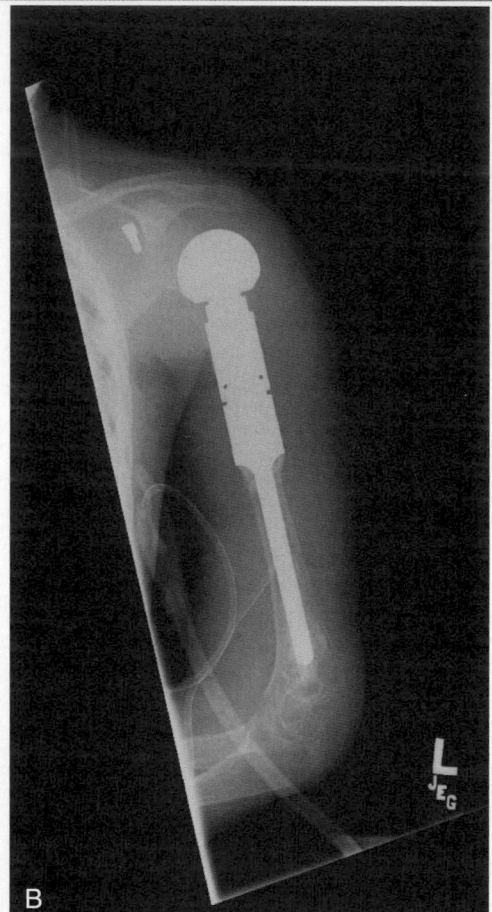

Figure 49-32 **A,** Intraoperative photograph of a metallic prosthesis used to reconstruct a patient with Ewing sarcoma who had a local recurrence after intercalary resection and allograft reconstruction. **B,** A postoperative radiograph of the prosthesis is shown. Active abduction is limited, but she has normal hand and elbow function.

be established. Response of pulmonary lesions to chemotherapy and radiotherapy is linked not only to the primary diagnosis but to the biologic subtype involved (i.e., favorable versus anaplastic Wilms tumor).

Second, the primary tumor must be controlled. A surgeon should not consider pulmonary metastasectomy before achieving local control of the primary lesion. However, biopsy to establish the presence of metastasis

is required in some settings, because it determines the intensity of therapy.

Third, the therapeutic benefit to surgical resection must be assessed, and this is clearly dependent on the specific tumor. Ideally, the cancer should be chemoresponsive so as to control residual micrometastases. The lack of effective adjuvant therapy may temper the enthusiasm for pulmonary metastasectomy.

Finally, the extent of the pulmonary resection required to remove all metastatic disease should be assessed. The extent of the resection must be balanced with the therapeutic benefit achieved. An aggressive resection creating pulmonary impairment is difficult to support in the presence of chemotherapy-resistant disease, particularly in the presence of multiple lesions. Some cancers (e.g., OSA, adrenocorticocarcinoma) require an aggressive operative approach to remove all gross evidence of disease because of limited chemotherapy response in an attempt to provide an improved overall and disease-free survival.

Metastasis Localization

Depending on the cancer involved, a combination of radiographic studies and nuclear imaging modalities are used to identify metastases, especially in the lungs. Multidetector CT (MDCT) is the mainstay of identifying pulmonary lesions, and nuclear imaging is used for osseous lesions. More than 80% of lesions greater than or equal to 3 mm can be readily identified with this imaging modality,[221,222] but increasing sensitivity comes with decreasing specificity. Many lesions identified on MDCT may not be

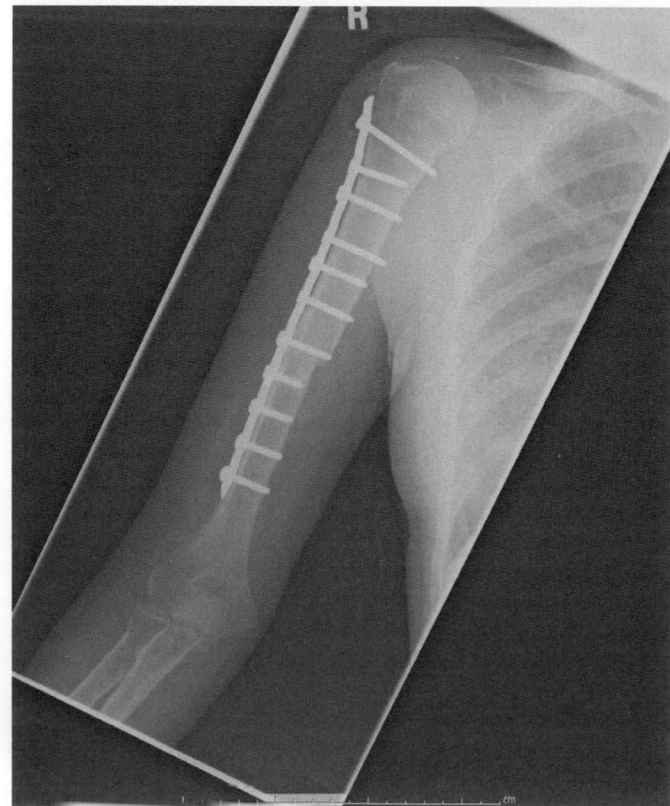

Figure 49-33 A proximal humeral osteoarticular allograft was used to reconstruct an intraarticular resection of the proximal humerus.

malignant. Although the appearance and location of the lesion may help, peripheral lesions that are smooth and well circumscribed are more likely to be malignant; biopsy is required for small lesions. Multiple lesions are also more likely to be malignant than isolated lesions.[223] Beyond this modality, nuclear medicine studies have been used for specific tumors with some success. Nuclear medicine studies exploit the biologic pathways of substrate molecules unique to specific tumors to identify these lesions as "hot spots" on subsequent whole-body scanning. These studies seldom stand alone as the only means to identify metastases, and they routinely act as corollary or confirmatory tests for lesions identified on MDCT. For example, a bone scintigraphy has been used to identify lesions in OSA,[220] but it is only taken up by large and biologically active lesions. Iodine[131] total body scans are routinely used in the evaluation and identification of pulmonary or osseous metastases in differentiated thyroid cancer, and it appears to be very sensitive and specific.[224-231] Finally, whole-body positron emission scanning utilizing fluorodeoxyglucose (18F-FDG PET) has been reported to have a sensitivity of 87% to 89% and a specificity of 100% in sarcomatous[232,233] and carcinomatous[233] pulmonary metastases, but this technique has limited assessment in pediatric primary malignancies, let alone metastases.

Biomarkers may be confirmatory tests for suspicious lesions found on MDCT or nuclear scintigraphy. Examples of tumor types with such markers that are routinely studied are adrenocortical carcinoma, differentiated thyroid carcinoma, germ cell carcinoma, and hepatoblastoma.

Technical Considerations

Pulmonary metastasectomy can be performed safely with minimal morbidity and a mortality rate of less than 1% documented in the International Registry of Lung Metastases.[233] The type of pulmonary resection can be either anatomic or nonanatomic ("wedge") despite early reports to the contrary,[234] but the vast majority of pulmonary metastasectomies performed are wedge resections that remove the lesion with a small rim of normal lung parenchyma (5 to 10 mm). Collective studies document the success of this procedure without the need for a formal lung resection along anatomic boundaries.[223,233, 235,236-238]

The use of MIS approaches for the resection of pulmonary lesions has been described in several studies.[239-244] Additionally, a recent report by Zaman and colleagues[245] analyzed various techniques—finger palpation, intraoperative ultrasound, hook-wire techniques, spiral-wire techniques, and fluoroscopic and/or radio guided detection—that can be used to assist in the localization of subcentimeter pulmonary nodules in conjunction with an MIS approach. Their conclusion was that radio guided techniques are superior to all others, especially finger palpation, which they recommended should be abandoned. MIS alone or in conjunction with other intraoperative localizing procedures has become an established technique except in the case of OSA, in which MDCT scanning has been shown to underestimate the number of lesions and formal thoracotomy has been recommended.[246] A cohort of patients with OSA and unilateral,

metachronous pulmonary metastases confirmed by MDCT within 2 years of the primary lesion were found to have occult metastases on the contralateral side in 78% of cases.[247] Therefore staged or sequential bilateral thoracotomies are recommended in patients with OSA by some authors, although this approach has not been shown in a prospective study to prolong either EFS or OS.

Select Pediatric Malignancies

Adrenocortical Carcinoma

Pulmonary metastases from adrenocortical carcinoma should be considered for complete surgical removal, because effective chemotherapy is not available. A recent review of the International Pediatric Adrenocortical Tumor Registry revealed that the mean age of patients at presentation was 3.2 years, and more than 90% of the lesions were functional tumors (84% virilizing).[248] The 5-year EFS was 54%, and the incidence of pulmonary metastases was 7% at presentation. Prognosis was improved for younger patients with completely resected, small (<200 g), early-stage tumors with virilizing symptoms. Separate analysis of the patients with lung metastases could not be performed because of the small number of patients. Isolated case reports in the literature document long-term survival in patients after pulmonary metastasectomy for adrenocortical carcinoma.[249,250] If one examines the adult studies addressing this question, the role for complete tumor excision becomes readily apparent. Kwauk and colleagues examined their series of 24 primarily adult patients with adrenocortical carcinoma and pulmonary metastases.[251] They noted that complete surgical excision of all metastatic disease achieved a 5-year survival rate of 71% versus 0% for those with unresected disease. Though their patient cohort was small and not randomized, they concluded that in the light of ineffective chemotherapy, complete pulmonary metastasectomy was not only indicated but mandatory to achieve long-term survival.

Schulick and colleagues echoed these results and sentiments when analyzing their institution's results with metastatic adrenocortical carcinoma in predominantly adult patients.[252] In fact, not only do they advocate for an initial pulmonary metastasectomy but for repeated resections as well. Some patients in their series had as many as seven resections for recurrent disease. Although this may seem overly aggressive, they note that for every reoperation, the median survival was longer for complete versus incomplete resection groups, which is probably a function of the biology of the tumor involved and anatomic limits of resection as opposed to the operation performed (Fig. 49-34). Furthermore the majority of metastatic resections performed were for pulmonary disease. Thus the data confirm the important role for surgery in the treatment of adrenocortical carcinoma metastatic to the lungs with resectable disease where increased survival and cure can be achieved.

Differentiated Thyroid Cancer

Pulmonary metastases from differentiated thyroid cancer should not be treated by surgical excision except in cases

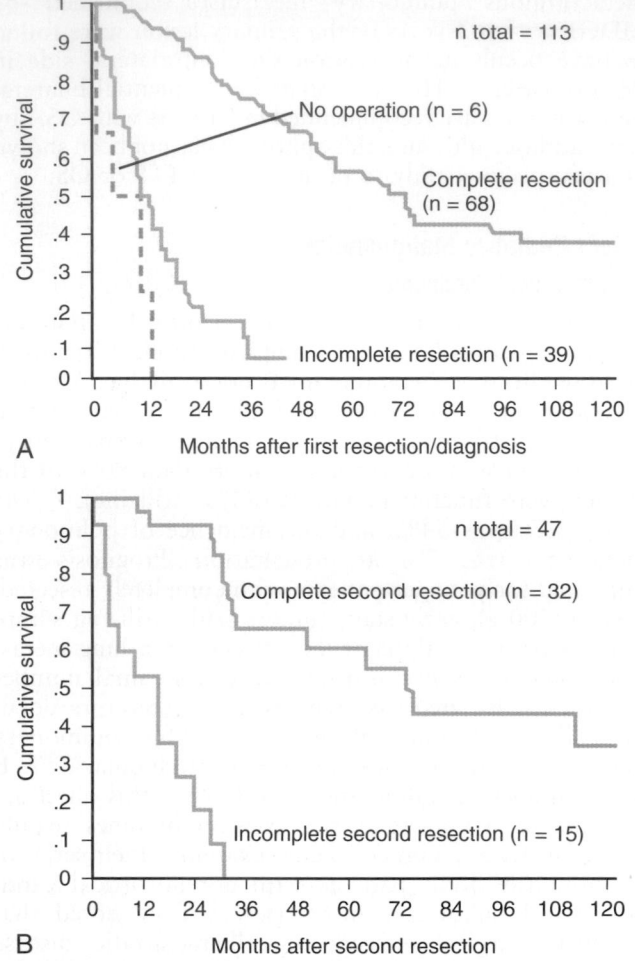

Figure 49-34 **A** and **B**, Disease-specific survival rates for patients undergoing complete versus incomplete primary resections for adrenocortical carcinoma. *(Modified from Schulick RD, Brennan MF: Long-term survival after complete resection and repeat resection in patients with adrenocortical carcinoma. Ann Surg Oncol 6(8):719–726, 1999.)*

in which there is indecision about the nature of the diagnosis, especially after treatment. Despite the presence of disseminated disease to the lungs, prognosis is still quite good. Unlike skeletal and pleural involvement, patients with pulmonary metastases have mortality rates from 0% to 6%.[226,227,229-231,252] Studies have reported the incidence of pulmonary metastases of 6% to 25%.[227,231,228,229-231] Interestingly, these studies have also documented that pulmonary metastases are very responsive to radioactive iodine treatment. They are seen more often in younger patients and can first appear more than 10 years from the initial diagnosis.

A recent comprehensive review of the treatment of thyroid cancer in children exposed to radiation from the Chernobyl nuclear power station comprises the largest series of pediatric thyroid carcinoma.[231] Seven hundred and forty cases of thyroid cancer occurred in 681 children with direct exposure to the accident. One hundred thirty-one cases (17.7 %) of pulmonary disease were diagnosed by radionuclide scan with a mean presentation of 19 months after the primary diagnosis. Only 2.3% of patients

diagnosed had pulmonary metastases that were found on chest radiograph; hence the authors recommended the use of radioactive iodine scanning as the procedure of choice because of its increased sensitivity and specificity. The risk factors for metastatic disease were female gender, a younger age at diagnosis, and the presence of clinical symptoms. Patients were treated with radioactive iodine for their initial pulmonary metastasis. With therapeutic radioactive iodine administration for pulmonary metastases, 28.9% had a complete response (negative nuclear imaging and thyroglobulin <1 ng/mL), 47.7% had a partial but stable response (negative nuclear imaging and thyroglobulin 1 to 10 ng/mL), and 23.4% had a partial response. The 5- and 10-year survival rates were 99.5% and 98.8%, respectively, with only 5 children dying of distant metastases (3 medullary, 1 follicular, and 1 papillary) with a mean follow-up period of 115 months. This study and others document the success of medical therapy. Surgery is required only for diagnosis if the lesions fail to take up iodine.

Germ Cell Tumors (Gonadal)

Pulmonary metastases from gonadal germ cell tumors should be biopsied only if their origin is in question. This tumor is very responsive to chemotherapy, so resection is performed only after treatment if radiographic abnormalities persist. Germ cell tumors comprise a broad range of tumors, 20% of which are malignant.[253] The malignant lesions are chemosensitive, and with the advent of cisplatin-based regimens long-term survival has increased to 90%.[254] However, residual disease after adjuvant therapies may harbor viable tumor,[254-258] with the lung being the most common site of distant metastasis.[255] Synchronous pulmonary metastases are found in 50% of patients with retroperitoneal lymphadenopathy and in 10% of patients without adenopathy.[254] Therefore the role of pulmonary metastasectomy is primarily to define the presence of viable tumor in residual lesions after chemotherapy. This would establish a basis for further therapy. Several groups have examined their data concerning the role and utility of pulmonary metastasectomy.

Cagini and colleagues examined their cohort of 141 patients over a 17-year period with both pulmonary and mediastinal involvement; 51% of patients had isolated pulmonary disease, 24% had pulmonary and mediastinal disease, and 24% had mediastinal disease alone.[254] Roughly, one third of patients had a single lesion, one third had 2 or 3 lesions, and one third had more than 3 lesions. Eighty-seven percent had a complete resection, and histological analysis revealed that 23% of the lesions had only necrosis or fibrosis, 45% had mature teratoma, and 32% were malignant. Biomarker analysis in these patients was not helpful, because 23% of patients with malignant disease had negative biomarkers. A second recurrence occurred in 47% of patients. The overall mortality rate was 19% for the entire group. Actuarial survival after pulmonary metastasectomy was 78% at 5 years, 76% at 10 years, and 66% at 15 years posttreatment. Statistically significant prognostic factors were the pathology of the specimen (complete necrosis or fibrosis of the specimen as opposed to the presence of viable tumor), presence of residual disease (mediastinal disease alone had a better outcome than pulmonary disease with or without mediastinal disease), and the number of resected lesions.

These results were echoed by Liu and colleagues who examined their cohort of 157 patients with isolated pulmonary metastases after chemotherapy over a 28-year period.[254] The majority of patients had multiple lesions (72%), and 89% of patients underwent nonanatomic resections. The mortality rate was 0.6%, and the morbidity rate was 6%. Pathologic analysis revealed viable tumor in 44% of the cohort, 37% of the cohort had a subsequent recurrence of disease in their chest, and 56% of these died. The overall mortality rate was 32%. Statistically significant negative prognostic factors were age older than 25 years, no cisplatin-based chemotherapy, the presence of viable tumor when the lesions were resected posttherapy, and the existence of metastatic disease outside of the thorax or retroperitoneum. The authors conclude that surgery plays a critical role in determining those patients who would benefit from further therapy. These results are also confirmed by other groups,[256-258] but patient selection is an important criteria. Ultimately, surgical salvage using pulmonary metastasectomy is a viable alternative to patients with residual, radiographically identifiable lesions to determine the chemoresponsiveness of these tumors and to provide for an increased long-term survival with complete surgical resection.

Hepatoblastoma

Pulmonary metastases from hepatoblastoma should be treated first with adjuvant chemotherapy, and only then any residual lesions should be resected. Data to support this concept have appeared over the last several decades with an initial report by Black and colleagues.[259] They reported four patients who were long-term survivors, and they stressed the need for complete local control and adjuvant chemotherapy. Furthermore they correlated the need to perform the pulmonary metastasectomy with the patient's α-fetoprotein levels, especially advocating early surgery for those patients with rising titers on appropriate therapy.

Feusner and colleagues[260] representing the CCG published their results, and they confirmed the premises outlined by Black and colleagues. Of their cohort of six patients with pulmonary recurrence, four had a complete remission and three had a survival of more than 5 years. Their approach was to combine adjuvant chemotherapy with aggressive pulmonary resections. Some caution is appropriate, however, when it is recognized that the OS or EFS of patients who have stage-IV disease in hepatoblastoma is 16%, and patients with relapse generally do worse having already received the primary therapies. Beyond these North American results, two reports from the SIOPEL have documented their results with hepatoblastoma and pulmonary metastases. The first report by Perilongo and colleagues[261] in 2000 documented the results of SIOPEL 1. 20% of patients with hepatoblastoma had pulmonary metastases, and they achieved a 5-year EFS rate of only 28%. A sustained remission of

26% of the cohort with metastatic pulmonary lesions was achieved from chemotherapy alone. Schnater and colleagues[90] analyzed the surgical approach in SIOPEL 1 and documented that 41% of patients who had pulmonary metastases were long-term survivors, but the four patients who underwent surgery and chemotherapy to treat their pulmonary metastases were alive at data analysis (minimum of 2.5 years posttreatment). In a nonrandomized study, the apparent difference in outcome may result from selection factors. Their data also suggest that recurrent pulmonary disease could be cured with surgery and chemotherapy as long as there was local control of the tumor. Thus these studies cumulatively support a possible role for pulmonary metastasectomy for hepatoblastoma in selected residual lesions.

Neuroblastoma

Pulmonary metastases from neuroblastoma are rare, and they should not be treated by surgical excision except in cases in which there is indecision about the nature of the lesion, especially after or during treatment. The incidence of pulmonary metastases from neuroblastoma has been reported to occur in fewer than 1% to 23% of cases[262-266]; however, most large studies report rates of 5% or less.[264-266] They can be synchronous or metachronous, and they are usually multiple, bilateral, subcentimeter, and peripheral. Patients with pulmonary metastases from neuroblastoma have a poor prognosis, a high association of unfavorable Shimada histology, MYCN amplification, and a lower EFS rate.[265,266] Hence the utility of performing resections except to confirm the diagnosis is not established.

Wilms Tumor

Pulmonary metastases from nephroblastoma should generally not be resected, and suspected lesions should only be biopsied, although some authors[236,267] have advocated for primary pulmonary metastasectomy to spare the effects of radiotherapy on patients.[268] North American centers under the protocols established by the NWTSG have demonstrated the efficacy of chemotherapy and radiotherapy in the treatment of pulmonary metastases over chemotherapy and surgical excision, regardless of pathologic subtype.[269-271] Specifically, Green and colleagues in 1991 examined patients enrolled in NWTSG studies 1 and 3 with pulmonary recurrences. Of the patients meeting study criteria, the resection of pulmonary metastases within 30 days of diagnosis did not affect 4-year survival outcomes in favorable or unfavorable histopathologic cohorts. Furthermore, Green and colleagues[271] reported results from NWTSG-4, in which pulmonary metastasectomy had almost no role in the treatment of patients with stage-IV disease patients. It was performed for residual lesions after chemotherapy and radiotherapy, but it did not affect the OS rates achieved of greater than 75% to 90%. The importance of biopsy for suspicious lesions, especially small lesions (<1 cm) found only on CT was confirmed recently by Erhlich and colleagues,[272] who reviewed the cases of those children enrolled in NWTSG-5. Thirty-three percent of those who received radiotherapy had a prior biopsy that was negative for tumor, and hence they were overtreated. These results were for patients with both isolated and multiple lesions. These studies collectively confirm the general success of combined chemotherapy and radiotherapy in the treatment of pulmonary metastases in nephroblastoma. Whether in fact those children with metastatic disease seen only on MDCT and resolved with chemotherapy need pulmonary radiotherapy remains an unanswered question. Finally, surgical intervention for pulmonary lesions in nephroblastoma should only be utilized to confirm the existence of malignancy in MDCT-defined masses before administering therapy.

Sarcomas

Pulmonary metastases from sarcomatous pediatric tumors should be biopsied at a minimum, and complete resections should be performed depending on the precise histologic subtype. The most comprehensive reports concerning this topic are by Temeck and colleagues from the National Cancer Institute, who published two reports in the 1990s that documented their results with initial[273] and recurrent pulmonary metastasectomies.[274] Their initial report examined 152 patients who underwent 258 thoracotomies over 18 years. The lesions included OSA (50%), nonrhabdomyosarcoma soft-tissue sarcomas (27%), EWS (18%), and rhabdomyosarcoma (3%). Eighty percent of patients had a complete resection, and the cohort had morbidity and mortality rates of approximately 6% and 1.3%, respectively. The highest median survival occurred in the OSA group (3.1 years), and the lowest was in patients with rhabdomyosarcomas (0.4 years). Statistically significant poor prognostic factors included the presence of three or more metastases, a diagnosis other than OSA, and an incomplete resection. Their follow-up study on recurrent lesions further documented the importance of histological subtypes, because no patients with rhabdomyosarcoma were eligible for evaluation. They also documented that CT missed 39% of lesions, 24% of which were found to be malignant, supporting the need for thorough evaluation of the thorax through an open approach. Furthermore they documented a complete resection rate of 77% with 5.6% morbidity rate and a 1% mortality rate. Finally they documented a statistically significant improved survival rate in those patients who underwent complete resections, regardless of the number of recurrences. In fact this survival advantage was eight to 20 times greater depending on the number of recurrences. These data, though encouraging for sarcomas as a whole, must be considered by individual histologic variants. The one sarcomatous variant that may benefit from pulmonary metastasectomy is OSA.

The utility of complete, recurrent pulmonary metastasectomy in OSA was ushered in with the report by Martini and colleagues describing their experience in 1971.[275] They reported a 45% survival rate in patients who had complete pulmonary metastasectomies, which is four times greater than that of chemotherapy alone. Reports from the last decade[†] have not only confirmed these

results but clarified the therapeutic approach to pulmonary metastases in OSA. First, OSA should be treated with a multiagent regimen that addresses synchronous pulmonary lesions at the time of local control. Second, pulmonary lesions should undergo repeated complete resections, because this is the best chance for long-term disease-free survival and OS. Third, extirpation of extrapulmonary metastases does not confer the same survival benefits as does pulmonary metastasectomy and is often less feasible, because many of these osseous. Fourth, CT imaging does not identify all pulmonary lesions, and most lesions are not calcified. Therefore staged bilateral thoracotomies are suggested by some for complete evaluation and resection of all pulmonary disease. Fifth, once metachronous lesions have been identified and treated surgically, a majority of patients will have at least one pulmonary recurrence, and most recurrences are within 12 months of the first resection. Therefore continued surveillance and frequent repeat imaging are essential. Finally, though tumor burden was and still is an important prognostic factor in the determination of outcome, several biologic features (e.g., disease-free interval and percentage of tumor necrosis on histopathologic evaluation) have become even more significant in recent reviews. Hence aggressive, repeated complete resection of pulmonary metastases is critical to the successful treatment of patients with OSA.

References available online at ExpertConsult.

KEY REFERENCES

2. Shamberger RC, Guthrie KA, Ritchey ML, et al: Surgery-related factors and local recurrence of Wilms tumor in National Wilms Tumor Study 4. *Ann Surg* 229(2):292–297, 1999.
   Cohort analysis of children treated on NWTSG-4 that demonstrates the clear association between tumor rupture at resection and failure to obtain lymph-node biopsies for staging with an increased occurrence of local relapse.

7. Weiner E, Anderson J, Ojimba J, et al: Controversies in the management of peri-testicular rhabdomyosarcoma: is staging retroperitoneal lymph-node dissection necessary for adolescents with resected peri-testicular rhabdomyosarcoma? *Semin Pediatr Surg* 10:146–152, 2001.
   Report of boys treated for paratesticular rhabdomyosarcoma on IRS-4. In this study CT scans were used for staging rather than retroperitoneal lymph-node biopsy. In the study, the diagnosis of retroperitoneal involvement was decreased by half, and the incidence of retroperitoneal relapse was increased fourfold as a result of decreased use of retroperitoneal radiotherapy and presumed understaging in a significant number of patients.

14. Shamberger RC, Holzman RS, Griscom NT, et al: Prospective evaluation by computed tomography and pulmonary function tests of children with mediastinal masses. *Surgery* 118(3):468–471, 1995.
   Prospective study of children and adolescents who had anterior mediastinal tumors. It demonstrated the efficacy of CT scans and pulmonary function tests to measure the tracheal area as a percentage of expected and the peaked expiratory flow rate as a percentage of expected. If patients' results were than 50% in both of these categories, there were no anesthetic complications.

21. Perger L, Lee E, Shamberger RC: Management of children and adolescents with a critical airway due to compression by an anterior mediastinal mass. *J Pediatr Surg* 43:1990–1997, 2008.
   Retrospective review of patients with a threatened airway caused by anterior mediastinal tumors. Based on the experience reported, a proposed treatment algorithm was proposed.

---

†References 239, 247, 276, 277, 278-288.

50. Lemerle J, Voute P, Tourade M, et al: Preoperative versus postoperative radiotherapy, single versus multiple courses of actinomycin D in the treatment of Wilms' tumor: preliminary results of a controlled clinical trial conducted by the International Society of Pediatric Oncology (SIOP). *Cancer* 38:647–654, 1976.

Report of the first randomized study of Wilms tumor by SIOP in which patients received either preoperative radiotherapy (920 Gy) or surgical resection. A significant decrease in the incidence of rupture at resection was seen in patients who had initial radiotherapy.

53. Lemerle J, Voute PA, Tournade MF, et al: Effectiveness of preoperative chemotherapy in Wilms' tumor: results of an International Society of Paediatric Oncology (SIOP) clinical trial. *J Clin Oncol* 1(10):604–609, 1983.

Second randomized study from SIOP compared preoperative radiotherapy (20Gy) and actinomycin D versus preoperative treatment with actinomycin D and vincristine. An equivalent low incidence of rupture during resection was seen.

54. Tournade MF, Com-Nougue C, Voute PA, et al: Results of the Sixth International Society of Pediatric Oncology Wilms' Tumor Trial and Study: a risk-adapted therapeutic approach in Wilms' tumor. *J Clin Oncol* 11(6):1014–1023, 1993.

Randomized study in which all patients received initial chemotherapy, and those who were stage II N0 (no evidence of lymphnode spread) were randomized between postoperative radiotherapy or no radiotherapy. Study was closed early after seven cases of local relapse occurred in the no-radiotherapy group compared with none in the radiotherapy group. Study suggested that posttherapy staging "downstaged" the disease, and the absence of abnormal pathology after chemotherapy was not a factor in patients best treated with radiotherapy.

56. Tournade MF, Com-Nougue C, de Kraker J, et al: Optimal duration of preoperative therapy in unilateral and nonmetastatic Wilms' tumor in children older than 6 months: results of the Ninth International Society of Pediatric Oncology Wilms' Tumor Trial and Study. *J Clin Oncol* 19(2):488–500, 2001.

Subsequent SIOP-randomized study comparing 4 and 8 weeks of initial therapy demonstrated no difference in "downstaging" between the two intervals or in the occurrence of operative rupture. The tumor was shown subsequently to have decreased in size between the 4- and 8- week intervals.

64. Nuchtern J, London W, Barnewolt C, et al: A prospective study of expectant observation as primary therapy for neuroblastoma in young infants: a Children's Oncology Group Study. *Ann Surg* 256(4):573–580, 2012.

Recent report from the Children's Oncology Group on a prospective study of expectant observation of infants with neuroblastoma with small adrenal primaries demonstrated that the major of patients could avoid resection and that tumor progression was rare.

73. Shamberger RC, Smith EI, Joshi VV, et al: The risk of nephrectomy during local control in abdominal neuroblastoma. *J Pediatr Surg* 33(2):161–164, 1998.

Retrospective review of infants and children treated for neuroblastoma demonstrated a lower incidence of nephrectomy in those treated initially with chemotherapy rather than radiotherapy.

74. Simon T, Haberle B, Hero B, et al: Role of surgery in the treatment of patients with stage 4 neuroblastoma age 18 months or older at diagnosis. *J Clin Oncol* 31(6):752–758, 2013.

German cooperative study of stage 4 neuroblastoma in children older than 18 months assessed patients treated with either preoperative or postoperative chemotherapy suggested that surgical resection did not affect the EFS, OS, or incidence of local relapse.

79. Malogolowkin MH, Katzenstein H, Meyers R, et al: Complete surgical resection is curative for children with hepatoblastoma with pure fetal histology: a report from the Children's Oncology Group. *J Clin Oncol* 29(24):3301–3306, 2011.

Intergroup study demonstrated that children with pure fetal histology hepatoblastoma had a high incidence of survival without adjuvant chemotherapy.

83. Reynolds M, Douglass E, Finegold M, et al: Chemotherapy can convert unresectable hepatoblastoma. *J Pediatr Surg* 27(8):1080–1084, 1992.

Report from this intergroup study demonstrated the efficacy of neoadjuvant chemotherapy to convert unresectable to resectable hepatoblastoma.

84. von Schweinitz D, Hecker H, Harms D, et al: Complete resection before development of drug resistance is essential for survival from advanced hepatoblastoma: a report from the German Cooperative Pediatric Liver Tumor Study HB89. *J Pediatr Surg* 30(6):845–852, 1995.

Prospective study demonstrated the occurrence of tumor chemotherapy resistance and regrowth of hepatoblastoma as early as after the fourth course of chemotherapy, emphasizing the continued need for early surgical resection.

91. Ortega J, Douglass E, Feusner J, et al: Randomized comparison of cisplatin/vincristine/fluorouracil and cisplatin/continuous infusion doxorubicin for treatment of pediatric hepatoblastoma: a report from the Children's Cancer Group. *J Clin Oncol* 18(14):2665–2675, 2000.

Report demonstrating equivalence of these two agents and excellent results from treatment combined with surgical resection.

92. Otte JB, Pritchard J, Aronson DC, et al: Liver transplantation for hepatoblastoma: results from the International Society of Pediatric Oncology (SIOP) study SIOPEL-1 and review of the world experience. *Pediatr Blood Cancer* 42(1):74–83, 2004.

Report of successful management of children with primary lesions too extensive for resection with orthotopic liver transplantation.

95. Crist W, Anderson J, Meza J, et al: Intergroup Rhabdomyosarcoma study-IV: results for patients with nonmetastatic disease. *J Clin Oncol* 19(12):3091–3102, 2001.

Report from the cooperative IRSG demonstrating the marked enhancement of survival of patients with rhabdomyosarcoma with multimodality therapy.

118. Picci P, Sangiorgi L, Rougraff B, et al: Relationship of chemotherapy-induced necrosis and surgical margins to local recurrence in osteosarcoma. *J Clin Oncol* 12:2699–2705, 1994.

Study demonstrates that extensive tumor necrosis postneoadjuvant chemotherapy and adequate surgical margins are prognostic of low risk for local recurrence in osteogenic sarcoma.

175. Fuchs B, Kotajarvi BR, Kaufman KR, et al: Functional outcome of patients with rotationplasty about the knee. *Clin Orthop Relat Res* 415:52–58, 2003.

Study demonstrates that a rotationplasty converts a high thigh amputation to a distal amputation with preservation of a "functional" knee joint.

182. Veenstra KM, Sprangers MA, van der Eyken JW, et al: Quality of life in survivors with a Van Ness-Borggreve rotationplasty after bone tumour resection. *J Surg Oncol* 73(4):192–197, 2000.

Report of the favorable physiologic and functional outcomes of rotationplasty.

196. Grier HE, Krailo MD, Tarbell NJ, et al: Addition of ifosfamide and etoposide to standard chemotherapy for Ewing's sarcoma and primitive neuroectodermal tumor of bone. *N Engl J Med* 348(8):694–701, 2003.

Very significant report of a prospective randomized study that demonstrated that the addition of ifosfamide and etoposide to the standard therapy for EWS had a significant enhancement in EFS and OS.

216. Otis JC, Lane JM, Kroll MA: Energy cost during gait in osteosarcoma patients after resection and knee replacement and after above-the-knee amputation. *J Bone Joint Surg Am* 67(4):606–611, 1985.

Study demonstrates that the energy cost of walking is lower for a patient with a prosthetic knee replacement than with an above knee amputation.

272. Ehrlich PF, Hamilton TE, Grundy P, et al: The value of surgery in directing therapy for patients with Wilms' tumor with pulmonary disease: a report from the National Wilms' Tumor Study Group. National Wilms' Tumor Study 5. *J Pediatr Surg* 41(1):162–167, 2006.

Study demonstrates the importance of surgical biopsy in patients with pulmonary lesions after therapy for Wilms tumor. It reveals that in some cases the small nodules were not malignant in origin or had no residual evidence of malignant elements posttherapy.

278. La Quaglia MP: Osteosarcoma: specific tumor management and results. *Chest Surg Clin North Am* 8(1):77–95, 1998.

Summary of the reports demonstrating the efficacy of surgical resection in the treatment of pulmonary metastases in osteogenic sarcoma.

HEMATOLOGIC MALIGNANCY

CHAPTER 50

Acute Lymphoblastic Leukemia

Alejandro Gutierrez and Lewis B. Silverman

CHAPTER OUTLINE

The acute leukemias of childhood are rare diseases that collectively represent about 30% of malignancies in children younger than age 15 years.[1] Approximately 3000 new cases of childhood leukemia occur annually in the United States, 80% of which are acute lymphoblastic leukemia (ALL). Between the 1960s and 1990s, the prognosis for children with ALL improved dramatically. With current multiagent chemotherapy regimens, 80% to 90% of children with ALL are long-term relapse-free survivors.[2,3,4] In this chapter, childhood ALL is reviewed with respect to classification, molecular pathogenesis, clinical presentation, laboratory findings, differential diagnosis, treatment strategies, prognosis, and late effects of therapy. Causative and epidemiologic considerations, including the incidence, prevalence, and life span of afflicted individuals, are discussed in Chapter 40. Discussion of the cytogenetic aspects of the leukemias appears in Chapter 45, and the molecular basis of human malignancy is further discussed in Chapter 33. Details concerning the various chemotherapeutic agents are provided in Chapter 46, and myelogenous leukemias and myeloproliferative disorders are discussed in Chapter 51.

CLASSIFICATION

The childhood leukemias can be classified as acute or chronic. *Acute leukemia* is characterized by clonal expansion of immature hematopoietic or lymphoid precursors, whereas *chronic leukemia* refers to conditions characterized by the expansion of mature marrow elements. *Congenital leukemia* refers to leukemias diagnosed within the first 4 weeks of life.

Acute leukemia is characterized by replacement of normal marrow elements with malignant blast cells, relatively undifferentiated cells with diffusely distributed nuclear chromatin, one or more nucleoli, and basophilic cytoplasm. A number of methods exist for characterizing malignant blast cells, including morphology, cytochemistry, and immunophenotype, as well as chromosomal and molecular genetic aberrations. Approximately 80% of cases of childhood acute leukemia are lymphoblastic.

Morphologic and Cytochemical Classification

The production of blast forms is part of the normal maturational sequence of hematopoietic and lymphoid elements. Blast cells are primitive precursors, lacking many of the features of differentiation. Under normal conditions, blast forms constitute fewer than 5% of the nucleated cells of the bone marrow. Blast cells are usually not observed in the peripheral blood, except during periods of profound overproduction of blood cells in response to infection or bleeding or from bone marrow invasion by granulomas, fibrosis, or tumor cells (leukoerythroblastosis). Leukemic blast cells can be difficult to distinguish morphologically from normal, nonmalignant blasts, although the finding of more than 5% blast forms in the marrow, or the presence of blast cells in the peripheral blood, should raise the suspicion of leukemia. In acute leukemia, patients often present with a marrow that is almost fully replaced by blast forms.

Once the diagnosis of leukemia is made, it is sometimes difficult to differentiate a lymphoid from a myeloid blast. The morphologic characteristics of lymphoblasts are shown in Figure 50-1. Wright-Giemsa–stained lymphoblasts have smooth, homogeneous nuclear material with indistinct nucleoli and only a small rim of light blue–staining cytoplasm, generally without granules. In contrast, myeloblasts differ from lymphoblasts in that the former have a lower nuclear-to-cytoplasmic ratio, more finely developed nuclear chromatin, and more distinct punched-out nucleoli. Cytoplasmic granules are often present in myeloblasts, and the detection of eosinophilic

Auer rods is pathognomonic. However, small myeloblasts may be confused with lymphoblasts morphologically, although they can usually be distinguished by flow cytometric or cytochemical studies.

A standardized morphologic classification system devised by the French-American-British (FAB) Cooperative Working Group is generally used to categorize the appearance of leukemic blasts.[5] In this system, ALL is subdivided into three morphologic categories: L1, L2, and L3 (see Fig. 50-1). L1 is the most common subtype, observed in about 90% of cases of childhood ALL. L1 lymphoblasts are small cells characterized by a high nuclear-to-cytoplasmic ratio. The pale blue cytoplasm is scanty and limited to a small portion of the perimeter of the cell. The cells have indistinct nucleoli and nuclear membranes that vary from round to clefted. Cells in the L2 category, found in 5% to 15% of pediatric cases, are larger than those classified as L1, show marked variability in size, and have prominent nucleoli and more abundant cytoplasm. They may be difficult to distinguish morphologically from the M1 variant of myeloid leukemia, and thus flow cytometric analysis of cell surface markers is essential to differentiate ALL from acute myelogenous leukemia (AML). L1 and L2 lymphoblasts do not differ significantly in terms of cell surface markers, genetic abnormalities, or prognosis.[6,7] Only 1% to 2% of

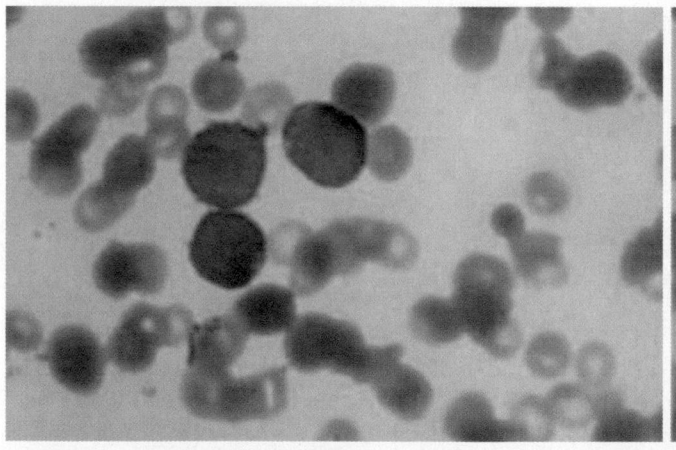

L1

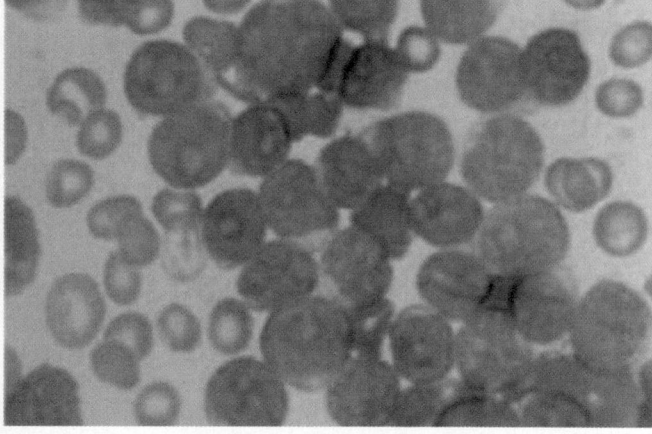

L2

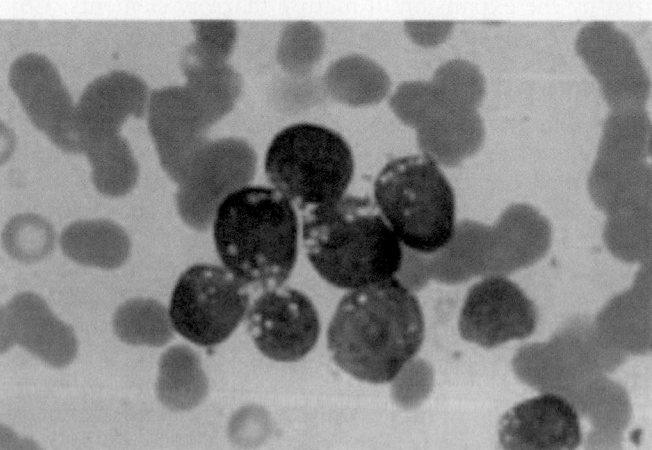

L3

Figure 50-1 The French-American-British (FAB) classification system of acute lymphoblastic leukemia. **L1,** Acute lymphoblastic leukemia (ALL). Note the high nuclear-to-cytoplasmic ratio and lack of distinct nucleoli. **L2,** ALL. Note the large nucleoli and increased amount of cytoplasm. **L3,** ALL. This subtype is associated with surface immunoglobulin. Note the dark blue cytoplasm and vacuoles. *(Courtesy Pearl Leavitt.)*

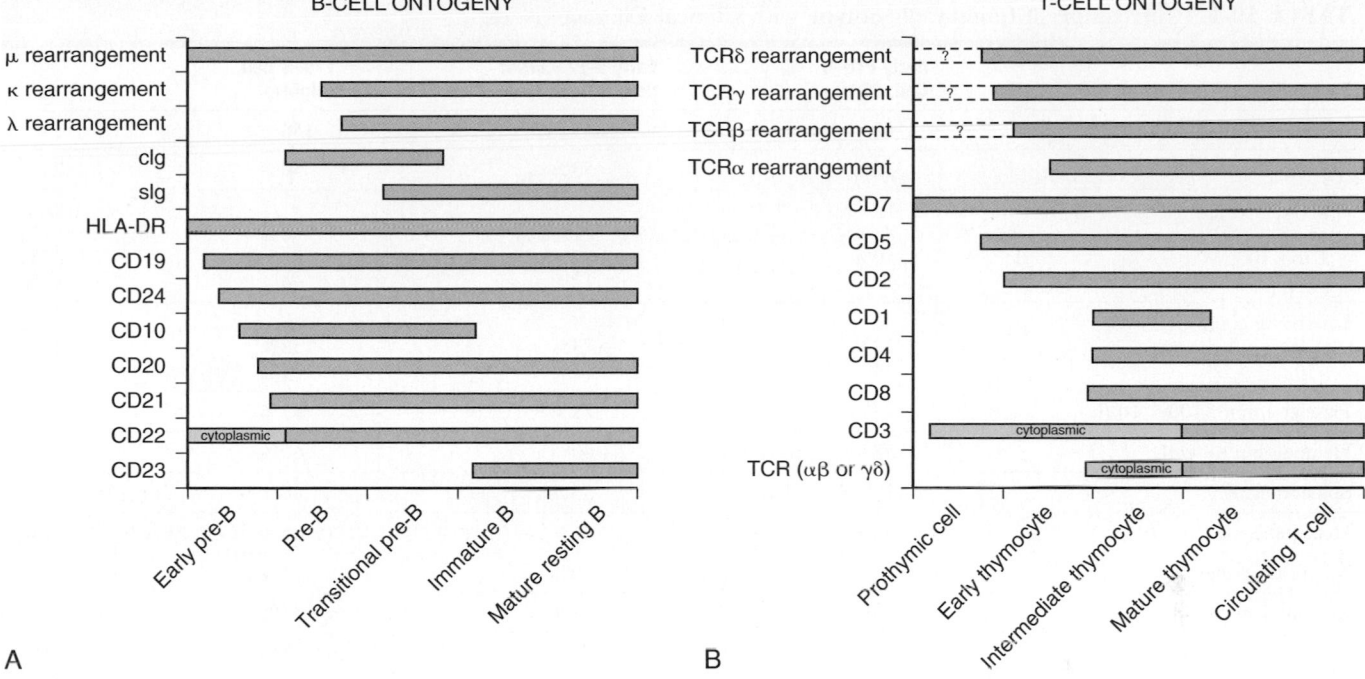

Figure 50-2 Schematic representation of human lymphoid differentiation. **A,** Hypothetical schema of marker expression and gene rearrangement during normal B-cell ontogeny. **B,** Hypothetical schema of marker expression and gene rearrangement during normal T-cell ontogeny. *(Modified from Pui CH, Behm FG, Crist WM: Clinical and biologic relevance of immunologic marker studies in childhood acute lymphoblastic leukemia.* Blood *82:343–362, 1993.)*

ALL pediatric patients have L3 lymphoblasts, which appear identical to Burkitt lymphoma cells, with deeply basophilic cytoplasm and prominent cytoplasmic vacuolization. L3 morphology is almost always associated with a mature B-cell phenotype (including expression of surface immunoglobulin) and translocations involving the *MYC* gene on chromosome 8; patients with these characteristics should be treated with regimens for advanced-stage Burkitt lymphoma rather than ALL.[8,9] Other morphologic variants of ALL, including ALL with hand mirror cells or granules, have been described but do not appear to have prognostic significance.[7]

Various cytochemical stains can distinguish ALL from AML. In approximately 80% of cases of ALL, lymphoblasts react positively with periodic acid–Schiff (PAS), which stains cytoplasmic glycogen.[10] Myeloid-specific stains, such as myeloperoxidase, specific and nonspecific esterase, and Sudan black (a cytoplasmic lipid stain), are usually negative in ALL. In contrast, myeloblasts are myeloperoxidase positive in 75% of patients. Terminal deoxynucleotidyl transferase (TdT), an enzyme that catalyzes the polymerization of deoxynucleoside monophosphates into a single-strand DNA primer, can be demonstrated in most cases of ALL but is rarely present in cases of myeloid leukemia.

Immunophenotype

ALL is subcategorized based on the expression of lineage- and maturation-specific antigens present on the cell surface and in the cytoplasm of lymphoblasts. In addition, immunophenotypic studies of lymphoblasts have

provided important insights into the differentiation and maturation of normal B and T lymphocytes. Because the leukemic blast represents the neoplastic expansion of a lymphoid progenitor cell, many phenotypic and genotypic features of the lymphoblast mimic those of the normal lymphoid cell counterpart of specific lineage and maturational stage.[11] Figure 50-2 depicts a schematic overview of lymphoid cell differentiation.[12]

Based on reactivity with a panel of lineage-associated antibodies, ALL has been subclassified into three broad categories: B-precursor cell, mature B cell, and T cell. The immunophenotypic subsets are associated with distinctive clinical features (Table 50-1).[13]

B-Precursor Cell ALL

The B-precursor cell phenotype is present in 80% to 85% of children with ALL. These leukemia cells are characterized by reactivity with monoclonal antibodies specific for B-cell–associated antigens (e.g., CD9, CD19, CD22, and CD79a) and are distinguished from mature B-cell ALL by the absence of surface immunoglobulin. In the vast majority (80% to 90%) of B-precursor cell ALL, the cells express CD10, also known as the common ALL antigen (CALLA).

Over 90% of cases of B-precursor cell ALL have evidence of immunoglobulin gene rearrangements, predominantly involving the immunoglobulin heavy chain (IgH).[14] Of note, T-cell receptor (TCR) gene rearrangements also may be observed in B-precursor cell ALL and IgH gene rearrangements have been observed in T-cell ALL.[15] These leukemia-specific clonal IgH and TCR gene

TABLE 50-1   Correlation of Immunophenotype with Clinical Characteristics

Parameter	Early Pro–B Cell, CD10–	Early B-Precursor Cell, CD10+	Pre–B Cell (cIgM+)	T Cell
No. of patients	52	635	156	124
Gender (% male)	39%	53%	50%	75%
Age (yr)				
<1	33%	1%	6%	1%
1 to <10	50%	82%	80%	62%
≥10	17%	17%	14%	37%
Leukocyte count (× 10⁹/L)				
≤20	38%	75%	53%	23%
>50	44%	11%	21%	57%
Platelet count ≤100 × 10⁹/L	77%	75%	81%	56%
Hemoglobin ≤8 g/dL	58%	40%	60%	15%
Splenomegaly*	50%	34%	46%	57%
Hepatomegaly*	56%	46%	48%	61%
Mediastinal mass	0%	0%	1%	72%
Lymphadenopathy	35%	36%	41%	78%
CNS-positive (CNS-3)†	10%	1%	1%	11%

From Reiter A, Schrappe M, Ludwig WD, et al: Chemotherapy in 998 unselected childhood acute lymphoblastic leukemia patients: results and conclusions of the multicenter trial ALL-BFM 86. Blood 84:3122–3133, 1994; and H. Riehm, personal communication, 1996.
cIgM+, Intracytoplasmic immunoglobulin M positive; CNS, central nervous system.
>4 cm below the costal margin.
†CNS-3, diagnostic cerebrospinal fluid specimen with five or more white blood cells/high-power field and lymphoblasts seen on cytospin preparation.

rearrangements have been used to quantify submicroscopic levels of residual leukemia in patients using polymerase chain reaction (PCR)-based assays.[15]

The presence of intracytoplasmic immunoglobulin (cIg) and various cell surface markers has been used to distinguish different subsets of B-precursor cell ALL based on their level of differentiation. These subsets include pro-B ALL (3% to 4% of pediatric patients), early pre-B ALL (60% to 70% of pediatric patients), and pre-B ALL (20% to 30% of pediatric patients):[16]

- Pro–B-cell ALL, believed to be derived from a very immature B-cell precursor, is characterized by CD10-negative immunophenotype and the absence of cIg. It is most frequently observed in infants with ALL, especially those with abnormalities involving chromosome 11q23 (*MLL* [also known as *KMT2A*] gene locus).[17,18]
- Early pre–B-cell ALL is the most common subtype of B-precursor cell ALL in children. It is believed to be derived from a more mature B-cell precursor than pro-B ALL. Early pre–B cells frequently express CD10 but still lack cIg. CD10 (CALLA)-positive leukemias without cytoplasmic immunoglobulin are also referred to as common ALL (c-ALL).[19]
- Pre–B-cell ALL is characterized by the presence of cIg.[20] It is believed to derive from an intermediate B precursor cell, more mature than those lacking cIg (early pre–B cells) but not as mature as those with surface immunoglobulin (mature B cells). Like early pre–B cells, pre–B lymphoblasts typically express

CD10 and human leukocyte antigen (HLA)-DR. Approximately 25% of cases of pre–B-cell (cIg+) ALL have the chromosomal translocation t(1;19) (q23;p13), which fuses the *TFPT* (formerly *E2A*) gene on chromosome 19 with the *PBX1* gene on chromosome 1.[20] This translocation is observed in only 1% of cases of early pre-B (or common) ALL.

Mature B-Cell ALL

Mature B-cell ALL accounts for 1% to 2% of childhood ALL cases.[21] It is characterized by the presence of surface immunoglobulin, most often IgM, which is monoclonal for κ or λ light chains. The cells generally express other B-cell antigens, including CD19, CD20, and HLA-DR. Morphologically, the blasts tend to be classified as FAB L3, with intensely staining cytoplasmic basophilia similar to that of erythroblasts. Cases of mature B-cell ALL without L3 morphologic features have been reported but are rare.[22] Almost all cases of mature B-cell ALL are associated with one of three non-random chromosomal translocations—t(8;14)(q24;q32) or, less commonly, t(2;8)(p12;q24) or t(8;22)(q24;q11).[23] The chromosomal breakpoints involve the *MYC* oncogene on chromosome 8 and the genes for the IgH (chromosome 14), κ light chain (chromosome 2), or λ light chain (chromosome 22). Mature B-cell ALL is clinically indistinguishable from disseminated Burkitt lymphoma and is much more successfully treated with regimens used for that disease than when treated with conventional childhood ALL therapy.[8,9]

T-Cell ALL

The T-cell immunophenotype is present in 10% to 15% of children with ALL.[24] Compared with B-precursor cell ALL, T-cell ALL is more frequently associated with older age at diagnosis, higher presenting leukocyte counts, and bulky extramedullary disease (including lymphadenopathy, hepatosplenomegaly, overt central nervous system [CNS] leukemia, and an anterior mediastinal thymic mass).[16] Historically, patients with T-cell ALL had an inferior outcome compared with those with B-precursor cell ALL, although this prognostic difference is not observed when more intensive regimens are used.[25] However, the time period in which relapses occur differs between the two immunophenotypic subtypes, with earlier relapses observed more frequently in T-cell ALL.[25]

T-cell ALL can be subclassified using monoclonal antibodies that recognize surface antigens expressed during discrete stages of normal T-cell development.[26] Most of the phenotypically defined subsets of T-cell ALL have limited clinical relevance.[27,28] However, gene expression profile studies have identified a biologically distinctive subset of T-cell ALL that, in retrospective analysis, was associated with a high risk for treatment failure.[29] These patients were noted to have a distinctive "early T-cell precursor" phenotype consisting of weak expression of CD5 and coexpression of stem cell or myeloid markers.[29] Similarly, another retrospective study using array comparative genomic hybridization (CGH) and quantitative DNA-PCR techniques identified the absence of V(D)J recombination at the TCRγ locus, a feature that is characteristic of early T-cell precursor cells, as a predictor of early treatment failure in patients with T-cell ALL.[30] Thus, T-cell ALL patients with features of development arrest at the earliest stages of T-cell development appear to have an inferior outcome.

Myeloid Antigen Coexpression

In some instances, individual leukemic cells simultaneously express lymphoid and myeloid surface antigens. Up to 20% of cases of ALL (i.e., with lymphoid surface antigen predominance) also coexpress myeloid antigens.[31,32] Myeloid antigen coexpression is associated with young age at diagnosis (<12 months), pro–B-cell (CD10−) immunophenotype, and certain chromosomal abnormalities, such as rearrangements of chromosome 11q23 (frequently observed in infants with ALL), the Philadelphia (Ph) chromosome [t(9;22)], and the ETV6-RUNX1 [t(12;21)] fusion.[33-35] Older studies suggested that patients with biphenotypic ALL had a worse prognosis,[36] but more recent reports have indicated that myeloid antigen coexpression lacks independent prognostic significance.[31-33] Cases of ALL with myeloid antigen coexpression should be distinguished from leukemia of ambiguous lineage, an uncommon entity in which the predominant lineage (lymphoid or myeloid) cannot be determined by immunophenotype and histochemistry. The World Health Organization classification system requires that cells express myeloperoxidase or evidence of monocytic differentiation, along with either T-cell antigen CD3 (cytoplasmic or surface) or B-cell surface antigens (CD19, CD79a, CD22, and CD10).[37]

MOLECULAR PATHOGENESIS

Lymphocytes arise from hematopoietic stem cells through a series of proliferation and differentiation steps that result in the formation of mature B or T lymphocytes, each expressing a specific immunoglobulin or TCR capable of responding to a narrow range of foreign antigens. The development of a fully competent adaptive immune system is dependent on the generation of a population of mature B and T lymphocytes with extraordinary diversity in antigen specificity, which collectively provide the ability to mount an effective immune response against a broad range of pathogens. This diversity in antigen receptor specificity is achieved through an elaborate process of somatic mutagenesis, including V(D)J recombination and somatic hypermutation, designed to introduce unique variations in the immunoglobulin or TCR gene structure of each individual developing lymphocyte. Despite their carefully regulated nature, these programmed mechanisms of somatic mutagenesis can go awry and introduce somatic mutations at other genomic loci. Mutations in oncogenes or tumor suppressors acquired during lymphocyte development can result in the aberrant proliferation and differentiation arrest that are characteristic of ALL.

Although a comprehensive review of the molecular pathogenesis of ALL is beyond the scope of this chapter, we highlight here select molecular lesions that have proven particularly informative to our understanding of the pathobiology of ALL and review in more detail the molecular pathogenesis of three particularly high-risk subtypes of ALL: BCR-ABL, hypodiploid, and early T-cell progenitor ALL.

Transcriptional Regulators

ETV6-RUNX1 Fusion Genes in B-Precursor Cell ALL

In 20% to 25% of childhood ALL cases a cryptic t(12;21) translocation results in expression of a fusion ETV6-RUNX1 (also known as TEL-AML1) translocation.[38] ETV6 and RUNX1 are transcription factors that are each required for normal hematopoiesis, and both are involved in other leukemia-related translocations. The t(12;21) translocation results in the fusion of the HLH domain of ETV6 to almost all of RUNX1. The mechanisms through which ETV6-RUNX1 fusions drive leukemogenesis remain incompletely understood, but recent work has shown that expression of this fusion oncoprotein in hematopoietic stem cells markedly increases their numbers and promotes their transformation after chemical mutagenesis.[39] Interestingly, ETV6-RUNX1 translocations can often be detected in prenatal blood specimens collected from children who went on to develop ETV6-RUNX1–rearranged ALL many years later, indicating that it is likely the initiating mutation in ALL.[40] However, this translocation is not sufficient for leukemogenesis because the incidence of detectable ETV6-RUNX1 fusions in normal neonatal blood is 100-fold greater than the incidence of leukemia with this translocation.[41] Several studies have shown that the presence of an *ETV6-RUNX1* translocation is associated with a favorable prognosis in childhood ALL.[42,43] Indeed, *ETV6-RUNX1* expression is associated with decreased expression of the *ABCB1* (also known as *MDR1*) multidrug resistance gene and of genes involved in purine metabolism, which may explain the particular sensitivity of these cases to mercaptopurine and methotrexate.[44,45]

MLL Fusion Genes in B-Precursor Cell ALL

Chromosomal translocations resulting in the fusion of the amino-terminus (N-terminus) of the *MLL* gene on 11q23 to the carboxy-terminus (C-terminus) of one of more than 60 different translocations partners occur in 70% of infant ALL, in 10% of AML, and in the majority of secondary AML cases that are induced by prior treatment with topoisomerase II inhibitors.[46] The presence of *MLL* translocations is associated with inferior outcomes despite aggressive chemotherapy in ALL, as discussed later in this chapter. *MLL* is the human ortholog of *Drosophila trithorax*, which positively regulates expression of multiple genes of the *HOXA* cluster and acts antagonistically to the polycomb group of proteins. The breakpoints of *MLL* translocations cluster between exons 5 and 11 of *MLL*, resulting in expression of fusion oncoproteins that retain the N-terminal domains of the protein that bind DNA in a sequence-nonspecific manner, whereas the C-terminal domains of MLL that mediate association of the wild-type protein with its endogenous chromatin modification complex and its Histone H3 lysine-4–specific N-methyltransferase activity are invariably lost.[47] Instead, the C-terminus of MLL fusion oncoproteins is provided by one of more than 60 different translocation partners, with common translocations such as the t(4;11), t(9;11), and t(11;19)(q23;p13.3) resulting in the in-frame fusion of *MLL* to the C-terminal domains of *AF4* (also known as *AFF1*), *AF9* (also known as *MLLT3*), and *ENL* (also known as *MLLT1*), respectively.[48,49] Expression of MLL fusion oncoproteins in murine hematopoietic precursors induces leukemia,[50-54] an effect that is dependent on MLL fusion oncoprotein–driven overexpression of several genes of the *HOXA* cluster.[55,56]

Until recently, the mechanism through which the C-terminal fusion partners of MLL contributed to leukemogenesis was unclear, because there were no apparent sequence similarities between the fusion partners involved. However, recent work has shown that several MLL translocation partners are functionally linked through their association in protein complexes that regulate transcriptional elongation.[47] MLL fusion oncoproteins bind at least three distinct complexes, including the polymerase-associated factor complex, the positive transcription elongator factor (pTEFb) complex, and the DOT1L histone methyltransferase complex.[57] The DOT1L methyltransferase is required for the maintenance of MLL-driven leukemias but appears to be less important for normal hematopoiesis, thus suggesting a therapeutic window for targeting DOT1L in MLL-rearranged ALL.[58-62] Indeed, a small molecule DOT1L inhibitor has recently been developed and demonstrates promising preclinical activity in murine models of MLL-rearranged leukemia, raising the possibility that such a therapeutic strategy could improve the prognosis for patients with MLL-rearranged ALL.[63]

MYC Translocations in Mature B-Cell ALL

Chromosome translocations that place the coding region of the *MYC* protooncogene under the control of gene regulatory elements of one of the immunoglobulin receptor genes, such as the t(8;14), t(2;8) or t(8;22), lead to aberrant overexpression of the *MYC* oncogenic transcription factor. *MYC* overexpression is potently oncogenic in a wide range of experimental systems. Although MYC has long been believed to be a traditional transcription factor that regulates a specific set of target genes, recent work has revealed that MYC accumulates at the promoters of essentially all transcriptionally active genes and acts as a nonlinear amplifier of existing gene expression programs.[64,65] Thus, rather than inducing expression of a specific gene expression program, these findings suggest that MYC instead acts to lock a cell's gene expression program into its existing form, which presumably can be oncogenic when it occurs in a cell that is in a highly proliferative state that normally should be transient. *MYC* translocations are characteristically found in mature B-cell leukemia, which is best considered a disseminated form of Burkitt lymphoma that responds poorly to standard ALL therapy. Outcomes for these patients are much improved with treatment regimens specifically designed for high-grade B-cell non-Hodgkin lymphomas.[8,9]

Activating *NOTCH1* Mutations in T-Cell ALL

NOTCH1 encodes an unusual cell surface receptor that, on activation by ligand binding to its extracellular domain, undergoes two distinct proteolytic cleavage events, culminating in release of the intracellular domain of NOTCH1 (ICN) into the cytoplasm. The ICN protein subsequently translocates to the nucleus, where it functions as a transcription factor that generally activates expression of its targets.[66] NOTCH1 is required at multiple stages of T-cell development, and its ectopic activation in murine T-cell progenitors is highly leukemogenic.[66-69] Although NOTCH1 can be activated by chromosomal translocations in very rare cases of T-cell ALL,[70] more than 50% of T-cell ALL cases harbor activating *NOTCH1* mutations, and these occur in all of the molecular subtypes of T-cell ALL.[71] Activating *NOTCH1* mutations typically occur either as missense mutations in the heterodimerization domain, where they promote ligand-independent proteolytic activation of the ICN domain, or as truncating or frameshift mutations in the C-terminal PEST domain of ICN, which lead to ICN protein accumulation as a result of impaired proteasomal degradation.[71,72] The pathogenic role of *NOTCH1* in T-cell ALL is mediated largely by its role as a transcriptional activator of two key downstream targets, *MYC* and *HES1*.[66,73-75]

One of the key proteolytic cleavage events required for NOTCH1 activation is mediated by the γ-secretase complex. Treatment of NOTCH1-mutant T-cell ALL cell lines with γ-secretase inhibitors leads to modest reductions in cell proliferation in a subset of cell lines,[71,76] but a number of NOTCH1-mutant T-cell ALL cell lines fail to respond to these inhibitors. The mechanisms of resistance to NOTCH1 inhibition have been an area of intense investigation, and recent work has revealed that inactivation of the *FBXW7* tumor suppressor, an E3 ubiquitin ligase that targets both ICN and *MYC* for proteasomal degradation, is one mechanism of resistance to γ-secretase inhibitors.[77,78] Additionally, resistance to inhibition of NOTCH1 or its downstream target *MYC* can be mediated by PTEN inactivation and resultant AKT activation in T-cell ALL, thus suggesting the potential therapeutic utility of AKT pathway inhibitors as a strategy to reverse resistance to γ-secretase inhibitor.[79,80] Moreover, glucocorticoid resistance in T-cell ALL has been shown to be reversible by γ-secretase inhibitors, and it appears that glucocorticoid therapy can ameliorate the intestinal toxicity of γ-secretase inhibitors.[81] Taken together, these findings provide a compelling rationale for clinical trials combining glucocorticoids with small molecule inhibitors of NOTCH1 and AKT.

Growth Factor Signaling
Cytokine Receptor Signaling

Cytokine receptor signaling plays key roles in normal lymphocyte development, with inactivating mutations in key cytokine receptor subunits (e.g., interleukin-2 receptor γ [*IL2RG*] and interleukin-7 receptor [*IL7R*]) or their downstream effector kinases (e.g., Janus kinase-3 [*JAK3*]), resulting in severe lymphopenia and the lack of a functional adaptive immune system characteristic of severe combined immunodeficiency. Conversely, aberrant activation of cytokine receptor signaling has recently been implicated in the molecular pathogenesis of ALL.

Cytokine receptor–like factor 2 (*CRLF2*) encodes a cytokine receptor subunit that heterodimerizes with IL7R to form the receptor for the cytokine TSLP (thymic stromal lymphopoietin), which is a proinflammatory cytokine secreted by endothelial cells that drives lymphocyte proliferation.[82] *CRLF2* rearrangements leading to aberrant overexpression have recently been described in B-precursor cell ALL, typically as a result of an intrachromosomal deletion leading to a *P2RY8-CRLF2* fusion, or translocations of the IgH locus to *CRLF2*.[83-85] *CRLF2* rearrangements are found in 5% to 10% of B-precursor cell ALL cases but in more than 50% of patients with Down syndrome–associated ALL, strongly suggesting that these collaborate with trisomy 21 in B-lymphoblast transformation. *CRLF2* rearrangements are often associated with activating mutations of Janus kinase 2 (*JAK2*), and CRLF2 overexpression and mutated JAK2 cooperate to induce cytokine-independent growth to Ba/F3 pro-B cells.

IL7R encodes a cytokine receptor subunit that can heterodimerize with the IL2Rγ (the common γc chain) to form IL7R, or with CRLF2 to form the TSLP receptor. Recent work has identified activating IL7Rα point mutations in 9% of cases of T-cell ALL, as well as in the "BCR-ABL–like" subset of B-precursor cell ALL (discussed in more detail later).[86,87] Interestingly, most of these mutations result in the introduction of a novel cysteine residue into the extracellular domain of IL7Rα, and aberrant signaling results because disulfide bond formation between these mutant cysteines can allow mutant IL7Rα proteins to aberrantly dimerize, leading to activation of downstream signaling pathways independent of ligand or of the common γc chain.[86,87] The potential therapeutic utility of targeting aberrant oncogenic signaling downstream of mutationally activated cytokine receptors is an area of active investigation.

PTEN and the PI3K-AKT Axis

The *PI3K-AKT* oncogenic pathway, which is negatively regulated by the *PTEN* tumor suppressor, mediates prosurvival and proliferative signaling downstream of activated growth factor receptors and is aberrantly activated in a broad range of human cancer subtypes.[88] Recent work has revealed that nearly half of T-cell ALL cases harbor mutational activation of oncogenic signaling through this pathway, most often as a result of truncating mutations or deletions of the *PTEN* tumor suppressor, but activating mutations of *PI3K* and *AKT* genes also occur.[79,89-91] *PTEN* deletions are a strong predictor of early treatment failure in T-ALL cases[86,89] and *PTEN* inactivation has been shown to induce resistance to NOTCH1 or *MYC* inhibition in zebrafish and murine models of T-cell ALL.[79,80] These findings highlight the potential application of small molecule inhibitors of the *PI3K-AKT* pathway for high-risk T-cell ALL.

Molecular Pathogenesis of Select High-Risk Subtypes
BCR-ABL and BCR-ABL–like ALL

The discovery of the Ph chromosome, which arises from the t(9;22)(q34;q11) translocation resulting in expression of a BCR-ABL fusion oncoprotein, was a major milestone in molecular oncogenesis that provided compelling support for the hypothesis, first put forth by Boveri in 1914, that cancer arises due to a genetic lesion in a single cell, resulting in outgrowth of a clonal population.[92,93] *BCR-ABL* translocations are pathognomonic of chronic myeloid leukemia and are also found in 4% to 5% of childhood and 25% of adult cases of B-precursor cell ALL.[38] The translocation underlying formation of the Ph chromosome results in expression of a BCR-ABL fusion oncoprotein with constitutively active tyrosine kinase activity, which transforms cells at least in part due to activation of the RAS-MAPK pathway, PI3K, and JUN-kinase pathways.[94] Although historically associated with an extremely poor prognosis, hematopoietic stem cell transplantation (HSCT) proved to be the first highly effective therapeutic modality for this high-risk subtype of ALL.[95] Additionally, the development of imatinib mesylate, a small molecule inhibitor of oncogenic signaling by the BCR-ABL kinase, has opened novel therapeutic opportunities for the management of Ph chromosome–positive ALL. Although single-agent therapy with imatinib leads to rapid development of resistance in Ph chromosome–positive ALL, pilot trials of the combination of conventional chemotherapy with imatinib or other tyrosine kinase inhibitors have been promising.[96,97]

Although the poor prognosis of BCR-ABL ALL was traditionally believed to be due to expression of the BCR-ABL oncoprotein, recent work has shown that this subtype of ALL is also characterized by inactivation of the DNA-binding protein Ikaros, which is encoded by the IKZF1 gene.[98] IKZF1 deletions have been identified in up to 15% of BCR-ABL–negative pediatric ALL cases and have been shown to be an independent predictor of adverse outcome.[99,100] These cases have been classified as "BCR-ABL–like" ALL on the basis of similarities in gene expression profiles with Ph chromosome–positive ALL.[99,100] Recent work has revealed that most of these "BCR-ABL–like" cases harboring Ikaros alterations, but lacking BCR-ABL translocations, commonly harbor mutational activation of tyrosine kinase signaling as a result of translocations or activating point mutations of receptor or cytoplasmic kinases, such as PDGFRB, CRLF2, EPOR, IL7R, FLT3, JAK2, and ABL1. Importantly, preclinical studies have demonstrated the potential therapeutic utility of targeting the aberrantly activated kinase involved for at least some of these cases.[101]

Hypodiploid ALL

The presence of hypodiploidy (<44 to 45 chromosomes) portends a poor prognosis in B-precursor cell ALL, with event-free survival (EFS) rates less than 40%.[102] Alterations in whole-chromosome number (aneuploidy) are very common in human cancer[103] and can be oncogenic.[104] However, the mechanisms through which hypodiploidy contributes to leukemogenesis in B-precursor cell ALL remain largely unknown.

A recent genomic study has shed key insights into the molecular pathogenesis of hypodiploid ALL.[105] Both copies of chromosome 21 were always retained in each of the 124 cases of hypodiploid ALL cases analyzed, which, given that trisomy 21 is one of the most common genetic alterations in B-precursor cell ALL, highlights the pathogenic role of additional copies of genes on chromosome 21 in B-precursor cell ALL.

Rather than representing a single subtype of ALL, hypodiploid ALL instead harbors distinct biologic subsets, including low hypodiploidy (32-39 chromosomes) and near haploidy (24-31 chromosomes), which differ strikingly on a molecular basis.

- *Near-haploid ALL (24 to 31 chromosomes):* Seventy percent of these cases are characterized by genetic lesions leading to activation of growth factor signaling pathways, including NRAS, KRAS, NF1, MAPK, FLT3, and PTPN11. Notably, deletions of tumor suppressors such as *NF1* and *PTPN11* were typically homozygous as a result of hypodiploidy, and loss of heterozygosity of tumor suppressors provides one mechanism through which hypodiploidy can contribute to oncogenesis. These data support the potential therapeutic utility of targeting these kinases, or their key downstream effectors, although such interventions await further preclinical investigation.
- *Low-hypodiploid ALL (32 to 39 chromosomes):* In marked contrast to near-haploid ALL, almost all cases of low-hypodiploid ALL harbored mutations

of the *TP53* tumor suppressor, whereas mutations of growth factor signaling pathways were rare in this subset. Mutations of *TP53* were present in remission bone marrow specimens in almost half of pediatric cases, strongly suggesting a germline origin consistent with the Li-Fraumeni syndrome; indeed, germline transmission was confirmed in one kindred.[105] Given that the induction of aneuploidy triggers *TP53*-dependent cell cycle arrest,[106] these data support a model in which *TP53* inactivation occurs early in the pathogenesis of low-hypodiploid ALL, thus allowing the subsequent acquisition of hypodiploidy to be tolerated by these cells. However, it remains entirely unclear why *TP53* mutations should be so rare in other ALL subtypes with striking degrees of aneuploidy, including near-haploid and hyperdiploid ALL. Low-hypodiploid cases were also associated with a high frequency of inactivating mutations of the *RB1* tumor suppressor, as well as a very high frequency of mutations involving Ikaros family members, particularly *IKZF2* (encoding Helios), which was mutated in more than 50% of cases.

A subset of cases with an apparently hyperdiploid chromosome complement was found to in fact represent "masked" hypodiploidy in which the hypodiploid genome has undergone reduplication, based on loss of heterozygosity apparent on the single-nucleotide polymorphism arrays performed. Although these cases might be classified clinically as hyperdiploid ALL (which has a favorable prognosis), masked hypodiploid ALL cases are indistinguishable from the respective hypodiploid ALL subtype (low-hypodiploid or near-haploid) based on gene expression profiling and pattern of oncogenic lesions, thus suggesting the need for clinical tests to distinguish this subtype from cases of "typical" hyperdiploidy, which has a favorable prognosis. Given that chromosomes 4 and 17 are lost in almost all cases of hypodiploid ALL, the presence of these trisomies may help to distinguish cases of true hyperdiploidy from masked hypodiploidy.[107]

Early T-Cell Progenitor T-Cell ALL

Recent work has revealed that differentiation arrest at the earliest stages of T-cell development, defined either by absence of biallelic TCRγ deletion (ABD; indicating failure to complete V(D)J recombination) or by an early T-cell progenitor gene expression profile pattern, identifies an overlapping subset of T-cell ALL cases at very high risk for treatment failure.[29,30] These cases are associated with aberrant oncogenic signaling through the RAS-MAPK, PI3K-AKT, and JAK-STAT pathways, typically owing to associated mutations in *RAS, FLT3, IL7R, BRAF,* and *JAK* kinases, as well as deletions of the *PTEN* tumor suppressor.[30,86] These cases are defined as T-cell ALL based on expression of cytoplasmic CD3 and harbor mutations in defining T-cell ALL oncogenes such as *NOTCH1*.[29,30] However, these cases also harbor additional mutations that are typically seen in AML, myelodysplastic, and myeloproliferative syndromes, such as *RUNX1, ETV6, EED, EZH2, SUZ12, DNMT3A, IDH1,* and *IDH2*.[29,108,109] Moreover, gene expression analyses have shown that early T-precursor T-cell ALL harbors similarities to normal hematopoietic stem cells and AML leukemic stem cells. The identification of effective targeted therapies is a subject of active investigation.

CLINICAL MANIFESTATIONS

ALL may present insidiously or acutely, as an incidental finding on a routine blood cell count of an asymptomatic child, or as a life-threatening hemorrhage, infection, or episode of respiratory distress. Common presenting symptoms include fever, pallor, bruising, petechiae, bone pain (presumably secondary to stretching of the periosteum or joint capsule by leukemic infiltration), and limp.

Although ALL is primarily a disease of the bone marrow and peripheral blood, any organ or tissue may be infiltrated by the abnormal cells. Such infiltration may be clinically apparent by physical examination. At initial diagnosis, 30% to 50% of children have enlargement of the liver or spleen, with organs palpable more than 4 cm below the costal margins (see Table 50-1). Lymphadenopathy caused by leukemic infiltration is an equally frequent presenting sign. Generally, the degree of organ infiltration correlates with peripheral blood blast count, thus reflecting the total leukemic mass. Leukemic invasion of tissues may, however, be occult and detectable only by histologic sampling.

Peripheral Blood

Clinical laboratory data often provide a broad spectrum of abnormal findings at the time of diagnosis of leukemia. Anemia, abnormal leukocyte counts and differential, and thrombocytopenia are common (see Table 50-1). However, some children with ALL may have normal peripheral blood cell counts at the time of diagnosis, even when the bone marrow is replaced by leukemic cells.

The red blood cells are usually normochromic and normocytic. Failure of erythroid production is manifested by a low reticulocyte count. Peripheral blood smear may reveal teardrop forms and nucleated red cells, consistent with marrow invasion.

Platelet counts may vary from normal to extremely low. Most children have fewer than 100,000 cells/mm³ at presentation, and the platelets are usually of normal size. In contrast to idiopathic thrombocytopenic purpura (ITP), thrombocytopenia at the time of ALL diagnosis is usually accompanied by other hematologic or physical manifestations of leukemia.[110]

There is a wide range of leukocyte counts observed at the time of diagnosis, from extremely low to more than 1 million cells/mm³. Approximately 20% of children with ALL present with leukocyte counts of more than 50,000 cells/mm³.[111] Even with high presenting leukocyte counts, absolute neutropenia is common. Blast forms may or may not be present on routine smears of peripheral blood. Even when present, peripheral blast cells may be misleading, and the definitive diagnosis of leukemia cannot be made from the morphologic examination of the peripheral blood. For example, myeloblasts may be detected in the peripheral blood when the marrow has been infiltrated by various disorders, including osteopetrosis,

myelofibrosis, granulomatous infections, sarcoidosis, metastatic tumor, and even ALL. Additionally, in patients with leukemia, the morphologic appearance of leukemic blast cells in the peripheral blood may differ from that of the marrow. Peripheral blood flow cytometry may be useful in distinguishing malignant blasts from "normal" myeloblasts, and differentiating ALL from AML, in patients with high presenting leukocyte counts.

Hypereosinophilia has been described in association with ALL.[112] The eosinophilia may precede the diagnosis of ALL, appear at presentation, and then disappear with successful remission induction.[112,113] Eosinophilia in B-precursor cell ALL has been associated with the t(5;14)(q31;q32) translocation, involving the IL3 gene on chromosome 5 and the IgH gene (IGH) on chromosome 14.[114,115]

In regard to hyperleukocytosis, approximately 10% of children with ALL present with extremely high leukocyte counts (>100,000 cells/mm³) (Table 50-2).[2,3,116] In patients with markedly elevated leukocyte counts, blood flow in the microcirculation can be impeded by intravascular clumping of the poorly deformable blasts. This may result in local hypoxemia, endothelial damage, hemorrhage, and infarction, especially in the CNS and lung. Clinically significant leukostasis, resulting in intracerebral hemorrhage or respiratory failure, is more common with hyperleukocytosis in AML than in ALL.[117] In one series, neurologic or pulmonary symptoms or both were observed in 5% to 10% of children with ALL and a

---

TABLE 50-2 Presenting Features by Age in 5181 Children and Adolescents with Acute Lymphoblastic Leukemia (ALL) Treated on ALL-BFM Trials (1986-1999)

| | Age (yr) | | |
Presenting Feature	<1 (2.5% of Patients)	1 to <10 (79% of Patients)	10-18 (18.5% of Patients)
Gender			
Male	52%	56%	61%
Female	48%	44%	39%
WBC count ≥100 × 10⁹/L	59%	10%	15%
Phenotype			
B-precursor cell	96%	90%	73%
T-cell	4%	10%	27%
CNS-positive*	21%	2.3%	3.9%
High hyperdiploidy†	1.5%	27%	15%
ETV6-RUNX1 fusion†	4.5%	27%	11%
t(9;22) BCR-ABL†	0%	2.2%	5.1%

Modified from Moricke A, Zimmermann M, Reiter A, et al: Prognostic impact of age in children and adolescents with acute lymphoblastic leukemia: data from the trials ALL-BFM 86, 90, and 95. Klin Padiatr 217:310–320, 2005.

CNS, Central nervous system; WBC, white blood cell.
*CNS-3, diagnostic cerebrospinal fluid specimen with five or more WBCs/high-power field and lymphoblasts seen on cytospin preparation.
†Results for B-precursor cases only.

presenting leukocyte count higher than 200,000 cells/mm³ and CNS hemorrhage was diagnosed in 2% of those patients (all of whom had leukocyte counts higher than $400 \times 10^9/L$).[117] Treatment of hyperleukocytosis consists of vigorous intravenous hydration. Red blood cell transfusions should be administered cautiously to avoid increasing whole blood viscosity and worsening symptoms. For patients with very high presenting leukocyte counts and symptomatic leukostasis, leukapheresis or exchange transfusion may prevent hyperviscosity and leukemia cell lysis–related problems.

Disseminated intravascular coagulation is infrequently observed in patients with ALL at diagnosis. It is more common in T-cell ALL as a result of thromboplastic substances released from T lymphoblasts.[118] It also has been reported in patients with the uncommon t(17;19) translocation, associated with the B-precursor cell immunophenotype.[119] Disseminated intravascular coagulation should be treated promptly with infusions of fresh-frozen plasma and cryoprecipitate.

Bone Marrow

Evaluation of the bone marrow by aspiration and biopsy is essential for making the diagnosis of leukemia. The marrow specimen is usually hypercellular and characterized by a homogeneous population of cells. In most cases of ALL, the marrow generally has more than 50% blasts.

A bone marrow aspirate may be difficult to obtain at the time of diagnosis. This is usually caused by the density of blast forms in the marrow, but it may be caused by marrow fibrosis or necrosis.[120,121] In such cases, a diagnosis can be made by bone marrow biopsy. "Touch preps" of the biopsy specimen can be helpful in elucidating morphology when aspiration is not successful.

Differences may occur in leukemic involvement found in marrow aspirates derived from widely separated sites. Patchy marrow involvement of leukemic infiltration has been reported at diagnosis and relapse.[122] If clinical findings suggest leukemia, but a single-site bone marrow specimen is nondiagnostic, the marrow should be sampled at additional sites.

The distinction between ALL with lymph node involvement and non-Hodgkin lymphoblastic lymphoma with bone marrow invasion (stage IV) is arbitrary. Commonly the disease is classified as ALL when there are more than 25% lymphoblasts in the marrow and as stage IV non-Hodgkin lymphoblastic lymphoma when there are fewer than 25% lymphoblasts in the marrow. Although the lymphoblasts of ALL and lymphoblastic lymphoma appear morphologically and immunophenotypically indistinguishable, gene expression profiling studies have suggested that there may be differences in underlying biology between these two diagnoses.[123] However, the distinction may not be clinically important because advanced-stage lymphoblastic lymphoma and ALL respond similarly to intensive ALL-type therapy.[124,125]

Extramedullary Leukemia

Although marrow replacement is the major cause of symptoms of leukemia, extramedulllary involvement may also contribute to presenting signs and symptoms.

CNS Manifestations

Up to 20% of children will have blast cells visible on a cytocentrifuged cerebrospinal fluid (CSF) specimen at diagnosis.[126,127] CSF lymphoblasts can usually be identified by the use of cytocentrifugation and Wright-Giemsa staining. Such morphologic evaluation is necessary to distinguish the pleocytosis of leukemic meningitis from that induced as a result of intrathecal chemotherapeutic agents (arachnoiditis) or from CNS infections.[128]

The vast majority of children with detectable CSF lymphoblasts at initial diagnosis do not have any symptoms related to CNS involvement. Symptomatic patients may present with diffuse or focal neurologic signs and symptoms, including manifestations of increased intracranial pressure (vomiting, headache, papilledema, and lethargy), seizures, and nuchal rigidity. Cranial nerve palsies can occur, with the facial nerve being the most frequently involved.[129,130]

Intracranial hemorrhage in patients with high presenting leukocyte counts is uncommon in ALL but can lead to severe and devastating neurologic consequences.[131] Clinically significant spinal cord involvement has been reported in ALL, manifesting as a localized epidural leukemic infiltrate compressing the cord.[132]

Anterior Mediastinal Mass

Leukemic infiltration of the thymus appears as an anterior mediastinal mass on a chest radiograph. It is observed in about 10% of newly diagnosed patients and is almost always associated with T-cell immunophenotype (see Table 50-1). Leukemic infiltration of the mediastinal structures may cause life-threatening tracheobronchial or cardiovascular compression. Pleural effusion may also be associated with thymic enlargement, which can exacerbate respiratory distress. Prompt initiation of systemic chemotherapy (e.g., corticosteroids) is necessary to handle such emergencies and, rarely, emergent radiation may be indicated.

Genitourinary Tract Manifestations

Testicular Enlargement. The clinical presentation of testicular ALL is a painless enlargement of one or both testes. Clinically detectable testicular leukemia is uncommon at diagnosis, occurring in 1% to 2% of boys, and does not appear to have prognostic significance.[133,134] Occult testicular involvement at diagnosis is more common, especially in the presence of a high tumor burden. In a study in which testicular biopsies were performed in boys with newly diagnosed ALL, approximately 20% had microscopic leukemic involvement.[135] However, this finding does not appear to have any prognostic significance, and routine testicular biopsies at the time of diagnosis to document occult disease are not recommended.

Other Genitourinary Tract Sites of Involvement. Ultrasonographically enlarged kidneys have been observed in children with ALL at the time of diagnosis and are believed to be primarily caused by leukemic infiltration.[136] Renal enlargement in acute leukemia also may be related to hyperuricemia, hemorrhage, and pyelonephritis. Hypertension is more commonly associated with the treatment of leukemia, especially with the prolonged use of corticosteroids, than with renal involvement. Occasionally, urolithiasis is observed at presentation or during therapy for ALL. Most renal stones in ALL patients are calcium-based in composition and occur most frequently during phases of therapy that include corticosteroids.[137]

Priapism is rare and usually associated with an elevated white blood cell count.[138] The pathogenesis may be caused by involvement of sacral nerve roots, or it may be related to mechanical obstruction of the corpora cavernosa and dorsal veins by leukemic infiltration or leukostasis.

Bone and Joint Manifestations

Bone pain, joint pain, and limp are common presenting symptoms in childhood ALL.[139,111] Bone pain may be the result of direct leukemic infiltration of the periosteum, periosteal elevation of underlying cortical disease, bone infarction, or expansion of the marrow cavity by the leukemic cells. Pain and swelling of the joint are less frequent but may be presenting manifestations of disease and can initially cause confusion in the diagnosis.[142] Migratory joint pain accompanied by swelling and tenderness can be misdiagnosed as juvenile rheumatoid arthritis (JRA) or rheumatic fever.[140,142]

Up to 25% of children with ALL have characteristic radiographic changes, such as osteopenia and fracture at diagnosis, including vertebral compression fractures.[140,141,143] Some patients have radiographic changes in the absence of bone pain, whereas others have bone pain unaccompanied by radiographic changes. Radiographic changes are most often seen in the long bones, especially around the areas of rapid growth (e.g., the knees, wrists, and ankles), and include subperiosteal new bone formation, transverse metaphyseal radiolucent bands, osteolytic lesions involving the medullary cavity and cortex, diffuse demineralization, and transverse metaphyseal lines of increased density (growth arrest lines).[144,145] The latter probably represent regions of growth arrest during active phases of the disease rather than direct infiltration by leukemic cells.

Gastrointestinal Manifestations

Hepatosplenomegaly is a common feature at the time of diagnosis. Severe hepatic dysfunction, manifested as hyperbilirubinemia, presumably from leukemic infiltration, has been observed at diagnosis in some children with ALL and can complicate initial therapy, because many induction agents are hepatically metabolized or hepatotoxic.[146,147] A short course of corticosteroid monotherapy before the initiation of multiagent induction chemotherapy may improve hyperbilirubinemia.[147]

Ocular Manifestations

Ophthalmic manifestations of leukemia can be observed in more than a third of all newly diagnosed patients.[148,149] Leukemia can involve almost all ocular structures. Retinal hemorrhages, the most frequent ocular abnormality, are presumably caused by thrombocytopenia or anemia.[150]

However, local infiltration of the capillary vessel walls with subsequent rupture and hemorrhage also may occur, especially in patients with very high leukocyte counts. Ocular motor palsies and papilledema are indicative of meningeal leukemia. Occasionally the optic nerve may be directly involved by leukemic infiltration.[151] In such situations visual acuity may be markedly affected and patients may present with monocular blindness. Prompt radiation therapy may be necessary to salvage useful vision. Leukemic infiltration of the anterior chamber with hypopyon and iritis has also been reported and can be the first manifestation of relapse.[152] Symptoms include conjunctival injection, photophobia, pain, blurring, and decreased vision.

Pulmonary Manifestations

Pulmonary leukostasis, which can lead to respiratory failure, can be seen at diagnosis, especially in patients with high presenting leukocyte counts.[117] This complication is more common in AML than in ALL. Radiographic distinction among infection, leukemic infiltration, and hemorrhage may be difficult.

Dermatologic Manifestations

Skin infiltration is uncommon in childhood leukemia, with the exception of congenital leukemia (both AML and ALL).[153] Leukemia cutis typically manifests as red or violaceous papules, nodules, or plaques.

DIFFERENTIAL DIAGNOSIS AND PROGNOSIS

A careful history and physical examination, together with an examination of the peripheral blood and bone marrow, result in a straightforward diagnosis of leukemia in the vast majority of cases. However, at times, ALL may present as the signs and symptoms of other conditions. These include ITP, aplastic anemia, JRA, infectious mononucleosis and other infections, and metastatic solid tumors.

Differential Diagnosis

Idiopathic Thrombocytopenic Purpura

ITP is the most common cause of the acute onset of petechiae and purpura in children. Patients with ITP usually present with isolated thrombocytopenia, often with large platelets seen on a blood smear, contrasting sharply to the more generalized blood cell abnormalities and small platelets typically observed in patients with ALL.[110] Physical findings in ITP are usually limited to bruising or bleeding associated with thrombocytopenia. An occasional patient develops modest splenomegaly, probably caused by a recent viral infection. In most cases, the leukocyte level and differential count are unremarkable and there is no anemia unless bleeding has been substantial or an unrelated anemia is present. Bone marrow examination is rarely necessary in uncomplicated cases of pediatric ITP (i.e., children with otherwise normal blood cell counts, consistent peripheral blood smear, and absence of adenopathy, hepatosplenomegaly, or other concerning findings on physical examination). However, if the diagnosis of ITP is in question or any of these concerning findings are present, clinicians should consider marrow evaluation to rule out leukemia before starting corticosteroids to avoid partially treating occult ALL.[154] The bone marrow aspirate is usually diagnostic because the marrow elements in ITP appear normal or show increased megakaryocytes.

Aplastic Anemia, Myelodysplasia, and Myeloproliferative Disorders

Like patients with leukemia, those with aplastic anemia, myelodysplasia, and myeloproliferative disease may present with pancytopenia and have fevers or infections associated with granulocytopenia. Lymphadenopathy and hepatosplenomegaly are unusual in aplastic anemia. Also, the radiographic skeletal changes sometimes seen in leukemia do not occur in aplastic anemia. To differentiate acute leukemia from these other disorders, marrow biopsy is mandatory and usually revealing.

Rarely, patients with ALL present with a transient pancytopenia preceding the leukemic phase.[155] The pancytopenic period may persist for a few days or weeks and be accompanied by high fevers. Spontaneous recovery with a period of normal blood cell counts often occurs before the onset of ALL.[155] In those cases, ALL typically becomes manifest several months after the period of aplasia. However, ALL may also develop after a period of aplasia, without any recovery of blood cell counts.[156] Distinguishing pre-ALL pancytopenia from aplastic anemia may be difficult. Repeated bone marrow aspirates or biopsies ultimately establish the correct diagnosis by demonstrating areas of marrow that are infiltrated with lymphoblasts. The pathogenesis of the preleukemic pancytopenia prodrome is unclear; in one case report, leukemia-associated genetic lesions were identified in the aplastic marrow when it was retrospectively analyzed.[157]

Juvenile Rheumatoid Arthritis and Connective Tissue Disease

Because ALL often presents primarily as joint or extremity complaints (especially limp, arthritis, or arthralgia), it may be confused with JRA or other autoimmune disorders.[142] Children with JRA can manifest fever, pallor, splenomegaly, and anemia, and patients with ALL can present with a positive test for antinuclear antibody, highlighting how difficult it may be to distinguish these conditions from each other.[142] Because of this difficulty, bone marrow aspiration should be considered before initiating corticosteroid therapy in children with presumed JRA.

Infectious Mononucleosis and Other Viral Infections

Childhood infectious mononucleosis and other viral illnesses can masquerade as leukemia. Patients may have generalized lymphadenopathy, splenomegaly, rash, fevers, and peripheral blood lymphocytosis. The atypical lymphocytes observed with acute Epstein-Barr virus (EBV) and other viral infections can sometimes be confused with peripheral leukemic blasts because they are larger than normal lymphocytes. Usually, viral infections can be differentiated from leukemia without bone marrow aspiration, but the procedure is sometimes necessary for accurate diagnosis. The detection of acute EBV infection in the blood by serology or PCR testing may be helpful in establishing the correct diagnosis.

Metastatic Solid Tumors

ALL and neuroblastoma may have similar presenting signs and symptoms, including fever, bone pain, and pancytopenia. Children with neuroblastoma frequently have malignant involvement of liver, lymph nodes, bone, or bone marrow; the marrow involvement may be extensive. In the bone marrow, neuroblasts tend to cluster and form pseudorosettes, in contrast to the diffuse involvement generally observed in ALL. Other solid tumors also rarely present as extensive marrow involvement, including rhabdomyosarcoma and Ewing sarcoma, and can initially be confused with leukemia. If questions remain after the examination of marrow morphology, other studies, such as immunophenotype and cytogenetics, may be helpful in distinguishing leukemia from a metastatic solid tumor.

Prognostic Factors

An array of clinical and biologic features have been identified as prognostically significant in childhood ALL, including age, presenting leukocyte count, immunophenotype, chromosomal abnormalities (ploidy, translocations), the presence of overt CNS leukemia at diagnosis, and the rapidity with which patients respond to initial induction chemotherapy.[111] Ultimately the prognostic significance of any factor is treatment dependent and the importance of a particular presenting feature in predicting outcome may vary, depending on the therapy delivered to that patient.

Age

The age of patients with ALL significantly correlates with clinical outcome. In childhood ALL, infants and adolescents have a worse prognosis than patients in the intermediate age group (aged 1 to 10 years).[116] ALL in infancy (<1 year at diagnosis) is associated with high presenting leukocyte counts, increased frequency of CNS leukemia at presentation, and a high incidence of rearrangements of the *MLL* gene on chromosome 11q23 (see Table 50-2).[17,18,116] Even when treated with intensified regimens, infants with *MLL* gene rearrangements have a dismal prognosis, with long-term EFS rates ranging from 10% to 40%.[116,158-161]

Adolescents (10 to 21 years of age) with ALL also have a less favorable outcome than children aged 1 to 10 years, although it is not as poor as that in infants. Adolescents with ALL more frequently present with "high risk" features at diagnosis, including T-cell immunophenotype, higher presenting leukocyte counts, and a lower incidence of cytogenetic abnormalities associated with a favorable prognosis, including high hyperdiploidy and the *ETV6-RUNX1* gene fusion (see Table 50-2).[116,162] Multiple retrospective studies have shown that adolescents fare better with pediatric ALL regimens than on treatments designed for adults with ALL.[162,163-165]

Leukocyte Count

The initial peripheral blood leukocyte count is a significant predictor of treatment outcome, with worsening outcomes as the leukocyte count increases.[111] Since 1996, based on the recommendation of the Cancer Therapy Evaluation Program of the National Cancer Institute (NCI), many investigators have considered a leukocyte count of 50,000 cells/mm^3 as the level separating patients with a higher risk for relapse from those with a more favorable prognosis.[111]

Immunophenotype

Historically, immunophenotype was considered an important prognostic factor, with inferior outcomes observed in patients with mature B-cell and T-cell disease. However, if they are treated with more intensive regimens, children with T-cell phenotype fare as well as those with B-precursor cell disease.[25] As noted earlier, mature B-cell ALL is more effectively treated with the same therapy used for advanced-stage Burkitt lymphoma.[8,9]

Some investigators have reported prognostic differences within subsets of patients with B-precursor cell ALL. Initial studies have suggested that patients with pre–B-cell ALL (cIg+) have a worse outcome than those with early pre–B-cell ALL (cIg–).[166] Subsequent reports indicated that the adverse outcome of patients with pre–B-cell ALL was caused by the subset with the t(1;19) translocation.[167] However, with greater treatment intensity, even patients with this cytogenetic abnormality do not appear to have an adverse prognosis.[168]

An early T-precursor phenotype is observed in 10% to 15% of cases of childhood T-cell ALL. This subset was initially indentified by gene expression profile analyses and is characterized by a distinctive immunophenotype (CD1a and CD8 negativity, with weak expression of CD5 and coexpression of stem cell or myeloid markers).[29] Retrospective analyses suggested that patients with early T-precursor cell ALL have a poorer prognosis.[29,169] In another retrospective study, patients with T-cell ALL with early T-precursor cell features were identified by ABD, indicating failure to complete V(D)J recombination at this locus.[30] Like early T-precursor cell ALL patients defined by immunophenotype, T-cell ALL patients with ABD were also found to have an inferior prognosis.

In 15% to 30% of patients with newly diagnosed ALL, flow cytometry reveals coexpression of at least one myeloid antigen on the cell surface of the lymphoblasts.[32,33,36] Myeloid antigen coexpression has been associated with several genetic abnormalities, including the ETV6-RUNX1 fusion [t(12;21)], MLL gene (11q23) rearrangements, and the Ph chromosome (BCR-ABL rearrangement), but is almost never observed in high hyperdiploid ALL (51 to 65 chromosomes).[33,35,170] Myeloid antigen coexpression was previously believed to be associated with an inferior outcome, but several more recent reports have indicated that it is not an independent prognostic factor.[33,171]

Chromosomal Abnormalities

Several recurrent chromosomal abnormalities are important prognostic factors in childhood ALL. Two abnormalities, high hyperdiploidy (51 to 65 chromosomes or a DNA index greater than or equal to 1.16) and the cryptic t(12;21) (ETV6-RUNX1 fusion), have been associated with a favorable prognosis.[43] High hyperdiploidy is observed in 25% to 30% of cases of childhood ALL and is more common in younger (noninfant) children with B-precursor cell phenotype and low leukocyte counts.[172] The most favorable outcomes in high hyperdiploid ALL patients have been associated with the presence of trisomies of chromosomes 4, 10, and 17.[107,173,174]

The ETV6-RUNX1 fusion, which is rarely detected by karyotypic analysis, has been identified in approximately 20% of children with ALL using other more sensitive techniques, such as fluorescence in situ hybridization and the reverse-transcriptase PCR assay.[175,176] Like high hyperdiploidy, the ETV6-RUNX1 fusion is more common in younger (noninfant) patients with low leukocyte counts and is observed almost exclusively in patients with B-precursor cell phenotype.[42,176] Up to 80% of children with B-precursor cell ALL diagnosed between the ages of 2 and 7 years have either high hyperdiploidy or the ETV6-RUNX1 fusion,[172] although almost never both; these two chromosomal abnormalities are almost always mutually exclusive.[172,177] Several studies have indicated that children with ETV6-RUNX1–positive ALL have favorable EFS rates.[42,43,176] When relapses are observed in children with ETV6-RUNX1–positive ALL, they tend to occur relatively late and may be more responsive to postrelapse salvage therapy.[176,178-180]

Chromosomal abnormalities associated with an adverse prognosis include hypodiploidy (fewer than 44 or 45 chromosomes),[102,181,182] rearrangements of the MLL gene on chromosome 11q23,[158,181,183] and the Ph chromosome [t(9;22)].[181,184-187] MLL gene rearrangements are more frequent in infants than in older children with ALL.[183] The incidence of Ph chromosome–positive ALL increases with age at diagnosis and is more common in adolescents and young adults.[184,186] Patients with Ph chromosome–positive ALL appear to fare better if treated with allogeneic hematopoietic stem cell transplantation (HSCT) in first remission[187]; recent work has suggested that favorable outcomes may also be achieved with the combination of tyrosine kinase inhibitors and intensive chemotherapy without transplant.[96,97]

Intrachromosomal amplification of the AML1 gene on chromosome 21 (iAMP21), detected in 1% to 2% of children with ALL, may also be associated with an inferior outcome.[188] Patients with this abnormality appear to fare better with more intensified "high risk" treatment than with less intensive regimens intended for patients with "standard risk" disease.[189,190] The t(1;19) translocation, observed in approximately 5% of cases of childhood ALL, had been previously associated with inferior EFS rates, but more recently conducted clinical trials have not found that this translocation is associated with an adverse prognosis. Some investigators have reported that patients with the t(1;19) translocation are at higher risk for CNS relapses,[191] but this finding has not been confirmed by others.[43,192,193] Chromosomal abnormalities in childhood ALL are reviewed in depth in Chapter 44.

Overt CNS Disease at Diagnosis

Lymphoblasts in the CSF can be detected in 15% to 20% of children who present with ALL.[126,127] Some children, such as those diagnosed within the first 12 months of life and those with T-cell ALL, have a higher incidence of CNS leukemia at diagnosis.[116]

Most investigators consider the presence of overt CNS disease at diagnosis to be an adverse prognostic indicator, and these patients are usually treated with more aggressive therapy. CNS status at presentation is usually classified as CNS-1 (no blast cells), CNS-2 (fewer than five leukocytes/μL with blast cells), and CNS-3 (five or more leukocytes/μL with blast cells or cranial nerve palsy).[111] Historically, CNS leukemia was defined as CNS-3 status (observed in approximately 5% of patients at diagnosis).[126,127] CNS-3 status at diagnosis is associated with a lower probability of EFS.[127] Several investigators have reported that patients with CNS-2 status also have a higher risk for relapse, although it does not appear to be as high as in patients with CNS-3 status at diagnosis.[126,127] Intensification of CNS-directed therapy (e.g., increasing the frequency of intrathecal chemotherapeutic treatments) may abrogate the adverse prognostic significance of CNS-2 status.[194] Thus patients with CNS-2 status at diagnosis usually receive extra doses of intrathecal chemotherapy without other changes in treatment whereas those with CNS-3 status are typically classified as higher risk and receive more intensive systemic and CNS-directed therapies.

Traumatic lumbar punctures with lymphoblasts on cytospin have also been associated with an adverse prognosis.[127,195] Like patients with CNS-2 status, those with traumatic lumbar punctures with lymphoblasts at diagnosis may also benefit from additional doses of intrathecal chemotherapy.[127]

Early Response to Induction Chemotherapy

The rapidity with which a patient responds to initial chemotherapy is a significant predictor of long-term outcome. Early response to therapy has been evaluated using morphologic measures (residual microscopic leukemia) and more sensitive techniques, such as PCR assay and flow cytometry.

Morphologic Response to Therapy. Patients who require two or more cycles of induction chemotherapy to achieve complete remission have a much worse prognosis than those who achieve complete remission within 1 month of diagnosis.[196-198] The Berlin-Frankfurt-Munster (BFM) group treats patients with 1 week of corticosteroid monotherapy (and one dose of intrathecal methotrexate) before beginning multiagent induction chemotherapy and has reported that poor peripheral blood response at the end of that week (defined as an absolute blast count of 1000/mm³) is an independent predictor of adverse outcome.[3] Others have reported that the rate of clearance of blasts from the peripheral blood after multiagent chemotherapy is also an independent predictor of relapse.[199-201] Similarly, the persistence of leukemia in bone marrow specimens obtained 7 or 14 days after beginning multiagent chemotherapy strongly correlates with poor outcome,[202] although intensification of therapy can abrogate the adverse prognostic significance of slow early response.[203]

Minimal Residual Disease. Minimal residual disease (MRD) evaluation involves the measurement of very low levels of leukemia using sensitive techniques, such as PCR assay or specialized multiparameter flow cytometry. Leukemic cells are identified using targets identified at diagnosis, including leukemia-specific immunophenotypes (for flow cytometry–based assays), chromosomal translocations, or lymphoblast-specific immunoglobulin or T-cell antigen receptor gene rearrangements (for PCR-based assays). Using these techniques, leukemia cells have been identified at levels as low as 1 in 1,000 to 1 in 100,000 cells.[204-207]

Many studies have demonstrated that MRD levels early in therapy are a significant and independent predictor of long-term outcome.[204,208-212] For patients achieving a morphologic remission at the end of induction therapy, those with higher levels of marrow MRD at that time point have a higher risk for relapse than those with lower or undetectable MRD.[204,208-210,212-214,215] The risk for relapse directly correlates with MRD level, that is, those with the highest MRD levels at the end of remission induction have the worst prognosis. High levels of MRD detected soon after beginning with postinduction therapy (weeks 12 to 14 of treatment) have also been associated with an increased risk for relapse,[215,216] as have high levels measured in the peripheral blood as early as day 8 and in the marrow at day 15 of induction therapy.[214,217]

Other Prognostic Factors

Gender and Race. Some investigators have reported that male patients fare worse than female patients.[218,219] This observation had been attributed, in part, to the risk for testicular relapse,[218] although higher relapse rates in males have been observed even when testicular relapse rates were low.[219] Race may also influence outcome, with lower EFS rates reported for African-American, Hispanic, and Native American patients, even after adjustment for differences in prognostically significant presenting features.[220-222] The reasons why patients of different race have varying responses to therapy on certain regimens have not been fully elucidated but may in part be related to differences in the biologic subtypes of ALL observed in different groups. For example, African-American children have a higher relative incidence of T-cell ALL and lower rates of high hyperdiploidy, a favorable genetic subtype of precursor B-cell ALL.[223] Hispanic children also have a lower frequency of *ETV6-RUNX1*–rearranged ALL[224] and, in one study, were noted to have a higher incidence of ALL with rearrangements of CRLF2, a subtype associated with an inferior prognosis.[225]

Pharmacogenomics. Several studies have suggested that outcome may be affected by how rapidly and effectively an individual patient metabolizes certain chemotherapeutic agents. Polymorphisms in genes involved in chemotherapy drug metabolism have been associated with risk for relapse.[226] More favorable long-term outcomes have been reported in patients with mutant thiopurine methyltransferase (TPMT) phenotypes involved in the metabolism of thioguanines, such as 6-mercaptopurine,[227,228] although such patients may also be at higher risk for developing significant treatment-related toxicities, including low blood cell counts, infection, liver dysfunction, and second malignancies.[229,230] Investigations of other genes, such as the glutathione S-transferase genes (encoding enzymes involved in the intracellular detoxification of various compounds)[231,232] and the folate metabolism genes (e.g., thymidylate synthase, methylenetetrahydrofolate reductase, and methylenetetrahydrofolate dehydrogenase)[233-235] have led to conflicting results, without clear consensus regarding the prognostic significance of various polymorphisms.

Treatment Adherence. Compliance with taking oral chemotherapy during the maintenance phase has been shown to impact outcome. In one study of pediatric ALL patients, nonadherence to 6-mercaptopurine (as assessed by electronic monitoring device that measured cap opening of the medication bottle) was associated with an inferior outcome. Adolescents and Hispanic patients were at higher risk for noncompliance. After adjusting for sex, NCI risk group, cytogenetics, ethnicity, and other factors, 6-mercaptopurine compliance was an independent prognostic factor, with a progressive increase in risk for relapse with decreasing levels of adherence.[236]

THERAPY

Historical Background

Over the past 50 years, there has been a dramatic improvement in the prognosis of children with ALL (Fig. 50-3). Prior to 1947, when the first complete remission in

TABLE 50-3 Outcome by Presenting Features of 491 Children and Adolescents (Ages 0 to 18 Years) Treated on Dana-Farber Cancer Institute ALL Consortium Protocol 95-01 (1996-2000)			
Presenting Feature	**No. of Patients**	**10-Year EFS (±SE)**	**10-Year OS (±SE)**
Overall	491	79 ± 2	89 ± 2
Age at diagnosis (yr)			
<1	14	42 ± 13	42 ± 13
1-9	385	82 ± 2	93 ± 1
≥10	92	75 ± 5	78 ± 4
WBC (× 10⁹/L)			
<10	239	83 ± 3	93 ± 2
10-49	155	80 ± 3	89 ± 3
50-99	43	70 ± 10	88 ± 5
≥100	54	66 ± 7	73 ± 6
Immunophenotype			
B-precursor cell	438	78 ± 2	89 ± 5
T-cell	52	85 ± 5	90 ± 4
Gender			
Male	274	78 ± 3	88 ± 2
Female	217	81 ± 3	91 ± 2
B-Precursor cell National Cancer Institute (NCI) risk group			
Standard	303	83 ± 2	94 ± 2
High	121	72 ± 5	82 ± 4

Modified from Silverman LB, Stevenson KE, O'Brien JE, et al: Long-term results of Dana-Farber Cancer Institute ALL Consortium protocols for children with newly diagnosed acute lymphoblastic leukemia (1985-2000). Leukemia 24:320–334, 2010.
EFS, Event-free survival; OS, overall survival; SE, standard error; WBC, white blood cell.

childhood ALL was attained by Farber and colleagues,[237] the median duration of survival from the time of diagnosis was 2 months.[238] During the 1950s, drugs such as 6-mercaptopurine, methotrexate, and corticosteroids were found to be active in leukemia-bearing mice and subsequently in human leukemias.[239,240] The first controlled clinical trials were conducted by Frei and associates,[241] who ushered in the era of single-agent (and soon thereafter combination-agent) antileukemic chemotherapy trials.[241,242] Active drugs introduced in the 1960s and 1970s included the anthracyclines (doxorubicin and daunorubicin), L-asparaginase, and the epipodophyllotoxins (etoposide and teniposide).[243-245]

With current regimens for the treatment of childhood ALL, more than 95% of patients achieve complete remission and approximately 80% are long-term event-free survivors (Table 50-3 and Fig. 50-4).[24,246,247] Overall survival, which includes patients who are salvaged after relapse, is now approximately 90%.[248] Improvement in outcome over the past 30 to 40 years occurred despite the fact that, with few exceptions, the drugs used for the treatment of ALL today were all available by the late 1960s and early 1970s. Improvement in cure rates can be attributed to many factors, including the development of complex chemotherapeutic regimens designed to achieve clonal eradication, improvements in

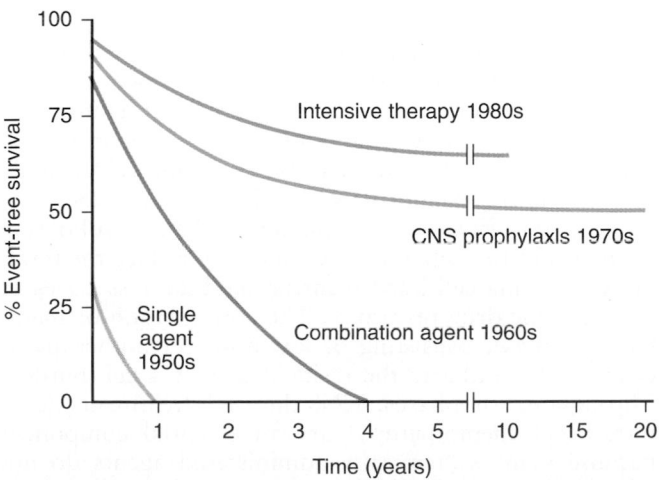

Figure 50-3 Historical perspective of the treatment of childhood acute lymphoblastic leukemia. The single-agent era resulted in few complete remissions and no cures. The combination-agent era without adequate central nervous system (CNS) treatment resulted in high complete remission rates but almost uniform mortality. Between the mid 1960s and 1970s, combination chemotherapy and CNS treatment resulted in prolonged, disease-free survival for approximately 50% of children. Intensive therapy in the 1980s and 1990s resulted in an event-free survival of 75% to 80% of children.

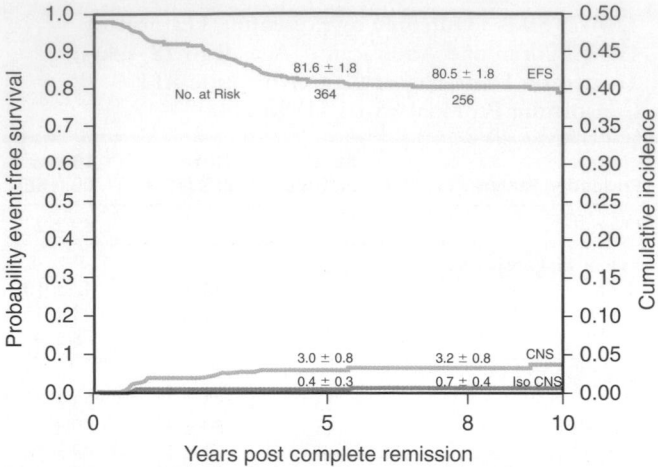

Figure 50-4 Event-free survival *(EFS)* and cumulative incidence of isolated or any central nervous system *(CNS)* relapse for 491 patients treated on Dana-Farber Cancer Institute ALL Consortium Protocol 95-01 (1996-2000). Median follow-up was 8.6 years. *(Modified from Silverman LB, Stevenson KE, O'Brien JE, et al: Long-term results of Dana-Farber Cancer Institute ALL Consortium protocols for children with newly diagnosed acute lymphoblastic leukemia [1985-2000]. Leukemia 24:320–334, 2010.)*

supportive care, recognition of the CNS as a sanctuary site, and application of risk-directed therapy.

Risk-Adapted Therapy

After the addition of CNS-directed therapy improved cure rates to approximately 50% in the 1970s, investigators compared presenting features in patients who were cured and those who relapsed to establish clinically relevant prognostic factors. Subsequent clinical trials used these prognostic factors to stratify therapy. More intensive therapy was administered to those patients considered to be at the highest risk for relapse. In contrast, some of the more morbid components of therapy were modified or eliminated for those children considered to have the best prognosis. The goal of risk-adapted therapy is to treat away adverse presenting features so that high-risk and low-risk patients have similar cure rates. For example, on Dana-Farber Cancer Institute (DFCI) ALL Consortium protocols, children with T-cell ALL (historically, a subgroup with an inferior prognosis) are treated as high-risk patients (receiving higher cumulative dosages of anthracycline and corticosteroid than lower-risk patients); with that therapy, their outcomes are as favorable as those with B-precursor cell disease.[25]

For many years, pediatric cooperative groups and institutions applied prognostic factors differently when defining risk categories for clinical trials. A more uniform approach to risk classification was proposed and agreed on at an NCI-sponsored workshop held in 1993.[111] For patients with B-precursor cell ALL, the standard-risk category was defined as age between 12 months and younger than 10 years and initial leukocyte count lower than 50,000/mm³. The remaining patients were considered to have high-risk ALL. Other characteristics used by the various cooperative groups to classify patients as high

risk include T-cell phenotype, CNS-3 status at diagnosis, and slow early response to initial therapy, including a high peripheral blood absolute blast count at the end of a 7-day prednisone prophase.[111] These various prognostic factors are discussed earlier.

Contemporary regimens have incorporated cytogenetic abnormalities and MRD levels into risk group stratification, and in some cases, only these factors are considered (and not more standard factors, such as age and leukocyte count) when assigning risk groups.[215] Patients with certain chromosomal abnormalities (e.g., *MLL* gene rearrangements and low hypodiploidy) are treated as high risk, regardless of other presenting features. Similarly, end-induction MRD is used by almost all groups as a factor determining the intensity of postinduction treatment, with patients found to have higher levels allocated to more intensive therapies.[215,249] On some protocols, MRD levels at a later time point (week 12) are also considered when risk-stratifying patients, because these have been shown to be prognostically important, especially in patients with T-cell ALL.[216]

MRD measurements, in conjunction with cytogenetics, have also been used to identify subsets of patients with an extremely low risk for relapse who may be successfully treated with less intensive therapies. The Children's Oncology Group reported a very favorable prognosis for patients with the B-precursor cell phenotype, NCI standard risk age/leukocyte count, CNS-1 status, and favorable cytogenetic abnormalities (either high hyperdiploidy with favorable trisomies or the *ETV6-RUNX1* fusion) who had low peripheral blood MRD levels at day 8 and low marrow MRD at end of induction.[214]

Ultimately, treatment is the most important prognostic factor, and those factors used to risk-stratify patients on one regimen may not be useful for patients treated on a different regimen.

Phases of Therapy

In general, treatment regimens for children with newly diagnosed ALL include three phases: remission induction, consolidation (or intensification), and continuation (or maintenance). The remission induction phase of therapy is designed to destroy measurable leukemia cells rapidly and minimize residual leukemia burden (i.e., the total number of leukemic cells in the body). The consolidation or intensification phase(s) is designed to reduce the total-body leukemia cell burden further and address issues of antileukemic drug resistance. The continuation or maintenance phase, consisting of low-dose chemotherapy, is designed to eradicate the residual leukemia cell burden. Throughout all phases, CNS-directed treatments (e.g., intrathecal chemotherapy) are an essential component because many systemically administered agents do not adequately penetrate the brain and spinal cord.

Remission Induction

After the diagnosis of ALL has been established and any urgent medical issues, such as metabolic imbalances, have been addressed, antileukemic chemotherapy should be initiated without delay. The initial phase of treatment, remission induction, is designed to reduce the leukemic cell burden to a clinically and hematologically undetectable level. *Hematologic remission* is defined as attainment of a normocellular bone marrow with 5% or fewer blasts and peripheral blood without lymphoblasts, with return of "normal" peripheral blood counts, that is, a granulocyte count exceeding 500 to 1000/mm³ and a platelet count exceeding 100,000/mm³. *Complete remission* is defined as achievement of these criteria along with the absence of any signs and symptoms of extramedullary leukemia. A complete remission must be induced before the next component of therapy is begun. The duration of most induction regimens is 4 to 6 weeks.

Clinical trials in the 1960s demonstrated that combinations of two agents were consistently superior to single agents for inducing complete remission in children with ALL. Vincristine and prednisone produced complete remission in approximately 90% of pediatric patients with ALL.[250,251] Addition of a third drug increased both the number of patients who achieved complete remission and the long-term relapse-free survival.[250,252] Current induction regimens, therefore, consist of at least three agents, most often L-asparaginase or an anthracycline, in addition to vincristine and prednisone.

Many groups have further intensified induction regimens to include four or more agents. In theory, these more intensive induction regimens may prevent the emergence of drug-resistant leukemic clones by an initial leukemic cell lysis of greater rapidity and magnitude.[253] The benefit in terms of long-term EFS of using four drugs during induction therapy (vincristine, prednisone, L-asparaginase, and an anthracycline) is widely accepted in higher-risk patients[254] but less clear in lower-risk patients.[255] Intensive induction regimens may enhance long-term EFS but can result in increased short-term morbidity, especially from infections during periods of granulocytopenia. However, even with four-drug induction regimens, few toxic deaths are reported (i.e., 1% to 2% of patients).[24,246,256]

The initiation of CNS treatment is an integral component of induction therapy. After the diagnosis of ALL has been established by bone marrow examination, a lumbar puncture is performed for diagnostic and therapeutic purposes. It is generally recommended that intrathecal chemotherapy be given with the first diagnostic lumbar puncture to reduce the theoretical risk for inadvertently seeding the meninges with peripheral blood lymphoblasts.[195] In addition to the diagnostic lumbar puncture, intrathecal chemotherapy is usually administered at least one more time during the first month of treatment. Patients with lymphoblasts present on their initial CSF specimen (CNS-2 or CNS-3 status, or traumatic lumbar puncture with blasts) typically receive more doses of intrathecal chemotherapy during the induction phase than those without any detectable CSF lymphoblasts (CNS-1 status).[127]

Failure to achieve remission after 1 month of therapy (induction failure) is uncommon, occurring in fewer than 5% of patients.[196,197] Induction failure is observed more commonly in patients with high presenting leukocyte counts or T-cell phenotype.[196,197] Successful treatment of refractory ALL has been reported with the use of drugs such as cytarabine, epipodophyllotoxins (e.g., etoposide, teniposide), and anthracyclines (e.g., idarubicin).[257-259] Nelarabine has been shown to induce remissions in patients with refractory T-cell ALL.[260,261] Ultimately, 80% to 90% of children with initially refractory disease are able to achieve a complete remission.[196,197] Despite this relatively high complete remission rate, overall survival for patients with a history of initial induction failure is poor (long-term overall survival rates of 20% to 30%).[196-198] Allogeneic HSCT in first remission may improve the outcome for patients with initial induction failure.[262] In a large retrospective series, a trend for superior outcome with allogeneic HSCT compared with chemotherapy alone was observed in patients with initial induction failure and either the T-cell phenotype (any age) or B-precursor cell phenotype and age younger than 6 years.[198] In that study, B-precursor cell ALL patients who were aged 1 to 5 years at diagnosis and did not have any adverse cytogenetic abnormalities (*MLL* translocation, *BCR-ABL*) had a relatively favorable prognosis, without any advantage in outcome with the utilization of HSCT compared with chemotherapy alone.

Consolidation (Intensification) Therapy

The goals of consolidation therapy are to reduce the disease burden further and to adjust the intensity of treatment based on the risk for subsequent relapse. A wide variety of agents and schedules have been used during postinduction consolidation in pediatric trials. In general, there has been an attempt in lower-risk patients to limit exposure to agents associated with significant acute and late toxicities while reserving the use of more intensive therapies for patients at higher risk for relapse.

A commonly used postinduction consolidation regimen was first introduced by the German BFM study group.[3] This consolidation scheme includes (1) a 4-week chemotherapy course (sometimes referred to as "consolidation" or "induction IB") immediately after the initial induction phase consisting of cyclophosphamide, low-dose cytarabine, and a thiopurine (mercaptopurine or thioguanine), followed by (2) an interim maintenance phase, which includes multiple doses of either high-dose or escalating doses of methotrexate with or without leucovorin rescue, and then (3) a reinduction course (or delayed intensification), which typically includes the same agents used during the initial induction/consolidation cycles. Augmentation of this regimen, including the use of two delayed intensification cycles instead of one, has led to improved outcomes for higher-risk patients, including those with a slow early morphologic response to initial induction therapy.[203,263-265] The DFCI ALL Consortium uses an alternative postinduction consolidation regimen that includes 20 to 30 weeks of L-asparaginase and, for higher-risk patients, additional doses of doxorubicin.[2]

Continuation Therapy

Almost all current treatment regimens for ALL include a phase of continuation or maintenance therapy, in which patients are treated with less-intensive chemotherapy to complete at least 2 years of therapy. Most continuation regimens consist of weekly low-dose methotrexate and daily oral 6-mercaptopurine. Some groups have added regular pulses of vincristine and corticosteroid to this regimen, although their benefit remains controversial.[266-268]

Several pharmacologic studies have documented highly variable bioavailability after oral administration of 6-mercaptopurine and methotrexate during the continuation phase.[269-273] This may have important prognostic implications, because lower intracellular levels of thioguanine nucleotides and methotrexate polyglutamates, the major metabolites of 6-mercaptopurine and methotrexate, have been correlated with a higher risk for relapse.[270,273,274] Variable bioavailability may be the result of various factors, including concurrent food, which may interfere with drug absorption.[272] Bioavailability of oral mercaptopurine appears to be improved if it is given in the evening, without food or milk.[272,275,276] Polymorphisms within genes involved in drug metabolism also affect rates of drug activation and clearance.[229] For example, patients with deficiency in the activity of TPMT, an enzyme that inactivates mercaptopurine, have higher rates of toxicity during continuation therapy (but also may have better survival) than patients with normal TPMT activity.[227,229] Most physicians attempt to compensate for the interindividual variations of bioavailability and metabolism by tailoring the dose of both drugs to the leukocyte count. Administration of maximally tolerated doses of methotrexate and 6-mercaptopurine during continuation therapy may improve outcome, as suggested by studies demonstrating that patients with lower leukocyte or neutrophil counts during continuation chemotherapy have lower relapse rates.[277,278] Lack of patient compliance with oral medications, as well as physician compliance with protocol dosages, may adversely affect the efficacy of continuation chemotherapy.[236,279,280]

6-Thioguanine is an alternative thiopurine that, unlike 6-mercaptopurine, does not rely on TPMT for its metabolism, resulting in higher intracellular levels of thioguanine nucleotides.[281] 6-Thioguanine also has been shown to be more potent than 6-mercaptopurine in inducing cell death of lymphoblasts in vitro.[282] The results of one randomized clinical trial comparing the two thioguanines indicated that 6-thioguanine was associated with a superior EFS (but not overall survival) in boys, primarily owing to a reduction in the frequency of CNS relapses.[283] However, other randomized trials comparing the two thiopurines did not confirm an EFS advantage for 6-thioguranine.[284,285] Additionally, the use of 6-thioguanine during the maintenance phase has been associated with significant hepatotoxicity, including veno-occlusive disease and cirrhosis, as well as higher remission death rates, primarily caused by infection.[283,284] Thus 6-mercaptopurine remains the thiopurine of choice during the continuation phase.

Several investigators have studied the relative efficacy and toxicity of two corticosteroids used during postinduction therapy: prednisone and dexamethasone. Interest in substituting dexamethasone for prednisone stems from studies suggesting that dexamethasone has more potent in vitro antileukemic activity, higher free plasma levels, and enhanced CSF penetration.[286-289] In several clinical trials conducted in the 1990s, the nonrandomized substitution of dexamethasone for prednisone appeared to affect outcome favorably.[290,291] This finding was confirmed in several randomized clinical trials that indicated that dexamethasone was associated with a superior 5-year EFS.[292-294] However, dexamethasone may also be associated with increased corticosteroid-related toxicities, including higher rates of fracture, osteonecrosis, and infectious complications, especially in older children and adolescents.[292-296] Thus the optimal corticosteroid preparation and dosing have yet to be determined and may differ based on presenting features (e.g., age) and risk for relapse.

Attempts to intensify continuation therapy by administering rotating pairs of non–cross-resistant drugs, including many agents not traditionally incorporated during the continuation phase, such as cyclophosphamide, epipodophyllotoxins, and cytarabine, have led to mixed results. In studies conducted by St. Jude Children's Research Hospital, this strategy resulted in improved outcomes for higher-risk but not lower-risk patients[297] but also was associated with high rates of toxicity, including secondary AML.[298] Based on this risk, these agents (especially epipodophyllotoxins) are, in general, no longer administered to most patients during the continuation phase.

CNS-Directed Therapies

In the 1960s, as systemic chemotherapy became more effective in prolonging the duration of hematologic remission in patients with ALL, the incidence of CNS leukemia as an initial site of relapse became progressively more common.[299,300] It was hypothesized that leukemia cells, even if subclinical, were present in the CNS in all patients and that these cells were protected by the blood-brain barrier from systemically administered chemotherapy. Thus, the concept of the CNS as a "pharmacologic sanctuary" (i.e., an anatomic space that is poorly penetrated by systemically administered chemotherapeutic agents) emerged. The introduction of radiation therapy to treat subclinical CNS leukemia in the 1970s was a pivotal step in boosting long-term disease-free survival rates in childhood ALL to 50%.[301] Although most pediatric patients are now treated without prophylactic cranial radiation, the importance of effectively treating subclinical CNS leukemia is undisputed for childhood ALL.

All successful treatment regimens for ALL include therapy directed at treating CNS leukemia. Options for CNS-directed therapies include cranial irradiation, intrathecal chemotherapy, and CNS penetrant systemic chemotherapy.

Radiation therapy was the first modality successfully used to prevent CNS relapses. The use of radiation for CNS treatment was based on experiments demonstrating that L1210 murine leukemia could be cured when cranial irradiation was added to systemic treatment with cyclophosphamide.[302] In the 1960s and 1970s, studies performed at St. Jude Children's Research Hospital documented the effectiveness of CNS radiation as preventive therapy in children with ALL.[303] In one study, patients were randomized to receive 2400 cGy of craniospinal radiation or no radiation. The difference in CNS relapse rates was striking: only 2 of 45 irradiated patients (4%) had their initial complete remissions ended by meningeal relapse, compared with 33 of 49 nonirradiated patients (67%).[304] Moreover, 31 of the patients who received prophylactic radiation remained alive after 18 to 20 years, compared with only 10 patients in the nonirradiated group. Subsequent studies demonstrated that 2400-cGy cranial irradiation with intrathecal methotrexate was as effective in preventing CNS relapse as 2400-cGy craniospinal irradiation without intrathecal chemotherapy.[305,306] Because craniospinal radiation was associated with increased toxicity, including excessive myelosuppression and spinal growth retardation, radiation directed only to the cranium administered with intrathecal chemotherapy became the standard form of CNS treatment in the 1970s.

Although 2400-cGy cranial irradiation (with intrathecal chemotherapy) effectively prevents CNS relapses in children with ALL, it is also associated with subsequent learning disabilities, growth and neuroendocrinologic abnormalities, and an increased risk for second malignant neoplasms. Thus many investigators have studied alternative CNS treatments, including lower doses of cranial radiation (1200 to 1800 cGy), systemically administered CNS-penetrant chemotherapy (i.e., agents known to achieve therapeutic levels in CSF), or intrathecal chemotherapy. Current regimens for childhood ALL include some or all of these CNS-directed therapies.

The proportion of patients receiving cranial radiation has decreased significantly over the past several decades; on current regimens, most pediatric patients are treated without radiation. When it is administered, cranial radiation is generally restricted to patients with a higher risk for relapse involving the CNS, especially those with T-cell disease, high presenting leukocyte counts, or CNS-3 status at diagnosis.[307] Doses lower than 2400 cGy have been shown to be effective, and therefore are typically used when cranial radiation is administered. For instance, CNS and marrow relapse rates were not significantly different when the dose of cranial radiation was lowered from 2400 to 1800 cGy in consecutive Children's Cancer Study Group trials.[308] The BFM and DFCI groups have successfully used 1200-cGy irradiation in the context of an intensive systemic regimen that included high-dose methotrexate (known to penetrate the CNS effectively).[294,309,310] Irradiated patients also typically receive intermittent intrathecal chemotherapy in addition to cranial irradiation as CNS preventive therapy.

Systemic therapy plays an important role in the prevention of CNS leukemia. Penetration of the CSF by drugs has been clearly demonstrated with the use of glucocorticoids[286] and high doses of methotrexate and cytarabine.[311,312] It has also been shown that systemically administered asparaginase, whose efficacy is a function of asparagine depletion, effectively lowers CSF asparagine levels.[313,314]

Intrathecal chemotherapy, used in conjunction with intensive systemic therapy and/or cranial irradiation, is an important component of CNS treatment. Many investigators have replaced cranial irradiation with frequent dosing of intrathecal chemotherapy, especially in lower-risk patients. The success of these efforts appears to depend on the frequency with which intrathecal chemotherapy is delivered, as well as the intensity and CNS penetration of the systemic chemotherapy administered. Investigators from the Children's Cancer Group demonstrated that administering intrathecal methotrexate throughout all phases of therapy was as effective in preventing CNS relapses in lower-risk patients as 1800-cGy cranial irradiation combined with only 6 months of intrathecal methotrexate, but only in the context of an intensified systemic regimen.[315] When a less-intensive systemic regimen was used, more CNS relapses were observed in nonirradiated patients. Similarly, in a DFCI ALL Consortium study, excessive CNS relapses were observed in standard-risk males when cranial irradiation was eliminated without increasing the frequency of intrathecal chemotherapy or the intensity of systemic chemotherapy.[316] However, in a subsequent study conducted by the same group, standard-risk patients who received more frequent doses of intrathecal chemotherapy had as low a CNS relapse rate as irradiated patients.[246] Some controversy exists regarding the relative efficacy of intrathecal methotrexate alone and "triple intrathecal chemotherapy" (intrathecal methotrexate, cytarabine, and hydrocortisone). In one randomized study in standard-risk patients, triple intrathecal chemotherapy was associated with a lower rate of isolated CNS relapse but there was no difference in overall EFS.[317] Randomized studies have also demonstrated that the use of dexamethasone instead of prednisone, which is believed to be less CNS penetrant, is associated with a lower rate of isolated CNS relapses in nonirradiated patients.[292,293] Thus those regimens that have successfully eliminated cranial radiation include extended and/or frequent dosing of intrathecal chemotherapy in conjunction with intensified, more CNS penetrant systemic therapy, including dexamethasone and/or high- or intermediate-dose methotrexate.[194,246,290,318-320]

Several clinical trials have been conducted on which cranial radiation was omitted for all patients, including high-risk subsets.[321-323] Most of these trials include multiple doses of either high-dose methotrexate or high-dose cytarabine and increased frequency of intrathecal chemotherapy. While the overall EFS on these trials was similar to that of contemporaneously conducted trials on which some patients received prophylactic radiation, some nonirradiated patient subsets had a significantly high risk for CNS relapse, including patients with T-cell phenotype or the presence of blasts in CSF at diagnosis. Additionally, some patients with high-risk features on these trials were treated with allogeneic SCT in first complete remission (which included total-body irradiation).[321]

The goal of eliminating cranial radiation in pediatric patients is to minimize long-term sequelae (see later). Although several studies have indicated that intrathecal chemotherapy and intensive systemic therapy can be as effective as cranial irradiation in preventing CNS relapses, the relative late neurocognitive toxicities of these CNS treatment strategies remains unsettled. Moreover, higher rates of acute neurotoxicity, including seizures, have been observed with regimens that included multiple courses of high-dose methotrexate and frequent doses of intrathecal chemotherapy.[324]

Cessation of Treatment

The optimal duration of therapy remains unknown. Most investigators continue to treat patients for 2 to 3 years, based on results of older studies, in which patients received therapy that was less intensive than in current regimens.[325] Randomized studies conducted by the Children's Cancer Group in the 1970s indicated that there was no significant difference in outcome when comparing 5 versus 3 years of therapy.[326,327] In the Childhood Leukaemia Trial UKALL VIII, a randomized study of 2 versus 3 years of continuation therapy conducted in the 1980s, the researchers observed no significant survival advantage with longer therapy. Patients receiving the shorter duration of therapy had a higher relapse rate, but this was counterbalanced by a higher remission death rate in those receiving 3 years of treatment.[328] Some early studies suggested that the optimal duration of therapy may be different for boys and girls, with boys benefiting from a more prolonged continuation phase,[329] although this finding may be less relevant with current regimens.

Even with more intensive regimens, attempts to shorten therapy duration from 2 years have not been successful. The BFM group randomized patients to receive 18 or 24 months of treatment and observed a higher relapse rate with patients who received the shorter course of treatment.[310] Similarly, high relapse rates were observed in a nonrandomized study conducted by the Tokyo Children's Cancer Study Group, in which patients received intensified therapy for only 12 months, suggesting that truncated therapy, even if intensive, is inadequate for most children with ALL.[330]

Treatment of Special Patient Subsets

Philadelphia Chromosome–Positive ALL Patients

The Ph chromosome, t(9;22)(q34;q11), which leads to fusion of the *BCR* and *ABL* genes, is detectable in approximately 5% of children and 20% of adults with ALL.[331] In pediatric ALL, it is more frequent in adolescents than in younger children.[116] When treated on regimens with conventional chemotherapeutic agents, these patients have a dismal prognosis, with long-term EFS rates ranging from 0% to 25%.[95,184-186] Allogeneic SCT in first remission has been shown to lead to more favorable outcomes and, prior to the availability of tyrosine kinase inhibitors, was considered the treatment of choice for children with Ph chromosome–positive ALL.[332] In one study, which reviewed the outcome of 610 children with Ph chromosome–positive ALL treated by 10 study groups in the pre–tyrosine kinase inhibitor era between 1995 and 2005, transplantation in first remission from an HLA-matched related or unrelated donor was associated with a higher likelihood of disease-free survival compared with chemotherapy alone.[187]

Imatinib mesylate is a selective inhibitor of the *BCR-ABL* tyrosine kinase. Phase I and II studies of single-agent imatinib in children and adults with relapsed or refractory Ph chromosome–positive ALL have demonstrated relatively high response rates, although these responses tended to be of short duration.[333,334] Results from pediatric trials have suggested that the administration of imatinib in combination with multiagent chemotherapy is feasible, without excessive toxicity.[96,97] In a pilot trial conducted by the Children's Oncology Group, patients treated with the combination of chemotherapy and imatinib (but without transplant) appeared to do at least as well as other patients on the same trial who underwent SCT in first remission.[96]

Infants

Patients diagnosed during the first year of life represent 2% to 4% of cases of childhood ALL.[335] The outcome of infants with ALL is significantly worse than that for older children, with reported long-term EFS rates of 20% to 40%.[160,336,337] The major cause of treatment failure is relapse, which tends to occur early, often in the first 1 to 2 years after diagnosis.[159,160,338-341] In vitro chemosensitivity assays have indicated that lymphoblasts from infants with ALL are relatively resistant to agents commonly used in childhood ALL regimens, such as corticosteroids and L-asparaginase.[342] Infants also appear to be more vulnerable to the toxic effects of therapy, especially severe infections.[160,339,343]

The poor outcome of infants appears to be related to the biologic distinctiveness of the disease observed in this age group. Up to 80% of infants with ALL present with molecularly detectable rearrangements of the *MLL* gene on chromosome 11q23.[17,18,160,161] The presence of a *MLL* gene rearrangement is an independent predictor of poor outcome in infant ALL, with the worst outcomes observed in *MLL*-rearranged patients who present at a very young age (<6 months at diagnosis) and with high presenting leukocyte counts.[160,161]

Because of their poor prognosis, infants with ALL are usually treated on separate protocols with intensified therapy. In vitro drug sensitivity testing and small, nonrandomized clinical trials have suggested that high-dose cytarabine, an agent more often used in AML, might benefit infants with ALL.[342-344] In the Interfant-99 trial, the largest clinical trial conducted for infants with ALL, a cytarabine-intensive regimen resulted in a 4-year EFS of 47%.[161]

The role of allogeneic SCT in first complete remission in infants with ALL remains controversial.[345,346] On the Interfant-99 trial, a subset analysis suggested that SCT in first remission may be beneficial in infants with high-risk features (*MLL* gene rearrangement, age younger than 6 months at diagnosis, and presenting leukocyte count at or above 300,000/µL); an EFS advantage for transplant was not demonstrated in other *MLL*-rearranged infants.[347]

Adolescents

Older children and adolescents (aged 10 to 18 years at diagnosis) have a less favorable outcome than children aged 1 to 10 years at diagnosis, and more aggressive treatments are generally administered to these patients. Adolescents present more frequently with adverse prognostic features, such as a high leukocyte count, T-cell immunophenotype, and the *BCR-ABL* translocation, and a lower frequency of favorable features, such as high hyperdiploidy and the *ETV6-RUNX1* fusion gene.[116,162,348] Adolescents also appear to be at higher risk than younger children for developing treatment-related complications, including osteonecrosis, pancreatitis, and thrombosis.[162,295,349] Several investigators have compared outcomes of older adolescents with ALL (aged 15 to 20 years) treated in pediatric or adult clinical trials, and all have found that these patients fare better with a pediatric regimen.[163-165,350] The superior outcome of older adolescents treated with pediatric ALL regimens may be related, in part, to the components of therapy; pediatric regimens tend to include higher cumulative dosages of vincristine, corticosteroid, and L-asparaginase than treatments designed for adults with ALL.[163]

Children with Down Syndrome

Children with Down syndrome have increased risk for developing both ALL and AML. Approximately one half to two thirds of cases of acute leukemia in children with Down syndrome are ALL. Although the vast majority of cases of AML in children with Down syndrome occur before the age of 4 years, ALL in children with Down syndrome has an age distribution similar to that of ALL in non–Down syndrome children.[351,352] Patients with ALL and Down syndrome almost always present with B-precursor cell phenotype and have a lower incidence of favorable and unfavorable cytogenetic abnormalities.[353-356] They appear to be at higher risk for developing treatment-related complications, especially those related to methotrexate, such as mucositis and myelosuppression.[357,358] Outcomes for children with Down syndrome and ALL have generally been reported to be less favorable than those of non–Down syndrome patients, which may be related to a higher incidence of treatment-related mortality because of infection and a lower frequency of favorable biologic features, such as high hyperdiploidy and the *ETV6-RUNX1* fusion.[352-356]

High expression of *CRLF2* occurs in 50% to 60% of cases of ALL in children with Down syndrome, compared with 5% to 10% of non–Down syndrome B-precursor cell ALL patients.[83,84,359] A higher frequency of activating mutations in *JAK2* has also been observed in Down syndrome ALL (~20% of cases)[360,361]; almost all patients with *JAK2* mutations also have *CRLF2* overexpression.[83,84,360] It does not appear that *CRLF2* genomic aberrations or *JAK2* mutations have independent prognostic relevance in Down syndrome ALL.[360] However, in one study, deletions of the *IKZF1* gene, observed in 35% of Down syndrome ALL cases (and frequently associated with *CRLF2* overexpression), was found to be a strong independent predictor of inferior EFS.[360]

COMPLICATIONS OF TREATMENT

At Diagnosis and during Treatment

At the time of diagnosis, the major clinical problems are the results of metabolic disturbances secondary to leukemia cell lysis, disrupted hematopoiesis leading to abnormal peripheral blood counts, and leukemic infiltration of nonhematopoietic organs. Initiation of chemotherapy may exacerbate these issues and lead to additional problems, including myelosuppression, bacterial and fungal infections, and mucosal toxicity.

Metabolic Complications

Rapid turnover of leukemia cells before and immediately after the initiation of chemotherapy leads to the release of intracellular contents, which can overwhelm the body's normal excretory mechanisms, especially in patients with high presenting leukocyte counts. The resultant metabolic disturbances include hyperkalemia, hyperuricemia, hyperphosphatemia, and hypocalcemia.[362,363] Patients with high levels of uric acid are at risk for the development of acute renal failure secondary to uric acid deposition in the kidney. To ensure that uric acid remains in solution in the renal tubule for optimal excretion, intravenous hydration should be instituted immediately after diagnosis to maintain dilute urine. In addition, administration of a xanthine oxidase inhibitor such as allopurinol, which prevents the formation of uric acid during cell lysis, should be started before the institution of antileukemic drugs. Recombinant urate oxidase, which catalyzes the breakdown of uric acid to the more soluble allantoin, may be used instead of allopurinol to decrease levels of uric acid rapidly, especially in patients presenting with high uric acid levels, high presenting leukocyte counts, or impaired renal function or in whom aggressive hydration is contraindicated.[364,365]

Hypercalcemia, although uncommon, has been reported in patients with ALL at diagnosis and appears to be related in many cases to elevated levels of parathyroid hormone–related peptide.[366] Hypercalcemia has also been associated with the t(17,19) translocation (*E2A-HLF* fusion), an uncommon chromosomal abnormality that also leads to disseminated intravascular coagulation.[366]

Infection

Life-threatening infection, observed at the time of diagnosis and during therapy, is one of the most frequent complications experienced by patients with ALL. Infections, most often bacterial and often associated with granulocytopenia, are the primary cause of treatment-related mortality in children receiving therapy for ALL.[256] Documented episodes of bacteremia have been reported in 15% to 30% of children receiving chemotherapy for ALL, and deaths caused by serious infection have been reported in up to 3% of patients.[3,256] Any febrile patient receiving therapy for ALL must be considered potentially bacteremic. Cultures should be obtained promptly, and the patient should be started immediately on broad-spectrum antibiotics with activity against bowel and respiratory organisms while awaiting culture results.[367]

As chemotherapy regimens have become more intensive, fungal disease, including invasive infections of *Candida* and *Aspergillus* species, have also been increasingly observed during the initial treatment of leukemia.[368,369] Viral infections can also cause significant morbidity in children with ALL. Varicella complicated by pneumonitis, hepatitis, or cerebritis can be particularly devastating.[370] Postexposure prophylaxis (within 72 hours) with varicella-zoster immunoglobulin and treatment with acyclovir once symptoms develop have reduced the frequency of severe disease.[371-373] However, even with these interventions, deaths from varicella have been reported in children undergoing therapy for ALL.[374] Rare cases of measles in children with ALL have been accompanied by a high incidence of morbidity and mortality.[375,376]

Pneumocystis jirovecii can cause a severe, often fatal interstitial pneumonitis in children receiving multiagent chemotherapy. The incidence of *P. jirovecii* increases with the degree and duration of immunosuppression and thus is usually observed during the later phases of ALL therapy, but it has been observed in the earlier phases as well.[377] Prophylaxis with trimethoprim-sulfamethoxazole markedly reduces the incidence of infection with *P. jirovecii* and is recommended for all children receiving therapy for ALL.[378]

The use of hematologic growth factors, such as filgrastim (granulocyte colony-stimulating factor), remains a matter of controversy. In prospective randomized studies, the use of filgrastim in children and adults receiving treatment for ALL was associated with a shorter duration of neutropenia and a tighter adherence to the planned treatment schedule.[379-382] However, although some investigators have reported a significantly decreased incidence in severe infections in patients treated with filgrastim during ALL therapy,[381,382] others have not confirmed this finding.[379,380] Also, filgrastim has not been shown to prolong survival or reduce the cost of supportive care for children with ALL.[380]

Typhlitis

A specific syndrome of right lower quadrant pain with rebound tenderness, abdominal distention, vomiting, and sepsis, referred to as typhlitis or necrotizing enterocolitis, can develop as a consequence of intensive chemotherapy, especially during the remission induction phase.[383,384] Findings on plain abdominal radiographs vary, but frequently show a paucity of air in the right lower quadrant.[383] Ultrasonography or computed tomography may reveal a characteristic thickening of the colonic mucosa.[384-386] The pathogenesis of typhlitis is most likely related to mucosal and bowel wall damage secondary to chemotherapy in the setting of prolonged neutropenia. It has rarely been observed before the institution of chemotherapy.[387,388] Management includes bowel rest, intravenous fluids, and broad-spectrum antibiotics. Surgery is usually not indicated, except in the rare case of perforation or uncontrolled bleeding.[389,390]

Acute Neurologic Toxicity

Intrathecal chemotherapy, high doses of systemic methotrexate, and cranial radiation, either alone or in combination, have been associated with acute neurotoxicity, including seizures.[324,391,392] Some of the highest rates of acute neurotoxicity have been observed in clinical trials that have used frequent dosing of intravenous and intrathecal methotrexate as a substitute for cranial radiation. For example, in a randomized trial conducted by the

Pediatric Oncology Group in children with lower-risk B-precursor cell ALL, the incidence of acute neurotoxicity was approximately 10% in patients receiving repeated courses of intermediate-dose intravenous methotrexate compared with 4% in those receiving low-dose oral methotrexate.[324]

A transient episode of somnolence, anorexia, lethargy, and fever often can be observed 6 to 8 weeks after cranial radiation.[393,394] This "somnolence syndrome" often is accompanied by electroencephalographic changes, CSF pleocytosis, and fever.[395] Most children recover uneventfully, and it is unclear whether there are any long-term neurologic implications.[395]

Peripheral and autonomic neuropathy secondary to vincristine is frequently seen in children receiving ALL therapy. Signs and symptoms vary in severity and include constipation, absent deep tendon reflexes, distal muscle weakness, gait abnormalities, parasthesias, and cranial nerve palsy.[396] Rarely, postural hypotension, bladder atony, and the syndrome of inappropriate secretion of antidiuretic hormone can occur.[396,397] Vincristine-associated neurotoxicity is usually reversible after therapy is completed, and long-term sequelae are rare.[396,398]

Other Acute Toxicities

Therapy with L-asparaginase is associated with pancreatitis in 5% to 10% of patients, and allergic reaction occurs in up to one third of children.[246,291] L-Asparaginase can also induce coagulopathy by inhibition of protein synthesis of clot-forming and clot-inhibitory proteins, including antithrombin III, plasminogen, and fibrinogen.[399-403] CNS and peripheral thromboses have been observed in 2% to 4% of patients receiving L-asparaginase for ALL.[246,291,404] The use of this agent has also been associated with transient hyperlipidemia.[405] Complications from corticosteroids include hypertension, hyperglycemia, myopathy, mood and behavioral problems, and an increased incidence of bone fractures.[293,295,406-408]

Late Effects of Treatment

With prolonged survival of children with ALL, late effects related to the disease and its treatment have become increasingly evident. The clinical magnitude of late effects is a function of treatment and host-related factors, such as age at diagnosis. Late effects include neurocognitive deficits, short stature, obesity, bony morbidity, cardiac dysfunction, and second malignant neoplasms.

CNS Sequelae

Historically, low and low-average intelligence quotients were frequent findings in survivors of ALL.[409-411] These learning disabilities were related to a slow speed of processing information, distractibility, and difficulty in dealing with complex or conceptually demanding material.[412,413] With contemporary therapy, neurocognitive late effects appear to be less severe and are related to treatment and patient characteristics. For example, younger children (<3 to 5 years old at diagnosis) are more vulnerable than older children[409,411,414] and, in some studies, girls are more vulnerable than boys.[412,415-417] Children with meningeal relapse who receive a second course of CNS treatment are at particularly high risk for significant and progressive intellectual loss.[418-420]

Most long-term neuropsychological effects have been attributed to cranial radiation.[409,410,413,417,421] The most severely impaired long-term survivors are those who received cranial radiation doses (24 to 28 Gy) that are higher than doses used in current treatment regimens (12 to 18 Gy).[422-424] Long-term survivors treated with 18 Gy of radiation (especially those who were 3 years or older at diagnosis) appear to fare relatively well, with less severe neurocognitive sequelae than children who had received higher doses of radiation. In some studies, this group of survivors does not demonstrate any significant cognitive deficits, although subtle effects are observed with detailed neuropsychological testing.[414,425]

The contribution of systemic and intrathecal chemotherapy to the development of neurocognitive sequelae has not been fully elucidated. There is evidence that cognitive deficits are present in long-term survivors treated without cranial radiation,[424-427] but these deficits do not tend to be severe, and overall neurocognitive function is generally within the normal range.[417,428] In most studies of long-term survivors, nonirradiated patients have fewer and less severe impairments than those who received cranial radiation,[411,421] although with current chemotherapy regimens and lower doses of radiation, the differences between the two groups may be subtle.[425] Systemic chemotherapy, including high-dose methotrexate and dexamethasone, may also contribute to neurocognitive late effects.[424,429,430]

Neuropathologic changes in the CNS have been identified in survivors of childhood ALL. Leukoencephalopathy, a relatively rare phenomenon, is characterized by multifocal demyelination visible on radiographic imaging (computed tomography or magnetic resonance imaging).[431] Patients may present with a wide range of neurologic and behavioral problems, including poor school performance, confusion, memory problems, personality changes, and, in its most severe form, progressive dementia and coma.[431] Risk factors for the development of leukoencephalopathy include large doses of cranial radiation (2400 cGy or higher) or high cumulative doses of systemic and intrathecal methotrexate.[378] In one study, the development of leukoencephalopathy was associated with escalating doses of weekly systemic methotrexate beyond 50 mg/m^2 in previously irradiated children.[432] Microcephaly has also been reported as a late effect of CNS treatment and was found to be dependent on the radiation dose.[433] Radiation-induced cavernous hemangiomas and other vasculopathies, sometimes leading to cerebral hemorrhage, have been reported in survivors of childhood ALL.[434,435]

Growth

In several studies, survivors of ALL are shorter than expected for their age.[436-440] Although all survivors of childhood ALL appear to be at increased risk for adult short stature, the greatest impact on final height has been noted in patients treated with 2400-cGy cranial irradiation, with less severe growth failure noted in patients whose CNS treatment included 1800-cGy or no cranial irradiation.[437,440,441] Young age and female gender are associated with more severe growth impairment.[437,439,440] Short stature in survivors of childhood ALL is occasionally associated with growth hormone deficiency,[442-444] suggesting that growth hormone replacement may have a potential therapeutic role in some patients.

Obesity is also prevalent among survivors of childhood ALL and, like short stature, is more frequently observed in girls and in those treated at a young age.[439,445-448] The cause of obesity is unclear; some investigators have reported an increased risk for obesity in survivors who received cranial radiation, especially at higher doses (>20 Gy),[448,449] whereas others have not observed any relationship between body mass index and prior radiation.[439,447,450] Corticosteroids may also play a role in the development of obesity, with increased rates of obesity associated with higher cumulative dosages.[447]

Bony Morbidity

Bony morbidity, including osteopenia, fractures, and osteonecrosis, has been reported to occur in up to 30% of survivors of childhood ALL and is primarily secondary to corticosteroids.[295] Several investigators have demonstrated that children with ALL have reduced bone mineral density during therapy,[451,452] resulting in an increased risk for fractures during and immediately after treatment.[407,453] However, it appears that bone mineral density improves once therapy is completed, although some degree of residual osteopenia may persist.[454-457] The clinical implications, if any, related to persistent osteopenia in long-term survivors have not yet been fully elucidated.

Osteonecrosis, also known as avascular necrosis, is a disabling bony toxicity, frequently involving multiple joints. Osteonecrosis can lead to significant pain and loss of function, sometimes necessitating total joint replacement.[458-460] Symptomatic osteonecrosis has been observed in 2% to 9% of children treated for ALL, with higher rates associated with higher cumulative dosages of corticosteroids.[295,349,461] Osteonecrosis occurs much more frequently in adolescents than in younger children.[294,349,461-463] Female sex has also been identified as a risk factor for the development of this complication.[349,462,463] In some studies, dexamethasone (when used instead of prednisone) has been associated with a higher risk for osteonecrosis.[294,462]

Cardiac Sequelae

Echocardiographic abnormalities, particularly increased afterload and decreased contractility, are well-characterized late effects of anthracycline therapy.[464,465] The mechanism of this toxicity is impairment of myocardial growth. The severity of cardiac dysfunction is correlated with higher cumulative doses of anthracycline and higher dose rates.[464-467] Patients treated at a young age, females, and those with Down syndrome appear to be more vulnerable to anthracycline-associated cardiac toxicity.[466,467] Over the past two decades, as patients have received lower cumulative dosages of anthracyclines, symptomatic congestive heart failure has become increasingly uncommon and now only rarely occurs in long-term survivors of childhood ALL.[465,467] In a randomized study of children with high-risk ALL, the cardioprotectant agent dexrazoxane was shown to reduce the incidence of doxorubicin-associated myocardial injury (as measured by cardiac troponin-T during treatment and echocardiographic measures of ventricular wall thickness and function 5 years after therapy) without affecting relapse risk or EFS.[468,469]

Sexual Development and Fertility

Ovarian and testicular function are relatively unaffected by most current childhood ALL regimens,[438,470,471] with the possible exception of programs that use high cumulative dosages of alkylating agents (e.g., cyclophosphamide).[472,473] Prophylactic gonadal radiation can also impair subsequent ovarian or testicular function,[473] but this treatment is no longer included in most regimens. Thus sexual development is normal and fertility is preserved in the vast majority of survivors of childhood ALL.[474] In a study of 949 female childhood ALL survivors, almost all experienced menarche within the normal range, although prior cranial radiation increased the risk for both early and late menarche.[475] In both genders, normal pubertal growth spurts may be blunted.[438,470] No evidence currently indicates that the progeny of survivors of childhood ALL are at increased risk for congenital abnormalities.[476,477]

Cataracts

Survivors of childhood ALL appear to be at increased risk for the development of posterior subcapsular cataracts.[478-480] In general, these cataracts are small and do not impair vision. Cataract formation is believed to be related to the administration of corticosteroids during ALL treatment,[480] although the incidence of cataracts may be higher in ALL survivors who also received cranial radiation.[479]

Second Malignancies

Long-term survivors of childhood ALL are at increased risk for developing second malignant neoplasms, including AML, brain tumors, non-Hodgkin lymphomas, and carcinomas of the parotid and thyroid glands.[481-485] The overall cumulative incidence of second malignant neoplasms reported in the literature ranges from 1% to 6%, depending on the treatment regimen and length of follow-up.[481-484,486] Compared with age-adjusted expected incidence in the general population, survivors of ALL appear to have a 6- to 14-fold increased risk for developing another cancer.[481-484,486] Risk factors for the development of secondary AML include treatment with epipodophyllotoxins and alkylating agents.[487-489] For example, the cumulative risk for secondary AML was 5% to 6% after treatment with epipodophyllotoxin-containing regimens[487,488] but less than 1% after therapy lacking both epipodophyllotoxins and alkylators.[486,490] Cranial and craniospinal radiation have been associated with an increased risk for secondary solid tumors, primarily malignant gliomas and meningiomas.[481-484] In several large studies, the long-term cumulative incidence rates of secondary brain tumors in previously irradiated patients ranged from 1.0% to 1.6%.[481,486,491] It is unclear whether

radiation dose is correlated with risk for secondary tumor, although, in one study, patients who had received 18 Gy of cranial radiation appeared to be at lower risk than those who had received 24 Gy of radiation.[482] The cumulative incidence of malignant glioma appears to plateau 15 to 20 years after diagnosis, although, even with 30 years of follow-up, a plateau in the incidence of meningiomas has not yet been observed.[483]

Other Sequelae

Abnormalities of dental and craniofacial development have been observed after cranial irradiation and appear to be related to the age of the patient at the initiation of therapy, with younger patients more severely affected.[492] Elevations of aminotransferase levels are common while patients are receiving therapy but are not associated with chronic liver disease once therapy is completed, and late-occurring hepatotoxicity is a rare phenomenon.[493,494] Chronic liver changes, including portal hypertension and cirrhosis, have been reported after the use of 6-thioguanine.[283,284,495]

RELAPSED ACUTE LYMPHOBLASTIC LEUKEMIA

Relapse subsequently occurs in 15% to 20% of children with ALL who achieve remission after initial induction chemotherapy. Several factors have been identified that influence the outcome of patients with relapsed ALL, including duration of initial remission, site of relapse, and immunophenotype.

Duration of initial remission is one of the most important prognostic factors, with significantly worse outcomes observed in patients who relapse early—defined as those occurring while on or within 6 months from completion of initial therapy—than in those with longer initial remissions.[496,497,498] T-lineage immunophenotype and age older than 10 years at initial diagnosis have also been associated with an adverse prognosis after relapse.[496-498]

Site of relapse also has prognostic importance, with superior outcomes observed for patients experiencing isolated extramedullary relapses compared with marrow relapses.[497,498] Some studies have suggested that patients with combined marrow and extramedullary relapses have a better prognosis than those with isolated marrow relapses,[496,498] although this has not been consistently demonstrated.[497]

By using these prognostic factors, investigators have identified subsets of relapsed patients with a relatively favorable prognosis (e.g., patients experiencing a late extramedullary relapse) who may be able to maintain durable second remissions with conventional-dose chemotherapy. Patients with a less favorable prognosis, such as those experiencing an early marrow relapse, are considered candidates for more intensive therapies, such as allogeneic SCT.

Marrow Relapse

Relapses involving the marrow account for the majority of recurrences of childhood ALL. Induction of second complete remission can be expected in 70% to 90% of children with relapsed B-precursor cell ALL but is lower in children with T-cell immunophenotype and those whose relapses occur early (<36 months from initial diagnosis).[496,499-501] After a second complete remission has been attained, subsequent treatment may include conventional-dose or high-dose chemotherapy with SCT.

Chemotherapy

Most trials of conventional-dose chemotherapy have been unsuccessful at producing long-term survival in the majority of patients who experience a marrow relapse. In large published series, overall survival rates for children treated with chemotherapy alone (without allogeneic SCT) have ranged from 25% to 40%.[496,502,503]

Duration of initial remission significantly predicts the outcome of children with a marrow relapse who receive chemotherapy alone as salvage therapy. In almost all reported chemotherapy trials, overall survival after an early relapse is less than 20%.[496,503-505] The most successful chemotherapy trial results have been achieved with patients whose initial complete remissions exceeded 30 to 36 months. With intensive chemotherapy regimens, the probability of EFS for this subset of patients has ranged from 40% to 60%.[496,497,503,506]

MRD levels may also help identify patients with late marrow relapses who might respond favorably to chemotherapy-only regimens after a marrow relapse. Several groups have demonstrated that MRD levels measured at the end of the first month of reinduction therapy predict long-term outcome in patients who have experienced a marrow relapse and are treated with chemotherapy only, with significantly higher survival rates associated with lower levels of MRD.[507,508] Patients with a late marrow relapse with high MRD levels at the end of reinduction fare much less with a chemotherapy-only approach. In a study conducted by the BFM group, allogeneic SCT was associated with an improved outcome (compared with historic controls treated with chemotherapy only) in late relapsing patients with high MRD levels at the end of reinduction.[509]

Allogeneic Stem Cell Transplantation

Allogeneic SCT is an important treatment option for children with relapsed ALL.[510-514] In most published reports, the most common cause of failure after allogeneic SCT is recurrence of leukemia.[512-514] Survival after HLA-matched sibling SCT appears to be better when total-body irradiation is included in the preparatory regimen.[506,515] Therapy-related toxicity, including infections and severe graft-versus-host disease, is also a major cause of death, occurring in 15% to 30% of patients.[510-513,515,516] In recent years, the incidence of treatment-related complications appears to be decreasing with improvements in supportive care.[506]

As has been demonstrated in chemotherapy trials for relapsed ALL, duration of initial remission is an important predictor of outcome after matched-sibling SCT, with improved survival observed in patients with longer initial remissions.[506,510] MRD levels, measured at the end of reinduction therapy and just before transplantation, also have been shown to predict outcome after matched-sibling allogeneic SCT, with poorer survival rates observed

for patients with higher levels of pretransplantation MRD.[517-519]

The indications for transplantation in second remission after marrow relapse remain controversial. Several studies have attempted to compare outcomes of patients treated with and without allogeneic SCT; however, there are many potential problems inherent in these analyses, including selection bias in terms of which patients receive a transplant. To address these issues, investigators have used matched-pair analyses and other statistical methods to control for time to transplantation and other important prognostic variables when comparing the two treatment modalities. In most of these reports, HLA-matched sibling SCT has been associated with a lower relapse risk and better survival rates compared with chemotherapy-only salvage regimens for patients with early marrow relapse.[506,510,511,514] However, these analyses have not clearly demonstrated that allogeneic SCT is associated with a survival advantage in patients with a late marrow relapse.[506,511] End-reinduction MRD may help to identify late-relapsing patients who might benefit from allogeneic SCT.[509]

HLA-matched siblings remain the donor of choice for allogeneic SCT for relapsed ALL. However, because over 80% of patients do not have histocompatible sibling donors, most patients needing allogeneic transplants rely on alternative donors. Other potential stem cell sources for transplantation include matched unrelated donors and umbilical cord stem cells. Historically, unrelated donor SCT in children with relapsed ALL was associated with a substantial risk for morbidity, with treatment-related mortality rates as high as 40% to 50% in some reports.[520,521] With improvements in supportive care and more accurate genomic typing of HLA antigens, treatment-related mortality after unrelated donor SCT has decreased significantly, making unrelated donor SCT a more viable treatment option.[522-524] Outcomes after unrelated donor SCT and unrelated cord blood SCT appear to be approaching those observed with HLA-matched sibling SCT.[524-526]

Autologous transplantation has also been investigated as an option for patients in second or subsequent complete remission who do not have a matched related donor. Autologous transplantation has been performed in conjunction with ex vivo purging of residual leukemia in harvested marrow via immunologic or pharmacologic techniques.[527-530] Relapse is the most common cause of treatment failure after autologous SCT, with a lower incidence of toxicity-related deaths than that observed after allogeneic SCT.[516] It does not appear that autologous SCT offers any advantage over chemotherapy[531] and, in general, should not be considered in pediatric patients with marrow relapses.

Isolated Extramedullary Relapses

Isolated extramedullary relapses, occurring either in the CNS or testis, are less frequent than marrow relapses in ALL. Such relapses may not actually be isolated; using sensitive molecular techniques, submicroscopic marrow disease can be demonstrated in most children at the time of an isolated extramedullary relapse.[532] The level of this submicroscopic marrow disease may predict response to postrelapse therapy.[532]

Isolated CNS relapse occurs in fewer than 10% of patients with ALL (see Fig. 50-4). Although CNS remission can be successfully induced in more than 90% of such patients with CNS-directed therapy, most patients treated without intensive systemic therapy will subsequently develop a bone marrow recurrence.[533,534] Thus, in addition to CNS-directed therapy, usually irradiation with intrathecal chemotherapy, patients with isolated CNS relapses are also treated with intensive systemic therapy. Several reports have indicated that intensive chemotherapy regimens in conjunction with cranial or craniospinal irradiation may provide adequate postremission therapy for patients with an isolated CNS relapse, with EFS rates as high as 70%.[535,536,537] From the limited published data, it is unclear that allogeneic SCT is associated with a survival advantage for patients with an isolated CNS relapse. In two published comparisons, outcomes after allogeneic SCT were similar to those achieved with chemotherapy and/or irradiation in children with an isolated CNS relapse.[538,539]

As with marrow relapses, patients experiencing late isolated CNS relapses have a better prognosis than those whose relapses occur earlier.[497,502,536,537] On two consecutive clinical trials conducted by the Pediatric Oncology Group, children with the B-precursor cell phenotype and a relatively late isolated CNS relapse (initial remission duration of at least 18 months) had EFS rates of 77% to 83% when treated with intensive chemotherapy and delayed cranial radiation, whereas patients with earlier relapses fared less well with the same regimen.[536,537] Some studies have indicated that patients whose initial CNS prophylaxis included cranial irradiation may have a worse prognosis after an isolated CNS relapse than previously unirradiated patients.[535]

Isolated testicular relapses are uncommon, occurring in 0.5% to 1% of boys with ALL.[24,246] For boys with isolated testicular relapses, systemic chemotherapy and testicular irradiation have resulted in prolonged second remissions in more than 80% of patients with late-occurring relapses.[540,541] This approach has been less successful in patients whose testicular relapses occurred during or soon after cessation of initial therapy, with long-term EFS ranging from 20% to 43%.[540,542]

Other rare sites of extramedullary relapse include eyes and ovaries. Case reports have indicated successful treatment of these patients with local irradiation and intensive systemic therapy.[543,544]

FUTURE DIRECTIONS

Although risk-adapted therapy has resulted in marked improvement in the outcome of children with ALL over the past few decades, molecular techniques may help identify biologic factors that may supplement or replace the currently applied clinical risk factors to identify those patients at highest risk for treatment failure. For example, using transcriptional profiling, single nucleotide polymorphism microarrays, transcriptional profiling, and other genomic assays, biologically distinctive

and prognostically relevant subtypes of ALL have been identified, including the BCR-ABL–like and early T-cell precursors (ETP) subsets.[29,99,100] In addition, research focused on germline genetic variation and pharmacogenomics may identify patient-related factors that affect outcome and help lead to more individualized therapy.[226,545]

New drug development is essential to improve outcomes. Newer cytotoxic agents, such as clofarabine and nelarabine, may help improve the outcome of some high-risk patients but, like currently available drugs, are associated with significant side effects.[260,546] Imatinib and other tyrosine kinase inhibitors have dramatically altered the therapeutic approach to patients with Ph-chromosome–positive ALL[96] and are the prototypes of a new type of antileukemic agent that is more specific and potentially less toxic than current chemotherapy. Such agents target molecules or pathways that are important in leukemogenesis or leukemic cell survival, and, like imatinib, potentially could be given with cytotoxic chemotherapy to improve outcomes in high-risk subsets. For example, bortezomib, a proteasome inhibitor, was shown to be synergistic with other chemotherapeutic agents in vitro and so was tested in multiply relapsed patients in the context of a standard reinduction treatment platform, with promising preliminary results.[547] Other potential therapeutic targets under investigation include the mammalian target of rapamycin (mTOR), Janus kinase (JAK) family members in CRLF2-overexpressing B-cell ALL, and NOTCH pathway inhibitors in T-cell ALL.[548-550] Additionally, epigenetic modifiers, including proteins that regulate chromatin remodeling, DNA cytosine methylation, and covalent histone modifications, are increasingly recognized as potentially important therapeutic targets in leukemia.[551]

In addition to cytotoxic and targeted therapies, there is increasing focus on the role of immune-based therapies in ALL. Novel approaches that aim to promote autologous T-cell lysis of lymphoblasts include: (1) genetic engineering of autologous T cells to express a chimeric antigen receptor specific for a B-cell surface antigen and (2) use of a bispecific monoclonal antibody that both simultaneously engages T cells and targets B-cell surface antigens.[552,553] Toxin-conjugated monoclonal antibodies directed toward leukemia cell surface antigens are also under investigation.[554]

As more children with ALL become long-term survivors, there is an increasingly important need to address issues of late sequelae and the physical and emotional costs of cure.[555,556] While awaiting the development of more specific antileukemic therapeutic modalities, the impact of currently available primary and salvage therapies must be better understood so that rational therapeutic decisions can be made, with the ultimate goal of improving survival and minimizing toxicity.

References available online at ExpertConsult.

KEY REFERENCES

3. Moricke A, Zimmermann M, Reiter A, et al: Long-term results of five consecutive trials in childhood acute lymphoblastic leukemia performed by the ALL-BFM study group from 1981 to 2000. *Leukemia* 24:265–284, 2010.

Most current treatment programs for childhood ALL are based on a regimen pioneered by the ALL-BFM study group from Germany. This report highlights results of clinical trials conducted by this group between 1981 and 2000 that provide the foundation for this commonly used treatment platform.

29. Coustan-Smith E, Mullighan CG, Onciu M, et al: Early T-cell precursor leukaemia: a subtype of very high-risk acute lymphoblastic leukaemia. *Lancet Oncol* 10:147–156, 2009.

    Investigators identified a new subtype of T-ALL with a gene expression profile highly related to that of immature T-cell progenitors. This subtype, characterized by a distinctive immunophenotype, appeared to have an inferior outcome compared with other cases of T-cell ALL.

43. Moorman AV, Ensor HM, Richards SM, et al: Prognostic effect of chromosomal abnormalities in childhood B-cell precursor acute lymphoblastic leukaemia: results from the UK Medical Research Council ALL97/99 randomised trial. *Lancet Oncol* 11:429–438, 2010.

    This study from the United Kingdom comprehensively characterizes the prognostic implications of the most commonly observed chromosomal abnormalities in childhood ALL in a large cohort of patients.

71. Weng AP, Ferrando AA, Lee W, et al: Activating mutations of NOTCH1 in human T cell acute lymphoblastic leukemia. *Science* 306:269–271, 2004.

    This article describes the discovery of activating NOTCH1 mutations, one of the most common genetic lesions in T-cell ALL and a potential therapeutic target.

86. Zhang J, Ding L, Holmfeldt L, et al: The genetic basis of early T-cell precursor acute lymphoblastic leukaemia. *Nature* 481:157–163, 2012.

    The authors used whole-genome sequencing to demonstrate that T-cell ALL cases with differentiation arrest at very early stages of T-cell development harbor a high frequency of mutations typically seen in acute myeloid leukemia and myelodysplastic syndromes, raising the possibility that this disease may represent a stem cell leukemia.

96. Schultz KR, Bowman WP, Aledo A, et al: Improved early event-free survival with imatinib in Philadelphia chromosome-positive acute lymphoblastic leukemia: a children's oncology group study. *J Clin Oncol* 27:5175–5181, 2009.

97. Biondi A, Schrappe M, De Lorenzo P, et al: Imatinib after induction for treatment of children and adolescents with Philadelphia-chromosome-positive acute lymphoblastic leukaemia (EsPhALL): a randomised, open-label, intergroup study. *Lancet Oncol* 13:936–945, 2012.

    References 96 and 97 are the first pediatric studies to demonstrate that the tyrosine kinase inhibitor imatinib can be feasibly combined with cytotoxic chemotherapy in patients with Philadelphia chromosome–positive ALL and that this combination appears to be associated with relatively favorable outcomes.

99. Mullighan CG, Su X, Zhang J, et al: Deletion of IKZF1 and prognosis in acute lymphoblastic leukemia. *N Engl J Med* 360:470–480, 2009.

    This manuscript was one of the first publications to describe a new, biologically distinctive high-risk subtype of ALL: cases with genomic characteristics of BCR-ABL that lack this translocation. Deletion of the IKZF1 gene was commonly seen in these BCR-ABL–like cases, and, in this series, was an independent predictor of poor outcome.

105. Holmfeldt L, Wei L, Diaz-Flores E, et al: The genomic landscape of hypodiploid acute lymphoblastic leukemia. *Nat Genet* 45:242–252, 2013.

    Using genomic profiling, the authors show that hypodiploid ALL, an uncommon chromosomal abnormality associated with a poor prognosis, is composed of two distinct biologic subtypes: near-haploid ALL (24-31 chromosomes), which is characterized by alterations of growth factor signal transduction pathways, and low-hypodiploid ALL (32 to 39 chromosomes), which is strongly associated with TP53 mutations that are often germline.

111. Smith M, Arthur D, Camitta B, et al: Uniform approach to risk classification and treatment assignment for children with acute lymphoblastic leukemia. *J Clin Oncol* 14:18–24, 1996.

    This manuscript established the NCI classification of age and leukocyte count for risk group stratification, which continues to be used in most clinical trials to risk-stratify patients.

161. Pieters R, Schrappe M, De Lorenzo P, et al: A treatment protocol for infants younger than 1 year with acute lymphoblastic leukaemia (Interfant-99): an observational study and a multicentre randomised trial. *Lancet* 370:240–250, 2007.

    This paper reports the results of an international collaborative clinical trial for infants with ALL. This is the largest trial for this group of patients and demonstrates their unique biology and relatively poor outcome. It also establishes prognostic risk groups based on age, leukocyte count, and chromosomal abnormalities.

163. Boissel N, Auclerc MF, Lheritier V, et al: Should adolescents with acute lymphoblastic leukemia be treated as old children or young adults? Comparison of the French FRALLE-93 and LALA-94 trials. *J Clin Oncol* 21:774–780, 2003.

    This study was one of the first to report that adolescents with ALL fare better when treated on a regimen designed for pediatric rather than for adult ALL patients. Since its publication, several other studies have confirmed this finding.

198. Schrappe M, Hunger SP, Pui CH, et al: Outcomes after induction failure in childhood acute lymphoblastic leukemia. *N Engl J Med* 366:1371–1381, 2012.

    This retrospective analysis of over 1000 pediatric patients with initial induction failure represents the largest study of this rare subset. This study confirmed the overall poor prognosis for this group of patients but also indicated that allogeneic stem cell transplant after complete remission is achieved may benefit some. It also identified a small minority of patients who appeared to do well despite initial induction failure for whom transplantion may not be indicated.

214. Borowitz MJ, Devidas M, Hunger SP, et al: Clinical significance of minimal residual disease in childhood acute lymphoblastic leukemia and its relationship to other prognostic factors: a Children's Oncology Group study. *Blood* 111:5477–5485, 2008.

    Using flow cytometric techniques, the Children's Oncology Group confirmed the prognostic importance of MRD levels early in treatment. Using these levels in combination with other factors (including age, leukocyte count, and chromosomal aberrations), researchers were able to identify groups of patients with an excellent prognosis.

215. Conter V, Bartram CR, Valsecchi MG, et al: Molecular response to treatment redefines all prognostic factors in children and adolescents with B-cell precursor acute lymphoblastic leukemia: results in 3184 patients of the AIEOP-BFM ALL 2000 study. *Blood* 115:3206–3214, 2010.

216. Schrappe M, Valsecchi MG, Bartram CR, et al: Late MRD response determines relapse risk overall and in subsets of childhood T-cell ALL: results of the AIEOP-BFM-ALL 2000 study. *Blood* 118:2077–2084, 2011.

    References 215 and 216 report the results of the AIEOP-BFM-ALL 2000 trial, the first clinical trial to incorporate MRD response (as assessed by PCR assay) into risk stratification. Taken together, these two manuscripts establish the prognostic significance of MRD and also indicate interpretation of MRD levels may be different between B-cell ALL and T-cell ALL.

236. Bhatia S, Landier W, Shangguan M, et al: Nonadherence to oral mercaptopurine and risk of relapse in Hispanic and non-Hispanic white children with acute lymphoblastic leukemia: a report from the Children's Oncology Group. *J Clin Oncol* 30:2094–2101, 2012.

    Although most studies focus on leukemia biology and presenting characteristics as outcome predictors, this study from the Children's Oncology Group indicated that adherence to oral mercaptopurine (a mainstay of the continuation phase of treatment in nearly all regimens) was also a significant predictor of outome, suggesting that strategies to improve home medication compliance may lead to improved outcomes.

248. Hunger SP, Lu X, Devidas M, et al: Improved survival for children and adolescents with acute lymphoblastic leukemia between 1990 and 2005: a report from the children's oncology group. *J Clin Oncol* 30:1663–1669, 2012.

    This report from the Children's Oncology Group demonstrates progressive improvement in overall survival rates in children and adolescents with ALL over the 15-year period between 1990 and 2005.

349. Mattano LA, Jr, Sather HN, Trigg ME, et al: Osteonecrosis as a complication of treating acute lymphoblastic leukemia in children: a report from the Children's Cancer Group. *J Clin Oncol* 18:3262–3272, 2000.

   This article reports that osteonecrosis, a potentially disabling skeletal toxicity related to corticosteroid treatment, is significantly more common in adolescent patients than younger children.

425. Waber DP, Turek J, Catania L, et al: Neuropsychological outcomes from a randomized trial of triple intrathecal chemotherapy compared with 18 Gy cranial radiation as CNS treatment in acute lymphoblastic leukemia: findings from Dana-Farber Cancer Institute ALL Consortium Protocol 95-01. *J Clin Oncol* 25:4914–4921, 2007.

   This study reports the long-term neurocognitive outcomes of pediatric ALL survivors who participated in a randomized comparison of 18-Gy radiation versus intrathecal chemotherapy only as CNS–directed therapy. The results of neurospychologic testing indicated that both groups of patients did not have significant impairments and also were similar to each other.

468. Lipshultz SE, Rifai N, Dalton VM, et al: The effect of dexrazoxane on myocardial injury in doxorubicin-treated children with acute lymphoblastic leukemia. *N Engl J Med* 351:145–153, 2004.

469. Lipshultz SE, Scully RE, Lipsitz SR, et al: Assessment of dexrazoxane as a cardioprotectant in doxorubicin-treated children with high-risk acute lymphoblastic leukaemia: long-term follow-up of a prospective, randomised, multicentre trial. *Lancet Oncol* 11:950–961, 2010.

   References 468 and 469 report the short- and long-term results of a clinical trial demonstrating that dexrazoxane prevents acute cardiac damage and long-term echocardiographic abnormalities in pediatric ALL patients treated with the anthracycline doxorubicin. Whereas cardiotoxicity was prevented by dexrazoxane, it did not have any impact on long-term EFS, suggesting that it can be safely used to prevent cardiac late effects without adversely impacting cure rates.

497. Gaynon PS, Qu RP, Chappell RJ, et al: Survival after relapse in childhood acute lymphoblastic leukemia: impact of site and time to first relapse—the Children's Cancer Group Experience. *Cancer* 82:1387–1395, 1998.

   This study from the Children's Cancer Group provides a good overview of the overall outcome and important prognostic factors in relapsed pediatric ALL.

509. Eckert C, Henze G, Seeger K, et al: Use of allogeneic hematopoietic stem-cell transplantation based on minimal residual disease response improves outcomes for children with relapsed acute lymphoblastic leukemia in the intermediate-risk group. *J Clin Oncol* 31:2736–2742, 2013.

   Previous studies had established that allogeneic SCT was associated with superior outcomes (compared with chemotherapy alone) in early-relapsing ALL, but its role in late-relapsing patients was unclear. This study demonstrates that allogeneic SCT in second complete remission may improve outcome for patients with late-relapsing ALL who have high levels of MRD at the end of the first month of reinduction chemotherapy.

536. Ritchey AK, Pollock BH, Lauer SJ, et al: Improved survival of children with isolated CNS relapse of acute lymphoblastic leukemia: a Pediatric Oncology Group study. *J Clin Oncol* 17:3745–3752, 1999.

537. Barredo JC, Devidas M, Lauer SJ, et al: Isolated CNS relapse of acute lymphoblastic leukemia treated with intensive systemic chemotherapy and delayed CNS radiation: a Pediatric Oncology Group study. *J Clin Oncol* 24:3142–3149, 2006.

   In two consecutive studies (references 536 and 537), the Pediatric Oncology Group demonstrated that patients with late isolated CNS relapse had favorable outcomes when treated with regimens that included high-dose CNS–penetrant systemic chemotherapy and delayed cranial radiation.

553. Grupp SA, Kalos M, Barrett D, et al: Chimeric antigen receptor-modified T cells for acute lymphoid leukemia. *N Engl J Med* 368:1509–1518, 2013.

   Chimeric angten receptor (CAR)-modified T cells represent a promising novel therapy for patients with relapsed, refractory ALL, as reflected in this report.

CHAPTER 51

Pediatric Myeloid Leukemia, Myelodysplasia, and Myeloproliferative Disease

Jason N. Berman and A. Thomas Look

CHAPTER OUTLINE

ACUTE MYELOGENOUS LEUKEMIA

Acute myelogenous leukemia (AML) comprises a heterogeneous group of disorders characterized by the malignant clonal transformation of a hematopoietic stem or progenitor cell. In recent years, deeper understanding has been gained into the chromosomal changes and specific genetic mutations that precipitate this transformation. AML is a relatively rare disorder in children, with between 500 and 600 newly diagnosed patients in the United States each year. Because of the heterogeneous nature of AML, it has proven difficult to find a treatment strategy that is effective for all patients; thus, overall cure rates for AML have improved only modestly in the past few decades, lagging behind those for acute lymphoblastic leukemia (ALL). Drawing from data from the Medical Research Council (MRC) trials, patients with AML are now risk stratified based on cytogenetic features and emerging data on the prognostic significance of minimal residual disease (MRD) early in therapy. Current ongoing clinical trials are attempting to minimize toxicity for patients with low-risk disease and intensify therapy for patients with high-risk disease. As the molecular genetics behind the biology of AML are better elucidated, there is a pressing need to develop new strategies for targeted therapy to improve outcomes in AML.

Epidemiology and Etiology

According to the National Cancer Institute (NCI) Surveillance Epidemiology and End Results (SEER) data, it was estimated that each year, from 2006 to 2010, 5.1 per 100,000 children younger than 14 years and 4.6 per

100,000 adolescents aged 15 to 19 years were diagnosed with cancer.[1,2] AML is less common than ALL: it comprises about 16% of childhood leukemias in children younger than 15 years but 36% of leukemias in adolescents 15 to 20 years, for a total of 500 to 600 new pediatric AML patients annually in the United States. AML has a bimodal distribution, occurring with higher incidence in children younger than 2 years and then again in adolescents 15 to 20 years old.

In ALL, boys are more commonly affected than girls; the incidence of AML is similar for all pediatric age groups, however, regardless of gender.[1,3] Similarly, although the incidence of childhood ALL is higher in white than in black children, the incidence of AML is comparable for both races across all pediatric age groups. With regard to ethnicity, there is a higher incidence of AML in Hispanic versus non-Hispanic children. Of interest, although the incidence of ALL for children younger than 15 years increased from 1977 to 1995, the incidence of AML did not change significantly over this time period.[3]

For a subset of patients with AML, a series of risk factors predisposing to the development of AML has been identified (Box 51-1) These risk factors fall into two general categories: exposures (environmental or toxic) and genetic predisposition. The best understood of the exposures is prior treatment with chemotherapy and radiation. Alkylating agents (e.g., nitrogen mustard, cyclophosphamide, ifosfamide, chlorambucil, and melphalan) are associated with the development of myelodysplastic syndrome (MDS) and secondary AML, with deletions of chromosomes 5 and 7.[4,5] Treatment with topoisomerase II inhibitors such as the epipodophyllotoxins has been linked to a specific type of AML with chromosome band 11q23 translocations, which produce fusion proteins involving the mixed-lineage leukemia (MLL) gene *(MLL)*.[6-10] Treatment with anthracyclines in adults with breast cancer, or in children for leukemias and sarcomas such as osteosarcoma, is associated with the development of secondary leukemias, including ALL, AML, and chronic myelogenous leukemia (CML).[11,12] Although therapy-related AML generally carries a worse prognosis than de novo AML, there have been reported cases of therapy-related AML harboring the better risk cytogenetic abnormalities: t(8;21), inv(16), t(16;16), and t(15;17), often in conjunction with other cytogenetic abnormalities.[13,14] In the case of therapy-related AML with inv(16) and t(16;16), a rare core-binding factor β *(CBFβ)*–myosin heavy chain 11 *(MYH11)* fusion transcript has been reported, with different breakpoints compared with the usual fusion transcript found in better-risk de novo AML.[14] Similarly, there is a case report of a patient with therapy-related AML with t(8;21), and the breakpoint at 21q22 was outside the *AML1* locus.[15]

Radiation exposure may be acquired from the environment or through medical procedures and is well documented to predispose to leukemia. The increased risk for AML and CML in survivors of nuclear blasts in Japan who were exposed to excessive doses of ionizing radiation has been well documented, and these patients have a higher rate of abnormalities of chromosomes 5 and

---

Box 51-1   Predisposing Factors for the Development of Acute Myelogenous Leukemia or Myelodysplastic Syndromes

PRENATAL EXPOSURES

Alcohol
Pesticides*
Foods naturally high in topoisomerase II inhibitors*
Viral infections

ENVIRONMENTAL EXPOSURES

Ionizing radiation
Chemotherapeutic agents
Alkylating agents
Epipodophyllotoxins
Anthracyclines
Organic solvents (e.g., benzene)
Radon*
Pesticides*
Viral infections*

HEREDITARY CONDITIONS

Down syndrome
Noonan syndrome
Neurofibromatosis
Fanconi anemia
Bloom syndrome
Severe congenital neutropenia (Kostmann syndrome)
Shwachman-Diamond syndrome
Klinefelter syndrome (XXY)*

GERMLINE PREDISPOSITION MUTATIONS

NF1 (for JMML)
RUNX1
CEBPA
GATA2
ANKRD26

ACQUIRED DISORDERS

Aplastic anemia
Paroxysmal nocturnal hemoglobinuria
JMML, Juvenile myelomonocytic leukemia.

*Conflicting or limited data.

7.[16-18] An increased risk for AML and ALL in children exposed to radiation in utero has been described, particularly in the past, when diagnostic radiographs were more common during pregnancy,[19,20] although a retrospective study of children with leukemia in Sweden did not confirm this finding.[21] Nuclear power plant workers have a higher risk for leukemia, although there does not appear to be a higher risk in residents living near such plants.[22-24] Air travel is a source of exposure to cosmic radiation, and studies have shown an increase in malignant melanoma and other skin cancers in flight crew members, an increase in breast cancer in female flight crew members, and an increase in AML in male cockpit crew members who logged more than 5000 flight hours annually.[25,26] Studies designed to measure the potential risk for malignancy from residential or occupational exposure to magnetic fields around high-voltage electrical lines have generated conflicting results, and a causal relationship with AML has not been conclusively established.[27-35]

There are several other environmental exposures with possible links to AML, some of which have yet to be proven definitively. Benzene exposure, which may occur occupationally or through tobacco smoking, has been shown to increase the risk for AML.[25,26,36,37] Several prenatal exposures have been studied as risk factors for the development of AML, particularly in children younger than 3 years. Maternal alcohol consumption during pregnancy was studied in a Children's Cancer Group (CCG) case-control study and found to have an association with increased rates of childhood AML in a dose-dependent matter, with an odds ratio of 2.64 overall and an odds ratio of 7.62 for classic French-American-British (FAB) classification category M1 (myeloblastic with minimal maturation) and M2 (myeloblastic with maturation) AML; other case-control studies have confirmed this finding.[38,39] Some early studies had suggested an association between maternal tobacco and marijuana use and childhood AML, but more recent analyses have not confirmed this association. A Children's Oncology Group (COG) case-control study looked at maternal consumption of foods such as soy, green and black tea, cocoa, red wine, and certain fruits and vegetables that are naturally high in DNA topoisomerase II inhibitors and found an odds ratio of 1.9 to 3.2 for the development of *MLL*-rearranged AML in the setting of high maternal consumption of these foods.[40] Some studies have suggested an increased risk for childhood AML after high exposure to pesticides, either prenatally or postnatally, up to 3 years of age.[41] There is interest in an association between viral infections and AML, but few data. One case-control study has suggested an increase in childhood AML in offspring of mothers who reactivated Epstein-Barr virus during pregnancy.[42] Parvovirus B19 is associated with pure red cell aplasia, and certain human leukocyte antigen (HLA)-DRB1 alleles seem to be associated with symptomatic infection.[43] One study of 16 leukemia patients suggested an association between parvovirus B19 infection and acute leukemia in 4 of the patients, including 1 patient with AML, all of whom carried these particular HLA-DRB1 alleles, although this association needs further investigation.[44] Several retrospective studies have suggested that breastfeeding may be protective against ALL and AML.[45-47] Risk related to indoor radon exposure is controversial. One French study showed a higher rate of AML in children with high exposure but other studies have showed no association.[48,49] Rarely used now, chloramphenicol use in children was formerly associated with an increased risk for AML.[50]

An increased incidence of AML has been observed for patients with certain hereditary disorders. Children with congenital disorders of myelopoiesis, such as Kostmann syndrome, Shwachman-Diamond syndrome, and Diamond-Blackfan anemia, are predisposed to AML.[51-58] Patients with inherited syndromes associated with chromosome fragility and impaired DNA repair mechanisms, such as Fanconi anemia[59-62] and Bloom syndrome,[63-65] also have an increased risk for development of AML. Neurofibromatosis type 1, which is caused by mutations in the neurofibromin tumor suppressor gene on chromosome 17, is associated with juvenile myelomonocytic leukemia (JMML).[66-68] Patients with certain constitutional chromosomal abnormalities carry a higher risk for AML.[69,70] Down syndrome is one of the most clinically prominent examples in this category. It is estimated that over 10% of infants with Down syndrome exhibit a transient myeloproliferative disease associated with a *GATA1* mutation.[71] Down syndrome patients have a 10 to 20 times higher than average risk for acute leukemia. In Down syndrome patients younger than 4 years, AML, usually acute megakaryoblastic (AMKL), is far more common than ALL: an estimated 1 in 500 Down syndrome patients develop AML.[71,72] In contrast to AMKL in the general pediatric population, which carries an extremely poor prognosis, this disease in Down syndrome patients is extremely sensitive to chemotherapy (see later).[71,72] Although early studies did not suggest a higher risk for AML in patients with Klinefelter syndrome (XXY), more recent data suggest that these patients may have a higher risk for hematologic malignancy, including AML.[73-75] More recently, a number of MDS/AML predisposition genes have been identified, including loss of function alterations affecting the key hematopoietic transcription factor genes *RUNX1*, *CEBPA*, and most recently *GATA2*.[76-80]

Although the predisposing risk factors and genetic conditions described may provide insight into the causative mechanisms that increase the risk for development of AML, most patients with de novo AML have no known predisposing exposures or conditions. Point mutations and chromosomal deletions and translocations occur at a background rate, even in healthy individuals, during hematopoietic stem and progenitor cell expansion. The extent to which inherited, expressed, single-nucleotide polymorphisms in the general population alter mutational rates during myelopoiesis and increase the risk for AML and other cancers remains an area of intense investigation.

Biology

Clonal Origin of Myeloid Leukemia Cells

Normal myelopoiesis is a complex differentiation program whereby primitive hematopoietic stem cells (HSCs) develop along a multistep pathway into fully differentiated, functionally active circulating blood cells.[81] This exquisitely controlled process is regulated by the intricate interactions among the expression levels of various transcription factors, growth factors and their receptors, cytokines, enzymes, and still unidentified novel molecules. A series of sequential genetic abnormalities perturbs this normal developmental progression and leads to AML. Although the relationships between specific morphologic subtypes of AML and their specific recurring genetic abnormalities have provided some insight into the mechanisms of leukemogenesis, understanding of the process whereby these fusion gene products interact with normal signal transduction pathways to subvert hematopoietic cell development is incomplete.[82]

Several strong lines of evidence support the hypothesis that AML progresses from a single transformed hematopoietic stem or progenitor cell. More than 30 years ago, studies were pioneered by Beutler and colleagues[83] and Fialkow[84] using X inactivation patterns in female patients to establish the clonal origin of human malignancies, including leukemia. By showing the presence of a single glucose-6-phosphate dehydrogenase (G6PD) isoenzyme in the leukemic myeloblasts of heterozygous females, the clonal origin of myeloid leukemia cells was demonstrated.[85-87] Females who are heterozygous at the G6PD locus express two isoforms of the enzyme. Approximately half of the cells in normal somatic tissue have randomly inactivated one of the X chromosomes, and approximately half of the cells should therefore express each isoform. Unlike normal somatic cells, AML cells of female patients heterozygous for G6PD expressed only one G6PD isoform, indicating cells of clonal origin.[86,87] In the 1980s, Vogelstein and coworkers[88,89] developed a strategy using X chromosome–linked DNA restriction length fragment polymorphisms to determine the clonal origin of human tumors. They established that maturing granulocytic cells arise from the malignant clone in patients with AML.[90] Later, X chromosome inactivation to determine clonality in malignancies was carried out using the polymerase chain reaction (PCR) assay to distinguish X-linked polymorphic genes.[91-93]

Transformation of Stem Cells with Self-Renewal Capacity

These earlier studies, and those performed by Bonnet and Dick and associates in the 1990s,[94,95] led to the insight that leukemia cell populations form a hierarchy in which leukemia stem cells or leukemia-initiating cells (LICs) are responsible for their own self-renewal and for the generation of the more differentiated progeny within the leukemic clone. This theory was in contrast to the stochastic model, which stated that malignant properties within cancer cell populations follow Gaussian distributions, resulting in the random or stochastic probability that individual cancer cells within the population are able to initiate malignant progression. Whereas AML was the first human cancer in which cancer stem cells were identified, the case has now been made in breast cancer,[96] brain tumors,[97-99] and colon cancer,[100] among others. In general, AML stem cells are believed to arise through the transformation of HSCs, which then retain the capacity for self-renewal, or through transformation of more differentiated hematopoietic progenitor cells that acquire the ability to self-renew by virtue of the particular transforming mutations, such as the formation of an *MLL* fusion gene.

AML is a heterogeneous disease in its clinical manifestations, response to therapy, and molecular genetics; thus insight into the cell of origin would have important ramifications regarding diagnosis and treatment. Moreover, refractory disease and relapse are often attributed to the presence of an LIC population that is resistant to chemotherapy; thus the ability to identify and target this subpopulation may be key to improving overall disease outcome.[101] In the 1990s, Dick's group produced a series of convincing papers[94,95,102] that strongly implicated the primitive, pluripotent HSC as the LIC in some types of AML. "Stemness," or the capacity to function as an LIC, includes self-renewal, proliferation, and differentiation and is tested in vitro by replating limiting dilution studies and in vivo by serial transplantation assays with the ability to regenerate a clonal leukemia in secondary and subsequent recipient animals. The HSC, with its inherent gene programs ensuring self-renewal, proliferation, and survival appears to be an ideal target to become sabotaged through a series of genetic events, leading ultimately to a fully transformed AML LIC that is capable of producing a clonal population of leukemia cells. According to this argument, different AML phenotypes often occur as a result of the gene(s) that are altered, leading to differentiation arrest within the progeny of the LIC, but not necessarily reflecting the degree of the commitment of the initially transformed cell. Support for this hypothesis initially came from several clonality studies in leukemic cells from patients with AML,[103-105] which demonstrated multiple-lineage involvement in a high proportion of cases, and implicated a multipotent HSC as the cell of origin.[104] More supportive evidence has come from studies looking at cytogenetic markers and characteristic cell surface antigen expression patterns.[106] Pluripotent HSCs express CD34 but do not express CD38 or HLA-DR, whereas more committed myeloid progenitor cells are CD34+, CD38+, and HLA-DR+.[81,106] Using fluorescence-activated cell sorting (FACS) of leukemic cell populations, the same two subpopulations, CD34+/CD38– and CD34+/CD38+, were isolated from the bone marrow of patients with different AML subtypes. The two subpopulations were then evaluated using fluorescence in situ hybridization (FISH) to determine the presence of cytogenetic abnormalities. The studies detected the same characteristic cytogenetic abnormalities in the CD34+/CD38– stem cell fraction as in the original leukemic bone marrow samples, implying origin in a very early HSC compartment.[107,108]

Further evidence supporting the stem cell origin model of AML was derived from transplantation experiments in which purified human AML cells were transplanted into mice with severe combined immunodeficiency (SCID). These experiments defined a SCID mouse leukemia–initiating cell (SL-IC) in the bone marrow of patients with AML and showed that these SL-ICs are CD34+/CD38– and that their engraftment produces large numbers of colony-forming progenitors. The CD34+/CD38+ and CD34– fractions did not engraft.[95] Similar results were obtained through transplantation studies in a modified SCID mouse, the nonobese diabetic mouse with SCID (NOD/SCID), with cells from patients with AML.[94] These studies identified and analyzed AML stem cells from samples of different FAB subtypes on the basis of their ability to initiate human AML after transplantation in NOD/SCID mice. These SL-ICs were able to proliferate and differentiate after transplantation, producing disease in the mice identical to that in the donor, as well as being able to renew themselves, reestablishing AML in secondary recipients, demonstrating that SL-ICs are capable of self-renewal. Again, the SL-ICs were found to reside in the CD34+/CD38– fraction and not in the CD34+/CD38+ or CD34– fractions. The SL-IC phenotype was consistent regardless of the FAB subtype (e.g., M1, M2, M4, M5). As few as 2 • 10^4 CD34+ cells were able to initiate the leukemic clone in recipient mice, whereas 100 times as many CD34– cells failed to engraft. Cells with the CD34 surface antigen were further fractionated on the basis of

CD38 expression. Only the CD34+/CD38− fraction contained SL-ICs.[94]

Whereas the transformation of the HSC provides an attractive mechanism to generate hierarchical myeloid leukemia cell populations, several studies have given new credence to a second mechanism through which committed progenitor cells along the pathway of myeloid differentiation are vulnerable to transforming mutations that confer self-renewal properties to progenitor cells that inherently lack this ability.[109-111] These transformation events create an LIC capable of generating a population of aberrant cells blocked at the differentiation state at which the initial transforming event occurred. Several translocations involving the *MLL* gene have been shown to initiate self-renewal in myeloid progenitor cells and to result in an AML phenotype.[110,112] A head-to-head comparison was conducted by retrovirally transducing the human AML-associated *MLL-ENL* fusion gene into murine HSC, common myeloid progenitors (CMPs), and granulocytic-monocytic–restricted progenitors (GMPs) and evaluating the relative transforming ability and resultant phenotype in each cell type. AML developed in mice transplanted with any of the three transduced cell populations and, in each case, displayed an identical myelomonocytic phenotype as assessed by morphology and flow cytometry.[110] Similarly, the *MOZ-TIF2* fusion gene was able to confer self-renewal properties to committed myeloid progenitor cells and resulted in AML when transplanted into irradiated mice.[111] Although the fusion genes *MLL-ENL* and *MOZ-TIF2* appear to impart leukemogenic capabilities to committed progenitor cells convincingly, other fusion genes such as *BCR-ABL* can induce leukemic transformation only when expressed in an HSC but not a more mature myeloid cell. Similarly, the potent oncogenic combination of *Hoxa9* and *Meis1* only resulted in AML when transduced into HSCs but not in more committed myeloid progenitors. In this case, expression of β-catenin was found to be the necessary factor for oncogenesis. Present in HSCs but absent in more committed progenitors, the addition of β-catenin to progenitors transduced with *Hoxa9* and *Meis1* was sufficient to lead to AML.[113] These findings point to the differing transforming abilities of different oncogenes that are likely cell-type and cell-context specific.[114] Hence both cell-of-origin hypotheses appear to be correct, depending on the specific oncogene or tumor suppressor that provides the initiating genetic lesion. Increased proliferation, survival, and self-renewal are all necessary attributes of a leukemia stem cell. Some genetic abnormalities, such as *MLL-ENL* and *MOZ-TIF2*, may be capable of inducing self-renewal and thus are able to transform a more differentiated myeloid cell into an LIC. By contrast, other oncogene fusions, such as *BCR-ABL*, or oncogenic transcription factor genes, such as *Hoxa9*, do not possess self-renewal capabilities and thus require a cell that inherently has this characteristic, namely, the HSC.

More recently, challenges to the cancer stem cell hypothesis have arisen out of a number of studies, predominantly in solid tumors such as melanoma, where the frequency of cells capable of giving rise to a new tumor in an immunocompromised host is of sufficient frequency to call into question whether the LIC represents a unique subpopulation or the original stochastic model of cancer progression holds true.[115] These studies have again called into question previously accepted tenets. CD34+/CD38+ populations, in addition to the CD34+/CD38−, have also been found to contain LICs when injected into more immune-deficient hosts that lack key components of the innate immune system.[116] These studies and additional syngeneic and cogenic transplant studies in mice as well as zebrafish[117-120] highlight the critical context of the recipient animal in determining the LIC. The heterogeneity of LICs in AML is further demonstrated by an increasing number of cell surface markers in addition to CD34 and CD38, including CD123, TIM3, and CD47.[121-123] Additionally, a number of studies have attempted to identify a specific LIC genetic signature, which has been found at least in some cases to independently predict prognosis. In this case, the LIC signature was reminiscent of the normal HSC, hearkening back to the original predictions of Dick's group highlighting the HSC as a putative LIC cell of origin.[124] However, although these findings are provocative, a consistent cadre of LIC genes has not yet been established. Clonality studies demonstrating the progressive acquisition of mutations in a given cell have also been put forward as an alternative to the cancer stem cell hypothesis.[125,126] Although seemingly at odds, these different concepts can be reconciled into a single integrated framework. Myeloid (and lymphoid) leukemia-initiating events may occur in both HSCs and committed progenitor cells, and each leukemia arises from a combination of multiple genetic abnormalities.[127] Secondary events subsequently are acquired in different subpopulations, generating unique clones with varying malignant potential depending on the genetic lesion and the self-renewal capacity of the cell in which these abnormalities occur. The number of genetic lesions necessary to cause frank AML is being defined based on next-generation sequencing studies recently published by the group at Washington University in St. Louis as well as other centers. The evolution of particular clones appears to determine the eventual phenotype of the AML cells documented at diagnosis (Fig. 51-1).[128,129]

These new discoveries have added additional complexity to our understanding of the contribution of LICs to AML pathogenesis by demonstrating that the heterogeneity inherent in this disease extends to the AML stem cells.[130] However, the identification of new LIC surface markers, genetic signatures, and gene-specific mutations hold out promise that LIC-targeted therapies will be realized in the coming years.

Molecular Genetics

Recent AML protocols have incorporated current knowledge regarding the significance of specific genetic abnormalities to direct risk-stratified approaches to treatment. Chromosomal abnormalities and, in particular, translocations identified on cytogenetic examination of the blast cells represent the initial genetic lesions incorporated into disease taxonomy and formed the basis of the World Health Organization (WHO) classification in 2008.[131-133] Careful analysis of these translocations and other recurring genetic abnormalities in leukemia patients has had a

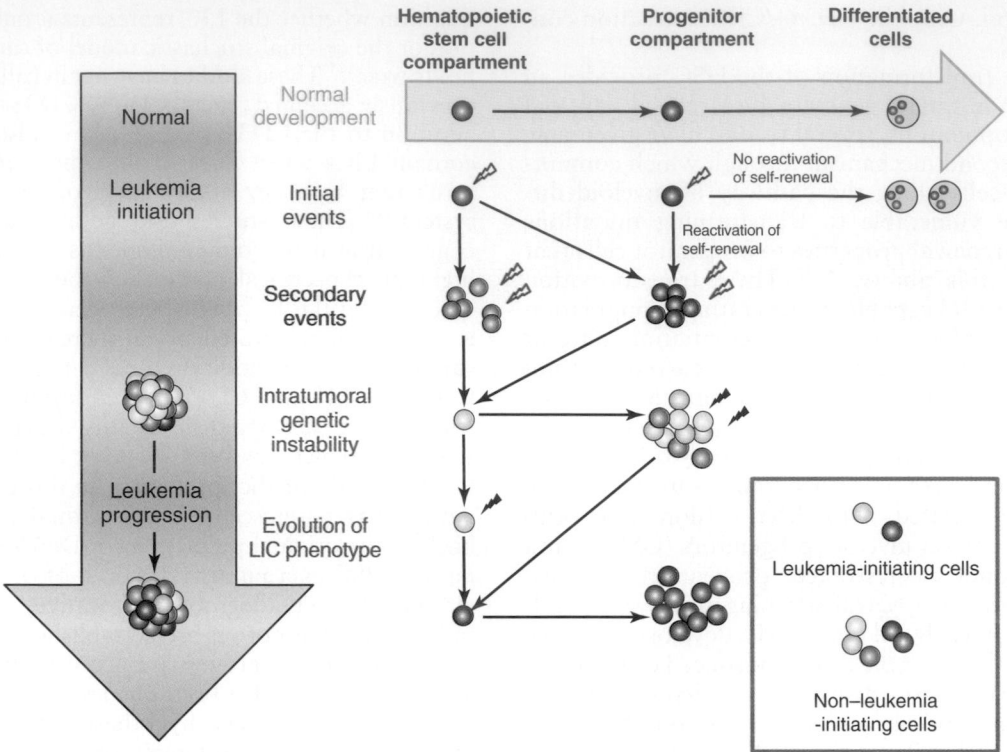

Figure 51-1 Integration of the leukemic initiating cell (LIC) and clonal evolution models of acute myelogenous leukemia pathogenesis. *(Modified from Dick JE: Stem cell concepts renew cancer research.* Blood *112:4793–4807, 2008.)*

profound impact on our understanding of the molecular genetic basis of leukemia (Fig. 51-2). Although many chromosomal abnormalities from AML blast cells have been identified and studied extensively, no single mutation has been shown to be sufficient to cause acute leukemia. These findings prompted Gilliland and colleagues[134-137] to propose what is now considered the classic "two-hit model" of AML pathogenesis. In this model, leukemic transformation results from distinct but collaborative sequential mutations in parallel molecular pathways that affect cell survival, proliferation, differentiation, and self-renewal. Class I mutations frequently involve an activated receptor or cytoplasmic-nuclear tyrosine kinase conferring a proliferative and/or survival ability to a specific cell but not affecting differentiation. By contrast, class II mutations specifically result in differentiation arrest and/or self-renewal and often involve key transcription factor oncogenes but alone do not confer a proliferative advantage. Although attractive, this model likely represents an oversimplification of AML pathogenesis. Initially, microarray studies and more recently, deep-sequencing approaches have revealed the presence of novel mutations and absence of tyrosine kinase lesions, particularly in normal karyotype AML, calling into question the general applicability of the "two-hit" model in all cases of AML. However, although the category of genetic lesions may not always subscribe to this classic paradigm, the number of "hits" required may be more universal. Genomic profiling of individual patient leukemias suggest that in some cases only two to three lesions are required for clonal evolution to frank AML,

with fewer "hits" necessary in pediatric AML than in its adult counterpart.[129,138] Regardless, the prevalence of lesions categorized by the "two-hit" model will be outlined here, followed by more recent discoveries of novel genes implicated in AML pathogenesis and the variable frequency of these lesions in pediatric versus adult AML.

Class I Mutations

Among the earliest examples of class I mutations, *RAS* mutations were described in the early 1980s. There are three functional *RAS* gene family members—*NRAS, KRAS,* and *HRAS*—that all act as guanosine nucleotide phosphate (GTP)-binding proteins.[136] Mutations of *NRAS* are the most prominent *RAS* mutations in AML and have been found in as many as 30% of adult patients with AML.[139] Mutations, most frequently in codons 12, 13, and 61, result in the retention of the RAS protein in its active GTP-bound state and lead to the constitutive activation of downstream effector proteins, which causes the transcriptional activation of various target genes that direct cellular differentiation, proliferation, and survival (Fig. 51-3).[140] RAS proteins may be alternatively activated by mutations in genes encoding a number of regulatory factors. Activating point mutations in the *SHP-2/ PTPN11* phosphatase provide a stimulatory signal through guanine nucleotide exchange factors, such as "Son of Sevenless" (SOS), resulting in increased RAS pathway signaling, as do inactivating mutations of neurofibromin 1 *(NF1),* which codes for a GTPase-activating protein (GAP) of the same name.[141,142] NF1, normally functions, at least in part, by increasing the

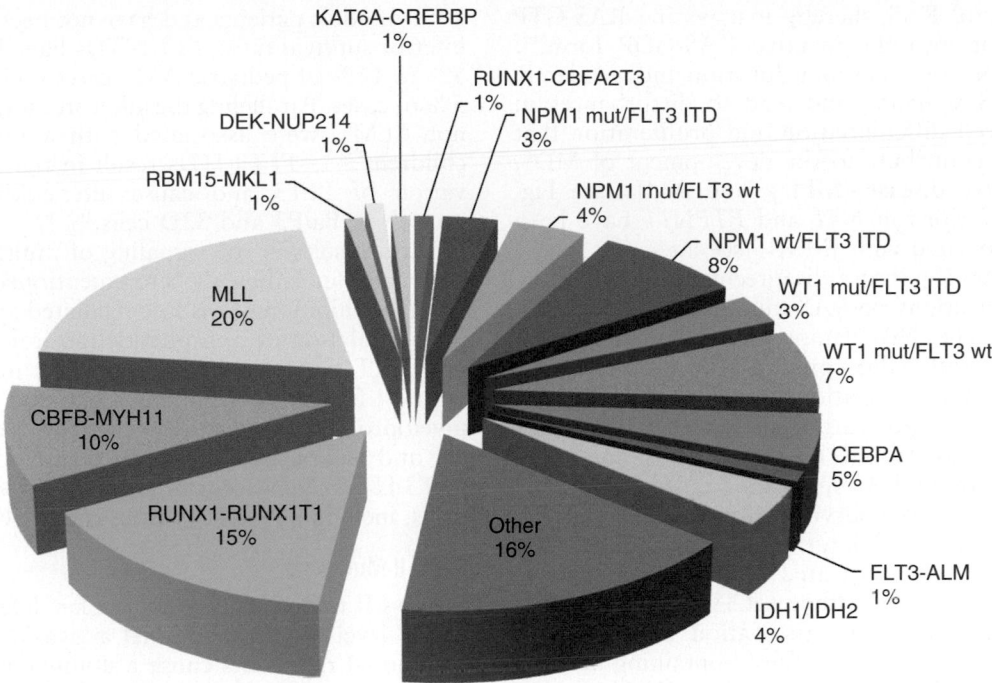

Figure 51-2 Approximate frequencies of recurrent genetic lesions in childhood acute myelogenous leukemia. *(Modified from Rubnitz J, Inaba H: Childhood acute myeloid leukemia. Br J Haematol 159:259–287, 2012.)*

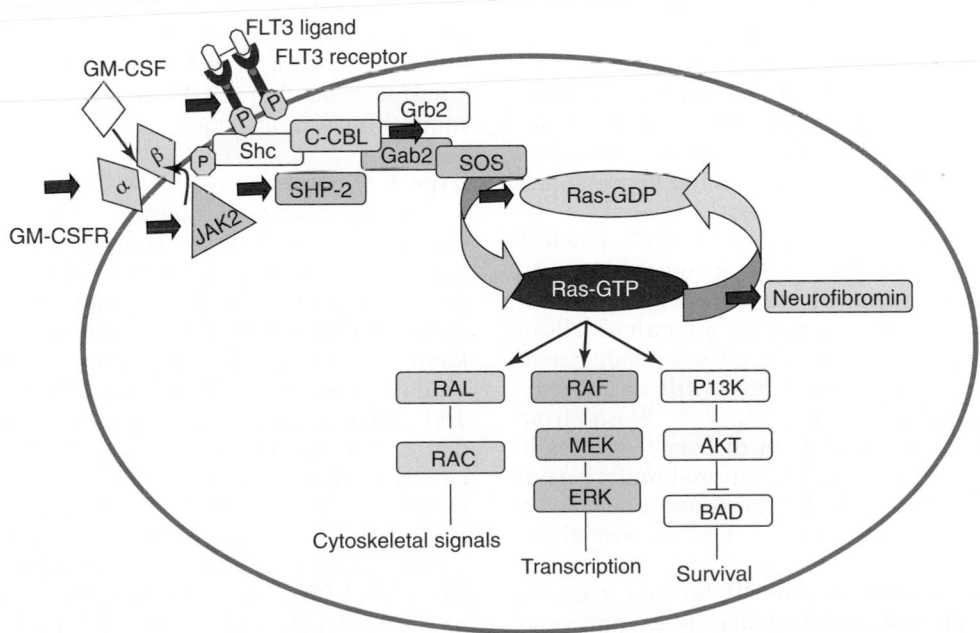

Figure 51-3 Constitutive activation of the RAS pathway is central to myeloid leukemogenesis. RAS pathway signaling may be constitutively activated via a number of mutually exclusive mechanisms *(horizontal red arrows)*. These include the following: mutations in the GM-CSF or FLT3 surface receptors, resulting in ligand independent activation (found primarily in de novo AML); activating mutations in JAK2 (found in PV, ET, and PM) or SHP-2, c-CBL (found in JMML); activating mutations in RAS itself (found in all types of AML); or inactivating mutations in neurofibromin (found in JMML). *PV*, polycythemia vera; *ET*, essential thrombocytosis; *PM*, primary myelofibrosis; *FLT3*, fms-like tyrosine kinase 3; *GM-CSF*, granulocyte-macrophage colony-stimulating factor; *JAK2*, Janus 2 kinase; *JMML*, juvenile myelomonocytic leukemia. *(Modified from Loh ML, Vattikuti S, Schubbert S, et al: Mutations in PTPN11 implicate the SHP-2 phosphatase in leukemogenesis. Blood 103:2325–2331, 2004; and Proytcheva M: Juvenile myelomonocytic leukemia. Semin Diagn Pathol 28:298–303, 2011.)*

GTPase activity of RAS, thereby inactivating RAS-GTP by converting it into the inactive RAS-GDP form.[143] These three types of mutations function independently to activate RAS signaling and lead to disturbances in hematopoietic cell differentiation and proliferation that may ultimately contribute to the development of MDS, myeloproliferative disease (MPD), and AML (see Fig. 51-3).[144-146] Mutations in NF1 and PTPN11 have been particularly associated with JMML (see later).[142,147]

There has been significant disagreement regarding the prognostic implications of RAS mutations in MDS and AML. Several studies have demonstrated that RAS mutations in patients with MDS confer a poor prognosis and increase the risk for progression to acute leukemia.[148-155] Other studies have reported no difference in survival in AML patients who carried RAS mutations compared with patients without RAS mutations,[152] whereas some have suggested improved survival in patients with AML and NRAS mutations.[153] A large study of more than 2500 patients with AML demonstrated no difference in prognosis in patients with or without RAS mutations. This study also demonstrated an association between RAS mutations and a leukemia karyotype containing inv(16), a class II mutation resulting in the CBFβ-MYH11 fusion protein and altered function of the core-binding factor (CBF) transcriptional complex.[156] A recent report from the COG examining 825 pediatric AML samples treated on two recent trials identified NRAS mutations in 10% of patients predominantly in codons 12 and 13, with no mutations in codon 61. Interestingly, most of these mutations were associated with good prognosis NPM1 mutations (see later) and not CBF alterations. However, multivariate analysis confirmed a lack of independent impact of NRAS mutations on prognosis.[157]

Another group of class I mutations involves constitutive activation of receptor or cytoplasmic-nuclear tyrosine kinases. The BCR-ABL translocation that is the sine qua non of CML is an example of a class I mutation causing the activation of the ABL tyrosine kinase. Similarly, receptor tyrosine kinase mutations activate the human protooncogenes KIT and FLT3 in AML. The KIT protein is activated by the binding of its ligand stem cell factor and is critical for the development and growth of mast cells, melanocytes, HSCs, and the interstitial cells of Cajal.[158] Mutations in KIT allow ligand-independent activation of KIT and confer factor-free growth and tumorigenicity in hematopoietic cell lines.[159,160] Blasts from patients with AML express KIT on their cell surfaces in most cases.[161-163] Deletional and insertional mutations of KIT have been identified in the blast cells of patients with AML, often in association with the CBF abnormalities inv(16) or t(8;21).[164]

The FLT3 gene encodes a class III fms-like receptor tyrosine kinase expressed in early hematopoietic progenitors. FLT3 mutations occur in two varieties, internal tandem duplications (ITDs) in the juxtamembrane region and activation loop mutations (ALMs), primarily at codons 835 and 836. The FLT3-ITD is one of the most frequent abnormalities in adult AML, documented in 25% to 30% of patients,[165-169] and generally confers a poor prognosis.[170,171] By contrast, ALMs occur in only 10% of adult patients and have not been associated with inferior survival rates. FLT3-ITDs have been observed in 5% to 16% of pediatric AML cases and ALMs in 2% to 5% of cases. Paralleling the adult studies, FLT3-ITDs, but not ALMs, were associated with a poor prognosis in children.[172-175] FLT3-ITDs result in the constitutive activation of FLT3 and cause interleukin-3–independent growth in Ba/F3 and 32D cells.[165,168,176] This activation, in turn, results in the signaling of multiple downstream pathways, including the aforementioned RAS pathway, and the inhibition of caspase-mediated apoptosis through the stimulation of phosphatidylinositol 3'-kinase (PI3K) and AKT (see Fig. 51-3). However, mice transplanted with FLT3-transformed hematopoietic cells develop a myeloproliferative disorder characterized by splenomegaly and leukocytosis but they do not develop AML.[177] FLT3-ITDs often occur in conjunction with other mutations, including NPM1 (see later) and WT1 (see later).[178]

Class II Mutations

In class II mutations, the molecular defect appears to be at the level of transcriptional activation, whereby transcriptional repressors cause a dominant negative inhibition of normal hematopoietic cell differentiation. AML can be subtyped based on the type of class II mutations in the blast cells of patients. The type 1 subset of class II mutations occurs in patients with de novo AML. These are typical chromosomal translocations resulting in chimeric oncoproteins that in some cases may cause the inhibition of differentiation. The type 2 subset of class II mutations usually are found in patients with AML arising after a prodrome of MDS and manifest more commonly in older adults or in patients who have received previous chemotherapy. Cytogenetic studies of the blast cell populations in these patients have complex karyotypes, lacking translocations but harboring deletions such as 5q–, monosomy 7, and 20q–.

Type 1 Mutations

Translocations Involving Core-Binding Factor Complex. Several of the translocations that have been identified in adult and childhood de novo AML involve the CBF complex. The CBF complex is the most frequent target of chromosomal translocations in the human leukemias. The CBF regulatory complex consists of a DNA-binding subunit, RUNX1 (also called CBFα or AML1) and CBFβ, a subunit that does not bind DNA independently but heterodimerizes with RUNX1 or one of its closely related family members.[179] Chromosomal translocations that modify the CBF complex in AML include the following: t(8;21)(q22;q22), which generates the AML1-ETO fusion protein, more recently referred to as RUNX1-RUNX1T1 (Fig. 51-4); t(3;21)(q26;q22), which gives rise to AML1-EVI1; and inv(16)(p13;q22), which fuses the CBFβ to smooth muscle myosin heavy chain (SMMHC), resulting in the CBFB-MYH11 fusion gene. The AML1 gene was inactivated in the germline of mice and was shown to be essential for definitive hematopoiesis of all cell lineages.[180,181] Homozygous animals die early in embryogenesis of central nervous system (CNS) hemorrhage, but they have normal morphogenesis and yolk sac hematopoiesis lineages.[180,181] Inactivation of the *CBFβ* gene in the mouse has shown a similar phenotype in the homozygous null mice.[179,182] These experiments have demonstrated that the AML1/CBFα complex is essential for normal hematopoiesis and that chromosomal rearrangements involving this complex may interfere with its regulatory function in ways that lead to disruption of cellular differentiation, and eventually malignant transformation.

Evidence primarily from knock-in studies in mice has supported the hypothesis that the AML1-ETO fusion protein functions as a dominant negative inhibitor of wild-type functions.[183-185] In these experiments, the *AML1-ETO* fusion gene is "knocked in" to the wild-type

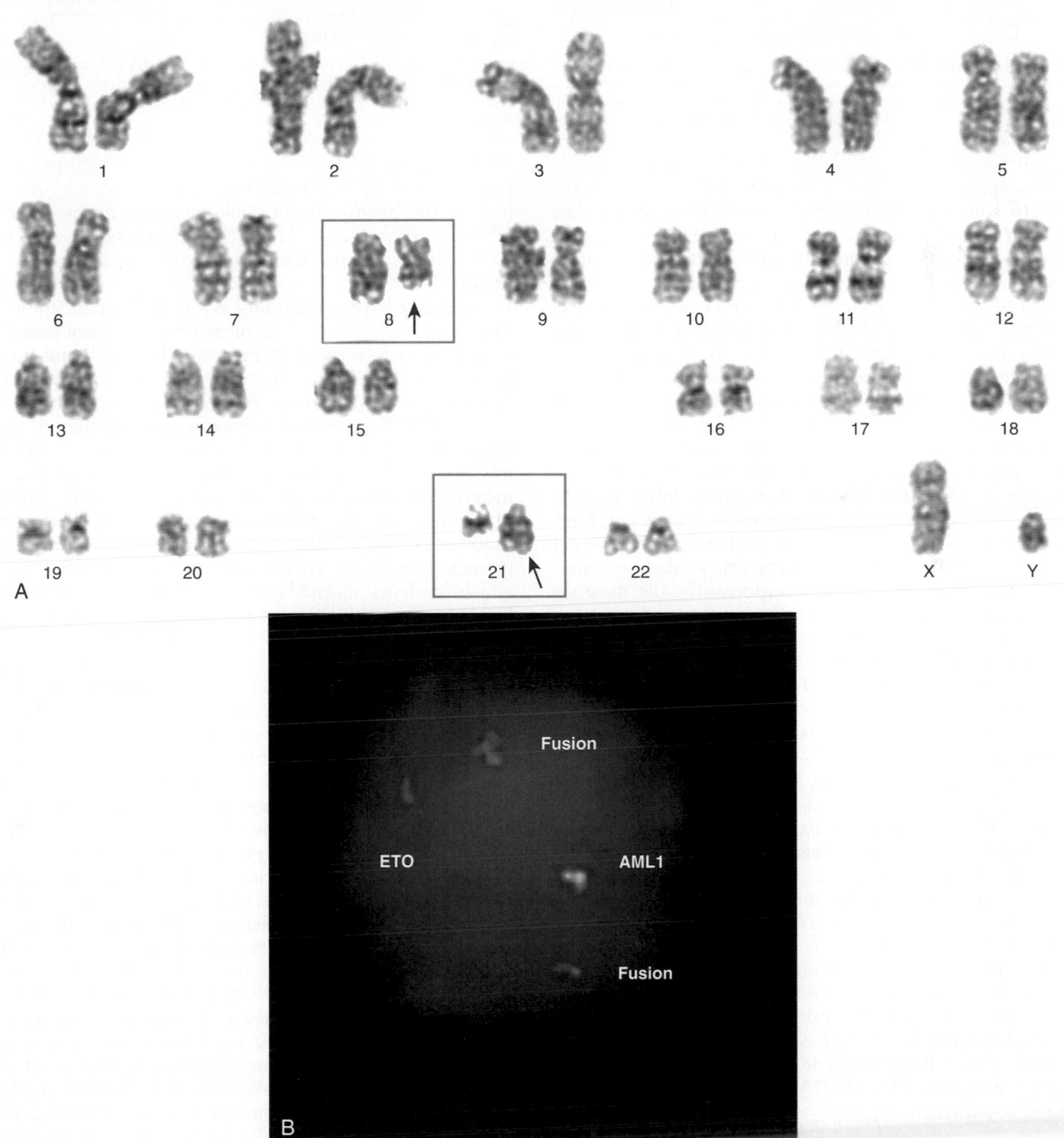

Figure 51-4 Consequences of the t(8;21) AML1-ETO (RUNX1-RUNX1T1) translocation. **A,** Karyotype demonstrating the reciprocal t(8;21)(q22;q22) translocation in an affected patient. **B,** Interphase fluorescence in situ hybridization (FISH) using the AML1/ETO dual-color, dual-fusion Vysis probe demonstrates the novel AML1-ETO fusion by the presence of linked green AML1 and red ETO signals.

Continued

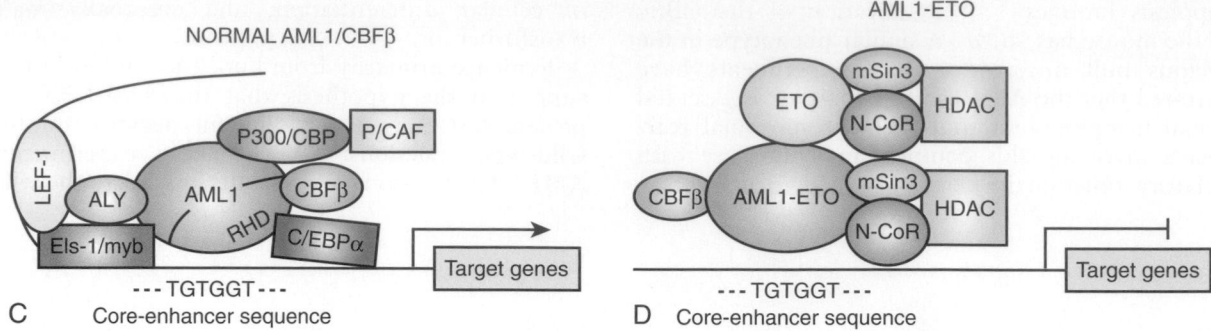

Figure 51-4, cont'd **C,** The normal AML1-CBFβ transcription factor complex. **D,** The molecular consequences of the AML1-ETO fusion; namely, transcription repression may occur in contexts in which the normal AML1/RUNX1-CBFβ acts as to transactivate gene expression. *(Courtesy of Dr. Barbara Morash, Cytogenetics, IWK Health Centre, Halifax, Nova Scotia, Canada; D modified from Downing JR: The core-binding factor leukemias: lessons learned from murine models. Curr Opin Genet Dev 13:48–54, 2003.)*

AML1 locus. The phenotype of these mice is identical to the *AML1* knockout; the mice die early in embryogenesis from CNS hemorrhage and lack any evidence of definitive hematopoiesis, although the rare cells that survive and express AML1-ETO have an increased capacity for self-renewal.[185] Biochemical experiments have shown that the ETO portion of the AML1-ETO chimeric protein recruits nuclear corepressor complexes to the CBF promoters, resulting in transcriptional inhibition of target genes normally activated by the AML1/CBFβ heterodimeric complex (see Fig. 51-4D).[186,187] Subsequent studies using inducible murine model systems to bypass the embryonic lethality of *AML1-ETO* overexpression have demonstrated that overexpression of this transgene at later developmental time points confers enhanced self-renewal capacity to bone marrow progenitors, as demonstrated by serial culture experiments. Importantly, the mice do not develop AML but appear to be predisposed to leukemogenesis. Thus after treatment with *N*-ethyl-*N*-nitrosourea (ENU), the mice developed rapid onset of AML compared with similarly exposed wild-type mice. Moreover, as noted, there is an association in myeloid leukemia of *AML1-ETO* translocations and mutant tyrosine kinases, such as KIT.[188] Interestingly, *AML1-ETO* transcripts may persist for a long time in patients with *AML1-ETO*–expressing AML in sustained remission.[189]

Translocations Involving the Retinoic Acid Receptor-α. Reciprocal chromosomal translocations involving the retinoic acid receptor-α *(RARA)* gene locus on chromosome 17 are the defining molecular features of acute promyelocytic leukemia (APL). Before the *RARA* translocations were described, retinoic acid was known to induce myeloid differentiation in vitro[190] and therapy with all-*trans*-retinoic acid (ATRA) in patients with APL was shown to induce complete remission (CR).[191] The intense investigation of the *RARA* gene triggered by these observations culminated in identification of the promyelocytic leukemia PML-RARA translocation breakpoint, t(15;17)(q22;q11), reported simultaneously by several groups.[192-197] Although most APL cases have the associated t(15;17), other reciprocal translocations involving the *RARA* gene have been identified in which the gene is fused to other gene partners. The most common of these

include the promyelocytic leukemia zinc finger *(PLZF)* gene on chromosome 11 in t(11;17)(p13;q11) and the nucleophosmin gene *(NPM)* on chromosome 5 in t(5;17) (q31;q11).[198,199]

Normally RARA functions as a ligand-dependent activator of transcription.[200] It forms a heterodimer with the related protein, retinoid X receptor (RXR),[201] and binds through its zinc finger domain to a specific promoter sequence; in the presence of the retinoic acid ligand, the RARA-RXR heterodimer activates transcription of retinoic acid–responsive genes.[194] This process is accomplished in concert with a coactivator complex that includes proteins such as p300 and pCAF. In the absence of retinoic acid, a corepressor complex is recruited, composed of N-CoR (nuclear receptor corepressor) or SMRT (silencing mediator of retinoid and thyroid receptors), which binds to another protein called Sin3 and then to HDAC1.[199,202-204] HDAC1 is a histone deacetylase protein, which epigenetically alters histones to keep DNA in an untranscribable form. The expression of retinoic acid–responsive genes is essential for normal myeloid development.[205]

Much evidence supports the hypothesis that the PML-RARA fusion protein functions as a dominant negative inhibitor of the PML protein and RXR. PML proteins are normally located in macromolecular nuclear organelles, called PML oncogenic domains (PODs).[206] The PML-RARA fusion protein disrupts the PODs, causing normal PML, RXR, and other nuclear proteins to disperse in an abnormal pattern.[207,208] ATRA and arsenic trioxide (As_2O_3)[209] have shown activity in APL blast cells and in patients with APL, and studies of these drugs have afforded important insights into the mechanisms of leukemogenesis in APL.[191,210-212] ATRA and As_2O_3 appear to act through different biochemical pathways, and promyelocytes resistant to ATRA are often sensitive to treatment with As_2O_3. Both drugs induce degradation of the PML-RARA fusion protein but through different mechanisms. Retinoic acid binding to wild-type retinoic acid receptors (RARs) in the cell nucleus causes degradation of the PML-RARA protein through the ubiquitin-proteosome and caspase systems, thus allowing for the terminal differentiation of leukemic promyelocytes.[213-215]

This binding also results in derepression whereby N-CoR is dissociated from the PML-RARA fusion protein and, subsequently, the nuclear coactivator complex is recruited to reverse histone deacetylase-mediated repression. PODs are relocated back to the normal nuclear pattern.[208,216] By contrast, As$_2$O$_3$ appears to target the PML portion of the PML-RARA fusion protein preferentially and causes its degradation by inducing apoptosis,[217] potentially through downregulation of the antiapoptotic factor BCL2.[213,218,219] The activity of these agents has led to the inferences that fusion proteins may interfere with normal myeloid cell development in several ways—through inhibitory effects on assembly of the PODs that contain PML or through dominant inhibitory effects on transcriptional targets of dimeric complexes with normal retinoid receptors, leading to arrest of differentiation at the promyelocyte stage.

Studies using transgenic mice have shown that the PML-RARA fusion product is involved in the development of leukemia. Transgenic mice generated with the PML-RARA fusion protein specifically expressed in the myeloid-promyelocytic lineage develop a myelodysplastic-like disorder during the first year of life.[220,221] A subset of these mice then develops a form of acute leukemia that closely mimics human APL and responds to ATRA. Given the relatively long latency period and the development of leukemia in only a fraction of the mice, it is likely that the PML-RARA translocation is insufficient by itself to cause APL and that second mutations are necessary for leukemic transformation.

Mixed-Lineage Leukemia Gene Translocations. Transcriptional coactivators and corepressors have been implicated in leukemogenesis.[134] An example is the myeloid-lymphoid or MLL protein, a large protein containing transcriptional activation and repression domains, which is believed to act epigenetically to modulate gene expression through its effects on chromatin structure and configuration. Wild-type MLL is required for normal hematopoiesis and HSC development.[222] Mice deficient in MLL die on embryonic day 10.5 and have numerous skeletal, neural, and hematologic deficits. Heterozygous mice have defects in embryonic segmentation and yolk sac hematopoiesis, and adults demonstrate a mild anemia and thrombocytopenia.[223,224] Chromosomal translocations of the MLL gene on chromosome segment 11q23 have been identified in human AML and ALL and confer a poor prognosis.[225,226] Many gene partners have been identified that are involved in these translocations, including AF4, AF9, ENL, AF6, ELL, and AF10. In most cases, the fusion proteins incorporate the 5′ end of MLL and the 3′ end of the partner.[227,228] Despite the number of different fusion partners, leukemias with MLL translocations tend to possess a distinct genetic signature compared with AML and ALL samples lacking an MLL translocation. This genetic signature includes the upregulation of a number of specific HOX family genes, including HOXA9, HOXA7, and MEIS1.[225,229-231] Wild-type MLL is known to play a major role in HOX gene transcriptional regulation.[232] In turn, HOX genes play critical roles in embryonic development and normal hematopoiesis. A number of studies have clearly demonstrated that overexpression of specific major HOX genes in mouse models and human bone marrow samples, whether by involvement in reciprocal translocations or by gene upregulation, is linked to the transformation of malignant HSCs in AML.[233-241] The mechanism whereby MLL fusion proteins upregulate HOX gene expression may differ, depending on whether the fusion partner encodes a nuclear partner with direct transcriptional activity or a cytoplasmic protein that results in MLL protein dimerization and subsequent transcriptional activation.[112]

Transcriptional control may be mediated through the modification of histone proteins, which function to maintain chromatin structure. Recently, the DOTL1 complex was identified as a critical factor in MLL-induced leukemogenesis.[242] DOT1L is a histone-3-lysine-79 (H3K79) methyltransferase, which was previously believed to play a fairly ubiquitous role in methylating gene targets in concert with transcription. However, Zhang and Armstrong's group definitively demonstrated through a series of elegant in vitro and in vivo experiments a specificity for DOT1L in the epigenetic regulation of MLL-translocated downstream targets. When DOT1L was knocked out or absent from MLL-AF9–transformed cell lines or transgenic mice, leukemia was prevented.[242-244] The MLL gene is rearranged in up to 20% of pediatric cases of AML.[245] Translocations of MLL are the single most common genetic alteration in infants with acute leukemia, regardless of phenotype, and account for approximately 70% of all cases of AML and ALL in infants.[246] In pediatric and adult cases of AML, the presence of the 11q23 translocation is generally associated with an unfavorable prognosis.[247]

Although less common than MLL translocations, the MLL gene can be altered by partial tandem duplications (PTDs) of particular exons. These PTDs occur in adult and pediatric AMLs with a normal karyotype, as well as those with trisomy 11. Similar to MLL fusions, the MLL-PTD tends to be associated with a poor prognosis and often with the presence of an FLT3 mutation. The mechanisms underlying MLL-PTD leukemogenesis have not yet been elucidated but appear to be different than those of MLL fusions.[228,248] Interestingly, MLL-PTD appears to repress wild-type MLL expression, which may be an important feature underlying the leukemogenic potential of this abnormality.[248]

Type 2 Mutations. The leukemogenic mutations discussed in the previous sections involve balanced translocations, duplications, or substitutions that appear to disrupt regulatory mechanisms controlling hematopoiesis and result in dysregulated cell differentiation. Another group of mutations involve unbalanced chromosome rearrangements, such as chromosome loss (e.g., monosomy 5, monosomy 7) or large chromosomal deletions (e.g., 5q–, 7q–, 20q–).[249,250] These mutations may lead to leukemic transformation by the loss of a tumor suppressor gene (or genes), which then confers a differentiation block and growth advantage to the mutated cells,[251] Identification of these putative tumor suppressor genes has been problematic because the deleted regions are usually large and include many candidate genes. Moreover, leukemogenesis is triggered by the gene's inactivation rather than by altered structure, making the abnormal gene difficult to identify. However, α-catenin has been identified by our group as a novel tumor suppressor gene on the proximal region of the long arm of chromosome 5.[252] Non–therapy-related AML with these chromosomal losses or deletions occurs most commonly in older patients and is often associated with the prodrome of MDS. In the pediatric population, this class of cytogenetic abnormality is uncommon and is also frequently preceded by MDS.[253] Monosomy 7 is the most frequent chromosomal abnormality documented in children with MDS and is sometimes the sole detectable cytogenetic abnormality.[254,255] Overall, chromosome loss represents about half of the chromosomal abnormalities identified in MDS.[253]

Therapy-Related AML. Chromosomal loss and large chromosomal deletions are common in therapy-related AML in the adult and pediatric populations. Although most cases of MDS and AML arise de novo, without evidence of any leukemogenic exposure, in 10% to 20% of patients the disease arises after previous exposure, particularly to topoisomerase II inhibitors, alkylating agents, and ionizing radiation.[256] The 11q23 translocations producing *MLL* gene fusions are common cytogenetic abnormalities in patients who develop AML after therapy with topoisomerase II inhibitors (e.g., epipodophyllotoxins).[6,7,257] AML developing after the use of topoisomerase II inhibitors has a short median latency period of 30 to 34 months, is usually FAB classification M4 or M5, and lacks the antecedent prodrome of MDS.[258] The blast cells of patients with AML or MDS occurring after exposure to alkylating agents often have large chromosomal losses or deletions and have a poor prognosis.[256,259,260] The most common chromosomal abnormalities in such cases involve chromosome 7 and chromosome 5. In contrast to the therapy-related AML with *MLL* fusion genes that develops after treatment with topoisomerase II inhibitors, MDS or AML related to therapy with alkylating agents typically develops after a longer median latency period, 3 to 5 years from the alkylator exposure. Mutations in the *TP53* tumor suppressor gene have been previously linked to therapy-related AML and were believed to be infrequent in de novo cases. However, more recently, *TP53* mutations have been found to be common in de novo AML with a complex karyotype. In both contexts there is an association with chromosome 5 and 7 copy number alterations.[261-264]

AML with a Normal Karyotype. Chromosomal abnormalities have provided some understanding of the mechanisms of malignant transformation in leukemia. However, in many cases of de novo leukemia, no chromosomal abnormality can be detected and the mechanism behind leukemogenesis in these cases is unknown. Because AML involves a block in myeloid differentiation, evidence for mutations in key transcription factors involved in normal myelopoiesis has been sought. Mutations in the early myeloid transcription factors PU.1 and CCAAT/enhancer-binding protein α (C/EBPα) have been identified in a number of AML subtypes and are generally not associated with a known chromosomal translocation.[265] Mouse models have demonstrated that the degree of transcription factor knockdown is critical to the

particular phenotype. Mice expressing PU.1 at 20% of normal levels develop AML, whereas those with complete knockdown or 50% of normal levels do not.[266] GATA1, a critical transcription factor for erythrocyte and megakaryocyte development, is mutated in nearly all cases of acute megakaryoblastic leukemia associated with Down syndrome (see later).[267]

Expression profiling using microarrays first used to distinguish prognostic tumor subclasses in breast carcinoma[268-271] and large B-cell lymphoma[272] has also been applied to leukemia.[233] Using this technology, a set of 50 genes was sufficient to discriminate ALL from AML. More recent validation of this technique in AML has demonstrated the correlation between gene expression profiling studies and the prognostic classification of human AML based on cytogenetic abnormalities.[273] Gene expression profiling has provided valuable new insights into the identification of prognostic subclasses in adult[274] and pediatric[275] AML with a normal karyotype.

Our understanding of the molecular mechanisms underlying de novo AML with a normal karyotype was advanced by the finding of mutations involving the *NPM* gene in 35% of cases of adult AML and 60% of cases with a normal karyotype.[276] This frequency supersedes the incidence of *FLT3* mutations and has established *NPM* mutations as the most frequent genetic abnormality in adult AML. The frequency of *NPM* mutations is lower in pediatric AML, occurring in only 6% to 8% of all pediatric patients with AML, but also occurs in a higher number of pediatric patients with a normal karyotype (approximately 27%).[277,278] The *NPM* gene on chromosome 5q was previously well known as a partner in a number of oncogenic translocations, including *NPM-ALK* (anaplastic lymphoma kinase) in anaplastic large cell lymphoma and *NPM-RARA* in APL. NPM is a molecular chaperone that shuttles between the cytoplasm and nucleus but is found most prominently in nucleoli. It has been shown to function in the prevention of protein aggregation in the nucleolus and the regulation of preribosomal particles through the nuclear membrane. It has also been shown to play a role in the regulation of the alternate reading frame (ARF)-TP53 tumor suppressor pathway. *NPM* mutations are heterogeneous but occur predominantly in exon 12, uniformly affecting the C-terminal of the protein and causing the formation of a neomorphic nuclear export signal in the resulting NPMc protein. This results in a shift of NPM localization, sequestering it exclusively to the cytoplasm. *NPM* mutations occur more frequently in children older than 10 years and, as is the case in adults, tend to be associated with a good prognosis. However, there has been a strong association established between patients with *NPM* mutations and *FLT3*-ITDs, which portend a poor prognosis. Patients with both these abnormalities do not fare as well as those with *NPM* mutations alone.

Similarly, mutations in *CEBPA* have been associated with a good outcome. *CEBPA* encodes the CCAAT/enhancer binding protein-alpha (C/EBPα), which functions as a transcription factor that plays a major role in terminal granulocytic differentiation as well as influencing proliferation. C/EBPα is a basic region leucine zipper transcription factor consisting of two amino-terminal transactivation domains, a basic DNA-binding region, and a carboxyl-terminal leucine zipper. Mutations in pediatric AML commonly occur in the amino-terminal domain and bZip domain of the leucine zipper, and many patients harbor both types of mutations.[279]

Mutations in the Wilms tumor 1 (WT1) transcription factor have been identified in approximately 10% of adult and childhood AML, predominantly in patients with a normal karyotype.[280-284] Mutations are common in exons 7, 8, and 9, comprising three of the four zinc fingers of WT1. WT1 mutations frequently occur together with FLT3-ITDs; however, in contrast to the adult studies, they do not independently confer a poor prognosis.[285] Recently, a number of large genomic studies using next-generation sequencing technology revealed novel frequent mutations in DNA methyltransferase 3A (DNMT3A) and IDH1 and IDH2 in adult normal karyotype AML.[128,286,287] In adult disease, these mutations confer a poor outcome. By contrast, these mutations are relatively rare in pediatric AML but similarly occur more commonly in patients with a normal karyotype, highlighting the different molecular spectrum of disease in adult and childhood counterparts.[288-290]

Morphology and Cytochemistry

The initial diagnosis of AML relies on accurate interpretation of the cellular morphology of the bone marrow smears. The diagnosis usually can be made based on the morphologic characteristics of the blasts in a Wright-Giemsa–stained bone marrow smear (Fig. 51-5). In addition to general morphology, the diagnosis can be confirmed in cases exhibiting Auer rods (thin, needle-shaped cytoplasmic deposits that stain pink with Wright-Giemsa and are strongly myeloperoxidase [MPO]-positive). In addition to examination of the morphology of the blasts, the Wright-Giemsa stain is also used to assess for dysplastic features in erythroid, myeloid, and megakaryocytic cell lines.

Additional cytochemical stains are important for the accurate diagnosis of AML. MPO and Sudan black B (SBB) are cytochemical stains for granulocyte, eosinophil, and monocyte lineages. Peroxidase is present in the primary granules of myeloid cells, beginning at the promyelocyte stage and throughout subsequent maturation. Typically, leukemic myeloblasts are also strongly peroxidase-positive. MPO staining of Auer rods is particularly robust in leukemic blasts and can demonstrate Auer rods not recognized using the Wright-Giemsa stain. By contrast, the MPO staining of monoblasts shows a fine granular pattern in the monoblast cytoplasm. The staining pattern of SBB is similar to that of peroxidase, particularly in myeloblasts and in the detection of Auer rods. Monoblasts either do not stain or show a weakly positive, diffuse pattern with SBB.

The esterase stains are useful for distinguishing granulocytic cells from cells of the monocytic lineage. Chloroacetate esterase is a specific stain for granulocytes and mast cells. Results of staining of early myeloblasts are often negative, but promyeloblasts and later granulocytic lineage cells stain strongly, as do Auer rods. Monoblasts do not stain with chloroacetate esterase. In contrast, the nonspecific esterases (NSEs) such as α-naphthyl butyrate esterase and α-naphthyl acetate esterase stain monoblasts and monocytes strongly. Granulocytic and lymphoid cells do not stain with the nonspecific esterases. The blast cells of AML-M4 (i.e., myelomonocytic leukemia) should demonstrate positive chloroacetate esterase activity and α-naphthyl butyrate esterase or α-naphthyl acetate activity; this finding is important for making the diagnosis. The periodic acid–Schiff (PAS) reaction is not as informative as the previously described stains, but it can be useful, particularly in the diagnosis of AML-M6 (i.e., erythroleukemia). Leukemic erythroblasts can stain strongly with PAS, whereas normal erythroid precursors generally demonstrate no PAS activity.

Immunophenotype

Since the 1980s, multiparameter flow cytometric analysis has become an important element in the diagnosis and classification of leukemia. More recently, multiparameter flow cytometry has been used as a tool to detect MRD in acute myeloid leukemia and is being incorporated into clinical trials to clarify prognostic groups and help make treatment decisions.[291-300] Immunophenotyping using a large panel of monoclonal antibodies to myeloid and lymphoid lineage and progenitor cell–associated antigens has been used to discriminate myeloid or lymphoid differentiation correctly in up to 98% of patients.[301,302] Monoclonal antibodies have been classified based on their reactivity with the lineage or differentiation-associated antigens on the surfaces of normal and malignant cells. Because the monoclonal antibodies are not leukemia cell–specific and most of the hematopoietic antibodies are not strictly lineage specific, it is necessary to use panels of antibodies on blast cell populations and to incorporate the immunophenotypic information with the clinical findings and other morphologic, cytochemical, and cytogenetic results for accurate leukemia cell classification.

Blasts of myeloid origin generally express HLA-DR, CD33, and CD34. Monocytic cells usually express HLA-DR at all stages of maturation, whereas promyelocytes and more mature cells of the granulocyte lineage do not. CD33 and CD13 are expressed on neutrophil and monocyte precursors, but CD33 is absent on mature neutrophils. CD14 is relatively specific for cells of the monocytic lineage. As myeloid differentiation continues, CD15 expression increases, whereas CD34 expression decreases. Megakaryocytic cells and platelets express CD41, CD42, and CD61.

Immunophenotyping has been particularly valuable for lineage assignment in undifferentiated leukemias (i.e., AML-M0), identification of acute megakaryocytic leukemia, and analysis of the lineage of leukemias with MLL gene translocations.[303-308]

Cytogenetics

Cytogenetic analysis is an essential component in the diagnosis and treatment of AML. The chromosomal aberrations detected by cytogenetic testing also have prognostic value and may be used as tumor markers. In

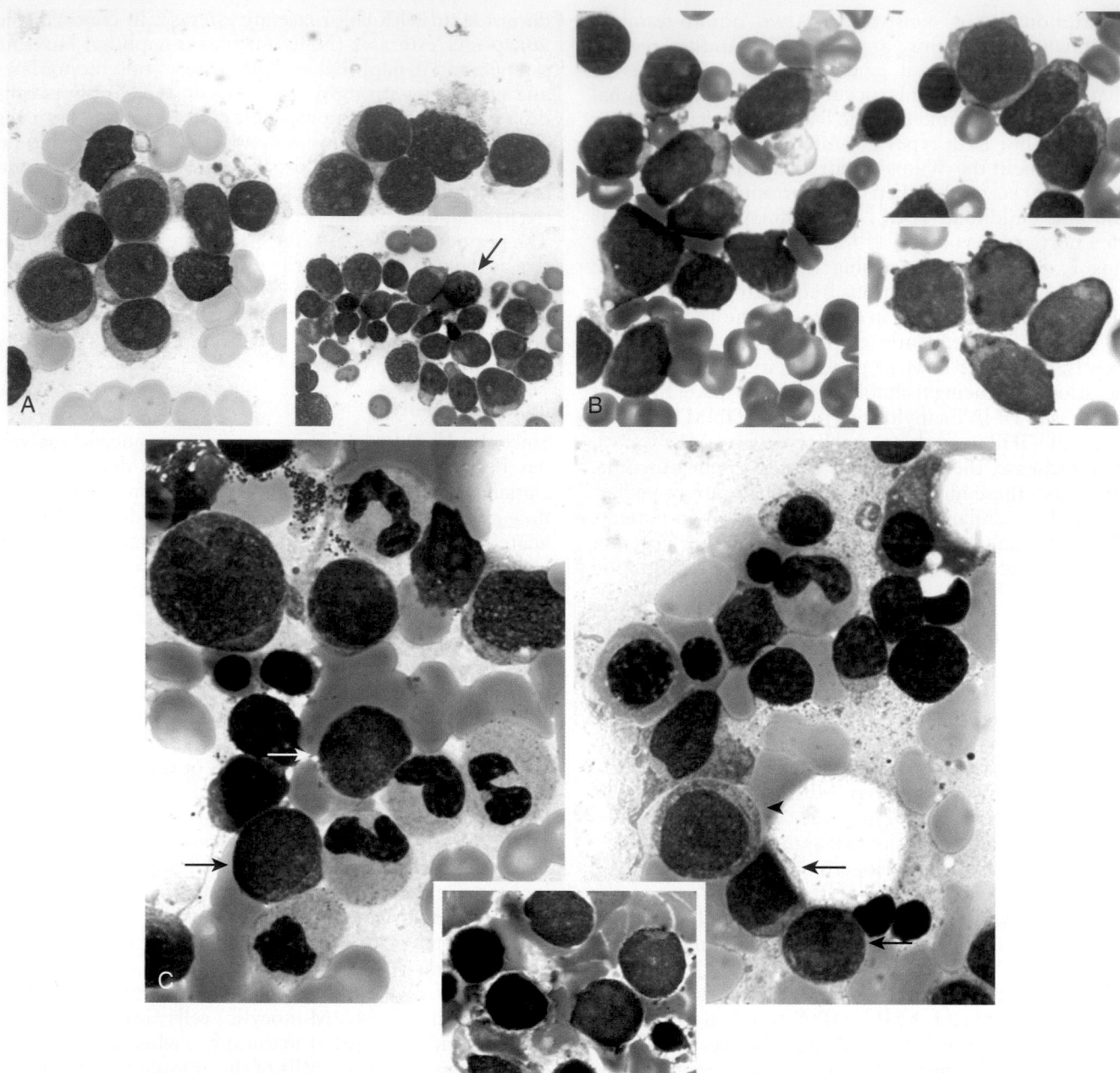

Figure 51-5 Subtypes of acute myeloid leukemia. All images are from Wright-Giemsa–stained bone marrow aspirate smears, except where otherwise designated. **A,** Acute myeloblastic leukemia, minimally differentiated. The blasts may vary in size but have round to oval nuclei, variably prominent single or multiple small nucleoli, and scant cytoplasm that is agranular. *Inset,* The blasts here show no reactivity for myeloperoxidase, although rare reactivity (<3% blasts) may be seen; a neutrophil *(arrow)* serves as a positive internal control. **B,** Acute myeloblastic leukemia, without maturation. Blasts generally predominate within the marrow and comprise 90% or more of nonerythroid cells. The blasts may contain cytoplasmic granules and occasional Auer rods or may resemble lymphoblasts. *Inset,* Myeloperoxidase positivity is present in more than 3% of blasts, although the reactivity itself is of varied intensity. **C,** Acute myeloblastic leukemia, with maturation. Blasts comprise 20% or more of marrow cellularity *(arrows),* whereas maturing neutrophils (e.g., promyelocytes, myelocytes, metamyelocytes, bands, and neutrophils) constitute 10% or more of nucleated elements. Dysmyelopoiesis may be evident. Auer rods are commonly present and may be long and tapered *(arrowhead). Inset,* Myeloperoxidase shows variable reactivity in a subset of the blasts (>3%) and strong reactivity in the maturing neutrophilic forms.

Continued on next page

the WHO classification of hematologic malignancies, specific cytogenetic abnormalities have been included in the diagnostic and prognostic criteria for differentiating subclasses of AML.[309]

Cytogenetic analyses of bone marrow samples have revealed chromosomal abnormalities in most patients with AML.[310-317] In the pediatric population, the incidence of cytogenetic abnormalities is even higher than that in adults.[245,310,318] However, the distribution of the specific cytogenetic abnormalities is different in the various age groups. In infants with AML, the most common chromosomal aberrations are translocations

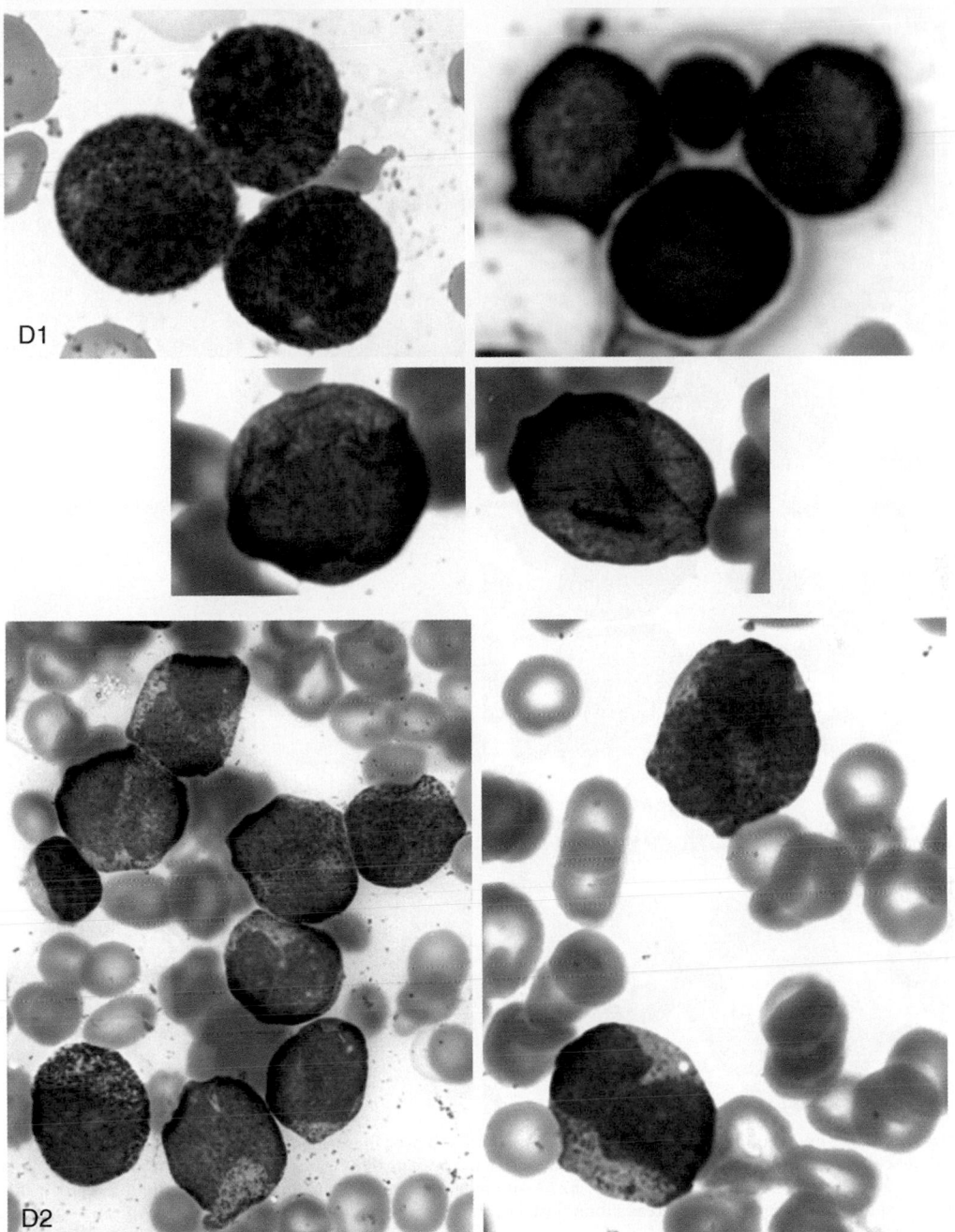

Figure 51-5, cont'd **D1,** Acute promyelocytic leukemia (hypergranular variant). Malignant promyelocytes have eccentric nuclei, prominent nucleoli, and abundant cytoplasm, with intense azurophilic granules. Varied numbers of promyelocytes may contain multiple Auer rods, a characteristic finding *(lower panels)*. Myeloperoxidase shows intense reactivity in the promyelocytes that largely obscures the nucleus *(upper right panel).* **D2,** Acute promyelocytic leukemia (microgranular variant). These malignant promyelocytes have a bilobed or butterfly-shaped nucleus, fine chromatin, variably prominent nucleoli, and abundant cytoplasm, with sparse to numerous azurophilic granules. Myeloperoxidase shows intense reactivity in these variants similar to that seen in the hypergranular forms.

Continued on next page

involving the *MLL* gene (band 11q23).[319-321] The incidence of 11q23 translocations is as high as 40% in AML blasts of children younger than 2 years. After age 2 years, the frequency of 11q23 translocations decreases with age, and the translocation is detectable in AML blasts from less than 10% of older children and adults.[132,245,310,318]

One rare chromosomal abnormality, the t(1;22)(p13;q13), is found almost exclusively in non–Down syndrome infants with acute megakaryocytic leukemia. In a published review of 39 patients with this translocation, 95% were younger than 2 years, and it was not identified in adults with AML.[322] This translocation is now known to

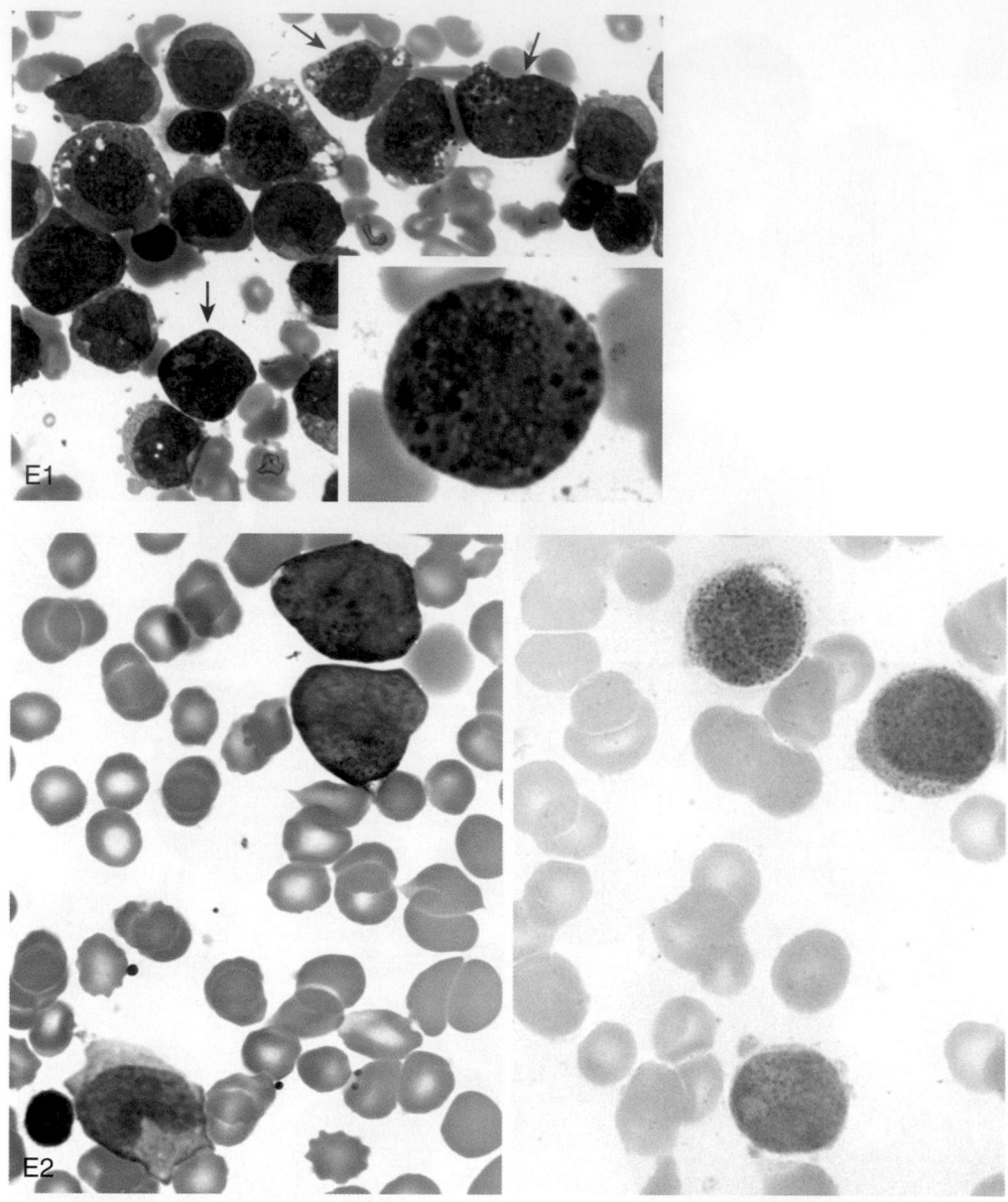

Figure 51-5, cont'd E1, Acute myelomonocytic leukemia with eosinophilia. Blasts, maturing neutrophils, and maturing monocytes each constitute 20% or more of marrow cellularity. Additionally, abnormal eosinophils are present in all stages of maturation and contain enlarged granules that are purple-violet as opposed to orangeophilic *(arrows; inset)*. E2, Acute myelomonocytic leukemia with eosinophilia (cytochemistries). At least 3% of blasts show myeloperoxidase reactivity *(left)*, whereas monoblasts, promonocytes, and monocytes exhibit nonspecific esterase reactivity that may be weak, as seen in this case *(right)*.

Continued on next page

result in aberrant expression of the *OTT-MAL* fusion gene.[323]

There are two classification systems for AML (see next section). The FAB classification is based exclusively on morphology. However, there are some morphologic subtypes such as M3 and M4eo that are always associated with particular cytogenetic changes, that is, *RARA* rearrangements for the former and inv(16) or t(16;16) in the latter. In addition, there are certain cytogenetic changes that are often (if not exclusively) associated with a particular subtype and that carry prognostic significance, such as the good prognosis t(8;21) often associated with the M2 subtype or *MLL* rearrangements often associated with the M5 subtype. The WHO classification system

takes this into account and has a category of "acute myeloid leukemia with recurrent genetic abnormalities," which includes t(8;21), inv(16) or t(16;16), t(15;17), and 11q23. The fusion proteins thus generated are discussed in more detail earlier (see "Acute Myelogenous Leukemia: Biology"). Some of the more common chromosomal abnormalities and their associated FAB and WHO subtypes are shown in Table 51-1 and Box 51-2. The prognostic significance of certain cytogenetic abnormalities is discussed later (see "Prognosis").

French-American-British Classification

In 1976, the FAB group proposed a system of classification of AML based on morphologic and cytochemical

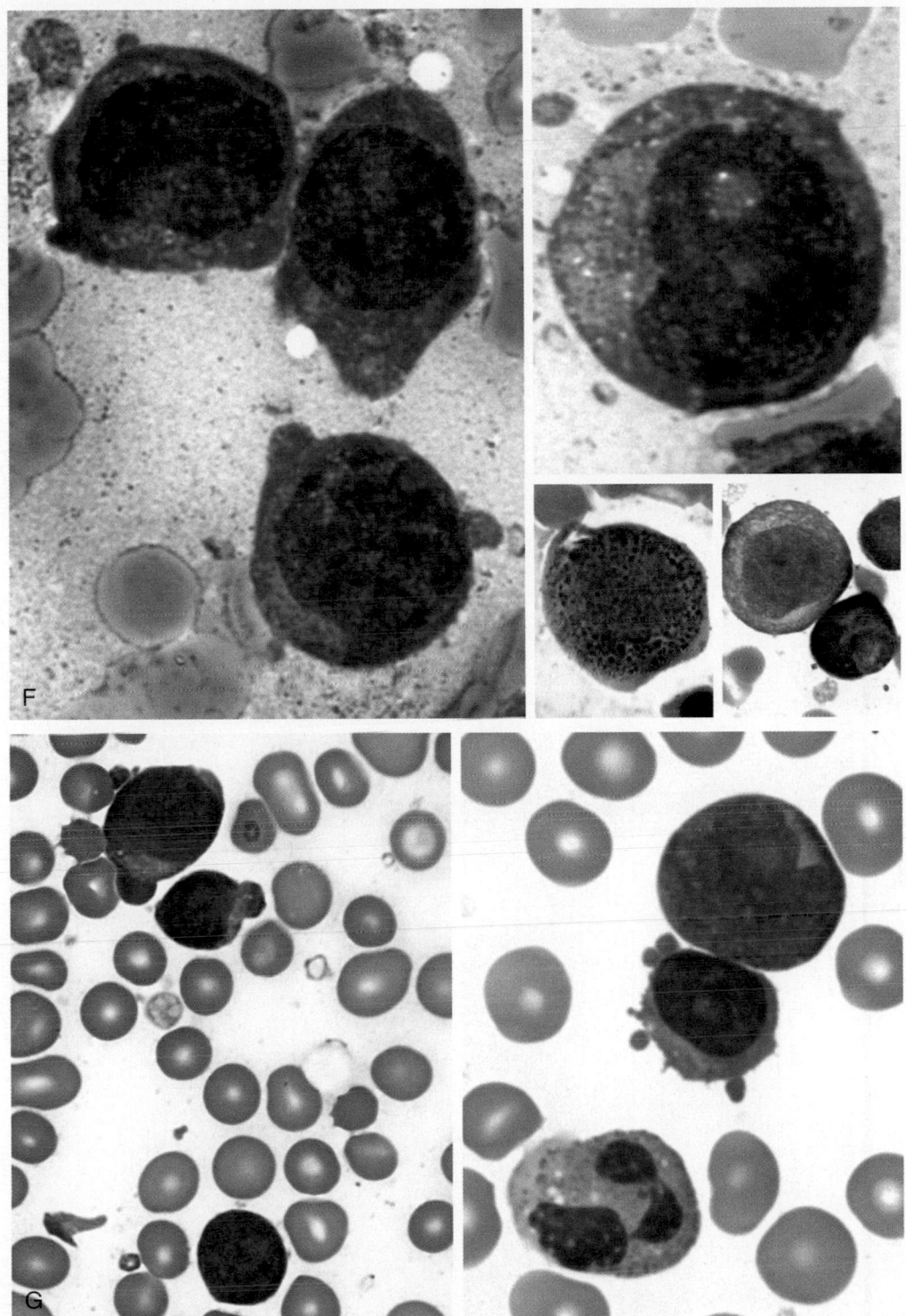

Figure 51-5, cont'd F, Acute monoblastic leukemia. Monoblasts are large and have round nuclei, prominent nucleoli, and abundant deeply basophilic cytoplasm, which may contain fine granules and/or vacuoles. Monoblasts show strong reactivity for nonspecific esterase *(lower right, left inset)* and are typically myeloperoxidase negative *(lower right, right inset)*. G, Acute megakaryoblastic leukemia. Megakaryoblasts are varied in size and have round, slightly indented or markedly irregular nuclear contours as well as fine chromatin, single to multiple small nucleoli, and scant to moderate basophilic (agranular or granular) cytoplasm, often with cytoplasmic blebs or pseudopod formation. *(Courtesy of Dr. Jo-Anne Vergilio, Assistant Professor in Pathology, Harvard Medical School.)*

TABLE 51-1   French-American-British (FAB) Classification of Acute Myelogenous Leukemia with Corresponding Cytogenetic and Immunophenotypic Characteristics

FAB Subtype	MPO	SBB	NSE	PAS	MYELOID CD11b	CD13	CD14	CD15	CD33	CD34	CD65	ERYTHROID Glycophorin A	CD41/61	MEGAKARYOCYTIC CD42	CD36	CD2	T-CELL LINEAGE CD3	CD4	CD7	CD56	OTHER HLA-DR	CD117	Translocations and Rearrangements	Genes Involved
M0	−	−	−	−	−	++	−	+	++	++	+	+	+	+	+	+	−	+−	+−	+	++	++	11q23; Trisomy 4, 8,13, −5, −7	MLL rearrangements
M1	+	+	−	−	−	+	−	+	+	+	−	−	−	+	−	+	−	+−	+	+	++	++	t(8;21)(q22;q22); t(9;22)(q34;q11); Trisomy 8, −5, −7	AML1-ETO; BCR-ABL
M2	+	+	−	−	+	+	−	++	++	++	−	−	−	+	−	+	−	−	+	+	++	+	t(8;21)(q22;q22); t(6;9); inv3(q21;q26), t(3;3) (q21;q26); Trisomy 8, −5, −7	AML1-ETO; DEK-CAN; EVI1
M3	+	+	−	−	−	+	−	+	+	+	−	−	−	−	−	+	−	−	+	+	+	+	t(15;17)(q22;q12); t(11;17)(q23;q12), t(5;17) (q32;q12)	PML-RARA; PLZF-RARA; NPM-RARA
M4	+	+	+	−	++	++	++	+	+	+	−	−	−	++	+	+	−	++	+	+	+++	+	t(6;9); inv3(q21;q26), t(3;3) (q21;q26); t(9;11)(p22;q23); 11q23	DEK-CAN; EVI1; AF9-MLL; MLL rearrangements
(M4eo)	+	+	+	+	++	++	+	+	+	+	+	−	−	++	−	+	−	−	+	+	+++	+	inv16(p13;q22), t(16;16)	MYH11-CBFβ
M5	−	−	+	+	++	++	++	++	+	++	−	−	−	++	+	+	−	++	+	+	+++	+	t(11;17)(q23;q21); 11q23; 11q23,t(9;11) (p22;q23) [M5a]; t(8;16), t(10;11) (p12;q23) [M5b]	MLL-AF17; MLL rearrangements; MLL, AF9-MLL; MOZ-CBP, AF10-MLL
M6	+	+	−	+	−	+	−	++	+	+	++	+	−	−	−	−	−	−	+	+	−	+	Trisomy 8, −5, −7	
M7	−	−	+	+	+	+	−	−	+	+	−	++	++	+, +	++	+	−	+	+	+	+	+	t(1;22)(p13;q13)	OTT-MAL
M7 (DS)	−	−	+	+	+	+	−	−	+	+	−	++	++	++	++	+	−	+	+	+	+	+	Trisomy 21	GATA-1

AML, Acute myelogenous leukemia; DS, Down syndrome; MLL, mixed-lineage leukemia; MPO, myeloperoxidase; NSE, nonspecific esterase; PAS, periodic acid-Schiff; SBB, Sudan black B.

features (see Table 51-1). The system divides AML into seven subtypes, M1 through M7.[305,324,325] An M0 subtype was later added to describe undifferentiated leukemia and, since 1976, immunophenotypic data have also been included.[304,305,326] In general, AML can be differentiated from ALL based on morphologic features and cytochemical stains. Cells of myeloid origin should stain with myeloperoxidase and SBB. Cells of monocytic derivation usually stain with NSE. AML blasts usually do not have PAS activity, except for erythroblasts in AML-M6 and eosinophils of the M4Eo subtype.

M0: Acute Myeloblastic Leukemia with Minimal Differentiation. In patients with AML-M0, the bone marrow is usually hypercellular and more than 90% of the cells are blasts. Most blast cells lack cytoplasmic granules, nucleoli, or Auer rods, and results with MPO and SBB stains are negative.[304] Immunophenotypic analysis shows the presence of myeloid or monocytic cell antigens (i.e., CD13, CD14, CD33, or CD34) that are detectable on the cell surface of most AML-M0 blasts, but some AML-M0 blasts express terminal deoxynucleotidyl transferase, an enzyme usually associated with ALL. AML-M0 is associated with a high incidence of cytogenetic abnormalities, most of which are complex and often involve chromosomes 5 and 7, trisomy 8, or MLL rearrangements.[302,327]

M1: Acute Myeloblastic Leukemia without Maturation. The bone marrow of patients with AML-M1 is hypercellular and filled with myeloblasts (more than 90% blasts). Most blasts stain with MPO and SBB. The blast cells in this subtype display minimal myeloid differentiation. Morphologically, the blast cells may contain scant gray-blue cytoplasm and few or no azurophilic granules or Auer rods. Prominent nucleoli are usually detectable. Flow cytometric analysis usually shows that the blast cells of AML-M1 express HLA-DR, CD13, CD33, and CD34. Cytogenetic abnormalities for this subclass often include monosomy 5 or 7 or trisomy 8.

M2: Acute Myeloblastic Leukemia with Maturation. The bone marrow of patients with AML-M2 usually shows evidence of some maturation beyond the myeloblast, with evidence of maturation beyond the promyelocyte stage in more than 10% of nonerythroid cells. Myeloblasts must represent more than 30% of the bone marrow cells but less than 90% of nonerythroid cells. The blasts generally have a few clusters of primary granules and stain with MPO and SBB. Auer rods and prominent nucleoli are common. Immunophenotypic expression of HLA-DR, CD13, CD33, CD11, and CD15 is typical. This subtype may exhibit monosomy 5 or 7, trisomy 8, t(8;21), t(6;9), or abnormalities of chromosome 3.

M3: Acute Promyelocytic Leukemia. There are two types of AML-M3. The more common type is the hypergranular variant, in which more than 30% of the blasts are promyelocytes and myeloblasts. Most promyelocytes have heavy granulation. Auer rods and Auer rod bundles are common. In the rare microgranular variant, the cells exhibit fine cytoplasmic granules, which are not distinguishable by light microscopy and nuclear morphologic irregularities (i.e., microgranular M3 or M3v). The cells of both subtypes stain strongly with MPO and SBB and also with chloroacetate esterase. The promyelocytes usually do not show PAS and NSE activity. The blasts express CD13, CD33, CD11, and CD15, but they are HLA-DR– and CD14–. This subtype exclusively exhibits *RARA* rearrangements, the vast majority of which are t(15;17) leading to *PML-RARA*.

M4: Acute Myelomonocytic Leukemia. The M4 subtype is defined by the presence of blast cells with both granulocytic and monocytic features. The bone marrow in these patients has more than 30% infiltration by immature myeloid precursors, and there is often extramedullary involvement and a peripheral blood monocytosis. The blasts are usually pleomorphic with regard to size, amount of cytoplasm, granularity, and nuclear morphologic features. Some Auer rods can be seen, and prominent nucleoli are usually present. Staining is variable, with some of the blast cells showing positivity for MPO, SBB, and NSE. M4 AML may be associated with t(6;9), abnormalities of chromosome 3, and *MLL* gene rearrangements, in particular t(9;11). A small proportion of patients with AML-M4 have a moderate eosinophilia in their bone marrow (M4Eo). The eosinophils are notable for the presence of basophilic and eosinophilic granules and stain with chloroacetate esterase and PAS. Cell surface antigen expression includes CD13, CD15, CD33, CD4, CD11c, CD14, CD64, and HLA-DR. M4eo AML exhibits an inv(16) or t(16;16).

M5: Acute Monocytic Leukemia. More than 80% of the nonerythroid bone marrow cells in patients with AML-M5 are monocytic. There are two subtypes: M5a (undifferentiated) and M5b (differentiated). In AML-M5a, more than 80% of the cells are monoblasts. Patients with AML-M5a tend to be younger, have higher presenting white blood cell (WBC) counts, and have a poorer prognosis. In AML-M5b, fewer than 80% of the monocytic cells are monoblasts, and most of the cells are recognizable as monocytes or promonocytes. The peripheral blood in patients with AML-M5b exhibits a profound monocytosis. In both subtypes, the blasts demonstrate strong NSE activity. MPO and SBB staining results are usually negative. Cell surface antigen expression includes CD13, CD15, CD33, CD4, CD11c, CD14, CD64, and HLA-DR. M5 AML often exhibits *MLL* gene rearrangements, t(9;11) or t(11;17) in M5a and t(10;11) in M5b.

M6: Acute Erythrocytic Leukemia. AML-M6 is an uncommon form of AML overall and is rare in children. This form of leukemia is defined by a more than 50% erythroblast infiltration of the bone marrow. M6 AML may exhibit monosomy 5 or 7 or trisomy 8.

M7: Acute Megakaryoblastic Leukemia. The bone marrow exhibits an infiltration with pleomorphic megakaryoblasts that often display cytoplasmic budding and may appear in clusters. Aspiration of the bone marrow

Box 51-2   **World Health Organization (WHO) Classification of Acute Myeloid Leukemia and Corresponding French-American-British (FAB) Subtype***

ACUTE MYELOID LEUKEMIA WITH RECURRENT GENETIC ABNORMALITIES (FAB)

t(8;21)(q22;q22); *(AML1/ETO; RUNX1-RUNX1T1)* **(M2)**
inv(16)(p13;q22) or t(16;16)(p13;q22); *(CBFβ/MYH11)* **(M4EO)**
t(15;17)(q22;q12) *(PML/RARA)* **(M3)**
AML with t(9;11)(p22;q23); *MLLT3-MLL*
AML with t(6;9)(p23;q34); *DEK-NUP214*
AML with inv(3)(q21q26.2) or t(3;3)(q21;q26.2); *RPN1-EVI1*
AML (megakaryoblastic) with t(1;22)(p13;q13); *RBM15-MKL1*

ACUTE MYELOID LEUKEMIA WITH MYELODYSPLASIA-RELATED CHANGES

Following myelodysplastic syndrome (MDS) or MDS/myeloproliferative disease (MPD)

THERAPY-RELATED MYELOID NEOPLASMS

ACUTE MYELOID LEUKEMIA (FAB)

Acute myeloid leukemia, minimally differentiated **(M0)**
Acute myeloid leukemia without maturation **(M1)**
Acute myeloid leukemia with maturation **(M2)**
Acute myelomonocytic leukemia **(M4)**
Acute monoblastic and monocytic leukemia **(M5)**
Acute erythroid leukemia **(M6)**
Acute megakaryoblastic leukemia **(M7)**
Acute basophilic leukemia
Acute panmyelosis with myelofibrosis

MYELOID SARCOMA

MYELOID PROLIFERATIONS RELATED TO DOWN SYNDROME

BLASTIC PLASMACYTOID DENDRITIC CELL NEOPLASM

Modified from Vardiman JW, Harris NL, Brunning RD: The World Health Organization (WHO) classification of the myeloid neoplasms. Blood 100:2292–2302, 2002; and Vardiman JW, Thiele J, Arber DA, et al: The 2008 revision of the World Health Organization (WHO) classification of myeloid neoplasms and acute leukemia: rationale and important changes. Blood 114:937–951, 2009.
*Shown in boldface.

may be challenging due to associated fibrosis. M7 blasts generally do not stain with MPO and SBB but show activity with PAS. Immunophenotyping is usually required to distinguish AML-M7 from ALL-L2, documenting the presence of the megakaryocytic antigens, glycoprotein Ib, glycoprotein IIb/IIIa, or factor VIII. Non–Down syndrome infants with M7 AML often exhibit a t(1;22). Down syndrome patients have a very high incidence of M7 AML with a particularly good prognosis, which is in contrast to the poor prognosis of M7 AML in non–Down syndrome children and adults.

World Health Organization Classification

The discovery of cytogenetic and molecular genetic abnormalities in malignant disease has had a significant impact on our understanding of malignant transformation. In myeloid malignancies, some genetic abnormalities have prognostic significance whereas others appear to define specific disease subtypes. The WHO has proposed a classification system for neoplastic diseases of the hematopoietic and lymphoid tissues that includes a classification for AML (see Box 51-2 and Fig. 51-5). This classification uses the traditional FAB-type morphologic

categories of disease and includes additional entities such as immunophenotype, molecular genetic, and clinical characteristics that make the system more clinically relevant for diagnosis, prognosis, and treatment.[328] The WHO classification system divides myeloid diseases into several major subtypes—myeloproliferative neoplasms; myeloid neoplasm associated with eosinophilia and abnormalities of *PDGFRA*, *PDGFRB*, or *FGFR1*; myelodysplastic-myeloproliferative neoplasms; MDS, AML and related neoplasms; and acute leukemias of ambiguous lineage. The 2008 revision of the WHO classification has expanded the category of AML to include AML with recurrent cytogenetic translocations, AML with myelodysplasia-related changes, therapy-related myeloid neoplasms, AML not otherwise specified, myeloid sarcoma, myeloid proliferations related to Down syndrome, and blastic plasmacytoid dendritic cell neoplasms.[329]

Within the subtype containing recurrent cytogenetic translocations, seven additional categories have been described:

AML with t(8;21)(q22;q22); *AML1-ETO*; *RUNX1-RUNX1T1*
AML with inv(16)(p13.1q22) or t(16;16)(p13.1;q22); *CBFB-MYH11*
APL with t(15;17)(q22;q12); *PML-RARA*
AML with t(9;11)(p22;q23); *MLLT3-MLL*
AML with t(6;9)(p23;q34); *DEK-NUP214*
AML with inv(3)(q21q26.2) or t(3;3)(q21;q26.2); *RPN1-EVI1*
AML (megakaryoblastic) with t(1;22)(p13;q13); *RBM15-MKL1*

AML with t(6;9)(p23;q34) and AML with inv(3) (q21q26.2) is relatively uncommon in children. Myeloid sarcomas, formerly called chloromas, may precede hematopoietic evidence of disease and so are now classified as a separate entity. The myeloid diseases of Down syndrome were incorporated into the revised WHO classification in 2008 and are described later in this chapter. Plasmacytoid dendritic cell neoplasms were formerly referred to as blastic NK-cell lymphomas, but the nomenclature has changed to reflect the origin of this myeloid malignancy in this subset of dendritic cells. This rare disease can manifest in children with skin lesions, adenopathy, and ultimately bone marrow involvement. Blast cells characteristically express CD4, CD43, CD56, and CD123 without expression of CD34 or CD117.[329]

The FAB standard used to define AML had been 30% replacement of the bone marrow by the blast cells, but later studies have shown that patients with 20% to 30% blasts (previously classified as refractory anemia with excess blasts in transformation [RAEB-T]) have a prognosis similar to that of patients with more than 30% blasts. The blast count for the diagnosis of AML in the WHO classification was therefore changed to 20%, and the category of RAEB-T was eliminated.

Certain specific and recurrent cytogenetic abnormalities are common in MDS, in alkylating agent–related AML, and in de novo AML with a poor prognosis. These abnormalities include 3q−, −5, 5q−, −7, 7q , +8, +9, 11q−, 12p−, −8, −19, 20q−, +21, t(1;7), t(2;11), and complex karyotypes. In the classification scheme, these cytogenetic abnormalities were considered to indicate a poor prognosis. Prior therapy with topoisomerase II inhibitors (i.e., epipodophyllotoxins and doxorubicin) was also associated with a poor prognosis. Typically, patients in whom AML develops after exposure to these agents have translocations involving 11q23 (*MLL*). The WHO classification includes these patients in the poor-prognosis category but distinguishes them from having alkylating agent–related secondary leukemia.

Patients may have MDS with unilineage or multilineage dysplasia, and these are reflected as distinct diseases in the most recent iteration of the WHO classification. Dysplasia is defined as being observed in greater than or equal to 10% of the cells of a given myeloid lineage. Children with 2% to 19% peripheral blasts or 5% to 19% bone marrow blasts can be classified according to the same criteria as adult MDS, but a new category of refractory cytopenia of childhood has been introduced to define children with persistent cytopenias and dysplasia of two or more lineages but less than 2% peripheral blasts or less than 5% bone marrow blasts.[329]

Clinical Presentation

The presenting signs and symptoms of AML result from leukemic blast cell infiltration of the bone marrow. The leukemia cells overwhelm the processes of normal hematopoiesis, resulting in anemia, thrombocytopenia, and neutropenia. It is rare for AML to be diagnosed incidentally on a routine medical evaluation, but there is considerable variability in the range of presenting signs and symptoms in patients with de novo AML. Usually, patients seek medical attention for fever, fatigue, pallor, skin or mucosal bleeding, bone pain, or infections not responding to appropriate antibiotic therapy.[330] Bone pain is a common symptom, and patients may present with a limp, rib pain, or back pain.[330]

The WBC count of patients with newly diagnosed AML can range from less than 1,000/μL to more than 500,000/μL.[330-332] The leukocyte count is more than 100,000/μL in approximately 25% of pediatric patients with AML, and an elevated count is more common in those with the M4 and M5 subtypes and in those with *FLT3*-ITD mutations.[174,175,330,333,334] The number of circulating granulocytes is often critically decreased, regardless of the total leukocyte count, and, because their function is usually impaired, the risk for overwhelming bacterial infection in patients with newly diagnosed AML is markedly increased. Patients with AML who have a fever require immediate treatment with broad-spectrum antibiotics after appropriate culture samples have been obtained. The hemoglobin level is occasionally normal but is usually less than 9 g/dL, and levels as low as 3 g/dL at diagnosis are not uncommon. About half of children with new-onset AML have platelet counts of 50,000/μL or less, which increases the risk for life-threatening bleeding.[330]

Disseminated intravascular coagulation (DIC) has been observed in patients with all FAB subtypes of AML but is most common in acute promyelocytic leukemia (APL; see later). Before the development of ATRA,

treatment with low-dose heparin during induction was initiated for patients with AML-M3 to prevent DIC.[335,336] The later addition of ATRA to induction therapy rapidly resolved DIC in patients with AML-M3 and markedly reduced early mortality.[191,337-340]

Patients with hyperleukocytosis have an increased risk for mortality from leukostasis, particularly in the brain or lung, and urgent leukapheresis or treatment with leukocyte-reducing agents such as hydroxyurea may be necessary (see "Complications").[341,342] Extramedullary leukemia occurs in 20% to 25% of children with AML and may include chloromas (tumor nodules), skin infiltration, CNS disease, gingival infiltration, hepatosplenomegaly, or testicular involvement.[330,343] Chloromas (e.g., myeloblastomas and granulocytic sarcomas) are solid tumors of myeloblasts that may occur in any area of the body but are most common in the orbit and epidural area.[344] Skin infiltration, or leukemia cutis, usually presents as slightly purple lesions (i.e., "blueberry muffin" spots), is more common in infants with monocytic leukemia, and may be the initial sign of disease.[345] CNS involvement at diagnosis is more common in AML than in ALL. Up to 15% of patients with AML have myeloblasts in the cerebrospinal fluid at diagnosis.[346-349] Gingival infiltration may present as hyperplasia, often accompanied by bleeding.[350] Severe extramedullary disease with massive hepatosplenomegaly is also a more common finding in infants.[345] Extramedullary involvement of the testes can also be documented but is less common than in ALL.[351,352] Extramedullary infiltration, particularly gingival involvement, is more common with the M4 and M5 (acute myelomonocytic and acute monoblastic and monocytic) leukemias.[350,353,354] Chloromas and CNS disease are more common in AMLs with t(8;21). Extramedullary infiltration in pediatric patients is not clearly associated with worse prognosis unless accompanied by a high presenting WBC count.

Treatment

As is true for any pediatric cancer, the goal of therapy for children with AML is to completely eradicate the disease while limiting treatment-induced toxicity. In general, therapy for AML includes immediate supportive care measures followed by intensive remission induction and consolidation chemotherapy. At any given time, several large, multicenter phase III clinical trials are ongoing, each aimed to improve overall survival (OS) through randomized comparisons of treatment options while minimizing short- and long-term toxicities.

Remission Induction

During the past 40 years, survival rates for patients with AML have risen from less than 10% to more than 50% of patients because of intensification of chemotherapy, use of hematopoietic stem cell transplantation (HSCT), and improved supportive care. The first phase of chemotherapy is termed *induction* and consists of two to four cycles of intensive chemotherapy with the goal of inducing remission. Morphologic remission is defined as the presence of fewer than 5% blasts visible on bone marrow aspirate obtained after recovery of counts. Patients may also achieve cytogenetic and FISH-negative remission, as defined by the absence of a previously detected leukemic clone–associated cytogenetic abnormality in the bone marrow cells. Remission is also now being defined by the absence of MRD, assessed by multiparameter flow cytometry that is designed to detect as few as 0.1% leukemic blasts in the marrow. The inclusion of MRD evaluation has not only identified children at risk for relapse who appeared to be in morphologic remission but has also revealed false-positive recovering marrows that had been deemed refractory disease.[355]

Induction chemotherapy should be initiated as soon as the diagnosis of AML is confirmed, preferably by morphologic, immunophenotypic, and cytogenetic studies of the bone marrow. In some cases, particularly in patients presenting with hyperleukocytosis, the patient's condition may be too unstable for bone marrow evaluation, in which case the diagnosis can often be confirmed on studies of the peripheral blood. Induction chemotherapy regimens consist of high-dose myelosuppressive cytotoxic agents that result in prolonged pancytopenia. The period of bone marrow hypoplasia generally lasts from 21 to 30 days from the initiation of therapy but may last considerably longer. During this period, patients have a high risk for life-threatening infection and bleeding. Aggressive supportive care is necessary (see later).

Historical North American Approaches to Treating AML. The basis of modern induction therapy for AML is a combination of cytarabine and an anthracycline. The classic combination therapy was the so-called 7 + 3 regimen, which consists of a continuous 7-day intravenous infusion of cytarabine at 100 to 200 mg/m²/day and 3 days of bolus infusions of daunorubicin at 45 to 60 mg/m²/day. Remission is achieved in 60% to 70% of patients with newly diagnosed AML using this regimen.[356-358] In children, several strategies have been used to intensify this regimen to achieve higher rates of CR. CCG trial 213 added etoposide, thioguanine, and dexamethasone to the traditional 7 + 3 regimen to create the five-drug Denver regimen. The Denver and 7 + 3 regimens were compared in a randomized fashion, and there was no significant difference in CR rate, with 79% of children achieving CR with 7 + 3 and 76% achieving CR with Denver regimen.[359]

In CCG trial 2891, the same drugs were used but the timing was intensified in an attempt to improve CR. The hypothesis was that leukemia cells may be recruited synchronously into the cell cycle after chemotherapy, and therefore reexposure at an earlier time point may affect cells while more of them are at a sensitive phase in the cell cycle. Thus the Denver regimen was modified into the five-drug DCTER regimen, again consisting of *d*examethasone, *c*ytarabine, *t*hioguanine, *e*toposide, and *R*ubidomycin (daunorubicin). Induction consisted of a total of four cycles of chemotherapy, and patients were randomized to standard or intensive timing. For standard timing, each cycle of induction began with count recovery from the previous cycle. With intensive timing, cycles 2 and 4 began at day 10 after the start of cycles 1 or 3, respectively, regardless of hematologic status. Not surprisingly, the intensive timing resulted in far greater toxicity, with 11% of patients in this arm of the trial dying of toxicity compared with only 4% of patients dying of toxicity in the standard timing trial arm.[360] Because of this, better supportive care measures were instituted for the intensive timing trial arm, including more aggressive empiric antibiotic and antifungal coverage and the use of granulocyte colony-stimulating factor (G-CSF). Interestingly, the CR rates were similar for the two arms in the trial—75% for intensive timing and 70% for standard timing—but the reason for failure to achieve remission was different, with 11% toxic death and only 14% resistant disease in the intensive timing arm versus only 4% toxic death but 26% resistant disease in the standard timing arm. The most dramatic results, however, came later, when it was shown that for patients who achieved a CR there was a 3-year disease-free survival (DFS) of 55% for those who had been treated in the intensive timing arm, versus a DFS of only 37% for patients who had received standard timing. For this reason, the standard timing arm of the trial was closed early and an intensive timing DCTER/DCTER schedule became the new standard combination therapy for newly diagnosed AML patients.

In the meantime, a comprehensive review of five randomized trials comparing idarubicin with daunorubicin as induction therapy for AML had shown improved remission induction rates and OS for patients receiving idarubicin.[361] For this reason, the CCG pilot trial 2941 tried to intensify therapy further by using idarubicin in place of daunorubicin in each cycle of the intensively timed regimen. Because of unacceptably high toxicity, with a toxic death rate of 14%, this was modified to idarubicin only in cycles 1 and 3, and more strict supportive care guidelines were put into place, including mandatory hospitalization during neutropenia, and stricter infection prophylaxis (see later, "Supportive Therapy at Diagnosis and during Therapy").[362] The addition of idarubicin showed no advantage in remission induction or event-free survival (EFS) but did show a decrease in marrow blasts at day 14 of induction. CCG trial 2961 continued to use the hybrid idaDCTER/DCTER intensive timing induction regimen resulting in induction remission rates of 89%, which were similar to historic controls. Most of the improvement was believed to be related to better supportive care rather than to the change in chemotherapy.

Medical Research Council Trials (MRC10, MRC12, and MRC15). During this period, data emerged from the British MRC trials that seemed to show better survival and less toxicity. MRC10 induction chemotherapy randomized DAT (daunorubicin, cytarabine, thioguanine) to ADE (cytarabine, daunorubicin, etoposide) in a 10-day cycle of chemotherapy followed by an 8-day cycle of the same drugs on WBC count recovery. The CR rate for children in this study was 93%, with a 4% rate of toxic death and a 3% rate of resistant disease.[363] Early data suggested a benefit for pediatric patients using ADE versus DAT, but the later data showed no difference in 10-year OS (DAT, 57%; ADE, 51%; P = .3), DFS (DAT,

53%; ADE, 48%; *P* = .3) or EFS (DAT, 48%; ADE, 45%; *P* = .5).[363,364] Because of the early results possibly favoring ADE, MRC12 compared ADE with MAE (mitoxantrone, cytarabine, etoposide) in a 10-day cycle followed by an 8-day cycle on count recovery. The CR rates were similar for the two groups (ADE, 92%; MAE, 90%; *P* = .3) with a slight increase in toxic deaths for the MAE group (ADE, 3%; MAE, 6%) but a lower relapse rate (ADE, 39%; MAE, 32%) and better DFS rate for the MAE group (ADE, 55%; MAE, 63%), although the 10-year EFS and OS rates were not significantly different (54% and 63%, respectively).[363,365] In MRC15 there were three randomized induction backbones—ADE; cytarabine and daunorubicin without etoposide, or idarubicin, fludarabine, cytarabine, and G-CSF (Ida-FLAG)—and three randomized consolidation backbones—amsacrine, cytarabine, and etoposide; cytarabine 1.5 g/m^2; or cytarabine 3 g/m^2 with and without the addition of gemtuzumab ozogamicin (GMTZ, GO, Mylotarg).[371] GMTZ, a recombinant humanized anti-CD33 monoclonal agent linked to the tumor antibiotic calicheamicin, was incorporated as a targeted therapy in these studies. Because CD33 is expressed on most AML cells but not on pluripotent HSCs or other tissues, this drug can target leukemia cells more specifically.[367,368] GMTZ was well tolerated overall, but no overall improvements in survival or relapse rate were observed regardless of the chemotherapy backbone in either induction or consolidation.[371]

Recent U.S. Trials. The next series of U.S. trials built on the data from these recent MRC studies. The COG has undertaken three therapeutic trials to date based on an MRC backbone. The COG AAML03P1 pilot and AAML0531 phase III groupwide study backbone included cytarabine/daunorubicin/etoposide (ADE 10+3+5) followed by ADE 8+3+5, cytarabine/etoposide (AE), mitoxantrone/cytarabine (MA), and, finally, high-dose cytarabine (Capizzi II) for children who did not go on to receive HSCT. The COG pilot trial AAML03P1 assessed the safety of adding a single dose of GMTZ to ADE 10+3+5 and MA cycles. Toxicity on this pilot study was acceptable, so GMTZ was added to these same two cycles on AAML0531 in a 1:1 randomization. Subsequent outcome data from the AAML03P1 trial demonstrated a 3-year EFS of 53% and OS of 66% with no increased treatment-related mortality over backbone chemotherapy.[369] Outcome data have not yet been released for AAML0531. However, after data were released from the Southwest Oncology Group (SWOG) Study 106, the U.S. Food and Drug Administration (FDA) removed GMTZ from the U.S. market because this adult-based study showed no benefit in outcome to the addition of GMTZ but an increase in induction deaths.[370] By contrast, subgroup analysis on the MRC 15 trial found that the addition of GMTZ to induction chemotherapy was of benefit to CBF AML and to intermediate-risk patients and did not contribute to increased toxicity.[371] Data from the COG AAML0531 trial demonstrated mixed results. GMTZ improved 3 year EFS and relapse risk for all patients but not OS. Interestingly, positive trends were seen for GMTZ in subgroup analysis, including OS in

high risk patients and relapse risk in low risk patients, although this was also associated with increased TRM in the low risk subgroup.[371a] Given this controversy regarding both toxicity and efficacy and the absence of data from the AAML0531 at the time of study initiation, GMTZ was not included on the current COG AAML1031 trial. However, other co-operative groups are planning future trials to examine the optimal dosing of GMTZ in pediatric AML (A. Gamis, personal communication, July 2014). The current COG trial risk stratifies patients into high- and low-risk AML based on cytogenetics and MRD and randomizes the addition of the proteosome inhibitor bortezomib as a potential AML stem cell targeted therapy. In addition, patients harboring the *FLT3*-ITD with sufficient allelic ratio have the option of being nonrandomly assigned to an MRC-based backbone arm with the addition of the FLT3 inhibitor sorafenib. Given recent MRC data that four cycles appear as effective as five cycles of therapy,[365] only four cycles are included on this protocol (ADE 10+3+5; ADE 8+3+5; cytarabine and etoposide; and mitoxantrone and cytarabine) for good responders. Patients with positive MRD after cycle 1, defined as more than 0.1% by multiparameter flow cytometry (MPFC) receive mitoxantrone and cytarabine instead of an additional ADE cycle, and high-risk patients receive high-dose cytarabine for cycle 4.

The St. Jude Children's Research Hospital (SJCRH) trial AML02 randomized patients to standard low- or high-dose cytarabine during the first cycle of induction together with etoposide and daunorubicin (ADE), although this was not found to impact remission rate, EFS, or OS.[372] Toxicity was generally similar in both arms of the trial, although patients treated on the high-dose arm had a greater incidence of serious fungal infections. The SJCRH trial incorporated MRD measurements during induction to guide therapy. MRD by MPFC was determined on a bone marrow sample obtained on day 22 of induction. Patients with MRD greater than 1% on day 22 received induction II before WBC count recovery. Patients with MRD greater than 1% at the end of the first month of induction I received GMTZ in addition to the second cycle of ADE. Patients with CNS-positive disease received triple intrathecal therapy. Patients who were MRD positive after induction I had a significantly worse outcome than patients who were MRD negative (3-year EFS, 43% vs. 74%). However, subgroup analysis revealed that this difference was only found in patients with high-risk AML at diagnosis (*FLT3*-ITD positive, monosomy 7, t(6;9), megakaryoblastic leukemia, therapy-related AML, or AML after MDS) or those with MRD levels greater than 1%. Low- and standard-risk AML patients or those with what was referred to in this study as low-level MRD (0.1% to 1%) did not demonstrate any outcome differences versus those with negative MRD. However, 20 patients who were MRD negative ultimately experienced relapse.[372] In the current SJCRH study, AML08, patients are randomly assigned to receive high-dose cytarabine, etoposide, and daunorubicin versus clofarabine and cytarabine in induction I. Low-risk patients (those with CBF leukemia with negative MRD after induction I) receive 4 courses of chemotherapy, whereas those at high risk for relapse—*FLT3*-ITD positive, monosomy 7, t(6;9), t(8;16), t(16;21), megakaryoblastic leukemia without t(1;22), treatment-related AML, AML after MDS, or MRD greater than 0.1% after induction II—receive two to three courses of chemotherapy followed by allogeneic HSCT. Standard-risk patients receive four courses of chemotherapy and are then eligible to receive one course of natural killer cell therapy if they have a killer cell immunoglobulin-like receptor (KIR)-mismatched haploidentical family member. Patients with *FLT3*-ITD receive sorafenib after each course of chemotherapy (J. Rubnitz, personal communication).

The BFM (Berlin-Frankfurt-Münster) trial for de novo AML, BFM-2010, is for all comers, including patients with APL. Patients are being randomized to ADE ± GMTZ in induction I with MRD measurements on day 8, 15 and 28. Induction II includes cytarabine and idarubicin (AI) for patients with inv(16) and APL (who also receive ATRA). Other favorable-risk patients, including those with t(8;21), *NPM1* mutations, and *CEBPA*, receive HAM (high-dose cytarabine 3 g/m² and mitoxantrone), and high-risk patients receive HAM plus targeted therapy, such as sorafenib if *FLT3*-ITD positive, or dasatinib if *KIT* mutant positive. The third course is hAM (high-dose cytarabine at 1 g/m²) for those who received AI and AI for low-risk patients who received HAM, with AI plus cladribine for the high-risk patients. Course 4 is hAM, except for the inv(16) and APL patients who receive cytarabine or cytarabine and etoposide as a final cycle. For all other patients, course 5 is high-dose cytarabine and etoposide. Liposomal daunorubicin, available in Europe, will be used in this trial. Prior studies have shown it to have equal efficacy in induction to idarubicin with less toxicity[373,374] (G. Kaspars, D. Reinhardt, and D. Johnston, personal communication, January 2013).

Postremission Therapy

Several randomized studies have demonstrated that without postremission therapy almost all patients with newly diagnosed AML suffer a relapse within 2 years.[375-377] The strategies for postremission therapy include autologous HSCT, allogeneic HSCT, or continued courses of chemotherapy. The CCG trials have shown no benefit to autologous HSCT over continued cycles of chemotherapy so, although that strategy continues to be used in some European trials, autologous HSCT is not included in current U.S. trials.[364,378-384] Most studies have shown a lower relapse rate for AML patients treated with matched related donor HSCT versus chemotherapy, but the OS is often no better because of the significant morbidity and mortality of HSCT.[381,383-396] For this reason, until the most recent trials, unrelated donor HSCT was believed to be too morbid for patients in first remission and thus trials used a genetic randomization, wherein all patients with a matched related donor proceeded to HSCT and all others proceeded with further cycles of chemotherapy.[383,385,386]

Based on the success of the MRC trials with chemotherapy alone using a combination of cytogenetic characteristics and response to therapy,[363,364,386,397] the COG and

SJCRH adopted risk-based criteria for HSCT. HSCT, even from a matched related donor, is not recommended for patients with low-risk disease. This was previously defined by COG as the presence of t(8;21) or inv(16) in the leukemic clone at diagnosis, but more recently the presence of a *CEBPA* or *NPM1* mutation has been added to this definition, based on the data revealing the better outcome for these patients.[279,398] The COG has classified high-risk disease as monosomy 7, −5/5q−, *FLT3*-ITD with high allelic ratio, MRD positive after induction chemotherapy, or more than 15% blasts in the marrow after one course of induction chemotherapy.* The incorporation of MRD after induction has enabled the COG to relegate normal karyotype patients to high- and low-risk groups, thereby dichotomizing patients and eliminating the intermediate-risk category. Therefore on the current AAML1031 protocol, high-risk patients will receive best available donor HSCT for consolidation, whereas good-risk patients will not go to transplant even if a sibling donor match is available. With recent advances in supportive care and improved therapy to prevent and treat graft-versus-host disease (GVHD), outcomes have improved for matched related and matched unrelated donor HSCT.[381,390,391,393] Therefore for patients with high-risk disease, both trials recommend HSCT in first CR with an unrelated donor if no matched family donor is identified. The optimal number of cycles of chemotherapy before HSCT to balance minimizing toxicity while minimizing MRD is variable, with the MRC10 trial using four cycles, the current SJCRH trial including two to three cycles, and the COG trial using three cycles before HSCT.[363,364]

For patients who do not proceed to HSCT there is controversy as to how many courses of chemotherapy are needed and what chemotherapy should be included. Several trials have shown that cycles of high-dose cytarabine after remission are associated with improved long-term survival.† MRC12 randomized patients to receive four versus five total cycles of chemotherapy, with early results suggesting that five cycles are superior; thus that strategy was subsequently used in the current U.S. trials.[397] However, more recent data from the MRC have shown that the fifth cycle added toxicity with no additional therapeutic benefit.[411] These findings are reflected in the current COG trial in which only four cycles of chemotherapy are used for good-risk patients with elimination of the high-dose cytarabine and asparaginase cycle (Capizzi II) that previously comprised the fifth cycle on AAML0531 and AAML03P1.[409,410,412,413] High-risk patients for whom a donor is not identified also only receive four cycles of chemotherapy, but they do receive Capizzi II as their last consolidation cycle. The SJCRH trial has tried to make up for the lack of amsacrine by tailoring the first postinduction cycle based on the patient's AML subtype and cytogenetics. On AML02, patients with t(9;11) or inv(16) AML receive cytarabine and cladribine, patients with M4/M5 AML receive cytarabine and etoposide, and patients with t(8;21) and all others receive high-dose cytarabine

---

*References 131, 255, 319, 321, 364, 399, 400, **401**, 402, **403**, 404, and 405.

†References 311, 316, 389, 394, and 406-410.

and mitoxantrone[311,414-419] followed by two courses consisting of cytarabine and asparaginase followed by cytarabine and mitoxantrone.[409,410,412,413] However, based on small subgroup numbers, AML08 uses a single backbone for all patients with the addition of sorafenib for patients with *FLT3*-ITD (J. Rubnitz, personal communication, January 2013). CNS leukemia in patients with AML is highly sensitive to chemotherapy, and the addition of cranial irradiation does not decrease CNS relapse compared with systemic and intrathecal chemotherapy. Therefore, cranial irradiation is no longer part of the therapy for patients with AML.[420] However, CNS-positive patients defined on the current COG AML study as having even one blast in the cerebrospinal fluid are treated with additional intrathecal cytarabine until the fluid is clear of blasts and for two additional intrathecal treatments beyond. Furthermore, in pediatrics, the addition of prolonged low-intensity maintenance therapy is associated with lower OS because of more resistant disease at relapse, so maintenance therapy is not used in the current U.S. trials.[421-423]

Supportive Therapy at Diagnosis and during Therapy

The diagnosis and treatment of childhood AML require a multidisciplinary approach involving pediatric oncologists, hematopathologists, pediatric surgeons, infectious disease specialists, pediatric intensivists, and pediatric nurses. While studies and procedures are initiated to make the diagnosis, special care must be taken to prevent and treat the life-threatening consequences of leukemia and accompanying pancytopenia. The most serious complications of leukemia at diagnosis are infection and bleeding with pancytopenia, tumor lysis syndrome, and leukostasis. The most common causes of death once remission is achieved are relapse, infection, hemorrhage, and cardiac events.[385,424] The improvement in OS of patients with AML over the past several decades is attributable as much to better supportive care efforts as to more effective treatment regimens.[425]

Infectious Complications. At the time of initial presentation, up to 40% of patients with leukemia exhibit fever, and most of these patients are neutropenic or have impaired neutrophil function.[330] During remission induction and subsequent cycles of chemotherapy, all AML patients experience profound prolonged neutropenia and are at high risk for life-threatening bacterial infections, particularly viridans group streptococcal infections.[424,426-428] Almost all AML patients experience at least one febrile neutropenic episode during therapy, and approximately 40% of these patients will have a documented infection; most commonly these are bacterial infections, followed by viral infections and then fungal infections. Infections account for nearly two thirds of deaths in patients in remission.[385,424,428] Therefore supportive care during induction and postremission therapy must pay particular attention to prophylactic, empiric, and treatment coverage for infectious complications. Several strategies are used to prevent infection or decrease mortality from infection. Some centers isolate patients receiving AML therapy in laminar airflow rooms during episodes of neutropenia.[424,429] The supportive

care guidelines for the CCG 2961 study included mandatory hospitalization for all patients, whether febrile or not, until the absolute phagocyte count had risen, and this rule has been strongly recommended in current COG trials. On CCG 2961, almost 50% of patients developed gram-positive infections and approximately 25% developed gram-negative infections across all phases of therapy. Infection-related mortality was 11%, including death from fungus. Bacterial agents included coagulase-negative staphylococci and α-hemolytic streptococci (including viridans streptococci) as well as *Klebsiella* and *Pseudomonas* species.[430] To decrease the rate of bacterial infections, some programs routinely prescribe the use of gut decontamination, mouthwashes, or prophylactic antibiotics.[385,425] A study by SJCRH demonstrated that initiation of antibiotics at the onset of neutropenia prevented sepsis, with the optimal regimen including both vancomycin and ciprofloxacin.[431] This remains an area of controversy because, in some studies, although prophylaxis may decrease the rate of bacterial infection it may also be associated with an increase in drug-resistant organisms. Further investigation is indicated in a prospective randomized fashion before it is widely adopted.[424,429,432-438] For example, in the SJCRH study, an earlier regimen of vancomycin and cefepime resulted in two cases of life-threatening resistant gram-negative bacteria and one of *Bacillus cereus*, leading to the change to ciprofloxacin for gram-negative coverage.[431] The COG is currently conducting a study of a related fluoroquinolone, levofloxacin, for bacterial prophylaxis in AML and patients with relapsed ALL. Patients will be randomized to receive levofloxacin versus no bacterial prophylaxis from the initiation of chemotherapy for two consecutive cycles. In contrast to the controversy regarding bacterial prophylaxis, there is broad agreement that patients who are febrile at initial presentation and patients who experience febrile neutropenia during therapy should be immediately started empirically on broad-spectrum antibiotics, including vancomycin, once cultures have been obtained.[439-441] In many centers, vancomycin is discontinued after 48 to 72 hours if there is no evidence of gram-positive bacteremia.[424] Typhlitis, or generalized bacterial infection of the cecum, is more common in children than in adults and is more common in patients treated with doxorubicin instead of daunorubicin.[442,443] Although this is a potentially life-threatening complication, conservative management with broad-spectrum antibiotics and nothing by mouth is generally preferable to surgical treatment in the setting of profound neutropenia.[444]

AML patients are at high risk for invasive fungal infection, which carries a high risk for mortality. The routine use of fungal prophylaxis is becoming more routine given the intensity of AML protocols. Data from the CCG 2961 study demonstrated *Candida* and *Aspergillus* infections in approximately 13% of patients across all phases of therapy and a strong association with infection-related mortality.[430] Some early studies have shown a decrease in some *Candida* species with fluconazole prophylaxis, but an increase in *Candida krusei* infections was documented, with no decrease in infection by invasive molds.[445-447] Two meta-analyses have concluded that there is a reduction in morbidity because of invasive fungal infections when prophylaxis is used for those with prolonged neutropenia and post-HSCT patients.[448,449] A randomized controlled trial of posaconazole versus fluconazole or itraconazole as fungal prophylaxis in neutropenic patients with AML or MDS has shown a lower rate of invasive fungal infections and improved OS in the posaconazole group.[450] However, posaconazole has not been studied in children younger than age 13 years and, owing to exclusively oral administration, may have limitations during administration of emetogenic AML chemotherapy. Voriconazole has been studied as a prophylactic agent that has activity against both yeast and aspergillus, but the incidence of invasive fungal infections was no different compared with fluconazole or itraconazole.[451-453] Voriconazole, similar to posaconazole, is metabolized through hepatic CYP450, leading to numerous interactions with other drugs and contributing further to a lack of enthusiasm in using either of these agents prophylactically. Thus fluconazole remains the most frequently used agent for fungal prophylaxis but lacks activity against *Aspergillus*.[451,454] Currently the COG is conducting a study randomizing patients with AML to caspofungin versus fluconazole for fungal prophylaxis. Caspofungin is from the echinocandin family of antifungal agents that functions by targeting fungal cell wall biosynthesis of β-1,3-glucan. It is effective against both *Candida* and *Aspergillus* species and has safety data in children as young as 3 months of age.[455-457] Caspofungin is given intravenously and is generally well tolerated but has minimal CNS penetration.

A test to detect galactomannan-containing *Aspergillus* antigens in the sera of immunocompromised patients has become commercially available. At this point, the galactomannan assay has been used most advantageously to follow the status of invasive aspergillosis and its response to therapy.[458,459] However, some centers do not use fungal prophylaxis during AML therapy but rather screen twice weekly with the galactomannan assay and use a low threshold for computed tomography (CT) to detect early invasive disease.[460,461] Whether or not fungal prophylaxis is used, empirical fungal therapy should be initiated for neutropenic patients who remain febrile for longer than 5 days, although some centers use a threshold of 72 hours. Patients who need empiric fungal therapy should be routinely scanned during neutropenia and after the recovery of circulating neutrophils be screened for evidence of fungal disease, and the diagnosis of fungal infection should be made by biopsy whenever feasible. Amphotericin has long been the antifungal agent of choice for empiric therapy, and the liposomal forms appear to be equivalent in efficacy and less toxic to renal function.[462,463] One prospective randomized trial has shown that caspofungin as empiric fungal therapy is as effective as liposomal amphotericin B and is generally better tolerated.[464] Whereas caspofungin is well tolerated with few drug interactions, as mentioned earlier, it does not cross the blood-brain barrier and thus is ineffective at treating suspected or proven CNS fungal infections. Voriconazole as empiric fungal therapy was compared with amphotericin in a prospective randomized trial and

found to provide comparable coverage with less renal toxicity but with more visual changes and hallucinations.[465] Voriconazole is seldom used empirically unless *Aspergillus* is highly suspected, such as in the case of prolonged febrile neutropenia with pulmonary lesions on imaging.

All patients undergoing AML therapy should receive prophylaxis against *Pneumocystis carinii* (now called *P. jirovecii*) pneumonia (PCP). The first-line agent in PCP prophylaxis is trimethoprim-sulfamethoxazole, but in some patients this is associated with significant allergic reaction or prolonged bone marrow suppression.[466-468] Dapsone is also effective as PCP prophylaxis in pediatric oncology patients but is associated with significant hemolysis and methemoglobinemia in some patients.[469] Atovaquone has been shown to be highly effective as PCP prophylaxis for pediatric leukemia patients, although it may be associated with gastrointestinal side effects, including pancreatitis.[470] Aerosolized pentamidine has also been shown to be effective as PCP prophylaxis in children with leukemia, although it may be associated with significant bronchospasm and can only be administered to children old enough to comply with the inhalational administration (usually >5 years).[471]

Viral infections can be a significant cause of morbidity and mortality in AML patients as well. CCG 2961 and COG AAML0531 advocate intravenous immune serum globulin (IVIG) administration for low IgG levels, and some centers also recommend respiratory syncytial virus (RSV) prophylaxis for infants. All blood products transfused should be leukoreduced and cytomegalovirus (CMV) negative whenever possible. Acyclovir may be required for patients with recurrent zoster or mucocutaneous herpes simplex.[472]

Growth factors, such as G-CSF and granulocyte-macrophage colony-stimulating factor (GM-CSF), have been used in the past, both as priming agents to synchronize the cell cycle before chemotherapy and as supportive care to decrease the duration of neutropenia after chemotherapy. Trials have shown that although G-CSF does shorten the duration of neutropenia its use does not lead to fewer episodes of febrile neutropenia, fewer microbiologically documented infections, less infection-related mortality, or improved OS.[425,473-476] Based on these data, most centers no longer advocate the routine use of growth factors as supportive care during AML therapy.

Bleeding Complications. Severe thrombocytopenia is not unusual in leukemia patients, and hemorrhage is one of the leading causes of early mortality in these patients.[477-479] AML patients who present with bleeding and thrombocytopenia should be treated with platelet transfusions. In patients who are thrombocytopenic but do not have active bleeding, concern still remains about spontaneous bleeding, particularly intracranial bleeding, which can be catastrophic and have irreversible sequelae. The level of thrombocytopenia that warrants prophylactic platelet transfusion to prevent bleeding, however, is controversial. Some early observations suggested that platelet counts less than 20,000/μL predispose to increased bleeding, and that number became a standard threshold for transfusion.[480] However, this was primarily in patients also receiving aspirin therapy, and subsequent studies have shown spontaneous bleeding occurs at a similar rate with platelet counts of less than 10,000 or 20,000/μL; and many centers have adopted 10,000/μL as the new threshold for transfusion.[481-487] The threshold for platelet transfusion in patients undergoing procedures such as line placement or lumbar puncture has also not been well studied, and the accepted standard threshold of 50,000/μL may be higher than necessary.[480,488] All blood products should be leukoreduced or CMV negative to prevent CMV infection, and irradiated to prevent transfusion-related GVHD.[489-491] Menstruating women may require hormonal menstrual suppression for the duration of therapy with expected platelet drops to less than 50,000/μL.

Patients with AML, particularly APL, may also present with DIC, and coagulation studies should be a routine part of the initial workup in a patient with AML.[492,493] In APL, overexpression of one of the plasminogen receptors, annexin A2, has traditionally been implicated as the cause of increased production of the fibrinolytic protein plasmin, which may be part of the cause of DIC in these patients.[494] However, recent in vitro studies performed in APL cell lines suggest that, in fact, a different plasminogen receptor, S100A10 (also known as p11), may actually be the culprit. Levels of S100A10 increased concomitantly with *PML-RARA* induction, and targeted inhibition of SA100A10 expression resulted in decreased fibrinolytic activity.[495] Patients whose leukemic cells are successfully treated will exhibit resolution of DIC with the reduction in blast cells but, while the blast count is decreasing, DIC should be treated with fresh-frozen plasma, cryoprecipitate, or recombinant factor VIIa as needed to prevent bleeding. For patients with APL, the initiation of ATRA before chemotherapy leads to rapid resolution of DIC and has markedly reduced the early mortality previously associated with APL.[338-340,496] Since the development of ATRA, patients with APL are no longer routinely treated with low-dose heparin to prevent DIC.[335,336]

Complications of Hyperleukocytosis. Patients with AML, particularly those with high presenting leukocyte counts, have an increased risk for tumor lysis syndrome. In patients with leukemia, the rate of blast cell turnover can exceed the body's ability to metabolize and excrete the contents of dying cells, leading to life-threatening metabolic derangements.[497] Hyperuricemia resulting from the metabolism of excessive amounts of released nucleic acids can cause renal failure. The ensuing hyperkalemia may lead to fatal cardiac arrhythmias, and hyperphosphatemia and hypocalcemia may cause seizures and worsen the renal failure. Elevated blood urea nitrogen levels cause platelet dysfunction, which may exacerbate an existing coagulopathy. Vigorous intravenous hydration and administration of bicarbonate and other agents, such as allopurinol or recombinant urate oxidase (rasburicase), should be started immediately to decrease formation and increase the solubility and renal excretion of insoluble urate.[498-500] Recombinant urate oxidase can

dramatically decrease uric acid levels within a few hours but, in patients with G6PD deficiency, it can cause methemoglobinemia and life-threatening hemolysis.[501,502]

Patients with WBC counts higher than 100,000/μL have an increased risk for leukostasis. Leukostasis causes intravascular clumping of blasts, leading to sluggish blood flow and subsequent hypoxia, hemorrhage, and infarction of tissue.[331,332,341,342,503] Leukostasis can be life threatening when it occurs in the organs at greatest risk, the brain and lungs. Patients with pulmonary leukostasis present with significant hypoxia and tachypnea, which may progress rapidly to respiratory failure. CNS leukostasis may produce symptoms of confusion, headache, and somnolence and can lead to coma, stroke, and death. Hydration and hydroxyurea are therapies that can be initiated immediately to decrease the blast count. Leukapheresis or exchange transfusion can reduce the number of circulating blasts quickly, although this effect is transient, and therapy with cytoreductive drugs should be started as soon as possible.[503] Routine pheresis for patients with a WBC count higher than 100,000/μL has resulted in lower mortality rates during induction compared with historic controls. In one study, patients who achieved a higher than 30% decrease in total WBCs through pheresis had a higher CR rate than those who achieved less than a 30% decrease.[341,504,505] Other retrospective reviews have shown a decrease in early mortality after leukapheresis but not an improvement in OS. Cytoreductive chemotherapy should be initiated as rapidly as possible because other measures to reduce leukemic blast numbers have only temporary effectiveness.[506,507]

Chemotherapy Complications. High-dose cytarabine is associated with chemical conjunctivitis, and dexamethasone or prednisolone eye drops were traditionally used to prevent this side effect.[508,509] However, recently owing to the unavailability of this steroid formulation, artificial tear products have been effectively substituted. High-dose cytarabine is also associated with neurotoxicity, including seizures and cerebellar dysfunction, which may not be reversible.[510-512] Patients should be monitored with frequent neurologic examinations, and high-dose cytarabine should be immediately discontinued if cerebellar signs develop. Cytarabine may also be associated with an impressive febrile response, which is difficult to distinguish from an infection-related fever.[513,514] AML chemotherapy is associated with significant nausea and vomiting, and aggressive antiemetic regimens should be instituted. However, because of the high risk for fungal infection in these patients, dexamethasone should be avoided as an antiemetic.[515-517] Mucositis is a significant toxicity during AML therapy, predominantly due to anthracyclines, and almost all patients require parenteral pain medication and nutrition. Malnutrition at the time of diagnosis appears to carry a worse prognosis in children with leukemia and, even in those who are well-nourished at diagnosis, weight loss during chemotherapy should be monitored closely, followed by the initiation of parenteral or enteral feedings in those who lose more than 10% of their initial body weight.[518]

Renal toxicity during AML therapy is common and may be caused by a combination of chemotherapy, tumor lysis syndrome, sepsis, or treatment with antibacterial, antifungal, and antiviral agents. A creatinine clearance or glomerular filtration rate should be checked in patients with abnormal creatinine clearance or prolonged use of medications with renal toxicity. For patients with a creatinine clearance lower than 60 mL/min/1.73 m^2, high-dose cytarabine, etoposide, and other renally cleared chemotherapy agents are usually given at reduced dosages. Significant liver toxicity can also be observed during therapy for AML, particularly for regimens containing the humanized anti-CD33 monoclonal antibody, GMTZ. GMTZ has been associated with sinusoidal obstructive syndrome and veno-occlusive disease, most commonly when used as a component of combination therapy or in patients who are heavily pretreated or who have undergone prior HSCT or undergo subsequent HSCT within 3 months of treatment with GMTZ.[519]

AML regimens rely heavily on anthracyclines and their derivatives. The cumulative anthracycline dose in these regimens is often 300 mg/m^2 or higher in daunorubicin equivalents and therefore carries a high risk for cardiac toxicity. Cardiac deaths are one of the top three causes of death in remission for AML patients.[385,425] All patients should undergo cardiac assessment before administration of chemotherapy cycles containing anthracyclines and yearly after chemotherapy is complete, until growth is completed in adulthood. However, recent pharmacogenomic studies suggest that certain genotypes, such as the rs7853758 variant within the SLC28A3 solute transporter, may particularly predispose children to developing anthracycline-induced cardiotoxicity.[520,521] In vitro evidence has suggested that the cardioprotectant dexrazoxane works synergistically, not antagonistically, with anthracyclines against AML blasts, and there is increasing interest in incorporating this medication into AML clinical trials.[522-524] On the current COG AML trial, use of dexrazoxane is permitted at the discretion of the treating physician and data will be collected to determine the impact on both cardiac outcome and secondary malignancy.

Extramedullary Disease

Between 20% and 40% of children with AML have evidence of extramedullary disease at the time of diagnosis.[350,353] The most common manifestations of extramedullary disease are skin infiltrates, soft tissue or bone involvement, gingival infiltration, and CNS involvement. Some patients, particularly infants, may have isolated extramedullary leukemia without other evidence of disease, but bone marrow infiltration invariably occurs in these patients without systemic therapy.

CNS Involvement. CNS involvement is more common in AML patients with high presenting WBC counts, favorable cytogenetic changes—t(9;11), t(8;21), and inv(16)—and children younger than 2 years.[346,420,525] One recent retrospective review of almost 1500 children enrolled on COG AML trials found an incidence of CNS disease (defined as CNS3 status >5 WBCs per high power field with the presence of blasts) of 11%.[526] AML patients with CNS disease at diagnosis have a higher risk for CNS relapse, but they often have a better overall prognosis because CNS disease is more common in the favorable-risk cytogenetic groups, which carry a lower risk for systemic relapse.[525,527] Specific CNS-directed therapy in AML may also be less important than in ALL because several AML chemotherapy agents, including high-dose cytarabine, have excellent CNS penetrance. Cranial radiation was previously used in AML patients as prophylaxis against CNS relapse, but because of concerns about the myriad side effects of CNS radiation, including secondary malignancy, endocrine and growth impairment, and neurocognitive toxicity, later trials attempted to minimize radiation.[528,529] In the BFM-87 study, all patients received intrathecal cytarabine, but the low-risk patients were randomized to additional therapy with cranial radiation or no further CNS treatment. An interim analysis demonstrated no increase in CNS relapse in the group that did not receive cranial radiation, so the radiation arm of the trial was closed early.[349] CNS radiation therapy is no longer routinely part of AML treatment protocols. Intrathecal chemotherapy with cytarabine alone, methotrexate alone, or triple intrathecal therapy with cytarabine, methotrexate, and hydrocortisone have been reported to be effective as CNS treatment and prophylaxis.[420,525,530,531] As prophylaxis for CNS-negative patients, COG study AAML0531 used intrathecal cytarabine alone at the start of each cycle, except for the Capizzi II cycle, which includes 3 g/m^2 of systemic cytarabine. For patients who had CNS disease at diagnosis, twice-weekly intrathecal therapy with cytarabine alone was used until the cerebrospinal fluid was clear, plus an additional two doses, with a minimum of four doses and a maximum of six doses. If more than six doses were required, the patient was taken off study for refractory CNS disease. These guidelines have been maintained on the current AAML1031 study. The SJCRH AML02 trial used a prophylaxis regimen of triple intrathecal chemotherapy with cytarabine, methotrexate, and hydrocortisone given at the start of each cycle but separated by at least 24 hours from systemic cytarabine dosages greater than or equal to 1 g/m^2 to prevent neurotoxicity. Patients with CNS disease at diagnosis receive once-weekly triple intrathecal chemotherapy for four doses. To decrease mucosal toxicity from the methotrexate, all patients receive leucovorin rescue at 24 and 30 hours after the intrathecal administration.

CNS relapse occurs in 2% to 8.8% of patients with AML.[409,420,532] Most AML patients who suffer a CNS relapse will simultaneously or soon thereafter develop a bone marrow relapse. Truly isolated CNS relapse is rare and is associated with age younger than 2 years, hepatosplenomegaly at diagnosis, elevated presenting WBC count, M5 AML, and chromosome 11 abnormalities.[527] For those with a truly isolated CNS relapse, the optimum treatment plan is unclear. There have been survivors reported after treatment with intrathecal chemotherapy alone, combined intrathecal and systemic chemotherapy, radiation therapy, and HSCT.[346,527]

Chloromas. Extramedullary infiltrations of the soft tissue, also known as chloromas, myelosarcomas, or granulocytic sarcomas, occur in 4% to 5% of children with AML.[344,350,533] They may also be documented in patients with CML, MDS, or rarely in ALL and may be initially confused with non-Hodgkin lymphoma.[534] Chloromas most often present simultaneously with AML or shortly before the systemic evidence of disease, but they may be isolated. The prognostic significance of extramedullary disease is not clear. Some groups have reported an unfavorable prognosis associated with chloromas,[382] but others have demonstrated a more favorable outcome.[407,532] Blast cells from patients with chloromas often exhibit the relatively favorable t(8;21).[353,354,535] Most studies from Europe, Saudi Arabia, Japan, and the United States have reported no influence of chloromas on the OS of children with AML,[343,350,382,387,409,536] and a recent review of four COG studies in fact demonstrated that children with orbital or CNS-based chloromas had significantly higher CR rates and OS compared with counterparts without chloromas treated on these same studies.[526] Accordingly, most centers treat patients who have chloromas with standard AML regimens, because there is no consistent evidence supporting more intensive therapy.[350] A beneficial role for radiation therapy in the treatment of chloromas has not been demonstrated.[536] In a CCG trial, patients with chloromas were treated with local irradiation in addition to systemic therapy. There was no difference in EFS or in the incidence of local recurrence compared with the chemotherapy-only regimen. However, chloromas arising in the orbit or CNS may cause loss of vision or cord compression, and emergency radiation therapy as well as chemotherapy is indicated in these situations.[536]

Prognosis

Although historically based exclusively on morphologic subtype, the ability to predict prognosis for patients with AML in the current genomic era derives from a composite of cytogenetic features, molecular subtype, and response to initial chemotherapy as evaluated by MRD. The recent integration of these features on the background of more intensive therapy with better supportive care has enabled a gradual improvement in pediatric AML outcome (Fig. 51-6). Classically, FAB subtype M0, which commonly harbors a complex karyotype, abnormalities of 5 or 7, or trisomy 8, is associated with a poor prognosis.[537] M7 AML (non–Down syndrome), often associated with monosomy 7, carries a poor prognosis.[538-542] M3 AML with the t(15;17) a group previously associated with a dismal prognosis, has emerged as a highly favorable subtype owing to responses with the addition of ATRA and As$_2$O$_3$ to chemotherapy regimens.[543-548] Similarly, CBF AML with t(8;21) or inv(16) and normal karyotype AML with either an isolated *CEBPA* or *NPM1* mutations are favorable subtypes.[403,549-551,552] By contrast, *FLT3*-ITD mutations with high allelic ratios are associated with a poor prognosis, as are patients without good risk molecular features who have significant residual MRD after induction therapy.[401-403,553]

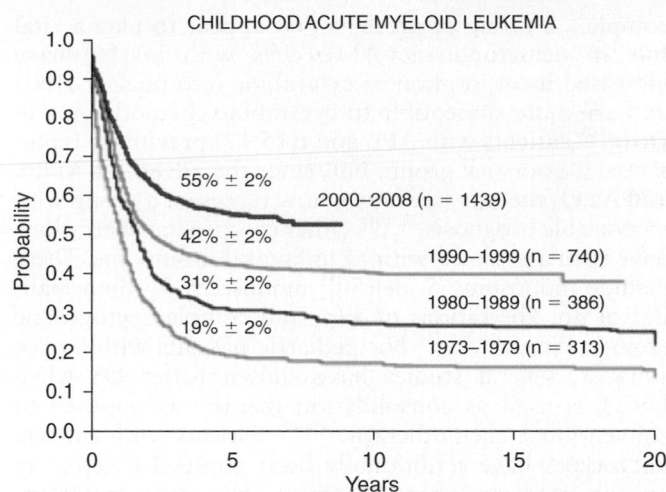

Figure 51-6 Overall survival for pediatric acute myeloid leukemia from 1973 to 2008. *(Modified from Rubnitz J, Inaba H: Childhood acute myeloid leukemia.* Br J Haematol 159:259–287, 2012.)

Demographic Risk Factors

Age older than 10 years was historically reported to carry a worse prognosis in clinical trials at SJRCH, as well as from the BFM and Japanese groups.[554-556] However, a recent report from the SJCRH AML02 study demonstrated comparable EFS and OS in children as old as age 21 years as in their younger counterparts, although these older children had higher toxic death rates predominantly of infectious etiology.[557] Race and ethnicity play a role in prognosis as well. Patients on CCG2891 who received chemotherapy alone had an OS of 48% for white children versus only 37% for Hispanic children (*P* = .016) and 34% for black children (*P* = .007).[558] On the SJCRH AML97, there was a trend toward inferior outcomes for black compared with white children (hazard ratio, 1.61; 95% confidence interval, 0.76 to 3.42; *P* = .22 with 5-year survival rates of 55.6% vs. 27.3%).[559] In these trials, there was no difference in other prognostic variables between the groups and these patients were hospitalized and received intravenous chemotherapy, received the same supportive care, and had the same compliance rates. Therefore, the observed differences may be attributable to pharmacogenomic differences that affect response to and toxicity from chemotherapy.[538,558] Patients who are overweight (body mass index ≥95th percentile) or underweight (≤10th percentile) also carry a worse prognosis and are less likely to survive and more likely to suffer treatment-related mortality.[560,561]

Cytogenetic Factors

Results of several large multicenter trials have confirmed the correlation between certain cytogenetic abnormalities and clinical outcome and have shown that karyotype in AML represents an independent prognostic variable for attainment of complete response and OS.[310,312,313,316,562] In children and adults, the highest complete response rates and longest survival times have been linked to association with t(8;21) and inv(16) or t(16;16).[403,549-552] These translocations result in modifications to the core-binding complex, a group of proteins that appear to play a vital role in hematopoiesis. AML cells with inv(16) have increased incorporation of cytarabine into nuclear DNA and are more susceptible to cytarabine chemotherapy in vitro.[563] Patients with APL and t(15;17) previously represented a poor-risk group, but, since the advent of ATRA and As$_2$O$_3$ therapy (see later), now represent a group with a favorable prognosis.[543-548] Other cytogenetic aberrations have been associated with an unfavorable outcome. These include monosomy 5, del(5q), monosomy 7, abnormalities of 3q, aberrations of 12p, and complex cytogenetic abnormalities.[310,315,564] For pediatric patients with monosomy 7, several studies have shown better OS when HSCT is used as consolidation therapy as opposed to conventional chemotherapy.[541-542] Patients with normal karyotypes have traditionally been grouped together in an intermediate-prognosis group, but now mutations such as the FLT3-ITD (poor prognosis) and NPM1 and CEBPA (good prognosis) have been demonstrated to alter prognosis sufficiently to influence the risk assignment of these patients at diagnosis on COG, SJCRH, BFM, and MRC trials. Abnormal karyotypes linked with an intermediate prognosis include del(7q), 11q23 translocations, +21, +8, +22, and del(9q).[310,565] Other karyotypes such as t(6;9)(p23;q34), t(8;16)(p11;p13), and t(16;21)(q24;q22) are uncommon but appear associated with a poorer prognosis.[557,566-568] While more studies with large numbers of patients undergoing cytogenetic evaluation are completed, certain groups of karyotype aberrations are showing heterogeneity in their prognostic significance. For example, all 11q23 translocations were previously grouped together in the intermediate- to poor-prognosis category. However, studies have shown that the 11q23 aberration may be subdivided into groups of lesser and greater prognostic risk.[569] Patients with the t(9;11) (p22;q23) have been found in some studies to have a longer EFS and OS than patients with other 11q23 translocations.[247,312,314,315,565,562] However, this was not found to be true in a recent review of outcome on MRC10 and 12 trials.[366] As new therapeutic agents are developed that target the specific molecular aberrations identified by cytogenetic analysis, accurate detection of these abnormalities becomes even more important.[565]

Molecular Genetic Factors

Analysis of molecular genetics is emerging as an invaluable tool in prognostic determination for patients with AML, as well as for providing insight into the pathogenesis of AML and elucidating possibilities for targeted therapy.[136] RAS mutations have been identified in pediatric AML patients, with NRAS mutations in 10% to 15% and KRAS mutations in 3% of patients.[570] HRAS mutations are rare in AML. In both adults and children these mutations are associated with favorable-risk AML. In adults, the association is with CBF leukemias and, in particular, inv(16).[570,571] Although some pediatric studies have also found a link between CBF AML and NRAS mutations,[570,571] others have found a distinct absence of NRAS with inv(16) and a unique correlation of NRAS and NPM mutations not seen in adult AML.[157] Independently, however, NRAS mutations have no significant

impact on prognosis.[153,572,570,573-576] Patients had similar 5-year EFS and OS, although patients with NRAS mutations were associated with increased treatment-related mortality on one study.[157] KIT mutations have been identified in 11.3% of pediatric AML patients,[570] predominantly in the CBF leukemias, ranging from 17% to 41% of patients.[178,577-580] The role of KIT mutations in prognosis has been unclear: in some series, the KIT mutations do not seem to have prognostic significance, in others, KIT mutations have been shown to confer worse prognosis in patients with t(8;21) but not in patients with inv(16) and, in still other trials, KIT mutations confer a worse prognosis in all subsets of CBF leukemias.[570,571,581,582] However, a recent review of more than 200 children with CBF AML enrolled on four COG AML trials concluded that KIT mutations do not alter prognosis.[178] Owing to their good outcome with chemotherapy alone, patients with CBF AML are currently nonrandomly assigned to chemotherapy without HSCT in CR1 even if a matched family donor is available. Based on these recent data, on current COG trials the presence of a KIT mutation does not alter risk stratification. This is in contrast to adult data which show that KIT mutations appear to confer an inferior outcome.[583-585] These prognostic differences in adult versus pediatric CBF AML may reflect more aggressive therapy in children and, potentially, an earlier cell of origin in the adult disease that contributes to increased resistance to therapy.

As noted, FLT3 mutations include ITDs in the juxtamembrane domain and point mutations in the activation loop (ALM). FLT3-ITDs have a worse prognosis, particularly when present in a high allelic ratio (>0.4),[174,586,587-590] whereas FLT3-ALMs seem to have no impact on prognosis.[174,586,589] Partial tandem duplications of the MLL gene have also been reported in 13% of pediatric AML patients and are associated with a worse prognosis in adult and pediatric patients.[228,586,591,592] Frameshift mutations in NPM1 lead to cytoplasmic localization of nucleophosmin and have been identified in 6% to 8% of all children with AML and 25% to 30% of pediatric AML patients with normal cytogenetics.[277,278] When identified as an isolated mutation in adults and children, it is associated with improved prognosis, but when found in conjunction with an FLT3-ITD, the poor prognostic impact of the FLT-ITD prevails.[277,278,593-595] With contemporary chemotherapy, children with AML with a normal karyotype and isolated NPM1 mutation have outcomes in keeping with CBF leukemia with OS greater than 80%; thus these children have been assigned to the low-risk arm on the current COG trial[557] (R. Aplenc, personal communication, June 2011). PTPN11 mutations are found in only 4% of pediatric patients with AML (4%), and 18% to 36% of the PTPN11 mutations are seen in M5 AML. In pediatrics, this mutation does not appear to have prognostic importance.[142,596] The Wilms tumor gene (WT1) is aberrantly expressed in AML; in adults, high expression levels of WT1 at diagnosis have been associated with a poor prognosis in many studies.[597-602] In pediatric patients, however, the available data have been contradictory. One small study of 47 patients has shown that low levels of WT1 at diagnosis are associated with good outcome,[603] whereas another small study of 41 patients has shown that high levels of WT1 are more commonly seen in association with the t(8;21) and inv(16) favorable prognosis cytogenetic findings, and therefore associated with a better prognosis.[604] Hollink and colleagues found an association between WT1 mutations and an inferior outcome.[282] More recently, a large study performed by the COG identifying 70 patients with WT1 mutations found that although there was significant overlap of the WT1 mutation with either CBF or FLT3-ITD, independently, WT1 mutations did not influence prognosis.[281] Interestingly, 28% of pediatric AML patients harbor a minor single nucleotide polymorphism (SNP) in exon 7 of WT1 (rs16754) that was found to result in an improved 5-year OS (62% vs. 44%) for patients treated on CCG 2961 compared with those with leukemic expression of the major WT1 allele.[289] Levels of expression of wild-type WT1 may also influence prognosis. However, at present, WT1 mutational status, presence of the minor SNP, and wild-type expression levels continue to be studied but are not being used to make treatment decisions. In addition to its role as a partner in the t(8;21) translocation, RUNX1 may also be mutated in approximately 5% of pediatric AML patients, specifically with point mutations in exons 3 and 8. Although typically associated with AML secondary to MDS, in de novo AML these patients had less organomegaly, a higher incidence of chloromas, and a trend toward improved outcome with modern intensive AML therapy.[605] However, RUNX1 mutations are not currently used for risk stratification.

CEBPA mutations have been found to be an independent prognostic marker conferring a good outcome in both pediatric and adult AML and, similar to that seen for CBF AML, at least in children.[279] Interestingly, pediatric patients with AML and CEBPA mutations tend to be older (age >10 years) and predominantly have a normal karyotype with an absence of other good- or poor-risk molecular abnormalities. Furthermore, patients with CEBPA mutations did not benefit from HSCT in first remission. Thus, in current studies, presence of a CEBPA mutation classifies a patient as low risk. Recent next-generation sequencing–based studies have revealed frequent mutations in the DNA methyltransferase gene, DNMT3A, the gene coding for the demethylating enzyme, TET2, and the genes IDH1 and IDH2, which code for proteins in the Krebs cycle. DNMT3A mutations are generally associated with a poor outcome and contribute to a worse prognosis when combined with FLT3 ITD. TET2 mutations are similarly associated with a poor prognosis, with or without corresponding FLT3 abnormalities. By contrast, IDH1/IDH2 mutations appear to be more positive prognostic features.[606,607] However, these abnormalities are generally rare in pediatric AML[608]; thus their impact cannot be easily determined, and at this time they have been excluded from any current pediatric AML risk stratification schemas.

Minimal Residual Disease

Early response to treatment, as assessed by MRD in the bone marrow and/or the peripheral blood after induction therapy, has been shown to be an independent and powerful prognostic factor in pediatric leukemia. MRD can be detected by molecular means such as PCR assay, which is beneficial for the monitoring of leukemias with fusion genes or recurrent mutations. Alternatively, the use of multiparameter flow cytometry (MPFC) is more universally applicable, but it may be user dependent and vary significantly based on technical aspects, threshold levels, and timing of evaluation.

PCR-based MRD evaluation requires that a cytogenetic abnormality or mutation present at diagnosis will be predictive of relapse or refractory disease. In CBF AML, persistence of the AML1-ETO t(8;21) or CBFB-MYH11 inv(16) transcripts long after completion of therapy has challenged the value of following these lesions either during or after completion of therapy.[557,609] However, a recent adult study[610] has suggested that at least in AML with inv(16), PCR analysis may have more predictive power. Negative bone marrow results of PCR assay for the CBFB-MYH11 transcript (<10 detectable copies per cell) early in consolidation with two subsequent negative PCR evaluations either in the bone marrow or peripheral blood later in consolidation and within 3 months of completing therapy were highly predictive of remaining in CR, with a high correlation between bone marrow and peripheral blood measurements during surveillance. In APL and CML (see later), levels of PML-RARA or BCR-ABL transcripts have been found to be extremely valuable for monitoring, although the site of monitoring has been somewhat controversial. Standardized monitoring for BCR-ABL levels in the peripheral blood is now accepted as the standard of care in CML, whereas the recently closed COG trial in APL has mandated bone marrow evaluations during maintenance and subsequent follow-up. A number of adult and pediatric studies have examined following FLT3, CEBPA, NPM1, MLL rearrangements/PTDs, or WT1 mutations in those patients harboring these abnormalities at diagnosis.[609,611-617] However, the utility of any of these mutations as a molecular MRD marker remains uncertain owing to stability of the mutation (FLT3-ITD) or normal background levels (WT1). Thus, although their presence at diagnosis may be indicative of response, persistence of these lesions is not being routinely used to evaluate disease response in pediatric AML.

By contrast, use of MRD by MPFC has proven to be a more broadly applicable component of risk stratification in both pediatric ALL[618] and AML.[403,404,619] Particularly in the large subset of intermediate-risk AML, MRD has allowed the distinction of standard- and high-risk groups, whereas the use of morphology alone proved insufficient.[355] The ability of MPFC MRD measurement to contribute to the evaluation of early treatment response and improve prognostic evaluation in pediatric AML was demonstrated for CCG 2961. OS for patients in morphologic remission after induction I was 41% if MRD was positive, compared with 69% for those who were MRD negative.[404] A strong impact of MRD was also apparent in AML patients who were in morphologic remission at the end of induction I on the recent AAML03P1 study. The 46 MRD-positive patients of the 188 patients deemed

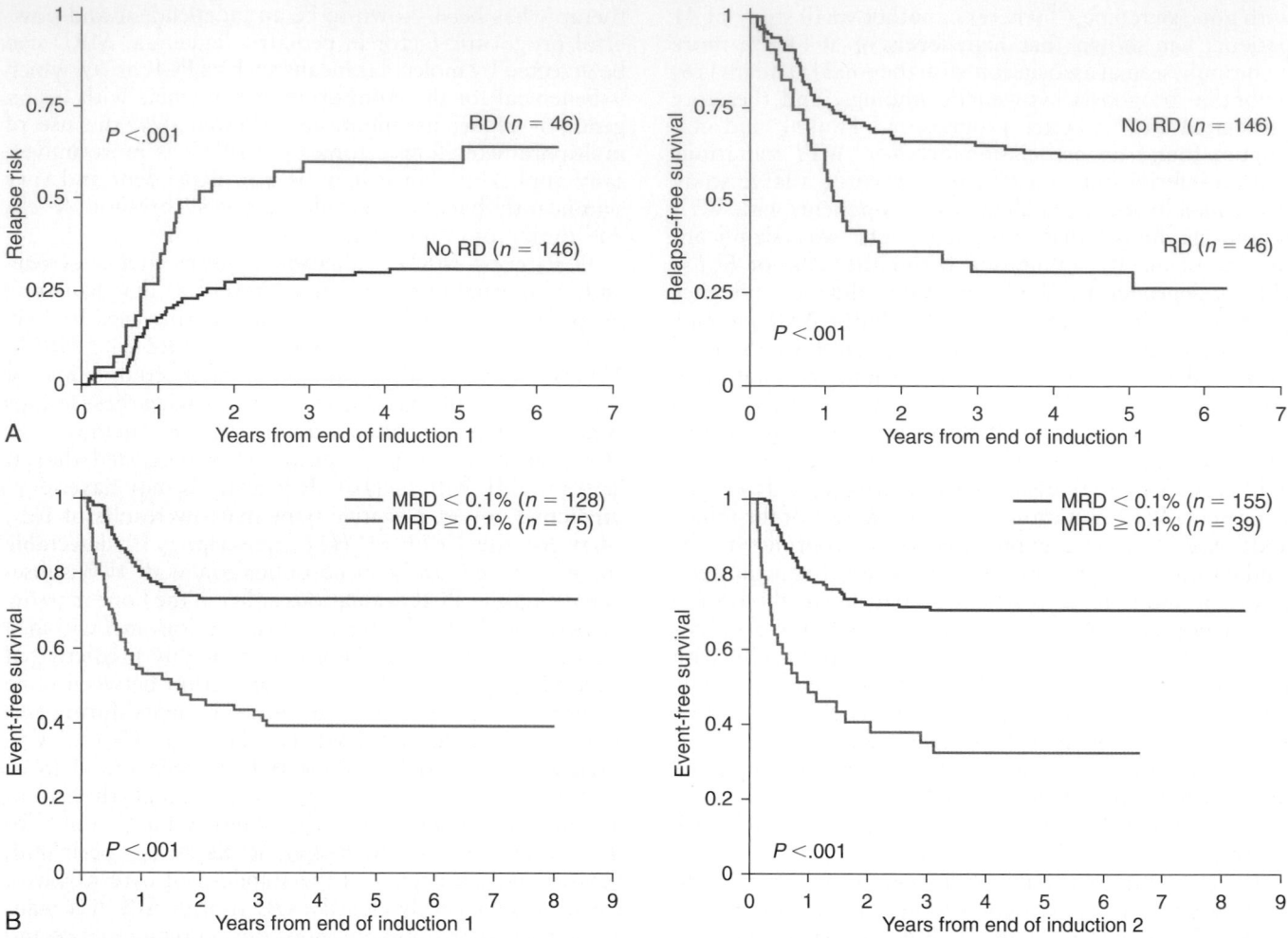

Figure 51-7 A, Minimal residual disease *(MRD)* by multiparameter flow cytometry (MPFC) can predict outcome for children with acute myeloid leukemia found to be in morphologic remission *(RD,* residual disease detected by MPFC). **B,** MRD levels less than 0.1% appear most predictive of event-free survival after induction therapy. *(Modified from Loken MR, Alonzo TA, Pardo L, et al: Residual disease detected by multidimensional flow cytometry signifies high relapse risk in patients with de novo acute myeloid leukemia: a report from the Children's Oncology Group. Blood 120:1581–1588, 2012; and Inaba H, Coustan-Smith E, Cao X, et al: Comparative analysis of different approaches to measure treatment responses in acute myeloid leukemia. J Clin Oncol 30:3625–3632, 2012.)*

in CR showed an increase in relapse risk (RR) at 3 years (60%, *P* <.001) and lower DFS (30%, *P* <.001) and OS (56%, *P* = .002) compared with those who were MRD negative (3-year RR, 29%; DFS, 65%; OS, 80%) (Fig. 51-7, *A*).[355] Not only did this study demonstrate the adverse prognostic value of positive MRD compared with morphology alone but, conversely, showed that 26% of patients deemed as having disease based on morphologic bone marrow evaluation were in fact MRD negative and had a good outcome.[355] Similar findings were identified by the SJCRH, confirming that recovering normal marrow blasts and leukemic myeloblasts can be challenging to distinguish morphologically even by the most experienced hematopathologist.[609] Multivariate analyses on COG and SJCRH studies confirmed positive MRD as an independent adverse prognostic factor, although the SJCRH study found that this was only significant for MRD levels greater than 1% after induction I, or greater than 0.1% after induction II,[403] whereas this distinction was not specifically identified in the COG studies.

Subsequent analysis by the SJCRH demonstrated that an MRD threshold of 0.1% was independently predictive of outcome both after induction I and induction II (see Fig. 51-7, *B*).[609] The impact of MRD was independently confirmed in recent MRC and Dutch trials.[619] Furthermore, COG studies found that MRD levels held their prognostic significance in normal karyotype AML. Based on these data, the COG has used MRD by MPFC to eliminate the intermediate-risk group of patients without prognostic cytogenetic or molecular features. Those patients with residual MRD at a threshold of 0.1% after the first induction cycle are deemed at high risk and relegated to more intensive therapy, whereas those with MRD levels below 0.1% are allocated to a low-risk study arm.

Relapsed or Refractory Disease

The prognosis is grave for children with disease refractory to induction chemotherapy or who have a disease relapse. Although 80% to 90% of pediatric patients with AML will achieve remission, 30% to 40% will later recur, and the OS remains only 40% to 60%.[363,530,531,538,620-624] The bone marrow is the most common site of relapse in AML, and isolated CNS relapse is an uncommon finding, but isolated CNS relapse has been associated with prior CNS involvement.[386,527,625]

Prognosis in Relapsed or Refractory Disease

A durable remission is less likely to be achieved and maintained in patients with relapsed or refractory AML than in patients with newly diagnosed AML, but the salvage rate in these patients has improved in recent years.[538,624,626] The single most important prognostic indicator after relapse is duration of first remission, with less than 1 year to relapse carrying an OS rate of 0% to 21% and longer than 1 year to relapse carrying an OS rate of 33% to 62%.[386,539,624,627-631] Other characteristics that have been associated with better prognosis after relapse are male gender, good-risk cytogenetic features of t(8;21) and inv(16), chemotherapy alone without HSCT as consolidation during first CR, and the use of HSCT as part of relapse therapy. The characteristics associated with worse prognosis after relapse are early recurrence, M5 or M7 morphology, poor-risk cytogenetics, and HSCT during first CR.

Conventional Therapy for Relapsed or Refractory Disease

There is no accepted standard therapy for adult or pediatric patients with relapsed or refractory AML. However, several researchers have demonstrated activity of high-dose cytarabine in patients with relapsed disease, even in those who had been exposed to cytarabine during prior treatment.[632] High-dose cytarabine has been used in combination with other agents, such as mitoxantrone, asparaginase, etoposide, fludarabine, cladribine, and clofarabine.[628,633-638] The combination of cytarabine and mitoxantrone was particularly effective as reinduction with a remission rate of 76%, but now that this regimen has been incorporated into the current standard first-line regimens, its use as a reinduction regimen may provide too much cumulative anthracycline for many patients.[628] Fludarabine, cladribine, and clofarabine are all deoxyadenosine analogues that have been used for the treatment of AML. Trials using high-dose cytarabine in combination with fludarabine and G-CSF (i.e., the FLAG regimen) have demonstrated a 70% remission rate in patients with relapsed AML, and this regimen is frequently used by many centers for patients who have experienced a relapse of their disease.[639-641] The addition of idarubicin to the FLAG regimen has resulted in longer-lasting remissions in some studies, but it has also been associated with more significant toxicity and for this reason is not frequently incorporated.[642-645] The combination of cytarabine and cladribine has been successful as a relapse regimen in some trials for adult patients and pediatric patients with de novo AML, particularly those with the M5 subtype.[417,646-651] However, this combination seems to be of little benefit in pediatric patients with relapsed or refractory AML.[652] Clofarabine was found to be effective as a single agent in relapsed ALL and AML and was subsequently approved by the FDA for use in relapsed ALL.[636,653] Clofarabine has been shown to be safe and effective in combination with cytarabine in regimens for adult patients, and this combination has been tested for pediatric patients with relapsed or refractory AML.[637,638,654] The recently closed COG study AAML0523 examined the combination of clofarabine and cytarabine for relapsed AML and ALL and found that a dose of 52 mg/m^2 of clofarabine was tolerated by patients with relapsed AML. Of the 46 patients who were evaluable, only 21% responded as evaluated by complete response or complete response with incomplete platelet recovery, which did not meet the predetermined statistical threshold for efficacy in overall response rate.[655] Based on these findings, this regimen has somewhat fallen out of favor compared with FLAG. However, as a result of compliance issues and failure to recognize complete response with incomplete count recovery as evidence of response, results from this study may in fact underestimate the efficacy of this combination therapy; thus clofarabine and cytarabine for relapsed AML as a bridge to HSCT (see later) may still be worthy of consideration. For patients who cannot tolerate high-dose cytarabine or further anthracyclines, one alternative regimen that has been used at the Memorial Sloan-Kettering Cancer Center is topotecan, vinorelbine, thiotepa, dexamethasone, and gemcitabine (TVTG), with 5 of 9 AML patients responding to this therapy.[656]

Long-term remission for patients with relapsed or refractory disease requires consolidation therapy with allogeneic HSCT.[359,644] Traditionally, this has included matched family members or matched unrelated donors, but the more recent use of alternative HSC sources, such as banked umbilical cord blood or haploidentical family donors, has increased the number of patients with a potential marrow source. A recent trend has been in using non–total-body irradiation (TBI)–based conditioning regimens for AML in first remission due to equal efficacy and less toxicity, but TBI may still be used in the conditioning of patients with relapsed AML.[657,658] It is possible to cure patients who have persistent, refractory disease at the time of allogeneic HSCT, particularly if they have less than 20% blasts in the marrow. Those patients with shorter remissions and higher blast percentages in their marrow have traditionally been associated with only a 25% chance of cure,[659-664] whereas for patients who have had a long first remission and proceed to HSCT in a second CR the OS rates are much better and may be as high as 40% to 62%.[538,624,664] However, although lower levels of MRD were associated with improved overall outcomes, investigators at the SJCRH found that with contemporary risk-adapted therapeutic regimens, allogeneic HSCT may be curative for patients with AML who continue to be MRD positive or even have persistent marrow blasts, with 5-year OS of 67% and 58%, respectively.[665] This analysis included patients with relapsed AML. These findings are in contrast to the impact of residual disease in ALL, which may be attributed at least in part to the graft-versus-leukemia (GVL) in AML.[615,665] This effect is difficult to measure directly but has been indirectly inferred from the presence of GVHD. The presence of acute and chronic GVHD has been associated with lower relapse rates in AML.[666-672] Donor lymphocyte infusions have been used successfully to induce GVL effect in patients with CML who experience relapse after allogeneic HSCT, but this strategy is much less effective in patients with AML who experience relapse after allogeneic HSCT.[673,674]

There can be GVL effect without GVHD, however, as evidenced by lower relapse rates in patients receiving HSCT from a matched sibling versus an identical twin, even in the absence of GVHD.[675] There is much interest in maximizing the GVL effect, and recent studies have concentrated on the role of alloreactive natural killer (NK) cells in this process. Donors who are mismatched at the KIR ligand produce NK cells that recognize and destroy host AML cells in response to the lack of expression of a self class I ligand on the AML cells.[676-678] Deliberate KIR mismatching through haploidentical HSCT has been shown in small studies to decrease the relapse rate without increasing GVHD, therefore resulting in improved long-term survival. This strategy is being used in clinical trials for patients with high-risk de novo AML or relapsed and refractory disease and is currently incorporated into ongoing pediatric trials of the COG and SJCRH.[677,679] The feasibility of engrafting haploidentical NK cells in children with AML in remission was recently demonstrated.[679]

Novel Agents and Targeted Therapy

Conventional therapy for AML is predominantly a "shotgun" approach in which leukemia cells, as well as normal hematopoietic stem and progenitor cells and many other normal tissues, are injured, with the hope that the normal cells will recover faster and more completely than the leukemia cells. As discussed earlier, this approach has not resulted in superior cure rates in AML and the intensity has been increased to the point that most patients suffer toxicity and treatment-related morbidity; a substantial fraction of patients suffer treatment-related mortality. While the molecular pathogenesis of AML has been elucidated, opportunities have appeared for the development of novel and targeted agents that preferentially destroy leukemia cells, with far less significant effects on normal hematopoietic cells and other normal tissues.[680,681] However, preclinical and adult clinical data, not to mention drug availability, are in rapid flux, given the growing interest in developing novel targeted therapeutics. Thus current therapeutic platforms for relapsed AML are moving to the model of having a standardized backbone to which novel agents can be rapidly inserted to be sufficiently nimble to adapt to the availability and promise of emerging drugs.

Antibody Therapy with Gemtuzumab Ozogamicin. Gemtuzumab ozogamicin (GMTZ, also discussed earlier in the induction chemotherapy section) is a recombinant, humanized anti-CD33 monoclonal antibody linked to the tumor antibiotic calicheamicin. CD33 is expressed on most AML cells but not on pluripotent HSCs or other tissues, thus making it possible to target leukemia cells more specifically.[367,368] GMTZ has been used successfully as a single agent for adults and children in relapse, with infusional side effects of fever and chills, hematologic toxicity resulting from pancytopenia, including some cases of prolonged thrombocytopenia, and hepatic toxic-

ity ranging from transient liver function abnormalities to fatal venoocclusive disease, particularly when used within 3 months of HSCT.[519,682-689] GMTZ as a single agent is not a particularly strong reinduction regimen, but it has now been used successfully in combination with cytarabine-mitoxantrone and cytarabine-asparaginase as part of a reinduction regimen.[558,681,688,690-694] Given the data from the United Kingdom on the limited efficacy of GMTZ in initial adult AML therapy,[370,371] current and future availability of this agent may be very limited. GMTZ may have a role specifically in relapsed APL, however (see later).

Receptor Tyrosine Kinase Inhibitors. *FLT3* (discussed in detail earlier) is a receptor tyrosine kinase that is upregulated in the AML cells of most patients. There are also two types of activating mutations in *FLT3* and, in pediatric patients with AML, ITDs are present in 5% to 16% and ALMs are present in 2% to 5% of cases.[172-175] Several small-molecule inhibitors of the FLT3 tyrosine kinase have been developed, some of which are effective against only the ITDs and some of which are effective against both the ITDs and the ALMs.[695,696] These inhibitors are now in various phases of clinical trials. Overall, they appear to be well tolerated and to induce a decrease in blasts, but as single agents they generally do not result in durable remissions.[172-175,697] The COG completed a pilot study of lestaurtinib in relapsed AML. The drug was well tolerated, but inadequate FLT3 inhibitory plasma concentrations were achieved and the study was closed prior to dose escalation, owing to concerns regarding drug availability. Quizartinib is a tyrosine kinase inhibitor that has shown promise in relapsed adult AML with *FLT3*-ITD with clearance of marrow blasts but incomplete count recovery.[698-700] Rapid resistance to quizartinib is an emerging problem but suggests that the short-term benefits observed are bona fide therapeutic responses. A phase I study conducted by the Therapeutic Advances in Childhood Leukemia and Lymphoma (TACL) consortium demonstrated the tolerability of quizartinib together with cytarabine and etoposide in relapsed and refractory AML and ALL, with remissions both with and without count recovery in four patients, including three with AML and *FLT3*-ITD.[701] Sorafenib is another tyrosine kinase inhibitor that has had documented activity as both a single agent and with cytotoxic therapy in relapsed AML,[702] although several of the mutations that are resistant to quizartinib are also resistant to sorafenib. Sorafenib is currently being incorporated upfront for de novo AML patients with *FLT3*-ITD and high allelic ratio on COG study AAML1031 and SJCRH AML08. With the use of these agents as frontline therapy, it is uncertain whether they will play a significant role in relapsed disease. However, in cases in which a patient without a prior *FLT3*-ITD at diagnosis develops such a lesion at relapse, FLT3 inhibitors should be considered as part of the reinduction-remission strategy. Finally, ponatinib is another new tyrosine kinase inhibitor with activity against *FLT3*-ITD, including those with mutations resistant to other inhibitors, and an impressive response rate in refractory CML harboring resistant *ABL* mutations.[700,703]

This agent may have more broad potential in pediatric myeloid disease; however, the drug has recently been issued a Black Box warning by the FDA due to an association with life threatening thromboses.

Farnesyltransferase Inhibitors. Mutations in *RAS* itself, as well as perturbations in the RAS pathway, are associated with AML. The RAS protein requires isoprenylation by farnesyltransferase to bind to the plasma membrane properly and be fully active. Several farnesyltransferase inhibitors have been developed with the goal of inhibiting upregulated or dysregulated RAS activity. Because these drugs do not specifically target a known mutation in *RAS* and have effect on other proteins that also require farnesylation, they can be effective in patients with or without *RAS* mutations. Tipifarnib (R115777, Zarnestra) as an oral agent has shown activity in adult patients with refractory AML and in older adult patients with de novo AML, with a few transient complete responses, even when used as a single agent.[704-707] The drug was generally well tolerated with toxicities of myelosuppression, neurotoxicity, and reversible renal toxicity.[704,706] In pediatrics, a phase I trial of tipifarnib for refractory solid tumors and neurofibromatosis type 1–related plexiform neurofibromas and a phase II trial for brain tumors both have shown that the drug was tolerated well overall, with dose-limiting toxicities of myelosuppression, rash, nausea, and vomiting; one patient also developed a seizure.[708,709] A phase I trial in patients with refractory leukemia was completed by COG in 2005. The drug has also been used safely in combination with capecitabine for children with advanced solid tumors. Currently, trials are ongoing combining tipifarnib with chemotherapy for adults with AML as well as a COG trial combining tipifarnib with *cis*-retinoic acid, cytarabine, and fludarabine with HSCT for children with JMML.[710] Two other farnesyltransferase inhibitors, lonafarnib (Sarasar, SCH66336) and BMS-214662 have also shown some promise in adults with myeloid disorders, but there are as yet no data for pediatric AML.[711]

Histone Deacetylase Inhibitors. Double-stranded DNA binds to histones to form compact nucleosomes when the DNA is not being actively transcribed. Acetylation of lysine residues by histone acetyltransferases allows the release of DNA from histones for transcription. Deacetylation by histone deacetylase (HDAC) reverses the process. Inappropriate recruitment of HDACs leading to gene silencing has been demonstrated in the CBF leukemic cells bearing translocations t(8;21) and inv(16), as well as in APL cells bearing t(15;17).[712-717] The use of HDAC inhibitors may allow for renewed expression of silenced genes that when activated can induce differentiation or cell death.[718,719] Several HDAC inhibitors have been tested in clinical trials in AML patients, including the antiseizure medication valproic acid. It has been used in clinical trials for adults with MDS or AML as monotherapy and in combination with ATRA, 5-aza-2'-deoxycytidine (DAC), as well as 5-azacytidine and ATRA together.[680,720,721] It was generally well tolerated, with toxicities of myelosuppression, neurotoxicity, and sedation. Some transient responses were seen, even when valproic acid was used

as monotherapy, but it was most effective when used in combination with ATRA and 5-azacytidine.[680,720,721] A more potent HDAC, depsipeptide, has been used in clinical trials and has had more toxicity, including fatigue, nausea, and constitutional symptoms. In these trials, it has shown some promise in T-cell lymphoma but thus far only modest antileukemia activity.[722,723] Vorinostat (suberoylanilide hydroxamic acid [SAHA]) is an HDAC inhibitor that has been under discussion for incorporation in pediatric relapse or refractory AML studies. Romidepsin is a newer HDAC inhibitor also under consideration (T. Cooper, personal communication, May 2013). HDAC inhibitors and DNA methyltransferase inhibitors as combination therapy are also being evaluated. In some trials this seems to be a safe and effective strategy,[724] but in at least one trial using decitabine and valproic acid the combination did not show an improved response rate versus decitabine alone and proved too toxic because of encephalopathy.[725] However, this approach may prove more fruitful in the combination of novel HDAC inhibitors and DNA methyltransferase inhibitors with less overlapping toxicities and in subsets of AML patients found to have particularly high levels of methylation and activity of methyl transferase enzymes. In particular, these therapeutic strategies may be specifically applicable for adult patients harboring *DNMT3A* and *TET2* mutations and *MLL* rearrangements in pediatric AML.

Apoptosis Inhibitors. BCL2 is an inhibitor of apoptosis that is highly expressed in some patients with AML and is associated with a poor prognosis.[726-728] A BCL2 antisense oligonucleotide has been tested as a single agent and shown to induce transient remission in some AML patients.[729] It has also been shown to be safe and effective in combination with cytarabine and daunorubicin.[730] This agent is now being used in clinical trials of AML through the Cancer and Leukemia Group B (CALGB) as part of combination therapy during induction and consolidation.[681] Specifically, a trial combining the pan-BCL2 inhibitor obatoclax with vincristine, doxorubicin, and dexrazoxane for relapsed solid tumors and leukemias has just been completed by the COG and results are pending.

Other Targeted Therapies. A number of new promising agents are emerging and being considered for introduction into relapsed AML trials. Some of these agents target recently emerging important molecular pathways in AML cells such as MK2206, which targets the PI3K-AKT pathway, or MK8776, which is a CHK1 inhibitor. AKT pathway activation may contribute to resistance to GMTZ[731] and may be particularly active in AML associated with Down syndrome[732] (see later). Phase I studies of MK2206 have been completed in adults, and a pediatric trial has just been completed. CHK1, or checkpoint kinase 1, regulates the G2 to M phase transition of the cell cycle and may be activated in the phase of DNA damage in AML cells.[733] CHK1-inhibiting agents have been evaluated in a number of adult phase I solid tumor studies[734] and may have efficacy in AML, particularly in children harboring complex karyotypes associated with the highest levels of DNA damage and CHK1 activity.[733]

CHK1 has been shown to suppress apoptosis mediated by caspase 2 in the context of DNA damage, and inhibition of CHK1 may restore apoptosis in AMLs with *TP53* mutations.[735] Another strategy is to interfere with the interaction of AML cells and their microenvironment through the use of drugs such as plerixafor. Plerixafor binds to and antagonizes the interaction of CXCL12 (also known as SDF1) and its receptor CXCR4 found on HSCs and potentially on LICs, affecting LIC mobilization from the stem cell niche and making these cells more accessible to cytotoxic chemotherapies. Thus this agent is believed to target the AML LIC and make these resistant cells more susceptible to conventional therapies. A recent phase I/II adult trial gave plerixafor prior to cytarabine, etoposide, and mitoxantrone for patients with relapsed AML and found that this combination was well tolerated and resulted in approximately 50% complete remission rates.[736]

ACUTE PROMYELOCYTIC LEUKEMIA

Pathobiology

APL or M3 AML is a subtype of AML defined by a specific morphology, a balanced translocation involving the *RARA* gene, and a characteristic coagulopathy.[173,283,737,738] Although most patients with APL have the classic t(15;17) resulting in the *PML-RARA* fusion gene, up to 8% do not. Approximately 5% of patients have a *PML-RARA* because of an insertion or other variant, 1% of patients have a t(11;17) resulting in a *PLZF-RARA*, another 1% have a t(5;17) resulting in an *NPM-RARA* or a t(11;17) resulting in a *NuMA-RARA* or a *STAT5b-RARA*, and 1% of patients do not have an identifiable *RARA* rearrangement.[739] APL provides a clear example of the classic two-hit model for AML (see earlier, "Molecular Genetics").[138] The fusion protein resulting from the pathognomonic translocation in APL, the PML-RARA protein, is an example of a class II mutation, resulting in a block in differentiation. As detailed earlier (see "Biology"), this protein has been shown to interfere with normal myeloid cell development through dominant inhibitory mechanisms as a potent transcriptional repressor that recruits a number of other corepressors to cause differentiation arrest at the promyelocyte stage.[211,740-743] Mutations in the receptor tyrosine kinase *FLT3* occur in up to 43% of cases of APL, and these mutations are classic examples of class I mutations, conferring a proliferative advantage.[744,745] At diagnosis, APL patients with *FLT3* mutations more often present with hyperleukocytosis, microgranular variant morphology, and the bcr3 PML breakpoint.[165,744-749] Although *FLT3*-ITDs clearly confer a worse prognosis in other subtypes of AML, their role in prognosis for APL is less clear. Some groups have reported a worse prognosis for APL patients with an *FLT3*-ITD, whereas other groups have found no statistically significant impact on the generally favorable risk outcome of this disease.[744,745,749-751] A recent report from the COG found *FLT3*-ITD or ALM mutations in 40% of children treated on the CALGB 9710 study and identified a strong correlation with higher WBC count and induction death rates in the *FLT3* mutant subgroup.[401]

Clinical Presentation and Risk Factors

APL is more common in girls and obese children, and obesity is associated with a higher rate of relapse and differentiation syndrome (see later).[561,752] Compared with adults, children with APL have a higher incidence of hyperleukocytosis at presentation, microgranular variant morphology, and *PML-RARA* isoforms bcr2 and bcr3.[753] Moreover, a recent retrospective review of two European studies demonstrated that children younger than age 4 years had a higher incidence of disease relapse than those age 5 to 12, whereas, by contrast, adolescents had higher OS than adults.[754] A presenting WBC count higher than 10,000/μL has been repeatedly shown to carry a worse prognosis,[543,755-757] as has a platelet count less than 40,000/μL, leading to the intensification of therapy with additional anthracycline, cytarabine, and/or ATRA for adult patients treated on recent French and Italian APL trials. Based on improved outcomes, on the recently completed COG trial AAML0631, patients with a WBC count greater than 10,000/μL were designated as high-risk patients who were relegated to additional consolidation cycle with high-dose cytarabine.[758] Before the 1970s, bleeding complications caused significant mortality for patients with APL. Measures that have been used successfully to manage the coagulopathy include platelet and cryoprecipitate transfusions, use of low-dose heparin, and prompt initiation of anthracycline-based chemotherapy.[335,336,354,738] However, the most dramatic decrease in early and induction-related deaths has been the result of the addition of ATRA to the induction regimen, which rapidly leads to the resolution of DIC, and therefore has markedly reduced early mortality.[191,337-340]

Treatment

All-*Trans*-Retinoic Acid

With the introduction of ATRA, the treatment and outcome of APL have changed dramatically. Although previously considered primarily a differentiation agent, a number of recent studies in *PML-RARA* expressing mice and cell lines containing the alternative *PLZF-RARA* fusion have uncoupled differentiation and leukemic cell death, suggesting that exclusive acceptance of a differentiation paradigm belies ATRA's true mechanism of action.[759] In keeping with these recent findings, while even low-dose ATRA induces differentiation in APL blasts in vivo and in vitro and induces remission in up to 90% of patients with newly diagnosed APL,[191,338,760-762] these affects are transient without additional chemotherapy or As$_2$O$_3$ (see later). Although ATRA therapy results in a lifting of the repression complex that inhibits APL blast differentiation, higher doses, As$_2$O$_3$, or chemotherapy is needed to degrade the PML-RARA fusion protein and halt the self-renewal process, ultimately eliminating the malignant clone. Elimination of PML-RARA may further result in more durable cures by targeting the LIC population in APL in which the initial t(15;17) occurred, as well as restoring the normal function of the intracellular PML bodies disrupted by the presence of the fusion protein.[211,759,763] Thus recent strategies combine ATRA with conventional chemotherapy, resulting in improved prognosis for patients with APL compared with chemotherapy alone.[545,764-768] A long-term analysis has demonstrated significantly higher actuarial EFS rates, lower relapse rates, and improved OS in the group treated with both ATRA and chemotherapy.[769] The addition of ATRA to the chemotherapy regimen has been particularly effective for pediatric patients. The APL93 trial used ATRA in combination with daunorubicin and cytarabine in induction, and the children in this trial had a complete remission rate of 97%.[770] The PETHEMA and GIMEMA-AIEOPAIDA groups have completed pediatric trials using ATRA and idarubicin as induction chemotherapy, with reported CR rates of 92% to 96%.[771,772] As such, this lower dose has become the standard for current North American APL studies in children. Current recommendations are to initiate ATRA therapy early, at the time when a diagnosis of APL first is suspected, to correct and prevent devastating consequences from an evolving coagulopathy.

One potentially life-threatening complication of ATRA therapy is the retinoic acid syndrome. This syndrome occurs in approximately 25% of patients and is characterized by fever, respiratory distress, pleural or pericardial effusions, edema, hypotension, and, in some cases, renal failure.[498,773-775] In most patients, the symptoms are preceded by an increasing WBC count.[761,774] Retinoic acid syndrome can be life threatening, and the mortality rate ranges from 8% to 15% in different reports.[765,766,774,776] The syndrome is also associated with a higher risk for bone marrow and extramedullary relapse.[773,777] The use of chemotherapy concurrently with ATRA therapy during induction, particularly in patients with high presenting WBC counts, results in a significantly lower incidence of fatal retinoic acid syndrome[778]; and given the dose dependence, ATRA syndrome now occurs less frequently with the use of 25 mg/m^2 as the standard therapeutic dosing (see later). The use of high-dose corticosteroids at the first sign of symptoms has also been shown to be effective in preventing ATRA syndrome and reducing its mortality rate. Another serious complication of ATRA therapy is pseudotumor cerebri, presenting as headache and papilledema. True pseudotumor cerebri is observed in up to 16% of children, and an additional 39% of children develop headaches without other signs of increased intracranial pressure.[770,772] Pseudotumor cerebri may require treatment with diuretics such as acetazolamide or serial lumbar punctures to reduce intracranial pressure; and, in some cases, discontinuation or dose reduction of ATRA is required.[779] Close follow-up with an ophthalmologist is advised because these patients may suffer visual loss, which in rare cases may be irreversible.[780] Because of the high rate of ATRA-related side effects, the AML-BFM study group studied dose reduction of ATRA during induction from 45 to 25 mg/m^2/day. They found that this dose was still effective, although in pediatric patients there was still a very high rate of CNS side effects, with 57% of children exhibiting headache, increased intracranial pressure, or frank pseudotumor cerebri.[781,782] The CALGB trial C9710 included pediatric patients and used the higher dose of ATRA, but recent data demonstrated no additional benefit and only increased toxicity compared

with 25 mg/m^2 dosing. Therefore this lower dose was incorporated into the recently closed first exclusively pediatric COG APL study, AAML0631, and this dose is now considered the standard of care in pediatric APL.

Arsenic Trioxide

Arsenic trioxide (As_2O_3,) has been used for decades in China as treatment for leukemia. The precise mechanism of action is actively being studied, but As_2O_3 appears to induce both differentiation and apoptosis of APL blasts and to degrade the PML-RARA fusion protein while not affecting transcriptional regulation per se.[213,218,783] As_2O_3 appears to induce nonterminal differentiation followed by apoptosis via the caspase pathway.[213,218,783-785] When As_2O_3 was used as a single agent in patients with APL, remission rates of 65% to 85% were reported and the 10-year survival was as high as 30%.[498] Later studies done in China and the United States showed favorable results, with moderate toxicity, using As_2O_3 in patients with relapsed APL who had previously received ATRA therapy.[210,784,786-788] Several studies have shown promising results using As_2O_3 in remission induction and consolidation therapy for patients with newly diagnosed APL.[789-791] One small series of 11 children with newly diagnosed APL treated with As_2O_3 as a single agent showed mild toxicity, including leukocytosis, skin changes, and mild neuropathy.[791] CR was induced in 91% of these patients, with 1 patient dying of cerebral hemorrhage during induction. With a relatively short median follow-up of 30 months, the DFS was 81% with only 1 relapse; the patient who experienced relapsed achieved a second CR, and thus the OS rate remains 91%.[791] On the U.S. phase I pediatric study of As_2O_3 for relapsed leukemia, 13 patients with relapsed APL received As_2O_3 intravenously daily at 0.15 mg/kg/dose for 5 days per week for 4 weeks with a 2-week break with maximum of 70 doses. A CR rate of 85% was observed after a median of 20 doses. Dose-limiting toxicities included rare vascular leak, anorexia, neuropathic pain, and QTc prolongation (see later).[792]

ATRA and As_2O_3 have been used safely together as induction therapy in children and adults.[213,218,783,793-795] The drugs may have a synergistic effect when used together; one study showed a shorter median time to CR in the group receiving the combination (40.5 days for ATRA alone, 31 days for As_2O_3 alone, 25.5 days for ATRA with As_2O_3).[795] The combination also provided longer duration of remission in this study. Because of these promising data, several groups have included As_2O_3 as part of induction or consolidation therapy for newly diagnosed pediatric patients with APL, with the hope of reducing the total cumulative dose of anthracycline exposure. As_2O_3 was used in a randomized fashion during consolidation in the CALGB 9710 trial that included pediatric patients through the COG and demonstrated a dramatic improvement in outcome. Patients 15 years of age and older who had the addition of As_2O_3 after a common ATRA and chemotherapy induction demonstrated significantly improved 3-year EFS (77% vs. 59%) and OS (86% vs. 77%) compared with patients who received ATRA and chemotherapy alone.[547] These results led to the nonrandom incorporation of As_2O_3 into the successor COG study

AAML0631, such that all patients nonrandomly received As_2O_3 in a dose of 0.15 mg/m² for 5 days a week for five courses during consolidation therapy.

As_2O_3 therapy is generally well tolerated, often with only minimal and reversible toxicity.[791,796,797] However, care must be taken with its use, because it can produce a prolonged QTc interval, which may be asymptomatic but can progress to torsades de pointes and fatal cardiac arrhythmia.[797-800] In one retrospective analysis, the rate of arrhythmia was significantly higher in African American patients (3 of 4) versus non–African-American patients (1 of 73).[801] QTc intervals should be followed closely by weekly electrocardiography during As_2O_3 treatment, and hypokalemia and hypomagnesemia should be meticulously avoided.[802] Because of the induction of cellular differentiation, As_2O_3 commonly results in a condition similar to retinoic acid syndrome, most often characterized by fluid retention and pleural and pericardial effusions.[803] This may be successfully treated in the same way as ATRA-induced retinoic acid syndrome. As_2O_3 can also cause a significant polyneuropathy, particularly when given in repeated courses.[804] Less dangerous side effects include skin changes with rash, hyperpigmentation, keratosis, and transient liver function test abnormalities. In a COG phase I study of As_2O_3 in children with refractory or relapsed acute leukemia, dose-limiting toxicities included prolonged QTc, pneumonitis, and neuropathic pain, whereas non–dose-limiting toxicities included elevated liver function test results, nausea, vomiting, abdominal pain, constipation, electrolyte changes, hyperglycemia, dermatitis, and headache.[805]

Owing to their synergistic effects, ATRA and As_2O_3 were both used upfront on the AAML0631 study and were generally well tolerated. Although used together with chemotherapy on this recently completed trial, the efficacy of this combination and recent adult studies demonstrating the ability of this combination therapy to lead to sustained remission without additional cytotoxic chemotherapy are likely to lead to future trials in which additional chemotherapy is significantly reduced or even eliminated to attain a first CR at least in standard patients. Most striking was the recent APL0406 study, which randomized adult APL patients to ATRA and As_2O_3 or ATRA and idarubicin in induction and found a 2-year EFS of 97% versus 86.7% in favor of the ATRA/As_2O_3 trial arm.[806,808] Thus the addition of anthracyclines and cytarabine may be reserved for APL patients designated high risk at diagnosis based on WBC count, those with more resistant disease (PML-RARA positive postconsolidation [see later]), or first recurrence.

Cytarabine

Although cytarabine is the backbone of induction chemotherapy for other subtypes of AML, its role in APL has been less clear.[340] The PETHEMA group completed a pediatric trial using ATRA and idarubicin as induction chemotherapy without cytarabine, and the CR rate was 92%.[771] The GIMEMA-AIEOPAIDA protocol also used ATRA and idarubicin during induction without cytarabine and showed a 96% CR rate in children.[772] However, this question was subsequently studied in a randomized

clinical trial in which patients younger than 60 years and with a presenting WBC count less than 10,000/µL were randomly assigned in induction to ATRA and daunorubicin, with or without cytarabine. CR rates were comparably high for the two groups—99% with cytarabine and 94% without; however, in the cytarabine arm, the relapse rate was significantly lower (4.7% vs. 15.9%; $P = .011$), the EFS higher (93.3% vs. 77.2%; $P =.0021$), and the OS higher (97.9% vs. 89.6%; $P = .0066$). Of note, the current trials all use high cumulative anthracycline doses to achieve excellent OS rates but there is concern about long-term cardiac toxicity, particularly in pediatric patients.[807] Considering the improved results with the addition of cytarabine to the induction and consolidation regimens, several groups have been studying the use of more cytarabine with less anthracycline in pediatric patients with APL. On AAML0631, 6 g/m² of cytarabine was given during the second consolidation cycle for all patients, with an additional 6 g/m² of cytarabine for high-risk patients. The cumulative anthracycline dose was decreased from 655 mg/m² on prior trials to 355 mg/m² for standard-risk patients and 405 mg/m² for high-risk patients.

Maintenance Therapy

Another difference between APL and other subtypes of AML historically has been an identified benefit from maintenance therapy. The APL93 trial randomized pediatric patients after consolidation to an arm with no further therapy or to arms with 2 years of intermittent ATRA, continuous chemotherapy with 6-mercaptopurine and methotrexate, or both ATRA and chemotherapy. Although 23% of pediatric patients in this trial experienced relapse, none of the patients who received both chemotherapy and ATRA during maintenance therapy did so.[770] In this trial, all patients with relapsed APL achieved a second CR. The 5-year EFS was 71%, and OS was 90%. The PETHEMA group also used ATRA plus 6-mercaptopurine and methotrexate during 2 years of maintenance therapy for pediatric patients and demonstrated a DFS of 82% and an OS of 87%.[771] Since these earlier studies, all recent trials for APL have included a maintenance phase of therapy. To be congruent with parallel European studies, the recently completed AAML0631 study included 2 years of maintenance therapy with ATRA, 6-mercaptopurine, and methotrexate, whereas the CALGB study only included a single year of maintenance with the same agents. However, the future of maintenance therapy in APL is uncertain. The need for chemotherapy versus ATRA alone in maintenance therapy has been raised. Preliminary results of upfront ATRA and As_2O_3 in both Italian and M.D. Anderson Cancer Center adult trials without inclusion of maintenance therapy have prompted consideration of elimination of maintenance therapy altogether.[808] Inclusion of maintenance therapy and whether any chemotherapy is necessary will be key therapeutic goals explored in upcoming trials.

Targeted Therapy

With the use of ATRA and As_2O_3, targeted therapy for APL has become a reality. Other targeted agents are also being used successfully in APL. GMTZ (see earlier) is a recombinant, humanized, anti-CD33 monoclonal antibody linked to the tumor antibiotic calicheamicin. APL cells express very high levels of CD33, making them an attractive target for GMTZ.[809] GMTZ has been used successfully as a single agent to induce remission in patients with multiply relapsed APL.[810,811] In a small series of 12 patients, GMTZ was used safely in combination with ATRA with or without idarubicin, depending on the extent of MRD, as induction therapy for patients with de novo APL with a CR rate of 84%.[812] Some groups are now studying the use of GMTZ as induction therapy in larger numbers of patients. Although not currently used initially for children with APL, GMTZ may be included for the management of high-risk patients and standard-risk patients who have a rise in their WBC count over 10,000/μL during induction therapy or, alternatively, as a strategy to induce remission after relapse in patients who have already received ATRA, As_2O_3, and cytotoxic chemotherapy.

As discussed earlier, mutations in FLT3 have been identified in up to 43% of patients with APL, making the use of FLT3 inhibitors an attractive option. Most FLT3 inhibitors are oral agents with little toxicity. In one mouse model of APL with the FLT3 mutation, treatment with doxorubicin alone had no impact on survival, but treatment with the FLT3 inhibitor SU11657, with or without doxorubicin, resulted in prolonged survival.[813] In another mouse model, treatment with ATRA and SU11657 resulted in the rapid regression of APL.[814] There is considerable interest in using FLT3 inhibitors in combination with ATRA and other targeted agents to improve therapy for patients with APL.

Hematopoietic Stem Cell Transplantation

Because the combination of chemotherapy and ATRA, and now ATRA and As_2O_3, results in such high cure rates for APL, HSCT is not recommended for patients in first CR, even with a matched sibling donor. There is evidence for prolonged remission without HSCT, even after relapse for patients treated with agents such as ATRA, As_2O_3, and GMTZ, especially when combined with chemotherapy.[210,784,786-788,810,811,815] Both autologous and allogeneic HSCT have been used successfully in patients with relapsed APL. For autologous HSCT to be successful, peripheral blood stem cells or bone marrow cells must be harvested once the patient has achieved negative MRD by PCR assay.[816,817] The GVL effect appears to play a role in the allogeneic HSCT treatment of APL, as evidenced by the fact that relapse rates are significantly lower after allogeneic HSCT compared with autologous HSCT and that patients who suffer a molecular relapse after allogeneic HSCT may achieve remission after the withdrawal of immunosuppression.[817-819] However, despite the lower relapse rate, because of significantly higher transplantation-related mortality (TRM) after allogeneic HSCT, OS in adults is higher after autologous HSCT than after allogeneic HSCT (postallogeneic HSCT: DFS, 92.3%; EFS, 52.2%; OS, 51.8%; TRM, 39%; and postautologous HSCT with negative preharvest PCR: DFS, 87.3%; EFS, 76.5%; OS, 75.3%; TRM, 6%).[817] In pediatric patients, allogeneic HSCT is much better tolerated. A retrospective analysis demonstrated no difference in OS after allogeneic

HSCT versus autologous HSCT, although the allogeneic HSCT group had a lower relapse rate and higher TRM (postallogeneic HSCT: RR, 10%; EFS, 71%; OS, 76%; TRM, 19%; and postautologous HSCT: RR, 27%; EFS, 73%; OS, 82%; TRM, 0%).[818] Given these data, in adults, autologous HSCT is usually the preferred choice versus allogeneic HSCT for patients in second CR, whereas in children, allogeneic HSCT is often the preferred choice, particularly if a fully matched sibling donor is available.

Central Nervous System Involvement

In patients with APL, CNS disease at the time of diagnosis is rare and, because of coagulopathy, diagnostic lumbar puncture prior to the initiation of therapy is not safe for most patients. Therefore if APL is suspected, lumbar punctures should not be performed until the coagulopathy is adequately corrected and ATRA initiated. In the pre-ATRA era, CNS relapse was rarely observed in APL patients. However, while the survival rate for APL improved dramatically with the introduction of ATRA, an increasing number of CNS relapses have been reported. Unlike other subtypes of AML, most APL regimens do not include CNS prophylaxis. CNS relapse is more common in patients with a presenting WBC count higher than 10,000/μL, with microgranular variant morphology, and with bcr3 PML-RARA isoform, all of which are also associated with the presence of an FLT3 ITD and all of which are more common in pediatric patients.[165,744-749,753,770,809,820,821] Although there was initially concern that ATRA itself was contributing to CNS relapses, it now seems that ATRA does not penetrate the CNS well and, with more patients surviving APL therapy, this likely contributes to the higher rate of CNS relapse currently observed.[820-823] Several groups have now initiated a screening lumbar puncture at the time of CR and use prophylactic intrathecal chemotherapy, usually with cytarabine and methotrexate, for patients at high risk for CNS relapse.[821,824] On AAML0631, prophylactic cytarabine was given intrathecally in consolidation 2, 3, 4 (for high-risk patients) and the first maintenance course but at a lower dose of 30 mg (25 mg for children >2 years of age but <3 years of age) compared with the 70-mg given as standard dosing in other subtypes of AML. Given the infrequency of CNS positivity in APL, future studies may eliminate intrathecal therapy entirely.

Minimal Residual Disease Monitoring

Detection of the PML-RARA fusion gene by reverse-transcriptase PCR (RT-PCR) has become a valuable tool for measuring MRD in APL. RT-PCR positivity at the end of induction does not seem to portend a higher risk for relapse and therefore should not be checked at that time point, but RT-PCR positivity after consolidation does carry a significantly higher risk for relapse. RT-PCR positivity during maintenance or after therapy is indicative of impending relapse in almost all patients.[772,825,826] MRD analysis is being used to identify high-risk groups that require more intensive therapy for cure.[772] When detected early by RT-PCR, molecular relapse may also be easier to treat than frank morphologic relapse because of the lower disease burden and the treatment of a healthier asymptomatic patient.[827] In many studies, RT-PCR analysis is carried out on bone marrow cells and evidence regarding analysis of peripheral blood is not as clear,[828] thus *PML-RARA* surveillance on AAML0631 mandated bone marrow samples. However, the frequency of relapse after therapy including As$_2$O$_3$ is so rare for standard-risk patients[829,830] that whether follow-up on future trials will require the invasiveness of bone marrow evaluations remains to be determined. There is also controversy regarding the threshold for a "positive" result; some groups do not consider a result a true positive unless there are two positive results separated by 2 to 4 weeks. However, in the event that suspicion is significant for recurrence based on a rising level of PML-RARA transcript in the peripheral blood, a bone marrow evaluation should be conducted to look for molecular, cytogenetic, and hematologic signs of relapse.

Relapsed Disease

In the current ATRA and As$_2$O$_3$ era, relapsed APL is a rare occurrence and there is limited experience on what therapeutic strategy to undertake in children who have already received ATRA, As$_2$O$_3$, and chemotherapy. Given their efficacy, reinduction with combination ATRA and As$_2$O$_3$ is a reasonable strategy if previously well tolerated, although it is unclear whether the addition of chemotherapy provides any further benefit or merely contributes to toxicity. Currently, patients with relapsed APL may have already seen a significant cumulative dose of anthracycline, such that additional anthracycline may push the normally accepted lifetime ceilings with which most clinicians are comfortable. However, the concomitant use of cardioprotectants, such as dexrazoxane, may provide the opportunity to provide further anthracycline therapy at relapse. Furthermore, if future studies show the initial use of chemotherapy and anthracyclines in particular may be significantly reduced owing to the efficacy of combination ATRA and As$_2$O$_3$, it may enable chemotherapy to be reserved for relapses and refractory cases. Regardless, particularly with early relapse, given the opportunity for GVL effect and the improvement in both high-resolution HLA typing and better supportive care, after reinduction, best available donor allogeneic transplant would be recommended by most experts.[831] However, on prior studies, TRM with allogeneic HSCT was higher than with autologous transplant, although there was no significant difference in 5-year OS or EFS,[818,832] so this decision should not be made lightly. With later relapses, the ability to induce a second sustained CR with ATRA, As$_2$O$_3$, and chemotherapy without HSCT may be a feasible alternative, although with small numbers of patients most of these data are anecdotal.[754]

DOWN SYNDROME WITH TRANSIENT DISORDER AND ACUTE MYELOGENOUS LEUKEMIA

Down Syndrome with Transient Myeloproliferative Disorder

Pathobiology

Down syndrome, characterized by trisomy 21, is the most common congenital chromosomal abnormality, occurring in an estimated 1 in 600 to 1000 live births.[833,834] Up to 10% of infants with Down syndrome are born with a transient myeloproliferative disorder (TMD) (also referred to as transient leukemia [TL] or transient abnormal myelopoiesis [TAM]). TMD is characterized by the presence of immature megakaryoblasts in the liver, bone marrow, and peripheral blood. The disorder usually spontaneously regresses within 3 months.[71,835-837] By morphology, TMD blasts are identical to AMKL blasts and, even though in most cases they regress, up to 30% of Down syndrome infants with TMD subsequently develop AMKL within 3 years.[838,839] Studies have shown that TMD blasts are clonal and that the same clone subsequently evolves into AMKL in a subset of patients.[840-843]

In 2002, Wechsler and colleagues[267] first reported mutations in exon 2 of *GATA1* in Down syndrome–associated AMKL. Soon thereafter, several groups reported that *GATA1* mutations were detectable in almost all patients with Down syndrome–associated TMD.[844-849] Interestingly, *GATA1* mutations have also been detected in approximately 10% of Down syndrome patients who have never been diagnosed with a hematologic abnormality.[850] It is not clear whether these patients have a history of subclinical TMD that regressed without detection or if the mutation simply did not result in the TMD phenotype in these cases. Normal GATA1 plays a vital role in the maturation of erythroid cells and megakaryocytes.[851] The *GATA1* mutations in Down syndrome TMD and AMKL result in GATA1s, a truncated protein lacking the amino-terminal activation domain.[847,852,853] GATA1s appears to be a normal isoform of GATA1 and has been detected in human hematopoietic cell lines and mouse fetal liver. However, because *GATA1* is an X-linked gene, only the truncated GATA1s is expressed in Down syndrome TMD and AMKL blasts. It has been hypothesized that the presence of a trisomy 21 in conjunction with a GATA1s allows abnormal proliferation of megakaryoblasts, but only in the fetal hematopoietic system (i.e., the fetal liver); thus TMD resolves with the loss of fetal hematopoiesis.[835,854] Although the combination of trisomy 21 and a *GATA1* mutation appears sufficient to result in TMD, this is not sufficient to result in frank leukemia, and only if additional mutations are accumulated over time will the disease progress to frank AMKL.

Wilms tumor gene *(WT1)* levels detected by PCR assay are elevated in patients with TMD. Levels normalized in four of five patients studied who had regression of TMD, with no further sequelae, but did not normalize in the fifth, who went on to develop AMKL at 11 months of age, making this an attractive marker for MRD and prognosis.[855] Both gain- and loss-of-function mutations in Janus kinase 3 *(JAK3)* have been identified in a subset of patients with TMD, although the prognostic relevance of this is not yet known.[856,857]

Clinical Presentation

Because Down syndrome infants with TMD are often asymptomatic, the incidence of 10% may be an underestimate, because many patients may have TMD that spontaneously regresses, without ever being detected.[846,858-861]

For this reason, many physicians obtain a routine screening complete blood cell (CBC) count at birth for all infants with known or suspected Down syndrome. However, some infants with Down syndrome have a dramatic presentation of TMD at or shortly after birth, with hydrops fetalis, pleural and pericardial effusions, ascites, and massive hepatosplenomegaly. These patients may rapidly progress to liver fibrosis or multisystem organ failure, both of which are most often fatal.[837,862-865] In the Pediatric Oncology Group (POG) trial 9481, 48 children with TMD were followed prospectively; 19% developed life-threatening disease with hepatic fibrosis or cardiopulmonary failure, with an overall mortality at 3 months of age of 10.4%.[837] Another retrospective analysis from Japan has shown that 22.9% of patients with TMD die before the age of 6 months, and the main causes of death were hepatic or cardiopulmonary failure.[866] In this study, early gestational age, WBC count greater than 100,000/μL, high percentage of peripheral blasts, elevated aspartate aminotransferase (AST), elevated direct bilirubin, and low Apgar score were significantly associated with poor survival. They noted that only 7.7% of term Down syndrome infants with a WBC count less than 100,000/μL died, whereas 54.5% of preterm infants with a WBC count higher than 100,000/μL died, suggesting that risk stratification may be possible to determine high-risk subgroups of patients who require earlier and more aggressive therapy.

Treatment

Because most patients with TMD will exhibit spontaneous regression, treatment often consists of supportive care only. Many groups, including COG protocols 2971 and 08B1, have recommended supportive care only for TMD patients unless they exhibit signs or symptoms of life-threatening disease, including hyperviscosity, with a total blast count higher than 100,000/μL, organomegaly causing respiratory compromise, congestive heart failure not caused by a congenital heart defect, hydrops fetalis, life-threatening hepatic dysfunction, defined as significant (grade 4 level toxicity) DIC, hyperbilirubinemia, ascites, or transaminitis.[837,867] For patients who require therapy, the choices include leukapheresis, exchange transfusion, or low-dose cytarabine.[862] Low-dose cytarabine has been effective when used early in critically ill patients.[868] In patients with hyperleukocytosis or who require therapy with cytarabine, treatment to prevent the consequences of rapid tumor lysis (see earlier) should be promptly initiated.

Down Syndrome with Acute Myelogenous Leukemia
Pathobiology

Children with Down syndrome have a markedly increased risk for leukemia during the first 10 years of life. Acute leukemia is 10 to 20 times more common in children with Down syndrome than in children in the general population, and leukemia in Down syndrome patients younger than 4 years is most commonly AML (specifically AMKL), whereas leukemia in older children with Down syndrome is most commonly ALL.[838,869-878] The ratio of ALL to AML is approximately 1:1 in children with Down syndrome, but in the first 4 years of life, AML is 100 times more common than ALL.[72] Although AMKL is a rare subtype of AML in the general population, it is the predominant form of AML in children with Down syndrome, making Down syndrome patients 500 times more likely than other children to develop AMKL. Unlike other children with AML, AMKL in children with Down syndrome often manifests after a period of myelodysplasia, usually characterized by months of thrombocytopenia and later by anemia.[72,879,880] Most cases of AMKL in Down syndrome patients are preceded by TMD (see earlier).[850,881] Several studies have confirmed that when there is a proven antecedent TMD, the same TMD clone subsequently evolves into AMKL.[844,846,882,883]

Also characteristic of AMKL in Down syndrome are GATA1 mutations (see earlier). Because GATA1 encodes a transcription factor essential for megakaryocyte development, samples from patients with AMKL were studied for evidence of GATA1 mutations.[267] Mutations in exon 2 of GATA1 were detected in AMKL blasts from Down syndrome patients but not in other subtypes of AML in Down syndrome patients or in AMKL blasts from non–Down syndrome patients. Several subsequent studies have confirmed GATA1 mutations leading to a premature stop codon in almost all cases of Down syndrome–associated AMKL.[844-849] GATA1 mutations have been identified in the blood spots of three of four Down syndrome patients with AMKL who had not been previously diagnosed with TMD, suggesting that in most cases of AMKL the mutation has been present since birth.[846,850,882,883] Down syndrome patients who develop AML after the age of 4 years do not usually have GATA1-mutated AMKL but have AML more typical of the general pediatric population (non–Down syndrome AML). This disease is not as sensitive to chemotherapy and does not carry the exceptionally good prognosis carried by Down syndrome AMKL (see later).[884-886]

Additional mutations beyond the GATA1 mutation in the presence of trisomy 21 are necessary to produce AMKL. The good-risk translocations common in other forms of pediatric AML, including t(8;21), t(15;17), inv(16), and t(9;11), are almost never seen in Down syndrome AMKL, although they are more commonly reported in Down syndrome patients who develop AML after the age of 4.[873,875,886-888] Other than trisomy 21, trisomy 8 is the most common cytogenetic abnormality in Down syndrome AMKL. Other translocations commonly reported in AMKL in the absence of Down syndrome, including t(1;22) and t(1;3), are only rarely documented in Down syndrome AMKL.[889] Monosomy 7, a widely accepted marker of pediatric and adult high-risk AML in the absence of Down syndrome, is also seen in 3.5% to 10% of patients with Down syndrome and AML and, although data are limited, it is generally associated with a worse outcome (see later).[890-892] Approximately 25% of patients have no cytogenetic abnormalities other than the constitutional trisomy 21, although some patients will exhibit tetrasomy 21. As in TMD, overexpression of WT1 and mutations in JAK3 have been reported in Down syndrome AMKL.[855-857] More recently, next generation sequencing approaches have identified a number of potential somatic mutational drivers that might contribute to the progression of TMD to AMKL including mutations in the cohesin complex; the epigenetic regulator, EZH2; as well as activating lesions in the RAS, WNT, mitogen activated protein kinase (MAPK) and phosphoinositide 3-kinase (PI3K) pathways.[892a,892b]

Clinical Presentation

Children with Down syndrome who develop AML present at a younger age than average for childhood AML, with 60% to 70% of patients diagnosed when they are younger than 2 years.[70,873,875,884,887,888] Down syndrome patients generally present with lower total WBC counts (median, 7,000 to 10,000/μL) and lower platelet counts (median, 25,000 to 30,000/μL) than other children. Hepatosplenomegaly is more common in Down syndrome patients with AML than in other children, whereas lymphadenopathy and CNS involvement are less common. Down syndrome AMKL is frequently preceded by TMD, which is almost absent in non–Down syndrome patients, or MDS, which is far less common in non–Down syndrome patients. Older Down syndrome patients with AML have presenting signs and symptoms that more closely mirror those of the general population, reflecting the virtual lack of AMKL with *GATA1* mutations in patients older than 5 years.

Treatment and Outcome

Many children with Down syndrome have been entered into large clinical trials since 1982, when legislation was passed that prohibits withholding medical intervention from children with disabilities.[72] In the early clinical trials that included patients with Down syndrome and AML, the outcome was poor because of excessive toxicity. The associated congenital abnormalities, increased susceptibility to infection, and altered drug metabolism in patients with Down syndrome made it challenging to find appropriate therapy for this group. However, while general medical care for children with Down syndrome has improved, the outcome for children with AML and Down syndrome has also improved. Multiple studies from around the world have consistently demonstrated that Down syndrome AML patients have a better overall prognosis than children with AML in the general population.[530,873,875,884,887,888,893] A remarkable feature of AML in children with Down syndrome is its extraordinary responsiveness to AML chemotherapy.[72,874] Compared with non–Down syndrome AML, leukemic blasts are 4.5-fold and 12-fold more sensitive in vitro to cytarabine (median half maximal inhibitory concentration [IC_{50}], 77.5 vs. 350.9 nM) and daunorubicin (median IC_{50}, 5.8 vs. 71.2 nM), respectively.[894,895] The increased sensitivity of Down syndrome AML blasts to cytarabine has been explained by a 5.2-fold greater accumulation of the active drug metabolite cytarabine-CTP compared with non–Down syndrome AML blasts.[896] Down syndrome AMKL blasts are significantly more sensitive to other chemotherapy agents, including amsacrine (16-fold), etoposide (20-fold), 6-thioguanine (3-fold), busulfan (5-fold), and vincristine (23-fold).[897] In addition to constitutionally

expressed genes encoded on chromosome 21, which modulate drug metabolism in Down syndrome AML blasts, such as cystathionine-β-synthase (CBS),[898-900] the expression of mutant GATA1 protein itself contributes to increased drug accumulation.[901,902] In addition, the cytidine deaminase (CDA) levels in Down syndrome AMKL blasts are low, leading also to increased sensitivity to cytarabine. The CDA promoter contains several binding sites for GATA1, suggesting that *GATA1* mutations may contribute to the sensitivity of these blasts.[900]

Observations of increased in vitro sensitivity of Down syndrome AMKL blasts to cytotoxic drugs have been complemented by pioneering studies in which very low doses of cytarabine, which were administered over a prolonged period of time (10 mg/m^2 subcutaneously for 12 hours for 7 days every 2 weeks for 2 years),[903,904] resulted in durable remissions in as many as 67% of cases (intention to treat analysis[903]). Although outcomes of the very-low-dose cytarabine regimen eventually did not match those of standard dose cytarabine,[904] the observation highlights a unique degree of drug sensitivity of Down syndrome AMKL blasts to cytarabine that is not encountered in pediatric non–Down syndrome AML. Recently, Japanese investigators showed that high-dose cytarabine could successfully be eliminated from a treatment protocol for Down syndrome AML while maintaining a 4-year EFS of 83%.[892] In parallel, studies maximizing dose intensity for the treatment of AML, although successful in the general pediatric population,[411,905] did not translate into any improvements in EFS for patients with Down syndrome and AML owing to excessive mortality during induction therapy in this group.[905] In the German collaborative AML-BFM93 protocol, children with Down syndrome fared worse than other patients because of an increased frequency of infectious complications, but none of the patients experienced relapse and EFS was approximately 70%.[886,906] Therefore, in the subsequent AML-BFM98 protocol, Down syndrome patients received a reduced intensity regimen and the EFS improved dramatically, to almost 90%. In the Nordic Society for Paediatric Haematology and Oncology-Acute Myeloid Leukaemia (NOPHO-AML) trials, the earlier, more intensive NOPHO-AML88 trial showed a high death rate from infectious complications for Down syndrome patients with AML, with an EFS of only 47%, compared with much better outcomes in the later, less-intensive NOPHO-AML93 trial, with an EFS of 85% (76% for those who received full-dose therapy and 92% for those who received reduced-dose therapy).[907] The MRC trials showed similar results with Down syndrome patients receiving the same standard therapy as other patients, resulting in a higher rate of death from toxicity but lower relapse rate when compared with other children.[908] Perhaps the most striking example comes from the CCG 2891 study. In this study, all children were randomly assigned to receive induction chemotherapy with intensive timing (i.e., proceeding with the second cycle, regardless of counts) versus standard timing (i.e., awaiting count recovery before initiating the second cycle). The Down syndrome patients in the intensive timing arm of the study suffered a 32% mortality rate compared with an 11% mortality rate for the remainder of the patients, prompting early closure of that study arm for Down syndrome patients.[875] Standard timing induction for Down syndrome patients resulted in an impressively high CR rate of 95% (2.4% with toxic death and 2.4% with resistant disease).[875] Postremission consolidation with allogeneic HSCT in this trial also resulted in an unacceptably high treatment-related mortality for Down syndrome patients, with only 33% survival at 4 years.[875] In this study, standard timing induction followed by consolidation with chemotherapy was clearly the superior treatment for Down syndrome patients, with a 4-year DFS of 88% compared with a DFS of only 42% for this regimen in the non–Down syndrome patients.[875] Given these collective data, COG trial A2971 used a less intensive approach for Down syndrome patients, with four cycles of standard timing low-dose cytarabine, daunorubicin, and thioguanine, followed by a cycle of high-dose cytarabine with asparaginase and then intrathecal therapy.[909] Five-year outcome data were comparable to those of CCG2891 with OS of 84% and EFS of 79%.[910]

The first toxicity to which DS-AML patients were identified as being particularly susceptible was cardiotoxicity. On the POG9421 AML study in which the total cumulative anthracycline equivalent dose was 535 mg/m^2, 21% of DS children developed congestive heart failure with diminished shortening fractions on echocardiogram requiring chronic diuretics and/or inotropes. Sixty percent of these patients had congenital heart defects, and a third of the patients with cardiac dysfunction died.[911] On both CCG2891 and A2971, the cumulative anthracycline dose was reduced to 350 mg/m^2, but together with the overall reduction in chemotherapy on A2971, grade 3 or higher cardiac toxicity occurred in only 4% of patients during induction and 2% of patients during intensification.[910] The most recent COG Down syndrome AML study, AAML0431, was designed to further reduce the cumulative dose of anthracycline based on A2971 and gave a cumulative dose of only 240 mg/m^2. The study closed in December 2011 and to date no significant cardiac toxicity has been reported (J. Taub, personal communication, June 2014). However, the second cycle of induction chemotherapy during which high-dose cytarabine is given resulted in the greatest number of adverse events, including longest median duration, longest period of myelosuppression, and highest rate of bacterial infections. These toxicities, together with prior data demonstrating the exquisite sensitivity of Down syndrome AMKL blasts to cytarabine, have prompted plans for elimination of high-dose cytarabine for the majority of patients on the upcoming COG Down syndrome AML trial.

Despite the overall favorable outcomes for AML in Down syndrome, 15% to 25% of patients do not achieve long-term survival with current treatment protocols, predominantly owing to relapse or refractory disease.[891,892,912] Lack of response to therapy is associated with very poor outcomes with survival rates of 20-26% even after HSCT.[912a,912b] Prognostic markers in AML in Down syndrome are few because many of the predictive genetic lesions discussed earlier for non–Down syndrome AML are very infrequent findings in Down syndrome patients. To date, age older than 4 years and monosomy 7 appear

the only known high-risk factors, both of which are relatively rare, and the outcome in patients harboring a monosomy 7 is still somewhat controversial. In the BFM-93 trial, 3 of 4 patients older than 4 years lacked the typical AMKL of Down syndrome and only 1 of the 3 survived.[886] In a combined analysis of European trials, 17 of 317 Down syndrome patients diagnosed with AML were older than 4 years.[885] DNA was available from blasts of 10 of these patients and, of these, 3 children younger than 7 years had the characteristic AMKL and 1 additional younger child had M0 AML with a GATA1 mutation. Of the 6 remaining patients without AMKL or a GATA1 mutation, all were 7 years of age or older and 4 experienced relapse. In CCG 2891, children older than 4 years of age ($n = 9$) had a significantly lower EFS at 6 years of only 33% ± 31%.[891] On A2971, patients younger than 4 years of age fared significantly better than older children (5 year EFS, 81% ± 7% vs. 33% ± 38%), although only 6 children older than age 4 years were included.[913] An international retrospective study of 451 Down syndrome patients with AML found monosomy 7 was associated with a moderately worse outcome, with a 5-year EFS of 69%. CCG studies 2891 and A2971, as well as a recent Japanese study,[892] found that only 11 of 16 patients with Down syndrome and AML and monosomy 7 were in complete clinical remission. These limited data suggest that older children with Down syndrome and AML, particularly given the absence of GATA1 mutations, have disease more reminiscent of non–Down syndrome AML and should be treated more aggressively. Similarly, the presence of monosomy 7 may contribute to an inferior outcome and justify more intensive therapy for this cohort. However, most children with Down syndrome and AML are younger than age 4 years and lack monosomy 7. For this group, similar to non–Down syndrome AML, MRD after induction may enable the ability to identify high-risk patients. These data will be forthcoming from the recently closed AAML0431 study and will inform future clinical trials.

MYELODYSPLASTIC SYNDROMES

The myelodysplastic syndromes are a heterogeneous group of clonal hematologic disorders characterized by ineffective hematopoiesis, progressive cytopenias, dysplastic transformation of hematopoietic cells, and a propensity for transformation into AML.[914] MDS is most common in patients older than 60 years, but at the same time it is an unusual but clinically important disease of childhood.

Diagnosis and Classification
Morphology

The morphologic features of MDS include bone marrow dysplastic changes involving all three cell lineages (i.e., trilineage dysplasia). A common theme underlying these features is asynchrony between the usual cytoplasmic and nuclear differentiation programs, so that nuclei appear abnormal and less mature than the features of the surrounding cytoplasm. Typical erythrocytic abnormalities

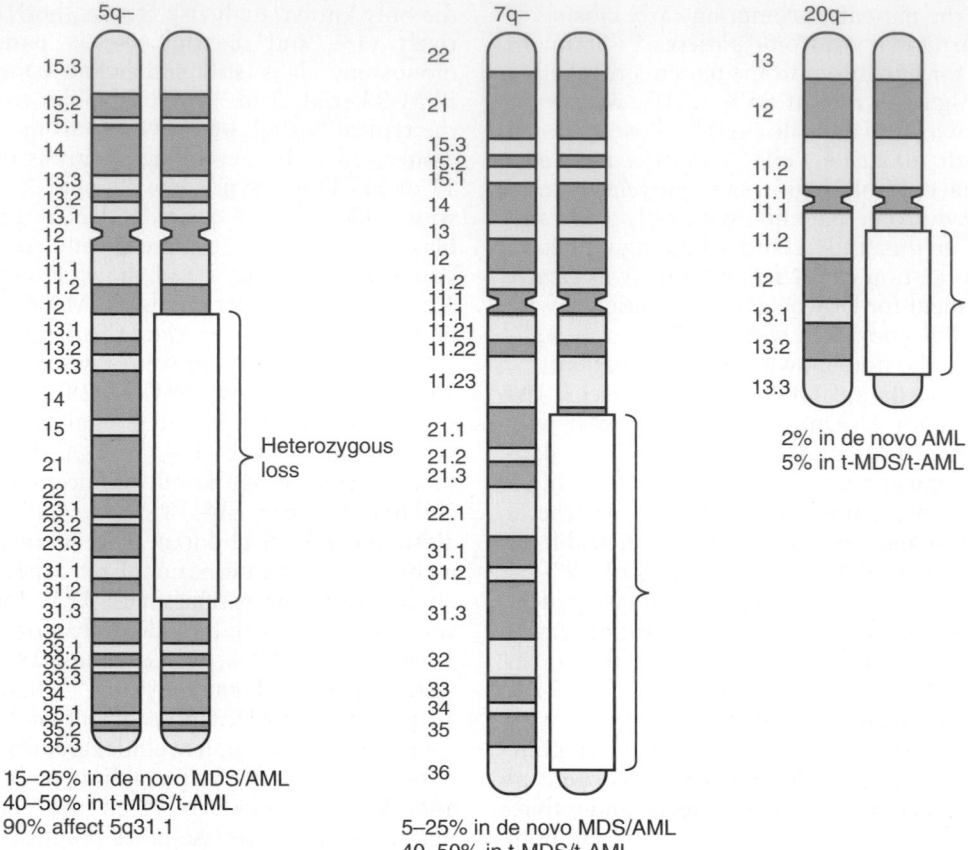

Figure 51-8 The hallmark of myelodysplastic syndrome (MDS) is the loss of specific chromosomal regions. Deletions of the long arm of chromosomes 5 and 7 (5q–, 7q–) occur in de novo MDS and acute myelogenous leukemia (AML) but much more frequently in therapy-related MDS and therapy-related AML after treatment with alkylating agents. 20q– abnormalities are less common but also occur in both de novo MDS and AML and after prior chemotherapy. *(Data from Heaney ML, Golde DW: Myelodysplasia. N Engl J Med 340:1649–1660, 1999; Hofmann WK, Lubbert M, Hoelzer D, et al: Myelodysplastic syndromes. Hematol J 5:1–8, 2004; Pedersen-Bjergaard J, Andersen MT, Andersen MK: Genetic pathways in the pathogenesis of therapy-related myelodysplasia and acute myeloid leukemia. Hematol Am Soc Hematol Educ Prog 2007:392–397, 2007.)*

include megaloblastoid changes, perinuclear ringlike deposits of iron (i.e., ringed sideroblasts), multinucleation, nuclear budding and fragmentation, and an increased percentage of immature forms. Dysmegakaryopoiesis is characterized by micromegakaryocytes, abnormal nuclei, and abnormal nuclear lobulation. The dysplastic features of the granulocytic cells comprise immature forms, hypogranulation, and the Pelger-Huët–type abnormality. Monocytic dysplasia includes increased numbers of bone marrow monocytes, abnormal granulation with increased azurophilic granules, hemophagocytosis, abnormal nuclei, and giant forms. Bone marrow cellularity is usually normal or increased, and the reticulin concentration is increased in most cases.

Patients with MDS may present initially with a single peripheral blood cytopenia, which usually progresses to pancytopenia with anemia, leukopenia, and thrombocytopenia. The anemia in MDS is caused by ineffective erythropoiesis with low reticulocyte counts and macrocytosis, teardrop cell formation, and moderate poikilocytosis. In addition, megaloblastoid circulating nucleated red blood cells are frequently detected. Peripheral blood dysgranulopoiesis manifests as circulating myeloblasts, progranulocytes, and Pelger-Huët cells. Thus early signs may

be a falling hematocrit with increasing mean corpuscular volume or unexplained thrombocytopenia. The peripheral blood may also exhibit increased numbers of monocytes and monoblasts.

Cytogenetics

Cytogenetic abnormalities are common in children with MDS and were reported in 59% of 227 children tested in one study.[915] Chromosomal deletions are the hallmark of MDS and frequently involve the long arms of chromosomes 5, 7, and 20 (Fig. 51-8). Other common cytogenetic abnormalities include trisomy 8, del(17p), +21, inv(1), and t(7;16).[253,916,917] These chromosomal abnormalities are accompanied by other complex karyotypic changes in many cases. Other abnormalities that have been reported in pediatric cases of MDS include +6, +9, and +11, whereas deletions of chromosomes 11, 12, and 13 and Y are rare.[918] Common balanced chromosomal translocations found in AML, such as t(8;21), t(15;17), and inv(16), are not usually detected in MDS.[919]

Classification

In 1982, the FAB cooperative group defined five categories for the adult myelodysplastic and myeloproliferative syndromes—refractory anemia (RA), RA with ringed sideroblasts (RARS), RA with excess blasts (RAEB), RA with excess blasts in transformation (RAEB-T), and chronic myelomonocytic leukemia (CMML).[324,325,920,921] Classification of childhood MDS into defined FAB subcategories is not always straightforward. Many children show overlapping features of MPD and MDS, particularly patients with JMML and infant monosomy 7 syndrome.[254] The classification of pediatric MDS is also complicated by the fact that some children develop MDS in the context of inherited predispositions such as neurofibromatosis type 1, severe congenital neutropenia, and Down syndrome.[254] Using the FAB system of classification, the most common subtypes of MDS in children are RAEB and RAEB-T, whereas RA and RARS are uncommon and CMML is rare.

The WHO proposed a revised classification of MDS in 1997. The WHO system includes the following changes to the FAB criteria: elimination of the RAEB-T subtype through a reduction in the marrow blast count to 20% for the diagnosis of AML and the division of the RAEB subtype into RAEB-I, consisting of 5% to 10% marrow blasts, and RAEB-II, comprising 11% to 20% blasts.[309,328,922] Other WHO recommendations include two new categories for patients with refractory cytopenias with multilineage dysplasia and a new category for unclassified MDS. In the new system, CMML is removed completely and reclassified as a myeloproliferative disorder.

A third classification system is used in parallel with the FAB and WHO systems, the IPSS Scoring System.[973] This system assigns a numeric value to each of the number of cytopenias, cytogenetic abnormalities, and percentage of bone marrow blasts, and a higher score is associated with a poor prognosis. The use of the IPSS in children is of somewhat limited value. The only factors found to be predictive were bone marrow blasts greater than 5% and platelet counts greater than 100,000/μL.[924,925]

Pathophysiology

Evidence for clonality in MDS comes primarily from nonrandom X-inactivation studies (see earlier) performed on the bone marrow cells of female patients with MDS. These studies have demonstrated clonal involvement of hematopoietic cells in this disorder.[926-928] The trilineage dysplasia that characterizes MDS strongly suggests that the cell of origin resides within the compartment containing early hematopoietic progenitors or stem cells with multilineage potential.[929] Early mutations in stem cells may cause a failure in myeloid cell maturation, as well as enhanced apoptosis, leading to dysplasia, whereas subsequent defects affecting myeloid cell proliferation and the development of antiapoptotic signals may cause the clonal expansion of aberrant cells and frank leukemia. An increased level of apoptosis has been documented in early MDS, which is followed by decreased blast cell apoptosis in patients whose disease transforms to AML. MDS cells have been found to overexpress certain cell surface death receptors and their ligands, which may be induced as a result of signals from inflammatory cells present in the hematopoietic microenvironment.[919]

Patients with more advanced MDS (FAB RAEB) have decreased levels of death receptor expression compared with early-stage MDS and increased expression levels of antiapoptotic factors, such as BCL2.[930,931]

The most common chromosomal abnormalities in childhood MDS involve large deletions, but little is known about the genes contained in the deleted segment[916,932-934] and whether these large genetic aberrations are inciting events leading to the development of MDS or represent secondary events. Ebert and colleagues[935] used an RNA interference screen to identify a putative gene deleted from the distal end of the long arm of chromosome 5 in 5q– syndrome, a subtype of MDS commonly encountered in older women but uncommon in pediatric patients. They found that haploinsufficiency of RPS14, a gene that codes for a component of the 40S ribosomal subunit, results in the characteristic phenotype of selectively diminished erythropoiesis, with preservation of megakaryocyte maturation. Moreover, the introduction of a lentiviral vector expressing RPS14 into the CD34+ cells of MDS patients demonstrates restored erythroid differentiation exclusively in those with a 5q– genotype. These elegant studies convincingly identified a specific genetic lesion underlying the 5q– syndrome and also established this ribosomal protein as critical in erythroid development.[935] This finding is in keeping with the elucidated role of other ribosomal proteins in a number of bone marrow failure syndromes, such as Diamond-Blackfan anemia.[936]

5q– syndrome has a reasonably favorable outcome because of its natural history of slower progression to AML and sensitivity to treatment with lenalidomide, an analogue of thalidomide.[937,938] In this select population, lenalidomide (Revlimid) reduces the need for red cell transfusions and induces significant cytogenetic responses, which has resulted in its recent approval by the FDA for the treatment of MDS patients with 5q– syndrome.[939] Although this therapy has demonstrated impressive efficacy in this condition, deletion of this distal region of 5q is relatively rare. Only a minority of MDS patients without this cytogenetic abnormality respond to lenalidomide, and responders possess no distinguishing clinical or laboratory characteristics compared with nonresponders.[940] However, other studies[941] suggest that responders have a unique genetic signature consisting of low expression levels of genes typically involved in terminal erythroid differentiation. These results imply that the restoration of normal red cell development underlies lenalidomide's mechanism of action, particularly in non-5q–, whereas in 5q– syndrome, lenalidomide may more directly suppress the malignant clone.[942] Clinically, this suggests that genetic profiling could be used to select a group of MDS patients without 5q– deletions who would be more likely to respond to this agent.

These large deletions also likely contain certain important tumor suppressor genes, the elimination of which contributes to MDS pathogenesis. For example, we completed a detailed analysis of the more proximally deleted region of the long arm of chromosome 5 and identified α-catenin as a novel tumor suppressor gene in MDS.[252] In both primary patient samples and AML cell lines with a deletion of 5q–, α-catenin expression levels were found to be specifically and substantially decreased through the combination of a deletion on one chromosome and epigenetic silencing by hypermethylation and histone deacetylation of the promoter of the second allele. Another group has identified the WT1 transcription factor, early growth response 1 (EGR1), as a putative candidate gene in this same region and demonstrated that haploinsufficiency of this tumor suppressor gene can result in MDS or MPD after treatment with an alkylating agent.[943]

In addition to gene deletions, a number of other genes have been found to contribute to MDS pathogenesis. Balanced translocations, such as those seen in de novo AML, are uncommon in MDS, but some of the same genes may be involved. Other genetic lesions appear to be specific for MDS. We and others have shown that certain HOX genes, most notably HOXA9, are overexpressed in the HSCs of patients with MDS.[944-946] Translocations involving HOX genes and the nucleoporin gene (NUP98) on chromosome 11, including NUP98-HOXA9[947] and NUP98-HOXA13,[948] have been found in rare patients with MDS. Certain genetic abnormalities are more characteristic after prior treatment with chemotherapy. Overexpression of the EVI1 transcription factor on chromosome 3, either through gene rearrangements or rare translocations, has been associated with MDS after chemotherapy.[949-951] Similarly, nucleophosmin and myeloid leukemia factor 1 (NPM-MLF1) fusion gene, formed as a result of a t(3;5) chromosomal translocation, occurs in rare cases of MDS or AML arising from MDS.[952,953] Mutations in RAS and FLT3, such as those seen in de novo AML, are found in patients with MDS, particularly those with 7q– and often after treatment with alkylating agents.[954] These patients may also have mutations in the AML1 gene, whereas the AML1-ETO translocation is rare in MDS.[955,956] Prior treatment with alkylators can also lead to MDS with 5q–, and these patients often have a mutation in TP53, a gene that is also frequently mutated in AML cases with a complex aberrant karyotype, which include a 5q deletion, but rarely in classic de novo AML.[955-957]

More recently, owing to responses in MDS to epigenetic regulating agents, such as DNA methyltransferase inhibitors, and the identification of a number of mutations in epigenetic regulating genes in AML, a series of studies using high-throughput genomic approaches have identified similar abnormalities in MDS. Mutations in TET2 occur in approximately 25% of adults with MDS,[958] whereas DNMT3A and IDH1 and IDH2 mutations were found in 3% to 10% of patients.[959-962] In addition, mutations have been found in histone modifying enzymes, including EZH2, which is rare in de novo AML,[963,964] and ASXL1, both associated with a worse outcome in adult MDS.[965,966] Finally, novel mutations in genes involved in the assembly of the spliceosome that removes introns from transcribed pre-mRNA have been identified. The genes most commonly involved include SF3B1 and U2AF1.[967-969] However, MDS is much rarer in children, and all of these mutations appear to be rare in pediatric MDS; thus their impact on pathogenesis and prognosis remain uncertain at this time.[970]

Inherited and Environmental Predisposing Factors

Several environmental exposures and inherited conditions are associated with an increased risk for MDS and AML. As noted, alkylating agents and topoisomerase II inhibitors can predispose to MDS and AML, which can occur as treatment-related second malignancies in patients treated for ALL and many other types of cancer. Secondary disease associated with alkylating agent chemotherapy tends to occur from 3 to 11 years after treatment, after which the incidence appears to plateau.[971-973] The disease often presents as MDS, and an underlying predisposition may involve defective DNA repair mechanisms. Commonly, there are deletions of chromosomes 5 or 7.[972] MLL gene rearrangements are often found in AML cases that arise after treatment with topoisomerase II inhibitors such as etoposide, but these patients tend to present with frank AML after a short latency of 1 to 3 years from therapy and without an MDS prodrome.[972,974]

A number of genetic conditions are associated with an increased risk for MDS and subsequent AML, particularly the bone marrow failure syndromes and chromosomal breakage disorders. Some disorders, such as Fanconi anemia, in which patients demonstrate both pancytopenia and increased sensitivity to DNA damage, suggest that impaired DNA repair may be a mechanism for malignant transformation. However, other marrow failure syndromes are not characterized by increased susceptibility to chromosomal breakage such as dyskeratosis congenita or may present predominantly as a single cytopenia, such as neutropenia in Shwachman-Diamond syndrome, anemia in Diamond-Blackfan anemia, and low platelets in amegakaryocytic thrombocytopenia. The evolution of MDS in these conditions is variable (10% to 20% in Shwachman-Diamond syndrome compared with 1% in Diamond-Blackfan anemia), and the mechanism remains elusive, although defective ribosomal processing may be involved, given the identified functions of the target proteins involved in a number of these conditions.[919,975] In addition, there are several MDS/AML predisposition genes that have been identified, including loss-of-function alterations affecting the key hematopoietic transcription factor genes, RUNX1, CEBPA, and, most recently, GATA2. Germline mutations in RUNX1 can result in familial platelet disorder with a propensity to myeloid malignancy (FPD/AML). These patients have thrombocytopenia or normal platelet numbers but abnormal platelet function and can evolve into MDS or AML.[76-79] A recently identified related disorder termed thrombocytopenia type 2 has been linked to mutations in a gene called ANKRD26 at 10p11.2-p12 in a number of Italian and American families with a progression to frank myeloid and lymphoid malignancies, with an MDS prodrome rarely described.[976] Deletions of the granulocyte-specifying gene CEPBA have been described in a small number of families resulting in an FAB M1 or M2 subtype AML; however, an MDS prodrome has not been described. The CEBPA mutations are autosomal dominant, similar to those involving RUNX1, but fully penetrant, in contrast to the highly variable penetrance observed for RUNX1 lesions.[78,977-979] Loss-of-function mutations or deletions involving *GATA2*, which plays a role in early blood, vascular, and lymphatic development, have been described as a cause of a familial MDS/AML syndrome. These patients may present with neutropenia, often with an associated monocytopenia[80] or with so-called mono-MAC syndrome/DCML deficiency associated with monocytopenia and dendritic, B-cell, and NK-cell lymphopenias with a predisposition to nontuberculosis mycobacterial infections. Some of these patients may also develop lymphedema.[80,980,981]

Clinical Presentation

Children with MDS generally present with the signs and symptoms associated with bone marrow failure. Abnormalities in the peripheral blood may also be detected on routine medical examinations in asymptomatic children. Symptomatic children often present with some degree of fatigue, fever, malaise, or infections. Physical examination frequently reveals pallor, easy bruising, and petechiae. Splenomegaly, hepatomegaly, and lymphadenopathy are uncommon findings. The peripheral blood cell counts usually reveal anemia, neutropenia, and thrombocytopenia.

Differential Diagnosis

With a careful history and physical examination, as well as the evaluation of peripheral blood and a bone marrow aspirate, biopsy, and cytogenetics, a diagnosis of MDS can be made. Severe nutritional deficiencies of vitamin B_{12} and folate should be excluded, because they may impart a megaloblastic appearance to the bone marrow. Other nutritional deficiencies such as thiamine, pyridoxine, iron, and riboflavin can also present as some degree of bone marrow dysplasia and should be considered in the differential diagnosis. Occasionally, severe aplastic anemia can be difficult to distinguish from MDS, although a bone marrow biopsy should resolve this question. Certain viral infections (e.g., human immunodeficiency virus, parvovirus B19, Epstein-Barr virus, human herpesvirus 6, cytomegalovirus) and exposures (e.g., irradiation, chemotherapy, organic solvents) are associated with bone marrow failure and should be considered before making the diagnosis of MDS. The bone marrow cell karyotype should be determined to identify any clonal abnormalities. In addition, evidence has suggested that whole-genome scan by SNP analysis may detect clonal abnormalities in some patients with a normal bone marrow cell karyotype.[982,983]

Treatment

The rarity and heterogeneity of MDS in children, the lack of consensus on nomenclature, and the need for a risk-based classification system specific for pediatric MDS have hindered the development of appropriate therapy for pediatric MDS. Most clinical trials studying MDS have enrolled adults, in whom the disease may be different, and there have been few meaningful trials enrolling children. Regardless of treatment, the overall clinical outcome of children with MDS is guarded.

The only proven curative treatment for MDS is allogeneic HSCT. AML-based chemotherapy without HSCT has resulted in poor survival in the 30% range.[984,985] Prior to HSCT, or if an appropriate donor was not available, treatment primarily consisted of supportive care with packed red blood cell or platelet transfusions, parenteral antibiotics, and hydration. Other noncytotoxic therapies, including hormone therapy (e.g., androgens, glucocorticoids), recombinant hematopoietic growth factors (e.g., G-CSF, GM-CSF, erythropoietin), and differentiating agents (e.g., 13-*cis*-retinoic acid, ATRA), have been used in adults and have shown minimal benefit.[986-996] Low-dose chemotherapy has been used in an attempt to promote differentiation of the malignant hematopoietic clone. Although studies using low-dose cytarabine have shown improvement in peripheral counts and decreased marrow blast percentages in some patients with MDS, the responses have not been sustained.[997] Other agents, such as melphalan, hydroxyurea, etoposide, topotecan, 6-mercaptopurine, and busulfan, have been used with only partial or temporary responses in small numbers of patients.

A number of new agents have emerged for the treatment of pediatric MDS after randomized clinical trials in adult patients. These therapies have evolved out of a growing interest in the field of epigenetics and the concept that the repression of key tumor suppressor genes in MDS may occur because of aberrant methylation and histone deacetylation, instead of or in concert with gene deletions and mutations.[252] Studies involving the *CDKN2B* (*p15^INK4B*) tumor suppressor gene have demonstrated evidence of methylated CpG islands in the promoter region, preventing gene transcription and leading to gene repression.[998,999] Since these initial studies, a number of other genes have been found to have reduced expression because of DNA methylation, thus prompting clinical trials of demethylating agents in MDS.[1000,1001] Based on the impressive response rates and delayed progression to AML compared with supportive care, two demethylating agents, 5-azacytidine and decitabine, have been approved by the FDA for the treatment of MDS in adults.[1002,1003] These agents have shown the greatest efficacy in low-risk MDS. They are given in a low-dosage schedule, and patients may need to be treated for several months before a clinical response is achieved. Although these agents have improved the time to progression in adult MDS, they cannot cure the disease. The role of these therapies in pediatric MDS is currently under active investigation. As indicated earlier, lenalidomide is now approved for the treatment of patients with MDS with the 5q– cytogenetic abnormality and appears to work best in those whose MDS clone lacks any other cytogenetic abnormalites.[937]

For children with MDS, allogeneic HSCT remains the treatment of choice. In the absence of a sibling donor, a matched unrelated donor should be sought. Children with lower-risk MDS are frequently treated with allogeneic HSCT without prior chemotherapy, particularly if a matched sibling is available, to avoid the need for large numbers of transfusions. In more advanced MDS (WHO RAEB1 and RAEB2), AML-type chemotherapy has been often administered to induce a remission or to reduce the disease burden before HSCT. A study from the Fred Hutchinson Cancer Research Center in Seattle in children with MDS demonstrated a 3-year survival rate of patients with lower-stage MDS of 74% compared with 68% for patients with more advanced disease.[1004] The European Working Group on MDS in Children (EWOG-MDS) reported a 55% 5-year EFS rate for 33 pediatric patients with MDS after HSCT.[1005] A recent pediatric study from the University of Minnesota demonstrated an OS of 53% and a DFS of 48% at 3 years for 37 pediatric patients with MDS who received allogeneic HSCT after myeloablative conditioning over a 20-year period ending in 2010. Earlier HSCT without preconditioning chemotherapy was associated with an improved outcome, suggesting that delaying transplant to reduce disease burden with AML-directed therapy is not warranted if an appropriate donor is available.[925] These results are in keeping with those found in a European study of pediatric MDS patients who received a myeloablative allogeneic HSCT in which the OS was 63% at 5 years.[984] This study similarly showed no benefit to pre-HSCT chemotherapy except for the group who had more advanced myelodysplasia-related AML, a subgroup not included in the prior study. A longer interval between diagnosis and HSCT was actually associated with less relapse but may have been confounded by the number of lower-risk MDS patients in this group.[984] TRM during transplant can be a significant issue, resulting in some groups attempting reduced-intensity conditioning regimens. These approaches have had variable success, with some studies reporting lower DFS rates.[925,1006]

MYELOPROLIFERATIVE DISORDERS

Juvenile Myelomonocytic Leukemia

JMML is a rare, clonal, myeloproliferative disorder of the stem cell that usually manifests in the first few years of life. It has also been referred to as juvenile chronic myelomonocytic leukemia (JCML), infantile monosomy 7 syndrome, or juvenile granulocytic leukemia. Although JMML, adult CML, and CMML have some similar features, JMML is a clinically and pathophysiologically distinct disorder of young children. An international consensus panel consisting of the JMML Working Group and the EWOG-MDS has established a set of clinical and laboratory criteria for the diagnosis of JMML (Box 51-3).[1007]

Pathobiology

The cause of JMML is unknown. Several recurrent chromosomal abnormalities have been associated with JMML, but their relevance to the pathogenesis of the disease is not well understood. For example, up to 20% of patients meeting the diagnostic criteria for JMML have abnormalities in chromosome 7 (e.g., monosomy 7, 7q−), and the genes involved and their contributions to disease pathogenesis remain an area of intense investigation.[540,1007] At the molecular level, one or more defects involving the NF1/RAS signal pathway have been demonstrated in studies of JMML cells, implicating this pathway in the development of the disease. Activating point mutations in NRAS and KRAS genes have been demonstrated in 15% to 30% of patients with JMML.[1008,1009] Other

---

Box 51-3   Recommended Diagnostic Criteria for Juvenile Myelomonocytic Leukemia

CATEGORY 1 (ALL OF THE FOLLOWING)

No Philadelphia chromosome or BCR-ABL rearrangement
Peripheral blood monocyte count higher than 1000/μL
Bone marrow blasts less than 20%
Splenomegaly

CATEGORY 2 (AT LEAST ONE OF THE FOLLOWING)

Somatic mutations in RAS, PTPN11, or CBL
Clinical diagnosis of neurofibromatosis type 1 or NF1 gene mutation
Monosomy 7

CATEGORY 3 (TWO OF THE FOLLOWING IF NO CRITERIA FROM CATEGORY 2)

Increased fetal hemoglobin level
Myeloid precursors in peripheral blood
White blood cell count greater than 10,000/μL
Clonal abnormalities (excluding monosomy 7)
Granulocyte-macrophage colony-stimulating factor hypersensitivity of myeloid progenitors in vitro

Modified from the World Health Organization criteria from the 2008 Juvenile Myelomonocytic Leukemia Symposium, Atlanta, Ga.

---

patients have loss of NF1, which codes for a RAS GTPase-activating protein involved in the GM-CSF signaling pathway.[68,1010] Mutations in PTPN11 encoding the SHP-2 phosphatase have also been found in patients with JMML.[1011,1012] Similar PTPN11 mutations have been found to cause Noonan syndrome, an autosomal dominantly inherited syndrome associated with short stature, cardiac abnormalities and characteristic facial features, and, occasionally, a JMML-like hematopoietic picture. More recently, studies using genome-wide SNP arrays have uncovered novel homozygous mutations in the E3 ubiquitin ligase gene, CBL, in patients with JMML without mutations in the other identified causative genes.[1013-1015] These mutations are all mutually exclusive. JMML cells grown in culture demonstrate a specific hypersensitivity to the growth factor GM-CSF that is not observed with other growth factors, such as interleukin-3.[1016] Knockout mice lacking expression of NF1 die at embryonic day 13 or 14, but hematopoietic progenitor cells from these embryos grown in culture also demonstrate a specific hypersensitivity treatment with GM-CSF.[144] Moreover, immunodeficient mice transplanted with these cells develop a myeloproliferative disorder similar to JMML.[146,1017]

An increasing body of evidence has suggested that JMML arises from a pluripotent HSC, but the molecular abnormalities underlying the transformation appear to be distinct from those in the adult-type myeloproliferative disorders.[1017] JMML cells maintain their clonality when grown in long-term culture-initiating assays, in contrast to Philadelphia chromosome–positive CML cells, which yield to polyclonal residual normal cells in similar culture assays. Marrow cells from patients with JMML grow in culture and generate granulocyte-macrophage colony-forming units (GM-CFUs) spontaneously, in the absence of added hematopoietic growth factors. In contrast, GM-CFUs from normal individuals and from patients with adult CML only grow when exogenous growth factors are added to the semisolid culture medium.

Clinical Presentation and Prognosis

The presenting signs and symptoms of JMML result from organ infiltration of malignant cells; the most common symptoms are fever, cough, infection, pallor, malaise, hepatosplenomegaly, lymphadenopathy, rash, bleeding, and failure to thrive.[1007] Splenomegaly has now been incorporated as a category 1 criterion because only 7% of patients with JMML do not have splenomegaly at diagnosis.[1018] Laboratory abnormalities usually include an elevated WBC count with monocytosis, anemia, thrombocytopenia, an elevated fetal hemoglobin level, and hypergammaglobulinemia.[1007]

JMML is a progressive and often rapidly fatal disease, particularly in older children. Children younger than 2 years may have a more indolent course and, in fact, the disease may spontaneously resolve, as has been observed in patients with Noonan syndrome (reminiscent of TMD in Down syndrome) and a proportion of JMML patients with *RAS* or *CBL* mutations.[1018,1019] However, patients with older age at diagnosis (>2 years), higher fetal hemoglobin level, and platelets less than 33,000/μL tend to present with more complex cytogenetic abnormalities and are predisposed to poorer outcome.[1020] Although some studies have not found any prognostic differences in the genetic cause, others have found *PTPN11* mutations to be associated with increased relapse after HSCT.[1021] The accelerated blast phase characteristic of adult CMML is unusual in children with JMML.

Treatment

Several treatment regimens have been used to improve survival, including low-dose chemotherapy, intensive AML-type therapy, and 13-*cis*-retinoic acid.[540,1022-1027] Although durable remissions have been reported in a minority of cases, the response to these agents is usually transient and the long-term survival is poor. The only known curative therapy for JMML is allogeneic HSCT, and neither pretreatment chemotherapy nor splenectomy has not been found to impact survival.[1018] When an HLA-matched related donor is available, HSCT is the recommended treatment for patients with newly diagnosed disease. Survival rates of 35% to 55% have been reported with HSCT, but treatment-related mortality and relapse rates remain high, particularly for patients who undergo unrelated donor HSCT.[1028-1031] Several issues remain controversial, including the management of patients without HLA-matched related donors, GVHD prophylaxis, pre-HSCT chemotherapy, and appropriate myeloablative therapy. Future therapies in JMML are aimed at targeting downstream pathways from RAS, including mTOR- and PI3K-inhibiting agents.

Chronic Myelogenous Leukemia Caused by the *BCR-ABL* Fusion Gene

In 1951, Dameshek first introduced the idea that CML, polycythemia vera (PV), essential thrombocythemia (ET), and primary myelofibrosis (PM) were related myeloproliferative syndromes, even though each has distinct clinical, laboratory, and biologic features.[1032,1033] A common feature is multilineage clonal proliferation involving the entire spectrum of myeloid cells, suggesting that transformation has occurred in a pluripotent stem cell. All these conditions, as well as systemic mastocytosis, hypereosinophilic syndrome, chronic eosinophilic leukemia, and chronic myelomonocytic leukemia, have been linked to a specific mutation or translocation resulting in the constitutive activation of a receptor tyrosine kinase. This accounts for the increased hematopoietic stem and progenitor cell proliferation with differentiation that characterizes these disorders. Patients may occasionally present with mixed manifestations rather than a distinct myeloproliferative disorder or, over the course of their illness, develop problems more typical of one of the other disorders.

Chronic myelogenous leukemia was first recognized as early as 1845, with several described cases of splenomegaly, anemia, and massive granulocytosis.[1034,1035] However, it was not until 1960, with the discovery of the Philadelphia chromosome, that the disease became better understood.[1036] CML constitutes 15% to 20% of all leukemias but accounts for only 1% to 3% of all childhood leukemias. In children, the disorder may present as one of two distinct clinical syndromes, adult-type CML (ACML), which is the same as the disease in older patients (and herein referred to as CML) and juvenile CML (JCML), now known as JMML, a syndrome described in the previous section that is restricted to children and has distinct clinical, laboratory, and cytogenetic characteristics (Table 51-2). The incidence of CML is less than 1 case/100,000 for patients younger than 20 years and 1 to 2 cases/100,000 for those 20 to 50 years, and it rises slowly thereafter. The median age at diagnosis is 67 years, and the male-to-female ratio is 1.8:1. It has been difficult to identify environmental factors associated with the pathogenesis of CML. Ionizing radiation is the only clearly identified risk factor for CML. A sevenfold increase has been documented in the survivors of the nuclear bomb–related exposure to radiation in Japan and, notably, the incidence of CML in this population was highest in young people, especially children younger than 5 years.[1037,1038]

Pathobiology

The diagnosis of CML is almost always associated with the t(9;22)(q34;q11) chromosomal translocation in bone marrow cells. This reciprocal translocation is detected by standard cytogenetic techniques in almost 90% of CML cases.[1036,1039] However, the presence of the Philadelphia chromosome in bone marrow cells is not pathognomonic for CML, because this chromosome is present at diagnosis in 25% to 50% of adult patients, 3% to 5% of children with ALL,[1040] and 2% of patients with AML. It is absent in 5% of patients with CML, although these patients' bone marrow cells may harbor a variant of the translocation detectable only by RT-PCR or FISH.[1041] The Philadelphia chromosome of CML involves a reciprocal translocation of the *ABL* gene from its normal position at the end of the q arm of chromosome 9 to a site on the q arm of chromosome 22 within the *bcr*

TABLE 51-2   Clinical Characteristics of Children with Juvenile Myelomonocytic Leukemia (JMML) versus Adult-Type Chronic Myelogenous Leukemia (CML)

Characteristics at Diagnosis	JMML	CML
Age (yr)	Usually <4	Usually >4
Lymphadenopathy	Common	Unusual
Skin lesions	Common	Unusual
Bleeding	Common	Unusual
Bacterial infection	Common	Unusual
White blood cell count >100,000/μL	Unusual	Common
Hemoglobin <12 g/dL	Common	Variable
Platelets	Usually decreased	Usually increased
Monocytosis	Common	Unusual
Circulating pronormoblasts	Common	Unusual
Increased fetal hemoglobin	Common	Unusual
Philadelphia chromosome	Absent	>90%
BCR-ABL fusion gene	Absent	Present
Leukocyte alkaline phosphatase decreased	Variable	Common
Clinical Course		
Median survival (yr)	1-2	Variable, >10 yr in chronic phase
Blast phase	Unusual	Common

region. The reciprocal t(9;22) chromosomal translocation creates a fusion *BCR-ABL* gene detectable in the bone marrow and peripheral blood by PCR assay. The chimeric gene encodes a dysregulated tyrosine kinase that is constitutively active, is expressed in the cytoplasm, and has increased activity compared with the normal ABL protein.[1042] In contrast to cytoplasmic BCR-ABL protein, normal ABL is a nuclear kinase, the activity of which is tightly regulated in vivo.[1043] Although the precise function of normal ABL is not known, available evidence suggests that it regulates pathways that mediate cell cycle arrest after genotoxic damage.[1044-1048] The main clinical manifestation of CML is an overabundance of mature myeloid cells from hyperproliferative progenitor cells. Evidence for the role of the *BCR-ABL* translocation in the pathogenesis of CML is confirmed by the observation that BCR-ABL proteins can also induce a CML-like syndrome in vivo in mice when they are expressed in hematopoietic progenitors.[1049-1052] Mechanistic studies of these fusion proteins have shown that RAS signaling is essential for transformation and that multiple accessory molecules, including the adapters GRB2, SHC, and CRKL, are used to couple the activated ABL kinase to RAS,

resulting in activation of Jun kinase.[1053-1055] Oncogenic signaling by BCR-ABL has also been shown to involve the cell cycle–regulated genes *MYC* and *cyclin D1*.[1056,1057] Thus, multiple signaling pathways are activated to mediate leukemic transformation by BCR-ABL. Transformation has also been shown to occur in the pluripotent stem cell. Murine experiments in which sorted HSCs were transduced with *BCR-ABL* and transplanted into irradiated recipients developed a CML-like phenotype, whereas the same experiment performed using more differentiated progenitor cells failed to induce a myeloproliferative disease.[111] Moreover, granulocytes, monocytes, erythroid cells, megakaryocytes, and lymphocytes from patients with this disease have been shown to be clonal progeny of a single cell and to harbor the Philadelphia chromosome.[1058-1060] Probably because of some persistent normal hematopoiesis in patients with CML and because of the long life span of some cell types, such as T lymphocytes, all patients do not have demonstrable involvement of all lineages.[1059] It is worth emphasizing that the *BCR-ABL* fusion gene is acquired somatically by an HSC and its expression is restricted to its clonal progeny, so the nonhematopoietic cells of the patient do not contain the translocation.[1061,1062]

Clinical Presentation

CML can present in one of three phases—chronic phase, accelerated phase, or blast crisis. Most patients present in the chronic phase and may be asymptomatic. When symptoms and signs are present, they are often mild and are caused by the accumulation of mature and immature granulocytic cells. Generalized malaise, weakness, weight loss, fever, pallor, and organomegaly, particularly splenomegaly, are frequent presenting symptoms. Abdominal pain from massive splenomegaly may also bring a patient to medical attention. CNS, retinal, and pulmonary dysfunction can occur, as well as arthritis and priapism. Occasionally, the diagnosis is made from a routine blood cell count.[1063] WBC counts usually exceed 100,000/μL, with the appearance of some circulating immature myeloid forms.[1064,1065] Basophilia and eosinophilia may also occur. In addition, platelet counts above 400,000/μL are frequently observed, although thrombocytopenia may also occur. The WBC and platelet counts in CML patients may fluctuate spontaneously and nonconcordantly, making it difficult to attribute changes to the effects of therapy.[1066] The presence of anemia is also variable in CML.[1067] Leukostasis, a syndrome caused by hyperleukocytosis and frequently presenting as neurologic symptoms, such as dizziness, confusion, and somnolence, or pulmonary symptoms, including tachypnea, dyspnea, and respiratory failure, is observed in AML and ALL secondary to high blast cell counts. However, symptoms of leukostasis are uncommon in adults with CML and are only slightly more common in childhood CML, even in patients with very elevated WBC counts.[1068] Skin nodules, representing extramedullary hematopoiesis, may also be present.[1069] The bone marrow in CML patients typically demonstrates normal myeloid maturation, with granulocytic hyperplasia and an increased myeloid-to-erythroid ratio. Megakaryocytic hyperplasia may also occur.[1063]

Dysplastic marrow basophils or eosinophils are common, and cells of these lineages may be increased in number. About one in six CML patients has lipid-laden macrophages, sometimes called sea-blue histiocytes, similar to Gaucher cells.[1070] Although an increase in reticulin may occur, myelofibrosis is unusual. By definition, in chronic phase CML, the blast cell percentages in both the peripheral blood and bone marrow are less than 10%, and an increase above these levels may indicate a transition from chronic phase to accelerated phase or blast crisis. Other abnormal laboratory findings in chronic phase CML include low leukocyte alkaline phosphatase (LAP) activity and increased vitamin B_{12} levels. The latter occurs because of the increased white blood cell mass, which produces WBC-derived vitamin B_{12}–binding protein. The cause of the low LAP is unclear but may involve imperfect maturation of CML granulocytes. With therapy, the level of vitamin B_{12} falls to normal, whereas changes in LAP are less predictable.[1071]

The accelerated phase is characterized by increased marrow or blood blast cell values of 10% to 19%, peripheral basophilia greater than 20%, persistent thrombocytopenia unrelated to therapy or thrombocytosis unresponsive to therapy, and increasing spleen size or WBC count. If marrow or blood blast cell percentages exceed 19% of total leukocytes, this signifies a transition to blast crisis, which may be myeloid, lymphoid, or mixed. Presentation in blast crisis can mimic an acute leukemia of lymphoid or myeloid lineage, and in this case the cells harbor the Philadelphia chromosome.

Differential Diagnosis

The differential diagnosis of an elevated WBC count (also known as a leukemoid reaction) includes severe infections, congenital heart disease, and metastatic cancer. In disorders other than CML, the peripheral blood rarely contains blasts and promyelocytes, the WBC count is usually somewhat lower, and the LAP scores and cytogenetic studies are normal. In general, patients with CML have a WBC count of more than $100,000/\mu L$, a WBC differential containing promyelocytes and myelocytes (the blood smear often appears similar to a marrow smear), a low LAP, a large spleen, and Philadelphia chromosome or molecular detection of the BCR-ABL transcript. Because CML patients can present in blast crisis, the patient with Philadelphia chromosome–positive ALL presents a problem in differential diagnosis. Determination of the size of the abnormal fusion protein (usually 210 kD in CML and 185 kD in Philadelphia chromosome–positive ALL) and the fusion transcript breakpoint by RT-PCR assay can help, as can the response to therapy. An important distinction is that in ALL the Philadelphia chromosome commonly disappears with intensive chemotherapy whereas in CML presenting in blast crisis the disease may revert to the chronic phase, with the Philadelphia chromosome persisting in the recovering bone marrow cells.[1072]

Clinical Course

Approximately 90% of patients are in the chronic phase at diagnosis. Prior to the advent of tyrosine kinase inhibitor therapy, patients sometimes enjoyed unimpaired lifestyles for periods of many months to years, with minimal therapy during the chronic phase of their disease. However, if untreated, most patients will experience progressive disease from 3 to 8 years after diagnosis. This is because of the development of the accelerated phase, which progresses to eventual blast crisis, usually within 3 months. Overall, blast crisis will develop in 75% to 85% of all untreated patients with CML. Blast crisis is a clinically high-risk form of CML that is difficult to control with chemotherapy and often leads to death within a short time, usually months.

Although BCR-ABL alone may be able to induce chronic-phase CML, evolution to accelerated phase or blast crisis is often accompanied by the acquisition of duplicated Philadelphia chromosome or additional cytogenetic abnormalities in the bone marrow, such as trisomy 8 or abnormalities involving chromosome 7, including the t7;11(p15;p15) that creates the NUP98-HOXA9 fusion.[1073] Transformation to blast crisis appears to follow many of the same multiple mutational steps involved in the molecular pathogenesis of de novo AML or ALL. LAP levels may also rise during the transition to blast crisis. Myeloid blast crisis is somewhat more common and carries a poorer prognosis than lymphoid blast crisis.[1072,1074-1076] About one third of patients have a lymphoblastic crisis, usually precursor B-cell by immunophenotype, although T-lymphoblastic crisis phenotypes can occur.[1077,1078] Patients with lymphoid blast crisis have a younger median age than patients with myeloid blast crisis.[1079] CML blast crisis can also contain subpopulations of blast cells with differing phenotypes (possibly subclones differentiated along both lymphoid and myeloid lineages, biphenotypic leukemias) and blast crisis in which individual cells simultaneously express features of more than one lineage (mixed-lineage leukemias).

Treatment

Historic Chemotherapy. Traditional chemotherapy for CML used busulfan or hydroxyurea.[1080] Busulfan is associated with infertility and, rarely, marrow aplasia and interstitial pneumonitis. Hydroxyurea is less toxic but only induces a decreased granulocyte count. Hydroxyurea does not induce cytogenetic remissions or change the natural history of the disease. Interferon-α (IFN-α) has demonstrated improved rates of hematologic remission over hydroxyurea, with evidence of hematologic control in 70% to 80% of patients and complete cytogenetic responses in 6% to 26% when given as a single agent in different series.[1081-1083] The normalization of bone marrow cytogenetics was shown to persist for many years in some patients, even after stopping the drug. Interestingly, these patients often remain PCR positive for the BCR-ABL transcript if sensitive techniques are used.[1084-1086] Despite the efficacy of IFN-α, unwanted side effects are common and include fatigue, myalgias, arthralgias, headaches, weight loss, depression, diarrhea, neurologic symptoms, memory changes, hair thinning, autoimmune diseases, and cardiomyopathy,[1087-1089] leading 14% to 26% of patients to discontinue therapy.[1090-1093] Thus although IFN-α demonstrated some promise in this disease, the toxicity profile made it intolerable to a large fraction of CML patients.

Tyrosine Kinase Inhibitors. The treatment of chronic phase CML has since been revolutionized with the advent of molecularly targeted therapy that specifically targets the BCR-ABL fusion protein. Imatinib mesylate, also known as STI-571 or Gleevec, is a tyrosine kinase inhibitor that blocks enzymatic activity of several tyrosine kinases, including mainly ABL, PDGFR, and KIT, by binding to the adenosine triphosphate (ATP) binding site. The promising results of phase I and II studies that produced impressive activity in patients who had already failed IFN-α[1094] led to the International Randomized Study of Interferon and STI571 (IRIS), which randomized patients to imatinib versus interferon with cytarabine as initial therapy for patients with CML.[1095] This study demonstrated better outcome with longer times to progression and to accelerated phase or blast crisis for patients initially treated with imatinib. Additionally, patients treated with imatinib had higher rates of hematologic and cytogenetic remission and, for the first time, molecular responses were obtained with an undetectable *BCR-ABL* fusion transcript. Treatment with imatinib effectively established new standards for response rates, including complete hematologic response (CHR), implying a normalization of peripheral blood cell counts; major cytogenetic response (MCyR), with the presence of Philadelphia chromosome in 1% to 35% bone marrow cells analyzed by metaphase spread; complete cytogenetic response (CCyR), with the absence of Philadelphia chromosome; and major molecular response (MMR), demonstrating a 3-log reduction in detection of the *BCR-ABL* transcript in bone marrow cell RNA compared with diagnostic levels. The 8-year follow-up of the IRIS study has now been published[1125] and has convincingly demonstrated the long-term benefit and tolerability of imatinib therapy, with increasing rates of MMR and CCyR over time. Imatinib has excellent oral bioavailability, with minimal systemic effects other than myelosuppression. Other side effects include peripheral and periorbital edema, muscle cramps, gastrointestinal intolerance, and rash. Cardiac complications, including congestive heart failure, are rare but have been reported.[1097] However, imatinib must be continued indefinitely because cessation of the drug is generally associated with an increase in bone marrow cell *BCR-ABL* transcript levels and, eventually, hematologic relapse. Given the success of imatinib therapy, a number of studies have strived to determine what cytogenetic or molecular milestones at what specific time points after initiation of imatinib are most predictive of response. CCyR is regarded as the gold standard and considered to correlate with a 2-log reduction of *BCR-ABL* transcript levels (expressed as 1% on the recently accepted international scale that establishes 100% as an initial transcript level). A recent study demonstrated that a transcript level of less than 10% at the 3-month mark had the greatest prognostic value in predicting outcome.[1098] Although current practice includes surveillance at later time points, this manuscript provocatively suggests that changes in management can effectively be made at this early juncture

and may preclude the need for further evaluations including invasive bone marrow evaluations. However, the counter argument is that bone marrow evaluations are important for examination of new collaborating cytogenetic abnormalities that may herald the evolution of a clonal population and accelerated disease.

Based on the success, promise, and safety profile of imatinib therapy in adults, studies to determine the efficacy of this drug in childhood CML have been undertaken. The COG published the results of a phase I trial of imatinib in children with Philadelphia chromosome–positive disease who had failed interferon therapy.[1099] Imatinib was well tolerated at escalating dose levels up to 570 mg/m^2 and CHR was demonstrated for all 14 chronic-phase patients within 1 month of starting therapy. Ten of 12 evaluated patients had achieved a CCyR by a median of 3 months. A phase II European pediatric study[1100] demonstrated equally encouraging results for children with chronic-phase CML who failed IFN-α therapy. These studies and extrapolation from adult data have resulted in imatinib becoming first-line therapy in children with chronic-phase CML. Confidence in this approach has been improved by evidence that prior imatinib therapy has no negative impact on the TRM after an allogeneic donor HSCT.[1101] Side effects of imatinib in children include gastrointestinal problems and rashes. If signs of leukostasis are present, more urgent therapy must be used. If the WBC count must be lowered quickly, leukapheresis and immediate chemotherapy with high-doses of hydroxyurea may be used. Proper hydration, alkalinization of the urine, and the use of allopurinol are imperative before the rapid lysis of cells is induced with chemotherapy.

Resistance to imatinib mesylate has been demonstrated.[1102-1106] Mechanisms of resistance include point mutations in *BCR-ABL*, amplification of the *BCR-ABL* gene, overexpression of the BCR-ABL protein, enhanced expression of the multidrug resistance gene, and excessive binding of imatinib by serum proteins. Analysis of a small number of blast crisis patients who experienced relapse while receiving imatinib has frequently shown either *BCR-ABL* gene amplification or *BCR-ABL* kinase domain mutations.[1103] These observations have indicated that resistance to imatinib as a single agent in the treatment of CML involves alterations of the BCR-ABL protein expression level or structure, allowing it to escape inhibition by the drug, rather than mutations in entirely different genes that might have reduced the malignant cells' dependence on BCR-ABL for transformation. A number of approaches have been suggested as interventions after the identification of imatinib resistance. High-dose imatinib has shown some promise for inducing cytogenetic remissions, despite a lack of efficacy of standard-dose therapy.[1107] Additionally, a number of new tyrosine kinase inhibitors have emerged and are more potent inhibitors of BCR-ABL than imatinib. Nilotinib is a structural derivative of imatinib and effective at lower concentrations.[1108] At doses of 300 mg to 400 mg twice daily, it is well tolerated in adults,[1108a] although it requires fasting before and after each dose, a requirement that potentially complicates its administration to children. Dasatinib has a completely different structure and binding configuration, making it active against most imatinib-resistant *BCR-ABL* mutations, as well as a host of other tyrosine kinases. Dasatinib has a higher incidence of thrombocytopenia than imatinib and is associated with a high incidence of pleural effusions in adult patients. Both dasatinib and nilotinib are FDA approved for the treatment of imatinib-resistant chronic-phase CML.[1107,1109,1110] More recently, head-to-head randomized control trials in adult patients with chronic-phase CML have demonstrated that both of these agents are more effective as frontline therapy at achieving CCYR by 1 year than imatinib.[1111,1112] The COG recently completed a phase I trial of dasatinib for imatinib-resistant leukemia and solid tumors. Nine CML patients who had experienced relapse were included and generally tolerated doses as high as 85 mg/m²; there was one case of hemangiomatosis, and cytogenetic responses were demonstrated in 5 patients (complete response in 3 and partial response in 2).[1113] These results have prompted studies in newly diagnosed patients with Philadelphia chromosome–positive ALL, combining dasatinib in doses of 60 mg/m² with intensive chemotherapy and a proposed COG study for dasatinib as a frontline agent in CML. Nilotinib is now being considered for a phase II study in pediatric CML resistant to imatinib or dasatinib.

Hematopoietic Stem Cell Transplantation. Of all malignancies, CML has the most extensive long-term data on the effectiveness of allogeneic HSCT. This approach can provide prolonged DFS in CML and is the only proven curative therapy. The effectiveness of allogeneic HSCT in CML is believed to be caused in part by the effects of the transplanted immune system, rather than solely the result of the high-dose total-body irradiation and chemotherapy in the conditioning regimen. The allogeneic graft creates a new immune system that plays an active role in eradicating CML cells. Immune-mediated antileukemic effects are suspected because patients may remain PCR positive for *BCR-ABL* transcripts for months after HSCT and yet appear to be cured of their disease and eventually convert to PCR negativity without further therapy. Furthermore, there is an extremely high relapse rate for autologous, syngeneic, and T-cell–depleted grafts with the same myeloablative conditioning regimens used for standard, non–T-cell–depleted grafts, a result that suggests alloreactivity is associated with lower relapse rates.[1114-1116]

The role of allogeneic HSCT in CML provides a moving target in the post–tyrosine kinase inhibitor era. The potential toxicity associated with allogeneic HSCT, especially from a matched unrelated donor, compared with the efficacy and tolerability of oral tyrosine kinase inhibitors has raised questions regarding the indications and timing for HSCT in CML patients. Although some patients may go on to long-term survival when HSCT is performed in accelerated phase or blast crisis of CML (15% to 30% of cases), results are substantially better when HSCT is performed in the chronic phase.[1117] If the procedure is performed while the patient is in chronic phase using a matched sibling donor, 1-year survival rates are 60% to 80%, with a 10-year DFS rate of approximately 50%.[1114,1118-1120] Some studies have demonstrated increased survival outcomes if the HSCT was performed within the first year of diagnosis.[1121-1123] Prior to imatinib therapy, these data prompted the initiation of allogeneic HSCT early in the course of treatment. However, HSCT has always been limited to patients who can medically tolerate the procedure and have appropriate donors— 30% have matched sibling donors, 5% have matches with additional family members, and 50% have matched unrelated donors in donor registries. Imatinib can be safely given pre-HSCT and has no impact on TRM.[1101,1124] Currently, most adult patients, including even those with sibling donors, are being maintained on imatinib until evidence of resistance develops, which then prompts a change in therapy and consideration of HSCT. In children, the timing of HSCT for CML is even more challenging. Although imatinib has now demonstrated impressive 8-year outcomes,[1125] will these be sustained for the many years that a child with CML would be required to take the drug? Allogeneic HSCT still remains the only curative therapy and is generally better tolerated by children, particularly with modern approaches to supportive care.

Between 10% and 15% of recipients of matched sibling HSCT and less than 5% of matched unrelated donor recipients experience relapse hematologically after allogeneic HSCT. Patients who experience relapse after HSCT may respond to interferon or withdrawal of immunosuppression.[1126-1129] Recent evidence has suggested that relapse rates may be reduced with the addition of imatinib therapy after HSCT whether or not the patient received imatinib before HSCT. However, the recommended duration of imatinib therapy after HSCT remains uncertain. Patients who experience relapse after HSCT may benefit from a second-generation tyrosine kinase inhibitor, such as dasatinib, a second HSCT, or donor-lymphocyte infusions. Sixty to 80 percent of patients who experience relapse cytogenetically or hematologically and return to chronic phase after HSCT can be salvaged by donor lymphocyte infusions without further cytotoxic chemotherapy.[674,1130-1132] Unfortunately, acute and chronic GVHD and marrow aplasia remain significant complications after donor lymphocyte infusion.[1133] Relapse occurs again in 5% to 15% of patients successfully treated with donor lymphocyte infusion, but remissions induced by this modality are durable in most patients.

Blast-Phase Chronic Myelogenous Leukemia

Blast-phase CML is generally resistant to chemotherapy.[1074] As in acute leukemia, leukostasis is more likely in patients with high blast counts, and rapid institution of therapy to lower the WBC count is indicated after initiating measures to protect the patient from tumor lysis syndrome. The blast cell morphology and surface markers should guide therapy in blast crisis of CML. Lymphoid blast morphology or surface markers predict a good initial response to drugs effective in ALL, such as prednisone and vincristine.[1063,1079,1134] However, patients whose blast cells have a myeloid morphology and immunophenotype respond poorly to most therapies. Median survival is only 2 months after transformation to myeloid blast crisis, compared with 6 months if the blast cells have lymphoblastic characteristics.[1135] Allogeneic HSCT in late-stage CML is associated with a poor outcome, primarily because of the high peri-HSCT mortality from regimen-related toxicity and an extremely high relapse rate.

Chronic Myelogenous Leukemia Caused by Other Translocations

Other chromosomal translocations have also been identified in CML. The *TEL* gene belongs to a large family of transcription factors referred to as the *ETS* family. These genes encode related proteins defined by a highly conserved, 90-amino acid, winged helix-turn-helix dimerization motif. This region appears to be an essential requirement for constitutive tyrosine kinase activity and transforming capacity of fusion proteins derived from chromosomal translocations involving *TEL*, generally partnered with a tyrosine kinase gene such as the *PDGF* receptor.[1136-1138] With the exception of the t(12;21)-associated *TEL-AML1* fusion gene exclusively associated with early B-cell lineage ALL, *TEL* gene rearrangements are rare in human leukemia. Because of the small numbers of patients with myeloid malignancy who have *TEL* gene fusions, there is insufficient clinical experience to determine their clinical implications. However, there is a trend toward an unfavorable outcome in patients with atypical CML or CMML accompanied by *TEL* gene rearrangements.

Polycythemia Vera

Polycythemia is defined as an increase in numbers of circulating erythrocytes, hemoglobin, and hematocrit. There are three types of polycythemia: (1) polycythemia vera (PV), or primary polycythemia; (2) secondary polycythemia; and (3) relative polycythemia.[1139] The first two types are associated with an increase in red blood cell mass, whereas in the third the red blood cell mass is normal and plasma volume is reduced. Secondary polycythemia can arise from a multitude of causes, including those that result in excessive erythropoietin production caused by decreased tissue oxygenation (physiologically appropriate), inappropriate erythropoietin secretion from a tumor, a mutant hemoglobin with abnormal oxygen affinity, and decreased erythrocyte diphosphoglycerate.

PV is a myeloproliferative disease caused by clonal expansion of an abnormal multipotent stem cell that produces erythroid progenitors that can proliferate in the absence of erythropoietin (EPO).[1140,1141] In contrast, normal fetal erythroid progenitors and those with mutations in the EPO receptor still require erythropoietin for their function. Growth of erythropoietin-independent erythroid colonies in serum-containing cultures can be a useful diagnostic test.[1141] Because this is an HSC disorder, aberrations in the WBC and platelet counts can accompany the increased red blood cell mass. The diagnosis of PV used to be a diagnosis of exclusion. One had to prove that the elevated red cell mass was not from a secondary cause, such as hypoxia or a high oxygen affinity hemoglobin, and that the *BCR-ABL* transgene was absent. However, in 2005, several groups simultaneously reported

the presence of a somatically acquired clonal *V617F* mutation in *JAK2* in more than 90% of cases of sporadic PV in adults.[1142-1145] This seminal discovery linked PV with the other myeloproliferative disorders, such as CML, by demonstrating a primary mutation in a tyrosine kinase as a causative factor and effectively established *JAK2* mutational analysis as a diagnostic test for PV. Interestingly, this same mutation was found in 50% of cases of essential thrombocythemia (ET; see later) and primary myelofibrosis (PM).[1142-1145] These three different phenotypes caused by the same genotype pose many questions, and scientists are currently investigating the role of gene dosage, modifying mutations, or genetic predisposition to account for the difference in disease phenotype. Some studies have suggested that patients with PV have at least a subpopulation of cells that are homozygous for the *JAK2* mutation whereas patients with ET are heterozygous.[1146,1147] Moreover, the *JAK2* mutation may be sufficient to induce PV but other mutations are likely required for the development of ET and PM. Rare cases of familial polycythemia may exhibit autosomal recessive or dominant inheritance, and erythropoietin levels can be low, normal, or elevated.[1148] Studies of these families have revealed that the *JAK2* mutation is acquired, suggesting that there is an inherited predisposition allele that has not yet been identified.[1149] In some of the families, a mutation in the negative regulatory domain of the erythropoietin receptor gene appears to be involved.[1150-1152] Several *JAK2-V617F*–negative patients with PV were found to have a number of different mutations involving exon 12 of *JAK2*.[1153]

The WHO previously established strict criteria for the diagnosis of PV, with recent suggestions for revisions to *JAK2* mutational evaluation.[1154-1156] Evaluation should include a careful history and physical examination, including examination for splenomegaly and measurements of oxygen saturation, a complete blood cell count, and serum erythropoietin level, *JAK2* mutational analysis, and bone marrow aspirate and biopsy, including cytogenetics to rule out *BCR-ABL* or other translocation-induced fusion genes.

PV is extremely uncommon in children. The median age at presentation is 60 years, and fewer than 1% of PV patients are younger than 25 years.[1139,1157,1158] Children with PV are also less likely than adults to exhibit the most prevalent *JAK2* mutation. Erythrocytosis can cause cardiac symptoms, such as dyspnea and hypertension, and symptoms of disturbed cerebral circulation, such as dizziness and paresthesias. Abnormal platelet function and thrombocytosis may lead to thrombosis and hemorrhage. Granulocytic proliferation can cause increased histamine turnover, resulting in gastrointestinal symptoms and pruritus. Hyperuricemia and hypermetabolic symptoms are common, including weakness and weight loss. Most patients have large spleens and may have large livers and increased blood pressure.[1139] The marrow shows hypercellularity, an increase in megakaryocyte number, and decreased iron stores. Serum erythropoietin levels are usually normal or decreased.[1159] A total of 10% to 25% of patients have a clonal chromosomal abnormality evident by cytogenetic analysis, most often a

---

Box 51-4 **Suggested Criteria for Childhood Polycythemia Vera***

MAJOR CRITERIA

Increased hemoglobin/hematocrit
Presence of *JAK2-V617F* mutation
No cause of secondary erythrocytosis, including:
  a. Absence of familial erythrocytosis (e.g., hereditary mutations of erythropoietin [EPO] receptor)
  b. No elevation of EPO caused by
    i. Hypoxia (PaO$_2$ <92%)
    ii. High oxygen affinity hemoglobin
    iii. Truncated EPO receptor
    iv. Inappropriate EPO production by tumor

MINOR CRITERIA

Spontaneous erythroid colony formation
Hypercellular bone marrow with trilineage proliferation
Low serum EPO levels

Modified from Vardiman JW, Harris NL, Brunning RD: The World Health Organization (WHO) classification of the myeloid neoplasms. Blood 100:2292–2302, 2002; Tefferi A, Thiele J, Orazi A, et al: Proposals and rationale for revision of the World Health Organization diagnostic criteria for polycythemia vera, essential thrombocythemia, and primary myelofibrosis: recommendations from an ad hoc international expert panel. Blood 110:1092–1097, 2007; Teofili L, Giona F, Martini M, et al: Markers of myeloproliferative diseases in childhood polycythemia vera and essential thrombocythemia. J Clin Oncol 25:1048–1053, 2007; Teofili L, Giona F, Martini M, et al: The revised WHO diagnostic criteria for Ph-negative myeloproliferative diseases are not appropriate for the diagnostic screening of childhood polycythemia vera and essential thrombocythemia. Blood 110:3384–3386, 2007; and Barbui T. How to manage children and young adults with myeloproliferative neoplasms. Leukemia 26:1452–1457, 2012.

*Requires the presence of both major and one minor criteria or two to three minor criteria in the absence of the JAK2 mutation.

20q– deletion. Box 51-4 lists suggested criteria for the diagnosis of pediatric PV.[1160,1161]

Prolonged survival after the diagnosis of PV is common, but spontaneous remission is rare.[1162] Vascular occlusive episodes related to high hematocrit levels are an important cause of morbidity and mortality, with Budd-Chiari syndrome being among the most common manifestations.[1163] Other life-threatening complications of polycythemia vera include bleeding, myelofibrosis with pancytopenia, and acute leukemia.[1164] A poorly defined spent phase may occur, characterized by a decrease in hematocrit (often because of increased plasma volume), variable depression of other blood cell counts, hepatosplenomegaly, and increased bone marrow reticulin and fibrosis.[1165,1166] The decision to treat children with PV who are otherwise asymptomatic is controversial, given the potential side effects and complications of the various therapeutic options. Some experts advocate for completing a thrombophilic workup to assist in determining factors that might contribute to the risk for developing significant thrombi and shift the risk-benefit balance in the direction of treatment.[1167,1168] Treatment includes phlebotomy, although isovolumic erythropheresis may be a safer procedure, but this requires specific resources and is not uniformly available.[1169] The highest risk for thrombotic or hemorrhagic complications is observed immediately after phlebotomy. Iron replacement therapy should

be given, because iron deficiency can lead to nonhematologic disturbances and an increase in blood viscosity.[1170] Low-dose aspirin is also recommended for adults with PV and has been adopted in the prophylaxis of thrombosis in children with PV.[1168,1171] Radioactive phosphorus or chemotherapy can also control the hematocrit in PV. However, these treatments have been associated with an increased risk for transformation to AML.[1164] Hydroxyurea, IFN-α, and anagrelide are all agents used in adults to control cell counts and may be useful in pediatric cases.[1172-1174] Hydroxyurea is simpler to administer and has fewer side effects than IFN-α, and the leukemogenic risk of hydroxyurea appears to be low, as demonstrated by a number of long-term studies in sickle cell anemia patients. However, the risk for transformation to AML is still higher in PV, because patients have a primary clonal stem cell disorder.[1175] The main toxicity from hydroxyurea is neutropenia. Anagrelide is a newer agent that inhibits the action of cyclic AMP phosphodiesterase and primarily targets megakaryocyte differentiation and proliferation. It has resulted in the disappearance of thrombocythemia-related symptoms in 80% of patients with PV.[1176] However, it has been found to be inferior to hydroxyurea in ET.[1177] Given their familiarity and experience with the agent, most clinicians would use hydroxyurea in children with PV deemed at higher risk for thrombosis, owing to extremely elevated hematocrit or prior thrombotic event or bleeding, due to features such as esophageal varices, which could be exacerbated by phlebotomy or therapy with acetylsalicylic acid. IFN-α, particularly newer pegylated versions, is both effective and better tolerated[366,1168] and thus a reasonable alternative. A number of JAK2- and combined JAK1/JAK2-inhibiting agents have been developed and have demonstrated some symptom relieve in PM (see later) but have not proven to be more effective than hydroxyurea, IFN-α, and anagrelide in PV.[1178,1179]

Essential Thrombocythemia

ET is a myeloproliferative disorder characterized by an increased platelet count not attributable to any other cause; Box 51-5 lists causes of thrombocytosis.[1157,1180-1184] Similar to the other myeloproliferative diseases, ET is a clonal stem cell disorder that also affects other hematopoietic lineages.[1185] The *JAK2 V617F* mutation is found in approximately 50% of cases, and other cases may be associated with a mutation affecting the genes encoding thrombopoietin or the thrombopoietin receptor (MPL).[1186-1188] ET may occur in childhood, but rarely,[1158,1186,1189-1191] and it may be familial in some cases.[1192] A number of families have been identified who have ET and/or other myeloproliferative diseases with or without acquisition of the *JAK2-V617F* mutation, demonstrating that other mutations are involved in the pathogenesis of the disease and that there is likely an underlying genetic predisposition that has not yet been elucidated.[1149,1193,1194] The requirements for ET are a platelet count greater than 450,000/μL (previously 600,000/μL), a hemoglobin concentration not exceeding 13 g/dL (normal red blood cell mass), normal iron stores, a lack of the Philadelphia chromosome by molecular or cytogenetic analysis, the absence of collagen

Box 51-5   **Causes of Thrombocytosis in Children**

NUTRITIONAL

Iron deficiency
Megaloblastic anemia
Vitamin E deficiency
Metabolic
Hyperadrenalism

INFECTIOUS

Viral factors
Bacterial
Mycobacterial

TRAUMATIC

Surgery
Fracture
Hemorrhage

INFLAMMATORY

Collagen vascular disease
Inflammatory bowel disease
Sarcoidosis
Any inflammatory condition

NEOPLASTIC

Myeloproliferative disease
Hepatoblastoma
Neuroblastoma
Histiocytosis
Lymphoma
Carcinoma

MEDICATION-RELATED

Corticosteroids
Vinca alkaloids
Citrovorum factor

MISCELLANEOUS

Splenectomy, congenital asplenia
Infantile cortical hyperostosis (Caffey disease)
Cerebrovascular accident
Hemolytic anemia

Data from Addiego JE, Jr., Mentzer WC, Jr., Dallman PR: Thrombocytosis in infants and children. J Pediatr 85:805–807, 1974; Heath HW, Pearson HA: Thrombocytosis in pediatric outpatients. J Pediatr 114:805–807, 1989; and Chan KW, Kaikov Y, Wadsworth LD: Thrombocytosis in childhood: a survey of 94 patients. Pediatrics 84:1064–1067, 1989.

fibrosis of the marrow, and no other identifiable cause of thrombocytosis.[1156,1180] Box 51-6 suggests criteria for the diagnosis of pediatric ET.

ET may be an incidental finding, or patients may present with venous or arterial thrombosis, bleeding, or symptoms of a hypermetabolic state. The bleeding is generally mild, and its cause is unknown, although platelet function is often abnormal.[1195,1196] Splenomegaly is common, as is mild leukocytosis. Bone marrow cytogenetics are usually normal. The clinical course is highly variable, and some patients have been followed up for 10 years without problems.[1184] In adults, 80% survive more than 100 months, with 5 of 95 patients ultimately experiencing a conversion to AML in one study.[1197] Patients with ET can also develop myelofibrosis. Children appear to have a more benign course than adults.[1158,1186,1198] Asymptomatic children do not need to be treated. Treat-

ment options are similar to those available for PV, including hydroxyurea, anagrelide,[1199-1201] or IFN-α.[1202,1203] Treatment is usually recommended to prevent thrombotic complications in patients with platelet counts higher than 1 million/μL or a prior history of thrombohemorrhagic episodes. Hemorrhage may paradoxically occur with these very high platelet counts as a result of an acquired von Willebrand disease.[1204,1205] A randomized clinical trial in adults of hydroxyurea and acetylsalicylic acid or anagrelide and acetylsalicylic acid has demonstrated equal efficacy of these combinations in lowering the platelet count but a higher incidence of arterial thromboses, significant hemorrhage, and transformation to myelofibrosis in the anagrelide-treated group.[1177] More recently, evaluation by the European LeukemiaNet revealed that although anagrelide increased response rates it did not impact OS.[1206] These results suggest that hydroxyurea should serve as frontline therapy, particularly because the theoretical risk for malignant transformation has not been seen.[366,1168] Acetylsalicylic acid has previously been considered to have value in primary prophylaxis for thrombosis, but its utility was called into question in a recent study demonstrating a preventative benefit only in patients with predisposing thrombotic risk factors (*JAK2* mutation or cardiovascular risk factors), where it otherwise increased bleeding risk.[1207] Thus prolonged use of acetylsalicylic acid may be falling out of favor for asymptomatic patients with ET.

Primary Myelofibrosis

PM is a myeloproliferative disease characterized by leukoerythroblastosis, myeloid metaplasia, and varying degrees of myelofibrosis.[1208-1210] The median age at

Box 51-6   **Suggested Criteria for Childhood Essential Thrombocythemia**

Sustained platelet count greater than 450,000/μL
Bone marrow biopsy specimen showing proliferation mainly of the megakaryocytic lineage, with increased numbers of enlarged mature megakaryocytes; no significant increase or left shift of neutrophil granulopoiesis or erythropoiesis
Not meeting World Health Organization criteria for polycythemia vera, primary myelofibrosis, chronic myelogenous leukemia, myelodysplastic syndrome, or other myeloid neoplasm (e.g., no Philadelphia chromosome or *BCR-ABL* fusion)
Demonstration of *JAK2-V617F* or of another clonal marker (e.g., *MPL* mutation) or, in the absence of a clonal marker, no evidence of reactive thrombocytosis

Modified from Vardiman JW, Harris NL, Brunning RD: The World Health Organization (WHO) classification of the myeloid neoplasms. Blood 100:2292–2302, 2002; Tefferi A, Thiele J, Orazi A, et al: Proposals and rationale for revision of the World Health Organization diagnostic criteria for polycythemia vera, essential thrombocythemia, and primary myelofibrosis: recommendations from an ad hoc international expert panel. Blood 110:1092–1097, 2007; Teofili L, Giona F, Martini M, et al: Markers of myeloproliferative diseases in childhood polycythemia vera and essential thrombocythemia. J Clin Oncol 25:1048–1053, 2007; and Teofili L, Giona F, Martini M, et al: The revised WHO diagnostic criteria for Ph-negative myeloproliferative diseases are not appropriate for the diagnostic screening of childhood polycythemia vera and essential thrombocythemia. Blood 110:3384–3386, 2007.

presentation is 60 years, and pediatric cases are rare.[1211] Approximately 22% of patients are younger than 56 years, and approximately 11% are younger than 46 years.[1212] Fewer than 100 cases have been reported in children, and many of these are in patients younger than age 3 years.[1168] Symptoms may include malaise, weight loss, night sweats, and discomfort from splenomegaly. Peripheral blood cell counts are varied, and the smears often show Pelger-Huët cells, leukoerythroblastosis, and teardrop formation, along with occasional immature WBC precursors.[1213] Bone marrow cells are difficult to aspirate, and biopsy specimens show fibrosis in most patients.[1213] Cytogenetic abnormalities are common in PM if enough marrow cells can be obtained for study.[260,1214] PM is a clonal disease involving all myeloid elements,[1214] and the cause of the associated myelofibrosis is unknown.[1215-1217] However, similar to PV and ET, the *JAK2-V617F* mutation has been found in approximately 50% of patients. Another 10% of patients have been found to have a *W515L* mutation in the thrombopoietin receptor.[1218] Because this disorder is very rare in children, other causes of myelofibrosis need to be ruled out. These causes include nutritional, inflammatory, infectious, and neoplastic disorders.[1219]

The natural history of PM can be variable, with patient survival varying from 1.5 to more than 5 years.[1220] Children with PM may have a more favorable natural history than adults.[1221,1222] Young adults tend to have less severe anemia, higher incidence of splenomegaly, lower frequency of thrombocytosis, and lower frequency of chromosomal abnormalities.[1212] Deletions of the long arm of chromosome 20 or 13—(del(20q) or del(13q)—or a normal karyotype have been associated with more favorable outcomes.[1168] Complications of this disease include bleeding, intercurrent infection, transformation to acute leukemia,[1223] and portal hypertension.[1220] Splenectomy will not cause a further reduction of blood cell counts and therefore should be considered only for mechanical problems, portal hypertension, refractory thrombocytopenia, and hemolytic anemia.[1224] The role of chemotherapy in PM is ill defined, although hydroxyurea, anagrelide, and IFN-α have been used, although none of these approaches is curative.[1225] Given the frequency of *JAK2* mutations in PM, a number of recent adult trials have examined the use of JAK2 or combined JAK1/JAK2 inhibitor in PM with evidence of some bona fide clinical responses, including reduction in splenomegaly and relief from constitutional symptoms, such as fatigue and pruritus.[1226,1227] Ruxolitinib, a combined JAK1/JAK2 inhibitor, was approved by the FDA for high- and intermediate-risk PM in 2011. However, none of these JAK inhibitors selectively targets the *JAK2-V617F* mutation, resulting in side effects such as myelosuppression. Moreover, the effectiveness of these agents in abrogating symptoms in PM appear more related to suppression of JAK-STAT pathway–mediated cytokine-related inflammation characteristic of PM than inhibition of the causative mutant clone.[1178] Thus at this time, allogeneic HSCT remains the only cure and should be considered for higher-risk patients with unfavorable cytogenetics or who are transfusion dependent.[1168]

Mastocytosis

Mastocytosis is a pathologic proliferation and accumulation of mast cells in various tissues in the body.[1228] Mast cells are myeloid cells derived from HSCs but, unlike other lineages, they exit the marrow before they are fully matured and complete their development in the tissues in which they eventually reside.[1229-1231] Given their role in allergic and inflammatory conditions, mast cells are commonly found in vascularized connective tissues such as the skin and the mucosal surfaces of the gastrointestinal tract and respiratory epithelium.[1232] The cutaneous form of mastocytosis is most common in children and may consist of an isolated mastocytoma or diffuse lesions termed *urticaria pigmentosa*.[1233] This is a generally benign condition, although in rare cases progression to systemic mastocytosis (SM) can occur. SM implies mast cell proliferation in an extracutaneous site, most commonly the bone marrow. SM is a clonal myeloproliferative disease frequently associated with a *D816V* point mutation in the gene encoding the KIT tyrosine kinase and presents as varying degrees of mast cell hyperproliferation and impaired differentiation, depending on the subtype.[1228] SM is further divided into subtypes— indolent systemic mastocytosis (ISM), systemic mastocytosis with an associated hematopoietic clonal non–mast cell lineage disease (SM-AHNMD), aggressive systemic mastocytosis (ASM), mast cell leukemia (MCL), mast cell sarcoma, and extracutaneous mastocytoma.[1234] Whereas the *KIT* mutations may be sufficient to result in the indolent form of the systemic disease, additional genetic abnormalities appear to be required for progression to the more aggressive forms of the disease.[1228] For example, the *TET2* mutation found in AML has also been identified in approximately 30% of cases of systemic mastocytosis[1235] and may be associated with more aggressive disease and poor prognosis.[1236] SM may also occur in conjunction with the generally favorable prognostic t(8;21) translocation *(AML1-ETO)* but, in this context, it confers a poor prognosis.[1237,1238] Similarly, MCL is associated with a poor outcome.[1234,1239] MCL occurs predominantly in adults, is frequently aleukemic, and may occur de novo or after localized or systemic mastocytosis, including in childhood.[1234] Patients with MCL may harbor the *KIT-D816V* point mutation, but a number of other novel *KIT* mutations have also been recently identified in these patients.[1234,1240,1241] Treatment strategies include combination therapy with steroids and IFN-α,[1239,1242] cladribine,[1243] and, more recently, tyrosine kinase inhibitors.[1244,1245] Imatinib mesylate, which is known to target the KIT tyrosine kinase in addition to BCR-ABL, has been used in patients with SM. Imatinib has shown preferential efficacy for the minority of patients who lack the *D816V* mutation[1246,1247] and has been approved by the FDA for this indication. Other tyrosine kinase inhibitors, including dasatinib[1248] and masatinib,[1240] have shown modest responses in aggressive mast cell diseases, whereas, more recently, midostaurin (PKC412) has shown some promise with improved responses in imatinib-resistant *D816V*-positive mastocytosis and MCL.[1249,1250]

CONCLUSION

Although considerable progress has been made in improving the remission induction rates in AML, remission is not attained in a significant number of children with newly diagnosed AML. The OS of patients with AML is still not optimal, and the toxicity of treatment is often excessive. Myeloid leukemias, myelodysplastic syndromes, and myeloproliferative disorders are heterogeneous in their molecular pathophysiologic course and are often difficult to treat effectively. With the tremendous improvements in outcome using paradigms of targeted approaches in the treatment of APL with ATRA and As_2O_3, and of CML with imatinib mesylate and other tyrosine kinase inhibitors, interest has grown in applying novel molecularly directed therapies to other types of myeloid disease. While more is understood about the molecular biology of the other types of myeloid malignancies, future studies will incorporate new agents that target malignant cells more specifically while sparing normal hematopoietic stem and progenitor cells. Moreover, recent genomic studies highlighting that the driving mutations in AML are likely few in number in any given patient, together with the evolution of more refined approaches to identify and define leukemic initiating cells, suggest that the ability to rationally apply targeted therapies to eliminate the source of the malignant clone may truly be realized. The incredible advancements in understanding the biology of myeloid diseases, coupled with the development of a large number of novel targeted agents, holds great promise to improve the outcome and reduce the toxicity for increasingly large subsets of patients afflicted by myeloid malignancies.

References available online at ExpertConsult.

KEY REFERENCES

94. Bonnet D, Dick JE: Human acute myeloid leukemia is organized as a hierarchy that originates from a primitive hematopoietic cell. *Nat Med* 3:730–737, 1997.
    One of the original reports showing that leukemia-initiating cells are relatively rare and have properties of stem cells, giving rise to a developmental hierarchy in AML.

113. Wang Y, Krivtsov AV, Sinha AU, et al: The Wnt/beta-catenin pathway is required for the development of leukemia stem cells in AML. *Science* 327:1650–1653, 2009.
    Demonstration that either endogenous or aberrant β-catenin pathway activation is critical for leukemic stem cell function.

125. Greaves MF, Wiemels J: Origins of chromosome translocations in childhood leukaemia. *Nat Rev Cancer* 3:639–649, 2003.
    Key review discussing the prenatal origin of some childhood leukemias.

138. Welch JS, Ley TJ, Link DC, et al: The origin and evolution of mutations in acute myeloid leukemia. *Cell* 150:264–278, 2012.
    Deep sequencing comparison of normal karyotype AML and promyelocytic AML expressing the PML-RARA fusion gene demonstrating the number of mutations that result in the clonal progression to frank disease.

157. Berman JN, Gerbing RB, Alonzo TA, et al: Prevalence and clinical implications of NRAS mutations in childhood AML: a report from the Children's Oncology Group. *Leukemia* 25:1039–1042, 2011.
    Children's Oncology Group study demonstrating conclusively that NRAS mutations have no independent prognostic value in childhood AML.

212. Ablain J, Leiva M, Peres L, et al: Uncoupling RARA transcriptional activation and degradation clarifies the bases for APL response to therapies. *J Exp Med* 210:647–653, 2013.
    Mechanistic studies demonstrating uncoupling of transcriptional activation and oncoprotein degradation due to all-trans-retinoic acid (ATRA) in acute promyelocytic leukemia.

244. Bernt KM, Zhu N, Sinha AU, et al: MLL-rearranged leukemia is dependent on aberrant H3K79 methylation by DOT1L. *Cancer Cell* 20:66–78, 2011.
    First demonstration of DOT1L as a key mediator of transformation and therapeutic target in MLL-rearranged leukemia.

279. Ho PA, Alonzo TA, Gerbing RB, et al: Prevalence and prognostic implications of CEBPA mutations in pediatric acute myeloid leukemia (AML): a report from the Children's Oncology Group. *Blood* 113:6558–6566, 2009.
    Children's Oncology Group study conclusively demonstrate CEBPA mutations as a favorable prognostic marker in childhood AML.

285. Ho PA, Kuhn J, Gerbing RB, et al: WT1 synonymous single nucleotide polymorphism rs16754 correlates with higher mRNA expression and predicts significantly improved outcome in favorable-risk pediatric acute myeloid leukemia: a report from the Children's Oncology Group. *J Clin Oncol* 29:704–711, 2010.
    Children's Oncology Group study examining the prognostic value of WT1 expression levels in childhood AML.

329. Vardiman JW, Thiele J, Arber DA, et al: The 2008 revision of the World Health Organization (WHO) classification of myeloid neoplasms and acute leukemia: rationale and important changes. *Blood* 114:937–951, 2009.
    The WHO classification of myeloid diseases that remains in current clinical use.

355. Loken MR, Alonzo TA, Pardo L, et al: Residual disease detected by multidimensional flow cytometry signifies high relapse risk in patients with de novo acute myeloid leukemia: a report from Children's Oncology Group. *Blood* 120:1581–1588, 2012.
    Children's Oncology Group study revealing the ability of multiparameter flow cytometry–based minimal residual disease (MRD) to improve prediction of relapse over morphologic evaluation alone in childhood AML.

360. Woods WG, Kobrinsky N, Buckley JD, et al: Timed-sequential induction therapy improves postremission outcome in acute myeloid leukemia: a report from the Children's Cancer Group. *Blood* 87:4979–4989, 1996.
    Landmark study by the Children's Cancer Group revealing that intensification of induction chemotherapy with consecutive cycles without waiting for bone marrow recovery improved disease-free survival.

363. Gibson BE, Wheatley K, Hann IM, et al: Treatment strategy and long-term results in paediatric patients treated in consecutive UK AML trials. *Leukemia* 19:2130–2138, 2005.
    Review of the MRC AML 10 and 12 studies demonstrating that inclusion of a fifth block of therapy (high-dose cytarabine and asparaginase) did not improve survival in children with AML, leading to four blocks of therapy on current UK and Children's Oncology Group trials.

398. Hollink IH, Zwaan CM, Zimmermann M, et al: Favorable prognostic impact of NPM1 gene mutations in childhood acute myeloid leukemia, with emphasis on cytogenetically normal AML. *Leukemia* 23:262–270, 2009.
    Key report demonstrating that NPM1 mutation without FLT3 activation is associated with a favorable outcome in childhood AML in keeping with associations identified in adult AML.

401. Kutny MA, Moser BK, Laumann K, et al: FLT3 mutation status is a predictor of early death in pediatric acute promyelocytic leukemia: a report from the Children's Oncology Group. *Pediatr Blood Cancer* 59:662–667, 2012.
    Evidence that the presence of an FLT3 mutation impacts remission-induction in childhood acute promyelocytic leukemia and thus serves as a biologic marker for risk stratification in this disease.

403. Rubnitz JL, Inaba H, Dahl G, et al: Minimal residual disease directed therapy for childhood acute myeloid leukaemia: results of the AML02 multicentre trial. *Lancet Oncol* 11:543–552, 2010.

Landmark study demonstrating the value of multiparameter flow cytometry–based minimal residual disease (MRD)as a predictive biomarker in childhood AML.

430. Sung L, Lange BJ, Gerbing RB, et al: Microbiologically documented infections and infection-related mortality in children with acute myeloid leukemia. *Blood* 110:3532–3539, 2007.
    Key publication from the Children's Oncology Group outlining the frequency and etiology of bacterial and fungal infections for children receiving intensive AML chemotherapy.

451. Maertens J: Evaluating prophylaxis of invasive fungal infections in patients with haematologic malignancies. *Eur J Haematol* 78:275–282, 2007.
    Review evaluating the relative benefits of different antifungal agents for prophylaxis in patients with leukemia.

526. Johnston DL, Alonzo TA, Gerbing RB, et al: The presence of central nervous system disease at diagnosis in pediatric acute myeloid leukemia does not affect survival: a Children's Oncology Group study. *Pediatr Blood Cancer* 55:414–420, 2010.
    One of the few studies to date specifically examining the impact of CNS disease in childhood AML.

551. Harrison CJ, Hills RK, Moorman AV, et al: Cytogenetics of childhood acute myeloid leukemia: United Kingdom Medical Research Council Treatment trials AML 10 and 12. *J Clin Oncol* 28:2674–2681, 2010.
    Report from the UK group demonstrating that their therapeutic strategy for the treatment of childhood AML was associated with equivalent outcomes to the Children's Oncology Group but with reduced toxicity, leading to the adoption of this approach in North America.

569. Balgobind BV, Raimondi SC, Harbott J, et al: Novel prognostic subgroups in childhood 11q23/MLL-rearranged acute myeloid leukemia: results of an international retrospective study. *Blood* 114:2489–2496, 2009.
    Demonstration in childhood AML that specific MLL fusion genes with different gene partners have different prognostic implications.

587. Zwaan CM, Meshinchi S, Radich JP, et al: *FLT3* internal tandem duplication in 234 children with acute myeloid leukemia: prognostic significance and relation to cellular drug resistance. *Blood* 102:2387–2394, 2003.
    Demonstration that FLT3-ITD is a high-risk prognostic feature in pediatric AML, similar to its role in adult AML.

732. Stankiewicz MJ, Crispino JD: AKT collaborates with ERG and Gata1s to dysregulate megakaryopoiesis and promote AMKL. *Leukemia* 27:1339–1347, 2013.
    A recent report demonstrating a role for the PI3K/AKT pathway in acute megakaryoblastic leukemia in children with Down syndrome.

735. Sidi S, Sanda T, Kennedy RD, et al: Chk1 suppresses a caspase-2 apoptotic response to DNA damage that bypasses p53, Bcl-2, and caspase-3. *Cell* 133:864–877, 2008.
    Landmark study defining a novel apoptotic pathway independent of TP53 and BCL2 family members that may represent a targeted therapeutic strategy in hematologic malignancies.

901. Ge Y, Dombkowski AA, LaFiura KM, et al: Differential gene expression, *GATA1* target genes, and the chemotherapy sensitivity of Down syndrome megakaryocytic leukemia. *Blood* 107:1570–1581, 2006.
    Microarray studies demonstrating a unique gene expression signature in Down syndrome acute megakaryoblastic leukemia cells that may account for increased sensitivity to chemotherapy.

910. Sorrell AD, Alonzo TA, Hilden JM, et al: Favorable survival maintained in children who have myeloid leukemia associated with Down syndrome using reduced-dose chemotherapy on Children's Oncology Group trial A2971: a report from the Children's Oncology Group. *Cancer* 118:4806–4814, 2012.
    Report from the Children's Oncology Group of the first clinical trial exclusively for AML in children with Down syndrome, which demonstrated that reduced intensity of therapy does not compromise the favorable outcome in this disease.

919. Corey SJ, Minden MD, Barber DL, et al: Myelodysplastic syndromes: the complexity of stem-cell diseases. *Nat Rev Cancer* 7:118–129, 2007.
    Comprehensive review on myelodysplastic syndromes emphasizing the roles of stem cell dysfunction, genetic instability, and dysregulated apoptosis.

984. Strahm B, Nollke P, Zecca M, et al: Hematopoietic stem cell transplantation for advanced myelodysplastic syndrome in children: results of the EWOG-MDS 98 study. *Leukemia* 25:455–462, 2011.
    Contemporary European multicenter study demonstrating the value of early allogeneic stem cell transplantation in pediatric MDS.

1015. Niemeyer CM, Kang MW, Shin DH, et al: Germline *CBL* mutations cause developmental abnormalities and predispose to juvenile myelomonocytic leukemia. *Nat Genet* 42:794–800, 2010.
    Recent identification of germline mutations in the E3 ubiquitin ligase, CBL, predisposing to the development of JMML.

1168. Barbui T: How to manage children and young adults with myeloproliferative neoplasms. *Leukemia* 26:1452–1457, 2012.
    Summary of a practical approach to using the current knowledge and risk factors in non-CML myeloproliferative diseases to manage children with these rare diagnoses.

CHAPTER 52

Infant Leukemias

Rachel Kobos, Neerav Shukla, and Scott A. Armstrong

CHAPTER OUTLINE

EPIDEMIOLOGY	Outcomes and Treatment
PRENATAL ORIGIN OF INFANT LEUKEMIA	Association with Down Syndrome
RISK FACTORS	Non–Down Syndrome–Associated Infant AMKL
BIOLOGY OF MIXED-LINEAGE LEUKEMIA TRANSLOCATIONS	**FUTURE DIRECTIONS IN INFANT ACUTE LEUKEMIA TREATMENT**
ACUTE LYMPHOBLASTIC LEUKEMIA	Targeting Epigenetic Mechanisms
Clinical and Biologic Features	Immunotherapy
Prognostic Factors and Outcomes	Modulators of Glucocorticoid Resistance
Treatment	FLT3 Inhibitors
ACUTE MYELOID LEUKEMIA	
Clinical and Prognostic Features	

The biologic features and clinical characteristics of infant leukemias differ significantly from those of leukemias in older children. Infant leukemias are distinguished not only by the young age of patients at diagnosis but by their unique morphologic, immunologic, clinical, and genetic presentation.[1] For example, acute lymphoblastic leukemia (ALL) and acute myeloid leukemia (AML) present in infants with a somewhat unique constellation of clinical features, including hyperleukocytosis, massive organomegaly, and central nervous system (CNS) involvement at diagnosis.[2,3] Biologically, the most notable feature distinguishing infant leukemia from leukemia in older children is the high incidence of rearrangements involving the mixed-lineage leukemia (MLL) gene* located on chromosome band 11q23.[2,4-7] In the case of infant ALL, unique clinical and biologic characteristics are accompanied by an exceptionally poor prognosis, which is in stark contrast to the cure rates achieved for older children with ALL. In this chapter, the epidemiologic, biologic, and clinical features and the treatment of infant ALL and AML will be discussed.

EPIDEMIOLOGY

The annual incidence of leukemia in the first year of life in the United States is approximately 40 cases per million children.[8] Infants account for 2.5% to 5% of ALL cases and 6% to 14% of AML cases in childhood.[9] Unlike in older children with leukemia, in whom the percentage of ALL cases is approximately four times that of AML, in infants the ratio of ALL to AML is approximately equal. Furthermore, in contrast to an excess of males among older children with leukemia, a slight female predominance is seen in infants with this disease.[8,10,11] Although neuroblastoma represents the most common neoplasm in infants, leukemia is the leading cause of death caused by neoplastic disease in this age group (Table 52-1).[1,8]

PRENATAL ORIGIN OF INFANT LEUKEMIA

The onset of leukemia in infancy strongly suggests a prenatal leukemogenic event, and significant molecular and epidemiologic evidence supports this hypothesis. Molecular studies of monozygotic twins with concordant ALL have demonstrated identical clonal, nonconstitutional rearrangements of the MLL gene and identical oligoclonal, heavy-chain immunoglobulin gene rearrangements in the peripheral blood of these infants.[12-15] This finding suggests the occurrence of a single in utero leukemogenic event in one twin with generation of a clone that is passed to the other fetus by intraplacental metastasis. Further evidence of oncogenesis in utero comes from reports of fetal deaths caused by AML with an MLL gene rearrangement.[16] Moreover, identical MLL gene fusions have been traced back to neonatal Guthrie

*In this chapter, *KMT2A* will be referred to as MLL. *ALL1* and *HRX* are also alternative names for this gene.

TABLE 52-1 Incidence of Cancer in Infants*

Histology	Incidence (per million)
Neuroblastoma	64.6
Leukemias	40.5
Central nervous system	29.7
Retinoblastoma	26.7
Wilms tumor	22.5
Germ cell	15.3
Soft tissue	15.2
Hepatic	9.5
Lymphomas	4.4
Epithelial	2.8
Other, unspecified	1.2
Bone	0.5

From Ries LAG, Smith M, Gurney JG, et al, editors: Cancer incidence and survival among children and adolescents: United States SEER Program 1975-1995 (NIH publication No. 99-4649). Bethesda, MD, 1999, National Cancer Institute.
*SEER Program, 1976-1984 and 1986-1994.

genetic screening cards of children who were diagnosed with ALL in their first 2 years of life.[12,17,18] Similarly, leukemia has been diagnosed in fetuses with Down syndrome as early as 33 weeks' gestation, and the characteristic GATA binding protein 1 (GATA1) gene mutation associated with megakaryocytic leukemia in young children with Down syndrome has been identified in the neonatal Guthrie genetic screening cards of children in whom leukemia later developed.[19,20]

RISK FACTORS

As with most cancers, the causes of infant leukemia remain largely unknown. However, several epidemiologic risk factors associated with an increased risk of leukemia in young children have been identified. Given the close temporal relationship between embryogenesis and the clinical diagnosis of cancer, most investigations have focused on maternal characteristics and in utero exposures. Maternal alcohol consumption during pregnancy has been correlated with an increased risk of infant AML.[21] Studies have also shown an increased incidence of infant leukemia, particularly ALL, in infants with birth weights higher than 4000 g.[22-24] It has been speculated that high levels of endogenous insulin-like growth factors associated with high birth weight may contribute to leukemogenesis.[9,25] Other proposed risk factors include maternal pesticide and solvent exposure, in utero radiation exposure, and an adverse maternal reproductive history.[26-31] However, given the rarity of infant leukemia, it has been difficult to connect the development of leukemia with any of these exposures or clinical features definitively.

Of particular interest is the potential relationship between maternal consumption of naturally occurring deoxyribonucleic acid (DNA) topoisomerase II inhibitors and the development of infant leukemia. MLL gene rearrangements, similar to those found in many infant leukemias, are common in secondary acute leukemias arising after exposure to DNA topoisomerase II inhibitors, including the epipodophyllotoxins (e.g., etoposide).[32-34] This relationship has led to the hypothesis that transplacental exposure to naturally occurring topoisomerase II inhibitors may be involved in the pathogenesis of infant leukemia.[35] This hypothesis is supported by the finding that both primary infant MLL gene–rearranged leukemias and therapy-related secondary acute leukemias have MLL gene break points that are similarly distributed within the MLL gene break point cluster region (BCR).[33] Furthermore, several dietary bioflavonoids, such as quercetin (found in certain fruits and vegetables) and genistein (found in soybeans) are known topoisomerase II inhibitors and have been shown to induce MLL gene cleavage in vitro.[36] In a study by the Children's Oncology Group (COG), it was found that increased maternal consumption of these and other naturally occurring topoisomerase II inhibitors such as catechins (found in red wine, tea, and cocoa) is associated with an increased risk of MLL gene–rearranged infant AML but not infant ALL.[22,37,38] This association, if true, likely only accounts for a small proportion of infant leukemia cases. Furthermore, the fact that many of these foods are commonly consumed and infant leukemia is rare suggests that this association is either weak or requires a combination of factors. Thus one cannot make recommendations to restrict certain foods to decrease the likelihood of the development of leukemia. Moreover maternal consumption of fruits and vegetables during pregnancy has been associated with a decrease rather than an increase in the risk of infant leukemia overall.[38]

Pharmacogenetic differences in the metabolism of topoisomerase II inhibitors have been hypothesized to modulate the relationship between exposure to these chemicals and the occurrence of MLL gene rearrangements. A common structural feature shared by many topoisomerase II inhibitors, including bioflavonoids, is a quinone moiety. Quinone metabolites generated as by-products of these compounds in the fetal liver have been shown to cleave the MLL gene.[36] Quinones are normally detoxified by reduced nicotinamide adenine dinucleotide phosphatase quinone oxidoreductase (NQO1). The presence of a low-activity variant of NQO1 has been associated with an increased risk of MLL gene–rearranged infant ALL.[39] However, a similar study has also demonstrated a relationship between this NQO1 polymorphism and infant ALL without MLL gene rearrangements.[40]

BIOLOGY OF MIXED-LINEAGE LEUKEMIA TRANSLOCATIONS

The MLL gene located on chromosome band 11q23 is commonly altered in infant leukemia in that it is rearranged in 80% of cases of infant ALL and 60% of cases of infant AML. These chromosomal abnormalities usually

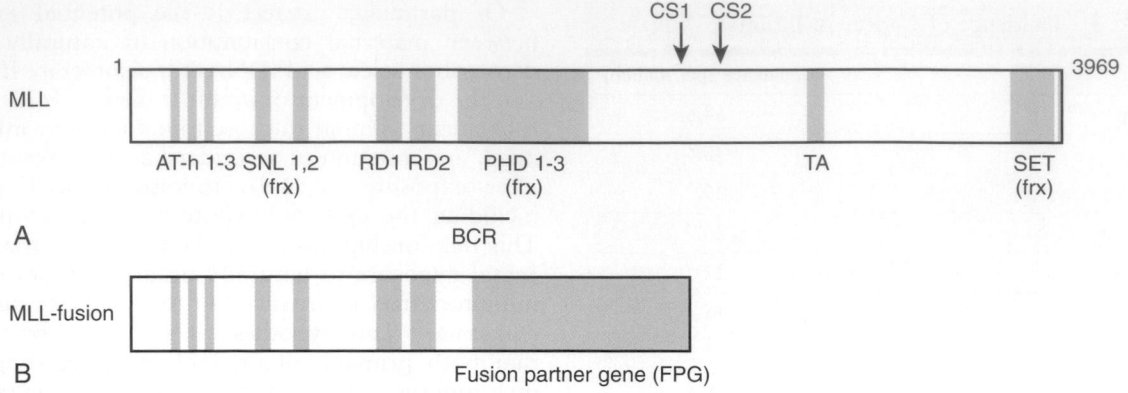

Figure 52-1 Schematic representation of the mixed-lineage leukemia *(MLL)* protein and MLL fusions. **A,** The MLL gene is approximately 89 kb long, consists of 37 exons, and encodes a 3969–amino acid nuclear protein with a complex domain structure (unique domains are highlighted). The N-terminus contains three short AT hook motifs *(AT-h 1-3),* which are thought to mediate binding to the minor groove of AT-rich genomic deoxyribonucleic acid (DNA) sequences. There are two nuclear localization sites (SNL1 and SNL2) immediately C-terminal to the AT hooks that are followed by a transcriptional repression domain *(RD)* consisting of two functional subunits, RD1 and RD2. RD1 contains a DNA methyltransferase homology domain. The plant homeodomains *(PHD)* zinc finger motifs may mediate binding to a number of different proteins or to chromatin. The transcriptional activation *(TA)* domain recruits the transcriptional coactivator CREB-binding protein and precedes a C-terminal Su(var)3-9, Enhancer of Zeste, Trithorax *(SET)* domain that possesses histone H3 lysine 4 (H3K4) methyltransferase activity. The breakpoint cluster region *(BCR)* spans exons 8 to 13. **B,** Structure of MLL fusion proteins generated by MLL translocations. A typical MLL fusion protein contains the N-terminus of MLL encoded by the first 8 to 13 exons and the C-terminus of one of more than 50 fusion partners. *CS,* Cleavage site.

involve reciprocal translocations, which encode chimeric transcripts that give rise to oncogenic fusion proteins with pronounced transforming potential.[41] A number of groups cloned the MLL-AF4 *(AFF1)* gene in the early 1990s.[42,43,44,45] The MLL-AF4 gene encodes a protein of 2304 amino acids, with the NH2-terminal 1439 amino acids derived from the MLL gene on chromosome 11 and COOH-terminal 865 amino acids derived from the AF4 gene on chromosome 4. Subsequently, close to 100 different translocations have been identified, all of which appear to produce a fusion protein possessing the NH2-terminus of MLL fused in-frame to the COOH-terminus of the fusion partner (Fig. 52-1).[41]

The MLL gene encodes a 3969–amino acid DNA-binding protein that possesses multiple recognizable protein motifs, including an NH2-terminal DNA binding domain, transcriptional activation and repression domains, and a COOH-terminal Su(var)3-9, Enhancer of Zeste, Trithorax (SET) domain that contains histone methyltransferase activity.[46,47] Biochemical studies have identified MLL as a member of a large multiprotein complex that contains members involved in chromatin modification and remodeling. Notably, the complex includes histone deacetylases and members of the switch/sucrose nonfermentable (SWI/SNF) chromatin remodeling complex.[47] Also MLL is recruited to the promoters of select cell cycle regulatory genes by the protein product of the multiple endocrine neoplasia 1 *(MEN1)* tumor suppressor gene, suggesting a role for MLL in tumor suppression and cell cycle control.[48,49] These data support the hypothesis that the MLL protein regulates gene expression via chromatin modification.[50]

Analysis of Mll knockout mice has suggested that Mll plays an important role in development and hematopoiesis through maintenance of appropriate homeotic (Hox) gene expression.[51,52] Detailed studies assessing the specific role of Mll in hematopoietic development have shown that Mll is necessary for definitive hematopoiesis and for the expansion of hematopoietic progenitors and stem cells found in the aorta-gonad-mesonephros region of the developing embryo.[53] The defect in hematopoietic progenitor expansion can be rescued by reexpression of Hox genes, confirming the importance of Mll-mediated Hox gene expression during hematopoiesis.

Multiple studies have demonstrated the ability of Hox genes to induce leukemia in mice,[54] and the t(7;11) (p15;p15) translocation found in some human acute myeloid leukemias results in a fusion of the homeobox A9 *(HOXA9)* gene to the nucleoporin 98kDa *(NUP98).*[55,56] Given the apparent importance of HOX genes in leukemogenesis, it seems likely that translocations involving MLL, a known regulator of HOX genes, alters expression of HOX genes that are important for leukemogenesis. Further support for HOX genes as central regulators of MLL gene–induced leukemogenesis comes from gene expression studies that have found multiple HOXA cluster genes more highly expressed in MLL gene–rearranged myelogenous and lymphoblastic leukemias compared with MLL gene germline leukemias.[57,58,59,60]

Gene expression studies of human MLL gene–rearranged B-precursor ALL have demonstrated that hundreds of genes are differentially expressed when compared with other B-precursor ALLs.[57-59,61] Based on the magnitude of the differences in gene expression, it appears that MLL gene translocations specify a unique lymphoblastic leukemia. Other large gene expression studies have also shown that ALLs with distinct chromosomal rearrangements have unique gene expression profiles, providing support for this hypothesis.[59] The genes that are relatively highly expressed in MLL gene–rearranged B-precursor ALL are those associated with hematopoietic progenitors and developing myeloid cells, whereas the genes expressed at lower levels are genes associated with lymphoid identity. Studies have also defined specific gene expression signatures associated with MLL gene translocations in pediatric—and in some cases infant—AML blasts.[60] It is of interest that even though clear differences exist in expression of lineage-associated genes between MLL gene–rearranged ALL and MLL gene–rearranged AML, a core gene expression profile appears to be found in all MLL gene–rearranged human leukemias, independent of the lineage markers.[60] Presumably, MLL fusion proteins directly regulate a subset of these genes. This theory is further supported by the fact that this MLL-associated signature consists of multiple highly expressed HOX genes.

The observation that leukemic cells bearing an MLL gene translocation often coexpress both myeloid and lymphoid markers raises the possibility that MLL fusion genes selectively transform hematopoietic stem cells (HSCs). If so, this HSC population would have an inherent self-renewal capacity that could be co-opted for leukemogenesis. Xenograft transplantation studies have demonstrated that a rare subpopulation of CD34+ and CD38– human myeloid leukemia cells are able to transfer the disease to immunodeficient mice, providing support for HSCs as the normal compartment from which leukemia-initiating cells (leukemia stem cells) might arise.[62] Alternatively, the translocation event between the MLL gene and a partner gene may affect a more committed population. In this scenario, the MLL fusion protein might confer a self-renewal and proliferative capacity to these short-lived progenitors and allow them to initiate leukemogenesis. Studies have suggested that Mll fusion proteins and potentially other translocation-associated fusion proteins are capable of inducing leukemia when expressed in fully committed myeloid progenitors, such as granulocyte-macrophage progenitors.[63,64] These findings are of particular importance because they suggest that products of chromosomal translocations found in human leukemias are able to induce a program of self-renewal that is not normally present in hematopoietic progenitors.

Multiple lines of evidence now point to a multistep pathogenesis of human acute leukemia. Elegant epidemiologic studies have suggested that childhood leukemias require at least two and probably more genetic events to occur for the development of leukemia. In particular, lymphoblastic leukemias with *ETV6-RUNX1 (TEL-AML1)* rearrangements appear to develop after a multistep process. TEL-AML1 rearrangements have been detected in blood taken at birth from a child in whom ALL then developed 3 to 5 years later. This finding suggests that TEL-AML1 rearrangements are the first genetic event but that other mutations also are required for the development of ALL.[65] Similar studies have been performed on blood spots from children in whom MLL gene–rearranged ALL subsequently developed, and the MLL gene translocations clearly develop in utero, even though the leukemias become apparent at some point during the first year of life.[12]

Receptor tyrosine kinases are attractive candidates as signaling molecules that may cooperate with translocation-associated fusion proteins during leukemogenesis. Ever-increasing evidence has suggested that activated kinases play a central role in the pathogenesis of leukemias and myeloproliferative syndromes.[66] The most dramatic evidence for such a role is activation of the Abelson (ABL) tyrosine kinase by the BCR-ABL fusion produced by t(9;22) and its inhibition by imatinib (Gleevec).[67,68] Other mutant kinases frequently identified in AML and subsets of ALL are the receptor tyrosine kinases fms-related tyrosine kinase–3 (FLT3), c-KIT, and platelet-derived growth factor receptor, among others.[66] Given the high level expression and recurrent mutation of FLT3 in MLL gene–rearranged ALL, studies are under way to assess FLT3 inhibitors in patients with MLL gene–rearranged ALL (discussed later). As approaches to target the rat sarcoma (RAS) signaling pathway are further developed, RAS inhibitors might also be considered in RAS-mutant cases.

Given the central importance of the MLL fusion protein generated by the MLL gene translocation, significant effort has been directed toward defining a unifying mechanism of oncogenesis, because it would facilitate pharmacologic targeting of shared leukemogenic mechanisms. Some broad patterns have emerged that have focused on mechanisms that control MLL target gene expression. The most commonly occurring MLL gene translocations generate chimeric fusion proteins that harbor the NH3-terminus of MLL fused to proteins that are normally part of nuclear complexes, the function for which is now emerging.[69] Nuclear proteins such as AF4, AF9, ENL, ELL, AF10, AF17, and AFF4—fusions of which together account for the vast majority of MLL leukemias—normally directly or indirectly associate with complexes that regulate gene expression.[70-75] A number of complexes linked to transcriptional elongation have been reported, often with overlapping protein components, such as the ENL-associated protein (EAP) complex,[72] the AF4/ENL/P-TEFb (AEP) complex,[75] the super elongation complex (SEC),[74] and the complex comprising the disruptor of telomeric silencing (DOT1)–like histone 3 lysine 79 (H3K79) methyltransferase (DOT1L; DOT1L containing complex [DotCom]; Fig. 52-1).[73] These data point to aberrant control of transcriptional elongation as critical for MLL fusion–mediated oncogenesis.

The histone methyltransferase DOT1 is a non-SET domain containing histone methyltransferase solely responsible for catalyzing the methylation of H3K79.[76] H3K79 methylation is associated with most genes that are highly expressed in hematopoietic cells and is believed to be involved either in activation or maintenance of gene expression. Thus a prominent hypothesis is that MLL fusion proteins induce aberrant gene expression via recruitment of DOT1L (among other protein complexes) to MLL target genes, including the HOXA cluster genes. Genome-wide studies have demonstrated elevated H3K79 methylation at MLL target genes in MLL gene–rearranged ALL and AML cells.[77-79] Several recent studies using conditional loss of function mouse models and ribonucleic acid (RNA) interference approaches have formally demonstrated a critical role for DOT1L in MLL fusion–driven leukemias.[79-82] These studies demonstrate that genetic inactivation of DOT1 leads to a decrease in MLL fusion target gene expression, including a rapid decrease in HOXA cluster gene expression that is correlated with an antiproliferative response. Remarkably, inactivation of DOT1L does not affect the transformation potential of a number of other leukemogenic oncogenes. Furthermore, microarray-based gene expression studies showed that MLL-fusion target gene expression is much more dependent on DOT1L than is gene expression broadly.[79] These studies highlight the importance of aberrant H3K79 methylation for the transforming activity of MLL fusion proteins including MLL-AF4, MLL-AF9, MLL-AF10, and MLL-ENL and show that DOT1L is required for continued HOXA cluster gene expression. These results potentially have profound clinical implications because these fusions comprise the vast majority of MLL gene–rearranged leukemias; small-molecule DOT1L inhibitors have been developed and are entering clinical trials (discussed later).

ACUTE LYMPHOBLASTIC LEUKEMIA

Clinical and Biologic Features

ALL in infants is characterized by a high leukocyte count at presentation, marked hepatosplenomegaly, and a relatively high incidence of CNS involvement.[2,3,83,84] The immunophenotype of infant ALL is usually that of an immature B-lineage precursor and is characterized by a lack of cluster of differentiation (CD)–10 expression, as well as by the coexpression of myeloid-associated antigens, such as CD14, CD15, and CDw65. Lack of CD10 expression and coexpression of myeloid markers correlates with the presence of an MLL gene rearrangement, which is present in 80% of infants who have ALL compared with only 2% to 4% of older children who have ALL.[4,6,85-87] MLL gene rearrangements are more frequent in younger infants, with approximately 90% of infants younger than 6 months at diagnosis having MLL gene rearrangements in their leukemic blasts compared with 30% to 60% of infants aged 6 to 12 months.[4,88,89] The most common MLL gene translocation observed in infant ALL is t(4;11)(q21;q23), resulting in the MLL-AF4 fusion. This translocation is found in approximately 70% of MLL gene–rearranged infant ALL cases. Other common translocations include t(11;19), resulting in the MLL-ENL fusion, and t(9;11), resulting in the MLL-AF9 fusion, which occur in 15% and 4% of MLL gene–rearranged infant ALL cases, respectively.[6,85-87,90] Cases of infant ALL without an MLL gene rearrangement generally resemble the more common B-precursor ALL phenotype (CD19+, CD10+) typical of older children with ALL. Chromosomal abnormalities known to be favorable in older children with ALL, such as high hyperdiploidy (51 to 65 chromosomes, or a DNA index more than 1.16) and the *TEL-AML1* fusion gene, are notably absent in infants.[84] The distinguishing presenting characteristics of infants with ALL are summarized in Table 52-2.

A striking feature of MLL gene–rearranged infant ALL is the paucity of secondary genomic alterations compared with older children who have pre–B-ALL.[91-94] A mutational profiling study of oncogenic RAS alterations in MLL gene–rearranged ALL samples identified mutations

in 15 of 109 samples (14%). Of the 38 samples with a t(4;11) MLL gene rearrangement, 9 (24%) were found to have RAS mutations. Identification of a RAS mutation was found to be an independent poor prognostic risk factor.[95]

Prognostic Factors and Outcomes

Despite extraordinary improvements in the cure rates for older children with ALL, the prognosis for infants with this disease remains poor. Historically, infants with ALL who were treated with standard regimens had a less than 20% event-free survival (EFS). During the past decade, intensified regimens designed especially for infants have resulted in improved rates of EFS ranging from 28% to 54% (Table 52-3).[84,85,87,89,97-104] In contrast, EFS rates are greater than 80% for older children with ALL.[105-108] Although 90% to 95% of infants with ALL achieve remission after initial induction chemotherapy, a favorable outcome is hampered by an exceedingly high relapse rate, typically within the first year after diagnosis.

Several closely related adverse prognostic factors have been identified for infants with ALL, including the presence of an MLL gene rearrangement, lack of CD10 expression, coexpression of myeloid markers, age less than 6 months at diagnosis, high white blood cell (WBC) count at presentation, CNS involvement, and poor early response to prednisone therapy.[87,97,109,111] In multivariate analyses, the presence of an MLL gene rearrangement, age younger than 6 months, and a poor early response to prednisone therapy consistently emerge as the most important adverse prognostic features.[89,102] In many studies, the presence of an MLL gene rearrangement is the most important independent predictor of outcome for infants.[88] Long-term EFS for infants with MLL gene–rearranged ALL has ranged from 13% to

TABLE 52-2 Presenting Characteristics of Infants and Older Children with Acute Lymphoblastic Leukemia

Characteristic	AGE (yr) 0-1 (%)	AGE (yr) 1-18 (%)
WBC* >100,000[84]	58	6.3
CNS-positive*[84]	14	1.5
Phenotype		
B lineage	96	86.5
T lineage	4	13.5
CD10-negative[84]	54.7	3.3
Myeloid antigen coexpression[96,97]	28	5
DNA index* >1.16[84]	1.5	24.7
TEL-AML1* rearrangement[84]	4.5	24.1
MLL rearrangement[85-87]	70-80	2-4

From Silverman LB: Acute lymphoblastic leukemia in infancy. Pediatr Blood Cancer 49:1070–1073, 2007.
MLL, Mixed-lineage leukemia; WBC, white blood cell.
*B-lineage patients only.

TABLE 52-3 Outcomes of Treatment Protocols for Acute Lymphoblastic Leukemia in Infants

Study	Publication Date	Patients Enrolled	CR Rate (%)	EFS Time Point (yr)	EFS (%)
DFCI (1985-1995)[90]	1997	23	96	4	54
Interfant-99[90]	2007	482	94	5	45
AIEOP-91, 95[109]	2006	52	96	5	45
BFM 86, 90, 95[84]	1999	129	95	8	43
CCG-1953[87]	2006	115	97	5	42
P9407[110]	2012	97	n/a	5	41
CCG-1883[101]	1999	135	97	4	39
CCG-107[101]	1999	99	94	4	33
UKALL-92[97]	2002	86	94	5	33
POG 8493[98]	1997	82	93	4	28

AIEOP, Associazione Italiana di Ematologia Oncologia Pediatrica; *BFM,* Berlin-Frankfurt-Münster; *CCG,* Children's Cancer Study Group; *CR,* complete remission; *DFCI,* Dana-Farber Cancer Institute; *EFS,* event-free survival; *POG,* Pediatric Oncology Group; *UKALL,* United Kingdom Acute Lymphoblastic Leukaemia.

34%, versus 52% to 95% for infants with germline MLL (Fig. 52-2).[4,6,87-89,97,99,102,112]

In addition to MLL gene status and age, early response to therapy has been shown to be an important predictor of outcome in infants with ALL. The Berlin-Frankfurt-Munster group has identified a poor response to prednisone as one of the strongest predictors of outcome for infants with ALL, regardless of MLL gene status.[97] Infants with ALL who have a poor response to a 7-day prednisone monotherapy prophase (defined as more than 1000 blasts/μL present in peripheral blood on day 8) had a 6-year EFS of only 15%, compared with a 6-year EFS of 53% for infants with a good response to prednisone. This finding was reproduced in the most recent clinical trial

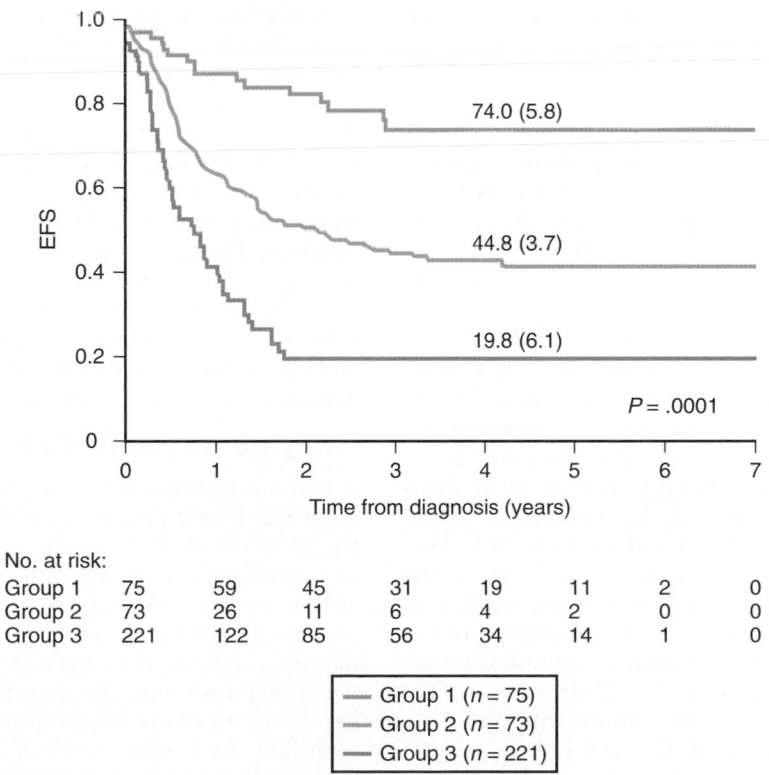

Figure 52-2 Event-free survival *(EFS)* for infants with acute lymphoblastic leukemia who were treated in the Interfant 99 trial.[103] Group 1 consisted of patients with the germline mixed lineage leukemia (MLL) gene. Group 2 consisted of patients with an MLL gene rearrangement, age younger than 6 months at diagnosis, and white blood cell count higher than 300 × 10⁹ cells/L at diagnosis. Group 3 consisted of all other patients. *(Modified from Pieters R, Schrappe M, De Lorenzo P, et al: A treatment protocol for infants younger than 1 year with acute lymphoblastic leukemia [Interfant-99]: an observational study and a multicentre randomized trial. Lancet 370:240–250, 2007.)*

conducted by the Interfant study group (Interfant 99), in which infants with a poor response to steroids had a 30% 4-year EFS, compared with a 56% 4-year EFS for good responders.[89] Similarly, the Children's Cancer Group found a threefold excess risk of treatment failure in infants whose bone marrows contained more than 5% leukemic blast cells after 14 days of multiagent chemotherapy.[102]

It has been suggested that the specific MLL gene fusion partner might also have prognostic significance for infants with ALL.[102,109] However, in a large retrospective study that included data from more than 200 cases of MLL gene–rearranged ALL in infants, no significant difference in outcome was found among cytogenetic subgroups, including t(4;11), t(9;11), t(11;19), and other 11q23 rearrangements.[90] The Interfant study group also failed to find any association between the specific MLL gene translocations and treatment outcome.[89] More recently, localization of the fusion break point has been identified as a potential prognostic biomarker, with break points within MLL intron 11 demonstrating poorer outcomes.[113] Gene expression profiling has also identified candidate prognostic markers. Analysis of 97 samples from P9407, a COG trial for infant ALL conducted between 1996 and 2006, identified patients with low FLT3 expression as having superior outcomes, which had previously been observed in patients enrolled in the Interfant 99 trial.[114] Patients with high FLT3 expression, in addition to either high iroquois homeobox 2 (IRX2) or high transforming, acidic coiled-coil containing protein 2 (TACC2) expression, had very poor 4-year EFS rates.[110]

Treatment

Attempts to improve clinical outcomes for infants with ALL have generally involved intensifying treatment regimens and incorporating chemotherapeutic agents more commonly used in AML therapy. An ongoing international trial, Interfant 06, is evaluating the outcome of patients randomly treated with either a standard consolidation approach using mercaptopurine, cyclophosphamide, and cytarabine or two consecutive AML-based cycles that include cytarabine, etoposide, and both daunorubicin and mitoxantrone. Several preclinical and clinical findings have also informed the development of treatment regimens for infants with ALL, including clinical response to prednisone therapy and in vitro drug sensitivity profiles of infant ALL lymphoblasts. When compared with cells from older children with ALL, leukemic blasts from patients with infant ALL are more often resistant to glucocorticoids (prednisone and dexamethasone) and L-asparaginase in in vitro assays. Importantly, both of these agents are central components of current ALL therapeutic regimens.[97,115-117] In vitro studies of sarcoma (Src) kinase inhibition demonstrated sensitization of MLL gene–rearranged ALL cell lines to glucocorticoids, highlighting this strategy as a possible future therapeutic option in these patients.[118,119] Given the prognostic significance of prednisone response in ALL, some infant ALL treatment groups now risk-stratify infants on the basis of prednisone response and other common prognostic factors, including MLL gene status, age, and diagnostic WBC count.[89]

Although infant ALL blasts are relatively resistant to some common ALL therapeutic agents, they are remarkably sensitive to cytosine arabinoside (ara-C; cytarabine), a drug commonly used in the treatment of AML.[115,116] This increased sensitivity may be related in part to elevated expression of the human equilibrative nucleoside transporter–1, which allows cytarabine to permeate the cell membrane at low to moderate concentrations.[120-123] Clinical data are accumulating to suggest that increased use of cytarabine may benefit infants with ALL.[89,99,102] Investigators from the Dana-Farber Cancer Institute ALL Consortium first reported an improved outcome in a small number of infants treated with intensified therapy that included high-dose cytarabine.[124] Subsequently the cooperative groups COG and Interfant incorporated high-dose cytarabine into their intensified therapeutic regimens, a strategy that is likely to have contributed to the improvements in EFS for infants with ALL observed during the past decade.

Hematopoietic Stem Cell Transplantation

The role of hematopoietic stem cell transplantation (HSCT) in first remission for infants with ALL is controversial. Small uncontrolled studies have suggested that HSCT may benefit infants with MLL gene rearrangements.[125-127] Although encouraging, these results must be interpreted with caution, given the small sample sizes, the failure to control for waiting time from diagnosis to transplantation, and the use of total body irradiation in cytoreduction, which many groups are avoiding given the significant morbidity associated with radiation in this age group.[128] The most recent Interfant study group trial (Interfant 99) identified a subgroup of high-risk patients who may benefit from HSCT, including those diagnosed before 6 months of age and who have either a poor steroid response or a high WBC count at diagnosis.[129] In contrast, a larger retrospective analysis did not confirm a benefit of HCST for infants with ALL.[90] Similarly, the COG found no benefit of transplantation compared with intensive chemotherapy alone.[87] Further studies are needed to adequately define the role for stem cell transplantation in infants with ALL.

Toxicity and CNS-Directed Therapy

A major consideration in the treatment of ALL in infants is the significant potential for short- and long-term toxicity, given the intensity of treatment regimens and the lack of pharmacokinetic and pharmacodynamic studies to ensure optimal dosing of chemotherapeutic agents in infants. Of particular concern is the risk of debilitating neuropsychological sequelae, especially in infants receiving cranial radiation. Severe neurologic deficits and learning disabilities have been reported in long-term survivors of infant ALL who received cranial radiation.[3,98,99] In almost all subsequent clinical trials, attempts have been made to reduce neuropsychological complications by minimizing, delaying, or eliminating cranial radiation. Currently most investigators favor eliminating radiation in infants with ALL, even those with CNS leukemia at diagnosis, relying instead on intensive systemic and intrathecal chemotherapy. Several observations have supported this approach, including outcomes from large cooperative group studies documenting very low CNS relapse rates (3% to 9%) with intensive systemic and intrathecal chemotherapy alone.[89,100,102]

ACUTE MYELOID LEUKEMIA

Clinical and Prognostic Features

Infant AML is characterized by a high incidence of myelomonoblastic (French-American-British [FAB] M4) or monoblastic (FAB M5) morphologic features, frequent CNS involvement, extramedullary disease (including skin involvement), and relatively high leukocyte counts at diagnosis.[2]

MLL gene rearrangements are found in about 60% of infant AML cases, with the most common translocation being t(9;11), resulting in the MLL-AF9 fusion, followed by t(11;19), resulting in the MLL-ENL fusion. MLL gene rearrangements in infant AML are associated with a FAB M4 or M5 morphology and hyperleukocytosis.[111,130,131] Other cytogenetic abnormalities in infant AML of the FAB M4 or M5 morphologic subtype include inv(16) and monosomy 7. Translocations commonly seen in older children with AML, such as t(8;21) and t(15;17), are rare in infants with AML.[132]

Unlike in infant ALL, the prognostic factors that predict outcome for infant AML are not clearly defined. Several studies have identified a variety of potential prognostic factors for infants with AML, including presenting WBC count, FAB M4 or M5 morphology, gender, and the presence of an MLL gene rearrangement, but the findings of these studies have varied widely and are often contradictory.[133-138] The difficulty in clearly identifying consistent prognostic factors in infant AML may point to more biologic heterogeneity in infant AML (compared with infant ALL), as well as significant variations in the definition of study groups and treatment regimens.

The prognostic significance of MLL gene rearrangements in infant AML is unclear. Several studies have found that MLL gene rearrangements lack prognostic significance in childhood AML, whereas at least one study has found a trend toward a worse outcome.[131,133,139-142] Alternatively, several groups have demonstrated that the presence of a specific translocation, t(9;11)(p22;q22) or MLL-AF9, confers a favorable prognosis.[138,143-146] For example, the investigators at St. Jude Children's Research Hospital found the presence of t(9;11) to be an important prognostic factor for patients treated in four consecutive pediatric AML trials. The 5-year EFS for infants whose leukemia cells carried t(9;11) was 70% versus 25% for those with other cytogenetic abnormalities, including other MLL gene rearrangements.[147]

The Berlin-Frankfurt-Munster Group recently reported on the clinical characteristics of 62 pediatric patients with AML who had t(8;16)(p11;p13) translocations. The average age of diagnosis was very young (1.2 years), with common features of erythrophagocytosis (70%), leukemia cutis (58%), and disseminated intravascular coagulation (39%). Strikingly, seven patients diagnosed within the first month of life underwent spontaneous remission of their disease, three of whom remained in remission at the time of publication.[148]

Outcomes and Treatment

Whereas age-associated treatment results are clearly evident in childhood ALL, with infants faring significantly worse, similar age-related differences in outcomes have not been routinely observed in AML. In large clinical trials in children with AML, EFS rates of 22% to 73% have been reported for infants, which do not differ significantly from outcomes achieved in older children (Table 52-4).[126,147,149-156] Given that treatment outcomes do not differ by age group, there has been no compelling clinical justification for the development of unique treatment strategies for infants with AML. Current therapeutic regimens for infants and older children focus on intensive remission induction and consolidation chemotherapy, with HSCT reserved for patients with matched sibling donors and those who have poor prognostic features. Although treatment regimens for infants with AML do not currently differ from those for older children, some potential differences have been proposed. The observation that t(9;11) may be a favorable prognostic factor in infants with AML has resulted in controversy with regard to whether bone marrow transplantation in first remission should be considered in this subgroup of patients. Another possible exception includes infants with megakaryoblastic leukemia who are harboring t(1;22) (p13;q13); these infants appear to have a particularly poor prognosis and may be candidates for more aggressive treatment or innovative experimental therapy.[157,158]

TABLE 52-4 Outcomes of Treatment Protocols for Acute Myeloid Leukemia in Infants

Study	Study Period	Patients Enrolled	EFS Time Point	EFS (%)
St. Jude (AML80-91)[138]	1980-1987	28	5	32
BFM (AML 93)[149]	1993-1998	112*	5	41
MRC (AML10, 12)[150]	1988-2002	151	5	58
POG (8821)[151]	1988-1993	122*	5	22
Nordic (NOPHO-93)[152]	1993-2001	57*	5	54
CCG 2891[153]	1989-1995	116	8	71
Japan (ANLL91)[154]	1995-1998	35	3	72
French (LAME 89, 91)[155]	1988-1998	42	5	37.3
FHCRC[156]	1995-1998	35*	3	72

AML, Acute myeloid leukemia; *ANLL*, acute nonlymphocytic leukemia; *BFM*, Berlin-Frankfurt-Münster; *CCG*, Children's Cancer Study Group; *EFS*, event-free survival; *FHCRC*, Fred Hutchinson Cancer Research Center; *LAME*, Leucémie Aiguë Myéloblastique L'Enfant; *MRC*, Medical Research Council; *NOPHO*, Nordic Society of Paediatric Haematology and Oncology; *POG*, Pediatric Oncology Group.
*Children 1 to 2 years of age were included.

Association with Down Syndrome

Several genetic syndromes including monosomy 7, del (7q) syndromes, Noonan syndrome, and neurofibromatosis type 1 are associated with an increased risk of developing myelodysplasia, myeloproliferative diseases, and myeloid leukemia in infancy. A striking example is the increased incidence of leukemia seen in children with Down syndrome. Persons with Down syndrome have a tenfold to twentyfold increased lifetime risk of developing leukemia, including ALL and AML. The most marked increase is observed in young children with Down syndrome in whom acute megakaryoblastic leukemia (AMKL; FAB M7) develops.[159] The risk of AMKL is estimated to be 500 times higher in children with Down syndrome than in the general population. A transient form of megakaryoblastic leukemia, known as transient leukemia, transient abnormal myelopoiesis, or transient myeloproliferative disorder (TMD), often precedes AMKL in newborn infants with Down syndrome (or trisomy 21 mosaicism). Although the true incidence of TMD is unknown, a small study has found that 10% of neonates with Down syndrome have evidence of TMD on examination of their peripheral blood smears.[160] The true incidence of TMD is likely to be higher, given that fetuses who develop TMD in utero may not be identified and neonates with subtle manifestations of TMD may go unnoticed.[161,162]

Clinically the presentation of TMD can be variable, ranging from asymptomatic, with an incidental finding of an elevated WBC count and circulating blasts in the peripheral blood, to fulminating life-threatening disease, with severe liver dysfunction and liver fibrosis, multiple effusions, and respiratory compromise. TMD has also been associated with intrauterine death and hydrops fetalis.[162,163] TMD usually has a relatively benign course, with spontaneous remission within the first 3 months of life. However, in 13% to 33% of infants who recover from TMD, AMKL will go on to develop by age 3 years.[164-166] Often the subsequent leukemia is preceded by a myelodysplastic phase, with progressive cytopenias and increasing marrow fibrosis. In a prospective study of neonates with TMD conducted by the COG, it has been found that 64% of infants with TMD experienced a spontaneous and continuous remission, 17% had an early death (predominantly because of liver failure), and 19% experienced a spontaneous remission but went on to develop AMKL at a mean age of 20 months.[166]

TMD and AMKL in persons with Down syndrome nicely illustrate the multistep process of leukemic transformation. Biologically, the blasts from TMD and AMKL are morphologically and immunophenotypically similar and consistent with megakaryoblastic progenitors.[167-169] Chromosomal abnormalities are more frequent in AMKL than in TMD, with the most common abnormality being trisomy 8.[160,170] The leukemic blasts of TMD and AMKL in patients with Down syndrome have been shown to harbor a unique mutation of the gene encoding the hematopoietic transcription factor *GATA1*.[171-174] These mutations are found exclusively in Down syndrome–associated TMD and AMKL and have not been found in non–Down syndrome–associated AMKL or in patients with Down syndrome who have ALL.[171,173,174] *GATA1* has essential functions during normal erythroid and megakaryocytic development.[175,176] Most *GATA1* mutations cluster within exon 2 and result in the expression of a truncated mutant protein, GATA1s, which retains its DNA binding zinc fingers but lacks the amino-terminal transcriptional activation domain. Studies in model systems have suggested that GATA1 possesses unique activity that leads to expansion of an early megakaryocyte progenitor in the fetal liver, perhaps explaining why *GATA1* mutations are only found in infant AMKL from patients with Down syndrome.[177] Several recent studies have demonstrated that although TMD is caused by constitutional trisomy 21 and *GATA1* mutations, progression to AMKL is caused by the acquisition of additional mutations. These mutations have been identified in multiple cohesin components and epigenetic regulators, as well as wingless type (WNT), Janus kinase–signal transducer and activator of transcription (JAK-STAT), and mitogen-activated protein kinase/phosphatidylinositol 3′-kinase (MAPK/PI3K) pathway genes.[178-180]

Another remarkable characteristic of AMKL in Down syndrome is its extraordinary responsiveness to AML therapy.[135,181-184] In early clinical trials, the outcomes for patients with AML and Down syndrome were not favorable, although poor outcomes were primarily the result of treatment-related toxicity rather than relapsed or refractory disease. Subsequently, patients with Down syndrome and AML who were treated in a series of large multicenter pediatric trials were found to have a better response to chemotherapy and better survival rates than were patients without Down syndrome. EFS rates for children with Down syndrome and AML treated by modern protocols range from 80% to 100%.[135,181,182,184-187] Current treatment protocols for patients with Down syndrome and AML favor less intensive regimens, which aim to maintain high cure rates while minimizing toxicity.

Non–Down Syndrome–Associated Infant AMKL

AMKL also occurs in a subset of infants who do not have Down syndrome. AMKL in these infants frequently harbors the t(1;22)(p13;q13) translocation.[157,158,188] The t(1;22)(p13;q13) translocation is found almost exclusively in infants and young children with AMKL. This disorder is typically accompanied by significant bone marrow fibrosis and organomegaly and has a poor prognosis, with a median survival of only 8 months. The t(1;22)(p13;q13) characteristic of this malignancy is associated with the fusion of RNA-binding motif protein–15 (*RBM15*), an RNA recognition motif-encoding gene, and megakaryoblastic leukemia–1 (*MKL1*), a gene encoding an SAP (scaffold attachment factor A and B [SAF-A/B], Acinus, and protein inhibitor of activated STAT [PIAS]) DNA binding domain.[189] The mechanism by which this fusion contributes to leukemogenesis is not yet fully understood, although it has been shown that Rbm15-Mkl1 can alter SET domain containing 1b (Setd1b) histone methyltransferase activity, leading to epigenetic dysregulation.[190] Alternate translocations have also been identified in non–Down syndrome AMKL. A recent genomic study of non–Down syndrome AML identified a novel cryptic translocation of chromosome 16 involving core-binding factor, runt domain, alpha subunit 2, translocated to 3 (CBFA2T3), a member of the eight-twenty-one (ETO) family of nuclear corepressors, and GLIS2, a GLI family transcription factor. This translocation was identified in 27% of studied cases and was associated with significantly poorer outcomes.[191] Translocations joining NUP98 on chromosome 11 to KDM5A (JARID1A) on chromosome 12 are found in approximately 10% of AMKL cases and are characterized by HOXA/B gene overexpression. Unique clinical or prognostic characteristics have not been identified in this subset of patients.[192]

FUTURE DIRECTIONS IN INFANT ACUTE LEUKEMIA TREATMENT

Although morphologic complete remission is achieved in the vast majority of infants with ALL, a favorable outcome is hampered by an exceedingly high relapse rate in the first year after diagnosis. To date, intensification of conventional chemotherapeutic agents has resulted in only incremental improvement in the prognosis of infants with ALL, emphasizing the need for novel, more effective therapies.[193]

Targeting Epigenetic Mechanisms

In the past few years we have seen an explosion in the understanding of the normal function of the MLL protein and the fusion proteins generated by MLL translocations. We now know that the wild-type MLL protein is a histone methyltransferase that influences the expression of important developmental genes such as the HOX genes. Indeed, these proteins that influence gene expression via modification of histones or other components of chromatin (known as epigenetic regulators) appear to be central to the development of a number of different leukemia subtypes and perhaps other cancers. Given that enzymes control many of the epigenetic processes, the possibility that a new generation of therapies that targets epigenetic regulators may be on the horizon is generating tremendous excitement. Histone deacetylase inhibitors and DNA hypomethylating agents may work through the modulation of either DNA or histone modifications, and such approaches are being considered in pediatric leukemias, including infant MLL gene–rearranged leukemias. Although a specific rationale does not exist as to why MLL gene–rearranged leukemias should be more sensitive to these approaches than other leukemias, it is worth considering these agents for clinical trials.

However, new data provide a potential rational approach to target MLL fusion proteins generated by MLL translocation. Recent studies have shown that leukemic transformation by MLL fusion proteins is highly, and somewhat uniquely, dependent upon the histone methyltransferase DOT1L that methylates histone H3 on lysine 79.[77-79] Remarkably, it appears that this enzyme is required for continued proliferation of most if not all MLL gene–rearranged leukemias, and thus a therapeutic agent targeting DOT1L might benefit patients with leukemia who are bearing any MLL translocation.[194] Preclinical studies using specific small molecule DOT1L inhibitors have been completed and demonstrate remarkable activity and minimal toxicity in animal models.[195,196] The phase I trials for such approaches are under way in adults with relapsed/refractory leukemia. The possibilities that this approach may represent are generating tremendous excitement. However, it will be important to thoroughly assess the toxicity of such approaches in adults and children given that this approach to cancer therapy is completely new.

Immunotherapy

Novel therapies directed at proteins on leukemic cells may offer further promise in treating infant leukemia. Three approaches to targeting CD19 for the treatment of pre–B-ALL exist. Blinatumomab is a bispecific antibody that binds both CD19 and CD3, thereby engaging T cells to attack leukemia cells. In a phase II trial of adult patients with persistent minimal residual disease (MRD), 80% of subjects achieved negative MRD after treatment with blinatumomab, and responses in children have already been reported.[197,198] The pediatric phase II trial is under way. Positive results using autologous chimeric antigen cells directed against CD19 have now been reported in both pediatric and adult patients, and further studies in patients with infant ALL will need to be pursued.[199,200] Finally, a novel antibody-drug conjugate, SGN-CD19a, which combines an anti-CD19 monoclonal antibody with an inhibitor of tubulin polymerization (monomethyl auristatin F), is being evaluated in patients with pre–B-ALL and may prove to be effective for treatment of infant ALL. All three therapies target the CD19 protein, which may be a limitation in MLL gene–rearranged infant ALL, given the existence of CD19-negative subpopulations in this leukemia.[201]

Relative to ALL, current options for immunotherapy in AML are fewer. SGN-CD33a, an antibody-drug conjugate in development, targets CD33 and utilizes a pyrrolobenzodiazepine dimer to create DNA damage. This drug is only recently entering into clinical trials but may be worth pursuing in future trials that assess novel infant AML therapy.[202]

Modulators of Glucocorticoid Resistance

Cellular drug resistance may significantly contribute to the poor prognosis of infant ALL.[193] Infants with ALL are more likely to have a poor in vivo response to prednisone than are older children with ALL.[97,117] In addition, leukemic blasts from infants with ALL are highly resistant to glucocorticoids in vitro.[115,116] Both in vivo and in vitro responses to prednisone are highly predictive of clinical outcome in childhood ALL, and thus the mechanisms of glucocorticoid resistance are attractive targets for novel therapeutic agents.[203,204] Gene expression profiling of steroid-resistant and steroid-sensitive lymphoblasts indicates that myeloid cell leukemia–1 (MCL1), an antiapoptotic member of the B-cell lymphoma–2 (BCL2) family, may be an important modulator of glucocorticoid resistance in ALL.[205,206] Furthermore, a gene expression–based chemical genomics screen has identified sirolimus (more commonly known as rapamycin), the mammalian target of rapamycin (mTOR) inhibitor, as an agent capable of reversing a gene expression signature associated with glucocorticoid resistance. It has also been shown that sirolimus sensitizes lymphoid cells to glucocorticoids via the modulation of MCL1 levels.[205] Other modulators of MCL1 have been identified, including honokiol, a naturally occurring compound, and the synthetic inhibitors Seliciclib (CYC202, or R-roscovitine) and R-etodolac (SDX-101).[207-210] The potential to overcome glucocorticoid resistance in infant ALL by compounds that modulate MCL1, or other antiapoptotic molecules such as BCL2, makes agents targeting the apoptotic pathway attractive candidates for further investigation as therapeutic approaches for the treatment of infant ALL.[211]

FLT3 Inhibitors

Lymphoblastic leukemias with rearrangements of the MLL gene display a unique gene expression profile that distinguishes them from other subgroups of ALL and AML.[57,59-61] This distinct gene expression profile has led to the identification of several potential therapeutic targets. One of the most highly expressed genes distinguishing MLL gene–rearranged ALL from other acute leukemias is *FLT3*, the gene encoding fms-like tyrosine kinase 3.[57,212] Activating *FLT3* mutations through internal tandem duplication (ITD) of the juxta-membrane domain (FLT3/ITD) occur in 11% to 17% of de novo pediatric AML cases and are associated with significantly poorer outcomes.[213-216] After identification of these activating mutations, numerous small-molecule FLT3 inhibitors were developed, and clinical trials are under way to evaluate the effectiveness of these compounds in the treatment of AML.[217-222] However, FLT3/ITD–positive AML is rare in infant AML, accounting for fewer than 2% of cases, and therefore may have very limited benefit in this population.[216] High levels of *FLT3* expression have also been demonstrated in MLL gene–rearranged ALL. FLT3 inhibitors have been shown to be active against MLL gene–rearranged cell lines that overexpress *FLT3*, as well as in primary MLL gene–rearranged lymphoblasts.[223-225] Additionally, results from in vitro experiments with MLL gene–rearranged cell lines have suggested that FLT3 inhibitors may work synergistically with several standard chemotherapeutic agents, including ara-C.[225,226] However, the sequence of administration of these agents appears to be important. In vitro studies have found that to achieve maximal synergistic cytotoxicity, the chemotherapeutic agent must be given immediately prior to the FLT3 inhibitor, whereas pretreatment with the FLT3 inhibitor followed by the chemotherapeutic agent results in antagonistic effects.[226,227] Furthermore, disruption of the stromal microenvironment through CXCR4 inhibition leads to increased sensitivity of MLL gene–rearranged ALL xenograft models to FLT3 inhibition.[228] The preclinical data demonstrating activity of FLT-3 inhibitors in infant ALL suggest that FLT3 inhibition may represent a novel therapeutic strategy for infant ALL, and clinical testing is under way. An ongoing COG study (trial AALL0631) is evaluating the benefit of the addition of the FLT3 inhibitor lestaurtinib to an intensive chemotherapy backbone for patients with infant ALL.

References available online at ExpertConsult.

KEY REFERENCES

12. Ford AM, Ridge SA, Cabrera ME, et al: In utero rearrangements in the trithorax-related oncogene in infant leukaemias. *Nature* 363:358–360, 1993.
    This report provides evidence that the leukemogenic events in infant leukemia originate in utero.
32. Felix CA, Hosler MR, Winick NJ, et al: ALL-1 gene rearrangements in DNA topoisomerase II inhibitor-related leukemia in children. *Blood* 85:3250–3256, 1995.
    This report associates mixed-lineage leukemia gene rearrangements with the majority of topoisomerase II inhibitor–associated leukemia.
42. Domer PH, Fakharzadeh SS, Chen CS, et al: Acute mixed-lineage leukemia t(4;11)(q21;q23) generates an MLL-AF4 fusion product. *Proc Natl Acad Sci U S A* 90:7884–7888, 1993.
43. Gu Y, Nakamura T, Alder H, et al: The t(4;11) chromosome translocation of human acute leukemias fuses the ALL-1 gene, related to Drosophila trithorax, to the AF-4 gene. *Cell* 71:701–708, 1992.
44. Tkachuk DC, Kohler S, Cleary ML: Involvement of a homolog of Drosophila trithorax by 11q23 chromosomal translocations in acute leukemias. *Cell* 71:691–700, 1992.
45. Ziemin-van der Poel S, McCabe NR, Gill HJ, et al: Identification of a gene, MLL, that spans the breakpoint in 11q23 translocations associated with human leukemias. *Proc Natl Acad Sci U S A* 88:10735–10739, 1991.
    References 42, 43, 44, and 45 describe the cloning of the t(4;11) translocation and identification of mixed-lineage leukemia.
52. Yu BD, Hess JL, Horning SE, et al: Altered Hox expression and segmental identity in Mll-mutant mice. *Nature* 378:505–508, 1995.
    This study establishes the role of mixed-lineage leukemia for normal homeobox gene expression.
57. Armstrong S, Staunton J, Silverman L, et al: MLL translocation specify a distinct gene expression profile that distinguishes a unique leukemia. *Nat Genet* 30:41–47, 2002.
    This study defines the gene expression program for mixed-lineage leukemia–rearranged (MLL-R) acute lymphoblastic leukemia (ALL) and is the first report of overexpression of fms-related tyrosine kinase-3 in MLL-R ALL samples.
59. Yeoh E, Ross M, Shurtleff S, et al: Classification, subtype discovery, and prediction of outcome in pediatric acute lymphoblastic leukemia by gene expression profiling. *Cancer Cell* 1:133–143, 2002.
    The initial characterization of gene expression profiles that differ across pediatric acute lymphoblastic leukemia cases.
75. Yokoyama A, Lin M, Naresh A, et al: A higher-order complex containing AF4 and ENL family proteins with P-TEFb facilitates oncogenic and physiologic MLL-dependent transcription. *Cancer Cell* 17:198–212, 2010.
    References 71 through 75 define the protein complexes associated with mixed-lineage leukemia fusion proteins.
77. Krivtsov AV, Feng Z, Lemieux ME, et al: H3K79 methylation profiles define murine and human MLL-AF4 leukemias. *Cancer Cell* 14:355–368, 2008.
    This study identifies aberrant H3K79 methylation in mixed-lineage leukemia–rearranged leukemias.
87. Hilden JM, Dinndorf PA, Meerbaum SO, et al: Analysis of prognostic factors of acute lymphoblastic leukemia in infants: report on CCG 1953 from the Children's Oncology Group. *Blood* 108:441–451, 2006.
    This analysis of 115 patients with infant acute lymphoblastic leukemia led to the identification of CD10 expression, age, and cytogenetics as the most significant factors associated with prognosis.

88. Pui CH, Behm FG, Downing JR, et al: 11q23/MLL rearrangement confers a poor prognosis in infants with acute lymphoblastic leukemia. *J Clin Oncol* 12:909–915, 1994.

    This clinical study established the presence of mixed-lineage leukemia gene rearrangements as a poor prognostic factor in infant acute lymphoblastic leukemia.

89. Pieters R, Schrappe M, De Lorenzo P, et al: A treatment protocol for infants younger than 1 year with acute lymphoblastic leukaemia (Interfant-99): an observational study and a multicentre randomised trial. *Lancet* 370:240–250, 2007.

    This is the largest clinical trial conducted to date for infant lymphoblastic leukemia. The protocol utilized a hybrid approach with acute myeloid leukemia–type therapy used during consolidations. The trial results were favorable. Age, white blood cell count, mixed-lineage leukemia–rearranged, and steroid response were identified as prognostic indicators.

91. Mullighan CG, Goorha S, Radtke I, et al: Genome-wide analysis of genetic alterations in acute lymphoblastic leukaemia. *Nature* 446:758–764, 2007.

    This study illustrates the paucity of additional genomic alterations in mixed-lineage leukemia–rearranged leukemias.

114. Stam RW, Schneider P, de Lorenzo P, et al: Prognostic significance of high-level FLT3 expression in MLL-rearranged infant acute lymphoblastic leukemia. *Blood* 110:2774–2775, 2007.

    This study provides evidence of poor prognosis associated with high levels of fms-related tyrosine kinase–3 expression in patients with mixed-lineage leukemia–rearranged infant acute lymphoblastic leukemia.

158. Carroll A, Civin C, Schneider N, et al: The t(1;22) (p13;q13) is nonrandom and restricted to infants with acute megakaryoblastic leukemia: a Pediatric Oncology Group study. *Blood* 78:748–752, 1991.

    A report of a novel translocation associated with acute megakaryoblastic leukemia.

171. Wechsler J, Greene M, McDevitt MA, et al: Acquired mutations in GATA1 in the megakaryoblastic leukemia of Down syndrome. *Nat Genet* 32:148–152, 2002.

    These studies reveal the role of GATA1 mutations in the leukemogenesis of acute myeloid leukemia in persons with Down syndrome.

212. Armstrong S, Kung A, Maban M, et al: Inhibition of FLT3 in MLL: validation of a therapeutic target identified by gene expression based classification. *Cancer Cell* 3:173–183, 2003.

    This study introduces fms-related tyrosine kinase–3 inhibition as a possible therapeutic intervention in mixed-lineage leukemia–rearranged acute lymphoblastic leukemia.

CHAPTER 53

Pediatric Lymphoma

Sarah Alexander and Adolfo A. Ferrando

CHAPTER OUTLINE

Lymphomas are neoplasms caused by the malignant transformation of the constituent cells of the immune system. Combined, Hodgkin and non-Hodgkin lymphomas are the third most common malignancies in children and adolescents, with Hodgkin lymphoma being the most common cancer in people between the ages of 15 and 18 years.

The treatment of children and adolescents with lymphoma is one of the important success stories in pediatric oncology. The transformation of what were uniformly fatal diseases to those in which cure is the expectation occurred first for those with Hodgkin lymphoma and more recently for the majority of children with non-Hodgkin lymphoma. The understanding of normal and abnormal lymphoid biology has been critical to the develop systems for classification and for the evolution of disease-specific therapy.

This chapter reviews the clinical and pathologic features, including molecular and cellular biology, of the most common pediatric lymphoma subtypes and reviews the current strategies for evaluation and treatment.

LYMPHADENOPATHY

The child with lymphadenopathy poses a relatively common diagnostic challenge for the pediatrician. Over one third of 5-year-old children seen for well-child care and two thirds evaluated for a sick visit have palpable adenopathy.[1,2] In most children, lymph-node enlargement results from transient, self-limited infectious processes that resolve without sequelae. However, serious, life-threatening benign and malignant diseases may present with lymphadenopathy as the first manifestation. Thoughtful decision making is critical regarding further investigation, including which children require biopsy of their nodes for pathologic evaluation.

Various definitions of adenopathy have been described, including specific measurements in the radiologic literature. In general, adenopathy is defined as any node greater than 1 cm in dimension. Epitrochlear nodes are considered enlarged if they are greater than 0.5 cm, and inguinal nodes are enlarged if they are greater than 1.5 cm. Lymphadenopathy is considered localized if it involves a single node or single nodal area and generalized if it involves more than 2 noncontiguous nodal groups and may include hepatosplenomegaly. Chronic adenopathy is variably defined but in general can be considered as enlargement that persists for longer than 3 weeks.

Enlargement of lymph nodes results from expansion and recruitment of normal lymph node cells, expansion of abnormal immune cells, or infiltration of extrinsic cells. Certain considerations narrow the diagnostic possibilities in evaluation of the child with lymphadenopathy. Not all masses in children that appear to be lymphadenopathy represent enlarged lymph nodes; non–lymph-node masses that may mimic cervical lymphadenopathy include thyroglossal duct cysts and branchial cleft cysts. Evidence of recent or current upper respiratory infection and the presence of tender cervical adenopathy suggest inflammation as the cause. The presence of associated systemic symptoms, the chronicity of the adenopathy, and whether the adenopathy is generalized or regional are important considerations in the differential diagnosis. In addition, the age of the patient is important in considering the differential diagnosis, especially as it relates to potential malignant conditions. An abbreviated list of common causes of lymphadenopathy is presented in Box 53-1. More complete listings have been published elsewhere.[3,4]

Approach to the Patient

The management of the child with lymphadenopathy should be focused on obtaining clues to a diagnosis from the history, physical examination, and noninvasive testing, with the goals of ascertaining whether the lymphadenopathy is likely to be a manifestation of a serious illness and determining as early as possible in the workup whether the child should undergo lymph node biopsy. The history should include the duration of the adenopathy, associated symptoms, evidence of recent infection in the regions drained by the involved lymph node, exposure to illnesses, cats, or rodents, and current medications. The physical examination should be focused on ascertaining the location and number of enlarged nodes, their size, and their texture. Involvement of supraclavicular lymph nodes suggests mediastinal pathology and is usually associated with a serious disease mandating a prompt workup including a chest radiograph. In contrast the involvement of upper cervical lymph nodes is more likely to be the result of an upper respiratory tract infection.

For the child with generalized lymphadenopathy initial evaluation to be considered should include a complete blood count and a chest radiograph. Testing for possible infectious pathogens including viruses, fungi, and bacterial and mycobacterial agents should be considered. If no clues emerge, lymph node biopsy is likely indicated.

The workup of a child with localized or regional lymphadenopathy must be tailored to the individual child. Retrospective studies have attempted to identify those children with adenopathy who are more likely to have an underlying malignancy. Of children who underwent node biopsies, predictive factors for the etiology being malignancy included age older than 10 years, node size greater than 2.5 cm, and supraclavicular site.[5,6] Additional factors that were possibly associated included persistence of the node for longer than 6 weeks, having the node be "fixed" by palpation, and having more than one nodal area involved. In asymptomatic children whose adenopathy does not have high risk features, observation with careful measurement of lymph node size and possibly an empirical trial of antibiotic therapy is a reasonable strategy. If the nodes increase in size or fail to decrease to normal size after several weeks of observation, a lymph-node biopsy should be considered.

Masses occurring in the mediastinum represent urgent and challenging diagnostic problems, whether the result of enlarged lymph nodes or of the involvement of extralymphatic tissues. Lymphomas account for a significant portion of anterior and middle mediastinal masses in children and adolescents. Their proximity to vital structures and their propensity to cause life-threatening symptoms from vascular or airway compromise mandate an expeditious, systematic approach involving close cooperation among the surgeon, radiologist, oncologist, anesthesiologist, radiotherapist, and pathologist. A differential diagnosis of mediastinal masses according to location within the mediastinum is shown in Box 53-2.

Box 53-1 Causes of Lymphadenopathy

INFECTION

Bacterial: *Staphylococcus aureus*, group A *Streptococcus*, *Bartonella henselae*, brucellosis, tularemia
Viral: Epstein-Barr virus, cytomegalovirus, human immunodeficiency virus, measles, rubella
Fungal: Histoplasmosis, coccidioidomycosis, *Cryptococcus*
Protozoan: Toxoplasmosis, malaria
Mycobacterial: Tuberculosis, atypical mycobacteria

AUTOIMMUNE DISEASE

Juvenile rheumatoid arthritis, systemic lupus erythematosus, serum sickness, autoimmune lymphoproliferative syndrome

STORAGE DISEASE

Niemann-Pick disease, Gaucher disease

DRUG REACTION

Phenytoin and others

MALIGNANCY

Lymphoma, leukemia, metastatic solid tumors, histiocytic disorders

MISCELLANEOUS

Sarcoidosis, Kawasaki disease, Kikuchi disease

Box 53-2 Differential Diagnosis of Mediastinal Masses

ANTERIOR MEDIASTINUM

Lymphoma
Thymic cyst
Thymic "hyperplasia"
Benign teratoma
Malignant germ-cell tumor
Thymoma

MIDDLE MEDIASTINUM

Lymphoma
Tuberculosis
Histoplasmosis
Sarcoidosis

POSTERIOR MEDIASTINUM

Neuroblastoma
Ganglioneuroma
Neurofibroma
Sarcoma
Duplication cyst

EMERGENCIES IN PATIENTS WITH NEWLY DIAGNOSED LYMPHOMA

Children with lymphoma can have life-threatening findings such as respiratory distress and superior vena cava (SVC) syndrome caused by a mediastinal tumor, bowel obstruction from large abdominal masses, cranial nerve palsies, and paraplegia in the case of central nervous system (CNS) involvement and, in rare cases, disseminated intravascular coagulation. Patients may exhibit the metabolic derangements of acute tumor lysis syndrome (ATLS), although more often this problem arises after the initiation of therapy. Invasive diagnostic measures, especially those requiring anesthesia, can create emergencies for children with lymphomas.

A mediastinal tumor can cause respiratory distress as a result of tracheal or other large-airway compression. Patients often have cough, shortness of breath, and orthopnea. If there is considerable respiratory impairment, then all invasive diagnostic procedures need to be completed expeditiously. In these patients general anesthesia carries potential for substantial risks including inability to ventilate the child because of airway compression as well as swelling of the tracheal mucosa secondary to intubation, which may lead to worsening of critical constriction. Diagnostic procedures often need to be completed with local anesthesia alone. The least invasive procedure that will allow for attainment of diagnostic tissue should be undertaken.[7] In emergent situations, completion of staging (e.g., diagnostic lumbar puncture) may need to be deferred. Once tissue has been obtained, then initiation of steroids can be considered until pathologic diagnosis is complete. Very rarely for the patient with impending respiratory failure empirical therapy without specific diagnosis may needed. Cytoreduction with prednisone 60 mg/m^2/day and cyclophosphamide 100 to 200 mg/m^2/day or mediastinal radiation with doses of 10 to 15 Gy may provide a life-saving intervention.

In addition to respiratory impairment, mediastinal tumors can cause SVC syndrome by compression of the SVC and subsequent venous congestion. Patients have dilated neck veins, facial swelling, and discoloration. The life-threatening risk is from CNS venous strokes, often presenting as confusion or somnolence and less often as seizures or focal neurologic deficits. The tempo of progression of SVC syndrome in children tends to be much quicker in children than in adults as a consequence of more rapidly growing tumors. Again, in these patients expeditious evaluation and initiation of therapy is of critical importance.

Patients who have cranial nerve palsies and especially those with signs of incipient paraplegia also require urgent care. As in other pediatric malignancies, interventions may include surgical decompression, radiation, and chemotherapy. In general for children with lymphomas, which tend to be highly and quickly responsive to chemotherapy, initiation of therapy with prednisone or dexamethasone with or without cyclophosphamide is often the best approach. Clinicians should be aware that lumbar puncture in patients with bulky CNS disease may carry the risk of brainstem herniation. Urgent imaging should be considered before the procedure.

ATLS describes the metabolic derangements that occur with tumor-cell breakdown and is characterized by various combinations of hyperuricemia, hyperkalemia, and hyperphosphatemia with or without hypocalcemia and can lead to seizures, arrhythmias, renal failure, and death.[8] ATLS can be present before the initiation of treatment but more commonly occurs immediately after the initiation of chemotherapy. The incidence of ATLS differs among tumor types and depends primarily on the growth fraction, tumor mass, and chemotherapeutic sensitivity of the tumor. Adult and pediatric risk stratification algorithms for ATLS syndrome has been made and includes age, malignancy type, stage/lactate dehydrogenase (LDH) level, and renal function as predictive factors.[8] Patients with non-Hodgkin lymphoma (NHL) are at high risk, particularly those with advanced stage Burkitt lymphoma (BL), Burkitt leukemia, or lymphoblastic lymphoma (LL) with LDH greater than twice normal.

Vigorous hydration, alkalinization, and the administration of allopurinol, an inhibitor of xanthine oxidase, have been considered mainstays of prevention and treatment of ATLS and are aimed at the reduction of uric acid production and prevention of its precipitation in the kidneys. Evidence supporting the use of alkalization is controversial, and some contemporary guidelines do not recommend its use.[8] For patients considered at low risk, no specific intervention is required. For those at intermediate risk, careful monitoring of fluid and electrolytes is critical. Hyperhydration and allopurinol are almost always sufficient.

For those with higher risk for tumor lysis or who have evidence of the syndrome before the initiation of therapy, rasburicase should be considered. This agent is a recombinant urate oxidase that catalyzes the conversion of uric acid to allantoin. Allantoin is an inactive metabolite that is five to ten times more soluble than uric acid, so renal excretion is facilitated. A single dose will result in the rapid reduction in uric acid levels in patients with hyperurecemia.[9] It is contraindicated in patients with a history of glucose-6-phosphate dehydrogenase (G6PD) deficiency because of substantial risks of precipitating severe hemolysis. In a systematic review of published randomized trials, rasburicase was highly effective at reducing elevated uric acid, although the impact on mortality and renal failure was unclear.[10] In a French study of children with advanced stage B-cell NHL that incorporated the use of rasburicase, the incidence of need for dialysis during the first days of treatment was only 2.6% compared with 16% and 23% in other cooperative studies using the same French protocol that used only allopurinol.[11]

In some patients, even with optimal ATLS care renal function is insufficient and early hemodialysis should be instituted. This situation may occur because of direct infiltration of the kidneys, obstruction of the urinary tract caused by lymphomatous compression, established urate or calcium phosphate nephropathy, or a combination of these conditions.

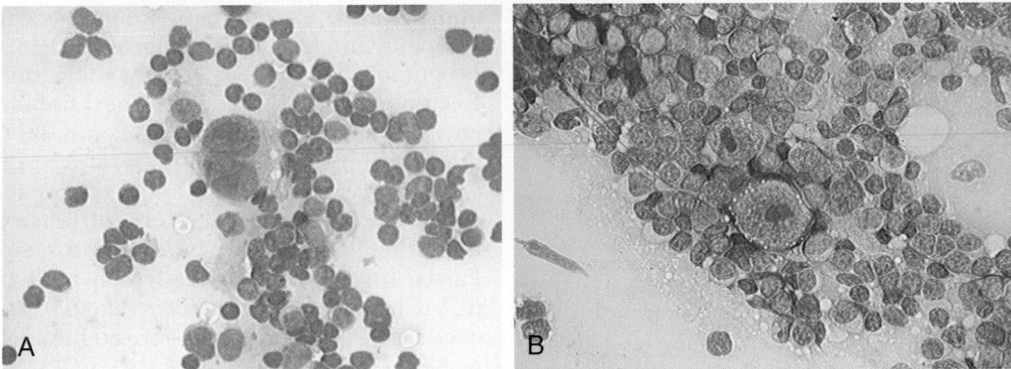

Figure 53-1 **A,** Reed-Sternberg cell. **B,** Hodgkin cell. Reed-Sternberg cells are large cells with abundant slightly basophilic cytoplasm and have at least two nuclear lobes or nuclei containing a prominent inclusion-like eosinophilic nucleolus. Mononuclear variants are known as Hodgkin cells and often have a more intense basophilic cytoplasm.

HODGKIN LYMPHOMA

Hodgkin lymphoma was first described in 1832 by Thomas Hodgkin as a disorder characterized by a peculiar enlargement of the absorbent (lymphatic) glands and spleen and was named in 1865 by Sir Samuel Wilks.[12,13] Sternberg and Reed, in 1898 and 1902, respectively, are credited with the first definitive and thorough description of the binucleate or multinucleated giant cells that when present, are considered pathognomonic of this disorder (Fig. 53-1).[14,15] The malignant nature of the disease was proven when Seif and Spriggs confirmed the clonal origin of the malignant cell by cytogenetic analysis.[16]

Before 1960 Hodgkin lymphoma was an almost uniformly fatal disease. In the 1960s investigators at Stanford and elsewhere developed the use of megavoltage radiotherapy and defined treatment fields including mantle, inverted Y, total nodal, and total lymphoid irradiation.[17] Subsequently in the late 1960s and early 1970s the first randomized trials were initiated.[18,19] Concurrently chemotherapy agents were being investigated. After the observation of the lympholytic effect of nitrogen mustard, this and other agents were used individually in the attempt to treat patients with leukemia and lymphoma. A major step forward toward the use of chemotherapy for Hodgkin lymphoma was the introduction of the four-drug combination of mechlorethamine, vincristine (Oncovin), procarbazine, and prednisone (the MOPP regimen), which led to substantial rates of cure in previously incurable patients.[20]

Over the next 20 years, standard therapy included clinical and surgical staging including laparotomy and splenectomy, as well as extended field radiation with doses of 36 to 44 Gy with or without combination chemotherapy. The probability of cure in children and adolescents using this strategy approached 90%.[21] Early on, however, late effects of therapy were noted. The first to be observed was the impact on musculoskeletal growth of young children receiving high-dose extended field radiation.[22] Subsequently, the long list of therapy-related late effects emerged to include second malignancies, serious cardiac and pulmonary compromise, infectious complications, and sterility.[23] For the last two decades the focus

of the development of care for patients with Hodgkin lymphoma has been to maximize the probability of long-term, disease-free survival but to do so while minimizing risks of late effects.

Unlike the complex evolution of classification systems for NHL, the systems used for Hodgkin lymphoma have been more straightforward. The Rye modification of the Lukes-Butler system of classification of Hodgkin disease was universally accepted for 25 years and formed the basis for the current World Health Organization (WHO) classification.[24,25] Studies of the biology and clinical course of the disease have shown that Hodgkin lymphoma should be subdivided into two entities, classic Hodgkin lymphoma (CHL) and nodular lymphocyte–predominant Hodgkin lymphoma (NLPHL) (Table 53-1). The two entities will be discussed separately in the next sections.

Classic Hodgkin Lymphoma
Pathologic Features

CHL is characterized by the presence of mononuclear Hodgkin and multinucleated Reed-Sternberg cells. Hodgkin and Reed-Sternberg cells are usually in the minority, residing in a reactive infiltrate of a variable mixture of nonneoplastic lymphocytes, eosinophils, neutrophils, plasma cells, fibroblasts, and collagen fibers present in response to cytokines produced by the tumor.[26] The Reed-Sternberg cells are large cells with abundant, slightly basophilic cytoplasm and have at least two nuclear lobes or nuclei containing a prominent inclusion-like eosinophilic nucleolus. Diagnostic Reed-Sternberg cells must have at least two nuclei in two separate lobes. Mononuclear variants are termed *Hodgkin cells* and often have a more intense basophilic cytoplasm. Microdissection techniques have enabled the isolation of Reed-Sternberg cells from frozen sections and the investigation of their lineage commitment. In more than 98% of cases, Reed-Sternberg cells are B cells, as defined by monoclonal immunoglobulin gene rearrangements.[27] Only a few cases have shown clonal T-cell receptor (TCR) gene rearrangement in the Reed-Sternberg cells, suggesting T-cell origin.[28] Reed-Sternberg cells of CHL express the B-lineage

TABLE 53-1   Pathologic and Clinical Features of Classic and Nodular Lymphocyte Predominant Hodgkin Lymphoma in Children and Adolescents

	CHL	NLPHL
Percentage of patients	92%-95%	5%-8%
Histologic hallmark	Reed-Sternberg cell	Lymphocyte-predominant cells (also called *popcorn cells*)
Immunophenotype	CD15 and CD30 common, CD20 rare	CD15 and CD30 rare, CD20 common
EBV association	Yes in 40%	Negative
Percentage male	50%	75%
Peak incidence	15-20 years	13 years
Disease at presentation	Majority with stage II or greater; mediastinal involvement common	Majority with stage IA or IIA; mediastinal involvement uncommon

Modified from Shankara A, Saw S: Nodular lymphocyte-predominant Hodgkin lymphoma in children and adolescents: a comprehensive review of biology, clinical course, and treatment options. Br J Haematol 159:288–298, 2012.
CHL, Classic Hodgkin lymphoma; *EBV,* Epstein-Barr virus; *NLPHL,* nodular lymphocyte-predominant Hodgkin lymphoma.

antigens CD20 and CD79a in variable proportions, whereas the B-cell–specific activator protein (BSAP), a product of the *PAX5* gene, is expressed in about 90% of cases.[29,30] Reed-Sternberg cells are almost invariably positive for the CD30 antigen[29] and usually express the CD15 antigen, whereas the expression of the epithelial membrane antigen (EMA) is rare. In Epstein-Barr virus (EBV)–positive cases of CHL, the Reed-Sternberg cells express the EBV latency type II pattern latent membrane (LMP) protein 1 and Epstein-Barr nuclear antigen (EBNA) 1, but without EBNA2.[31]

Based on the characteristics of the reactive infiltrate and the morphology of the Reed-Sternberg cells, four subtypes of classic Hodgkin lymphoma are distinguished in the WHO classification[25,32]: lymphocyte-rich Hodgkin lymphoma (LRHL), lymphocyte-depleted Hodgkin lymphoma (LDHL), mixed-cellularity Hodgkin lymphoma (MCHL), and nodular sclerosis Hodgkin lymphoma (NSHL). The immunophenotypic and genetic features of the Reed-Sternberg cells are identical in these histologic subtypes, whereas they differ in clinical features and association with EBV. CHL is associated with overexpression and an abnormal pattern of cytokines and chemokines and their receptors by Reed-Sternberg cells and the cells of the reactive background.[33,34] The abnormal cytokine and chemokine expression most likely accounts for the abundant admixture and pattern of inflammatory cells in CHL lesions as well as for distinct clinical features.

The NSHL subtype is characterized by a nodal growth pattern with collagen bands that surround at least one nodule, the formation of clusters of Reed-Sternberg cells, and so-called *lacunar cells* (mononuclear Hodgkin cells with only moderately prominent nucleoli).[26,35] NSHL can be grade 1 or 2, mainly depending on the number of Reed-Sternberg cells in distinct nodules.[36] The EBV-encoded LMP1 antigen is less commonly expressed than in other subtypes.

The MCHL subtype is characterized by scattered classic Reed-Sternberg cells in a diffuse or vaguely nodular mixed inflammatory background without sclerosis. Partial involvement of the lymph node can be observed in MCHL, described as *interfollicular disease.* The EBV-encoded LMP1 antigen is more commonly expressed than in NSHL.

The LRHL and LDHL subtypes are relatively rare in children.[37,38] The LRHL subtype contains scattered Reed-Sternberg cells and a nodular or diffuse background of small lymphocytes but with an absence of neutrophils and eosinophils. The LDHL subtype is a diffuse form of CHL, rich in Reed-Sternberg cells and/or depleted of non-neoplastic lymphocytes and is often sarcomatoid in appearance.

In some patients, distinction between true Hodgkin lymphoma and certain subtypes of NHL can be difficult. Grey-zone lymphomas are those that do not fit into a single disease entity. The WHO classification includes the entity of "B-cell lymphoma, unclassifiable with features intermediate between diffuse large B-cell lymphoma (DLBCL) and classic Hodgkin lymphoma," although this entity is exceptionally rare in children.[25]

Molecular and Cellular Biology

The cell of origin of the malignant cells in CHL was long a matter of controversy because of the low incidence of Reed-Sternberg cells in the tumors and their unusual immunophenotype in that they lack expression of immunoglobulins and other B-cell markers; rather, they express markers characteristic of dendritic cells, granulocytes, monocytes, and T cells.[40] However, the identification of immunoglobulin gene rearrangement[27,41,42] and somatic hypermutation in microdissected Reed-Sternberg cells in almost all cases of CHL has demonstrated that these cells derive from postgerminal B cells. In addition these studies have demonstrated that about 25% of CHL cases carry crippling immunoglobulin-gene rearrangements that destroy the function of the immunoglobulin protein.[27,41] These nonfunctional rearrangements typically induce rapid apoptosis in normal B cells, suggesting that Hodgkin lymphoma may originate from germinal-center B cells that have escaped apoptosis. Analysis of TCR rearrangements has shown that despite the common expression of T-cell markers, CHL originates from T cells in only 1% to 2% of cases.[28]

In NLPHL, the malignant popcorn cells show expression of B-cell markers such as CD20 and CD79a, suggesting a B-cell origin for these tumors as well. As in CHL, the analysis of immunoglobulin genes in microdissected tumors has shown clonal and somatically mutated gene rearrangements.[27,43] In addition, 50% of cases have shown evidence of ongoing somatic hypermutation, which strongly suggests that they derive from germinal center B cells.[27]

Mechanisms of Transformation. EBV has been associated with the pathogenesis of CHL, which shows EBV infection of the Reed-Sternberg cell in 40% of the cases in the Western world and 90% in Central America.[44-46] Importantly, EBV can immortalize human B cells in vitro, and Reed-Sternberg cells are clonally infected by EBV, which suggests that viral infection occurs early in the pathogenesis of the disease.[47] EBV positive Reed-Stenberg cells express EBNA1, LMP1, and the *LMP2a* viral gene, which is characteristic of the viral latency II stage. Mechanistically, LMP1 mimics an active CD40 receptor and can activate the nuclear factor κB (NF-κB) pathway, which is constitutively active in Hodgkin lymphoma (see later).[48] LMP2, a second viral gene product, mimics B-cell receptor signaling and might play a role in rescuing Reed-Sternberg cells from apoptosis with immunoglobulin-crippling mutations.[49] Cytogenetically, Reed-Sternberg cells often show ancuploidy and chromosomal abnormalities, with 20% of the cases harboring chromosomal translocations involving the immunoglobulin loci, a hallmark of many B-cell lymphomas.[50,51]

The most prominent molecular abnormality found in Hodgkin lymphoma is the constitutive activation of the NF-κB pathway. NF-κB functions as an important survival-signaling pathway in B cells in response to the activation of members of the tumor necrosis factor (TNF) receptor family (CD30, CD40). In Hodgkin lymphoma, somatic mutations in different elements of the NF-κB pathway keep it constitutively activated. Thus the *REL* gene, which encodes an NF-κB component, is amplified in the of 30% of the cases.[52,53] Gains of NF-κB–inducing kinase (NIK), a positive regulator of the alternative NF-κB pathway, are also commonly found in Reed-Sternberg cells,[54,55] and translocations and amplifications resulting in overexpression of the *BCL3* gene in Reed-Sternberg cells has been described.[56] Moreover, mutations of the gene-encoding NF-κB inhibitors IKBA and IKBE are found in 10% to 20% of cases of Hodgkin lymphoma.[57-59] Most significantly *TNFAIP3*, which encodes A20, a ubiquitin-modifying enzyme involved in the negative regulation of NF-κB signaling, harbors loss of function mutations and deletions in almost 45% classic Hodgkin lymphomas.[60,61] Notably, *TNFAIP3* mutations and deletions are more common in EBV-negative tumors and are rarely found in lymphocyte-predominant Hodgkin lymphomas.[61,62] Finally, activation of TNF signaling by the microenvironment and activation of NF-κB by the LMP1 EBV oncogene may also contribute to aberrant NF-κB signaling.

Gene amplifications involving the *JAK2* locus have been described in about 20% of CHL cases, suggesting a role for *JAK2* activation in the pathogenesis of this disease.[63] In addition, rearrangements of *JAK2* including a recurrent *SEC31A–JAK2* translocation have been described in rare cases of Hodgkin lymphoma.[64] Moreover, loss of function mutations in *SOCS1*, a negative regulator of Janus kinase (JAK)–signal transducer and activator of transcription (STAT) signaling are present in about 50% of classic and lymphocyte-predominant Hodgkin lymphomas and are associated with increased levels of JAK signaling.[65,66]

Translocations involving the major histocompatibility complex (MHC) class II transactivator gene *CIITA*, resulting in impaired MHC class II expression, are found in 15% of CHL cases[67] and seem to be associated with unfavorable prognosis.[68] In contrast to CHL, the malignant cells of the lymphocyte-predominant type of Hodgkin lymphomas are always EBV-negative, and there is little information on the molecular lesions implicated in the pathogenesis of this group. Chromosomal translocations involving the *BCL6* oncogene can be detected in 30% of cases.[69] *BCL6* is a zinc-finger transcription repressor that functions as a master regulator of germinal-center formation and drives B-cell transformation. Thus *Bcl6*-null mice fail to generate germinal centers in response to immunization, and deregulated expression of *Bcl6* induces B-cell lymphomas in mice.[70] Mechanistically, aberrant expression of *BCL6* in lymphoma hijacks the role of *BCL6* in the control of B-cell activation, differentiation, deoxyribonucleic acid (DNA) damage response, cell-cycle arrest, and apoptosis.[70] Finally, about 40% of lymphocyte-predominant Hodgkin lymphoma tumors show mutations in *SOCS1*,[66] but mutations in *TNAIP3* and *NFKBIA* are rare despite strong NF-κB activity.[62,71]

Cellular Microenvironment: Cytokines and Chemokines. The cellular and cytokine microenvironment surrounding the lymphoid cells in Hodgkin lymphoma plays an essential role in the pathogenesis of this disease. In particular, the expression of soluble factors and their receptors by malignant cells and the reactive microenvironment seems not only to mediate the inflammatory characteristics observed in the histology of Hodgkin lymphoma, but also to contribute to the proliferation and survival of the malignant clone. Thus the cellular microenvironment supports and is supported by a network of cytokines secreted in autocrine and paracrine loops that are essential for the proliferation of Reed-Sternberg cells and the maintenence of a favorable inflammatory environment rich in regulatory T cells (Tregs) and eosinophils.

Both interleukin (IL) 13 and the IL-13 receptor IL-13RA1 are expressed in Hodgkin lymphoma and constitute an important autocrine loop for Reed-Sternberg cells.[72,73] Other cytokines expressed in Hodgkin lymphoma and thought to influence survival of these cells include IL-4, IL-6, IL-7, IL-9, and IL-15.[33,34]

The vast majority of cells in a tumor biopsy of Hodgkin lymphoma are not malignant cells but represent an inflammatory-like cellular infiltrate composed mainly of CD4+ T lymphocytes intermixed with macrophages, eosinophils, plasma cells, and fibroblasts. Most lymphocytes present in this infiltrate are Tregs, which play an important role in protecting the tumor's Reed-Sternberg cells from cytotoxic T cells involved in antitumor immune surveillance.[49]

In contrast with the abundance of Tregs, Th1 CD4+ T cells and CD8+ cytotoxic T cells are rare in Hodgkin lymphoma biopsies and are not detected in the immediate proximity of Reed-Sternberg cells. The recruitment of cells involved in immune tolerance and the exclusion

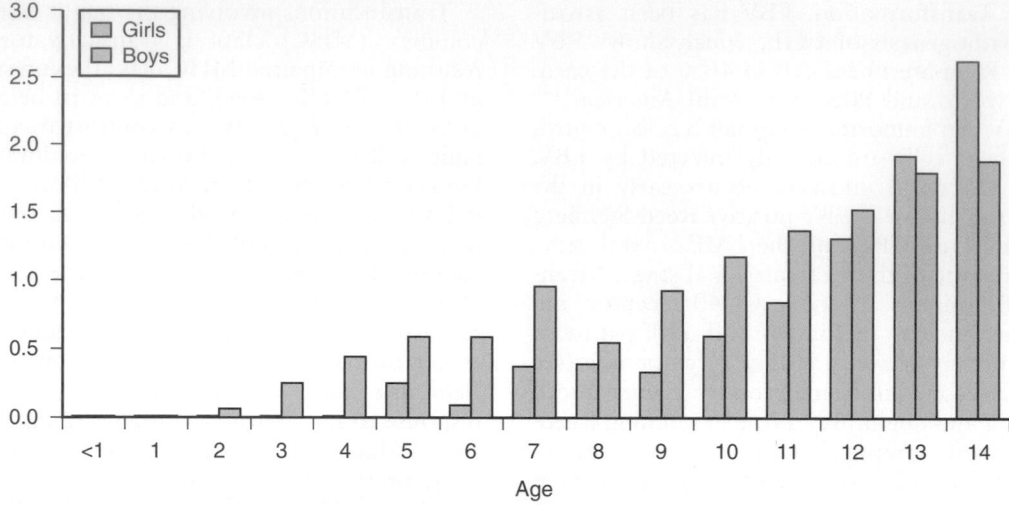

Figure 53-2 Age- and gender-specific incidence rates (per 100,000) of Hodgkin lymphoma during childhood in Germany, 2000 to 2004. *(Modified from Kaatsch P, Spix C: Annual report, 2005: German Childhood Cancer Registry, Mainz, Germany, 2007, Institut für Medizinische Biometrie, Epidemiologie, und Informatik, p 52.)*

of lymphoid cells responsible for antitumor immune responses are explained by the expression of Reed-Sternberg cells of pro-Th2–associated cytokines, such as IL-4 and IL-13, and anti-Th1 or CD8 cytokines, such as IL-10 and transforming growth factor (TGF) β.[49] The secretion of these immunosuppressive cytokines creates an immune-privileged microenvironment, allowing the tumor cells to avoid immune surveillance and T-cell–mediated apoptosis.

One of the most prominent features of Reed-Sternberg cells is the expression of CD30. Although coexpression of CD30 and its respective receptor CD153 initially suggested an autocrine mechanism promoting the proliferation of Reed-Sternberg cells via NF-κB, it is now well established that the activation of CD30 is primarily a CD153-independent process.[74] Two additional members of the TNF receptor family, CD40 and receptor activator of nuclear factor κB (RANK), are expressed in Reed-Sternberg cells. Activation of CD40 seems to be mediated by the expression of CD40 ligand (CD40L) on T lymphocytes surrounding the Reed-Sternberg cell.[75,76] Importantly, soluble CD40L induces proliferation and blocks CD95-induced apoptosis in Reed-Sternberg cells.[75-77] Other factors that help rescue Hodgkin and Reed-Sternberg cells from an immunologic attack include the expression of the PD1 ligand and secretion of IL-10, TGF-β, and galectin 1 by the Reed-Sternberg cell,[78-82] as well as inhibition of cytotoxic T cells by regulatory T cells (Tregs).[78] Activation of RANK and osteoprotegerin, a member of the TNF-receptor superfamily, is triggered by the autocrine expression of RANK ligand (RANKL) in Reed-Sternberg cells.[83] Activation of RANK promotes NF-κB activation and contributes to the maintenance of an inflammatory microenvironment by promoting interferon gamma (IFN-γ) and IL-13 secretion.[49] Overall, the activation of TNF receptors by different mechanisms seems to play an important role in promoting the survival of the Reed-Sternberg cell.

Epidemiology and Causative Factors

The epidemiology of Hodgkin lymphoma is complex, with variation across geographic regions and with age, sex, and socioeconomic status. Data from cancer incidence surveys conducted in five continents have suggested that Hodgkin lymphoma has a bimodal peak at ages 15 to 34 years and a second peak in those older than 60 years.[84] In Asian populations the overall incidence is only half that of the incidence in Europe.[85,86] In all regions, Hodgkin lymphoma occurs rarely in children younger than 5 years of age (Fig. 53-2).

Hodgkin lymphoma occurring in patients younger than 15 years of age, referred to as *childhood Hodgkin lymphoma,* has several unique features compared with the more common disease of older adolescents and young adults. In childhood disease there is a 2 to 3:1 male preponderance, whereas in older patients the disease is almost equal in males and females.[87] Within the younger age group, mixed cellularity and nodular lymphocyte-predominant histologies are more common.[88] In addition, in childhood Hodgkin lymphoma increasing family size and lower socioeconomic status are risk factors for disease. Conversely, in Hodgkin lymphoma in adolescents and young adults, higher socioeconomic status and smaller family size are risk factors for disease.[89,90]

The role of EBV as an etiologic agent for Hodgkin lymphoma has been the source of much study.[91] In 1966 MacMahon[92] was the first to suggest an infectious cause of Hodgkin lymphoma, and in 1974 Rosdahl and colleagues[93] reported an increased risk of Hodgkin lymphoma in people with a history of infectious mononucleosis.[87] Molecular studies identified monoclonal EBV genomes in Reed-Sternberg cells, implying that they were infected before malignant transformation.[94,95] Subsequent studies showed EBV genome sequences associated with Reed-Sternberg cells in 59% of cases.[96] The proportion of EBV-positive Hodgkin lymphoma cases varies, however, according to geographic region, age, and histologic subtype. The proportion of EBV-positive Hodgkin lymphoma cases is higher in children than adults. It is most prevalent in mixed cellularity histology and more common in boys. The incidence is higher in the developing world including parts of Africa, Asia, and South America, with an incidence of EBV-positive Hodgkin lymphoma as high as 90% in Peru.[97]

Familial aggregation of Hodgkin lymphoma was first described by Razis and coworkers in 1959[98] and is now well documented.[99-102] The familial risk of Hodgkin lymphoma ranks among the highest in the population-based Swedish Family Cancer Database.[103] In an analysis of 28 reports of familial Hodgkin lymphoma there is only one major peak between 15 and 34 years of age for familial Hodgkin lymphoma instead of the classic bimodal age distribution of sporadic Hodgkin lymphoma.[104] This corresponds to the findings of two large studies of an increased sevenfold risk in siblings of cases diagnosed at ages younger than 45 and 35 years of age, respectively, but little or no increased risk in siblings of cases diagnosed at older ages.[105,106] Strong evidence for a role for genetic susceptibility was provided by the finding that monozygotic twins of patients with Hodgkin lymphoma have a 99-fold increased risk, whereas no increased risk in dizygotic twins was observed.[99]

Familial aggregation of Hodgkin lymphoma may in part reflect inherited abnormalities of the immune response. A familial or personal history of autoimmune conditions and sarcoidosis is associated with an increased risk for Hodgkin lymphoma.[107,108] A 51-fold increased risk for Hodgkin lymphoma was found in kindreds predisposed to autoimmune lymphoproliferative syndrome, a disorder of lymphocyte homeostasis usually associated with germline *FAS* gene mutations.[109] In patients with ataxia-telangiectasia mutation (ATM), the risk of Hodgkin lymphoma was increased, but its risk was much lower than the risk of NHL.[110] In 1975 Svejgaard and coworkers first described an association of certain human leukocyte antigen (HLA) loci with an increased risk of Hodgkin lymphoma, suggesting a disease susceptibility gene within or near the histocompatibility region on chromosome 6.[111,112] Since then, numerous studies have confirmed the association of particular HLA loci in the susceptibility to Hodgkin lymphoma, including HLAs A1, B5, B8, B15, B27, B35, and B37.[113] In a large study on familial Hodgkin lymphoma, Chakravarti and colleagues[114] have found strong evidence for a recessive mode of inheritance for susceptibility to Hodgkin lymphoma, and approximately 60% of associations were caused by an HLA-linked susceptibility gene. Recent genetic studies have identified disruption of *KLHDC8B* in the germline of a family with several cases of Hodgkin lymphoma[115] and a germline frameshift mutation in the *NPAT* gene in a family with four cases of NLPHL.[116] Finally a genome-wide association study has identified risk loci at 2p16.1 (*REL*), 8q24.21 (*PVT1*), and 10p14 (*GATA3*) and confirmed the strong HLA association with this disease.[117]

Clinical Characteristics

The most common clinical presentation of Hodgkin lymphoma in children and adolescents is a persistently enlarged node in the cervical or supraclavicular region. Characteristically the lymph nodes involved with Hodgkin lymphoma are not painful and have a "rubbery" firmness on palpation. Enlarged nodes have often been present for weeks or months, increasing and decreasing in size irrespective of whether antibiotic therapy has been given. Although the majority of patients have painless cervical adenopathy, the clinical presentation varies considerably, ranging from life-threatening airway compression to the coincidental detection of an enlarged node during an otherwise routine examination. Approximately 80% of children have disease in one or both sides of the upper or lower neck. Of those with cervical adenopathy, more than two thirds have intrathoracic disease, most commonly in the anterosuperior mediastinum, paratracheal, and tracheobronchial lymph node groups. Pulmonary parenchymal involvement is rarely observed in the absence of hilar disease. Pleural effusions are uncommon; they are usually an indication of lymphatic obstruction from bulky central disease rather than a sign of advanced-stage disease. Pericardial effusion may occur in cases with pericardial involvement and occurs most often in the setting of bulky mediastinal disease.[118] Hodgkin lymphoma has a strong tendency for contiguous spread along adjacent lymph-node regions. Although about 30% of patients have supradiaphragmatic and infradiaphragmatic disease, Hodgkin lymphoma limited to infradiaphragmatic sites is rare.[38]

Systemic symptoms including fatigue and anorexia are common in patients with Hodgkin lymphoma. At the time of diagnosis, approximately 30% of patients have constitutional signs referred to as *B symptoms* and defined as the presence of fever (temperature higher than 38°C [100.4°F]) for 3 consecutive days, drenching night sweats and unexplained body weight loss of 10% or more over the preceding 6 months. Classically the fever associated with Hodgkin lymphoma, called the *Pel-Epstein fever*, occurs in the evening and becomes more pronounced with time. Severe and unexplained pruritus is associated with Hodgkin lymphoma, sometimes preceding the development of adenopathy. A poorly understood and relatively unusual sign of Hodgkin lymphoma is pain at the sites of disease with alcohol ingestion.

Laboratory findings are often nonspecific with mild anemia and elevated erythrocyte sedimentation rate (ESR) being the most common findings. Nonspecific hematologic laboratory findings include neutrophilia, monocytosis, lymphopenia, and eosinophilia. Acute-phase reactants including C-reactive protein, ferritin, and serum copper may be elevated. High levels of alkaline phosphatase can be associated with bone involvement.

Rarely patients with Hodgkin have findings suggestive of paraneoplastic syndromes such as nephritic syndrome, polymyositis, idiopathic cholestasis and autoimmune hemolytic anemia, neutropenia, and thrombocytopenia, or combinations of these. Limbic encephalitis or subacute cerebellar degeneration have also been reported as very rare paraneoplastic syndromes in patients with Hodgkin lymphoma.[119]

At the time of diagnosis patients may exhibit altered immune function characterized by reduced cellular immunity, whereas humoral immunity is usually relatively intact.[120] The nature of the immune defect is unclear. The severity of the impairment increases with advanced stage, disease progression, and recurrence and after treatment with radiotherapy and chemotherapy. T-cell deficits may persist for a prolonged period in successfully treated patients.

Diagnosis and Staging

Biopsy to provide pathologic tissue for examination is required for the diagnosis of Hodgkin lymphoma. Excisional biopsy of an enlarged node is preferred. Samples from needle biopsies are often insufficient for the diagnosis of Hodgkin lymphoma because of the importance of the information provided by the nodal architecture and background stroma, as well as the need to identify the relatively rare Reed-Sternberg cell. In a case series, one third of children who ultimately were diagnosed with Hodgkin lymphoma and who underwent core needle biopsies of their mediastinal masses were not able to be diagnosed from these initial samples.[121] Needle biopsy should be restricted to situations in which surgery and general anesthesia may carry undue risks for the patient. If needle biopsy is performed, multiple biopsy samples should be taken to augment diagnostic potential.

The purpose of a staging evaluation is to identify all sites and characteristics of Hodgkin lymphoma in each patient to permit accurate stratification of therapy based on risk, the definition of areas to be included in potential radiation fields, and to inform follow-up imaging studies. Table 53-2 gives an overview of suggested evaluations.

A plain film of the chest is useful in providing preliminary information about mediastinal involvement and is an essential evaluation in a patient who will undergo anesthesia for cervical node biopsy (Fig. 53-3). Computed tomography (CT) of the neck, chest, abdomen, and pelvis are standard initial staging evaluations.[122] In the past, imaging of the neck was considered not necessary given the ability to detect cervical node by physical examination. Imaging of the neck, however, can be of significant importance to current care, because it allows for the most accurate radiation field planning, avoiding potential overtreatment of the neck, and providing baseline data for the measurement of disease response.[23] CT of the chest provides detailed information about sites of disease involvement including the mediastinum, pulmonary parenchyma, pleura, and pericardium. Sites of disease in the abdomen and pelvis are visualized with CT done with oral and intravenous (IV) contrast. Alternatively, magnetic resonance imaging (MRI) or ultrasound can also be used for staging abdominal and pelvis disease.

Functional nuclear imaging is an important component to initial staging though perhaps has an even more significant role in assessment of disease response (see later). Gallium-67 imaging has largely been replaced by 18-fluorodeoxyglucose positron emission tomography (FDG-PET) because of increased sensitivity and specificity.[123,124] Increased 18F-FDG uptake in lymphoma is based on elevated glycolysis and the longer residence time of 18F-FDG in malignant cells compared with most normal

TABLE 53-2	Recommended Investigations in Children and Adolescents with Hodgkin Lymphoma
Laboratory studies	1. Complete blood count (CBC) 2. Erythrocyte sedimentation rate (ESR) 3. Renal and liver function studies 4. Albumin 5. Lactate dehydrogenase (LDH) 6. Alkaline phosphatase
Imaging	1. Chest x-ray 2. Computed tomography (CT) of neck and chest 3. CT or ultrasound or magnetic resonance imaging (MRI) of the abdomen and pelvis 4. Positron emission tomography (PET) (if available) 5. Bone scan (if no PET available and focal bony pain or advanced stage disease)
Other investigations	1. Bone marrow biopsy, except stage 1A and 2A, and possibly those without evidence of bone-marrow involvement by PET (see below) 2. Selective biopsy for sites of potential involvement that are ambiguous and whose clarification is important for staging and treatment planning
Other pretherapy considerations	1. Assessment of pulmonary function 2. Assessment of cardiac function 3. Assessment of thyroid function 4. Consideration of fertility preservation (sperm banking) 5. Consideration for need of stable intravenous access

tissues.[125] Numerous studies in adults with Hodgkin lymphoma have demonstrated that PET is able to detect an additional number of Hodgkin lymphoma lesions compared with conventional imaging studies, in particular CT and bone marrow biopsy, resulting in a modification of staging in 15% to 20% of patients, with an impact on disease management in 5% to 15% of cases.[126] The data in children are more limited.[127,128] A review of a single-center experience showed that the findings from the diagnostic FDG-PET were more sensitive than conventional imaging and that the findings altered the involved-field radiation treatment fields in 17% of patients.[129] Prospective studies are required to assess whether FDG-PET done at the time of diagnosis has on impact on outcome or on treatment burden.

Historically, surgical staging including splenectomy was considered standard for patients with Hodgkin lymphoma. Staging splenectomy is associated with significant risks. In the German-Austrian experience of 1181 children with Hodgkin lymphoma, the survival was poorer for children younger than age 10 years because of episodes of infection and death caused by sepsis in splenectomized children.[130,131] With the availability of cross-sectional imaging techniques, routine staging laparotomy has now been abandoned. In the relatively rare circumstance of imaging findings that are ambiguous in defining

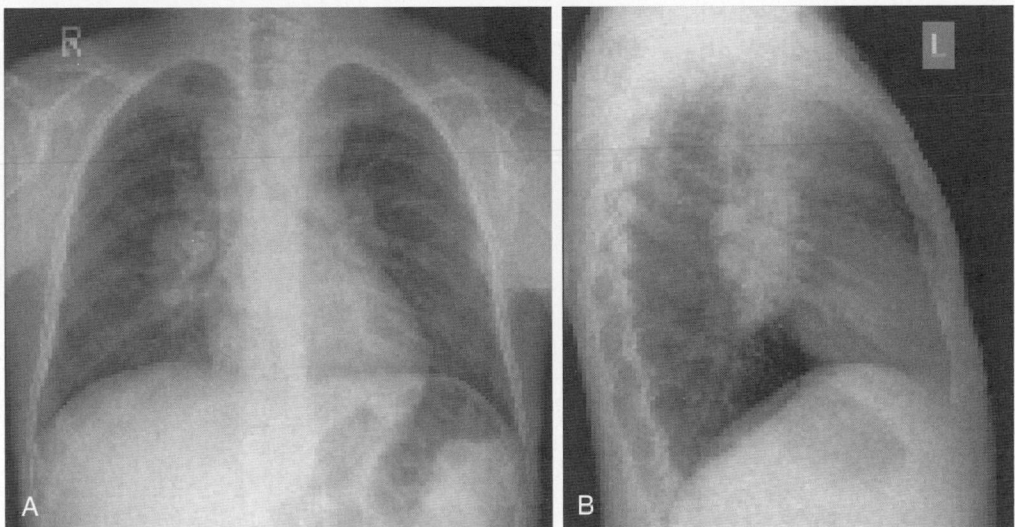

Figure 53-3 Chest x-ray of a patient with Hodgkin lymphoma and involvement of the mediastinal nodes and hilum.

disease involvement or noninvolvement, and when this information affects therapeutic decision making and in particular radiation fields, then staging biopsy may still be warranted.

Until recently bone marrow biopsy has been considered a standard component of the initial staging evaluation for any child with cytopenias at presentation and all patients except for those with stage 1A or 2A disease. Retrospective investigations have suggested that the impact of the findings from diagnostic bone marrow biopsies had a minimal effect on patient-risk assignment and subsequent therapy.[132] FDG-PET is a sensitive and specific method for detection of bone marrow disease. Two recent studies provide data to support the idea that FDG-PET can replace bone marrow biopsies for staging purposes[133,134] in an analogous fashion to cross-sectional imaging of the abdomen replacing staging laparotomy in the past.

The Ann Arbor staging classification for Hodgkin lymphoma, adopted in 1971, was based on the recognized orderly spread of the disease between contiguous lymph nodes, which predominates until late in the course of the disease (Table 53-3).[135] The distinct lymph node regions recognized by the Ann Arbor classification system are shown in Figure 53-4. The substage classifications A, B, and E amend each stage based on distinct features. Stage A designates asymptomatic disease; B indicates the presence of any one of the three B symptoms as defined in Table 53-3; and extralymphatic disease is designated as E, referring to limited extranodal extensions that easily can be encompassed within a radiotherapy portal. Extralymphatic disease is further designated as L (lung), P (pleura), and O (osseous) according to this system. The decision to classify extralymphatic disease either as substage E or as stage IV is based on the clinician's judgment and often depends on whether the extralymphatic disease can be adequately covered in a radiotherapy treatment portal. Multiple E lesions are automatically considered to be stage IV.

Treatment

Centers treating children with Hodgkin lymphoma should have extensive experience and a dedicated multidisciplinary team, including a pediatric surgeon, radiation oncologist, pediatric oncologist, pathologist, and diagnostic radiologist. If such a team is not available at the

TABLE 53-3   Ann Arbor Staging Classification for Hodgkin Lymphoma

Stage	Description
I	Involvement of a single lymph-node region (I) or a single extralymphatic organ or site (I_E)
II	Involvement of two or more lymph node regions on the same side of the diaphragm (II) or localized contiguous involvement of only one extralymphatic organ or site and its regional lymph node(s) on the same side of the diaphragm (II_E)
III	Involvement of lymph-node regions on both sides of the diaphragm (III), which may also be accompanied by involvement of the spleen (III_S) or by localized contiguous involvement of an extralymphatic organ or site (III_E) or both (III_{SE})
IV	Diffuse or disseminated involvement of one or more extralymphatic organs or tissues, with or without associated lymph-node involvement
Designations Applicable to Any Stage	
A	No B symptoms
B	B symptoms, defined as presence of fever (>38°C [100.4°F]) for 3 consecutive days, drenching night sweats, or unexplained loss of 10% or more of body weight in the preceding 6 months
E	Involvement of a single extranodal site that is contiguous or proximal to the known nodal site

Modified from Carbone PP, Kaplan HS, Musshoff K et al: Report of the Committee on Hodgkin's Disease Staging Classification. Cancer Res 31:1860–1861, 1971.

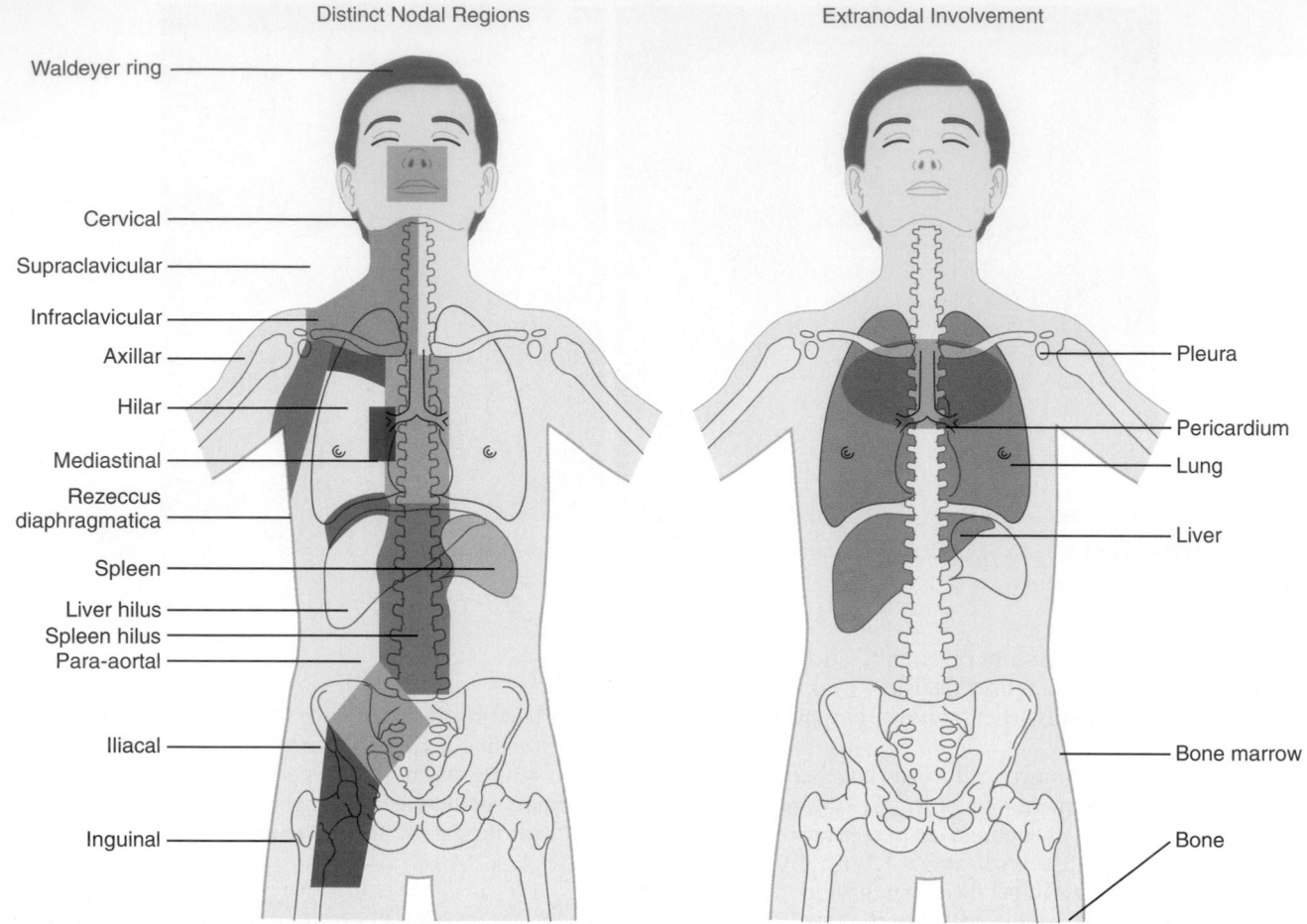

Figure 53-4 Distinct nodal regions according to the Ann Arbor staging classification for Hodgkin lymphoma. *(Modified from Dörffel W, Schellong G: Morbus Hodgkins. In Gadner H, Gaedicke G, Niemeyer C, Ritter J, editors:* Paediatrische Haematologie und Onkologie, *Heidelberg, Germany, 2006, Springer, p. 770–776.)*

facility at which the child is initially seen, prompt referral to a comprehensive childhood cancer center is essential.

Prognostic Factors/Stratification of Treatment. As with other malignancies, prognostic factors are useful as tools for defining risk groups for stratification of treatment intensity. For patients with Hodgkin lymphoma this translates into both the choice of chemotherapeutic regimen and the use of radiotherapy. The stage of disease is a strong prognostic factor and widely used for risk stratification that has been used in all major cooperative groups.[37,130,136] Apart from the stage of disease, a number of factors have been reported to be associated with the risk of treatment failure, including the presence of B symptoms, histologic subtype, bulky disease, gender, anemia, ESR, and evidence of latent EBV infection, some of which have lost significance with improvements in therapy.[137,138] The prognostic value of these variables has not been consistent across studies, in part related to treatment prescribed. For example, mediastinal bulky disease—defined as a mass larger than one third of the maximum chest diameter—was associated with increased risk for relapse in some studies but not in the German-

Austrian trial DAL-HD90. However, in this protocol patients with a larger residual mass at the end of chemotherapy received a boost dose in addition to the involved field irradiation.[130,139] Similarly, male gender had an adverse impact on outcome in that trial. For boys, however, procarbazine was partially replaced by etoposide, and girls received a full dose of procarbazine. Race and ethnicity have been identified as risk factors in some pediatric cancers. In a single-center retrospective review, African-American children had an inferior event-free survival (EFS) rate but an identical overall survival (OS) as compared with white children.[140]

The risk-group definitions used in selected clinical trials are described in Table 53-4. In general in addition to stage, disease bulk and presence of B symptoms are the factors used. The kinetics of disease response to chemotherapy, measured by CT and/or PET scan is used in many cooperative group trials as an important additional tool for the stratification of treatment intensity including the use of radiation (see below).

Treatment and Outcome. In the 1960s extended-field radiation with doses of 35 to 44 Gy were shown to be curative in a significant portion of patients with Hodgkin

TABLE 53-4   Risk Group Definitions in Clinical Trials of Pediatric Hodgkin Lymphoma

Study Group	Stage		
	Low Risk	Intermediate Risk	High Risk
DAL-HD90[130]	IA, IB, IE, IIA	IIEA, IIB, IIIA	IIEB, IIIEA, IIIB, IIIEB, IV
GPOH-HD2002[148]	IA, IB, IIA	IE, IIEA, IIB, IIIA	IIEB, IIIEA, IIIB, IV
CCG 5942[161]	I + IIA, without*	I + II with* IIB, III	IV
Stanford, St. Jude, Boston Consortium[159]	I, II, without†	"Unfavorable" I, II with† III, IV	
POG[160]	I, IIA, IIIA1	"Unfavorable" IIB, IIIA₂, IIIB, IV	
COG[157,158]	IA, IIA without‡	IA+IIA with bulk, IB+IIB, IIIA, IVA	IIIB + IVB

CCG, Children's Cancer Study Group; COG, Children's Oncology Group; DAL-HD, Deutsche Arbeitsgemeinschaft fir Leukamiefarschung-Hodgkin disease; GPOH-HD, German Society for Pediatric Oncology and Hematology-Hodgkin disease; POG, Pediatric Oncology Group.
*Adverse disease features (one or more of the following): hilar adenopathy, more than four nodal regions, mediastinal tumor >33% of chest diameter, node or nodal aggregate with diameter >10 cm.
†Presence of one or more of the following: bulky disease, peripheral nodal disease 6 cm or larger, and/or mediastinal tumor one third of intrathoracic diameter or more, and B symptoms.
‡No bulk or extranodal extension.

lymphoma.[141,142] In children, the negative sequelae of high-dose extended-field radiation quickly became apparent.[143] Soon thereafter the MOPP combination was created by Devita and coworkers[20] to treat patients with Hodgkin lymphoma. The basic rationale was to combine single drugs with proven efficacy but different mechanisms of action and resistance that had few overlapping toxicities to maximize antitumor effect and limit side effects caused by use of moderate doses of the individual drugs. The second important combination chemotherapy regimen for the treatment of Hodgkin lymphoma was doxorubicin (Adriamycin), bleomycin, vinblastine, and dacarbazine (ABVD), which was developed by Bandanna and coworkers.[144] Variations of these two regimens have formed the cornerstone of almost all subsequent chemotherapy regimens.

Combined-modality therapy using both chemotherapy and radiation has emerged as the standard of care for most children and adolescents diagnosed with Hodgkin lymphoma. The use of six cycles of MOPP chemotherapy combined with involved-field radiotherapy (IFRT) was pioneered by the Stanford investigators in children with pathologically staged disease.[145] This pivotal trial has served as the model for combined-modality treatment programs in children.

Subsequent studies evaluated regimens with modifications incorporated designed to minimize risks of late effects while maintaining efficacy. Changes have included both the substitution of drugs the use of which is associated with lower risks of specific long term toxicities as well as limiting the cumulative dose of drugs that are associated with risks of late sequelae in a dose dependent manner. Some modifications have been gender specific. Table 53-5 gives an overview of chemotherapy combinations. With most of these multiagent combinations, comparable high disease-free survival rates have been achieved.[37,38,130,145,146,147]

The balance of efficacy and late risk of the combined-modality of chemotherapy and radiotherapy adopted by the German-Austrian study group has been investigated over a series of trials (Table 53-6). Modifications investigated have included reduction of the cumulative dose of alkylating agents and replacement of mechlorethamine of MOPP with doxorubicin (vincristine [Oncovin], prednisone, procarbazine, and doxorubicin [OPPA]) and cyclophosphamide (cyclophosphamide, vincristine [Oncovin], procarbazine, and prednisone [COPP]); reduction of radiotherapy (volume, dose, and number of patients who receive radiotherapy); and replacement of procarbazine by etoposide for boys. The seventh of the sequential studies built on findings of the previous six trials.[148] In this study the primary aim was to evaluate modifications of therapy to maintain good outcomes for boys but to do so with less gonadotoxic therapy. In this study procarbazine was replaced with higher dose etoposide in the first two cycles and with dacarbazine in the subsequent two to four cycles. The outcomes for boys and girls on this study were superimposable, supporting the efficacy of this regimen.

The second strategy that is of critical importance in trying to maximize efficacy and minimize toxicity is the stratification of treatment intensity based on the patient's risk for relapse. Cooperative group trials of pediatric and adolescent Hodgkin lymphoma have generally divided patients into low-, intermediate-, and high-risk groups (see Table 53-4). In addition to stratification by stage, studies have also evaluated modifications of therapy based on early disease response. Many reports from these therapeutic studies are confined to a distinct risk group of patients. Comparisons among trials confined to patient subsets need to be done with caution, because the risk group definitions vary both based on the patient characteristics at the time of initial staging and the criteria of disease response.

TABLE 53-5   Combination Chemotherapy Courses for Treatment of Hodgkin Lymphoma

Course	Drugs	Dosage and Route	Days
MOPP[21]	Mechlorethamine	6.0 mg/m², IV	1, 8
	Vincristine (Oncovin)	1.4 mg/m², IV	1, 8
	Procarbazine	100 mg/m², PO	1-15
	Prednisone	40 mg/m², PO	1-15
MOPP Derivatives			
COPP[607]	Cyclophosphamide	600 (500) mg/m², IV	1, 8
	Vincristine (Oncovin)	1.4 mg/m², IV (max 2 mg)	1, 8
	Procarbazine	100 mg/m², PO	1-15
	Prednisone	40 mg/m², PO	1-15
COMP[608]	Cyclophosphamide	600 mg/m², IV	1, 8
	Vincristine (Oncovin)	1.4 mg/m², IV (max 2 mg)	1, 8
	Methotrexate	40 mg/m², IV	1, 8
	Prednisone	40 mg/m², PO	1-15
COP[609]	Cyclophosphamide	600 mg/m², IV	1, 8
	Vincristine (Oncovin)	1.4 mg/m², IV (max 2 mg)	1, 8
	Procarbazine	100 mg/m², PO	1-14
ABVD[144]	Doxorubicin (Adriamycin)	25 mg/m², IV	1, 15
	Bleomycin	10 U/m², IV	1, 15
	Vinblastine	6 mg/m², IV	1, 15
	Dacarbazine	375 mg/m², IV	1, 15
MOPP-ABVD Hybrids and Derivatives			
OPPA[148]	Vincristine (Oncovin)	1.5 mg/m², IV (max 2 mg)	1, 8, 15
	Procarbazine	100 mg/m², PO	1-15
	Prednisone	60 mg/m², PO	1-15
	Doxorubicin (Adriamycin)	40 mg/m², IV	1, 15
OPA[608]	Vincristine (Oncovin)	1.5 mg/m², IV (max 2 mg)	1, 8, 15
	Prednisone	60 mg/m², PO	1-15
	Doxorubicin (Adriamycin)	40 mg/m², IV	1, 15
OEPA[130]	Vincristine (Oncovin)	1.5 mg/m², IV (max 2 mg)	1, 8, 15
	Etoposide	125 mg/m², IV	3-6
	Prednisone	60 mg/m², PO	1-15
	Doxorubicin (Adriamycin)	40 mg/m², IV	1, 15
ChlVPP[610]	Chlorambucil	6 mg/m², PO	1-14
	Vinblastine	6 mg/m², PO	1, 8
	Procarbazine	100 mg/m², PO	1-14
	Prednisone	40 mg/m², PO	1-14
VAMP[145,159]	Vinblastine	6 mg/m², IV	1, 15
	Doxorubicin (Adriamycin)	25 mg/m², IV	1, 15
	Methotrexate	20 mg/m², IV	1, 15
	Prednisone	40 mg/m², PO	1-14
VBVP[147]	Vinblastine	6 mg/m², IV	1, 8
	Bleomycin	10 mg/m², IV	1
	Etoposide (VP-16)	100 mg/m², IV	1-5
	Prednisolone	40 mg/m², PO	1-8
COPP-ABV[161]	Cyclophosphamide	600 mg/m², IV	0
	Vincristine (Oncovin)	1.4 mg/m², IV	0
	Procarbazine	100 mg/m², PO	0-6
	Prednisolone	40 mg/m², PO	0-13
	Doxorubicin (Adriamycin)	35 mg/m², IV	7
	Bleomycin	10 U/m², IV	7
	Vinblastine	6 mg/m², IV	7

TABLE 53-5   Combination Chemotherapy Courses for Treatment of Hodgkin Lymphoma (Continued)

Course	Drugs	Dosage and Route	Days
ABC[161]	A		
	Cytarabine	3 g/m², IV over 3 hr, q12h	0, 1
	Etoposide	200 mg/m², IV over 1 hr, q12h	0, 1
	G-CSF	5 µg/kg, SC	Starting on day 2
	B		
	COPP-ABVD	See COPP/ABVD	21-27
	G-CSF	5 µg/kg, SC	Starting on day 28
	C		
	Vincristine	1.4 mg/m², IV	42
	Cyclophosphamide	1200 mg/m², IV	42-43
	Doxorubicin	25 mg/m²/day, continuous infusion	42-44
	Methylprednisolone	250 mg/m², IV q6h	42
	Prednisone	60 mg/m², PO	43-46
	G-CSF	5 µg/kg, SC	Starting on day 46
BEACOPP[157]	Bleomycin	10 U/m², IV	8
	Etoposide	200 mg/m², IV	1-3
	Doxorubicin (Adriamycin)	35 mg/m², IV	1
	Cyclophosphamide	1200 mg/m², IV	1
	Vincristine (Oncovin)	2 mg/m² (max 2 mg), IV	8
	Procarbazine	100 mg/m², PO	1-7
	Prednisone	40 mg/m², PO	1-14
DBVE[611]	Doxorubicin	25 mg/m², IV	1, 15
	Bleomycin	10 mg/m², SC	1, 15
	Vincristine	1.5 mg/m² (max,] 2 mg), IV	1, 15
	Etoposide	100 mg/m², IV over 1 hr	1-5
Stanford V[612]	Mechlorethamine	6 mg/m², IV	1
	Vinblastine	6 mg/m², IV	1, 15
	Doxorubicin	25 mg/m², IV	1, 15
	Etoposide	60 mg/m², IV	15, 16
	Vincristine	1.4 mg/m² (max 2 mg), IV	8, 22
	Bleomycin	5 U/m², IV	8, 22
	Prednisone	40 mg/m², PO	Every other day
ABVD-PC[158]	Doxorubicin (Adriamycin)	25 mg/m² IV	1, 2
	Bleomycin	10 IU/m²* IV	1, 8
	Vincristine	1.4 mg/m² IV (max 2.8)	1, 8
	Etoposide	125 mg/m² IV	1-5
	Prednisone	40 mg/m², PO	1-7
	Cyclophosphamide	800 mg/m² IV	1
	G-CSF	5 µg/kg SC	Starting day 6

G-CSF, Granulocyte colony-stimulating factor; *IV*, intravenous; *PO*, per os; *SC*, subcutaneous
*Modified to 5 IU/m² on day 0 mid-study.

Table 53-7 summarizes treatment strategy and results of therapeutic studies in the patient subgroup defined as low risk. Patients at low risk in general are those with stage I and II disease without B symptoms and without bulky disease. These patients have been shown to have excellent outcomes with sequential trials using two to four cycles of multiagent chemotherapy and low-dose involved-field radiation.[38,145,147] These regimens have been designed to minimize exposure to anthracyclines, alkylators, and epipodophyllotoxins in order to minimize risks of cardiac dysfunction, infertility, and secondary acute myelogenous leukemia (AML), respectively.

Table 53-8 summarizes the treatment strategy and results of selected therapeutic studies in patients considered to have intermediate- or high-risk disease. Chemotherapy for these groups generally consists of combinations of ABVD and MOPP or hybrid regimens. Most regimens contain four to six cycles of chemotherapy followed by involved-field radiation with some including high-dose radiation to bulky or residual sites of disease.

Prognostic information for patients with Hodgkin lymphoma is based on information available at the time of the child's initial evaluation. Additionally the importance of the kinetics of disease response to chemotherapy has been shown to be a predictive factor for this disease, as it has been for pediatric leukemias.[149] The premise is that those with more robust responses to initial chemotherapy have more favorable disease and that responsiveness can be included in the factors that are used to decide the intensity of therapy, including whether irradiation is indicated. The definition of a favorable response to chemotherapy, including the timing of assessment of response, the intensity of the chemotherapy regimen used to get the response, and the tools used to measure response have

TABLE 53-6　Development of Treatment Strategy and Outcome for Children and Adolescents with Hodgkin Lymphoma in Seven Sequential Trials of the German-Austrian Multicenter Study Group

Study	No. of Patients (EFS)	Therapy Group 1			Therapy Group 2			Therapy Group 3		
		Stages (% of patients) EFS	Chemotherapy	Radiotherapy	Stages (% of patients) EFS	Chemotherapy	Radiotherapy	Stages (% of patients) 5-yr EFS	Chemotherapy	Radiotherapy
DAL-HD78[607]	170 (92%)	I, IIA (43%) 95%	OPPA ×2	EF, 36-40 Gy	>IIA (57%) 89%	OPPA ×2 COPP ×4	EF, 36-40 Gy	Included in TG2		
DAL-HD82[613]	203 (96%)	I, IIA (49%) 99%	OPPA ×2	IF, 35 Gy	IIB, IIIA (26%) 96%	OPPA ×2 COPP ×2	IF, 30 Gy*	IIIB, IV (25%) 87%	OPPA ×2 COPP ×4	25 Gy*
DAL-HD85[613]	103 (77%)	I, IIA (58%) 59%	OPA ×2	IF, 35 Gy	IIB, IIIA (20%) 62%	OPA ×2 COMP ×2	IF, 30 Gy*	IIIB, IV (22%) 62%	OPA ×2 COMP ×4	25 Gy*
DAL-HD87[614]	204 (85%)	I, IIA (51%) 84%	OPA ×2	IF, 30 Gy*	IE, IIEA IIB, IIIA (17%) 82%	OPPA ×2 COPP ×2	25 Gy*	IIIB, IV (28%) 89%	OPPA ×2 COPP ×4	25 Gy*
DAL-HD90[130]	578 (91%)	I, IIA (46%) 94%	OPPA ×2[†] OEPA ×2[‡]	IF, 25 Gy*	IE, IIEA IIB, IIIA (21%) 93%	OPPA ×2[†] COPP ×2 OEPA ×2[‡] COPP ×2	25 Gy*	IIEB, IIIEA IIIB, IV (31%) 86%	OPPA ×2[†] COPP ×4 OEPA ×2[‡] COPP ×4	20 Gy*
GPOH-HD95[38]	1018 (88%)	I, IIA (40%) 94%	OPPA ×2[†] OEPA ×2[‡]	CR: no RT (28%)[§]; non-CR: IF, 20 Gy*	IE, IIEA IIB, IIIA (26%), 87%	OPPA ×2[†] COPP ×2 OEPA ×2[‡] COPP ×2	CR: no RT (19%)[§]; non-CR: IF 20 Gy*	IIEB, IIIEA; IIIB, IV (33%) 83%	OPPA ×2[†] COPP ×4 OEPA ×2[‡] COPP ×4	CR: no RT (17%)[§]; non-CR: IF, 20 Gy*
GPOH-HD02[148]	573 (89%)	1A/B, IIA (34%) 92%	OPPA ×2[†] OE*PA ×2[‡]	CR: no RT (33%)[§]; non-CR: IF, 20 Gy*	IE, IIEA, IIB, IIIA (24%) 93%	OPPA ×2[†] COPP ×2 OEPA ×2[‡] COPDAC ×2	20 Gy*	IIEB, IIIEA; IIIB, IV (42%) 87%	OPPA, ×2[†] COPP ×4 OEPA ×2[‡] COPDAC ×4	20 Gy*

COMP, Cyclophosphamide, vincristine (Oncovin), methotrexate, and prednisone; COPDAC, cyclophosphamide, vincristine (Oncovin), prednisone, and dacarbazine; COPP, cyclophosphamide, vincristine (Oncovin), procarbazine, and prednisone; CR, complete remission; DAL-HD, Deutsche Arbeitsgemeinschaft für Leukämieforschung-Hodgkin disease; EF, extended field; EFS, event-free survival; GPOH-HD, German Society for Pediatric Oncology and Hematology-Hodgkin disease; IF, involved field; OEPA, vincristine (Oncovin), etoposide, prednisone, and doxorubicin (Adriamycin); OE*PA, vincristine (oncovin) etoposide, prednisone and doxorubicin (adriamycin); OPA, vincristine (Oncovin), prednisone, doxorubicin (Adriamycin); OPPA, vincristine (Oncovin), prednisone, procarbazine, and doxorubicin (Adriamycin); RT, radiotherapy; TG2, therapy group 2.

*Boost to residual tumor to 30-35 Gy.
†Female.
‡Male.
§Percentage of patients in the treatment subgroup who did not receive radiotherapy.

TABLE 53-7 Combined-Modality Treatment Strategy and Results for Low-Risk Patients with Hodgkin Lymphoma in Selected Multicenter Trials

Group or Institution	No. of Patients	Stage	Chemotherapy*	Radiation (Gy), Field	EFS or RFS Overall (%)	Survival (%)
GPOH-HD95[38]	281	I, IIA	Female: OPPA ×2 Male: OEPA ×2	CR[†]: no RT (22%); non-CR: IF, 20 Gy; residual tumor, 30-35 Gy	94	NR
GPOH-HD02[148]	195	IA/B, IIA	Female: OPPA ×2 Male: OE*PA[‡] ×2	CR[†]: no RT (33%); no-CR: IF, 20 Gy; residual tumor, 30-35 Gy	92	99
French Society of Pediatric Oncology[147]	202	I, II I, II	4 VBVP, good responders; 4 VBVP + 1 or 2 OPPA, poor responders	20, IF 20, IF	91 and 78[§]	97.5
Stanford-St. Jude-Boston Consortium[159]	88	1, II[‖]	4 VAMP	CR post 2 cycles, no IF No CR: 25.5 Gy	90 (2 yr)	99
CCG5942[161]	294	I + IIA without[¶]	COPP-ABV × 4	CR,** random: IF 21 Gy vs. no RT; PR, 21 Gy IF	95 (3 yr)	100
POG9226[611]	51	I, IIA, IIIA1	4 DBVE	25, IF	91(6 yr)	98

CCG, Children's Cancer Study Group; COPP-ABV, cyclophosphamide, vincristine (Oncovin), procarbazine, and prednisone–doxorubicin (Adriamycin), bleomycin, and vinblastine; CR, complete remission; DBVE, doxorubicin, bleomycin, vincristine, etoposide; EFS, event-free survival; GPOH-HD, German Society for Pediatric Oncology and Hematology–Hodgkin disease; IF, involved field; NR, not reported; OEPA, vincristine (Oncovin), etoposide, prednisone, and doxorubicin (Adriamycin); OPPA, vincristine (Oncovin), prednisone, procarbazine, and doxorubicin (Adriamycin); POG, Pediatric Oncology Group; PR, partial remission; RFS, relapse-free survival; RT, radiotherapy; VAMP, vinblastine, doxorubicin (Adriamycin), methotrexate, and prednisone; VBVP, vinblastine, bleomycin, etoposide (VP-16), prednisolone.
*For the composition of combination chemotherapy courses, see Table 53-8.
[†]CR defined as reduction of tumor volume of >95% and residual mass <2 mL.
[‡]OE*PA includes higher dose of etoposide than OEPA.
[§]For good and poor responders respectively.
[‖]Less than 3 nodal sites, no B symptoms, no mediastinal bulk, no extranodal extension.
[¶]Peripheral nodal disease, <6 cm, mediastinal tumor smaller than one third of intrathoracic diameter, absence of extranodal involvement.
**CR defined as >70% reduction of initial tumor volume and gallium-negative if initially gallium-positive.

varied widely between study groups and over time. Table 53-9 describes the criteria for disease response evaluations in recent cooperative group trials.

Cross-sectional imaging can define response based on a percentage decrease in size. In Hodgkin lymphoma, a significant proportion of patients have residual masses at the time of disease response assessment and at the end of therapy. Functional imaging methods such as gallium scanning and PET are able to assess metabolically active tissue associated with residual disease (Fig. 53-5). A series of studies primarily performed in adults with Hodgkin lymphoma where therapy was not changed based on interim radiographic results have shown that PET scans performed after two cycles of chemotherapy are highly predictive of outcome.[150-153] The accuracy of PET to predict treatment outcome is higher early in the course of treatment as compared with the end of chemotherapy.[151,154,155] Both the German-Austrian study GPOH-HD2002 and the Children's Oncology Group (COG) studies of intermediate- and high-risk disease addressed the strength of early PET obtained after two cycles of chemotherapy; however the results are still pending.[156]

Several cooperative group studies have focused on modifications of regimens to avoid gender-specific toxicities. The COG evaluated a strategy of stratifying patients with high-risk disease based both on response and gender.[157] All patients received escalated bleomycin, etoposide, doxorubicin (Adriamycin), cyclophosphamide, vincristine, procarbazine, and prednisone (BEACOPP) therapy for 4 cycles. Patients with a rapid early response, defined as a 70% tumor reduction and having a negative gallium scan after four cycles, were then assigned to subsequent therapy based on gender. Boys received two additional cycles of ABVD designed to minimize risks of infertility and involved field radiation. Girls received four cycles of COPP/doxorubicin (Adriamycin), bleomycin, and vinblastine (ABV) and no radiation in order to avoid the risks of secondary breast cancer. Those with disease that met the criteria for slow early response received an additional 4 cycles of BEACOPP. Seventy-seven percent of girls avoided radiotherapy, whereas 68% of boys avoided alkylating agents during consolidation. The EFS and OS rates remained excellent.

The German GPOH-HD2002 study also evaluated sex-based modifications of therapy but did not use patient response for treatment allocation.[148] Boys received two cycles of dose-intensified vincristine, etoposide, prednisone, and doxorubicin (Adriamycin; OEPA) therapy

TABLE 53-8   Combined-Modality Treatment Strategy and Results for Patients with Intermediate- and High-Risk Hodgkin Lymphoma in Selected Multicenter Trials

Group or Institution	No. of Patients	Stage	Chemotherapy	Radiation (Gy), Field	EFS at 5 years	Overall Survival (%)
DAL-HD90 (high risk)[130]	179	IIEB, IIIEA, B, IIIB, IVA, B	2 OEPA-OPPA + 4 COPP	IF, 20-25 Gy residual tumor 30-35 Gy	86%	94%
GPOH-HD95 3-5 ABVD-PC[38]	265	IIEA, IIIEA, B, IIIB, IVA, B	2 OPPA/OEPA + 4 COPP	CR*: no RT (22%); non-CR: IF, 20 Gy; residual tumor, 30-35	79% DFS no IFRT 91% DFS with IFRT	NR
GPOH-HD02[148] (intermediate risk)	139	IAE, IB, IIAE, IIB, IIIA	2 OPPA + 2 COPP† 2 OE*PA +2 COPAD‡	IF, 20 Gy; residual tumor, 30-35	93%	98%
GPOH-HD02[148] (highest risk)	239	IIBE, IIIAE, IIIB, IVA, IVB, IVE	2 OPPA + 4 COPP† 2 OE*PA + 4 COPAD‡	IF, 20 Gy; residual tumor, 30-35	87% EFS	95% 5 yrs
Stanford-St. Jude-Boston Consortium[609]	159	I-II unfavorable,§ III, IV	3 VAMP/3 COP	15-25.5 Gy,‖ IF	76 at 5 yr	93% at 5 yr
POG[160]	179	IIB, IIIA2, IIIB, IV	4 MOPP, 4 ABVD	21 Gy total nodal	79%	92%
POG[138]	216	IB, IIA/IIIA with bulk, IIB, IIIB, IV	3-5 ABVD-PC	21 Gy IF	84% at 5 yr	95% at 5 yr
CCG[37]	394	I/IIB, IIB, III	6 COPP-ABV	CR: randomized to 21 Gy vs. no IFRT, no CR 21 Gy IFRT	87%	95%
CCG[37]	141	IV	COPP-ABV + CHOP + Ara-C	CR: randomized to 21 Gy vs. no IFRT, no CR 21 Gy IFRT	90%	100%
COG[157]	98	IIB with bulk,¶ IIIB with bulk, IV	BEACOPP × 4 then one of: COPP/ABV × 4‡ ABVD × 2† BEACOPP × 4#	Female, RER**: no RT Male or SER: 21 Gy Residual tumor, 35 Gy	94% EFS	97% 5 yr

ABV, Doxorubicin (Adriamycin), bleomycin, and vinblastine; *ABVD*, doxorubicin (Adriamycin), bleomycin, vinblastine, and dacarbazine; *Ara-C*, cytarabine; *BEACOPP*, bleomycin, etoposide, doxorubicin (Adriamycin), cyclophosphamide, vincristine, procarbazine, and prednisone; *CCG*, Children's Cancer Study Group; *CHOP*, cyclophosphamide, doxorubicin (hydroxydaunorubicin), vincristine (Oncovin) and prednisone; *COG*, Children's Oncology Group; *COPAD*, cyclophosphamide, vincristine (Oncovin), prednisolone, and doxorubicin; *COP*, cyclophosphamide, vincristine, prednisone; *COPP*, cyclophosphamide, vincristine (Oncovin), procarbazine, and prednisone; *CR*, complete remission; *DAL-HD*, Deutsche Arbeitsgemeinschaft fir Leukamiefarschung-Hodgkin disease; *DFS*, disease-free survival; *EFS*, event-free survival; *GPOH-HD*, German Society for Pediatric Oncology and Hematology–Hodgkin disease; *IF*, involved field; *IFRT*, involved-field radiotherapy; *MOPP*, mechlorethamine, vincristine (Oncovin), procarbazine, and prednisone; *NR*, not reported; *OEPA*, vincristine (Oncovin), etoposide, prednisone, and doxorubicin (Adriamycin); *OE*PA*, vincristine (oncovin) etoposide, prednisone and doxorubicin (adriamycin); *OPPA*, vincristine (Oncovin), prednisone, procarbazine, and doxorubicin (Adriamycin); *PC*, prednisone, cyclophosphamide; *POG*, Pediatric Oncology Group; *RER*, rapid early responder; *RT*, radiotherapy; *SER*, slow early responder; *VAMP*, vinblastine, doxorubicin (Adriamycin), methotrexate, and prednisone

*CR defined as reduction of tumor volume of >95% and residual mass <2 mL.

†Males.

‡Females.

§Defined as presence of one or more of the following: bulky disease, peripheral nodal disease 6 cm or larger, and/or mediastinal tumor one third of intrathoracic diameter or larger; and B symptoms.

‖15 Gy for nonbulky sites and complete response after two cycles of chemotherapy.

¶Bulk defined as mediastinal mass greater than intrathoracic diameter at level of T5 or extrathoracic nodal mass greater than 10cm.

#Slow early responders.

**SER, partial response not meeting criteria for RER; RER, >70%reduction in tumor volume and gallium negative post 4 cycles.

TABLE 53-9 Definitions of Favorable Response to Therapy in Selected Multicenter Trials in Children and Adolescents with Hodgkin Lymphoma

Study	Definition of Favorable Response	Timing of Assessment	Treatment Modification for Those with Favorable Response
CCG5942[37]	>70% reduction in initial tumor volume and gallium negative	At completion of chemotherapy	Randomized to IFRT or no IFRT
GPOH-HD02[148]	≥95% reduction in tumor volume	After 2, 4, or 6 cycles of chemotherapy depending on disease group	No IFRT for patients with low-stage disease only (TG1)
Stanford-St. Jude-Boston Consortium[609]	≥75% reduction in perpendicular diameters of measurable lesions, or return no normal size and gallium or PET negative	After 2 cycles of VAMP	No IFRT
COG[158]	Disappearance of all clinical and disease-related symptoms and PET negative	After 2 cycles of ABVD-PC	All get IFRT; Less than good response: chemo intensified with additional 2 cycles ifos/vinolebine

ABVD-PC, Doxorubicin (Adriamycin), bleomycin, vinblastine, and dacarbazine–prednisone, cyclophosphamde; *CCG,* Children's Cancer Study Group; *COG,* Children's Oncology Group; *GPOH-HD,* German Society for Pediatric Oncology and Hematology–Hodgkin disease; *IFRT,* involved-field radiotherapy; *PET,* positron emission tomography; *TG1,* therapy group 1; *VAMP,* vinblastine, doxorubicin (Adriamycin), methotrexate, and prednisone.

followed by two (for those with intermediate-risk disease) or four (for those with high-risk disease) cycles of cyclophosphamide, vincristine (Oncovin), prednisone, and dacarbazine (COPDAC) designed to attempt to limit gonadal toxicity. Girls received the same number of cycles but of OPPA followed by COPP. EFS and OS rates did not differ between the two sexes with the regimens employed.

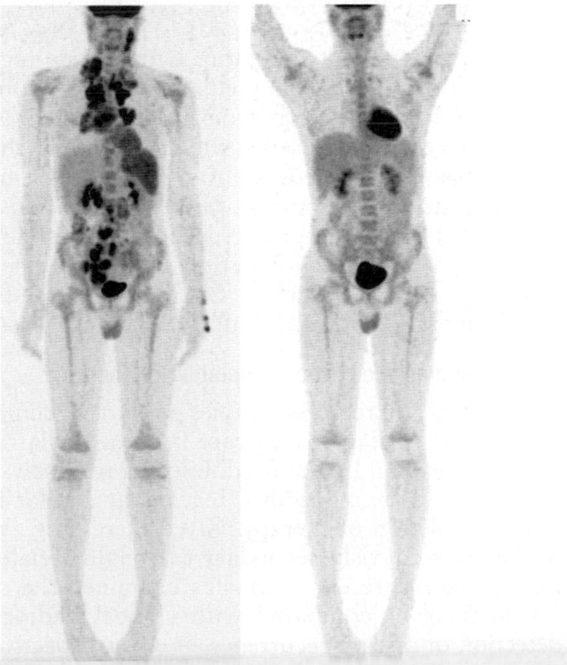

Figure 53-5 PET scan at diagnosis and after two cycles of ABVD-PC chemotherapy in an adolescent with advanced-stage Hodgkin lymphoma.

The Pediatric Oncology Group (POG) evaluated response-based modifications of therapy without modifications for sex in patients with intermediate- and high-risk disease.[158] In this study patients were evaluated for response after three cycles of therapy. Those with a rapid early response defined as a greater-than-70% reduction in disease and gallium negative, received 21 Gy IFRT. Those who were slow responders received an additional two cycles followed by radiation. With this strategy the 5-year EFS rate was the same in both groups, and the OS rate was 95%.

Whether radiotherapy can be omitted from treatment for at least some children and adolescents with Hodgkin lymphoma is one of the important questions in recent and ongoing clinical trials. Three cooperative group trials in the low-risk group each evaluated the removal of IFRT in a subset of patients with largely successful results. In the Stanford-St.Jude-Boston protocol, patients with a complete response, defined as greater than 75% reduction of the sum of the perpendicular of all lesions after two cycles of vinblastine, doxorubicin (Adriamycin), methotrexate (methotrexate), and prednisone (VAMP) chemotherapy were nonrandomly assigned to no radiation. All patients received four cycles of VAMP chemotherapy. Fifty three percent of patients met criteria for complete response. The 2-year EFS rates of this group were no different from those who did receive radiation, at 89% and 92% respectively.[159] The GPOH-HD 2002 study also nonrandomly assigned patients at low risk with a complete response after two cycles, defined as more than 95% volume reduction, to no radiation. Thirty three percent of patients met this criterion, did not receive radiation, and had an outcome identical to those who did receive IFRT, with EFS rates at 5 years of 93% and 91% respectively.[148] The Children's Cancer Group (CCG) study 5942 randomly assigned patients who obtained a complete remission (CR), defined as 70% mass reduction

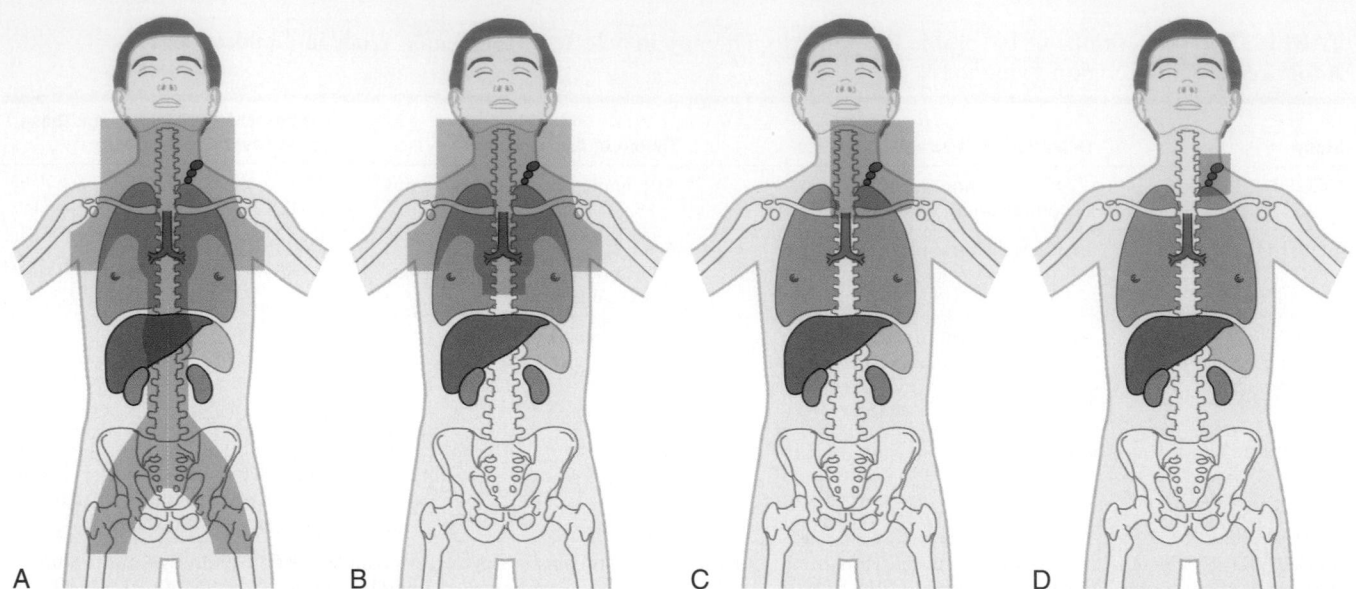

Figure 53-6 Radiation fields for treating Hodgkin lymphoma. **A,** Total nodal irradiation. **B,** Mantle field. **C,** Involved field. **D,** Radiation field individualized to the patient's local disease, taking into account the tolerance of involved or adjacent extranodal organs. *(Courtesy of Dr. W. Dörffel, Berlin, Germany.)*

of tumor volume and negative gallium scan, to radiation or no radiation after four cycles of COPP/ABV therapy. The EFS rates for randomized patients at 3 years were significantly different at 97% versus 91%; however, the OS rate at 3 years in both groups was 100%.[37]

Omission of radiation has also been investigated in subgroups of patients with intermediate- and high-risk disease with mixed results. In the POG trial 8725, patients with stages IIB, IIIA2, IIIB, and IV were randomized to receive eight alternating cycles of MOPP/ABVD chemotherapy followed by total nodal irradiation (21 Gy) or no radiotherapy in cases of CR.[160] There was no difference in EFS or OS between patient groups who did or did not receive radiation. In the GPOH-HD95 trial patients who achieved a complete response received no further therapy, whereas those who did not received 20 to 35 Gy of IFRT.[38] In the intermediate- and high-risk groups, omission of radiation was associated with a significantly decreased EFS rate of 77% for those treated with chemotherapy only versus 92% for those who received combined modality therapy.

The CCG5942 trial included subjects with all disease stages. Based on their risk-group assignment, patients received either four or six cycles of COPP/ABV or six cycles of the mutiagent ABC regimen chemotherapy.[37] Patients with at least a 70% tumor-volume reduction and negative gallium scan at the completion of chemotherapy were randomized to receive or not receive IFRT with 21 Gy. This randomized trial was stopped because of a significantly higher number of relapses in the no-IFRT arm. Most of the relapses were at sites of initial disease. Patients who did not receive IFRT had an EFS rate at 3 years from the time of randomization of 87% compared with 92% (P = .057) for patients treated with IFRT in the intent-to-treat analysis. Importantly, longer term follow-up study of this cohort has shown that the

OS in the two arms is no different. At 10 years postrandomization, the EFS of those treated or not treated with IFRT were 91.2% and 82.9% (P = .004), respectively, whereas the OS of the two groups were 97.2% and 95.5% (P = .5), respectively.[161]

Radiation remains a critical component of therapy for the majority of children and adolescents with Hodgkin lymphoma. Radiotherapy planning involves decision making about both dosage and field, with the goals of maximizing efficacy but limiting late effects. Radiation fields have evolved over time (Fig. 53-6). IFRT, used in the majority of contemporary protocols, generally involves radiation of the entire lymph-node region that includes the pathologically enlarged node.[23] One major implication of the change from mantle-field radiation to IFRT for cervical disease is the exclusion of the axilla, which significantly reduces the exposure of lung and breast tissue. Investigations of further limitations to radiation fields are ongoing. The dosages in most contemporary studies used in combination with chemotherapy are generally no greater than 21 Gy, with some studies using higher dosages to sites of bulky or residual disease.

Disease Surveillance after Completion of Therapy

Driven both by required studies as part of clinical trials and as part of standard of care in some pediatric oncology settings, children and adolescents routinely undergo surveillance imaging with CT scans at regular intervals after completion of therapy. Given increasing awareness of the potential risks secondary to imaging-related radiation exposure, recent work has examined the utility of CT imaging as compared with clinical findings in the detection of disease recurrence.[162] A retrospective review of patients treated in a POG study showed that the majority of relapses occurred within the first year and were detected by clinical findings. For the patients with late relapse, detection by either by clinical symptoms or surveillance imaging did not change the OS rate.[163] These authors suggest limiting surveillance-CT imaging to the first 12 months after completion of therapy. FDG-PET scanning, which has utility in staging newly diagnosed patients and in the assessment of disease response (see above) has no established role in off-therapy surveillance.[164] More widespread use of MRI as a replacement for CT may also allow for reduction of radiation exposure in lymphoma patients in the future.[165]

Nodular Lymphocyte-Predominant Hodgkin Lymphoma

Pathologic Features

NLPHL is a monoclonal B-cell neoplasm.[35,166] The histology is characterized by effacement of the lymph node architecture by a nodular or nodular and diffuse infiltrate of small lymphocytes, with an associated follicular dendritic network and scattered or clustered large cells referred to as *lymphocytic and histiocytic (L&H) cells*.[26,35] NLPHL corresponds to Hodgkin paragranuloma of the classification of Jackson and Parker from 1947[167] and to lymphocyte-predominant Hodgkin lymphoma of the Rye modification of Lukes and Butler.[24] Differentiation of NLPHL from the lymphocyte-rich subtype of classic Hodgkin lymphoma can be difficult in some cases. However, the phenotype of L&H cells (also termed *popcorn cells* because of their often multilobed nuclei) is different than classic Reed-Sternberg cells of the CHL subtypes in that they express CD45 and usually retain most normal markers of B-cell differentiation, such as CD20, CD79a, and the B-cell specific transcription factors BOB.1 and Oct-2, but do not express CD30 and CD15 (see Table 53-1).[26,35] Also, markers of EBV infection are consistently absent from L&H cells of NLPLH.[166] In some patients with NLPHL, progressively transformed germinal centers are observed in association with NPLHL. However, it remains uncertain whether these lesions are truly preneoplastic, because most patients with such lesions in reactive lymph-node hyperplasia do not develop a lymphoma.[168]

Clinical Features

NLPHL comprises between 5% and 8% of Hodgkin lymphoma in children and adolescents and accounts for an even higher percentage of prepubertal patients.[169] Unlike in patients with CHL, there is a significant male preponderance in those with NLPHL. The disease course is more indolent, and a higher proportion of patients have low-stage disease, most often presenting as localized peripheral adenopathy, most commonly in the neck and less commonly in the inguinal area. Mediastinal involvement is relatively rare.[170] Unlike CHL, where contiguous nodal spread is the norm, in NLPHD noncontiguous spread is observed in those with high-stage disease. The pattern of relapse of disease also differs from CHL, with relapses occurring late and often repeatedly.[171,172] An additional unique feature of NLPHL is the increased risk of transformation to NHL occurring in 5% to 12% of cases, whereas this is very rarely observed in CHD.[173]

Diagnostic evaluation should include excisional node biopsy. Fine-needle aspirate is often inadequate and can lead to the misdiagnosis of reactive nodal tissue.[174] Staging of patients with NLPHL uses the Ann Arbor system as used for CHL, and staging evaluations to be considered are the same as those for a patient with CHL except that bone marrow biopsies are rarely indicated. The only consistent prognostic factor for patients with NLPHL is stage of disease, although some data suggest that a ratio of lymphocyte count to monocyte count at the time of diagnosis may also have prognostic value.[175,176]

Treatment and Outcomes

Historically patients with NLPHL have been included in most therapeutic studies of childhood and adolescent Hodgkin lymphoma. Uncertainty remains about optimal therapy for these patients. Given the favorable prognosis and the burden of late effects from therapy, the evaluation of less intensive regimens has been undertaken.[177]

The majority of patients with NLPHL have low-stage disease, which is sometimes amenable to complete resection. One of the unique features of NLPHD is that a portion of children with low-stage disease treated with resection alone are cured of their disease. Studies of patients treated in this fashion have reported relapse-free survival rates of 67% to 100%.[178-181] All of the recurrences in patients with relapse were low stage, and the OS has been reported as 100%.[180] For pediatric patients with NLPHD, a watchful waiting approach for those who are in CR after initial surgery is appropriate. However, a careful postoperative staging and meticulous follow-up observation is essential. Other strategies for patients with low-stage disease are the use of radiotherapy alone[175] or low-intensity alkylator-based chemotherapy regimens.[182,183]

Data to evaluate the best therapy for patients with advanced stage NLPHL are relatively scarce. Outcome of these patients is similar to those with CHL, and the usual recommendation is that they receive therapy similar to those with advanced-stage CHL. Investigation of the possible role for therapy with rituximab as a single agent or as part of combination therapy for this disease are ongoing.

Treatment of Relapsed Hodgkin Lymphoma

Although the success of primary therapy for children and adolescents is high, approximately 10% of patients develop relapsed disease.[184] The outcome for those with relapsed disease is variable. The two strongest predictive factors are time to relapse and response to reinduction chemotherapy.[185-187] Time to relapse can be subdivided into three prognostic groups: 1) patients with primary refractory disease or recurrent disease within the first 3 months have the worst outcomes; 2) those with disease relapse within 12 months of diagnosis form an intermediate group; and 3) those with relapses occurring longer than 12 months from diagnosis have the most favorable outcome.[188] Patients who have no response to reinduction therapy have a dismal prognosis, as do those with active disease immediately before autologous stem cell transplantation (SCT).[189,190] Additional prognostic factors include the intensity of primary therapy, stage, and B symptoms at relapse.

There is no consensus on optimal salvage therapy for children with relapsed disease. The options include chemotherapy with or without radiation, autologous SCT, allogeneic SCT, or novel therapies. Data to support treatment choices can be difficult to interpret because there is a lack of randomized trials evaluating these therapeutic options in children; the majority of studies in patients with relapse have been single-arm trials with varying inclusion criteria.

Patients with late relapse who have responsive disease to reinduction therapy have a favorable prognosis with treatment with chemotherapy and radiation.[188] Chemotherapy regimens have been evaluated in this setting including ifosfamide, carboplatin, and etoposide (ICE)[188]; carmustine (BCNU), etoposide, cytarabine (ara-C), and melphalan (miniBEAM)[191]; cytarabine, cisplatinum, and etoposide (APE)[192]; as well as newer regimens including gemcitabine and vinorelbine (GV)[193] among others. Information that should be considered in choosing a salvage regimen should include knowledge of the frontline therapy used, in part to avoid toxicities with cumulative drug exposure.

For patients with high-risk relapsed disease, intensifying therapy with autologous SCT should be considered, although controversy about which patients are likely to benefit from this therapy remains. In a prospective randomized trial of the German Hodgkin Lymphoma Study Group, adults with chemotherapy-sensitive disease had a significantly higher failure-free survival probability when treated with two cycles of dexamethasone, carmustine (BCNU), etoposide, cytarabine (ara-C), and melphalan (Dexa-BEAM) followed by autologous SCT compared with patients receiving four cycles of Dexa-BEAM without SCT.[194] For childhood Hodgkin lymphoma there are very few prospective or randomized trials. In a retrospective study of 51 pediatric patients with recurrent Hodgkin lymphoma treated with different salvage regimens, there was a beneficial impact of autologous SCT on survival only for patients refractory to first-line therapy, but sensitive to second-line therapy disease.[195] The outcome of children with disease that is unresponsive to chemotherapy who undergo autologous SCT is dismal.[184]

The European trial for children with relapsed Hodgkin lymphoma, EuroNet-PHL-C1, divides patients into low-, intermediate- and high-risk groups based on time to relapse and early response assessment. Patients with low-risk disease are treated with chemotherapy and radiation. Those with high-risk disease have their therapy intensified with autologous SCT. Those with intermediate-risk disease have therapy allocated based on response, with those with a good response receiving chemotherapy and radiotherapy only.

The use of allogeneic transplant in relapsed Hodgkin lymphoma, with the hopes of making use of graft-versus-lymphoma effects has been investigated including myeloablative SCT, reduced intensity SCT, and reduced intensity SCT after autologous SCT.[196,197] In this very–high-risk group, both relapsed disease and transplant-related mortality limit the adoption of this therapy except for those patients with adequate performance status and limited curative options.[184]

Novel therapies for relapsed disease are needed. One agent that shows significant promise is the antibody-drug conjugate brentuximab vedotin (also known as SGN-35), which combines an anti-CD30 monoclonal antibody with the antimicrotubule agent, monomethyl auristatin E. In a phase 2 study of patients with very–high-risk disease (71% had primary refractory disease, and 100% of patients had previously been treated with autologous SCT), the overall response rate was 75%, with 34% of patients achieving a CR and with a high percentage of these patients remaining without evidence of relapsed disease at 1.5 years. The median age of the patients in this trial was 31 years, with the youngest being 15 years old. Toxicity of the agent was relatively mild, including neuropathy and cytopenias.[198] The safety and effectiveness of adding this agent to standard chemotherapy as well as including it in front-line therapy is being investigated by several cooperative groups.

Late Effects of Therapy

Given the high rate of cure in children and adolescents with Hodgkin lymphoma, the risks of long-term effects of treatment are very important. In the scientific literature, the number of reports on late sequelae after successful treatment of pediatric Hodgkin lymphoma patients has exceeded that of reports on prospective therapeutic trials. Many of these reports document late sequelae associated with earlier treatment approaches. The treatment for pediatric Hodgkin lymphoma has evolved because of a continuous process of attempting to maximize efficacy while limiting the long-term risks of therapy. Therefore many of the reports of sequelae of therapy administered several decades ago may not accurately reflect the risks of late effects associated with current treatment strategies.

Some late effects of Hodgkin lymphoma therapy can be attributed to a distinct treatment modality or a single drug; others may have a multifactorial pathogenesis. Table 53-10 lists late effects that have impact on morbidity and mortality, as well as those that affect the quality of life for survivors.

In two large, single-center series of patients with pediatric Hodgkin lymphoma treated over several decades, the long-term cumulative risk of death from treatment-related sequelae such as infections, cardiac disease, and second cancers approached that of the risk of death from relapsed Hodgkin lymphoma.[199,200] Data from 2742 patients treated between 1970 and 1986 who were under the age of 21 at the time of diagnosis, who were alive longer than 5 years posttherapy, and who were in the Childhood Cancer Survivor Study (CCSS) has delineated the risks and causes of excess mortality.[201] With a median follow-up length of greater than 20 years, of the 500 observed deaths in the cohort, 35% were from Hodgkin lymphoma, 23% from second malignant neoplasms (SMNs), and 14% from cardiovascular disease. The 30-year OS rate from diagnosis was 74%.

SMNs are devastating sequelae of therapy for Hodgkin lymphoma. In the U.S. Childhood Cancer Survivor

TABLE 53-10 Late Effects of Treatment of Children and Adolescents with Hodgkin Lymphoma

Late Effect	Radiotherapy	Chemotherapy
Musculoskeletal growth impairment[201]	X	
Cardiomyopathy[216]		Anthracyclines
Coronary artery disease, valvular disease, and pericardial disorders[214,218]	X	
Stroke[201]	X	
Infections (postsplenectomy or splenic radiation)[219]	X	
Thyroid dysfunction[222]	X	
Female gonadal dysfunction[227-229]	X	
Male infertility[223-226]	Inguinal, pelvic irradiation	Alkylating agents; procarbazine
Lung dysfunction[220]	X	Bleomycin; BCNU; CCNU; busulfan
Second cancer (hematologic)[202-210]		Alkylating agents; topoisomerase II inhibitors
Solid tumors[202-213]	X	

BCNU, Carmustine; CCNU, lomustine.

Cohort consisting of more than 13,000 survivors of childhood cancers, patients treated for Hodgkin lymphoma were at the highest risk to develop an SMN.[202] Patients treated with full-dose radiation are at significant risk for SMNs with a cumulative incidence of greater than 25% after 30 years of follow-up study.[203,204] Fifteen years postdiagnosis of Hodgkin lymphoma, the second leading cause of mortality after death from the primary disease is death from an SMN.[205] Breast cancer makes up the largest component of the excess solid tumors in female patients.[203]

Contemporary therapy no longer uses high-dose extended-field radiation. The impact of lowering radiation dosage and the use of combination chemotherapy on risks of SMN continues to be investigated. In a cohort study including both children and adults treated for Hodgkin lymphoma, 459 second malignancies were described in 5798 patients.[206] These patients were treated between 1963 and 2001. All received chemotherapy, and 3432 also received radiation. Of those who received chemotherapy only, there remained significantly increased risks of second malignancies including leukemia, NHL, and lung cancer with the peak period of risk between 5 and 9 years posttherapy. For those who received combined modality therapy including radiation, the absolute risk of an SMN was significantly higher and included a wider arrays of malignancies; the period of risk extended

to 25 years and longer. In a small cohort of 112 pediatric patients treated at a single institution between 1970 and 1990 with combined modality therapy including 15 to 25.5 Gy IFRT, the rate of SMN including sarcomas and breast and thyroid carcinomas was similar to that reported in studies of patients who had received higher doses of radiation.[207] Other studies have suggested that low-dose radiation and limiting cumulative alkylator exposure may have a protective effect in adult patients but not in children.[208] Still others have shown that patients who received less than 23 Gy of mediastinal radiation had a lower incidence of breast cancer, which may in part be related to the transition from extended-field radiation to IFRT.[209] The cumulative incidence of second leukemias ranges from 0.6% to 2.1% and reaches a plateau after 10 to 14 years.[131,200,204,210,211] The risk of second leukemias is associated with the cumulative dose of alkylating agents and is almost absent in patients treated with radiotherapy alone.[200,204] The risk of developing thyroid cancer is clearly related to radiotherapy and is highest in young children.[203,204,212] Almost all thyroid tumors arise within the radiation field.[204] A recent study analyzing the genetic factors that may contribute to radiation-induced tumors in survivors of Hodgkin lymphoma has identified variants at chromosome band 6q21, implicating the *PRDM1* gene in the etiology of secondary malignancies.[213]

Cardiovascular disease contributes significantly to the morbidity and mortality of patients who are survivors of Hodgkin lymphoma.[201] Damage to the heart after full dose radiotherapy includes coronary artery disease, valvular pathology, and pericardial disease.[214] Cardiomyopathy with ventricular dysfunction can result from anthracycline therapy.[215] Risks of late anthracycline cardiotoxicity are higher in young children, in girls, and with higher cumulative doses.[216,217] In long-term follow-up observation of a cohort of patients from a single-center combination of exposure to mediastinal radiation and anthracycline was associated with the highest risk of cardiac morbidity.[218] Data regarding the long-term cardiac risks associated with contemporary therapy using low-dose IFRT and chemotherapy regimens that generally limit cumulative anthracyclines exposure to less than 250 mg/m² are needed.

Death from overwhelming infections related to splenectomy was a major risk that has been significantly reduced since splenectomy was abandoned from staging procedures.[131,199] Irradiation of the spleen may also induce functional impairment of the spleen, at least if dosages of 20 Gy or more are used.[219]

Chronic lung disease can result from irradiation of the lung and exposure to several chemotherapy agents used in Hodgkin lymphoma regimens, including bleomycin and the nitrosourea derivatives BCNU and lomustine (CCNU). The cumulative dose of these drugs is the most crucial determinant for chronic lung injury. Very young age may be an additional risk factor for possible fatal lung toxicity from BCNU and CCNU.[220] The combination of radiotherapy and drugs with lung toxicity contributes to increased risk of long-term lung impairments. This is of special concern in patients requiring salvage treatment for recurrent Hodgkin lymphoma that includes high-dose chemotherapy.

Survivors of pediatric Hodgkin lymphoma are at increased risk for thyroid malfunction—mainly hypothyroidism but also hyperthyroidism, benign and malignant thyroid nodules, and Graves disease.[221] The risk increases with the dose of neck irradiation, younger age at treatment, and female gender.[222]

Musculoskeletal growth impairment was one of the first sequelae recognized to be a consequence of high-dose radiotherapy for children with Hodgkin lymphoma.[143] Prepubertal children treated with 40 Gy of mantle irradiation would have predictable sequelae of lack of growth of the bone and soft tissues of the neck and clavicles, leading to orthopedic complications as well as significant cosmetic effects. This complication is ameliorated by low-dose IFRT used in most contemporary regimens.

The primary risk factor for gonadal toxicity is exposure to alkylating agents, primarily cyclophosphamide and procarbazine.[223,224] Historically mechlorethamine was the primary cause of chemotherapy-related sterility in males. Dose-dependent testicular damage from germ-cell depletion and Leydig-cell dysfunction has also been documented in prepubertal and postpubertal boys after MOPP; chlorambucil, vinblastine, procarbazine and prednisone (ChlVPP); and OPPA-COPP chemotherapy.[225,226] The ABVD regimen appears to be less toxic to germ cells.[227] Results from the German-Austrian studies on pediatric Hodgkin lymphoma have shown clearly that with moderate doses of cyclophosphamide, male infertility correlates with the cumulative dose of procarbazine. Historically in girls, the most substantial risk of infertility was from pelvic lymph node irradiation and was ameliorated to some extent by ovarian transposition.[143,228] The risks of early menopause for females receiving contemporary therapy is likely fairly low, and small studies have shown no measurable impact of ABVD therapy on fertility in women.[229]

Follow-up care of survivors of Hodgkin lymphoma should follow a structured plan such as that described in the *COG Long-Term Follow-up Guidelines*.[230,231] Availability of a detailed and accurate treatment summary is imperative to determining appropriate care and surveillance investigations in follow-up observation.

NON-HODGKIN LYMPHOMA

NHLs are a diverse collection of malignant neoplasms of lymphoid cell origin, including all the malignant lymphomas that are not classified as Hodgkin lymphoma. They account for 7% of all cancers in those younger than 20 years old.[232] NHLs are heterogeneous in their pathology, clinical features, and responsiveness to therapy. With improved understanding of biology and data from sequential disease-based clinical trials as well as better supportive care, the outcome of children with NHL has improved dramatically over the last several decades. With conventional therapy, depending on subtype and stage, the majority of children with NHL can be cured of their disease.

The classification of NHL has been and continues to be a topic of scientific discussion and a source of confusion for clinicians. The Rappaport system used growth patterns (diffuse vs. nodular) and cytology (undifferentiated vs. differentiated) as the basic criteria for disease definitions.[233] The Lukes Collins classification system was based primarily on splitting the lymphocytic system into T and B lymphocytes.[234] The Kiel classification system attempted to translate information about how the lymphatic system is organized into a classification system for NHL, in which the lymphoma cells were related morphologically and immunophenotypically to the normal cell categories of the immune system.[235,236] The National Cancer Institute Working Formulation for Clinical Usage, established in 1982, did not intend to constitute another classification of NHL; rather it was to be a common language to translate between existing classifications.[237] It took into consideration the clinical course of patients and resulted in a grading of NHL into low-grade, intermediate-grade, and high-grade NHL. This system was widely used by clinicians in North America. In Europe and Asia, the Kiel classification was more broadly used. The use of different classification systems hampered or even made it impossible to compare results of clinical trials. In the 1990s, the International Lymphoma Study Group undertook a major effort to overcome this confusion and to create a uniform classification of NHL based on biologic principles. The result was the Revised European-American Classification of Lymphoid Neoplasms (REAL) classification, which then lead to the WHO Classification of Tumors of the Hematopoietic and Lymphoid Tissues produced in 2002 and revised in 2008.[25] The basic principles of the WHO classification system include subdivision of neoplasms according to the lineage (B, T, or natural killer [NK] cell) and the definition of distinct subtypes within each lineage according to a combination of morphology, immunophenotype, genetic features, and clinical features.

The revisions of the WHO classification system in 2008 included diseases that overlap between entities, such as B-cell lymphomas with features intermediate between DLBCL and BL and B-cell lymphomas with features intermediate between DLBCL and Hodgkin lymphoma. In addition, age-specific factors defined several new disorders including pediatric type follicular lymphoma (FL) and systemic EBV-positive T-cell lymphoproliferative disease of childhood.[238]

Combination chemotherapy is the cornerstone of successful treatment of children and adolescents with NHL. A key moment in the development of current treatment concepts was the recognition that different NHL subtypes require different chemotherapeutic strategies. In children and adolescents with NHL, three main disease groups account for the vast majority of the diagnoses. The three are LL, mature B-cell neoplasms (including BL and DLBCL), and anaplastic large-cell lymphoma (ALCL; Fig. 53-7). In the era of solid organ and SCT, posttransplant lymphoproliferative diseases are becoming more common.

Epidemiology and Causative Factors

There is significant variation in incidence rates according to geographic areas, gender, age, and ethnicity in

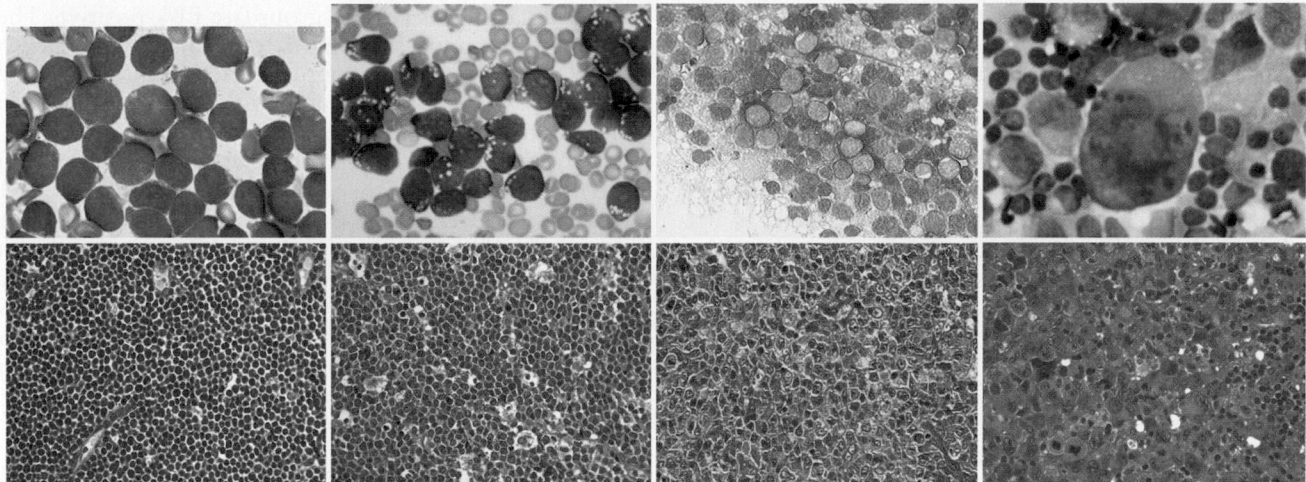

Figure 53-7 Morphology, immunophenotype, and specific cytogenetics of main non-Hodgkin lymphoma subtypes of childhood and adolescence.

childhood NHL. The comparison of incidence rates of NHL in childhood and adolescence in different geographic areas is limited because of a paucity of true population-based registries, different degrees of completeness of data, and the use of various disease classification systems over time. The reported incidence rates range from 6.6 per million population in the United Kingdom to 12.5 per million in Japan. Specific subtypes of NHL, however, occur at a much higher rate in particular regions. Endemic BL accounts for 74% of all childhood malignancies in equatorial Africa, whereas all NHLs combined account for 7% of pediatric cancer in North America.[239-241]

In all registries the incidence rates of NHL are higher in males than in females, usually by a factor of 2.[242-246] The male-to-female ratio varies considerably among different NHL subtypes. Whether male predominance in most NHL subtypes reflects hormonal differences rather than loss of an X-chromosome–linked tumor suppressor

gene remains to be determined. The incidence of NHL and of the various subtypes varies widely by age, with substantial differences between children and adults. Among patients younger than 18 years of age there is also considerable variability (Fig. 53-8).[247] NHL as a whole in children younger than 3 years of age is extremely rare. BL or leukemia is the predominant subtype in younger children. The incidence of DLBCL and ALCL increases in those older than 15 years of age.

In the U.S. Surveillance, Epidemiology, and End Results (SEER) program, the incidence rate in Caucasian children is higher as compared with African American children.[242,248] In adults, an increased risk for NHL has been described in first-degree relatives of patients with hematopoietic malignancies.[101,249] Except for classic known hereditary immunodeficiency syndromes predisposing for NHL, only a few specific genes have been associated with risks of childhood NHL. Biallelic mutations in mismatch repair genes have been associated in a series of families

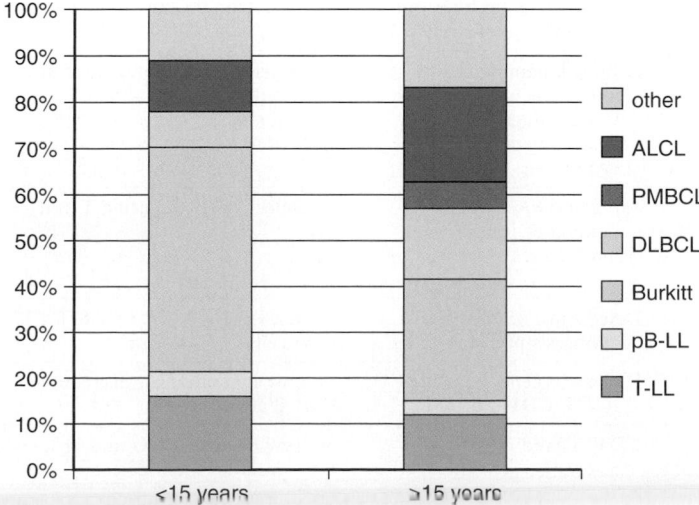

Figure 53-8 Distribution of non-Hodgkin lymphoma subtypes by age. *(Modified from Burkhardt B, Oschlies I, Klapper W et al: Non-Hodgkin's lymphoma in adolescents: experiences in experiences in 378 adolescent NHL patients treated according to pediatric NHL-BFM protocols.* Leukemia 25:153–60, 2011.)

with several types of childhood malignancies including T-cell lymphomas.[250]

Conclusive data to support the association of environmental factors and risk of childhood NHL are extremely limited. Conversely, data to support the role of infection in a subset of NHLs has been long established. Denis Burkitt not only recognized and described BL as a new disease entity but also established the epidemiologic basics for the current view of its association with EBV, malaria, and possibly arbovirus infections and described the lymphoma belt of Africa."[240,251] In 1964, Epstein and associates[252] described viral particles—later referred to as EBV—in BL samples from African patients. Subsequently the EBV genome was found to be incorporated into 96% of endemic BL cases in the African lymphoma belt, whereas in France and Germany, only 10% to 15% of cases are EBV-positive.[253] It was postulated that EBV infection in addition to exposure to malaria and possibly arboviral infections early in life may be crucial for the pathogenesis of endemic EBV-positive BL.[240,241,254-256] In addition to endemic BL, lymphoproliferative disease, and lymphomas in children with acquired or congenital immunodeficiency are often EBV positive.

Inherited and acquired immunodeficiency is a strong risk factor for developing NHL during childhood.[257] Table 53-11 presents the most common inherited immunodeficiencies associated with lymphoproliferative disorders and lymphoma.[258] For patients with these inherited (also called *primary*) immunodeficiencies, the chance of dying of lymphoma is 10 to 200 times the expected rate for age-matched unaffected children. Many of the lymphomas in this patient group are EBV-positive. There is a male preponderance, partly explained by the fact that some of the inherited immunodeficiencies are X-linked disorders.[259] Children infected with human immunodeficiency virus (HIV) have more than 150 times the risk of developing NHL in comparison with general population rates.[260,261] NHLs are the most common neoplasms occurring in children with HIV, and most are of B-cell lineage.[262,263] For some children NHL may be the first defining condition for acquired immunodeficiency syndrome (AIDS).[262,263] The introduction of highly active antiretroviral therapy has been associated with a significant decrease the incidence of some HIV-related malignancies, such as Kaposi sarcoma, but the effect on the incidence of NHL appears to be more modest.[264]

Initial Evaluation and Staging

As is the case for patients with HL, the most common symptom of childhood NHL is painless lymphadenopathy. In contrast to Hodgkin lymphoma, the nodes may enlarge more rapidly because of a much higher growth fraction of NHL. The variety of presenting features of childhood NHL is even larger than that for Hodgkin lymphoma, ranging from a single painless enlarged lymph node, an asymptomatic asymmetrical enlarged tonsil, or a harmless-looking skin papule to a life-threatening condition. Almost any organ, tissue, and anatomic area can be involved. The most common disease sites are the cervical lymph nodes, abdomen (including the liver and spleen), mediastinum, and head and neck region. Lesions in the head and neck area may involve the tonsils, Waldeyer ring, paranasal sinuses, and any bone structure

TABLE 53-11   Inherited Immunodeficiency Syndromes Associated with Lymphoma in Children

Syndrome	Genetics/Pathogenesis	Immune Defect	Malignancy
Ataxia telangiectasia	*ATM*; impaired DNA repair	Progressive decline in T cells, abnormal immunoglobulins	T-cell ALL and T-cell LL, CHL, BL, DLBCL
Wiskott-Aldrich syndrome (WAS)	*WASP*; abnormal cytoskeletal architecture of hematopoietic cells	Defects in T cells, B cells, neutrophils, macrophages	EBV-associated DLBCL, Hodgkin, lymphomatoid granulomatosis
Severe combined immunodeficiency (SCID)	X-linked: gamma chain mutations with defective IL signaling; *ADA*: defective adenosine deaminase	Dependent of subtype but in general low or absent T and NK cells, nonfunctional B cells	EBV-associated lesions
X-linked lymphoproliferative disease (XLP)	*SH2D1A*; *SAP*, which modulates B- and T-cell interactions	Defective EBV-specific T and NK cells	EBV-associated hematophagocytic lymphohistiocytosis, B-cell lymphoproliferative disease
Autoimmune lymphoproliferative syndrome (ALPS)	Defects in *FAS*-mediated apoptosis pathway	Increased CD4 and CD8 T cells	LPHL, CHL, DLBCL, BL
Common variable immunodeficiency (CVID)	Defects in genes encoding *ICOS*, CD19, *BAFFR*	Low IgG and IgA, decreased B cells	EBV-associated lesions, DLBCL, Hodgkin
X-linked hyperimmunoglobulin M syndrome	CD40 ligand mutation leading to defective B cells	Low or absent IgG and IgA, variable T-cell defects	EBV-associated lesions, DLBCL, Hodgkin

Modified from Tran H. Immunodeficiency associated lymphomas. Blood Rev 22 261-381, 2008.
ALL, Acute lymphoblastic leukemia; *BL,* Burkitt lymphoma; *CHL,* classic Hodgkin lymphoma; *DLBCL,* diffuse large B-cell lymphoma; *DNA,* deoxyribonucleic acid; *EBV,* Epstein-Barr virus; *Ig,* immunoglobulin; *IL,* interleukin; *LL,* lymphoblastic lymphoma; *LPHL,* lymphocyte-predominant Hodgkin lymphoma; *NK,* natural killer.

including the skull and cranial base. Other sites are bone, soft tissue, kidneys, and skin. Testicular involvement occurs in fewer than 5% of boys and usually manifests as painless unilateral or bilateral enlargement of the testicle. Involvement of ovaries is diagnosed in fewer than 5% of females. The pancreas, adrenal glands, thyroid gland, and salivary glands are rarely affected.

The presenting clinical features, largely based on the site of disease leading to symptoms, vary considerably between different NHL subtypes. Because of the variety of clinical patterns of sites in childhood NHL, careful history and physical examination is essential and should focus on signs and symptoms associated with possible emergent problems such as respiratory compromise from a mediastinal mass or bowel obstruction from abdominal disease. Because CNS involvement is not uncommon in B-cell NHL and LL, careful neurologic examination is necessary to detect signs of cranial nerve involvement, paresis, or increased intracranial pressure. Special attention should be directed to the examination of the skin because of the relatively common involvement, especially in patients with ALCL.

Basic laboratory studies include peripheral blood counts, serum concentrations of LDH, basic coagulation parameters, liver and renal function tests, and serum electrolyte levels. Chest x-ray is critical before anesthesia for invasive procedures to evaluate for mediastinal disease. Other imaging studies vary based on clinical presentation and pathologic information but almost always include CT of the chest. Imaging of the abdomen can be done by CT, although in some centers this is done by ultrasound or MRI. Cranial and spinal imaging is mandatory in any patient for whom there are concerns of possible neurologic impairment. Determination of sites of metastatic disease, except for bone marrow and cerebrospinal fluid (CSF), is largely based on clinical and imaging findings. The use of additional biopsy for staging purposes should be restricted to cases where the findings are uncertain and involvement or noninvolvement would alter treatment.

The involvement of bone marrow and the CNS affects treatment of all subtypes of childhood NHL and therefore needs special attention. Historically, bone-marrow involvement was diagnosed if more than 5% blasts are present in a representative bone-marrow aspiration smear detectable by morphology alone. With the use of flow cytometry and polymerase chain reaction (PCR) for detection of disease-specific genetic alterations, smaller percentages of disease cells in the bone marrow can be routinely detected. A generally agreed upon convention regarding the threshold of detection for allocation of patients as bone marrow-positive or not is lacking. With modern immunophenotyping techniques the additive value of bone-marrow biopsies is somewhat unclear.

There is no internationally standardized definition of CNS involvement in childhood NHL. The definition of CNS involvement includes those patients with an intracerebral mass and/or lymphoma cells in the CSF.[265-269] Opinions differ on how patients with cranial nerve paralysis and paraspinal involvement should be classified, and these patients have been allocated to both CNS-positive and CNS-negative groups in different cooperative group studies.

Despite its increasing use, the role of FDG-PET in the initial evaluation and staging of children with NHL is unclear. FDG-PET is highly sensitive and specific for the detection of sites of disease involvement.[270,271] In adult patients there is evidence of clinical benefit for the use of FDG-PET in disease-response assessment for those patients with Hodgkin lymphoma and DLBCL; however its use for initial staging and for disease response assessment in those with other histologies is less clear.[272] As is true with the introduction of any new, more sensitive testing modality, the risk of its use is "upstaging" patients with the consequence of them receiving potentially unnecessary intensive therapy. Prospective studies are required to evaluate and verify the diagnostic role of FDG-PET in staging and to assess whether the findings of FDG-PET compared with conventional imaging translate into different staging, and more importantly, whether this affects patients' outcomes. The use of FDG-PET as a tool for evaluation of the kinetics of response to therapy as a prognostic marker in children with NHL also requires careful investigation. For this indication, pretreatment FDG-PET is indicated, at least for distinct NHL subtypes with variable FDG uptake.[126]

Skeletal scintigraphy (either FDG-PET or bone scan) can detect bone involvement. Skeletal involvement was not found to be a prognostic factor in several analyses, and therefore bone imaging with skeletal scintigraphy to detect clinically occult bone foci is unnecessary.[273-276] Specific imaging procedures may be indicated in patients with symptoms of bone involvement such as pain and swelling. Larger bone lesions are almost always symptomatic and can be imaged using simple x-ray and evaluated further with MRI if needed.

Obtaining tissue for accurate disease diagnosis is critical. If a malignant lymphoma is suspected, it is important to determine whether the diagnosis can be confirmed with minimally invasive tests. Many children have advanced-stage disease at diagnosis, including bone marrow disease and/or malignant effusions. In many of these cases, correct diagnosis can be made by cytology, immunophenotyping by flow cytometry, and genetic evaluation of bone marrow or effusion samples. A diagnostic surgical procedure should be performed if a definitive diagnosis cannot be achieved by less invasive means. If surgery is to be performed, the procedure should be minimally invasive and should only be used to provide enough biopsy material to characterize the disease fully. A complete resection of a small, localized lymphoma may be beneficial for patients with mature B-cell NHL. However, resections at the expense of functional deficits or risks of significant surgical morbidity, including delay in initiating systemic chemotherapy, are not justified.

With the available routine diagnostic tools, a needle aspiration of a pathologically enlarged node is generally not adequate to provide sufficient material for complete pathologic examination and should be reserved for exceptions, such as when a more invasive procedure would represent an undue risk for the patient.

TABLE 53-12   St. Jude Staging System for Pediatric Non-Hodgkin Lymphoma

Stage	Definition
I	A single tumor (extranodal) or involvement of a single anatomic area (nodal), with the exclusion of the mediastinum and abdomen
II	A single tumor (extranodal) with regional node involvement Two or more nodal areas on the same side of the diaphragm Two single (extranodal) tumors, with or without regional node involvement on the same side of the diaphragm A primary gastrointestinal tract tumor (usually in the ileocecal area), with or without involvement of associated mesenteric nodes, that is completely resectable
III	Two single tumors (extranodal) on opposite sides of the diaphragm Two or more nodal areas above and below the diaphragm Any primary intrathoracic tumor (mediastinal, pleural, or thymic) Extensive primary intraabdominal disease Any paraspinal or epidural tumor, whether or not other sites are involved
IV	Any of the above findings with initial involvement of the central nervous system, bone marrow, or both

Modified from Murphy SB: Classification, staging and end results of treatment of childhood non-Hodgkin's lymphomas: dissimilarities from lymphomas in adults. Semin Oncol 7:332–339, 1980.

The aim of staging procedures is to identify all disease sites to inform therapeutic decisions, response assessment, and follow-up monitoring. The St. Jude staging system, developed in the late 1970s, is widely accepted for the staging of childhood NHL (Table 53-12).[277] The St. Jude staging system is primarily based on the clinicopathologic features of the main NHL subtypes of childhood LL and BL. It takes into account the different patterns of disease spread of these disorders as compared with Hodgkin lymphoma, especially the more common extranodal involvement. The definition of stages is determined by the number and anatomic pattern of disease sites, their resectability, and the involvement of the bone marrow and CNS. Lymphoblastic neoplasms are considered to be acute lymphoblastic leukemia (ALL) if there are 25% or more lymphoblasts in the bone marrow. For BL, infiltration of the bone marrow with more than 25% lymphoma cells is characterized as B-cell or Burkitt-cell leukemia, also referred to as *B-ALL*. The St. Jude staging system has proven useful for the stratification of therapy intensity for the treatment of these entities. For other entities, such as ALCL, its usefulness for treatment stratification is less well defined.

Lymphoblastic Lymphoma

Neoplasms of the precursor B and T cells occur in two different clinical patterns, as ALL or as LL. Conventionally, ALL and LL are separated by the degree of bone marrow involvement. Cases with at least 25% lympho- blasts in the bone marrow with or without extramedullary disease are diagnosed as ALL, whereas those with extramedullary manifestations and less than 25% bone marrow lymphoblasts are referred to as LL. The WHO classification system categorizes the disease as T-lymphoblastic leukemia/lymphoma and B-lymphoblastic leukemia/lymphoma, with multiple subtypes based on recurrent genetic abnormalities.[25] About 80% of children with T-cell ALL and 90% of those with T-cell LL have a mediastinal tumor at presentation. In a minority of cases, T-cell ALL occurs as bone-marrow disease alone, and 10% of T-cell LL cases have no mediastinal tumor.

Pathologic Features

T-cell LL and B-cell LL are morphologically indistinguishable. The neoplastic cells are uniform in size, with scanty or indistinct cytoplasm and nuclei larger than those of small lymphocytes with finely distributed chromatin. They are historically referred to as the *L1* and *L2 types* according to the French-American-British (FAB) Classification of Acute Leukemias.[278] Nuclear membranes may possess subdivisions of varying prominence, giving rise to a distinction between convoluted and nonconvoluted variants of LL.[237] This distinction may be merely a histopathologic nuance, however,[279] and is not included in the WHO classification.

Both precursor B-cell and precursor T-cell LLs may coexpress myeloid CD13, CD33, and rarely, CD117. A useful marker to distinguish LL of precursor B and T cells from mature B-cell and T-cell neoplasms is terminal deoxyribonucleotidyl transferase (TdT). TdT adds single nucleotides to double-strand DNA breaks during the process of immunoglobulin gene and TCR gene recombination, respectively, a process essential during precursor B-cell and T-cell differentiation.[280,281] TdT is only expressed during this process and thus is a specific marker for neoplasms of precursor B and T cells but not for mature T- and B-cell neoplasms.

ALL cases can be further subdivided according to the maturational stages of the leukemic cells, defined by the sequence of expression of antigens into pro-B, common ALL, and pre-B in the precursor B-cell ALL category and into pro-T, pre-T, thymus cortex type, and thymus medullary type in the precursor T-cell category.[282] Few data exist about whether the same subdivision is possible for LL cases.

Molecular and Cellular Biology

Few data are available on genetic findings in LL, mainly because of the lack of fresh tumor tissue appropriate for cytogenetic and molecular studies. As a result, most molecular and cytogenetic data available are derived from the study of T-cell ALL cases. Globally, xome sequencing and array comparative genomic hybridization analyses of pediatric T-cell ALL shows a broad heterogeneity in the mechanisms of T-cell transformation and a low mutation load with an average of 8.2 coding mutations per sample.[283-285]

Role of T-Cell Receptor Translocations. Classic recurring chromosomal rearrangements found in T-cell ALLs and LLs involve the *TCRB* locus (7q34) or the *TCRA/D* locus (14q11) and are generated from mistakes in the recombination process that generate functional TCRs during the development of normal thymocytes.[286-288] These translocations typically induce the aberrant expression of transcription factor oncogenes in T-cell progenitors, activating an irregular transcriptional program that interferes with normal T-cell development and contributes to leukemic transformation. Transcription factor oncogenes involved in these T-cell ALL-specific translocations include members of the basic helix-loop-helix (bHLH) family (*MYC, TAL1, TAL2, LYL1,* and *BHLHB1*),[289-294] the LIM- domain only (LMO) protein genes (*LMO1* and *LMO2*),[295] homeodomain genes (*TLX1/HOX11, TLX3/HOX11L2,* and *HOXA9*),[296-299] *MYB,*[300,301] and *NOTCH1.*[302]

Importantly, a number of chromosomal rearrangements that do not involve the TCR loci are also involved in the aberrant expression of some of these oncogenes. Thus *MYB* can be activated by a t(6;7)(q23;q34) translocation[300] or alternatively by a small intrachromosomal duplication selectively affecting the *MYB* locus in the long arm of chromosome 6.[301] The TAL1d rearrangement, a small intrachromosomal deletion that places the *TAL1* gene under the control of the promoter of the nearby *SIL* gene, is found in about 25% of T-cell ALL cases.[303] Similarly, *LMO2* can be activated by small intrachromosomal deletions in the short arm of chromosome 11.[304] Both *TAL1* and *LMO2* are often expressed biallelically in T-cell ALL cases without known alterations in their respective loci, suggesting that activation of upstream regulatory mechanisms controlling the expression of these genes may also participate in the pathogenesis of T-cell ALL.[305,306]

NOTCH1 Activation. The most characteristic molecular lesion associated with the pathogenesis of T-cell lymphoblastic leukemias and lymphomas is the aberrant activation of the NOTCH1 signaling pathway. The NOTCH signaling pathway plays a critical role in the hematopoietic system by participating at multiple stages of T-cell development.

During early hematopoiesis, NOTCH signaling is required for the commitment of multipotent hematopoietic progenitors to the T-cell lineage.[307-309] Conversely, mice harboring a conditional deletion of *Notch1* in hematopoietic progenitors fail to develop T cells and show ectopic B-cell development in the thymus.[309] In some systems, this occurs between CD4 and CD8 lineages.[310-313]

Mature NOTCH receptors (NOTCH1 through 4) are transmembrane heterodimeric proteins generated from a precursor polypeptide that is postranslationally cleaved by a furin protease in the trans-Golgi network. This first cleavage generates both N-terminal and C-terminal NOTCH fragments, which in the absence of a NOTCH signaling stimulus form a heterodimeric transmembrane protein. The N-terminal fragment of the receptor contains multiple epidermal growth factor (EGF) repeats involved in ligand interaction followed by a series of Lin12-NOTCH repeats (LNRs) that in the absence of ligand, stabilize the heterodimeric association between the N-terminal and C-terminal NOTCH fragments. The latter (membrane-bound) fragment of the receptor contains a transmembrane proximal RBPJ-associated molecule (RAM) domain followed by a series of ankyrin repeats, both of which participate in the interaction with the DNA-binding factor RBPJ, and a carboxy-terminal proline, glutamic acid, serine, and threonine (PEST) sequence responsible for the proteosomal degradation of the activated receptor in the nucleus.

The NOTCH signaling pathway is normally triggered by the interaction of a NOTCH receptor in one cell with a NOTCH Jagged 1,2 and Delta-like 1,3,4 (DSL) ligand expressed in the surface of a neighboring cell. This ligand–receptor interaction induces two consecutive proteolytic cleavages at the cell surface that release the cytoplasmic intracellular domain of NOTCH (ICN1) of the receptor from the cell membrane.[314,315] The first of these ligand-induced cleavages is mediated by extracellular metalloproteases of the A disintegrin and metalloproteinase (ADAM) family. Two ADAM proteases (ADAM10 and ADAM17) have been implicated in the activation of the NOTCH signaling pathway in different organisms.[314,315] After S2 cleavage, the resultant activated membrane-bound form of NOTCH is further processed by the γ-secretase complex that catalyzes the final endomembrane cleavage step and releases the intracellular domains of NOTCH from the membrane.

After γ-secretase cleavage, the consequent activated form of NOTCH rapidly translocates to the nucleus, where it interacts with the RBPJ DNA-binding protein. In the absence of NOTCH signals, the RBPJ transcription factor binds to the DNA in NOTCH target promoters, where it recruits transcription inhibitory factors to form a multiprotein transcriptional corepressor complex.[315] Binding of ICN1 to RBPJ displaces these repressors and recruits the MAML1 coactivator to the complex, thereby switching the activity of RBPJ from repressor to activator and inducing the transcriptional activation of NOTCH-RBPJ target genes.

The human *NOTCH1* receptor gene was originally identified as part of the t(7;9)(q34;q34.3), a rare chromosomal translocation that moves the *NOTCH1* gene next to the *TCRB* locus, leading to the aberrant expression of a truncated and constitutively active form of *NOTCH1* in about 1% of human T-cell ALLs.[302] Despite evidence that NOTCH signaling plays a major role in the development of the T-cell lineage and that aberrant NOTCH1 signaling can transform T-cell progenitors, the significance of activated *NOTCH1* in human T-cell ALL seemed limited to rare human T-cell ALLs harboring the t(7;9). This perception was quickly revised after the identification of activating mutations in *NOTCH1* in 50% of human primary T-cell ALL and LL samples and more than 80% of human T-cell ALL cell lines.[316,317,318]

Activating mutations in *NOTCH1* in human T-cell ALL are concentrated in exons 26 and 27, which encode the homodimerization (HD) domain in the extracellular portion of the receptor and in exon 34, which encodes the PEST domain in the C-terminal region of the protein. In addition, *NOTCH1* juxtamembrane expansion (JME) mutations resulting from small in-frame insertions in exon 28 introduce extra amino acids in the extracellular juxtamembrane region of the receptor in about 5% of T-cell ALLs.[319] NOTCH1 HD and JME mutations probably operate by inducing ligand-independent activation of NOTCH1, whereas PEST mutations are predicted to result in increased levels of intranuclear active NOTCH1 by impairing its degradation by the proteasome.[320,321] Thus both types of mutations result in increased NOTCH1 activity (five- to tenfold over baseline). Importantly, double-mutant alleles harboring both HD and PEST mutations are often found in T-cell ALL samples and increase the activation of NOTCH1 tenfold more than HD or PEST mutations alone (50-fold over baseline).[316]

Aberrant activation of NOTCH1 signaling in hematopoietic progenitors drives commitment to the T-cell lineage and promotes malignant transformation by inducing deregulated cell growth, proliferation, and survival. Genomic studies on the identification of NOTCH1 direct target genes and pathways in T-cell ALL have uncovered a major role for oncogenic NOTCH1 as a critical regulator of cell growth and metabolism in T-cell lymphoblasts.[322] Thus NOTCH1 directly binds the promoters of numerous genes involved in protein biosynthesis and anabolic pathways through RBPJ.[322] In addition, oncogenic NOTCH1 controls the expression of MYC, which further increases the expression of cell-growth genes.[321-324]

The relevance of the NOTCH-MYC regulatory axis in T-cell transformation is further supported by the identification of mutations in FBXW7 in about 15% of T-cell ALL and LL cases.[317,318,325] This -box protein mediates the proteosomal degradation of activated NOTCH1, MYC, JUN, and cyclin E.[326] FBXW7 mutations found in T-cell ALL are clustered in three critical arginine residues involved in the interaction with its target proteins. Thus mutant FBXW7 works as a dominant negative factor to promote the stability of activated NOTCH1, mimicking the effect of NOTCH1-PEST mutations.[325] In addition mutant FBXW7 also stabilizes MYC, which further enhances the NOTCH-MYC axis (see earlier) and blocks the degradation of cyclin E, which may contribute to T-cell ALL transformation by promoting cell-cycle progression.[326]

The identification of activating NOTCH1 mutations present in patients with T-cell ALL and LL has created great interest in developing anti-NOTCH therapies as treatment of this disease.[316] These include γ-secretase inhibitors (GSIs), which block the release of activated NOTCH1 (ICN1) from the membrane, and have been proposed as potential targeted therapy in T-cell ALL and T-cell LL[316,327,328]; stapled peptides targeting the NOTCH transcriptional complex[329]; and NOTCH1-specific inhibitory antibodies that have been proposed as alternative anti-NOTCH1 therapies for the treatment of T-cell ALL and LL.[330] Notably, blocking NOTCH1 signaling with γ-secretase inhibitors can reverse glucocorticoid resistance in some T-cell ALL and LL tumors, and glucocorticoid treatment abrogates the intestinal secretory-cell metaplasia and gastrointestinal toxicity associated with systemic inhibition of NOTCH signaling, supporting the use of anti-NOTCH1 therapies and glucocorticoids in combination in the clinic.[327,328]

MYC. The c-MYC oncogene has been implicated in the pathogenesis of T-cell ALL by the t(8;14)(q24;q11) translocation that induces aberrantly high levels of MYC expression in T-cell progenitors.[331,332] Furthermore the prominent role of MYC in T-cell transformation is reinforced by the identification of MYC as an important direct transcriptional target of NOTCH1[322-324] and by the identification of FBXW7 mutations that contribute to increased MYC levels by blocking the proteosomal degradation of the MYC protein.[325,326]

TAL1, TAL2, LYL1, and BHLHB1 bHLH Factors and LMO1 and LMO2 Transcriptional Oncoproteins.

TAL1 is a class II bHLH factor gene aberrantly expressed in more than 60% of T-cell ALL cases.[333] TAL1 activation can occur by means of chromosomal translocation of the TAL1 locus in the vicinity of TCR genes[334] or by a small intrachromosomal deletion that places the TAL1 gene under the control of the nearby SIL locus, present in 25% of T-cell ALL cases.[291] In addition, sporadic cases of T-cell ALL harbor chromosomal rearrangements that place TAL1-related genes such as TAL2, LYL1, and BHLHB1 in the vicinity of the TCR loci.[292-294] Class II bHLH factors heterodimerize with the class I bHLH proteins E12, E47, HEB, and E2-2 and modulate their transactivating activities.[335] T-cell tumors expressing TAL1 contain TAL1-E47 and TAL1-HEB heterodimers.[336] In addition, E2A-deficient mice develop T-cell lymphomas,[337,338] suggesting that TAL1 and related bHLH proteins TAL2, LYL1, and BHLHB1 may contribute to leukemia by interfering with E protein function. However, recent genome-wide mapping of TAL1 binding sites in the leukemia genome and TAL1-regulated genes shows a more complex scenario in which TAL1 antagonizes both activating and repressing functions of E2A in T-cell ALL.[339]

Loss of function of E2A and HEB is also believed to be the mechanism of transformation in tumors with chromosomal translocations involving the LMO protein genes, LMO1 and LMO2.[304] LMO1 or LMO2 are frequently coexpressed with TAL1[333] in T-cell ALL, and TAL1-LMO2-E2A complexes are detected in human T-cell ALL cells.[340,341] Furthermore, aberrant expression of LMO2 accelerated the leukemogenic process in transgenic mice expressing TAL1 in the thymus.[342]

TLX1(HOX11), TLX3(HOX11L2), and HOXA9 Homeobox Genes.

Homeobox (HOX) genes constitute an evolutionarily conserved family of transcription factors that are expressed in specific patterns during embryogenesis and are responsible for the regulation of various developmental processes in vertebrates.[343] The TLX1 (HOX11) family of HOX genes includes TLX2 (HOX11L1) and TLX3 (HOX11L2),[344] which are characterized by the presence of a threonine in the third helix of the homeodomain; this confers specific DNA-binding properties. Both TLX1 and TLX3 have been linked to the pathogenesis of T-cell ALL through their identification as genes activated by chromosomal translocations. In contrast, HOX11L1 is normally expressed in T-cell progenitors and does not seem to play a role in the transformation of normal thymocytes.[333]

TLX1 was originally isolated at the breakpoints of the recurrent t(10;14)(q24;q11) in T-cell ALL[296,297,345,346] and is aberrantly expressed in 5% of pediatric and up to 30% of adult T-cell ALL cases.[333,347-349] Like other *HOX* genes, *TLX1* plays an important role during embryonic development and acts as a master transcriptional regulator necessary for the genesis of the spleen.[350,351]

Several possible mechanisms through which aberrant *TLX1* expression might lead to malignant transformation have been proposed. In particular, the TLX1 protein is believed to function as a transcriptional regulator, a hypothesis supported by the presence of both a 61-amino acid, helix-turn-helix, DNA-binding domain (or homeodomain) and by the localization of *TLX1* in the cell nucleus.[344] In addition, *TLX1* has been shown to bind to a protein serine-threonine catalytic subunits of phosphatase 2A (PP2AC) and phosphatase 1 (PP1C). Both PP2A and PP1 are targets for oncogenic viruses and chemical tumor promoters. Thus inactivation of PP2A by *TLX1* could contribute to the transformation of T-cell progenitors.[352]

A second *HOX11* family member, *TLX3*, has been implicated in the pathogenesis of human T-cell ALL through characterization of the t(5;14)(q35;q32), a cryptic chromosomal translocation detectable only by fluorescence in situ hybridization (FISH) and chromosome-painting techniques.[298] This translocation leads to the ectopic expression of *TLX3*, possibly by bringing it under the influence of regulatory elements in the *BCL11B* gene, which is highly expressed during T-lymphoid differentiation.[298,353] In contrast to the predominance of *TLX1* expression in adult T-cell ALL cases, both t(5;14) and *TLX3* expression are present in 20% to 25% of pediatric cases but in only 5% of adult T-cell ALL cases.[347,349,354,355] As is the case for *TLX1*, *TLX3* plays an important role during embryonic development when it is essential for the normal development of the ventral medullary respiratory center.[356]

The TLX1 and TLX3 proteins are closely related in structure and possess a high degree of sequence identity at the amino-acid level, especially in the HOX domain, where their sequences only differ in three amino acids. The high level of structural homology in their DNA binding domains supports the hypothesis that TLX1 and TLX3 may induce T-cell ALL through the regulation of the same transcriptional targets. Gene expression profiling studies analyzing the expression signatures associated with *TLX1* and *TLX3* expressing T-cell ALLs and detailed characterization of a transgenic mouse model of T-cell ALL induced by forced expression of TLX1 in developing T cells have shown a remarkable overlap in the gene expression programs and direct transcriptional targets controlled by TLX1 and TLX3 in T-cell ALL.[357] Moreover, these studies have revealed a transcriptional repressor role for TLX1 and TLX3 in the control of gene expression and uncovered the *BCL11B* and *RUNX1* genes as prominent tumor suppressor genes downregulated by TLX1 and TLX3 in the pathogenesis of T-cell ALL.[358] Additionally, *TLX1* has been implicated in the development of aneuploidy via disruption of mitotic checkpoint mechanisms[357] and in

blocking T-cell development via inhibition of *TCRA* recombination.[359]

MYB. The translocation t(6;7)(q23;q34) is a rare recurrent rearrangement that juxtaposes the *TCRB* and *MYB* loci in very young pediatric T-cell ALL cases (median age, 2.2 years).[300] The pathogenic role of *MYB* in T-cell ALL is further supported by the identification by molecular cytogenetic techniques of a short somatic duplication, which includes the *MYB* locus in 15% of T-cell ALL cases.[300,301] These abnormalities induce increased *MYB* expression, particularly in the case of the *TCRB-MYB*–rearranged leukemias. The MYB transcription factor is essential for primitive and adult hematopoiesis, including the T-cell lineage, and the *MYB* locus is a common site of retroviral insertional mutagenesis-induced leukemias; however, the specific mechanisms that mediate *MYB*-induced transformation in T-cell ALL remain to be elucidated. Notably, *MYB* is upregulated downstream of *HOXA9* and *MLL-ENL* T-cell oncogenes and is required for *HOXA9*- and *MLL-ENL*-induced leukemic transformation.[360]

CALM-AF10. The t(10;11)(p13;q14-21) is a recurrent chromosomal translocation found in patients with AML and T-cell ALL. The product of this translocation is a chimeric oncogene resulting from the fusion of clathrin assembly lymphoid myeloid leukemia gene (*CALM*) and AF10.[361,362]

CALM is a ubiquitously expressed protein containing an epsin N-terminal homologous domain involved in the interaction with clathrin during endocytosis.[363] AF10 is a ubiquitously expressed transcription factor originally identified as a partner of *MLL* in AML.[364,365] *CALM-AF10* rearrangements are present in 5% to 10% of T-cell ALL cases and seem to be particularly common in tumors with a very early block in T-cell development or those expressing TCRad.[366,367] Gene-expression profiling studies have demonstrated that *CALM-AF10* expression is associated with high levels of *HOXA* genes, including *HOXA9*.[299,368]

MLL-ENL. Rearrangements of *MLL*, located on human chromosome 11q23, are common in infant and therapy-related leukemias and can occur in AML and ALL. These rearrangements typically generate a fusion oncogene containing the N-terminus part of *MLL* and various protein domains from more than 50 different fusion partners. The *MLL-ENL* fusion oncogene is found in rare cases of T-cell ALL and, in contrast with *MLL* rearrangements in other hematologic tumors, is associated with a favorable prognosis.[333] *MLL* is normally responsible for the maintenance of gene expression at the *HOX* paralog groups. *MLL*-fusion oncogene products disrupt the normal function of MLL and result in aberrant expression of *HOX* genes.[369,370] *MLL*-rearranged T-cell ALL cases have high levels of expression of *HOX* genes, including *HOXA9* and *HOXA10*.[333,370]

Transcription Factor Tumor Suppressors. *BCL11B* encodes for a transcription factor critically required for normal T-cell development.[371] Loss-of-function mutations and heterozygous deletions of the *BCL11B* are recurrently found in T-cell ALL, suggesting that *BCL11B* haploinsufficiency is an important pathogenetic event in T-cell leukemogenesis.[357,372] In addition, the Wilms tumor suppressor gene 1 (*WT1*) is deleted and mutated in about 10% of T-cell ALLs.[373,374] Similarly, monoallelic or biallelic deletions involving the *LEF1* locus and mutations in the *LEF1* gene are recurrently present in T-cell ALL cases.[375] Finally, *ETV6*, *RUNX1*, and *GATA3* loss-of-function mutations are characteristically present in a fraction of early-immature T-cell ALLs, a leukemia group characterized by a very early arrest in T-cell development and poor prognosis.[358,376-378]

Cell Cycle Regulators. Deletions of chromosome bands 9p21-229 involving the $p16^{INK4A}$, $p14^{ARF}$, and $p15^{INK4B}$ tumor suppressor genes are the most common abnormality found in T-cell lymphoblastic tumors.[379,380] p15 and p16 are involved in cell-cycle regulation by inhibiting cyclin-CDK complexes, whereas $p14^{ARF}$ is a negative regulator of TP53. Thus loss of these tumor suppressors affects both the control of cell proliferation and cell survival.

Chromosomal translocations targeting the cyclin D2 (*CCND2*) locus at chromosome band 12p13 and the *TCRB* or *TCRAD* loci result in high levels of *CCND2* overexpression. *CCND2* expression is normally confined to early (double-negative) stages of thymocyte differentiation and is replaced by *CCND3* in more mature (double-positive) cells, suggesting that sustained expression of *CCND2* in *CCND2*-rearranged T-cell ALL cases is oncogenic.[300]

Chromatin Remodeling Tumor Suppressor Genes. The polycomb repressive complex 2 (PRC2) is the "writer" of lysine 27 trimethylation on Histone 3 (H3K27me3), a major chromatin mark associated with transcriptional silencing. Loss-of-function mutations and deletions of *EZH2* and *SUZ12* genes encoding two critical components of the PRC2 complex are found in about 25% of T-ALLs.[377,381] In addition, *PHF6*, a plant homeodomain (PHD)–containing factor involved in epigenetic regulation of gene expression is mutated and deleted about 16% of pediatric T-cell ALL cases.[382]

Genetic Alterations Driving Activation of Oncogenic Signaling Pathways. The *PTEN* tumor suppressor gene, which encodes a central negative regulator of the PI3K–AKT pathway, is mutated and deleted in 5% to 10% of T-cell ALL cases,[383] and prototypical activating mutations in *NRAS*-activating mutations are common in early immature T-cell ALLs.[376,377,384] In addition, deletions and mutations in the neurofibromatosis type 1 (*NF1*) gene, which encodes a negative regulator of Ras signaling, are found in 3% of T-cell ALLs.[385] Aberrant JAK signaling drives T-cell transformation in T-cell ALLs harboring the t(9;12)(p24;p13) translocation, a rare rearrangement encoding a constitutively active *ETV6-JAK2* oncoprotein.[386] Moreover, activating mutations in *JAK1* and *JAK3* and the *IL7R* gene resulting in constitutive activa-

tion of the JAK-STAT signaling are present in approximately 15% of T-cell ALLs.[377,387-390]

Other Genetic Alterations. Numerous additional genes and pathways whose mechanism of action remains to be fully clarified are altered in T-cell ALL. Among these, recently identified genetic-lesion mutations affecting the ribosomal proteins RPL5, RPL11, and RPL10 including recurrent alterations of Arg98 in RPL10 are particularly intriguing and suggest a role for disruption of ribosomal function in T-cell transformation.[283]

Clinical Characteristics

Children and adolescents with LL most commonly show signs and symptoms of mediastinal disease such as cough, shortness of breath, or orthopnea. Patients may have severe distress that is sometimes made worse by the effects of pleural or pericardial effusions. Patients may also have painless adenopathy, most often cervical or supraclavicular, although the disease can be widely disseminated and involve the liver and spleen. Those with B-cell LL more often show limited-stage disease of skin, isolated node, or bone. Disease limited to the skin most commonly involves the scalp.[391] Patients may have symptoms related to CNS disease, including signs associated with increased intracranial pressure such as headache, nausea and vomiting, and visual changes or with cranial nerve palsies.[267] Many who are subsequently found to have CNS will not have had preceding symptoms. By definition, patients with LL have less than 25% bone marrow involvement. Most patients therefore do not exhibit signs or symptoms associated with severe pancytopenia, and most commonly the complete blood count (CBC) is normal or near normal.[392] Involvement of the testes for patients with LL is relatively rare. Table 53-13 describes the clinical features at the time of diagnosis in patients with LL in selected cooperative group studies.

Treatment and Outcomes

The treatment of children and adolescents with LL is largely based on the strategies and protocols developed for the treatment of ALL. Outcomes for selected

TABLE 53-13   Presenting Features in Children and Adolescents with T-Cell Lymphoblastic Lymphoma

	% Male	% with Mediastinal Mass	% with CNS Disease	% with Bone Marrow Disease
EORTC-CLG58881[605]	62	81	3	NR
NHL-BFM90[394]	77	89	3	15
NHL-BFM95[403]	63	78	4	26
POG 9404[399]	77	89	4	NR

CNS, Central nervous system; *EORTC-CLG,* European Organization for Research and Treatment of cancer–Children's Leukemia Group; *NHL-BFM,* Non-Hodgkin Lymphoma–Berlin-Frankfurt-Munster; *NR,* not reported; *POG,* Pediatric Oncology Group.

TABLE 53-14 Treatment Protocols and Results in Recent Multicenter Studies of Childhood and Adolescent Lymphoblastic Lymphoma

Protocol	Stages	Immunophenotype	No. of Patients	Duration of Therapy	Cranial Radiation	EFS	Outcome
NHL-BFM90[244,394]	I-IV	T only	105	24 months	12 Gy prophylaxis 24 Gy if CNS+	90% (5 years)	Excellent outcome with ALL-like therapy and prophylactic cranial radiation, no local radiation
EORTC-CCG58881[605]	I-IV	T only	121	24 months	none	77% (6 years)	No increase in CNS relapse rate observed without cranial radiation, response to prephase therapy predictive of outcome.
POG9404[399]	III-IV	T and B	137	25 months	18 Gy all patients	85% (5 years)	Addition of high-dose methotrexate did not improve outcome for patient with LL (although it did for those with T-cell ALL)
NHL-BFM95[403]	I-IV	T and B	198	24 months	No prophylaxis 18 Gy if CNS +	80% (5 years)	In patients with stage III and IV CNS-positive disease and good response to induction, prophylactic cranial radiation can be avoided
COG A5971[400]	I-IV	T and B	257	24 months	No prophylaxis 18 Gy if CNS +	83% (3 years)	For patients with stage III + IV CNS-negative disease, neither high-dose methotrexate nor intensified anthracycline/cyclophosphamide improved outcome

ALL, Acute lymphoblastic leukemia; *CNS*, central nervous system; *COG*, Children's Oncology Group; *EORTC-CCG*, European Organization for Research and Treatment of cancer–Children's Cancer Study Group; *LL*, lymphoblastic lymphoma; *NHL-BFM*, Non-Hodgkin Lymphoma–Berlin-Frankfurt-Munster; *NR*, not reported; *POG*, Pediatric Oncology Group.

cooperative groups trials are presented in Table 53-14. Considerations for therapy include immunophenotype, stage including CNS involvement, and more recently, the impact of the presence of minimal disease involvement of the bone marrow at the time of diagnosis.[393] Other clinical factors such as age, gender, and LDH as well as tumor response were not found to be prognostic in the Berlin-Frankfurt-Munster (BFM) studies. Patients with low-stage disease have survival rates that exceed 90%, whereas the rate for those with stage 3 or 4 disease approaches 80%.[394,395]

Patients with stage 1 and 2 disease account for a minority of patients with LL. Approximately 75% of the low-stage group has B-lineage disease.[395] Early studies of localized NHL evaluating 9 weeks versus 8 months of therapy showed that those with LL had a significantly worse outcome than other NHL phenotypes, with evidence of some benefit for longer therapy in this subgroup.[396] Studies that have included patients with all

stages of LL have consistently reported favorable outcomes for those with limited disease with EFS rates of 73% to 100%.[397] The largest series of patients with stage 1 and 2 LL disease treated in a uniform manner comes from the COG study A5971. Patients were assigned to a CCG-BFM–like ALL regimen that included 24 months of therapy, intensive intrathecal therapy, and no radiation.[395,398] Seventy five percent of the patients had pre-B immunophenotype, and the majority had disease in their head and neck region, involving skin and nodal tissue with a minority who had isolated bone disease. The 5-year EFS and OS rates were 90% and 95%, respectively.

The majority of patients with LL have advanced-stage disease at diagnosis and have the T-cell phenotype. The most effective regimens for this group of patients are based on regimens adopted from the treatment of children with ALL. Most treatment protocols include corticosteroids, vincristine, anthracyclines, L-asparaginase, and cyclophosphamide; and methotrexate, cytarabine, 6-mercaptopurine, and 6-thioguanine; and some include epipodophyllotoxins. Most involve induction, consolidation, and maintenance phases of chemotherapy and prolonged treatment lasting approximately 2 to 3 years. Radiotherapy to sites of disease outside the CNS is not generally used in contemporary treatment protocols.

In the context of multidrug therapy, isolating the importance of specific agents is challenging. There is mixed evidence that the use of high-dose methotrexate is important in the treatment of children with advanced-stage disease. The BFM90 trial, which included 4 courses of 5 gm/m^2 of methotrexate in consolidation, had excellent outcomes with a 5-year EFS rate of 90% to 95%.[394] The POG9404 study evaluated the addition of high-dose methotrexate to an intensive ALL backbone for patients with T-cell ALL and T-cell LL. The 5-year EFS rate was better for those who received high-dose methotrexate in patients with T-cell ALL but there was no measurable difference for those with T-cell LL.[399] A recent COG study evaluating the impact of induction intensification and the use of high-dose methotrexate in consolidation found no benefit to either intervention.[400] Evidence for the efficacy of L-asparaginase in patients with T-cell LL can be derived from a randomized study conducted by the former POG.[401] Patients with T-cell LL receiving weekly L-asparaginase after induction had a higher EFS rate than controls. Dexamethasone instead of prednisone in induction resulted in improved outcome of children suffering from ALL at the expense of higher toxicity.[402] Randomized BFM-based trials as to whether dexamethasone in induction can also further improve the EFS rate of patients with T-cell LL are ongoing.

Oral 6-mercaptopurine and methotrexate are basic elements of maintenance therapy during remission; they are administered for a treatment duration of 18 to 24 months from the start of chemotherapy. With the exception of the BFM strategy, additional agents (vincristine and steroids) and multiple intensification pulses of different composition are used in many study protocols. When comparing overall results of studies, there is little evidence for a beneficial effect of intensification of maintenance.

CNS-directed chemotherapy including high-dose methotrexate and intrathecal therapy without prophylactic cranial irradiation is sufficient for prevention of CNS relapse in patients with advanced-stage LL without overt CNS disease.[399,403,404,405] In the NHL BFM 95 study, including high-dose methotrexate (5 g/m^2 IV, four times daily) and 11 doses of intrathecal methotrexate but no cranial radiotherapy (CRT), both disease-free and CNS relapse–free survival rates of patients were not significantly inferior to the historic control group of the preceding NHL BFM86 and BFM90 trials, in which patients received prophylactic CRT.[403] High-dose methotrexate therapy also appears efficacious to prevent relapse in the testes.[394]

For patients with overt CNS disease, 18 to 24 Gy CRT, in addition to aggressive systemic chemotherapy, is highly effective in preventing CNS recurrences.[265,394,397] In the BFM studies, patients with CNS-positive LL had EFS rates comparable to patients who were CNS-negative

when receiving high-dose methotrexate (5 g/m^2 IV infusion) over 24 hours and intrathecal therapy followed by CRT with 18 Gy.[265]

Therapy for Patients with Relapsed Disease

The outcome for patients with relapsed LL is poor.[406] The general strategy for these patients includes intensive reinduction therapy, and for those patients with responsive disease, ideally a second CR to proceed to SCT. One of the main reasons for poor outcomes is the failure of disease, once it has relapsed, to respond to further therapy. There is no standard reinduction regimen. Various combinations have been described including ifosfamide, carboplatin, and etoposide (ICE)[407] and dexamethasone, etoposide, cisplatin, cytarabine, and L-asparaginase (DECAL).[408]

Nelarabine, a nucleoside analogue, has been shown to have activity as a single agent in children with relapsed and refractory T-cell malignancies.[409] Nelarabine in combination with etoposide and cyclophosphamide has been described in a small case series as being safe and effective. In this series seven of the seven patients had some evidence of disease response and five of seven obtained CR.[410] Nelarabine, in addition to T-cell ALL backbone therapy, is being tested for safety and efficacy in the current phase III randomized trial for children with newly diagnosed high-risk T-cell ALL and T-cell LL within the COG.

The data for SCT in patients with relapsed LL are limited. Unlike for other types of NHL, there is no clear role for autologous SCT in patients with relapsed LL.[411] In a report from the BFM, no patient with relapsed LL who did not proceed to allogeneic SCT was a long-term survivor. The majority of patients did not undergo SCT because of nonresponsive disease. Of the nine patients who were able to undergo allogeneic SCT, four remain in second CR.[406]

Mature B-Cell Neoplasms

Of the numerous subtypes of neoplasms of mature B cells, only two commonly occur during childhood and adolescence, BL and DLBCL. All others are rare in children. Combined, these two entities account for approximately 60% percent of NHL in children and adolescents.

Pathologic Features: Burkitt Lymphoma

Classic BL is composed of monomorphic medium-sized cells with deep basophilic cytoplasm and round to ovoid nuclei, with granular dispersed chromatin and multiple nucleoli corresponding to L3 morphology according to the FAB classification.[278] Lipid vacuoles are commonly present in the cytoplasm and the nuclei but are not mandatory. Numerous mitotic and apoptotic cells are usually seen. On histomorphology, a "starry sky" pattern is usually present, created by the intercalation of numerous macrophages that have ingested apoptotic cells. Using proliferation-associated markers such as Ki67, the growth fraction is high and can be up to 100%.[39]

BL cells invariably express the B-lineage antigens CD19, CD20, CD22, and CD79a and surface immunoglobulin and are negative for CD5, CD23, and TdT.[26] The expression of the germinal center markers BCL6 and CD10 points to a germinal center origin of BL cells.[412]

The 2008 WHO classification eliminated the category of Burkitt-like lymphoma.[238] Two provisional diagnostic groups were added: B-cell lymphoma, unclassifiable, with features intermediate between DLBCL and BL and B-cell lymphoma, unclassifiable, with features intermediate between DLBCL and CHL[39] that account for disease whose morphologic, immunologic and molecular phenotype lies between classic disease groups.

Molecular and Cellular Biology. BL is universally characterized by a characteristic gene expression signature that includes the aberrant expression of MYC.[413] This cellular oncogene encodes a helix-loop-helix transcription factor involved in the control of multiple cellular processes that contribute to cellular transformation, including cell growth, division, death, metabolism, adhesion, and motility. Chromosomal translocations characteristic of BL juxtapose the c-MYC locus in chromosome band 8q24 with strong enhancers from the immunoglobulin genes and drive high levels of MYC expression.[414,415] In 80% of BL cases, the t(8:14)(q24;q32) translocation places MYC in the vicinity of the IGH locus.[416] In 15% of cases, the translocation partner is the IGK locus at chromosome 2p11, whereas the remaining 5% of cases involve the IGL locus at chromosome 22q11. BL exhibits a distinct gene-expression profile characterized by the high-level expression of MYC target genes, which allows accurate differentiation of BL from other NHL subtypes such as DLBCLs.[413,417]

Tumors with the t(8;14) show differences in the location of the breakpoints relative to the MYC gene and the IGH genes, which are strongly associated with the geographic origin of the patient.[418-422] In endemic BL, the chromosome 8 breakpoints are found up to 100 kb 5′ from the MYC exon 1, whereas the chromosome 14 breakpoints occur most often in the IGH joining regions (J_Hs). In contrast, in sporadic and AIDS-associated BL, the chromosome 8 breakpoints are most often located between MYC exons 1 and 2, and those in chromosome 14 are found in the IGH $S\mu$ switch region. In cases with MYC rearrangements involving the light-chain immunoglobulin genes, the breakpoints on chromosome 8 are located at variable distances from the 3′ of the MYC locus,[423,424] and the breakpoints on chromosomes 2 and 22 are located 5′ from the constant region of the IGK and IGL genes. These findings suggest that in sporadic and AIDS-associated BLs with the t(8;14), the chromosome 14 breakpoints are generated during immunoglobulin-class switch recombination. This supports a germinal center B-cell origin for these tumors. In contrast, in endemic BL, the breakpoints on chromosome 14 originate during RAG-mediated variable-diversity-joining (V[D]J) recombination, suggesting that these tumors most probably derive from pre-B cells, which normally express RAG genes, or from germinal center B cells undergoing RAG gene reexpression.[425] In addition, the breakpoints of the translocation t(8;14) also differ between EBV-positive and EBV-negative cases, with breakpoints outside the MYC locus on chromosome 8 associated with EBV positivity and breakpoints within the MYC locus being identified in EBV-negative cases.[419] Notably, immunoglobulin gene analysis has revealed two distinct cells of origin for EBV-positive and EBV-negative cases, irrespective of the subtype (endemic, sporadic, or immunodeficiency-associated BL), suggesting that EBV status rather than the geographic distribution determines the biology of the disease.[426]

The first exon and first intron of c-MYC contain negative transcription regulatory sequences.[427,428] These negative regulators of MYC expression are removed in sporadic BL, with t(8;14) breakpoints located in MYC intron 1. In contrast, in endemic BL and sporadic BL with light-chain gene translocations, the chromosomal breakpoints are located 5′ or 3′ to the MYC locus, respectively. However, in these tumors, the MYC exon 1 and intron 1 are often mutated and show loss of the negative transcriptional regulatory elements located in these regions.[429,430] Thus even though the immunoglobulin enhancers drive high levels of MYC ribonucleic acid (RNA) expression, MYC levels are further increased in BL by the deletion and/or mutation of negative regulatory sequences within the MYC locus.

Additionally, BL tumors often show mutations of MYC at codon 58. These mutations stabilize the MYC protein by disrupting a critical threonine phosphorylation site involved in the proteosomal degradation of this transcription factor.[431-434]

Other Recurrent Genetic Abnormalities. Recent genomic studies have uncovered novel, highly prevalent, genetic alterations involved in the pathogenesis of BLs.[54,435-437] Most prominently, 70% of sporadic and immunodeficiency-associated BLs and 40% of endemic tumors show somatic mutations that activate the transcription factor TCF3 or disrupt the activity of its negative regulator ID3, highlighting a major role for TCF3 activation in B-cell transformation. ID3 mutations (38% to 68%) are more common than TCF3 mutations (11%). Mechanistically, TCF3 modulates essential genes for germinal center function and can activate the prosurvival PI3K pathway by intensifying B-cell receptor signaling. In addition, about 40% of sporadic BLs and a minority of endemic tumors show mutations in the CCND3 cell-cycle regulator, resulting in highly stable CCND3 isoforms that drive cell-cycle progression. These studies also confirmed the presence of mutations in the TP53 tumor-suppressor gene in about 30% of BLs.[438,439] Notably, MYC overexpression can induce apoptosis by TP53-dependent and TP53-independent mechanisms.[440-442] Thus the loss of TP53, which has prominent roles in the control of programmed cell death, may enhance the transforming effects of MYC. Additional highly prevalent mutant genes in BL include those encoding the DDX3X RNA helicase, the SMARCA4 SWI/SNF chromatin regulator, the NCOR2 transcriptional corepressor, the PDCD11 ribosomal RNA maturation factor and the GNA13 G protein signaling factor.

Role of Epstein-Barr Virus. EBV infection is present in 90% of endemic BL cases, 20% of sporadic BL cases, and about 40% of HIV-associated BL cases.[423] Although molecular data have indicated that EBV infection precedes or occurs concomitantly with B-cell transformation,[443] the specific mechanisms whereby EBV infection contributes to the pathogenesis of BL have not been fully elucidated. However, the virally encoded *EBNA-1* gene may play an important role, because it can induce B-cell lymphomas in transgenic mice[444] and has been shown to be essential for EBV-induced B-cell transformation in vitro.[445,446]

Pathologic Features: Diffuse Large B-Cell Lymphomas

DLBCLs are composed of large, transformed lymphoid cells derived from germinal-center and postgerminal-center B cells.[39] DLBCL cells consistently express pax5, CD79a, and CD20, whereas expression of all other B-lineage markers varies. Morphologically, DLBCLs are diverse and can be subdivided into three distinct variants. The centroblastic variant is composed of medium-sized to large cells with basophilic cytoplasm, oval to round nuclei, and two to four membrane-bound nucleoli. The immunoblastic variant has a preponderance of immunoblasts with centrally located nucleoli and basophilic cytoplasm. The anaplastic variant has very large, round, oval, or polygonal cells with bizarre pleomorphic nuclei, which may resemble Reed-Sternberg cells and commonly express CD30. However, this variant is biologically unrelated to ALCL. The centroblastic variant is the most common histiologic type of DLBCL in children.

Other subtypes of DLCBL have been described, including T-cell and histiocyte-rich large B-cell lymphoma. Most cells of this type are nonneoplastic T cells, with or without histiocytes; fewer than 10% of the infiltrate are neoplastic B cells, which resemble immunoblasts, centroblasts, Hodgkin cells, or L&H cells of NLPHL. Because of the predominance of reactive cells, this variant may be misdiagnosed as representing a reactive lymph node. Also, the distinction from NLPHL may be difficult, and an overlap between both cannot be completely excluded.[39]

Complex cytogenetic abnormalities are observed in DLBCL. So far, no entity-specific, nonrandom chromosomal translocations have been described for this subgroup, which may reflect its heterogeneity. In many cases, translocations, including the *c-MYC* locus 8q24, are observed, as well as abnormalities in 3q27, where the protooncogene *BCL6* is located.[447] Based on gene expression profiling, two main subtypes of DLBCL can be distinguished: germinal center B-cell–like (GCB) DLBCL and activated B-cell–like (ABC) DLBCL.[448] The subdivision of DLBCL cases into GCB and ABC subtypes by gene expression analysis could be reproduced by means of immunohistochemistry, applying the germinal-center cell markers CD10 and BCL6, and the postgerminal center marker MUM1.[449] CD10 expression assigned cases to the GCB type independently of *MUM1* expression, but in CD10-negative cases, *BCL6* positivity and negativity for *MUM1* were associated with GCB type. Although indistinguishable from adult DLBCL cases in terms of morphology, DLBCLs in children appear to comprise a biologically distinct subgroup of germinal center B-cell lymphomas.[450] In contrast to adult DLBCL, pediatric DLBCL is predominantly of germinal center origin (6:1) but differs from adult DLBCL of the GCB type in that it

invariably lacks t(14;18).[451] Chromosomal abnormalities in 8q24 including *MYC* rearrangements and gain or amplification of *MYC* are present in 31% and in 50% of pediatric DLBCL cases.[451,452] Additional common chromosomal alterations include losses at 3q and 6q and gains at 1q and 12q.[451,452] In addition, although array-based comparative genomic hybridization (aCGH) analysis has identified genetic lesions shared between adult and pediatric DLBCL (+12q15, +19q13, and −6q), these studies have also highlighted abnormalities unique to the pediatric cases (−4p14, −19q13.32, and +16p11.2).[451]

Clinical Characteristics

In 1958 Denis Burkitt described a "sarcoma involving the jaw in African children," which a short time later was shown by O'Connor to be a lymphoma. Burkitt recognized the endemic nature of the disease.[251] In 1964 viral particles subsequently known as *EBV* were identified in the tumor.[252] Most NHL cases in children in North America and Europe were morphologically indistinguishable from BL. Because there was no geographic limitation and most cases were not associated with EBV infection, they were referred to as *sporadic BLs,* in contrast to the endemic BL of central Africa. According to the WHO classification, three clinical subtypes are recognized. These are morphologically indistinguishable but differ in clinical presentation and biology and include endemic BL, sporadic BL, and immunodeficiency-associated BL.[39] Endemic BL occurs in equatorial Africa, Papua New Guinea, and equatorial regions of South America. In up to 95% of endemic BL cases, the tumor cells carry the EBV genome.[453] Sporadic BL occurs throughout the world in much lower incidence rates as compared with endemic BL. Nevertheless in industrialized countries, BL lymphoma is the most common subtype of NHL in childhood and adolescence and the most common of the mature B-cell neoplasms. In contrast to areas with endemic BL in central Europe, only 10% to 15% of patients with pediatric BL carry the EBV genome.[253,254] Immunodeficiency-associated BL occurs most often in patients with HIV infection but also in patients after solid organ transplantation. The incidence of EBV infection in immunodeficiency-associated BL in North American patients is less than 40%. The incidence of immunodeficiency-associated BL has fallen somewhat with the use of antiretroviral therapy.[416]

The pattern of disease at presentation varies between sporadic and endemic BL and DLBCL. The most common site of disease at presentation for patients with sporadic BL is the abdomen.[454] Common presenting symptoms include abdominal distension, nausea and vomiting, gastrointestinal bleeding, and abdominal pain. A classic although relatively rare presentation of patients with BL is intussusception, where ultrasound imaging reveals evidence of a tumor as a "lead point mass" in the small bowel.[455] Other common sites include the head and neck including cervical nodes, tonsils, and sinuses.

Patients with Burkitt leukemia most often present as a leukemic disease in combination with large tumors.[456] However, in some cases the disease can be confined to the bone marrow without any extramedullary involvement.

In children with Burkitt leukemia, the peripheral blood may show prominent vacuolate lymphoblasts. However, in contrast to pediatric early B-cell ALL, the blast count in the peripheral blood rarely exceeds 30,000/L. In general the degree of anemia and thrombocytopenia is less severe compared with other types of pediatric leukemia, reflecting a lesser degree of bone-marrow invasion.

Patients with endemic BL have classically presenting symptoms of jaw disease, most commonly found in younger children. In addition periorbital findings and abdominal involvement are common. The incidence of symptomatic CNS disease, particularly paraplegia, is much higher than that in the developed world.[265] In low-income countries the majority of patients present with advanced disease, and many are malnourished at the time of diagnosis.[457] By contrast, patients with DLBCL most often have symptoms of nodal disease including involvement of peripheral nodes as well as those in the abdomen and mediastinum. The majority have advanced stage disease, although CNS and bone marrow involvement is rare.

Treatment and Outcome of Mature B-Cell Neoplasms

In adult patients therapy for those with DLBCL and those with BL differs. In children the chemotherapy regimens developed and utilized for patients with BL, who make up of the majority of patients, have proven to be equally effective for those with DLBCL. Hence in the majority of contemporary pediatric protocols the two diseases are treated identically.

Chemotherapy for BL was pioneered in Africa, where Denis Burkitt achieved remission in children with BL with single or few doses of cyclophosphamide, low-dose methotrexate, or vincristine.[458] He recognized that children with a small tumors were more likely to achieve CR than those with large tumors, which suggests a relationship between tumor mass and response.[459] The next important step was the introduction of the combination chemotherapy of cyclophosphamide, vincristine, methotrexate, and cytarabine, which proved not only efficacious for African children with endemic BL but also for American patients with sporadic BL.[460,461] The high incidence of CNS relapses and the failure of cranial irradiation to prevent them was described by this group, leading to the introduction of combined intrathecal chemotherapy.[460,462,463] Based on the African experience, Ziegler and colleagues first explored the principle of dose intensity and achieved CRs with high-dose chemotherapy in American patients with BL that was unresponsive to lower dose therapy.[464]

In the 1980s, treatment strategies were further improved by the emerging information about the peculiar biologic features of BL. A most important characteristic regarding therapeutic strategy is its high proliferation activity. BL cells cycle extremely rapidly, with an estimated generation time of only 25 hours.[465] It can be estimated that within 48 to 72 hours, every Burkitt cell is likely to traverse the cell cycle, thereby encompassing a period of greatest sensitivity to cytotoxic treatment.[466-468] Based on this knowledge, combination chemotherapy courses were designed based on the principle of maintaining—by means of frac-

tionated administration or continuous infusion—cytotoxically active drug concentrations for the length of time needed to affect as many lymphoma cells as possible during the vulnerable active cell cycle.[469-472] Therapeutic regimens that adhere to the principle of rapidly repeated cycles of dose-intensive combination chemotherapy have resulted in a dramatic increase in the cure rate over the last several decades from less than 40% to greater than 85%.[473]

Although there are few randomized trials testing the impact of individual drugs there is considerable evidence that cyclophosphamide and methotrexate may be key agents. Monotherapy with methotrexate or with cyclophosphamide, with or without low-dose methotrexate and vincristine can induce durable remissions in BL.[458,461,474] The important role of methotrexate can be extrapolated from the effect of different dosages. In patients with stage III disease and high tumor mass (LDH >500 U/L, approximately twice or more the upper limit of normal for age), and in patients with Burkitt leukemia, a 10-fold increase of the dose of methotrexate from 0.5 to 5 g/m^2 resulted in significantly improved outcome.[456,475] Similarly, the elevation of the dose of methotrexate from 3 to 8 g/m^2 in the Societe Francaise d'Oncologie Pediatrque-Lymphoma Maligancy B (SFOP-LMB) protocols resulted in an excellent outcome of patients with advanced-stage BL, including those with CNS involvement.[266,476,477] Comparatively little evidence exists as to the role of corticosteroids and anthracyclines. In a CCG study of the 1980s, addition of daunomycin to the combination of cyclophosphamide, vincristine, methotrexate, and prednisone (COMP) did not improve the outcome of patients with advanced-stage non-LL as compared with COMP alone.[478]

The therapeutic strategies used for children with mature B-cell lymphomas are associated with significant short-term toxicity including severe mucositis and risks of infections. The mucosal toxicity is caused primarily, but not solely, by high-dose methotrexate. In patients with significant mucositis together with the severe neutropenia, risks of bacteremia (often from intestinal flora) are high. Patients with advanced disease stages are at the greatest risk. For these patients, the rate of toxicity-induced death is up to 5%, even in the most recent treatment studies.[266,475] Postchemotherapeutic application of granulocyte colony-stimulating factor (G-CSF) had no effect on treatment-related toxicity, as demonstrated in a randomized trial.[479] Toxicity and the risk of toxic death is greatest during and after the first treatment course.

Risk stratification for patients with BL and DLBCL is of critical importance, allowing for allocation to the most appropriate treatment regimen. Treatment regimens vary in intensity based on the number of drugs used, their dosage, and the number of treatment courses that have obvious implications for both short- and long-term toxicities. Criteria used to stratify patients include stage, LDH level, and CNS involvement but have differed somewhat between cooperative groups (Table 53-15). Other prognostic factors include poor response to "reduction therapy" with cyclophosphamide, prednisone, and vincristine; poor-risk cytogenetics; and mediastinal disease.[473,480] The genetic changes detectable by karyotype associated

TABLE 53-15   Treatment Stratification and Results in Two Large Multicenter Trials of Pediatric Mature B-Cell Neoplasms

Group	Definition	Patients, N (% of all patients)	EFS (%)	Chemotherapy Courses (Randomized Study Questions)	Outcome
FAB-LMB96 Trial[269,483,606]					
A	Stage I, resected; stage II, abdominal, resected	132 (12%)	98 (4 year)	COPAD-COPAD	2 courses of therapy and no intrathecal treatment is curative in patients with resected localized disease.
B	Stage I + II not resected; Stage III Stage IV with bone-marrow blasts <25%	657 (67%)	90 (4 year)	COP-COPADM1-COPADM2-CYM-CYM-M1 (randomization for complete responders after COPADM1 to therapy reduction verus standard)	Therapy reductions of 50% dose reduction of cyclophosphamide and omission of M1 was equally as efficacious as the standard regimen.
C	>25% bone-marrow blasts and/or CNS+ nonresponder to COP of group B	235 (21%)	79 (4 year)	COP-COPADM1-COPADM2-CYVE1-CYVE2-M1-M2-M3-M4 (randomization for complete responders after COPADM1 + M2)	Therapy reductions of reduced intensity "mini-CYVE" and omission of M2, M3, and M4 resulted in inferior outcome.
NHL-BFM95[484]					
R1	Stages I + II, resected	48 (10%)	94	A-B (randomization: methotrexate IV over 24 hr vs. 4 hr)	Methotrexate over 4 hr less toxic, equally efficacious
R2	Stages I + II, not resected; stage III, LDH <500/U/L	233 (46%)	94	p-A-B A-B (randomization: methotrexate IV over 24 hr vs. 4 hr)	Methotrexate over 4 hr less toxic, equally efficacious
R3	Stage III, LDH 500-999 U/L Stage IV and LDH <1000U/L and CNS–	82 (16%)	85	p-AA-BB-CC-AA-BB (randomization: methotrexate in AA, BB IV over 24 hr vs. 4 hr)	Methotrexate over 4 hr less toxic but in this group less effective
R4	Stage III + IV and LDH ≥1000 U/L and/or CNS+	142 (28%)	81	p-AA-BB-CC-AA-BB-CC (randomization: methotrexate in AA, BB IV over 24 hr vs. 4 hr)	Methotrexate over 4 hr less toxic but in this group less effective

COP, Cyclophosphamide, vincristine, prednisone; *COPAD,* cyclophosphamide, vincristine (Oncovin), prednisolone, and doxorubicin; *CYM,* cytarabine, methotrexate; *CYVE,* cytarabine, etoposide; *EFS,* event-free survival; *FAB-LMB,* French-American-British–lymphoma malignancy B; *LDH,* lactate dehydrogenase; *M,* maintenance; *NHL-BFM,* Non-Hodgkin Lymphoma–Berlin-Frankfurt-Munster.

with an inferior outcome are +7q and deletion (13)q.[452] The presence of minimal disseminated disease in the bone marrow at diagnosis has also been found to be associated with a worse prognosis.[481] The use of bone marrow monitoring for assessment of responses to therapy and persistence of minimal residual disease may be of importance in the future.[482] Within pediatric protocols neither age (older or younger than 15 years) or histology (BL versus DLBCL) is prognostic.

Patients with localized disease have excellent outcomes with an EFS rate approaching 100%. The international study FAB-LMB96 enrolled patients of all disease stages. One hundred and thirty two patients with resected stage I or completely resected abdominal stage II disease were treated with two courses of cyclophosphamide, vincristine, prednisolone, and doxorubicin (COPAD) without intrathecal therapy. The 4-year EFS and OS rates were 98.3% and 99.2%, respectively.[483] In the NHL-BFM95 study, 48 patients with completely resected stage I or II disease were treated with two courses of therapy which

include dexamethasone, vincristine, ifosfamide, cytarabine, etoposide, cyclophosphamide, doxorubicin, and methotrexate in addition to intrathecal triple therapy and had a 3-year EFS rate of 94%.[484]

Patients defined as having intermediate-risk disease according to the FAB-LMB protocols, the "group B" patients (see Table 53-15) compromise the largest group. These are individuals with unresected stage I or II disease, those with stage III or IV disease without CNS involvement, or those with bone marrow disease meeting criteria for Burkitt leukemia. This patient group also has an excellent outcome with modern intensive therapy. Patients in the FAB-LMB96 study were randomized in a 2-×-2 factorial design to evaluate two-dose reduction questions, reduction of cyclophosphamide dose, and removal of a maintenance cycle of therapy. Six hundred and fifty seven patients with intermediate-risk disease were randomized. The 4-year EFS and OS rates were 90.9% and 93.4%, respectively, with no significant difference across study arms. Patients in the NHL-BFM95 study with stage I or

II unresected disease or those with stage III disease with a low LDH who received four courses of chemotherapy also had a similarly favorable outcome with 3-year EFS rate of 94%.[484]

The use of LDH for stratification of treatment intensity is a major difference between the FAB-LMB and the NHL-BFM studies (see Table 53-15). The serum concentration of LDH, considered a proxy for tumor mass, may vary largely in patients at the same stage, especially for those with stage-III BL. Although not used prospectively for risk assignment on the FAB-LMB study, analysis of patients enrolled showed that LDH greater than two times the institutional upper limit of normal was a significant risk factor for an inferior outcome.[480] The current international study of childhood B-cell lymphoma, InterB-NHL 2010 Ritux defines a group of patients with high-risk disease in part based on LDH.

Patients with high-risk disease in the LMB studies have been defined as those with CNS disease (parenchymal brain involvement, cranial nerve palsies, or CSF disease) or those with Burkitt leukemia (bone marrow with >25% blasts). BL accounts for 70% to 80% of the patients in this group. The EFS and OS rates of this patient group approaches 80%. Reduction of therapy in patients with high-risk disease has not been successful, as it has been for the low- and intermediate-risk groups. In the FAB-LMB96 study the 4-year EFS rate for all patients with high risk was 79%.[269] For those who had responsive disease and therefore were eligible for randomization, the EFS was 90% for those receiving standard therapy and 80% for those receiving reduced intensity therapy. This difference led to the closure of the randomization and assignment of subsequent patients to the standard therapy arm. The NHL BFM95 evaluated the reduction of high-dose methotrexate-related toxicity by shortening the infusion time. Unlike in patients with lower risk where shorter infusion times had similar disease control but less toxicity, in patients with high risk changing the infusion time for the high-dose methotrexate from the standard 24 hours to only 4 hours resulted in an excess of tumor failures in patients with advanced disease.[484] The 3-year EFS rate for R3 and R4 groups (groups described in Table 53-15) overall were 85% and 81%, respectively. Combined, the R3 and R4 groups who received a shorter (4-hour) methotrexate infusion had an EFS rate of 77% versus 93% for those who received the longer (24-hour) infusion.

The group of patients with the worst outcome with current therapy is that of patients with CNS disease, defined by blasts in the CNS, cranial nerve palsies, or an intracranial mass. Among these patients the subgroup with the least favorable prognosis is those with blasts detectable in the CSF at the time of diagnosis, with EFS of 70% to 75% in FAB and BFM trials.[269,484]

Rituximab, the monoclonal chimeric anti-CD20 antibody, when added to conventional chemotherapy for adults with mature B-cell NHL, significantly improves outcomes.[485-487] For children and adolescents it is not part of standard therapy, primarily based on lack of evidence of efficacy in this patient group. Given the favorable outcome of children with conventional chemotherapy, the significant differences between chemotherapy regimens used in children and adults and the biologic difference in pediatric B-cell NHL, the adoption of the data from adult studies cannot be simply applied to pediatric care. Rituximab has shown to be active as a single agent when given upfront in a window trial before conventional therapy for children with B-cell NHL.[488] The COG has established the safety of combining rituximab with FAB-LMB96 therapy in a single-arm pilot trial of patients with high-risk disease.[489] The current international phase III trial for patients with high-risk B-cell NHL, InterB-NHL_2010_ritux will randomize patients to therapy based on the FAB backbone with or without rituximab to gather the needed data regarding efficacy.

Primary Central Nervous System DLBCL. Primary CNS NHL is exceptionally rare in children and adolescents. Most primary CNS NHLs of childhood are of the diffuse large B-cell subtype, though other histologies have been described.[265,490] In a large cohort of 2170 patients of the NHL-BFM studies, only 10 patients were observed with primary CNS lymphoma.[265] The estimated incidence in children in North America is 15 to 20 cases per year.[491] Most cases present with unifocal or multifocal intraparenchymal masses but some patients have meningeal disease only or combinations of both. The clinical features resemble those of brain tumors characterized by signs of increased intracranial pressure with headache, nausea and vomiting, and visual changes, as well as cranial nerve palsies, personality changes, and endocrinologic disturbances.

As with other rare tumors, optimal therapy in children and adolescents with primary CNS lymphoma is not clear. Treatment analogous to what patients who have CNS involvement as a component of more disseminated disease would receive has been effective in the BFM series.[265] The largest case series of pediatric patients with isolated CNS disease included 29 patients treated in various regimens with the majority receiving methotrexate-based regimens and one third receiving radiation in addition to chemotherapy. The 2-year OS rate was 82%.[492] The use of intrathecal rituximab combined with intrathecal methotrexate in adult patients with recurrent B-cell CNS lymphoma in a phase-I trial showed it to be feasible and active, although results have not been reported in children.[493]

Therapy of Relapsed Disease

Given the effectiveness of primary therapy, relapses are relatively rare. When they do occur, patients with BL generally relapse within 6 months from the time of completion of therapy. The period of risk is somewhat longer for those with DLBCL. Patients with primary refractory or relapsed B-cell NHL have a dismal prognosis. In a cohort of patients diagnosed with BL between 1977 and 1997, only 12% of those with relapsed disease survived.[494] There is no standard reinduction regimen for these patients. Commonly used regimens have included ICE as well as ifosfamide, etoposide and high-dose cytarabine.[416] A COG study evaluated the effectiveness of rituximab in addition to ICE therapy and showed a response rate of 60%. Six of the 20 patients were able to proceed in to

SCT. The OS rate at 3 years was 37%, with a majority of the survivors having received either an autologous or allogeneic SCT.[495] Retrospective data from the Center for International Blood and Marrow Transplant Research (CIBMTR) between 1990 and 2005 showed similar outcomes for both autologous and allogeneic SCT for patients with relapsed BL (31% and 27%, respectively) and DLCBL (50% and 52%, respectively).[411]

Anaplastic Large-Cell Lymphoma

ALCL accounts for 10% to 15 % of childhood NHL.[496] ALCL was first described by Stein and colleagues[18] in 1985, followed by the discovery of the nonrandom translocation of t(2:5) (p23; q35), causing the fusion of nucleophosmin (NPM) to the anaplastic lymphoma kinase (ALK) in a majority of the cases.[497,498] The disease has multiple features that are unlike other pediatric NHL subtypes, including the sites of involvement of disease at diagnosis and the responsiveness of relapsed disease to therapy as well as unique biologic features.

Pathologic Features

ALCL is characterized by large pleomorphic cells of a T/null immunophenotype. The morphology is variable but includes cells with eccentric horseshoe-shaped nuclei, called the *hallmark cells*.[39] A number of histologic variants have been described, including the common variant, characterized by sheets of large lymphoid cells; the lymphohistiocytic variant, characterized by a large number of reactive histiocytes that may even mask the anaplastic tumor cell population and can therefore be misdiagnosed as reactive histiocytic disease or malignant histiocytosis[40]; the small-cell variant, characterized by a predominant population of small to medium sized neoplastic cells with irregular nuclei[499,500]; and other rare variants including the giant cell variant, sarcomatoid variant, and neutrophil-rich variant. In some cases, mixtures of histologic subtypes are observed in one lesion, whereas in other patients different subtypes can be seen in different lesions.[500] In addition, in patients with relapsed disease the morphology of disease at relapse may be a different variant than was present at initial diagnosis.[501]

ALCL is CD30-positive on the cell membrane, particularly on large cells and in the Golgi region.[29] ALK detection is reliably measured by immunohistochemistry.[502] Cells express T-cell markers including CD2, CD5, and CD4, although the null-cell phenotype may not express several pan–T-cell antigens.[39]

ALK-negative ALCL is a unique disease category in the WHO classification. It is morphologically indistinguishable from the ALK-positive disease but lacks the expression of the ALK protein.[25] It accounts for less than 10% of pediatric disease and unlike in adult patients, has not been found to be associated with a worse prognosis in children.[273,274,500,503,504]

Molecular and Cellular Biology

The clonal nature of ALCL has been confirmed by the detection of the nonrandom chromosomal translocation t(2;5)(p23;q35) in malignant cells.[497,505,506] This translocation causes the NPM gene located at 5q35 to fuse with

a gene at 2p23 encoding the receptor tyrosine kinase ALK.[498] The production of monoclonal antibodies directed against fixative-resistant epitopes of ALK allows its detection by immunohistochemistry.[507,508] Although the translocation t(2;5)(p23;q35) is the most common, more than 10 other chromosomal translocations juxtaposing the ALK gene at chromosome 2p23 to a partner gene have been detected. The partner gene of ALK determines the immunohistochemical ALK staining pattern. Only the NPM-ALK fusion protein is detectable in the cytoplasm and the nucleus because of the heterodimerization of the NPM portion with normal NPM, which functions in the nuclear shuttling of proteins.[509] All other fusion-gene products lacking the NPM portion are detectable only in the cytoplasm. Conversely, the ALK staining pattern, cytoplasmic and nuclear versus extranuclear, distinguishes the NPM-ALK translocation from all others.[510] In children, more than 90% of ALCL cases are ALK-positive.[273]

The cellular origin of ALCL is still not completely clarified. The vast majority express T-lineage antigens, have clonally rearranged TCR genes, and express the cytotoxic molecules perforin, granzyme B, and T-cell–restricted intracellular antigen (TIA) 1.[511] However, findings of plasmablastic B-cell lymphoma carrying the translocation t(2 ;5) and expressing NPM-ALK transcripts have suggested that the translocation involving ALK may not be restricted to ALCLs of T-cell lineage.[512] In a minority of cases, the expression of the natural killer (NK) cell–associated marker CD56 and the lack of detectable TCR gene rearrangements suggest an origination from NK cells rather than cytotoxic T cells.[511,513,514]

In most cases, ALCL occurs as a de novo malignant lymphoma. On rare occasions, however, ALCL appears as a secondary lymphoma that evolves from a low-grade or high-grade malignant T-cell lymphoma, Hodgkin lymphoma, or lymphomatoid papulosis.[515-518]

As mentioned, the most characteristic molecular feature of ALCL is the presence of gene rearrangements involving the ALK locus in chromosome band 2p23. ALK is a transmembrane receptor tyrosine kinase of the insulin receptor superfamily normally expressed only in cells of neural origin. ALCL translocations lead to the aberrant expression and constitutive activation of ALK.[519] The most common of these translocations present in 80% of ALCL cases is the t(2;5)(p23;q35).[520,521] In this translocation, the 5' region of the NPM gene on chromosome 5q35 is fused to the ALK gene.[498,521-523] NPM is a ubiquitously expressed nucleolar phosphoprotein involved in the shuttling of ribonucleoproteins between the nucleus and cytoplasm.[524] The NPM-ALK fusion oncogene resulting from the t(2;5)(p23;q35) translocation encodes a constitutively active form of ALK,[521] which promotes cell transformation in vitro[509,525] and in vivo[526] by phosphorylating and activating important mediators in a number of critical signaling pathways such as PLCG, PI3K-AKT-mTOR, JAK2, STAT3, STAT5, and MEK-ERK.[519,522,527]

In addition to the t(2;5)(p23;q35) rearrangement, several other chromosomal translocations involving the ALK gene have been found in 20% of ALK-positive ALCL cases. All these rearrangements result in the fusion of the catalytic domain of ALK with different partners, such as tropomyosin (TPM) 3 and TPM4, TGF, ATIC, clathrin heavy chain, moesin, AL017, TSPYL2, KIAA1618, VCL, KIF5B, and MYH9,[519,527] and result in constitutively active ALK phosphorylation and activation.[521,528] All partners except MYH9 provide dimerization domains, leading to the dimerization of the fusions and to the constitutive activation of the kinase.[528] The importance of the elucidation of constitutively active ALK as a major mechanism in the transformation of ALCL is highlighted by the development of specific ALK inhibitors. These may provide a targeted therapeutic strategy for treatment of this disease.[529]

In addition to ALK rearrangements, ALCLs also show other chromosomal alterations; however, few recurrent somatic lesions have been reported. About 25% of ALCLs display recurrent deletions affecting the 17p13.3-p12 region where the TP53 gene is located, and 19% of cases show losses of 6q21 encompassing the PRDM1 and ATG5 genes.

Clinical Features

Most children and adolescents with ALCL have presenting symptoms of advanced stage disease. Almost all have lymphadenopathy at diagnosis, but 60% also have extranodal disease, most often involving soft tissue and skin followed by bone and lung.[274,503,504,530-532] Patients may have an indolent phase consisting of lymphadenopathy, which in some instances may be waxing and waning and sometimes associated with a history of illness including fever and other B symptoms.[516,533] Soft-tissue involvement may occur as multiple tumors in the subcutaneous tissue and muscles, or as a single larger tumor resembling a soft-tissue sarcoma. Bone manifestations vary from small osteolytic lesions to large tumors simulating bone tumors. Skin lesions may be single or multiple bluish-colored cutaneous or subcutaneous nodules, large ulcerated lesions or multiple or disseminated papillomatous lesions of a red-yellow color.

Compared with patients with BL or LL, the incidence of microscopically detectable bone-marrow disease at the time of diagnosis is lower. Occasionally, marked hemophagocytosis by macrophages can be observed in the bone marrow of patients with ALCL. In rare cases, disseminated intravascular coagulation of yet unknown pathogenesis has been observed as a paraneoplastic syndrome.[534] CNS disease is rare in patients with ALCL, affecting 1% to 4% of children.

Treatment and Outcomes

Prognostic Factors. Prognostic factors based on standard on clinical information used for informing treatment decisions have been less well-defined for patients with ALCL compared with other pediatric lymphomas. As with other NHLs, lower-stage disease is thought to be favorable. In the BFM90 study, nine patients with stage I and II resected disease had an EFS rate of 100% at 5 years with three courses of therapy.[274] A report including 36 patients with stage I disease on the ALCL99 study showed that those who had completely resected disease and received short-course chemotherapy also had an EFS

rate of 100%, whereas those with incompletely resected disease had a relapse rate of 30%, similar to patients with higher-stage disease.[535]

A study that combined patients from three cooperative groups found that poor prognostic risk factors included disease involving the mediastinum, visceral involvement (lung, liver, or spleen), or skin lesions. Factors not significant in multivariate analysis included stage, B symptoms, and level of LDH.[536] In contrast to adults with ALCL, the ALK1 positivity or negativity had no significant impact on outcome for children and adolescents.[273,274] However, this may be partly related to the relatively rarity of ALK-negative disease in children and therefore there is limited power to detect outcome differences.

Two specific tests, both unique to patients with ALK-positive ALCL and both done at the time of diagnosis, have been found to have prognostic significance in children with ALCL: the titer of anti-ALK antibodies in blood and copy number of NPM-ALK transcripts measured by quantitative PCR of bone marrow. Patients with ALK-positive ALCL often have measurable autoantibodies to ALK at the time of presentation with disease.[508] In a study of 95 uniformly treated pediatric patients with ALK-positive ALCL, an increased level of ALK autoantibodies in the patient's serum from the time of diagnosis correlated with a significantly lower incidence of relapse, suggesting that a preexisting immune response to the antigen product of the disease-specific translocation was protective from the risk of relapse.[537] Patients with morphologic involvement of their bone marrow make up a small proportion of those with ALCL. In a study of 80 pediatric patients with ALK-positive ALCL, only eight had morphologic evidence of bone-marrow involvement, but by assessing these samples with PCR, it was determined that 47.5% had detectable NPM-ALK transcript in these bone marrow samples. Using quantitative PCR it was found that those with a higher level of NPM-ALK transcript detection had a significantly higher rate of relapse.[538] When the two tests were combined from three patients groups treated in similar though not identical ways, three risk groups could be identified with dramatically different rates of progression survival. Twenty percent of patients had evidence of minimal disseminated disease as determined by PCR and had low or negative antibody titers. This high-risk group had a progression-free survival (PFS) rate of 28%. Conversely those who were negative for minimal disseminated disease and had high antibody titers, 31% of the patients, had a PFS rate of 93%. The intermediate-risk group, which included all others and accounted for 48% of the patients, had a PFS rate of 68%.[539] Replication of these findings and use in patient stratification are components of current and planned cooperative group trials.

Treatment. There is no consensus on optimal therapy for ALCL. Some groups have used brief intensive therapy, similar to that used for mature B-cell disease, whereas others have investigated more prolonged repeated pulse chemotherapy. EFS rates are very similar across studies even with the use of these variable chemotherapy regimens (Table 53-16).

TABLE 53-16   Prospective Randomized Trials of Childhood and Adolescent Anaplastic Large-Cell Lymphoma

Study Protocol (years)	No of Patients	Description of Therapy	Primary Study Question and Design	EFS at 3-5 Years	Primary Study Outcome
NHL-BFM90 (90-95)[274]	89	Short-pulse B NHL-type therapy: Stage I/II resected, 3 courses; Stage II non resected, stage III, 6 courses; Stage IV, 6 intensified courses; 2-5 months	Effectiveness of therapeutic regimen in nonselected group of uniformly treated patients, non randomized	76%	Short-pulse B NHL therapy is effective in ALCL.
POG (94-00)[530]	180	APO-based therapy for patients with large-cell lymphoma, both ALCL and DLBCL 12 months	Evaluation of intensified therapy with intermediate dose methotrexate and high-dose Ara-C, randomized between two regimens postinduction	71%	Intensification of therapy did not improve EFS and increased toxicity.
EICNHL (99-05)[504]	352	Short-pulse B NHL-type therapy; 5 months	Evaluation of modification of methotrexate dose and infusion time with or without intrathecal therapy, of efficacy of therapy with 3 g/m^2 over 3 hours versus 1 gm/m^2 over 24 hours	74% at 2 years	Methotrexate at 3 g/m^2 over 3 hours was as effective and less toxic than a lower dosage with prolonged infusion plus intrathecal therapy. Addition of vinblastine in maintenence delayed relapse but did not impact 2-yr EFS.
ALCL99 (99-06)[503]	110	Short-pulse B NHL-type therapy; 5 months	Evaluation of addition of vinblastine in maintenence versus no maintenence	70%-73% at 2 years	Addition of vinblastine in maintanence delayed relapse but did not impact 2-yr EFS.
COG[542]	125	APO-based therapy; 12 months	Evaluation of vincristine versus vinblastine in postinduction	76% at 3 years	No benefit was found with the use of vinblastine compared with vincristine; vinblastine administration was limited by myelotoxicity.

ALCL, Anaplastic large-cell lymphoma; *APO,* doxorubicin, vincristine, prednisone, 6-mercaptopurine, and low-dose methotrexate; *Ara-C,* cytarabine; *COG,* Children's Oncology Group; *DLBCL,* diffuse large B-cell lymphoma; *EFS,* event-free survival; *EICNHL,* European Intergroup for Childhood Non-Hodgkin Lymphoma; *NHL,* non-Hodgkin lymphoma; *NHL-BFM,* Non-Hodgkin Lymphoma–Berlin-Frankfurt-Munster; *POG,* Pediatric Oncology Group.

Analysis of patients from three consecutive BFM trials showed that the use of B-cell NHL short-pulse therapy was effective for the ALCL group, with a 5-year EFS rate of 76%.[540] In the BFM90 trial, 89 patients with ALCL were treated. In this trial patients were divided into three groups based on stage: K1, stage I and II resected; K2, stage II nonresected and stage III; and K3, stage IV or those with multifocal bone involvement. All groups received a prephase treatment and then 3 to 6 cycles of therapy lasting 2 to 5 months, with the K3 group's therapy intensified primarily by higher dose methotrexate. With this regimen the OS rate at 5 years for the whole group was again 76%.[274] Of the patients that did relapse, the vast majority did so within 15 months of the completion of therapy. Relapses occurred at both original and new sites.

After the BFM90 trial, a large randomized study, ALCL99, was conducted by the European Intergroup for Childhood Non-Hodgkin Lymphoma (EICNHL) and designed to address two questions in patients with ALCL. The first task was to assess the safety and efficacy of two methotrexate regimens (3 g/m^2 over 3 hours with no intrathecal therapy versus 1 g/m^2 over 24 hours with intrathecal therapy). The 2-year EFS rate was identical in the two arms at 74%, although the shorter high-dose methotrexate arm was associated with less toxicity. There was no difference in CNS relapses. Again in this trial it was noted that almost all of the relapses occurred within 2 years from completion of therapy.[503]

The second question addressed in ALCL99 included only the high-risk patients, defined as those with mediastinal, lung, liver, spleen, or skin involvement. Eligible patients were randomized to receive vinblastine concurrent with intensive therapy and as a single-drug maintenance regimen for a total duration of therapy of 1 year versus the standard backbone therapy and no maintenance.[503] At 1 year from the time of randomization the EFS rate for those receiving vinblastine was superior (91% versus 74%), but by 2 years the difference was no longer present with an EFS rate of 73% and 70% respectively. The conclusion was that vinblastine delivered in this manner delayed recurrences but did not impact the overall outcome.[503]

In North America POG performed a series of clinical trials evaluating modifications of the APO therapy backbone.[530,541] APO therapy involves the use of doxorubicin, prednisone, and vincristine in addition to 6-mercaptopurine, low dose methotrextae and intrathecal therapy given as multiple cycles over 2 years in the outpatient setting. This therapy includes a cumulative anthracycline dose of 300 mg/m². Patients in these earlier studies included those with advanced-stage disease and with both DLBCL and T-cell phenotype large-cell lymphoma. In these studies, neither intensifying therapy with cyclophosphamide or with intermediate-dose methotrexate and high-dose cytarabine had an impact of EFS, with no statistical difference in outcome between randomized arms in either study. The 4-year EFS rate for the subgroup of ALCL patients, irrespective of randomized therapy, was 71%.[530] Analogous to the pattern in the European trails, the majority of relapses occurred within 2 years of diagnosis.

Subsequent to these studies and analogous to the ALCL99 trial, the COG investigated the impact of vinblastine in the context of APO therapy. In the trial, patients were randomized between treatment with vincristine or vinblastine as part of multiagent maintenance therapy based on the APO backbone. No benefit was found with the use of vinblastine compared with vincristine, although the ability to administer the vinblastine at the originally planned doses was hampered by cytopenias.[542]

The incidence of CNS relapse in patients who are initially CNS-negative is very low, with therapy protocols that involve corticosteroids and systemic methotrexate therapy with or without intrathecal therapy.[265,273,274,516] Prophylactic cranial irradiation is unnecessary. In the European intergroup trial ALCL99 based on the treatment strategy of the NHL-BFM90 study, including dexamethasone as a corticosteroid, it was shown that systemic methotrexate, 3 g/m², given as an IV infusion for 3 hours, is sufficient CNS protection for patients without overt CNS disease at diagnosis, and additional intrathecal chemotherapy is not necessary.[534] Because of the small numbers of patients with overt CNS disease at diagnosis, no conclusions can be drawn about optimal treatment in this circumstance. Therapeutic cranial irradiation with doses of 18 to 24 Gy, depending on age, may be efficacious in addition to high-dose methotrexate and high-dose cytarabine combined with triple-drug intrathecal therapy.[273,274]

Treatment of Relapsed Anaplastic Large-Cell Lymphoma

One of the unique features of ALCL compared with other pediatric NHLs is its sensitivity to chemotherapy after recurrence. Of particular interest is the experience of maintenance of prolonged second remissions with single-agent vinblastine. A report of 41 children with relapsed disease enrolled in three consecutive French Society of Pediatric Oncology trials described outcomes with various second-line therapies.[543] Thirty-six of 41 patients (88%) were able to achieve a second complete response. The overall and disease-free survival rates were 69% and 44%, respectively, at 3 years. In this series it was noted that eight of 13 patients had long-lasting remissions with single-agent vinblastine therapy alone. A second report described the experience with 30 patients treated with single-agent vinblastine most commonly given at a dose of 6 mg/m² weekly, for varying durations, at varying time points in the patient's disease course, although the majority were treated for first of second relapse.[504] Fifty percent of the patients had a preceding SCT before their vinblastine therapy. The CR rate for the whole group was 83%. The 5-year EFS and OS rates for the whole group were 30% and 65%. Of note, 30% of those treated with vinblastine only remained in CR.

ALCL is characterized in part by its expression of CD30. Monoclonal antibody therapy directed at CD30 has shown to be safe but with limited activity in early phase studies in adult patients.[544] Brentuximab vedotin (SGN-35) is an antibody drug conjugate combing an anti-CD30 antibody with a potent microtubule inhibitor, monomethylauristatin E (MMAE). A phase-II study in adult patients with primary refractory or relapsed ALK-positive or ALK-negative ALCL showed very encouraging results.[545] Eighty-six percent (50/58) of heavily pretreated patients had a response to therapy, and 57% obtained complete response to monotherapy with brentuximab vedotin. Toxicity was modest, including cytopenias and peripheral neuropathy. Studies evaluating the safety and efficacy of this agent in children and in combination with conventional chemotherapies as part of initial therapy and therapy for relapsed disease for patients with both Hodgkin lymphoma and ALCL are being undertaken.

Another extremely exciting agent for the treatment of children and adolescents with ALK-positive ALCL is crizotinib, a small-molecule inhibitor of ALK tyrosine kinase. Two adult patients with refractory ALK-positive ALCL were able to obtain a complete response with crizotinib.[546] In the pediatric setting it is being investigated in early-phase studies for patients with ALK-positive disease including ALCL and neuroblastoma.[547] Given the early indications of safety of the drug and of efficacy in patients with ALCL, plans for evaluating crizotinib in conjunction with standard chemotherapy in newly diagnosed patients are being pursued by the COG.[232]

Rare Lymphomas in Children and Adolescents

LL, mature B-cell lymphomas, and ALCL account for the vast majority of NHLs diagnosed in children and adolescents; however approximately 10% of cases are made up of an array of much rarer entities, some of which are much more commonly seen in adults. A discussion of some of these rare tumors is included below.

Primary Mediastinal (Thymic) Large B-Cell Lymphoma

Primary mediastinal (thymic) large B-cell lymphoma (PMBCL) is a DLBCL with unique clinical, histologic, and genetic characteristics that have justified its being identified as a unique entity in the WHO classification system for lymphomas.[39] Microscopically a prominent compartmentalizing sclerosis dominates the histologic appearance. The malignant cells are of putative thymic B-cell origin and are large, often pleomorphic, lymphoid cells with abundant pale cytoplasm. The cells express CD45 and B-lineage markers such as CD19, CD20, and CD79a, but surface immunoglobulin is usually absent. Contrary to DLBCL, PMLBL cells do not express CD10 or *BCL6* and *BCL2*.[548] The neoplastic cells may express CD30, although usually less strongly than in Hodgkin lymphoma.

PMBCL usually presents with symptoms emanating from the effects of a large mediastinal mass such as cough, shortness of breath, and signs and symptoms of SVC syndrome. The tumor generally spreads locally with invasion into the pleura, pericardium, and lungs but may also involve the liver.[549] Bone-marrow and CNS involvement is exceptionally rare.[550]

The prognosis for pediatric patients with PMBCL has been less favorable than for the other mature B-cell lymphomas. Multiple pediatric international cooperative group studies have reported remarkably consistent outcome data with a 5-year EFS rate of 66% to 67% and an OS rate of 73% to 79%.[551,552] The best results reported to date are from a case series of adult patients treated with rituximab in addition to the combination chemotherapy regime of dose-adjusted etoposide, prednisone, vincristine (Oncovin), cyclophosphamide, and doxorubicin (hydroxydaunorubicin) (EPOCH).[553] The importance of radiotherapy in this group of patients is controversial, with some adult studies reporting improved outcome with IFRT, whereas its impact on patient outcomes in the combined pediatric data showed no advantage.[551,554] The international pediatric B-cell study (interB NHL-ritux-2010) will evaluate the use of dose-adjusted EPOCH with rituximab in a single-arm phase-II component of the larger trial.

Juvenile Follicular Lymphoma

FL is a common diagnosis in adults with NHL but is very rare in children, accounting for fewer than 2% of all pediatric cases. In the 2008 WHO classification of lymphomas, pediatric FL is identified as a unique entity based on patient age but also on the unique biologic features including lack of *BCL2* expression and absence of t(14:18) in the majority of cases.[39] Pediatric FL tends to be of higher grade than its adult counterpart.[555] Children with FL generally have a presentation of low-stage disease, most often involving cervical nodes, other peripheral nodes, Waldeyer ring, or isolated testicular disease. The outcome for children with FL is very favorable including a small number of patients successfully treated with surgical resection alone, although the majority of patients have been treated with brief courses of multiagent chemotherapy.[556-558] Unlike in adult patients, the use of rituximab in the treatment of pediatric FL has not been investigated.[559]

Peripheral T-Cell Lymphomas

Peripheral T-cell lymphomas (PTCLs) other than ALCLs are rare in childhood and account for fewer than 1% of cases. They represent a heterogeneous group of neoplasms, with the most common histology among pediatric patients being PTCL, not otherwise specified. The clinical features, histology, and genetic features are variable by subtype.[39]

Data in children and adolescents with non-ALCL PTCL are limited to several case series and a number of case reports but suggest that the outcome of these patients is inferior compared with that of the more common pediatric NHL histologies.[560-563] Patients with lower-stage disease have a more favorable outcome, although the majority of patients have presenting symptoms of advanced stage disease. The optimal therapy for patients with non-ALCL PTCL is unclear, with some groups suggesting B-cell NHL–type therapy and others T-cell leukemia/lymphoma–like therapy, and with some data supporting specific therapies based on specific histology. In addition, the role of high-dose therapy and autologous or allogeneic transplant in the management of pediatric patients remain unclear.

Late Effects of Therapy

In contrast to pediatric Hodgkin lymphoma, few reports are available on late effects in long-term survivors of childhood and adolescent NHL. The risk of second cancer for survivors of childhood and adolescent NHL appears to be much lower compared with patients with Hodgkin lymphoma. In the CCSS, the excess risk for second cancers was among the lowest for children treated for NHL as compared with all other malignancies, with a cumulative risk for SMN of 1.9% after 20 years.[202,564] However, only events occurring 5 years or later from diagnosis of NHL were included in that analysis, and therefore secondary AML, which usually has a short latency, may have been underestimated in that study. In a single-center study of 497 former pediatric NHL patients, AML was reported to be the most common second malignancy.[565] In that study, the cumulative incidences of SMN at 10 and 20 years were 2.1% and 4.8%, respectively. Seven of 16 SMNs observed were AML with exposure to epipodophyllotoxins a significant risk factor. Another analysis of 103 patients treated as children for NHL, major late effects observed were cardiac toxicity and hepatitis C virus (HCV) infection, the latter presumably resulting from blood transfusions before HCV screening was introduced.[566] Cardiotoxicity was observed in patients who received anthracycline doses of more than 400 mg/m^2. Fertility was not greatly impaired. In long-term survivors of pediatric NHL, the risk for limitations on physical performance and daily activities was among the lowest compared with survivors of other childhood cancers, although higher compared with healthy siblings.[567]

POSTTRANSPLANTATION LYMPHOPROLIFERATIVE DISEASE

Lymphoproliferative disorders are the most common malignancies in children and adolescents with iatrogenic impaired immune function after solid-organ transplantation (SOT) or allogeneic hematopoietic SCT.[568]

Posttransplantation lymphoproliferative disease (PTLD) represents a spectrum of clinically, morphologically, and biologically heterogeneous disorders defined as any lymphoid proliferation or lymphoma developing as a consequence of pharmacologic immunosuppression after SOT or hematopoietic SCT. The initial clinical presentation is extraordinarily broad, ranging from a single, small, asymptomatic lymphomatous tumor, an infectious mononucleosis-like syndrome, and unexplained fever to a widespread disseminated disease with a rapid fatal course. Any organ can be involved by interstitial infiltration of lymphocytes or tumorous lesions, including meninges and the CNS. Occasional spontaneous regression is observed and may be a feature intrinsic to the nature of the disorder as a result of a disturbed balance of immune surveillance. Especially in patients who have had hematopoietic SCT, PTLD may even go unrecognized until autopsy because of the lack of localized tumors and may be clinically misdiagnosed for graft-versus-host disease (GVHD) or infection.[569] In post-SOT PTLD, the malignant cells are almost invariably of recipient origin, whereas in postallogeneic SCT the cell of origin is more commonly of donor origin.

Classification and Epidemiology

According to the WHO classification of hematologic malignancies, PTLD is divided into four subtypes: early lesions, polymorphic PTLD, monomorphic PTLD (classified according to the lymphomas they resemble), and classic Hodgkin lymphoma–type PTLD (Box 53-3).[26,39] In the vast majority of cases, PTLD cells are of B-cell lineage, with a wide spectrum of phenotypes.[570] The B-lineage antigen CD20 is expressed in most cases but not all.[571] In rare cases a T-cell phenotype of PTLD is observed.[572] PTLD can be polyclonal, oligoclonal, or monoclonal, and polymorphic and monomorphic lesions

can be observed concurrently in the same patient.[573] Of post-SOT PTLD cases, 70% to 80% are associated with EBV, whereas almost all posthematopoietic SCT PTLD cases are EBV-positive.[26]

The incidence of PTLD in post-SOT varies widely. The two most significant risk factors for PTLD are the organ recipient being EBV-negative at the time of transplant and the degree of immunosuppression.[574] Degree of immunosuppression varies with type of SOT, and consequently risks of PTLD vary with organ type, with the incidence highest in patients who have had heart-lung or intestinal transplants, intermediate for those who have had heart or liver transplants, and lowest for patients after kidney transplant. Children have a higher incidence than adults, explained in part by the increased rate of EBV negativity at the time of organ transplant. Risk of PTLD after allogeneic SCT is increased in those with a T-cell–depleted stem-cell source and in patients whose conditioning regimen included antithymocyte globulin.

Treatment and Outcomes

Preemptive strategies for PTLD in patients with SOT have had mixed results. In contrast to cytomegalovirus (CMV), the prophylactic or preemptive use of antiviral drugs such as acyclovir or ganciclovir appears not to be efficacious to prevent EBV-related disease in transplant recipients.[575] Serial quantitative measurements of EBV DNA by real-time PCR in the blood of patients receiving transplants is a sensitive but not specific marker for the risk of development of PTLD.[576-580] The combined testing for EBV viral load and the amount of EBV-specific T cells that are CD8- and/or CD4-positive in transplant recipients increases significantly the accuracy to predict the risk of PTLD.[581,582] The use of preemptive rituximab may prove to be of benefit.[583]

The mortality of PTLD remains high with survival at 2 years ranging between 54% and 89%,[584-587] with deaths attributed both to progressive disease as well as to graft loss. Principles of therapy include early recognition, risk stratification for therapeutic decisions, and considerations for restoring host immunocompetence.

Reduction of immunosuppression (RIS) should be considered in all newly diagnosed patients. The success of RIS varies widely with increased likelihood of response found in those patients with polymorphic histology, localized nonbulky disease, and a normal LDH.[588-590] Patients with localized disease who undergo complete surgical excision and tolerate RIS have a very good outcome.[588,590] The average time to response has been reported as 3 weeks.[589] For patients with monomorphic or disseminated disease as well as those for whom RIS is initiated but then show evidence of progressive disease or organ rejection, additional interventions need to be undertaken. The utility of RIS in PTLD posthematopoietic SCT is unknown.

Monotherapy with the anti-CD20 agent rituximab has been investigated in patients who are unresponsive to RIS or with recurrent disease. Response rates range from 44% to 85% percent with approximately 2 out of 3 of patients having durable responses.[591,592] A single study of

---

Box 53-3   Classification of Posttransplantation Lymphoproliferative Disease

EARLY LESIONS

Plasmacytic hyperplasia
Infectious mononucleosis-like lesion

POLYMORPHIC POSTTRANSPLANTATION LYMPHOPROLIFERATIVE DISEASE

MONOMORPHIC POSTTRANSPLANTATION LYMPHOPROLIFERATIVE DISEASE

B cell neoplasms:
  Diffuse large B-cell lymphoma
  Burkitt lymphoma
  Plasma-cell myeloma
  Plasmacytoma-like lesions
  Other
T-cell neoplasms
  Peripheral T-cell lymphoma, not otherwise specified
  Hepatosplenic T-cell lymphoma
  Other

CLASSIC HODGKIN LYMPHOMA–TYPE POSTTRANSPLANTATION LYMPHOPROLIFERATIVE DISEASE

Modified from Swerdlow SH, Campo E, Harris NL et al: WHO classification of tumours of haematopoietic and lymphoid tissues, IARC Press, 2008, Lyon.

patients with posthematopoietic SCT PTLD strongly favored rituximab, with none of those who did not receive it alive at day 180 versus 46% of those who did.[593] A strategy of "risk-stratified sequential approach" with the use of rituximab and RIS for 4 weeks. Those achieving CR had an additional 4 weeks of rituximab, and those with less than a CR received to rituximab plus cyclophosphamide, doxorubicin (hydroxydaunorubicin), vincristine (Oncovin) and prednisone (CHOP) chemotherapy. All had excellent outcomes with a 1-year progression free survival rate of 93%.[594]

Therapy with low-dose chemotherapy regimens have been investigated using cyclophosphamide and prednisone with or without rituximab with evidence of durable responses in approximately 70% of patients.[595,596] Patients with fulminant PTLD, defined as those with fever, hypotension, and disseminated disease, have a worse prognosis that may be improved by the addition of rituximab to low-dose regimens.[596]

Standard intensive lymphoma therapy should be considered for patients who are unresponsive to low-dose regimens, have EBV-negative PTLD, and for those with Burkitt pathology.[597] Patients with CNS involvement of their PTLD have significantly inferior survival rates. For these patients the addition of high-dose methotrexate should be considered. Responses to intrathecal rituximab have been reported.[598,599] The optimal treatment for the rare patient with T-cell PTLD is unknown, although regimens similar to those used for T-cell ALL have been used.

There is no standard therapy for patients with PTLD after SCT. A number of reports have described the efficacy of rituximab in this setting.[591,600,601] Others have reported responses to donor lymphocyte infusions.[602,603] The adoptive transfer of EBV-specific T-effector cells offers a promising option to treat and or even prevent PTLD.[604]

CONCLUSION AND FUTURE DIRECTIONS IN PEDIATRIC LYMPHOMA

Insights into the pathogenesis and cellular biology have dramatically improved, as have the outcomes for children and adolescents treated for lymphoma. Widely accepted classification systems have allowed for clearer description and comparison of data between investigators. Nevertheless, important issues remain. Knowledge of causative factors is still limited. Although lymphomas were among the first human malignancies for which an infectious cause was hypothesized, definitive clarification of the role of infectious agents in the pathogenesis of childhood lymphoma is still evolving. BL and Hodgkin lymphoma, as well as PTLD, are all associated with EBV and account for a considerable proportion of childhood malignancies worldwide. Thus the clarification of an interaction of genetic predisposition and infectious agents in their pathogenesis merits ongoing efforts. For those lymphomas where curative therapy is now the expectation, investigations into reduction of the treatment burden while maintaining efficacy are warranted. In addition, exploration of new treatment options based on more refined

understanding of biology and the availability of targeted therapy such as ALK inhibitors or novel monoclonal antibodies has the potential to change the nature of lymphoma therapy. Refining prognostic indicators such as kinetics of disease response by functional imaging or measurement of minimal disseminated and residual disease may allow for more informed decisions regarding treatment intensity. The outcome of children and adolescents with lymphoma has changed dramatically in the past 50 years. The hope and expectation is that progress will continue in the basic scientific understanding and in its translation to clinical care to continue to improve the outlook for these patients.

References available online at ExpertConsult.

KEY REFERENCES

7. Garey CL, Laituri CA, Valusek PA, et al: Management of anterior mediastinal masses in children. *Eur J Pediatr Surg* 21:310–313, 2011.
   This article provides a succinct review of the important aspects of the management of children with anterior mediastinal masses.
8. Cairo MS, Coiffier B, Reiter A, et al: Recommendations for the evaluation of risk and prophylaxis of tumour lysis syndrome (TLS) in adults and children with malignant diseases: an expert TLS panel consensus. *Br J Haematol* 149:578–586, 2010.
   This paper summarizes the current classification and therapy for patients with risk of tumor lysis syndrome.
20. Devita VT, Jr, Serpick AA, Carbone PP: Combination chemotherapy in the treatment of advanced Hodgkin's disease. *Ann Intern Med* 73:881–895, 1970.
   This paper was a landmark study describing combination chemotherapy and radiation for the treatment of patients with Hodgkin lymphoma.
146. Donaldson SS, Link MP, Weinstein HJ, et al: Final results of a prospective clinical trial with VAMP and low-dose involved-field radiation for children with low-risk Hodgkin's disease. *J Clin Oncol* 25:332–337, 2007.
   This study describes long-term outcomes of the early pediatric combination treatment for patients with Hodgkin lymphoma.
148. Mauz-Korholz C, Hasenclever D, Dorffel W, et al: Procarbazine-free OEPA-COPDAC chemotherapy in boys and standard OPPA-COPP in girls have comparable effectiveness in pediatric Hodgkin's lymphoma: the GPOH-HD-2002 study. *J Clin Oncol* 28:3680–3686, 2010.
   This study describes favorable outcomes with a Hodgkin regimen designed in part to decrease the likelihood of late effects of therapy.
150. Gallamini A, Rigacci L, Merli F, et al: The predictive value of positron emission tomography scanning performed after two courses of standard therapy on treatment outcome in advanced stage Hodgkin's disease. *Haematologica* 91:475–481, 2006.
   This paper is one of a series of papers describing the utility of PET for evaluation of disease response to therapy and subsequent prognostic value.
172. Nogova L, Reineke T, Brillant C, et al: Lymphocyte-predominant and classical Hodgkin's lymphoma: a comprehensive analysis from the German Hodgkin Study Group. *J Clin Oncol* 26:434–439, 2008.
   This article provides contemporary data on outcomes of children with both lymphocyte predominant and classical Hodgkin lymphoma.
180. Mauz-Korholz C, Gorde-Grosjean S, Hasenclever D, et al: Resection alone in 58 children with limited stage, lymphocyte-predominant Hodgkin lymphoma: experience from the European network group on pediatric Hodgkin lymphoma. *Cancer* 110:179–185, 2007.
   This paper describes the outcomes of children with low-stage lymphocyte-predominant Hodgkin lymphoma treated with resection alone.

184. Daw S, Wynn R, Wallace H: Management of relapsed and refractory classical Hodgkin lymphoma in children and adolescents. *Br J Haematol* 152:249–260, 2011.
    This paper provides an overview of contemporary therapies for children with relapsed or refractory Hodgkin lymphoma.

198. Younes A, Gopal AK, Smith SE, et al: Results of a pivotal phase II study of brentuximab vedotin for patients with relapsed or refractory Hodgkin's lymphoma. *J Clin Oncol* 30:2183–2189, 2012.
    This paper provides insights into the efficacy and safety of single agent brentuximab vedotin in patients with relapsed or refractory Hodgkin lymphoma.

201. Castellino SM, Geiger AM, Mertens AC, et al: Morbidity and mortality in long-term survivors of Hodgkin lymphoma: a report from the Childhood Cancer Survivor Study. *Blood* 117:1806–1816, 2011.
    This paper provides a succinct review of current knowledge of late effects of therapy for Hodgkin lymphoma.

394. Reiter A, Schrappe M, Ludwig WD, et al: Intensive ALL-type therapy without local radiotherapy provides a 90% event-free survival for children with T-cell lymphoblastic lymphoma: a BFM group report. *Blood* 95:416–421, 2000.
    This paper describes a highly effective treatment regimen for children with T-cell lymphoblastic lymphoma.

404. Sandlund JT, Pui CH, Zhou Y, et al: Effective treatment of advanced-stage childhood lymphoblastic lymphoma without prophylactic cranial irradiation: results of St Jude NHL13 study. *Leukemia* 23:1127–1130, 2009.
    This paper shows that, in the context of St. Jude NHL therapy, patients with lymphoblastic lymphoma can be effectively treated without prophylactic cranial radiation.

483. Gerrard M, Cairo MS, Weston C, et al: Excellent survival following two courses of COPAD chemotherapy in children and adolescents with resected localized B-cell non-Hodgkin's lymphoma: results of the FAB/LMB 96 international study. *Br J Haematol* 141:840–847, 2008.
    This study describes excellent outcomes in children with low-stage B cell NHL with minimal therapy including no intrathecal therapy.

489. Goldman S, Smith L, Anderson JR, et al: Rituximab and FAB/LMB 96 chemotherapy in children with stage III/IV B-cell non-Hodgkin lymphoma: a Children's Oncology Group report. *Leukemia* 27:1174–1177, 2013.
    This pilot study describes the safety of the addition of rituximab to intensive multiagent B-cell–lymphoma therapy.

503. Le Deley MC, Rosolen A, Williams DM, et al: Vinblastine in children and adolescents with high-risk anaplastic large-cell lymphoma: results of the randomized ALCL99-vinblastine trial. *J Clin Oncol* 28:3987–3993, 2010.
    This study showed that the addition of vinblastine as a maintenance therapy for children with advanced stage ALCL delayed but did not decrease relapse risk.

539. Mussolin L, Damm-Welk C, Pillon M, et al: Use of minimal disseminated disease and immunity to NPM-ALK antigen to stratify ALK-positive ALCL patients with different prognosis. *Leukemia* 27:416–422, 2013.
    This study showed that these two tests done at the time of patient's diagnosis with ALCL were able to provide powerful prognostic information.

543. Brugieres L, Quartier P, Le Deley MC, et al: Relapses of childhood anaplastic large-cell lymphoma: treatment results in a series of 41 children—a report from the French Society of Pediatric Oncology. *Ann Oncol* 11:53–58, 2000.
    This paper describes the treatment of children with relapsed disease including a cohort of children with long-term disease remission treated with vinblastine alone.

545. Pro B, Advani R, Brice P, et al: Brentuximab vedotin (SGN-35) in patients with relapsed or refractory systemic anaplastic large-cell lymphoma: results of a phase II study. *J Clin Oncol* 30:2190–2196, 2012.
    This paper describes significant activity of this monoclonal antibody directed at CD30 in adult patients with ALCL.

546. Gambacorti-Passerini C, Messa C, Pogliani EM: Crizotinib in anaplastic large-cell lymphoma. *N Engl J Med* 364:775–776, 2011.
    This paper describes two patients with dramatic disease response to therapy with the tyrosine kinase inhibitor crizotinib for relapsed relapsed Alk-positive ALCL.

596. Gross TG, Orjuela MA, Perkins SL, et al: Low-dose chemotherapy and rituximab for posttransplant lymphoproliferative disease (PTLD): a Children's Oncology Group Report. *Am J Transplant* 12:3069–3075, 2012.
    This study provides outcome information for children with PTLD treated with relatively limited chemotherapy in addition to rituximab.

SOLID TUMORS

CHAPTER 54

Neuroblastoma

Suzanne Shusterman and Rani E. George

CHAPTER OUTLINE

Neuroblastoma is an embryonal tumor of the sympathetic nervous system arising from the neural crest. It is a common extracranial solid tumor of childhood and is a disease distinguished by its clinical and biologic heterogeneity. The prognosis for persons with neuroblastoma is variable and largely dependent on tumor biology. Patients with localized disease and favorable tumor biology may be successfully treated with surgery alone or with minimal therapy with an estimated 5-year survival rate of 90%.[1] However approximately half of all patients present with metastatic disease, adverse tumor-specific biologic features, or both. For these children with "high-risk" disease features, cure rates remain poor, with estimated 5-year survival rates of 30%.[1] The development of resistance to chemotherapy and radiation is the cause of most treatment failures, and neuroblastoma accounts for 10% of

childhood cancer mortality. This chapter summarizes our current understanding of neuroblastoma biology and pathogenesis and how this rapidly evolving insight has affected current and future treatment strategies.

EPIDEMIOLOGY

Neuroblastoma accounts for 7% of all childhood cancer diagnoses, with more than 650 new cases diagnosed in the United States each year.[2] The incidence of neuroblastoma is 10.5 per million children younger than 15 years of age per year.[2] It is the most commonly diagnosed cancer of infancy.[2] The median age of diagnosis is 19 months, with a peak incidence in children younger than 4 years.[3] There is no racial preponderance, although African Americans are more likely to have high-risk

1675

disease and a fatal outcome.[4,5] Large-scale genetic studies to investigate how this likelihood may influence the disease phenotype revealed that a single nucleotide polymorphism (SNP) within the sperm-associated antigen 16 (*SPAG16*) gene had a higher risk allele frequency in the African reference population and contributed to the ethnic disparities in high-risk disease and survival.[6]

The cause of neuroblastoma is largely unknown. The embryonal origin of the tumor, as well as the young age of onset, suggest that prenatal and perinatal exposures may be important. Studies have investigated a variety of prenatal exposures including tobacco, alcohol, pesticides, and maternal medication or drug use, as well as birth characteristics, including small size for gestational age and maternal history of fetal loss.[7-10,11] The findings from these studies have been inconsistent, and none of these associations has been confirmed in large studies.

Because the majority of neuroblastomas produce catecholamine metabolites that can be detected in the urine, infant screening programs have been conducted to see if it is possible to decrease the mortality from high-risk neuroblastoma by diagnosing cases earlier. In Japan, starting in 1985, a nationwide mass screening program for neuroblastoma was conducted in 6-month-old infants. Results showed that the incidence rate of neuroblastoma increased two- to threefold as a result of the screening, implying that without screening, many of these tumors would have regressed spontaneously and would never have been diagnosed clinically. In addition, the majority of patients had low-stage disease and biologically favorable features, and screening did not decrease overall neuroblastoma mortality.[12-17] Through the Quebec Neuroblastoma Screening Program, infants were screened at 3 weeks and 6 months; the findings confirmed the Japanese results[18,19] and showed a significant complication rate in patients undergoing treatment for tumors found by screening.[20] In the German Neuroblastoma Screening Study, investigators looked at postponing screening until 10 to 19 months of age.[21,22] They found less "overdiagnosis" of neuroblastoma and a greater frequency of patients with unfavorable clinical and biologic features. However, no decrease in the mortality of the patients with unfavorable features was documented. Because of these results, mass screening efforts for neuroblastoma in infants have largely been abandoned.

PATHOGENESIS

Embryology

Neuroblastoma arises during development from neural crest cells committed to the sympathoadrenal lineage.[23,24] The two predominant cell types comprising neuroblastoma are neuroblasts and Schwann cells. Neuroblasts derive from pluripotent cells that arise in the neural crest and eventually form various components of the sympathetic nervous system: the sympathetic ganglia, the chromaffin cells of the adrenal medulla, and the paraganglia, which are typical sites where neuroblastic tumors can arise. What causes persistence of these embryonal cells that develop into peripheral neuroblastic tumors is unclear. Genes that dictate neural development could be altered, causing defects in the normal differentiation and programmed cell death pathways, leading to uncontrolled proliferation and aberrant cell survival.

Microscopic neuroblastic nodules have been reported in fetal adrenal glands during development, peaking at around 17 to 20 weeks' gestation and regressing by birth or within the first few months of postnatal life.[25,26] Beckwith and Perrin[27] (1963) termed these nodules, which were histologically identical to neuroblastoma, "neuroblastoma in situ," which they noted during postmortem examinations of infants younger than 3 months of age who died of other causes. These lesions were detected with a frequency fiftyfold higher than the expected incidence of primary adrenal neuroblastoma and were initially thought to be neuroblastomas that regressed spontaneously. However, with new insights into the development of the adrenal gland, it is clear that these are remnants from normal fetal development.[27] Indeed, the genetic profiles of normal developing neuroblasts and malignant neuroblastomas are similar in many respects, as shown by messenger ribonucleic acid (mRNA) expression profiling of sympathetic neuroblasts from human fetal adrenal glands.[28]

Development of the Sympathetic Nervous System

The sympathetic nervous system is derived from the neural crest, a multipotent embryonic structure that appears early in development and is made up of a transient population of cells that migrate from the neural tube to the region of the dorsal aorta during development.[29-31] These cells develop into sympathetic, parasympathetic, enteric, or sensory neurons governed by transcriptional regulators and growth factors as they exit from the neural tube, during migration or at sites where these cells differentiate. Development of the sympathetic phenotype is summarized in Figure 54-1.[32] Premigratory neural crest cells are specified by the expression of several markers, including FoxD3 and SOX10. *Foxd3* is required for sublineage fate specification, migration, and survival. Zebrafish homozygous for *foxd3* inactivating mutations have nearly a complete loss of sympathetic neurons and their precursor populations.[33] *Sox10* is responsible for the multipotency of neural crest–derived cells and is required for sympathetic nervous system and melanocyte development.[34] At the dorsal aorta, prespecified *SOX10*-positive sympathetic progenitors that are under the influence of extrinsic factors, bone morphogenetic proteins, start the process of differentiation into noradrenergic neurons.[35] The basic helix-loop-helix (bHLH) transcription factor *Ascl1* and the homeodomain transcription factor *Phox2b* are the first transcription factors that are expressed upon initiation of differentiation of sympathoadrenal precursors.[36-40] *Phox2a*, a homolog of *PHOX2B*, is expressed downstream of both *Phoxb* and *Ascl1*,[36,40,41] but its role in the initial stages of the sympathetic lineage remains undefined. Further neuronal differentiation occurs under the influence of the transcription factors *Hand2*,[42,43] *Gata2/3*,[44] and *Tfap2a*,[45,46] which interact in a complex regulatory network to ultimately induce the expression of tyrosine hydroxylase (TH) and dopamine beta hydroxylase. These two enzymes are required for

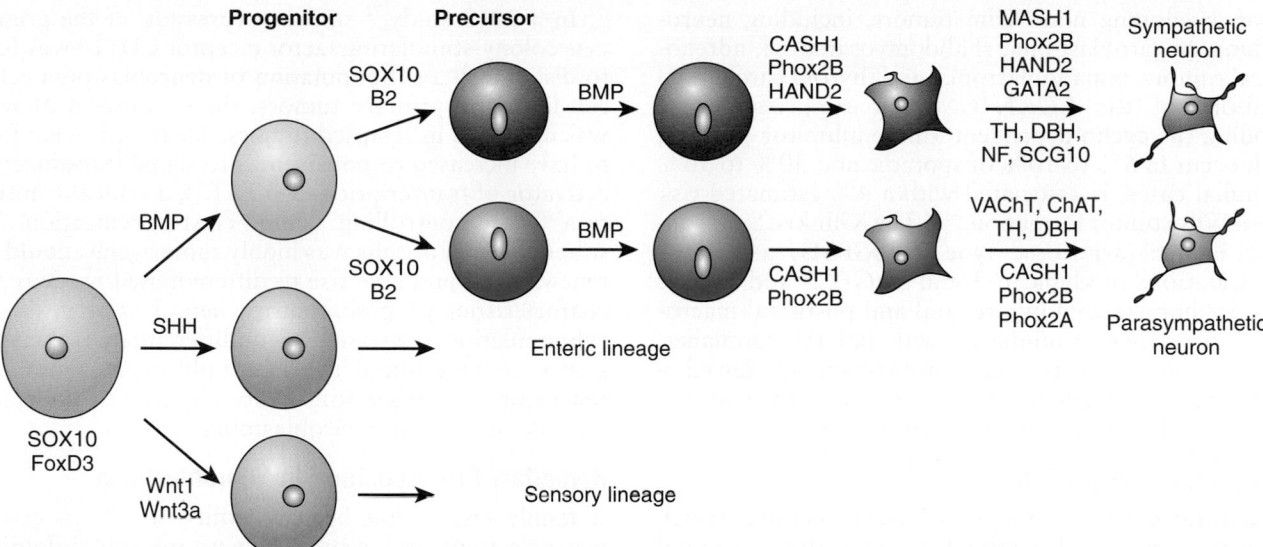

Figure 54-1 The development of the autonomic nervous system. A series of growth factors and transcriptional regulators affect different stages of neurogenesis of neural crest–derived progenitor cells. Neural crest cells segregated from the neuroepithelium can be identified by the expression of forkhead box D3 *(FoxD3)* and sex-determining region Y box–10 *(SOX10)*, among other markers. Progenitor cells differentiate into sympathetic, parasympathetic, enteric, or sensory neurons that are in part dependent upon instructive signals encountered early at or near the time of egress from the neural tube. Additionally, extrinsic cues encountered during migration or at sites where neural crest–derived cells differentiate influence patterns of gene expression. *(Modified from Howard MJ. Mechanisms and perspectives on differentiation of autonomic neurons. Dev Biol 277:271–286, 2005.)*

catecholamine production and serve as markers of terminal sympathetic neuronal differentiation.[47,48] *Hand2* appears to have more of a role in noradrenergic cell proliferation than differentiation. A massive reduction in sympathetic ganglion size occurs after elimination of Hand2 in the neural crest of model organisms because of a nearly complete block in proliferation of immature sympathetic neurons.[49] Thus different members of the gene regulatory network appear to have selective functions, some in proliferation and others in differentiation.[30]

Neural crest cells from the cranial region migrate from the neural folds into the pharyngeal arches and heart, where they play essential roles in septation of the single outflow of the heart (the truncus arteriosus) and in the formation of the conotruncal portion of the ventricular septum.[50] It follows that coexistence of neuroblastoma with anomalies of other neural crest–derived structures is biologically plausible because of the shared roles of regulatory and developmental genes. For example, ablation of the cardiac neural crest results in congenital cardiovascular malformations in the chick embryo.[50] Indeed, a significantly increased incidence of congenital cardiac malformations, especially those that involve neural crest–derived tissues, was noted in patients with neuroblastoma compared with other malignancies, such as leukemia.[51] These cardiac anomalies were seen primarily in patients with neuroblastoma who were younger than 1 year and had lower stage tumors. Menegaux et al.[52] (2005) confirmed the association of neuroblastoma with conotruncal cardiac anomalies, as well as with various urogenital anomalies; other studies have shown varying results.[53-55] Although the malignant transformation of neuroblasts

and the disruption of normal cardiogenesis are likely to be multistep processes, it is possible that shared initiating genetic lesions occur very early in development, causing derangement of common developmental pathways.

Genetic Disorders Associated with Neuroblastoma

Neuroblastoma may occur rarely in association with chromosomal anomalies. In addition to the increased incidence of neuroblastoma in girls with Turner syndrome,[56] neuroblastoma has also been noted to occur in patients with Noonan syndrome.[57] The gene encoding the protein phosphatase PTPN11 is mutated in 50% of patients with Noonan syndrome and is associated with an increased risk of leukemia[58] and neuroblastoma.[57,59] Other neuro-cardio-facial syndromes such as Costello syndrome have been associated with neuroblastic tumors. Mutations in the neurofibromatosis type 1 *(NF1)* gene have been detected in neuroblastoma cell lines,[60,61] and the literature includes one case report of a patient with a germline *NF1* mutation and neuroblastoma who had a homozygous deletion of the *NF1* gene in the tumor.[62] However, germline inactivation of *Nf1* does not predispose to neuroblastoma in the mouse.

Persons affected with overgrowth disorders such as Beckwith-Weidemann syndrome are at risk for embryonal tumors, including neuroblastoma. The increased risk is mainly during the first 4 years of life, and current recommendations include quarterly evaluation with abdominal ultrasound until age 8 years.[63] The molecular aberrations that predispose to neuroblastoma in particular are unknown, although maternal differentially methylated region 2 (DMR2) loss of methylation that occurs in 50% to 60% of cases is thought to confer a 1% to 5%

risk of developing non–Wilm tumors, including neuroblastoma, hepatoblastoma, rhabdomyosarcoma, adrenocortical tumors, gonadoblastoma, and thyroid carcinoma. Mutations of the *CDKN1C* tumor suppressor gene (encoding the cyclin-dependent kinase inhibitor p57[KIP2]), which occur in 5% to 10% of sporadic and 30% to 50% of familial cases, is associated with a 4% estimated risk of non–Wilm tumor formation.[63,64] The X-linked Simpson-Golabi-Behmel syndrome type 1 (SGBS1), associated with mutations in glypican 3 and 4 *(GPC3 and GPC4)* genes, is characterized by prenatal and postnatal macrosomia, distinctive craniofacies with palatal anomalies, congenital heart defects, and neuroblastoma (reviewed in reference 65). Surveillance is recommended for embryonal tumors starting in the newborn period.[65]

Neuroblastoma Stem Cells

The natural course of high-risk neuroblastoma, which results in relapse and a refractory state after an initial good response, suggests the likely existence of cancer stem cells (CSCs) in these tumors. CSCs are a subpopulation of cells within a tumor with the ability to self-renew, generate differentiated progeny, and reproduce a heterogeneous cancer population.[66] These cells have enhanced tumorigenicity, resistance to chemotherapy, and the ability to establish metastatic foci. Hansford et al.[67] (2007) demonstrated that dissociated cells from neuroblastoma tumors and bone marrow metastases grow as spheres and are capable of self-renewal. Spheres generated from the tumors underwent differentiation under neurogenic conditions to form neurons. Neuroblastoma stem cells from high-risk tumors expressed markers of neural crest stem cells and clinical markers of neuroblastoma, exhibited a higher self-renewal rate than those from low-risk tumors, and formed metastatic tumors that could be serially passaged in xenograft models.[67] Compounds that selectively targeted these tumor-initiating cells (TICs)—DEC14 and rapamycin—were identified; they induced regression of TIC tumor models in vivo and markedly decreased self-renewal or tumor initiation capacity.[68] Moreover, compounds that targeted PI3K/Akt, PKC, aurora kinase, ErbB2, Trk, and polo-like kinase–1 (PLK1) emerged from a small molecule inhibitor library screen designed to identify signaling pathways important for the survival and self-renewal of neuroblastoma TICs. Genetic and chemical inhibition of PLK1 caused regression of TIC tumor models both singly and in combination with irinotecan, suggesting that this kinase may regulate TIC growth and survival.[69]

Cluster of differentiation (CD)–133, in addition to being a marker of hematopoietic stem cells, is also a marker of TICs in several human cancers. CD133-positive subpopulations of cells with tumor-initiating and metastatic properties have been identified in neuroblastoma tumors.[70] Similarly, the stemness-related polycomb repressive complex–1 (PRC1) protein BMI1 is thought to have a role in tumor sphere formation. BMI1 is thought to inhibit neuroblastoma differentiation by repressing expression of the tumor suppressor in lung cancer 1 (TSLC1) and kinesin family member 1B (KIF1B) in these cells.[71]

In a 2013 study,[72] surface expression of the granulocyte colony-stimulating factor receptor CD114 was found to distinguish a subpopulation of neuroblastoma cells in cell lines and primary tumors, the proportion of which was increased in relapsed tumors. These cells were found to have increased responsiveness to signal transducer and activator of transcription–3 (STAT3), a critical transcription factor controlling neural crest specification. This subpopulation of cells was highly tumorigenic, could self-renew, and could give rise to differentiated progeny with characteristics of premigratory neural crest cells. This subpopulation possessed an undifferentiated phenotype similar to that found in early multipotent neural crest precursors.[72] Further studies are required to understand the role of CSCs in neuroblastoma.

Hereditary Predisposition to Neuroblastoma

A family history has been identified in 1% of cases of neuroblastoma and is suggestive of autosomal-dominant inheritance.[73] In these children, neuroblastoma develops at an earlier age and often manifests as multiple primary tumors.

PHOX2B Mutations

The first predisposition mutation identified in neuroblastoma was in *PHOX2B*.[74,75] *Phox2b* is a key regulator of autonomic neuron development, because its complete absence leads to embryonic lethality in mice as a result of the failure of sympathetic nervous system formation.[38,76] This gene is transiently expressed in murine primary sympathetic neuron progenitors from E10.5 to E13[76] and regulates their differentiation.[77-79] *Phox2b* also has growth inhibitory effects, because its overexpression promotes cell cycle exit and inhibits the proliferation of cultured sympathetic neurons.[80,81]

Heterozygous germline mutations of the *PHOX2B* gene occur in pedigrees and are associated with neuroblastoma, ganglioneuroblastoma, congenital central hypoventilation syndrome, and Hirschsprung disease.[74,75,82-85] The human *PHOX2B* gene maps to chromosome 4p13 and consists of three exons encoding a highly conserved 314–amino acid protein with two polyalanine repeats of 9 and 20 residues C-terminal to the homeodomain. Whereas the *PHOX2B* variants in congenital central hypoventilation syndrome largely involve expansions of the second polyalanine repeat within the C-terminus of the protein,[86-88] those associated with neuroblastic tumors are nearly always frameshift and truncation mutations.[74,75,85,86,89] More recently, whole-allele deletions resulting in the reduction of the protein have been reported.[90] Proposed mechanisms contributing to neuroblastoma predisposition include partial loss of function with the preserved ability to suppress cellular proliferation but not to promote differentiation,[83] complete loss of function due to functional haploinsufficiency,[91] and both dominant-negative and gain-of function effects.[81,92,93] Mutated *PHOX2B* also suppresses proliferation in vitro; heterozygous insertion of two frameshift variants, 931del5 and 693del8, into the mouse *Phox2b* locus resulted in impaired proliferation of sympathetic ganglion progenitors and biased differentiation toward the glial lineage.[93] Aberrant *Phox2b* expression in the zebrafish models has been shown to cause an arrest in the normal maturation of sympathetic neurons, leading to immature cells that are resistant to retinoic acid-induced differentiation.[94] Allelic deficiency of *PHOX2B* causes a decrease in the terminal differentiation markers *th* and *dbh* in sympathetic ganglion cells.[94] The neuroblastoma-associated frameshift mutations 676delG and K155X—but not the R100L missense mutation—functioned dominant negatively to impede differentiation.[94] Thus a reduced dosage of *PHOX2B* during development, through either a heterozygous deletion or dominant-negative mutation, imposes a block in the differentiation of sympathetic neuronal precursors, resulting in an immature cell population that is likely to be susceptible to secondary transforming events. The block in differentiation of immature sympathetic neurons caused by certain *PHOX2B* variants could be due to their inability to bind to interacting proteins critical to this process.[95] The neuronal calcium sensor protein HPCAL1 (VILIP-3) exhibits strong binding to wild-type *PHOX2B*, but only weakly or not at all to neuroblastoma-associated frameshift and truncation variants leading to impaired subcellular localization of HPCAL1 and impaired differentiation in vitro.

Anaplastic Lymphoma Kinase Mutations

Dominant mutations in the anaplastic lymphoma kinase (ALK) tyrosine kinase receptor have been identified in approximately 50% of familial neuroblastoma cases.[96,97] Several distinct germline mutations have been described to date—R1275Q, R1192P, T1151R, and G1128A—with R1275Q being the most frequent (Table 54-1). ALK germline mutations generally occur in the context of multifocal tumors, although in one study, affected patients

TABLE 54-1   ALK Mutations in Neuroblastoma

Mutation	Tumor/Cell Line	Effect of Mutation	ALK Domain	Reference(s)
ALKΔ2-3	T/C	GOF, can occur in amplified ALK	Δ224-318	586
ALKΔ4-11	T/C	GOF, can occur in amplified ALK	Δ318-782	587
K1062M	T/C	GOF	JMR	154
G1128A*	T	GOF	P-loop	96, 588
M1166R*	T	Ligand dependent or GOF	αC helix	96, 589
I1171N*	T	GOF	αC helix	96, 588
F1174I*	T	GOF	αC helix	96, 200, 589
F1174L/S*	T/C	GOF	αC helix	96, 154, 155, 200, 590
R1192P*	T	GOF	β4 strand	96, 588
F1245C*	T	GOF	C-loop	96, 155, 588
R1275Q*	T/C	GOF	A-loop	96, 97, 154, 155, 200
T1087I	T	Ligand dependent	JMR	154, 589
D1091N	T/C	Ligand dependent	β1 strand	96, 155, 589
A1099T	T	Ligand dependent	β2 strand	589
T1151M*	T	Ligand dependent	β3 strand	155, 589
A1234T*	T	Ligand dependent	αE helix	155, 589
1464STOP	T	Ligand dependent	C-terminal to kinase domain	589
I1250T*	T	Kinase dead	C-loop	96, 591
R1061Q	T	Unknown	JMR	184
T1151R*	T	Unknown	β3 strand	592
I1170T/S*	T	Unknown	αC helix	186
F1174C/V*	T	Unknown	αC helix	154
R1231Q*	T	Unknown	αE helix	184
L1240V*	T	Unknown	αE helix	186
F1245I/L/V*	T/C	Unknown	C-loop	96, 155, 200
R1275L*	T	Unknown	A-loop	97
Y1278S*	T	Unknown	A-loop	97

ALK, Anaplastic lymphoma kinase; *A-loop,* activation loop; *C-loop,* catalytic loop; *GOF,* gain of function; *JMR,* juxtamembrane region; *P-loop,* phosphate-binding loop.
*Mutations within the kinase domain (aa 1122-1376).

did not necessarily have younger age of onset. Further guidelines on screening need to be derived from a consensus analysis of inherited cases, but it would seem that in addition to a family history, the presence of multifocal tumors would call for genetic screening. In fact, in the United States, genetic testing for *ALK* and *PHOX2B* mutations is recommended for every newly diagnosed patient with a family history of neuroblastic tumors.

Germline Susceptibility Variants

Genome-wide association studies have identified SNPs within or adjacent to genes that predispose to sporadic neuroblastoma: *BARD1* (BRCA1-associated RING domain 1), *LINC00340* (long intergenic nonprotein coding RNA 340, *CASC15*), *LMO1* (LIM domain only 1), *DUSP12* (dual-specificity phosphatase 12), *DDX4/IL31RA* (DEAD box polypeptide 4/interleukin [IL]31 receptor A), *HSD17B12* (hydroxysteroid [17-beta] dehydrogenase 12), *LIN28B* (lin-28 homolog B), and *HACE1* (HECT domain and ankyrin repeat containing E3 ubiquitin protein ligase–1).[98-102] The *BARD1* SNP effect at chromosome 2q35 has been confirmed in African-American children,[5] and the *BARD1β* isoform[103] and *LIN28B*[104] are oncogenic in neuroblastoma. Patients with neuroblastoma who were homozygous for the risk alleles were more likely to have metastatic disease, amplification of *MYCN* (v-myc avian myelocytomatosis viral oncogene neuroblastoma-derived homolog), and disease relapse.[105] However, the absolute risk conferred by the susceptibility allele is extremely small,[105] and the risk that neuroblastoma may recur in families with these risk alleles is estimated to be very low.[106] A common copy number variation at 1q21.1 was also associated with neuroblastoma, the significance of which is uncertain.[99] The mechanisms through which these risk alleles and associated genes contribute to neuroblastoma initiation and/or maintenance require further investigation.

Genetic Aberrations in Sporadic Neuroblastoma

DNA Ploidy

Neuroblastomas are classified into those with diploid modal chromosomal content (with a deoxyribonucleic acid [DNA] index of 1) or hyperdiploid modal chromosomal content (DNA index greater than 1). Hyperdiploidy is associated with whole chromosome gains and overall favorable biology, whereas diploidy is associated with segmental chromosomal rearrangements and unbalanced translocations. Such segmental chromosomal aberrations seem to affect certain chromosomes—1p, 11q, and 17q—although the biologic significance is unclear at present.[107] Hyperdiploid tumors are often localized and have a favorable outlook, whereas diploid tumors not only tend to have a poor prognosis but also are associated with other high-risk genetic aberrations and *MYCN* amplification. Originally, infants (those younger than 1 year) with a hyperdiploid modal chromosome number were found to respond well to conventional therapy, whereas those with advanced stage disease with diploidy failed to respond to conventional therapy.[108,109] Subsequent studies have shown that tumor cell ploidy predicts responsiveness to therapy in children up to 18 months of age with advanced stage neuroblastoma without MYCN amplification.[110]

MYCN Amplification

MYCN, the first oncogene proven to be of clinical significance in neuroblastoma and gene amplification, occurs in approximately 20% to 30% of primary tumors and 90% of cell lines.[111,112] *MYCN* amplification is generally associated with advanced disease, poor outcome, and rapid tumor progression in neuroblastoma.[112,113] It occurs in 5% to 10% of early stage tumors and in half of the tumors of patients with advanced stage disease.[114,115] The detection of *MYCN* gene amplification in tumor cells at diagnosis is used by most cooperative groups to stratify patients to more intensive therapy. *MYCN* copy number appears to be consistent throughout the natural course of the disease, that is, at diagnosis and relapse and between primary and metastatic tumors in individual patients.[116] The Children's Oncology Group (COG) currently classifies *MYCN* amplification as more than 10 copies per diploid cell; it is unclear whether lower levels of gain (i.e., *MYCN* copy number between 3 and 10) confer an adverse outcome. A correlation usually exists between amplification and increased *MYCN* expression, and tumors with *MYCN* amplification generally express higher levels of MYCN than do nonamplified tumors; however, it has been reported that high expression is not linked to outcome.[117] MYC deregulation is common in high-risk tumors without *MYCN* amplification,[118] suggesting that MYC signaling could contribute to the high-risk phenotype.

Amplification manifests cytogenetically as double minutes or homogeneously staining regions; the latter occur mainly in tumors and the former in cell lines (Fig. 54-2).[119-121] However, there is no difference in clinical outcome whether *MYCN* amplification is manifested as double minutes or homogeneously staining regions in tumor samples obtained at diagnosis.[122] The genomic region amplified with *MYCN* is around 500 to 1000 kb, and several genes have been shown to be coamplified with *MYCN* in neuroblastoma. These genes include *DDX1* (DEAD box helicase 1),[123-125] *NAG* (*NBAS* [neuroblastoma amplified sequence]),[126,127] and *NCYM* (*MYCNOS*—*MYCN opposite strand*),[125,128,129] and it is possible that coamplification of these genes may contribute to the tumor phenotype.

Role of MYCN during Development. *MYCN* is a highly conserved bHLH leucine zipper transcription factor located on chromosome 2p24.3 and a member of the *myc* family of oncogenes. The coding regions of both *MYC* and *MYCN* are highly homologous, with each having long 5′ and 3′ untranslated regions and gene products of similar sizes.[130,131] Both dimerize with Max and bind DNA at consensus E-box sequences (CANNTG; reviewed in reference 132).[132] Mice homozygous for disrupted MYCN die at around 10 days of gestation and have multiple organ defects, including tissues of the central and peripheral nervous systems, mesonephros, lung, gut, and heart.[133,134]

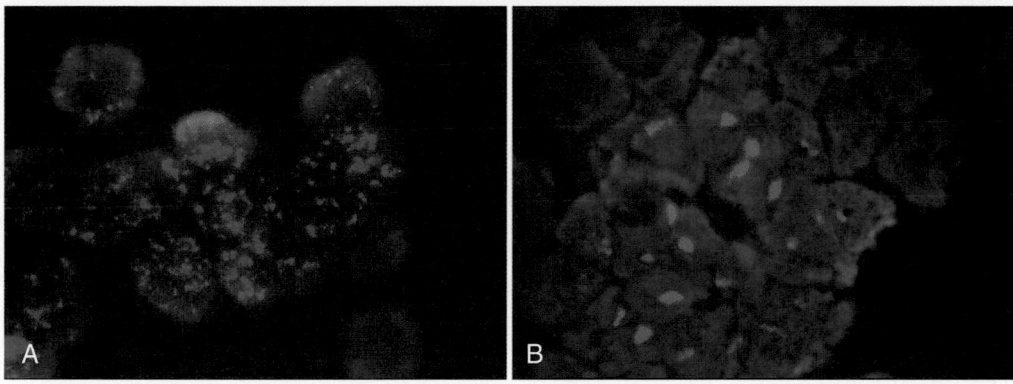

Figure 54-2 V-myc avian myelocytomatosis viral oncogene neuroblastoma-derived homolog *(MYCN)* amplification in neuroblastoma. A fluorescence in situ hybridization image of neuroblastoma tumors depicting *MYCN* amplification manifested as **(A)** double minutes and **(B)** homogeneously staining regions.

MYCN is highly expressed in fetal and neonatal development, specifically in the forebrain, hindbrain, and kidney, but not in adult tissues.[135] MYCN is expressed in the fetal brain up to the onset of differentiation and is also present at high levels in neuroblasts migrating from the neural crest through the adrenal cortex.[136] MYCN regulates overlapping stem-related gene expression programs in neuroblastoma and neural stem cells. MYCN induces a stemlike state by blocking differentiation pathways and activating self-renewal and pluripotency factors such as KLF2 and KLF4 (Kruppel-like factor 2 and 4) and LIN28B.[137,138]

Role of MYCN in Tumorigenesis. Suppression of MYCN expression in neuroblastoma cell lines results in a more differentiated phenotype.[139] Indeed downregulation of MYCN occurs in neuroblastoma cells induced to differentiate with chemical agents, and MYCN overexpression can block retinoic acid–induced differentiation.[140,141] Deletion of MYCN in neural progenitor cells showed decreased brain size and an increase in neuronal differentiation.[142] Enhanced expression of MYCN and the mutant H-*ras* gene cause tumorigenic conversion of primary rat embryo fibroblasts, and these transformed cells elicit tumors in athymic mice and isogenic rats.[143,144] Targeted expression of MYCN to the neuroectoderm of mice using a tyrosine hydroxylase promoter resulted in neuroblastoma tumors with chromosomal copy number abnormalities syntenic to those found in human tumors.[145,146] The prolonged latency together with the additional chromosomal anomalies in these tumors suggests that additional genetic mutations are required for neuroblastoma formation.

MYCN is involved in all aspects of tumor cell metastasis: adhesion, motility, and invasion (reviewed in reference 132). It downregulates integrins α1 and β1 to allow invasion.[147,148] MYCN-amplified tumors have increased angiogenesis: overexpression of MYCN is associated with proangiogenic factors such as angiogenin and vascular endothelial growth factor (VEGF) through the PI3K/mTOR (mammalian target of rapamycin) pathway.[149]

Role of MYCN in Altered Tumor Metabolism. Similar to other cancers, neuroblastomas require abnormally high amounts of glucose and other macromolecules to enable their continued unchecked proliferation. These needs are met through alterations in key metabolic pathways that can potentially be harnessed for the development of new anticancer therapies.[150]

Normal cells generate adenosine triphosphate (ATP) from glucose through oxidative phosphorylation when oxygen is abundant. During oxygen deprivation, which occurs commonly in solid tumors, including neuroblastoma, ATP generation occurs through glycolysis (the Warburg effect). Genes involved in glycolysis are selectively activated by hypoxia-inducible factor–1α (HIF1a), which is upregulated in hypoxic states. HIF1a is preferentially expressed in MYCN-amplified neuroblastoma cells; moreover, high levels of MYCN have been shown to override HIF1a inhibitory effects on cell cycle progression, thus enabling continued proliferation under hypoxic conditions.[151] Therefore both deregulated MYCN and HIF1a cooperate to contribute to the Warburg effect in neuroblastoma cells. Moreover, expression of glycolytic genes phosphoglycerate kinase 1 *(PGK1)*, hexokinase 2 *(HK2)*, and lactate dehydrogenase A *(LDHA)* were higher in MYCN-amplified neuroblastoma than in those without MYCN amplification, with depletion of LDHA inhibiting tumorigenesis in vivo, suggesting that these metabolic pathways could be targeted therapeutically.

MYCN-amplified cells have also been shown to depend on exogenous glutamine for their survival. MYCN-amplified neuroblastoma cells overexpress high-affinity glutamine transporters and other glutaminolytic enzymes that correlate with poor prognosis. Glutamine depletion in MYCN-amplified neuroblastoma cells led to apoptosis through p53-independent PUMA (p53-upregulated modulator of apoptosis) and NOXA induction,[152] an effect that is mediated by activation of the activating transcription factor–4 (ATF4). ATF4 has both context-dependent prosurvival and proapoptotic effects. In MYCN-amplified cells, it appears to have a prodeath role, because ATF4 agonists and glutaminolysis inhibitors potently induced apoptosis in vitro and inhibited tumor growth in vivo, suggesting that ATF4 agonists could be potential therapeutics for MYCN-amplified neuroblastomas.[152]

MYCN in Immune Surveillance. MYCN is also important in immune surveillance in that it represses several chemoattractant proteins that are required for recruitment of natural killer T cells (NKTs).[153] NKTs are important for producing proinflammatory cytokines to recruit immune cells, stimulate the maturation of dendritic cells, and generate antigen-specific T cells to target the tumor. Patients with MYCN-amplified neuroblastoma with bone marrow metastases had fewer bone marrow NKTs. One such protein repressed by MYCN is monocyte chemoattractant protein–1/chemokine (C-C motif) ligand 2 (MCP-1/CCL2).[153] Deletion of MYCN in MYCN-amplified cells rescues MCP-1 production and NKT recruitment. Therefore avenues to improve NKT function are being explored as therapeutic modalities in neuroblastoma.

ALK Amplification and Mutation

The identification of somatic mutations in the ALK receptor in neuroblastoma represents the first therapeutically targetable genetic aberration in this disease.[96,97,154,155] ALK, a cell surface tyrosine kinase receptor of the insulin receptor superfamily, is located in humans at chromosome 2p23 and contains an extracellular ligand-binding domain, a transmembrane domain, and an intracellular tyrosine kinase domain (reviewed in reference 156).[156,157] Ligand binding leads to receptor dimerization and activation via trans-autophosphorylation of tyrosine residues.[158] The 177-kDa polypeptide encoded by the human *ALK* gene undergoes posttranslational modification, such as N-glycosylation, to generate a mature protein doublet of 220 and 190 kDa.[158] ALK is preferentially expressed in the central and peripheral nervous systems during development (i.e., thalamus, hypothalamus, midbrain, cranial ganglia and olfactory bulb, and dorsal root ganglia).[159] ALK levels decrease postnatally, so that in adults ALK expression is restricted to rare scattered neural cells, endothelial cells, and pericytes in the brain.[159-161] The physiologic function of ALK is not clear, although its predominant expression in the nervous system during development suggests that it likely plays an important role in the development of the nervous system. Homozygous ALK-null mice are viable and develop without obvious anatomic abnormalities and a normal life span,[162] other than increased basal dopaminergic signaling within the prefrontal cortex and an age-dependent increase in basal hippocampal progenitor proliferation,[162] as well as mild behavioral phenotypes.[163,164] In *Drosophila melanogaster*, the receptor is important for the development of visceral gut musculature because absence of dALK leads to the loss of mesodermal founder cells responsible for gut development.[165] The zebrafish alk ortholog is expressed at high levels in the developing nervous system.[166] Ectopic expression of alk during early neurogenesis results in increased cell proliferation and aberrant neurogenesis in the central nervous system (CNS), leading to mispositioning of differentiated neurons and activation of the MEK/ERK pathway. Morpholino-mediated and pharmacologic depletion of alk, however, did not affect neuron progenitor formation, but it did cause compromised neuronal differentiation and survival in the CNS.[166]

Signaling by the Wild-Type ALK Receptor. Pleotropin (PTN) and midkine (MK) have been reported as candidate ligands of mammalian ALK.[167,168] Whether PTN and MK are true ligands of ALK remains controversial because some groups have failed to reproduce the binding and activation of ALK by PTN.[169-171] Signaling by these two molecules may trigger dimerization and phosphorylation of ALK, leading to activation of downstream signaling pathways. In *D. melanogaster* and *Caenorhabditis elegans*, the ALK ligands are Jelly belly (Jeb)[172] and hesitation behavior 1 (HEN1),[173,174] respectively, with Jeb being structurally different from either PTN or MK.[175] Ligand activation of ALK has been implicated in the inhibition of apoptosis and induction of neuronal cell differentiation through the mitogen-activated protein kinase (MAPK) pathway.[176-178] Signaling through the phospholipase Cγ (PLCγ) pathway by activated ALK, leading to transformation of NIH 3T3 cells, has also been reported.[179]

ALK Mutations in Neuroblastoma. In human tumors the most common mechanism of constitutive ALK activation involves chromosomal translocations that result in the generation of oncogenic *ALK* fusion genes, such as nucleophosmin *(NPM1)-ALK* in anaplastic large cell lymphoma[180] and echinoderm microtubule-associated protein like 4 *(EML4)-ALK* in non–small cell lung cancers (NSCLCs),[181] among others.[182] ALK translocations have not yet been reported in neuroblastomas, apparently because the ALK receptor is normally expressed by sympathetic neuroblasts, and a heterologous promoter does not need to be provided through translocation. Rather, ALK aberrations take the form of point mutations, amplification, and copy number gain. Activating mutations in ALK occur in 7% to 8% of sporadic neuroblastomas.[154,155,97,183-186] ALK is also amplified in neuroblastoma, although always in combination with MYCN amplification, and amplified ALK appears to mediate overexpression alone in that the affected ALK allele does not harbor activating point mutations.[155]

Altogether 12 different residues are known to be affected by ALK mutations (Table 54-1).[156] Mutations range from silent to activating, with the two major mutational hot spots being R1275 and F1174; the R1275Q mutation is found in both familial and sporadic neuroblastoma, whereas the F1174L mutation is restricted to sporadic tumors, presumably because it is embryonic lethal. Activating ALK mutations are associated with constitutive phosphorylation of ALK and that of downstream targets such as ERK, STAT3, and AKT.[156] These ALK variants are for the most part retained intracellularly in the endoplasmic reticulum and Golgi and exhibit impaired maturation with defective N-linked glycosylation.[187] Moreover, the constitutive activity of these variants does not require receptor dimerization.[187] Their oncogenic potential has been demonstrated by cytokine-independent growth,[155,184] transformation of NIH-3T3 fibroblasts in soft agar colony formation assays,[154] and tumor formation in nude mice.[154] Knockdown of ALK in ALK-mutant neuroblastoma cell lines led to significant inhibition of cell proliferation and induction of cell death, further emphasizing the strong oncogenic "addiction" of these cells to mutationally activated ALK.[155]

Elucidation of the crystal structure of ALK in its inactive conformation and mapping of neuroblastoma-associated mutations has shown that many of the ALK residues that become mutated in neuroblastoma play structural roles in autoinhibition of ALK.[188,189] Mutations allow unrestricted mobility of the alphaC helix, phosphate-binding loop, and N-terminal lobe, leading to kinase activation. Both the F1174L and R1275Q mutants show accelerated catalytic efficiency compared with wild-type ALK, with R1275Q exhibiting approximately fourfold increased catalytic efficiency and F1174L exhibiting approximately eightfold increased catalytic efficiency compared with the wild-type enzyme. This increased catalytic efficiency is at least partly due to the enhanced ATP binding affinity of these mutations for both ATP and peptide substrate.[189,190]

The ALK mutants show varying degrees of transformation capabilities. ALK^{F1174L} is considered the most aggressive of all ALK mutations in neuroblastoma, possessing higher transforming potential and kinase activity.[184] Importantly, ALK^{F1174L} also arises secondarily as a mechanism of resistance after an initial response to crizotinib in patients with ALK-rearranged cancers.[191] Moreover, the F1174L mutation cosegregates with MYCN amplification in patients with neuroblastoma, and this combination is associated with a particularly poor prognosis.[184] ALK^{F1174L} potentiates the oncogenic activity of MYCN in vitro[192,193] and in vivo,[194-196] although by itself, ALK^{F1174L} appears to be insufficient to cause the malignant transformation of neural crest–derived stem cells.[194,195] When crossed with MYCN transgenic mice, mice overexpressing ALK^{F1174L} in neural crest–derived cells gave rise to doubly transgenic progeny that developed aggressive neuroblastoma with 100% penetrance and a very short latency period.[194] ALK^{F1174L}/MYCN tumors exhibited increased MYCN dosage due to ALK^{F1174L}-induced activation of the PI3K/AKT/mTOR and MAPK pathways, coupled with suppression of MYCN pro-apoptotic effects.[194] Similarly, coexpression of ALK^{F1174L} and MYCN in zebrafish markedly increased the frequency of tumor formation and accelerated the time of onset.[195] MYCN overexpression induces adrenal sympathetic neuroblast hyperplasia, blocks chromaffin cell differentiation, and ultimately triggers a developmentally timed apoptotic response in the hyperplastic sympathoadrenal cells. Coexpression of activated ALK with MYCN provides prosurvival signals that block this apoptotic response and allow continued expansion and oncogenic transformation of hyperplastic neuroblasts, thus promoting progression to neuroblastoma.[195]

ALK mutations show no predilection for particular clinical stages of tumor progression.[185] With the exception of F1174L mutations that occur preferentially in MYCN-amplified tumors, somatic ALK mutations do not appear to be associated with survival,[184] although a more recent study reported that mutation-positive cases had a decreased overall survival (OS) probability.[197] However, ALK overexpression in the absence of mutation or amplification does appear to be associated with OS.[186,198] ALK RNA and protein overexpression is detectable in approximately 90% of primary tumors[199] and in some reports is associated with activation of downstream signaling.[200,201] The significance of this phenomenon, as well as the mechanism underlying activation of ALK, is presently unclear. Passoni et al.[198] (2009) argue that it is the level of expression that dictates oncogenicity, based on the fact that constitutive phosphorylation of ALK was observed in cells with high expression, whereas those with low expression lacked activation. This observation, plus the fact that genetic knockdown of wild-type ALK caused a decrease in cell proliferation,[97] suggest that overexpression of wild-type ALK may have some degree of proproliferative activity. Other studies have shown that neuroblastoma with elevated expression of wild-type ALK had clinical and molecular phenotypes similar to those of tumors with mutated ALK gene expression.[186] These data suggest that mechanisms other than mutation and amplification can lead to ALK activation.

ALK Amplification. ALK is amplified in around 2% to 3% of primary neuroblastoma cases.[184] Amplification tends to coexist with MYCN amplification; in fact, ALK amplification has been detected in up to 15% of primary neuroblastomas with MYCN amplification.[155,169,202] ALK amplification does not appear to have any independent prognostic value in neuroblastoma. ALK copy number gain appears to be more common than mutation or amplification, occurring in 15% to 20% of cases,[184,185] and usually involves whole chromosome 2 gain. Such chromosome 2p gains are associated with significantly increased ALK expression, correlating with poor survival.[97,184,198]

ALK Signaling in Neuroblastoma. Constitutively activated ALK as a result of ALK amplification binds to the activated Src homology 2 domain–containing adaptor protein ShcC and thereby activates downstream signaling.[169] Inhibition of this binding impairs survival, differentiation, and motility of neuroblastoma cells through blockage of the MAPK and PI3K/AKT pathways and impairs the induction of apoptosis.[201] Gain-of-function ALK mutations also commonly signal through the MAPK, PI3K/AKT/mTOR, and STAT pathways to regulate cell growth, transformation, and antiapoptotic signaling (reviewed in references 156 and 157).

ATRX Mutations

The alpha thalassemia/mental retardation syndrome X-linked (ATRX) gene is mutated primarily in 44% of neuroblastoma tumors in adolescents and young adults, which largely have an indolent tumor phenotype compared with that in children and infants.[203,204] These loss-of-function mutations are associated with absence of the ATRX protein in the nucleus and telomere lengthening, the mechanism of which is unclear. ATRX is involved in the regulation of ATP-dependent chromatin remodeling, nucleosome assembly, and telomere maintenance. ATRX also plays a role in epigenetic regulation of gene expression by controlling the deposition of histone H3.3 at transcriptionally silent regions of the genome, which may potentially lead to increased expression of oncogenes in tumors with ATRX mutations. ATRX mutations correlate with older age at diagnosis (age >5 years) and chronic or indolent disease. The ATRX gene is present on the X chromosome, and both males and females were affected. These mutations are not thought to be associated with MYCN amplification, although further studies are required to validate this supposition.[204]

Chromosomal Abnormalities in Neuroblastoma
Chromothripsis

Chromothripsis is a phenomenon that has been recently identified in 18% of high-stage neuroblastomas.[203] Chromothripsis[205] is a local shredding of chromosomes with subsequent random reassembly of the fragments. These structural alterations recurrently affected ODZ3 (TENM1 [teneurin transmembrane protein 1]), PTPRD (protein tyrosine phosphatase, receptor type, D), and CSMD1 (CUB and Sushi multiple domains 1) genes involved in neuronal growth cone stabilization.[203] ODZ3 and PTPRD encode transmembrane receptors expressed in the developing nervous system localizing to axon and axonal growth cones.[206] Chromothripsis-related structural aberrations were associated with amplification of MYCN or cyclin-dependent kinase–4 (CDK4) and loss of heterozygosity (LOH) of chromosome 1p.[203]

1p Loss of Heterozygosity

LOH of the short arm of chromosome 1p is a common occurrence in neuroblastoma.[207] The common region of LOH is within 1p36.2-1p36.3.[208-210] However, this region may be much larger, extending from 1p35 to the terminal end.[211-213] This abnormality has been reported not only in neuroblastoma but also in melanoma, pheochromocytoma, and medullary thyroid carcinoma, all of which are neural crest–derived tumors.[214-216] LOH of 1p occurs in 30% to 40% of neuroblastomas[217] and is positively correlated with older age, advanced stage, MYCN amplification, and a poor outcome.[218] When MYCN amplification and 1p LOH are present together, they define a genetically distinct and very aggressive subset of neuroblastoma.[219] Because cases with MYCN amplification represent a subset of patients with 1p deletion (because MYCN amplification is rarely found in the absence of 1p deletion), it is believed that 1p deletion may precede the development of MYCN amplification. Although 1p loss is also present in almost all samples with MYCN amplification, it is also found in high-risk cases without MYCN amplification.[217]

Therefore it follows that loss or inactivation of a gene or genes on 1p would be critical for the development or progression of neuroblastoma. This scenario has been suggested by reports of constitutional 1p36 alterations in patients with neuroblastoma.[220] Transfection of chromosome 1p into a neuroblastoma cell line restores a differentiated phenotype and abrogates tumorigenicity.[221] In addition, cell fusion experiments between MYCN amplified and single copy cells have resulted in abrogation of MYCN expression, suggesting than MYCN could be regulated by a gene located on 1p.[213] Several candidate tumor suppressor genes have been identified, including CHD5 (chromodomain helicase DNA binding protein 5),[222-224] KIF1B (kinesin family member 1B),[225,226] TP73 (tumor protein p73),[227] MIR34A (microRNA 34A),[228] CAMTA1 (calmodulin binding transcription activator),[229] and CASZ1 (castor zinc finger 1).[230]

CHD5. CHD5, a member of the CHD family of proteins involved in chromatin remodeling, is preferentially expressed in the nervous system and maps to a small region of deletion on 1p36.3 in neuroblastomas.[224] Expression of CHD5 has been found to be low or absent in cell lines and tumors with 1p deletion. Low expression of CHD5 is also highly correlated with MYCN amplification, advanced stage, and unfavorable histology.[224,231] When CHD5 was expressed in neuroblastoma cell lines with low or absent expression, clonogenicity and tumor growth were abrogated.[223] Mouse models with loss of a region corresponding to human 1p36 implicated CHD5 as a tumor suppressor that controls proliferation, apoptosis, and senescence via the p19^{Arf}/p53 pathway.[222] CHD5 mutations, however, are rare in neuroblastoma,[224] although it is now becoming clear that complete inactivation of the gene does not appear to be necessary for malignant transformation. Rather, gene dosage may be another mechanism that regulates tumor suppressor activity as shown for some PHOX2B mutations.[94] In a study by Bagchi et al.,[222] (2007) increased dosage of CHD5 (as in wild-type or three copies) led to tumor-suppressive properties, whereas decreased dosage (as in heterozygous 1p deletion) enhanced immortalization, spontaneous foci formation, and sensitivity to oncogenic transformation. In addition, it has been suggested that almost complete inactivation of the second allele may occur by an epigenetic phenomenon because the CHD5 promoter was found to be highly methylated in two cell lines that lacked CHD5 expression.[223]

KIF1B. The kinesin family member, KIF1B, is located on 1p36.2 and is thought to function as a tumor suppressor gene in neuroblastoma and pheochromocytoma.[226] Germline loss-of-function mutations have been detected in patients with neuroblastoma, leading to abrogation of the apoptosis that is a requisite to normal neuronal developmental culling when nerve growth factor (NGF) becomes limiting. Neuroblastoma cells have been shown to undergo apoptosis when NGF is withdrawn, which is mediated through the EglN3 prolyl hydroxylase. KIF1B acts downstream of EglN3.[232,233] Similar to the case with CHD5, KIF1B haploinsufficiency may be sufficient for loss of its tumor suppressor activity, especially if combined with loss or abnormalities of other genes on 1p36 such as CHD5.[222] In support of this theory, when KIF1B levels were decreased to 50% using short hairpin (sh)RNA knockdown, inhibition of apoptosis was observed.[226]

CASZ1. Deletion of CASZ1, a neuronal differentiation gene, has been implicated in neuroblastoma tumorigenesis.[229,234-236] CASZ1 is the human homologue of the *Drosophila* zinc finger transcription factor, castor.[237] Low expression of CASZ1 via LOH or epigenetic suppression is associated with poor prognosis in patients with neuroblastoma.[234,238] Moreover, the restoration of CASZ1 in neuroblastoma cells suppresses cell proliferation by activation of pRB in G1 and inhibition of the G2/M regulators cyclin B1 and Chk1 and induces cell differentiation.[234,235] Decreased CASZ1 expression in neuroblastoma is thought to be due to upregulation of one of the three core subunits of the polycomb repressor complex 2, EZH2 (enhancer of zeste 2).[238] This methyltransferase regulates trimethylation of histone H3 on lysine 27 (H3k27me3 [histone H3 trimethyl lysine 27]), which is associated with gene silencing. Analysis of expression data sets revealed that patients with neuroblastoma who have a poor prognosis have increased levels of EZH2 expression.[238] Silencing of EZH2 leads to decreased H3K27me3 and increased expression of CASZ1. Thus a model has been suggested in which one allele of CASZ1 could be lost by 1p LOH, with the remaining allele epigenetically silenced by EZH2-mediated H3k27me3. Moreover, EZH2 also was found to silence a number of tumor suppressors that control differentiation in neuroblastoma, such as clusterin *(CLU)*, runt-related transcription factor–3 *(RUNX3)*, and nerve growth factor receptor *(NGFR)*. Genetic and pharmacologic inhibition of EZH2 inhibited neuroblastoma cell growth and induced differentiation.[238]

MIR34A. The microRNA (miRNA)-34a *(MIR34A)* on 1p36.23 is expressed at lower levels in primary tumors and cell lines with 1p deletion and is also thought to function as a tumor suppressor gene.[228,239,240] Reintroduction of this miRNA into neuroblastoma cell lines with 1p deletion causes a dramatic reduction in cell proliferation through the induction of a caspase-dependent apoptotic pathway and by reducing levels of E2F3, a transcriptional inducer of cell-cycle progression. *MIR34A* also increases during retinoic acid–induced differentiation of neuroblastoma cells.[239,241] Indeed, targeted delivery of miRNA-34a using nanoparticles conjugated to an anti-GD2 antibody that is expressed on the surface of virtually all neuroblastoma cells was shown to result in decreased tumor growth in orthotopic xenograft models, highlighting its therapeutic potential.[242] In addition, *MIR34A* has also been found to directly target and downregulate MYCN and B-cell lymphoma–2 (BCL2).[240] *MIR34A* causes significant suppression of cell growth through increased apoptosis and decreased DNA synthesis in neuroblastoma cell lines with MYCN amplification.[228]

ARID1 Mutations. Deletions and sequence alterations in the chromatin-remodeling genes *ARID1A* and *ARID1B* (AT-rich interactive domain 1A and 1B) have been reported in 11% of tumors.[243] These mutations were associated with early treatment failure and decreased survival. ARID1 family genes are integral components of the switch/sucrose nonfermentable (SWI/SNF) neural

progenitor-specific chromatin-remodeling BRG1-associated factor (BAF) complex that is essential for the self-renewal of multipotent neural stem cells.[244] ARID1A was affected by insertional and point mutations predicted to result in premature termination of the protein and deletion of the other allele at 1p36, largely leading to biallelic inactivation.[243] Hemizygous deletions encompassing the whole coding sequence, intragenic hemizygous deletions, and splice-site and missense mutations targeting ARID1B were also reported in this study. High expression of members in the neural progenitor BAF complex correlated with a high-risk neuroblastoma phenotype, whereas high expression of components of the neuron-specific BAF complex or downstream neuritogenesis target genes correlated with low-risk neuroblastoma.[243] Thus it is possible that disrupted BAF complex signaling preserves an undifferentiated progenitor state, although this preservation has not as yet been demonstrated.

LIN28B Overexpression

Overexpression of the *LIN28B* gene that encodes a protein that binds small RNAs has been reported in neuroblastoma.[104] Lin28b is highly expressed in stem cells and developing tissues and regulates germ cell development, skeletal myogenesis and neurogenesis, and glucose metabolism. It is a master regulator of pluripotency in embryonic stem (ES) cells, and in combination with *NANOG* (Nanog homeobox), *OCT4* (organic cation transporter–4), and *SOX2* (sex-determining region Y box–2), it can reprogram differentiated cells to pluripotent stem cells.[245-247] High LIN28B expression was found to be an independent risk factor for adverse outcome in persons with neuroblastoma. In neuroblastoma cells, *LIN28B,* through repression of the let-7 miRNA family, caused elevated MYCN expression and inhibition of normal neuroblast and neuroblastoma differentiation, whereas overexpression of LIN28B in nonmalignant neuroblasts drives proliferation. Targeted expression of LIN28B in the sympathetic adrenergic lineage induced development of neuroblastomas marked by low let-7 miRNA levels and high MYCN protein expression. Mechanisms underlying the overexpression of LIN28B in neuroblastoma are currently unclear.[104] *LIN28B* has also been identified in a genome-wide association study of patients with neuroblastoma as influencing susceptibility to neuroblastoma, and high expression was associated with worse OS.[248]

Chromosome 17q Gain

Gain of chromosome 17q is the most common cytogenetic abnormality in neuroblastoma; it occurs in more than 60% of neuroblastomas and is associated with an unfavorable prognosis[249] and metastatic disease.[250] Gain usually takes the form of one to three extra copies. The break points vary, but in general, gain of a region from 17q22-qter is observed. Partial gain often results from unbalanced translocation of 17q21-25 to another chromosome. Unbalanced 1;17 translocations occur in primary neuroblastoma and result in loss of distal 1p with gain of 17q material.[251] Unbalanced 17q gain is associated with MYCN amplification and most likely harbors an oncogene that contributes to neuroblastoma tumorigenesis. However, 17q translocation break points are not uniform and can involve other partner chromosomes, especially 11q.[252] The break point positions on 11q were found to be variable, whereas all break points on 17q appeared to cluster proximal to position 43.1 Mb on the DNA sequence map.[253]

Isogenic cell lines derived from MYCN-driven murine tumors in transgenic mice showed gains of regions syntenic with human 17q.[254] One of the candidate genes on 17q is survivin, the expression of which is significantly associated with a poor prognosis.[255] Other candidate genes in the 17q region are nm23-H1 and nm23-H2, which are both targets of MYCN. Nm23-H1 binds to Cdc42, which is encoded on 1p36 and prevents neuroblastoma cell differentiation. Overexpression of Nm23 due to gain of 17q and induction by MYCN combined with decreased expression of Cdc42 due to loss of 1p36 can block neuroblastoma tumor differentiation.[256]

Chromosome 11q LOH

Allelic loss of 11q occurs in 35% to 45% of primary tumors.[257,258] Chromosome transfer experiments involving transfer of an intact chromosome 11 into a neuroblastoma cell line induces differentiation.[221] The common region of deletion has been mapped to 11q23, indicating that this could be a location for a neuroblastoma suppressor gene.[259] Chromosome 11q loss is associated with multiple chromosomal breaks, possibly reflecting an underlying DNA repair defect.[260] Chromosome 11q LOH occurs mainly in tumors *without* MYCN amplification and identifies a high-risk subset of patients with advanced stage, older age, and disease with unfavorable histologic features. Unbalanced deletion of 11q occurs in 15% to 20% of cases and is associated with a poor event-free survival (EFS) in patients with otherwise low-risk and intermediate-risk disease (Fig. 54-3).[261]

Chromosome 14q LOH

Deletion of 14q has also been reported in 25% of neuroblastomas,[262-264] with a common region of deletion within 14q23-qter.[265] LOH for 14q is inversely related to 1p36 LOH, MYCN amplification, and 11q LOH.
Other areas of chromosomal gain noted especially in tumors with an aggressive clinical phenotype, but not MYCN amplification, include gain of 1q and 12q.[266] Chromosomal regions that have been deleted are 3p,[267] 4p,[217] 9p,[268] and 18q,[269] but these regions are all less common.

Neurotrophin Receptors in Neuroblastoma

Tropomyosin receptor kinase (TRK) receptors, when activated by their respective neurotrophins, mediate the survival and differentiation of neurons during development (reviewed in reference 270).[270] NGF-induced dimerization of TRKA (NTRK1) or brain-derived neutrotrophic factor (BDNF)–induced dimerization of TRKB receptors leads to activation of the tyrosine kinase domain, which facilitates binding of SHC and phospho tyrosine binding (PTB) domain protein adaptors and PLCγ protein binding, respectively, leading to activation

of the major growth factor–regulated signaling pathways—the Ras/MAPK pathway and PI3K/3-phosphoinositide–dependent protein kinase–1 (PDK1)/AKT pathway—and to increases in Ca++ release and activation of the PLCγ pathway. The main ligand for TRKA, NGF, promotes survival and induces differentiation in developing sympathetic neuroblasts. Neuroblastoma tumor cells with high levels of TRKA expression differentiate in the presence of NGF in vitro but will undergo apoptosis in its absence.[271] Depending on the tumor microenvironment, therefore, TRKA signaling could induce differentiation or regression of favorable neuroblastomas. During normal development, depletion of NGF occurs in sympathetic neurons, causing TRKA signaling to activate predetermined apoptotic pathways. It has been postulated that spontaneous regression of neuroblastomas is but a delay in this normal developmental pattern.[92] A neurodevelopmentally regulated splice variant of TRKA, TrkAIII, has been identified that antagonizes the antioncogenic NGF/TRKA signaling and promotes neuroblastoma tumor growth.[272] High levels of TRKA expression are associated with a good prognosis in neuroblastoma and are strongly correlated with favorable tumor stage, younger age, and nonamplified MYCN. Patients with hyperdiploid tumors with favorable outcome identified by mass screening were also shown to have very high TRKA expression.[271]

The TRKB (NTRK2) transcript is expressed primarily in highly aggressive MYCN-amplified tumors.[273] The ligand for TRKB is BDNF, and activation of TRKB by BDNF leads to enhanced proliferation, migration, angiogenesis and resistance to chemotherapy in neuroblastoma.[274] Neuroblastoma cells that survive repeated exposures to cytotoxic agents express increasing levels of BDNF, suggesting that this pathway contributes to a multidrug-resistant phenotype.[275] Moreover, hypoxia induces increased TrkB expression and may contribute to a phenomenon in the tumor microenvironment where autocrine activation of the BDNF/TrkB signaling enables survival of residual tumor cells after repeated rounds of chemotherapy.[276] The full-length TRKB, which is expressed in about one third of tumors tested, is expressed primarily in those with MYCN amplification, whereas the truncated form resulting from alternative splicing, which lacks the tyrosine kinase domain, is expressed in ganglioneuromas and ganglioneuroblastoma.[273] The truncated TRKB is thought to sequester BDNF and thus prevent TRKB signaling.[277-279] Studies have shown that survival of neuroblastoma cells exposed to cytotoxic drugs is mediated partly by activation of the Trk receptor via PI3K,[280] activation of Akt,[281] and inactivation of glycogen synthase kinase–3 beta (GSK3B).[282] Thus the response of neuroblastoma cells to chemotherapeutic agents depends on the levels of BDNF; tumor cells expressing low levels of TrkB exhibit minimal effects on exposure to cytotoxic agents in the setting of a BDNF-rich environment. BDNF/TrkB-induced increases in HIF1a may lead to increased VEGF and angiogenesis in neuroblastoma.[283] Thus hypoxia associated increases in neuroblastoma cell invasiveness can be blocked by inhibition of TrkB.[284] Activation of the BDNF/TrkB signaling pathway stimulates

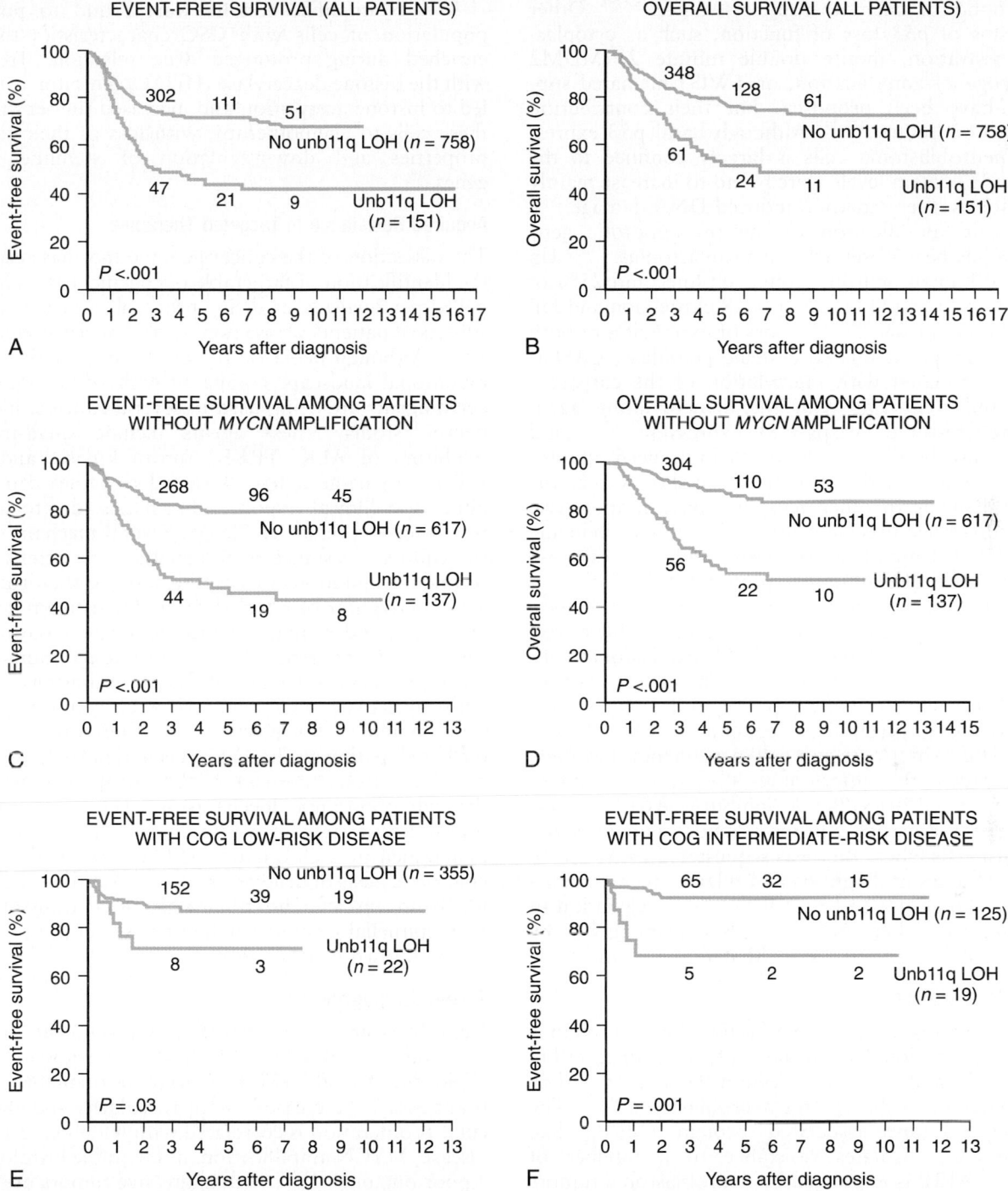

Figure 54-3 Survival according to unbalanced 11q loss of heterozygosity *(unb11q LOH)*. The rates of event-free and overall survival are shown for all patients (**A** and **B**), for patients whose tumors did not have v-myc avian myelocytomatosis viral oncogene neuroblastoma-derived homolog *(MYCN)* amplification (**C** and **D**), and event-free survival for those with low-risk disease (**E**) and intermediate-risk disease (**F**) as defined by the Children's Oncology Group *(COG)*. The numbers of patients at risk for an event are shown along the curves. *(From Attiyeh EF, London WB, Mosse YP, et al: Chromosome 1p and 11q deletions and outcome in neuroblastoma.* N Engl J Med *353:2243–2253, 2005.)*

tumor cell survival and angiogenesis and contributes to chemotherapy resistance and anoikis.[270]

TRKC, like TRKA, is involved in the biology of favorable neuroblastomas, and expression corresponds to lower stages.[285] Although its expression is found in 25% of primary neuroblastomas, it does not have independent prognostic significance, because all tumors with TRKC expression also have TRKA expression.

Apoptosis

In contrast to most human tumor types, the *p53* gene is very rarely mutated in neuroblastoma at diagnosis[286-289] but is found in chemotherapy resistance.[287,286] Other mechanisms of *p53* loss of function, such as cytoplasmic sequestration, mouse double minute 2 (MDM2 protooncogene) amplification, or TWIST-mediated suppression have been proposed, but their contribution appears to be limited.[290-292] Although basal p53 expression in neuroblastoma cells is largely confined to the cytosol, p53 protein levels were found to increase mainly in the nucleus after radiation-induced DNA damage.[293]

Epigenetic modification of the pro-apoptotic gene caspase-8 has been observed in neuroblastomas.[294,295] Up to 70% of human neuroblastoma cell lines and 25% of primary tumors tested lack caspase-8 expression and fail to undergo apoptosis.[294,296,297] Loss of expression of both caspase 8 (apoptosis-related cysteine peptidase, *CASP8*) alleles is correlated with methylation of the caspase-8 gene,[294] and treatment with the demethylating agent decitabine restored caspase-8 expression[296,298] and increased susceptibility to doxorubicin-induced apoptosis.[294] In addition, methylation has been shown to be the mode of silencing of other genes involved in apoptosis: the four tumor necrosis factor–related apoptosis-inducing ligand (TRAIL) apoptosis receptors and the caspase-8 inhibitor FLICE-like inhibitory protein (FLIP).[296,299]

Overexpression of BCL2, an inhibitor of apoptosis, has been found to be associated with unfavorable histology and MYCN amplification.[300] Neuroblastoma cells and tumors are primed for death with sequestration of BIM, a direct activator of apoptosis, either by the pro-survival BCL-2 or myeloid cell leukemia–1 (MCL-1) proteins.[301] This pattern of survival dependency has been shown to predict the pattern of response to Bcl-2 antagonists. The Bcl-2/Bcl-xl/Bcl-w inhibitor ABT-737 was active against Bim:Bcl-2 primed tumor xenografts but not against cells where Bim was sequestered by Mcl-1. In isogenic cell lines at diagnosis and relapse, therapy resistance was shown not to be mediated by upregulation of Bcl-2 family members or loss of Bim priming but by repression of Bak and/or Bax-mediated apoptosis.[301]

Therapy Resistance

The multidrug resistance gene encoding P-glycoprotein is thought to function by causing enhanced drug efflux from the cell, and its overexpression has been found to predict outcome of therapy for neuroblastoma.[302,303] The multidrug resistance-associated protein (MRP), like P-glycoprotein, mediates resistance to a number of drugs.[304,305] MRP is expressed by neuroblastoma tumors of all stages. Tumors with *MYCN* amplification have been shown to have significantly higher expression levels of MRP than do those with normal *MYCN* copy numbers. Reduced MRP expression levels correlate with differentiation of neuroblastoma cells in vitro.[306] In addition, an association has been found between high levels of MRP expression and poor outcome, which is independent of *MYCN* amplification.[307] It is possible that both multidrug resistance protein–1 (MDR1) and MRP function together with several other factors that confer resistance to drug therapy in neuroblastoma such as *MYCN* amplification, TRKB signaling, or loss of p53 expression.[274,308]

MYCN-amplified tumors were found to possess a population of cells with CSC characteristics that was enriched during prolonged drug selection. Treatment with the histone deacetylase (HDAC) inhibitor vorinostat led to histone acetylation and increased the sensitivity of these cells to chemotherapy, with loss of their stemness properties and downregulation of stemlike marker genes.[309]

Acquired Resistance to Targeted Therapies

The dissection of the cancer genome that has resulted in the identification of targetable oncogenic drivers has propelled personalized medicine protocols aimed at treating subsets of patients whose tumors harbor sensitizing mutations. Although pediatric tumors have a relatively silent mutational landscape compared with adult tumors, targeted agents are being used in several cancers, including neuroblastoma. These agents include small-molecule inhibitors of ALK, TRKB, aurora kinase, and PI3K/mTOR, to name a few. Targeted therapies can induce impressive clinical responses, but relapse due to acquired resistance is a major challenge. Several mechanisms lead to acquired resistance to targeted agents: acquisition of secondary mutations or amplification of the drug target itself, activation of alternative or downstream signaling pathways, and changes in drug efflux or bioavailability (reviewed in reference 310).[310] Secondary mutations in the target gene such as gatekeeper mutations preserve pathway activity and confer resistance by interfering with drug binding. Engagement of alternative receptor–mediated pathways has also been reported as causing resistance. Resistance to targeted therapy can also occur through nongenetic mechanisms, such as a reversible drug-tolerant state in a subpopulation of cells that is maintained by a chromatin modification, implicating an epigenetic basis of drug resistance.[311] Another mechanism involves transdifferentiation or histologic transformation with epithelial to mesenchymal transition in the absence of any known genetic mechanism.[312]

Tumor Angiogenesis

Neuroblastoma is characterized by prominent angiogenesis, and neuroblastoma cells have been shown to induce angiogenesis in the chick embryo chorioallantoic membrane assay.[313] Increased tumor vascularity and microvascular proliferation is correlated with widely disseminated disease, MYCN amplification, unfavorable histology, and a poor outcome.[314-316] Such aggressive tumors are associated with high expression of VEGF, basic fibroblastic growth factor, and platelet-derived growth factor A[299,314] and integrins, which are markers of active angiogenesis.[317] The presence of angiogenesis appears to be influenced by the cellular composition of the tumor in that in highly aggressive stroma-poor neuroblastoma, angiogenesis is present as a result of the secretion of angiogenic stimulators, whereas in stroma-rich tumors, numerous angiogenic inhibitors secreted by Schwann cells appear to maintain the inhibitory phenotype.[318] The Schwann cells in neuroblastoma tumors have been shown to have very low tumor vascularity with production of angiogenesis inhibitors, such as tissue inhibitor of matrix metalloproteinase–2 (TIMP-2), pigment epithelium-derived factor, and SPARC (secreted protein acidic and rich in cysteine), a calcium-binding matricellular glyco-protein.[117,314,319] SPARC expression has been found to be inversely correlated with the degree of malignant progression in neuroblastoma tumors, and neutralizing SPARC with antibodies reverses the antiangiogenic activity of Schwann cell–conditioned media.[319]

Metastasis

Metalloproteinases such as matrix metalloproteinase–9 (MMP9), along with CD44 and NM23-H1, which regulate tumor cell adhesion and migration, may play a role in metastasis.[320-322] Overexpression of MMP2 and MMP9 is associated with tumor invasion and metastasis in many types of cancer, whereas inhibitors of MMPs have been shown to suppress tumor invasion and angiogenesis. An association between increased levels of MMP2 and MMP9 and advanced-stage tumors has been observed in neuroblastoma. Caspase-8 has also been shown to be a metastasis suppressor gene.[323] Decreased caspase-8 expression has been shown to occur during the establishment of neuroblastoma metastases in vivo, and reconstitution of caspase-8 expression in deficient neuroblastoma cells suppressed these metastases. Caspase-8 selectively potentiated apoptosis in metastasizing cells, and loss of caspase-8 allowed cellular survival in the stromal microenvironment and promoted metastases.[323,324] In the TH-MYCN mouse model of neuroblastoma, caspase-8 was associated with increased metastasis, specifically to the bone marrow, possibly caused by upregulation of genes involved in epithelial-mesenchymal transition (EMT), decreased cell adhesion, and increased fibrosis.[325]

PATHOLOGY

Neuroblastomas arise from primitive sympathetic precursors of the neural crest and belong to the family of small round blue cell tumors. The histopathology of the tumor cells correlates with stages of sympathetic nervous system development. Tumors are composed of small blue round cells that are uniformly sized and contain dense, hyperchromatic nuclei and scant cytoplasm. Surrounding the neuroblasts is stroma, known as Schwannian stroma. A typical feature of neuroblastoma is the presence of neuropil, which is made up of neuritic processes and is found in the majority of neuroblastomas. One of the pathognomonic features of neuroblastoma is the Homer-Wright pseudorosette, a collection of neuroblasts surrounding areas of neuropil, which occurs in up to half of cases (15% to 50%; Fig. 54-4, A).[326]

Neuroblastoma manifests as a spectrum of three histologic patterns ranging from neuroblastoma to ganglioneuroblastoma to ganglioneuroma, based on the degree of tumor cell differentiation. Neuroblastomas are composed of mostly small immature blue round cells with scanty cytoplasm, little evidence of differentiation, and high mitotic activity. Ganglioneuroblastomas are tumors with differentiated ganglion cells admixed with neuroblastic tissue. These tumors may vary from predominantly neuroblastic with rare ganglion cells to predominantly maturing cells with rare undifferentiated components, such as neuroblastic cells. If less than 50% of the cells are maturing cells, the tumor is termed a "maturing neuroblastoma," and if more than 50% of the cells are maturing cells, it is termed a "ganglioneuroblastoma." Ganglioneuroblastomas can also be focal or diffuse, and both types can exist within a single tumor. Two forms of ganglioneuroblastoma exist: (1) the intermixed variety, in which cells in various stages of differentiation are interspersed with small nests of neuroblasts, predicting a good outcome, and (2) the nodular type, in which hemorrhagic areas and macroscopic nodules are present, which is associated with a worse prognosis. Ganglioneuromas are fully differentiated tumors consisting entirely of maturing ganglion cells, neuropil Schwannian stroma, and nerve fibers.[327,328]

Primary histologic diagnosis may be enabled by hematoxylin and eosin staining and light microscopy. Other techniques also help distinguish neuroblastomas from other small round blue cell tumors of childhood, such as immunohistochemistry with use of antibodies for neural markers, such as neurofilament protein, synaptophysin, neuron-specific enolase, ganglioside GD2, chromogranin A, and tyrosine hydroxylase. Electron microscopy studies may exhibit dense core-membrane–bound neurosecretory granules and microfilaments and parallel arrays of microtubules within the neuropil.[329]

Tumor histology in neuroblastoma has traditionally been determined by the Shimada classification system.[330] Tumors are classified as favorable or unfavorable based on three features: amount of stroma, degree of neuroblastic cell differentiation, and the mitosis-karyorrhexis index (MKI; the percentage of tumor cells in mitosis versus karyorrhexis). This system had one drawback in that it was age-linked, and age itself is a strong independent prognostic feature in neuroblastoma. The Joshi system was simpler in that it examined the presence of calcification and mitotic rate (less than or equal to 10 mitoses per 10 high-power fields) and was designed to be independent of age and stage; however, it did not have the same prognostic power as the Shimada system.[331] Subsequently a unified classification, the International Neuroblastoma Pathology Classification (INPC), was established in 1999[332] and revised in 2003.[333] This classification schema was formulated on the basis of the natural history of neuroblastoma of involution and maturation as described by Beckwith and Perrin (1963).[27] In other words, it is based on the age-dependent normal ranges of morphologic features such as Schwannian stroma, degree of neuroblastic differentiation, and MKI and seeks to divide neuroblastic tumors into those with favorable and unfavorable histology (Fig. 54-4, B).[334]

The INPC has four main morphologic categories (Table 54-2).The first category is neuroblastoma (Schwannian-stroma poor), which is a tumor with nests of neuroblastic cells interspersed with little or minimal stroma. There are three subtypes, based on grade of differentiation: (a) undifferentiated, (b) poorly differentiated (some neuropil and <5% of cells exhibiting differentiation), and (c) differentiating (abundant neuropil and >5% of cells showing differentiation toward ganglion cells).

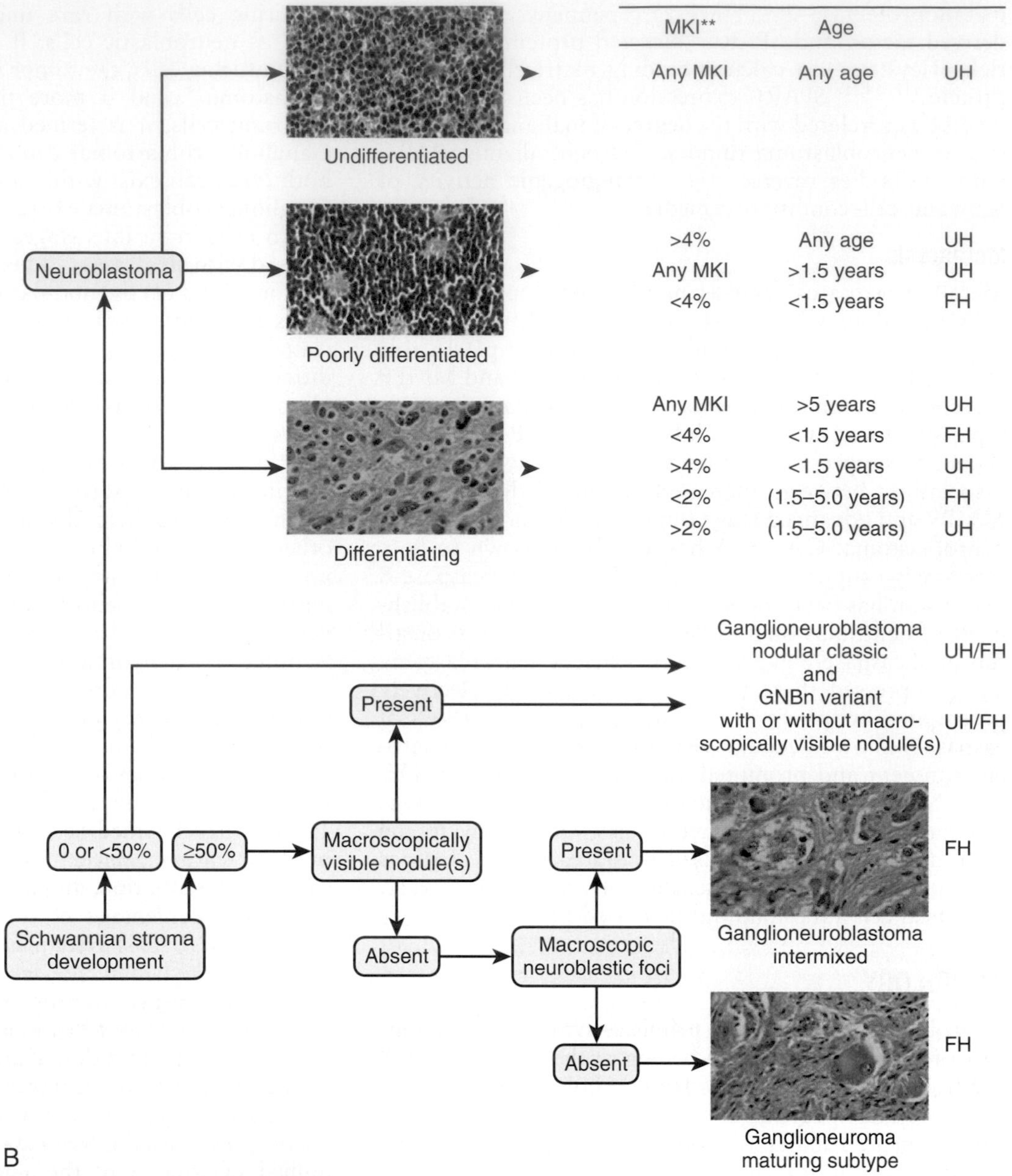

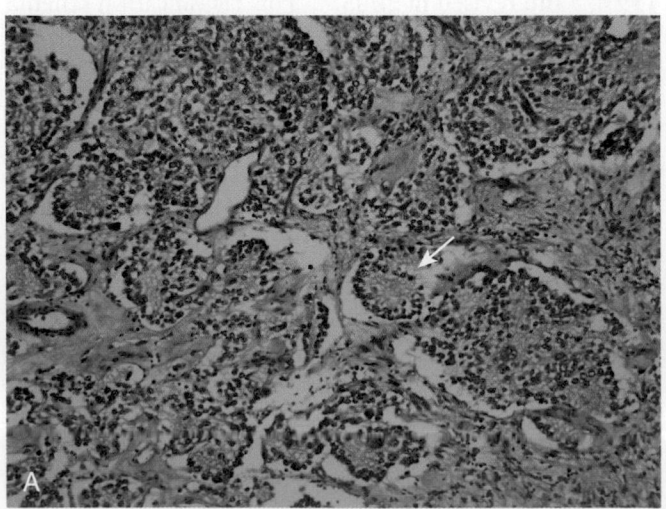

MKI**	Age	
Any MKI	Any age	UH

Undifferentiated

>4%	Any age	UH
Any MKI	>1.5 years	UH
<4%	<1.5 years	FH

Poorly differentiated

Any MKI	>5 years	UH
<4%	<1.5 years	FH
>4%	<1.5 years	UH
<2%	(1.5–5.0 years)	FH
>2%	(1.5–5.0 years)	UH

Differentiating

Neuroblastoma

Ganglioneuroblastoma
nodular classic   UH/FH
and
GNBn variant
with or without macro-   UH/FH
scopically visible nodule(s)

Present

Macroscopically
visible nodule(s)

0 or <50%   ≥50%

Schwannian stroma
development

Absent

Present

Macroscopic
neuroblastic foci

Absent

Ganglioneuroblastoma
intermixed   FH

Ganglioneuroma
maturing subtype   FH

B

Figure 54-4 Neuroblastoma pathology. **A,** Neuroblastoma tumor showing that aggregates of tumors are composed of small immature blue round cells, uniformly sized, containing dense, hyperchromatic nuclei and scant cytoplasm. Homer-Wright pseudorosettes, which are rings of neuroblasts surrounding eosinophilic neuropil, are seen *(arrowhead)*. **B,** The International Neuroblastoma Pathology Classification. *FH,* Favorable histology; *GNBn,* ganglioneuroblastoma; *MKI,* mitosis-karryorhexis index; *UH,* unfavorable histology. *(From Park JR, Eggert A, Caron H: Neuroblastoma: biology, prognosis, and treatment.* Pediatr Clin North Am *55(1):97–120, x, 2008.)*

TABLE 54-2 International Neuroblastoma Pathology Classification

International Neuroblastoma Pathology Classification		Original Shimada Classification	Prognostic Group
Neuroblastoma Favorable <1.5 yr	Schwannian Stroma-poor* Poorly differentiated or differentiating and low or intermediate MKI tumor	Stroma-poor Favorable	Favorable
1.5-5 yr	Differentiating and low MKI tumor		
Unfavorable <1.5 yr 1.5-5 yr ≥5 yr	1. Undifferentiated tumor† 2. High MKI tumor 1. Undifferentiated or poorly differentiated tumor 2. Intermediate or high MKI tumor All tumors	Unfavorable	Unfavorable
Ganglioneuroblastoma -Nodular	Composite Schwannian stroma rich/stroma dominant with stroma poor	Stroma-rich nodular (Unfavorable)	Unfavorable
Ganglioneuroblastoma-intermixed	Schwannian stroma rich	Stroma rich intermixed (Favorable)	Favorable
Ganglioneuroma Maturing Mature	Schwannian stroma dominant	Well differentiated (Favorable) Ganglioneuroma	Favorable‡

Shimada H, Ambros IM, Dehner LP, et al: The International Neuroblastoma Pathology Classification (Shimada) System. Cancer 86:364–372, 1999.

MKI, Mitosis-karyorrhexis index.

*Subtypes of neuroblastoma are described in detail elsewhere.[332]

†Rare subtype, especially diagnosed in this age group. Further investigation and analysis are required.

‡Prognostic grouping for these tumor categories is not related to patient age.

The second category is ganglioneuroblastoma, intermixed (Schwannian stroma-rich), which is a tumor that contains well-defined microscopic nests of neuroblastic cells intermixed in ganglioneuromatous stroma. The nests are composed of neuroblastic cells in various stages of differentiation, but they are primarily composed of differentiating neuroblasts and maturing ganglion cells in a background of neuropil. The third category is ganglioneuroblastoma, nodular (composite Schwannian stroma-rich/stroma-dominant and stroma-poor). This tumor is composed of biologically different clones, an aggressive clone composed of grossly visible, hemorrhagic neuroblastic nodules (stroma-poor component), and a nonaggressive clone comprising ganglioneuroblastoma, intermixed (stroma-rich component), or with ganglioneuroma (stroma-dominant component). The fourth category is ganglioneuroma (Schwannian-stroma–dominant), of which there are two subtypes, maturing and mature. The maturing subtype is composed predominantly of ganglioneuromatous stroma with scattered differentiating neuroblasts or maturing ganglion cells, as well as fully mature ganglion cells. The mature subtype is composed of ganglion cells and Schwannian stroma.

In the new and revised International Neuroblastoma Risk Group (INRG) classification schema, tumor histology will be classified independent of age and will primarily be based on degree of differentiation and the MKI.

CLINICAL PRESENTATION

Neuroblastomas are tumors of sympathetic nervous system and can arise anywhere along the sympathetic chain or in any sympathetic ganglia. Most primary tumors occur in the abdomen (65%), and half of abdominal tumors occur in the adrenal gland. Other common sites of disease origin include the chest, neck, and pelvis, although rarely a primary tumor cannot be found. Because the sites of origin of neuroblastoma are so diverse, the signs and symptoms of disease at presentation vary widely and depend on both the location of the primary tumor and the degree of disease dissemination.

Localized Disease

Approximately 40% of patients present with localized disease.[335] Primary abdominal disease can present as an asymptomatic abdominal mass or with abdominal pain and fullness. Symptoms of obstruction can occasionally be seen, along with renin-mediated hypertension caused by compression of the renal vasculature.[336] Abdominal or pelvic tumors can also occasionally cause compression of lower extremity venous and lymphatic drainage, leading to lower extremity and scrotal swelling. Rarely abdominal tumors spontaneously hemorrhage, and patients with such hemorrhage present with a sudden, dramatic enlargement of an abdominal mass with increased distension and pain. Lower thoracic tumors are usually identified incidentally when a chest radiograph is obtained for unrelated reasons. Occasionally large thoracic tumors are associated with mechanical obstruction and resultant superior vena cava syndrome. Upper thoracic or cervical tumors may cause Horner syndrome.[337] Congenital tumors arising in this site can also cause hematochromia of the iris as a result of decreased pigmentation of the iris on the affected side.[338] Neuroblastoma arising from the paraspinal ganglia in the chest, abdomen, or pelvis can grow through the intervertebral foramina and compress the spinal cord. Patients may be asymptomatic or present with pain or neurologic deficits resulting from spinal cord compression, which requires emergent treatment as detailed later in this chapter.

Metastatic Disease

Metastatic spread of neuroblastoma occurs through the lymphatics or hematogenously. Regional lymph node metastases are seen in one third of patients with apparently localized tumors, and half of patients present with hematogenous metastases.[335] Hematogenous spread occurs most frequently to the bone, bone marrow, and/or liver; rarely, metastasis to the lungs and brain occurs, usually at relapse rather than at presentation. Classic signs of metastatic neuroblastoma include proptosis and periorbital ecchymoses (commonly referred to as "raccoon eyes") due to tumor infiltration of the periorbital bones. Patients also frequently present with limping and irritability due to bone pain from bone and bone marrow disease, as well as nonspecific symptoms including fever and failure to thrive. The presence of fever is usually associated with extensive bone metastases. Signs and symptoms of bone marrow replacement are also sometimes seen—most frequently pallor (which may also be caused by bleeding within the primary tumor), as well as bruising and increased risk of infection as a result of a low white blood cell count.[339]

Stage 4S Neuroblastoma

Stage 4S (S = special) is a unique presentation of neuroblastoma seen in infants; it was originally described by D'Angio, Evans, and Koop in 1971.[340] Infants with stage 4S neuroblastoma often present with massive hepatomegaly caused by diffuse liver metastases and nontender, bluish subcutaneous nodules as a result of skin nodules. Stage 4S disease accounts for 7% to 12% of neuroblastoma diagnoses and is historically defined as the presence of a small, localized primary tumor with metastases isolated to the liver, skin, and/or bone marrow in an infant younger than 12 months.[341] This special neuroblastoma often spontaneously regresses, although infants younger than 2 months can present with respiratory compromise due to a rapidly enlarging liver and may require cancer-directed treatment.[342] Based on an analysis of a large cohort of international patients diagnosed with neuroblastoma between 1990 and 2002, the INRG Task Force has extended the definition of 4S neuroblastoma to include patients up to the age of 18 months and those with primary tumors crossing the midline.[343]

Paraneoplastic Syndromes

Opsoclonus-myoclonus syndrome (OMS) and vasoactive intestinal peptide syndrome, which are well-described paraneoplastic syndromes associated with neuroblastoma, are detailed in this section, along with a newly described syndrome known as rapid-onset obesity with hypothalamic dysfunction, hypoventilation, and autonomic dysregulation (ROHHAD). Patients with these syndromes usually have localized tumors with favorable biology, perhaps because the syndrome causes early detection of tumor or, more likely, because of a correlation between the syndrome and the tumor biology.

OMS is observed in 2% to 3% of children with neuroblastoma[344] and is usually diagnosed between the age of 1 and 3 years.[345] It is often referred to as "dancing eyes, dancing feet syndrome" and is characterized by the acute onset of rapid eye movements, ataxia, myoclonic jerking of the limbs and trunk, and behavioral disturbances.[345] Although children with neuroblastoma and OMS generally have favorable tumor prognostic features and a high survival rate,[346-348] 70% to 80% experience long-term neurologic sequelae that can include global developmental delay, speech and/or motor delay, behavioral disturbances, and cognitive deficits that can seriously affect quality of life.[344,347,349,350] OMS in children is associated with neuroblastoma more than half of the time.[345] After exclusion of CNS pathology, all children with OMS should be evaluated for neuroblastoma with imaging of their chest and abdomen, an iodine 123–metaiodobenzylguanadine (MIBG) scan, and urine catecholamines.[351] Traditional methods to detect neuroblastoma may be insensitive in patients with OMS,[352,353] and therefore high-resolution computed tomography (CT) or magnetic resonance imaging (MRI) of the chest and abdomen should be considered, even in patients with negative catecholamines or negative results of an MIBG scan, to screen for small tumors.

OMS and its sequelae are thought to be immune mediated and are likely caused by the presence of an antineural antibody that cross-reacts with a common antigen on both neuroblastoma and normal nervous system tissue.[345] Improvement in symptoms can be seen after tumor removal in some cases, but generally immunosuppression with glucocorticoids or adrenocorticotropic hormone is used to relieve acute symptoms.[345,347,354] However more than 80% of patients will have a relapse of symptoms with steroid weaning or in association with a viral syndrome,[351] and more than half of patients will need prolonged steroid treatment, necessitating additional treatment approaches. Intravenous immune globulin has also been used in the treatment of OMS, either with or without steroids, with varying success.[355,356] Case reports have shown efficacy of other immunomodulating strategies including plasmapheresis, rituximab, and mycophenolate.[357-361] Although often effective in treating acute symptoms, none of these treatments has been consistently correlated with improved long-term outcome. Interestingly, a report from the Pediatric Oncology Group (POG) suggested that patients who received chemotherapy to treat their neuroblastoma had a more favorable neurologic outcome.[344] This benefit may be due to the immunosuppressive effects of chemotherapy or to less severe activation of the immune system in patients with more advanced stages of tumor.[345] The same benefit was not observed in a similar review performed by the Children's Cancer Group (CCG),[347] and the benefit of chemotherapy for the treatment of OMS needs to be investigated further. The COG recently conducted a trial for OMS in which patients with low-risk neuroblastoma who would not otherwise receive chemotherapy were treated with cyclophosphamide in addition to steroids. Long-term outcome of these patients compared with historic control subjects should provide insight regarding the role of chemotherapy for the treatment of OMS.

Further investigation is needed to determine the best treatment approach for OMS.[362] Regardless of treatment, physicians caring for patients with OMS should anticipate long-term neurologic abnormalities and use early intervention to help minimize these deficits.

Tumor secretion of vasoactive intestinal peptide can cause a syndrome of chronic watery diarrhea and failure to thrive. Most tumors secreting vasoactive intestinal peptide are histologically mature. Surgical removal of the tumor usually results in complete resolution of symptoms.[363]

ROHHAD syndrome is characterized by rapid-onset obesity, hypothalamic dysfunction, hypoventilation, and autonomic dysregulation.[364] Tumors of neural crest origin have been found in more than one third of cases[364,365] and are usually differentiated (ganglioneuromas or ganglioneuroblastomas).[366] ROHHAD syndrome most commonly affects otherwise normal children between 2 and 4 years of age and typically presents first with rapid weight gain and obesity followed at varying time intervals by autonomic dysfunction and hypoventilation. The prognosis is poor, and at least 25% of children die because of respiratory failure. A genetic cause has been suggested because of the constellation and consistency of symptoms and the reported occurrence in siblings,[366] but several candidate genes (including *PHOX2B*, *ASCL1* [achaete-scute family bHLH transcription factor–1], *NTRK2* [*TRKB*], and *BDNF*) have been sequenced in affected patients and have not been informative.[364,366] Monozygotic twins discordant for ROHHAD have recently been reported,[367] although this in itself should not preclude a genetic cause because modifier genes or epigenetic variation may play a role in the variable phenotype. Because of the association with neuroblastic tumors and the finding of extensive infiltrates of lymphocytes and histiocytes in the hypothalamus of some patients,[368,369,370] a paraneoplastic cause has been postulated. Immune-modulating agents including intravenous immunoglobulin, rituximab, and cyclophosphamide have been tried in small series of patients with varying success,[367,370a] and collaborative studies are needed to determine the cause of this rare disorder. Surveillance for tumors in patients with this constellation of features is recommended.

DIAGNOSIS AND EVALUATION

Diagnosis

The diagnosis of neuroblastoma is usually established from histopathologic evaluation of primary tumor tissue.[371] In most cases, especially if features of neuronal differentiation are present, a tissue diagnosis of neuroblastoma can be made on the basis of conventional hematoxylin and eosin staining. However, in cases in which there is little differentiation and only small round blue cells are evident, immunohistochemical staining for neuron-specific enolase, chromogranin A, and/or synaptophysin, as well as cytogenetic and molecular analysis, can help differentiate neuroblastoma from other small round blue cell tumors of childhood.[357-359]

In addition to establishing the diagnosis, primary tumor material is essential for risk stratification and prognosis, particularly in children younger than 18 months with locoregional or metastatic spread. In cases in which primary tumor tissue cannot be obtained safely, the diagnosis of neuroblastoma can also be made by demonstrating unequivocal neuroblastoma cells in a bone marrow aspirate or biopsy in conjunction with increased urinary catecholamines. Urinary catecholamine metabolites are increased in 90% to 95% of neuroblastomas using sensitive detection techniques such as high-performance liquid chromatography[372,373] and can be helpful in establishing a diagnosis, as well as in monitoring disease activity and response to therapy in patients who are known to excrete the metabolites. In sympathetic cells the catecholamine precursor 3,4-dihydroxyphenylalanine (DOPA) is converted to dopamine by DOPA decarboxylase, which is converted to norepinephrine and then to epinephrine by the enzyme phenylethanolamine-N-methyltransferase, which is not present in neuroblastoma cells.[374] Instead the enzymes catechol-O-methyltransferase and monoamine oxidase convert DOPA and dopamine to homovanillic acid and norepinephrine and epinephrine to vanillylmandelic acid, both of which are inactive metabolites that are excreted in the urine. Both urinary homovanillic acid and vanillylmandelic acid should be measured for diagnostic purposes. For undifferentiated tumors, urinary dopamine may also be useful.[371] Despite this catecholamine production, symptoms of catecholamine excess such as hypertension, flushing, and sweating are rarely seen in persons with neuroblastoma, likely because of the relatively low concentrations of active catecholamines in the circulation.

Clinical Disease Assessment

The primary tumor and the extent of disease should be evaluated using imaging techniques both at diagnosis and to evaluate response to treatment. Either CT or MRI are routinely used to evaluate the extent and origin of the primary tumor, as well as possible solid organ metastases.[375] CT is more widely available and can rapidly capture images, reducing the need for sedation, but it is associated with substantial radiation exposure. Ionizing radiation is not used to perform MRI but it has a longer imaging acquisition time, making sedation necessary in most young children. Currently no consensus exists with regard to which imaging technique is optimal for evaluating tumors and metastases in the abdomen, pelvis, or mediastinum. Availability and clinical factors, including the risks of sedation, should be taken into account. MRI is preferred for assessing paraspinal lesions, particularly those with possible intraextension and spinal cord impingement. Although abdominal ultrasonography is not as useful for assessing tumor volume and anatomy, it may be useful as a noninvasive method for following tumor response or surveying for disease relapse. Brain imaging is only recommended if clinically indicated by symptoms or examination.

Bone and bone marrow should also be evaluated by imaging to look for the presence and extent of metastatic disease. MIBG is a norepinephrine analogue that is selectively concentrated in more than 90% to 95% of neuroblastomas and can be combined with either the iodine 131 or ^{123}I isotopes for scanning purposes. MIBG scintigraphy is highly sensitive and specific for detecting osteomedullary disease and can also be used to assess the primary tumor, as well as occult soft tissue disease (Fig. 54-5). The ^{123}I isotope provides enhanced image resolution and is the isotope of choice when it is available. MIBG scans are essential for the initial staging of neuroblastoma and should be performed prior to primary tumor resection. International guidelines are available for patient preparation, radiotracer administration, and imaging techniques.[376] A bone scan using technetium 99m–diphosphonate scintigraphy is a relatively sensitive but less specific method to detect bony metastases in patients with neuroblastoma. Bone scans are recommended in cases in which the primary tumor is not MIBG avid, or in cases in which tumor uptake of MIBG cannot be confirmed (i.e., in cases in which the primary tumor is removed prior to imaging for metastatic disease).[375] Fluorine 18–labeled deoxyglucose positron emission tomography (FDG-PET) can also be used to evaluate metastatic disease in persons with neuroblastoma.[377-379] Its sensitivity and specificity in comparison with MIBG scintigraphy is still being evaluated, with studies suggesting that MIBG is more sensitive than FDG-PET for the detection of bone lesions and skull-based lesions, and that FDG-PET is more sensitive than MIBG for the detection of small soft tissue tumors and nodal metastases.[380] The routine use of FDG-PET is not currently recommended, but it may be a helpful tool to follow-up patients with metastatic disease who do not have MIBG-avid tumors.

Bone marrow aspirates and biopsies from both iliac crests are recommended to assess for the presence of bone marrow disease using standard histologic analysis.[371,381] Both immunocytochemical and polymerase chain reaction–based technologies can be used to increase sensitivity of marrow detection. Immunocytochemical analysis of bone marrow aspirates with monoclonal antibodies directed against neural-specific antigens (e.g., GD2 and NCAM, neural cell adhesion molecule) increases the sensitivity of detecting marrow involvement to 1:100,000 nucleated cells.[382] Reverse-transcriptase polymerase chain reaction methodologies that target the expression of neuroblastoma-specific messages such as tyrosine hydroxylase, protein gene product 9.5, or GD2 synthase can enhance sensitivity further.[383-388] However, the clinical and prognostic significance of this enhanced detection, remains to be determined, and these studies are generally only recommended within the context of a clinical study.

Staging

The International Neuroblastoma Staging System (INSS) was established in the 1990s to replace three major staging systems used throughout the world in an effort to provide international uniformity so that clinical trials and biology studies performed by different groups in different countries could be compared.[371,381] The INSS (Table 54-3) is largely based on the surgical assessments of a patient at diagnosis and has been used nationally and internationally for more than 20 years. However, because surgical approaches are not uniform, the INSS stage for patients with locoregional disease can vary considerably depending on the degree of initial tumor resection, making comparison of clinical trials conducted in different parts of the world difficult. To address this problem, the INRG Task Force developed a new staging system based on tumor imaging rather than extent of surgical resection.[389] This staging system (known as the INRG staging system) uses radiologic characteristics of the primary tumor to predict surgical risk and resectability (Tables 54-4 and 54-5).[390] Using this approach, in INRG staging, locoregional disease is classified as stage L1 or L2 on the basis of whether the tumor is locally invasive by imaging at the time of diagnosis. Stage M indicates metastatic disease that is assessed in the same

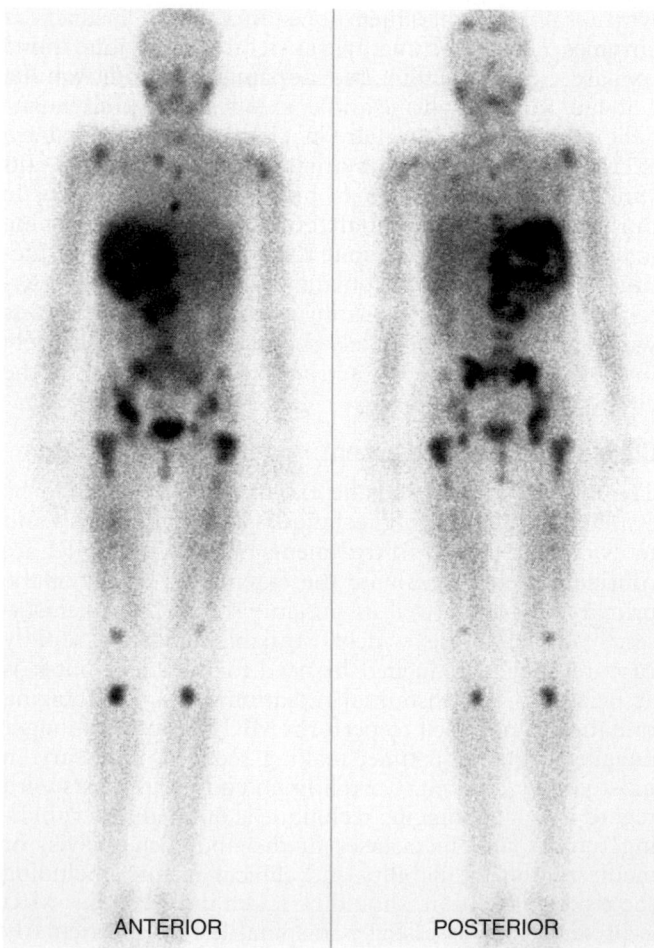

ANTERIOR   POSTERIOR

Figure 54-5 Metaiodobenzylguanidine scan. Primary tumor uptake (right adrenal gland), as well as bone/bone marrow metastases, are visualized. *(Courtesy of F. Grant, MD, Division of Nuclear Medicine, Children's Hospital, Boston, Mass.)*

TABLE 54-3   International Neuroblastoma Staging System[371,381]

Stage	Description
1	Localized tumor with complete gross excision, with or without microscopic residual disease; representative ipsilateral lymph nodes negative for tumor microscopically (nodes attached to and removed with the primary tumor may be positive)
2A	Localized tumor with incomplete gross excision; representative ipsilateral nonadherent lymph nodes negative for tumor microscopically
2B	Localized tumor with or without complete gross excision, with ipsilateral nonadherent lymph nodes positive for tumor; enlarged contralateral lymph nodes must be negative microscopically
3	Unresectable unilateral tumor infiltrating across the midline,* with or without regional lymph node involvement; *or* localized unilateral tumor with contralateral regional lymph node involvement; *or* midline tumor with bilateral extension by infiltration (unresectable) or by lymph node involvement
4	Any primary tumor with dissemination to distant lymph nodes, bone, bone marrow, liver, skin and/or other organs (except as defined for stage 4S)
4S	Localized primary tumor (as defined for stage 1, 2A, or 2B), with dissemination limited to skin, liver and/or bone marrow† (limited to infants younger than 1 year of age)

Multifocal primary tumors (i.e., bilateral adrenal primary tumors) should be staged according to the greatest extent of disease, as previously defined, followed by a subscript "M" (e.g., 3_M).
*The midline is defined as the vertebral column. Tumors originating on one side and "crossing the midline" must infiltrate to or beyond the opposite side of the vertebral column.
†Marrow involvement in stage 4S should be minimal, that is, less than 10% of total nucleated cells identified as malignant on bone marrow biopsy or aspirate. More extensive marrow involvement would be considered to be stage 4. The metaiodobenzylguanidine scan (if done) should be negative in the marrow.

way it was assessed by INSS criteria, via both imaging and pathology.

The INRG system also differs from the INSS system in that the midline and lymph node status are not included in the staging criteria. In addition, INRG stage MS includes patients up to 18 months of age and those with L2 tumors, whereas INSS stage 4S has an upper age limit of 12 months and includes only patients with stage 1 or 2 primary tumors.

Because imaging can be retrospectively reviewed, the INRG staging system should provide data that are more uniform than the INSS system. The INRG staging system is currently used in Europe and will be adopted into the COG studies as well.

TABLE 54-4   Image-defined Risk Factors in Neuroblastic Tumors[375,593]

Anatomic Region	Description
Multiple body compartments	Ipsilateral tumor extension within two body compartments
Neck	Tumor encasing carotid artery, vertebral artery, and/or jugular vein Tumor extending to skull base Tumor compressing trachea
Cervicothoracic junction	Tumor encasing brachial plexus roots Tumor encasing subclavian vessels, vertebral artery, and/or carotid artery Tumor compressing trachea
Thorax	Tumor encasing aorta and/or major branches Tumor compressing trachea and/or principal bronchi Lower mediastinal tumor infiltrating costovertebral junction between T9 and T12 vertebral levels
Thoracoabdominal junction	Tumor encasing aorta and/or vena cava
Abdomen and pelvis	Tumor infiltrating porta hepatis and/or hepatoduodenal ligament Tumor encasing branches of the superior mesenteric artery at the mesenteric root Tumor encasing the origin of the celiac axis and/or the origin of the superior mesenteric artery Tumor invading one or both renal pedicles Tumor encasing the aorta and/or vena cava Tumor encasing the iliac vessels Pelvic tumor crossing the sciatic notch
Intraspinal tumor extension	Intraspinal tumor extension provided that more than one third of the spinal canal in the axial plane is invaded, the perimedullary leptomeningeal spaces are not visible, or the spinal cord signal intensity is abnormal
Infiltration of adjacent organs and structures	Pericardium, diaphragm, kidney, liver, duodenopancreatic block, and mesentery

TABLE 54-5　International Neuroblastoma Risk Group Staging System[389]

Stage	Description
L1	Localized tumor not involving vital structures as defined by the list of image-defined risk factors and confined to one body compartment
L2	Locoregional tumor with the presence of one or more image-defined risk factors
M	Distant metastatic disease (except stage MS)
MS	Metastatic disease in children younger than 18 months with metastases confined to skin, liver, and/or bone marrow

Patients with multifocal primary tumors should be staged according to the greatest extent of disease as defined in the table.

RISK STRATIFICATION

Neuroblastoma is a tumor in which biologic factors are consistently used to influence disease risk stratification and treatment. In 1998 the COG established a risk-stratification system that stratifies patients into low-, intermediate-, or high-risk categories based on prognostic features including age at diagnosis, stage, tumor histology, DNA index (ploidy), and MYCN amplification status (Table 54-6). Treatment recommendations are based on this risk grouping, as described in the next section, and prognosis is distinct for each risk group (Fig. 54-6).

In an effort to unify risk stratification internationally and facilitate comparison of clinical trials performed in different parts of the world, the INRG Task Force was formed with representatives from the major pediatric cooperative groups. The INRG Task Force retrospectively analyzed the prognostic effect of 13 variables in a cohort of 8800 patients diagnosed with neuroblastoma between 1990 and 2002 with respect to EFS. Based on these analyses, a consensus INRG classification scheme was created using the most statistically significant and clinically relevant factors, which include INRG stage, age, histology, grade of tumor differentiation, MYCN and 11q status, and tumor ploidy (Table 54-7).[343] The significance of the risk factors used in both the INRG and COG stratification systems is described later.

Clinical Variables

Age is an important prognostic factor in neuroblastoma. Traditionally it was thought that infants (those younger than 1 year or 365 days of age) had a more favorable outcome, whereas children older than 1 year had a

TABLE 54-6　Current Children's Oncology Group Risk Group Classification

INSS	Age	MYCN*	Ploidy	Shimada[†]	Risk Group
1	Any	Any	Any	Any	Low
2	Any	Not amp	Any	Any	Low
2	Any	Amp	Any	Any	High
3	<547 days	Not amp	Any	Any	Intermediate
3	≥547 days	Not amp	Any	FH	Intermediate
3	≥547 days	Not amp	Any	UH	High
3	Any	Amp	Any	Any	High
4	<365 days	Amp	Any	Any	High
4	<365 days	Not amp	Any	Any	Intermediate
4	365 - <547 days	Not amp	>1	FH	Intermediate
4	365 - <547 days	Any	1	Any	High
4	365 - <547 days	Any	Any	UH	High
4	365 - <547 days	Amp	Any	Any	High
4	≥547 days	Any	Any	Any	High
4S	<365 days	Not amp	1	FH	Low
4S	<365 days	Not amp	1	Any	Intermediate
4S	<365 days	Not amp	Any	UH	Intermediate
4S	<365 days	Amp	Any	Any	High

Courtesy of the Children's Oncology Group.

FH, Favorable histology; *MYCN,* v-myc avian myelocytomatosis viral oncogene neuroblastoma derived homolog; *INSS,* International Neuroblastoma Pathology Classification; *UH,* unfavorable histology.
*MYCN amplification status: *Amp,* amplified; *non-amp,* not amplified.
[†]International Neuroblastoma Pathology Classification.

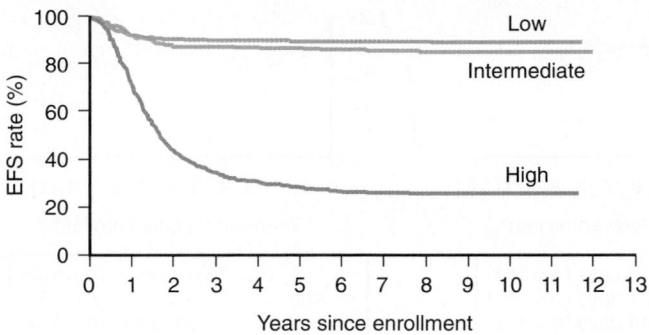

Figure 54-6 Event-free survival *(EFS)* of patients with neuroblastoma stratified according to risk group. *(Courtesy of W. B. London, PhD, Children's Oncology Group.)*

much more dismal outcome, especially those with metastatic disease at diagnosis.[391,392] However, recent studies of a large series of cases have demonstrated that age is a continuous prognostic variable in neuroblastoma, and 18 months has been identified as the age under which patients with stage 3 and 4 disease share the same favorable outlook as those younger than 1 year of age (Fig. 54-7).[3,110,393] Whether children aged between 12 and 18 months who have advanced stage disease but otherwise favorable biologic features can be cured with less aggressive therapy is currently under investigation. Fewer than 5% of cases of neuroblastoma are diagnosed in children older than 10 years. Experience suggests that older patients with high-risk–type disease can have a more indolent course but ultimately a dismal outcome, implicating a unique tumor biology.[394-397] Age older than

10 years is not currently used in risk stratification but may be in the future when the biology is more clearly understood.

Stage has always been considered an important prognostic factor, with low stage or localized disease having a better outcome than high stage or metastatic disease; the overall prognosis for patients with stage 1, 2, and 4S disease is 80% to 90%, whereas patients with disease between stages 3 and 4 have a 2-year survival rate of 20% to 40%.[374] As described previously, the INRG staging system, which determines local-regional disease extent based on image-defined risk factors rather than surgical risk factors, is in the process of being adopted internationally.

Pathologic features are also used to classify neuroblastomas. The Shimada classification divides tumors as having "favorable" and "unfavorable" histology by incorporating age with tumor differentiation, MKI, and Schwannian stroma.[330] However, because age itself is a strong independent prognostic variable, new classification systems such as the INRG examine MKI and differentiation as independent variables, along with established clinical and biologic variables.

Biologic Variables

Biologic factors currently used for neuroblastoma risk stratification include *MYCN* copy number by fluorescence in situ hybridization,[397a] DNA ploidy by flow cytometry,[108] and tumor histology using the INPC.[332] *MYCN* amplification automatically stratifies children into the high-risk category in a majority of cases, except for completely resected INSS tumors, which remains controversial. DNA index or ploidy is considered prognostic

TABLE 54-7 International Neuroblastoma Risk Group Consensus Pretreatment Classification[343]

INRG Stage	Age (mo)	Histologic Category	Grade of Tumor Differentiation	MYCN	11q Aberration	Ploidy	Pretreatment Risk Group
L1/L2		GN maturing; GNB intermixed					A Very low
L1		Any, except GN maturing or GNB intermixed		NA Amp			B Very low K High
L2	<18	Any, except GN maturing or GNB intermixed		NA	No Yes		D Low G Intermediate
	≥18	GNB nodular; neuroblastoma	Differentiating	NA	No Yes		E Low H Intermediate
			Poorly differentiated or undifferentiated	NA Amp			N High
M	<18 <12 12 to <18 <18 ≥18			NA NA NA Amp		Hyperdiploid Diploid Diploid	F Low I Intermediate J Intermediate O High P High
MS	<18			NA Amp	No Yes		C Very low Q High R High

AMP, Amplified; *GN,* ganglioneuroma; *GNB,* ganglioneuroblastoma; *INRG,* International Neuroblastoma Risk Group; *NA,* not amplified.

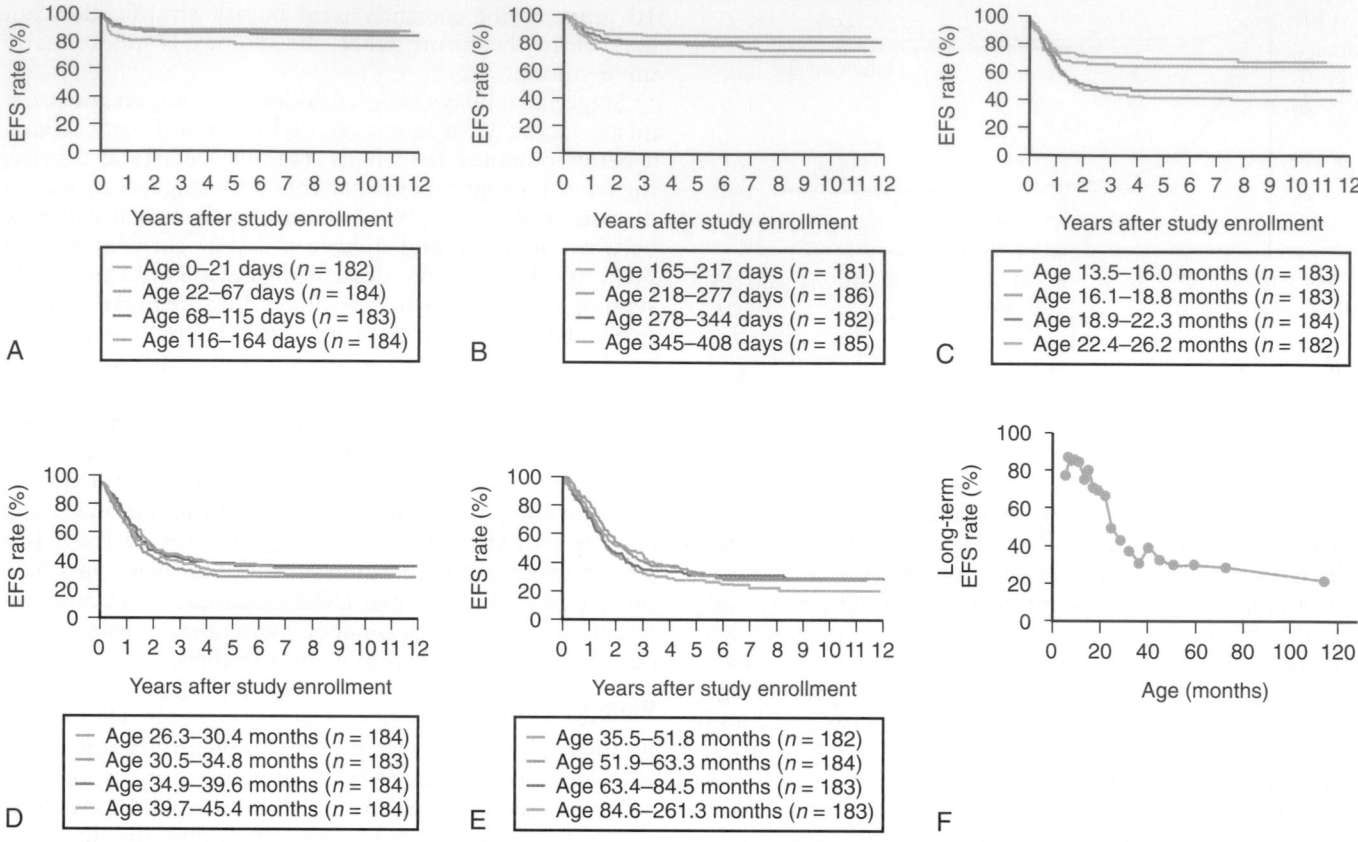

Figure 54-7 Kaplan-Meier event-free survival *(EFS)* curves by age group. **A,** 0 to 164 days. **B,** 165 to 408 days. **C,** 13.5 to 26.2 months. **D,** 26.3 to 45.4 months. **E,** 35.5 to 261.3 months. **F,** Long-term EFS rate by age group (not a Kaplan-Meier curve). *(From London WB, Boni L, Simon T, et al: The role of age in neuroblastoma risk stratification: the German, Italian, and Children's Oncology Group perspectives. Cancer Lett 228:257–266, 2005.)*

in children up to 18 months of age.[110] Neuroblastoma tumors are classified as diploid (DNA index [DI] = 1) and hyperdiploid (DI > 1). In the COG schema, a DI of 1 would stratify a patient to the high-risk group if the patient was between 12 and 18 months of age with stage 4 disease, regardless of *MYCN* amplification status or histology. Diploid DNA content in infants (<12 months) with *MYCN* nonamplified, stage 4S disease will signify intermediate risk, regardless of tumor histology.

Other genetic features such as evaluation for LOH of 1p36 and 11q23[261] were used to stratify therapy in prior studies and could be important for stratification of non–high-risk patients with neuroblastoma. In patients with neuroblastoma whose tumors did not have MYCN amplification, the prognostic impact of the three most common segmental chromosomal alterations—1p deletion, 11q deletion, and/or 17q gain—was studied.[107] Segmental chromosomal anomalies were more frequent in children older than 18 months and with stage 4 disease. In multivariate analysis, the presence of a segmental genotype significantly correlated with a poorer EFS, although age and stage were still more significant; therefore the utility of such a segmental genomic profile for prognostic risk assessment is questionable, given that age and stage were still more significant in this study (*P* < .0001 and

P = .0002, respectively, vs. *P* = .01 for the segmental genotype).[107]

APPROACH TO TREATMENT

The modalities used in the treatment of neuroblastoma include surgery, chemotherapy, radiotherapy, and biotherapy, as well as observation alone in a small subset of patients. The determination of treatment is largely based on prognostic factors and subsequent risk group assignment, as previously described. A major goal of ongoing neuroblastoma clinical trials is to prospectively validate the existing risk group assignments, as well as to evaluate newer prognostic markers for future refinement of risk stratification and treatment assignment. The general principles of therapy for each of the current risk groups are detailed below.

Treatment of Low-Risk Disease

Low-risk neuroblastoma is defined as INSS stage 1 disease in patients of any age, INSS stage 2 in infants 365 days of age or older with any MYCN status and histology, INSS stage 2 in children older than 365 days with MYCN of any status and favorable histology, and INSS stage 4S MYCN—not amplified, favorable histology, and hyperdiploid. For patients with INSS stage 1 disease, surgical resection is almost always the only treatment required, and these patients have an excellent OS rate. The COG study P961 prospectively evaluated 915 eligible patients with low-risk neuroblastoma. The 453 patients with INSS stage 1 disease had a 5-year EFS and OS of 93% ± 2% and 99% ± 1% with surgery as their primary treatment, which is consistent with findings of previous studies.[398] The same COG study showed that chemotherapy can be omitted for most patients who have biologically favorable but incompletely resected localized tumors (INSS stage 2A and 2B). Patients with asymptomatic INSS stage 2 disease were observed after surgery and had 5-year EFS and OS of 87% ± 2% and 96% ± 1%, respectively. The EFS was significantly better for patients with stage 2A disease compared with stage 2B disease (92% ± 3% and 85% ± 3%; P = .0321), but the OS did not differ. The majority of patients with INSS stage 2B disease had unfavorable histology and/or diploid tumors, which independently had a significant impact on EFS and OS. Similar results were published by the International Society of Pediatric Oncology neuroblastoma group.[399] For low-risk disease, chemotherapy should only be used in cases in which the tumor is causing organ- or life-threatening symptoms or in cases of recurrent of progressive disease not amenable to surgery. Although disease recurrence is rarely seen, it usually occurs within a year of diagnosis, and the majority of recurrences are local.[400-402] Local recurrences in low-risk patients can usually be managed with second surgeries. Metastatic recurrences are rare but are often salvageable with more intensive systemic therapy.

Neuroblastoma is known to have one of the highest rates of spontaneous regression among malignant tumors, which has been well documented in patients with stage 4S disease.[403] Data from mass screening studies in Japan show a two- to threefold higher incidence of neuroblastoma in areas with screening programs.[404] This increase in the rate of diagnosis supports the hypothesis that a subset of non–stage 4S neuroblastomas in young infants can undergo spontaneous regression as well. The German Society of Pediatric Oncology and Hematology reported a prospective trial supporting this hypothesis.[405] Ninety-three infants with localized neuroblastoma were observed without use of surgery or chemotherapy. Spontaneous regression was seen in 44 of the 93 infants (47%), and 17 infants had a complete regression. The 3-year EFS (56% ± 5%) was low because approximately half of the infants required an intervention, but the overall survival remained excellent (99% ± 1%). This study included patients with locally invasive disease and any tumor biology except for MYCN amplification. The COG recently completed an observation study for perinatally detected adrenal tumors to further explore the hypothesis of spontaneous regression in young infants with localized tumors.[406] This study had more restricted eligibility than did the German study, limiting enrollment to patients 6 months of age or younger with tumors limited to the adrenal gland, but biopsies were not performed to confirm diagnosis and determine tumor biology. Parents could choose observation or immediate surgical resection at enrollment. Eighty-seven eligible patients were enrolled, and for 83 patients, the parents elected observation. For the observation arm, 56 patients completed observation and 27 discontinued observation (13 were lost to follow-up). The majority of the patients who completed observation had a decrease in the volume of their adrenal mass, and 27 patients (48%) had no residual mass at the end of the observation period. Sixteen observation patients had surgery (one at the end of the observation period); 10 patients had neuroblastoma, 2 had low-grade adrenal cortical neoplasms, 2 had adrenal hemorrhages, and 2 had extralobar pulmonary sequestrations. Nine of the patients with neuroblastoma underwent surgery as a result of progression, seven had INSS stage 1 disease, one had INSS stage 2B disease, and one had INSS stage 4S (neither of the latter two patients required further treatment). For the overall cohort, the 3-year EFS for a neuroblastoma event was 97.7% ± 2.2%, and the 3-year OS was 100%. The results of this study confirm that expectant observation results in excellent survival rates and spares surgery in a majority of infants with adrenal masses. The COG has plans to extend observation to all L1 tumors in infants in a future clinical trial.

The optimal treatment of the rare patient with MYCN-amplified, localized neuroblastoma is controversial. Most studies have demonstrated a worse outcome for patients with localized tumors with MYCN amplification. A CCG prospective analysis of 374 patients with Evans stage I and II disease showed that four of seven patients (four with stage I disease and three with stage II disease) who had MYCN amplification experienced a relapse (in three cases, the disease was metastatic) between 2 and 22 months from diagnosis, and three of these patients died as a result of disease progression.[400] A POG analysis of 329 patients with stage A neuroblastoma showed that 4 of 11 patients with MYCN amplification remained disease free 22 months to 68 months after initial surgery. Additional treatment of four of seven patients with recurrent disease was successful. In the COG P9641 study previously described, 10 patients with INSS stage 1 disease had MYCN amplification. Five-year EFS was 93% ± 2% and 70% ± 17%, and OS was 99% ± 1% and 80% ± 15% for MYCN nonamplified and MYCN-amplified tumors, respectively (P < .001).[398] Although these results clearly support a worse outcome for MYCN-amplified localized disease, they also show (based on a small sample size) that a subset of patients may achieve long-term remission with surgery alone.[401] A retrospective review of 600 patients (32 with MYCN-amplified tumors) who had localized neuroblastoma and were enrolled in a POG neuroblastoma biology study from 1990 to 1999 suggests that ploidy might be useful for further risk stratification of these rare patients. In this study ploidy was significantly correlated with outcome for patients with MYCN-amplified localized disease (7-year OS 87% + 9% for patients with hyperdiploid tumors vs. 38% + 12% for patients with diploid/hypodiploid tumors).[407] The same outcome was found in a retrospective analysis of the INRG database, which contains 2600 patients with low-stage neuroblastoma, known MYCN status, and available follow-up data. In this database 87 patients had low-stage disease with MYCN-amplified tumors, and they had a less favorable outcome compared with patients who had nonamplified tumors (5-year OS 72% ± 7% vs. 98% ± 1%).[408] As in the POG analysis, the outcome of patients with hyperdiploid tumors was significantly better than in patients with diploid tumors (5-year OS 94% ± 11% vs. 54% ± 15%). Further prospective evaluation is needed to determine a consensus treatment strategy for these patients.

Cord compression from intraspinal tumor extension can occur in children who otherwise would be considered low risk and is an oncologic emergency requiring rapid intervention. The choice of emergent therapy is somewhat controversial, with pediatric oncologists favoring chemotherapy and neurosurgeons favoring laminectomy with spinal cord decompression.[409] Retrospective analyses show similar neurologic outcomes for patients treated with chemotherapy versus laminectomy.[410-413] The severity of motor impairment at diagnosis seems to be the strongest predictor of short-term response to treatment and the development of long-term functional outcome. Studies have also shown that because of the young age of most of these patients, laminectomy can result in significant long-term orthopedic problems.[414] For these reasons, intermediate-risk–type chemotherapy is preferred in most cases for emergent treatment of spinal cord compression. Neurosurgery should be reserved for patients with rapid neurologic deterioration or those in whom worsening symptoms develop while they are receiving chemotherapy. Radiation therapy can also be used but is usually reserved for patients with progressive neurologic abnormalities despite chemotherapy and surgical decompression because of the long-term morbidity of spinal irradiation in infants and young children.[409]

Most patients with INSS stage 4S disease have favorable biologic features (single-copy MYCN, hyperdiploid, and favorable Shimada histology) and are categorized as having low-risk disease. The POG reviewed 110 patients with stage D(S) neuroblastoma diagnosed between 1987 and 1996 and found a 3-year OS rate of 85% ± 4% with a significantly worse prognosis for infants younger than 2 months of age or those with tumor cell diploidy, unfavorable histology, or MYCN amplification.[341] A report from the CCG showed similar results for 80 infants with a 5-year OS of 92%.[342] Patient with suspected INSS stage 4S neuroblastoma should undergo biopsy of the primary tumor or an accessible metastatic site (such as a subcutaneous nodule) to establish the diagnosis and to determine biologic features of the tumor. Patients with favorable biologic features usually do not require therapy and should be observed closely.[340] Resection of the primary tumor is not necessary to achieve an excellent outcome in these patients.[341] Patients with progressive or symptomatic disease and those who are too ill to undergo a biopsy at diagnosis are generally treated with moderately intensive chemotherapy, such as that currently recommended for intermediate-risk disease.[341,342] Patients with hepatomegaly that progresses despite chemotherapy and causes respiratory compromise are treated with small doses of radiation—450 to 600 cGy in 150-cGy fractions. The rare patient with INSS stage 4S disease who has unfavorable ploidy and/or histology tumors should be treated with intermediate-risk–type therapy. Patients with INSS stage 4S disease who have MYCN amplification should be treated with high-risk–type therapy.

Treatment of Intermediate-Risk Disease

The intermediate-risk classification group includes a wide spectrum of disease. The current approach to treatment utilizes a combination of moderate-dose multiagent chemotherapy and surgery with an expected OS of greater than 90%. The CCG 3881 study was one of the first to prospectively stratify patients according to risk group. In this study intermediate-risk patients (defined by MYCN status, age, histology, and ferritin level) were treated with moderately dose-intensive chemotherapy (cyclophosphamide, doxorubicin, cisplatin, and etoposide), along with local radiation for any gross residual disease after surgery. Patients who had favorable biology (i.e., MYCN that was not amplified, a favorable Shimada classification, and a low serum ferritin level) had an OS of 92% to 100% depending on stage, and infants with unfavorable features had an OS of 93%.[415,416] After this study, in the COG A3961 study, investigators attempted to reduce acute and long-term toxicity of the CCG regimen by substituting carboplatin for cisplatin and decreasing total cumulative doses of chemotherapy while maintaining dose intensity and eliminating radiation therapy in all patients except those with unresectable primary tumors and unfavorable biologic features at the end of chemotherapy. This study used the COG risk stratification described previously and enrolled 479 eligible patients between 1997 and 2005. Intermediate-risk neuroblastoma was defined as INSS stage 3 or 4 disease in an infant (<365 days of age) without MYCN amplification; stage 3 disease and favorable histopathologic features in a child (≥365 days of age); and stage 4S disease with unfavorable histopathologic features and/or a diploid DNA index. Patients received four to eight cycles of chemotherapy depending on risk factors. Among all patients, 3-year EFS and OS were 88% ± 2% and 96% ± 1%, proving that therapy could be substantially reduced for the majority of intermediate-risk patients.[417] The outcome for patients with INSS stage 4 disease (for 176 patients, EFS and OS 81% ± 3% and 93% ± 2%, respectively) was inferior to that of patients with INSS stage 3 or 4S but did reach the overall study goal of maintaining a 3-year OS greater than 90% for all patients. Ploidy was significantly associated with outcome for patients of all ages. This study was followed in the COG by a study that prospectively used 1p and 11q status to further stratify patients and reduce therapy for patients whose tumors lack LOH at 1p and 11q and who have other favorable biologic factors.[261] The results of this study are still pending, but early reports suggest that excellent OS can be maintained despite the reduction of therapy in intermediate-risk patients who have favorable risk factors.

Existing data suggest that adjuvant therapy could be further reduced despite the presence of gross residual tumor in patients with locoregional tumors who have favorable biology. Traditionally, patients receive chemotherapy with the goal of facilitating surgical resection.

Experience from Memorial Sloan Kettering Cancer Center showed that patients with non–stage 4, non–*MYCN*-amplified disease who had gross residual disease after initial surgery could be safely observed and could maintain an excellent survival rate without use of cytotoxic therapy.[418] In this report only 1 of 22 patients required chemotherapy, and 4 of 13 patients with gross residual disease required a second surgery. This outcome is also supported by the European experience. In the German neuroblastoma 97 protocol, infants who had stage 2 or 3 MYCN nonamplified tumors with incomplete resections were observed postoperatively without use of adjuvant chemotherapy. Regression without further treatment was seen in 32 of 55 patients, and salvage therapy was effective for patients who progressed or experienced a recurrence, with a 3-year OS rate of 98%.[405] On the basis of this information, the most recent COG intermediate-risk study used partial response as the treatment end point in patients with favorable biology and INSS stage 2 or 3 disease.

Treatment of High-Risk Disease

Treatment of disseminated neuroblastoma remains one of the greatest challenges in pediatric oncology. High-risk neuroblastoma represents more than half of all newly diagnosed neuroblastoma cases and is the cause of most of the mortality associated with the disease. Treatment approaches that utilize a combination of intensive induction therapy, myeloablative consolidation therapy with stem cell support, and biologic therapy for minimal residual disease have improved 5-year survival rates from less than 15% to 30% to 40%.[259,419] This modest improvement in survival, however, has come at the cost of increased doses of both chemotherapy and radiotherapy, significantly increasing treatment-related morbidity in disease survivors.

Induction Therapy

The goal of induction therapy is to maximally reduce the overall tumor burden by using a combination of chemotherapy, surgery, and radiation therapy. High-risk neuroblastoma is generally sensitive to initial chemotherapy, even in cases with MYCN amplification. A retrospective meta-analysis of 44 trials showed that a correlation existed between dose intensity and treatment efficacy, including improved response and survival.[420] Induction chemotherapy for high-risk neuroblastoma generally consists of five to seven alkylator and platinum-based cycles using agents selected to reduce cross-resistance. A number of combinations have been used in the United States and Europe, including a regimen developed at Memorial Sloan-Kettering Cancer Center that has been widely used. This regimen consists of cycles of cyclophosphamide, vincristine, and doxorubicin alternating with cycles of cisplatin and etoposide. In a single-institution study of this regimen, Kushner et al.[421] reported a complete response rate of 63% and a complete plus very good partial response rate of 87% in 24 patients. The French Society of Pediatric Oncology Neuroblastoma Study Group used this induction regimen in a multiinstitution study of 47 patients and found a complete response rate of only 45%.[422] Similar results were obtained in the COG A3973 phase III trial, where 242 of 477 patients (51%) attained a complete or very good partial response, suggesting that chemotherapy resistance during induction remains an obstacle to cure.[423]

One strategy to improve induction response is to decrease treatment intervals during induction to lead to more rapid cell death with less chance of drug resistance. Pearson and colleagues[424] (2008) reported a European randomized clinical trial comparing treatment of 262 patients with stage 4 neuroblastoma using rapid-timing chemotherapy (i.e., a cycle every 10 days) versus standard-timing chemotherapy (i.e., a cycle every 21 days) using the same cumulative doses of five chemotherapeutic drugs given over 10 weeks or 18 weeks. The rapid regimen, also known as COJEC (cisplatin, vincristine, carboplatin, etoposide, and cyclophosphamide) was feasible without markedly increased toxicity. Complete or very good partial responses were achieved in 53% of patients assigned to conventional treatment and in 71% of patients assigned to rapid treatment ($P = 0.002$), although no significant difference in OS was found between the two regimens.

The COG piloted an alternative strategy of using non–cross-resistant chemotherapeutic agents to further improve induction response rates. Topotecan is a topoisomerase-1 inhibitor that has shown antineuroblastoma activity in both phase I and II trials with a limited toxicity profile, including dose-limiting myelosuppression and mild to moderate nausea, vomiting, and mucositis.[425,426] Thirty-one patients were enrolled in a COG feasibility trial that incorporated high-dose topotecan into the Memorial Sloan-Kettering backbone.[427] The induction regimen was well tolerated, without unexpected toxicities. Fifteen of 31 patients (48%) achieved a complete or very good partial response. This regimen was recently studied by the COG in a large phase III trial in a large patient population to more accurately access efficacy; the results are pending.

A growing body of evidence suggests that the quality of induction response correlates with outcome. Ladenstein and colleagues[428] performed a multivariate analysis of 549 patients with high-risk neuroblastoma included in the European Bone Marrow Transplantation Solid Tumor Registry and showed that persistent cortical bone lesions ($P = .004$) and bone marrow involvement ($P = .03$) were the only independent adverse prognostic factors. This report included patients treated over a 14-year period, leading to significant interpatient treatment variability. More recent smaller retrospective studies have shown that MIBG response at the end of induction assessed by semiquantitative scoring methods directly correlates with EFS after myeloablative therapy.[429-431] Yanik and colleagues[432] assessed a semiquantitative MIBG score using the Curie scoring system for patients with INSS stage 4 disease who were treated in the COG A3973 trial at diagnosis ($n = 280$) and at the end of induction ($n = 237$). They found that patients who had a Curie score greater than 2 at the end of induction ($n = 52$) had a significantly decreased EFS compared with patients who had Curie scores of 2 or less (3-year EFS 15.4% ± 5.3%

vs. 44.9% ± 3.9%, $P < .001$). Patients who had MYCN amplification with a Curie score greater than 2 ($n = 6$) at the end of induction were particularly affected, with a 3-year EFS of 0% compared with 44.2% ± 6.9% for patients with MYCN amplification who had a Curie score of 2 or less ($n = 65$). These results support previous studies that showed that residual disease at the end of induction measured using Curie scoring of MIBG scans is clearly associated with a worse outcome in patients with high-risk disease. Efforts to further improve survival may need to include response-based end-of-induction treatment stratification, and alternative treatment strategies should be strongly considered for patients with Curie scores greater than 2.

Local Control

Patients with high-risk disease usually have large and locally invasive primary tumors that chemotherapy alone is unlikely to eradicate. Local control is obtained using a combination of surgery and local radiation therapy. Definitive surgery on the primary tumor is usually performed near the end of induction therapy after four to five cycles of chemotherapy. Delaying surgical resection until after chemotherapy has been shown to improve resectability and may reduce the surgical complication rate.[433,434] However, the benefit of complete resection in the treatment of high-risk neuroblastoma remains controversial because the impact of aggressive treatment of the primary tumor site on EFS is unclear in the face of metastatic disease. Several retrospective studies have shown contradictory results. La Quaglia and colleagues[435] reviewed 141 patients treated at Memorial Sloan-Kettering Cancer Center with sequential protocols between 1979 and 2002 and showed evidence of a significant improvement in survival with a gross total resection. Similarly, Adkins and colleagues[433] reviewed the 210 patients (out of 539 total patients) entered in the CCG 3891 study who achieved a complete response by resection and showed a trend toward improved 5-year EFS and OS. However, a report from St. Jude Children's Research Hospital that examined the extent of resection compared with outcome in 107 children older than 1 year with stage 4 neuroblastoma treated with one of four consecutive protocols between 1984 and 2001 showed no evidence of association between survival and the extent of surgery.[436] In addition, Von Allmen and colleagues[437] reported on the local control of 76 patients treated at two institutions using the same treatment protocol with a consistent surgical approach. They found that aggressive surgery followed by local radiation provided excellent local tumor control with no isolated local occurrences in patients who had greater than 90% resection (60 of 76 patients). However the completeness of resection was not correlated with a difference in EFS or OS. Further prospective evaluation of the role of surgery in high-risk neuroblastoma is needed. It is likely that resectability is a surrogate for tumor biology. Gross total resection with nodal resection should be the goal to provide adequate local control, but it should not be performed if it is done at the cost of vital organs or significant postoperative morbidity that would lead to a delay in further therapy.

Neuroblastoma is a highly radiosensitive tumor, and local radiation directed at the primary tumor site in persons with high-risk disease has been shown to decrease the risk of local recurrence.[377,438,439] The total dose generally used in the United States is 2160 cGy in daily 180-cGy fractions to the postinduction chemotherapy, preoperative primary tumor volume. Local radiation is generally used either at the end of induction or after recovery from consolidation chemotherapy. Patients whose radiation field includes their liver may be at higher risk of veno-occlusive disease if radiation is used prior to stem cell transplant.[440] To reduce the possibility of local recurrence after an incomplete surgical resection, the most recent COG study investigated giving patients who have an incomplete resection of the primary tumor an additional boost of 1440 cGy to the gross residual volume in addition to the standard 2160 cGy (for a total dose of 3600 cGy to the gross residual tumor volume). Results of this intervention are still under analysis.

Proton therapy, which can result in improved sparing of normal tissue, is becoming more widely available for pediatric patients. Preliminary studies show no difference in local control compared with photons.[441,442] Assessment in regard to improvement in late toxicity will require long-term follow-up of a large group of patients.

Consolidation Therapy

The goal of the consolidation phase of therapy for patients with high-risk neuroblastoma is to consolidate the response obtained during induction by eliminating any remaining tumor cells using myeloablative chemotherapy and stem cell rescue. The role of dose intensification to overcome tumor drug resistance mechanisms followed by bone marrow or peripheral blood stem cell support has been investigated for more than 20 years. Early nonrandomized studies suggested a survival advantage compared with historic control subjects but may have been influenced by selection bias.

The CCG conducted a randomized study from 1991 to 1996 to test the hypothesis that consolidation with myeloablative chemotherapy followed by purged autologous bone marrow rescue would improve EFS probability compared with nonmyeloablative consolidation chemotherapy.[443] A total of 539 eligible patients were enrolled in this clinical trial, and 379 patients were randomly assigned to myeloablative therapy (consisting of carboplatin, etoposide, melphalan, and 1000 cGy of total body irradiation) with autologous marrow rescue ($n = 189$) or continuation chemotherapy ($n = 190$). An intent-to-treat analysis showed a significant improvement in 3-year EFS for the patients assigned to myeloablative therapy (34% ± 4% vs. 22% ± 4%; $P = 0.03$; Fig. 54-8, A). A follow-up report of this study assessing long-term outcomes confirmed the benefit of myeloablative therapy, with a 5-year EFS of 30% ± 4% for patients treated with myeloablative chemotherapy versus 19% ± 3% for patients treated with conventional chemotherapy.[444] The German Society of Pediatric Oncology showed similar results in a randomized study of 295 patients receiving either myeloablative therapy with autologous stem cell rescue ($n = 149$) or consolidation with oral maintenance chemotherapy

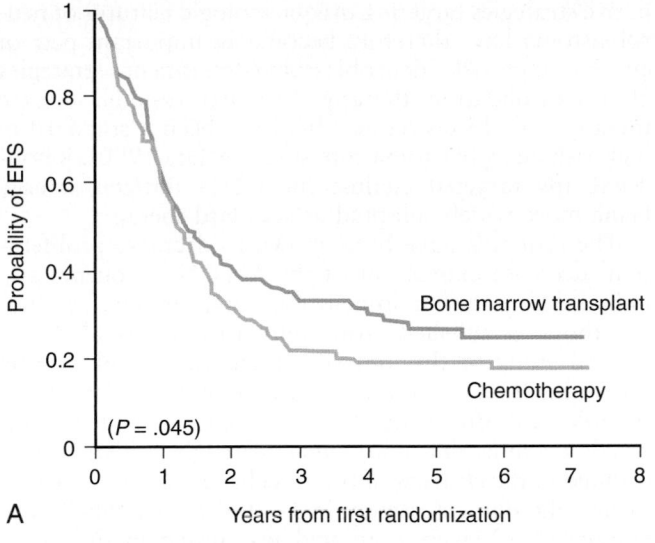

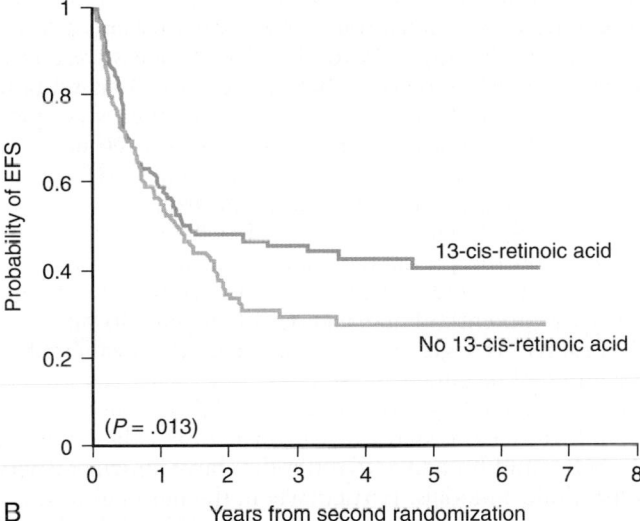

Figure 54-8 Children's Cancer Group study 3891 showing that autologous bone marrow transplant (ABMT) and 13-cis-retinoic acid improve event-free survival for patients with high-risk neuroblastoma. Patients were treated with identical induction chemotherapy, then randomized to ABMT or continuation chemotherapy and then further randomized to receive 13-cis-retinoic acid or no further therapy. **A,** Event-free survival *(EFS)* from time of randomization for patients randomized to ABMT (*n* = 189) or continuation chemotherapy (*n* = 180; *P* = .03). **B,** EFS from time of randomization to 13-cis-retinoic acid (*n* = 130) or no further therapy (*n* = 128; *P* = .03). *(Modified from Matthay KK, Villablanca JG, Seeger RC, et al: Treatment of high-risk neuroblastoma with intensive chemotherapy, radiotherapy, autologous bone marrow transplantation, and 13-cis-retinoic acid. Children's Cancer Group. N Engl J Med 341:1165–1173, 1999.)*

(*n* = 146). An intent to treat analysis again showed an improvement in 3-year EFS for patients assigned to myeloablative therapy (47%, 95% confidence interval [CI] 38-55, vs. 31%, 95% CI 23-39).[445]

Early myeloablative regimens for high-risk neuroblastoma used bone marrow as rescue with allogeneic marrow showing no survival advantage compared with autologous marrow.[446,447] The use of peripheral blood stem cells results in more rapid engraftment and less transplant-related morbidity.[448,449] In addition, peripheral blood stem cells may be less likely to contain contaminating tumor cells.[450] Peripheral blood stem cells are now the standard for myeloablative autotransplant regimens and are typically harvested after two to four cycles of induction chemotherapy.

An important concern relating to autotransplant is potential tumor cell contamination of the stem cell product contributing to relapse. Strategies to purge tumor cells from harvested marrow or peripheral blood stem cells include ex vivo immunomagnetic purging based on neural-specific antigens or CD34+ selection of hematopoietic progenitor cells.[449,451] A randomized clinical trial designed to test the efficacy of ex vivo purging of immunocytochemically negative peripheral blood stem cell products was performed by the COG. No difference in survival was seen in patients who received immunomagnetic purged stem cells compared with patients who did not receive these stem cells (5-year EFS 40% vs. 36% and 5-year OS 50% vs. 51%).[423]

Given the improvement in EFS observed with single transplant myeloablative strategies, tandem and even triple transplant regimens have been evaluated in limited institution and cooperative group pilot studies. The theoretic advantages to multiple transplants include exposure to multiple non–cross-resistant therapies at maximal doses in a relatively rapid sequence and possible modulation of the tumor microenvironment during the first transplant, potentiating cell killing with subsequent transplant(s).[449] Grupp and colleagues[449] and George and colleagues[452] treated 97 patients with high-risk neuroblastoma between 1994 and 2002 with a tandem rapid sequence myeloablative consolidation regimens using peripheral blood stem cell support in a limited institution single-arm study. They showed that tandem transplant was feasible with rapid myeloid cell recovery and low treatment-related mortality (five treatment-related deaths; 82 patients completed two transplants). The progression-free survival (PFS) rate at 5 years from diagnosis was 47% (95% CI, 36% to 56%), and the PFS at 7 years was 45% (95% CI, 24% to 55%) and the overall survival rate at 5 and 7 years, respectively, was 60% (95% CI, 42% to 64%) and 53% (95% CI, 40% to 64%; Fig. 54-9). This study and several others[453-455] suggest that further intensification of consolidation therapy may affect survival of patients with high-risk neuroblastoma. The COG recently completed a large randomized trial of single versus tandem myeloablative consolidations to further evaluate the true impact of a tandem high-dose myeloablative consolidation strategy, the results of which are still pending.

Using different chemotherapy for myeloablation is an alternative strategy that is being explored for high-risk consolidation therapy. A recent European high-risk neuroblastoma trial randomly compared two myeloablative regimens—busulfan and melphalan versus carboplatin, etoposide, and melphalan. Randomization was stopped early because of an interim analysis that showed that the regimen containing busulfan had a superior outcome (a 3-year EFS of 49% vs. 33% and a 3-year OS of 60% vs. 48%).[456] In this study the rapid COJEC induction regimen

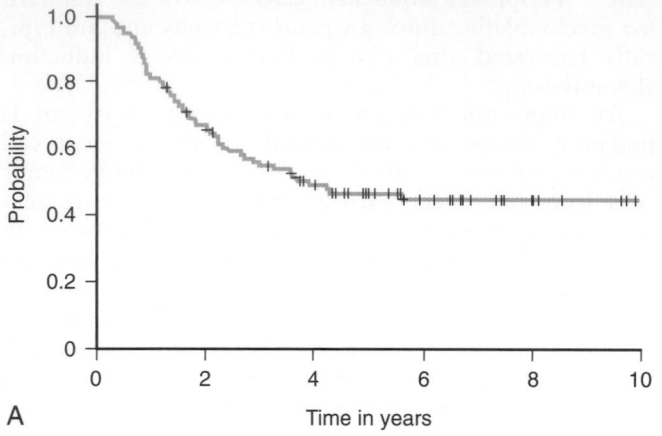

PROGRESSION-FREE SURVIVAL FROM DIAGNOSIS
FOR ALL PATIENTS (n = 97)

A   Time in years

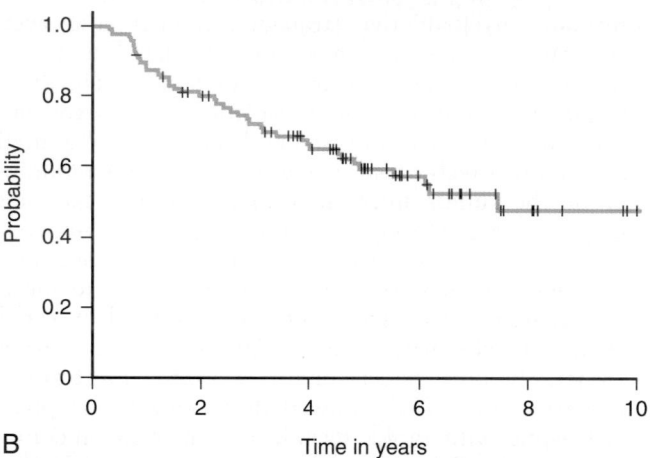

OVERALL SURVIVAL FROM DIAGNOSIS
FOR ALL PATIENTS (n = 97)

B   Time in years

Figure 54-9 Tandem transplant for high-risk neuroblastoma. Progression-free survival (**A**) and overall survival (**B**) from diagnosis of 97 patients. *(From George RE, Li S, Medeiros-Nancarrow C, et al: High-risk neuroblastoma treated with tandem autologous peripheral-blood stem cell-supported transplantation: long-term survival update. J Clin Oncol 24:2891–2896, 2006.)*

was used for all patients.[457] The high cumulative dose of platinum in this regimen may help explain the lower-than-expected survival for the arm containing carboplatinum, etoposide, and melphalan. Although results are still being analyzed, conditioning with busulfan and melphalan had less associated acute toxicity. The COG is running a pilot study to determine the feasibility of using busulfan and melphalan as consolidation therapy after the COG induction used in the last randomized trial. If feasible, this regimen will likely be used in the next COG phase III high-risk study.

Treatment of Minimal Residual Disease

Even when a complete remission is obtained after myeloablative therapy and stem cell rescue, relapse remains a significant problem, suggesting the presence of highly chemotherapy-resistant minimal residual disease. Alter-

native strategies targeting unique biologic features of neuroblastoma have therefore become an important part of current high-risk neuroblastoma treatment strategies after consolidation therapy. Minimal residual disease therapy with 13-cis-retinoic acid has been a standard in high-risk neuroblastoma care since the late 1990s. Immunotherapy targeted against the GD2+ antigen is now being more widely adopted as standard therapy.

The retinoids have been shown to decrease proliferation, decrease expression of the MYCN oncogene, and induce differentiation in neuroblastoma cell lines, including those established from refractory tumors.[458,459] A phase I study of children with high-risk neuroblastoma showed that an intermittent schedule of high-dose 13-cis-retinoic acid after transplant had minimal toxicity (primarily cheilitis, dry skin, and hypertriglyceridemia) and resulted in the clearing of tumor cells in the bone marrow by morphologic assessment in 3 out of 10 patients.[460] The efficacy of 13-cis-retinoic acid was tested in the previously mentioned CCG randomized trial using a factorial design after randomization to myeloablative or continuation chemotherapy.[443] A total of 130 patients were randomly assigned to receive either six cycles of 13-cis-retinoic acid or no further therapy. The cohort of patients assigned to receive posttransplant therapy with 13-cis-retinoic acid had a significantly improved EFS probability ($46\% \pm 6\%$ vs. $29\% \pm 6\%$ from second randomization; $P = .03$; see Fig. 54-8, *B*). Ongoing studies of 13-cis-retinoic acid are focusing on the pharmacokinetics and proper dosing of 13-cis-retinoic acid, particularly in the youngest patients, as well as potential late toxicities of chronic dosing.[461,462]

Another biologic strategy that has been evaluated in the minimal residual disease phase of therapy is antibody therapy directed against the GD2 disialoganglioside that is uniformly expressed on neuroblastoma cells. Murine, chimeric, and humanized antibodies have shown activity in preclinical models, particularly in the minimal residual disease setting,[463-465] as well as phase I and II clinical trials.[377,466-468] The COG completed a randomized clinical trial testing the efficacy of ch14.18 with IL-2 and granulocyte-macrophage colony-stimulating factor and 13-cis-retinoic acid versus 13-cis-retinoic acid alone after myeloablative chemotherapy. The results showed a significant improvement in 2-year EFS and OS in the immunotherapy group compared with the patients who received isotretinoin alone (EFS, $66\% \pm 5\%$ vs. $46\% \pm 5\%$, and OS, $86\% \pm 4\%$ vs. $75\% \pm 5\%$[469]; Fig. 54-10). A nonrandomized trial of ch14.18 given alone that was performed by Simon and colleagues[470] showed no benefit of antibody therapy, suggesting that cytokine-mediated activation of antibody-dependent cell-mediated toxicity may be necessary. GD2 has restricted distribution in normal tissue to neurons, skin melanocytes, and peripheral sensory nerve fibers, and thus the toxicities usually associated with chemotherapy are not seen with immunotherapy. Instead, neuropathic pain can be a significant adverse effect in addition to cytokine-mediated capillary leak and hypersensitivity reactions associated with either the antibody or cytokines. Ongoing studies are exploring alternative antibodies, as well as alternative methods of cytokine delivery, as discussed later.

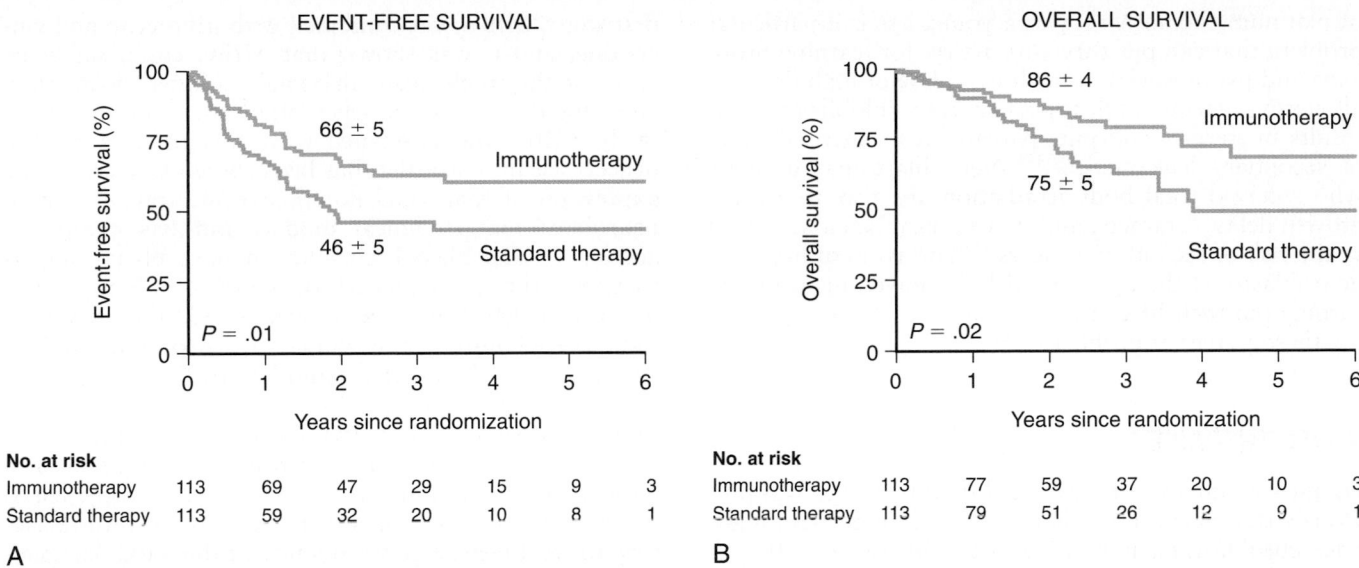

Figure 54-10 Children's Oncology Group study showing the efficacy of chimeric antiGD2 antibody and immunocytokine in high-risk patients. Kaplan-Meier Estimates of survival for patients randomly assigned to immunotherapy versus standard therapy (13-cis-retinoic acid alone). **A,** Event-free survival. **B,** Overall survival. *(From Yu AL, Gilman AL, Ozkaynak MF, et al: Anti-GD2 antibody with GM-CSF, interleukin-2, and isotretinoin for neuroblastoma. N Engl J Med 363:1324–1334, 2010.)*

Assessment of Response to Treatment

For neuroblastoma, response to treatment is assessed using the International Neuroblastoma Response criteria, which are detailed in Table 54-8.[371] Determination of overall response requires assessment of both primary and metastatic sites. This assessment should be made using the same modalities that were used at diagnosis. The timing of response assessments varies according to protocol and risk group, but they are generally performed at the end of induction, before and after surgical procedures, and at the end of treatment. In addition to these response criteria, semiquantitative scoring systems for evaluating MIBG-positive disease have been developed.[429,471] As previously mentioned, the Curie scoring system has prognostic significance in patients with high-risk neuroblastoma. The ability to objectively quantify MIBG response is also useful in clinical trials for relapsed disease. Patients who have had a relapse often have only bone and/or bone marrow disease that can be seen with a MIBG scan but cannot be measured by CT or MRI using standard response criteria.

Late Effects of Therapy

Improvements in survival of patients with high-risk neuroblastoma during the past 20 years has come at the cost of intensification of therapy, putting these patients at increased risk of experiencing late effects of treatment. Hearing loss caused by exposure to high cumulative doses

TABLE 54-8 Definitions of Response to Treatment[371,381]

Response	Primary*	Metastases*	Markers*
1. CR	No tumor	No tumor (chest, abdomen, liver, bone, HVA/VMA bone marrow, nodes, etc.)	HVA/VMA normal
2. VGPR	Reduction >90% but <100%	No tumor (as above except bone); no new bone lesions, all preexisting lesions improved	HVA/VMA decreased >90%
3. PR	Reduction 50%-90%	No new lesions; 50-90% reduction in measurable sites; 0-1 bone marrow samples with tumor; bone lesions same as VGPR	HVA/VMA decreased 50%-90%
4. MR	No new lesions; >50% reduction of any measurable lesion (primary or metastases) with <50% reduction in any other; <25% increase in any existing lesion†		
5. NR	No new lesions; <50% reduction but <25% increase in any existing lesion†		
6. PD	Any new lesion; increase of any measurable lesion by >25%; previous negative marrow positive for tumor		

CR, Complete response; *HVA,* homovanillic acid; *MR,* mixed response; *NR,* no response; *PD,* progressive disease; *PR,* partial response; *VGPR,* very good partial response; *VMA,* vanillylmandelic acid.
*Evaluations of primary and metastatic disease as outlined in the text.
†Quantitative assessment does not apply to marrow disease.

of platinum chemotherapy at a young age is a particular problem that can put survivors at risk for learning problems and psychosocial difficulties.[472] Use of high doses of alkylating agents and topoisomerase inhibitors often results in sterility and puts patients at an increased risk of secondary leukemias.[473,474] Neuroblastoma survivors who received total body irradiation are also at risk for growth delay, cataracts, and thyroid insufficiency, as well as the risk of secondary cancers.[475] Survivors of high-risk neuroblastoma therapy should be followed-up regularly throughout their lifetimes with anticipatory management for these potential problems.[476]

NOVEL THERAPIES

Despite the intensive multimodal treatment that was previously described, more than half of children with high-risk neuroblastoma have a 5-year EFS of less than 50%.[343] Currently no standard treatment regimen exists for patients with relapsed neuroblastoma. Cytotoxic chemotherapy regimens for relapsed neuroblastoma are typically based on the camptothecin derivatives topotecan and irinotecan. Topotecan has been combined with both cyclophosphamide and with vincristine and doxorubicin in phase II studies.[477,478] Irinotecan is most commonly given with temozolamide[479] and is being used more frequently in the United States now that topotecan is being used in induction therapy for high-risk patients in the COG. Neither topotecan nor irinotecan-based therapies led to ultimate cure. Using novel strategies that are targeted to tumor-specific genetic alterations up front in conjunction with standard chemotherapeutic agents may improve cure rates without increased toxicity. Several of these targeted therapies are in clinical or preclinical development, as described later.

Targeted Radiotherapy

In addition to its use for staging and response evaluations, MIBG can be labeled with ^{131}I and used to deliver targeted radiotherapy. ^{131}I-MIBG has undergone extensive single-institution and, more recently, cooperative group clinical trials for the treatment of refractory neuroblastoma.[416,32] The results from a phase II study of 164 patients show that MIBG is active against refractory neuroblastoma with an objective response rate of 36% and disease stabilization in 34% of patients with frequent palliation of pain.[480] Treatment-related toxicity, even at substantial doses, is usually minimal. The most significant reported toxicity is hematologic with prolonged thrombocytopenia, which is most marked in patients with tumor in the bone marrow, and myelosuppression, both of which can be abrogated by autologous stem cell infusion.[480,481] Nonhematologic toxicities include brief nausea and vomiting, transient hepatic dysfunction, and chemical hypothyroidism. More recent clinical trials have focused on combining MIBG with potential radiosensitizing agents with known activity in neuroblastoma to enhance efficacy. The New Approaches to Neuroblastoma Therapy (NANT) consortium completed two phase I studies combining MIBG with a radiosensitizer. In the first study, MIBG was combined with irinotecan and vincristine, and it was shown that MIBG could safely be given at the single-agent maximal tolerated dose along with standard doses of chemotherapy.[482] In the other study, MIBG was combined with vorinostat, a histone deacetylase inhibitor that has been shown to increase the expression of functional norepinephrine transporters in neuroblastoma preclinical models and has completed accrual.[483] The NANT consortium next plans on performing a three-way phase II comparison of both combinations and MIBG as a single agent. In addition to MIBG, radiolabeled anti-GD2 antibodies are also under investigation to provide targeted radiotherapy.[484]

A phase I dose escalation study of ^{131}I-MIBG followed by myeloablative carboplatin, etoposide, and melphalan with stem cell rescue showed a response rate of 27% in patients who were refractory to standard therapy. Based on these promising results in patients who were refractory to treatment, a phase II study at the maximal tolerated dose was completed.[485,486] The COG is currently performing a pilot study to determine the feasibility of giving ^{131}I-MIBG prior to consolidation therapy in newly diagnosed high-risk patients.

Immunotherapy

As previously discussed, a monoclonal antibody directed against the GD2 antigen in combination with cytokines has been shown to significantly improve survival and is now being used as a standard part of the minimal residual disease phase of treatment in newly diagnosed high-risk patients. Current research is focusing on enhancing efficacy and making the regimen less toxic. To this end, the chimeric anti-GD2 antibody is being piloted with subcutaneous (rather than intravenous) IL-2[487] and with lenolidomide, which has been shown to enhance NK cell–mediated antibody dependent cellular cytotoxicity in preclinical models.[465,488] Humanized antibodies are also being developed that are designed to cause less hypersensitivity-type reactions and have increased tumor specificity. One of these antibodies, hu14.18K332A, has a single amino acid mutation that limits its ability to fix complement and thereby reduced the pain associated with ch14.18 while retaining the antibody-dependent cellular toxicity capabilities.[488a] Additionally, preclinical studies have shown that antibody efficacy can be enhanced by creating a fusion protein consisting of antibody linked to a cytokine such as IL-2.[463] A phase II study of a humanized GD2 antibody fused to IL-2 (hu14.18-IL2) showed a complete response in 5 of 24 patients with MIBG and/or bone marrow disease with tolerable toxicity, warranting further investigation.[489]

One limitation of monoclonal antibody therapy in patients with neuroblastoma is that it seems to be most active in the setting of minimal residual disease, with questionable benefit in patients who have bulky disease. More active immunotherapy strategies are also being developed to try to address this problem. These strategies include use of immunostimulatory antibodies such as ipilimumab (anti-cytotoxic T-lymphocyte antigen 4) and vaccination with anti-idiotype antibody or dendritic cells.[490-492] In addition, engineered cytolytic T lymphocytes that are directed against tumor-associated antigens (chimeric antigen receptor T cells) are under development with encouraging preliminary results.[493,494]

Molecular Targeting

Several large-scale sequencing efforts have concluded that sequence alterations are not represented in neuroblastoma in a major way, especially those that can be readily targeted therapeutically. However strategies focused on targeting genetic pathways relevant to proliferation of neuroblastoma cells hold promise. Additionally, alterations in chromatin remodeling and other epigenetic regulators may provide novel avenues for therapeutic intervention.

ALK

ALK mutations have been established as oncogenic drivers in neuroblastoma and offer bona fide therapeutic targets.[495] ALK small molecule inhibitors may be beneficial not only to 10% to 12% of patients with neuroblastoma who have mutation and amplification, but also to the proportion whose tumors overexpress the wild-type, phosphorylated ALK receptor and that appear to respond to genetic and chemical ALK depletion by undergoing apoptosis (Fig. 54-11).[186,198]

Small Molecule Inhibitors. The first ALK inhibitor to be developed was NVP-TAE684 (Novartis), a 5-chloro-2, 4-diaminophenylpyrimidine compound that induces significant cytotoxicity in neuroblastoma cells expressing different ALK mutations (Fig. 54-12).[155,496,497] This highly selective ATP-competitive inhibitor was identified by screening a kinase-targeted small molecule library against Ba/F3 cells expressing oncogenic kinases, specifically NPM-ALK.[496] TAE684 is especially selective for ALK because the orthomethoxy group of TAE684 projects into a small groove located between the side chains of residues L258 and M259 of the NPM-ALK kinase domain; bulkier amino acids at the L258 position (which are seen in other kinases) would lead to a steric clash with TAE684.[496] Treatment of neuroblastoma cells harboring the F1174L and the R1275Q ALK mutations induces rapid inhibition of phosphorylated ALK and its downstream signaling, leading to apoptosis and cell cycle arrest.[155,497] However TAE684 could not be taken forward to clinical development because it tends to form an extensive number of reactive adducts upon metabolic oxidation, which creates the potential for significant toxicity.[498] Nevertheless, it remains a valuable compound for preclinical studies of ALK kinase inhibition.

Crizotinib (PF-2341066; Xalkori), an orally bioavailable, 2,4-pyrimidinediamine derivative, is an ATP-competitive dual inhibitor of MET and ALK.[499,500] Crizotinib binds to the inactive conformation of both MET and ALK[501] and has shown striking efficiency against ALK-rearranged tumors, both in mouse models

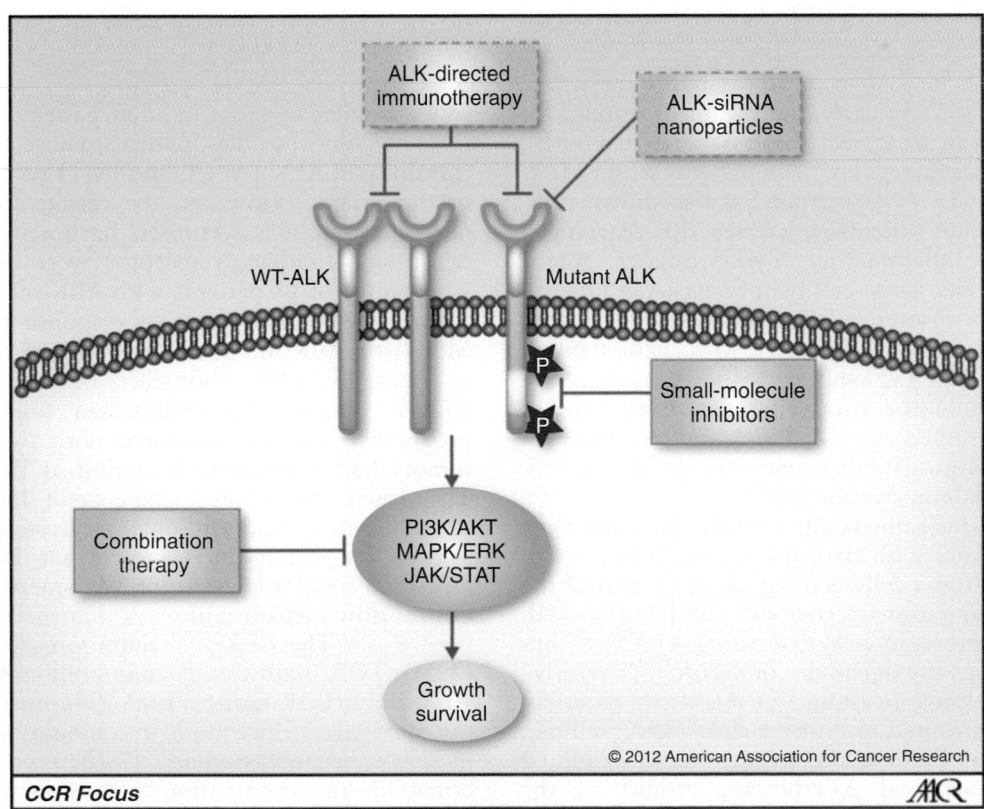

Figure 54-11 Current and future prospects for targeting anaplastic lymphoma kinase (ALK) in neuroblastoma. *JAK/STAT,* Janus kinase/signal transducer and activator of transcription; *MAPK/ERK,* mitogen-activated protein kinase/extracellular signal-regulated kinase; *PI3K,* phosphoinositide-3-kinase; *siRNA,* small interfering ribonucleic acid; *WT,* wild-type. *(From Matthay KK, George RE, Yu AL: Promising therapeutic targets in neuroblastoma.* Clin Cancer Res *18(10):2740–2753, 2012.)*

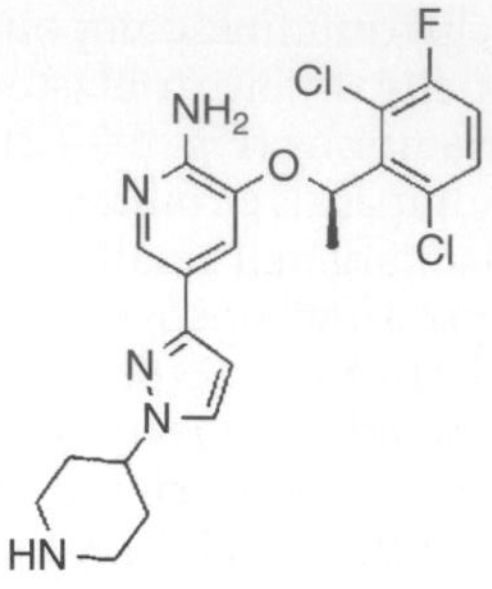

Figure 54-12 Chemical structures of representative anaplastic lymphoma kinase inhibitors.

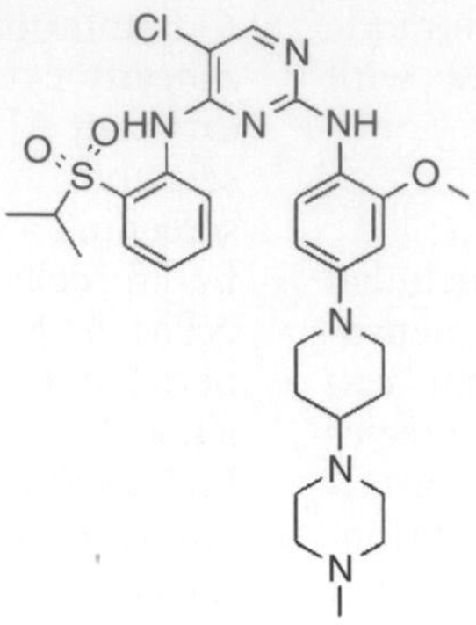

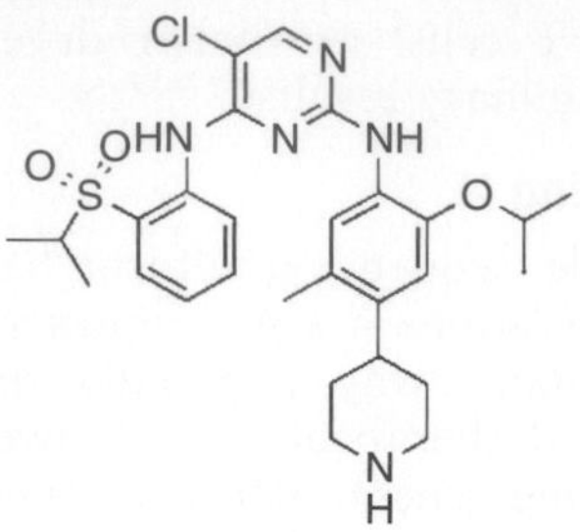

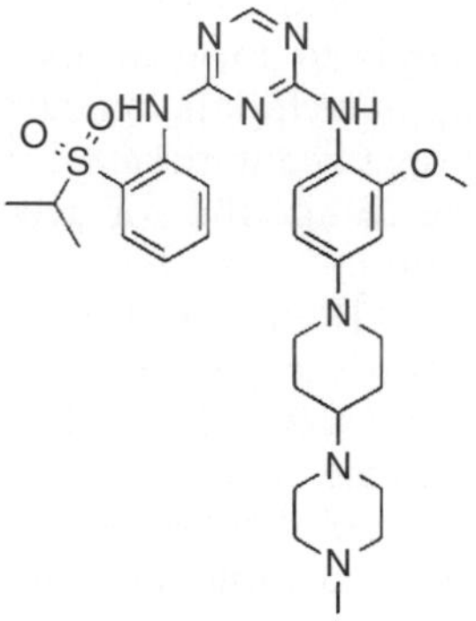

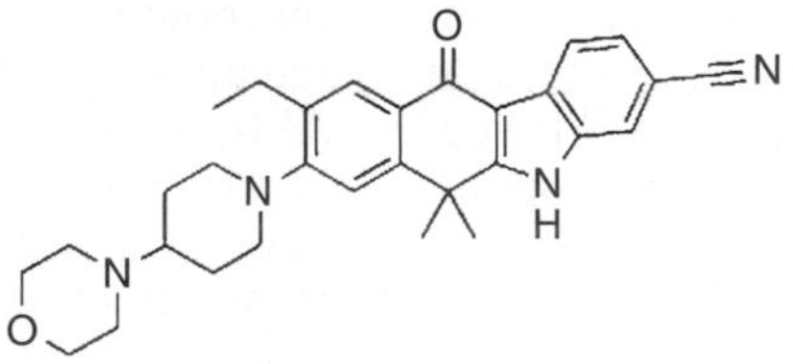

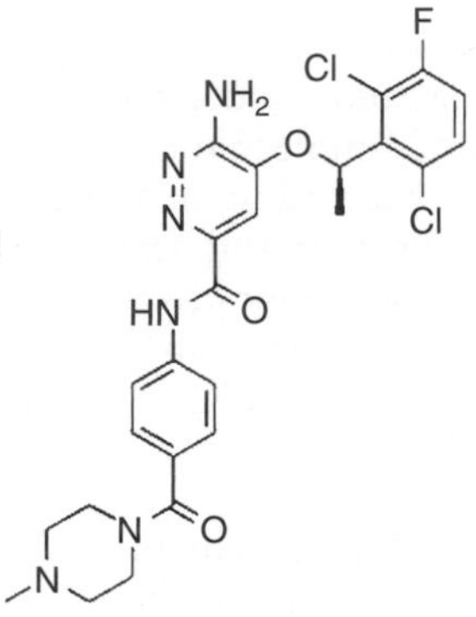

and in the clinic.[500,502] In early-phase clinical testing, for example, at a mean treatment duration of 6.4 months, the overall response rate was 57% in patients with EML4-ALK–positive NSCLC.[502] Crizotinib has also shown striking responses in adult patients with other ALK-rearranged cancers such as inflammatory myofibroblastic tumor (IMT) and anaplastic large-cell lymphoma (ALCL).[503,504] A phase III trial showed a superior PFS and overall response rate for crizotinib compared with chemotherapy in patients with NSCLC who had disease progression after standard chemotherapy.[505] Because of this result, crizotinib was granted approval for the treatment of patients with ALK-positive metastatic NSCLC by the U.S. Food and Drug Administration (FDA).

Unfortunately, the same positive results have not been observed in patients with neuroblastoma. When tested against neuroblastoma cells bearing either of two of the more common mutations, crizotinib inhibited growth and induced apoptosis in cells expressing ALK^{R1275Q} but failed to inhibit the growth of ALK^{F1174L}-positive cells.[194,506] The relative resistance of ALK^{F1174L} to crizotinib has been attributed to either lack of direct contact with the crizotinib-binding site within the ATP-binding pocket or the increased ATP-binding affinity of the mutant, with complete inhibition of constitutively active ALK attainable only at very high doses of the drug.[191] Crizotinib was tested in a COG phase I trial that included patients whose tumors expressed aberrant ALK. With

results similar to those in adult patients and as expected from preclinical studies, patients whose tumors expressed translocated ALK (ALCL and IMT) responded very well to the drug.[507] However, the results for patients with neuroblastoma whose tumors harbored point mutations within the full-length receptor were less encouraging, with only 1 of 11 patients with ALK-mutated neuroblastoma showing an objective response to this agent.[507] Moreover, ALK mutations exhibit differential sensitivity to crizotinib. In this study, three of the four patients with ALK^{F1174L}-positive neuroblastoma tumors experienced progressive disease, compared with two of five whose tumors had a missense mutation at the R^{1275} locus.[507] Therefore crizotinib as a single agent does not appear to be sufficient to induce tumor regression in neuroblastoma. Other studies have shown that the cytotoxicity of crizotinib could be significantly enhanced by targeting the critical downstream pathways that mediate ALK signaling.[194,508,509] The ALK^{F1174L} mutation signals through the PI3K/mTOR pathway,[156] and combined inhibition of ALK and mTOR induces tumor regression and prolongs the survival of mice both in xenografts and transgenic models of neuroblastoma.[194,509] Therefore clinical trials of crizotinib in combination with downstream pathway inhibitors may enhance the antitumor activity of the former, and in particular, their ability to overcome the resistance of ALK^{F1174L}-mutated neuroblastoma cells to crizotinib.

Several other compounds are in development or are even in early-phase trials in adults with ALK-aberrant cancers.[498,510] LDK378 (Novartis Pharmaceuticals, Basel, Switzerland), which is derived from TAE684,[496] is an orally active inhibitor of the ALK kinase. In cellular assays, LDK378 inhibits ALK at an inhibitory concentration of 50% of 40 nM against wild-type ALK and of 22 nM against NPM-ALK. It also has an excellent pharmacokinetic profile in rodents, with an oral bioavailability of greater than 50%. LDK was shown was shown to induce a response rate of 80% in patients with NSCLC who had experienced disease progression after an initial response to crizotinib, and therefore this drug has received "breakthrough therapy" designation from the U.S. FDA for patients with ALCL or metastatic NSCLC whose disease progressed while being treated with crizotinib or who are intolerant to it. LDK is currently in phase II trials for NSCLC. It is currently being tested in phase I trials in pediatric patients (NCT01283516, ClinicalTrials.gov), and it may hold promise for the treatment of patients with neuroblastoma who have mutated ALK.

Other ALK inhibitors in development include CH5424802 (Roche/Chugai Pharmaceuticals, Ltd., Tokyo, Japan),[510] an orally available inhibitor that was shown to potently inhibit the growth of neuroblastoma cells expressing amplified ALK. This agent also displayed in vitro inhibitory activity against neuroblastoma cells expressing ALK^{F1174L}, which was shown to be comparable to that achieved in cells with wild-type ALK.[510] Whether CH5424802 will show efficacy for in vivo models of neuroblastoma with mutated ALK remains to be seen. Other ALK inhibitors in phase I/II clinical trials include ASP3026 (Astellas Pharma, Northbrook, Ill.),[511] CEP-28122 (Cephalon Inc., Frazer, Pa.),[512] AP26113 (ARIAD, Cambridge, Mass.), a small molecule that has exhibited activity as a potent dual inhibitor of ALK and epidermal growth factor receptor,[513] and X-396 (Xcovery, West Palm Beach, Fla.).[514]

ALK-Based Immune Therapy. The abundant expression of ALK on the surface of most neuroblastoma tumor cells and its restricted tissue expression in normal tissues render it an ideal tumor-associated antigen.[199] Treatment of neuroblastoma cell lines with ALK-specific monoclonal antibodies has been shown to induce enhanced immune cell-mediated cytotoxicity with inhibition of cell proliferation and cell death.[515] Moreover exposure to crizotinib induced accumulation of ALK on the cell surface, thus increasing the accessibility of the antigen for antibody binding. If validated in vivo, this strategy may be useful in cases of neuroblastoma that constitutively express ALK, either alone or in combination with small-molecule inhibitors. Other avenues such as treatments with an ALK-based chimeric antigen receptor are being actively explored.

RNA Interference-Based Therapeutic Strategies. Nanoparticles carrying ALK small interfering RNA have been shown to be effective in inducing antitumor activity in ALK-expressing neuroblastoma models.[516] In this study,

the use of a special anti-GD2 targeted liposomal formulation of nanoparticles ensured the death, as well as specific and nontoxic delivery, of ALK-small interfering RNA GD2 expressing neuroblastoma cells. Although still far removed from the clinic, these preliminary results have the potential to be developed into therapies for children with neuroblastoma.

Resistance to ALK Inhibitors. One issue with molecularly targeted agents is the inevitable development of resistance, as has been observed with crizotinib.[508,517] Even if the small-molecule inhibitor is potent enough to block tumor growth once a tumor has acquired additional aberrations, this strategy generally becomes ineffective, leaving the patient with static disease that begins to progress once treatment is stopped.[518] Resistance to targeted agents usually develops as a result of the development of secondary mutations or activation of compensatory signaling pathways. Secondary mutations are frequently acquired in the "gatekeeper" position, where the presence of amino acids with bulky side chains such as methionine interferes with the binding of the kinase inhibitor. The ALK L1196 mutation has been identified in a patient with lung cancer with an EML4-ALK tumor translocation, after an initial response to crizotinib.[517] The F1174L mutation that occurs de novo in neuroblastoma also developed in a patient with IMT bearing the RAP2-ALK translocation who experienced a relapse after therapy with crizotinib that was initially successful.[191] Another mechanism by which cancer cells with activated mutant kinases evade treatment with kinase inhibitors is to switch to alternative signaling pathways. Thus NSCLC cells with MET gene amplification develop resistance to crizotinib by overexpressing the epidermal growth factor receptor.[519] Preclinical models of resistance will enable prediction of resistance mechanisms to newer ALK inhibitors and aid in the design of drug combinations to delay or even prevent resistance.

Targeting Amplified MYCN

Because deactivation of MYCN in MYCN-expressing neuroblastoma tumors causes proliferative arrest and tumor regression, treatment strategies focused on silencing MYCN would be expected to affect an appreciable proportion of patients with high-risk neuroblastoma. Yet direct targeting of MYCN has proved difficult because (1) it lacks an obvious "druggable" domain, and (2) its requirement in normal cells imposes a high risk of prohibitive nonspecific toxicity. However, it is possible to target MYCN indirectly through the molecules that regulate MYCN activation or stability either at the mRNA or protein level. These strategies include inhibition of epigenetic proteins such as BRD4,[520,521] decreasing MYCN protein stability through inhibition of aurora kinase,[522] or targeting molecules that are synthetic lethal to the growth and proliferative activity of MYCN.[523] Other methods include activation of p53-induced apoptosis,[524] differentiation induction,[141] and inhibiting MYCN-dependent metabolic dependencies.[525,526] A major consideration in thinking about strategies to inhibit MYCN regulation and function is to have a therapeutic window sufficient for antitumor activity without inducing severe toxicity to normal tissues.

BET Bromodomain Inhibitors. The bromodomain and extraterminal (BET) family of transcriptional coactivators are epigenetic reader proteins that recognize and bind to covalent modifications of chromatin[527] to promote gene activation. BET proteins BRD2, BRD3, and BRD4 have been found to be critical in promoting transcription of MYC and MYCN through their recognition of lysine side-chain acetylation on histone tails.[520,528] JQ1 is a novel thienotriazolo-1,4-diazepine compound that displaces BET bromodomains from chromatin by competitively binding to the acetyl lysine recognition pocket.[528] JQ1 suppresses the growth of MYCN-amplified neuroblastoma in both orthotopic models and transgenic *TH-MYCN-MYCN* models, with a significant increase in survival. Tumors showed increased apoptosis and decreased proliferation concomitant with decreased expression of MYCN.[520] JQ1 displaces BRD4 from the MYCN promoter, with depletion of MYCN mRNA and protein after its administration. Downregulation of the MYCN transcriptional program was induced in JQ1-treated cells, with genes involved in proliferation, apoptosis, neural crest stemness, and cellular differentiation being particularly affected. Therefore BET bromodomain inhibition may be a promising option for patients with MYCN-amplified neuroblastoma, and clinical trials are being developed.[520] Similar results were also seen with another BRD4 inhibitor GSK1324726A (I-BET726), which induced potent growth inhibition and cytotoxicity in most neuroblastoma cell lines tested irrespective of MYCN copy number or expression level.[521]

Although MYCN amplification predicted sensitivity to BRD4 inhibition in these two studies, cell lines that were sensitive to JQ1 did not always have MYCN amplification, suggesting that MYC or MYCN is not the sole predictor of sensitivity to BET inhibition. Wyce et al.[521] (2013) reported that BRD4 inhibition led to direct suppression of BCL2 in addition to MYCN, although neither protein fully accounted for the sensitivity of I-BET726 in neuroblastoma cells.

Aurora Kinase Inhibitors. The aurora serine/threonine protein kinase–A is critical for the stabilization of MYCN. Aurora kinase A (AURKA) associates with MYCN and prevents its Fbxw7 ubiquitin ligase-mediated proteosomal degradation.[522,529] AURKA also plays an important role in centrosome maturation and spindle formation during mitosis.[530] AURKA overexpression has been reported in MYCN-amplified neuroblastoma[531]; these cells depend on high levels of this protein for maintaining MYCN function.[522,531] The Aurora-A inhibitors, MLN8054 and MLN8237, have shown promising activity in neuroblastoma models.[529,532,533] These agents disrupt the MYCN-AURKA complex and promote degradation of MYCN. The disruption of the complex inhibits MYCN-dependent transcription, correlating with tumor regression and prolonged survival in a transgenic MYCN neuroblastoma model.[529] Additionally, additive effects have been observed with the combination of MLN8237

and vorinostat, an HDAC inhibitor.[534] AURKA inhibition has also been shown to inhibit angiogenesis in neuroblastoma.[535] MLN 8237 is currently in phase II trials in patients with neuroblastoma (NCT01154816).

PI3K inhibition. Small-molecule inhibitors of PI3K have been shown to block the growth of transgenic neuroblastoma models, and they also induce cell cycle arrest and apoptosis in human neuroblastoma cells with MYCN amplification.[536,523] MYCN is a critical target for PI3K inhibitors.[523] The MYCN protein is stabilized through PI3K signaling,[537] and blockage of PI3K and mTOR can destabilize MYCN, leading to decreased MYCN protein levels and blocked proliferation of tumors driven by TH-MYCN.[536,538] In addition to promoting MYCN degradation, PI3K/mTOR inhibitors have been shown to induce secondary paracrine blockage of angiogenesis. The PI3K inhibitor NVP-BEZ235 improved survival in both human (highly pretreated MYCN-amplified orthotopic xenograft) and transgenic mouse models of MYCN-driven neuroblastoma.[523] Clinical trials of the mTOR inhibitor temsirolimus, in combination with irinotecan and temozolomide, have shown tolerability in patients with relapsed or refractory solid tumors, including neuroblastoma,[539] and phase II trials of the combination are ongoing.

p53-Pathway Inhibition. Another way of inhibiting the effects of MYCN is by targeting the p53-dependent apoptotic pathway activated by MYCN. MDM2, an E3 ubiquitin ligase, mediates p53 degradation, as well as cytoplasmic localization and transcriptional inactivation. Deregulation of the ARF/MDM2 pathway is seen in neuroblastoma tumors, resulting in high MDM2 activity and subsequent p53 deactivation.[540] Uncoupling p53 from MDM2 with small molecules that compete for respective docking sites may offer another avenue for targeted therapy by activating gp53. Nutlin-3, a cis-imidazoline small molecule that mimics a p53-binding peptide, has been shown to interfere with MDM2 binding to p53 and has proven effective in reducing growth and inducing apoptosis in neuroblastoma cells.[541,542] Nutlin-3 has also been shown to prevent tumor metastasis in xenograft models[540] with accumulation of p53 protein, as well as induction of p53 target gene expression. Synergy has been shown between nutlin-3 and DNA-damaging chemotherapeutic agents,[543] as well as with the pan CDK inhibitor roscovitine (Seliciclib)[544] and the anti-VEGF antibody bevacizumab.[545] Nutlin-3 has also been shown to be effective in relapsed neuroblastoma by inhibiting drug efflux activities of P-glycoprotein and multidrug resistance–associated protein 1.[546] Thus nutlin agents may offer benefit in patients with neuroblastoma.

Polyamines. A number of genes involved in polyamine homeostasis are known to be MYCN or c-MYC targets, and the expression of others is linked to *MYCN* status.[525,526] Approaches that target the polyamine pathway may be effective in treating high-risk neuroblastoma, especially those with MYCN amplification. Polyamines are positively charged multifunctional polycations that are critical for cell growth, differentiation, and survival. Polyamine depletion leads to growth arrest, whereas overexpression is cytotoxic; therefore tight regulation of intracellular levels is critical (reviewed in reference 547).[547] Polyamines are elevated in neuroblastoma cells and the gene encoding ornithine decarboxylase–1 (ODC1), the rate-limiting enzyme in polyamine biosynthesis, is a direct transcriptional target of MYCN. ODC1 is coamplified or overexpressed with MYCN and is associated with a poor prognosis in MYCN-amplified tumors.[525] a-difluoromethylornithine (DFMO), which acts as a specific inhibitor of ODC1 and is the most widely studied inhibitor of polyamine metabolism, serves both as a chemotherapeutic and a chemopreventive agent.[548] DFMO treatment in neuroblastoma cell lines inhibited proliferation and increased tumor latency and overall survival in MYCN-driven transgenic neuroblastoma models.[525] It also enhances the effects of the cytotoxic chemotherapeutic agents cyclophosphamide and cisplatin[525] and induces synergistic and antiproliferative effects when combined with the cyclooxygenase 2 inhibitors celecoxib and sulindac.[549] A phase I clinical trial coordinated by the NANT consortium for the treatment of refractory neuroblastoma using high-dose DFMO and celecoxib in combination with standard chemotherapy (cyclophosphamide and topotecan) is under way. Polyamine enhancement is also seen in nonamplified tumors and is associated with high-risk disease, and therefore these strategies may also be effective in the latter group as well.[525,550]

Retinoids

Fenretinide (N-[4-hydroxyphenyl] retinamide; 4-HPR) is a synthetic retinoid that is cytotoxic to neuroblastoma cells in vitro. Unlike 13-cis-retinoic acid, it does not induce tumor differentiation of cells but is cytotoxic by a variety of other mechanisms.[551-553] Its mechanism of action is thought to be through de novo ceramide synthesis induction,[554-556] generation of reactive oxygen species,[557] angiogenesis inhibition,[558,559] and increased NK cell activity.[560] Fenretinide has been tested in preclinical and early phase clinical studies and showed wide interpatient variability of plasma levels with suggested antitumor activity in relapsed disease.[23-26] To improve plasma levels, an oral powder in an organized lipid complex was developed that increased 4-HPR levels in plasma and tissues.[560a] A phase I trial of this formulation of fenretinide confirmed attainment of higher plasma levels with minimal toxicity. Complete tumor responses were observed in patients with tumor involvement limited to bone marrow and/or bone metastasis, suggesting that relapsed patients who commonly present with similar disease may benefit most from this agent.[561]

TRKB Inhibitors

In animal models, CEP-701 (lestaurtinib), a small-molecule inhibitor, has shown activity against the TRKB tyrosine kinase,[562,563] which acts as an oncogenic kinase in a subset of neuroblastomas. In animal models, lestaurtinib alone significantly inhibited tumor growth, and it also enhanced the antitumor efficacy of the cyclophosphamide/topotecan combination.[564] Lestaurtinib was tested in a phase I trial and was found to be well tolerated, with evidence of tolerability of a dose level sufficient to inhibit phospho-TRKB activity in plasma. Additionally, lestaurtinib in combination with 13-cis-retinoic acid was found to be additive or synergistic in neuroblastoma cells.[565]

CDK4/CDK6 Inhibitors

The cyclin D/CDK4/CDK6/RB pathway is hyperactive in many cancers.[566] CDK4 and CDK6 encode serine threonine kinases that complex with D-type cyclins to phosphorylate or inactivate the RB protein. This in turns induces the release of RB from E2F transcription factors, thus allowing progression of G1-S phase progression and cell proliferation. Moreover, CDK4/CDK6 also suppresses senescence through the forkhead box M1 (FOXM1) transcription factor.[566a] Genomic amplification of cyclin D1 and CDK4 has been reported in a subset of neuroblastomas.[567-571] Others have evaluated CDK4/CDK6 inhibitors in neuroblastoma and have shown sensitivity to inhibition, with sensitivity attributed to G1 arrest and cellular senescence. Treatment with the Novartis inhibitor LEE011 reduced proliferation in 12 of 17 lines, although the mean inhibitory concentration of 50% was in the 300-nM range in sensitive lines. It caused cell cycle arrest and cellular senescence that was attributed to dose-dependent decreases in phosphorylated RB and FOXM1, respectively. Treatment resulted in delay of subcutaneous tumor xenografts.[572] Given that CDK4/CDK6 inhibition causes a cytostatic response, it is unclear what the effects would be if it were used in combination with conventional cytotoxic agents that rely on S-phase DNA replication,[573] and further studies may be required to provide elucidation. Therefore CDK4/CDK6 inhibition may be most effective in postchemotherapy maintenance treatment.

HDAC Inhibitors and Demethylating Agents

It is becoming increasingly clear that not only in other cancers but also in neuroblastoma, a large portion of the cancer genome undergoes DNA methylation and histone modification, leading to silencing of tumor suppressor genes. Methylation of caspase-8[294] and that of the tumor suppressor gene CHD5 on chromosome 1p,[223] for example, have been reported in neuroblastoma. HDAC agents have also shown preclinical activity against neuroblastoma[280,574] and are of potential therapeutic benefit because they cause apoptosis of human neuroblastoma cells, with an enhanced inhibitory effect when combined with retinoic acid.[574-577] It is thought that HDAC inhibitors potentiate the derepression of retinoid responsive genes in the presence of ligand.[578] Vorinostat, an oral class 1 and II HDAC inhibitor, has shown efficacy in solid tumor models with additive or synergistic preclinical and/or clinical activity in combination with the demethylating agent 5-aza-2-deoxycytidine (decitabine)[579] and 13-cis-retinoic acid.[580] In pediatric phase I trials, no objective responses were seen, although a complete response was seen in one patient with neuroblastoma who received the combination of retinoic acid and vorinostat.[581] Increased acetylated-H3 histones in peripheral blood lymphocytes were identified as a surrogate marker of drug target activity.[581] Based on preclinical evidence that low-dose decitabine is sufficient to induce demethylation and subsequent expression of caspase-8 in neuroblastoma cells,[582] decitabine was tested in combination with cytotoxic chemotherapy in a phase I trial.[583] Although this dose resulted in caspase-8 promoter demethylation and gene expression in bone marrow samples, the dose of decitabine capable of producing clinically relevant biologic effects were not well tolerated with cytotoxic chemotherapy in these patients. Demethylation and reexpression of melanoma antigen-encoding gene (MAGE)–1 in peripheral blood mononuclear cells as a marker of demethylation was seen in the majority of patients.[583] Decitabine has also been shown to increase the expression of other cancer/testis antigens—MAGE-A3 and NY-ESO-1—on neuroblastoma cells, facilitating cytotoxic T-lymphocyte–mediated tumor cell killing,[490,584] and forms the basis of a cancer antigen vaccine therapy for patients with relapsed neuroblastoma (NCT01241162).

EZH2 Inhibitors

MYCN has been shown to induce EZH2 expression and activity,[237,585] and therefore inhibition of EZH2 could potentially cause reexpression of tumor suppressor genes that are suppressed as a result of stimulation of EZH2 by MYCN. In neuroblastoma cells, inhibition of MYCN expression causes decreased EZH2 protein levels, which is accompanied by a decrease in global H3K27me3.[237] EZH2 inhibition was shown to cause induction of genes having tumor suppressive or differentiation-inducing capacity. Inhibition of EZH2 using small hairpin RNA knockdown or a small-molecule inhibitor of EZH2, 3-Deazaneplanocin A, led to decreased growth and induction of neurites and induction of cell death as a result of increased activated caspase-3/7 activity.[237] The small-molecule inhibitor also inhibited the growth of neuroblastoma xenografts, suggesting that this may be a potential avenue to investigate in neuroblastoma.

CONCLUSIONS AND FUTURE DIRECTIONS

The clinical heterogeneity of neuroblastoma is clearly correlated with tumor biology. The significant progress to date in understanding neuroblastoma biology has led to the ability to stratify patients and adapt treatment according to prognostic variables, resulting in a significant reduction in therapy for low- and intermediate-risk patients and the intensification of treatment for high-risk patients. A remaining challenge for low- and intermediate-risk disease is to better understand the biology of the small subset of patients who have a poor outcome and tailor their therapy accordingly. High-risk disease remains a significant clinical problem. We have likely reached the limits of dose intensification, and innovative approaches are needed to improve survival and decrease treatment-related morbidity. Future progress will likely be made by translating new discoveries regarding the underlying pathobiology of neuroblastoma into targeted therapies

that can then be integrated into current treatment strategies for newly diagnosed patients. The challenge will be to determine how these individually targeted agents can be combined with cytotoxic chemotherapy, whether up front, concomitantly, or in the setting of minimal residual disease. Finally, an understanding of relapsed high-risk tumors can be achieved only by analysis of the molecular aberrations that have developed during the evolution of resistance either by direct examination of relapsed tissue or through the validation of surrogate markers.

References available online at ExpertConsult.

KEY REFERENCES

74. Trochet D, Bourdeaut F, Janoueix-Lerosey I, et al: Germline mutations of the paired-like Homeobox 2B (PHOX2B) gene in neuroblastoma. *Am J Hum Genet* 74(4):761–764, 2004.
75. Mosse YP, Laudenslager M, Khazi D, et al: Germline PHOX2B mutation in hereditary neuroblastoma. *Am J Hum Genet* 75(4):727–730, 2004.
    References 74 and 75 provide the first reports of germline paired-like homeobox–2b (PHOX2B) mutations causing predisposition to neuroblastoma.
96. Mosse YP, Laudenslager M, Longo L, et al: Identification of ALK as a major familial neuroblastoma predisposition gene. *Nature* 455(7215):930–935, 2008.
97. Janoueix-Lerosey I, Lequin D, Brugieres L, et al: Somatic and germline activating mutations of the ALK kinase receptor in neuroblastoma. *Nature* 455(7215):967–970, 2008.
    References 96 and 97 provide the first reports of anaplastic lymphoma kinase (ALK) as a familial neuroblastoma predisposition gene.
108. Look AT, Hayes FA, Nitschke R, et al: Cellular DNA content as a predictor of response to chemotherapy in infants with unresectable neuroblastoma. *N Engl J Med* 311(4):231–235, 1984.
    The first report of the importance of deoxyribonucleic acid ploidy in neuroblastoma prognosis.
111. Schwab M, Alitalo K, Klempnauer KH, et al: Amplified DNA with limited homology to myc cellular oncogene is shared by human neuroblastoma cell lines and a neuroblastoma tumour. *Nature* 305(5931):245–248, 1983.
    The first report of the identification of v-myc avian myelocytomatosis viral oncogene neuroblastoma derived homolog (MYCN) amplification in neuroblastoma.
112. Brodeur G, Seeger RC, Schwab M, et al: Amplification of N-myc in untreated human neuroblastomas correlates with advanced disease stage. *Science* 224:1121–1124, 1984.
113. Seeger RC, Brodeur GM, Sather H, et al: Association of multiple copies of the N-myc oncogene with rapid progression of neuroblastomas. *N Engl J Med* 313:1111–1116, 1985.
    References 112 and 113 are the first articles describing the clinical impact of v-myc avian myelocytomatosis viral oncogene neuroblastoma derived homolog (MYCN) amplification in neuroblastoma.
145. Weiss WA, Aldape K, Mohapatra G, et al: Targeted expression of MYCN causes neuroblastoma in transgenic mice. *EMBO J* 16(11):2985–2995, 1997.
    This article describes a transgenic mouse model of neuroblastoma generated by targeted expression of v-myc avian myelocytomatosis viral oncogene neuroblastoma-derived homolog (MYCN) to the neural crest.
154. Chen Y, Takita J, Choi YL, et al: Oncogenic mutations of ALK kinase in neuroblastoma. *Nature* 455(7215):971–974, 2008.
155. George RE, Sanda T, Hanna M, et al: Activating mutations in ALK provide a therapeutic target in neuroblastoma. *Nature* 455(7215):975–978, 2008.
    References 154 and 155 provide the first reports of the identification of anaplastic lymphoma kinase (ALK) mutations in sporadic tumors.
261. Attiyeh EF, London WB, Mosse YP, et al: Chromosome 1p and 11q deletions and outcome in neuroblastoma. *N Engl J Med* 353(21):2243–2253, 2005.

A study describing the prognostic impact of chromosome 1p and 11q deletions in neuroblastoma.

332. Shimada H, Ambros IM, Dehner LP, et al: The International Neuroblastoma Pathology Classification (Shimada) System. *Cancer* 86:364–372, 1999.

333. Peuchmaur M, d'Amore ES, Joshi VV, et al: Revision of the International Neuroblastoma Pathology Classification: confirmation of favorable and unfavorable prognostic subsets in ganglioneuroblastoma, nodular. *Cancer* 98(10):2274–2281, 2003.
References 332 and 333 provide descriptions of the current pathologic classification system used in risk group analysis for neuroblastoma.

341. Katzenstein HM, Bowman LC, Brodeur GM, et al: Prognostic significance of age, MYCN oncogene amplification, tumor cell ploidy, and histology in 110 infants with stage D(S) neuroblastoma: the pediatric oncology group experience—a pediatric oncology group study. *J Clin Oncol* 16(6):2007–2017, 1998.

342. Nickerson HJ, Matthay KK, Seeger RC, et al: Favorable biology and outcome of stage IV-S neuroblastoma with supportive care or minimal therapy: a Children's Cancer Group study. *J Clin Oncol* 18(3):477–486, 2000.
References 341 and 342 show prognostic factors in infants with stage 4S neuroblastoma.

371. Brodeur GM, Pritchard J, Berthold F, et al: Revisions of the international criteria for neuroblastoma diagnosis, staging, and response to treatment. *J Clin Oncol* 11(8):1466–1477, 1993.
This article describes the international neuroblastoma staging system (INSS) that is currently used in the United States.

389. Monclair T, Brodeur GM, Ambros PF, et al: The International Neuroblastoma Risk Group (INRG) staging system: an INRG Task Force report. *J Clin Oncol* 27(2):298–303, 2009.
The International Neuroblastoma Risk Group Task Force recommendation of a new staging system to improve comparison of international studies.

393. Schmidt ML, Lal A, Seeger RC, et al: Favorable prognosis for patients 12 to 18 months of age with stage 4 nonamplified MYCN neuroblastoma: a Children's Cancer Group study. *J Clin Oncol* 23(27):6474–6480, 2005.
The report of a study showing that age is a continuous prognostic variable and that the traditional cutoff of 1 year can be extended in some patients.

398. Strother DR, London WB, Schmidt ML, et al: Outcome after surgery alone or with restricted use of chemotherapy for patients with low-risk neuroblastoma: results of Children's Oncology Group study P9641. *J Clin Oncol* 30(15):1842–1848, 2012.
A Children's Oncology Group study confirming that surgery alone is adequate treatment for low-risk neuroblastoma.

405. Hero B, Simon T, Spitz R, et al: Localized infant neuroblastomas often show spontaneous regression: results of the prospective trials NB95-S and NB97. *J Clin Oncol* 26(9):1504–1510, 2008.

406. Nuchtern JG, London WB, Barnewolt CE, et al: A prospective study of expectant observation as primary therapy for neuroblastoma in young infants: a Children's Oncology Group study. *Ann Surg* 256(4):573–580, 2012.
References 405 and 406 show the feasibility of observation in infants with localized neuroblastoma.

417. Baker DL, Schmidt ML, Cohn SL, et al: Outcome after reduced chemotherapy for intermediate-risk neuroblastoma. *N Engl J Med* 363(14):1313–1323, 2010.
The first large study showing that excellent overall survival can be maintained with reduced therapy in patients with intermediate-risk neuroblastoma.

423. Kreissman SG, Seeger RC, Matthay KK, et al: Purged versus non-purged peripheral blood stem-cell transplantation for high-risk neuroblastoma (COG A3973): a randomised phase 3 trial. *Lancet Oncol* 14(10):999–1008, 2013.
A phase III randomized study showing that ex-vivo purging of stem cells does not improve outcome in patients with high-risk neuroblastoma.

432. Yanik GA, Parisi MT, Shulkin BL, et al: Semiquantitative mIBG scoring as a prognostic indicator in patients with stage 4 neuroblastoma: a report from the Children's Oncology Group. *J Nuclear Med* 54(4):541–548, 2013.
A study showing the prognostic importance of residual metaiodobenzylguanidine (MIBG)-avid disease in a large group of high-risk patients treated with a single protocol.

443. Matthay KK, Villablanca JG, Seeger RC, et al: Treatment of high-risk neuroblastoma with intensive chemotherapy, radiotherapy, autologous bone marrow transplantation, and 13-cis-retinoic acid. Children's Cancer Group. *N Engl J Med* 341(16):1165–1173, 1999.

444. Matthay KK, Reynolds CP, Seeger RC, et al: Long-term results for children with high-risk neuroblastoma treated on a randomized trial of myeloablative therapy followed by 13-cis-retinoic acid: a Children's Oncology Group study. *J Clin Oncol* 27(7):1007–1013, 2009.
The first randomized study showing efficacy of myeloablative therapy in patients with high-risk neuroblastoma (ref 443) and a follow-up study on long-term results (ref 444).

456. Ladenstein RL, Poetschger U, Luksch R, et al: Busulphan melphalan as a myeloablative therapy (MAT) for high-risk neuroblastoma: results from the HR-NBL1/SIOPEN trial (Abstract 2). Presented at the 2011 American Society of Clinical Oncology Annual Meeting, June 3-7, 2011, Chicago, IL.
An abstract showing the superiority of Busulphan-melphalan conditioning compared with standard conditioning in a Society of Paediatric Oncology European Neuroblastoma Network (SIOPEN) trial.

469. Yu AL, Gilman AL, Ozkaynak MF, et al: Anti-GD2 antibody with GM-CSF, interleukin-2, and isotretinoin for neuroblastoma. *N Engl J Med* 363(14):1324–1334, 2010.
A randomized phase III study showing clear efficacy of anti-GD2 therapy in patients with high-risk neuroblastoma in a minimal residual disease setting.

480. Matthay KK, Yanik G, Messina J, et al: Phase II study on the effect of disease sites, age, and prior therapy on response to iodine-131-metaiodobenzylguanidine therapy in refractory neuroblastoma. *J Clin Oncol* 25(9):1054–1060, 2007.
A large phase II study showing the efficacy of metaiodobenzylguanidine (MIBG) in patients with relapsed and refractory disease.

CHAPTER 55

Pediatric Renal Tumors

Jeffrey S. Dome, Elizabeth A. Mullen, and Pedram Argani

CHAPTER OUTLINE

Pediatric renal tumors account for approximately 5% of malignancies in children younger than 15 years old and 3.6% of malignancies in children younger than 20 years old.[1] Among 9731 patients registered with the National Wilms Tumor Study Group (NWTSG) (1969–2002), Wilms tumor (WT) composed the vast majority of childhood renal tumors (92%), followed by clear cell sarcoma of the kidney (3.4%), congenital mesoblastic nephroma (1.7%), malignant rhabdoid tumor (1.6%), and rare miscellaneous neoplasms, including primitive neuroectodermal tumor, synovial sarcoma, neuroblastoma, and cystic nephroma (1.1%). Although not historically included on NWTSG studies, renal cell carcinoma accounts for 8% of renal tumors in children from birth to 19 years, according to data from the Surveillance, Epidemiology, and End Results (SEER) program.[1]

The study of pediatric renal tumors has had a significant impact on the field of oncology. WT has provided a paradigm for multidisciplinary treatment approaches and the conduct of cooperative group studies. WT investigators took the lead in establishing one of the leading biologic-sample banks, which now contains several thousand annotated tumor, blood, and urine samples. Tenets of cancer biology, including Knudson's two-hit model and loss of imprinting in tumorigenesis, were pioneered in WT. This chapter reviews the pathology, epidemiology, genetics and biology, and treatment of pediatric renal tumors.

PATHOLOGY OF PEDIATRIC RENAL TUMORS

Staging

Stage is the major determinant of prognosis and therapy for all pediatric renal neoplasms. Two staging systems are widely used (Table 55-1). The Children's Oncology Group (COG) staging system reflects tumor extent after surgery

TABLE 55-1   Staging Systems for Pediatric Renal Tumors

	Children's Oncology Group (COG) (Prechemotherapy)	International Society of Pediatric Oncology (SIOP) (Postchemotherapy)
I	Tumor is limited to kidney and is completely resected Renal capsule intact, not penetrated by tumor No tumor invasion of veins or lymphatics of renal sinus No nodal or hematogenous metastases No prior biopsy Negative margins	Tumor is limited to kidney and is completely resected Renal capsule may be infiltrated by tumor, but tumor does not reach the outer surface Tumor may protrude or bulge into the pelvic system or ureter, but does not infiltrate Vessels of renal sinus not involved
II	Tumor extends beyond kidney but completely resected • Tumor penetrates renal capsule • Tumor in lymphatics or veins of renal sinus • Tumor in renal vein with margin not involved • No nodal or hematogenous metastases • Negative margins	Tumor extends beyond kidney but completely resected • Tumor penetrates the renal capsule into perirenal fat • Tumor infiltrates the renal sinus or invades blood and lymphatic vessels outside renal parenchyma (or both) but is completely resected • Tumor infiltrates adjacent organs or vena cava but is completely resected
III	Residual tumor or nonhematogenous metastases confined to abdomen • Involved abdominal nodes • Peritoneal contamination or tumor implants • Tumor spillage of any degree occurring before or during surgery • Gross residual tumor in abdomen • Biopsy of tumor (including fine needle aspiration) before removal of kidney • Resection margins involved by tumor	Incomplete excision of the tumor which extends beyond the resection margins (gross or microscopic residual) • Involved abdominal lymph nodes, including necrotic tumor or chemotherapy-induced changes • Tumor rupture before or intraoperatively • Tumor has penetrated the peritoneal surface • Tumor thrombi present at resection margins • Surgical biopsy before resection (does not include needle biopsy)
IV	Hematogenous metastases or spread beyond abdomen	Hematogenous metastases or spread beyond abdomen
V	Bilateral renal tumors Each side should be substaged separately according to the preceding criteria (e.g., stage V, substage II [right], substage I [left])	Bilateral renal tumors Each side should be substaged separately according to the above criteria (e.g., stage V, substage II [right], substage I [left])

before chemotherapy is given. By contrast, the International Society of Pediatric Oncology (SIOP) system reflects tumor extent after 4 to 6 weeks of chemotherapy and surgery. The COG and SIOP staging systems are applied to all pediatric renal tumors except renal cell carcinoma, for which the TNM (tumor, nodes, metastasis) system is used.[2]

The COG staging schema is very similar to that used in the National Wilms Tumor Study 5 (NWTS-5), although one change distinguishes the current COG staging criteria from the prior NWTS-5 criteria.[3,4] Localized spillage or rupture, or any form of biopsy before removal of the kidney, is no longer considered stage II but instead is considered stage III. The SIOP system was recently revised to classify tumors with local and regional lymph node involvement as stage III. Previously lymph node involvement was considered stage II, with separate designations for node-positive and node-negative disease.[5]

Wilms Tumor (Nephroblastoma)

Gross Features

WT typically presents as a unicentric, spherical mass that is sharply demarcated from the renal parenchyma.[6] Approximately 10% of WTs are multicentric, a finding that is associated with an increased likelihood of WT formation in the contralateral kidney. Approximately 5% to 6% of WTs are bilateral at presentation.

The cut surface of WT is generally pale gray and uniform, but hemorrhage, necrosis, and cyst formation are common. The texture is usually soft and friable, but stroma-rich neoplasms may have a dense, myomatous consistency. Calcification is relatively uncommon. Prominent septa frequently impart a multinodular appearance.

WT may arise anywhere in the cortex or medulla, frequently compressing and distorting renal parenchyma around its margin. Rarely exophytic tumors connected to the renal surface by a narrow stalk mimic extrarenal WT. Polypoid masses in the pelvicalyceal lumen may occur either as extensions from the primary intrarenal neoplasm or as separate neoplasms arising within the pelvic wall. The renal vein and its branches not uncommonly are filled by tumor thrombus that can extend via the inferior vena cava into the right atrium.

Cystic Variants of Wilms Tumor

Scattered cysts are commonly encountered in conventional WT, but rarely the encapsulated, well-delineated neoplasm is composed entirely of cystic spaces and delicate septa, without an expansile solid component. For neoplasms that are entirely composed of mature cells, the term is cystic nephroma (CN). If the septa contain embryonal cell types, the designation cystic, partially differentiated nephroblastoma (CPDN) is appropriate. In contrast, cystic WT is distinguished by the presence of solid, expansile regions that replace or distort the cystic spaces, rather than being passively molded by the cysts. This distinction is best made by careful examination of the gross specimen.[7]

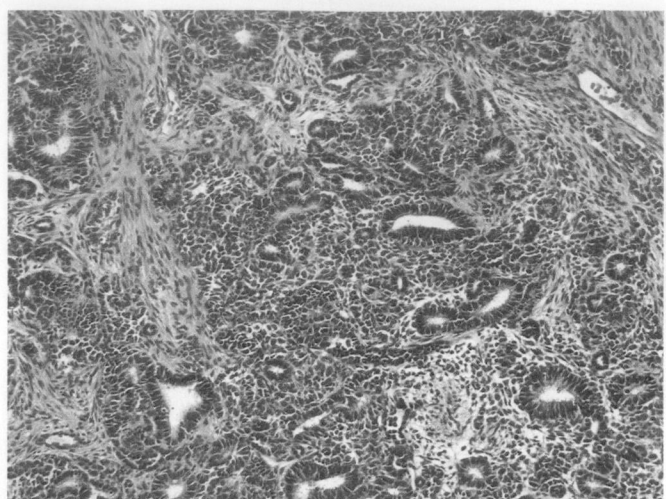

Figure 55-1 Wilms tumor, favorable histology, triphasic pattern.

CPDN has traditionally been thought to be a transitional stage in a continuum ranging from CN to WT. However recent studies show that CN is associated with *DICER1* mutations, whereas such mutations are not observed in CPDN. This suggests that the two cystic renal tumors are distinct entities.[8] The distinction of CN from CPDN has little clinical importance when the lesion has been completely resected because both lesions are curable by resection alone.

Microscopic Features

WTs are surpassed only by teratomas in their diversity of cell and tissue types and degrees of differentiation. Most WTs exhibit, at least focally, the so-called triphasic appearance, including cells of blastemal, stromal, and epithelial lineage (Fig. 55-1). However monophasic and biphasic WTs are relatively common, consisting of only one or two of these cell lineages. Each of the three major cell types can demonstrate a spectrum of patterns and degrees of differentiation, accounting for the remarkable diversity of appearances characterizing various WTs.

Blastemal Patterns. The blastemal cells of WT are small, tightly packed cells with a high nucleus-to-cytoplasm ratio, demonstrating little or no evidence of differentiation toward epithelial or stromal cell types at the light-microscopic level. Their nuclei are usually round or oval, with moderately coarse chromatin, and mold to one another in the same fashion as do the nuclei of small cell carcinoma of the lung. Nucleoli are relatively inconspicuous. Blastemal cells form several distinctive aggregation patterns, which can be divided into two broad categories, diffuse and nested, depending on their structure and degree of invasiveness. Monomorphous, relatively dyscohesive sheets of blastemal cells with aggressively invasive margins characterize the diffuse blastemal pattern. This is the most consistently aggressive pattern of WT. Stage I WTs rarely show this pattern; the majority of diffuse blastemal WT present at advanced stage, stage III or IV. Fortunately most neoplasms with the diffuse blastemal pattern are highly responsive to modern therapeutic pro-

tocols, so this pattern remains in the "favorable histology" category.[9] The diffuse blastemal pattern can be readily confused with other small blue cell tumors of childhood, and ultrastructural or other special studies may be required to establish the correct diagnosis (Fig. 55-2).

Nested blastemal patterns are characterized by sharply outlined clusters of blastemal cells in a myxoid mesenchymal background. They usually lack the invasive behavior seen with the diffuse blastemal pattern, and these neoplasms have sharply defined margins at their advancing edge. Several nested patterns may be seen. The serpentine blastemal pattern features long, serpiginous, anastomosing cords of blastemal cells in a loose, stellate, spindled stroma. This is a highly distinctive pattern of WT and helps distinguish WT from other small blue cell neoplasms of childhood. The nodular blastemal pattern resembles the serpentine pattern but has rounded blastemal nests instead of long cell cords. The basaloid blastemal pattern resembles the serpentine or nodular patterns, except that the blastemal cell clusters are outlined by a palisaded layer of cuboidal or columnar cells, reminiscent of the architecture of cutaneous basal cell carcinoma.

Epithelial Patterns. Epithelial differentiation in WT produces a variety of cell types and degrees of differentiation. Most of these recapitulate events in normal nephrogenesis (homologous differentiation). Others, such as squamous differentiation or mucinous differentiation, do not occur in the normal kidney at any stage of development (heterologous differentiation). Tubular differentiation is the most frequent epithelial pattern. This ranges from vague hints at tubular formation in blastemal foci (which may resemble rosettes) to highly differentiated tubules resembling those of the mature kidney. WTs in which tubular differentiation is predominant tend to be less aggressive, and most of these present at stage I. Although not usually invasive, tubular-predominant WTs often grow rapidly, and it is not uncommon to find huge tumors that remain confined to the kidney. Glomerular

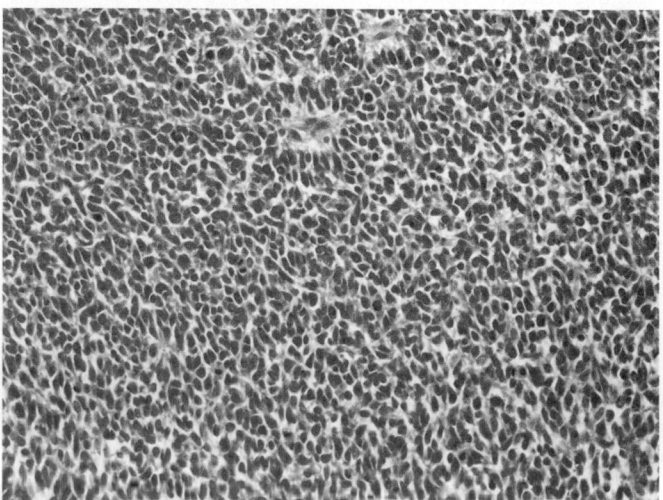

Figure 55-2 Wilms tumor, favorable histology, diffuse blastemal pattern.

differentiation, present in many WTs, ranges from simple papillary formations barely suggesting glomerulogenesis to mature tumor glomeruli closely resembling those of normal developing kidneys.

Stromal Patterns. Immature myxoid and spindled mesenchymal cells are the most common stromal cell types seen in WTs. Skeletal muscle is the most common heterologous cell type. The presence of skeletal muscle (rhabdomyoblastic differentiation) in WT must not be confused with renal rhabdoid tumor, which is discussed later in this chapter. In fact, the presence of skeletal muscle in a pediatric renal neoplasm is very strong evidence supporting the diagnosis of WT.

Anaplasia: the Sign of Unfavorable Histology in Wilms Tumor

Approximately 5% of WTs demonstrate anaplastic nuclear change, the only criterion of "unfavorable histology."[10] All WTs lacking this feature are designated as having "favorable histology." Anaplasia is almost never seen in WT diagnosed during the first year and is rare in the second year of life. The relative frequency of anaplasia increases after that age, and it is found in approximately 10% of WTs diagnosed after the age of 5 years. Anaplastic nuclear change reflects extreme polyploidy and is usually apparent under low magnification (10× objective). The features of anaplasia include (a) markedly enlarged tumor cell nuclei with increased chromatin content (hyperchromasia) and (b) multipolar mitotic figures (Fig. 55-3). The former criteria reflect polyploidy, whereas the latter criterion helps exclude degenerative nuclear changes, as are commonly seen in cells showing skeletal muscle differentiation, from the anaplastic category. Anaplasia is tightly correlated with the presence of *TP53* gene mutations.[11,12] Whereas favorable-histology WT virtually never harbors *TP53* mutations, the majority of anaplastic WTs do. At a practical level, p53 protein overexpression by immunohistochemistry correlates well but not perfectly with morphologically defined anaplasia.[13]

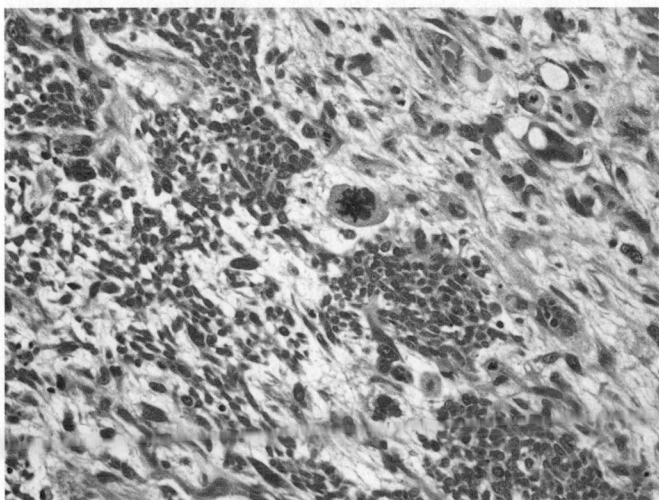

Figure 55-3 Wilms tumor, anaplastic.

Focal and Diffuse Anaplasia. Initially the presence of anaplastic nuclear changes in any region of a WT was considered prognostically unfavorable. It subsequently was suggested that anaplasia is an indicator of increased resistance to adjuvant chemotherapy and not necessarily a marker of increased tumor aggressiveness; therefore stage I anaplastic WT and WT with limited intrarenal foci of anaplasia (focal anaplasia [FA]) would be predicted to have an excellent prognosis. This concept implies that the prognosis for a patient with anaplastic WT is determined by the completeness of surgical removal of anaplastic cells.[14] However recent data on patients with stage I anaplastic WT have challenged this concept.[15] Regardless the definition of FA includes only those WTs meeting the following criteria:

1. Anaplasia is confined to one or more discrete sites within the primary tumor and is not present in extrarenal sites.
2. Tumor cells outside anaplastic foci show no "nuclear unrest" (nuclear or mitotic abnormalities that approach, but do not quite attain, the degree of severity required for a designation of anaplasia).

Any WT not meeting this definition of FA is designated as having diffuse anaplasia (DA). Any of the following situations merits assignment to the DA category:

1. Nonlocalized anaplastic change
2. Anaplastic change or nuclear unrest in invasive sites or any extrarenal deposits
3. Localized anaplastic change in a tumor that also has severe nuclear unrest elsewhere
4. Anaplasia in a random biopsy specimen
5. Anaplasia involving the edge of one or more sections, and the site(s) from which the sections were taken cannot be determined. (The latter emphasizes the importance of mapping the sections taken from a WT, best done on a photograph of a cut section of the tumor.)

Anaplastic foci are usually clearly demarcated from adjacent nonanaplastic tumor. Most cases in the FA category have a single focus of anaplasia. Anaplastic foci are usually only a few millimeters in diameter but can be larger if their localized nature can be convincingly documented.

The SIOP Postchemotherapy Histologic Classification System

Patients treated on SIOP studies receive several weeks of chemotherapy before undergoing nephrectomy. Chemotherapy usually affects necrosis of immature and actively proliferating cell types in WT, whereas slowly replicating and differentiated cell types are usually unaffected. For example, tumors composed mostly of mature skeletal muscle or renal tubules show little clinical regression with chemotherapy because so few cells are proliferating. The microscopic appearance of the tumor after chemotherapy has prognostic significance. Approximately 5% to 10% of WTs are completely necrotic after chemotherapy, a finding associated with a 98% 5-year relapse-free survival rate.[16] By contrast, WTs with a predominance of blastemal cells after chemotherapy, defined as viable cells in more than one third of the tumor mass and blastemal cells in

TABLE 55-2 Comparison of COG and SIOP Histologic Risk Classification Schemas

Children's Oncology Group (COG)	International Society of Pediatric Oncology (SIOP)
Favorable-histology Wilms tumor • No evidence of anaplasia Focal anaplastic Wilms tumor • Anaplasia confined to one or more discrete sites within the primary tumor with no extrarenal involvement • No nuclear unrest outside anaplastic foci Diffuse anaplastic Wilms tumor • Nonlocalized anaplasia • Anaplasia in invasive sites or extrarenal deposits • Localized anaplasia with severe nuclear unrest elsewhere • Anaplasia in a random biopsy specimen. • Anaplasia involving the edge of one or more sections Non–Wilms renal tumors not included in this classification schema	Low risk • Mesoblastic nephroma • Cystic partially differentiated nephroblastoma • Completely necrotic Wilms tumor Intermediate risk • Wilms tumor of epithelial, stromal, mixed, or regressive types • Focal anaplastic Wilms tumor High risk • Blastemal-type Wilms tumor • Diffuse anaplastic Wilms tumor • Clear cell sarcoma of the kidney • Rhabdoid tumor of the kidney

at least two thirds of the viable component, have relapse rates of nearly 40%.[5,17] Based on these observations, the SIOP histologic risk classification schema divides renal tumors into three risk categories: low risk, intermediate risk, and high risk. The COG and SIOP histologic classification systems are compared in Table 55-2.

Ultrastructural and Immunohistochemical Studies

Ultrastructural study is rarely necessary to establish a diagnosis of WT but can occasionally be very helpful in distinguishing blastemal WT from other undifferentiated neoplasms.[18,19] The diversity of differentiation in WT creates a correspondingly varied profile of immunohistochemical results. Blastemal cells may or may not label for vimentin and cytokeratin, whereas various differentiating elements will label according to their patterns of differentiation. For example, primitive rhabdomyoblasts within a tumor will label for the myogenic transcription factor myogenin and for cytoskeletal proteins such as actin and desmin. WT blastemal cells characteristically label for desmin but not for actin, myogenin, or other muscle markers.[20] Immunoreactivity for WT1 protein is typically limited to the blastemal and epithelial components of WT, with the stroma being negative.[21] Hence absence of labeling for WT1, particularly in a stroma-rich tumor, does not exclude the diagnosis of WT. Although WT1 immunoreactivity may help distinguish WT from PNET, it should be noted that desmoplastic small round cell tumor typically labels for WT1. Although useful, WT1 immunoreactivity cannot in and of itself establish or disprove a diagnosis of WT.

Nephrogenic Rests and Nephroblastomatosis

In more than 30% of kidneys resected for WT, the renal parenchyma contains one or more regions of persistent embryonal tissue, representing potential precursors of WT. These lesions have been given many names in the past; however, the term suggested by Dr. J. Bruce Beckwith, nephrogenic rests (NRs), is the currently accepted terminology.[22,23] The presence of multiple or diffusely distributed NRs is called nephroblastomatosis. This term is most commonly applied when the NRs are in an active state of cellular proliferation and are large enough to be apparent on imaging studies.

NRs have a dynamic life history that can yield a variety of appearances. Dr. Beckwith's classification is based on the assumption that the structure of NRs reflects both the dynamic state and the history of an individual rest. A brief summary is provided here.

Two fundamental categories of NRs are recognized, based on their topographic relation to the renal lobe. These are designated perilobar nephrogenic rests (PLNRs) and intralobar nephrogenic rests (ILNRs). ILNRs may occur anywhere in the renal lobe, including the peripheral cortex. They may also occur within the renal sinus, including in the walls of the pelvicalyceal system. ILNR have a more varied structure than do PLNRs and typically intercolate between nephrons, whereas PLNRs usually are discrete structures that are well delineated from adjacent nephrons. Rests of either major category may be further classified on the basis of their developmental fates. An individual NR may undergo any of the following fates, several of which often occur sequentially over time:

1. It may remain unchanged in size or composition, even for many years, as a tiny, microscopic blastemal focus (dormant NR).
2. It may undergo maturation, sclerosis, and eventual disappearance (sclerosing NRs and obsolescent NRs). This is the most common fate of NRs.
3. It may undergo hyperplasia, or coordinated proliferation of all susceptible cells of the rest, as distinguished from a clonal neoplastic process originating in a single cell of the rest. Hyperplastic NR may produce large, actively growing masses that have numerous mitotic figures, and a section from the interior of a hyperplastic NR may be indistinguishable from WT. Several features do help make this distinction. First diffuse hyperplastic growth, involving all or most cells of a rest, tends to preserve the original shape of the rest. When PLNRs form a continuous layer of embryonal cells at the lobar surface, hyperplastic proliferation will produce a thick "rind" of abnormal tissue at the renal surface. Ovoid and lenticular masses result from hyperplasia of NRs that originally had these shapes. An irregular-shaped, multinodular appearance will result if only some of the cells are capable of proliferation. In contrast, WT, a neoplasm presumably arising from a single cell, tends to form spherical masses. The second important feature distinguishing actively hyperplastic NRs from WT is the usual

absence of a pseudocapsule at the interface between hyperplastic NRs and the renal parenchyma.

4. Neoplastic induction is assumed to represent a clonal event originating in single cells of a rest, resulting in WT or benign adenomas. As mentioned previously rapidly growing tumors originating at a single point (or cell) will tend to grow equally in all directions, forming spherical, expansile nodules with compressed rest remnants often present at the periphery.

5. Very rarely, anaplasia may develop in nephrogenic rests.[24]

An individual rest commonly progresses through several of these processes sequentially. For example, an incipient or dormant rest may undergo hyperplasia, followed by phases of growth arrest and maturation. This will result in a large but inactive-appearing lesion. Ultimately, one or more cells within the regressing rest may be induced to form a WT.

ILNRs are most often found at the tumor-kidney interface, where they can be misinterpreted as infiltrating tumor cells or effaced by tumor compression. A helpful feature distinguishing ILNRs at the edge of a WT is the poorly defined, irregular outer border of the ILNR, which contrasts with the sharp, pushing interface between the WT and the rest within which it arose. Also ILNRs are usually less cellular than the adjacent WT that they surround.

The presence of NRs in a kidney removed for WT is correlated with an increased risk for subsequent WT formation in the remaining kidney. The type of rest and the age of the patient modify this risk.[25] When a carefully sampled kidney is free of rests, the risk of contralateral WT is extremely low. The possibility of subsequent WT developing in the remaining kidney should be considered in planning the follow-up of patients whose nephrectomy specimen reveals the presence of NRs in addition to WT.

Differential Diagnosis of Wilms Tumor

Triphasic Wilms Tumor. The triphasic pattern rarely presents a problem in diagnosis, except when small biopsies are obtained from large retroperitoneal masses of uncertain origin. In this setting other mixed neoplasms might deserve consideration, including teratoma, hepatoblastoma, pancreatoblastoma, teratoma, mesothelioma, synovial sarcoma, and intraabdominal desmoplastic small round cell tumor. In the absence of nephrogenic differentiation or the distinctive nested blastemal patterns described previously, ancillary studies such as immunohistochemistry, molecular biology, or electron microscopy may be required to distinguish some of these lesions from WT. WT with extensive heterologous differentiation ("teratoid WT") is easily confused with immature teratoma. Renal teratomas are extremely rare, and some of the reported cases likely represent teratoid WT.

Blastemal Wilms Tumor Versus Other Small Blue Cell Tumors of Childhood. The problem of distinguishing blastemal WT from other small blue cell tumors is most likely to arise when dealing with biopsies from metastatic sites or from large abdominal tumors of uncertain

origin. The distinctive aggregation patterns of blastemal WT, the presence of nuclear molding, or the focal presence of tubular differentiation will often reveal the diagnosis. Early tubular differentiation in WT lacks lumens and therefore can sometimes be confused with rosettes of neuroblastoma or primitive neuroectodermal tumor (PNET). The presence of true lumens even focally confirms tubular differentiation, whereas neurofibrils are diagnostic of a neuroblastic pseudorosette. Neuroblastic rosettes do rarely occur in WT, but usually only in teratoid WTs, which are not likely to be confused with neuroblastomas or PNETs. Immunohistochemistry, electron microscopy, molecular diagnostic techniques, cytogenetics, circulating tumor markers, and other special studies are often required to confirm the nature of a small blue cell tumor.

Epithelial Predominant Wilms Tumor Versus Papillary Renal Cell Carcinoma. The challenge of distinguishing epithelial predominant WT from papillary renal cell carcinoma (PRCC) is most often encountered in tumors from adolescents or adults. Papillary adenoma, the benign precursor of PRCC, may resemble epithelial predominant NRs, and epithelial predominant WTs can have a predominantly papillary architecture. Sometimes PRCCs have a predominant tubular or solid component. Molecular or cytogenetic studies may be helpful because PRCC characteristically contains increased copies of chromosomes 7 and 17 and, in tumors from male patients, deletion of Y.[26] Unequivocal glomerular differentiation, characteristic blastemal aggregation patterns, or the presence of heterologous cell types can confirm the diagnosis of WT. Immunoreactivity for cytokeratin 7 has been advocated as a useful marker for PRCC, but focal positive labeling for this marker occurs in many WTs. Only when diffusely positive is cytokeratin 7 labeling likely to be discriminatory. Nuclear labeling for WT1 protein may distinguish WT, NRs, and metanephric adenoma from PRCC, insofar as only the latter does not label.[27]

Clear Cell Sarcoma of the Kidney
Gross Appearance

Clear cell sarcoma of the kidney (CCSK) is always unicentric, with a distinct tumor-kidney junction. Tumors are usually relatively large, with a mean specimen diameter of approximately 11 cm.[28] The cut surface is often glistening and gelatinous. Cysts are almost always present and may be so prominent as to suggest cystic nephroma on gross examination or imaging studies.

Microscopic Appearance

Under low magnification, most CCSKs appear monomorphous, without the prominent lobulation usually seen in WT. CCSK usually has a scalloped border that appears fairly sharp under low power. Under higher magnification, the border appears less sharply defined because of the penetration of neoplastic cells a short distance into the surrounding kidney or the tumor capsule. This growth pattern tends to surround and isolate individual single nephrons, which is rarely if ever seen with WT. The entrapped tubules are usually confined to the peripheral 2 to 3 cm of a CCSK. Their epithelium commonly shows embryonal metaplastic changes similar to those entrapped in congenital mesoblastic nephroma, and the resultant basophilic epithelium creates confusion with WT. Dilation of these entrapped tubules produces intratumoral cysts that may mimic cystic nephroma. CCSK may show a wide variety of morphologic patterns, described in the subsequent sections.[28-31]

Classic Pattern. The hallmark of the classic pattern is an evenly distributed network of vascular septa, which has a branching, "chicken-wire" pattern similar to that seen in myxoid liposarcoma or oligodendroglioma. These fibrovascular septa subdivide the tumor into a conspicuous pattern of cords and nests, averaging six to ten cells in width, composed of polygonal cells that usually lack distinct cytoplasmic borders. Cells within the cords are less densely packed than those of blastemal WT, and overlapping nuclei are less frequent. Nuclear chromatin is usually finely granular, with inconspicuous nucleoli (Fig. 55-4). In well-fixed specimens, the fine nuclear chromatin pattern is the most helpful clue to the diagnosis. However, it is influenced markedly by the timing and type of fixation. Mitotic figures are variable in number but are usually less numerous than those in WT. The cytoplasm usually lacks distinct borders and is surrounded by extracellular mucopolysaccharides, which creates the illusion of clear cytoplasm.

CCSK is easily confused with other neoplasms because the classic pattern is often modified, presenting alterations that mimic other neoplasms to a sometimes striking degree. Fortunately the classic pattern of CCSK predominates in most specimens and is present at least focally in more than 90% of tumors. However the pathologist who is unaware of these variant patterns is likely to diagnose CCSK as another neoplasm, with different therapeutic and prognostic implications. These variant patterns are described in the subsequent sections.[28-30]

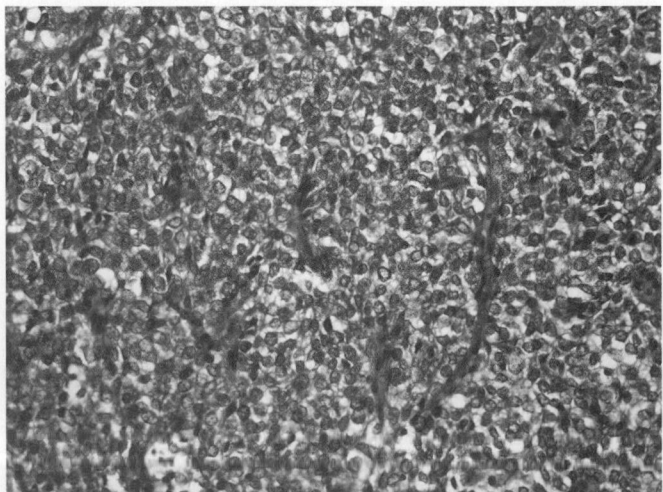

Figure 55-4 Clear cell sarcoma of the kidney.

Epithelioid Patterns. Condensation of cord cells of the classic CCSK pattern creates striking epithelioid arrangements in approximately 15% of cases.[28] These condensations usually form trabeculae or rosettes. These epithelioid formations conform to the pattern of the original cell cords and can be either straight or undulating in configuration. The epithelioid variants of CCSK are most likely to be mistaken for WT. In all of the examples analyzed by immunohistochemistry, these epithelioid formations have been negative for epithelial markers, in contrast to the epithelial cells of WT.

Spindle Cell Patterns. Spindle cell patterns are observed in approximately 10% of cases and result from two mechanisms.[28] Proliferation of septal cells produces wide spindle cell septa that compress or obliterate the cell cords. Intersections of these hyperplastic septal cells often resemble the storiform patterns seen with fibrohistiocytic neoplasms. Spindled transformation of cord cells yields a spindled pattern with preservation of thin fibrovascular septa.

Myxoid and Sclerosing Patterns. Most CCSKs contain abundant mucopolysaccharide, apparently produced by the cord cells.[28] This material separates cord cells and creates the appearance of clear cytoplasm. In approximately 30% of cases, mucopolysaccharide occupies more volume than the neoplastic cells themselves and forms large pools or cystic spaces.[28] While it accumulates, the tumor cells become progressively more isolated and eventually degenerate. In time the mucoid material becomes denser, eosinophilic, and hyaline in appearance. Hyaline sclerosis is found in 35% of CCSK. Complete replacement of cell cords by hyaline sclerosis preserves the original cord pattern with retention of the vascular septa, preserving the chicken-wire appearance. More diffuse zones of dense stromal sclerosis surrounding individual tumor cells may create an osteosarcoma-like appearance. Dense stromal sclerosis is relatively uncommon in untreated WT, and this finding can be a clue to the diagnosis of CCSK or rhabdoid tumor in limited biopsy material.

Palisading (Verocay-Body) Pattern. Nuclear palisading resembling schwannoma is focally prominent in approximately 10% of CCSK specimens.[28] Unlike schwannomas, these areas are not immunoreactive for S-100 protein.

Monstrocellular (Anaplastic) Pattern. Approximately 3% of CCSK contain foci with enlarged, pleomorphic nuclei and bizarre mitotic figures, resembling the appearance of anaplastic WTs or pleomorphic sarcomas. This is the only pattern of CCSK that frequently overexpresses p53 protein.[28]

Posttherapy Patterns. Recurrences of CCSK after therapy may have a deceptively hypocellular and bland appearance, suggesting low-grade fibromatosis or myxoma. A lump appearing anywhere in a child with a history of CCSK should be viewed as a potential metastasis until proven otherwise.

Ultrastructure, Immunohistochemistry, and Cytogenetics

Ultrastructural studies yield few clues as to the putative cell of origin of CCSK.[32] The tumor cells are characterized by a high nuclear-to-cytoplasmic ratio, with nuclear shapes that are more irregular and variable than would be expected from light microscopy. The cytoplasm is usually tenuous, with elongated, irregular processes surrounding abundant intercellular matrix. This latter feature is responsible for the vacuoles often seen with the light microscope. The cytoplasm tends to be poor in organelles. Immunohistochemistry has afforded little new insight into the histogenesis of CCSK, except to exclude various potential lines of differentiation for this enigmatic neoplasm. Vimentin is positive in nearly all specimens and BCL2 in some, but other markers are consistently negative. These include stains for epithelial markers (cytokeratins and epithelial membrane antigen [EMA]), neural markers (S-100 protein), neuroendocrine markers (chromogranin, synaptophysin), muscle markers (desmin), CD34, CD117 (c-kit), and CD99 (MIC2).[28] A subset of CCSK harbor a t(10;17)(q22;p13) chromosome translocation, resulting in a *YWHAE-FAM22* gene fusion.[33]

Differential Diagnosis of Clear Cell Sarcoma of the Kidney

The distinction of CCSK from other renal neoplasms can be extremely difficult, even for those with extensive experience in pediatric renal neoplasm pathology. The distinction of CCSK from rhabdoid tumor of the kidney is covered in the section on the latter. The major differential diagnostic concerns are discussed in the text that follows.

Clear Cell Sarcoma of the Kidney Versus Wilms Tumor. Some blastemal WT are richly vascular, and the vascular pattern may perfectly mimic that of CCSK. Several features help in this differential diagnosis. First, under low magnification, blastemal WTs often show distinctive nested patterns, whereas CCSKs are not typically nested. Second, blastemal WTs are more densely cellular than are CCSKs. When cells are closely packed, most nuclei are overlapping, and nuclei mold to one another, WT is more likely than CCSK. Third, heterologous tissues such as skeletal muscle are never seen in CCSK. The presence of a focus resembling CCSK in an otherwise unequivocal WT can safely be ignored. Fourth, multicentricity is common in WT, whereas multicentric and bilateral CCSKs have not been reported. Fifth, sclerotic, hyalinized stroma in an untreated tumor favors CCSK over WT. Finally, a fine nuclear chromatin pattern favors a diagnosis of CCSK over WT, although this feature is susceptible to fixation and processing artifacts.

Clear Cell Sarcoma of the Kidney versus Congenital Mesoblastic Nephroma. Cellular congenital mesoblastic nephroma (CMN) may resemble spindled variants of CCSK, and the age ranges of these two entities overlap. Small foci resembling CCSK may occur in CMN, but CMN lacks the diversity of morphologic patterns that typifies CCSK. The absence of the t(12;15) chromosome translocation that is characteristic of cellular CMN in all

CCSKs examined to date indicates that these two neoplasms are unrelated.

Congenital Mesoblastic Nephroma
Gross Appearance

CMN arises unicentrically and usually appears to have arisen deep within the medial parenchyma, near the renal sinus. The renal sinus and adjacent structures on the medial side of the kidney are major sites of extrarenal spread of CMN. Surgeons and pathologists must pay particular attention to the medial margin of the CMN resection specimen. However because of the predominance of freely mobile fat in this location and retraction artifact, the medial specimen margin is notoriously difficult to evaluate, and it is rarely possible to be certain that it is free of involvement by CMN.

The appearance of the sectioned surface of CMN is variable and depends on the subtype. Classic CMNs have a tough, whorled appearance resembling that of leiomyoma, but cellular CMNs may be soft, friable tumors. Hemorrhage, necrosis, and cyst formation are present to some degree in a majority of cellular CMNs.

Microscopic Appearance

CMN is a low-grade fibroblastic sarcoma of the infantile kidney. The classic type of CMN has a fibrous, whorled gross appearance. Morphologically, classic CMN is identical to infantile fibromatosis; it is composed of bland fibroblastic or myofibroblastic cells, arranged in fascicles that dissect into the native kidney (Fig. 55-5).[34] Mitoses are usually rare, and necrosis is absent. The leading edge of the tumor characteristically induces angiomatous vascular proliferation where it abuts perirenal fat. Entrapped renal tubules may acquire a primitive appearance (embryonal metaplasia), which may cause confusion with true neoplastic tubular differentiation that would suggest a diagnosis of biphasic stromal-epithelial WT. In contrast, the cellular variant of CMN typically has a softer, more fleshy and hemorrhagic appearance with necrosis and cystification. Microscopically, cellular CMN is identical to infantile

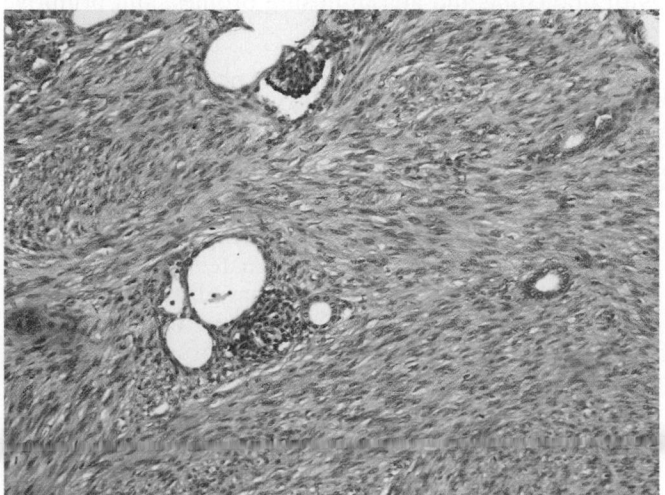

Figure 55-5 Congenital mesoblastic nephroma, classic type.

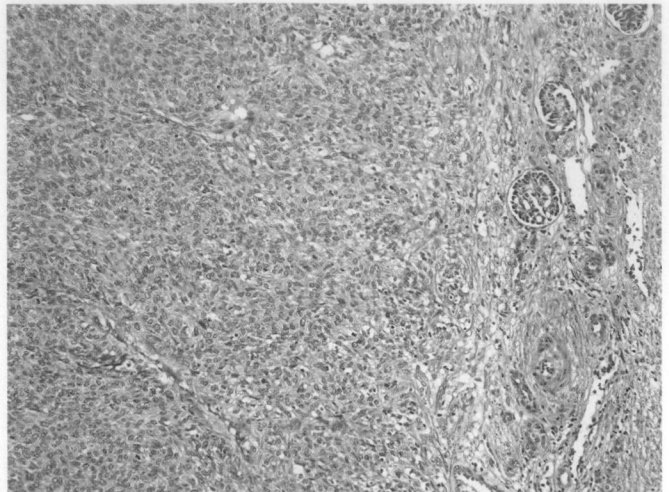

Figure 55-6 Congenital mesoblastic nephroma, cellular type.

fibrosarcoma (IFS).[35] Compared with the classic variant, cellular CMNs more often have a "pushing" border, demonstrate sheetlike growth patterns, are less often fascicular, are more cellular, and have a higher mitotic rate (Fig. 55-6). Tumor cells may be polygonal with well-demarcated pink cytoplasm and nuclei with vesicular chromatin and prominent nucleoli; this raises the differential diagnosis of rhabdoid tumor of the kidney. Alternatively the tumor cells may be thinner, primitive, and spindled, yielding a more embryonal "blue cell" appearance. Mixed CMNs have areas identical to both cellular and classic CMN in varied proportions within the same tumor.

Immunohistochemistry and Ultrastructure

Immunohistochemistry is of limited value in the diagnosis of CMN. The cells of CMN label in a fashion consistent with fibroblasts or myofibroblasts.[36] Whereas actin may be focally positive, desmin and CD34 are typically negative (P. Argani, unpublished observations). INI1 protein is retained. Ultrastructural studies also reveal features consistent with fibroblasts or myofibroblasts.[37] Most CMN cells show abundant rough endoplasmic reticulum with branching and anastamosing profiles, and primitive cell junctions are often found.

Differential Diagnosis of Congenital Mesoblastic Nephroma

The differential diagnosis for CMN includes stromal-predominant WT, CCSK, metanephric stromal tumor (MST) and malignant rhabdoid tumor (MRT). These distinctions are crucial because most children with CMN do not require adjuvant chemotherapy, whereas those with WT, CCSK, and MRT are treated on specific chemotherapy protocols. Features that distinguish CCSK and MRT from CMN are covered in the sections on CCSK and MRT, respectively. The features that distinguish CMN from WT and MST are expanded on in the subsequent sections.

Congenital Mesoblastic Nephroma Versus Wilms Tumor. As mentioned previously, embryonal metaplastic changes in nephrons surrounded by CMN cells are sometimes misinterpreted as tubular or papillary elements in a WT. Rarely untreated WT will be composed predominantly of stromal cells. In most of these the presence of immature or mature skeletal muscle readily excludes the diagnosis of CMN. Specimens removed after chemotherapy are particularly challenging. Treatment often ablates the embryonal, proliferating elements of a WT but tends to spare stromal cells. The resulting appearances can readily be confused with CMN. The following features are helpful in the differential diagnosis:

1. A diagnosis of CMN should be considered suspect in a patient who has received prior therapy, unless the clinical and pathologic features are characteristic.
2. Most CMNs are diagnosed in the first 3 months of life, whereas WT is relatively uncommon at this age. Only 10% of CMNs are diagnosed after 1 year, and virtually none are diagnosed after 2 years.
3. Most WTs express a diversity of cell types and tissue patterns. In contrast blastemal foci do not occur in a CMN, and skeletal muscle is never seen. However nodules of entrapped cartilage and squamous pearls may occur in CMN (likely reflecting coexisting renal dysplasia), and this should not be taken as evidence for WT.
4. The interdigitating, irregular border of classic CMN distinguished it from most WTs. However, cellular CMN often has a sharp, pushing border, similar to that of most WTs.
5. Bilaterality or the presence of NRs (or both) strongly favors WT over CMN.

Congenital Mesoblastic Nephroma Versus Metanephric Stromal Tumor. Many tumors previously considered to be CMNs in children older than age 3 years are in fact distinct from CMN and represent the newly recognized entity MST.[38] MST is identical to the stromal component of metanephric adenofibroma [39] (previously known as nephrogenic adenofibroma),[40] a biphasic tumor containing an epithelial component that is identical to metanephric adenoma. MST is a benign lesion composed of spindled to stellate cells featuring thin hyperchromatic nuclei and thin indistinct cytoplasmic extensions. Several of the characteristic features of MST distinguish it from CMN. MST characteristically surrounds and entraps renal tubules and blood vessels to form concentric "onion-skin" rings or collarettes around these structures. Most MSTs induce angiodysplasia of entrapped arterioles, consisting of epithelioid transformation of medial smooth muscle and myxoid change. One fourth of MSTs feature juxtaglomerular cell hyperplasia within entrapped glomeruli, which may occasionally lead to hypertension associated with hyperreninism. Finally, unlike CMNs, MSTs are typically immunoreactive for CD34, but labeling may be patchy.

Malignant Rhabdoid Tumor of the Kidney
Gross Appearance

Most MRTs are relatively small because metastasis occurs early in the evolution of the neoplasm. On gross

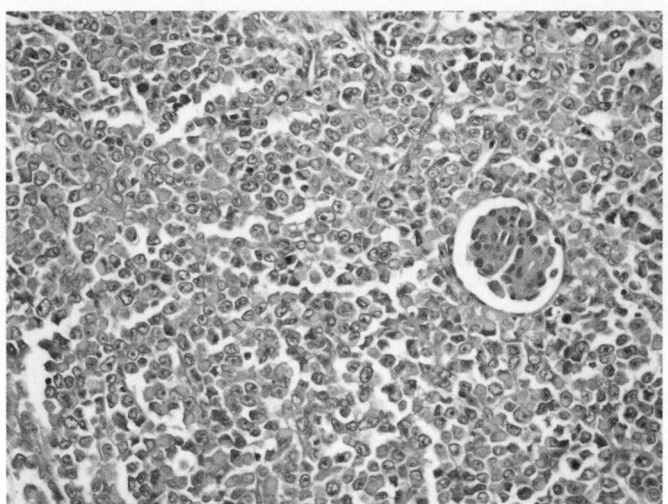

Figure 55-7 Malignant rhabdoid tumor of the kidney.

examination MRTs are typically fleshy or hemorrhagic neoplasms, with ill-defined borders and frequent satellite nodules that reflect the tumor's highly invasive nature.[41]

Microscopic Appearance

MRT was so named because of the resemblance of the tumor cells to rhabdomyoblasts. However this highly lethal infantile neoplasm does not demonstrate muscle differentiation. Microscopically these neoplasms typically engulf native renal elements at their periphery and demonstrate extensive vascular invasion. MRT classically consists of sheets of monotonous cells featuring a characteristic cytologic triad: vesicular chromatin, prominent nucleoli, and hyaline cytoplasmic inclusions (Fig. 55-7). These features are variably well developed within a given tumor, which means that it may be necessary to examine multiple microscopic fields from many sections to find them.

Ultrastructure and Immunohistochemistry

Ultrastructurally the cytoplasmic inclusions correspond to whorled intermediate filaments.[42] The whorled filaments may trap antibodies used for immunohistochemistry, yielding a nonspecific polyphenotypic pattern. With this caveat, strong vimentin and focal EMA labeling are characteristic immunohistochemical findings. Recently, an immunohistochemical assay for INI1 protein has become available. Loss of INI1 protein expression reflects *INI1* genetic status and, within the kidney, is a sensitive and nearly specific marker for MRT.[43]

Differential Diagnosis of Rhabdoid Tumor of the Kidney

The diagnosis of MRT is often challenging because a wide variety of renal and extrarenal tumors of adult and children may feature fully developed "rhabdoid" cytology, at least focally.[44,45] In the pediatric kidney these include cellular CMN (of the plump cell type), CCSK, blastemal WT, PNET, renal medullary carcinoma, and rhabdomyosarcoma.[44] In general, thorough sampling of such tumors is most helpful, insofar as it typically reveals specific differentiation that excludes MRT. Additionally, the age of

the patient is very helpful because MRT is not seen outside of early childhood. Finally, in the kidney loss of INI1 protein expression by immunohistochemistry is highly specific for MRT or renal medullary carcinoma.[46] Several specific differential diagnoses are covered in the subsequent sections.

Malignant Rhabdoid Tumor Versus Wilms Tumor. Both blastemal and myogenic elements of WT may contain cytoplasmic inclusions resembling those of MRT. A distinctive serpentine blastemal pattern, other distinctly nephrogenic features, or heterologous cells such as skeletal muscle supports the diagnosis of WT. The prominent nucleoli characteristic of MRT are not typically seen in WT, with the exception of some anaplastic specimens.

Malignant Rhabdoid Tumor Versus Cellular Congenital Mesoblastic Nephroma. The plump cell variant of cellular CMN often has vesicular nuclei with prominent nucleoli, and a rare CMN contains foci with hyaline cytoplasmic inclusions. A predominance of spindled patterns and a less invasive tumor periphery favor a cellular CMN over a rhabdoid tumor. Cytogenetic or molecular analysis (or both) may be invaluable in this setting; demonstration of chromosome 22q loss or loss of INI1 protein expression by immunohistochemistry supports MRT, whereas the presence of the ETV6-NTRK3 gene fusion supports cellular CMN.

Malignant Rhabdoid Tumor Versus Clear Cell Sarcoma of the Kidney. CCSK may rarely show prominent nucleoli, which can lead to difficulty in distinguishing CCSK from MRT. The presence of classic cytologic features of CCSK elsewhere and the presence of characteristic CCSK patterns are the major clues to the correct diagnosis in such instances. CCSKs lack the extreme invasiveness of MRTs and are generally more subtly invasive neoplasms.

Renal Carcinomas in Children

All of the common renal cell carcinomas (RCCs) of adulthood (clear cell, papillary, chromophobe, and collecting duct) may occasionally affect the pediatric kidney, but the clinical and differential diagnostic considerations differ in this setting. Children with von Hippel-Lindau syndrome are predisposed to develop conventional (clear cell) RCC. Children with tuberous sclerosis are at increased risk for developing both RCC and epithelioid angiomyolipoma,[47] and immunohistochemical analysis may be needed to distinguish these two. As discussed previously, PRCC may overlap morphologically with epithelial predominant WT or metanephric adenoma. However most pediatric RCCs represent distinctive neoplastic entities. Four of these entities are described in the subsequent sections.

Xp11.2 Translocation Renal Cell Carcinomas

RCCs with chromosome translocations involving Xp11.2 and resulting gene fusions involving the *TFE3* transcription factor gene were officially recognized in the 2004 World Health Organization Renal Tumor Classification.[48] Although this subtype of RCC is relatively uncommon on

TABLE 55-3   MiTF/TFE Translocation Neoplasms

Gene Fusion	Chromosome Translocation	Age (Years)	Tumor
ASPL-TFE3	der(17)t(X;17) (p11.2;q25)	5-40	ASPS
ASPL-TFE3	t(X;17)(p11.2;q25)	2-68	RCC
PRCC-TFE3	t(X;1)(p11.2;q21)	2-70	RCC
PSF-TFE3	t(X;1)(p11.2;p34)	5-68	RCC
NoNo-TFE3	inv(X)(p11;q12)	39	RCC
CLTC-TFE3	t(X;17)(p11.2;q23)	14	RCC
Alpha-TFEB	t(6;11)(p21;q12)	6-53	RCC

ASPS, Alveolar soft part sarcoma; *RCC,* renal cell carcinoma.

a percentage basis in adults, it most likely accounts for the majority of pediatric RCCs. One distinctive subtype bears a t(X;17)(p11;q25), which results in the identical *ASPL-TFE3* gene fusion, as was initially identified in alveolar soft part sarcoma (ASPS), and has been designated the *ASPL-TFE3* RCC.[49] Other subtypes are listed in Table 55-3.

Xp11.2 translocation RCCs closely resemble conventional (clear cell) renal carcinomas on gross examination, usually being tan-yellow and often necrotic and hemorrhagic. A papillary carcinoma composed of clear cells is the most distinctive histopathologic appearance (Fig. 55-8), because this combination is uncommon in other defined types of renal carcinomas. However the Xp11.2-translocation RCCs often have nested architecture and often contain cells with granular eosinophilic cytoplasm. The histologies of Xp11-translocation RCC associated with different *TFE3* gene fusions differ. The *ASPL-TFE3* RCCs feature cells with voluminous, clear to eosinophilic cytoplasm, discrete cell borders, vesicular nuclear chromatin, and prominent nucleoli. In contrast, the *PRCC-TFE3* RCCs, characterized by a t(X;1)(p11.2; q21),

typically have less abundant cytoplasm; fewer psammoma bodies; fewer hyaline nodules; and a more nested, compact architecture.[50]

Renal carcinomas with Xp11.2-associated translocations characteristically underexpress epithelial immunohistochemical markers such as cytokeratin and epithelial membrane antigen. Only approximately one half of cases will be positive with these markers, and the labeling is often focal. Vimentin immunoreactivity is also often focal compared with that of the adjacent blood vessels; this also differs from conventional RCCs, which are diffusely positive. Rare Xp11.2-translocation carcinomas, especially ones with variant gene fusions such as *PSF-TFE3* and *CLTC-TFE3*,[51] express melanocytic markers HMB45 and Melan A, creating confusion with epithelioid angiomyolipoma. Cathepsin K, a serine protease normally expressed in osteoclasts, is expressed in approximately 50% of translocation RCC but no other subtype of RCC.[52,53] The most distinctive immunohistochemical feature of these neoplasms is nuclear labeling for TFE3 protein using an antibody to the C-terminal portion of TFE3, which is retained in the gene fusions. Nuclear labeling for TFE3 is a common feature of all Xp11.2-translocation RCC and ASPS but does not occur in other RCCs (Fig. 55-9). Because native TFE3 is known to be ubiquitously expressed but is not detectable in normal tissues by immunohistochemistry, it is postulated that the different *TFE3* gene fusions consistently lead to overexpression of the fusion protein relative to native TFE3, such that the protein becomes detectable by this assay.[54] However TFE3 immunohistochemistry is difficult to optimize in the setting of variable fixation, and a break-apart fluorescence in situ hybridization (FISH) assay for *TFE3* gene rearrangements is a more reliable assay in formalin-fixed, paraffin-embedded tissue.[55]

When analyzed by electron microscopy, Xp11.2-associated carcinomas feature cell junctions, microvilli, intracytoplasmic fat, and glycogen and thereby most closely resemble conventional renal carcinomas. However a subset of cases demonstrates distinctive ultrastructural

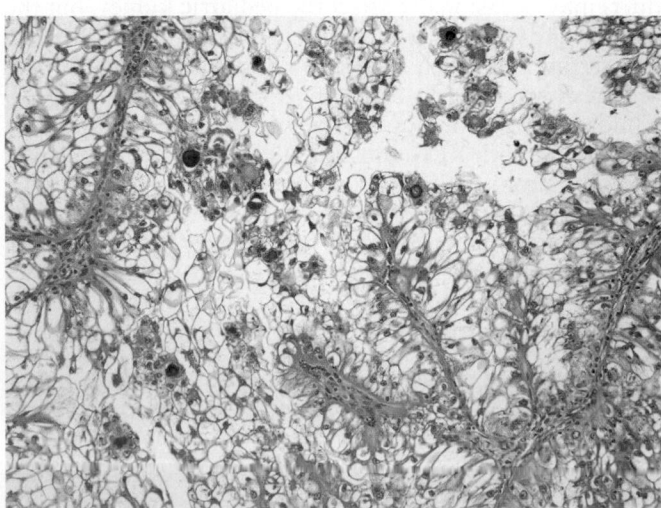

Figure 55-8 Xp11.2 translocation renal cell carcinoma.

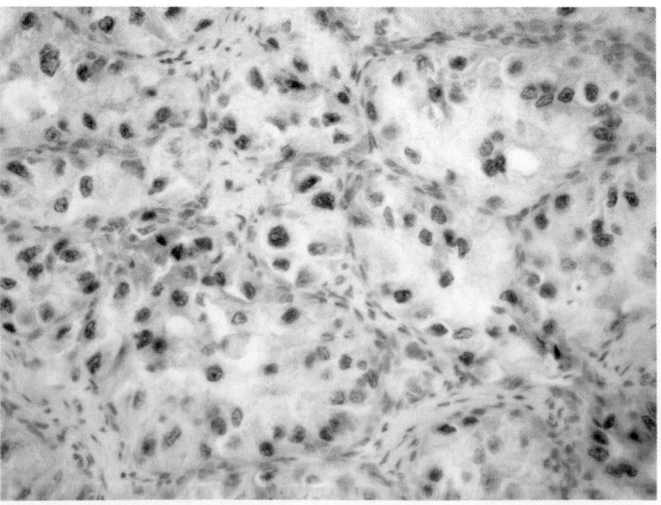

Figure 55-9 Xp11.2 translocation renal cell carcinoma, TFE3 immunohistochemistry.

features. Most of the *ASPL-TFE3* RCCs contain membrane-bound cytoplasmic granules, and a few have membrane-bound rhomboidal crystals that are identical to those seen in soft tissue ASPS. Some *PRCC-TFE3* RCCs have had distinctive intracisternal microtubules similar to those seen in malignant melanoma and extraskeletal myxoid chondrosarcoma.

t(6;11)(p21;q12) Renal Cell Carcinomas

Another distinctive type of RCC bears a t(6;11)(p21;q12). The distinctive clinicopathologic features of these neoplasms were not described until 2001.[56] On microscopic examination these neoplasms usually feature nests and tubules of polygonal epithelioid cells, separated by thin capillaries. Some cases have had papillary formations. The majority of the tumor cells have abundant clear to granular eosinophilic cytoplasm, well-defined cell borders, and round nuclei with small nucleoli. However a second population of smaller epithelioid cells is also characteristic, typically (but not always) clustered around nodules of hyaline basement membrane material within larger acini (Fig. 55-10). The cases examined have generally been negative for cytokeratins by immunohistochemistry, but almost all have labeled at least focally for HMB45, Melan A, and Cathepsin K, again creating confusion with epithelioid angiomyolipoma.

The t(6;11)(p21;q12) has been shown to result in a fusion of the intronless, untranslated *Alpha* gene with *TFEB*, a gene belonging to the same transcription factor family as *TFE3*.[57,58] The consequence of the *Alpha-TFEB* fusion is dysregulated expression of the normal full-length TFEB protein. Along these lines, the t(6;11) RCCs (also known as *Alpha-TFEB* RCCs) demonstrate specific nuclear labeling for TFEB protein by immunohistochemistry (IHC), whereas other neoplasms and normal tissues do not (Fig. 55-11). Hence nuclear labeling for TFEB is a sensitive and specific diagnostic marker for this neoplasm with a *TFEB* gene fusion, just as nuclear labelling for TFE3 is a sensitive and specific marker for neoplasms

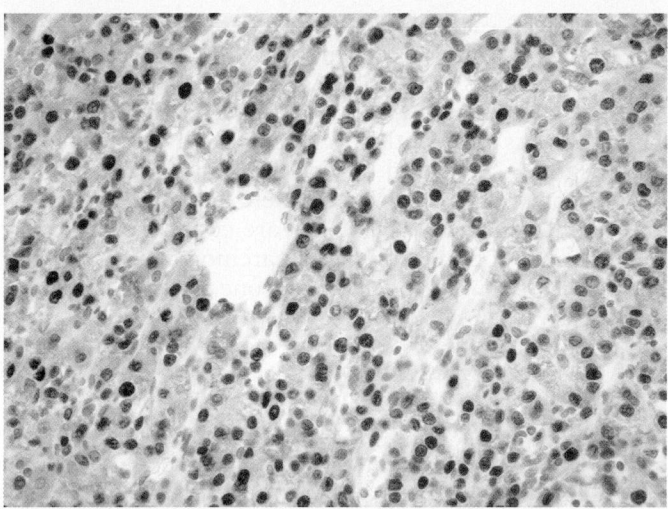

Figure 55-11 Renal cell carcinoma with t(6;11) (p12:q12) translocation, transcription factor EB immunohistochemistry.

bearing *TFE3* gene fusions.[59] A break-apart FISH assay for *TFEB* gene rearrangements has recently been developed for formalin-fixed, paraffin-embedded tissue and is proving to be more sensitive than TFEB IHC assay.[60]

Renal Medullary Carcinoma

Renal medullary carcinoma (RMC) was first described in 1995 by Davis and colleagues as "the seventh sickle cell nephropathy."[61] These tumors characteristically affect young patients (mean age, 22 years) with sickle cell trait. Tumors are typically centered in the renal medulla but demonstrate an aggressively infiltrative growth pattern with frequent vascular permeation. The tumor cells feature vesicular chromatin and prominent nucleoli, frequently associated with hyaline intracytoplasmic inclusions, therefore imparting a rhabdoid cytologic appearance. The tumor cells of RMC demonstrate diffuse (sheetlike), cribriform, gland-forming, microcystic, or reticular growth patterns, the latter two simulating yolk-sac tumor (Fig. 55-12). The stroma is typically desmoplastic and

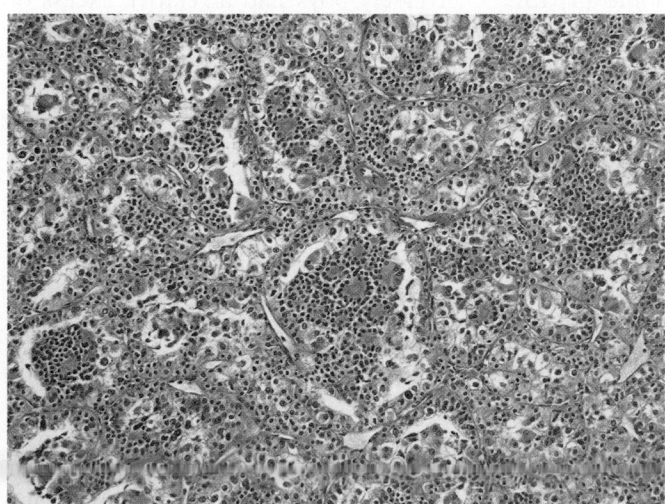

Figure 55-10 Renal cell carcinoma with t(6;11) (p12;q12) translocation.

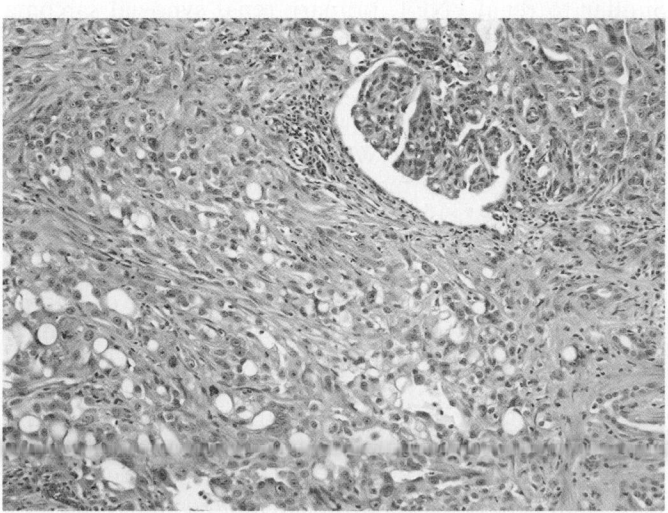

Figure 55-12 Renal medullary carcinoma.

infiltrated by neutrophils, and close examination of extravasated red blood cells may reveal sickling. However, hemoglobin electrophorosis is more reliable than the latter for determining that the patient has sickle cell trait. These tumors frequently present at high stage and are highly lethal; Davis and colleagues reported a mean survival of only 15 weeks. Given their medullary epicenter and high-grade cytology, RMCs are considered by some to be variants of collecting duct carcinoma, although the latter entity is a notoriously elusive one to define. As noted previously, RMCs consistently show loss of expression of INI-1 protein by IHC, similar to RTK.

Oncocytic Renal Carcinomas in Neuroblastoma Patients

Meideros and coworkers have described oncocytic renal carcinomas arising in children who had previously had neuroblastoma.[62] The genetic alterations identified in these lesions did not match those of known renal carcinomas, suggesting that these are another distinctive entity.

Primitive Neuroectodermal Tumor of Kidney

Primary renal PNET should be considered in the differential diagnosis of any undifferentiated blue cell tumor of the kidney. This neoplasm is encountered mainly in adolescent and young adult patients and tends to present at advanced stage.[63] Tumors consist of sheets of undifferentiated small blue cells with frequent necrosis and occasional rosettes. Renal PNETs are frequently mistaken for blastemal WTs of adolescent or adult patients and might account for some of the adverse prognosis attributed to "adult WT." Compared to WT, tumor cell nuclei are less hyperchromatic and more evenly placed. Molecular detection of the EWS-FLI1 gene fusion that results from the characteristic and specific t(11;22)(q24;q12) chromosome translocation is a useful way to confirm the diagnosis of PNET in suspected cases.[64] Also helpful is immunohistochemical labeling for CD99; the characteristic membrane staining pattern observed in PNETs is rarely if ever observed in WT blastemal cells or cellular CCSKs, which are the main differential diagnosis.[65]

Synovial Sarcoma of the Kidney

Similar to renal PNET, primary renal synovial sarcoma has been established as a distinctive neoplastic entity by demonstration of its specific chromosome translocation and gene fusion.[66,67] Genetically confirmed cases have affected young adults. Many have previously been classified as adult blastemal WT, embryonal sarcoma of the kidney, adult cellular mesoblastic nephroma, or sarcoma arising in cystic nephroma. Renal synovial sarcomas are typically large and often cystic, and they present at advanced stage. The typical appearance is that of a monomorphic, highly cellular neoplasm composed of plump, spindled cells growing in short fascicles. Tumor cells have ovoid nuclei and minimal cytoplasm and may be associated with sclerosis. Grossly identified cysts are lined by mitotically inactive polygonal eosinophilic cells with apically oriented nuclei ("hobnailed epithelium"), and the cellularity of their walls may be deceptively low, creating confusion with cystic nephroma in limited biopsy samples. Overall, the appearances are best conceptualized as monophasic spindle-cell synovial sarcoma encircling native renal collecting ducts. True epithelial differentiation yielding a biphasic synovial sarcoma may occur, but this is less common. Immunohistochemically, tumor cells label focally for epithelial markers (EMA more likely than cytokeratin), but many cases are completely negative for all epithelial markers. Many cases have labeled for CD99. The diagnosis can be confirmed in such cases by molecular demonstration of the SYT-SSX gene fusion that results from the t(X;18)(p11;q11) that is characteristic of this neoplastic entity. As with renal PNET, renal synovial sarcoma is more aggressive than WT and also may account for some of the adverse prognosis attributed to "adult WT."

WILMS TUMOR (NEPHROBLASTOMA)

Epidemiology

The age-adjusted incidence of pediatric renal tumors in the United States is 7.5 per million children younger than 15 years of age and 6 per million children younger than 19 years of age.[1] Although WT is the most common renal tumor overall, its relative frequency compared with other pediatric renal neoplasms varies according to patient age. Between 0 and 1 month of life, CMN is more common than WT, and after age 14 years RCC surpasses WT as the most prevalent renal cancer.[1,68] In North America the average age of diagnosis for unilateral WT is 42 months for boys and 47 months for girls.[69] Children with clinical malformations, genetic abnormalities, and tumor predisposition syndromes have a significantly earlier median age of diagnosis of WT.[70] For bilateral WT the average age of diagnosis is 30 months for boys and 33 months for girls.[69] The younger age of presentation for bilateral WT is due to genetic predisposition, an observation that provided the basis for Knudson's two-hit model.[71] The reason for the later age of presentation in girls is more elusive. An analysis from the NWTSG revealed that, compared with boys, girls had a relative excess of PLNRs, WT precursor lesions associated with genetic alterations of the Beckwith-Wiedemann syndrome locus at chromosome 11p15.[72] Conversely boys had a relative excess of ILNRs, distinct precursor lesions associated with mutations of the WT1 gene at chromosome 11p13. ILNR-associated WTs arise at an earlier age than PLNR-associated WTs, partially explaining the gender difference in age distribution. However even in the absence of NRs, girls presented with WTs a few months later, on average, than boys. In North America there is a slight preponderance of WT in girls compared with boys, with a female-to-male ratio of 1.1 to 1.

There also are racial and ethnic differences in the predisposition to WT.[69] Most Caucasian populations have an age-adjusted incidence of six to nine cases per million children annually. Black populations in North America and some parts of Africa exceed 10 cases per million children annually. In Japan, the Philippines, and China, the incidence is fewer than four cases per million children per year. Interestingly, in these East Asian populations, there is an excess of male subjects with WTs, the age at diagnosis is earlier than in North America, and PLNRs are rarely seen.[73] There may also be biologic differences associated with racial differences in WT. A small study of WT in 15 Kenyan children demonstrated differences in molecular signature by imaging mass spectrometry and immunostaining compared with histology and age-matched North American controls. The Kenyan tumors exhibited more aggressive histology and worse outcome, although it is difficult to distinguish truly biologic aggressive disease from inadequate care related to resource limitations.[74]

Several studies have uncovered maternal and paternal environmental associations with WT. Maternal exposures that have been associated with WT include cigarettes, coffee or tea, oral contraceptives, hormonal pregnancy tests, hair-coloring products, hypertension, household pesticide use, and vaginal infections.[75,76] However none of these factors was confirmed by subsequent case-control studies conducted by the NWTSG.[77,78] In a COG study breastfeeding was found to be associated with reduced risk of WT, although the effect was restricted to mothers with less than a college education.[79] On the paternal side the occupations of machinist, welder, and other jobs involving exposure to hydrocarbons or lead were associated with increased risk of WT.[80,81] A subsequent case-control study found an association with the paternal occupations of vehicle mechanics, auto-body repairmen, and welders, although no unifying exposure could be established.[82] A correlation of a low Apgar score (0-5) with a higher risk (46%) of cancer diagnosis was found in a nationwide population-based study in Denmark and Sweden that followed 5,091,188 children from age 0 to 14 years from 1978 to 2006 (excluding children with birth defects). The potential impact of the low Apgar score and cancer diagnosis was largely confined to children diagnosed with cancer before 6 months of age, and the highest risk was observed for the occurrence of WT.[83]

Molecular Biology and Genetics

Retinoblastoma and WT were the original tumors used by Knudson to establish the two-hit hypothesis of oncogenic transformation.[71] Unlike retinoblastoma, in which alterations of a single gene (*Rb*) account for the vast majority of tumors, several genes have been implicated in the genesis of WT, and a sizable proportion of WTs have indeterminate genetic etiology. The genes that are most commonly mutated or epigenetically altered in sporadic WTs are *WT1, IGF2,* β-catenin (*CTNNB1*), *WTX,* and *TP53*. These five genes are discussed in detail in the subsequent sections, whereas other genes and loci implicated in WT are summarized in Table 55-4.

WT1

WT1 was the first gene found to be specifically mutated in WT.[84-86] The gene was originally identified via study of patients with the WAGR syndrome. Children with WAGR suffer from the constellation of WT, *a*niridia, *g*enitourinary abnormalities, and mental *r*etardation. Chromosomal analysis of these patients revealed heterozygous constitutional deletions at 11p13. Subsequent investigation of the genes contained within these deletions identified disruption of the *PAX6* gene as the basis of aniridia

and *WT1* as the key tumor suppressor. The remaining allele of *WT1* is mutated in the WTs from these patients.

WT1 encodes an approximately 45-kd DNA-binding protein that contains domains rich in glutamine and proline in the amino terminus and four zinc fingers in the carboxy terminus, collectively suggesting that it acts as a transcription factor. The *WT1* gene is quite complex insofar as it encodes numerous distinct isoforms and contains an evolutionarily conserved cryptic splice site that can result in the insertion of three amino acids, lysine, threonine, and serine (KTS), between zinc fingers 3 and 4. Notably distinct functions have been identified for the different KTS isoforms. Patients with Frasier syndrome, characterized by male pseudohermaphroditism, progressive glomerulopathy, and an increased risk of WT, have a congenital donor splice-site mutation in *WT1* that results in loss of the +KTS isoform.[87] Furthermore mice that express only the +KTS or only the −KTS isoform have distinct phenotypes.[88]

Congenital point mutations in *WT1* are also the basis of Denys-Drash syndrome.[89] Patients with this syndrome suffer from renal failure, pseudohermaphroditism, and a susceptibility to WT. Denys-Drash syndrome is caused by missense mutations in *WT1* that disrupt zinc finger binding to DNA. The phenotype of patients with Denys-Drash is quite severe, and evidence suggests that these mutations may lead to a dominant-negative protein that impairs function of the normal protein encoded by the remaining allele. Nonetheless the remaining *WT1* allele is mutated in the WTs that arise in these patients, suggesting that mutation of both alleles is required for tumor formation. Notably whereas mutations in *WT1* are the basis of several syndromes that predispose to the formation of WT, *WT1* is mutated in only 10% to 20% of sporadic tumors.[90] Mouse models have provided insight into the contributions of *WT1* to development and tumor suppression. *WT1* is expressed at high levels in the developing kidney, gonads, spleen, and mesothelium and at lower levels in several other tissues. Mice deficient for *WT1* die midgestation with abnormalities of the metanephric blastema, gonads, mesothelium, heart, and lungs.[91] Cells from the metanephric blastema in these mice undergo apoptosis, and consequently the metanephric kidney never develops. Based on these data it has been postulated that the WT1 protein regulates gene expression pathways required for morphogenesis of the kidney, and that its disruption results in aberrant stimulation of tissue-specific growth. This role in differentiation may also explain why WT is largely a disease of early childhood insofar as kidney morphogenesis is initiated in utero and is completed in early postnatal life. Indeed the level of *WT1* plummets within a few weeks after birth in mice. Whereas $WT1^{-/-}$ mice are not viable, $WT1^{+/-}$ mice live but do not develop WTs. This differs from the human condition in which individuals with germline *WT1* deletions or mutations have a greatly increased risk for developing WT compared with the general population.

β catenin (CTNNB1)

The Wnt signaling pathway regulates the cellular processes of proliferation, differentiation, motility, and

TABLE 55-4 Genes and Loci Associated with Wilms Tumor

Locus	Gene	Gene Function	Comments	Key References
11p13	WT1	Transcription factor	WAGR, Denys-Drash, and Frasier syndromes associated with WT predisposition; somatic mutations in 10% to 20% of WT	84-86, 90
11p15	WT2 (IGF2/H19)	Insulin-like growth factor pathway	Beckwith-Wiedemann syndrome associated with WT predisposition; somatic genetic or epigenetic alterations seen in 70% of WT	113-115
Xq11	WTX (AMER1/FAM123B)	Wnt signaling pathway	Osteopathia striata congenita with cranial sclerosis syndrome has not been associated with WT predisposition but somatic mutations seen in 20% to 30% of WT	97-99
3p21	CTNNB1 (β-catenin)	Wnt signaling pathway	Somatic mutations seen in 15% of WT; strong correlation with WT1 mutations	93, 94
17q12-q21	FWT1	Unknown	Locus associated with familial WT; gene not identified	305, 306
19q13	FWT2	Unknown	Locus associated with familial WT; gene not identified	307
17p13	TP53	Cell cycle checkpoint and apoptosis	Li-Fraumeni syndrome associated with WT predisposition; somatic mutations seen in 75% of anaplastic WT but uncommon in favorable-histology WT	11, 12, 120
13q12	BRCA2 (FANCD1)	DNA repair	Fanconi anemia; biallelic mutations associated with WT predisposition	308, 309
16p12	PALB2 (FANCN)	DNA repair	Fanconi anemia; associated with WT predisposition	310
15q26	BLM	DNA helicase	Bloom syndrome; associated with WT predisposition	311-313
15q15	BUB1B	Mitotic spindle checkpoint	Mosaic variegated aneuploidy; associated with WT predisposition	311, 314
Xq26	GPC3	Wnt signaling pathway	Simpson-Golabi-Behmel syndrome; associated with WT predisposition	311, 315-318
2q37	DIS3L2	Micro-RNA processsing	Perlman syndrome; associated with WT predisposition	319
7p14-15	POU6F2	Transcription factor	None	320, 321
1q25-q32	HRPT 2 (parafibromin)	RNA processing; histone modification	Hyperparathyroidism-jaw tumor	322
6q21	HACE1	Ubiquitin ligase	None	323, 324
2p24	MYCN	Transcription factor	Somatic gene amplification seen in 5% to 10% of WT	325
4q31	FBXW7	Ubiquitin ligase	Somatic mutations seen in 4% of WT; germline mutation described	326

WAGR, Constellation of Wilms tumor, *a*niridia, genitourinary abnormalities, and mental *r*etardation; *WT,* Wilms tumor.

survival. Central to the pathway is the transcriptional activator β-catenin, which is actively degraded in the absence of Wnt signaling.[92] Activating mutations in the *β-catenin (CTNNB1)* gene occur in approximately 15% of WTs.[93,94] Interestingly mutations in *β-catenin* occur predominantly in tumors in which *WT1* is also mutated, suggesting that these two events cooperate in the genesis of WT.[94,95] In the developing kidney *Wnt4* is an inducer of the mesenchymal to epithelial transition that underlies normal nephron development; disruption of normal renal development may be the means by which *β-catenin* mutation contributes to the formation of WT.[96]

WTX (AMER1/FAM123B)

WTX was discovered by an array comparative genomic hybridization screen that identified deletions of the Xq11.1 locus in male patients with WT. Further investigation found deletions and mutations in girls. Intriguingly *WTX* is inactivated by a single hit affecting either the sole *WTX* copy in male subjects or the copy located on the active X chromosome in female subjects.[97] According to the initial report, *WTX* was deleted or mutated in approximately one third of WTs, although other groups have reported a lower mutation frequency.[97-99] Germline *WTX* mutations have been observed in individuals with osteopathia striata congenita with cranial sclerosis, a rare slerosing bone dyspasia.[100] Individuals with osteopathia striata congenita with cranial sclerosis do not have increased risk for WT or other cancers, but NRs have been observed in one individual with a germline *WTX* mutation.[101]

WTX is alternatively spliced to encode two isoforms of a protein with disparate functions.[100] The short isoform of the protein is nuclear and forms a complex with β-catenin, AXIN1, APC, and β-TrCP2, ultimately promoting ubiquitination and degradation of β-catenin, thereby acting as a negative regulator of the WNT signaling pathway.[102] The full-length WTX protein binds to the adenomatous polyposis coli protein and regulates its distribution between microtubules and the plasma membrane.[103] WTX also interacts with WT1 protein and enhances its function as a transcriptional activator.[104] It was recently shown to bind p53 and modulate p53 function through its activator CBP/p300.[105]

Although *WT1* and *β-catenin* mutations are highly concordant, there is no clear association between *WT1* and *WTX* mutations.[97,98] This suggests that *WTX* and *β-catenin* mutations are not functionally equivalent even though both proteins reside within the WNT pathway.

IGF2

Cytogenetic analyses have long suggested the presence of an additional WT gene at 11p15 distinct from the *WT1* locus at 11p13.[106] Loss of heterozygosity (LOH) at 11p15 occurs in some cases of sporadic WT. Additionally, this locus is linked to Beckwith-Wiedemann syndrome (BWS), an overgrowth disorder associated with macroglossia, umbilical hernia, gigantism, neonatal hypoglycemia, and predisposition to WT and other cancers. BWS arises from alterations in several different genomically imprinted genes at the 11p15 locus.[107] Genomic imprinting is the preferential expression of a gene from either the maternal or paternal allele. The molecular basis of genomic imprinting is epigenetic modification, most notably DNA methylation. The 11p15 locus has two imprinting domains (Fig. 55-13). The telomeric domain (domain 1) includes the genes *insulin-like growth factor 2 (IGF2)* and *H19*. *IGF2* encodes a growth factor expressed at high levels in the developing kidney and WT.[108,109] *H19* encodes a biologically active untranslated RNA that may function as a tumor suppressor.[110] In normal cells these genes are oppositely expressed such that *IGF2* is expressed only from the paternal allele and *H19* is expressed only from the maternal allele. The centromeric imprinting domain (domain 2) contains several imprinted genes, including *KCNQ1 (KvLQT1)*, *KCNQ1OT1 (LIT1)*, and *CDKN1C (p57KIP2)*. *KCNQ1* encodes a subunit of a voltage-gated potassium channel that is implicated in several cardiac arrhythmia syndromes, including long-QT syndrome 1. *KCNQ1OT1* encodes a noncoding RNA with antisense transcription of *KCNQ1*. *CDKN1C* encodes a member of the cyclin-dependent kinase inhibitor family of proteins that negatively regulates cell proliferation and is a tumor suppressor. Molecular subgroups of BWS include those with (1) loss of methylation in domain 2, which is associated with decreased expression of *CDKN1C* (~50%); (2) duplication of domains 1 and 2 of the paternal allele with no maternal contribution (uniparental isodisomy) (~20%); (3) mutation of CDKN1C (~10%); (4) gain of methylation of domain 1, resulting in increased IGF2 expression and decreased H19 expression (~2% to 7%); 5) small duplications or chromosome rearrangements (<2%); and (5) unknown genetic etiology (~13% to 15%).[107] Interestingly, the Silver-Russell syndrome, associated with growth retardation, is caused by loss of methylation at domain 1 and maternal 11p15 duplication (i.e., the opposite of BWS).[111,112]

In the past decade correlations between BWS genotypes and cancer predisposition have emerged. Uniparental isodisomy and gain of methylation at domain 1 carry the highest risk of WT. Loss of methylation at domain 2 is associated with omphalocele, macrosomia, and a distinct lack of WT, although these individuals develop other tumor types.[113-115] A common thread in the patients most susceptible to WT is increased expression of *IGF2*.

Wilms Tumor Subsets Defined by Genetic and Epigenetic Features

A traditional model of WT development purports that WTs fall into two discrete subtypes: type I and type II.[72,116] Type I WT is caused by *WT1* mutation, resulting in intralobar NRs, which then accumulate second hits

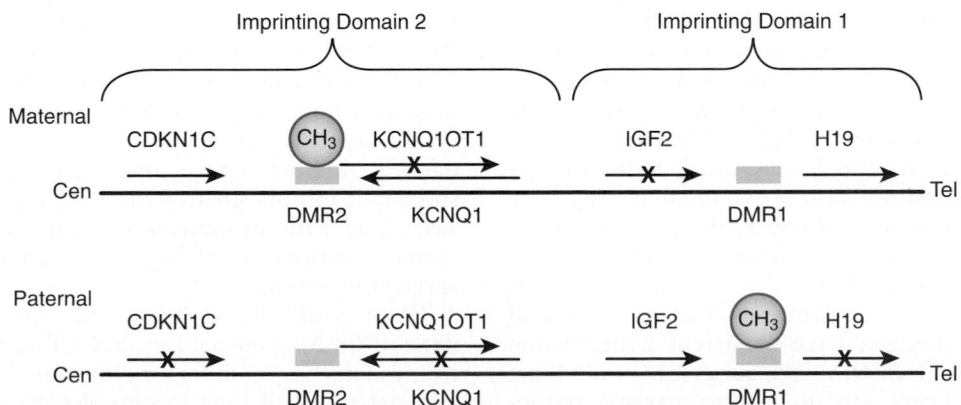

Figure 55-13 The Beckwith-Wiedemann syndrome locus. The chromosome 11p15.5 locus contains several imprinted genes clustered in two imprinting domains: centromeric *(cen)* and telomeric *(tel)*. Each domain has a differentially methylated region *(DMR)* that controls expression of surrounding genes. In normal individuals the DMR of domain 1 is methylated in the paternal allele, resulting in expression of *IGF2* and silencing of *H19*. In normal individuals the DMR of domain 2 is methylated in the maternal allele, resulting in expression of *CDKN1C (p57)* and *KCNQ1* and silencing of *KCNQ1OT1 (LIT1)*. Beckwith-Wiedemann syndrome can arise from decreased methylation of domain 2, increased methylation of domain 1, duplication of the paternal 11p15 allele with no contribution of the maternal allele (uniparental isodisomy), or small deletions or rearrangements. Increased methylation of domain 1 and uniparental isodisomy carry the greatest risk of Wilms tumor.

such as Wnt activating mutations (β-catenin or WTX mutations). Type II WT is caused by genetic or epigenetic changes in the 11p15 locus that result in IGF2 overexpression, perilobar NRs, and presumably other second-hit genetic changes that lead to WT. Comprehensive mutation analyses of WT1, β-catenin, WTX, and the 11p15 locus in WT samples indicate that whereas some tumors fit the classic paradigm, other tumors have evidence of both *IGF2* overexpression and *WT1* mutation. Indeed transgenic mice with *Igf2* overexpression and *Wt1* deletion developed WT, whereas neither genetic abnormality alone was sufficient to cause WT.[117] Other WTs lack evidence of either *IGF2* or *WT1* alteration. The requirement for coexisting mutations likely depends on the developmental stage of the cell of origin of a particular tumor.[118]

TP53

Constitutional mutations of the *TP53* gene are responsible for Li-Fraumeni syndrome (LFS), which predisposes carriers to cancer.[119] *TP53*, one of the most commonly mutated genes in human cancer, encodes a transcription factor that is a master regulator of cell cycle arrest, apopotosis, and DNA repair in response to a variety of stimuli. Although WT is not a defining criterion for LFS, several LFS families with WT have been identified.[120] It is important to note that *TP53* mutations are associated with the anaplastic histology subtype of WT; approximately 75% of anaplastic WTs have detectable *TP53* mutations, whereas *TP53* mutations are uncommon in favorable histology tumors.[11,121,122] Several lines of evidence suggest that anaplastic WT arises from the acquisition of a *TP53* mutation in a favorable histology WT. First, patients with bilateral WT often have discordant histologies between contralateral tumors.[15] Second, some WTs have favorable histologic features at diagnosis but are found to have anaplastic histology at relapse.[121] Finally, microdissected WTs were found to have *TP53* mutations restricted to areas of anaplasia within the tumor tissue.[12]

Clinical Presentation and Diagnostic Evaluation

The most common presenting signs and symptoms of WT are abdominal mass (75%), abdominal pain (28%), hypertension (26%), gross hematuria (18%), microscopic hematuria (24%), and fever (22%).[123] The hypertension, which can be severe, may be due to ectopic renin production by the tumor, compression of the renal artery by the tumor with resulting physiologic renin production, or ectopic adrenocorticotropic hormone production. An analysis of 31 patients with WT with hypertension at diagnosis found increased plasma renin levels in 81% of patients.[124] Some patients have persistent hypertension after the tumor has been removed, suggesting underlying renal pathology. There are no tumor markers pathognomic for WT, although associated laboratory findings include hematuria and anemia. An association between WT and acquired von Willebrand disease has been described.[125]

WT can spread locally or hematogenously. Locally the tumor has the potential to spread into structures surrounding the kidney and can occasionally invade other organs such as the liver. If the tumor ruptures, peritoneal tumor deposits can be detected. WT also spreads to lymph nodes near the renal hilum and in the paraaortic chain. Between 6% and 8% of WTs spread through the renal vein and form a tumor thrombus in the inferior vena cava, which can propagate into the heart.[126,127] The most common sites of distant metastasis are the lung and liver. There are reports of WT spread to brain or bone, but this is very uncommon. About 7% of patients have synchronous or metachronous bilateral tumors, and 10% have unilateral multifocal tumors.[69]

Radiologic evaluation of WT focuses on the identification of local and distant sites of spread. A computed tomography (CT) scan of the abdomen and pelvis is recommended to visualize the primary tumor, the contralateral kidney, lymph nodes, and intraabdominal or pelvic tumor deposits. CT also provides information valuable to surgical planning. Assessment of the diagnostic performance of CT in identifying the presence or absence of preoperative rupture found moderate specificity but relatively low sensitivity when CT findings were compared to operative notes or pathologic examination. The single best indicator of rupture was the finding of ascites beyond the cul-de-sac, followed by perinephric fat stranding and retroperitoneal fluid.[128] Doppler ultrasound has historically been used as a complementary test to evaluate for tumor thrombus in the renal vein and inferior vena cava. The detection of tumor thrombus by CT versus ultrasound was compared in a study population drawn from the first 1015 patients enrolled on the COG AREN03B2 Renal Tumor Biology and Risk Classification study. CT scans from 62 children with and 111 children without tumor thrombus identified at nephrectomy were reviewed. Comparable sensitivity and specificity of CT and ultrasound were found for detection of cavoatrial thrombus. These findings suggest that CT can adequately identify tumor thrombus that will affect surgical approach and that Doppler ultrasound evaluation is not a diagnostic requirement.[129] CT imaging can also aid in surgical planning by allowing an estimation of tumor weight before surgery.[130,131] In the COG AREN03B2 risk-stratification process, tumors less than 550 gm are considered for treatment with observation only, and preoperative weight estimation can be used in determining the appropriateness of central line placement at time of nephrectomy. On the other end of the spectrum, tumors greater than 1000 gm have also been associated with an increased risk of intraoperative spill; therefore estimation of larger size can also be a factor in surgical planning.[132]

Chest x-rays have historically been used to assess patients for lung metastases, but CT scans are more sensitive in detecting nodules or effusions.[133,134] On NWTS-5, 129 patients had lung lesions detected on CT scan but not chest x-ray. Forty-two of these patients with "CT-only" nodules had lung biopsies, and tumor was confirmed in 31 patients (73.8%).[135] Retrospective studies of the prognostic significance of CT-only lung nodules have yielded conflicting results.[133,136-139] The largest analysis to date included 186 patients with CT-only nodules from

NWTS-4 and -5. These patients were treated heterogeneously (+/– doxorubicin, +/– lung radiation) because the treatment decisions were left to the discretion of the local physicians. Outcome analysis found that patients with CT-only nodules who were treated with doxorubicin had superior relapse-free survival compared with patients who did not receive doxorubicin, but the study found no impact on overall survival. The use of lung radiation did not have a significant effect on outcome.[140,141] Based on these findings, the first generation of COG renal tumor studies recommended CT scans, but not chest x-rays, for the diagnostic staging evaluation for WT. Lung nodules are considered to contain tumor unless biopsy proves otherwise.

Bone scan and brain magnetic resonance imaging are not routinely recommended in the evaluation of patients with newly diagnosed WT. Fluorodeoxyglucose (FDG) positron emission tomography (PET) scanning is not a routine part of the WT workup. Initial experience with PET scans indicates that most WTs are FDG avid.[142,143] Correlations of PET avidity and measures of standardized uptake value with histology and treatment response have been reported in small patient series. These studies suggest that FDG PET may have value in assessing response to chemotherapy as well as a role in identifying tumor viability in lesions with no radiologic evidence of change.[144-146]

Treatment

The treatment approach to WT has evolved along two distinct pathways. The NWTSG, which became the Renal Tumor Committee of COG in 2002, advocates the upfront nephrectomy approach whenever surgically and medically feasible, followed by chemotherapy. This approach provides for accurate histologic diagnosis and staging information. In contrast, SIOP uses preoperative chemotherapy, which shrinks the tumor, thereby reducing the risk of surgical complications such as intraoperative tumor spillage. It is difficult to compare the two approaches side by side because of differences in the staging systems and treatment plans, but both approaches produce excellent outcomes. Regardless of the timing of initial surgery, the three pillars of WT treatment are surgery, chemotherapy, and radiation therapy.

Surgery

In the SIOP treatment protocols, patients 6 months of age or older receive chemotherapy before surgery unless there is evidence of tumor rupture, in which case they undergo immediate nephrectomy. Open or needle biopsy is not routinely performed. Infants younger than 6 months old are treated with upfront nephrectomy because non-Wilms renal tumors, such as mesoblastic nephroma or malignant rhabdoid tumor, are prevalent in this age group.

In the COG treatment protocols, all patients are considered candidates for immediate surgery, although there are several indications to give preoperative chemotherapy: (1) bilateral WT; (2) tumor thrombus in the inferior vena cava above the level of the hepatic veins; (3) tumors that invade adjacent organs such that resection of the tumor would involve resection of the other structures (except the adrenal gland); (4) tumors that, in the surgeon's judgment, would result in significant morbidity or mortality if resected before chemotherapy; and (5) respiratory distress resulting from extensive pulmonary metastatic disease. If preoperative chemotherapy is given, it is recommended not to delay definitive surgery beyond week 12 of treatment.

A generous transabdominal, transperitoneal, or thoracoabdominal incision is recommended for adequate exposure. An increased rate of rupture and complication is associated with a midline laparotomy.[147] Complete exploration of the abdomen should be performed, followed by a radical nephrectomy, dividing the ureter as distally as possible. Routine exploration of the contralateral kidney is not recommended if imaging is satisfactory and does not suggest a bilateral process because the chance of detecting a contralateral kidney tumor during surgery that is undetected with modern imaging techniques is less than 1%, and the outcome of these patients is excellent.[148] An important component of WT surgery is lymph node sampling, even if the nodes appear normal. NWTS-4 showed that patients with positive lymph nodes had better outcomes than patients whose lymph nodes were not sampled, indicating that some patients who did not undergo lymph node sampling were understaged and undertreated.[149] Another important facet of surgery is to remove the tumor en bloc, avoiding tumor spillage. Intraoperative spillage was shown to increase the risk of tumor recurrence.[149] In a review of the first 2000 patients enrolled on COG Biology and Risk Stratification study AREN03B2, an intraoperative rupture rate of 9.7% was found in 1131 primary nephrectomies for unilateral WT. Risk factors for intraoperative spill were diameter (>12 cm) and laterality (right).[150]

Surgical resection or biopsy of lung nodules plays an important role in the diagnosis of metastatic WT. Current COG renal tumor studies consider circular lung nodules, regardless of size, to be metastatic disease unless proven benign by biopsy. The resection of lung metastases may also provide a therapeutic benefit. In the SIOP protocols, patients whose lung nodules are resected completely do not receive pulmonary radiation therapy (XRT). The COG AREN0533 study tested a new strategy for favorable-histology WT with lung metastases. Lung nodules were assessed after 6 weeks of chemotherapy and XRT omitted for patients with a complete response. With this approach it is appropriate not to resect all lung nodules upfront to assess chemosensitivity.

Radiation Therapy

Radiation therapy is a mainstay of WT treatment. Initially used in all patients with WT, successive studies from the NWTSG and SIOP demonstrated that only patients with stage III or IV disease require radiation therapy (Table 55-5). Among these patients radiation doses have been reduced over time, thereby decreasing the potential for late adverse effects.

The radiation guidelines for favorable-histology WT that were used in NWTS-5 are commonly applied as standard practice in North America. Patients with positive lymph nodes, positive tumor margins after surgery,

TABLE 55-5   Key Findings of National Wilms Tumor and SIOP Studies

NWTS Study	Key Findings	SIOP Study	Key Findings
NWTS-1 (1969-1973)	Group I: XRT not beneficial for patients <2 years of age treated with AMD Group II/III: VCR/AMD superior to either agent alone; anaplastic histology strongly predictive of adverse outcome	SIOP 1 (1971-1974)	Preoperative XRT reduces the number of tumor ruptures and produces more low-stage tumors
NWTS-2 (1974-1978)	Group I: reduction of chemotherapy duration from 15 to 6 months did not adversely affect RFS; XRT not needed for this group Group II: inferior outcome for those with lymph node involvement Groups II-IV: addition of DOX to VCR/AMD improved outcome	SIOP 2 (1974-1976)	9 months of VCR/AMD equivalent to 15 months Reduction of tumor ruptures in preoperative treatment group confirmed
NWTS-3 (1979-1986)	Stage I FH: RFS similar whether duration of VCR/AMD was 10 or 26 weeks Stage II FH: Addition of DOX to VCR/AMD did not improve RFS; XRT not necessary Stage III FH: • Without DOX, 20 Gy flank XRT superior to 10 Gy • Addition of DOX to 10 Gy flank XRT improved RFS • Addition of DOX to 20 Gy flank XRT did not improve RFS Stage IV FH: Addition of CYCLO did not improve RFS Stage II to IV diffuse anaplasia: Addition of CYCLO appeared to improve RFS	SIOP 5 (1977-1979) SIOP 6 (1980-1987)	Preoperative chemotherapy equivalent to XRT in preventing tumor ruptures Stage I: 17 weeks VCR/AMD equal to 38 weeks Stage IIN0: Withholding XRT triggered stopping rule because of abdominal relapses; however, DFS and OS were not affected by withholding XRT Stage IIN+/III: DOX improved DFS but not OS
NWTS-4 (1986-1994)	Stage I to IV FH: No difference in RFS when AMD was given as a single dose rather than as 5 doses; toxicity profile and cost better with single dose Stage III to IV FH: No difference in RFS when DOX given as a single dose rather than as 3 doses; toxicity profile and cost better with single dose Stage II to IV FH: No difference in RFS between 6 and 15 months of therapy Stage II to IV diffuse anaplasia: Improved RFS with addition of CYCLO confirmed	SIOP 9 (1987-1991)	4 weeks of preoperative VCR/AMD is equivalent to 8 weeks in terms of % of stage I tumors, EFS, and OS
NWTS-5 (1995-2002)	Stage I FH, age <2 years, tumor <550 gm: Without chemotherapy, 2-year RFS rate was only 86% but OS was 100% Stage I to IV FH: LOH at 1p and 16q predict decreased RFS and OS Stage I anaplasia: RFS and OS inferior to stage I FH Stage II-IV diffuse anaplasia: Best reported outcomes to date using VCR/DOX/CYCLO/ETOP	SIOP 93-01 (1993-1999)	Patients with stage I WT do just as well with 4 weeks of postoperative VCR/AMD as with 18 weeks Postchemotherapy histology predictive of relapse: complete necrosis = low risk; blastemal predominance = high risk

AMD, Dactinomycin; *CYCLO,* cyclophosphamide; *DFS,* disease-free survival; *DOX,* doxorubicin; *EFS,* event-free survival; *ETOP,* etoposide; *FH,* favorable histology; *LOH,* loss of heterozygosity; *NWTS,* National Wilms Tumor Study; *OS,* overall survival; *RFS,* relapse-free survival; *SIOP,* International Society of Paediatric Oncology; *VCR,* vincristine; *WT,* Wilms tumor; *XRT,* radiation therapy.

or tumor spillage receive 10.8 Gy to the flank. Patients with diffuse tumor spillage or peritoneal seeding receive 10.8 Gy to the whole abdomen. Sites of gross residual disease after surgery receive a boost of 10.8 Gy. Early reports from the NWTSG demonstrated that XRT delay beyond 9 days from surgery was an adverse prognostic factor.[151,152] NWTSG studies recommended that radiation commence by day 9 after surgery. However a retrospective analysis of NWTS-3 and -4 did not detect a difference in local recurrence rate between patients who received radiation within 9 days and patients whose radiation was delayed beyond day 9, although very few patients had XRT delayed much beyond day 10.[153] To allow for real time central review and risk stratification, COG renal tumor therapeutic protocols allow up to 14 days from surgery to initiation of abdominal or flank radiation.

Patients whose tumors are initially unresectable have radiation therapy delayed until after definitive surgery.

The local radiation doses that the SIOP treatment protocols use are higher than those in COG studies. Patients with stage III intermediate-risk histology receive 14.4 Gy to the abdomen or flank rather than 10.8 Gy. Patients with stage II or III high-risk histology receive 25.2 Gy.

The radiation guidelines for patients with distant metastatic disease are evolving. The most common metastatic site is the lung. In the NWTSG studies all patients with lung metastases received whole lung radiation to a dose of 12 Gy at the beginning of treatment, yielding 16-year relapse-free survival rates of 80%.[154] In SIOP studies patients whose lung nodules resolve with chemotherapy and surgery did not receive lung XRT. A number of studies using this approach have showed varied outcome.

With this approach the 4-year survival rate was 83%.[155] However the United Kingdom Wilms Tumor Study used the SIOP approach and observed a 6-year survival rate of only 65%.[156] In the SIOP 93-01 protocol, patients were treated with 6 weeks of three-drug (vincristine/dactinomycin/doxorubicin) preoperative chemotherapy. Patients in complete remission (CR) after 6 weeks of chemotherapy +/− surgical metastasectomy did not receive pulmonary radiation and continued with three-drug therapy. Patients without CR at 6 weeks received intensified chemotherapy with etoposide/carboplatin and ifosfamide/doxorubicin. If after 9 weeks of this therapy, CR was obtained, no pulmonary radiation was given. If CR was not obtained, patients received 15 Gy of lung radiation with a boost to residual disease. In the study 84% of patients were in CR after the initial 6 weeks of therapy, 17% requiring metastectomy. Only 14% of patients received radiation as front-line therapy. Patients in CR after chemotherapy only or chemotherapy and metastectomy had good overall survival rates (88% and 92%), whereas patients with residual pulmonary metastatic disease had a significantly lower overall survival rate of 48%. This disparity may relate to differences in patient populations and treatment, but it raises the question of whether more stringent selection criteria should be used for withholding lung XRT.

The COG AREN0533 Higher Risk Favorable Histology Wilms Tumor study also stratified therapy according to the lung nodule response after 6 weeks of three-drug chemotherapy. The study asked whether XRT can be omitted without compromising event-free survival for patients whose lung nodules disappear after 6 weeks of chemotherapy and whether outcomes can be improved by intensifying chemotherapy therapy for patients whose lung nodules do not resolve. Patients without pulmonary complete response received 1200 cGy (1050 cGy for ages younger than 12 months) of pulmonary XRT and an intensified chemotherapy with cyclophosphamide/etoposide added to the three-drug therapy. That study closed in 2013 after reaching accrual of 395 patients, and results have not yet been published.

Chemotherapy

In the mid-1950s Farber and colleagues pioneered the use of dactinomycin as an adjunct to surgery and radiation therapy for the treatment of WT. With the introduction of dactinomycin, unprecedented survival rates were observed, particularly in patients with metastatic disease.[157] In the early 1960s the Southwest Oncology Group found that vincristine produced regression of metastatic WT and that the response to vincristine plus XRT was similar to that reported for dactinomycin.[158] In 1969 the first National Wilms Tumor Study (NWTS-1) found the combination of vincristine and dactinomycin to be superior to either agent alone for groups II and III tumors.[159] Since then vincristine/dactinomycin has been the backbone of WT therapy worldwide, although subsets of patients with stage I disease fare well with vincristine alone or even surgery only, as discussed later. In the early 1970s the third stalwart of WT chemotherapy regimens, doxorubicin, was introduced. NWTS-2 demonstrated the

benefit of doxorubicin for patients with groups II to IV disease, and NWTS-3 showed that radiation doses can be reduced when doxorubicin is used.[160,161] NWTS-4 refined how dactinomycin and doxorubicin are given. Both agents were as effective when delivered as a single dose rather than as separate doses over 5 (dactinomycin) or 3 (doxorubicin) days.[162] Not only was this "pulse-intensive" dosing more convenient and cost-effective, but it also was associated with less hematologic toxicity.[163,164] The key findings of the NWTSG studies are summarized in Table 55-5.

By the end of NWTS-4 the survival rate for patients with favorable histology WT was approximately 90%. Given this success the priority for NWTS-5 was to identify novel prognostic markers to help stratify patients into risk-appropriate treatment groups. Pilot data from NWTS-3 and -4 showed that LOH at chromosomes 1p and 16q was associated with adverse outcome in patients with WT.[165] Following this lead NWTS-5 prospectively evaluated the prognostic significance of LOH in more than 2000 patients.[166] There was no significant association between LOH and outcome in patients with anaplastic WT, CCSK, or MRT. However LOH at 1p and 16q was associated with increased risk of relapse and death in patients with favorable-histology WT, with the greatest effect seen in tumors with LOH at both loci (Table 55-6).

A second objective of NWTS-5 was to determine whether therapy can be reduced in selected populations of patients with truly outstanding outcomes. Earlier studies suggested that young patients with small stage I tumors with favorable histology have excellent outcomes, so NWTS-5 asked if these patients could be treated with

TABLE 55-6   Effect of Loss of Heterozygosity on Patient Outcome (NWTS-5)

Stage	4-Year RFS (%)	RR	P	4-Year OS (%)	RR	P
Favorable Histology Stage I/II						
No LOH	91.2	1.0		98.4	1.0	0.02
LOH 1p only	80.4	2.19	0.02	91.2	4.03	0.6
LOH 16q only	82.5	1.91	0.01	98.1	1.40	0.01
LOH 1p and 16q	74.9	2.88	0.001	90.5	4.25	
Favorable Histology Stage III/IV						
No LOH	83.0	1.0		91.9	1.0	0.36
LOH 1p only	89.0	0.69	0.37	97.6	0.52	0.76
LOH 16q only	85.3	0.89	0.67	92.0	0.88	0.04
LOH 1p and 16q	65.9	2.41	0.01	77.5	2.66	

LOH, Loss of heterozygosity; NWTS-5, National Wilms Tumor Study 5; OS, overall survival; RR, relative risk, with group with no LOH as a baseline; RFS, relapse-free survival.

TABLE 55-7   NWTS-5: Treatment Overview

Tumor Histology and Stage	Chemotherapy Regimen	Radiation Therapy
Favorable-histology Wilms tumor		
Stage I/II	VCR/AMD × 18 weeks	None
Stage III/IV	VCR/AMD/DOX × 18 weeks	Flank/abdomen if local stage III and to metastatic sites
Focal anaplastic Wilms tumor		
Stage I	VCR/AMD × 18 weeks	None
Stage II-IV	VCR/AMD/DOX × 18 weeks	Flank/abdomen and to metastatic sites
Diffuse anaplastic Wilms tumor		
Stage I	VCR/AMD × 18 weeks	None
Stage II-IV	VCR/DOX/CYCLO/ETOP × 24 weeks	Flank/abdomen and to metastatic sites
Clear cell sarcoma of the kidney		
Stage I-IV	VCR/DOX/CYCLO/ETOP × 24 weeks	Flank/abdomen and to metastatic sites
Malignant rhabdoid tumor		
Stage I-IV	CARBO/ETOP/CYCLO × 24 weeks	Flank/abdomen and metastatic sites

AMD, Dactinomycin; *CARBO,* carboplatin; *CYCLO,* cyclophosphamide; *DOX,* doxorubicin; *ETOP,* etoposide; *LOH,* loss of heterozygosity; NWTS-5, National Wilms Tumor Study 5; *VCR,* vincristine.

surgery alone, without adjuvant chemotherapy and radiation therapy.[167] Among 75 patients treated with surgery only, eight patients relapsed and three patients developed metachronous tumors in the contralateral kidney.[168] The 2-year disease-free survival rate was only 86%, which triggered a stopping rule, and the study was discontinued. However 74 of the 75 patients survived, suggesting that the nephrectomy-only approach should be revisited. Although the standard treatment for stage I favorable-histology WT in North America is 18 weeks of vincristine and dactinomycin, the United Kingdom WT group treated with 10 weeks of vincristine only and the SIOP 93-01 study demonstrated that 4 weeks of postoperative treatment is equivalent to 18 weeks.[169,170] The treatment regimens from NWTS-5 are summarized in Table 55-7, and the corresponding outcomes are summarized in Table 55-8.

With the foundation of the findings from the NWTS studies, the first COG renal tumor studies (opened 2006) aimed to further refine the treatment of favorable-histology WT. For entry into any COG Renal Tumor Therapeutic study, patients first had to enroll in the COG Renal Tumor Biology and Risk Stratification study AREN03B2, which continued the NWTSG tradition of central pathology and surgery review and tumor banking. More than 4000 patients enrolled in the first 6 years of the study, with a steady accrual of 600 patients annually. Submission of pathology slides, radiology images, operative reports, and tumor and blood samples for analysis was required within 7 days of surgery to meet enrollment deadlines stipulated by the therapeutic studies. Central pathology review for histology and stage, radiology review for presence of bilateral lesions and pulmonary metastases, and surgical review for operative stage were completed electronically by a panel of expert reviewers. An Initial Risk Assignment was made by the study chairs on the basis of the multidisciplinary central reviews. Final Risk Assignments included LOH status of 1p and 16q for patients with favorable-histology WT, and response of pulmonary metastases for patients with stage IV favorable-histology WT. Real-time central review was shown to be

feasible, with a median time to Initial Risk Assignment of 8 days from initial surgical procedure.

The AREN0532 study for the treatment of Very Low and Standard Risk Favorable-Histology WT reassessed the feasibility of surgery without adjuvant therapy for patients younger than 2 years old with stage I favorable-histology WTs less than 550 grams. Participation in this study arm required a real-time central review with verification of lymph node sampling confirmed negative for tumor, and the patient could not have an underlying predisposition syndrome, contralateral rests, or multifocal tumors. The study completed accrual of 116 patients with very low-risk disease in August 2013, and outcome data are pending. AREN0532 also assessed the benefit of therapy augmentation for patients with stage I and II favorable-histology WT with LOH at 1p and 16q. Instead of receiving the standard therapy with vincristine and dactinomycin, patients with LOH receive vincristine, dactinomycin, and doxorubicin. Likewise, the AREN0533 study (higher-risk favorable-histology WT) augmented therapy for patients with stage III and IV favorable-histology WT with LOH at 1p and 16q. Instead of receiving vincristine, dactinomycin, and doxorubicin, these patients received a new regimen that added four cycles of cyclophosphamide and etoposide to the standard treatment. AREN0533 also introduced a new approach to patients with lung metastases. Patients whose lung nodules responded completely after 6 weeks of vincristine, dactinomycin, and doxorubicin chemotherapy did not receive lung radiation therapy (see previous section on radiation therapy). By contrast, patients whose lung nodules did respond completely received radiation therapy and augmented chemotherapy with vincristine, dactinomycin, doxorubicin, cyclophosphamide, and etoposide.

The SIOP 2001 study aimed to evaluate whether doxorubicin is necessary for patients with stage II and III intermediate-risk tumors; patients were randomized to receive vincristine and dactinomycin with or without doxorubicin. Preliminary analysis showed equivalent 5-year overall survival of 96% in both treatment groups.[171] The study also adjusted chemotherapy according to

TABLE 55-8   NWTS-5: Treatment Results

Stage	4-Year Relapse-Free Survival Rate (%)	4-Year Overall Survival Rate (%)
Favorable Histology without LOH 1p		
I (<24 months/tumor weight <550 g)	95.6	100
I (≥24 months/tumor weight ≥550 g)	94.2	98.4
II	86.2	97.7
III	86.5	94.4
IV	76.4	86.1
V	64.8	87.1
Focal Anaplastic Histology		
I	67.5	88.9
II	80.0	80.0
III	87.5	100
IV*	61.4	71.6
V	76.2	87.5
Diffuse Anaplastic Histology		
I	68.4	78.9
II	82.6	81.5
III	64.7	66.7
IV	33.3	33.3
V	25.1	41.6
Clear Cell Sarcoma[†]		
I	100	100
II	86.8	97.3
III	73.8	86.9
IV	35.6	45.0
Malignant Rhabdoid Tumor[‡]		
I	—	33.3
II	—	46.9
III	—	21.8
IV	—	8.4

LOH, Loss of heterozygosity; NWTS-5, National Wilms Study 5.
*Results are for patients who received preoperative chemotherapy because very few patients in this group had upfront nephrectomy.
[†]Results are reported as 5-year relapse-free and overall survival.
[‡]Results are combined results for NWTS 1-5.

histologic response to preoperative treatment. Patients with stage I blastemal predominance after 4 weeks of preoperative chemotherapy received a regimen containing doxorubicin instead of just vincristine and dactinomycin. Patients with stage II and III blastemal predominance received a regimen of alternating cyclophosphamide and doxorubicin with carboplatin and etoposide.

Anaplastic Wilms Tumor

In 1978 Beckwith and Palmer published a detailed histopathologic review of the patients entered in the first NWTSG.[172] Approximately 6% of the WT specimens contained anaplasia, as defined in the pathology section

of this chapter. The presence of anaplasia was prognostically significant; 11 of 25 (44%) patients with anaplasia died as a result of tumor, whereas only 26 of 364 (7.1%) patients without anaplasia died as a result of tumor. Subsequent National Wilms Tumor Studies, as well as SIOP and the United Kingdom Wilms Tumor Study, confirmed the adverse prognostic significance of anaplastic histology.[156,173,174]

The first NWTSG trial to stratify patients with anaplastic WT into a distinct treatment group was NWTS-3. In this study and in NWTS-4, patients received 15 months of vincristine, dactinomycin, and doxorubicin and were randomized to receive or not receive cyclophosphamide. Patients with stages II through IV diffuse anaplastic WT had a 4-year relapse-free survival rate estimate of 27.2% when treated without cyclophosphamide, compared with 54.8% when treated with cyclophosphamide ($P = .02$).[175] Patients with all stages of focal anaplastic histology and stage I diffuse anaplastic histology had excellent outcomes regardless of treatment regimen.[161,162]

On the basis of these results, cyclophosphamide was incorporated into the treatment plan of NWTS-5 for patients with stages II and IV diffuse anaplastic WT. Patients received a regimen consisting of vincristine, doxorubicin, and cyclophosphamide alternating with cyclophosphamide and etoposide for 24 weeks of treatment and flank radiation therapy to a dose of 10.8 Gy.[15] With this regimen the 4-year relapse-free survival rate and overall survival rate compared favorably with historic data from NWTS-3 and -4 (see Table 55-8). Patients with stage I diffuse anaplastic histology were treated with vincristine and dactinomycin according to the regimen used for favorable-histology WT. With this approach the 4-year event-free survival was only 68.4%, significantly worse than that seen for stage I favorable-histology tumors.[15] Patients with stage II through IV focal anaplastic WT were treated with vincristine, doxorubicin, dactinomycin, and radiation therapy and had outcomes intermediate between favorable histology and diffuse anaplasia (see Table 55-8).

AREN0321, the COG study for high-risk renal tumors, sought to build on the NWTS-5 experience by adding carboplatin to the treatment regimen for diffuse anaplastic WT. Patients were scheduled to receive 31 weeks of alternating vincristine, doxorubicin, and cyclophosphamide, and cyclophosphamide, carboplatin, and etoposide with flank radiation therapy. Because of the poorer-than-expected outcomes for stage I anaplastic WT, the AREN0321 study treated such patients with vincristine, dactinomycin, doxorubicin, and radiation therapy instead of just vincristine and dactinomycin. Patients with stage IV diffuse anaplastic WT had a 4-year relapse-free survival rate estimate of only 33% in NWTS-5. For this group the priority was to identify new chemotherapy combinations. The AREN0321 study included a phase 2 "window" study to evaluate the antitumor activity of vincristine and irinotecan. This combination was selected on the basis of preclinical and clinical data showing activity of the camptothecins (topotecan and irinotecan) against WT.[176] The study was opened in 2006 and permanently closed to accrual in 2013. Outcome results are pending.

Bilateral Wilms Tumor

Between 4% and 6% of patients with WT have tumor involvement of both kidneys at initial presentation (synchronous bilateral WT).[69] These patients pose a dual challenge, with the need to eradicate the tumor cells while preserving renal function. Although renal failure occurs in fewer than 1% of patients with unilateral WT, the long-term incidence of renal failure in patients with bilateral WT has been reported to range from 11% to 20%.[177] Historically synchronous bilateral WT was managed with surgical resection followed by chemotherapy. Typically a unilateral nephrectomy of the more involved kidney was performed with biopsy or partial nephrectomy of the contralateral kidney, followed by adjuvant therapy. With the recognition that chemotherapy could decrease tumor volume and facilitate partial nephrectomy, preoperative chemotherapy has become the standard approach to treatment. Data from the NWTSG showed no difference in outcome whether the tumor was resected at the time of diagnosis or after preoperative chemotherapy.[178-180] Despite the effectiveness of preoperative chemotherapy, approximately 60% of patients continue to undergo nephrectomy of at least one kidney. In NWTS-4 only 19% of patients underwent bilateral nephron-sparing procedures, but more recent data from single-institution series suggest that more patients are candidates for bilateral partial nephrectomies.[181-183] NWTS data also showed that children with bilateral WT or WT and contralateral NRs who had complete radiologic resolution lesions in a kidney after initial treatment did well without surgical intervention to that kidney.[184] An aim of the current COG AREN0534 study for bilateral WT is to decrease the percentage of patients who require nephrectomy.

Chemotherapy regimens for bilateral WT use the same agents as for unilateral WT. In the NWTSG and SIOP studies, patients started treatment with vincristine and dactinomycin therapy and doxorubicin was reserved for patients known to have distant metastatic disease, locally advanced disease, or poor response to therapy. With this treatment approach long-term survival rates for patients with synchronous bilateral WTs were approximately 70% to 80%.[178-180] The COG AREN0534 study for bilateral WT treats all patients with vincristine, dactinomycin, and doxorubicin before surgery to promote improved local control. Given the high likelihood of bilateral renal lesions representing WT and the known limitations of biopsy, upfront biopsy or resection is discouraged in this study. However open biopsy or definitive surgical resection is mandated by week 12 for all patients in the study. Review of the NWTS-4 cohort of patients with synchronous bilateral WT identified 38 patients with progressive or nonresponsive disease, who had a median of 7 months of therapy before surgery. Pathology at eventual surgery revealed histologic subtypes (anaplasia or rhabdomyomatous or differentiated stromal tumors) that could have benefited from earlier surgery.[185] In the patients with bilateral WT with anaplasia from the NWTS-4, core needle biopsy did not identify anaplasia in seven of seven children, whereas open biopsy or complete nephrectomy identified anaplasia in 10 of 18 at initial diagnosis. In 20 of 24 there was discordance in histology between kidneys.[186] In the AREN0534 study chemotherapy after surgery is tailored according to histologic response, on the basis of the postchemotherapy risk classification schema developed by the SIOP group.

Recurrent Wilms Tumor

Approximately 10% of patients with favorable-histology WT and 50% of patients with anaplastic WT develop recurrent disease. The survival rate after recurrence depends on several factors, including histology, time from diagnosis to recurrence, initial stage and treatment regimen, and site of recurrence.[187,188] The NWTS-5 study included treatment of recurrent WT. Patients with favorable-histology WT whose initial treatment consisted of vincristine and dactinomycin received vincristine, doxorubicin, cyclophosphamide, etoposide, and radiation therapy as salvage therapy, resulting in 4-year event-free and overall survival estimates of 71.1% and 81.8%, respectively.[189] Patients whose initial treatment was vincristine, dactinomycin, doxorubicin, and radiation therapy received a salvage regimen of alternating cyclophosphamide and etoposide, and carboplatin and etoposide, resulting in 4-year event-free survival rates and overall survival rates of 42.3% and 48.0%, respectively.[190] Interestingly female patients had better event-free survival rates and overall survival rates (54.7 and 58.7%) than male patients (28.6% and 38.0%). Other studies have demonstrated the efficacy of ifosfamide, carboplatin, and etoposide chemotherapy in the treatment of recurrent WT.[191,192] A phase II trial of topotecan demonstrated a response rate of 48% in patients with multiply recurrent favorable-histology WT.[176] The outcomes of patients with recurrent anaplastic WT are poor, with salvage rates on the order of 10%. Because upfront therapy for anaplastic WT involves the known active agents, patients with recurrent disease are candidates for phase 1 and 2 studies.

An unresolved question is whether high-dose chemotherapy with autologous stem cell rescue provides a benefit for patients with recurrent WT. Several series have reported survival rates of approximately 60% in patients with recurrent WT using single or tandem transplants.[193-195] However similar results have been attained without high-dose therapy, so the benefit of high-dose therapy remains undefined.[196] Efforts toward a randomized clinical trial to answer this question have been hampered by patient numbers. A meta-analysis of 100 patients from six studies attempted to determine characteristics of patients that predict survival with high-dose therapy and autologous stem cell rescue, comparing these patients to the published outcomes of the patients in the NWTS-5 relapse study who were treated for relapse without autologous stem cell transplant. The 4-year survival rate in the group of patients who underwent transplant was 54%. Patients who relapsed in the lung only who underwent transplant had a significantly higher 4-year survival rate (77.7%) than those with relapse in other locations or multiple relapses (4-year survival rate: 41.6%) who were treated with high-dose therapy and stem cell transplant. In comparison with the NWTS-5 cohort, 4-year survival rates were higher for stages I and II patients treated with salvage chemotherapy rather than with transplant, but the outcomes for patients with stages III through IV disease were comparable with both treatment approaches.[197] A second meta-analysis divided patients with relapse WT into three risk groups. Only patients who received four or more drugs for initial therapy or for previous relapse seemed to benefit from high-dose therapy and stem cell rescue.[198]

Most WT relapses occur within 2 years from diagnosis, but a small number of patients experience late relapse.

A review of children registered in 10 national or international cooperative clinical trials identified 70 of 13,330 with relapse more than 5 years after initial diagnosis. The median time to diagnosis of this group was 13.2 years. Outcome after late relapse was most influenced by site of relapse, with an 87% survival rate in the 15 patients with relapse in the contralateral kidney and 47% for all other patients.[199]

Late Effects of Wilms Tumor Treatment

The excellent relapse-free survival rate for favorable-histology WT heightens the importance of minimizing long-term effects of treatment. Follow-up of the NWTSG cohort has identified several treatment-related effects that current studies are aiming to minimize.

One of the most feared complications of WT therapy is cardiotoxicity. The cumulative frequency of congestive heart failure in patients treated in NWTS-1 through -4 was 4.4% at 20 years for patients treated initially with doxorubicin and 17.4% for patients treated with doxorubicin for recurrent disease.[200] The risk for congestive heart failure was strongly associated with female sex (relative risk 4.5 compared with male subjects), cumulative doxorubicin dose (relative risk 3.3 for each 100 mg/m^2); lung radiation (relative risk 1.6), and left abdominal radiation (relative risk 1.8).[201]

A second major complication of WT therapy is second malignant neoplasms (SMNs). The 15-year cumulative incidence of SMN in WT survivors treated in NWTSG studies between 1969 and 1991 was 1.6% and increasing steadily.[202] The SMNs observed in this series were sarcomas, carcinomas, leukemias, lymphomas, and brain tumors. Although no cases of leukemia or lymphoma were seen after 8 years, the risk of developing a solid tumor continued to increase with time. Abdominal radiation increased the risk of SMNs, with doxorubicin potentiating the effect. Each 10 Gy of abdominal radiation therapy was estimated to increase the SMN incidence by 22% without doxorubicin and by 66% with doxorubicin. An international cohort of North American, British, and Nordic subjects between 1960 and 2004 found similar results, with a standardized incidence ration of 5.1 and 5 for solid tumors and leukemias, respectively. The leukemia risk was highest in the first 5 years after treatment, but the solid tumor risk increased with age after diagnosis. Leukemia rates were highest for those diagnosed after 1990, and rates of solid tumors were lower for those diagnosed after 1980. This may reflect the increase in intensity of chemotherapy regimens and decreased use of radiation therapy.[203]

Renal failure is a concern for WT survivors because patients undergo nephrectomy or partial nephrectomy as part of their treatment. However the cumulative incidence of end-stage renal disease (ESRD) at 20 years after WT diagnosis is only 0.6% among patients with nonsyndromic unilateral WT.[177] A small cohort of patients followed up to 5 decades after nephrectomy for childhood unilateral renal tumor demonstrated mild to moderate renal function loss, increasing from the third to fifth decade.[204] The cumulative incidence of ESRD is much higher for patients with unilateral WT and WAGR syndrome (36%), Denys-Drash syndrome (74%, but this is probably an underestimate due to inaccurate classification of the syndrome), and isolated genitourinary anomalies (7%).[177] The cumulative incidence of ESRD is also high among patients with non-syndromic bilateral WT (12%). The high rate of renal failure among patients with bilateral WT is related mainly to bilateral nephrectomies performed for tumor control.[205] However the renal failure seen with WAGR and Denys-Drash syndromes is caused by underlying renal pathology.[206,207] In the follow-up of 173 children enrolled in NWTS who developed ESRD, treatment and outcomes were very different in the 55 patients who developed ESRD from progressive bilateral WT than in the 118 who had ESRD from other causes (grouped as chronic kidney disease).[208] Of the 55 subjects with PBWT, 25 died while on initial ESRD treatment with dialysis, all but four of these as a result of WT. Only 47% of these patients had a renal transplant at 5 years. In the 118 patients with ESRD from chronic kidney disease, 77% had received a transplant at 5 years, and the survival at 10 years was 73%. Once renal transplant had been performed, the differences in outcome between the patients with progressive bilateral WT and those with chronic kidney disease were markedly reduced, suggesting that renal transplant should be considered earlier for some patients rather than waiting the 1- to 2-year tumor-free interval, as is commonly recommended.

A review of pregnancy outcomes in patients treated in NWTS-1 through -4 revealed that fetal malposition and early or threatened labor were more frequent among women who received abdominal irradiation compared with unirradiated women.[207] There were an excessive number of infants born before 36 weeks of gestation to women who received flank radiation and an excessive number of infants with birth weight below 2500 g. Most of the birth weights were appropriate for gestational age. Congenital malformations were more frequent among the offspring of women who received flank radiation compared with those of unirradiated women. Fertility was related to the dose and field of radiation therapy.[209] In general fertility is preserved in WT survivors after upper abdominal radiation that does not include the pelvis and flank, rather than whole-abdominal radiation.

Dental abnormalities (e.g., root stunting, enamel hypoplasia, microdontia) in excess of the expected incidence in control patients were observed in WT survivors.[210] A small study of 49 WT survivors revealed osteopenia in 27%.[211] Stature loss has been observed in WT survivors, with a predicted height deficit at age 18 years of 1.8 cm for children treated with 10 Gy to the flank at age 4 years.[212] Height deficits were negatively correlated with age (greater deficit with younger age of irradiation) and positively correlated with radiation dosage. Unlike cardiac effects or second malignancies, doxorubicin did not exacerbate reduction in stature.

Additional late effects were assessed in the Childhood Cancer Survivor Study, through the 25-year follow up of childhood WT.[213] This study assessed chronic health conditions, health status, health care utilization, socio-economic status, SMNs, and mortality of WT survivors diagnosed from 1970 to 1986. In this cohort there was a cumulative incidence of all and severe chronic health conditions of 65.4% and 24.2% at 25 years. WT survivors reported more adverse general health status than the sibling group, but mental health status, socioeconomic outcome, and health care utilization were similar. There was a 3% cumulative incidence of SMN and 6.1% incidence of mortality. Radiation exposure increased the likelihood of congestive heart failure (with and without doxorubicin), as well as occurrence of SMN and death.

CLEAR CELL SARCOMA OF THE KIDNEY

Epidemiology

The average age of onset of CCSK in the NWTSG experience was 36 months, with a range of 2 months to 14 years. In contrast to WT, a male predominance was noted, with a male-to-female ratio of 2 to 1. In a review of published series and cases reports of CCSK, no familial cases were described, and only three cases were bilateral. Because these were all in patients with widely disseminated disease, they may have represented metastatic disease rather than second primary tumors.[28,214]

Molecular Biology and Genetics

The genetic etiology of CCSK is poorly understood. Most cases of CCSK have normal karyotypes, although a recurrent t(10;17) translocation has been identified in 10% to 15% of CCSK, resulting in a fusion transcript of the YWHAE and FAM22 genes.[33] Although the TP53 gene is located at the 17p13 breakpoint of these translocations, p53 is not thought to play a prominent role in the pathogenesis of CCSK because most CCSK tumors lack detectable p53 protein by immunostaining,[28,215,216] TP53 mutations are infrequently detected by sequencing analysis,[216] and CCSK primary cell cultures have a functional p53 pathway in response to DNA damage.[217] Other recurrent abnormalities detected by either conventional karyotyping or comparative genomic hybridization include chromosome 14q deletion (two cases) and 1q gain (three cases).[217-219]

Gene expression analysis of CCSK tumors has revealed frequent upregulation of neural markers with activation of the sonic hedgehog and phosphoinositide-3-kinase/Akt pathways.[220] Among the upregulated members of the Akt signaling pathway was the epidermal growth factor receptor (EGFR) gene. A subsequent study found EGFR protein immunoreactivity in 12 of 12 CCSK samples, EGFR gene amplification in 1 of 12 samples, and a somatic EGFR mutation in one sample.[221] Two samples had mutations of PTEN, a negative regulator of the Akt pathway.[221] These results provide a rationale for evaluating EGFR inhibitors in patients with CCSK that is refractory to current treatment modalities.

Clinical Presentation and Diagnostic Evaluation

Although CCSK has been termed the "bone-metastasizing renal tumor of childhood," metastatic disease at the time of initial presentation is distinctly uncommon. Only 4% of patients have distant metastatic disease at diagnosis, with bone, lung, and liver as the most common sites.[28] However approximately 30% of patients who undergo local lymph node sampling are found to have tumor involvement in the renal hilar and periaortic lymph nodes.[28] The value of bone scan versus skeletal survey to detect bone metastases has been addressed. Most lesions are detectable by both modalities, but some lesions are seen by only one of the two modalities.[222] Despite the predilection of this tumor to bone, bone marrow involvement is uncommon and bone marrow aspiration is no longer recommended as part of the staging workup.

Treatment

Although considered one of the unfavorable-histology renal tumors, significant progress has been made in the treatment of CCSK. Data from NWTS-1, -2, and -3 suggested that the addition of doxorubicin to the combination of vincristine and dactinomycin improved the 6-year relapse-free survival rate percentage.[223] The beneficial effect of doxorubicin was confirmed in a retrospective review of 351 cases, including 182 cases from NWTS-1 through -4.[28] NWTS-3 demonstrated no improvement in outcomes of patients with CCSK when cyclophosphamide was added to the combination of vincristine, dactinomycin, and doxorubicin.[223] However, the cyclophosphamide was delivered at a relatively low dosage and intensity. NWTS-4 asked whether the duration of therapy affects outcome for patients with CCSK. Compared with 6 months of vincristine, dactinomycin, and doxorubicin therapy, 15 months of therapy was associated with a trend toward improved 8-year relapse-free survival rate (87.8% versus 60.6%, $P = .08$), although there was no difference in 8-year overall survival rate (87.5% vs. 85.9%).[224] NWTS-5 treated patients with 6 months of a combination of vincristine, doxorubicin, and cyclophosphamide alternating with a combination of cyclophosphamide and etoposide. Preliminary analysis showed 5-year event-free and overall survival estimates of 79% and 89%, respectively.[225] Interestingly 14 patients had stage I disease, and none of these patients relapsed. An aim of the COG AREN0321 study was to assess whether the outstanding outcomes for stage I patients can be maintained without flank radiation therapy. This study closed to accrual in 2013, and outcome data are pending.

The treatment and outcomes of 191 patients with CCSK were reported from the SIOP 93-01 and SIOP 2001 protocols.[226] Significant discordance in initial pathology diagnosis and SIOP panel pathology diagnosis was noted. Of the CCSK patients 27% were initially diagnosed as a different renal tumor type, and seven cases of CCSK were changed to another tumor type by panel pathologists. Of 191 subjects, 169 received SIOP preoperative chemotherapy (recommended therapy vincristine and dactinomycin for 4 weeks for localized disease and vincristine, dactinomycin, and doxorubicin for 6 weeks for metastatic disease). Through evaluation with Response Evaluation Criteria In Solid Tumors (RECIST) criteria, 21% had a partial response after preoperative chemotherapy, 15% had minor response,

31% had stable disease, and 33% had progressive disease. All patients underwent total nephrectomy, and 189 of 191 received postoperative chemotherapy. Recommended postoperative chemotherapy was a three- or four-drug therapy regimen. Abdominal radiation therapy (mean dose of 25.2 Gy) was given to 85 patients, 2 of 71 stage 1 patients, 33 of 43 stage II patients, 44 of 50 stage III patients, and 4 of 13 stage IV patients. Five-year event-free survival and overall survival rates were 78% and 86%, respectively. The brain and lung were the most common sites of relapse, followed by bone and primary site. Five-year event-free survival and overall survival rates varied by stage as follows: stage I 79% and 87%, stage II 92% and 91%, stage III 69% and 82%, stage IV 58% and 73%. The timing of full staging in patients varied, insofar as almost all received preoperative chemotherapy for a presumed diagnosis of WT, and bone scans and brain imaging were not done routinely before starting therapy. Patients younger than 12 months were noted to have worse outcomes, with five-year event-free survival and overall survival rates of 49% and 61%.

An interesting observation on recent CCSK trials has been a shift in the site of recurrent disease. Although CCSK is associated with bone metastases, the brain has now surpassed bone as the most common site of recurrence in North American and European studies.[225,227,228] The reason for this shift is unclear, but it is possible that improved disease control outside the central nervous system has uncovered the brain as a sanctuary site for tumor cells.

MALIGNANT RHABDOID TUMOR

Epidemiology

MRT occurs primarily in infants, with a mean age of diagnosis of 15 months.[229] However, older children and rare adults with MRT have been reported. MRT is associated with mutations of the *SNF5* gene at chromosome 22q11.1, and familial MRT has been described.[230] A recent report of three individuals with MRT whose parents shared a common site of employment raises the possibility of an environmental etiology.[231]

Molecular Biology and Genetics

MRTs most frequently occur in the kidney, where they are referred to as *rhabdoid tumor of the kidney*, and the central nervous system, where they are referred to as *atypical teratoid/rhabdoid tumors*, but they can also occur in soft tissues throughout the body, where they are generally referred to as *extrarenal rhabdoid tumors*. It had long been debated whether renal, central nervous system, and extrarenal rhabdoid tumors are distinct cancers that possess similar histologic appearances or whether they are the same cancer in different anatomic locations. This issue was largely resolved when the majority of rhabdoid tumors from all anatomic sites were found to have specific biallelic inactivating mutations in *SMARCB1* (also known as *INI1*, *BAF47* and *HSNF5*).[232,233] Inactivating mutations in both copies of *SMARCB1* occur in 70% of MRT and an additional 20% to 25% of the tumors do not express SMARCB1 protein even though a specific mutation cannot be identified.[234] Whereas loss of SMARCB1 occurs in the majority of MRTs, mutation of other genes such as SMARCA4(BRG1) account for a minority of cases.[235,236]

Constitutional mutation in one allele of SMARCB1 is the basis of familial MRT, a condition termed *rhabdoid predisposition syndrome*.[237,238] Carriers have a markedly increased risk for MRT in all sites and can present with more than one primary tumor. Invariably, the second SMARCB1 allele has been inactivated in these cancers. Constitutional mutation also accounts for the approximately 15% of patients who, after treatment for MRT, develop a second primary MRT. The frequency of germline mutations in patients presenting with new onset rhabdoid tumor is somewhat unclear. It has been reported to be present in as many as 33% (16 of 49) of cases, although this number is likely inflated by selection bias.[234] Patients who carry a germline SMARCB1 mutation typically present with early onset rhabdoid tumor. Most, but not all, of these individuals are diagnosed before 1 year of age. Given the relatively high frequency of germline SMARCB1 mutations, patients with new-onset MRT should have their brain and kidneys imaged to rule out additional tumors. Sequencing the *Smarc* gene from the peripheral blood of newly diagnosed patients should also be considered to rule out a constitutional mutation. If a constitutional mutation is identified, other family members should be screened for this mutation. Notably although familial studies have identified cancer-free carriers, three families with multiple siblings affected by SMARCB1 mutant MRT have been identified in which neither of the parents carried a SMARCB1 mutation. This suggests that gonadal mosaicism in a parent can be the basis of familial cases. Consequently the absence of a constitutional mutation in the parents of a patient with a germline SMARCB1 mutation does not fully exclude the possibility that siblings may be affected.

SMARCB1 encodes a core member of the SWI/SNF chromatin remodeling complex. Tightly compacted chromatin provides an organizational structure for DNA but constitutes a significant barrier to gene expression. Nucleosomes, consisting of 147 base pairs of DNA wrapped around an octamer of histones, are a fundamental unit of chromatin. The SWI/SNF complex regulates transcription of specific targets by using the energy of adenosine triphosphate hydrolysis to mobilize nucleosomes and thereby control access of the transcriptional machinery to promoters. Mice heterozygous for *Snf5* are predisposed to the formation of rhabdoid tumors that display a histologic appearance essentially indistinguishable from human MRT.[239-241] Further, conditional inactivation of both Snf5 alleles leads to the extremely rapid formation of cancer, with 100% of mice developing either lymphoma or MRT at a median onset of only 11 weeks. Because the SWI/SNF complex regulates expression of many genes, the precise genes involved in the development of MRT remain to be elucidated. Evidence suggests that the cyclinD1/p16INK4a, aurora kinase A, interferon, and sonic hedgehog pathways are downstream of SMARCB1 and are dysregulated in MRT.[242-248]

Clinical Presentation and Diagnostic Evaluation

Children with MRT of the kidney present with signs and symptoms related to an intrarenal mass. Because of the young age at presentation, it is difficult to assess pain, yet most parents report fussiness. About 60% of patients have gross hematuria, which contrasts with WT in which only 20% have hematuria.[249] Fever is a presenting feature in 50% of patients, and hypertension is seen in up to 70%. Because MRT of the kidney can be associated with involvement of the central nervous system, patients may present with focal neurologic signs or signs of increased intracranial pressure.

The diagnosis of MRT must be made by histologic confirmation, although several laboratory features are suggestive of MRT. Approximately 25% of patients have hypercalcemia and 55% have hemoglobin levels less than 9g/dL. Gross or microscopic hematuria is evident in 75% of patients. The most common sites of MRT metastasis are the lung, bone, and brain. Many of the central nervous system lesions likely represent second primary tumors rather than metastatic disease. The staging evaluation for MRT therefore includes a CT scan of the chest, abdomen, and pelvis; ultrasound of the abdomen to evaluate for tumor thrombus; bone scan; and magnetic resonance imaging of the brain. Bone marrow aspirates and biopsies are not routinely required.

Treatment

MRT is one of the most lethal and aggressive pediatric cancers. Patients with rhabdoid tumor of the kidney historically were treated in NWTSG trials with vincristine, dactinomycin, and doxorubicin, with or without cyclophosphamide. The outcomes attained with these agents were poor (see Table 54-8).[229,250] In an attempt to improve on these results, NWTS-5 tested a treatment regimen consisting of carboplatin and etoposide, alternating with cyclophosphamide, but this regimen did not yield improved survival rates compared with previous regimens.[229] Case reports have highlighted patients with metastatic rhabdoid tumor who had durable survival after treatment with various combinations of ifosfamide, etoposide, carboplatin, vincristine, doxorubicin, and cyclophosphamide.[251-254] Survivors treated with high-dose therapy and autologous stem cell rescue have also been reported,[254] but it is unclear whether this provides a benefit compared with intensive regimens of standard-dose chemotherapy. On the basis of this limited experience, the COG AREN0321 study aimed to test the efficacy of the combination of cyclophosphamide, carboplatin, and etoposide alternating with vincristine, doxorubicin, and cyclophosphamide. The protocol opened in 2006 and accrued 39 patients with MRT of the kidney before permanent closure in 2013. Outcome data are still pending. A window phase of treatment with vincristine and irinotecan was trialed on this protocol for stage IV MRT, but it did not demonstrate activity in these patients. SIOP reported survival data on 107 patients with MRT treated on the SIOP 93-01 and 2001 (1993-2005).[255] Of these patients 22% had surgery performed at time of diagnosis, 62% received vincristine/dactinomycin (VA) therapy for 4 weeks prior to surgery, and 38% received vincristine/dactinomycin/doxorubicin (VAD) for 6 weeks before surgery. Postoperative treatment recommendations included four-drug therapy with etoposide, carboplatin, cyclophosphamide or ifosfamide, and doxorubicin or epirubicin. Five-year event-free survival and overall survival rates were 22% and 26%. Most patients demonstrated evidence of chemosensitivity with marked tumor reduction with initial chemotherapy, but this did not correlate with increased survival. The median time from diagnosis to relapse was 8 months, and survival after relapse was markedly poor (4 of 60, 1 to 5 years from relapse). Advanced tumor stage and young patient age were significant poor prognostic factors.

The lack of treatment uniformity among reported patients makes it difficult to determine if radiotherapy is effective for MRT. In NWTS-1 through -5, radiation therapy was given to the flank or abdomen at total doses of 1080 to 3500 cGy, yet no relationship was observed between dose and outcome.[229] Radiation therapy is a cornerstone of treatment for central nervous system rhabdoid tumors, and some suggest that the high doses delivered to the posterior fossa improve patients' outcomes.

RENAL CELL CARCINOMA

Epidemiology

Two European registries of childhood RCC revealed that the median age of diagnosis in children and adolescents was 10 to 11 years, with a male-to-female ratio of 1 to 1.1.[256,257] Among the first 3250 patients enrolled in the COG Renal Tumor Biology Study AREN03B2, 3.8% had RCC. In adults clear cell RCC, associated with mutations of the von Hippel Lindau gene, is the predominant type of RCC. In children the clear cell subtype is uncommon.[258,259] An association between oncocytoid RCC and a previous history of neuroblastoma has been described.[62,260] Translocation RCC, associated with translocations involving the *TFE3* (chromosome Xp11.1) or *TFEB* (chromosome) genes, has been associated with previous exposure to chemotherapy.[261] The evolving characterization of translocation RCC revealed that a large percentage (up to two thirds) of pediatric RCC falls within this subtype.[258,259]

Molecular Biology and Genetics

The molecular pathogenesis of the Xp11.2 and t(6:11) translocation carcinomas is an area of active study.

Xp11.2 and t(6:11) (p21:q12) Translocation Carcinomas

The fusion partners of *TFE3* have variable functions. *PSF* and *NonO* are splicing factor genes.[262] *PRCC* and *ASPL* are novel genes of unknown function, but the former may also be involved in splicing.[263-266] The clathrin heavy chain gene (*CLTC*) trimerizes with a single light chain to form clathrin, the major protein constituent of the coat that surrounds organelles (cytoplasmic vesicles) to mediate selective protein transport.[267] All TFE3 fusion proteins retain the C terminal portion of TFE3, including its leucine-zipper dimerization domain, nuclear localization signal, and DNA binding domain. It is likely that the genes fused 5' to *TFE3* contribute strong promoters that cause overexpression of the chimeric protein, as suggested by results with TFE3 immunohistochemistry. Both PRCC-TFE3[268] and ASPL-TFE3 fusion proteins[269] localize to the nucleus and can act as aberrant transcription factors. PRCC-TFE3 may also interfere with splicing and mitotic checkpoint control through protein-protein interactions.[270]

Both ASPS and the t(X;17) renal carcinomas feature one of two types of *ASPL-TFE3* fusion transcript, in which the *ASPL* gene is fused to *TFE3* exon 4 (type 1 fusion) or *TFE3* exon 3 (type 2 fusion). Four types of *PRCC-TFE3* fusion transcripts have been described. Significant differences in clinicopathologic features between cases with different fusion types have yet to be established. Both *ASPL-TFE3* and *PRCC-TFE3* fusion transcripts are readily detected by conventional RT-PCR using appropriate primers, as described in detail elsewhere.[49,50]

A recent gene expression study has identified several novel genes that are differentially expressed between the Xp11 translocation carcinomas and conventional renal carcinomas and has shown that Xp11 translocation carcinomas may be more similar to ASPS than to conventional renal carcinomas.[271] Additionally gene expression profiling has identified potential therapeutic targets in the Xp11 translocation RCC. For example the ASPL-TFE3 fusion protein transactivates the promoter of the MET receptor tyrosine kinase, leading to MET protein overexpression. Inhibition of the MET receptor tyrosine kinase may therefore be a potential avenue of targeted therapy for these RCCs.[272]

The characteristic t(6;11)(p21;q12) translocation fuses the *Alpha* gene, an intronless gene of unknown function at 11q12, with the first intron of the *TFEB* transcription factor gene at 6p21. The breakpoint on *TFEB* is just upstream of the *TFEB* initiation ATG codon, which results in retention of the entire *TFEB* coding region in the fusion. Although the *Alpha* promoter drives expression of the fusion gene, the *Alpha* gene does not contribute to the open reading frame. Therefore the consequence of the *Alpha-TFEB* fusion is dysregulated expression of the normal full-length TFEB protein. These findings explain why the t(6;11) renal carcinomas demonstrate specific nuclear labeling for TFEB protein by IHC whereas other neoplasms and normal tissues do not. The association of both the Xp11.2 and the t(6;11) renal translocation carcinomas with exposure of the child to prior chemotherapy raises the possibility that the *TFE3* and *TFEB* loci may be particularly susceptible to DNA damage that promotes chromosome translocations.[261]

It is now thought that the t(6;11) renal carcinomas are related to the Xp11-translocation carcinomas based on the following findings:

1. Their clinical predilection to affect young patients is similar.
2. Their morphology is similar. Both neoplasms are composed of nests of predominantly clear to eosinophilic epithelioid cells, typical of a conventional RCC on routine hematoxylin and eosin sections.

3. Their immunohistochemical profiles are similar. Given their epithelioid morphology, both tumors underexpress epithelial IHC markers (cytokeratins, EMA). Several Xp11-translocation carcinomas (specifically, those with PSF-TFE3 and CLTC-TFE3 fusions) have expressed melanocytic markers by IHC, just as the t(6;11) renal neoplasms characteristically do. Both RCCs express cathepsin K in contrast to other RCC subtypes. Both RCCs overexpress proteins in the MiTF/TFE transcription factor family (TFE3 fusion proteins or native TFEB), and in each case a routine IHC assay detects this overexpression in a highly sensitive and specific fashion.

4. Their molecular pathologies are related. TFEB, TFE3, TFEC, and Mitf are members of the microphthalmia subfamily of basic helix-loop-helix transcription factors, which have homologous DNA binding domains and in fact bind to a common DNA sequence.[273] Members of the MiTF/TFE transcription factor family homodimerize and heterodimerize in all combinations to bind similar or identical DNA sequences. Therefore it seems likely that the transcription factors that are overexpressed in these two tumors (TFE3 fusion proteins and native TFEB) have similar downstream targets. Most of these targets remain to be determined; however, genes normally expressed in melanocytic differentiation may be one such example. In cell line transfection assays, overexpression of TFE3 activates the promoter of the tyrosinase gene, whereas both TFEB and TFE3 activate the promoter of the tyrosinase-related protein 1 gene.[274] The genes encoding tyrosinase and tyrosinase-related protein 1 are normally expressed in melanocyte differentiation, where they are regulated by another MiTF/TFE family member, MiTF. These results suggest that aberrant overexpression of TFEB may be responsible for the expression of melanocytic markers, a characteristic and distinctive feature of the t(6;11) renal carcinomas, and that some specific TFE3 fusion proteins may do so as well. Mouse knockout studies provide further evidence that MiTF family members may functionally overlap in certain cell types. In these studies severe osteopetrosis occurs in mice with combined TFE3 and MiTF inactivation, but there is no effect of TFE3 or MiTF loss individually on osteoclasts.[275]

Therefore, based on the preceding facts, it has been suggested that the t(6;11) renal carcinomas and the Xp11.2 translocation carcinomas should be classified as members of the "MiT translocation carcinoma family."[276] This suggestion was adopted by the 2012 International Society of Urologic Pathology Consensus Conference in Vancouver, British Columbia.

Clinical Presentation and Diagnostic Evaluation

The most common presenting signs and symptoms of pediatric RCC are flank or abdominal pain, hematuria, fever, nausea and vomiting, abdominal mass, anemia, pallor, and malaise.[256,257] It is unusual for children to present with the typical adult RCC triad of abdominal mass, hematuria, and hypertension. Approximately 20% of patients have locoregional lymph node metastases, and as many as 30% have distant metastatic disease at initial presentation. The lung, mediastinum, and liver are the most common sites of distant spread, but osseous, central nervous system, and other soft tissue metastases are also possible.[257,277] The imaging workup for pediatric RCC therefore includes CT of the chest, abdomen, and pelvis, with consideration of a bone scan and magnetic resonance imaging of the head. The role of PET scan has not been fully determined, but some forms of pediatric RCC have been found to be PET active. CT imaging has been demonstrated to have a high specificity but relatively low sensitivity for detection of local lymph nodes in pediatric RCC, underlining the importance of lymph node sampling at surgery, insofar as pathologically confirmed nodal disease can be observed even with small primary tumors (COG AREN03B2 study, unpublished observations).

Treatment

Several series of pediatric RCC have demonstrated stage-for-stage outcomes that mirror outcomes observed in adult patients.[256,257,277] Survival rates for patients with stage I, II, III, and IV disease are about 92%, 85%, 73%, and 13%, respectively.[277] A difference between adult and pediatric RCC is the prognostic significance of local lymph node involvement in the absence of distant metastases.[277] Whereas the survival rate for adult patients with local lymph node involvement is in the 20% to 30% range, approximately 75% of children with local lymph node involvement survive.[257,277] This difference likely reflects the disparate histologies between adult and pediatric RCC. Given the good outcomes of children with localized RCC and the lack of agents with known efficacy, the COG AREN0321 study recommended treating such patients without adjuvant therapy. Patients with metastatic RCC are treated according to the physician's professional judgment. The study was open from 2006 to 2013, and outcome data are pending.

Historically, the only therapy with proven benefit for metastatic RCC was immunotherapy using interleukin-2, interferon-alpha, or a combination of these agents. However immunotherapy produces tumor responses in only 10% to 20% of patients, most of whom achieve a transient response and experience substantial toxicity.[278] With the development of drugs targeted to signal transduction and tumor-related angiogenesis, multiple trials have response rates and impact on progression-free survival in adult RCC. Agents that have demonstrated benefit in some studies of adult RCC include vascular endothelial growth factor pathway inhibitors (sorafenib, sunitinib, pazopanib, axitinib, and bevacizumab) and mTOR inhibitors (temsirolimus and everolimus). In the wake of these studies, molecularly targeted therapy has become the frontline treatment for advanced RCC in adult patients. However in considering treatment of pediatric RCC, the clinician must remember that childhood and adult RCC are distinct entities. Most of the patients enrolled in adult studies had the clear cell subtype of RCC, whereas the majority of pediatric RCC patients have the translocation or papillary subtypes. A retrospective series from the Juvenile RCC Network indicated that tyrosine kinase inhibitors, most notably sunitinib, have produced objective responses or disease stabilization in translocation RCC.[279] A prospective trial of tyrosine kinase inhibition therapy for metastatic or recurrent translocation RCC is under development by the COG.

A category of pediatric RCC with a distinctly poor outcome is renal medullary carcinoma, which is observed in patients with sickle cell trait.[61] Patients with renal medullary carcinoma almost always present with metastatic disease and have fatal outcomes. Transient responses have been observed after chemotherapy treatment with a combination of methotrexate, vinblastine, doxorubicin, and cisplatin[280-282] and a combination of platinum, gemcitabine, and taxane.[283,284] Agents that target the ABL tyrosine kinase may be considered for investigation in renal medullary carcinoma because these tumors have been reported to have ABL gene amplification and BCR-ABL rearrangements.[281,282] A tumor also recently was found to have a translocation involving the ALK gene.[285] A patient with renal medullary carcinoma was shown to have a complete tumor response after treatment with the proteosome inhibitor bortezomib.[286]

CONGENITAL MESOBLASTIC NEPHROMA

Epidemiology

The average age of diagnosis of CMN is 3.4 months. The vast majority of cases are diagnosed in infancy, but in rare cases children up to 9 years of age have been diagnosed. Congenital malformations accompanied 14% of CMN cases, including genitourinary and gastrointestinal anomalies, polydactyly, and hydrocephalus.[287] There is a strong correlation of age at diagnosis and histologic subtype; the cellular type is seen more commonly in children older than 3 months of age.[288]

Molecular Biology and Genetics

IFS and cellular CMN have much in common. The two neoplasms have virtually indistinguishable morphology and affect the same young age group. Both also are associated with a prognosis that is better than that expected given their ominous-appearing morphology; both IFS and cellular CMN only rarely metastasize. There had also been molecular hints of a relationship between IFS and cellular CMN, insofar as both tumors are characterized by polysomies, particularly of chromosomes 11, 17, and 20.[289,290]

A major advance occurred in 1998, when it was discovered that IFS is characterized by a specific t(12;15) (p13;q25). The t(12;15) results in fusion of the ETV6 gene on chromosome 12 with the NTRK3 gene on chromosome 15.[291] The ETV6 (TEL) gene had previously been implicated in the t(12;21)(p13;q22) of pediatric precursor B-cell acute lymphoblastic leukemia and encodes a transcription factor with a helix-loop-helix protein dimerization domain. NTRK3 is a receptor tyrosine kinase that is activated by ligand-dependent dimer-

ization and is involved in neural development. The chimeric ETV6-NTRK3 protein is postulated to be constitutively dimerized and therefore to affect constitutively active tyrosine kinase growth pathway signaling. Significantly, neither infantile fibromatosis nor adult-type fibrosarcomas, two entities in the histologic differential diagnosis of infantile fibrosarcoma, contain this gene fusion.

Given the clinicopathologic similarities of IFS and cellular CMN, the question arose as to whether cellular CMN bore the same chromosome translocation and gene fusion. Two studies have conclusively proven this to be true.[292,293] Of 11 cellular CMNs studied, 10 contained the fusion transcript, whereas all five classic CMNs (the renal counterpart of infantile fibromatosis) did not. Hence it is tempting to consider cellular CMN to be essentially an IFS of the renal sinus. Indeed there is no clinical, morphologic, histopathologic, or genetic reason to think otherwise. Additionally these studies highlight the fact that classic and cellular CMNs are molecularly distinctive neoplasms, not just two morphologic patterns of one neoplasm, as their names would suggest. The data on mixed CMN is conflicting, but most recent studies have found an absence of the ETV6-NTRK3 gene fusion in mixed CMN.[67,289,294]

Further studies have addressed the function of the ETV6-NTRK3 fusion gene. Wai and colleagues have shown that ETV6-NTRK3 chimeric tyrosine kinase is capable of transforming NIH3T3 cells.[295] Tognon and colleagues have subsequently shown that this requires activation of both the Ras-Raf1-Mek1-ERK1/2 mitogenic pathway and the phosphatidylinositol 3'-kinase (PI3K)-Akt cell survival pathway, such that inhibition of either pathway abolishes transformation.[296] These findings raise the possibility that MEK or PI3K inhibitors could be potentially useful in treating the minority of patients who develop metastatic disease. Jin and coworkers have shown that the ETVG-NTRK3 chimeric tyrosine kinase suppresses transforming growth factor(TGF) β tumor suppressor activity by binding to the type II TGF-β receptor.[297] Finally the ETV6-NTRK3 gene fusion has also been found to be consistently present in secretory carcinoma of the breast, a rare epithelial cancer that tends to affect young people, and mammary analogue secretory carcinoma of the salivary gland.[298,299] Rare cases of acute myeloid leukemia have been shown to bear the same gene fusion.[300,301] Hence the ETV6-NTRK3 gene fusion is remarkable in that it may apparently transform cells of the mesenchymal, epithelial, and hematopoietic lineages.

Clinical Presentation and Diagnostic Evaluation

A palpable abdominal mass is the most common presenting symptom in infants with CMN. Other signs and symptoms at presentation include hematuria (18%), hypertension (4%), anemia (4%), and vomiting (6%).[287] Hypercalcemia has been reported as a presenting feature of CMN.[302] Patients with CMN do not present with metastatic disease, although the cellular histologic type has the potential to metastasize to the lung and, rarely, the brain later in the course of the disease. A baseline chest, abdomen, and pelvis CT scan is recommended.

Treatment

Outcomes for patients with CMN are generally excellent without adjuvant therapy, with overall survival rates of 95%.[287,303] The few tumors that recur are almost exclusively the cellular type of the CMN. In addition to cellular histologic subtype, age greater than 3 months and stage III disease have been associated with relapse.

The standard therapy for all stages of classic CMN (noncellular) and stage I and II cellular CMN is surgical resection followed by observation with serial imaging studies. It remains to be established whether patients with stage III cellular CMN benefit from adjuvant chemotherapy. In a series published by the German Pediatric Oncology Group, two of five patients with stage III cellular CMN developed recurrent disease, whereas only one of the remaining 45 patients experienced recurrence.[303] Experience with presurgical treatment of CMN shows that most of these tumors respond to a combination of vincristine and dactinomycin therapy.[303] Recurrent cellular CMN tumors are responsive to combinations of vincristine, doxorubicin, and dactinomycin; vincristine, dactinomycin, and cyclophosphamide; vincristine, doxorubicin, and cyclophosphamide; and ifosfamide, carboplatin, and etoposide.[304] There is no established role for radiation therapy in the treatment of CMN.

FUTURE DIRECTIONS

A broad view of the field of pediatric renal tumors provides cause for both celebration and trepidation. Treatment of favorable-histology WT has been a terrific success, with cure rates in the 90% range. Remarkably the success has been coupled with a diminishment in treatment, thereby sparing patients of acute and long-term adverse effects. Clinicians have a more complete understanding of renal tumor biology than ever before, with the discovery of several new genes (WTX, BRCA2, INI1, TFE3, and others) and increased understanding of previously identified genes (WT1 and the 11p15 locus). The availability of a new pipeline of molecularly targeted agents provides the opportunity to advance renal tumor therapies beyond the traditional cytotoxic agents.

On the other hand challenges remain. Outcomes for children with anaplastic WT, bilateral WT, recurrent WT, RCC, and MRT remain suboptimal (all with survival rates of less than 75%). For some of these tumor types, such as anaplastic WT and MRT, increased chemotherapy doses and intensity are approaching the maximum level of patient tolerance. Novel treatment approaches, such as molecularly targeted agents, differentiating agents, or immunotherapy, are required. A pitfall to the introduction of new agents is that the patient populations are small, so clinical trials take years to execute. New initiatives for international collaboration between the COG and SIOP will facilitate the conduct of clinical research on the uncommon pediatric renal tumors. For tumor types such as pediatric RCC, the tumor biology and natural clinical history have only recently begun to

be understood. Broad support for pediatric renal tumor research is essential for further progress.

References available online at ExpertConsult.

KEY REFERENCES

5. Vujanic GM, Sandstedt B, Harms D, et al: Revised International Society of Paediatric Oncology (SIOP) working classification of renal tumors of childhood. *MedPediatr Oncol* 38:79–82, 2002.
   This was the first article to describe the SIOP histologic classification system for pediatric renal tumors. This system is based on postchemotherapy histologic changes, including the percentage of the tumor that is necrotic and the predominant cell type (blastemal, epithelial, or stromal) after chemotherapy. By contrast, the COG system is based on prechemotherapy histology and uses only anaplasia as a histologic prognostic factor.

8. Doros LA, Rossi CT, Yang J, et al: DICER1 mutations in childhood cystic nephroma and its relationship to DICER1-renal sarcoma. *Mod Pathol* 2014 [epub ahead of print].
   This study found loss-of-function DICER1 mutations in 14 of 20 (70%) cystic nephromas evaluated, whereas none of six CPDNs had DICER1 mutations. CPDN previously was considered to lie on a spectrum between cystic nephroma and WT, but these data suggest that the two cystic renal tumors are distinct entities. The authors also describe sarcomas developing within cystic nephromas, analogous to the progression from the cystic type 1 pleuropulmonary blastomas to the solid and sarcomatous type PPBs, also associated with DICER1 mutations.

11. Bardeesy N, Falkoff D, Petruzzi MJ, et al: Anaplastic Wilms' tumour, a subtype displaying poor prognosis, harbours p53 gene mutations. *Nat Genet* 7:91–97, 1994.
    This study first showed an association between TP53 mutations and anaplastic histology WT. Several lines of evidence indicate that anaplastic WT arises on a background of favorable-histology WT. About 75% of anaplastic WTs have TP53 mutations. Studies are under way to assess whether prognosis and biology differ between anaplastic WTs based on their TP53 mutation status.

15. Dome JS, Cotton CA, Perlman EJ, et al: Treatment of anaplastic histology Wilms' tumor: results from the fifth National Wilms' Tumor Study. *J Clin Oncol* 24:2352–2358, 2006.
    This study demonstrates that patients with stage II through IV diffuse anaplastic WT had improved survival rates compared with historic controls using a new regimen consisting of vincristine, doxorubicin, and cyclophosphamide alternating with cyclophosphamide and etoposide. The study indicates that although anaplastic WT is relatively resistant to therapy compared with favorable-histology WT, outcomes were improved with a more intensive chemotherapy regimen. The study also showed that patients with stage I anaplastic WT fared significantly worse than patients with stage I favorable-histology WT, contrary to the previous belief.

17. Weirich A, Leuschner I, Harms D, et al: Clinical impact of histologic subtypes in localized non-anaplastic nephroblastoma treated according to the trial and study SIOP-9/GPOH. *Ann Oncol* 12:311–319, 2001.
    This was the first study to correlate postchemotherapy histologic changes with prognosis in WT. The work here formed the basis of the SIOP histologic classification schema for pediatric renal tumors (see Reference 5).

22. Beckwith JB, Kiviat NB, Bonadio JF: Nephrogenic rests, nephroblastomatosis, and the pathogenesis of Wilms' tumor. *Pediatr Pathol* 10:1–36, 1990.
    This classic paper describes the natural history of NRs, clusters of embryonal renal cells that persist abnormally into childhood and represent precursor lesions to WT.

28. Argani P, Perlman EJ, Breslow NE, et al: Clear cell sarcoma of the kidney: a review of 351 cases from the National Wilms Tumor Study Group Pathology Center. *Am J Surg Pathol* 24:4–18, 2000.
    This seminal paper describes the clinicopathologic features and treatment results of a large series of CCSK.

49. Argani P, Antonescu CR, Illei PB, et al: Primary renal neoplasms with the ASPL-TFE3 gene fusion of alveolar soft part sarcoma: a distinctive tumor entity previously included among renal cell

carcinomas of children and adolescents. *Am J Pathol* 159:179–192, 2001.

This paper describes molecular genetic abnormality seen in the majority of cases of childhood RCC. "Translocation-type" RCC is now recognized as a distinct RCC subtype by the World Health Organization.

68. van den Heuvel-Eibrink MM, Grundy P, Graf N, et al: Characteristics and survival of 750 children diagnosed with renal tumors in the first seven months of life: a collaborative study by the SIOP/GPOH/SFOP, NWTSG, and UKCCSG Wilms tumor study groups. *Pediatr Blood Cancer* 50:1130–1134, 2008.

This large international series of 750 infants with renal tumors describes the epidemiology and treatment results for this patient subgroup.

69. Breslow N, Olshan A, Beckwith JB, et al: Epidemiology of Wilms tumor. *Med Pediatr Oncol* 21:172–181, 1993.

This classic paper contains valuable data on age, tumor laterality, gender, ethnicity, and congenital malformations in WT.

71. Knudson AG, Strong LC: Mutation and cancer: a model for Wilms' tumor of the kidney. *J Nat Cancer Inst* 48:313–324, 1972.

Knudson first described the "two-hit" model of mutagenesis and cancer using retinoblastoma as a model. This paper, published 1 year after the retinoblastoma paper, applied the same principles to WT. Many of the observations made in this seminal paper hold true today, although we now recognize that more than two hits are required and that several distinct pathways are involved in Wilms tumorigenesis.

84. Bonetta L, Kuehn SE, Huang A, et al: Wilms tumor locus on 11p13 defined by multiple CpG island-associated transcripts. *Science* 250:994–997, 1990.

85. Call KM, Glaser T, Ito CY, et al: Isolation and characterization of a zinc finger polypeptide gene at the human chromosome 11 Wilms' tumor locus. *Cell* 60:509–520, 1990.

86. Gessler M, Poustka A, Cavenee W, et al: Homozygous deletion in Wilms tumours of a zinc-finger gene identified by chromosome jumping. *Nature* 343:774–778, 1990.

The preceding three papers describe the initial identification of the WT1 gene and provide the first insights into its function as a transcription factor. Subsequent papers indicate that there are multiple splice variants of this gene with differing functions.

90. Huff V: Wilms tumor genetics. *Am J Med Genet* 79:260–267, 1998.

This is an excellent survey of germline and somatic WT1 mutations in WT and genotype-phenotype relationships.

93. Koesters R, Ridder R, Kopp Schneider A, et al: Mutational activation of the β-catenin proto-oncogene is a common event in the development of Wilms tumors. *Cancer Res* 59:3880–3882, 1999.

94. Maiti S, Alam R, Amos CI, et al: Frequent association of beta-catenin and WT1 mutations in Wilms tumors. *Cancer Res* 60:6288–6292, 2000.

The preceding two papers are the first to describe β-catenin (CTNNB1) mutations in WT. There is a strong correlation between β-catenin mutations and WT1 mutations, suggesting that the two pathways collaborate in Wilms tumorigenesis.

97. Rivera MN, Kim WJ, Wells J, et al: An X chromosome gene, WTX, is commonly inactivated in Wilms tumor. *Science* 315:642–645, 2007.

This is the first paper to describe a relatively new WT gene, WTX. The gene encodes a protein that acts in the WNT signaling pathway. The biology of this tumor supressor is unconventional because only one hit is required based on its location on the X chromosome.

108. Scott J, Cowell J, Robertson ME, et al: Insulin-like growth factor-II gene expression in Wilms' tumour and embryonic tissues. *Nature* 317:260–262, 1985.

109. Reeve AE, Eccles MR, Wilkins RJ, et al: Expression of insulin-like growth factor-II transcripts in Wilms' tumour. *Nature* 317:258–260, 1985.

The preceding two papers establish the link between the 11p15/Beckwith-Wiedemann syndrome locus and IGF2 overexpression in WT. How these alterations relate to other genetic changes observed in WT was described more recently (see Reference 118).

117. Hu Q, Gao F, Tian W, et al: Wt1 ablation and Igf2 upregulation in mice result in Wilms tumors with elevated ERK1/2 phosphorylation. *J Clin Invest* 121:174–183, 2010.

WT has traditionally been categorized into two subtypes: those associated with WT1 mutations and those associated with alterations of the Beckwith-Wiedemann 11p15/IGF2 locus. It is now clear that the lines are blurred between the two subtypes. This paper describes one of the first genetically engineered mouse models of WT obtained by combined Wt1 ablation and Iff2 upregulation.

118. Gadd S, Huff V, Huang CC, et al: Clinically relevant subsets identified by gene expression patterns support a revised ontogenic model of Wilms tumor: a Children's Oncology Group Study. *Neoplasia* 14:742–756, 2012.

This paper describes a detailed analysis correlating gene expression patterns with WT1 mutations, 11p15 copy number and methylation, CTNNB1 (β-catenin) mutations, and WTX mutations in more than 300 WT samples. The analysis led to a revised ontogenic model of WT consisting of five subsets with distinct clinical and biologic features.

141. Grundy PE, Green DM, Dirks AC, et al: Clinical significance of pulmonary nodules detected by CT and not CXR in patients treated for favorable histology WT on National Wilms Tumor Studies-4 and -5: a report from the Children's Oncology Group. *Pediatr Blood Cancer* 59:631–635, 2012.

This paper describes the largest study to date on the significance of WT lung nodules detected by CT scan but not chest x-ray. The findings suggest that so-called CT-only nodules have clinical significance because patients treated with only two-drug therapy (vincristine and dactinomycin) had a significantly lower event-free survival rate compared with patients treated with three-drug therapy (vincristine, dactinomycin, and doxorubicin). The overall survival rate, however, was not different between the two groups.

149. Shamberger RC, Guthrie KA, Ritchey ML, et al: Surgery-related factors and local recurrence of Wilms tumor in National Wilms Tumor Study-4. *Ann Surg* 229:292–297, 1999.

This study emphasizes the contribution of surgery-related factors to clinical outcomes in WT. The findings illustrate the importance of lymph node sampling in assigning appropriate therapy: patients with lymph nodes positive for WT fared better than patients with no lymph nodes sampling at all.

166. Grundy PE, Breslow NE, Li S, et al: Loss of heterozygosity for chromosomes 1p and 16q is an adverse prognostic factor in favorable-histology Wilms tumor: a report from the National Wilms Tumor Study Group. *J Clin Oncol* 23:7312–7321, 2005.

This is the primary paper reporting outcomes for favorable-histology WT in the NWTS-5. It describes a prospective analysis of LOH at 1p and 16q as a prognostic marker. Combined LOH at both loci was found to predict inferior event-free and overall survival in all stage groups. These findings influenced the risk stratification schema for WT on the most recent generation of COG studies.

168. Green DM, Breslow NE, Beckwith JB, et al: Treatment with nephrectomy only for small, stage I/favorable histology Wilms' tumor: a report from the National Wilms' Tumor Study Group. *J Clin Oncol* 19:3719–3724, 2001.

One of the primary objectives of the NWTS-5 was to assess whether young patients with small stage I favorable-histology WT can be treated with surgery only, without adjuvant chemotherapy. The study closed early after the predefined stopping rule for number of relapses was reached. However the salvage rate after recurrence exceeded expectations, so the overall survival rate with this approach was outstanding. This question was revisited in the recently completed COG AREN0532 study.

171. Pritchard Jones K, Graf N, Bergeron C, et al: Doxorubicin can be safely omitted from the treatment of Stage II/III intermediate risk histology Wilms Tumour: results of the SIOP 2001 randomized trial. *Pediatr Blood Cancer* 57:741, 2011.

Although published only in abstract form at the time this chapter was written, these results are important because they will lead to a reduction in therapy for a large group of patients. The study found that withholding doxorubicin does not affect overall survival in patients with stage II and III intermediate-risk WT. It is important to recognize that these findings cannot be applied to patients treated in COG studies because the staging and histologic classification systems differ.

172. Beckwith JB, Palmer NF: Histopathology and prognosis of Wilms tumor. *Cancer* 41:1937–1948, 1978.

   This is the first paper to associate anaplastic histology with adverse prognosis in WT. Despite the remarkable expansion of knowledge on the molecular genetics of WT, anaplasia remains the most powerful predictor of outcome.

189. Green DM, Cotton CA, Malogolowkin M, et al: Treatment of Wilms tumor relapsing after initial treatment with vincristine and actinomycin D: a report from the National Wilms Tumor Study Group. *Pediatr Blood Cancer* 48:493–499, 2007.

190. Malogolowkin M, Cotton CA, Green DM, et al: Treatment of Wilms tumor relapsing after initial treatment with vincristine, actinomycin D, and doxorubicin. A report from the National Wilms Tumor Study Group. *Pediatr Blood Cancer* 50:236–241, 2008.

   The preceding two papers describe the outcomes of patients with relapsed WT treated in NWTS-5. Two primary prognostic categories emerged. Patients who were treated initially with only two-drug therapy had overall survival rates after relapse af approximately 80%. Patients treated initially with three drugs or more had overall survival rates of approximately 50% with a more intensive salvage regimen. Initial treatment overshadowed other prognostic factors for survival after recurrence, including site of recurrence and time to recurrence.

197. Presson A, Moore TB, Kempert P: Efficacy of high-dose chemotherapy and autologous stem cell transplant for recurrent Wilms' tumor: a meta-analysis. *J Pediatr Hematol Oncol* 32:454–461, 2010.

198. Ha TC, Spreafico F, Graf N, et al: An international strategy to determine the role of high dose therapy in recurrent Wilms' tumour. *Eur J Cancer* 49:194–210, 2013.

   An unresolved question about the management of recurrent WT is whether high-dose therapy with autologous stem cell rescue provides benefit. Because no randomized clinical trials have been conducted, two groups conducted meta-analyses to address this question. Both analyses agree that high-dose therapy is not beneficial for relapses that occur after initial therapy with only two drugs. The greatest benefit for transplant appears to be within the group of patients who received four or more drugs before

transplant—that is, those with anaplastic histology or those with multiply recurrent favorable-histology WT.

229. Tomlinson GE, Breslow NE, Dome J, et al: Rhabdoid tumor of the kidney in the National Wilms' Tumor Study: age at diagnosis as a prognostic factor. *J Clin Oncol* 23:7641–7645, 2005.

   One of the largest series of rhabdoid tumor of the kidney demonstrated the lack of progress over the years treating this aggressive malignancy. Young age was established as an adverse prognostic factor.

232. Versteege I, Sevenet N, Lange J, et al: Truncating mutations of hSNF5/INI1 in aggressive paediatric cancer. *Nature* 394:203–206, 1998.

   This classic paper establishes the association between SMARCB1/INI1/SNF5 mutations and MRT. This work shows that rhabdoid tumors arising at different sites—renal, brain, and extrarenal or extra central nervous system—have a common molecular etiology.

258. Bruder E, Passera O, Harms D, et al: Morphologic and molecular characterization of renal cell carcinoma in children and young adults. *Am J Surg Pathol* 28:1117–1132, 2004.

   This paper describes the histologic subtypes of RCC in children and adolescents. It illustrates that childhood RCC is distinct from adult RCC.

291. Knezevich SR, McFadden DE, Tao W, et al: A novel ETV6-NTRK3 gene fusion in congenital fibrosarcoma. *Nat Genet* 18:184–187, 1998.

292. Knezevich SR, Garnett MJ, Pysher TJ, et al: ETV6-NTRK3 gene fusions and trisomy 11 establish a histogenetic link between mesoblastic nephroma and congenital fibrosarcoma. *Cancer Res* 58:5046–5048, 1998.

293. Rubin BP, Chen CJ, Morgan TW, et al: Congenital mesoblastic nephroma t(12;15) is associated with ETV6-NTRK3 gene fusion: cytogenetic and molecular relationship to congenital (infantile) fibrosarcoma. *Am J Pathol* 153:1451–1458, 1998.

   The preceding three papers describe ETV6-NTRK3 translocations as a feature of the cellular type of CMN. These papers also establish a histogenetic link between CMN and congenital infantile fibrosarcoma. Whereas recurrence is exceedingly rare in CMN without the translocation, 20% to 25% of cases of stage III disease with the translocation experience recurrence.

CHAPTER 56

Retinoblastoma

Carlos Rodriguez-Galindo, Matthew W. Wilson, and Michael Dyer

CHAPTER OUTLINE

Retinoblastoma is the most frequent neoplasm of the eye in childhood and the third most common intraocular malignancy in all ages, following malignant melanoma and metastatic carcinoma. Retinoblastoma represents 2.5% to 4% of all pediatric cancers but 11% of cancers in the first year of life.[1] The average age-adjusted incidence rate of retinoblastoma in the United States and Europe is 2 to 5 per million children (approximately one in 14,000 to 18,000 live births).[2,3] Thus retinoblastoma develops in an estimated 8000 children each year worldwide.[4]

Retinoblastoma is a cancer of the very young; two thirds of all cases of retinoblastoma are diagnosed before 2 years of age, and 95% of cases are diagnosed before 5 years of age.[1] For these reasons, in addition to cure of the disease, therapeutic approaches require consideration of the need to preserve vision with minimal long-term adverse effects.

Retinoblastoma presents in two distinct clinical forms. The first form is bilateral or multifocal and heritable (occurring in 25% of all cases of retinoblastoma); it is characterized by the presence of germline mutations of the retinoblastoma-1 (RB1) gene. Multifocal retinoblastoma may be inherited from an affected survivor (25%), or it may be the result of a new germline mutation (75%). The second form is unilateral (representing 75% of all cases); about 85% to 90% of the cases are nonhereditary, and the remainder carry a germline RB1 mutation.

EPIDEMIOLOGY

The incidence of retinoblastoma is not distributed equally around the world. It appears to be higher (6 to 10 cases per million children) in Africa[2,5] and India[6] and among children of Native American descent in the North American continent.[7,8] The increased incidence in those groups occurs primarily at the expense of unilateral cases. Whether these geographic variations are due to ethnic or socioeconomic factors is not known. However the fact that even in industrialized countries an increased incidence of retinoblastoma is associated with poverty and low levels of maternal education[9] suggests a role for the environment. Differences in the incidence of embryonal tumors between countries and ethnic groups have been consistently reported during the past decades, particularly for retinoblastoma[2]; however the deficiencies inherent to suboptimal cancer registries in low-income countries have made proper estimates difficult. In a country as ethnically diverse and socioeconomically heterogenous as Brazil, De Camargo and colleagues[10] calculated the age-adjusted incidence rates (AAIR) of retinoblastoma in 20 population-based cancer registries and noted higher AAIRs than those of developed countries. The AAIR for children 0 to 4 years of age was as high as 15 and 27 in Salvador and Bahia, respectively, two of the most deprived states in the country (versus 10 to 12 in the United States and Europe).[10] In a broader study testing the differences in incidence for embryonal tumors and their correlation with socioeconomic status, the same group documented an inverse correlation between the incidence of retinoblastoma and socioeconomic index. A similar phenomenon has been reported in Mexico, where a higher incidence of retinoblastoma has been documented, particularly in deprived states such as Chiapas.[11,12]

Decreased dietary intake of vegetables and fruits during pregnancy, resulting in decreased intake of nutrients such as folate and carotenoids, which are necessary for deoxyribonucleic acid (DNA) methylation and synthesis and for retinal formation, has also been associated with an increased risk of unilateral sporadic retinoblastoma.[13] In a case-control study, the risk of developing retinoblastoma was associated with a maternal polymorphism in dihydrofolate reductase (DHFR 19bpdel), particularly in women taking prenatal synthetic folic acid supplements.[14]

It is well known that exposure to certain toxic agents during gestation increases the frequency of germinal mutations in animals. The vast majority of germline mutations in sporadic heritable retinoblastoma are paternally derived,[15] and studies have suggested an association between paternal age[9,16,17] and occupation[18] with the occurrence of sporadic heritable retinoblastoma. Reports have also suggested an association between retinoblastoma and increased sunlight exposure,[19,20] air toxins from gasoline and diesel combustion,[21] or in vitro fertilization.[22-24] In a case-control study of sporadic retinoblastoma, radiologic studies of the abdomen leading to scattered radiation exposure of the gonads was associated with an increased risk of bilateral retinoblastoma in the child.[25]

Retinoblastoma tumors arise from fetal retinal cells that have lost function of both allelic copies of the RB1 gene, the first of the tumor suppressor genes to be cloned. The first event may be either a germline or a somatic mutation, but the second and subsequent events are always somatic. Not all tumors have mutations in RB1, suggesting that there is either another gene or alternate mechanisms for inactivation of RB1 function.[26,27] For example, the RB1 gene can be epigenetically silenced through hypermethylation of the promoter.[28,29] In recent years, studies have suggested a role for human papillomaviruses (HPVs) in the pathogenesis of retinoblastoma. The viral oncoprotein E7 of high-risk HPV types has been shown to bind to and inactivate the RB1 gene product. Therefore it is plausible that HPV infection could be functionally equivalent to the biallelic loss of RB1.[30] Transgenic mice expressing HPV16 E6 and E7 proteins develop retinoblastoma.[31] Presumably exposure to HPV would occur peripartum from genital infection of the mother. In this regard the use of barrier methods of contraception is associated with a reduced incidence of both retinoblastoma and HPV infection,[9,32] and studies have also shown a correlation with sexually transmitted diseases during pregnancy.[17] Interestingly an overlap occurs between countries in which the relative incidence of retinoblastoma is greatest and those in which the incidence of cervical carcinoma is highest.[32] High-risk HPV sequences have been detected in 28% to 36% of tumors in some populations.[32,33]

BIOLOGY OF RETINOBLASTOMA

Cellular Origins of Retinoblastoma

It is widely believed that the molecular and cellular features of a tumor reflect its cell of origin and can thus provide clues about treatment targets. Since 1897 when Wintersteiner first proposed that rosettes in retinoblastoma are reminiscent of photoreceptor differentiation,[34] the cell of origin and the cellular features of retinoblastoma have been debated. Initially the focus was on the cellular features that could be identified by histologic analyses, such as the presence of rosettes. With advances in molecular biology and biochemistry, the debate about the retinoblastoma cell of origin has been revisited, with a strong predilection toward photoreceptors being the cell of origin.[35-43] In addition to photoreceptors, a number of independent studies suggested that retinoblastomas may also have features of progenitor cells or interneurons such as amacrine cells.[38,44,45,46,47-51] The possibility of tumor cells with a hybrid molecular/cellular phenotype was not considered in those previous studies.

In a recent study of the molecular, cellular, neuroanatomic, and neurochemical features of mouse and human retinoblastoma, it was shown that they have features of multiple cell classes, principally amacrine/horizontal interneurons, retinal progenitor cells, and photoreceptors.[52] Indeed, single-cell gene expression array analysis showed that these multiple cell type-specific developmental programs are coexpressed in individual retinoblastoma cells, which creates a progenitor/neuronal hybrid cell. It is widely believed that the initiating genetic lesion in the RB1 gene occurs in proliferating retinal progenitor cells during fetal development. Retinal progenitor cells may be the cell of origin for retinoblastoma, and the multiple differentiation programs that are found in human and mouse retinoblastomas may reflect the multipotent competence of retinal progenitor cells. Indeed in single-cell gene expression array analyses of mouse retinal progenitor cells, photoreceptor and interneuron genes were often expressed in proliferating retinal progenitor cells.[53]

The finding that retinoblastoma tumor cells express multiple neuronal differentiation programs that are normally incompatible in development suggests that the pathways that control retinal development and establish distinct cell types are perturbed during tumorigenesis. This discovery underscores the challenges of assigning cell-of-origin status without first establishing the full molecular and cellular signature of a tumor. It is important to emphasize that these studies do not necessarily indicate that a photoreceptor, interneuron, or progenitor cell is the cell of origin for retinoblastoma. Detailed cell-lineage studies combined with live imaging approaches will be required to definitively identify the cell of origin for retinoblastoma. Nonetheless, this detailed characterization of the neuronal pathways that are deregulated in retinoblastoma may provide novel targets for therapeutic intervention. This example highlights the importance of comprehensive molecular, cellular, and physiologic characterization of human cancers with single-cell resolution as we incorporate molecular targeted therapy into treatment regimens.

Retinoblastoma Tumor Cell Differentiation

Many of the previous studies on retinoblastoma tumor cell differentiation have focused on photoreceptor features, including a recent study linking the origin of retinoblastoma to cone photoreceptors.[43] As previously described, a detailed cross-species gene expression array analysis indicated that retinoblastomas express molecular features of photoreceptors and that the rod signature is more robust than the cone signature.[52] However morphometric and neuroanatomic studies of mouse and human retinoblastomas showed few cellular features of photoreceptors, which raises the possibility that the gene regulatory network that controls photoreceptors is deregulated in human retinoblastomas. Interestingly a large number of photoreceptor genes are also expressed in medulloblastomas[54,55] despite their distinct cellular origins, which may indicate that the transcriptional pathways involved in photoreceptor differentiation are nonspecifically deregulated in a variety of tumors of the central nervous system (CNS). It is not known if this "photoreceptor signature" has any prognostic or therapeutic significance in retinoblastoma or other tumors of the CNS.

Human and mouse retinoblastomas have molecular, morphometric, neuroanatomic, and neurochemical features of interneurons, including amacrine and horizontal cells.[52] Indeed, the cell-type specific features that are most common across human and mouse retinoblastomas are those related to amacrine cell differentiation. As previously discussed, the tumor's cell of origin may be completely independent of amacrine interneurons, and because tumor suppressor or oncogenic pathways are deregulated during tumorigenesis, the amacrine differentiation program may be aberrantly activated during retinoblastoma tumorigenesis.

Nonetheless, the amacrine differentiation of human and mouse retinoblastoma may be functionally significant for tumor survival and progression. The most striking evidence for amacrine differentiation at the cellular level came from the identification of dense core vesicles in human and mouse retinoblastomas in electron micrographs. Retinoblastomas produce catecholamines and other monoamines,[56-58] and several of the receptors for monoamines are expressed, as are the genes involved in the biosynthesis of monoamines. When monoamine receptors were blocked with pharmacologic agents, retinoblastoma growth was reduced in culture and in vivo. In contrast, agents that block the other major neurotransmitter signaling pathways (γ-aminobutyric acid, glycine, and glutamate) had no effect on retinoblastoma, nor did the inhibition of selective reuptake of catecholamines with pharmacologic agents. One interpretation of these data is that retinoblastoma cells are engaged in an autocrine induction of the catecholamine-signaling pathway. All of the major catecholamine/monoamine receptors are G-protein–coupled receptors and signal through adenyl cyclase–mediated cyclic adenosine monophosphate induction. This pathway can directly or indirectly stimulate the mitogen-activated protein kinase pathway and provide an important mitogenic signal for retinoblastoma. It may also explain why retinoblastomas form in the retina. That is, this tissue is uniquely susceptible to tumorigenesis because the amacrine-differentiation pathway can be co-opted for mitogenic signaling after RB1 gene inactivation. Additional studies will be required to determine whether catecholamine signaling influences survival and growth through the mitogen-activated protein kinase pathway or if it is required for some other aspect of tumorigenesis.

Retinoblastoma Genomics and Epigenomics

Most retinoblastomas initiate with biallelic loss of the RB1 gene.[59] RB1 inactivation confers limitless replicative potential to retinoblasts, and these preneoplastic cells can progress to retinoblastoma by acquiring additional somatic mutations that contribute to the acquisition of new cellular properties, including evasion of cell death and senescence, sustained angiogenesis, and activation growth–signaling pathways. Several different mechanisms have been proposed to explain the rapid progression of retinoblastoma after RB1 inactivation. In a series of studies using genetically engineered murine cells and immortalized human cells, it was shown that RB1 may play an important role in maintaining genomic stability.[60-62] Thus in some cellular contexts, inactivation of the RB1 gene could lead to chromosome instability, allowing secondary and tertiary mutations in key cancer pathways to be rapidly acquired. Alternatively RB1 has also been implicated in a variety of epigenetic processes, so it is also possible that perturbations in the epigenetic landscape may contribute to tumorigenesis in the retina. In support of an epigenetic mechanism, recent whole-genome sequencing and integrated epigenetic analysis of human retinoblastoma revealed that the tumors have relatively stable genomes, and several cancer genes were epigenetically deregulated.[63] At least one of those epigenetically deregulated genes (spleen tyrosine kinase; SYK) is required for retinoblastoma tumor cell survival in vivo (discussed later).[63] These two alternative mechanisms (genome instability and epigenetic deregulation) of retinoblastoma progression are not necessarily mutually exclusive, and some tumors may show evidence of both chromosomal instability and epigenetic deregulation.

Although epigenetic deregulation of key cancer pathways has been shown to be directly relevant for retinoblastoma tumor progression, the functional significance of recurrent secondary genetic lesions is still poorly understood. During the 27 years since the *RB1* gene was cloned, researchers have focused on identifying genetic lesions in retinoblastoma that contribute to tumor progression after *RB1* inactivation.[64] Cytogenetic and array comparative genome hybridization studies have led to the identification of regions of the genome that are gained or lost in retinoblastomas and may contribute to tumorigenesis.[64] Those studies have led to the identification of candidate oncogenes and tumor suppressor genes whereby copy number variations (CNVs) correlate with changes in gene expression.[65,66] However the major limitation of those studies is their relatively small number of tumors analyzed and the modest effects on gene expression for tumors with CNVs versus those without the corresponding lesion. Even for the most common recurrently mutated gene in retinoblastoma, BCL6 corepressor *(BCOR)*, there have been no direct in vivo studies showing that it contributes to tumorigenesis.

Carefully designed in vivo experiments to explore the role of putative oncogenes and tumor suppressor genes in retinoblastoma tumorigenesis are important for advancing our understanding of the molecular mechanisms of retinoblastoma progression. For example, a recent study showed that in a small proportion (1.5%) of human unilateral nonfamilial retinoblastomas, no *RB1* gene mutations are present and they have v-myc avian myelocytomatosis viral oncogene neuroblastoma derived homolog *(MYCN)* amplification (≥10 copies).[27] The authors suggested that in those patients, *MYCN* amplification may initiate tumorigenesis.[27] This observation was recently validated and extended in an independent study with a separate cohort of patients.[67]

Recent whole-genome sequencing of human retinoblastomas and their matched germline DNA demonstrated that at least some retinoblastomas have relatively stable diploid genomes with few CNVs or somatic nucleotide variations,[63] and thus genome instability may not be required for retinoblastoma progression. One of the most common misconceptions related to cancer genomics is that tumors with few CNVs have stable genomes and tumors with more CNVs have unstable genomes. Chromosome instability is a dynamic process that cannot be accurately measured at a single time point because it involves the acquisition of sequential chromosomal lesions over time. It is important to distinguish between such dynamic processes that reflect the continuous accumulation of genetic lesions versus more acute genomic events such as multiple chromosome trisomies as seen in hyperdiploid acute lymphoblastic leukemia (ALL), multiple chromosome loss as seen in hypodiploid ALL, and the more recently described process of chromothripsis.[68,69] The best way to directly analyze chromosome instability is to sample the same tumor at multiple time points and perform a comprehensive analysis of the genetic

landscape at each time point. Orthotopic xenografts of human retinoblastoma in immunocompromised mouse eyes have proved to be very useful for analysis of chromosome instability in retinoblastoma because the genomic landscape can be analyzed sequentially over time.[63] Clearly this does not preclude the possibility that some retinoblastomas have unstable genomes, but genome instability is not a universal hallmark of *RB1*-deficient retinoblastomas, nor is it required for rapid tumor progression.

In the most recent genomic analysis of retinoblastoma, single nucleotide polymorphism 6.0 analysis was performed on 94 human retinoblastomas and matched normal germline DNAs. These data were used to identify regions of loss of heterozygosity and copy number changes, including whole chromosomes, regional changes, and focal changes (<3 Mb). Specifically, the majority (70%) of retinoblastomas have relatively few (≤10 per tumor) chromosomal, regional, or focal CNVs.[67] No correlation was found between the number of CNVs and the heritable or sporadic form of disease, nor was there any relationship between the type of *RB1* mutation and the number of lesions.[67] A much larger study will be required to determine if more subtle associations exist between the clinicopathologic features of retinoblastoma and the rate of CNVs.

The overall low rate of CNVs was consistent with the paucity of focal recurrent lesions in genes. As reported previously, inactivation of the *RB1* gene and the *BCOR* gene were the most common deletion events, and amplification of the *MYCN* gene was the most common focal recurrent gain.[63] In this most recent study, a new recurrent focal amplification of orthodenticle homeobox 2 *(OTX2)* was discovered in 3% of retinoblastomas. *OTX2* is a homeobox gene that is involved in photoreceptor and retinal pigment epithelium development.[70-73] Retinoblastomas express a variety of rod and cone photoreceptor genes,[38,52] and in future studies, it will be important to determine if OTX2 plays a role in modulating the photoreceptor differentiation program in retinoblastoma.

One of the most important aspects of the study was analysis of the relationship between mutations in *MYCN*, *BCOR*, and *OTX2* and the mechanism of *RB1* inactivation by sequencing all 27 exons of *RB1* in the cohort.[67] In total, 10 tumors were identified that had no single nucleotide variations or insertions or deletions in the coding region of *RB1*. Whole-genome sequencing on those 10 tumors and their matched normal germline DNA led to the identification of one tumor with a wildtype *RB1* gene and *MYCN* amplification. That tumor sample showed robust RB1 nuclear protein expression, suggesting that retinoblastoma can initiate in the absence of *RB1* mutation. Gene expression array analysis showed that the tumor with wild-type *RB1* was indistinguishable from all other retinoblastomas with *RB1* mutations. Those data confirm a previous report from the Gallie laboratory that a small subset of retinoblastomas (~1% to 2%) have wild-type *RB1*.[27] More importantly this larger more recent genomic analysis also identified three tumors that had focal chromothripsis, disrupting the *RB1* gene and leading to loss of RB1 protein expression. The chromothriptic lesions are not detected by routine genetic analyses because all the exons are present in the genome. This is the first example of chromothripsis in the *RB1* gene in human cancer and the first clear example of chromothripsis as a mechanism for tumor initiation in a well-defined developmental cancer—retinoblastoma. Whole-genome sequencing combined with break-apart fluorescence in situ hybridization analysis of the *RB1* locus and RB1 immunohistochemistry (IHC) can be used to identify this unique subset of retinoblastoma tumors.

Retinoblastoma Preclinical Models

Mouse models of cancer have become increasingly important in the fields of cancer genetics and translational research. The importance of mouse models is particularly true for pediatric cancers because the patient population is relatively small and preclinical models are essential for validating the efficacy of new combinations of chemotherapy before initiating clinical trials in children. In addition, animal models of cancer can provide important new insight into the molecular, cellular, and genetic mechanisms underlying tumor initiation and progression.

One challenge of modeling pediatric cancer in mice is that these tumors initiate in the context of developing tissues that change rapidly, and the cells that give rise to the tumors can display an extraordinary degree of plasticity and heterogeneity. This situation is further complicated by the fact that many tumor suppressor genes and protooncogenes play essential roles in regulating cell-fate specification and differentiation during development. Specifically, the genetic lesions that contribute to tumor initiation and progression may also alter the intrinsic cell-fate specification and differentiation programs in the tumor cells, thereby making it very difficult to infer the cell of origin for that tumor.

Retinoblastoma is a relatively simple tumor that initiates with a common genetic lesion (*RB1* inactivation) and progresses rapidly in children. Moreover many features of retinal development are also conserved across species, making retinoblastoma an ideal tumor for cross-species comparison.

During the past decade a series of knockout mouse models of retinoblastoma have been generated by conditionally inactivating multiple Rb family members in the developing retina.[52,74,75] Knockout mouse models of retinoblastoma have also been valuable for studying the contribution of other tumor suppressor pathways such as the p53 pathway[74] and for testing novel therapeutic agents for the treatment of retinoblastoma.[76,77] In one study six different strains of mice that developed retinoblastoma were analyzed side by side using the same retinal progenitor–specific Cre transgene (*Chx10-Cre*) to inactivate tumor suppressor genes in the developing retina.[52] Histopathologic analysis, gene expression profiling, and morphometric, neuroanatomic, and neurochemical analyses[52] showed that mouse retinoblastomas faithfully recapitulate the molecular and cellular features of human retinoblastomas. However whereas the timing of retinoblastoma initiation was indistinguishable across the six strains, tumor penetrance and the rate of progression varied dramatically.[52] These data raise the possibility that the genetic and epigenetic changes that accompany human retinoblastoma progression may not be faithfully recapitulated in the mouse, despite the remarkable interspecies similarities at the molecular and cellular level.

To more directly assess the similarities and differences across species for retinoblastoma, a recent study analyzed the aneuploidy, CNVs, somatic nucleotide variations, and epigenetic landscape of murine retinoblastoma. Similar to human retinoblastoma, mouse tumors have a low rate of single-nucleotide variations in genes.[78] However mouse retinoblastomas have a higher rate of aneuploidy and regional and focal copy number changes, and this is dependent on the genetic lesions that initiate tumorigenesis in the developing murine retina.[78] In addition the epigenetic landscape in mouse retinoblastoma was significantly different from human tumors, and some pathways that are candidates for molecular targeted therapy for human retinoblastoma such as SYK or myeloid cell leukemia–1 are not deregulated in genetically engineered mouse models (GEMMs). Taken together these data suggest that important differences exist between mouse and human retinoblastomas with respect to the mechanism of tumor progression, and those differences can have significant implications for translational research to test the efficacy of novel therapies for this devastating childhood cancer.

In fact, preclinical testing of combination chemotherapy (etoposide, carboplatin, and vincristine) showed dramatic differences in response between GEMMs and human orthotopic xenografts; virtually all of the GEMMs were cured of their disease, whereas no improvement was seen in progression-free survival or overall survival in the orthotopic xenograft model.[79] It is possible that such species-specific differences could be further amplified when testing molecular targeted therapeutics directed toward processes important for maintaining genomic stability or the epigenetic landscape of retinoblastoma or targeting pathways such as SYK/myeloid cell leukemia–1 that are not deregulated in murine retinoblastoma. A careful assessment of the pathways that are deregulated in murine retinoblastomas is essential to make an accurate evaluation of the efficacy of novel therapeutics in preclinical studies focused on selecting the most promising new drugs for testing in clinical trials.

Understanding the intra- and interspecies differences is paramount when choosing the right model for the study of retinoblastoma. Unlike orthotopic xenograft models, genetic mouse models present the advantage of understanding the developmental processes that support tumor formation arising from a single cell and provide an ideal tool for genetic characterization of the contribution of individual pathways in retinoblastoma progression. On the other hand, orthotopic xenografts from patients faithfully recapitulate the mechanisms by which gene deregulation occurs in the human disease and can be more accurate for testing novel therapeutics. As a result, orthotopic xenografts are an important tool for target identification and target validation during preclinical trials, and GEMMs are important for understanding tumor initiation and progression in the developing retina.

Retinoblastoma Translational Research

Worldwide retinoblastoma is diagnosed in approximately 8000 children each year, including 250 to 300 patients in the United States. In developed countries more than 90% of patients with localized retinoblastoma disease are cured using a combination of chemotherapy, focal therapies, surgery (enucleation), and radiation therapy.[80-85] However many patients in developing countries present with advanced intraocular or metastatic disease. Although mortality is low with aggressive multimodal therapy, partial or full loss of vision occurs in approximately 50% of patients with advanced bilateral retinoblastoma.[86] In addition, significant late effects of therapy occur, including facial deformities and increased incidence of secondary malignancies.[87,88] A vigorous effort is now under way to develop targeted therapies to improve ocular salvage and vision preservation and reduce late effects of therapy without compromising therapeutic outcomes.[63,89]

Major advances have recently been made in understanding the biology of retinoblastoma, including identification of several molecular targets such as the inhibition of the MDM4-p53 interaction, SYK, histone deacetylase (HDAC), and the B-cell lymphoma–2 (BCL2) family of proteins. MDM4 is overexpressed in most human retinoblastomas and has been shown to contribute to tumor formation by suppressing p53. Consequently specific inhibition of the MDM4-p53 interaction represents a promising drug target for retinoblastoma treatment. The small-molecule MDM2/MDM4 antagonist nutlin-3a has been shown to efficiently induce p53-mediated cell death in retinoblastoma cells and mouse models of retinoblastoma.[79] Subsequent characterization of the genetic and epigenetic landscapes of retinoblastoma revealed profound increases in expression of the protooncogene *SYK*. Although *SYK* is not expressed in the normal human retina, it is upregulated in all retinoblastomas analyzed to date.[63] *SYK* is also expressed at high levels in metastatic and posttreatment retinoblastomas (Brennan and Bahrami, unpublished data). Many small-molecule *SYK* inhibitors with diverse physiochemical properties are in development for rheumatoid arthritis and oncology applications, and some of these novel therapeutics may eventually benefit patients with retinoblastoma.[90-93] Moreover, previous studies of *SYK* inhibition have implicated a number of downstream signaling molecules, including the BCL2 family of proteins, as mediators of the *SYK* survival signal.[94] Thus small-molecule BCL2 inhibitors currently in development for other cancers, such as Obatoclax, ABT-737, and TW-37,[95] may also prove to be effective therapeutic agents for retinoblastoma. Retinoblastomas are also highly sensitive to HDAC inhibition, and many HDAC inhibitors are currently in clinical trials.[96]

Retinoblastoma is unique because several well-established routes of drug delivery exist that provide flexibility when considering novel therapeutics. Systemic routes can be used for some drugs but are typically limited by poor penetration across the blood-retinal barrier (BRB) and systemic toxicity concerns.[89] Local ocular delivery routes include topical (transcorneal), periocular (transcleral), intravitreal (direct injection) and intraarterial infusion. However all routes are not amenable to all compounds because of the physiochemical property of the compounds, the effects on normal tissues, and the schedule of drug administration. Some chemotherapy drugs such as topotecan effectively cross the BRB, and equivalent intraocular pharmacokinetic (PK) profiles result from either systemic or local topotecan.[77,97] Topotecan is routinely administered daily for 5 days in children with cancer, providing repeat tumor exposure in an outpatient setting. In contrast carboplatin and nutlin-3a[79,98] cannot be administered systemically because of insufficient penetration of the BRB, and in these cases, subconjunctival injections have been a significantly more effective delivery route. However subconjunctival injections are only performed during examination with use of an anesthetic once every 3 weeks, precluding the opportunity for repeat dosing of the drug. Moreover reports of significant and dose-limiting local ocular toxicities of carboplatin have prevented widespread use of subconjunctival delivery for children with retinoblastoma. These studies highlight the importance of pharmacokinetics and toxicokinetics in drug-specific route selection for intraocular targets.

Because of the young age of the patient population and the relatively rarity of the disease, preclinical testing is a critical component of developing retinoblastoma therapeutics. A standardized approach for evaluating efficacy and safety using mouse genetic models of retinoblastoma and human orthotopic xenograft models has been developed, but the large number of potential compounds, routes, and formulations precludes preclinical testing of all possible combinations. Previous work suggests that, given the unique challenges of drug delivery to the eye, one way to streamline the candidate selection process is to determine which route and formulation achieve optimal PK before conducting preclinical studies. When administered using the routes and formulations that, according to PK studies, achieved target intraocular exposure, topotecan, nutlin-3a, and carboplatin were all efficacious. In contrast, despite promising in vitro cytotoxicity, subconjunctival delivery of a SYK inhibitor failed to provide efficacy in preclinical studies; this failure was related to insufficient exposure. However alternative formulations and routes of local delivery did improve PK compared with systemic delivery; intraocular concentration never reached levels required for cytotoxicity.

In conclusion, effective translational research for retinoblastoma is built on a foundation of outstanding basic research to advance our understanding of the pathways that are deregulated in this devastating childhood cancer. From there, suitable targets for therapy are identified, such as MDM4, HDAC, or SYK, and small molecules that disrupt signaling through those pathways are identified and tested for in vitro cellular effects. Next pharmacokinetic, pharmacodynamic, and toxicokinetic studies are combined with approaches to optimize formulation of the drugs for the different routes of delivery. Finally when suitable exposure is achieved with minimal toxicity, comprehensive preclinical testing using validated preclinical models is performed to compare efficacy of the new combination with current standard of care and other possible novel therapeutic approaches. Variations in schedule and integration with upfront standard of care therapy can also be tested at this stage to achieve an optimal route, dose, and schedule for a new retinoblastoma clinical trial.

GENETIC COUNSELING FOR FAMILIES WITH RETINOBLASTOMA

Retinoblastoma is a unique neoplasm in that the genetic form imparts a predisposition to developing tumor in an autosomal-dominant fashion with almost complete penetrance (85% to 95%).[99] The majority of such children acquire the first mutation as a new germline mutation, with only 15% to 25% having a positive family history. However some families display an inheritance pattern characterized by reduced penetrance and expressivity.[26] These low-penetrance retinoblastoma mutations either cause a reduction in the amount of normal protein produced or result in a partially functional mutant protein.[100] An MDM2 polymorphism has also been shown to modify the clinical penetrance of the RB1 mutation, either by enhancing RB1 haploinsufficiency or by increasing resistance to p53-mediated apoptosis.[101] Also the *RB1* gene mutation can occur at a late stage of embryogenesis, resulting in a variable expression depending on the tissue, causing mosaicisms in 10% to 15% of the patients or their progenitors.[102] In general, however, based on the inheritance pattern and considering the existence of mosaicisms, the following risk estimates can be made,[99] which may be refined on the basis of DNA sequence analysis of the *RB1* gene in the patient with retinoblastoma and his or her offspring or siblings.

1. Risk for offspring of survivors of retinoblastoma:
   a. The risk of retinoblastoma arising in the offspring of survivors of bilateral disease is 45%.
   b. In the case of patients with unilateral disease, investigators have estimated the risk of retinoblastoma overall to be 2.5%. However this estimate includes offspring of survivors of unilateral retinoblastoma who have a positive family history and whose risk is similar to that of bilateral cases—45%. If the family history is negative and genetic screening has not been performed, the actual risk is probably less than 2%.
2. Risk for siblings of patients with retinoblastoma: In the case of siblings of bilaterally affected children whose parents are also affected, the risk of developing retinoblastoma is 45%; if the sibling is unilaterally affected, the risk is 30%. For cases without a family history, the empirically derived risk is 2% for siblings of bilateral cases and 1% for siblings of unilateral cases.

Genetic counseling is of the utmost importance to assist parents in understanding the genetic consequences of each form of retinoblastoma and to estimate the risk in relatives. Counseling is relatively straightforward when a parent is affected, or when the child presents with bilateral disease; these patients all have the heritable form. For children without an affected parent who have only a single tumor, there is always a question about whether they carry the mutated gene. Children with unilateral disease who are older than 2 years at the time of diagnosis are not likely to be gene carriers, but we recommend that all children with retinoblastoma be screened for mutations in *RB1*, regardless of laterality and age at diagnosis. With the refinement in methods of mutational analysis during the past decade, detection rates have increased from 20% to 30%,[103,104] to 70% to 80%,[105,106] to greater than 90% at present.[26] Given the heterogeneity in the site and type of gene defects, no single technology will be sensitive and effective, and a multistep approach must be taken. More than 80% of the mutations can be detected with sequencing of the 27 exons of the *RB1* gene using a quantitative multiplex polymerase chain reaction.[26,105] However 10% to 20% of the defects are due to large deletions,[104,105] and therefore deletion scanning and Southern blotting is required for cases with no detectable mutations by quantitative multiplex polymerase chain reaction. Finally a small proportion of cases (probably less than 5%) may result from gene inactivation by promoter methylation, and therefore screening for constitutional[26,105] methylation should be considered if the other methods do not reveal a mutation. Finally 1% to 2% of retinoblastomas have germline *RB1*, and in these cases *MYCN* amplification and chromothripsis of the *RB1* gene may be the initiating events.[27]

With the recent improvements in the detection rates, genetic testing could be performed in the offspring of retinoblastoma survivors who are known to have the mutated gene (detection of the mutation is relatively easily accomplished if the parental mutation is known), and screening can be tailored appropriately. Even if genetic screening is negative for the mutation, newborn siblings of children with retinoblastoma should be examined periodically until they are about 2 years of age, because inherited retinoblastoma would be extremely rare beyond that age. In the future if the false-negative rate is negligible, one might expect that molecular diagnosis of mutations would lead to earlier treatment and better health outcomes for patients with retinoblastoma, with lower cost than conventional surveillance for children at risk.[26]

PATHOLOGY OF RETINOBLASTOMA

Retinoblastoma arises from the photoreceptor elements of the inner layer of the retina and usually extends into the vitreous cavity as a fleshy nodular mass (endophytic retinoblastoma).[107] Less frequently it extends externally, causing a secondary retinal detachment, in which case there is no localized visible vitreous nodule (exophytic retinoblastoma). Macroscopically retinoblastoma is soft and friable and it tends to outgrow its blood supply, with resulting necrosis and calcification. Because of its friability, dissemination within the vitreous and retina in the form of small, white nodules (seeds) is common. In those cases it may be difficult to distinguish a multicentric primary tumor from a disseminated tumor.

Microscopically the appearance of retinoblastoma depends on the degree of differentiation. Undifferentiated retinoblastoma is composed of small, round, densely packed cells with hypochromatic nuclei and scant cytoplasm. Several degrees of photoreceptor differentiation have been described and are characterized by distinctive arrangements of tumor cells. Homer-Wright rosettes are composed of irregular circlets of tumor cells arranged around a tangle of fibrils with no lumen or internal limiting membrane. They are infrequently seen in retinoblastoma and are most often seen in other neuroblastic tumors such as neuroblastoma and medulloblastoma. Flexner-Wintersteiner rosettes, on the other hand, are specific for retinoblastoma. These structures consist of a cluster of low columnar cells arranged around a central lumen that is bounded by an eosinophilic membrane analogous to the external membrane of the normal retina. The lumen contains an acid mucopolysaccharide similar to that found around normal rods and cones. These rosettes are seen in 70% of tumors. The fleurettes are less often seen. In this case the cells exhibit even more ultrastructural characteristics of photoreceptor differentiation. They are composed of larger cells with abundant eosinophilic cytoplasm arranged in a distinctive fleur de lis pattern. Especially well-differentiated tumors composed almost entirely of fleurettes have been called retinomas or retinocytomas. Ultrastructurally retinoblastoma cells also demonstrate photoreceptor differentiation with the presence of the 9-0 microtubule doublet pattern, abundant cytoplasmic microtubules, synaptic ribbons, and neurosecretory granules.[108,109]

Dissemination of retinoblastoma occurs via several routes. Choroidal invasion provides access to a rich vascular network that serves as a potential route for distant metastases. In advanced cases direct extension occurs through the sclera into the orbit. Retinoblastoma can also invade the iris and the ciliary body and metastasize to the regional lymph nodes. Finally retinoblastoma can extend along the optic nerve, gaining access to the subarachnoid space and intracranial cavity. In cases of disseminated disease, positive cone-rod homeobox (CRX) staining may help differentiate retinoblastoma from other common small, blue, round cell malignancies of childhood.[110] The typical macroscopic and microscopic characteristics of retinoblastoma are depicted in Figure 56-1. Guidelines for processing and evaluation of the enucleated eye have been published.[111]

CLINICAL MANIFESTATIONS OF RETINOBLASTOMA

Retinoblastoma is by definition a tumor of the young child, and the age at presentation correlates with laterality. Patients with bilateral retinoblastoma tend to present at a younger age (usually before 1 year) than do patients with unilateral disease (often in the second or third year of life).[99,112] Half of the cases of retinoblastoma diagnosed during the first year are bilateral, compared with fewer than 10% of cases diagnosed after 1 year of age.[1] It is rare for retinoblastoma to be diagnosed during the first month of life, except in familial cases in which examination has been recommended early, however, regardless of the family history, in more than 90% of neonatal cases, either bilateral disease is present at presentation or asynchronous bilateral retinoblastoma will develop.[107]

In more than half of cases the presenting sign is leukocoria, which occasionally is first noticed after a flash photograph (Fig. 56-2). Strabismus, the second most common presenting sign, usually correlates with macular involvement. Very advanced intraocular tumors may become painful as a result of secondary glaucoma.[112] Other childhood diseases that can present with leukocoria must be considered, such as persistent hyperplastic primary vitreous, retrolental fibrodysplasia, Coats disease, congenital cataracts, toxocariasis, and toxoplasmosis. In some series these nonmalignant conditions account for a significant proportion of enucleated eyes.[113,114] In familial cases, the diagnosis is usually made through screening, although almost 50% of familial cases are diagnosed later in life, when patients present with the typical signs of retinoblastoma, underscoring the importance of genetic counseling.[112]

The successful management of retinoblastoma depends on the ability to detect the disease while it is still intraocular. Disease stage correlates with delay in diagnosis.[115,116] In developing countries, late referrals are strongly associated with orbital and metastatic disease (Fig. 56-2).[116-118] For this reason, eye assessment should be performed in all newborns and at all subsequent health supervision visits by the primary care provider.[119] Eye assessment is encouraged in all newborns and at subsequent health visits. The consensus guidelines by the American Academy of Pediatrics and Bright Futures for Pediatric Preventive Care include health supervision visits at birth and at 3 to 5 weeks of life, at 1, 2, 4, 6, 9, and 12 months during the first year, at 15, 18, and 24 months during the second year, and at 30 months and 3, 4, and 5 years of life. Importantly evaluation of vision and ocular health, including red reflex examination, is a component of each health supervision visit. Mass screening is also being considered, especially where the tumor presents in advanced stages, such as in areas of South America and Asia. Photoscreening is a system by which a photograph is produced by a calibrated camera under prescribed lighting conditions, which shows a red reflex in both pupils. A trained observer can identify ocular abnormalities by recognizing characteristic changes in the photographed pupillary reflex. This technique is fast, efficient, and reproducible, but it is still evolving.[120]

Most patients with bilateral retinoblastoma carry a germline mutation of the RB1 gene. However a small proportion (5% to 6%) carry a deletion involving the 13q14 locus, which is large enough to be detected by karyotype analysis, either as a deletion or as part of a balanced translocation, most typically t(X;13).[121] In those cases retinoblastoma is part of a more complex syndrome resulting from the loss of additional genetic material. Patients with the 13q deletion syndrome are characterized by typical facial dysmorphic features, subtle skeletal abnormalities, and different degrees of mental retardation and motor impairment.[122-124] Dysmorphic features more consistently found include thick anteverted ear lobes, a high and broad forehead, a prominent philtrum, and a short nose.[122,123] A proportion of patients also

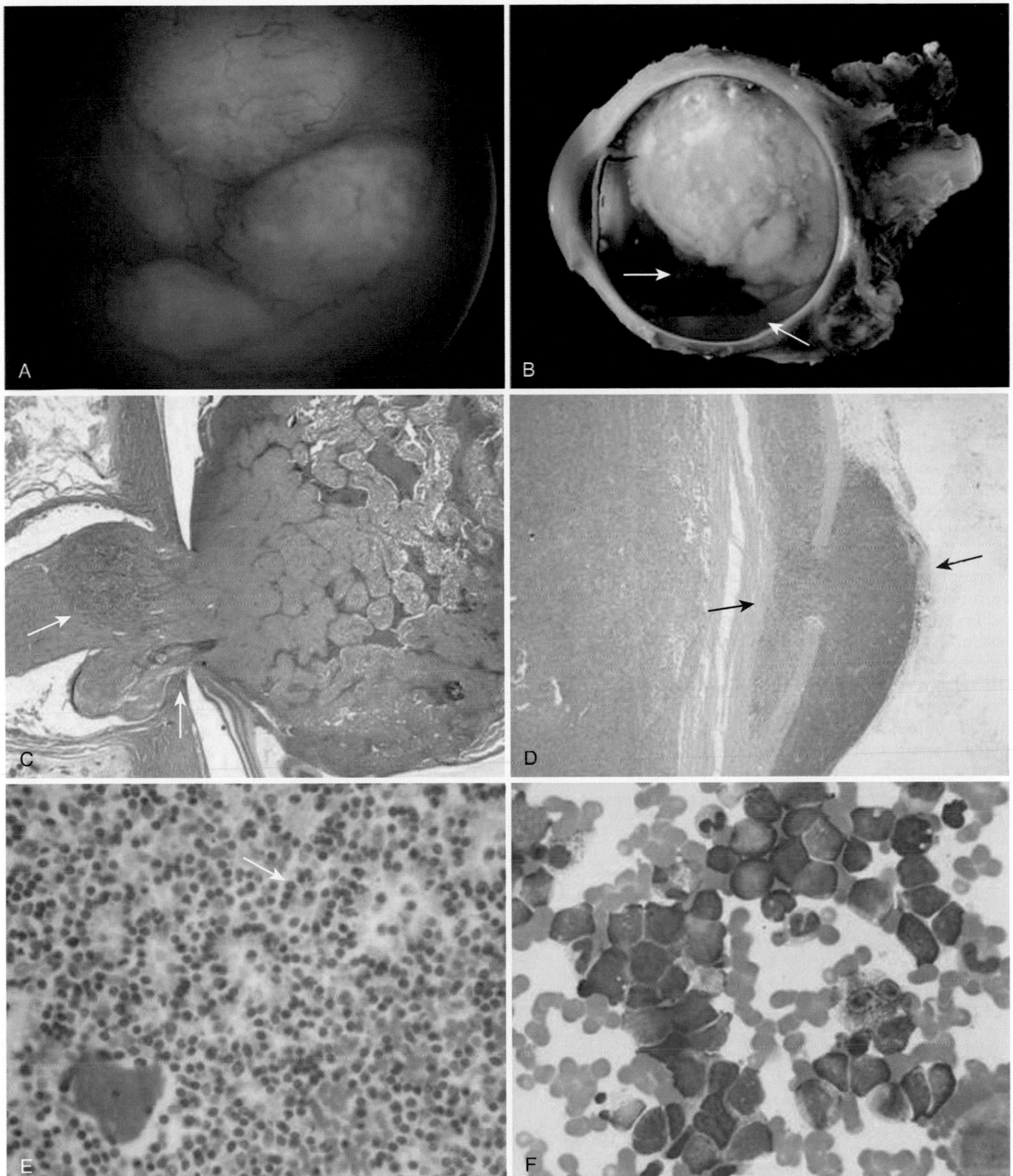

Figure 56-1 Pathology of retinoblastoma. **A,** Dilated eye examination of a group E retinoblastoma. **B,** Gross appearance of an enucleated eye showing a large retinoblastoma filling the posterior chamber, vitreous seeds and retinal detachment *(arrows)*. **C,** Retinoblastoma invasion of the optic nerve *(arrow)*. **D,** Transscleral invasion *(arrows)*. **E,** Microscopic appearance of retinoblastoma showing distinctive rosettes *(arrow)*. **F,** Metastatic retinoblastoma to the bone marrow.

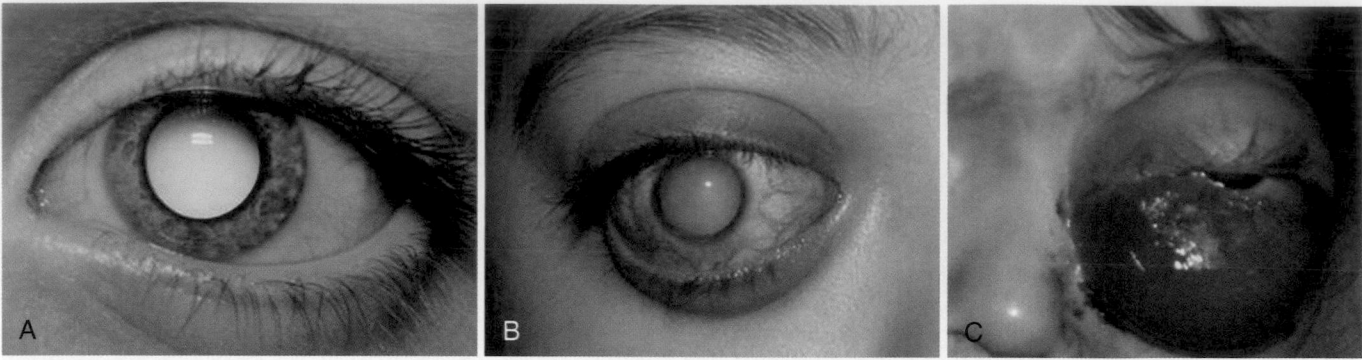

Figure 56-2 Clinical presentation of retinoblastoma showing progressive delay in diagnosis and referral. Retinoblastoma usually presents as leukocoria (**A**), but as disease advances, patients present with buphthalmos (**B**) and extraocular disease (**C**).

have overlapping fingers and toes, microcephaly, and delayed skeletal maturation. The severity of the deficits correlate with the size of the deletion; normal psychomotor development may be seen in patients in whom the deletion is restricted to the 13q14 band.[122]

Trilateral retinoblastoma refers to the association of bilateral retinoblastoma with an asynchronous intracranial tumor (Fig. 56-3).[125-127] Tumors comprising trilateral retinoblastoma are primitive neuroectodermal tumors (PNETs) exhibiting varying degrees of neuronal or photoreceptor differentiation, suggesting an origin from the germinal layer of primitive cells.[128] This association can occur in 3% to 9% of patients with the heritable form and appears to be more common in familial cases. Until recently the prognosis has been almost uniformly fatal; trilateral retinoblastoma has been the principal cause of death from retinoblastoma during the first decade of life in the United States.[129] The majority of these tumors are pineal region PNETs (pineoblastomas), but in 20% to

25% of cases, the tumors are suprasellar or parasellar. Rare cases of quadrilateral retinoblastoma have been reported, in which bilateral retinoblastoma is associated with both pineal region and suprasellar intracranial primary PNETs.[130] In most cases, the intracranial PNETs in association with retinoblastoma resemble undifferentiated retinoblastomas with the more frequent formation of Homer-Wright rosettes. The median age at diagnosis of trilateral retinoblastoma is 23 to 48 months,[125,126,129,131] and the interval between the diagnosis of bilateral retinoblastoma and the diagnosis of the brain tumor is usually more than 20 months.[127,131] Suprasellar tumors are usually diagnosed earlier,[127] and in 15% to 20% of cases, the intracranial tumor antecedes the diagnosis of retinoblastoma.[126] In recent years with the more widespread use of chemoreduction treatments and the decrease in the use of radiation therapy for patients with bilateral retinoblastoma, the incidence of trilateral retinoblastoma has decreased dramatically.[132,133] However pineal cysts

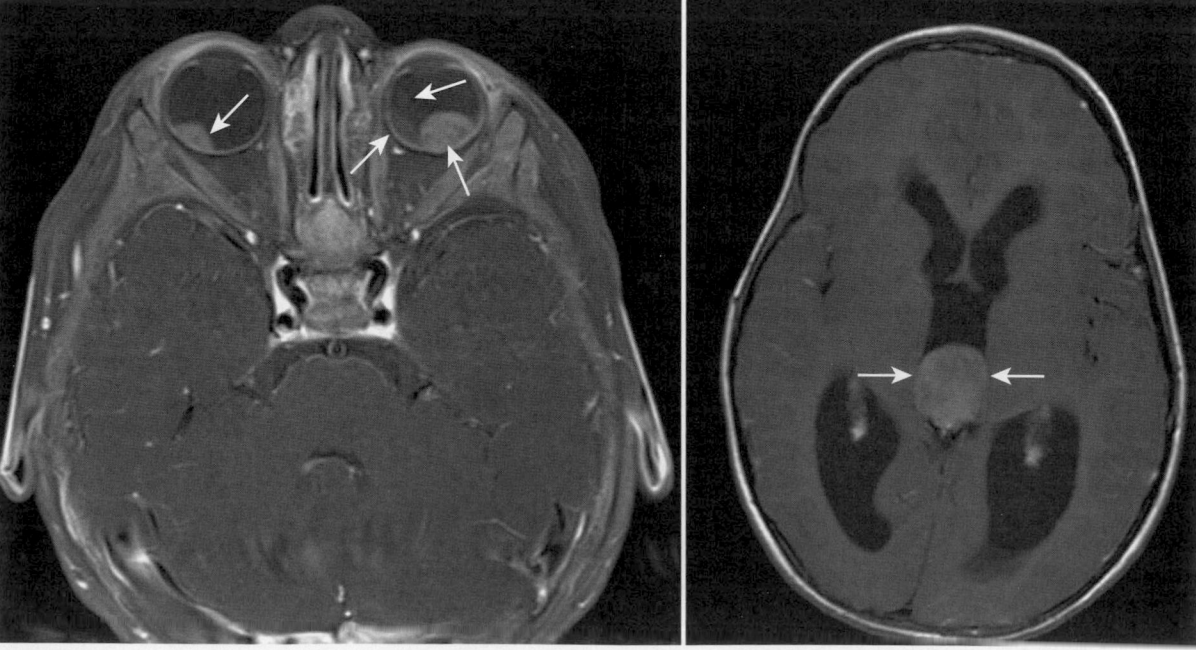

Figure 56-3 A, An axial T1-weighted magnetic resonance image showing bilateral intraocular masses in an 8-month-old infant with retinoblastoma *(arrows)*. **B,** A pineal gland tumor *(arrow)* in a 3-year-old child with a history of bilateral retinoblastoma and presenting with hydrocephalus.

develop in approximately 5% to 8% of patients with bilateral disease; these cysts appear to be a forme fruste of trilateral retinoblastoma.[133,134,135]

DIAGNOSIS AND EXTENT OF DISEASE EVALUATIONS IN RETINOBLASTOMA

The diagnosis of intraocular retinoblastoma is usually made without pathologic confirmation. An examination with use of an anesthetic with a maximally dilated pupil and scleral indentation is required to examine the entire retina. A careful examination of the iris and the anterior chamber is first performed, and the intraocular pressure is measured. Retinoblastoma usually appears as a mass projecting into the vitreous, although the presence of retinal detachment or vitreous hemorrhage may make its visualization difficult. Endophytic tumors are those that grow inward to the vitreous cavity. Because of its friability, endophytic retinoblastoma may seed the vitreous cavity (Fig. 56-4, D). Exophytic retinoblastoma grows into the subretinal space, thus causing progressive retinal detachment and subretinal seeding (Fig. 56-4, C). Exophytic tumors frequently resemble Coats disease. Less frequently retinoblastoma can adopt an infiltrative pattern without an obvious mass; this infiltrative pattern appears to be more frequent among older children. A very detailed documentation of the number, location, and size of tumors, the presence of retinal detachment and subretinal fluid, and the presence of vitreous and subretinal seeds must be performed. Wide-angle real-time retinal imaging systems such as RetCam (Clarity Medical Systems, Pleasanton, Calif.) provide a 130-degree field of view and digital recording, facilitating diagnosis and monitoring.

Additional imaging studies that aid in the diagnosis include bidimensional ultrasound, computerized tomography (CT), and magnetic resonance imaging (MRI). These imaging studies are particularly important to evaluate extraocular extension and to differentiate retinoblastoma from other causes of leukocoria. CT is very helpful to detect calcifications, although it is generally avoided to limit radiation exposure, particularly in children with bilateral disease, and MRI is very helpful in considering the differential diagnosis of Coats disease and other inflammatory conditions, along with persistent fetal vasculature of hyperplastic primary vitreous (Fig. 56-3).[136] In the absence of extraocular disease, MRI is not useful in the estimation of microscopic or optic nerve involvement.[137-139]

Evaluation for the presence of metastatic disease also needs to be considered in a subgroup of patients. Metastatic disease occurs in approximately 10% to 15% of patients, and it usually occurs in association with distinct intraocular histologic features, such as massive choroidal and scleral invasion, or with involvement of the iris or ciliary body and optic nerve beyond the lamina cribrosa.[140] In these cases additional staging procedures must be performed, including bone scintigraphy, bone marrow aspirates and biopsies, and lumbar puncture. In as many as one third of high-risk patients, the synthase of ganglioside GD2 messenger ribonucleic acid may be detected in the cerebrospinal fluid by reverse transcriptase-polymerase chain reaction, and it appears to correlate with massive involvement of the optic nerve, the presence of glaucoma at diagnosis, and a high risk of cerebrospinal fluid relapse.[141] In general in the absence of high-risk disease in patients undergoing enucleation, and in patients with intraocular disease who are undergoing ocular salvage therapies, a metastatic workup is usually not necessary. In patients with extraocular disease the use of immunocytology with GD2 or CRX staining may increase the yield for detection of small clumps of metastatic cells.[142,110]

STAGING OF RETINOBLASTOMA

The Reese-Ellsworth (R-E) grouping system has been generally accepted as the standard for intraocular disease. This grouping system was initially designed to predict the outcome after external beam radiation therapy (EBRT). It divides eyes into five groups on the basis of the size, location, and number of lesions and the presence of vitreous seeding (Box 56-1).[143] However developments in the conservative management of intraocular retinoblastoma have made the R-E grouping system less predictable of eye salvage and less helpful in guiding treatment.[85,144] A new staging system (International Classification of Retinoblastoma) has been developed, with the goal of providing a simpler, more user-friendly classification that is more applicable to current therapies. This new system is based on the extent of tumor seeding within the vitreous cavity and subretinal space rather than on tumor size and location, and it seems to be a better predictor of treatment success (Box 56-2; Fig. 56-4).[144,145]

For patients undergoing enucleation, pathologic staging that incorporates other features known to influence the modality of treatment and the prognosis, such as choroidal and scleral involvement, optic nerve extension, and the presence of metastatic disease, is used.

Box 56-1 Reese-Ellsworth Grouping for Suitability for Treatment of Retinoblastoma by Radiation Therapy

GROUP I. VERY FAVORABLE

Ia. Solitary tumor smaller than 4 dd at or behind the equator
Ib. Multiple tumors, none larger than 4 dd, all at or behind the equator

GROUP II. FAVORABLE

IIa. Solitary tumor, 4 to 10 dd, at or behind the equator
IIb. Multiple tumors, 4 to 10 dd, at or behind the equator

GROUP III. DOUBTFUL

IIIa. Any lesion anterior to the equator
IIIb. Solitary tumor larger than 10 dd behind the equator

GROUP IV. UNFAVORABLE

IVa. Multiple tumors, some larger than 10 dd
IVb. Any lesion extending anteriorly to the ora serrata

GROUP V. VERY UNFAVORABLE

Va. Massive tumors involving more than half the retina
Vb. Vitreous seeding

From Reese AB, Ellsworth RM: The evaluation and current concept of retinoblastoma therapy. Trans Am Acad Ophthalmol Otolaryngol 67:164–172, 1963.

dd, Disk diameter.

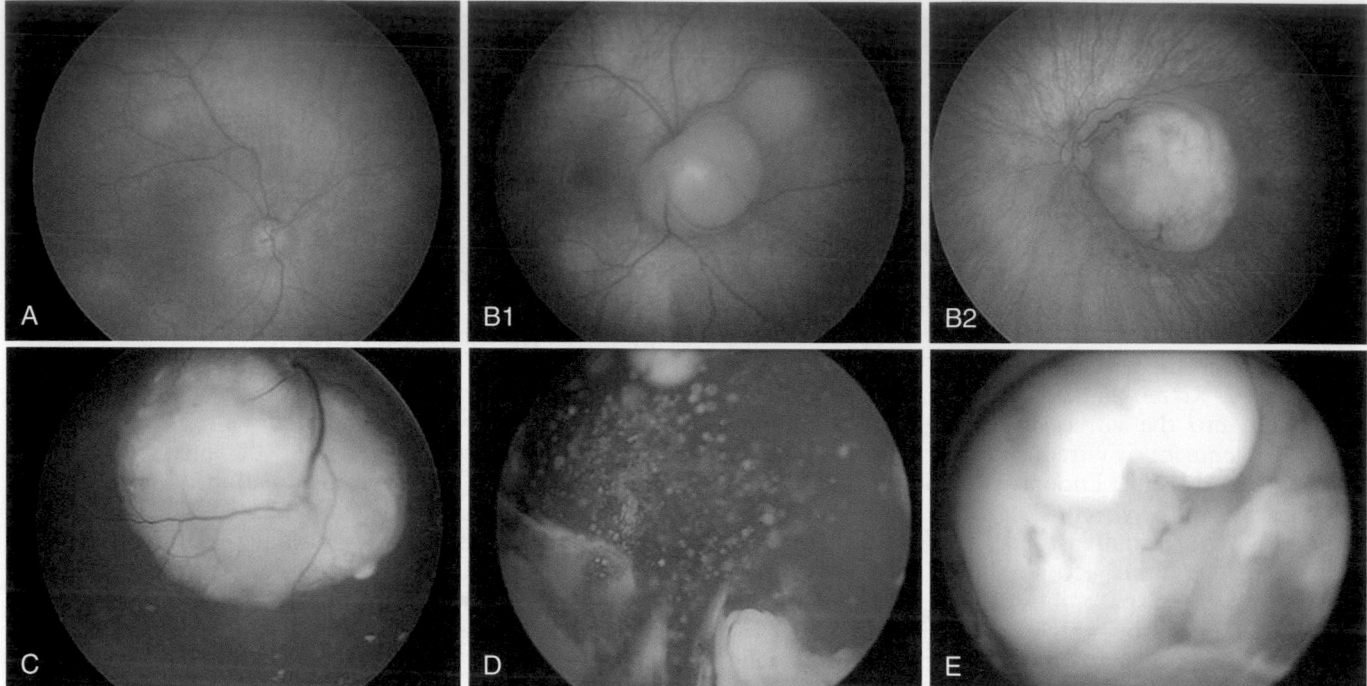

Figure 56-4 International Classification for Intraocular Retinoblastoma. **A,** A small tumor confined to the retina and distant from the foveola and the optic nerve (group A). **B1,** Two small tumors confined to the retina but adjacent to the optic nerve (group B). **B2,** Tumor with a small amount of subretinal fluid and no subretinal seeding (group B). **C,** Exophytic retinoblastoma with subretinal fluid and seeding (group C). **D,** Endophytic retinoblastoma with massive vitreous seeding (group D). **E,** Large retinoblastoma filling more than two thirds of the globe (group E).

Growth and invasion occur as a sequence of events, and extraretinal extension occurs only after the tumor has reached large intraocular dimensions.[146] As part of this process, retinoblastoma extends into the ocular coats (choroid and sclera), the optic nerve, and the anterior segment. Extraocular disease is the next step in this progression; locoregional dissemination occurs by direct extension through the sclera into the orbital contents and preauricular lymph nodes, and extraorbital disease manifests as intracranial dissemination and hematogenous metastases. Different staging systems have been classically used, including the Grabowski-Adamson,[147] the St. Jude Children's Research Hospital,[148] the American Joint

Committee on Cancer (AJCC),[149] and the International Retinoblastoma Staging System (IRSS).[150] The IRSS is a newly proposed staging system developed by an international consortium of ophthalmologists and pediatric oncologists that incorporates the most important elements of the older systems (Box 56-3). The IRSS (Box 56-3) and AJCC (Box 56-4) systems appear to be the most reliable for grouping patients according to their risk of extraocular relapse.[151]

Although the clinical significance of extraocular extension is obvious, there is no uniform agreement on the prognostic implications of the different histologic characteristics, resulting in the use of different staging

---

Box 56-2   International Classification for Intraocular Retinoblastoma

GROUP A

SMALL TUMORS AWAY FROM THE FOVEOLA AND DISC

- Tumors ≤3 mm in the greatest dimension confined to the retina, *and*
- Located at least 3 mm from the foveola and 1.5 mm from the optic disc

GROUP B

ALL REMAINING TUMORS CONFINED TO THE RETINA

- All other tumors confined to the retina not in group A
- Subretinal fluid (without subretinal seeding) ≤3 mm from the base of the tumor

GROUP C

LOCAL SUBRETINAL FLUID OR SEEDING

- Local subretinal fluid alone >3 to <6 mm from the tumor
- Vitreous seeding or subretinal seeding ≤3 mm from the tumor

GROUP D

DIFFUSE SUBRETINAL FLUID OR SEEDING

- Subretinal fluid alone >6 mm from the tumor
- Vitreous seeding or subretinal seeding >3 mm from the tumor

GROUP E

PRESENCE OF ANY OR MORE OF THESE POOR PROGNOSIS FEATURES

- More than two thirds of the globe is filled with tumor
- Tumor in the anterior segment
- Tumor in or on the ciliary body
- Iris neovascularization
- Neovascular glaucoma
- Opaque media from hemorrhage
- Tumor necrosis with aseptic orbital cellulitis
- Phthisis bulbi

From Linn Murphree AL: Intraocular retinoblastoma: the case for a new group classification. Ophthalmol Clin N Am *18:41–53, 2005.*

Box 56-3   **International Retinoblastoma Staging System**

Stage 0. Patients treated conservatively
Stage I. Eye enucleated, completely resected histologically
Stage II. Eye enucleated, microscopic residual tumor
Stage III. Regional extension
   a. Overt orbital disease
   b. Preauricular or cervical lymph node extension
Stage IV. Metastatic disease
   a. Hematogenous metastasis (without CNS involvement)
      1. Single lesion
      2. Multiple lesions
   b. CNS extension (with or without any other site of regional or metastatic disease)
      1. Prechiasmatic lesion
      2. CNS mass
      3. Leptomeningeal and CSF disease

From Chantada G, Doz F, Antonelli CBG, et al. A proposal for an international retinoblastoma staging system. Pediatr Blood Cancer 47:801–5, 2006.
CNS, Central nervous system; CSF, cerebrospinal fluid.

systems. Even in the absence of extraocular disease, a variable risk of developing metastatic disease exists.[152-160] Many studies have attempted to evaluate the risk associated with the different histologic variables. Two thirds of patients have exclusive retinal disease, and invasion of the anterior segment, choroid, and optic nerve occur in variable proportions and combinations in the remaining patients. Extension of tumor into the sclera and across the line of transection of the optic nerve are associated with elevated mortality and by definition are considered to represent extraocular disease.[157,159,160] The question arises when interpreting the other variables, because the risk associated with each variable is confounded by the lack of standardized grading methods and biased by the use of adjuvant chemotherapy.

Optic nerve involvement is common (occurring in 25% to 45% of all cases), but its impact on outcome appears to be limited to the involvement beyond the lamina cribrosa (where the meninges insert) and to the extension up to the transection line.[152,153,159-164] The mortality rates for untreated patients with those features are 40% to 60% and greater than 80%, respectively.[153-156,159,160]

Choroidal involvement is found in up to 40% of patients, although massive invasion occurs in fewer than 10% of cases.[156,158,161,164,165] This distinction is important, because although choroidal invasion might have prognostic implications,[140,152,162,166] its impact appears to be limited to cases with massive replacement by tumor.[158,161] However contrary to optic nerve evaluation, criteria for determining the extent of choroidal disease are more subjective, and the grading of invasion is seldom reported. Consensus criteria for definition of massive or significant choroidal invasion include a maximum diameter (thickness or width) of invasive focus of tumor of 3 mm or more in any diameter and reaching the inner fibers of the sclera. A tumor focus of less than 3 mm and not reaching the sclera is considered focal choroidal invasion.[111]

Evaluating the risk for each histologic variable individually is insufficient; different combinations of simultaneously occurring factors are very frequent.[146,167] When choroidal invasion is present, half the cases will also show optic nerve involvement, whereas optic nerve invasion is uncommon (20%) if the choroid is intact.[152,155,168] Conversely, when the optic nerve is invaded, 30% to 40% of cases will have choroidal replacement (more than 80% if the tumor has spread to the transection line), but significant choroidal invasion is quite rare (less than 20%) if the optic nerve is free of tumor.[152,154,155,167,168] Therefore the risk associated with each histologic variable can only be estimated in the light of its association with others. Most available data support the notion that choroidal invasion alone is not associated with increased risk of extraocular spread, although massive choroidal replacement by tumor may be an exception.[158,161] Similarly retrolaminar optic nerve invasion appears to be of prognostic significance only when there is concomitant significant choroidal invasion,[155,159,165,168,169] but this represents fewer than 20% of cases.[152,155] The significance of other histologic features, such as invasion of the anterior segment or grade of differentiation, remains unclear.[161,162] The presence of extensive tumor necrosis appears to correlate with high-risk histologic features, such as postlaminar optic nerve involvement and choroidal invasion.[170]

Clinical presentation correlates with disease only in cases of advanced intraocular disease; group E eyes, and those presenting with increased intraocular pressure or buphthalmos, have a higher frequency of high-risk histology.[164,171]

PRINCIPLES OF TREATMENT OF RETINOBLASTOMA

Treatment of retinoblastoma aims to save life and preserve useful vision, and thus it needs to be individualized. Factors that need to be considered include laterality of the disease and *RB1* germline status, potential for preserving vision, and intraocular and extraocular staging. For patients presenting with intraocular disease, particularly those with bilateral eye involvement, a conservative approach consisting of tumor reduction with intravenous or ophthalmic artery chemotherapy coupled with aggressive focal therapy may result in high ocular salvage rates. Radiation therapy, one of the most effective treatments in retinoblastoma, is usually reserved for cases of intraocular or extraocular disease progression.

Surgery

Enucleation is indicated for large tumors filling the vitreous for which there is little or no likelihood of restoring vision, and in cases of tumor present in the anterior chamber or in the presence of neovascular glaucoma. This corresponds to group E eyes and a significant proportion of group D eyes; upfront enucleation should be offered to those patients. Enucleation should be performed by an experienced ophthalmologist. The eye must be removed intact, without seeding the malignancy into the orbit and avoiding globe perforation. For optimal staging, a long section (10 to 15 mm) of the optic nerve needs to be removed with the globe. An orbital implant is usually fitted during the same procedure, and the extraocular muscles are attached to it. In the past, orbital

---

Box 56-4   American Joint Committee on Cancer Staging System

CLINICAL CLASSIFICATION (cTNM)

PRIMARY TUMOR (T)

TX	Primary tumor cannot be assessed
T0	No evidence of primary tumor
T1	Tumors no more than 2/3 the volume of the eye with no vitreous or subretinal seeding
T1a	No tumor in either eye is greater than 3 mm in largest dimension or located closer than 1.5 mm to the optic nerve or fovea
T1b	At least one tumor is greater than 3 mm in largest dimension or located closer than 1.5 mm to the optic nerve or fovea. No retinal detachment or subretinal fluid beyond 5 mm from the base of the tumor
T1c	At least one tumor is greater than 3 mm in largest dimension or located closer than 1.5 mm to the optic nerve or fovea, with retinal detachment or subretinal fluid beyond 5 mm from the base of the tumor
T2	Tumors no more than 2/3 the volume of the eye with vitreous or subretinal seeding. Can have retinal detachment
T2a	Focal vitreous and/or subretinal seeding of fine aggregates of tumor cells is present, but no large clumps or "snowballs" of tumor cells
T2b	Massive vitreous and/or subretinal seeding is present, defined as diffuse clumps or "snowballs" of tumor cells
T3	Severe intraocular disease
T3a	Tumor fills more than 2/3 of the eye
T3b	One or more complications present, which may include tumor-associated neovascular or angle closure glaucoma, tumor extension into the anterior segment, hyphema, vitreous hemorrhage, or orbital cellulitis
T4	Extraocular disease detected by imaging studies
T4a	Invasion of optic nerve
T4b	Invasion into the orbit
T4c	Intracranial extension not past chiasm
T4d	Intracranial extension past chiasm

REGIONAL LYMPH NODES (N)

NX	Regional lymph nodes cannot be assessed
N0	No regional lymph node involvement
N1	Regional lymph node involvement (preauricular, cervical, submandibular)
N2	Distant lymph node involvement

METASTASIS (M)

M0	No metastasis
M1	Systemic metastasis
M1a	Single lesion to sites other than CNS
M1b	Multiple lesions to sites other than CNS
M1c	Prechiasmatic CNS lesion(s)
M1d	Postchiasmatic CNS lesion(s)
M1e	Leptomeningeal and/or CSF involvement

PATHOLOGIC CLASSIFICATION (pTNM)

PRIMARY TUMOR (pT)

pTX	Primary tumor cannot be assessed
pT0	No evidence of primary tumor
pT1	Tumor confined to eye with no optic nerve or choroidal invasion
pT2	Tumor with minimal optic nerve and/or choroidal invasion:
pT2a	Tumor superficially invades optic nerve head but does not extend past lamina cribrosa *or* tumor exhibits focal choroidal invasion
pT2b	Tumor superficially invades the optic nerve head but does not extend past lamina cribrosa *and* exhibits focal choroidal invasion
pT3	Tumor with significant optic nerve and/or choroidal invasion:
pT3a	Tumor invades optic nerve past lamina cribrosa but not to surgical resection line *or* tumor exhibits massive choroidal invasion
pT3b	Tumor invades optic nerve past lamina cribrosa but not to surgical resection line *and* exhibits massive choroidal invasion
pT4	Tumor invades optic nerve to resection line or exhibits extra-ocular extension elsewhere
pT4a	Tumor invades optic nerve to resection line but no extra-ocular extension identified
pT4b	Tumor invades optic nerve to resection line and extra-ocular extension identified

REGIONAL LYMPH NODES (pN)

pNX	Regional lymph nodes cannot be assessed
pN0	No regional lymph node involvement
pN1	Regional lymph node involvement (preauricular, cervical)
N2	Distant lymph node involvement

METASTASIS (pM)

cM0	No metastasis
pM1	Metastasis to sites other than CNS
pM1a	Single lesion
pM1b	Multiple lesions
pM1c	CNS metastasis
pM1d	Discrete mass(es) without leptomeningeal and/or CSF involvement
pM1e	Leptomeningeal and/or CSF involvement

From American Joint Committee on Cancer: Retinoblastoma. In Edge SB, Byrd DR, Compton CC, et al, editors: AJCC Cancer Staging Manual, ed 7, New York, 2010, Springer, p. 562–63.
CNS, Central nervous system; CSF, cerebrospinal fluid.

---

implants were avoided because it was believed that they would interfere with the palpation of the socket and clinical detection of orbital recurrence. However with improved understanding of the histologic risk factors and the availability of better imaging techniques to detect orbital disease, implants should be placed at the time of the enucleation. Different orbital implants are available, including polymethylmethacrylate, polyethylene, and coralline and bovine hydroxyapatite spheres. A tissue wrap to the implant is placed, which will allow the four rectus muscles to be anatomically reattached, thus providing implant motility with little resistance in the orbit. The size and type of implant are important to stimulate orbital growth. A ceramic false eye is later fitted in the orbital socket. Orbital exenteration is very seldom indicated, although it should considered in cases of tumor recurrence after radiation. For patients presenting with orbital disease, a judicious use of chemotherapy, surgery, and radiation therapy will result in effective tumor control, avoiding the need for orbital exenteration.

Focal Therapies

Focal treatments are used for small tumors (less than 3 to 6 mm) and in combination with chemotherapy.[172] In this setting of a patient undergoing chemotherapy for cytoreduction, focal treatments should be applied to tumors that fail to calcify; it is usually recommended to allow maximal reduction in tumor size with one or two cycles of chemotherapy prior to proceeding with aggressive focal consolidation to minimize the damage to the surrounding retina, particularly when the tumor is close to visually critical structures, such as the fovea and the optic nerve.[173] The focal therapies available to treat retinoblastoma include argon green laser, diode laser, cryotherapy, and brachytherapy. The use of each modality depends on the tumor location and size. Lasers are more commonly used to treat posterior tumors, whereas more anterior tumors are easily accessed with cryotherapy. Brachytherapy is reserved for tumors that cannot be consolidated with either of those two approaches, usually because of their size.[172]

Two wavelengths of light are used to treat retinoblastoma. The argon green laser, with a wavelength of 532 nm, photocoagulates tissue by inducing a temperature in excess of 65°C; it has been traditionally used to treat the retina edge surrounding a tumor in an effort to deprive the tumor of its blood supply and subsequently induce tumor regression, and for the treatment of retinal neovascularization due to radiation therapy.[172,174] Using an indirect ophthalmoscope, a double row of white burns is used to encircle the tumor, and powers of 250 to 350 mW and burn durations of 0.3 to 0.5 seconds are used.[172,175] This technique is limited to tumors measuring no greater than 4.5 mm in base and no greater than 2.5 mm in thickness. Debate exists as to whether the tumor surface should be directly treated for fear of releasing tumor cells into the vitreous. Newer generations of the 532-nm laser permit continuous delivery similar to that of the diode laser; such modalities have led some persons to advocate its use in the treatment of retinoblastoma.[172] If the tumor surface is treated, the desired end point remains a subtle whitening of the treated areas. Laser energy should be kept at the lowest possible level necessary to achieve the desired end point; powers in excess of 500 mW will result in tumor disruption and should be avoided. As with all focal therapies, treatment should be continued until the residual fish-flesh tumor regresses into a flat chorioretinal scar. Typically treatment with lasers is administered every 3 to 4 weeks. The optimal indication for direct treatment with the argon green laser is a residual fish-flesh mass overlying a largely calcified tumor. In such situations, the uptake of the diode laser is unpredictable. With use of the argon green laser, a whitening of the tumor can be seen, ensuring an adequate treatment. The argon laser has both direct and indirect cytotoxic effects. Photocoagulation directly kills tumor cells, and the thermal spread from the laser may have secondary hyperthermic effects that act synergistically with ongoing chemotherapy. Argon laser photocoagulation should not be performed if there is a retinal detachment overlying the tumor.[172]

The diode laser, with a wavelength of 810 nm, was adapted for the treatment of retinoblastoma based on its success in the treatment of choroidal malignant melanoma. The laser energy is readily absorbed by melanin pigment and proved successful in the treatment of small melanocytic tumors.[172] Low-power settings coupled with a large spot size (2 to 3 mm) and prolonged delivery achieved hyperthermia (45°C to 65°C) at subphotocoagulation temperatures. The end result was a sustained penetrant burn with direct cytotoxic effects.[172] The term *transpupillary thermotherapy*, or TTT, was coined to describe this technique.[176,177] The methods of TTT were subsequently adapted to treat retinoblastoma. The infrared laser is focused directly on the tumor surface using either an ophthalmic microscope adapter or a large spot size indirect ophthalmoscope adapter. When using the indirect ophthalmoscope for TTT, it is important to ensure that the correct adapter is being used, because adapters designed for diode photocoagulation will not provide a continuous wavelength delivery necessary for hyperthermia.[172,178] For small tumors the underlying retinal pigment epithelium aids in absorption and transfer of the heat to the tumor. The desired end point is a subtle whitening of the tumor free of hemorrhage. Powers are titrated based on the tumor size and pigmentation of the underlying retinal pigment epithelium but should not exceed 600 mW when there is visible uptake by the surrounding retinal pigment epithelium. Tumors with significant elevation or residual elements that rest on adjacent calcified tumor do not readily whiten with TTT. Prolonged treatment sessions of 5 to 10 minutes using powers of 600 to 800 mW may be needed to achieve a therapeutic effect. Even with such prolonged treatment, a visible change in the tumor may not be seen until follow-up examination 3 to 4 weeks later. If available the argon green laser may provide a more effective treatment.[172] The sequential administration of thermotherapy with carboplatin enhances the antitumor effect by increasing the platinum-DNA adducts, for which reason thermochemotherapy is becoming a very important component in the treatment of intraocular retinoblastoma.[81,83]

Cryotherapy is used for the treatment of small equatorial and peripheral lesions, measuring no more than 3.5 mm in base and no more than 2 mm in thickness.[172,179,180] Cryotherapy is directly cytotoxic, causing cell lysis by disruption of the cell membrane that occurs after the formation of cytoplasmic ice crystals. Nitrous oxide gas is used to deliver a transscleral freeze via a cryoprobe under direct visualization. The lesion to be treated is visualized with an indirect ophthalmoscope, and the scleral underlying the tumor is indented with a cryoprobe. A succession of three freezes with three intervening thaws is applied to the tumor. An "ice ball" should be seen to encompass the tumor and adjacent vitreous with each freeze. Treatment should be limited to the area of the tumor to minimize damage to adjacent normal retina. Multiple tumors may be treated at one examination, but extensive treatments should be avoided. Aggressive cryotherapy may cause serous retinal detachments and iatrogenic retinal breaks. Although each cryotherapy unit may vary, we target a freezing temperature of −70°C during treatment. Treatments should be repeated at 3- to 4-week intervals until the lesion regresses to a flat chorioretinal scar. Posterior tumors can also be treated with cryotherapy. The conjunctiva is opened in the quadrant of the tumor to be treated. The curved cryoprobe is passed along the curvature of the eye and the tumor is indented. Once the tumor has been identified, the triple freeze-thaw is applied. This "cut-down" cryotherapy is usually reserved for recurrent posterior tumors not amenable to laser treatment.[172] Also in addition to its effect on tumor control, cryotherapy contributes to increase the intraocular penetration of chemotherapy agents, presumably through disruption of the blood-vitreous barrier.[181,182] In general local control rates of 70% to 80% can be achieved.[174,180,83] Complications of focal treatments include transient serous retinal detachment, retinal traction and tears, and localized fibrosis.[179]

Chemotherapy

Chemotherapy is indicated in patients with extraocular disease, in the subgroup of patients with enucleated eyes with intraocular disease and high-risk histologic features, and in patients with bilateral disease in conjunction with aggressive focal therapies. Agents with documented efficacy include microtubule inhibitors (vincristine and paclitaxel), platinum compounds (cisplatin and carboplatin), topoisomerase II inhibitors (teniposide and etoposide), alkylating agents (cyclophosphamide and ifosfamide), anthracyclines (doxorubicin and idarubicin), and topoisomerase I inhibitors (topotecan).[183,184] The first clinical experience with chemotherapy in the treatment of retinoblastoma was reported with the use of nitrogen mustard in 1953.[185] Institutional experiences in the management of extraocular retinoblastoma were reported subsequently, usually applying regimens modeled after the treatment regimens for metastatic neuroblastoma.[186,187] Since then the role of chemotherapy has continued to expand, and it is now a main component in the management of intraocular disease.

Ocular Pharmacokinetics

Application of new therapeutic possibilities for cancer treatment involves drug delivery in many forms, but ocular drug delivery is hampered by the barriers protecting the eye. The eye is protected from the xenobiotics of the bloodstream by blood-ocular barriers. The anterior blood-eye barrier (blood-aqueous barrier) is constituted by the endothelial cells in the uvea. This barrier limits access of hydrophilic drugs from plasma into the aqueous humor; however, inflammation may disrupt the integrity of this barrier, causing unlimited drug distribution to the anterior chamber. The posterior blood-eye barrier (BRB) is formed by the neural retina, the retinal pigment epithelium (RPE), and the tight walls of retinal capillaries. The inner border of the neural retina faces the vitreous, and the outer border is next to the RPE. The neural retina is composed of nine layers, and the RPE is composed of a monolayer of polarized cells. The blood supply to the inner two thirds of the retina is from retinal vessels; the retinal endothelial cells have basal lamina, and they are surrounded by pericytes, thus forming tight junctions. The blood supply to the outer third of the retina and the RPE comes from the choroidal circulation. Unlike the retinal capillaries, the vasculature of the choroid has extensive blood flow and leaky walls; drugs easily gain access to the choroid extravascular space, but thereafter distribution into the retina is limited by the RPE and retinal endothelia.[188,189] Lipophilicity, molecular weight, and protein binding (It is believed that only unbound drugs can pass through the BRB) are the main factors for penetration through the barrier. Inflammation and trauma

also have important roles in breaking the BRB by disrupting tight junctions, increasing transendothelial vesicles, and increasing pinocytosis.[190] It is possible that a similar phenomenon occurs in retinoblastoma.

Ocular Drug Transporters

The BRB restricts the movements of substances after systemic and periocular administration to the retina. The tight junctions form the penetration barrier to hydrophilic substances, thereby limiting the transfer of compounds both inward (blood to vitreous) and outward (vitreous to blood). The RPE has many important features essential for normal retinal function, such as transport of nutrients and waste products, regulation of ion, and fluid balance. RPE thus expresses many transporters and channels related to these physiologic functions. Among those the RPE and the endothelial cells also express efflux transporters such as P-glycoprotein, multidrug resistance–associated protein–1, –4, and –5, and breast cancer resistance protein. This efflux protein activity restricts movements of certain drugs to the retina. In most cases this is an important protective system for the retina, but it also limits drug delivery to the posterior eye segment.[188] Many antineoplastic agents are known substrates of efflux proteins.

Mechanisms for Transscleral Drug Delivery

Transscleral drug delivery is a potential solution to the need to achieve high intraocular concentrations of chemotherapeutic agents. Traditionally subconjunctival, subtenon, and retrobulbar injections have been used to administer drugs such as steroids and local anesthetic agents. The high permeability of the sclera to macromolecules has revived the interest in this route of drug administration.[191] For transscleral drug delivery, the drug is placed into a periocular space (subconjunctival, subtenon, peribulbar, retrobulbar, or posterior juxtascleral), and it may permeate from the periocular space into the vitreous via the anterior chamber, via a direct penetration pathway across the sclera, or through the systemic circulation. In the anterior chamber route, the drug reaches the aqueous humor either directly across the sclera and ciliary body or indirectly via the tear fluid and cornea, and it subsequently diffuses to the posterior chamber and into the vitreous. In the direct penetration pathway, the drug permeates into the vitreous through the underlying tissues; in the anterior eye, the drug may diffuse through the ciliary body and then to the posterior chamber and vitreous, whereas in the posterior eye, the drug has to permeate across the choroid, retinal pigment epithelium, and neural retina to reach the vitreous. Finally a small proportion of the drug enters the general circulation via conjunctival, episcleral of choroidal vessels and returns into the eye with the systemic blood flow.[189] The relative importance of each route to vitreal drug delivery has been investigated in animal models. The direct penetration pathway is the most important route in the vitreal delivery of most compounds with widely differing physicochemical properties.[191]

The drug must permeate across several tissues, and some of the barriers are different in the anterior and posterior eye. The RPE is the rate-limiting permeation barrier in the retinal delivery of hydrophilic drugs and macromolecules through the transscleral route. Permeability in RPE is determined both by physical-chemical factors (e.g., molecular weight, lipophilicity, and charges) and affinity to active transporters. The transporters may decrease or increase the drug transfer across the RPE depending on the type of transporter (influx or efflux) and its location (vitreal or blood side). The permeating drug also faces active barriers such as the clearance via choriocapillaris blood flow. The choroidal blood flow is higher than in any other tissue (relative to the tissue weight), and choriocapillaris walls contain large fenestrations. Large macromolecules are able to diffuse through the fenestrations in rabbit choriocapillaris. In a rabbit model for administration of triamcinolone acetonide, elimination of the blood flow with cryotherapy did not result in improved penetration of the drug after subtenon administration.[61,192] The orbital and conjunctival vasculature and lymphatics seem to have a larger role in drug clearance than does the choroid. The elimination of conjunctival lymphatic and blood flow by incising a small window in the conjunctiva was more effective in increasing the vitreous concentration than was the elimination of the choroidal blood flow. When considering the orbital clearance, the posterior subtenon location appears to be the best periocular route, because it is closer to the sclera and farther from the orbital vasculature.[193] After periocular injection, the drug must penetrate across the sclera, which is more permeable than the cornea. However for the drug to reach the retina, it must pass across the choroid and RPE (a tighter barrier than the sclera), at which point drugs may be cleared significantly to the bloodstream.[194]

The sclera has a large surface area (16.3 cm^2), and scleral permeability shows no dependence on lipophilicity but dependence on molecular radius. The sclera is composed of collagen and proteoglycan fibers with few protein-binding sites. Drugs permeate through the aqueous intercellular media of the sclera, occupying the pores between the collagen fibers. Pore diameter and intercellular space are important determinants of transscleral drug delivery, particularly for drugs such as large hydrophilic peptides and oligonucleotides. Scleral permeability is affected by an increase in intraocular pressure.[190] Scleral permeability may be enhanced in several ways. Treatment of many ocular diseases incorporates the use of transscleral depots, either as scleral implants (used for antiinflammatory agents) or collagen matrix and fibrin sealants, or the use of microspheres and other nanoparticles.[190,195]

Periocular Chemotherapy in Retinoblastoma

Control of the intraocular tumor burden requires achieving high levels of chemotherapeutic agents in all the intraocular compartments, including the vitreous, the subretinal space, and the ocular coats. Although it is effective systemic administration of chemotherapy is limited by the blood-ocular barriers previously described. In recent years methods to increase the intraocular concentrations of chemotherapeutic agents have been extensively investigated, and periocular administration of carboplatin has been incorporated into most regimens for the treatment of advanced intraocular retinoblastoma. In the transgenic murine retinoblastoma treated with intravitreous injections of carboplatin, inhibition of tumor growth occurs in a dose-dependent manner,[196] thus suggesting that higher intraocular levels of chemotherapy would be desirable. In this retinoblastoma model, subconjunctival administration of carboplatin resulted in tumor control in a dose-dependent manner,[197] suggesting good intraocular penetration of this agent when given periocularly. Pharmacokinetic studies performed in the rabbit eye have validated this method.[198] Mendelsohn and colleagues[199] compared the intraocular concentrations of agents after local or systemic administration in primates. Intravenous carboplatin was given at the standard dose used in humans (18.7 mg/kg), and systemic and intraocular pharmacokinetics were compared with peribulbar and episcleral injections of 10 mg of carboplatin. The intravenous administration resulted in higher levels in the aqueous humor than did peribulbar or episcleral injections. However vitreous levels were significantly higher when carboplatin was administered periocularly. Importantly systemic absorption after periocular administration was minimal; plasma levels of carboplatin were 3% of those achieved after intravenous administration. In the same study no etoposide was detected in the aqueous or vitreous humor when given systemically. Etoposide is a protein-bound drug, and it likely stays in the plasma and thus has limited penetration. Studies in the mouse model have also shown little intravitreal penetration of etoposide when given intravenously. The vitreous/plasma ratios when measured as area under the curve concentrations were 0.59 for carboplatin and 0.07 for etoposide.[76] However these models may not recapitulate the natural history of retinoblastoma because the blood-vitreous barrier is likely disrupted by tumor. In fact intraocular carboplatin concentrations in the human eye with retinoblastoma are higher after intravenous administration than what the primate eye model shows; levels in the vitreous are much higher than what the animal studies would predict and are similar to levels measured in unaffected animals when the drug is given after cryotherapy.[200] The periocular route has also been explored in animal models for topotecan[97,201] and for new investigational agents such as SYK and MDM4 inhibitors.[63,79]

Given the promising preclinical data, periocular administration of carboplatin has been progressively incorporated into the clinical practice. Patients tolerate the administration of 2 mL of the 10 mg/mL solution, although acute orbital toxicity is significant. In the only phase II study reported, responses were seen in three of the five eyes with vitreous disease and in two of the five eyes with retinal tumors.[202] The role of this form of administration in the management of retinoblastoma is still being evaluated. Patients with advanced intraocular disease (particularly those with massive vitreous or subretinal seeding) are candidates to receive up to three doses of periocular carboplatin concomitantly with systemic chemotherapy to maximize intraocular levels of the agent. However great caution should be exerted if periocular carboplatin is administered; acute toxicities (e.g., periorbital edema and inflammation) and long-term toxicities (e.g., orbital fat necrosis, soft tissue and muscle fibrosis, and optic neuritis) are common.[203,204] Although periocular carboplatin has a very limited role as a single agent, it may lead to long-term disease control when combined with other treatment modalities (Box 56-4).[205] Topotecan has also been used via periocular administration, although its intraocular penetration may be lower[97,201] and its potential role in therapy may be more limited.[206] In the animal model periocular administration of topotecan reached potentially active levels of its active lactone moiety without significant toxicity.[97] However systemic absorption was significant. A recently completed phase I study has documented the feasibility of administering 2 mg of topotecan periocularly, although no significant responses were seen.[160]

Although effective in increasing intraocular levels, subconjunctival administration of carboplatin or topotecan in aqueous media has many limitations. Most of the drug delivered is dispensed quickly throughout the subconjunctival space and surrounding orbit, thus exposing extraocular tissues to high transient concentrations of the drugs and potential toxicities. Methods for improving periocular delivery while minimizing toxicity include the use of a collagen matrix or fibrin sealants. Studies have shown that carboplatin may enhance fibrin clot formation.[207] One benefit of the sealant is that the anhydrous form of carboplatin can be overloaded beyond its solubility limit to provide higher levels of drug for extended periods. The scleral drug exposure is maximized, extending the duration of therapeutically significant intraocular drug penetration, and decreasing the need for repeated periocular injections.[208] However in the animal models, as the intraocular levels increase, so does the risk of retinal toxicity.[196,208,209]

Intravitreal and Intraarterial Chemotherapy for Intraocular Retinoblastoma

Administration of chemotherapy drugs directly into the tumor vasculature is a common practice in oncology. A small, localized tumor such as retinoblastoma would be an excellent candidate for such an approach. Japanese investigators have pioneered the administration of intravitreal and intraarterial melphalan for patients with advanced or recurrent intraocular retinoblastoma.[210,211] Preclinical data suggest that retinoblastoma is very sensitive to melphalan and that there is a synergistic effect with thermotherapy[212] and with other agents such as topotecan.[213] Direct delivery to the ocular vasculature has been limited by the technical difficulties in the cannulation of the retinal artery. Kaneko and Suzuki[210] initially reported the feasibility of injecting melphalan into the ipsilateral carotid artery, with documented efficacy. The technique was later perfected by Suzuki and colleagues[211] and Mohri[214] using a balloon catheter that allowed for selective injection into the ophthalmic artery. More recently Abramson and colleagues[215] reported a variation of this technique that includes a direct cannulation of the ophthalmic artery using a microcatheter (supraselective). Successful catheterization and delivery of chemotherapy

can be achieved in 98% of cases,[216,217] although in 16% of patients an alternative vascular route is required—often the orbital branch of the middle meningeal artery.[218] This approach has also been documented as being feasible as tandem therapy in patients with bilateral disease.[219]

Although melphalan has remained the most commonly used agent and the most effective agent, it is often combined with topotecan or carboplatin when responses are suboptimal or the intraocular disease is very advanced.[216,217,220-223] The doses of the chemotherapeutic agents are determined by patient age (and ocular volume) and by the angioanatomy; doses reported to result in a significant antitumor effect and limited toxicity are 2.7 to 7.5 mg for melphalan, 0.3 to 0.6 mg for topotecan, and 25 to 50 mg for carboplatin.[216,220,221,223,224] In pigs, the infusion of 7 mg of melphalan or 1 mg of topotecan to the ophthalmic artery results in peak vitreous levels higher than the inhibitory concentration of 50%, and with limited systemic exposure.[213,225] In children a large variability of systemic exposure occurs, and patients receiving tandem administrations of melphalan have a higher risk of the development of neutropenia, which correlates with plasma levels.[213]

Patients typically receive one to six (median, three) intraarterial administrations of chemotherapy including melphalan alone or in combination, and responses are usually seen immediately after the first administration. For patients with treatment-naive eyes, the 2-year radiation-free ocular survival rate is 80% to 90%.[216,220,223] Similar outcomes are also being reported with single-agent carboplatin and in combination with topotecan.[221] Outcome correlates with the intraocular burden; patients with early intraocular disease (group B and C eyes) have an excellent outcome and may be treated with single-agent therapy.[221,222] Eyes with significant vitreous or subretinal seeding have a worse outcome, with radiation-free survival rates of 80% for eyes with subretinal seeding and 65% for eyes with vitreous seeding.[226] For patients with very advanced intraocular disease, an alternative is the use of systemic chemotherapy followed by consolidation with intraarterial melphalan.[227] The presence of massive retinal detachment is not a contraindication to intraarterial chemotherapy; studies have shown that this approach promotes retinal reattachment and may result in ocular salvage rates in excess of 85%.[228] Ocular salvage rates when intraarterial chemotherapy administration is used as salvage for patients with recurrent or progressive disease are consistently lower, with globe survival rates of 50% to 60%.[216,217,223,226] However the use of a more intensive three-drug regimen with melphalan, topotecan, and carboplatin in patients whose disease has progressed after undergoing standard systemic and focal therapies has been reported to result in radiation-free ocular salvage rates of 75% at 2 years.[224]

Patients with bilateral disease can receive tandem administrations.[219] In those circumstances patients are at a higher risk of systemic toxicity as a result of melphalan exposure,[213] and single-agent carboplatin may be used to treat the eye with less advanced disease during the tandem procedure.[229] For neonates and very young infants for whom the cannulization of the ophthalmic artery is not feasible, a "bridge" treatment with single-agent systemic carboplatin until the baby is 3 months old or weighs 6 kg followed by consolidation with intraarterial chemotherapy has been shown to be very effective, with 1-year radiation-free ocular survival of 95%.[230]

Direct administration of high doses of chemotherapy to a sensitive organ such as the eye of a young child is not devoid of complications. In the nonhuman primate model, treatment with three cycles of melphalan or carboplatin results in a significant inflammatory response, with leukostasis and retinal arteriole occlusion with ultrastructural changes in the endothelial cells and surrounding pericytes. Eyes also show nerve fiber infarcts and optic nerve hemorrhage and leukostasis, central retinal artery thrombosis, choroidal inflammation, and birefringent intravascular foreign bodies.[231] Similar histopathologic evidence of vasculopathy is seen in enucleated eyes of children with retinoblastoma after intraarterial chemotherapy.[232] Clinically a transient chorioretinal ischemia has been documented during the procedure, the impact of which is not fully understood.[233,234] However approximately 15% of the eyes show a long-term sectorial choroidal atrophy, and 15% have delayed vitreous hemorrhage leading to enucleation.[222,235] The impact of the intraocular vascular changes on vision has not been fully assessed because of the young age of the first cohorts of patients treated. The majority of patients do not have substantial electroretinographic changes,[236] and preservation of central vision has been reported.[237] However in patients with heavily pretreated eyes, intensive intraarterial chemotherapy may result in worsening of retinal function.[224]

Acute and usually transient adverse events include mild eye edema, blepharoptosis, and orbital congestion with temporary dysmotility.[221,222,238] Systemic effects are minimal; grade III neutropenia develops in only 10% of patients,[216] although this proportion is higher in children with bilateral disease who undergo tandem therapy.[213] Major vascular complications are very rare; no strokes or significant acute neurologic events have been reported when the procedure is performed at a state of the art treatment center.[211,216,217] However stenosis of the ophthalmic artery and occlusion of the retinal artery have been documented.[238] The risk of thrombosis is significantly increased in children with thrombophilia.[239]

One additional risk associated with intraarterial chemotherapy is the exposure to ionizing radiation during fluoroscopy. In very experienced hands, the mean fluoroscopy time per procedure is 7 minutes.[240] Radiation doses per procedure can be as high as 191 mGy to the affected eye and 35 mGy to the contralateral eye,[241] although doses as low as 1 mGy per procedure have been reported by the center with the most experience in performing the procedure.[240] After multiple procedures, cumulative doses can reach 0.1 to 0.2 Gy, which can be cataractogenic and potentially carcinogenic in this susceptible population.[241] Long-term outcome data reported by Japanese investigators seem to indicate that no increase occurs in the incidence of second malignancies[211], however, longer follow-up will be required to fully ascertain the risks associated with the procedure.

To achieve the maximum concentrations of chemotherapy close to the tumor and in the vitreous, investigators have attempted direct intravitreal delivery. This approach was pioneered by Swedish investigators in the 1960s.[242,243] Thiotepa was the agent selected in those initial studies, and repeated injections of 1 to 1.5 mg were administered, often in conjunction with EBRT. Regressions were obtained, but long-term control of the intraocular disease was generally not possible. This approach was rekindled by Seregard et al.[244] in three patients with bilateral disease with recurrent retinoblastoma in a single remaining eye. Patients received repeated intravitreal injections of thiotepa, followed by vitrectomy and weekly injections, for a total cumulative dose of 10 to 14 mg of thiotepa; no obvious clinical responses were observed.

Direct administration of melphalan into the vitreous is a promising approach for patients with vitreous disease. Clinical responses in patients with progressive retinoblastoma were obtained with use of intravitreal melphalan followed by hyperthermia,[210] and more recent data seem to indicate that intravitreal chemotherapy may have a role in the management of patients with progressive vitreous disease.[245,246] This approach is currently being explored in combination with systemic chemotherapy for patients with advanced intraocular disease.

Radiotherapy

Retinoblastoma is a very radiosensitive tumor. Radiotherapy in combination with focal treatments can provide excellent tumor control.[247,248,249] However because radiation therapy increases the risk of second malignancies, contemporary management of intraocular retinoblastoma is designed to avoid or delay its use. The role of irradiation is mainly as salvage management for eyes that have failed to respond to chemotherapy and focal treatments, usually because of progression of vitreous and subretinal seeding.[250] Because most patients with intraocular retinoblastoma who undergo radiotherapy have multifocal disease, the entire retinal surface needs to be irradiated to a uniform dose. Several techniques can be used, usually through lateral or anterior fields.[247-249] Recommended total doses are 40 to 45 Gy, in 180 to 200 cGy fractions, although doses of 36 Gy and even lower may be effective in conjunction with other techniques.[82,251-253] Radioactive plaque technique is useful when treating localized tumors, both because the procedure time is short and because a high dose of irradiation is delivered to the areas of interest while minimizing irradiation effects in extraocular structures.

Episcleral Plaque Brachytherapy

Indications for plaque therapy include solitary tumors with a diameter ranging between 6 and 15 mm, tumor thickness of 10 mm or less, and location of the lesion more than 3 mm from the optic disc or fovea.[250] Since the early use of cobalt-60 plaques in the 1950s, the field has evolved to the more common use of iodine-125, iridium-192, and ruthenium-106.[254-258] In combination with appropriate use of chemotherapy and focal consolidation, brachytherapy can be very effective, even in the presence of focal vitreous seeding overlying the tumor.[250,259]

The most commonly used radioisotope is [125]iodine, a low-energy γ-ray emitter (27 to 35 keV; half-life, 60 days) that is readily available in encapsulated form, allowing custom fabrication of gold plaques of varying sizes.[254] [125]Iodine seeds are loaded within the wells of the plaque to achieve the dose and distribution desired based on the size and location of the tumor; lesions of up to 10 to 12 mm in height and 10 to 15 mm in diameter can be treated using this approach. [192]Iridium and [106]ruthenium are alternative isotopes of higher energy (295 to 612vkeV and 3.5 MeV, respectively) and longer half-life (74 and 374 days, respectively), which makes dosimetry calculations and safety measures more complex. The dose is prescribed to reach the tumor apex and overlying localized vitreous seeds if present. For [125]iodine the target dose is usually 40 Gy at the apex at 40 to −80 cGy per hour; the dose at the tumor base may approximate 120 Gy. Tumor control using this approach may be close to 80%. In approximately 25% of the eyes, long-term complications may occur, including nonproliferative retinopathy, papillopathy, and nonproliferative maculopathy.[254,260] Similar results are achieved with [106]ruthenium.[255]

External Beam Radiation Therapy

EBRT is commonly used as consolidation therapy in conjunction with chemotherapy for intraocular retinoblastoma when the disease is not responding well to conservative management, usually because of the presence of vitreous or subretinal seeding or progression of the retinal tumors, and in the management of extraocular disease.[250] Traditionally the opposed "D" fields have been used to treat bilateral retinoblastoma, with the isocenter placed 2 to 3 mm behind the lens; with this approach, aimed at sparing the lens, the retina anterior to the equator may be relatively underdosed.[261,262] Currently the use of conformal and intensity-modulated radiation therapy (IMRTs) can provide coverage of the entire retina and vitreous cavity while limiting the dose to the lacrimal gland and soft tissues and orbital bones.[262,263] The standard EBRT dose is 40 to 45 Gy, delivered in 180 to 200 cGy fractions; doses higher than 45 Gy do not seem to be associated with an increased benefit.[261] One study also showed the potential role of low-dose (26 Gy) EBRT to consolidate advanced intraocular retinoblastoma upon completion of chemotherapy, in the absence of disease progression.[253] IMRT may be superior to three-dimensional (3D) conformal radiation therapy and conventional two-dimensional irradiation in terms of the dose delivered to normal orbital and extraorbital tissues.[264] However although increasing the conformity of the treatment results in a sharp decline of the dose-volume curve at the higher doses, this gain still comes at the expense of increasing the volume of normal tissue that receives the lowest doses. Even with optimal IMRT planning, 50% of the orbit receives 50% of the prescribed dose.[250] The use of fractionated stereotactic radiation therapy may allow for a significant decrease in the orbital volume exposed.[265] Proton beam therapy allows for exquisite dosimetry, thus providing a theoretic advantage in sparing radiation exposure to orbital tissues.[263,266] A proton beam has exquisite stopping power and may produce essentially no lateral scatter, and thus protons can be used to control tumors at any depth without the entrance and exit doses associated with photon beam irradiation that are responsible for the complications associated with radiation therapy in patients with retinoblastoma.[266] In a study comparing protons with conformal therapy, electron therapy, and IMRT, protons had the best orbital bone-sparing dose distribution. Only 10% of the bone exceeded 5 Gy, compared with 25% for 3D–conformal radiation therapy electrons, 69% for IMRT, 41% for a single 3D lateral beam, 51% for a 3D anterolateral beam with a lens block, and 65% for a 3D anterolateral beam without a lens block.[250,266] Very importantly preliminary long-term data seem to indicate that the cumulative incidence of second malignancies in the irradiated field is significantly lower with protons when compared with standard photon therapy.[267]

Radiation therapy is indicated for extraocular retinoblastoma and after enucleation when high-risk features are present (e.g., transscleral involvement and involvement of the cut end of the optic nerve). The target volume is the orbit and may extend to include regional sites and lymph nodes based on clinical and imaging evidence of tumor extension. The dose typically used for treatment of the orbit or regional extraocular sites is 45 Gy. Radiation therapy may be indicated for patients with metastatic disease based on response to chemotherapy. In most treatment protocols, patients with hematogenous metastases or CNS involvement who achieve a complete response to induction chemotherapy do not undergo irradiation; however, patients with an incomplete response usually undergo irradiation at the completion of therapy, which often includes consolidation with high-dose chemotherapy and autologous hematopoietic stem-cell rescue. This sequence is also recommended for patients who require craniospinal irradiation. Based on age older patients who require craniospinal irradiation should receive 36 Gy to the neuraxis and 45 Gy to residual disease. Younger patients should receive at least 23.4 Gy to the neuraxis. Evidence suggests that clinically defined disease has limited microscopic tumor infiltration so that the clinical target volume surrounding the clinically identifiable residual tumor (gross tumor volume) may be as small as 5 mm.[250]

TREATMENT OF INTRAOCULAR RETINOBLASTOMA

Treatment of retinoblastoma is tailored to the intraocular and extraocular disease burden, disease laterality and germline status, and potential for vision (Fig. 56-5).

Unilateral Retinoblastoma

In the absence of extraocular disease, enucleation alone is curative for 85% to 90% of children with unilateral retinoblastoma.[113,161,165,268] The outcome for patients with unilateral disease that has been enucleated is excellent, with good functional results and minimal long-term effects.[269] However in view of the success in the treatment of bilateral intraocular disease with systemic or intraarterial chemoreduction and focal treatments, more patients

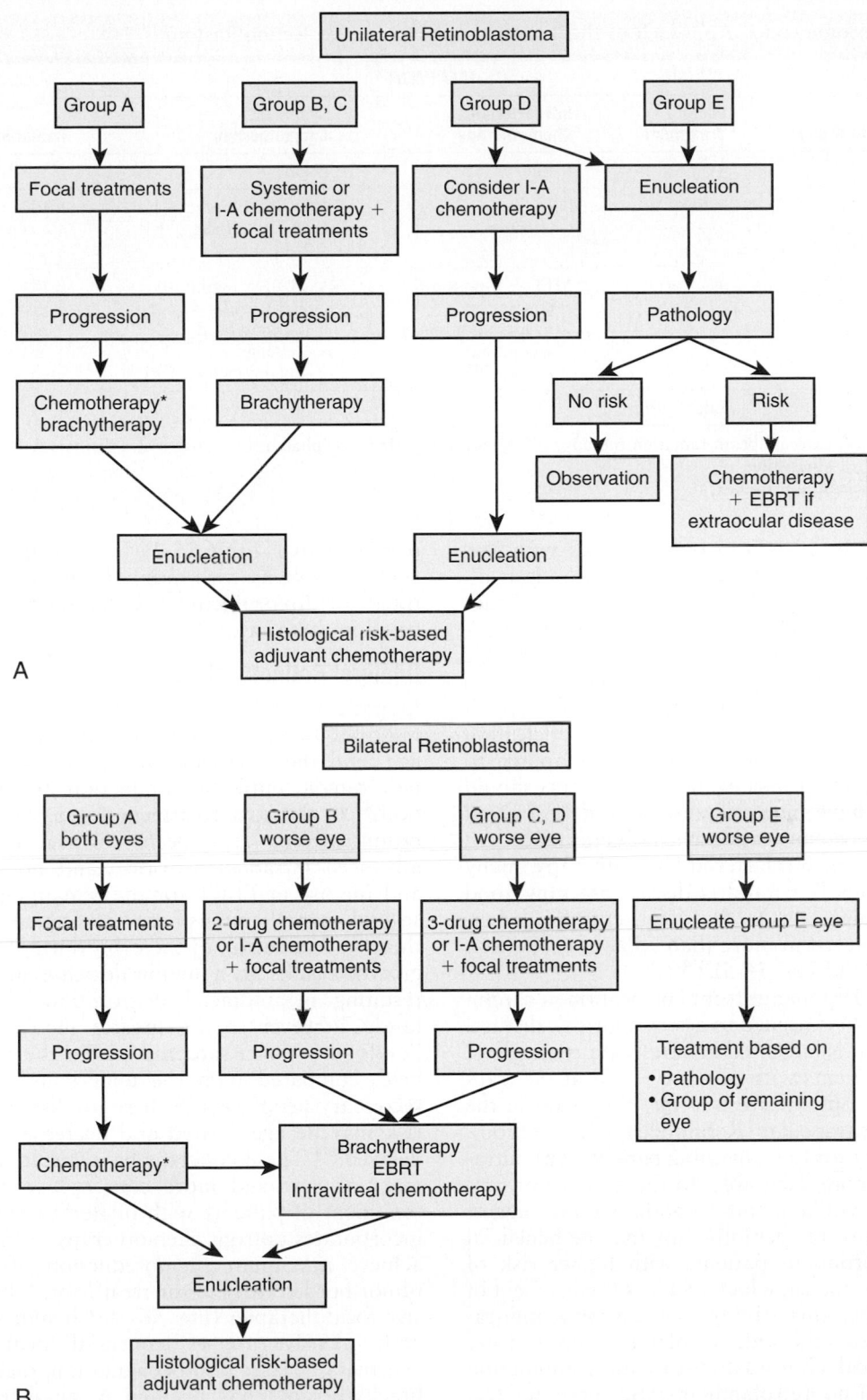

Figure 56-5 Algorithms for the management of unilateral (**A**) and bilateral (**B**) retinoblastoma. *EBRT,* External beam radiation therapy; *I-A,* intra-arterial. *Systemic or I-A.

are considered candidates for ocular preservation treatments. This is particularly important in very young children in whom metachronous bilateral disease may develop. Using the standard three-drug regimen (vincristine, carboplatin, and etoposide) and aggressive focal consolidation, more than two thirds of patients with unilateral disease do not respond to therapy and ultimately require either enucleation or radiation therapy.[270] Therefore the use of upfront systemic chemotherapy in this group of patients with unilateral disease needs to be

TABLE 56-1 Recommended Approach to the Treatment of Intraocular Retinoblastoma

R-E Group	ABC Group	TREATMENT			
		Focal Treatment	Intraarterial Chemotherapy	Systemic Chemotherapy	Radiation
I-II	A	+	If PD	If PD	If PD
I-III	B	+	MEL 3-5 mg × 3-6 courses	VCR 0.05 mg/kg d 1 CBP 18.6 mg/kg d 1 × 2-6 courses	If PD
IV-V	C-D*	+	MEL 3-5 mg × 3-6 courses Consider addition of second agent (TOP, CBP)	VCR 0.05 mg/kg d 1 CBP 14 mg/kg d 1, 2 ETO 6 mg/kg d 1, 2 × 6 courses ± subconjunctival CBP	If PD Consider early EBRT if massive vitreous seeding at completion of chemotherapy
V b	E	Enucleation			

CBP, Carboplatin; EBRT, external beam radiation therapy; ETO, etoposide; MEL, melphalan; PD, progressive disease; R-E, Reese-Ellsworth; TOP, topotecan; VCR, vincristine.
*Consider upfront enucleation if unilateral.

considered very judiciously and only in cases with low intraocular disease and when focal consolidation is available. Preenucleation chemotherapy results in downstaging with underestimation of extraretinal and extraocular disease, leading to an increased risk of metastatic spread.[271] However patients presenting with group E eyes and buphthalmos, in whom enucleation might be associated with surgical risks, may benefit from preenucleation chemotherapy; in these cases, given the inability to perform proper histologic risk evaluation, patients should be considered to have high-risk disease and be treated accordingly with postenucleation chemotherapy.[164,171]

With the advent of intraarterial chemotherapy, many patients with groups B, C, and D disease are now good candidates for ocular salvage, and long-term eye preservation may be achieved in more than 75% of cases (Box 56-4, Table 56-1, and Fig. 56-5).[216]

For patients undergoing upfront enucleation, a careful histologic evaluation is needed to assess high-risk disease. Adjuvant treatment is indicated in cases with transscleral invasion and in patients with positive tumor at the transection line of the optic nerve (see the discussion in the "Treatment of Extraocular Retinoblastoma" section). Adjuvant treatment for the remaining patients with intraocular disease is more debatable. In the absence of randomized studies, available information would suggest that the use of adjuvant chemotherapy may be beneficial for the selected group of patients with higher risk of extraocular dissemination, which includes involvement of the anterior chamber, ciliary body, or iris, massive infiltration (>3 mm) of the choroid, retrolaminar optic nerve infiltration, or focal choroidal disease in combination with any degree of nonretrolaminar optic nerve involvement (Table 56-2 and Fig. 56-5).[146,156,157-159,161,165,167,272] Adjuvant chemotherapy is not indicated for patients with isolated prelaminar involvement[156,251] or isolated focal choroidal involvement.[158,161,165,251,268] Different chemotherapy regimens have been proposed. Six-month treatment with vincristine, cyclophosphamide, and doxorubicin; vincristine, carboplatin, and etoposide; or a hybrid with alternating courses of both regimens appears

to be effective (Table 56-2). Idarubicin is also an effective agent in persons with retinoblastoma and can be substituted for doxorubicin.[273] Radiation therapy is not indicated in these cases.

Bilateral Retinoblastoma

In patients with germline mutation of the RB1 gene, multiple, bilateral retinoblastomas develop at an earlier age, and these patients are at risk of development of new tumors until the completion of retinal differentiation.[87] In the past treatment for patients with bilateral retinoblastoma has been enucleation of eyes with advanced intraocular disease and no visual potential, and the use of EBRT for the remaining eyes. However, several complications are associated with radiation therapy. Irradiation of the orbit during a period of rapid growth results in a major decrease in orbital volume, resulting in midfacial deformities.[274,275] More importantly however is the greatly increased risk for the development of a sarcoma within the radiation therapy field, compared with the underlying increased risk of secondary neoplasms in these predisposed persons. This risk may be age related and decreases as irradiation is delayed.[276] These concerns have resulted in the development of new and more conservative approaches. The treatment of patients with bilateral retinoblastoma now incorporates upfront chemotherapy, which is intended to achieve maximum chemoreduction of the intraocular tumor burden early in the treatment, followed by aggressive focal therapies (Fig. 56-5). Chemoreduction coupled with intensive use of sequential focal therapies (e.g., cryotherapy, laser photocoagulation, thermotherapy, and brachytherapy) has resulted in an increase in the eye salvage rates and in a decrease (and delay) in the use of radiation therapy. Intraocular retinoblastoma is extremely chemosensitive, and disease progression during treatment is rarely seen. Noticeable responses are seen in more than 90% of the eyes; these responses are maximum after two cycles, and tumor regression after subsequent cycles is less pronounced (Fig. 56-6).[134,277,278] However chemotherapy alone can only save fewer than 10% of

TABLE 56-2 Adjuvant Chemotherapy for Retinoblastoma with High-Risk Histology

Regimen	Drugs	Doses	Comments
COG-ARET0332 protocol	VCR	0.05 mg/kg day 1	6 cycles
	CBP	18.6 mg/kg day 1	
	ETO	5 mg/kg days 1, 2	
Chantada et al.[165]	VCR	0.05 mg/kg day 1	Cycles 1, 3, 5, 7
	CYC	65 mg/kg day 1	
	IDA	10 mg/m^2 day 1	
	CBP	18.7 mg/kg (<10 kg) days 1, 2	Cycles 2, 4, 6, 8
		560 mg/m^2 (≥10 kg) days 1, 2	
	ETO	3.3 mg/kg (<10 kg) days 1, 2, 3	
		100 mg/m^2 (≥10 kg) days 1, 2, 3	
SJCRH*	VCR	0.05 mg/kg (<12 mo) day 1	Cycles 1, 3, 5
		1.5 mg/m^2 (≥12 mo) day 1	
	CYC	40 mg/kg (<12 mo) day 1	
		1,200 mg/m^2 (≥12 mo) day 1	
	DOX	1.5 mg/kg (<12 mo) day 1	
		45 mg/m^2 (≥12 mo) day 1	
	VCR	0.05 mg/kg (<12 mo) day 1	Cycles 2, 4, 6
		1.5 mg/m^2 (≥12 mo) day 1	
	CBP	AUC 6.5 mg/mL/min day 1	
	ETO	3.3 mg/kg (<12 mo) days 1, 2, 3	
		100 mg/m^2 (≥12 mo) days 1, 2, 3	

AUC, Area under the curve; *CBP,* carboplatin; *CYC,* cyclophosphamide; *DOX,* doxorubicin; *ETO,* etoposide; *IDA,* idarubicin; *SJCRH,* St. Jude Children's Research Hospital; *VCR,* vincristine.
*SJCRH regimen from Sullivan EM, Wilson MW, Billups CA, et al: Pathologic risk-based adjuvant chemotherapy for unilateral retinoblastoma following enucleation. *J Pediatr Hematol Oncol* 36:e335–40, 2014.

the eyes.[134] Macular tumors are more sensitive to chemotherapy, probably because of the richer vascular supply that maximizes exposure to chemotherapy. Up to two thirds of macular tumors can be controlled with chemotherapy alone,[23,279] and with the addition of thermotherapy, this proportion may increase to greater than 80%.[23,24,279,280] Chemoreduction coupled with intensive use of sequential focal therapies (e.g., cryotherapy, laser photocoagulation, thermotherapy, and brachytherapy) has resulted in an increase in eye salvage rates and in the decrease (and delay) in the use of radiation therapy.

Different chemotherapy combinations are used, although the best results are achieved with a combination of vincristine, carboplatin, and etoposide (or tenipo-

side).[80,83,281-283] An alternative chemotherapy regimen includes the addition of cyclosporin to the three-drug regimen.[284] The rationale for the use of cyclosporin originates from the documentation of the presence of the P-glycoprotein efflux pump in a significant proportion of retinoblastomas, an expression that appears to correlate with treatment failure.[285] The concurrent administration of cyclosporin could potentially abrogate the efflux of drugs from the cancer cell. However the expression of P-glycoprotein does not always seem to predict response,[286] and cyclosporin adds toxicity. For patients with early intraocular stages (R-E groups I to III or International group B), a less intensive regimen with vincristine and carboplatin alone appears to be effective (Box 56-4 and Figs. 56-5 and 56-6).[134,287]

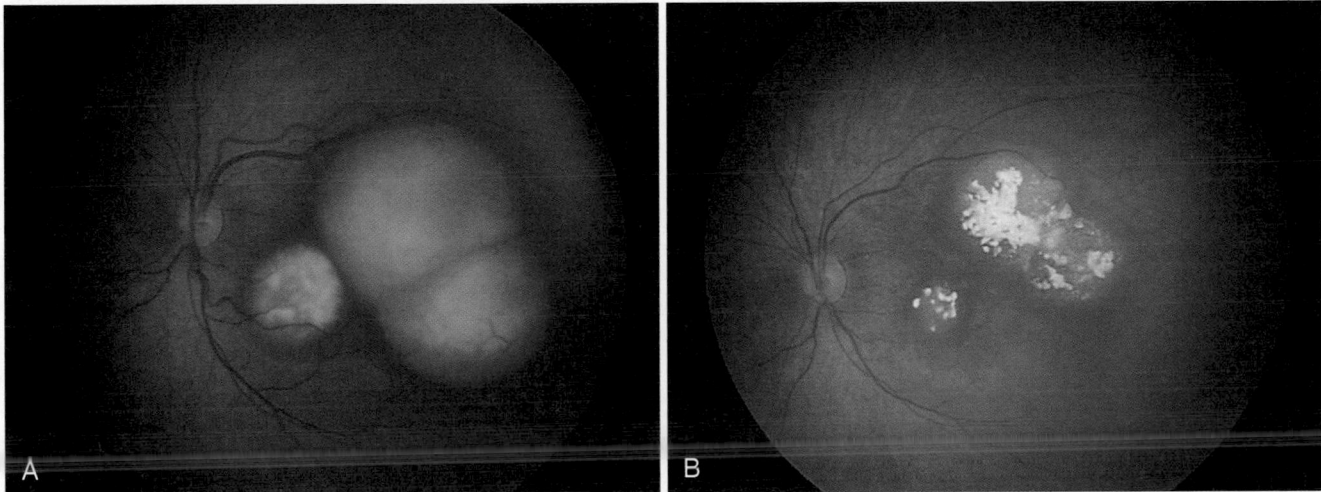

Figure 56-6 Response of a group B retinoblastoma (**A**) to two courses of vincristine and carboplatin (**B**).

Salvage rates for eyes classified as R-E groups I to III approaches 100% with use of these techniques. For patients with advanced intraocular tumors (International groups C and D), ocular salvage rates are not better than 50% to 70% when systemic chemoreduction is used, and EBRT is usually required.[281] However the use of radiation therapy is usually delayed for several months, which allows for better orbital growth and a decrease in the risk of second malignancies. A major proportion of failures occur because of progression of tumor in the vitreous, or as subretinal implants, two areas of difficult access for antineoplastic agents.[80] For these patients, if systemic chemotherapy is used, the addition of periocular carboplatin may be beneficial.[205]

Thus the treatment of patients with advanced intraocular disease (R-E groups IV and V or International groups C and D) remains a major challenge. Although randomized studies have not been performed, compared with radiation therapy and focal treatments alone, chemoreduction does not seem to improve overall ocular salvage significantly for patients with very advanced intraocular disease.[247-249] Chemotherapy intensification appears to correlate with outcome, and better results are obtained with protocols that include at least six courses of vincristine, etoposide, and carboplatin.[281,288,289] Central retinal tumors usually respond better to chemotherapy than tumors in the peripheral retina,[290] but large central tumors may be associated with subretinal seeds, which ultimately may cause treatment failure.[291] Despite the addition of aggressive sequential focal therapies, globe retention is still no better than 50% for patients with group D eyes, and most patients eventually require irradiation. A major proportion of failures occur because of progression of tumor in the vitreous or as subretinal implants, two areas of difficult access for antineoplastic agents.[80] Radiation therapy appears to be the only valid alternative for these patients, and with the incorporation of lower doses of irradiation (26 Gy) early in the treatment, in a situation of minimal disease, before disease progression occurs, ocular salvage rates for International group D eyes may improve.[253]

New agents with better intraocular penetration are under investigation. Topotecan, a topoisomerase-I inhibitor with well-documented efficacy against pediatric tumors, is a promising alternative. Studies performed in the animal model have shown that topotecan has excellent intraocular penetration and antitumor effect.[76] In a phase II study using an upfront window of vincristine and topotecan in patients with advanced bilateral disease, responses were documented in 90% of the patients.[292]

Direct administration of chemotherapy drugs into the ophthalmic artery to maximize drug exposures is a very effective approach and has become the standard of care at many centers, particularly for children with advanced bilateral disease, with ocular survival rates in excess of 80% (as previously discussed).

New Tumor Formation during Treatment with Chemotherapy

In the natural history of patients with germline *RB1* mutation, new tumors continue to form after diagnosis. It is not clear whether the use of chemotherapy may alter this process. Several authors have evaluated the impact of primary systemic chemotherapy on the rate of new tumor formation in patients with hereditary retinoblastoma. For patients receiving treatment with the standard two- or three-drug regimens that include six to eight cycles of chemotherapy, the cumulative incidence of new tumors after the start of chemotherapy is 10% to 24%,[293,294] although higher incidences have also been reported.[295] However most new tumors develop after chemotherapy is discontinued.[134,294] The incidence of new tumors is higher if a regimen of shorter chemotherapy duration is used or only focal treatments are administered.[296-298] Younger age at diagnosis, a family history of retinoblastoma, and lower grouping at diagnosis are factors that significantly increase the likelihood of new tumor formation.[293-295] These risk factors are intrinsically tied together; patients with a family history are more likely to be screened early and be diagnosed at a younger age, early in the natural history of the disease. Importantly the majority of the new tumors after the start of chemotherapy develop in the equatorial or peripheral retina, and fewer than 20% of the tumors form in the macula.[293] This tumor distribution is likely tied to retinal development rather than to the use of chemotherapy, but it is possible that small tumors in the richly vascularized central retina are effectively treated with chemotherapy before they become visible. New tumors may still retain sensitivity to the drugs used, because they likely represent new somatic mutations that occur after the start of treatment. With the recent implementation of intraarterial chemotherapy as primary treatment for patients with bilateral disease, a similar preventive phenomenon has been observed.[299] All in all these data seem to suggest that small tumors undetectable by ophthalmoscopy may be present at diagnosis that can be effectively treated before becoming apparent.

TREATMENT OF EXTRAOCULAR RETINOBLASTOMA

Extraocular dissemination of retinoblastoma bears a close relationship with the socioeconomic conditions that result in delayed diagnosis and treatment. In Europe and the United States, fewer than 5% of patients present with extraocular disease,[152,300,301] in contrast to 12% to 20% in South America,[268,302] 25% to 40% in Mexico and India,[118,303,304] and more than 50% in less developed countries.[305]

Four patterns of extraocular disease have been recognized: (1) locoregional dissemination, including orbital disease, tumor extending to the cut end of the optic nerve, and lymphatic spread to the preauricular lymph nodes; (2) CNS dissemination; (3) metastatic retinoblastoma; and (4) trilateral retinoblastoma (Figs. 56-2 and 56-3).

Orbital and Locoregional Retinoblastoma

Orbital retinoblastoma occurs as a result of progression of the tumor through the emissary vessels and sclera. For this reason, scleral disease is considered to be extraocular and should be treated as such. Orbital retinoblastoma is isolated in 60% to 70% of cases; lymphatic, hematogenous, and CNS metastases occur in the remaining patients.[306] Treatment should include systemic chemotherapy and radiation therapy; with this approach, 60% to 85% of patients can be cured. Because most recurrences occur in the CNS, regimens using drugs with well-documented CNS penetration are recommended. Different chemotherapy regimens have proven to be effective, including vincristine, cyclophosphamide, and doxorubicin, platinum- and epipodophyllotoxin-based regimens, or a combination of both.[307,308,309-311] For patients with macroscopic orbital disease, it is recommended that surgery be delayed until response to chemotherapy has been obtained (usually with two or three courses of treatment). Enucleation should then be performed, and an additional four to six courses of chemotherapy should be administered. Local control should then be consolidated with orbital irradiation (4000 to 4500 cGy). Using this approach, orbital exenteration is not indicated.[312,313] Similar management should be followed for patients with scleral disease, including radiation therapy, although good outcomes without irradiation have also been reported.[302] Patients with isolated involvement of the optic nerve at the transection level should also receive similar systemic treatment, and irradiation should include the entire orbit (3600 cGy) with a 1000 cGy boost to the chiasm (for a total of 4600 cGy). Also because metastases in parameningeal bones have been associated with intracranial dissemination,[307] irradiation fields should be adjusted carefully. The preauricular and cervical lymph nodes should be explored carefully, because 20% of patients with orbital retinoblastoma have lymphatic metastases.[306] Lymphatic dissemination does not carry a worse prognosis, provided that the involved lymph nodes are also irradiated.[301,312,314] Patients with spontaneous or accidental ocular perforation and patients with intraocular surgery for unsuspected retinoblastoma should be considered to have orbital disease by definition and treated accordingly.

Central Nervous System Disease

Intracranial dissemination occurs by direct extension through the optic nerve, and its prognosis is dismal.[308,315,316] Treatment for these patients should include platinum-based intensive systemic chemotherapy and CNS-directed therapy. Although traditionally intrathecal methotrexate (with or without cytosine arabinoside) has been used, no preclinical or clinical evidence exists to support its use.[317] Other intrathecal agents with documented effect against retinoblastoma include topotecan[76,292,318] and thiotepa.[314,319] However no evidence indicates that their use can have an impact on outcome. Although the use of irradiation in these patients is controversial, responses have been observed with craniospinal irradiation, with a dose of 2500 cGy to 3500 cGy to the entire craniospinal axis, and a boost (1000 cGy) to sites of measurable disease.[307,311,312,314,315] Therapeutic intensification with high-dose, marrow-ablative chemotherapy and autologous hematopoietic progenitor cell rescue has been explored,[307] but its role is not yet clear. Despite the intensity of the treatment and the documented responses of the intracranial disease,[316] most patients succumb to their disease, and reports of survivors are anecdotal.[307,309]

Trilateral Retinoblastoma

The prognosis for patients with trilateral retinoblastoma is very poor; most patients die of disseminated neuroaxis disease in less than 9 months.[125,127,131] The rare survivors are usually those diagnosed with screening imaging and treated with intensive chemotherapy with or without craniospinal irradiation.[67,131] Pineal primary neuroectodermal tumors (PNETs; pineoblastoma) occurring in patients without retinoblastoma are also associated with a poor prognosis in younger patients. However with an appropriately aggressive multimodal approach, these patients can be cured. PNETs are chemosensitive tumors, and they appear to have a steep dose-response curve for alkylating agents. Studies in older patients with pineoblastoma have recently shown that a treatment with complete resection and intensive alkylator- and cisplatin-based therapy, followed by craniospinal irradiation (3600 cGy with a boost to the pineal gland to 5900 cGy) and consolidation with high-dose, myeloablative chemotherapy and autologous hematopoietic progenitor cell rescue, may produce survival rates in more than two thirds of patients.[320] It is therefore possible that similar treatment guidelines could be used for trilateral retinoblastoma. However one must consider the serious long-term toxicities of such doses of irradiation in the very young child. Therefore current strategies are directed toward avoiding irradiation and instead using intensive chemotherapy followed by consolidation with myeloablative chemotherapy and autologous hematopoietic progenitor cell rescue, an approach similar to those being used in the treatment of brain tumors in infants. With use of the Head Start regimen, which takes this approach, improved outcomes have been reported in young children who have supratentorial PNETs, including pineoblastomas.[321]

Because of the poor prognosis of trilateral retinoblastoma, screening neuroimaging is a common practice. One fourth of the cases in the literature correspond to cases found during screening.[131] Given the short interval between the diagnosis of retinoblastoma and the occurrence of trilateral retinoblastoma, routine screening might detect the majority of cases within 2 years.[131] Although it is not clear whether early diagnosis can have an impact on survival,[322,323] it is usually recommended that neuroimaging be performed every 6 months until 5 years of age.[127,131,323,324]

(Extracranial) Metastatic Retinoblastoma

Hematogenous metastases may develop in the bones, bone marrow, and, less frequently, in the liver.[302,308,311,312,315,325,326] Although long-term survivors treated with conventional chemotherapy have been reported,[326] these cures should be considered anecdotal; metastatic retinoblastoma is not curable with conventional chemotherapy.[302,312] In recent years, however, small series of patients have shown that metastatic retinoblastoma can be cured with use of high-dose, marrow-ablative chemotherapy and autologous hematopoietic progenitor cell rescue (Table 56-3).[307,308,311,315,325,327,328] The approach is similar to that used with metastatic neuroblastoma; patients receive short and intensive induction regimens that usually contain alkylating agents, anthracyclines, etoposide, and platinum

TABLE 56-3   Recommended Chemotherapy Regimen for Metastatic Retinoblastoma

Phase	Drugs	DOSES		Days
		<36 months	>36 months	
Induction (4 cycles)	VCR	0.05 mg/kg	1.5 mg/m²	1, 8, 15
	CDDP	3.5 mg/kg	105 mg/m²	1
	CYC	65 mg/kg	1950 mg/m²	2, 3
	ETO	4 mg/kg	120 mg/m²	2, 3
Consolidation	CBP	AUC 7 (maximum 16.7 mg/kg)	AUC 7 (maximum 500 mg/m²)	−8, −7, −6
	TT	10 mg/kg	300 mg/m²	−5, −4, −3
	ETO	8.3 mg/kg	250 mg/m²	−5, −4, −3

From Dunkel IJ, Khakoo Y, Kernan NA, et al: Intensive multimodality therapy for patients with stage 4a metastatic retinoblastoma. Pediatric Blood Cancer 55:55–59, 2010.

AUC, Area under the curve; CBP, carboplatin; CDDP, cisplatin; CYC, cyclophosphamide; ETO, etoposide; TT, thiotepa; VCR, vincristine.

compounds, and consolidation is then performed with marrow-ablative chemotherapy and autologous hematopoietic cell rescue. With use of this approach, the outcome appears to be excellent. As with any "megatherapy" consolidation, the agents selected may be important. In general recurrences are intracranial, and for this reason, agents with proven efficacy in intracranial retinoblastoma should be used. In this regard the combination of carboplatin and etoposide has been shown to be effective against CNS disease,[316] and for this reason it should be part of the regimen. In one of the largest series, seven patients underwent consolidation with the CARBOPEC combination (i.e., carboplatin, 1250 to 1750 mg/m²; etoposide, 1750 mg/m²; and cyclophosphamide, 6.4 g/m²). Five of these patients were cured, and the regimen failed in two patients because of CNS relapse. In two other series a thiotepa-based consolidation regimen has been used (i.e., thiotepa, 900 mg/m²; etoposide, 750 to 1200 mg/m²; and carboplatin, 1500 mg/m²). A strong rationale exists for using thiotepa: retinoblastoma is responsive to alkylating agents such as thiotepa, a group of agents for which dose escalation is shown to overcome resistance. Furthermore thiotepa has excellent CNS penetration.[308,315,329] An interesting observation is that patients with distant bone metastases (i.e., outside the orbit and skull) that show good response to induction chemotherapy may not require radiation therapy when they are treated with marrow-ablative chemotherapy.[307,327]

LONG-TERM EFFECTS OF RETINOBLASTOMA AND ITS TREATMENT

Retinoblastoma is a cancer of the very young, and patients are very susceptible to the long-term effects that the disease and the treatments administered may have with regard to organ development and function. More importantly patients with bilateral retinoblastoma are born with a germline mutation of the RB1 gene, probably the most potent tumor suppressor gene, and are at risk of the development of cancers throughout their lives; in this regard, retinoblastoma may be just the beginning.

Second Malignancies

The cumulative incidence of second cancers in patients with germline mutations of the RB1 gene increases steadily with age, to up to 30% to 60% at 40 to 50 years of age, although more recent studies estimate a considerably lower risk.[87,330-333] Second malignancies are responsible for an excess risk of mortality in survivors of bilateral disease;[334] up to 50% of the deaths of survivors are due to second cancers.[333] The type of mutation, whether de novo or inherited, appears to influence the risk of second cancers—patients with a family history of the disease have a higher cumulative incidence of second neoplasms when compared with survivors of bilateral retinoblastoma who do not have a family history of the disease.[335] Patients with nonhereditary retinoblastoma are not at increased risk. Most information on second malignancies in retinoblastoma survivors is derived from the prospective follow-up of a cohort of 1601 survivors of retinoblastoma who were diagnosed between 1914 and 1984 at institutions in Boston and New York. The sequential updated analyses of this cohort have provided (and continue to provide) the most reliable description of cancer risk in this population.[87,335-337]

In the most recent analysis, the median follow-up for patients with hereditary and nonhereditary retinoblastoma was 25.2 years and 29.5 years, respectively.[87] The standardized incidence ratio (SIR) in these studies was calculated as the ratio of the observed number of cancers to the expected number from the Connecticut Tumor Registry. The incidence of second cancers was significantly elevated in survivors of hereditary retinoblastoma (SIR, 19 vs. 1.2 in patients with nonhereditary retinoblastoma), and almost any neoplasm has been described in this population[87,338]; similar data have been reported using population-based registries.[333] For hereditary retinoblastoma, the greatest risk (SIR >100) was for neoplasms of bone, connective, and soft tissue, eye and orbit, and nasal cavities. An increased risk (SIR >10) was also noted for pineoblastoma, melanoma, CNS malignancies, and neoplasms of the buccal cavity and corpus uteri. The lowest risk (SIR <10) was seen for neoplasms of the lung, breast, and colon (Table 56-4).

The cumulative incidence of a second neoplasm after 30 years from diagnosis of retinoblastoma is greater than 30%.[87,330,331,333,338] Reports differ on the risk, and cumulative incidences in excess of 50% have been reported.[331,338] The more accurate data probably derive from the Boston–New York cohort, which illustrates the changes in cancer

TABLE 56-4 Risk and Type of New Cancers in 963 Survivors of Hereditary Retinoblastoma

Cancer Site	Observed (%)	SIR (95% CI)
All sites	260 (100)	19 (16-21)
Bone	75 (28.8)	360 (283-451)
Soft tissue	34 (13)	122 (84-170)
Nasal cavities	32 (12.3)	1111 (760-1569)
Melanoma	29 (11.1)	28 (18-40)
Eye and orbit	17 (6.5)	266 (155-426)
Brain	10 (3.8)	13.6 (6.5-25)
Breast	10 (3.8)	3.96 (1.9-7.3)
Corpus uteri	7 (2.7)	20 (8.0-41)
Buccal cavity	7 (2.7)	20 (8.2-42)
Lung	5 (1.9)	5.94 (1.9-14)
Pineoblastoma	5 (1.9)	90.8 (29-212)
Colon	3 (1.1)	6.28 (1.3-18)
Hodgkin lymphoma	3 (1.1)	3.4 (0.7-10)
Bladder	2 (0.7)	6.15 (0.7-22)
Thyroid	2 (0.7)	3.34 (0.4-12)
Leukemia	2 (0.7)	2.25 (0.3-8.1)

Modified from Kleinerman RA, Tucker MA, Tarone RE, et al: Risk of new cancers after radiotherapy in long-term survivors of retinoblastoma: an extended follow-up. J Clin Oncol 23:2272–2279, 2005.

CI, Confidence interval; SIR, standardized incidence ratio.

risk estimates with longer follow-up. The cumulative incidence of second cancers at 50 years in survivors of hereditary retinoblastoma was estimated to be 51% in the analysis reported by Wong et al.[331] in 1997. This figure decreased to 36% in the analysis of the same cohort reported by Kleinerman et al.[87] in 2005, probably reflecting the lower doses of scatter radiation received by patients treated in more recent eras. Although patients have a lifetime risk of developing additional malignancies, the second malignancy usually occurs in the first decades after the diagnosis of retinoblastoma. The median age at diagnosis of a second neoplasm is 15 to 17 years.[276,331] However survivors of retinoblastoma continue to have an increased risk of second malignancy–associated death throughout their life.[333,337] Furthermore survivors of a second neoplasm appear to have an increased risk of developing a third and a fourth malignancy, which occur at shorter intervals. The cumulative incidence of a third neoplasm is 22% at 10 years from the time of diagnosis of the second cancer, and it occurs at a median of 5.8 years.[339]

Radiation therapy plays a major role in the risk of second neoplasms in patients with hereditary retinoblastoma. The second tumorigenic event ("second hit") is usually chromosomal in nature, often as a result of mitotic recombination errors.[100,340] This second hit is very sensitive to environmental factors such as ionizing radiation, thus explaining the increased risk of radiation-induced malignancies in survivors of retinoblastoma.[341] Radiation results in a significant increase in the incidence of second cancers in patients with hereditary disease; the cumulative probability of developing a second malignancy is 38% in patients who have been treated with radiation versus 21% in patients who have not been treated with radiation.[87] The greatest risk (SIR >100) is for neoplasms of bone, soft tissues, nasal cavities, and orbits, and for pineoblastoma. The risk of second cancer appears to correlate as well with timing of radiation; children receiving radiation therapy during their first year may have a higher risk of developing a second cancer.[276,337] However the need for earlier radiation may also be an indication of a biologically and clinically more aggressive disease. Changes in radiation techniques over the years are having an impact on cancer risk. As shown in the cohort reported by Kleinerman and colleagues,[87] the use of orthovoltage prior to 1960 was associated with a higher risk of second malignancies than radiation techniques used in subsequent decades; the cumulative incidence of second cancers at 40 years was 32.9% and 26.3%, respectively. With the evolving treatment approaches for intraocular retinoblastoma, which may decrease the overall need for external beam radiation, and the development of newer radiation techniques, such as conformal, intensity-modulated, and proton-beam radiation, it is likely that a further decrease in cancer risk will be observed. In a cohort of British retinoblastoma survivors born before 1950, prior to the routine use of radiation therapy, fewer than 15% of second tumors were sarcomas, highlighting the important role of radiation therapy in the development of those malignancies.[338] Population-based studies have shown a significant decline in the use of radiation therapy during the past decades, from 30.5% of patients in the 1980s to less than 3% after 1999.[333] This change in practice is likely to lead to a further decline in the risk of second cancers in this population.

Traditionally an excess risk has been attributed solely to the use of radiation therapy; the added risk of the use of chemotherapy is not fully understood. In survivors of childhood cancer, an increased risk of second malignancies has been documented, particularly osteosarcoma, which is associated with the combined use of chemotherapy and radiation therapy.[342] A similar phenomenon may occur in retinoblastoma survivors, and the most recent analyses suggest a synergistic effect in carcinogenic risk with the use of chemotherapy. The overall risk of cancer for persons with hereditary retinoblastoma who received radiation and chemotherapy was 25, compared with 19 for persons who received only radiation. Most of this difference was accounted for by the higher risk noted for osteosarcomas; the SIR was 539 for combined treatment and 302 for radiation only.[87]

Sarcomas of bone and soft tissues account for more than 40% of all second neoplasms, followed by neoplasms of the nasal cavities and melanoma (Table 56-4).[87,331] Sarcomas in general and osteosarcoma in particular are cancers of the young retinoblastoma survivor; 76% of all cancers in the irradiated patients occurring at less than 25 years are sarcomas versus 33%

in nonirradiated patients. Conversely 76% of cancers diagnosed at less than 25 years of age are sarcomas, whereas sarcomas represent fewer than 50% of cancers in older patients; in irradiated patients not treated with radiation, the proportion was 33% in persons younger than 25 years and 8% in persons older than 25 years.[87,338]

The role of imaging screening for the early detection of second malignancies has not been fully addressed. One study using whole-body MRI concluded that although this approach had good specificity, its sensitivity was low (66.7%).[343] However age- and disease-specific screening methods may need to be evaluated.

Osteosarcoma

Osteosarcoma as a second malignancy is often associated with retinoblastoma. In the general population only 7% of osteosarcomas follow other malignancies, and almost half of these cases occur in retinoblastoma survivors.[344] Similarly although multifocal osteosarcoma accounts for only 4% of all osteosarcomas, 25% of those occur in retinoblastoma survivors.[345] Osteosarcoma is the most common malignancy in survivors of retinoblastoma, both in the irradiated and the nonirradiated areas, and account for 25% to 40% of all second malignancies.[87,276,337,346-348] One half to two thirds of osteosarcomas occur in the irradiated fields of the skull and face,[87,276,346-348] one third of tumors develop in the extremities, and fewer than 10% develop in the trunk.[87] The SIR is 360; it is higher in irradiated fields (SIR 406), but it is still significantly increased in nonirradiated fields (SIR 69). Osteosarcoma occurring in patients with retinoblastoma who have been treated with radiation therapy accounts for 30% of all osteosarcomas of the head and neck.[349]

The clinical presentation is similar to that of conventional osteosarcoma, and the clinical behavior does not seem to be different; fewer than 20% of the cases are metastatic.[350] Osteosarcomas occur in young patients, both in irradiated and nonirradiated fields, usually peaking during the adolescent years.[276,346,350] However osteosarcomas that occur during the first decade of life are usually in the irradiated fields.[350] With appropriate multidisciplinary treatment, secondary osteosarcoma occurring in retinoblastoma survivors is curable.[351,352] However a major limitation is the common occurrence in the head and neck, which are sites where local control is challenging.[347-349]

Ewing sarcoma, although rare, has also been described in retinoblastoma survivors. It accounts for 15% to 25% of all bone tumors, almost always occurring outside the radiation field.[330,348] Ewing sarcoma in retinoblastoma survivors accounts for approximately 16% of cases of Ewing sarcoma that occur as a second malignancy.[353]

Soft Tissue Sarcomas

Soft tissue sarcomas are the second most common malignancy in retinoblastoma survivors, with an SIR of 122, and they account for approximately 10% to 15% of all second malignancies.[337,354,355,356] Soft tissue sarcomas are closely associated with the use of radiation; the SIR is much higher in irradiated fields (140) than in nonirradiated fields (23). In the Boston–New York cohort, the cumulative risk for soft tissue sarcomas at 50 years after radiation therapy was 13.1%.[354,356] Approximately 10% of all secondary sarcomas in children surviving cancer occur in retinoblastoma survivors.[355]

As with osteosarcoma, most soft tissue sarcomas occur in the irradiated fields; sarcomas of the head and face account for 70% of the cases, with the remaining being in the trunk (20%) and limbs (<5%).[276,346-348,354,356] A very characteristic spectrum of histologies has been described (Table 56-5). Leiomyosarcoma is the most common subtype, accounting for approximately one third of the cases, followed by fibrosarcoma, malignant fibrous histiocytoma, rhabdomyosarcoma, nonspecified sarcomas, and liposarcoma. When compared with the normal population, SIR is significantly elevated for leiomyosarcoma (390), fibrosarcoma (398), and rhabdomyosarcoma (279), but it is also higher for malignant fibrous histiocytoma (100) and liposarcoma (99).[356] A correlation exists between radiation exposure and histologic subtype; fibrosarcoma, rhabdomyosarcoma, malignant fibrous histiocytoma, and nonspecified subtypes almost always occur

TABLE 56-5   Risk and Type of Soft Tissue Sarcomas in 963 Survivors of Hereditary Retinoblastoma

| | TREATMENT | | | | | |
| | All Treatments | | Radiation | | No Radiation | |
Histology	Observed (%)	SIR (95% CI)	Observed	SIR (95% CI)	Observed	SIR (95% CI)
Total	69 (100)	184 (143-233)	66	212 (164-270)	3	47 (9.4-137)
Soft tissue sarcoma NOS	10 (14.5)	96 (46-177)	10	115 (55-211)	0	0.0 (0.0-218)
Fibrosarcoma	13 (18.8)	398 (211-681)	13	475 (253-813)	0	0.0 (0.0-691)
Malignant fibrous histiocytoma	12 (17.4)	100 (52-175)	11	110 (55-197)	1	51 (0.66-284)
Liposarcoma	3 (4.3)	99 (20-286)	3	120 (24-351)	0	0.0 (0.0-329)
Leiomyosarcoma	23 (33.3)	390 (247-585)	22	476 (298-720)	1	78 (1.0-436)
Rhabdomyosarcoma	8 (11.6)	279 (120-551)	7	281 (112-578)	1	271 (3.5-1510)

Modified from Kleinerman RA, Tucker MA, Abramson DH, et al: Risk of soft tissue sarcomas by individual subtype in survivors of hereditary retinoblastoma. J Natl Cancer Inst 99:24–31, 2007.
CI, Confidence interval; NOS, not otherwise specified; SIR, standard incidence ratio.

in the irradiated fields. Conversely leiomyosarcoma and liposarcoma commonly arise in the nonirradiated fields. Although secondary sarcomas in childhood cancer survivors are associated with increasing doses of anthracyclines or alkylators,[357] the use of chemotherapy does not appear to increase the risk of soft tissue sarcomas in retinoblastoma survivors; however the combined use of radiation and chemotherapy appears to increase the risk for leiomyosarcoma when compared with radiation alone.[356]

Soft tissue sarcomas are a malignancy of the young survivor, and more than half of the tumors are diagnosed in the first 30 years after retinoblastoma diagnosis.[276,346,356] Fibrosarcoma, rhabdomyosarcoma, rhabdomyosarcoma, and malignant fibrous histiocytoma predominantly occur 10 to 20 years from retinoblastoma diagnosis, whereas nonspecified sarcomas occur across all time intervals. An exception to the rule is leiomyosarcoma, which more commonly (78%) occurs after 30 years from retinoblastoma diagnosis, and typically outside the irradiated fields; the SIR for this subtype after 30 years is 435.[28] Very common locations for leiomyosarcoma are the uterus and bladder,[330,337,354,356,358,359] and these tumors may also occur as a radiation-induced malignancy in the paranasal sinuses.[352]

The liposarcoma risk also increases with age.[356] Alteration of the *RB1* gene has been demonstrated in both lipomas and liposarcomas. An interesting observation is the increased incidence of lipomas in survivors of hereditary retinoblastoma. Lipomas were present in 3.6% of patients with hereditary retinoblastoma, compared with only 0.6% in patients with sporadic disease.[360] The incidence of a second neoplasm appears to be higher in patients with lipomas; 30% of patients with lipoma experienced a second malignant neoplasm, compared with 12% of patients without lipoma. These data suggest that the presence of lipomas could be a clinical marker of susceptibility to second neoplasms.[360]

Sarcoma risk and location do not seem to differ by sex, except for leiomyosarcomas. In males, 64% of primaries were in the face, whereas for females, 58% of tumors were in the pelvic area, highlighting the relevance of uterine primary tumors.[356]

Skin Cancers

Skin cancers account for 16% to 19% of all second cancers in survivors of hereditary retinoblastoma, and they occur both inside and outside the irradiated fields, usually within the first three decades of life.[276,330,337,354] The highest risk is for melanoma, but basal cell and squamous cell carcinomas are also common. The SIR for melanoma is 28 in the radiation field and 15 outside the irradiated areas. The risk of developing melanoma is higher in survivors with a family history, compared with persons with de novo mutations.[335] Skin cancer also accounts for approximately one third of all third tumors.[276]

Lung Cancer and Other Common Cancers of Adulthood

In recent years with improvements in treatment that have resulted in longer survival rates, it has become apparent that patients with hereditary retinoblastoma are also at risk of developing epithelial cancers late in adulthood.[337,338] The SIR is elevated for lung, breast, colon, buccal cavity, bladder, and corpus uteri cancers (see Table 56-4).[354] Lung cancer appears to be one of the most common second neoplasms that occur in adulthood, which is not surprising because somatic mutations of the *RB1* gene are known to contribute to the development of lung cancer.[332,361] Compared with the general population, hereditary retinoblastoma survivors have a higher mortality from lung cancer and all other epithelial cancers combined (standard mortality ratio 7.01 and 3.29, respectively).[338] Rather than being epithelial, most bladder and uterine cancers (and a large proportion of colon neoplasms) are probably leiomyosarcomas.[354,356] An increased incidence of breast cancer occurs in patients who have been treated with radiation therapy, but this increased risk is similar for patients with hereditary and nonhereditary retinoblastoma; the dose to the breast from scatter radiation is approximately 0.4 Gy. New reported excess risks include carcinomas of the salivary glands and tongue; low doses of radiation (<5 Gy) have been associated with secondary salivary cancers.[354] It is possible that most of the excess cancer risks might be preventable by limiting exposure to agents that damage the DNA, such as tobacco and ultraviolet light.

Hematologic Malignancies

Patients with hereditary retinoblastoma have a slightly increased risk of developing hematologic malignancies, with an SIR of 2.25 (and an SIR of 1.27 in nonhereditary cases).[354] The use of etoposide and other topoisomerase-II inhibitors such as anthracyclines may add an additional risk to this patient population.[362] However the cumulative doses of those agents are relatively low, and it is therefore assumed that the risk of treatment-related leukemia is minimal. Therapy-related acute myeloid leukemia after the treatment of retinoblastoma has been reported, although its occurrence does not appear to be higher than in other patients receiving etoposide.[363,364]

Trilateral Retinoblastoma

Trilateral retinoblastoma refers to the association of bilateral retinoblastoma with an asynchronous intracranial tumor (Fig. 56-3).[126,129,131] The SIR for trilateral retinoblastoma is 90.8, and it seems to be associated with the use of radiation therapy (SIR is 0 in patients who have not been treated with radiation therapy). Tumors comprising trilateral retinoblastoma are PNETs that exhibit varying degrees of neuronal or photoreceptor differentiation, suggesting an origin from the germinal layer of primitive cells.[128] This association can occur in 3% to 9% of patients with the genetic form and appears to be more common in familial cases. The prognosis is almost uniformly fatal. Trilateral retinoblastoma was the principal cause of death from retinoblastoma during the first decade of life in the United States.[129] The majority of these tumors are pineoblastomas, but in 20% to 25% of the cases, the tumors are suprasellar or parasellar. The association of bilateral retinoblastoma with a tumor in the pineal gland and a fourth primary tumor of suprasellar location is called "quadrilateral retinoblastoma."

In most cases trilateral retinoblastoma resembles undifferentiated retinoblastomas, with the more frequent formation of Homer-Wright rosettes. The median age at diagnosis of trilateral retinoblastoma is 23 to 48 months,[125,126,129,131] and the interval between the diagnosis of bilateral retinoblastoma and the diagnosis of the brain tumor is usually more than 20 months.[127,131] Suprasellar tumors are usually diagnosed earlier,[42,127] and in 15% to 20% of the cases, the intracranial tumor antecedes the diagnosis of retinoblastoma.[126] In recent years with the more widespread use of chemoreduction treatments for patients with bilateral retinoblastoma and a decrease in the use of radiation, the incidence of trilateral retinoblastoma has decreased dramatically, to the point that patients with the genetic form of retinoblastoma are now considered to be almost protected against this fatal complication.[132] However pineal cysts develop in approximately 5% to 8% of patients with bilateral disease; these cysts appear to be a forme fustre of trilateral retinoblastoma.[133,134,135]

The prognosis for patients with trilateral retinoblastoma is dismal—patients die of disseminated neuroaxis disease in fewer than 9 months.[125,127,131] The rare survivors are usually those diagnosed with screening imaging and treated with intensive chemotherapy with or without craniospinal radiation.[131] Because of the poor prognosis of trilateral retinoblastoma, screening neuroimaging is a common practice. One fourth of the cases in the literature correspond to cases found during screening.[131] Given the short interval between the diagnosis of retinoblastoma and the occurrence of trilateral retinoblastoma, routine screening might detect the majority of cases within 2 years.[131] Although it is not clear whether early diagnosis can have an impact on survival,[322] it is usually recommended that neuroimaging be performed every 6 months until 5 years of age.[127,131,323,324]

OTHER LONG-TERM EFFECTS

Orbital Growth and Facial Asymmetry

Because their orbital growth is still in progress, children treated for retinoblastoma are at risk of functionally and cosmetically significant bony orbital abnormalities. These sequelae become evident by early adolescence, when orbital growth is largely complete, and results in the "hourglass facial deformity."[274] Both enucleation, which causes orbital contraction, and radiotherapy, which induces arrest of bone growth, adversely affect orbital growth. In children treated for bilateral retinoblastoma, the impact of enucleation in orbital development is not different from that of irradiation. Final orbital volumes after enucleation correlate with the size of the prosthetic implant, but there are no differences in final orbital volumes based on the type of implant.[275,365]

Delay of radiation therapy should therefore be a goal when designing treatment for children with bilateral retinoblastoma. Studies show that the therapeutic strategy of chemoreduction and aggressive focal treatments can successfully delay the use of radiation therapy for at least 6 or 7 months (median age, 21 months).[134,281] In addition to theoretically decreasing the risk of second cancers, delaying radiation therapy may also allow more complete facial and orbital growth to occur, thus reducing the degree of midfacial deformities.[274,275] However with the use of a multidisciplinary approach, the dose of radiation needed for disease control may also be reduced.[82]

Visual Outcome

Visual outcome is frequently good in children treated for retinoblastoma[366]; however maculopathy and deficits in acuity, visual fields, dark adaptation, and visuomotor integration have been reported for many patients.[269,366] Visual outcome correlates with the intraocular stage and, more importantly, tumor location. Visual acuity of 20/40 or better can be achieved in 90% of eyes with extramacular tumors and in 24% of eyes with macular tumors. Overall a final visual acuity of 20/40 or better may be achieved in half of the eyes, and two thirds have a visual acuity of 20/200 or better.[367] However visual outcome is not always easily predicted on the basis of the initial presentation.[368] These findings suggest that visual function in survivors of retinoblastoma is influenced by more distal elements of the visual system, including the primary visual cortex. Because retinoblastoma affects the visual system at an age at which the CNS is still developing,[369] differences in visual outcome among patients with retinoblastoma may be due, at least in part, to disease- or treatment-induced differences in visual field development in the primary visual cortex. New imaging technology such as functional MRI and diffusion tensor imaging may be used to evaluate changes in the visual pathways and the primary visual cortex.[370,371]

Cognitive and Functional Development of Patients with Retinoblastoma

Patients with retinoblastoma may experience a restriction in their development because of their visual limitations. However few studies have addressed the development of these young children. Interestingly the earliest articles describing cognitive development in this population suggested that children with retinoblastoma might have above average or superior intelligence.[372-375] These findings were based on a small number of patients and were never confirmed or unconfirmed, but the idea of superior intelligence became part of the "lore" among clinicians working with the retinoblastoma population. In the report of Ek and colleagues,[366] a population-based study from Sweden, 22 children with retinoblastoma were assessed at 4 and 6 years of age. Patients with both bilateral and unilateral disease showed above-average developmental quotients, with the bilateral group showing higher scores in the superior range. Only two children in the cohort demonstrated below-average development, and both of these patients had bilateral disease and received radiation therapy in the first month of life. The authors concluded that bilateral retinoblastoma is associated with superior cognitive capacities. The other recent series involved 54 patients who were assessed prior to the age of 42 months with the Bayley Scales of Infant Development.[269] No indication of superior intelligence was found in this cohort, but neither was there an indication of increased difficulties. The average mental and motor development scores were in the normal range and did not differ from population norms. Thus although children with retinoblastoma do not appear to be at-risk developmentally, questions regarding the developmental trajectory for this population remain.

Other Late Effects

Platinum compounds are commonly used to treat retinoblastoma. Although the effects of cisplatin on hearing are well documented, evidence is conflicting with regard to the potential ototoxic effects of carboplatin. Although it is usually assumed that carboplatin ototoxicity is extremely rare, very few studies have investigated the cumulative incidence of and prognostic factor for ototoxicity as a result of the use of this platinum agent. In two of the studies reported, no cases of carboplatin-induced hearing loss were documented.[376,377] However infants younger than 6 months appear to be at a higher risk of hearing loss.[378] Thus very careful age-appropriate evaluations of hearing function, including tympanometry, otoacoustic emission measurement, and visual reinforced audiometry, must be performed.[376,379]

References available online at ExpertConsult.

KEY REFERENCES

4. Chantada GL, Qaddoumi I, Canturk S, et al: Strategies to manage retinoblastoma in developing countries. *Pediatr Blood Cancer* 56:341–348, 2011.
   This article provides good guidelines for the development of retinoblastoma programs in countries with limited resources.

14. Orjuela MA, Cabrera-Muñoz L, Paul L, et al: Risk of retinoblastoma is associated with a maternal polymorphism in dihydrofolate reductase (DHFR) and prenatal folic acid intake. *Cancer* 118:5912–5919, 2012.
   This recent epidemiologic study is a good example of the potential interplay between ethnic, paternal, and environmental factors in the pathogenesis of retinoblastoma.

45. Donovan SL, Schweers B, Martins R, et al: Compensation by tumor suppressor genes during retinal development in mice and humans. *BMC Biol* 4:14, 2006.
   In humans, inactivation of retinoblastoma 1 (RB1) is sufficient for retinoblastoma formation. In mice, Rb1 and one of the other family members must be inactivated. In this article, the investigators show that mice require inactivation of two retinoblastoma gene family members because of species-specific intrinsic genetic compensation in the developing retina.

46. Johnson D, Zhang J, Frase S, et al: Neuronal differentiation and synaptogenesis in retinoblastoma. *Cancer Res* 67:2701–2711, 2007.
   This article provides a detailed neuroanatomical characterization of retinoblastoma using electron microscopy.

52. McEvoy J, Flores-Otero J, Zhang J, et al: Coexpression of normally incompatible developmental pathways in retinoblastoma genesis. *Cancer Cell* 20:260–275, 2011.
   Single cell gene expression array analysis of human retinoblastomas shows coexpression of photoreceptor, interneuron, and progenitor programs in individual cells. The conclusion from this study was that the cell of origin cannot be inferred from the gene expression profile of the tumors.

62. Manning AL, Longworth MS, Dyson NJ: Loss of pRB causes centromere dysfunction and chromosomal instability. *Genes Dev* 24:1364–1376, 2010.
   This article provides data showing that in retinal pigment epithelial cells, when retinoblastoma 1 is knocked down, defects occur in sister chromatid cohesion.

63. Zhang J, Benavente CA, McEvoy J, et al: A novel retinoblastoma therapy from genomic and epigenetic analyses. *Nature* 481:329–334, 2012.
   In this study, epigenetic deregulation of spleen tyrosine kinase and other cancer genes was demonstrated in human retinoblastoma, suggesting that epigenetic processes contribute to tumorigenesis.

67. McEvoy J, Nagahawatte P, Finkelstein D, et al: RB1 inactivation by chromothripsis in human retinoblastoma. *Oncotarget* 5:438–450, 2014.
   This article provides independent validation that approximately 1% of human retinoblastomas have wild-type retinoblastoma 1 (RB1) and v-myc avian myelocytomatosis viral oncogene neuroblastoma derived homolog (MYCN) amplification. It also shows for the first time that the RB1 gene can be inactivated by chromothripsis in a small subset of tumors.

74. Laurie NA, Donovan SL, Shih CS, et al: Inactivation of the p53 pathway in retinoblastoma. *Nature* 444:61–66, 2006.
   This article shows that the p53 pathway is silenced by MDM4 overexpression in retinoblastoma.

75. Zhang J, Schweers B, Dyer MA: The first knockout mouse model of retinoblastoma. *Cell Cycle* 3:952–959, 2004.
   This article describes the first genetically engineered mouse model of retinoblastoma with inactivation of retinoblastoma and p107.

78. Benavente CA, McEvoy JD, Finkelstein D, et al: Cross-species genomic and epigenomic landscape of retinoblastoma. *Oncotarget* 4:844–859, 2013.
   This article shows that despite remarkable similarities between mouse models and human retinoblastomas, fundamental differences exist in their chromosomal and epigenetic landscapes.

87. Kleinerman RA, Tucker MA, Tarone RE, et al: Risk of new cancers after radiotherapy in long-term survivors of retinoblastoma: an extended follow-up. *J Clin Oncol* 23:2272–2279, 2005.
   This article analyzes the long-term risk of second malignant neoplasms in survivors of retinoblastoma and describes the pattern of second tumors.

88. Fletcher O, Easton D, Anderson K, et al: Lifetime risks of common cancers among retinoblastoma survivors. *J Natl Cancer Inst* 96:357–363, 2004.
   This article shows that survivors of retinoblastoma are also at increased risk of developing the common cancers of adulthood.

101. Castera L, Sabbagh A, Dehainault C, et al: MDM2 as a modifier gene in retinoblastoma. *J Natl Cancer Inst* 102:1805–1808, 2012.
   This article shows that polymorphisms in mouse double minute 2 (MDM2) may influence the penetrance and clinical presentation in patients with the hereditary form of retinoblastoma.

111. Sastre X, Chantada GL, Doz Fo, et al: Proceedings of the Consensus Meetings from the International Retinoblastoma Staging Working Group on the Pathology Guidelines for the Examination of Enucleated Eyes and Evaluation of Prognostic Risk Factors in Retinoblastoma. *Arch Pathol Lab Med* 133:1199–1202, 2009.
   This consensus article provides guidelines for processing of enucleated eyes and for defining high-risk features.

133. Ramasubramanian A, Kytasty C, Meadows AT, et al: Incidence of pineal gland cyst and pineoblastoma in children with retinoblastoma during the chemoreduction era. *Am J Ophthalmol* 156:825–829, 2013.
   This article shows that children with retinoblastoma commonly develop pineal cysts, which need to be distinguished from the more aggressive pineoblastomas of the trilateral form.

134. Rodriguez-Galindo C, Wilson MW, Haik BG, et al: Treatment of intraocular retinoblastoma with vincristine and carboplatin. *J Clin Oncol* 21:2019–2025, 2003.
   This article shows that for patients with early intraocular disease, a two-drug regimen with vincristine and carboplatin coupled with aggressive focal treatments is effective.

141. Laurent VE, Sampor C, Solernou Vn, et al: Detection of minimally disseminated disease in the cerebrospinal fluid of children with high-risk retinoblastoma by reverse transcriptase-polymerase chain reaction for GD2 synthase mRNA. *Eur J Cancer* 49:2892–2899, 2013.
   This article shows that reverse transcriptase–polymerase chain reaction for GD2 is a promising tool for the evaluation of minimal residual disease in patients with high-risk retinoblastoma.

145. Linn Murphree AL: Intraocular retinoblastoma: the case for a new group classification. *Ophthalmol Clin N Am* 18:41–53, 2005.

This article provides the description of the current international classification of intraocular retinoblastoma.

211. Suzuki S, Yamane T, Mohri M, et al: Selective ophthalmic arterial injection therapy for intraocular retinoblastoma: the long-term prognosis. *Ophthalmology* 118:2081–2087, 2011.

This article reports on the largest series of patients with retinoblastoma treated with intraarterial chemotherapy by the pioneers of the technique.

216. Gobin Y, Dunkel IJ, Marr BP, et al: Intra-arterial chemotherapy for the management of retinoblastoma: four-year experience. *Arch Ophthalmol* 129:732–737, 2011.

This article shows that the use of direct ocular administration via the ophthalmic artery has provided a new means for control of advanced intraocular disease and has established a new treatment paradigm.

235. Munier F, Beck-Popovic M, Balmer A, et al: Occurrence of sectoral choroidal occlusive vasculopathy and retinal arteriolar embolization after superselective ophthalmic artery chemotherapy for advanced intraocular retinoblastoma. *Retina* 31:566–573, 2011.

This article shows that the use of intraarterial chemotherapy is associated with vasculopathy; this potential adverse effect must be considered when choosing this technique in patients with bilateral retinoblastoma in whom vision preservation is a priority.

245. Munier FL, Gaillard M-C, Balmer A, et al: Intravitreal chemotherapy for vitreous disease in retinoblastoma revisited: from prohibition to conditional indications. *Br J Ophthalmol* 96:1078–1083, 2012.

This article shows that direct injection of chemotherapy into the vitreous may provide a very good alternative to the treatment of patients with advanced or refractory vitreous disease.

266. Lee CT, Bilton SD, Famiglietti RM, et al: Treatment planning with protons for pediatric retinoblastoma, medulloblastoma, and pelvic sarcoma: how do protons compare with other conformal techniques? *Int J Radiat Oncol Biol Phys* 63:362–372, 2005.

This article shows that proton therapy offers the possibility of significantly decreasing the exposure of normal orbital structures to radiation during the treatment of patients with retinoblastoma.

267. Sethi RV, Shih HA, Yeap BY, et al: Second nonocular tumors among survivors of retinoblastoma treated with contemporary photon and proton radiotherapy. *Cancer* 120:126–133, 2014.

This article shows that treatment of intraocular retinoblastoma with proton therapy is associated with a significantly decreased risk of second malignancies in survivors of hereditary retinoblastoma.

308. Dunkel IJ, Khakoo Y, Kernan NA, et al: Intensive multimodality therapy for patients with stage 4a metastatic retinoblastoma. *Pediatr Blood Cancer* 55:55–59, 2010.

This article shows that patients with metastatic retinoblastoma may be cured with intensive chemotherapy and consolidation with high-dose chemotherapy and autologous hematopoietic stem cell transplantation.

356. Kleinerman RA, Tucker MA, Abramson DH, et al: Risk of soft tissue sarcomas by individual subtype in survivors of hereditary retinoblastoma. *J Natl Cancer Inst* 99:24–31, 2007.

This article analyzes the risk of development of soft tissue sarcomas and describes the distribution of the different histologies and their associated risks.

378. Qaddoumi I, Bass JK, Wu J, et al: Carboplatin-associated ototoxicity in children with retinoblastoma. *J Clin Oncol* 30:1034–1041, 2012.

This article shows that the risk of hearing loss associated with treatment with carboplatin is not negligible. Children younger than 6 months appear to be at higher risk of hearing loss with this treatment.

CHAPTER 57

Tumors of the Brain and Spinal Cord

Mark W. Kieran, Susan N. Chi, Peter E. Manley, Adam L. Green, Pratiti Bandopadhayay, Guillaume Bergthold, Nathan J. Robison, Andres E. Morales La Madrid, Nadine P. Sauer, Sanjay P. Prabhu, Keith L. Ligon, Liliana C. Goumnerova, Karen Jean Marcus, and Rosalind A. Segal

CHAPTER OUTLINE

Tumors of the central nervous system (CNS) account for approximately 25% of pediatric cancer but are now the leading cause of cancer-related mortality in children. The complexities of tumors in this site are related to the large number of different histologies within the CNS and a historic nomenclature that is confusing, even to those in this field. With the need to modify therapies to spare important neurocognitive function in the youngest patients and the presence of the blood-brain barrier (BBB), which restricts the delivery of effective therapies, improvement in outcome has lagged well behind that of many other cancers, especially childhood leukemia. The molecular revolution offers the chance to begin classifying tumors by the signals that drive their phenotype rather than by their appearance under the microscope.[1]

In this chapter we will discuss the different types of brain tumors in children, their diagnoses, and their treatments, while incorporating the expanding knowledge of tumor biology.

Although clinical studies often focus on progression-free survival (PFS) and overall survival (OS), successful therapy incorporates much more. Accepting a lower overall cure rate but preserving neurocognitive function is the norm for many types of brain tumors, especially those of infants and young children. Optimization of outcome requires expertise in multiple subspecialties that play a role in the care of these children. The skill of the neurosurgeon, the sophistication of the radiation planning, and the safe administration of chemotherapy are all important factors in improving the long-term outcome

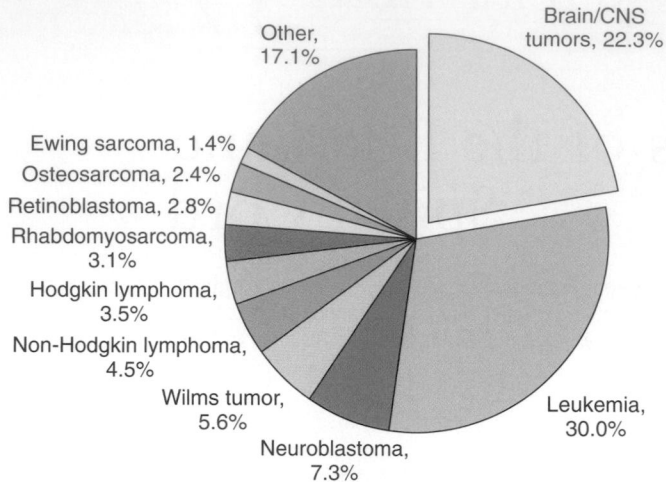

Figure 57-1 Incidence of pediatric cancer. *CNS,* Central nervous system. *(Data from American Cancer Society:* American Cancer Society Cancer Facts & Figures, 2007, *Atlanta, Ga, 2007, American Cancer Society.)*

for these patients.[2] In fact, many centers now use neurooncologists who have completed additional training in outcome optimization. When combined with a large number of subspecialty services (e.g., endocrinology, neurology, neuropsychology, social work, back to school, and physical and occupational therapy), truly optimal care is now possible for this patient population. Needs of the family continue to evolve as patients transition from diagnosis to treatment to posttherapy follow-up.[3,4] A comprehensive understanding of pediatric neurooncology and the delivery of comprehensive care to these patients and their families will be the focus of this chapter.

To assist the reader, a number of important review articles summarizing different aspects of the care of children with CNS tumors are referenced.[5-18]

EPIDEMIOLOGY

Primary CNS (PCNS) tumors rank second behind leukemia as the most common pediatric cancer diagnosed in the United States each year (Fig. 57-1). Brain tumors are the most common form of solid tumors in children and are now the leading cause of death from solid tumors in children. The spectrum of adult brain tumors[19] based on location, histology, and outcome differs significantly from that in pediatrics, suggesting that the causative events are different from those for pediatric brain tumors. No single standard classification system has been implemented for pediatric brain tumors, although development of a standardized platform for epidemiologic studies has been attempted.[20,21] The 2013 Central Brain Tumor Registry of the United States Statistical Report included primary nonmalignant (1.93 per 100,000 children) and malignant (3.33 per 100,000 children) pediatric brain and CNS tumors with a total incidence of 5.26 per 100,000 children.[22] Similarly in the 2013 National Cancer Institute Surveillance Epidemiology and End Results (SEER) Cancer Statistics Report, the annual age-adjusted inci-

dence rate of pediatric malignant brain and other nervous system tumors was listed as 3.1 cases per 100,000 children.[23] The rate is higher in males (3.2 per 100,000) compared with females (2.9 per 100,000). Approximately 4100 new cases of childhood PCNS tumors are diagnosed in the United States each year. Of these, an estimated 3007 will be in children younger than 15 years. The incidence for all brain tumors is highest among 0- to 4-year-olds (5.77 per 100,000) and lowest among 10- to 14-year-olds (4.78 per 100,000), results that are similar to those reported in 2005.[21] The age-adjusted mortality rate for pediatric CNS tumors in 2010 was 0.6 per 100,000 children, resulting in an estimated 500 deaths per year in the United States for those aged 0 to 19 years. The prevalence rate for all malignant and benign pediatric CNS tumors (ages 0 to 19 years) is estimated at 9.5 per 100,000, with more than 26,000 children estimated to be living with this diagnosis in the United States in 2000. However the prevalence rate for patients with only malignant brain tumors was 7.9 per 100,000, with more than 21,000 children estimated to be living with a diagnosis of primary malignant CNS tumor in the United States in 2000.[24] The distribution of pediatric brain tumors by site is presented in Figure 57-2. Different brain tumor histologies have different age distributions (Fig. 57-3). The most common histologies in the younger age group (ages 0 to 14 years) include pilocytic astrocytomas (PAs) and medulloblastomas, which account for 20% and 16% of cases, respectively. The broad category of glioma accounts for 56% of tumors in children younger than 15 years. The most common histologies in adolescents ages 15 to 19 years include PA and pituitary tumors, which account for 15% and 14% of cases, respectively. The broad category of glioma accounts for 45% of tumors in adolescents ages 15 to 19 years. The rates among boys are slightly higher than those in girls, and brain tumors are more common in whites (4.7 per 100,000) than in blacks (3 per 100,000).

The histologic-specific differences in brain and CNS tumor distribution by age and gender suggest that childhood tumors have different mechanisms whereby normal cells, possibly somatic CNS stem cells, are susceptible to oncogenic mutation. Although certain histologic subtypes can also differ by race,[25,26] the overall concordance of tumor histologies among different ethnic groups and different locations suggest that specific local environmental factors are not the cause of most cancers in children.[27-29] The incidence of common pediatric brain tumors such as medulloblastoma, malignant gliomas, and diffuse pontine glioma do not differ significantly in industrialized versus nonindustrialized countries, in vegetarian versus meat-eating societies, and in areas where smoking and drinking are permitted versus where they are not permitted. Similarly death rates for children with CNS tumors between different ethnic groups within the United States (Hispanics, Asians, blacks, and whites) do not differ significantly for most CNS tumor types.[30]

In the mid 1990s an increase in the incidence of childhood brain cancer appeared to occur compared with that in the previous two decades. This increase is now thought to reflect the introduction and widespread use of

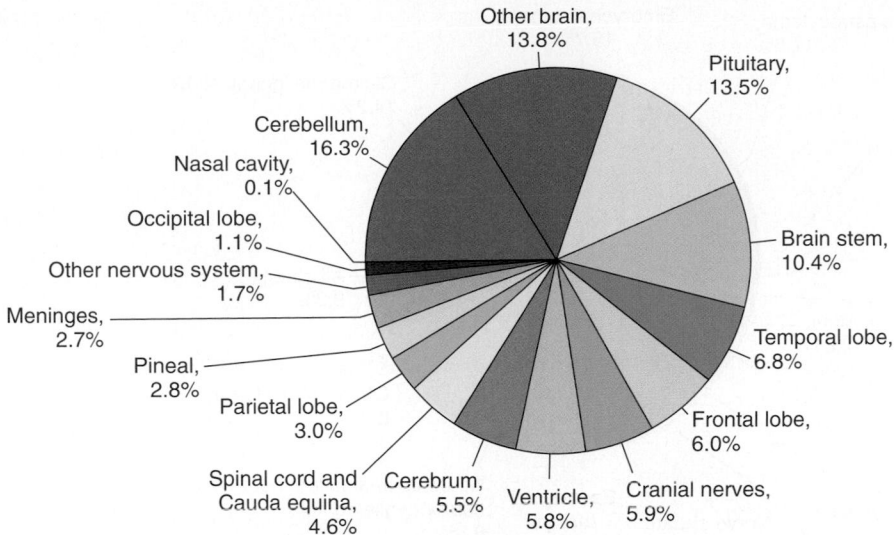

Figure 57-2 Distribution of childhood (ages 0 to 19 years) primary brain and central nervous system tumors by site (*n* = 21,512). (*Data from Ostrom QT, Gittleman H, Farah P, et al: CBTRUS Statistical Report: Primary Brain and Central Nervous System Tumors Diagnosed in the United States in 2006-2010. Neuro Oncol 15[Suppl 2]:ii1–ii56, 2013; and Central Brain Tumor Registry of the United States: 2007-2008 Statistical Report: Primary Brain Tumors in the United States Statistical Report, 2000-2004 [Years of Data Collected], Chicago, Ill., 2008, University of Illinois at Chicago School of Public Health.*)

magnetic resonance imaging (MRI) technology in the mid 1980s, resulting in improved detection and reporting of pediatric brain tumors. More precise classification of brain tumors and diagnostic capabilities, such as stereotactic biopsy, also may have contributed to the increase in incidence. The rise in incidence was followed by the establishment of a new baseline that has remained stable. Mortality rates have not mirrored the increase in incidence.[31]

PCNS tumors develop from an accumulation of genetic changes. Such changes can result from inherited mutations or develop from exposure to chemical, physical, or biologic agents that damage deoxyribonucleic acid (DNA). Unlike in adults, for whom lifetime exposure is significant, most pediatric tumors are believed to be the result of random genetic mutations that occur during normal cellular proliferation. Today molecular biologic techniques are used to unravel the complex genetic errors that lead to the development of CNS tumors. To date most pediatric brain tumors have demonstrated a limited number of mutations, even in highly aggressive tumors, suggesting that their presence during development or within the stem cell compartment is an important aspect of tumorigenesis in pediatric patients.[32]

The search for causative factors that place children at risk for developing CNS tumors has not yielded clear answers.[33] Numerous epidemiologic studies have evaluated potential risk factors. Similar to most pediatric cancers, no specific risk factor explains more than a small proportion of tumors.[34] Factors studied but not conclusively found to increase risk include exposure to tobacco and smoke,[35] alcohol, traffic-related air pollution, electromagnetic fields, pesticides, and occupational and industrial chemicals; diet; drugs and medications; infections and viruses; epilepsy; and consumption of cured meats during pregnancy.[36-45] The dramatic increase in the use of

cellular telephones has generated concerns about the potential risk for the development of brain tumors. A meta-analysis of nine case-control studies concluded that cellular phone users have no overall increased risk of brain tumors. The potential risk after long-term cellular phone use awaits analysis in future studies.[46] A seasonal variation unique to medulloblastoma incidence by month of birth may provide evidence for an environmental exposure cause, although further studies are needed.[47] An association between atopic disease and a reduced risk of glioma has been observed in adult epidemiologic studies, with the implication that heightened immune surveillance decreases the risk of brain tumor development.[33,48] Prenatal multivitamin use has been associated with a protective effect in the development of pediatric brain tumors in a large meta-analysis.[49] Confirmation of this result in a prospective trial is needed.

The role of viruses in the pathogenesis of tumors has been documented in experimental animals, and adenovirus serotypes have been shown to induce tumors in rodents. Adenoviral sequences were evaluated in more than 500 tumors derived from 17 different pediatric cancer entities. Although most leukemias and solid tumors were negative for the presence of adenoviral sequences, tumor material from 25 of 30 glioblastomas, 22 of 30 oligodendrogliomas, and 20 of 30 ependymomas, as well as normal brain, were positive by polymerase chain reaction assay for adenoviral gene sequences. This finding raises important questions about the contribution of this infectious agent to pediatric brain tumorigenesis.[50] In contrast, tests for polyomavirus sequences in adult and pediatric CNS tumors were rarely positive.[51]

Ionizing radiation, immunosuppression, and certain hereditary genetic disorders are the only factors that have been proven thus far to increase a child's risk for CNS malignancy. Ionizing radiation exposure is a

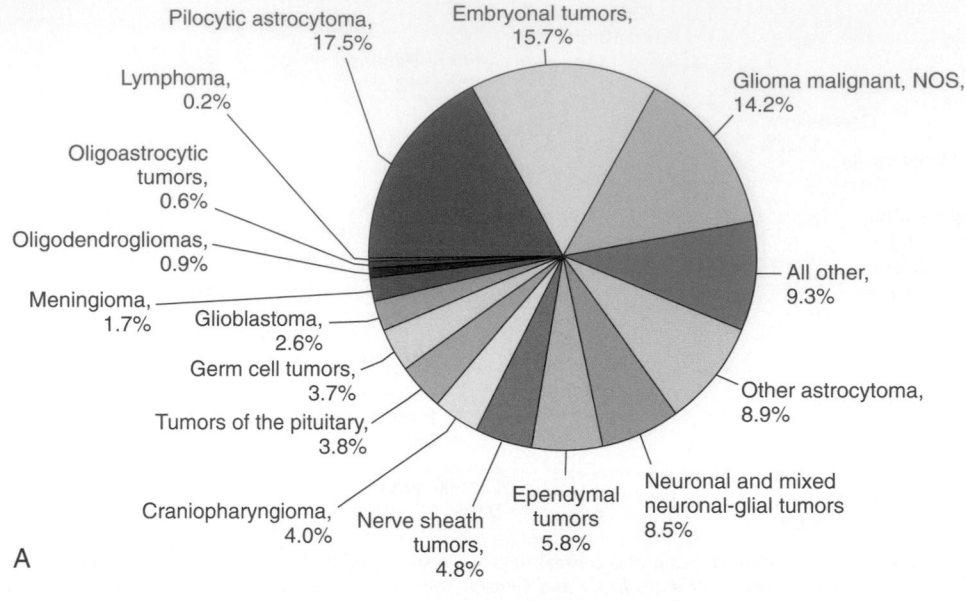

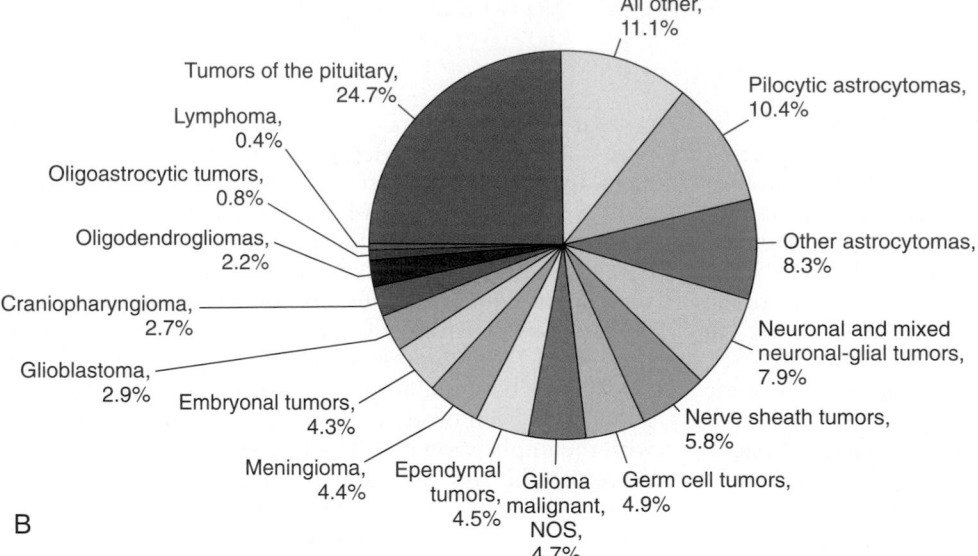

Figure 57-3 A, Distribution of childhood primary brain and central nervous system (CNS) tumors by histology and age (ages 0 to 14 years; *n* = 15,398). **B,** Distribution of childhood primary brain and CNS tumors by histology and age (ages 15 to 19 years; *n* = 6114). *NOS,* Not otherwise specified. *(Data from Ostrom QT, Gittleman H, Farah P, et al: CBTRUS Statistical Report: Primary Brain and Central Nervous System Tumors Diagnosed in the United States in 2006-2010. Neuro Oncol 15:ii1–ii56, 2013.)*

well-documented cause of brain tumors.[52] Children who undergo therapeutic irradiation to the CNS for the treatment of malignancy are at risk for development of a second tumor, specifically meningioma, high-grade glioma (HGG), or sarcoma. Since its introduction in the 1970s, computed tomography (CT) has become an essential tool in the diagnosis and monitoring of disease. The growing use of CT scans has raised concerns about potential risks. Pediatric CT scans may result in a small but not negligible increased lifetime risk for cancer mortality.[53]

Immunocompromised children are at increased risk for PCNS lymphoma. The risk for developing CNS lymphoma is 1% to 5% higher for adults and children undergoing transplantation and for those with congenital immunodeficiencies. The risk is 2% to 6% higher for persons with acquired immunodeficiency syndrome (AIDS). This risk will probably increase with longer survival because of improved AIDS treatment.

In summary although a few environmental factors are associated with an increased risk of developing a pediatric CNS tumor, the vast majority of patients have no easily identifiable risk factors. For a small percentage, inherited genetic mutations contribute to the onset of these tumors, but for the remainder, CNS tumors are likely the result of spontaneous mutations.

NEURODEVELOPMENT

Our understanding of the steps in hematopoietic development, together with the pathways and markers that distinguish precursors along each blood cell lineage, has been instrumental in allowing better classification and subsequently better treatment of leukemias. In the same way that leukemias can be viewed as deregulated expansion of hematopoietic precursor cell pools, pediatric brain tumors may similarly be considered as the proliferation of neuropoietic precursors. Thus knowledge of the steps and intermediates in neural development may help us understand and treat pediatric brain tumors. A current schema for neuropoiesis relies heavily on models for hematopoiesis but introduces two additional aspects of developmental regulation, the first of which is the importance of regionalization. During neural development a rostral-caudal gradient delineates distinct zones for proliferation and differentiation, while the orientation of proliferating cells relative to the dorsal-ventral axis provides the basis for determining the progeny of each proliferative event.

The second aspect of neuropoiesis is the concept of mitogenic niches. Although hematopoietic stem cells can proliferate and give rise to the entire array of blood cell types when exposed to the environment of the immature or mature bone marrow, neural stem cells use a number of distinct niches, some of which are eliminated before birth, some that persist through early childhood, and some that remain extant into adult life. These niches provide important cues for proliferation and differentiation but may also provide an environment that fosters the growth of tumor cells.

Neural Tube

The nervous system develops as a specialized zone of the epithelium. In the third week after fertilization, the midline zone of the epithelium becomes specialized as the neural plate. This distinctive zone extends from the caudal to the rostral portion of the embryo. While the embryo turns, the neural plate grows and folds (Fig. 57-4). Subsequent fusion of the folds creates a discrete neural tube that zips up from both the top and bottom. The two last places where the fold fuses are the hindbrain (the incipient cerebellum) and the lumbar spine. Cells at the crest of the developing neural tube are the neural crest cells, which give rise to the peripheral nervous system, including sympathetic ganglia, dorsal root ganglia, and Schwann cells, as well as to melanocytes in the developing skin. The neural crest cells are the precursors to neuroblastomas,[54] neurofibromas,[55] and melanomas.[56]

After the neural tube fuses, rapid expansion of cell number continues, but this expansion occurs very differently along the rostral-caudal axis. The dramatic expansion of cell number in the rostral neural tube provides the building blocks for the brain, whereas the more caudal regions undergo more limited growth and engender the spinal cord.

Development of Brain Structures

Along the rostral-caudal axis of the neural tube, three outpouchings can be seen at the end of the fourth week after fertilization—the forebrain, midbrain, and hindbrain (Fig. 57-5). Subsequent branching of the forebrain forms two lateral protrusions that are destined to become the left and right cortex, and the midline portion of the forebrain gives rise to the thalamus. The midbrain does not undergo much expansion, but the hindbrain undergoes massive proliferation to give rise to the cerebellum and underlying pons, as well as the medulla. Cerebral cortical tumors, including supratentorial primitive

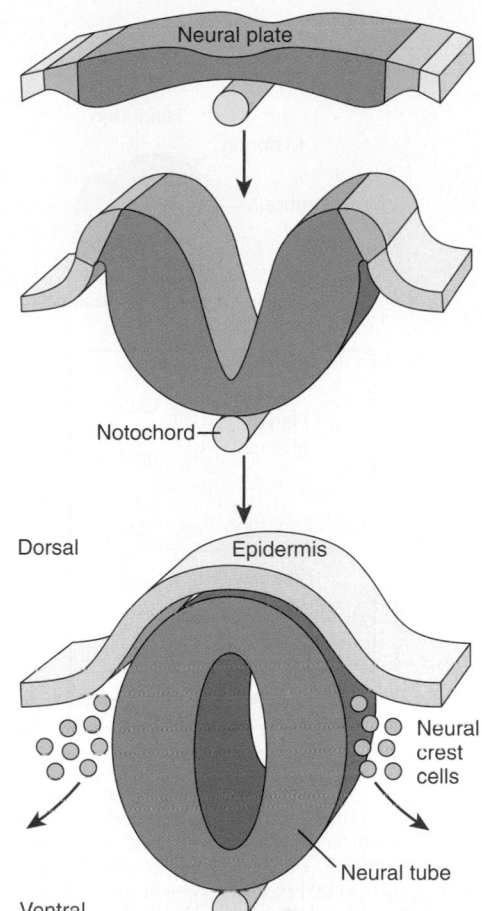

Figure 57-4 Growth and folding of the neural plate.

neuroectodermal tumors (CNS PNETs) and cortical and subependymal astrocytomas, all derive from the forebrain. Posterior fossa tumors, including the distinctive pontine gliomas, medulloblastomas, and cerebellar PAs, all derive from the hindbrain. Thus the areas of the brain that undergo rapid expansion in early life engender most pediatric brain tumors. Along the dorsal-ventral plane of the neural tube, greater proliferation of neural tube precursors occurs in the dorsal part of the tube than in the ventral tube. Proliferation of more dorsal precursors gives rise to the multilayer structures of the cerebral and cerebellar cortex; these areas are also the regions that give rise to many pediatric brain tumors.

Forebrain and Cerebral Cortex

In the forebrain the open spaces within the lateral outpouchings of the neural tube become the lateral ventricles, and proliferation largely occurs adjacent to the ventricular zone (VZ) in the medial and lateral ganglionic eminences, in the subventricular zone (SVZ) or subependymal zone. Early in development, neural stem cells/precursors divide extensively to provide the cellular elements of the cerebral cortex, thalamus, and basal ganglia (see Fig. 57-5, A).

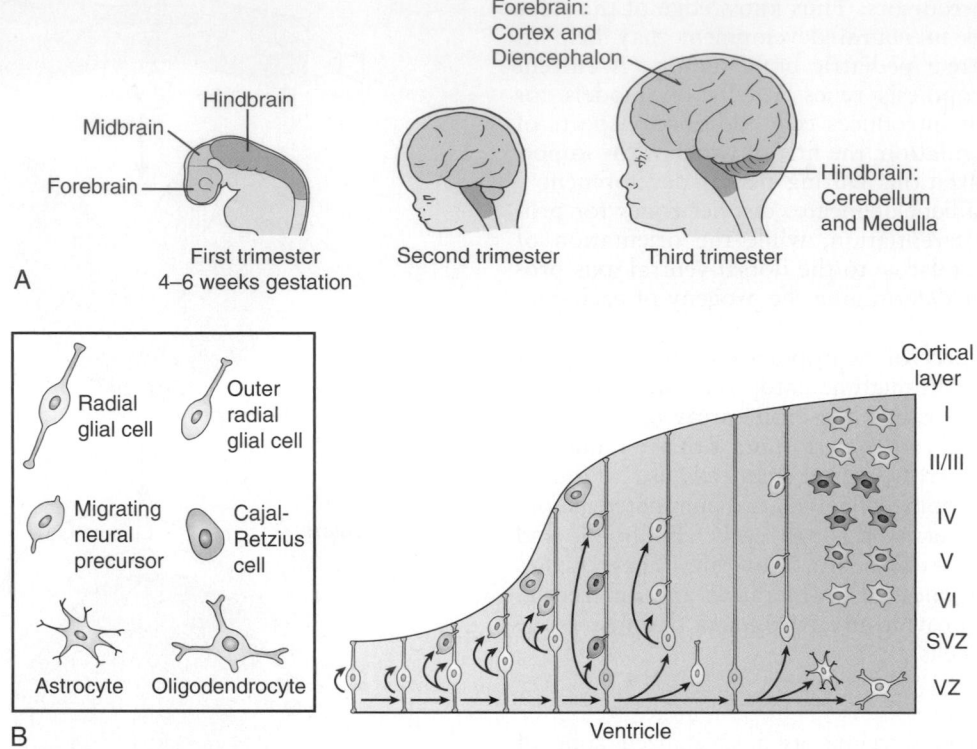

Figure 57-5 A, Outpouching of the neural tube. **B,** Cortical Development process. Radial Glia (RG) function as neural stem/precursor cells. Initially, the population of RG expands by proliferation, and the early RG produce a largely transient population of Cajal-Retzius cells. RG continue to proliferate and produce: (1) outer RG located in the Subventricular zone *(SVZ),* (2) more RG, and (3) early cortical neurons. Neurons produced by the RG and the outer RG migrate along the RG to the cortex. Neurons are generated in an inside-out pattern so that the earliest neurons are found in the deep cortical layers. After most of the neurons have been generated, RG give rise to astrocytes and oligodendrocytes. The cell of origin for astrocytomas may be residual RG, outer RG, or astrocytes.

Although the VZ in the forebrain initially contains the dividing neural stem/progenitor cells, during development the size of the VZ progressively decreases while the adjacent SVZ increases in size. The early generated cells migrate radially from the VZ and SVZ to become the neurons of the innermost cortical layer (layer VI), and later mitoses give rise to neurons that also migrate radially and occupy increasingly superficial layers. Inhibitory neurons are derived from precursors in the medial ganglionic eminence. They migrate tangentially throughout the cortex. Thus the cortex develops in an inside-out pattern. Toward the end of the prenatal neurogenic phase, the precursors of the VZ and SVZ generate glial cells, including astrocytes, oligodendrocytes, and ependymal cells.[57,58]

A small population of precursors remains in the SVZ, just above the ependymal cells, throughout life. These neural stem cells continue to generate glial cells and oligodendrocytes and also continue to give rise to a limited number of neuronal cells through adult neurogenesis. An additional zone of adult neurogenesis is located in the hippocampus, adjacent to the granular zone. Thus the neural stem cell represents a common precursor for glial

and neuronal cells. Accumulating data suggest that many, if not most, brain tumors arise from such stem cells or their early derivatives.

Cerebellar Cortex

The cerebellar cortex develops in a way that has some similarities to, but some differences from, the pattern in the cerebral cortex. The hindbrain is the site where the neural tube closes last. While closure occurs, the neural folds pucker to form the rhombic lips. These two protrusions will give rise to many cell types of the cerebellum and pons. Cells in the VZ of the upper rhombic lip proliferate and then begin an unusual migration pattern. The precursor cells of the rhombic lip migrate over the top of the rhombic lip and disperse by moving from the caudal aspect of the pucker to cover the rhombic lip or incipient cerebellum. The rhombic lip–derived precursors settle in a zone that covers the developing cerebellum, which is called the external granule cell (external germinal cell [EGL]) layer. This layer constitutes a site of extensive postnatal proliferation and is a specialized mitogenic niche where precursors divide and give rise almost exclusively to cerebellar granule cells, the most numerous neuronal cells in the brain. This secondary proliferative zone may be necessary to generate this vast number of granule cells. To generate the 60 to 80 billion granule cell neurons, the granule cell precursors in the EGL undergo many rounds of cell divisions, beginning in the ninth week after fertilization and continuing through the first 18 months of life in humans. Other stem/precursors in the VZ follow distinct differentiation paths. Radial glia adjacent to the cerebellum provide one source of these multipotential stem/precursors. Some VZ stem/precursors migrate toward the cerebellar white matter, where they can give rise to cerebellar interneurons and glia. Others migrate past the cerebellar white matter and form the Bergmann glia of the cerebellar cortex.

It has been suggested that four distinct subtypes of cerebellar stem/precursors each give rise to a distinct subtype of medulloblastoma. A great deal of evidence has indicated that the granule cell precursors of the EGL are a cell of origin for the sonic hedgehog (SHH) subtype of medulloblastoma.[59] First, in very young children, medulloblastomas are often continuous with the EGL, and an intermediate zone of dysplastic cells can sometimes be seen to join the EGL and tumor tissue. Second, the appearance and pattern of gene expression of the granule cell precursors resemble those of SHH-type medulloblastoma. Finally, SHH signaling pathways that normally regulate proliferation of granule cell precursors are constitutively active in one type of medulloblastoma (discussed later).

The precursor cells adjacent to the ventricle that resemble radial glia have been suggested to be the cells of origin of Wingless (Wnt)-subtype medulloblastomas. In mouse models, activation of the Wnt pathway and/or activation of phosphoinositide 3′ kinase (PI3K) in these radial glial precursors can mimic this group of medulloblastomas.

The cellular origin and the oncogenic mutations responsible for initiating other medulloblastoma subtypes have also been identified. For example, it has been suggested that the stem cells of the white matter and earlier stem cells may provide the cellular origin for group III and IV medulloblastomas, respectively.[60] It has been suggested that less specialized stem cells can give rise to medulloblastomas. Indeed molecular characterization of medulloblastomas suggests that genetically distinct tumor types exist that may represent the oncogenic transformation of cerebellar precursor cells at different locations and stages.[61,62] This scenario would be analogous to leukemias, in which oncogenic transformation of hematopoietic precursors at distinct developmental stages leads to distinct types of leukemias.

Cancer Stem Cells

Brain tumors have predominantly been classified as neuronal or glial in nature. The neuronal tumors include CNS PNETs, pineoblastomas, and medulloblastomas, as well as ganglion cell tumors. Glial tumors include many different gliomas, such as juvenile PA, subependymal giant cell astrocytoma, other low-grade astrocytomas, pontine glioma, malignant astrocytoma (including glioblastoma multiforme), and tumors that resemble other glial cell types, such as oligodendroglioma and ependymoma. Although this classification schema remains useful, it appears that many brain tumors are generated by oncogenic mutations in neural stem–precursor cells, rather than more mature cell types. Furthermore although cancers traditionally have been viewed as clonal, increasing evidence indicates that this is not the case. Instead the concept of the existence of a subpopulation of cancer stem cells has developed—distinctive cells within the tumor that are uniquely capable of regenerating the cancer.[63] Recent studies of brain tumors have identified cluster of differentiation (CD)-133–positive cells as radioresistant, slowly proliferating cancer stem cells that are particularly prevalent in high-grade tumors, such as glioblastoma multiforme. The ability of these cancer stem cells to survive surgical resection, radiation, and cytotoxic chemotherapy is a major reason for the difficulty in curing high-grade brain tumors.

Genetic and Signaling Pathways Implicated in Development and in Pediatric Tumors

Inherited disorders that cause a familial propensity for brain tumors have provided an important method for identifying genetic pathways that contribute to these cancers.[64-68] Neurofibromatosis, tuberous sclerosis, Gorlin syndrome, Turcot syndrome, Cowden syndrome, and the *SMARCB1* (switch/sucrose nonfermentable [SWI/SNF]–related, matrix-associated, actin-dependent regulator of chromatin, subfamily b, member 1) mutation all represent heritable disorders associated with an increased risk of brain tumors (Table 57-1).[69]

Neurofibromatosis Type 1

Neurofibromatosis type 1 (NF-1) is an autosomal-dominant neuroectodermal disorder characterized by café-au-lait spots and fibromatous tumors of the skin. Additional clinical features that can be seen in NF-1 (Box 57-1) include Lisch nodules in the iris, scoliosis, cognitive problems, and epilepsy.[70-72] Several tumors occur with greater frequency in persons with this disorder, including pheochromocytoma, ependymoma, meningioma, and glioma; this characteristic may relate to dysregulation of specific stem cell populations.[73] Among these tumors, gliomas of the optic pathway are the most common tumors seen.[74] The unique biology of these tumors is slowly being elucidated through studies of the role of NF-1 in the development of the optic pathway in animal models.[75] Neurofibromatosis is caused by heterozygous mutations in neurofibromin, and the cancers observed in this disorder result from loss of heterozygosity at chromosome 17q11.2, leaving only the mutant NF-1 allele.[76] Although this disorder is inherited as an autosomal-dominant disease, as many as 50% of patients represent new germline mutations and therefore do not have a family history of the disorder.

The neurofibromin protein is a 250-kD tumor suppressor that functions as a guanosine triphosphatase activator for the small G protein Ras.[77] In this way, active neurofibromin decreases the ratio of guanosine triphosphate–bound (active) to guanosine diphosphate–bound (inactive)

TABLE 57-1 Common Chromosomal Abnormalities Associated with Pediatric Central Nervous System Tumors

Chromosomal Abnormality	Tumor
Monosomy 22	Atypical teratoid-rhabdoid tumor Acoustic neuromas Meningioma Ependymoma
1p and/or 22q loss	Oligodendroglioma
Isochrome i17	Medulloblastoma
9q22 loss (*PTCH1* gene)	Medulloblastoma
Loss of chromosome 10, 9p, 17p	Progression to high-grade glioma

Ras or Ras-like protein. While activated Ras stimulates mitogen-activated protein kinases (MAPKs) and PI3Ks, the change in Ras activity leads to unregulated proliferation and survival (Fig. 57-6).[78] Although the incidence of brain tumors, particularly optic nerve gliomas, is significantly increased in persons with NF-1 (approximately 5% to 15%), the tumors that develop in these patients tend to be less aggressive than other gliomas. These tumors are more susceptible to chemotherapeutic interventions and thus can be treated differently than other gliomas. In fact many tumors stop growing spontaneously. The unique developmental environment of the optic pathways may account for the differential occurrence of these tumors in patients with NF-1, as well as their increased responsiveness.[79] In addition to optic pathway gliomas (OPGs), non-OPGs occur at frequencies 100 times greater than expected, with the most common sites being the brainstem (49%), cerebral hemispheres (21%), and basal ganglia (14%). Other MRI signal abnormalities within the brain are often observed in patients with NF-1.[80,81] The most characteristic abnormality is the unidentified bright object.[82] Unlike low-grade gliomas (LGGs), these lesions are bright on T2-weighted imaging, do not demonstrate contrast enhancement, and usually produce neither mass effect nor symptoms. They often come and go and should not be biopsied or treated. The varied intracranial localization of lesions and variable need for neurosurgical intervention in a subset of children with NF-1 suggests that radiologic surveillance should be based on careful and regular neurologic and ophthalmologic examinations.[83]

Box 57-1 Diagnostic Criteria of Neurofibromatosis Type 1*

Six or more café-au-lait spots ≥1.5 cm in postpubescent individuals or >0.5 cm in prepubescent individuals
Two or more neurofibromas or one or more plexiform neurofibromas
Freckling in the axillae or groin
Optic glioma
Two or more Lisch nodules
Dysplasia of the sphenoid bone or dysplasia or thinning of the cortex of long bones
A first degree relative with neurofibromatosis type 1

*The diagnosis of neurofibromatosis type 1 requires any two or more of these criteria.

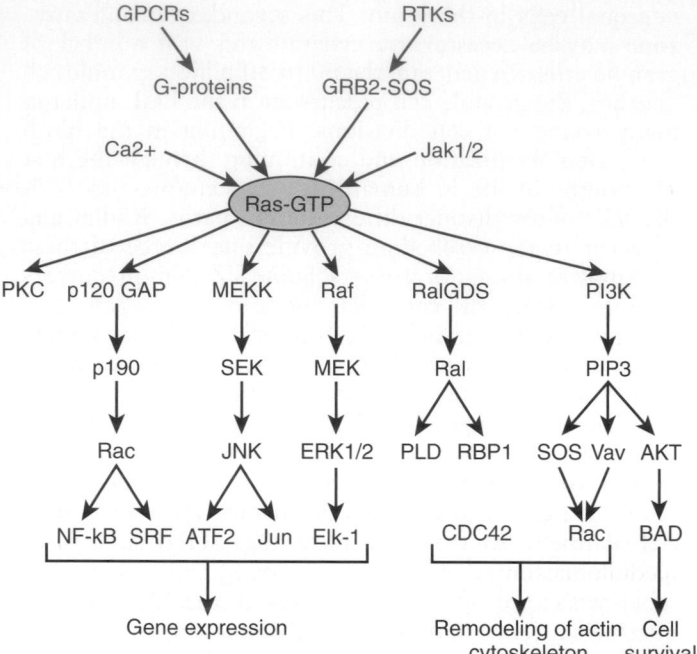

Figure 57-6 Ras and downstream pathway. *AKT*, V-Akt Murine Thymoma Viral Oncogene Homolog; *ATF2*, activating transcription factor 2; *Bad*, bcl-2-associated death promoter; Ca2+, Calcium; *CDC42*, cell division cycle 42; *Elk-1*, ETS domain-containing protein; *GPCRs*, G-Protein Coupled Serpentine Receptors; *G proteins*, guanosine nucleotide-binding proteins; *GRB2-SOS*, Growth Factor Receptor-Bound Protein-2—Son of Sevenless; *Jak1/2*, Janus kinase inhibitor1/2; *JNK*, c-Jun N-terminal kinases; *Jun*, jun proto-oncogene; *MEK*, mitogen-activated protein kinase kinase 1; *ERK1/2*, Extracellular Signal-Regulated Kinase 1/2; *MEKK*, mitogen-activated protein kinase kinase kinase 1, E3 ubiquitin protein ligase; *NF-KappaB*, Nuclear Factor-KappaB; *PI3K*, phosphatidylinositol 3-kinase, catalytic subunit type 3; *PIP3*, Phosphatidylinositol (3,4,5)-trisphosphate (PtdIns(3,4,5)P3); *PKC*, Protein Kinase-C; *PLD*, Phospholipase D; *p120 GAP*, Ras GTPase activating protein; *p190*, RhoGAPp190; *Rac*, ras-related C3 botulinum toxin substrate 2 (rho family, small GTP binding protein Rac2); *Raf*, v-raf murine sarcoma 3611 viral oncogene homolog; *Ral*, v-ral simian leukemia viral oncogene homolog B (ras related; GTP binding protein); *RalGDS*, Ral Guanine Nucleotide Dissociation Stimulator; *Ras-GTP*, v-Ki-ras2 Kirsten rat sarcoma viral oncogene homolog guanosine triphosphate (GTP); *RBP1*, Retinoblastoma binding protein1; *RTKs*, Receptor tyrosine kinases; *SEK*, Dual specificity mitogen-activated protein kinase kinase 4; *SOS*, son of sevenless homolog 1; *SRF*, serum response factor (c-fos serum response element-binding transcription factor); *Vav*, vav 3 guanine nucleotide exchange factor.

Patients with NF-1 appear to be at increased risk of moyamoya syndrome,[84,85] and this risk becomes especially high after cerebral radiation therapy. Patients with NF-1, even in the absence of a brain tumor, are also affected by a number of other problems as a result of their disease, in particular neurocognitive impairment, which can range from mild to severe.[78]

Neurofibromatosis Type 2 (Merlin)

Neurofibromatosis type 2 (NF-2) is characterized by familial, bilateral acoustic neuromas and is caused by mutations in the gene that encodes merlin, or schwannomin, localized to chromosome 22q12.2.[86,87] Merlin interacts with cytoskeletal components and appears to be important in adhesion-dependent growth control. Persons with germline mutations also have skin tumors with both peripheral schwannomas and neurofibromas and have a propensity to develop intracranial meningiomas or, more rarely, gliomas and spinal tumors.[88] The onset of symptomatic tumor growth is uncommon in childhood, and in most patients the condition is identified in adulthood.

Tuberous Sclerosis

A third neurocutaneous disorder associated with an increased propensity for brain tumors is tuberous sclerosis (TS). This condition can be caused by mutations in either of two genes, *TSC1* (hamartin, at chromosome 9q34)[89] or *TSC2* (tuberin, at chromosome 6p), and it is characterized by hamartomata in multiple organs. The most common clinical manifestations include epilepsy, cognitive and behavioral problems, and characteristic skin lesions. The white leaf-shaped skin lesions can best be seen under a Wood light; adenoma sebaceum (facial angiofibroma) can also be seen. Renal manifestations include angiomyolipomas, renal cysts, and, more rarely, renal cell cancer. Brain tumors develop in between 5% and 14% of patients, the most common being the subependymal giant cell astrocytoma (SEGA); other gliomas and ependymomas are also relatively frequent. Careful serial evaluations are required because of the possibility of additional tumor development in this patient population.[90] Cortical tubers can cause seizures and require specialized neurosurgical approaches in children.[91] Resection of tubers does not always control seizures and suggests that extratuberal epileptogenic brain abnormalities may be present that require more specialized imaging.[92]

The phenotypic similarity of mutations in Tsc1 and Tsc2 is explained by the finding that these two proteins interact directly with one another.[89] This complex acts as a guanosine triphosphatase–activating protein for Ras homolog enriched in brain (Rheb). The decreased activity of Rheb inhibits the mammalian target of rapamycin (mTOR) and p70 ribosomal S6 kinase–1. As a result there is diminished translation by eukaryotic translation initiation factor 4E-binding protein–1 (EIF4EBP1; 602223). The hamartin-tuberin complex thereby regulates growth and proliferation of subependymal and subventricular neural stem cells. The Tsc-mTOR pathways may normally be regulated by Wnt and insulin-like growth factor (IGF) ligands during development. Patients with TS who have SEGA or LGGs have demonstrated responses to mTOR inhibitors, confirming the clinical relevance of these findings.[93]

Gorlin Syndrome

Gorlin syndrome (also known as basal cell nevus syndrome or nevoid basal cell carcinoma syndrome) is characterized by multiple basal cell carcinomas or basal cell nevi before the age of 30 years, odontogenic keratocysts or polyostotic bone cysts, and palmar and plantar pits. Other manifestations include rib or vertebral anomalies, large head circumference with frontal bossing, cardiac or ovarian fibroma, and lymphomesenteric cysts.[94] Gorlin syndrome is caused by mutations in PTCH1 (chromosome 9q22.3), the receptor for the SHH ligand.[95-100] Medulloblastoma develops in approximately 4% to 10%

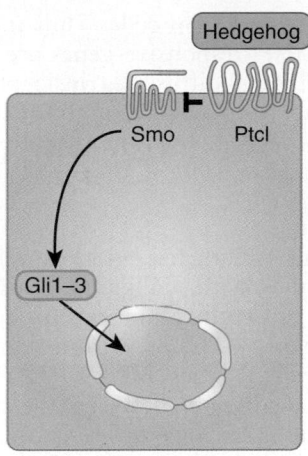

Figure 57-7 The PTCH1 gene product functions as both a receptor and negative regulator of signaling initiated by sonic hedgehog or the related ligands, Indian hedgehog and desert hedgehog. These ligands initiate an unusual and incompletely understood signaling pathway that culminates in Gli1-3 initiating transcription of cell cycle genes, including cyclin D1 and D2. *Smo,* Smoothen.

of persons with Gorlin syndrome. This syndrome also predisposes to other tumors, such as rhabdomyosarcoma and meningioma.[101,102]

The PTCH1 gene product functions as both a receptor and negative regulator of signaling initiated by SHH or the related ligands, Indian hedgehog and desert hedgehog. These ligands initiate an unusual and incompletely understood signaling pathway (Fig. 57-7). When a hedgehog ligand binds to Ptc, this alters the activation state of smoothened, or Smo, a seven-transmembrane protein. Normally Ptc represses the activity of Smo; however, when a ligand binds to Ptc, this derepresses Smo activity. Active Smo translocates to a distinctive subcellular organelle known as a primary cilium. Here active Smo enables the dissociation of a signaling complex containing suppressor of fused homolog (SUFU) and Glioma-associated Oncogene Homolog (Gli) transcription factors. The dissociation of this complex results in the nuclear relocalization of Gli family members and increased expression of Gli family members, as well as the expression of v-myc avian myelocytomatosis viral oncogene neuroblastoma derived homolog (MYCN), D-type cyclins, and the stem cell–associated chromatic complex component, B lymphoma Mo-MLV insertion region 1 homolog (Bmi-1). The active pathway thereby potentiates proliferation and inhibits apoptosis.

Good evidence indicates that constitutive activity of the SHH pathway can cause medulloblastoma. Gorlin syndrome is associated with increased incidence of medulloblastoma, as is the analogous mutation in mice. Activating mutations in Smo, or mutations in suppression of fused (SuFu), can also lead to these brain tumors. Recent studies have suggested that specific inhibitors of Smo may provide valuable biologic therapies for medulloblastoma.

The value of understanding developmental pathways that normally regulate neural precursor proliferation to decipher the mechanisms that cause pediatric brain tumors is reinforced by data showing that SHH ligand stimulates and regulates proliferation of granule cell precursors and neural stem cells. Thus it is perhaps not surprising that SHH-responsive genes are also expressed in gliomas, including diffuse intrinsic pontine gliomas (DIPG) and glioblastoma. Thus inhibitors of SHH signaling may play a role in treating several types of brain tumors.[103]

Turcot Syndrome

Turcot syndrome is characterized by familial polyposis of the colon, together with malignant brain tumors. This disorder can be caused by mutations in the adenomatous polyposis coli gene (*APC*, on chromosome 5q21) or in the mismatch repair genes *MLH1* (120436) or *PMS2* (600259). The distinction between the clinical entities that result from mutations in *APC* and mutations in repair genes[104] include the nature of the brain tumors seen; the characteristic brain tumors seen are medulloblastomas or astrocytomas, respectively.[105] APC is a large protein whose activity is critical in the Wnt signaling pathway. Therefore inactivating mutations of *APC* result in the aberrant accumulation of β-catenin and increased transcription of transcription factor 4 (Tcf4)-dependent genes, including *c-myc*. Mutations in β-catenin and in APC have also been reported in sporadic medulloblastoma,[104] highlighting the importance of this pathway for this malignant cerebellar tumor.

Wnts constitute a family of ligands that can act through two distinct signaling pathways. The canonical Wnt pathway is initiated when Wnt proteins bind to cell-surface receptors of the Frizzled family. This binding leads to activation of Dishevelled (DSH) family proteins. When DSH becomes activated, it inhibits a protein complex that includes axin, glycogen synthase kinase–3

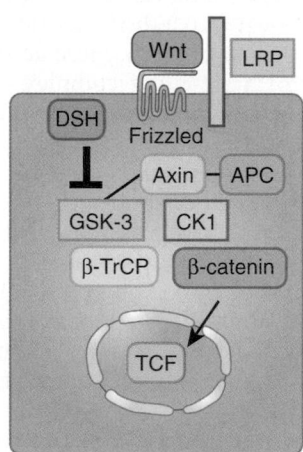

Figure 57-8 Wnts are a family of ligands that can act through two distinct signaling pathways. The canonical Wnt pathway is initiated when Wnt proteins bind to cell-surface receptors of the Frizzled family, which leads to activation of Dishevelled family proteins. When Dishevelled *(DSH)* is activated, it inhibits a protein complex that includes axin, glycogen synthase kinase 3 *(GSK-3)*, and adenomatous polyposis coli *(APC)*. The axin/GSK-3/APC complex usually promotes degradation of β-catenin. After this β-catenin destruction complex is inhibited, cytoplasmic β-catenin becomes stabilized so that it is able to enter the nucleus. Nuclear β-catenin interacts with the transcription factor *(TCF)* family transcription factors to promote expression of a gene program that includes cyclin-D and thereby stimulates cell cycle progression. *CK1,* Casein kinase 1; *LRP,* lipoprotein receptor-related protein; *β-TrCP,* beta-transducin repeat containing protein.

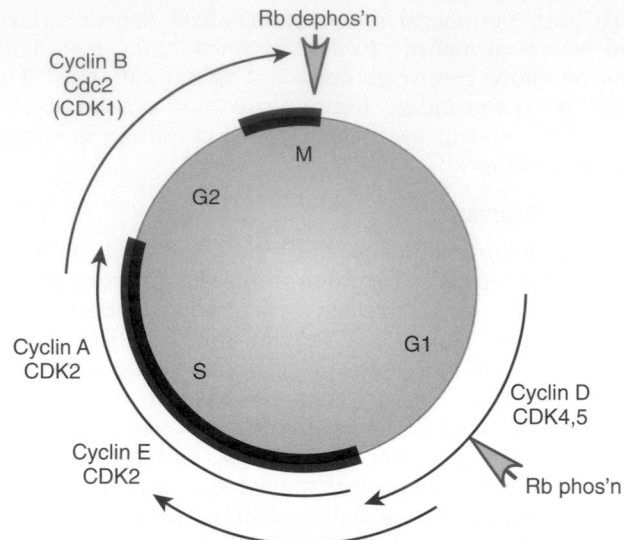

Figure 57-9 Cell cycle diagram. Oncogenic events can increase cyclin-D (i.e., hedgehog or Wnt signals) or alter other cell cycle regulators. *Cdc2,* Cell division cycle protein 2 homolog; *CDK,* cyclin-dependent kinase; *Rb dephos'n,* retinoblastoma 1 dephosphorylated; *Rb phos'n,* retinoblastoma 1 phosphorylated.

(GSK3), and APC (Fig. 57-8). The axin–GSK3–APC complex promotes the proteolytic degradation of β-catenin. After this β-catenin destruction complex is inhibited, cytoplasmic β-catenin becomes stabilized and β-catenin is then able to enter the nucleus. Nuclear β-catenin interacts with TCF-LEF (lymphoid enhancer-binding factor 1) family transcription factors to promote the expression of a gene program that includes c-myc, N-myc, and cyclin D1 and thereby stimulate cell cycle progression (Fig. 57-9). It is not clear whether the noncanonical Wnt pathway, which does not involve APC, also contributes to brain tumors.

As is the case for SHH signaling, the ability of the deregulated Wnt pathway to cause medulloblastomas highlights the relevance of understanding neurodevelopment. In the absence of Wnt1, the cerebellum does not form properly.[106] The Wnt and SHH pathways cooperate during normal development to generate normal cerebellar neurons. It is likely that these pathways also synergize in tumor formation, particularly during medulloblastoma oncogenesis.

Lhermitte-Duclos Disease, Cowden Syndrome, and *PTEN* Mutation

Activation of PI3K results in phosphorylation of phospholipids at the 3′ position; this phosphorylation is removed by the phosphatase and tensin homolog *(PTEN)* phosphatase. Therefore mutations in *PTEN* result in excess and/or incorrectly localized activation of the PI3K pathway. PI3K is critical in several signaling pathways that regulate proliferation, survival, migration, and cell size. The multiplicity of functions explains the diverse spectrum of disorders seen in *PTEN* mutations, including neurologic, cutaneous, and oncologic syndromes.

Molecular studies on Lhermitte-Duclos disease (LDD) tissue have revealed *PTEN* gene mutations in 83% of cases, with immunostaining showing lost or reduced *PTEN* expression in 78% of cases. As a consequence, Akt phosphorylation is increased.[107] Initially Cowden syndrome was described as a familial predisposition for breast cancers, thyroid cancers, brain tumors, and other neoplasia. This syndrome was subsequently recognized as a spectrum of disorders that includes LDD and Bannayan-Ruvalcaba-Riley syndrome. The diagnosis of LDD depends on characteristic hamartomas of the cerebellum. These lesions in the cerebellar cortex exhibit thickened cerebellar folia, with misplaced cerebellar granule cells and enlarged size of the cerebellar neuronal cell bodies. In addition to cerebellar ataxia, these hamartomas can cause hydrocephalus and herniation. Another manifestation of the *PTEN* mutations is seen in Bannayan-Ruvalcaba-Riley syndrome, with macrocephaly, seizures, cognitive dysfunction, and autistic behaviors. Different manifestations of the mutation can be observed even within a family, and thus a careful consideration of family history is warranted.

RB1 Mutations

The retinoblastoma gene was the first tumor suppressor gene identified. In addition to the retinal tumors seen in persons with germline mutations in *Rb1*, "trilateral" retinoblastoma has been described. In these persons, bilateral retinoblastoma is accompanied by a pineal tumor (pineoblastoma) with similar characteristics to retinoblastoma. The other secondary tumors that occur in patients with retinoblastoma are osteosarcomas. The Rb1 protein is required for the G1 checkpoint, and studies on this pathway have provided key insights into the mechanisms of growth regulation.

Atypical Teratoid Rhabdoid Tumor

Mutations in the sucrose nonfermentable 5/integrase interactor 1 (SNF5/INI1) component of the SWI-SNF DNA remodeling complex cause rhabdoid tumors. These tumors include renal and soft tissue tumors and brain tumors. In the CNS, these brain tumors, called atypical teratoid rhabdoid tumors (ATRTs), are characteristically found in the cerebellopontine angle or in supratentorial locations. Prior to the identification of deletions or mutations of the *SMARCB1* gene on chromosome 22, these tumors were historically grouped with medulloblastomas and PNETs. However their histology is distinct, with a mixture of atypical spindle cells, poorly differentiated small round blue cells, and rhabdoid cells with prominent cytoplasmic inclusions, large eccentric vesicular nuclei, and adjacent whorls of intermediate filaments. The nature of the cell of origin for these tumors, and why they predominantly arise in very young children, is as yet poorly understood.

CONCEPTUAL ORGANIZATION OF PEDIATRIC BRAIN TUMORS

Leukemias are considered in the context of their lineage and stage of development, whereas neuroblastoma is evaluated by the extent of spread, age of the child, and molecular phenotype. Neither of these approaches is well suited to CNS tumors. Although brain tumors share an anatomic site, a number of unique cell types, significant heterogeneity in distribution, and differences in the consequence of therapy differ according to the age of the patient and location within the CNS. These factors, combined with a complicated historic nomenclature, require a different approach to understanding these tumors.

The CNS is made up of three major elements, and therefore three major groups of tumors are commonly observed:

1. Glial cells—responsible for structural support and maintenance of the CNS, and composed of three cell subtypes:
   a. Astrocytes—structural support for the CNS → astrocytoma
   b. Ependymocytes—help regulate homeostasis of the CNS → ependymoma
   c. Oligodendrocytes—myelination for the neural axons → oligodendroglioma
2. Neurons—electrical activity → medulloblastoma, pineoblastoma, CNS PNETs
3. Choroid plexus—production of cerebrospinal fluid (CSF) → choroid plexus carcinoma (CPC)

Tumors arising from glia, neurons, or the choroid plexus account for approximately 90% of all pediatric CNS tumors. The remaining 10% of pediatric brain tumors arise from cells that are derived from extracranial sources but become entrapped in the developing CNS during embryogenesis (Fig. 57-10).

4. Germ cells, which arise in the primordial gonadal ridge and normally migrate down to their final resting place in the abdomen (ovaries) or scrotum (testes), can occasionally migrate upward and become enveloped in the developing brain → germinoma, nongerminomatous germ cell tumor (NGGCT)
5. Cells from the Rathke pouch, which normally gives rise to structures of the head and neck, can become trapped within the developing brain → craniopharyngioma

Two additional tumor types that are rare in children but account for approximately 80% of CNS tumors in

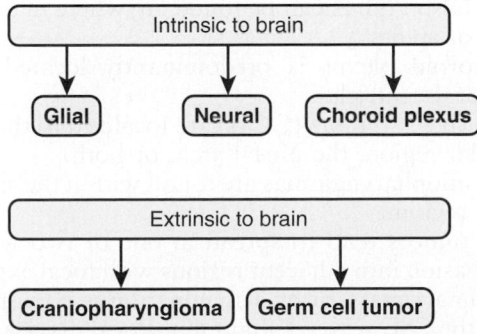

Figure 57-10 Most pediatric brain tumors can be classified into one of five different categories, based on cell of origin. Glial, neuronal, and choroid plexus tumors account for those that derive from cells within the central nervous system (CNS), while germ cell tumors and craniopharyngiomas arise from cells that are enclosed in the developing CNS in early development as a result of abnormal migration.

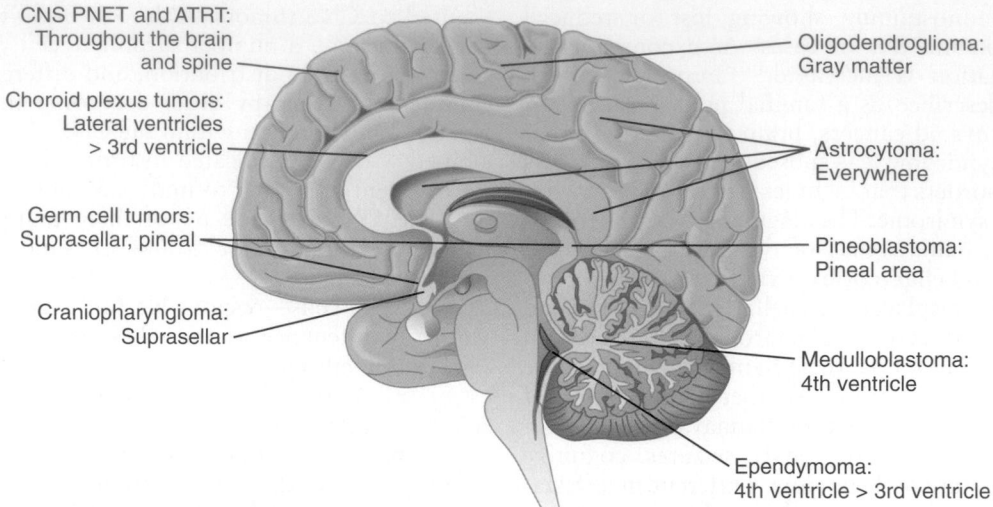

Figure 57-11 Common distributions of different pediatric central nervous system *(CNS)* tumor histologies. *ATRT,* Atypical teratoid/rhabdoid tumor; *CNS PNET,* primitive neuroectodermal tumor.

adults include metastatic carcinoma, especially of the breast, colon, lung, and prostate. Metastatic lesions to the brain in pediatric patients are exceptionally rare, and when they occur, they are usually in the context of end-stage disease.[108-110] Meningiomas are the other common adult brain tumor that is rarely observed in children.

The five primary cell types of the brain are not evenly distributed in the CNS (Fig. 57-11):

1. Glia.
   a. Astrocytes are found throughout the entire brain and spine.
   b. Ependymocytes line each of the ventricles, and hence these cells are most predominant in the 4th ventricle > 3rd ventricle.
   c. Oligodendrocytes are found around the junction of the gray-white matter.
2. Neural tumors are defined by location rather than histology; molecular characterization indicates that these distinctions based on location are biologically important.
   a. Medulloblastoma is found within the posterior fossa.
   b. Pineoblastoma is found within the pineal region.
   c. CNS PNETs can be found anywhere in the brain or spine.
3. Choroid plexus is predominantly located in the lateral ventricles.
4. Germ cell tumors (GCTs) are localized to the suprasellar region, the pineal area, or both.
5. Craniopharyngiomas are found within the suprasellar region.

Brain tumors tend to spread in one of two ways, by direct invasion into adjacent regions with focal expansion of the primary mass, or by dissemination (seeding) of cells through the CSF, with resultant multifocal disease. Of the five tumor types listed, glial tumors and craniopharyngiomas tend to grow by direct extension and the other three tend to grow by seeding cells into the CSF. The workup of patients with newly diagnosed brain tumors will therefore require MRI of the involved area for glial tumors and craniopharyngioma, and craniospinal imaging and CSF cytology will be needed for seeding tumors (neural, choroid plexus, and germ cell).

Three major treatment strategies are considered for all CNS tumors: (1) surgery, (2) radiotherapy, and (3) chemotherapy. Certain general principles can be applied to their use (Table 57-2):

1. Surgery is important for making the diagnosis, achieving rapid reduction in tumor size, and relieving elevated pressure from obstructive hydrocephalus.
2. Radiotherapy is effective for a wide range of tumors but has significant morbidity on the developing CNS, which frequently limits its applicability. In general focal tumors (gliomas and craniopharyngiomas) are treated with focal radiation therapy, whereas seeding tumors (medulloblastomas, pineoblastomas, CNS PNETs, CPCs, and GCTs) are treated with craniospinal radiotherapy with a boost to the primary site and areas of metastatic disease, particularly in children 3 years and older.
3. Chemotherapy is effective for most seeding tumors and has become part of the initial therapy for these tumors (neural, choroid plexus, and germ cell). By contrast chemotherapy has had limited success for most focal tumors (malignant gliomas and craniopharyngiomas).

The classification of tumors based on their histologic characteristics is important to provide prognostic information, although the unique environment of the brain makes the classification of benign versus malignant less important than for most other sites in the body. The brain and spine are critical for the control of basic autonomic response, as well as higher order function, and therefore limit the ability to obtain complete resection with a wide margin in most cases. Even benign tumors located in critical and inoperable structures may result in death if their growth cannot be stopped or slowed. Conversely many highly malignant World Health Organization (WHO) grade IV brain tumors (defined histologically)

TABLE 57-2 Common Types of Treatment for Pediatric Central Nervous System Tumors*

Type of Tumor	Method of Spread	Attempted Surgery	Type of Radiation Therapy†	Chemotherapy
Glial	Local	Yes	Focal	No‡
Neuronal	Seeding	Yes	CSI	Yes
Choroid	Seeding	Yes	CSI	Yes
Germ cell	Seeding	Yes	CSI	Yes
Cranio	Local	Yes	Focal	No

CSI, Craniospinal irradiation.

*Tumors that exhibit focal growth receive attempted resection and focal radiation therapy. Tumors that are at high risk for early dissemination are treated with focal surgery, CSI, and chemotherapy.

†Radiation therapy is often deferred in children younger than 3 years.

‡Symptomatic unresectable low-grade gliomas are treated with chemotherapy to delay radiation therapy.

that are responsive to radiation treatment (CNS germinoma) or radiation and chemotherapy (medulloblastoma) have an excellent prognosis. Because patients and their parents have preconceived notions about the importance of benign versus malignant, clarifying these terms early can be important.

The presenting symptoms for patients with CNS tumors can usually be categorized into one of two patterns: (1) direct compression of nerves or (2) obstructive hydrocephalus. The location of the tumor, histologic subtype, and age of the patient are major determinants in the length of clinical symptoms before the diagnosis is made.[111] Although dependent on the location and rapidity of growth, the time to diagnosis for many children may range from 3 to 8 months, and multiple visits to primary care providers is not infrequent.[112] For younger children who cannot verbalize their symptoms and for whom fine motor coordination, speech, and gait are still developing, even greater delays may result.

Symptoms related to the direct compression of adjacent nerves by a tumor will cause a unique constellation of symptoms that can be localized to an area as a result of the highly organized structure of the CNS.

- The posterior fossa contains the brainstem, 12 cranial nerves, and the descending and ascending fibers connecting the upper and lower aspects of the CNS, in addition to the cerebellum, which is responsible for movement and balance. Tumors in this area result in cranial nerve dysfunction such as diplopia, choking, or facial asymmetry. Tumors of the brainstem can compress the descending motor tracts, resulting in lower motor deficits. Compression of the cerebellum will lead to ataxia or dysmetria.
- The thalamus is the major relay station of coordinated function from the motor strip and other areas of the cortex. Tumors in this area will often lead to significant hemiparesis.
- The frontal lobe regulates mood and behavior and contains the motor cortex. Patients with tumors in

this area will often present with changes in behavior (more aggressive or more passive), worsening school performance, or specific motor deficits (except those controlled by the cranial nerves).[113,114] In some patients, more subtle signs of frontal lobe dysfunction such as fatigue, lack of interest, or decreased energy can be mistaken for the behaviors frequent in adolescence.

- The parietal lobe possesses the centers for sensory function. Tumors in this area can often compress a specific area of the sensory cortex, resulting in a focal sensory deficit that does not follow classic dermatomal or peripheral nerve patterns.
- The hypothalamus and suprasellar regions contain the area that coordinates endocrine function (i.e., growth hormone, regulation of salts, pubertal development, and stress hormones). This area is near the optic nerves and chiasm. Tumors in this area often present as a change in growth (accelerated or delayed), hormonal dysfunction, or change in vision.
- The occipital lobe organizes and interprets vision. Tumors in the occipital lobe will present with homonymous defects in vision.
- The pineal area sits adjacent to the centers of upward gaze (supranuclear tectal or pretectal areas). Lesions in this area can result in Parinaud syndrome (paresis of upward gaze, enlarged pupils that are poorly reactive to light, and poor or limited convergence).
- The spinal cord possesses all the ascending and descending tracks for sensory and motor function to all areas innervated from that segment of the cord and below. Mass lesions in this area will reduce the motor and/or sensory activity of those areas below the lesion and can consist of motor, sensory, temperature, position, and vibration abnormalities.
- Gray matter is where neuron bodies are concentrated. Lesions in the gray matter of the frontal, parietal, temporal, and occipital lobes can result in seizure activity.[115] Although initially focal in nature, seizures can rapidly become generalized, obscuring the initial presenting focality.
- White matter tracts are the myelinated axons of neurons. Lesions in white matter tracts typically result in focal neurologic deficits that correspond to the tracts compressed.

The differential diagnosis of a new tumor of the CNS should be developed using the preceding information. Symptoms will help localize the probable site of the tumor. In turn the site will assist in developing a limited differential diagnosis of possible tumors at that site. Staging and treatment can then be considered in the context of focal versus seeding tumors. Although this exercise will not obviate the need for a definitive biopsy, it can help organize the large array of CNS tumors and ensure that appropriate presurgical planning and staging have been completed.

Obstructive Hydrocephalus and Raised Intracranial Pressure

The brain and spinal cord are supported in the cranium and spinal canal by the CSF, which is largely localized to

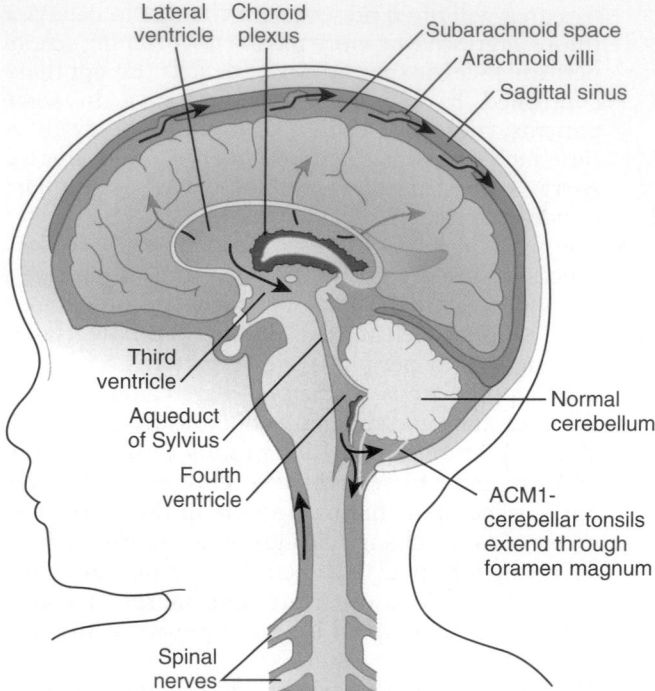

Figure 57-12 Normal flow of cerebrospinal fluid. *Blue arrows* show compression of cortex as a result of obstructive hydrocephalus. *ACM1,* Arnold-Chiari Malformation Type 1.

the subarachnoid space. CSF is initially made by the choroid plexus in the lateral ventricles and, to a lesser degree, in the third and fourth ventricles. The production of CSF is not linked to its passage from the lateral and third ventricles to the fourth ventricle and, finally, through the foramen of Magendie or foramen of Luschka, where it is eventually reabsorbed by the arachnoid villi (Fig. 57-12). The ventricles hold approximately 50 mL of CSF and, with approximately 500 mL of CSF produced each day, any failure to remove old CSF in the context of continued production will cause the fluid-filled ventricles to expand like water balloons in the closed cranium. Obstruction anywhere above the exit from the ventricles to the subarachnoid space (posterior fossa or above) will therefore result in obstructive hydrocephalus. The speed with which the accumulation of fluid occurs will in part determine the rapidity of the symptoms, as well as their severity. Obstructive hydrocephalus is considered a medical emergency because progressive expansion of the ventricular volume will force the brain to be compressed in all directions, including downward, resulting in tonsillar herniation.

The three common symptoms of obstructive hydrocephalus include headaches, often severe in nature, that are thought to arise as a result of stretching of vessels and the pial surfaces. These headaches can often be worsened by changes in body position or head motion. They can be dull, aching, or stabbing in nature. Because of the prevalence of headaches in the general population, it is their persistence and worsening in the context of other symptoms (e.g., morning vomiting and focal neurologic deficits) that usually trigger further investigation. Patients will often have vomiting (often associated with a headache), especially early in the morning upon wakening. Whether this symptom results from hydrostatic pressure changes when first getting up, resulting in compression of the area postrema, or changes in CNS homeostasis upon wakening as a result of more rapid breathing and carbon dioxide release is unknown. Unfortunately the significance of morning vomiting is often overlooked and thought to be related to school avoidance or the flu. Many patients present with prolonged histories of intermittent morning vomiting and headache, suggesting that this process can be partial and relieved by the vomiting, which itself causes raised intraabdominal pressure and equilibration of the CSF pressure gradient. A third common symptom in children with hydrocephalus is blurring of the optic discs, related to the increase in intracranial pressure (ICP). Patients often report blurring or double vision, as well as difficulty in upward gaze. These symptoms likely result from a constellation of factors, including compression of the brainstem and cranial nerves, as well as edema and swelling of the optic discs (papilledema) and pathways leading to vision. The final common symptom of obstructive hydrocephalus is the presence of lower motor deficits, likely because of compression of motor tracts within the brainstem and difficulties with balance and gait related to pressure on the cerebellum.

The symptoms of obstructive hydrocephalus differ in infants, in whom the presence of open sutures permits the head to expand. This expansion relieves the buildup of pressure and thus the associated symptoms. While their head size expands, infants may begin to show some signs of delay in gaining milestones. Careful attention to head circumference changes will help identify these infants early, independent of the cause of the obstruction.

CT imaging of the brain is a rapid method for confirming the presence of obstructive hydrocephalus. Images (without the need for contrast material) will demonstrate enlargement of the ventricles above the area of obstruction. Increasing concerns of radiation dose regarding repeat CT imaging in young children has resulted in a shift to rapid-sequence MRI vent checks.[116] These images are performed without contrast material and are not useful for assessing changes in the tumor. However they have the advantage of assessing changes in fluid within the CNS and without exposure of the child to ionizing radiation.[117,118] MRI will show large ventricles on T1- and T2-weighted images. Best seen on fluid-attenuated inversion recovery (FLAIR) sequences, the presence of a bright signal around the ventricles is suggestive of transependymal flow, which is thought to result from the backward transduction of pressure from the ventricle to the brain parenchyma (Fig. 57-13).[119] Obstructive hydrocephalus is a surgical emergency and requires urgent intervention. For posterior fossa tumors such as medulloblastoma, ependymoma, or low-grade astrocytoma, relief from obstruction can be achieved with resection of the tumor in most patients, thus avoiding the need for a separate CSF diversion procedure.[120]

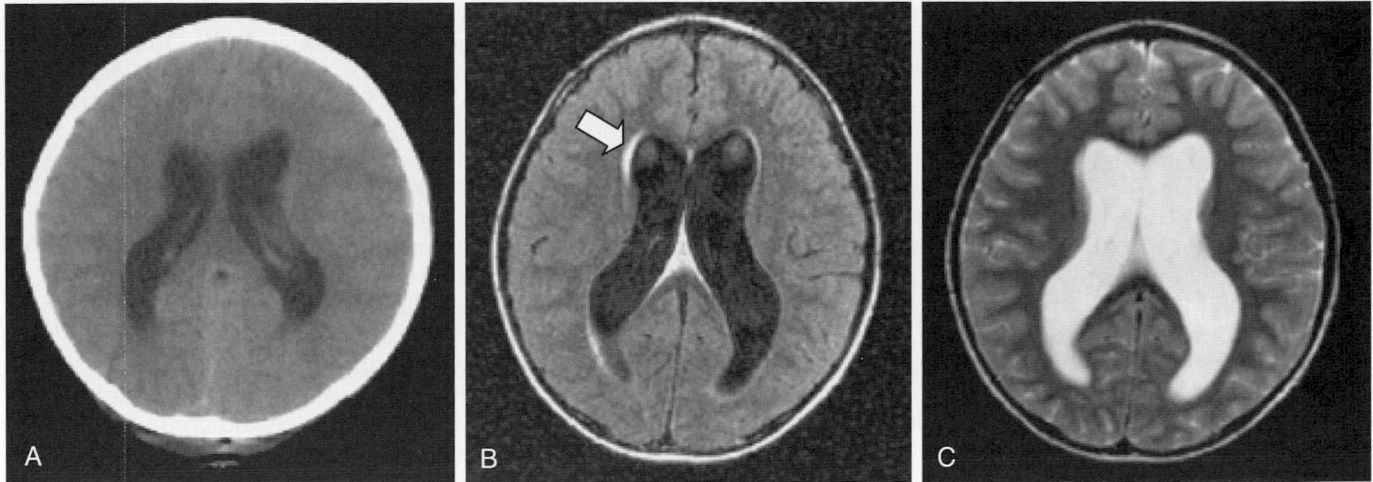

Figure 57-13 Hydrocephalus. **A,** An axial computed tomography noncontrast scan demonstrating significant enlargement caused by obstructive hydrocephalus. **B,** An axial fluid-attenuated inversion recovery image demonstrates enlarged ventricles and transependymal flow *(arrow)*, suggestive of raised intracranial pressure. **C,** An axial T2-weighted magnetic resonance image demonstrating enlarged ventricles.

IMAGING STUDIES

Neuroimaging

Imaging of brain tumors entails determining the size and site of origin of the lesion, establishing primary diagnosis, and planning treatment. Neuroimaging is critical for the appropriate placement of catheters for stereotactic biopsy, resection, planning of radiation, guided application of experimental therapeutics, and delineation of tumor from functionally important neuronal tissue. After treatment, imaging is used to quantify response and the extent of residual tumor. At follow-up imaging helps determine tumor progression and differentiate recurrent tumor growth from treatment-induced tissue changes, such as radiation necrosis.[121]

Imaging brain tumors in children presents unique challenges not encountered in adult imaging, including the need for sedation and consideration of the long-term effects on a growing child. Cranial CT and MRI remain the main modalities for the primary diagnosis of brain tumors. However several other techniques are being increasingly used in the evaluation of this patient population, including positron emission tomography (PET), MR perfusion and diffusion, and MR spectroscopy (MRS). Assessment of response in pediatrics is a critical component in the appropriate treatment of patients, as well as in identifying active regimens. Recently adult neurooncologists have adopted a new series of guidelines (developed by the International Radiologic Assessment in Neuro-Oncology Committee) to aid in better differentiating tumor progression from pseudoprogression and similarly tumor response from pseudoresponse. Although some of these adult criteria will be useful in pediatrics, the types of tumors common in the pediatric population will require some modifications to the adult approach. Currently an International working group is developing recommendations for children with brain tumors (Radiologic Assessment in Pediatric Neuro-Oncology).[122]

CT is a rapid and inexpensive modality for assessing fluid, blood, and calcification in the central CNS. As such it has typically been the first imaging procedure in children with a presumed intracranial bleed or raised ICP that might require immediate neurosurgical intervention. Other than for lesions arising from the skull vault and to assess calcified tumors, CT scans are used less frequently for routine surveillance of pediatric patients because of an increase in long-term cancer risk caused by CT imaging.[53,116]

MRI is currently the modality of choice for localization and assessment of the size of brain tumors. MRI provides valuable information about secondary phenomena such as mass effect, edema, hemorrhage, necrosis, and signs of increased ICP. In addition MRI provides excellent tissue contrast and high spatial resolution. Standard T1- and T2-weighted MRI sequences detect brain tumors with high sensitivity. Varying acquisition parameters such as T1 or T2 weighting, techniques such as diffusion- and perfusion-weighted images, and FLAIR sequences reveal a characteristic pattern of each tumor, depending on tumor type and grade.[123] Susceptibility-weighted MRI is useful for detecting areas of hemorrhage, calcifications, and increased vascularity associated with brain tumors.[124] Recently rapid-sequence MRI for the assessment of bleeds or hydrocephalus has been developed, which can avoid the radiation doses associated with CT scans and, like CT scans, can be performed without sedation, even in young children.[117,118,125] However it should be noted that these studies are limited in evaluation of the tumor burden and should only be used to assess for acute findings.

MRS can also be helpful for the initial characterization of tumors[126,127]; it can also be used to differentiate tumor tissue from other tissue in children with CNS tumors in certain circumstances.[128] MRS has continued to evolve, and the development of multivoxel and two-dimensional techniques has resulted in improved spatial resolution, thereby supplying additional information regarding tumor heterogeneity and intratumoral metabolite distribution. Although MRS is a sensitive technique, it still lacks specificity as a stand-alone technique in the clinical setting. In a recent study, brain proton MRS biomarkers were shown to predict survival of children with CNS tumors better than standard histopathology. More accurate prediction using this noninvasive technique represents an important advance and may suggest more appropriate therapy, especially when a diagnostic biopsy is not feasible.[129] In general, decreased N-acetylaspartate (NAA) and creatine concentrations and increased choline concentrations correlate with tumor grade. Reduction of NAA is likely because of neuronal death or damage, although the reduction in creatine is likely to be a result of changes in cell energetics. The increase in choline is believed to reflect increased membrane synthesis. Increases in lipid and lactate concentrations have been observed in some gliomas. Lactate accumulation is believed to be a result of central tumor necrosis.

Diffusion-weighted MR pulse sequences enable a quantitative and reproducible assessment of the diffusion changes, not only in areas exhibiting signal abnormality in conventional MRI but also in areas of normal signal.[130] MR diffusion using predominantly echoplanar techniques has been useful in the characterization of tissue, tumor cellularity, tumor grading, tumor response to treatment, and distinction of tissue types.[131,132] Diffusion tensor imaging (DTI) provides visualization of fiber bundle direction and integrity, with in vivo characterization of the rate and direction of white matter diffusion. DTI is useful for presurgical planning or coregistration of tractography data with radiosurgical planning and functional MRI data.[133] Fractional anisotropy using DTI may prove helpful for the assessment of treatment-induced white matter changes in children.[134,135]

The usefulness of diffusion-weighted imaging (DWI) for characterizing intracranial cystic or cystlike lesions has been demonstrated in a number of studies.[136-139] DWI has long been used to differentiate between epidermoid and arachnoid cysts.[139,140] Arachnoid cysts are characterized by free diffusion, whereas epidermoids have an apparent diffusion coefficient similar to that of brain parenchyma, thereby demonstrating restricted diffusion.[137] The usefulness of DWI in the distinction between ring-enhancing cerebral lesions such as brain abscesses, cystic or necrotic HGG, or metastasis has been shown in multiple studies during the past decade, although this differentiation continues to be a challenge.[141] The ring enhancement of a brain abscess can be indistinguishable from that of a cystic or necrotic HGG or metastasis. Other lesions that may also have a similar appearance are subacute ischemic infarction, resorbing hematoma, and demyelinating disease.[130] Abscesses demonstrate high signal on DWI and a reduced apparent diffusion coefficient (ADC) in a cystic ring-enhancing cerebral lesion.[140,141] ADC values have been assessed between tumor types; however, considerable overlap exists between certain tumor types, requiring additional evaluations.[132,142] Authors of a retrospective study of ADC values of 275 adult and pediatric brain tumors have reported a significant negative correlation between ADC and WHO astrocytic tumor grades II through IV.[142] Other comparisons included a higher ADC in dysembryoplastic neuroepithelial tumors (DNETs) than in astrocytic grade II tumors (100% accuracy) or other glioneuronal tumors, a lower ADC in malignant lymphomas compared with glioblastomas and metastatic tumors, a lower ADC in CNS PNETs compared with ependymomas, and a lower ADC in meningiomas compared with schwannomas. The ADC of craniopharyngiomas was higher than that of pituitary adenomas, whereas the ADC of epidermoid tumors was lower than that of chordomas. In meningiomas the ADC was not indicative of malignant grade or histologic subtype. DWI has also been used to obtain additional information regarding tumor type and grade. The reduction in extracellular space, as well as high nuclear-to-cytoplasmic ratios of some cancer cells, causes a relative reduction in ADC values.[131,143] In some studies overlap was seen in ADC values of HGGs and LGGs.[132] The presence of glycosaminoglycans such as hyaluronan in the extracellular space of some HGGs may decrease water content and cause a reduction in ADC values.[144] In addition, one pitfall of DWI is that high-grade tumors that may exhibit necrosis can lead to higher ADC values.[145]

DWI and proton MRS have been evaluated as diagnostic tools, and in a study of children with posterior fossa lesions in which these techniques were combined, MRI was successful in correctly identifying the histologic diagnosis in every case.[146] Although this approach does not replace the pathologic diagnosis, it demonstrates the increasing accuracy of biologic-based imaging.[147,148] Similar results have been reported for ADC analysis.[149,150] DWI may also be helpful in differentiating postsurgical changes from tumor recurrence.[148] DWI can also detect acute changes in white matter from methotrexate administration, which must be differentiated from progressive disease.[151]

Determination of the tumor margins is considered by many investigators to be extremely important for the management of brain tumors. Complete resection of tumors with minimal neurologic deficit is the ultimate goal of surgical resection. In some studies DWI has been shown to discriminate among tumor, infiltrating tumor, peritumoral edema, and normal brain parenchyma.[152,153] However other studies have not found DWI to be helpful for evaluating tumor margins.[132,154]

MR diffusion imaging has also been assessed as a biomarker for early prediction of treatment response in patients with brain tumors. Recent studies have indicated the possibility of using functional diffusion map analysis as an early biomarker for treatment response preceding decrease in tumor size.[155,156] Increasingly MR perfusion imaging is being used to evaluate cerebral perfusion dynamics by analysis of the hemodynamic parameters of relative cerebral blood volume (CBV), regional cerebral blood flow (CBF), and mean transit time. CBV is the parameter most commonly quantified in brain tumors.[157] CBV is defined as the volume of blood in a region of brain tissue, commonly measured in milliliters per 100 g of brain tissue. CBF refers to the volume of blood/unit time passing through a given region of brain tissue, measured in milliliters per minute per 100 g of brain tissue. Mean transit time refers to the average time it takes blood to pass through a given region of brain tissue and is commonly measured in seconds.[158] Perfusion imaging techniques include T2-weighted dynamic susceptibility techniques, arterial spin labeling (ASL) techniques, and T1-weighted dynamic contrast-enhanced perfusion techniques. These techniques use exogenous tracer agents, such as paramagnetic contrast material, or endogenous tracer agents, such as magnetically labeled blood (arterial water).[159] The most common method currently performed in the clinical setting is dynamic contrast-enhanced perfusion MRI with an exogenous tracer, such as gadopentetate dimeglumine. It is assumed that the tracer is restricted to the intravascular compartment and does not diffuse into the extracellular space. Imaging is performed dynamically (rapid imaging over time during a bolus injection) using echoplanar imaging–based spin echo or gradient echo sequences. It is thought that the spin echo sequences are more sensitive to capillary level blood vessels, whereas gradient echo techniques are more sensitive to the larger vessels.[160] Although gradient echo sequences are associated with more magnetic susceptibility artifacts, particularly in the posterior fossa, they are the more common of the two techniques. For young children and infants, challenges exist relating to intravenous (IV) access, smaller intravenous catheters, and limitations of the contrast medium dose.

DTI is an adaptation of DWI and is performed by acquiring diffusion data in six or more directions, enabling determination of the direction and magnitude of water diffusion. Connecting the directions of diffusion in each voxel to those of neighboring voxels using a variety of mathematical algorithms enables creation of a three-dimensional (3D) white matter tract map, termed "tractography." This technique is used to delineate important white matter tracts affected by tumor[161] and help guide surgical resection. In conjunction with functional MRI, tractography can be used to predict possible postoperative deficits resulting from white matter tract damage.

Dynamic T1-weighted contrast imaging can be used to assess microvascular permeability (measured as the transendothelial transfer constant, or Kps) in brain tumors.[162] Kinetic modeling of the dynamic signal changes can yield estimates of regional fractional blood volume and Kps, which is an indicator of BBB disruption and correlates with angiogenesis. This technique can be successfully performed in children, and applications of this technique may be useful for monitoring antiangiogenic therapies in pediatric patients with brain tumors.[163-165] ASL is an MR perfusion technique that does not use an IV contrast agent.[166] The perfusion contrast in the image results from the subtraction of two successively acquired images, one with and one without proximal labeling of arterial water spins, with a magnetic gradient used to invert the magnetization of inflowing blood.[167] The signal-to-noise ratio, anatomic coverage, and shorter imaging time are currently better for the dynamic contrast perfusion techniques compared with ASL. However ASL may have a future role in the imaging of pediatric brain tumors,

particularly because it relies on a noninvasive endogenous contrast agent.[168,169]

The use of PET and single-photon emission CT (SPECT) imaging continues to improve[170] and can be important in helping to differentiate treatment effect from tumor recurrence.[171-174] The usefulness of PET imaging is especially evident when a baseline evaluation is performed so that postoperative changes can be evaluated in the context of the pretherapy PET avidity, thus requiring consideration of nuclear imaging early in the workup of these patients.[175,176]

Standardization of neuroimaging parameters for children with CNS tumors and the testing of novel sequences that can be adapted to specific molecular inhibitors now being evaluated in this population are being developed.[130,177]

A further advance in MRI of brain tumors has occurred with the availability of intraoperative scanners. These scanners enable preoperative guidance for stereotactic biopsy and for planning tumor resection, and they provide a review of the resection site for residual tumor prior to closure of the craniotomy.[178] Intraoperative DTI has been proposed to aid in the preservation of fiber tracts and to minimize postoperative deficits.[179]

Somatostatin receptor scintigraphy has been used to differentiate the presence of residual or recurrent tumor from scar and necrosis and is better than MRI scans for a number of pediatric tumor types.[180,181] Molecular imaging is likely to play an expanding role in neurooncology as more pathway-specific inhibitors become available.

Posterior reversible leukoencephalopathy (PRES) is increasingly identified in children with brain tumors, particularly in children with episodes of hypertension. Patients present with headaches that are usually severe, mental and visual status changes, and seizures concurrent with hypertension and characteristic MRI findings, including T2 signal abnormalities.[182] MRI findings are those of vasogenic edema with T2 and FLAIR hyperintensities involving predominantly the parietal and occipital regions bilaterally (Fig. 57-14). The diffusion changes in PRES are traditionally thought to be represented by higher ADC values, consistent with vasogenic edema. Focal areas of restricted diffusion (likely representing infarction–tissue injury with cytotoxic edema) are uncommon (11% to 26%) and may be associated with an adverse outcome.[183-187] Hemorrhage (focal hematoma, isolated sulcal-subarachnoid blood, or protein) is seen in approximately 15% of patients.[188,189] The parietal and occipital lobes are most commonly affected, followed by the frontal lobes, the inferior temporal-occipital junction, and the cerebellum.[188] Lesion confluence may develop as the extent of edema increases.

The mechanism of PRES remains controversial, although the hypertension-hyperperfusion theory is favored because of the common presence of elevated blood pressure and perceived response to hypertension management. Key issues remain problematic, including PRES in normotensive patients with pressures rarely reaching autoregulatory limits, and brain edema that is lower in patients with severe hypertension. Hypertensive

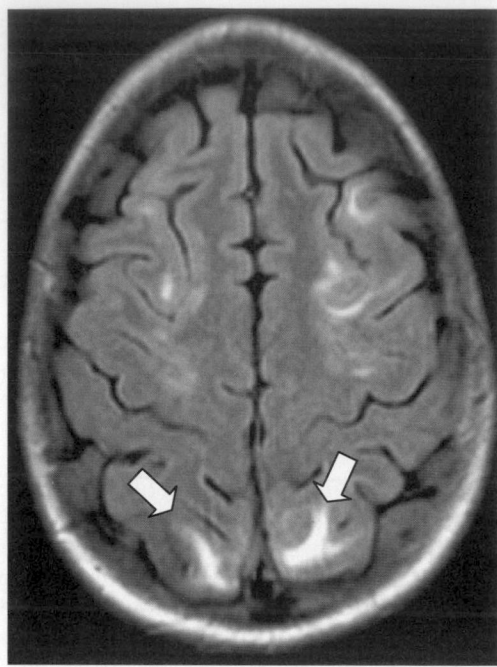

Figure 57-14 An axial fluid-attenuated inversion recovery image in a patient after radiation therapy with new-onset seizure and hypertension with bilateral hyperintense signal in the occipital lobes *(arrows)*. Also note increased signal to a lesser extent in the frontal lobe.

encephalopathy animal models do not reflect the systemic toxicity that is present, and hyperperfusion has not conclusively been demonstrated in patients.

Intracranial vasospasm has been seen with conventional and MR angiography, suggesting vasospasm as a possible pathophysiologic mechanism for the observed findings.[190] MR DWI was instrumental in establishing and consistently demonstrating that the areas of abnormality represent vasogenic edema. Prompt treatment with antihypertensive therapy or discontinuation of immunosuppressive agents can lead to complete recovery in some cases. However, if untreated, permanent neurologic deficits or even death may occur as a result of cerebral infarctions or hemorrhages,[191] and 20% to 40% of patients with PRES can be normotensive.[192,193] PRES can be associated with a number of inciting events, including chemotherapy, radiation therapy, and antiangiogenic drugs.[194] This latter group of drugs may cause PRES as a result of their direct effect on vascular endothelial growth factor (VEGF) and raised blood pressure. Rapid recognition of this entity is critical to prevent permanent damage from occurring.

Surveillance Imaging

The role and usefulness of surveillance imaging for patients with a brain tumor remain controversial and depend on a number of factors, such as the age of the patient, histology of the tumor, time from diagnosis, and type of treatment. For example, in one study only nine of 318 imaging encounters identified an asymptomatic recurrence.[195] Other studies have demonstrated the cost-effectiveness of surveillance imaging,[196] recognizing that decisions are often made on the basis of insurance coverage. A common practice has been imaging every 3 months while the patient is undergoing therapy (to assess continued response while undergoing therapy), and then every 3 months for the first year after the completion of therapy. Beginning in the second year, scans are performed every 6 months for a year and then annually afterward. With time the risk of tumor recurrence will go down, although the risks of radiation-induced vasculopathy and second tumors begin to increase. Modification of these guidelines for children with tumors at low risk of recurrence (e.g., completely resected craniopharyngioma or low-grade astrocytoma) or those who did not receive radiation therapy can be made on a case-by-case basis.

NEUROPATHOLOGY

The neuropathologic classification of pediatric brain tumors has evolved greatly during the past century. Categorizing tumors is helpful to guide therapy and estimate prognosis. A number of outstanding reviews on the classification of CNS tumors have been written.[197-206] When attempting to determine the treatment and/or prognosis of a tumor based on published reports or meeting abstracts, the classification schema used in those reports will become critical before applying this information to other patients.

Most current classification systems are based on the pioneering work of Cushing and Bailey almost 100 years ago. The major premise of this approach was to define tumors by their presumed cell of origin and cell lineage based on morphologic similarity to normal immature or mature brain cells. This system was adapted by Kernohan when he proposed that certain tumors, especially those with a glial appearance, such as astrocytomas, ependymomas, and oligodendrogliomas, could be further classified by the degree of anaplasia, which related to prognosis. Most current systems now use these two criteria—presumed cell lineage and degree of anaplasia—as the primary basis for classification of adult and pediatric CNS tumors. In spite of the usefulness of this classification schema, it is becoming progressively clear that most brain tumors do not derive from mature cell types but rather from primitive precursors or stem cells that can differentiate down many different pathways, obscuring the cell lineage. In comparison with their adult counterparts, pediatric brain tumors are exceptionally diverse in their morphologic appearance and therefore represent a particular challenge for classification by morphologic criteria alone. This diversity likely stems from the fact that pediatric brain tumors are derived from a wide spectrum of proliferative cell types at many developmental stages not present in adult brains.

Significant advances have been made in the field of neuropathology. The WHO classification of CNS tumors has been recently revised, with a number of important modifications based on histopathologic recognition of new pediatric brain tumors.[207] A synopsis of the WHO 2007 classification system is provided in Table 57-3. Increasingly the field has begun to include use of molecular alterations for many tumors and the use of highly specific immunohistochemical markers.[198-201,206,208-212] When

TABLE 57-3 Simplified World Health Organization Classification of Pediatric Central Nervous System Tumors

Type	Subtype	Example(s)	Grade
Glial tumors	Astrocytic tumors	Pilocytic astrocytoma	I
		Subependymal giant cell astrocytoma	I
		Pilomyxoid astrocytoma	II
		Pleomorphic xanthroastrocytoma	II
		Diffuse (fibrillary) astrocytoma	II
		Anaplastic astrocytoma	III
		Glioblastoma multiforme	IV
		Gliosarcoma	IV
		Gliomatosis cerebri	III-IV
	Oligodendroglial tumors	Oligodendroglioma	II
		Oligoastrocytoma	II
		Anaplastic oligodendroglioma	III
		Anaplastic oligoastrocytoma	III
	Ependymal tumors	Subependymoma	I
		Myxopapillary ependymoma	I
		Ependymoma	II
		Anaplastic ependymoma	III
Neural/embryonal tumors		Medulloblastoma	IV
		Pineocytoma	I
		Pineal parenchymal tumor of intermediate differentiation	II-III
		Papillary tumor of the pineal region	II-III
		Pineoblastoma	IV
		Primitive neuroectodermal tumor (medulloepithelioma, ependymoblastoma)	IV
		Atypical teratoid-rhabdoid tumor	IV
Choroid plexus tumors		Choroid plexus papilloma	I
		Atypical choroid plexus papilloma	II
		Choroid plexus carcinoma	III
Germ cell tumors	Germinoma		III
	Nongerminoma	Embryonal carcinoma	III
		Yolk sac tumor	III
		Choriocarcinoma	III
		Mature teratoma	0
		Teratoma	I
		Immature teratoma	III
		Teratoma with malignant transformation	III
Craniopharyngioma	Craniopharyngioma	Adamantinomatous	I
		Papillary	I
Other	Mixed glial neuronal tumor	Ganglioglioma	I
		Gangliocytoma	I
		Anaplastic ganglioglioma	III
		Dysembryoplastic neuroepithelial tumor	I
		Desmoplastic infantile astrocytoma	I
		Central neurocytoma	II
		Extraventricular neurocytoma	II
	Neuroepithelial	Astroblastoma	—
	Nerve tumors	Schwannoma	I
		Neurofibroma	I
		Malignant peripheral nerve sheath tumor	II-IV
	Meningeal	Meningioma	I
		Atypical meningioma	II
		Anaplastic meningioma	III
		Hemangioblastoma	I

combined with immunohistochemical analysis and the increasing use of cytogenetic classification and molecular profiling, the classification of tumors continues to become more reproducible and predictive of clinical outcomes. A simplified overview of the chromosomal abnormalities associated with pediatric brain tumors is presented in Table 57-1. For many large consortium-based studies in both Europe and North America, molecular profiling of tumors to ensure proper classification is now required, especially for medulloblastoma and ATRTs.

The immunohistochemical patterns used to classify CNS tumors require considerable experience on the part of the neuropathologist, as well as appropriate control subjects. Most markers lack specificity and can be identified in a wide array of histologies, requiring correlation with other clinical or molecular data.[213] Common

TABLE 57-4 Immunohistochemical Markers of Pediatric Central Nervous System Tumors

Marker	Tumor
Glial fibrillary acidic protein	Astrocytoma, oligodendroglioma, ependymoma, choroid plexus papilloma, PNET, ATRT
Synaptophysin/NeuN	PNETs, ganglial tumor, neurocytoma
MIB1/Ki-67	Measures all cells not in G0
Mitotic rate	Measures cells in mitosis
Neurofilament proteins	Ganglial tumor, PNET, neurocytoma, subependymal giant cell tumor, ATRT
S-100 and neuron-specific enolase	Normal and neoplastic glial and neuronal in origin
Retinal S-antigen	Pineal parenchymal tumor, PNET, retinoblastoma
Desmin	Muscle tumor, teratoma, PNET
Smooth muscle actin	Muscle tumor, ATRT
Cytokeratin	Chordoma, choroid plexus tumor, meningioma, some malignant gliomas, nongerminomatous germ cell tumor, PNET, ATRT
Epithelial membrane antigen	Meningioma, ependymoma, teratoma, ATRT
Vimentin	Mesenchymal tumor, meningioma, sarcoma, melanoma, ependymoma, astrocytoma, chordoma, schwannoma, PNET, ATRT
Alpha-fetoprotein	Embryonal carcinoma, endodermal sinus (yolk sac) tumor
Human chorionic gonadotropin	Germinoma, choriocarcinoma
Placental alkaline phosphatase	Germ cell tumor
INI-1	ATRT

ATRT, Atypical teratoid/rhabdoid tumor; *PNET,* primary neuroectodermal tumor.

markers used to classify pediatric CNS tumors are provided in Table 57-4. Four commonly used immunohistochemical markers are the oligodendrocyte lineage transcription factor 2 (OLIG2)[214] and glial acidic fibrillary protein (GFAP), which stain glial cells (Fig. 57-15); synaptophysin, which stains neurons (Fig. 57-16); and Ki-67, which stains cells that have left G0 cell cycle and are at some stage of cellular division (Fig. 57-17).

TREATMENT STRATEGIES

Neurosurgery

The neurosurgeon is often the first of the specialized team of caregivers called to see a child with a brain tumor, with

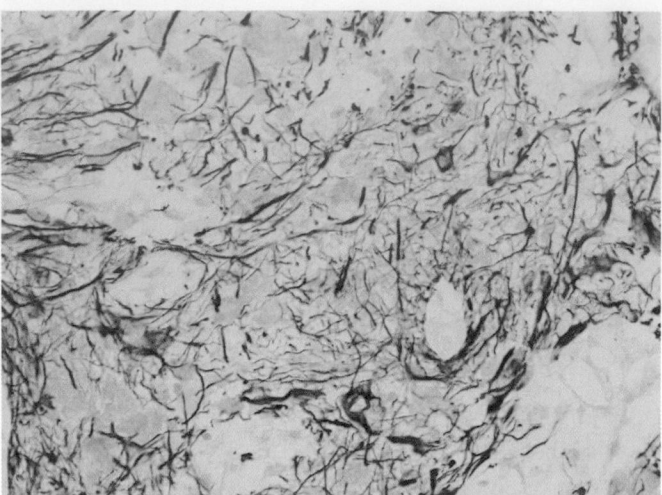

Figure 57-15 Glial acidic fibrillary protein staining of astrocytic cells in a child with glioblastoma multiforme (×400).

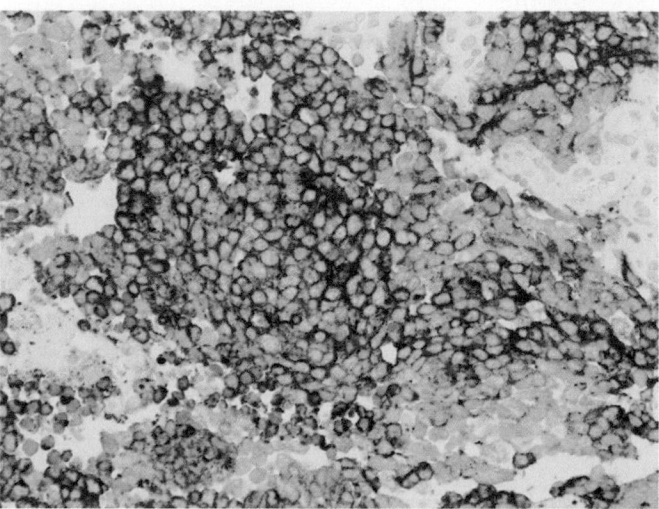

Figure 57-16 Synaptophysin immunohistochemical staining of medulloblastoma (×400).

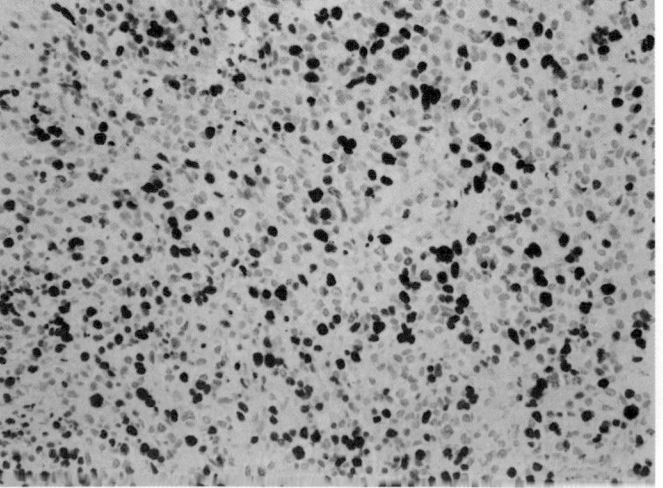

Figure 57-17 Ki-67 immunohistochemical staining in glioblastoma multiforme (×200).

the call frequently coming from the emergency department or radiology department. The initial evaluation consists of acute management—that is, assessment of the patient's clinical condition with respect to neurologic stability and the possibility of acute neurologic decompensation requiring immediate intervention, and subsequent to that the development of a plan that includes surgical interventions geared toward obtaining tissue for pathologic diagnosis, resection of tumor as part of the overall management of the tumor, and dealing with the secondary effects of the tumor.[215-217]

In the field of neurosurgery remarkable advances have occurred in technology, from intraoperative microscopes, robotics, and computer-assisted navigation to intraoperative MRI, endoscopic techniques, and minimally invasive techniques.[218,219] Each of these advances has been instrumental in reducing the morbidity of neurosurgical procedures while ensuring maximal surgical resections.

Acute Management Issues

Hydrocephalus. Hydrocephalus is the most common clinical presentation of posterior fossa brain tumors, which are the most common pediatric brain tumors. Historically the initial evaluation of children suspected of harboring a posterior fossa brain tumor has been via CT scan. However with improved technologies and more recent concerns regarding the long-term effects of radiation exposure, there is a trend toward less utilization of CT scans. If possible the initial assessment should be an MRI of the brain, which can provide the dual information regarding the brain tumor and the extent of hydrocephalus. The cause of the hydrocephalus is obstruction to the CSF flow as a result of the tumors in and around the fourth ventricle. The evaluation should consist of assessing the severity of the hydrocephalus (via the presence of periventricular capping/edema and tonsillar herniation) and the need for immediate intervention. High-dose steroids will often produce significant relief in symptoms as peritumoral edema is suppressed, and they are often utilized as a temporary measure for symptom relief. In infants, hydrocephalus can be asymptomatic and only evidenced by a rapidly enlarging head circumference. Supratentorial brain tumors can also produce hydrocephalus by causing mass effect on the ventricles, as well as by obstructing CSF flow through the ventricular system. Patients with suprasellar tumors can also have inadequate cortisol production or electrolyte disturbances, which need to be addressed as quickly as possible and often in concert with preparation for surgery.[220]

Raised ICP is a medical emergency. Immediate relief can be accomplished by temporary placement of a catheter (drainage tube) in the ventricles, although this step is rarely needed, primarily because of the fact that steroids in the preoperative period followed by surgery to remove the tumors within 24 to 48 hours after diagnosis usually relieves the obstruction. Permanent techniques of hydrocephalus treatment include the placement of a ventriculoperitoneal (VP) shunt that drains CSF around the obstruction into the peritoneal space via a permanently implanted tube and more recently via an endoscopic third ventriculostomy (ETV).[221,222] The latter has become the treatment of choice in the management of obstructive hydrocephalus and is not associated with the long-term complications of shunt revisions and infections.[223] Most pediatric centers with sufficient expertise now routinely perform ETVs as the primary management of hydrocephalus in children with brain tumors.[224] In addition the overall incidence of shunting for brain tumors has decreased during the past two decades.[225,226] Like all complex procedures, rare but significant neurologic risks are associated with this procedure in approximately 1% of cases.[227] The possibility of closure of a third ventriculostomy and resultant acute hydrocephalus requires long-term follow-up with neurosurgery, as with all children who have had placement of shunts for the management of the hydrocephalus.

Visual and Endocrine Evaluation. Children with tumors in the sellar and suprasellar area can present with blindness, which rarely can be acute in onset. In those circumstances, although extremely rare, it is possible to obtain some recovery of vision by immediate treatment of the tumor. If a large mass or cyst is causing compression, acute drainage in conjunction with steroid administration can lead to some recovery of vision. Tumors in this location can also interfere with endocrine function and may lead to electrolyte disturbances and decreased steroid production, and these effects can be critical if they are unrecognized, especially if acute surgical intervention is indicated.

Surgical Management

Surgical management after treatment of hydrocephalus consists of obtaining tissue for diagnosis and resecting the tumor. The decision to perform these procedures depends on the location of the tumor, the known biology, and the goals of treatment management.

Certain tumors do not require routine biopsy or attempted resection at diagnosis (e.g., diffuse pontine gliomas, classic optic pathway tumors in children with NF-1, and some suprasellar or pineal lesions with positive serum or CSF tumor markers). Tectal gliomas are rare tumors centered in the tectum with a classic radiographic appearance and presentation of hydrocephalus and, rarely, neurologic deficits. Their management consists solely of treatment of the hydrocephalus via ETV and radiographic and clinical follow-up.

The leading factor in the outcome of a child with a brain tumor is not the presenting symptoms, age of the child, or the final disease. Rather it is the experience of the neurosurgeon performing the operation and the number of similar procedures performed during the prior few years.[228] With increasing cure rates in children with CNS tumors, careful consideration of the neurosurgical morbidity, which can often be lifelong, needs to be taken into account while a treatment plan is developed.[229]

Advances in Surgical Techniques. Recent advances in image-guided neurosurgical techniques have been considerable. Endoscopic procedures provide minimally invasive techniques to address not just obstructive hydrocephalus but also biopsy or resection of intracranial masses, with minimal morbidity in experienced hands.[230] New techniques using intraoperative ultrasound have been developed and are being used in pediatric patients.[231] 3D laser-guided maps can assist in the orientation and surrounding environment of the tumor during a procedure. More recently intraoperative MRI facilities now allow surgeons to use MRI procedures with the same magnet strength as that used for diagnostic imaging while operating.[232] Real-time MRIs can assist the neurosurgeon in the detection of residual disease or hemorrhage before closure of the resection site.[233]

The surgical approach used by the neurosurgeon will depend on a number of factors that must balance the need for diagnosis with the potential risks of operating in a given area.[234] While the relative risks of general anesthesia and neurosurgical procedures continue to diminish with improving techniques, it is now common to perform staged operations in which a limited resection is performed to confirm the diagnosis. Based on the pathologic results obtained, decisions about more complicated or risky surgery can be considered for lesions in which complete resection is a critical component of improved outcome and can be deferred in lesions in which additional resection would not significantly alter prognosis but could cause significant morbidity. Specialized techniques such as endonasal endoscopic approaches can allow a minimally invasive approach, with excellent outcome in centers that have expertise in this approach.[235]

The need of neurosurgeons to be aware of the evolving treatment strategies for children reinforces the role of the multidisciplinary team. During the past 5 years this need has become even more important, because many pediatric brain tumors now require molecular classification to guide therapy. For example in spite of their similar appearance, the treatment of posterior fossa medulloblastoma now differs significantly from posterior fossa ATRT. Treatment on national protocols therefore requires submission of fresh-frozen material obtained at the time of surgery for proper stratification on the basis of therapy protocols. As our molecular classification of pediatric brain tumors expands and newer and better molecular inhibitors of specific pathways become available, the role of the neurosurgeon and neuropathologist in ensuring the proper processing of these samples will continue to expand.

Perioperative Issues. A number of factors must be considered for a child after a tumor-based procedure has been completed. The rate of weaning steroids after an operation will depend on many factors, including the histology, degree of resection, postsurgical edema, and patient status. Although most patients can be weaned off steroids rapidly after an operation, it is important that the members of the team have a coordinated structure so that as children pass from neurosurgical care to the radiation therapist or oncologist, overall management of these issues is seamless. A similar discussion holds true for anticonvulsant agents. Whereas many patients will receive preoperative or perioperative anticonvulsant therapy, most can be weaned rapidly, and communication among team members will therefore be required.

Seizures can be a presenting symptom for many patients with brain tumors or a result of electrolyte disturbances in the perioperative period. Management includes anticonvulsant agents and surgical resection geared not only toward the tumor but also toward dealing with the seizures. Intraoperative electrocorticography is particularly useful in the management of temporal and frontal lobe tumors with seizures and requires a multidisciplinary approach, which can lead to excellent overall outcomes. Choices of antiepileptic drugs (AEDs) are important because some may interfere with metabolism of chemotherapeutic agents, which requires a comprehensive approach toward the management of the patient's seizures and tumor.

Hyponatremia is a common problem that can occur after neurosurgical intervention and requires immediate recognition.[236] Two common conditions, both resulting in hyponatremia but needing different interventions, can occur. Cerebral salt wasting (CSW) occurs because of excess renal loss of sodium with volume depletion and has been associated with abnormally high atrial natriuretic peptide or brain natriuretic peptide levels, which block all stimulators of zona glomerulosa steroidogenesis, resulting in mineralocorticoid deficiency.[237] CSW usually occurs 1 to 2 days after neurosurgical intervention, and patients typically demonstrate polyuria, dehydration, a serum sodium level less than 130 mEq/L, and excess urine sodium or urine osmolarity. Duration of CSW was 1 to 9 days in a study of 12 pediatric patients.[238] CSW is generally treated with salt repletion, although fludrocortisone supplementation has also been successful.[239] Syndrome of inappropriate diuretic hormone (SIADH), by contrast, results when water is preferentially retained, causing dilution of serum sodium. Patients present with hyponatremia and an elevated urine sodium level.[240] The major clinical difference between CSW and SIADH is that in the former, dehydration is common, whereas in SIADH, symptoms of dehydration are lacking. SIADH is treated with water restriction. CSW was much more common than SIADH in one study of 30 patients.[241]

Posterior fossa syndrome (or cerebellar mutism syndrome) is a complex and heterogeneous disorder that tends to occur 24 to 48 hours after resection of a posterior fossa tumor,[242] usually medulloblastoma, ependymoma, or low-grade astrocytoma. Posterior fossa syndrome will develop in up to 25% of patients undergoing surgical resection in the posterior fossa and, in most patients, it will be severe.[242] The pathophysiologic basis for this syndrome is unclear, with many hypotheses proposed. It is likely related to pressure effects on the deep cerebellar nuclei and is more frequently associated with large tumors extending into those areas. Gross total resection (GTR) of most posterior fossa brain tumors is associated with better long-term outcomes, and it is thought that the more aggressive surgical resections for those reasons are associated with the perceived increase in the frequency of this syndrome. The exact clinical patterns of posterior fossa syndrome can vary among patients both in constellation and severity. Usually the disorder includes loss of speech in patients who were capable of talking immediately after surgery. Other symptoms include irritability, which may relate to difficulties in communication, emotional withdrawal, and motor difficulties with ataxia.[242] In a review of 450 children from two large Children's Cancer Group (CCG) protocols for high-risk and standard-risk medulloblastoma, 107 patients (24%) had posterior fossa syndrome. It was classified as severe in 43%, moderate in 49%, and mild in 8%. As with many neurologic insults, most patients demonstrated significant improvement, although neurologic abnormalities persisted in a large proportion of patients.[243] No uniform diagnostic criteria exist for posterior fossa syndrome, and radiologic imaging with SPECT has failed to define a specific controlling neurologic region.[244]

Venous thrombosis in adults with brain tumors is common, especially when compared with adults undergoing operations for causes not related to brain tumors,[245,246] and typically requires therapy. A similar predilection to significant symptomatic thrombosis in children with CNS tumors has not been identified.[247] Because of the risks of spontaneous hemorrhage in patients taking anticoagulants, their routine use is discouraged for pediatric patients.[248] When thromboses in this patient population are identified, other precipitating factors such as the presence of a central venous access device[247] are usually evident.[249] CNS hemorrhage is rare in pediatric patients undergoing tumor resection. Use of recombinant factor VIIa has been used successfully when bleeding was difficult to control.[250]

Long-Term Follow-Up

Long-term follow-up is extremely important because neurosurgical sequelae of the treatment of brain tumors exist. The management of hydrocephalus is lifelong, and all survivors of childhood brain tumors who have treated hydrocephalus should undergo frequent evaluations by a neurosurgeon and radiographic evaluation of the patency of the ETV (via specialized MRIs) or of their shunt systems.

A relatively rare but significant complication of radiation therapy and surgery for tumors in the sellar/suprasellar area is moyamoya disease. This condition is manifested by the development of occlusive vascular disease at the base of the skull with subsequent ischemic events and stroke. The management includes surgical revascularization, which is effective in stopping the clinical symptomatology and preventing new ischemic events and is performed in centers with specialized interest in this condition and expertise in the surgical procedure.

Radiotherapy

A detailed section on the fundamentals of radiation oncology is included elsewhere in this text (see Chapter 48). The primary goal of this brief discussion is to focus on radiation therapy issues that are specific to pediatric neurooncology.[251] An understanding of the basic principles of radiation therapy is critical because it remains one of the most effective, albeit toxic, therapies for this patient population.

Like chemotherapy, radiation therapy targets dividing cells, one of the hallmarks of cancer therapy. Unlike chemotherapy, however, delivery of radiation therapy is not limited by the BBB. The biologic effects of ionizing radiation are the result of damage to cellular DNA, primarily through irreparable double-strand breaks. Photon radiation can cause damage through direct interaction with DNA or through the formation of free radicals, which damage the DNA. Charged particles can cause damage through direct interactions with the nucleus. This damage results in complex cascades of molecular events, affecting cell cycle checkpoints, apoptosis, DNA damage response, and DNA repair. Tumor cells have lost the regulation required to repair DNA damage before entering cell replication. In contrast normal adjacent cells that receive radiation therapy will repair the damage between fractions. After weeks of continued radiation therapy, normal cells will have repaired themselves, although the repair process is not perfect and accounts for the toxicity to normal brain caused by radiation therapy. Tumor cells, on the other hand, will have accumulated significant damage, leading to cell death. The concept of fractionation is the hallmark of radiation therapy.

Technical Aspects of Radiation Therapy

Radiation therapy technology has advanced continually since the discovery of x-rays. The most commonly used modalities in the treatment of CNS tumors are photon radiotherapy and proton radiotherapy. Both these forms of irradiation provide the same treatment dose to the tumor tissue, and therefore their differences are not related to efficacy. Rather the differences in the therapeutic beams and the physical properties associated with them result in different dose distributions. The major clinical difference between the two techniques relates to potential toxicities to the normal brain.

Photon Therapy. Photons are packets of high energy that enter tissue, depositing their energy as they pass through both normal tissue and the tumor, eventually exiting the brain. The presence of an exit dose is one of the major differences between this modality and proton therapy. The generation of photon beams is easily achieved with a large array of commercially available machines and, with more than 60 years of clinical experience, photon radiotherapy remains the most widely used form of radiation therapy. Significant advances in this modality have occurred through the development of better imaging (MRI and functional imaging such as PET and metaiodobenzylguanidine), planning algorithms, and machine delivery that has allowed the radiation oncologist to target tumors more accurately and to minimize the dose delivered to normal tissue.

Opposed Lateral Fields. Used largely before 1990, opposed lateral fields typically rely on two wide beams, usually one from the left and the other from the right. This approach is no longer considered the standard of care in children with a brain tumor because of excessive toxicity to normal brain tissue. At a minimum conformal fields should be used.

Conformal Radiation Therapy. The conformal radiation technique uses the principle of tumor volume definition through MRI and CT scans. In the treatment of CNS tumors, the anatomic localization of the bony structures of the skull using CT scans are fused to the MRI with specialized fusion software. This technique allows accurate tumor definition and submillimeter accuracy in treatment. Radiation therapists choose beam placement to maximize tumor coverage while avoiding normal brain tissue. With 3D conformal radiation therapy, conformal beams are used to shape the dose delivered to the target, and wedges or compensators can be used to optimize the dose distribution. With 3D conformal radiation therapy, variable field weighting and use of different energies (higher beam energies are more penetrating) are additional tools that enable optimization of the dose distribution. With the development of more rapid and powerful computers, the ability to generate a large number of different beam orientations has allowed for diffusion of the radiation dose over normal tissue, thus reducing long-term damage while ensuring complete coverage of the tumor volume.[252]

Stereotactic Radiotherapy. Stereotactic radiotherapy is a further improvement on 3D conformal therapy by ensuring improved head immobility so that beam configuration may be further reduced without having to worry about head position and tumor location.[253] In the normal delivery of the radiation beam, some head movement may occur; therefore, the target volume must be expanded in all directions to ensure that at no time is part of the tumor outside the targeted area. To overcome this difficulty, a series of techniques have been developed that use head immobilization to ensure less head movement and consequently smaller target volumes. Options for such immobilization include frames bolted to the skull and then fixed to the radiation device, which is the standard procedure for stereotactic radiation surgery (discussed later). The major limitation of this procedure, however, is that radiation therapy is delivered over approximately 6 weeks, and bolting screws into the skull for this length of time is not practical. A second option is the use of a head mask made for each patient, which fits around the face and skull and can sometimes use the ear canals or palate to ensure exact and reproducible fits. A new development is the use of real-time CT scans that constantly reevaluate the position of the skull, with computer software that corrects for changes in head position to reset the beams accordingly. In children the additional dose of radiation therapy from CT scans is not trivial and needs to be considered in the choice of method.

Intensity-Modulated Radiation Therapy. Intensity-modulated radiation therapy (IMRT) gives radiation therapists the opportunity to modulate the intensity of a radiation beam so that instead of uniform dosing throughout a volume, areas of decreased intensity may spare critical structures.[254] For example if a critical nerve runs through or adjacent to a tumor, IMRT allows the radiation therapist to spare the middle, like a doughnut, while still treating the entire surrounding tumor. IMRT is a device that fits onto the gantry of a radiation machine and moves small metal slots in and out of the beam path as it moves in arcs to deliver the required fields. Large metal (macroleaf) and small metal (microleaf) pieces are available. The microleaf collimators allow for a more refined shaping of the field. An important limitation of this technique is the development of hot spots in areas within the field. As a general rule this technique can be added to 3D conformal and stereotactic radiation therapy treatment plans.

Stereotactic Radiosurgery. Stereotactic radiosurgery (SRS) techniques (e.g., gamma knife, cyber knife, or X-knife) use a single fraction (or occasionally several fractions) rather than the prolonged treatment courses that are standard with radiation therapy. As the names imply in these techniques, all develop a focused beam of energy that covers a tight volume and causes the cells within the volume to die.[255] Unlike traditional radiation therapy, in which normal cells recover between successive doses while tumor cells do not, the principle for this technique is similar to focusing sunlight with a magnifying glass to burn a small area. Because of the significant toxicities possible with a technique designed to kill a targeted area, a specific volume that excludes normal adjacent structures is critical. To achieve this requirement, after induction of general anesthesia, the head is often bolted into a metal head frame, and then the metal frame is bolted to the radiation device. In this way no additional or unintended movement can occur that would result in the targeted beam missing part of the tumor and damaging uninvolved adjacent normal brain tissue. New methods that can avoid the need for fixed head localization are being developed.[256]

Proton Radiotherapy. The use of proton beam radiation therapy as an alternative to high-energy x-rays (photons) has the potential to limit some of the late effects of radiation therapy by reducing the exposure of normal tissue to the radiation.[257,258] Physically, photon beams deliver their maximum radiation dose near the surface, followed by a continuously reducing dose with increasing depth. Tissues outside the target area receive an exit dose of the radiation beams. For example when a single posterior field is used to treat the spinal axis, critical organs along the path such as the heart, lung, bowel, and ovaries may receive significant exposure. In contrast in proton beam radiotherapy, while the charged particles—namely, protons—move through tissue, they ionize particles and deposit their radiation dose along the path. The maximal dose, called the Bragg peak, occurs shortly before the point of greatest tissue penetration, which is dependent on the energy of the proton beam. Because the energy can be precisely controlled, the Bragg peak can be placed within the tumor targeted to receive the radiation dose. Because the protons are absorbed at this point, normal tissues beyond the target receive little irradiation.[259] Proton beam radiotherapy is becoming more readily available but remains a more limited and costly modality. Children most likely to benefit from proton beam treatment are those with favorable or curable brain tumors such as craniopharyngiomas, medulloblastomas, LGGs, ependymomas, and GCTs. With the increasing complexity of radiation planning, a dedicated pediatric radiation oncology team is required to ensure appropriate care for the pediatric patient.[260-262]

Toxicity of Radiation Therapy

Even with the significant advances in the highly precise delivery of radiation therapy, a number of circumstances limit its usefulness for children. Humans achieve their maximum number of brain cells shortly after birth. From that time forward, a steady loss of cells continues throughout life. While we age our neurocognitive development is related to the development of new connections and interactions between cells, not the addition of cells. For reasons that are poorly understood, irradiation can affect not only the proliferation of new cells in infancy but also the ability of cells already present to form or maintain connections in children and adolescents.

Late effects of radiotherapy in the treatment of children with brain tumors include neurocognitive sequelae, ototoxicity, hormonal dysfunction, vascular complications, growth disturbance, and secondary malignancies.[263-273] The severity of these effects depend upon many factors. The three major factors that determine the severity of the impairment after radiation therapy are the age of the patient, the volume of the brain to be irradiated, and the dose of radiation therapy required.

1. *Age.* Because the age of the patient at diagnosis is not mutable, simply withholding radiation therapy until a child has had an opportunity to grow older would reduce the long-term morbidity, but this approach may allow a tumor to recur. As such, the decision between accepting toxicity or foregoing efficacy is not uncommon in pediatric practice.
2. *Volume.* Although neurocognitive development is most active from birth until the age of 3 years, significant development occurs up to the age of 10 years and even into adulthood, which implies that radiation therapy to large parts of the brain can cause detrimental effects on cognition throughout life. Because the volume of brain to be irradiated is determined by the extent of tumor spread, radiation therapists must treat the required volumes with all the associated long-term morbidity or reduce the volume to be treated with a corresponding reduction in the efficacy that radiation provides.
3. *Dose.* The third factor related to radiation toxicity is the dose used. Because most brain tumors require the use of maximal tolerated doses to have a significant clinical impact on outcome, reducing the dose would again require a tradeoff between toxicity reduction and efficacy reduction.

Further discussion of the toxicities of radiation therapy is found in Chapter 47.

Chemotherapy

The approach and use of chemotherapy, like radiation therapy, does not differ significantly for most children with brain tumors when compared with children with other cancers. Similarly the effects of antiseizure medications on chemotherapy mirror those of other patient populations, and agents susceptible to altered metabolism by enzyme-inducing anticonvulsants, such as irinotecan, require appropriate dose adjustments or a switch to a nonenzyme-inducing anticonvulsant.[274-276] This requirement has resulted in the development of many pediatric treatment regimens modified from adult studies.[277] The increasing recognition of the unique nature of pediatric tumors in general and pediatric brain tumors specifically has led to the development of pediatric-specific preclinical models of cancer.[278-281] Incorporation of information from these models is likely to be slow as different combinations of chemotherapy, biologic therapies, and radiation therapy undergo evaluation. The need for drugs to cross into the brain raises questions about agents that showed no activity in prior clinical trials. Although the routine approach was to discard such agents as inactive, the ability to modify such agents to improve their CNS penetration has resulted in the need to retest some of these chemotherapeutic classes.[282-284]

Blood-Brain Barrier

The BBB results from the tight junctions of endothelial cells and astrocytic projections surrounding the brain that limit the penetration of substances, especially infections and inflammatory responses, from gaining access to the CNS. A slightly different barrier exists between the blood and CSF (called the blood-CSF barrier), although the primary role of the two systems remains the same—to isolate the brain from the entry of as many foreign chemicals and pathogens as possible.

While tumors develop, they grow and invade normal structures, which can disrupt the BBB. Tumors also need to secure a blood supply, which can be achieved through the secretion of a large number of cytokines, of which the best characterized is VEGF. Before its discovery in stimulating angiogenesis, this molecule was initially discovered as vascular permeability factor (VPF) because of its ability to open up endothelial junctions, allowing for changes in fluid shifts. The secretion of VEGF (VPF) by tumors is responsible for significant peritumoral edema and leakage of the BBB. For reasons that remain poorly understood at present, many tumors, or areas within tumors, do not demonstrate disruption of the BBB, making their detection on contrast-enhanced MRI scans more difficult.

General principles of chemotherapy administration in tumors of the CNS are similar to those of other tumors of the body. The CNS lacks a lymphatic system and, because of the presence of the BBB, extraneural metastases are uncommon. Thus the goal of treatment remains focused on the brain and spine. Some agents may not fully penetrate through the BBB,[285,286] depending on the characteristics of the drug and local breakdown of the BBB. Although the chemical structure of compounds should be an important consideration in their predicted ability to penetrate the BBB, and thus have the potential for clinical activity, many hydrophilic drugs have demonstrated activity in brain tumors. However some hydrophobic agents, which should easily traverse the BBB, do not traverse it. Even with extensive knowledge of the hydrophobicity of a drug, one cannot predict with certainty whether it will have activity in CNS tumors. The platinum drugs, for example, which would not be predicted to penetrate into the brain significantly, are active agents for various tumors in the brain and spine. This outcome may in part relate to the breakdown of the BBB around tumors, resulting in penetration of drugs into restricted areas. One important variable that can significantly affect BBB penetration is the degree of protein binding. To overcome this problem of drug delivery, direct application of drugs into surgical cavities or cysts is possible. Hydrostatic pressure gradients moving from tissue into an empty cavity draw most of the drugs away from the tumor and likely account for the limited activity of chemotherapeutic agent–impregnated wafers along the resection margin.

Intrathecal or Intra-Ommaya Chemotherapy

Intrathecal administration of chemotherapy can overcome the blood-CSF barrier and is of importance in tumors with a predilection to seeding of the brain and spine. This technique is not safe in patients with obstructed CSF flow, but for patients without this problem who also lack diversional shunts that would draw the drugs out of the CSF spaces, high concentrations can be delivered.[287] Because repeated access to the lumbar spine can be uncomfortable, insertion of an Ommaya or Rickham reservoir may reduce the difficulties of repeated administration. To assist in the delivery of chemotherapeutic agents into the CSF, insertion of reservoirs that sit on top of the skull or in the subcutaneous tissue of the abdomen or flank can make repeated administration more practical. Although a number of new agents have been investigated for intrathecal or intra-Ommaya/Rickham administration, including busulfan, etoposide, and mafosfamide,[288-291] overall a limited number of agents may be safely administered to this compartment, including standard intrathecal agents used in leukemia (e.g., methotrexate and cytarabine), etoposide,[292] topotecan,[293] and liposomal cytarabine.[294,295]

An important approach to increasing the penetration of chemotherapy into the brain has been the use of high-dose systemic therapy followed by stem cell rescue. The efficacy of this approach and management of the associated toxicities continue to be an area of significant study (discussed later).

Newer methods of targeting penetration of drugs into the CNS include BBB disruption agents. These agents are in clinical trial and are designed to temporarily open up the tight junctions protecting the CNS.[296] They are typically administered just before the active anticancer agent is administered. Although this approach is promising and deserving of additional evaluation, a common problem to date has been the opening of the BBB in normal areas of the brain, resulting in greater toxicities to uninvolved areas. In a similar approach new lipophilic carrier molecules have been designed to help transport drugs across the BBB, and further advances in these areas are expected.

Convection-Enhanced Delivery

With the movement of fluids away from areas of high interstitial pressure to areas of low interstitial pressure, passive diffusion of drugs deep into tumors is unlikely to occur in sufficient concentrations to be effective. To overcome this problem developments in convection-enhanced

delivery have been reported. These techniques require the implantation of small catheters that can be tunneled under the scalp, which then penetrate the solid tumor parenchyma or adjacent brain. By injecting drugs under high pressure, these agents move through the interstitial space between cells, giving the drugs an opportunity to kill tumor cells, even in critical areas of the CNS such as the pons.[297] Because tumors usually penetrate along the pathway of least resistance, similar to fluids under pressure, this technique allows the drug to spread out in a fashion similar to that of the infiltrating tumor. A number of candidate molecules designed for convection-enhanced delivery are being developed. This technique should be equally well suited to small-molecule inhibitors, chemotherapeutic agents, biologic drugs (including large protein molecules), and gene vectors. Advances in drug packaging may permit control of drug delivery, improving the activity of this approach.[298]

Novel Chemotherapeutic and Biologic Agents

The revolution in the molecular classification of adult and pediatric tumors has significantly advanced our understanding of pathways implicated in tumor initiation, progression, and metastases. These pathways have also become important targets for new therapy approaches that are included in the realm of chemotherapy but differ in many fundamental ways. The unique mechanism of action of these inhibitors, and their lack of typical chemotherapy-related toxicity (e.g., myelosuppression) make them ideally suited for combination with traditional chemotherapy and radiation therapy.[5,299] In addition to classic cytotoxic agents, the use of agents that modulate the epigenome, such as histone deacetylases, which modify DNA methylation, a process critical in gene regulation, may allow apoptotic or differentiation genes to be reactivated while turning off proliferative pathways.[300,301]

The development of new formulations of old drugs also deserves comment. Many drugs that were tested in children with tumors of the CNS did not demonstrate activity, which may have been the result of poor penetration or unknown pharmacokinetics. Modifications to older agents such as doxorubicin by pegylation and liposomal encapsulation will require additional clinical testing.[302] Even vincristine, which is commonly used in pediatric patients with CNS tumors despite a lack of clear data demonstrating its activity in these diseases, is being redeveloped to improve its potential activity.[284,303]

Numerous targeted agents are now available, and each will require some early pediatric clinical experience regarding dosing and tolerability.[304] Unfortunately most biologic agents are unlikely to possess significant single-agent activity or resistance will develop, although some exciting responses have been observed in a number of different pathways, including SHH and BRAF.[305] Many of these drugs may be better at slowing tumor progression and will need to be used in combination with other molecular inhibitors, radiation therapy, and chemotherapy. These targets may also have important roles as prognostic markers, as well as therapeutic targets.[306,307]

Small-Molecule Inhibitors. The sequencing of the human genome and the identification of a number of critical signaling pathways, especially the receptor tyrosine kinases, have provided the basis for a whole new class of anticancer agents.[308] Normal cells transmit signals from the external environment to the nucleus via receptor tyrosine kinases. These molecules sit on the cell surface and homodimerize or heterodimerize in the presence of ligand, which results in a conformational change in the intracellular domain of the receptor. This process allows a phosphorylation event on the cytoplasmic component of the receptor that begins a complex cascade that results in the alteration of cell function. Many tumors use these receptors or their pathways to drive cell proliferation and migration, as well as decouple cell repair and apoptosis.[309]

The activation of receptor tyrosine kinases results from the phosphorylation of a tyrosine residue in the intracellular domain of the receptor. This process can be blocked by the steric interference of small molecules designed to fit into the phosphorylation pocket. By carefully designing the shape of these molecules, the ability to define the specificity of these drugs to related receptors means that some inhibitors can disrupt only a single receptor or entire families of receptors. A number of experimental studies of these inhibitors have been tested in children with brain tumors, including those targeting the platelet-derived growth factor receptor (PDGFR)[310] and ras pathways.[311] One problem with small-molecule inhibitors, as with other agents targeting the CNS, is the need to get drugs across the BBB; small molecules are ideally suited for this purpose, but efflux pumps are present that may expel the agents, resulting in limited activity.[312] Unfortunately this mechanism must be evaluated on a drug-by-drug basis.

Immunotherapy

Although the brain and spine are considered immunologically privileged sites, the presence of lymphocytic infiltrates in many brain tumors suggests that activation of the immune system is possible. Significant attempts to activate the immune system against these tumors,[313] especially malignant gliomas, have followed two main approaches. Some groups have attempted to increase the immune activation of lymphocytes by cytokine stimulation of the innate immune system. In the second approach a patient's own tumor is required to generate tumor-specific immune-activated cells.[314] While more is learned about how immune cells interact with and are activated by tumors, opportunities to develop immunotherapies may become more feasible,[315,316] and some early encouraging results are already being reported.[317,318]

Gene Therapy

The use of gene vectors for the treatment of brain tumor allows for the expression of a large array of different molecules.[319] Many experimental approaches have focused on modulators of the immune response.[320] An important component in the expansion of these approaches will be the identification of different vectors,[321] as well as improvement in direct delivery of large molecules directly into the brain to bypass the BBB.[322]

Antiangiogenic Agents

During the past few decades the role of angiogenesis in the development of cancer has evolved from a novel hypothesis to a fundamental area of research and therapeutic intervention. Although not brain tumor–specific, angiogenesis has been a hallmark of the progression of malignant gliomas. A large number of antiangiogenic inhibitors are now in clinical trials and have focused on targeting the cytokine vascular endothelial growth factor,[323,324]; other inhibitors of the angiogenic cascade are being tested as well.[325,326] Although bevacizumab has been extensively tested in adults with malignant gliomas, its role in pediatric tumors remains unclear.[327,328] A developing area ideally suited for pediatric patients has been the use of oral antiangiogenic chemotherapy.[329-331] The principle behind this approach is the use of very-low-dose chemotherapy that targets dividing endothelial cells rather than tumor cells. A number of low-dose chemotherapy approaches are being tested, and preliminary results are encouraging.[226,332-336]

Suppression of Tumor Resistance

The innate resistance of many tumors to cytotoxic agents, especially those of glial origin, is well documented by the near-complete and rapid progression of HGGs after upfront radiation and chemotherapy.[337] Tumors can use a number of pathways to avoid cell death when confronted with DNA-damaging agents. Temozolomide has become widely used in conjunction with radiation therapy in adults and has demonstrated clear activity in these patients. Although this combination has demonstrated prolongation in time to progression of the disease, in the vast majority of patients the disease will eventually progress as resistance mechanisms are activated. To help overcome this problem recent clinical trials have begun testing molecules that can bind and inactivate the enzymes responsible for resistance. One such example is O(6)-benzylguanine (O(6)-BG), a small molecular compound that can bind the enzyme O(6)-methylguanine-DNA methyltransferase (MGMT), which functions to remove the methyl group on the O(6) position of guanine after temozolomide treatment.[338] By treating the patient in advance with O(6)-BG, all free MGMT can be consumed, at which point administration of temozolomide can damage the DNA. Although still early in pediatric testing, this approach offers considerable opportunity.[339,340] Additional resistance pathways have been identified in pediatric and adult brain tumors that may guide therapeutic approaches, as well as the development of new inhibitors of the resistance pathways.[341,342] For example mutations within the *PMS2* mismatch repair gene, which can lead to tumorigenesis and treatment resistance, may be influenced by the addition of retinoic acid.[343]

High-Dose Chemotherapy with Stem Cell Rescue

The principles of high-dose chemotherapy and stem cell rescue are similar to those for other malignant diseases. Many brain tumors, especially those of primitive neuroectodermal origin, such as medulloblastoma and CNS PNETs, have demonstrated dose-dependent chemotherapy responses.[344-346] This technique has therefore been used extensively in children with relapsed disease after standard upfront therapy[347-349] and in young children and infants.[350-353] In light of the long-term neurocognitive effects of radiation therapy for young children, particularly for diseases that require craniospinal radiation therapy, high-dose chemotherapy with autologous stem cell rescue (ASCR) currently serves as the backbone treatment in many infant protocols around the world. Although the conditioning regimens, disease histologies, and patient characteristics have differed across multiple clinical trials and retrospective studies, this approach has demonstrated positive results in patients who could achieve minimal residual disease prior to transplant.[354-356] The addition of this modality with other therapies remains to be tested and may influence the utility of this approach in persons without minimal residual disease or the ability to maintain the disease-free state.[357] The role of high-dose chemotherapy with stem cell rescue is debatable, however, in the recurrent setting.[358] The evaluation of patients after transplantation can be complicated by the presence of therapy-related signal changes on MRI scan, including heterogeneously enhancing lesions, often causing clinical symptoms related to their location. Although these lesions can appear consistent with disease progression early after transplantation, they do not progress and need to have long-term follow-up with regard to their clinical significance.[359]

PEDIATRIC BRAIN TUMORS

Gliomas

Glial tumors are usually classified according to the type of glial cell that constitute the tumors—astrocytomas, ependymomas, and oligodendrogliomas. Each is further divided by morphologic features, degree of invasiveness, and location and is assigned a grade ranging from I to IV as the features of malignancy increase. In pediatrics, the grading of astrocytomas has been defined by the WHO or St. Anne-Mayo system and is predictive of patient survival.[213,360] In pediatrics, the modified WHO classification of CNS tumors[197] has become the standard classification system (see Table 57-3). Astrocytomas can be classified as low grade (WHO grades I and II) or high grade (WHO grades III and IV). LGGs may consist of relatively pure tumors such as a juvenile pilocytic (grade I) or fibrillary (grade II) astrocytoma or mixed populations of both glial and neuronal lineages, such as ganglioglioma or glioneurocytoma. The classification of several other subtypes is still being debated. Although the differentiation of HGG from LGG is universally used and based on degree of atypia, mitoses, necrosis, and vascular proliferation, with greater molecular definition of astrocytic tumors, the need to separate grade I from II and grade III from IV tumors regarding treatment and prognosis is increasing. Pediatric gliomas can also be discussed in the context of location, rather than grade. This approach recognizes some of the unique aspects of the environment in which tumors of similar histologies can grow and its effect on treatment and prognosis (Box 57-2).

Box 57-2 Histologic Classification of Low-Grade Gliomas

Astrocytic tumors
  Pilocytic astrocytoma
  Pilomyxoid astrocytoma
  Diffuse astrocytomas (fibrillary, protoplasmic, gemistocytic)
  Pleomorphic xanthoastrocytoma
  Subependymal giant cell astrocytoma
Oligodendroglial and mixed glial tumors
  Oligodendrocytoma
  Oligodendroglioma
  Oligoastrocytoma
Mixed glial-neuronal tumors
  Gangliocytoma
  Ganglioglioma
Dysembryoplastic infantile astrocytoma and dysembryoplastic infantile ganglioglioma
Dysembryoplastic neuroepithelial tumor
Special locations that are often not biopsied
  Optic pathway gliomas
  Tectal gliomas
Cervicomedullary gliomas

Low-Grade Glioma

Supratentorial, Cerebellar Pilocytic, and Other Low-Grade Astrocytomas. LGGs represent the most frequent group of brain tumors that develop during childhood. According to the latest statistical report from the Central Brain Tumor Registry of the United States,[22] the annual incidence of pediatric LGGs in the United States is 2.1 per 100,000 persons. PAs, which make up the majority of LGGs, are well-circumscribed tumors classified as WHO grade I.[361] These tumors were formally referred to as juvenile PAs but are now classified simply as PAs. Grade I tumors are the most common LGGs found in children, representing 20% to 30% of all childhood brain tumors. PAs typically appear in the first two decades, with no clear gender predominance. They usually grow slowly, although their presentation can occur as acute deterioration as a result of obstructive hydrocephalus. NF-1 is the best example of a condition associated with an increased risk of PA in up to 15% of these patients.[362] The localization of PAs in the context of NF-1 and their improved long-term prognosis is well established,[363,364] although the molecular basis for this difference is unclear. Other predisposing factors such as common cytogenetic abnormalities are uncommon.[365] Low-grade astrocytomas typically lack epidermal growth factor receptor (EGFR) amplification,[366] although defects in the BRAF pathway have recently been reported and are present in the majority of cases.[367]

Clinical Presentation. Low-grade astrocytomas in children have a varied course, ranging from dissemination and persistent recurrence to spontaneous regression without therapy, and they behave differently from low-grade astrocytomas in adults.[368,369] The biologic factors that account for these differences remain investigational, although telomere length may play an important role.[370] PAs commonly occur throughout the brain, including the optic pathways, optic chiasm–hypothalamus, thalamus and basal ganglia, cerebral hemispheres, cerebellum, and brainstem (dorsally exophytic brainstem glioma). PAs of the spinal cord are less common.

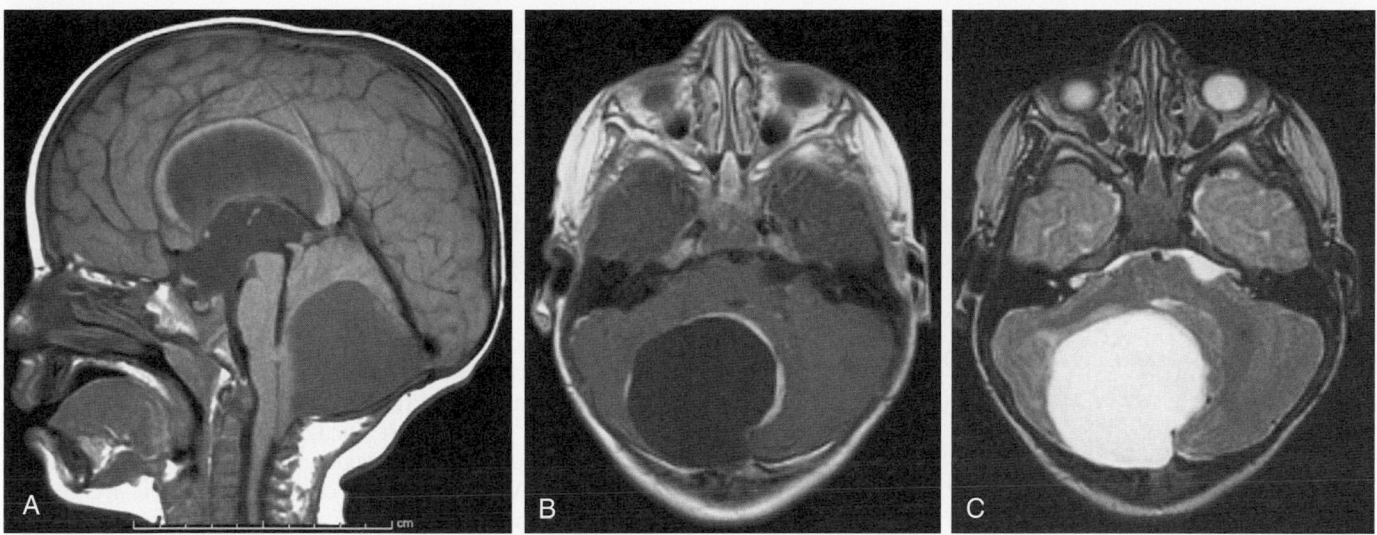

Figure 57-18 Posterior fossa pilocytic astrocytoma (juvenile pilocytic astrocytoma). **A,** A sagittal T1-weighted image without use of contrast material. **B,** An axial T1-weighted image with use of contrast material. **C,** An axial T2-weighted image.

The spectrum of clinical manifestations of a PA depends on the site of origin, its size, the age of the patient, and the presence of raised ICP. Cerebellar PAs and dorsally exophytic brainstem PAs usually present with symptoms of increased ICP, such as headache, nausea, and vomiting. Children may also present with a relatively long history of progressive focal neurologic deficits, including gait disturbance, and infants may present with progressive secondary macrocephaly. Signs of chronicity such as bone remodeling, scoliosis, or hemihypertrophy may be present, depending on the primary tumor location. The diencephalic syndrome is unique to low-grade astrocytomas, both PA and pilomyxoid astrocytoma, is typically seen in infants whose tumors arise from the hypothalamus or optic pathways, and consists of emaciation, emesis, euphoria, and normal linear growth.[371,372] Although many other deep-seated low-grade glial tumors cannot be resected, patients with diencephalic syndrome appear to have a worse prognosis, suggesting that subtle biologic differences among these tumors and other PAs may exist. Leptomeningeal dissemination is associated at diagnosis in 3% to 5% of cases.[373,374]

Imaging and Histology. The typical MRI appearance of a grade I astrocytoma is that of an intensely homogeneous, well-circumscribed, contrast-enhancing lesion with minimal surrounding edema. Lesions are typically bright on both T1- and T2-weighted images. Tumoral cysts are more prevalent in the cerebellum than in the cerebrum (Fig. 57-18) and often possess a contrast-enhancing mural nodule. Apparent diffusion coefficient imaging may be useful in differentiating PAs from higher grade astrocytomas.[375] Imaging characteristics can help with the differential diagnosis of low-grade lesions preoperatively but are not specific enough to be used without biopsy confirmation.[376]

Histologic examination reveals a biphasic pattern, with a compacted component containing bipolar cells (Fig. 57-19) and Rosenthal fibers and a loose cellular array containing microcysts and eosinophilic granular bodies. Rosenthal fibers and eosinophilic granular bodies are pathologic hallmarks of pilocytic astrocytomas, although they can be observed in other diseases of the CNS. Rosenthal fibers are brightly eosinophilic, hyaline masses composed of alpha-B-crystalline and are best seen on tumor smear preparations (Fig. 57-20). Eosinophilic granular bodies are globular aggregates within astrocytic processes and are also best visualized with smear preparations. PAs stain intensely with the GFAP immunoreagent. Invasion of the overlying meninges and adjacent brain parenchyma is commonly observed. Mitoses are rare, and the MIB1 labeling index is usually lower than 4%.[377] Although the pathologic criteria for anaplastic astrocytoma include the identification of mitoses, their presence in PAs does not indicate a higher grade.

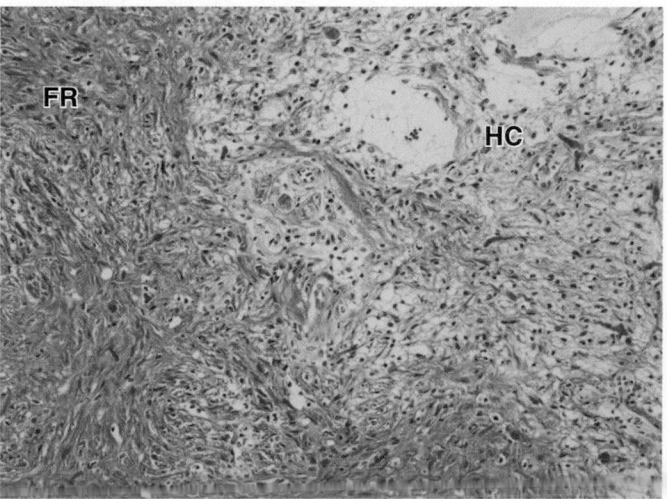

Figure 57-19 Pilocytic astrocytoma. Shown is a biphasic pattern of compact, fiber-rich *(FR)* tumor and hypocellular *(HC)* areas with microcysts (×200).

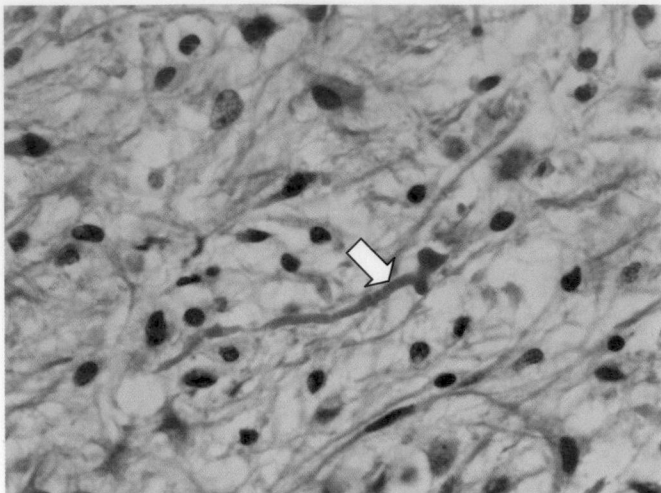

Figure 57-20 Rosenthal fiber *(arrow)* in a pilocytic astrocytoma (hematoxylin and eosin; ×1000).

Inexperienced pathologists can often misinterpret these mitoses, resulting in a diagnosis of a malignant rather than an LGG. Similarly PAs can have vascular proliferation, a hallmark of glioblastoma multiforme (grade IV astrocytoma), although, again similar to that of the presence of mitoses, this does not indicate transformation to a more malignant phenotype. Rarely PAs can present with diffuse leptomeningeal dissemination, especially in the variant of pilomyxoid astrocytoma.[378-381] Characteristic of the unique biology of PAs, each of the metastatic lesions continues to behave as a low-grade astrocytoma with a slow, indolent course. These tumors therefore are not difficult to treat as a result of their metastatic phenotype but rather as a result of their slow, persistent recurrences.

Molecular and Genetic Characteristics of Pediatric LGGs. Recent efforts in the characterization of genomic alterations in pediatric LGGs have significantly expanded our understanding of the biology of those tumors.[210] Genomic alterations of the *BRAF* gene, resulting in alteration of the MAPK pathway, are prominent in pediatric but not adult LGGs.[382] Other genomic alterations affecting PI3K/AKT, EGFR, PDGFRa, FGFR1, TrkB, MybL1 and VEGF signaling pathways have been described in a subset of pediatric LGGs.[383,384]

Importantly pediatric LGGs present distinct molecular alterations compared with adult LGGs. Tumor protein p53 *(TP53)* mutations are frequent in adult LGGs (up to 60% to 70%)[385] but are rare in pediatric LGGs.[386-388] Deletion of 1p and 19q is the most frequent copy number alteration in adult oligodendrogliomas.[389,390] In contrast very few 1p-19q codeletions have been reported in pediatric LGGs.[391,392] IDH1 and IDH2 mutations occur in about 70% of adult LGG,[393] whereas these mutations are very rarely described in the pediatric population.[394,395]

BRAF Truncation-Duplication. The high incidence of LGGs in patients with NF-1 prompted initial investigation into the role of the MAPK pathway in pediatric LGG

tumorigenesis.[396] Early comparative genomic hybridization studies performed on pediatric LGGs, especially PAs, identified a significant recurrent gain of the 7q34 region containing the BRAF locus. This region is amplified in 50% to 90% of pediatric PAs, with the highest frequency in tumors of the posterior fossa and of the hypothalamic/chiasmatic region and less frequently in fibrillary astrocytomas and oligodendroglial tumors,[397-399] and they are thought to have a better prognosis than other LGGs.[400] Further genomic studies found that the 7q34 gain corresponded to a *BRAF* duplication and *KIAA1549* insertion.[401,402] In vitro validation showed that this gene product is constitutively active, leading to downstream upregulation of effectors of the MAPK pathway, MEK and ERK.[403] One short form of the *KIAA1549-BRAF* fusion induces anchorage independent growth in vitro.[404,405] Also short-term cultured pediatric LGG lines showed significant diminution of cell proliferation rate using pharmacologic inhibitors of MEK1 and MEK2.[401] Other partners of BRAF fusion have recently been identified that involve either SRGAP3 or FAM131B, all causing MAPK pathway activation.[404-408] Although break points between *BRAF* genes differ in those variants, they all result in the loss of the N-terminal inhibitory domain of *BRAF*, leading to the constitutive activation of the BRAF kinase. Recent functional studies using BRAF fusion variants have highlighted the importance of the context in which this genomic alteration drives tumor growth. Kaul et al and colleagues[409] demonstrated that in vivo transfection of the BRAF fusion transcript in mature astrocytes was not able to induce glioma tumors, whereas transfected neural stem cells were able to develop tumors. Another recent study comparing the overexpression of the BRAF-KIAA transcript in neural stem cells of different regions within the brain showed that tumors appeared only in neural stem cells located in the third ventricular region.[73]

BRAF V600E Point Mutation. BRAF V600E mutation has been described in a variety of cancer subtypes including melanoma, colorectal cancers, papillary thyroid carcinoma, non–small-cell lung carcinoma, and leukemia. This mutation enhances BRAF kinase activity and leads to the constitutive activation of the MAPK pathway. In contrast to BRAF truncation-duplication, which is strongly associated with grade I histology, the BRAF V600E mutation occurs more frequently in grade II pediatric LGGs (PLGGs), especially fibrillary astrocytomas, gangliogliomas, pilomyxoid astrocytomas, and pleomorphic xanthoastrocytomas (PXAs).[388,410-413] V600E mutation was also described as transforming fibroblasts in vitro,[405] suggesting that this specific genomic alteration drives cell proliferation in a subset of PLGGs. Interestingly a recent study showed that BRAF V600E mutation promotes neural stem cell transformation followed by senescence, which may parallel the natural history of PLGGs.[414]

Other Genomic Alterations Affecting Key Pathways. In addition to the MAPK pathway, other pathways such as PI3K/AKT/mTOR, EGFR, SHH, and VEGF have been described to be altered in PLGGs. Although PTEN deletions and p16 deletions were previously identified in anaplastic astrocytomas and therefore associated with a more aggressive phenotype of astrocytic tumors,[415] a recent study of 32 PLGGs showed that 44% had PI3K/Akt/PTEN/mTOR activation, mostly through PTEN promoter methylation.[416] Additionally BRAF fusion transcript transfection in vivo is associated with mTOR pathway activation through the S6-kinase cascade.[409] EGFR amplification, assessed by genomic hybridization and fluorescence in situ hybridization, was described in a subset of disseminated PLGGs, suggesting that the EGFR pathway may play a role in a fraction of invasive LGGs.[374] Evidence of WNT pathway activation in a subset of PAs, especially in young children, has been highlighted by a recent study showing that the patched (PTCH1) gene, coding for the PTCH receptor, was highly expressed in a subset of PAs, especially in patients younger than 10 years.[417] PAs might also carry abnormal function of the VEGF pathway, supported by the observation that vessel architecture of those tumors is often immature and unstable, comparable with that of HGGs.[418] The active phosphorylated forms of the VEGF receptors 1, 2, and 3 have been shown to be highly expressed in tumor vasculature in PAs.[419]

Recently genomic alterations of the transcriptional activator MYB, a known oncogene in other tumor subtypes, especially T-cell acute lymphoblastic leukemia,[420] have been identified in PLGGs. MYB amplification and focal deletions have been described in fibrillary astrocytomas and in angiocentric gliomas, respectively.[384,421]

Management. Surgery is the mainstay of therapy for most pilocytic and other low-grade astrocytomas.[422] GTR is often curative, even though residual microscopic disease may often be left behind.[423,424] Radiation therapy and chemotherapy are typically not required as part of upfront therapy after a complete resection.[425] Surgery is also an effective method of seizure control in patients with LGGs, especially those of the temporal lobes.[426,427] PLGGs in more eloquent areas may not be amenable to surgical resection. Because the OS even of nonresectable PLGG is very high, surgical resection should not be attempted when a significant risk of morbidity exists.[428] Unfortunately even in patients with complete resection, the presence of a tumor and surgical intervention can be associated with some long-term adverse effects.[429] PAs of the optic pathway in patients with NF-1 do not require surgical confirmation unless atypical radiographic or clinical features are present.[430] Patients with tectal gliomas require CSF diversion but do not benefit from biopsy; they can be diagnosed on the basis of the presence of hydrocephalus and MRI appearance of the lesion alone. In the largest prospective series of patients with PLGG stratified to observation, chemotherapy, or radiation therapy, the overall outcome of these patients was similar to that of patients reported in other independent series and is an important milestone in the assessment of more than 1000 patients with PLGG.[431]

Progressive or unresectable PAs, or those arising in infants or children that cause alterations of vision or other neurologically relevant symptoms, may require adjuvant treatment.[432] Chemotherapy is assuming an increasingly important role in the management of unresectable and/or progressive LGGs, diencephalic LGGs in younger patients, and other unresectable tumors (Table 57-5). Various combination regimens, such as carboplatin and vincristine or thioguanine, procarbazine, lomustine (CCNU), and vincristine (TPCV) have produced consistent, durable responses,[433-435] reviewed by Perilongo.[436] Monthly carboplatin is more easily administered but may have less activity[437-439] and requires additional study.

With multiagent combinations, stabilization of tumor occurs in almost 50% of patients, and radiographic response is observed in an additional 40%. Median time to progression is approximately 3 years, and up to 60% of patients will eventually demonstrate tumor growth. The Children's Oncology Group (COG) recently completed a prospective randomized phase III clinical trial examining outcomes of children younger than 10 years treated with vincristine and carboplatin versus TPCV. The TPCV arm showed a trend toward a superior 5-year event-free survival (EFS) compared with the vincristine and carboplatin arm (52% vs. 39%, respectively), although no statistically significant difference was found.[440] The ability to retreat these patients with multiple regimens has allowed most patients to avoid radiation therapy, especially early in life when the long-term morbidity of this modality is greatest. Although the time to progression may appear short and the overall progression rate of 50% to 60% appears high, these chemotherapy regimens are well tolerated, with few long-term complications. This outcome is in contrast to radiation therapy, which demonstrates a significantly improved response rate (85% response or stable disease) and duration of disease control (longer than 10 years)[441]; however, radiotherapy also entails significant long-term morbidities, such as neurocognitive, vascular, hormonal, and second tumor risks. Because most children with LGGs will be long-term survivors, this is exactly the population that would benefit from the avoidance of the late effects of radiation therapy.[442] To reduce the volume of normal tissue, stereotactic conformational external radiotherapy,[443] stereotactic radiosurgical techniques,[444] and proton radiotherapy[445] have been evaluated in the treatment of recurrent and progressive PLGG tumors. However more focused delivery of radiation in patients with PLGGs only marginally mitigates the long-term sequelae, which include malignant transformation and second malignancy, vascular injury, and, depending on location, neurocognitive decline, endocrinopathies, and other neurologic deficits. These significant and largely irreversible iatrogenic sequelae, conferred in the treatment of a disease whose natural history is self-limiting in most cases, provide an argument in favor of a radiation-avoidance strategy for children with PLGG.

The overall improved outcome for patients with NF-1 has also been confirmed,[440] indicating that these tumors may have a unique biologic phenotype. Temozolomide (TMZ), an orally active alkylating agent with a favorable adverse effect profile, has been shown to have some activity as monotherapy for adult LGGs.[446] Although it has not been widely studied, it appears to have a low response rate in LGGs in children, with a median time to

TABLE 57-5   Chemotherapy for Pediatric Low-Grade Gliomas

Treatment	No. of Patients	Objective Response, % (CR + PR)	Overall Response, % (CR + PR + SD)	EFS or OS
Carboplatin[437]	80	2 CR, 17 PR	2 CR, 17 PR, 4 MR, 46 SD	72% 3-yr EFS in patients with NF-1; 62% 3-yr EFS in patients without NF-1
Carboplatin[1911]	12 ND	4 PR	4 PR, 6 SD	
Carboplatin[1912]	4 ND, 2 PD		6 SD	
Carboplatin[1913]	13 ND/PD	1 CR/PR		
Iproplatin[1913]	15 ND/PD	1 CR/PR	1 CR/PR, 9 SD	
Cyclophosphamide[449]	15 ND	1 CR	1 CR, 9 SD	
Cyclophosphamide[1914]	1 PD, 3 ND with leptomeningeal dissemination		2 PR/MR, 2 SD	
Ifosfamide[1915]	6	1 PR	1 PR, 3 SD	
Temozolomide[1916]	21 PD	1 PR	1 PR, 20 SD	
Temozolomide[447]	13 PD	2 CR, 3 PR	2 CR, 3 PR, 3 MR, 4 SD	57% 3-yr EFS
Temozolomide[1917]	10 ND, 20 PD	3 PR	3 PR, 1 MR, 25 SD	51% 2-yr PFS and 17% 4-yr PFS
Temozolomide[1918]	2 PD		2 SD	
Methotrexate[1919]	10 PD	2 PR	2 PR, 5 SD	
Topotecan[1920]	2 PD	1 PR	1 PR, 1 SD	
Topotecan[1921]	11 PD		5 SD	
Etoposide[1922]	14 PD	1 CR, 4 PR	1 CR, 4 PR, 3 SD	
Etoposide[1923]	12 ND		6 PR/SD	
Vincristine–actinomycin-D[1924]	24 ND	3 PR	3 PR, 6 MR, 15 SD	
Vincristine-carboplatin[489]	123 ND		105/123 CR, PR or SD	61% 5-yr PFS
Vincristine-carboplatin[433]	78 ND	4 CR, 22 PR	4 CR, 22 PR, 18 MR, 29 SD	68% 3-yr PFS
Vincristine-carboplatin[434]	24 PD	7 PR	7 PR, 5 MR, 5 SD	
Carboplatin-etoposide[1925]	13 ND	1 CR	1 CR, 3 MR, 6 SD	69% patients alive at mean of 30 mo
Cisplatin-etoposide[469]	31 ND, 3 PD	1 CR, 11 PR	1 CR, 11 PR, 12 MR, 11 SD	3-year PFS 100% in patients older than 5 yr, 66% in patients younger than 5 yr
Vincristine-etoposide[1926]	11 ND, 9 PD	1 PR	1 PR, 4 MR, 9 SD	
Tamoxifen-carboplatin[1927]	12 ND, 1 PD	2/13 PR	2/13 PR, 9/13 SD	47% 3-yr PFS, 69% 3-year OS
6-Thioguanine, vincristine, CCNU, dibromodulcitol, procarbazine (TPDCV)[435,492]	15 ND (4 patients were treated with other therapy and are not included), 42 ND	11 PR, 15 CR/PR	11/15 PR, 15 CR/PR + 25 SD	Median TTP not reached at 79 wk,[312] median TTP at 132 wk[313]
Procarbazine, carboplatin, vincristine, etoposide, cisplatin, cyclophosphamide[1928]	85 ND	36/85	74/88; 36 CR or PR, 15 MR, 23 SD	34% 5-yr PFS, 89% 5-yr OS

TABLE 57-5   Chemotherapy for Pediatric Low-Grade Gliomas (Continued)

Treatment	No. of Patients	Objective Response, % (CR + PR)	Overall Response, % (CR + PR + SD)	EFS or OS
Carboplatin, etoposide, cyclophosphamide, vincristine, CCNU, procarbazine[460]	7 ND, 3 PD	2/10	70% CR + PR + MR; 100%, including SD	70% PFS at 5.6 yr
5-Fluorouracil, vincristine, cyclophosphamide, etoposide[450]	13 (12 ND, 1 PD)	6/13, 1 CR, 5 PR	8/13, 1 CR, 5 PR, 2 SD	6-yr PFS 67%
Vinblastine[332]	9 (ND with carboplatin allergy; nonprogressive at time of therapy)	2/9	9/9; 1 CR, 1 PR, 5 MR, 2 SD	Median follow-up of patients, 10 mo
Thioguanine, procarbazine, CCNU, vincristine[491]	9 (5 ND with carbo allergy; nonprogressive at time of therapy, 4 PD)	0/9	7/9; 7 SD	78% progression-free at 13 mo
Cisplatin, etoposide, vinblastine[1929]	16 ND	4/16 4 PR	9/16 4 PR, 5 SD	5-yr PFS 56%

Modified from Perilongo G: Considerations on the role of chemotherapy and modern radiotherapy in the treatment of childhood low-grade glioma. J Neurooncol 75:301–307, 2005.

CR, Complete remission; EFS, event-free survival; MR, minor response; ND, newly diagnosed; NF-1, neurofibromatosis type 1; OS, overall survival; PD, progressive disease; PFS, progression-free survival; PR, partial remission; SD, stable disease; TTP, time to progression.

progression of 6.7 months, although many patients appear to have prolonged stable disease.[447,448] Responses with TMZ in disseminated low-grade astrocytomas have also been reported,[378] although another alkylator, cyclophosphamide, when given every 3 weeks, lacked significant activity.[449] The role of TMZ in combination with vincristine and carboplatin for PLGGs is currently being investigated. Other investigators have successfully used novel combinations containing 5-fluorouracil.[450] The metronomic application of vinblastine, a mitotic inhibitor, has resulted in some clinical responses or stable disease in children with LGGs who are unable to tolerate carboplatin.[332] Vinblastine is also being evaluated alone[451] and in combination with carboplatin in newly diagnosed patients. Although more information on the activity of these approaches is needed, responses in refractory LGGs have been reported with other metronomic-based chemotherapy approaches,[326] suggesting that angiogenesis may be an important pathway in these tumors. Antiangiogenic approaches, such as bevacizumab, have also been tested with some responses,[452-455] which is also consistent with the presence of vascular proliferation observed in these tumors. Chemotherapy may also allow for improved surgical resection of previously unresectable lesions and therefore should be continuously reevaluated as a therapeutic option.[456] Tumors treated with chemotherapy, even if they are not smaller, can be easier to resect because of less bleeding and a firmer texture at the time of the procedure. The recent identification of BRAF mutations in the majority of PLGGs offers the potential for targeted approaches to these patients. Phase II studies of the downstream inhibitor of mTOR, called everolimus, have recently been completed in this patient population with encouraging activity. In addition BRAF V600E small-molecule inhibitors are also being evaluated for patients

with this specific mutation. Importantly the majority of patients with LGGs have the truncated fusion of BRAF (often referred to as the KIAA1549 fusion because this is the most common translocation). Treatment with a BRAF drug such as sorafenib or other V600E targeted agents would be expected to stimulate tumor growth as a result of a complex feedback loop, not to inhibit tumor growth.[457,458] Patients with truncated fusions will require therapy that accounts for this biologic pathway, and MEK inhibitors are just entering clinical trials for this patient population.

Although most chemotherapy regimens for LGGs have been reserved for children younger than 10 years, older children seem to derive equal benefit with the use of these regimens, potentially avoiding radiation therapy and the risks of second tumors, vasculopathy, and hormonal dysfunction.[459] The use of dose-intensive chemotherapy has been pilot tested in a small series of children, with results similar to those observed using standard doses.[460]

Radiotherapy is considered to be contraindicated in children with NF-1 and is usually deferred in children with PAs and other LGGs, especially in diencephalic and optic pathway tumors. Even highly focused radiation therapy in these locations cannot avoid the potential cognitive, endocrine, or vascular risks associated with radiation therapy. In spite of this highly focused radiation therapy is effective for LGGs and is without significant marginal failures, suggesting that these lesions have not deeply penetrated into surrounding brain.[461] Long-term concerns about second tumors, hormone dysfunction, and cognitive impact, however, still make this approach questionable for children.[462,463] Additional late effects of radiation therapy when used in younger children with diencephalic gliomas may include strokes related to a moyamoya-like syndrome.[85,464,465]

Prognosis. The prognosis for surgically resectable tumors is excellent after GTR. For patients with PAs whose tumors can be completely surgically resected, depending on location, the 10-year PFS approaches 90%.[380,466,467] Even in patients with incompletely resected lesions, treatment is not always required and, depending on the patient and clinical scenario, observation can be considered unless tumor or symptom progression is documented.[468] The most critical variable in the treatment of PAs is the anatomic location of the tumor. Complete resections are most difficult for tumors located in the brainstem, spinal cord, optic pathways, thalamus, and hypothalamus. As such, the PFS of children with centrally located tumors (e.g., in the optic chiasm, thalamus, or hypothalamus) is less than 50%.[467] Given the favorable toxicity profile of chemotherapy versus radiation therapy in young children, chemotherapy is preferred as the first therapeutic modality in young patients with tumors not amenable to gross total resection.[433] The use of chemotherapy as initial treatment in patients with centrally located or unresectable lesions allows for the delay of radiation therapy until the child is less likely to incur the serious developmental and neuropsychological sequelae of radiation therapy. Patients demonstrating radiographic response to chemotherapy have PFS similar to those whose tumors remained stable.[434,469] Ultimately the quality of survival depends on multiple factors, including the tumor location, the extent to which the tumor can be resected, timing of any radiotherapy, and adverse effects of surgery, chemotherapy, and radiotherapy.[470] Transformation of PAs into higher grade malignant gliomas is highly unusual.[471]

Optic Pathway Gliomas

Optic pathway gliomas (OPGs) represent approximately 4% to 6% of all primary pediatric brain tumors; the incidence is higher when asymptomatic lesions in patients with NF-1 are also included.[472] OPGs are evenly distributed between boys and girls. These tumors may involve various parts of the optic pathway, such as the optic nerves, chiasm, optic tract, and optic radiations. They may also infiltrate the adjacent hypothalamus and temporal lobes. Optic nerve gliomas are strongly associated with NF-1, although sporadic lesions are not uncommon. OPGs in patients with NF-1 have a more indolent course than those arising in patients without NF-1[473] and likely represent a different biology than sporadic tumors.[75,474] Although OPGs may be considered a subset of PAs, their unique features and management necessitate a separate discussion.[475,476]

Clinical Presentation. Most OPGs consist of PAs (WHO grade I).[477] The clinical course of OPGs can vary considerably, from an indolent mass in a child with NF-1 to a relatively aggressive, invasive, and expansile diencephalic tumor. Unilateral optic nerve gliomas often present with the classic triad of visual loss, proptosis, and optic atrophy. Optic nerve tortuosity, which can be present alone or in the context of OPGs in children with NF-1, does not necessarily define the presence of disease or the need for therapy.[478] Chiasmatic involvement may lead to unilateral or bilateral visual loss, a bitemporal visual field

defect, and obstructive hydrocephalus as the tumor grows dorsally to obstruct CSF flow in the third ventricle. Further invasion into brain parenchyma may result in more pronounced visual field deficits, as well as hemiparesis. Chiasmatic tumors in infants present as large suprasellar masses that may also extend into the hypothalamus and third ventricle, producing hydrocephalus and endocrine abnormalities. In cases of hypothalamic extension, in addition to nystagmus, visual loss, and hydrocephalus, the diencephalic syndrome may occasionally be seen. This syndrome consists of hyperkinesia, euphoria, and emaciation, with preserved normal linear growth.[372] Failure to thrive is a common presentation of this syndrome, but in the context of a number of other conditions that may also cause failure to thrive during infancy, a delay in diagnosis of a brain tumor is not uncommon.[371] Endocrine deficiencies commonly accompany PAs in this location, and these tumors are more likely to have CSF dissemination in association with diencephalic syndrome, in spite of their histopathologic classification as benign.[479] Many patients with NF-1 will have long-standing, subtle ophthalmologic abnormalities, and thus regular visual evaluation is required. For these patients routine surveillance MRI scans are not indicated because many asymptomatic and clinically irrelevant tumors will be diagnosed, creating a treatment dilemma.[480]

Imaging and Histology. The clinical diagnosis of an OPG is suspected when a child presents with visual impairment, nystagmus, and/or optic atrophy. MRI of the brain or orbits typically shows a solid, cystic, or mixed type of tumor, with strong gadolinium enhancement. The imaging characteristics of LGGs of the optic pathway are similar to those of low-grade astrocytomas in other locations. The typical MRI appearance of a grade I astrocytoma is an intensely homogeneous, well-circumscribed, enhancing lesion with minimal surrounding edema (Fig. 57-21). Lesions are typically bright on both T1- and T2-weighted images. A higher ADC may predict a greater chance of progression.[481] MRI studies and clinical presentation may distinguish an OPG from other childhood tumors that arise in the suprasellar location, such as a GCT or craniopharyngioma. Histologically OPGs are usually grade I PAs or, less frequently, grade II fibrillary astrocytomas. Mixed LGGs have been reported in this region, but the overall therapeutic approach is not altered, because most of these lesions are not resectable at diagnosis. Tumors with an elevated MIB1 labeling index of more than 1% and p53 expression were more likely to be WHO grade II and had a worse outcome compared with tumors with an MIB1 and p53 labeling index less than 1%, all of which were PAs. PAs with a more aggressive behavior had an MIB1 labeling index of 2% to 3% but retained a low p53 labeling index of less than 1%.[477] Like LGGs in other locations, patients with sporadic OPGs have both BRAF V600E and truncated fusion KIAA1549 abnormalities.[399,482,483] BRAF abnormalities are rare in patients with NF-1 because of the existence of constitutive activation of the ras/raf/mek/MAPK pathway.

Management. The unpredictable clinical course of patients with optic pathway tumors has led to controversy

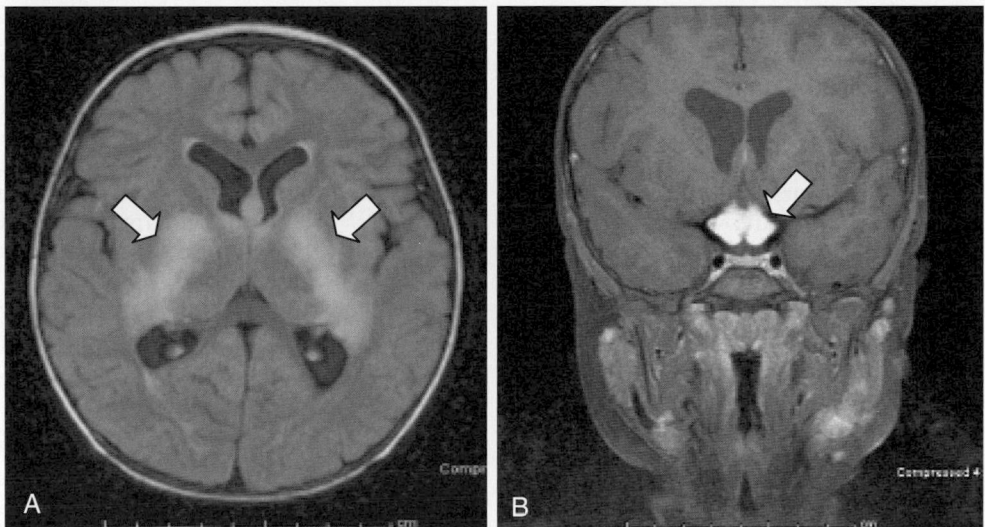

Figure 57-21 A large optic pathway glioma in a 2-year-old boy who does not have neurofibromatosis type 1. **A,** An axial T2-weighted fluid-attenuated inversion recovery image that demonstrates bilateral involvement of the optic tracts posterior to the chiasm *(arrows)*. **B,** A T1-weighted gadolinium-enhanced coronal image demonstrating the enhancing tumor expanding the optic chiasm *(arrow)*. The patient has no functional vision and is legally blind.

regarding the optimal management of these tumors. The clinical course, age of onset, severity of symptoms, size and extent of the tumor, and presence of NF-1 may all affect management decisions. Treatment is frequently started promptly in younger patients, in patients with progressive symptoms, and in those with more extensive CNS involvement, with the paramount concern being preservation of vision. Although progression can be easily quantified on an MRI scan, correlation between MRI findings and visual outcome is poor.[484] The initial treatment of choice is chemotherapy (see Table 57-5),[436] which may cause stabilization or regression[485] even in older children and adolescents[486] and is not associated with the neurocognitive decline observed with radiation therapy.[487] Surgery can be used upfront in selected cases, but the tumor may not be removed from the optic nerve without sacrificing vision.[488] Combination therapy with carboplatin and vincristine[433,489,490] or with TPCV[491] has been considered to have comparable beneficial effects. TPCV should not be used in children with NF-1 because of the increased risks of secondary tumors associated with alkylator-based treatment. When progression of the tumor occurs after treatment with vincristine and carboplatin, vincristine and actinomycin can be considered for patients with NF-1 to avoid further risks of alkylator therapy.[492,493] As for other LGGs, a number of new chemotherapy regimens are being developed (see Table 57-5) and can include bevacizumab and irintoecan,[452] vinblastine,[451] metronomic therapy,[335] and low-dose cisplatin and etoposide.[494] Current clinical trials targeting the mTOR pathway are under way, as is a phase II trial of lenalidomide.[495] Although delaying radiation therapy is paramount in young children, older patients may also benefit from these chemotherapy approaches and from delaying or avoiding radiation therapy.[459]

A randomized phase III COG study comparing the two regimens, carboplatin and vincristine versus TPCV

for the treatment of progressive low-grade astrocytoma in children younger than 10 years, closed to accrual in 2005.[440] The results have shown that both regimens are well tolerated and can delay or obviate the need for radiation therapy in most patients, and that some patients will show improvement in vision with therapy.[496,497] Newer chemotherapy clinical trials for OPGs combine a number of agents such as TMZ with vincristine and carboplatin, and vinblastine and carboplatin. Although a definitive role for radiotherapy exists for the management of OPG,[498,499] current trends in treatment favor a delay in the initiation of radiotherapy in young patients.[500] Newer surgical techniques with direct administration of radiotherapy are also being explored and have demonstrated usefulness for selected patients.[501] Unlike LGGs in other areas, optic pathway tumors affect vision directly, and changes in visual fields and acuity can be a better determinant of both disease response or progression than are changes on MRI. Recent consensus criteria for the assessment of visual function in patients with NF-1 have been reported, and these criteria should provide a useful platform for the assessment of therapies that target OPGs.[502]

Prognosis. Although optic pathway tumors are almost always of low-grade histology, their location often results in serious morbidity. In patients with significant visual deterioration, progressive vision loss can continue for many years after the tumor has become stable on routine surveillance imaging.[503] The growth rate of these tumors, however, often slows during late childhood so that by adulthood, tumors may become quiescent and do not require further therapy.[442] Children with NF-1 have been shown to have a better PFS, although an age of younger than 1 year is clearly associated with a higher risk of tumor progression.[504] Patients with NF-1 appear to be at high risk for the development of moyamoya disease,[84] as well as radiation-induced second malignancies.[505] Patients with NF-1–associated optic nerve gliomas may remain stable for several years. Close observation and symptomatic management are recommended for these patients.

Low-Grade Astrocytomas of the Brainstem

Although most brainstem tumors are DIPGs, approximately 20% of brainstem tumors are low-grade astrocytomas involving the medulla, midbrain, tectum, or cervicomedullary, pontomedullary, or midbrain-pontine junction. Although 20% of nonpontine tumors in these locations can be classified as grade III or IV malignant gliomas, 80% are low-grade glial lesions with a much better prognosis.[506] These lesions differ from diffuse pontine gliomas by their clinical presentation and their imaging characteristics. Early identification of the type of brainstem lesion is critical in the workup, especially for consideration of neurosurgical intervention.[507]

Presentation. Patients with brainstem lesions can present with various clinical symptoms, depending on the location of the tumor. Medullary tumors are more common than midbrain tumors, and the male to female ratio is approximately 1 : 1.[508] In spite of the eloquent function of the brainstem, most patients with low-grade astrocytomas in this location have an indolent course with subtle neurologic findings. Most commonly patients present with cranial nerve dysfunction or head tilt. Lower motor weakness with subtle hemiparesis is also seen. Most parents have difficulty defining the start of the symptoms and refer to their child as having always been clumsy or weak. Rarely these tumors can be multifocal in nature.[509]

Histology and Imaging. Most low-grade brainstem tumors are either grade I or II astrocytomas; fewer than 20% are malignant astrocytomas. Imaging characteristics are similar to those of other LGGs; PAs (grade I) tend to be bright on T1- and T2-weighted images and enhance after administration of contrast material. Edema tends to be minimal. Fibrillary astrocytomas (grade II), by comparison, enhance to a lesser degree after administration of contrast material. The considerable overlap and variability in the imaging characteristics of grade I versus grade II astrocytomas, however, prevents accurate diagnosis based on MRI characteristics alone. The histologic features of brainstem low-grade astrocytomas are identical to grades I and II astrocytomas in other locations.

Management. Brainstem low-grade astrocytomas that remain focal can often be surgically resectable if they possess a plane between the brainstem and tumor.[510] If the tumor is completely resected, these patients are unlikely to need additional therapy. Given the good long-term outcome of this patient population, aggressive surgery should not risk damage in areas with poor tumor boundaries.[511] Incompletely resected brainstem low-grade astrocytomas have a high recurrence rate, and most of these patients will need additional therapy,[512] usually chemotherapy rather than radiation therapy, given the good long-term prognosis of these patients (see Table 57-5).[436] White matter tracts are often displaced by these tumors,

and preoperative DTI can assist the neurosurgeon regarding the optimal approach to maximize resection while minimizing morbidity in this patient population.[513] Although postsurgical morbidity such as problems with swallowing can be significant, many patients eventually recover function, although this process can take many months and requires extensive physical and occupational therapy.[514] The chemotherapy options for these tumors are identical to those for low-grade astrocytomas in other locations and include vincristine and carboplatin or TPCV chemotherapy. Recurrence and need for retreatment are common, but most tumors will eventually stop growing while these patients enter adulthood.

Prognosis. Because most patients with a low-grade brainstem glioma will be long-term survivors,[510] it is important that the workup and treatment of these patients be adapted with this likely outcome in mind. Differentiation from DIPGs is usually easily made on the basis of imaging and clinical criteria. Surgical intervention must be based on the expectation that minimal long-term morbidity will result, given the large number of other treatment options available for these patients.

Low-Grade Thalamic Astrocytomas

Thalamic tumors are rare in pediatric patients, accounting for fewer than 5% of intracranial tumors. Most thalamic tumors are unilateral, and approximately 50% are low-grade astrocytomas.[515,516] Thalamic tumors occur at a slightly older age than do many other LGGs of childhood. Low-grade thalamic tumors present as unilateral or bithalamic in location, which appears to have prognostic significance.

Clinical Presentation. Thalamic tumors can present with a number of different clinical findings.[517] Raised ICP, tremors, motor deficits, seizures, and mood changes are the most commonly observed presenting symptoms.[518] Unlike in adult tumors, dementia is a rare presenting symptom.[519]

Imaging and Histology. Imaging characteristics of thalamic tumors are similar to those of gliomas in other locations (Fig. 57-22). Low-grade and high-grade histologies are approximately equally distributed, although pathologic classification of these tumors can be influenced by sampling error from small biopsy specimens.[520] The use of PET or SPECT imaging can help identify areas to be biopsied.[521] Although astrocytic histologies predominate, oligodendroglial tumors have also been identified.[516]

Management. The presence of tumor in the thalamus presents a number of management difficulties. Because of their location, complete resection is difficult,[519] although surgery can result in symptom improvement in selected cases.[522] Even attempts at biopsy can result in significant morbidity. The small amount of surgical material often raises concerns of sampling error in attempting to determine the histopathologic grade of the tumor. Biopsy of the most malignant component of these deep-seated

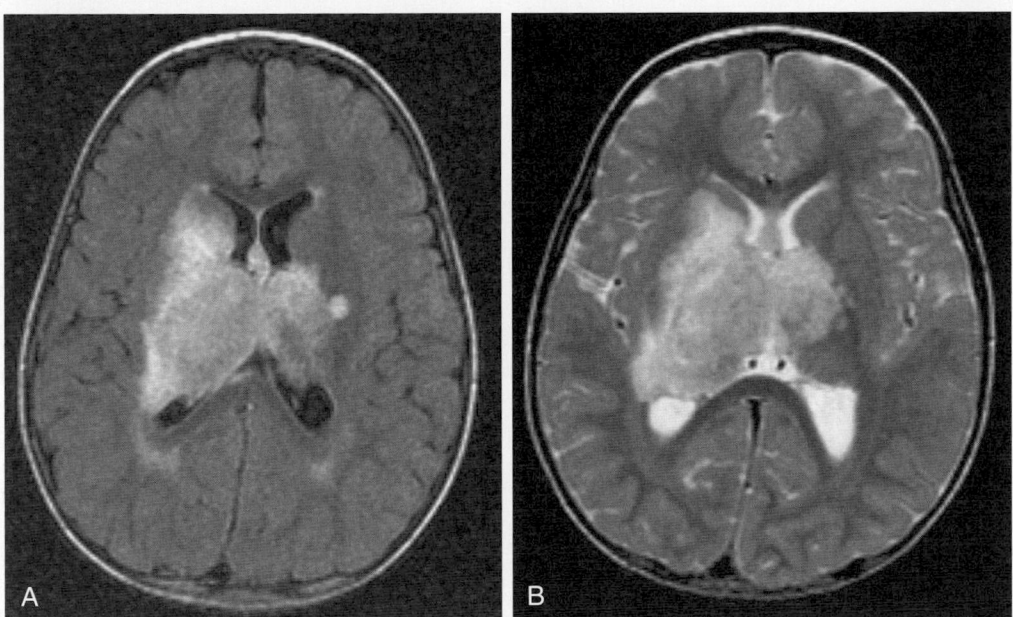

Figure 57-22 Bithalamic astrocytoma. **A,** An axial fluid-attenuated inversion recovery image. **B,** An axial T2-weighted image.

lesions can be guided with PET imaging.[521] This guidance is particularly important for astrocytic tumors, for which samples of sufficient size and content are needed to define the elements of tumor grade. In the analysis of children with thalamic lesions, most tumors are unilateral in nature, and approximately 50% to 60% are low-grade astrocytomas; the remaining 40% are high-grade lesions.[515] Some tumors are amenable to significant resection.[523,524] The response of low-grade thalamic tumors to chemotherapy and radiation is not known to be different from that of similar tumors in other locations. Thus younger patients are often treated initially with chemotherapy used for other low-grade astrocytomas (Table 57-5).[436] In those with rapid progression or histologic verification of high-grade features, radiotherapy can be used, although a significant portion of the brain will receive a substantial dose, resulting in long-term toxicity for survivors.

Prognosis. Contrary to some reports of very poor outcome for bithalamic astrocytomas of any grade,[525] five of nine patients were long-term survivors in one retrospective series.[515] Part of the difficulty in assigning an accurate prognosis to these tumors is the limited biopsy material available for assessment. With a number of reports of survivors now available, even in the context of bilateral disease, all young patients should be given a trial of chemotherapy.

Low-Grade Diencephalic Astrocytomas (Diencephalic Syndrome)

Diencephalic tumors remain a unique and poorly understood subtype of PLGGs. They typically occur in young infants, although a few patients have presented late in the first or second decade of life.[526] A high incidence of dissemination throughout the neural axis has been

recognized[509] and may relate to the increased frequency of the pilomyxoid variant in this location. The presence of failure to thrive in infants often leads to an extensive and prolonged workup for gastrointestinal abnormalities before the correct cause is identified.[527] The presence of diencephalic tumors with early age of onset and the propensity to disseminate suggest that unique biologic differences may exist among these tumors and other low-grade astrocytomas, although no specific abnormalities have yet been documented.

Clinical Presentation. Diencephalic low-grade astrocytomas are differentiated from other LGGs in children by their presence around the hypothalamus–optic chiasm and a unique constellation of symptoms, including the three "E's"—emaciation, emesis, and euphoria. In spite of severe failure to thrive that is often seen, most infants retain normal growth rates and maintain normal pituitary secretion prior to surgical resection.[526] Although an accurate clinical picture for these patients continues to be defined, because many lack the typical constellation,[372] their management is difficult because of the deep-seated nature of these lesions and the frequent presence of leptomeningeal dissemination at diagnosis.[528] As such, these patients require full craniospinal imaging at diagnosis, along with CSF analysis. Any patient presenting with symptoms of spinal disease needs to undergo immediate restaging.

Imaging and Histology. The imaging characteristics of diencephalic LGGs do not differ from those of low-grade astrocytomas in other locations. Lesions are centered around the hypothalamus and chiasm, are bright on T2-weighted images, and usually show homogeneous enhancement after administration of contrast material.[529] The lesions are typically PAs or fibrillary astrocytomas, although the pilomyxoid variant can also be observed in this location.[520] These tumors cannot be differentiated by mutational status of BRAF because some patients have the BRAF V600E mutation, some have the BRAF truncated fusion KIAA1549, and other patients have neither.[413]

Management. The approach to therapy follows that used for other low-grade astrocytomas. Because of the young patient age and deep location of these tumors, radiation therapy is usually contraindicated and will result in significant cognitive impairment over the long term.[464] Most patients undergo maximal safe surgery, followed by chemotherapy with vincristine and carboplatin or TPCV (see Table 57-5).[436] Radiographic response or stable disease accompanied by weight gain is common.[371,530,531] High-dose chemotherapy has also been used successfully[532] as an investigational approach. Radiographic responses and improvement is weight have also been reported with bevacizumab and irinotecan.[452]

Prognosis. In spite of the low-grade nature of diencephalic tumors, patients with these tumors do less well than do patients with similar tumors located in the optic pathway, brainstem, or cerebellum.[431] In addition to the continued progression of these tumors, which leads to compression of vital structures, patients are at high risk for surgery-induced hypothalamic damage resulting in obesity.

Fibrillary Astrocytomas

Fibrillary (WHO grade II) astrocytomas are low-grade astrocytomas that are distinct from PAs. Precise determination of the incidence of fibrillary astrocytomas is difficult because many tumors, particularly those in deep structures of the diencephalon or brainstem, cannot be resected sufficiently to provide the material required to classify the tumor accurately. Thus the terms "fibrillary astrocytoma" and "low-grade astrocytoma" are often used interchangeably. Although all fibrillary astrocytomas are LGGs, most LGGs are PAs. Many tumors are classified as grade II astrocytoma with piloid features because a biopsy specimen may have been too small to identify all the elements required for classification as a grade I PA. Similarly the histologic term "pilocytic astrocytoma with fibrillary features" is used to indicate tumors that have all the components of grade I pilocytic astrocytomas but with areas of infiltration suggesting that they could be grade II. Other LGGs include pilomyxoid astrocytomas, oligodendrogliomas, and gangliogliomas. Fibrillary astrocytomas localized to the posterior fossa represent 3% to 15% of cerebellar tumors[533]; their incidence is lower in the remainder of the brain and spine. No gender predilection exists, and the peak age at diagnosis is 6 to 10 years. Genetic abnormalities in LGGs are uncommon.[365] The reported incidence of LGGs has increased during the past several years. Although an association with paternal workplace exposure in the chemical and electrical industries is purported, a more likely explanation is the increased use and availability of MRI and the diagnosis of presymptomatic lesions.[19,534]

Clinical Presentation. The initial symptoms of fibrillary astrocytomas vary, depending on the location of the tumor. Patients with medullary tumors may present with a long history of dysphagia, hoarseness, ataxia, and hemiparesis. Cervicomedullary tumors may cause medullary or upper cervical symptoms such as neck discomfort, weakness or numbness of the hands, and an asymmetrical quadriparesis. Patients with midbrain tumors such as a tectal glioma often present with signs and symptoms of raised ICP. Other symptoms include diplopia and hemiparesis. In children with dorsally exophytic brainstem glioma, a component of the tumor arises in the medulla and expands in a dorsal direction, resulting in noncommunicating hydrocephalus. Supratentorial fibrillary astrocytomas more commonly present with seizures, although thalamic lesions present with motor deficits. Hypothalamic lesions can present as diencephalic syndrome.[520] Low-grade astrocytomas in the brainstem are usually focal rather than diffuse. They tend to arise in the midbrain, cerebellar peduncles, medulla, or cervicomedullary region. Because of the slow rate of progression of these lesions, most patients have subtle neurologic changes that only become evident over a long period. Unlike adult fibrillary astrocytomas, with which degeneration to malignant gliomas is common, pediatric fibrillary astrocytomas remain low grade, even after multiple recurrences.[515,535] Symptoms may exist for months to years prior to the diagnosis of a low-grade astrocytoma.

Imaging and Histology. Most low-grade fibrillary astrocytomas appear isodense on CT without significant contrast enhancement. The tumors are hypointense on T1-weighted and hyperintense on T2-weighted MRI, with minimal or no gadolinium enhancement (Fig. 57-23) except for dorsally exophytic brainstem tumors. This appearance is in contrast to that of most PAs, in which homogeneous contrast enhancement is common. Pathologic examination may demonstrate some cellular pleomorphism, but no mitoses, necrosis, or endothelial proliferation are present (i.e., no histologic features of malignancy are present). Although PAs are usually well-circumscribed lesions with a biphasic pattern of areas of bipolar cells and Rosenthal fibers and other areas with microcysts, fibrillary astrocytomas have greater cellularity and infiltrating boundaries.[536] In contrast to grade III or IV astrocytomas, fibrillary astrocytomas must lack features of malignancy, such as significant atypia and pleomorphism, mitoses, vascular proliferation, and palisading necrosis. A number of other subtypes of grade II astrocytomas have been identified, including the lipoastrocytic,[537] protoplasmic, gemistocytic,[538] and xanthomatous types.[536] These subtypes are much less common in pediatric patients compared with adults, and may have a worse outcome compared with fibrillary astrocytomas and PAs. The rarity of these lesions prevents formal studies of these subtypes.

Management. Management of most fibrillary astrocytomas is similar to that of PAs and depends on the clinical prodrome, age, and location of the primary tumor.[539]

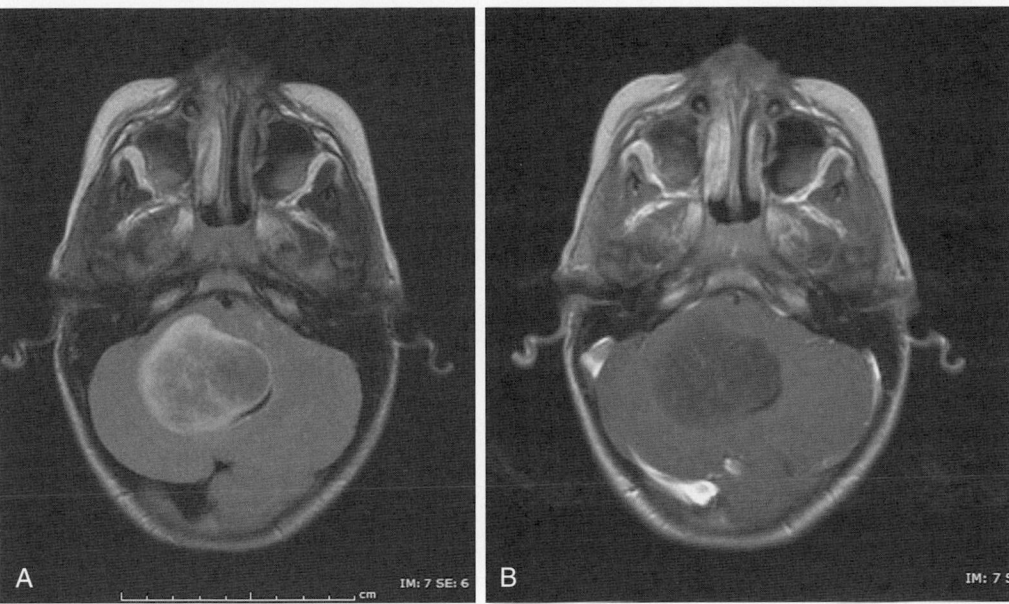

Figure 57-23 Grade II fibrillary astrocytoma. **A,** An axial fluid-attenuated inversion recovery image. **B,** An axial T1-weighted image with use of contrast material showing a noncontrast-enhancing fibrillary tumor.

Rapidly evolving clinical symptoms in the setting of an operable tumor usually warrant prompt neurosurgical intervention. On the other hand, a lesion with a long history of indolent and mild symptoms is often managed with close MRI and clinical surveillance.[468] In patients who subsequently show progressive neurologic symptoms and for whom MRI studies suggest tumor growth, therapeutic intervention is required.[540] Diffuse fibrillary astrocytomas in eloquent locations such as the thalamus or motor regions are often biopsied to confirm the diagnosis and to exclude higher grade glial tumors. They do not lend themselves to radical resections, as is commonly performed for PAs. However in certain cases, such as dorsally exophytic brainstem astrocytomas, radical resection can often confer a long symptom-free outcome. In cases in which resection is not feasible, chemotherapy or radiotherapy may be indicated.[432] As in the case of progressive or unresectable PAs, chemotherapy is the preferred first approach for patients (see Table 57-5).[491,436,541-543] Patients respond well to either vincristine and carboplatin or TPCV chemotherapy. A recent randomized clinical trial of grades I and II astrocytomas has been completed in which these two treatment regimens were compared.[440] Although recurrences occur in most patients, necessitating retreatment with other chemotherapeutic agents, the overall prognosis remains good. Experience with novel combinations of agents[469,450] or high-dose chemotherapy is limited.[460] Radiotherapy is reserved for older children or younger patients whose tumors progress and are refractory to chemotherapy. Reduced radiation doses to adjacent normal tissue, with equivalent tumor control to that of standard photon therapy, can be achieved with conformal proton therapy.[498] Radiation therapy delivered at the time of initial diagnosis does not appear to provide additional benefit for OS.[425]

Prognosis. The long-term survival rate for completely resected pediatric supratentorial low-grade astrocytomas is excellent, especially when compared with similar tumors in adults.[369] Even partially or unresected fibrillary astrocytomas may remain stable for many years. An example of this is the focal midbrain or tectal glioma, which is rarely biopsied or resected.[544,545] Response to chemotherapy appears to be similar to that observed in PAs, although most patients will experience one or more episodes of progression, requiring retreatment with additional chemotherapy.[546,547] However children with primary tumors arising in the pons or thalamus have a worse prognosis.[506,548] The presence of a gemistocytic component characterized by a predominance of large astrocytes, with thick processes and dramatic accumulation of GFAP, represents a histologic variant of low-grade fibrillary (grade II) astrocytoma. This variant may be associated with p53 mutations and may also convey a higher predisposition to malignant transformation.[549,550]

Although most patients with low-grade astrocytomas will survive,[442] patients with fibrillary astrocytomas have a poorer outcome than patients with grade I astrocytomas.[551] Because PAs are more focal and easier to resect than are fibrillary astrocytomas, prognosis may be related to the ease of resection rather than to biologic differences between these histologic variants. Overall survival after chemotherapy of children and adolescents with low-grade astrocytomas at 10 years is 70% to 80%.[425,489,459] The role of MIB1 expression in the prognosis of low-grade astrocytomas is not established as a prognostic factor, after age and degree of resection are excluded.[552] Survivors of low grade astrocytomas still have a number of limitations.[470,553] Future treatment efforts for these tumors therefore will need to combine effective therapy with improved quality of survivorship in these patients.

Tectal Gliomas

Tectal gliomas are typically hamartomas or low-grade astrocytomas, and patients present with acute hydrocephalus in most cases. These tumors appear to represent a unique variant of low-grade tumors, based on their positive long-term outcome, with relief of hydrocephalus as the sole therapeutic intervention. Because biopsy or surgical resection of these lesions is rarely required, little is known about the pathways that drive their activation. No known genetic syndromes give rise to these tumors.

Presentation. Most patients with tectal gliomas present with the symptoms of obstructive hydrocephalus because of expansion of these lesions adjacent to the periaqueductal space. When the presence of these tumors is picked up incidentally, many patients will demonstrate prolonged periods of stability and do not require treatment.

Imaging and Histology. The radiographic appearance of most tectal gliomas is similar to that of other LGGs. Most tumors lack contrast enhancement (Fig. 57-24). Based on their location and presenting symptoms, histologic verification is not required to make the diagnosis and can cause significant morbidity if attempted.

Management. Biopsy or resection of tectal gliomas is usually not required. Rather, most patients require immediate CSF diversion through a third ventriculostomy.[554,555] Failures of third ventriculostomies have been reported, even many years after the initial procedure, necessitating the proper education of families regarding symptoms that should precipitate immediate evaluation.[556] Reduction in ventricular size is often incomplete and the ventricular size continues to change during the first year after diversion.[557] Rarely tectal gliomas larger than 10 cm at presentation will continue to progress over time and may require surgical debulking and chemotherapy.[558] Tumors that have atypical radiographic features, rapid progression, or repeated recurrence may require a biopsy. Tumors with asymptomatic progression can often be observed carefully.[559] When treatment is required, approaches similar to those used for other low-grade astrocytomas are recommended. Chemotherapy is usually initiated. Radiation therapy is not required for most patients, and continued progression of these lesions into adulthood is rare.

Prognosis. The long-term outcome for patients with tectal gliomas remains excellent, which is surprising given the unresectable nature of the lesion and the absence of therapy for most patients. Overall survival approaches 100% in this population,[560] and thus avoidance of unnecessary surgical or radiation-related long-term morbidity is critical.

Pilomyxoid Astrocytomas

Pilomyxoid astrocytomas are a newly stratified group of grade II pediatric tumors in the 2007 WHO classification[207,361] that were previously grouped together with PAs.[561,562] Although no specific molecular pathway responsible for these tumors has yet been identified, the presence of defects in the *BCR* gene on chromosome 17[563] provides possible clues that require further analysis. Other chromosomal aberrations have also been identified.[564] Pilomyxoid astrocytomas are found most commonly in the midline of the brain and spine.[565] These tumors are usually identified in infants and young children, although their presence in adults has been

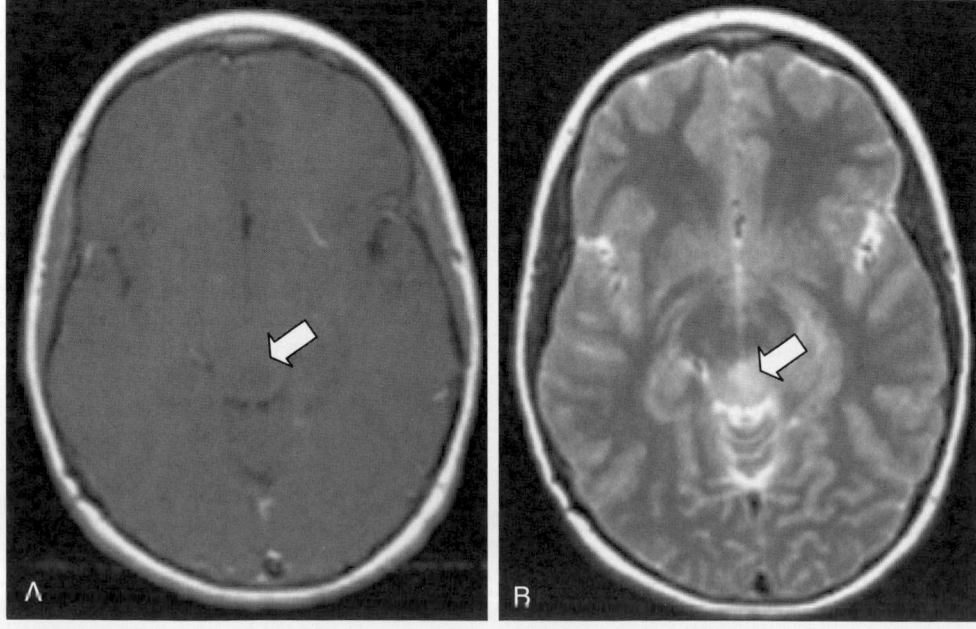

Figure 57-24 Tectal glioma. **A,** An axial T1-weighted image with use of contrast material showing a noncontrast-enhancing tectal tumor *(arrow)*. **B,** An axial T2-weighted image shows T2 hyperintense lesion in the tectum *(arrow)*.

reported.[566] At recurrence, tumors can appear as classic PAs, suggesting a developmental relationship between the two types of tumors.[567]

Clinical Presentation. Although pilomyxoid astrocytomas present in a manner similar to that of other LGGs, the incidence of metastatic disease at presentation appears higher and requires a full workup, including spinal MRI and CSF for cytologic evaluation. Patients with pilomyxoid astrocytomas may be at greater risk for spontaneous hemorrhage at the time of diagnosis or resection or during follow-up.[568,569]

Imaging and Histology. On MRI pilomyxoid astrocytomas appear similar to PAs, with well-circumscribed margins and little peritumoral edema.[570] They are usually found in the midline, including the brainstem[571] and spine,[572] and can be solid or solid and cystic. They are usually bright on T1- or T2-weighted and FLAIR sequences, and they enhance with administration of contrast material.[573] In approximately 50% of cases, the contrast enhancement is heterogeneous.[574,575] Adjacent areas of brain can demonstrate elevated choline-to-creatinine ratios suggestive of an infiltrative margin.[575] Although their location, young patient age, and increased presence of dissemination provide clues to the diagnosis before a biopsy is performed, imaging characteristics do not clearly differentiate these tumors from other LGGs in the pediatric population.[576] Histologically these lesions lack many features of PAs, such as Rosenthal fibers and a biphasic pattern. Rather a monophasic pattern and myxoid background is seen, with strong GFAP and synaptophysin staining.[577] Like other glial tumors, mixed lineages may also be possible for pilomyxoid astrocytoma.[578] The variable histologic appearance compared with PAs,[579] MRS signal changes,[580] and a higher incidence of progression and dissemination support their distinction from PAs.[561] A predilection for younger age appears to exist when the tumor is localized to the pituitary-hypothalamic region.[581]

Management. Because of the more aggressive nature of these tumors compared with PAs, pilomyxoid astrocytomas are now classified as grade II gliomas. Treatments typically follow those of other LGGs, including vincristine and carboplatin and TPCV chemotherapy. Other therapies used for PLGGs have also been used for patients with pilomyxoid astrocytomas (Table 57-5).[582,583] Upfront chemoradiation therapy combinations have also been tried for these tumors.[584] Formal clinical trials for this rare subtype are not possible, however. Because of the young age of the patient and the deep location of these tumors in many patients, radiation-based strategies will lead to significant long-term morbidity in most survivors. Many patients with pilomyxoid astrocytomas are infants and have diencephalic syndrome with dissemination, and thus complete surgical resection is not possible. Thus most patients will start with LGG chemotherapy. The use of intrathecal therapy for patients with disseminated disease who are unable to receive craniospinal radiation can be considered.

Prognosis. Without well-defined studies, the prognosis of pilomyxoid astrocytoma is difficult to assess with certainty. Confounding issues of deep-seated lesions, especially around the hypothalamic region in which surgical options are limited, along with the young age of these patients and the presence of metastatic disease, likely affect the overall poor prognosis. A mean OS of 60 months for patients with pilomyxoid astrocytoma versus 220 months for patients with grade I PAs has been reported.[581] Whether their unique biology affects survival is unknown, although these tumors can recur as typical grade I pilocytic astrocytomas.[567] As in other LGGs, nestin expression may correlate with a worse prognosis.[585]

Ganglioglioma and Glial-Neuronal Tumors

Gangliogliomas are low-grade (WHO grade I) glioneuronal tumors. These tumors represent 4% to 8% of primary brain tumors in children, with 80% occurring before age 30 years and at a mean age less than 10 years.[586] These tumors are frequently associated with seizures and tend to grow slowly. Gangliogliomas can occur throughout the CNS,[587,588] although most are localized to the temporal and parietal lobes.[586] A significant proportion of these tumors have the BRAF V600E mutation,[388,411,413,589] which is now being targeted in open international clinical trials. The presence of this oncogenic mutation may result is a more aggressive behavior and worse outcome.[590]

Clinical Presentation. Seizures are the first manifestation in 50% of cases of ganglioglioma, and many patients have a prolonged history of seizures of longer than 2 years.[586] Complex partial seizures are common because gangliogliomas are frequently located in the temporal lobe, particularly the temporomesial region,[591] although they can occur anywhere in the brain or spine.

Imaging and Histology. Gangliogliomas are typically contrast-enhancing cystic lesions on CT scans. The MRI appearance of these tumors can be variable but is frequently hypointense on T1-weighted sequences and hyperintense on T2-weighted images. Gadolinium enhancement varies in intensity from absent to significant and can be nodular, solid, or circumferential.[592] An infantile variant of ganglioglioma, desmoplastic infantile ganglioglioma (DIG), can occur (discussed later). Pathologic studies show synaptophysin and neuronal nuclear antigen (NeuN)–positive ganglion cells, as well as a GFAP-positive astrocytic component.[593] Lesions associated with the ganglion cell but lacking the astrocytic component are called gangliocytomas. Gangliogliomas are frequently WHO grade I tumors, although some may show anaplastic features in the glial or neural component.[594,595] MIB1-positive cells are usually localized to the astrocytic component.[596] Glial-neuronal tumors likely represent a spectrum of LGGs that include gangliogliomas and may also have PI3K pathway activation.[597]

Management. Complete or near-total resection is the treatment of choice[591] and, in most cases, can eliminate or significantly improve seizure frequency in this patient population.[598,599] Recurrent or unresectable tumors may be treated with radiation therapy,[586,600,601] although these lesions may respond to LGG chemotherapy, and thus patients may avoid some of the long-term toxicity of radiation.[459] In the case of recurrent or unresectable ganglioglioma, response to LGG chemotherapy has been demonstrated.[586] Treatment for recurrent or unresectable gangliogliomas is included in current LGG chemotherapy trials. It should be noted that these tumors have been shown to undergo malignant transformation over time, usually involving the astrocytic component. Clinical trials of BRAF V600E inhibitors are under way for persons with this mutation, and significant durable responses have been reported.[305]

Prognosis. GTR is often curative, making tumor location and extent of resection the most important prognostic factors.[591] Most patients are rendered seizure-free after GTR.[599] Gangliogliomas of the posterior fossa have also been reported, and their outcomes appear to be similar to those for supratentorial lesions. Patients whose tumors can be fully resected to remove the enhancing components are likely to remain disease free, although persons with subtotal resected disease often require additional resection, chemotherapy, and/or radiation therapy.[587] The uncommon presentation of these tumors in the infratentorial location and the limited sample sizes in case reports limit the confidence with which therapeutic approaches can be recommended. Spinal cord ganglioglioma appear to have an indolent course. Patients with subtotal resection can remain stable for prolonged periods. Therefore treatment should be deferred until lesions show clear evidence of progressive disease.[602] Very rarely, gangliomas and glial neuronal tumors can degenerate into a CNS PNET (the neural component) or into a malignant glioma (the astrocytic component).

Desmoplastic Infantile Gangliogliomas

DIGs are supratentorial tumors involving the leptomeningeal surface and are identified predominantly in children younger than 2 years,[603] although reports in older children are available.[604] These lesions are often very large, in part because of the presence of cysts, and they frequently involve the dura. Although precise estimates of their incidence are lacking, they make up fewer than 1% of pediatric brain tumors. A number of chromosomal abnormalities have been reported, although only in a small number of cases, particularly at chromosome 7q31 (corresponding to *MET* gene). One case containing the BRAF V600E mutation was also noted in this series[605] and was reported in two other patients in a different analysis.[606]

Clinical Presentation. Most patients present with increasing head circumference, bulging fontanelle, and lethargy. Older patients present with focal motor deficits.

Imaging and Histology. DIGs are large cystic structures on CT scans, with contrast enhancement of the solid component. T1-weighted MRI sequences demonstrate an isointense tumor; T2-weighted intensity of the tumor is variable. The tumors usually enhance after administra-

tion of contrast material. Peritumoral edema is uncommon. DIGs possess a desmoplastic stromal background, with neoplastic neurons and astrocytes. They often have areas with an elevated MIB1 labeling index, although this characteristic does not usually represent transformation to a more malignant phenotype.[607] Tumors lacking the neural component are called desmoplastic infantile astrocytomas.

Management. Cure can be achieved with complete resection. Many patients have remained progression-free after total resection without additional treatment.[608] Chemotherapy, as for other low-grade astrocytomas, can be considered for patients with symptomatic or progressive cases for whom surgical removal is not feasible.[593,609]

Prognosis. Most patients will be long-term survivors if a complete resection is achieved.[608] Lesions that are more deep-seated may have a poorer outcome, and initiation of chemotherapy may be considered at the first signs of progression in these unresectable tumors.[603,610] Metastatic lesions have been reported, suggesting that in rare cases, a more malignant phenotype can occur.[593,611]

Dysembryoplastic Neuroepithelial Tumors

DNETs are recently described tumors that may comprise as many as 1% of all brain tumors in patients younger than 20 years.[612] Two thirds of all DNETs are located in the temporal lobe, and DNETs are found in 5% to 15% of temporal lobe resections for intractable epilepsy. These lesions are classified as WHO grade I tumors.[613] Thought to be developmental in nature, they are treated with surgery. They are considered to have limited proliferative potential, suggesting that complete surgical resection is not required for long-term disease control[614]; nonetheless, recurrences can occur.[615]

Clinical Presentation. The diagnosis of DNET should be a consideration in children and young adults with new-onset seizures or a long history of epilepsy. Patients with these tumors typically present with a long history of complex partial seizures, with an average age of onset of 9 years. In many patients the seizures are refractory to anticonvulsant medications. The superficial cortical location of DNETs may account for the high risk of seizures.

Imaging and Histology. Contrast-enhanced cranial MRI typically shows a temporal or frontal lobe lesion, absent peritumoral edema, and only minimal, if any, gadolinium enhancement. The tumors are bright on T2-weighted sequences and hypointense on T1-weighted images (Fig. 57-25). Mass effect is minimal to absent. Although routine fluorine 18–labeled deoxyglucose–PET imaging has not been helpful in the preoperative identification of these lesions, Carbon 11–methionine–PET was able to distinguish these lesions from other low-grade lesions.[616] The pathologic findings include a specific glioneuronal element manifested by GFAP-negative oligodendroglia-like cells and neurons in a mucinous eosinophilic background that give the appearance of floating neurons.[617] Because

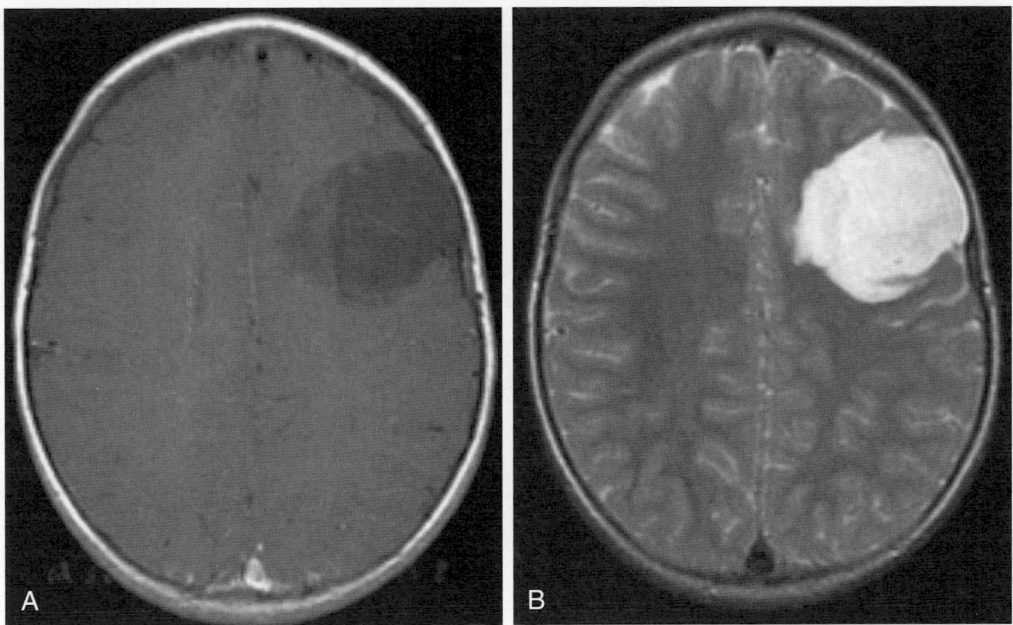

Figure 57-25 Left frontal dysembryoplastic neuroepithelial tumor. **A,** An axial T1-weighted image with use of contrast material showing a large nonenhancing tumor. **B,** An axial T2-weighted image.

oligodendrocytes, astrocytes, or both are found on histopathologic analysis, the pathologic differential diagnosis often includes oligodendroglioma, mixed oligoastrocytoma (OA), and ganglioglioma. Like gangliogliomas and PXAs, DNETs have been reported to have the BRAF V600E mutation in approximately 30% of cases.[618] Differentiation of DNETs from other LGGs can be difficult.

Management. Although these tumors have a benign course, the associated seizures may be refractory to antiepileptic drugs because of the increased expression of multidrug transporters.[619] Gross total resection is often curative and typically alleviates the seizures, especially if the areas of cortical dysplasia can also be removed,[620] although some case series have shown a significant number of patients who continue to have residual seizures.[614,615] Adjuvant chemotherapy or radiation therapy is not recommended. Rare cases of malignant transformation of DNETs after radiation and chemotherapy have been reported.[621]

Prognosis. The stable behavior of these tumors over time results in an excellent prognosis after gross total or partial resection.[614] Patients often have improved seizure control after surgery, especially if a complete resection was achieved,[622] and some improvement in neuropsychologic functioning has been observed.[623]

Pleomorphic Xanthoastrocytomas

Pleomorphic xanthroastrocytomas (PXAs) are uncommon grade II cortical tumors that mainly occur in children and adolescents and account for fewer than 1% of CNS tumors. The median age at the time of diagnosis is 14 years. The molecular pathogenesis of these tumors is poorly understood, and no causative chromosomal

abnormalities have been identified. The BRAF V600E activating mutation has been detected in more than 50% of cases, and drugs targeting this mutation are now in clinical trials.[412,413] A recent analysis of 50 PXAs by comparative genomic hybridization, however, has revealed that loss of chromosome 9 is the most common chromosomal lesion.[624] A few reports of PXA in conjunction with NF-1 may implicate the Ras pathway in this disease.[625]

Clinical Presentation. PXAs are typically large and superficially located, especially in the temporal lobes. Seizures are the most common presenting feature. For tumors of the cerebellum, pineal region, or spine, direct nerve compression results in focal deficits, and obstruction of CSF flow results in raised ICP.[626] Rare cases of dissemination have been reported.[627,628]

Imaging and Histology. PXAs typically manifest enhancement on MRI, with occasional intratumoral cysts and calcification (Fig. 57-26). Peritumoral edema is uncommon. Tumors usually extend to the meninges. The typical histopathologic picture includes a pleomorphic appearance of the astrocytic component, with significant cellular atypia and bizarre multinucleated giant cells with intracellular lipid accumulation. The proliferative indices are usually low, although necrosis, endothelial proliferation, and mitoses have been described. PXA can be confused with glioblastoma multiforme[629] because of the presence of multinucleated cells and occasional foci of necrosis.[630] The expression of CD34 on most tumors may be useful in the histologic classification of difficult or atypical cases.[631] Prognosis appears to correlate with MIB1 expression.[632] In lesions with mitoses, an elevated MIB1 labeling index, and necrosis, the term "pleomorphic xanthoastrocytoma with anaplastic features" is used.

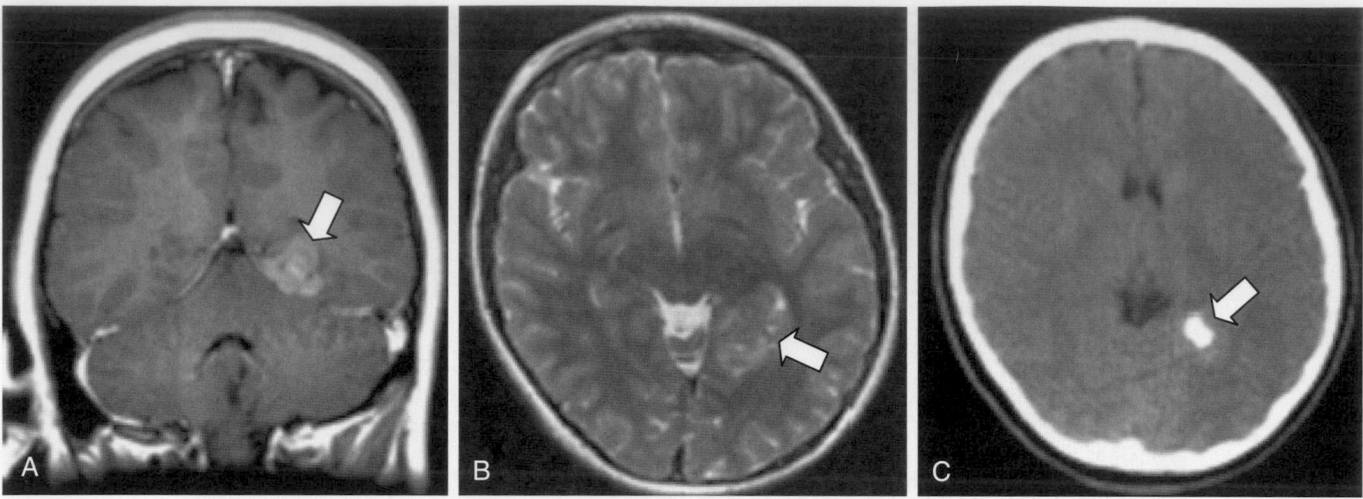

Figure 57-26 Pleomorphic xanthoastrocytoma. **A,** A coronal T1-weighted image with use of contrast material *(arrow)*. **B,** An axial T2-weighted image *(arrow)*. **C,** A noncontrast computed tomography image *(arrow)*.

Management. The clinical diagnosis of PXA should be suspected in children who present with new-onset seizures, focal deficits, and a large, enhancing cortical mass on brain imaging. The goal of surgery is to achieve a GTR, which is usually curative.[633,634] Adjuvant therapy can be deferred, although the patient should be followed expectantly. Tumors that recur and incompletely resected lesions with anaplastic features may be treated with chemotherapy[635] or radiotherapy,[636] although significant activity for these modalities has not been demonstrated. Few formal clinical trials for this rare subtype have been performed.

Prognosis. Several series have reported a 5-year PFS of greater than 70%. However the presence of mitoses, endothelial proliferation, or necrosis on the pathologic specimen, although rare, may significantly alter the clinical behavior and prognosis.[632] Cases of anaplastic PXA with subsequent malignant transformation have been reported.[637,638] Radiation therapy does not alter the poor outcome in these cases.

Subependymal Giant Cell Astrocytomas

SEGAs usually originate in the ependymal walls of the lateral ventricles and are associated almost exclusively with TS, an autosomal-dominant disorder.[639] Patients with TS have hamartomas and benign tumors of multiple organs, including the brain. The CNS manifestations include cortical tubers (hamartomas), subcortical glioneuronal hamartomas, subependymal glial nodules, and subependymal giant cell astrocytomas.[640] Two genetic defects, one in the *TSC1* gene on chromosome 9q and the other in the *TSC2* gene on chromosome 16p, account for TS. Sporadic cases are rare.[641]

Clinical Presentation. SEGA is sometimes the presenting feature of TS in patients without the typical physical stigmata of the syndrome. Because of the variable phenotype of TS, a consensus on diagnostic criteria has been developed. Presentation in older children and adolescents is common. Although patients with TS typically have multiple periventricular SEGAs, those that produce symptoms of hydrocephalus arise in close proximity to the foramen of Monro, although lesions around the pineal gland can also result in symptoms.[642] Most patients with known TS are followed up with regular neuroimaging and the SEGAs are removed serious neurologic syndromes, such as headaches, altered sensorium, or weakness are present.[324] Of note, patients with TS may have other significant neurologic symptoms, such as seizures and cognitive deficiency related to cortical tubers.[643]

Imaging and Histology. CT and MRI are essential for early and accurate diagnosis. Although CT is superior to MRI for detecting small calcified lesions, MRI is superior to CT for identifying areas of gliosis, heterotopia, and SEGAs, which have the typical radiographic appearance of candle dripping.[644] SEGAs typically show diffuse contrast enhancement on CT and MRI studies (Fig. 57-27).[90] SEGAs are considered grade I astrocytomas. They are well-circumscribed tumors that are positive for GFAP, neurofilament, neuron-specific enolase, and synaptophysin.[645,646] Mitoses can be identified but do not indicate a higher grade or more malignant phenotype. They can occasionally be associated with bleeding.[647]

Management. The management of patients with TS is complex and requires adherence to recent consensus conference guidelines.[648] GTR is the treatment of choice for SEGAs that are progressive, and cause obstructive hydrocephalus[649] or seizures.[650,651] The major risk of surgery is injury to the forniceal columns, resulting in memory disturbance. The benign behavior of these tumors warrants reoperation in the case of recurrence or progression after subtotal resection. Inhibition of the mTOR pathway in SEGAs has resulted in a very high response rate, and mTOR inhibitors have now been approved for the treatment of these lesions.[93,652]

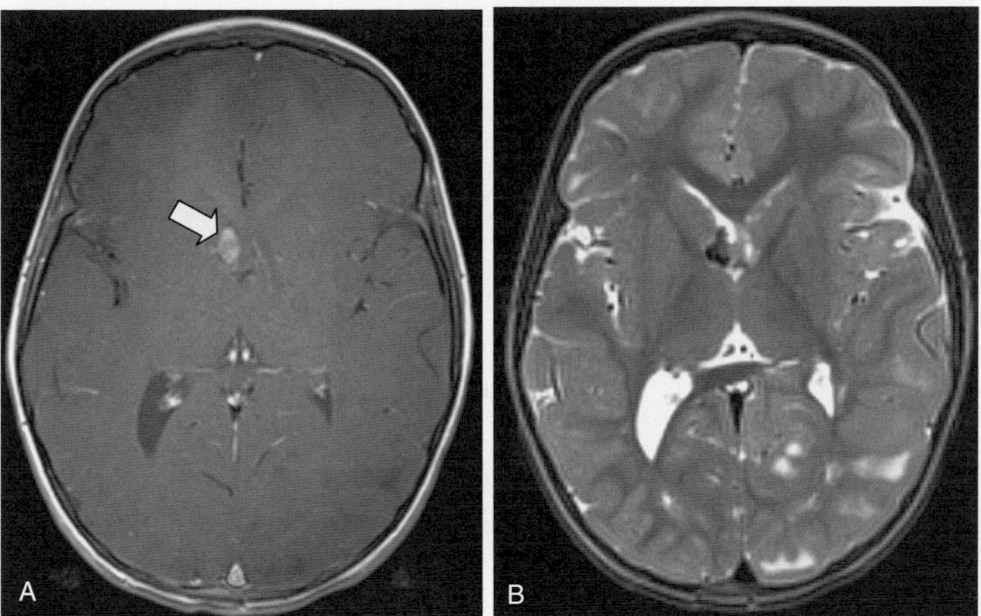

Figure 57-27 Subependymal giant cell astrocytoma. **A,** An axial T1-weighted image with use of contrast material showing an enhancing tumor *(arrow)*. **B,** An axial T2-weighted image showing an area of dark signal corresponding to tumor.

Prognosis. SEGAs are essentially benign tumors, and gross total resection is generally curative. However multiple tumors may arise in some patients with TS, requiring ongoing radiologic surveillance.[90] The overall prognosis for patients with TS is good, despite increased susceptibility to other tumor types, including rhabdomyomas of the myocardium and angiomyomas of the kidney, liver, adrenals, and pancreas.[653]

Hemangioblastomas

Hemangioblastomas are WHO grade I lesions associated with von Hippel-Lindau (VHL) disease. They occur primarily in adults and are centered in the cerebellum, brainstem, and spinal cord.[654] Although sporadic tumors can arise, pediatric cases are usually associated with the inherited syndrome. Cases associated with VHL disease can be single or multifocal, although most sporadic cases involve isolated nodules. Hemangioblastomas are highly vascularized lesions, although the genetic defect is localized to the stromal elements rather than the vasculature.[655] Tumor development appears to be related to the deregulation of VEGF. Patients with hemangioblastomas need to undergo complete genetic evaluation for VHL disease and, for those with the inherited disease, careful lifelong screening is necessary.[656]

Clinical Presentation. Obstruction of CSF flow is the primary reason for symptomatology in patients with VHL disease who are diagnosed with hemangioblastomas. Headaches, morning vomiting, and long tract signs are therefore common. Ataxia and cranial nerve dysfunction can also be observed.[657]

Imaging and Histology. Hemangioblastomas are typically well-circumscribed cystic lesions with a solid tumor nodule. The solid component tends to enhance brightly with contrast and is usually located peripherally within the cyst (Fig. 57-28). Flow voids are commonly observed on MRI and can be well delineated with angiography. Peritumoral edema is commonly observed. Tumors are usually composed of two elements—the stromal cells, which express vimentin and VEGF, and the endothelial cells, which express the VEGF receptor VEGFR2. Hemangioblastomas typically have low proliferative levels based on MIB1 immunoreactivity and are considered grade I tumors.

Management. The management of these tumors requires specialized neurosurgical expertise because of the high risk of bleeding. The primary approach to these lesions, which tend to occur most commonly in the posterior fossa and cervicomedullary area, is maximal surgical resection.[656] This approach provides long-term control in most patients,[658] although, because of the underlying genetic predisposition, new tumors may continue to develop throughout the life of the patient. Embolization can reduce the intraoperative risks of bleeding.[659,660] Radiosurgery can successfully treat the mural component of these tumors, although control is negatively influenced by the presence of the cysts.[661] VEGF inhibitors have been tested in this population with initial encouraging results, although follow-up of these reports is still pending.[662] A case of prolonged stable disease with thalidomide treatment was reported, although whether this outcome was related to its antiangiogenic or immune modulatory effects is unknown.[663]

Prognosis. Because of the genetic basis of these lesions, recurrences are common and likely represent new tumors rather than recurrences of previously resected ones, which

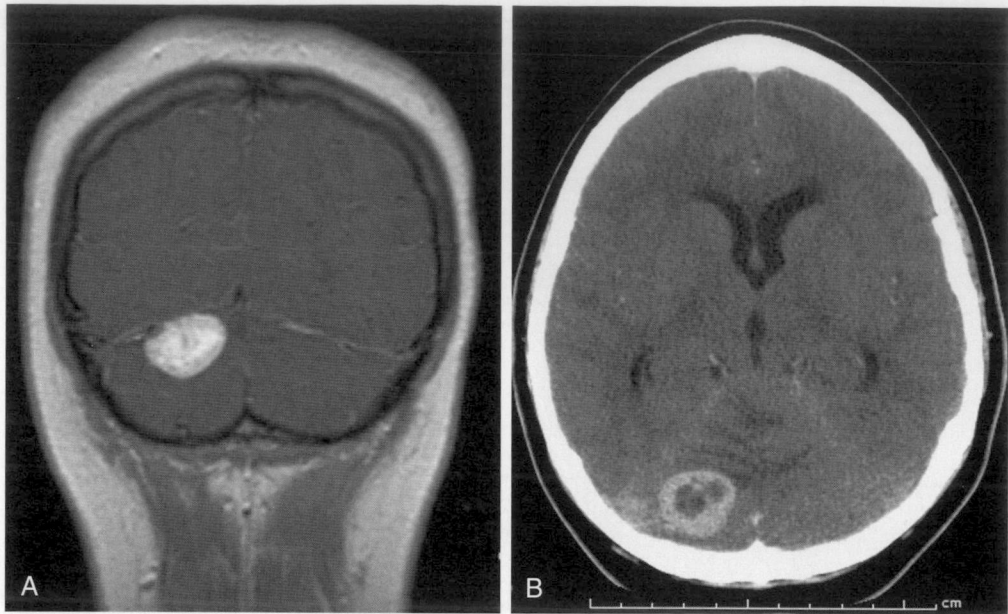

Figure 57-28 Cerebellar hemangioblastoma. **A,** A coronal T1-weighted image with gadolinium. **B,** A computed tomography image.

indicates the importance of continued careful evaluation in this patient population.

Rare LGGs

Tanycytic Astrocytomas. Tanycytic astrocytomas are rare and poorly characterized tumors. They are most common in adults and usually occur in the hypothalamic region.[664] Their malignant potential is not well defined, although recurrences after complete resection have been observed. One reported case occurred in the context of an adolescent with NF-2.[665]

Lipoastrocytomas. Lipoastrocytomas are rare cortical tumors that, as the name suggests, possess fat droplets that give them the appearance of adipocytes in the context of a low-grade astrocytic lesion. These tumors express GFAP.[537] Recurrences can occur and are treated with resection. Malignant transformation has not been reported in this tumor type, although one case was identified on autopsy in a patient with diffuse intrinsic pontine glioma.[666]

Dysplastic Cerebellar Gangliocytomas. Dysplastic cerebellar gangliocytomas are rare tumors of the cerebellum and fourth ventricle region that are of limited proliferative potential. They have a characteristic imaging pattern on MRI, with an abnormal laminated pattern in the cerebellum, although this pattern is not pathognomonic and can be mimicked by medulloblastoma. As such biopsy is recommended to differentiate the two entities.[667] Dysplastic cerebellar gangliocytomas do not typically require therapeutic intervention, although seizure activity can occur as a result of their presence.[668]

Disseminated Oligodendroglial-Like Leptomeningeal Tumor of Childhood. Disseminated oligodendroglial-like leptomeningeal tumor of childhood is a newly described entity that typically demonstrate leptomeningeal enhancement on MRI and associated cystic or nodular T2 hyperintense lesions within the spinal cord/brain along the subpial surface. A discrete intraparenchymal lesion, usually in the spinal cord, is found in the majority of cases. These tumors are thought to have a greater risk of malignant transformation.[669]

High-Grade Astrocytomas

High-grade astrocytomas (HGAs) encompass anaplastic astrocytoma (WHO grade III) and glioblastoma (previously glioblastoma multiforme, WHO grade IV) of the brain and spinal cord. This category also includes as a subgroup DIPG, even though these tumors occasionally show lower grade histology. HGAs, unlike LGGs, are much less common in children than adults. Whereas more than 30% of all pediatric brain tumors are LGGs, non-DIPG HGAs represent only 6% to 12% of all primary pediatric brain tumors, and DIPGs represent another 10%. In the past several years, many key discoveries have been made about the biology of these tumors, and increasingly, important distinctions from adult HGA biology are being found.[670] Unfortunately major treatment advances have not yet followed the biologic discoveries, and most children with these tumors eventually succumb to their disease. Because of key differences between DIPGs and other pediatric HGAs, most notably in prognosis and management, DIPG is discussed separately from the remainder of tumors in this category.

Supratentorial HGAs (Excluding DIPG). Although adult and pediatric HGAs are similar histologically, increasing evidence indicates key biologic differences, even within shared pathways of tumorigenesis. Common pathways include the overexpression or mutation of EGFR,[671] although both changes are less frequent in pediatrics,[672] activation of the PI3K signaling pathway via silencing of the PTEN tumor suppressor,[673-675] most often by methylation in pediatrics,[676] and the MGMT DNA repair pathway, which is commonly methylated in adult HGAs but is more often overexpressed in pediatric tumors,[677,678] perhaps helping to explain TMZ resistance in children with HGAs.[342]

Recent findings have also demonstrated involvement of new pathways and features of pediatric HGA, further distinguishing them from adult tumors. These new pathways include overexpression of PDGFRα[679,680] and novel histone mutations in *H3F3A* (observed in a minority of these tumors vs. a majority of DIPGs).[681,682] Comprehensive profiling of HGA genetics has shown gains in chromosome 1q in pediatric HGA on copy number analyses,[683,684] which is unusual in adults; fewer cases show chromosome 7 gain and 10q loss, two features seen in the majority of adult HGAs.[684] One study appeared to show two distinct gene expression profiles in pediatric HGA, one that is similar to adult HGA, and one that is divergent.[685] The PARP DNA repair pathway is also overexpressed in many pediatric HGAs,[686] and this feature is associated with a poor prognosis[687]; PARP inhibitors may be useful as radiosensitizers.[687] Aurora kinase B is overexpressed in a majority of pediatric HGAs.[688] Unlike in adults, *IDH1* mutations have not been found in pediatric HGAs.[689] Pediatric tumors have demonstrated abnormalities in the Ras and Akt pathways, as well as Y-box protein-1.[690,691] Microsatellite instability, which has been associated with a number of adult tumors, is very rare in pediatric HGAs.[692-694]

Overexpression of many proteins distinguish pediatric HGAs from LGGs, including the DNA repair protein insulin-like growth factor binding protein 2 (IGFBP2),[695] the cancer-testis antigen and possible immunotherapy target NY-ESO-1,[696] the p53 inhibitor HDMX,[697] the angiogenic marker endoglin,[698] and the catalytic subunit of human telomerase reverse transcriptase (HTERT)[699]; the differentiation marker NF1A is underexpressed in pediatric HGA compared with LGG.[700] In the CCG study of children with malignant HGGs (CCG945), p53

status was an important independent prognostic variable, with a 5-year PFS of 44% in tumors expressing a low level of p53 versus 17% in those overexpressing p53.[701] Finally new epigenetic findings in pediatric HGAs include hypermethylation of the LIM homeobox 9 (LHX9) transcription factor,[702] downregulation of class II and IV histone deacetylases (HDACs),[703] acetylation of histone H3.3,[703] and a decrease in adenosine deaminase, ribonucleic acid (RNA)-specific, 2 (ADAR2)–mediated RNA editing.[704]

Clinical Presentation. The clinical manifestations of HGAs depend on the anatomic location and the age of the patient. The clinical prodrome is usually short and rapidly evolving, with signs and symptoms of elevated ICP and focal neurologic deficits. A protracted course may evolve in the usual case of malignant transformation of a low-grade glioma,[705] but in general, transformation of low-grade gliomas to high-grade gliomas is extremely rare in children, unlike in adults. Dissemination of HGA into the cerebrospinal fluid is less common than for medulloblastoma and other neural tumors but is being recognized more frequently,[706] particularly as patients survive longer. Approximately 3% of pediatric patients with an HGA will have CNS metastatic disease at presentation.[707]

Imaging and Histology. Typical HGAs have an MRI appearance of heterogeneous enhancement or diffuse nonenhancing tumor with significant edema on the T1-weighted image, compressing or displacing adjacent ventricular structures and occasionally causing hydrocephalus. The T2-weighted signal is often more diffuse, consistent with both infiltrative tumor and edema (Fig. 57-29). MRS demonstrates a markedly elevated choline-to-NAA ratio; a 40% increase in choline over normal brain tissue indicates an HGA with 90% sensitivity and specificity. Lesions tend to be ^{18}F-labeled deoxyglucose–PET avid, although ^{18}F-fluoro-ethyl-tyrosine (FET)–PET may be superior for treatment planning and distinguishing between LGGs and HGAs.[708,709] Technetium 99m–sestamibi SPECT (MIBI SPECT) imaging can also detect

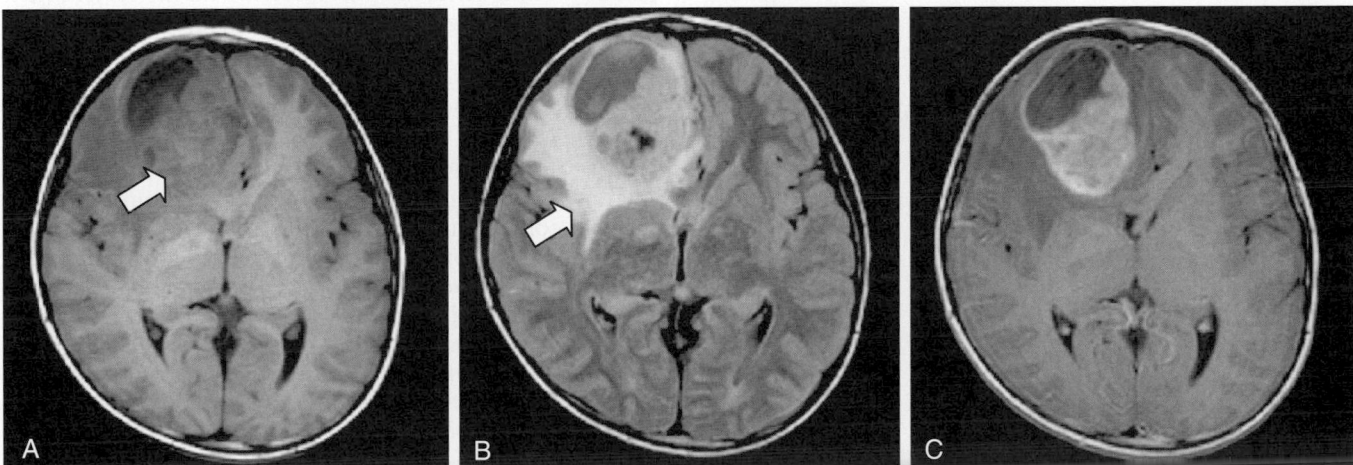

Figure 57-29 Right frontal glioblastoma. **A,** An axial T1-weighted image without use of contrast material showing the tumor *(arrow).* **B,** An axial fluid-attenuated inversion recovery image showing peritumoral edema and infiltrating tumor *(arrow).* **C,** An axial T1-weighted image with use of contrast material.

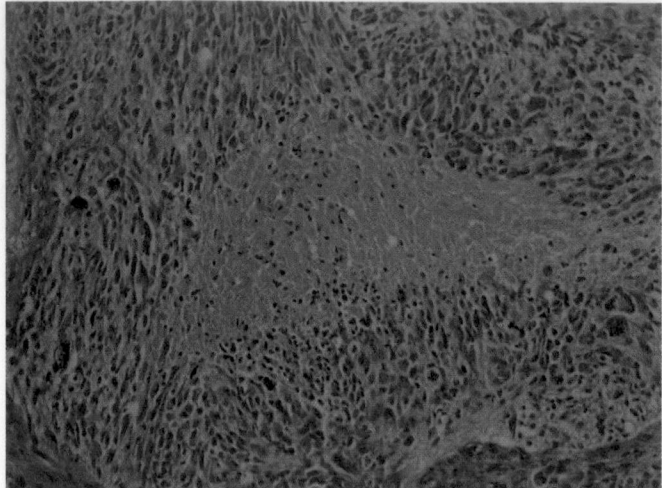

Figure 57-30 Palisading necrosis in a child with glioblastoma (hematoxylin and eosin; ×400).

HGAs and can be used to follow up for response or recurrence,[174] as can serial diffusion weighted assessment.[710] Areas of hemorrhage within pediatric HGAs at diagnosis are not uncommon.[711] The presence of an HGA within the volume of a previously irradiated field is difficult to differentiate from a radiation-induced high-grade transformation of a low-grade astrocytoma, although preliminary studies have identified some molecular differences distinguishing radiation-induced glioblastoma.[712] Malignant features on histopathologic examination of HGA include nuclear pleomorphism, mitoses, palisading necrosis (Fig. 57-30), endothelial proliferation (Fig. 57-31), and a high Ki-67 or MIB1 labeling index (see Fig. 57-17), although high interobserver variability exists between pathologists in judging these features.[713] Most pediatric HGAs are nestin-positive on immunohistochemistry.[714] Distinguishing between grade III and IV tumors relies on differences in histologic features; all HGAs must demonstrate nuclear atypia and mitoses, whereas grade IV

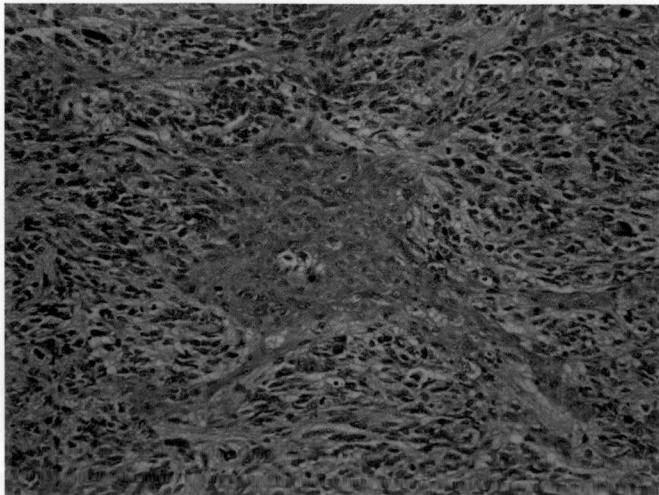

Figure 57-31 Vascular proliferation with a glomeruloid tuft in a child with glioblastoma (hematoxylin and eosin; ×400).

tumors must also show either endothelial proliferation, necrosis, or both. It has now been shown that a proportion of CD133+ HGA cells costain for CD105 (endoglin), an angiogenesis marker, suggesting that vasculogenic mimicry occurs in pediatric HGAs, which may help increase angiogenesis in HGA through the formation of fluid-conducting vessels of tumor cells. CD105 staining is an unfavorable prognostic marker.[698]

Management. The initial management of pediatric HGA after neuroimaging is to administer high-dose corticosteroids to achieve symptomatic relief. Subsequently the goals of neurosurgery include establishing a histologic diagnosis and, whenever possible, achieving GTR.[715] GTR is often not possible given the infiltrative properties of HGA, but even subtotal resection that achieves internal decompression or debulking makes subsequent radiotherapy more tolerable and probably more effective, given the lower tumor burden. Resection also diminishes the duration of corticosteroid therapy.[716] Intraoperative MRI appears to increase the likelihood of GTR.[717] The role of radiation therapy in the treatment of older children has been clearly established during the past 30 years,[718,719] and the current standard in patients 3 years of age and older is a conformal dose of 5400 cGy to the primary tumor volume with a boost to 5940 cGy in the tumor bed.

Ever since the first national randomized trial comparing radiation versus radiation with chemotherapy in pediatric HGAs (CCG-943) showed a survival benefit for patients treated with chemotherapy, the use of adjuvant chemotherapy has been standard in the treatment of pediatric HGAs.[720] However subsequent trials have failed to show a similar benefit, and the role of chemotherapy in the disease remains unclear. One area of recent focus has been the use of TMZ, which has become the standard of care in adult HGA. However a primary pediatric HGA phase II trial of concomitant TMZ and radiation therapy, followed by adjuvant TMZ, failed to show an improvement in overall or EFS compared with historic control subjects.[721] Other phase II trials of the mTOR inhibitor temsirolimus,[722] the VEGF inhibitor bevacizumab,[723] and TMZ in combination with the DNA repair inhibitor O6-benzylguanine,[338] all in recurrent or progressive pediatric HGA, also failed to meet their aims. Radiosensitizers, including inhaled carbogen, have also failed to show efficacy.[724] A strategy that has shown potentially more promise is multiagent chemotherapy, with or without ASCR. Multiagent, multicourse chemotherapy with radiation therapy improved survival over historic control subjects in patients with primary HGA who had undergone GTR.[725] Another trial of multiagent chemotherapy given over a long period showed promise in delaying radiation therapy for patients with HGA who were younger than 3 years, given the especially severe neurodevelopmental effects of radiation in this age group.[726] Treatment with high-dose chemotherapy and ASCR has also been attempted in this group.[727,728] The risk-benefit ratio is still under investigation,[729] with initial reports of a 23% overall response but a mortality rate of 16%.[730] A trial of high-dose thiotepa and carboplatin followed by ASCR produced one long-term survivor out of four children treated for recurrent or progressive HGA; remission at the time of treatment appeared to be a key positive prognostic factor in this trial, which also included children with high-grade nonastrocytic brain tumors.[507]

Clearly, further study of the role of chemotherapy in pediatric HGAs is needed, as are new strategies. A current COG trial is comparing three potential chemotherapy regimens (the HDAC inhibitor vorinostat, TMZ, and bevacizumab) to be given with radiation therapy, followed by maintenance chemotherapy with TMZ and bevacizumab. Recent phase I trials have used the EGFR inhibitor erlotinib[731] and a prolonged dosing schedule of TMZ.[732] An autologous dendritic cell–based vaccine has shown potential efficacy.[733] Oral valproic acid has shown some effect retrospectively and is well tolerated, making it an attractive potential additive agent for future trials.[734] New mouse models of pediatric HGA inspire hope for more effective preclinical testing that could help bring more novel treatments to clinical trials.[735,736]

Prognosis. The prognosis for children with HGA is poor but is better than for adults.[737-739] The degree of surgical resection is associated with better PFS.[740,741] Patients with anaplastic astrocytoma have a more favorable prognosis than those with glioblastoma.[742,743] A report from the CCG[740] showed that the 5-year PFS rates for anaplastic astrocytoma were 44% ± 11% and 22% ± 6% for children who underwent GTR versus other types of surgery, respectively. The 5-year PFS rates for glioblastoma were 26% + 9% and 4% ± 3% for children who underwent GTR versus other types of surgery, respectively. Patients younger than 3 years appear to have a survival advantage compared with older patients.[744] One study showed worse PFS for patients initially treated with dexamethasone, raising the question of whether tumor inflammation may be important to treatment.[745] Poor performance at diagnosis on the FMH health status scale correlates with a worse prognosis.[746] The size of the treating medical center has no effect on prognosis.[747] In terms of biologic markers, PTEN expression[748] and MGMT methylation[749] favorably affect survival, whereas p53,[701] endoglin,[698] and PARP[686] positivity are negative prognostic markers. MIB1 staining is usually elevated in pediatric HGA and correlates with grade and prognosis. Patients with MIB1 levels greater than 36% had a 5-year PFS of 11% compared with 33% in persons with MIB1 levels less than 18%.[742]

SPECIAL CASES. HGAs occur more commonly in persons with certain genetic syndromes. These syndromes include hereditary nonpolyposis colorectal carcinoma[104] and Li-Fraumeni syndrome, a dominantly inherited syndrome involving mutations of the p53 tumor suppressor protein.[750] *TP53* mutations are rare in sporadic pediatric CNS tumors lacking a typical family history.[751] HGAs may also arise in persons with NF-1, although low-grade lesions are far more common; in one large case series, HGAs developed in 0.5% of patients.[752]

Cases of de novo congenital HGAs have been observed at birth or within the first 3 months of life and show similarities in gene expression profiling compared with both pediatric and adult HGA.[753] Prognosis, however, appears to be far better. Long-term survival, occasionally even without treatment,[754] occurs in the majority of these patients and supports the unique characteristics of these otherwise fatal tumors.[738,755-759]

Thalamic gliomas can occur as high-grade or low-grade lesions.[516] Poor prognostic factors in these patients include a short interval of symptoms, poor early response to chemoradiotherapy, high-grade histology, and inability to resect the lesion.[515,760] For spinal HGA the median age of presentation is 4 years. Positive prognostic factors include age younger than 5 years, anaplastic astrocytoma histologic features, lack of hemorrhage, and GTR.[761] Multimodality treatment may have some effect.[762] Another rare subtype of pediatric glioblastoma is giant cell glioblastoma. Although time to progression in this variant may be slightly longer, overall prognosis is not significantly better than in other pediatric HGAs.[763]

Gliosarcomas are glioblastomas with a sarcomatous component that can affect children of any age but seem to be most frequent in infants and toddlers, as well as patients who have received prior radiation therapy. They most often present with increased ICP and are located in the cerebrum. Gliosarcoma also carries a poor prognosis.[764] Optic nerve gliomas show HGA features on pathologic examination in approximately 17% of patients. School-aged children are most often affected. The 5-year OS rate is approximately 20% with high-grade histologic features, apparently irrespective of treatment with radiation or surgery.[765]

Diffuse Intrinsic Pontine Gliomas

Tumors of the brainstem occur in approximately 10% of pediatric patients with CNS tumors. The majority of these tumors, approximately 80%, are classified as DIPG and are infiltrative, expansile lesions of the pons. Most of these tumors are anaplastic astrocytoma or glioblastoma on histopathologic examination, although grade II DIPG has been reported; the dismal prognosis is not affected by grade.[766,767] This diagnosis must be distinguished from other pediatric brainstem tumors[768] that are usually WHO grade I, well circumscribed as opposed to infiltrative, and carry a much improved prognosis. The median age at diagnosis of DIPG is 5 to 9 years, but these tumors may occur throughout childhood.

Lack of understanding of DIPG biology was a major roadblock in the past, mostly because researchers had minimal tissue to study because these tumors were rarely biopsied; the procedure was believed to be highly morbid. In addition many samples that were obtained were from areas at the periphery of the tumor and included normal cells and reactive gliosis. Even autopsy specimens were rare. However in more recent years, two major trends have emerged. First, researchers determined that obtaining DIPG tissue by autopsy was feasible, and provided an opportunity that families of these children generally greatly appreciated and did not regret.[769-772] This tissue, generally preirradiated, led to new DIPG culture lines[769] and biologic studies. Second, new neurosurgical techniques emerged, along with targeted therapies based on initial biologic studies,[773] that could be offered to families who consented to upfront biopsy so that patients' tumors could be tested for susceptible genetic changes.

With tissue available, studies of DIPG biology have emerged at a rapid pace. One theme across several studies is amplification of the region containing PDGFR alpha (PDGFRA),[684,774] and protein expression analysis has confirmed the importance of PDGFRA deregulation in DIPG.[684] Thirty-six percent of DIPG samples in another study had PDGFRA amplification, far more than in pediatric and adult HGA.[775] Another key finding has been the discovery of novel mutations in *H3F3A*, encoding histone H3.3, or histone cluster 1, H3b *(HIST1H3B)*, encoding histone H3.1.[776] These mutations were isolated by whole genome sequencing of DIPG samples. Of note, the *H3F3A* mutation was also found in 22% of nonbrainstem pediatric HGAs but was not found in adult HGAs. In a subsequent study in which investigators looked for these mutations in a targeted manner, it was found that the H3.3 mutation occurred in 71% of DIPGs.[681] Although the biologic consequences of this mutation are not yet clear, it does seem to correlate negatively with prognosis.

Other new findings have included overexpression of Aurora kinase B,[688] WEE1 G2 checkpoint kinase (WEE1),[777] B7-H3 (CD276),[778] and interleukin (IL)-13Rα2.[779] Common mutations have been found in TP53, PI3K catalytic subunit (PI3KCA),[780] and EGFR, which surprisingly showed expression of the vIII mutant in a majority of cases, although confirmation of this finding is needed.[781] Authors of one study suggested two biologic subgroups of DIPG, one driven by proangiogenic changes and one driven by PDGFRA amplification or mutation; this latter group seemed to have more deaths before 10 months from diagnosis.[782] Finally, with establishment of a plausible cell of origin that depends on the hedgehog pathway,[783] as well as development of new preclinical models including mouse intracranial xenograft models,[784,785] further understanding of the disease should be forthcoming.

Clinical Presentation. The clinical presentations of children with brainstem tumors appear to fall into two groups. Patients with fewer than 3 months of symptoms, multiple cranial neuropathies (unilateral or bilateral), long tract signs (e.g., Babinski sign, hyperreflexia, and weakness), and cerebellar signs (e.g., ataxia, dysmetria, and dysarthria) are likely to have DIPG. Symptomatic hydrocephalus is present in fewer than 10% of patients with DIPG at presentation. Although the pons is not typically associated with behavior changes, pathologic laughter or separation anxiety have been symptoms noted in persons with DIPG.[786] In contrast children with low-grade brainstem gliomas tend to manifest a more insidious history of isolated cranial nerve palsy or weakness, usually for longer than 3 months.

Imaging and Histology. The diagnosis of DIPG may be made on the basis of the classic MRI appearance of a diffusely expanded pons with encirclement of the basilar artery.[707] Most DIPGs appear to be hypointense on T1 weighted MRI and hyperintense on T2-weighted imaging. A prominent edema signal is common (Fig. 57-32). The ventral pons may appear swollen and infiltrated. Contrast enhancement is variable, from homogeneous rim enhancement to patchy enhancement to complete absence of enhancement. In contrast to DIPGs low-grade focal lesions of the brainstem present with a more circumscribed appearance and associated contrast enhancement that occupies less than 50% of the axial diameter of the brainstem. These tumors may be composed of cystic and solid components. Leptomeningeal dissemination at diagnosis and recurrence may be more common in DIPGs than previously understood,[788] and given the negative effect on prognosis, spine MRI at diagnosis should be considered. Diagnosis by imaging alone puts DIPG in a unique category, apart from nearly every other pediatric tumor, and some studies showing variability in reading of MRIs have called the practice into question.[789] Another study of MRI-biopsy correlation showed that all diffuse, nonenhancing tumors were DIPG pathologically, whereas the diagnosis was more variable with focal or enhancing tumors.[790]

New MRI techniques have been found to have specific roles in diagnosing DIPGs. DTI is helpful in differentiating DIPG from demyelinating disease when the diagnosis is in question.[791] Susceptibility-weighted imaging appears to be the best technique for detecting hemorrhages in DIPGs, which appear to be present in 47% of patients at diagnosis, although most hemorrhages are petechial and asymptomatic.[792] MRS has identified a specific spectrum consistent with the malignant potential of DIPG. More importantly this method can detect positive responses in patients after radiation therapy, as well as changes indicative of progression in advance of MRI changes.[793] The Cho:NAA ratio and lactate measurement on MRS appear to correlate with the length of survival.[794,795] Elevated tumor perfusion on MRI after radiation therapy appears to predict a longer OS, and perfusion has been shown to decrease prior to clinical progression.[796] Serial measurement and estimation of response may be best achieved with FLAIR imaging,[797] although no radiologic methodology is optimal for disease assessment or response. Time to progression or OS, rather than radiographic response, may therefore be the best determination of treatment activity in clinical trials for this population.[798] Ventriculomegaly without obstruction appears to be a common finding after radiation therapy in persons with DIPG, suggesting communicating hydrocephalus.[799]

The histologic appearance of DIPG is similar to that of other HGAs.[800] Most biopsy samples show evidence of atypia and mitoses and qualify as grade III anaplastic astrocytomas. Differentiation between anaplastic astrocytoma and glioblastoma in the pons is not relevant because all these patients appear to have an equally poor outcome.

Management. During the past 30 years, little progress has been made in the treatment of DIPG.[801] Radiation therapy has improved the median OS from weeks to months, but it can at best be considered palliative therapy. Despite many clinical trials, no chemotherapeutic agent has shown an improvement compared with radiation alone. Few patients survive more than 2 years.[802]

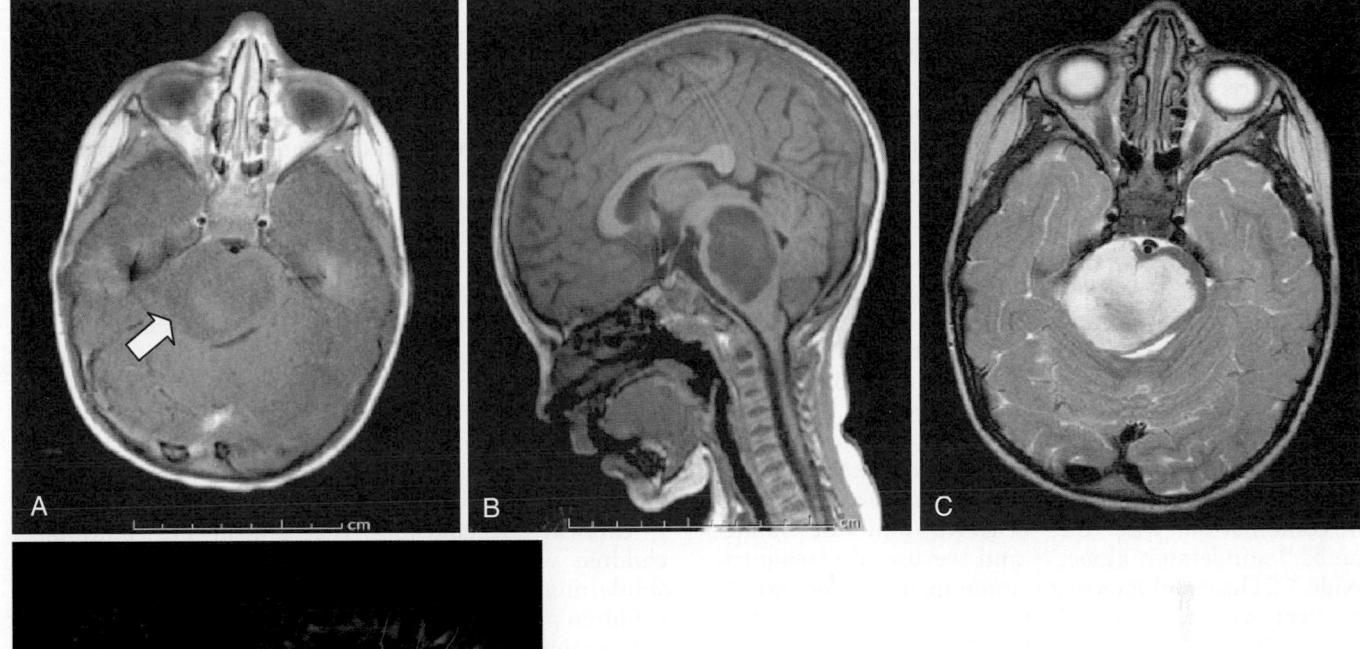

Figure 57-32 Diffuse intrinsic pontine glioma. **A,** An axial T1-weighted image with use of contrast material with minimal enhancement *(arrow)*. Note the tumor encroachment around the basilar artery. **B,** A sagittal T1-weighted image without use of contrast material. This is a large, diffusely expanding, low T1-weighted lesion of the pons with little encroachment into the midbrain or medulla. **C,** An axial T2-weighted image with little to no edema. **D,** Axial and sagittal diffusion tensor imaging showing posterior displacement of the corticospinal tract *(blue color* and *arrows)*.

Corticosteroids are generally started at the time of diagnosis, because peritumoral edema may contribute significantly to symptoms, and steroids may therefore offer some relief. Patients with DIPG often require steroids for a long duration, and investigation of agents that can offer relief from peritumoral edema without the adverse effects of steroids is ongoing.

The tide is clearly shifting toward diagnostic biopsy in patients with suspected DIPG. Several retrospective studies of open and stereotactic biopsy showed that the procedure is feasible and safe.[803-805] A prospective trial of 24 patients undergoing stereotactic biopsy showed that transient cranial nerve palsies in two children were the only complications, with tissue obtained in all patients, including two for whom the biopsy results changed the management approach.[806] A consensus statement in support of biopsy on behalf of a large group of DIPG experts has now been published.[807] The procedure still carries risk, however, and should be performed at experienced centers by experienced neurosurgeons. The ideal locations for stereotactic biopsy appear to be areas of focal anaplasia, represented by T2 hypointensity, contrast enhancement, and diffusion restriction.[808]

Radiation therapy remains the mainstay and standard treatment for DIPG. The tumor volume and a 1- to 2-cm volume of surrounding brainstem are generally included in the field, and conventional doses range from 5400 to 5940 cGy given over 6 weeks. This treatment is generally effective at decreasing tumor size, decreasing symptoms, and allowing patients to stop taking steroids, but these effects generally last only a matter of months, and the treatment is still considered palliative instead of curative. Multiple studies have attempted hyperfractionation techniques, ranging from 6600 to 7800 cGy, without improvement in survival[809-815]; this outcome may relate to the inherent resistance of these tumors.[816] More recently in an attempt to reduce the impact of the radiation therapy schedule for these children with a limited life span, hypofractionation schedules have been tested, usually 3900 to 4500 cGy over 3 to 4 weeks, with a noninferior response rate and duration.[817,818] Reirradiation is also the only therapy that has shown any potential efficacy at recurrence: two retrospective reports showed transient responses of some patients to reirradiation doses of 1800 to 2000 cGy, with children who had a prolonged duration of response from initial radiation therapy most likely to benefit.[819,820]

Many adjuvant chemotherapy agents and strategies have been tried and have failed to improve outcomes in patients with DIPG compared with radiation therapy alone. Many recent phase II trials have centered on the use of TMZ, given that this agent is now standard of care in adults with HGG. However three phase II trials of TMZ given with radiation therapy, followed by TMZ alone, have failed to show an increase in survival time compared with historic standards from radiation therapy alone,[721,821,822] and the addition of TMZ worsened toxicity. Other recent phase II trials have shown no benefit of tamoxifen,[823] pegylated interferon α-2b,[824] a regimen of cisplatin, etoposide, ifosfamide, vincristine, and valproate,[725] and inhaled carbogen as a radiosensitizer.[724] Other past failed agents and strategies have included preirradiation multiagent chemotherapy,[825,826] topotecan as a radiosensitizer,[827,828] etanidazole as a radiosensitizer,[829] chemotherapy concurrent with radiation therapy including thalidomide,[830] trofosfamide and etoposide,[831] carboplatin,[832] carboplatin and etoposide,[833] TMZ and cis-retinoic acid,[834] chemotherapy with BBB disruption,[835] intraarterial bevacizumab injection,[836] and a postradiation high-dose chemotherapy regimen.[837] New strategies that have been the subject of recent phase I reports include the use of the PDGFR inhibitor dasatinib in combination with the VEGFR2 inhibitor vandetanib,[838] vandetanib alone,[839] and the use of arsenic trioxide.[840] The development of nonhuman primate models of direct drug delivery into the brainstem opens another avenue for developing improved therapies for these tumors.[841,842]

Prognosis. DIPG remains the most challenging of pediatric tumors to cure. Despite all approaches most survival curves are superimposable with regard to OS.[843] Meta-analyses of numerous clinical reports indicate that median PFS ranges from 5 to 9 months, with a median OS of 6 to 16 months. One-year and 2-year survival ranges from 17% to 50% and 7% to 29%, respectively, with less than 10% survival at 3 years.[843,844] Neither MRI characteristics nor WHO grade has an impact on prognosis in persons with DIPG.[845] Poor performance at diagnosis on the FMH health status scale correlates with a worse prognosis.[746] The size of the treating medical center has no effect on prognosis.[747] One report indicated an improved prognosis for patients with DIPG who are younger than 3 years,[846] although questions of misclassification of patients with low-grade brainstem glioma as having DIPG inevitably arise with reports of improved survival—yet another reason for the use of diagnostic biopsy. Very few cases of neonatal DIPG have been reported, and outcomes in these reports have been inconsistent, ranging from spontaneous regression to death within weeks.[847-849] Retrospective studies have shown worse prognoses for patients initially treated with dexamethasone or rofecoxib, raising the question of whether tumor inflammation may be important to treatment.[745,850] Patients with leptomeningeal dissemination at diagnosis appear to have a shorter PFS than do patients who do not have this finding.[788] It is hoped that with time, the greatly improved understanding of DIPG biology and promising preclinical models will soon lead to successful clinical trials and an improved outlook for patients afflicted with this terrible disease.

Gliomatosis Cerebri

Although much more common in adults, gliomatosis cerebri has also been identified in children.[851] Similar to adults, in children these lesions are often grade III astrocytomas that diffusely infiltrate the brain and appear to favor white matter tracts,[852] and they can easily cross the corpus callosum. In spite of the widespread presence of disease, often involving both hemispheres and multiple lobes, a large primary focal mass is usually absent. All parts of the brain and spine can be involved. The overall prognosis is very poor by virtue of the disease's diffuse nature and unresectability.[853] Patients can be kept alive with palliative care for longer than would be expected for widely diffuse lesions, suggesting a different biology from that of typical grade III astrocytomas.[854] Genetic aberrations, including loss of chromosomes 13q and 10q or gains of chromosome 7q, have been shown to be markers of poor outcome.[855] Some tumors demonstrate abnormalities in the p53 pathway.[856,857] Recently IDH1 mutations have also been found in adult but not pediatric gliomatosis cerebri.[858]

Clinical Presentation. The clinical presentation of children with gliomatosis cerebri is varied and often subtle, mimicking a number of neurologic conditions.[859,860] Children present more frequently than adults with refractory seizures that can be palliated with surgical intervention.[861] Other presentations of this disease include raised ICP and cognitive impairment.[862] Tumors involving the brainstem can result in cranial nerve deficits, and those in the optic pathway can present with visual field deficits.

Imaging and Histology. Gliomatosis cerebri is diagnosed on MRI scan and demonstrates a characteristic diffuse infiltrative pattern.[863] T1-weighted sequences are usually isointense to hypointense and underestimate the extent of disease, whereas T2-weighted sequences are hyperintense and highlight the full extent of the disease (Fig. 57-33). Signal abnormality usually involves multiple lobes.[864] The presence of contrast enhancement is strongly correlated with a poorer prognosis in both adult and pediatric patients.[854,855] A solid area of tumor is usually not evident. MRS demonstrates elevation of choline and a decrease in NAA levels.[865] Although the hallmark of gliomatosis cerebri is an infiltrative astrocytic tumor, areas of oligodendroglial cells are not uncommon for adult and pediatric patients.[866,867] Most tumors are consistent with grade III histology, and mitoses are often present. MIB1 staining can vary considerably. The absence of mitoses is more likely to be because of sampling error. GFAP and S-100 can be positive or negative. Nestin and vimentin can be positive.[868] Because of their infiltrative growth and co-opting of existing blood vessels, these tumors lack the abundant neovascularization observed in other malignant gliomas,[869] which suggests that they will not be effectively treated with antiangiogenic agents.

Management. Currently patients with gliomatosis undergo biopsy to confirm the diagnosis. Given the diffuse nature of these tumors, complete resection is rarely feasible. The mainstay of therapy is irradiation to the involved region, which, for pediatric patients, may require almost complete whole-brain therapy. In addition to significant morbidity, large-volume radiation therapy for

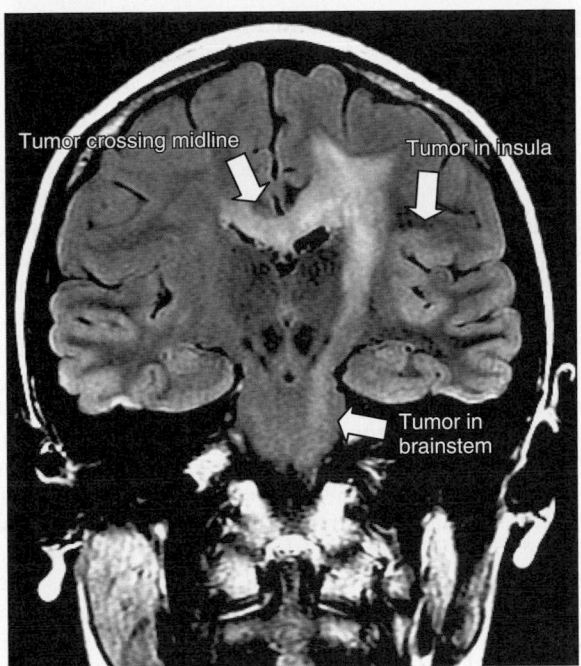

Figure 57-33 Gliomatosis cerebri. This coronal fluid-attenuated inversion recovery image demonstrates the diffuse infiltration. Note that a solid uniform mass is absent.

gliomatosis cerebri has not been proven to be effective,[867] although it may delay the time to progression.[870] Objective responses to TMZ have been documented in adults[871,872] and, in oligodendrogliomas, correlate with chromosome 1p and/or 19q loss.[873] The impact of MGMT expression on response and outcome has not yet been determined.

Prognosis. Pediatric patients with gliomatosis cerebri have a poor outcome.[853,854] In a large series of pediatric and adult patients, a median survival of 14.5 months was demonstrated. Younger age, lower grade histology, and chemoresponsiveness were associated with slightly longer survival times.[874] Although long-term survival is unlikely, adults whose tumors have chromosomal 1p and/or 19q loss can show more chemoresponsiveness to agents such as TMZ.[855] Similar activity in pediatric patients has not been reported because of the rarity of these tumors in this population.

Ependymomas

Ependymomas are glial tumors that arise from ependymal cells that line the ventricles in the CNS. Ependymal cells play an essential role in the transport of CSF. Experimental evidence has indicated that these cells may be derived from radial glia.[875,876] Ependymal tumors represent approximately 10% of all childhood intracranial neoplasms, constituting the third most common pediatric brain tumor, after astrocytomas and medulloblastoma. They are equally distributed between males and females, and the median age at diagnosis is approximately 6 years. They are significantly less common in blacks than whites.

Ninety percent of pediatric ependymomas are intracranial, with 66% to 75% arising from the posterior fossa.[877] Supratentorial ependymomas are often located in the brain parenchyma, away from the ependymal surface, in contrast to infratentorial ependymomas, which are usually located in relation to the fourth ventricle. Spinal cord ependymomas represent fewer than 10% of pediatric intramedullary spinal tumors. In contrast ependymomas represent more than 50% of intramedullary spinal tumors in adults.[878]

The WHO classification system[879] recognizes four major types: subependymoma and myxopapillary ependymoma (WHO grade I), classic ependymoma (WHO grade II), and anaplastic ependymoma (WHO grade III). Differentiation of grade II and grade III ependymoma does not clearly have an influence on outcome,[880] in contrast to the grade in astrocytic tumors. Subependymomas are well circumscribed, slow-growing, and often asymptomatic intraventricular neoplasms that are usually found incidentally in middle-aged and older adults or at autopsy. Myxopapillary ependymomas (WHO grade I) are also slow-growing tumors of the conus medullaris, cauda equina, and filum terminale and manifest primarily in young adults. They account for approximately 10% of all ependymomas and portend an overall good prognosis with surgery-only approaches.

Recent advances in molecular studies have found that ependymomas from different compartments of the brain and spine have unique molecular signatures with distinct patterns of gene expression,[881] chromosomal changes, and protein expression.[882] Deletion of tumor suppressor P16INK4A (located at chromosome 9p21.3) was frequently observed in supratentorial ependymoma. Witt et al[883] analyzed the transcriptome of 177 patients with posterior fossa ependymoma and proposed two distinct subtypes of posterior fossa ependymoma based on different clinical and molecular characteristics (i.e., age, tumor location, degree of genomic instability, alterations in molecular pathways, and prognosis). The "pediatric" subgroup (median age of 2.5 years), designated as group A in the study, showed relatively less genomic instability but commonly harbored chromosome 1q gain and 22q loss. A balanced genomic profile and chromosome 1q amplification have been previously described as two of three defining molecular features of posterior fossa ependymoma.[884,885] The older subgroup (median age of 20 years), designated as group B, exhibited a much higher degree of genomic instability and extensive cytogenetic aberrations. Interestingly a balanced genomic profile, seen in the pediatric subgroup, was paradoxically associated with a worse prognosis. Posterior fossa ependymomas in young children were much more likely to recur, metastasize, or result in mortality. Even accounting for whether GTR was achieved, group A tumors exhibited worse PFS and OS compared with group B (18% 5-year PFS and 52% OS in group A vs. 91% 5-year PFS and 100% OS in group B; $P < .0001$).[882,883] The identification of immune markers in these analyses may provide important opportunities for the development of immunotherapy-based treatments.[886] Chromosome 22q loss is commonly associated with spinal ependymoma in adults and children.[887,888]

The most consistent genetic defects in ependymoma are monosomy 22 or structural abnormalities of chromosome 22q,[889] which raises the possibility that a tumor suppressor gene may be located on chromosome 22.[890-892] As previously noted, comparative genomic hybridization has demonstrated significant differences between infant and childhood ependymoma, suggesting that the pathogenesis of this disease differs by age[893] and location.[894] A number of other molecular defects have been described in ependymomas, including the abnormal expression of ERBB2 and ERBB4 receptors,[895] defects in the p53 homologue p73,[896] increased expression of the VEGF protein,[897] Nestin expression,[898] PI3K activation,[899] immune targets such as EphA2, IL-13Rα2, and Survivin,[900] amplification or overexpression of the p53 regulator MDM2,[901] overexpression of cyclooxygenase-2 (COX-2),[902] the presence of telomerase activity,[903,904] and expression of protein 4.1.[905] Other molecules implicated in the pathogenesis of ependymoma have been reported by using micro RNAs[906] and proteomic fractionation of tumor tissue. Future studies will be required to determine the significance of these molecules and their potential use as diagnostic markers and targets for therapy.[306]

Significant progress has also been made in the use of these markers in attempting to understand and characterize the putative ependymoma stem cell[907,908] with expression of OLIG2.[909] The role of telomerase may also be an important factor in the recurrence of ependymomas,[910,911] and additional markers are being developed.[891,912] The advances in assessment of the epigenome of ependymoma have also recently been reported and give important clues about the role of DNA methylation in the genesis and possibly targets of ependymoma.[913-915] Finally, the presence of JC (John Cunningham) viral sequences identified in 5 of 18 ependymomas (but 0 of 32 medulloblastomas) raises the possibility that this agent is associated with ependymal tumorigenesis.[916] Simian virus 40 (SV40) viral, large, T-antigen sequences have also been identified in ependymomas and choroid plexus papillomas (CPPs)[917] but are negative in adjacent normal brain.[918] Although these results have generated significant discussion, they have not been confirmed.[919,920] Further studies will be needed to validate these findings.

In myxopapillary ependymoma, a WHO grade I ependymoma that is confined to the conus medullaris-cauda equina-filum terminale of spinal cord, upregulation of 20 members of the homeobox (HOX) family that are not typically observed in intracranial ependymoma has been described.[921] EGFR has also been identified in ependymomas of the brain[922] and myxopapillary ependymoma and correlates with progression.[923]

Persons with NF-2 have an increased susceptibility to intramedullary spinal cord ependymomas.[924] Although the NF2 gene is located at chromosome 22q12, mutations in NF2 (Merlin) are rarely found in sporadic ependymomas.[925,926] A recent microarray analysis of pediatric ependymomas has identified a cluster of genes distinct from NF2 that may be involved in ependymoma tumorigenesis.[891] Expression profiling has indicated that histologically similar ependymomas from different parts of the CNS are molecularly and clinically distinct disease subgroups.[875,927] Certain familial colon cancer syndromes may also be associated with an increased incidence of ependymoma in offspring.[928]

Clinical Presentation. The presenting symptoms of infratentorial ependymomas are a result of their origin from ependymal tissue lining the fourth ventricle. Hydrocephalus results when the tumor fills the fourth ventricle, causing obstruction of the normal spinal fluid flow and subsequent development of headache, irritability, nausea, vomiting, and ataxia. Papilledema can often be found on physical examination. Tumors that extend out of the foramen of Luschka may compromise lower cranial nerve function and cause hearing impairment, hoarseness, and/or dysphagia. If the tumor extends through the foramen of Magendie, the patient may report neck discomfort or be noted to have torticollis. The most common signs of the tumor in infants are irritability, decreased oral intake, vomiting, ataxia, head pain, lethargy, and increased head circumference.[929] Supratentorial ependymomas which represent approximately one third of ependymomas, are more common in older children and adults. These patients present with focal neurologic deficits and seizures. Spinal ependymomas are typically located in the cervical region. The most common presenting symptom is pain or motor deficits localized to the level of the spinal cord lesion. The pain is typically described as being worse at night, presumably because of congestion of the spinal venous plexus that occurs when the patient is in the recumbent position. The second most common symptom is radicular dysesthesias, and a late manifestation of this symptom is progressive spastic quadriparesis. Thoracic ependymomas are associated with scoliosis. Myxopapillary ependymomas of the conus medullaris and filum terminale may cause low back pain, radicular pain, saddle anesthesia, and sphincter dysfunction.[930] When these tumors disseminate, they usually remain in the spine,[931] although cranial metastases have been reported; therefore craniospinal imaging at diagnosis should be undertaken.[932] Pediatric myxopapillary ependymoma may have a higher propensity to spread compared with adult tumors.[932]

Imaging and Histology. A typical MRI appearance of a fourth ventricular ependymoma is that of a homogeneously enhancing well-circumscribed solid mass, extending out one of the foramina of Luschka or Magendie with obstructive hydrocephalus. These tumors classically wrap around the brainstem or herniate through the foramen magnum (Fig. 57-34). Hemorrhage and calcifications can be observed and are more common in supratentorial lesions. Ependymomas may occasionally spread via CSF, seeding the leptomeninges or ventricles, either at diagnosis or at recurrence.[933] Careful attention to staging of patients is therefore important.

The characteristic microscopic feature of a classic ependymoma is that of dense cellularity, intermixed with perivascular pseudorosettes consisting of tumor cells and surrounding a neoplastic blood vessel (Fig. 57-35). True ependymal rosettes representing abortive canals are relatively uncommon.[934] Histologically the anaplastic variant is recognized by the presence of mitoses, necrosis, and

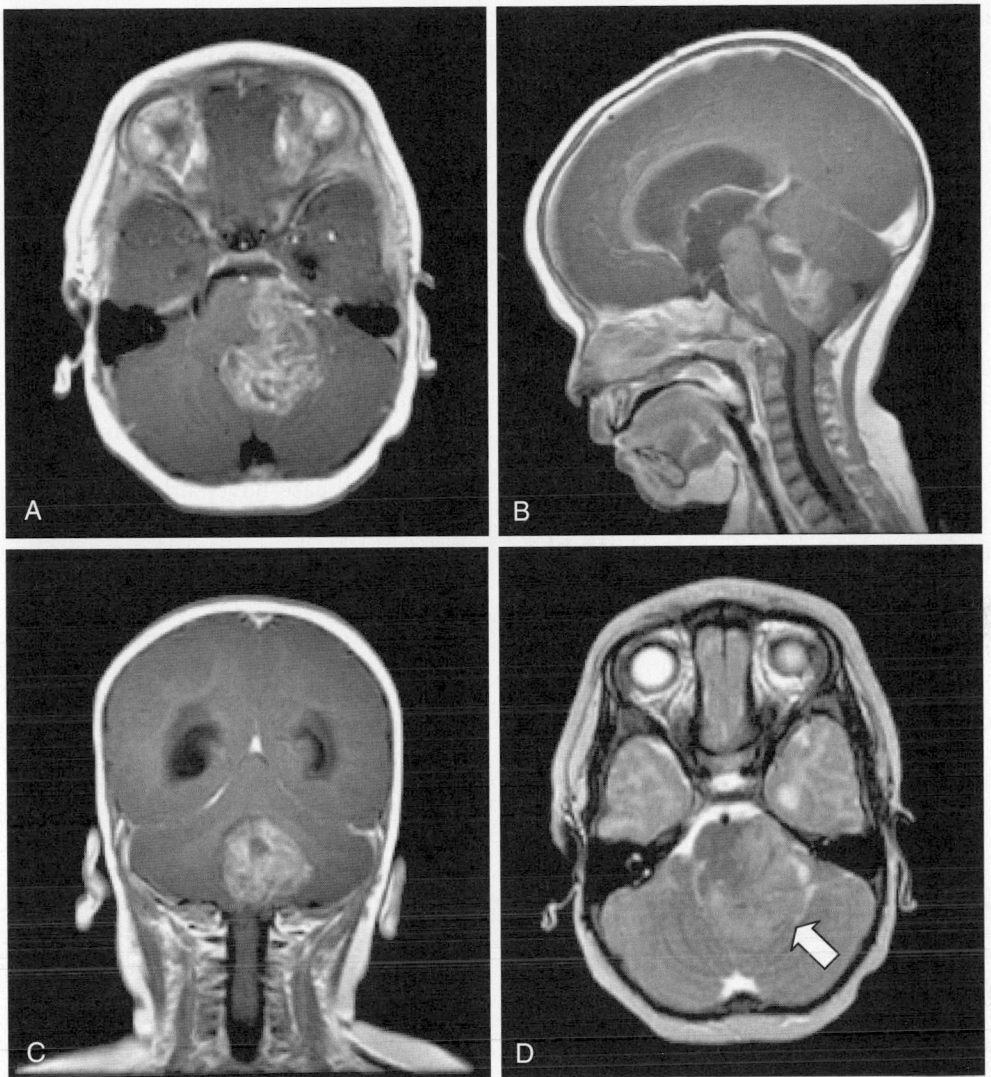

Figure 57-34 Posterior fossa ependymoma. **A,** An axial T1-weighted image with use of contrast material. **B,** A sagittal T1-weighted image with use of contrast material. **C,** A coronal T1-weighted image with use of contrast material. **D,** An axial T2-weighted image showing a T2 isodense lesion *(arrow)*.

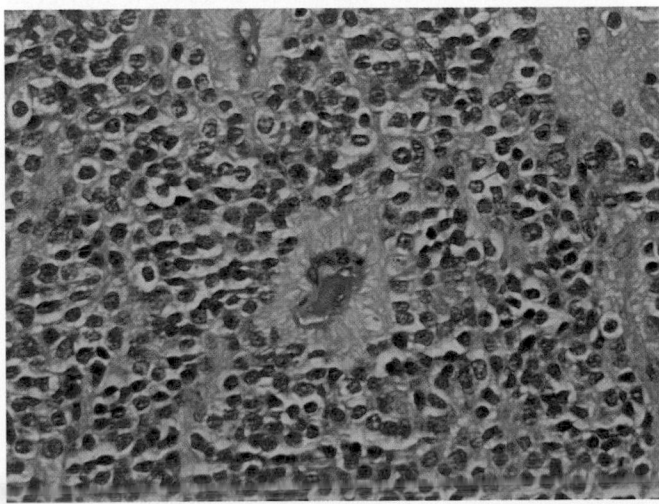

Figure 57-35 Ependymal pseudorosette (hematoxylin and eosin; ×600).

vascular proliferation. They tend to be more cellular than grade II ependymomas but usually remain well demarcated. MIB1 rates greater than 5% in incompletely resected tumors or greater than 15% in completely resected tumors correlate with more aggressive behavior.[935] GFAP and S-100 are positive in most ependymomas, and epithelial membrane antigen (EMA) stains are positive in anaplastic variants. The presence of perivascular elastic fibers may also be a diagnostic feature of these tumors.[936] In patients in whom the diagnosis of ependymoma is indeterminate, electron microscopic analysis of cilia structure and junctional complexes, which are found in most ependymomas, can be used to confirm or exclude the diagnosis. Myxopapillary ependymomas have a mucinous appearance and arise almost exclusively in the cauda equine.[930] Their MIB1 labeling index is typically low. Tanycytic ependymomas are a rare subtype of ependymoma that can occur throughout the brain or spine.[664,937] Other rare subtypes include cellular ependymoma, papillary ependymoma,[938] and clear cell ependymoma[939] variants.

Management. Evaluation of patients at diagnosis or recurrence should include an MRI of the brain and spinal cord, as well as cytologic evaluation of the CSF, usually performed at least 14 days after the operation.[940] Attempting CSF analysis during the surgery or shortly after could give false-positive results. The usefulness of CSF sampling in patients may not be particularly sensitive.[941,942] A number of factors have been associated with an unfavorable outcome, including younger age at diagnosis, subtotal resection, and a high MIB1 labeling index. Anaplastic histology remains controversial as a negative prognostic factor. Of these factors the single most important factor in the determination of prognosis appears to be whether a complete resection can be accomplished.[943]

The first line of treatment is surgery with the goal of GTR. If a complete resection with clear margins of a grade II spinal cord or supratentorial ependymoma can be achieved, adjuvant therapy can be deferred in some patients.[944] Technologic advances such as the operating microscope, Cavitron ultrasonic aspirator, intraoperative ultrasound, and intraoperative MRI, as well as electrophysiologic monitoring, have facilitated the safety of resections of intraaxial spinal cord tumors while reducing operative morbidity.[945] Overall, spinal cord ependymomas are more easily resectable than astrocytomas because of the presence of a better demarcated cleavage plane. Tumors with an infiltrative boundary, or those with anaplastic histology, require adjuvant therapy. All posterior fossa tumors, independent of grade and degree of resection, should also receive adjuvant treatment. Spinal myxopapillary ependymomas with a complete surgical resection have an excellent prognosis[946] and do not usually require adjuvant therapy even in the presence of drop metastases in the thecal sac.[947] Given the overall good prognosis of these tumors, the need for radiation in incompletely resected disease is unclear, and careful surveillance imaging is needed.[948] Early radiation therapy is not always routinely used but is recommended by some persons.[949,950]

Regarding radiation therapy, there is a long history of deferring radiation therapy for infants and young children who have posterior fossa ependymomas, with use of various conventional chemotherapy regimens instead. Previous treatment recommendations included radiation therapy for patients in whom gross resection was not achieved or for patients with recurrent disease. However partially resected tumors almost invariably recur, requiring further surgery, radiotherapy, and conventional chemotherapy. As such, in the United States the current strategy for ependymoma is to recommend deferral of adjuvant therapy in persons with completely resected supratentorial ependymoma, use of radiotherapy in the involved fields alone for completely resected posterior fossa ependymoma, and use of multiagent chemotherapy for subtotally resected ependymoma, followed by second-look surgery and involved field radiation therapy.[951-953] The benefit of hyperfractionation has not been established.[954] Wide-field pulsed reduced dose rate radiotherapy is currently being evaluated.[955] Craniospinal radiation therapy does not appear to be superior to focal radiation therapy.[877] Several studies have suggested that radiotherapy prolongs PFS after subtotal resection of an ependymoma. Deferral of radiation therapy after initial complete resection can result in reduced cure, even when complete resection is achieved a second time.[956] Proton radiation therapy appears to have equal efficacy when compared with photon therapy; it can reduce the potential long-term toxicity by decreasing the volume of normal brain tissue that is also targeted and is therefore recommended over photon therapy if it is available locally.[957,958]

Until recently there was no clear role for chemotherapy in the management of ependymomas outside of clinical trials.[959] Several small series in newly diagnosed and recurrent disease have shown objective responses to the following drugs: carboplatin, cisplatin, ifosfamide, and etoposide.[960] Chemotherapy is more often used for infants and younger children with incompletely resected or disseminated disease.[961-963] Encouraging results have been reported from the most recent cooperative group clinical trial involving preirradiation chemotherapy,[964] which showed a 40% complete response (CR) rate in patients who received preirradiation chemotherapy for residual postoperative tumor.[965,966] The two factors associated with a favorable outcome were the achievement of a complete resection and supratentorial disease. Chemotherapy should therefore be used to achieve a CR or improve the chances of a complete surgical resection at second-look surgery. It is not highly effective as sole treatment for this disease, and recurrences occur relatively rapidly in a significant percentage of patients if radiotherapy is not administered early. Infants may be more responsive, and 23% to 40% can be cured with chemotherapy alone.[967,968] The use of high-dose chemotherapy and stem cell rescue in infants with ependymoma has failed to demonstrate a significant advantage compared with standard modalities in most,[969] although not all, studies.[970] Although uncommon, up to 10% of patients can have leptomeningeal spread of ependymoma. Response to intrathecal liposomal cytarabine has been reported.[961]

Recurrences of intracranial ependymoma can occur throughout the first decade after initial therapy, although most recur within the first few years.[971] Surveillance scanning is important because it allows smaller asymptomatic tumors to be identified that may be more amenable to reresection. Most recurrences are within the original radiation field[972] and do not appear to be related to marginal failures.

Prognosis. The most important prognostic factors for intracranial and spinal cord[973] ependymoma are age, tumor grade,[974] extent of surgical resection, and delivery of radiation therapy with doses of at least 5400 cGy.[975-980] Children younger than 3 years, those with WHO grade III disease, or those with less than a GTR have been shown to have lower survival rates.[981] The 5-year PFS and OS for patients with subtotal versus total resection of posterior fossa ependymomas is 25% and 66%, respectively. The prognosis of patients with disseminated disease is worse.[539,976,982] Patients with a supratentorial nonanaplastic ependymoma can be treated with surgery only if the tumor can be completely resected. Recently a molecular assay for HTERT expression has been shown to predict the likelihood of progression and survival of pediatric intracranial ependymoma.[910] Additional studies on the molecular profile of ependymomas will likely lead to improved stratification and prognostication of patients as previously discussed.[891,912] Patients with an elevated MIB1 labeled index of more than 5% in incompletely resected ependymomas or of more than 15% in completely resected ependymomas were reported to have a worse prognosis in one study.[935] Patients with a deletion of 6q15.3 appear to have an improved outcome.[983] Molecular profiling has identified that the group A ependymomas (posterior fossa, infants) have a more aggressive biologic behavior and worse prognosis when compared with the group B ependymomas (supratentorial),[882] although this classification is not currently being used to guide therapy intensity at the present time.

Most patients with completely resected ependymoma followed by focal radiation therapy will be long-term survivors. Consideration of advanced radiation planning and the type of radiation delivered (i.e., proton vs. photon) are critical to minimize long-term neurocognitive morbidity in this population.[984]

At the time of recurrence, no standard salvage regimen has been proven to be effective.[985] Reoperation to achieve a complete resection has been curative in some patients and is typically the first modality considered[986]; this approach can be combined with reirradiation.[987,988] SRS has also been used with some success for focal recurrences of ependymoma.[989,990] Patients with metastatic disease or infiltration into the brainstem or other critical structures have a poor salvage rate, presumably because of the lack of good therapies for recurrent disease and the inoperable nature of the lesions. Oral etoposide alone[991] or in combination as a metronomic therapy combination has demonstrated responses in this disease.[341,335] Bevacizumab in combination with irinotecan did not show any significant activity.[992] A single case report of a response to the mTOR inhibitor sirolimus has also been published.[993]

Recurrence of myxopapillary ependymoma can occur after complete resection and can be associated with dissemination. Although cranial metastases have been reported, most cases result in regional metastases of the spine but not beyond the foramen magnum.[994] Many of these patients can undergo salvage therapy with radiation. Consequently frequent surveillance scanning of patients with myxopapillary ependymoma is recommended to identify recurrent disease early.

Oligodendrogliomas

Oligodendrogliomas are rare brain tumors in children, representing fewer than 1% of all pediatric brain tumors.[995,996] The mean age at diagnosis is approximately 10 to 13 years, with a male predominance.[997,998] The WHO grading system recognizes two grades for oligodendroglial tumors: well-differentiated grade II oligoden-

droglioma and grade III anaplastic oligodendroglioma.[999] As with other glial tumors, higher grade is a predictor of decreased OS. Other reported markers in oligodendrogliomas include deletions of the cyclin-dependent kinase inhibitor 2A (CDKN2A) gene on chromosome 9p, mutations in TP53 and PTEN, and amplification of the EGFR.[1000,1001] However it is not known whether these factors are predictive of outcome in pediatric patients. Unlike adult tumors, pediatric oligodendrogliomas do not typically have the chromosome 1p or 19q deletions or mutations in TP53 or IDH1.[382]

Clinical Presentation. Oligodendrogliomas are diffusely infiltrating tumors that tend to occur in the white matter of the cerebral hemispheres. Patients frequently present with seizures, although higher-grade tumors may present with evidence of increased ICP because of more rapid growth.[1002] Other symptoms at presentation can include headache, visual field defect, paresis, and cranial nerve palsy.[998] Although uncommon, oligodendrogliomas can also occur throughout other areas of the brain, including the posterior fossa, brainstem, and spine.[1003-1007]

Imaging and Histology. MRI evaluation of oligodendrogliomas typically reveals increased T2-weighted signal and decreased T1-weighted signal.[1002] Gadolinium contrast enhancement is more common in tumors that grow as solid masses and less common in purely infiltrative tumors. Contrast enhancement is also more common in grade III than in grade II oligodendrogliomas.[1008] Although oligodendrogliomas bear morphologic similarity to oligodendrocytes, the cellular origin of these tumors has remained difficult to prove. Histologic examination of fixed specimens of oligodendrogliomas reveals a monotonous pattern of cells with round nuclei and clear perinuclear halos (a "fried egg" appearance). This appearance is an artifact of formalin fixation and is not seen in frozen sections or tumor smears. Higher-grade anaplastic oligodendrogliomas (WHO grade III) are characterized by increased nuclear variability, increased mitotic activity, and/or microvascular proliferation. These features can occur diffusely throughout the tumor or in discrete foci. The differentiation between oligodendrogliomas and other diffuse gliomas such as astrocytomas and OAs is difficult because of a lack of reliable molecular markers that distinguish oligodendroglial tumors from astrocytic tumors. Mature oligodendrocyte-specific markers such as myelin basic protein, 2'3'–cyclic-nucleotide 3'-phosphodiesterase, and myelin-associated glycoprotein are not expressed in oligodendrogliomas, although astrocytic markers such as GFAP and S-100β are expressed in both astrocytomas and oligodendrogliomas.[999] More recently the lineage markers OLIG1 and OLIG2 have been evaluated in the hope that they may enable specific identification of oligodendroglial tumors.[1009] However despite the restriction of OLIG2 expression to normal oligodendrocytes and their precursors, OLIG2 stains all diffuse gliomas and precludes specific immunohistochemical classification of these tumors.[1010] The loss of chromosome 1p and/or 19q is commonly seen in adult oligodendrogliomas and correlates strongly with chemotherapy responsiveness and outcome.[1011] Pediatric oligodendrogliomas have a much lower incidence of chromosomes 1p and/or 19q deletions.[1012,1013] Even in children in whom these deletions are identified, the greater chemoresponsiveness observed in adults is less evident.

Management. Treatment of pediatric oligodendrogliomas, like other glial tumors, involves surgical resection, radiation therapy, and chemotherapy. The goal of surgery is to facilitate accurate diagnosis and to remove as much of the tumor as safely possible. In the adult literature, there is uncertainty as to whether the extent of resection correlates with OS. Although some larger case series have shown no prognostic value in the extent of resection,[1011] most evidence seems to indicate that the extent of resection may be associated with better prognosis.[1014,1015] In pediatric patients, it appears that the extent of resection is a sensitive predictor of outcome.[547] Fewer pediatric low-grade oligodendroglial tumors progress to high-grade tumors, so it is possible that patients with subtotally resected tumors may still have a good outcome. For example in one series of 20 patients with oligodendrogliomas treated with surgery only, 70% remained progression-free at a median of 5 years.[1016]

Despite the fact that oligodendroglial tumors are radiosensitive,[1017] the use of adjuvant radiation therapy in asymptomatic children with incompletely resected oligodendrogliomas is not favored because of the well-described late effects of radiation therapy.[425] Children who are symptomatic, who have tumors in critical locations such as the brainstem, or who have progressive disease despite resection and/or chemotherapy may benefit from radiotherapy.[466] However it is now clear that a subset of these children can be effectively treated with chemotherapy, allowing for a delay in, or avoidance of, radiation therapy.[1018] The combination of carboplatin and vincristine chemotherapy has demonstrated activity in various low-grade astrocytomas, regardless of histologic subtype. This therapy should therefore be considered for patients with oligodendroglioma.[433] Older children may also benefit from chemotherapy.[459] Based on overlapping activity in children with low-grade astrocytomas, the combination of TPCV might also be of use in patients who do not respond to or have disease progression after vincristine and carboplatin therapy. The combination of procarbazine, lomustine, and vincristine or TMZ monotherapy could also be considered based on the responses seen in adults, but these treatments have not yet been adequately tested in children.[492,1019,1020]

In patients with anaplastic oligodendroglioma or progressive disease, despite surgery and adjuvant chemotherapy, the risks of radiation therapy may be offset by the risk of further tumor growth. A recent survey of adult neurooncologists has found that the most commonly recommended treatment for anaplastic oligodendroglioma is the use of concurrent TMZ and radiotherapy followed by adjuvant TMZ.[1021] In rare cases of dissemination, the overall prognosis for these patients is poor, although transient chemotherapy responsiveness can be achieved.[1022] Patients with oligodendroglial gliomatosis cerebri have a very poor prognosis.

Prognosis. Overall long-term survival from low-grade oligodendrogliomas appears comparable with that of other LGGs.[1023] It should be noted, however, that only limited numbers of case series are available, making comparisons among studies difficult. Bowers and colleagues[1016] have reported an OS of at least 5.5 years in a series of 20 patients with low-grade oligodendrogliomas treated initially with surgical resection alone. Six of 20 patients in this series had disease progression at a median of 2.2 years after initial resection. Other studies have reported 5-year OS rates of 65% to 84.4%,[997,998] although the proportion of patients treated with radiation therapy and/or chemotherapy differed among these studies. Children younger than 3 years and children with incompletely resected tumors may do worse.[1024] The rarity of anaplastic oligodendroglioma in children makes specific estimates of survival in pediatric patients difficult. Oligodendrogliomas that are more centrally located do not appear to do as well as those located more peripherally in the cortex.[997]

A number of studies from adult patients have indicated that allelic losses at chromosomes 1p and 19q, typically involving the entire chromosomal arm at both sites, correlate with histologic classification, response to treatment, and prognosis.[1025] Loss at chromosome 1p is a predictor of chemosensitivity, and loss at combined chromosomes 1p and 19q is associated with both chemosensitivity and longer recurrence-free survival.[1026] Recent evidence has indicated that loss at chromosomes 1p and 19q is associated with MGMT promoter methylation and lower expression of MGMT.[1027] Interestingly these chromosomal features appear to be less common in pediatric oligodendrogliomas.[1011,1012] One study has reported the lack of allelic loss in children younger than 9 years, although a modest number of tumors from children older than 9 years had losses of chromosome 1p (45%) and/or 19q (27%).[1013] Nevertheless the incidence of chromosomal losses is significantly less than that seen in adults (50% to 90%). Taken together these studies suggest that the oncogenesis of these tumors is distinct from their adult counterparts.

Oligoastrocytomas

OAs are tumors containing a mixture of two distinct neoplastic cell types that morphologically resemble the tumor cells of oligodendrogliomas and diffuse astrocytomas. These tumors correspond histologically to WHO grade II. The demography of OAs and anaplastic OAs (WHO grade III) is difficult to ascertain because of a high variability in the histopathologic criteria used for classification of these tumors. Clinically these tumors present with signs and symptoms similar to those of astrocytomas and oligodendrogliomas. Tumors arise most frequently in the cerebral hemispheres and lack any neuroradiologic features that would facilitate distinguishing them from oligodendrocytomas. Histologic diagnosis requires the recognition of the two different glial components, both of which must be neoplastic.[1028] Anaplastic OAs are WHO grade III oligoastrocytomas with histologic features of malignancy, including high cellularity, high mitotic activity, and increased nuclear atypia and pleomorphism. Currently treatment for OAs and anaplastic OAs is similar to that for other grade II and III glial lesions—surgical resection with adjuvant chemotherapy and/or radiation therapy for higher grade or progressive lesions.

Embryonal Tumors

Embryonal tumors represent a large and important fraction of pediatric brain tumors, both for their clinical impact and the importance of the scientific insights gained through their study. The most common embryonal tumors include medulloblastoma, pineoblastomas, and CNS PNETs. A number of other tumors are grouped into this category, such as ATRTs, ependymoblastomas, and medulloepitheliomas (see Table 57-6). Recent advances in gene expression array technologies have facilitated a new understanding of the molecular features of tumors within this set of diseases.[1029] The grouping of these tumors into the larger category of CNS PNETs will continue to evolve while a better understanding of their origin progresses. Currently all these tumors share a common property: high risk of dissemination and therefore the need to treat the entire craniospinal axis. It is expected that new technologies will soon allow for a better understanding of the cell of origin of the different tumor types. These considerations are no longer intellectual exercises. Gene-based classification systems may

be the key to improved stratification and management and will likely augment, if not replace, the current histopathology-based classification system that underlies current treatment protocols.

The history of small round blue cell tumors is a fascinating story that spans the evolving approach to cancer during the past century. Histopathology was, and remains, the cornerstone of all classification schemas. Tumors from different sites that appeared the same under microscopic examination were assumed to be similar tumors arising from different organs. With the introduction of immunohistochemical techniques of pathologic specimens, pathologists began to define important differences among populations. Small round blue cell tumors within the body were now divided into unique categories based on the presumed cell of origin. Tumors such as lymphoma, neuroblastoma, Ewing sarcoma, rhabdomyosarcoma, and others became easily differentiated. The classification of small round blue cell tumors of the brain, by contrast, took a different direction. Medulloblastoma, a small round blue cell tumor of the cerebellum, was previously differentiated from other similarly appearing tumors based on its location within the posterior fossa,[1030] but some investigators thought that this arbitrary separation was unwarranted. Hart and Earle[1031] attempted to classify all embryonal tumors based on the expanding array of immunohistochemical markers and variations in the patterns of staining among these tumors. Rather than clarifying the classification of embryonal tumors, further blurring of the understanding of these tumors resulted. One contributing factor involved differing definitions for the grouping of embryonal tumors. For some investigators, medulloblastoma was considered a PNET and thus was lumped with pineoblastomas and sPNETs, whereas for other investigators, medulloblastoma remained a separate category. Another factor was the considerable variability in the quality of the staining pattern and heterogeneity within different areas of a single tumor and within different tumors of the same type. With advances in molecular pathology, classification has moved away from the simple microscopic appearance of a tumor to one that incorporates the pathways active in the tumor. Molecular signatures for these different tumors have been demonstrated; these signatures have shown that the tumors arise from different cell populations and, as a result, these tumors will likely require different treatments. Many prior treatment protocols grouped all these heterogeneous tumors together, which has confounded the true efficacy of the therapy under consideration and the prognoses for this heterogeneous group of tumors.

Medulloblastomas

Medulloblastomas represent approximately 15% of all pediatric brain tumors and approximately one third of posterior fossa tumors.[1032,1033] In addition medulloblastoma accounts for more than 50% of pediatric embryonal intracranial tumors. The incidence in males is twice that of females, and the median age at diagnosis is 5 to 7 years, with most cases diagnosed in the first decade of life.[1034] The current standard of care for children diagnosed with medulloblastoma involves maximal surgical

TABLE 57-6 Classification of Embryonal Tumors

Tumor Location	Histologic Classification	Histologic Subtype
Fourth ventricle	Medulloblastoma	Classic or nondesmoplastic Desmoplastic Anaplastic Large cell Melanotic
	Cerebellar neuroblastoma*	
	Atypical teratoid-rhabdoid tumor	
Pineal	Pineocytoma Pineoblastoma Atypical teratoid-rhabdoid tumor	
Supratentorial or intratentorial	Primitive neuroectodermal tumor* Cerebral neuroblastoma Atypical teratoid-rhabdoid tumor Ependymoblastoma†	

*The nomenclature for neuroblastoma and primitive neuroectodermal tumor (PNET) in the central nervous system results from the historic grouping of these tumors with other small round blue cell tumors of the body. Primary cerebral or cerebellar neuroblastoma are unrelated to similarly named tumors in the body and do not possess the abnormalities in the N-Myc pathway. Similarly central nervous system PNET is unrelated to Ewing sarcoma PNET and does not possess the classic chromosome 11;22 translocation.

†Ependymoblastomas were previously grouped with ependymomas but are now differentiated from this group as a result of their embryologic development and patterns of spread.

resection and adjuvant therapy with radiotherapy and chemotherapy. Radiation therapy involves a boost to the tumor site with craniospinal prophylaxis. Chemotherapy is administered both concurrently with radiation therapy and as multiagent maintenance chemotherapy after the completion of radiation therapy. Approximately 80% of children with medulloblastoma are cured,[1035] but current treatment strategies result in significant long-term morbidity.

With recent advances in transcriptome and genomic profiling of medulloblastoma, it has become apparent that medulloblastoma encompasses a heterogenous group of tumors with distinct pathologic features and clinical outcomes.[1036-1039] These findings represent exciting prospects for the development of novel tumor-directed therapies and treatment strategies that are stratified according to the genetic profiles of the individual medulloblastoma.

Different subtypes of medulloblastoma are thought to originate from distinct germinal zones within the cerebellum—the EGL, which contains committed granule cell precursors, and the ventricular zone, which contains multipotent stem cells that give rise to most cerebellar neurons. Several cancer predisposition syndromes carry an increased risk of medulloblastoma, including nevoid basal cell carcinoma syndrome or Gorlin syndrome, Turcot syndrome, and Li-Fraumeni syndrome.[1040-1042] Gorlin syndrome, although rare, is an important factor that must be considered in the treatment of these patients, because they are at high risk for the development of nevoid basal cell carcinoma, especially within the involved radiation fields.[1043] In addition Gorlin syndrome provided the first clues as to potential pathways that may be involved in the pathogenesis of medulloblastoma, with the finding of mutations in SHH pathway members, such as *PTCH1*, increase the risk of tumorigenesis.[1044]

Recent cooperative studies have comprehensively profiled the biology of medulloblastoma to reveal four distinct subgroups of tumors.[1036-1039] The groups are distinguishable from each other on the basis of gene expression, methylation, copy number, and mutation profiles.[1045-1049] These groups have been designated as Wnt-positive medulloblastoma, SHH-positive medulloblastoma, and group 3 and group 4 medulloblastoma.[1037] Wnt-positive medulloblastomas are characterized by mutations of β-catenin, resulting in activation of Wnt pathway signaling. Children with Wnt-positive medulloblastoma rarely have metastatic disease and have an excellent overall prognosis. The SHH group is characterized by tumors that carry mutations of the SHH pathway, with resultant pathway activation. The types of SHH pathway mutations differ between infants, children, and adults and may affect the use of targeted therapies for this group.[1050] These tumors can encompass multiple histologic subtypes, although nodular desmoplastic medulloblastomas are more likely to carry SHH pathway mutations. Group 3 medulloblastomas carry a poor prognosis and are largely characterized by amplification of *MYC* or amplification/overexpression of the *OTX2* oncogene. Group 4 medulloblastomas carry an intermediate prognosis and are likely to have isochrome of 17q, and gene expression studies show enrichment of genes

involved in neuronal differentiation and development. *TP53* mutations have been described to be enriched in the SHH subgroup of medulloblastoma, and when present, they are associated with inferior responses to therapy.[1051] Profiling studies of recurrent medulloblastomas have revealed that the subgroup determinations are stable, with recurrent tumors maintaining the same subgroup profile as they were at diagnosis.[1052]

In addition to the driver genomic alterations identified in medulloblastoma, evidence is growing that epigenetic dysregulation may play a role in the pathogenesis of these tumors.[1045] This belief is supported by the observation of enrichment in genomic alterations of chromatin modifiers in large-scale profiling projects for medulloblastoma.[1049,1053,1054] These alterations include inactivating mutations of the histone methyltransferase genes MLL2 and MLL3,[1055] *KDM1A* a histone demethylase[1056] and *SMARCA4*, a member of the SWI/SNF chromatin remodeling complex.[1053,1057] Mutations and aberrant hypermethylation of the telomerase reverse transcriptase (TERT) promoter have also been recently described in large-scale sequencing projects of medulloblastoma.[1058] Mutations in TERT promoters have been found to be particularly enriched in the SHH subtype of medulloblastoma.[1059] In addition altered expression of genes regulated by the polycomb repressor complex have also been described in medulloblastoma.[1060,1061] Alterations in chromatin modifiers have been described in medulloblastoma, and novel agents that target chromatin modification are being investigated as potential therapeutic for medulloblastoma. These agents include drugs that suppress expression of the MYC isoforms by inhibiting bromodomain containing 4 (BRD4), a bromodomain and extraterminal (BET)–containing protein,[1062] and inhibitors of enhancer of zeste 2 (EZH2).[1060]

Alterations in genes involved in cell cycle regulation have also been described in medulloblastoma.[1049] These alterations include amplification of cyclin-dependent kinase (CDK)/cyclin D genes[1063] and loss of the cell cycle inhibitor p27Kip1.[1063] Inhibition of *CDK6* has been shown to reduce cell proliferation in medulloblastoma cell lines,[1059] and small molecule CDK inhibitors may have a potential therapeutic role in this disease. In addition strategies that target G2-M regulators have also been investigated in model systems of SHH medulloblastoma using Aurora and Polo-like kinase inhibitors.[1064,1065]

No specific single environmental factor has been demonstrated to be associated with the development of medulloblastoma, although the nonrandom occurrence of disease detected in children born in the fall raises the possibility that some environmental or infectious pathogen may be implicated.[47] The association between the development of medulloblastoma and viruses remains controversial. Multiple reports implicating polyomaviruses (including JC[1066] and SV40[1067,1068] virus in animal models) as a causative agent in medulloblastoma have been published. Human medulloblastoma samples have been found to possess JC and SV40 viral sequences.[918,1069,1070] However independent confirmation of JC and SV40 sequences in human tumors could not be duplicated.[51,920] Prematurity was identified as a significant risk factor in one study.[1071] Whites are affected 42% more often than blacks.[1072] In contrast several genetic syndromes (e.g., nevoid basal cell carcinoma syndrome or Gorlin syndrome, Turcot syndrome, and Li-Fraumeni syndrome) are associated with a significantly increased risk for the development of medulloblastoma.[1040-1042] Gorlin syndrome, although rare, is an important factor that must be considered in the treatment of these patients, because they are at high risk for the development of nevoid basal cell carcinoma, especially within the involved radiation fields. Children of African-American descent require especially careful skin evaluation for the early detection of these lesions.[1043]

Clinical Presentation

Many of the clinical manifestations of medulloblastoma are similar to those of other tumors that arise in the fourth ventricular region and are related to obstructive hydrocephalus. Headache, nausea, and vomiting, characteristically in the morning, are the most common initial symptoms and usually precede diagnosis by 4 to 8 weeks, although longer intervals are not uncommon, especially if the headaches and vomiting caused by obstructive hydrocephalus are intermittent.[1073] Interestingly it appears that the duration of presenting symptoms may correlate inversely with disease state at the time of presentation; patients with low-stage disease were shown in one series to have a longer median duration of symptoms than were patients with high-stage disease.[1074-1076] Personality changes (irritability) are an early feature but may be difficult to recognize as a sign of a brain tumor. Other features that can lead to diagnosis include lethargy, diplopia, head tilt, and truncal ataxia. The common signs found on physical examination are papilledema, ataxia, dysmetria, and cranial nerve involvement. Abducens nerve (cranial nerve VI) palsy as a result of raised ICP may cause diplopia and head tilt. Torticollis can be a sign of cerebellar tonsil herniation. Less commonly, intratumoral hemorrhage may lead to acute onset of confusion, headache, and loss of consciousness. The presentation in infants may include an abnormal rate of increase in head circumference. Other presenting symptoms can include loss of previously achieved milestones and failure to thrive. With regard to metastatic disease, at the time of diagnosis, although lumbar CSF analysis or MRI-visualized leptomeningeal metastases occur in 20% to 30% of children with medulloblastoma,[1077,1078] clinical manifestations of metastases are uncommon. Back pain and radicular pain may indicate the rare complication of spinal canal dissemination. Attention to the clinical manifestation of posterior fossa tumors is important because the presenting signs mimic many other common ailments in children, including viral infections and stress. Because tumors have a significant propensity to metastasize early, careful evaluation of associated neurologic signs (e.g., papilledema and diplopia) can help identify children in need of referral for imaging sooner.

Imaging and Histology

Most medulloblastomas arise in the cerebellar vermis and extend into the fourth ventricle, resulting in obstructive hydrocephalus. The remainder are localized to the cerebellar hemisphere, especially in older patients and those with the desmoplastic subtype.[1079] The signs and symptoms of obstructive hydrocephalus, such as severe headache, morning vomiting, long tract signs, and papilledema, can be a medical emergency and require immediate evaluation. CT scanning of the head or rapid sequence MRI is the immediate choice of imaging to rule out an obstructive mass. This rapid study provides good differentiation between the fluid cavities and brain and will be sufficient to allow the neurosurgeon to determine whether immediate action is required. Often CSF diversion can be avoided if tumor resection is immediately possible. When required third ventriculostomy is preferred to VP shunts. All patients will require high-quality MRI scans of the brain and spine, including the entire thecal sac at the base of the spine. Lumbar puncture for CSF cytologic examination in newly diagnosed patients should be deferred if any possibility of elevated ICP exists; lumbar puncture is usually better performed after the tumor has been resected and CSF flow has been restored.

The MRI findings may differentiate between medulloblastoma types,[1080] as well as from other cerebellar tumors, such as ependymoma and pilocytic astrocytoma, and may be helpful before surgical resection.[1081] However atypical appearances of these three tumors can also occur, and thus a diagnosis based solely on imaging characteristics currently is not feasible. The appearance of a vermian location, hypercellularity (often demonstrated as dark areas of tumor on T2-weighted imaging), and intratumoral hemorrhage is more compatible with a cellular medulloblastoma or an ependymoma. A tumor that fills the fourth ventricle and extends through the foramina of Luschka and Magendie is more likely to be an ependymoma, although one with a large cyst and mural nodule (with a small area of solid tumor) is more consistent with a PA. PAs typically arise in the cerebellar hemisphere and are imaged on T2-weighted MRI as areas of homogeneous high-signal intensity, with the fluid collections defining the less intense tissue components of the tumor.

Medulloblastoma has T1-weighted MRI signal characteristics more similar to those of gray matter, reflecting hypercellularity and typically resulting in a relatively homogeneous image. On T2-weighted images these tumors can appear to be hyperintense or, more frequently, they can display mixed signal characteristics indicative of small intratumoral cysts, calcification, or small areas of hemorrhage.[1082,1083] The background signal intensity of medulloblastoma on T2-weighted images is characteristically lower than in other tumor types, indicating a dense packing of cells and a high nuclear-to-cytoplasmic ratio. Because medulloblastoma typically arises in the roof of the fourth ventricle, a cleft of CSF beneath the tumor in the fourth ventricle helps distinguish this tumor from ependymoma. Tumors are typically enhanced with administration of gadolinium (Fig. 57-36). The presence of characteristic gyriform morphology and a well-circumscribed appearance on an MRI scan suggest the presence of the nodular subtype of medulloblastoma.[1084] Functional imaging with PET and SPECT are helpful for the improved diagnosis of medulloblastoma. A number

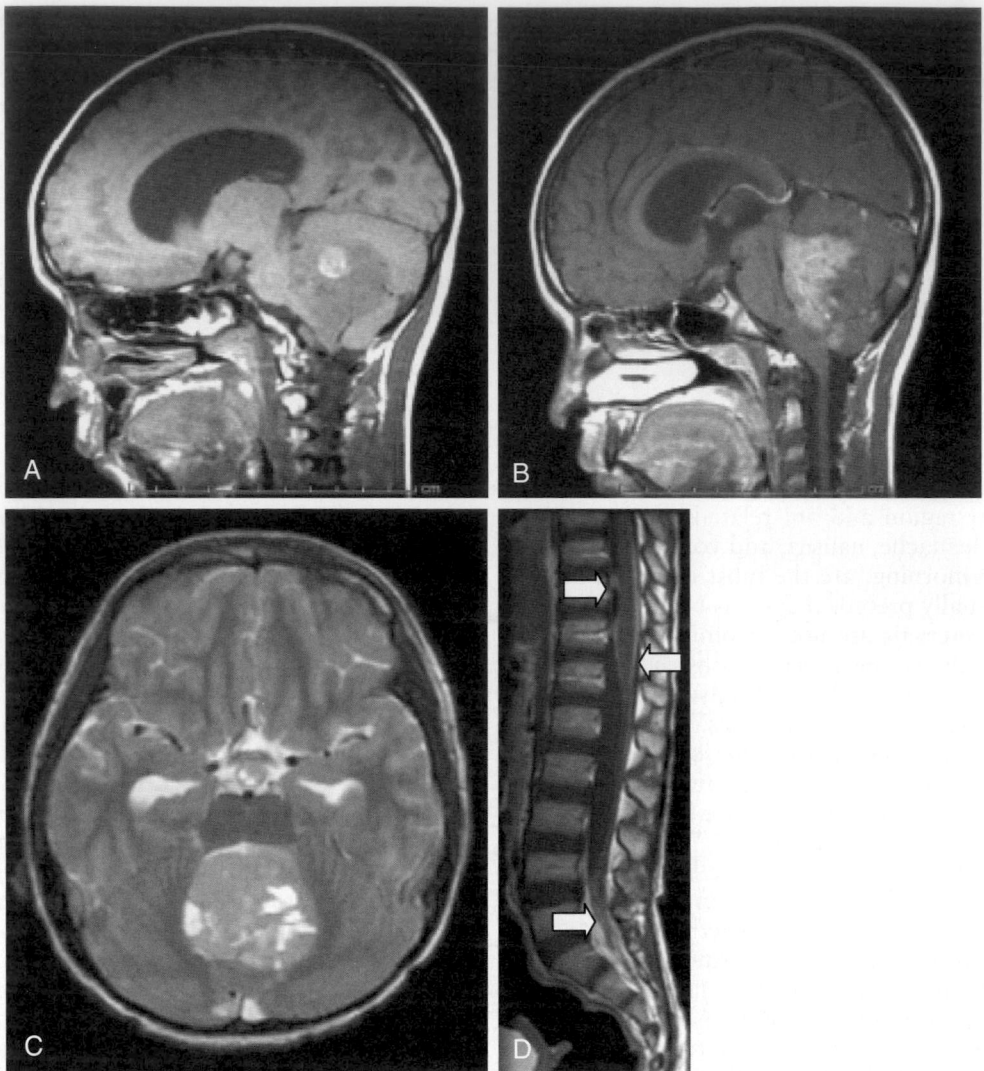

Figure 57-36 Medulloblastoma. **A,** A sagittal T1-weighted image without use of contrast material. An area of hemorrhage is present. **B,** A sagittal T1-weighted image with contrast of a medulloblastoma. **C,** An axial T2-weighted image. The areas of low T2 signal suggest a cellular lesion. **D,** A saggital T1-weighted image with use of contrast material. The lumbar-sacral-enhancing nodules *(arrows on left)* and leptomeningeal coating *(arrow on right)* represent metastatic disease.

of agents such as oxidronate (OctreoScan) can directly assess for the presence and activity of certain cellular constituents, which helps differentiate recurrent disease from scarring.[1085]

Histopathologic analysis of resected tumor specimens is essential for diagnosis and treatment planning. It should be noted that the histopathologic classification and nomenclature of medulloblastoma, within the broader context of embryonal tumors, has long been controversial and even today shows signs of continued evolution.[1086] The most current WHO classification schema considers medulloblastoma to be an independent entity in the group of embryonal tumors,[1040] separate from sPNET (now called CNS PNET in the revised WHO classification[207]). Within medulloblastoma, it is also clear that these tumors are not a homogeneous entity from a histopathologic viewpoint. At present five main histologic subtypes are recognized—classic, desmoplastic-nodular, anaplastic,

large cell, and medulloblastoma with extensive nodularity. In addition any of these five variants of medulloblastoma can have areas of myogenic or melanotic differentiation.[1087] Classic (nondesmoplastic) medulloblastoma is the most common subtype, with approximately two thirds of tumors being classified as such, followed by the desmoplastic subtype (25%). This distribution is not uniform and is influenced by factors such as age and the presence of Gorlin syndrome. Individual tumors are often heterogeneous with regard to the extent of desmoplasia.[1088,1089]

Classic medulloblastoma consists of uniform sheets of densely packed small round blue cells with round to oval hyperchromatic nuclei and scant cytoplasm[1040] (Fig. 57-37). Desmoplastic medulloblastoma is characterized by so-called pale islands, or reticulin-free nodules, that are surrounded by reticulin-producing proliferating cells. Desmoplastic medulloblastoma is linked to the

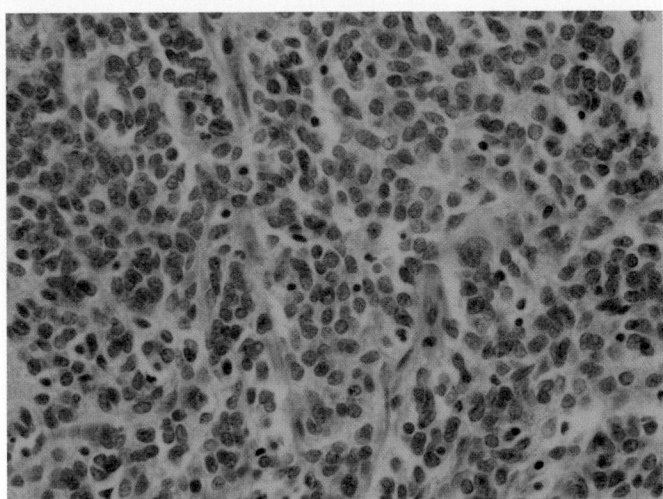

Figure 57-37 Nonanaplastic medulloblastoma. Lesions consist of sheets of homogeneous-appearing undifferentiated tumor cells (hematoxylin and eosin; ×600).

nevoid basal cell carcinoma (Gorlin) syndrome, caused by mutations in the *PTCH1* gene and leading to dysregulation of SHH signaling. Only recently have the large-cell and anaplastic variants of medulloblastoma been identified. These variants are defined by light microscopic findings of prominent nuclei with a high degree of pleomorphism, high mitotic indices, increased cytoplasm, and a higher rate of necrosis than in other variants.[1090] These tumors are uniformly positive for synaptophysin and are generally positive for chromogranin. Anaplastic and large-cell medulloblastomas tend to have higher rates of metastasis at presentation, loss of chromosome 17p13.3, and *MYC* amplification, and both have relatively poor prognoses.[1091] These two variants can occur together and contain cells with markedly increased nuclear atypia and/or large nuclei with prominent nucleoli (Fig. 57-38).[1091-1093]

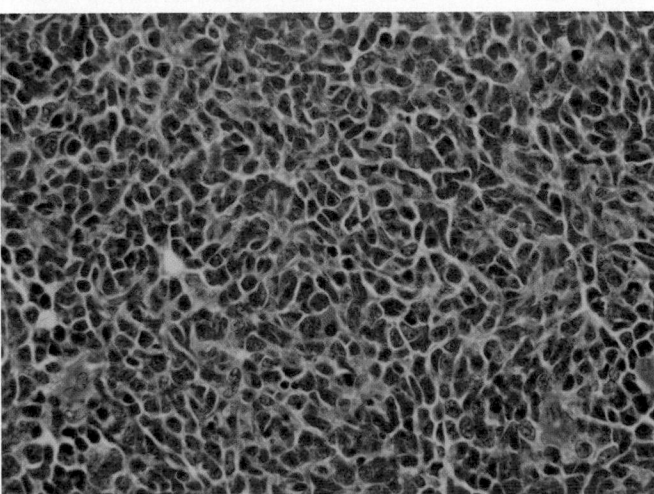

Figure 57-38 Anaplastic medulloblastoma. Tumor cells are pleomorphic with atypia, increased nuclear size, nuclear molding, and cell-cell wrapping (hematoxylin and eosin; ×600).

Wnt-positive medulloblastomas are usually classic histology. SHH group tumors include classic histology tumors, and nodular desmoplastic medulloblastomas most commonly belong in this group. Group 3 and 4 tumors have higher rates of MYC or MYCN amplification and isochrome 17q.

One of the cardinal features of medulloblastoma is its tendency to differentiate along one or more pathways, most commonly neuronal, astrocytic, and ependymal lineages. Synaptophysin expression, a characteristic feature of medulloblastomas, indicates neuronal lineage.[1094] The expression of certain intermediate filament proteins, such as nestin, vimentin, and GFAP, can also be seen in medulloblastomas.[1095] Medulloblastoma is divided into five variants:

1. Nondesmoplastic (classic) medulloblastoma may be strongly immunoreactive for vimentin. Although GFAP expression is typically restricted to developing and mature astrocytes, most classic medulloblastomas contain GFAP-positive cells, which could indicate astrocytic differentiation.[1040]
2. Nodular-desmoplastic medulloblastoma has been shown to have an increased degree of reticulin staining,[1096] with reticulin-free areas that can be identified throughout the lesion or only focally. The nodules represent regions of neuronal maturation.[1040] This rare subtype makes up only 5% of medulloblastomas but accounts for 57% of medulloblastomas in infants[1089] and accounts for the particularly good outcome in this age group.[1097]
3. Anaplastic medulloblastoma has marked nuclear pleomorphism, a high mitotic rate, apoptotic cells, and significant atypia. If only small areas of anaplasia are identified, the tumor does not meet the diagnostic criteria for the anaplastic subtype. Experienced pediatric neuropathologists are therefore required for difficult cases. Anaplasia may be related to abnormalities in *c-Myc*.[1098,1099]
4. Large-cell medulloblastoma is a rare subtype with abundant mitoses and apoptotic bodies.[1093] The name derives from the large nuclei that are present.[1100] It often contains areas of anaplasia, possibly related to specific aberrant signaling pathways,[1101] and thus many refer to these two variants as large-cell/anaplastic medulloblastoma.
5. Medulloblastoma with extensive nodularity, previously called cerebellar neuroblastoma, is typically identified in infants and has very large reticulin-free zones in comparison with desmoplastic medulloblastoma.[1102]

Medulloblastoma with myogenic differentiation refers to the presence of rhabdomyoblastic elements[1103,1104] and can be seen with any of the five variants of medulloblastoma discussed earlier (classic, desmoplastic, anaplastic, large cell, and medulloblastoma with extensive nodularity).[1105] The historic term for medulloblastoma with rhabdomyoblastic elements was *medullomyoblastoma*,[1106] although this latter term is no longer recommended. Similarly medulloblastoma with melanotic differentiation refers to the presence of melanin and does not represent an additional unique variant of the disease.[1107,1108] Rather

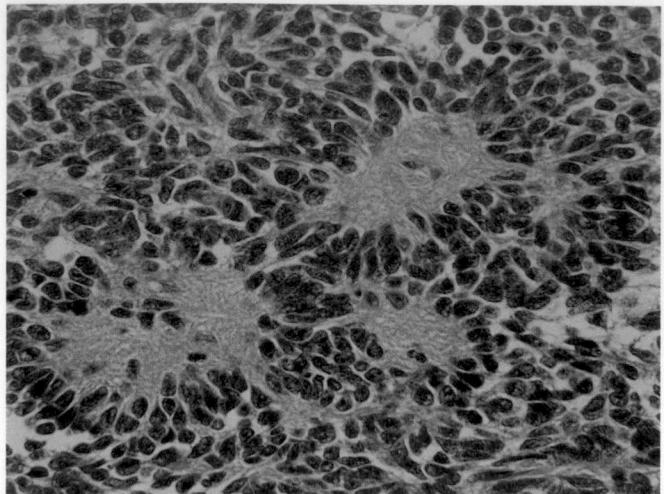

Figure 57-39 Homer-Wright rosettes (hematoxylin and eosin; ×600).

melanotic differentiation can occur with the other recognized variants. This tumor type was previously called "melanocytic medulloblastoma."

Mitoses and other markers of proliferation such as the MIB1 labeling index are common features of these tumors and do not alter the prognosis.[1109] A mitotic index of 0.5% to 2%, an MIB1 index higher than 20%, and the presence of Homer-Wright rosettes, that is, cells arranged around a central lumen or hub (Fig. 57-39),[1110] are often associated with increased atypia and mitotic activity and are seen in approximately one third of cases. Pseudorosettes—that is, cells arranged around a central clearing with a vessel in the middle—are a common feature of medulloblastoma but are variable; they are not prognostic. Vascular proliferation and necrosis are uncommon.

Determining the cellular origin of medulloblastoma may be a key to the proper stratification and management of these tumors.[1111] As noted earlier current evidence indicates that patients with the desmoplastic variant, which is thought to originate from cerebellar granule cell precursors, have a better prognosis than patients with the classic or large-cell/anaplastic variants.[1112] Similarly patients with the large-cell and anaplastic variants appear to have a worse prognosis, and our developing understanding of the unique pathways involved will likely allow better classification and therapy in future studies.

Historic Perspective

Like most other treatments, the development of our current approaches to multimodality therapy for medulloblastoma is the result of a series of overlapping clinical trials. It is beyond the scope of this chapter to give a detailed recounting of the progression to our current understanding of medulloblastoma therapy. Rather a few key events will provide some idea of why we do what we currently do and indicate some of the weaknesses on which our current assumptions are based.

For decades after the first description of medulloblastoma was published by Bail and Cushing in 1925, the prognosis for this highly malignant tumor was extremely poor. Cushing's development of neurosurgical techniques to remove tumors of the fourth ventricle, coupled with a dramatic decline in surgical morbidity, was critical to the development of effective therapies.[1113] With the introduction of radiation therapy and further refinements in neurosurgical techniques between 1950 and 1970, significant improvements in survivorship were achieved. For the first time patients with standard-risk disease had a 5-year EFS approaching 50%, whereas those with high-risk disease were estimated to have a 5-year EFS of approximately 20%. It was demonstrated that radiation therapy could cure a significant percentage of patients, thus securing its place in the standard approach for these tumors. The craniospinal dose for all patients at that time was 3600 cGy (craniospinal irradiation; CSI), with a posterior fossa boost to an approximate total of 5400 cGy. The promise of EFS was tempered, however, by the poor functioning levels seen in surviving patients.

Based on these outcomes and late effects, treatments were modified on the basis of risk categories. For high-risk patients, chemotherapy was added to full-dose 3600 cGy craniospinal radiotherapy, and the resulting improvement in outcome was easily measured, with 3- and 5-year EFS rates of approximately 60%. By contrast the approach to patients with standard-risk disease was to reduce the dose of craniospinal radiotherapy from 3600 to 2400 cGy to spare neurocognitive function, while maintaining the boost to the posterior fossa of 5400 cGy. A national clinical trial in the United States was undertaken, but as the study progressed, there was concern that the number of recurrences in the 2400-cGy treatment arm was greater than that for the 3600-cGy treatment arm. Consequently the study was terminated early. With further follow-up, however, the survival curves for the two treatment arms began to approach one another, such that no statistical difference in outcome was identified, and the early termination of the trial hindered the determination of the statistical conclusion. The results from these treatment studies suggest that chemotherapy in combination with craniospinal radiation therapy could positively affect outcome. The strategy for standard-risk disease thus became the lower-dose radiation therapy of 2400 cGy CSI with the addition of chemotherapy. In follow-up studies of these combinations, PFS of 86% and 79% at 3 and 5 years, respectively, was achieved for standard-risk patients.[1114] The two approaches for high- and standard-risk disease have now become the basis of most North American treatment trials.

Current Treatment

Management. A high level of clinical suspicion is critical for an early diagnosis of medulloblastoma. Neuroimaging is usually the first step, with CT or MRI scanning of the brain frequently performed in the acute setting. MRI of the brain and spine should be performed as soon as is feasible. In children in whom the diagnosis of medulloblastoma is suspected, an MRI of the spine should be obtained because the incidence of CSF dissemination at diagnosis ranges between 20% and 30%.[1077] Corticosteroids are usually used to control increased ICP. A lumbar

---

Box 57-3   Modified Chang Staging System in Medulloblastoma

Stage M0: No evidence of subarachnoid or hematogenous metastases

Stage M1: Microscopic tumor cells found in the cerebrospinal fluid

Stage M2: Gross nodular metastatic seeding in the subarachnoid space or ventricular system distant from the primary site of disease

Stage M3a: Gross nodular seeding in the spine subarachnoid space without evidence of intracranial seeding

Stage M3b: Gross nodular seeding in the spinal subarachnoid space, as well as intracranial seeding

Stage M4: Extraneural metastases

---

puncture should be deferred until after intracranial hypertension has been relieved by surgery. Because extraneural spread of medulloblastoma is possible, bone marrow aspiration and biopsy should be considered for the complete evaluation of patients with medulloblastoma,[1115] although these procedures are no longer required for participation in cooperative clinical trials. Although the exact incidence of extraneural metastases is evolving, current estimates suggest that such metastases occur in fewer than 5% of patients. Because patients will require general anesthesia for insertion of a central line for the administration of chemotherapy, bone marrow samples and a baseline lumbar sample can be easily obtained with minimal trauma to the child or family. CSF obtained from the ventricular or cisternal fluid is not considered an adequate sample upon which to base staging decisions; thus lumbar sampling is recommended for all patients in whom such sampling is not contraindicated pretherapy.[1116]

At present risk stratification and treatment assignment are based primarily on clinical factors, although this will change with greater reliance on molecular profiling.[1111] Recently histology has been added in the risk assignment of medulloblastoma. The modified Chang criteria[1117] are based on the extent of tumor and the degree of metastasis (Box 57-3). After completion of the staging evaluation (i.e., MRI of the brain and spine, CSF cytology, and bone marrow studies), histology, and degree of resection, patients are stratified to the standard-risk, high-risk, or infant-risk groups. The major determinants of clinical risk categorization are age at diagnosis (younger than 3 years vs. 3 years or older),[1072] metastasis or M stage (M0 versus higher than M0), volume of residual postoperative disease (less than 1.5 cm³ residual disease vs. greater than 1.5 cm³ residual disease),[1118] and histology (anaplastic–large cell versus other).[1119] Although these criteria are widely used in the staging of medulloblastoma, the role of complete resection versus less than 1.5 cm³ residual disease, the age of the patient, and the significance of anaplastic histology are still in question, and entry criteria may vary from those indicated.

Histology has just recently begun to be considered in risk stratification. Most prior published series of patients with medulloblastoma had incorporated patients with anaplasia–large cell medulloblastoma into standard-risk treatment if they met the other criteria for standard risk. The recognition that infants with the desmoplastic variant may do better than infants with the nondesmoplastic variant may provide an opportunity to deescalate therapy in this particular group. Newer protocols are now incorporating these variables. Tolerability of therapy has also recently come to light as more adult programs begin to treat older patients with regimens similar to those that have produced significant advances in pediatric patients. Older patients, including adolescents, do not tolerate therapy as well as younger children or infants, which provides an argument for dose modifications in this group.[1120]

ATRTs of the posterior fossa often resemble medulloblastomas. In prior cooperative group studies, up to 30% of patients with ATRTs were misclassified as having a medulloblastoma. With the use of INI1 immunohistochemical analysis of the tumor sample, rapid differentiation of these two histologies is required because the treatment for ATRT differs from that of medulloblastoma in most large cooperative groups.

Treatment

Surgery. Treatment of medulloblastoma, as well as of other embryonal tumors, is multimodal, consisting of surgery, radiation therapy, and chemotherapy, with current therapies guided primarily by age and stage at diagnosis. The initial goal of surgery is to control raised ICP, if present. Once the safety of the patient is ensured, consideration of tumor resection becomes the next objective. If metastatic tumor is already known to be present, immediate aggressive surgery within the posterior fossa will not reduce the need for more intensive radiation therapy and chemotherapy. Rather the goal of surgical resection should be to achieve maximal tumor volume reduction without significant damage to adjacent areas. In balance it is more important for the neurosurgeon to preserve function rather than to maximize resection. Given the excellent prognosis for patients with medulloblastoma, even with metastatic disease, damage to the brain in a high percentage of patients means a high percentage of survivors with permanent neurologic damage.[1121] A third ventriculostomy (preferred) or VP shunt should be deferred prior to initial surgery but may be necessary if sufficient resection to reopen CSF flow is not achieved.

A number of surgical approaches are possible to optimize resection of posterior fossa and cerebellar tumors. Most fourth ventricular lesions will require interruption of the cerebellar vermis, although resections through the vermis using horizontal or vertical incisions have both been associated with posterior fossa syndrome. Even attempts at going under rather than through the vermis have been associated with this morbidity. The brainstem must also be protected while removing medulloblastomas within the fourth ventricle. Because these tumors can invade the brainstem, intraoperative decisions regarding the aggressiveness of resection must be made. Similarly resection must protect the nearby cranial nerves. New neurosurgical techniques are now available that allow for greater guidance in resection and in physiologic monitoring so that damage to important anatomic structures can be avoided. The use of intraoperative MRIs has improved the neurosurgeon's ability to ensure adequate yet safe resection.[1122,1123]

Potential complications of surgery in this location, regardless of tumor type, include cerebellar mutism (also called posterior fossa syndrome)[1124] and aseptic meningitis. The posterior fossa syndrome, or cerebellar mutism, occurs in approximately 10% to 20% of cases, although it is being reported in an increasing percentage of patients as more attention is given to the quality of survivorship. The characteristics are reduced speech output or mutism, personality changes, hypotonia, ataxia, and reduced oral intake. Symptoms typically appear 1 or 2 days after surgery, may range between mild to severe, and may last from days to months with varying degrees of recovery.[1125]

Radiation Therapy. Radiotherapy has become an important modality in the long-term outcome of patients with medulloblastoma. During the past 20 years, a great deal of effort has been focused on the reduction of craniospinal doses as a result of significant long-term neurocognitive damage, as well as secondary tumor risk and stroke. Radiotherapy is currently risk adapted, and additional modifications to dose and volume continue.[1126] For standard-risk patients, 5400 to 5580 cGy are administered to the tumor bed. This volume continues to evolve, from inclusion of the entire posterior fossa, even when the tumor is small and focal, to more limited fields that encompass only structures in contact with the tumor and a small margin. Previous standard-radiation therapy included craniospinal doses of 3600 cGy. A national clinical trial evaluating standard-risk patients with a craniospinal dose of 2400 cGy demonstrated equal efficacy to historic reports, although this study did not randomize between the two CSI doses; 2400 cGy has been accepted as the new standard for this patient population.[1127] An important conclusion from this study was the poor outcome of patients with high-risk disease treated with lower dose craniospinal radiotherapy, reinforcing the importance of proper staging and radiation planning for all patients. A COG clinical trial for patients with standard-risk medulloblastoma is ongoing; this trial randomizes children younger than 8 years to receive either 2400 or 1800 cGy CSI and randomizes all children to receive either a full posterior fossa boost or an involved field boost. This trial will help define the dose and field of radiation therapy required for this population.

For patients with high-risk disease that is caused either by the presence of bulk unresectable disease within the posterior fossa or by the presence of metastatic disease, treatment remains 3600 cGy to the craniospinal axis and a focal dose to the involved posterior fossa of 5400 to 5940 cGy. Although this dose to the entire brain and spine increases the morbidity of therapy, it is an important component of effective treatment, as noted in the previously described randomized trial for standard-risk patients who, on central review, were found to have high-risk disease. A number of cooperative group trials are currently evaluating drugs combined with radiotherapy (radiation sensitizers) to augment the activity of radiation therapy in children with high-risk medulloblastoma.

Infants with medulloblastoma (and other CNS PNETs) continue to pose the greatest therapeutic dilemma. Even in the presence of standard-risk disease, the contraindication for craniospinal radiation therapy limits the treatment options for this group and their long-term prognoses. The omission of craniospinal radiotherapy has required the acceptance of a lower cure rate but a much higher functionality for those who do survive.[1128] The use of treatment protocols that rely only on surgery and chemotherapy demonstrate a relatively poor outcome for this group in all but a select group (e.g., those with nodular desmoplastic medulloblastoma[1097]), again supporting the importance of radiation therapy for the treatment of medulloblastoma. Because many relapses occur locally, many centers have tested focal radiotherapy to the posterior fossa, forgoing the craniospinal component of therapy.[727,1129] This approach attempts to improve local control to the cerebellum, which is thought to be an area less important for neurocognitive development than the cortex. However in a recently completed COG study (trial P9934) that pilot-tested focal radiation therapy to the posterior fossa, it was noted that many recurrences occurred in sites that were outside the radiation field.[1130]

Hyperfractionation of radiotherapy—that is, twice-daily dosing of radiation therapy—has not demonstrated significant improvement in outcome,[1131] although one pilot trial has reported such an improvement.[1132] By contrast a significant delay in the completion of the radiation therapy appears to negatively affect survival.[1133,1134] Proton radiation therapy is increasingly used for children with medulloblastoma. Although its efficacy is similar to that of conventional photon radiotherapy, the absence of an exit dose can reduce radiation exposure to areas uninvolved with tumor. The limited number of proton beam facilities, however, restricts the wider application of this technique. Other more readily available radiation therapy options include IMRT. In particular, tighter margins within the posterior fossa and better 3D conformal planning with IMRT-based techniques can help avoid the auditory apparatus and thus long-term hearing impairment.

The potential use of chemotherapy before delivery of craniospinal radiotherapy has been pilot tested[1134,1135] and has been shown to be associated with inferior EFS and OS.[1135] A national clinical trial with randomization between standard-dose radiation therapy (3600 cGy) and reduced-dose (2340 cGy) CSI in patients with low-stage (M0) disease who were not receiving adjuvant chemotherapy resulted in an increased rate of recurrence outside of the posterior fossa.[1136] However it should be noted that no statistically significant difference was found between the two groups at 6 to 7 years after treatment.

Chemotherapy. The chemosensitivity of medulloblastoma and the benefits of adjuvant chemotherapy in treatment regimens have been demonstrated by a number of studies.[1137-1139] During the past 20 years studies have shown a nearly 20% to 30% improvement in EFS and OS by using chemotherapy during and/or after radiation therapy. Most regimens have included vincristine, cisplatin, etoposide, and an alkylator (cyclophosphamide or CCNU). Although platinum-containing regimens are considered important components of the treatment of medulloblastoma, the ultimate cumulative dose required for optimal activity while minimizing renal and audiologic impairment remains to be defined.[1140] Chemotherapy is currently a standard adjuvant therapy in children. Similarly infant studies with chemotherapy alone have shown the importance of chemotherapy as an effective strategy for patients with medulloblastoma. For most of these infant studies the removal of CSI has had a negative effect on survival, although a significant proportion of survivors can achieve cure.[1097] Recently methotrexate has been added into multiagent chemotherapy for medulloblastomas and other PNETs with excellent tumor response. In one phase II study consisting of four cycles of carboplatin, etoposide, and methotrexate, CR and partial response (PR) rates of 71% and 81% were achieved in patients younger than 3 years and older than 3 years, respectively.[1141]

The concurrent use of craniospinal radiation therapy and multiagent chemotherapy for medulloblastoma can result in significant impairment of nutrition during therapy for these patients.[1142] Patients who present with persistent vomiting likely initiate therapy in a negative nutritional state. A large proportion of patients will require nutritional support through a nasogastric tube or gastric tube. Constant surveillance of nutrition is important because this issue is often dismissed early and is only recognized when severe weight loss has occurred.

Impairment in hearing function continues to be a major concern in survivors of medulloblastoma. The overlap between posterior fossa radiation therapy and the use of ototoxic drugs such as cisplatin has resulted in significant toxicity for this patient population. Conformal radiation planning with tighter margins, the use of IMRT, and the use of proton beam radiation therapy can all significantly reduce the damage to the auditory apparatus. Recent medulloblastoma treatment protocols have also reduced the cumulative doses of cisplatin. The use of amifostine continues to be controversial, with some studies showing efficacy at protecting hearing and other studies not showing efficacy.[1143,1144] Concerns about protecting the tumor from the chemotherapy remain, and only a well-controlled randomized trial will resolve this question.

STANDARD-RISK DISEASE. The components of combination chemotherapy used during and after CSI continue to evolve. A large national clinical trial involving 2400 cGy CSI with a boost to 5400 cGy to the posterior fossa and randomizing between vincristine, cisplatin, and either CCNU or cyclophosphamide (COG trial A9961) demonstrated that both treatment arms have approximately similar activity. The OS for both groups was approximately 90%, with only a slight difference in EFS between the two chemotherapy regimens (85% for patients who received CCNU vs. 83% for those who received cyclophosphamide).[1035] The emphasis in the ongoing clinical study has been to reduce the CSI dose further in a randomized fashion for children younger than 8 years (i.e., those most at risk for the severe neu-

rocognitive impact of radiation therapy) while combining the CCNU and cyclophosphamide agents to reduce the total exposure to each. The safety of 1800 cGy craniospinal radiotherapy was pilot tested in 10 patients with standard-risk medulloblastoma, and in this small cohort, the survival outcome appeared equally effective to that for 2400-cGy therapy and with less neurocognitive impairment.[1145] Radiation- and chemotherapy-adapted approaches are especially important for younger patients given the significant dose-dependent neurocognitive impact of radiation therapy in this population.[1146] A large European cooperative group trial of standard versus hyperfractionated radiation therapy showed no significant outcome difference between these two approaches and has led to the adoption of daily fractionated radiation therapy as the standard for children with medulloblastoma.[1147]

HIGH-RISK DISEASE. Treatment strategies for this population have focused on the addition of new agents, including radiosensitizing agents and novel biologic inhibitors, targeting pathways important for these tumors in the hopes of further improving outcome.[1148] It should be noted that the sequence of treatment has been shown to be of major importance, with the best survival rates being achieved if radiation therapy is not delayed,[1149] although a recent study (Pediatric Oncology Group [POG] trial 9031) reported no difference in EFS in children who received radiation therapy first compared with those who received chemotherapy first in the presence of high-risk disease.[1150]

INFANT CHEMOTHERAPY. Patients younger than 3 years at diagnosis are considered to have higher risk disease at all stages and degrees of resection, related to the limitations of delivering craniospinal radiation therapy to this group. There is also an increased frequency of leptomeningeal dissemination at the time of diagnosis in young children (27% to 43%) versus older children (20% to 25%) with similar histologic diagnoses.[1151] After surgical resection, infants with medulloblastoma are often treated with chemotherapy alone or chemotherapy with involved field radiotherapy in an effort to reduce the high incidence of developmental and neuropsychological sequelae caused by craniospinal irradiation. It is clear that the risks of craniospinal radiation therapy in infants and young children are significantly greater than the benefits of therapeutic response in terms of neurocognitive development.[1152] Currently several chemotherapy regimens designed to delay or eliminate the need for whole-neuraxis radiation therapy are being investigated, including regimens using intraventricular chemotherapy.[1097] In addition high-dose regimens have been found to be feasible and effective for young children with disseminated medulloblastoma.[1153] The relative merits and risks of conventional multiagent chemotherapy compared with high-dose submyeloablative or myeloablative chemotherapy with stem cell support is under investigation.[348,728] An important finding in a recent study for infants with medulloblastoma is the particularly good outcome in infants with the desmoplastic variant, even without radiation therapy,[1097] suggesting that nodular desmoplastic medulloblastoma may represent a low-risk group that does well with less intensive therapy. These tumors are also commonly of the SHH subtype, and it is possible that integration of novel agents targeting this pathway may have a potential therapeutic role. Ongoing studies to confirm this finding are under way but raise the possibility that desmoplastic medulloblastoma may form a new low-risk group.

Prognosis

Patients with standard-risk medulloblastoma have a 5-year survival of approximately 75% to 90%, whereas 5-year survival in patients with high-risk medulloblastoma remains at between 40% and 60%.[1035,1129,1154] Infants with metastatic disease or bulky unresectable disease continue to do poorly, with a 3-year EFS of less than 40%, except in those with the desmoplastic variant. Patients with other rarer subtypes of medulloblastoma, including the large-cell, anaplastic, large-cell/anaplastic, and melanotic variants, continue to do poorly, even with maximal upfront therapy.[1092] Various histologic features associated with improved prognosis have been evaluated, of which nodular appearance appears to be most important.[1088] The presence of dissemination is the single most important factor that correlates with poor outcome.[1155] Lifelong repeated surveillance imaging is required in anticipation of radiation-induced secondary malignancies, such as a meningioma or HGG.[1156] Radiotherapy, particularly in young children, can also cause significant adverse late effects in neurocognitive development, growth, and endocrine function.[1146,1157,1158] Gene profiling of medulloblastoma was an accurate method of predicting outcome, even when evaluated in the context of clinical data. Variables such as age, M stage, and degree of resection did not significantly improve the predictive ability of this independent data set.[1159]

Relapsed Medulloblastoma

Relapses occur as failures at the primary site, at distant sites, or both. MRI is not always accurate when lesions are identified, and pathologic correlation is important in avoiding toxic therapy for patients whose disease has not actually progressed.[1160] Tumors occurring at the primary site within the posterior fossa may have a greater chance for salvage. Patients treated without upfront radiation therapy (infants, in particular) also have a good salvage rate.[1161] Retrieval therapy is rarely curative, but long-term disease control may occur with high-dose myeloablative chemotherapy in a small proportion of patients.[348,1162] Past experience has shown that patients entering high-dose chemotherapy without chemotherapy-responsive disease, or with residual disease at the time of transplantation, are unlikely to benefit from this approach. A large number of new intrathecal,[1163] biologic, and antiangiogenic agents are being evaluated for patients with relapsed medulloblastoma.[335,1164-1166] Although these agents are likely to be more effective when moved up early in the upfront setting, additional testing is still required. Most exciting are preliminary results with SHH inhibitors in this subgroup of patients.[1167] Given the distribution of mutations within the SHH pathway that differ between infants, children, and adults,[1050] as

well as concerns for premature bone closure in infants and children taking these inhibitors, careful selection of patients and a balance of prognosis versus toxicity is required.

Future Directions

The recent discovery of genetic alterations defining different subtypes of medulloblastoma presents novel and exciting opportunities for the development of targeted therapies for children with medulloblastoma. Trials examining the efficacy of SHH inhibitors for those of the SHH subtype are currently under way, and novel agents that target the *MYC* transcription factor or activation pathways also are currently being investigated for MYC or MYCN amplified tumors. In addition studies that determine potential mechanisms by which medulloblastomas may acquire resistance to targeted agents are also important to provide insights into potential combination therapies.[1052,1168] Conversely treatment strategies that minimize long-term therapy-related morbidity in children with Wnt-positive medulloblastoma are also being investigated. The challenge in the coming era will be to develop strategies that incorporate risk stratification and biologically targeted agents in the upfront treatment strategy for children with medulloblastoma.

Pineocytomas and Pineoblastomas

Tumors of the pineal region are often grouped together based on their location rather than on their cellular origins and behavior. Embryonal tumors of the pineal region include pineocytoma, pineal parenchymal tumor of intermediate differentiation (PPTID), pineoblastoma, and papillary tumor of the pineal region (PTPR). Together they account for less than 5% of all pediatric CNS tumors. Other pineal-based lesions include GCTs and, less commonly, astrocytic tumors.[642] GCTs are discussed in a separate section. In a recent series of children diagnosed with pineal parenchymal tumors, the extent of surgical resection has been reported to be a significant prognosticator.[1169]

Pineocytomas

Pineocytomas arise from the pinocyte, the primary function of which appears related to photoreceptor activity and neuroendocrine function.[1170] They are classified as low-grade (grade I) neoplasms that are most common in adults and in late adolescence, although they can be observed in young children. They account for approximately 50% of the tumors of pineal origin, although pineal region neoplasms account for only 1% to 5% of all pediatric CNS tumors.[1171]

Clinical Presentation. Like other pineal region lesions, pineocytomas often present with a constellation of symptoms related to their location. This constellation includes obstructive hydrocephalus and Parinaud syndrome,[1172] a cluster of abnormalities of eye movements and papillary dysfunction characterized by paralyzed upgaze, pseudo–Argyll Robertson pupils, convergence-retraction nystagmus, eyelid retraction, and a conjugate downgaze "sunsetting" sign. Impairment of hypothalamic-pituitary, brainstem, and cerebellar function is also possible. Unlike malignant pineoblastomas, metastases are rare.

Imaging and Histology. On neuroimaging, pineocytomas are typically small focal lesions that can contain cysts and/or calcifications; they are best seen by CT. They are similar to other low-grade tumors on MRI, with strong contrast enhancement, hypointensity on T1-weighted sequences, and high signal intensity on T2-weighted sequences. Surgically these tumors tend to be well demarcated from surrounding tissue. Areas of hemorrhage are not uncommon. Microscopically pineocytomas are made up of small, round, mature-looking cells that have maintained features of pinocytes, including rosettes.[1173] These tumors demonstrate characteristic pineocytomatous rosettes that differentiate them from pineoblastomas. Mitoses are rare, as are other features of malignancy. Pineocytomas are usually strongly synaptophysin and neuron-specific enolase (NSE)–positive. If areas of pineoblastoma are identified with a pineocytoma, treatment is dictated by the most malignant element (i.e., pineoblastoma).

Management. Surgery remains the mainstay of the therapeutic approach for these lesions. Treatment directed at the hydrocephalus with third ventriculostomy may provide an opportunity to obtain a biopsy before aggressive and potentially morbid surgical resection is attempted.[1174,1175] Tumors with persistent growth can be irradiated, although the benefit of this treatment has not been clearly demonstrated. A role for chemotherapy has not been defined. Patients with incompletely resected tumors do not require therapy unless clear progression is demonstrated. Even patients with metastatic disease can remain untreated. The overall benign course observed with pineocytomas is in stark contrast to that of pineoblastomas.

Prognosis. The long-term prognosis remains excellent, even with incompletely resected disease. Conservative management should be followed with regard to attempted surgical resection and radiation therapy. Because almost all patients with pineocytomas will be long-term survivors, the need to avoid toxicity is paramount.

Pineal Parenchymal Tumor of Intermediate Differentiation

PPTIDs are tumors of the pineal region that occur at all ages, although they are frequent in middle age, and are classified as grade II or III, depending on pathologic features. They account for 20% of pineal region tumors and were formally identified in 1993. Although reports are limited, there appears to be a slight female preponderance. Genetic evaluation has demonstrated a large number of abnormalities.[1176]

Clinical Presentation. The presentation of patients with PPTID is similar to that of pineocytomas and includes obstructive hydrocephalus, as well as Parinaud syndrome,[1172] a cluster of abnormalities of eye movements and papillary dysfunction characterized by paralyzed upgaze, pseudo–Argyll Robertson pupils, convergence-retraction nystagmus, eyelid retraction, and conjugate downgaze. Impairment of hypothalamic-pituitary, brainstem, and cerebellar function is also possible. Unlike pineocytomas, metastatic disease appears to be slightly more frequent.

Imaging and Histology. Imaging characteristics are similar to those of other lesions of pineal origin. They are cellular lesions with moderate nuclear atypia and a low mitotic index.[1177] Because of sampling error, diagnosis can be difficult with limited tissue, especially tissue obtained via third ventriculostomy.

Management. Because of the increasing degree of malignant potential when compared with pineocytomas, attempts at surgical resection should be considered. Although formal pediatric studies are lacking, radiation therapy and chemotherapy should be considered. Intensity of treatment can be based on the localization of the tumor (focal, invasive, or disseminated), as well as the proportion of mitoses, necrosis, atypia, and possibly neurofilament protein expression.[1178]

Prognosis. A definite prognosis for PPTID has not been clearly established. Grade is likely to play an important part in the long-term outcome of patients, as is the size and metastatic stage of patients.[1179] Because these tumors span all age groups, large homogeneous studies are difficult to perform.

Pineoblastoma

Unlike pineocytomas, pineoblastomas are highly malignant embryonal tumors. Like other small round blue cell tumors, these lesions are considered WHO grade IV and have a high propensity to metastasize. Typically they are observed in children younger than those seen with pineocytomas, although considerable overlap exists. Pineoblastomas can be associated with the genetic form of retinoblastoma and in such cases are often referred to as trilateral retinoblastomas.[1180] In a recent study of 408 patients with retinoblastoma, pineoblastoma was detected in 1% of all patients.[1181] An association with familial adenomatous polyposis has also been reported.[1182] Little is known about the molecular classification of these tumors with respect to their genesis or their association with other neural tumors of the CNS (PNET or medulloblastoma).[1183] Defects in *TP53* have not been reported.

Clinical Presentation. Presenting symptoms of pineoblastoma are virtually identical to those for pineocytomas, although the duration of symptoms may be shorter than that seen for other tumors in this location. Pineoblastomas often present with a constellation of symptoms related to their location, including obstructive hydrocephalus in most patients,[1184] as well as Parinaud syndrome,[1172] a cluster of abnormalities of eye movements and papillary dysfunction, as previously described. Impairment of hypothalamic-pituitary, brainstem, and cerebellar function is also possible. Pineoblastomas have a much greater propensity to metastasize and thus may demonstrate symptoms beyond the pineal region.

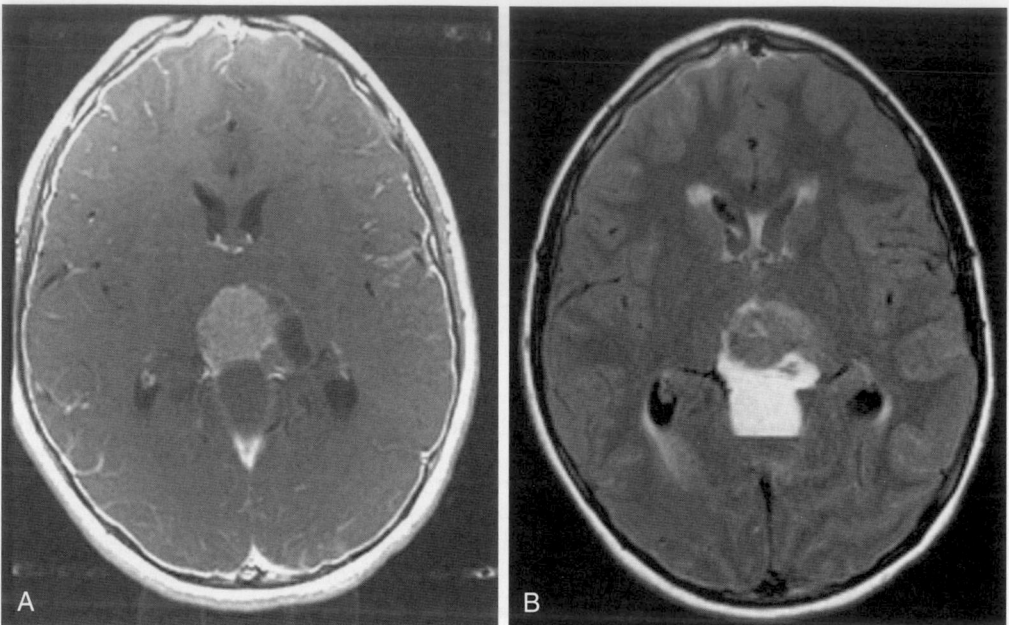

Figure 57-40 A large contrast-enhancing pineoblastoma. **A,** An axial T1-weighted image with use of contrast material. **B,** An axial fluid-attenuated inversion recovery image demonstrating a bright T2-weighted signal.

Imaging and Histology. The neuroimaging characteristics of pineoblastomas are not pathognomonic for these tumors, but they are differentiated from pineocytomas by a significant increase in the volume of the tumor and the presence of much less distinct boundaries. MRI characteristics include low signal on T1-weighted sequences and heterogeneous areas of contrast enhancement (Fig. 57-40).[1185] T2-weighted signals may be lower than in pineocytomas because of the higher nuclear-to-cytoplasmic ratio evident in these more malignant tumors.[1186] On histologic analysis these tumors are similar to other small round blue cell tumors, composed of sheets of cells but lacking the characteristic pineocytomatous rosettes of pineocytomas.[1187] Pineoblastomas are typically synaptophysin- and NSE-positive and other markers, including those for photoreceptor pathways, can be present, consistent with the developmental role of the pineal gland.[1178,1188] Homer-Wright rosettes (i.e., cells with a central zone of cytoplasm; see Fig. 57-39) and Flexner-Wintersteiner rosettes (i.e., cells with a central zone of cytoplasm and a central space; Fig. 57-41) are common, but these rosettes can be seen in a large number of other embryonal tumors. These tumors often have significant atypia, and mitotic activity can be high. When additional pathways of differentiation are present (e.g., melanin, cartilage, and muscle), the tumors are called pineal anlage tumors. Regions of pineoblastoma can also be identified as part of a pineocytoma and are treated as a pineoblastoma. Although sporadic pineoblastoma has no clear genetic association, patients with hereditary (bilateral) retinoblastoma have a significant incidence of pineoblastoma (trilateral retinoblastoma). The clinical course of retinoblastoma associated pineoblastoma can differ from that of sporadic pineoblastoma.[1189]

Recent profiling of genomic alterations have reported copy number alterations observed in pineoblastoma. These alterations include loss of chromosome 16q and amplification of PCDHGA3, and FAM129A.[1169] In addition DNA copy number profiles have reported more similarities between sPNETs and pineoblastoma than between these tumors and the lower grade tumors of the pineal region.[1190] The development of pineoblastoma has also been reported in a young patient with a germline mutation of *DICER1*, which is also associated with the development of pleuropulmonary blastoma.[1191]

Management. The therapeutic approaches for pineoblastoma have followed those of other embryonal seeding

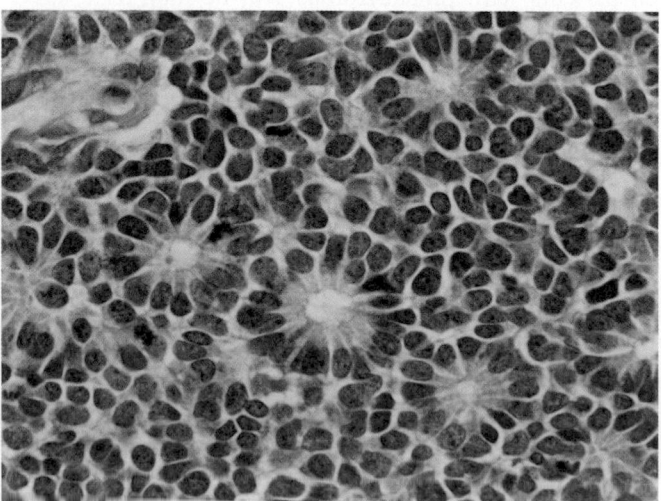

Figure 57-41 Flexner-Wintersteiner rosette in a patient with pineoblastoma (hematoxylin and eosin; ×600).

tumors of the CNS. The workup of patients with pineo-blastoma includes immediate intervention for obstructive hydrocephalus and assessment of risk for herniation. A rapid CT or MRI scan, in conjunction with the examination and presenting history, will permit the neurosurgeon to assess these risks. If urgent CSF shunting is not required, then completion of the imaging baseline workup, including MRI of the brain and spine, can be performed and surgical resection can be planned. Unlike medulloblastoma, the location of pineoblastomas with adjacent vascular structures makes exploratory surgery much more risky, and referral to a highly specialized center should be considered. A third ventriculostomy or VP shunt should be deferred prior to initial surgery but may be necessary if sufficient resection with reestablishment of CSF flow is not achieved. In many patients an endoscopic biopsy of the tumor to confirm the diagnosis and concurrent third ventriculostomy can be performed with a planned open craniotomy and resection once the patient is clinically stable, the disease has been defined, and possible presurgical chemotherapy has been provided.[1174] Patients with metastatic disease at diagnosis should not undergo upfront aggressive surgery because adjuvant therapy will be required. For patients with focal disease at diagnosis based on initial MRI and documentation of negative results of a lumbar puncture, complete removal of the tumor ultimately will be an important component of long-term prognosis[1192] but should not be undertaken at any costs. Consideration for staged surgeries (second- and even third-look approaches) may be equally effective without causing permanent neurologic damage.

As with other embryonal seeding tumors of the CNS, craniospinal radiotherapy is an important modality in treating microscopic metastatic disease at presentation. Unlike medulloblastoma, pineoblastomas do not have a standard-risk category. All patients require aggressive therapy, including a craniospinal dose of 3600 cGy and a focal boost to the primary site of 5400 to 5940 cGy. Sites of metastatic disease require radiation boosts as well. Even with focal resectable disease, the prognosis for pineoblastoma falls significantly below that of medulloblastoma.[1184] In persons with disseminated disease, especially diffuse leptomeningeal spread, and infants, for whom craniospinal radiotherapy is contraindicated, the prognosis remains especially poor. The use of SRS or other similar modalities to deliver single-fraction ablative radiation therapy may provide added disease control of unresectable tumor, although these approaches are limited to small areas of disease.

Chemotherapy is an important modality for patients with pineoblastoma, and significant responses to chemotherapy have been observed, including in patients with trilateral retinoblastoma.[1193] Results from infant studies, which deferred radiotherapy, demonstrated that although chemotherapy can be effective at reducing bulk disease, few patients are long-term survivors with this modality alone.[1194] Because of the rarity of this entity most protocols have combined these patients with patients who have other embryonal tumors, including CNS PNETs and, occasionally, medulloblastoma. Specific estimates of sur-vival from different therapies have therefore been difficult to determine. Current approaches continue to include initial craniospinal radiotherapy in combination with chemotherapy, followed by postradiation chemotherapy. Most regimens have used combinations of vincristine, cyclophosphamide, cisplatin, and etoposide.[1192] Because of the chemoresponsiveness of these tumors, pilot clinical trials with high-dose chemotherapy with stem cell transplantation have also been undertaken. The results of the German HIT2000 clinical trial, which included children with CNS PNET and pineoblastoma, recently reported 5-year EFS and OS of 24% ± 10% and 40% ± 12%, respectively, with multiagent chemotherapy and radiation therapy.[1195] Children with high-risk disease received intensified therapy.

The concurrent use of craniospinal radiation therapy and multiagent chemotherapy for pineoblastoma has resulted in a significant impairment of nutrition during therapy for these patients.[1142] A large number of patients will require nutritional support through a nasogastric tube or, more commonly, a gastric tube. Constant surveillance of nutrition is important because these issues are often dismissed early and are only recognized when severe weight loss has occurred. Patients with persistent vomiting usually initiate therapy in a negative nutritional state.

Prognosis. The outcome of patients with pineoblastoma remains poor. Patients with focal disease that can be completely resected have 3- and 5-year EFS of approximately 50%.[1184,1192] Infants, patients with incompletely resected disease by the end of therapy, or patients with metastatic disease continue to do poorly, with 3- and 5-year EFS estimates of 20% or lower. Progression tends to occur early and can occur at the primary site, throughout the CNS, or both. A recent study of recurrence patterns in children with embryonal intracranial tumors noted a high rate of relapses that involved the spine in children with pineoblastoma.[1196] Extracranial metastases are uncommon. Some patients with metastatic disease, however, are long-term survivors.[1192] After recurrence, no standard therapy has been documented to be effective, and most patients will succumb to their disease, usually within months.

Papillary Tumors of the Pineal Region

PTPRs are rare tumors of children and adults that were separated from other pineal tumors in 2003.[207,1197] As the name implies these neuroepithelial lesions possess papillary structures and are thought to be derived from specialized ependymal cells. Because of their varied appearance, they can be confused with ependymomas, choroid plexus tumors, and pineocytomas.[1198] PTPRs appear to fall into the WHO grade II or III category.

Clinical Presentation. The clinical presentation of PTPRs is similar to that of other lesions of the pineal area. Hydrocephalus is present in almost all patients, and Parinaud syndrome[1172] is common. Impairment of hypothalamic-pituitary, brainstem, and cerebellar function is also possible. Metastatic disease does not appear to be as prevalent as in pineoblastomas.

Imaging and Histology. PTPRs are well-circumscribed, often cystic lesions. They are hyperintense on T1- and T2-weighted sequences and enhance with administration of contrast material.[1199,1200] Histologically these tumors stain strongly for keratins and are usually negative or weakly positive for GFAP (in contrast to ependymomas) and synaptophysin.[1201] Most of the tumor cells show strong expression of NSE, cytokeratins (particularly CK18), S-100 protein, and vimentin. The mitotic index and MIB1 labeling index are intermediate but of unclear prognostic significance.[1202]

Management. In spite of their differentiated appearance, PTPRs are aggressive tumors that are not highly responsive to therapy.[1203] In a recent report of 31 patients, 21 of whom achieved a gross total resection, adjuvant radiation therapy alone resulted in a PFS rate of only 27%.[1204] The ability of achieve a gross total resection has been reported in some studies to be associated with improved PFS.[590,1203]

Prognosis. In spite of complete resection and focal radiation therapy, local recurrences are common,[1205] although patients with complete removal of these tumors may do better.[1206] Dissemination appears rare, and craniospinal radiation therapy therefore does not appear to be required. Patients with an elevated MIB1 labeling index or mitotic rate may tend to do worse.[1207]

Supratentorial or Central Nervous System Primitive Neuroectodermal Tumors

Supratentorial or CNS PNETs are tumors of neuroepithelial origin.[1208] The classification of CNS PNET (previously called sPNET) as separate from medulloblastoma and other embryonal tumors, which was initially proposed in 1973,[1031] has not been without controversy. Historically these tumors have been called by various names, including cerebral medulloblastoma, cerebral neuroblastoma, and cerebral ganglioneuroblastoma. Rorke[1209] (1983) proposed that these tumors are the supratentorial equivalent of medulloblastoma, another common embryonal neoplasm. Although these tumors are histologically similar to medulloblastoma, they respond poorly to medulloblastoma-specific therapy. Part of the confusion in the approach to CNS PNETs has been in the nomenclature—the overlap in the term "PNET" for tumors of the body as well. These tumors do not share the molecular pathways,[1183] metastatic sites, or treatment responses of the extracranial PNET tumors. Even within the CNS, PNETs likely represent a heterogeneous group of tumors.[1029] According to the WHO classification schema,[1210] a number of subtypes of PNET are recognized: classic PNET, PNET with neuronal differentiation (called cerebral neuroblastoma), and, if ganglion cells are present as part of the tumor, cerebral ganglioneuroblastoma. Neither of the latter two entities is related to classic neuroblastoma, which is typically identified around the adrenal gland and shares a common name as a result of historical nomenclature only. New molecular determinants associated with PNETs of the brain have been identified using molecular and proteomic analysis and will, it is hoped, be useful for better subclassification of the diseases that fall into this broad category of tumors.[306,1211-1213] Recently gene expression and genomic profiling efforts of CNS PNETs have confirmed that this disease entity is heterogenous and consists of multiple different tumor types. Copy number analyses of PNETs have in general revealed a complex karyotype with frequent copy number alterations.[1190] In addition these efforts have highlighted the inherent difficulty in classifying tumors based on histology. Molecular profiles have been found to match those of other tumor types, including ATRT (characterized by loss of INI1) and HGGs (characterized by the presence of mutations in the histone genes). Importantly, clustering of profiles have revealed that tumors have distinct profiles based on the underlying lineage of the tumor, including primitive neural, oligoneural, and mesenchymal lineages.[1214] These groups are associated with differences in clinical courses and prognosis, with tumors with an underlying primitive neural profile exhibiting the worse prognosis. Further, these profiling studies have shed light on other genes that may be involved in the pathogenesis of these brain tumors and thus may represent candidates for targeted therapies. These therapies include amplification of genes involved in cell cycle regulation.[1063]

CNS PNETs are relatively rare, occurring at a rate that is approximately 10% to 20% that of medulloblastoma.[1215] Precise statistics regarding incidence are difficult to ascertain because of historically different views regarding classification and nosology. These tumors are more common in early childhood, with most patients diagnosed before the age of 10 years,[1216] and white persons make up most of the reported cases. Most cases are identified in early childhood, but they span all ages. Although they are classified as supratentorial in nature, these tumors have been identified in the infratentorial and spinal compartments. A better term has recently been adopted by WHO[207]—*CNS PNET*.

Clinical Presentation

Presenting features of CNS PNETs depend on the location of the lesion. Those adjacent to the ventricular flow path will usually include signs and symptoms of raised ICP as a result of obstructive hydrocephalus. Specific neurologic signs are dependent on the anatomic structures adjacent to the tumor and can include seizures, mood changes, or hemiparesis. Metastases are frequent in CNS PNETs, and clinical symptoms unrelated to the primary site of disease require investigation.

Imaging and Histology

CNS PNETs appear similar, independent of location within the CNS. As in medulloblastoma and pineoblastoma, these tumors can have areas of cyst or necrosis evident on CT or MRI. Lesions are dark on T1-weighted sequences unless hemorrhage is present and dark on T2-weighted sequences, reflecting their high nuclear-to-cytoplasmic ratio.[1217] CNS PNETs are usually contrast-enhancing after administration of gadolinium (Fig 57-42). Edema, as evident on T2-weighted or FLAIR sequences, is often prominent. All CNS PNETs are

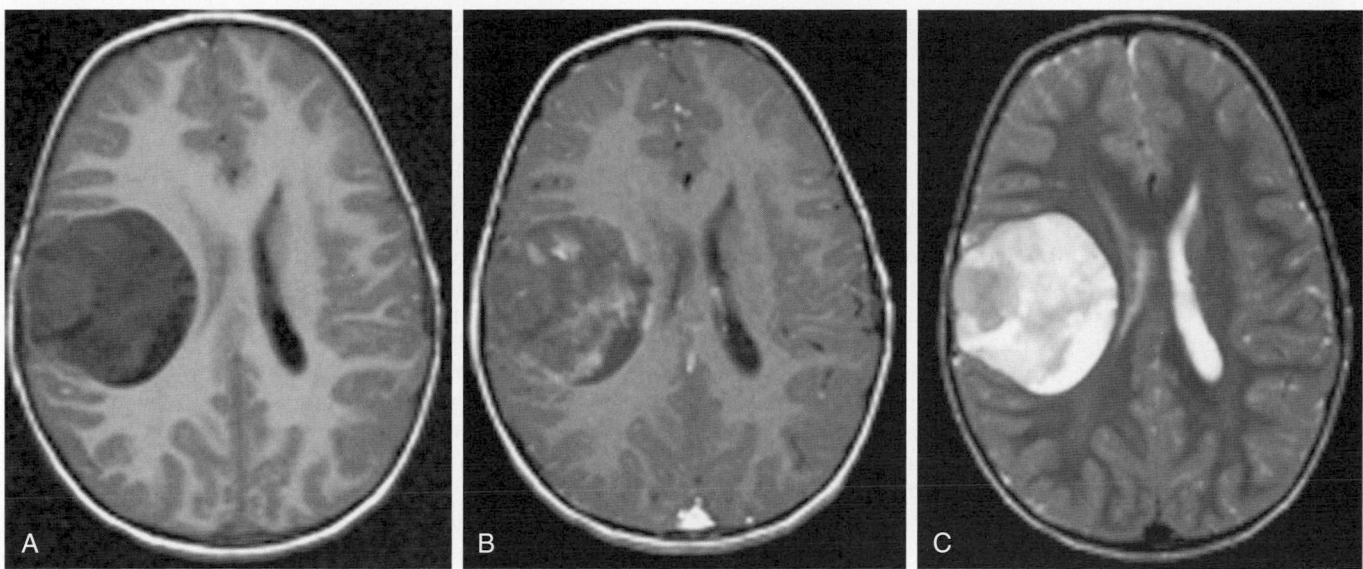

Figure 57-42 Primitive neuroectodermal tumor. **A,** An axial T1-weighted image without use of contrast material. **B,** An axial T1-weighted image with use of contrast material. **C,** An axial T2-weighted image.

considered WHO grade IV. The light microscopic features of CNS PNETs can be similar to those of medulloblastoma or pineoblastoma. Tumors are characterized by the presence of neuroepithelial cells. Many CNS PNETs have evidence of differentiation along glial, neuronal, ependymal, or oligodendroglial lines, although most (approximately 60%) appear undifferentiated.[1218]

Immunohistochemical markers of CNS PNETs include synaptophysin, B-tubulin, and S-100. Occasionally GFAP can be identified in these tumors and indicates their ability to undergo divergent differentiation. Mitotic rates are often high and, although variable, the MIB1 labeling index is usually abundant. Mutations of p53 are rare[1219] and were identified in only 3 of 28 cases of CNS PNET in one study, although many tumors had overexpression of wild-type p53, which correlated with a poor prognosis.[1220] Specific markers for CNS PNETs that distinguish them from medulloblastoma do not exist. Other features, such as Homer-Wright rosettes and perivascular pseudorosettes (i.e., cells around a central blood vessel) are observed in many different tumors (see Figs. 57-35 and 57-39). ATRTs may resemble PNETs, but the presence of cells that stain positively for myosin but lack the protein produced by the *SMARCB1 (hSNF5/INI1)* gene are diagnostic features for ATRT.[1221,1222]

Medulloepitheliomas, Ependymoblastomas, and Embryonal Tumors with Abundant Neuropile and True Rosettes

Historically medulloepitheliomas, ependymoblastomas, and embryonal tumors with abundant neuropile and true rosettes (ETANTRs) have been considered distinct subtypes of CNS PNETs. However recent genomic and gene expression profiling efforts, including genome-wide DNA methylation and copy number profiling, have revealed similarities in genomic profiles, suggesting that they may represent spectrums of the same biologic entity.[1223] In this study, which included 97 tumor samples, all tumors were found to strongly express LIN28A, which had previously been described in ETANTRs.[1224,1225] No difference in clinical features was observed, and unsupervised hierarchical clustering did not reveal subgroups for 41 tumors with sufficient material to perform the analysis, while as a group the tumors clearly separated from other pediatric brain tumors. Finally 95% of tumors were found to harbor amplification of chromosome 19q13.42, previously associated with embryonal tumors with multilayered rosettes.[1226-1228] This study suggests that these entities share the same biology and can be considered spectrums of the same disease. However we will describe the traditional classification and clinical features of these tumors, in keeping with the current WHO classification.

CNS PNET tumors that have re-created features of the neural tube, called medulloepitheliomas, are typically found in very young children[1229] and have even been reported in newborns. They can occur throughout the brain, spine, and optic tract[1230] and can also occur outside the CNS. Their imaging characteristics differ somewhat from other CNS PNETs, with bright appearance on T2-weighted imaging.[1231] They tend to be large on macroscopic imaging. Additional immunohistochemical markers include nestin and vimentin staining.[1210] As with other CNS PNETs, maximal surgical resection, chemotherapy, and radiation therapy are the cornerstone of therapy.[1232] The predilection for young age in this subset of PNETs limits the use of craniospinal radiation.

PNET tumors with ependymoblastic rosettes are called ependymoblastomas and have features that overlap other CNS PNETs.[1223] These tumors predominate in infants and young children[1233] and can be found throughout the CNS, although most are associated with the ventricular system.[1210] Dissemination throughout the CNS is common,[1234] and symptoms include obstructive hydrocephalus, enlarging head circumference in infants, and focal neurologic deficits. The MRI appearance is similar to that of other PNETs, and edema is commonly observed.[1235] Treatment mirrors that of other CNS PNETs. Maximal resection is paramount, followed by multiagent chemotherapy. Although craniospinal radiation therapy is likely important for outcome, the prevalence of ependymoblastoma in infants precludes its use. Prognosis is poor, with rapid disease progression in most patients.

ETANTR is another rare CNS PNET tumor with a spectrum of histologic features and chromosomal abnormalities.[1210] These lesions can be large, cystic, and calcified and come to clinical presentation as a result of mass effect.[1236] Their rarity makes treatment recommendations difficult, although most are approached in a manner similar to that of other PNETs of the brain. The presence of isochrome 17[1237] in only a few cases suggests that they are biologically distinct from medulloblastoma.[1238] Various cytogenetic abnormalities have been defined.[1239]

Cerebral Neuroblastomas

PNETs with neuronal differentiation are called cerebral neuroblastomas and are rare tumors of infancy and childhood. They are unrelated to the more prevalent peripheral sympathetic nervous system form of neuroblastoma and predominate in young infants,[1240] occurring in both the cerebrum[1241] and posterior fossa.[1242] Lack of immunohistochemical staining with IGF2 and IGF type 1 receptor, which is positive in many other infant CNS tumors, can help with the diagnosis.[1210,1243]

A related entity of cerebral neuroblastoma is termed *ganglioneuroblastoma*, which has the presence of ganglion cells in addition to the neuronal component.[1210] These tumors cannot be differentiated from other malignant seeding tumors of infancy by MRI characteristics.[1244] Unlike most other CNS PNETs, cerebral neuroblastoma and CNS ganglioneuroblastoma may have a better prognosis[1245] with surgery and chemotherapy.

Treatment Strategies

A number of treatment protocols based on the successful therapeutic approaches of medulloblastoma have been applied to CNS PNETs.[1148] Repeated studies using maximal surgery, high-dose craniospinal radiotherapy to 3600 cGy with a boost to the primary site of at least 5400 cGy, and multiagent chemotherapy have not fared as well for CNS PNETs[1246,1247] as for high-risk medulloblastoma, with 4-year survival of approximately 40% in one retrospective series.[1216] In one study of 55 patients treated with maximal surgery, craniospinal radiation therapy, and CCNU, vincristine, and prednisone versus 8-in-1 chemotherapy sandwiched in the middle, OS and EFS were comparable. The 3-year EFS was approximately 50% in the two groups and thus appeared similar to that reported in other studies. Poor prognostic variables included the presence of metastases and age younger than 2 years. Patients with pineoblastoma did better, with an estimated 3-year PFS of 65%.[1247] Compared with medulloblastoma, CNS PNETs often respond poorly to medulloblastoma-specific therapy, despite the fact that they are histologically similar.[1248] The use of high-dose chemotherapy with stem cell rescue has been successful for some young children in eliminating the need for radiation therapy, with 5-year EFS of 39%.[1249] The exact conditioning regimen and number of cycles of intensive chemotherapy remain under investigation.[1250] Recurrences are often disseminated,[1248,1251] even when craniospinal radiation therapy is delivered upfront, and the salvage rate for these patients is exceedingly poor. In spite of these overall poor results, there have been reports of survivors after surgery, especially GTR, and radiation therapy.[1252] In one study patients treated with surgery, radiation therapy, and high dose stem cell–supported chemotherapy were reported to have a 5-year EFS of 75% ± 17% and an OS of 88% ± 13%.[1253] For patients with high-risk metastatic disease, the use of adjuvant carboplatin with radiation therapy as a radiosensitizer has been pilot tested in a phase I/II trial with promising results[1254] and is currently undergoing further investigation by the COG.

The concurrent use of craniospinal radiation therapy and multiagent chemotherapy for CNS PNETs has resulted in a significant impairment of nutrition during therapy for these patients.[1142] Therapy is intensive, and supportive care is important. A large number of children will require nutritional support through a nasogastric tube or, more commonly, a gastric tube. Constant surveillance of nutrition is important because these issues are often dismissed early and are only recognized when severe weight loss has occurred. Patients with persistent vomiting may initiate therapy in a negative nutritional state.

Prognosis

Although the prognosis of CNS PNET is well below that of medulloblastoma, 40% of patients will be long-term survivors. The most important variable for prolonged survival is the ability to achieve a complete resection in patients with nonmetastatic disease, followed by CSI and multiagent chemotherapy. The success of salvage therapy in patients who have had a relapse is exceedingly poor, even with high-dose chemotherapy and stem cell rescue.[1255,1256]

Atypical Teratoid Rhabdoid Tumors

ATRTs are uncommon, highly malignant tumors seen primarily in infants and in young children,[1257-1259] with a peak incidence between birth and 3 years. Cases throughout childhood[1260] and in adults have been reported,[1261] however, as has hereditary transmission of the susceptibility gene, resulting in congenital disease.[1262] Although CNS ATRTs account for approximately 1% to 2% of childhood brain tumors, they represent almost 10% of CNS tumors in infants.[1263,1264] Rhabdoid tumors may arise anywhere in the body but are most common in the kidney, CNS, and soft tissues. CNS ATRTs are most commonly identified in the posterior fossa (60%) at the cerebellopontine angle, although supratentorial ATRTs are also frequently seen.[1265] Pineal, spine, and suprasellar area ATRTs have also been reported. This tumor has a strong male preponderance, and metastases at diagnosis are common.[1265]

ATRTs have a spectrum of morphologic and molecular variants,[1266] but the hallmark of this disease is the loss of the *SMARCB1* (also known as *INI1*, *SNF5*, and *BAF47*) gene product on chromosome 22 as a result of biallelic inactivating mutations.[1267] Since the original description of monosomy 22 in ATRTs, this tumor suppressor gene has been cloned from this region[1268] and encodes a core subunit of the SWI/SNF chromatin remodeling complex.[1267] Recent publications have reported on the absence of other canonical pathway mutations and the extremely low mutation rates found in these tumors, thus demonstrating the remarkably simple genome of malignant rhabdoid tumors.[1269,1270]

Mutations and loss of the *SMARCB1* gene and protein expression may not be confined to ATRTs alone because reports on choroid plexus carcinoma, CNS PNET, and medulloblastoma have been reported,[1257] along with a recently identified entity, cribriform neuroepithelial tumor.[1271] Whether these later reports represent other diseases with *SMARCB1* mutations or atypical cases of rhabdoid tumors is controversial. Other diseases such as familial schwannomatosis, multiple meningiomas, epithelioid sarcomas, and extraskeletal myxoid chondrosarcomas are known to have loss of SMARCB1.[1272-1275] In addition, mutations in other subunits of the SWI/SNF chromatin remodeling complex (AT rich interactive domain 1A [ARID1A], polybromo 1 [PBRM1], and BRG1) have also recently been identified in neuroblastoma and ovarian, kidney, and lung cancers.[1276-1280]

Clinical Presentation

Presenting symptoms are dependent on the age and location of the tumor. In persons with posterior fossa tumors, obstructive hydrocephalus with headaches, morning vomiting, and long tract signs is common. Because most patients are young, irritability, lethargy, or failure to thrive may be evident. In patients without closed fontanelles, rapidly enlarging head circumference is observed. Cranial nerve dysfunction is common, resulting in head tilt and diplopia. Patients with supratentorial tumors will often have obstructive hydrocephalus because of the rapid growth and concurrent cysts that obstruct CSF flow. Additional symptoms can be referred to direct compression of neural structures adjacent to the tumor and thus are dependent on location.[1265,1281] Although uncommon spinal ATRT can occur and present with focal motor deficits. Because of the high incidence of metastatic disease, patients with symptoms related to a specific area away from the primary tumor site require thorough investigation. Although rare constitutional loss of the *SMARCB1* gene (or the *INI1* gene; the nomenclature is interchangeable) can occur,[1263] resulting in intracranial and metachronous extraneural disease. Patients should therefore undergo CT evaluation of the chest, abdomen, and pelvis.

Imaging and Histology

Imaging characteristics are similar to those of other neuroectodermal tumors (medulloblastoma and PNET) of the CNS,[1282] including isointense appearance on T1-weighted MRI and heterogeneity on FLAIR and T2-weighted sequences.[1283,1284] Cystic areas are common. Tumors are usually heterogeneously enhancing with contrast administration. Because of their high cellular composition,

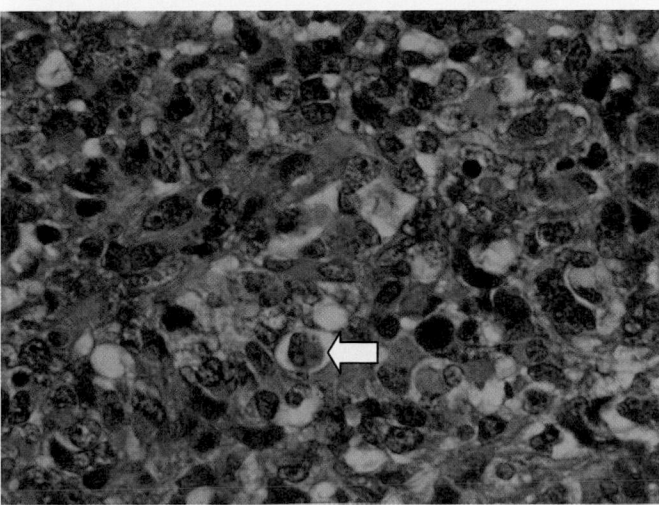

Figure 57-43 An atypical teratoid rhabdoid tumor *(arrow)* demonstrating prominent nucleoli and eosinophilic globular cytoplasmic inclusions (hematoxylin and eosin; ×600).

restricted diffusion is often observed. The presence of hemorrhage and calcifications is not uncommon.[1285]

ATRT has been recognized as a distinct pathologic entity, and it is differentiated from medulloblastoma and other CNS PNETs.[1286] This distinction has been supported by findings of deletions or loss at chromosome 22q11.2, the identification of the tumor suppressor gene *SMARCB1*, and the finding of germline and somatic mutations of *SMARCB1* in approximately 75% of cases of CNS ATRTs,[1287] although ATRTs based on morphologic criteria with normal expression of *SMARCB1* have been identified.[1288] Rhabdoid cells have the characteristic appearance of an eccentric nucleus, prominent eosinophilic nucleoli, and abundant cytoplasm, with an eosinophilic globular cytoplasmic inclusion (Fig. 57-43).[1289] These cells stain with EMA and vimentin. GFAP and synaptophysin can also be positive.

SMARCB1 (also known as *INI1* or *BAF47*) staining is routinely used to confirm the diagnosis and has become a standard assessment tool for making the diagnosis of ATRT in atypical cases.[1222] The expression of this nuclear protein, which remains expressed in endothelial cells, is characteristically lost in tumor cells (Fig. 57-44). Tumors without the presence of rhabdoid cells but with loss of *SMARCB1* staining are still considered ATRTs.[1288] Whether choroid plexus tumors can have loss of *SMARCB1* expression or whether these tumors represent actual ATRTs is controversial.[1221,1290] ATRTs are classified as WHO grade IV[1289] lesions with an elevated MIB1 labeling index and are composed of primitive neuroepithelial, epithelial, and mesenchymal components. Large areas of small round blue cells can predominate, resulting in the misdiagnosis of medulloblastoma or CNS PNET. In a review of 55 cases from a POG study, the small round blue cell component resembled medulloblastoma,[1291] and ATRT was misclassified as medulloblastoma in more than 50% of cases.[1257] These findings emphasize the need for confirmatory testing with *SMARCB1* immunohistochemical staining or fluorescence in situ hybridization to look

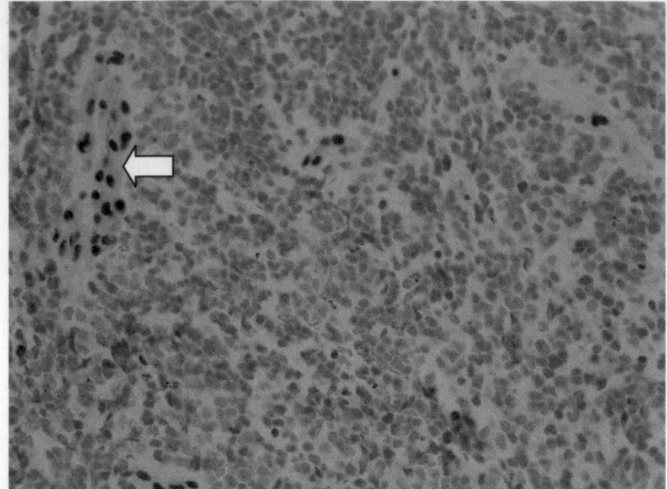

Figure 57-44 An atypical teratoid rhabdoid tumor with absence of switch/sucrose nonfermentable–related, matrix-associated, actin-dependent regulator of chromatin, subfamily b, member 1 (SMARCB1; INI1) immunoreactivity in the tumor cells. Normal endothelial cells within the blood vessels have normal SMARCB1 expression *(arrow;* SMARCB1 immunostaining; ×400).

for monosomy chromosome 22 to help confirm or exclude the diagnosis of ATRT.[1291] Similarly a central pathology review of 227 of 284 eligible infants with brain tumors from a CCG clinical trial for infant patients (trial 9921) showed that ATRT is a significant component of the tumors in this population and that frequent misdiagnoses occur.[962] Given the predominance of *SMARCB1* loss of expression in ATRT, it is now standard practice to evaluate *SMARCB1* expression for treatment stratification onto the appropriate disease-specific protocols.

Management

Multimodality protocols developed for the treatment of medulloblastoma have not been effective for ATRTs. Some success has been achieved by using treatment protocols based on therapy for children with rhabdomyosarcoma[1281,1292] and high-dose myeloablative chemotherapy.[1265,1293,1294] Currently the optimal therapy for pediatric ATRT remains maximal surgical resection, multiagent chemotherapy, and radiation therapy.[1260,1295] Older patients appear to have a better prognosis and, with complete surgical resection, multiagent chemotherapy, and craniospinal radiotherapy, they have 2-year EFS and OS of 78% and 89%, respectively. In contrast children younger than 3 years have a dismal outcome with EFS and OS of 11% and 17%, respectively.[1260] A recent risk-adapted treatment protocol in which patients received maximal surgery, multiagent chemotherapy, both systemic and intrathecal, and focal radiation therapy in children younger than 3 years and CSI in older patients has demonstrated encouraging results. The 2-year EFS and OS in this group of patients, most of whom were younger than 3 years, was 53% and 70%, respectively.[1295] These results indicate that ATRT can be effectively treated and that even patients with metastatic disease can be long-term survivors. The need for radiation therapy in the treatment of ATRT remains

controversial, especially for the youngest patients, although some centers have encouraged its use.[1296] The overall positive outcomes seen in infants treated with 3D-conformal therapy, as well as those treated with high-dose chemotherapy and a stem cell transplantation approach without radiation therapy, suggest that craniospinal radiotherapy is not needed in all patients. The identification of a radiation-resistant CD31-positive stem cell may explain some of the innate resistance of this tumor to current therapies.[1297] It is hoped that the continued discovery of the function of the *SMARCB1* tumor suppressor gene, coupled with an improved understanding of the pathways aberrant in these tumors, will lead to more specific targeted therapies.[1298]

Prognosis

Until recently estimates of survival rates for ATRT ranged from 6 to 11 months.[962,1291,1299,1300] CNS ATRT tumors tend to have specific mutational hotspots in the *SMARCB1 (INI1)* gene,[1301] although treatment response and outcome are not known to be influenced by specific mutations. Although tumors tend to be initially responsive to chemotherapy, recurrence rapidly occurs, both locally and with metastatic disease.[1287] However the prognosis for patients with ATRT may be improved dramatically with intensive multimodality treatment.[1260,1295] Although survival is extremely uncommon, some survivors of relapsed disease have been reported.[1281]

Neurocytomas

Central neurocytomas are rare tumors, comprising between 0.25% and 0.5% of all brain tumors.[1302,1303] First described in 1982 by Hassoun and colleagues, neurocytomas typically occur in adolescents and young adults. These tumors are of neural lineage based on the expression of neuronal markers such as βIII-tubulin, neural cell adhesion molecule, NSE, and synaptophysin.[1304,1305] A gene expression profile comparison of central neurocytoma cells with normal adult VZ progenitors has demonstrated significant overlap, indicating that central neurocytoma is most consistent with proneural cells and that these neurocytoma cells differ from progenitor cells by the increased expression of IGF2 and receptors and effectors of the canonical Wnt signaling pathway and *PDGFR*.[1306] Neurocytomas usually arise in the lateral ventricles, especially in proximity to the third ventricle and foramen of Monro, and are called central neurocytomas. Those localized to the brain parenchyma are called extraventricular neurocytomas. Historically neurocytomas have been frequently described as benign lesions because of the positive outcome of patients with complete surgical resections, although aggressive behavior and poor outcome are not uncommon.[1307,1308] Furthermore numerous reports have been made of tumors with MIB1 labeling indices greater than 3%[1309] and/or atypical histologic features such as increased mitotic activity, vascular proliferation, and/or focal necrosis.[1310] The mean age at presentation in adults is 28 to 29 years, with most patients between the ages of 20 and 40 years,[1302] and a male-to-female ratio of 3:2.[1311] A review of neurocytoma in 60 children younger than 18 years, compiled primarily from reports in the medical literature, has demonstrated a median age of 16 years, with a similar male predominance (61%).[1312]

Clinical Presentation

Most neurocytomas are located in the ventricular system,[1313,1314] specifically the anterior portion of the lateral ventricles near the foramen of Monro, although extraventricular tumors have been described.[1308,1315] Symptoms of raised ICP are common as a result of tumor obstruction of CSF flow at the level of the foramen of Monro or cerebral aqueduct.[1307,1314] Patients with neurocytoma typically present with symptoms including headache, visual changes, nausea, and vomiting.[1316] Focal neurologic deficits are less common presenting signs. Hemorrhage can result in acute symptoms, leading to the diagnosis. Primary disease in the fourth ventricle[1317] or spinal cord has been reported in children.[1318]

Imaging and Histology

The typical MRI appearance of central neurocytoma is that of a well-circumscribed lobulated mass in the anterior portion of the lateral ventricles, making it difficult to distinguish from other intraventricular neoplasms such as ependymomas, astrocytomas, and oligodendrogliomas. Tumors often have an isointense or slightly hypointense signal relative to the cerebral cortex on T1-weighted images and a hyperintense signal on T2-weighted images with enhancement upon administration of gadolinium (Fig. 57-45).[1319-1321] Proton MRS and DWI have recently been described as a possible diagnostic tool in central neurocytoma.[1322] A characteristic MRS appearance of a high choline peak, a low NAA peak, and a glycine peak at 3.55 ppm is seen in a subset of patients.[1323,1324]

Histopathologic analysis of neurocytomas often reveals benign-appearing tissue composed of uniform round cells. Neurocytomas are classified as WHO grade II.[1325] Features such as large fibrillary areas, calcifications, and perivascular pseudorosettes are commonly observed.[1326] Routine hematoxylin and eosin staining of a neurocytoma can reveal the presence of cells with perinuclear halos suggestive of oligodendroglioma. However the reactivity with immunohistochemical staining for neuronal markers such as synaptophysin, βIII-tubulin, neural cell adhesion molecule, and NSE helps establish the diagnosis of a neurocytoma.[1327] As noted earlier atypical forms with mitoses, necrosis, and endothelial proliferation have been reported.[1328,1329] In tumors lacking synaptophysin or Neu-N staining, electron microscopy can assist in confirming the diagnosis.[1330] An MIB1 labeling index is useful for prognostic purposes. Patients with an MIB1 labeling index greater than 2% to 3% are referred to as having atypical neurocytoma and have a worse prognosis for local control and survival.[1309,1310,1328,1329] Subtotal resection, atypical histologic features, and older patient age have been associated with an increased risk of recurrence.[1331,1332]

Management

GTR can be curative for central neurocytomas and is the treatment of choice for pediatric patients.[1333,1334] A review of 73 children younger than 18 years pooled from multiple studies has shown an OS of 100% at 10 years for children who underwent a GTR.[1335,1336] Local failure was demonstrated in approximately 15% of patients who underwent complete resection alone versus 0% in patients who underwent complete resection with adjuvant radiation therapy. However given the absence of survival

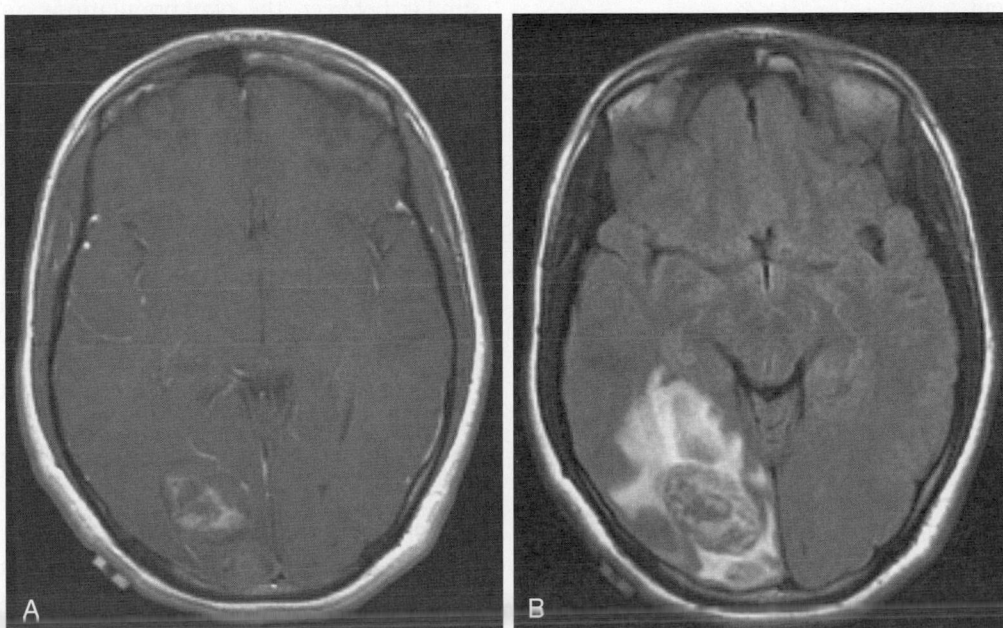

Figure 57-45 Right occipital extraventricular neurocytoma. **A,** An axial T1-weighted image with use of contrast material. **B,** An axial fluid-attenuated inversion recovery image. This tumor is an isointense to hyperintense extraventricular neurocytoma with surrounding edema.

difference and the potential neurocognitive toxicities, adjuvant radiation therapy is not recommended as initial treatment.[1312] Children with incomplete resections have a significantly higher risk of recurrence (mean, 100 months) and a lower OS (82%). Adjuvant radiation therapy has been shown to reduce the risk of recurrence but not the risk of death.[1312] In the case of incomplete resection, radiotherapy may be beneficial at a dose of 5400 cGy,[1337] although it should be noted that the number of patients available for evaluation in these studies is small. Radiotherapy should be more seriously considered for atypical neurocytomas, such as those with a high MIB1 labeling index (higher than 3%). A recent meta-analysis has shown that patients with lesions that have an MIB1 labeling index less than 3% have less than a 15% risk of recurrence and a 95% 5-year OS, compared with 38% and 66%, respectively, for patients with tumors that have an MIB1 labeling index higher than 3%.[1309,1310] In a review of 85 adult and pediatric patients, Rades and colleagues[1338] have demonstrated a marked difference in 5-year survival for incompletely resected atypical neurocytoma (43%). The addition of adjuvant radiation therapy increased 5-year survival rates to 78%. Complete resection was again found to be the best treatment, with 5-year survival rates of 93%. Adjuvant radiotherapy held no additional benefit in cases of completely resected atypical neurocytomas. Stereotactic radiosurgery has been explored as a potential first-line treatment for neurocytoma, but only in limited numbers of adult and pediatric patients,[1339] and it requires careful attention to the radiation therapy margins.[1340] Historically the use of chemotherapy for central neurocytoma has been limited, with only case reports and small case series being reported.[1341] Brandes and associates[1342] have described three adult patients with progressive neurocytoma treated with etoposide, cisplatin, and cyclophosphamide, which led to disease stabilization in two patients and complete remission in one patient.

Prognosis

Complete surgical resection and an MIB1 labeling index of less than 2% are the most important prognostic markers.[1309] Even with extraventricular location and atypical features, most patients will be long-term survivors. Thus judicious use of therapeutic modalities that can lead to significant long-term morbidity, such as radiation therapy, is indicated.

Choroid Plexus Tumors

Choroid plexus tumors usually arise from the epithelium of the choroid plexus in the lateral or fourth ventricles, where the choroid plexus is found. Although choroid plexus lesions represent only 3% of pediatric brain tumors, they comprise 10% to 20% of tumors that develop in the first year of life and account for a considerable percentage of in utero diagnoses.[1343] The median age at diagnosis for choroid plexus tumors is younger than ten years.[1344] Three histologic choroid plexus variants have been described: papillomas, atypical papillomas, and carcinomas.[1345] CPPs outnumber CPCs by a ratio of at least 5:1. Both tumors typically arise in the lateral

ventricles in 50% of cases and in the fourth ventricle in 40% of cases. Tumors arising from multiple ventricles represent only 5% of cases. Because of their rarity, little is known about the molecular abnormalities that give rise to these tumors,[1346] although their strong association with the Li-Fraumeni p53 cancer susceptibility gene is well established.[1347] A significant percentage of choroid tumors will have abnormalities on array comparative genomic hybridization analysis.[889] The presence of normal SMARCB1 staining in these tumors can be used to exclude ATRTs, which share many histologic features with choroid plexus tumors.[1221]

Little is known at present about the developmental or molecular biology of choroid plexus tumors, although a number of markers have been identified using gene array analysis.[1348,1349] Recent findings have implicated the transcription factor, TWIST1, notch3 signaling pathway, and tumor necrosis factor–related apoptosis-inducing ligand.[1350,1351] Patients with Li-Fraumeni syndrome who have a germline mutation of p53 are at increased risk for CPCs.[1347] Epigenetic analysis looking at DNA methylation patterns has shown increased methylation in CPC.[1352] DNA sequences from sporadic papillomas may harbor the human neurotropic JC virus.[916] The role of SV40 (another polyomavirus) in the development of pediatric CNS tumors, particularly ependymomas and choroid plexus, is an interesting one. SV40 sequences have been found in the tumor tissue of up to 50% of patients but not in adjacent areas of normal brain. SV40 is known to induce brain tumors in preclinical models, and SV40 can transform human cells in vitro, which may support a causative role for this polyomavirus in choroid plexus tumors.[917] Polio vaccines used in certain countries in the 1950s and 1960s were contaminated with SV40. In countries that have used uncontaminated vaccines, the identification of SV40 sequences in choroid plexus tumors is rare. However the incidence of choroid plexus tumors is similar between the two populations and thus appears independent of both SV40 exposure and SV40 detection within the tumors.[919,1353] Because of the strong association of Li-Fraumeni syndrome and p53 mutations with CPC, patients need a comprehensive family history to ascertain the incidence of associated cancers and assist in the screening of family members. The presence of a p53 germline mutation may affect the choice of radiation therapy as a therapeutic option and would indicate the need for genetic counseling in other family members.[1347] Additional mutations in the TP53 gene have been discovered that lead to an increased incidence of CPC and can have an impact on the survival of patients with choroid plexus tumors.[1354-1356] The presence of PDGFR expression in a high percentage of cases (87%) is a rationale for the use of targeted inhibitors of this pathway in the context of a clinical trial.[1357]

Clinical Presentation

Initial symptoms are usually secondary to elevated ICP and hydrocephalus and include headaches, nausea, and vomiting, with papilledema. Other possible manifestations include lethargy, seizures, and failure to thrive. Because these tumors tend to arise in infants who retain

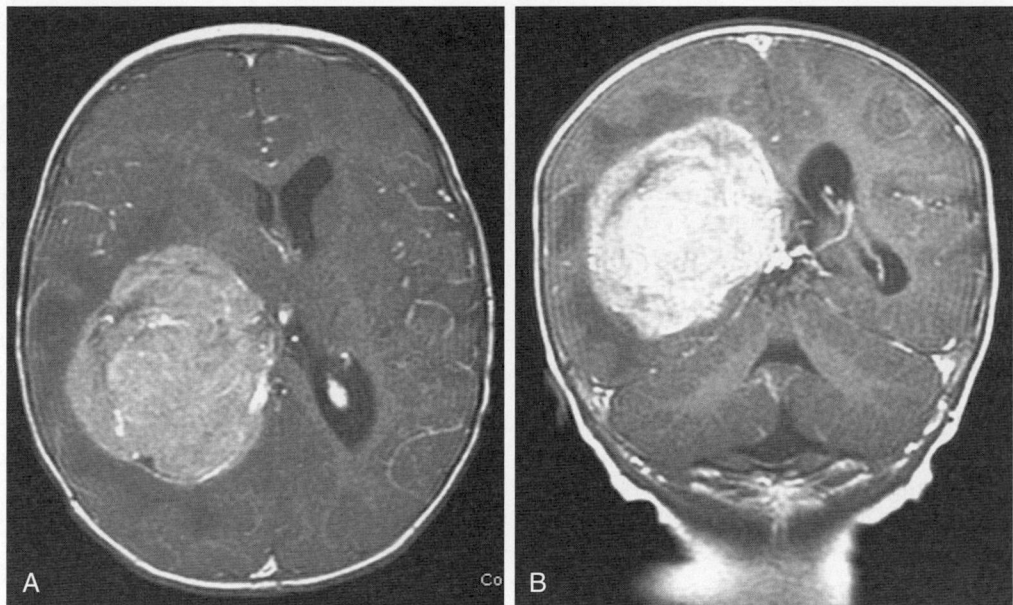

Figure 57-46 Choroid plexus carcinoma. **A,** An axial T1-weighted image with use of contrast material. **B,** A sagittal T1-weighted image with use of contrast material.

open sutures, the presentation may be relatively delayed, and the tumors may reach an exceptional size. Infants typically demonstrate irritability, lethargy, vomiting, a tense fontanelle, and macrocephaly, with splayed sutures. Although most choroid plexus tumors arise in the lateral ventricles, predominantly in infants, fourth ventricular choroid plexus tumors occur in persons of all ages, including adults. Metastatic disease can occur in CPPs, although these patients still have a good prognosis and many of the tumors will not progress. Leptomeningeal dissemination is common with CPCs and is a poor prognostic marker because of the limited use of craniospinal radiation therapy in this very young population. Dissemination through a VP shunt has been reported.[1358]

Imaging and Histology

A choroid plexus tumor should be suspected when a large enhancing tumor in the lateral ventricle is visualized on gadolinium-enhanced MRI (Fig. 57-46). Multilobular, calcified, well-delineated contrast-enhancing intraventricular masses are characteristic of choroid plexus tumors. Tumors are usually isodense on T1-weighted images and bright on T2-weighted images.[1359] CPCs often have more heterogeneous enhancement and edema signal on FLAIR than is routinely seen with CPPs.[1360] Unique characteristics of MRS can differentiate CPP from CPC at diagnosis although, for most patients, this differentiation will not obviate the need for surgery because of the high incidence of CSF flow obstruction in these patients, necessitating neurosurgical intervention.[1361]

CPPs (WHO grade I) have the lowest proliferative rate and are composed of fibrovascular fronds covered by a single layer of epithelial cells. They closely resemble the normal choroid plexus. Cytokeratin, S-100 protein, podoplanin, and vimentin are typically expressed on immunohistochemistry. GFAP, which is typically not seen

in the normal choroid plexus, is found in approximately 25% to 50% of CPPs. In rare cases CPPs can transform into CPCs.[1362] In contrast CPCs (WHO grade III) manifest higher cell density, nuclear pleomorphism, frequent mitoses (more than 5 of 10 high-power fields), high nuclear-to-cytoplasmic ratios, necrosis, and invasive appearance (i.e., blurring of the papillary structures). Up to 20% of CPCs can be positive for GFAP.[1363] Atypical CPPs (WHO grade II) refer to cases in which a CPP has increased mitotic activity. Clear diagnostic criteria for these atypical tumors have not been established. These tumors can possess greater pleomorphism, increased cellularity, and areas of necrosis, but these elements are not required for diagnosis. However it appears that the presence of mitotic activity (2 mitoses or more per 10 high-power fields) is the sole atypical histologic feature independently associated with recurrence.[1363] Atypical CPPs accounted for approximately 15% of all CPPs in one large series.[1363]

Management

After diagnostic neuroimaging studies, high-dose corticosteroids are often administered when elevated ICP or tumor edema is suspected. Because the extent of surgical resection is the single most important factor that determines the prognosis in choroid plexus tumors, the goal of the neurosurgeon is to perform a GTR.[1364] In patients with CPP, complete resection is usually sufficient therapy.[1365] Achieving complete resection may require more than one surgical procedure but appears to improve outcome.[1366] One obstacle to the surgical removal of choroid plexus tumors is the rich vascular network that is often located within the tumor. The choroid plexus receives its blood supply from the anterior and posterior choroidal arteries, branches of the internal carotid artery, and the posterior cerebral artery. Achieving a GTR in cases of CPP and atypical papilloma is often curative, and adjuvant therapy may be deferred after normal results of a restaging evaluation are found.

Because most children diagnosed with CPC are younger than 3 years, chemotherapy is the treatment of choice in those for whom a complete resection cannot be achieved.[1194,1344] Various multiagent chemotherapy regimens have been explored, and preliminary evidence suggests that CPCs are chemosensitive tumors. Currently an International Society for Pediatric Oncology protocol exists that is exploring different chemotherapeutic options. Agents such as carboplatin and etoposide have shown good activity. In addition, intrathecal therapy has been incorporated into treatment with ara-C and etoposide. The role of radiotherapy is controversial and is usually reserved for children older than 3 years who have had a subtotal resection, malignant features within the tumor, or dissemination of the tumor along the neuraxis.

Prognosis

GTR is often curative for CPP. Even in patients with a subtotal resection, 50% of the residual tumor will not demonstrate progression.[1367] The 5- and 10-year PFS and OS rate for patients with papillomas are 81% and 77%, respectively, versus 41% and 35%, respectively, for persons with carcinomas.[1344] Atypical CPP can recur, and thus careful follow-up is needed. The long-term prognosis for this group of patients remains excellent.[1363] Patients with dissemination at diagnosis do less well. Several adjuvant platinum-based chemotherapy regimens have been used with some measure of success,[1368] but at present no standard protocol has been established for CPC. Development of an international protocol for the prospective treatment and outcome of choroid papilloma, atypical CPP, and CPC is under way.

Germ Cell Tumors

CNS GCTs are the most prevalent tumors of the pineal region and represent approximately 3% to 5% of intracranial childhood malignances in the United States. These tumors are much more common in Asia, particularly in Japan.[1369,1370] The reason for this geographic variability is unknown. Most GCTs occur in early adolescence, and males are affected significantly more often than are females.[1371] Males are much more likely to have both pineal and suprasellar GCTs, with a reported male to female ratio of approximately 14:1.[1372] Germinomas are much more common than nongerminomas.[1373] Histologically these tumors resemble the GCTs that arise in the gonads.

Most (95%) GCTs arise in midline sites such as the infundibular region (40%) and pineal region (50%), although 5% arise simultaneously in both regions without an apparent connection.[1374] Occasionally they are isolated to the basal ganglia[1375] but can be approached in a similar fashion to those in the pineal or suprasellar area.[1376] CNS GCTs are presumed to result from the abnormal migration of primitive germ cells early in embryogenesis within the gonadal ridge.[1377,1378] Occasionally metachronous lesions at both sites are detected at the time of diagnosis.[1377,1379] CNS GCTs are divided into

two clinical groups, which reflect sensitivity to cytotoxic therapies—pure germinomas (60%) and NGGCTs (40%).[1369,1380] NGGCTs include yolk sac tumors (endodermal sinus tumors), embryonal carcinomas, choriocarcinomas, immature teratomas, teratomas with malignant transformation, and mixed GCTs. Mixed GCTs are defined as tumors that contain any two of the elements previously listed and can include mixtures of germinoma and nongerminoma. Germinomas are the most common GCT of the pineal region,[1372] although NGGCTs and germinomas arise with equal frequency in the suprasellar region. A male predominance occurs in pineal region tumors, although both genders are equally affected by tumors in the suprasellar region. Mature teratomas of the brain causing significant mass effect have been reported.[1381] Their peak age of occurrence is in the second and third decade of life.

No clear genetic predisposition to CNS GCTs has been identified other than males with Klinefelter syndrome (47XXY).[1382] Of interest a number of CNS GCTs have an abnormal karyotype, including gain of chromosome X, which raises the possibility that patients with Klinefelter syndrome are uniquely at risk because of the presence of their additional X chromosome. A number of cases of GCTs in patients with Down syndrome have also been reported.[1383,1384]

Clinical Presentation

The clinical presentation between suprasellar and pineal region GCTs can differ. Patients diagnosed with suprasellar GCTs often have a long prodrome, often several years in duration.[1385] The earliest symptoms usually involve endocrine dysfunction, most frequently symptoms of diabetes insipidus (DI).[1386] This presenting symptom can also be observed in other lesions of the pituitary region, such as lymphocytic hypophysitis.[1387] In some patients with DI, a mass is not identified on MRI scan but over time a mass becomes evident, leading to the diagnosis. Eventually other endocrine manifestations may occur, such as growth impairment, delayed puberty, and hypothyroidism. Visual loss and symptoms of raised ICP are late manifestations when the tumor has reached appreciable size or spread in a periventricular distribution. Even in patients without MRI evidence of pituitary or hypothalamic involvement of tumor, endoscopic evaluation can often detect subtle areas of tumor.[1388] It is not yet clear whether patients with endoscopically identified regional disease should be considered to have metastatic disease.

Tumors arising in the pineal region often produce headache, nausea, and vomiting because of obstructive hydrocephalus. Limitation of vertical gaze, convergence nystagmus, impaired pupillary reflexes, and double vision may occur because of tectal compression (Parinaud syndrome). Atypical presentations occur when GCTs arise in unusual locations such as the basal ganglia, when they present with widespread leptomeningeal metastases, or when they diffusely infiltrate deep white matter structures.

GCTs can cause precocious puberty because of release of β-human chorionic gonadotropin (β-HCG).[1389,1390] Atypical presentations, such as movement disorders or

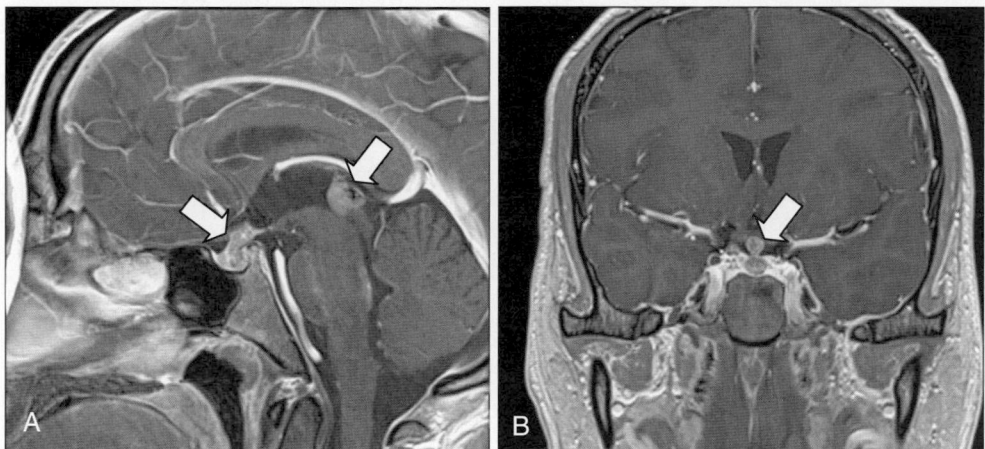

Figure 57-47 Pituitary and pineal germinomas. **A,** A sagittal T1-weighted image with use of contrast material showing two lesions, one in the pituitary and one in the pineal region. A coronal T1 fat-saturated image. **B,** A coronal T1-weighted image with use of contrast material showing the same pituitary/suprasellar lesion.

depression as the presenting symptom, can result in significant delays in diagnosis.[113,1385]

Imaging and Histology

GCTs can have a heterogeneous appearance on CT and MRI and can differ between the pineal and suprasellar regions.[1391] Most are contrast-enhancing solid lesions, with isointense signal on T1-weighted sequences and a bright signal on T2-weighted sequences (Fig. 57-47).[1392] Cysts are commonly observed, especially in nongerminomas.[1393] These signal characteristics overlap with other common tumors of the pineal region and require biopsy or hormone marker analysis for accurate diagnosis.[1380,1394] An important exception is CNS teratoma. These lesions are composed of all three mature tissue elements and therefore will demonstrate calcified areas with adjacent cysts and low-density regions of fat. Areas of bright signal on T1-weighted images, consistent with hemorrhage, are suggestive of choriocarcinoma.[1393]

The NGGCTs are unique among CNS tumors in that they can be diagnosed solely on the basis of expression of tumor markers.[1395,1396] Either β-HCG, a normal product of syncytiotrophoblasts, α-fetoprotein (AFP), a normal product of yolk sac endoderm, or both can be detected in the blood and CSF of patients with NGGCTs. β-HCG is associated with choriocarcinoma, although low levels can also be associated with germinomas. CSF levels tend to be higher than levels in the serum.[1397] AFP is expressed by yolk sac tumors, although low immunohistochemical expression can be observed in some teratomas. Although placental alkaline phosphatase (PLAP) and lactate dehydrogenase isoenzymes and CSF c-kit have been used as markers of germinoma,[1395,1398-1400] immunohistochemical staining for these markers is more commonly used for diagnosis. Because AFP is normally expressed in newborns, considerable attention must be given to interpretation of these levels in infants.[1401]

The histologic identification of CNS GCTs is critical for proper therapeutic assignment and prognostic counseling. Seven major categories are recognized by the WHO.[1402] Clinically mixed GCTs are encountered in most patients, except those with pure germinomas or mature teratomas, and the most malignant component typically dictates the type and intensity of the therapy.

Germinoma is the most common CNS GCT encountered and is considered the equivalent of the testicular seminoma. The appearance of these large cells on hematoxylin and eosin staining, frequent mitoses, and lymphocytic infiltrates is characteristic and can easily be observed on smear preparations. Cells stain brightly for both c-kit and octamer-4.[1403,1404] Placental alkaline phosphatase has been less reliable. SALL4 has been studied as a novel marker and appears sensitive in the diagnosis of CNS GCT.[1405] Even pure germinomas can possess syncytiotrophoblastic giant cells, resulting in low-level expression of β-HCG, which does not upstage their classification to the more malignant choriocarcinoma.[1390]

NGGCT is typically used to refer to one of three different malignant germ cell tumor variants, as well as teratomatous elements with atypical or malignant degeneration. The first, yolk sac tumor (endodermal sinus tumor), is an epithelial tumor that can mimic the appearance of germinomas but highly expresses AFP throughout the cytoplasm. Embryonal carcinoma is an epithelial-derived tumor that has a characteristic appearance with abundant mitoses and diffuse presence of cytokeratin. This latter feature can help differentiate these tumors from germinomas because both can express PLAP and octamer-4. Lastly, choriocarcinoma is a trophoblastic tumor of extraembryonic origin. It requires the identification of cytotrophoblastic elements and syncytiotrophoblastic giant cells. Hemorrhagic necrosis is a common feature of this tumor, and the giant cells stain brightly for β-HCG.

Teratoma refers to a group of three lesions that have evidence of differentiation along the three embryonic germ cell layers—ectoderm, endoderm, and mesoderm:

1. Mature teratoma possesses fully differentiated tissue elements of all three layers. The ectodermal components often contain skin, brain, and/or choroid plexus. The mesodermal component can frequently include cartilage, bone, fat, and/or

muscle, although the endodermal component often contains respiratory or gastrointestinal cysts lined by epithelium. Teratomas usually have an absent or low mitotic index.

2. Immature teratoma is similar to mature teratoma but possesses some elements from one or more of the germ cell layers that are not fully differentiated. Most commonly seen are mitotically active stromal elements or neuroectodermal cells. These immature elements are at considerable risk for malignant degeneration and thus require additional therapy unless a complete resection has been performed.[1406]

3. Teratomas with malignant transformation are rare lesions in which an area of malignant cells of any histologic type is observed. Rhabdomyosarcoma or undifferentiated sarcoma is the most commonly seen, although almost any tumor can occur in the context of teratomas because teratomas already possess all three germ cell layers.[1407]

The diagnosis of an intracranial GCT is suspected in any patient with acquired DI or Parinaud syndrome. Although the location of the primary tumor on neuroimaging studies and certain features of the clinical presentation are supportive of the diagnosis of a CNS GCT, the diagnosis must be confirmed by histology or CSF tumor markers (Table 57-7). Patients with a thickened pituitary stalk with DI are more likely to have an infiltrative tumor process than Langerhans cell histiocytosis or hypophysitis, and the appropriate workup should be initiated.[1408] Histologic confirmation may not be necessary in patients with elevated serum and/or CSF concentrations of tumor markers (AFP or β-HCG) consistent with an NGGCT.[1395,1396]

The tumor markers β-HCG and AFP are useful in not only confirming the presence of a CNS GCT but also in monitoring response to therapy and in suspecting earlier recurrence. Elevation of AFP alone suggests yolk sac (endodermal sinus tumor), whereas a high level of β-HCG suggests choriocarcinoma. Pure germinomas may have modest elevations of CSF β-HCG, usually lower than 50 mIU/mL (100 mIU/mL at some institutions). Lactate

dehydrogenase isoenzymes, the soluble c-kit oncogene product, and PLAP are also detectable in the CSF of patients with a germinoma.[1395,1399,1400] Serum markers of β-HCG at diagnosis can be negative, even in the presence of significantly elevated CSF levels, demonstrating the importance of a comprehensive workup for this patient population, including MRI of the spine and CSF for markers and cytology.[1395,1409] Proper prospective studies using ventricular CSF rather than lumbar CSF have not been completed and therefore should not be used for staging at present.[1116]

Management

Preoperative evaluation should include contrast-enhanced brain and spine MRI, serum and CSF tumor markers (if lumbar puncture can be safely performed), CSF cytology, assessment of endocrine function and visual acuity, and visual field examinations for suprasellar disease. In the absence of elevated lumbar CSF tumor markers, a biopsy should be performed. Aggressive resection leading to morbidity is neither necessary nor advisable in cases of germinoma because of the tumor's exquisite sensitivity to cytotoxic and radiation therapies. Thus less invasive neurosurgical procedures to obtain a tissue sample, such as an endoscopic or stereotactic biopsy, are used more frequently.[1174,1388,1410] A third ventriculostomy is frequently performed at the same time as an endoscopic biopsy in patients with noncommunicating hydrocephalus and a pineal region tumor.[1411] Radical resections of an NGGCT may be easier to accomplish after several courses of chemotherapy.[1412]

Patients with germinomas have a number of nonsurgical treatment options.[1413,1414] With radiation therapy alone for pure germinoma, the 5-year OS rate has approached 90% to 95% in clinical series[1415]; however, radiation therapy alone is inadequate for NGGCT, with 5-year OS ranging from 0% to 30%.[1416,1417] Several new treatment strategies are under investigation in an attempt to minimize some of the late effects of radiation therapy, as seen in long-term survivors of CNS germinomas.[1418] Administering an intermediate radiation dose of

TABLE 57-7   Common Marker Analysis in Central Nervous System Germ Cell Tumors*

Type of Tumor	Placental Alkaline Phosphatase	Oct-4	c-kit	AFP	β-HCG	Cytokeratin	Cerebrospinal Fluid Marker Positivity
Germinoma	+	+	+	−	+	−	c-kit, low level of β-HCG[†]
Yolk sac tumor	−	−	−	+	−	+	AFP
Embryonal carcinoma	−	−	−	−	−	+	−
Choriocarcinoma	−	−	−	−	+	+	β-HCG
Mature teratoma	−	−	−	−	−	−	−
Immature teratoma	−	−	−	−	−	−	−
Teratoma with malignant transformation	−	−	−	−	−	−	−

AFP, α-Fetoprotein; β-HCG, β-human chorionic gonadotropin; Oct-4, octamer-4.
*The common staining patterns provided do not include positive reactions in small subsets of cells.
[†]Germinomas can express low concentrations of β-HCG (50-100 mIU/mL), depending on institutional preference.

approximately 4000 to 5000 cGy encompassing the brain and ventricles is curative treatment for most patients with localized intracranial germinomas. Craniospinal radiation therapy is no longer routinely used for this population. Although whole-brain radiotherapy (WBRT) has been used in the past, whole ventricular fields are now recommended to spare the outer margin of the cortex without increasing the risk of recurrence. Typically 3000 cGy is administered to the whole ventricular region and the primary tumor receives an additional 1500 cGy. This therapy is effective, with 10-year EFS in excess of 90% and distant recurrences such as spinal metastases rarely occurring.[1419] Concurrent pineal and pituitary tumor locations represent regional rather than metastatic disease and can also be adequately treated with whole ventricular radiation therapy.[1420] Like other patients with brain tumors receiving radiation therapy, these children often experience late consequences of radiation therapy, such as cognitive and endocrine deficiencies and radiation therapy–induced secondary tumors.[1418] This outcome has led to the development of treatment regimens using adjuvant chemotherapy followed by response-based radiotherapy to permit a selective reduction in dose (from 4500 to 3000 cGy) in patients whose tumors completely disappear after two to four courses of chemotherapy.[1421-1424] A similar approach has been used with success by the Japanese cooperative group, including an intermediate-risk group of germinomas with elevated β-HCG.[1425] Decreasing the volume from whole ventricle to involved field is not sufficient because a number of failures have been noted with this approach.[1426,1427] The optimal dose and field of radiation and the best combination of chemotherapy are still being investigated and will require further follow-up to confirm efficacy and decreased toxicity. Proton radiation therapy is favored over photon therapy when it is available because efficacy seems equivalent but potential toxicity may be reduced.[1428] In one study attempts at treating patients with chemotherapy alone have demonstrated significant responses but a recurrence rate of approximately 50%.[1429,1430] Although these patients had an excellent salvage rate with radiation therapy, a higher craniospinal dose of 3600 cGy is then required. For this reason chemotherapy alone is not used for germinomas outside of formal clinical trials.

Relapse germinoma is rare, but patients who have a relapse may still respond well to treatment, including additional radiation, chemotherapy, and high-dose chemotherapy with autologous transplant.[356,1431]

For patients with NGGCT, more aggressive chemotherapy, radical tumor resection, and high-dose and high-volume radiotherapy are required for survival.[1421,1432-1435] NGGCTs are highly responsive to chemotherapy, as was seen in one study with 16 of 17 patients achieving a CR or PR with two cycles of cisplatin and cyclophosphamide-based therapy, one third of whom were long-term survivors.[1432] The use of consolidation with high-dose chemotherapy and stem cell rescue is being developed in patients with residual disease[348] and appeared to further improve outcome in a small pilot series.[1106] It is not clear if patients with focal NGGCT require CSI, and this question is currently being evaluated in a large prospective

cooperative group trial. Many patients initially treated with chemotherapy who have progressive disease can undergo salvage therapy with high-dose chemotherapy and craniospinal radiation therapy.[1437] Immature teratomas are classified as NGGCTs but can often be treated with a more conservative approach. A complete resection may be sufficient therapy, and the prognosis is good. Patients with incomplete resection likely require adjuvant therapy.[1406]

After treatment GCTs can demonstrate significant progressive growth on an MRI scan with concurrent clinical decline in the setting of normal tumor markers (β-HCG and/or AFP). Although a nonsecreting germ cell recurrence cannot be excluded, most of these cases represent growing teratoma syndrome.[1438,1439] These lesions are nonmalignant progression of the teratomatous component of lesions that, when resected, will relieve the clinical symptoms.[1438,1440] Patients with growing teratomatous syndrome are not considered to have progressive disease, in spite of the dramatic increase in the size of the lesion on MRI. Neither radiation therapy nor chemotherapy should be discontinued in these patients.

Prognosis

Patients with germinoma have an excellent prognosis because of the tumor's sensitivity to radiation and chemotherapy. For these patients the major treatment challenge is maximizing the quality of life and limiting long-term sequelae of therapy. The COG is currently conducting a randomized phase III study comparing standard radiation therapy alone versus chemotherapy followed by response-dependent reduced-intensity radiation therapy, in which the primary outcome measures are PFS, OS, and quality of life. For patients with germinoma who progress after radiation therapy, many can undergo salvage therapy with high-dose chemotherapy, with or without stem cell transplantation, followed by a higher dose and volume of radiation therapy.[1441,1442] Chemotherapy and radiation therapy for patients not previously treated with radiation therapy can also lead to a high salvage rate.[1437]

Nongerminomas have a less favorable prognosis and thus clinical trials are evaluating conventional multiagent chemotherapy followed by dose-intensive myeloablative chemotherapy and second-look surgery for poor responders, followed by high-dose craniospinal radiation therapy. A small fraction of these patients will respond to high-dose chemotherapy and stem cell rescue,[1442] and long-term survival will improve, particularly if they can be brought back to a state of minimal residual disease.[1443] The response rate of recurrent NGGCT to second-line chemotherapy is poor. Poor prognostic factors in NGGCTs include degree of resection, presence of hemorrhage, and metastases.[1444] A rise in CSF β-HCG can be a sensitive marker of pending relapse and was identified well in advance of elevated levels in the serum.[1397]

Craniopharyngiomas

Craniopharyngiomas are benign nonglial tumors in children and account for 3% to 5% of all pediatric brain tumors, with a peak age ranging between 6 and 14 years.

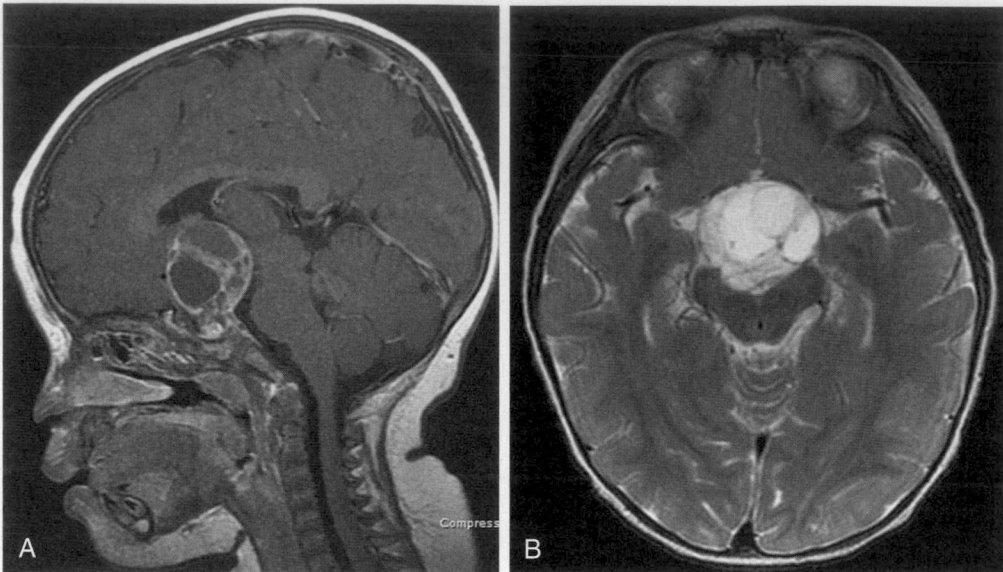

Figure 57-48 Craniopharyngioma with multiple cysts. **A,** A sagittal T1-weighted image with use of contrast material. **B,** An axial T2-weighted image.

These tumors arise from Rathke pouch epithelium and are classified as WHO grade I tumors.[1445] Craniopharyngiomas are slow-growing tumors that arise in the sella and parasellar regions; they are composed of both solid and cystic components, which often extend into the parasellar cisterns and occasionally invade adjacent cortical and vascular structures.[1446] Calcification is a common finding of these lesions,[1447] although it is not pathognomonic for these tumors. Compression of critical intracranial structures can lead to pituitary, hypothalamic, and optic dysfunction. As a result these patients often have complicated medical courses and long-term sequelae. Nigerian and Japanese children appear to have a greater risk for these tumors.[1370,1448] A strong association between β-catenin mutations and adamantinomatous craniopharyngioma has been identified.[1449,1450]

Clinical Presentation

The typical onset of craniopharyngioma is insidious and can extend over several years. The diagnosis is often made in retrospect upon recognizing one or more slowly evolving symptoms, such as progressive visual loss, delay in sexual maturation, growth failure, weight gain, and DI.[1451] Eventually clinical recognition is heralded by a change in mental status as enlargement of the cystic component causes obstructive hydrocephalus. More than 70% of children have growth hormone deficiency, obstructive hydrocephalus, short-term memory deficits, and/or psychomotor slowing at the time of diagnosis. The presenting feature in young adults also includes other symptoms of hypopituitarism, such as galactorrhea or amenorrhea in females and impotence in males. The differential diagnosis of a suspected craniopharyngioma is limited because of the characteristic radiographic findings of these lesions.[1452] Congenital craniopharyngioma associated with a paraneoplastic expression of parathyroid hormone–related protein expression has been reported.[1453]

Imaging and Histology

MRI features (Fig. 57-48) usually include a multicystic and solid enhancing suprasellar mass.[1454] The T1-weighted signal is usually isointense. The chiasm is often stretched over the suprasellar mass and, if dorsal extension is sufficient, hydrocephalus will be apparent.[1455] A classic neuroimaging distinction of craniopharyngiomas from other suprasellar tumors such as a diencephalic glioma or GCT is the presence of calcifications on a noncontrast CT scan. With use of contrast material, the solid components of craniopharyngiomas are usually bright on CT. Transcranial Doppler can also be used in the diagnosis and surveillance of these tumors.[1456]

Histologically craniopharyngiomas are divided into adamantinomatous and papillary subtypes. Adamantinomatous craniopharyngiomas are the more common variant in adults and children and typically consist of cystic and solid areas, with frequent calcifications. Papillary tumors, which are seen almost exclusively in adults, are predominantly solid, without calcification, and are less infiltrative. The cysts seen in craniopharyngioma usually contain a dark liquid with the consistency of machine oil. The diagnosis of adamantinomatous craniopharyngioma requires the presence of squamous epithelium bordered by palisading columnar epithelium.[1445] Gliosis and Rosenthal fibers can be observed but rarely result in misdiagnosis because of the other characteristic features of craniopharyngioma. Palisading columnar cells can have a high MIB1 labeling index rate ranging from 0% to 15%, but this finding does not correlate with a poorer outcome than for patients with a low MIB1 labeling index rate.[1457,1458]

Management

Surgical resection remains the standard approach for craniopharyngioma in many centers, both through an

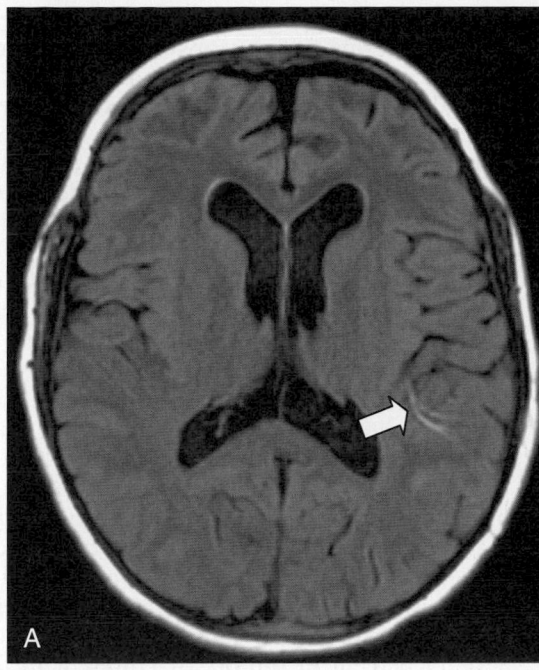
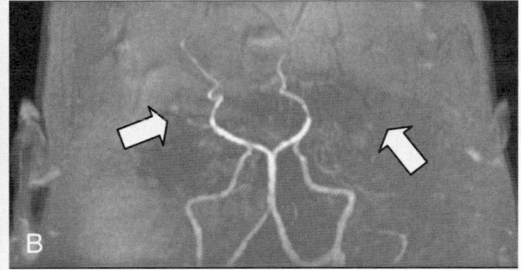

Figure 57-49 Radiation-induced moyamoya disease. **A,** An axial fluid-attenuated inversion recovery image showing the "IVY" sign of slow flow *(arrow)*. **B,** Coronal reconstruction from a maximal intensity projection image from magnetic resonance angiography demonstrating missing lateral vessels *(arrows)*.

open approach and via an endoscopic endonasal approach.[1452,1459,1460] When the child presents with acute raised ICP, the initial management will relate to measures to alleviate this condition with high-dose corticosteroids and monitoring in the intensive care unit. Because patients may have unappreciated panhypopituitarism, baseline hormonal and electrolyte levels should be obtained and the child should be given empiric stress-dose steroids.

Although it is somewhat controversial, a complete microsurgical resection of the entire tumor is the treatment of choice for newly diagnosed craniopharyngiomas.[1461] A multistaged operative approach may be planned, including a combination of transsphenoidal, pterional, and transcallosal approaches, depending on the extent and location of the tumor. Many tumors are adherent to adjacent structures, which will either limit the degree of resection or result in potentially significant postsurgical morbidity.[1446]

Despite the surgical accessibility of many of these tumors, radical resection does not guarantee recurrence-free survival, and the 3-year EFS after a GTR is 60%.[1462] Aggressive resection can result in more extensive hypothalamic deficiencies and visual complications,[1459,1463] even in patients without evidence of hypothalamic involvement at diagnosis.[1464] Careful management of DI can be required immediately after surgical resection in these patients,[1465] which may lead to a permanent condition. Postoperative behavioral sequelae include altered regulation of appetite and weight control, impulsivity, hypersexuality, and changes in memory.

An alternative treatment strategy for the long-term control of craniopharyngiomas is subtotal resection[1466] followed by high-dose radiotherapy of the involved field.[1467-1469] Whether this approach is superior in terms of tumor control and preservation of quality of life remains to be established, but several studies have reported comparable or even improved PFS and OS statistics in retrospective, uncontrolled institutional series.[1462,1470-1473] In patients with recurrent craniopharyngioma, an attempt at a complete resection can be considered, although the need for focal radiation therapy will be required for most of these patients. Proton therapy, based on the lack of an exit dose, is considered the preferred method of radiation therapy if it is available locally.[1474,1475] Long-term complications of radiation therapy include secondary malignancies, optic neuropathy, and vascular injury leading, rarely, to moyamoya disease (Fig. 57-49).[85,1476-1478] The recent identification of the BRAF V600E activating mutation in almost all papillary craniopharyngiomas, which are usually seen in adults,[1479] offers this patient population the option of targeted therapy.[1480] The adamantinomatous subtype, which is found predominantly in children and is characterized by mutations in B-catenin, will need to await development of improved inhibitors of this pathway.

A temporizing approach to control the cystic components of the tumor is the intracystic instillation of sclerosing agents such as bleomycin or phosphorus-32.[1481-1483] The use of intralesional bleomycin has also been shown to help delay the need for aggressive surgery or radiation therapy, although prospective clinical trials of this approach are needed.[1484] This procedure has the risk of leakage of the bleomycin from the cyst into adjacent brain tissue and should be reserved for patients for whom all other management approaches have failed.[1485] However the solid tumor usually continues to grow and make new cysts, thus making subsequent resections more difficult. In addition subsequent external beam radiotherapy treatment planning may be difficult because of the unpredictable dosimetry of ^{32}P.[1482] Recently pegylated interferon alpha 2b has been used to stabilize cystic progression in patients with craniopharygioma.[1486]

Recurrent or progressive craniopharyngiomas may be treated with surgery, radiosurgery, fractionated radiotherapy, or chemotherapy. Responses to chemotherapy have been reported with interferon, vinblastine, cisplatin, pegylated interferon,[1487] and other agents,[1471,1488-1493] although well-designed studies to test different agents for craniopharyngioma are lacking.[1494]

Prognosis

The most important factors that correlate with PFS are the extent of resection and postoperative radiation therapy. Larger tumors and those with cysts are more likely to recur.[1495] In a surgical series, recurrence or progression occurred in 7% to 15% of cases after total resection and in 50% of cases after subtotal resection.[1496] The recurrence rate of 15% is observed when subtotal resection is followed by radiation therapy.[1497] The outcomes between adult and pediatric patients does not appear to be different.[1498] Recurrences along the surgical tract have been reported but are thought to be related to the procedure rather than representing metastatic disease and are treated with surgery and focal irradiation, if needed.[1499] Unfortunately many long-term survivors experience significant morbidity related to panhypopituitarism,[1500] cognitive impairment, sleep pattern disturbance, and obesity.[1498,1501-1505] Growth hormone deficiency is present in 100% of patients,[1506] but the early use of growth hormone in these patients is not thought to be contraindicated.[1507,1508] Although narcolepsy is uncommon,[1509] control of weight and regulation of sleep can be difficult because their circadian rhythms are disrupted and melatonin production is severely diminished.[1510] The use of stimulants has been investigated, with preliminary positive results,[1511] although clear efficacy for these interventions is lacking.[1512-1514] Although still in the early stages, attempts to regulate obesity in these patients have also demonstrated some success.[1515] Finally, psychosocial problems can be significant in this patient population, and a comprehensive team approach is beneficial.[1516]

Infant Tumors

Infants and young children with brain tumors present specific therapeutic challenges because of the morbidity associated with current treatment strategies. As a group infants and young children with brain tumors have poor outcomes, with 5-year EFS and OS rates as low as 19% and 25%, respectively.[1517] This poor prognosis can be related to unique characteristics of the tumors in this age group, as well as the significant limitations with regard to therapy. Evidence from numerous sources has suggested that neural development extends from the embryonic period through adolescence and is especially prominent during the first 3 years of life, making young children most susceptible to neurotoxic insults.[1518] These findings are in keeping with early observations that the

most devastating consequences of radiotherapy in children, in terms of neuropsychological sequelae, were greatest in children younger than 3 years.[1519] Although early observations have led to the arbitrary age limit of 3 years as the cutoff for introduction of radiation therapy, numerous subsequent studies have shown that even older children can experience cognitive, endocrine, behavioral, and many other medical problems after undergoing radiation therapy.[1520,1521] Consequently several strategies have emerged to delay or eliminate radiotherapy through the use of chemotherapy in an attempt to preserve cognitive, neurologic, and endocrine function in younger children.[1522,1523]

A significant proportion of pediatric brain tumors occur in infants and young children. Data from the Childhood Brain Tumor Registry of the United States from 2000 to 2004 have shown that approximately 28% of childhood brain tumors occur in children younger than 4 years[1524] and 18% of brain tumors occur in children younger than 2 years.[1525] Tumor location in infants and young children is different from that in the older child, with a predominance of supratentorial tumors.[1525-1527] Seventy percent of tumors that present in the first week of life are also located supratentorially[1528] compared with 56% for the pediatric population.[1529] The male to female ratio in this age group is also different in that there is a lower male predominance in this age group[1526] when compared with childhood brain tumors overall. Histopathologic subtypes in infants and young children are also different from those in the older child, but accurate determination of this difference has been difficult because early epidemiologic data collected by the traditional data collection agencies such as the SEER registry and National Brain Tumor Registry did not have standardized histologic subtype information. For example PNET was not previously recognized as a separate entity in the SEER Registry. In the large cooperative groups brain tumors were categorized differently, and thus the POG excluded medulloblastoma from PNET protocols, although the CCG routinely included medulloblastoma in PNET protocols.[1522] The distribution of tumor types treated in the infant POG clinical trial ("Baby POG") was medulloblastoma, followed by ependymoma, PNET, and malignant glioma.[1530] However in a review of 1289 patients aged younger than 1 year reported in the literature, astrocytoma was the most common diagnosis, comprising 31% of cases (of which 75% were low grade and 25% were reported as high grade), followed by medulloblastoma at 12%, ependymoma at 11%, choroid plexus tumors at 11%, sPNET at 7%, and teratoma at 5%.[1526] Astrocytoma and medulloblastoma remain the most common in the young age group, although a peak of ependymoma is seen within the first 2 years of life, along with an increased incidence of PNET.[1517] A recent analysis of the SEER database has revealed that the incidence of brain tumors in infants and young children has remained stable since 1986. The most common histologies in the dataset were glioma, medulloblastoma, and sPNET and ependymomas.[1531]

Two important histologic diagnoses in infants include teratomas and ATRTs, which account for 4.9% and

0.3%, respectively, of infant brain tumors.[1526] Briefly, ATRT is a rare tumor of childhood (see the earlier section on ATRT), which has only recently been recognized as a separate entity; 75% of these tumors carry a unique chromosome 22q11.2 cytogenetic abnormality.[1291] An initial description of malignant rhabdoid tumors of the kidney,[1532] followed by the description of the simultaneous appearance of renal and CNS tumors with similar histologic features,[1533] eventually resulted in the recognition that this unique histology represents a separate entity.[1257,1300] ATRT primarily affects young children at a mean age of 17 to 24.5 months, with 75% occurring in children younger than 3 years.

Clinical Presentation

The clinical presentation of brain tumors in infants and young children is most often associated with the symptoms of obstructive hydrocephalus, which in this age group manifests as persistent vomiting, irritability, lethargy, abnormal gait and coordination difficulties, failure to thrive, bulging and splayed fontanelles, seizures, and loss of developmental milestones. In a meta-analysis of 13 studies reported in the literature consisting of 332 children younger than 4 years presenting with intracranial tumors, increasing head circumference and macrocephaly was reported as the most common presentation (41%). Other presentations included focal motor weakness, head tilt, squint, abnormal eye movements, altered levels of consciousness, and hemiplegia.

Management

The historic approach to treating infants and young children with brain tumors had focused on the use of surgery and radiation. In the late 1960s serious functional and neurocognitive sequelae that were incompatible with a normal productive life, especially for children younger than 2 years, were recognized.[1519] As a result several different strategies to delay or exclude radiotherapy from the treatment of young children with brain tumors were developed and were centered on the use of chemotherapy.[1522,1523,1534,1535] van Eys and coworkers[1536] (1985) treated 12 young children with medulloblastoma using mechlorethamine, Oncovin (vincristine), procarbazine, and prednisone chemotherapy without radiotherapy and found that 8 of 12 patients were long-term survivors. This strategy led to other clinical trials, including those investigated by the POG, which worked on the premise of giving chemotherapy until the child achieved an age at which radiotherapy was accepted as less detrimental and its benefits could still be realized.[1522,1523] The "Baby POG" protocol, initiated in 1986, enrolled 198 children, 132 of whom were younger than 24 months, who were treated with chemotherapy for 2 years, and an additional 66 children between the ages of 24 and 36 months were enrolled, who received chemotherapy for 1 year prior to receiving radiotherapy.[1530] Chemotherapy consisted of two 28-day cycles of cyclophosphamide plus vincristine followed by one 28-day cycle of cisplatin and etoposide; these cycles were given for 1 or 2 years, depending on the age of the child at diagnosis or until there was disease progression, after which radiotherapy was administered.

After two cycles of cyclophosphamide and vincristine, 39 of 109 evaluable patients showed a CR or PR, although patients with brainstem glioma and PNET did poorly. The PFS at 1 year for children diagnosed between the ages of 24 to 36 months and PFS at 2 years in children diagnosed at younger than 24 months were 41% and 39%, respectively. The 5-year PFS was reported as 30% ± 5%, and the 5-year OS was 39% ± 4%. The single most important predictor of survival was the degree of surgical resection, because children with a GTR had a 5-year OS of 62% ± 7% compared with those with a subtotal resection, whose 5-year survival was only 31% ± 5%. Of great importance in this landmark study was its demonstration that a small subset of children could achieve disease control without radiotherapy, and that even a delay of 1 or 2 years did not adversely affect outcome in all patients.[1522,1523,1534] Other study groups have adopted a similar approach of delaying radiotherapy through use of chemotherapy. The national CCG-9921 clinical trial for infants with medulloblastoma, CNS PNET, and ependymoma used upfront chemotherapy for 1 year followed by focal radiotherapy to the involved site or craniospinal radiotherapy.[1537] This was an "8-drugs-in-1-day" clinical trial that included 46 children with medulloblastoma who were younger than 18 months at the time of diagnosis, most of whom had gross total resections and were able to avoid radiotherapy; 22% were progression-free at 3 years.[1537] The German Pediatric Brain Tumor Study Group pilot tested an intensive chemotherapy regimen consisting of procarbazine, ifosfamide, cisplatin, cytarabine, vincristine, and high-dose methotrexate for children to delay or avoid radiotherapy (trial HIT-SKK87). A direct comparison to the results of Baby POG cannot be made because the results of HIT-SKK87 have not yet been published. The United Kingdom Children's Cancer Study Group piloted a Baby Brain protocol in 1989 using weekly alternating cycles of myelosuppressive and nonmyelosuppressive chemotherapy consisting of vincristine and carboplatin, vincristine and methotrexate, vincristine and cyclophosphamide, and cisplatin to delay or avoid radiotherapy. Although only 28 children were treated with the protocol, the 4-year OS was 35%.[1538]

The overall results of these "Baby" chemotherapy protocols were thus somewhat disappointing, with EFS rates of 20% to 40%, although the ability to defer radiation therapy in this patient population was an important advance. Given the high response rate for infants treated according to these protocols, strategies centered on high-dose chemotherapy with ASCR were developed to improve the response rates already being observed.[728,1535] The French Society of Pediatric Oncology used this approach of high-dose chemotherapy with autologous bone marrow rescue (ABMR) in their BBSFOP protocol in an attempt to extend survival of young children with relapsed or progressive disease who received conventional chemotherapy. Twenty children (median age, 23 months) with medulloblastoma in whom progressive disease developed while they were treated with conventional chemotherapy were then treated with high-dose busulfan and thiotepa followed by ASCR. Of these patients 75% demonstrated a radiographic response to chemotherapy.

For patients with initial local relapses only, an EFS rate of 50% and a median survival rate of 39.5 months were achieved.[1539] A follow-up report of this study demonstrated a 69% 5-year OS in patients with local relapse while eliminating the need for craniospinal radiotherapy in 30% to 50% of patients. The need for a complete resection limits use of this strategy for many patients, especially those with metastatic disease.[1534]

Another chemotherapy-based approach has been the "Head Start" protocols, in which conventional induction chemotherapy followed by high-dose chemotherapy with autologous stem cell transplantation is used in the newly diagnosed setting to delay or defer radiation therapy in infants and young children. "Head Start I" consisted of five induction cycles of cisplatin, vincristine, etoposide, and cyclophosphamide. After this treatment patients with no radiologic evidence of disease, or after second-look surgery or reresection of tumor, underwent myeloablative therapy with carboplatin, thiotepa, and etoposide with ABMR. Radiotherapy was deferred in patients who achieved complete remission. Of 62 children enrolled (median age, 30 months), 37 patients proceeded to ABMR, of whom 15 patients were free of disease and required no further treatment; this outcome resulted in a 3-year EFS and OS of 40% and 25%, respectively. Seven deaths occurred as a result of treatment-related complications. These results are similar to those noted earlier and again demonstrate that a subset of patients can be effectively treated with chemotherapy and avoid radiotherapy.[1540] Head Start II further intensified the induction regimen with the addition of high-dose methotrexate for the patients with the highest risk, specifically patients with high-risk tumors (nonmedulloblastoma) or those presenting with evidence of metastatic spread. A total of 21 patients with disseminated medulloblastoma were treated, 17 of whom had a CR yielding a 3-year EFS and OS of 49% and 60%, respectively.[1153] In this cohort of patients, 13 had a GTR and 10 patients received radiotherapy as part of their upfront or salvage therapy; six patients avoided radiotherapy altogether. For patients with CNS PNETs, this approach appears to confer an improved 5-year EFS and OS of 39% and 49%, respectively.[1249] Patients with nonpineal CNS PNET fared better than those with pineal-based tumors, although metastatic disease at diagnosis, age, and extent of resection were not significant prognostic factors; 60% of survivors were able to avoid radiotherapy. In contrast, this approach has not demonstrated equivalent results for patients with ependymoma with an estimated 5-year EFS and OS of 12% and 38%, respectively, with younger age as the only significant prognostic factor.[969] In this cohort of 29 children with ependymoma, 22 were younger than 36 months and only 8% of patients were radiation-free at 5 years.

To further increase chemotherapy dose intensity, other investigators have followed induction chemotherapy with tandem cycles of high-dose chemotherapy with stem cell rescue. In a small series of 15 infants between 4 and 38 months old with varied histologies, including five medulloblastomas, four CNS PNETs, five malignant gliomas, and one ependymoma, patients were treated with induction chemotherapy. This treatment consisted of three cycles of cisplatin, cyclophosphamide, and etoposide followed by three cycles of tandem high-dose therapy with carboplatin and etoposide and ASCR.[1541] Although the follow-up period was short, the 2-year PFS and OS rates of 52% and 72%, respectively, is encouraging. Furthermore, of the 10 patients who were alive, only five received local radiotherapy, and only one patient with M1 stage medulloblastoma received craniospinal radiotherapy.[1541] Similar results have also been reported by the French Society for Pediatric Oncology in a small series of seven patients with medulloblastoma and CNS PNET using high-dose therapy with busulfan and melphalan.[1542] Although three patients received additional treatment with thiotepa and two patients received additional treatment with topotecan, all patients were able to avoid radiotherapy. The PFS was 71% ± 17%, although longer follow-up will be needed.

With regard to the long-term benefits of adjuvant chemotherapy strategy of delaying or deferring radiotherapy, authors of one infant study evaluated their neuropsychological outcomes in a follow-up report. Of the six children who did not receive radiotherapy, all had intelligence quotient (IQ) scores within the normal range, with a mean of 101, although the five children who had received radiation therapy had lower IQs, with a mean of 85 at 5.8 years and a continued decline to a mean of 63 by 10 years.[1543]

In addition to the use of intensive chemotherapy to defer or omit radiation therapy, radiation techniques themselves have also been optimized in attempts to minimize long-term morbidity. This optimization includes the administration of involved field radiation for infants with brain tumors[291,1130,1535] and the use of proton beam radiation therapy.[261,1544] The Pediatric Brain Tumor Consortium also completed a pilot study to assess the feasibility of adding intrathecal mafosfamide to multisystemic chemotherapy followed by conformal radiation therapy.[291] This study included 93 newly diagnosed infants with embryonal CNS tumors and resulted in a 5-year OS rate of 51% ± 11%.

Specific Management Issues in Infants and Young Children

A more detailed description of the diagnosis and management of individual disease categories was provided earlier, but management issues specific to infant tumors are described here.

Infant Medulloblastoma. Despite significant improvements in the treatment of standard-risk medulloblastoma in older children, the outcome of infants and young children with medulloblastoma remains poor, mainly because of limitations in the use of radiotherapy to the developing brain, increased risk of metastatic disease at presentation, and difficulty in achieving a complete surgical resection in infants.[1545] Although the strategies of delayed radiotherapy with chemotherapy and intensification of treatment with stem cell rescue have shown some promising results in infants and young children, the small number of patients, heterogeneous histologies, and varied staging limit their immediate widespread adaptation.[1153,1541,1542] Salvage therapy in infants and young children has also been shown to be feasible in up to 50% of patients but requires the use of radiotherapy. Thus some cognitive impact and compromise will be required in these patients if disease control is to be achieved with this modality.[1546] Attempts at reduction in radiotherapy dose to reduce neurodevelopmental damage can significantly compromise OS.[1547] Alternative therapeutic strategies are therefore needed in the treatment of medulloblastoma of the infant and young child.

With increasing understanding of the biology of medulloblastoma, it has been recognized that the frequency of different histologic subgroups varies with different stages of development. The nodular-desmoplastic subtype of medulloblastoma occurs most frequently in infants and young children and has been found to be most frequently associated with the SHH subtype and is associated with favorable prognosis.[1548] It has also been reported that children younger than 3 years of age who have nodular-desmoplastic medulloblastoma have a high frequency of germline mutations in the negative regulator of SHH pathway signaling, SUFU.[1549] Although SHH-positive desmoplastic medulloblastomas also occur in adults, those that occur in infants have been found to be molecularly distinct to their adult counterparts.[1550] Desmoplasia is not prognostic in the adult tumors, which have an inferior outcome compared with those that occur in infants.

The incorporation of high-dose methotrexate in chemotherapy regimens has been investigated. In the German HIT-SKK study, intrathecal methotrexate and systemic methotrexate were administered to 43 children younger than 3 years who had medulloblastoma, including 26 patients with M+ disease. The 5-year OS for patients with completely resected tumors, residual tumor, and macroscopic metastases was 93% ± 6%, 56% ± 14%, and 38% ± 15%, respectively, an improvement compared with historic control subjects.[1097] Only 38% of survivors received radiotherapy. Of note desmoplastic histology was highly predictive of good outcome, with an OS of 95% ± 4% versus an OS of 41% ± 11% for patients with classic histology; histology was found to be an independent prognostic marker, along with age younger than 2 years. Although outcomes for children with localized disease or favorable histology was excellent without the use of radiation therapy, the poor outcomes of patients with metastatic disease or unfavorable histology led to the inclusion of involved-field radiation therapy to this treatment protocol.[1551] High-dose methotrexate has also been investigated in the "Head Start II" protocol and was shown to be particularly effective for young patients with high-risk medulloblastoma.[1153] The major concern with the use of methotrexate is that this agent has been associated with white matter changes on MRI, especially when methotrexate is administered after radiation therapy.[1552,1553] In spite of this finding the use of methotrexate continues to be investigated, given the overall poor prognoses for this subset of patients. Stratification of risk groups through better histologic diagnosis, together with an improved understanding of the biology of medulloblastoma, may help improve survival in this age group.[1545,1554]

A recent study that included a cohort of 12 patients with medulloblastoma assessed outcomes of infants and very young children treated with surgery, with adjuvant high-dose chemotherapy followed by proton beam radiation.[1544] Longer-term follow-up of this cohort is required to document both survival outcomes and long-term morbidity. In COG study P9934, children were treated with induction chemotherapy after surgery, followed by age- and response-adapted conformal radiation therapy to the posterior fossa and maintenance chemotherapy.[1130] Four-year EFS and OS were 50% ± 6% and 69% ± 5.5%, respectively. Consistent with other infant studies, children whose histologies were desmoplastic medulloblastoma had superior outcomes compared with those without desmoplasia. Of note the children who experienced recurrence after administration of conformal radiation therapy had progression of their disease outside the radiation field.

Infant CNS PNETs and Pineoblastoma. CNS PNET is a neuroepithelial tumor similar to medulloblastoma but with a significantly worse prognosis.[1210,1555] The most recent WHO classification clarifies the nomenclature of this heterogeneous group of tumors. It was traditionally referred to as sPNET and is now called CNS PNET, not otherwise specified, and includes biologically similar tumors that can also be found in the brainstem and spinal cord.[207] Even though medulloblastoma and CNS PNET are classified together as embryonal tumors, cytogenetic[1238,1239] and molecular evidence from microarray analyses[1079] suggests that biologic differences exist between these tumors. Pineoblastomas are also tumors of embryonal origin with a clinically aggressive course.[1187]

CNS PNETs are the fourth most common brain tumors of infants[1526] and account for approximately 10% of all brain tumors occurring in children younger than 3 years.[1556] It is also the most common malignant brain tumor in the first year of life[1525] and, according to SEER data, has a dismal OS of 19% in this age group.[1517] In a national clinical trial, POG 8633, 13 patients with nonpineal CNS PNET who were younger than 3 years were treated. These patients presented with large, well-demarcated tumors with limited edema. In this study CNS PNET was the most common supratentorial tumor in this age group. Presenting symptoms included seizures, nausea, vomiting, lethargy, irritability, headache, focal motor weakness, and increased head circumference; 12 of 13 subjects had symptoms for less than 1 month at the time of presentation.[1557] For unknown reasons, younger children with CNS PNETs and pineoblastomas present with more aggressive disease and a higher frequency of leptomeningeal disease.[1558,1559] Whether this manifestation is inherent to the biology of the disease or related to clinical factors remains controversial. In a retrospective review of 50 patients with CNS PNET, metastatic disease at diagnosis, extent of initial resection, and tumor site did not affect OS, although it was affected by age younger than 2 years and the use of radiotherapy and chemotherapy.[1216] Similar findings were also reported in 46 patients with CNS PNET registered in the CCG-9921 study; treatment regimen, M stage, extent of resection, and age were not found to be significant prognostic factors.[962] In contrast in the "Baby POG" study, 28 patients with CNS PNET, including 11 with pineoblastoma, were treated, all of whom received chemotherapy and delayed radiotherapy.[1522] This study showed a considerable difference in the 3-year survival between the four patients in whom GTR was achieved (100% survival) compared with the nine patients with a subtotal resection (11% survival). Authors of this study also concluded that chemotherapy did not provide benefit.[1522] No benefit from chemotherapy was seen in the French BBSFOP protocol for 25 patients with supratentorial embryonal tumors, which included 17 patients with CNS PNET treated with chemotherapy in order to delay or omit radiotherapy. Of the five patients with CNS PNET who survived, four underwent salvage therapy with high-dose chemotherapy and/or surgery and radiotherapy.[1560] Results from the Head Start studies have also suggested a benefit from intensification of chemotherapy because 60% of this cohort of 43 patients with CNS PNET avoided radiotherapy and achieved an estimated 5-year EFS and OS of 39% and 49%, respectively.[1249] Interestingly metastasis at diagnosis, age, and extent of resection were not significant factors, although numbers were small and the interpretation of individual subgroups is limited.

Pineoblastoma in infants has been associated with a dismal outcome. In the "Baby POG" study 11 patients were treated, ranging from 1 to 35 months (eight patients were younger than 12 months), and all patients had local recurrences, the majority with metastatic disease. All children died 4 to 13 months from the time of diagnosis, despite the use of radiotherapy in six patients.[1194] Similar dismal results have been reported in the CCG 921 protocol in which eight infants with predominantly nonmetastatic, subtotally resected tumors all had progression of their disease within 3 to 14 months (median, 4 months), with a median time to death of 10 months.[1561] Similarly five children younger than 3 years with pineoblastoma, treated according to the German Pediatric Oncology Group HIT-SKK87 and HIT-SKK92 protocols, all had progression of their disease within 6 months and had a median overall survival of 0.9 year.[1558] Although there have been reports of better survival rates in patients with pineal region PNETs, these patients tended to be older and more often received radiotherapy.[1192,1561]

A treatment strategy for infants and young children with CNS PNETs may involve intensification of treatment, as demonstrated by the "Head Start I and II" experience in which 5-year EFS and OS rates of 39% and 49%, respectively, were achieved.[1249] High-dose chemotherapy and ASCR have also been reported to be successful in a series of newly diagnosed children and adults, which included two infants who avoided radiotherapy. The 4-year PFS and OS rates of 69% and 71%, respectively, were observed.[1562] In contrast the German HIT-SKK87 and HIT-SKK92 studies had PFS and OS rates of only 15% and 17%, respectively, for 29 children between the ages of 3 and 37 months who were treated with chemotherapy to delay radiotherapy. A positive impact on survival was seen in patients who were able to achieve complete resection and those who received radiother-

apy.[1563] The use of radiotherapy in some of these patients may improve survival, but radiation therapy diminishes the quality of survivorship.[1564] Findings from the CCG 921 study showed that all children with CNS PNET who received radiotherapy and were younger than 9 years experienced significant developmental delays.[1561] The current recommendations for infants with CNS PNETs include maximal safe surgery, multiagent chemotherapy, consideration of high-dose chemotherapy with stem cell rescue, and focal 3D conformal radiation therapy, if permitted by the field size and tumor location.

Infant Ependymoma. Ependymoma is the third most common tumor of infants and young children and the second most common CNS malignancy in children younger than 3 years who are referred for treatment.[1530] Approximately 43% of ependymomas occur in children younger than 2 years.[1233,1517] Unlike adult ependymoma, most ependymomas in infants and young children occur intracranially and, unlike other infant brain tumors, are predominantly infratentorial.[1565] Negative prognostic factors from several studies have demonstrated the importance of the extent of resection (less than GTR or biopsy) and young age (younger than 3 years at diagnosis).[981,1566,1567] Another prognostic factor that has been reported includes anaplastic histology. However the heterogeneity of anaplasia seen in tumors and the differences in the diagnostic criteria for anaplastic histology by pathologists, which have ranged from 7% to 89%, have made a full prognostic assessment of this factor difficult.[943] An MIB1 or Ki-67 index rating of 20 or higher[1568] may also be a negative prognostic marker.[1569] Although the 5-year OS for children with ependymoma has been estimated at 55% to 66%,[976,978] the 5-year survival for infants and young children remains around 25% and is worse if radiotherapy is delayed or a complete resection is not achieved.[963] The role of chemotherapy remains controversial in this population, even though cisplatin is an active agent against ependymoma.[1570] Several studies incorporating chemotherapy have shown lack of efficacy,[1570] including those with dose escalation such as in "Head Start."[969] In the "Head Start III" protocol, which consisted of maximal surgical resection followed by five cycles of induction chemotherapy with a myeloablative consolidation, excellent outcomes were reported only for infants with supratentorial ependymomas. Infants with infratentorial ependymomas had poor outcomes in the absence of radiation therapy.[1571] POG study 9233 ("Baby POG 2") reported improvement in PFS in infants with ependymoma after the administration of dose-intensified chemotherapy, but no difference in OS was observed.[968]

The importance of radiotherapy in the treatment of ependymoma has been clearly established, and stereotactic radiation therapy administration has been demonstrated to be safe and effective.[461] A phase II study of conformal radiotherapy treating 88 young children, many of whom were younger than 18 months (after chemotherapy and maximal surgical resection were completed), yielded a PFS of 75% + 6% and reduced early neurocognitive deficits, even though younger patients received 5400 cGy of conformal radiotherapy, supporting the use of the modality in these patients.[951] Although long-term neurocognitive follow-up of this younger population is not yet known, this study formed the basis for the COG clinical trial of conformal radiotherapy, including short-duration chemotherapy in the subset of patients who achieved only subtotal resections. A previous CCG clinical trial (study 9942), in which children with incompletely resected ependymoma received upfront chemotherapy before radiation therapy, has also been completed. Experience from the United Kingdom Children's Cancer Study Group–International Society of Pediatric Oncology collaboration for patients with ependymoma has suggested some benefit from the administration of alternating courses of nonmyelosuppressive chemotherapy with myelosuppressive chemotherapy in patients with incomplete resections who do not have metastatic disease.[1572] In this series of 89 children younger than 3 years, in which nine patients had metastatic disease, preirradiation chemotherapy resulted in a 5-year EFS and OS of 42% and 63%, respectively. In addition the 5-year cumulative incidence of freedom from radiotherapy was 42% in the nonmetastatic cohort. Also patients who received the highest dose intensity had a 5-year OS of 76% compared with those with the lowest dose intensity, who had a 5-year OS of 52%.[1572] All patients with metastatic disease in this study experienced a relapse, and the 5-year OS in this group was approximately 25%.[1572] The outcome of patients with metastatic disease at presentation compared with those with localized disease has ranged from no difference in outcome[963,978] to relapse and death in all patients within 2 years of surgery.[1573] Fortunately fewer than 10% of patients with ependymoma present with metastatic disease, although this rate is slightly higher in infants.[963,978] In a retrospective meta-analysis of prognostic factors of 40 patients with metastatic ependymoma, including 29 children younger than 3 years, those in whom GTR was achieved had the best 5-year EFS and OS of 35% ± 13% and 59% ± 13%, respectively, compared with the 5-year EFS and OS of 25% ± 9% and 32% ± 10%, respectively, for those who did not have GTR.[1574] The EFS for patients who received radiotherapy was 57% ± 19%, and it was 40% ± 22% for those who received combined chemoradiotherapy. For patients treated with chemotherapy alone, the EFS was 20% ± 9%. Because no statistical difference was found in the 5-year OS between patients with M1 and M3 disease (51% ± 16% and 40% ± 9%), even patients with bulky disease can be treated if a GTR can be achieved.[1574]

Infant Glioma. Astrocytoma is the most common tumor in children younger than 3 years,[1556] as well as in infants younger than 1 year, and constitutes 30% of the total, of which 75% are low-grade tumors and 25% are reported as high-grade tumors.[1526] Management of these tumors in infants and young children mirrors the approaches used in older children, including observation for patients with completely resected low-grade lesions, chemotherapy for patients with symptomatic, progressive low-grade tumors, and chemotherapy and radiotherapy for patients with high-grade lesions. One major difference between young children and adults with HGGs is the improved prognosis observed in infants. In the "Baby POG series," 18 children younger than 3 years who were diagnosed with HGG (13 of whom were younger than 12 months) had 5-year PFS and OS rates of 43% ± 23% and 50% ± 14%, respectively.[758] Four survivors completed the 24 months of therapy but did not undergo irradiation because of parental refusal and remained without evidence of recurrence. Similar results have been reported in the French BBSFOP trial, in which 21 children younger than 5 years (13 with WHO grade III tumors and 8 with grade IV tumors) received postoperative chemotherapy and had 5-year PFS and OS rates of 35% and 59%, respectively. Of the 12 survivors, 10 did not receive radiotherapy at the time of reporting.[739] Another retrospective review of 16 patients younger than 3 years showed similar results, with 5-year EFS and OS rates of 29% (standard error [SE], 12%) and 66% (SE, 12%), respectively, although six patients received upfront radiation therapy and an additional six patients received radiation therapy at the time of progression.[1575] In the CCG-945 trial for children with newly diagnosed HGGs, children younger than 3 years were treated with the intent to avoid radiation therapy, including 49 children younger than 3 years. In this cohort of 49 children, the 10-year EFS and OS rates were 29% ± 6% and 37.5% ± 7%, respectively.[1576]

Infant CPC. Choroid plexus tumors account for 1% to 3% of childhood brain tumors, and approximately 30% to 40% are CPCs,[1577] with 70% occurring before the age of 2 years.[1578] Because of the association with Li-Fraumeni syndrome, analysis for the presence of *TP53* mutations is recommended.[1356] GTR has been shown to be prognostic[1579] although technically difficult to achieve because of the highly vascular nature of these lesions.[1526] The role of radiotherapy for the treatment of this highly invasive tumor is controversial.[1580,1581] In the "Baby POG" study it was reported that eight patients had choroid plexus tumors, two of whom were alive without use of radiotherapy.[1579] Other investigators have also reported long-term survival without use of radiotherapy in this group.[1582] Because the number of patients with this rare disease is so small, international collaboration is needed to determine the best treatment strategy for this group of patients. Currently maximal safe surgery and adjuvant chemotherapy constitutes a reasonable approach to avoid or delay radiotherapy,[1526] and salvage therapy is possible, not necessarily including craniospinal radiation therapy.[1583]

Other Tumors

Meningiomas

Meningiomas are rare pediatric tumors that are often seen in conjunction with either NF-2 or after radiation therapy[1584]; they account for 1% to 3% (range, 0.4% to 4.1%) of all childhood tumors of the CNS.[1585,1586] Familial meningiomas have been reported, and thus a detailed family history is required.[1587] In one study of children who received radiation therapy to the CNS for childhood leukemia, meningiomas were found in 20% upon routine

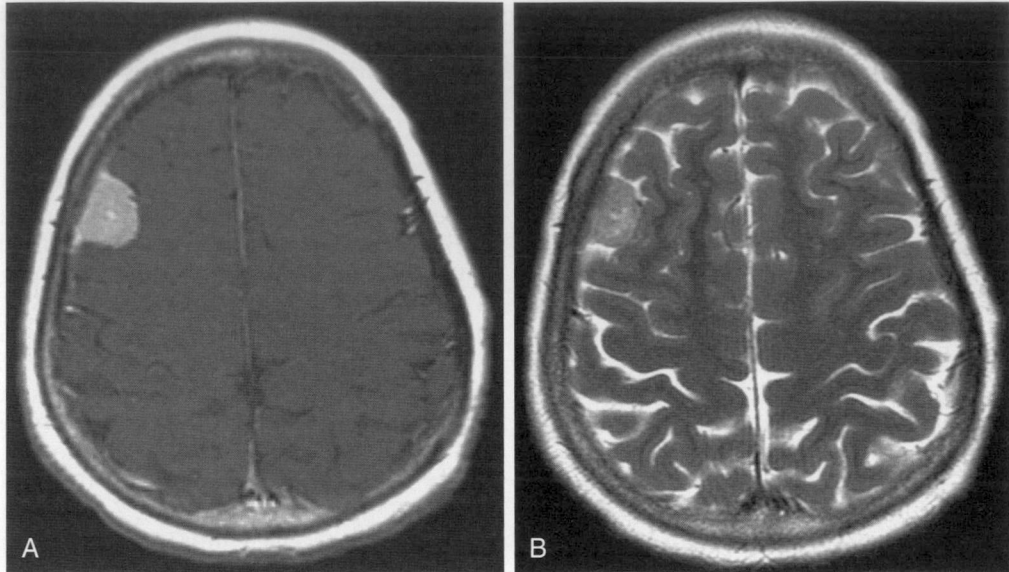

Figure 57-50 Peripheral contrast-enhancing meningioma. **A,** An axial T1-weighted image with use of contrast material. Note the dural tail. **B,** An axial T2-weighted image—bright T2 signal of a right frontal meningioma.

surveillance imaging.[1588] Although meningiomas are uncommon in pediatric patients, they are the second most common primary brain tumor in adults, after gliomas. Meningiomas are frequently identified as an incidental finding at autopsy, suggesting that many of these tumors remain small and asymptomatic. Molecular differences between symptomatic lesions and those that remain asymptomatic suggest that they may be distinct entities.[1589] Meningiomas are known to express hormone receptors, and a number of cell cycle pathways have been implicated in their dysregulated growth.[1590] In a review of the literature, radiation-induced meningiomas were the second most common radiation-induced malignancy after malignant glioma in children treated for a primary malignant neoplasm, with a mean latency of 21.1 and 13.7 years for atypical and benign meningiomas, respectively.[1591] Similarly in a cohort of children with acute lymphoblastic leukemia (ALL) who received cranial radiotherapy (1800 to 2400 cGy) and were monitored by serial scans, meningiomas were the most common tumor, with a mean latency of 21 years.[1588] In one study of patients who were treated with radiation therapy to the CNS for childhood leukemia, 20 years after treatment, it was reported that the incidence of meningioma was as high as 47%.[1592]

Clinical Presentation. The most common clinical presentations in children are seizures (33%), headaches (13%), ataxia (10%), and hemiparesis (10%). Tumor locations are primarily supratentorial (64%), with the remainder distributed infratentorially (16%), intraventricularly (12%), and in the spinal cord (8%).[1585] A few small series have indicated that the location and behavior of meningiomas in children may differ from those in adults, with a greater male preponderance, intraventricular location, increased multiplicity on first presentation,

and increased atypical or anaplastic subtypes (15% in childhood).[1586,1593,1594]

Imaging and Histology. Meningiomas are usually well-circumscribed dural lesions on CT and MRI. Areas of calcification are common and are best seen on CT scans. Tumors tend to have low T1-weighted and bright T2-weighted and FLAIR signals. They are usually brightly contrast-enhancing and can be associated with edema.[1595] A "dural tail" is a common finding on MRI scans in which there is dural thickening, tailing away from the lesion (Fig. 57-50). This finding does not indicate a greater propensity of the tumor to invade.[1596] Although most pediatric meningiomas are low-grade lesions (WHO grade I), a higher number of pediatric meningiomas have features of atypia or anaplasia (WHO grades II and III) compared with adult patients, especially in spontaneously arising tumors. This trend can be more pronounced with younger age.[1584] In adult meningiomas good correlation exists between histologic atypia, recurrence, and staining for the Ki-67 monoclonal antibody, a marker of proliferation. Such correlation is not seen in pediatric meningiomas, suggesting that the aggressiveness of pediatric meningioma is not related to proliferation alone.[1597] A number of histologic variants of meningioma can occur in children.[1598-1601] Most meningiomas stain for EMA and vimentin. Loss of chromosome 22 is commonly observed in grade I meningiomas. Loss of heterozygosity of chromosomes 14 and 18 has been associated with tumor grade.[1602] Additional chromosomal abnormalities can be observed in atypical and anaplastic meningioma. In patients without NF-2, a high incidence of mutations in this gene are still detected.[1603] A subset of meningiomas lacking NF-2 mutations have recurrent oncogenic mutations in AKT1 (E17K) and SMO (W535L).[1604]

Management. The management of pediatric meningiomas is difficult to define because of their rare occurrence and association with other mitigating factors, such as prior radiation therapy or association with NF-2.[1584] Treatment guidelines from cooperative groups such as the British Children's Cancer and Leukemia Group are beginning to emerge.[1605]

Meningiomas that are asymptomatic are usually left untreated and followed up carefully for the development of neurologic sequelae, radiologic progression, or radiologic evidence of transformation, at which point neurosurgical intervention should be considered. GTR is usually curative, although the appearance of other lesions is not uncommon. In patients with progressive or symptomatic lesions, radiotherapy can be delivered and can often stop tumor progression. For small unresectable lesions, SRS is also being used with increasing frequency. Meningiomas that develop after radiotherapy in the pediatric population can take on a more malignant phenotype, and early surgical resection should therefore be considered, which may lead to a better outcome, especially if a GTR can be achieved.[1588] The role of chemotherapy in the treatment of meningiomas is limited. Recurrent malignant and atypical meningiomas are difficult to treat successfully, and treatment with chemotherapy has been unsuccessful. Brachytherapy has been proposed for the treatment of patients who have had a relapse, but with high accompanying morbidity.[1606] Partial responses of refractory meningiomas to hydroxyurea[1607,1608] and tamoxifen[1609] have been reported in the literature but need to be confirmed in larger clinical trials.[1610,1611] A phase II trial of combination therapy of imatinib and hydroxyurea in adult patients with relapsed or refractory meningioma demonstrated only modest activity.[1612] A number of new molecularly targeted therapies for meningiomas are now being developed and tested.[1613]

Prognosis. Because of the peripheral nature of many of these lesions, complete resection is achieved in a high percentage of cases. Surgery remains the primary modality of treatment of these tumors and is a major determinant of outcome.[1586] Histologic grade is a further determinant of EFS.[1585] Even though the OS of patients with meningioma has been reported to be close to 90%, length of follow-up is limited or unknown.[1614] In one series extending between 1935 and 1984, long-term survival of 35% in children was reported, with a mean follow-up of 10 years after diagnosis.[1615] The true extent of the morbidity and mortality of this tumor in children is not accurately known[1614] and needs to be the subject of a prospective study by national and international cooperative groups.

Pituitary Adenomas

Although infrequent in pediatric patients compared with adults, pituitary adenomas account for approximately 2.7% of pediatric brain tumors.[1616] The differential diagnosis of pituitary fossa tumors includes craniopharyngioma, GCTs, and Langerhans cell histiocytosis. The vast majority of childhood pituitary adenomas are hormone-secreting or functional, meaning that they produce active hormones, including adrenocorticotropic hormone (ACTH), prolactin, growth hormone, thyroid-stimulating hormone (TSH), luteinizing hormone (LH), or follicle-stimulating hormone (FSH).[1617] Nonfunctioning adenomas account for only 3% to 6%.[1618,1619] Depending on the series, the two most commonly secreted hormones are prolactin and ACTH, followed by growth hormone,[1618,1620-1623] and finally TSH, LH, and FSH.[1617,1624]

Clinical Presentation. The main clinical manifestations of pituitary adenomas are determined by their location and function and usually consist of headaches (with or without signs of raised ICP), visual field defects, endocrine dysfunction, and menstrual irregularities. Other endocrine-specific presentations can be related to hyperprolactinemia, causing secondary amenorrhea and galactorrhea. Cushing disease resulting from ACTH oversecretion presents with hypertension, weight gain, and occasionally diabetes, although gigantism and acromegaly are rarely observed as a result of growth hormone oversecretion. Hypopituitarism can manifest as hypogonadism with delayed or arrested puberty, amenorrhea, and hypoadrenalism, which can manifest as fatigue, hypoglycemia, and/or weight loss. Short stature or growth failure can result from growth hormone deficiency. Hypothyroidism with a low thyroxine and a low-normal TSH level can also be a manifestation, although hyperthyroidism from a thyrotropinoma is a rare finding in childhood.[1624] Nonfunctioning tumors can also have endocrine manifestations, but these manifestations are typically related to pituitary insufficiency.[1625]

Imaging and Histology. The diagnostic workup and management of these tumors includes MRI of the pituitary region with and without contrast, although a CT scan can be useful in extensive disease or in an emergency to rule out local invasion or hemorrhage.[1626] Loss of the pituitary bright spot can indicate compression of the pituitary stalk.[1627] Microcystic and macrocystic structures are also easily identified on MRI (Fig. 57-51).[1627] A detailed biochemical workup in conjunction with an endocrinologist is vital to making a diagnosis and should include determination of serum prolactin, thyroxine and TSH, LH, FSH, serum urea, electrolyte, and morning cortisol levels. Determination of growth hormone, IGF1 and its binding partner IGF-BP3, and urine-free cortisol levels and a low-dose dexamethasone suppression test may be indicated if a growth hormone–secreting tumor or Cushing disease is suspected. Occasionally bilateral inferior petrosal sinus sampling for ACTH may be necessary for the diagnosis of Cushing disease.[1628] Visual field testing should be performed as part of a baseline assessment, and serum β-HCG and AFP should also be part of an initial assessment to rule out a GCT.

Management. Elevated secretion of prolactin can be associated with hyperplasia of TSH and prolactin-secreting cells but without the presence of a pituitary adenoma. Hypothyroidism should be managed before surgical intervention in cases in which hyperplasia may be evident.[1629] In terms of managing patients with

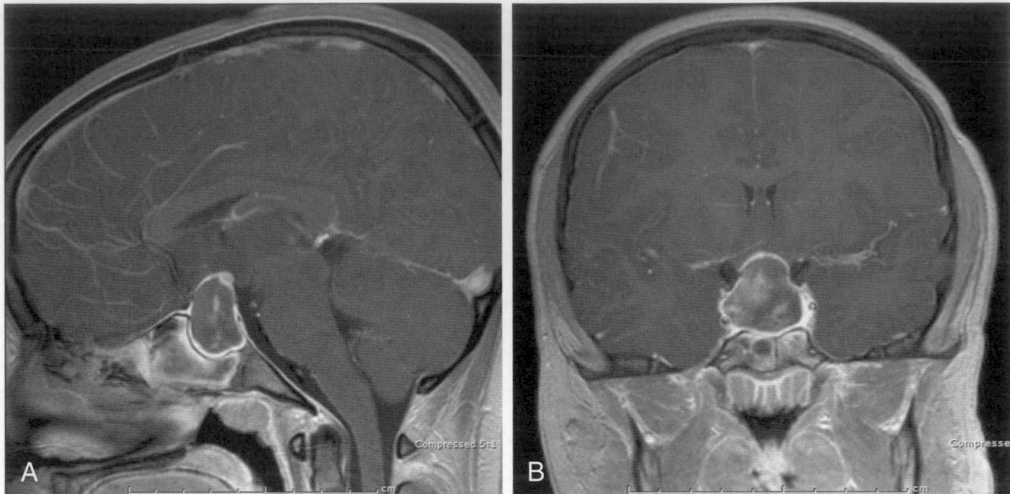

Figure 57-51 Large hemorrhagic pituitary adenoma. **A,** A sagittal T1-weighted image with use of contrast material. **B,** A coronal T1-weighted fat-saturated image.

pituitary adenoma, medical management alone with agents such as bromocriptine or similar analogues may be all that is needed for persons with prolactinoma.[1630] Transsphenoidal surgical resection is typically used for the treatment of growth hormone–secreting and ACTH-secreting tumors,[1631] although a potential role for somatostatin analogs such as octreotide has been proposed for the medical treatment of acromegaly.[1632] Multimodal therapy with medication, surgery, or radiotherapy may be necessary where initial therapy has failed.[1623,1624] Fortunately endocrinologic remission can be achieved in most patients with growth hormone- and ACTH-secreting tumors.[1622]

Multiple endocrine neoplasia type I (MEN1) is an autosomal-dominant disorder characterized by hyperparathyroidism, enteropancreatic tumors, pituitary adenomas, and, rarely, carcinoid, adrenal adenoma, and lipoma. Pituitary adenomas are observed at first presentation in 10% of cases.[1633] Familial isolated pituitary adenoma, characterized by familial pituitary adenomas in the absence of other tumors, is associated with germline mutations in the aryl hydrocarbon receptor-interacting protein gene *(AIP)*.[1634] The prevalence of germline mutations in *MEN1* or *AIP* in seemingly sporadic cases of pituitary adenoma in the pediatric population is high. One study demonstrated that 22% of patients younger than 18 years with sporadic pituitary adenoma had either *MEN1* or *AIP* germline mutations.[1635] In another study *AIP* mutations were reported in 20% of patients younger than 30 years who had pituitary adenomas.[1636] Although formal guidelines are lacking, because there is an increased incidence of genetic disorders such as MEN1 in pituitary tumors in children compared with adults,[1637] the families of index cases of childhood pituitary adenoma should be referred for screening and long-term follow-up.

Prognosis. The long-term prognosis of children with pituitary adenomas is excellent. Remission from abnormal hormone secretion is common; in one review it was achieved in 100% of patients with Cushing disease and 89% of patients with growth hormone secretion.[1622] Although disease control can be achieved in most patients with surgery, 40% may require radiation therapy.[1638] Given the central location of these tumors, this patient population must be carefully followed up for neurocognitive impact, radiation-induced tumors, and additional endocrinopathies because of pituitary dysfunction and radiation-mediated vascular damage.

Hamartomas

Hamartomas are an excessive but focal growth of cells and tissues native to the organs within which they occur. They have been described in the brain, eye, liver, lung, kidney, pancreas, heart, and gastrointestinal tract and in the lymphatic and vascular systems. Although they are benign lesions, hamartomas are regarded by pathologists as a link between developmental malformations and neoplasia. Because of the difficulty in distinguishing these two entities, hamartomas can sometimes be tenuously and variously interpreted as benign neoplasms.[1639] However despite their benign histology, their location and dysregulated growth in the brain can be the source of great morbidity, causing intractable seizures, obstructive hydrocephalus, and developmental delay.

Among the best-known conditions associated with hamartomas in the CNS are NF-1 and TS.[1640] NF-1–associated Lisch nodules are pigmented hamartomas in the iris and are found in more than 95% of affected adults and children older than 6 years; they are thought to be virtually pathognomonic for the condition.[1641] Although Lisch nodules remain asymptomatic and do not usually interfere with vision, they are important as a diagnostic criterion for NF-1. These lesions may be associated with unidentified bright spots seen in patients with NF-1[1642] and have been hypothesized ultimately to be related to neurofibromin levels.[1643] NF-2 results from loss of the tumor suppressor merlin and is characterized by predisposition to the development of multiple tumors, including schwannoma (particularly of the vestibular nerve), meningioma, and spinal cord glioma. Although not a commonly described association, combined pigment epithelial and retinal hamartoma have also been reported in patients with NF-2, although as a rare finding.[1644-1646] Their clinical significance is not clear. TS, like NF-1 and NF-2, results from the loss of the *TSC1* and *TSC2* tumor suppressor genes, which encode for hamartin and tuberin, respectively. These act by downregulating the Akt-mTOR pathway,[1647] as well as by regulating transcription through cross-talk with the Wnt signaling pathway through the ability of TSC1 and TSC2 to form a β-catenin degradation complex.[1648] A pathologic feature of TS within the CNS is the formation of cortical tubers, which are hamartomatous growths, in addition to subependymal nodules and the propensity to develop SEGAs. The clinical manifestation of this disorder is often seizures, cognitive disability, and other systemic manifestations, including dermatologic and visceral changes.[1640]

Several other rare inherited syndromes are associated with hamartomatous lesions in the brain, including Cowden disease, Bannayan-Zonana syndrome, Bannayan-Riley-Ruvalcaba syndrome, and LDD. In considering other conditions that are associated with hamartomatous lesions in the brain, Cowden disease (Online Mendelian Inheritance in Man [OMIM] 158350) is important because it is characterized by the familial predisposition to multiple benign hamartomas. These patients are also at increased risk of malignant lesions in all three germ layers involving most major organs, including the brain, mucocutaneous tissue, breast, thyroid, and uterus,[1649] with multiple tricholemmomas or benign neoplasms of the hair follicle, which are considered pathognomonic.[1650] The gene responsible for Cowden disease on chromosome 10 was cloned by linkage analysis and found to be a phospholipid phosphatase *PTEN* (phosphatase tenascin).[1651,1652] It is mutated in the germline in 80% of patients with Cowden disease, as well as in the Bannayan-Zonana syndrome.[1653] The same gene is also mutated in

60% of patients with Bannayan-Riley-Ruvalcaba syndrome (OMIM 153480), which is manifested by macrocephaly, developmental delay, and intestinal hamartomas. Several authors have reported mutations in the *PTEN* gene in patients with Proteus or Proteus-like syndrome; hamartomatous growths develop in both syndromes. Although rare LDD is associated with hamartomas of the brain resulting in ataxia, increased ICP, and seizures. The underlying lesion is a dysplastic gangliocytoma of the cerebellum, which is thought to be a hamartomatous overgrowth of Cowden disease.[1654,1655] In fact adult-onset of LDD is considered pathognomonic for Cowden disease by the National Comprehensive Cancer Network Guidelines.[1640,1649] Some authors have suggested that these familial hamartomatous syndromes be clustered with Cowden disease and the Bannayan-Riley-Ruvalcaba syndrome into a new category called PTEN hamartoma tumor syndrome, although this suggestion remains controversial.[1656] Recently a consortium was established, which published revised diagnostic criteria for PTEN hamartoma tumor syndrome to address this issue.[1657]

Imaging and Histology. Considerable variability exists in the imaging characteristics and pathologic appearance of hamartomas in the brain. Certain commonly observed features include areas of calcification on CT scan. On MRI scan, most lesions tend to be hypointense to isointense on T1-weighted sequences and bright on T2-weighted sequences and FLAIR (Fig. 57-52).[1658] Hamartomas of the brain are normally noncontrast-enhancing, which can help differentiate them from low-grade astrocytomas. The load of signal abnormality can be correlated with the severity of the symptoms and prognosis in many patients, such as those with TS.[1659] Using magnetoencephalography and concurrent SPECT imaging, precise tuber localization can be achieved and can assist in surgical planning.[1660,1661] Histologic features of hamartomas are highly dependent on their location.

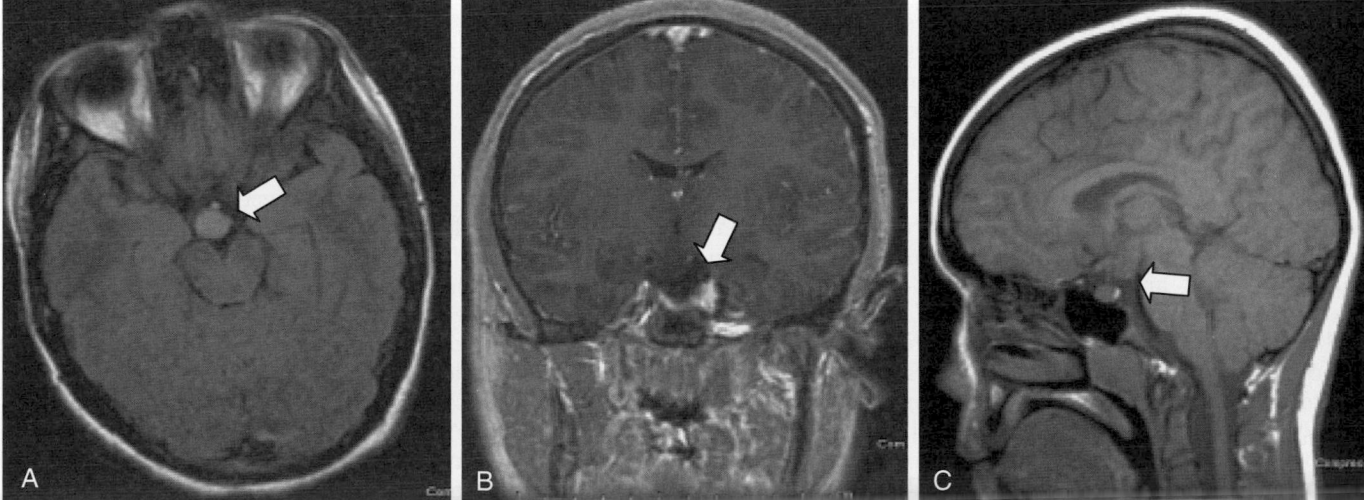

Figure 57-52 Hypothalamic hamartoma. **A,** An axial fluid-attenuated inversion recovery (FLAIR) image of a FLAIR bright lesion *(arrow)*. **B,** A coronal T1-weighted image with use of contrast material demonstrates little contrast enhancement *(arrow)*. **C,** A sagittal T1-weighted image without use of contrast material with hypointensity to isointensity *(arrow)*.

Management. The detailed management of tumors arising from the hamartoma conditions of LDD and Cowden disease, tuberous sclerosis, and neurofibromatosis is beyond the scope of this text. Multidisciplinary team management involving input from the geneticist, neurologist, neurooncologist, neurosurgeon, and affiliated specialists such as the neuropsychologist is highly recommended to provide comprehensive care. Molecular testing of patients and tumor tissues is also mandatory as targeted therapies with new agents emerge. Rapamycin and its analogs and derivatives specifically target mTOR, which is downstream from the PTEN/PI3K/Akt pathway and is common to neurofibromatosis and TS.[1647] Everolimus has been shown in a randomized phase III trial to be effective for the treatment of subependymal giant cell astrocytomas in patients with TS.[1662] Similar therapeutic agents are also available for targeting Ras through the inhibition of farnesyltransferase and are the subject of ongoing clinical trials for progressive plexiform neurofibromas.[1663] Pallister-Hall syndrome, which results in hypothalamic hamartomas, involves abnormalities in the SHH–Gli 3 pathway,[1664] and a number of new molecular inhibitors of this pathway are beginning to undergo clinical investigation.[1665]

Optimal management of hamartomatous lesions of the CNS is typically directed at the presenting symptoms.[1666] Seizures are a common presenting symptom, and treatment with antiepileptic agents is the first approach. Hamartomatous lesions are often refractory to these medications, even when multiple drugs are coadministered. Complete resection of hamartomas is not always required to improve seizure control, because disconnection of the epileptiform focus without gross surgical resection has resulted in significant clinical improvement in hypothalamic hamartomas.[1667]

Prognosis. Although isolated hamartomatous lesions that can be resected have a good prognosis, patients usually present with a number of comorbid symptoms related to the hamartomas and to the underlying associated genetic syndrome. Mental retardation, autism, and behavioral issues can persist. Seizures are not always amenable to surgical intervention, especially in deep structures of the diencephalon. Even in patients who are treated successfully, their underlying genetic susceptibility places them at risk for the development of new lesions.

Astroblastoma

Astroblastoma is a rare glial tumor of the CNS that accounts for 0.45% to 2.8% of all primary brain gliomas[1668] and approximately 0.92% of all pediatric brain tumors.[1669] The tumor was first described by Bailey and Cushing in their 1924 classification of brain tumors,[1030] but some persons argue that the term *astroblastoma* is confusing because the tumor is neither overtly astrocytic nor blastic in nature.[1670] The current widely accepted pathologic description of astroblastoma is that of a generally solid, well-circumscribed mass that is histologically defined by the presence of astroblastic pseudorosettes and perivascular hyalinization.[1671] Ependymoma is an important differential diagnosis because of the

clinical and histopathologic similarity between these tumors, which includes perivascular orientation, pseudorosette formation, and immunohistochemical staining with GFAP and EMA. These histopathologic similarities have led to the suggestion that the tanycyte, or ependymal cell, may be a common precursor of ependymoma and astroblastoma.[1672] Even though astroblastoma does have some distinctive features, including broader tapering perivascular processes, lack of fibrillarity, and perivascular hyalinization, which is not seen in ependymoma, this rare tumor continues to be classified under "other neuroepithelial" tumors in the latest WHO classification of CNS tumors.[1673]

Clinical Presentation. The clinical presentation of astroblastoma is usually in children and young adults in the first three decades of life,[1670] with several reports in children 5 years or younger,[1669,1674-1677] as well as a congenital form.[1668] Several case series have shown a female preponderance.[1670,1678,1679] Presenting signs and symptoms are usually of headache and raised ICP because of mass effect or obstruction of CSF flow. The site of the tumor is most often supratentorial, peripherally located in the brain.

Imaging and Histology. Radiologically, astroblastomas appear as large, well-circumscribed, heterogeneous, lobulated, solid and cystic masses, with little vasogenic edema disproportional to their size. This lack of edema is a feature that can also help distinguish astroblastoma from ependymoma and HGGs. The solid component of the mass is described as bubbly, and the MRI T2-weighted signal is isointense with gray matter. Enhancement of the solid component is seen in 75% of cases, and punctate calcification is occasionally seen.[1678,1679]

The histopathologic features of astroblastoma include strong immunoreactivity for S-100, GFAP, and vimentin, with focal staining with EMA.[1673] Histologic grade is considered as either well differentiated, which correlates with the ability to achieve a GTR,[1670] or malignant, with features of anaplasia, which is a poor prognostic marker.[1677] MIB1 immunoreactivity has been observed over a wide range (1% to 18%), although it is unclear whether an increasing MIB1 index rating is related to a poorer outcome.[1670] A formal WHO grade has not yet been assigned.[1673]

Management. Treatment of these tumors includes maximal surgical resection followed by focal or WBRT, especially when features of anaplasia are present. The role of TMZ,[1680,1681] intensive chemotherapy in younger children,[1677] or other forms of chemotherapeutic agents[1669] has not been determined. The establishment of an international registry to gain more information on treatment responses and a detailed understanding of the biology of these tumors has been proposed to optimize treatment approaches for this rare tumor.[1682] To this end studies of chromosomal abnormalities, such as gains of chromosome 20q and chromosome 19[1670] or loss of heterozygosity of chromosome 9p,[1683] are important and help distinguish this tumor from ependymomas. The description of variants of astroblastoma that have rhabdoid features and a better prognosis[1680,1684] warrants further study of this rare tumor.

Prognosis. The prognosis of astroblastoma is in part dependent on the histologic features. Anaplastic lesions do less well than those with low-grade features.[1671,1677] Complete resection is important for long-term survival and may be sufficient therapy for most patients, including some lesions with more of an anaplastic appearance.[1670]

Primary CNS Lymphoma

CNS lymphoma is a rare group of tumors that can arise in the CNS. Although primarily associated with immunosuppression from human immunodeficiency virus (HIV) or other immunodeficiency states, CNS lymphoma has also been detected in patients lacking a prior infectious or immunocompromised history. These tumors are often very responsive to therapy, including radiation therapy and/or chemotherapy.[1685]

PCNS lymphoma in childhood and young adults is an extremely rare tumor, accounting for about 1.2% to 1.5% of all brain tumors,[1686,1687] with an annual incidence rate of 0.02 per 100,000 based on data collected by the Childhood Brain Tumor Trust between 2000 and 2004. These data suggest that approximately 16 new cases per year are expected in the United States.[1032] Children with congenital immunodeficiency syndromes face an inherent 4% overall risk of developing cancer, which is 10,000 times higher than the expected rate. The highest risk groups are ataxia-telangiectasia and common variable immunodeficiency.[1688] Data collected by the Immunodeficiency Cancer Registry have shown a median age of presentation in this group of children to be 10 years, and more than 50% of the cases consist of non-Hodgkin lymphoma, 30% of which were extranodal.[1689] Patients with Wiskott-Aldrich syndrome have the highest proportion of CNS lymphoma among the congenital immunodeficiencies, which is estimated at approximately 3%,[1690] followed by immunoglobulin (Ig)A deficiency, hyper-IgM syndrome, and severe combined immunodeficiency.[1691] Immunodeficiency after organ transplantation also carries a risk of between 1% and 5% for PCNS lymphoma, and increasing rates are being observed in renal, cardiac, lung, and liver transplant recipients.[1692] AIDS, particularly HIV-AIDS in adults, was responsible for a peak in CNS lymphoma in the mid 1990s, with 2% to 13% of adult patients with AIDS affected.[1693] In one study of pediatric patients with AIDS, the Centers for Disease Control and Prevention reported 18 of 6209 patients presenting with CNS lymphoma.[1694,1695] The overall risk of CNS lymphoma was estimated at 17% to 42% in pediatric patients with AIDS.[1688,1696,1697] Subsequent reporting by the SEER program has not shown an increase in the rate of PCNS lymphoma in the 0- to 19-year-old age group, unlike in adults, whose rates have fallen dramatically since the peak in the 1990s.[1698] This finding is probably attributable to the introduction of multiantiretroviral therapies (e.g., highly active antiretroviral therapy) and other therapeutic improvements.[1699]

Although patients with immunodeficiencies are at higher risk of developing PCNS lymphoma, most adult and pediatric patients in whom this malignancy develops are immunocompetent.[1685,1692,1700] The pathogenesis of PCNS lymphoma in the immunocompetent host is unknown. One hypothesis is that systemic inflammatory cells have become trapped in the brain and subsequently transform, isolated from the remainder of the immune system by virtue of the immunologic sanctuary status of the brain. This hypothesis does not fully explain the fact that normally only T lymphocytes traffic through the CNS, although most cases of PCNS lymphoma are of B-cell origin.[1701]

Clinical Presentation. Although the clinical presentation of PCNS lymphoma is in keeping with the diffuse infiltrative growth seen in adult patients and is dominated by cognitive dysfunction, psychomotor slowing, behavioral changes, raised ICP, and seizures,[1702,1703] most pediatric patients present with symptoms of increased ICP, hemiparesis, ataxia, and cranial nerve dysfunction.[1685,1686,1700]

Imaging and Histology. Radiologic features of PCNS lymphoma include enhancing unifocal or multifocal lesions, usually in the periventricular area, although cortical lesions are not uncommon. MRI is the best modality to use because these lesions are characteristically hypointense on T1-weighted sequences and T2 hyperintense tumor with evidence of peritumeral edema.[1702] Most tumors are brightly enhancing upon administration of contrast material. PET and SPECT imaging can also help confirm the presence of lymphomas and identify metastases in the CNS and outside of the brain.[1704-1706] Using the Revised European American Lymphoma classification system, the diffuse large B-cell phenotype accounts for most cases, followed by the small, noncleaved Burkitt phenotype.[1707] Anaplastic large T-cell lymphoma is rare.[1700,1703] Pediatric patients with AIDS, on the other hand, have been found to have small noncleaved B-cell tumors, both of the Burkitt and non-Burkitt types, and are more frequently associated with Epstein-Barr virus infection.[1688,1708]

Management. The treatment of PCNS lymphoma has followed the adult practice because pediatric-based studies to define optimal therapy have not been conducted. Although PCNS lymphomas are aggressive tumors and require intensive treatment, they are responsive to radiation therapy and chemotherapy. Historically treatment for adults with CNS lymphoma consisted of radiotherapy alone, but these patients also had high relapse rates, which led to the introduction of combination chemotherapy using high-dose methotrexate (greater than 1 g/m^2), a treatment that has proven to be effective.[1709] The role of WBRT as part of consolidation therapy in adults is controversial given its toxicity, especially in older adults and when given in combination with high-dose methotrexate. Some persons consider it to be an essential part of therapy and believe it should be excluded only in persons of advanced age or with neurocognitive impairment.[1710] In contrast to the data with high-dose methotrexate, evidence suggests that consolidation with WBRT and high-dose cytarabine or high-dose cytarabine alone does not improve survival in patients who achieve complete remission with high-dose methotrexate-based combination treatment.[1711] With effective salvage regimens such as re-treatment with high-dose methotrexate or treatment options with TMZ, rituximab, and other agents,[1709] a compelling argument exists to exclude WBRT as part of first-line treatment.

Although pediatric patients have been successfully treated with WBRT alone,[1685,1686] this treatment is often too toxic, especially in younger children. In a multicenter retrospective review of 12 pediatric patients who had a 5-year EFS of 70% and OS of 75% (median follow-up of 79 months), only two patients received radiotherapy, and one patient was treated with high-dose chemotherapy and ASCR, confirming that radiotherapy can be excluded from the upfront therapy of these patients.[1700] Most patients in this study received multiagent chemotherapy including high-dose methotrexate (8 g/m^2), high-dose cytarabine, and steroids, with patients having been treated according to the French-American-British LMB-96 protocol (group C for persons with CNS disease). All patients in this retrospective study had received intrathecal chemotherapy, with the exception of one immunocompromised patient who was treated with hydroxyurea only. Similar results have been reported in a recent single-institution retrospective analysis of six pediatric patients with PCNS lymphoma.[1712] All patients were treated with systemic, methotrexate-based chemotherapy and intrathecal chemotherapy. The estimated 5-year survival rate was 83.3% in this cohort. Organ transplantation patients can be treated with multimodality therapy, as discussed earlier, in addition to a decrease in their immunosuppressive regimens,[1713] although care must be taken to protect their grafts.

Prognosis. A recent, relatively large ($n = 29$) multicenter retrospective analysis of pediatric patients with PCNS reported a 3-year OS of 82%.[1714] It should be noted that these results are based on a cohort of mixed immunocompetent and immunocompromised patients. Further improvements in treatment outcome will require a large prospective multinational study that separates immunocompetent and immunocompromised patients with PCNS lymphomas to determine optimum therapy for this rare malignancy.

Dermoid, Epidermoid, and Arachnoid Cysts

A vast array of cysts can occur throughout the CNS,[1715-1717] and although they are not classified as tumors, these CNS lesions can cause significant morbidity and often require surgical intervention. If they are completely removed, recurrences are uncommon, although incompletely resected lesions can lead to a reaccumulation of fluid, resulting in recurrence of symptoms and necessitating further resection[1718] or cyst drainage.[1719]

The benign cysts of the CNS are often divided into two main categories. The first are those that arise from tissue within the CNS, including porencephalic cysts, arachnoid cysts, ependymal cysts, and hemangioblastomas. The second group of cysts consists of those that arise from extracranial tissue and includes teratomas, dermoid and epidermoid cysts, craniopharyngioma, and endodermal, colloid, enterogenous, and Rathke cleft cysts.[1715] Cysts may also arise from infectious origins, such as cysticercosis or toxoplasmosis.

Arachnoid Cysts. Arachnoid cysts are CSF-filled cavities lined by arachnoid cells[1720,1721] that arise from the arachnoid layer of the meninges. They account for approximately 1% of all intracranial space-occupying lesions and are more common in boys.[1716] They are usually congenital and occur in early infancy[1722] but can also occur as a result of inflammation in older children. Arachnoid cysts usually occur in the supratentorial compartment, arising in areas that are rich in arachnoid tissue, with 50% occurring in the Sylvian fissure,[1723] although they can occur anywhere in the CNS.[1724] Arachnoid cysts are often incidental findings on CT or MRI scans obtained for unrelated symptoms. Although usually isolated in their occurrence, multiple arachnoid cysts can be part of inherited syndromes such as the acrocallosal syndrome (a mutation in the *GLI3* gene, OMIM 200990) or the Chudley-McCullough syndrome (OMIM 604213), both of which are associated with agenesis of the corpus callosum. A familial pattern associated with cysts in multiple family members has been reported, one of which includes abnormalities on chromosome 16.[1725] Arachnoid cysts need to be distinguished from cysts associated with malignant primary or metastatic brain tumors, which are thought to develop as a result of a disrupted BBB as a result of the malignant process.[1726]

Clinical Presentation. In infants and children, arachnoid cysts tend to present with increasing head circumference or hydrocephalus, seizures, headaches, and psychomotor retardation.[1716] In the suprasellar region, 90% of patients present with obstructive hydrocephalus,[1727] although precocious puberty has also been recognized.[1728] In this location, it may be necessary to distinguish arachnoid and Rathke cleft cysts from craniopharyngioma, especially because the clinical management of craniopharyngioma differs significantly. Although differentiating these lesions can be difficult, arachnoid and Rathke cleft cysts are usually uniformly cystic and lack a solid component. In contrast craniopharyngiomas are solid in 10% of patients and solid and cystic in 43% of patients. Another distinguishing feature is the presence of calcification in approximately 90% of craniopharyngiomas, a finding that is rare in arachnoid cysts.[1729] Although the neurologic presentation of craniopharyngioma and arachnoid cysts can be similar, 95% of craniopharyngiomas have accompanying endocrine dysfunction, which is usually absent in patients with arachnoid cysts.

Imaging and Histology. The radiologic appearance of arachnoid cysts is usually nonenhancing, and they appear hypodense on CT and isointense to CSF on MRI (Fig. 57-53).[1730] Several theories have been proposed to explain the expansion of arachnoid cysts, which vary from the pulsatile movement of CSF into cyst cavities to osmotic gradients between cysts and CSF.[1716] Analysis of cyst fluid confirms that it is CSF, although the protein content tends to be elevated.[1731]

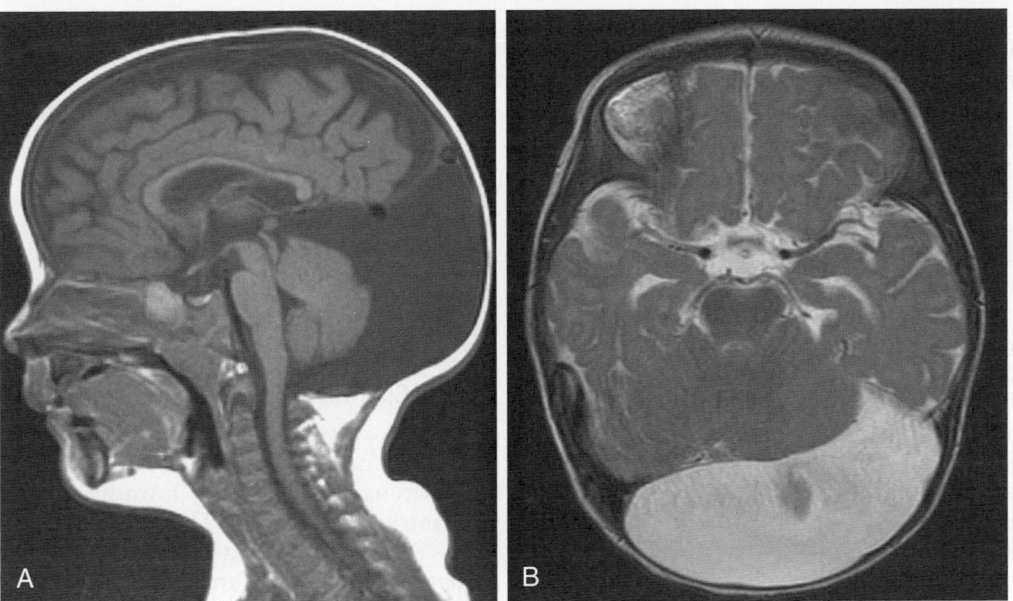

Figure 57-53 Arachnoid cyst. **A,** A sagittal T1-weighted image without use of contrast material. **B,** An axial T2-weighted image.

Management. The management of arachnoid cysts is usually conservative, especially if the patient is asymptomatic.[1732] However approximately 6% of patients with arachnoid cysts will experience complications, including cyst rupture or hemorrhage. Risk factors for cyst rupture or hemorrhage include large cyst size (greater than 5 cm) and head trauma.[1733] A clearly expanding lesion or worsening signs and symptoms will necessitate surgical intervention with cyst fenestration[1728,1734] or cystoventricular shunting.[1719] Newer surgical approaches with endoscopic management have been developed and have been successful.[1727,1735] Retrospective analysis of 1324 cases of pediatric arachnoid cysts demonstrated that open craniotomy for cyst excision or fenestration, endoscopic fenestration, and cystoperitoneal shunting have similar outcomes.[1736] Most patients will have resolution of their presenting symptoms after surgical intervention, although approximately 20% will not experience resolution.[1737,1738] Potential postsurgical complications include infections, subdural hygroma, and CSF leak.[227]

Prognosis. The long-term prognosis of children with arachnoid cysts is excellent. Because fluid reaccumulation can recur, repeat surgical procedures will be required in approximately 20% of patients.[1738] Patients requiring shunting from the ventricles or cysts may require additional procedures as they grow.[227,1739,1740] Seizure control can require lifelong anticonvulsants, especially if complete surgical resection of the lesion is not feasible. Patients with a history of arachnoid cysts may be at increased risk of chronic subdural hematomas.[1741]

Dermoid and Epidermoid Cysts. Dermoid and epidermoid cysts account for 0.5% and 0.8%, respectively, of all intracranial space-occupying lesions[1742] and result from the intrusion of nonnervous tissue, mainly epithelia, into the neuraxis at the time of closure of the neural tube, between the third and fifth weeks of embryonic life.[1718,1743,1744] These cysts are most often located in the major subarachnoid cisterns of the brain—namely, the suprasellar cistern, pineal region, and cerebellopontine angle cistern.[1715] Although benign and slow growing, these lesions can be problematic if they cause local mass effect or obstructive hydrocephalus, and they have a tendency to recur if they are not completely resected or are complicated by secondary infection. In general dermoid cysts are primarily located in the midline in the suprasellar, frontobasal, and cisterna magna areas, although epidermoid cysts can also be found in the suprasellar area. Epidermoid cysts are more common in the lateral skull base around the cerebellopontine angle and are rare in the brain parenchyma or intraventricular region. Both dermoid and epidermoid cysts can occur in the brainstem and spinal cord.[1717,1718,1742,1745]

The presentation of intracranial dermoid cysts occurs in younger patients (10.5 years) compared with epidermoid cysts, which present in adulthood with a mean age of 27 years.[1717] Although usually sporadic in their presentation, intracranial dermoid cysts can have a familial predisposition affecting several generations (OMIM 600679).[1746] Unlike arachnoid cysts, which have a more clearly defined association with intracranial syndromic malformations such as Aicardi syndrome, dermoid and epidermoid cysts do not appear to follow the same pattern. However patients with dermoid cysts can also have associated CNS malformations, such as agenesis of the corpus callosum (OMIM 600679).[1747,1748] In Goldenhar syndrome, which is composed of oculoauricular dysmorphic features and hemifacial microsomia, associated epibulbar dermoid cysts have been reported (OMIM 164210) but do not have a link with cancer predisposition. In contrast Gardner syndrome, a variant of familial adenomatous polyposis with associated predisposition to colorectal carcinomas, includes hyperostosis of the skull and subcutaneous and intraabdominal dermoid cysts (OMIM 175100). Turcot syndrome is characterized by familial polyposis coli with a predisposition to the development of malignant neuroepithelial tumors[1042] and is also associated with mutations in the APC and mismatch repair genes.[1749,1750] The coexistence of Gardner and Turcot syndromes in a family,[1751,1752] coupled with the report of an intracranial epidermoid cyst in a patient with Gardner syndrome,[1753] has suggested that dermoid and epidermoid cysts may share a common pathogenesis. Finally, epidermoid cysts can present as a late effect of a lumbar tap.[1754]

Clinical Presentation. Dermoid and epidermoid cysts can present with a wide array of symptoms, including recurrent fevers, headaches, signs of raised ICP, cerebellar ataxia, behavioral changes, seizures, cranial nerve palsies, increased head circumference, Parinaud syndrome, deafness, long tract signs, visual loss, and cord compression.[1717,1718,1742,1755]

Imaging and Histology. The MRI appearances of dermoid and epidermoid cysts are of well-circumscribed lesions with an accompanying sinus tract that is often visualized on imaging. They produce moderate mass effect but no perilesional edema. They are usually hypointense on T1-weighted imaging and hyperintense on T2-weighted imaging, with enhancement of the solid component (Fig. 57-54).[1718] In a recent study of intraparenchymal epidermoid cysts, the imaging characteristics were similar to extracerebral epidermoid cysts with isointensity to CSF on both T1- and T2-weighted images, with additional diagnostic information from DWI.[1756] Histologically dermoid and epidermoid cysts show overlap consistent with their ectodermal origin. Both are lined by squamous epithelium and some degree of keratin deposition and both lack features of invasion. In addition dermoid cysts can have skin adnexa present in the cyst wall, including hair follicles, sebaceous glands with sebum, and keratin flakes in the cyst fluid.[1717,1757]

Management. The management of dermoid and epidermoid cysts is surgical when intervention is required. Maximal safe resection should be attempted but can be complicated by adherence of the cyst wall to vital structures, limiting the resection.[1718] Subtotal resection is associated with a high rate of recurrence, requiring repeated surgery.[1746] Potential complications include aseptic meningitis in cases of spillage of cyst contents and even malignant transformation.[1743]

Prognosis. Dermoid and epidermoid cysts can recur and continued surveillance is required, especially for lesions that are incompletely resected.

Spinal Cord Tumors

Spinal cord tumors of infants and children are rare and account for 1% to 10% of all tumors of the CNS. They can occur as extradural, intradural but extramedullary, or intramedullary.[1758] There is a slight male predominance, with 58% of cases occurring in males.[1759] Approximately 80% of tumors are low-grade neoplasms. Predominant histologies in the spine from one large series include ependymoma (19%), schwannoma (neurilemmoma; 17%), and astrocytoma[565] (15%).[27] Benign cysts are also common in this location.[1760] Rare histologies identified in this region include neuroblastic tumors,[1761] oligodendroglioma,[1003] gangliogliomas,[602] anaplastic ganglioglioma,[588] nongerminomatous germ cell tumor,[1762] teratoma,[1763] cavernous angioma,[1764] clear cell meningioma,[1765] lipoma,[1766] PNET,[1767] and ATRT.[1768] In a review of 164 patients with spinal cord tumors undergoing resection, the median age was 8.6 years.[1769]

Clinical Presentation. The clinical symptomatology of pediatric spinal cord tumors relates to neurologic impairment concordant with the level of the lesion. Because most spinal tumors grow along the cord, a number of segments are commonly involved. Each segment of the

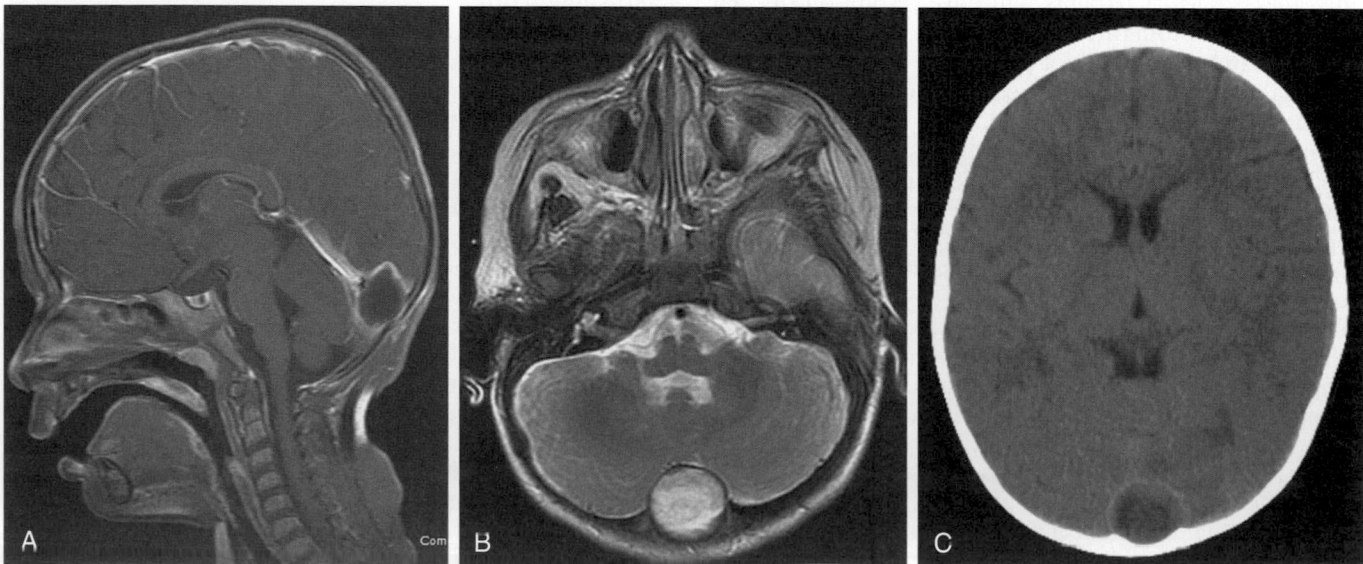

Figure 57-54 Occipital dermoid cyst. **A,** A sagittal T1-weighted image with use of contrast material. **B,** An axial T2-weighted image. **C,** A computed tomography noncontrast image.

spinal cord (cervical, thoracic, lumbar, and sacral) can be involved by tumors, and no histologic type is localized to a single area except myxopapillary ependymomas, which are predominantly found in the conus medullaris and filum terminale. Common symptoms of spinal cord tumors include pain (the most common symptom and identified in up to 80% of cases in most series), motor weakness, sensory loss, torticollis, and bladder and bowel incontinence.[1770-1773] Delay in diagnosis is common because of the nonspecific nature of the symptoms early in the disease process.[1774] Patients with evidence of a cerebral mass and spinal cord symptoms must undergo spinal imaging for metastatic disease.

Imaging and Histology. MRI is important in differentiating the location of tumors in the spine (extradural, intradural extramedullary, and intramedullary), as well as differentiating the possible histologies.[1775] As a general rule the imaging characteristics of spinal cord lesions are similar to those of the same histology in the brain. Histologic evaluation of spinal cord tumors follows that of the same lesions in the brain.

Management. Complete or near-complete resection of intraspinal tumors can be achieved in a significant majority of patients. In one large series of 164 patients, a greater than 95% resection was obtained in 76% (125 patients).[1769] Because most spinal tumors are low-grade tumors and can be cured with complete resection, having an experienced neurosurgeon perform the procedure is of utmost importance in achieving a complete resection. Other adjuvant therapies may be considered on the basis of the histology of the tumor. Myxopapillary ependymomas are best managed with complete surgical resection, which is achievable in most patients. Radiation therapy is administered to patients with progressive disease.[947] Patients with spinal ependymoma may have better outcomes than those with similar tumors of the posterior fossa in that many children can be treated effectively with surgery alone, without the need for radiation therapy. In a group of 20 children, a complete resection was achieved in 14 patients, and 6 patients had subtotal resections. None of these six patients received radiation therapy, and yet three remained without progressive disease.[1776] Children with high-grade astrocytomas of the spine who are treated with radiation therapy do as poorly as those with supratentorial tumors.[1777] Low-grade astrocytomas of the spine generally respond to vincristine and carboplatin[1778] or focal radiotherapy.[1779] Chemotherapy (irinotecan and cisplatin) has been used in infants with astrocytomas to delay the need for radiation therapy, with good results in three patients.[1780] Radiotherapy should be reserved for those in whom a complete resection cannot be obtained.[1781] Gangliogliomas are often cured with resection alone; patients with incomplete resection or recurrence can be treated with LGG therapy or focal radiotherapy.[602]

Prognosis. The long-term outcomes for patients with spinal cord tumors are not significantly different from those with brain tumors of the same histology and degree of resection. The morbidities of the tumor and therapies, however, may be significant. Direct neurologic consequences of spinal cord tumors include pain and motor and sensory deficits, as well as urinary and bowel incontinence. Many patients will demonstrate significant improvement in these deficits after treatment. Negative predictive factors for prolonged or permanent motor deficits include older age, unilateral symptoms, preoperative urinary symptoms, and other preoperative deficits.[1782] High-grade astrocytic histology and a short history of symptomatology can also be poor prognostic markers.[1783] Patients who present with sensory deficits do worse than those without this symptom at presentation.[1783] In the case of spinal cord ependymomas, location can effect prognosis, with lesions in the lower half of the spinal cord carrying a poorer prognosis.[1784] Persons with symptoms related to cyst enlargement are most likely to regain function.[945] More than one fourth of patients (27%) experience long-term spinal deformity as a result of their initial laminectomy.[1785,1786] Chronic pain can be particularly difficult in this patient population and requires aggressive management.[1787]

Patients with radiation therapy to the cervical spine can experience paresthesias a few months after therapy that are often described as a feeling of electric shock in the spine. This phenomenon, called Lhermitte sign, is related to transient demyelinization from radiation therapy.[1788] Patients are treated symptomatically, and the sensations typically resolve without the need for intervention.

Chordomas

Chordomas are rare tumors of the skull base that are thought to derive from remnants of the primitive notochord.[1789] Although most cases arise in adults, they can be observed at all ages, including in infants.[1790] Whites appear to be more commonly affected than are African Americans, and males are affected more often than are females.[1791,1792]

Clinical Presentation. Chordomas can present along the axial skeleton, including the skull base, spine, and sacral area. Skull-based lesions typically present with headaches and diplopia. Spinal lesions often result in pain, motor weakness, or sensory deficits. Although initially minor these symptoms tend to progress and eventually result in referral for imaging. Rarely metastatic disease identified on CSF cytology is detected and provides an argument for complete staging of patients, particularly those with atypical or poorly differentiated disease.[1793]

Imaging and Histology. Chordomas are well-circumscribed lesions on CT imaging that can demonstrate areas of calcification. They are hypointense on MR T1-weighted images and bright on T2-weighted images and FLAIR sequences (Fig. 57-55). Chordomas can brightly enhance after administration of gadolinium.[1791] The histologic appearance of chordomas can vary.[1794] Although conventional chordomas (58%) predominated in one pediatric series of 73 cases, 23% were chondroid chordomas and

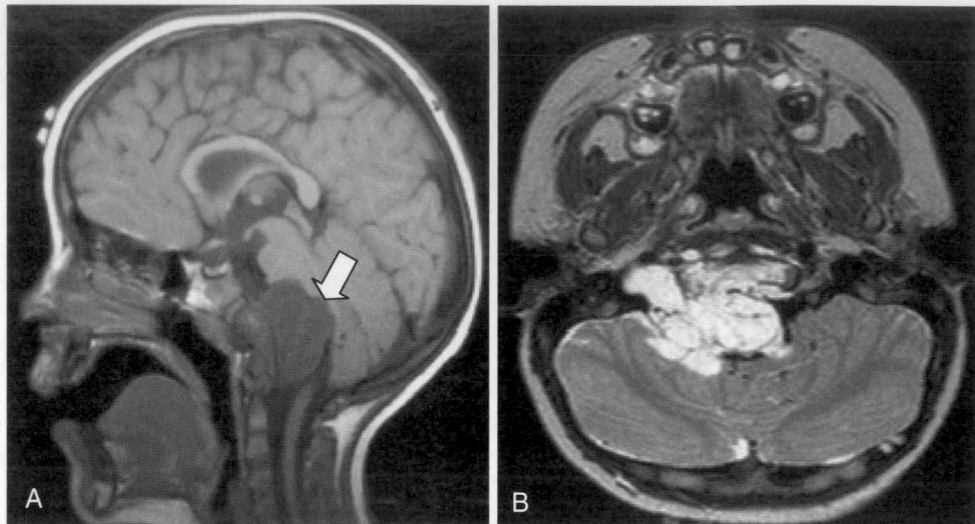

Figure 57-55 A large skull-based chordoma. **A,** A sagittal T1-weighted image without use of contrast material showing a hypointense lesion *(arrow).* **B,** An axial T2-weighted image.

an additional 19% had high cellularity.[1795] Tumors stained positively for keratin, EMA, S-100, and vimentin. Mitoses and necrotic areas were also commonly observed.[1795]

Management. Radiation therapy can be effective in the treatment of chordomas. In addition to reducing the toxicity of photon radiation therapy to normal structures,[1796] proton beam radiation therapy in combination with IMRT can provide excellent delivery of a high dose to the lesion.[1797] Chordomas are largely resistant to chemotherapy. In patients with more aggressive lesions, or for those refractory to radiation therapy, chemotherapy can be offered. Response to ifosfamide and doxorubicin was reported in one patient with metastatic disease in conjunction with triple intrathecal therapy (cytarabine, hydrocortisone, and methotrexate).[1798] The use of a combination of actinomycin D, cyclophosphamide, and methotrexate or cisplatin and 5-fluorouracil demonstrated no activity in this report.[1798] A retrospective review of six pediatric patients with clival chordomas reported some success with ifosfamide and regimens containing etoposide.[1799] Repeat irradiation with proton therapy and SRS have also been used as salvage therapy in patients who have had a relapse.[1800,1801]

The recent identification of PDGFR-α and PDGFR-β in tumor cells and concurrent expression of the receptors in adjacent stromal cells suggest a possible role for therapeutic intervention with imatinib mesylate.[1802,1803] Another molecular target identified in these tumors includes EGFR; one patient with metastatic disease achieved a partial response with cetuximab and gefitinib.[1804] Modest activity in recurrent chordomas has also been observed with 9-nitrocamptothecin.[1805]

Prognosis. Patients who have chordomas with poorly differentiated features have a worse prognosis than those with classic forms of the disease. Complete resection remains an important prognostic factor. In one large pediatric series, 81% of patients were alive at a median of 7

years after treatment with proton beam radiation therapy.[1795] An elevated MIB1 rating has also been reported as an important predictor of recurrence and OS.[1806]

LATE EFFECTS OF TREATMENT

The long-term and late effects of therapy are a critical concern in pediatric neurooncology.[1807,1808] The developing nervous system is uniquely vulnerable to the long-term effects of radiation therapy, and these effects can become apparent and progressive throughout the life span of the child into adulthood.[1809] Although much of the interest about late effects has refocused on the consequences of radiation therapy, increasing evidence indicates that the presence of the tumor compressing the brain, the surgery needed to remove it, and the chemotherapy provided to treat it all add to the experience of late effects by survivors of pediatric brain tumors.[1810,1811] The improving prognoses of patients with CNS tumors means that more children will be at risk of developing a wide range of late effects of therapy,[1812] including secondary malignancies.[1813] Of particular importance is the focus on the cognitive outcome of children treated for CNS tumors as we shift from the number of survivors to the number of functioning survivors. In association with cognitive deficits, patients can experience depression, anxiety, and social isolation. Survivors have increased risk for suicidal ideation and increased need for psychosocial intervention, and all patients should have follow-up with psychosocial providers to ensure that psychosocial symptoms are not having a significant impact on their lives.[1814,1815] This need for follow-up has required the development of specialized neurocognitive assessment tools[1816-1820] and will also require the development of markers to identify which patients are at risk for late effects from different therapies. Genetic constitution, pharmacogenomics, and individualized pharmacokinetics will need to be assessed when therapy is planned, and appropriate modifications will need to be made to adapt to the unique variables of each individual patient.[1821]

Not all late effects result solely from therapy. Many late effects are the direct result of the tumor or the raised ICP at presentation. For example seizures can occur as a function of the location of the tumor, the therapy, or both. The occasional breakthrough seizure that is relatively well-controlled and not a major concern in childhood can become a significant problem with respect to work and driving while the survivor enters adulthood.[1822] The effect of having had a brain tumor on body image can also be significant. Facial asymmetry caused by tumor infiltration of the brainstem, visual impairment from tumors in the optic pathway, or gait abnormalities from involvement of the motor cortex provide daily reminders to patients that they continue to live with the effects of having had a brain tumor. Raised ICP can also lead to significant vision loss.[1823]

Late Effects of Surgery

Although GTR is the goal of surgery for most types of brain tumors, the consequences of cerebellar or brainstem injury after resection of posterior fossa tumors or the behavioral and endocrine alterations after resection of suprasellar tumors may have a serious impact on the long-term quality of life for a patient. Many surgical morbidities may be acute and can improve over time but other deficits may persist, directly affecting the quality of life for survivors.[1824] The association between surgical dissection of the vermis for tumors involving the fourth ventricle and cerebellar mutism (posterior fossa) syndrome has been well documented, although a precise mechanism has yet to be elucidated. In a report from two large cooperative clinical trials for patients with medulloblastoma, up to 25% of patients were retrospectively identified as having cerebellar mutism syndrome and 92% of cases were deemed moderate or severe. More concerning, 1 year after surgery a significant proportion of these patients were reported to have continued nonmotor speech, language, and neurocognitive deficits, and/or ataxia.[242] Changes in respiratory function related to cerebellar dysfunction can also persist.[1825] Long-term balance problems after posterior fossa surgery remains a major issue for patients and, although this adverse effect may be improved with sparing of the deep cerebellar nuclei when resecting posterior fossa lesions, a significant proportion of children will still have residual deficits.[1826]

The increasing use of third ventriculostomies to treat hydrocephalus has helped reduce the need for prolonged VP shunt management. Patients with VP shunts will need long-term assessment of shunt function and, for patients who were very young at the time of VP shunt placement, repeat surgery to reposition and lengthen tubing may be required. Patients must be aware of the risks of shunt failure (both VP shunts and third ventriculostomies) throughout their lives.

Children with brain tumors who undergo surgical resection as their sole treatment—many with benign histologies—are expected to have few long-term effects from their tumor or treatment. However detailed neuropsychiatric and neurocognitive assessments have revealed that these patients often demonstrate significant abnormalities, including mood, behavioral, and academic difficulties.[429,1827] These results indicate that all brain tumor survivors, including those receiving minimal intervention, require long-term evaluation and support.

Late Effects of Radiation

Radiation therapy can produce acute, subacute, and late effects on the CNS.[1828] The subacute effects of radiation therapy typically become evident 2 to 6 months after treatment and include the radiation somnolence syndrome (RSS), Lhermitte sign, and radiation necrosis.

RSS typically follows within 1 to 2 months of large-volume cerebral irradiation. In a series of 19 adult patients treated with radiation therapy for their CNS tumors, 16 experienced RSS.[1829] Patients typically become lethargic and anorexic and may report fever and headaches. Drowsiness and inability to concentrate are also common.[1829] Many of the symptoms recapitulate those at presentation of the initial tumor and can be very distressing to patients and their parents. The syndrome spontaneously resolves within 1 month in most cases, but occasionally low-dose corticosteroids are required.[1830]

Lhermitte sign is described by patients as an electric shock sensation traveling down the spine on neck flexion, usually arising within several months of cervicothoracic spinal irradiation.[1788] Occurrence after administration of chemotherapy, especially cisplatin, has also been reported.[1831] It is estimated to occur in 3% to 13% of adults[1832] but has not been well studied in the pediatric population. It usually resolves spontaneously within 2 to 3 months, although a few rare cases of prolonged sensory symptoms have been reported.[1832]

Radiation necrosis (Fig. 57-56) frequently occurs within months of treatment, although it can be observed

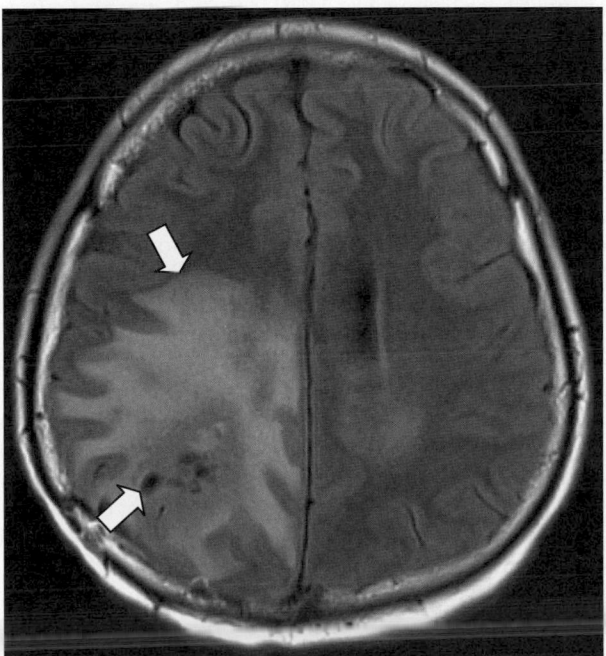

Figure 57-56 Radiation-induced necrosis demonstrating edema (*anterior arrow*) and central necrosis and blood products (*posterior arrow*).

even years later; a median of 9 months for onset was reported in one retrospective series.[1833] The incidence can increase in association with chemotherapy.[1834] Common findings on MRI include an enlargement of the tumor region, with a central area of necrosis and strong edema signal best demonstrated on T2-weighted or FLAIR sequences. Because of the overlapping symptoms and MRI appearance of radiation necrosis with tumor progression, surgery is sometimes required to confirm the diagnosis and to relieve symptoms. A number of newer imaging modalities are being evaluated to better differentiate tumor necrosis from tumor progression; these modalities include perfusion MRI,[1835] DTI,[1836] and ^{11}C-methionine or ^{13}N-NH3-PET imaging.[1837,1838] On histopathologic examination, if a biopsy is performed, a significant lymphocytic infiltration can be observed.[1839] The occurrence of radiation necrosis is associated with increasing doses of radiation therapy and is most common with doses greater than 6000 cGy and fraction sizes greater than 180 cGy. It is commonly associated with SRS, especially in highly cellular tumors. Small round blue cell tumors of the CNS and glioblastoma multiforme are at particular risk. The treatment of radiation necrosis has historically relied on the use of high-dose steroids to suppress the inflammatory response and resulting edema. More recently the use of antiangiogenic agents has demonstrated activity in this regard. VEGF (initially identified as vascular permeability factor) regulates endothelial cell integrity. Thus agents that target VEGF signaling may become important therapeutic options in this regard.[1840,1841]

The late effects of radiation therapy can occur over a wide time range, and patients have an increase in mortality rate as adults as a result of secondary malignancies, recurrence, and vasculopathy.[1842,1843] On MRI transient T2-weighted signal abnormalities have been identified in patients approximately 1 year after radiation and chemotherapy. These lesions are smaller than 1 cm, and patients are generally asymptomatic. They occur in the high-dose radiation volumes and typically resolve on subsequent MRIs.[1844] These MRI findings can be a cause of concern for tumor recurrence but will usually resolve without therapy.

Late consequences of CNS radiotherapy include subtle or symptomatic, progressive, cognitive deficiencies in areas such as attention[1845] and memory impairment; learning disabilities become apparent[1158] and are related to the dose and volume delivered.[1846] Younger age at the time of radiation therapy is a critical variable. Patients younger than 3 years are at severe risk; those aged 3 to approximately 10 years can anticipate some cognitive decline. Even older children and adults will demonstrate some cognitive deficits after large-volume, high-dose cranial irradiation. It is unclear whether this effect reaches a plateau. Abnormal patterning of the hippocampus in patients undergoing radiation therapy have been observed and may account for some of the memory difficulties in this group of survivors.[1847] Similarly distinct patterns of volume loss in the posterior components of the corpus callosum in patients treated for medulloblastoma have also been reported and follow the radiation dosimetry in these regions.[1848] A detailed evaluation and assessment of the neurocognitive effects caused by therapy requires standardized and validated tools.[1820,1849]

Leukoencephalopathy has been described in children with ALL who received intrathecal and intravenous methotrexate[1850] and whole-brain irradiation.[1851] Similar findings are reported in association with high-dose cytarabine. Leukoencephalopathy may manifest subtle but progressive cognitive decline, as well as seizures. In its severe form, the child becomes demented and incapacitated. MR and CT imaging show diffuse periventricular leukomalacia, with patchy necrosis and calcification. The administration of high-dose intravenous methotrexate after craniospinal irradiation may lead to an especially high risk of leukoencephalopathy and transverse myelitis, and this sequence of treatments should be avoided. Myelopathy may arise as a late consequence of spinal irradiation. Changes in white matter as a result of radiation therapy can have a dramatic impact on cognitive function later in life, and serial assessment of these changes may be used to guide survivorship issues and intervention.[1852,1853] Many patients with significant cognitive decline after radiation therapy, particularly of the temporal lobes, may not demonstrate specific white matter or vascular changes to explain the clinical deterioration.[1854]

Radiation injury to vascular endothelium may lead to ischemic strokes.[1855,1856] If the process is slowly progressive, multiple small collateral vessels may arise consistent with a moyamoya pattern, as seen on MRI or angiogram. Patients with NF-1 are particularly at risk.[1828] This damage to vascular structures of the brain can result in long-term cerebrovascular problems, even decades later,[1857] ranging from acute hemorrhages and cavernous angiomas[1858] to slow and progressive loss of the vasculature and compensatory development of new vessels. The new vessels associated with moyamoya, however, are insufficient to replace the damaged ones.[85] When diagnosed, moyamoya can be corrected with a procedure called pial synangiosis and is well tolerated.[1859,1860]

Secondary malignancies including HGGs, atypical meningiomas,[1861] osteosarcomas,[1862] thyroid carcinoma,[1863] cavernous malformations, and schwannomas have been observed within the treatment field several years after the completion of radiation therapy (Fig. 57-57). Most radiation-induced tumors are not observed before 5 years and can often occur in the marginal areas that received intermediate doses (Fig. 57-58). From a molecular basis, radiation-induced secondary tumors in children do not appear significantly different than those that arise de novo. The prognoses for secondary HGG, atypical meningiomas, and osteosarcomas remains exceedingly poor,[712] thus arguing for the judicious use of radiation therapy, especially for patients with low-grade tumors.[621] Patients with Turcot syndrome, Gorlin syndrome, and NF-1 are more likely to have a secondary malignant glioma after radiation therapy compared with patients who do not have these conditions.[1864]

Pediatric patients with CNS tumors are at high risk for various endocrinologic abnormalities as a result of their tumor[1865] if they needed surgery (especially for pituitary region tumors) or radiation therapy that involves the

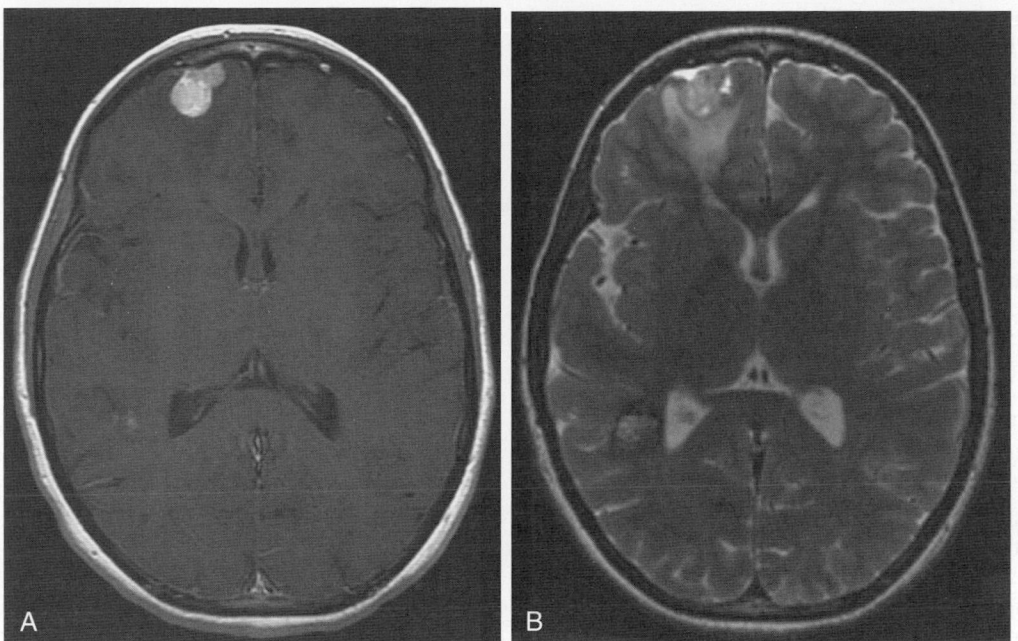

Figure 57-57 Radiation-induced meningioma and cavernous malformation. **A,** An axial T1-weighted image with use of contrast material. **B,** An axial T2-weighted image.

hypothalamus and/or pituitary region.[1866,1867] Growth retardation is usually multifactorial.[1868] Radiation to the pituitary gland may affect the production and release of growth hormone.[1869] Pituitary function may also be impaired by direct invasion of the gland by adjacent tumor. Obesity can be a direct result of radiation therapy on the hypothalamus.[1870] In addition spinal radiation (as part of craniospinal treatment) affects the growth of the vertebral bones and overall bone density, within the radiation field and throughout the body.[1871] Ovarian function can be protected with laparoscopic oophoropexy preirradiation therapy in prepubertal girls in whom the ovaries are likely to be near the midline.[1872] Growth failure after treatment requires active and continued participation by endocrinologists as the cause of growth failure changes from chemotherapy-induced cachexia to radiation-mediated growth hormone deficiency.[1873] Although many patients are discouraged from initiating growth hormone replacement because of concerns for reactivation of the primary tumor or a second malignancy, no evidence exists that these phenomena occur.[1874,1875] In contrast the morbidity related to not replacing growth

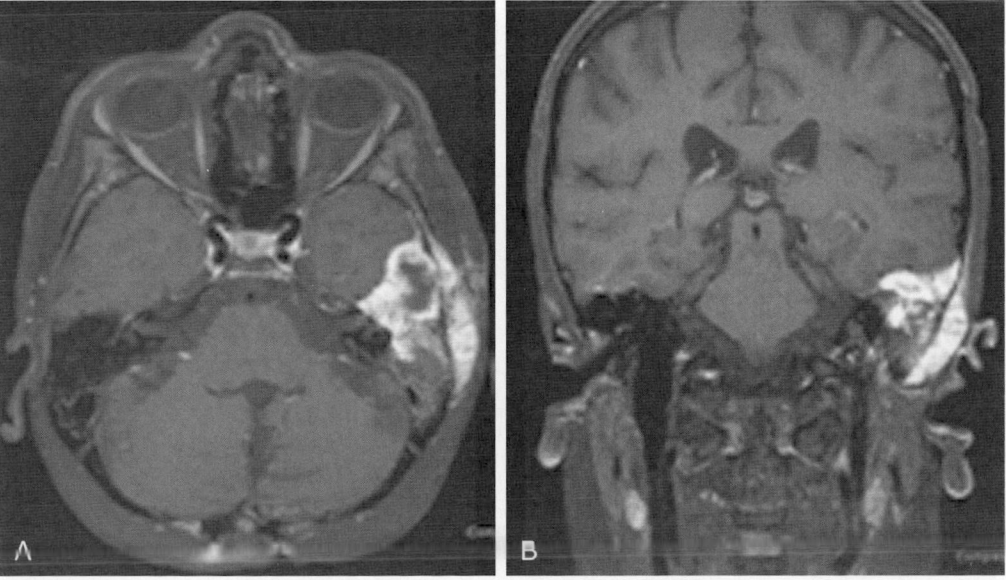

Figure 57-58 A radiation-induced left cranial osteosarcoma. **A,** An axial T1-weighted image with use of contrast material, with fat suppression. **B,** A coronal T1-weighted image with use of contrast material, with fat suppression.

hormone for persons who are deficient can be severe and lifelong.[1876] Although most centers start growth hormone 1 year after completion of therapy, no evidence suggests that earlier treatment would increase the risk of tumor recurrence. Sleep problems and daytime fatigue[1503,1877] are also highly prevalent, and hypothyroidism and adreno-cortical dysfunction can augment these problems and need to be corrected before any additional interventions are initiated.

Proton beam radiation therapy is becoming more common, and children needing radiation therapy for treatment should be evaluated for proton beam radiation therapy if possible because of the decrease in exit dose that would further minimize exposure of normal tissue to radiation.[1878]

Late Effects of Chemotherapy

Although most chemotherapy-related toxicities occur acutely, a number of long-term adverse effects are well recognized. Many of the neurologic effects of chemo-therapy become evident at the time of drug administration and will improve after cessation of the drug. In some patients, however, these toxicities can become long-term issues. Peripheral neuropathy is a common late effect of several chemotherapy agents,[1879] particularly vincris-tine.[1879] Cisplatin and carboplatin mainly affect proprio-ception and spare pain and temperature sensation. The usual presenting symptoms are painful dysesthesias and tingling sensations in the toes and later in the fingers. Motor fibers are spared. In contrast vincristine produces sensorimotor neuropathies. The first symptoms are usually tingling in the toes and fingers. Loss of ankle reflexes is typically the first objective sign. Continued treatment with the drug leads to loss or decrease in reflexes and motor weakness involving the dorsiflexors of the feet. Patients with preexisting neuropathies may become quadriparetic after treatment with vincristine. Cerebellar syndromes of acute onset may be seen with high-dose cytarabine and occasionally with 5-fluorouracil. These complications are usually reversible within 2 weeks, but severe irreversible damage to Purkinje cells may occur if the drug is given for several months or if the drug is reintroduced at a later time.[1880] Transverse myelopathy is seen with prolonged treatments with intrathecal metho-trexate or cytarabine. The risk is higher when combined with spinal irradiation.

Speech, language, and hearing are important compo-nents of daily functioning and can often be significantly impaired as a result of the brain tumor itself and its treat-ment.[1881] Many patients can have significant impairment that requires early and aggressive diagnosis and manage-ment.[1882] Radiation therapy can cause long-term hearing impairment,[1883] but platinum agents such as cisplatin and, to a lesser extent, carboplatin can cause significant sen-sorineural hearing loss in a dose-dependent manner. Although the higher frequencies of hearing, those above the normal hearing range, are usually affected initially, progressive loss can occur over time, including frequen-cies within the normal range. In one retrospective insti-tutional study, 4% of patients treated with carboplatin and 57% of patients treated with cisplatin experienced

significant hearing loss.[1884] The question of whether agents such as amifostine can reduce cisplatin-mediated hearing loss is controversial.[1143,1144] Patients at risk for hearing loss should therefore be followed up regularly by audiologists so that early corrective action (e.g., dose reduction of platinum agents and hearing aids) can be instituted.[1885]

Renal dysfunction is a rare complication of cisplatin toxicity; it can lead to lifelong proteinuria and salt wasting.[1886] Various electrolytes can be lost with renal impairment and may require daily oral supplementation.

Secondary malignancies are a rare but significant late effect of chemotherapy. In children acute myelogenous leukemia is the most common type of secondary malig-nancy induced by chemotherapy, and it is most frequently caused by intravenous etoposide.[1887] The risk of acute myelogenous leukemia appears to be dependent on the frequency and dose administered and is highest when etoposide is administered weekly, is less when adminis-tered monthly, and is very low when given daily in low-dose oral administration. These leukemias tend to occur 3 to 5 years after etoposide administration. Alkylating agents and platinum-based drugs are less commonly implicated. The transient genotoxic damage to chromo-somes by chemotherapy may account for this risk.[1888]

A critical measure of the effectiveness of treatment of pediatric brain tumors is the patient's quality of life. Although this broad measure is difficult to define across all heterogeneous tumor types, age at presentation, and presenting morbidities, a greater emphasis on under-standing how to optimize each child's potential has become the focus of many treatment protocols. The development of new assessment tools will also be impor-tant as new therapies are evaluated based on their efficacy and the quality of life.[1889]

Survivors have indicated the constant stress they feel after the medical team, family, and friends have declared success in curing them and their brain tumors.[1890] They recognize their own impaired social functioning much of the time[1891] and yet can also be unaware of important psychosocial and behavioral issues evident to others.[1892] Depression is a frequent and often poorly recognized outcome in these patients.[1893] Even patients with excellent prognoses, such as those with a history of LGGs, dem-onstrate chronic medical problems, as evidenced in one report of 87 patients in which 100% of patients had such issues.[1894] Declines in attention and concentration in sur-vivors of pediatric brain tumors are a major problem,[1895] even when compared with other populations that have received therapy directed toward the CNS, such as survi-vors of childhood ALL.[1896] Part of this effect likely reflects the dosimetry of radiation used for patients with brain tumors, which increases neurocognitive impairment.[1897] Verbal memory difficulties associated with the treatment of tumors in the third ventricular region are significantly greater than those seen in patients with posterior fossa tumors, in whom attention difficulties predominate.[1898] The development of models to assist in the risk assess-ment of having a poor outcome is needed.[1899] These issues become particularly acute for this population, especially when they reach adulthood, when they are often faced with insurance barriers preventing them from receiving much-needed therapy.[1900]

Given the broad issues faced by brain tumor survivors, it is difficult to develop a single all-encompassing guideline for follow-up care. Multidisciplinary care in dedicated survivor programs can focus resources needed to identify and address issues in this patient population. From the imaging standpoint, many centers have adopted the standard of scanning patients who have completed therapy every 3 months for the first year, every 6 months for the second year, and then yearly thereafter. Routine surveillance of renal and audiologic assessments depends on the field and dose of radiation therapy, as well as the cumulative dose of platinum chemotherapy agents. The frequency of cardiac and pulmonary assessments also depends on particular agents previously used and their cumulative doses. Continued radiologic and blood chemistry surveillance is recommended for most patients as the risk of tumor recurrence decreases and is replaced by increased second tumor risk.

PALLIATIVE CARE

Although clinicians and caregivers focus a great deal of attention on attempts to eradicate disease, a significant proportion of patients with pediatric brain tumors will not survive and, in the process, many often suffer. The early introduction of palliative services, including discussions on the management of all symptoms[1901] and resuscitative measures (e.g., do not resuscitate orders),[1902] can allow patients and families in the terminal phase of care a more peaceful and dignified death.[1903-1905] Early and aggressive management of pain must be anticipated and the necessary expertise put in place.[1906] Children can often participate in discussion of end-of-life care.[1907] Decisions about where the child will die, either at home or in the hospital, as well as other aspects of terminal care must be addressed with the family and caregivers and require institutional support and resources.[1908] Finally, the discussion about the possibility of autopsy is never an easy one. The more time that patients, parents, and families have to consider an autopsy, separated in time from the actual death and grieving, the more likely they are to be able to make a decision that is right for themselves and their families. To understand the patient's disease better so that other children might be spared the same fate is comforting to families who consent to an autopsy.

Although limited by local governing policy, there is a low risk of transmission of cancer via transplanted organs from children with primary CNS tumors because of their infrequent spread outside the brain and spine. Given the severe shortage of organs, consideration of this option should be presented to the patient, family, and transplantation team.[1909]

Many families have expressed the importance of their relationship with the caregiving team. Many families actually feel abandoned after the child has died when communication and interaction with the medical team suddenly ends.[3] A number of palliative care programs and the expanding literature in this area are now available to help parents and caregivers through the grieving period.

References available online at ExpertConsult.

CHAPTER 58

Hepatoblastoma and Other Liver Tumors in Children

Gail E. Tomlinson

CHAPTER OUTLINE

INTRODUCTION AND EPIDEMIOLOGY

Liver tumors in children account for approximately 1.1% of all malignancies in children younger than 20 years of age according to the National Cancer Institute's Surveillance, Epidemiology, and End Results (SEER) reports. The age-adjusted incidence rate of liver tumors is approximately 11 per million in infants younger than the age of 1 year and approximately 6 per million in children between 1 and 4 years of age.[1] This translates to approximately 100 to 150 new cases of liver cancer annually in children in the United States.

Liver malignancies in children can be divided into three broad classifications: hepatoblastoma, which accounts for two thirds of malignant liver cancers and the predominant malignant tumor type in young children; hepatocellular carcinoma (HCC), the predominant tumor type in adolescents; and other rare hepatic malignancies of childhood. A spectrum of benign tumor histologies broadens the differential diagnosis of the infant or child with a liver mass.

In an early meta-analysis of eleven separate series totaling 1256 primary liver tumors in children reported by Weinberg and Finegold, 43% were hepatoblastoma,

23% HCC, 13% benign vascular tumors, 6% mesenchymal hamartomas, 6% sarcomas, 2% adenomas, 2% focal nodular hyperplasia, and 5% other tumors.[2] Rare tumors of the liver also include rhabdoid tumors and hepatic germ cell tumors. An international working group recently provided guidelines regarding the histologic classification of pediatric liver tumors.[3]

Most liver tumors in childhood are more common in boys than girls. The male-to-female ratio observed for hepatoblastoma in cooperative group trials has ranged from 1.5 to 1 to 2 to 1; a combined analysis of multiple studies suggests that the male-to-female ratio in hepatoblastoma is 1.65,[4-7,8] consistent with SEER data.[1]

Hepatoblastomas have a unique age distribution (Fig. 58-1). Two peak ages occur, one at birth or within the first month of life and a second broad peak between 16 and 20 months of age. Ninety percent of hepatoblastomas occur in children younger than 4 years of age, and 95% of hepatoblastomas occur by age 5. Although rare, hepatoblastoma has been seen in adults, as described in multiple sporadic case reports.[9-31] A systematic review of hepatoblastoma in adults suggests that these tumors are associated with a particularly poor prognosis, although the time frame over which these cases were gathered

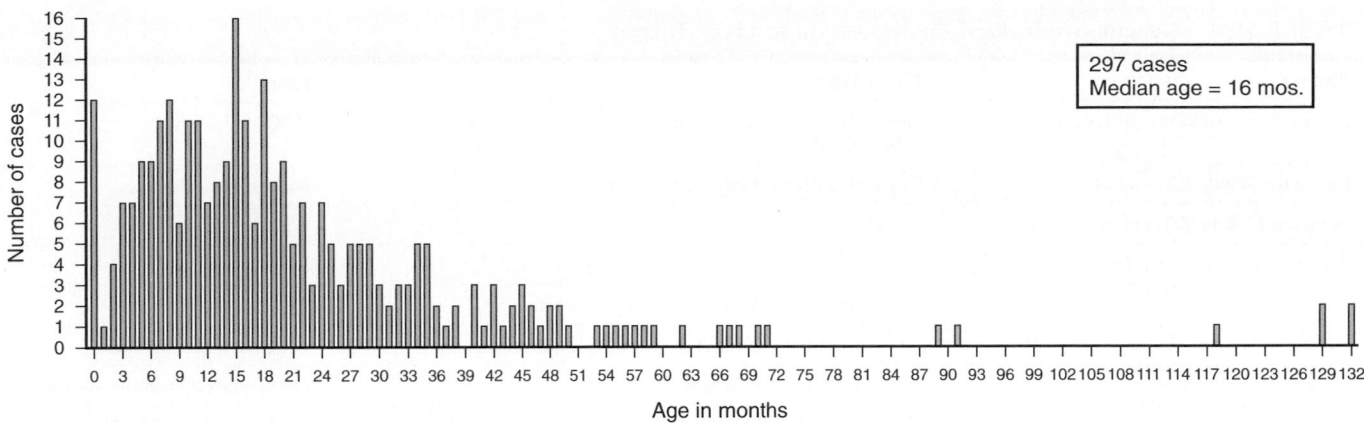

Figure 58-1 Age distribution of hepatoblastoma derived from 256 sequential cases representing all stages and histologies of hepatoblastoma. An initial peak is seen at birth, reflecting tumors developing during gestation. The median age of all children with hepatoblastoma is 18 months, and the oldest age is 78 months. In 99% of cases hepatoblastoma was apparent by 5 years of age.

spanned multiple decades.[32] In contrast hepatoblastomas diagnosed very early in life (i.e., in the neonatal period) are associated with a favorable outcome.[33]

Hepatoblastoma in children older than 5 years of age is often more aggressive than the typical hepatoblastoma, has characteristics of HCC, and has been termed *transitional liver cell tumor*.[34] More recently pathologists prefer to designate this poorly understood entity as *hepatocellular tumor, not otherwise specified*, pending a much-needed and more thorough understanding of the biology of these tumors with features of both hepatoblastoma and HCC.[3] HCCs make up the bulk of liver tumors seen after age 10 years and throughout adolescence and adulthood. As with hepatoblastoma, HCC is more common in male subjects than female subjects.[35-37] The fibrolamellar variant of HCC is a notable exception, with equal occurrence in male and female subjects.[38,39,40]

The incidence of liver tumors has increased over recent decades, perhaps more than any other type of childhood tumor. During a single decade the incidence rates of hepatic tumors in infants younger than 1 year of age increased from 4 to 8 per million.[41] The increase in rates was especially pronounced in female infants, in whom rates of hepatic cancer increased from 2 to 12 per million in a single decade. Ross and Gurney estimated that the average annual percentage change in incidence of hepatoblastoma between 1973 and 1992 was 5.2% for males and 8.2% for females.[42] The rise in incidence of hepatoblastoma has been estimated to be 4% per year between 1992 and 2004[43] and continues to rise in recent years compared with even recent SEER data.[1,44] The largest contributing factor to the increased incidence is thought to be the increased survival rates of premature infants who are at markedly increased risk of hepatoblastoma, as discussed in subsequent sections of this chapter.

ORIGINS OF HEPATOBLASTOMA

Hepatoblastoma has long been thought to have prenatal origins,[45,46] and increasing evidence points to prematurity, prenatal exposures, and overgrowth in early infancy

as factors contributing to hepatoblastoma. It has long been presumed that embryonal tumors derive from primitive cells and that hepatoblastoma, as an embryonal tumor of the liver in which cells morphologically resemble cells in the developing embryonal and fetal liver, derives from a primitive hepatic cell. In rodents immature oval cells that proliferate after exposure to hepatocarcinogens express both biliary and hepatocytic markers.[47] These cells are characterized by staining with OV-1 and OV-6 markers. Ruck and colleagues demonstrated the existence of a similar cell type in hepatoblastoma on the basis of marking with OV-1 and OV-6 in a small population of cells within the tumor.[48-50] These OV-1 and OV-6 staining cells account for fewer than 1% of the cells within the tumor and provided evidence to support the existence of a population of stem cells in hepatoblastoma. Fiegel and coworkers analyzed hepatoblastomas for stem cell markers including CD34, Thy1, and c-kit and demonstrated the co-occurrence of these stem cell markers with hepatobiliary markers in ductal cells phenotypically resembling stem cells, which suggests that stemlike cells play a role in the histogenesis of hepatoblastoma.[51] Other markers of hepatic progenitor cells including epithelial cell adhesion molecule (EpCAM), cytokeratin 19 (CK19), octamer-binding transcription factor 3/4 (Oct-3/4), and delta-like 1 homologue (DLK1) have been shown to be expressed in hepatoblastoma tumor cells.[52] NOTCH2, which peaks in the second half of fetal development and then declines toward birth, is expressed in most hepatoblastomas.[53] CITED1, expressed in embryonic mouse liver and a marker of hepatic progenitor cells, is shown to be present in hepatoblastoma, providing another similarity of hepatoblastoma to hepatic precursor stem cells.[54]

GENETIC PREDISPOSITION AND LIVER TUMORIGENESIS

Most cases of childhood liver malignancy are not associated with an apparent major genetic syndrome. However numerous syndromes have been observed in association with hepatoblastoma or HCC, as well as some benign

TABLE 58-1   Genetic Syndromes' Predisposition to Liver Tumors

Disease	Tumor Type	Gene
Familial adenomatous polyposis	Hepatoblastoma, adenoma, hepatocellular carcinoma, biliary adenoma	APC
Beckwith-Wiedemann syndrome	Hepatoblastoma, hemangioendothelioma	Multiple candidates
Simpson-Golabi-Behmel syndrome	Hepatoblastoma	GPC3
Trisomy 18	Hepatoblastoma	No single gene
Li-Fraumeni syndrome	Hepatoblastoma, undifferentiated sarcoma	TP53
Glycogen storage disease types I-IV	Hepatocellular adenoma, carcinoma hepatoblastoma	Glucose-6-phosphatase
Hereditary tyrosinemia	Hepatocellular carcinoma	Fumarylaceto-acetate hydrolase
Alagille syndrome	Hepatocellular carcinoma	JAGGED-1, NOTCH2
Other familial cholestatic syndromes	Hepatocellular carcinoma	FIC1, ABCB11
Neurofibromatosis	Hepatocellular carcinoma, malignant schwannoma, angiosarcoma	NF-1
Ataxia—telangiectasia	Hepatocellular carcinoma	ATM
Fanconi anemia	Hepatocellular carcinoma, fibrolamellar cancer, adenoma	FAA, FAC, others (20%)
Tuberous sclerosis	Angiomyolipoma	TSC1, TSC2

hepatic tumors. A complete summary of genetic syndromes and liver tumors in children is provided in Table 58-1. The major genetic syndromes associated with childhood liver tumors are discussed in the subsequent sections.

Familial Adenomatous Polyposis

Familial adenomatous polyposis (FAP) is caused by germline mutation of the *APC* gene,[55] FAP is best characterized by the presence of colonic polyps, which without intervention are associated with the virtual certainty that adenocarcinoma of the colon will develop. Germline mutation of the *APC* gene is, however, also associated with a marked increased risk of hepatoblastoma. The risk of hepatoblastoma in children in FAP kindred is estimated to be 800-fold.[56] The risk that a parent with an *APC* mutation will have a child with hepatoblastoma is 0.4%.[57] Because FAP is an autosomal dominant disorder, genetic testing should demonstrate a predisposing mutation in 50% of offspring, such that the risk of hepatoblastoma in an infant who is a documented mutation carrier would be slightly less than 1%. Within a series of consecutive hepatoblastoma patients for whom family histories were obtained, approximately 8% of sequential cases of hepatoblastoma have a family history suggestive of FAP, and abnormalities of the *APC* gene were detectable in all cases.[58]

Also reported in children from FAP kindreds, albeit less commonly, are other liver tumors, including HCCs.[59-62] A benign precursor lesion, hepatocellular adenoma has been reported in a patient with a germline *APC* mutation and colonic polyps.[63] Within resected liver tissue from children with germline *APC* mutations and hepatoblastoma, multiple hepatic nodules were consistent with precursor lesions with potential to progress to either

hepatoblastoma or HCC.[64] Presumably the timing of additional mutations or key developmental processes could determine the resulting histologic tumor type in the predisposed liver.

Significantly of nine reported cases of hepatoblastoma in siblings, at least four were in families with FAP;[65-68] Of the remaining reported sibling pairs, one was affected with type 1a glycogen storage disease,[69] and two sibling pairs had no apparent familial syndrome,[70,71] and one recent report of a sibling pair with hepatoblastoma demonstrated an *APC* mutation in only one of the siblings.[72] These reports suggest that whereas *APC* mutation accounts for a significant percentage of familial cases of hepatoblastoma, additional predisposition genetic changes may exist either as a distinct underlying cause of hepatoblastoma or as a modifying factor in infants with an existing *APC* mutation.

The percentage of sporadic hepatoblastoma patients (those without an obvious family history) who carry a germline mutation of the *APC* gene is not well defined. However it has been suggested both that children with hepatoblastoma be screened for germline *APC* mutations and that asymptomatic children in families with known polyposis be screened for hepatoblastoma.[73] Within the *APC* gene genotype-phenotype correlations suggest regions of the gene that predict both the severity of polyposis as well as the presence of extracolonic manifestations. The literature suggests that germline mutations in FAP families with children who are affected by hepatoblastoma can occur throughout the gene (Fig. 58-2) and can also include whole gene deletions or chromosome rearrangements such that the site or type of the individual *APC* mutation cannot be used to predict the occurrence of hepatoblastoma.[58,65,74] This finding implies a risk to all *APC* mutation carriers.

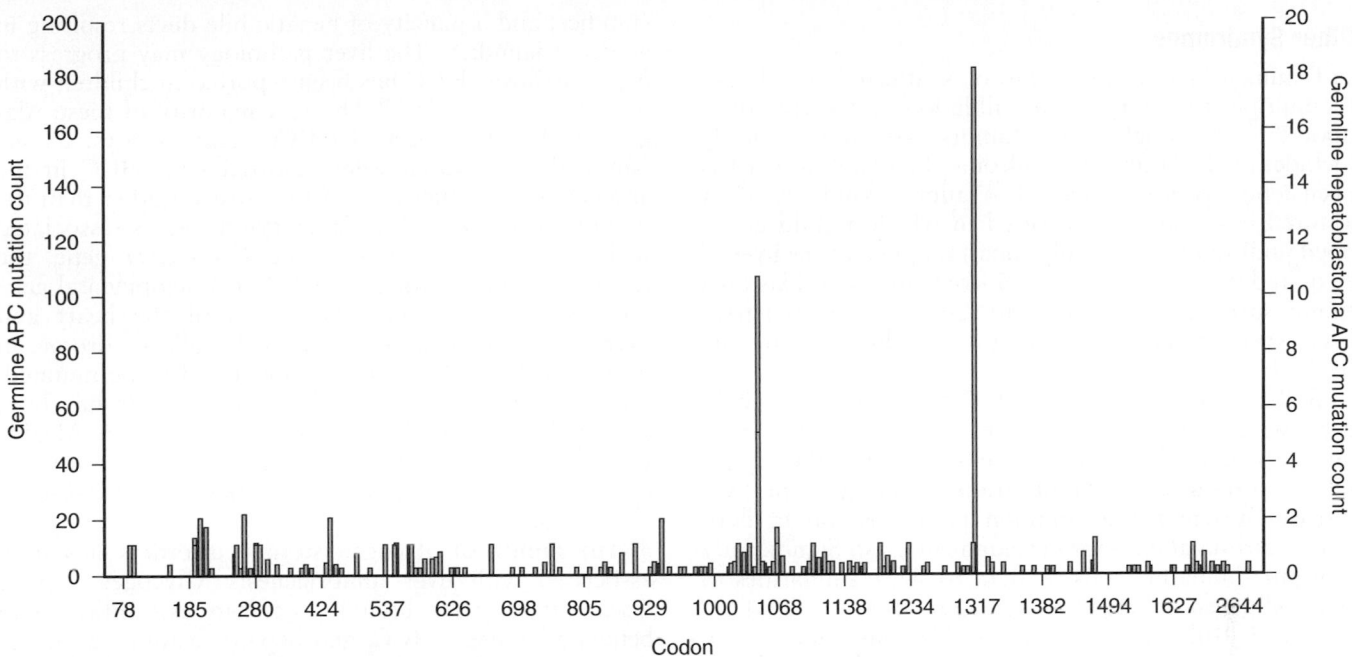

Figure 58-2 Frequency histogram of mutations in the adenomatous polyposis coli *(APC)* gene. Left axis and black lines represent all known APC germline mutations. Right axis and orange lines represent APC germline mutations in children with hepatoblastoma. Germline mutations associated with hepatoblastoma are observed throughout the gene. *(From Hirschman B, Pollock B, Tomlinson G: The spectrum of APC mutations in children with hepatoblastoma from familial adenomatous polyposis kindreds.* J Pediatr 147:263–266, 2005.*)*

Overgrowth Syndromes and Hepatoblastoma

Beckwith-Wiedemann syndrome (BWS) is an overgrowth disorder classically characterized by large birth weight, macroglossia, omphalocele, and visceromegaly.[75,76] It is associated with a markedly increased risk of all embryonal tumors, including Wilms tumors, hepatoblastoma, neuroblastoma, and adrenal cortical adenoma.[75,77,78] A registry of children with BWS followed at the National Cancer Institute determined that the relative risk of hepatoblastoma in children with BWS was 2280, higher than the relative risk of any other type of cancer in BWS.[79] Unlike hepatoblastoma and FAP, hepatoblastoma has not been seen in siblings with BWS, despite the extraordinarily high relative individual risk in a patient with BWS. Presumably, this is because of the low incidence of familial occurrence of BWS.

BWS maps to chromosome 11p15, a region known to show loss of alleles in hepatoblastoma[80,81] as well as parental-specific expression of genes (i.e., imprinting), including *IGF2* and *H19*. Molecular subtyping demonstrated that genetic alterations underlying BWS include mutations, epigenetic events involving imprinted genes, or uniparental disomy and that imprinting defects are of two types—those with imprinting defect at the imprinting control element 1 (IC1) at distal 11p15.5 and involving IGF2 and H19 hypermethylation and those with a defect at the imprinting control element (IC2), which is more proximal and involved imprinting changes of KvDMR1 and KCN11OT1.[82,83] One series demonstrated that significantly more neoplasia is noted with either uniparental disomy or imprinting defects at IC1,[82] although hepatoblastoma has been observed in BWS patients with mutations at the IC2 locus.[83] Although differences may exist specific to the type of underlying genetic alteration, it is not possible at this time to tailor screening recommendations to genetic subtype. Present screening recommendations involve periodic ultrasonography of the abdomen and measurement of serum alpha-fetoprotein (AFP).[84-86] In a series of tumors detected in children with BWS who underwent such surveillance, all tumors were small and resectable at diagnosis.[84] Because hepatoblastoma has been noted to occur in the early neonatal period in BWS, some experts recommend screening at an early age.[87] Even though AFP levels are normally very high in the neonatal period, screening with AFP should confirm a downward trend in the absence of tumor.

Simpson-Golabi-Behmel syndrome (SGBS) is an X-linked syndrome characterized by overgrowth with clinical features reminiscent of BWS, including an increased risk of embryonal tumors. Individual cases of SGBS with hepatoblastoma have been reported.[88-90] The underlying gene for SGBS, *GPC3*, is highly expressed in hepatoblastoma compared with normal liver, which is consistent with a potential role in the tumorigenesis of hepatoblastoma.[91-93] Although no longitudinal tumor surveillance studies have been carried out for SGBS, the overlap in tumor types observed suggests that surveillance similar to that used for BWS may be appropriate.

Sotos syndrome, an overgrowth syndrome that has clinical features overlapping with BWS and is associated with a predilection for tumors, has been reported in a child with hepatoblastoma.[94,95] No large series have been reported, however, and the benefit of screening is unclear at this time.

Other Syndromes

Li-Fraumeni syndrome predisposes affected individuals to multiple tumor types in childhood and early adulthood.[96,97] Although liver tumors are not typically included in Li-Fraumeni syndrome, hepatoblastoma has been reported in two Asian Li-Fraumeni kindreds.[98,99] A kindred has also been reported in which a child developed undifferentiated (embryonal) sarcoma of the liver.[100] Acquired mutations of the TP53 gene in hepatoblastoma tumor specimens, however, are rare or absent but have been reported in the undifferentiated embryonal sarcoma of the liver.[101-103]

Both hepatoblastoma and HCC have occurred in children with primary biliary atresia.[104,105] However it is unclear whether liver tumor development in children with biliary atresia is a complication resulting from liver disease or whether a common predisposition to both biliary atresia and tumor development exist. Significantly the same immature cells thought to share similarities to stem cells seen in hepatoblastoma are also seen in biliary atresia.[106] Multiple cases of hepatoblastoma and trisomy 18 have been reported.[107-113] This is somewhat notable in that trisomy of chromosome 18 is not seen as an acquired event despite the observation of multiple other recurring trisomies.[114]

Hepatoblastoma has been reported in a female subject with monosomy 7 myelodysplasia, a predisposition syndrome not previously seen with hepatoblastoma.[115] Hepatoblastoma has also been reported in neurofibromatosis type 1, although it is not characteristic of this disorder.[116]

A recent report has noted a possible association of hepatoblastoma with prune-belly syndrome, a congenital disorder of lax abdominal musculature and urogenital abnormalities.[117] A review of data from the Children's Oncology Group (COG) demonstrated a significant association with kidney and bladder congenital abnormalities.[118]

Genetic Syndromes and Hepatocellular Carcinoma

HCC, in contrast to hepatoblastoma, is seen in genetic syndromes that are characterized by hepatic cirrhosis. Progressive familial intrahepatic cholestasis, a condition marked by neonatal hepatic cirrhosis, is associated with liver tumor development in children. Both HCC and cholangiocarcinoma are known to occur in this disorder. The disorder, also known as Byler disease, is a heterogeneous syndrome.[119] The underlying genetic etiology is a germline mutation of the ABCB11 gene, which encodes a bile salt export pump.[120] In a series of 11 cases of HCC in children younger than 5 years with neonatal hepatitis with clinical characteristics of familial intrahepatic cholestasis, 10 had immunohistochemical evidence of a deficiency in bile acid transporter bile salt export pump.[121] In all patients in whom genotyping was possible, a germline mutation of the ABCB11 gene encoding bile salt export pump was detected.

Alagille syndrome is an autosomal-dominant disorder characterized by a characteristic facies, congenital heart disease, intrahepatic cholestasis with neonatal jaundice, and a paucity of hepatic bile ducts resulting in neonatal jaundice. The liver pathology may progress to frank cirrhosis. HCC has been reported in children with Alagille syndrome.[122-127] The vast majority of these Alagille syndrome–associated HCCs occur in boys. In one family three children were reported with HCC in the absence of any other type of liver disease other than the Alagille syndrome.[123] Alagille syndrome is associated with germline mutations in the JAGGED1 gene, the endogenous ligand for NOTCH2, a developmental gene involved in controlling maturation of the heart and liver.[128] In a minority of cases of Alagille syndrome, in which the JAGGED1 gene is not found to be mutated, the NOTCH2 gene itself is mutated.[98,129] It has been shown that the mechanism of liver disease in Alagille syndrome may relate to an increased expression in hepatocyte growth factor in cells that carry JAGGED1 mutations.[130]

The family of glycogen storage disorders has been associated with liver tumorigenesis. Glycogen storage disease type I has been reported in association with benign adenomas, HCC, and hepatoblastoma, although the latter has been reported only in adolescents.[69,131,132] Similarly glycogen storage disorder type III has been associated with HCC,[133] and type IV has been associated with hepatocellular adenoma.[134] Because HCC is known to occur in diseased liver, with long-term follow-up HCC may be considered a complication of increased survival of patients with glycogen storage disease.[132,135]

Hereditary tyrosinemia type 1, characterized by the deficiency of fumarylacetoacetate hydrolase is likewise associated with HCC in the setting of severe liver disease.[136]

Fanconi anemia is associated with liver tumors, although the association has been almost always reported in association with the use of androgenic steroid treatment.[137-143] In a review of 1301 reported cases of Fanconi anemia, 2.8% of subjects were reported to have a liver tumor.[144] The most common type of liver tumor reported in Fanconi anemia is HCC, but adenomas are also seen in these patients. The incidence appears to increase with age and does not appear to plateau. In multiple instances liver malignancy was seen in patients with Fanconi anemia who also had a diagnosis of leukemia. The extent of the associated androgen treatment with development of hepatic malignancy versus the effect of the underlying genetic defects in DNA repair as manifested by chromosome breakage in Fanconi anemia is unclear, but a review of the association of androgens and liver tumors suggests that patients with Fanconi anemia develop liver tumors after smaller and briefer androgen exposure than do individuals without Fanconi anemia.[145] It is also unclear whether there is a difference among the genetic subtypes of Fanconi anemia with regard to the predisposition to hepatic and other malignancy.[146]

Genetic Syndromes and Other Benign Liver Tumors

In addition to syndromes predisposing to malignant liver tumors, several syndromes are associated with benign liver tumors. Tuberous sclerosis has been linked to development of benign hepatic angiomyolipomas.[117,118]

Although these hepatic growths are not as common as renal angiomyolipomas, which may develop in as many as 80% of patients with tuberous sclerosis, the hepatic lesions are evident in imaging studies in approximately 13% of patients with tuberous sclerosis, according to one study.[149]

PREMATURITY AS A RISK FACTOR

One of the most intriguing aspects of hepatoblastoma is its association with premature or low-birth-weight infants. This association was initially reported by Japanese investigators who analyzed patient diagnoses and birth weights in the Japan Children's Cancer Registry over the 9-year period from 1985 to 1993.[150] It was found that 3.9% of patients with hepatoblastoma were of very low birth weight. Moreover it was observed that when data were subdivided over 4-year periods, the percentage of hepatoblastoma cases of low birth weight rose from 0.7% in 1985 to 1989 to 8.6% in 1990 to 1993 and demonstrated a linear increasing trend. The risk of hepatoblastoma has also been shown to be inversely proportional to birth weight.[151] The relative risk for an infant between 2000 and 2999 grams is 1.21, whereas the relative risk for an infant of less than 1000 grams is 15.64.

Data from the Children's Cancer Group survey confirmed the preponderance of former premature infants in a series of 76 patients with hepatoblastoma.[152] A second confirmation in the United States comes from the California population-based cancer registry, which also reported an elevated risk of hepatoblastoma in children of very low birth weight.[153] This study also pointed out that the age of diagnosis of hepatoblastoma in children of low birth weight was actually older than that of children of normal birth weight, which could partly be explained by gestational age.

It has been speculated that the increase in the percentage of low-birth-weight infants among children with hepatoblastoma may be partially caused by the increased survival rates of low-birth-weight infants. It is also believed that the increase in survival rates of premature infants at risk for hepatoblastoma may contribute to the overall increase in childhood liver tumors.

Indeed the rise in the rate of hepatoblastoma has been found to be consistent with the risk in births of low-birth-weight infants.[154] However whether the pathways by which low-birth-weight infants develop hepatoblastoma involve key exposures in the newborn period, increased sensitivity of the liver in premature infants to potential carcinogens, disruption of the normal process of liver development by premature birth, or a combination of these factors has yet to be defined. One small single-institution study, in which treatment records of five infants who developed hepatoblastoma were compared with those of infants of similar birth weights who did not develop hepatoblastoma, suggests that perinatal intensive long-term treatments contribute to the development of hepatoblastoma.[155] A somewhat larger study comparing 12 hepatoblastoma cases and 75 birth weight–matched controls suggests that the duration of oxygen therapy, use of furosemide, and length of time taken to regain body weight at birth were factors in predicting the likelihood that hepatoblastoma would develop in premature infants.[156] A study from the United Kingdom reported that polyhydramnios and either eclampsia or preeclampsia are more common in children with hepatoblastoma compared with those without hepatoblastoma, and that the eclampsia or preeclampsia observed was also associated with low birth weight.[157]

A recent case-control study of 600 COG patients with hepatoblastoma (AEPI04C1) has examined exposures in low-birth-weight and other infants with hepatoblastoma and has not found an association with maternal illness or medication use during pregnancy or infertility treatment and hepatoblastoma.[158,159] Previously use of assisted reproductive technology was postulated to be a contributing factor, although it is thought that it may contribute to hepatoblastoma development only through the associated risk of BWS and assisted reproductive technology (ART), but not as an independent risk factor.[159,160]

ENVIRONMENTAL EXPOSURES AND HEPATOBLASTOMA

An early epidemiologic case-control study of risk factors for hepatoblastoma by Buckley and colleagues, based on parental interviews, revealed an association of hepatoblastoma with maternal occupational exposure to metals, such as those used in welding or soldering (odds ratio [OR] = 8); petroleum products such as lubricating oils or greases (OR = 3.7); and paints or pigments (OR = 3.7). There was also a significant association with paternal occupational exposure to metals (OR = 3, P = .01) and a marginally significant association with paternal occupational exposure to petroleum products (OR = 1.9).[161] Although the aforementioned study did not find an association of parental smoking with hepatoblastoma, this has been reported in several subsequent studies.[162-164] The risk of hepatoblastoma in children of parents who smoked was approximately double in all three studies. Indeed in 2009 the International Agency of Research on Cancer declared that parental smoking is a carcinogen in the developing liver. Subsequent findings have been variable, however. A recent report from COG, the largest etiologic study to date, reported no association between smoking and hepatoblastoma. Variability among studies, however, could be based on small numbers and differences in reporting and overall smoking prevalence in the different populations. Although alcohol clearly plays a role in cirrhosis of the liver and HCC in adults, the COG study reported no association with parental alcohol use and hepatoblastoma in offspring.

VIRAL HEPATITIS AND LIVER TUMORS IN CHILDREN

Viral hepatitis infection has historically accounted for a large percentage of HCC cases. Before the introduction of the hepatitis B vaccine in Taiwan, HCC accounted for 80% of cases of liver tumors in children.[165] With the introduction of the hepatitis B vaccination in 1984, rates of liver tumors in Taiwanese children older than 6 years dropped significantly, from 0.70 per 100,000 from 1981 to 1986 to 0.36 per 100,000 between 1990 and 1994.[166] The decrease in rates of HCC after introduction of the vaccine was more pronounced in boys than in girls. In fact the incidence of HCC decreased in boys but not in girls.[167] The male-to-female incidence of HCC in Taiwan steadily decreased from 4.5 per 100,000 in 1981 to 1986 to 1.9 per 100,000 in 1990 to 1996, 6 to 12 years after the introduction of the vaccine. The reasons for these sex-related differences in responses to the vaccine are not known.[168] It has been demonstrated that among children with hepatitis B the presence of a deletion of the pre-S region of the hepatitis B virus was an additional risk factor for the development of HCC (OR = 36.69).[169]

PRESENTATION AND EVALUATION OF THE CHILD WITH A LIVER MASS

Aside from patients with known genetic syndromes (discussed in the preceding sections), most cases of hepatoblastoma occur in otherwise well children who present with an abdominal mass, often with some degree of abdominal discomfort.

Isosexual precocious puberty has been observed in some boys as a presenting finding in hepatoblastoma and occurs secondary to tumor production of chorionic gonadotropin.[170-182] In one study of 48 children, the incidence of precocious puberty in children with liver tumors was 6%.[183] To the authors' knowledge, there are no known cases of precocious puberty associated with hepatoblastoma in girls.

Laboratory evaluation of the child with a liver mass should include a complete blood count and liver function tests, as well as AFP and β-human chorionic gonadotrophin tumor marker levels. The platelet count is often high in hepatoblastoma but is not diagnostic of hepatoblastoma among children with liver tumors.[184] This thrombophilia is associated with high serum levels of thrombopoietin (TPO), also known as c-Mpl ligand. Normally synthesized in the liver, TPO has also been shown to be expressed in hepatoblastoma tumor tissues and is present at higher than normal levels in the serum of patients with hepatoblastoma.[185] In a large series of patients of various ages (13 to 84 years) who had hepatic tumors, thrombocytosis was noted in 2.7%. The high platelet count was correlated with higher serum TPO levels.[186] Other components of the complete blood count are usually normal insofar as bone marrow involvement with liver tumors has not been reported.

AFP is the primary serum marker that is used diagnostically and prognostically, as well as in surveillance. A sample should be obtained in the initial evaluation of any child with a liver mass.[187] AFP levels are markedly elevated in more than 90% of hepatoblastomas and more than 50% of HCCs. Care should be taken in interpreting AFP levels in the young infant because levels are normally very high at birth and decline to less than 10 ng/dL over the first year of life. Of note is that some liver malignancies—notably the small cell undifferentiated subtype of hepatoblastoma as well as the fibrolamellar variant of HCC—are not associated with elevation of the AFP.[188,189] Likewise, sarcomas and rhabdoid tumors are not associated with elevated AFP. The International Society of Oncology Epithelial Liver Group (SIOPEL) has demonstrated that hepatoblastomas with low AFP levels at diagnosis (less than 100 ng/mL) tend to present at a higher stage and are associated with a poor outcome.[188] A low AFP level has also been noted to be a marker of poor outcome across multiple studies compiled and analyzed by the Children's Hepatic Tumor International Consortium (CHIC) group.[190] The β-human chorionic gonadotrophin level is only occasionally elevated in hepatoblastoma, usually in cases that present with precocious puberty. The β-human chorionic gonadotrophin level is also elevated in the rare choriocarcinoma of the liver, as well as teratomas.

Evaluation of a child with a liver tumor should include a thorough family history to document specific cancers in relatives, with notation made of any early-onset colon cancers or colectomies, in addition to the presence of thyroid cancers or medulloblastoma, which can be part of FAP syndrome. Testing for germline mutation of the APC gene may be indicated; if performed, it should include appropriate genetic counseling. These patients with hepatoblastoma and germline APC mutations will require long-term surveillance for colonic polyps and tumor development.

In addition the medical history should note the birth weight, history of prematurity, and presence or absence of stigmata of neonatal overgrowth, including omphalocele and hemihypertrophy, which would suggest BWS and a risk for other embryonal tumors.

STAGING

Although North American trials have traditionally used a postsurgical diagnostic staging group, applied after the initial surgical procedure (biopsy or resection), the European system, based on the appearance by imaging before chemotherapy and surgical resection (PRETEXT), is being adopted worldwide. PRETEXT stages I through IV reflect the number of sectors that are involved with tumor. Other components of the staging system reflect extension into the vena cava, extension into the portal vein, extrahepatic abdominal disease, or distant metastases. The SIOPEL staging is shown schematically in Figure 58-3. A comparison of the prior North American staging and the current SIOPEL staging is shown in Table 58-2.

Figure 58-4 demonstrates a small hepatoblastoma tumor image that was initially diagnosed by surveillance ultrasound in a patient with BWS. This tumor involved two sectors and as such is classified as PRETEXT II, but because it was completely surgically excised after diagnosis, it would be stage 1 using the North American staging system. Figure 58-5 demonstrates a multifocal hepatoblastoma that involves all four sectors and had metastatic lesions in the lung; therefore it is PRETEXT IV by the North American staging system. If the patient had not had metastatic lesions, the tumor would be stage 3 according to the North American system but still PRETEXT IV.

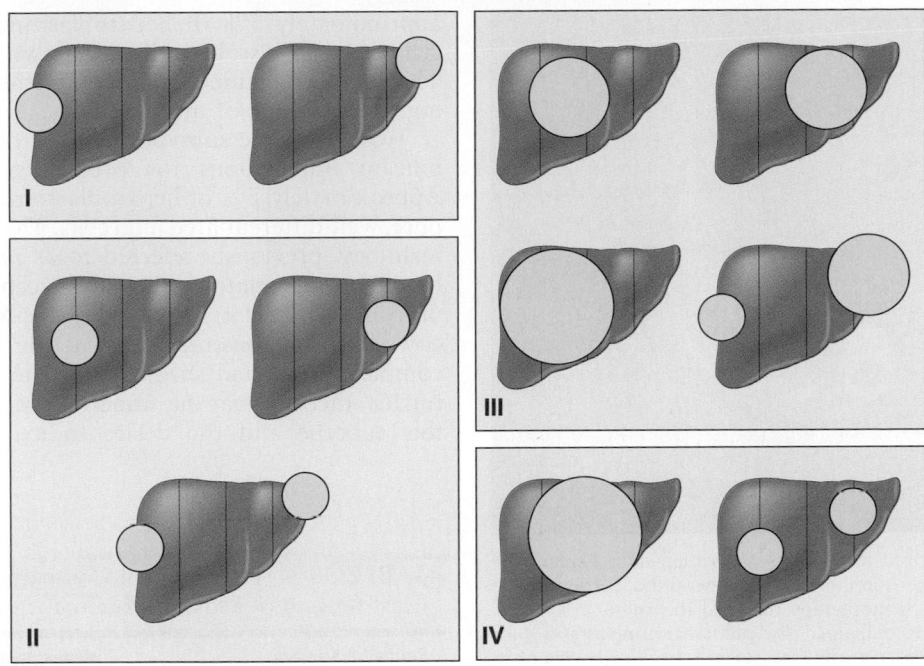

Figure 58-3 Pretreatment imaging-defined staging protocol presurgical staging system used by the International Society of Pediatric Oncology to predict outcome. The liver image is divided into four sectors, and tumor stage is defined as the number of free sectors. In this system, stage is further defined by extension of tumor beyond the liver as *V* indicating extension into the vena cava or all three hepatic veins (or both), *P* indicating extension into the main or both left and right branches of the portal vein, *E* indicating extrahepatic disease proved by biopsy, and *M* indicating the presence of distant metastases.

TABLE 58-2   North American Postsurgical Staging Versus European Presurgical Staging

	North American Staging	European Staging SIOPEL/PRETEXT
	Postsurgical Staging	Presurgical Staging
Stage 1	No metastases; tumor completely resected	Tumor involves only one quadrant; three adjoining liver quadrants free of tumor
Stage 2	No metastases, tumor grossly resected with microscopic residual disease (i.e., positive margins, tumor rupture, or tumor spill at the time of surgery)	Tumor involves two adjoining quadrants; two adjoining quadrants are free of tumor
Stage 3	No distant metastases, tumor unresectable or resected with gross residual tumor, or positive nodes.	Tumor involves three adjoining quadrants or two nonadjoining quadrants; one quadrant or two nonadjoining quadrants are free of tumor
Stage 4	Distant metastases regardless of the extent of liver involvement.	Tumor involves all four quadrants; there is no quadrant free of tumor

PRETEXT, Pretreatment Imaging-Defined Staging Protocol; *SIOPEL*, International Society of Pediatric Oncology Epithelial Liver Group.

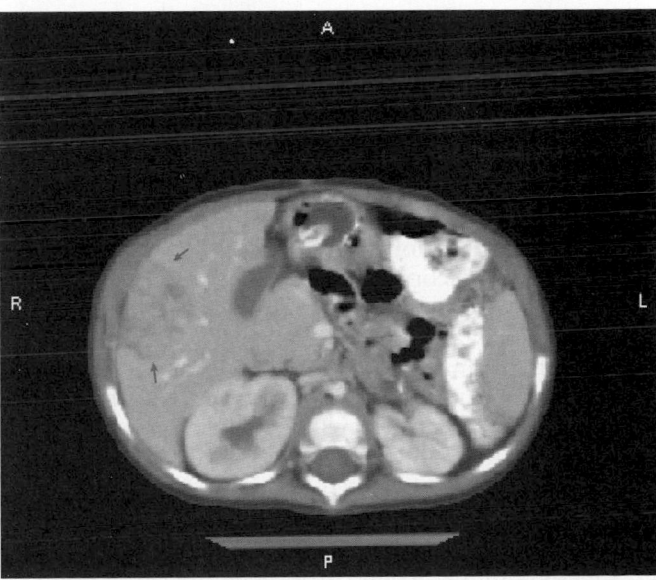

Figure 58-4 Computerized tomography scan of a low-stage hepatoblastoma detected by periodic surveillance with ultrasound in a patient at high risk of hepatoblastoma because of Beckwith-Wiedemann syndrome. The tumor was fully resected and classified as stage 1. *(Courtesy of Children's Medical Center, Dallas, Tex.)*

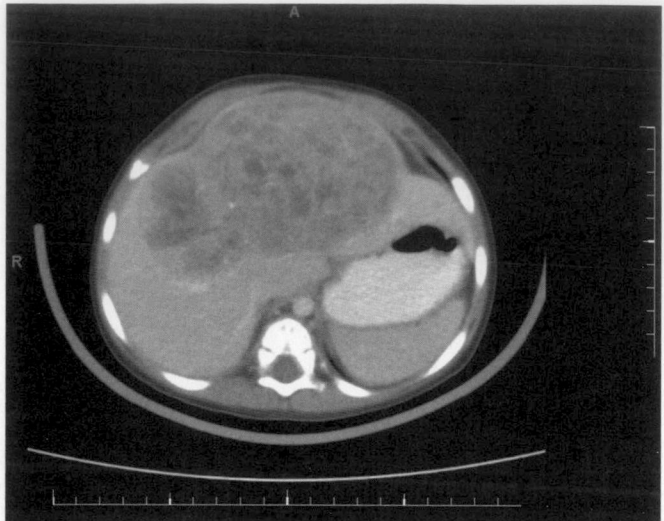

Figure 58-5 Computerized tomography of a high-stage hepatoblastoma. The tumor occupies most of the left lobe and a portion of the right lobe. Preoperative chemotherapy rendered this tumor resectable. This tumor was also accompanied by pulmonary metastases (not shown) and therefore was classified as stage 4 by North American staging system. *(Courtesy of Children's Hospital, Boston, Mass.)*

Both staging systems have been shown to have prognostic significance, but it is difficult to compare studies using different staging systems.[191] In the future the PRETEXT system will be used by most groups internationally.

PATHOLOGY OF HEPATOBLASTOMA AND HEPATOCELLULAR CARCINOMA

Grossly hepatoblastomas occur as single expansile masses, usually in the right lobe of the liver. A series of international discussions originating at the Los Angeles COG International Pathology Liver Tumors Symposium in 2011 resulted in a consensus classification of liver tumors in children, summarized in Table 58-3. A description of immunohistochemical properties currently recommended to aid in the classification of pediatric liver tumors is provided in Table 58-4.

A representative resected hepatoblastoma tumor is shown in Figure 58-6. Hepatoblastomas are composed primarily of epithelial cells that resemble different stages of the developing liver. Most hepatoblastomas are a mixture of cells resembling fetal cells and cells resembling embryonal cells. A typical hepatoblastoma of fetal and embryonal histology is shown in Figure 58-7, *A*. Because hepatoblastomas derive from immature cells that may retain the potential to differentiate, tumors often have foci of other types of more differentiated cells, including hematopoietic cells, as demonstrated in Figure 58-7, *B*. A subset of hepatoblastomas are characterized by cholangiocyte-like cells, which suggest the differentiation of the neoplastic cells along the cholangiocyte lineage as opposed to the hepatocyte lineage.[192] When the epithelial cells are aligned in thick cordlike structures, the tumor is described as having macrotrabecular features. In

approximately 5% of hepatoblastomas, only fetal-type cells are seen histologically, as shown in Figure 58-7, *C*. These fetal-only tumors are now further classified according to the degree of mitoses.[3]

Two histologic subtypes of hepatoblastoma have significant implications for predicting clinical outcome. Approximately 7% of hepatoblastomas are composed of pure, well-differentiated fetal cells. The well-differentiated histology, previously referred to as *pure fetal histology*, has been associated with an exceptionally favorable outcome. A recent COG study by Malogolowkin and coworkers demonstrated that if the hepatoblastoma is completely resected surgically at the time of diagnosis, further therapy may be unnecessary.[193] The presence of this subtype and the desire to avoid the toxicity of

TABLE 58-3   International Consensus Classification of Pediatric Tumors

Epithelial Tumors	Mesenchymal tumors
Hepatocellular	Benign
Benign and tumor-like	Vascular tumors
conditions	Infantile hemangioma
Hepatocellular adenoma	Mesenchymal hamartoma
Focal nodular hyperplasia	PEComas
Macroregenerative nodule	
Premalignant lesions	
Dysplastic nodules	
Malignant	Malignant
Hepatoblastoma	Embryonal sarcoma
Epithelial variants:	Rhabdomyosarcoma
Pure fetal with low	Vascular tumors
mitotic activity	Epithelioid
Fetal, mitotically active	hemangioendothelioma
Pleomorphic, poorly	Angiosarcoma
differentiated	Other malignancies
Embryonal	Tumors of uncertain origin
Small-cell	Malignant rhabdoid tumor
undifferentiated	INI1-negative (or
INI1-negative	documented *INI1*
INI1-positive	mutation)
Epithelial mixed (any/all	Nested epithelial stromal
above)	tumor
Cholangioblastic	Germ cell tumors
Epithelial	Teratoma
macrotrabecular	Yolk sac tumor
Mixed epithelial and	Desmoplastic small round
mesenchymal:	cell tumor
Without teratoid	Peripheral primitive
features	neuroectodermal tumor
With teratoid features	
Hepatocellular carcinoma	
Classic	
Fibrolamellar	
Hepatocellular neoplasm not	
otherwise specified	
Biliary	
Benign—bile duct adenoma/	
hamartoma	
Malignant	
Cholangiocarcinoma	

From Lopez-Terrada D, Alaggio R, de Davila MT, et al: Towards an international pediatric liver tumor consensus classification: proceedings of the Los Angeles COG liver tumors symposium. Mod Pathol 27:472–91, 2014.

TABLE 58-4   Immunohistochemical Evaluation of Pediatric Liver Tumors

	Fetal WDF	Fetal with Mitoses	Pleomorphic	Embryonal	Small Cell Undifferentiated	Mesenchymal	Cholangioblastic
GPC3	Finely granular	+++ Coarse	++ Coarse	+++ Coarse/rare –	–, Rare+cell	–	–
β-cat	Variably +/+++ nuclear or normal	+/+++ Nuclear	+/+++ Nuclear	+/+++ Nuclear, can be–	+++ Nuclear	+++ Nuclear on osteoid/blastema/neg in teratoid elements	Variable/positive nuclei
GS	+++	+++	Variable	Variable, can be neg	–	–	–
Hep Par	+++	+++	Variable	Usually –	–	–	–
Cyclin D1	–	+/++	+/+++	+/+++	+/++	Variable/neg in teratoid	
CK7	–	–		–	–/+	Variable/weak in blastema	+++
CK19	–	–	–	–	+/++ Variable	Neg/weak in blastema	+++
CD34	+ Endo	+ Endo					
Vimentin	–		–	–	+/++	+++	Usually –
INI1	+++	+++	+++	+++	Negative in pure SCU; variable when mixed	+++	+++

From Lopez-Terrada D, Alaggio R, de Davila MT, et al: Towards an international pediatric liver tumor consensus classification: proceedings of the Los Angeles COG liver tumors symposium. Mod Pathol 27:472–91, 2014.

chemotherapy remain compelling reasons to pursue upfront resection whenever possible.

The small cell undifferentiated variant accounts for approximately 5% of hepatoblastoma and also carries clinical significance. Histologically the cells are small and pleomorphic and show high mitotic rates, as shown in Figure 58-7, D. There are several reports in small cell undifferentiated hepatoblastoma of unique chromosome translocations involving chromosome 22q12, the region of *SMARCB/INI1*, the gene most often associated with rhabdoid tumors and atypical teratoid tumors. Emerging evidence suggests that from histologic, cytogenetic, molecular genetic, and clinical perspectives these tumors resemble rhabdoid tumors to varying degrees.[194] Immunohistochemistry demonstrated loss of the INI1 protein in the small cell undifferentiated variant, and it is now recommended that INI1 staining be performed as part of the histologic characterization (see Table 58-4).[3] Mounting evidence suggests that the small cell variant is associated with a poor outcome.[188,194,195]

HCCs consist of cells that are well-differentiated and resemble normal hepatocytes. A typical HCC is shown in Figure 58-8. The fibrolamellar variant of HCC is characterized by larger, polygonal cells mixed with fibrous stroma and often eosinophilic cytoplasm, occasionally with cystic degeneration (Fig. 58-9).[196-198] In contrast to hepatoblastoma, the adjacent liver tissue in patients with HCC is often marked by cirrhosis. The fibrolamellar variant is an exception in which surrounding liver tissue is usually noncirrhotic.

ACQUIRED GENETIC CHANGES IN HEPATOBLASTOMA

Karyotypic changes in hepatoblastomas can be classified into two broad categories: numeric changes and structural changes of individual chromosomes, the most common of which involve translocations of chromosome

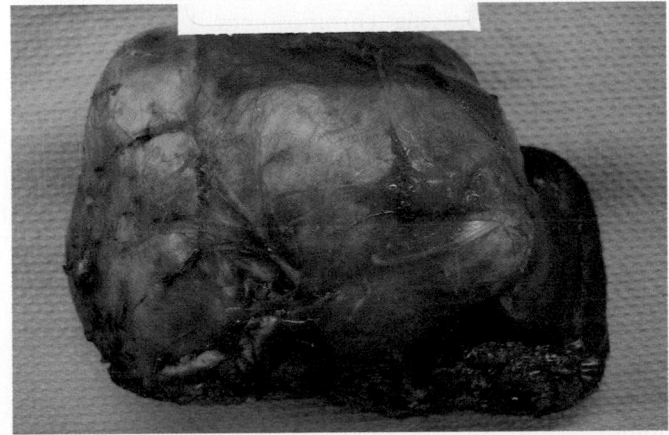

Figure 58-6 Gross pathology of resected hepatoblastoma tumor specimen. Tumor appears as a large expansile mass. The tumor has a whitish appearance compared with the darker adjacent liver in background. The cut surface is shown at the bottom of the image and has a variegated appearance. (*Courtesy of Victor Saldivar, MD, Children's Hospital of San Antonio, Tex.*)

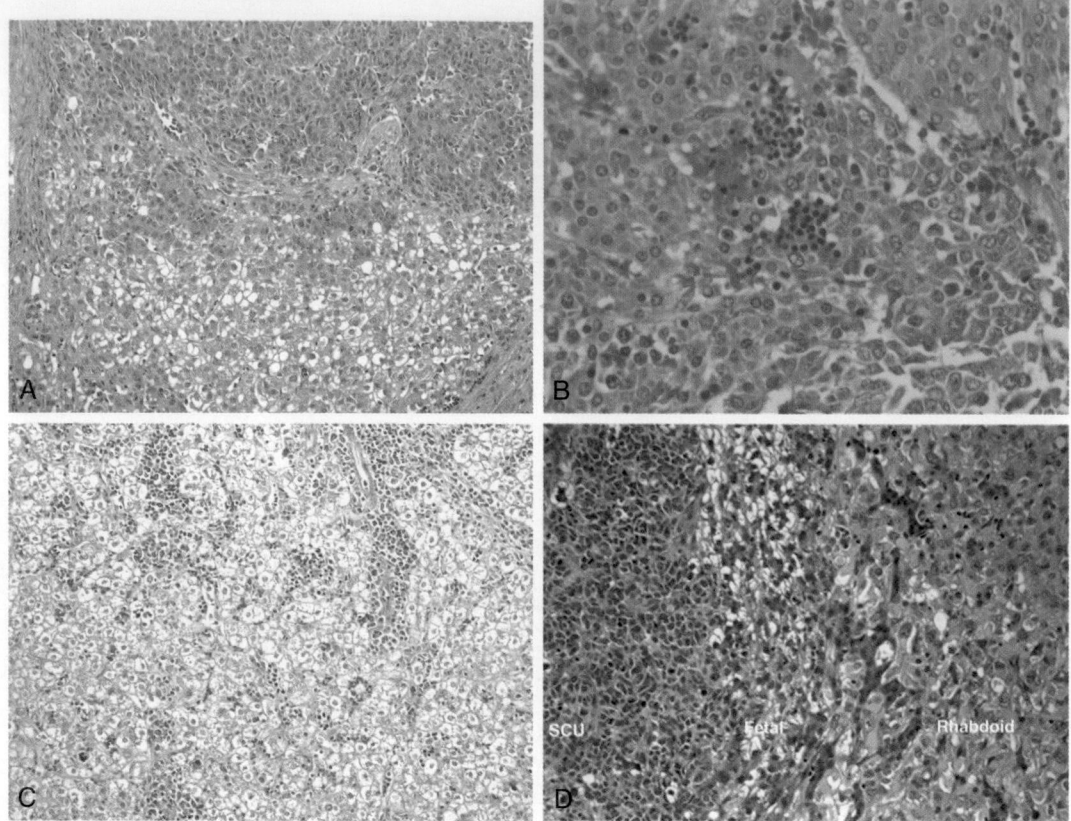

Figure 58-7 A, Mixed fetal and embryonal epithelial hepatoblastoma. This hepatoblastoma shows two different morphologic patterns. The fetal pattern, seen in the lower part of the image, is composed of uniform, small cuboidal cells with distinct cell membranes, whereas the embryonal pattern, seen in upper part of the image, consists of smaller angulated cells with hyperchromatic nuclei, higher nuclear-to-cytoplasmic ratios, and indistinct cell membranes. This is the most common histologic pattern of hepatoblastoma. **B,** Hepatoblastoma with extramedullary hematopoesis. As is often observed in hepatoblastoma, islands of hematopoietic cells are observed as clusters of small dark cells with prominent nuclei within surrounding tumor tissue. **C,** Pure fetal epithelial hepatoblastoma. This is composed of relatively uniform, small cuboidal cells. The cells have a small round nucleus with inconspicuous nucleolus, abundant cytoplasm that may be clear or finely granular, and distinct cell membranes. The pure fetal variant accounts for approximately 5% of all hepatoblastomas and is associated with a favorable outcome. **D,** Small cell undifferentiated hepatoblastoma. The central portion shows cells resembling fetal hepatoblastoma. On the *left*, cells appear undifferentiated with round nuclei and minimal cytoplasm and fail to form tubules. At *right*, cells are more typical of rhabdoid-like histology. *(A, Courtesy of Dinesh Rakheja, MD, Children's Medical Center, Dallas, Tex.; B, Courtesy of Victor Saldivar, MD, Children's Hospital of San Antonio, Tex.; C, Courtesy of Dinesh Rakheja, MD, Children's Medical Center, Dallas, Tex.; D, Courtesy of Milton Finegold, MD, Texas Children's Hospital, Houston, Tex.)*

1.[114] The initial recurring translocation described was the translocation involving chromosomes 1 and 4, t(1;4) (q12;q34).[199,200] It has since been reported in a large series that hepatoblastoma is characterized by a family of chromosome translocations with similar breakpoints on either chromosome 1q12 or 1q21.[114] Each such translocation observed is unbalanced, resulting in a gain of the long arm of chromosome 1, and is also frequently associated with numerous whole chromosomal gains.

Most of the numeric aberrations result in addition of whole chromosomes, but occasionally they result in loss of chromosomes. The specific numeric changes are nonrandom. Trisomies of chromosome 2, 8, and 20 are the most common recurring numeric aberrations. The most commonly observed chromosomal losses are chromosomes 4 and 18. Although these whole chromosome changes have been described previously by classical karyotype analysis, they can perhaps be better visualized by whole genome comparative genomic hybridization, as shown in Figure 58-10. The clinical significance of these chromosomal abnormalities is not yet known..

HCC is also characterized also by chromosomal gains and losses, with loss of the Y chromosome a notable finding.[201] Duplication of chromosome 1q is also seen in HCC with increased expression of numerous chromosome 1 genes.[202,203] Cytogenetic data on the fibrolamellar variant of HCC is sparse, but one childhood fibrolamellar carcinoma has been characterized by a hypertriploid karyotype with clonal evolution and multiple additional chromosomal gains as well as loss of the Y chromosome.[204]

MOLECULAR ABERRATIONS

The most common genetic alteration in hepatoblastoma is alteration of the Wnt signaling pathway. *CTNNB1* alteration is detected in the vast majority of hepatoblastomas, either as a point mutation in exon 3 or a large gene deletion.[205,206] Less commonly alterations are observed in other members of the Wnt signaling pathway, including *APC* and *AXIN* genes.[207] *CTNNB1* accumulates in the nucleus of tumor cells with alterations of the Wnt signaling pathway.

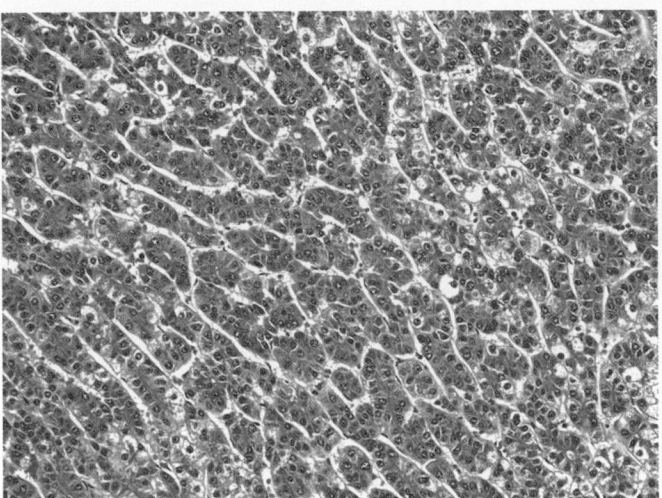

Figure 58-8 Hepatocellular carcinoma. This well-differentiated hepatocellular carcinoma is composed of two- to four-layer thick cords or trabeculae of cells resembling normal hepatocytes. Sinusoidal-like spaces lined by endothelial cells are present between the trabeculae, further mimicking the architecture of normal liver. No portal tracts are present. *(Courtesy of Dinesh Rakeja, MD, Children's Medical Center, Dallas, Tex.)*

In a preliminary whole exome study by Trevino and colleagues, mutation of the *NFE2L2* gene was present in approximately 6% of hepatoblastoma tumors.[208] Of note, this same gene mutation is observed in 6% of HCCs in adults.[209]

Cairo and coworkers have demonstrated that upregulation of MYC in conjunction with Wnt signaling aberration is a hallmark of aggressive hepatoblastoma and have described a 16-gene signature in a posttreatment resected specimen that was associated with a more aggressive clinical behavior.[210] These and other molecular findings will need to be examined in a prospective study to determine the impact on patient risk stratification and management.

TREATMENT: CHEMOTHERAPY IN HEPATOBLASTOMA

Chemotherapy has been used extensively in the management of hepatoblastoma to reduce tumor bulk and thereby render tumors resectable and to treat microscopic disease after resection. Surgical resection, as discussed later, is essential for all malignant liver tumors to achieve cure. Although great strides have been made in the development of chemotherapeutic approaches for hepatoblastoma, challenges remain in eradicating unresectable disease as well as in determining new effective agents for refractory disease. Success in the past three decades has been obtained primarily through the four major cooperative groups based in North American (COG and its predecessors), Europe (SIOPEL), Germany (Cooperative German Paediatric Liver Tumor Study), and Japan (Japanese Study Group for Pediatric Liver Tumor [JPLT]). The legacy North American cooperative group approach has been to resect, if possible, before the administration of chemotherapy, whereas the European approach has been

to use neoadjuvant chemotherapy with initial biopsy to shrink tumors before therapy. Regimens used in the treatment of hepatoblastoma have centered largely on platinum agents and doxorubicin. Other agents studied and incorporated into protocols have included vincristine, 5-fluorouracil, ifosfamide, etoposide, and recently irinotecan. A summary of results of published treatment regimens is given in Table 58-5.

Early reports documented the effectiveness of vincristine as a single agent,[211,212] and subsequent Pediatric Oncology Group and Children's Cancer Group trials used vincristine along with 5-fluorouracil and cisplatin. Doxorubicin was shown to be effective in a phase II trial of refractory pediatric solid tumors, including hepatoblastoma, using either a 4-day course of 15 to 20 mg/m^2 daily or a 3-day course of 30 mg/m^2 daily.[213]

A study from St. Jude Children's Research Hospital reported a response to cisplatin (DDP) at a dose of

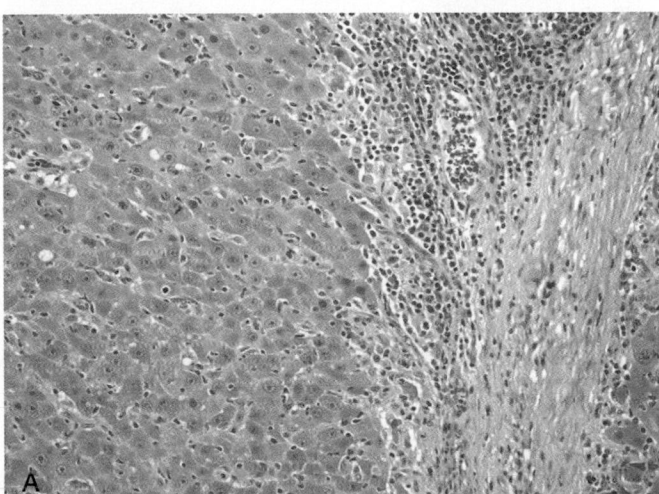

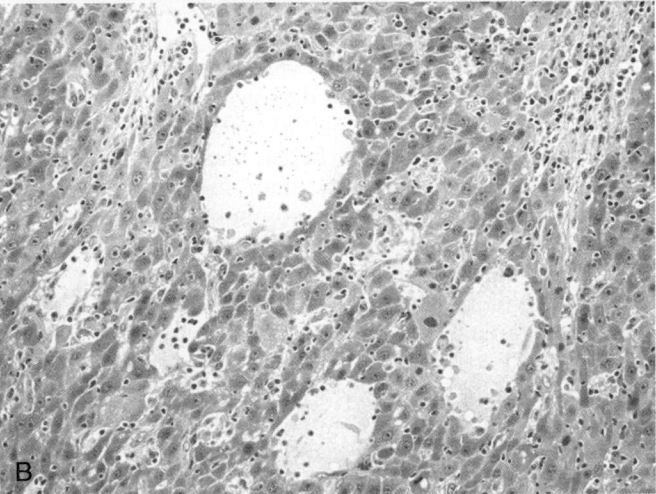

Figure 58-9 Fibrolamellar hepatocellular carcinoma. Fibrolamellar hepatocellular carcinoma is composed of sheets of polygonal tumor cells that are larger than normal hepatocytes and have a deeply eosinophilic cytoplasm, a large nucleus with prominent eosinophilic nucleolus. As shown prominently in **A**, the cells are embedded in collagenous stroma, and variably thick fibrous septa course through the tumor. Often there are focal infiltrates of mononuclear inflammatory cells. **B**, Foci of cystic degeneration (pseudogland formation) are apparent. *(Courtesy of Dinesh Rakeja, MD, Children's Medical Center, Dallas, Tex.)*

TABLE 58-5   A Summary of Recent Cooperative Group Studies in Europe and North America

Study Protocol	Presurgical chemotherapy	Chemotherapy agents	N =	Outcome	Reference
POG—#8697	No	Cisplatin, vincristine, fluorouracil (C5V)	73	3-year EFS: stage I (UH) / II: 91% stage III: 67% stage IV 12.5%	305
COG—#9645	Yes	C5V vs. intensified platinum*	33	5-year EFS: stage III: 73% stage IV: 27%	306
INT—0098	Selected patients	C5V vs. cisplatin and doxorubicin	182	5-year EFS: stage I (UH) / II: >90% stage III/IV: >50%	4
HB—89	Yes	Ifosfamide, cisplatin, doxorubicin	72	3-year EFS: stage I: 100% stage II: 50% stage III: 74% stage IV: 29%	225
HB—94	Selected patients	Ifosfamide, cisplatin, doxorubicin	69	3-year EFS: stage I: 96% stage II: 100% stage III: 76% stage IV: 36%	226
SIOPEL—1	Yes	cisplatin, doxorubicin	154	5-year OS: 75%	222
SIOPEL—2	Yes	Cisplatin/carboplatin, doxorubicin—risk stratified	150	3-year OS[†] SR: 90% HR: 78%	7
SIOPEL—3	Yes	Cisplatin/ carboplatin	151 (HR)[‡]	3-year OS: 69% (HR)	223
SIOPEL—4	Yes	Cisplatin—dose dense	61 (HR)	3-year OS = 83% (HR)	224

COG, Children's Oncology Group; EFS, event-free survival; HR, high risk; OS, overall survival; POG, Pediatric Oncology Group; SIOPEL, Childhood Liver Tumours Study Group; SR, standard risk; UH, unfavorable histology.

*Only Stage II and IV patients enrolled.

[†]SR: Standard risk. Defined as hepatoblastoma confined to the liver and involving no more than three hepatic sectors.

[‡]HR: High risk. Defined as hepatoblastoma extending into all four sectors or lung metastases or extrahepatic involvement (or a combination thereof).

90 mg/m^2 in 10 of 11 patients with hepatoblastoma.[214] A subsequent study at MD Anderson Cancer Center used high-dose cisplatin (150 mg/m^2 as a single dose) in patients with unresectable hepatoblastoma, showing a marked response in primary tumor size as well as metastatic disease.[215] Platinum compounds subsequently emerged as the most effective means to treat hepatoblastoma, although treatment has been associated with considerable toxicity. Ototoxicity was observed in 37% of children receiving platinum agents, according to a European study that included 120 children with cancer diagnosed at a median age of 2.6 years, including 11 patients with hepatoblastoma; the ototoxicity was most severe in patients younger than 36 years of age at diagnosis and was progressive over time.[216]

The use of doxorubicin and cisplatin together in the treatment of hepatoblastoma has long been shown to be effective. The first report of this combination described a 15-month-old girl with unresectable hepatoblastoma of mixed histology who received doxorubicin and cisplatin.[217] Quinn and colleagues reported four patients with hepatoblastoma, three of whom had unresectable tumors that were treated with cisplatin and doxorubicin.[217a]

The successful combination of cisplatin with doxorubicin was further studied in Toronto. In this study 15 children were treated with cisplatin (20 mg/m^2 daily for 5 days) in combination with doxorubicin (25 mg/m^2 daily for 3 days), with unresectable disease in 13 of the original 15.[8] A second report, also from Toronto, documented success in administering similar doses of cisplatin and doxorubicin simultaneously as a continuous infusion in an attempt to further increase cell kill while minimizing toxicity.[218] Significant tumor reduction allowing surgical resection was attained in all six of the patients studied, with five surviving over the long-term and one child dying perioperatively as a result of surgical complications.

The Children's Cancer Study Group undertook a study administering cisplatin at a dose of 100 mg/m^2 daily together with continuously infused doxorubicin and reported efficacy in initially unresectable hepatoblastoma.[219] Building on this successful combination of doxorubicin and cisplatin, the two North American cooperative groups designed an intergroup study to determine the efficacy and safety of this regimen in a large number of patients. The doxorubicin and cisplatin regimen was

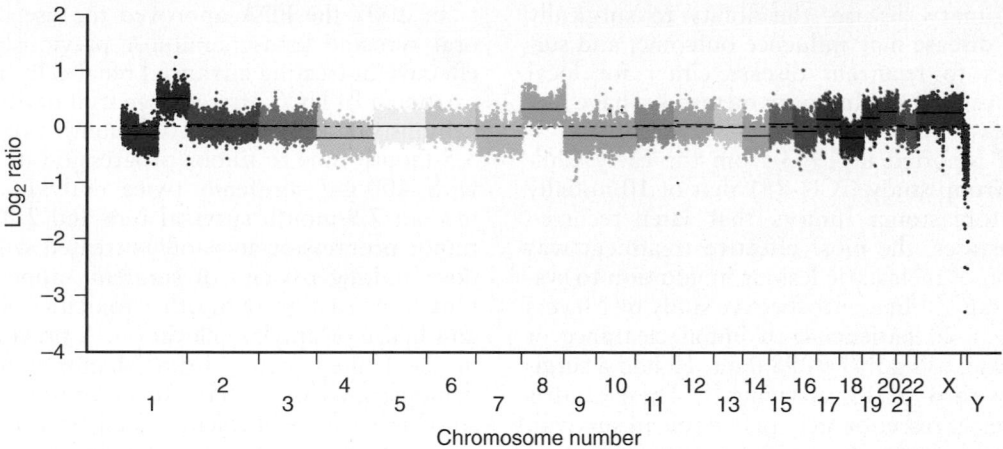

Figure 58-10 Genome-wide copy number comparative genomic hybridization (CGH) scan of hepatoblastoma tumor compared with standard normal male control DNA. Hepatoblastoma is characterized by whole chromosome gains and losses as well as unbalanced translocations of chromosome 1 resulting in duplication of the long arm of chromosome 1q. This CGH plot demonstrates increased copy number of chromosome 8, 17, 19, and 20 as well as whole chromosome losses of chromosomes 4 7, 9, 10, 14, and 18. In addition a duplication of chromosome 1q and loss of chromosome 1p is observed. Numeric aberrations of X and Y reflect the female sex of the child rather than tumor-specific changes.

found to be as effective as the cisplatin, vincristine, and 5-fluorouracil regimen (C5V); however toxicity was greater, particularly in infants, in the patients treated with the doxorubicin and cisplatin regimen.[4] Subsequent studies in North America have omitted doxorubicin and concentrated on platinum-based regimens.

The use of alternating platinum analogues cisplatin and carboplatin without concomitant use of other agents was attempted in a randomized trial conducted by the Pediatric Oncology Group P9645, but this resulted in a dismal outcome of a 37% event-free survival rate compared with a 57% event-free survival rate for patients receiving the C5V regimen. In addition, patients randomized to receive intensified platinum therapy only experienced more toxicity and a greater need for transfusions. Therefore the standard of care in North America returned to the C5V regimen, with the recent trials (AHEP0731) re-incorporating the use of doxorubicin in addition to C5V in intermediate-risk patients. This trial also explored the efficacy of irinotecan as an upfront window in the patients at highest risk.

Because early reviews suggested that tumors of pure fetal histology had a more favorable outcome,[220,221] a concentrated effort has been made to reduce therapy in this group. The first attempt to reduce therapy in this subset of tumors was in the intergroup study POG 8945/ CCG 8881, in which patients with stage 1 tumors of pure fetal histology were treated with four courses of doxorubicin only, compared with patients with other tumors, which were treated with multiagent therapy. In the recent AHEP0731 study, tumors of pure fetal histology, if fully resected, received no further therapy. The ability to avoid chemotherapy in this select group of tumors, based on pathology, argues strongly for the need for histologic characterization before embarking on any course of chemotherapy.

The Europe-based SIOPEL group also used a regimen of cisplatin and continuous infusion of doxorubicin in the SIOPEL-1 study, with 5-year survival rates of PRETEXT I, II, III, and IV disease observed to be 100%, 83%, 56%, and 46%, respectively.[222] SIOPEL-2 used cisplatin for standard-risk patients and cisplatin alternating with carboplatin and doxorubicin in higher-risk patients.[7] SIOPEL-3 demonstrated notable improvement in patients with metastatic disease, with a 5-year survival rate of 56% following intensive treatment of 10 cycles of cisplatin alternating with carboplatin and doxorubicin.[223] The recent SIOPEL-4 study used a dose-dense cisplatin-based regimen that also included doxorubicin for high-risk patients (i.e., those with extrahepatic abdominal disease, major vascular invasion, tumor rupture, tumor in all segments, or metastatic disease). The overall survival rate at 3 years was 83%, a significant improvement over past regimens; however moderate to severe ototoxicity occurred in 50% of patients.[224] Given the efficacy of cisplatin along with the frequent occurrence of ototoxicity now documented in multiple studies, families of children currently treated for hepatoblastoma should be advised of the risk of hearing loss, and children should be closely monitored during treatment and for years afterward. A current priority is the development of therapies that are less toxic.

Exploration of treatment by the German cooperative groups has included the use of ifosfamide in conjunction with cisplatin and doxorubicin (IPA). The overall survival rate was 75%, which is comparable to that of SIOPEL and North American studies and indicates a possible alternative approach. However the combination of etoposide, ifosfamide, and carboplatin used in stage IV tumors had a survival rate of 21%, a dismal result similar to those of previous regimens.[225,226]

Treatment of Recurrent or Refractory Disease

Despite the often successful treatment of newly diagnosed hepatoblastoma, treatment of recurrent hepatoblastoma remains a significant therapeutic challenge. The relative rarity of tumor recurrence poses additional challenges to retrieval protocol development strategies. As with the treatment of primary disease, the ability to surgically resect recurrent disease may influence outcome, and surgical approaches to recurrent disease either for local hepatic recurrence or for pulmonary metastases have met with some success.

Feusner et al reported in 1993 from the early Children's Cancer Group study CCG-881 that of 10 initially low-stage hepatoblastoma tumors that later recurred with lung metastases, the most effective treatment was surgical resection of metastatic lesions in addition to systemic chemotherapy.[227] In a retrospective study by Meyers and colleagues of 20 patients with initial clearance of pulmonary disease, using INT-0098 data, 13 had a surgical approach, with 4 of 13 surviving.[228] These studies suggest that surgical resection may play a role in survival, but they also underscore the need for better systemic therapies to control metastatic disease. The SIOPEL group reported 59 patients from SIOPEL studies 1,2, and 3.[229] All of these patients received doxorubicin as part of their initial therapy. Retrieval strategies were attempted in 52 patients and varied, including chemotherapy plus surgery in 25 (42%), chemotherapy alone in 21 (36%), and surgery alone in 7 (12%). Palliative care only was provided in five cases. Slightly more than half of the patients achieved a second complete response, but the 3-year event-free survival rate was only 34 %. Factors associated with successful outcome included PRETEXT group I through III at diagnosis and the use of both surgery and chemotherapy as a retrieval strategy.

High-dose chemotherapy with stem cell rescue has been attempted for hepatoblastoma with little success, as summarized elsewhere.[230] The Japanese Study Group for Pediatric Liver Tumor, JPLT-2, has also reported limited success with high-dose chemotherapy and stem cell transplant.[231]

TREATMENT OF HEPATOCELLULAR CARCINOMA

Compared with the successes in treating hepatoblastoma with chemotherapy, the progress in treating HCC has been for the most part disappointing in both children and adults. Although an early study indicated that doxorubicin induced remission in HCC in 14 of 44 (32%) patients[232] subsequent studies with doxorubicin in HCC have been disappointing. Within the cooperative groups, because of the small numbers seen, HCC has been treated similarly to hepatoblastoma, with acknowledgment that it is a distinct entity. Survival for initially unresectable HCC has remained dismal. When patients treated with regimens of cisplatin, vincristine, and 5-fluorouracil were compared to patients treated with continuously infused cisplatin and doxorubicin using the same regimens shown to be effective in hepatoblastoma[4] the results demonstrated that less than 20% of stage III and IV patients survived.[37] However among eight patients with HCC that was resected at diagnosis, the long-term survival rate was 88%. This is the largest treatment study of HCC in children. Thus early resectability is an important factor in predicting the likelihood of survival in children who have HCC, which is similar to that observed in adults with HCC.

In 2007 the FDA approved the use of sorafenib, an oral tyrosine kinase inhibitor previously shown to be effective in treating advanced renal cell carcinoma, in the treatment of HCC after a large trial of 602 adult patients demonstrated a median 10.7-month survival rate and a 5.5-month time to tumor progression in patients treated with 400 mg sorafenib twice daily compared with a median 7.9-month survival rate and 2.8-month time to tumor progression in patients treated with placebo. The dose-limiting toxicity of sorafenib appears to be hand-foot skin reaction with other toxicities, such as diarrhea and lipase or amylase elevation. A previous recent study in the United States, from Memorial Sloan Kettering, demonstrated in a phase II, nonrandomized study that sorafenib was well-tolerated, albeit with a modest efficacy, which would suggest an indication for its future inclusion in multiagent trials for HCC.[233] Interestingly this study also performed gene expression microarray analysis on tumors treated with sorafenib and placebo and determined a pattern of gene expression that correlated with a response to sorafenib; this information could conceivably serve as a means of treatment stratification in future trials. Further exploration of the role of sorafenib in pediatric liver tumors is warranted.

SURGICAL ASPECTS OF LIVER TUMORS

Surgical resection is an important component in the management of both benign and malignant liver tumors. In the case of benign lesions such as adenoma, focal nodular hyperplasia, and mesenchymal hamartoma, complete resection of the tumor is usually curative. Resection may involve anatomic lobectomy when necessary or nonanatomic wedge resection in the case of smaller peripheral lesions. In the case of hemangiomas or other vascular malformations of the liver, specific diagnosis is essential to avoid unnecessary surgical intervention or inappropriate use of steroids or chemotherapy agents.[234]

In the assessment of hepatoblastoma for resectability, a high-quality computed tomography (CT) scan or magnetic resonance imaging (MRI) is essential, especially in the adoption of the PRETEXT staging system, which relies on presurgical imaging.[235-238] These studies should be performed with particular attention to the vascular anatomy of the liver. A dual-phase CT scan with both arterial and venous phases may be used to assess vascular involvement and resectability. MRI, sometimes supplemented with magnetic resonance angiography, provides an excellent depiction of vascular anatomy.[238]

Although the PRETEXT staging system is a useful guide for deciding whether a lesion is resectable, the ultimate decision regarding surgical management rests with the surgeon. If possible primary resection should be undertaken for PRETEXT I or II tumors if there is no vascular involvement. Involvement of all three hepatic veins or both branches of the portal vein will usually preclude surgical resection. However a PRETEXT III or IV lesion that appears unresectable at the time of diagnosis may respond very well to chemotherapy, and repeat imaging after two or three cycles of chemotherapy might demonstrate adequate regression of the tumor from vital vascular structures, enabling resection. Very rarely will arterial or biliary involvement preclude tumor resection. In some cases of extensive tumor involving the bifurcation of the bile ducts, biliary reconstruction may be necessary. At the time of surgical resection, any suspicious porta hepatis, hepatic artery, celiac, or periaortic lymph nodes should be sampled. When complete tumor resection is not feasible despite adequate chemotherapy, liver transplantation should be performed.[239-242] Therefore early referral of patients with PRETEXT III or IV tumors to a center that performs liver transplantation is essential.

Surgery remains the mainstay of treatment for HCC given the poor response to chemotherapy and other modalities, including chemoembolization, radiofrequency ablation, and cryotherapy. When HCC develops in the context of cirrhosis, surgery may be limited by the lack of liver physiologic reserve.[243] In these cases transplantation may be the only safe option even for early-stage disease. In the fibrolamellar variant, the remaining adjacent liver is usually normal and therefore resection is more often possible even with extensive disease; this may be a factor contributing to the impression that fibrolamellar HCC has a better prognosis than standard HCC, although stage for stage, fibrolamellar HCC is not different from other types of HCC and depends on resectability for cure.[39,244] Other malignant tumors of the liver, including angiosarcoma, embryonal sarcomas, rhabdoid tumors, and rhabdomyosarcoma, like other malignant liver tumors, require complete resection if there is to be any hope for cure.[245-255]

Transplantation has become increasingly common in the treatment of unresectable hepatoblastoma. In most cases involving malignant liver tumors, complete surgical resection is a necessary component of therapy. Whether benign or malignant, when complete surgical resection by way of partial hepatectomy is not possible because of the extent of disease or lack of hepatic reserve, liver transplantation is the only remaining option. Approximately 2% of children undergoing liver transplants received the livers as treatment for hepatoblastoma,[256] although clearly this number is increasing in recent years. Although liver transplantation for malignant disease was used during the early years of liver transplantation, the survival rate was poor because of transplantation complications as well as recurrent disease. More recent data demonstrate significantly improved survival rates in select patients after transplantation to treat both hepatoblastoma and HCC.[257,258-262] The combined experience of SIOPEL studies was quite favorable: 25 patients with otherwise unresectable hepatoblastoma confined to the liver underwent transplantation after chemotherapy, with the survival rate for patient and graft at 100% after 1 year for living related donor transplants (N = 7) and 91% for cadaveric transplants (N = 18). At 10 years after transplant, the survival rate was 77.6% for cadaveric transplants and 83% for living related donor transplants.[263] In a recent overview of SEER data involving patients younger than 20 years of age undergoing surgery for hepatoblastoma, of a total of 318 patients with hepatoblastoma, 16.7% underwent transplant; of 80 patients with HCC, 25% underwent transplant. The survival rate at 5 years

was 86.5% for hepatoblastoma and 85.3% for HCC.[264] PLUTO (Pediatric Liver Unresectable Tumor Observatory) is an international registry established to capture data, including detailed clinical parameters and outcome statistics, and will be a source of additional information on transplantation of pediatric liver tumors.[265]

In the planning of therapy for patients with advanced hepatoblastoma that may require liver transplantation, early referral to a liver transplant center is key. Options for transplantation include the more traditional deceased donor whole organ or donor split liver transplants and also, more recently, living-donor transplants.[256] Although there are no data to suggest optimal timing for transplantation, most centers will administer at least two rounds of chemotherapy before transplantation in an attempt to shrink the tumor and determine whether resection without transplantation may be an option. Given the small window of opportunity to perform a transplant between cycles, close communication between the oncology team and the transplant team is critical. Evaluation by an experienced transplant team should take place as soon after diagnosis as possible. Current United Network for Organ Sharing (UNOS) liver allocation policy prioritizes children who require liver transplantation for hepatoblastoma. A child listed for transplantation with a diagnosis of hepatoblastoma is automatically assigned 30 PELD (Pediatric End-Stage Liver Disease) points, with the opportunity to be upgraded to status 1B after 30 days. This high priority listing allows patients a reasonable chance of receiving transplants between cycles when hematologic counts are not prohibitive. In the case of living-donor transplantation, the surgery can be scheduled electively. At the time of transplant an initial early abdominal exploration to rule out metastatic disease is required. If intraabdominal metastatic disease is discovered and is not completely resectable, transplantation should be aborted.

Liver transplantation for HCC has evolved significantly over the past several years, and as stated previously, SEER data indicate an 85% 5-year survival rate for HCC patients younger than 20 years undergoing liver transplantation.[264] Centers have used the Milan criteria to select patients for liver transplantation; these criteria allow for increased MELD (Model for End-Stage Liver Disease) points in patients with stage II disease.[260] However data from the University of California San Francisco (UCSF) group demonstrate acceptable patient survival rates after transplantation for patients who exceed the Milan criteria, generally established for adult patients.[266]

LESS COMMON MALIGNANT TUMORS OF THE LIVER

Embryonal sarcoma of the liver, also termed *undifferentiated embryonal sarcoma of the liver* (UESL), is the third most common malignant liver tumor in children.[100] UESL was first recognized as a distinct entity in 1978.[267] Histologically these tumors are composed of mixtures of cells with histiocytoid, fibrohistiocytoid, myofibroblastic, and undifferentiated (primitive mesenchymal) morphologies.[268] They share a chromosome translocation similar to that seen in mesenchymal hamartoma (discussed later) and are thought to arise from the benign mesenchymal hamartoma as a malignant counterpart.[252,269-273] UESL can be distinguished from biliary tract rhabdomyosarcomas by several immunohistochemical stains, including myogenin and MyoD1, which are negative in UESL and positive in rhabdomyosarcoma.[274] UESL differs from rhabdomyosarcoma of the liver in that the median age of UESL is 10.5 years, compared with 3.6 years for rhabdomyosarcoma.

The male-to-female ratio in UESL is 1:1. USEL is considered an aggressive malignancy that should be treated with multiagent regimens used for soft tissue sarcomas of other sites.[275] A European Cooperative Group study from Italy and Germany treated a series of 17 patients with UESL with chemotherapy, conservative surgery, and (in two patients) radiotherapy. Of the 17 patients 12 survived (70%), and all of those who underwent complete resection survived.[276] A more recent series reported 10 patients with UESL, all receiving both combination chemotherapy and surgery, three with upfront resection, and seven with resection after neoadjuvant chemotherapy. Nine of the ten (90%) survived.[277]

True rhabdomyosarcomas, when they are seen in the hepatobiliary system, occur in the biliary tract. These tumors are mesenchymal in origin and histologically resemble rhabdomyosarcomas of other sites with prominent myoblastic cells that stain for myogenin.[274] The tumors may have a botryoid appearance.[278,279] Obstructive jaundice is the usual presenting sign, with or without abdominal distention.[279,280] In an early report from the Intergroup Rhabdomyosarcoma Study, only 4 of 10 patients with biliary tract tumors survived.[280] However additional reports cite better long-term survival rates with chemotherapy regimens and without the need for extensive surgery.[281,282]

Angiosarcomas of the liver are rare but aggressive high-grade malignancies derived from endothelial cells.[246,248,283] Angiosarcoma of the liver in children was previously known as *infantile hemangioendothelioma type 2*.[284] Fewer than 40 cases have been reported. Some cases have been preceded by a diagnosis of infantile hepatic hemangioendotheliomas.[246,285,286] In contrast to other malignant liver tumors in children, angiosarcomas are more common in girls than boys. The pathology of pediatric angiosarcoma is distinct from angiosarcomas in adults in that kaposiform spindle cells are present. The overall prognosis is poor.[246] Although liver transplantation had been reported as successful in one child, a recent European study indicated an overall exceptionally poor outcome in a series of angiosarcomas after liver transplantation.[287,288]

Choriocarcinoma of the liver is an extremely rare tumor. Most cases of infantile choriocarcinoma are actually metastases from gestational choriocarcinoma of the placenta that spreads to the child; however, primary tumors of the liver have been reported. This can be an aggressive and devastating tumor, and although the overall outcome has been historically poor, there are recent reports of cures with chemotherapy, including one case with liver transplant.[289-292] Other primary germ cell tumors of the liver have been reported but are extremely rare.[293]

BENIGN TUMORS OF THE LIVER

Hepatic mesenchymal hamartoma (HMH) is a benign tumor with an age distribution similar to hepatoblastoma, with almost all cases occurring by 5 years. Patients with these tumors present with an enlarged abdomen. Clinical presentation can resemble that of hepatoblastoma, although the serum AFP level is not elevated.[294] As with hepatoblastoma, the majority of HMHs arise in the right side of the liver. HMHs are characterized by the presence of cysts, which are less characteristic of hepatoblastoma. Figure 58-11 demonstrates the cystic appearance on imaging. These benign tumors are characterized by massive growth and cause morbidity by compressing adjacent structures. Occasionally these tumors are diagnosed prenatally and can be a cause of fetal demise.[294] Microscopically HMH consists of spindle cells in a myxoid background with occasional areas of extramedullary hematopoiesis similar to that seen in hepatoblastoma. Figure 58-12 demonstrates the histologic pattern characteristic of HMHs with fluid-filled cystic areas. Cytogenetically these tumors are characterized by translocations involving 19q13.4, as described in multiple cases.[252,271,295-297] The breakpoints involved in one such translocation have been characterized.[273] An interstitial deletion at 19q13.4 has also been reported.[298] HMH can show malignant transformation into malignant mesenchymoma or embryonal sarcoma.[270,299] Treatment of HMH is usually surgical removal. Long-term follow-up of patients after resection is generally favorable.[300]

Hemangioendothelioma is a term that has been used to denote a type of benign vascular tumor. Previously

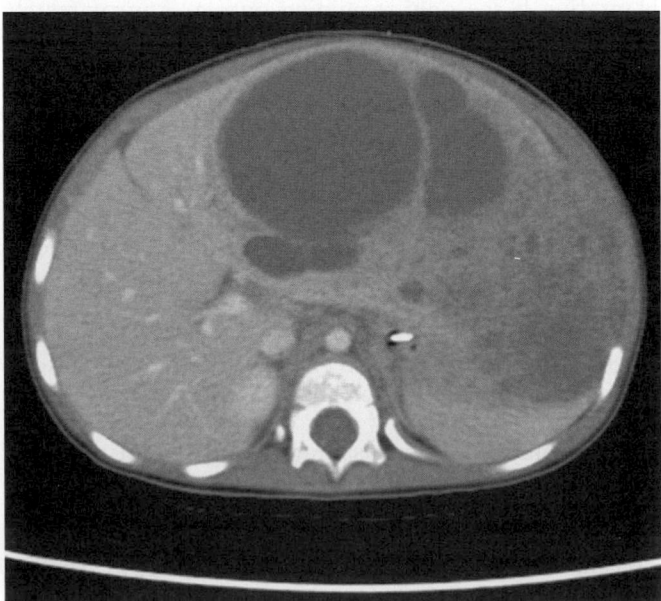

Figure 58-11 Computerized tomography image of an child with mesenchymal hamatoma. Note the multiple cysts with little solid component.

activity.[301] Figure 58-13 demonstrates these two benign hepatic vascular disorders. Patients with hepatic hemangioendothelioma usually exhibit abdominal enlargement with or without congestive heart failure. Hemangioendothelioma may be distinguished from hepatoblastoma by imaging studies, particularly Doppler flow studies.[302] Many hepatic hemangioendotheliomas involute without intervention. Although steroids have been used in the past, propranolol has been used successfully to treat some hemangiomas of the liver, although the precise indications for its use have not yet been well-defined.[303,304]

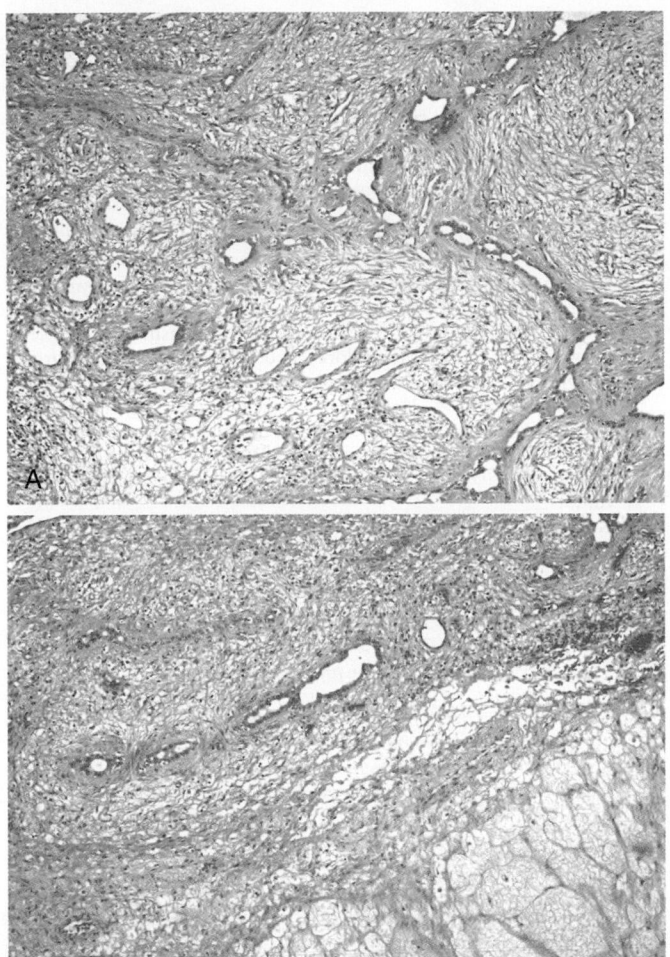

Figure 58-12 Mesenchymal hamartomas. Mesenchymal hamartoma is composed of haphazardly arranged and architecturally distorted elements that are normally found in the liver. In **A,** dilated and serpentine biliary ducts, each surrounded by a variably thick cuff of collagen, are apparent. The bile ducts are lined with low cuboidal epithelial cells without cytologic atypia. The second image (**B**) also shows fluid-filled lymphatic-like cystic spaces. All of these elements are embedded in a myxoid and edematous mesenchyme containing delicate fibroblasts. *(Courtesy of Dinesh Rakheja, MD, Children's Medical Center, Dallas, Tex.)*

grouped together as *infantile hepatic hemangioendothelioma,* the pediatric benign hepatic vascular tumors have recently been shown to be at least two different lesions—hepatic infantile hemangioma and congenital hepatic vascular malformation with associated capillary proliferation. One type (infantile or juvenile hemangioma) often manifests as multiple masses that usually involute and regress. The other type, which has been called a vascular malformation, is usually a large single mass that often undergoes central infarction, does not regress, and may be associated with consumption coagulopathy caused by platelet trapping in the abnormal vasculature. GLUT1 endothelial reactivity distinguishes the two entities histologically, with hepatic infantile hemangiomas staining positively for GLUT1 whereas the hepatic vascular malformations do not exhibit GLUT1 immunore-

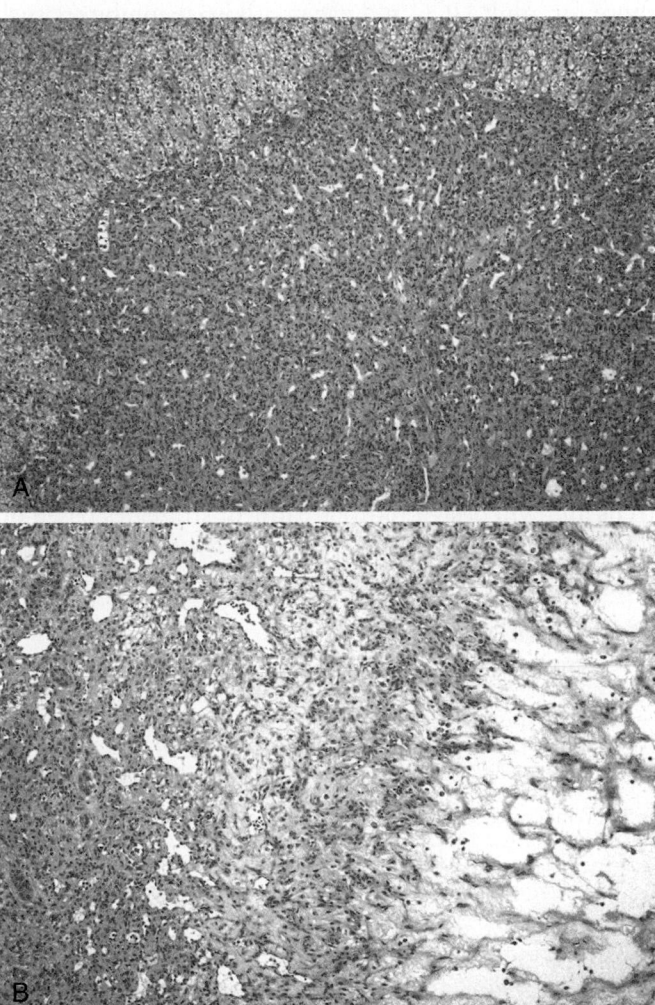

Figure 58-13 Benign hepatic vascular tumors. Previously grouped together as infantile hepatic hemangioendothelioma, the pediatric benign hepatic vascular tumors have recently been identified as at least two different lesions. Hepatic infantile hemangioma can be distinguished from congenital hepatic vascular malformation with associated capillary proliferation by the presence or absence of GLUT1 staining. The infantile or juvenile hemangioma, shown in **A,** often presents as multiple masses that usually involute and regress. Microscopically the lesions are sharply demarcated lobules composed of closely packed capillary-sized vessels that stain for the glucose transporter GLUT1. The other type, also known as hepatic vascular malformation, is usually a large single mass that often undergoes central infarction, does not regress, and may be associated with consumption coagulopathy. As shown in B, the area of infarct is surrounded by variably dilated thin-walled vessels with entrapped bile ducts and hepatocytes. The lesional vessels are negative for GLUT1. *(Courtesy of Dinesh Rakheja, MD, Children's Medical Center, Dallas, Tex.)*

FUTURE CHALLENGES IN TREATMENT OF PEDIATRIC LIVER TUMORS

Although cure rates for liver tumors, particularly hepatoblastoma, have increased over recent decades, many significant challenges remain. The rarity of these malignancies has contributed to the difficulty in the design and implementation of clinical trials, and each treatment hypothesis proposed may take many years to test. Agents of current interest for clinical application for hepatoblastoma include irinotecan and incorporation of sorafenib. Clinical trials for childhood HCC will likely parallel those for adult HCC and use multikinase inhibitors such as sorafenib in addition to chemotherapy.

Additional biologic markers for predicting prognosis and stratifying risk are needed. Although several molecular pathways have been identified in pediatric liver tumors, the integration of molecular characteristics in disease risk stratification and prognosis needs to be developed. In addition, more therapies specifically targeting relevant pathways are needed, with the additional goal of limiting toxicities.

The recently formed Children's Hepatic International Consortium will foster an exciting international collaboration in the analysis of risk factors and outcomes in hepatoblastoma, as well as accelerating new clinical approaches to the treatment of liver tumors in children.[190] This consortium has to date established a series of prognostic risk factors based on a compilation of international trials and will design future treatment strategies based on these classifications.

References available online at ExpertConsult.

KEY REFERENCES

1. *SEER Cancer Statistics Review, 1975–2010*, 2013, National Cancer Institute. At http://seer.cancer.gov/csr/1975-2010/. Accessed April 2013.
   The latest epidemiologic data on disease etiology and outcome by site and age, as compiled by the National Cancer Institute, is presented.
2. Weinberg A, Finegold M: Primary hepatic tumors of childhood. *Hum Pathol* 14:512–537, 1983.
   A classic article describing the spectrum of primary liver tumors in children in two large institutions, including discussion of etiologic factors and histologic characteristics of hepatoblastoma, HCC, and the less common liver tumors of childhood. An observation is made regarding the association of pure fetal histology and favorable outcome.
3. Lopez-Terrada D, Alaggio R, de Davila MT, et al: Towards an international pediatric liver tumor consensus classification: proceedings of the Los Angeles COG liver tumors symposium. *Mod Pathol* 27:472–491, 2014.
   A recent update of the classification of liver tumors in childhood from an international working group of pediatric pathologists. The classification described here will be used in upcoming international treatment protocols.
7. Perilongo G, Shafford E, Maibach R, et al: Risk-adapted treatment for childhood hepatoblastoma. Final report of the second study of the International Paediatric Oncology—SIOPEL 2. *Eur J Cancer* 40:411–421, 2004.
   This article describes treatment outcomes for standard risk (three sectors or less) and high risk (four or more sectors or metastatic). Standard-risk patients were given dose-intense cisplatin with a reported 97% subsequent resection rate and a 91% overall survival rate. High-risk patients were treated with dose-dense cisplatin alternating with carboplatin, with 67% subsequent resection rate and 53% overall survival rate.

32. Wang YX, Liu H: Adult hepatoblastoma: systemic review of the English literature. *Dig Surg* 29:323–330, 2012.
   Prior reports of hepatoblastoma in adults consisted primarily of single case reports. This represents a compilation of 36 prior reports of 40 cases, indicates a one-year survival rate is 29%, and underscores the importance of resection in obtaining cure.
33. Trobaugh-Lotrario AD, Chaiyachati BH, Meyers RL, et al: Outcomes for patients with congenital hepatoblastoma. *Pediatr Blood Cancer* 60:1817–1825, 2013.
   Congenital hepatoblastoma, once thought to have a poor outcome, was suggested to have a survival rate of 86% from this meta-analysis from U.S. and German series as well as a review of multiple published studies.
34. Prokurat A, Kluge P, Koscieza A, et al: Transitional liver cell tumors (TLCT) in older children and adolescents: a novel group of aggressive hepatic tumors expressing beta-catenin. *Med Pediatr Oncol* 39:510–518, 2002.
   This study observes that older children with hepatoblastoma may have more aggressive tumors that have characteristics of both HCC and hepatoblastoma—hence the term transitional liver cell tumor.
37. Katzenstein H, Krailo M, Malogolwkin M, et al: Hepatocellular carcinoma in children and adolescents: results from the Pediatric Oncology Group and the Children's Cancer Group intergroup study. *J Clin Oncol* 20:2789–2797, 2002.
   The results presented in this report from the Pediatric Intergroup Hepatoma Protocol INT-0098 treating childhood HCC according to chemotherapy protocols similar to those used for hepatoblastoma in North America demonstrate a dismal overall survival rate of 19% in HCC. Initial surgical resection was associated with a good prognosis.
39. Katzenstein H, Krailo M, Malogolowkin M, et al: Fibrolamellar hepatocellular carcinoma in children and adolescents. *Cancer* 97:2006–2012, 2003.
   This study reports no difference in 5-year survival rates for patients with fibrolamellar variant of HCC compared with the typical HCC, the although the median survival rate is longer. Unlike other liver tumors, the fibrolamellar HCCs occur equally in male and female patients.
56. Giardiello F, Offerhaus G, Krush A, et al: Risk of hepatoblastoma in familial adenomatous polyposis. *J Pediatr* 119:766–768, 1991.
   The data presented in this study from the Johns Hopkins Registry of 197 families with FAP covering 1220 person-years demonstrate that the relative risk of hepatoblastoma in children 0 to 4 years of age is a remarkable 846.
57. Hughes LJ, Michels VV: Risk of hepatoblastoma in familial adenomatous polyposis. *Am J Med Genet* 43:1023–1025, 1992.
58. Hirschman B, Pollock B, Tomlinson G: The spectrum of APC mutations in children with hepatoblastoma from familial adenomatous polyposis kindreds. *J Pediatr* 147:263–266, 2005.
   This study reports that in patients with hepatoblastoma who reported a family history of FAP, the spectrum of mutations found occurred throughout the gene, and there is no "hotspot" mutation in the APC gene for hepatoblastoma.
79. DeBaun M, Tucker M: Risk of cancer during the first four years of life in children from children from the Beckwith-Wiedemann Syndrome Registry. *J Pediatr* 132:398–400, 1998.
   National Cancer Institute data demonstrate the relative risk of hepatoblastoma in Beckwith-Wiedemann syndrome to be 2280, a higher relative risk than for any other embryonal tumor.
84. Clericuzio C, Chen E, NcNeil E, et al: Serum alpha-fetoprotein screening for hepatoblastoma in children with Beckwith-Wiedemann syndrome or isolated hemihyperplasia. *J Pediatr* 143:270–272, 2003.
   This study demonstrates in five patients that screening of children with Beckwith-Wiedemann syndrome or isolated hemihyperplasia with AFP as well as ultrasonography led to early detection in each case.
114. Tomlinson G, Douglass E, Pollock B, et al: Cytogenetic analysis of a large series of hepatoblastoma: numerical aberrations with recurring translocations involving 1q12-21. *Genes Chromosomes Cancer* 144:177–184, 2005.
   Cytogenetic analyses in a large series demonstrate that numeric aberrations of whole chromosomes are the most common feature of hepatoblastoma. In addition, a family of unbalanced

translocations involving chromosomal breakpoints at proximal chromosome 1q is described.

121. Knisely A, Strautnieks S, Meier Y, et al: Hepatocellular carcinoma in ten children under five years of age with bile salt export pump deficiency. *Hepatology* 44:478–486, 2006.
    This study shows an interesting association of HCC and bile salt export pump deficiency and associated germline mutation.

151. Tanimura M, Matsui I, Abe J, et al: Increased risk of hepatoblastoma among immature children with a lower birth weight. *Cancer Res* 1998:3032–3035, 1998.
    Data from the Japanese Children's Cancer Registry show an increase in hepatoblastoma in low-birth-weight children born after 1988, when survival rates among low-birth-weight children began to increase. The relative risks of hepatoblastoma in low-birth-weight infants compared with infants weighing more than 2500 g vary inversely with birth weight, with the highest relative risk calculated as 15.64 for infants born at less than 2500 g.

158. Musselman JR, Georgieff MK, Ross JA, et al: Maternal pregnancy events and exposures and risk of hepatoblastoma: a Children's Oncology Group (COG) study. *Cancer Epidemiol* 37:318–320, 2013.
    A Children's Oncology Group study of maternal events and hepatoblastoma risks found little evidence of illness or medication during pregnancy affecting risk of hepatoblastoma.

160. Williams CL, Bunch KJ, Stiller CA, et al: Cancer risk among children born after assisted conception. *N Engl J Med* 369:1819–1827, 2013.
    A large cohort study from the United Kingdom demonstrated no definitive over all risk of childhood cancer after assisted conception, although a very small increased risk of hepatoblastoma was reported.

166. Chang M, Chen C, Lai M, et al: Hepatitis B vaccination in Taiwan and the incidence of hepatocellular carcinoma in children. Taiwan Childhood Hepatoma Study Group. *N Engl J Med* 336:1855–1859, 1997.
    A demonstration that universal hepatitis B vaccination resulted in a decline in the incidence of childhood hepatocellular carcinoma in Taiwan.

190. Czauderna P, Lopez Terrada D, Hiyama E, et al: Hepatoblastoma state of the art: pathology, genetics, risk stratification, and chemotherapy. *Curr Opin Pediatr* 26:19–28, 2014.
    A very recent overview of the emerging international trends in hepatoblastoma collaborative research and a look toward future therapeutic trial design.

193. Malogolowkin MH, Katzenstein HM, Meyers RL, et al: Complete surgical resection is curative for children with hepatoblastoma with pure fetal histology: a report from the Children's Oncology Group. *J Clin Oncol* 29:3301–3306, 2011.
    As predicted, the North American Children's Oncology Group trial demonstrates that outcome is excellent for children with hepatoblastoma of pure fetal histology who undergo surgery alone.

194. Trobaugh-Lotrario AD, Tomlinson GE, Finegold MJ, et al: Small cell undifferentiated variant of hepatoblastoma: adverse clinical and molecular features similar to rhabdoid tumors. *Pediatr Blood Cancer* 52:328–334, 2009.
    The results of this study, which combined histologic, immunochemical, and molecular array data on hepatoblastomas with features of the small cell undifferentiated variant, along with clinical outcome data, suggest that this variant has much in common with rhabdoid tumors.

195. Haas JE, Feusner JH, Finegold MJ: Small cell undifferentiated histology in hepatoblastoma may be unfavorable. *Cancer* 92:3130–3134, 2001.

199. Schneider N, Cooley L, Finegold M, et al: The first recurring chromosome translocation in hepatoblastoma: der(4)t(1;4)(q12;q34). *Genes Chromosomes Cancer* 19:291–294, 1997.
    Report of the first recurring translocation in hepatoblastoma t(1;4) resulting in duplication of the long arm of chromosome 1, later found to be part of a family of translocations.

200. Sainati L, Leszl A, Stella M, et al: Cytogenetic analysis of hepatoblastoma: hypothesis of cytogenetic evolution in such tumors and results of a multicentric study. *Cancer Genet Cytogenet* 104:39–44, 1998.

205. Koch A, Denkhaus D, Albrecht S, et al: Childhood hepatoblastomas frequently carry a mutated degradation targeting box of the beta-catenin gene. *Cancer Res* 59:269–273, 1999.
    The initial report of β-catenin mutation in hepatoblastoma; β-catenin alteration has subsequently been shown to be one of the major molecular alterations in hepatoblastoma.

206. Lopez-Terrada D, Gunaratne PH, Adesina AM, et al: Histologic subtypes of hepatoblastoma are characterized by differential canonical Wnt and Notch pathway activation in DLK+ precursors. *Hum Pathol* 40:783–794, 2009.
    This study emphasizes the prevalence of mutation of β-catenin and the important role of canonical Wnt pathway in hepatoblastoma.

207. Taniguchi K, Roberts LR, Aderca IN, et al: Mutational spectrum of beta-catenin, AXIN1, and AXIN2 in hepatocellular carcinomas and hepatoblastomas. *Oncogene* 21:4863–4871, 2002.

210. Cairo S, Armengol C, De Reynies A, et al: Hepatic stem-like phenotype and interplay of Wnt/beta-catenin and Myc signaling in aggressive childhood liver cancer. *Cancer Cell* 14:471–484, 2008.
    An extensive molecular study of hepatoblastoma emphasizing the role of Wnt and Mcy signaling and proposing a 16-gene signature correlating with tumor aggressiveness.

222. Brown J, Perilongo G, Shafford E, et al: Pretreatment prognostic factors for children with hepatoblatoma—results from the International Society of Pediatric Oncology (SIOP) Study SIOPEL 1. *Eur J Cancer* 36:1418–1425, 2000.
    The PRETEXT staging system explained in terms of its role in predicting outcome in hepatoblastoma.

223. Zsiros J, Maibach R, Shafford E, et al: Successful treatment of childhood high-risk hepatoblastoma with dose-intensive multiagent chemotherapy and surgery: final results of the SIOPEL-3HR study. *J Clin Oncol* 28:2584–2590, 2010.

224. Zsiros J, Brugieres L, Brock P, et al: Dose-dense cisplatin-based chemotherapy and surgery for children with high-risk hepatoblastoma (SIOPEL-4): a prospective, single-arm, feasibility study. *Lancet Oncol* 14:834–842, 2013.
    The final outcome of the dose-dense chemotherapy regimen used in SIOPEL-4 proves highly efficacious, with the most notable side effect being ototoxicity.

238. McCarville MB, Roebuck DJ: Diagnosis and staging of hepatoblastoma: imaging aspects. *Pediatr Blood Cancer* 59:793–799, 2012.
    A comprehensive review of imaging techniques in hepatoblastoma.

258. Otte JB, de Ville de Goyet J: The contribution of transplantation to the treatment of liver tumors in children. *Semin Pediatr Surg* 14:233–238, 2005.
    A nice review of the increasing role in liver transplantation as a means of treating pediatric liver cancers.

264. McAteer JP, Goldin AB, Healey PJ, et al: Surgical treatment of primary liver tumors in children: outcomes analysis of resection and transplantation in the SEER database. *Pediatr Transplant* 17:744–750, 2013.

265. Otte JB, Meyers RL, de Ville de Goyet J: Transplantation for liver tumors in children: time to (re)set the guidelines? *Pediatr Transplant* 17:710–712, 2013.
    The preceding two papers present a retrospective review of SEER data regarding transplantation and an interesting commentary based on the current state of the art.

282. Spunt SL, Lobe TE, Pappo AS, et al: Aggressive surgery is unwarranted for biliary tract rhabdomyosarcoma. *J Pediatr Surg* 35:309–316, 2000.
    An extensive review of the role of surgery in conjunction with chemotherapy in biliary rhabdomyosarcoma, a rare cancer of the hepatobiliary tract in children.

283. Nazir Z, Pervez S: Malignant vascular tumors of liver in neonates. *J Pediatr Surg* 41:e49–e51, 2006.

301. Mo JQ, Dimashkieh HH, Bove KE: GLUT1 endothelial reactivity distinguishes hepatic infantile hemangioma from congenital hepatic vascular malformation with associated capillary proliferation. *Hum Pathol* 35:200–209, 2004.
    GLUT1, an important immunohistochemical study distinguishing subtypes of infantile hepatic hemangiomas.

CHAPTER 59

Rhabdomyosarcoma

Richard B. Womer, Frederic G. Barr, and Corrine M. Linardic

CHAPTER OUTLINE

PATHOLOGIC CLASSIFICATION OF RHABDOMYOSARCOMA

The term *rhabdomyosarcoma* (RMS) comprises a heterogeneous family of soft tissue cancers that are related in poorly understood ways to the skeletal muscle lineage. Some of these tumors occur in the vicinity of skeletal muscle, but others occur in areas without obvious skeletal muscle; thus these cancers cannot be defined solely as tumors of skeletal muscle. Instead, this family is derived from unknown mesenchymal precursors and is characterized by a shared program of skeletal myogenesis. Despite this shared program, some precursors may intrinsically undergo myogenesis whereas others may have developed this ability aberrantly.

Histopathologic classification has evolved over time, but two principal histopathologic subtypes have been recognized consistently in children: alveolar RMS (ARMS) and embryonal RMS (ERMS).[1] The criteria for these categories were refined over time as these subtypes were associated with clinically distinct phenotypes. As described in detail later, ARMS more often occurs in the extremities and axial musculature in older children and is associated with a less favorable prognosis whereas ERMS tends to occur in the head, neck, and genitourinary tract of younger patients and is associated with a favorable prognosis. ARMS and ERMS account for 20% to 30% and 70% to 80% of RMS cases, respectively.

The diagnosis of RMS is often difficult because of the paucity of features of striated muscle differentiation. A variety of pediatric solid tumors, including RMS, neuroblastoma, Ewing sarcoma, and non-Hodgkin lymphoma, can present as collections of poorly differentiated cells (small round blue cell tumors). To detect more subtle evidence of myogenic differentiation, immunohistochemical reagents are used to identify muscle-specific proteins, such as MYOD, myogenin, desmin, myoglobin, and skeletal muscle-specific actin.[2] In addition, the detection of myofilaments by electron microscopy provides further evidence of the myogenic phenotype.

In ARMS, the tumor cells are small blue round cells with only small amounts of cytoplasm (Fig. 59-1, A).[3] The prominent round nuclei generally have monotonous, coarse chromatin, and central nucleoli are often present. These tumor cells form highly cellular aggregates separated by fibrovascular septa. Within these aggregates,

discohesive areas tend to form, resulting in spaces or clefts lined by rhabdomyoblasts. ARMS was named for these open spaces, which have an appearance reminiscent of pulmonary alveoli. In addition to these features, the tumor cells tend to align along septa in a "picket-fence" pattern and tumor giant cells are often present. In a subset of cases there is a paucity of fibrovascular stroma, no evidence of spaces, and the predominance of a highly cellular small round cell population with cytologic features similar to the classic alveolar pattern; such cases are referred to as the solid variant of ARMS.

ERMS is so named because of its histologic similarity to developing skeletal muscle. The tumor cells show varying degrees of differentiation along the myogenic spectrum, from small primitive round cells to larger oblong cells with eccentric oval nuclei and varying amounts of eosinophilic cytoplasm (see Fig. 59-1, B).[3] ERMS nuclei are often notable for a relatively bland chromatin pattern. These differentiated cells can elongate to assume a strap-like appearance and occasionally show cross-striations and multinucleation. In addition to the characteristic cytology, ERMS tumors classically have variable cellularity, in which areas of hypercellularity alternate with areas of hypocellularity in a loose myxoid stroma.

Within the ERMS category, there are several histologic variants. In sclerosing RMS, there is abundant desmoplasia and the tendency to form microalveolar tumor cell nests within the desmoplastic areas[4]; in some cases, this microalveolar appearance has been mistaken for ARMS. In a second variant, there are dense clusters of ERMS cells that can be confused with the solid variant of ARMS[5]; this dense ERMS variant can be distinguished based on cytologic features and other special studies. Finally, two variants of ERMS have been associated with

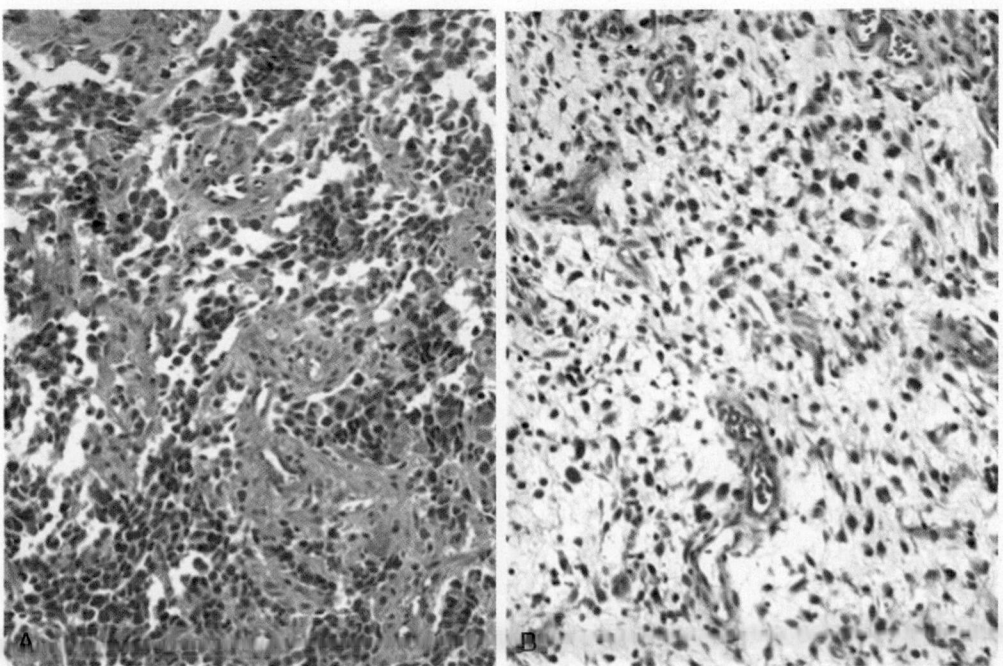

Figure 59-1 Histopathology of RMS subtypes. **A,** Alveolar rhabdomyosarcoma (hematoxylin-eosin, original magnification ×100). **B,** Embryonal rhabdomyosarcoma (hematoxylin-eosin, original magnification ×100). *(Courtesy Dr. Bruce Pawel, Children's Hospital of Philadelphia.)*

an improved prognosis.[3] Botryoid RMS typically occurs in the lumen of a hollow viscus, such as the urinary bladder, vagina, or extrahepatic bile ducts, and grossly has multiple polypoid nodules. At the microscopic level, this tumor typically has a dense cambium layer of tumor cells under an intact epithelial surface. Spindle-cell RMS has dense bundles or whorls of spindle-shaped cells that resemble smooth muscle. In children, these lesions commonly occur in the paratesticular region, but in adults, in whom the prognosis is worse, these lesions tend to occur in the head and neck and are often associated with a sclerosing pattern. In both of these latter two variants, the tumors cells can show marked rhabdomyoblastic differentiation.

Another small subset of RMS cases demonstrates discrete areas with ERMS-like histology and separate discrete areas with ARMS-like histology.[5] The ERMS-like and ARMS-like areas can have any one of the various histologic patterns described earlier. Although these cases

were previously diagnosed as ARMS or ERMS based on prevailing histopathologic criteria, these cases are currently classified as mixed RMS.

A final RMS subset shows features similar to anaplastic Wilms tumors.[6] Although the anaplasia can be seen in both ARMS and ERMS, it is more prevalent in the latter. Anaplastic RMS tumors have large, lobated hyperchromatic nuclei and atypical mitoses. In some cases anaplastic cells are scattered in small patches (focal anaplasia), whereas other cases have larger clusters or sheets of anaplastic cells (diffuse anaplasia).

RHABDOMYOSARCOMA IN CANCER PREDISPOSITION SYNDROMES

The majority of RMS cases arise as sporadic nonheritable tumors, but a small fraction of cases are associated with heritable genetic syndromes (Table 59-1). In some cases the proband with RMS inherited a mutant gene as part

TABLE 59-1   Familial Cancer Predisposition Syndromes Associated with Rhabdomyosarcoma

Cancer Syndrome	Locus	Gene	Nonneoplastic Findings	Characteristic Tumors	Frequency of RMS
Costello syndrome	11p15.5	HRAS	Facial anomalies, cardiac hypertrophy, cognitive defects, developmental delay	*Benign:* skin papillomas *Malignant:* RMS, neuroblastoma, bladder cancer	7%
Li-Fraumeni syndrome	17p13.1 22q12.1	TP53 CHEK2	None	Sarcoma, breast cancer, brain tumor, adrenocortical cancer, leukemia	6%
Hereditary retinoblastoma	13q14	RB1	None	Retinoblastoma, osteosarcoma	2%
Neurofibromatosis type 1	17q11.2	NF1	Café au lait spots, skinfold freckling, Lisch nodules, cognitive deficits	*Benign:* neurofibroma *Malignant:* MPNST, AML	1%
Constitutional mismatch-repair-deficiency syndrome	7p22.2 and others	PMS2, MLH1, MSH2, MSH6	Café au lait spots	hematologic cancers, brain tumors, colorectal cancer	1%
Beckwith-Wiedemann syndrome	11p15.5	Unknown	Macrosomia, macroglossia, hemihyperplasia, visceromegaly	Wilms tumor, hepatoblastoma	<1%
Nevoid basal cell carcinoma syndrome	9q22	PTCH	Macrocephaly, skin cysts, palmar and plantar pits, rib anomalies	Basal cell carcinoma, medulloblastoma	<1%
Rubinstein-Taybi syndrome	16p13.3	CREBBP	Mental retardation, facial anomalies, and broad thumbs	Leukemia, brain tumors	<1%
Noonan syndrome	12q24 and others	PTPN11, SOS1, RAF1, and others	short stature, facial anomalies, congenital heart defects	Neuroblastoma, ALL, glioma, RMS	<1%
DICER1 syndrome (formerly PPB family tumor and dysplasia syndrome)	14q32	DICER1	None	PPB, cystic nephroma	Unknown

ALL, Acute lymphoblastic leukemia; *AML,* acute myelogenous leukemia; *MPNST,* malignant peripheral nerve sheath tumor; *PPB,* pleuropulmonary-blastoma; *RMS,* rhabdomyosarcoma.

of an established familial syndrome, and in other cases a new germline mutation occurred in one germ cell that ultimately produced the proband. The penetrance of RMS in individuals with new or inherited germline mutations varies from as high as approximately 7% in Costello syndrome to 0.1% to 1% in other syndromes. Although there are rare cases of RMS found in association with other syndromes, the determination that such syndromes increase predisposition to RMS is limited by the overall low frequency of these syndromes. In a similar way, the small contribution of known RMS susceptibility syndromes to the overall incidence of RMS is related to the low incidence of these syndromes in the general population. Neurofibromatosis type 1 has the highest prevalence, occurring in approximately 1 in 3500 individuals and accounting for about 1% of all RMS cases.[7,8] Although TP53 germline mutations occur less frequently (~1 in 20,000 individuals), there is a higher prevalence of RMS in these mutation carriers; thus this susceptibility syndrome has been reported to occur in up to 10% all RMS cases.[9]

Among the syndromes predisposing to RMS, three syndromes (termed RASopathies) are caused by alterations of the RAS signaling pathway. Costello syndrome is caused by mutations in HRAS codons 12 or 13.[10] These same mutations commonly occur in many types of sporadic tumors, have transforming activity in cell culture, and thus are gain-of-function alleles. Similarly, Noonan syndrome is caused by activating mutations of one of several oncogenes encoding downstream RAS pathway components with growth stimulatory function.[11] In contrast, neurofibromatosis type 1 is caused by inactivating mutations of the NF1 tumor suppressor gene, which encodes neurofibromin, a guanosine triphosphatase–activating protein that negatively regulates RAS signaling.[12] The presence of a common affected signaling pathway is also indicated by the significant overlap in nonneoplastic phenotype in both Costello and Noonan syndromes. In contrast, neurofibromatosis type 1 is associated with different nonneoplastic phenotypic features. Analysis of these heritable syndromes has thus shown that activation of RAS signaling by one of several genetic changes leads to a low and variable frequency of RMS susceptibility.

The RMS tumors associated with these hereditary predisposition syndromes display a number of notable properties. In many of these syndromes, the RMS tumors occur at a younger age than sporadic RMS tumors, which is in accord with the two-hit tumor susceptibility gene model.[13] Of note, RMS cases in hereditary retinoblastoma occur at a later age but are associated with radiation treatment of the primary retinoblastoma, thus suggesting the need for a postnatal DNA damage event for RMS in this setting.[14] From a pathology perspective, most of these syndromic RMS tumors are diagnosed as ERMS, the subtype that is not associated with the PAX3-FOXO1 and PAX7-FOXO1 gene fusions (described later).[11] In the few cases in which tumors are described as ARMS, such as in hereditary retinoblastoma or Beckwith-Wiedemann syndrome, molecular testing reveals that these RMS tumors are fusion negative.[15,16]

GENETICS OF SPORADIC RHABDOMYOSARCOMA

Gene Fusions Generated by Chromosomal Rearrangements

Cytogenetic studies established that nonrandom chromosomal translocations distinguish most ARMS tumors from ERMS and other pediatric solid tumors (Fig. 59-2). A translocation involving chromosome 2 and 13, t(2;13) (q35;q14), was found in 56% of 99 published ARMS cases, and a variant translocation involving chromosome 1 and 13, t(1;13)(p36;q14), was identified in 6% of cases (http://cgap.nci.nih.gov/Chromosomes/Mitelman). This latter fraction is probably an underestimate because the 1;13 translocation is usually followed by an amplification event (see later). In contrast to ARMS, the 2;13 and 1;13 translocations were found in 3% and 0% of 77 published ERMS cases, respectively. Such rare translocation-positive ERMS cases may represent tumors with mixed histology or misdiagnosed ARMS tumors.

At the molecular level, the 2;13 and 1;13 translocations break and rejoin portions of transcription factor–encoding genes to generate fusion genes expressed as fusion transcripts (see Fig. 59-2). The rearranged genes on chromosomes 2 and 1 are PAX3 and PAX7, which encode related members of the paired box family.[17,18] The chromosome 13 locus in these translocations is FOXO1 (FKHR), which encodes a member of the forkhead family.[19] Although two reciprocal fusion genes, PAX3-FOXO1 and FOXO1-PAX3 (or PAX7-FOXO1 and FOXO1-PAX7), are formed by these translocations, the higher and more consistent expression of PAX3-FOXO1 or PAX7-FOXO1 supports the premise that the PAX3-FOXO1 or PAX7-FOXO1 products are involved in ARMS pathogenesis.

The PAX3-FOXO1 and PAX7-FOXO1 fusion transcripts are translated into novel chimeric transcription factors (see Fig. 59-2).[18,19] The wild-type PAX3, PAX7, and FOXO1 genes encode transcription factors organized with an amino-terminal (N-terminal) DNA-binding domain and a carboxy-terminal (C-terminal) transcriptional activation domain. The translocations break within PAX3 or PAX7 intron 7 and maintain an intact DNA-binding domain but separate it from an essential part of the transactivation domain. In addition, the translocations break within FOXO1 intron 1 and disrupt the DNA-binding domain but maintain an intact transactivation domain. In the chimeric transcripts, the 5′ PAX3 (or 5′ PAX7) and 3′ FOXO1 coding sequences are fused in-frame to generate a 2508- or 2484-nucleotide open reading frame encoding an 836- or 828-amino acid fusion protein, respectively. These fusion proteins contain the first seven exons of PAX3 or PAX7, including an intact DNA-binding domain, and the last two exons of FOXO1, including an intact transactivation domain. A functional fusion protein cannot be created by other combination of PAX3 and FOXO1 exons because of incompatible reading frames or loss of functional domains. These rearrangements of PAX3 or PAX7 intron 7 and FOXO1 intron 1 thus appear to be selected because of functional constraints related to genomic organization of PAX3, PAX7, and FOXO1.

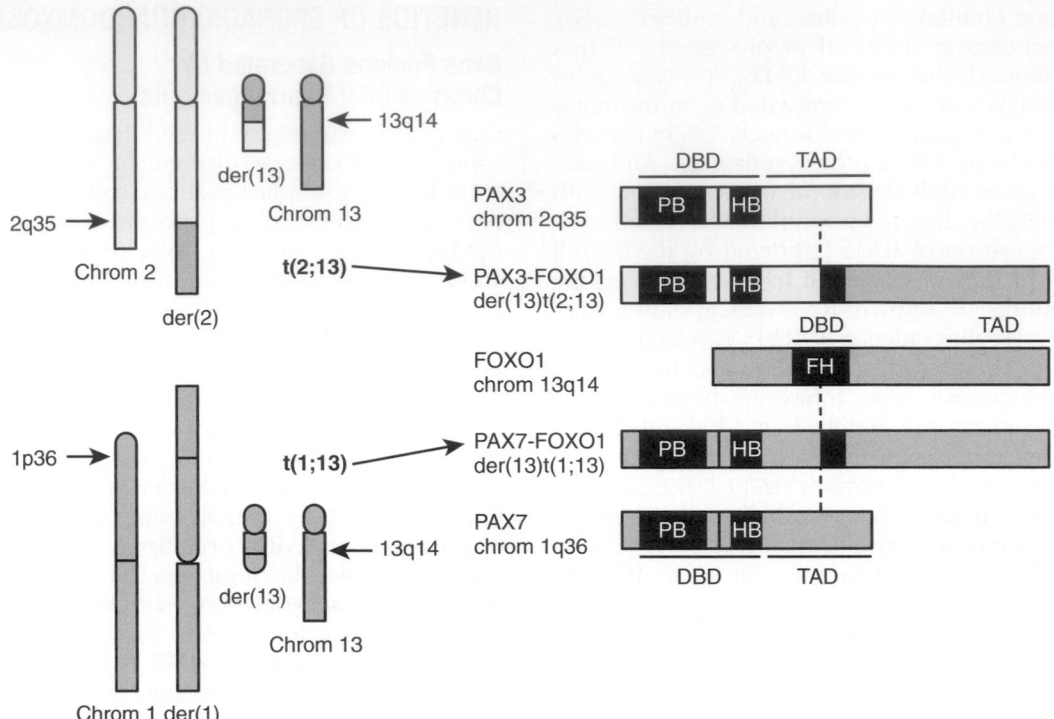

Figure 59-2 Diagrams of 2;13 and 1;13 chromosomal translocations and associated fusion products. A schematic representation of the normal and derivative chromosomes associated with t(2;13) and t(1;13) is shown on the left. The translocation breakpoints are indicated by *short horizontal arrows* with the location of involved chromosomal region. The wild-type and fusion products associated with 2;13 and 1;13 translocations are shown on the right. The paired box (PB), octapeptide, homeobox (HB), and forkhead (FH) domains are indicated as *dark purple boxes*, and transcriptional domains (DBD, DNA binding domain; TAD, transcriptional activation domain) are shown as *solid bars*. The *vertical dashed line* indicates the translocation fusion point.

There are changes in both function and expression caused by the fusion events in ARMS. The chimeric transcription factors activate transcription from PAX3/PAX7-binding sites but are much more potent as transcriptional activators than the wild-type PAX3 and PAX7 proteins.[20,21] This difference in transcriptional activity appears to be caused by a decreased sensitivity of the FOXO1 activation domain to the inhibitory effects of N-terminal PAX3 (or PAX7) domains, when compared with the effect of these N-terminal domains on the PAX3 (or PAX7) activation domain. The fusion proteins may also have a relaxed capability to bind and activate target genes owing to increased structural flexibility in the N-terminal DNA-binding domain.[22] In addition to changes in transcriptional function, the PAX3-FOXO1 or PAX7-FOXO1 fusion products are expressed in ARMS tumors at higher levels compared with the corresponding wild-type PAX3 or PAX7 products.[23] The gene-specific mechanisms for this enhanced fusion product expression are described later. Therefore these chromosomal changes result in high levels of chimeric transcription factors that inappropriately activate transcription of genes with PAX3/PAX7 DNA-binding sites. These biologic effects contribute to tumorigenesis by modulating myogenic differentiation, altering growth and apoptotic pathways, and stimulating motility and other metastatic pathways.

Several methodologies, including reverse-transcriptase polymerase chain reaction (RT-PCR) assay and fluorescent in situ hybridization (FISH), were applied to detect the *PAX3-FOXO1* and *PAX7-FOXO1* fusions in clinical material.[24-27] A single large study of RMS cases from the Intergroup Rhabdomyosarcoma Study (IRS) IV protocol showed that all 93 cases of RMS or undifferentiated sarcoma with a diagnosis other than ARMS were fusion negative, whereas 77% of the 78 ARMS cases were fusion positive.[28] Of these ARMS cases, 55% expressed *PAX3-FOXO1*, 22% expressed *PAX7-FOXO1*, and 23% were fusion negative.[28] These findings were confirmed by several other large cooperative group studies. In other studies of mixed RMS, most but not all cases were fusion negative.[27,29] Furthermore, when areas with ARMS-like and ERMS-like histology were individually examined by FISH, there was concordance for fusion status among the regions in a single tumor.

These molecular pathology studies establish that there is a significant subset (~20%) of ARMS cases that do not express either the *PAX3-FOXO1* or *PAX7-FOXO1* fusion. The IRS IV protocol and subsequent cooperative group studies used centralized pathology review and uniform tissue banking, and thus these fusion-negative results cannot be explained by inaccurate histopathologic diagnosis or suboptimal tissue samples. Subsequent analysis of these fusion-negative cases revealed that a small subset have variant fusions of *PAX3*, *PAX7*, or *FOXO1* with other genes, including fusion of *PAX3* with the *FOXO1*-related locus *FOXO4 (AFX1)* and fusion of *PAX3* with *NCOA1* or *NCOA2*, which encode two similar transcription factors unrelated to the forkhead family.[30,31] However, these variant fusions are uncommon; most fusion-negative ARMS cases do not have any rearrangements of *PAX3, PAX7,* or *FOXO1* and thus appear to represent true fusion-negative cases with respect to these loci.

Although genetic studies have not revealed any chromosome rearrangements that occur in most ERMS cases, gene fusions have been identified in a small number of ERMS cases. In particular, rearrangements of the *NCOA2* gene in the 8q11-13 chromosomal region were detected in four ERMS tumors.[31,32] The pathologic subtype in three of the four cases was a spindle cell variant of ERMS. Furthermore, all four cases occurred in infants younger than 1 year of age and thus are characterized as congenital/infantile RMS. Further analysis of three cases demonstrated fusions to different partners in each case—*PAX3* (2q35), *SRF* (8q11), and *TEAD1* (11p15). Finally, there is a report of an unrelated fusion, *EWSR1-DUX4,* in an ERMS in a 19-year-old patient.[33]

Chromosome Copy Number Changes

Various studies, including classic cytogenetics (http://cgap.nci.nih.gov/Chromosomes/Mitelman), chromosome-based comparative genomic hybridization (CGH), and DNA-based microarrays established that a second set of differences between the RMS histopathologic subtypes is at the level of whole chromosome gains and losses.[34,35-37] ERMS tumors have multiple numerical changes of whole chromosomes. The most frequent chromosome change in ERMS involves gains of chromosome 8. This change is characterized by polysomy, or multiple copies, of chromosome 8 and occurs in 50% to 90% of ERMS tumors but only 10% to 20% of ARMS tumors. This chromosome gain results in elevated expression of genes along chromosome 8 and cannot be localized to any specific chromosomal region. Additional common gains in ERMS involve chromosomes 2, 7, 11, 12, 13, and 20. In contrast to chromosome 8 gains, each of these latter changes is often a low-level gain, most likely a trisomy, and occurs in 20% to 50% of ERMS cases. Several of these gains, such as chromosome 2, 11, and 13, occur at significantly lower frequencies (2- to 10-fold) in ARMS tumors. Whole chromosome losses in ERMS commonly involve chromosomes 6, 9, 10, 14, 15, and 16 and occur in 15% to 25% of ERMS tumors. A study of intermediate-risk ERMS reports higher frequencies of these chromosome losses, suggesting that these events may vary among RMS risk groups.[35] There are also quantitative differences in chromosome losses between ERMS and ARMS, but these differences are not as striking as the differences involving gains.

Although the chromosome gains and losses are not prevalent in the ARMS cases as a group, the fusion-negative ARMS subset has a pattern of gains and losses that is much more similar to ERMS than to the fusion-positive ARMS subset.[37] The most striking finding involves chromosome 8; these events occur in more than 50% of fusion-negative ARMS tumors but not in fusion-positive ARMS tumors. As a second example, chromosome 11 gains occur in 30% of fusion-negative ARMS tumors but only 10% of fusion-positive ARMS tumors.

TABLE 59-2 Frequently Amplified Chromosomal Regions in Rhabdomyosarcoma

Chromosome Region	Genes Involved	FREQUENCY		
		PAX3-FOXO1	PAX7-FOXO1	Fusion-negative
1p36	*PAX7*	0%	>90%	0%
2p24	*MYCN*	20%	20%	0-6%
12q13-14	*CDK4* and others	24	<5%	<5%
13q14	*FOXO1*	<10%	>90%	0%
13q31	*MIR17HG*	<10%	70%	<10%

Amplification of Specific Chromosomal Regions

CGH and DNA-based microarray studies revealed that ARMS has significantly more genomic amplification events than ERMS. In CGH studies, one or more amplification events were detected in 47 of 84 ARMS cases (56%) compared with 7 of 43 ERMS cases (16%).[34,38,39] The most common amplicons in ARMS tumors were derived from chromosomal regions 1p36, 2p24, 12q13-q14, 13q14, and 13q31 (Table 59-2).[38,40-42] The pattern of changes in the fusion-negative ARMS subset was again more similar to the pattern in ERMS than that in fusion-positive ARMS.[37] This difference is exemplified by the finding of 12q13-q14 amplification in 24% of fusion-positive ARMS, 4% of fusion-negative ARMS, and 0% of ERMS. In addition to differences between fusion-positive and fusion-negative tumors, many of these high-frequency amplicons have a marked preference for either the *PAX3-FOXO1*– or *PAX7-FOXO1*–positive subset.

The amplification events at 1p36 and 13q14 generally occur in the same cases and are indicative of *PAX7-FOXO1* amplification (see Table 59-2).[41] In particular, *PAX7-FOXO1* is amplified in more than 90% of *PAX7-FOXO1*–positive cases whereas *PAX3-FOXO1* is amplified in less than 10% of *PAX3-FOXO1*–positive cases. As a further difference, there is a higher number of cells containing the amplicon in amplified *PAX7-FOXO1*–positive cases than in amplified *PAX3-FOXO1*–positive cases. At the expression level, the fusion transcript is expressed at higher levels in *PAX7-FOXO1*–positive cases than in *PAX3-FOXO1*–positive cases. Despite these differences, both fusion products are expressed in ARMS tumors at higher levels than the corresponding wild-type *PAX3* or *PAX7* products.[23] This high expression is postulated to generate a fusion product level above a critical threshold for oncogenic activity. Although there is a common feature of fusion overexpression in fusion-positive ARMS, the mechanism of overexpression differs between the two subtypes. In *PAX7-FOXO1*–positive tumors, the fusion is generally overexpressed because of genomic amplification, a copy number–dependent mechanism. In contrast, *PAX3-FOXO1* is generally overexpressed by a copy number–independent increase in transcriptional rate.

For amplification of the 2p24 chromosomal region, the minimal amplified region contains the *MYCN* protooncogene (see Table 59-2).[40] This genomic region corresponds to the same region that is frequently amplified in neuroblastoma. In ARMS there is a comparable incidence of 2p24 amplification (20%) in *PAX3-FOXO1*– and *PAX7-FOXO1*–positive tumors. In contrast, this amplification occurs very infrequently in ERMS and fusion-negative ARMS tumors (0% to 6% of cases).[37] In addition to amplification, low copy number gains, which may be explained in part by whole chromosome 2 gains, were found in 50% to 60% of ARMS and ERMS cases.[43] In fusion-positive tumors, 2p24 amplification generally results in high expression of the *MYCN* transcript and an increase in MYCN protein expression. The lower-level gains may also be associated with moderate increases in *MYCN* expression.

Amplification of the 12q13-q14 chromosomal region was found in numerous cancers, including bone and soft tissue sarcomas (e.g., osteosarcoma and liposarcoma), brain tumors (mostly glioblastoma), and carcinomas (including breast cancer).[44] In ARMS, the minimal amplified region was localized to a 0.5-Mb region containing more than 20 genes, including CDK4, which encodes a cell cycle regulatory protein (see Table 59-2).[40] The 12q13-q14 region is amplified preferentially in *PAX3-FOXO1*–positive cases; there is a 24% and 4% frequency of 12q13-q14 amplification in *PAX3-FOXO1*– and *PAX7-FOXO1*–positive cases, respectively. This amplification also occurs at a low frequency in fusion-negative RMS tumors. In fusion-positive RMS tumors, 12q13-q14 amplification is associated with increased expression of multiple (but not all) genes in the minimal amplified region. Of note, the nearby 12q15 region (containing *MDM2*) is independently amplified at a low frequency in both fusion-positive and fusion-negative RMS tumors.[40,45-47]

The 13q31 amplification event was localized to a 150-kb region surrounding the *MIR17HG* gene (see Table 59-2).[42] This gene contains the miR-17-92 cluster, and the transcript expressed from the *MIR17HG* gene is processed to six microRNAs (miRs). This 13q31 region is also amplified in diffuse large B-cell lymphoma and small cell lung carcinoma.[48] In RMS, this region is preferentially amplified in *PAX7-FOXO1*–positive cases; this amplicon is present in 70% of *PAX7-FOXO1*–positive cases and less than 10% of *PAX3-FOXO1*–positive RMS and fusion-negative RMS cases. In RMS tumors with 13q31 amplification, five of the six microRNAs in the cluster (miR-17, miR-19a, miR-19b, miR-20a, and miR-92a) are expressed at high levels. Transcripts from a number of tumor suppressor genes are targets of these microRNAs, and thus these microRNAs are postulated to be oncogenic by decreasing tumor suppressor expression.

Allelic Loss Events

RMS studies using polymorphic markers to distinguish between the two alleles at a locus reveal that allelic loss (or conversion to homozygosity) occurs commonly in ERMS tumors.[49] With the use of DNA-based arrays with polymorphic markers, the genome-wide incidence of allelic loss (termed *fractional allelic loss*) was twofold higher in ERMS compared with ARMS tumors.[50] Furthermore, the fusion-negative ARMS subset demonstrated a fractional allelic loss similar to that of ERMS tumors that was more than twofold higher than that of fusion-positive ARMS tumors.

In ERMS, chromosome 11 is most commonly affected by allelic loss, and the smallest region of consistent allelic loss is 11p15.5 (Fig. 59-3).[51] This 11p15.5 allelic loss is also detected in a small subset (24%) of fusion-positive ARMS tumors but is much more common (77%) in ERMS and fusion-negative ARMS tumors.[50,52] The probable presence of a tumor suppressor gene in this region, which is inactivated in RMS, is supported by several pieces of evidence. First, the gene or genes responsible for Beckwith-Wiedemann syndrome (which predisposes to several cancers, including RMS) were localized to this chromosomal region.[53] Second, transfer of wild-type copies of chromosome 11 or fragments containing the 11p15 region suppresses growth of ERMS cells.[54,55]

Determination of the parent of origin of the two alleles from the 11p15.5 region revealed that ERMS tumors preferentially maintain the paternal allele and lose the maternal allele (see Fig. 59-3).[56] This preference suggests the action of genomic imprinting, a normal epigenetic developmental process that selectively inactivates expression of alleles in a gamete-of-origin–dependent process. Several genes in the human 11p15 chromosomal region and the corresponding mouse region show imprinting.[53] For example, *IGF2*, encoding an embryonic growth factor, is preferentially expressed from the paternal allele, whereas *CDKN1C*, which encodes a cyclin-dependent kinase inhibitor (p57/KIP2) that negatively regulates cell-cycle progression, is preferentially expressed from the maternal allele. Two additional genes with preferential maternal expression and tumor suppressor function derive from opposite strands of the *H19* locus, which produces the nontranslated H19 RNA, and the HOTS nucleolar protein.[57] These combined studies of allelic loss in the 11p15.5 region suggest that ERMS tumorigenesis frequently involves inactivation of an imprinted tumor suppressor by allelic loss of the active maternal allele and retention of the inactive paternal allele.

Oncogene and Tumor Suppressor Gene Mutations in Rhabdomyosarcoma

The earlier-described studies of RMS patients with cancer predisposition syndromes revealed genes that are mutated and corresponding pathways that are altered in the pathogenesis of rare RMS cases. In particular, RMS cases occurred in syndromes in which the RAS pathway was activated whereas other cases occurred in syndromes in which the RB1 or TP53 signaling pathway was inactivated. The corresponding pathways thus are strong candidates for alterations in sporadic tumors, either by mutating the same genes that are altered in the predisposition syndromes or mutating other genes in these pathways.

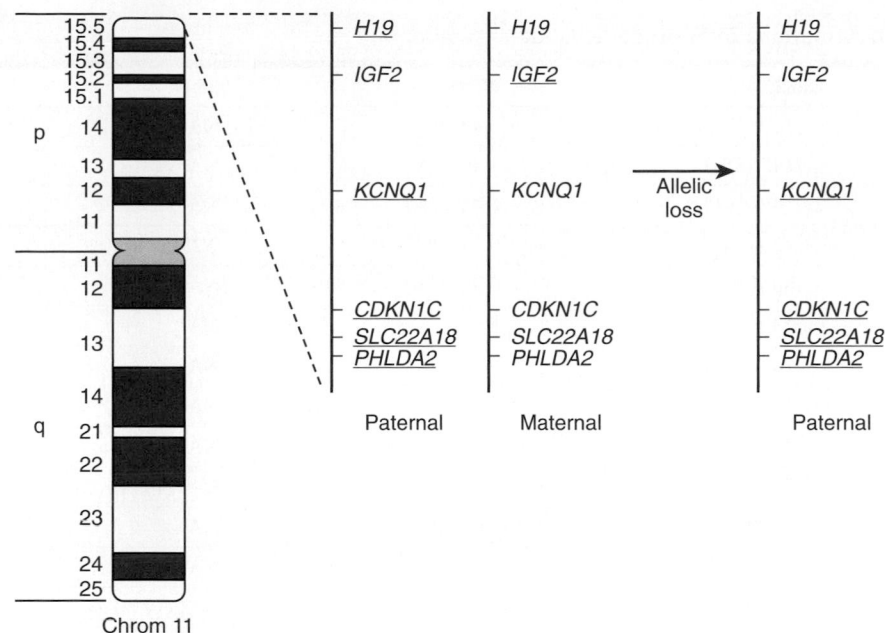

Figure 59-3 Allelic loss of imprinted region at 11p15.5 in RMS. In the 11p15.5 chromosomal region, there is parent of-origin-specific expression (imprinting) of multiple genes, such that *underlining* indicates an expressed allele and lack of underlining indicates an unexpressed allele. In many cases of ERMS, a few cases of ARMS, and other tumors, the maternal alleles in the 11p15.5 region (and variable amounts of contiguous regions) are lost by one of a variety of genomic mechanisms in a process termed *allelic loss, loss of heterozygosity,* or *conversion to homozygosity.*

Several studies suggest that small mutations are more common in ERMS than ARMS. In a recent next-generation sequencing (NGS) study of 147 RMS cases (53 fusion-positive and 94 fusion-negative), the mean rate of verified nonsynonymous mutations was fourfold higher in fusion-negative tumors (17.8 mutations/tumor) compared with fusion-positive tumors (6.4 mutations/tumor).[58] Recurrent deleterious point mutations involving known genes were found in more than 50% of fusion-negative RMS cases compared with less than 5% of fusion-positive cases. Of note, only two recurrent point mutations (*PIK3CA* and *BCOR*) were found in the 48 fusion-positive ARMS cases whereas three recurrent point mutations were found in 11 fusion-negative ARMS cases. These overall findings in this NGS study were very similar to a second smaller NGS study[59] as well as a directed mutation study.[60] In this latter directed mutation study of 31 genes, mutations were detected in 14 of 57 (25%) ERMS cases compared with 1 of 21 (5%) ARMS cases.[60] Except for one ERMS case with two mutations, the other 13 ERMS cases had only one mutation per case from this panel of 31 genes. An insufficient number of cases was examined to comment on mutation frequency in the fusion-negative ARMS subset.

The RAS pathway is frequently activated in sporadic ERMS tumors by mutations in one of several genes (Table 59-3). In recent studies analyzing 147 ERMS cases, *RAS* family genes were mutated in 20% of ERMS cases.[35,60-63] More than half of these *RAS* family mutations (19/31, 61%) occurred in the *NRAS* gene and the majority (15/19, 79%) of these *NRAS* mutations involved codon 61. In contrast, only one *RAS* family gene mutation (in *KRAS*) was detected in 41 cases of ARMS (2%). Of various other RAS pathway components, *PTPN11* and

BRAF mutations were found in 3% and 1% of ERMS cases but not in any ARMS cases.[60-65] In 1 of 12 ERMS cases (8%), a mutation was also found in the *SPRY1* gene, which encodes a modulator of RAS signaling.[63] Finally, homozygous deletions involving the *NF1* locus were found in 15% of ERMS cases.[35] The *RAS*, *PTPN11*, and *BRAF* point mutations as well as the *NF1* deletions are mutually exclusive, consistent with the premise that these changes activate the same pathway. Therefore, one of several components in the RAS pathway can be altered to activate this pathway in more than 40% of sporadic ERMS cases but in very few (<5%) sporadic ARMS cases.

Alterations in genes encoding RB1 or proteins regulating RB1 function occur in sporadic ERMS and ARMS tumors, providing several mechanisms to alter RB1 signaling. Although small *RB1* mutations were not conclusively investigated in sporadic RMS, homozygous deletions were found in 22% (6/27) of ERMS and 10% (2/20) of ARMS cases (see Table 59-3).[66] A higher frequency of *RB1* gene alterations in ERMS is suggested by the finding of significantly lower RB1 expression in ERMS compared with ARMS tumors. As described earlier, 12q13-q14 amplification in a subset of ARMS cases results in overexpression of CDK4, which phosphorylates RB1 and contributes to RB1 functional inactivation. In another subset of RMS cases, homozygous deletions and/or point mutations occur in *CDKN2A* and *CDKN2B*, which encode inhibitors of CDK4 and CDK6.[35,67-69] These alterations occur in both ARMS and ERMS, with an overall homozygous deletion frequency of 13% (11/82) and a mutation frequency of 7% (6/88).

There is also evidence for genetic changes that alter the TP53 pathway in sporadic RMS tumors (see Table 59-3). In multiple studies examining a total of 159 RMS cases,

TABLE 59-3A   Point Mutations in Sporadic Rhabdomyosarcomas*

Gene	ERMS	ARMS	Other[†]	All RMS
HRAS	5/147[‡] (3%)	0/41 (0%)	NA	5/188 (3%)
KRAS	7/147 (5%)	1/41 (2%)	NA	8/188 (4%)
NRAS	19/147[‡] (13%)	0/41 (0%)	NA	19/188 (10%)
BRAF	1/93 (1%)	0/31 (0%)	0/29 (0%)	1/153 (1%)
MAP2K1	0/80 (0%)	0/21 (0%)	NA	0/101 (0%)
MAP2K2	0/23 (0%)	NA	NA	0/23 (0%)
PTPN11	3/108 (3%)	0/31 (0%)	NA	3/139 (2%)
SPRY1	1/12 (8%)	0/7 (0%)	NA	1/19 (5%)
SOS1	0/20 (0%)	NA	NA	0/20 (0%)
CDKN2A	0/27 (0%)	0/17 (0%)	6/44 (14%)	6/88 (7%)
CTNNB1	2/57 (4%)	0/21 (0%)	NA	2/78 (3%)
DICER1	4/57 (7%)	NA	NA	4/57 (7%)
FGFR4	11/112 (10%)	2/47 (4%)	2/12 (17%)	15/171 (9%)
PIK3CA	3/57 (5%)	0/21 (0%)	1/12 (8%)	4/90 (4%)
TP53	2/50 (4%)	0/41 (0%)	10/68 (15%)	12/159 (8%)

ARMS, Alveolar rhabdomyosarcomas; *ERMS*, embryonal rhabdomyosarcomas; *NA*, not available.
*RMS cell lines were not included in this compilation.
[†]Other includes Botryoid, pleomorphic, mixed, and unclassified cases.
[‡]In one ERMS case, both a HRAS and a NRAS mutation were detected.

12 missense mutations (8%) were detected in the *TP53* gene.[46,47,70-72] Although many cases were not subclassified for histopathologic subtype, mutations were found in both ARMS and ERMS.[46,47,71,73] Homozygous deletions involving *TP53* were also detected in a few cases.[73,74] In addition to these direct changes in *TP53*, changes in the TP53 pathway may be caused by *MDM2* gene amplification (described earlier), which encodes a protein that binds to and inactivates TP53. Finally, deletion of the *CDKN2A* locus (described earlier) also eliminates expression of p14ARF, which is a protein that normally blocks MDM2 function and stabilizes the TP53 protein.[69]

Activation of several additional signaling pathways is also implicated in sporadic RMS tumors (see Table 59-3). Mutation in the tyrosine kinase domain of the membrane receptor fibroblast growth factor receptor 4 *(FGFR4)* was detected in 15 of 171 (9%) RMS tumors, including 11 in 112 (10%) ERMS and 2 in 47 (4%) ARMS cases.[35,60,75] These mutations activate downstream signaling from FGFR4 and increase proliferation, invasion, and metastatic potential in mutation-bearing cells. Other genes in which mutations were found only in ERMS tumors include *PIK3CA* (3/57, 5%) and *CTNNB1* (2/57, 4%); these mutations will activate phosphatidylinositol-3-kinase and Wnt signaling pathways, respectively.[60,64] Although activation of the Hedgehog signaling pathway has been noted in a substantial subset of ERMS tumors, point mutations were not found in genes encoding several classic pathway components.[76-78] As a possible alternative explanation of this increased Hedgehog signaling, low-level gains of the *GLI1* locus were found in numerous ERMS cases.[35] Finally, *DICER1* mutations have been detected in 2 of 52 (4%) sporadic ERMS tumors and result in deregulated microRNA processing.[79,80]

Hypermethylation as an Alternative Mechanism of Gene Inactivation in Rhabdomyosarcoma

In a final set of genomic changes in RMS, genetic loci can be silenced by epigenetic events involving tumor-specific hypermethylation of CpG islands. The cytosine residues in CpG dinucleotides are ordinarily unmethylated in normal cells but can become methylated during

TABLE 59-3B   Homozygous Deletions in Sporadic Rhabdomyosarcomas*

Gene	ERMS	ARMS	Other[†]	All RMS
CDKN2A/B	8/32 (25%)	1/6 (17%)	2/44 (5%)	11/82 (13%)
NF1	4/26 (15%)	NA	NA	4/26 (15%)
RB1	6/27 (22%)	2/20 (10%)	NA	8/47 (17%)
TP53	1/4 (25%)	0/2 (0%)	1/31 (3%)	2/37 (5%)

ARMS, Alveolar rhabdomyosarcoma; *ERMS*, embryonal rhabdomyosarcoma; *NA*, not available.
*RMS cell lines were not included in this compilation.
[†]Other includes Botryoid, pleomorphic, mixed, and unclassified cases.

tumorigenesis, thereby altering the nearby chromatin structure and silencing transcription of associated genes. Studies of small numbers of RMS cases indicated that several genes often hypermethylated in other tumor types, such as CDKN2A, are not affected in a significant subset of RMS cases. However, hypermethylation of the CpG islands in the RASSF1A, HIC1, and CASP8 genes was detected in both ARMS and ERMS tumors.[81-83] In contrast, there is evidence of differential methylation of the CpG islands in the MYOD and PAX3 genes such that hypermethylation occurs in most ERMS cases and hypomethylation occurs in most ARMS cases.[84,85] A genome-wide approach also identified 140 promoter regions hypermethylated in at least four of ten RMS tumors compared with skeletal muscle, including genes implicated in development and tumorigenesis, such as GATA6 and HES5.[86] Unsupervised hierarchical cluster analysis indicates that DNA methylation pattern correlates with RMS subtype. These hypermethylation events are generally associated with loss of expression of the corresponding proteins, providing an alternative nonmutagenic mechanism for inactivating genes and altering associated pathways.

APPLICATIONS OF MOLECULAR GENETIC APPROACHES TO DIAGNOSIS AND PROGNOSIS

Detection of Recurrent Gene Fusions

As described earlier, RT-PCR and FISH methodologies were developed to detect the PAX3-FOXO1 and PAX7-FOXO1 gene fusions in clinical material.[24-27] In contrast to Southern blot approaches, both RT-PCR and FISH can be applied to detect these fusions in small amounts of input tissue. Furthermore, both RT-PCR and FISH approaches have been developed for formalin-fixed paraffin-embedded tissues as well as fresh and frozen tissues. Another favorable feature of the RT-PCR assays is high technical sensitivity, which permits detection of micrometastatic spread of rare fusion-positive cells to tissues such as bone marrow.[87] Although FISH has lower technical sensitivity, a break-apart FOXO1 FISH assay has simplified detection of FOXO1 rearrangements resulting from either PAX3-FOXO1 or PAX7-FOXO1.[41] In addition, break-apart PAX3 and PAX7 assays facilitate detection of variant fusions in ARMS cases that do not contain either of the two usual fusions.[27]

Pathologic and Clinical Differences between Fusion Subtypes

Clinical-molecular correlative studies revealed several differences between fusion-negative and fusion-positive tumors. In comparisons of outcome among the fusion subsets, the fusion-negative ARMS cases have a failure-free survival (FFS) and overall survival (OS) similar to ERMS cases and significantly better than fusion-positive ARMS cases.[37,88] There is a similar frequency of other parameters, such as unfavorable sites and metastasis, in ERMS and fusion-negative ARMS, and this frequency is lower in fusion-negative ARMS than in fusion-positive ARMS. Finally, in an examination of histopathologic

parameters, nearly half of fusion-negative cases lack cystic foci and show totally "solid alveolar" architecture.[89]

Although there are no detectable histopathologic differences between PAX3-FOXO1– and PAX7-FOXO1–positive cases,[89] there are clinical differences between these two fusion-positive subsets. The OS rate in the PAX7-FOXO1–positive subset is superior to that in the PAX3-FOXO1–positive subset and similar to the OS rate in the ERMS and fusion-negative ARMS categories.[41,88,90] In contrast, failure free survival in the two fusion-positive subsets is similar. In addition to OS, there are other clinical differences between these two fusion-positive subsets. In particular, the PAX7-FOXO1–positive tumors are typically diagnosed at a younger age, more often present with an extremity primary tumor, and are associated with a lower frequency of local invasion and nodal metastasis.[28,41] A multivariate analysis of the contributions of prognostic parameters found that fusion status was an independent predictor of OS. A risk-based stratification incorporating fusion status, stage, and age has potential utility for stratifying the Children's Oncology Group (COG) intermediate-risk group into distinct subgroups.[90]

Gene Expression Profiling with Microarrays

Microarray-based analyses of genome-wide gene expression compared RMS with other pediatric tumors included in the differential diagnosis of small blue round cell tumors. Cases were clustered based on differences and similarities in expression patterns. Statistical analyses identified lists ranging from 20 to 93 genes that can correctly classify all tumors.[91-94] These lists contain genes specifically expressed in each tumor category, including muscle-specific and myogenesis-related genes that are specifically expressed in RMS. With the use of minimization strategies, the criteria needed for classification were reduced in size to lists ranging from 7 to 31 genes. To extend these findings, 39 genes were selected to design a multiplex RT-PCR assay, which generates findings comparable to the microarray platform.[95]

Microarray studies also developed classifiers for subsets within the RMS family. With the use of clustering algorithms, it was shown that the PAX3-FOXO1– and PAX7-FOXO1–positive subsets of ARMS cluster together, indicating no major expression differences between the two fusion-positive subsets.[37,50,96,97] In contrast, there was a striking difference in expression pattern between the fusion-positive and fusion-negative ARMS cases. There were four published cases with variant fusions: two clustered with fusion-positive tumors and two clustered with the fusion-negative tumors. These analyses also demonstrated a striking difference in expression pattern between ERMS and fusion-positive ARMS cases. Comparison of ERMS and fusion-negative ARMS cases did not reveal any recurrent expression differences between these two groups of fusion-negative RMS cases. Therefore, based on expression pattern, RMS cases can be divided into two major categories: the fusion-positive and fusion-negative cases. Furthermore, when viewed on a multidimensional scaling plot, the fusion-positive group showed a dense cluster whereas the fusion-negative group showed a cluster with more heterogeneous spread.

The fusion-negative RMS category is proposed to be further divisible into three novel subsets, which are related to expression of muscle differentiation and chromosome 11 genes.[50] A well-differentiated RMS subset expressed both gene sets, whereas a moderately differentiated RMS subset expressed the chromosome 11 genes with decreased levels of muscle differentiation genes. A final subset containing approximately 25% of ERMS tumors as well as undifferentiated sarcomas and non-RMS soft tissue tumors (NRSTS) did not express either gene set. In addition, tumors in this last subset had a fractional allelic loss (including 11p loss) similar to that in fusion-positive RMS tumors and twofold lower than that in the well-differentiated and moderately differentiated subsets. The significance of these subsets is highlighted by the finding of good, intermediate, and poor outcomes in well-differentiated, moderately differentiated, and undifferentiated sarcoma/NRSTS categories, respectively.

For prospective diagnosis of fusion-positive or fusion-negative RMS, genes differentially expressed between the two fusion subsets were identified to generate initial signatures ranging from 121 to 534 genes.[37,50,96,97] The genes preferentially expressed in fusion-positive tumors were overrepresented in PAX3-FOXO1 downstream targets (including genes involved in neurogenesis) and chromosome 6 genes, whereas the genes preferentially expressed in fusion-negative tumors were overrepresented in chromosome 8 genes. Additional statistical approaches identified minimal signatures consisting of 10, 5, or even 2 genes with predictive accuracy of 95% or greater.[50,97,98] To develop an assay applicable to formalin-fixed paraffin embedded samples, biomarkers were identified that correspond to differentially expressed genes with commercially available antibodies suitable for immunohistochemistry.[50,99] These efforts identified epidermal growth factor receptor (EGFR), fibrillin-2, and high-mobility group AT-hook 2 (HMGA2) as markers expressed in fusion-negative RMS cases and transcription factor AP-2β (TFAP2B) and P-cadherin as markers expressed in fusion-positive RMS cases. The combination of two markers for each RMS subset achieved specificity of 90% or greater and a sensitivity of 60% or greater.

Several microarray and other genomic approaches were used to identify fusion protein downstream targets. In one approach, transduction of PAX3-FOXO1 or PAX7-FOXO1 in an ERMS cell line modulated expression of 334 genes (266 increased and 68 decreased); 81 of these genes (24%) were also differentially expressed between fusion-positive and fusion-negative RMS tumors.[100] In the second approach, siRNA-mediated downregulation of PAX3-FOXO1 in an ARMS cell line decreased expression of 1834 genes after 24 hours of treatment; only 51 (3%) of these genes overlapped the differential expression signature in RMS tumors.[101] In a final approach, ChIP-Seq analysis identified 1463 genomic regions bound to the fusion protein in ARMS cells; these genomic regions correspond to 24% of genes expressed at higher levels in fusion-positive RMS and 6% of the genes expressed at higher levels in fusion-negative RMS.[102] These findings indicate that only a fraction of expression differences between fusion-positive and fusion-negative tumors is directly attributable to the fusion protein; many of the expression differences may result from other genetic and environmental differences between these RMS subsets.

Microarray analysis also elucidated genes whose expression predicts outcome in RMS patients. In particular, Cox regression proportional hazards modeling of OS with RMS microarray expression data identified 15 or 34 gene sets whose aggregate pattern of expression was correlated with OS.[90,103] The performance of these two gene sets was high in the initial patient cohort and lower but still significant in a validation cohort. For the 34 gene set, this expression-based stratification of RMS cases was related to the current COG risk classification system. In addition, this expression-based stratification for both the 15- and 34-gene sets was also correlated with PAX3-FOXO1 and PAX7-FOXO1 fusion status. Multivariate analysis showed that these 15- or 34-gene sets were not independent predictors of outcome.

A hypothesis was also proposed that fusion protein downstream targets may predict outcome.[100] Starting with 81 target genes that were both modulated by exogenous fusion protein in ERMS cells and differentially expressed between the fusion-positive and fusion-negative tumors, Cox regression modeling elucidated a 28-gene predictor. An aggregate score calculated from expression of these 28 genes is predictive of OS in ARMS and independent of known prognostic variables. This finding suggests that modulation of downstream fusion protein target expression is associated with differences in biologic aggressiveness of ARMS.

Detection of Rhabdomyosarcoma in Sites Other Than Primary Tumor

Molecular markers in conjunction with high-sensitivity detection methodologies have been applied to screen for RMS dissemination in accessible and commonly involved sites such as bone marrow, peripheral blood, and lymph nodes (Table 59-4). In general, these approaches screen for molecular markers within cells to identify cases that are not detected by conventional radiology or pathologic examination. One strategy for minimal disseminated disease detection focuses on tumor-specific markers, such as PAX3-FOXO1 and PAX7-FOXO1.[87,104] A second strategy, which is broadly applicable to all RMS subtypes, assays lineage-specific markers, such as myogenic markers of determination and differentiation (including MYOD1 and MYOG).[104-106] In a third strategy, sites of disease spread were assayed for proteins involved in metastatic pathways, such as CXCR4 and MET.[107] RT-PCR assays were developed to detect several of these markers and demonstrate analytical sensitivity in the range of one positive cell per 10^4 to 10^5 normal cells.[87,104,105] More recent PCR protocols use real-time technology to quantify the extent of disseminated disease and can thus monitor changes in disease load over time and compare results to an empirically determined clinical threshold. In addition to PCR assays, antibodies have been used to

TABLE 59-4   Assays for Detecting RMS in Sites Away from Primary Tumor

Marker	Molecule	Target	Assay
ACHRA	mRNA	Tumor cells	RT-PCR
ACHRG	mRNA	Tumor cells	RT-PCR
PAX3/PAX7-FOXO1	mRNA	Tumor cells	RT-PCR
MYOD1	mRNA protein	Tumor cells	RT-PCR Immunocytology
MYOG	mRNA protein	Tumor cells	RT-PCR Immunocytology
CXCR4	Protein	Tumor cells	Immunocytology
MET	Protein	Tumor cells	Immunocytology
CD45/CD56	Protein	Tumor cells	Flow cytometry
miR-206	miRNA	Plasma/serum	RT-PCR
IGFBP2	Protein	Plasma/serum	ELISA
VEGF-A	Protein	Plasma/serum	ELISA

ELISA, Enzyme-linked immunosorbent assay; *mRNA*, messenger ribonucleic acid; *RT-PCT*, reverse-transcriptase polymerase chain reaction assay.

detect various protein markers in immunocytochemical or flow cytometry assays.[106,107] These assays also have a high level of analytical sensitivity ($\sim 10^{-4}$), which is significantly better than conventional morphology-based evaluation.

These minimal disseminated disease assays were applied to clinical material from RMS patients in several different settings (see Table 59-4). Multiple studies addressed the feasibility of detecting occult disease in bone marrow.[87,104,105] These studies showed that histologically positive bone marrows are consistently detected, regardless of the methodology or marker. For histologically negative marrows, various methodologies and markers detected submicroscopic disease, with the frequency tending to be higher for ARMS relative to ERMS. In ARMS, which often metastasizes to the bone marrow, the frequency of a positive result in a histologically negative marrow ranges from 15% to 60%. In ERMS, in which bone marrow is not a common site of metastasis, the frequency of a positive result in a histologically negative marrow ranges from 7% to 33%. The presence of these marrow-infiltrating RMS cells is not consistently associated with subsequent overt marrow involvement, suggesting that the marrow can act as a transitory reservoir for disseminated RMS cells.[107] Despite this finding, a significant association was found between poor outcome and detection of RMS cells in bone marrow; marrow involvement was associated with a significantly higher risk for recurrence (50% vs. 11%, $P = .011$) and poorer OS rate (47% vs. 92%, $P = .01$).[106] In addition to bone marrow, studies also evaluated peripheral blood samples at diagnosis, during treatment, and after treatment.[105,108] Comparison with outcome revealed that a positive result at the end of treatment was associated with poor outcome,

and persistent positive results preceded a metastatic relapse.

Recent studies also examined expression of molecular markers in the serum or plasma. These markers include miR-206 and other muscle-specific miRNAs (see section below on microRNAs), which were measured by RT-PCR, and RMS-associated proteins, such as insulin-like growth factor–binding protein 2 (IGFBP2) and vascular endothelial growth factor (VEGF)- A (VEGF-A), which were assessed by enzyme-linked immunosorbent assay (ELISA).[109-111] The finding of higher abundance of these markers in the plasma or serum of RMS patients relative to normal controls indicates a possible use in noninvasive diagnosis. Furthermore, an application in disease monitoring is suggested by the finding of decreased levels after treatment. Finally, an association of plasma IGFBP2 levels with metastatic RMS suggests a potential role in patient stratification for risk-based therapy.

MOLECULAR AND CELLULAR BIOLOGY OF RHABDOMYOSARCOMA

Myogenic Pathways in the Tumorigenesis of Rhabdomyosarcoma

Based on the premise that RMS is related to the skeletal muscle lineage, the expression pattern of muscle-specific proteins has been extensively examined in RMS. In particular, many studies have focused on the family of myogenic transcription factors (MyoD, Myf5, myogenin, and MRF4) that are responsible in part for the determination of stem cells into myoblasts and then differentiation into myocytes. Assays of the corresponding genes detected RNA expression of *MYOD* and *MYF6* in all ARMS and ERMS tumors and RNA expression of *MYOG* (myogenin) and *MYF5* in all ARMS and most ERMS tumors.[112] Antibodies directed to MyoD and myogenin have proved to be suitable for immunohistochemistry on paraffin-embedded, formalin-fixed tissues.[113] With the use of these antibodies the vast majority of RMS cases (about 97% in a study of 956 cases) showed positive nuclear immunostaining for each protein.[2] Because positive staining also occurred in multiple cases of pleuropulmonary blastoma, the specificity of these reagents was estimated to be between 90% and 91%. There are differences between ARMS and ERMS tumors in the myogenin staining patterns such that most cells within an ARMS tumor stain positive, whereas fewer cells within an ERMS tumor stain positive. This differential staining between ARMS and ERMS has also been shown for MyoD. There is a statistical difference in the extent of MyoD or myogenin expression among the RMS subtypes, but there is still overlap. Hence the immunohistochemical pattern of these myogenic proteins is not sufficient to classify cases but may be helpful in selecting cases for further testing.

Functional studies in RMS cell lines determined that MyoD is not an active transcription factor in the RMS environment (Fig. 59-4).[114] In particular, although MyoD is able to bind DNA at its specific binding sites in RMS cells it is not capable of acting as a transcriptional activator on model genes with these DNA-binding sites. These

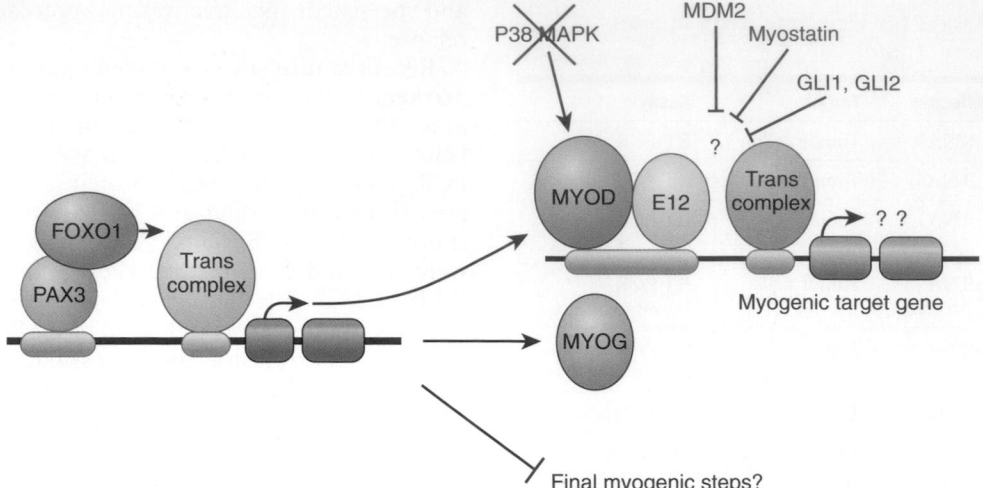

Figure 59-4 Influences on myogenic differentiation in ARMS. A model *PAX3-FOXO1* target gene is shown on the left, with PAX3-FOXO1 binding to a positive acting *cis*-element and interacting with the transcriptional machinery at the promoter to upregulate transcription of mRNA and ultimately increase production of the target protein. Two such targets are postulated to be MYOD and myogenin (MYOG). In turn, MYOD and its binding partner E12 bind to *cis*-elements of myogenic target genes and stimulate the transcriptional machinery to upregulate transcription of the corresponding mRNAs. In alveolar rhabdomyosarcoma (and embryonal rhabdomyosarcoma), various upstream changes can influence the transcriptional activity of the MYOD protein and thereby inhibit myogenic differentiation.

effects may contribute to the failure of RMS cells to undergo terminal differentiation. Various factors may contribute to this inhibition of transcriptional activation by MyoD. Experiments fusing RMS cell lines to a second normal cell line resulted in some instances in which the transcriptional activation block was overcome, suggesting that the RMS line was deficient in a *trans*-acting factor. In other instances, the block was not overcome by this cell fusion, suggesting a dominant-acting inhibitory factor. As an example of the former recessive scenario, the p38 mitogen-activated protein kinase (MAPK) pathway is deficient in some RMS cell lines, resulting in the absence of an essential activator of MyoD during myogenic differentiation.[115] Examples of the latter dominant scenario include amplification of *MDM2* in an RMS cell line that inhibited MyoD activity by a mechanism involving competition for the transcription factor Sp1[116,117] and upregulation of musculin and a novel splice variant of E2A that inhibited MyoD activity by competing for heterodimer formation and preventing formation of functional MyoD:E-protein heterodimers, required for the switch to differentiation.[118] In addition, increased expression of the negative muscle growth regulator myostatin, which is found in both ERMS and ARMS, is also capable of inhibiting MyoD-mediated transcriptional activity, possibly via Smad3 interactions.[119] In RMS associated with activation of the Hedgehog pathway, expression of the transcription factor GLI1 or GLI2 inhibits MyoD-mediated transcriptional activation by reducing heterodimerization with its partner E12 and DNA binding.[120] Finally, as discussed in the later section "Epigenetic Regulation," MyoD activity can also be inhibited by decreased expression associated with KMT1A methyltransferase activity.[121]

The identification of *PAX3-FOXO1* and *PAX7-FOXO1* gene fusions in ARMS also highlight PAX3 and

PAX7 as important proteins in normal and aberrant myogenic transcriptional control. In murine systems, both Pax3 and Pax7 are involved in early embryonic development of cells giving rise to axial musculature, and Pax3 also has a necessary role in the early embryonic development of the limb musculature.[122-124] In the adult mouse, Pax7 has an important role in the development of the major population of myogenic satellite cells and Pax3 is expressed in satellite cells in a subset of muscles.[125,126] This developmental biology of *PAX3* and *PAX7* is relevant to ARMS tumors, which express *PAX3* or *PAX7* as a fusion with *FOXO1*,[127] and to ERMS tumors, which express wild-type *PAX3*, *PAX7*, or both.[128]

The wild-type and fusion PAX proteins can variably affect the myogenic status of the cells expressing them. When wild-type Pax3 is introduced into explanted embryonic tissues, it can activate the myogenic program as shown by expression of MyoD, Myf5, and myogenin as well as myogenic differentiation products.[129] In contrast, Pax3 could not induce this myogenic program in NIH 3T3 murine fibroblasts, suggesting that this murine fibroblast represents a less permissive environment.[130] Studies of the PAX3-FOXO1 fusion protein have demonstrated a range of activities on the myogenic program (see Fig. 59-4). First, studies focusing on the *MyoD* and *myogenin* promoters provide evidence that both of these genes are transcriptional targets of PAX3-FOXO1. Of two studies of NIH 3T3 cells, one indicated that PAX3-FOXO1 induced the myogenic program, including the upstream products MyoD, myogenin, Six1, and Slug as well as downstream myogenic products, such as troponins and myosin light chain.[130] However, a second study of NIH 3T3 cells demonstrated induction of the upstream products MyoD, myogenin, and desmin but no induction of the downstream product myosin heavy chain.[131] In contrast to these findings, transduction of *PAX3-FOXO1* into two additional murine fibroblast lines (10T1/2 and Plus) resulted in expression of both upstream and downstream myogenic products and fusion into multinucleated myotubes. In contrast, introduction of PAX3 or PAX3-FOXO1 into two myogenic cell lines, C2C12 myoblasts and MyoD-expressing 10T1/2 cells, inhibited terminal myogenic differentiation after stimulation of differentiation by growth factor withdrawal.[132] PAX3-FOXO1 was more potent than wild-type PAX3 in this phenotypic activity. Finally, repression of PAX3-FOXO1 expression in human ARMS cell lines with RNA interference (small interfering RNA [siRNA] or short hairpin RNA [shRNA] constructs) results in decreased proliferation without apparent apoptosis, decreased motility and invasion, and increased differentiation as demonstrated by morphologic and myogenic gene and protein expression.[101,133,134] This finding indicates that PAX3-FOXO1 normally represses expression of this myogenic pathway in this cell type.

The finding of both stimulatory and inhibitory effects of PAX proteins on myogenic events may be explained by the hypothesis that these wild-type or fusion PAX proteins facilitate entry into the myogenic pathway and variably inhibit the final steps of the pathway depending on the cellular environment. In support of this hypothesis, data suggest that PAX3-FOXO1, by inducing MyoD expression but attenuating its activity, and inducing FGFR expression to block differentiation, simultaneously stimulates but blocks completion of myogenesis.[135] This intermediate commitment to differentiation may be partially explained by recent studies in which expression of PAX3-FOXO1 in muscle satellite cells did not inhibit expression of MyoD but did inhibit expression of MyoD target genes.[136]

MicroRNAs

Although decades of study shed light on the intrinsic cellular signaling pathways and extrinsic microenvironmental stimuli that control skeletal muscle differentiation during embryogenesis, postnatal life, and muscle repair, it was not until 2005 that another layer of control was identified. In work examining the spatiotemporal control of cardiogenesis, it was discovered that specific microRNAs were expressed in cardiac and skeletal muscle and served to balance proliferation and differentiation of muscle precursor cells.[137] Since that time, a great deal of information on these small noncoding RNAs that enable the regulation of protein dosage through binding to 3′ ends of mRNA and affecting stability or translation to protein has been gathered and understood not only in the framework of normal skeletal myogenesis but also in tumors related to the skeletal muscle lineage such as RMS.

MicroRNAs influencing skeletal myogenesis can generally be divided into myomirs (miRs specific to skeletal and cardiac muscle) and nonmyomirs (miRs expressed in nonmuscle tissue but that can also be found in muscle.) The myomirs (nomenclature miR-1 to miR-206, which includes the miR-133 group) are encoded in bicistronic clusters on chromosomes 6, 18, and 20 and control such diverse developmental processes as somite organization, muscle precursor cell migration, survival, differentiation,

fusion, and cross talk with epigenetic processes that control differentiation (see next section). Similar to other human cancers, RMS tumors are noted to have lost expression of miRs and their tumor suppressive properties. When miR-206 is expressed in human RMS cells, xenograft growth is halted and accompanied by differentiation,[138] presumably by the orchestrated downregulation of hundreds of miR-206 target genes,[139] including MET.[138] Mir-206 expression levels also correlate with clinical behavior of RMS.[140] Regarding the nonmyomirs, the reader is referred to two reviews on microRNAs and their role in RMS.[141,142] For example, miR-185 suppresses RMS tumor growth and progression by targeting the Six1 oncogene[143] (see later discussion under "Metastatic Pathways in Rhabdomyosarcoma").

Finally, as was discussed in the section on "Rhabdomyosarcoma in Cancer Predisposition Syndromes," germline or somatic mutations of DICER1, the enzyme that cleaves pre-microRNA to mature microRNA, have been found associated with ERMS.[80,144,145] To date these mutations appear to be in the RNase IIIb domain, resulting in a decrease in its activity.

Epigenetic Regulation

Although the block to myogenic differentiation in RMS cells has been apparent for decades, only recently is there insight into some of the epigenetic changes enforcing this inhibition. As mentioned earlier, whereas the muscle-specific transcription factor MyoD can bind DNA in RMS, some targets fail to activate. For example, although MyoD binds similarly at the genome-wide level in both normal and RMS (in this case the human embryonal RMS cell line RD was studied), in RMS there is a subset of genes to which MyoD binds poorly and thus does not activate.[146] This subset includes the transcription factors MEF2C, RUNX1, JDP2, and NFIC, found expressed at lower levels in RMS compared with normal muscle cells. There was also differential DNA accessibility, including changes in DNA methylation status. Therefore it has become clear that epigenetic changes contribute as much to RMS as changes in the DNA sequence itself. Below are summarized some of the epigenetic changes found in RMS, including changes in DNA methylation (introduced earlier in "Hypermethylation as an Alternative Mechanism of Gene Inactivation in Rhabdomyosarcoma"), changes in histone methylation, and changes in nucleosome positioning.

Methylation of gene promoters at CpG islands by DNA-specific methyltransferases serves to silence expression of target genes. Thus it would follow that tumors should demonstrate different DNA methylation profiles compared with nonmalignant tissue, and indeed a study of the genomes of RMS compared with normal skeletal muscle showed this to be the case.[147] In both ERMS and ARMS, genes involved in development and differentiation were hypermethylated compared with normal skeletal muscle. However, there were also differences between ERMS and ARMS, with ARMS showing more hypermethylation of Polycomb target genes (see later.) As methods to improve the speed and resolution of the detection of DNA methylation patterns improve, further changes are expected to be identified.

Methylation of lysine residues in histones by Polycomb group remodeling complexes (known as PRC1 and PRC2) also serves to silence chromatin, by influencing nucleosome formation and function. Although this process occurs in a carefully controlled manner during development, if Polycomb complexes are inappropriately recruited to target genes or inappropriately activated due to component mutation, impaired commitment to cell lineage or a frank block in differentiation can ensue, resulting in a primitive cellular phenotype. For example, in both ERMS and ARMS the NF-κB-YY1-mir-29 regulatory circuit that ordinarily controls skeletal myogenesis is usurped; YY1 recruits PRC2 to silence target genes including *MIR29*, so that muscle differentiation cannot occur.[148] In ARMS, PAX3-FOXO1 transcriptionally activates JARID2 expression, which recruits PRC2 to the promoter regions of target genes including *MYOG* and *MYL1*, again impairing differentiation.[149] Recently, there has been some focus on the catalytic component of PRC2 known as the EZH2 methyltransferase. EZH2 was found upregulated at the protein level in RMS tumors[150]; and in loss-of-function studies in RD cells, silencing of EZH2-induced MyoD activation and partial reversal of the tumorigenic phenotype.[151]

There are also methyltransferases independent of Polycomb group remodeling complexes that appear dysregulated in RMS. For example, the histone methyltransferase KMT1A (formerly known as Suv39h1), which methylates histone H3 on the lysine 9 residue, represses myogenic gene expression directed by MyoD.[152] In ARMS this keeps the cells in an undifferentiated state. In support of its presumed oncogenic role, suppression of KMT1A by siRNA decreases ARMS cell and xenograft growth.[121] In independent studies, a screen for tumor suppressors in a Kras- driven model of zebrafish ERMS revealed that point mutations in KMT1A suppress RMS formation.[153]

Regarding the epigenetic changes that occur in response to nucleosome repositioning, components of the SWI/SNF chromatin remodeling tumor suppressor complex have been found mutated in RMS. An early hint of the involvement of the SWI/SNF complex was in the study of TPA-mediated differentiation of RD cells, which was shown to work by recruiting proteins including BRG1 (a subunit of SWI-SNF) to the myogenin promoter,[154] driving differentiation. Later work showed that the BAF53a subunit of SWI/SNF is not downregulated in RMS and thus contributes to a differentiation block.[155]

Role of Insulin-like Growth Factors in Rhabdomyosarcoma

Insulin-like growth factor 2 (IGF-2) is an important growth factor during the fetal period and is highly expressed in fetal skeletal muscle but not detectably expressed in adult skeletal muscle.[156] High-level IGF-2 expression in murine myoblasts results in an increased proliferative rate, impaired myogenic differentiation, and anchorage independence, indicating a potential role of IGF-2 in neoplasia of the myogenic lineage.[157] In accord with these findings, IGF-2 is highly expressed by both ERMS and ARMS tumors as well as in derived RMS cell

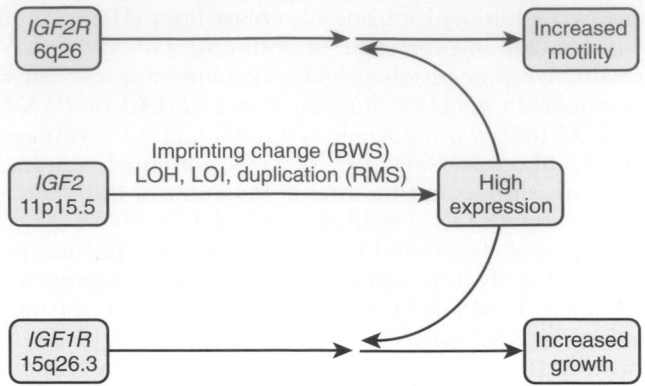

Figure 59-5 Changes in IGF pathway and associated phenotypic consequences in RMS. The three involved genes and their chromosomal locations are shown on the *left*. Genetic or epigenetic changes are indicated above the *horizontal arrows*. Changes in expression or phenotype are indicated on the *right*. *BWS*, Beckwith-Wiedemann syndrome; *LOH*, loss of heterozygosity; *LOI*, loss of imprinting.

lines[158] (Fig. 59-5). In addition to the growth factor, both RMS subtypes express the IGF-1 receptor (IGF-1R), which is a cell surface receptor for IGF-2 as well as IGF-1. This simultaneous expression of growth factor and receptor creates an autocrine loop that stimulates the growth and motility of RMS cells. No mutations have been detected in these genes; hence this autocrine situation may reflect the fetal muscle expression pattern that is maintained or induced by the other genetic alterations. The growth response is mediated through IGF-1R, whereas the motility response is mediated through the distinct IGF-2/mannose-6-phosphate receptor.[159] Numerous studies have explored different strategies for interfering with the action of IGF-1R. These strategies include an antibody directed to this receptor, a kinase-deficient mutant that acts as a dominant negative, and an antisense construct directed to this receptor.[160-162] Each of these strategies decreases the response of the cells to IGF-2 stimulation, inhibits cell growth and anchorage independence in culture, and inhibits tumorigenicity in vivo. Exploitation of this downregulation for preclinical and clinical studies is described in "Preclinical Investigation of Emerging Drug Targets for Rhabdomyosarcoma" and "Clinical Research in Rhabdomyosarcoma".

As described earlier, the *IGF2* gene is located in the 11p15.5 chromosomal region, which is implicated in allelic loss events that occur in RMS tumors and in genetic alterations in the inherited disorder BWS, which predisposes to malignant tumors, including RMS.[49,52,53] The *IGF2* gene is part of an imprinted region and is preferentially expressed from the paternally inherited alleles. The result of the allelic loss events and genetic changes in BWS is loss of the nonexpressed maternal allele and maintenance or gain of the expressed paternal allele. In addition to these genetic changes, other alterations of 11p15 involving the *IGF2* locus have been identified in both ARMS and ERMS tumors. In one study of 11 RMS tumors (including 4 ARMS tumors, 6 ERMS tumors, and 1 RMS tumor of uncertain classification), 1 ARMS and 3 ERMS cases demonstrated evidence of duplication of an *IGF2* allele.[163] Furthermore, although *IGF2* is normally expressed from only one allele, loss of imprinting can occur and result in a biallelic expression pattern. In RMS, loss of imprinting at the *IGF2* locus has been observed in 5 of 12 ERMS and 9 of 16 ARMS cases.[163-165] These duplication or imprinting changes increase the number of active *IGF2* alleles and may thereby contribute to the high expression of *IGF2* mRNA and protein found in RMS tumors.

In mammalian cells, the subcellular localization of the wild-type FOXO1 (previously FKHR) and related FOXO3 and FOXO4 proteins is regulated by a PI3K-AKT (PKB-dependent) signaling pathway that is activated by survival- and growth-related signals such as IGF-2.[166] In this signaling pathway, AKT-mediated phosphorylation of FOXO proteins leads to protein transfer from the nucleus to the cytoplasm and thus inactivates transcriptional function. Of the three AKT phosphorylation sites in FOXO1, two are retained in PAX3-FOXO1 and PAX7-FOXO1. If the fusion proteins are regulated by this pathway, the high level of IGF-2 in ARMS cells would cause these proteins to be phosphorylated and sequestered in the cytoplasm. However, experiments show that PAX3-FOXO1 is retained in the nucleus and is transcriptionally active in cultured cells in the presence of active AKT and in ARMS cells.[167] All studies performed to date find that PAX3-FOXO1 is constitutively nuclear, even in the presence of activated AKT.[167,168] However, whereas one transfection study did not find any changes in PAX3-FOXO1 transcriptional activity in the presence of activated AKT, a more recent study of a murine model of ARMS found that AKT hyperactivation results in PAX3-FOXO1 phosphorylation and decreased transcriptional activity. Studies in human ARMS cells are needed to resolve these issues and discern whether AKT activation has any effect on PAX3-FOXO1 function.

Modulation of Growth and Apoptotic Pathways by Fusion Oncoproteins

Gene transfer experiments have investigated specific functions of the PAX3-FOXO1 and PAX7-FOXO1 fusion proteins and suggest that these proteins exert an oncogenic effect through multiple pathways. In initial studies of growth control, transduction of PAX3-FOXO1 into murine NIH 3T3 or chicken embryo fibroblasts resulted in transforming activity, whereas wild-type Pax3 did not transform these cells.[169,170] In a complementary study, a protein consisting of the N-terminal region of PAX3 fused to the KRAB transcriptional repression domain reverted the transforming activity of ARMS cells in culture and suppressed tumor formation of ARMS cells in mice.[171] In mutagenesis analyses, the homeodomain but not the paired box is needed by PAX3-FOXO1 for transformation; thus target genes with paired box binding sites may not be required for cellular transformation. In addition, transforming activity is activated when the VP16 activation domain is substituted for the C-terminal domain of PAX3, suggesting that other activation domains can mimic the effect of the C-terminal FOXO1 domain.[172]

More recent studies indicate that there is an antagonistic balance between transforming activity and growth-suppressive or toxic activity in many cell types in which PAX3-FOXO1 is expressed.[173,174] Transforming activity is optimally exerted at low expression levels of exogenous fusion protein. In contrast, at higher expression levels, comparable to the levels in human ARMS tumors, PAX3-FOXO1 causes cell death or growth suppression in various nontransformed cell lines. Therefore human ARMS cells can tolerate these high "physiologic" expression levels, whereas the non-ARMS cells do not tolerate these higher levels. The hypothesis proposed is that additional genetic alterations are necessary in ARMS to attenuate the toxic and growth-suppressive effects of the fusion protein. One such event may be inactivation of the *CDKN2A* tumor suppressor gene that collaborates with PAX3-FOXO1 to permit primary human skeletal muscle cell precursors to bypass the senescent growth arrest checkpoint.[175] It is noteworthy that mutation studies show that the growth suppressive and toxic activity is at least partly dependent on an intact paired box but does not require an intact homeodomain.[173] These findings suggest that there may be two separate sets of target genes mediating the transforming and toxic phenotypes as a result of the complex function of the PAX3-FOXO1 DNA-binding domain.

Despite the ability of PAX3-FOXO1 to induce toxic effects when introduced into many cultured cells, an important function of the PAX3-FOXO1 oncoprotein in ARMS cells is maintenance of cell viability by inhibiting apoptosis. Treatment of ARMS cells with either an antisense oligonucleotide directed against the *PAX3* translational start site or with siRNAs directed against the 5′ *PAX3* region resulted in a decrease in PAX3-FOXO1 protein expression.[101] This expression change was associated with a significant decrease in cell number as well as with morphologic and biochemical characteristics of apoptosis. Similarly, expression of a tamoxifen-inducible PAX3-KRAB construct in ARMS cells demonstrated evidence of apoptosis when induced in low serum conditions or tumor xenografts.[176] One downstream transcriptional target of PAX3-FOXO1 that at least partially mediates this apoptotic function is the gene that encodes the transcription factor TFAP2B.[101] The functional role of TFAP2B is indicated by the induction of apoptosis in ARMS cells when this gene is downregulated by siRNA and by the prevention of apoptosis mediated by siRNA directed against the 5′ *PAX3* region when a construct constitutively expressing TFAP2B is introduced into ARMS cells.

Metastatic Pathways in Rhabdomyosarcoma

Early studies of RMS metastasis examined subclones of the RD ERMS cell line. The metastatic capacity of different subclones did not correlate with the tumorigenic or proliferative capability of the subclones.[177] After exposure to conditions that stimulate myogenic differentiation, some subclones showed increased differentiation manifested by an increased fraction of myosin-positive cells.[178] Although proliferative capability did not correlate with this in vitro differentiation, the metastatic efficiency was reduced in subclones demonstrating differentiation.

Additional studies with the RD line showed that its metastatic efficiency is affected by alterations of cell surface molecules. In the case of the cell surface glyco-protein NCAM (neural cell adhesion molecule), this protein is posttranslationally modified by the addition of polysialic acid on its extracellular domain.[179] When the enzyme endoneuraminidase-N was injected intraperito-neally to cleave the polysialic acid from the surface of intraperitoneally implanted RD cells, there was a decrease in the frequency of lung and liver metastases. When the integrin VLA-2 ($\alpha2\beta1$) that is not normally expressed by RD cells was introduced into these cells, there was increased adhesion to collagen and laminin in vitro and more metastatic foci in mice after either intravenous or subcutaneous injection.[180]

Among the various RMS subtypes, there are differences in matrix metalloproteinase (MMP) expression that may contribute to differences in metastatic behavior. Immunohistochemical analysis of 5 MMPs in 33 RMS cases found higher expression of MMP1, MMP2, and MMP9 in ARMS than in ERMS cases.[181] After confirming the higher MMP2 expression in ARMS in a comparison of ARMS and ERMS cell lines, the high MMP2 expression was correlated with more invasive behavior in the ARMS cell lines.[182] In a human RMS cell line with spontaneous metastatic progression, there was upregulation of MMPs and downregulation of tissue inhibitors of metalloproteinases.[183] Finally, attachment of RMS cells to fibronectin results in increased MMP2 expression and in vitro invasive behavior along with increases in COX-2 expression and prostaglandin E_2 production.[184] Treatment with exogenous prostaglandin E_2 can recapitulate this effect and increase MMP2 expression at the level of the MMP2 promoter. In contrast, treatment of cells with COX-2 inhibitors can reverse the fibronectin effects on

MMP expression and invasive behavior. Another soluble factor released by RMS cells is heparanase, which is found upregulated in several human RMS cell lines. Heparanase cleaves heparan sulfates, thus releasing and likely making more bioactive heparan-bound growth factors. shRNA-mediated suppression of heparanase in RD and Rh30 cells (a commonly studied human ARMS cell line) inhibited their invasive properties as assessed by Matrigel invasion assays. Parallel studies examining heparanase mRNA expression in human tumor samples and human serum in order to validate the upregulation were suggestive but not statistically significant because total numbers were small and error bars wide, thus suggesting that further studies will be required.[185]

Three cell surface receptors, MET, CXCR4, and LIFR, are expressed in RMS and function in signaling pathways that impact metastatic behavior[186-188] (Fig. 59-6). Although *MET* and *CXCR4* genes are downstream targets of the PAX3-FOXO1 fusion protein, all three genes are expressed in both ARMS and ERMS tumors. CXCR4 is a G-protein–coupled chemokine receptor whose ligand is stromal derived factor-1 (SDF1), whereas MET is a member of the tyrosine kinase family of receptors whose ligand is hepatocyte growth factor/scatter factor (HGF/SF). Finally, leukemia inhibitory factor (LIF) binds to a heterodimeric membrane receptor composed of the LIF-specific LIFR and the gp130 receptor chain, which is also used as the receptor for interleukin (IL)-6, oncostatin M, and several other cytokines. All three ligands are secreted by the bone marrow, an important site of ARMS metastasis. The CXCR4-SDF1 signaling pathway is involved in the homing of normal cells to hematopoietic sites, and the MET-HGF/SF signaling pathway is involved in the

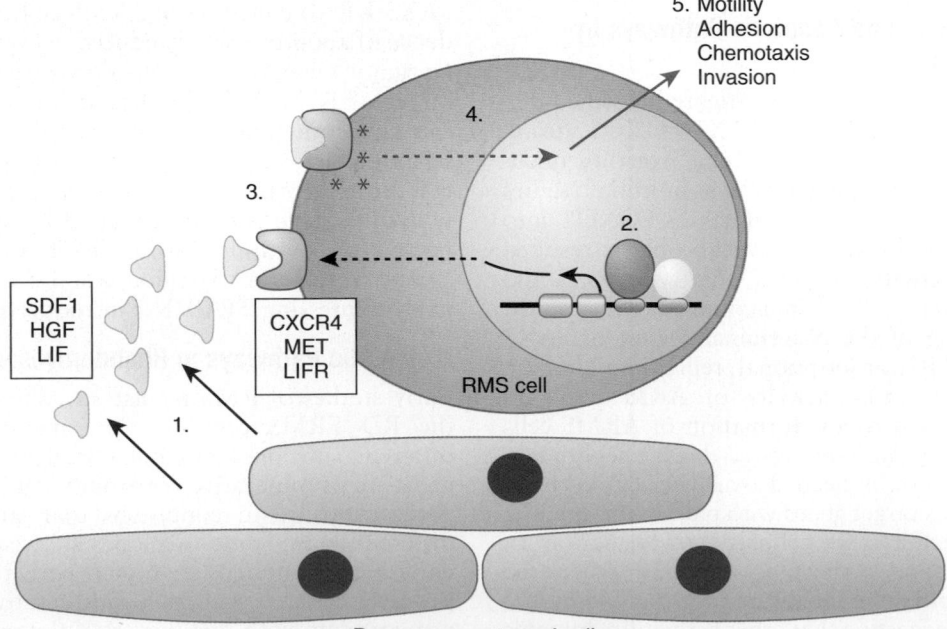

Figure 59-6 Role of secreted protein mediators in metastatic behavior of RMS cells. Bone marrow stromal cells secrete various protein mediators, including SDF1, HGF, and LIF (step 1). The RMS cells transcribe genes and then express cell surface receptors for these protein mediators (step 2). Binding of protein mediators to cognate receptors (step 3) activates various signaling pathways in the RMS cells (step 4). These signaling pathways ultimately modulate expression pathways in the nucleus that result in phenotypic changes (step 5).

proliferation and motility of various cell types. The LIF-LIFR signaling pathway has a variety of roles in multiple tissues, including proliferation of hematopoietic cells and muscle satellite cell production. For these reasons, usurpation of these signaling pathways has been proposed in the metastasis of various cancers.

Cell culture studies have explored the influence of CXCR4-SDF1, MET-HGF/SF, and LIFR-LIF signaling on the metastatic behavior of ARMS cells. SDF1, HGF, or LIF treatment of RMS cell lines induced cell culture changes in relevant properties, including motility, adhesion, chemotaxis, and invasion. In an in vivo experiment, more ARMS cells than ERMS cells are chemoattracted to and seed lethally irradiated bone marrow in association with the upregulation of HGF and SDF1 in irradiated bone marrow stroma. In addition, a selected ARMS subclone that preferentially responds to LIF demonstrates increased seeding of bone marrow, liver, and lymph nodes after intravenous injection and increased cells in bone marrow and lung 6 weeks after intramuscular injection. Recently, another receptor for SDF-1 called CXCR7 has been identified. This receptor binds not only SDF-1 but also interferon-inducible T-cell α chemoattractant (ITAC) chemokine. It is expressed in both ARMS and ERMS cells and appears to be independent from CXCR4, suggesting that CXCR4-SDF-1 axis targeting alone may not be enough.[189] Finally, as models of pathway-specific potential therapeutic strategies, a CXCR4-specific inhibitor blocked SDF1-directed adhesion and chemotaxis in ARMS cells, an siRNA directed against LIFR inhibited in vivo metastasis of ARMS cells, and suppression of MET receptor by shRNA in RMS cells decreased the migratory response in vitro.[190]

Recently, three additional cell surface receptors including IL-4 receptor-α (IL-4Rα), FGFR4 (discussed in "Oncogene and Tumor Suppressor Gene Mutations in Rhabdomyosarcoma"), and cannabinoid receptor 1 (CNR1) have been implicated in RMS metastasis. IL-4Rα is found upregulated in human and murine ARMS, and blockade by a neutralizing antibody inhibited both lymphatic and hematogenous metastasis in a genetically engineered murine model of ARMS.[191] Because there are neutralizing antibodies to IL-4R (and cognate ligands IL-4 and IL-13) in clinical use for nononcologic human diseases, this may be a feasible approach toward blocking RMS metastasis. FGFR4 gain of function (K535 and E550 tyrosine kinase domain) mutants enhanced the metastatic phenotype when expressed in both murine RMS cell lines and NIH 3T3 cells, as assessed by lung metastasis burden in xenograft assays.[75] Lastly, CNR1, which is also a PAX3-FOXO1 target, was shown to be dispensable for PAX3-FOXO1–driven cell proliferation and transformation but required for invasion and metastasis. In transformed primary mouse myoblasts expressing PAX3-FOXO1, either genetic or pharmacologic suppression of CNR1 reduced cell invasion in vitro and lung metastasis in vivo.[192]

Studies of a murine metastatic RMS model system elucidated an important pathway involving the *Vil2* (encoding Ezrin) and *Six1* genes. In this model system, RMS tumors developed in transgenic mice that were deficient in *CDKN2A (Ink4/Arf)* and overexpressed *HGF/SF*.[193] In a comparison of gene expression profiles of highly and poorly metastatic cell lines derived from this system, 44 differentially expressed genes were identified (28 overexpressed and 16 underexpressed in highly metastatic cells), including the overexpressed genes *Vil2* and *Six1*.[194] Ezrin is an adhesion molecule and member of the ERM family that promotes cytoskeletal reorganization in pathways linked to survival, motility, invasion, and adherence. Six1 is a homeodomain-containing transcription factor involved in the development of several lineages, is a downstream target of PAX3-FOXO1 in NIH 3T3 cells, and is expressed by ARMS cells.[130] Furthermore, the gene encoding Ezrin is a direct transcriptional target of Six1.[195] These gene expression relationships were confirmed by RMS tumor studies in which both genes were generally expressed at higher levels in fusion-positive RMS tumors than in fusion-negative RMS tumors.

Expression of *Vil2* and *Six1* in RMS tumors was correlated with clinical stage, which is consistent with a role in tumor progression and metastatic behavior.[194] There is direct proof of this role: transfer of either gene into low metastatic RMS lines from the HGF transgenic system caused increased metastatic activity. Similarly, when expression of either protein was suppressed by shRNA or repressed by a dominant-negative inhibitor, metastatic activity in the highly metastatic lines decreased. Finally, Ezrin is needed for Six1 to exert its metastatic function, thus further confirming that Ezrin acts downstream of Six1.[195] These studies provide the framework of a pathway that leads from the fusion proteins to Six1 to Ezrin to metastatic activity.

There are surely additional genes and proteins supporting the metastatic phenotype in RMS, and to this end a European collaborative group evaluated in RMS the expression of genes known to support metastasis using an Affymetrix approach.[196] After examining 19 primary human RMS tumor samples, they focused on two genes known as *LMO4* and *FOFOXF1*. Although they did not evaluate for expression of the protein products of these genes in RMS samples, they did assess their role in metastasis by showing that siRNA suppression of these genes in RD and Rh30 cells decreased migration as assessed by Matrigel invasion.

PRECLINICAL INVESTIGATION OF EMERGING DRUG TARGETS FOR RHABDOMYOSARCOMA

Preclinical Models to Study Rhabdomyosarcoma Tumorigenesis

Human Tumor Cell Xenografts in Immunodeficient Mice

Although the identification of mutations and/or dysregulated signaling in RMS is accelerating, the value of these entities as therapeutic targets must be evaluated in preclinical models before application in humans. The original models to study cancer treatments other than in cell lines were xenograft models, in which human cell lines were injected as xenografts into immunocompromised mice. Historically for RMS this began at St. Jude's Research Children's Hospital in the 1980s and has evolved into the Pediatric Preclinical Testing Program (http://pptp.nchresearch.org/). This program is a large-scale effort to systematically evaluate new agents against a panel of human RMS and other pediatric cancer cell lines by testing novel drugs against not only classic oncogene and tumor suppressor pathways including TP53 and receptor tyrosine kinases (RTKs) but also against newly identified targets found dysregulated in childhood cancer. Recently, the feasibility of adding radiation therapy to the Pediatric Preclinical Testing Program was demonstrated, using RMS as a pilot.[197]

There are obvious advantages to examining the efficacy of novel agents against pediatric tumor cell lines, including that they are of human origin and have been validated in prior biologic studies. But there are disadvantages as well, including that many cell lines have been passaged in culture for decades, acquiring genetic changes not representative of the original tumor. There is also the practical problem of cell line annotation[198]; however, with the development of methods to fingerprint cell lines, identification has been more reliable. Finally, the intrinsic property that enables evaluation of human cell lines in a whole murine organism— their immunodeficient state—does not permit the evaluation of the role of the immune system in tumorigenesis, a problem that can be overcome by the use of genetically engineered mouse models.

Genetically Engineered Murine Models of RMS

With the advent of genetic manipulation of the murine genome, it is now possible to examine the genesis and pathophysiology of RMS at the organism level. Indeed there are more than two dozen genetically engineered murine models that give rise to RMS. The earliest models were serendipitously discovered, for example that ERMS occurs in TP53 knockout mice or SV40 transgenic mice. Later models were deliberate in their design and incorporated genetic lesions found in RMS, including overexpression of the cMET signaling pathway or PAX3-FOXO1 fusion gene. These and others are reviewed elsewhere.[199] More recently, sophisticated models have emerged in which Cre-Lox (or Flp-Frt) recombinase technology has been harnessed to turn on or turn off expression of specific genes or negative regulatory components such as shRNAs. This has been especially useful in examining the cells of origin of RMS, which may range from an undifferentiated mesenchymal stem cell to the myonucleus of a differentiated myofiber.[200] These approaches have led to some surprising discoveries, such as the finding that RMS can arise from the adipocyte lineage[201] and that ERMS is on a continuum with a common adult sarcoma known as undifferentiated pleomorphic sarcoma.[202] Last, these genetically engineered mouse models have also been useful as additional models for preclinical studies, such as the PAX3-FOXO1–based ARMS model.[203]

Lower Eukaryote Models of RMS

Although murine models have been the mainstay of modeling human cancer including RMS, lower organisms including zebrafish (Danio rerio) and the fruitfly (Drosophila melanogaster) are more amenable to genetic manipulation

and screening and contribute a unique understanding of RMS genesis and metastasis. For example, zebrafish models of ERMS[204] have been useful for in vivo imaging of tumor-propagating cells and their properties[205] and understanding the impact of oncogenic RAS expression at different stages of muscle development.[206] Drosophila models of ARMS have provided insight into the pathophysiology of PAX-FOXO1 fusion genes[207] and the role of defective myoblast fusion in RMS.[208]

A comprehensive listing of RMS animal models and their utility is available.[199] Along with the xenograft and genetically engineered mouse models, these models have enabled testing of pharmacologic agents in a preclinical fashion before to moving to phase I clinical trials. Below are listed some examples of agents that have been tested in a variety of in vivo preclinical models.

Inhibitors of Receptor Tyrosine Kinases

RTKs are embedded in the cellular plasma membrane and transmit signals from the environment to the cell interior. When a ligand binds to an RTK, dimerization occurs and this leads to internal phosphorylation events and signaling through a variety of canonical intracellular signaling pathways such as AKT, MAPK, mammalian target of rapamycin (mTOR), and many others. Because RTKs are at the cell surface, they can be blocked with interfering antibodies (or their ligands can be inhibited with neutralizing antibodies). Given the expansion in our understanding of the RTKs that are dysregulated or upregulated in RMS,[209] there are several monoclonal antibodies that have been evaluated in RMS. The prototype was a monoclonal targeting IGFR-1, known as figitumumab (previously CP-751871).[210] This agent not only blocked binding of ligand to the IGFR-1 but also downregulated the receptor, suppressed signaling to AKT, inhibited tumor-derived VEGF, and synergized with rapamycin. Several other studies followed, including testing of other anti–IGFR-1 monoclonal antibodies,[211,212] some of which advanced to clinical trials. However, tumor cells were able to activate bypass routes, rendering resistance to IGFR-1 blockade. Bevacizumab, a monoclonal antibody to VEGF, has been evaluated in a phase II clinical trial for RMS (see "Clinical Research in Rhabdomyosarcoma"). Still in development and preclinical testing are monoclonal antibodies to FGFR4[213] and NCAM,[214] both upregulated in a significant percentage of RMS tumors and implicated in RMS metastasis (see "Metastatic Pathways in Rhabdomyosarcoma"). Other new agents are also being considered for RMS.[215]

Given their enzymatic activity, RTKs can also be inhibited with small molecules. In a manner similar to the prototype small molecule imatinib, which was developed to inhibit the BCR-ABL fusion protein in chronic myelogenous leukemia,[216] there are also small molecule inhibitors being evaluated for RMS-associated RTKs. An early example was BMS-754807, an oral small molecule inhibitor of IGFR-1,[217] which showed intermediate efficacy in RMS. Later examples include sunitinib, cediranib, and pazopanib, which are small molecules that inhibit the kinase activities of platelet-derived growth factor receptor (PDGFR) and other RTKs, VEGF receptors 1 to

3 (VEGFR1 to VEGFR3), and VEGFR1 to VEGFR3 and other RTKs, respectively.[209] Given the known resistance that emerges with RTK monotherapy, these small molecules are now being tested in conjunction with traditional chemotherapeutic agents. For example, pazopanib has been tested in combination with topotecan, and in Rh30 xenografts this combination inhibits tumorigenesis.[218] Indeed, this has supported the incorporation of pazopanib into human clinical trials (see "Clinical Research in Rhabdomyosarcoma"). Whereas the upregulation of a specific RTK in RMS warrants investigation of that RTK as a drug target, not all RTK inhibitors have efficacy. For example, although EGFR is found upregulated in some RMS tumors, erlotinib (an EGFR inhibitor) had no effect on blocking tumorigenesis in a genetically engineered mouse model of ARMS.[219]

In addition to inhibiting RTKs, whether through monoclonal antibodies or small molecules, there are also efforts to inhibit heparanases (discussed in "Metastatic Pathways in Rhabdomyosarcoma"). Pharmacologic inhibition of heparanases using SST0001, a chemically modified heparin, in RD and Rh30 xenografts showed inhibition of tumor growth. The precise mechanism is not clear, but there was evidence of decreased angiogenic factors secreted from the RMS cell lines in the in vitro studies.[220]

Inhibitors of Intracellular Signaling Pathways

Regarding downstream signaling pathways, it is clear that blockade of only one pathway is not durably antitumorigenic because of compensatory upregulation of other pathways. Therefore there are ongoing efforts to simultaneously block two or more pathways. Dual blockade of the PI3K/AKT/mTOR and RAS/MEK/ERK pathways with small molecules synergistically inhibits RMS cell growth in vivo.[221] Similarly, treatment of RMS xenografts with rapamycin was shown to block tumor growth by inhibiting not only the mTOR pathway but also Hedgehog signaling,[222] and indeed rapamycin analogues are in human clinical trials (see "Clinical Research in Rhabdomyosarcoma"). Attesting to the power of utilizing lower eukaryotes for target discovery, a screen performed in an oncogenic RAS-driven model of zebrafish RMS identified dual MEK and mTOR/S6K1 inhibition as effective.[223]

Finally, there is RAS itself, which is found mutated in a significant portion of ERMS tumors (see previous section, "Oncogene and Tumor Suppressor Gene Mutations in Rhabdomyosarcoma"). Targeting the RAS protein has proven difficult. However, silencing of Sprouty1, an upstream modulator of RAS that is also found in ERMS tumors and associated with upregulated ERK signaling, using shRNA triggers complete regression of ERMS xenograft tumors carrying a mutated oncogenic RAS gene,[224] suggesting that there will be alternate ways to block RAS signaling in the future.

Inhibitors of Developmental Pathways

Pharmacologic blockade of RTK signaling by small molecule inhibitors became possible because of a deep structural understanding of their enzymatic activity. As the role of the evolutionarily conserved developmental pathways (e.g., Hedgehog, Notch, Wnt, transforming growth factor-β [TGF-β]) in RMS tumorigenesis has become apparent,[225] it has become similarly imperative to understand the molecular basis for their dysregulation. For the most part, it appears that in RMS these pathways, which during normal development and tissue homeostasis direct myogenesis by promoting myogenic stem cell maintenance, expansion, and tight control of differentiation, are usurped and prevent proper myogenic lineage progression. In this regard, agents developed to inhibit members of these pathways must be evaluated for unanticipated effects on normal tissue, especially considering the continual growth and development of pediatric patients. Studies in *Ptch* mutant mice, which through increased Hedgehog signaling develop both medulloblastoma and RMS, showed that combined dosing with the epigenetic drugs 5-aza-2′-deoxycytidine and valproic acid inhibited tumor formation when treated early.[226] In human RMS xenografts, treatment with betulinic acid (a naturally occurring plant product), GANT61 (a Gli antagonist), or forskolin (also derived from a naturally occurring plant product) suppressed Hedgehog signaling and RMS tumor growth.[227-229] Recently, several additional small molecule inhibitors of Smoothened and Gli have been developed, raising the expectation that blockade of Hedgehog signaling will be possible in human cancers.[230]

Regarding Notch signaling, given its critical role in normal muscle development and the upregulation of many components of this pathway in RMS, this pathway has gained attention, and several Notch pathway genes and proteins have been suppressed using genetic (shRNA) or pharmacologic (γ-secretase inhibitors) approaches and when suppressed shown to inhibit the growth of RMS xenografts, including Notch1, Notch3, RBPJ, and Hey1.[231-233] Although as important in skeletal muscle development as Notch, the Wnt pathway is not as well understood in the pathobiology of RMS and therefore in vivo preclinical studies using genetic or pharmacologic approaches to target the Wnt pathway are lagging. Finally, regarding TGF-β signaling, this pathway, too, is under investigation in RMS. However, recently a miR that is suppressed by TGFB1 known as miR 450b-5p, when overexpressed in RMS cells inhibits cell growth in vitro and tumor xenografts in vivo and promotes myogenic differentiation.[234]

Inhibitors of Other Cellular Processes That Support Rhabdomyosarcoma Tumorigenesis

Apoptosis

In addition to specific signal transduction pathways, there are efforts to target specific cellular processes. For example, as described earlier, RMS cells can resist apoptosis (programmed cell death) through upregulation of anti-apoptotic proteins or the suppression of pro-apoptotic proteins. Therapeutic approaches therefore may include inhibiting anti-apoptotic signaling, for example through neutralizing Bcl-2 family proteins (although caution must be taken because some Bcl-2 family members have pro-survival roles), or activating pro-apoptotic signaling, for example through stimulation of the extrinsic apoptotic pathway via members of the tumor necrosis factor (TNF)-related apoptosis-inducing ligand (TRAIL) receptors.[235] Drozitumab is a monoclonal antibody to death receptor 5 that supports assembly of death-induced signaling complexes and has shown efficacy in RMS xenografts.[236] It may also be possible to reestablish normal function of mutated pro-apoptotic pathways. For example, in ARMS xenografts the MDM2 inhibitor RG7112 interferes with MDM2-TP53 binding, releasing TP53 from negative control and permitting its normal cell surveillance function.[237] Finally, although apoptosis has historically been the major focus of inducing cell death, the process of necroptosis (nonapoptotic cell death) has been found to be induced in RMS cells via obatoclax, which inhibits BCL2.[238]

Although involved not only in avoidance of apoptosis but also many other pro-tumorigenic processes, it is important to note that MYCN has been proven targetable through the use of antigene therapy in which a peptide nucleic acid oligonucleotide (tethered to a nuclear localization signal peptide and targeted against the antisense strand of MYCN exon 2) was delivered to ARMS cells. This antigene therapy caused a decrease in proliferation and an increase in apoptosis in vitro and eliminated 75% of tumors in Rh30 RMS xenografts, with 25% showing a reduction in tumor.[239]

Cell Cycle

Although apoptosis is a cellular event that can be triggered by many distinct stimuli, direct manipulation of the cell cycle and its checkpoints also provides opportunities for pharmacologic manipulation and treatment of RMS. Of long-standing interest are antimitotic agents, which interfere with transit through mitosis, including spindle assembly, chromosome positioning, and chromosome separation. Classic chemotherapy agents such as vincristine, which is a backbone of RMS therapy, interfere with the mitotic spindle by binding tubulin. Indeed, a more potent synthetic antitubulin agent, eribulin, which is distinct from the Vinca alkaloids in how it binds tubulin, has shown some complete responses in RMS xenografts.[240] More recently, kinases and kinesin motor proteins that control mitosis are now able to be pharmacologically targeted and agents blocking these proteins are being evaluated against human cancer panels, including RMS. The agents MLN8237 and B16727, Aurora A, and Pololike kinase inhibitors, respectively, have both demonstrated some response in RMS xenograft studies.[241,242] The kinesin spindle protein inhibitor ispinesib was toxic and ineffective in inhibiting RMS xenograft growth,[243] whereas the CENP-E kinesin inhibitor GSK923295A showed some efficacy.[244]

Regulation of Protein Stability and Turnover

The heat shock and ubiquitin-proteasome systems, which contribute to homeostasis of protein stability and turnover, have also been mined for their potential as anticancer targets. 17-DMAG, a first-in-class derivative of geldanamycin that inhibits Hsp90, showed some antitumor activity in xenograft models of ARMS,[245] whereas a non-geldanamycin Hsp90 inhibitor, AT13387, showed no objective tumor responses.[246] Bortezomib, which is approved by the U.S. Food and Drug Administration (FDA) for the treatment of several human diseases, showed activity in ERMS and ARMS xenografts in vivo.[247] MLN4924, a first-in-class NEDD8-activating enzyme inhibitor that affects the ubiquitin-proteosome pathway also showed efficacy in RMS.[248]

Epigenetic Modifiers

Currently there are two groups of agents under study that qualify as epigenetic modifiers. The first group of agents is composed of histone deacetylase (HDAC) inhibitors. Agents in the second group inhibit DNA methylation and include 5-aza-2′-deoxycytidine. Although results of early in vitro studies were promising,[249,250] there are few in vivo studies demonstrating inhibition of RMS tumorigenesis in response to epigenetic modifiers. As mentioned earlier, combined dosing with the epigenetic drugs 5-aza-2′-deoxycytidine and valproic acid, which target Dnmt and HDAC, respectively, in a genetically engineered mouse model of Ptch-mutant mice inhibited tumor formation, but only when the mice were treated early during tumorigenesis.[226] Additionally, drugs that target proteins involved in epigenetic regulation can have unanticipated protumorigenic effects, as in the case of the HDAC inhibitor trichostatin A and DNA demethylating agent (5-Aza), which reactivated the expression of Ezrin, a known prometastatic protein in RMS.[251]

Immunotherapy for Rhabdomyosarcoma

In addition to pharmacologic agents, there are efforts to stimulate or harness the immune system to target and kill RMS tumor cells. However, like most other cancers, RMS is remarkably successful at evading the immune system. One approach to overcome this evasion is isolation and expansion of natural killer cells obtained from normal healthy donors, which can kill human sarcoma cells in vitro and Ewing sarcoma xenografts in vivo.[252] Recently, IL-15 cytokine–induced killer cells from donors were shown to be active in xenograft models of RMS.[253] Another novel approach is chimeric antigen receptor therapy, which although still in early phases has been effective in the treatment of leukemias. Thus there is hope that this approach can be similarly used in solid tumors. To prepare for these efforts, a recent study identified candidate cell surface proteins on pediatric tumors including RMS that could be future therapeutic targets for immunotherapy.[254] Finally, there are ongoing efforts to develop vaccines to solid tumors including RMS. Given the specific expression of the PAX3-FOXO1 fusion protein in ARMS, an epitope-enhanced peptide bearing the PAX3-FOXO1 breakpoint was designed and generated. Because this peptide represents a neoantigen exclusively found in ARMS, the immune system should recognize it as such; and, indeed, dendritic cells pulsed with this peptide generated a CTL line that lysed human ARMS tumor cells in vitro.[255] Similar proposals have been made to use the fetal acetylcholine receptor and other antigens for RMS immunotherapy.[256,257]

CLINICAL RESEARCH ON RHABDOMYOSARCOMA

RMS may be the most clinically complex tumor in pediatric oncology. In addition to its histologic and biologic diversity, RMS has a remarkable variety of sites and clinical behaviors.

Much of our clinical knowledge of RMS has come from well-organized multiinstitutional clinical trials in North America and Europe. In the United States and Canada (and later Australia, New Zealand, and Switzerland) the first Intergroup Rhabdomyosarcoma Study (IRS-I) opened in 1972 and closed in 1978, recruiting patients from the pediatric division of the Southwest Oncology Group (SWOG) and the Children's Cancer Study Group (CCSG). There were five further IRS studies (II, III, IV-pilot, IV, and V), during which the pediatric division of SWOG became the Pediatric Oncology Group (POG) and the CCSG became the Children's Cancer Group (CCG). Finally, the IRS, POG, CCG, and the National Wilms Tumor Study merged to form the Children's Oncology Group (COG), and that group's Soft Tissue Sarcoma Committee completed the IRS-V studies before launching its own ARST series. Publications from the first generation of COG RMS studies (ARST series) are beginning to appear.

Meanwhile, in Europe, the International Society of Pediatric Oncology (SIOP) has conducted a series of Malignant Mesenchymal Tumor studies (SIOP 75 and MMT-84, MMT-89, and MMT-95). The German CWS (*Cooperative Weichteilsarkom Studie*) conducted four trials, CWS 81, 86, 91, and 96. The Italian Rhabdomyosarcoma Group had two clinical trials, RMS 79 and 88, before joining the CWS studies. Limited patient numbers made randomized controlled trials difficult, so the Europeans joined to form the European Paediatric Soft Tissue Sarcoma Study Group (EpSSG), which has launched a randomized controlled trial for patients with localized RMS (RMS-2005). Unfortunately, the loss of Germany for regulatory reasons has slowed accrual, and the results of many of the earlier European studies have never been published.

INCIDENCE AND EPIDEMIOLOGY

RMS accounts for about half of the soft tissue sarcomas in children and adolescents and about 3% of childhood cancer cases. This varies with age, so that they are 60% of soft tissue sarcomas in patients aged younger than 5 years and 23% in the 15- to 19-year age group.[258] They occurred in 4.6 children per million per year in 1996 to 2003 according to the Surveillance, Epidemiology and End Results (SEER) database,[259] and in the period 1973 to 2005 the incidence increased at a mean annual rate of 0.58%.[260] The highest incidence (8.4 per million children) is in the 1- to 4-year age group, after which the incidence is stable at about 4 per million children per year. SEER data show that the incidence of ERMS peaks at about age 3 and then declines until about age 10, whereas the incidence of ARMS is fairly constant from birth to age 19.[261] Most studies report a slight male preponderance (about 5:4); recent analyses of SEER data found no

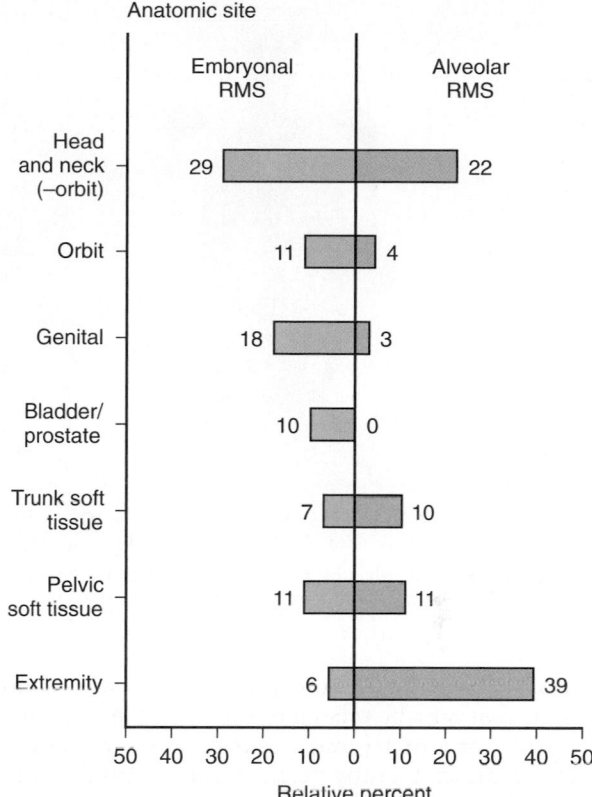

Figure 59-7 Primary sites of embryonal and alveolar RMS, percent of distribution by histology. *(From Gurney JG, Young JL, Roffers SD, et al: Soft Tissue Sarcomas, SEER Pediatric Monograph, Bethesda, Md., 1999, National Cancer Institute, p. 116.)*

significant differences in incidence by race[260] or a slightly higher incidence in black children.[261]

CLINICAL PRESENTATION AND EVALUATION

RMS occurs in virtually all parts of the body outside the central nervous system (although they may involve it). ERMS often occurs in areas where there is very little skeletal muscle, such as the orbit, pharynx, sinuses, vaginal wall and paratesticular tissues. ARMS has a greater tendency to occur where there is skeletal muscle, such as in the trunk and limbs (Fig. 59-7).

The clinical presentations of either histology are myriad and vary with the primary site. For example, tumors of the parameningeal region (e.g., the sinuses and pharynx) may have cranial nerve deficits as initial symptoms, orbital tumors often produce proptosis and diplopia, and tumors of the bladder base and prostate usually cause urinary retention. Often, however, the tumor is a painless mass without associated symptoms. Usually it is hard or firm, smooth, fixed to surrounding tissues, and not tender. There may be palpable regional lymphadenopathy and, occasionally (with alveolar histology tumors), distant involved nodes and metastases to the skeleton or marrow.

The initial evaluation of a patient with a suspected RMS has three components: the evaluation of the extent and anatomic relationships of the primary tumor; the

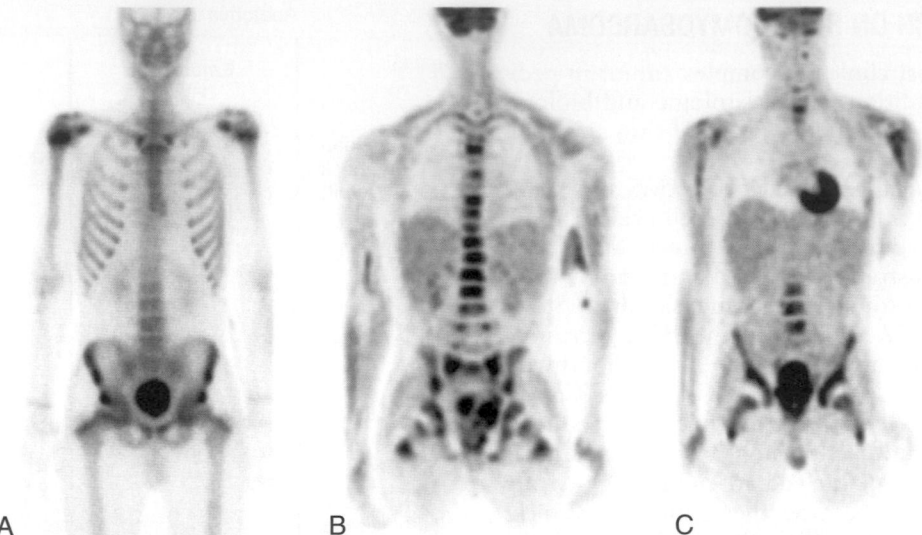

Figure 59-8 Metastatic alveolar rhabdomyosarcoma. Radionuclide bone scan (**A**) and two images from a tomographic coronal PET scan (**B** and **C**). The abnormalities in the bone scan are few and subtle; the PET scan clearly shows multiple skeletal metastases.

detection of metastases; and the identification of other problems that may be related to the tumor (e.g., a cranial nerve palsy or urinary retention) or that are unrelated but could affect therapy (e.g., a cancer predisposition syndrome).

The most appropriate time for referral to a pediatric oncology center is at the first suspicion of a malignancy. Experienced radiologists should perform the imaging of the primary tumor before a biopsy has produced local hemorrhage and edema, using equipment that can share images with computerized radiation therapy planning systems. If possible, the surgeon who will perform the definitive excision of the tumor should perform, or at least supervise, the diagnostic biopsy of a suspected sarcoma. Violation of tissue planes or neurovascular structures with inexpertly placed biopsy tracts (whether open or closed) may limit excision and reconstruction options, prevent limb salvage procedures, or increase the chances of local recurrence. Because sarcomas are often very heterogeneous and contain large areas of necrosis and because molecular techniques are increasingly important in diagnosis, generous fresh specimens are important, with frozen section confirmation of specimen adequacy before the procedure is declared complete. Many passes of the needle (10 or more) are usually required if closed techniques are used. Fine-needle aspirates do not provide the tissue architectural information currently necessary for pediatric sarcoma diagnosis or sufficient tissue for advanced diagnostic techniques.

For evaluation of the primary tumor, the current standard of care is magnetic resonance imaging (MRI) with contrast enhancement, encompassing the primary tumor and regional lymph nodes. Traditionally, patients have also undergone a spiral chest computed tomographic (CT) scan without administration of a contrast agent (although contrast enhancement is necessary to find hilar or mediastinal adenopathy or to distinguish a mass from a surrounding pleural effusion) and a radionuclide bone

scan to detect skeletal metastases, as well as bilateral bone marrow aspirates and biopsies. However, a recent analysis indicates that these studies are unnecessary in patients with noninvasive tumors without regional node involvement (T1N0), which are about one third of cases.[262]

The use of fluorodeoxyglucose-18–labeled positron emission tomography (FDG-PET) is particularly promising for the detection of involved regional nodes and distant metastases[263,264] and skeletal and marrow disease not revealed by conventional techniques (Fig. 59-8). The combination of PET and CT (PET/CT) can help discern the extent of tumor versus peritumoral edema or whether a remote mass is a tumor. A retrospective study of 23 RMS patients showed that side-by-side evaluation of PET/CT and conventional imaging (primary site MRI, bone scintigraphy, marrow biopsy, chest CT) provided more accurate staging than either conventional imaging or PET/CT alone.[265] A larger single-institution study of 30 pediatric RMS patients retrospectively compared the findings of conventional imaging (MRI, chest CT, bone scintigraphy), marrow aspirates and biopsies, biopsies of selected possible metastases, and PET/CT. For regional nodes, PET/CT was equally sensitive to conventional imaging but much more specific (95% v. 14%); for bone and marrow disease PET/CT was more sensitive (detecting 4 of 4 patients with bone or marrow disease, versus 1 of 4 with bone scintigraphy); and PET/CT detected soft tissue metastases not visible on conventional imaging in 2 patients. Chest CT revealed more nodules than PET/CT (seven nodules in 6 patients vs. one nodule in 1 patient).[266] A retrospective comparison of PET/CT and conventional imaging in 35 pediatric and adult RMS patients (two thirds with alveolar histology) similarly found PET/CT more sensitive and specific for both regional node and metastatic assessment.[267] The potential role of PET/CT in assessing response to therapy will be discussed later.

Whole-body MRI for detection of metastasis was tested in several single-institution studies. In particular, a large single-institution study compared whole-body MRI, FDG-PET, and bone scintigraphy in the detection of skeletal metastases in 39 pediatric patients with a variety of tumors (including Ewing sarcoma, RMS, osteosarcoma, lymphoma, melanoma, and Langerhans cell histiocytosis), with biopsy of all detected lesions for histologic confirmation. PET had the highest sensitivity (90%), followed by whole-body MRI (82%), and bone scintigraphy (71%), although all three modalities had both false-positive and false-negative results that varied with anatomic location (for example, the high glucose uptake in the brain made PET relatively insensitive in the skull). The greatest sensitivity (96%) came from combining any two imaging modalities.[268] A recent large multicenter study enrolled a cohort of 188 children with soft tissue sarcoma, lymphoma, or neuroblastoma. With a complex system of central review, the investigators compared the findings of whole-body MRI with those of CT and disease-appropriate scintigraphy (metaiodobenzylguanidine, gallium, or [in some patients] FDG-PET). Whole-body MRI detected more skeletal metastases per patient, but this did not change the staging of any patient's tumor; and it was less sensitive than conventional imaging in detecting liver and lung metastases. The investigators concluded that whole-body MRI "is not justified" as "the initial study of choice" for staging pediatric cancers.[269]

RISK GROUP CLASSIFICATION

RMS varies tremendously in prognosis, from almost 100% survival (for orbital embryonal tumors) to virtually no prospect of survival (for disseminated alveolar tumors). There has been a variety of schemes for classifying RMS to try to match treatment intensity to prognosis. Some of the schemes are prospective, relying on tumor characteristics before any therapy, whereas others are dynamic, subject to change based on response to surgery or chemotherapy. We will consider individual prognostic variables and then the ways in which they have been combined.

Histology and Fusion Status

Patients with ARMS are less likely to survive than patients with ERMS, even if all other factors are equal. Alveolar tumors are also more likely to be regionally or metastatically disseminated at the time of diagnosis and are more likely to be invasive (Table 59-5) The difficulties in classifying tumors with alveolar histology that lack a *PAX-FOXO1* gene fusion and the differences between alveolar tumors with fusions involving *PAX3* and *PAX7* have already been discussed. So far, histology has taken precedence over fusion status, but this appears to be changing with accumulating evidence that fusion status is the key determinant of clinical behavior.[270,271]

Site

The clinical behavior and prognosis of RMS varies greatly with the site of the primary tumor, independently of histology. For example, an ERMS of the orbit is almost

TABLE 59-5   Clinical Features of Embryonal and Alveolar Rhabdomyosarcoma

	Embryonal Tumors	Alveolar Tumors
Age	Younger	Older
Location	Central, not muscular	Peripheral, muscular
Invasiveness	Low/moderate	High
Metastases	Lung	Everywhere
Prognoses	40% to 90% + PFS	0 to 60% PFS

PFS, Progression-free survival.

always curable whereas an ERMS arising in the ethmoid sinus, just a few centimeters away, carries about 25% mortality despite more intense therapy. The favorable sites for RMS are the orbit, superficial head and neck, biliary tree, vagina, and paratestis; all other sites are considered unfavorable. The biologic basis for this variability remains mysterious, with many different hypotheses (size at diagnosis, access to lymphatics, ploidy, and many others) having been explored and discarded.

Age

The prognosis for patients with RMS is best in preschool and middle childhood and worse for infants, adolescents, and adults. An analysis of data from the IRS-III, IRS-IV pilot, and IRS-IV (spanning 1984 through 1997) showed that when infants younger than 1 year of age are assigned a risk of treatment failure of 1.0, the relative risk for older children is 0.4 to 0.6 and that for adolescents (≥10 years) is 0.8.[272] Although other prognostic variables such as histology, nodal status, stage, site, and clinical group differed between the three age groups, the impact of age remained when all other factors were controlled. A more recent analysis of infants enrolled in the IRS-IV and COG D9602 and D9803 studies largely confirmed these findings and noted that the outcome for infants with group III tumors (gross residual disease at the beginning of chemotherapy) have a particularly poor outcome, perhaps related to fewer than half receiving protocol-assigned radiation therapy. Overall, FFS at 5 years was 57%, 81%, and 67% for patients aged younger than 1, 1 to 9 years, and 10 years and older, respectively.[273] Prognosis varies with age gradually, however, so the 1- and 10-year boundaries are somewhat arbitrary.

Adults with RMS have a much worse prognosis than children and adolescents. The SEER registry analyzed the records of 2600 RMS patients diagnosed from 1973 to 2005. The OS rate of patients younger than age 19 was 61% at 5 years versus 27% for patients older than 19. Hazard ratios for death increased steadily with increasing age past 19 years; on multivariate analysis the other significant independent variables were histology, primary site, and extent of tumor (local, regional, metastatic).[274] A multicenter study of 169 pediatric and adult RMS diagnosed between 1977 and 2009 (ages birth to 73 years) identified through the Dutch National Histological Database System considered a variety of tumor, host, and treatment variables, many of which were significantly associated with outcome in univariate analysis. On multivariate analysis, increasing age was the most important factor influencing relapse-free survival (RFS), with histology the only other factor retaining significance.[275]

Invasiveness and Size (Tumor Stage)

Invasive tumors, those that cross tissue planes or extend beyond the organ of origin (designated T2 in the TNM system), have a worse prognosis that noninvasive tumors (T1). Similarly, patients with tumors 5 cm in diameter or larger (Tb) have a worse prognosis than those with tumors less than 5 cm (Ta). The International Rhabdomyosarcoma Workshop pooled data from four studies conducted in the late 1970s and 1980s (IRS-II, CWS-81, SIOP RMS 75, and the Italian Cooperative Group study) to examine prognostic factors in 951 patients with localized disease. In multivariate analysis, site and invasiveness were the surviving factors.[276] Histology was not among the variables considered, but it is closely related to site and invasiveness. European studies have used invasiveness for risk classification, but North American clinical trials have not, largely because a definition that would be usable in a large cooperative group has been elusive.

Size is highly correlated with invasiveness in multivariate analyses[276] and is much simpler to measure. The current COG risk classification uses stage, which depends on both site and size (Table 59-6).

Clinical Group

The extent of tumor when chemotherapy begins determines the clinical group (see Table 59-6). It is not a true staging system, because it depends on the initial surgery;

stage and group only overlap in patients with metastases (stage 4, group IV). IRS-I showed clinical group to be a powerful prognostic variable, but it is a complex one: site, invasiveness, the aggressiveness of the surgeon, the attitude of the family toward mutilating surgery, and the confidence of the treating team in chemotherapy and radiation therapy can all influence whether a tumor is excised with negative margins at diagnosis (group I) or only sampled (group III).

Lymph Node Involvement

Lymph node positivity is variably defined as clinical involvement on physical examination or imaging or histologic involvement at biopsy; some reports provide no definition. The International Rhabdomyosarcoma Workshop found lymph node involvement (undefined) to be a prognostic factor in univariate analysis but not as strong as tumor stage, size, or site.[276] Clinical involvement of local or regional lymph nodes was prognostically significant among IRS-III and IRS-IV patients with stage 3, group III ARMS (5-year OS of 66% with negative nodes vs. 34% for positive nodes, $P = .01$), but not for patients with embryonal tumors.[277] A later study using IRS-IV cases with localized tumors or single metastatic sites came to the same conclusion about ERMS, but for ARMS multivariate analysis showed nodal positivity (whether by physical examination, imaging, or histology) to be a potent adverse factor, with N0 and N1 5-year FFS rates of 73% and 43%, respectively.[278] The investigators also found that 80% of N1 primary ARMS overexpressed immune-related genes such as β_2-microglobulin, immunoglobulins, complement, and histocompatibility complex components.

Metastases at Diagnosis

Patients with metastases at diagnosis fare poorly, and there has been little change over the years. Patients with group IV tumors had a 5-year OS of 20% in IRS-I, 23% in IRS-II, 20% in CWS-86, and 23% in MMT-98 and across a range of IRS studies beginning with IRS-III.[279-283] However, they are not a uniform population. Patients younger than the age of 10 years with metastatic ERMS were classified as intermediate-risk (rather than high-risk) patients in the IRS-V series of studies because of a 51% FFS rate in the previous three studies.[272,284] An analysis of patients with metastases at diagnosis in IRS-IV found that the number of metastatic sites and histology defined two risk groups: patients with one or two metastatic sites, or three metastatic sites with embryonal histology, had a 3-year OS of 43% to 47%, but patients with three or more metastatic sites and alveolar histology had a 3-year survival of only 5%.[285] After pooling 788 patients with metastatic RMS from nine cooperative group studies (IRS, SIOP MMT, and Italian), a multivariate analysis identified four unfavorable prognostic factors: unfavorable site, bone or marrow metastases, age younger than 1 or older than 9 years, and three or more metastatic sites. Applying these factors divided the population into two groups: the first had none to one unfavorable factor, accounted for 42% of the patients, and had an event-free survival (EFS) of 44%; the second had two or more

TABLE 59-6   Comparison of IRS Clinical Group and Stage for Rhabdomyosarcoma

GROUP I: Complete excision No gross or microscopic residual disease	STAGE 1: Favorable site Orbit, superficial head and neck, biliary tree, paratestes, vagina
GROUP II: Microscopic residual disease	STAGE 2: Unfavorable site, diameter ≤5 cm, and nodes clinically negative or unknown
IIa: Microscopically positive excision margins	All sites except the favorable ones above are unfavorable.
IIb: Excision margins negative; involved nodes but completely excised; most distant node negative	
IIc: Microscopically positive margins at primary site or grossly excised nodes; or most distant node positive	
GROUP III: Gross residual disease Biopsy only or incomplete excision	STAGE 3: Unfavorable site and diameter >5 cm or clinically involved nodes
GROUP IV: Distant metastases	STAGE 4: Distant metastases

factors, accounted for 58% of the patients, and had an EFS of 14%.[286]

Interactions

All of these variables interact, which complicates classification. For example, large extremity primary tumors are usually alveolar histology, often have involved regional nodes, and often occur in teenagers, and ARMS are usually invasive.

A recent multivariate analysis of 1164 CWS study patients, enrolled between 1980 and 2002, identified histology, age (≤10 years vs. >10 years), tumor size (5-cm cutoff), clinical group, site, and the use of radiation therapy in treatment as significant factors. Further distillation led to three groups of patients, those with (1) embryonal tumors 5 cm or less, whose 5-year EFS was 76%, whose relapses were only 19% systemic, and whose postrelapse survival was 46%; (2) embryonal tumors larger than 5 cm, with an EFS of 64%, whose relapses were 32% systemic, and postrelapse survival was 18%; and (3) alveolar tumors, with an EFS of 46%, systemic relapse rate of 52%, and postrelapse survival of 13%.[287]

Many different risk classification schemes exist for RMS, and they change from one clinical trial to another. In the system used by the COG for current studies, stage (which depends on site and size), clinical group, and histology are combined to produce a three-way risk classification (Fig. 59-9 and Table 59-7). The system used in the current European studies assigns patients to four risk groups (low, standard, high, and very high) based on histology, clinical group (referred to as stage), site, nodal involvement, tumor size, and age; these four risk groups are then divided into eight subgroups based on clinical group, nodal status, age, and tumor size (Table 59-8). In

TABLE 59-7 Children's Oncology Group Risk Stratification for Rhabdomyosarcoma

	Low Risk	Intermediate Risk	High Risk
Metastases	No	No	Yes
Histology	Embryonal	Any	Any
Stage	Any if group I or II; 1 if group III	1, 2, or 3 if alveolar histology; 2 or 3 if embryonal histology	4
Group	I, II, or III if stage 1; I or II if stage 2 or 3	III if stage 2 or 3; I, II, or III if alveolar histology	IV

view of recent information on the overarching importance of *PAX-FOXO1* fusion status,[271] risk classifications are likely to change in the next generation of cooperative group studies.

TREATMENT

Before the advent of chemotherapy for RMS, survival was rare—a retrospective review of 64 CCSG RMS cases with "complete" surgical excisions revealed a survival rate of less than 8%.[288] The dramatic progress in treatment and survival of RMS patients over the past 40 years has flowed mostly from multidisciplinary care, in which surgeons, oncologists, radiologists, radiation oncologists, and pathologists approach treatment in a planned, coordinated fashion. Such care, which was pioneered in the late 1960s,[289] has been the foundation for clinical trials in RMS in the United States and Europe.

Chemotherapy

Systemic chemotherapy for all patients with RMS began with a Children's Cancer Study Group randomized controlled trial, which ran from 1967 to 1971. Patients with complete excisions (group I) were randomly assigned to chemotherapy with vincristine and dactinomycin (actinomycin D) for 6 to 13 nine-week cycles or to observation only, whereas patients with microscopic residual disease were nonrandomly assigned to the chemotherapy arm of the trial. RFS at 4 years was 82% in the chemotherapy group and 47% in the control group (*P* = .03); RFS was 90% in group II.[288] This trial established the role of chemotherapy in treating RMS and also established the feasibility and importance of coordinated multidisciplinary care on a national, multiinstitutional scale.

Cyclophosphamide

Cyclophosphamide was part of combination chemotherapy for RMS from some of the earliest trials, based on its efficacy as a single agent in patients with advanced RMS.[289,290] The vincristine-dactinomycin (actinomycin D)-cyclophosphamide (VAC) combination has been in continuous use since IRS-I[280] and the first European

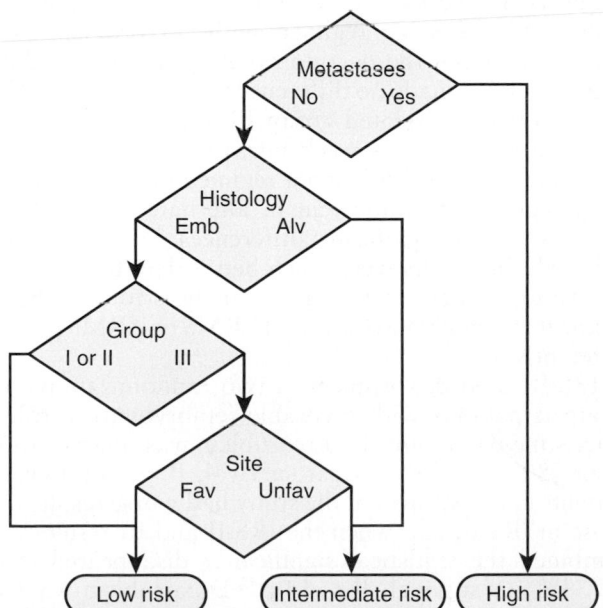

Figure 59-9 Risk group assignment algorithm for the first generation of Children's Oncology Group ARST studies (ARST0331, ARST0431, ARST0531). The results of those studies and the use of molecular rather than histologic criteria for alveolar RMS are likely to change this considerably. *Alv,* Alveolar; *Emb,* embryonal.

TABLE 59-8 European Paediatric Soft Tissue Sarcoma Study Group Risk Stratification for Rhabdomyosarcoma

Risk Group	Subgroups	Pathology	Postsurgical Stage (IRS Group)	Site	Node Stage	Size and Age
Low risk	A	Favorable	I	Any	N0	Favorable
Standard risk	B	Favorable	I	Any	N0	Unfavorable
	C	Favorable	II, III	Favorable	N0	Any
	D	Favorable	II, III	Unfavorable	N0	Favorable
High risk	E	Favorable	II, III	Unfavorable	N0	Unfavorable
	F	Favorable	II, III	Any	N1	Any
	G	Unfavorable	I, II, III	Any	N0	Any
Very high risk	H	Unfavorable	I, II, III	Any	N	Any

cooperative group trials. The standard North American chemotherapy combination for patients with intermediate-risk tumors is still the VAC regimen. The exact composition of the VAC regimen has varied considerably over time (Table 59-9), but no randomized controlled trial has shown any combination to be more effective.

In IRS-I, patients with group II tumors were randomized between 2-year regimens consisting of vincristine-dactinomycin (VA) (with six doses of vincristine and 5 consecutive days of dactinomycin per 9-week cycle) or VAC (12 weekly doses of vincristine at the start of therapy only, dactinomycin every 12 weeks, and daily oral cyclophosphamide). There was no significant difference between the two study arms,[280] but the design of the comparison allows one to conclude only that cyclophosphamide could substitute for 60 doses of vincristine and three cycles of dactinomycin.

The IRS-II study addressed the role of cyclophosphamide in two randomizations. In group I patients, the VAC regimen from IRS-I (for 2 years) was compared with the VA regimen alone for 1 year, with the same 12 initial weekly doses of vincristine and dactinomycin every 12 weeks. The VAC regimen provided a statistically insignificant advantage in disease-free survival (DFS) but no advantage in OS. For group II patients there was a randomization between two 1-year regimens: the VA regimen with 9-week cycles incorporating six weekly doses of vincristine and one 5-day series of dactinomycin doses per cycle and a VAC modification with 4-week cycles each containing a single dose of vincristine, a single 5-day series of dactinomycin injections, and intravenous cyclophosphamide. The contest was a draw,[281] and because the VA regimen had three times the vincristine and half the dactinomycin of the cyclophosphamide-containing regimen, inferences regarding the role of cyclophosphamide are impossible.[291] There is evidence that cyclophosphamide (or ifosfamide) can allow omission of radiation therapy for some patients with vaginal RMS, however (discussed later).

There is also no evidence of a relationship between the dose of cyclophosphamide and its efficacy. For intermediate-risk patients getting the VAC regimen, IRS-III prescribed the equivalent of 900 mg/m^2 per 3-week cycle in regimen 34[292]; IRS-IV used 2.2 g/m^2 per cycle in its VAC regimen[293]; and a pilot IRS study tried 3.6 g/m^2

of cyclophosphamide per cycle (a dose of 4.5 g/m^2 proved too toxic).[294] However, there was no change in FFS rates across these three trials despite a fourfold increase in cyclophosphamide dose and dose intensity,[293,294] and the most recent COG ARST studies use 1200 mg/m^2 of cyclophosphamide in their VAC arms.

Doxorubicin

Doxorubicin is probably the single most effective agent against sarcomas generally, but its role in RMS remains been both unclear and controversial despite three decades of study. Concern about its cardiotoxicity (especially in young patients) has limited its use. The value of doxorubicin in treating RMS, and particularly its relative efficacy against embryonal and alveolar tumors, remain open questions.

The investigators of the IRS tried doxorubicin in a variety of ways. In IRS-I, patients with group III and IV tumors were randomized between VAC (with dactinomycin every 12 weeks and continuous oral cyclophosphamide) and the same regimen with doxorubicin doses halfway between the dactinomycin cycles. The addition of doxorubicin made no difference to either DFS or OS.[280] The IRS-II study treated group III and IV patients with more modern, every-4-week intravenous regimens, randomizing between VAC and a regimen in which doxorubicin replaced dactinomycin in alternate cycles. Again, there were no significant differences in DFS or OS, although the results were much better than those of IRS-I.[281] Unfortunately there was no analysis to see whether doxorubicin might have affected ERMS or ARMS patients differently.[291]

IRS-III used doxorubicin in two randomizations. For group II patients with favorable (embryonal) histology, vincristine-dactinomycin-doxorubicin was superior to VA alone (89% vs. 54% 5-year survival, P = .03); however, patients in the VA arm of the study had worse results than those in IRS-II, and when the IRS-II and III results were combined the statistical significance disappeared (89% vs. 73% for survival, P = .14).[292] Doxorubicin was also part of all three randomized regimens for clinical group III and IV patients in complex ways that make its contribution to the results impossible to assess.[291]

The COG compared six "phase II window" regimens to IRS-III in 420 patients with group IV (metastatic)

TABLE 59-9 Evolution of Vincristine/Dactinomycin (Actinomycin D)/Cyclophosphamide (VAC) Chemotherapy

	VCR Dose	VCR Schedule	AMD Dose	AMD Schedule†	CPM Dose	CPM Schedule	Duration	Total VCR	Total AMD	Total CPM
IRS-I	2 mg/m²; max: 2 mg	Weekly × 12	0.015 mg/kg/day × 5 days; max: 0.5 mg/dose	q12 wk	2.5 mg/kg	Daily PO	2 yr	12 doses	10 cycles	51.5 g/m²
IRS-I*	2 mg/m²; max: 2 mg	Weekly × 12, then q4 wk	0.015 mg/kg/day × 5 days; max: 0.5 mg/dose	q4 wk	10 mg/kg/day × 3	× 1, q3-4 wk	1 yr for group II, 2 yr for others	35 doses	24 cycles	27 doses, 24.3 g/m²
IRS-II	1.5 mg/m²; max: 2 mg	Weekly × 12, then q3-4 wk	0.015 mg/kg/day × 5 days; max: 0.5 mg/dose	q3-4 wk	10 mg/kg/day × 3	× 1, q3-4 wk	2 yr	36 doses	21 cycles	27 doses, 24.3 g/m²
IRS-IVP	1.5 mg/m²; max: 2 mg	Weekly × 12, then q3 wk with q1 wk intervals	1.35 mg/m² (1 dose)	q3 wk	3600 to 4500 mg/m² (first four cycles), then 2200 mg/m² IV	× 1, q3 wk	38 wk	32 doses	11 doses	13 doses, 34.2 to 37.8 g/m²
IRS-IV	1.5 mg/m²; max: 2 mg	Weekly × 12, then q3 wk with q1 wk intervals	0.015 mg/kg/day × 5 days; max: 0.5 mg/dose	q3 wk	2200 mg/m² IV	× 1, q3 wk	44 wk	32 doses	9 cycles	12 doses, 26.4 g/m²
IRS-V	1.5 mg/m²; max: 2 mg	Weekly × 12, then q3 wk with q1 wk intervals	1.5 mg/m²; max: 2 mg	q3 wk	2200 mg/m² IV	× 1, q3 wk	40 wk	30 doses	12 doses	14 doses, 30.8 g/m²
COG ARST‡	1.5 mg/m²; max: 2 mg	Weekly × 12, then q3 wk with q1 wk intervals	0.045 mg/kg (max 2.5 mg)‡	q3 wk	1200 mg/m² IV	× 1, q3 wk	40 wk	30 doses	12 doses	14 doses, 16.8 g/m²

AMD, Actinomycin (dactinomycin); *ARST*, Rhabdomyosarcoma and Soft Tissue; *CPM*, cyclophosphamide; *IV*, intravenously; *PO*, orally; *VCR*, vincristine.
*Repetitive-pulse VAC.
†Except during radiation therapy.
‡Lower doses for infants.

RMS. Patients receiving the doxorubicin-ifosfamide and ifosfamide-etoposide combinations and the IRS-III treatment did best in terms of FFS; there was no ultimate difference in OS, however.[279] Again, this analysis failed to shed any specific light on the role of doxorubicin.

In Europe, doxorubicin was part of the vincristine-doxorubicin (Adriamycin)-cyclophosphamide/dactinomycin (actinomycin D) (VACA) and vincristine-doxorubicin (Adriamycin)-ifosfamide-dactinomycin (actinomycin D) (VAIA) regimens of CWS-81 and CWS-86, respectively, was part of retrieval regimens for poor responders in MMT-84, and was widely used in the Italian RMS 79 and RMS 88 studies, but there were no randomized comparisons.[282,295] The addition of epirubicin (a doxorubicin analogue) along with carboplatin and etoposide proved to be no improvement over ifosfamide-vincristine-dactinomycin (actinomycin D) (IVA) in EFS or OS in the MMT-95 study of patients with incompletely excised RMS of unfavorable sites; and the six-drug regimen was considerably more toxic.[296] We still do not know the value of doxorubicin (or other anthracyclines) in treating RMS.

Ifosfamide

DeKraker and Voute reported promising phase II results for the combination of vincristine and ifosfamide and went on to substitute ifosfamide for cyclophosphamide in the VAC combination in an study of 18 previously untreated patients.[297] The German CWS-86 study substituted ifosfamide for cyclophosphamide to change its VACA combination to VAIA, and the results were slightly improved[282]; however, it was not a randomized controlled trial. A randomized controlled comparison of cyclophosphamide and ifosfamide had to await IRS-IV; 457 patients were randomly assigned to either VAC (with cyclophosphamide as a single 2.2 g/m^2 dose) or VAI (with ifosfamide as five daily doses of 1.8 g/m^2 each); the Kaplan-Meier plots of FFS were identical.[293] Thus, although the IVA regimen has long been the European standard for intermediate-risk RMS, there are no data demonstrating its superiority to VAC; and ifosfamide has more urothelial, renal, and neurologic toxicity than cyclophosphamide.[298,299]

Etoposide

A phase II study of etoposide showed some activity in RMS.[300] The IRS-III had a three-way randomization for intermediate-risk patients that included a comparison of VAC with VAC plus cisplatin, plus or minus etoposide. Neither the cisplatin nor the cisplatin-etoposide combination added to the efficacy of VAC.[292]

In a comparison of "phase II window" regimens for patients with metastatic disease at diagnosis, in contrast, ifosfamide-etoposide was significantly superior to the IRS-III combination therapy, ifosfamide-doxorubicin, irinotecan, vincristine-melphalan, topotecan, or topotecan-cyclophosphamide in producing FFS. Survival of the ifosfamide-etoposide–treated patients was also longer, although the proportion surviving at 5 years was not improved.[279]

The combination of ifosfamide and etoposide produced complete or partial responses in 9 of 13 patients with recurrent or refractory RMS in a phase II National Cancer Institute study,[301] a remarkable level of activity. In the IRS-IV study, intermediate-risk patients were randomly assigned to chemotherapy with vincristine-ifosfamide-etoposide, VAC, or VAI; the three regimens had almost identical efficacy.[293] This showed that not only cyclophosphamide and ifosfamide are interchangeable (as given in the trial) but so are etoposide and dactinomycin. Because dactinomycin can be given in a single dose rather than three to five daily doses, and because all four patients who developed myeloid leukemia or myelodysplasia as a second malignancy in IRS-IV had received etoposide,[293] VAC was carried forward as the control regimen for the IRS-V study.

Oral etoposide as a single agent, given daily for 21 days in every 28-day cycle, produced stable disease after two cycles in 3 of 11 patients with refractory or relapsed RMS or other soft tissue sarcoma in a British phase II trial.[302] Responses to oral etoposide appeared to be independent of previous etoposide exposure. A Turkish phase II study of a similar regimen included 4 patients with RMS; 1 had a durable complete response (87+ months), and another had a partial response lasting 10 months.[303] There have been no reports of regimens incorporating oral etoposide into initial therapy or any combination regimens using it in RMS or other pediatric sarcomas.

Topotecan

Topotecan is a camptothecin analogue and as such is a topoisomerase I poison that appeared to be active against a variety of pediatric solid tumors in preclinical trials. In a phase II Pediatric Oncology Group study, the topotecan-cyclophosphamide combination produced complete or partial responses in 10 of 15 patients with RMS.[304] The IRS-COG conducted a "phase II window" study of topotecan alone,[305] and then topotecan with cyclophosphamide,[306] in patients with group IV (metastatic at diagnosis) RMS, but neither distinguished itself in either EFS or OS.[279] More patients with alveolar histology responded to topotecan alone,[305] but the ERMS and ARMS patients responded similarly to topotecan-cyclophosphamide.[304,306]

The IRS-V intermediate-risk study randomized 516 patients between VAC and VAC alternating with vincristine-topotecan-cyclophosphamide. There were no differences in EFS or OS between the two regimens and no differences in toxicity apart from a slightly higher incidence of febrile neutropenia in the VAC arm of the study.[307]

Irinotecan

Irinotecan is another topoisomerase I poison with promising preclinical activity against pediatric solid tumors in preclinical models.[308] A British-French phase II study of irinotecan given as a single bolus dose every 3 weeks to patients with relapsed RMS produced only one complete response and three partial responses among 35 patients.[309] The results of a COG phase II study were similar, with one partial response among 18 RMS patients using a "daily times five" schedule (5 consecutive days of treatment every 3 weeks).[310] A "daily times five times two" schedule (5 days of treatment, 2 days off, then 5 more days of treatment, repeated every 3 weeks) was shown to be promising in both a xenograft model and children with refractory solid tumors in a phase I study,[311] but in an Italian phase II study only 2 of 12 RMS patients had a complete or partial response.[312]

Vincristine and topotecan appeared to be synergistic in mouse xenografts,[313] inspiring a combination of vincristine and irinotecan in an IRS (later COG) study.[314] In the first part of the study, which enrolled patients with RMS metastatic at diagnosis, patients received 6 weeks (two cycles) of irinotecan using the "daily × 5 × 2" schedule, followed by VAC; in the second part patients were treated with vincristine-irinotecan. The response rate for the irinotecan window was 42%, but 32% had progressive disease; and the response rate to the combination vincristine-irinotecan window was 70%, with only 8% having progressive disease. Initial responses did not translate into improved survival, however: patients who declined "phase II window" therapy received VAC alone and had a similar response rate and FFS (23%) to patients receiving vincristine-irinotecan.

A subsequent COG study randomized patients with relapsed or refractory RMS between the "daily × 5 × 2" schedule (10 doses over 2 weeks) and a "daily × 5 × 1" schedule (five doses in 1 week) and found no significant differences in response or toxicity; the authors recommended carrying the more-convenient shorter regimen forward.[315] The most recent COG study for patients with intermediate-risk RMS randomized patients between VAC and alternating 6-week blocks of vincristine-irinotecan and VAC; results are anticipated soon.

Other Agents

Despite good results when the cisplatin-etoposide combination was tested in a phase II study,[316] cisplatin was shown not to add to the efficacy of VAC in intermediate-risk patients in IRS-III, either alone or in combination with etoposide (see earlier). There has been no evaluation of carboplatin in a phase III study, but the addition of carboplatin to the ifosfamide-etoposide combination (the ICE regimen) in a phase II study produced 51% complete and partial responses in patients with a variety of relapsed sarcomas,[317] which was very similar to the response rate to ifosfamide-etoposide, and with greater toxicity. The SIOP MMT-98 study included a "phase II window" of carboplatin in 16 RMS patients with metastases at diagnosis. Five patients had complete or partial responses after two cycles (31%), but 4 (25%) had progressive disease,[318] and the carboplatin-treated patients had significantly worse 3-year EFS than those treated with doxorubicin "window" therapy or those treated with standard four-drug initial therapy.[283] These results, along with the prolonged myelosuppression it produces, have limited enthusiasm for carboplatin.

Melphalan with vincristine was a "phase II window" combination in an IRS-IV trial for patients with metastases at diagnosis; however, it produced an unimpressive response rate and more toxicity than ifosfamide/etoposide.[279,319]

Combinations

Two attempts to improve outcome for patients with intermediate- or high-risk RMS with intense combinations of several agents have failed in randomized controlled trials. IRS-III compared VAC with the same drugs plus doxorubicin and cisplatin, etoposide, or both; the outcomes were identical for the three arms of the study.[292] The MMT-95 study randomly assigned similar patients to IVA or IVA plus carboplatin, epirubicin, and etoposide; the EFS and OS were the same at 3, 5, and 10 years, although the toxicity of the intensified regimen was significantly greater and it was associated with twice as many second malignancies.[296]

The success of alternating vincristine-doxorubicin-cyclophosphamide and ifosfamide-etoposide (VDC-IE) in Ewing sarcoma inspired a limited-institution trial of that therapy in 46 patients with intermediate-risk RMS and a comparison with the results with similar patients in IRS-IV. FFS for VDC-IE and IRS-IV were 82% and 72%, respectively (P = .26), and OS at 5 years was 76% for both. However, a comparison of the VDC-IE patients in a stratified analysis with 346 IRS-IV patients matched for site, histology, age, and clinical group showed a relative risk of failure of 0.5 with VDC-IE (P = .06).[320] The COG has completed a study of interval-compressed VDC-IE combined with vincristine and irinotecan in patients with metastatic RMS (ARST0431), but the results are not yet available.

Alternating topotecan-cyclophosphamide with VAC did not improve outcomes in patients with intermediate-risk RMS in the COG D9803 study[307]; and the results of the ARST0531 study comparing VAC with VAC alternating with vincristine-irinotecan are awaited.

A French phase II study of vinorelbine and continuous oral cyclophosphamide in relapsed pediatric soft tissue sarcomas showed an overall response rate of 36% among 50 patients with RMS.[321] This combination is under study in a phase III EpSSG study (see later).

Duration of Chemotherapy

The IRS-I, II, and III studies prescribed 2 years of treatment for most patients; in IRS-IV the duration of treatment was trimmed to 44 weeks for patients with intermediate-risk tumors and 32 weeks for patients with low-risk tumors.[293] In contrast, the European MMT-84 and CWS-81 and CWS-86 studies used 30 to 56 weeks of therapy.[282,322] The recent COG trials used only 22 weeks of therapy for patients with the lowest-risk tumors and 42 and 51 weeks for intermediate- and high-risk patients respectively. Although there have been no apparent adverse consequences of shorter durations of therapy, there have been no systematic controlled comparisons.

The current EpSSG study is testing the efficacy of 24 weeks of "maintenance" therapy with vinorelbine and oral cyclophosphamide after 26 weeks of intense cyclic chemotherapy for high-risk patients who achieve a complete response.

Treatment Strategies

There have been three broad approaches to the treatment of RMS: the SIOP MMT studies have used intense initial chemotherapy and then SIOP tried to tailor primary tumor treatment according to responses to initial chemotherapy, so as to minimize the use of surgery and radiation (with their accompanying late effects). The Intergroup Rhabdomyosarcoma Studies in North America (now the Soft Tissue Tumor Committee of the COG) has sought to maximize EFS through the use of chemotherapy, surgery, and radiation therapy in almost all patients. The German-Italian CWS studies have taken an intermediate approach. The European groups established a joint European Paediatric Soft Tissue Sarcoma Study Group (EpSSG), which has launched a protocol for localized RMS (RMS-2005), although the Germans have withdrawn from the consortium.

These different philosophies are illustrated in the groups' treatments for orbital RMS. The MMT-84 and MMT-89 studies treated patients with intense multiagent chemotherapy and no radiation therapy for those achieving a complete response. The IRS gave all patients radiation therapy (45 to 55 Gy, depending on the study) and evolving chemotherapy that was either relatively mild (vincristine and dactinomycin) or intense (the IRS-IV randomization between VAC, VIE, and IVA). The CWS studies modulated the radiation dose according to the response to intense multiagent chemotherapy: 40 or 50 Gy in CWS-81 and the Italian ICG-88 study and 32 or 54.4 Gy in CWS-86 for good and poor responders, respectively. Although the three approaches led to very different EFS rates at 10 years (57% for MMT to 86% for IRS, $P < .001$), the OS rates were almost identical (85% and 88%, $P = .67$). The incidence of radiation-associated late effects was higher in the IRS patients than in the MMT patients, although the total burden of therapy in the MMT approach includes the treatment of relapse in 37% of patients.[323]

A recent comparison of Intergroup Rhabdomyosarcoma Study Group (IRSG), SIOP MMT, Italian ICG, and German CWS approaches to bladder-prostate RMS reflected similarly divergent treatment philosophies. Forty-eight percent of SIOP-ICG patients received radiation as part of their initial therapy, compared with 85% of IRSG-CWS patients. However, there were no significant differences in FFS and OS between the groups.[324]

A comparison of RMS of all sites treated on MMT-89 and IRS-IV gave a considerable advantage to the IRS approach, however. Overall, IRS-IV had higher EFS and OS than MMT-89 (78% vs. 57% and 84% vs. 71%, respectively). For some sites there was no difference (e.g., genitourinary tract, not including bladder and prostate: IRS-IV vs. MMT-89 83% vs. 82% EFS, 90% vs. 94% OS), but for others the difference was large (e.g., limbs, IRS-IV vs. MMT-89 64% vs. 35% EFS, 71% vs. 46% OS). For patients with ERMS, the IRS approach had a small advantage for OS (87% vs. 78%) but a large advantage for patients with ARMS (71% vs. 38%), orbital tumors (100% vs. 85%), and nonparameningeal head and neck tumors (89% vs. 64%).[325] Another review found that the four major RMS clinical trial groups enjoyed roughly equal success in preventing metastatic relapse, but there were considerable differences in local relapse, ranging from 13% for the IRS to 30% for the

MMT; the CWS and Italian groups were in the middle, with 19% and 22%.[287]

Response Assessment

Recent results call into question the CWS strategy of modifying treatment according to primary tumor response assessed by conventional imaging (CT or MRI). A review of group III patients treated on IRS-IV demonstrated no relationship between response to the first 8 weeks of therapy (complete, partial, or none) and 5-year FFS. This was true for patients who were initially treated with chemotherapy alone, as well as for those with parameningeal tumors with intracranial extension who received early radiation therapy. The only statistically significant difference found was among patients with ARMS, in whom patients with no response had better FFS (81%) than patients with complete (71%) or partial (39%) responses ($P = .04$).[264] More recently, a review of imaging and second-look surgery results from IRS-IV patients with group III tumors showed a weak relationship between imaging response and histologic response at second-look surgery, with tumor viability at second-look surgery associated with better FFS.[326]

FDG-PET imaging might prove to be useful, because it can differentiate between viable tumor and a residual mass of necrosis or fibrosis.[327] A single-institution retrospective study reviewed RMS patients who had PET/CT performed at diagnosis, after initial chemotherapy, and after radiation therapy. For the 68 patients who had scans at all three times, PET negativity after initial chemotherapy was weakly associated with better local RFS (97% vs. 81% at 3 years, $P = .06$), although the association was stronger for postirradiation PET negativity (94% vs. 75%, $P = .02$). Among patients with a complete response by CT, PET response predicted better local RFS (97% vs. 43%, $P = .01$); but among patients with a residual mass on CT, PET response was not useful (3-year local RFS 80% vs. 64%, $P = .72$).[328]

Current Practice and Protocols

Most RMS patients in North America are enrolled on COG studies, when they are open for accrual. Patients are classified as of low, intermediate, or high risk based on whether there are metastases, the tumor stage, histology, and clinical group (see Table 59-7). Low-risk patients were treated with four cycles of VAC (using a single 1200-mg/m^2 dose of cyclophosphamide), followed by vincristine-dactinomycin for a total of 6 months or 1 year of chemotherapy. Patients with group II or III tumors receive radiation therapy. Intermediate-risk patients were randomized on the COG ARST-0531 study between the standard therapy of VAC for 1 year, or a regimen in which blocks of vincristine-irinotecan therapy alternate with blocks of VAC; results are pending. The results of treatment in high-risk patients are poor enough that it is difficult to designate any treatment as "standard"; the COG recently completed a single-arm study using vincristine-irinotecan and interval-compressed (every-2-week) vincristine doxorubicin-cyclophosphamide alternating with ifosfamide and etoposide, but the data are not yet available.

The EpSSG is using a complex algorithm to classify patients without metastases into eight risk groups and subgroups, with further treatment subdivisions based on response to initial chemotherapy (see Table 59-8). Low-risk patients are being treated with eight cycles of vincristine-dactinomycin. Standard-risk patients are receiving regimens including IVA and vincristine-dactinomycin, whereas high-risk patients are being enrolled in two randomized controlled trials, one evaluating the role of doxorubicin added to IVA and the other exploring "maintenance" chemotherapy with vinorelbine and cyclophosphamide. "Very high risk" patients (those with alveolar histology and involved nodes; EpSSG excludes patients with metastases) are being treated with IVA, doxorubicin, and maintenance vinorelbine-cyclophosphamide. All patients except those with group I ERMS are also receiving radiation therapy.

Primary Tumor Treatment

When only local therapy with surgery and irradiation was available, the survival rate of RMS patients was dismal. Chemotherapy has dramatically improved survival, and it has also changed the surgical and radiotherapeutic approaches, with minimization of late effects becoming a new priority. Optimal outcomes require multidisciplinary care.

Surgery

The surgeon is often involved with an RMS patient from the time of initial biopsy. This is best done at the cancer center where treatment will occur and where a full complement of diagnostic tools (including molecular techniques) is available. The biopsy needs careful planning and execution, because diagnosis, treatment, and late effects can all depend on it.

The earliest classification system for RMS, the IRS clinical grouping system, is based on the amount of tumor remaining after the first surgical intervention, be it a complete excision with clear margins (group I) or only a biopsy with gross residual disease remaining (group III) (see Table 59-5). IRS-I showed that the clinical group is a powerful predictor of survival[280] and established the role of surgery in the treatment of RMS in the chemotherapy era. Although initial complete surgical excision can involve disfigurement or loss of function, it may have a smaller late effects burden than primary tumor treatment with radiation in some patients, so multidisciplinary consultation is essential.

When a patient's initial excision leaves microscopically positive margins (group II), or when the initial excision was performed outside the pediatric cancer center, there may be value in a "primary reexcision" before chemotherapy begins. An analysis of patients with trunk or limb RMS in IRS-I and IRS-II showed that group II patients converted to group I had the same survival as patients who were rendered group I in their initial procedure. Patients who were referred as group I patients and had primary reexcisions had superior outcomes to those who did not.[329]

Regional lymph node sampling is important in limb primary tumors, which often have alveolar histology and a predilection for nodal involvement. Patients age 10 years or older with paratesticular RMS also have an increased risk of paraspinal nodal relapse and should have node sampling. Otherwise, lymph node sampling may be limited to nodes that are suspicious by physical examination or imaging.[330,331]

Traditional surgical teaching is that an attempt at excision is not valuable unless the patient can be left with microscopic residual disease at most (group I or II). Among patients with unresectable tumors (group III), debulking surgery may be beneficial even if the patients remain in clinical group III. In a retrospective study of IRS patients treated between 1984 and 1991 with large (≥ 5 cm) group III or IV retroperitoneal tumors, patients with embryonal histology who underwent debulking surgery before chemotherapy fared better than those who did not (FFS 72% vs. 39% at 4 years, $P = .03$); too few patients with alveolar histology tumors had debulking surgery to permit analysis.[332] It is not yet clear whether this principle applies only to retroperitoneal tumors or whether it is generally applicable. However, a retrospective analysis of the Italian RMS-79, RMS-88, and RMS-96 protocols that compared the fate of 323 patients with biopsy only and 71 patients with debulking surgery (defined as more than 50% excision but still group III) found no overall benefit. One subgroup, patients 10 years or older, appeared to benefit from debulking surgery (EFS 73% vs. 50%, $P = .04$; OS 83% vs. 62%, $P = .06$), but no other subgroup defined by site, size, histology, invasiveness, or response to initial chemotherapy did so.[333]

In patients with gross residual disease when chemotherapy begins (group III and IV), second-look operations and delayed excision of residual tumor masses, even after radiation therapy and chemotherapy, may improve the chances for survival. In a retrospective study of second-look operations in IRS-III, 12% of patients clinically believed to have had a complete response had residual viable tumor and three fourths of patients clinically believed to have had a partial response or no response either had no viable tumor or were converted to a complete response at surgery. These "converted" patients had the same 3-year survival as those whose complete responses were confirmed at second-look surgery (73% and 80%, respectively).[331] A single-institution study of 48 group III patients showed that those who had a delayed complete surgical excision (n = 22) had superior RFS and OS to those who did not (approximately 90% vs. 60% RFS, $P = .013$).[334] Patient numbers were too small to permit a multivariate analysis, however, and histology and nodal status were also significant variables on univariate analysis.

Radiation Therapy

Because RMS can often occur in sites that are not amenable to surgery, radiation therapy has a key role in primary tumor treatment. Advances in radiation therapy techniques are reducing the acute and late morbidities of treatment. However, there are large gaps in our knowledge of how best to use radiation to treat RMS.

The first knowledge gap is to determine who needs radiation therapy. A retrospective analysis of 439 group

I patients in IRS-I, IRS-II, and IRS-III found no benefit from irradiation for patients with embryonal tumors for OS (95% at 10 years for both groups, $P = .83$). For alveolar and undifferentiated tumors, however, each of the IRS studies showed a benefit from radiation therapy, analyzing by treatment received.[335] Subsequently, an analysis of IRS-III and IRS-IV data found no EFS or OS advantage for radiation therapy in alveolar stage 1 and 2 tumors but it remained important for patients with stage III tumors.[336]

A retrospective analysis of the CWS-81, CWS-86, CWS-91, and CWS-96 studies showed that the use of radiation therapy roughly halved the risk for death for patients with embryonal tumors smaller than 5 cm ($P = .02$) and for patients with larger embryonal tumors ($P = .001$) but had a smaller effect for patients with alveolar tumors (risk of death ratio 0.7, $P = .09$).[287] Another analysis of the same studies focused on 203 patients with group II tumors (microscopic residual disease at diagnosis). It compared the 110 patients who received radiation therapy with the 93 who did not (for a variety of reasons). The two groups of patients differed significantly in histology (more irradiated patients had alveolar tumors), site (more extremity and parameningeal tumors, and fewer vaginal-paratesticular tumors, among the irradiated patients), and age (fewer infants among the irradiated patients). All patients received combination chemotherapy according to one of several regimens. Despite the greater number of unfavorable characteristics among the irradiated patients, their local control was better (83% vs. 65%, $P < .04$), and their EFS was better (76% vs. 58%, $P < .005$), although the OS rates of the irradiated and unirradiated patients were similar (84% and 77%).[337] In the IRS studies I through IV there were 37 patients with group II tumors who did not receive radiation; their FFS was 69%, and OS 85%, which was very similar to the 73% and 78%, respectively, for the entire cohort.[338] Thus radiation therapy probably confers an advantage to group II patients but it is far from indispensable for local control and survival.

The management of patients with initially unresected tumors (Group III) who have delayed excisions is also a contentious issue. The IRS and subsequent COG protocols have required radiation therapy for these patients, although European protocols have not. A single institution study of 48 patients with group III RMS identified 22 who had complete excisions at second-look surgery, of whom 13 were treated with subsequent radiation and 9 were not. One patient in each group experienced relapse ($P = .67$), neither at the primary site.[334] In the MMT-89 study, 58% of the 289 survivors with "incomplete" initial surgery or biopsy only had either chemotherapy alone or chemotherapy plus "conservative" local therapy (defined as no functional deficits and no external-beam irradiation).[339] Unfortunately, these patients are not classified by stage or site, but radiation therapy was not indispensable for cure. Similarly, the CWS-86 study had 31 group III patients who did not receive radiation therapy (16 because of age <3 years), again not classified by site or histology. All but 1 had a complete response to chemotherapy and surgery. The local relapse rate was 27%, versus 10% for patients receiving radiation ($P = .2$), and the overall relapse rate was 40%, versus 28% for irradiated patients ($P = .001$).[282] Thus, although radiation therapy seems to reduce the local recurrence risk and improves the survival rate for patients with group III tumors, it is not indispensable.

Assuming the use of radiation therapy, the question becomes how much radiation the different presentations of RMS require to maximize the chances for cure. At the low side of the dose-response curve, it is unclear how much radiation is advisable. A single-institution study of 32 patients with IRS group II RMS (all but two embryonal histology) used chemotherapy (vincristine, doxorubicin, actinomycin, cyclophosphamide, with or without methotrexate, bleomycin, and carmustine) and from 30 to 60 Gy of radiation. Nineteen patients received 40 Gy or less, with only one local relapse; 14 received 36 Gy or less, with the same single local failure.[340] The CWS-86 study compared 67 group III patients who received 25 to 35 Gy (mean 31.6 Gy) with 49 patients who received 40 to 67 Gy (mean 52 Gy); 31% of the lower-dose group and 26% of the higher-dose group experienced relapse, although a higher proportion of the relapses in the higher-dose group were metastatic rather than local or regional.[282] In this study, the higher doses of radiation seem to have reduced the risk for local recurrence. The COG D9602 study of low-risk RMS used lower doses of radiation for selected patients: 36 Gy for patients with microscopic residual, N0 disease (41.4 Gy in earlier studies), and 45 Gy for patients with orbital tumors (had been 50.4 Gy). The local relapse rates were higher than in IRS-IV, but changes in chemotherapy for orbital and vaginal tumors (elimination of cyclophosphamide or ifosfamide) complicated the analysis. The authors concluded that the lower radiation doses do not lead to poorer local control, provided that cyclophosphamide is part of the chemotherapy.[341,342]

At the high side of the dose-response curve, IRS-IV randomized patients with group III tumors between 50.4 Gy by conventional fractionation (180 cGy/day) and 59.4 Gy by hyperfractionation (110 cGy twice daily). The hyperfractionated regimen was designed to allow a higher dose without an increase in late effects. There was no difference in any outcome measure between the two regimens (FFS, OS, local relapse, distant relapse) and no difference according to histology.[293] This indicates that 50.4 Gy is sufficient to control most gross residual RMS; less radiation may be equally efficacious.

In an effort to spare normal tissues from radiation, some institutions have used brachytherapy at the time of second-look surgery.[343-346] This technique usually involves the placement of catheters in the tumor or tumor bed during surgery; the catheters are subsequently loaded with radioactive pellets and then removed when the dose is complete. The brachytherapy dose often needs to be supplemented with external-beam radiation, and we have found that intensity-modulated radiation therapy (IMRT) and proton therapy have largely replaced brachytherapy.

Some institutions have also used intraoperative radiation therapy (IORT), which involves the delivery of a single large fraction of external-beam radiation with the tumor or tumor bed surgically exposed. Generally, larger radiation fractions decrease the therapeutic index, especially for late effects, and this may be the case in pediatric IORT. One series of seven children treated with IORT for neuroblastoma followed for 4 to 143 months (median 38 months) after irradiation; all 7 had hypertension, 5 had vascular stenosis in the radiation field, and 2 patients died in remission (one of mesenteric artery stenosis and bowel ischemia and another of massive ascites).[347] Similarly, of eight surviving patients in another series treated for a variety of pediatric solid tumors, 2 patients required surgery for hydronephrosis and small bowel obstruction, a third developed severe renovascular hypertension and superior mesenteric artery stenosis, and 2 developed neuropathies.[348] In another series, 3 of 14 children treated with IORT for recurrent brain tumors developed radiation necrosis within 6 to 12 months.[349] However, the largest reported series of IORT-treated children (n = 59) who had a variety of malignancies, recorded no long-term toxicities among the 14 long-term survivors.[350]

Proton therapy minimizes the irradiation of normal tissues surrounding the target, and its resulting potential to decrease late effects makes it particularly attractive for treating children. Proton therapy is currently available only at a small (but growing) number of centers, and there are few systematic evaluations. A comparison of conformal radiation, IMRT, and proton plans for a patient with parameningeal RMS calculated that protons reduced the risk for a second malignant neoplasm by a factor of two or more.[351] A retrospective study of 17 consecutive children with parameningeal RMS found 4 with local recurrences (of whom 3 had had intracranial extension at diagnosis), and late effects that were similar to or less frequent than those reported in other studies.[352] Ten of those patients had both proton and IMRT plans, and a comparison of them showed that the two techniques provided equally good coverage of the target volumes but the proton fields greatly reduced the irradiation of normal tissues (by factors of twentyfold to over fiftyfold for median doses to contralateral structures), except for the ipsilateral cochlea and mastoid.[353] Another study compared the proton and three-dimensional conformal radiotherapeutic plans of seven patients treated with protons for orbital RMS. Proton therapy reduced the radiation dose to the hypothalamus, pituitary, temporal lobes, and optic chiasm by 82% to 94% and reduced the dose to the ipsilateral lens by 65%.[354] Similarly, an analysis of 7 consecutive patients with bladder-prostate RMS showed that proton therapy statistically significantly reduced radiation doses to the bladder, testes, femoral heads (sixfold), growth plates, pelvic bones, and bone volume compared with IMRT. Rectal, prostatic, and bowel doses were not significantly affected.[355] More patients, longer follow-up, and application of objective criteria will be necessary to determine whether the lower doses lead to fewer or milder late effects.

The last radiation therapy variable is timing, which has been most controversial in parameningeal RMS. Different IRSG and COG protocols have called for radiation for parameningeal RMS to begin at times ranging from the first week of treatment to the twelfth. Earlier radiotherapy was associated with better survival in IRS-II and IRS-III, although there were so many other changes in treatment that its role cannot be isolated.[291] A recent analysis of consecutive studies has settled the question. In IRS-IV, patients with parameningeal RMS and cranial nerve palsies or cranial base bony erosion had irradiation during the first week, and similar patients in COG D9803 had irradiation beginning in the twelfth week; patients with no such risk factors had irradiation beginning at weeks 6 to 9 in IRS-IV and week 12 in COG D9803. For all parameningeal RMS patients, the 5-year local failure rate, FFS, and OS were almost identical in the two studies (19% local failure in both, $P = .67$; FFS 70% vs. 67%, $P = .32$; OS 75% vs. 73%, $P = .45$). There were also no statistically significant or consistent differences in local failure rates within the groups of patients with and without intracranial extension or cranial nerve palsies.[356] There appears to be no advantage to earlier radiation therapy in RMS; in fact, there may be an advantage to later irradiation through reduction of late effects. A single-institution study of 22 patients with parameningeal RMS showed that the use of delayed irradiation with a shrinking field technique reduced the mean treated area by half, from 99 cm² before chemotherapy to 48 cm² after chemotherapy, with no apparent effect on RFS.[357]

Special Situations
Infants and Toddlers

Infants with RMS differ from older children in the characteristics of their tumors, their treatment, and their responses to treatment and outcomes. An analysis of 76 infants (age <1 year) treated on IRS-IV and IRS-V showed fewer embryonal and more undifferentiated and other histologies in infants than in older children (ages 1 to 9 years). Infants also had more tumors of the limbs, trunk, bladder-prostate, and abdomen and fewer tumors of the parameningeal sites and orbit.[273]

Treating small children with unresectable (group III) tumors without devastating late effects can be difficult, because tissues irradiated to the doses used for RMS will not grow. Results with very young patients treated without radiation challenge the dogma that radiation therapy is essential for cure of all but group I patients. In the CWS-86 study, 30 patients with stage III (equivalent to group III) tumors, about half of them younger than age 3 years, were treated without radiation therapy, having achieved a complete response with chemotherapy and surgery. Twelve of the 30 (40%) experienced relapse, and 8 (27% of the 30 patients) had local recurrences, for a progression-free survival (PFS) rate of about 60%.[282] Although this was similar to the EFS rate for stage III patients with a complete response to initial therapy in this study, the patients are not classified according to other risk factors (such as site), and the numbers are too small for statistically meaningful comparison. In the IRS-IV and IRS-V analysis, 23 of 72 infants with group III tumors received no radiation; their 5-year FFS was inferior to that of the group receiving radiation (32 vs. 47%, $P = .17$), but the OS was similar (58% vs. 63%, $P = .49$).[273]

Infants and toddlers also appear to tolerate aggressive chemotherapy less well than older children. In the COG D9803 intermediate-risk study, which used VAC with a single dose of dactinomycin and 2.2 g/m^2 of cyclophosphamide, there were 18 cases of hepatopathy resembling sinusoidal obstructive syndrome, 4 of them fatal.[358] The total incidence of hepatopathy among 339 eligible patients was 6%, but it was 14% for patients younger than 36 months and only 4% for older patients. A modification of dactinomycin and cyclophosphamide doses for young patients ameliorated the problem. Cooperative group protocols have varying schemes for calculating infant chemotherapy doses (such as using a weight basis rather than a surface area basis), but none has a foundation in data.

The effects of these compromises on outcome is unclear. A retrospective analysis of IRS-COG studies from 1984 through 1997 (IRS-III, IRS-IV pilot, and IRS-IV) found that patients younger than 1 year of age have a much lower FFS than patients aged 1 to 9 years and one similar to that of adolescents (age ≥ 10 years) (53% v. 72% vs. 52%, $P < .001$)[272]; the infants with nonmetastatic RMS in IRS-IV and IRS-V did similarly.[273] In contrast, the SIOP MMT-84 and MMT-89 studies compared infants (<1 year of age) with localized RMS to children aged 1 to 9 years and adolescents 10 years and older and found identical EFS and OS rates between the infants and older children, both of whom did better than the adolescents (EFS 57% vs. 58% vs. 42%; OS 72% vs. 72% vs. 59%, $P < .001$ between adolescents and the other groups).[359] The infants more often had alveolar histology than older children and also more often had bladder-prostate and limb primary sites. In the earlier IRS study and the MMT studies there was no analysis of deviations from protocol therapy, whereas the later COG analysis showed many deviations from protocol-prescribed radiation therapy but few from prescribed chemotherapy. It remains unclear how reductions in therapy and biologic differences contribute to the inferior outcomes.

Bladder and Prostate Tumors

Because RMS can occur anywhere in the pelvis, and because pelvic tumors are often very large at the time of diagnosis, the exact primary site may be difficult to determine. One should not assume that a pelvic RMS is arising from the bladder or prostate without definitive imaging or cystoscopy. Bladder-prostate tumors usually produce urinary symptoms and are rarely alveolar histology, so one should be especially suspicious that tumors without these characteristics are arising in nongenitourinary pelvic sites. This distinction can have large implications for primary tumor treatment.

The evolution of approaches to bladder-prostate RMS can be traced through the IRS trials. Early approaches included extensive surgery (often complete or partial pelvic exenteration) in addition to chemotherapy. In IRS-I, more than half of the patients with bladder-prostate RMS had initial excisions (group I or group II), often involving anterior exenteration or cystectomy. At 5 years the DFS rate was 67% and the OS rate was 76%. The

effectiveness of chemotherapy led to efforts to use initial chemotherapy and postpone and reduce surgery in favor of radiation therapy in hopes of preserving genitourinary anatomy and function. When this approach was taken in IRS-II, the proportion of group I or II patients decreased to 5%. However, the DFS rate declined substantially (to 51%), although the OS was comparable (71%). The new approach had no effect on the proportion of patients alive and with intact bladders, however, which were 23% in IRS-I and 22% in IRS-II.[360] The IRS-III study used more intense chemotherapy (all patients receiving VAC plus doxorubicin, cisplatin, and etoposide), radiation therapy beginning at week 6, and second-look surgery at week 20. The fraction of patients retaining their bladders rose to 60%, with PFS and OS rates improving to 74% and 83%, respectively.[292,361] IRS-IV used different chemotherapy, moved the radiation therapy from week 6 to week 9, and encouraged second surgical procedures short of complete cystectomy or prostatectomy unless there was biopsy-proven residual tumor at the end of therapy or progression. The OS rate of the 88 reviewed patients was 82%, the FFS rate was 77%, and 63% of patients retained their bladders.[362] A retrospective study of 63 CWS patients produced similar results, with an approach that varied the radiation dose and fractionation for group II and III patients according the response to initial chemotherapy.[363] As discussed previously, a comparison of results from the Italian, SIOP MMT, German CWS, and IRS/COG studies showed statistically insignificant variations in EFS despite the groups' different approaches, and no difference in OS (range, 79% to 85%; $P = .93$).[324]

There have been two problems with these bladder-preserving strategies: often the bladders do not work very well, and the collateral side effects can be considerable. Radiation therapy can cause fibrosis of the bladder and sphincters, leading to limited bladder capacity, dribbling, or incontinence. Radiation therapy to the pelvis limits bony growth, and even with modern IMRT techniques it can be difficult to avoid irradiation of the hip joints, leading to future orthopedic problems. A review of IRS-I and IRS-II patients, which involved asking physicians whether their patients' urinary function was normal, found "normal" urinary function in 73% of the 52 patients who had retained all or part of their bladders; the remaining 27% had incontinence, frequency, or nocturia. Radiation therapy and cyclophosphamide (before mesna's availability) combined to produce hematuria after completion of treatment in 20%. Outside the urinary tract, spontaneous reporting disclosed 4 patients with colostomies to repair fistulas or relieve strictures and 6% with fecal incontinence, chronic diarrhea, or rectal stenosis. Eight percent had orthopedic problems, including slipped femoral epiphyses, and pelvic fibrosis or hypoplasia.[364]

A more recent study of IRS-IV patients used routine follow-up forms and questionnaires to physicians. Of 55 patients with preserved bladders, two thirds were reported to have normal urinary function while the balance had late diversions, dribbling, incontinence, enuresis, hydronephrosis, or strictures. Interestingly, no differences in relapse rate or pattern could be found between patients who had protocol-specified radiation therapy and those who had major deviations in radiation therapy (including 9 who received none), although 2 irradiated patients developed second malignancies.[362]

The cooperative group data may underestimate the frequency and severity of late effects in this population, however. A single-institution study of 26 girls cured of pelvic RMS (including nonbladder sites) found that 23 (88%) had grade III or IV late effects at a median of 20 years follow-up, with over half requiring surgery for these complications. The most common problems were musculoskeletal hypoplasia, recurrent urinary tract infections, incontinence, urinary reflux, and short stature. There were three secondary solid tumors in radiation fields. Radiation therapy was associated with more late effects per patient ($P = .002$), and patients treated since 1984 had about twice as many late effects per patient than patients treated earlier (12.5 vs. 6.5, $P = .041$).[365]

None of these studies used urodynamics to measure bladder function objectively. One single-institution study that did so had 11 patients with pelvic RMS (7 with tumors of the bladder or prostate) and found that all 7 patients who had received radiation therapy had markedly reduced bladder capacity (11% to 48% of age norms) and abnormal voiding patterns; 4 had upper tract abnormalities, and 2 had severe bilateral hydronephrosis.[366]

Bladder-prostate RMS is unusual in that one can monitor the tumor easily with cystoscopy and biopsy. In view of the considerable late effects of radiation therapy in particular, some centers use cystoscopic and histologic monitoring to delay and minimize the use of irradiation, moving in the direction of the SIOP MMT studies.[367] This requires expert pathologic interpretation, however, because distinguishing between viable RMS and harmless differentiated rhabdomyoblasts can be very difficult, especially in the field of previous surgery or radiation therapy.[367,368]

Vaginal Tumors

Excellent survival rates make the female genitourinary tract a favorable site in RMS trials but one fraught with anatomic, late effects, and emotional difficulties. In the young girls in whom this tumor most often occurs, the vagina is very small, very thin-walled, deep in the pelvis, and sandwiched between the urethra (and bladder, if distended with tumor) and the rectum. The late effects of complete or partial excision are severe, as can be the effects of radiation therapy (on both the soft tissues and nearby hips). The use of chemotherapy and conservative surgery alone is thus very attractive.

A retrospective survey of female genitourinary RMS patients on the MMT-84 and MMT-89 studies, which used the SIOP strategy of relying on chemotherapy (IVA regimen) and avoiding local therapy whenever possible, included 38 patients. Four had initially complete excisions with conservative surgery and survived event free; 13 had incomplete excisions and chemotherapy with no further local therapy and were event-free survivors; and 17 required local therapy for microscopic or gross residual tumor after initial chemotherapy. This was radical

surgery in 6 patients, radiation in 10, and conservative surgery in 1. Although it is extremely difficult to trace the 38 patients through their treatment, the data showed that about half of girls with genitourinary RMS were cured with the IVA chemotherapy regimen without radical surgery or irradiation.[369]

More recently, the COG reviewed vaginal RMS treated on the consecutive low-risk studies D9602 and ARST0331. On the former study, group I and IIA (microscopic local disease) patients received 45 weeks of vincristine-dactinomycin, whereas patients with regional nodal involvement or gross residual tumor (groups IIB, IIC, and III) received 45 weeks of VAC. In ARST0331, patients received four cycles of VAC (with a lower dose of cyclophosphamide; see Table 59-9) and then VA to a total of 24 weeks (groups I and IIA) or 46 weeks (all others). Local therapy was based on response assessments beginning at week 11 to reduce or avoid radiation. Of 37 group IIA or III patients, only 4 received radiation; 4 had tumor progression before local treatment. However, the local recurrence rates were 26% and 43% on D9602 and ARST0331, respectively, and there appeared to be a strong relationship between total cyclophosphamide dose and risk of local recurrence. Therapy after recurrence was not collected systematically, but OS was excellent despite the local recurrences (100% on D9602 and 94% on ARST0331).[370] Successful treatment of vaginal RMS without mutilating surgery or irradiation appears possible using alkylating agent–containing chemotherapy (VAC or IVA regimens) and careful local surveillance. Fortunately, females are much less likely than males to be sterilized by alkylator chemotherapy.

Parameningeal Tumors

The parameningeal sites include the nasal cavity and nasopharynx, parapharyngeal space, paranasal sinuses (ethmoid, maxillary, and sphenoid), the pterygopalatine and infratemporal fossae, and the middle ear and mastoid sinuses. Parameningeal RMS has a tendency to invade the cranium and intracranial contents, either by eroding through the skull base or by extending through a foramen. Curiously, tumors arising in the orbits are much less aggressive. Complete excision of parameningeal tumors at diagnosis is almost never possible, so that they are at best stage II, group III in the IRS-COG staging system. The vast majority are of embryonal histology.

In the IRS-I study, 5-year OS was only 47%[280]; it was identical in CWS-81.[371] The IRS-II study intensified therapy for patients with parameningeal tumors with craniospinal radiation and intrathecal chemotherapy (methotrexate, cytarabine, and hydrocortisone) beginning immediately after diagnosis, and OS improved to 67%.[281,372] IRS-III substituted whole-brain for craniospinal radiation therapy and began it early only for patients with cranial nerve palsies or intracranial extension or base-of-skull erosion on imaging; chemotherapy was also considerably more intense. Survival improved again, to 73%, but 5 patients (3.4%) developed ascending myelitis, which was fatal in 3.[373] In IRS-IV, intrathecal chemotherapy was eliminated, and the radiation field was reduced to the involved area with a 5-cm margin, with no loss of efficacy found on a retrospective analysis of 611 IRS II-IV patients.[372]

A univariate analysis of parameningeal RMS patients in IRS II and IRS-IV identified age between 1 and 9 years; site in the nasal cavity, nasopharynx, parapharynx, middle ear, or mastoid; and lack of bony erosion or intracranial extension as favorable features.[372] Patients with entirely favorable features had a 92% OS at 5 years, compared with 57% for those with entirely unfavorable features. Size and histology were not statistically significant factors.

Results in Europe lagged far behind, with 5-year OS 55% in SIOP, 47% in Germany, and 39% in Italy.[374] An international workshop in 1994 combining the American and European experience recommended routine use of MRI to define the extent of the tumor; treatment of all parameningeal RMS patients with radiation therapy (in the SIOP-84 study 18 of 44 had not been irradiated, with only 5 surviving); a minimum dose of 50 Gy with a 2-cm margin; and routine external quality control of radiation.[374]

Recent results have largely settled the long-running controversy over the timing of radiation in parameningeal RMS, as discussed in an earlier section.

Relapsed Rhabdomyosarcoma

The prognoses of patients whose RMS relapses are highly variable, but mostly depend on initial tumor characteristics and treatment. An analysis of survival after relapse in 605 IRS-III, IRS-IV pilot, and IRS-IV patients showed 5-year survival rates ranging from 3% (for patients with alveolar histology and originally group II through group IV tumors) to 72% (for patients with originally stage I or group I tumors and embryonal histology).[375] The median survival for all relapsed patients was 9.8 months, and OS was 17% at 5 years. Postrelapse survival for patients with embryonal histology was far better than for those with alveolar or undifferentiated tumors, but other prognostic factors were different for the two histologic groups.

An analysis of relapsed patients from Italian RMS studies (n = 125) identified metastatic relapse, unfavorable primary site, alveolar histology, and relapse or progression during initial therapy to be unfavorable features. When each of those was used as a risk factor, the 5-year survival ranged from 72% with no risk factors to nil with three or four factors.[376] The analysis only included patients with initially localized tumors, which may be why the median survival after relapse (15.4 months) and 5-year OS (28%) were better than those observed in the IRSG study.

The most sophisticated analysis of postrelapse survival was based on nonmetastatic patients who experienced relapse after treatment on the SIOP MMT-84, MMT-89, and MMT-95 studies (n = 474). Two thirds of the relapsed patients had not had irradiation as part of their original treatment, reflecting the philosophy behind the studies. In a multivariate analysis, the prognostic variables were the type of chemotherapy (2, 3, or 6 drugs), histology, nodal status, primary site, original size, metastatic or local recurrence, radiation therapy as part of initial treatment, and time to recurrence. These eight variables were combined into a nomogram, permitting estimation of prognosis for an individual patient.[377] The remarkably high OS rate (36% at 5 years) reflects the exclusion of patients whose tumors were metastatic at diagnosis, and the omission of initial radiation therapy in a large proportion of patients.

For treatment of relapsed RMS, after a COG trial in patients with metastases at diagnosis demonstrated that vincristine-irinotecan was superior to vincristine alone,[314] the COG conducted a randomized controlled trial in relapsed patients of two schedules of vincristine-irinotecan "window" therapy followed by five-drug alternating chemotherapy (vincristine-doxorubicin-cyclophosphamide/ifosfamide-etoposide). This showed that a 5-day schedule with irinotecan 50 mg/m²/day was less toxic, and at least as effective, as a "daily × 5 × 2" schedule that used 20 mg/m²/day irinotecan for 5 days on 2 consecutive weeks. Unfortunately, the median survival remained dismal at 1.3 and 1.4 years, as did FFS (14% and 15% at 3 years).[315] The most recent COG study (ARST0921) was a randomized phase II trial comparing bevacizumab and temsirolimus added to concurrent vinorelbine and cyclophosphamide. The results are pending.

Megatherapy for Metastatic and Recurrent Rhabdomyosarcomas

A perennial question in the treatment of patients with metastases at diagnosis, or who have experienced relapse, is the role of megatherapy: high-dose chemotherapy, with or without total-body irradiation, with autologous (occasionally allogeneic) stem cell or marrow transplantation. The analytic problems are large: there are vast differences between different populations of patients with metastases, with 3-year survivals ranging from 5% to 47% and an even wider range of prognoses for patients with relapsed RMS (see earlier). There are also wide variations in entry criteria for megatherapy studies, ranging from having a complete response to initial salvage chemotherapy, to failing to achieve a complete response to initial chemotherapy. Often, the entry criteria and key terms (e.g., "high risk") remain undefined. For all these reasons, reports of results of megatherapy in RMS merit careful scrutiny (see the excellent review by Meyers[378]).

Two recent systematic reviews of high-dose therapy in metastatic RMS could find no randomized controlled trials, and only two historically controlled trials, each with serious methodologic limitations and potential biases. The reviews concluded that there is no evidence to justify the use of megatherapy in metastatic RMS patients outside a controlled clinical trial.[379,380] Until randomized controlled trials are performed, the role of megatherapy in RMS will remain dubious.

FOLLOW-UP AFTER TREATMENT

Surveillance and Patterns of Recurrence

Examination of Kaplan-Meier plots of many studies of newly diagnosed RMS shows that the vast majority of failures (progression or relapse) occur in the 3 years after diagnosis, although they can occur even 9 years after diagnosis. The complex nature of RMS persists as complex patterns of failure, varying by primary site and histology, and being local, regional (lymph nodes), metastatic, or any combination. In IRS-III, for example, local failures outnumbered distant ones by 7:1 among patients with orbital primary tumors; but among patients with extremity primary sites, distant and combined failures outnumbered local ones by almost 7:1. Among patients with embryonal histology tumors, local failures outnumbered combined and distant failures by about 2:1; but among patients with alveolar and "other" histology, combined and distant failures were more common.[381]

In the same analysis of failure patterns in IRS-III, univariate analysis identified N1 (clinically positive) nodal status as the key risk factor for local or combined local and regional or distant failure; N1 nodal status was, in turn, associated with older age, alveolar histology, large (>5 cm) tumors, and unfavorable primary sites.[381] Distant failure was most likely in patients with N1 nodes and primary tumors in limbs.

A review of IRS-IV data showed that achievement of a complete response at the end of therapy (no residual tumor present on examination and conventional imaging) appears to have no effect on prognosis in group III RMS patients; nor does it influence local, regional, or distant failure rates (e.g., complete vs. partial or no response 13.5% vs. 13.5% for local failure). Similarly, resection of a residual mass at the end of therapy did not appear to improve outcome.[382]

Failure patterns appear to have changed across the first three IRS studies, but this may be due to shifts in definitions and classifications. Attention to definitions is again necessary when assessing reports, because, for example, failures in regional lymph nodes may be considered local (if they were within the radiation therapy field), regional, or distant.

The follow-up intervals and procedures prescribed in COG RMS protocols reflect the changes in risk over time. They include a history, physical examination, and chest imaging (radiograph or CT) every 3 months during the first year off therapy, every 4 months during the second and third years, and every 6 months during the fourth year, with primary site imaging depending on the site and the primary tumor treatment used. During and annually after this follow-up for tumor recurrence, monitoring for late effects of treatment is also necessary, especially for tissues in a radiation field.

Late Effects

The late effects of childhood cancer and its treatment are discussed thoroughly in Chapter 71. In patients treated for RMS, most observed late effects are from the tumor itself (e.g., cranial nerve palsies from parameningeal tumors), surgery, and radiation therapy. Radiation therapy sequelae are particularly problematical because of the young ages of many of the patients and the locations of their tumors.

Chemotherapy late effects particularly relevant to RMS include late hemorrhagic cystitis from cyclophosphamide and ifosfamide and secondary myelodysplasia or leukemia. Ifosfamide may cause a nephropathy, which is occasionally progressive.[383] Relatively few patients treated on current protocols receive anthracyclines (with their attendant risk of late heart disease) or cisplatin (with its hearing loss and renal dysfunction). Sterility in males and early menopause in females may result from the high doses of alkylating agents used.

FUTURE DIRECTIONS

Among ERMS there is an enormous range of clinical behavior that varies with site and age. Fusion-bearing ARMS is a highly aggressive tumor, with the PAX7-FOXO1–bearing variant perhaps being less so. However, we remain far from having molecularly based classification of RMS that correlates with, much less explains, the enormous variations observed in clinical behavior, especially among embryonal (fusion-negative) tumors. Techniques such as gene expression profiling, application of epigenetic analyses, and increasingly sophisticated evaluation of combined clinical and laboratory data may allow us to discern the combinations of tumor and host variables that make, for example, a paratesticular ERMS much more aggressive in a teenager than in a preschooler.

More sophisticated classification opens opportunities for "tailoring" chemotherapy but also presents the challenge of smaller populations of patients for study. In the COG, it is already barely statistically feasible to carry out randomized controlled trials with intermediate-risk patients in 5 years. International collaboration has the benefit of providing larger patient numbers, but having fewer studies means that fewer ideas are tested. The bureaucratic and regulatory barriers are also formidable. The path through these obstacles is not obvious.

Therapeutically, there are two challenges: identifying promising new agents and integrating them into existing therapy. One cannot predict which of the many newly discovered biochemical pathways and small molecule inhibitors will lead to improvements in outcome in RMS patients. The numbers of patients are too small to provide an attractive market for the pharmaceutical industry, so an agent that would, for example, specifically block the action of the PAX-FOXO1 fusion proteins is unlikely to become available. Downstream of the fusion proteins lay potential pharmacologic targets that may well be commercially interesting, however. Immunotherapy is a possibility for the future if appropriate antigens can be found and paired with the appropriate technology.[384]

The quest for new targets and agents is very unlikely to lead to a "magic bullet" that makes current therapy obsolete. Thus we must continue our efforts with "traditional" chemotherapy and carefully integrate new agents. The closest to clinical application are probably the tyrosine kinase inhibitors (particularly pazopanib) and "rapalog" mTOR inhibitors, but the former have only been tested in mice, and one of the latter is in a phase II trial in combination with chemotherapy. Large improvements in outcome have occurred in the leukemias in the past decade, with a collection of drugs that are at least 25 years old; one of the advantages of that disease system is easy evaluation of response through marrow aspiration. Good early response markers (perhaps PET) could extend the same advantage to RMS and other solid tumors.

References available online at ExpertConsult.

KEY REFERENCES

5. Rudzinski ER, Teot LA, Anderson JR, et al: Dense pattern of embryonal rhabdomyosarcoma, a lesion easily confused with alveolar rhabdomyosarcoma: a report from the Soft Tissue Sarcoma Committee of the Children's Oncology Group. *Am J Clin Pathol* 140:82–90, 2013.
   This article refines the histopathologic diagnosis of ERMS and ARMS.
10. Quezada E, Gripp KW: Costello syndrome and related disorders. *Curr Opin Pediatr* 19:636–644, 2007.
   A summary is presented of the finding of HRAS mutations in Costello syndrome, which increases susceptibility to ERMS development.
19. Galili N, Davis RJ, Fredericks WJ, et al: Fusion of a fork head domain gene to PAX3 in the solid tumour alveolar rhabdomyosarcoma. *Nat Genet* 5:230–235, 1993.
   This article elucidates the molecular genetic basis of the 2;13 chromosomal translocation in ARMS.
23. Davis RJ, Barr FG: Fusion genes resulting from alternative chromosomal translocations are overexpressed by gene-specific mechanisms in alveolar rhabdomyosarcoma. *Proc Natl Acad Sci U S A* 94:8047–8051, 1997.
   This discussion reveals that the PAX3-FOXO1 and PAX7-FOXO1 fusion products are overexpressed in ARMS by fusion gene-specific mechanisms.
32. Mosquera JM, Sboner A, Zhang L, et al: Recurrent NCOA2 gene rearrangements in congenital/infantile spindle cell rhabdomyosarcoma. *Genes Chromosomes Cancer* 52:538–550, 2013.
   This article describes a novel set of gene fusions in a subset of ERMS tumors.
35. Paulson V, Chandler G, Rakheja D, et al: High-resolution array CGH identifies common mechanisms that drive embryonal rhabdomyosarcoma pathogenesis. *Genes Chromosomes Cancer* 50: 397–408, 2011.
   The authors used array-based CGH analysis to perform a comprehensive analysis of the chromosomal and focal copy number changes in ERMS.
36. Weber-Hall S, Anderson J, McManus A, et al: Gains, losses, and amplification of genomic material in rhabdomyosarcoma analyzed by comparative genomic hybridization. *Cancer Res* 56:3220–3224, 1996.
   The authors used chromosomal-based CGH to distinguish chromosomal and focal copy number changes between ARMS and ERMS and establish the higher frequency of gene amplification in ARMS.
37. Williamson D, Missiaglia E, de Reynies A, et al: Fusion gene-negative alveolar rhabdomyosarcoma is clinically and molecularly indistinguishable from embryonal rhabdomyosarcoma. *J Clin Oncol* 28:2151–2158, 2010.
   This article reveals that the clinical outcome in fusion-negative ARMS is similar to that in ERMS and distinct from the behavior in fusion-positive ARMS.
58. Shern JF, Chen L, Chmielecki J, et al: Comprehensive genomic analysis of rhabdomyosarcoma reveals a landscape of alterations affecting a common genetic axis in fusion-positive and fusion-negative tumors. *Cancer Discov* 4:216–231, 2014.
   These researchers used next-generation sequencing to provide a comprehensive evaluation of the somatic changes in ARMS and ERMS.
96. Wachtel M, Dettling M, Koscielniak E, et al: Gene expression signatures identify rhabdomyosarcoma subtypes and detect a novel t(2;2)(q35;p23) translocation fusing PAX3 to NCOA1. *Cancer Res* 64:5539–5545, 2004.
   Expression profiling is used to identify distinct genome-wide expression patterns in ARMS and ERMS. The expression pattern of fusion-negative ARMS is more similar to ERMS than that of fusion-positive ARMS.

114. Tapscott SJ, Thayer MJ, Weintraub H: Deficiency in rhabdomyosarcomas of a factor required for MyoD activity and myogenesis. *Science* 259:1450–1453, 1993.
   This article describes the deficiency of MyoD in promoting skeletal muscle differentiation in RMS.
125. Seale P, Sabourin LA, Girgis-Gabardo A, et al: Pax7 is required for the specification of myogenic satellite cells. *Cell* 102:777–786, 2000.
   The critical role of the transcription factor Pax7, which is expressed in ERMS and as the fusion gene PAX7-FOXO1 in ARMS, is identified in the lineage development of skeletal muscle satellite cells.
129. Maroto M, Reshef R, Munsterberg AE, et al: Ectopic Pax-3 activates MyoD and Myf-5 expression in embryonic mesoderm and neural tissue. *Cell* 89:139–148, 1997.
   The critical role for the transcription factor Pax3, which is expressed in ERMS and as the fusion gene PAX3-FOXO1 in ARMS, is identified as upstream of the myogenic factors MyoD and Myf-5.
138. Taulli R, Bersani F, Foglizzo V, et al: The muscle-specific microRNA miR-206 blocks human rhabdomyosarcoma growth in xenotransplanted mice by promoting myogenic differentiation. *J Clin Invest* 119:2366–2378, 2009.
   The authors identify deficiencies of some microRNAs in RMS and demonstrates that reexpression of miR-206 downregulates cMET, stimulates myogenic differentiation, and blocks RMS xenograft growth.
148. Wang H, Garzon R, Sun H, et al: NF-kappaB-YY1-miR-29 regulatory circuitry in skeletal myogenesis and rhabdomyosarcoma. *Cancer Cell* 14:369–381, 2008.
   The authors identify a molecular circuit that recruits the Polycomb group remodeling complex PRC2 to DNA to epigenetically repress myogenic differentiation during muscle and RMS development.
193. Sharp R, Recio JA, Jhappan C, et al: Synergism between INK4a/ARF inactivation and aberrant HGF/SF signaling in rhabdomyosarcomagenesis. *Nat Med* 8:1276–1280, 2002.
   The authors used a genetically engineered mouse model of ERMS to identify a role for the HGF-cMET axis in RMS.
203. Nishijo K, Chen QR, Zhang L, et al: Credentialing a preclinical mouse model of alveolar rhabdomyosarcoma. *Cancer Res* 69: 2902–2911, 2009.
   The use of a genetically engineered mouse model of ARMS for preclinical screening of active agents in ARMS is validated.
223. Le X, Pugach EK, Hettmer S, et al: A novel chemical screening strategy in zebrafish identifies common pathways in embryogenesis and rhabdomyosarcoma development. *Development* 140: 2354–2364, 2013.
   This article highlights the use of a lower eukaryotic model of RMS (in this case zebrafish ERMS) in high-throughput screens to identify pathways common to both normal development and RMS.
239. Tonelli R, McIntyre A, Camerin C, et al: Antitumor activity of sustained N-Myc reduction in rhabdomyosarcomas and transcriptional block by antigene therapy. *Clin Cancer Res* 18:796–807, 2012.
   The authors describe the development and evaluation in xenograft models of a peptide nucleic acid oligonucleotide directed to exon 2 of MYCN, an oncogene commonly upregulated in RMS.
255. van den Broeke LT, Pendleton CD, Mackall C, et al: Identification and epitope enhancement of a PAX-FKHR fusion protein breakpoint epitope in alveolar rhabdomyosarcoma cells created by a tumorigenic chromosomal translocation inducing CTL capable of lysing human tumors. *Cancer Res* 66:1818–1823, 2006.
   This article is a discussion of the use of the unique breakpoint epitope of PAX3-FOXO1 to generate an immune reponse to kill ARMS cells.
262. Weiss AR, Lyden ER, Anderson JR, et al: Histologic and clinical characteristics can guide staging evaluations for children and adolescents with rhabdomyosarcoma: a report from the Children's Oncology Group Soft Tissue Sarcoma Committee. *J Clin Oncol* 31.3226 3232, 2013.
   This is an analysis of more than 1600 IRS/COG patients, showing that about one third do not require the traditional staging studies (chest computed tomography, bone marrow

studies, bone scans) and providing an algorithm to steer the clinical evaluation.

271. Missiaglia E, Williamson D, Chisholm J, et al: *PAX3/FOXO1* fusion gene status is the key prognostic molecular marker in rhabdomyosarcoma and significantly improves current risk stratification. *J Clin Oncol* 30:1670–1677, 2012.
     This is why the presence or absence of the fusion gene is likely to supplant histology as a key risk classification and prognostic factor in rhabdomyosarcoma.

276. Rodary C, Gehan EA, Flamant F, et al: Prognostic factors in 951 nonmetastatic rhabdomyosarcoma in children: a report from the International Rhabdomyosarcoma Workshop. *Med Pediatr Oncol* 19:89–95, 1991.
     This is the first report of a series of international workshops that have compared different approaches to treating rhabdomyosarcoma.

307. Arndt CA, Stoner JA, Hawkins DS, et al: Vincristine, actinomycin, and cyclophosphamide compared with vincristine, actinomycin, and cyclophosphamide alternating with vincristine, topotecan, and cyclophosphamide for intermediate-risk rhabdomyosarcoma: Children's Oncology Group study D9803. *J Clin Oncol* 27:5182–5188, 2009.
     This reports the results of the IRS-V intermediate-risk study and illustrates both the frustrations of trying to improve the outcomes for these patients and the principle that more is not necessarily better.

323. Oberlin O, Rey A, Anderson J, et al: Treatment of orbital rhabdomyosarcoma: survival and late effects of treatment—results of an international workshop. *J Clin Oncol* 19:197–204, 2001.
     The SIOP emphasis on chemotherapy and minimization of radiotherapy leads to more local recurrences but the same overall survival as the IRS/COG approach using less chemotherapy and more radiation.

324. Rodeberg DA, Anderson JR, Arndt CA, et al: Comparison of outcomes based on treatment algorithms for rhabdomyosarcoma of the bladder/prostate: combined results from the Children's Oncology Group, German Cooperative Soft Tissue Sarcoma Study, Italian Cooperative Group, and International Society of Pediatric Oncology Malignant Mesenchymal Tumors Committee. *Int J Cancer* 128:1232–1239, 2011.
     This is the third in a series of international workshops and refines risk factors and compares outcomes resulting from different approaches to treatment.

352. Childs SK, Kozak KR, Friedmann AM, et al: Proton radiotherapy for parameningeal rhabdomyosarcoma: clinical outcomes and late effects. *Int J Radiat Oncol Biol Phys* 82:635–642, 2012.
     This series of 17 consecutive patients graphically depicts the sparing of normal tissues with proton radiotherapy and compares results with those using photon radiation.

356. Spalding AC, Hawkins DS, Donaldson SS, et al: The effect of radiation timing on patients with high-risk features of parameningeal rhabdomyosarcoma: an analysis of IRS-IV and D9803. *Int J Radiat Oncol Biol Phys* 87:512–516, 2013.
     After many years of debate about whether earlier or later radiotherapy leads to better survival, this paper addressed the question with data and shows that local control rates are no different.

377. Chisholm JC, Marandet J, Rey A, et al: Prognostic factors after relapse in nonmetastatic rhabdomyosarcoma: a nomogram to better define patients who can be salvaged with further therapy. *J Clin Oncol* 29:1319–1325, 2011.
     A valuable analysis of a large number of patients with relapsed rhabdomyosarcoma that culminates in a nomogram that allows one to estimate the probability of survival for a particular patient.

380. Peinemann F, Kroger N, Bartel C, et al: High-dose chemotherapy followed by autologous stem cell transplantation for metastatic rhabdomyosarcoma—a systematic review. *PLoS One* 6:e17127, 2011.
     This is a very careful review of available data on this controversial topic.

CHAPTER 60

Nonrhabdomyosarcoma Soft Tissue Sarcomas and Other Soft Tissue Tumors

Ian J. Davis, Antonio R. Perez-Atayde, and David E. Fisher

CHAPTER OUTLINE

Soft tissue sarcomas of childhood and adolescence constitute a heterogeneous group of tumors that exhibit features of mesenchymal differentiation (Tables 60-1 and 60-2). From a pediatric oncology perspective, the various types of rhabdomyosarcoma, the most common soft tissue sarcoma in younger children, are grouped separately such that the remainder of these tumors are collectively termed the *nonrhabdomyosarcoma soft tissue sarcomas* (NRSTS). This term seems an odd eponym, defining a category of soft tissue sarcoma by exclusion

and grouping together widely disparate clinicopathologic entities distinguished by clinical features, molecular pathogenesis, and biologic behavior. However, the term *NRSTS* carries a unique value in pediatric oncology, enabling the study of significant cohorts of children with uncommon tumors. Sarcomas in children represent a somewhat distinct set of tumors that diverge in both incidence and histology from those in adults. The types of sarcomas that develop in adolescents and young adults are similar to those seen in older individuals; however,

TABLE 60-1 World Health Organization Classification of Soft Tissue Tumors: Intermediate (Rarely metastasizing) and Malignant

	Intermediate (Rarely Metastasizing)	Malignant
Adipocytic		Dedifferentiated liposarcoma Myxoid liposarcoma Pleomorphic liposarcoma Liposarcoma, not otherwise specified
Fibroblastic/Myofibroblastic	Solitary fibrous tumor Dermatofibrosarcoma protuberans (fibrosarcomatous and pigmented) Inflammatory myofibroblastic tumor Low-grade myofibroblastic sarcoma Myxoinflammatory fibroblastic sarcoma (including atypical) Infantile fibrosarcoma	Adult fibrosarcoma Myxofibrosarcoma Low-grade fibromyxoid sarcoma Sclerosing epithelioid fibrosarcoma
So-Called Fibrohistiocytic	Plexiform fibrohistiocytic tumor Giant cell tumor of soft tissues	
Smooth Muscle		Leiomyosarcoma (excluding skin)
Pericytic (Perivascular)		Malignant glomus tumor
Skeletal Muscle		Embryonal rhabdomyosarcoma Alveolar rhabdomyosarcoma Pleomorphic rhabdomyosarcoma Spindle cell/sclerosing
Vascular Tumors	Retiform hemangioendothelioma Papillary intralymphatic angioendothelioma Composite hemangioendothelioma Pseudomyogenic (epithelioid-like) hemangioendothelioma Kaposi sarcoma	Epithelioid hemangioendothelioma Angiosarcoma of soft tissue
Chondroosseous		Extraskeletal mesenchymal chondrosarcoma Extraskeletal osteosarcoma
Nerve Sheath Tumors		Malignant peripheral nerve sheath tumor Epithelioid malignant nerve sheath tumor Malignant triton tumor Malignant granular cell tumor Ectomesenchymoma
Gastrointestinal Stromal Tumors		Gastrointestinal stromal tumors, malignant (AFIP groups 3b, 5, 6a, 6b)
Uncertain Differentiation	Ossifying fibromyxoid tumor Myoepithelioma Parachordoma	Synovial sarcoma (including spindle cell and biphasic) Epithelioid sarcoma Alveolar soft part sarcoma Clear cell sarcoma of soft tissue Extraskeletal myxoid chondrosarcoma Extraosseous Ewing sarcoma Desmoplastic small round cell tumor Extrarenal rhabdoid tumor Neoplasms with perivascular epithelioid cell differentiation (PEComa) (includes clear cell myomelanocytic tumor Intimal sarcoma
Undifferentiated/Unclassified		Undifferentiated spindle cell sarcoma Undifferentiated pleomorphic sarcoma Undifferentiated round cell sarcoma Undifferentiated epithelioid sarcoma Undifferentiated sarcoma, not otherwise specified

Modified from Fletcher CD, Bridge JA, Hogendoorn PCW, et al, editors: World Health Organization classification of tumors of soft tissue and bone, *Lyon, 2013, IARC Press.*
AFIP, Armed Forces Institute of Pathology.

TABLE 60-2   World Health Organization Classification of Soft Tissue Tumors: Benign and Intermediate (Locally Aggressive)

	Benign	Intermediate (Locally Aggressive)
Adipocytic	Lipoma Lipomatosis Lipomatosis of nerve Lipoblastoma/lipoblastomatosis Angiolipoma Myolipoma Chondroid lipoma Extrarenal angiomyolipoma Extraadrenal myelolipoma Spindle cell/pleomorphic lipoma Hibernoma	Atypical lipomatous tumor/ well-differentiated liposarcoma
Fibroblastic/Myofibroblastic	Nodular fasciitis Proliferative fasciitis Proliferative myositis Myositis ossificans Fibroosseous pseudotumor of digits Ischemic fasciitis Elastofibroma Fibrous hamartoma of infancy Fibromatosis coli Juvenile hyaline fibromatosis Inclusion body fibromatosis Fibroma of tendon sheath Desmoplastic fibroblastoma Mammary-type myofibroblastoma Calcifying aponeurotic fibroma Angiomyofibroblastoma Cellular angiofibroma Nuchal-type fibroma Gardner fibroma Calcifying fibrous tumor	Palmar/plantar fibromatosis Desmoid-type fibromatosis Lipofibromatosis Giant cell fibroblastoma
So-Called Fibrohistiocytic	Tenosynovial giant cell tumor (localized and diffuse types and malignant) Deep benign fibrous histiocytoma	Plexiform fibrohistiocytic tumor Giant cell tumor of soft tissues
Smooth Muscle	Deep leiomyoma	
Pericytic (Perivascular)	Glomus tumor (and variants) Myopericytoma	
Skeletal Muscle	Rhabdomyoma (adult, fetal and genital types)	
Vascular Tumors	Hemangioma (synovial, venous, arteriovenous hemangioma/ malformation, lymphangioma) Epithelioid hemangioma Angiomatosis Lymphangioma	Kaposiform hemangioendothelioma
Gastrointestinal Stromal Tumors	Benign gastrointestinal stromal tumor (AFIP prognostic groups 1, 2, 3a)	
Nerve Sheath Tumors	Schwannoma Melanotic schwannoma Neurofibroma (including variants and plexiform neurofibroma) Perineuroma (malignant perineuroma) Granular cell tumor Dermal nerve sheath myxoma Solitary circumscribed neuroma Ectopic meningioma Nasal glial heterotopia Benign triton tumor Hybrid nerve sheath tumors	
Chondroosseous	Soft tissue chondroma	
Uncertain differentiation	Acral fibromyxoma Intramuscular myxoma Juxtaarticular myxoma Deep ("aggressive") angiomyxoma Pleomorphic hyalinizing angiectatic tumor Ectopic hamartomatous thymoma	Hemosiderotic fibrolipomatous tumor

Modified from Fletcher CD, Bridge JA, Hogendoorn PCW, et al, editors: World Health Organization classification of tumors of soft tissue and bone, *Lyon, 2013, IARC Press.*
AFIP, Armed Forces Institute of Pathology.

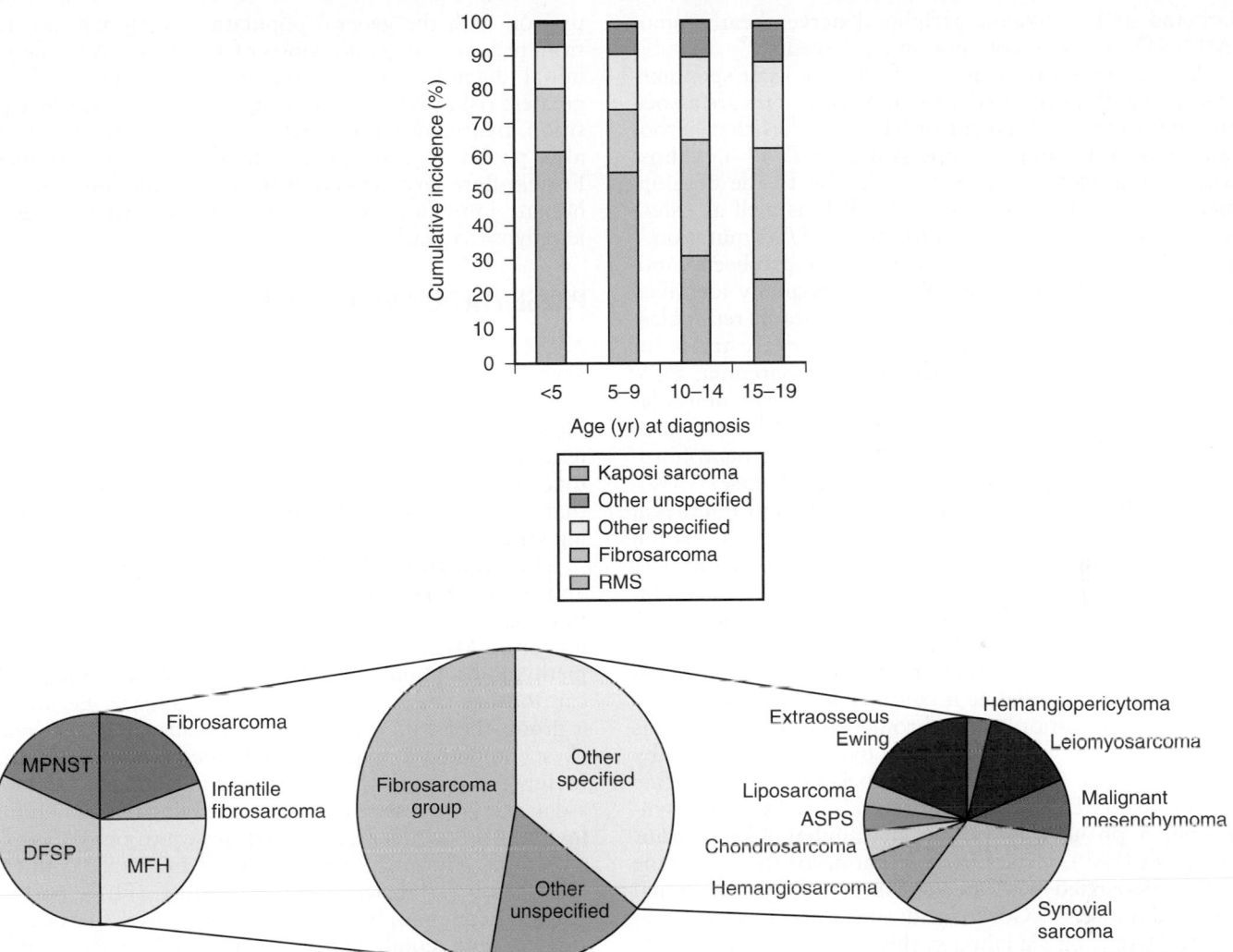

Figure 60-1 Incidence and distribution of pediatric soft tissue sarcomas. **A,** Age-adjusted incidence for soft tissue sarcomas of childhood grouped according to the International Classification of Childhood Cancer. **B,** Depiction of age-adjusted incidence for the specific tumors that comprise the major classifications of NRSTS. *ASPS,* Alveolar soft part sarcoma; *DFSP,* dermatofibrosarcoma protuberans; *MFH,* malignant fibrous histiocytoma; *MPNST,* malignant peripheral nerve sheath tumor; *RMS,* rhabdomyosarcoma. *(Data from Kramarova E, Stiller CA: The International Classification of Childhood Cancer. Int J Cancer. 68:759–765, 1996; and Gurney JG, Young JL, Jr., Roffers SD, et al: Soft tissue sarcomas. In Ries LAG, Smith MA, Gurney JG, et al, editors: Cancer incidence and survival among children and adolescents: United States SEER Program 1975–1995. NIH publication No. 99-4649, Bethesda, Md., 1999, National Cancer Institute, p. 111–124.)*

the relative incidence and response to therapy may differ.[1] In addition, the term *NRSTS* permits the flexibility to include undifferentiated tumors and tumors that, based on treatment, are typically excluded from other groupings (e.g., desmoplastic small round cell tumor [DSRT]). Finally, by evoking those tumors prevalent in the pediatric population, the term *NRSTS* also permits consideration of the unique toxicities specific to children when evaluating treatment approaches and designing clinical trials.

NRSTS are often characterized by distinct, consistent cytogenetic, transcriptional, and intracellular signaling changes. Exploring these molecular alterations may offer insights into the biology of mesenchymal development and the pathogenesis of these tumors, thus leading to the development of new treatment strategies.

EPIDEMIOLOGY

In children younger than 5 years, rhabdomyosarcoma constitutes the most frequent type of soft tissue sarcoma (STS), however by late school age and continuing into adolescence the incidence of NRSTS rises to exceed that of rhabdomyosarcoma (Fig. 60-1). The total incidence for STS in children and adolescents younger than 20 years is approximately 11 per million, which represents 7.4% of cancer in this population.[2] NRSTS constitute about one half of these cases or 3% to 4% of childhood malignancies. Within the class of NRSTS, specific tumor types demonstrate a strong age association. Although the median age at diagnosis is approximately 13 years, NRSTS prevalent in younger children include infantile fibrosarcoma and rhabdoid tumor, whereas synovial sarcoma and malignant peripheral nerve sheath tumor (MPNST) are more common in adolescents.[3-9]

Although the vast majority of NRSTS occur spontaneously, several cancer predisposition syndromes are associated with the development of STS. Families that harbor mutations of the tumor suppressor gene *TP53* (i.e., those with Li-Fraumeni syndrome) are prone to the development of many types of cancer.[10,11] STS as well as osteosarcoma can be associated with germline *TP53* mutation.[12] The cell cycle regulatory protein RB has also been implicated in STS development. *RB* was originally identified as the locus deleted in hereditary and sporadic retinoblastoma.[13] However, retinoblastoma survivors are at risk for the development of STS, including fibrosarcoma, pleomorphic sarcoma, and leiomyosarcoma, and molecular analysis of these tumors may demonstrate homozygous *RB* deletion.[14,15] In addition to other tumors, neurofibromatosis type 1 (NF1, von Recklinghausen disease) is associated with the development of MPNSTs and multifocal gastrointestinal stromal tumors (GISTs).[16,17] Radiation therapy for optic nerve glioma in patients with NF1 increases the risk for subsequent MPNST development.[18,19] Carney triad is associated with multifocal GIST (as well as paragangliomas and pulmonary chondromas).[20,21] Individual Carney triad tumors are associated with specific nongermline mutations, although a possible common association with chromosome 1 changes has been reported.[22] Carney-Stratakis dyad, characterized by paraganglioma and GISTs, is associated with germline mutations in *SDHA, SDHB,* or *SDHC.*[23-25] Gardner syndrome, a phenotypic variant of familial adenomatous polyposis (FAP), results from mutation of the *APC* gene and is associated with an increased risk for abdominal desmoid tumor.[26-30] Gorlin syndrome, caused by mutation of the Hedgehog signaling pathway regulator *PTCH,* is associated with undifferentiated sarcoma.[31] Werner syndrome is caused by mutations of the deoxyribonucleic acid (DNA) helicase gene *RECQL2* or nuclear lamin gene *LMNA* and is associated with several cancers, including STS in early and middle adulthood.[32-34] Typically resulting from mutations in *TSC1* or *TSC2,* dominantly inherited tuberous sclerosis is associated with spontaneously resolving cardiac rhabdomyomas in infants and renal angiomyolipoma, including the malignant epithelioid variant, as well as pulmonary lymphangiomyomatosis.[35-38] Pleomorphic sarcoma in adults has infrequently been associated with Lynch syndrome, which is characterized by mutations in the DNA mismatch repair genes *MLH1* and *MLH2.*[39]

In addition to cancer predisposition syndromes, environmental exposures have been linked to sarcoma development. Although osteosarcoma predominates, radiation exposure is associated with NRSTS, including fibrosarcoma and pleomorphic sarcoma, with an incidence associated with the dose of radiation.[40-43] Of the several environmental chemical exposures that have been linked to the development of sarcomas in adults, vinyl chloride exposure demonstrates the strongest association to the development of angiosarcoma.[44] Childhood cancer survivors also appear to be at ninefold higher risk for the development of sarcomas (particularly NRSTS) in comparison with the general population, with a mean time from primary cancer diagnosis of 11 years.[45] Although an initial diagnosis of sarcoma was associated with the greatest risk, perhaps indicating an underlying predisposition, treatment with radiation or alkylating agents was also positively associated with sarcoma development. Epstein-Barr virus infection in individuals infected with human immunodeficiency virus (HIV) predisposes to leiomyosarcoma.[46]

PRESENTATION AND EVALUATION

NRSTS typically presents as a persistent or enlarging, asymptomatic mass. Although NRSTS may arise in any location, extremities constitute the most common sites. However, within the first year of life, soft tissue tumors tend to develop in the trunk and head and neck.[3] A significant fraction of tumors may be associated with pain that likely indicates invasion or compression of surrounding structures.[7]

The evaluation of NRSTS is typically initiated with appropriate imaging then followed by biopsy. For most tumors, plain radiography and magnetic resonance imaging (MRI) are justified. Technetium-99m–labeled methyldiphosphonate (^{99m}Tc MDP) nuclear scintigraphy can localize sites of bony metastatic disease. Because as a group these tumors tend to metastasize to the lungs, chest computed tomography (CT) is commonly indicated. Imaging may narrow the differential diagnosis and will aid in assessing resectability by identifying tumor margins, involved tissue planes, and relationship to neurovascular structures. Fluorine-18 (^{18}F)-labeled fluorodeoxyglucose (FDG) or ^{18}F-labeled fluorothymidine (FLT) positron emission tomography (PET) has been used for sarcoma staging, and combined PET/CT can identify primary tumors as well as metastatic spread and may detect metastatic lesions missed by bone scintigraphy.[47] However, small lesions (<1 cm) are difficult to visualize by PET. FLT-PET has been used to distinguish between low- and high-grade sarcomas.[48]

Accurate tissue diagnosis is critical to establish a treatment plan and to predict prognosis.[5] Because of the diverse range of sarcoma subtypes as well as their rarity, arriving at a definitive diagnosis can be challenging.[49] The complexity of NRSTS diagnosis and grading requires the integration of histopathology with immunohistochemical, ultrastructural, cytogenetic, and molecular studies (Table 60-3). Advance communication between the surgeon or interventional radiologist, pathologist, and pediatric oncologist can help ensure that sufficient material is obtained and suitably processed. Fine-needle aspiration often generates an inadequate specimen to yield a specific diagnosis. Multiple core needle biopsies may be sufficient to initiate the evaluation, with additional tissue resulting from eventual resection. Although sentinel lymph node biopsy is not a standard component of NRSTS evaluation, it could be considered for high-grade sarcomas such as clear cell sarcoma, synovial sarcoma, vascular sarcomas, and undifferentiated sarcomas.[50-52]

In general, sarcomas can be classified as those with a recognizable recurrent chromosomal rearrangement

TABLE 60-3 Diagnostic Studies in the Evaluation of Nonrhabdomyosarcoma Soft Tissue Sarcomas

Tumor	Immunohistochemical Markers	RECURRENT CYTOGENETIC CHANGES	
		Associated Karyotype	Genes Implicated
Alveolar soft part sarcoma	TFE3, MyoD1 (cytoplasmic), desmin (50%), S100 protein (25%), MSA (in some)	der(17)t(x;17)(p11;q25)	*ASPSCR1 (ASPL, TUG, RCC17), TFE3*
Angiomatoid fibrous histiocytoma	Vimentin, desmin (50%), CD68 (50%), CD99 (50%), EMA (40%)	t(2;22)(q33;q12) t(12;16)(q13;p11) t(12;22)(q13;12)	*EWSR1, CREB1* *FUS, ATF1* *EWSR1, ATF1*
Angiosarcoma	ERG, factor VIII–associated (VWF), CD34, FLI1, CD31		
Congenital infantile fibrosarcoma	Vimentin, actins (30%), desmin (20%), cytokeratins (20%)	t(12;15)(p13;q25)	*ETV6, NTRK3 (TRKC)*
Clear cell sarcoma	MITF, HMB45, S100, melan A	t(12;22)(q13;q12) t(2;12)(q32.3;q12)	*EWSR1, ATF1 EWSR1, CREB1*
Dermatofibrosarcoma protuberans	CD34, apolipoprotein D	t(17;22)(q22;q13)	*COL1A1, PDGFB*
Desmoplastic small round cell tumor	WT1 (carboxy terminus), desmin (dotlike), EMA, cytokeratin, vimentin	t(11;12)(p13;q12)	*EWSR1, WT1*
Desmoid-type fibromatosis	Vimentin, actins, β-catenin (nuclear)	+8, +20	
Ectomesenchymoma	S100 protein, synaptophysin, GFAP, neurofilament protein, rhabdomyosarcoma markers (MSA, desmin, myogenin, MyoD1)	+2, −6, +11, +20	
Epithelioid sarcoma	Cytokeratins, EMA, vimentin, CD34 (60%), CA-125		
Epithelioid hemangioendothelioma	VWF, CD31, CD34 Cytokeratins (25% weak)	t(1;3)(p36.3;q25) t(X;11)(p11.23;q22.1)	*WWTR1, CAMTA1* *YAP1,TFE3*
Extraosseous Ewing sarcoma	CD99 (membranous), NSE, vimentin, cytokeratins (25%), FLI1 (nuclear)	t(11;22)(q24;q12) t(21;22)(q21;q12) t(7;22)(p22;q12) t(17;22)(q12;q22) t(2;22)(q36;q12)	*EWSR1, FLI1* *EWSR1, ERG1* *EWSR1, ETV1* *EWSR1, ETV4 (E1AF)* *EWSR1, FEV*
Extrarenal rhabdoid tumor	Vimentin, cytokeratins, EMA, CD99, NSE, synaptophysin	Abnormalities of 22q11	*SMARCB1 (hSNF5, INI1, BAF47)*
Gastrointestinal stromal tumor	CD117 (KIT), CD34		
Extraskeletal myxoid chondrosarcoma	S100 protein (50%), CD117 (KIT, 30%), cytokeratin (focal), EMA (30%) Neuroendocrine markers (chromogranin, NSE, synaptophysin) in t(9;17) tumors	t(9;22)(q22;q12) t(9;17)(q22;q11) t(9;15)(q22;q21)	*EWSR1, NR4A3 (TEC, CHN, CMSF, NOR1)* *TAF15 (RPB56, TAF2N), NR4A3* *TCF12 (HTF4), NR4A3 (TEC)*
Giant cell angioblastoma	Actins, vimentin		
Inflammatory myofibroblastic tumor	ALK, vimentin, actins, desmin (50%), cytokeratins (focal), CD68 (25%)	Multiple translocations involving 2p23	*ALK*, multiple partners
Kaposiform hemangioendothelioma	D2-40, CD31, CD34, FLI1, SMA, D2-40		
Kaposi sarcoma	D2-40, CD31, CD34, FLI1, HHV-8 (KSHV) (in situ hybridization)		
Leiomyosarcoma	SMA, desmin, h-caldesmon	Complex	

Continued on following page

TABLE 60-3   Diagnostic Studies in the Evaluation of Nonrhabdomyosarcoma Soft Tissue Sarcomas (Continued)

Tumor	Immunohistochemical Markers	RECURRENT CYTOGENETIC CHANGES	
		Associated Karyotype	Genes Implicated
Lipoblastoma	S100 protein, desmin	del(8)(q12;q24),r(8) t(7;8)(p22;q13)	HAS2, PLAG1 COL1A2, RAD51L1
Low-grade fibromyxoid sarcoma	Vimentin, actins (focal)	t(7;16)(p33;p11)	FUS, CREB3L1, CREB3L2 (BBF2H7)
Malignant peripheral nerve sheath tumor	S100 (50-90%), GFAP (50%-90%), CD57 (50%), myelin basic protein (40%), TP53	Numerical and structural abnormalities of chromosomes 1, 4, 7, 11, 12, 14, 16, 17, and 22	
Mesenchymal chondrosarcoma	S100 protein (cartilaginous component) NSE, CD57, CD99 (membranous) (undifferentiated component)	Complex cytogenetics alterations del(8)(q13.3;q21.1)	HEY1, NCOA2
Myxoid liposarcoma	S100 protein	t(12;16)(q13;p11) t(12;22)(q13;q12)	FUS (TLS), DDIT3 (CHOP) EWSR1, DDIT3 (CHOP)
Plexiform fibrohistiocytic tumor	CD68, actins (70%), EMA (30%), BCL2 (30%)		
Solitary fibrous tumor	STAT6 (nuclear), CD34, CD99 (cytoplasmic)		NAB2, STAT6
Synovial sarcoma	EMA, cytokeratins, S100 protein (30%), CD99 (cytoplasmic), BCL2, TLE1	t(x;18)(p11;q11)	SS18 (SYT), SSX1 SS18 (SYT), SSX2
Undifferentiated round cell and spindle cell sarcomas			EWSR1, NFATC2, PATZ1, POU5F1, SMARCA5, SP3 CIC, DUX4

EMA, Epithelial membrane antigen; GFAP, glial fibrillary acidic protein; HHV-8, human herpesvirus 8; MITF, microphthalmia-associated transcription factor; MSA, muscle-specific actin; NSE, neuron-specific enolase; VWF, von Willebrand factor.
Note: Immunohistochemical markers and cytogenetic changes found in a large percent of tumors. Less common abnormalities are not listed.

(typically translocation) and those without. The identification of cytogenetic abnormalities, many of which are highly specific of certain pediatric and young adult NRSTS, is helpful in arriving at or confirming a diagnosis (see Table 60-3). However, the same gene can be translocated in different tumor types. For example, the EWSR1 gene is rearranged in DSRT, clear cell sarcoma, myxoid liposarcoma, and a subset of undifferentiated sarcomas in addition to Ewing sarcoma. In contrast, the rearrangement of certain genes is highly restricted, such as SS18 (SYT) rearrangement in synovial sarcoma. Molecular studies (e.g., polymerase chain reaction [PCR] assay and interphase fluorescence in situ hybridization [FISH]) may be required to evaluate for specific cytogenetic abnormalities, especially if there a high index of suspicion and standard cytogenetics are unavailable or unremarkable.[53] High-throughput DNA sequencing and other comprehensive genomic approaches have rapidly emerged as strategies to identify genetic alterations in sarcomas. Ongoing efforts to systematically identify mutations in select STS include the Pediatric Cancer Genome Project and the Cancer Genome Atlas. Although translocations can be detected relatively easily when sequencing the whole genome, owing to significant expense and technical considerations, most current high throughput sequencing applications focus on exonic sequence variation and consequently are not designed to detect intronic breakpoints. However, RNA sequencing as well as whole exome and targeted sequencing of cancer-associated genes offers the potential to identify individuals with specific and therapeutically actionable mutations. To take advantage of emerging techniques for molecular analyses and biomarker identification, additional tumor material, if possible, should be preserved at −70° C for DNA or ribonucleic acid (RNA) analysis. For those sarcomas that may metastasize to the bone marrow, aspiration and biopsy may be performed to complete the evaluation for distant spread.

STAGING AND GRADING

As with all cancers, appropriate recommendations for therapy depend on accurate predictions of clinical course and prognosis. Clinically informative classification schemes will accurately predict tumor outcome and will aid in the development and interpretation of multicenter trials necessary to study these uncommon cancers. Studies of adult extremity STS suggest that grade followed by tumor depth and size are of independent prognostic value for the rates of distant metastases and tumor mortality.[54] However, the clinicopathologic classification of pediatric NRSTS poses unique challenges. The low incidence of these tumors results in grouping potentially disparate tumors in clinical trials. Patient age may influence outcome. For some tumors, high grade does not predict clinically aggressive behavior, whereas other tumors behave

TABLE 60-4 Children's Oncology Group Histologic Grading System

Grade	Description
1—Low	Myxoid and well-differentiated liposarcoma Well-differentiated or infantile (≤4 years old) fibrosarcoma Well-differentiated or infantile (≤4 years old) hemangiopericytoma Well-differentiated malignant peripheral nerve sheath tumor Extraskeletal myxoid chondrosarcoma
2—Intermediate	Sarcomas not specifically included in grade 1 and 3 and in which: • <15% of the surface area shows necrosis • Mitotic count is ≤5/10 high-power fields using a 40× objective • Absence of marked nuclear atypia* • Tumor is not markedly cellular*
3—High	Pleomorphic or round cell liposarcoma Mesenchymal chondrosarcoma Extraskeletal osteosarcoma Malignant triton tumor Alveolar soft part sarcoma Sarcomas not included in grade 1 with >15% of surface area with necrosis or ≥5 mitoses/10 high-power fields using a 40× objective

Modified from Parham DM, Webber BL, Jenkins JJ, III, et al: Nonrhabdomyosarcomatous soft tissue sarcomas of childhood: formulation of a simplified system for grading. Mod Pathol 8:705–710, 1995; and Khoury JD, Coffin CM, Spunt SL, et al: Grading of soft tissue sarcoma in children and adolescents. Cancer 116:2266–2274, 2010.

*Secondary criteria. Tumor diagnoses specified in grade 1 or 3 are excluded from grade 2.

TABLE 60-5 Surgical-Pathologic Grouping System of the Intergroup Rhabdomyosarcoma Study

Group	Definition
Low-Stage	
I	Localized disease, completely resected
II	Total gross resection with evidence of regional spread
IIa	Grossly resected tumor with microscopic residual disease
IIb	Regional disease with involved nodes, completely resected with no microscopic residual disease
IIc	Regional disease with involved nodes, grossly resected but with evidence of microscopic residual disease and/or histologic involvement of the most distal regional lymph node from the primary site in the dissection.
High-Stage	
III	Incomplete resection with gross residual disease
IV	Distant metastatic disease present at onset

Modified from Meza JL, Anderson J, Pappo AS, et al: Analysis of factors in patients with nonmetastatic rhabdomyosarcoma treated on Intergroup Rhabdomyosarcoma Studies III and IV: the Children's Oncology Group. J Clin Oncol 24:3844–3851, 2006.

sification system for pediatric tumors (Table 60-6).[62-64] STS may also be classified according to the American Joint Commission on Cancer (AJCC) or Enneking staging systems, which integrate tumor size, location relative to the superficial fascia, regional lymph node status, presence of distant metastases, and histologic grade (Table 60-7).[65,66]

NRSTS most commonly spread locally and hematogenously but may exhibit regional lymph node metastases. The lung is the most common site for distant metastases, but with less frequency these tumors can metastasize to

aggressively regardless of histologic appearance. To address these issues, the Pediatric Oncology Group (POG) grading system incorporates histology, cytologic features, and age to classify NRSTS as low, intermediate, or high grade (Table 60-4).[55] Low grade is defined by histologic type, whereas intermediate grade takes into account necrosis and mitosis with secondary consideration of nuclear atypia and tumor cellularity. High-grade tumors include those of specific histologies as well as tumors with more than 15% necrosis or five or more mitoses/10 high-power field. The National Cancer Institute (NCI) and Fédération Nationale des Centres de Lutte Contre le Cancer (FNCLCC) grading specifications are alternative methodologies validated on sarcomas in adults.[56-59] Similar to the POG system, they take into consideration mitotic index, necrosis, and histologic type or tumor differentiation. The POG and FNCLCC perform similarly in their ability to correlate with outcome.[60] Gene expression signatures have also been used to predict outcomes in non–translocation-associated sarcomas in adults.[61]

Pediatric multicenter studies also make use of the surgical-pathologic grouping system of the Intergroup Rhabdomyosarcoma Study (IRS) (Table 60-5), which incorporates tumor spread and outcome of surgical resection, or the International Society of Pediatric Oncology (SIOP)-International Union Against Cancer TNM clas-

TABLE 60-6 SIOP-UICC TNM Soft Tissue Sarcoma Clinical Staging System

Stage	Description
I	T1—Tumor confined to organ or tissue of origin N0—No evidence of regional lymph node involvement M0—No evidence of distant metastasis
II	T2—Tumor involving one or more contiguous organs or tissues or with adjacent malignant effusion N0 M0
III	Any T N1—Evidence of regional lymph node involvement M0
IV	Any T Any N M1—Evidence of distant metastases

Modified from Rodary C, Flamant D, Donaldson SS; the SIOP-IRS Committee: An attempt to use a common staging system in rhabdomyosarcoma: a report of an international workshop initiated by the International Society of Pediatric Oncology (SIOP). Med Pediatr Oncol 17:210–215, 1989.

TABLE 60-7   American Joint Committee on Cancer Staging

Primary Tumor (T)		Regional Lymph Nodes (N)	
TX	Primary tumor cannot be assessed	NX	Regional lymph nodes cannot be assessed
T0	No evidence of primary tumor	N0	No regional lymph node metastasis
T1	Tumor 5 cm or less in greatest dimension*	N1	Regional lymph node metastasis[†]
T1a	Superficial tumor		
T1b	Deep tumor		
T2	Tumor more than 5 cm in greatest dimension*		
T2a	Superficial tumor		
T2b	Deep tumor		

Distant Metastasis (M)		Histologic Grade (G)	
M0	No distant metastasis	(FNCLCC System Preferred)	
M1	Distant metastasis	GX	Grade cannot be assessed
		G1	Grade 1
		G2	Grade 2
		G3	Grade 3

Anatomic Stage/Prognostic Groups

Stage IA	T1a	N0	M0	G1, GX
	T1b	N0	M0	G1, GX
Stage IB	T2a	N0	M0	G1, GX
	T2b	N0	M0	G1, GX
Stage IIA	T1a	N0	M0	G2, G3
	T1b	N0	M0	G2, G3
Stage IIB	T2a	N0	M0	G2
	T2b	N0	M0	G2
Stage III	T2a, T2b	N0	M0	G3
	Any T	N1	M0	Any G
Stage IV	Any T	Any N	M1	Any G

From American Joint Committee on Cancer: AJCC cancer staging manual, 7th ed. New York, 2002, Springer-Verlag.

*Note: Superficial tumor is located exclusively above the superficial fascia without invasion of the fascia; deep tumor is located either exclusively beneath the superficial fascia, superficial to the fascia with invasion of or through the fascia, or both superficial yet beneath the fascia.

[†]Note: presence of positive nodes (N1) in M0 tumors is considered Stage III.

bone or brain. Metastatic spread at the time of diagnosis likely occurs in alveolar soft part sarcoma, high-grade MPNST, clear cell sarcoma, high-grade angiosarcoma, and epithelioid sarcoma.[5]

Several factors have been shown to be prognostic for tumor-associated mortality. In both univariate and multivariate analyses of patients with grossly resected tumors, tumor invasion into contiguous structures and size (>5 cm) are the most highly predictive of decreased 5-year event free survival (EFS) and overall survival (OS). Other factors that correlate with poor outcome including female sex, older age, high-grade tumors, high-grade MPNST histology, and tumors in nonextremity locations.[5]

TREATMENT

Surgical resection constitutes the mainstay of treatment of localized tumors. Complete resection for large tumors may result in significant functional compromise, and amputation should be considered for those patients in whom limb-sparing surgery would leave residual tumor. Radiation therapy is typically reserved for those tumors for which complete resection is not possible. However, the high radiation dose required for sarcoma therapy is associated with significant growth-associated side effects in children. Although surgery with or without radiation results in good outcome for localized and low-grade disease, high-grade disease is associated with significant morbidity and mortality. With the exception of synovial sarcoma and extraskeletal Ewing sarcoma, the role of conventional chemotherapy remains ill defined. However, in pediatric NRSTS, responses can be observed and may reduce tumor burden prior to surgical resection. Biologically targeted therapies have altered the management of individual tumor types (e.g., GISTs in adults), and their roles are evolving as they enter clinical trial.

Local Control

Surgical resection is typically the initial therapy for operable nonmetastatic NRSTS. Complete resection of small (<5 cm) NRSTS results in a 5-year OS in excess of 80%.[60,67-69,70] However, large, high-grade or incompletely resected tumors have a significant chance of local recurrence. Tumor location (e.g., abdomen vs. extremity) and invasion may limit the ability to perform a wide local excision necessary to achieve tumor-free margins. For these patients, external-beam radiation therapy has been used to reduce the risk for local recurrence based on adult studies.[71-73] Pediatric studies seem to confirm that radiation therapy reduces the risk for local recurrence associated with an inability to achieve a wide surgical margin (>1 cm) for high-grade disease.[74] The impact of postoperative radiation therapy may be most significant for IRS group II patients, although grade and size may mitigate this effect.[75] Higher radiation doses are associated with increased rates of local control in NRSTS.[76,77] However, these doses are associated with abnormalities of bone development, complicating the delivery of this modality to growing children.

Brachytherapy—interstitial, intercavitary or surface placement of radioisotopes—constitutes an alternative approach to deliver radiotherapy.[78,79] Brachytherapy can precisely deliver high doses of radiation to the tumor or resection site while sparing normal tissue. Brachytherapy can also be administered concurrently with external-beam radiation, and a study of adult STS suggests that the combination may result in increased rates of local control when surgical margins are positive.[80] Other techniques to augment local control include radiofrequency ablation, cryoablation, and embolization.[81-83] Strategies for local control that incorporate site-directed chemotherapy include intralesional chemotherapy followed by electroporation at accessible sites and intraperitoneal chemotherapy infusion.[84]

Chemotherapy

Because complete resection of NRSTS is associated with a high rate of cure, chemotherapy is principally employed when tumors are unresectable, incompletely resected, or metastatic. The infrequency of each of the heterogeneous tumors that constitute the class of NRSTS makes clinical trials of chemotherapy particularly challenging. To enable multicenter groups to accrue sufficient subjects, the nonselective inclusion of NRSTS complicates the interpretation and extrapolation of most trials. Nonetheless, several consistent themes emerge. In contrast to the striking successes of chemotherapy for Ewing sarcoma and rhabdomyosarcoma, NRSTS tend to be relatively chemoresistant, with synovial sarcoma and extraosseous Ewing sarcoma as exceptions.[5,69,85,86] For patients with fully resected tumors, the inclusion of chemotherapy fails to increase survival.[87,88] The impact of chemotherapy may be most significant for patients harboring tumors with the highest risk for metastatic spread. For high grade, grossly resected tumors, chemotherapy was associated with a 5-year metastasis-free survival of 49.5% compared with 0% for untreated patients.[89] Chemotherapy may also be beneficial for patients with unresectable tumors. For both chemotherapy-sensitive and chemotherapy-resistant tumors, neoadjuvant treatment may permit the subsequent surgical resection of initially nonresectable tumors.[85] Patients with unresected or metastatic tumors have a poor outcome, although 40% to 50% of patients with advanced disease demonstrate some response (partial + complete response) to a regimen containing either ifosfamide and doxorubicin or cyclophosphamide and doxorubicin.[86,88,90] Treatment with doxorubicin, cyclophosphamide, and vincristine alternating with ifosfamide and etoposide together with aggressive local control for incompletely resected tumors or those metastatic at presentation, resulted in a partial + complete response of 80%.[90] Approximately 40% of children and adolescents with NRSTS responded to ifosfamide and doxorubicin, results similar to those for cyclophosphamide and doxorubicin.[86,88] Based on the principle that advanced sarcomas may respond to intensive therapies, the feasibility of dose-intensified neoadjuvant chemotherapy has been an end point of several trials using doxorubicin, ifosfamide, and dacarbazine in adults and doxorubicin, cyclophosphamide, ifosfamide, etoposide, and vincristine in children.[86,91-94] However, evidence in support of high-dose chemotherapy with autologous stem cell infusion remains limited.[95]

Regarding specific chemotherapeutic agents, topoisomerase 1 inhibitors may also have activity against these tumors. Topotecan with high-dose cyclophosphamide as well as irinotecan demonstrated limited efficacy against recurrent NRSTS, and the effect of irinotecan together with temozolomide is currently being studied.[96-99] The combination of vinorelbine with low-dose cyclophosphamide may also have activity against these tumors.[100] Gemcitabine and docetaxel, both of which have some activity against adult sarcomas, were more effective together than gemcitabine alone in adult patients with metastatic sarcoma.[101] In adults, advanced disease may also respond to the combination of gemcitabine and vinorelbine.[102] In children, however, the efficacy of gemcitabine or docetaxel administered individually in the setting of relapsed pediatric solid tumors seems small.[103-105] As previously mentioned, synovial sarcoma is considered an exception to the general chemoresistance of NRSTS. Children and adolescents exhibit a 5-year EFS of about 70% with decreased EFS, progression-free survival (PFS), and OS associated with tumor size (>5 cm), local invasion, and IRS grouping (III and IV).[106-108,109] Another exception is extraosseous Ewing sarcoma, which is generally grouped with bony Ewing sarcoma for treatment purposes (see Chapter 61, "Ewing Sarcoma").

Insights regarding the biology of STS are beginning to identify novel targetable pathways. The management of GISTs in adults has been altered by treatment with KIT and PDGFR-targeted tyrosine kinase inhibitors. Multitargeted tyrosine kinase inhibitors have demonstrated efficacy in nonadipocytic STS in adults, and sorafenib has activity against desmoid tumors.[110,111] Insulin-like growth factor 1 (IGF-1) inhibition has demonstrated efficacy in a fraction of patients with DSRT.[112] Targeting the mammalian target of rapamycin (mTOR) pathway demonstrated a significant, although brief, delay in disease progression in a large adult trial of sarcomas previously treated with cytotoxic chemotherapy.[113]

GENERAL BIOLOGIC FEATURES

STS can be classified into two groups based on cytogenetics. Tumors that occur in children and young adults tend to reveal relatively simple karyotypes often characterized by an easily recognizable and frequently pathognomonic reciprocal chromosomal translocation. In contrast, STS of adults typically demonstrate complex karyotypes without recurrent cytogenetic abnormalities. Cellular mechanisms for telomere maintenance may correlate with translocation status. Tumors harboring single translocations tend to have normal to short telomeres, suggestive of active telomerase, whereas tumors with complex karyotypes have longer telomeres, suggesting the use of alternative mechanisms of telomere lengthening.[114-118] Although other cellular changes, in addition to translocations, are likely to be necessary for sarcoma development, the difference between sarcomas of children and young adults and those of older individuals may reflect divergent cellular origins. Experimentally, haploinsufficiency of the nonhomologous end-joining DNA repair pathway in the context of *Ink4a/Arf*-deficient mice leads to the development of sarcoma with varied histology and karyotype.[119] Although the tumors that develop in these mice demonstrate translocations, amplifications, and deletions, the translocated regions are not recognizably syntenic with known human translocations suggesting that these sarcomas more closely reflect adult sarcomas. This finding also highlights the issue of whether complex cytogenetic abnormalities themselves result in oncogenesis or are a manifestation of genomic instability associated with the loss of cell cycle and DNA repair checkpoints.

ADIPOCYTIC TUMORS

Liposarcoma is the most common of the STS in adults.[120] In children, however, approximately 95% of adipose tumors are benign lipomas and lipoblastomas with liposarcomas accounting for the remainder.[121] Lipoblastomas tend to occur in children younger than 3 years of age, whereas liposarcomas predominate in older school-aged children and adolescents. Liposarcoma is classified into three morphologic types: well-differentiated/dedifferentiated, myxoid/round cell, and pleomorphic.[122] Morphologic types correspond to a developmental progression bearing similarities to that seen during induced mesenchymal differentiation into adipocytes.[123] Dedifferentiated/well-differentiated and pleomorphic liposarcomas occur predominantly in the retroperitoneum, whereas myxoid/round cell histology tends to occur in the extremities.[124] High-grade, dedifferentiated liposarcomas carry the highest risk for recurrence and metastasis.[125,126] In contrast to adults, most children present with the myxoid variant.[127,128] Myxoid liposarcoma is histopathologically characterized by proliferation of round to spindled primitive mesenchymal cells and scattered lipoblasts in an abundant faintly eosinophilic, homogeneous myxoid matrix (Fig. 60-2). A network of delicate straight and curvilinear capillaries is distinctive. The presence of a

round cell component may increase the risk for disease progression.[129] Complete resection is associated with prolonged tumor-free survival. When margins are microscopically positive, the addition of radiation therapy may increase disease-free survival. The histologic variants of liposarcoma are associated with differences in response to chemotherapy. Myxoid liposarcoma demonstrates the highest likelihood of response to a doxorubicin and ifosfamide regimen.[130] Myxoid liposarcoma also exhibits sensitivity to trabectedin (ecteinascidin-743; ET-743), a DNA minor groove–binding small molecule.[131,132]

Myxoid and round cell liposarcomas share recurrent chromosomal translocations that distinguish them from other liposarcoma histologies. t(12;16)(q13;p11) results in fusion of *FUS* (also known as TLS, an abbreviation for translocated in liposarcoma) with the transcription factor *DDIT3 (CHOP),* and t(12;22)(q13;q11) fuses *EWSR1* with *DDIT3.*[133-135] DDIT3 is a member of the b-ZIP family of transcriptional regulatory proteins and seems to function as a negative transcriptional regulator. Chimerism with both EWSR1 and FUS (TLS) suggests that the retained domains of EWSR1 and FUS confer similar activities to the DNA-binding domain of *DDIT3.* Ectopic expression of either FUS-DDIT3 or EWSR1-DDIT3 in NIH-3T3 cells resulted in characteristics of oncogenic transformation, including growth in soft agar and tumor formation in immunocompromised mice.[136] Furthermore, implantation of mice with primary murine mesenchymal progenitor cells transduced with FUS-DDIT3 led to the development of tumors that morphologically and immunohistochemically resemble human myxoid liposarcoma.[137]

Well-dedifferentiated liposarcomas are associated with complex karyotypes. However, a frequent finding is amplification of 12q, which includes *MDM2* and *CDK4.*[138,139] MDM2 binds TP53 to inhibit its activity. In the context of wild-type *TP53,* inhibition of MDM2 by the small molecule nutlin3 results in increased apoptosis in liposarcoma cell lines.[140,141] Transgenic mice expressing FUS-DDIT3 in mesenchymal progenitor cells developed sarcomas only in the absence of TP53. Interestingly, treatment of these mice with trabectidin resulted in adipocytic differentiation, which was increased by concurrent treatment with the peroxisome proliferator-activated receptor γ (PPARγ) agonist rosiglitazone.[142] Comprehensive genomic analysis of several sarcomas demonstrated *TP53* and *NF1* mutation in a subset of pleomorphic liposarcomas whereas *PIK3CA* was mutated in nearly 20% of myxoid/round cell liposarcomas.[143]

Chromosomal rearrangements of 8q12 are found in lipoblastoma, and their detection can aid in diagnosis. These rearrangements have implicated the zinc finger DNA-binding protein PLAG1. In lipoblastoma, translocation places the PLAG1 coding exons under the transcriptional control of the *HAS2, COL1A2,* or *RAD51L1* promoters.[144,145] PLAG1 was originally identified based on its translocation in pleomorphic adenoma of the salivary gland.[146] In contrast to lipoblastoma, *PLAG1* is translocated near *CTNNB1, CHCHD7* or *TCEA1* in pleomorphic adenoma.

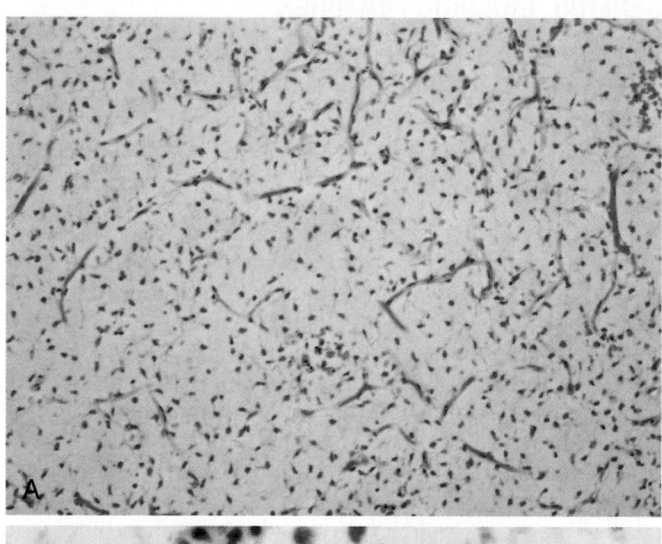
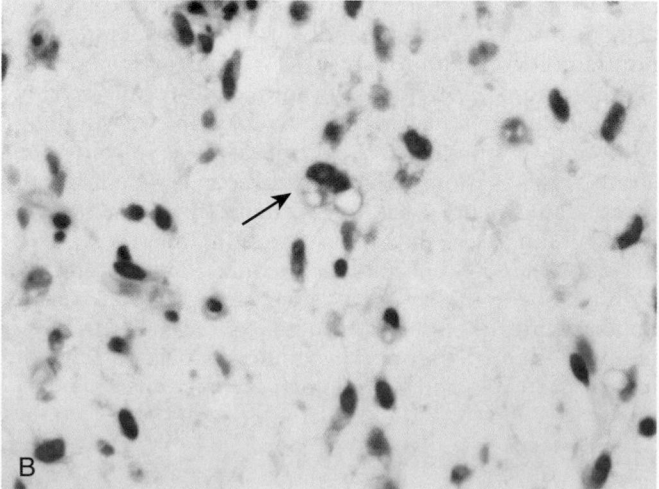

Figure 60-2 Myxoid liposarcoma. **A,** Uniform stellate and spindled cells in a prominent myxoid stroma and with characteristic branching capillaries. **B,** Primitive tumor cells and scattered lipoblasts *(arrow)* in a myxoid background.

FIBROBLASTIC AND MYOFIBROBLASTIC TUMORS

Desmoid Tumor

Desmoid tumor, also known as deep musculoaponeurotic fibromatosis, presents from infancy through adulthood with a median age at diagnosis in the early 30s and a twofold higher incidence in women. Although most tumors occur spontaneously, FAP patients, and in particular those with Gardner syndrome, have reported incidences of desmoid tumors ranging from 3.5% to 32%.[27,147] Desmoid tumors in the pediatric population tend to occur in the second decade and are located in the extremities and head and neck, in contrast to the adult population in whom abdominal and truncal sites are common.[148,149] Abdominal desmoids are more common in FAP patients, whereas limb and trunk locations predominate in non-FAP patients.[150]

The tumors consist of an infiltrating, uniform, spindled cell proliferation lacking nuclear pleomorphism and mitotic activity (Fig. 60-3). Although desmoid tumors have a high potential for local invasion and recurrence, they never metastasize. Surgery is the primary treatment; however, tumors have a significant chance of local recurrence even if negative margins can be achieved.[149] Achieving negative margins without severe disfigurement or functional impairment may be impossible. In these circumstances, preoperative chemotherapy or partial resection and postoperative chemotherapy should be considered, although, given a highly variable clinical course, close observation may be justified. Multiple drug regimens have been shown to shrink or stabilize desmoid tumor growth. These include methotrexate with vinblastine or tamoxifen with diclofenac.[151-154] Other potentially active treatments include the combination of doxorubicin, vincristine, dactinomycin, and cyclophosphamide or the combination of doxorubicin and dacarbazine.[155-157] Responses to imatinib and sorafenib have been observed in about half of desmoid patients.[111,158,159]

Although most desmoid tumor cells are karyotypically diploid, abnormalities of the Y chromosome and 5q and gains in chromosome 8 and 20 may be noted.[160-163] Abnormalities have been identified in a subset of tumor cells, and the finding of trisomy 8 may suggest an increased risk for recurrence.[161] Gardner syndrome, which is associated with colonic polyposis and abdominal desmoid tumors, is a phenotypic variant of FAP, which is caused by mutation of APC. APC regulates β-catenin, the downstream mediator of WNT signaling. Stabilized β-catenin forms a multiprotein complex with members of the T-cell factor/lymphoid enhancer factor family (TCF-LEF) resulting in transcriptional activation of TCF-LEF target genes.[164-167] APC mutations resulting in increased β-catenin or stabilizing mutations in the β-catenin gene (CTNNB1) have been implicated in the proliferation of sporadic desmoid tumors.[168-170] Eighty-five to 90 percent of sporadic desmoid tumors are associated with somatic mutation of CTNNB1.[171] Mice expressing either mutant APC or stabilized β-catenin develop aggressive fibromatoses.[172,173]

Infantile Myofibroma/Myofibromatosis and Hemangiopericytoma

In recent World Health Organization (WHO) classifications of soft tissue tumors, the term *hemangiopericytoma* is no longer used; instead, a majority of these tumors are currently classified as solitary fibrous tumors.[174,175] Infantile hemangiopericytoma, recognized as a distinct category of benign hemangiopericytoma by Enzinger, is currently regarded in the category of infantile myofibroma/myofibromatosis.[176] Infantile myofibromatosis is a benign proliferation of myofibroblastic cells affecting almost exclusively young children. The tumors are solitary or multicentric and may involve the skin, muscle, viscera, or bone. Sixty percent are noted at birth, and 88% occur before the age of 2.[177] More commonly found in males, solitary lesions typically develop in the soft tissues of the head and neck and trunk. In contrast, the multicentric form is more common in females and in addition to affecting soft tissues it can develop in bones and viscera. Histopathologically, infantile myofibroma and myofibromatosis have similar features. They are multinodular and biphasic with alternating hemangiopericytoma-like,

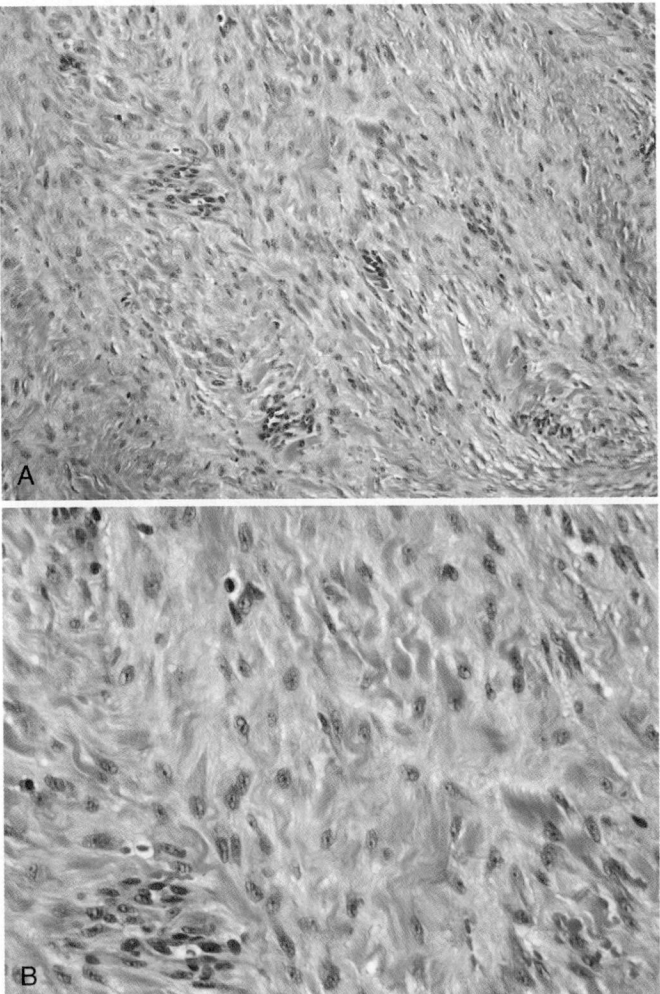

Figure 60-3 Desmoid tumor. **A,** Spindle cell neoplasm with prominent collagenization. **B,** Tumor cells are histopathologically bland with ovoid uniform nuclei, open chromatin, and single small nucleolus. Some cells have abundant eosinophilic cytoplasm.

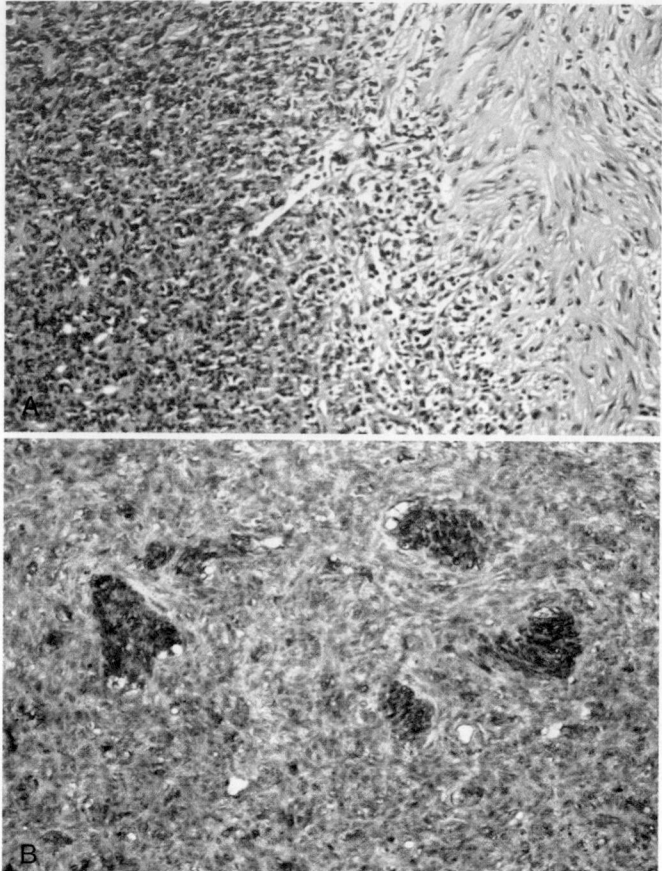

Figure 60-4 Infantile myofibromatoses. **A,** Biphasic tumor with an area of bland smooth musclelike proliferation *(right)* sharply demarcated from an area of cellular hemangiopericytoma-like tumor. **B,** Characteristic nests of strongly actin-immunoreactive cells *(red)* are scattered through a cellular hemangiopericytoma-like area.

densely cellular areas and less cellular areas with smooth muscle differentiation immunoreactive to actin (Fig. 60-4). Solitary lesions can rarely recur. Multicentric lesions undergo spontaneous regression; however, multiple visceral lesions may increase in size and number prior to regression, compromising vital structures and, rarely, leading to death.[178] Optimal initial therapy involves complete surgical excision. Life-threatening multifocal disease has been treated successfully with low-dose vincristine and dactinomycin or low-dose vinblastine and methotrexate.[179] Urinary basic fibroblast growth factor has been shown to be elevated in an infant during the proliferative phase, and connective tissue growth factor is expressed in both tumor and stromal cells.[180,181] An autosomal dominant pattern of inheritance has been associated with mutations in the growth factor receptor PDGFRB.[182-186]

Infantile myofibroma/myofibromatosis should be distinguished from pericytoma with t(7;12), a distinct tumor with histologic, immunohistochemical, and ultrastructural features of pericytic differentiation and a translocation involving t(7;12)(p22;q13).[187] Although typically developing in soft tissue, this entity can develop in bone.[188] The translocation brings together the β-actin gene *(ACTB)* with the zinc finger transcription factor *GLI1*.[189] Originally identified based on amplification in human glioma, GLI1 is activated by Sonic hedgehog signaling through the transmembrane receptor *PTCH*.[190-192] In t(7;12) pericytoma the carboxyl terminus of GLI1 is fused with the amino-terminal domain of ACTB. Intriguingly, *GLI1* has also been found to be amplified in a subset of rhabdomyosarcoma and osteosarcoma that lack typical markers of differentiation.[193]

Infantile Fibrosarcoma

Infantile (congenital) fibrosarcoma is one of the most common NRSTS in young children.[194] In contrast to fibrosarcoma in adults, this low-grade tumor displays a benign clinical behavior and is typically cured by surgical excision. However, large tumors for which surgical excision would result in significant morbidity may be treated with preoperative chemotherapy (Fig. 60-5, *A*). Regimens with activity against these tumors include vincristine and dactinomycin alone or together with either cyclophosphamide, ifosfamide, or doxorubicin.[195-202]

Histopathologically, the tumor is characterized by intersecting bundles with a herringbone pattern composed of cellular spindle to ovoid cells with a high proliferative rate, frequent mitoses, and areas of necrosis (see Fig. 60-5, *B* and *C*). Some tumors may have a hemangiopericytoma-like pattern of growth. Scattered chronic inflammatory cells are frequently present. Tumor cells have a fibroblastic and myofibroblastic ultrastructure (see Fig. 60-5, *D*) and immunophenotype with variable positivity for desmin and actin. Aberrant cytokeratin expression is observed in 15% to 20% of the tumors.

Infantile fibrosarcoma is characterized by t(12;15) (p13;q25).[203] This translocation fuses the amino-terminal helix-loop-helix oligomerization domain of the ETV6 transcription factor (also known as *TEL*) with the carboxyl-terminal tyrosine kinase domain of the neurotrophic tyrosine kinase receptor, type 3 (*NTRK3*, also known as *TRKC*). The detection of ETV6-NTRK3 by reverse-transcriptase PCR is highly specific and can distinguish infantile fibrosarcoma from more aggressive spindle cell sarcomas.[204] Intriguingly, the same translocation also occurs in congenital mesoblastic nephroma, secretory breast carcinoma, and acute myeloid leukemia.[205-208]

Chimerism results in constitutive activation by autophosphorylation of NTRK3 tyrosine residues. Translocation also results in aberrant *NTRK3* expression. *ETV6* is widely expressed whereas *NTRK3* is normally restricted to neuronal cells and fetal kidney.[209-211] ETV6-NTRK3 expression can transform NIH3T3 cells as assayed by growth in soft agar and in xenografts in immunocompromised mice.[212] ETV6-NTRK3 is associated with several signaling pathways that may be important in oncogenesis. ETV6-NTRK3 activates both the MAPK and AKT pathways, with AKT activation mediated by direct interaction of ETV6-NTRK3 with SRC.[213,214] Activation of signaling also leads to phosphorylation of YAP1 and WWTR1, Hippo pathway transcriptional coactivators, and a characteristic transcriptional profile.[215] ETV6-NTRK3–mediated fibroblast transformation also requires the insulin-like growth factor receptor (IGF1R) possibly

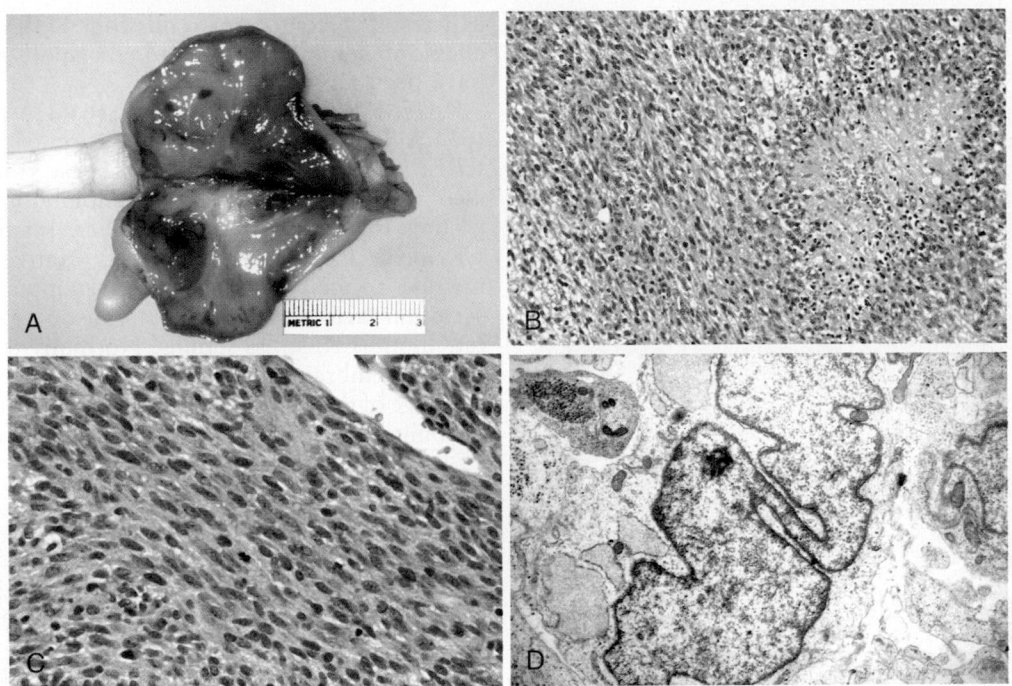

Figure 60-5 Infantile fibrosarcoma. **A,** Partial amputation of the hand in an infant with a rapidly growing soft tissue mass. On cut section the mass is fleshy and soft with areas of hemorrhage and necrosis. **B,** Histopathology shows a cellular spindle cell sarcoma with frequent mitoses, apoptosis, and confluent areas of necrosis. **C,** At higher magnification, nuclei appear uniform and hyperchromatic and cytoplasm is elongated and pink. Scattered inflammatory cells are also present. **D,** Ultrastructurally, tumor cells have the features of fibroblasts with prominent secretory-type rough endoplasmic reticulum.

through directly interacting with the IGF1R substrate IRS-1.[216-218] The ETV6-NTRK3 fusion may also act by suppressing transforming growth factor-β (TGF-β) signaling through interaction with the type II TGF-β receptor.[219]

Fibrosarcoma Arising in Dermatofibrosarcoma Protuberans and Giant Cell Fibroblastoma

Dermatofibrosarcoma protuberans (DFSP) is a rare cutaneous fibrohistiocytic tumor characterized by locally aggressive behavior. DFSP may begin as a plaquelike, raised red-blue lesion followed by a rapid growth phase that may be associated with the development of one or more nodules. DFSP appears as a cellular, spindle cell proliferation, frequently with a distinct storiform pattern that infiltrates the surrounding dermis and subcutaneous fat (Fig. 60-6, *A*). Tumor cells are typically immunoreactive for apolipoprotein D and CD34 (see Fig. 60-6, *B*). The Bednar tumor refers to an uncommon DFSP variant with scattered dendritic cells containing melanin.[220] The majority of the tumors develop on the trunk and upper extremity. Although typically diagnosed during the fourth and fifth decades, DFSP may occur in children and adolescents.[221] Inadequate resection of the tumor is associated with a significant risk for local recurrence.[222] Radiation therapy can be used effectively as an adjuvant for the treatment of resection sites with positive margins.[223-225] Rarely, DFSP can evolve into a high-grade fibrosarcoma often associated with a loss of CD34 staining and an increased risk for metastasis (Fig. 60-7, *A* and *B*).[226] Giant cell fibroblastoma, a rare tumor predominantly of males younger than 10 years of age, is in the

spectrum of DFSP. Histopathologically, giant cell fibroblastoma is composed of variably cellular spindle or stellate cells often in a myxoid background containing pseudovascular spaces and multinucleated giant cells (see Fig. 60-7, *C*).[227-229]

Like DFSP, giant cell fibroblastoma is characteristically immunoreactive for CD34 and apolipoprotein D.[230] Both lesions also harbor a pathognomonic translocation between the collagen, type I, alpha 1, gene *(COL1A1)* and the platelet-derived growth factor-β gene *(PDGFB)*.[231-233] In contrast to the other sarcoma-associated translocations, the translocated *COL1A1-PDGFB* locus may be present as a low-level amplification on a ring chromosome. Detection of the resulting *COL1A1-PDGFB* transcript can provide confirmation of the diagnosis.[234] The fusion of *PDGFB* with *COL1A1* preserves the full coding region of *PDGFB*, and the resulting chimeric polypeptide is subject to intracellular processing that results in the secretion of a native PDGFB molecule that is capable of activating its receptor, PDGFR.[235,236] Although the mechanisms for autocrine-activated PDGFR signaling are not known, it may function through STAT3 and ERK activation.[237] Presumably through the inhibition of autocrine PDGFR activation, the growth of xenografted primary human DFSP cells can be inhibited with the kinase inhibitor imatinib (Gleevec).[238] Treatment with imatinib has also been shown to be effective in children and in patients with metastatic or unresectable disease.[239-245] Imatinib-resistant DFSP may respond to sorafenib or sunitinib.[246,247] Response to vinblastine and methotrexate has also been reported.[248]

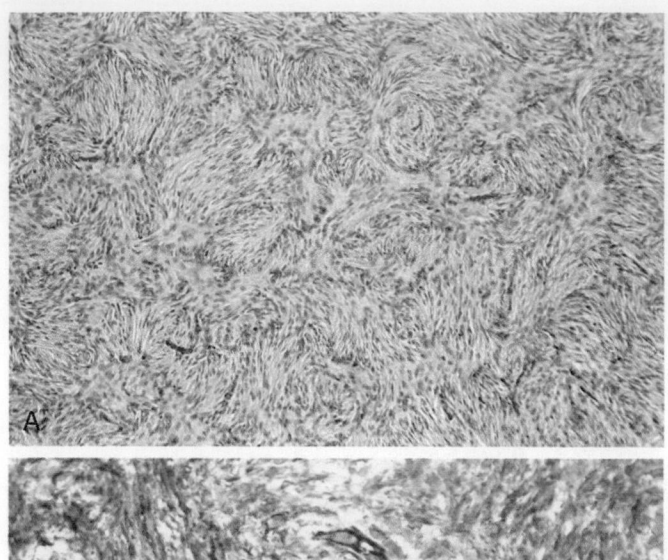

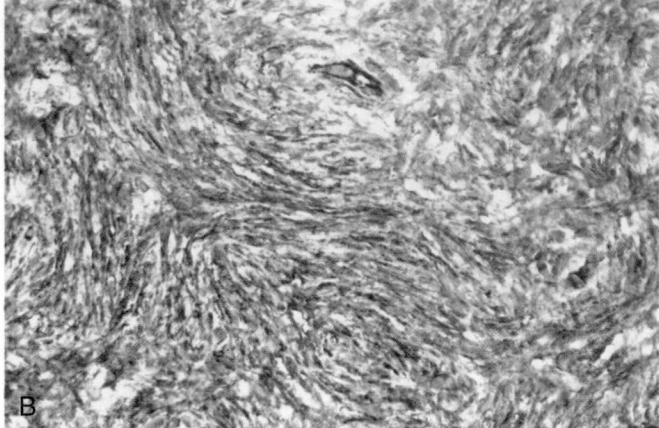

Figure 60-6 Dermatofibrosarcoma protuberans. **A,** Cellular spindle cell neoplasm with distinct storiform (cartwheel) pattern of growth. **B,** Tumor cells are diffusely immunoreactive with CD34.

Low-Grade Fibromyxoid Sarcoma

Low-grade fibromyxoid sarcoma (LGFMS) typically develops in the lower extremities of young adults and occasionally in adolescents (Fig. 60-8). Described by Evans in 1987, it is characterized by bland, uniform spindle cells with a short fascicular or whorly pattern of growth in a dense collagenous or variably myxoid stroma (Fig. 60-9).[249,250] An abrupt transition between cellular myxoid and hypocellular collagenous areas is frequently present. Dense collagenous areas mimic desmoid tumor. Myxoid areas contain characteristic arcades of curvilinear vessels that may be sclerotic or be surrounded by more densely cellular spindle cells. Mitotic count is characteristically low. Occasionally there are giant collagenous rosettes (hyalinizing spindle cell tumor with giant rosettes). Vimentin is the only constant marker present in tumor cells. Some tumors may be focally immunoreactive for actin, CD34, cytokeratins, or epithelial membrane antigen (EMA). MUC4 reactivity is common in LGFMS and can distinguish it from other histologically similar tumors.[251] A superficial location occurs more frequently in children.[252] Although primary resection typically results in disease control, local recurrences and pulmonary metastases can develop in 5% to 10% of patients after many years.[253,254] However, resection of recurrent disease

can result in long-term remission. LGFMS seems to be chemoresistant, although limited responses to trabectedin have been reported.[255,256]

LGFMS is associated with t(7;16)(q34;p11) or t(11;16) (p11;p11), which results in the fusion of *FUS (TLS)* with *CREB3L2* or *CREB3L1*.[257-260] These translocations are also found in sclerosing epithelioid fibrosarcoma, suggesting that these tumors may be related.[261] *EWSR1-CREB3L1* has also been noted.[262] Native CREB3L2 is a member of the CREB basic leucine zipper family of transcription factors and acts as a transducer of endoplasmic reticulum (ER) stress signals. Normally tethered through a transmembrane domain to the ER, ER stress results in cleavage of the cytoplasmic amino terminal b-ZIP domain, enabling it to translocate to the nucleus and to activate

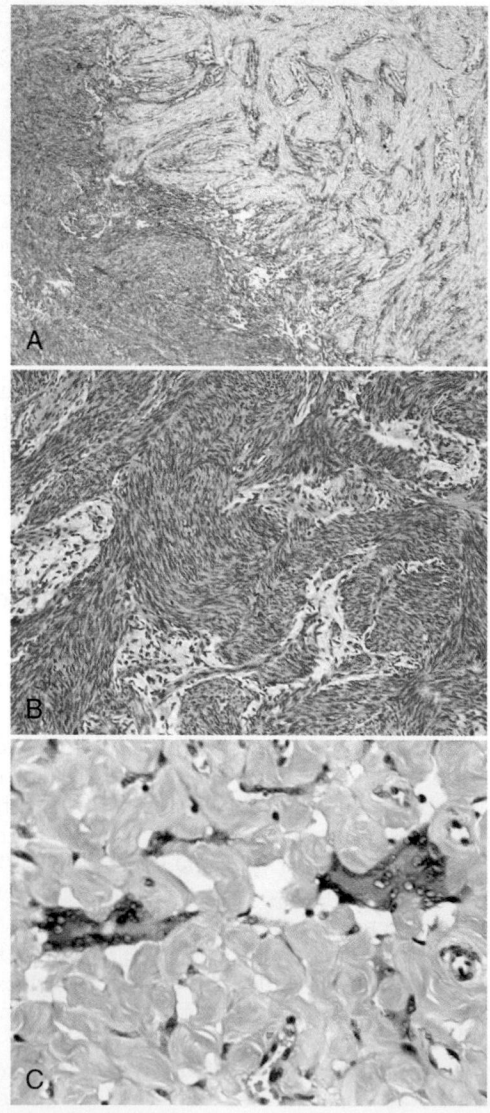

Figure 60-7 Fibrosarcoma in dermatofibrosarcoma protuberans/giant cell fibroblastoma. **A,** Loss of CD34 immunoreactivity in dedifferentiated fibrosarcoma area, which appears sharply demarcated from adjacent CD34-positive dermatofibrosarcoma protuberans *(lower left corner)*. **B,** Highly cellular fibrosarcoma with fascicular pattern and numerous mitoses. **C,** Giant cell fibroblastoma with characteristic multinucleated giant cells and spindled cells with collagenization.

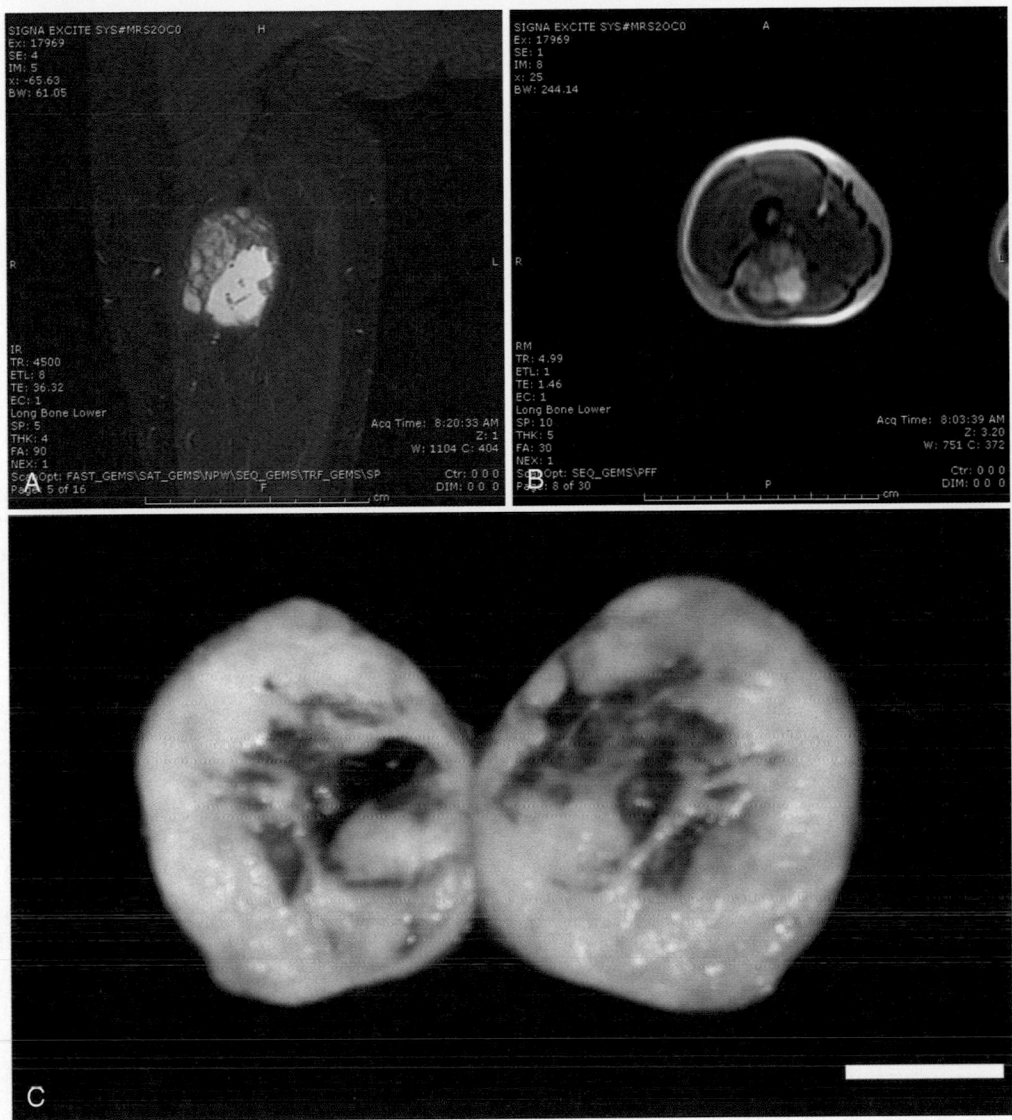

Figure 60-8 Low-grade fibromyxoid sarcoma. **A** and **B,** MR images of enhancing well-delineated heterogeneous thigh mass. **C,** Grossly the tumor is well circumscribed and shows a soft white and tan cut surface with areas of hemorrhage and cystification.

transcription from cyclic adenosine monophosphate (AMP)–responsive elements.[263] Chimerism with FUS, a translocation partner with CHOP in myxoid liposarcoma, likely deregulates CREB3L2 transcriptional activity.[264] PCR-based identification of the fusion gene product from paraffin sections can be used to confirm the diagnosis.[261] LGFMS is associated with a gene expression profile that distinguishes it from similar tumors and is marked by the expression of *FOXL1*.[265]

Myxofibrosarcoma

Myxofibrosarcoma (MFS) is one of the most common sarcomas of the elderly but has been reported in adolescents and young adults.[266,267] Typically developing in the sixth and seventh decades of life, MFS exhibits a predilection for the dermal or subcutaneous tissues of the extremities.[260,270] MFS may be alternatively referred to as low-grade myxoid malignant fibrous histiocytoma or fibrosarcoma, myxoid type. Histopathologically, it is characterized by a multinodular growth of spindled or stellate cells in a myxoid stroma (Fig. 60-10). MFS grading has prognostic value and is based on cellularity, nuclear pleomorphism, and mitotic activity.[271] Resection is typically curative for low- or intermediate-grade tumors; however, recurrent tumors may show morphologic and molecular multistep tumor progression.[272,273] Large tumor size, necrosis, and decreased myxoid stroma in low-grade tumors are associated with a significant risk for local and distant recurrence.[274] Intermediate- and high-grade tumors have a significant risk for recurrence and metastasis.[275] In a study of adults, 23% of patients with intermediate- or high-grade tumors developed metastases, most commonly to the lung and lymph nodes and rarely to the brain. A subset of intermediate- or high-grade tumors exhibiting an epithelioid morphology seems to behave more aggressively than other high-grade histologies.[276] In addition to grade, an initial incomplete resection and infiltrative MRI T2-weighted signal

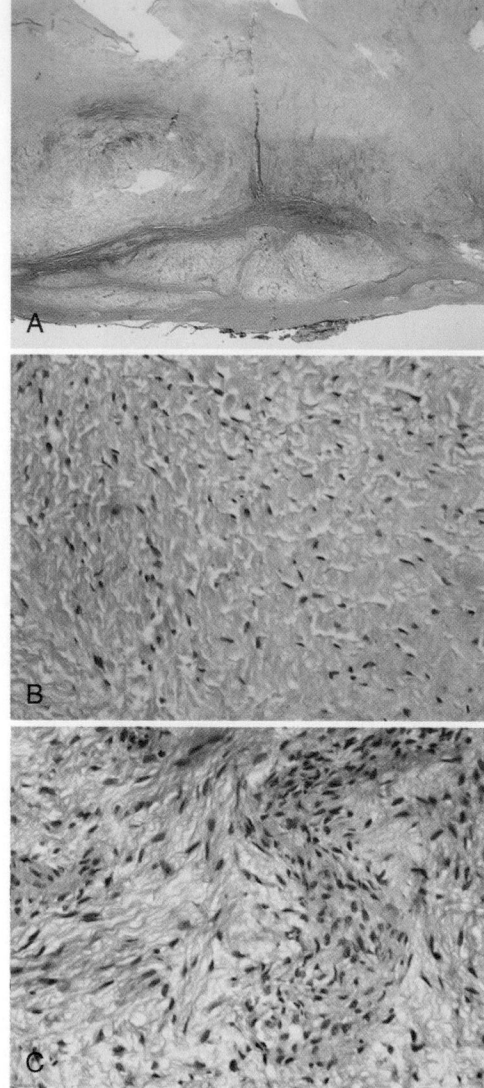

Figure 60-9 Low-grade fibromyxoid sarcoma. **A,** Multinodular, infiltrative growth at the tumor periphery and a variably myxoid stroma. **B,** Fibromatosis-like area with bland spindled cells immersed in a collagenous background. **C,** Characteristic curvilinear blood vessels, bland spindled cells, and myxoid background.

correlates with an increased risk for local recurrence.[277] Combined chemotherapy and irradiation has efficacy for MFS.[278] Cytogenetically, MFS may be diploid but is typically complex. Numerous chromosomal gains and losses as well as ring chromosomes have been observed.[273,279] Large-scale 7q gains were associated with increased expression of the hepatocyte growth factor receptor MET and CDK6, and increased expressed of these proteins was associated with lower metastasis-free survival.[280,281] Ezrin expression also correlates with decreased metastasis-free survival.[282] Isolated chromosomal translocations have been noted.[283,284]

Solitary Fibrous Tumor

Solitary fibrous tumor (SFT) is a fibroblastic tumor that was originally described in the pleura but can occur at other sites, most frequently the abdomen and pelvis.

Most of the tumors formerly classified as hemangiopericytomas are currently categorized as SFT. SFT can be classified as classic, malignant, or dedifferentiated.[285,286] Five to 10 percent of soft tissue SFTs are malignant. SFT may be associated with hypoglycemia owing to synthesis by tumor cells of insulin-like growth factor 2 (IGF-2).[287,288] The histopathology is described as a patternless proliferation of spindle cells with a hemangiopericytoma-like growth (Fig. 60-11). Areas of sclerosis and hyalinization are characteristic. Mitotic count is generally low. Although the behavior of SFTs cannot be always predicted by histopathology, the presence of frequent mitoses, hypercellularity, pleomorphism, and necrosis is generally associated with malignant behavior. Large tumors and those with a mitotic index greater than 4 indicate an increased risk for recurrence locally or, more frequently, metastatically, even in the presence of negative resection margins.[289] Tumor cells are immunoreactive with CD34 and CD99 (see Fig. 60-11, *inset*). Some tumors also express EMA, actin, BCL2, apolipoprotein D, or nuclear β-catenin.[290-292] Recurrent NAB2-STAT6 fusions have

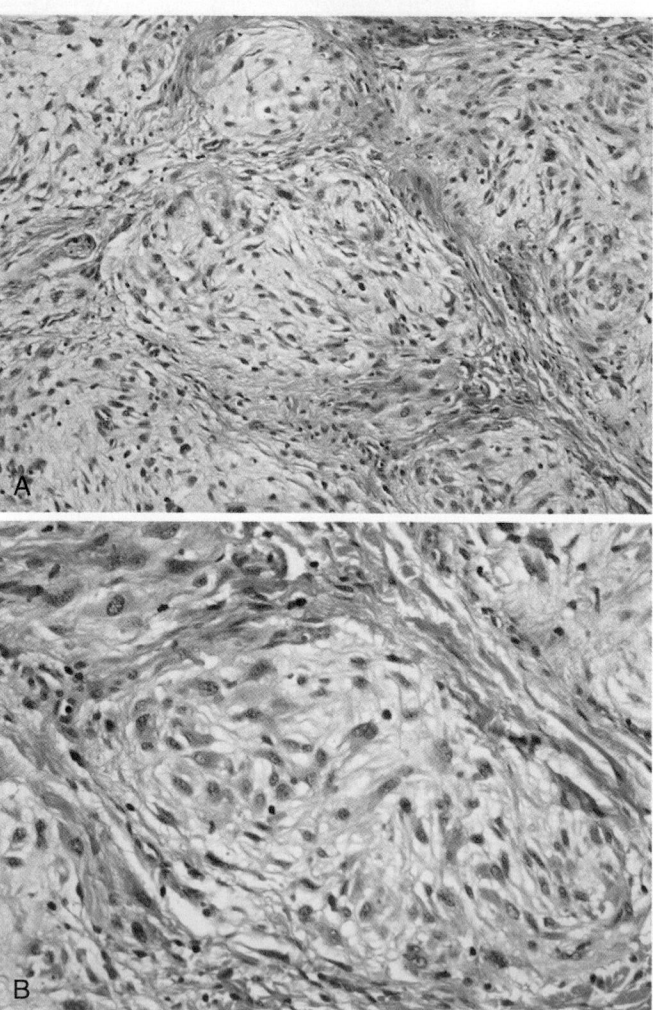

Figure 60-10 Myxofibrosarcoma. **A,** Multinodular growth pattern and prominent myxoid stroma. Numerous curvilinear vessels are present at the periphery of the nodules. **B,** Atypical myofibroblasts with large mildly pleomorphic nuclei and abundant cytoplasm.

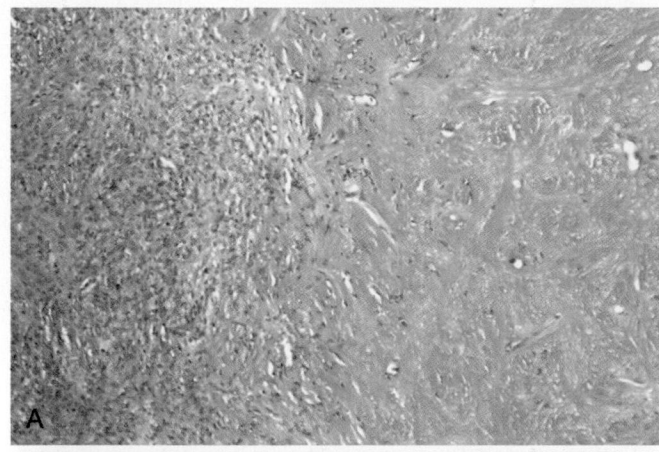

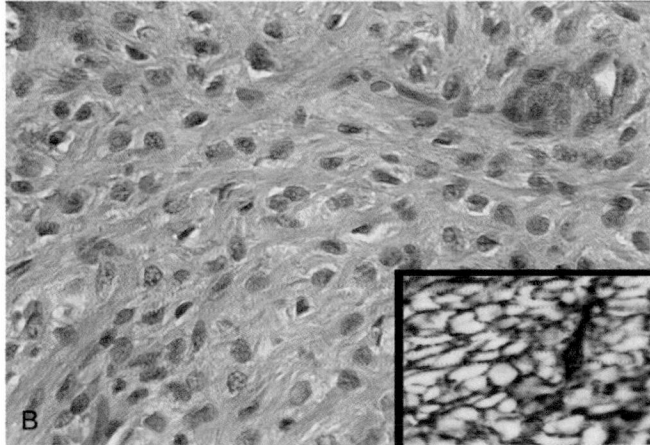

Figure 60-11 Solitary fibrous tumor. **A,** Spindle cell tumor with a prominent area of sclerosis. **B,** Patternless proliferation of spindled cells with uniform, ovoid nuclei, inconspicuous nucleoli, and eosinophilic cytoplasm with poorly defined borders. Tumor cells are strongly immunoreactive with CD34 (inset).

been identified in the majority of SFTs regardless of the site of origin or SFT classification.[293,294] In this fusion protein, NAB2 contributes an amino-terminal EGR1 binding domain and STAT6 contributes a carboxyl terminal transcriptional activation domain with or without an associated DNA-binding domain. The resulting protein may cooperate with EGR1 to activate growth factor pathways. Based on this chromosomal rearrangement, virtually all SFTs demonstrate nuclear expression of STAT6 by immunohistochemistry.[295] Dacarbazine has demonstrated efficacy in SFTs as has treatment with bevacizumab or one of several tyrosine kinase inhibitors, including sorafenib, sunitinib, and pazopanib.[110,296-300]

Inflammatory Myofibroblastic Tumor

Inflammatory myofibroblastic tumors (IMTs) occur primarily in the viscera and soft tissue (particularly lungs) of children and young adults with a mean age of 13.2 years.[301] Of intermediate biologic potential, these tumors often recur locally but rarely metastasize. They are characterized by a proliferation of myofibroblastic spindled cells and an inflammatory, predominantly lymphoplasmacytic infiltrate (Fig. 60-12, A). Approximately half of

IMTs show immunoreactivity for anaplastic lymphoma kinase (ALK) (see Fig. 60-12, B). ALK-positive IMTs are more common in younger patients and seem less likely to metastasize than ALK-negative disease, although local recurrence occurs with equal frequency.[301]

Clonal cytogenetic changes that activate ALK occur in 50% to 70% of IMTs.[302] The most common chromosomal translocation results in a fusion of the ALK receptor tyrosine kinase with the amino-terminal coiled domain of tropomyosin 3 or tropomyosin 4 (TPM3 and TPM4). ALK may also be fused to the amino-terminal domains of clathrin heavy chain (CTLC), cysteinyl-tRNA synthetase, RAN-binding protein 2 (RANBP-2), SEC31L1, or PPFIBP1.[303-307] ALK rearrangements were first identified in anaplastic large cell lymphoma, in which the fusion of ALK with nucleophosmin is most common, although chimerism with CTLC has also been observed.[308,309] Possibly based on ALK hyperactivation, the ALK/MET inhibitor crizotinib has demonstrated activity, although the response may be limited by mutation-associated resistance.[310-312] IMTs frequently demonstrate expression of MYC, cyclin D1, and MCL1 regardless of ALK status. Cyclooxygenase 2 inhibitors may be effective for IMT.[313,314]

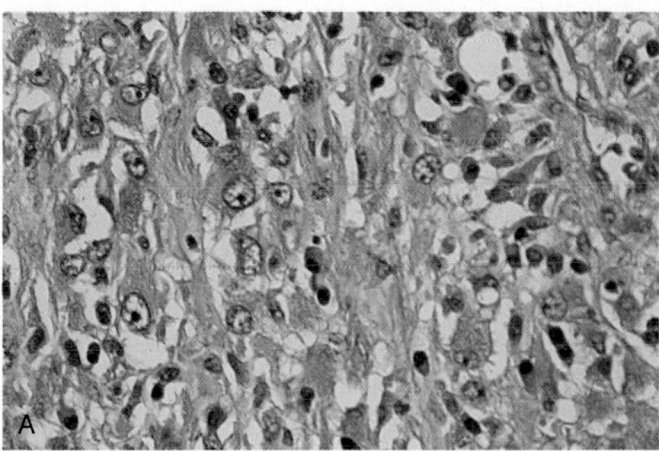

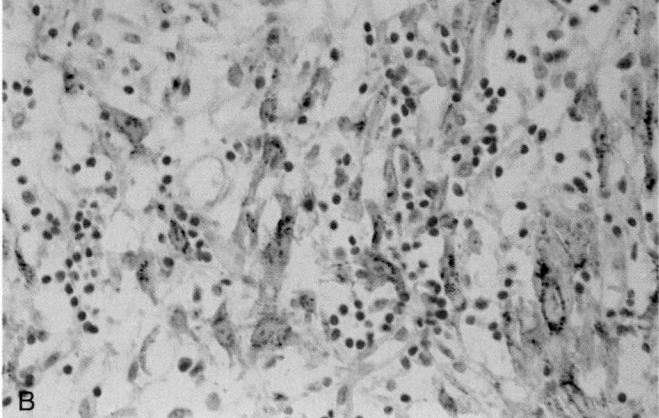

Figure 60-12 Inflammatory myofibroblastic tumor. **A,** Spindled and plump myofibroblasts with abundant eosinophilic cytoplasm, round to ovoid nuclei, and prominent single nucleolus. Intermingled are numerous lymphocytes and plasma cells. **B,** Neoplastic myofibroblasts show cytoplasmic immunoreactivity for anaplastic lymphoma kinase.

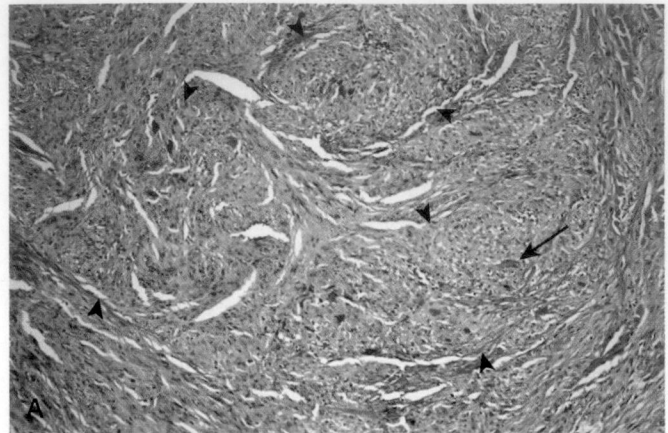

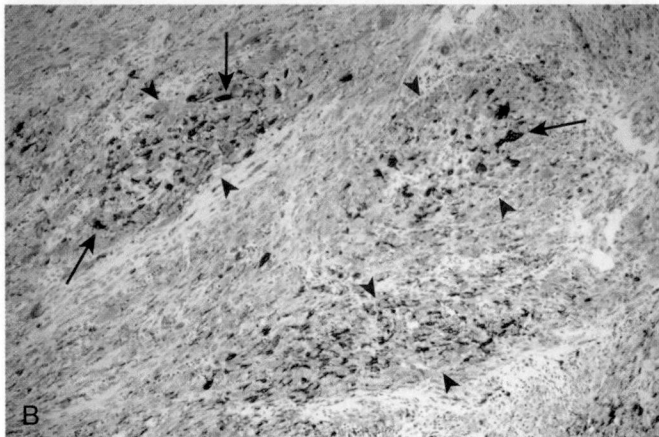

Figure 60-13 Plexiform fibrohistiocytic tumor. **A,** Multiple micronodules *(between arrowheads)* of fibrohistiocytic cells and multinucleated giant cells separated by collagenous stroma. **B,** Strong CD68 immunoreactivity of multinucleated giant cells *(arrows)* within micronodules *(between arrowheads).*

SO-CALLED FIBROHISTIOCYTIC TUMORS

Plexiform Fibrohistiocytic Tumor

Plexiform fibrohistiocytic tumor is a fibrohistiocytic neoplasm of intermediate malignant potential with a multinodular (plexiform) pattern of growth that occurs in the deep dermis and subcutaneous tissue primarily in children, adolescents, and young adults, with a mean age of 14.5 years.[315,316] Histopathologically these tumors are characterized by a plexiform growth of small nodules composed of mononuclear histiocyte-like cells, fibroblasts, and multinucleate giant cells (Fig. 60-13). Mitoses are infrequent, and pleomorphism is minimal. Immunohistochemical findings reflect the proportion of histiocytic to fibrous elements, with CD68 marking osteoclast-like multinucleated giant cells and smooth muscle actin (SMA) focally marking the fibrous component.[317] These tumors are histologically similar to some neurothekomas, but immunohistochemical staining for microphthalmia-associated transcription factor (MITF) may discriminate these entities.[318,319] This tumor has a tendency to locally recur and in about 5% of cases may metastasize, particularly to regional lymph nodes.[320] Cytogenetic abnormalities in the few cases reported are heterogeneous.

SMOOTH MUSCLE TUMORS

Sporadic Leiomyosarcoma

Leiomyosarcoma (LMS) is one of the most common STS in adults.[321] LMS can develop in uterus, bowel, vascular structures, and skin, as well as soft tissue and bone.[322,323] In children, LMS most commonly develops in the gastrointestinal tract and skin. In infants, intestinal LMS can present as perforation and obstruction.[324,325] In the head and neck, trunk, and extremities LMS has an equal incidence and tends to exhibit a more low-grade morphology and a clinical behavior comparable to that in adults.[326,327] Secondary LMS may develop in the radiation field of childhood cancer survivors.[328] Histopathologically, LMS is characterized by intersecting fascicles of spindle cells with prominently eosinophilic cytoplasm and elongated cigar-shaped nuclei (Fig. 60-14). In some tumors, nuclear pleomorphism and hyperchromatism are present. Mitoses are usually easily found, and their frequency is often uneven throughout the tumor. Tumor cells are immunoreactive for SMA, desmin, and h-caldesmon.

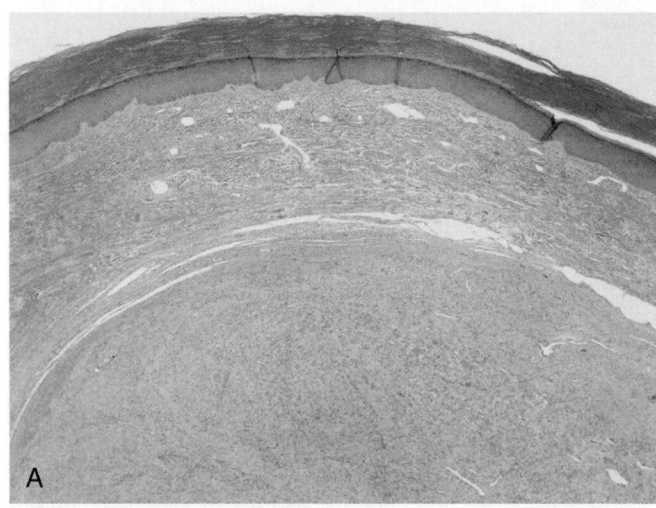

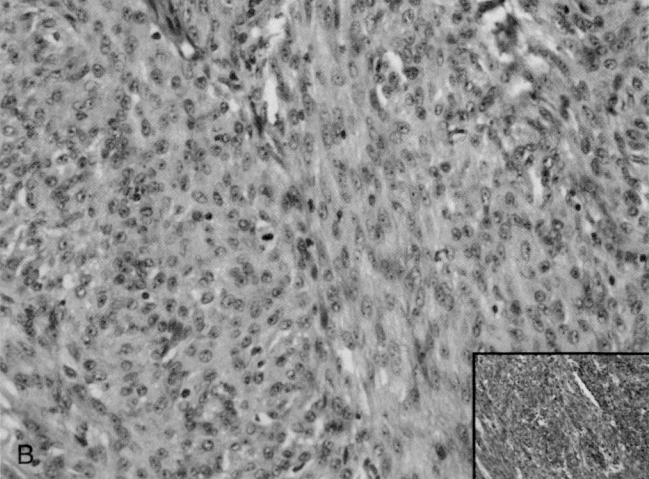

Figure 60-14 Leiomyosarcoma. **A,** Large tumor nodule is centered in the deep dermis and subcutaneous tissue. **B,** Tumor cells are spindled and have brightly eosinophilic cytoplasm and prominent nuclei with distinct centrally located nucleoli. Note strong and diffuse immunoreactivity for smooth muscle actin *(inset).*

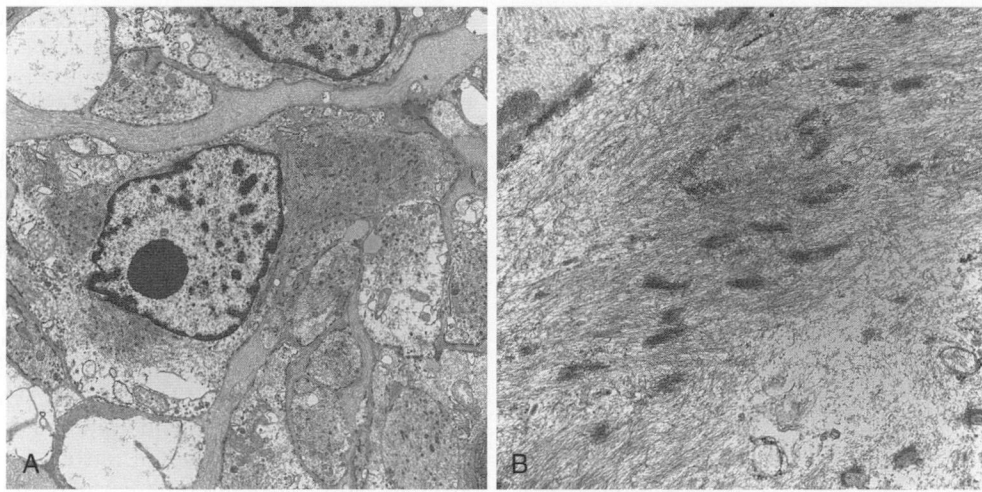

Figure 60-15 Leiomyosarcoma, electron microscopy. **A,** Tumor cells are individually invested by a continuous, well-developed basal lamina, and the abundant cytoplasm is filled with smooth muscle–type filaments. **B,** At higher magnification, note actin-type filaments with uniformly distributed dense bodies, typical of smooth muscle.

Ultrastructurally, tumor cells are invested by a continuous basal lamina and have subplasmalemmal densities and their cytoplasms contain abundant smooth muscle–type myofilaments with evenly distributed dense bodies (Fig. 60-15). Owing to the morphologic continuum of smooth muscle tumors, mitotic activity is the most reliable way to distinguish a leiomyoma from an LMS.

LMS has been treated with doxorubicin or ifosfamide as a single agent but with limited efficacy.[329,330] Patients with unresectable LMS treated with gemcitabine together with docetaxel demonstrated an overall response rate of 53%.[331] In recurrent or progressive STS, including LMS, the combination of gemcitabine and docetaxel was superior to gemcitabine alone.[101] Gemcitabine with docetaxel followed by doxorubicin in uterus-limited LMS resulted in a 57% PFS at 3 years.[332] When vinorelbine or dacarbazine is combined with gemcitabine the response rates have been reported as 15% to 20%.[102,333] Treatment with bendamustine resulted in stable disease in 40% of patients with LMS refractory to other agents.[334] Treatment with trabectedin is associated with disease stabilization in a significant fraction of patients in several clinical trials, including in pretreated LMS patients.[132,335-338] The multikinase inhibitor pazopanib also has limited disease-stabilizing activity in LMS.[110,339]

Germline mutation of the fumarate hydratase gene *(FH),* resulting in fumarate hydratase deficiency, is associated with a cancer predisposition syndrome with an increased risk for renal cell carcinoma, benign leiomyomas of the skin and uterus, and uterine leiomyosarcoma.[340,341,342] These tumors exhibit complex and unbalanced karyotypes. Genome-wide examination of DNA copy number variation and gene expression segregates a class enriched in the conventional LMS histologic subtypes with chromosome 10 and 13 losses and gains at 17p11-12. The remainder exhibit gene expression and copy number variation patterns similar to those of undifferentiated pleomorphic sarcomas and MFS.[343,344] *MED12,* which is mutated in the majority of uterine leiomyomas, is

occasionally mutated in leiomyosarcoma.[345,346] MED12 is a component of the mediator transcriptional complex and can regulate TGF-β receptor signaling, influencing cellular responses to tyrosine kinase inhibition.[347] Vascular endothelial growth factor (VEGF) overexpression detected by immunohistochemistry was associated with a significantly shorter survival, suggesting a mechanism for the activity of pazopanib.[348] Tissue and expression microarray-based studies comparing uterine LMS with uterine leiomyoma demonstrated increased expression of CDKN1A, TP53, PDGFR, KIT, and CDKN21A.[349-354] Approximately 20% of transgenic mice expressing teratocarcinoma-derived growth factor 1 (also known as CRIPTO) from an MMTV promoter developed uterine leiomyosarcoma.[355,356] Chromosome 10q deletion is associated with *PTEN* loss and hyperactivation of the phosphatidylinositol 3′-kinase/serine–threonine kinase (PI3K/AKT) pathway. Consistent with the importance of this pathway in LMS, conditional *Pten* inactivation in smooth muscle led to the development of abdominal LMS in mice.[357] Decreased tumor growth after treatment with the rapamycin derivative everolimus suggested the importance of mTOR activation in this model. However, clinical trials failed to demonstrate significant treatment responses to mTOR inhibition by temsirolimus or ridaforolimus in LMS.[113,358,359]

Leiomyosarcoma Associated with Epstein-Barr Virus

Immunosuppression associated with solid transplantation and HIV infection can result in EBV-associated LMS, particularly in children and young adults.[46] Multicentricity is common. The histopathologic, immunohistochemical, and ultrastructural features are similar to the sporadic ones (Fig. 60-16). In situ hybridization with EBV-encoded RNA shows nuclear positivity in nearly all tumor cells (see Fig. 60-16, *inset*). EBV can infect smooth muscle cells, resulting in expression of latent and replicative viral products and production of infectious virus.[360] Reducing immunosuppression can lead to long-term remission.[361-363]

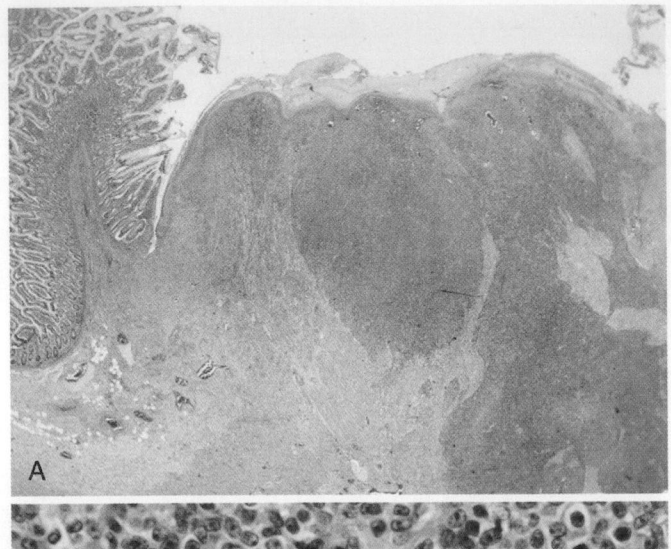

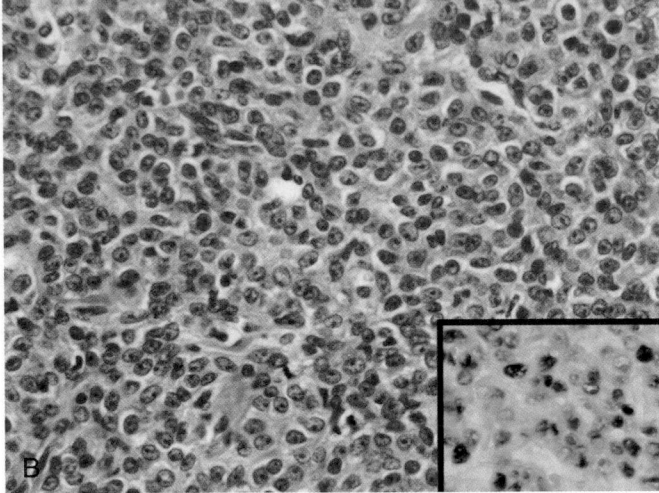

Figure 60-16 Epstein-Barr virus–associated smooth muscle tumor. **A,** Small intestine with large ulcerating and infiltrative submucosal mass. **B,** The tumor is cellular with spindled and round tumor cells with uniform nuclei and a distinct single nucleolus. Diffuse nuclear positivity for EBV-EBER is seen by in situ hybridization *(inset)*.

VASCULAR TUMORS

Epithelioid Hemangioendothelioma

Epithelioid hemangioendothelioma (EHE) is a vascular tumor that most commonly develops in superficial or deep soft tissue of the extremities.[364] Other sites include the liver, bone, lung, skin, lymph nodes, and central nervous system.[365-370] EHE often seems to arise from a medium to large vein. Unlike epithelioid hemangioma, vascular differentiation in EHE is primitive with a solid growth pattern or in strands (Fig. 60-17). The stroma is usually myxoid. Tumor cells are large with abundant eosinophilic cytoplasm. Intracellular vacuoles are characteristic and represent early lumen formation sometimes containing erythrocytes. Occasionally there are associated eosinophils and lymphocytes. Focal cellular spindling, atypia, and necrosis are associated with a more aggressive course; however, a bland-appearing lesion may also metastasize.[371] The differential diagnosis includes metastatic carcinoma, melanoma, or various sarcomas with epithelioid appearance, in particular, epithelioid angiosarcoma and epithelioid sarcoma. Tumor cells are immunoreactive with vascular markers, such as CD31, factor VIII–related antigen, and CD34. Ultrastructurally, tumor cells reveal vascular differentiation with prominent cytoskeletal intermediate filaments, Weibel-Palade granules, pinocytosis, and basal lamina. Two translocation-associated gene fusions have been reported in EHE. t(1;3) (p36.3q25) in EHE results in the *WWTR1-CAMTA1* gene fusion.[372-374] CAMTA1 is a member of a family of calmodulin-binding transcriptional regulatory proteins, and WWTR1 (also known as TAZ) is a component of the Hippo pathway. Interestingly, this pathway has been implicated in infantile fibrosarcoma. In t(1;3)-negative tumors, RNA sequencing identified a *YAP1-TFE3* gene fusion.[375] *TFE3* translocation has also been described in alveolar soft part sarcoma (ASPS) and translocation-associated renal cell carcinoma, although with different fusion partners.

Extended periods of stable disease as well as partial spontaneous resolution have been noted.[376] Lower-grade lesions can be conservatively resected, whereas malignant lesions likely justify radical surgical resection. Although surgical resection can result in cure, about one third of patients will develop a local recurrence or distant metastasis, most commonly to the lung. Although EHE is considered to be chemoresistant, responses to carboplatin with etoposide and carboplatin with paclitaxel for aggressive pulmonary disease and to interferon-alfa 2 (IFN-2α) for multifocal or disseminated liver disease have been reported.[377-381] Targeting the VEGF pathway with sorafenib and bevacizumab has shown limited efficacy.[382-384] Thalidomide and lenalidomide have also demonstrated activity.[385,386]

Giant Cell Angioblastoma

Giant cell angioblastoma is a rare neonatal vascular tumor. Although the tumor grows slowly, it can be locally

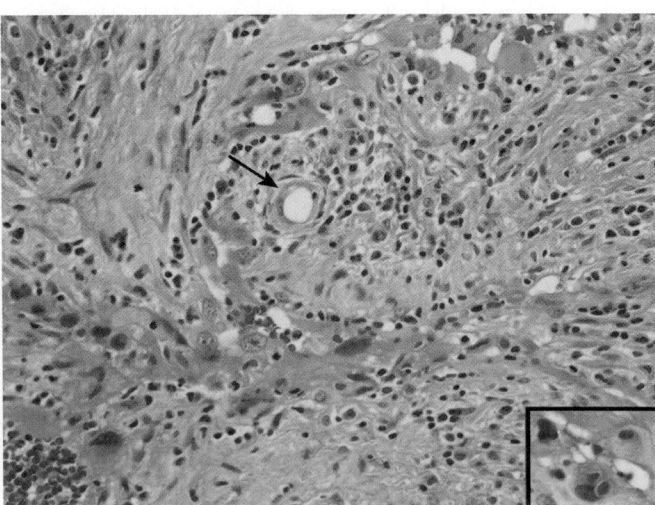

Figure 60-17 Epithelioid hemangioendothelioma. Poorly formed vascular channel lined by large epithelioid cells in an inflammatory stroma. Tumor cells have cytoplasmic vacuoles *(arrow)*. Red blood cells can be seen within cytoplasmic vacuoles *(inset)*.

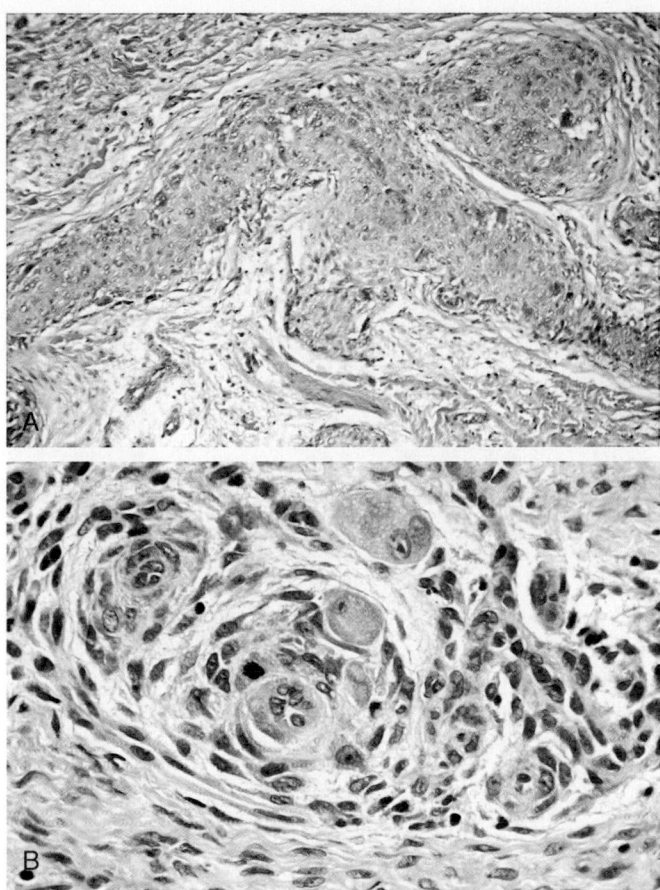

Figure 60-18 Giant cell angioblastoma. **A,** Nodular and plexiform aggregates of oval to spindle cells, mononuclear cells, and multinucleated giant cells in a perivascular distribution. **B,** Perivascular giant, spindled, and epithelioid cells.

invasive and highly destructive.[387,388] Histopathologically it consists of nodular and plexiform aggregates of oval to spindle cells, mononuclear cells, and multinucleated giant cells in a perivascular distribution. Like epithelioid sarcoma, this tumor mimics granulomatous inflammation (Fig. 60-18). Based on previous success with hemangiomas, two patients have been effectively treated with IFN-α2b.[389]

Kaposiform Hemangioendothelioma

Kaposiform hemangioendothelioma (KHE), a vascular tumor of infancy and childhood, occurs in either superficial or deep soft tissue. Large lesions, particularly in the retroperitoneum, are aggressive and present as consumption coagulopathy and thrombocytopenia (Kasabach-Merritt syndrome).[390] The lesions usually develop postnatally with a mean age at diagnosis of 3 years, 9 months. The lesions are multinodular, often with desmoplasia and vasoformative spindling of tumor cells resembling Kaposi sarcoma and glomeruloid structures (Fig. 60-19). Droplets of hyalin, fragmented erythrocytes, hemosiderin granules, and fibrin thrombi are characteristic. A lymphatic component is usually present. A majority of tumor cells are immunoreactive to CD31, CD34,

and D2-40.[391] In contrast to infantile hemangiomas, GLUT1 is negative.[392] Tumors can spread locally but do not metastasize distantly.[393]

The mortality rate associated with KHE approaches 30%, typically resulting from Kasabach-Merritt phenomenon, which presents as consumption coagulopathy characterized by moderate microangiopathic hemolytic anemia, severe thrombocytopenia, and hypofibrinogenemia.[394] Although Kasabach-Merritt phenomenon is believed to be a consistent association with KHE, smaller lesions (<8 cm) may not result in sufficient platelet trapping to cause thrombocytopenia.[395] Large and invasive lesions are more likely to be associated with platelet trapping.[396] Surgical resection may be effective for superficial lesions. Unresectable tumors may respond to sirolimus, propranolol, ticlopidine, IFN-α, corticosteroids, vincristine, embolization, or low-dose radiation therapy.[397-402] For extensive disease, combination therapy with vincristine, cyclophosphamide, and dactinomycin with or without methotrexate may result in long-term remission.[403,404]

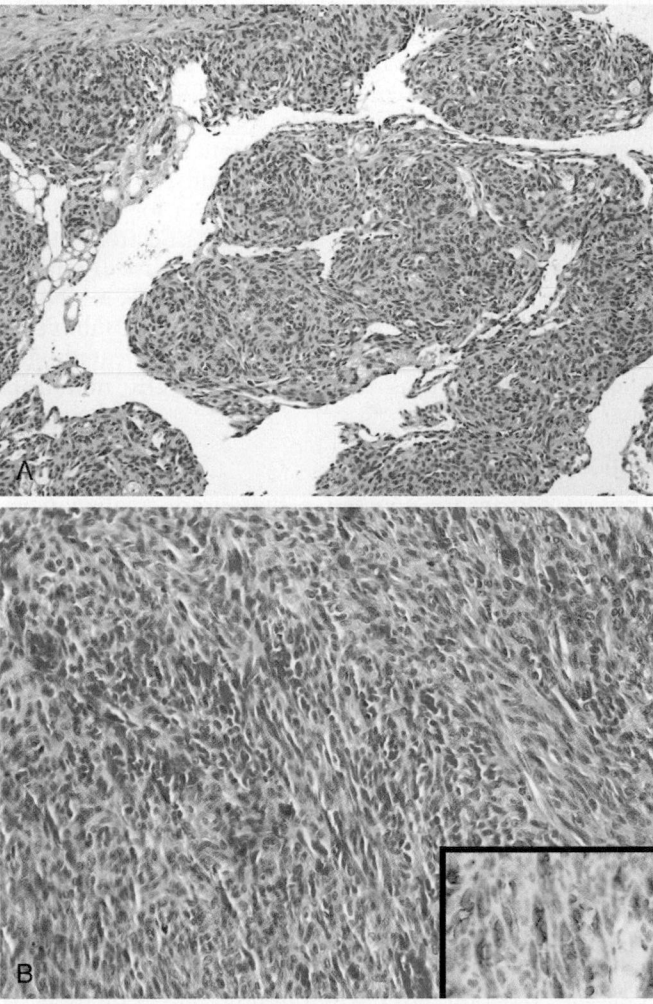

Figure 60-19 Kaposiform hemangioendothelioma. **A,** Irregular nests of tumor with spindled cells and glomeruloid structures. **B,** Kaposi-like area with cellular spindled cell growth and erythrodiapedesis. Spindled cells are immunoreactive with D2-40, a marker associated with lymphatic differentiation *(inset).*

Kaposi Sarcoma

Kaposi sarcoma (KS) is an endothelial cell malignancy that results from transformation by human herpesvirus 8 (HHV-8, also known as Kaposi sarcoma herpesvirus).[405-407] KS can be multifocal and represent clonal or oligoclonal disease.[408,409] Four clinicoepidemiologic variants of KS are recognized: African (endemic), classic, acquired immunodeficiency syndrome (AIDS)-related (epidemic), and immunosuppression associated. Immunosuppression-associated KS can develop after solid-organ or bone marrow transplantation.[410] The incidence of AIDS-related KS has significantly decreased, likely owing to improvements in anti-HIV therapies.[411] KS in immunosuppressed individuals tends to behave aggressively, presenting as multifocal skin lesions and involvement of mucosal surfaces with spread to lymph nodes, brain, lung, gastrointestinal tract, and bones.[412-415]

The lymphadenopathic form of KS is most common in children; it is characterized by replacement of lymph nodes by a monotonous spindled cell proliferation, variable presence of slitlike vascular channels, and a lymphoplasmacytic infiltrate (Fig. 60-20, A). Spindled cells show striking nuclear reactivity for HHV-8 by in situ hybridization (see Fig. 60-20, B). HHV-8, like EBV, is a gammaherpesvirus, and, similar to immunosuppression-related EBV-associated lymphoproliferative disorder, KS may respond to reduced immunosuppression. KS also responds to pegylated liposomal doxorubicin and pegylated INF-2α.[416-419] Radiation therapy is effective for cutaneous disease.[420] Bevacizumab treatment was associated with an approximately 50% response rate in a phase II trial.[421] Preclinical evidence supports a role for mTOR inhibition acting through VEGF secretion and HSP90 inhibition acting through the viral latency-associated nuclear antigen (LANA).[422,423] Clinical responses to mTOR inhibitors have been observed.[424,425]

Angiosarcoma

Angiosarcomas are aggressive high-grade malignancies with endothelial differentiation that constitute approximately 2% of vascular tumors in children.[426] Angiosarcomas typically develop in skin or soft tissues.[427] In young children, angiosarcomas tend to occur in soft tissues and internal organs, including the liver, spleen, heart, and testes, and may be associated with Aicardi and Klippel-Trenaunay-Weber syndromes.[428-431] In adults, angiosarcoma development is associated with chronic lymphedema, prior radiation exposure, and exposure to vinyl chloride, arsenic, and thorium oxide.

Angiosarcomas are aggressive tumors with a 5-year survival of 20% to 40%.[432-435] Complete surgical resection is associated with survival.[436] Angiosarcomas have a high rate of local and distant recurrence and can metastasize to the regional lymph nodes, lungs, soft tissue, bones, liver, and brain.[427] Although tumors are typically resistant to chemotherapy and radiation, a partial response by unresectable tumors to chemotherapy may facilitate resection.[437] Docetaxel with radiation, paclitaxel, liposomal doxorubicin, vinorelbine, and metronomic trofosfamide may have efficacy in the treatment

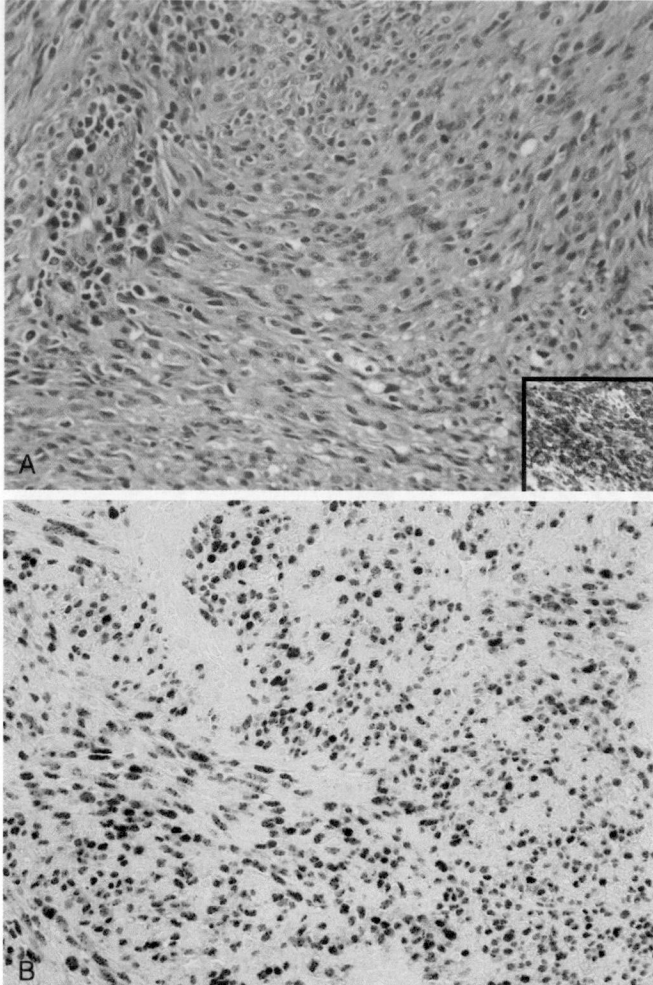

Figure 60-20 Kaposi sarcoma. **A,** Fascicles of monomorphic spindle cells and clusters of inflammatory cells, particularly lymphocytes and plasma cells. Spindled cells are strongly immunoreactive for D2-40 a lymphatic marker *(inset).* **B,** The majority of tumor cells show nuclear staining for human herpesvirus 8 by in situ hybridization.

of these tumors.[438-442] Sorafenib or bevacizumab may be transiently effective for a subset of patients.[443,444] Radiation therapy is associated with decreased incidence of local recurrence.[433] Liver transplantation for hepatic angiosarcoma does not seem to result in increased survival, although long-term survival after transplantation has been reported for type II infantile hepatic hemangioendothelioma, which is considered a form of angiosarcoma.[445]

Angiosarcomas are vasoformative tumors with varying degrees of differentiation (Fig. 60-21). Tumor cells stain positive for factor VIII, CD31, CD34, and ERG, supporting an endothelial nature.[446,447] The cellular target of the antiangiogenic compound angiostatin, annexin II, is expressed in angiosarcoma.[448] Chromosomal gains at the *MYC* and *FLT4* loci can be detected in radiation-associated angiosarcoma.[449,450] Angiosarcomas are consistently positive for TEK (Tie2), and this kinase may serve as a therapeutic target.[451,452]

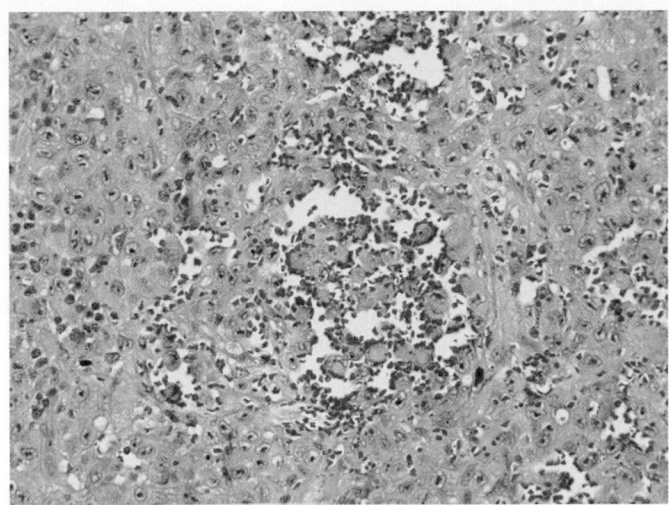

Figure 60-21 Angiosarcoma. High-grade angiosarcoma composed of large epithelioid cells with large pleomorphic nuclei, inclusion-like nucleoli, and abundant eosinophilic cytoplasm. There is vasoformation and hemorrhage.

CHONDROOSSEOUS TUMORS

Mesenchymal Chondrosarcoma

Mesenchymal chondrosarcoma is a rapidly growing, highly metastatic cartilaginous tumor. Although the majority develop in bone, more than 30% can develop in extraskeletal sites.[453] In contrast to most chondrosarcomas, mesenchymal chondrosarcoma tends to occur in young adults and, infrequently, children. Histopathologically, mesenchymal chondrosarcoma has two components: one consists of well-differentiated cartilage and the other of small cells resembling Ewing sarcoma (Fig. 60-22). Transition between these two components is usually abrupt. The small cell component frequently shows a hemangiopericytoma pattern of growth. The small cell component is immunoreactive with CD99, and the islands of cartilage are immunoreactive with S100 protein. Given its malignant behavior, patients with this tumor have a 38-month median survival with 5- and 10-year survival rates of 54.6% and 28%, respectively.[454,455] SOX9 expression can distinguish mesenchymal chondrosarcoma from small round blue cell malignancies.[456] Chromosomal translocation results in *HEY1-NCOA2* gene fusion in the majority of mesenchymal chondrosarcoma but not in other types of chondrosarcoma.[457] *HEY1* encodes hairy/enhancer of split, a component of the Notch signaling pathway. *NCOA2* encodes a transcriptional coactivator that functions with nuclear hormone receptors. *NCOA2* is a relatively promiscuous translocation partner contributing a carboxyl-terminal domain to gene fusion partners *ETV6 (TEL)* and *MYST3 (MOZ)* in a small number of leukemias, to *PAX3* in alveolar rhabdomyosarcoma, and to *AHRR* in soft tissue angiofibroma.[458-461] t(1;5)(q42;q32), resulting in *IRF2BP2-CDX1* fusion, has also been described.[462]

Extraskeletal Myxoid Chondrosarcoma

Rare in children and adolescents, extraskeletal myxoid chondrosarcoma (EMC), also known as chordoid sar-

coma, typically develops in older adults, with a peak incidence in the fifth or sixth decade.[463-465] EMC is a slowly growing, occasionally painful, deep mass commonly in the extremities. Histopathologically, it exhibits a multinodular growth pattern with a prominent chondroid appearance. Tumor cells are uniform, are arranged in cords or strands, and are ovoid. The cytoplasm is usually eosinophilic and rarely has rhabdoid-type inclusions. Tumor cells are consistently immunoreactive to vimentin. About half weakly express S100 protein, and a lesser proportion are immunoreactive to cytokeratins, synaptophysin, and EMA.[466-469] SMARCB1 (INI1, SNF5) is deficient in about 10% of EMCs, and these tumors can be difficult to discriminate histologically for extrarenal rhabdoid tumor.[470] Like other STS, EMC has a significant propensity for late recurrences and pulmonary metastases.[471,472] Responses to sunitinib have been observed.[473]

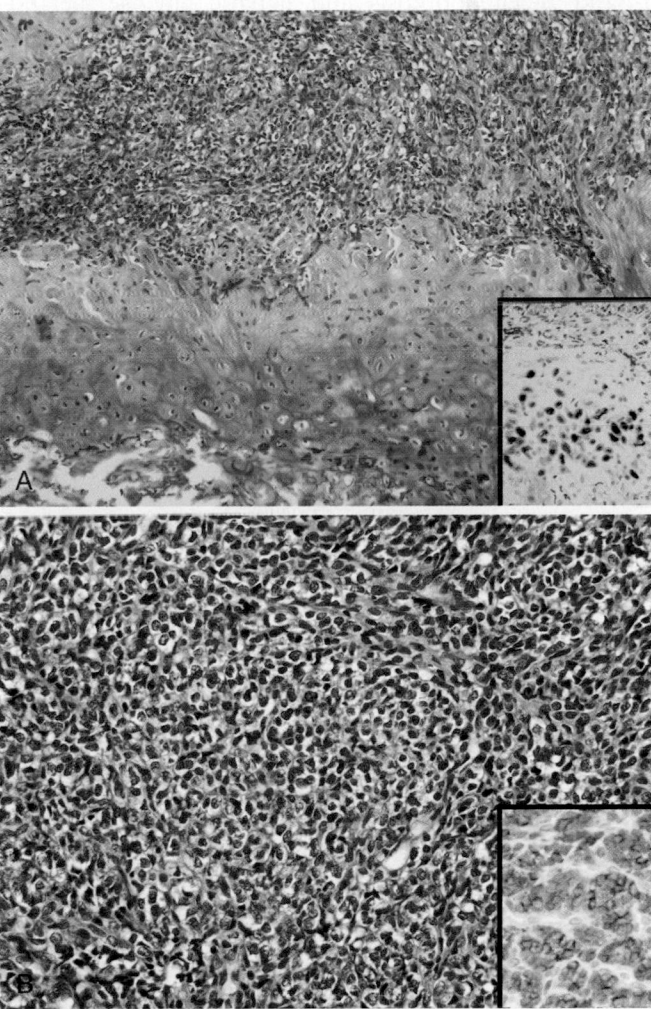

Figure 60-22 Mesenchymal chondrosarcoma. **A,** Biphasic tumor with a small cell Ewing sarcoma–like component at the top of the photograph and well-differentiated cartilage at the bottom. Cartilage component is strongly immunoreactive to S100 protein *(bottom of inset)*. **B,** The small cell component is shown at higher magnification demonstrating undifferentiated small cells with membranous CD99 immunoreactivity *(inset)*.

EMC is characterized by several recurrent clonal translocations. Approximately 75% harbor t(9;22)(q22;q12), which brings together the Ewing sarcoma gene *EWSR1* with *NR4A3 (CHN, TEC, NOR-1, MINOR)*.[474,475] Other translocations fuse *TAF15 (TAF2N, TAFII-68, RBP56)* and *TCF12* with *NR4A3*.[476-478] In contrast to EWSR1 and TAF15, which are ubiquitously expressed RNA binding proteins and translocated in many sarcomas, TCF12 is a basic helix-loop-helix transcription factor that contributes its DNA-binding domain to the *NR4A3* fusion.[479,480] NR4A3 is a member of a family of orphan nuclear receptors that includes NUR77 (NR4A1) and NURR1 (NR4A2).[481-484] In contrast to typical nuclear receptors such as the estrogen receptor that require binding to a ligand for activity, the NR4A family of transcription factors regulate transcription in a ligand independent fashion.[485] Their activity is controlled by regulated expression and posttranslational modification by phosphorylation.[486-490] The NR4A family has been implicated in a variety of cellular processes, including T- and B-cell apoptosis and hepatic glucose metabolism.[491-493] Mice deficient for both *Nr4a1* and *Nr4a3* develop acute myeloid leukemia in the early postnatal period.[494] The fusion of *EWSR1* with *NR4A3* results in an increase in transactivation activity over the native *NR4A3*.[495] Targets of the oncogenic fusion are not known; however, expression profiling of EMC with differing histologies and translocations demonstrated a consistent RNA profile distinct from that of myxoid liposarcoma (which is characterized by an *EWSR1-DDIT3* fusion).[496] *PPARG* and *NDRG2* have been identified as transcriptional targets for EWS-NR4A3.[497]

TUMORS OF UNCERTAIN DIFFERENTIATION

Synovial Sarcoma

Synovial sarcoma typically originates in proximity to major articular structures, bursae, and tendon sheaths, particularly of the proximal lower extremity. In spite of its name, a true relationship with synovium is no longer believed and intraarticular location is exceptional. Other sites for synovial sarcoma development include the trunk, head and neck, and mediastinum.[498-500] Synovial sarcoma is classified into two histologic subtypes, the more common monophasic spindle cell morphology subtype and a biphasic subtype (Fig. 60-23). Both subtypes exhibit an undifferentiated spindled cell component. In addition, the biphasic subtype has a variable degree of epithelial differentiation in the form of glandular structures or clusters of poorly organized epithelial cells. A small proportion of cases are characterized by small round cells with an organoid, hemangiopericytomatous pattern mimicking Ewing sarcoma (see Fig. 60-23, C). This group is associated with a worse prognosis. Glandular structures, epithelial clusters, and focally the spindle cell component show intense immunoreactivity for keratin and EMA.

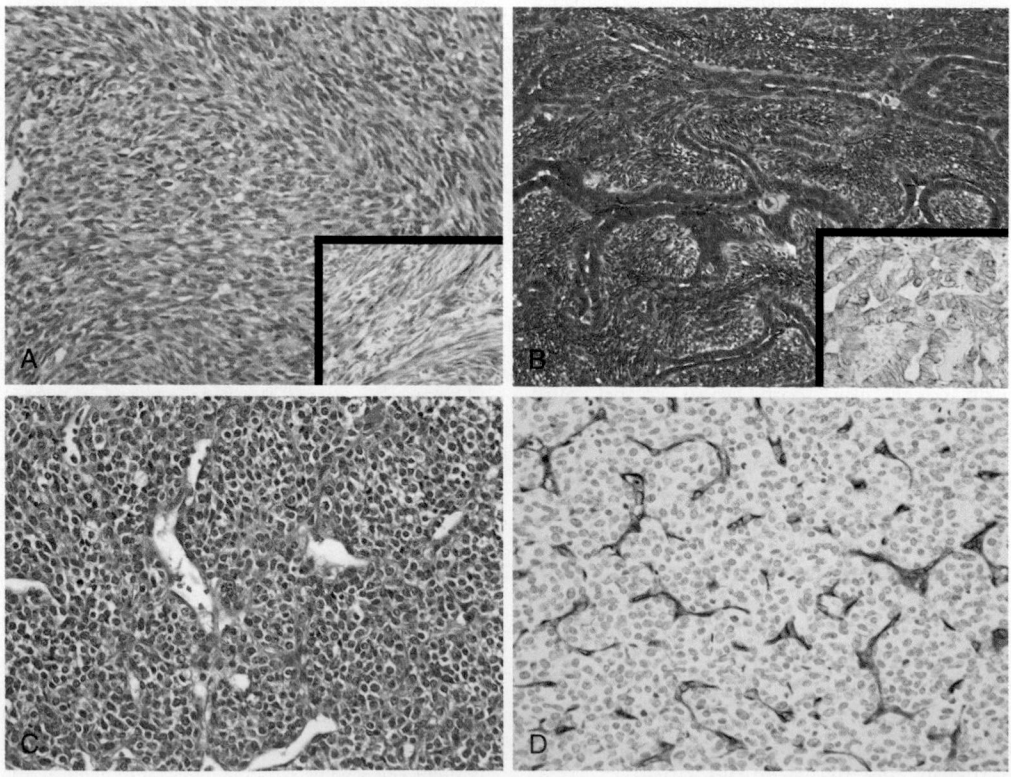

Figure 60-23 Synovial sarcoma. **A,** Monophasic synovial sarcoma composed of cellular undifferentiated spindled cells. Focal immunoreactivity for epithelial membrane antigen *(inset)*. **B,** Biphasic synovial sarcoma with prominent slitlike glandular component and intervening undifferentiated spindled cells. The glandular component is strongly immunoreactive to cytokeratins *(inset)*. **C,** Small round cell synovial sarcoma with a hemangiopericytoma-like pattern mimicking a malignant primitive neuroectodermal tumor. **D,** Malignant primitive neuroectodermal tumorlike synovial sarcoma showing characteristic vessels highlighted by CD34-immunoreactive endothelium.

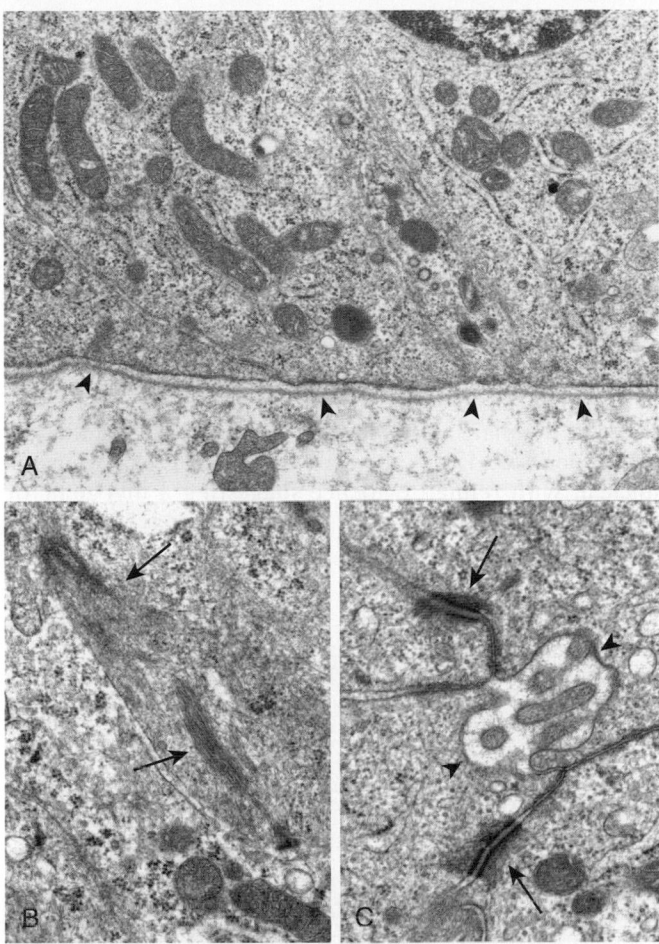

Figure 60-24 Synovial sarcoma. **A,** Groups of tumor cells are invested by a well-formed, continuous basal lamina *(arrowheads).* **B,** Well-developed cytoplasmic tonofilaments *(arrows).* **C,** Rudimentary intercellular lumen with microvilli *(arrowheads)* and well-developed desmosomes *(arrows).*

chimeras demonstrate nuclear localization in a speckled distribution.[516,517] SS18 is an integral component of the SWI/SNF (BAF) chromatin remodeling complex.[518-521] SS18-SSX competes with normal SS18, resulting in an aberrant BAF complex lacking SMARCB1 (SNF5). The aberrant *BAF* complex activates *SOX2,* and *SS18* overexpression displaces *SS10-SSX* binding, decreasing *SOX2* expression and cell proliferation.[521] SS18-SSX–associated SWI/SNF disruption places synovial sarcoma in a class of tumors that share aberrancy of this large multiprotein complex, including malignant rhabdoid tumors (see later) and a growing number of epithelial cancers. Moreover, an increasing number of proteins have been found to be components of the mammalian SWI/SNF complex, increasing the number of tumors in which mutations in the genes that encode for these proteins have been identified.[522] Gene expression studies in human pluripotent stem cells expressing SS18-SSX indicated that expression changes virtually always represented gene activation.[523] Intriguingly, only half of the genes are regulated by SS18-SSX in mesenchymal stem cells, supporting an emerging theme in chromatin biology that cell lineage–specific epigenetic differences are critical in determining the gene expression consequences. Human synovial sarcoma likely derives from an early stem cell because tumors and cell lines consistently express stem cell marker genes *OCT3/4, NANOG,* and *SOX2.*[524] SS18 was also found to interact with a nuclear coactivator (SIP/CoAA) that shares regional homology with EWS and TLS/FUS.[525,526] The SS18-SSX1 fusion demonstrates transforming activity in a rat fibroblast cell line not shared by SS18 or SSX1 alone.[527] Tissue-specific activation of *SS18-SSX2* fusion controlled by the ubiquitous ROSA26 promoter in a conditional knock-in system by myoblast Myf5-activated Cre results in tumor development in 100% of surviving mice between 3 and 5 months of age (100% penetrance).[528] The mouse tumor shares histopathology with human synovial sarcoma, exhibiting both monophasic and biphasic components, and it has been shown that some mouse tumors shared gene expression profiles. Intriguingly, the timing of SS18-SSX2 expression plays a critical role in the resulting phenotype. Expression of SS18-SSX2 in early embryos was lethal, whereas expression in developing myocytes resulted in myopathy.

Several studies have attempted to identify pathologic and clinical differences between tumors harboring the most common fusions. Pathologically, tumors harboring the *SSX1* fusions demonstrate biphasic morphology and increased Ki67 staining, whereas those with the *SSX2* fusions are monophasic.[529,530] Although a large multicenter study comparing the outcome of patients with tumors harboring the *SS18-SSX1* fusion to those with the *SS18-SSX2* fusion demonstrated that the *SSX1* fusion predicted a worse outcome,[531,532] a more recent multicenter study failed to confirm this finding but demonstrated that histologic grade was a strong predictor of survival.[533,534] An analysis of cell cycle–related proteins demonstrated that tumors with the *SS18-SSX1* fusion express higher levels of cyclin A and D1 relative to those with *SSX2* fusion.[535,536] Although there are biologic and

Ultrastructurally there is evidence of epithelial differentiation with basal lamina, cell junctions, and microvilli in both glandular and spindle cell components (Fig. 60-24).

Cytogenetically, more than 95% of synovial sarcomas are characterized by t(X;18)(p11;q11), which results in the fusion of *SS18* (also known as *SYT*) with *SSX1, SSX2,* or *SSX4.*[501-506] A variant fusion of the SS18-related gene *SS18L1* at 20.q13.3 with *SSX1* has also been reported.[507] Identification of the fusion by RT-PCR assay in paraffin-embedded tissue is an important diagnostic tool with a sensitivity of 95% and a specificity of 100%.[508-512] Nuclear immunostaining of SS18 in paraffin-embedded tissue has a sensitivity of 85%.[513]

SSX1, SSX2, and *SSX4* are distinct genes that are located in proximity on the X chromosome.[514] SSX1 and SSX2 are highly conserved proteins characterized by acidic carboxyl and amino termini with homology to the Kruppel-associated box (KRAB), which, in the context of a DNA-binding protein, has been implicated in transcriptional repression.[515] The translocations found in synovial sarcoma encode nearly full-length *SS18* fused to the carboxyl terminus of SSX.[506] SS18 and the SS18-SSX epidemiologic differences between these fusions, these differences are likely to be subtle.

In addition to the *SSX* fusions, other genes have been associated with synovial sarcoma biology. The expression of IGFR1 has been shown to correlate with a high incidence of lung metastases.[537] A significant fraction of synovial sarcoma also express hepatocyte growth factor (HGF) and/or its receptor MET.[538] Expression of HGF or coexpression of MET and HGF were associated with large, high-grade and high-stage tumors and correlated with decreased survival.[539] Synovial sarcoma–specific gene expression patterns have been identified. Compared with undifferentiated pleomorphic sarcoma, synovial sarcoma shows increased expression of several growth factors and receptors, notably insulin-like growth factor–binding protein 2 (IGFBP2), the receptor tyrosine kinase HER2 (ERBB2), IGF-2, and fibroblast growth factor receptor 3 (FGFR3).[540] Activation status of AKT/mTOR correlates with decreased EFS.[541] Compared with other STS, synovial sarcoma demonstrated increased expression of genes involved in the Wnt or notch signaling pathway, including *TLE1,* which was shown to immunohistochemically discriminate synovial sarcoma from other sarcomas.[542,543] SS18-SSX mediates Wnt signaling by interacting with β-catenin in the nucleus, and small molecule inhibition of Wnt signaling in transgenic mice resulted in decreased tumor growth.[544,545]

Recent studies have begun to explore the role of immune-directed therapy for synovial sarcoma based on the consistent expression of the tumor antigen NY-ESO-1.[546,547] However, a pilot study of the anti-CTLA4 antibody ipilimumab was discontinued owing to disease progression.[548]

Alveolar Soft Part Sarcoma

ASPS is a malignant tumor that usually presents in the thigh and trunk of young adults but can develop in the orbit or tongue in children.[549-551] Unusual primary locations include breast, heart, bladder, vagina, and uterine cervix.[552-556] About 25% of patients present with metastatic disease.[557] Because ASPS can metastasize to the brain in addition to lung and bone, the staging evaluation should include head CT. Complete surgical resection is associated with long-term survival.[558,559] ASPS is generally considered to be resistant to chemotherapy, although a small fraction of patients may respond.[557] Although pulmonary metastases may demonstrate response to treatment with vincristine, cyclophosphamide, and doxorubicin alternating with etoposide and ifosfamide, chemotherapy does not seem to extend survival.[560] Although considered an indolent tumor, ASPS carries a poor prognosis, given the insidious propensity for late metastases. Despite localized disease at presentation, subsequent distant recurrence results in a 77% survival at 2 years, 60% at 5 year, 38% at 10 years, and 15% at 20 years in adults.[561,562] Long-term survival in the pediatric population is significantly better with 5- and 10-year OS of 87% and 78%, respectively.[557] Given the protracted course of ASPS, metastatic disease can be palliated by resection of metastatic disease to lung and brain.[563-565] ASPS seems particularly responsive to VEGF-directed therapy, an observation

consistent with gene expression profiling demonstrating elevated expression of several genes associated with angiogenesis.[566] Becvacizumab, sunitinib, and cediranib have efficacy in advanced ASPS.[567-571] Trabectedin may also be effective.[572,573]

Histologically, ASPS is characterized by an organoid, pseudoalveolar proliferation of large polygonal cells that range from eosinophilic to clear (Fig. 60-25). Intravascular tumor growth is often present. A characteristic of these tumors is the presence of cytoplasmic periodic acid–Schiff-positive crystalline structures visible on light and electron microscopy. Ultrastructurally these membrane-bound crystals consist of a latticework with distinctive periodicity (Fig. 60-26). The crystals are composed of monocarboxylate transporter protein MCT1 and its chaperone CD147.[574] The cell of origin for ASPS remains unclear, with refuted evidence suggesting a myogenic or neural crest derivation.[575,576] Tumor cells may show focal

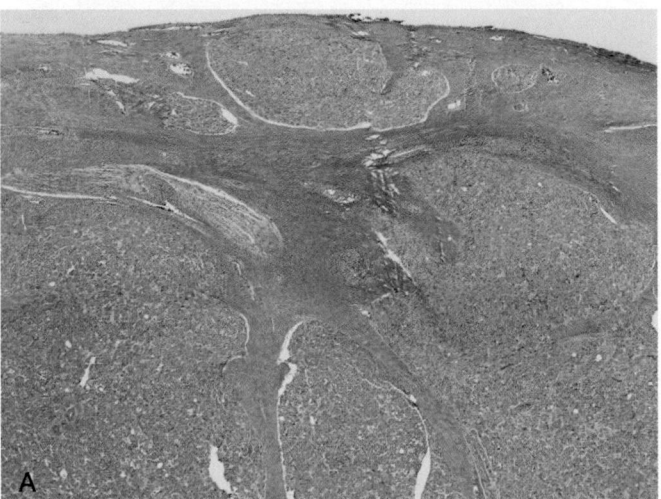

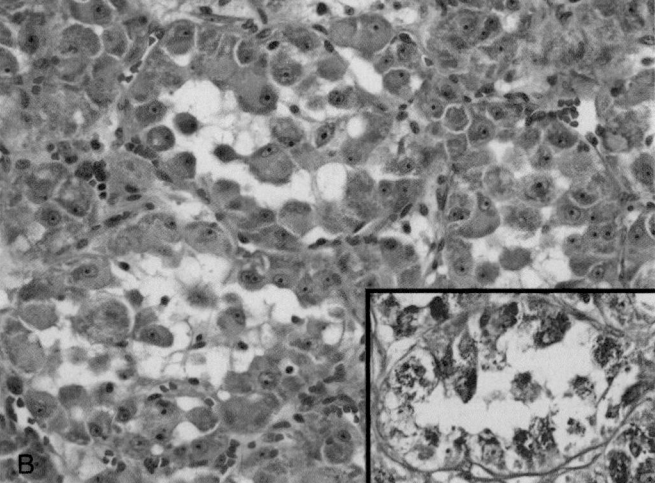

Figure 60-25 Alveolar soft part sarcoma. **A,** Multinodular growth with intervening fibrous septa. **B,** Large tumor cells with abundant eosinophilic cytoplasm are arranged with pseudoalveolar structures. Nuclei are large and round and contain a single prominent nucleolus. Note characteristic cytoplasmic periodic acid–Schiff-positive diastase-resistant inclusions *(inset).*

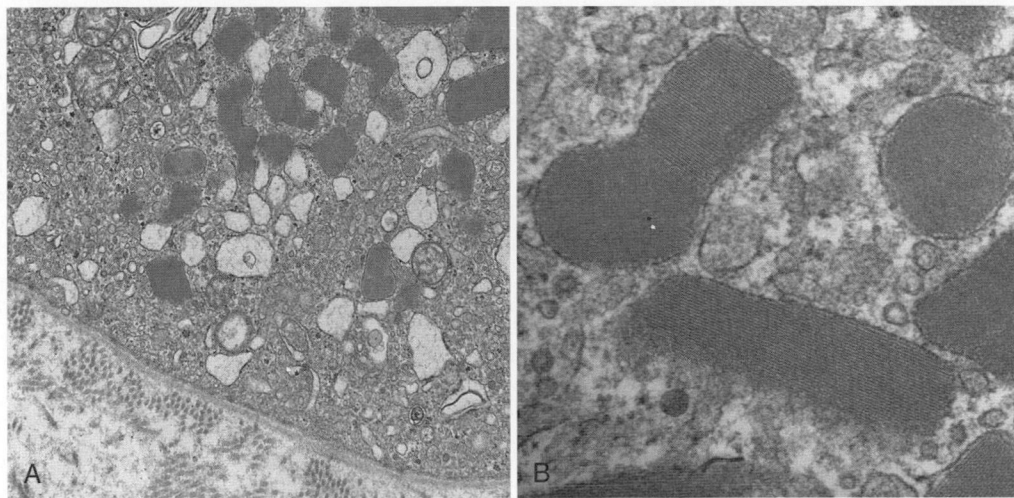

Figure 60-26 Alveolar soft part sarcoma. **A,** Pseudoalveoli are invested by a well-developed basal lamina, and tumor cells contain prominent endoplasmic reticulum cisternae filled with dense proteinaceous material. **B,** At higher magnification, proteinaceous material shows a paracrystalline periodicity, typical of this tumor.

positivity for actin or desmin, but these markers are not muscle specific.

ASPS is characterized by a unique chromosomal translocation, t(X;17)(p11;q25).[577,578] The translocation is frequently unbalanced, consistently resulting in the fusion of *TFE3* with *ASPSCR1* (also known as *ASPL*).[579] *TFE3* is a member of the MiT basic helix-loop-helix leucine zipper transcription factor family.[580,581] ASPSCR1 is not well characterized. However, amino acid sequence similarity suggests that ASPSCR1 may be the human homolog of mouse Tug, a protein that regulates intracellular trafficking of the glucose transporter GLUT4.[582] The *ASPSCR1-TFE3* translocation may dysregulate *TFE3* expression by placing it under the control of the ubiquitous *ASPSCR1* promoter. Alterations in the *TFE3* locus can be detected cytogenetically, by FISH or PCR assay. In addition, nuclear immunoreactivity for TFE3 provides a sensitive and possibly specific marker.[583] ASPSCR1-TFE3 likely functions by altering target gene transcription. *ASPCR1-TFE3* translocation can also be found in pediatric translocation-associated renal carcinoma, and *TFE3* can also be translocated in perivascular epithelioid cell neoplasm and epithelioid hemangioendothelioma.[375,584,585] One potential target gene with therapeutic potential is the receptor tyrosine kinase MET, although a clinical trial of tivantinib demonstrated modest effect.[586,587] TFE3 fusions may also regulate the mTOR pathway, suggesting activity of inhibitors of this pathway.[588] The biologic importance of aberrant *TFE3* in ASPS classifies it together with a growing number of other MiT family–associated tumors, including clear cell sarcoma (see later), translocation-associated renal carcinoma, and melanoma.

Clear Cell Sarcoma

Clear cell sarcoma (CCS) is a slowly growing soft tissue tumor that typically arises in the tendons, aponeuroses, and fascial structures of the extremities of adolescents and young adults.[589,590] It often presents as a small (<5 cm)

painful nodule around the ankle or foot. CCS has a propensity for late metastasis, regionally to lymph nodes and distantly to lungs and bone. Overall, CCS is associated with a 5-year survival of 40% to 70%, with children faring somewhat better than adults.[591-594] Aggressive surgical management is critical to achieve disease control. In a pediatric population, fully resected and small tumors (<3 cm) are associated with a 5-year EFS of 90% to 100% whereas larger tumors (>10 cm) result in a 20% 5-year EFS.[593] Postoperative radiation therapy is probably not necessary for fully resected CCS but may result in improved local control when negative margins cannot be achieved, a situation that frequently arises because complete surgical excision with wide margins at common locations is often not feasible without amputation. Unresectable, metastatic, relapsed CCS is refractory to conventional chemotherapy; however, postoperative chemotherapy may be of benefit for localized resectable disease.[85,595] Responses to sorafenib and sunitinib have been observed.[596,597] Although MET activation by HGF was demonstrated in clear cell sarcoma, clinical trials of tivantinib have had limited efficacy.[587,598]

Clear cell sarcoma has an infiltrative, nesting and fascicular pattern of growth (Fig. 60-27). The nesting pattern is highlighted by a reticulin framework. Tumor cells are usually ovoid or spindle with ovoid to elongated nuclei and distinct prominent eosinophilic nucleoli. CCS shares several histologic, immunophenotypic, and ultrastructural similarities with cutaneous melanoma, leading to the frequent designation of this tumor as "malignant melanoma of the soft parts."[590] Melanocytic differentiation of CCS is demonstrated by the expression of melanoma markers, including MITF, HMB45, S100, neuron-specific enolase (NSE), and melastatin.[599,600] Furthermore, about 70% of CCSs reveal melanin pigment by hematoxylin and eosin or Fontana stains and, ultrastructurally, they may contain premelanosomes and melanosomes.[600-602] By microarray expression analysis, CCS segregates from other sarcomas based on a

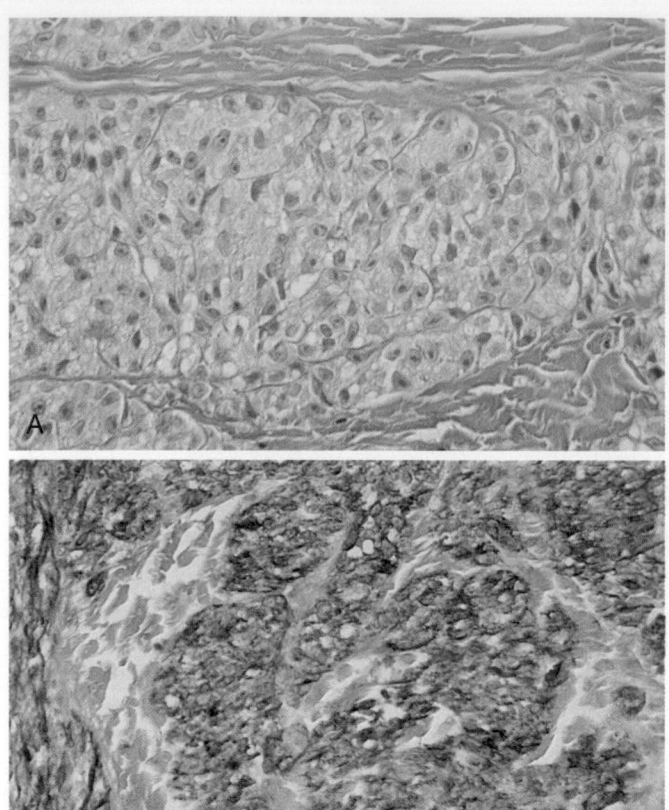

Figure 60-27 Clear cell sarcoma. **A,** Well-defined nest of tumor cells surrounded by fibrous septa. Tumor cells have abundant pale-staining cytoplasms and rounded vesicular nuclei with prominent single centrally located nucleolus. **B,** Tumor cells are strongly immunoreactive for HMB45, a melanoma marker. Strong staining for S100 protein is also characteristic of clear cell sarcoma *(not shown)*.

melanocytic expression pattern.[603,604] However, clinically and cytogenetically, CCS and cutaneous melanoma are distinct. CCS presents as isolated masses in deep soft tissue, often originating from tendons and aponeuroses. CCS rarely shows the degree of anaplasia or microsatellite instability associated with melanoma and, unlike with melanoma, *BRAF* is not mutated.[605-607] The vast majority of CCS tumors are distinguished by t(12;22)(q13;q12) that results in fusion of the Ewing sarcoma gene *EWSR1* with the CREB transcription factor family member *ATF1*.[608] The *EWSR1-CREB1* gene fusion is less commonly observed in soft tissue CCS but is more common in gastrointestinal CCS. These translocations are not found in cutaneous melanoma. Native ATF1 is regulated by serine phosphorylation in response to cyclic AMP levels by protein kinase A.[609,610] In CCS, translocation dysregulates ATF1 activity by replacing the kinase-inducible domain of *ATF1* with the amino-terminal region of *EWSR1*.[611] *Ewsr1-Atf1* expression in mice resulted in the high penetrance development of tumors that shared histologic and immunohistochemical features with the human tumor.[612,613]

Induction of MITF expression by EWSR1-ATF1 links the melanocytic phenotype of CCS with tumor proliferation/survival.[607] MITF, a member of the MiT basic helix-loop-helix leucine zipper transcription factor family, is the master regulatory factor of melanocyte differentiation and survival.[581,614] EWS-ATF1 coopts the typically melanocyte-stimulating hormone (MSH)-regulated cyclic AMP response element in the *MITF* promoter, aberrantly activating *MITF*. A critical transcriptional target, MITF mediates both the survival and proliferation of the melanocytic phenotype of CCS. TFE3 and TFEB, other members of the MiT transcription factor family, can rescue the effect of inhibited MITF expression in CCS.[607] This functional redundancy places CCS among a family of tumors that share aberrant MiT transcription factor family expression, including cutaneous melanoma, ASPS, and translocation-associated renal cell carcinoma. A gastrointestinal form of CCS is associated with a translocation that brings together *EWSR1* with *CREB1*.[615] Despite the related activity of *CREB1* with *ATF1*, this form of clear cell sarcoma does not express MITF or markers of melanocytic differentiation. Microarray expression profiling of the gastrointestinal CCS demonstrates a pattern that clusters more closely with angiomatoid fibrous histiocytoma (AFH) than soft tissue CCS (see later).[616]

Epidermal growth factor signaling may be important for CCS development. Clear cell sarcoma cell lines express ERBB3 and either ERBB2 or ERBB4.[603,617] Furthermore, ERBB3 is constitutively phosphorylated in cells, expressing its ligand neuregulin (NRG1), and can be activated by exogenous neuregulin in those cells that are not activated in an autocrine fashion. Treatment with the pan-ERBB inhibitor CI-1033 decreases cell proliferation.[617]

Desmoplastic Small Round Cell Tumor

Desmoplastic small round cell tumor (DSRT) typically arises in intraabdominal soft tissues. It has a strong predilection for males. Although its most common site is the peritoneum, DSRT can arise in kidney, testes, ovaries, pleura, scalp, ethmoid sinuses, and pancreas.[618-622] DSRT usually presents as abdominal pain and weight loss and is frequently locally or distantly metastatic at the time of diagnosis. The diffuse paraserosal spread of DSRT may prevent resection with negative margins. A high tumor response rate in untreated DSRT and previously treated DSRT to high-dose cyclophosphamide, doxorubicin, and vincristine (HD-CAV) alternating with ifosfamide and etoposide may cytoreduce bulky disease, permitting surgical resection and radiation therapy, if necessary.[623] Although the results are mixed, patients with high-risk disease may benefit from consolidation with high-dose chemotherapy and autologous stem cell rescue.[624,625] Relapsed disease may respond to irinotecan and temozolomide or low-dose cyclophosphamide and vinorelbine.[626,627] Because DSRT tends to develop and spread widely in the peritoneum, based on its efficacy for peritoneal carcinomatosis, the use of continuous hyperthermic peritoneal infusion of chemotherapy is being studied, although initial results do not appear promising.[626,628] Multimodality therapy was associated with a 3-year

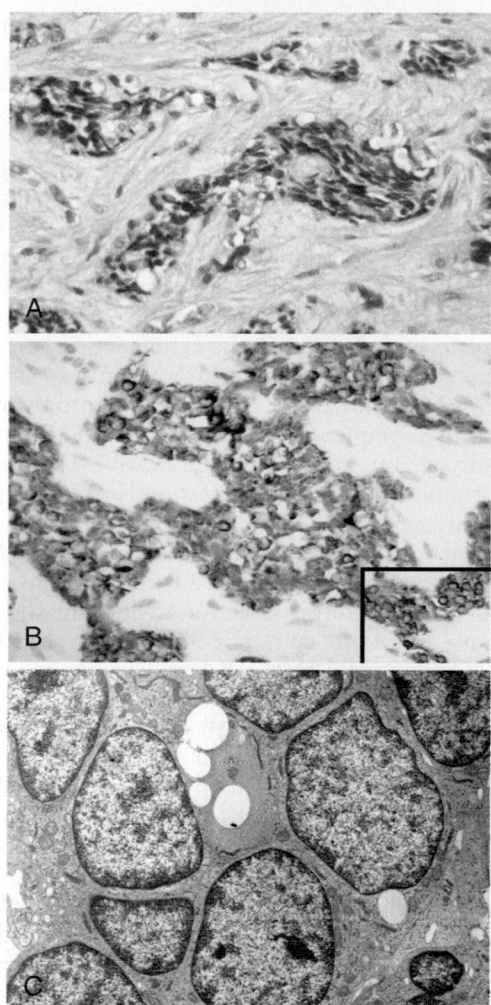

Figure 60-28 Malignant desmoplastic small round cell tumor. A, Infiltrative growth of elongated nests of variable size immersed in a densely collagenous stroma. Tumor cells are small and round or ovoid with hyperchromatic nuclei and poorly defined cytoplasmic borders. B, Tumor cells show strong diffuse and dotlike cytoplasmic immunoreactivity for desmin and diffuse cytoplasmic immunoreactivity for cytokeratin *(inset)*. C, Ultrastructurally, a cluster of undifferentiated small tumor cells with uniform round nuclei and occasional cytoplasmic whorls of intermediate filaments is evident.

survival of 55% compared with 27% when all three modalities were not used. Gross tumor resection was associated with a 58% 3-year survival compared with no survivors in the nonresection control.[629] However, despite multimodality therapy, long-term survival remains very low.

As the name implies, DSRT appears histologically as malignant undifferentiated small round cells typically associated with a prominent desmoplastic reaction (Fig. 60-28).[630] Desmoplastic stroma, however, is not always present, and location of the tumor may play a role in this regard. For example, DSRT originating in the kidney characteristically lacks desmoplastic stroma.[618] Some tumors have glandular or rosettelike epithelial differentiation. Nuclei are usually hyperchromatic with little pleomorphism, dispersed chromatin, and small nucleolus. The scant cytoplasm is poorly outlined. A rhabdoid-type

cytoplasmic inclusion can be observed focally in about half of the cases. Areas of necrosis and frequent mitoses are common. Multiphenotypic differentiation is characteristic immunohistochemically. Most cases show immunoreactivity for cytokeratin, EMA, vimentin, and desmin. Desmin and vimentin often show a dotlike intracytoplasmic pattern corresponding to the rhabdoid-type inclusion. Nuclear WT1 expression with antibodies to the carboxyl terminus is usually observed. Ultrastructurally, tumor cells are primitive, are organelle poor, and may show paranuclear whorls of intermediate filaments (see Fig. 60-28, C). Cell junctions including desmosomes may be observed focally.

Molecularly, DSRT is characterized by t(11;22) (p13;q12), which fuses the Ewing sarcoma gene *EWSR1* with *WT1*.[631-634] Although there is variability in the structure of the resulting chimera, the most common fusion includes *EWSR1* exons 1 to 7 and *WT1* exons 8 to 10.[634,635] WT1 is a $Cys_2\text{-}His_2$ zinc finger DNA-binding protein that shares a high degree of homology and DNA recognition motif with the growth factor–stimulated zinc finger DNA-binding protein EGR1.[636-639] The most common translocations result in *EWSR1-WT1* chimeras that preserve three of the four zinc finger motifs; however, owing to molecular heterogeneity, chimeras may lack *EWSR1* or *WT1* exons.[635] The *EWSR1-WT1* fusion has been detected in two intraabdominal tumors with histologic features of epithelioid leiomyosarcoma but lacking desmoplastic stroma, suggesting either a variant DSRT or another tumor type marked by *EWSR1-WT1*.[640] Based on the paradigm of the other transcription factors fused to the Ewing sarcoma gene, *EWSR1-WT1* is believed to exert its oncogenic activity through transcriptional mechanisms, and several putative transcriptional targets have been identified. The EWSR1-WT1 fusion activates platelet-derived growth factor alpha (PDGFA), T-cell acute lymphoblastic leukemia–associated antigen 1 (TALLA-1), and interleukin-2/15 receptor expression.[641-643] DSRTs stain positive for PDGF and IGF-2.[644] As a mitogen potentially acting on tumor-associated fibroblasts, PDGF seems a plausible cause for the desmoplastic reaction characteristic of these tumors. However, immunohistochemical analysis demonstrated an inverse correlation of PDGF expression with desmoplasia.[645] Although PDGF expression might suggest therapeutic PDGFR inhibition, imatinib demonstrated little to no activity as a single agent for DSRT.[646] About one third of DSRTs stain positive for androgen receptor, and androgen blockade may result in some response.[647]

Angiomatoid Fibrous Histiocytoma

Angiomatoid fibrous histiocytoma (AFH) was first described by Enzinger.[648] Histopathologically, it consists of a nodular fibrohistiocytic proliferation that is usually surrounded by lymphoid follicles and a lymphoplasmacytic infiltrate (Fig. 60-29). The lesion often undergoes focal cystification and hemorrhage. In contrast to the more common (and similar sounding) adult tumor malignant fibrous histiocytoma (currently classified as high-grade undifferentiated pleomorphic sarcoma [see later]), the current WHO classification of STS no longer

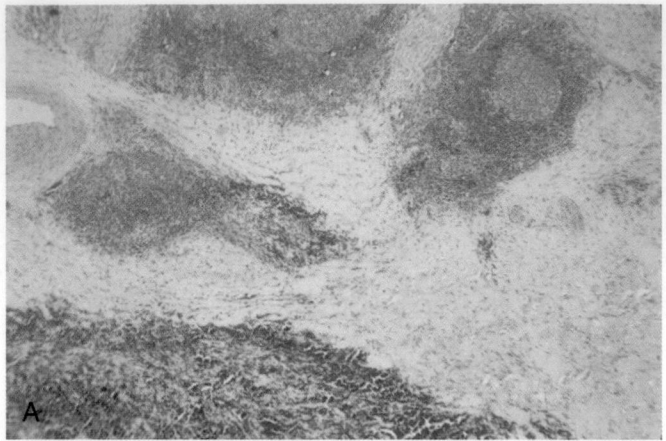
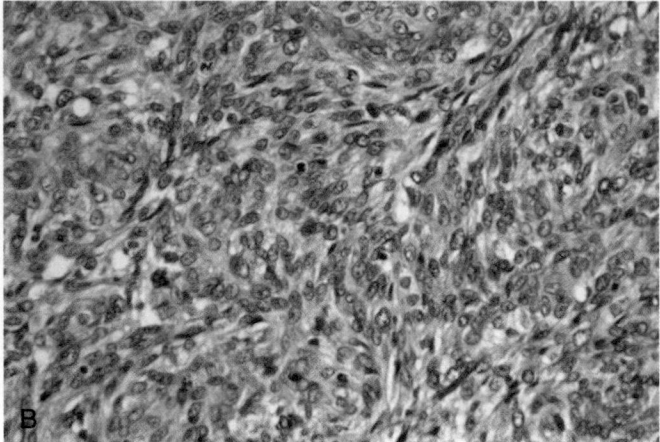

Figure 60-29 Angiomatoid fibrous histiocytoma. **A,** Nodular spindle cell proliferation with hemorrhage *(bottom)* and peripheral fibrous tissue with well-formed lymphoid follicles. **B,** Histiocyte-like cells and fibroblasts poorly arranged in short fascicles.

considers AFH a malignancy. Surgery is considered curative treatment. However, incomplete resection is associated with a significant rate of local recurrence. Metastases to lung and brain have been reported in a single case in an adult with a large tumor.[649]

AFH is associated with a translocation of *EWSR1* or its related protein FUS1 with *CREB1* or the related CREB family member *ATF1*.[616,650,651] These translocations are also characteristic of clear cell sarcoma (see earlier) and have been reported in primary pulmonary myxoid sarcoma.[652] In contrast to typical CCS, these tumors do not express markers of melanocytic differentiation, including MITF. Because *SOX10* is required for *CREB1/ATF1*-mediated *MITF* activation, the differences in expression may reflect the absence of *SOX10* in AFH.[607]

Extrarenal Rhabdoid Tumor

Soft tissue rhabdoid tumor is a high-grade malignant tumor that occurs almost exclusively in infants and children. A subset is congenital, and some of these may be disseminated at presentation.[653-655] Similar to its counterpart of renal origin, extrarenal rhabdoid tumor is an aggressive tumor with a very high rate of distant metastases, most commonly to the lung, lymph nodes, and liver.[656] Soft tissue rhabdoid tumors usually occur in the deep soft tissue, particularly in the paraspinal and neck regions. Some tumors arise adjacent to cutaneous benign mesenchymal lesions.[657,658] Tumor cells have little cohesiveness and grow in sheets or in a pseudoalveolar pattern, often mimicking alveolar rhabdomyosarcoma. Tumor cells are of medium size and are rounded with large eccentric nuclei and a prominent eosinophilic nucleolus. Typically, the cytoplasm contains a paranuclear eosinophilic inclusion. Although extrarenal and renal rhabdoid tumors in children form a discrete entity, soft tissue rhabdoid tumors in adolescents and adults are a heterogeneous group without consistent cytogenetic aberrations.

A majority of tumor cells are immunoreactive for vimentin, EMA, and cam5.2. CD99, synaptophysin, and NSE are also frequently positive. Actin, S100 protein, desmin, myogenin, and CD34 are negative. Ultrastructurally, the rhabdoid inclusion corresponds to a paranuclear whorl of intermediate filaments.

Cytogenetic analysis of rhabdoid tumor consistently demonstrates abnormalities of 22q11.[659] These changes include deletions and translocations. Mapping the deleted region in rhabdoid tumor cell line implicated the *SMARCB1 (hSNF5, INI1, BAF47)* gene, which was found to be mutated and truncated in other tumors.[660,661] SMARCB1 is a component of the multiprotein SWI/SNF adenosine triphosphate (ATP)-dependent chromatin remodeling complex. Mutations that disrupt SWI/SNF function have been identified in a growing number of human cancers in children and adults.[522] Loss of SMARCB1 results in polyploidization and chromosomal instability of rhabdoid cells. Expression of wild-type SMARCB1 results in cell cycle arrest, possibly through restoration of DNA damage-responsive cell cycle checkpoints or replicative senescence, processes mediated by CDKN2A and CDKN1A.[662,663] For further discussion of rhabdoid tumor of the kidney and central nervous system atypical teratoid/rhabdoid tumor, see Chapters 55 and 57.

Epithelioid Sarcoma

Epithelioid sarcoma is a distinctive high-grade soft tissue neoplasm that arises most commonly in the distal extremities of adolescents and young adults, particularly in the fingers, wrists, and hands. In young children, the tumor is more likely to arise in the head and neck as well as the pelvis.[664-667] The tumor can present as a superficial ulcerated lesion or a deep, often painful, mass. Dermis, subcutaneous tissue, fascia, and tendons can be involved, and on recurrence the tumor has a propensity for local spread along fascial planes and neurovascular bundles, resulting in the formation of proximal tumor satellites. Histologically, these tumors may resemble MPNSTs, synovial sarcoma, CCS, rhabdoid tumor, and melanoma.[668] The occurrence of intravenous extension or lymph node involvement is predictive of a very high rate of pulmonary metastases.[669,670] In adults, epithelioid sarcoma demonstrates a 77% risk for local recurrence and a 45% risk for metastatic disease.[671] Survival in children with epithelioid sarcoma exceeds that in adults.[672] In children, epithelioid sarcoma is associated with a 5-year EFS of 61% and an OS that declines from 92.4% at 5 years to 86.9%

and 72% at 10, and 15 years, respectively, indicating the propensity for late recurrence.[673] A small series of children with epithelioid sarcoma demonstrated that after lymphadenectomy with or without irradiation, all patients were free of disease approximately 10 years after diagnosis.[6] Tumor size is the best predictor of prognosis, with tumors larger than 5 cm associated with a worse prognosis.[673,674] Wide local excision with negative margins provides no advantage over primary amputation for patients with localized disease or regional metastases.[675] In a palliative setting, systemic chemotherapy offers a limited and brief response, although an extended response was observed with navelbine.[676,677] Disease stabilization with sunitinib has been described.[678]

Histologically, the more aggressive "proximal" type variant exhibits a distinct rhabdoid phenotype with a pattern of growth that is more sheetlike than nodular.[679] Nodular aggregates consist of medium-sized to large epithelioid and plump spindled cells with central necrosis and collagenization simulating granulomas or metastatic carcinoma (Fig. 60-30, A).[680] Immunohistochemically, tumor cells are commonly positive for keratin 8 and 19, EMA (see Fig. 60-30, B), vimentin, and CD34.[681,682] Tumor cells are typically diploid, although deletions of the long arm of chromosomes 22 and 1, monosomy 21,

and isochromosome 8q as well as gains at 22q have been noted.[683-688] t(8;22)(q22;q11) and t(6;8)(p25;q11.2) have been reported in isolated cases of epithelial sarcoma.[689,690] As in malignant rhabdoid tumors, the majority of epithelioid sarcoma lose SMARCB1, which is located at 22q12, through homozygous deletion, although this loss may be less common in pediatric cases.[691-694] Epidermal growth factor receptor (EGFR) overexpression has been noted in epithelioid sarcoma, and one cell line derived from a recurrent malignant tumor demonstrates interleukin-6 secretion and receptor expression, suggesting autocrine activation.[695-697] In preclinical studies, EGFR modulation affected tumor cell proliferation and motility and combined EGFR and mTOR inhibition decreased tumor cell growth.[698] Autocrine MET activation by HGF production has been speculated based on detection of both proteins by immunohistochemistry.[538]

Extraosseous Ewing Sarcoma

Although more commonly associated with an osseous origin, extraosseous Ewing sarcoma (peripheral primitive neuroectodermal tumor) can arise in many locations, including the small intestines, kidney, and spinal epidural space. Like its osseous counterpart, extraosseous Ewing sarcoma consists of undifferentiated small round cells with minimal neuronal differentiation. It is characterized by membranous immunoreactivity for CD99 and harbors rearrangement of the EWSR1 gene on chromosome 22 with a variety of partner genes, but most commonly with FLI1 on chromosome 11. Other partner genes include ERG, ETV1, EIAF, and FEV. EWSR1 break-apart FISH can be diagnostic. Extraosseous Ewing sarcoma is treated similarly to the osseous form.[699,700] Given differences in treatment and prognosis, care should be made to distinguish central nervous system Ewing sarcoma from central primitive neuroectodermal tumors. For a more complete discussion of Ewing sarcoma see Chapter 61, "Ewing Sarcoma."

Gastrointestinal Stromal Tumor

Most commonly originating from the stomach or small intestine, GISTs are mesenchymal neoplasms that can develop throughout the gastrointestinal tract. Typically, GISTs occur in middle-aged to older adults; however, approximately 3% of GISTs are identified in patients younger than 21 years of age.[701,702] Congenital GIST has been reported.[703,704] In children, the majority of tumors are identified in girls. Although isolated GIST predominates, multifocal epithelioid GIST is associated with Carney triad and together with paraganglioma in Carney-Stratakis syndrome.[702] GIST is also associated with NF1 patients in whom small multifocal but indolent tumors tend to be located in the small intestine.[705] Pediatric GIST typically presents as gastrointestinal hemorrhage that can result in anemia. Although the majority of tumors identified in children are surgically resectable and associated with a good prognosis, GIST is frequently metastatic. The most common sites of metastases at the time of presentation or recurrence are the liver and omentum.[706]

The cell of origin for GIST is uncertain, but the observation that tumor cells have immunohistochemical[548] and

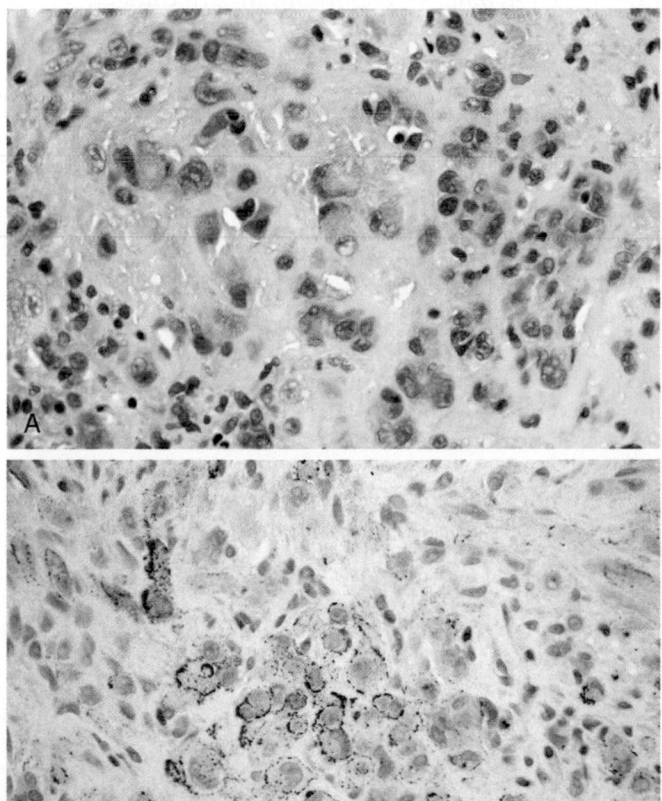

Figure 60-30 Epithelioid sarcoma. **A,** Granuloma-like cluster of large atypical cells (some with rhabdoid morphology), scattered inflammatory cells, and collagenization. **B,** Tumor cells are strongly immunoreactive for epithelial membrane antigen *(membranous pattern).*

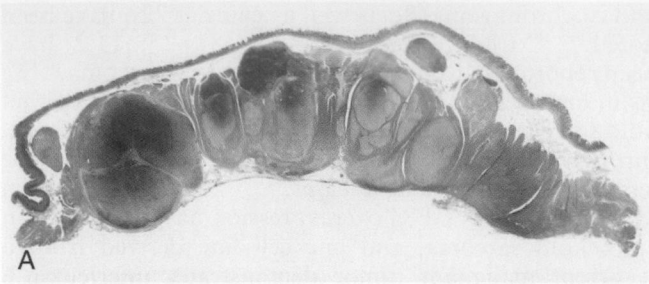

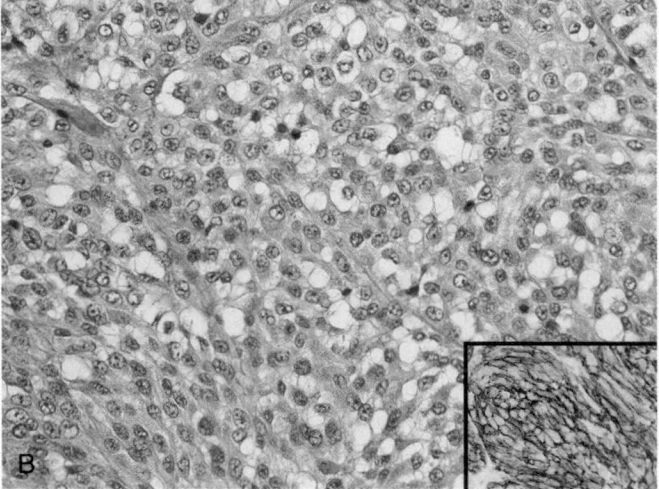

Figure 60-31 Gastrointestinal stromal tumor. **A,** Gastric antrum showing multifocal GISTs centered within the muscularis propria. **B,** Nests of tumor are composed of spindled and epithelioid cells, diffusely immunoreactive for *KIT (inset).*

ultrastructural[707,708] similarities to the interstitial cells of Cajal led to the proposition that GIST derives from these cells.[707,708] Histopathologically, most GISTs are composed of spindled cells with blunt-ended, elongated nuclei and moderately abundant cytoplasm (Fig. 60-31). They resemble smooth muscle or peripheral nerve sheath tumors. Unlike these tumors, however, immunohistochemistry of GIST in adults and children almost uniformly demonstrates the presence of the receptor tyrosine kinase KIT (CD117) (see Fig. 60-31, *B inset*) and, less frequently, CD34.[709,710]

Several molecular features distinguish adult and pediatric GIST. Whereas GIST in adults is often associated with chromosomal losses of 1p, 14q, and 22q with additional chromosomal gains and losses in metastatic tumors, pediatric GIST typically lacks cytogenetic aberrancy.[711-713] GIST in adults is frequently associated with activating mutations identified in multiple regions of the stem cell factor (also known as mast cell growth factor) receptor *KIT*.[714-716] Mutations include in-frame deletions and amino acid substitutions. A significant fraction of tumors that lack *KIT* mutations harbor activating mutations in *PDGFRA*.[717] The ETS family transcription factor ETV1 is highly expressed in GIST and cooperates with activated KIT.[718] Strikingly, in pediatric GIST, *KIT* and *PDGFRA* are infrequently mutated.[702,713,720] GIST in children and young adults is more commonly associated with mutations that affect the succinate dehydrogenase (SDH)

complex.[23,721] The SDH complex, located in the mitochondrial inner membrane, consists of four proteins and catalyzes the oxidation of succinate to fumarate in the citric acid cycle, and mutations significantly decrease complex activity.[24,722] Loss of SDH activity leads to accumulation of fumarate and succinate, which inhibits α-ketoglutarate–dependent processes, including histone demethylases and the TET family of 5-methylcytosine hydroxylases that may alter chromatin in tumors.[723] In addition, SDH loss can increase oxidative stress and promote DNA mutagenesis.[724] Mutations in *SDHB, SDHC,* and *SDHD* have been associated with GIST as well as paraganglioma and pheochromocytoma.[725-729] Mutation in *SDH* genes have been also associated with other tumors, including renal cell carcinoma. IGF1R is frequently expressed in *SDH* mutation–negative tumors, and IGF1 and IGF2 expression seems to correlate with disease-free survival.[730,731]

Historically, nonmetastatic GIST was managed surgically.[732] However, treatment with the KIT and PDGFR targeted inhibitor imatinib demonstrates a significant and durable response in a majority of patients harboring *KIT*- and *PDGFR*-activating mutations.[733,734] Although a significant fraction of tumors progress owing to acquired resistance to imatinib, they may respond to second-line treatment with sunitinib.[735,736] Consequently, *KIT* and *PDGF* genotyping is important in determining initial treatment. For localized tumors without *KIT* or *PDGF* mutation, surgical resection should be performed. For asymptomatic patients with unresectable or metastatic disease, frequent surveillance is reasonable, with resection reserved for disease progression or development of clinical symptoms.[737] In children, the demonstration of KIT activation in the absence of mutation suggests that KIT inhibition may be effective.[713]

Ectomesenchymoma

Ectomesenchymoma is a rare tumor that affects primarily young children. Histopathologically, ectomesenchymomas are composed of a mixture of embryonal rhabdomyosarcoma, ganglioneuroma, and other neuroectodermal or mesenchymal components.[738-740] These tumors are believed to derive from neural crest cells. Treatment of these tumors typically involves surgical resection followed by sarcoma- or rhabdomyosarcoma-directed chemotherapy.[739,741]

NEUROECTODERMAL TUMORS

Malignant Peripheral Nerve Sheath Tumors

MPNSTs are sarcomas that ultrastructurally and immunohistochemically demonstrate nerve sheath differentiation.[742] An origin from a nerve or within a benign nerve sheath tumor or ganglioneuroma as well as a history of NF1 are also important in the diagnosis of this tumor. Previously referred to as malignant schwannomas and neurofibrosarcoma, the term MPNST is preferred given the heterogeneity of tumor cell morphology. MPNSTs typically arise in the deep soft tissues of the extremities, head and neck, and trunk and may present as a mass or symptoms of nerve compression, including

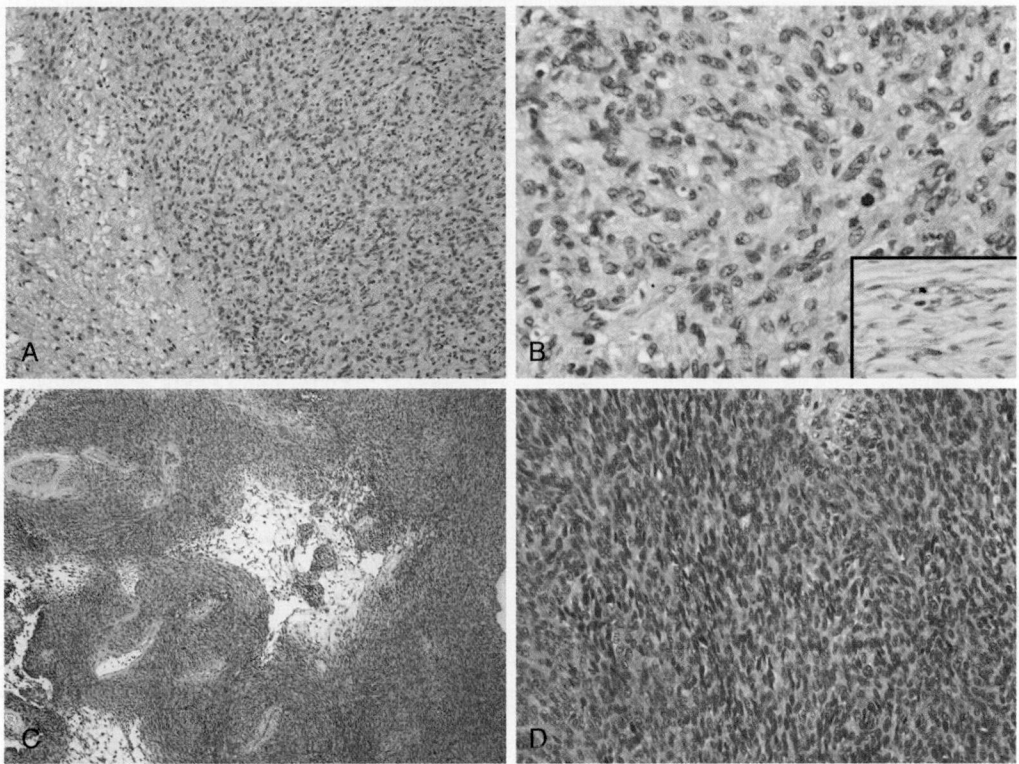

Figure 60-32 Malignant peripheral nerve sheath tumor. **A,** Low-grade MPNST showing a cellular area *(at right)* sharply demarcated from a less densely cellular component *(left).* **B,** At higher magnification, low-grade MPNST showing mild atypia and occasional mitoses. Low-grade MPNST shows focal strong nuclear and cytoplasmic immunoreactivity for S100 protein *(inset).* **C,** High-grade MPNST showing densely cellular spindled cell tumor. **D,** At higher magnification, tumor cells in high-grade MPNST are densely arranged and have hyperchromatic nuclei and scattered mitoses and apoptosis.

pain, dysesthesia, or motor disturbance.[742,743] Fifty to 80 percent of MPNSTs develop spontaneously. Patients with NF1 have a lifetime incidence of MPNSTs between 2% and 29%.[16,18,744-747] In a pediatric population, MPNSTs in NF1 patients tend to develop at an older age and tumors tend to be larger, less likely to be resectable, and less likely to respond to chemotherapy than those that develop spontaneously.[743] MPNST is associated with a 5-year OS of 40% to 50% and a PFS of 35% to 37%.[743,748] However, IRS grouping strongly predicts both OS and PFS with complete surgical resection associated with an OS of 80% at 10 years. Histologically, MPNST is composed of fascicles of spindled cells with oval to wavy, slender nuclei with tapering poles and a pale cytoplasm with a poorly defined border (Fig. 60-32).[742] Perivascular hypercellularity and abrupt changes from dense cellular areas to zones containing abundant myxoid matrix are features that suggest nerve sheath differentiation. Pleomorphic, hyperchromatic nuclei are frequently present. Mitoses are usually frequent except in low-grade tumors arising in preexisting neurofibromas in patients with neurofibromatosis (see Fig. 60-32, *A* and *B*). High-grade MPNSTs are densely cellular with frequent mitoses and areas of necrosis (see Fig. 60-32, *C* and *D*). MPNST with rhabdomyoblastic differentiation is referred to as malignant triton tumor and has a worse prognosis than the typical MPNST. Osteosarcomatous or glandular differentiation may also occur. Immunohistochemically, MPNST may show focal positivity for S100 protein, EMA, and glial fibrillary acidic protein (GFAP). For unresectable or metastatic disease or for large tumors, chemotherapy with doxorubicin and ifosfamide or ifosfamide alone can be of limited benefit.[743] Radiation therapy can be beneficial for higher-grade lesions and incomplete resections and is often administered concurrently with chemotherapy. MPNST in the context of NF1 tends to be more refractory to chemotherapy and more likely to recur locally.

The development of MPNST is associated with loss of the tumor suppressor *NF1* at 17q11.2, which encodes neurofibromin. Neurofibromin is a guanosine triphosphatase (GTPase)-activating protein that modulates RAS signaling.[749-753] MPNSTs also frequently harbor mutations of *TP53* and the *CDKN2A/CDK2AP2* (*p16^{INK4a}/ p14^{ARF}*) locus affecting both the TP53 and RB pathways in 75% of tumors.[754] *CDKN2A* or *CDK2AP2* promoter inactivation by CpG island methylation may also downregulate expression.[755] Mice with homozygous *Tp53* and heterozygous *Nf1* deficiency develop predominantly MPNST and malignant triton tumor–appearing sarcomas, and these tumors demonstrate loss of heterozygosity at the *Nf1* locus.[756,757] Multiple signaling pathways appear to be involved in MPNST development. EGFR is consistently expressed in MPNST and MPNST-derived cell lines, and 26% of MPNSTs demonstrate amplification of the *EGFR* locus.[758,759] *IGF1R* is amplified in 24% of tumors and expression correlates with survival.[760]

Enforced EGFR expression in transgenic mice results in Schwann cell hyperplasia with rare tumor development, whereas EGFR haploinsufficiency in *Nf1+/−*, *Tp53+/−* mice significantly reduces tumor formation.[761] Mutagenesis screening in mice identified Wnt/β-catenin as well as PI3K/AKT/mTor pathway alterations in MPNST.[762,763] PTEN, which modulates PI3K signaling, is involved in malignant transformation.[764]

Melanotic Neuroectodermal Tumor of Infancy

Melanotic neuroectodermal tumor (retinal anlage tumor, melanotic progonoma) is a dysembryoplastic tumor that recapitulates embryonic retinal development. Most cases occur in the head and neck region, particularly in the maxilla, and usually affect male children younger than 1 year of age. The tumors are typically benign but grow rapidly, invade locally, and may metastasize in about 5% of cases.[765] Although complete surgical resection is required for cure, chemotherapy has been shown to decrease tumor mass, thus improving resectability.[766,767] Local recurrence after resection is common, with virtually all recurrences within 4 months and justifying close follow-up.[768] Balancing the desire for negative margins with disfigurement supports a staged surgical approach, and multiple resections may be required to ultimately establish disease control.

The tumor is classified in the family of neuroblastic tumors, and rare cases are associated with elevated urinary levels of vanillylmandelic acid. The histopathology is characteristically biphasic with a component of neuroblast-like cells with neuropils arranged in nests and an epithelioid melanocyte-like component containing melanin (Fig. 60-33). The melanocyte-like cells are usually arranged at the periphery of the neuroblastic-like cells, forming pseudoglandular or pseudoalveolar structures in a densely fibrous stroma. Both cellular components are immunoreactive with neuroectodermal markers such as synaptophysin, GFAP, and Leu7. Melanocyte-like cells are also immunoreactive with HMB45 and cytokeratins.

UNDIFFERENTIATED TUMORS

Undifferentiated Pleomorphic Sarcoma and Undifferentiated Round Cell and Spindle Cell Sarcoma

Advances in immunophenotyping, microscopy, and molecular-based techniques have resulted in improved classification of soft tissue tumors. Historically, for the purposes of therapeutic trials in childhood cancers, undifferentiated sarcoma had been grouped with rhabdomyosarcoma. However, the application of MyoD1 and myogenin immunohistochemistry enabled segregation of rhabdomyosarcoma from undifferentiated sarcoma. A similar reclassification also occurred for adult undifferentiated sarcomas. Many of the tumors previously described as malignant fibrous histiocytoma have been reclassified to specific categories on the basis of immunohistochemistry, electron microscopy, and molecular genetics.[769-771] However, as a diagnosis of exclusion, undifferentiated sarcomas represent a collection of tumors that lack identifiable morphologic, immunohistochemical, or genetic changes, thus permitting classification as a specific subtype

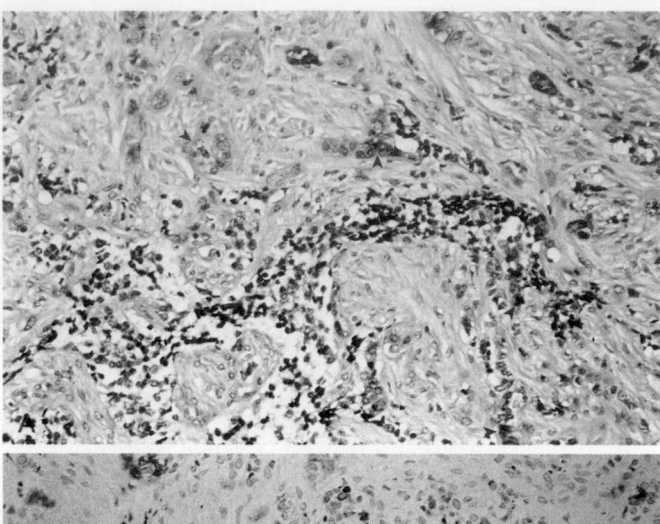
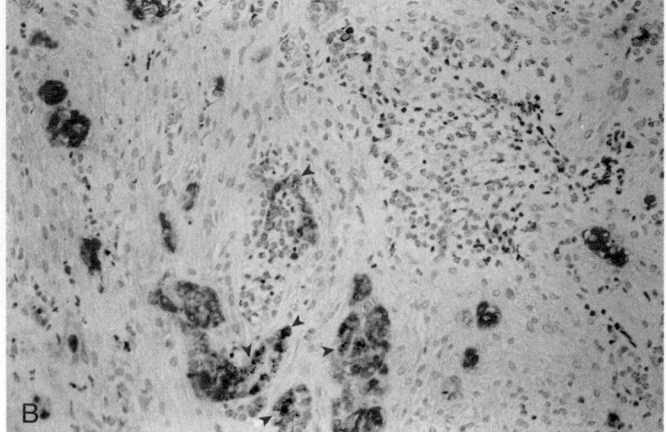

Figure 60-33 Retinal anlage tumor (progonoma). **A,** Biphasic tumor with a component of neuroblastic-like cells with neuropil arranged in nests and an epithelioid melanocyte-like cell component containing melanin *(arrowheads).* The melanocyte-like cells arranged at the periphery of the neuroblastic-like cells form pseudoglandular or pseudoalveolar structures in a densely fibrous stroma. **B,** Strong cytokeratin immunoreactivity in melanocyte-like cells *(red).* The dark cytoplasmic granules represent melanin pigment *(arrowheads).*

of sarcoma using currently available technologies (Fig. 60-34). Classification of these otherwise undifferentiated tumors rests exclusively on their histology, including undifferentiated round cell and spindle cell sarcoma and undifferentiated pleomorphic sarcoma.

In infants younger than 1 year of age, undifferentiated sarcoma constitutes the most common nonrhabdomyosarcoma malignant mesenchymal tumor. Surgery and chemotherapy result in a 10-year OS of 75%.[8] Undifferentiated pleomorphic sarcoma constitutes a common soft tissue tumor of older adults, with a peak incidence in the seventh decade, and rarely occurs in children or adolescents.[772] A high-grade malignancy, this tumor demonstrates a significant incidence of local and distant recurrence. Pulmonary and lymph node metastases are most common. In a trial of docetaxel and gemcitabine compared with docetaxel alone in metastatic sarcoma, undifferentiated pleomorphic sarcoma was among the most responsive tumor type and demonstrated superior response to both agents in combination.[101]

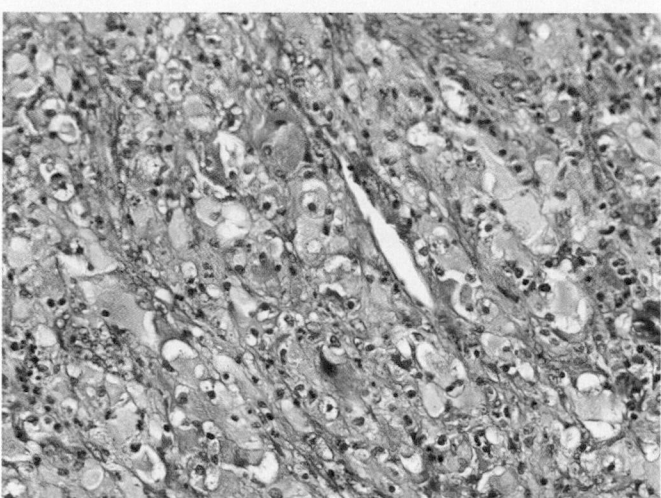

Figure 60-34 High-grade undifferentiated sarcoma. Undifferentiated, pleomorphic sarcoma composed of large highly anaplastic tumor cells. Immunohistochemistry, electron microscopy, and cytogenetics defied further classification.

Pediatric undifferentiated sarcomas may express vimentin, KIT, and VEGF.[773] Hierarchical clustering of adult STS based on messenger RNA expression array profiling revealed an undifferentiated sarcoma class, distinct from, among other tumors, fibrosarcoma and liposarcoma.[542] Expression analyses performed by other groups have also clustered undifferentiated sarcomas but with intermingling of liposarcoma and leiomyosarcoma to varying degrees.[774,775] Cytogenetic studies have also demonstrated that a subset of undifferentiated sarcoma share some features with liposarcoma, but tumors with 12q14-15 amplification, which includes MDM2 and CDK4, are now classified as dedifferentiated liposarcoma.[61,776] Murine modeling suggests that some undifferentiated pleomorphic sarcomas exist on a developmental continuum with embryonal rhabdomyosarcoma and arise from muscle satellite cells.[777]

Undifferentiated round cell and spindle cell sarcomas are occasionally characterized by *EWSR1* translocations and fusion with genes other than those of the ETS transcription factor family typical in Ewing sarcoma. Gene partners include *PATZ1, POU5F1 (OCT3/4), SMARCA5, NFATC2,* and *SP3.*[778] Although the involvement of *EWSR1* as a translocation partner in these tumors suggests that they constitute Ewing sarcoma variants, genomic targeting of these fusions would be expected to differ from the ETS transcription factor containing fusions characteristic of Ewing sarcoma.[779] Other translocations include *CIC-DUX4* and *BCOR-CCNB3*. WNT signaling seems to play a central role in undifferentiated sarcoma development. DKK1, the secreted inhibitor of WNT signaling, is expressed in undifferentiated sarcoma, and it inhibits differentiation by blocking Wnt2/β-catenin signaling.[780] Conversely, treatment of an undifferentiated sarcoma cell line with either exogenous Wnt2 or Wnt5a induced markers of adipogenic or osteogenic differentiation. JUN deregulation may also play a role in undiffer-

entiated sarcoma. *JUN* and *JNK* can be amplified in undifferentiated sarcoma, and JUN can inhibit adipogenic differentiation.[781]

References available online at ExpertConsult.

KEY REFERENCES

55. Parham DM, Webber BL, Jenkins JJ, 3rd., et al: Nonrhabdomyosarcomatous soft tissue sarcomas of childhood: formulation of a simplified system for grading. *Mod Pathol* 8:705–710, 1995.
    This report describes the development of the grading system used for childhood NRSTS.
60. Khoury JD, Coffin CM, Spunt SL, et al: Grading of nonrhabdomyosarcoma soft tissue sarcoma in children and adolescents: a comparison of parameters used for the Fédération Nationale des Centers de Lutte Contre le Cancer and Pediatric Oncology Group Systems. *Cancer* 116:2266–2274, 2010.
    This study compares FNCLCC with POG grading systems for NRSTS and demonstrates that both systems perform similarly while proposing a system that incorporates histology-based grading as well as incorporation of mitotic figures for intermediate-risk clinical grouping.
69. Pratt CB, Pappo AS, Gieser P, et al: Role of adjuvant chemotherapy in the treatment of surgically resected pediatric nonrhabdomyosarcomatous soft tissue sarcomas: a Pediatric Oncology Group Study. *J Clin Oncol* 17:1219, 1999.
    This study demonstates that for children with completely resected tumors, chemotherapy offers limited additional benefit.
70. Horowitz ME, Pratt CB, Webber BL, et al: Therapy for childhood soft-tissue sarcomas other than rhabdomyosarcoma: a review of 62 cases treated at a single institution. *J Clin Oncol* 4:559–564, 1986.
    This single-institution study reaffirms that complete resection of NRSTS results in the best prognosis, justifying aggressive surgery and re-resection.
75. Paulino AC, Ritchie J, Wen BC: The value of postoperative radiotherapy in childhood nonrhabdomyosarcoma soft tissue sarcoma. *Pediatr Blood Cancer* 43:587–593, 2004.
    For incompletely resected NRSTS, the incorporation of postoperative radiation therapy can improve overall survival.
85. Cecchetto G, Alaggio R, Dall'Igna P, et al: Localized unresectable non-rhabdo soft tissue sarcomas of the extremities in pediatric age: results from the Italian studies. *Cancer* 104:2006–2012, 2005.
    This retrospective study indicates that complete delayed resection after neoadjuvant chemotherapy is particularly important even for nonchemosensitive NRSTS.
108. Ferrari A, Gronchi A, Casanova M, et al: Synovial sarcoma: a retrospective analysis of 271 patients of all ages treated at a single institution. *Cancer* 101:627–634, 2004.
    A large study of patients with synovial sarcoma demonstrates a benefit to chemotherapy, particularly in older adolescents.
113. Demetri GD, Chawla SP, Ray-Coquard I, et al: Results of an international randomized phase III trial of the mammalian target of rapamycin inhibitor ridaforolimus versus placebo to control metastatic sarcomas in patients after benefit from prior chemotherapy. *J Clin Oncol* 31:2485–2492, 2013.
    This large study of adults with advanced sarcomas demonstrated a small benefit to treatment with ridaforolimus, an mTOR inhibitor.
123. Matushansky I, Hernando E, Socci ND, et al: A developmental model of sarcomagenesis defines a differentiation-based classification for liposarcomas. *Am J Pathol* 172:1069–1080, 2008.
    Comparing gene expression changes during mesenchymal stem cell differentiation and across various liposarcoma histologies suggests that liposarcomas share a developmental progression.
143. Barretina J, Taylor BS, Banerji S, et al: Subtype-specific genomic alterations define new targets for soft-tissue sarcoma therapy. *Nat Genet* 42:715–721, 2010.
    Although not focused on sarcomas common to children, this study describes the approach to integrative genomic analysis for sarcomas.

231. Simon MP, Pedeutour F, Sirvent N, et al: Deregulation of the platelet-derived growth factor B-chain gene via fusion with collagen gene *COL1A1* in dermatofibrosarcoma protuberans and giant-cell fibroblastoma. *Nat Genet* 15:95–98, 1997.

   The identification of translocation-directed growth factor activation in NRSTS offers a rationale for the therapeutic use of kinase inhibitors.

341. Tomlinson IP, Alam NA, Rowan AJ, et al: Germline mutations in FH predispose to dominantly inherited uterine fibroids, skin leiomyomata and papillary renal cell cancer. *Nat Genet* 30:406–410, 2002.

   This study, as well as those studying succinate dehydrogenase, demonstrates that alteration in cellular metabolism increases the risk for various forms of cancer, including sarcomas.

521. Kadoch C, Crabtree GR: Reversible disruption of mSWI/SNF (BAF) complexes by the SS18-SSX oncogenic fusion in synovial sarcoma. *Cell* 153:71–85, 2013.

   By linking the product of one of the genes translocated in synovial sarcoma to the SWI/SNF complex, this study adds this sarcoma to the exceptionally broad range of cancers associated with aberrant chromatin regulation.

607. Davis IJ, Kim JJ, Ozsolak F, et al: Oncogenic MITF dysregulation in clear cell sarcoma: defining the MiT family of human cancers. *Cancer Cell* 9:473–484, 2006.

   This study, as well as others, contributes to the growing range of cancers in which dysreguation of various members of the MiT family of transcription factors plays a key role.

734. Joensuu H, Roberts PJ, Sarlomo-Rikala M, et al: Effect of the tyrosine kinase inhibitor STI571 in a patient with a metastatic gastrointestinal stromal tumor. *N Engl J Med* 344:1052–1056, 2001.

   Although not specifically relevant to pediatric gastrointestinal stromal tumors, this report demonstrated the efficacy of tyrosine kinase inhibitors targeted toward specific genetic alterations in sarcomas.

774. Baird K, Davis S, Antonescu CR, et al: Gene expression profiling of human sarcomas: insights into sarcoma biology. *Cancer Res* 65:9226–9235, 2005.

   Microarray-based gene expression analysis of a broad range of sarcomas demonstrates the variation between types of sarcomas.

777. Rubin BP, Nishijo K, Chen HI, et al: Evidence for an unanticipated relationship between undifferentiated pleomorphic sarcoma and embryonal rhabdomyosarcoma. *Cancer Cell* 19:177–191, 2011.

   Using conditional mouse models, this study demonstrates the relationship between embryonal rhabdomyosarcoma and undifferentiated pleomorphic sarcomas.

779. Patel M, Simon JM, Iglesia MD, et al: Tumor-specific retargeting of an oncogenic transcription factor chimera results in dysregulation of chromatin and transcription. *Genome Res* 22:259–270, 2012.

   Protein chimerism with EWSR1, a feature of a wide range of sarcomas, offers a mechanism for transcription factors to acquire chromatin-remodeling activity.

CHAPTER 61

Ewing Sarcoma

Steven G. DuBois, Holcombe E. Grier, and Stephen L. Lessnick

CHAPTER OUTLINE

In 1921 James Ewing described the cancer that came to carry his name: a primary bone tumor composed of small round blue cells and devoid of the malignant osteoid that characterizes osteosarcoma.[1] Subsequently, pathologists described other clinicopathologic entities initially thought to be distinct, such as peripheral primitive neuroectodermal tumor (PNET) of bone or soft tissue or the Askin tumor of the chest wall.[2] However, biologic study and clinical responses to chemotherapy have now linked these tumors into one entity or family of tumors, a grouping that also includes extraosseous Ewing sarcoma. Commonly used terms for this tumor include Ewing sarcoma, Ewing tumors, and Ewing sarcoma family of tumors. In this chapter the World Health Organization–approved term, Ewing sarcoma, is generally used. When appropriate, specific characteristics that differentiate Ewing sarcoma, PNET, and Askin tumors are described.

The chapter begins with a discussion of the epidemiology of Ewing sarcoma. Next, the current understanding of the cellular and molecular features of these tumors is reviewed. An overview of the clinical presentation and prognostic features of patients with this disease are presented. This overview is followed by a discussion of the management of patients with Ewing sarcoma. The chapter concludes with a review of the late effects seen in patients treated for these tumors.

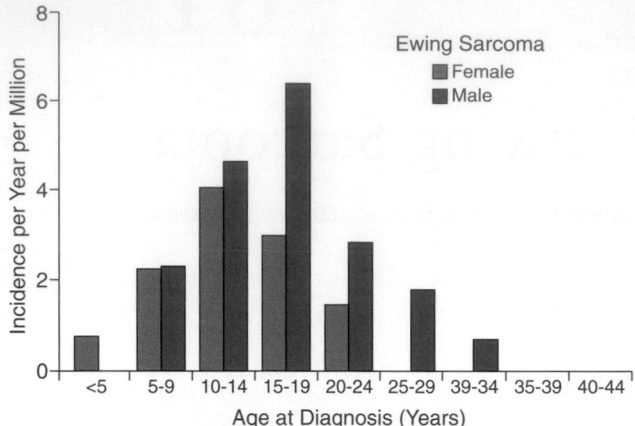

Figure 61-1 Incidence of Ewing sarcoma for male and female subjects according to age at initial diagnosis. *(From Mascarenhas L, Siegel S, Spector L, et al., Malignant bone tumors. In Cancer epidemiology in older adolescents and young adults 15 to 29 years of age, including SEER incidence and aurvival 1975-2000. Bleyer A, O'Leary M, Barr R, and Ries L, Editors. 2006, National Cancer Institute: Bethesda. p. 98–109.)*

EPIDEMIOLOGY

Ewing sarcoma is the second most common type of primary bone cancer in the United States and Europe, accounting for approximately 25% to 34% of malignant bone tumors.[3-5] Approximately 250 new cases of Ewing sarcoma are diagnosed in the United States each year.[4,5] In the United States Ewing sarcoma has had a relatively stable average incidence of 2.5 to 3 cases per million per year from 1975 to 2000.[4,6] A similar age-adjusted incidence has been noted in Europe.[3] As shown in Figure 61-1, the peak incidence occurs during adolescence, with an average incidence of 4.6 cases per million per year for the 15- to 19-year age range.[4] Younger children are affected less frequently, and the disease is distinctly uncommon in adults older than 35 years of age. A male predominance has been noted, with a male-to-female ratio of approximately 1.25 : 1.[5,7] However, one study reported a female predominance in patients younger than 3 years of age at initial diagnosis.[8] There is no seasonal variation in the appearance of this disease.[7,9]

The incidence of Ewing sarcoma varies markedly among races and countries, with the highest frequency reported from Australia and Sao Paolo, Brazil.[10] People of African ancestry appear to have the lowest incidence of this disease. Figure 61-2 demonstrates the dramatically lower incidence of these tumors in the U.S. African-American/Black population.[55] A similar low incidence in sub-Saharan Africa has been reported and suggests a possible genetic difference in the risk of developing Ewing sarcoma.[10,11] Patients of African ancestry with Ewing sarcoma have higher rates of soft tissue tumors and an older age distribution compared with patients of European ancestry, indicating that racial differences in this disease extend beyond differences in incidence.[12] Ewing sarcoma also appears to be uncommon in people of East Asian ancestry, based on data from China, Japan, and Thailand.[10,13,14] Data from the Middle East, North

Africa, and the Indian subcontinent suggest that Ewing sarcoma is at least as common in these populations as in people of European ancestry.[10,15-17] In small studies from Kuwait and Bombay, for example, Ewing sarcoma was identified as the most common primary malignant bone tumor.[16,17]

Based on these geographic differences in the incidence of Ewing sarcoma, several groups have investigated the genetic epidemiology of this disease. One group reported differences between African and European populations in the number of Alu repeat sequences in intron 6 of the *EWSR1* gene, upstream of the breakpoint region involved in translocations at this locus seen in most cases of Ewing sarcoma.[18] Two studies further focused on this possibility that differences in the incidence of Ewing sarcoma may be due to differences in polymorphisms in the *EWSR1* locus that could result in different rates of translocation.[19,20] Both studies each identified a different single nucleotide polymorphism with low-level statistical association with Ewing sarcoma, although the effect of each polymorphism on the risk of Ewing sarcoma was small. Another study investigated the incidence of other tumors that harbor *EWSR1* translocations across racial groups and observed higher rates of desmoplastic small round cell tumor in the U.S. African-American population compared with the U.S. European-American population.[21] This finding of higher rates of an *EWSR1*-associated tumor in a population with a lower rate of Ewing sarcoma provides additional evidence that differential susceptibility to translocation at the *EWSR1* locus does not account for racial differences in the incidence of Ewing sarcoma. More recently, a genome-wide association study identified and validated polymorphisms in three loci, 1p36, 10q21, and 15q15, associated with increased risk of

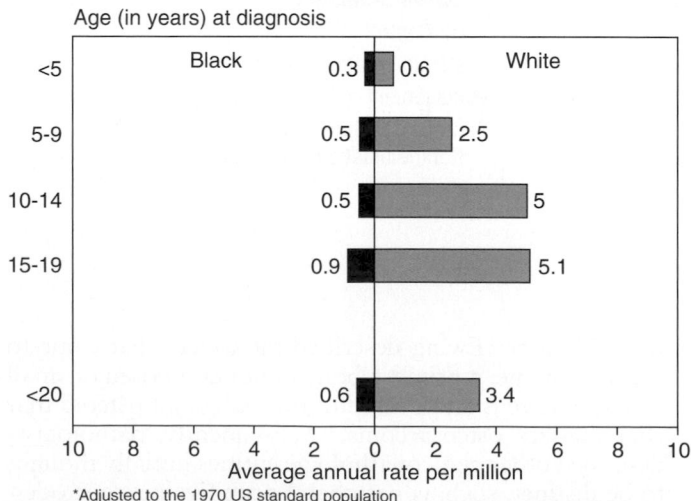

Figure 61-2 Incidence of Ewing sarcoma by age according to race, demonstrating the marked rarity of the disease in the United States African-American/Black population. *(From Gurney JG, Swensen AR, Bulterys M: Malignant bone tumors, in cancer incidence and survival among children and adolescents: United States SEER Program 1975-1995. Ries LAG, Smith MA, Gurney JG, et al, editors. National Cancer Institute, SEER Program, NIH Pub. No. 99-4649, Bethesda, MD, 1999, p. 99–110.)*

Ewing sarcoma. These risk variants are present at lower frequencies in African populations, providing one potential explanation for the lower rates of Ewing sarcoma in this population.[22]

The etiology of Ewing sarcoma remains largely obscure. These tumors are not generally believed to be familial, although rare cases of sibling pairs with Ewing sarcoma have been reported.[23-25] First- and second-degree relatives of patients with Ewing sarcoma do not appear to have an increased overall risk of cancer, although a higher rate of stomach cancer, melanoma, renal cancer, and brain tumors has been reported.[26,27]

Patients with Ewing sarcoma appear to have an increased incidence of specific congenital anomalies. The most consistent finding has been an association between Ewing sarcoma and congenital hernias, particularly inguinal hernias.[28-30] A pooled analysis of the available literature has confirmed this association, with an odds ratio of developing Ewing sarcoma of 2.8 for children with congenital hernias compared with children without congenital hernias.[31] Whether a common hormonal or environmental mechanism underlies the development of both congenital hernias and Ewing sarcoma remains unclear. Patients with Ewing sarcoma have also been noted to have an increased incidence of bone anomalies, particularly rib and vertebral anomalies.[30,32,33] Other congenital anomalies, including cataracts and genitourinary anomalies, have been reported in patients with Ewing sarcoma.[30,32,34] These anomalies occur at a low incidence in these patients and without a consistent pattern, suggesting that their occurrence with Ewing sarcoma may be coincidental.

Various parental exposures have been associated with the risk of developing Ewing sarcoma. The most consistent finding has been an association between parental farm exposure around the time of conception through birth and the subsequent development of Ewing sarcoma. This association has been reported in a series of case-control studies and affirmed in a meta-analysis, with an increased risk if either parent was involved in farming.[28,35-38] Specific exposures related to agricultural work that have been suggested as driving this increased risk include parental fertilizer, pesticide, solvent, and wood dust exposure.[36,37,39] Less consistently reported associations include an increased risk of Ewing sarcoma with parental cigarette smoking and parental occupation in manual labor.[28,36] Family income does not appear to be associated with the risk of Ewing sarcoma.[28,37]

Additional attention has focused on features of physical growth and development that might distinguish patients with Ewing sarcoma. Differences in birth weight between patients with Ewing sarcoma and controls have not been observed.[40] Given its peak incidence during adolescence, some groups have investigated differences in the onset of puberty between patients with Ewing sarcoma and controls. One group reported that boys with Ewing sarcoma began shaving earlier than boys without Ewing sarcoma.[29] Other differences related to development of secondary sex characteristics have not been observed.[29,40] At the time of diagnosis, patients with Ewing sarcoma do not seem to be taller than their peers.[40-42]

Several viruses have been suggested as playing a role in the pathogenesis of Ewing sarcoma. One group reported that the adenovirus *E1A* gene could specifically induce the chromosomal translocation characteristic of these tumors.[43] Follow-up studies failed to corroborate this finding.[44-47] Based on increased Epstein-Barr virus titers in patients with Ewing sarcoma, other groups evaluated Ewing tumors for Epstein-Barr virus infection and found no viral involvement.[48,49] Both BK and SV40 viral sequences have been variably identified in cases of Ewing sarcoma, but the functional importance of these findings remains unknown.[50-52]

Ewing sarcoma rarely develops as a second malignancy. Several case reports describe the development of Ewing sarcoma years after the successful treatment of children with a range of hematologic malignancies and solid cancers.[53-58] More formal studies indicate that Ewing sarcoma as a second malignancy occurs only infrequently. In a population-based study, 2.1% of all Ewing sarcoma cases arose as second malignancies.[59] In a large institutional review, only 1.3% of second malignancies following treatment of pediatric cancer were Ewing sarcoma or PNET.[60] Several large series of patients with secondary bone sarcomas have reported only a small number of patients with Ewing sarcoma.[61-64] These secondary Ewing tumors do not appear to be radiation-related.[59] In addition, the wide range of primary malignancies described in these patients suggests that these tumors do not arise as part of a specific cancer predisposition syndrome.

BIOLOGIC FEATURES

Chromosomal Rearrangements in Ewing Sarcoma

In the mid-1980s the presence of a recurrent reciprocal chromosomal translocation, t(11;22)(q24;q12), was reported in Ewing sarcoma tumors and cell lines.[65,66] The same translocation was also identified in PNET, supporting the hypothesis that these two tumors represented the same disease exhibiting varying levels of differentiation along a neuronal pathway.[67] Subsequent studies demonstrated that t(11;22)(q24;q12) was present in approximately 83% of Ewing sarcomas.[68]

The early analysis of translocations in Ewing sarcoma demonstrated that the derivative chromosome 22 was always maintained as these tumors and cell lines undergo clonal evolution, whereas the derivative chromosome 11 could be lost.[66] This indicated that the "22;11" derivative is the key chromosomal abnormality, whereas the reciprocal "11;22" is unnecessary. The t(11;22)(q24;q12) is a tumor-specific or somatic mutation because it is not found in the germline DNA of patients.[66]

In addition to the t(11;22)(q24;q12) rearrangement (and related translocations with similar molecular consequences, discussed later), other chromosomal abnormalities have also been reported in Ewing sarcoma.[66,69-75] A careful analysis of these sometimes complex karyotypes has revealed a small group of recurrent, nonrandom chromosomal abnormalities. Gains (usually trisomies) of chromosome 8 may be observed in up to 50% of cases, and gains of chromosomes 12 and 1q are seen in approximately 25% of cases.[69,73,74,76,77] Gains in chromosome 20 have also been reported in 10% to 20% of cases.[78] Interestingly, a chromosomal translocation that is unrelated to the t(11;22)(q24;q12) has been observed in approximately 20% of cases: der(16)t(1;16).[69,73,74,76,77] This translocation is often found as an unbalanced rearrangement and thus results in partial gains (trisomies and occasionally tetrasomies) of 1q and losses (monosomies) of 16q.[69,73,74,76,77] The breakpoints of this translocation appear to be variable and range from q11 through q32 on chromosome 1 and from q11.1 through q24 on chromosome 16.[69,73,74,76,77] This suggests that the translocation does not alter particular target genes at the breakpoint but rather introduces gains of 1q and losses of 16q. Finally, losses at 1p36 have also been observed.[75] More recent high-resolution copy number studies have identified copy number alterations in specific genes or regions of the genome, although the role of specific genomic gains or losses has yet to be determined.[79-82] There has also been a report of genomic instability, as measured by microsatellite instability and loss of heterozygosity, in Ewing sarcoma.[83] This finding, however, is somewhat controversial, insofar as a second group was not able to replicate the microsatellite instability findings.[84]

The Cloning of EWS/FLI

A major advance in the understanding of the pathogenesis of Ewing sarcoma occurred when the breakpoint of the (11;22)(q24;q12) translocation was cloned in 1992.[85] The translocation breakpoint was localized roughly in the middle of two genes: *EWSR1* and *FLI1*. *EWSR1* had not been previously identified and so was named on the basis of its involvement in the Ewing sarcoma translocation breakpoint (*Ew*ing *s*arcoma *r*earrangement domain *1*).[85,86] *FLI1* had been previously identified in mice as the *F*riend *L*eukemia Virus *i*ntegration site.[87] As a result of the translocation event, these two genes become fused and the expressed transcript encodes the EWS/FLI fusion protein (Fig. 61-3).[85]

Wild-Type EWS Protein

EWSR1 encodes the EWS protein (see Fig. 61-3).[85] Wild-type EWS contains 656 amino acids and appears to be ubiquitously expressed.[85,88,89] EWS is primarily localized to the nucleus,[90-92] although it has also been detected in the cytoplasm[93] and on the cell surface.[94] The amino terminus of EWS (sometimes referred to as NTD-EWS) contains 285 amino acids consisting of 31 pseudorepeats rich in tyrosine, glutamine, serine, threonine, glycine, alanine, and proline.[85] This region bears some similarity to the carboxyl-terminal domain (CTD) of RNA polymerase II.[85] This similarity suggested that the region could modulate RNA transcription. The carboxyl terminus of EWS contains an RNA recognition motif (an RRM domain), as well as three arginine-glycine-glycine (RGG) domains that are often found in RNA binding proteins. Indeed, it has been demonstrated, in vitro, that EWS can bind to RNA.[89,95] These findings suggest that wild-type EWS may be involved in RNA transcription or processing. The carboxyl-terminal region also contains a potential C_2C_2 zinc finger of uncertain significance.[96] There is evidence that EWS may undergo posttranslational

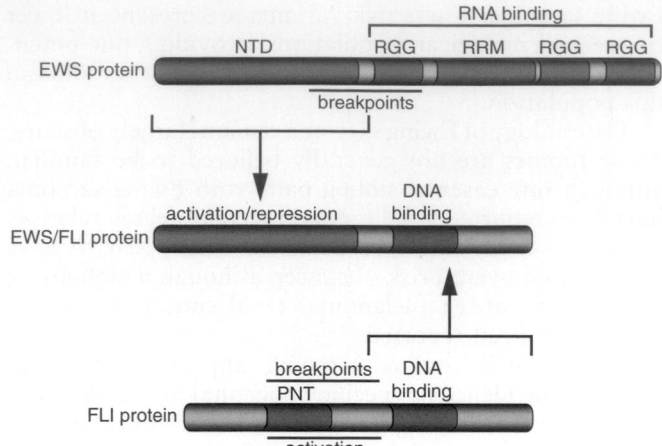

Figure 61-3 Fusion of EWS and FLI produces the EWS/FLI protein. Wild-type EWS is characterized by an amino-terminal domain *(NTD)*, along with three RGG regions and an RNA recognition motif *(RRM)* that confer RNA-binding properties to the protein. Wild-type FLI contains a pointed domain *(PNT)* that overlaps with a transcriptional activation domain and an ETS-type DNA-binding domain. The translocation breakpoint regions of each protein are shown. After a translocation event, EWS/FLI is formed. EWS/FLI maintains the NTD of EWS (which functions as both a strong transcriptional activation domain and a transcriptional repression domain in this context), and the DNA-binding domain of FLI.

modifications, but the significance of these alterations is not well understood.[94,95,97-100]

EWS is closely related to two additional sarcoma-associated translocation partners, TLS (*t*rans*l*ocated in *s*liposarcoma; also called FUS) and TAF15 (also known at TAF$_{II}$68, TAF2N, and RBP56), as well as to a *Drosophila melanogaster* protein named cabeza (also known as SARFH; originally called P19).[96,101-104] TLS was first identified in human myxoid liposarcoma in the context of the t(12;16)(q13;p11) translocation, which encodes a TLS/CHOP fusion protein (Table 61-1).[102,104] TAF15 is a member of the TFIID general transcription complex.[101] It is found fused to NR4A3 (also called CHN, TEC, CSMF, or NOR1) in extraskeletal myxoid chondrosarcomas and to ZNF384 (also called CIZ or NMP4) in acute leukemias (see Table 61-1).[105-107] TAF15 also has significant homology and domain organization to EWS and TLS.[101,103] The three human proteins are sometimes described as the TET family of proteins (*T*LS, *E*WS, *T*AF15) or the FET family (*F*US, *E*WS, *T*AF15). Although the normal function of these proteins is not completely understood, some evidence suggests that they may be involved in RNA splicing, gene expression, microRNA processing, and formation of RNA-containing intracellular granules.[90,101,108-125] Interestingly, constitutional mutations in TLS result in familial amyotrophic lateral sclerosis (ALS), and mutations in TAF15 may also be associated with the disease.[126,127]

Wild-Type FLI Protein

FLI is a member of the ETS family of transcription factors.[128] This family is defined by the presence of an ETS type DNA-binding domain and consists of 27 different members in humans.[129] As with most transcription

TABLE 61-1 Translocations in Ewing Sarcoma, Ewing Sarcoma-Like, and Other Tumors that Contain *EWSR1*, *TLS* (also called *FUS*), or *TAF15* Family Members*

Tumor Type	Translocation	Fusion Gene
Ewing sarcoma	t(11;22)(q24;q12)	*EWSR1/FLI1*
	t(21;22)(q22;q12)	*EWSR1/ERG*
	t(7;22)(p22;q12)	*EWSR1/ETV1*
	t(17;22)(q12;q12)	*EWSR1/ETV4*
	t(2;22)(q35;q12)	*EWSR1/FEV*
	t(16;21)(p11;q22)	*TLS/ERG*
	t(2;16)(q35;p11)	*TLS/FEV*
Ewing-like sarcoma	t(20;22)(q13;q12)	*EWSR1/NFATC2*
	(NB: can occur in ring chromosome and may be amplified)	*EWSR1/POU5F1*
	t(6;22)(p21;q12)	*EWSR1/SMARCA5*
	t(4;22)(q31;q12)	*EWSR1/ZSG*
	Submicroscopic inv(22) in t(1;22) (p36.1;q12)	
	t(2;22)(q31;q12)	*EWSR1/SP3*
	t(4;19)(q35;q13)	*CIC/DUX4*
	inv(X) (p11.4;p11.22)	*BCOR/CCNB3*
Clear cell sarcoma	t(12;22)(q13;q12)	*EWSR1/ATF1*
Desmoplastic small round cell tumor	t(11;22)(p13;q12)	*EWSR1/WT1*
Extraskeletal myxoid chondrosarcoma	t(9;22)(q22;q12)	*EWSR1/NR4A3*
	t(9;17)(q22;q11)	*TAF15/NR4A3*
	t(9;15)(q22;q21)	*TCF12/NR4A3*
Myxoid liposarcoma	t(12;16)(q13;p11)	*TLS/DDIT3*
	t(12;22)(q13;q12)	*EWSR1/DDIT3*
Angiomatoid fibrous histiocytoma	t(12;16)(q13;p11)	*TLS/ATF1*
Low grade fibromyxoid sarcoma	t(7;16)(q33;p11)	*TLS/CREB3L2*
Acute myelogenous leukemia	t(16;21)(p11;q22)	*TLS/ERG*
Acute myelogenous, lymphoblastic, or undifferentiated leukemia	t(12;22)(p13;q12)	*EWSR1/ZNF384*
	t(12;17)(p13;q11)	*TAF15/ZNF384*

*Gene names are provided rather than their corresponding protein names.

factors, ETS family members have a modular architecture with separate domains that contribute DNA binding and transcriptional functions.[130] The DNA-binding ETS domain of FLI is present in the carboxyl-terminal portion of the protein (see Fig. 61-3).[128] Most ETS family members (including FLI) bind to sequences containing a GGAA or GGAT core sequence.[129,130] In addition to DNA-binding function, FLI contains two separate transcriptional activation domains, one in the amino terminus and a second in the carboxyl terminus (distal to the ETS DNA-binding domain; see Fig. 61-3).[131] Wild-type FLI also contains a PNT (pointed) domain in the amino terminal portion of the protein.[132] PNT domains are thought to mediate protein-protein interactions.[133]

The normal role of FLI appears to be primarily in the hematopoietic lineage, where it regulates megakaryocytic development.[134,135] Knockout of murine Fli-1 results in abnormal megakaryocytic differentiation and a loss in vascular integrity that results in embryonic lethality from central nervous system hemorrhage.[136,137] Hemizygous deletion of FLI is found in patients with Paris-Trousseau or Jacobsen thrombocytopenia syndromes.[136,138,139] FLI also appears to be important for vascular development in the mouse and zebrafish.[136,140] FLI is also expressed in neural crest–derived mesenchyme in both the mouse and quail.[141,142] This finding is particularly interesting in light of the neural crest phenotype of Ewing sarcoma.

FLI itself can function as an oncogene, at least in the hematopoietic context. Indeed, the murine *Fli* locus was first defined as a predominant Friend *mu*rine *l*eukemia *v*irus (F-MuLV) insertion site.[87] Thus insertion of F-MuLV at the *Fli* locus results in upregulation of the *Fli* gene and subsequent development of erythroleukemia.[87,128] The oncogenic activity of FLI appears to be limited to the hematopoietic system as introduction of the protein into other models of oncogenesis, such as the NIH3T3 cell model, does not result in the transformed phenotype.[90]

EWS/FLI and Other TET/ETS Fusions in Ewing Sarcoma

EWS/FLI consists of the amino terminus of EWS fused, in frame, to the carboxyl terminus of FLI (see Fig. 61-3).[85] The EWS portion retained in the fusion contains the pseudorepeat domain that harbors a strong transcriptional activation function as well as a transcriptional repression function.[85,90,119,143] The RNA-binding domain of EWS is lost in the fusion protein and instead is replaced by the portion of FLI that contains its ETS DNA-binding domain.[85]

EWS/FLI functions as an oncoprotein. EWS/FLI can induce NIH3T3 cells (an immortalized mouse fibroblast cell line) to exhibit both anchorage independent growth and growth as tumors when injected subcutaneously into immunodeficient mice.[144-146] Conversely, blockade of EWS/FLI expression or function (via antisense RNA, dominant-negative blocking alleles, or RNA interference) causes Ewing sarcoma cells to lose their transformed phenotype.[147-155] These data demonstrate that EWS/FLI expression is required for the oncogenic phenotype of Ewing sarcoma. Interestingly, it has been reported that after therapy-induced neural differentiation of Ewing sarcoma, EWS/FLI expression may also be lost.[156] Although these data support an important role for EWS/FLI expression in Ewing sarcoma proliferation and transformation, they do not address whether EWS/FLI formation is the first step in Ewing sarcoma development or whether other oncogenic events occur first and are followed by EWS/FLI formation.

There are three main consequences of the t(11;22)(q24;q12) rearrangement. First, it places the transcriptional regulation of the EWS/FLI fusion under the control of the *EWSR1* promoter. This is important because the activity of the *FLI1* promoter is limited to hematopoietic (and perhaps neural crest) lineages, whereas the *EWSR1* promoter appears to be active in most, if not all, cell types (see previous sections). Second, the translocation results in a loss of one wild-type *EWSR1* allele and one wild-type *FLI1* allele. Loss of one *FLI1* allele is probably of no consequence because wild-type *FLI1* is not expressed in Ewing sarcoma.[155] Whether loss of one *EWSR1* allele is important in Ewing sarcoma development is not known. The third consequence of the translocation is that it creates the EWS/FLI fusion protein. This is important because although EWS/FLI functions as an oncoprotein, neither wild-type EWS nor wild-type FLI could induce transformation of NIH3T3 cells, thus demonstrating a gain of function for the EWS/FLI fusion.[90] Structure-function analyses of EWS/FLI demonstrated that both the amino terminal EWS domain and the ETS DNA-binding domain of FLI were required for oncogenic transformation of NIH3T3 cells and Ewing sarcoma cells.[143,144] These results indicate that the fusion protein functions as an aberrant transcription factor. Comparisons of EWS/FLI with wild-type FLI demonstrated that the EWS domain included in the fusion protein could function as a much stronger transcriptional activation domain than the domain of FLI that was lost in the fusion.[90] These results suggested that EWS/FLI induced oncogenic transformation by binding to target genes through its ETS DNA-binding domain and upregulating the expression of those genes through its EWS domain.

The mechanisms by which the EWS portion of the fusion functions as a transcriptional activation domain are only now beginning to be understood. Because wild-type EWS has been shown to interact with TFIID, RNA polymerase II, or the p300/CBP coactivators, it appears likely that these interactions are also important for EWS/FLI function.[109,111,116,117] RNA helicase A (RHA) has also been shown to be important for the transcriptional activity of EWS/FLI.[157] Thus RHA may also function as a coactivator for gene expression mediated by the fusion protein.

More recently, it has been appreciated that EWS/FLI also functions as a transcriptional repressor. For example, analysis of the transcriptional program triggered by EWS/FLI in Ewing sarcoma cells has revealed that more genes are downregulated by the fusion than are upregulated.[152,155] Additional analysis has demonstrated that EWS/FLI functions as a direct transcriptional repressor at some target genes, like *LOX* and *TGFBR2*.[143,158] The mechanism of repression appears to be through binding of a transcriptional corepressor complex called NuRD, that includes nucleosome remodeling function, as well as histone deacetylase and histone lysine-specific demethylase activities.[143] Both transcriptional activation and repression functions are required for the oncogenic activity of EWS/FLI in Ewing sarcoma cells.[143]

Analysis of EWS/FLI binding sites in the human genome revealed that the fusion protein binds to sites that contain "classic" ETS-type high-affinity sequences (e.g., ACCGGAAGTG).[159-161] However, a more interesting and unusual finding was that EWS/FLI was also found to bind to GGAA-containing microsatellite sequences.[159-162] EWS/

FLI binds to these microsatellites and uses them as response elements to activate the expression of target genes, and the transcriptional function is proportional to the length of the microsatellite.[159,162,163] This raises the intriguing possibility that polymorphisms in GGAA-microsatellites associated with key EWS/FLI target genes (e.g., *NR0B1*, *CAV1*, or *GSTM4*) may alter susceptibility to Ewing sarcoma or perhaps outcome in patients with the disease.[162,164,165] It has also been suggested that the lack of GGAA-microsatellites near critical EWS/FLI target genes, such as *NR0B1*, in organisms other than humans might be the reason that only humans develop Ewing sarcoma.[159,162]

In addition to EWS/FLI, other less frequent Ewing sarcoma translocation breakpoints were cloned and revealed a very similar structural organization (see Table 61-1). As described, approximately 83% of Ewing sarcoma tumors contain an (11;22)(q24;q12) translocation.[66-68] Approximately 10% of cases demonstrate an alternate translocation, t(21;22)(q22;q12).[166] Cloning of the breakpoint of this rearrangement revealed that EWS was fused, in frame, to another member of the ETS family, ERG.[166] As in the case of EWS/FLI, the EWS/ERG fusion contains the amino terminus of EWS fused to the carboxyl terminus of ERG, which harbors its ETS DNA-binding domain.[166] Interestingly, the ETS DNA-binding domains of FLI and ERG are 98% identical at the amino acid level.[166,167] Subsequent investigations demonstrated that EWS/ERG also functioned as an oncoprotein in the NIH3T3 cell model.[146,168] In subsequent years additional translocations were identified in Ewing sarcoma, including a t(7;22)(p22;q12), t(17;22)(q12;q12), and t(2;22)(q33;q12).[169-172] Cloning of transcripts from these translocations demonstrated that in each case EWS was fused to another member of the ETS family.[169-172] Currently, five EWS/ETS fusions have been described (see Table 61-1).[85,166,169-173] It is assumed that all EWS/ETS fusion proteins bind similar (if not identical) target genes to induce oncogenic transformation.[173]

Overall, most cases of Ewing sarcoma appear to harbor fusions between EWS and various ETS family members. Rarely, fusions between TLS and ETS family members may be present in Ewing sarcoma instead, as shown by the identification of TLS/ERG fusions in four patients with Ewing sarcoma and the identification of a TLS/FEV fusion in another case (see Table 61-1).[174,175] These findings highlight the similarities across the TET family and across the ETS family. Perhaps the most generic manner of describing the fusion proteins in Ewing sarcoma would be as "TET/ETS fusions."[173] Because EWS/FLI is the most common fusion identified in Ewing sarcoma, most of the experimental work has been performed using this fusion protein. Experimental findings based on EWS/FLI have only occasionally been confirmed using other Ewing sarcoma fusion proteins.

In addition to variability of fusion partners, variability also exists in the exonic structure of some of the fusion proteins (Fig. 61-4). The breakpoints found in Ewing sarcoma translocations occur in the introns of *EWSR1* and *FLI1* (and presumably the other ETS factors as well, although in most cases this has not been experimentally

Genomic structures:

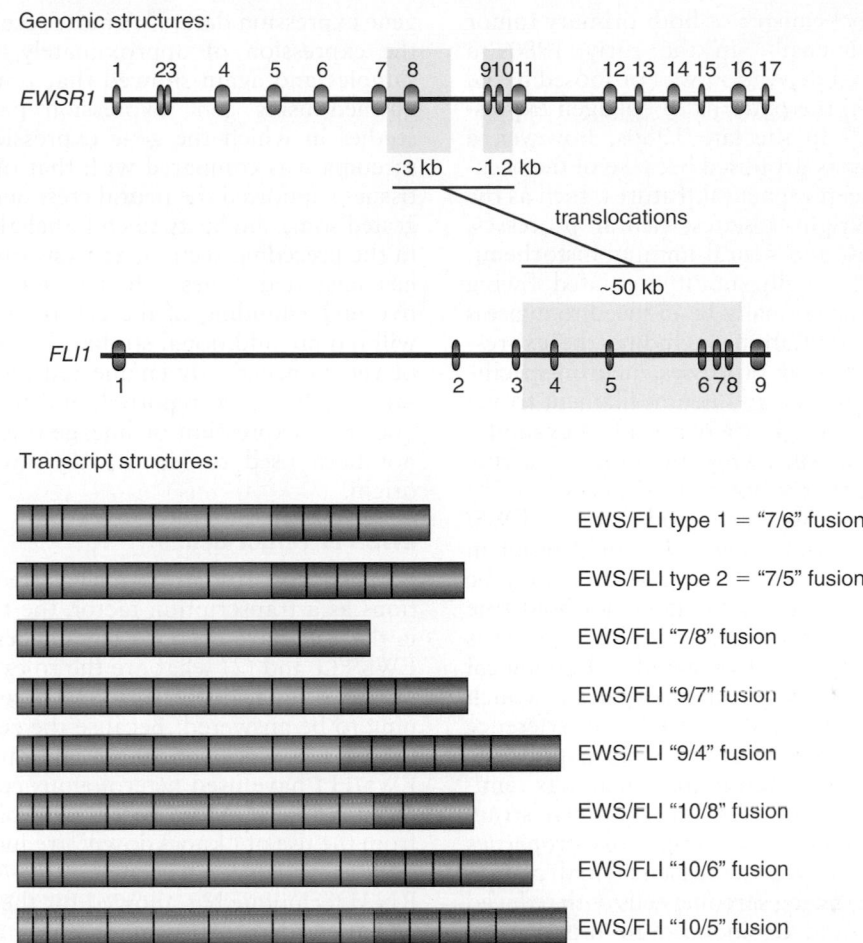

Figure 61-4 Translocation breakpoints may occur within one of two portions of a 6-kb region of the *EWSR1* gene and in a 50-kb region of the *FLI1* gene. This variety results in the observed heterogeneity of EWS/FLI fusion transcripts, as indicated.

confirmed).[85,86,176,177] The breakpoints in the *EWSR1* gene are found in one of two regions (3 kb and 1.2 kb in size) present in an approximately 6 kilobase (kb) region that includes four of the gene's 16 introns.[85,86,176] The breakpoints in *FLI1* occur over an approximately 50-kb region, which includes six of eight *FLI* introns.[85,86,176] Splicing events join adjacent exons together in the fusion transcript.[85,86,176,177] As a result of this variability in breakpoint and subsequent RNA splicing, at least 10 different EWS/FLI isoforms are generated (see Fig. 61-4).[85,86,144,176-178]

The most common Ewing sarcoma translocation fuses exon 7 of *EWSR1* to exon 6 of *FLI1*.[85,177] This "7/6" fusion is commonly referred to as a "type 1" EWS/FLI fusion and accounts for approximately 50% to 60% of EWS/FLI fusions.[177,179] A "type 2" fusion joins exon 7 of *EWSR1* to exon 5 of *FLI1* and is the second most common EWS/FLI fusion, accounting for approximately 20% to 30% of EWS/FLI fusions.[85,177,179] Laboratory studies suggested that the type 1 EWS/FLI fusion was a weaker oncoprotein than the type 2 fusion, and originally it was thought to have prognostic significance.[180,181] However, these functional differences were not reflected on changes in gene expression between type 1 and type 2 fusions, and large-scale clinical cor-

relative data did not indicate a prognostic difference based on fusion subtype.[182-184]

Although there is general agreement regarding the designation of the type 1 and type 2 fusions, there is no generalized nomenclature for the remaining fusions, and so these are best described in terms of which exons are fused to one another. In addition to variability in the EWS/FLI breakpoint, EWS/ERG has also been reported to demonstrate variability based on fusion points, with at least four fusions reported.[166,177] Because the other fusions are so rare, there is only minimal information as to whether they also show similar levels of breakpoint heterogeneity.

Ewing Sarcoma Cell of Origin

The cell of origin of Ewing sarcoma is unknown, and the subject has generated intense debate.[185] The original description by James Ewing in 1921 suggested that this "round cell sarcoma" was of endothelial origin and hence properly referred to as a "diffuse endothelioma of bone."[1] Dr. Ewing later suggested that it may arise from perivascular lymphatic endothelium.[186] A hematologic origin was proposed in the early 1970s following an in-depth evaluation of light and electron microscopic characteristics and cytochemistry of both primary tumor and cell culture specimens.[187] In the early 1980s a fibroblastic-mesenchymal derivation was proposed based on, among other things, the patterns of collagen expression of the tumor.[188,189] In the late 1980s, however, a neural crest derivation was proposed because of the occasional identification of certain neural features, such as the presence of Homer Wright rosettes, neural processes, neurosecretory granules, and neural immunohistochemical markers.[190-195] Additionally, undifferentiated Ewing sarcoma cell lines can occasionally be induced to express markers of neural differentiation, including the expression of neuritelike elongated processes, neuron-specific enolase (NSE), cholinesterase, and neural filament triplet protein.[191,193,196-199] Interestingly, there are a few examples of neural differentiation of Ewing sarcoma occurring after therapy, which further supports this theory.[156,200-202] More recently, it was shown that introduction of EWS/FLI into murine mesenchymal stem cells could result in oncogenic transformation, suggesting that these may be the cell of origin (although the same does not hold true for human mesenchymal stem cells).[203,204] This hypothesis was further supported by microarray and cell biological studies performed on Ewing sarcoma cell lines in which EWS/FLI expression was reduced using RNA interference techniques.[205,206] In the absence of EWS/FLI expression, these cells had a gene expression pattern that was reminiscent of mesenchymal stem cells and a cellular structural organization and adhesive and migratory properties that were also consistent with a mesenchymal phenotype.[205,206] Furthermore, Ewing sarcoma cells with reduced EWS/FLI expression could be induced to differentiate into other mesenchymal cell types, such as fat and bone.[205] This is a characteristic that is shared by mesenchymal stem cells.

It is important to note, however, that the phenotype of Ewing sarcoma (at least the neural crest component) may be a *consequence* of the (11;22) translocation rather than being related to the tumor's cell of origin. Introduction of EWS/FLI into NIH3T3 murine fibroblasts induces a phenotype that is highly similar to Ewing sarcoma, including the small round blue cell morphology and features of neural differentiation.[145,146] Similarly, expression of EWS/FLI in human rhabdomyosarcoma cells, neuroblastoma cells, or even normal human fibroblasts causes those cells to express genes that are similar to the genes expressed in Ewing sarcoma.[207-209] This suggests that EWS/FLI may cause transdifferentiation of its target cells. Thus the neural crest phenotype of Ewing sarcoma may be induced by EWS/FLI.

Transcriptional profiling experiments (e.g., those using oligonucleotide or complementary DNA microarrays and, more recently, RNA sequencing) in Ewing sarcoma tumors and cell lines have allowed for a comprehensive analysis of the gene expression patterns associated with this disease. One of the earliest studies compared Ewing sarcoma tumors and cell lines with other small round cell tumors of childhood, including neuroblastoma, non-Hodgkin lymphoma, and rhabdomyosarcoma.[210] These studies demonstrated that these histologically similar tumors could be distinguished from one another using

gene expression data.[210] A more recent analysis compared the expression of approximately 180 sarcoma tumor samples and again showed that tumors could be distinguished using gene expression patterns.[211] Additional studies in which the gene expression pattern of Ewing sarcoma was compared with that of a variety of normal tissues supported the neural crest derivation but also suggested some similarity to endothelial cells.[212] As discussed in the preceding section, analysis of some model systems has suggested a mesenchymal stem cell origin. A definitive understanding of the cell of origin of these tumors will require additional studies. It should be noted that as of yet no genetically engineered mouse model of Ewing sarcoma has been reported, and therefore tissue-specific oncogene expression or lineage-tracing approaches have not been used to identify the Ewing sarcoma cell of origin.

EWS/FLI Target Genes

Because most studies have suggested that EWS/FLI functions as a transcription factor, the two biggest questions in the field have been (1) what genes are dysregulated by EWS/FLI and (2) what are the roles of these gene targets in oncogenic transformation? These questions are beginning to be answered. Because the cell of origin of Ewing sarcoma is unknown, most laboratory-based studies of EWS/FLI have used heterologous cell types with varying results.[155,213-218] More recent approaches have benefited from the use of "knockdown" (reduction) of gene expression using RNA interference (RNAi).[152,154,155,219-222] The RNAi technique has allowed for the analysis of EWS/FLI in patient-derived Ewing sarcoma cell lines themselves, thus avoiding the concerns associated with using heterologous cell types.[152,154,155,219-222]

Gene expression analysis of Ewing sarcoma cells in which EWS/FLI has been knocked down has allowed a comprehensive identification of the thousands of genes that are modulated by the fusion protein.[152,155,219,221] For example, increased expression of NKX2.2 and NR0B1 are required for the oncogenic phenotype of Ewing sarcoma, although the specific mechanisms by which these transcriptional regulators facilitate the transformed phenotype remains poorly understood.[155,221,223,224] Similarly, repression of TGFBR2 (the receptor for transforming growth factor β) and lysyl oxidase (LOX) by EWS/FLI are also required for tumorigenicity of Ewing sarcoma cells.[143,158]

Gene expression studies also demonstrated that EWS/FLI represses the expression of the insulin-like growth factor binding protein 3 (IGFBP-3).[152] IGFBP-3 appears to be involved in Ewing sarcoma apoptosis, and thus decreased expression of this protein appears to prevent apoptosis.[152] These data complement a growing body of literature that supports a critical role for IGF-1 signaling in Ewing sarcoma development. For example, it was shown that Ewing sarcoma tumors and cell lines express IGF-1 and IGF receptors.[225,226] IGF-1 and its receptor appear to function in an autocrine/paracrine fashion in Ewing sarcoma, and disruption of this signaling pathway blocks various functions that contribute to tumorigenesis.[225,227-232] This occurs both in Ewing sarcoma cell lines as well as in model systems.[225-239] Indeed, disruption of this pathway has shown some efficacy as a molecularly targeted therapeutic approach for this disease (discussed later).

NPY1R was identified as an EWS/FLI target gene through microarray analysis.[155] Neuropeptide Y (NPY) is a small polypeptide neurotransmitter with diverse functions.[240,241] Engagement of NPY receptors by NPY in Ewing sarcoma cell lines is growth inhibitory, suggesting a potential therapeutic role for these receptors.[241,242] This result was surprising, insofar as Ewing sarcoma cells also express the NPY ligand.[241,242] It appears likely that Ewing sarcomas are protected from the growth-inhibitory effect of NPY/NPY1R interactions by the expression of dipeptidyl peptidase IV, which cleaves NPY into a form that is unable to bind NPY1R.[243,244] This cleaved form, NPY_{3-36}, functions as an angiogenic factor by binding to NPY2R receptors on endothelial cells, thus providing a likely explanation for the maintenance of this growth-inhibitory autocrine pathway in Ewing sarcoma cells.[243]

Another protein that has been shown to be upregulated by EWS/FLI is vascular endothelial growth factor (VEGF).[208,245] VEGF levels are increased in Ewing sarcoma cell lines and xenografts.[246] VEGF levels are also increased in the blood of patients with Ewing sarcoma and VEGF has been shown to be expressed in 55% of Ewing sarcoma tumor samples by immunohistochemistry.[245,247,248] In the case of Ewing sarcoma, VEGF may induce not only angiogenesis but also vasculogenesis.[249,250] Blockade of VEGF function in Ewing sarcoma model systems prevents tumor growth.[246,250-252] These preclinical studies demonstrate the potential for VEGF inhibition as a therapeutic strategy for Ewing sarcoma.

Most, but not all, studies of Ewing sarcoma have shown that these tumors typically express telomerase activity.[253-256] Interestingly, it appears that hTERT, the catalytic subunit of the telomerase holoenzyme, is upregulated by EWS/ETS proteins.[245,257,258] This upregulation appears to be caused by specific binding of the ETS portion of the fusion to the *TERT* promoter.[245,258,259] These data suggest that EWS/ETS fusions regulate telomerase activity by direct activation of the *TERT* promoter.

One key protein whose expression may be regulated by EWS/FLI is CD99 (also called MIC2).[208] In human fibroblasts engineered to express EWS/FLI, the expression of CD99 closely mimicked that of the fusion protein.[208] In the early 1990s it was found that CD99 is expressed at high levels in Ewing sarcoma cells but is uncommonly found on other tumor types.[260-262] The CD99 antigen is recognized by a variety of monoclonal antibodies, including 12E7, HBA71, and O13, and these antibodies have an important role in the diagnosis of Ewing sarcoma (discussed later).[260-269] The CD99 antigen is a membrane glycoprotein that plays a role in T-cell development and activation and migration of monocytes through endothelial junctions.[270-279] In Ewing sarcoma CD99 inhibits neural differentiation and thus contributes to oncogenic transformation.[280] Significantly, emerging data suggest that antibody-mediated engagement of CD99 may eventually be exploited as a new therapeutic approach

to Ewing sarcoma.[281,282] CD99 engagement in Ewing sarcoma results in apoptosis of the tumor cells.[281,282] This effect enhances tumor cell killing by chemotherapeutic agents.[281,283] Gene expression studies of CD99-mediated apoptosis suggested a role for the cytoskeletal protein zyxin in this process, and this finding was confirmed through functional studies.[284] The identification of zyxin in this process was interesting in light of subsequent studies demonstrating that zyxin acts as a tumor suppressor in Ewing sarcoma.[285] Taken together, these studies suggest that CD99 may be an effective therapeutic target in Ewing sarcoma by modulating cytoskeletal actin function.

Cooperative Pathways in Ewing Sarcoma Oncogenesis

Multiple potentially cooperating mutations in addition to TET/ETS fusions have been identified in Ewing sarcoma. The most widely assessed are mutations in the p53 and RB pathways. The p53 pathway includes proteins such as p14[ARF] and MDM2, as well as p53 itself.[286-290] When expressed in some heterologous systems, such as primary human fibroblasts, EWS/FLI induces the expression of p53.[208] This finding suggests that there is selective pressure to inhibit the p53 pathway. This hypothesis appears to be at least partially true. Deletions in the *CDKN2A* locus (commonly called the *INK4a* locus encoding both the p14[ARF] and p16[INK4a] proteins; note that p14[ARF] is involved in the p53 pathway, whereas p16[INK4a] is involved in the RB pathway) have been identified in approximately 10% to 30% of primary Ewing sarcoma tumors and more than 50% of Ewing sarcoma cell lines.[291-293] Amplifications or overexpression of *MDM2* is occasionally seen in Ewing sarcoma.[294-297] Mutations in p53 are found in 5% to 20% of Ewing sarcomas.[293,294,297-299] Taken together, mutations in the p53 pathway may be present in nearly 70% of Ewing sarcomas, and these mutations may have prognostic significance in this disease (discussed later). Because there are likely additional components of the pathway yet to be identified or analyzed, the frequency of alterations in this pathway may be even higher.

The RB pathway regulates the cell cycle and includes proteins such as CDK4, D-type cyclins, and p16[INK4a].[300-302] Mutations have been found in RB itself, and deletions of the *INK4a* locus have been documented as well in Ewing sarcoma.[291,292,303] As was observed in the case of the p53 pathway, mutations in the RB pathway also appear to be relatively common in this disease.[291,292,303]

Whereas mutations in the p53 and RB pathways are relatively common in Ewing sarcoma, mutations in other genes or pathways have only rarely been identified. For example, mutations in BRAF (which is also a member of the RAS/MAPK pathway) have been identified in 1 of 22 cell lines examined.[304] No mutations in other components of the pathway, including RAS or receptor tyrosine kinases, have been identified, as of yet. This suggests that the RAS/MAPK pathway is only rarely activated by mutation in this disease.

Although the RAS/MAPK pathway does not appear to be frequently activated by mutation, there is some evidence for a requirement of pathway activation in Ewing sarcoma tumor development. In the NIH3T3 model system, it was shown that expression of EWS/FLI induced phosphorylation of the ERK1 and ERK2 proteins (downstream members of the MAPK pathway).[305] This effect may result from autocrine stimulation of these transformed cells by PDGF-C, which was also shown to be induced by EWS/FLI expression in the NIH3T3 model, and expressed in Ewing sarcoma cell lines and tumor specimens.[215,306] There is some controversy as to whether PDGF-C plays a role in the human disease, as PDGFR-α, which is required for PDGF-C responsiveness, is not expressed in Ewing sarcoma.[307] Although PDGF-C may not be involved in Ewing sarcoma, inhibition of the MAPK pathway does block oncogenic transformation mediated by EWS/FLI in the NIH3T3 model.[305] This finding was not replicated in Ewing sarcoma cells, thus raising the question as to whether this is an NIH3T3-specific pathway.

Many members of the Wnt signaling pathway are expressed in Ewing sarcoma, including soluble Wnt ligands, Wnt receptors (frizzled), and Wnt coreceptors (LRP5/6).[308] Additionally, microarray analysis of EWS/FLI target genes has demonstrated downregulation of the Wnt inhibitor DKK1 and upregulation of various Wnt signaling components.[155,207,221] These data suggest that Wnt signaling occurs in Ewing sarcoma. In contrast, analysis of the pathway in Ewing sarcoma cell lines in tissue culture has not demonstrated evidence of active Wnt autocrine signaling.[207,308] If the pathway is involved in Ewing sarcoma, it seems likely that it is important for processes such as migration and metastasis, rather than proliferation and transformation.[308] Current studies have not addressed this possibility.

Finally, genes involved in chromosomal stability or chromatin remodeling have also been implicated in Ewing sarcoma. For example, the STAG2 protein helps regulate chromosomal separation during mitosis and was found to be deleted in a number of human tumor types, including Ewing sarcoma.[309] It was suggested that this may be a mechanism of chromosomal instability in Ewing sarcoma and other tumors.[309] Deletion of *SMARCB1* (encoding the SMARCB1/INI1/SNF5 protein) was found in approximately 10% of Ewing sarcoma cases.[81] SMARCB1 is a member of the SWI/SNF chromosome remodeling complex whose deletion is tightly associated with atypical teratoid/rhabdoid tumor.[310] Whether SMARCB1-deleted Ewing sarcoma tumors represent a unique subset of Ewing sarcoma or instead indicate that alterations in chromatin remodeling complexes are widespread in Ewing sarcoma is currently unknown. Interestingly, a newly identified chromosomal rearrangement, t(4;22)(q31;q12), encodes an EWS/SMARCA5 fusion protein in tumors that appear consistent with Ewing sarcoma, supporting the idea that alterations in this chromatin remodeling complex may indeed be widespread in this disease.[311] Another possibility is that the EWS/SMARCA5 fusions are found in tumors that are similar, but not identical, to Ewing sarcoma.[173] Indeed, the most recent World Health Organization guidelines have named these (and other non-TET/ETS translocation-bearing tumors that have similar appearance to Ewing sarcoma; see Table 61-1) as *Ewing-like sarcomas*.[312]

Apoptotic Pathways in Ewing Sarcoma

As described previously, mutations in the p53 pathway are relatively common in Ewing sarcoma. These mutations likely confer resistance to the growth effects of TET/ETS fusions in the disease and may also protect against apoptosis.[208,313,314] Whereas p53 is an important mediator of apoptosis, other signaling pathways are involved as well. These other pathways have been evaluated in Ewing sarcoma in a number of studies.

Both Fas and the Fas ligand (FasL) are expressed in the majority of Ewing sarcomas.[315-317] The status of the FasL in Ewing sarcoma is somewhat controversial; one study reported soluble FasL in Ewing sarcoma–conditioned media,[317] whereas another study reported that the FasL is only found intracellularly and thus is not accessible to cell surface receptor.[315] In terms of the receptor, Fas at the cell surface can be functional, but Ewing sarcoma cells can be divided into Fas-sensitive, Fas-inducible, and Fas-resistant groups.[315] Fas-sensitive lines are killed by coincubation with a FasL-expressing effector cell.[315] Fas-inducible lines are killed by this effector cell line only after pretreatment with interferon-γ (IFN-γ) or cycloheximide (or both).[315] The Fas-resistant lines were resistant regardless of pretreatment.[315] The differences between sensitive and resistant cells are not completely known but may involve differences in Fas expression or expression of proapoptotic or antiapoptotic mediators, such as BAD and BAR.[315,318] Strategies to improve Fas-mediated killing of Ewing sarcoma cells have been investigated, such as allowing for accumulation of more FasL through the use of metalloproteinase inhibitors[319] and upregulation of Fas by administration of interleukin-12.[320,321]

In addition to Fas/FasL, evaluations of tumor necrosis factor–related apoptosis-inducing ligand and tumor necrosis factor α as inducers of Ewing sarcoma apoptosis have also been conducted, in vitro and in vivo, alone and in combination with other agents.[322-333] Taken together, these data support a potential use of proapoptotic ligands in the treatment of Ewing sarcoma. However, the variability of the effects seen demonstrate the need for an ongoing mechanistic evaluation of these pathways in this disease.

Biological Features Summary

The identification of t(11;22)(q24;q12) and subsequent cloning of the EWS/FLI fusion protein represented a major advance in the understanding of the pathogenesis of Ewing sarcoma. EWS/FLI appears to function primarily as an aberrant transcription factor to dysregulate gene targets involved in the development of this disease. Multiple gene targets and cooperating molecular pathways have been identified. These represent a wide array of functions, including growth factor signaling, survival and apoptosis pathways, angiogenesis, cellular immortalization, and cellular differentiation. Despite these myriad molecular functions, a unified mechanistic understanding of Ewing sarcoma development has not yet been reached. Similarly, the cell of origin of the disease has not yet been clearly identified. Nonetheless, there is great hope that a detailed understanding of the molecular mechanisms involved in Ewing sarcoma development will lead to new diagnostic, prognostic, and therapeutic approaches for this disease.

CLINICAL PRESENTATION AND DIAGNOSIS

Clinical Presentation

The most common presenting symptoms of Ewing sarcoma are pain, a palpable mass, or both. In one series 89% of patients with Ewing sarcoma reported pain at the time of initial presentation.[334] Pain does not necessarily occur at night; this pattern was reported in only 19% of patients in one series.[334] Patients may report that their pain began at the same time as a minor musculoskeletal injury. This presentation, reported in approximately 25% of patients, may delay the diagnosis.[334] Unlike patients with osteosarcoma, patients with Ewing sarcoma may report constitutional symptoms such as fever and weight loss. Approximately 15% to 20% of patients have fever at presentation.[335-337] Other symptoms depend on the site of disease. For example, 40% to 94% of patients with paraspinal tumors have presenting symptoms of spinal cord compression.[338-341] Patients with large pelvic tumors may complain of an alteration in voiding. Extensive bone marrow metastatic disease may cause symptoms related to anemia, thrombocytopenia, or neutropenia. Patients may have symptoms for many weeks or months before seeing a physician for evaluation, with most studies reporting an average time from symptom onset to diagnosis of 3 to 5 months.[342-344]

Ewing sarcoma can arise from any bone but has a predilection for pelvic bones and long bones of the leg. Approximately 45% of Ewing sarcomas develop in the axial skeleton. More than half of these axial tumors arise from pelvic bones, and a quarter of axial tumors arise from a rib.[4,5] Up to 30% of Ewing sarcomas arise from long bones in the leg, and up to 15% of tumors develop in long bones in the arm.[4,5] Tumors of the hands, feet, and head develop only rarely, accounting for 10% or fewer of all tumors.[4,5] The distribution of primary tumor site does not vary among racial groups.[10] Soft tissue tumors may arise in any location, although axial sites predominate.[345,346]

Laboratory studies in patients with newly diagnosed Ewing sarcoma may reveal nonspecific abnormalities. More than a third of patients have an elevated erythrocyte sedimentation rate (ESR) at the time of diagnosis.[337,347] Similarly, serum lactate dehydrogenase (LDH) levels are elevated in approximately one third of patients.[336,347-349] Laboratory manifestations of tumor lysis syndrome are uncommon with these tumors. Unlike osteosarcoma, alkaline phosphatase is not typically elevated in patients with Ewing sarcoma of the bone. Patients with advanced bone marrow metastatic disease may have anemia, thrombocytopenia, and neutropenia detected on a complete blood count. In one large series 12% of patients had anemia even in the absence of metastatic disease.[336]

Box 61-1 summarizes the differential diagnosis of Ewing sarcoma. In most cases of Ewing sarcoma of the bone, the main alternative diagnosis is osteosarcoma.

Box 61-1   Clinical Differential Diagnosis of Ewing Sarcoma

EWING SARCOMA OF BONE

Osteosarcoma
Primary bone lymphoma
Ewing-like sarcoma
Langerhans cell histiocytosis
Osteomyelitis
Metastasis of an extraosseous malignancy
Benign bone tumor
Osteoblastoma
Chondrosarcoma
Giant cell tumor of the bone

EWING SARCOMA OF SOFT TISSUE

Rhabdomyosarcoma
Nonrhabdomyosarcoma soft tissue sarcoma
Lymphoma
Benign soft tissue tumor
Ewing-like sarcoma
Neuroblastoma
Malignant germ cell tumor

Table 61-2 displays features that may help differentiate Ewing sarcoma of the bone from osteosarcoma. Compared with osteosarcoma, Ewing sarcoma is more likely to occur in the axial skeleton. Those Ewing tumors that arise in long bones have a greater tendency to occur in the diaphysis, compared with the tendency of osteosarcoma to arise in the metaphysis of long bones.[350] Patients with Ewing sarcoma are more likely to report constitutional symptoms than are patients with osteosarcoma. Other malignant tumors in the differential diagnosis of Ewing sarcoma of the bone include primary bone lymphoma, giant cell tumor of the bone, and bone metastasis of an extraosseous malignancy. The differential diagnosis of Ewing sarcoma arising from the soft tissues is more broad because the site of origin for these tumors is not restricted to the bone. The site of origin may help narrow the differential diagnosis. Paraspinal tumors may be confused with neuroblastoma, particularly in younger patients. Pelvic tumors may suggest rhabdomyosarcoma or malignant germ cell tumor. Lymphoma and other soft tissue sarcomas can arise at any site and should be included in the differential diagnosis.

Reports from several cooperative group studies have defined the metastatic behavior of Ewing sarcoma. Approximately 25% of patients exhibit distant metastases at presentation.[351,352] Rates of metastatic disease do not appear to differ between patients with skeletal tumors and those with soft tissue primary tumors.[346] Patients with pelvic primary tumors have an increased incidence of metastatic disease at initial diagnosis.[353] The lung is the most common metastatic site, with pulmonary dissemination reported in 50% to 60% of patients with metastatic disease.[354,355] Patients with isolated pulmonary metastasis represent between 26% and 36% of cases of metastatic disease.[354,356] Patients usually have multiple lung nodules identified in both lungs.[351]

The bone is the next most common metastatic site at presentation. One group reported cortical bone metastases in 43% of patients with metastatic disease.[355] A large

TABLE 61-2   Clinical Differentiation of Ewing Sarcoma of Bone from Osteosarcoma

	Ewing Sarcoma	Osteosarcoma
Age distribution	Peak in adolescence Occurs in young children Very rare in adults >40 years	Peak in adolescence Very rare in children <5 years Occurs in older adults
Racial distribution	Rare in patients of African or East Asian ancestry	No racial predilection
Predisposing factors	Not associated with radiation No known familial predisposition	Radiation exposure Li-Fraumeni syndrome History of retinoblastoma
Constitutional symptoms	Yes	No
Involved bones	Both flat and long bones	Long bones more common
Location in long bones	Diaphyseal more common	Epiphyseal/metaphyseal more common
Type of periosteal reaction	Laminated/layered "Onion-skinning"	Spiculated "sunburst"
Laboratory findings	Normal alkaline phosphatase Abnormal CBC if marrow disease	Elevated alkaline phosphatase Normal CBC
Histologic findings	Small round blue cells No malignant osteoid	Malignant spindle cells Malignant osteoid

CBC, Complete blood count.

cooperative group reported that the bone marrow is involved in approximately 19% of metastatic patients at initial diagnosis.[355] A smaller series noted bone marrow involvement in 52% of patients with metastatic disease.[357] This group performed up to 10 bone marrow aspirates on patients at initial presentation, suggesting that routine sampling may underestimate the incidence of bone marrow involvement. Brain metastasis at initial diagnosis appears to be extremely uncommon. In two series of patients with brain metastasis from Ewing sarcoma, all cases were reported at the time of disease recurrence and not at initial presentation.[358,359]

Fewer than 10% of patients have lymph node involvement at initial diagnosis.[360] The incidence of node involvement is higher in patients with soft tissue rather than bone primary tumors.[355,360,361] In one population-based study, the incidence of regional node involvement among patients with soft tissue tumors was 12.4% compared with 3.2% in patients with bone primary tumors.[360] The incidence of regional node involvement is also higher among patients with distant metastatic disease.[360]

This metastatic pattern helps determine the appropriate staging evaluation for patients with Ewing sarcoma (Box 61-2). In addition to computed tomography (CT)

or magnetic resonance imaging (MRI) scans of the primary tumor, all newly diagnosed patients should be evaluated with a chest CT scan. Assessment for bone metastasis has conventionally been with radiolabeled-technetium bone scan. More recent data indicate that positron emission tomography (PET) scans are superior for this indication (discussed later), prompting wider adoption of PET imaging at initial diagnosis.[362] At least bilateral bone marrow aspirates and biopsies should routinely be performed in newly diagnosed patients, with biopsy more sensitive for detection of marrow involvement compared with aspirate.[363] Attention to regional nodes on imaging studies is particularly warranted in patients with soft tissue primary tumors. These evaluations will indicate whether a patient has metastatic or nonmetastatic Ewing sarcoma at initial diagnosis. This distinction serves as the main staging classification in practice for these patients. Although a staging classification for musculoskeletal tumors has been devised by Enneking, this system is not routinely used in the clinical care of patients with Ewing sarcoma.[364]

Imaging Features

Most patients with Ewing sarcoma of the bone are initially evaluated with a plain radiograph. Two representative radiographs are shown in Figure 61-5. These tumors typically appear as poorly circumscribed lesions arising from the bone, but with an associated soft tissue mass.[350] Both lytic and sclerotic areas may be seen within the bony component of the tumor. Given the aggressive nature of these tumors, periosteal reaction is commonly observed. A layered or laminated periosteal reaction is most typical, often giving an onion-skin appearance (see Fig. 61-5, A).[350,365] A spiculated "sunburst" periosteal reaction is more commonly associated with osteosarcoma but may be occasionally observed in Ewing sarcoma (see Fig. 61-5, B).[350] Codman triangle, a triangular area forming under the periosteum in the setting of a rapidly growing bone lesion, may also be seen in some cases. Cortical thickening is present in approximately 20% of tumors.[350] Pathologic fractures occur in 15% of patients with Ewing sarcoma of bone.[337,350,366]

CT scans and MRI scans are used to better define the extent of local tumor in patients with both osseous and

---

Box 61-2   Recommended Evaluations for Newly Diagnosed Patients with Ewing Sarcoma

ASSESSMENT OF PRIMARY TUMOR

Magnetic resonance imaging (MRI) scan and/or
Computed tomography (CT) scan

EVALUATION FOR METASTATIC DISEASE

CT scan of the chest
Whole body fluorodeoxyglucose positron emission tomography scan or radiolabeled-technecium bone scan
Bone marrow aspirate and biopsy

EVALUATION BEFORE INITIATING CHEMOTHERAPY

Echocardiogram
Serum creatinine (with formal creatinine clearance if renal function in question)

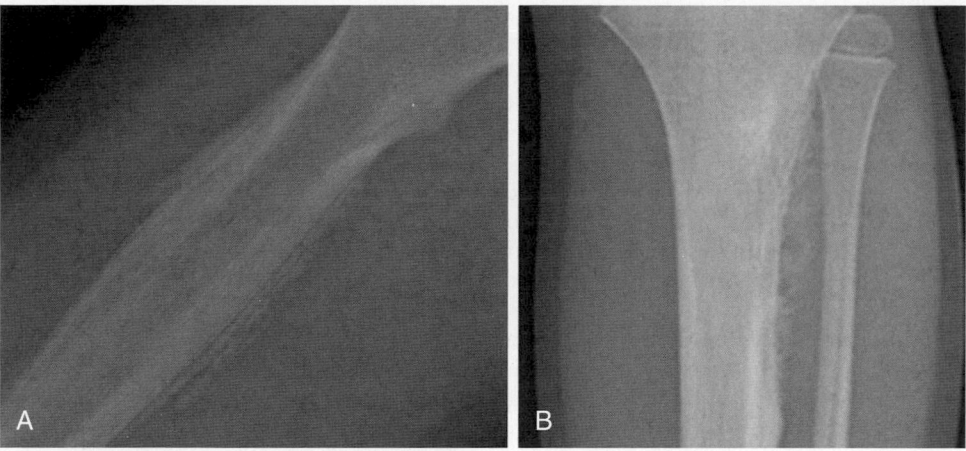

Figure 61-5 **A**, Plain radiograph of a femoral Ewing sarcoma demonstrating a laminated periosteal reaction, resulting in an "onion-skin" appearance. **B**, Plain radiograph of a tibial Ewing sarcoma with a spiculated periosteal reaction.

extraosseous tumors. CT scans most commonly demonstrate a heterogeneous mass with heterogeneous contrast enhancement.[367-371] The soft tissue component generally has lower attenuation than muscle on non-enhanced CT scans.[367,369,372] MRI scans typically reveal a mass that is heterogeneous with respect to both signal intensity and gadolinium contrast enhancement.[370,371,373] Typically T1- and T2-weighted MRI scans demonstrate areas of increased signal intensity of the soft tissue component compared with skeletal muscle.[367,370,371] Although both CT and MRI are able to delineate the soft tissue component of the tumor, MRI may be better able to determine the extent of bone marrow extension and the degree of growth plate involvement.[374]

Emerging evidence suggests that fluorodeoxyglucose PET (FDG-PET) may play an increasing role in the management of patients with Ewing sarcoma. In one series all 32 patients with Ewing sarcoma evaluated by FDG-PET imaging before initiation of chemotherapy had FDG-avid tumors.[375] Figure 61-6 demonstrates an FDG-PET scan of a patient with widely metastatic Ewing sarcoma at initial presentation. A group of studies has evaluated the role of FDG-PET imaging in screening for metastatic disease and for disease recurrence. Several groups have demonstrated that FDG-PET imaging has superior sensitivity and specificity compared with conventional bone scans for detecting bone metastases in patients with Ewing sarcoma.[376-378] In contrast, FDG-PET appears to be inferior to spiral CT scans in screening for pulmonary metastases in these patients.[379] In screening patients with Ewing sarcoma for overall disease recurrence at any site, FDG-PET imaging may have lower sensitivity but higher specificity compared with conventional imaging.[380] Finally, one group has reported that a decrease in FDG-avidity in response to neoadjuvant chemotherapy correlates with improved progression-free survival.[375]

Pathologic Diagnosis

Once imaging studies have localized the tumor, diagnostic tissue must be obtained. The current pathologic diagnosis of Ewing sarcoma depends on tumor morphology, immunohistochemistry findings, and demonstration of a Ewing sarcoma–specific translocation (by standard cytogenetics, fluorescence in situ hybridization [FISH], or reverse transcriptase polymerase chain reaction assays [RT-PCR]).[381] In planning for biopsy, the physician must ensure that adequate tissue will be available to perform each of these tests. For example, one series reported successful cytogenetic analysis in only 59% of fine needle aspirations performed for Ewing sarcoma.[382] The biopsy should be planned with an eye toward ultimate local control of the tumor. If surgical resection is ultimately planned, the biopsy tract should be included in the resected specimen.[383]

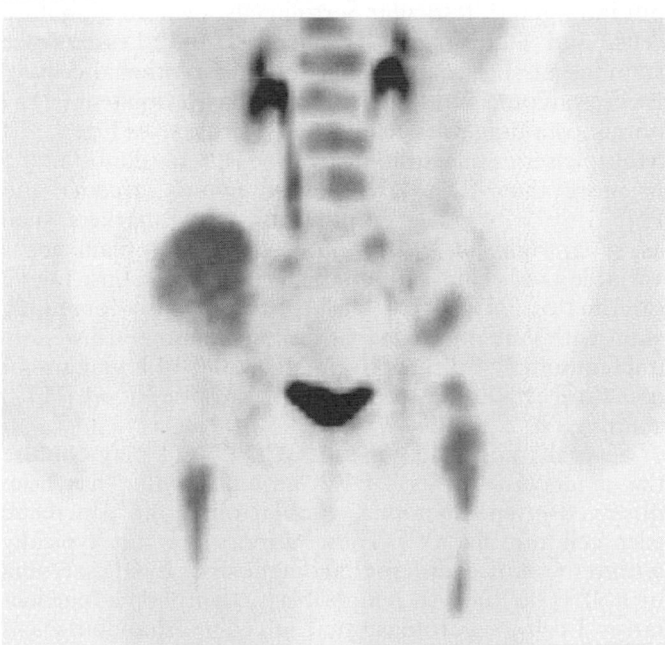

Figure 61-6 Whole-body fluorodeoxyglucose positron emission tomography (FDG-PET) scan of a patient with widely metastatic Ewing sarcoma at initial diagnosis. FDG uptake is evident in bones, soft tissue, and bone marrow.

Ewing sarcoma and PNET form a morphologic continuum ranging from tumors with no apparent neural differentiation to tumors with evidence of early neural differentiation. Of note, the histologic classification of these tumors does not imply site of origin because tumors with either histology may arise in the bone or soft tissue. Ewing sarcoma appears as relatively monomorphic small round blue-staining cells with scant cytoplasm (Fig. 61-7).[384,385] The nuclei tend to be round without prominent nucleoli.[384,385] These cells demonstrate positive periodic acid–Schiff staining owing to cytoplasmic glycogen.[381,385] Electron microscopy may reveal these glycogen stores.[381,385] The tumor cells grow in sheets without additional structure.[384-386] A large cell or atypical Ewing sarcoma subset has been described with large irregular nuclei and more conspicuous nucleoli.[384-386] As many as 30% of tumors with Ewing sarcoma histology arise in soft tissues rather than bone.[384,386] PNETs typically display primitive Homer Wright pseudorosette formation.[384,386] Electron microscopy may reveal additional features suggestive of neural differentiation, such as neurosecretory granules.[381,385,387] Tumors without pseudorosette formation may also be classified as PNETs if they express two or more neural markers (discussed later).[386] Approximately 50% of tumors with PNET histology arise in bone.[384,386] Despite these morphologic differences, Ewing sarcoma and PNET are now viewed as the same biological entity.

Immunohistochemistry plays a key role in differentiating Ewing sarcoma and PNET from other small round cell tumors of children and young adults. The most useful antigen in the diagnosis of Ewing sarcoma appears to be CD99. This protein product of the *MIC2* gene is expressed in a limited number of normal tissues, including strong staining of ependymal cells, pancreatic islet cells, anterior pituitary gland, testicular Sertoli cells, ovarian granulosa cells, and maturing T lymphocytes.[261,388] Less intense staining has been noted in scattered endothelial cells.[261] Ewing sarcoma and PNET both display prominent CD99 immunostaining in a membranous pattern (see Fig. 61-7). Multiple series have found strong CD99 immunostaining in more than 90% of cases of Ewing sarcoma and PNET.[261-263,268,269,388-391] Staining for neural markers, such as synaptophysin, S-100, NSE, and neurofilament, is variable and helps to characterize tumors as Ewing sarcoma or PNET.[381,384-386] These tumors also commonly stain with vimentin, whereas desmin staining is distinctly uncommon.[384,386,392] Approximately 30% of Ewing sarcomas and PNETs demonstrate diffuse c-kit (CD117) staining.[393-395]

Several tumors also express CD99 and may confuse the diagnosis. Strong CD99 immunostaining has been observed in ependymoma, glioblastoma, and pancreatic islet cell tumors.[261,388] These tumors are not typically within the clinical differential diagnosis of Ewing sarcoma or PNET. In contrast, lymphoblastic lymphoma (particularly T-cell), neuroblastoma, alveolar rhabdomyosarcoma, synovial sarcoma, and desmoplastic small round cell tumor may demonstrate variable levels of CD99 staining and are frequently considered in the differential diagnosis of these tumors.[261,392,396-400] Whereas both Ewing

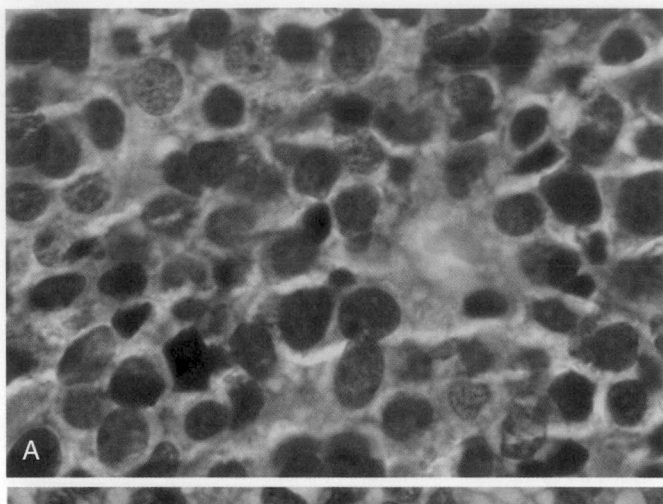
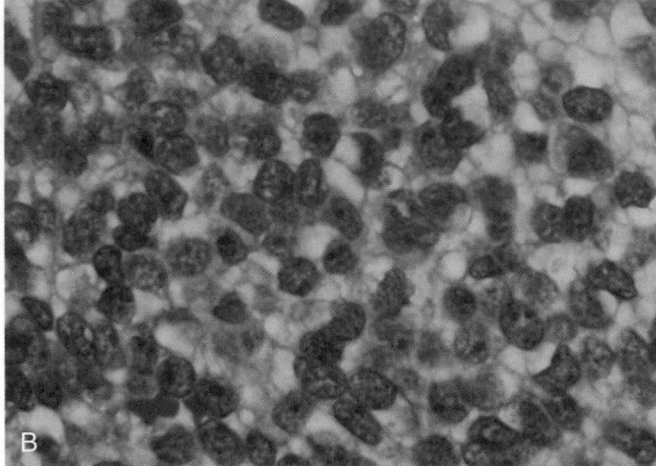
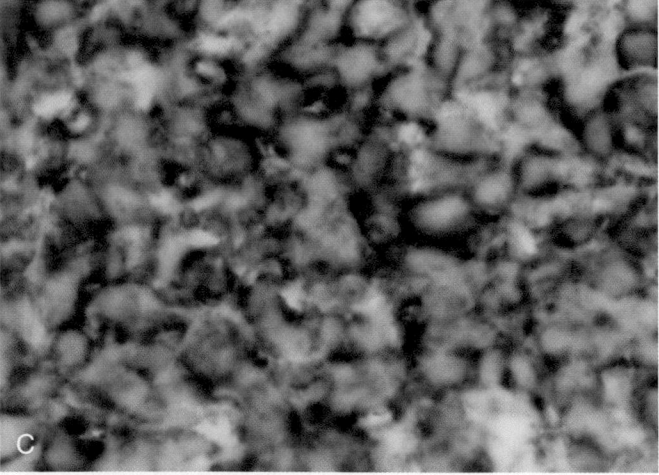

Figure 61-7 A, Characteristic morphology of Ewing sarcoma with monomorphic small round blue cells without pseudorosette formation. B, Morphologic features of a primitive neuroectodermal tumor (PNET), including a pseudorosette formation in the center of the panel. C, The characteristic strong membranous CD99 immunohistochemical staining of Ewing sarcoma. *(Courtesy Dr. Antonio Perez-Atayde, Department of Pathology, Children's Hospital, Boston, Mass.)*

sarcoma and lymphoblastic lymphoma may demonstrate strong CD99 staining, Ewing sarcoma and PNET should be negative for lymphocyte markers, particularly leukocyte common antigen and terminal deoxynucleotidyl transferase.[386,392,398] Ewing sarcoma and PNET are also more likely to demonstrate strong vimentin staining compared with lymphoblastic lymphoma.[392] The immunohistochemical differentiation of Ewing sarcoma and PNET from neuroblastoma is typically more straight-forward largely because CD99 staining in neuroblastoma, if present, is weak and patchy.[261,397] Neuroblastomas commonly demonstrate strong staining with NSE, whereas Ewing sarcoma and PNET occasionally will show weak to moderate NSE staining.[263,397] Poorly differentiated synovial sarcoma and desmoplastic small round cell tumor may both also demonstrate CD99 staining and morphologically be difficult to differentiate from Ewing sarcoma and PNET.[396,399,400] In both cases strong membranous staining is more consistent with Ewing sarcoma and PNET. In contrast, weak staining for CD99 and strong staining for cytokeratin and epithelial membrane antigen suggest synovial sarcoma.[396,399] Desmoplastic small round cell tumors reliably demonstrate nuclear staining for WT1, whereas Ewing sarcoma and PNET typically do not stain with WT1.[400] Nuclear staining for FLI1 may also help differentiate these tumors from other pediatric CD99 small round cell tumors. Most cases of Ewing sarcoma and PNET demonstrate nuclear FLI1 staining, whereas synovial sarcoma, neuroblastoma, and rhabdomyosarcoma only rarely show positive nuclear FLI1 staining.[384,401,402] Significantly, however, a high proportion of lymphoblastic lymphomas also exhibit nuclear FLI1 staining.[401] Finally, a number of small round cell tumors of bone harboring novel translocations have been described (see Table 61-1). These have recently been classified as Ewinglike sarcomas.[312] As an example, a BCOR/CCNB3-containing tumor has recently been described. This entity has a gene expression profile that is distinct from that of Ewing sarcoma, demonstrates membranous CD99 positivity in only a minority of cases, and can be identified by intense immunohistochemical staining for CCNB3.[403]

The combination of characteristic morphology and immunohistochemistry typically allows an experienced pathologist to render the diagnosis of Ewing sarcoma or PNET. The identification of recurrent chromosomal translocations and their associated oncoproteins in these tumors has allowed for the incorporation of molecular testing into their diagnosis. These methods play a role as confirmatory tests in the setting of typical morphology and immunohistochemistry. In more unusual cases these molecular tests may serve as the key feature on which the diagnosis is based. Although these molecular approaches have been very effective, it is worth recognizing their strengths and weaknesses when interpreting diagnostic studies.

Karyotypic analysis is one approach to confirming the diagnosis of Ewing sarcoma. The presence of one of the characteristic translocations can be considered strong supportive evidence for the diagnosis.[66-68,404,405] It is important to recognize that false-negative results may occur from a number of sources, including overgrowth of nonmalignant elements during culture, complex translocations in which the characteristic Ewing-associated rearrangement is partially masked by the presence of an additional fusion partner,[68,406-408] and cryptic rearrangements in which the translocation cannot be identified using typical techniques.[407,409] FISH can be very helpful as a complementary technique to demonstrate that the EWSR1 locus is "split," which suggests a translocation event.[407,410-414] FISH for the FLI1 and/or ERG loci that demonstrates a split signal from either of these genes or fusion between EWSR1 and FLI1 or ERG signals provides additional strong evidence for involvement of these genes in the rearrangement.[407,410-414] A false-negative FISH result may occur when the fusion involves a rarer translocation partner, such as TLS (in lieu of EWS) or ETV1, ETV4, or FEV (in lieu of FLI or ERG).[169-172,175] These rare translocations are not typically included in the molecular diagnostic evaluation of these tumors.

A positive EWSR1 "split" FISH assay is not specific for the diagnosis of Ewing sarcoma because of the presence of EWSR1 rearrangements in tumor types other than Ewing sarcoma (see Table 61-1). For example, clear cell sarcoma (also called malignant melanoma of the soft parts) usually harbors a t(12;22)(q13;q12) rearrangement.[415] This translocation fuses EWS to the ATF1 protein to form the EWS/ATF1 protein.[415] Similarly, desmoplastic small round cell tumor harbors a t(11;22)(p13;q12) rearrangement.[416] This fuses the EWS protein to the Wilms tumor suppressor WT1 to form the EWS/WT1 protein.[416] EWS or TAF15 can join the NR4A3 orphan nuclear receptor to form EWS/NR4A3 and TAF15/NR4A3 fusion proteins in extraskeletal myxoid chondrosarcoma.[107,417-420] EWS is occasionally fused to DDIT3 (also called CHOP) to form EWS/DDIT3 in t(12;22)(q13;q12) positive myxoid liposarcoma.[421] An EWS/ZNF278 fusion was identified in a small round cell sarcoma as a result of a t(1;22)(p36;q12) rearrangement.[422] In some cases there may be diagnostic confusion between some of these tumor types and Ewing sarcoma, and thus the presence of a rearranged EWSR1 locus may not be adequate for diagnostic purposes. In rare instances tumors may show biphenotypic differentiation with both neural and myogenic patterns. At least some of these express EWS rearrangements (EWS/FLI or EWS/ERG fusions) as well as the classic PAX3/FKHR fusion protein associated with alveolar rhabdomyosarcoma.[423-425]

The use of RT-PCR may provide greater specificity in the diagnosis of Ewing sarcoma. RT-PCR is a useful method for detection of EWS/ETS fusions.[414,426-428] As with any PCR-based method, false-positive results may occur from contamination. False-negative results may occur because of degradation of the RNA, alternate fusion partners, or because an RT-PCR primer pair may be designed to detect some EWS/FLI transcripts but not others.[426-428] False-negative results may also occur when biopsies do not capture viable tissue or primarily include nonmalignant elements. Despite their shortcomings, molecular techniques have become an important addition to the diagnostic approach for Ewing sarcoma.

PROGNOSTIC FACTORS

A number of clinical and molecular features have been identified as prognostic variables in patients with Ewing sarcoma. The presence of metastatic disease at initial diagnosis is widely regarded as the most important adverse clinical prognostic feature. In the largest analysis of prognostic features in this disease, patients with metastatic disease at presentation had a 5-year relapse-free survival rate of 21% compared with 55% for nonmetastatic patients.[353] Patients in this analysis received therapy according to several sequential treatment protocols. Patients with metastatic disease treated in the North American study INT-0091 had a similar 5-year event-free survival rate of 22% regardless of their chemotherapy regimen.[352] Patients with isolated lung metastases have a better outcome than patients with dissemination to other sites or with dissemination to lungs plus other sites.[351,353,356,429] Within this group of patients, patients with unilateral lung metastases may fare better than patients with bilateral lung metastases.[351] Dissemination to regional lymph node is also an adverse prognostic factor, even among patients with otherwise localized disease.[360]

Tumor size has long been recognized as a predictor of outcome in patients with Ewing sarcoma. Patients with larger tumors are at increased risk for having metastatic disease at initial diagnosis. For example, a pooled analysis of German patients treated in the European Intergroup Cooperative Ewing's Sarcoma Study (EICESS) and Cooperative Ewing's Sarcoma Study (CESS) indicated that tumor volume greater than 100 mL was an independent predictor of metastatic disease at initial diagnosis.[430] The effect of tumor size on outcome does not depend entirely on this increased risk of metastatic disease, however. Tumor size appears to be prognostic even among patients with initially nonmetastatic tumors. The CESS-81 study demonstrated that tumor volume greater than 100 mL was a significant adverse prognostic factor for patients treated with either surgery or radiation.[431] The follow-up CESS-86 study found that tumor volume greater than 200 mL was a major adverse prognostic feature for patients with localized Ewing sarcoma.[432,433] The North American INT-0091 study reported that nonmetastatic patients with tumors greater than 8 cm in maximal dimension had an inferior outcome compared with patients with smaller tumors.[352] The French EW88 study reported that tumor size, using either tumor volume or longest dimension, was prognostic only among patients who received radiotherapy alone as the mode of local control.[347] Although some smaller studies have not observed this effect of tumor size on outcome,[434] most investigators consider tumor size prognostic. Indeed, a large pooled analyses of prognostic factors in Ewing sarcoma identified large tumor volume as an independent predictor of poor outcome.[353]

Tumor site is also widely considered a prognostic factor in Ewing sarcoma, with axial tumors carrying a worse prognosis. The Intergroup Ewing Sarcoma Study 1 (IESS-1) established pelvic site as an unfavorable prognostic feature.[435] Several other cooperative group studies have confirmed this finding and indicated that patients with axial tumors generally have a worse outcome compared with patients with nonaxial tumors.[343,352,436,437] In many of these studies, patients with pelvic primary tumors have been shown to have a particularly poor outcome compared with patients with other axial locations.[343,352,436] However, the inferior outcomes in patients with pelvic tumors may be confounded by a higher incidence of both large tumor size and metastatic disease.[353,430] For example, in the CESS-86 trial, axial tumor location was a significant adverse prognostic feature on univariate analysis.[433] After controlling for tumor size and chemotherapy response, however, the prognostic impact of axial site became insignificant. Several groups evaluated only patients with nonmetastatic tumors and found that patients with pelvic tumors still had an inferior outcome compared with patients with nonpelvic tumors.[352,435,436] Two other groups used multivariate methods to evaluate the prognostic impact of axial tumor location in nonmetastatic patients.[336,353] Both groups reported that axial tumors have an inferior outcome compared with extremity tumors, even after controlling for potential confounders. Neither analysis controlled for tumor size, however. Therefore whether axial tumor location portends poor outcome independent of large tumor size remains unclear.

The prognostic impact of soft tissue rather than bone primary tumor origin remains unclear. In one population-based study, soft tissue origin was independently associated with improved outcomes compared with bone origin.[346] In contrast, a cooperative group clinical trial that included both patients with soft tissue and bone tumors showed equivalent outcomes.[438] As more trials include patients with soft tissue tumors, the prognostic impact of tumor origin will become clearer.

A number of groups have specifically evaluated histologic response to neoadjuvant chemotherapy as a predictor of outcome. Patients with a favorable chemotherapy response (typically 90% to 100% tumor necrosis depending on the grading scale used) at the time of surgery have been found to have a decreased risk of disease recurrence compared with patients who exhibited less necrosis.[255,347,431,433,439-442] For patients with nonmetastatic tumors of the extremity, chemotherapy response is prognostic independent of age and tumor size.[440] Despite these results, grading of chemotherapy response in Ewing sarcoma has not yet become routine practice, perhaps at least in part because this variable is not evaluable in those patients who receive definitive radiotherapy as their mode of local control. An alternative to histologic grading is radiographic grading of chemotherapy response. Two groups have reported that favorable radiographic response to chemotherapy is a predictor of favorable outcome.[433,437,439] Evaluation of radiographic response may also not be possible in all patients, particularly in patients with tumors confined to bone without an associated soft tissue mass.

Age at initial diagnosis has been increasingly recognized as an important prognostic feature in Ewing sarcoma. Several studies have indicated that younger patients have an improved outcome compared with older patients.[336,348,352,353,434,435] Older patients have an increased risk of presenting with large tumors, but interestingly they do not have a higher incidence of metastatic disease at initial diagnosis.[430] Even controlling for these potential confounders, age has been identified as an independent predictor of outcome in a number of studies.[336,348,436]

Most studies have used a single cut-point in the 12- to 15-year age range. One study divided patients into three groups (younger than 10 years, 10 to 17 years, and 18 years or older) and found that nonmetastatic patients 18 years of age or older at initial diagnosis had a particularly poor outcome (44% 5-year event-free survival rate).[352] A number of studies have focused on outcomes in older adolescents and adults with Ewing sarcoma. These studies have typically identified the same adverse prognostic features (metastatic disease, large size, axial location, and poor chemotherapy response) in older patients that have been identified in larger studies in patients at a wide range of ages.[443-446] The mechanism underlying these differences in outcome with age remains unclear. Possible explanations include biological differences in tumor and host as well as health care delivery differences in compliance and dose intensity. For example, at least two reports have noted higher rates of soft tissue tumors in adults older than 40 years of age at initial diagnosis, which suggests biological differences in this disease when it arises in older patients. Another series noted lower treatment intensity and inferior outcomes in older patients,[447,448] whereas another series reported similar treatment intensity and outcomes in older patients.[448,449] These results highlight the importance of optimizing treatment intensity to maximize outcomes in adults with this disease.

Serum LDH at initial diagnosis also appears to be prognostic. Several early studies reported that patients with elevated serum LDH levels at diagnosis had an increased risk of disease recurrence.[450-452] More recent studies have confirmed this finding and have found that the negative prognostic impact of an elevated LDH remains even after controlling for other possible confounding variables.[336,348,453] A meta-analysis evaluating a range of tumor markers in Ewing sarcoma also concluded that elevated LDH at diagnosis is associated with inferior outcomes.[454] Presumably, elevated LDH levels indicate greater tumor cell turnover and therefore more aggressive clinical behavior.

A variety of other clinical and demographic features at diagnosis have been variably reported to be prognostic in Ewing sarcoma. Two groups have reported that female sex is an independent predictor of favorable outcome.[336,348] Other groups have not corroborated this finding.[352,353,432] Other studies have demonstrated superior outcomes among the U.S. white, non-Hispanic population compared with members of other racial and ethnic groups.[12,455,456] A greater degree of neural differentiation has been reported as an unfavorable marker by some groups but not by others.* Fever, anemia, leukocytosis, elevated erythrocyte sedimentation rate, and hypoalbuminemia at initial diagnosis have also been suggested as unfavorable prognostic features, but their prognostic value has not yet been validated.[336,347,453,462]

The nature of the Ewing sarcoma–specific translocation does not appear to provide prognostic information. One group has demonstrated that patients with any type of EWS/FLI translocation have similar outcomes to

patients with any type of EWS/ERG translocation.[463] Previous studies suggested that patients with a type 1 EWS/FLI translocation had better outcomes compared with other types of EWS/FLI or EWS/ERG translocations.[179] However, two large cooperative group trials both demonstrated that translocation subtype does not affect survival in the setting of modern therapy.[183,184]

Several studies have measured EWS/FLI fusion transcripts in the peripheral blood or bone marrow to predict outcome. These studies use RT-PCR techniques to identify occult metastatic disease, with 25% of clinically nonmetastatic patients noted to have detectable EWS/FLI fusion transcripts in blood or bone marrow in one early study.[464] The results of studies correlating these findings to clinical outcome have been mixed. In one report patients with clinically localized disease but positive peripheral blood EWS/FLI RT-PCR at diagnosis had a higher risk of relapse compared with patients with negative peripheral blood EWS/FLI RT-PCR.[465] A second study evaluating bone marrow EWS/FLI RT-PCR at diagnosis was not able to confirm this finding.[466] Patients in this study had follow-up EWS/FLI RT-PCR performed on blood or bone marrow (or both). Patients with positive blood or bone marrow EWS/FLI RT-PCR at their last evaluation had a significantly increased risk of clinical disease recurrence.[466] The utility of this methodology for predicting outcome in patients with Ewing sarcoma will require further prospective evaluation.

Chromosomal changes beyond the characteristic TET/ETS translocations may also provide prognostic information. Although it is the most common additional karyotypic abnormality in Ewing sarcoma, at least three groups have reported that trisomy 8 does not appear to influence outcome.[467-469] A small series of 21 patients reported that all three patients with gain of chromosome 1q died as a result of disease.[470] Another study of 88 patients with complete cytogenetic data did not observe an association between 1q gain and poor outcome, although only 12 patients had 1q gain.[469] A larger study of 124 patients with Ewing sarcoma included 26 patients with gain of chromosome 1q and found that patients with gain of chromosome 1q have a worse outcome.[467] One study reported that more global karyotypic anomalies may also be prognostic, including complex karyotypes (more than five chromosomal anomalies) or hyperdiploidy (more than 50 chromosomes).[469]

Aberrations in p53 and p16 have also been correlated with outcome in patients with Ewing sarcoma. The 10% to 15% of patients with mutations in the TP53 gene (encoding the p53 protein) have consistently been shown to have a significantly worse outcome compared with patients who have wild-type TP53, even after controlling for other prognostic factors.[293,471] Additional work has suggested that mutations or deletions of the CDKN2A/INK4A gene may also confer a poor outcome in these patients.[292,293,472] For example, aberrant TP53 or CDKN2A/INK4A gene status in one study was shown to be an independent negative prognostic feature.[293] However, another study focused exclusively on CDKN2A/INK4A deletion failed to show an association with prognosis.[473] A formal meta-analysis of this issue concluded

---

*References 194, 263, 361, 385, 386, 433, 457-461.

that *CDKN2A/INK4A* aberration is a strong negative prognostic factor.[474]

A number of other molecular markers have been proposed to have prognostic impact in Ewing sarcoma. In one study telomerase activity in the peripheral blood during follow-up, but not at initial diagnosis, was strongly associated with disease recurrence.[255] None of the patients in this study with low telomerase activity during follow-up had disease recurrence. CD56 co-expression has been reported to be a favorable prognostic indicator in one series.[475] One report suggested that serum IGF-1R levels were prognostic,[476] although two other studies found no prognostic impact of IGF-1R levels.[477,478] Two studies identified expression of the genes encoding glutathione S-transferases, enzymes involved in chemotherapy metabolism, as novel prognostic factors.[165,479]

TREATMENT OF PATIENTS WITH NONMETASTATIC EWING SARCOMA

Local Control

Patients with nonmetastatic Ewing sarcoma require aggressive multimodality therapy to achieve long-term disease control. Local control of the primary tumor plays a key role in modern treatment for these patients. Historically, patients received radiation therapy alone as local control. Surgical local control was less commonly used because therapy was generally viewed as palliative. With improved outcomes thanks to chemotherapy, however, the late effects of radiotherapy on long-term survivors of Ewing sarcoma became apparent. In addition, limb-salvage surgical techniques became more advanced. As a result, surgical local control of resectable tumors has become the standard of care. Radiotherapy for local control of the primary tumor is now generally reserved for unresectable tumors or tumors that have been resected with inadequate margins. This section reviews the principles of radiotherapy and surgical resection in the care of patients with Ewing sarcoma.

Surgical resection is generally recommended for those tumors deemed completely resectable with wide or radical margins. For extremity tumors, surgical resection may take the form of an amputation or a limb-sparing procedure. Rotationplasty is another option for patients with femoral tumors.[383] Technical advances, such as expandable implanted prostheses, have made limb-sparing procedures increasingly appealing.[383,480] However, the choice of a limb-sparing procedure over other surgical options must not compromise the adequacy of the resection.[383] Tumor infiltration of surrounding neurovascular structures, muscle, or skin should raise concern that a limb-sparing procedure will not result in the desired wide resection.[383] Often neoadjuvant chemotherapy will produce sufficient response to allow for limb salvage when this option did not appear feasible at initial presentation.[383] In a cooperative group analysis of chest wall tumors, resection after neoadjuvant chemotherapy was associated with higher rates of negative margins compared to initial resection.[461] However, data from a single institution suggested that neither the likelihood of an adequate margin nor the overall outcome differs between patients who had surgical resection at initial diagnosis compared with patients who had surgical resection after a period of neoadjuvant chemotherapy.[482,483] Nevertheless, most available data support the current standard approach of neoadjuvant chemotherapy before planned surgical resection.

Investigators from the CESS group and the Rizzoli Institute evaluated the impact of surgical margins on outcome in Ewing sarcoma in two retrospective case series.[484,485] These groups both reported the rate of obtaining an adequate surgical margin as approximately 75%, among those patients selected for planned definitive resection.[484,485] Both groups observed that an adequate margin is more difficult to obtain in axial tumors. For example, the Rizzoli group reported that approximately one quarter of the extremity tumors treated with a limb-salvage procedure had inadequate margins. In contrast, none of the paraspinal or sacral tumors in their large series of surgically treated patients had an adequate margin.[484] The Rizzoli group observed that the 5-year event-free survival rate was higher for patients with an adequate surgical margin, although this finding may reflect improved outcome with smaller, more resectable tumors.[484] In both series a small group of patients with inadequate surgical margins did not receive postoperative radiotherapy. Only 14% to 21% of these patients experienced a local recurrence.[484,485] However, the risk of local recurrence was diminished by the addition of postoperative radiotherapy, which is the current standard practice.

Radiation therapy alone can provide adequate local control in Ewing sarcoma. In fact, the radiosensitivity of these tumors was one of the early characteristics that distinguished Ewing sarcoma from osteosarcoma.[1] Local control rates with definitive radiation therapy in large series have been reported to range from 53% to 86%.[486] For patients treated with radiation therapy alone, axial tumors (particularly pelvic tumors) have a higher rate of local failure than extremity tumors.[436,487-489] One group reported that patients with metastatic disease treated with radiation alone or surgery plus radiation have a higher rate of local failure compared with patients who have nonmetastatic disease.[490]

Several studies have evaluated the appropriate treatment volume, dose, timing, and schedule of radiotherapy in Ewing sarcoma. The IESS-1 study group reported on their experience with radiotherapy.[488] All patients received radiotherapy as the mode of local control in this study. Across the range of doses administered (30 Gy to more than 60 Gy), no differences in local failure rates were observed, although very few patients received less than 40 Gy. Most patients received radiation to the whole bone involved with tumor, but some patients were treated with more limited fields. Patients who received radiotherapy to the primary tumor plus a 5-cm margin had the same local failure rate as patients treated with whole bone radiotherapy (8% for both groups). Patients treated with less than a 5 cm margin had an inferior local control rate.

The Pediatric Oncology Group conducted a study from 1983 and 1988 with the specific aim of determining the appropriate radiation volume for patients with Ewing sarcoma of the bone.[487] Patients with tumors in expendable bones were recommended for surgical resection. Other patients were randomized to receive whole bone irradiation or involved field radiation. Patients treated with whole bone irradiation received 39.6 Gy to the entire bone containing tumor plus a boost to 55.8 Gy to the tumor with a 2-cm margin. Patients treated with involved field radiation received 55.8 Gy to the tumor with a 2-cm margin. Because of enrollment issues, 20 patients were randomized to whole bone radiation and 20 patients to involved field radiation. An additional 54 patients were nonrandomly assigned to involved field radiation. The 5-year event-free survival rate did not differ between patients randomized to whole bone radiation and patients randomized to involved field radiation (37% and 39%, respectively). The local control rate was 53% in both treatment arms. Of note, patients who received radiotherapy according to protocol guidelines for dose and volume had a superior local control rate (80%) compared with patients with major deviations (16% local control rate) or minor deviations (48% local control rate). Deviations in treatment volume seemed to be more critical. These results indicate that involved field radiation is an acceptable mode of local control for these patients but that treatment to the initial tumor volume plus an adequate margin is necessary.

Several retrospective single-institution case series have evaluated the impact of radiation dose on local control in Ewing sarcoma.[490-492] In one series patients treated with less than 49 Gy had a 5-year local control rate of 37% compared with 89% for patients treated with 49 Gy or more.[491] In this study higher doses seemed particularly important for larger tumors. In another series patients with larger tumors had a uniform local failure rate regardless of radiation dose, whereas patients with smaller tumors treated with more than 40 Gy had a higher local control rate compared with patients who had smaller tumors treated with less than 40 Gy.[492] A third case series reported no difference in outcome between patients treated with radiation doses above and below 54 Gy.[490] The CESS-81 trial randomized extremity tumors to receive 46 Gy or 60 Gy. The local failure rate was similar in these two groups.[431]

Three studies have specifically commented on the use of lower-dose radiotherapy.[462,493,494] The first study administered approximately 30 Gy in patients mainly in conjunction with some type of surgical resection, although five patients received radiotherapy only.[493] No local failures were noted in this group. The other two studies administered 30 to 36 Gy as definitive local control to patients with an objective response to neoadjuvant chemotherapy.[462,494] This strategy resulted in an unacceptably high local failure rate.

The timing of radiotherapy may be important for patients receiving definitive radiotherapy and not for patients receiving radiotherapy after surgery. A retrospective analysis of patients treated with surgery followed by radiation therapy in the CESS-86 and EICESS-92 trials demonstrated that the interval between surgery and radiation did not affect the local control rate or event-free

survival rate, even up to intervals beyond 90 days.[495] In contrast, a retrospective analysis of patients with pelvic Ewing sarcoma suggested that initiating definitive radiotherapy earlier may result in a lower local failure rate.[496] A pooled analysis has also suggested that longer periods (15-18 weeks) of neoadjuvant chemotherapy before starting radiation therapy may have a negative impact on the overall survival rate.[497]

Two retrospective case series evaluated hyperfractionated radiotherapy in the management of Ewing sarcoma.[490,498] Both series concluded that local control rates were not improved by hyperfractionation. One group reported better functional results with the hyperfractionated schedule.[498] The CESS-86 trial randomized patients to conventional or hyperfractionated radiation schedules.[499,500] Patients on the conventional schedule had chemotherapy held during radiotherapy, while patients on the hyperfractionated schedule continued to receive chemotherapy during radiation. For patients treated with radiotherapy alone, the local control rate was 82% for patients on the conventional schedule and 86% for patients on the hyperfractionated schedule. The radiation schedule did not affect overall or relapse-free survival rates. The radiation schedule did not affect disease control in patients treated with surgery followed by radiation.[500]

On the basis of this experience with radiotherapy for Ewing sarcoma, current practice is for patients with unresectable tumors to receive definitive radiotherapy after 4 to 6 cycles of chemotherapy. Most groups administer 54.4 to 60 Gy as definitive radiotherapy. Patients typically receive treatment as 45 Gy to the pretreatment volume plus a safety margin of at least 2 cm followed by a boost to full-dose radiotherapy to the treatment volume remaining after neoadjuvant chemotherapy.[486] Tumors with soft tissue extension, but not infiltration, into the chest or pelvic cavities often receive treatment to the postchemotherapy volume plus a safety margin. Some centers advise full-dose preoperative radiotherapy to tumors that may become fully resectable with such therapy. Patients with inadequate surgical margins are recommended to receive postoperative radiation. The EURO-EWING group also recommends postoperative radiotherapy for patients with adequate surgical margins and a poor histologic response to chemotherapy, although this practice is not standard in North America. The EURO-EWING group recommends a hyperfractionated schedule of radiotherapy, whereas the standard in North America remains conventional fractionation.

Several groups have compared the three available modes of local control: surgery, definitive radiation, and surgery plus radiation. Several studies have clearly documented that patients who undergo surgical resection have higher local control rates or improved overall outcomes (or both) compared with patients who receive definitive radiotherapy only.* These studies must be interpreted with caution because of the presence of confounding by indication. For example, because small extremity tumors

---

*References 336, 343, 347, 348, 352, 484, 485, 487, 500, 501.

are typically selected for surgery and large axial tumors are typically managed with radiotherapy alone, the outcome between these two groups might be expected to differ on account of reasons other than the chosen mode of local control. Indeed, not all studies have concluded that surgery provides superior disease control compared with radiation. A retrospective single-institution study of 76 patients with nonmetastatic Ewing sarcoma concluded that the overall survival rate and the rate of local control were equivalent between patients who received local control as surgery, radiation, or surgery plus radiation, although the power to detect a difference may have been limited by the small size of this study.[502] A secondary analysis of data from the United Kingdom Children's Cancer Study Group (UKCCSG) ET-2 trial reached the same conclusion.[503] In addition, the overall rate of disease recurrence did not differ between local control groups. In the SE 91-CNR Italian cooperative group trial, the 3-year event-free survival rates did not differ between patients who received surgery alone and those who received radiotherapy alone.[434]

Although a randomized trial might resolve the issue of optimal mode of local control, such a randomization would be untenable to patients. Instead, several analyses have evaluated this issue by attempting to control for the known confounding factors influencing both outcome and choice of local control modality. An analysis from the Rizzoli Institute showed that patients treated with definitive radiotherapy had inferior event-free survival rates compared with patients who received surgery alone, even after controlling for age, tumor size, and serum LDH level.[484] This group did not control for tumor site in this analysis. Two similar previous analyses by this same group controlled for tumor site, among other factors.[336,348] In these analyses patients treated with radiotherapy did not have an increased risk of relapse. The EICESS/CESS experience with local control has also been retrospectively reviewed in several analyses.[500,501] On univariate analyses, these studies have demonstrated that patients treated surgically have improved local control compared with patients treated with definitive radiotherapy. Although this group has not reported a multivariate analysis of outcome based on local control, they have reported a subgroup analysis based on tumor size (above and below 100 cm³) and site (axial versus appendicular).[501] Patients treated with radiation alone had inferior local control for all combinations of tumor size and site except small central tumors. However, patients treated with surgery appeared to have a higher rate of systemic failure compared with patients treated with radiation alone, such that the overall rate of disease recurrence was the same between groups.[485,501] This finding has not been reported by other groups. An analysis of 220 patients treated at St. Jude Children's Research Hospital also demonstrated that surgical resection was associated with lower rates of local failure, even after controlling for tumor size and year of treatment.[504] This analysis did not control for tumor site, however. Significantly, this analysis and a prospective randomized trial demonstrated lower rates of local failure in patients treated with more modern

TABLE 61-3   Major Chemotherapy Regimens Evaluated for Ewing Sarcoma

Abbreviation	Regimen
VAC	Vincristine, actinomycin-D, and cyclophosphamide
VACA	Vincristine, actinomycin-D, cyclophosphamide, and doxorubicin
VDC	Vincristine, doxorubicin, and cyclophosphamide
IE	Ifosfamide and etoposide
VAI	Vincristine, actinomycin-D, and ifosfamide
VDI	Vincristine, doxorubicin, and ifosfamide
VAIA	Vincristine, actinomycin-D, ifosfamide, and doxorubicin
VIDE	Vincristine, ifosfamide, doxorubicin, and etoposide

chemotherapy regimens that included ifosfamide and etoposide.[352,504]

Systemic Treatment with Chemotherapy

The use of chemotherapy for patients with Ewing sarcoma has revolutionized the care of these patients. Before the 1970s, standard therapy for this disease consisted solely of local control directed at the primary tumor. Most patients treated in this manner ultimately died from local or systemic recurrent disease.[505-507] In one series patients treated with local control alone had a median survival rate of 11 months.[506] In the 1960s and 1970s, evidence emerged that systemic chemotherapy could prevent recurrent disease in a substantial number of patients with Ewing sarcoma. This section reviews the development of modern chemotherapy regimens for this disease. Table 61-3 lists major chemotherapy regimens evaluated for Ewing sarcoma along with abbreviations for these regimens. Table 61-4 summarizes the major cooperative group trials that have contributed to current treatment approaches to this disease.

Early Improvements with Vincristine, Actinomycin-D, Doxorubicin, and Cyclophosphamide

Given the poor outcomes observed with local control alone, investigators began using single-agent chemotherapy for Ewing sarcoma. Although single-agent therapy did not substantially improve the long-term outcomes for these patients, these studies did identify a group of drugs capable of inducing tumor regression. Some of the most effective agents included vincristine, actinomycin-D, doxorubicin, and cyclophosphamide. Very quickly, investigators began to evaluate the use of these drugs in combination for patients with Ewing sarcoma.

One group evaluated two different combinations: vincristine with cyclophosphamide given in 8-week cycles for five cycles and vincristine, actinomycin-D, doxorubicin, and cyclophosphamide (VACA) given in weekly components for 18 months.[506] Most patients received

TABLE 61-4 Outcome for Patients with Localized Ewing Sarcoma of Bone in Cooperative Group Trials of Nonmyeloablative Therapies

Trial	Years	Regimen(s)	5-year EFS or RFS	Reference(s)
VACA Trials				
IESS-1	1973-1978	VACA	60%	435
		VAC + WLI	44%	
		VAC	24%	
IESS-2	1978-1982	High dose VACA	73% nonpelvic	513
		Protracted VACA	55% pelvic	531
			56% nonpelvic	513
First French	1978-1984	VACA	52% (4 year)	437
UKCCSG ET-1	1978-1986	VACA	41%	343
CESS-81	1981-1985	VACA	55%	431
French EW88	1988-1991	Protracted VACA	58%	347
VACA/IE Trials				
Second French	1984-1987	VAI/VDI	52%	335
CESS-86	1986-1991	VAIA for high risk	53% (10 year)	433
		VACA for low risk	49% (10 year)	
UKCCSG ET-2	1987-1993	VAI/VDI	62%	436
INT-0091	1988-1992	VACA/IE	69%	352
		VACA	54%	
SSG IX	1990-1996	VDI/PDI	58%	344
Italian SE 91-CNR	1991-1997	VACA/IE	69%	434
French EW-93	1993-1999	VACA for low risk	70%	519
		VACA/IE for intermediate risk	54%	
EICESS-92	1992-1999	VAIA for low risk	68%	520
		VACA for low risk	67%	
		VAIA for high risk	44%	
		VAIAE for high risk	52%	
Dose Intensified VACA/IE Trials				
INT-0154	1995-1998	VACA/IE standard	72%	438
		VACA/IE intensified	70%	
AEWS0031	2001-2005	VACA/IE 3-week	65%	522
		VACA/IE 2-week	73%	
EURO-EWING 99	Ongoing	VIDE	Ongoing	
AEWS1031	Ongoing	VDC/IE 2-week	Ongoing	
		VDC/IE/TC 2-week		

EFS, Event-free survival; *PDI,* cisplatin, doxorubicin, and ifosfamide; *RFS,* relapse-free survival; *TC,* topotecan and cyclophosphamide; *VAIAE,* vincristine, actinomycin-D, ifosfamide, doxorubicin, and etoposide; *WLI,* whole lung irradiation. See Table 61-3 for additional abbreviations.

radiotherapy as the mode of local control. In both regimens chemotherapy and radiotherapy started simultaneously at the initiation of treatment. Patients who received either regimen had a statistically significant improvement in outcome compared with historical controls who received only local control, suggesting that the VACA regimen resulted in better outcomes than the vincristine-cyclophosphamide regimen.

Another group reported on 30 patients with nonmetastatic Ewing sarcoma treated with 10 months of vincristine, doxorubicin, cyclophosphamide, and procarbazine.[507] Chemotherapy and radiotherapy were given concurrently

at the start of therapy. The 6-year disease-free survival rate was 49%, which was a substantial improvement on outcomes in historical controls treated with radiotherapy alone.

The Memorial Sloan Kettering Cancer Center treated 20 patients with localized Ewing sarcoma with 18 to 20 months of VACA as adjuvant therapy.[508] The cumulative dose of doxorubicin used in this study typically exceeded 500 mg/m^2, higher than in most other studies. The 5-year disease-free survival rate was 75%, perhaps highlighting the sensitivity of Ewing sarcoma to doxorubicin. The cardiotoxicity associated with these doses of doxorubicin resulted in a reduction in the cumulative doxorubicin exposure in subsequent studies by this group.[509]

The St. Jude Children's Research Hospital evaluated the use of neoadjuvant therapy with cyclophosphamide and doxorubicin for five cycles. An early report of this regimen reported that 19 of 23 evaluable patients had a complete response to therapy.[510] After these five cycles of neoadjuvant therapy, patients received local control, usually with radiotherapy. With the start of local control, patients began adjuvant therapy with vincristine and actinomycin-D for approximately 11 weeks followed by an additional six cycles of cyclophosphamide and doxorubicin. At the time of a follow-up report of 50 evaluable patients with nonmetastatic disease treated in this manner, 17 patients had developed recurrent disease.[462] A larger cooperative group study evaluating radiotherapy in Ewing sarcoma used a similar chemotherapy regimen and reported a 5-year event-free survival rate of 51% in patients with nonmetastatic disease.[487]

The Rizzoli Institute performed a series of trials evaluating both adjuvant (after local control) and neoadjuvant (before local control) VACA regimens. In the first trial patients received adjuvant therapy with vincristine, doxorubicin, and cyclophosphamide (VDC) for 2 years.[505] At the time of diagnosis, patients began chemotherapy in concert with local control of the primary tumor. In the 85 patients with localized disease treated in this manner, the 5-year event-free survival rate was 34%.[342] In contrast, only 5% of historical controls treated with local control only remained continuously free of disease.[505] The successor study treated 59 patients with localized disease with 18 months of VACA.[511] In this study the 5-year event-free survival rate was 59%, suggesting a benefit to the addition of actinomycin-D. The next study by this group evaluated VDC given as three neoadjuvant cycles followed by VACA chemotherapy after local control for a total of 15 months.[342,512] The 5-year event-free survival rate for the 108 patients with localized disease treated in this study was 49%. Compared to VACA given exclusively as adjuvant therapy, this result suggests that the change to neoadjuvant therapy did not improve outcomes for these patients.

Based on these promising results, several cooperative groups set out to evaluate vincristine, actinomycin-D, and cyclophosphamide (VAC) and VACA regimens in large groups of uniformly treated patients. IESS-1 was the first randomized study in patients with Ewing sarcoma.[435] This study enrolled patients from 1973 and 1978. The 342 patients with nonmetastatic Ewing sarcoma were randomized to one of three treatment arms. Patients in the first and second treatment arms received VAC, with patients in the second treatment arm also receiving prophylactic whole lung irradiation. Patients in the third treatment arm received VAC plus doxorubicin. Patients in this arm received doxorubicin every 12 weeks and actinomycin-D every 12 weeks, such that they received one of these agents every 6 weeks. Patients in the VAC arms received actinomycin-D every 12 weeks. All patients received radiotherapy to the primary tumor. Patients who received doxorubicin had a 5-year relapse-free survival rate of 60% compared with only 24% for patients who received VAC only. Patients who received VAC with whole lung irradiation had an intermediate 5-year relapse-free survival rate of 44%. These results indicated that the addition of doxorubicin to VAC significantly improved outcomes compared with either VAC alone or VAC with whole lung irradiation. The contribution of increased dose intensity in the doxorubicin arm to this improved outcome is not clear. Subgroup analysis showed that outcomes were inferior for patients with pelvic primary tumors and did not differ by treatment arm for these patients. Doxorubicin performed as well as whole lung irradiation in preventing lung metastasis. Based on these results, four-drug therapy with VACA became the standard chemotherapy approach for patients with Ewing sarcoma.

The IESS-2 study expanded on these results by randomizing patients with nonmetastatic disease not involving the pelvis to two different VACA dosing schedules.[513] Patients on one schedule received cycles of therapy every 3 weeks, and patients on the other schedule received more moderate doses of the same drugs at more frequent intervals. All patients received treatment for approximately 20 months. A total of 214 patients were enrolled in this study from 1978-1982. The 5-year relapse-free survival rate for patients with nonpelvic tumors who received higher-dose intermittent VACA was 73%, compared with 56% for patients who received more protracted VACA. Overall survival rate results showed a similar pattern. These results indicated a significant survival advantage for the higher-dose intermittent dosing schedule, at least for patients with tumors arising outside the pelvis.

The first German cooperative group trial for this disease (CESS-81) also used VACA administered in 3-week cycles.[431] This trial enrolled 93 patients with nonmetastatic disease from 1981 to 1985. Treatment duration was only 10 months, which was shorter than treatment on the IESS protocols. The 5-year disease-free survival rate was 55%, including patients with pelvic tumors. This result is similar to the outcome of VACA-treated patients on IESS-1, which also included patients with pelvic tumors. This result suggested that a shorter treatment duration using higher-dose regimens every 3 weeks does not compromise outcome.

The first Ewing sarcoma study of the United Kingdom Children's Cancer Study Group (UKCCSG ET-1) sought to standardize the treatment of newly diagnosed Ewing sarcoma using VACA-based chemotherapy.[343] This nonrandomized trial enrolled 142 patients from 1978 to 1986. Patients received one or two induction cycles of chemotherapy with VDC. Local therapy, with a preference for definitive radiotherapy, occurred next while patients received weekly cyclophosphamide and vincristine. Patients then received cycles of VDC alternating every 3 weeks with VAC for a total of 1 year of therapy. The 5-year relapse-free survival rate was 41%, and the 5-year overall survival rate was 44% for patients with nonmetastatic disease. The study authors suggest that the inferior outcome in this trial compared with that of other VACA-based trials at the time may have been due in part to decreased early doxorubicin dose intensity.[343]

The first French cooperative group study of Ewing sarcoma also used VACA-based chemotherapy as well as radiotherapy as the preferred mode of local control.[437] This study enrolled 95 patients between 1978 and 1984. Patients received cycles of VDC alternating with VAC for a total of 16 months of treatment. The 4-year disease-free survival rate for patients with nonmetastatic disease was 52%.

A follow-up French cooperative group study (EW88) enrolled 141 patients with nonmetastatic disease from 1988 to 1991.[347] This study administered cyclophosphamide in a more protracted manner, following a regimen piloted at St. Jude's Children's Research Hospital in the 1970s. Patients received initial chemotherapy with cyclophosphamide given daily for 7 days followed by doxorubicin on day 8. Patients received five cycles of this therapy before proceeding to local control. Surgery was recommended when possible. Radiotherapy was reserved for patients with unresectable tumors, incompletely resected tumors, or tumors with more than 5% viable tumor after initial chemotherapy. Following local control, patients received vincristine and actinomycin-D for 12 weeks followed by six additional cycles of cyclophosphamide and doxorubicin using the same schedule used neoadjuvantly. Administering these standard four drugs in this manner resulted in a 5-year disease-free survival rate of 58%.

Addition of Ifosfamide and Ifosfamide with Etoposide to VACA-Based Therapy

An initial report from the U.S. National Cancer Institute (NCI) demonstrated a response rate of 45% in 20 patients with recurrent Ewing sarcoma treated with a 5-day course of ifosfamide.[514] A follow-up study by this group evaluated ifosfamide combined with etoposide (IE) for patients with recurrent pediatric tumors.[515] Of the 17 evaluable patients with recurrent Ewing sarcoma included in the preliminary report, 16 patients had a partial response to therapy, for a response rate of 94%. A larger cooperative group study sponsored by the Pediatric Oncology Group included 55 patients with recurrent Ewing sarcoma treated with ifosfamide and etoposide.[516] The response rate in this study was 25%. Based on these promising results in patients with recurrent disease, the St. Jude Children's Research Hospital evaluated IE in patients with newly diagnosed high-risk disease.[517] This group gave three cycles of IE as an initial window before proceeding with doxorubicin and cyclophosphamide chemotherapy. Only 1 of 26 patients failed to respond to IE, for a response rate of 95%.

A number of single-institution studies incorporated ifosfamide and etoposide into the VACA backbone of therapy for newly diagnosed patients. One study from the NCI administered IE alternating with VDC or VAC for a total of 18 3-week cycles.[518] Ifosfamide was administered both before and after local control. A total of 31 patients with nonmetastatic disease were treated and had a 5-year event-free survival rate of 64%. This outcome was significantly better than historical controls with nonmetastatic disease treated with VDC and total body irradiation with stem cell rescue. Two studies from the Rizzoli Institute introduced ifosfamide at different times and reached different conclusions. In the REN-2 study, patients with localized disease received ifosfamide for the first time after local control.[512] The cumulative ifosfamide dose was 54 grams/m². The 5-year event-free survival rate for the 82 patients treated was 51%. This result was not different from historical controls treated with VACA-based therapy. In the REN-3 study, ifosfamide was introduced before local control with the cumulative dose held constant at 54 grams/m².[342] The 157 patients with nonmetastatic disease had a 5-year event-free survival rate of 71%, which was significantly better than any of the previous chemotherapy regimens evaluated at their center. These results suggest that early introduction of ifosfamide may improve outcome.

Several cooperative group studies have evaluated the efficacy of ifosfamide both with and without etoposide. One of the first cooperative group studies incorporating ifosfamide was the second French cooperative group study of Ewing sarcoma.[335] Patients enrolled from 1984 to 1987 and received initial therapy with alternating 3-week cycles of vincristine, actinomycin-D, and ifosfamide (VAI) and vincristine, doxorubicin, and ifosfamide (VDI) for a total of six cycles. Patients then underwent local control, with a preference for complete surgical resection. All patients were to receive radiotherapy, with the dose dependent on the extent of surgical resection. During radiotherapy patients received two cycles of vincristine with doxorubicin and two cycles of vincristine with ifosfamide. Following local control, patients received alternating 3-week cycles of VAI and vincristine with doxorubicin to complete a total of 1 year of therapy. The 5-year disease-free survival rate was 52% for 95 patients with nonmetastatic disease. This result prompted this group to conclude that substituting ifosfamide for cyclophosphamide did not improve outcomes. In addition, patients in this study had a higher than expected incidence of diminished cardiac function, prompting early closure of the study.

The CESS-86 trial was the first cooperative group attempt to risk-stratify patients and alter therapy based on risk.[433] Patients with small (less than 100 mL tumor volume) extremity tumors received VACA given as 3-week cycles for 36 weeks. Patients with large (100 mL or greater) tumors or axial tumors received identical therapy except ifosfamide was substituted for cyclophosphamide (VAIA). For the 301 nonmetastatic patients treated on this study, the ten-year event-free survival did not differ between patients who received VACA or VAIA (49% and 53%, respectively). However, multivariate analysis demonstrated that, controlling for tumor size and site, VACA chemotherapy was less effective than VAIA.

The French EW-93 study prescribed doxorubicin and cyclophosphamide for all patients with localized disease and reserved IE for patients with a poor response to three cycles of that therapy.[519] Patients with less than 50% regression of soft tissue mass on first evaluation were nonrandomly assigned to receive two cycles of IE before surgical resection. Of 214 patients, 33 received IE, and only eight of these refractory patients responded to IE before local control measures.

The UKCCSG ET-2 study evaluated the substitution of ifosfamide for cyclophosphamide in newly diagnosed patients.[436] This nonrandomized trial enrolled 243 patients from 1987 to 1993. Patients received VDI for four 3-week cycles before undergoing local control. In contrast to ET-1, ET-2 suggested a preference for surgery as mode of local control. Following local control, patients received VAI to complete 1 year of therapy. Patients received a cumulative doxorubicin dose of 420 mg/m^2 and cumulative ifosfamide dose of 114 grams/m^2. The 5-year relapse-free survival rate was 62% for patients with nonmetastatic disease. These results demonstrate a substantial improvement over the results of the UKCCSG ET-1 study. These improvements may be due to increased doxorubicin dose intensity, use of ifosfamide, preference for surgery as local control, or a combination of these factors.

An Italian cooperative group study (SE 91-CNR) enrolled 160 evaluable patients with nonmetastatic Ewing sarcoma from 1991 to 1997.[434] Patients treated on this protocol received initial therapy with alternating 3-week cycles of VDC and VAI. After 24 weeks of therapy, patients received alternating 3-week cycles of IE and VAC to complete 36 total weeks of therapy. Surgery was the preferred mode of local control for resectable tumors. The 5-year event-free survival rate was 69.4%.

A Scandinavian Sarcoma Group trial (SSG IX) enrolled patients with metastatic and nonmetastatic Ewing sarcoma from 1990 to 1996.[344] All patients received 35 weeks of chemotherapy given as 3-week cycles. Patients received cycles of VDI every 3 weeks, with cisplatin, doxorubicin, and ifosfamide substituted at cycles 2, 5, 8, and 11. Surgery was the preferred mode of local control. The 5-year metastasis-free survival rate was 58% for the 73 patients with initially nonmetastatic disease. The 5-year overall survival rate for these patients was 70%. The 5-year overall survival rate for patients presenting with metastatic disease was 28%. These results compare favorably to those from other contemporary trials.

Two randomized cooperative group trials have directly compared VACA-based chemotherapy to ifosfamide-containing chemotherapy. The North American intergroup study INT-0091 enrolled 518 patients with metastatic and nonmetastatic Ewing sarcoma from 1988 to 1992.[352] The standard arm on this study consisted of 3-week cycles of VDC. The experimental arm consisted of 3-week cycles of VDC alternating with IE. In both treatment arms, actinomycin-D was substituted for doxorubicin after a cumulative doxorubicin dose of 375 mg/m^2. All patients received 17 cycles of therapy, for a total study duration of 49 weeks. Local control occurred at week 12 of the therapy, with mode of local control determined on an individualized basis. The addition of IE significantly improved the outcome for patients with nonmetastatic disease, with a 5-year event-free survival rate of 69% compared with 54% for patients receiving VDC only. The incidence of local failure was also lower for patients who received IE, indicating that improved systemic therapy also improves local control. Based on these results, the combination of VDC and IE has become the standard therapy for patients with nonmetastatic Ewing sarcoma treated in North America.

The EICESS-92 study represents a collaborative effort between the UKCCSG and German cooperative groups. This trial enrolled 647 patients with either localized and metastatic Ewing sarcoma from 1992 to 1999. Patients with small (less than 100 mL tumor volume) localized tumors were deemed standard risk. These patients received initial chemotherapy with VAIA given as 3-week cycles followed by a randomization between continued VAIA or VACA. All other patients were deemed high risk and were randomized to receive VAIA or VAIA plus etoposide. Among standard-risk patients there were no statistically significant differences in event-free or overall survival rates between the randomized arms, although it is important to note that all patients received ifosfamide before randomization.[520] Among high-risk patients there were trends suggesting improved outcomes with the addition of etoposide to VAIA, although no statistically significant differences were found.

Dose-Intensified VACA/IE Regimens

The next generation of chemotherapy regimens emphasizes increasing the dose intensity of known active agents in this disease. The P6 protocol from the Memorial Sloan Kettering Cancer Center used an augmented dose of cyclophosphamide given in combination with vincristine and standard-dose doxorubicin.[521] Patients received a total of seven cycles of alternating VDC and IE along with local control of the primary tumor. The 4-year event-free survival rate for the 44 patients with localized disease was 82%, suggesting an improvement in outcome with higher-dose cyclophosphamide.

Two recent North American cooperative group studies have investigated strategies for dose-intensifying therapy. The first trial, known as INT-0154, included 478 eligible patients with nonmetastatic Ewing sarcoma diagnosed from 1995 to 1998.[438] Patients were randomized at study entry to receive alternating 3-week cycles of VDC and IE using either a dose-intensified or standard-dose approach. The standard-dose arm emulated the therapy given to patients assigned to the experimental arm of INT-0091. Patients in the dose-intensified arm received higher individual doses of the alkylating agents than patients in the standard-dose arm, but cumulative drug doses were approximately equivalent between arms. Patients in the dose-intensified arm completed therapy in 30 weeks, whereas patients in the standard-dose arm completed therapy in 48 weeks. Dose-intensified treatment did not improve event-free or overall survival rates and was associated with increased toxicity, such that this approach is not recommended for this population.

In Children's Oncology Group (COG) protocol AEWS0031, 568 patients with nonmetastatic Ewing sarcoma were randomized at study entry to receive cycles of standard-dose VDC and IE alternating every 3 weeks or every 2 weeks.[522] Individual and cumulative drug doses were equivalent between treatment arms. All patients received 14 cycles of therapy, requiring 42 weeks in standard arm and 28 weeks in the interval compression arm. Interval compression was feasible, with a median cycle length of 15 days in the interval compression arm. Patients randomized to the interval compression arm had a superior event-free survival rate compared with patients randomized to the standard arm (73% versus 65% at 5 years). Toxicity was equivalent between both arms. Based on these findings, this approach has been adopted in North America as a standard practice for patients with localized Ewing sarcoma.

Several groups have evaluated chemotherapy regimens that combine multiple active agents given together during a cycle of therapy. In a protocol at St. Jude Children's Research Hospital, 51 patients with Ewing sarcoma received ifosfamide, etoposide, cyclophosphamide, and doxorubicin given together for three cycles before local control.[523] Patients then received alternating cycles of IE and cyclophosphamide with doxorubicin for a total of 41 weeks of therapy. The doses of ifosfamide, etoposide, and cyclophosphamide given after local control were higher than in previous studies. Patients were able to complete the planned neoadjuvant therapy, but myelosuppression limited the ability of patients to receive the planned adjuvant therapy on schedule. Specifically, only 66% of patients received all planned chemotherapy, and only 25% of patients received all planned chemotherapy on schedule. Despite difficulties in achieving the desired degree of dose intensification, outcomes remained favorable. The 3-year event-free survival rate for patients with localized disease was 78%.

A British group has piloted the use of vincristine, ifosfamide, doxorubicin, and etoposide (VIDE) as neoadjuvant therapy for this disease.[524] In this study 30 patients with newly diagnosed Ewing sarcoma were treated with six 3-week cycles of VIDE. Because of hematologic toxicity, etoposide was dose reduced or omitted from 50% of the planned cycles. All attempts at collecting peripheral blood stem cells after a cycle of VIDE were successful. Of the 24 patients evaluable for radiographic response, only one patient had progressive disease. Patients in this pilot study received additional therapy following local control. The final results of this study are not yet available.

The European cooperative groups have initiated a combined trial known as EURO-EWING 99 that relies on VIDE as neoadjuvant therapy. All patients receive initial treatment with six 3-week cycles of VIDE. This trial then tailors therapy according to risk. Patients with small (less than 200 mL tumor volume) nonmetastatic tumors with good chemotherapy response are randomized to receive additional therapy with seven cycles of VAC or VAI. Patients with large tumors, pulmonary metastases, or poor chemotherapy response are randomized to receive additional therapy with seven cycles of VAI or high-dose therapy with stem cell rescue (discussed later). This randomized trial is ongoing.

Two nonrandomized trials have reported on the use of high-dose chemotherapy as a consolidation strategy for patients with localized Ewing sarcoma and adverse prognostic factors. In the French EW93 trial, patients with localized Ewing sarcoma were considered high risk if they had either a 30% or greater viable tumor at time of surgical resection or a 50% or less reduction in tumor volume by imaging for patients not candidates for surgical resection.[519] These patients were nonrandomly assigned to receive high-dose chemotherapy with busulfan and melphalan. There were 48 patients who were classified as high risk, 34 of whom received high-dose chemotherapy. For the entire cohort of patients with high-risk disease, the 5-year event-free survival rate was 48%. A joint Italian-Scandinavian protocol adopted a similar approach, with busulfan and melphalan high-dose chemotherapy prescribed for patients with localized disease and macroscopic foci of tumor at the time of surgery or incomplete regression of soft tissue masses in patients not candidates for surgical resection.[525] Outcomes for the 126 patients with these poor risk features who received high-dose therapy were similar to those of patients without poor risk features who did not receive high-dose therapy. Given the nonrandomized study designs and risk of selection bias for patients who proceeded to high-dose therapy in these two trials, the role of this approach in patients with localized Ewing sarcoma remains unclear.

Management of Tumors Arising at Special Sites
Pelvic Ewing Sarcoma

Ewing sarcoma frequently arises in the pelvis. These pelvic tumors tend be large and associated with crucial viscera, nerves, and bones (particularly of the acetabulum), making complete surgical resection difficult. The local failure rate for patients with pelvic primary tumors ranges from 15% to 27%, which is higher than the local failure rate typically reported in appendicular tumors.[526-530] In one large series, even after exclusion of patients with a local relapse, the outcome for patients with pelvic primary tumors was still inferior to outcomes at other sites.[527] This result suggests that both systemic control and local control are inadequate for these patients.

Recognizing the poor outcome of patients with pelvic primary tumors, the IESS-2 trial nonrandomly assigned patients to the higher-dose intermittently scheduled VACA arm of that study.[531] In addition, an increased emphasis was placed on surgical control of pelvic tumors. With this strategy, patients with pelvic tumors had a 5-year relapse-free survival rate of 55% compared with only 23% for patients in the IESS-1 trial. Because the higher dose VACA arm resulted in better outcomes in the randomized nonpelvic patients treated in IESS-2, the improvements in outcome seen in patients with pelvic tumors may have been attributable to better systemic control, better local control, or both. Indeed, patients with pelvic tumors in IESS-2 were more likely to undergo complete surgical resection and had a lower local failure rate compared to patients with pelvic tumors in IESS-1. Compared with patients who did not have a complete resection, complete resection did not improve the overall or relapse-free survival rate in these patients in IESS-2.[531]

The optimal mode of local control for pelvic tumors has been difficult to determine with rigorous studies. A report from the Mayo Clinic found that patients with pelvic Ewing sarcoma treated with surgery had a statistically significant superior overall survival rate compared with patients treated without surgery.[532] In several other series of patients with pelvic primary tumors, the mode of local control has not clearly been shown to affect outcome,[527-529,533] although some trends have suggested improvements in survival rates among patients treated surgically.[528,529,533] Some groups have also reported a trend toward a lower local recurrence rate in patients treated surgically,[496,527,528,532] although not all groups have reported this trend.[529] The results of these studies are often difficult to evaluate insofar as patients treated with complete surgical resection typically have small resectable tumors. However, two groups have attempted to control for this and other confounding factors. The French cooperative group reported on 53 patients with pelvic Ewing sarcoma.[534] After controlling for size and other potential confounding factors, researchers found that patients treated with radiotherapy alone had an increased risk of recurrence and death compared with patients who received surgery or surgery with radiotherapy. The COG retrospectively analyzed 75 patients with pelvic primary tumors treated on INT-0091.[530] In contrast to the results of the French group, the mode of local control did not affect event-free survival or local failure rates after controlling for confounding factors such as size. As observed in the main analysis of all tumor sites, patients with pelvic tumors who were randomized to receive VACA plus IE on this study had a lower risk of local failure compared with patients randomized to receive VACA alone.[530] Given this uncertainty and the risk of second tumors from radiotherapy, many groups choose to resect pelvic tumors that can be resected without functional consequences. For tumors that cannot be resected without functional consequences, options include either definitive radiotherapy alone or preoperative radiotherapy with the possible addition of wide resection.

Chest Wall Ewing Sarcoma

Chest wall tumors also require specialized management, particularly insofar as these tumors often invade the pleura or have associated pleural effusions. Some data suggest that surgical resection of chest wall tumors provides superior local control, although these analyses do not account for differences in tumor size that influence resectability.[535,536] Indeed, other analyses have not shown a difference in outcome based on mode of local control for chest wall tumors.[481,537,538] Results from INT-0091 and INT-0154 indicate that neoadjuvant chemotherapy before attempted resection of a chest wall tumor increases the likelihood of obtaining negative margins compared with results from attempted resection before chemotherapy.[481,538] Delayed resection at this site therefore decreases the need for postoperative radiotherapy in these patients.[481,538] Avoiding chest wall radiation is particularly appealing given the added pulmonary and cardiac toxicities associated with this therapy.

Whereas several reports have suggested that an associated pleural effusion did not worsen outcome, patients with chest wall tumors and pleural effusions were often recommended to receive hemithorax irradiation in these studies.[536,537,539] Indeed, a report from the French cooperative group suggested that patients with rib primary tumors and an associated pleural effusion had an increased risk of local relapse without radiotherapy.[537] In the EICESS/CESS studies, patients who received hemithorax irradiation had more unfavorable features than patients who did not receive hemithorax irradiation.[540] Despite this difference, the rate of local relapse was the same in both groups, whereas the rate of systemic relapse was higher in the group of patients who did not receive hemithorax irradiation.[540] This result may be interpreted as evidence of the direct benefit of hemithorax irradiation in preventing dissemination of residual tumor cells from the pleural space. Alternatively, hemithorax irradiation may reduce the volume of lung at risk for subsequent relapse, because the IESS-1 researchers noted that whole lung irradiation can prevent lung metastasis in patients with initially nonmetastatic disease. Patients with chest wall primary tumors and positive pleural fluid cytology or pleural-based nodules treated according to the most recent COG protocol received hemithorax radiation.

Ewing Sarcoma of the Spine

Management of patients with tumors arising along the spinal column requires careful planning by a multidisciplinary team, including oncologists, radiation oncologists, orthopedic surgeons, general surgeons, and neurosurgeons. Small case series have suggested that local control and overall outcomes for patients with primary tumors at this site do not differ from outcomes for patients with tumors arising from other sites.[341,541] One group reported that sacral primary tumors fare less well than other vertebral tumors,[340] although this result was not replicated in other series.[338,339,341] The largest reported experience with vertebral Ewing sarcoma comes from the EICESS/CESS studies.[542] A total of 116 patients had tumors arising from cervical, thoracic, or lumbar vertebrae. Given the difficulties in obtaining a complete resection at this site, all but four patients received radiotherapy as part of local control of the tumor. The local failure rate for patients treated with radiotherapy alone was not significantly different from that of patients treated with surgery plus radiotherapy (22.6% and 18.7%, respectively). Local relapses typically occurred within the radiation field, suggesting that inadequate selection of radiotherapy fields was not to blame for these local relapses. Despite the fact that the spinal cord limits radiotherapy dosing at this site, the local failure rate for patients with vertebral tumors treated with radiotherapy alone was not higher than the local failure rate for patients with tumors of any location treated with radiotherapy alone.[501,542] This effect may result from the generally smaller size of paraspinal tumors compared with that of other tumors selected for local control with definitive radiotherapy. It should be noted, however, that patients with a vertebral tumor treated with radiotherapy who experience local recurrence often have few local control options because additional radiotherapy may compromise the spinal cord.[542]

Soft Tissue Ewing Sarcoma

Historically, patients with soft tissue Ewing sarcoma were not included in cooperative group clinical trials for patients with Ewing sarcoma of bone. Instead, patients with soft tissue Ewing sarcoma have often been included in protocols designed for patients with other soft tissue sarcomas, including rhabdomyosarcoma.[543,544] More recent work suggests that these patients should receive treatment following Ewing sarcoma protocols. For example, one study compared patients treated according to International Society of Paediatric Oncology (SIOP) protocol MMT89 without doxorubicin to patients treated on the French EW93 protocol with doxorubicin.[543] Although it was a nonrandomized comparison, baseline patient characteristics were similar between both groups, but event-free and overall survival rates were superior for patients treated according to the EW93 protocol. In North American study INT-0154, patients with soft tissue disease had outcomes equivalent to those of patients with skeletal primary tumors.[438] These results support the current practice of including these patients in modern trials for Ewing sarcoma.

Summary of Outcomes for Patients with Nonmetastatic Ewing Sarcoma

Patients with Ewing sarcoma have shown great improvements in outcome over the past 4 decades. For patients with localized tumors, expected survival rates have increased to greater than 70% with modern multimodality therapy. Figure 61-8 demonstrates these improvements graphically, using Surveillance, Epidemiology, and End Results (SEER) data from 1975 to 2000.[5,545] A similar pattern of steady improvement over time has also been reported using data from a large European registry.[546]

TREATMENT OF PATIENTS WITH METASTATIC EWING SARCOMA

Systemic Therapy

Despite the recognition that these patients have a poor prognosis, early studies often treated patients with metastatic disease with the same combined modality therapy used for nonmetastatic patients. Because the outcomes for these patients have not improved in concert with the gains seen in nonmetastatic patients, more aggressive strategies have been added to this backbone. These strategies are discussed here.

Attempts to improve outcomes for these patients through changes in chemotherapy regimens have been largely unsuccessful. The IESS-2 study attempted to improve on the 30% 5-year overall survival rate for metastatic patients treated on IESS-1.[355] This group added 5-fluorouracil to the VACA backbone of IESS-1. As in IESS-1, radiation to all metastatic sites was prescribed. The 5-year overall survival rate was 28% despite the addition of 5-fluorouracil.[355] Single-institution studies suggested that the addition of IE to VACA did not improve the outcome for patients with initially metastatic disease.[518,521,523] The INT-0091 study confirmed these disappointing results.[352,356] INT-0091 also included a nonrandomized arm in which patients with newly diagnosed metastatic disease received dose-intensified VDC and IE.[547] Patients received higher doses of doxorubicin, cyclophosphamide, and ifosfamide compared with patients treated in the randomized portion of INT-0091. Although this was a nonrandomized comparison, the 60 patients treated with dose-intensified therapy had similar outcomes to patients with metastatic disease treated with standard-dose therapy on INT-0091. The Pediatric Oncology Group and Children's Cancer Group conducted a phase II study of alkylator-intensive chemotherapy for patients with newly diagnosed metastatic disease.[548] Patients in this study received topotecan (N=36) or topotecan and cyclophosphamide (N=37) in an upfront window. After the window phase, patients received IE alternating with VDC, with higher doses of ifosfamide and cyclophosphamide used than in standard protocols. This strategy did not improve the outcomes for these patients. A regimen developed in Seattle combines vincristine, doxorubicin, cyclophosphamide, ifosfamide, and etoposide given together each cycle.[549] All five patients with metastatic Ewing sarcoma and evaluable disease obtained a complete radiographic response to this therapy. Only one of these patients remains free of disease 33 months from initial diagnosis.

Patients with metastatic disease at initial diagnosis are candidates for novel approaches to the treatment of Ewing sarcoma. COG evaluated the addition of metronomic chemotherapy with vinblastine and celecoxib to the VACA/IE backbone used in INT-0091 in 35 patients with metastatic disease.[550] This approach used an antiangiogenic approach together with known active cytotoxic chemotherapy in an attempt to improve the outcome for these patients. This approach was feasible, although small patient numbers precluded conclusions about the impact of vinblastine and celecoxib on disease control.

Patients with metastatic disease who do not respond to initial therapy may receive second-line chemotherapy (described later, in the section on patients with recurrent disease). These patients may also be candidates for other investigational therapies, including high-dose therapy with hematopoietic stem cell rescue (discussed later).

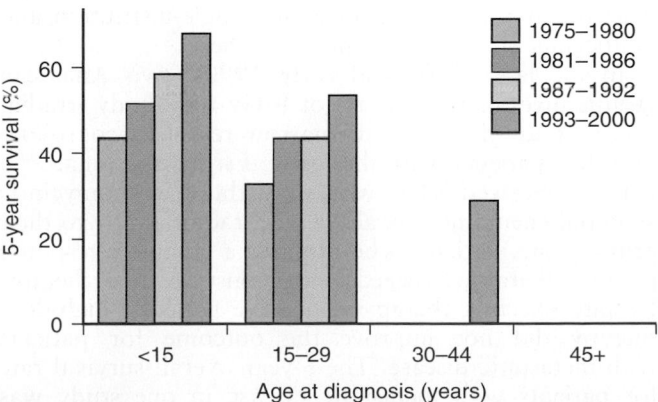

Figure 61-8 Overall survival rates at 5 years from initial diagnosis of Ewing sarcoma according to age at initial diagnosis and treatment era. (*Gurney JG, Swensen AR, Bulterys M: Malignant bone tumors. In Ries LAG, Smith MA, Gurney JG, et al, editors:* Cancer incidence and survival among children and adolescents: United States SEER Program 1975-1995, *Bethesda, MD. 1999, National Cancer Institute, SEER Program, NIH Pub. No. 99-4649, p. 99–110.*)

Role of Surgery and Radiation in Patients with Metastatic Disease

Patients presenting with metastatic disease typically receive local control of their primary tumor. Because of their disseminated disease and poor prognosis, the local control strategy for these patients tends to differ from that of patients with nonmetastatic disease. In particular, patients with metastatic disease are more likely receive definitive radiotherapy for local control because they often require radiotherapy to other sites of disease. Indeed, at least one analysis has demonstrated the importance of local control measures directed against both primary and metastatic sites of disease in improving outcomes for this high-risk patient population.[551]

Whole lung irradiation appears to be an effective therapy for patients with lung metastases. The St. Jude Children's Research Hospital reported on patients at their center with lung metastases at initial diagnosis. Patients in this series received whole lung irradiation if they had residual lung metastases after initial chemotherapy. Patients in this series who received whole lung irradiation for residual lung metastases had an outcome equivalent to that of patients whose lung metastases resolved with initial chemotherapy and who did not receive whole lung irradiation.[552] The authors argue that the patients with residual lung metastases after initial chemotherapy would have had an even worse outcome without the addition of whole lung irradiation. Data from the CESS studies suggest that a dose-response relationship may exist for whole lung irradiation.[553] This group reported that patients with initial lung metastases who remained in clinical remission had received higher doses of whole lung irradiation than patients who relapsed. The number of patients reported in this series was small, but the group reported that four of ten patients who received 12 to 16 Gy remained in remission compared with five of six patients who received 18 to 21 Gy. Only one of six patients who did not receive whole lung irradiation remained in clinical remission.[553]

The strongest evidence in favor of whole lung irradiation for patients with lung metastases comes from the EICESS group. This group reported on 100 evaluable patients with isolated lung metastases, 75 of whom received 15 to 18 Gy whole lung irradiation as part of their combined modality therapy.[351] The risk of pulmonary recurrence was significantly decreased with the addition of whole lung irradiation. Moreover, the overall risk of disease recurrence diminished with this intervention. The 5-year event-free survival rate for patients treated with whole lung irradiation was 38%, compared with 27% for patients who did not receive whole lung irradiation. This result is even more striking in light of the fact that the indication for whole lung irradiation in this trial was residual lung metastasis after chemotherapy. Although whole lung irradiation was not prescribed in a randomized manner, potential confounding variables appeared to be balanced between patients who received whole lung irradiation and patients who did not receive whole lung irradiation. In addition, a Cox regression model indicated that whole lung irradiation improved the event-free survival rate after controlling for potential confounding variables.[351] An additional report from the EICESS group indicated that whole lung irradiation improves the outcome even for patients with lung metastases combined with metastases at other sites.[354] Currently, whole lung irradiation is commonly being employed for patients with lung metastases at initial presentation regardless of the radiographic response to initial chemotherapy. Patients with bone metastases also typically receive radiotherapy directed to these sites, although data supporting this strategy are lacking.

Pulmonary metastasectomy plays little role in the management of patients with lung metastases at initial diagnosis. One small case series suggested that pulmonary metastasectomy might improve the outcome for these patients, although this result was confounded by the fact that only patients with resectable lung metastases underwent resection.[554] Surgical resection of pulmonary metastases was not shown to improve outcomes in patients treated by the EICESS group who had residual lung metastases after initial chemotherapy.[351]

Role of High-Dose Therapy with Hematopoietic Stem Cell Rescue for Metastatic Disease

Patients with initially metastatic Ewing sarcoma may be candidates for high-dose therapy with stem cell rescue. The role of high-dose therapy for these patients remains unclear, with most studies relying on comparisons with historical controls consisting of patients treated without high-dose therapy. For example, a study using data from a bone marrow transplant registry observed similar outcomes between patients treated with and without high-dose therapy.[555] Numerous groups have demonstrated the feasibility of delivering myeloablative therapy as consolidation therapy after initial chemotherapy and local control in these high-risk patients. No completed studies have evaluated high-dose therapy in a randomized manner. As such, studies suggesting a benefit from this modality are subject to selection bias in which only patients with good overall physical condition who attain a certain level of disease control are considered for high-dose therapy. Results from larger single-institution and multicenter studies are summarized here.

In the late 1980s and early 1990s, two American groups investigated the use of 8 Gy total-body irradiation with autologous bone marrow rescue as consolidation for patients with high-risk Ewing sarcoma.[556,557] Patients received VDC with or without actinomycin-D as initial chemotherapy along with radiotherapy to their primary site. Patients who attained a complete response to this therapy proceeded to consolidation therapy. Despite selecting therapy-responsive patients, high-dose therapy did not improve the outcome for patients with metastatic disease. The 6-year overall survival rate for patients with metastatic disease in one study was only 14%.[557]

Two EICESS centers evaluated 12 Gy total-body irradiation combined with melphalan and etoposide as consolidation therapy in patients with bone metastases or early relapsed disease.[558,559] Patients in this series received either autologous or allogeneic transplant if they had responded favorably to initial chemotherapy. Although an initial report showed a relapse rate of only 52%, a follow-up report indicated that the event-free survival rate from the time of transplant for this cohort of patients was 24%. The outcomes did not differ significantly between patients who received autologous stem cells and those who received allogeneic stem cells, although patients who underwent allogeneic transplant had a higher rate of complications. A follow-up study from this same group evaluated two consolidation courses of myeloablative melphalan and etoposide in 17 patients with bone metastases.[560] The 5-year event-free survival rate for these patients was 21%.

A later Children's Cancer Group study evaluated melphalan, etoposide, and 12 Gy total-body irradiation for patients with newly diagnosed Ewing sarcoma with bone or bone marrow metastases.[561] These patients received VDC alternating with IE for five cycles along with radiotherapy to their primary tumor and bone metastases. Patients with a complete response or very good partial response to initial therapy received the planned myeloablative therapy. The 2-year event-free survival rate for all 32 patients enrolled in this study was 20%. For the group of patients who were able to receive myeloablative therapy, the 2-year event-free survival rate was 24%. The outcome did not differ from a cohort of historical controls treated in protocol INT-0091. As such, the authors concluded that myeloablative therapy did not improve the outcome for patients with bone and bone marrow metastases.

A French multicenter trial prospectively evaluated the role of high-dose therapy in patients with newly diagnosed metastatic disease.[429] Patients in this trial received initial chemotherapy with cyclophosphamide and doxorubicin alternating with IE. Of the 97 patients enrolled in the study, 75 had a favorable response to initial therapy and proceeded to consolidation therapy with busulfan and melphalan followed by stem cell rescue. The 5-year event-free survival rate was 37% for all 97 patients and 47% for the 75 patients who received high-dose therapy. Much of the improvement after high-dose therapy appeared to be in patients with isolated lung metastases. These patients had a 5-year event-free survival rate of 52% compared with 24% for patients with metastases involving other sites.

A joint Italian and Scandinavian trial treated 102 patients with newly diagnosed metastatic disease, the majority of whom had isolated pulmonary metastatic disease.[562] Patients initially received multiagent chemotherapy and local control measures followed by high-dose chemotherapy with busulfan and melphalan. Patients with lung metastasis at study entry also received 12 to 15 Gy whole lung radiation. High-dose chemotherapy was administered to 79 patients, and the primary reason that the remaining patients did not receive high-dose chemotherapy was early disease progression. The 5-year event-free survival rate for the entire study population was 43%. For patients with isolated pulmonary metastatic disease who were able to receive high-dose chemotherapy and whole lung radiation, the 5-year event-free survival rate was 53%.

A report of 171 patients treated by the EICESS group indicated that high-dose therapy did not improve the outcome among patients with metastatic disease at initial diagnosis.[354] Further analysis suggested that patients with multiple sites of metastases require some form of intensified therapy, either as high-dose therapy or whole lung irradiation. The 4-year event-free survival rate for patients with multiple metastatic sites treated with high-dose therapy, whole lung irradiation, or both modalities was 27% compared with 0% for patients who did not receive at least one form of intensified therapy.[354]

The only randomized study comparing high-dose therapy with other treatment for high-risk patients is ongoing. This trial, known as the EURO-EWING 99 study, randomizes newly diagnosed high-risk patients to receive consolidation therapy with busulfan and melphalan followed by stem cell rescue or continuation chemotherapy. Patients with isolated pulmonary metastases are randomized to consolidation therapy with high-dose chemotherapy and stem cell rescue or to continuation chemotherapy followed by whole lung irradiation. Patients with metastases beyond the lung are nonrandomly assigned to high-dose chemotherapy with stem cell rescue. Of note, patients with nonmetastatic disease with poor response to neoadjuvant chemotherapy are also randomized to high-dose chemotherapy or to continuation chemotherapy. Results of the randomized portion of this trial will not be available for several years. However, patients with extrapulmonary metastatic disease were nonrandomly assigned to receive high-dose chemotherapy and their outcomes have been reported.[563] Of 281 enrolled patients, 169 patients went on to receive high-dose therapy, mainly with busulfan and melphalan conditioning. The event-free survival rate at 3 years for the entire cohort of 281 patients was 27%. The selected group of patients in complete remission at the time of high-dose therapy had a 3-year event-free survival rate of 57%, compared with 32% and 24% for patients with partial response or stable disease/progressive disease, respectively. These results indicate the importance of remission status if high-dose therapy is to be considered in this high-risk patient population.

The use of autologous stem cell infusion raises the concern of re-infusion of Ewing cells contaminating the stem cell product. Several groups have investigated this issue using PCR techniques with mixed results. The incidence of tumor cell contamination ranges from 6% to 100% of pheresis products, depending on the study.[564-567] The largest and most recent evaluation of this issue studied 88 patients with high-risk Ewing sarcoma treated with high-dose therapy with stem cell rescue.[567] Only seven patients had tumor cell contamination of their infused product. The outcome of these seven patients did not appear to differ from the outcome of patients without tumor cell contamination of their infused product.

Summary of Outcomes for Patients with Metastatic Ewing Sarcoma

Despite improved outcomes for patients with nonmetastatic disease over time, patients with initially metastatic disease have not been as fortunate. Most reports suggest that no more than 30% of patients with metastatic Ewing sarcoma are long-term survivors, although this number may be slightly higher for patients with isolated lung metastases.[351,356] Even with combined modality therapy, many patients never attain a complete remission. One recent study reported a complete response rate of only 43% after these patients received chemotherapy, surgery, radiation, and combinations thereof.[548] As such, a number of these patients have treatment-refractory disease. Among patients who do attain a complete remission, disease recurrence remains a major barrier to durable cure.

RECURRENT EWING SARCOMA

Location and Timing of Disease Recurrence

Among patients whose disease recurs, recurrence involving distant sites is more common than isolated local recurrence. Isolated distant relapse accounts for 48% to 71% of recurrences,[568,569] although this appears to be more common in patients with initially metastatic disease.[570-573] Another 10% to 29% of recurrences are combined local plus distant recurrences, and estimates of isolated local recurrence vary widely among studies, ranging from 11% to 35%.[352,570-573] Most initial distant relapses involve the lung, the bones, or both.[571,572]

Most episodes of disease recurrence occur after patients have completed their planned initial therapy. Disease recurrence within 2 years of initial diagnosis is more common than later recurrence, with more than 70% of relapses occurring during this time frame in two large analyses.[568,569] The median time to disease recurrence across several series ranges from 17 to 27 months.[570-573] Patients with initially metastatic disease that recurs have a shorter time to recurrence compared with patients who have initially localized disease that recurs.[569] An analysis of data from the UKCCSG ET-1 and ET-2 studies indicated that patients have a relatively stable rate of death during the first 2 years after diagnosis.[574] Between 2 and 5 years after diagnosis, the rate of death is lower but remains relatively constant during this interval. Only after 5 years from initial diagnosis does the risk of death plateau at an even lower rate that remains constant with extended follow-up. However, Ewing sarcoma can recur very late. In one series 5 of 31 patients who remained disease free for 5 years from the time of initial diagnosis later recurred.[575] In another report 25 of 326 patients who had been in complete remission for 5 years from initial diagnosis experienced late disease recurrence.[576] Other series of patients with recurrent disease include patients with disease recurrence beyond 10 years from initial diagnosis.[570,571,576,577] For example, a report from the Childhood Cancer Survivor Study observed that 26% of late relapses (beyond 5 years from initial diagnosis) occurred 10 or more years from initial relapse.[577] These results highlight the need for extended follow-up in patients with this disease.

General Approach to Patients with Recurrent Ewing Sarcoma

Patients with progressive or recurrent disease after initial therapy present a particular challenge to the clinical team.

The time to disease recurrence provides an important indication of the likelihood of long-term survival for these patients (discussed later). More than one quarter of patients with late (more than 2 years from initial diagnosis) recurrence may achieve long-term disease control with aggressive therapy.[568-573] Most clinicians initiate systemic chemotherapy for these patients to assess their sensitivity to the chosen chemotherapy regimen. For patients with chemotherapy-responsive disease, the use of surgery or radiation (or both) for sites of recurrence is often considered. For a local recurrence another attempt at local control may be undertaken with surgery, radiation, or both. For patients with pulmonary recurrence, many clinicians will recommend whole lung irradiation. Patients who respond well to second-line therapy may also be candidates for high-dose therapy with stem cell rescue, although this approach remains unproved (discussed later). Patients with late recurrent disease that does not respond to initial chemotherapy are managed as for poor-risk recurrent disease, according to the strategies outlined in subsequent paragraphs.

For patients with an early (less than 2 years from initial diagnosis) recurrence, the likelihood of long-term disease control is less than 10%.[570-573] Given these data, the appropriate treatment for these patients must be highly individualized, with a clear understanding of the patient's and family's goals for therapy. A variety of strategies are considered for these patients, ranging from palliative measures to aggressive multimodality therapy with curative intent. These patients often receive treatment with the second-line chemotherapy regimens described later in this chapter and are also candidates for investigational phase I and phase II clinical trials. For patients with chemotherapy-responsive disease, more aggressive measures can then be considered.

Systemic Therapies for Recurrent Ewing Sarcoma

Historically, very few chemotherapy options existed for patients with recurrent Ewing sarcoma. As such, patients with late-relapse disease were often treated with agents that they had received at initial diagnosis. In one small series a substantial number of patients who relapsed when they were off therapy responded again to the same agents they received as initial therapy; some of these patients had a durable second remission.[578] Another group reported on 35 patients with disease recurrence after ifosfamide-containing chemotherapy, of whom 34% responded to higher-dose ifosfamide (15 grams/m^2/course).[579] Nevertheless, because of concerns regarding resistance to previously used agents, most clinicians now use newer chemotherapy regimens for patients at the time of relapse. However, for patients who experience late relapses, some clinicians will incorporate previously used active agents into an overall treatment plan that also includes newer second-line regimens. Some of these more common second-line regimens are reviewed here.

Camptothecin-containing regimens have demonstrated efficacy for patients with relapsed Ewing sarcoma. Topotecan monotherapy appears to have limited activity against Ewing sarcoma, with objective response rates of 0% to 10%.[580,581] In contrast, topotecan in combination with cyclophosphamide has a response rate of approximately 30% in patients with relapsed or refractory disease.[582,583] Patients with disease that was refractory to standard alkylator-containing therapy responded to this regimen, which suggests that this response rate was not attributable solely to cyclophosphamide but rather to the combination of topotecan with cyclophosphamide. Patients with newly diagnosed metastatic disease treated in an upfront window study had a response rate of 57% to topotecan and cyclophosphamide.[548] On the basis of this activity, the combination is being evaluated in a COG trial for patients with newly diagnosed localized disease (AEWS1031).

A second camptothecin-containing regimen has shown promise in patients with Ewing sarcoma. An initial phase I study of irinotecan and temozolomide found that this well-tolerated regimen induced one complete response and one partial response among seven patients with Ewing sarcoma treated in this study.[584] A follow-up report that included these seven patients plus seven additional evaluable patients reported an objective response in four patients (28%), although an additional four patients had a mixed response or stable disease.[585] A single-institution series of this same regimen reported a 63% response rate in 19 evaluable patients, confirming the activity of this combination in patients with relapsed disease.[586]

Two carboplatin-based regimens have benefited patients with relapsed or refractory Ewing sarcoma. One group reported a 26% response rate among 39 patients treated with carboplatin, cyclophosphamide, and etoposide.[587] A second group evaluated carboplatin, ifosfamide, and etoposide in patients with a range of relapsed or refractory sarcoma.[588] Of the 21 patients with Ewing sarcoma, 48% had an objective response. The contribution of carboplatin to these responses is unclear because both regimens contain first-line agents that are also effective in the treatment of this disease (ifosfamide, etoposide, and cyclophosphamide).

The combination of docetaxel and gemcitabine has also been tested in patients with recurrent Ewing sarcoma, with limited success. In three retrospective case series that included 11 patients with relapsed disease, only one patient had a partial response to standard doses of this combination.[589-591] A formal phase II study of this same regimen demonstrated a 14% response rate in 14 patients with relapsed disease.[592] One group used higher doses of gemcitabine and docetaxel and observed a 66% response rate, suggesting that if there is activity of this combination, dose intensity may be critical.[593]

A number of novel therapies have been evaluated in patients with recurrent Ewing sarcoma. Of these, the most promising and consistent results have been with monoclonal antibodies targeting the IGF-1R. In initial phase I studies, an early signal of objective responses emerged in a subset of patients with relapsed disease.[594,595] Follow-up phase II studies of several different IGF-1R monoclonal antibodies confirmed this activity, with response rates of approximately 10% to 15% between studies.[596-598] Another study evaluated an IGF-1R monoclonal antibody together with an mTOR inhibitor in 17 patients with Ewing sarcoma and reported tumor regressions greater than 20% in 29% of patients.[599] Follow-up studies are necessary to evaluate these agents in combination with cytotoxic chemotherapy and to identify predictors of response to IGF-1R inhibition.

Role of Surgery and Radiation for Recurrent Ewing Sarcoma

Patients with recurrent Ewing sarcoma typically must respond to systemic therapy for long-term disease control to be possible. However, surgery and radiation also play a role at the time of disease recurrence. One study reported that patients who received surgery for local recurrence had a superior outcome compared with patients who did not receive surgery, although this analysis did not control for the size of the recurrent tumor.[570] This same study reported that whole lung irradiation may benefit patients with isolated pulmonary recurrence.[570] Radiotherapy also plays an important role in controlling pain for patients with refractory Ewing sarcoma.

Pulmonary metastasectomy at relapse has a much more limited role in Ewing sarcoma compared with other diseases, such as osteosarcoma. One group reported that pulmonary metastasectomy did not improve the outcome for patients with Ewing sarcoma and isolated pulmonary relapse.[570] Two groups compared patients who underwent pulmonary metastasectomy and patients with lung metastases that were not resected.[554,600] Both groups suggested that metastasectomy improved the outcome for these patients. However, in both studies patients were selected for resection only in the presence of resectable disease, such that the comparison group may have had a greater burden of disease. Another center described 12 patients with isolated pulmonary relapse treated with surgery alone.[601] Five of these patients remained disease free for at least 3 years. The authors noted that these 12 patients were selected for resection alone on the basis of favorable characteristics, such as a small number of pulmonary nodules and a long period of time from diagnosis to relapse. Whether this strategy would benefit a less favorable group of patients remains to be demonstrated. Currently, pulmonary metastasectomy at relapse is considered mainly for diagnostic purposes and only rarely for therapeutic purposes.

Role of High-Dose Therapy with Hematopoietic Stem Cell Rescue for Recurrent Disease

Some clinicians recommend high-dose therapy as consolidation therapy for patients with recurrent Ewing sarcoma who respond favorably to salvage therapy. Data supporting this approach are relatively limited, particularly because many of the reported studies include both patients with metastatic disease and patients with recurrent disease. Although most studies do not report specific outcomes for patients with recurrent disease, the EICESS group reported that patients treated with high-dose therapy for early relapse had a 5-year event-free survival rate of approximately 45%.[560]

Two reports retrospectively evaluated the impact of high-dose therapy on outcome in patients with recurrent disease. In one series of 64 patients with relapsed disease, seven patients received high-dose therapy with stem cell rescue.[573] The outcomes for these seven patients did not differ from outcomes for patients who received other types of relapse therapy. These results differ from a single-institution report of 55 patients with relapsed Ewing sarcoma, of whom 13 received high-dose therapy with busulfan, melphalan, and thiotepa.[572] Patients who received high-dose therapy had a 5-year progression-free survival rate of 61% compared with 7% for other patients. Because high-dose therapy was offered only to patients who responded to second-line therapy, this report also compared the outcomes of patients who received high-dose therapy and those of patients who had responsive disease but did not receive high-dose therapy. In this analysis high-dose therapy resulted in improved 5-year progression-free survival rate over other therapy (61% versus 21%). A multivariate analysis confirmed that high-dose therapy was an independent predictor of favorable outcome.

Outcomes for Patients with Recurrent Ewing Sarcoma

The outcome for patients with recurrent disease is generally poor. The median overall survival rate from the time of recurrence is 9 to 14 months with current therapies.[568,573] Estimates of 5-year overall survival rates from the time of disease recurrence range from 8% to 23%.[570-573] For patients with recurrent disease, the most widely recognized determinant of outcome is time to disease recurrence. An initial single-institution study noted that four of five patients with relapse more than 5 years from diagnosis were salvaged compared with only 2 of 44 patients with earlier relapses.[575] Follow-up studies have all confirmed this association, including two large cooperative group analyses that both demonstrated that time to relapse was the strongest independent predictor of outcome after first relapse.[568-573] Estimates of 5-year progression-free survival rate for patients with recurrence more than 2 years from initial diagnosis were approximately 30% compared with 7% for earlier relapses.[568,569] Another common finding is that patients with a combined local and distant relapse fare poorly compared with patients who experience either isolated local failure or isolated systemic failure.[568,569] Metastatic site at recurrence has not consistently been associated with outcome after relapse.[568-573]

LATE EFFECTS IN PATIENTS TREATED FOR EWING SARCOMA

Given the nature of the therapy required to treat Ewing sarcoma, patients treated for this disease have an increased risk of developing second cancers. In one large European cohort study, patients with Ewing sarcoma had a thirty-fold increased cumulative risk of developing a solid second cancer 25 years from initial diagnosis.[602] The relative risk that patients will develop a second solid cancer or a bone cancer after Ewing sarcoma was second only to that of patients with an initial primary cancer diagnosis of retinoblastoma.[61,602] In another series survivors of Ewing sarcoma had a risk of second malignancy that was second only to that of survivors of Hodgkin lymphoma.[603] A number of groups have reported that the risk of

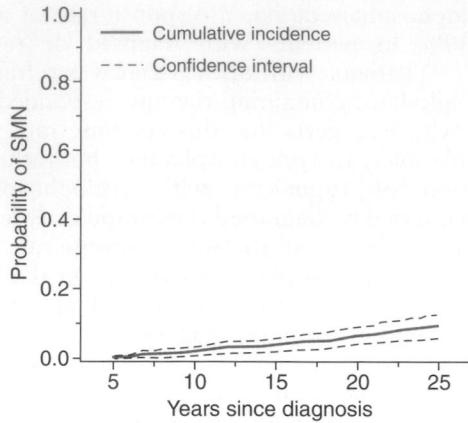

Figure 61-9 Cumulative incidence of second malignancies in patients treated for Ewing sarcoma. *(Ginsberg JP, Goodman P, Leisenring W, et al: Long-term survivors of childhood Ewing sarcoma: report from the childhood cancer survivor study.* J Natl Cancer Inst 102:1272–83, 2010.)

developing any second cancer continues to increase with increasing time from initial diagnosis of Ewing sarcoma. Estimates of the cumulative incidence of developing any second malignancy from the time of initial diagnosis range from 0.7% to 0.9% at 5 years, 2.9% to 6.5% at 10 years, 4.7% at 15 years, 4.7% to 12.7% at 20 years, and 9% at 25 years.[604-608,609-611] Figure 61-9 demonstrates this trend in one representative report from the Childhood Cancer Survivor Study.[609]

Radiation-induced sarcomas and chemotherapy-induced acute leukemia constitute the majority of second malignancies seen in these patients. Osteosarcoma accounts for approximately 25% of the secondary sarcomas, with a variety of other bone and soft tissue sarcomas also observed.[604,606,607,612] Estimates of the cumulative incidence of secondary solid cancers are 1.7% to 1.8% in 10-year survivors and 6% to 22% in 20-year survivors.[61,605,606,611,613] This wide range likely results from variations in sample size, follow-up time, and second malignancy surveillance programs between studies. In almost all cases, these secondary sarcomas arise in the initial radiation field. One group has reported that the incidence of these secondary sarcomas increases with increasing radiation dose, with no cases of secondary sarcoma reported in those patients who received less than 48 Gy.[606]

Secondary acute leukemia occurs significantly earlier than secondary sarcomas in these patients.[604,612] Reported mean latency periods from initial diagnosis of Ewing sarcoma to onset of acute leukemia range from 2.3 to 4.8 years, although some patients have developed secondary acute leukemia while still receiving chemotherapy for Ewing sarcoma.[604,612,614,615] Most of these cases of secondary acute leukemia are acute myeloid leukemia or myelodysplastic syndrome. In one large clinical trial, the cumulative incidence of secondary acute myeloid leukemia or myelodysplastic syndrome was approximately 2% 7 years from the initial diagnosis of Ewing sarcoma, with no additional cases observed beyond that time.[614] These cases are characterized by high frequencies of monosomy

5, monosomy 7, and abnormalities at 11q23.[614,615] These cytogenetic findings suggest a role for alkylating agents (cyclophosphamide and ifosfamide associated with monosomy 5 and monosomy 7) and topoisomerase II inhibitors (doxorubicin and etoposide associated with 11q23 abnormalities) in the pathogenesis of these cases. Interestingly, in protocol INT-0091, the incidence of secondary leukemia, including leukemias with the 11q23 abnormality, did not increase with the addition of ifosfamide and etoposide to the regimen of vincristine, doxorubicin, and cyclophosphamide.[614] However, a report from a single institution suggested that the risk of secondary leukemia was increased with more modern treatment protocols that included etoposide.[611] Increased rates of secondary acute myeloid leukemia have been reported in patients with Ewing sarcoma who received augmented doses of alkylating agents and anthracyclines compared with patients who received conventional doses.[614,615] By way of contrast, in protocol INT-0154 increasing the dose rate of alkylating agents while holding the cumulative dose constant did not increase the rate of secondary leukemias.[438]

Patients treated for Ewing sarcoma are at risk for a variety of late effects in addition to second cancers. Cardiac toxicity from anthracycline therapy can result in significant morbidity and mortality rates for these patients. In one small series 6 of 30 Ewing sarcoma survivors developed echocardiographic shortening fractions less than 20% compared with only 1 of 26 patients with soft tissue sarcomas treated with anthracyclines.[616] Both groups of patients received the same mean doxorubicin dose, but patients with Ewing sarcoma received higher individual doses of doxorubicin at shorter intervals. The addition of ifosfamide to chemotherapy regimens for Ewing sarcoma has resulted in the development of chronic renal tubular dysfunction in a subset of these patients.[617] Patients treated with radiation therapy to the bone are at risk for fractures in the radiation field, with an incidence of approximately 20% in one series of Ewing sarcoma survivors.[618] Use of whole lung radiation for patients with lung metastases may result in acute and late pulmonary toxicity, with one series reporting a 7% incidence of severe pulmonary complications.[619] Patients treated for Ewing sarcoma may have hematologic changes after treatment, including mild thrombocytopenia and macrocytosis.[615] Fertility is impaired among survivors of Ewing sarcoma. In one study 29.7% of female survivors reported a pregnancy compared with 40.1% of female sibling controls.[609] The impact of fertility in male survivors may be even greater, with this same series reporting 11.3% of male survivors siring a pregnancy compared with 33.2% of male sibling controls.[609] Indeed, among 23 male survivors of Ewing sarcoma who underwent sperm analysis, 13 were azospermic, 8 were oligospermic, and only 2 were normospermic.[610]

Several studies have evaluated the psychosocial ramifications of treatment for bone sarcomas, including Ewing sarcoma. A study from the Childhood Cancer Survivor Study reported that survivors of lower-extremity bone tumors overall have excellent self-reported orthopedic function and quality of life.[620] Approximately 5% of these patients reported severe or complete disability. Long-term function and quality of life do not appear to differ between patients who underwent amputation and patients who underwent limb-salvage procedures.[620,621] In another report from the Childhood Cancer Survivor Study, survivors of lower-extremity bone tumors were less likely to be married than sibling controls.[622] In addition, adolescents who underwent amputation were less likely to complete high school and were more likely to have difficulties with health insurance issues compared with sibling controls. Some of these findings were replicated in a single-institution study specific to Ewing sarcoma survivors.[623] In this study survivors had lower rates of employment and marriage than sibling controls, although educational attainment and insurance access did not differ between the two groups. All these studies highlight the importance of evaluation for late effects in survivors of Ewing sarcoma.

FUTURE DIRECTIONS

Remarkable gains have been achieved in the treatment of patients with Ewing sarcoma over the past 40 years. During this same period the understanding of the biology of these tumors has also greatly progressed. Future improvements in the management of this disease will require taking advantage of this improved understanding of the events involved in Ewing sarcoma tumorigenesis. Specific avenues of investigation should include therapies directed at key targets in Ewing sarcoma, including IGF-1R, CD99, mTOR, PARP, and EWS/FLI itself. These therapies will likely be attempted first in those patients with the worst prognosis: patients with metastatic disease and patients with early relapse. Effective targeted therapies in these populations will then be applied to patients with lower-risk disease. Targeted therapy holds the promise not only of improving outcomes for patients with Ewing sarcoma but also of reducing exposure to conventional chemotherapy and the late effects of that therapy. For now, further study of the clinical and molecular prognostic features of this disease is required so that current active agents may be applied in a more risk-adapted approach.

References available online at ExpertConsult.

KEY REFERENCES

1. Ewing J: Diffuse endothelioma of bone. *Proceedings of the New York Pathological Society* 21:17–24, 1921.
   This reference is the original description of Ewing sarcoma and is of historic interest.
5. Gurney JG, Swensen AR, Bulterys M: Malignant bone tumors. In Ries LAG, Smith MA, Gurney JG, et al, editors: *cancer incidence and survival among children and adolescents: United States SEER Program 1975-1995*, Bethesda, MD, 1999, National Cancer Institute, SEER Program, NIH Pub. No. 99-4649, pp 99–110.
   This monograph provides a comprehensive overview of the clinical epidemiology of Ewing sarcoma.
22. Postel-Vinay S, Veron AS, Tirode F, et al: Common variants near TARDBP and EGR2 are associated with susceptibility to Ewing sarcoma. *Nat Genet* 44(3):323–327, 2012.
   This reference reports the outcome of the first genome-wide association study investigating the genetic origins of Ewing sarcoma.

85. Delattre O, Zucman J, Plougastel B, et al: Gene fusion with an ETS DNA-binding domain caused by chromosome translocation in human tumours. *Nature* 359(6391):162–165, 1992.
    This reference describes the original cloning of the EWS/FLI oncoprotein.

143. Sankar S, Bell R, Stephens B, et al: Mechanism and relevance of EWS/FLI-mediated transcriptional repression in Ewing sarcoma. *Oncogene* 32:5089–5100, 2013.
    This is the first biochemical explanation for the transcriptional repressive function of EWS/FLI and suggests that histone deacetylase or lysine-specific demethylase inhibitors could be a therapeutic approach for Ewing sarcoma.

144. May WA, Gishizky ML, Lessnick SL, et al: Ewing sarcoma 11;22 translocation produces a chimeric transcription factor that requires the DNA-binding domain encoded by FLI1 for transformation. *Proc Natl Acad Sci U S A* 90(12):5752–5756, 1993.
    This is the first demonstration that EWS/FLI functions as an oncoprotein.

155. Smith R, Owen LA, Trem DJ, et al: Expression profiling of EWS/FLI identifies NKX2.2 as a critical target gene in Ewing's sarcoma. *Cancer Cell* 9(5):405–416, 2006.
    This paper provides a description of the EWS/FLI expression profile in Ewing sarcoma cells and first identifies NKX2.2 as a critical downstream target gene.

159. Gangwal K, Sankar S, Hollenhorst PC, et al: Microsatellites as EWS/FLI response elements in Ewing's sarcoma. *Proc Natl Acad Sci U S A* 105(29):10149–10154, 2008.
    This paper first describes the GGAA microsatellite as an EWS/FLI binding site and response element.

166. Sorensen PH, Lessnick SL, Lopez-Terrada D, et al: A second Ewing's sarcoma translocation, t(21;22), fuses the EWS gene to another ETS-family transcription factor, ERG. *Nat Genet* 6(2):146–151, 1994.
    This is the first description of an "alternate" fusion protein in Ewing sarcoma, EWS/ERG.

205. Tirode F, Laud-Duval K, Prieur A, et al: Mesenchymal stem cell features of Ewing tumors. *Cancer Cell* 11(5):421–429, 2009.
    This paper provides the first experimental data that Ewing sarcoma could be a tumor derived from a mesenchymal stem cell origin.

210. Khan J, Wei JS, Ringner M, et al: Classification and diagnostic prediction of cancers using gene expression profiling and artificial neural networks. *Nat Med* 7(6):673–679, 2001.
    This report provides the first microarray gene expression profile of Ewing sarcoma.

225. Yee D, Favoni RE, Lebovic GS, et al: Insulin-like growth factor I expression by tumors of neuroectodermal origin with the t(11;22) chromosomal translocation. A potential autocrine growth factor. *J Clin Invest* 86(6):1806–1814, 1990.
    This paper first suggested an autocrine insulin-like growth factor pathway in Ewing sarcoma.

291. Kovar H, Jug G, Aryee DN, et al: Among genes involved in the RB dependent cell cycle regulatory cascade, the p16 tumor suppressor gene is frequently lost in the Ewing family of tumors. *Oncogene* 15(18):2225–2232, 1997.
    This report demonstrates loss of the p16INK4a tumor suppressor in Ewing sarcoma.

294. Kovar H, Auinger A, Jug G, et al: Narrow spectrum of infrequent p53 mutations and absence of MDM2 amplification in Ewing tumours. *Oncogene* 8:2683–2690, 1993.
    This report demonstrates mutation of p53 in Ewing sarcoma.

351. Paulussen M, Ahrens S, Craft AW, et al: Ewing's tumors with primary lung metastases: survival analysis of 114 (European Intergroup) Cooperative Ewing's Sarcoma Studies patients. *J Clin Oncol* 16(9):3044–3052, 1998.
    This report describes the positive impact of whole lung radiotherapy for patients with pulmonary metastatic Ewing sarcoma.

352. Grier HE, Krailo MD, Tarbell NJ, et al: Addition of ifosfamide and etoposide to standard chemotherapy for Ewing's sarcoma and primitive neuroectodermal tumor of bone. *N Engl J Med* 348(8):694–701, 2003.
    This report describes the outcome of a randomized phase III clinical trial that established the positive impact of the use of ifosfamide and etoposide on outcomes in patients with localized Ewing sarcoma.

353. Cotterill SJ, Ahrens S, Paulussen M, et al: Prognostic factors in Ewing's tumor of bone: analysis of 975 patients from the European Intergroup Cooperative Ewing's Sarcoma Study Group. *J Clin Oncol* 18(17):3108–3114, 2000.
    This report describes the largest evaluation of clinical prognostic factors in patients with Ewing sarcoma.

356. Miser JS, Krailo MD, Tarbell NJ, et al: Treatment of metastatic Ewing's sarcoma or primitive neuroectodermal tumor of bone: evaluation of combination ifosfamide and etoposide—a Children's Cancer Group and Pediatric Oncology Group study. *J Clin Oncol* 22(14):2873–2876, 2004.
    This reference reports that patients with metastatic Ewing sarcoma randomized to receive ifosfamide and etoposide added to standard chemotherapy did not have improved outcomes compared with patients randomized to receive standard chemotherapy.

435. Nesbit ME, Jr, Gehan EA, Burgert EO, Jr, et al: Multimodal therapy for the management of primary, nonmetastatic Ewing's sarcoma of bone: a long-term follow-up of the First Intergroup study. *J Clin Oncol* 8(10):1664–1674, 1990.
    This reference reports the outcome of the first cooperative group randomized clinical trial for patients with Ewing sarcoma. This report demonstrated the impact of doxorubicin on outcomes with this disease.

438. Granowetter L, Womer R, Devidas M, et al: Dose-intensified compared with standard chemotherapy for nonmetastatic Ewing sarcoma family of tumors: a Children's Oncology Group Study. *J Clin Oncol* 27(15):2536–2541, 2009.
    This report describes similar outcomes for patients with localized Ewing sarcoma randomized to receive standard-dose chemotherapy or dose-intensified chemotherapy. This was the first cooperative group trial to include patients with soft tissue Ewing sarcoma.

487. Donaldson SS, Torrey M, Link MP, et al: A multidisciplinary study investigating radiotherapy in Ewing's sarcoma: end results of POG #8346. Pediatric Oncology Group. *Int J Radiat Oncol Biol Phys* 42(1):125–135, 1998.
    This reference describes the results of a randomized clinical trial investigating radiation fields in Ewing sarcoma of the bone. This trial established that involved field radiotherapy provided acceptable local control compared with radiotherapy directed to the entire bone.

501. Schuck A, Ahrens S, Paulussen M, et al: Local therapy in localized Ewing tumors: results of 1058 patients treated in the CESS 81, CESS 86, and EICESS 92 trials. *Int J Radiat Oncol Biol Phys* 55(1):168–177, 2003.
    This report describes the largest evaluation to date of local control measures in Ewing sarcoma.

513. Burgert EO, Jr, Nesbit ME, Garnsey LA, et al: Multimodal therapy for the management of nonpelvic, localized Ewing's sarcoma of bone: intergroup study IESS-II. *J Clin Oncol* 8(9):1514–1524, 1990.
    This reference reports the results of a randomized clinical trial that demonstrates improved outcomes with the use of chemotherapy administered as discrete, intermittent cycles compared with protracted administration.

520. Paulussen M, Craft AW, Lewis I, et al: Results of the EICESS-92 Study: two randomized trials of Ewing's sarcoma treatment—cyclophosphamide compared with ifosfamide in standard-risk patients and assessment of benefit of etoposide added to standard treatment in high-risk patients. *J Clin Oncol* 26(27):4385–4393, 2008.
    This reference reports the outcomes of the largest randomized clinical trial conducted to date for patients with Ewing sarcoma. This trial used a risk-adapted approach to guide therapy for patients with low- and high-risk disease.

522. Womer RB, West DC, Krailo MD, et al: Randomized controlled trial of interval-compressed chemotherapy for the treatment of localized Ewing sarcoma: a report from the Children's Oncology Group. *J Clin Oncol* 30(33):4148–4154, 2012.
    This report describes superior outcomes for patients with localized Ewing sarcoma randomized to receive interval compressed chemotherapy administered every 2 weeks compared with outcomes for patients randomized to receive chemotherapy administered with standard timing every 3 weeks.

561. Meyers PA, Krailo MD, Ladanyi M, et al: High-dose melphalan, etoposide, total-body irradiation, and autologous stem-cell reconstitution as consolidation therapy for high-risk Ewing's sarcoma does not improve prognosis. *J Clin Oncol* 19(11):2812–2820, 2001.

This report describes the first cooperative group trial evaluating myeloablative therapy for patients with metastatic Ewing sarcoma. The report concluded that outcomes were no different from those of historical controls treated with standard chemotherapy.

568. Leavey PJ, Mascarenhas L, Marina N, et al: Prognostic factors for patients with Ewing sarcoma (EWS) at first recurrence following multi-modality therapy: a report from the Children's Oncology Group. *Pediatr Blood Cancer* 51(3):334–338, 2008.

This report describes the North American experience with outcomes after recurrent Ewing sarcoma and demonstrates improved outcomes with recurrence after 2 years from initial diagnosis.

569. Stahl M, Ranft A, Paulussen M, et al: Risk of recurrence and survival after relapse in patients with Ewing sarcoma. *Pediatr Blood Cancer* 57(4):549–553, 2011.

This report describes the European experience with outcomes after recurrent Ewing sarcoma and demonstrates outcomes with recurrence after 2 years from initial diagnosis.

594. Tolcher AW, Sarantopoulos J, Patnaik A, et al: Phase I, pharmacokinetic, and pharmacodynamic study of AMG 479, a fully human monoclonal antibody to insulin-like growth factor receptor 1. *J Clin Oncol* 27(34):5800–5807, 2009.

This report provides the first clinical response of Ewing sarcoma to an IGF-1R monoclonal antibody. Subsequent phase II clinical trials confirmed this activity.

609. Ginsberg JP, Goodman P, Leisenring W, et al: Long-term survivors of childhood Ewing sarcoma: report from the childhood cancer survivor study. *J Natl Cancer Inst* 102(16):1272–1283, 2010.

This report provides a comprehensive overview of the burden of late effects in patients treated for Ewing sarcoma.

CHAPTER 62

Osteosarcoma

Katherine Janeway

CHAPTER OUTLINE

Osteosarcoma is the most common primary bone tumor. There are approximately 600 cases/year in the United States.[1] The term *osteosarcoma* was first used in the early 1800s by Alexis Boyer,[2] the imperial family surgeon for Napoleon. Although low-grade forms of osteosarcoma do exist, more than 90% of osteosarcomas are high-grade malignant lesions. Low-grade osteosarcomas will be discussed, but most of what follows pertains to high-grade osteosarcomas.

Osteosarcoma usually occurs in adolescents and young adults. Presenting symptoms can include tumor-related pain with or without a mass, a painless mass, and a pathologic fracture. The distal femur is the most frequent site of primary disease, followed by the proximal tibia and then the proximal femur, hip, and proximal humerus.[3] As early as 1818 it was recognized that untreated patients with osteosarcoma often developed metastatic disease.[2] The most common site of metastasis is the lungs, followed by bone. Metastatic disease is present in approximately 15% of patients at the time of diagnosis.[4]

Prior to the 1970s, when chemotherapy was first used to treat osteosarcoma, overall survival (OS) was approximately 20%. With modern chemotherapy and surgical control, the 10-year OS of patients with localized osteosarcoma is around 70%.[5] The OS is much worse for patients with metastases at diagnosis and for those with relapsed disease. In both groups, the 5-year OS rate is approximately 25%.[4,6,7] The most active chemotherapy agents in osteosarcoma are doxorubicin (Doxo), cisplatin (CP), and high-dose methotrexate (HDMTX). Ifosfamide and etoposide are also active against osteosarcoma and are typically used in addition to Doxo, CP, and HDMTX in patients with metastatic disease and in patients with recurrence.

In the past three decades, a number of discoveries have led to a better understanding of osteosarcoma biology. For example, the tumor suppressor gene *TP53* and the retinoblastoma gene *RB1* are altered in osteosarcoma. Oncogenes, including *MYC, MET,* and *FOS,* have also been implicated in osteosarcomagenesis. These tumor suppressors, oncogenes, and other biologic factors will be discussed in detail. Unlike most childhood cancers, there has been minimal improvement in OS over the past three decades.[8,9] Consequently, one of the research priorities in osteosarcoma is the identification of additional active therapies.

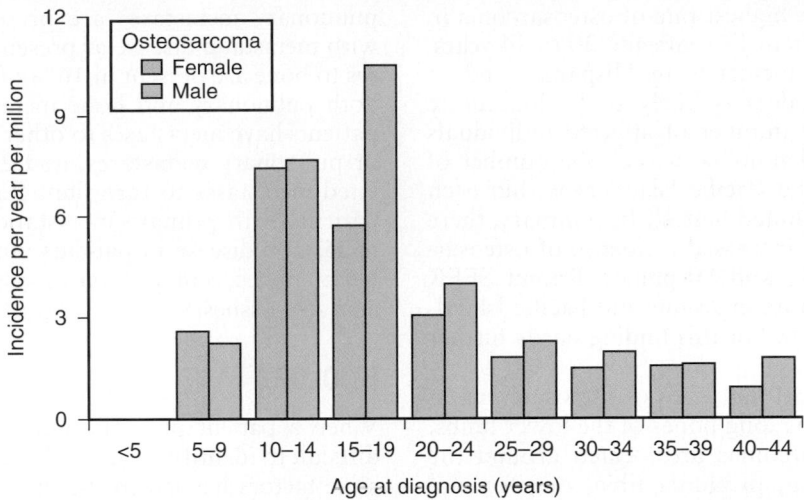

Figure 62-1 Age Distribution of osteosarcoma based on U.S. cases between 1975 and 1999. *(Data from Bleyer A, O'Leary M, Barr R, et al, editors: Cancer epidemiology in older adolescents and young adults 15 to 29 years of age, including SEER incidence and survival: 1975-2000. NIH publication No. 06-5767. Bethesda, Md., 2006, National Cancer Institute.)*

EPIDEMIOLOGY

Osteosarcoma is the most common primary bone tumor in children.[1] The average annual incidence of osteosarcoma in children younger than 20 years in the United States is 4.8/million. Approximately 3% of all malignancies in this age group are osteosarcomas. In 2000, the most recent year for which data are available, there were 410 cases of osteosarcoma in children from birth to 19 years of age in the United States. There were an additional 135 cases in young adults aged 20 to 29.[1] Internationally, incidence rates approximate the U.S. rate, with the exception of a higher incidence in some African countries. In Sudan and Uganda, the osteosarcoma incidence in children younger than 14 years is 5.3 and 6.4/million respectively, compared with an incidence of between 2 and 3/million in this age group in the United States, Europe, and Asia.[10,11]

Osteosarcoma occurs rarely in children younger than 5 years. After age 5, the incidence increases steadily, reaching a peak at age 15 years.[12] After the adolescent peak, the rate of osteosarcoma steadily declines, leveling off at a rate of 1 to 2/million. A second peak in incidence, approximately half the magnitude of the adolescent peak, occurs in the sixth to seventh decade.[13,14] Osteosarcoma in older patients is associated with Paget disease and prior radiation therapy, although approximately half of older patients with osteosarcoma have neither condition.[15] The adolescent peak occurs at age 13 years in girls and between ages 15 and 17 years in boys (Fig. 62-1). The age at peak incidence corresponds to the age of greatest growth velocity in each gender. This association contributes to the evidence supporting a role for growth in the cause of osteosarcoma (see "Etiology"). Osteosarcoma is slightly more common in males, particularly in the 15- to 19-year-old age group.

In the United States, osteosarcoma is slightly more common in African Americans, Hispanics, and Asians and Pacific Islanders (Fig. 62-2). Several studies have reported that rates of osteosarcoma in black children younger than 14 years are about twice those in white children of the same age.[16,17] In the most recent report on osteosarcoma from the Surveillance, Epidemiology, and End Results (SEER) Program of the National Cancer Institute, U.S. blacks younger than 20 years continue to have a slightly higher rate of osteosarcoma.[12] As shown in Figure 62-2, for the age group 15 to 29 years, the racial group with the highest rate of osteosarcoma is Hispanic. The relative risk of developing osteosarcoma for Hispanic children younger than 14 years of age, based on data collected between 1975 and 2003, is 1.3.[18] Asians and

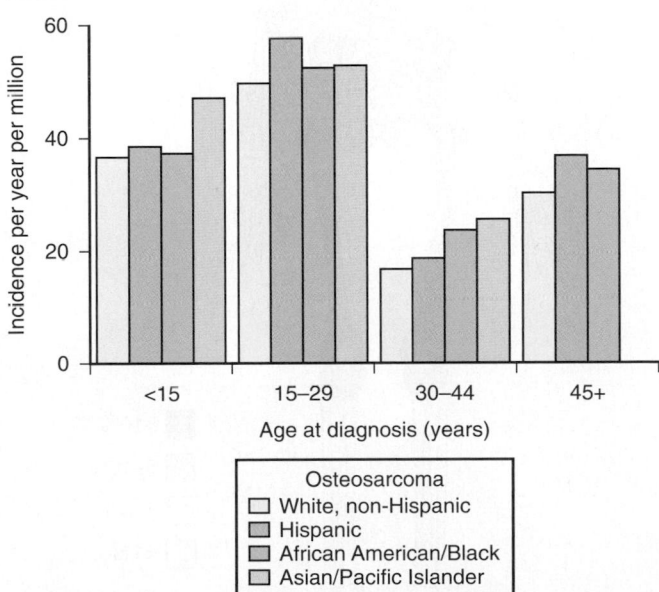

Figure 62-2 Incidence of osteosarcoma by racial group based on U.S. cases between 1990 and 1999. *(Data from Bleyer A, O'Leary M, Barr R, et al, editors: Cancer epidemiology in older adolescents and young adults 15 to 29 years of age, including SEER incidence and survival: 1975-2000. NIH publication No. 06-5767. Bethesda, Md. 2006, National Cancer Institute.)*

Pacific Islanders have the highest rate of osteosarcoma in the age groups younger than 15 years and 30 to 44 years. However, the reported incidence in Hispanics and in Asians and Pacific Islanders is likely to be inaccurate given the small absolute number of affected individuals and uncertainty in the denominator (i.e., the number of Hispanics and Asians and Pacific Islanders within each age group living in the United States). In summary, there is evidence for a slightly increased incidence of osteosarcoma among U.S. blacks and Hispanics. Recent SEER data show an increased rate in Asians and Pacific Islanders younger than 15 years, but this finding needs further investigation.

The most common anatomic sites of osteosarcoma at initial presentation are the long bones of the lower limbs. Fifty percent of osteosarcomas are located around the knee, in the distal femur, proximal tibia, or proximal fibula (Fig. 62-3). Approximately 10% of tumors occur in the mid or proximal femur, and 9% occur in the proximal humerus.[3,12] Of patients with osteosarcoma, 10% to 20% have metastatic disease at initial presentation. The most common site of metastasis is the lungs. Isolated pulmonary metastases are present in 61% of patients with metastatic disease at presentation. Isolated metastases to bone are present in 16% of patients, and 14% have both pulmonary and bone metastases. Seven percent of patients have metastases to other rare sites plus bone and/or pulmonary metastases, and 2% of patients have isolated metastases to rare sites. Rare sites of metastasis in patients with primary metastatic disease, as opposed to metastatic disease in patients with recurrent disease, are lymph nodes, central nervous system, liver, adrenal gland, and soft tissues.[4]

ETIOLOGY

When a patient presents with osteosarcoma, it is often difficult to identify a cause. However, recognition of causative factors has led to the discovery of biologic mechanisms of transformation, as in the case of predisposition to osteosarcoma in Li-Fraumeni syndrome, or the identification of exposures to be avoided, as in the case of radiation-induced osteosarcoma. Inherited syndromes in which there is an increased occurrence of osteosarcoma are hereditary retinoblastoma and Li-Fraumeni, Rothmund-Thomson, Bloom, and Werner syndromes. There is a clear association between the risk for osteosarcoma and prior radiation therapy or treatment with alkylating chemotherapy. Epidemiologic studies and clinical observation have suggested that increased height may be a risk factor for the development of osteosarcoma. Finally, environmental exposures to radium and beryllium likely increase the risk for osteosarcoma, but exposure to high doses of these agents is rare.

As noted, peak rates of osteosarcoma coincide with the period of maximal linear growth during puberty. Most osteosarcomas occurring in the adolescent age group are in the long bones of the axial skeleton, the bones in which the most active growth occurs. These clinical observations have led to the hypothesis that the hormonal milieu during maximal linear growth encourages the development of osteosarcoma and that, by extension, osteosarcoma would be more common in taller adolescents. Multiple epidemiologic studies have addressed this question,[19-24] but results are contradictory. Approximately 50% of the studies have found that osteosarcoma patients are taller at diagnosis than age-matched controls or the normal population.[22-24] The remaining studies have not supported an association between height and the occurrence of osteosarcoma.[19-21] The larger studies[23] and those with more reliable sources of height data[22] have shown a positive association between tall stature and osteosarcoma. These data, in part, have led to the investigation of the insulin-like growth factor axis in osteosarcoma (see "Biology").

Approximately 1% of patients develop secondary bone tumors after treatment of a primary pediatric malignancy[25]; of these secondary bone tumors, 50% to 80% are osteosarcomas. On the other hand, secondary Ewing sarcoma is rare.[25,26] The relative risk of secondary osteosarcoma increases greatly with radiation doses to the bone higher than 1000 cGy. In patients who received between 3000 and 5000 cGy to the bone during

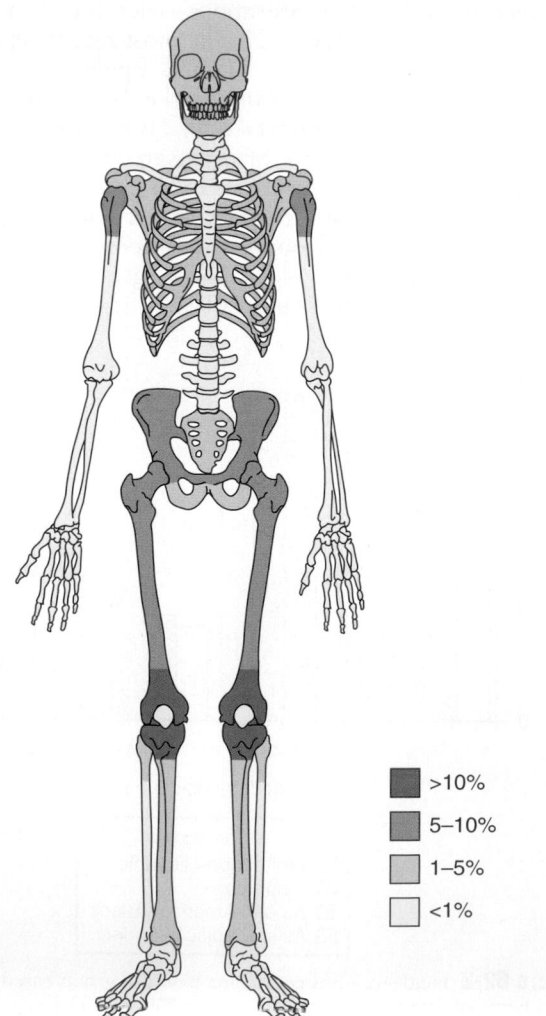

Figure 62-3 Anatomic sites of osteosarcoma at initial presentation. *(Modified from Dahlin DC, Unni KK: Osteosarcoma of bone and its important recognizable varieties. Am J Surg Pathol 1:61–72, 1977.)*

>10%

5–10%

1–5%

<1%

treatment of their primary pediatric malignancy, the relative risk of secondary osteosarcoma was variably reported, but it may be as high as 100.[25,27] A study in patients with primary Ewing sarcoma has concluded that only higher radiation doses increase the risk for secondary sarcomas, with no tumors developing in patients who had received less than 4800 cGy. The highest risk, 130 cases/10,000 person-years of observation, was observed among patients who had received 6000 cGy or more.[28] In the 92 published cases of secondary osteosarcoma for whom radiation dose was reported, the median radiation dose delivered was 4500 to 5400 cGy.[29] The average time between diagnosis of the primary malignancy and development of secondary osteosarcoma is 10 years.[26] Another factor that increases the likelihood that survivors of a primary cancer will develop secondary osteosarcoma is treatment with alkylating agents. This class of chemotherapy increases the relative risk of secondary osteosarcoma by a factor of 5.[25]

Data regarding an increased risk for cancer in people exposed to low levels of radiation from the atomic bombs in Hiroshima and Nagasaki have led to increased concern about the risk of diagnostic imaging with x-rays and computed tomographic (CT) scans, particularly in pediatric patients.[30] However, current evidence does not suggest that osteosarcoma risk would be increased from commonly used imaging modalities.[31] In particular, the radiation dose of a CT scan is approximately 6 cGy and the risk for bone cancer in pediatric cancer survivors who received less than 1000 cGy to the bone is not increased.[25]

Osteosarcoma is seen in a number of inherited cancer predisposition syndromes. These syndromes have often illuminated mechanisms of transformation in sporadic osteosarcoma. Children with hereditary retinoblastoma have a germline heterozygous, inactivating deletion, and/or a frameshift or point mutation of the tumor suppressor gene retinoblastoma 1 (RB1). Affected children develop retinoblastoma usually in one or both eyes. The cumulative incidence of a nonretinoblastoma malignancy in hereditary retinoblastoma is 51%, and approximately 40% of these second malignancies are osteosarcomas.[32] Both osteosarcomas and retinoblastomas in these patients have loss of heterozygosity of the RB1 allele, resulting in a complete loss of RB1 function. As discussed later (see "Biology"), loss of RB1 function also occurs in sporadic osteosarcomas.[33,34]

In the Li-Fraumeni syndrome, patients carry a heterozygous inactivating mutation of the tumor suppressor gene TP53. Affected individuals have a greatly increased cancer risk at a young age. The most common malignancies are breast cancer and bone and soft tissue sarcomas, brain tumors, and leukemia.[35] Slightly more than 10% of the malignancies in patients with Li-Fraumeni syndrome are osteosarcomas. Among patients with Li-Fraumeni syndrome, mutations in the TP53 DNA-binding domain (as compared with mutations outside the DNA-binding domain or null mutations) are associated with early sarcomas.[36] Patients with osteosarcomas and other cancers that develop in Li-Fraumeni syndrome have loss of the normal TP53 allele consistent with the tumor suppressor function of the TP53 gene product. Loss of TP53 function

by TP53 mutation or amplification of MDM2 or COPS3 is also present in most sporadic osteosarcomas (see "Biology").[37]

Rothmund-Thomson, Bloom, and Werner syndromes are members of a family of autosomal recessive disorders caused by mutations in one of the RECQ DNA helicases. Rothmund-Thomson syndrome, caused by mutations in the RECQL4 gene, is characterized by rash, skeletal dysplasias, and sparse hair. Up to 30% of patients with Rothmund-Thomson syndrome develop osteosarcoma at a slightly younger age than in sporadic osteosarcoma.[38,39] Bloom syndrome, caused by mutations in the BLM (RECQL2) gene, is characterized by short stature, telangiectasia, and an increased risk for developing a wide variety of cancers at a young age.[40] Unlike in Rothmund-Thomson syndrome, only a small percentage of cancers occurring in affected individuals are osteosarcomas. Werner syndrome is caused by a mutation in the WRN (RECQL3) gene. Patients have scleroderma-like skin changes, premature aging, and a typical body habitus with short stature, long spindly limbs, and a stocky trunk. Like in Bloom syndrome, the risk for developing cancer at a young age is increased in Werner syndrome. Also like in Bloom syndrome, osteosarcoma constitutes fewer than 10% of the malignancies occurring in patients with Werner syndrome.[41] For a further discussion of the role of RECQ DNA helicases in osteosarcoma, see "Biology".

The risk for developing osteosarcoma is increased in adults with Paget disease. In Paget disease, which affects up to 1% of adults older than the age of 40 years, bone resorption by osteoclasts is increased. As a result, there is a compensatory increase in osteoblast activity and bone formation.[42] Osteosarcoma develops in less than 1% of patients with Paget disease, but this represents a higher rate than that seen in the general population. The average age of patients with Paget disease–related osteosarcoma is 70 years.[15]

A single genome-wide association study has been conducted in osteosarcoma. There are two susceptibility loci achieving statistical significance in osteosarcoma. One locus occurs in a gene desert and the other, at 6p21.3, implicates GRM4, a glutamate receptor gene involved in inhibition of the cyclic adenosine monophosphate (AMP) cascade.[43]

Previously, some believed that trauma may cause osteosarcoma. However, modern epidemiologic studies have not supported a relationship between trauma and osteosarcoma.[20] Prior observations linking trauma and osteosarcoma were likely the result of the fact that a traumatic event may result in a previously existing osteosarcoma being brought to medical attention.

Environmental exposures, other than ionizing radiation, for which there is evidence of an association between exposure and osteosarcoma risk, include exposure to radium and beryllium. Radium is a radioactive element that is variably present in well water. When ingested, radium retained in the body is deposited in bone. Studies of those exposed to high levels of radium while painting dials on clocks in the 1920s strongly indicated that exposure to high doses of radium causes osteosarcoma.[44] The risk for osteosarcoma from exposure to low levels of radium in drinking water is less clear. Two studies have shown a slight increase in risk for bone sarcoma or osteosarcoma in those born in areas with drinking water containing relatively high concentrations of radium.[45,46] Conversely, two studies have shown no link between mean levels of radium in water and osteosarcoma.[46,47] Beryllium is a metallic element with limited use in the production of aerospace structural material, x-ray tubes, and nuclear reactors. Although intravenous injection of beryllium salts causes osteosarcoma in rabbits, there is limited evidence of an increased risk for osteosarcoma caused by beryllium exposure in humans.[48] Case-control studies have failed to identify other environmental or occupational exposures that increase the risk for osteosarcoma.[24] Because fluoride can stimulate bone formation there has been concern about a possible relationship between fluoride in drinking water and osteosarcoma. This is a very difficult question to study adequately given that multiple factors beyond water fluoridation may impact fluoride intake. So far, there is no substantial evidence to support a causative association between fluoride exposure and osteosarcoma.[49]

CLINICAL PRESENTATION AND EVALUATION

Clinical, laboratory, and radiologic findings are often highly suggestive of osteosarcoma but are not pathognomonic. Biopsy is always required for diagnosis. Atypical imaging characteristics, including a benign appearance in

Box 62-1   Differential Diagnosis of Osteosarcoma
OTHER MALIGNANT PRIMARY BONE TUMORS
Ewing sarcoma
Chondrosarcoma
Fibrosarcoma
Langerhans cell histiocytosis
OTHER MALIGNANCIES PRESENTING AS BONE TUMOR(S)
Lymphoma
Neuroblastoma
Metastatic rhabdomyosarcoma
Metastatic melanoma
BENIGN BONE TUMORS
Aneurysmal bone cyst
Osteoblastoma
Osteoid osteoma
Giant cell tumor
Unicameral bone cyst
INFECTION
Osteomyelitis

high-grade osteosarcoma, have been described.[50] The differential diagnosis of osteosarcoma includes benign and malignant bone tumors (Box 62-1; Fig. 62-4).

Clinical Manifestations

Clinical symptoms of osteosarcoma are nonspecific; 25% of patients have pain and a palpable mass at presentation,

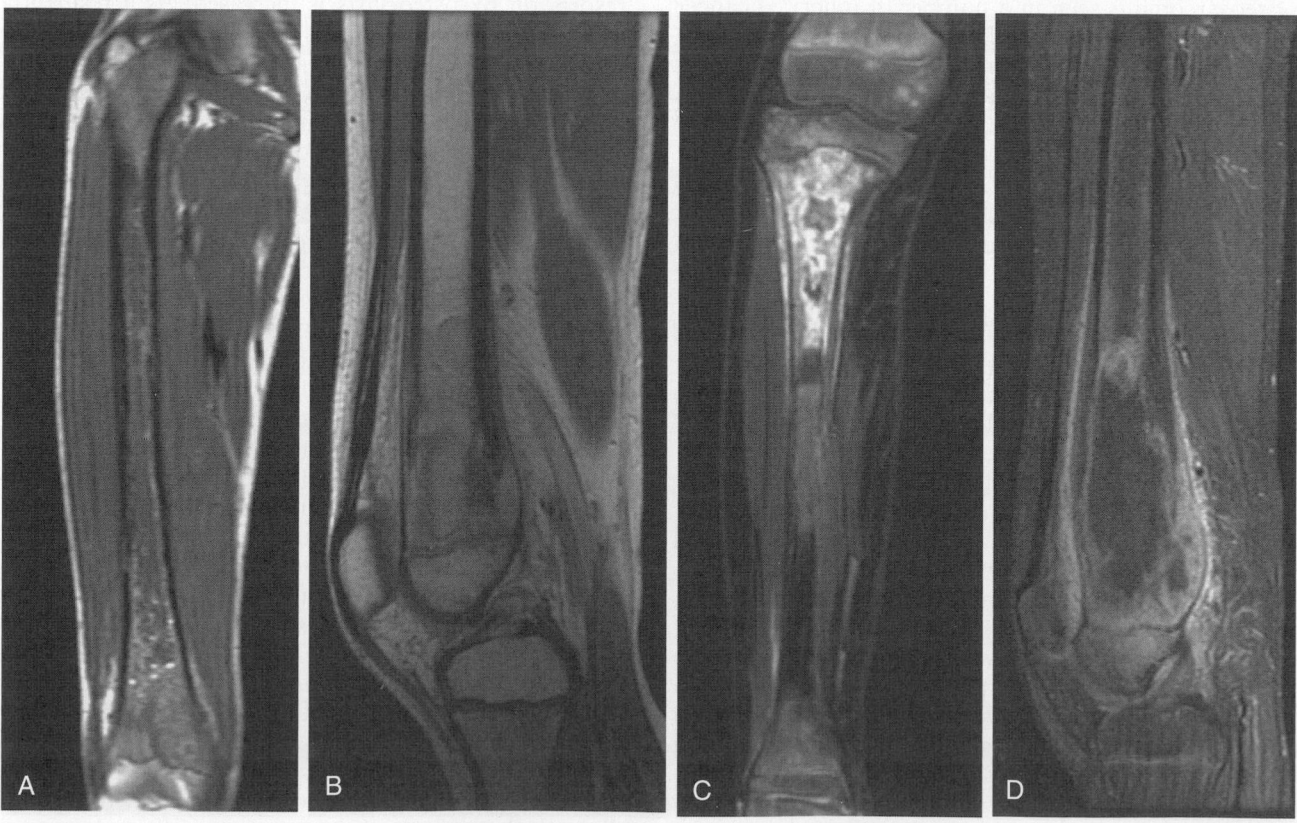

Figure 62-4 MRI appearance of osteosarcoma and lesions that can be confused with osteosarcoma in clinical presentation and radiographic appearance. **A,** Osteomyelitis of the femur. **B,** Lymphoma of the distal femur. **C,** Ewing sarcoma of the proximal tibia. **D,** Osteosarcoma of the distal femur.

and 70% of patients present with pain as their only complaint. Pain tends to be intermittent and exacerbated by activity. The remaining patients present with a painless mass.[51] The duration of symptoms before diagnosis ranges from 1 day to 5 years, with a median of about 2½ months. In approximately 10% of patients, symptom duration is longer than 6 months.[52] A pathologic fracture is present in 8% of patients at the time of diagnosis.[53]

Radiologic Evaluation

Radiologic evaluation in osteosarcoma informs the initial diagnostic impression, aids in the determination of the best approach for biopsy, facilitates surgical resection, and identifies sites of metastatic disease, if present. The recommended imaging studies for osteosarcoma at the time of diagnosis are plain radiography and magnetic resonance imaging (MRI) of the primary tumor site to evaluate the extent of local disease, a bone scan to screen for bony metastases, and a CT scan of the chest to determine whether pulmonary metastases are present. Whenever possible, these imaging studies should be performed before diagnostic biopsy because postsurgical atelectasis interferes with evaluation of the lung parenchyma. MRI of the primary tumor should include the entire bone from which the tumor arises and the closest adjacent joint to

screen for skip metastases properly. An additional MR image should be obtained after neoadjuvant chemotherapy has been given but before definitive resection to determine the best plan for the surgical approach.

A plain radiograph of the primary tumor has usually been obtained before referral to an oncologist or orthopedist. Most appendicular osteosarcomas are located in the metaphyseal portion of the long bone. Both lytic destruction of bone and sclerotic irregular new bone formation can occur. Osteosarcoma usually has a mixed pattern of bone lysis and sclerosis, but one of these patterns can predominate. Regardless of the predominant pattern, the boundary between tumor and normal bone is usually irregular. The bone cortex is often disrupted by tumor growth into the surrounding soft tissue. Osteoid formation within the tumor results in areas of calcification visible in the bony and soft tissue components of the tumor. Periosteal new bone formation in osteosarcoma can be irregular or can occur in a sunburst pattern. "Sunburst" refers to linear new bone growth that is perpendicular to the bony cortex and arranged in a fanlike pattern (Fig. 62-5).[54] In contrast, in Ewing sarcoma, periosteal new bone growth typically occurs in an onionskin pattern in which linear new bone is oriented parallel to the bony cortex.[3] Periosteal new bone formation in

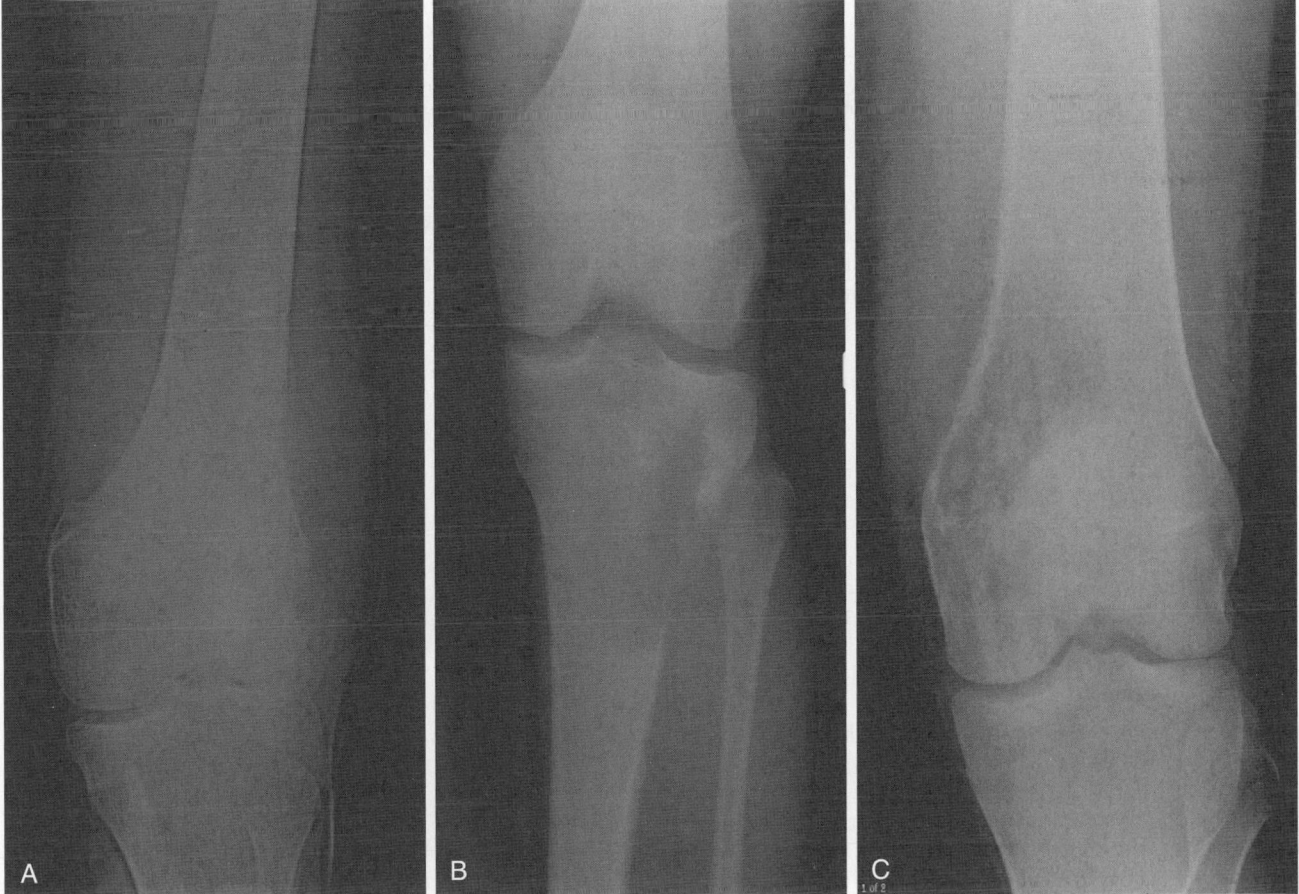

Figure 62-5 Three typical patterns observed in plain radiographs of osteosarcoma. **A,** Predominantly sclerotic pattern in an osteosarcoma of the distal femur with sunburst periosteal new bone formation. **B,** Predominantly lytic pattern in an osteosarcoma of the proximal tibia. **C,** Mixed lytic and sclerotic pattern in an osteosarcoma of the distal femur.

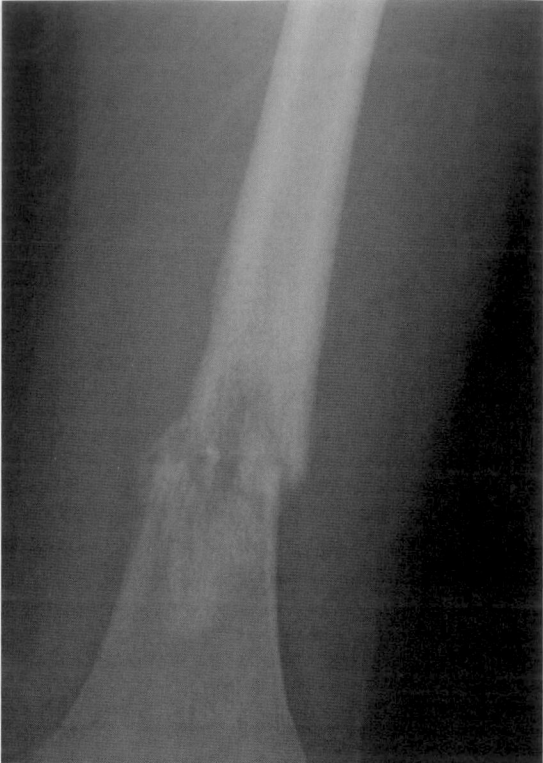

Figure 62-6 Pathologic fracture in an osteosarcoma of the distal femur.

osteosarcoma can also be present at the edge of the preserved cortex, resulting in the Codman triangle. Plain radiographs also assist in the diagnosis of pathologic fractures (Fig. 62-6).

Although plain radiographs of the primary tumor are informative, MRI is preferable for local staging, presurgical planning, and identification of skip metastases. CT is an acceptable alternative to MRI, but most orthopedic surgeons and oncologists prefer MRI. In two studies directly comparing preoperative CT and MRI results with pathologic findings in patients with osteosarcoma, MRI was found to be superior to CT in defining the longitudinal extent of intraosseous tumor,[55,56] extension into adjacent muscle compartments, and involvement of the neurovascular bundle. The two modalities were equivalent in their ability to define cortical bone and joint involvement. However, a more recent study in a larger patient population did not find a statistically significant difference between CT and MRI in their ability to predict the involvement of bone, muscle, joints, and the neurovascular bundle.[57] One possible explanation for the contradictory results is improvements in CT quality during the interval between the studies. In addition, the later study grouped all primary bone tumors together for analysis but, given that 60% of the bone tumors were osteosarcoma, results would likely be similar for osteosarcomas alone. In comparison to CT and technetium-99 m (^{99m}Tc) bone scanning, MRI more accurately predicts the intraosseous extent of osteosarcoma.[56] The presence of significant edema has been associated with inaccurate assessment of the margins of tumor on MRI. Because edema can

resolve with chemotherapy, imaging performed for the purpose of surgical planning should be obtained after the administration of neoadjuvant chemotherapy.[58]

A *skip metastasis* is defined as a smaller distinct focus of osteosarcoma that is either within the same bone as the primary tumor or on the other side of the joint adjacent to the primary tumor.[59] There must be normal structures not involved with tumor present between the primary tumor and skip metastasis. Skip metastases are synchronous with the primary tumor and thus are present at initial presentation. Diagnosis of skip metastases is of critical importance for prognostication and because complete surgical remission in osteosarcoma with skip metastases requires complete resection of both the primary tumor and skip metastases. Over 80% of skip metastases are visible on MR images (Fig. 62-7). In contrast, skip metastases are visible on bone scan, CT scans, and plain radiographs in only 46%, 45%, and 36% of cases, respectively.[60] Interestingly, a common reason for failure to identify skip metastases by bone scanning is merging of the signal from the primary tumor with the signal from the skip metastasis.[61] To ensure that skip metastases are identified, MRI of the primary tumor should include the entire bone and adjacent joint. Bony metastases that are not skip metastases are best identified with a ^{99m}Tc bone scan (Fig. 62-8).[61] The usefulness of ^{18}F-labeled fluorodeoxyglucose positron emission tomography (FDG-PET) in osteosarcoma has not yet been adequately evaluated. Results of preliminary studies have suggested that FDG-PET is more useful for assessing tumor response to chemotherapy and for posttherapeutic

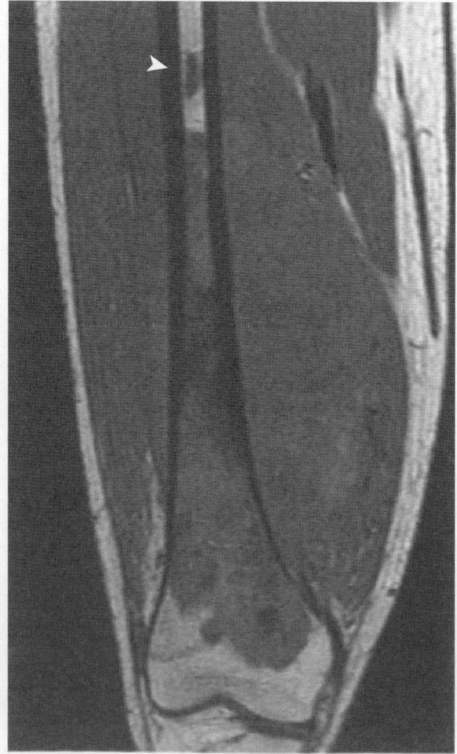

Figure 62-7 Skip metastasis *(arrowhead)* of an osteosarcoma of the distal femur as seen on T1-weighted MR image.

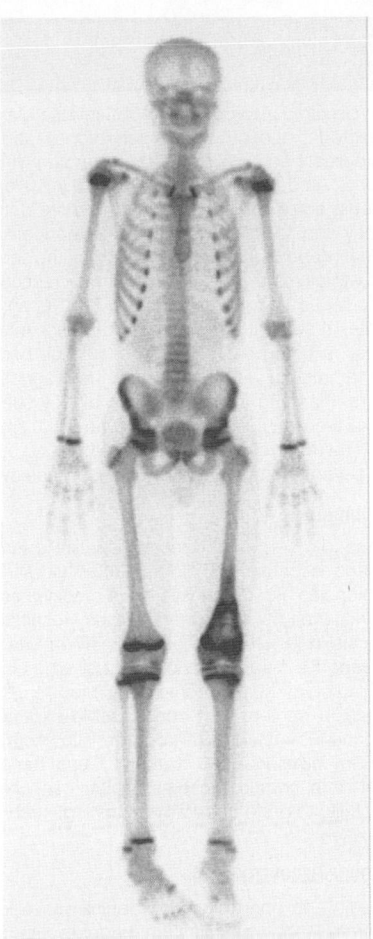

Figure 62-8 Technetium-99 m bone scan showing an osteosarcoma of the distal femur without distant bony metastases.

monitoring for recurrence than for assessing the initial tumor.[62] Because edema can resolve with chemotherapy, imaging performed for the purpose of surgical planning should be performed after the administration of neoadjuvant chemotherapy.[58]

CT of the chest is the most sensitive radiologic study for detection of pulmonary metastases. A generally accepted definition of definitive pulmonary metastatic disease is three or more lesions 5 mm or larger or one lesion 1 cm or larger.[63] The interpretation of very small lesions (<5 mm) and solitary lesions between 5 mm and 1 cm detected by high-resolution CT can be difficult. In some cases, it is not possible to determine whether such CT findings represent metastatic disease or a nonmalignant lung process, and biopsy may be needed. Compared with a CT scan, a plain radiograph of the chest has a sensitivity of 57% and a ^{99m}Tc bone scan has a sensitivity of 41%.[64] Although CT is highly sensitive, evaluation at the time of thoracotomy usually reveals more pulmonary metastases than are appreciated on the CT scan.[65] Importantly, chest CT scans should be obtained before biopsy of the primary tumor because postanesthesia atelectasis makes chest CT scans more difficult to interpret.

Whole-body MRI screening as a method of surveillance in patients with cancer predisposition is currently being evaluated. In a small group or individuals (n = 25) with hereditary retinoblastoma, whole-body MRI detected two cases of osteosarcoma. An additional individual was diagnosed with osteosarcoma due to symptoms.[66] A screening protocol including whole-body MRI utilized in individuals with Li-Fraumeni syndrome detected no cases of osteosarcoma but did detect one case of malignant fibrous histiocytoma.[67]

Biopsy

Traditionally, bone tumor tissue for pathologic examination was obtained by open biopsy. However, percutaneous core needle biopsies have become more common as the availability and sophistication of interventional radiology services have increased. A number of retrospective series have reported on the diagnostic yield and accuracy of core needle biopsies in osteosarcoma.[68-73] Although none specifically studies pediatric osteosarcoma, all series that provide patient age included children. In these published series, core needle biopsy resulted in a definitive, correct diagnosis in 78% to 94% of cases. The more recently published series have reported a diagnostic accuracy of 90% or greater.[69,73] However, even those percutaneous biopsies that yield sufficient tumor material for a diagnosis often do not yield sufficient tumor specimen for other biologic studies.

The outcome of percutaneous biopsy varies depending on the provider, technique, and patient population. In the published series reporting a high diagnostic yield, biopsies were performed by experienced interventional radiologists in consultation with orthopedic surgeons in tertiary or referral centers with considerable expertise in the diagnosis and management of bone tumors. In the more recent series, patients underwent conscious sedation or were given general anesthesia. Specific techniques included the use of fluoroscopic, CT, or ultrasound guidance and use of at least a 14-gauge needle. The tumor component targeted for biopsy was the soft tissue mass, if present, followed by the lytic aspect of an intraosseous lesion.

The most common reason for failure to obtain diagnostic tissue by core needle biopsy is the presence of a highly sclerotic tumor.[70,71] Of the various types of osteosarcoma, telangiectatic osteosarcoma most often results in a nondiagnostic specimen or is misdiagnosed.[69,70] Development of osteosarcoma in a percutaneous biopsy tract has been reported.[74] Therefore, it is important that the biopsy site be located so that it can be resected en bloc with the primary tumor. Because fine-needle aspiration has a diagnostic yield lower than core needle biopsy[68] and does not obviate the need for sedation in the pediatric population, it is not a recommended approach for diagnosis.

Surgical or open biopsy of bone tumors can be incisional or excisional. Excisional biopsy is almost never performed in osteosarcoma because neoadjuvant chemotherapy can decrease tumor edema and, in doing so, simplify resection. In addition, time is required for adequate surgical planning, especially for younger children in whom placement of a growing prosthesis is being considered. Complications of open biopsy include anesthesia-related events, infection, bleeding, and tumor seeding in the biopsy tract.[75] In addition, disruption of anatomic compartments and incorrect localization of the biopsy incision can lead to a more complex or more extensive tumor resection and can occasionally result in an amputation that would not have otherwise been necessary.[76] As with percutaneous biopsy, the incision for an open biopsy should be placed and oriented in a way that allows it to be excised en bloc with the primary tumor. Complications of open biopsy, including those that result in more extensive resections, are unusual when the biopsy is performed at a center specializing in the diagnosis and treatment of malignant bone tumors.[77]

In summary, the percutaneous and open biopsy routes are both acceptable. Given the implications for ultimate surgical resection of a poorly performed biopsy, biopsy should be performed or planned by an orthopedic surgeon with bone tumor expertise, ideally by the same orthopedic surgeon who will perform the ultimate resection. Percutaneous biopsies should only be performed by experienced interventional radiology staff working in conjunction with an experienced orthopedic surgeon. If the percutaneous route is recommended, it is important to counsel patients and families about the possible risks of core needle biopsy, including the potential for an inconclusive specimen. For a further discussion of the debate regarding the correct route for bone tumor biopsy, see Box 62-2.

Laboratory Evaluation

Laboratory test results are often normal in osteosarcoma. When laboratory abnormalities are present, they are nonspecific, having many other potential causes. The serum alkaline phosphatase level is elevated in approximately 50% of patients presenting with osteosarcoma.[78,79] A higher percentage of patients with metastatic disease have a high alkaline phosphatase level, but this is not a reliable test of metastatic disease, because some patients with metastatic disease will have a normal result. As will be discussed later, alkaline phosphatase elevations are associated with a poorer prognosis. Lactate dehydrogenase (LDH) is elevated in approximately 30% of osteosarcoma patients.[80] The erythrocyte sedimentation rate is generally not elevated in patients with osteosarcoma, whereas it is often elevated in those with Ewing sarcoma.

PATHOLOGY AND STAGING

Pathology

On gross examination, osteosarcoma usually presents as a large mass located in the metaphysis (Fig. 62-9) arising in the medullary cavity and crossing the bony cortex, with invasion into the adjacent soft tissues. Microscopically, the malignant cells are pleomorphic but spindle cells typically predominate. Epithelioid, small round cells, multinucleated giant cells, and plasmacytoid cells may also be present and occasionally are the predominant morphology.[81] Osteoid, which can be plentiful or sparse, is currently essential for the diagnosis of osteosarcoma. Sometimes, it is not present in the initial biopsy sample but is seen in the definitive resection specimen. If not

---

Box 62-2 Controversies in Osteosarcoma: Open vs. Core Needle Biopsy

There are two possible approaches to obtaining a diagnostic specimen in suspected osteosarcoma—open biopsy and core needle biopsy. Considerable controversy exists regarding which diagnostic approach is best. An open biopsy is performed in the operating room by an orthopedic surgeon. As discussed in more detail in the text, an open biopsy should be performed by orthopedic surgeon with experience treating bone tumors and ideally by the same orthopedic surgeon who will ultimately perform the tumor resection. In a core needle biopsy, while imaging the tumor with CT, an interventional radiologist obtains several needle cores of tumor material. As with an open biopsy, a core needle biopsy should be performed by an interventional radiologist with expertise in the diagnostic evaluation of bone tumors. Planning for core needle biopsy should include a discussion with the orthopedic surgeon who will ultimately perform the resection. The relative merits of core needle and open biopsy as they relate to several core issues are discussed below:

1. DEFINITIVE DIAGNOSIS

Because orthopedic surgeons directly visualize a tumor during an open biopsy and because pathologists often view frozen sections during open biopsies, nondiagnostic open biopsies are uncommon. In retrospective series,[68-73] core needle biopsy results in a definitive, correct diagnosis in 78% to 94% of cases. The more recently published series report a diagnostic accuracy of 90% or more.[69,73] The interventional radiology-guided core needle biopsies in these studies were performed in centers with considerable experience with the diagnosis of bone tumors and similar diagnostic accuracy would not be expected in inexperienced centers. Less tumor material is obtained from core needle biopsies, which can compromise the pathologist's ability to perform additional testing, such as cytogenetics, in some cases.

2. POSTPROCEDURE RECOVERY

Both core needle and open biopsies require general anesthesia in children. In general, open biopsies are longer procedures, requiring a greater length of general anesthesia. Open biopsies are also more invasive and result in a longer postprocedure recovery.

3. IMPACT ON ULTIMATE RESECTION

Whether the biopsy approach is core needle or open, definitive surgical treatment of osteosarcoma, which is essential for cure, requires excision of the biopsy tract or site en bloc with the primary tumor. A poorly placed biopsy can convert a tumor amenable to limb-sparing surgery into one that requires amputation. This impact on ultimate resectability is one of the greatest potential negative aspects of core needle biopsy. Because interventional radiologists are less knowledgeable about surgical approaches for definitive tumor resection in osteosarcoma, the risk of a poorly placed biopsy is potentially higher with a core needle biopsy. However, supporters of core needle biopsy argue that this risk can be reduced through discussion of the biopsy with the patient's treating orthopedic surgeon.

4. IMPACT ON BIOLOGIC STUDIES OF OSTEOSARCOMA

Although the availability of tumor material for the study of osteosarcoma biology is not an important issue from the perspective of the individual patient with osteosarcoma, it is an important issue from the perspective of researchers and future patients who could benefit from research discoveries. Because tumor resection occurs after the administration of chemotherapy, osteosarcoma resection specimens are often not suitable for laboratory investigation. After open biopsy there is usually sufficient prechemotherapy tumor material available for biologic studies after the diagnosis is made. This is not the case with core needle biopsies. Thus, progress in osteosarcoma research would likely be negatively affected if the majority of centers were to perform core needle biopsies.

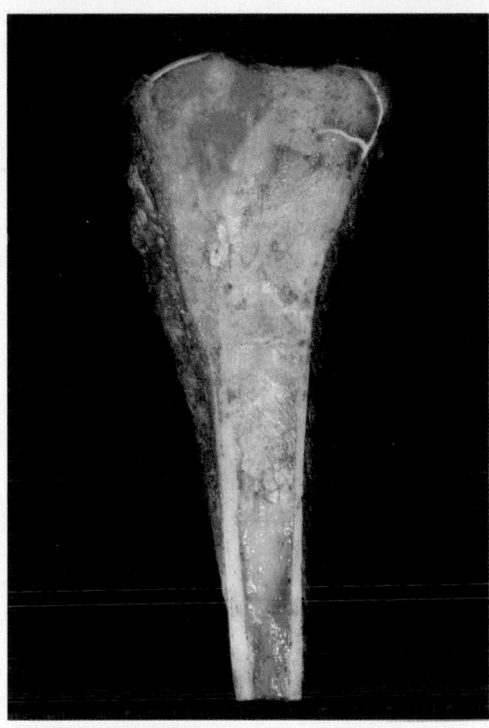

Figure 62-9 Osteosarcoma: gross pathologic appearance.

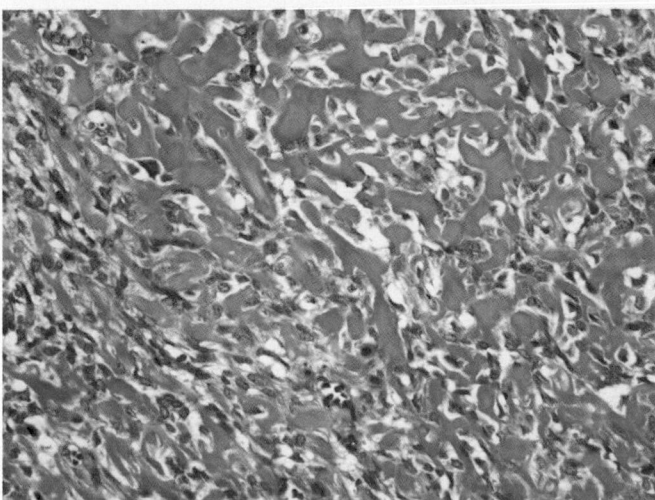

Figure 62-10 High-grade osteosarcoma composed of malignant-appearing tumor cells having a high nuclear-to-cytoplasmic ratio, hyperchromatism, and prominent nucleoli and an abundant eosinophilic osteoid matrix.

present in either, the diagnosis of osteosarcoma cannot be made with certainty. The histologic appearance of osteoid is dense, pink, and amorphous. Classic or conventional osteosarcoma comprises 70% to 80% of cases of osteosarcoma.[79] A number of other types of osteosarcoma are distinguished from classic osteosarcoma based on clinical or pathologic features (Table 62-1).

Classic osteosarcoma has a highly malignant appearance, with prominent anaplasia and frequent mitoses. There is variability in the histologic appearance of conventional osteosarcoma. To facilitate pathologic diagnosis and best describe this variability in appearance, classic osteosarcoma is divided into three subtypes based on the predominant matrix produced by the malignant cells.[79] In the first, 50% of typical osteosarcoma is osteoblastic osteosarcoma, in which osteoid is the predominant matrix (Fig. 62-10). Next, 25% of typical osteosarcoma is chondroblastic osteosarcoma in which cartilaginous islands are the predominant matrix. This subtype is differentiated from chondrosarcoma by the presence of osteoid. Because osteoid can be sparse in chondroblastic osteosarcoma, distinguishing chondroblastic osteosarcoma from chondrosarcoma can require extensive biopsy material, which may necessitate rebiopsy. Sixty-one percent of chondrosarcomas have mutations in the isocitrate dehydrogenase 1 and 2 genes (*IDH1* and *IDH2*). Mutations in these genes have not been seen in osteosarcoma. Therefore, the identification of an *IDH1* or *IDH2* mutation in a malignant bone tumor with a chondroid matrix would strongly suggest a diagnosis of chondrosarcoma.[82,83] The remaining 25% of typical osteosarcoma is fibroblastic. In fibroblastic osteosarcoma, osteoid is minimal and spindle cells grow in a herringbone pattern.[3]

TABLE 62-1   Pathologic Features and Relative Frequency of Osteosarcoma Subtypes

Type	Pathology	Approximate % (of all Osteosarcoma)
Classic	Anaplastic, numerous mitoses	70-80
Osteoblastic	Predominant matrix osteoid	35
Chondroblastic	Predominant matrix chondroid	18
Fibroblastic	Spindle cells in herringbone pattern	18
Jaw	Similar to classic osteosarcoma	3-7
Secondary	Similar to classic osteosarcoma	7
Telangiectatic	Cysts and septa, scant osteoid, giant cells present	4-10
Small cell	Small round malignant cells, osteoid present but quantity variable	1-4
Low-grade intramedullary	Minimal atypia, few mitoses	1-2
Parosteal	Located on bone surface, low grade, matrix osteoid and, in 50%, cartilage	4
Periosteal	Located on bone surface, intermediate grade, predominant matrix cartilage	1-2

Many osteosarcomas have a mixture of different histologies, but in mixed histology cases one histology usually predominates. Of note, the subtypes of typical osteosarcoma were originally designated for the purpose of diagnosis, and their prognostic significance is uncertain. A better histologic response to chemotherapy in fibroblastic osteosarcoma and a poorer histologic response to chemotherapy in chondroblastic osteosarcoma have been consistent findings in several studies.[80,84,85] Telangiectatic osteosarcoma also has a better histologic response to chemotherapy (see later). Whether these differences in histologic response to therapy are correlated with differences in OS is not entirely clear. In the largest study to evaluate this question, there was a slight, statistically significant 5-year OS advantage in patients with fibroblastic osteosarcoma. Unlike other types of osteosarcoma, histologic response to chemotherapy may not be correlated with outcome in chondroblastic osteosarcoma.[85]

The remaining 20% to 30% of osteosarcomas that are not classic osteosarcomas are divided into secondary (occurring in Paget disease or after irradiation), jaw, telangiectatic, small cell, parosteal, periosteal, and low-grade intramedullary osteosarcoma. Telangiectatic osteosarcoma accounts for 4% to 11% of all osteosarcoma cases.[79,86-88] The age and gender distribution are the same as in conventional osteosarcoma. Pathologic fracture is more common, occurring in 15% to 25% of cases.[79,87,88] Radiographically, a lytic pattern is present because of the presence of large or small cystic areas and minimal osteoid formation. Microscopically, cysts are divided by septa that are lined with malignant cells producing scant osteoid. Cysts are also lined by benign, multinucleated giant cells. The presence of cysts and multinucleated giant cells can lead to misdiagnosis as an aneurysmal bone cyst or giant cell tumor, both benign bone tumors.[79] Although case series published prior to the modern era of multi-agent chemotherapy had reported that telangiectatic osteosarcoma has an adverse prognostic implication, more recent studies have reported a better histologic response to therapy and improved survival as compared with typical osteosarcoma.[85-87]

Small cell osteosarcoma is a rare but histologically distinct variant representing 1% to 4% of osteosarcomas.[89,90] The clinical and epidemiologic characteristics are the same as conventional osteosarcoma. Microscopically, tumors are composed of small round cells that produce variable amounts of osteoid. Differentiation from Ewing sarcoma and lymphoma can be difficult.

Osteosarcomas of the jaw, located in the maxilla or mandible, deserve specific mention. Even when secondary osteosarcomas are excluded, the mean age of patients with osteosarcoma in this location is the mid-30s, which is older than in classic osteosarcoma.[79,91,92] These tumors are more often low grade; approximately 50% are low grade in most series.[92,93] Histologically, the appearance is similar to that of classic osteosarcoma but a larger proportion of tumors are chondroblastic. In concordance with the greater proportion of low-grade tumors, prognosis is better for osteosarcoma of the jaw. Although local recurrence does occur, especially when the initial resection is inadequate, metastasis is unusual.

Low-grade intramedullary osteosarcoma is relatively rare, making up 1% to 2% of all osteosarcomas. Patients developing this form of osteosarcoma tend to be older than those with conventional osteosarcoma, with 30 years being the mean age at diagnosis. Microscopic examination reveals spindle cells permeating bony trabeculae, with minimal atypia and few mitoses. A variable amount of osteoid is present. Recurrence and metastasis are rare. With adequate resection, chemotherapy is generally not indicated.[94,95]

Parosteal osteosarcoma is another low-grade osteosarcoma distinguished from low-grade intramedullary osteosarcoma by its location on the cortical surface of the bone. It is generally a sclerotic tumor attached to the bone by a broad base. Microscopically, the stroma is sparsely populated by minimally atypical spindle cells. The matrix contains osteoid and, in 50% of cases, cartilage.[96] A limited degree of medullary involvement is seen in 25% of cases. Areas of dedifferentiation can be present at diagnosis or at the time of recurrence and portend a poorer prognosis. Of patients with dedifferentiation, 31% will die of disease, usually with pulmonary metastasis.[97] Parosteal osteosarcoma makes up approximately 4% of all osteosarcomas. Like intramedullary low-grade osteosarcoma, parosteal osteosarcoma occurs in slightly older patients than conventional osteosarcoma and recurrence and metastasis are rare in adequately resected cases without dedifferentiation.[98]

Parosteal osteosarcoma must be distinguished from periosteal osteosarcoma. Periosteal osteosarcoma also arises from the surface of the bone but is an intermediate- or high-grade lesion. Periosteal osteosarcoma has an age distribution similar to that of typical osteosarcoma but almost all tumors arise in the proximal tibia. The appearance on plain radiography is highly characteristic and suggests the diagnosis. Histology is of a spindle cell neoplasm with osteoid and cartilaginous islands present, usually in large amounts. The prognosis is better than in conventional osteosarcoma but probably not as good as in parosteal osteosarcoma without dedifferentiation or intermedullary low-grade osteosarcoma.[99] There is controversy regarding the need for chemotherapy for periosteal osteosarcoma. The entity is too rare to permit conduct of prospective randomized controlled trials. Interpretation of retrospective series is difficult because variability in chemotherapy administration likely correlates with variability in clinicopathologic features related to outcome.[100,101]

Secondary osteosarcoma arises in previously irradiated bone or in patients with Paget disease. In both cases, patients are older than those with conventional osteosarcoma. Pathology is similar to conventional osteosarcoma. Prognosis is poorer in Paget disease than in conventional osteosarcoma.[84] There is some evidence that radiation-induced osteosarcomas have similar outcomes to de novo osteosarcoma if standard osteosarcoma chemotherapy is given.[102,103]

Staging

Staging of osteosarcoma follows the Enneking[104] or musculoskeletal society staging system (Table 62-2). The

TABLE 62-2 Enneking Staging System for Osteosarcoma: Distribution of Osteosarcoma and Indicated Treatment by Stage

Stage	Grade	Site	Metastasis	% of Patients[107]	Surgical Margin	Chemotherapy	Representative Subtype
IA	G1	T1	M0	5	Wide	No	Parosteal
IB	G1	T2	M0	3	Wide	No	
IIA	G2	T1	M0	5	Wide	Yes	Periosteal
IIB	G2	T2	M0	74	Wide	Yes	Classic
III	G1, G2	T1, T2	M1	13	Variable	Yes	Classic

Modified from Enneking WF, Spanier SS, Goodman MA: A system for the surgical staging of musculoskeletal sarcoma. Clin Orthop Relat Res *(153):106–120, 1980.*
G1, Low grade, characterized by few mitoses and a relatively well-differentiated appearance; G2, high grade characterized by higher mitotic rate and a less differentiated appearance; M0, no distant metastases present; M1, distant metastases present; T1, tumor is intracompartmental or confined to the anatomic compartment of origin; T2, tumor is extracompartmental or extends beyond the anatomic compartment of origin.

TNM system is not used for several reasons. The TNM system lacks biologic relevance in that osteosarcoma seldom metastasizes to lymph nodes. In addition, it is more complex than needed for predicting outcome, because patients in different TNM stages have overlapping prognoses.[104]

The Enneking staging system is based on tumor grade (G), site (T), and metastasis (M). Low-grade (G1) tumors are well differentiated and have few mitoses, corresponding to Broders grades I and II.[95] Osteosarcoma is high grade (G2) if it is poorly differentiated and has numerous mitoses, corresponding to Broders grades III and IV. As noted, most osteosarcomas are high grade (G2). Surgical site (T) is determined by whether the tumor is contained within its anatomic compartment of origin (T1) or extends beyond its compartment of origin (T2). For example, a typical osteosarcoma that arises in the medullary space and extends through the cortex into the soft tissue is T2. A parosteal osteosarcoma that does not extend from the bone surface, its site of origin, into the medullary space and does not invade the surrounding soft tissue is T1. Most classic osteosarcomas are T2. Metastases are absent (M1) or present (M2). Stages IA and IB are low-grade (G1) tumors. Stages IIA and IIB are high-grade tumors. Stage IA tumors are low-grade osteosarcomas that are T1 or lack extension beyond the compartment of origin. Stage IB tumors are low-grade osteosarcomas that are T2 or demonstrate extension beyond the compartment of origin. Similarly, stage IIA tumors do not have extracompartmental extension, whereas IIB tumors do. Stage III osteosarcomas are tumors of any grade and any site that have distant metastases.[104-106] The vast majority of osteosarcomas are stage IIB. The next most common stage for osteosarcoma at presentation is stage III. Stages IA, IB, and IIA are uncommon, with 3% to 5% of osteosarcomas falling into each of these categories.[107]

NATURAL HISTORY AND PROGNOSIS

The most significant predictor of survival in osteosarcoma is the presence of residual disease caused by incom-plete resection of primary tumor in localized osteosarcoma, local recurrence, or the presence of metastases. Consequently, the natural history, prognosis, and prognostic factors of localized, relapsed, and metastatic osteosarcoma differ significantly.

Localized Disease
Natural History

Prior to the use of chemotherapy for osteosarcoma, the OS of patients with localized disease who had a complete resection was 20%. Death was almost always caused by complications of pulmonary metastases.[79,108] With wide or radical surgical margins, local recurrence was rare. The development of pulmonary metastases in 80% of patients treated with only complete resection of the primary tumor has been interpreted as evidence of the presence of micrometastatic foci in the lungs at the time of diagnosis[109] and was one rationale for adjuvant chemotherapy.

Five-year event-free survival (EFS) and OS of localized osteosarcoma in the era of modern therapy are 65% to 75% and 70% to 80%, respectively.[110,111-113] Approximately 80% of relapses are pulmonary either alone or, in 25% of patients, with a second disease site, which is most often bone. Bone, distant from the initial resection, is the initial relapse site in 8% of patients; 1% to 2% of patients have recurrence isolated to unusual sites such as brain, kidneys, heart, or liver.[6,7,114] Local recurrence is seen in 2% to 8% of patients, despite having had adequate surgical margins.[53,115,116] Most relapses occur during the first 2 years after completion of chemotherapy. However, relapses occur as late as 10 years and the EFS decreases slowly between 2 and 10 years. In the few studies reporting long-term follow-up data, EFS decreases to 60% at 10 years from 65% at 5 years.[115,117]

Prognostic Factors

The most consistent predictor of outcome in localized, fully resected osteosarcoma is the extent of tumor necrosis after neoadjuvant chemotherapy.[52,53,118-121] When investigators at the Memorial Sloan-Kettering Cancer

TABLE 62-3 Grading of Histologic Response to Neoadjuvant Chemotherapy

Response	Grade	Histology
Poor	I	Necrosis minimal or absent
	II	Necrosis is <90% of the tumor but greater than minimal
Good	III	Scattered areas of viable tumor but >90% of tumor necrotic
	IV	No viable tumor

Modified from Rosen G, Caparros B, Huvos AG, et al: Preoperative chemotherapy for osteogenic sarcoma: selection of postoperative adjuvant chemotherapy based on the response of the primary tumor to preoperative chemotherapy. Cancer 49:1221–1230, 1982.

Center first gave neoadjuvant, or preoperative, chemotherapy to facilitate surgical resection without amputation, they noted varying degrees of necrosis on pathologic examination of resected tumor specimens.[122] It was later observed that patients with significant necrosis had a better EFS and OS than those with lesser degrees of necrosis.[123] However, tumor response is not a true prognostic factor because it cannot be determined until after the initiation of chemotherapy.

The generally accepted grading system for tumor necrosis (Table 62-3) assigns higher grades to tumors with greater evidence of necrosis. In most studies, grades III and IV, in which more than 90% of the tumor is necrotic, define the group of patients whose tumors have a good response to chemotherapy. Patients whose tumors have a poor response have 10% or more viable tumor, corresponding to grades I and II. Patients with a poor response have disease-free survival (DFS) rates of 40% to 50%, whereas those with a good response have DFS rates of 70% to 80% (Fig. 62-11).[111,124-126] An improved outcome for poor responders is an objective

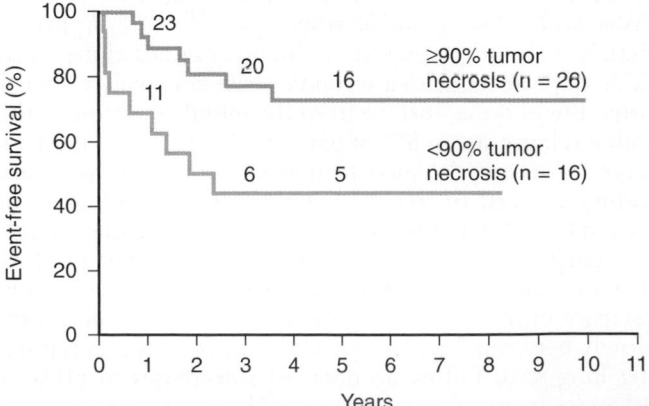

Figure 62-11 Representative event-free survival curve of patients with localized osteosarcoma greater than or equal to 90% *(blue line)* or less than 90% *(green line)* tumor necrosis after neoadjuvant chemotherapy. *(Modified from Goorin AM, Schwartzentruber DJ, Devidas M, et al: Presurgical chemotherapy compared with immediate surgery and adjuvant chemotherapy for nonmetastatic osteosarcoma: Pediatric Oncology Group Study POG-8651. J Clin Oncol 21:1574–1580, 2003.)*

of past and current trials (see "Chemotherapy for Localized Disease").

Radiographic parameters have been investigated for correlation with tumor necrosis and outcome. A decrease in FDG-PET standard uptake value (SUV) before and after neoadjuvant chemotherapy is correlated with histologic response. Neither the change in SUV nor absolute SUV after neoadjuvant chemotherapy has a statistically significant association with OS in localized osteosarcoma. The lack of statistical significance may be due to investigation in only a small population of patients,[127] and larger studies are needed to determine whether FDG-PET responses are predictive of outcome in osteosarcoma. Various MRI techniques including dynamic contrast-enhanced MRI[128] and diffusion-weighted MRI[129] show promise for potential to predict histologic response.

Additional prognostic factors have been identified in localized osteosarcoma. In many cases these factors are not consistently demonstrated to be statistically significant across studies. This may be due to a small effect size and, as a result, the need for large studies to identify a factor as being statistically related to outcome. In other cases, differences in measurement or categorization contribute to variable results across studies.

Tumor size has been identified as a significant prognostic factor by multivariate analysis in several studies.[52,53,113,120] However, other studies have not found this patient variable to be predictive of outcome.[118,130-132] One possible explanation for this conflict is variability in the definition of tumor size and measurement techniques. Some studies evaluate absolute tumor length, others use relative (to the entire bone) tumor length, and still others base analyses on tumor volume. Most studies showing size to be a significant predictor of outcome on multivariate analysis have measured tumor volume.[53,113,120] However, the volume that distinguishes small, low-risk tumors from large, high-risk tumors varies among studies. In summary, further studies using standard measurement techniques and risk criteria need to be conducted before tumor size can be used as a clinically significant predictor on which to counsel patients or base therapeutic decisions. The prognostic significance of tumor size might be caused by the influence of tumor size on resectability. In other words, larger tumors may confer a poorer prognosis because it is less likely that the tumor will be completely resected with wide margins.

Several studies have found an association between tumor site and outcome, with axial and proximal appendicular primary tumors having a worse prognosis than distal extremity tumors.[52,53,110,113,120,133-136] However, there are potential interactions between tumor site and other osteosarcoma prognostic factors. In particular, site and size are likely to be associated. A distal extremity osteosarcoma is likely to be noticed at a smaller size because of the relative lack of soft tissue. More importantly, the higher risk sites, such as axial skeleton, are also those for which a complete resection is less likely.

Elevated LDH and alkaline phosphatase levels at the time of diagnosis are associated with a poorer prognosis.[53,118,119] In one study,[118] the EFS of patients with a normal alkaline phosphatase level at diagnosis was 88%, whereas it was 46% for patients with an elevated alkaline phosphatase level. There are several issues that limit the usefulness of LDH and alkaline phosphatase as prognostic indicators. First, elevated levels are not consistently associated with a poorer prognosis in all studies. Second, elevations in LDH and alkaline phosphatase levels confer only a modestly increased relative risk (1.5 for LDH and 2 for alkaline phosphatase) of a poor outcome.[119]

Other prognostic factors that have been reported to be significant in a limited number of studies are age and gender, with older age and male gender being associated with a worse outcome.[52,53,137,138] Chemotherapy toxicity, represented by grade 3 or 4 mucositis, has been found to be correlated with improved OS.[138,139] A single study from the Children's Oncology Group (COG) identified a high body mass index at the time of diagnosis as a risk factor for inferior survival.[140]

As noted earlier, histologic subtype may be a prognostic factor. P-glycoprotein positivity, loss of heterozygosity at the RB1 locus, and high ezrin expression have been identified as possible biology-based predictors of a poor outcome.[141,142] These prognostic factors are discussed more extensively (see "Biology").

In summary, the extent of tumor necrosis is the most reliable prognostic indicator in localized, completely resected osteosarcoma. Additional factors correlated with a poorer outcome include older age, less chemotherapy toxicity, larger tumor size, axial tumor site, elevated LDH and alkaline phosphatase levels, and high body mass index. However, for prognostic factors other than tumor necrosis to be utilized for risk stratification, further validation is required in large populations who received uniform therapy. Identification of reliable prognostic factors available at the time of diagnosis is a research priority in osteosarcoma. Biologic efforts such as TARGET (see "Genomics" under "Biology") and further investigation of imaging characteristics are most likely to provide robust predictors of outcome.

Metastatic and Relapsed Disease

The OS for patients with relapsed disease is poor, with most series showing a 25% OS at 5 years.[6,7,114] As with primary osteosarcoma, the most significant prognostic factor for postrelapse survival is the ability to achieve complete resection of all disease sites. In one report of 162 patients with initially localized osteosarcoma who developed recurrent disease, the 5-year projected OS was 39% for those who had complete resection of all disease and 0% for those who did not.[6] With isolated pulmonary metastases, prognosis is significantly influenced by the number of pulmonary nodules and whether there is unilateral or bilateral pulmonary disease.[6,7,114] In particular, having more than one pulmonary nodule at relapse conveys a worse prognosis. An additional prognostic factor is the duration of remission. Patients experiencing relapse less than 24 months after initial diagnosis have a worse outcome.[6,114] Finally, use of chemotherapy is associated with a slightly improved postrelapse prognosis,[7] particularly in patients with unresectable disease.[6] Patients who experience second and subsequent recurrences have

a 5-year OS rate of about 15%. As with the initial recurrence, the duration of relapse-free interval, the number of lesions at recurrence, and the ability to resect recurrent disease are all associated with outcome.[143]

Local recurrence warrants special mention because of its dismal prognosis. The 5-year DFS is 0% to 15%.[115,116,144,145] Local recurrence is almost always associated with concurrent or delayed pulmonary metastasis.[115] In one series, the outcome of patients with local recurrence was strongly influenced by the presence or absence of systemic metastases at the time of local recurrence. The 5-year DFS was 25% for patients without systemic metastases at the time of local recurrence, and it was 0% for those with systemic metastases.

The outcome and prognostic factors for metastatic disease present at diagnosis are similar to those for relapsed disease. The 5-year OS of patients presenting with primary metastatic disease is 20% to 30%.[4,146] One exception to the poor prognosis for patients with metastatic disease is skip metastases. In patients with skip metastases, OS is 50%, even when pulmonary metastases are also present.[60] Higher OS has been reported in some chemotherapy trials, possibly because of therapy efficacy or shorter periods of follow-up.[147] An important predictor of a poor outcome is the inability to achieve complete surgical remission. Similarly, patients with metastases to more than one site or more than one organ are at increased risk for death from disease.[4,146] Lymph node metastasis at the time of diagnosis is uncommon, occurring in less than 5% of patients. Lymph node involvement at the time of diagnosis is associated with larger tumor size and an extraskeletal primary lesion. OS at 5 years for those with lymph node metastasis at diagnosis is 10%.[148] In one study, an alkaline phosphatase level higher than 500 IU/L was significantly associated with poor prognosis on multivariate analysis.[146]

BIOLOGY

Structural chromosomal alterations, loss of tumor suppressor function, and oncogene amplification have all been described in osteosarcoma. In addition, alterations in specific proteins contribute to chemotherapy resistance and metastatic behavior. A summary of genes altered in osteosarcoma is presented in Table 62-4.

Cell of Origin

Genetically engineered murine models of osteosarcoma have helped define the cell of origin for osteosarcoma. Lineage-specific models have demonstrated that osteosarcoma can arise from mesenchymal stem cell progenitors, osteoblast progenitors, and osteoblasts. In these lineage-specific genetically engineered mouse models, osteosarcoma develops with the highest penetrance and shortest latency when derived from osteoblast progenitors whereas mesenchymal stem cell progenitors give rise to a larger proportion of poorly differentiated soft tissue sarcomas.[149] A case report of osteosarcoma arising from donor cells after allogeneic stem cell transplantation suggests that mesenchymal stem cells can give rise to osteosarcoma in humans as well.[150]

TABLE 62-4   Genes Implicated in Osteosarcoma Pathogenesis and Biologic Progression

Gene	Alteration	Gene Function	% of Sporadic Osteosarcoma
RB1	Deletion, inactivation	Cell cycle control	70
TP53	Mutation, inactivation	Apoptosis Response to DNA damage Cell cycle control	50
MDM2	Gene amplification	TP53 regulation	10-15
COPS3	Gene amplification	TP53 regulation	25
CDKN2A	Deletion, promoter methylation	Cell cycle control through inhibition of CDK4-CCND1	15-20
MET	Increased expression	Motility Invasion	60
FOS	Increased expression	Proliferation Possibly, differentiation	60
MYC	Gene amplification	Proliferation	40
ABCB1	Increased expression	Efflux of chemotherapeutic agents	25-45
DHFR	Increased expression	Folate metabolism; MTX target	60% relapsed tumors
ERBB2	Increased expression	Growth factor receptor	40
Ezrin	Increased expression	Membrane cytoskeleton linker, facilitates metastasis	92
FAS	Decreased expression	Apoptosis	60% pulmonary metastases lack FAS
Reduced folate carrier	Decreased expression	MTX transport	65
IGF1R	Increased expression	Growth factor receptor, proliferation	Unknown

MTX, Methotrexate.

Genomics

Osteosarcomas contain complex genomic aberrations, suggesting the involvement of multiple genes in osteosarcoma development. Copy number abnormalities, changes in ploidy, and structural rearrangements are seen in all high-grade osteosarcomas. It is a tumor type in which chromothripsis has found to occur frequently.[151] Homogeneously staining regions and marker, double-minute, and ring chromosomes are seen in most tumors.[152,153] A representative karyotype and Circos plot are shown in Figure 62-12. Nonclonal changes, often superimposed on clonal aberrations, are present in many tumor specimens.[81] Several comprehensive next-generation sequencing projects are underway, including one being conducted as part of the National Cancer Institute sponsored Therapeutically Applicable Research to Generate Effective Treatments (TARGET) project. The nonclonal complex nature of the osteosarcoma genome makes the interpretation of genomic data difficult and the identification of candidate genes implicated in a significant proportion of osteosarcomas challenging.[154,155]

Osteosarcoma DNA ploidy ranges from diploid to hexaploid.[152] Spectral karyotyping (SKY) of osteosarcomas reveals an average of 39 chromosomal rearrangements/tumor.[156] Chromothripsis is the simultaneous occurrence of multiple somatic rearrangement events during one

single cellular episode. In nine osteosarcoma samples, three (33%) had evidence of chromothripsis.[151] Chromoplexy is a related mechanism of chromosomal rearrangement in which series of interrelated rearrangements affect multiple chromosomes.[157] Preliminary results of an ongoing comprehensive next-generation sequencing study found evidence of chromoplexy in most osteosarcoma samples studied.[158] Pilot studies have demonstrated the feasibility of using detection of patient-specific translocations to track disease burden in patients with osteosarcoma and other solid tumors.[159] Whether this method for detection of minimal residual disease burden will have prognostic implications in osteosarcoma as it has in leukemia remains to be determined.

Multiple genomic techniques have been applied to the assessment of copy number alterations in osteosarcoma. Traditional and spectral karyotype permitted the initial identification of genomic complexity and copy number alterations in osteosarcoma. More sophisticated techniques such as array comparative genomic hybridization (CGH) and single nucleotide polymorphism (SNP) arrays have permitted the identification of recurrently amplified and deleted regions.[154] In almost all CGH analyses, gains are more common than losses.[160-164] Amplified regions consistently seen in a significant proportion of tumors and across studies include 1q21-q24, 6p11.2-p12, 8q21.3-q24, 17p11.2-p12 (high-level amplification), 1p, 1q21,

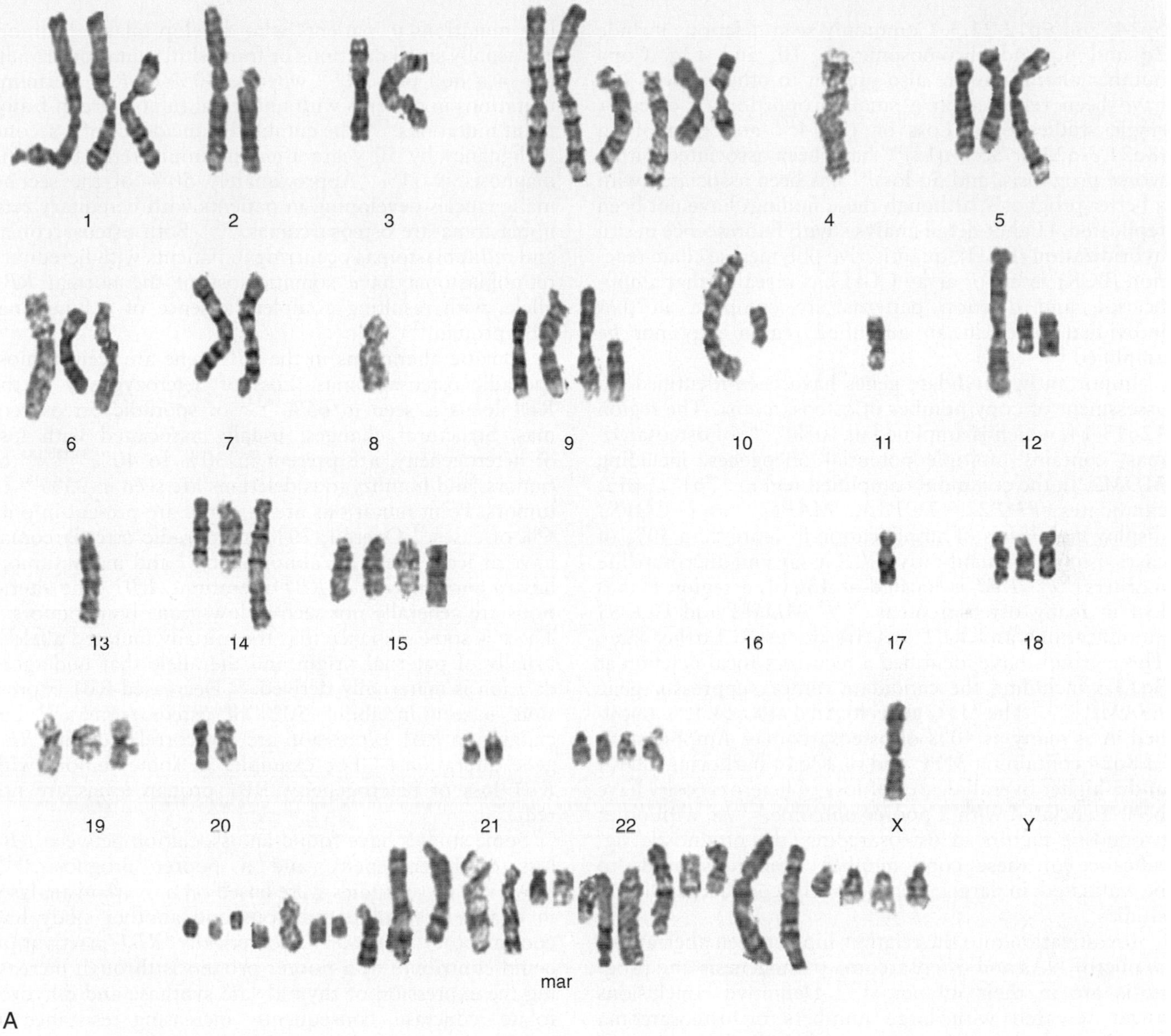

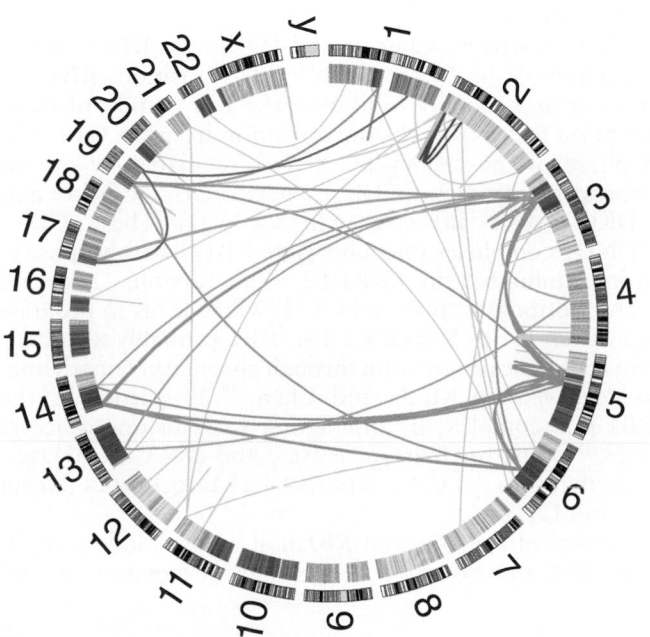

Figure 62-12 **A,** Representative osteosarcoma karyotype showing chromosome 16 loss, multiple marker chromosomes, monosomies, trisomies, and tetrasomies. **B,** Circos plot from whole-genome sequencing of an osteosarcoma sample.

5p14, and 6p12-21.3. Commonly seen deletions include 2q and 6q and chromosomes 9, 10, and 13q. Copy number alterations are also present in other regions but have been reported in a small proportion of cases or single studies only. Loss of 13q14[161] and gain of 8q (8q21.3-q22 or 8cen-q13)[160] have been associated with a worse prognosis, and 5q loss[161] has been associated with a better prognosis, although these findings have not been replicated. Higher-detail analysis with fluorescence in situ hybridization (FISH), quantitative polymerase chain reaction (PCR) assay, or array CGH has revealed that amplification and deletion patterns are complex, in that individual genes in an amplified region may not be amplified.[165]

Importantly, candidate genes have been identified via assessment of copy number in osteosarcoma. The region 12q13-14, which is amplified in 10%[160,162] of osteosarcomas, contains multiple potential oncogenes, including *MDM2*. In the commonly amplified region 17p11.2-p12, candidates *PMP22, TOP3A, MAPK7,* and *COPS3* display high levels of amplification in more than 50% of cases using semiquantitative PCR assay and microsatellite markers.[166,167] *RB1* is located at 13q14, a region that is lost in many osteosarcomas.[152,153] *MDM2* and *COPS3* amplifications and *RB1* loss are discussed further later. Three groups have identified a recurrent focal deletion at 3q13.3 including the candidate tumor suppressor gene *LSAMP*.[168-170] The *MYC* gene, located at 8q24.1, is amplified in as many as 40% of osteosarcomas. Amplification of 8q24 containing *MYC* and of 12q14 harboring CDK4 and a higher overall degree of loss of heterozygosity have been associated with a poorer outcome.[171] As with other prognostic factors in osteosarcoma, the prognostic significance of these copy number alterations needs to be validated in larger, prospectively conducted clinical studies.

Investigation into the relationship between aberrations in microRNAs and osteosarcoma pathogenesis and prognosis are in their infancy.[172-174] Definitive conclusions await research with large numbers of osteosarcoma samples and more robust statistical methodologies.

Tumor Suppressors

RB1

The retinoblastoma gene *RB1*, located at 13q14, was the first tumor suppressor gene identified and is one of the most frequently altered genes in osteosarcoma. As noted earlier (see "Etiology"), the second most common tumor in patients with hereditary retinoblastoma who carry germline *RB1* mutations[33] is osteosarcoma. *RB1* abnormalities are also present in most sporadic osteosarcomas. *RB1* inactivation is believed to contribute to osteosarcoma tumorigenesis through its role in cell cycle control and possibly through its regulation of differentiation and apoptosis.

Hereditary retinoblastoma is a condition in which individuals with a heterozygous germline *RB1* mutation develop retinoblastoma, a malignant tumor of the embryonal neural retina, with 90% penetrance.[175] Germline *RB1* mutations can be sporadic or inherited. *RB1* germ-

line mutations in patients who develop bilateral tumors are usually small deletions or frameshift mutations resulting in a null protein,[176] whereas 40% of *RB1* germline mutations in patients with unilateral tumors are in-frame point mutations.[176] The cumulative incidence of a second malignancy by 50 years after the initial retinoblastoma diagnosis is 51%. Approximately 50% of the second malignancies developing in patients with hereditary retinoblastoma are osteosarcomas.[32,177] Both osteosarcomas and retinoblastomas occurring in patients with hereditary retinoblastoma have somatic loss of the normal *RB1* allele, with resulting complete absence of a functional RB1 protein.[33,178,179]

Somatic alterations in the *RB1* gene are seen in most sporadic osteosarcomas. Loss of heterozygosity at the *RB1* locus is seen in 65%[34,142] of sporadic osteosarcomas. Structural changes, usually associated with loss of heterogeneity, are present in 30% to 40%[34,180,181] of tumors, and homozygous deletions are seen in 23%[182] of tumors. Point mutations are rare and are present in only 6% of cases.[34] Overall, 70% of sporadic osteosarcomas have at least one *RB1* abnormality,[34] and many tumors have a combination of *RB1* alterations. *RB1* gene alterations are generally not seen in low-grade bone tumors.[34] There is some evidence that the initially mutated allele is usually of paternal origin and the allele that undergoes deletion is maternally derived.[183] Decreased RB1 expression is seen in about 50% of osteosarcomas,[184] but changes in RB1 expression are not correlated with *RB1* gene alterations.[34] For example, in some tumors with *RB1* loss of heterogeneity, RB1 protein levels are not reduced.

Some studies have found an association between *RB1* loss of heterogeneity and a poorer prognosis.[34,142] However, these studies were based on univariate analyses in relatively small populations and another study had contradictory results.[185] Theoretically, *RB1* inactivation could contribute to a poorer prognosis through increasing the expression of thymidylate synthase and dihydrofolate reductase, consequently increasing resistance to antimetabolites,[186] an important component of osteosarcoma therapy.

As reviewed by Classon and Harlow,[187] RB1 is a key regulator of the G1 to S cell cycle transition. RB1, by binding and thereby inhibiting the E2F family of transcription factors, blocks the transition from the G1 to the S phase of the cell cycle. RB1 is regulated by cyclin-dependent kinases (CDKs), particularly CDK4 and CDK6, which interact with CCND1. These CDK-CCND1 complexes phosphorylate RB1. RB1 phosphorylation inhibits the RB1-E2F interaction, allowing transcriptional activation by E2F, which leads to progression from G1 to S (Fig. 62-13). RB1 probably also controls cell cycle progression through chromatin remodeling, as reviewed by Khidr and Chen.[188] In particular, the RB1-E2F complex, by interacting with histone deacetylases, histone methyltransferases, and DNA methylases, contributes to the inactivation of E2F target genes during G0 and G1.

Genetically engineered *Rb1* null mouse models implicate Rb1 in regulation of cellular differentiation and

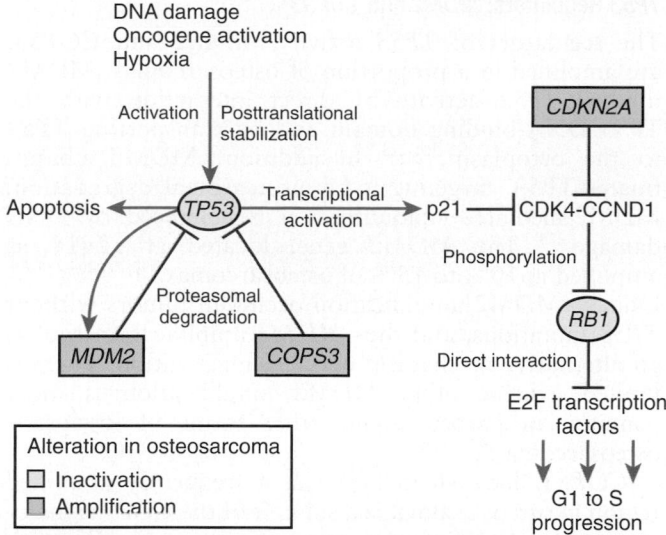

Figure 62-13 Selected regulators and effectors of *TP53* and *RB*. Alterations present in osteosarcoma are highlighted in *yellow* and *blue*.

apoptosis. *Rb1* deletion in mice results in embryonic lethality due to a placental defect.[189] When rescued from the placental defect, abnormal bone development is noted, and this appears to be due to increased proliferation in osteoblast cells combined with a failure in terminal osteoblastic differentiation.[190] Through interaction with CBFA1, a key transcriptional regulator in osteoblasts, RB1 induces osteogenic differentiation.[191] Loss of RB1 in osteoblast precursors appears to result in dedifferentiation, as demonstrated by an increased propensity for adipogenic differentiation.[192] The significance of RB1 differentiation and apoptosis roles in tumorigenesis in general and osteosarcomagenesis in particular is not clear.

TP53

There is convincing evidence that abnormal TP53 function is one of the central events in osteosarcomagenesis. Patients with Li-Fraumeni syndrome, who carry heterozygous germline *TP53* mutations, are predisposed to osteosarcoma. Somatic alterations in the *TP53* gene are found in a significant percentage of sporadic osteosarcomas. Furthermore, several different transgenic mouse models, with altered or absent TP53 function, develop osteosarcoma. Finally, components of the TP53 regulatory and effector pathways, *MDM2* (murine double-minute 2), *CDKN2A* (cyclin-dependent kinase inhibitor 2A), and *COPS3* (COP9 constitutive photomorphogenic homolog subunit 3) are also frequently perturbed in osteosarcoma, particularly in tumors lacking *TP53* mutations.

Of cancers arising in patients with Li-Fraumeni syndrome, 10% are osteosarcoma, making osteosarcoma the second most common tumor in Li-Fraumeni syndrome.[33] In addition to osteosarcoma, patients with Li-Fraumeni syndrome are predisposed to breast cancer, various soft tissue sarcomas, brain tumors, and various carcinomas. *TP53* germline mutations are present in 7% of osteosar-

coma patients who have a personal history of multiple cancers but who do not meet Li-Fraumeni diagnostic criteria.[193] Individuals with Li-Fraumeni syndrome have germline mutations in *TP53* located throughout the gene, although approximately 75% of the mutations are in exons 5 to 8,[194] which encode the DNA-binding domain of the TP53 protein. Tumors arising in patients with Li-Fraumeni syndrome typically have loss of the normal *TP53* allele.[195]

Somatic alterations of the *TP53* gene are present in 20% to 50% of sporadic osteosarcomas.[37,196-204] Despite the prevalence of somatic *TP53* mutations in sporadic osteosarcomas, germline *TP53* mutations are rare in patients with sporadic osteosarcoma without a personal or family history of multiple cancers.[205,206] The wide range in the reported frequency of somatic *TP53* alterations in sporadic osteosarcoma is the result of small study size, differences in techniques of ascertainment, and varying definitions of an abnormal result. *TP53* point mutations are present in 20% to 30% of osteosarcomas.[37,197,200-202] As with *TP53* mutations in other cancer types, missense mutations constitute approximately 75% of osteosarcoma point mutations.[207] Point mutations are present throughout the *TP53* coding sequence, although, as with Li-Fraumeni syndrome germline mutations, approximately 73% occur in exons 5 to 8.[201] The initial *TP53* abnormality to be recognized in osteosarcoma was gross rearrangements of the *TP53* gene.[199] Gross rearrangements are present in 15% to 25% of cases.[197,198,200] Studies that evaluated *TP53* for both point mutations and gross gene rearrangements have found that almost 50% of osteosarcomas examined have aberrant *TP53*.[200,203] Because mutant TP53 protein usually accumulates in cells because of an increased half-life,[208] TP53 immunohistochemistry has been used to screen for *TP53* mutations in osteosarcoma. By immunohistochemistry, 15% to 25% of osteosarcomas have TP53 abnormalities,[196,204] reflecting the fact that immunohistochemistry has a relatively low sensitivity for detecting *TP53* mutations. Approximately 50% of osteosarcomas with *TP53* point mutations have loss of the normal allele.[201]

Several genetically engineered mouse models with dysfunctional or absent *Tp53* develop osteosarcoma. In a genetically engineered mouse model in which *Tp53* and *Rb1* deletion is restricted to osteoblasts, osteosarcoma develops with a high penetrance and short latency.[209,210] Mice homozygous for null *Tp53* develop a variety of tumors. Although lymphoma and hemangiosarcoma are the most common tumor types seen, 4% of the mice develop osteosarcoma.[211] Mice heterozygous for null *Tp53* develop tumors at 25% the rate and at an older age than homozygous null mice, but 25% of the tumors that develop are osteosarcomas.[212] Osteosarcomas are much more common in mice genetically engineered to be heterozygous for a common cancer-associated *Tp53* mutation, R172H. Almost 50% of these mice develop osteosarcoma, usually associated with hematogenous metastases.[213] Several other mouse models heterozygous for mutant *Tp53* develop osteosarcoma at a rate of 20% to 30%. Metastases are common in these models as well.[214,215] Transgenic mice expressing the SV40 T antigen from different promoters[216,217] develop osteosarcoma at a rate of approximately 70%. The mechanism of transformation in the SV40 T antigen–expressing models probably involves the inactivation of Tp53 and Rb1.

In other cancers, *TP53* mutation status has been associated with proliferation, response to chemotherapy, and outcome. In osteosarcoma, the response to chemotherapy is equivalent in *TP53* mutant and *TP53* wild-type osteosarcomas.[218] Several studies have examined the impact of *TP53* mutation on survival in osteosarcoma. Only one study, in 30 patients, showed a worse survival in patients whose tumors had *TP53* mutations.[203] The remainder of the studies did not show a relationship between *TP53* mutation status and outcome.[196,200,218,219] Finally, *TP53* mutations are not more common in metastatic disease than in localized disease.[201] Actually, the *TP53* mutation status of primary and metastatic tumors tends to be concordant.[201]

As reviewed by Levine[208] and Vogelstein and colleagues,[220] *TP53* mutations and structural alterations lead to transformation by interfering with TP53 tumor suppressor functions and, possibly, by producing a TP53 protein that has gained oncogenic function. TP53 tumor suppressor activities include cell cycle control and induction of apoptosis. Several forms of cellular stress, including DNA damage, hypoxia, shortened telomeres, and oncogene activation lead to TP53 posttranslational stabilization and TP53 activation. After activation, TP53 binds DNA and promotes the transcription of several genes, including *CDKN1A* and *MDM2*. As in other tumor types, the *TP53* mutations seen in sporadic osteosarcomas and Li-Fraumeni syndrome are concentrated in the DNA-binding domain and interfere with the transcriptional activity of the protein.[207] TP53 prevents progression from the G1 phase to the S phase of the cell cycle through the actions of one of its target genes, *CDKN1A*. The CDKN1A protein inhibits the CDK4-CCND1 complex, which in turn keeps RB1 in an unphosphorylated state. Unphosphorylated RB1 binds E2F transcription factors, preventing progression into the S phase (see Fig. 62-13).[220] TP53 also plays a regulatory role in the G2 to M cell cycle checkpoint. Another inhibitor of CDK4-CCND1 is CDKN2A. CDKN2A abnormalities are also seen in osteosarcoma (see later).

As with TP53-mediated cell cycle control, TP53-mediated apoptosis is triggered by DNA damage. In addition, oncogene overexpression and *RB1* inactivation stimulate TP53-mediated apoptosis. The pathways involved in TP53-mediated apoptosis are not fully understood. However, they likely involve proapoptotic proteins whose genes are targets of TP53 transcriptional activation, including *BAX*, *PMAIP1*, and *TP53AIP1*.[220]

TP53 inactivation allows cells to progress through the cell cycle and escape apoptosis, despite the presence of DNA damage. Consistent with this observation, the presence of a *TP53* mutation in osteosarcoma is significantly correlated with a greater level of genomic instability.[37] Thus promotion of genomic instability and the resultant accumulation of secondary mutations in oncogenes or tumor suppressors is yet another mechanism of transformation in *TP53* mutant tumors.

TP53 Regulators: *MDM2* and *COPS3*

The regulators of *TP53* activity, *MDM2* and *COPS3*, are amplified in a proportion of osteosarcomas. MDM2 inhibits TP53 activity by direct interaction with the TP53 DNA-binding domain and by transporting TP53 to the cytoplasm.[221-223] In addition, MDM2 ubiquitinates TP53, targeting it for proteasomal degradation. MDM2-mediated ubiquitination is enhanced by DNA damage.[224] The *MDM2* gene, located at 12q14, is amplified in 10% to 15% of osteosarcomas.[197,203,204,225-227] Usually, *MDM2* amplification occurs in tumors without *TP53* mutations, and thus *MDM2* amplification acts as an alternative mechanism of TP53 inactivation. There is limited evidence that *MDM2* amplification is more common in parosteal and other forms of low-grade osteosarcoma.[165,228,229]

COPS3, located at 17p11.2, a frequently amplified region in osteosarcoma, is a subunit of the COP9 signalosome. The COP9 signalosome interacts directly with TP53 and, through phosphorylation, targets TP53 for interaction with MDM2 and degradation by the 26S proteasome.[230] *COPS3* gene amplification is present in 25% to 30% of osteosarcomas.[231,232] Increased COPS3 expression through alternative mechanisms is present in some tumors lacking *COPS3* gene amplification.[231] Like *MDM2* amplification, COPS3 overexpression may be an alternative mechanism of *TP53* inactivation. *TP53* mutations are present in a small proportion of *COPS3*-amplified osteosarcomas.[231,232]

CDKN2A and *CDKN2D*

As described earlier, CDKN2A, like the TP53-inducible protein CDKN1A, is an inhibitor of the CDK4-CCND1 complex. As with CDKN1A, inhibition of CDK4-CCND1 by CDKN2A prevents progression from the G1 to the S phase. Ten to 20 percent of osteosarcomas have *CDKN2A* homozygous deletion,[197,202,203,233] and in another 5% to 10% the *CDKN2A* promoter is methylated. Similarly, by immunohistochemistry, 16% of osteosarcomas lack CDKN2A protein expression.[234] *CDKN2A* deletions appear to be more common in osteosarcomas grown in cell culture[235] but seem to be less common in osteosarcomas with *RB1* abnormalities, possibly because the two alterations have a similar effect on cell cycle control.[233] Few studies have evaluated the coexistence of *TP53* mutations and *CDKN2A* deletions in osteosarcomas. There is limited evidence that the two abnormalities occur simultaneously.[203]

CDKN2D is an alternatively spliced product of the gene encoding *CDKN2A*. CDKN2D inhibits MDM2 by direct binding.[236] Thus loss of CDKN2D leads to increased MDM2-mediated TP53 degradation. As a consequence of the gene structure, the 10% to 20% of osteosarcomas with *CDKN2A* homozygous deletion also lack functional CDKN2D.

RECQ DNA Helicases

As noted earlier, osteosarcoma incidence is increased in three autosomal recessive cancer predisposition syndromes caused by RECQ DNA helicase mutations, Rothmund-Thomson syndrome, Werner syndrome, and

Bloom syndrome. The overlapping but distinct clinical features and specific nature of osteosarcoma predisposition in these syndromes has already been discussed (see "Etiology"). Whereas germline *RECQL4* mutations predispose patients with these syndromes to osteosarcoma, somatic *RECQL4* mutations are not present in sporadic osteosarcomas.[237]

Patients with Rothmund-Thomson syndrome caused by mutations in *RECQL4*[238] develop osteosarcoma with a prevalence of approximately 30% and probably do not have an increased susceptibility to other types of cancer.[239] Interestingly, osteosarcoma occurs only in the 60% of patients with Rothmund-Thomson syndrome who have truncating or inactivating *RECQL4* mutations.[38] On the other hand, patients with Bloom and Werner syndromes, caused by mutations in *RECQL2* and *RECQL3*, respectively,[240,241] are prone to a wide variety of cancers, and osteosarcoma represents less than 10% of the cancers occurring in these patients.[40,41] Why *RECQL4* mutations, in contrast to *RECQL2* and *RECQL3* mutations, specifically increase the risk for osteosarcoma is unknown.

The mechanism whereby loss of function of RECQ DNA helicases results in tumor development generally and in osteosarcoma in particular are not well understood. Proposed RECQ functions that could be related to tumor formation include participation in DNA recombination, maintenance of chromosome stability, recovery from DNA replication collapse, initiation of DNA replication, and telomere processing. The three RECQ DNA helicases mutated in cancer predisposition syndromes have overlapping but not identical functions. In vitro cell culture and mouse models of *RECQL4* mutant Rothmund-Thomson syndrome display increased chromosomal instability with high rates of aneuploidy.[242] Bloom and Werner syndrome models have abnormally high rates of homologous recombination events, with accumulation of recombination intermediates.[243] Studies with the *Xenopus RECQL4* homologue have suggested that RECQL4 participates in the initiation of DNA replication.[244] Several lines of evidence have indicated that the RECQ helicases likely play an essential role in reestablishing DNA replication after disruption of the replication fork.[243] Finally, WRN may be involved in telomerase-independent telomere maintenance.[243,245]

WWOX

WWOX encodes a WW domain containing oxoreductase. This class of proteins has a wide variety of functions including regulation of protein degradation, transcription, and splicing. There is evidence from other cancers that *WWOX* can act as a tumor suppressor. Mice carrying a homozygous deletion of *Wwox*[246] develop osteosarcoma at a rate of 30% prior to premature death at 4 weeks postnatal age.[246] Thirty percent of human osteosarcoma samples have *WWOX* deletions, and 60% have reduced or absent WWOX expression. WWOX interacts directly with RUNX2, a regulator of osteoblast differentiation. In osteosarcoma cell lines deficient in WWOX expression, forced WWOX expression results in decreased RUNX2 expression, decreased proliferation, decreased invasion, and a reduction in xenograft viability.[247,248]

Developmental Pathways and Stem Cell Programs

Wnt Pathway

The Wnt pathway is active in bone development. Activating mutations in *LRP5* (low density lipoprotein receptor–related protein 5), which encodes an Wnt coreceptor (with frizzled4), cause high bone mass whereas inactivating *LRP5* mutations result in decreased bone mass. Despite multiple investigations into Wnt pathway activity in osteosarcoma, it remains unclear how and whether perturbations in Wnt pathway activity contribute to osteosarcomagenesis.[249] The majority studies conclude that overactive Wnt signaling contributes to osteosarcoma formation. For example, deletion of the Wnt inhibitory factor, *Wif1*, in mice increased osteosarcoma formation after irradiation.[250] However, there are conflicting reports such as a genome-wide expression study finding downregulation of the Wnt pathway in osteosarcoma.[251]

USP1

USP1 encodes a deubiquitinating enzyme that deubiquitinates inhibitor of DNA-binding/differentiation (ID) proteins, preventing their degradation. ID proteins or inhibitors of DNA binding are basic helix-loop-helix transcription factors that have been shown to inhibit differentiation and maintain a stemlike state. In a small group of osteosarcoma tumors, expression of USP1 and ID2 were correlated and 7 of 14 tumors had high USP1 and ID2 expression. In U2OS and 143B osteosarcoma cell lines USP1 knockdown decreased ID1, ID2, and ID3 protein levels; decreased expression of the stem cell markers e-cadherin and fibronectin; and increased expression of markers of mature osteoblasts. *USP1* knockdown decreased the number of cells in S phase of the cell cycle and decreased xenograft formation.[252] If the results of this single study are validated, USP1 inhibition is a potential therapeutic avenue for osteosarcoma. Development of USP1 inhibitors is of interest owing to potential for activity in a wide variety of cancers, including lung cancer.[253,254]

Oncogenes

Multiple cell surface receptor oncogenes are expressed and activated in osteosarcoma. It appears as though coexpression and coactivation of multiple cell surface receptors is a feature of osteosarcoma cell lines.[255,256] Whether this phenomenon is also present in primary osteosarcoma tumors is not yet known. *MET*, *FOS*, *ERBB2*, and *MYC* are oncogenes that have been extensively investigated in osteosarcoma.

MET

MET, a receptor tyrosine kinase, was first identified and noted to be oncogenic in a transformed human osteosarcoma cell line. In the 1970s, Rhim and colleagues[217] treated a human osteosarcoma cell line with N-methyl-N′-nitronitrosoguanidine (MNNG), a chemical carcinogen. MNNG treatment resulted in a morphologic change and the acquisition of in vivo tumor-forming capacity. Subsequent studies have shown that the transforming event is formation of a fusion oncogene, *TRP-MET*, which leads to high levels of MET expression.[257,258]

MET is highly expressed in human osteosarcomas and osteosarcoma cell lines. The exact proportion of osteosarcomas that have high MET expression varies, depending on the detection method used. By Western blotting, 60% to 88% of osteosarcoma tumor specimens and 100% of osteosarcoma cell lines display high levels of MET protein.[259,260] Immunohistochemical analysis yields more variable results, with 35% to 75% of osteosarcomas highly expressing MET.[261,262] The quantitative PCR assay also demonstrates elevated MET expression in all osteosarcoma tumor specimens and cell lines studied.[263] Of note, the benign bone tumors osteoblastoma and nonossifying fibroma do not express MET but chondroblastoma and giant cell tumors do express MET.[259,260,262] When primary and metastatic tumors from the same patient are compared, metastatic tumors have higher MET expression than the primary tumors, suggesting a role for MET in osteosarcoma metastasis.[259,261,264] The mechanism of elevated MET expression in osteosarcoma is not known. When evaluated, *MET* gene amplification does not appear to be present in osteosarcoma.[259]

Functional studies in cell lines have contributed to the understanding of MET-transforming roles in osteosarcoma. Expression of MET carrying an activating mutation or overexpression of MET by lentiviral transfection transforms normal osteoblasts.[263] Despite a high level of MET expression, MET is not activated in the absence of its ligand, hepatocyte growth factor (HGF).[265] An autocrine-paracrine loop may cause MET activation in human osteosarcomas in vivo.[260] Addition of HGF to MET-expressing osteosarcoma cell lines results in MET activation, activation of downstream signaling intermediates MAPK and AKT, and increased invasive growth.[265,266] MET-HGF interaction in other model systems induces proliferation and enhances motility, cellular changes that frequently precede metastasis.[267]

As reviewed by Trusolino and Comoglio,[267] the MET receptor, and HGF, turn on cellular programs that lead to invasive growth. Downstream mediators of MET activity include cadherins, integrins, and metalloproteinases. The ultimate outcome of MET activation includes loss of cell-cell adhesion, increased cell motility, and extracellular matrix degradation. Physiologic requirements for invasive growth include organogenesis, tissue regeneration, and wound healing. Inappropriate activation in cancer cells leads to tissue invasion and metastasis.

FOS

FOS was initially identified as osteosarcomagenic through investigation of the FBJ murine virus. Mice inoculated with FBJ murine virus develop osteosarcomas that are pathologically similar to human tumors.[268] The viral protein responsible for transformation after infection with FBJ murine virus has almost complete homology with the murine c-Fos protein expressed from the murine Fos gene.[269] Transfection of a functional, highly expressed *FOS* gene transforms fibroblasts.[270]

Further evidence that c-Fos overexpression can induce osteosarcomas has been provided by transgenic mouse models. Transgenic mice in which *Fos* is expressed from a major histocompatibility complex (MHC) class I promoter develop osteosarcoma with 100% penetrance.[271] In these mice, *Fos* is highly expressed in both osteoblasts and osteosarcomas. Transgenic mice in which the gene is expressed from a different universally expressed promoter, human metallothionein, also develop osteosarcomas but at a much lower frequency,[272] suggesting that there is a dose-response relationship between the extent of FOS overexpression and the development of osteosarcoma.

FOS is overexpressed in human osteosarcoma tumor specimens. By immunohistochemical analysis, 50% to 60% of human osteosarcomas express high levels of FOS protein.[273,274] Only 20% of benign bone tumors have immunohistochemical positivity for FOS, and the level of FOS immunohistochemical staining in benign tumors is not as high as in osteosarcomas.[234] When compared with normal tissues and nonosteosarcomatous lesions, FOS expression, as assessed by immunohistochemistry, is 150%.[274] FOS RNA levels are increased in 40% of osteosarcomas.[275] One study has found an association between FOS expression and the occurrence of metastasis or recurrence,[275] but another did not.[273]

Although it is known that FOS, a member of the AP1 transcription factor complex, is an important mediator between extracellular signaling and transcriptional activation in normal bone development, it is not known exactly how FOS overexpression contributes to osteosarcomagenesis. Induction of *Fos* expression in osteoblasts alters CCND1 levels and increases entry into the S phase.[276] Wagner[277] has noted that AP1 complex activity is regulated by vitamin D, transforming growth factor β, and parathyroid hormone, all of which are important factors influencing bone formation, growth, and healing. In particular, FOS appears to play an essential role in enchondral ossification. *Fos* null mice have significant osteopetrosis, suggesting that FOS activity is required for normal osteoclast function.[278,279]

Insulin-like Growth Factor

As noted earlier (see "Etiology"), there is epidemiologic evidence for a link between normal bone growth and osteosarcoma, including the coincidence of osteosarcoma peak incidence with maximal linear growth in adolescence and the higher rate of osteosarcoma in larger dog breeds.[280] The observed epidemiologic links between osteosarcoma and bone growth could have alternate explanations. Osteosarcoma in large-breed dogs could be caused by the underlying genetics of breed founders rather than by rates of bone growth. Nevertheless, as central mediators of normal linear bone growth and cellular proliferation in general, insulin-like growth factor 1 (IGF-1) and its receptor, insulin-like growth factor 1 receptor (IGF1R), have been investigated in osteosarcoma. In vitro and in vivo data have supported a possible role for IGF-1 and IGF1R in osteosarcoma proliferation and invasion.

IGF-1 and IGF1R are members of the family of insulin-like growth factors and insulin-like growth factor receptors. The other ligands in the IGF-1 family are IGF-2 and insulin. There are three tyrosine kinase receptors in the family, IGF1R, IGF2R, and the insulin receptor. IGF1R is the primary target of IGF-1 and the most thoroughly studied insulin-like growth factor receptor in osteosarcoma. IGF2R also appears to be highly expressed across a number of osteosarcoma cell lines.[256] Other key modulators of IGF1R activity are the insulin-like growth factor binding proteins (IGFBPs).[281] Knockout mice lacking IGF-1 or IGF1R are approximately half the size of normal mice and have delayed formation of their ossification centers.[282] Several humans with fetal growth restriction and postnatal short stature were found to have mutations in IGF1R.[283,284]

Competitive binding assays, affinity labeling experiments, and Northern and Western blot studies have demonstrated expression of IGF1R by osteosarcoma cell lines.[285,286] IGF-1 expression is variable across osteosarcoma cell lines.[287] Although less thoroughly studied than IGF-1, IGF-2 appears to be expressed by osteosarcoma cells.[286,288] There has been limited investigation into IGFBPs in osteosarcoma, but one study has shown that IGFBP3 transcription is augmented in MG-63 osteosarcoma cells in response to IGF-1.[289]

In osteosarcoma cell lines, IGF1R is not activated in the absence of its ligand.[290] Addition of IGF-1 to osteosarcoma cells in culture results in IGF-1R activation,[291] activation of IGF-1R downstream signaling, including AKT and ERK activation,[291] and increased proliferation[285,287,288] One study has shown that IGF-2 is also mitogenic for osteosarcoma cell lines and that this effect is mediated by binding to IGF2R.[288]

Multiple mechanisms of IGF1R inhibition in vitro and in vivo suppress osteosarcoma growth and invasion. In a number of different osteosarcoma cell lines, antibodies to IGF1R decrease osteosarcoma proliferation in a dose-dependent manner.[285,287,288,292] In some cases, antibody treatment causes 100% inhibition of IGF-1–induced proliferation. Forced expression of IGFBP5 or IGFBP3 by genetic or chemical mechanisms results in decreased IGF-1 expression, increased expression of differentiation markers, and decreased proliferation of osteosarcoma cells.[293,294] In vivo interruption of growth hormone by hypophysectomy or growth hormone–releasing hormone antagonism leads to a dramatic decrease in osteosarcoma xenograft tumor size and metastasis.[248,256,286,295]

IGF-1 and IGFBP3 levels in patients with osteosarcoma are different than established age- and gender-matched normal values, with 68% of patients having low IGF-1 levels. IGF-1 and IGFBP3 levels are not correlated with clinical variables such as metastasis and outcome.[296] Phase I studies of octreotide pamoate, a growth hormone antagonist, in patients with osteosarcoma have shown a 50% decrease in serum IGF-1 levels. However, there were no clinical responses to octreotide pamoate. There are several possible explanations that could reconcile these clinical findings, with evidence suggesting an important role for the IGF axis in osteosarcoma. The behavior of IGF-1 and IGF1R in osteosarcoma models may not accurately represent osteosarcoma in patients. More likely, IGF-1 may act in a paracrine rather than endocrine manner, so that IGF-1 serum levels are not representative of the tumor milieu. Alternatively, IGF1R activation in osteosarcoma in vivo may be mediated by IGF-2 or the extent of IGF1R activation may not be determined by ligand concentration. Finally, osteosarcoma biology is likely to be heterogeneous, with the IGF axis being important in some tumors but not in others. Early phase IGF1R antibody trials included an insufficient number of osteosarcoma patients to determine whether these drugs are effective in osteosarcoma.[297] It is not clear whether IGF1R antibodies will continue to be developed given lack of activity of these drugs in carcinomas. IGF1R kinase inhibitors continue to be developed.

ERBB2

The ERBB2 protooncogene encodes the human epidermal growth factor receptor 2, a receptor tyrosine kinase in the epidermal growth factor receptor family. ERBB2 is amplified in 20% of breast cancers,[298] and ERBB2 protein is expressed in a similar proportion of breast cancers.[299] In breast cancer, ERBB2 amplification or ERBB2 expression is associated with a poorer prognosis. Trastuzumab, an anti-HER2 therapeutic antibody, improves survival in patients with ERBB2-amplified tumors.[300]

ERBB2 protein levels are increased in 30% to 40% of osteosarcomas.[196,301-303] Initial studies raised the possibility of an association between ERBB2 expression and a worse prognosis, but this finding was not confirmed in later studies.[304] Some investigators have found evidence of ERBB2 gene amplification in osteosarcoma,[302] but others have not.[301,305,306] As discussed later (see "Treatment"), these findings led to a COG study, AOST 0121, that evaluated the feasibility of adding trastuzumab to multiagent chemotherapy. Eligible patients were those with high-risk metastatic osteosarcoma whose tumors were ERBB2 positive. Outcome in ERBB2-positive patients was similar to that of historical controls, suggesting limited activity of trastuzumab in ERBB2-positive osteosarcoma.[303]

MYC

The MYC gene, located at 8q24.1 is amplified in 7% to 10% of osteosarcomas when assessed by Southern blotting.[275,307] The more sensitive technique, array CGH, detects MYC amplification in 44% of osteosarcomas.[164,275,307,308] MYC mRNA and protein levels are increased in a similar proportion of osteosarcomas, and MYC expression might be correlated with metastasis. MYC, when complexed with MAX, activates the transcription of a number of genes, perhaps as many as 15% of all genes. Downstream effects of MYC transcriptional activation include proliferation, cell growth, inhibition of differentiation, and apoptosis. Exactly how MYC regulates these diverse cell processes and how MYC amplification leads to cancer is an area of active investigation.[309,310] One percent of mice with conditional *Myc* overexpression from the EµSRa promoter develop osteosarcoma.[311] With the recent development of BET bromodomain inhibitors, MYC has become a potential therapeutic target.[312]

Determinants of Metastasis

One of the defining features of osteosarcoma is its tendency to metastasize early, hence the need for systemic chemotherapy in all patients. Metastasis is a complicated process that involves motility, migration, degradation of extracellular matrix, extravasation, survival during transit through vasculature, invasion, and growth. Given the complicated nature of the process, many factors are likely to play a role in metastases, but it is difficult to decipher the specific contribution of each. Several of the factors that have been more extensively studied in the context of osteosarcoma will be discussed.

Chemokine ligand 12 (CXCL12) is a cytokine-like protein expressed on the surface of vascular endothelial cells. Through binding to its chemokine receptor, CXCR4, it plays a role in cytoskeleton rearrangement, adhesion to endothelial cells, and chemotaxis.[313,314] Involvement of the CXCR4/CXCL12 pathway has been implicated in the metastatic potential of several cancers, including rhabdomyosarcoma and lymphoma.[315-317] CXCR4 mRNA has been shown to be expressed in osteosarcoma and associated with the presence of metastases at the time of diagnosis.[318-320] In vitro assays have shown that migration of osteosarcoma cells expressing CXCR4 follows an CXCL12 gradient and that their adhesion to endothelial and bone marrow stromal cells is promoted by CXCL12 treatment.[320] This study also provided a rationale for the propensity of osteosarcoma to metastasize to the lung, where CXCL12 concentration is high, and demonstrated prevention of pulmonary metastasis in a murine model by the administration of a CXCR4 inhibitor, suggesting molecular strategies inhibiting this axis as a therapeutic target.[320]

Ezrin is a membrane-cytoskeleton linker protein that allows direct cellular interactions with the microenvironment, facilitating signal transduction through growth factor receptors and adhesion molecules, thereby regulating cell migration and metastasis, among other processes.[141] In an orthotopic model of murine osteosarcoma, ezrin expression was threefold higher in the more aggressive K7M2 cell line, which correlated with its metastatic potential when compared with the less aggressive K12 cell line.[321,322] In follow-up experiments, ezrin expression was found to provide an early survival advantage for pulmonary metastatic osteosarcoma, which is in part mediated by AKT.[141] Ezrin exists in phosphorylated (active) and unphosphorylated (inactive) states.[323] Establishment of osteosarcoma metastases in a mouse model is dependent on fluctuation between the active and inactive forms of ezrin.[324] Ezrin phosphorylation at threonine 567 is mediated in part by protein kinase C in osteosarcoma cell lines. The identification of protein kinase C as a mediator of ezrin phosphorylation and the discovery of small molecules that inhibit ezrin phosphorylation make ezrin a potential therapeutic target for osteosarcoma.[325]

A significant correlation between high ezrin expression and poor outcome in osteosarcoma has been shown, with shorter DFS and higher risk for metastatic relapse, supporting the animal model data.[141]

Overexpression of MET and its ligand hepatocyte growth factor, in osteosarcoma cell lines suggests a role for MET in its metastatic phenotype. Binding of the ligand to the MET ligand receptor stimulates both cell proliferation and motility, features associated with metastasis.[259,326] In a study of 17 osteosarcoma tumor samples, 60% expressed the MET ligand receptor at high levels.[259] When primary and metastatic tumors from the same patient are compared, metastatic tumors have higher MET expression than the primary tumors, indicating its role in potentiating the metastatic phenotype of osteosarcoma.[259-261]

FAS is a transmembrane receptor that activates the extrinsic cell death pathway on stimulation by its ligand, FASL. There is increasing evidence that a variety of tumor types that escape from apoptosis may enhance the ability of tumor cells to metastasize.[327] Studies in an osteosarcoma murine xenograft model with a high rate of pulmonary metastasis have suggested that decreased FAS expression enhances osteosarcoma metastasis. Therapies enhancing FAS expression inhibit the development of metastases in this model system. However, evidence that perturbations in FAS are a generalized mechanism of enhanced metastatic potential in osteosarcoma is limited.

The SAOS2 LM6 cell line was produced by serially passaging a human osteosarcoma cell line, SAOS2, through immunodeficient mice until pulmonary metastasis developed reliably and rapidly after tail vein injections. FAS protein and mRNA levels are lower in the SAOS2 LM6 metastasis–producing cell line compared with the seldom-metastasizing parental cell line SAOS2.[328] Furthermore, when SAOS2 LM6 FAS expression is increased through transfection, the number and size of pulmonary metastases developing after tail vein injection decrease.[329] FAS expression can also be induced by interleukin-12 (IL-12).[328] Intrapulmonary aerosolized IL-12 gene therapy after SAOS2 LM6 tail vein injection increases FAS expression in metastatic tumors and inhibits the development of pulmonary metastases.[330-333] Interestingly, ifosfamide and IL-12 display a synergistic relationship when used together in this model system, possibly because of ifosfamide-induced expression of FASL.[330]

FAS expression has been evaluated in human osteosarcoma pulmonary metastases from 28 patients. FAS was not expressed in 60% of the tumors, and the remaining 40% had only weak FAS expression.[334] Further study is needed to confirm that decreased FAS expression contributes to the metastatic potential of osteosarcoma occurring in humans and in osteosarcoma models other than the SAOS2 LM6 model.

Other factors that likely play a role in osteosarcoma metastases include expression of matrix metalloproteinases[335] and other degradative enzymes. The expression of these enzymes is necessary to degrade the extracellular matrix, permitting extravasation into the vasculature.

Biologic Markers of Response to Chemotherapy

The response of osteosarcoma to chemotherapy is evident in the change in patient survival resulting from its administration. Defining "response" is somewhat more difficult. Chemotherapy response in osteosarcoma is typically used to refer to the degree of necrosis in the definitive surgical resection specimen. The degree of necrosis seen in that specimen is a consistent predictor of patient survival across studies, as described elsewhere in this chapter. In the original description of the grading system, a grade I response was considered indicative of no histologically visible response to chemotherapy. Subsequently, this was specified as being less than 50% necrosis, because untreated osteosarcomas could have as much as 25% spontaneous necrosis. It was therefore believed that necrosis more than double this amount would be attributable to a chemotherapy effect. Numerous biologic studies have been performed correlating a particular marker with the necrosis grading. In some of these studies, the necrosis grading was used as a surrogate for EFS, with the anticipation that these will correlate. The advantage of necrosis grading in this context is that the data are available much sooner than mature EFS data. In other contexts, the necrosis grading is used as a marker of chemotherapy response. Complicating these analyses, the standard of care in osteosarcoma is multiagent chemotherapy. Factors that only affect responsiveness to a single agent may not be predictive in the context of multiagent chemotherapy. Given these limitations, relating a genetic alteration to necrosis grading may provide a more robust relationship with chemotherapy response than survival, because survival may be influenced by many factors other than chemotherapy response. Similarly, necrosis grading may be a better marker of response than radiographic response in osteosarcoma, because the mineralized matrix of an osteosarcoma prevents radiographically visible shrinkage of the tumor.

Because chemotherapy has had a dramatic effect on the outcome of osteosarcoma, it is perhaps intuitive to assume that genetic alterations that produce drug resistance would be associated with inferior chemotherapy response and patient survival. Along these lines, perhaps the most extensively studied prognostic marker is the expression of P-glycoprotein (PGP) or multidrug resistance protein 1 (MDR1). This is a transmembrane adenosine triphosphate–dependent efflux pump protein encoded by the multidrug resistance gene (ABCB1, formerly MDR1), which is responsible for the efflux of numerous chemotherapeutic agents from the malignant cell. In the context of osteosarcoma, the most important drug that can be effluxed by MDR1 is doxorubicin, although etoposide is also a substrate. Immunohistochemistry and reverse-transcriptase (RT)-PCR quantification studies have explored MDR1 and ABCB1 expression in osteosarcoma and demonstrated overexpression of MDR1 in 23% to 45% of tumors, with decreased survival reported for patients with MDR1-positive tumors[336-341] in initial studies. Of interest, although many of these studies demonstrated a correlation with outcome, several key studies did not demonstrate a relationship with the

necrosis grade. This suggests that use of necrosis grading as an early marker of outcome may not always be appropriate in the context of some biologic markers. A meta-analysis has proposed that MDR1 is associated with an increased risk for disease progression.[342] Although the early literature suggested that MDR1 may be a marker of drug resistance and aggressiveness in osteosarcoma, this finding has not been verified consistently across studies.[336-339,341] In addition, a prospective clinicopathologic cooperative group study has concluded that there is no correlation between MDR1 expression and percentage of osteosarcoma tumor necrosis after induction chemotherapy or EFS in localized osteosarcoma.[343] Overexpression of ABCB1 has also been explored with regard to its prognostic relevance. Although a small pilot study has shown a trend toward a worse outcome in patients exhibiting high levels of ABCB1 expression,[344] a larger prospective investigation did not identify a correlation between ABCB1 messenger RNA expression and prognosis in osteosarcoma patients, with patients with either very low or very high levels of ABCB1 having a relatively poor outcome.[345]

High-dose methotrexate (HDMTX) with leucovorin rescue is a major component of current protocols for the treatment of osteosarcoma.[110,346] HDMTX is vastly more effective than conventional dose methotrexate in the treatment of osteosarcoma, a finding that is not observed in other malignancies treated with MTX, implying a mechanism of intrinsic MTX resistance within osteosarcoma tumor cells.[347] In experimental systems, resistance to methotrexate can occur through a variety of mechanisms, including impaired intracellular transport of the drug via the reduced folate carrier, upregulation of dihydrofolate reductase, and diminished intracellular retention caused by decreased polyglutamylation. Studies have demonstrated that impairment of drug influx as a result of decreased expression and mutations in the reduced folate carrier gene is the major basis of intrinsic resistance; 65% of osteosarcoma tumor samples were found to have decreased reduced folate carrier expression at the time of initial biopsy.[347] In contrast, dihydrofolate reductase overexpression was seen relatively infrequently at initial biopsy, in only 10% of tumor samples, compared with 62% of the tumors examined at the time of definitive surgery or relapse, suggesting dihydrofolate reductase overexpression as the major mechanism of acquired MTX resistance in osteosarcoma.[347]

In vitro induction of HMGB1 expression in osteosarcoma cells prevented apoptosis. HMGB1 is a chromatin-binding nuclear protein that may be involved in chemotherapy resistance in other cancers.[348] Evaluation of HMBG1 in human osteosarcoma samples has not been performed. Other potential mechanisms of drug resistance include alterations in multidrug resistance protein expression, topoisomerase II, glutathione S-transferases, DNA repair, DNA damage response, drug metabolism or inactivation, and reduced intracellular delivery. Few studies have been performed in osteosarcoma to indicate whether these processes play a role in defining chemotherapy response.

In other studies, necrosis after chemotherapy has been used as a marker of response, and investigators have attempted to identify genetic signatures predictive of response. In each of these studies, a large number of genes were required to define a profile of response. The studies reported using 60 genes,[349] 104 genes,[350] and 45 genes[351] to distinguish between responders and nonresponders. This may be related to the small sample sizes used in each of these studies. Alternatively, the lack of robust clustering may be caused by the heterogeneity of osteosarcoma itself. Lack of robust clustering on gene expression profiling appears to be a property of non–translation–associated sarcomas, a result of their high levels of genetic complexity.

Translational Science

Bone metabolic pathways are of interest in osteosarcoma given that this is a tumor arising from osteoblasts and osteoblast precursors. Zoledronate is a nitrogen-containing bisphosphonate and the most potent of its class. It inhibits the development of osteolytic and osteoblastic bone lesions.[342,352] Preclinical models have shown cytotoxicity against osteosarcoma cell lines.[353,354] In vivo models in mice inoculated intravenously with the spontaneous murine osteosarcoma cell line POS-1 have shown prolonged survival when treated with single-agent zoledronate.[355] Moreover, combination with ifosfamide has shown more activity than either agent alone in preventing tumor recurrence, improving tissue repair, and increasing bone formation.[356] Bisphosphonates may also improve bone integrity after limb salvage surgery.[357,358]

Receptor activator of nuclear factor κB ligand (RANKL, also known as tumor necrosis factor ligand superfamily member 11 [TNFSF11]) and its receptor RANK have the physiologic function of regulating bone turnover. In response to RANKL-RANK binding, osteoclast precursors differentiate and become activated resulting in bone resorption.[359] An antibody against RANKL, denosumab, has been approved by the U.S. Food and Drug Administration (FDA) for treatment of osteoporosis. RANK is expressed in 57% of human osteosarcomas, most human osteosarcoma cell lines, and 70% of canine osteosarcomas, including two of two canine osteosarcoma skin metastases.[360,361] RANKL is expressed in 75% of human osteosarcoma tumor specimens, and the strength of expression is associated with prognosis.[362] In osteosarcoma cell lines, RANKL activates downstream signaling and modulates gene expression.[361,363] Further evidence supporting activity of the RANK-RANKL pathway in osteosarcoma is provided by a transgenic mouse model of osteosarcoma. In an osteosarcoma mouse model created by expression of the SV40 T/t antigen from the osteocalcin promoter, heterozygous deletion of *Prkar1a* accelerates development of osteosarcoma via increased *Rankl* gene expression. A subset of human osteosarcomas have low *PRKAR1A* expression and high *RANKL* expression.[365] In vivo studies of denosumab are limited by the fact that the antibody does not recognize murine or canine Rankl. To circumvent these limitations, in vivo studies have utilized other approaches to inhibit

Rankl activity, including Rank gene therapy, which creates a decoy receptor for Rankl, RANK-Fc, a chimeric protein that efficiently binds Rankl, or SiRNA directed against Rankl. In a murine orthotopic OS model, Rank gene therapy decreased primary and metastatic tumor burden: mice receiving this therapy did not develop osteosarcomatous lung metastases whereas 80% of control mice developed lung metastases.[365] A study by the same group using RANK-Fc confirmed these original findings.[366]

The phosphatidylinositol 3′ kinase/mammalian target of rapamycin (PI3K/mTOR) pathway is a central signaling pathway contributing to proliferation and survival in many cancers. The pathway has been recognized to contribute to proliferation, drug resistance, and metastasis in osteosarcoma. Expression of mTOR and p70S6K, an indicator of mTOR activation, is present in 70% to 80% of osteosarcomas, and the level of expression has been correlated with overall and disease free survival.[367] Activation of PI3K-AKT signaling is downstream of several biological processes involved in osteosarcoma metastasis such as Ezrin expression.[368] Micro-RNA-221, expressed at high levels in osteosarcoma targets PTEN, increases cell survival, decreases apoptosis, and induces cisplatin resistance.[369] The dual PI3K/mTOR inhibitor BEZ235 and the alpha selective PI3K inhibitor BYL719 induce cell cycle arrest and decrease tumor formation in vivo.[370,371] The clinical trial experience with mTOR inhibition in osteosarcoma is limited, and PI3K inhibitors have not been evaluated in this disease. There have been rare but dramatic responses to mTOR inhibition in patients with advanced, refractory osteosarcoma.[372] In a study using a sequenom assay to identify cancer-associated mutations in osteosarcoma, 3 of 89 tumors were found to have mutations in *PIK3CA*, the PI3K catalytic subunit.[373] A comprehensive next-generation sequencing study of 59 osteosarcoma samples thus far presented only in abstract form, identified PI3K/mTOR pathway alterations in 25% of osteosarcomas.[158]

GD2 is a cell surface sialic acid containing glycosphingolipid expressed normally in the central nervous system, peripheral nerves, and melanocytes. In neuroblastoma, anti-GD2 antibody given with cytokines to promote antibody-dependent cell-mediated cytotoxicity significantly improves EFS and OS.[374] More than 90% of osteosarcomas express GD2, and the intensity of expression, in most samples, is greater than that seen in neuroblastoma.[375,376] In the phase I/Ib trial of the murine anti-GD2 antibody, 14.2G2a, plus interleukin-2, one of two osteosarcoma patients treated had a complete response persisting for 8 months.[377]

There is mixed evidence regarding the role for immunotherapy in osteosarcoma. Completed clinical trials utilizing general immune stimulation with interferon α (IFN-α)[378] and inhaled granulocyte-macrophage colony-stimulating factor (GM-CSF)[379] did not demonstrate significant activity of either approach. Dendritic cell therapy has shown anti-osteosarcoma activity in one mouse model, particularly when pulsed in vitro with irradiated tumor and administered in a minimal residual disease setting.[380] However, in a clinical study of dendritic cell vaccination there was a lack of T-cell response and no evidence of clinical benefit.[381] Immune surveillance by T cells may delay or prevent the development of metastasis, as seen in a mouse model.[382] In a single study in a murine xenograft model, chimeric antigen receptor T cells expressing interlukin-11Rα treatment resulted in regression of pulmonary metastases.[383]

TREATMENT

Local Control

Definitive surgical treatment of osteosarcoma (discussed more extensively in Chapter 49 "Pediatric Surgical Oncology") has two components: tumor resection and reconstruction. Tumor resection is essential for cure of osteosarcoma. Ten-year survival in patients with macroscopic residual tumor is less than 15%, even with multiagent chemotherapy.[52,384] Tissue margins on the resection specimen should be wide. Although the exact tissue margin required is not known, wide margins are generally defined as 2 to 5 mm for soft tissue and 2 to 3 cm for bone marrow. Marginal and intralesional margins are associated with a poor outcome and an increased risk for local recurrence.[53,385] As noted earlier (see "Natural History and Prognosis"), an additional factor increasing the risk for local recurrence and poor outcome is a poor histologic response to chemotherapy. In one study, inadequate margins and a poor histologic response to therapy were independent predictors of local recurrence.[386] In this study, having both a poor histologic response to therapy and inadequate margins dramatically increased the risk for local recurrence.[386]

Options for limb reconstruction include limb-sparing techniques that use allografts or fixed or expandable endoprostheses. Currently, 75% to 80% of patients with nonaxial tumors are treated with limb-sparing surgery.[110,115] As long as the resection margins are adequate, limb-sparing techniques do not change EFS or OS.[119,132] Because of the significant cosmetic impact, amputation and rotationplasty are often reserved for those patients whose tumors are not amenable to limb-sparing techniques. Occasionally, however, patients will opt for amputation or rotationplasty because of their advantages, which include a lower incidence of repeated surgical revisions and a greater ability to participate in high-impact activities.[387] Benefits of endoprostheses over allografts include a shorter postoperative recovery time and a lower incidence of perioperative complications. Allografts have the important advantage of allowing preservation of the growth plate. The relative strengths and weaknesses of the various surgical options are discussed further later (see "Complications of Therapy") and in Chapter 49, "Pediatric Surgical Oncology."

The optimal surgical approach should be determined by a multidisciplinary team that includes a radiologist, oncologist, and orthopedic surgeon with experience in the treatment of bone tumors. Adequate imaging, usually MRI, is required to determine which surgical procedures will produce sufficient margins. Finally, a good understanding of the patient's and family's priorities is needed to provide appropriate counseling.

Chemotherapy for Localized Disease

The use of neoadjuvant and adjuvant chemotherapy has increased the OS of patients with localized high-grade osteosarcoma from 20% to 70% to 75%. The most active chemotherapeutic agents for localized osteosarcoma are HDMTX with leucovorin rescue, doxorubicin (Doxo), and cisplatin (CP). In addition, ifosfamide and etoposide have demonstrated efficacy in metastatic osteosarcoma. Institutional and cooperative group studies have attempted to identify the optimal combination of active agents, the most effective drug dosing, and the impact of dose intensity and schedule on outcome and toxicity (Tables 62-5 and 62-6). Much has been learned from these studies. However, important questions remain, including the ability to improve high-risk disease outcomes through chemotherapy intensification, the role of immune modulators in osteosarcoma therapy, and whether there is additional benefit of adding ifosfamide and etoposide to first-line therapy for localized disease.

Chemotherapy and Outcome

It has not always been clear that chemotherapy is effective in osteosarcoma. Successful treatment of osteosarcoma with chemotherapy was first reported in the literature in the early 1970s. Jaffe and colleagues[109] treated 20 patients with adjuvant HDMTX and vincristine (VCR). They noted 1 death in 20 patients compared with 14 expected deaths, based on historical controls. In 12 patients with completely resected primary tumors, there was 1 death, which was 6 fewer than predicted by historic controls.[109] Cortes and colleagues[388] saw similar dramatic improvements in OS and EFS in 21 patients treated with surgery and Doxo. The Memorial Sloan-Kettering Cancer Center (MSKCC) has reported an OS of 75% with neoadjuvant HDMTX containing multiagent chemotherapy.[123] Other groups reported improved survival compared with historical controls with adjuvant CP and Doxo[389] or adjuvant multiagent chemotherapy containing Doxo.[390] However, in other studies, chemotherapy did not appear to improve outcome. Lange and colleagues[391] treated 20 patients with completely resected nonmetastatic osteosarcoma with HDMTX, VCR, and Doxo and observed an OS of only 26%, a rate similar to that of untreated historical controls.

Randomized controlled trials comparing chemotherapy and observation have been conducted for several reasons, despite the positive results of some early chemotherapy studies. First, the improved outcome observed with chemotherapy could have been caused by an improved outcome for all patients unrelated to chemotherapy. Advances in diagnosis and surgical approach could have improved outcome, irrespective of other therapies provided. Results of a randomized controlled trial at the Mayo Clinic,[134,392] in which the EFS was 42% in both treated and untreated patients, supported this theory. Second, because of the lack of a control group, the favorable results of these early chemotherapy trials could have been caused by patient selection.[393]

Two randomized controlled trials published in the mid-1980s confirmed the effectiveness of chemotherapy

TABLE 62-5   Randomized Controlled Trials of Chemotherapy for Nonmetastatic Osteosarcoma

Group	Year	Regimen(s)	No. Patients	EFS/ DFS	Primary Objective(s)	Results/Conclusions
Mayo[134]	1984	HDMTX/VCR vs. observation	38	42%	Demonstrate superior outcome with adjuvant chemotherapy.	1. EFS and OS equivalent in chemo and observation arms. 2. EFS/OS in observation arm better than historic controls. 3. Power inadequate to detect a difference. 4. Natural history may be improving.
POG[394]	1986	HDMTX/Doxo/BCD vs. Observation	36	66% 17%	Demonstrate superior outcome with adjuvant chemotherapy.	1. Adjuvant chemotherapy improves outcome. 2. Natural history is not improving.
UCLA[395]	1987	HDMTX/VCR/Doxo/BCD vs. Observation	59	55% 20%	Demonstrate superior outcome with adjuvant chemotherapy.	1. Adjuvant chemotherapy improves outcome. 2. Natural history is not improving.
EORTC-SIOP[450]	1988	HDMTX/Doxo/CTX + adjuvant HDMTX/Doxo/CP vs. HDMTX/Doxo/CTX + adjuvant pulmonary XRT	205	40%	Compare efficacy of adjuvant chemotherapy vs. adjuvant pulmonary XRT.	1. EFS and OS equivalent in all arms. 2. Pulmonary XRT less toxic than chemotherapy.
MSKCC (T10)[412]	1982	HDMTX/BCD/Doxo ±VCR Good response: Continue same Poor response: −HDMTX, +CP, ± VCR	57	93% 96% 91%	Evaluate the effect of VCR on EFS.	1. Improved EFS compared with historic controls 2. VCR has no impact on EFS.
COSS[125]	1988	MTX/Doxo/CP Good response: Continue same Poor response: ifosfamide/CP/ BCD vs. IFN-α MTX/BCD Good response: Continue same Poor response: Doxo/CP	141	58% 49%	Improve survival or decrease toxicity by altering chemotherapy intensity based on tumor response.	1. Lower intensity therapy results in a reduced EFS. 2. Higher-intensity therapy for poor responders does not result in an increased EFS (compared with historic controls).
Rizzoli[118]	1990	MTX/CP Good responders: Continue same Fair response: + Doxo Poor response: + Doxo/BCD HDMTX: 7500 mg/m² vs. MDMTX: 750 mg/m²	127	58% 42%	Compare efficacy of HDMTX and MDMTX.	1. EFS worse in patients receiving MDMTX although result is not statistically significant. 2. Lower intensity therapy for good responders results in a reduced OS of 20%.
EOI[126]	1992	HDMTX/Doxo/CP vs. Doxo/CP	198	41% 57%	Compare efficacy of multiagent regimen and two-agent regimen.	Two-drug regimen as efficacious as multiagent regimen.
EOI[422]	1997	HDMTX/VCR/BCD/Doxo/CP vs. Doxo/CP	407	44%	Compare efficacy of multiagent, prolonged (44 wk) regimen and two-agent shorter (18 wk) regimen.	1. EFS and OS equivalent in both arms. 2. Compliance better in shorter, two-agent regimen.

TABLE 62-5   Randomized Controlled Trials of Chemotherapy for Nonmetastatic Osteosarcoma (Continued)

Group	Year	Regimen(s)	No. Patients	EFS/ DFS	Primary Objective(s)	Results/Conclusions
MSKCC (T12)[112]	1998	HDMTX/BCD Poor response: + Doxo/CP Good response: + Doxo vs. Neoadj.: HDMTX/BCD/Doxo/CP Poor/good response: Continue	73	73% 78%	Improve outcome by intensifying preoperative chemotherapy.	1. Preoperative chemotherapy intensification increases percentage of good responders. 1. EFS is equivalent in both arms. 2. Intensifying preoperative chemotherapy does not increase DFS.
POG[111]	2003	Neoadj.: None Adj: HDMTX/BCD/Doxo/CP vs. Neoadj.: HDMTX/Doxo/CP Adj.: + BCD	106	65%	Compare outcomes of patients treated with or without neoadjuvant chemotherapy.	1. Neoadjuvant chemotherapy does not improve or worsen EFS. 2. Limb salvage rates are similar in both arms.
COG[5,110]	2005	HDMTX/Doxo/CP ⊥ MTPPE ± Ifosfamide	667	63%	Improve outcome by intensifying chemotherapy with ifosfamide, MTPPE or both.	1. OS and EFS were not statistically different between arms on initial analysis. 2. On follow-up analysis OAS is slightly better in patients receiving MTPPE.
EOI[423]	2007	Doxo/CP q3 wk cycles vs. Doxo/CP q2 wk cycles (w/G-CSF)	497	39% 41%	Improve survival by increasing dose intensity.	1. EFS/OAS equivalent in both arms. 2. Toxicity equivalent in both arms. 3. Outcome with two agent, shorter regimen (this study) significantly worse than with multiagent prolonged regimen (other studies).

Adj., Adjuvant; *BCD,* bleomycin, cyclophosphamide, and dactinomycin; *CP,* cisplatin; *DFS,* disease-free survival; *Doxo,* doxorubicin; *EFS,* event-free survival; *G-CSF,* granulocyte colony-stimulating factor; *HDMTX,* high-dose methotrexate; *IFN-α,* interferon-α; *MDMTX,* moderate-dose methotrexate; *MTP-PE,* muramyl tripeptide phosphatidylethanolamine; *Neoadj.,* neoadjuvant; *OS,* overall survival; *VCR,* vincristine; *XRT,* radiation therapy.

TABLE 62-6   Nonrandomized, Uncontrolled Trials of Chemotherapy in Nonmetastatic Osteosarcoma

Group	Date	Regimen(s)	No. Patients	EFS
CHOP[391]	1982	HDMTX/VCR/Doxo	20	26%
CCG[132]	1997	Neoadj.: HDMTX/VCR/BCD Good responders: Doxo Poor responders: Doxo/CP	268	53% 81% 46%
COSS[133]	1998	Low-risk: HDMTX/Doxo/CP High-risk: HDMTX/Doxo/CP/I	171	66%
Rizzoli[115]	2000	Neoadj.: HDMTX/Doxo/CP Good response: Continue same Poor response: + IE	164	61%
St. Jude[405]	2001	HDMTX/Doxo/I	69	72%
SSG[404]	2003	Neoadj.: HDMTX/Doxo/CP Good response: Continue same Poor response: + I/E	113	63%
ISG/SSG[113]	2005	HDMTX/Doxo/CP/I	182	64%

BCD, Bleomycin, cyclophosphamide, and dactinomycin; *CP,* cisplatin; *Doxo,* doxorubicin; *EFS,* event-free survival; *HDMTX,* high-dose methotrexate; *I,* ifosfamide; *IE,* ifosfamide and etoposide; *Neoadj.,* neoadjuvant; *VCR,* vincristine.

and an unchanged osteosarcoma natural history. In a multiinstitutional study, 36 patients with nonmetastatic fully resected osteosarcoma were randomized to observation or treatment with HDMTX, Doxo, and a regimen of bleomycin, cyclophosphamide, and dactinomycin (BCD).[394] The EFS was 66% in the group treated with chemotherapy but only 17% in the observed patients. Investigators at the University of California, Los Angeles, randomized 59 patients to a similar chemotherapy regimen or observation and obtained almost identical results.[395] Of treated patients, 55% were free of disease at 2 years whereas only 20% of observed patients remained free of disease. Statistically significant improvement in EFS and OS with chemotherapy has remained after long-term follow-up of this study population.[396]

Chemotherapeutic Agents

Cisplatin. In addition to the initially identified agents, HDMTX and Doxo, CP was identified as an active anti-osteosarcoma drug in the late 1970s[397] and was rapidly incorporated into multiagent protocols. Adjuvant CP, in combination with Doxo, results in DFS rates at least as high as those seen with adjuvant HDMTX and Doxo.[389] In the past, it was theorized that intraarterial administration of cisplatin directly to the primary tumor might improve local control and survival. However, several randomized trials have failed to show survival gains from the intraarterial administration route,[133,398] despite an increased proportion of tumors with a good histologic response in some studies. Thus, it is now generally accepted that intraarterial administration of cisplatin is not of sufficient benefit to be worth the increased risk and inconvenience, although countervailing opinions remain.[399] Carboplatin has successfully replaced cisplatin in the treatment of some other cancers, but it may be less efficacious than CP in osteosarcoma. In a Pediatric Oncology Group study, presurgical carboplatin produced pathologic tumor responses in only 1 of 37 chemotherapy-naïve patients with metastatic osteosarcoma.[400] On the other hand, patients enrolled on a single-arm St. Jude Children's Research Hospital study in which chemotherapy consisted of carboplatin, ifosfamide, and Doxo[401] had similar outcomes compared with historical populations treated with CP-containing chemotherapy regimens. Carboplatin may have adequate activity in osteosarcoma when combined with some chemotherapy regimens, particularly those containing ifosfamide.

A recently published trial conducted by the Société Française d'Oncologie Pédiatrique (SFOP)[402] has underscored the importance of CP in osteosarcoma therapy. This study had two arms, with different preoperative chemotherapy regimens. In one arm, preoperative chemotherapy was HDMTX and Doxo, and patients in the other arm received HDMTX and combined ifosfamide and etoposide (IE). Patients with a poor histologic response to preoperative chemotherapy in the HDMTX-IE arm received postoperative CP-Doxo and had an EFS of 60%, whereas patients with a poor histologic response in the HDMTX-Doxo arm received postoperative IE without CP and had an EFS of 49%.

Ifosfamide and Etoposide. After demonstration of anti-osteosarcoma activity in unresectable or metastatic disease,[403] ifosfamide was incorporated into multiagent treatment protocols for localized disease with the goal of improving outcome[113,115,133,404] or minimizing toxicity.[405] In two separate nonrandomized studies, one conducted at the Rizzoli Institute (Italy) and one by the Scandinavian Sarcoma Group (SSG), patients with a poor histologic response were treated with the IE regimen. In both studies, outcome was improved in patients with a poor response when compared with historical controls.[115,404] However, in a follow-up joint study by the SSG and the Italian Sarcoma Group (ISG), ifosfamide was given to all patients regardless of tumor response and the outcome was similar to that of historical controls.[113] Because none of these trials was randomized, a definitive conclusion regarding the additional benefit gained by adding IE to first-line therapy of localized disease is not possible. In a randomized controlled COG trial, the addition of ifosfamide to Doxo, CP, and HDMTX for patients with localized osteosarcoma did not increase survival.[110] Of note, in this trial, patients were treated with ifosfamide not in combination with etoposide, and ifosfamide was administered in a relatively low dosage (9 g/m²/course). In another approach to incorporating ifosfamide into osteosarcoma regimens, the ISG conducted the ISG/OS-1 trial in which ifosfamide was administered to all enrolled patients in the neoadjuvant period. The use of ifosfamide in the neoadjuvant period did not improve the proportion of patients with a good histologic response or EFS or OS when compared with appropriate historical populations.[406]

A meta-analysis of osteosarcoma trials found that three-drug regimens, most of which do not contain ifosfamide, and four-drug regimens, most of which do contain ifosfamide, produce equivalent EFS and OS. This outcome does not eliminate a potential role for ifosfamide in osteosarcoma chemotherapy regimens.[407] Ifosfamide may be utilized to decrease the cumulative dose of other chemotherapy agents such as Doxo to decrease toxicity. In addition, studies conducted to date have not adequately addressed whether there is a role for ifosfamide in improving outcomes in high-risk patients. An international, multigroup study, the European and American Osteosarcoma Study Group (EURAMOS), is examining the efficacy of the addition of postoperative IE for improving EFS in patients whose tumors have a poor histologic response to chemotherapy.

Methotrexate. In early protocols, MTX was administered at dosages between 3 and 7.5 g/m².[109,123,131] However, methotrexate pharmacokinetics in children result in lower peak MTX levels for a given dosage per kilogram of body weight partly because of faster renal clearance.[408] Since this information became known, most regimens have used a MTX dosage of 12 g/m².[110,111] Several retrospective studies have shown a correlation between higher peak methotrexate levels (700 to 1000 µmol/L) and tumor necrosis[80] and DFS.[409] At a methotrexate dosage of 12 g/m², more than 90% of patients achieve peak methotrexate levels above 1000 µmol/L.[409,410] However, the only study directly comparing 7.5 g/m² and 12 g/m² did not demonstrate improved survival with the higher dosage.[411] Moderate MTX dosages (600 to 750 mg/m^2) do not seem to be as effective as high MTX dosages.[118,130] Alkaline intravenous fluids and leucovorin are administered with HDMTX, and MTX levels should be monitored after MTX administration.

Microtubule Inhibitors Vincristine and Eribulin. VCR was used in combination with MTX in the initial chemotherapy study by Jaffe and colleagues[109] because of preclinical data suggesting that VCR potentiated cellular MTX uptake. It is no longer used because a randomized controlled trial has shown no effect on EFS compared with MTX alone.[412] Eribulin is a synthetic analogue of a natural product, halichondrin B, and has a novel mechanism of action when compared with other microtubule inhibitors. Unlike other antimicrotubule drugs that suppress the shortening and growth phases of microtubule dynamic instability, eribulin works by inhibition of microtubule growth.[413,414] When evaluated by the Pediatric Preclinical Testing Program (PPTP), a platform for assessing the activity of novel agents in xenografts of common pediatric malignancies, eribulin had significant activity in osteosarcoma xenografts. Three of six patients with osteosarcoma receiving xenografts had a complete response, one had stable disease, and the remaining two had progressive disease. In a preclinical study with the osteosarcoma cell line U2OS, eribulin affected mitotic spindle centromere dynamics.[415] On the basis of these promising preclinical results, a phase II trial of eribulin in recurrent osteosarcoma is planned.

Bleomycin, Cyclophosphamide, and Dactinomycin. The combination of bleomycin, cyclophosphamide, and dactinomycin (BCD) was initially used by investigators at MSKCC[123] in combination with other active agents. BCD was included in a number of other treatment regimens in a nonrandomized fashion. However, in a direct comparison of BCD and CP in combination with HDMTX, VCR, and Doxo conducted by the Cooperative Osteosarcoma Study Group (COSS), the results of therapy with BCD were equivalent to those with CP.[124] In addition, BCD does not cause tumor regression in patients with previously treated metastatic disease.[416] Because of the equivalency with CP, lack of demonstrated efficacy in metastatic disease, and potential pulmonary toxicity, BCD is no longer included in most osteosarcoma chemotherapy regimens.

Immune Modulators. In vitro, IFN-α decreases the proliferation of osteosarcoma cell lines.[417] In vivo, growth of mouse osteosarcoma xenografts is inhibited by IFN-α.[418] Based on these preclinical data, investigators at the Karolinska Institute in Sweden gave IFN-α monotherapy to patients with localized fully resected osteosarcoma. The EFS was 53%.[419] Because of the impressive EFS in this study, a randomized trial evaluating IFN-α as maintenance after multiagent chemotherapy was conducted by EURAMOS. Results of this study have been presented, and IFN-α maintenance therapy did not improve EFS or OS.[378]

Another immunomodulatory therapy that might have activity in osteosarcoma is muramyl tripeptide phosphatidylethanolamine (MTP-PE). MTP-PE is a liposomal encapsulated bacille Calmette-Guérin cell wall component. It activates macrophages and, in mouse xenografts, induces tumoricidal activity.[420] Adjuvant treatment of osteosarcoma in dogs with MTP-PE alone led to a significantly increased DFS.[421] The addition of MTP-PE to HDMTX, Doxo, and CP was evaluated in a COG randomized controlled trial.[110] In the initial analysis of this study, neither EFS nor OS was statistically significantly improved in patients treated with the addition of MTP-PE or MTP-PE and ifosfamide to standard three-drug HDMTX, CP, and Doxo when compared with those treated with the three-drug combination of HDMTX, CP, and Doxo alone. Interpretation of the study results remains controversial, especially in light of a recently published follow-up analysis of the study data. In this analysis, the addition of MTP-PE to the standard three-drug regimen of HDMTX, CP, and Doxo significantly improved 6-year OS from 70% to 78% but did not significantly improve EFS.[5] At present, the FDA application for approval of MTP-PE is pending and MTP-PE is therefore not currently available.

Neoadjuvant Chemotherapy

Neoadjuvant chemotherapy is an approach in which some of the chemotherapy cycles are given prior to tumor resection and the remaining cycles are given postoperatively. Neoadjuvant chemotherapy in osteosarcoma has several potential benefits. Theoretically, neoadjuvant chemotherapy could increase DFS and OS through earlier treatment of microscopic metastatic foci.[123] From a practical perspective, neoadjuvant chemotherapy provides sufficient time for custom endoprosthesis preparation and other surgical planning. In addition, if sufficient tumor shrinkage occurs, neoadjuvant chemotherapy could make a patient who would have required amputation eligible for limb-sparing surgery. Postoperative healing could also be improved by neoadjuvant chemotherapy because there is less urgency to resume chemotherapy.

Theoretically, the greatest benefit of neoadjuvant chemotherapy is that it permits evaluation of tumor response to chemotherapy, the only clear predictor of outcome in osteosarcoma. Identifying patients with a poorer prognosis combined with subsequent therapeutic interventions could improve outcome. However, at present, there are no known therapeutic interventions that improve outcomes for patients with a poorer prognosis based on histologic response to chemotherapy. If therapeutic interventions that improve outcomes in patients with a poor tumor response to chemotherapy are not identified, the value of neoadjuvant chemotherapy will be diminished.

Neoadjuvant chemotherapy was initially used in MSKCC protocols.[123,412] The OS in patients treated with the MSKCC neoadjuvant protocols was 75% to 93%. Because an OS of 93% was significantly better than outcomes reported with adjuvant chemotherapy, there was initial excitement that neoadjuvant therapy would improve survival. However, a COSS protocol using the neoadjuvant approach, COSS-80, had an EFS of 68%, similar to EFS in ongoing studies of adjuvant chemotherapy.[124] Nevertheless, essentially all protocols after 1980 included, in a nonrandomized fashion, neoadjuvant chemotherapy. In general, EFS in these neoadjuvant protocols was similar to EFS seen in protocols giving only adjuvant therapy.

In the only randomized controlled trial comparing adjuvant and neoadjuvant chemotherapy,[111] OS and EFS were not significantly different for patients receiving adjuvant or neoadjuvant chemotherapy. Other than allowing the identification of a group of patients with a poorer prognosis, there did not appear to be significant additional benefits to neoadjuvant chemotherapy. The number of limb salvage procedures was the same in the adjuvant and neoadjuvant groups. Surgical complications were not reduced by neoadjuvant chemotherapy. Several patients had progression of the primary tumor during neoadjuvant chemotherapy, and a few of these patients developed pulmonary metastasis. Thus patients with clearly documented tumor progression during neoadjuvant chemotherapy should proceed to resection without completing the planned course of neoadjuvant therapy. This is especially true in the case of proximal tumors at risk for becoming inoperable (e.g., a proximal humeral lesion crossing the shoulder joint). On the other hand, chemotherapy-induced swelling of the tumor can sometimes be difficult to distinguish from progressive disease.

Response-Based Therapy

Multiple protocols have attempted to improve outcome in patients with a poorer prognosis by intensifying chemotherapy for this group of patients. In general, poor histologic tumor response after neoadjuvant chemotherapy has been used to stratify patients into an intensified treatment arm. Treatment intensification has generally been through the addition of one or two agents in the adjuvant phase not given during the neoadjuvant phase. For example, in Children's Cancer Group, Rizzoli Institute, and COSS protocols using neoadjuvant therapy consisting of HDMTX and BCD, adjuvant treatment was intensified by adding CP and Doxo.[118,125,132] Similarly, in the MSKCC T10 protocol, CP was administered to intensify therapy after neoadjuvant treatment with HDMTX, BCD, and Doxo.[412] With the exception of the T10 protocol, patients in the poor responder group had a similar outcome to historical controls (who did not get intensified chemotherapy), despite chemotherapy intensification.

In protocols in which both Doxo and CP are given neoadjuvantly, ifosfamide with or without etoposide has been used to intensify adjuvant chemotherapy for patients with a poor histologic response.[113,115,125,404] In the SSG protocol SSGVIII[404] and a recent Rizzoli protocol,[115] HDMTX, Doxo, and CP were given neoadjuvantly and IE was given adjuvantly to poor responders. In the Rizzoli trial, patients did not have a better outcome than historical controls (who did not receive IE intensification), whereas in the SSGVIII trial, outcome was better than historical controls, with an OS of 70% in patients with a poor histologic response.

In a different approach to chemotherapy intensification, COSS divided patients into high-risk and low-risk groups based on tumor size, pathologic subtype, and clinical response to neoadjuvant chemotherapy, measured by results of a bone scan. Patients in the high-risk group were treated with additional ifosfamide, added to the HDMTX, Doxo, and CP therapy. High-risk patients achieved the same outcome as low-risk patients. These results can be interpreted either as an indication that ifosfamide is effective at improving survival in high-risk patients or as indicating that the factors used to define the high-risk group do not actually convey a worse prognosis.[133] In summary, there is no convincing evidence that intensifying adjuvant chemotherapy for patients whose tumors have a poor histologic response results in an improved outcome. The lack of randomized studies addressing this question prevents a definitive conclusion about the usefulness of this approach.

On the other hand, there is fairly clear evidence that attempting to decrease toxicity for low-risk patients whose tumors have a good chemotherapy response by de-intensifying chemotherapy results in a worse prognosis.[118,125] In one arm of COSS-82, neoadjuvant chemotherapy consisted of HDMTX and BCD and, during adjuvant therapy, a lower dose of Doxo (30 mg/m^2 × 2 days) was given than had been used in previous protocols. The EFS was 41% in this arm of the study, which was significantly less than in both the other study arms and in historical controls. In a trial at the Rizzoli Institute, after neoadjuvant therapy with HDMTX and CP, patients with a good response received only further HDMTX and CP. These patients had an EFS of only 27%.

The conclusion of a series of studies by the European Osteosarcoma Intergroup (EOI)[126,422,423] is that a two-drug regimen of Doxo and CP is inferior to regimens that include three or more drugs. In the first and second randomized studies, outcomes in patients treated with CP and Doxo and those treated with regimens containing at least the three drugs were equivalent.[117] However, in these two studies and a third study, in which all patients were treated with Doxo and CP, EFS was approximately 40%, a lower rate than is seen in studies of multidrug regimens conducted by other groups.

Non–Risk-Based Chemotherapy Intensification

There are gains to be made in outcome for all osteosarcoma patients, not just those with high-risk disease. With this in mind, some groups have evaluated the impact of intensifying chemotherapy for all patients. The MSKCC T12 trial randomized patients to a more- or less-intensive neoadjuvant chemotherapy regimen. Patients randomized to the more-intensive study arm received HDMTX, BCD, Doxo, and CP neoadjuvantly and adjuvantly, whereas patients randomized to the less-intensive arm received HDMTX and BCD neoadjuvantly, with adjuvant therapy based on tumor response. Doxo was continued for patients with a good response, with Doxo and CP used for poor responders. EFS was 73% for patients in the less-intensive arm of the study and 78% for those in the more-intensive arm of the study,[110] a difference that is neither clinically nor statistically significant.

The COG conducted a randomized trial to evaluate the impact of adding adjuvant ifosfamide and/or MTP-PE to the initial HDMTX, Doxo, and CP. As noted earlier, in the initial analysis of this trial, neither the addition of ifosfamide nor the addition of MTP-PE significantly improved survival.[110] However, in a follow-up analysis, MTP-PE was shown to improve 6-year OS significantly, by a small margin.[5] As noted, interpretation of these data remain uncertain. As with chemotherapy intensification for poor responders, randomized controlled trials are needed to determine whether additional benefit can be gained from adding ifosfamide, etoposide, or other active agents such as immunomodulators to the core anti-osteosarcoma agents HDMTX, Doxo, and CP.

Dose Density

The most recent EOI study has evaluated the impact on toxicity and survival of shortening the interval between CP and Doxo courses from 3 to 2 weeks. In this randomized trial, patients on the every-2-week arm were supported with granulocyte colony-stimulating factor (G-CSF) between chemotherapy cycles. The EOI found that the shortened interval dosing was equivalent in both toxicity and outcome to the longer interval dosing.[423]

Current Approach to Therapy

Most of the osteosarcoma research groups, COG, SSG, COSS, and the EOI, have collaborated on an international trial, EURAMOS 1. The chemotherapy administered to all patients in the trial initially is neoadjuvant and adjuvant HDMTX, Doxo, and CP (Table 62-7). The objectives of this randomized trial are the following. (1) to determine whether the postoperative addition of IE improves EFS of patients with a poor response to neoadjuvant chemotherapy; and (2) to evaluate whether the postoperative addition of IFN-α after neoadjuvant chemotherapy improves outcome in patients with a good histologic response. All patients will receive a total of 10 weeks of neoadjuvant chemotherapy with HDMTX (four cycles) and Doxo and CP (two cycles). Patients with a poor response will be randomized to continue HDMTX, Doxo, and CP or to continue HDMTX, Doxo, and CP with the addition of IE. Patients with a good response will be randomized to continue HDMTX, Doxo, and CP or to continue HDMTX, Doxo, and CP, with the addition of IFN-α. The results of the good histologic response study arm were reported at the American Society of Clinical Oncology Annual Meeting in 2013. There was no difference in event free or overall survival between those who received IFN-α and those who did not. Only 55% of enrolled patients completed IFN-α therapy per protocol; 45% stopped early due to toxicity. The conclusion of this arm of the study is that, when given as tolerated, IFN-α does not improve outcome in osteosarcoma. The results of the poor histologic response study arm are still not available.[423a]

Initially Metastatic Osteosarcoma

As noted earlier (see "Natural History and Prognosis"), the presence of metastatic disease at the time of initial diagnosis is the most unfavorable prognostic feature. In view of the unfavorable outlook of these patients, strategies that included higher toxicity regimens have been used in an effort to improve patient outcome. The Pediatric Oncology Group (POG)[400] administered carboplatin, 1 g/m^2 as a 48-hour continuous infusion, to patients with initially metastatic osteosarcoma as initial therapy. Only 1 patient had an overall partial response. After researchers separately analyzed the primary and metastatic sites of disease, they found that 3 patients had a partial response of their primary tumor (2 had histologic evaluation of the tumor at definitive surgery, showing between 50% and 90% necrosis), 3 had complete responses, and 1 had partial response of their pulmonary disease. However, 20 of 37 patients had unequivocal progressive disease while receiving carboplatin. After induction, multiagent chemotherapy was administered with a combination of high-dose methotrexate, ifosfamide (2.4 g/m^2/day for 5 days, as a single agent), CP, and Doxo, for a total of 40 weeks. Overall outcome was poor, with an EFS of 24% and OS of 40% at 3 years. Patients with isolated pulmonary metastasis had a more favorable outlook, as in the COSS series, with a 44% 3-year survival. Those with unresectable bony metastases had a particularly poor outcome, 6% survival at 3 years.

A subsequent POG study began therapy with two cycles of high-dose ifosfamide (3.5 g/m^2/day for 5 days) and etoposide (100 mg/m^2/day, also for 5 days).[147] This was based on a prior phase I study of etoposide with escalating dosage of ifosfamide, in which 6 of 13 patients with recurrent osteosarcoma responded to therapy with higher dosage levels of ifosfamide.[424] Induction with ifosfamide and etoposide was followed by multiagent chemotherapy with high-dose methotrexate, CP, and Doxo, as well as three additional cycles of a slightly lower dosage of ifosfamide, 2.4 g/m^2/day for 5 days, and etoposide, 100 mg/m^2/day for 5 days. Surgery of the primary and resectable metastatic sites was encouraged. Of 41 evaluable patients, 2-year progression-free survival was 43%, with an OS probability of 55%. In the limited number of patients studied, survival was similar for

---

TABLE 62-7 Schema of Typical Administration Scheduled for Doxorubicin (A), Cisplatin (P), and High-Dose Methotrexate (M) Therapy for Osteosarcoma

Week*	1	4	5	6	9	10	11	12†	15	16	17	20	21	22	24	25	26	28	29
Therapy	A, P	M	M	A, P	M	M	Surgery		A, P	M	M	A, P	M	M	A	M	M	A	M	M

*Weeks 2, 3, 7, 8, 13, 14, 18, 19, 23, and 27 no therapy scheduled.
†Week 12 chemotherapy is administered after adequate postoperative healing has occurred.

patients with isolated pulmonary metastases, 52% at 2 years, as compared with patients with bone metastases, with or without lung metastases, 58% at 2 years. Toxicity was significant, however, with two toxic deaths, one from gram-negative sepsis and the second from congestive cardiac failure. Eighty-three percent of patients experienced severe neutropenia, with sepsis in 10% (including the septic death) and other bacterial infections in an additional 7%.

In view of the relatively favorable outcome of the IE-containing regimen, it served as the model for the core regimen in the COG study AOST 0121. The ifosfamide dosage utilized was one level lower (2.8 g/m^2/day for 5 days), along with etoposide 100 mg/m^2/day for 5 days because of toxicity observed on the previous trial, and the ordering of the cycles was slightly different. As noted earlier (see "Biology"), the presence of ERBB2 expression in osteosarcoma was believed to confer an unfavorable prognosis and to represent a tumor target. Trastuzumab is a humanized antibody that binds specifically to the ERBB2 protein. Preclinically, it was found to antagonize the function of the growth-signaling properties of the ERBB2 system, signal immune cells to attack and kill tumor targets, and augment chemotherapy-induced cytotoxicity.[425-429] A pivotal randomized phase III trial in women with previously untreated ERBB2-positive metastatic breast cancer has shown a significantly improved response rate and survival for those who initially received trastuzumab along with chemotherapy.[300] Trastuzumab increased the risk for cardiotoxicity when given with anthracyclines. However, trastuzumab cardiotoxicity appears to be reversible on discontinuation of the drug.[430] In view of the possible increased risk for cardiotoxicity, entry into AOST 0121 was limited to the highest-risk patients—those with bone metastases, bilateral lung metastases, or unilateral lung metastases with at least four nodules. In addition, dexrazoxane was administered as a cardioprotective agent prior to bolus doxorubicin. Approximately one third of patients had tumors that expressed ERBB2, and only these patients received trastuzumab. Toxicity data demonstrated that it is feasible to combine trastuzumab with multiagent chemotherapy in osteosarcoma. Clinically significant cardiac events did not occur. Outcome in ERBB2-positive patients was similar to that for ERBB2-negative patients treated with chemotherapy alone and to that for historical controls, suggesting limited activity of trastuzumab in ERBB2-positive osteosarcoma.[303]

More recently the COG conducted a study in patients with initially metastatic osteosarcoma incorporating zoledronate into the same background chemotherapy utilized in AOST 0121. The study assessed the feasibility and safety of adding zoledronate to multiagent chemotherapy. Zoledronate could be successfully combined with chemotherapy. Similar results were obtained in a related study in which pamidronate was combined with chemotherapy.[431] The 5-year EFS and OS in patients with metastatic osteosarcoma treated with chemotherapy and zoledronate were 45% and 62%, respectively.[432] Because of differences in study populations these outcomes could not be compared with prior prospectively studied patients

and thus determining the effectiveness of inhibiting bone turnover in osteosarcoma will require additional studies. A trial being conducted by the SFOP may shed some light on this question.

The trial evaluating the addition of MTP-PE to chemotherapy also enrolled patients with metastatic disease (see "Immune Modulators" under "Chemotherapy for Localized Disease"). As in patients with localized osteosarcoma, the 5-year OS in patients with metastatic osteosarcoma randomized to receive MTP-PE plus chemotherapy was slightly better than in those randomized to receive chemotherapy alone. However, this result was not statistically significant.[433] Therefore, as with MTP-PE in localized osteosarcoma, the results of this initial randomized study of MTP-PE are not conclusive. An additional clinical trial of MTP-PE would help clarify the role of this therapy in metastatic osteosarcoma.

In the absence of positive results from any of the clinical trials that have been conducted in the metastatic patient population, the standard approach to chemotherapy in patients with metastatic osteosarcoma is to use treatment protocols utilized in patients with localized disease. Some clinicians will intensify therapy such as by adding ifosfamide and etoposide to a HDMTX, Doxo, and CP based regimen as was done for the COG studies AOST 0121[303] and AOST 06P1.[432]

As with localized osteosarcoma, complete resection of all gross disease, when feasible, is an important part of therapy in metastatic osteosarcoma. For patients with isolated pulmonary metastases, metastasectomy of all pulmonary disease improves prognosis.[4] The surgical technique to best accomplish resection of pulmonary metastases in osteosarcoma has not been investigated with clinical trials and is a question open to debate. Because CT has been demonstrated to have less sensitivity for presence of pulmonary metastases than surgical exploration, some researchers believe that the surgical standard of care for osteosarcoma with isolated pulmonary metastases should be open thoracotomy with resection of all palpable pulmonary disease.[434] However, others argue a video-assisted thoracoscopic surgery approach is adequate in some cases.[435]

Recurrent Osteosarcoma

The recurrence of osteosarcoma is an unfavorable event, with subsequent outcome most influenced by the time to recurrence, burden of disease at the time of recurrence, and resectability of the recurrent disease. In a series from the COSS group,[7] 576 of an initial 1702 patients developed recurrent disease at a median time of 1.6 years (range, 0.1 to 14.3 years). EFS was 0.13 (standard error [SE], 0.01) at 5 years and 0.11 (SE, 0.02) at 10 years, with an OS of 0.23 (SE, 0.02) at 5 years and of 0.18 (SE, 0.02) at 10 years. The most important factor associated with survival was achievement of a second surgical complete remission. The ability to achieve second surgical complete remission was likely related to the number and bilaterality of pulmonary lesions, as well as pleural disruption by the pulmonary metastasis. Patients with multiple lesions, bilateral lesions, and lesions that disrupted the pleura fared less well. Chemotherapy was of limited benefit, with multiagent therapy probably more effective than single-agent therapy.

Similar results have been reported from the Rizzoli Institute[6] in a study of 175 patients. Again, achievement of a second surgical remission was key to survival and was more readily accomplished in patients with recurrence limited to the lungs (97 of 125 [75%] of those with isolated pulmonary recurrence as compared with 21 of 37 [57%] of those with other than lung metastasis). EFS was 16%, with postrelapse survival of 39% at 5 years for those who achieved a second complete surgical remission but 0% among those who did not. A longer initial relapse-free interval (>24 months) and the presence of only one or two lung metastases were favorable prognostic indicators in patients with isolated pulmonary metastases who achieved a second complete surgical remission. Chemotherapy slightly prolonged survival in those who did not achieve a second surgical complete remission and possibly in those with three or more pulmonary nodules who underwent resection. Other groups have reported comparable findings in smaller numbers of patients.[114,431,435,437] Aggressive and, if necessary, repeated thoracotomies have also been advocated by many.[438-441]

As discussed earlier (see "Determinants of Metastasis" under "Biology"), the development of pulmonary metastasis may be facilitated by the absence of FAS on the malignant cell surface. Tumor cells expressing FAS are eliminated by the lung endothelium, which constitutively expresses FASL. The metastatic potential of osteosarcoma cells in model systems has been shown to be inversely related to FAS expression, and metastatic osteosarcoma samples often lack FAS expression.[334,442,443] It was hypothesized that the administration of GM-CSF by the inhalation route may enhance FAS expression on osteosarcoma cells. A study at the Mayo Clinic in 40 patients with pulmonary metastases from a variety of malignancies has shown benefit in at least 50%.[444] Dose escalation in patients with melanoma has shown melanoma-specific T cells at the higher dosage levels of 1750 and 2000 μg administered by the inhalation route twice daily, 1 week on and 1 week off (S. Markovic, personal communication, 2008). A COG study (AOST 0221) investigated the feasibility of inhaled GM-CSF monotherapy in patients with recurrent osteosarcoma, with biologic end points including analysis of the FAS pathway and study of infiltrating dendritic cells. Metastatic nodules resected after inhaled GM-CSF did not display induction of FAS expression and had limited evidence of dendritic cell infiltrate.[379]

Chemotherapy administration via the inhalation route is one approach being considered for both recurrent and primary metastatic osteosarcoma. Advantages of inhaled delivery include the ability to circumvent first pass metabolism in the liver, decreased systemic absorption, and, consequently, decreased systemic symptoms. A phase Ib/IIa study of inhaled lipid cisplatin demonstrated this therapy to be feasible and to have minimal systemic toxicity. Activity in patients with gross pulmonary metastases was limited.[445] An ongoing phase II study is evaluating the activity of this therapy in patients with recurrent osteosarcoma limited to the lungs whose pulmonary nodules have been completely resected.

In a phase II study of the pan-kinase inhibitor sorafenib in 35 patients with recurrent osteosarcoma with measurable disease, 3 patients (8%) had a partial response according to RECIST (Response Evaluation Criteria in Solid Tumors) and progression-free survival at 4 months was 46%.[446] The mechanism of action of sorafenib in osteosarcoma is not known. Data from preclinical models suggests sorafenib inhibits angiogenesis, which is not unexpected given that sorafenib is a potent inhibitor of vascular endothelial growth factor receptors (VEGFRs).[369] This hypothesis is supported by the observation of partial responses in osteosarcoma patients enrolled on phase I trials of potent VEGFR inhibitors cediranib[447] and regorafenib.[448] Sorafenib may also function via inhibition of ERK1/ERK2 signaling.[369]

In summary, recurrent osteosarcoma carries a grave prognosis. Cure is most likely in the minority of patients who have a limited number of metastases that are completely resected, leading to a second complete surgical remission, especially if the first remission was of relatively long duration. The role of adjuvant therapy for patients with recurrent osteosarcoma is uncertain. Enrollment of such patients in clinical trials should be encouraged.

Radiation Therapy

Radiation therapy is relatively ineffective against osteosarcoma, especially when compared with the combination of adequate surgery and multiagent chemotherapy. In vitro studies comparing osteosarcoma with other human cell lines have demonstrated that osteosarcoma cells are more resistant to irradiation.[449] In addition, those osteosarcomas with loss of TP53 function would be expected to survive radiation-induced DNA damage.[208,220]

Adjuvant pulmonary radiation therapy has been compared in a randomized fashion with adjuvant VCR plus HDMTX.[450] Although outcomes were the same in patients receiving chemotherapy and those receiving pulmonary irradiation, DFS in both arms of the study was much lower (at 24%) than with the current standard approach of wide surgical resection and multiagent chemotherapy.[110] In addition, 14% of patients receiving adjuvant pulmonary irradiation experienced decreased pulmonary function. Thus adjuvant pulmonary irradiation is not recommended.

Radiation therapy has been used for local control of osteosarcoma. When radiation therapy is the only local control measure (i.e., no operation is performed), the local recurrence rate is almost three times greater than is seen with surgical resection.[450] Nevertheless, when surgical resection of the primary lesion is not an option, there may be a role for radiation therapy. Machak and colleagues[451] have reported a 5-year OS survival of 60% in 31 patients who refused surgical resection of the primary tumor and were treated instead with local irradiation and multiagent chemotherapy. Similarly, patients with osteosarcoma of the spine who had intralesional margins or no surgery tended to have a better outcome if they received local irradiation plus multiagent chemotherapy than chemotherapy alone, although the difference was not statistically significant.[452] Proton-based radiotherapy used in the setting of incomplete or no resection produced reasonable local control rates, but only 35% of patients in the series had high-grade osteosarcoma.[453] Contrasting results have been presented by Hug and associates,[454] who saw local failures in 2 of 3 patients who did not undergo surgical resection of the primary tumor but were treated with local irradiation and multiagent chemotherapy.

Preoperative irradiation, in combination with neoadjuvant multiagent chemotherapy, has been given in an attempt to increase the rate of limb salvage surgery.[455] Although this approach has resulted in a higher percentage of limb salvage procedures compared with historical controls, local complications were also increased. Given the increased rate of local complications, this approach is not recommended.

Whether postoperative irradiation is useful when inadequate surgical margins are present is controversial. There are no randomized trials comparing postoperative irradiation with observation in patients whose tumor resection specimens had marginal or intralesional surgical margins. Studies that have compared such patients with similar historical controls show an improved local control rate and OS in patients treated with local postoperative irradiation.[452,456] However, a great diversity of tumor burden is present in patients with intralesional and marginal tumor margins, and chemotherapy regimens have changed over time. Thus, comparison with historical controls might not be valid.

Samarium 153-labeled ethylenediaminetetramethylene phosphonate ([153]Sm-EDTMP) is a pharmaceutical radioisotope that is efficiently and specifically taken up by bone. Patients with osteosarcoma bone metastases treated with [153]Sm-EDTMP experience a rapid decrease in pain symptoms.[457] At high doses of [153]Sm-EDTMP, peripheral blood stem cell rescue is required.

Complications of Therapy and Late Effects

Patients receiving osteosarcoma therapy can experience acute complications from chemotherapy and surgery. As noted, the usual initial osteosarcoma chemotherapy comprises HDMTX, Doxo, and CP. Ifosfamide and etoposide are also given in many protocols. The acute toxicities of HDMTX, Doxo, and CP combination chemotherapy with and without ifosfamide have been well documented in numerous osteosarcoma treatment protocols.[111,113,133,404,422,423] The most common acute side effects, occurring in 75% of patients, are grades 3 or 4 leukopenia and neutropenia. Significant nausea and vomiting are also common and occur in 60% to 70% of patients, particularly during Doxo-CP cycles; 20% to 30% of patients experience mucositis. A similar percentage develops significant infections. Reversible aminotransferase elevations occur in about 15% of patients, usually because of HDMTX. Renal toxicity, which occurs in 1% to 2% of patients, presents as renal insufficiency or tubular dysfunction, with accompanying electrolyte abnormalities. Renal dysfunction can be acute or chronic. Neurologic toxicity presenting as seizures, headache, or radiologic changes is rare. The rate of therapy-related mortality varies from 0% to 4%, with most protocols reporting a 1% to 2% rate of therapy-related mortality, usually caused by infection and, less frequently, by cardiotoxicity.

A potential complication of HDMTX therapy in all disease settings is renal damage from insoluble MTX metabolites. Because MTX is primarily excreted by the kidneys, renal damage can lead to delayed MTX clearance, which in turn worsens renal dysfunction and further delays MTX clearance. Delayed MTX clearance, even in the setting of adequate leucovorin rescue, can lead to severe mucositis and prolonged myelosuppression. With adequate hydration, alkalinization, and monitoring of drug levels, the incidence of severely delayed MTX clearance is low. Delayed MTX clearance can be treated with increased hydration, adjustments in leucovorin dosing, hemodialysis, or carboxypeptidase (glucarpidase), an enzyme that converts MTX to inactive metabolites that are readily excreted in the urine.[458]

Acute complications of osteosarcoma primary resection surgeries are reviewed extensively in Chapter 49, "Pediatric Surgical Oncology." Limb salvage procedures have a much higher rate of perioperative complications than amputations. In one study, 41% of limb-sparing procedures had wound complications compared with only 13% of amputations.[111] Acute complications of surgery include infection, flap necrosis, damage to the neurovascular bundle, and venous thrombosis.[111,459]

Late effects of chemotherapy in patients with osteosarcoma include cardiac dysfunction, hearing loss, secondary malignancy, and decreased fertility.[115] Guidelines regarding posttreatment monitoring for late effects and relapse are presented in Table 62-8. Many osteosarcoma protocols use a cumulative doxorubicin dosage of 450 mg/m^2. Published rates of cardiac toxicity after treatment for osteosarcoma range from 0% to 5%.[111,120,404,423] Cardiac dysfunction caused by Doxo is irreversible and can be severe enough to cause death or require transplantation. Doxo-related cardiotoxicity is more common in women and is more likely with higher cumulative Doxo dosages.[460] Younger children treated with Doxo may develop delayed cardiac failure during rapid somatic growth in adolescence, and women may similarly develop cardiac failure as a result of the increased cardiac workload presented by pregnancy. The long-term cardiac outcome of patients treated with Doxo especially at a relatively high cumulative dosage remains to be defined. Administration of dexrazoxane in conjunction with Doxo in pediatric sarcoma patients has led to preservation of left ventricular function, without any change in outcome, compared with placebo control in an initial small clinical trial.[461] Recently, dexrazoxane administration in patients receiving therapy for Hodgkin disease has been associated with an increased risk for subsequent acute myeloid leukemia and myelodysplastic syndrome.[462] It is uncertain whether these findings pertain to patients with other disease types.

Second malignancies occur at an increased rate in osteosarcoma survivors compared with the general population or patients with benign bone tumors.[463,464] The incidence of second malignancies ranges from 2% to 4%.

TABLE 62-8 Typical Monitoring after Completion of Therapy*

Routine Monitoring for Tumor Recurrence (also imaging for symptoms, as indicated)

First Year	
Primary site	Plain radiograph every 3 months
Site(s) of bone metastases	Plain radiograph film every 3 months
Chest	Chest CT every 3 months
Second Year	
Primary site	Plain radiograph every 6 months
Site(s) of bone metastases	Plain radiograph every 6 months
Chest	Chest CT every 6 months
Third Year	
Primary site	Plain radiograph every 6 months
Site(s) of bone metastases	Plain radiograph every 6 months
Chest	Chest radiograph every 6 months
Fourth and Fifth Years	
Primary site	Plain radiograph every 12 months
Site(s) of bone metastases	Plain radiograph every 12 months
Chest	Chest radiograph every 6 months
Sixth to Tenth Years	
Primary site	Plain radiograph every 12 months
Site(s) of bone metastases	Plain radiograph every 12 months
Chest	Chest radiograph every 12 months

Monitoring for Late Effects of Chemotherapy

Cardiac	Echocardiogram every 12 months for 2-3 years then at the time of pubertal growth spurt and pregnancy
Nephrotoxicity	Monitor electrolytes, blood urea nitrogen, creatinine every 12 months
Ototoxicity	Audiology at end of therapy
Secondary malignancy	Complete blood cell count every 12 months
Fertility	Semen analysis offered to postpubertal males
All	Physical examination every 3 months × 1 year, every 6 months until 5 years after completion of therapy then yearly

CT, Computed tomography.

*Recommendations for posttreatment surveillance vary. For further reading see references 475 to 477.

Because a number of genetic cancer syndromes increase osteosarcoma risk, it is difficult to determine whether second malignancies are caused by an underlying genetic predisposition or a complication of osteosarcoma therapy. Certainly some of the osteosarcoma survivors who develop a second malignancy have no family history of cancer. No particular type of secondary malignancy predominates.

Ototoxicity as a result of osteosarcoma therapy is predominantly caused by CP. In some patients, aminoglycoside treatment of infectious complications of chemotherapy may be a contributing factor. Mild ototoxicity, which does not involve the frequencies of audible speech, is relatively common. Significant ototoxicity involving the audible speech frequencies is rare, reported in 1% or fewer patients.[465] Amifostine, administered concurrently with CP, has been tested in a small group of pediatric osteosarcoma patients. Compared with untreated controls, patients receiving amifostine had less severe myelosuppression but the incidence of renal and ototoxicity was not decreased by amifostine therapy. Amifostine was emetogenic but was otherwise well tolerated.[466]

Azoospermia is known to be caused by alkylating agents and is common in osteosarcoma patients treated with ifosfamide. Azoospermia has also been seen in patients who were treated with HDMTX, Doxo, and CP; and it is likely that this is chemotherapy related.[467] Data on female infertility after osteosarcoma therapy are limited. In one study, 6% of female patients treated with HDMTX, Doxo, and CP plus ifosfamide had early menopause.[468]

Long-term orthopedic complications, which depend on the type of surgical resection performed, are discussed further in Chapter 49, "Pediatric Surgical Oncology." Patients who have limb-sparing operations are more likely to have late orthopedic complications. Most late complications are caused by endoprosthesis or allograft failure, although late infections also occur.[459] Thirty percent of endoprostheses will require surgical revision or replacement by 10 years after the initial surgery.[469] Other problems that arise in patients undergoing limb-sparing surgery include poor joint mobility and leg-length discrepancy, both of which can impair limb function. Although limb-sparing procedures have a higher complication rate, the functional outcome is superior when assessed by oxygen consumption during walking. Functionally, rotationplasty is equivalent to a below-knee amputation.[459] In long-term follow-up studies, quality of life did not differ in those who had an amputation when compared with those who underwent a limb-sparing procedure. Poorer lower limb function does have an adverse impact on quality of life, and failure of a limb-sparing procedure had an impact on body image.[470] Compared with survivors of other childhood cancers and their siblings, survivors of osteosarcoma have greater activity limitations.[471,472] Despite these limitations, those who are long-term survivors after osteosarcoma appear to have similar social and occupational outcomes as their siblings.[473]

CONCLUSION AND FUTURE DIRECTIONS

Osteosarcoma treatment and prognosis have not changed significantly during the past 2 decades. The standard basic chemotherapy for localized osteosarcoma—Doxo, CP, and HDMTX—has remained the same. Consequently, outcomes in patients with localized osteosarcoma are similar today to outcomes 20 years ago. New therapies, particularly ifosfamide and etoposide, have been used for patients with metastatic and recurrent disease, and there are early indications that this may result in a slight improvement in outcome. In contrast, surgical approaches have changed significantly over the past 20 years. Previously, amputations were common; currently, many patients have limb-sparing surgeries. In addition, there has been increasing recognition of the ability to increase survival via complete resection of pulmonary metastases.

This relatively slow rate of progress in treatment of osteosarcoma is partly the result of the biologic complexity of the disease. There have been a number of biologic insights over the past 2 decades, but none has revealed obvious drug targets that are of central relevance in a large proportion of osteosarcomas. An additional factor slowing the rate of progress in osteosarcoma is the small patient population available for clinical studies.

Several ongoing clinical studies should provide important clinical insights in the next 5 to 10 years. It is hoped the results of the international cooperative study EURAMOS1 will determine whether the postoperative addition of ifosfamide and etoposide improves the EFS of patients with a poor response to neoadjuvant chemotherapy.

Identification of new therapeutic agents with activity in osteosarcoma is a major research priority. Several novel agents are likely to be evaluated in phase II clinical trials in osteosarcoma in the next several years. The Sarcoma Alliance for Research through Collaboration (SARC) is studying an SRC inhibitor in patients with metastatic osteosarcoma. Phase II studies of the microtubule inhibitor eribulin, of the anti-GD2 antibody CH14.18, and of the RANKL antibody denosumab have been proposed by the COG.[474]

Breakthroughs in the understanding of osteosarcoma biology are likely in the next 10 years as the number and sophistication of tools and techniques for biomedical research continue to increase. For example, improved transgenic mouse models of osteosarcoma are likely to be developed, and these models will facilitate basic and applied studies. Results of comprehensive next-generation sequencing studies are expected at the time of publication. Genomic and proteomic techniques requiring minimal amounts of tumor tissue will continue to facilitate the study of human osteosarcoma samples, which are in limited supply. It is hoped the combination of these new techniques, with the proliferation of new drug compounds and the recently established international collaboration for clinical studies, will lead to significant advances in osteosarcoma in the near future.

References available online at ExpertConsult.

KEY REFERENCES

1. Bleyer A, O'Leary M, Barr R, et al, editors: *Cancer epidemiology in older adolescents and young adults 15 to 29 years of age, including SEER incidence and survival: 1975-2000.* NIH publication. No. 06-5767, Bethesda, MD, 2006, National Cancer Institute.

Incidence data and survival characteristics including bone malignancies within the vulnerable age group.

2. Dahlin DC, Unni KK: Osteosarcoma of bone and its important recognizable varieties. *Am J Surg Pathol* 1:61–72, 1977.

Description of diagnostic subclassification for key osteosarcoma subtypes.

3. Kager L, Zoubek A, Potschger U, et al: Primary metastatic osteosarcoma: presentation and outcome of patients treated on neoadjuvant Cooperative Osteosarcoma Study Group protocols. *J Clin Oncol* 21:2011–2018, 2003.

Review of clinical features including outcomes for metastatic osteosarcoma treated on neoadjuvant-based clinical trials.

4. Meyers PA, Schwartz CL, Krailo MD, et al: Osteosarcoma: the addition of muramyl tripeptide to chemotherapy improves overall survival—a report from the Children's Oncology Group. *J Clin Oncol* 26:633–638, 2008.

Impact of muraml tripeptide combination therapy with cytotoxic chemotherapy in COG clinical trial.

5. Ferrari S, Briccoli A, Mercuri M, et al: Postrelapse survival in osteosarcoma of the extremities: prognostic factors for long-term survival. *J Clin Oncol* 21:710–715, 2003.

Description of factors associated with survival following relapse in patients with osteosarcoma of the extremities.

6. Kempf-Bielack B, Bielack SS, Jurgens H, et al: Osteosarcoma relapse after combined modality therapy: an analysis of unselected patients in the Cooperative Osteosarcoma Study Group (COSS). *J Clin Oncol* 23:559–568, 2005.

Analysis of relapse-associated characteristics for osteosarcoma patients after multimodality-based therapy.

7. Mirabello L, Troisi RJ, Savage SA: Osteosarcoma incidence and survival rates from 1973 to 2004: data from the Surveillance, Epidemiology, and End Results Program. *Cancer* 115:1531–1543, 2009.

SEER incidence and survival data for osteosarcoma for the interval 1973-2004.

52. Bielack SS, Kempf-Bielack B, Delling G, et al: Prognostic factors in high-grade osteosarcoma of the extremities or trunk: an analysis of 1,702 patients treated on neoadjuvant cooperative osteosarcoma study group protocols. *J Clin Oncol* 20:776–790, 2002.

Characterization of prognostic features for high-grade osteosarcomas treated on neoadjuvant-containing cooperative group clinical trials.

65. Kayton ML, Huvos AG, Casher J, et al: Computed tomographic scan of the chest underestimates the number of metastatic lesions in osteosarcoma. *J Pediatr Surg* 41:200–206, 2006.

Analysis of CT scan in estimating pulmonary metastasis numbers in osteosarcoma patients.

106. Wolf RE, Enneking WF: The staging and surgery of musculoskeletal neoplasms. *Orthop Clin North Am* 27:473–481, 1996.

Review of staging and surgical approach for malignancies including osteosarcoma.

111. Goorin AM, Schwartzentruber DJ, Devidas M, et al: Presurgical chemotherapy compared with immediate surgery and adjuvant chemotherapy for nonmetastatic osteosarcoma: Pediatric Oncology Group Study POG-8651. *J Clin Oncol* 21:1574–1580, 2003.

Analysis of the role for neoadjuvant therapy for treatment of nonmetastatic osteosarcoma in a POG study.

143. Bielack SS, Kempf-Bielack B, Branscheid D, et al: Second and subsequent recurrences of osteosarcoma: presentation, treatment, and outcomes of 249 consecutive cooperative osteosarcoma study group patients. *J Clin Oncol* 27:557–565, 2009.

Characteristics of recurrences and associated features, beyond initial relapse of osteosarcoma.

147. Goorin AM, Harris MB, Bernstein M, et al: Phase II/III trial of etoposide and high-dose ifosfamide in newly diagnosed metastatic osteosarcoma: a Pediatric Oncology Group trial. *J Clin Oncol* 20:426–433, 2002.

Combination etoposide and high-dose ifosfamide as initial therapy for nonlocalized osteosarcoma in a POG trial.

149. Janeway KA, Walkley CR: Modeling human osteosarcoma in the mouse: from bedside to bench. *Bone* 47:859–865, 2010.

Review of preclinical models of osteosarcoma and their applications.

154. Sandberg AA, Bridge JA: Updates on the cytogenetics and molecular genetics of bone and soft tissue tumors: osteosarcoma and related tumors. *Cancer Genet Cytogenet* 145:1–30, 2003.
    Use of genomics related technologies for osteosarcoma diagnostics and molecular classification.

155. Kuijjer ML, Hogendoorn PC, Cleton-Jansen AM: Genome-wide analyses on high-grade osteosarcoma: making sense of a genomically most unstable tumor. *Int J Cancer* 133:2512–2521, 2013.
    Use of deep genomic-based technologies to examine oncogenic events in osteosarcoma formation.

195. Malkin D, Li FP, Strong LC, et al: Germline *p53* mutations in a familial syndrome of breast cancer, sarcomas, and other neoplasms. *Science* 250:1233–1238, 1990.
    Identification of mutations in TP53, "guardian of the genome" within germline of families affected by multiple cancers.

394. Link MP, Goorin AM, Miser AW, et al: The effect of adjuvant chemotherapy on relapse-free survival in patients with osteosarcoma of the extremity. *N Engl J Med* 314:1600–1606, 1986.
    Major report describing the impact of postsurgical chemotherapy on producing long-term survival from extremity osteosarcoma.

437. Goorin AM, Delorey MJ, Lack EE, et al: Prognostic significance of complete surgical resection of pulmonary metastases in patients with osteogenic sarcoma: analysis of 32 patients. *J Clin Oncol* 2:425–431, 1984.
    Use of surgical resection of lung metastases in patients with metastatic osteosarcoma.

438. Briccoli A, Rocca M, Salone M, et al: Resection of recurrent pulmonary metastases in patients with osteosarcoma. *Cancer* 104:1721–1725, 2005.
    Use of surgical resection of lung metastases in patients with metastatic osteosarcoma.

474. Gorlick R, Janeway K, Lessnick S, et al: Children's Oncology Group's 2013 blueprint for research: bone tumors. *Pediatr Blood Cancer* 60:1009–1015, 2013.
    Cooperative Group coordinated efforts toward understanding and improving outcomes for bone sarcomas including osteosarcoma.

477. Meyer JS, Nadel HR, Marina N, et al: Response to "imaging guidelines for children with Ewing sarcoma and osteosarcoma: a report from the Children's Oncology Group Bone Tumor Committee. *Pediatr Blood Cancer* 51:839–840, 2008.
    Guidelines and associated challenges in the management of pediatric bone tumor patients.

CHAPTER 63

Pediatric Germ Cell Tumors

A. Lindsay Frazier, Deborah Billmire, and James Amatruda

CHAPTER OUTLINE

Germ cell tumor (GCT) is the designation given to neoplasms arising from the cells of the germline—the cells that are destined to become either the egg or the sperm. A number of unique features of these tumors including their bimodal and wide age distribution, remarkable phenotypic diversity, and varying biologic behavior make GCTs a particular challenge for the surgeon, pathologist, and oncologist. Successful treatment regimens developed over the last several decades have focused current clinical research on ways to maintain efficacy and minimize toxicity for most patients and intensify treatment for patients who fail first-line therapy. Recent advances in understanding the underlying aberrations in germline development shed light on the genesis of these tumors and may provide insight into new avenues for treatment.

DEVELOPMENT OF THE GERMLINE

The pathogenesis of GCTs can best be understood through an analysis of the mechanisms of germline development.[1] The role of the germ cell is to ensure the continuation of a species by producing the gametes, cells that will give rise to the next generation. Reflecting this unique role, germ cells are set aside from somatic cells very early in development. In humans, germ cells arise in an extraembryonic position and must migrate to the site at which the gonads will form. The pluripotency of germ cells is reflected in the wide histopathologic diversity of GCTs.

Specification of Primordial Germ Cells

Much of what is known about early molecular events in the mammalian germline comes from examination of germ-cell development in the mouse.[2-5] Similar molecular mechanisms of germ cell development appear to operate in humans, based on studies of human embryos and human embryonic stem cells differentiating into germ cells in vitro.[6-10] Development of the germline begins at the time of blastocyst implantation, when the extraembryonic ectoderm and the visceral endoderm send signals to cells in the proximal epiblast, also known as the *embryonic ectoderm* (Fig. 63-1). The major inductive signals are the bone morphogenetic proteins (BMPs), which are members of the transforming growth factor β (TGF-β) superfamily.[11-14] In response to BMPs, some of the epiblast cells begin to express the marker *fragilis*,

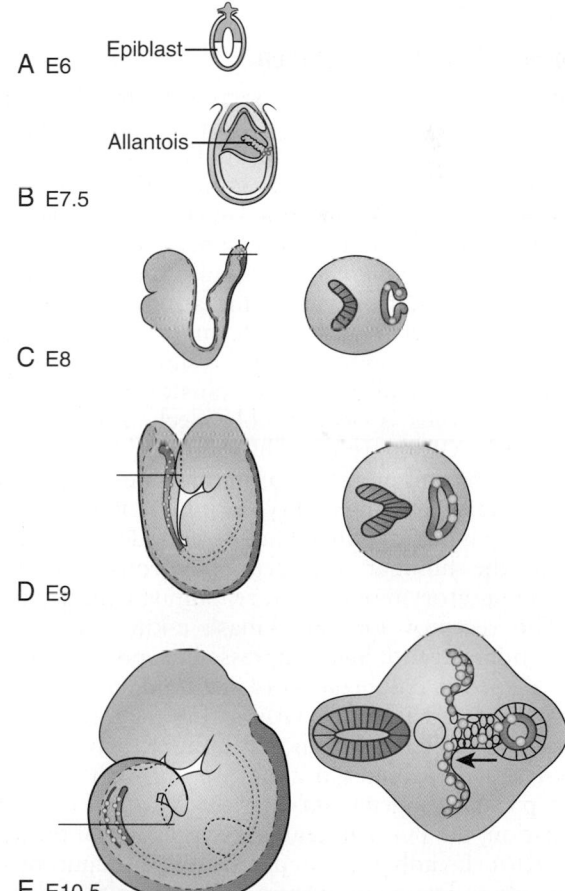

Figure 63-1 Development and migration of PGCs. Stages of embryonic development and primordial germ cell (PGC) migration in the mouse. **A,** At E6 the epiblast *(white)* and extraembryonic tissue *(gray)* are discernable. **B,** By E7.5 the allantois has developed and the PGCs *(yellow)* appear. **C,** At E8 the neural tube *(blue)* and hindgut[70] can are visible. In cross-section *(right side)*, the PGCs can be seen colonizing the hindgut. **D,** At E9 the embryo has turned and the posterior section is to the left; the PGCs are migrating through the hindgut. **E,** At E10.5 the PGCs begin exiting the hindgut and migrate through the dorsal mesentery *(white cells)* to enter the genital ridges *(green)*. The equivalent stages of human embryonic development are: **A,** Weeks 1 and 2; **B,** Week 2.5; **C,** Week 3; **D,** Week 4; **E,** Week 5. *(Modified from Starz-Gaiano M, Lehmann R: Moving towards the next generation. Mech Dev 105:5–18, 2001.)*

A E6 — Epiblast
B E7.5 — Allantois
C E8
D E9
E E10.5

signaling their competence to become germ cells.[2,15] Of these *fragilis*-expressing cells, a few begin to express the transcriptional repressor *Blimp1/Prdm1*.[16] These cells, in which expression of somatic genes such as *Hoxb1, T/Brachyury,* and *Snail* is repressed, will become the primordial germ cells (PGCs). Unlike other epiblast-derived cells, PGCs regain or maintain expression of certain genes associated with pluripotency such as *STELLA, OCT3/4,* and *NANOG*.[2,17-25] Certain pluripotency genes can be reactivated in GCTs and may contribute to malignant potential; for example, *NANOG* and *OCT3/4* have been used as sensitive markers of malignant germ cells in studies of GCTs.[26-30] In humans, PGCs can be identified in the wall of the yolk sac by their intrinsic alkaline phosphatase activity beginning at about day 24. The PGCs begin to proliferate as they migrate out of the yolk sac into the embryo.[31]

Primordial Germ Cell Migration

In humans, as in many other organisms, the PGCs arise in an extraembryonic location, distant from the eventual site at which the gonad will form. This physical separation may serve to insulate the germ cells from various proliferation and differentiation signals in the developing embryo or to enforce a quality control by selecting for healthy PGCs capable of successfully navigating to the developing gonad. Proper PGC migration is critical to the survival of the germ cells and formation of the gonad, and failure of this migration can result in ectopic germ cells. Persistence and malignant transformation of these ectopic germ cells is one possible mechanism by which extragonadal GCTs are thought to arise.[32]

Toward the end of gastrulation, morphogenetic movements in the developing embryo bring the PGCs in proximity to the hindgut.[31] Invading the endoderm, the PGCs colonize the hindgut and begin vigorous, apparently random migratory movements, remaining confined to the gut. The receptor tyrosine kinase c-kit, expressed in PGCs, and its ligand, Steel, expressed in somatic cells, are required for the colonization of the hindgut and for the survival and migration of PGCs within the gut.[33-36] Wylie and co-workers have shown that in mice, PGCs deficient in c-kit signaling undergo apoptosis through the action of the p53-target gene, *Bax*.[36-39] At 5 to 6 weeks after fertilization, the PGCs upregulate expression of the adhesion factor E-cadherin[40] and exit the hindgut on the dorsal side to begin colonization of the genital ridge primordia. The genital ridges are bilateral swellings of mesenchyme covered by coelomic epithelium and situated on either side of the dorsal aorta on the posterior wall of the embryo in the lower thoracic and lumbar regions.[41] The genital ridges appear to attract the PGCs because of their expression of stromal cell–derived factor 1 (SDF-1, or CXCL12), which is a ligand for the chemokine receptor CXCR4, which is expressed in the PGCs.[42,43] As the PGCs exit the hindgut, they divide into two lateral streams to colonize the genital ridges. PGCs that fail to colonize the ridges and remain in the midline are eliminated by apoptosis, as the midline cells downregulate expression of Steel.[39] Once they have entered the genital ridges, PGCs become much less motile but continue several more rounds of division. This proliferation is dependent on continued Steel/c-kit signaling.[31,38,39,42,44]

Erasure of Imprinting

Imprinting refers to the epigenetic modification of certain genes (typically by cytosine methylation) such that only the maternal or paternal allele of the gene is expressed.[45-47] Lineage-specific patterns of imprinting are established in different tissues, including the germline, around the time of gastrulation.[46,48] Upon entering the gonadal ridges, however, PGCs actively erase these genomic methylation patterns. This erasure is necessary in order to allow the maternal and paternal imprinting patterns to be established in the oocytes and sperm, respectively. Imprinting is reestablished in sex-specific patterns during gonadogenesis.[49-51] GCTs exhibit partial or total erasure of imprinting, implying their origin from early germ cells.[1]

Gonadogenesis

Beginning shortly before the arrival of the PGCs in the genital ridges, the coelomic epithelium begins to proliferate and invade the underlying mesenchyme, forming the primitive sex cords. Migrating PGCs entering the gonad are surrounded by the cords. At this early stage, the appearance of the developing gonad is identical in males and females, and the tissue is referred to as the *indifferent gonad*. Subsequently, changes occur in both the germ cells and the gonadal somatic cells according to the genetic sex of the embryo. In genetic males, sex determination occurs under the influence of the testis-determining *SRY* gene on the Y chromosome.[52,53] After the initial rounds of cell division, male germ cells enter a mitotic arrest that persists until after birth.[14] In males, the primitive sex cords proliferate and penetrate deeper into the mesenchyme, forming the testis or medullary cords, which connect proximally to form the rete testis. By the fourth month of development, the cords consist of germ cells and the supporting Sertoli cells, which are derived from the surface epithelium of the genital ridge. The cords remain solid until puberty, when they form lumens to become seminiferous tubules. By the eighth week of development the mesenchyme of the gonadal ridge gives rise in males to Leydig cells, which secrete testosterone. Secretion of antimüllerian hormone by the Sertoli cells and testosterone by the Leydig cells leads in males to degeneration of the paramesonephric ducts and the development of the mesonephric ducts into the vas deferens and epididymis. Testosterone is also necessary for male differentiation of the external genitalia.

Female gonadal development proceeds along different lines. In the absence of the Y chromosome, the sex cords initially degenerate and are replaced by a new set of cortical sex cords derived from the surface epithelium. By the fourth month the cortical sex cords have become isolated clusters with each cluster surrounding a single germ cell. In females the primitive germ cells, called *oogonia*, continue rapid proliferation, reaching maximal numbers by the seventh month. After that point, most of the oogonia degenerate; the remaining cells, now called *primary oocytes,* enter meiosis and arrest at the diplotene stage of the first meiotic prophase. Granulosa cells (derived from the surface epithelium) and thecal cells (derived from the mesenchyme) together form the follicle cells that surround each primary oocyte. Beginning at adolescence, groups of oocytes periodically resume meiosis. In females, the paramesonephric (müllerian) ducts develop into the oviducts, uterus, cervix, and upper part of the vagina. The mesonephric ducts degenerate.

In summary, development of the germline requires the proper specification of PGCs and their migration through the embryo to the gonadal ridges, where the gonads are formed through interactions of the germ cells with somatic cells. Concomitant with this process, the inherited pattern of genomic imprinting is erased, and a new, sex-specific pattern is formed. The complex process of gonadal organogenesis is subject to both genetic and environmental influences. Abnormal development of the gonads during the embryonic and fetal periods leads to defects such as cryptorchidism and gonadal dysgenesis, which are strongly associated with the risk of developing GCTs.

HISTOPATHOLOGY OF GERM CELL TUMORS

GCTs are a heterogeneous group of neoplasms with a wide variety of histopathologic features. This variety reflects the pluripotent nature of the PGCs from which GCTs arise.[1,54] Adding to the complexity of this tumor type, GCTs with apparently similar histopathology can have very different biologic behaviors when presenting at different ages or anatomic sites. The five major histologic subtypes of GCTs are teratoma, yolk sac tumor (YST), germinoma, embryonal carcinoma, and choriocarcinoma. The World Health Organization (WHO) classification of GCTs is presented in Boxes 63-1 and 63-2.

Overview of Testicular Germ Cell Tumors

Before puberty in infants and children, teratoma and/or YST account for the vast majority of GCTs.[55-57] *Seminoma* (the term used for a testicular germinoma), embryonal carcinoma, and choriocarcinoma are very rare in this age group. GCTs of the prepubertal testis differ from their adult counterparts not only in the distribution of histologic subtypes, but also in their spectrum of cytogenetic abnormalities. After the early peak of testicular YST and teratoma in the 0-to-4–years age group, testicular tumors are relatively rare until the onset of puberty. Between ages 10 and 40 years, there is a second peak in testicular tumor incidence, comprised of seminoma and nonseminomas (including embryonal carcinoma, teratoma, YST, and choriocarcinoma). Postpubertal tumors demonstrate a wider array of histopathologic differentiation than do the GCTs of the prepubertal testis. Moreover, adolescent and adult GCTs share a common precursor cell of origin (the carcinoma in situ [CIS] or intratubular germ cell neoplasia, unclassified [IGCNU]), as well as characteristic cytogenetic abnormalities including the near-universal presence of amplifications of chromosome 12p. These histopathologic and molecular cytogenetic differences have lent support to the hypothesis that different pathogenic mechanisms underlie juvenile and adult testicular GCTs.[58-60]

Overview of Ovarian Germ Cell Tumors

In neonates and infants, the most common ovarian lesions are ovarian cysts.[61] Cysts can occur any time from late gestational stages onwards, and they occur at a greater rate in babies of mothers with diabetes, preeclampsia, and Rh immunization. Ovarian cysts in children often resolve

---

Box 63-1   World Health Organization Classification of Germ Cell Tumors: Male

GERM CELL TUMORS

Intratubular germ cell neoplasia, unclassified
Other types

TUMORS OF ONE HISTOLOGIC TYPE

Seminoma
  Seminoma with syncytiotrophoblastic cells
  Spermatocytic seminoma
  Spermatocytic seminoma with sarcoma
Embryonal carcinoma
Yolk sac tumor
Trophoblastic tumors
  Choriocarcinoma
  Trophoblastic neoplasms other than choriocarcinoma
    Monophasic choriocarcinoma
    Placental site trophoblastic tumor
Teratoma
  Dermoid cyst
  Monodermal teratoma
  Teratoma with somatic type malignancies

TUMORS OF MORE THAN ONE HISTOLOGIC TYPE

Mixed embryonal carcinoma and teratoma
Mixed teratoma and seminoma
Choriocarcinoma and teratoma/embryonal carcinoma
Others

SEX CORD/GONADAL STROMAL TUMORS

PURE FORMS

Leydig cell tumor
Malignant Leydig cell tumor
Sertoli cell tumor
  Sertoli cell tumor lipid rich variant
  Sclerosing Sertoli cell tumor
  Large cell calcifying Sertoli cell tumor
Malignant Sertoli cell tumor
Granulosa cell tumor
  Adult type granulosa cell tumor
  Juvenile type granulosa cell tumor
Tumors of the thecoma/fibroma group
  Thecoma
  Fibroma
Sex cord/gonadal stromal tumor, incompletely differentiated
Sex cord/gonadal stromal tumor, mixed forms
Malignant sex cord/gonadal stromal tumor
Tumors containing both germ cell and sex cord/gonadal stromal elements
  Gonadoblastoma
  Germ cell-sex cord/gonadal stromal tumor, unclassified

Box 63-2   World Health Organization Classification of Germ Cell Tumors: Female

GERM CELL TUMORS

Dysgerminoma
Yolk Sac Tumor
  Polyvesicular vitelline tumor
  Glandular variant
  Hepatoid variant
Embryonal carcinoma
Polyembryoma
Nongestational choriocarcinoma
Mixed germ cell tumor

BIPHASIC OR TRIPHASIC TERATOMA

Immature teratoma
Mature teratoma
  Solid
  Cystic
    Dermoid cyst
  Fetiform teratoma

MONODERMAL TERATOMA AND SOMATIC-TYPE TUMORS ASSOCIATED WITH
DERMOID CYSTS

Thyroid (Struma ovarii)
Carcinoid
Neuroectodermal
Carcinoma

Melanocytic
Sarcoma
Sebaceous tumors

GERM CELL SEX CORD-STROMAL TUMORS

Gonadoblastoma
  Variant with malignant germ cell tumor
Mixed germ cell sex cord-stromal tumor
  Variant with malignant germ cell tumor

SEX CORD-STROMAL TUMORS

Granulosa-stromal cell tumor
  Granulosa cell tumor
    Adult type granulosa cell tumor
    Juvenile type granulosa cell tumor
Tumors of the thecoma/fibroma group
  Thecoma
  Fibroma
Sertoli-stromal cell tumors
  Sertoli cell tumor
  Stromal-Leydig cell tumor
Sex cord-stromal tumors of mixed or unclassified types
Steroid-cell tumors
  Leydig cell tumor
  Steroid cell tumor, not otherwise specified

spontaneously without intervention.[62] GCTs account for 75% of ovarian tumors in the first 2 decades of life and up to 90% of ovarian tumors in premenarchal girls. The majority of these (95%) are benign, mature teratomas, mostly commonly "desmoid" tumors.[63] Five percent of ovarian GCTs are malignant; these include dysgerminomas, immature teratomas, mature teratomas with somatic malignancies, YSTs, choriocarcinoma, embryonal carcinoma, polyembryoma, and mixed GCTs. Finally, gonadoblastoma is a mixed germ cell–sex cord stromal tumor occurring in cases of mixed gonadal dysgenesis with ambiguous genitalia, or 45,X Turner syndrome with Y chromosome material.[64-67] The histopathology of ovarian GCT types is similar to that of their testicular counterparts. After the third decade of life, ovarian GCTs occur rarely, and carcinomas derived from the coelomic epithelial covering of the ovary are much more common.[68]

Intratubular Germ Cell Neoplasia, Unclassified

IGCNU,[69] also called *testicular CIS*,[70] is considered the precursor for all invasive testicular GCTs (TGCTs) of postpubertal males[59,71-76] except spermatocytic seminoma.[77] According to one source, if left untreated IGCNU has a up to a 50% probability of progressing to invasive TGCT, either seminoma or nonseminoma, within 5 years.[74] Nonseminomas can be composed of embryonal carcinoma (the stem cell component), teratoma (somatic differentiation), and YST and choriocarcinoma (extraembryonic lineages). In IGCNU, germ cells with abundant vacuolated cytoplasm; large, irregular nuclei; and prominent nucleoli are found within the seminiferous tubules, showing similarities to PGCs and early gonocytes.[69] IGCNU is found in 1% of cases of male infertility and in 2% to 4% of cryptorchid testes in adults.[69,73,76,78-81] In men with a TGCT, the prevalence of IGCNU is about 80% in the ipsilateral testis (range, 63% to 99%),[79,82] predominantly in men with nonseminomas,[83] and 5% in the contralateral testis.[71,84,85] Various markers such as placental alkaline phosphatase (PLAP), c-kit, transcription factor AP-2γ, OCT3/4 (POU5F1), and testis-specific protein Y-encoded (TSPY) have been extensively used for immunohistochemical detection of IGCNU.[26,30,79,86-93] All these markers are also found in PGCs and/or gonocytes, which supports the model that IGCNU derives from PGCs or gonocytes.[1,30,94]

Whether an identifiable precursor lesion exists for GCTs of children is much less clear. In prepubertal children, the incidence of IGCNU appears to be very low,[58,95,96] although several cases have been reported.[94,97-99] These data must be interpreted with caution, however, because of the difficulty of distinguishing IGCNU in the developing gonad, in which primitive germ cells normally express markers such as *OCT3/4* and *c-KIT*.[94] The precursor lesion for the teratomas and YSTs of neonates and infants is yet to be identified. These pediatric tumors show partially erased imprinting, suggesting that the cell of origin is most likely a germ cell at an earlier development stage than that of IGCNU.[100-102]

IGCNU has been reported in a high percentage of gonadal biopsy specimens from children with disorders of sexual development (DSDs) who are at risk for the development of germ cell malignancies.[103,104] These disorders include gonadal dysgenesis,[105,106] partial androgen insensitivity syndrome (AIS),[107] and less often, complete AIS.[66,108-110] Development of these tumors in patients with DSDs is linked to the presence of a specific fragment of the Y chromosome, known as the *GBY region*.[29,93,111-114] For these patients with an increased risk of germ cell malignancy, prophylactic gonadectomy is often indicated.[103,115] However, overdiagnosis of IGCNU is possible

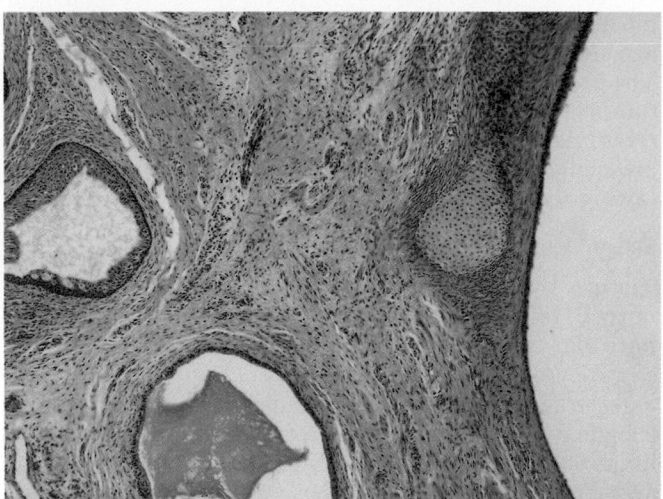

Figure 63-2 Mature teratoma. Low-power view showing cystic tumor with areas of cartilaginous differentiation.

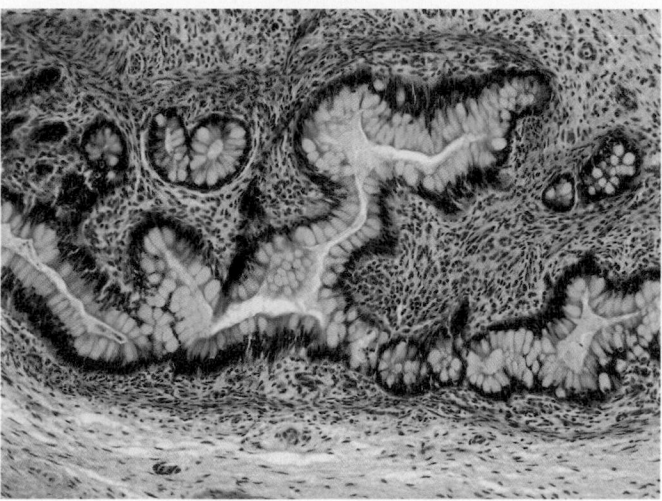

Figure 63-3 Mature teratoma with glandular differentiation.

in this setting because of the common maturation delay of germ cells in patients with DSDs, resulting in retained presence of *c-kit*-positive germ cells.[21,116,117] Therefore careful examination of the distribution pattern of OCT3/4-positive cells and their position within the seminiferous tubule are essential to making the diagnosis of IGCNU.[66,110,116]

TERATOMA

Histopathology of Teratoma

Teratomas are tumors composed of multiple tissues that are normally foreign to, and able to proliferate in excess of, the site in which they occur.[118] In the usual definition of *teratoma,* tissue elements of all three germ layers (endoderm, mesoderm, and ectoderm) are present; however, teratomas also occur in which only one or two of the germ layers are present (referred to as *monodermal* or *bidermal teratomas,* respectively). The clinical and biologic behavior of teratomas varies significantly with differing anatomic location, degree of maturity of the tumor tissue, and age of onset. Grossly, teratomas are nodular and heterogeneous with solid and cystic areas depending on the types of differentiated tissue present. Cartilage, bone, hair, and pigmented areas may be recognizable (Fig. 63-2). At the histopathologic level, ectodermal derivatives such as neuroepithelium, skin, and hair are the most common tissues in teratomas of infants and children. However, practically any tissue type can be seen, including muscle, bone, cartilage, and well-differentiated glands (Fig. 63-3).

Mature teratomas are typically cystic and contain differentiated adult-type tissue from one or more of the germ layers. The term *dermoid cyst* refers to the common finding in mature teratomas of tissue resembling the adult epidermis and its appendages. Immature teratomas are those in which embryonal-appearing tissue is present, typically in the form of neuroepithelial rosettes and tubules and often mixed with mature tissue (Fig. 63-4). A loose, myxoid stroma of immature mesenchyme with

focal differentiation into osteoid, fat, cartilage, and rhabdomyoblasts may be present.[119] Hypercellularity, increased mitotic index and nuclear atypia can be present. The prognostic significance of these findings is different for ovarian and testicular teratomas,[56] and these are discussed separately in the next sections.

Testicular Teratoma

Testicular Teratoma in Infants and Children

In most series, testicular teratoma is the second most common GCT of the prepubertal testis, representing about 35% of GCTs.[56,60,120-123] However, the actual incidence may be higher, because prepubertal testicular teratomas are uniformly benign and thus may be underreported to tumor registries.[122-125] Histologically, 85% of prepubertal testicular teratomas are mature, and 15% are immature. Unlike the case of ovarian teratomas, the

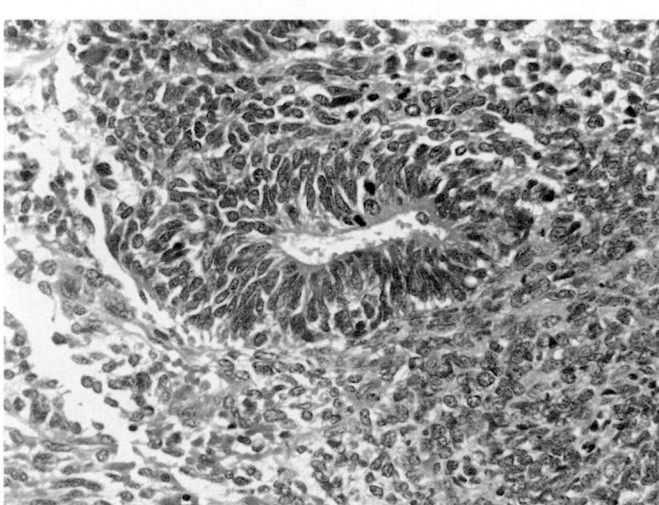

Figure 63-4 Immature teratoma. Immature teratomas are graded according to their content of primitive neuroepithelium. In this high-power view, the rosette formation characteristic of these tumors can be seen.

degree of histologic immaturity of childhood testicular teratoma does not carry prognostic significance. In this age group, pure testicular teratomas lack metastatic potential and have not been found to recur after surgical removal of the tumor.[56,126-129] A review of cases of immature teratoma from Pediatric Oncology Group (POG)/ Children's Cancer Study Group (CCG) protocols concluded that the presence of microscopic foci of YST, rather than the grade of immature teratoma, is the only valid predictor of recurrence in pediatric immature teratoma at any site.[130] The benign nature of these tumors has permitted the widespread use of testis-sparing enucleation surgery for prepubertal testicular teratomas.[58,124,131-133] In agreement with the benign clinical behavior of pure teratomas of the prepubertal testis, these tumors display normal karyotypes and normal results from comparative genomic hybridization (CGH).[123,134,135] Epidermoid cysts are rare tumors in the prepubertal testis and are most likely monodermal teratomas showing ectodermal differentiation.[63,124,136,137] These tumors, which have a characteristic ultrasonographic appearance, are hormonally inactive and do not produce α-fetoprotein (AFP);[124] as with other teratomas of the prepubertal testis, they are managed conservatively with testis-sparing surgery.[124,136,138] In the prepubertal testis, the seminiferous tubules surrounding the teratoma may contain germ cells with atypical features such as enlarged nuclei. However, these features are distinct from the seminoma-like changes of IGCNU, and do not signify malignant transformation of the germ cells.[139,140]

Testicular Teratoma in Adolescents and Adults

Teratoma occurs as a component of 50% of mixed nonseminomas in the postpubertal testis. Pure teratoma is rare, accounting for only 2% to 3% of postpubertal TGCTs.[141,142] Testicular teratomas in adolescents and adults may spread, giving rise to teratomatous and nonteratomatous metastases.[55,69,133] Furthermore, adult testicular teratomas typically are associated with IGCNU and exhibit characteristic cytogenetic abnormalities such as isochromosome 12p that are also found in seminomas and in other types of nonseminomatous TGCTs. Based on these findings, Ulbright proposed that teratomas in the adult testis arise from a germ cell that has already undergone malignant transformation; thus the histogenesis of adult teratoma is distinct from that of teratomas arising in the ovary or the prepubertal testis.[133,143] Postpubertal teratomas may contain syncytiotrophoblastic giant cells, and patients with teratoma may have gynecomastia[144] or elevated serum β-human chorionic gonadotropin (β-HCG) or AFP.[145,146]

Ovarian Teratoma

Teratoma is the most common GCT of the ovary, comprising more than 95% of all ovarian GCTs.[63] Ovarian teratomas differ in important ways from testicular teratomas. Teratomas in the prepubertal testis are uniformly benign. In adolescents and adults, testicular teratomas are nearly always malignant and occur as a component of mixed malignant GCTs (MGCTs), the exception being dermoid cysts of the testis. In the ovary, in contrast, the phenotype of teratomas does not vary as strikingly by age, and ovarian teratomas are usually pure tumors.[147,148] The great majority of ovarian tumors are mature, benign tumors (often referred to as *dermoid cyst* or *mature cystic teratoma*).[133,143,149,150] Less than 5% of ovarian teratomas are malignant; these are discussed separately in the following sections.

Benign, Mature Ovarian Teratoma

Mature ovarian teratomas are diploid, cytogenetically normal tumors.[123,151-154] This contrasts to postpubertal testicular teratomas, which are aneuploid and demonstrate cytogenetic abnormalities such as i12p. Interestingly, when polymorphic molecular markers are assayed, a high percentage of mature ovarian teratomas show a homozygous pattern, indicating that these tumors can arise from a germ cell that has completed meiosis I but not meiosis II.[107,134,151,155-159] Mature ovarian teratomas are usually cystic, though solid tumors can occur, especially in the first two decades.[160,161] Other characteristics of mature ovarian teratomas include a well-ordered, "organoid" appearance to the differentiated tissues within the teratoma, and the absence of cytologic atypia.[162] Mature ovarian teratomas are uniformly benign, except in the rare case of postteratomatous "malignant degeneration" of a dermoid cyst.[133,162,163]

Malignant Ovarian Teratoma

In children, immature teratoma is the most common type of malignant ovarian teratoma. Also in this category are other tumors that are rare in children, such as monodermal teratomas with malignant elements (e.g., papillary thyroid carcinoma in struma ovarii), dermoid cysts with malignant degeneration, and the rare case of mixed malignant ovarian GCT (MOGCT) with a teratoma component.

Immature Teratoma

The term *immature teratoma* refers to teratomas containing immature-appearing tissues, principally neuroepithelium.[164] Additionally, foci of mitotically active glia may be present. A grading system has been developed for immature teratomas based on the amount of neuroepithelial tissue present.[119,165] Mature teratomas containing only fully differentiated tissue are considered grade 0, and immature teratomas range from grade 1 (comprised of less than 10% immature neuroepithelium) to grade 3 (more than 50% immature neuroepithelium present). A two-component grading system (low grade and high grade) has also been proposed and shown to have improved reproducibility.[166] In adult ovarian teratomas, the finding of grade 2 or 3 immature teratoma predicts the likelihood of metastasis and confers a worse prognosis.[119,160,166,167] In children, however, it is not clear that the same relationship of grade to outcome of immature teratomas holds true. A POG study concluded that surgery alone was curative in children and adolescents with stage I immature teratomas of any grade and that chemotherapy should be reserved for cases of relapse.[130,168]

Immature teratomas may be associated with implants of glial tissue on the peritoneum, known as *gliomatosis peritonei.*[169-171] If the implants are composed solely of mature tissues, the presence of gliomatosis peritonei does not "upstage" the patient.[172,173] Interestingly, data suggest that the implants arise from metaplastic transformation of pluripotent müllerian stem cells in the peritoneum or underlying mesenchyme, rather than representing metastasis of the teratoma tissue.[174-176]

Monodermal Teratomas

Monodermal teratomas consist largely or exclusively of a single type of tissue, such as thyroid, carcinoid, and neuroectodermal tissues.[63,177-180] Monodermal teratomas with neuroectodermal differentiation include indolent types such as ependymoma and poorly differentiated forms such primitive neuroectodermal tumor (PNET), as well as anaplastic tumors resembling glioblastoma.[123,181-185] These tumors are rare in children.

Teratoma with Malignant Transformation

Teratoma with malignant transformation makes up 0.2% to 1.4% of mature cystic tumors of the ovary.[133,163,186] In these tumors, more commonly seen in older women, somatic-type malignancies are seen among the individual tissues in the teratoma. Squamous cell carcinomas are the most common tumor type,[187,188] but others including melanoma, adenocarcinoma, small cell carcinoma, sarcomas (including PNET), and malignant glioma may also occur.[133,162]

YOLK SAC TUMOR

Histopathology of Yolk Sac Tumor

YST is the most common malignant GCT in infancy and childhood.[56,57,118,122,189] The differentiation of the tumor cells is predominantly along endodermal lines and can take the form of both intraembryonic endodermal derivatives, such as primitive gut and liver, and extraembryonic structures such as allantois and yolk sac. There are many synonyms for YST, including *orchioblastoma, Teilum's tumor,* and *clear cell adenocarcinoma.* Although *endodermal sinus tumor* is commonly in use as a synonym for YST, some consider the term problematic, because the endodermal sinus is not a component of normal human embryogenesis.[190] In macroscopic appearance, YSTs are yellowish, with multiple cysts and areas of hemorrhage, necrosis, and liquefaction.[162] Microscopically, YSTs display a loose, myxoid stroma containing a reticulated pattern of microcystic spaces (Fig. 63-5). The cysts are lined by a flattened, periodic acid-Schiff (PAS)–positive, diastase-resistant epithelium. About 20% of YSTs exhibit characteristic Schiller-Duval bodies (a clustering of cells around a small, central blood vessel) (see Fig. 63-5). In addition to the microcystic/reticular pattern, several variant histologies of YST are described, including the solid, polyvesicular, and parietal types (corresponding to primitive endoderm and extraembryonic structures such as the allantois and yolk sac) and the glandular and hepatic types (corresponding to the intraembryonic endodermal derivatives, primitive lung and liver).

YSTs are typically cytokeratin-positive, which can help differentiate the solid YST variant from germinomas.[162]

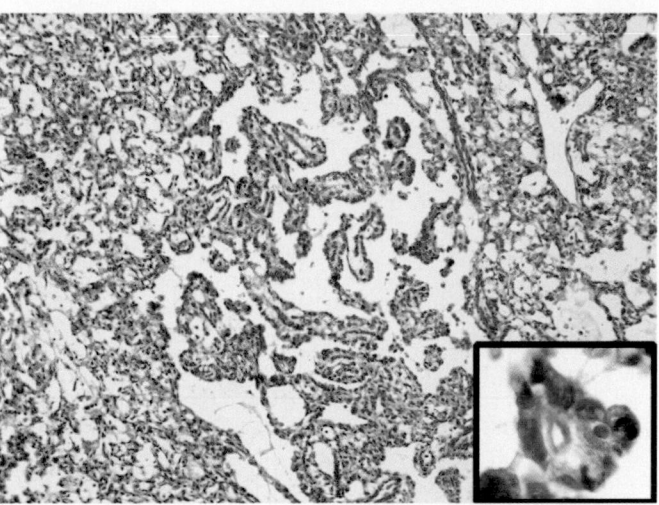

Figure 63-5 YST. A loose, myxoid stroma is filled with a labyrinthine network of cysts lined by clear, flattened epithelial cells. *Inset,* Schiller-Duval body.

Alpha-fetoprotein (AFP) expression is characteristic of these tumors, and AFP is a valuable tumor marker. Neonates and infants have high physiologic levels of AFP in serum, which can confound the use of serum AFP levels for diagnosis of YST or for monitoring therapy. Tables of normal serum AFP levels in neonates and infants have been published (Fig. 63-6).[191-193] In addition, at least 70% of YSTs have detectable AFP expression by immunohistochemical assays.[194-198]

Testicular Yolk Sac Tumor

Testicular Yolk Sac Tumor in Infants and Children

YST[199] is the most common malignant GCT in infants and children, comprising approximately 65% of prepubertal testicular GCTs.[121,200] YST is most common in males aged 0 to 2 years and can occur in pure form or as a malignant component of teratoma.[56] Histologically, prepubertal YSTs show the same spectrum of patterns as their adult counterparts: pseudopapillary, reticular, polyvesicular vitelline, and solid, with the pseudopapillary pattern being most common in children.[201] IGCNU is not a feature of childhood YST, and it is unlikely that P53 mutations play a role in pathogenesis.[95,96,135] Unlike childhood teratomas, YSTs in children are aneuploid, with characteristic, nonrandom chromosomal abnormalities including gains at 3p and losses at 1p and 6q.[135,202,203] Immunohistochemistry detects AFP expression in more than 90% of YSTs, and in most cases the serum AFP level is also elevated.[56,195,198,204-208]

Testicular Yolk Sac Tumor in Adolescents and Adults

YST in the adolescent and adult testis is extremely rare in the pure form but occurs in approximately 40% of mixed TGCTs.[209] In one series of primary mediastinal GCTs, YST was present in nearly 50% of the tumors.[210] As in childhood YST, hematogenous metastases are common, especially to the liver. The majority of tumors

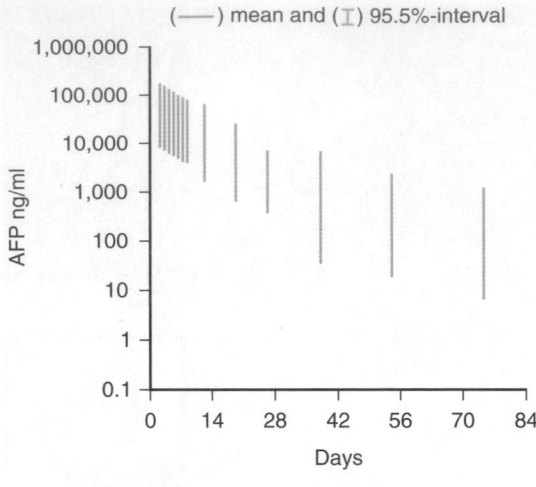
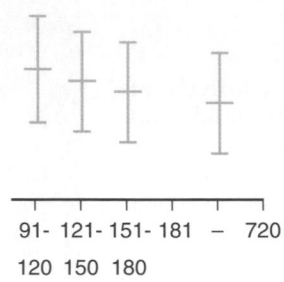

(——) mean and (I) 95.5%-interval

AFP ng/ml

Days

91- 121- 151- 181 — 720
120 150 180

Figure 63-6 Serum AFP values in term babies, mean *(–)* and 95.5% interval *(I)*. *(From Blohm ME, Vesterling-Horner D, Calaminus G, Gobel U: Alpha 1-fetoprotein [AFP] reference values in infants up to 2 years of age.* Pediatr Hematol Oncol *15:135–142, 1998.)*

stain positive for AFP, and serum AFP is commonly elevated.[211]

Ovarian Yolk Sac Tumor

YST of the ovary is a clinically aggressive tumor that often presents at advanced stages with metastasis to lymph nodes or peritoneal structures. The tumors are rarely bilateral.[118,196,212,213] The median age at diagnosis is 18 to 19 years.[61,214-216] In a series of 26 pediatric patients, reticular type was the most common histology identified.[196]

SEMINOMA AND DYSGERMINOMA

Histopathology of Seminoma and Dysgerminoma

Seminomas are a class of GCTs in which the tumor cells resemble primitive, undifferentiated germ cells, both in morphology and in expression of pluripotency genes such as *OCT3/4, NANOG,* and *STELLAR/DPPA3.*[28,30,91,217-219] These tumor are referred to as *germinomas* when arising in extragonadal locations (such as the pineal gland, the mediastinum, or the retroperitoneum), *dysgerminomas* when arising in the ovary, and *seminomas* when arising in the testis. The histology of seminoma is identical regardless of the site in which the tumor occurs. Grossly, these are rounded, nodular tumors, separated into lobules by fibrous bands. Microscopically, seminomas are characterized by a monotonous proliferation of large, uniform cells with large central nuclei and prominent nucleoli (Fig. 63-7). The cytoplasm is clear or granular and often PAS-positive because of high glycogen content. A lymphocytic infiltrate is a typical feature of seminomas.

Seminoma

Seminoma is extremely rare in children. In the postpubertal testis, seminoma can occur in pure form or as a component of mixed GCT.[69,143,220] The peak age of onset of seminoma is 34 to 45 years, slightly later than that of nonseminomatous tumors.[69,221] Several distinct variants of seminoma have been recognized. Up to 7% of classic seminomas contain syncytiotrophoblastic giant cells, and almost 25% of seminomas contain foci that stain positive

for β-human chorionic gonadotropin (HCG).[222-225] These tumors may be accompanied by an elevation in serum β-HCG; however, the presence of syncytiotrophoblasts or elevated β-HCG does not worsen the prognosis.[226-228] Marked elevations of β-HCG or persistently elevated β-HCG after orchiectomy may indicate the presence of choriocarcinoma.[229] *Anaplastic* or *atypical seminoma* is the designation used for seminomas displaying increased mitotic activity, nuclear pleomorphism, and sparse lymphocytic infiltrate on histologic examination.[230-233] Whether these aggressive features portend a worse prognosis or a higher likelihood of metastasis remains controversial. Whereas some studies have suggested that anaplastic seminomas are clinically more aggressive tumors,[234,235] others have found no evidence of a worse prognosis when these features are present.[226,230,236]

Dysgerminoma

Dysgerminoma is the most common MOGCT of children and adolescents, and makes up one third of

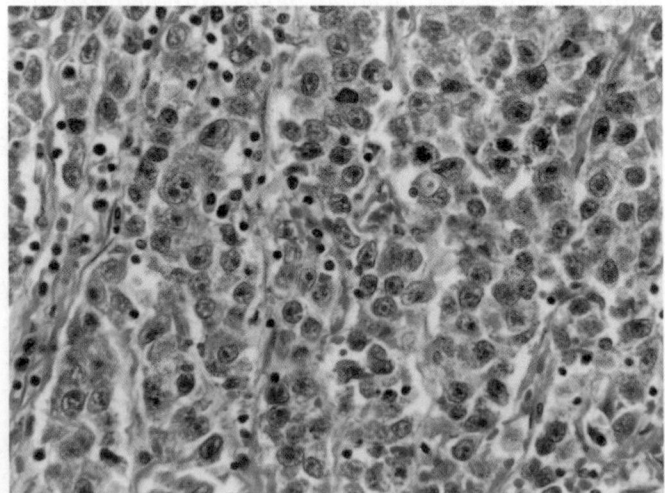

Figure 63-7 Dysgerminoma. Germinomas consist of sheets of large, uniform cells with clear or granular cytoplasm, large central nuclei and prominent nucleoli. A lymphocytic infiltrate is a typical feature of germinomas. The histologies of ovarian dysgerminoma, testicular seminoma, and extragonadal germinoma are identical.

MOGCTs.[237-239] Pathologically, dysgerminoma is the ovarian counterpart of the seminoma of the testis and the germinoma of extragonadal sites. Unlike seminomas of the testis, which are rare in the prepubertal period, dysgerminomas can occur at any age, though the peak incidence is age 15 to 19 years.[239-242] Also unlike seminomas, which develop from IGCNU, dysgerminomas do not appear to arise from a precursor cell.[162] Dysgerminomas stain positively for *OCT4* on immunohistochemistry, which can be useful for distinguishing these tumors from nondysgerminomas.[243,244] As with seminomas, the majority of dysgerminomas also stain positive for *c-KIT*.[245]

EMBRYONAL CARCINOMA

Histopathology of Embryonal Carcinoma

Embryonal carcinoma is very rare in infants but can occur in prepubertal females and adults of both sexes. Embryonal carcinomas commonly have areas of hemorrhage and necrosis and can be locally invasive into the epididymis and spermatic cord in males.[69,162] At the microscopic level, the tumors consist of large, epithelial-appearing cells that resemble the early embryonic cells of the inner cell mass (Fig. 63-8). The tumor cells may grow in solid, papillary, and reticular patterns, forming many clefts and glandlike structures. The tumors are typically cytokeratin and CD30-positive, but negative for epithelial membrane antigen (EMA), carcinoembryonic antigen, and vimentin.[162,246] Syncytiotrophoblast cells, when present in the tumor, can produce β-HCG and cause precocious pseudopuberty in premenarchal girls or vaginal bleeding in older women.[194]

Testicular Embryonal Carcinoma in Adolescents and Adults

Embryonal carcinoma is the most common pure non-seminomatous TGCT in adults, representing about 2% to 10% of cases in this age group. Additionally, 80% of

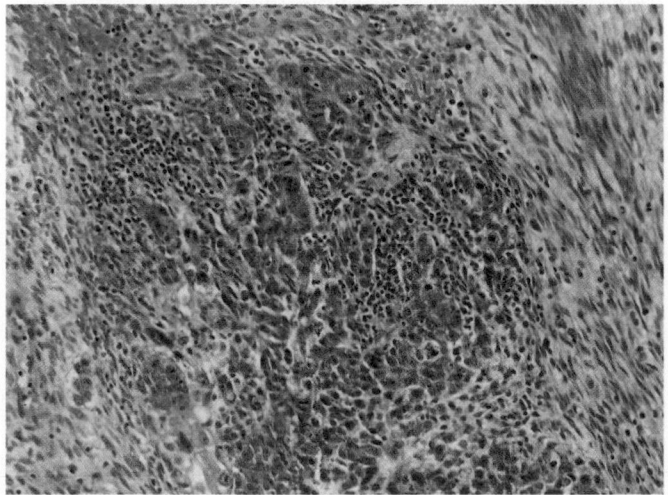

Figure 63-8 Embryonal carcinoma. Embryonal carcinomas consist of large, irregular epithelial-like cells with indistinct borders. The designation *embryonal carcinoma* derives from the resemblance of the tumor cells to the early embryonic cells of the inner cell mass.

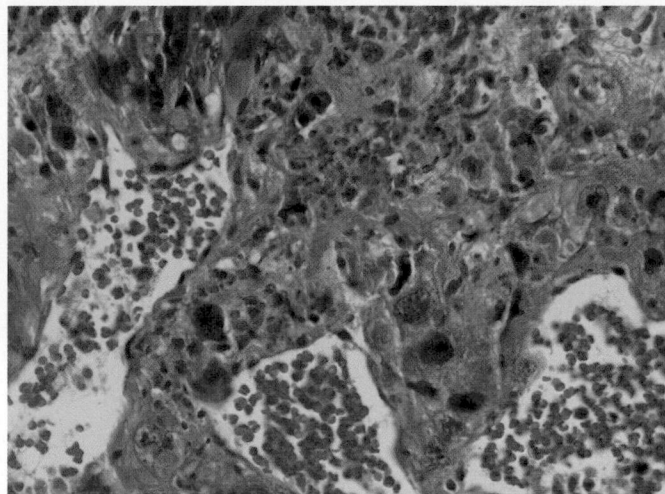

Figure 63-9 Choriocarcinoma. Choriocarcinomas are characterized by a mixture of syncytiotrophoblastic, cytotrophoblastic, and intermediate trophoblastic cells, with multiple areas of hemorrhage.

mixed malignant TGCTs contain embryonal carcinoma as one component.[247,248]

Ovarian Embryonal Carcinoma

Embryonal carcinoma occurs in the ovary less commonly than in the testis, accounting for 4% of malignant ovarian tumors.[194,196] The median age at diagnosis is 14 years, somewhat younger than ovarian YST. Ovarian embryonal carcinoma is more often associated with β-HCG production and with hormonal manifestations such as precocious puberty, amenorrhea, and hirsutism.[194] Owing to the totipotent nature of embryonal carcinoma cells, differentiation into various histologies may be seen including teratomas and syncytiotrophoblastic giant cells resembling choriocarcinoma. Polyembryoma is a rare tumor in which appear multiple embryoid bodies resembling presomite stage embryos. Polyembryoma is considered by some to be an organoid variant of embryonal carcinoma,[162] though others describe it as one component of mixed GCTs.[249,250]

CHORIOCARCINOMA

Choriocarcinoma is a rare tumor composed of cytotrophoblast, syncytiotrophoblast, and extravillous trophoblast. The tumor can cause anemia and bleeding symptoms, as well as pseudoprecocious puberty because of expression of β-HCG by the tumor cells.[118] Choriocarcinomas are usually large tumors with prominent foci of hemorrhage. The histopathology of choriocarcinoma is a mixture of syncytiotrophoblastic, cytotrophoblastic, and intermediate trophoblastic cells, often mixed in random fashion surrounding areas of hemorrhage and necrosis (Fig. 63-9).[69] Vascular invasion is a common feature of choriocarcinomas.

Testicular Choriocarcinoma in Adolescents and Adults

Choriocarcinoma, like YST, is rare in pure form but occurs in approximately 8% of mixed TGCTs in adults.[247,251]

Ovarian Choriocarcinoma

Primary (nongestational) choriocarcinoma occurs rarely as a pure tumor and more often as a component of mixed ovarian GCT, usually in association with teratoma.[238] Choriocarcinoma in infants may arise as a primary tumor in the lung, liver, brain, kidney, or other location.[118,252,253] Treatment of infantile choriocarcinoma is a medical emergency (see "Infantile Choriocarcinoma: A Rare but Rapidly Fatal Condition if Not Recognized.") Gestational choriocarcinoma arises in the placenta and may metastasize widely in the mother; case reports describe metastasis of gestational choriocarcinoma to the infant.[254] In patients in the reproductive years, deoxyribonucleic acid (DNA) analysis to detect the presence of paternal sequences can be helpful in determining the placental origin of gestational choriocarcinoma.[255,256]

MIXED OVARIAN GERM CELL TUMOR

Mixed ovarian GCTs are composed of two or more of the malignant germ cell histologic subtypes. These tumors comprise 8% of malignant GCTs of the ovary in children and adolescents and 20% of ovarian malignant GCTs overall.[61,257,258] Mixed GCTs thus represent only about 1% of all ovarian GCTs in contrast to the postpubertal testis, in which one third of GCTs are of the mixed type.[63,69,143] Dysgerminoma, YST, and teratoma are the most common germ cell components, with embryonal carcinoma and choriocarcinoma more rarely present.[63,216]

Pathology of Mixed Germ Cell-Sex Cord Tumors

Gonadoblastoma

Gonadoblastomas contain mixtures of two cell types: large cells resembling primitive germ cells and smaller cells, similar to immature Sertoli and granulosa cells (Fig. 63-10). It occurs most exclusively in cases of mixed gonadal dysgenesis with ambiguous genitalia, or 45,X Turner syndrome with Y chromosome material.[64,65,67,110] Gonadoblastoma can occur as single or multiple nodules; foci of calcification are a characteristic finding.[118] Microscopically, nests of germ cells within basement membrane material are surrounded by supportive cells (i.e., Sertoli-granulosa cells). The stroma may have elements resembling Leydig or luteinlike cells.[259] The presence of gonadoblastoma substantially increases the risk that a malignant GCT will develop in a dysgenetic gonad. From several studies, the average incidence of GCTs in gonadal biopsy specimens from patients with mixed gonadal dysgenesis is 12%.[66] Gonadoblastoma gives rise most often to dysgerminoma, and less commonly to embryonal carcinoma, teratoma, YST, and choriocarcinoma. The germ cells in dysgenetic gonads abnormally retain their embryonic characteristics, as demonstrated by their marker expression profile, including OCT3/4 and TSPY. These cells give rise to gonadoblastoma in areas of undifferentiated gonadal tissue within the dysgenetic gonad, whereas IGCNU arises in regions with testicular differentiation.* Thus just as IGCNU is the

---

*References 21, 26, 29, 30, 66, 110.

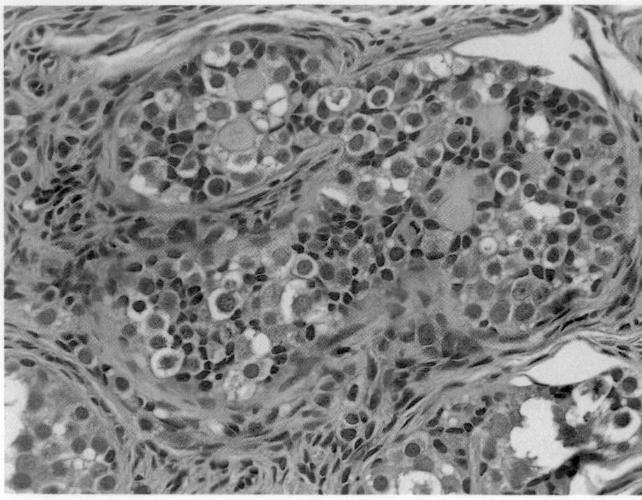

Figure 63-10 Gonadoblastoma. Gonadoblastomas are mixed germ cell-stromal tumors consisting of nests of primitive germ cells surrounded by immature-appearing Sertoli and Leydig cells.

precursor lesion for invasive TGCTs, gonadoblastoma can be considered a precursor lesion to the invasive GCTs of dysgenetic gonads.

SUMMARY OF PATHOLOGY

The five major histologic subtypes of GCTs are teratoma, YST, germinoma, embryonal carcinoma, and choriocarcinoma. In infants and children, teratoma and YST are the most common GCTs. YSTs occurring at any age are malignant tumors. Teratomas are benign in the prepubertal testis; in the postpubertal testis teratomas occur as one component of nonseminomatous GCTs and are uniformly malignant. Most ovarian teratomas are benign; however, ovarian teratomas with a significant immature component are considered malignant. Germinomas in the ovary are known as dysgerminomas and may occur in children and adults. The testicular counterpart is known as seminoma and occurs exclusively in the postpubertal setting. Extragonadal germinomas can occur in both sexes, typically in the midline of the retroperitoneum or mediastinum or in the pineal gland. The remaining tumor types (embryonal carcinoma and choriocarcinoma) are very rare in children but can occur in the testis or the ovary in adolescents and adults, either as pure tumors or as one component of a mixed GCT.

EPIDEMIOLOGY OF PEDIATRIC GERM CELL TUMORS

Incidence

Pediatric GCTs account for only a small proportion of all cancer diagnosed in children under age 20, but incidence fluctuates dramatically with age. Teratomas, which are benign, are the most common neoplasm of the newborn. However, there are malignant forms of GCT that arise in early childhood between the ages of 0 and 4 years, particularly extragonadal GCT in girls and TGCT in boys.[260]

During adolescence, rates of GCT rise substantially for both males and females. Whereas in children younger than 15 years old, GCTs represent only 3.5% of all cancer diagnoses, during adolescence between ages 15 and 19 years, GCTs represent 16% of the total cancer burden. The incidence of testicular GCTs continues to rise throughout young adulthood, peaking in the third decade, and are the most common malignancy in men between the ages of 15 and 34 years of age.[261] Approximately 8300 cases of testicular cancer are diagnosed among adult males annually.

Extrapolating data from the Surveillance, Epidemiology, and End Results (SEER) cancer registry of childhood cancer collected between 1976 and 2006, it is estimated that in the United States, approximately 850 children and adolescents under the age of 20 are diagnosed with a gonadal or extragonadal malignant GCT each year (see Tables 63-1 and 63-2).[260] Incidence of GCT in childhood has a bimodal distribution; there is a peak in diagnosis at birth and up to age 4, and then a second peak after the onset of puberty. Histology varies dramatically with age. YST is the predominant histology in newborns and younger children, whereas tumors that arise in the peripubertal period contain a wider range of histologies, including YST, embryonal carcinoma, and choriocarcinoma, as well as germinomatous tumors (testicular seminoma and ovarian dysgerminoma).

The site of GCT varies by gender. Under age 10 years, the overall rates are similar between boys and girls, but the extragonadal site is much more common in girls than boys. Over age 10 years, incidence increases in both males and females, but the magnitude differs. Rate increases sixfold in boys but only 2.5 fold in girls. Site, however, is primarily gonadal in both sexes after puberty.

Incidence rates vary dramatically by race as well. Non-white boys have higher rates than white boys under age 10, but over age 10, African-American men have much lower rates than white males. In contrast, the rates of GCT are higher among African-American women at all ages. These striking differences in rates of diagnosis by race persist into adulthood; adult African-American males also have a very low likelihood of being diagnosed with testicular cancer.[262]

Incidence not only varies by race and ethnicity, but the overall incidence of GCT has been steadily increasing over the last several decades. Among pediatric patients, incidence rates between 1975 and 2006 increased among boys ages 10 to 19 years (annual percentage change, 1.2; 95% confidence interval [CI], 0.4 to 2.1) and among girls ages birth to 9 years (annual percentage change, 1.9; 95% CI, 0.3 to 2.5). In England and Wales from 1962 to 1990, investigators examined trends in cancer registry data for testicular cancer in males younger than 15 years of age and reported that on average incidence increased 1.3% per annum over the interval.[263] German investigators also report an increase in the incidence of pediatric GCTs over the last several decades.[264,265]

An increase in testicular cancer has also been noted in adult males in many of the countries of the developed world since at least 1940. In the most recent analysis of U.S. data, the incidence of testicular GCTs in adult men rose 44% between 1973 and 1998, with a more pronounced rise in seminoma (64%) than in nonseminoma (24%).[266] In a study of 22 European countries, incidence was noted to be increasing between 1% (Norway) to 6% per year (Spain and Slovenia).[267] The fact that similar trends in incidence have been observed in both young children and adults strengthen the hypothesis that it is exposures that occur either prenatally or in

TABLE 63-1   Average Annual Aged-Adjusted* Incidence Rates per Million for Germ Cell Trophoblastic and Other Gonadal Cancers by Sex And Subtype, Age <20 All Races, SEER, 1986-95

ICCC Group X, a-e	Description	Total	Males	Females
	Germ cell trophoblastic and other gonadal tumors	11.6	12	11.1
Xa	Intracranial and intraspinal GCTs	1.6	2.3	0.9
Xb	Other and unspecified nongonadal GCTs (This category includes the tumors of infants and young children that originate in the sacrococcygeal region as well as mediastinal tumors primarily developing in older children.)	1.6	1.5	1.8
Xc	Gonadal GCTs	6.7	8	5.3
	Testis	4.1	8	—
	Ovary	2.6		5.3
Xd	Gonadal carcinoma	1.4	0.1	2.9
	Ovary	1.3	—	2.6
	Other	0.1	0.1	0.03
Xe	Other and unspecified malignant gonadal tumors	0.2	0.1	0.3

GCT, Germ cell tumor; SEER, Surveillance, Epidemiology, and End Results.
*International Childhood Cancer Classification (ICCC).

TABLE 63-2   Average Annual Age-Adjusted* Incidence Rates per Million for Germ Cell Trophoblastic and Other Gonadal Cancers by Race, Sex, and Subtype Age <20, SEER, 1975-95

ICCC Group X	ICCC Germ cell Tumor Category	White Male	Black Male	White Female	Black Female
X a-e	All	12.3	3.2	9	10.8
Xc	Gonadal GCTs	9.1	1.2	4.5	5.6
	Testis	9.1	1.2	—	—
	Ovary	—	—	4.5	5.6
Xa,b,d,e	Other than gonadal GCTs	3.2	2	4.5	5.2

GCT, Germ cell tumor; *ICCC*, International Childhood Cancer Classification; *SEER*, Surveillance, Epidemiology, and End Results.
*Adjusted to the 1970 U.S. standard population.

early childhood that are responsible for this increase in incidence.

Possible Environmental Etiologies

Given the worldwide increase in testicular cancer of almost 100% in the last 3 decades, and the concomitant rise in pediatric GCTs, there has been significant interest in identifying potential environmental exposures that could be implicated. The parallel rise among both children and young adults has pointed to early life exposures as likely being related to development of GCTs.

One of the primary hypotheses has been that induction of GCTs occurs in the setting of prenatal exposure to high levels of maternal estrogens that could affect gonadal development.[268] Several lines of evidence suggest this is a plausible hypothesis. When diethylstilbestrol (DES) is administered to pregnant mice, it causes maldescent of the testes and testicular hypoplasia. Male offspring of women who took DES during pregnancy have higher rates of cryptorchidism, a known risk factor for TGCT in humans. Maternal use of DES has also been directly associated with increased risk of testicular cancer in some but not all studies.[269]

The fetus is also exposed to high levels of endogenous maternal estrogens during pregnancy (versus exogenous sources such as DES or oral contraceptives). Several conditions of pregnancy are known to be associated with higher levels of serum estrogens and have also been linked to increased risk of GCT, including hyperemesis gravidum and preeclampsia. Testicular cancer is more common among first-born males and twins, especially dizygotic twins, and again, both conditions of pregnancy are known to be associated with higher levels of circulating estrogens.[268,270-273] Increased birthweight, which has been associated with higher risk of testicular cancer, is also associated with higher estradiol and estriol levels in both the first and third trimesters of pregnancy.[274] Maternal weight gain is a predictor of higher birthweight and is also associated with higher insulin levels, leading to lower sex hormone–binding globulin levels, which thereby increases levels of bioavailable estrogens.

Furthering the hypothesis of the importance of early life exposures playing a role in testicular carcinogenesis, it has been noted that men born during World War II in Norway, Sweden, and Denmark have a decreased risk of testicular cancer compared with men born before or after the war. Lack of maternal weight gain during wartime may explain in part this temporal association. Rationing during WWII in Norway resulted in a 15% to 20% energy restriction and a resultant decrease in maternal weight in the period from 1941 to 1945.[275] Height, determined in part by childhood nutrition, has been found to be strongly associated with risk of testicular cancer in two case-control studies.[276,277]

Because GCTs are rare in children, the number of case-control studies conducted among children has been quite limited. The Children's Cancer Group (CCG) conducted an epidemiologic study that included all children with cancer registered for treatment with CCG between 1982 and 1989.[278] Parents were asked to complete a 22-page self-administered questionnaire. Approximately 50% of those with children who had eligible cancer cases completed the questionnaire; controls were obtained through a random-digit–dialing procedure. Among all the cases, there were 105 cases of children younger 15 years of age with a malignant GCT and 639 controls. In this study, several factors were associated with risk of GCT. Birthweight of more than 4000 g was related to 2.4-fold increase in risk (CI, 1.0 to 5.8) compared with a birthweight of less than 3000 g after adjustment for gestational age. Pregnancy conditions such as nausea and vomiting or hypertension or eclampsia were not associated with risk. An inverse association between maternal smoking and risk was noted; among mothers who smoked more than 15 cigarettes per day, risk of GCT was reduced by 70%. Among mothers who ever reported being exposed to chemicals or solvents or to plastic and resin fumes, an increased risk was observed (odds ratio [OR] 4.6; CI, 1.9 to 11.3); (OR 12.0; CI, 1.9 to 75).

A more in-depth follow-up study that specifically focused on GCTs in children was conducted under the aegis of the Children's Oncology Group (COG).[279] The study included 278 cases and 423 controls identified through random-digit dialing. Subjects completed a self-administered questionnaire, a telephone interview, and a medical record review of the maternal records before and during the index pregnancy. The study did not confirm a relationship between maternal exposure to exogenous hormones (either DES or oral contraceptives) and risk of pediatric germ tumor. None of the pregnancy-related conditions including birthweight, hyperemesis, preeclampsia, pregnancy-induced hypertension, or maternal weight gain that can alter circulating levels of endogenous estrogen were related to risk.[279] The study also failed to replicate the finding from the prior case-control study in CCG that showed a relationship between maternal smoking and decreased risk of GCT[280]; neither environmental or occupational exposure to pesticides and other chemicals increased risk of GCT in offspring.[281]

Predisposing Syndromes

Cryptorchidism and Testicular Cancer

Many studies have shown a definitive relationship between cryptorchidism and testicular cancer with relative risks that range from 2.1 to 17.6.[282] Of note, cryptorchidism is three to four times more common in white males than African-American males, which mirrors the difference in incidence by race. The etiology of the relationship between cryptorchidism and testicular cancer remains unclear. It has been suggested that exposure of the testis to higher temperatures in the abdomen as compared to in the scrotum in some way promotes cancer growth. In this case, orchiopexy should minimize risk, especially if it is done before the hormonal stimulation and proliferation of puberty. Others have suggested that the etiology of the undescended testicle and the cancer is the same, and in this case, orchiopexy should not significantly decrease risk. It has been observed that there is an increased risk of testicular cancer in the descended contralateral testicle, which supports this hypothesis for a common etiology. In a case-control study from Kaiser-Permanente of 183 patients with testicular cancer matched to 551 controls, there were 20 men who had had a cryptorchid testes.[283] Interesting, if orchiopexy had been performed successfully by age 11, there was no increase in risk of testicular cancer. However, among men whose cryptorchid testis was not treated until after their eleventh birthday, who had a failed orchiopexy, or who had never had treatment, the odds of testicular cancer were increased 32 fold. Although the study was limited by small numbers, it would suggest that orchiopexy in early childhood before puberty may obviate the risk of subsequent testicular cancer. In the case in which an abdominal testes is discovered after the onset of puberty, an orchiectomy may be the most prudent procedure.

Turners Syndrome and Gonadoblastoma

Turner syndrome, the most common sex-chromosome abnormality in girls (1:2000 live births), is caused by partial or total loss of an X chromosome, resulting in a 45,XO karyotype. Most girls with Turner syndrome have short stature and many have primary amenorrhea. Approximately two thirds of girls have only the remnant of an ovary or "streak gonad." In these dysgenetic and often nonfunctional ovaries, there is a high risk of developing a gonadoblastoma, particularly in girls who also retain a portion of the Y chromosome. Gonadoblastoma is itself a benign lesion, but some of these tumors undergo malignant degeneration, and therefore gonadectomy is usually recommended, although this recommendation has become more controversial. In a Danish study that examined 114 girls with Turner syndrome, presence of the Y chromosome was documented in 13 girls (12%).[284] In the 10 girls with Y-chromosome material who subsequently underwent gonadectomy, gonadoblastoma was present in only one specimen. Therefore the authors suggest that close follow-up examination by ultrasound may be sufficient for monitoring rather than routine gonadectomy but urged that more prospective data is necessary.

Klinefelter Syndrome

Klinefelter syndrome, a condition present in between 1:500 and 1:1000 males, is caused by an extra X chromosome resulting in the 47, XXY karyotype. Men with Klinefelter syndrome have abnormal testicular development and are usually infertile. Men with Klinefelter syndrome also have a substantially increased risk of developing GCTs, particularly mediastinal GCTs, beginning in early adolescence.[285]

Androgen Insensitivity Syndromes

Mutations either in the androgen receptor itself or its downstream effectors results in phenotypic females with an XY karyotype. The prevalence of this disorder is estimated to be approximately 1:20,000 females. Oftentimes, these patients do not come to medical attention until they undergo evaluation of primary amenorrhea. Patients with complete androgen insensitivity have little to no axillary or pubic hair, no uterus, and serum testosterone levels of a male. Testes are abdominal or inguinal but can also present on rare occasions as labial masses. These cryptorchid testes are at high risk for development of gonadoblastoma and/or more malignant GCTs and gonadectomy is advised.

MOLECULAR BIOLOGY OF GERM CELL TUMORS

Analysis of the GCT genome and transcriptome has begun to yield insight into the pathogenesis of these tumors in recent years. Genome-wide association studies (GWAS) comparing GCT cases with unaffected controls have identified a number of loci linked to GCT susceptibility. Several different types of analyses, described in the following sections, lend support to the idea that prepubertal and postpubertal GCTs arise from different molecular mechanisms. In the coming years, identification of specific gene expression signatures, mutations, copy number aberrations, and other abnormalities in different subclasses of GCTs will undoubtedly help refine risk stratification in newly diagnosed patients, as well as provide new targets for novel therapies, especially in chemotherapy-resistant disease.

The GCT Transcriptome

In the last decade studies have begun to illuminate the messenger ribonucleic acid (mRNA) expression pattern of TGCTs in adult men.[218,286-290] These analyses have revealed gene signatures distinguishing GCTs from other types of malignancies and further identified differences in gene expression among different histologic subtypes of GCTs. A major unresolved question of whether pediatric GCTs exhibited the same gene expression patterns was addressed by Palmer, Coleman, and co-workers in an investigation of the pediatric GCT transcriptome, the largest such study to date.[291] This study demonstrated striking differences in the gene expression repertoire of malignant YSTs compared to seminomas, with the former enriched for genes associated with the self-renewing or pluripotent phenotype and the latter enriched for genes associated with differentiation and proliferation. In addition, Palmer et al compared gene expression in childhood GCTs with that in adult TGCT, as described in a study by Korkola et al.[292] The analysis of Palmer and colleagues showed clear differences between the transcriptional profile of pediatric and adult GCTs, even within the same histologic subtype (Fig. 63-11, A and B).

A key additional question is whether particular gene expression patterns are associated with clinical outcome in GCTs, a point addressed by some studies of adult TGCT.[287,293] A study by Korkola and co-workers identified and validated a prognostic mRNA gene expression signature that defined 5-year overall survival in both a training and validation cohort of nonseminomatous TGCTs.[293] Further work will be required to translate this finding into a robust, clinically useful prediction tool.

Noncoding RNAs

Micro RNAs (miRs) are short, 21-nucleotide, noncoding RNAs that have major roles in regulating gene expression and are often misexpressed in cancer.[294] A seminal study in 2006 identified miR-372 and miR-373 as oncogenes in TGCTs—one of the first demonstrations that miRs play a role in human cancer.[295] In childhood GCTs, Palmer and co-workers demonstrated that relative to normal gonadal tissue, MGCTs overexpress miRs from the miR-371~373 and miR-302 clusters, regardless of histologic subtype, patient age, or gonadal vs. extragonadal origin.[296] This study also demonstrated that expression of these miRs causes specific downregulation of their target miRs in GCTs. In a subsequent study, Murray et al. further defined miRs with differential expression that distinguished YSTs from germinomatous GCTs and identified a core set of transcription factors that may be regulated by these miRNAs and contribute to the specific cellular phenotypes of different subtypes of GCT.[297]

Micro RNAs have been shown to be shed from tumor cells into the circulation.[298] The translational significance of the finding that miR-371~373 and miR-302 family members are universally overexpressed in GCTs became clear with the demonstration that these same miRs were present at elevated levels in the serum of a child with YST at diagnosis and fell in parallel with declining AFP levels during treatment.[299] Further studies have confirmed that serum levels of these miRs are increased in patients with GCT at diagnosis, regardless of age group, tumor histology, or location (Fig. 63-12).[300,301] This is a particularly important finding, since many patients with GCT do not manifest elevation of serum tumor markers such as AFP, HCG, or lactate dehydrogenase (LDH).[302] Serum miRs may thus represent sensitive and specific new tumor markers for MGCTs.

Chromosomal Constitution and Copy Number Aberrations

The analysis of tumor karyotypes and genomic copy number aberrations (CNAs) in GCTs provides some of the most important evidence for distinct pathogenic mechanisms of GCT in children compared with adolescents and adults.[60,154,202,303-305] In addition, the gain or loss

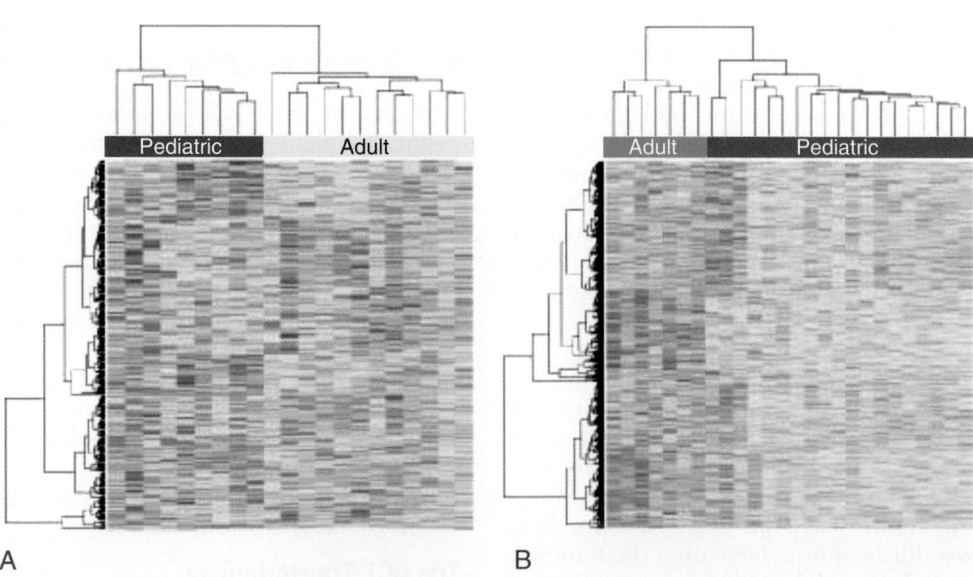

A   B

Figure 63-11 Pediatric and adult germ cell tumors (GCTs) display different gene expression patterns. Heat maps comparing the transcriptomes of 27 pediatric GCTs with that of pure histologic diagnosis adult TGCTs. **A,** Seminomas. **B,** YSTs. *Red* represents relative overexpression and *blue* represents underexpression. *(Modified from Palmer RD, et al: Pediatric malignant GCTs show characteristic transcriptome profiles. Cancer Res 68:4239–4247, 2008.)*

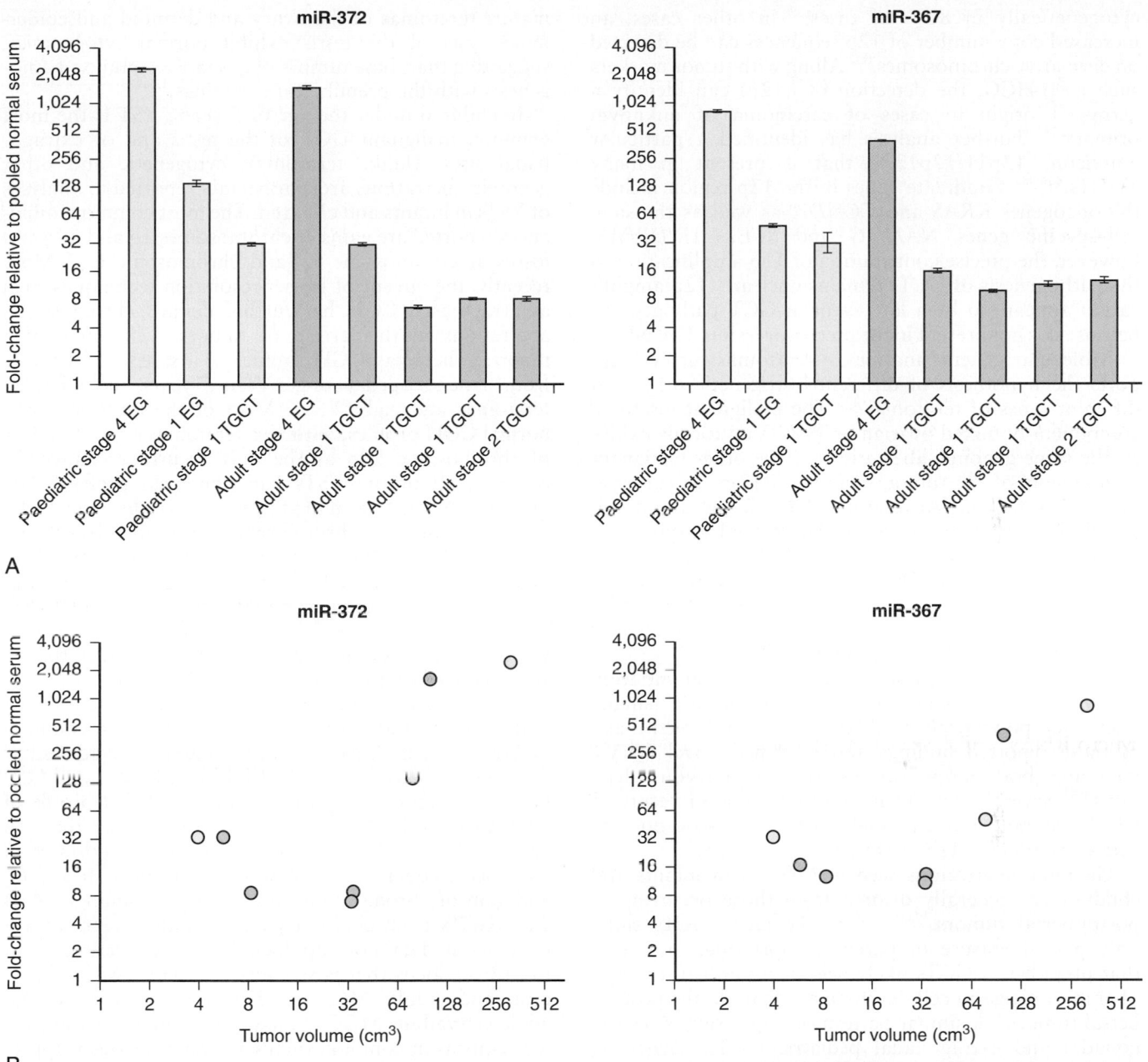

Figure 63-12 MiRs as serum biomarkers of malignant germ cell tumors (GCTs). **A,** Relative levels of miR-372 *(left)* and miR-367 *(right)* in the serum of patients with GCTs at diagnosis, compared with levels in control serums. MiR-372 and miR-367 are elevated in all patients regardless of age, site or tumor histology. **B,** Serum expression of miR-372 and miR-367 at diagnosis correlates to volume of the primary tumor. *(Modified from Murray MJ, Coleman N: Testicular cancer: a new generation of biomarkers for malignant germ cell tumours. Nat Rev Urol 9:298–300, 2012.)*

of specific chromosomal regions may provide important clues as to the molecular mechanisms of germ-cell tumorigenesis.[1,69,94]

Adolescent and adult malignant TGCTs are universally aneuploid, and polyploidization of germ cells has been emphasized as an early event in testicular germ-cell tumorigenesis.[306,307] IGCNU and seminoma cells are hypertriploid, whereas nonseminomas of all histologic types are hypotriploid. TGCTs consistently exhibit biallelic expression of imprinted genes.[102,308-312] Erasure of parental imprinting occurs in mammalian embryonic germ cells,[313,314] implying the origin of TGCTs from an early germline cell.[1]

The most common cytogenetic aberrations in TGCTs are relative loss of all or parts of chromosomes 4, 5, 11, 13, 18, and Y and gain of material from chromosomes 7, 8, 12, and X.[307,315-321] Of these, the most consistent chromosomal aberration in adolescent/adult malignant GCTs is the overrepresentation of chromosome 12p, which is found in all histologic subtypes and primary sites (ovarian, testicular, and extragonadal).[322-331] A characteristic isochromosome 12p (i[12p]) can be detected cytogenetically in 80% of cases;[59] in other cases, an increased copy number of 12p sequences can be detected on derivative chromosomes.[332] Along with tumor markers such as β-HCG, the detection of i(12p) can identify a germ-cell origin in cases of carcinoma of unknown primary.[333] Further analysis has identified a particular amplicon, 12p11-12p12.1, that is present in many TGCTs.[334,335] Candidate genes in the 12p region include the oncogenes KRAS and CCND2, as well as the stem cell–specific genes NANOG and STELLAR/DPPA3; however, the precise contribution of 12p amplification to the pathogenesis of GCTs remains unclear.* 12p amplification appears to be a late event in GCT pathogenesis, because it is not present in the precursor lesion, IGCNU.[342]

Molecular genetic analysis of teratomas further supports the hypothesis of different histogenetic origins of different types of teratomas.[133] The malignant teratoma component of mixed ovarian or TGCTs uniformly exhibits the same genomic aberrations as the other malignant components of the tumor, including i(12)p. In contrast, mature, cystic ovarian teratomas and dermoid and epidermoid cysts of the testis exhibit normal karyotypes.† Based on these observations, Ulbright has proposed that mature ovarian teratomas develop directly from transformed germ cells, whereas the post-pubertal testicular teratomas develop through a malignant IGCNU stage, as do the other malignant post-pubertal TGCTs.[133]

A recent study of genome-wide copy number variation (CNV) in seminomas using high-resolution single-nucleotide polymorphism (SNP) arrays confirmed many of these reported findings and identified novel CNVs, including both amplifications and homozygous deletions.[344] Several genes identified in regions of recurrent CNV are potential candidate seminoma susceptibility genes, including FAT3, EDNRB1, and RASSF8.

Genomic aberrations seen in MGCTs of infants and children are generally distinct from those occurring in postpubertal tumors.[19,60,154,202,303] Pediatric GCTs show only partial erasure of parental imprinting, indicating that prepubertal GCTs likely arise from an earlier stage of embryonic germ cell development than do the postpubertal tumors.‡ A similar pattern of imprinting is seen in gonadal and extragonadal pediatric GCTs, suggesting that gonadal and nongonadal tumors share a common pathogenesis and cell of origin.[100,102,154,305,346]

In analyses of chromosomal structure and copy number imbalances, differences between the pediatric and adolescent/adult GCTs are again consistently found. In the prepubertal period, pure teratomas of the testis or of extragonadal sites nearly always exhibit a normal profile in genomic analyses, including classical cytogenetics, fluorescence in situ hybridization, loss-of-heterozygosity analysis, and array CGH.§ These data contrast sharply with the universally abnormal cytogenetic profile of postpubertal teratomas arising as a component of a mixed malignant GCT. In adolescents and adult GCTs, only

mature teratomas of the ovary and dermoid and epidermoid cysts of the testis exhibit normal cytogenetics, suggesting that these tumors may share a common pathogenesis with the prepubertal teratomas.[123,133]

In children under the age of 5 years, YST is the most common malignant GCT of the testis and of extragonadal sites. Unlike teratomas, cytogenetic and other genomic aberrations are consistently reported in analyses of YSTs in infants and children. The most common imbalances reported are gains at chromosomes 1q and 20q and losses at chromosome 1p and chromosome 6q.¶ More recently, the advent of higher-resolution techniques such as array-based CGH has further defined chromosomal aberrations in this group of tumors. Veltman et al[203] reported the array CGH profiles of a series of 24 GCTs from patients aged younger than 5 years, including 16 teratomas and eight YSTs. Most of the teratomas had normal CGH profiles, with two teratomas exhibiting loss of chromosome 20p as the only recurrent change. In contrast, all of the YSTs had abnormal profiles. The recurrent changes, seen in at least three of the eight YSTs, included gains of chromosomes 1q (1q32-1qter), 3p (3p21-pter), and 20q (20q13) and loss of chromosomes 1p (1p35-pter), 6q (6q24-qter), and 18q (18q21-qter). In the Veltman et al study, only one tumor from a child aged younger than 5 years exhibited gain of chromosome 12p, whereas five of seven cases from children older than 5 years showed gains at chromosome 12 p. Most of these tumors occurred in the ovary, supporting the hypothesis that ovarian and testicular MGCTs have a common pathogenesis, at least in older children and adults.[1,353] Another study from the U.K. Children's Cancer and Leukaemia Group examined the metaphase CGH profile of 34 malignant GCTs in children aged younger than 16 years.[354] This study supported the previous reports of an increased frequency of loss of chromosomes 1p and 6q and gain of chromosome 3p in YSTs. Intriguingly, 4 of 14 MGCTs from children younger than 5 years of age demonstrated gain of 12p, including in two cases gain of the 12p11 locus that is strongly associated with adolescent and adult MGCTs. Therefore childhood and adolescent/adult MGCTs may share more pathogenic mechanisms in common than has been previously appreciated based on the analysis of a relatively small number of cases.

Loss of chromosomes 1p and 6q correlates with loss-of-heterozygosity analysis indicating true allelic loss in these regions in pediatric GCTs.[349,355] However, the most common chromosomal aberrations of pediatric GCTs 1p−, 1q+, 6q−, and 20q+ are not highly specific for GCTs but are seen in other cancers of childhood, including neuroblastoma and Wilms tumor, as well as carcinomas.[356,357] Deletion of chromosome 1p is associated with MYCN amplification and poor prognosis in neuroblastoma,[358,359] which has led to the speculation that one or more genes in this interval may act as a tumor-suppressor in neuroblastoma.[360] Several candidate genes have been proposed, including CHD5, TNFRSF25, CAMTA1, and

---

*References 1, 6, 94, 219, 243, 311, 336-341.
†References 123, 151, 152, 183, 203, 328, 331, 343.
‡References 100, 102, 123, 154, 305, 345, 346.
§References 123, 134, 153, 203, 347-349.

¶References 91, 134, 135, 154, 303, 304, 348, 350-352.

AJAP1.[361] *CHD5* was shown to act as a tumor-suppressor in vivo.[70] Whether these or other genes in the 1p and 6q deleted regions play a pathogenic role in pediatric MGCTs is not known.

Genome-Wide Association Studies

A number of genome-wide studies have used SNP arrays to analyze the constitutional (germline) DNA of men with TGCT, resulting in the identification of a large number of novel GCT susceptibility loci. In 2009 two groups reported strong linkage of GCT susceptibility to loci on chromosomes 5, 6, and 12, suggesting roles for *SPRY4* and *KITLG*, both components of receptor tyrosine kinase signaling, as well as for the proapoptotic *BAK1* gene.[362,363] A follow-up study by Turnbull and co-workers identified additional susceptibility loci near the *DMRT1*, *TERT*, and *ATF7IP* genes.[364] The studies have subsequently been replicated in other patient populations.[365-367] More recently, further GWAS studies have identified new candidate GCT susceptibility loci, including genes with potential roles in telomere regulation, such as *PITX1*, or germ-cell development, such as *TEX14*, *RAD51C*, *PRDM14,* and *DAZL*.[368,369]

The Role of Developmental Signaling Pathways in Germ Cell Tumor Pathogenesis

Compared with many other solid malignancies, relatively few somatic mutations have been described in GCTs. The most commonly reported mutated gene is *KIT*, a tyrosine kinase growth factor receptor that plays important roles in germ cell development.[199,243,370-373] Mutations have also been reported in *NRAS* and *KRAS*, signaling components of the mitogen-activated protein (MAP) kinase pathway that act downstream of *KIT*.[374-377] Interestingly, somatic mutations in *BRAF*, another MAP kinase pathway member, have been associated with cisplatin resistance in adult TGCTs[378]; however, *BRAF* mutations appear to be rare in pediatric GCTs.[379]

Large-scale genomic profiling projects, now underway in several centers, will be required to fully delineate the mutational landscape of MGCTs. Other mechanisms impairing normal gene expression in GCTs such as CNV and aberrant miR expression are being explored (described previously), as is differential methylation. Epigenetic modulation of gene expression through promoter DNA methylation is commonly found in adult and pediatric GCTs. Smiraglia and co-workers first reported that seminomas are globally hypomethylated compared to nonseminomas,[380] whereas Netto et al. extended these observations to show that IGCNU cells, like seminomas, appear globally hypomethylated. Other groups have examined the potential contributions of differential methylation to TGCT susceptibility[381] or cisplatin resistance.[382] Two recent studies examined global DNA methylation patterns specifically in pediatric GCTs. Jeyapalan and co-workers found that pediatric YSTs exhibited a "methylator" phenotype, perhaps attributable to higher expression of DNA methyltransferase 3B in these tumors. Among the genes predicted to be silenced were several associated with caspase-8–dependent apoptosis.[383] Amatruda et al. found a similar pattern of differential methylation comparing YSTs to seminomas and further identified effects on the expression of genes associated with stem cell pluripotency and Wnt/β-catenin signaling.[384]

In addition to these efforts, many studies have focused on understanding how aberrant control of normal developmental pathways may play a role in GCT pathogenesis. Fritsch and co-workers showed that pediatric YSTs and teratomas express active Wnt/β-catenin signaling and Wnt target gene expression.[385] Pediatric YSTs express high levels of *BMP2*, a component of the BMP signaling pathway,[291] and expression of *BMP7* is associated with poor outcome in TGCTs.[293] The importance of BMP was further revealed in the analysis of zebrafish bearing inactivating mutations in a cell-surface BMP receptor, which develop GCTs strongly resembling human seminomas.[386] Thus the state of BMP signaling distinguishes undifferentiated tumors such as seminomas from the more differentiated nonseminomas.[387]

Another key developmental pathway concerns the pluripotency gene *LIN28*, which is universally expressed in GCTs.[388-390] Whereas *LIN28* expression is critical for normal embryonic development, prolonged or aberrant *LIN28* expression in germ cells may be pathogenic, owing to *LIN28*'s ability to block maturation of the let-7 family of tumor-suppressing miRs.[390] Let-7 normally regulates a number of genes associated with proliferation such as *MYCN*, *RAS*, *AURKB*, and *CCNF*, and Murray et al. have shown that *LIN28* expression drives the upregulation of many of these oncogenes in GCT cells.[391]

Although the above studies have begun to yield important insight into the mechanisms by which perturbations in the Wnt, BMP and *LIN28*/let-7 pathways may contribute to GCT pathogenesis, strategies to target these defects are still at fairly early stages of development. There may potentially be more immediate translational impact from the finding that GCTs express cell-surface proteins that have been successfully targeted by monoclonal antibodies in other solid tumors, including *ERBB2/ Her-2*, *CD30*, and epithelial cell adhesion molecule (EpCAM).[392-396]

DIAGNOSIS AND STAGING OF PEDIATRIC GERM CELL TUMORS

In this section, the clinical presentation of GCTs, evaluation of the patient for metastatic disease, and the use and interpretation of the tumor markers in the diagnosis and staging of GCTs will be discussed. The surgical approach, for purpose of both diagnosis and staging, will also be delineated.

Clinical Presentation of Pediatric Germ Cell Tumors

The clinical presentation of a pediatric GCT is determined by the site of origin. Site of origin varies by age. Gonadal tumors, particularly testicular tumors, do present during infancy but are more common after the onset of puberty. The site of the extragonadal GCT also varies as a function of age at diagnosis. Sacrococcygeal tumors, much more common in females than males, present either at birth (typically mature/immature teratomas) or between 6 months and 4 years of life (typically

MGCT with a large component of YST). Mediastinal tumors are rare in infancy; incidence begins to rise at onset of puberty, particularly among males. Site-specific features of the presentation are discussed in the sections that follow.

Presentation of Testicular Germ Cell Tumors

Testicular GCTs most often present with painless generalized swelling of the scrotum. Gynecomastia and infertility are rarely present,[220] though subfertile and infertile men do appear to have an increased risk of developing TGCT.[397,398] Local extension to the spermatic cord and the epididymis may occur, and the presenting symptoms can be mistaken for epididymitis. Symptoms of metastasis, including back or abdominal pain, cough or dyspnea, are present at diagnosis in about 10% of adult patients.[69]

An initial testicular ultrasound that shows the lesion to be intratesticular with areas of microcalcification is often helpful in clarifying the differential diagnosis, which includes lymphoma and paratesticular rhabdomyosarcoma. Eighty-five percent of children younger than age 4 have a tumor that is confined to the testes (stage I), as compared with only 35% of adults.[399]

Choriocarcinoma is the most aggressive histologic subtype of testicular GCT, with a propensity to hematogenous metastasis. Patients may have an occult primary tumor and few or no testicular complaints but rather symptoms caused by hemorrhage of visceral metastases, such as hemoptysis or neurologic symptoms resulting from brain metastases. Because of the risk of hemorrhage, the suspected diagnosis of metastatic choriocarcinoma is a medical emergency that requires prompt initiation of treatment, often without confirmatory biopsy and just on the presumption of the diagnosis given the presenting signs, symptoms, radiologic appearance, and markedly elevated β-HCG. However, it has been hypothesized that chemotherapy may actually precipitate hemorrhage, and therefore patients need very careful monitoring; some have advocated initiation of chemotherapy in an intensive care–unit (ICU) setting. With the extreme elevation of the serum β-HCG that can be seen in choriocarcinoma, occasional patients manifest thyrotoxicosis or gynecomastia resulting from the cross-reactivity of β-HCG with the thyroid and luteinizing hormone receptors.[220,400-404]

Presentation of Ovarian Germ Cell Tumors

Ovarian GCTs typically present with abdominal pain and a palpable pelvic-abdominal mass (85%).[405] Symptoms of acute abdomen occur in about 10% to 25% of patients and are usually caused by rupture, hemorrhage, or torsion of the ovarian tumor that requires immediate surgical exploration.[258] Other less common presenting symptoms include abdominal distension (35%), fever (10%), and vaginal bleeding (10%). Rarely, patients can experience precocious puberty resulting from the production of β-HCG by the tumor. Not uncommonly, a young girl with an abdominal/pelvic mass and and an elevated β-HCG is assumed to be pregnant. This assumption is especially distressing for young females who are peripubertal and have not yet have initiated sexual intercourse.

If the diagnosis of dysgerminoma is made, it is important to recognize that 10% to 15% of cases are bilateral; therefore the finding of dysgerminoma on frozen section during surgical exploration of an ovarian mass generally warrants close inspection and sometimes biopsy of the contralateral ovary.[406-409] Most dysgerminomas present as stage I (disease confined to the ovary),[406-409] but lymphatic metastasis of these tumors to pelvic, paraaortic, mediastinal, and supraclavicular lymph nodes can occur.[216,410,411] Five percent of dysgerminomas arise in dysgenetic gonads of girls with 46XY (Sweyer syndrome or testicular feminization) or who have 45X/46XY mosaicism.[412] For this reason, karyotyping should be considered for all girls with a prepubertal pelvic mass.[216] If dysgenetic gonads and/or the presence of Y-chromosome material are detected, removal of both of the gonads is indicated because of the 25% to 50% risk of developing malignancy such as a gonadoblastoma or dysgerminoma in the contralateral ovary.[66,110,413,414] See "Epidemiology of Pediatric Germ Cell Tumors" for more information.

Presentation of Sacrococcygeal Germ Cell Tumor

Sacrococcygeal teratomas (SCTs) occur predominately in females. In Altman's classic 1974 review of 405 clinical cases, 74% occurred in females.[415] However, even though SCTs are much more common in females, rate of malignancy does not vary by gender. Of note, 18% of patients with SCT had associated congenital anomalies. The most prevalent defects were in the musculoskeletal system, but other organ systems that were involved included renal, cardiovascular, gastrointestinal, and central nervous systems. More than half of the patients were diagnosed on the first day of life, but approximately 10% were diagnosed after 1 year of age.

Altman classified sacrococcygeal tumors by the degree of internalization vs. externalization of the tumor (Fig. 63-13).[415] An "Altman type I" SCT is a tumor that is entirely external; an Altman type IV SCT is entirely internal. Altman was the first to note the correlation between rate of malignancy, age at diagnosis, and degree of internalization. At younger than 2 months of age, 7% of girls and 10% of boys had malignant tumors, whereas after 2 months of age, more than half of the tumors were malignant (48% of SCT in girls and 67% of SCT in boys).[415]

Most neonatal SCTs have a significant external component (Altman type I or II) and can be completely excised in the neonatal period. Over 90% are benign lesions (either mature or immature teratoma) that do not require further therapy. Recurrence rates after resection of neonatal mature or immature teratoma have been estimated to range from 4% to 21% with a malignancy rate of 50% to 70%.[192,416] The reason that a fraction of neonatal tumors do recur could either be because of oversight of a malignant element during the initial pathologic review, such as a microscopic foci of YST, or because malignant transformation of a small benign remnant left in situ after the initial procedure. Presacral tumors that are predominately internal present later in infancy through age 4 years. Usual presenting symptoms of an internal lesion are either constipation or a buttock/abdominal mass; probability is quite high that these lesions are malignant.

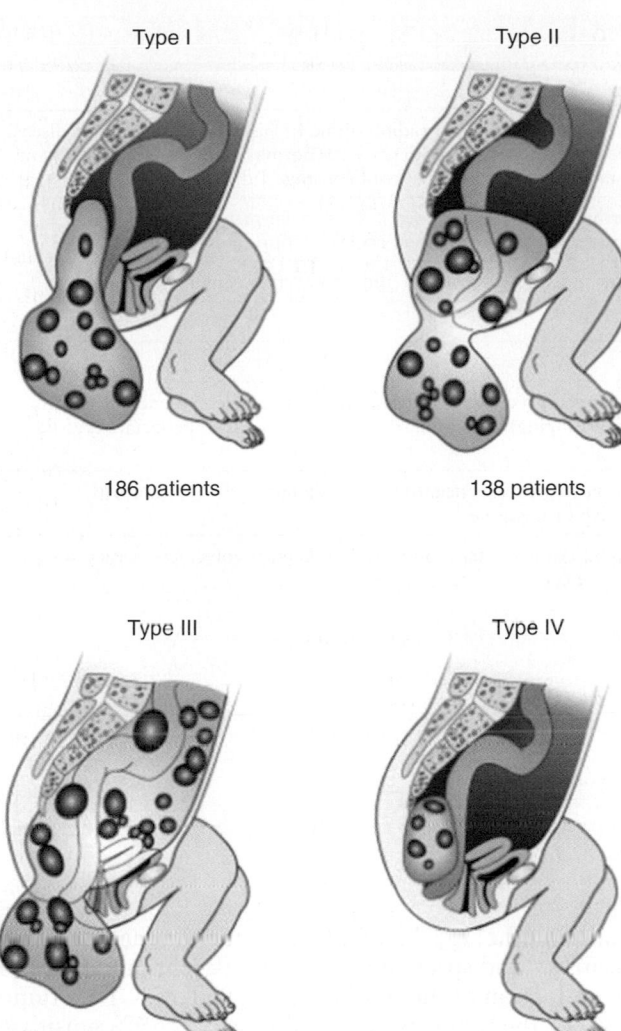

Type I

186 patients

Type II

138 patients

Type III

35 patients

Type IV

39 patients

Figure 63-13 Altman classification of sacrococcygeal germ cell tumors. SCTs are classified according to their degree of internalization. Type I tumors are nearly entirely external; in type II tumors the mass extends equivalently into and external to the pelvis. Type II tumors have only minimal external component, and Type IV tumors are entirely internalized. The numbers of patients with each type of tumor in this series of 398 patients is shown. *(From Altman RP, Randolph JG, Lilly JR: Sacrococcygeal teratoma: American Academy of Pediatrics Surgical Section Survey, 1973. J Pediatr Surg 9:389–398, 1974.)*

Presentation of Mediastinal Germ Cell Tumors

In a series of patients with mediastinal GCTs registered on the German MAKEI protocols, chest pain or respiratory symptoms such as cough or dyspnea were the most common presenting clinical symptoms.[417] Other presenting clinical scenarios included discovery of the mass as an incidental finding on fetal ultrasound or during a workup for pneumonia that did not resolve with standard antibiotics. In the MAKEI experience, all mediastinal tumors that presented at younger than 1 year of age (n = 9) were either mature or immature teratomas.[417] Mediastinal tumors presenting after infancy but before puberty were either pure YSTs or had predominant yolk sac components. Embryonal carcinoma was more prevalent after

the age of 10 years. Mediastinal seminoma was not diagnosed before age 10 years.

Presentation of Extragonadal Germ Cell Tumor at Other Sites

Extragonadal GCTs are the most common fetal and neonatal neoplasm; perinatal teratomas present at wide array of sites. In a review of all perinatal GCTs reported in the literature from 1965 through 2004, the author identified 534 cases.[56] The sacrococcygeal site is the most common (40%), but perinatal GCTs have also been reported in the cervical area (30%), in the oropharynx and nasopharynx (8%), and in other sites including cardiac (7.5%), gastric (2.6%), orbital (2.4%), facial (1.5%), mediastinal (2.6%), and placental (1.5%) locations. In addition, there were 17 teratomas reported in other sites, including tongue, tonsil, liver, retroperitoneum, ileum, mesentery, vulva, and the anorectal area. In addition, 25 cases of fetus in fetu were reported. Most common reasons for diagnosis included detection of a mass on prenatal ultrasound, polyhydramnios, or respiratory distress. Other symptoms were specific to site; for instance, pericardial effusion and tamponade were the most common signs in neonates with intracardiac teratomas. The vast majority of perinatal GCTs are benign, either mature or immature teratomas. Overall the incidence of YST within the neonatal teratoma was 5.8%; the highest rate of YST (10%) was documented in SCTs. Teratomas detected antenatally had three times the mortality rates as those diagnosed postnatally. Fetal survival rate was 53%; neonatal survival rate was 85%. Cause of death was most commonly either because of prematurity or to hydrops. Survival rate was only 7% among those patients whose tumors were diagnosed as a result of fetal distress before 30 weeks of gestation.

Evaluation for Metastatic Disease

The current system for staging pediatric GCTs in use by the COG is shown in Table 63-3.[418] All patients suspected of having a GCT should have a radiologic evaluation of the extent of the disease including either an ultrasound (if testes is the primary site), computed tomography (CT), or magnetic resonance imaging (MRI) of the primary site; abdominal/pelvic CT if the tumor is likely to drain to the lymph nodes of the retroperitoneum and abdomen; and a chest CT. Radiologic staging is preferably obtained preoperatively so that the clinician does not have to differentiate between malignant involvement and postoperative changes (i.e., atelectasis on the chest CT or postoperative lymph node enlargement after surgery). GCTs can also metastasize to brain and bone. Although bone and brain metastases are generally considered quite rare, German investigators reported that up to 10% of patients have bone metastasis, and that incidence was as high as 26% among stage IV patients.[419] On the last combined U.S. intergroup GCT study, 6% of patients overall had bone metastases, but the incidence increased among stage IV patients, of whom 13% had bone metastases at diagnosis.[420] Brain metastases are present in about 4% of adults with GCT. In a review of the St. Jude experience in 206 cases of pediatric GCT from 1962 to 2002, 16 patients in the series had brain metastases at some point

TABLE 63-3   Staging of Testicular, Ovarian, and Extragonadal Tumors

Testicular	
I	Limited to testis, completely resected by high inguinal orchiectomy; no clinical, radiographic or histologic evidence of disease beyond the testis; tumor markers normal after appropriate half-life decline: patients with normal or unknown markers at diagnosis must have negative ipsilateral retroperitoneal lymph node sampling to confirm stage I disease.
II	Transscrotal orchiectomy; microscopic disease in scrotum or high in spermatic cord (<5 cm from proximal end): retroperitoneal lymph node involvement (<2 cm) and/or increased tumor markers after appropriate half-life decline
III	Tumor-positive retroperitoneal lymph node(s) >2 cm diameter: no visceral or extra abdominal involvement
IV	Distant metastases that may include liver
Ovarian	
I	Limited to ovary, peritoneal washings negative for malignant cells; no clinical, radiologic, or histologic evidence of disease beyond the ovaries (gliomatosis peritonei did not result in upstaging): tumor markers negative after appropriate half-life decline
II	Microscopic residual or positive lymph nodes (<2 cm); peritoneal washings negative for malignant cells (gliomatosis peritonei did not result in upstaging); tumor markers positive or negative
III	Gross residual or biopsy only; tumor-positive lymph node(s) >2 cm diameter; contiguous visceral involvement (omentum, intestine, bladder); peritoneal washings positive for malignant cells
IV	Distant metastases that may include liver
Extragonadal	
I	Complete resection at any site; coccygectomy included as management for sacrococcygeal site; negative tumor margins
II	Microscopic residual; lymph nodes negative
III	Gross residual or biopsy only; regional lymph nodes negative or positive
IV	Distant metastases that may include liver

during treatment.[421] Only two patients (1%) had brain metastases at diagnosis. Twelve patients were diagnosed at relapse, and 2 patients were discovered to have brain metastases at autopsy. Most patients with brain metastases had clinical symptoms (12/16) and also had concurrent pulmonary metastases (14/16). The data may overestimate the incidence of brain metastases, however, because 11/16 were diagnosed before 1982 when cisplatin-based chemotherapy was not routine. Risk factors for the development of brain metastases in the St. Jude's study included extragonadal site ($P = .013$), advanced stage ($P = .02$) and choriocarcinoma ($P < .001$). In comparison, in a more recent cohort of the patients treated from 1990 through 1996 in the U.S. pediatric intergroup study, only three out of 299 patients were diagnosed with brain metastases; two of these patients were stage IV at diagnosis.[420] All patients had other sites of metastatic disease; the histology of all three patients included choriocarcinoma. Two of three patients are alive and well; one was treated with PEB alone and one patient received bleomycin, etoposide, and cisplatin (PEB) plus x-ray therapy (XRT). Therefore a bone scan should be obtained in all patients with advanced stage disease (stage III or IV), but head CT or brain MRI are recommended only for patients with stage IV disease, particularly in patients who have choriocarcinoma.

The use of fluorodeoxyglucose F 18 positron emission tomography (PET) has not been systematically evaluated in pediatrics, but its use is becoming more routine among adult patients with GCTs in the setting of a residual mass postchemotherapy. In a German study that compared the sensitivity and specificity of three different modalities for the evaluation of the residual mass, PET vs. CT vs. tumor markers, the results were as follows: PET, 59% sensitivity and 92% specificity; CT, 55% sensitivity and 86% specificity; and tumor markers, 42% sensitivity and 100% specificity.[422] The positive and negative predictive values for PET were 91% and 62%, respectively. Teratomas are not PET-avid. The authors concluded that PET did not add to the preoperative inference in the setting of a mass in which viable tumor was suspected by CT and tumor marker, but it was a useful adjunct in the setting in which tumor markers had normalized or the patient had marker-negative disease at diagnosis. PET-negative masses also require resection because of the possibility of residual teratoma that is PET-negative.

Tumor Markers

Specific subtypes of GCTs secrete proteins that can be used as markers of tumor presence. The pattern of these tumor markers and degree of elevation provide an indication of the likely histology (Table 63-4).[423] AFP is a glycoprotein that is synthesized by the fetal liver and yolk sac. AFP is elevated in patients with YST,[199] although low levels of AFP (generally <100 IU) are often observed in immature teratoma (perhaps because of occult microscopic foci of YST within the tumor). When an elevated AFP level is detected, one must consider other reasons for an elevated AFP in the differential diagnosis, including synthesis by a liver tumor, such as a hepatoma

TABLE 63-4   Histologic Subtype and Tumor Marker Levels

Term	Synonym	Comments*	Incidence Pre- vs. Post-Puberty	Tumor Marker
Seminoma	Dysgerminoma, germinoma	Seminoma-testes tumor; dysgerminoma-ovarian tumors; germinoma-extragonadal tumors	Post	Low levels of AFP; low levels of β-HCG in dysgerminoma caused by presence of multinucleated syncytiotrophoblastic giant cells
Endodermal Sinus Tumor	Yolk sac tumor	Most common form before puberty, besides teratoma	Pre	AFP +++
Embryonal Carcinoma			Post	AFP + β-HCG +++
Choriocarcinoma		Pure forms rare; most commonly one component of mixed GCT	Post	β-HCG +
Teratoma			Pre and Post	
Immature Teratoma			Pre and Post	≈⅓ of immature teratoma produce low levels of AFP
Dermoid cyst				
Polyembryoma				AFP +; β-HCG +
Mixed GCT		Tumors with more than one component are categorized by the most malignant component, not by the most common component	Pre and Post	Depends on the components

AFP, α-Fetoprotein; GCT, germ cell tumor; HCG, human chorionic gonadotropin.
*Much of the therapy for pediatric GCTs has been gleaned from experience treating testicular GCTs in adult males. An excellent guide for the workup and treatment of adult testicular tumors is the National Comprehensive Cancer Network (NCCN) Practice Guidelines in Oncology (http://www.nccn.org/).

or hepatoblastoma, or other disease states such as hypothyroidism, folate deficiencies, autoimmune disorders, acquired immunodeficiency syndrome (AIDS), congenital heart defects, cystic fibrosis, and platelet aggregation disorders. β-HCG is a peptide hormone produced in pregnancy, that is made by the embryo soon after conception and later by the syncytiotrophoblast (part of the placenta). Its role is to prevent the disintegration of the corpus luteum of the ovary and thereby maintain progesterone production that is critical for a pregnancy in humans. In tumors that originate in extraembryonic tissues, like choriocarcinoma, β-HCG can be significantly elevated. β-HCG is also sometimes mildly elevated in seminoma/dysgerminoma (<50 IU/L).

Interpretation of AFP levels must incorporate knowledge of age-related norms (see Fig. 63-6).[191,192] AFP is elevated in all infants at birth because there of continued synthesis of AFP by the fetal liver. Over the course of the first 2 years of life, AFP declines in normal infants as the synthesis in the liver ceases. To establish normal values for infants, Blohm et al analyzed data on 414 full-term infants, 90 preterm infants, and 259 children up to age 2 years from the University Hospital Düsseldorf (Germany).[192] Using regression analysis, the authors estimated that the half-life of AFP increases with age over the first 2 years of life. From birth to day 28, the half-life is estimated to be 5.1 days. The half-life of AFP increases thereafter to 14 days at 1 to 2 months of age, 28 days

from 2 to 4 months of age, and 42 days from 4 to 6 months of age. The increase in the half-life of AFP with age also results in a "shouldering" of the AFP curve during the first 2 years of life. Not all children have adult levels of AFP by 2 years of age. In the Blohm study, the mean AFP at age 2 was 8 ng/mL; however, the 95% range extended between 0.8 and 87 ng/mL. Similar results were reported in an earlier and smaller study by Wu et al.[191] Values of AFP obtained in children under age 2 ought to be plotted on the nomogram developed by Blohm et al to determine whether the value falls within the normal range.[192]

Tumor markers may also be prognostic. In adult males with testicular cancer, the prognostic significance of postoperative tumors markers is well established. An international consortium pooled data on over 5000 men with testicular cancer and used multivariate analysis to investigate prognostic factors that created the International Germ Cell Consensus Classification (IGCCC), which divided patients into good, intermediate, and poor risk groups based on the extent of elevation of tumor markers, the presence of nonpulmonary visceral metastases or a nontesticular primary site of disease.[424] Although elevated tumor markers are one of the primary variables that determine risk group assignment in adult men, evaluation of the prognostic significance of tumor markers in pediatrics has been limited. In adult males, the failure of tumor markers to decline appropriately among poor-risk patients has also been shown to be a poor prognostic feature. Further discussion can be found in "Prognostic Factors at Diagnosis of Pediatric Germ Cell Tumors."

Tumor markers are also used prospectively to differentiate between stage I and II tumors. For patients with gonadal GCTs who have had all disease completely removed surgically and in whom no evidence of further disease is noted on pathologic or radiologic staging evaluations a watch-and-wait strategy is often recommended. However, if tumor markers fail to decline according to the expected half-life, the patient by definition has occult metastatic disease. The patient should be upstaged to stage II and therapy commenced.

There is one situation in which tumor markers may increase and not be cause for alarm. During the first cycle of chemotherapy, it has been observed that tumor markers can increase transiently. However, levels should have declined to the expected level by the start of the second cycle of chemotherapy.

SURGERY AND GERM CELL TUMOR

Surgery is an integral part of the management of GCTs. For benign tumors, complete excision is curative. For malignant tumors, proper staging and appropriate timing of excision are important for optimal outcome. At all sites, primary excision should be considered if the tumor can be safely removed without significant risk of morbidity. For tumors that pose risk to adjacent structures or expectation of incomplete excision, biopsy should be performed for diagnosis and neoadjuvant chemotherapy should be given. Reduction in tumor size allows greater expectation of safe and complete excision. Evidence is mounting that delayed resection of extragonadal tumors does not just decrease morbidity but also more importantly may increase survival, because of the ability to achieve complete resection at the time of the delayed surgery. In the case of expected malignancy, a child should be referred to a center with surgeons with experience in oncologic surgery, preferably a site that participates in COG clinical trials so that the proper staging can be done to allow for trial entry.

Surgical Approach to Sacrococcygeal Tumors

Over 90% of neonatal sacrococcygeal tumors are benign (mature or immature teratoma), and require complete excision at diagnosis should be attempted without harming adjacent structures. There is a 9% to 14% risk[425,426] of malignant recurrence in benign tumors, and long-term follow up care is important. Beyond the neonatal period, the risk of malignancy increases, and the tumor configuration is more likely to have an internal component (Altman types III and IV; see Fig. 63-13). Children with a large sacrococcygeal tumor suspected to be malignant should be evaluated for feasibility of resection. Gastrointestinal and genitourinary complications are far more common than lower extremity neurological sequelae, with up to 41% patients affected in one study.[39] Long-term follow up observation is mandatory in these children to ensure that normal bowel, bladder, and sensory-motor function is preserved.[40] If a problem is

encountered, these children are best cared for by a multidisciplinary team that simultaneously initiates symptom management (such as management of constipation) with investigational studies including functional evaluations such as anorectal manometry and urodynamic studies (including direct electromyography [EMG] evaluation of the urinary sphincters) to define the extent of the problem at discovery as well as any progress (or lack thereof) in response to the prescribed interventions.[427] One final note is recognition of the recommendation by Ozkan and colleagues,[41] who suggest the need for defining the extent of neurologic, gastrointestinal, and genitourinary dysfunction before any intervention so as to better categorize any impairment of function at baseline and not just after surgery.[428] This suggestion is especially valuable for those patients whose tumors are discovered outside of the neonatal period.

Therefore an initial biopsy with a delayed resection must be seriously considered if morbidity is likely to be reduced.[429] In patients whose lesions involve the rectum or extend into the sacral bone or in patients already shown to have metastatic disease, biopsy rather than resection is the more appropriate initial surgical approach. If a needle biopsy is used to obtain diagnostic material, multiple passes should be obtained because of the histologic heterogeneity of these tumors and the possibility that the malignant foci will not be found in every sample. The histologic diagnosis should also be evaluated in the context of the information from tumor markers. A benign histologic diagnosis in the setting of elevated tumor markers should lead one to question whether there was a sampling error in the sample obtained or in the pathologic review. Lin28 is a new histochemical reagent that can be used to detect YST in the specific and sensitive way that should be used to detect occult YST.[388]

Delayed resection of a SCT has been definitively demonstrated not to adversely affect survival. In fact, German investigators have shown that patients with locally advanced and metastatic tumors actually had better overall survival when treated with chemotherapy before tumor resection. Overall survival for patients with delayed resection was 83%, whereas overall survival for patients who had an initial resection was only 45% (P = 0.01).[419] Preoperative chemotherapy allowed for more complete primary resection of the tumor; 19 of 31 patients had a complete resection after preoperative chemotherapy vs. only 11 of 35 patients who had a complete resection when definitive surgery was attempted before chemotherapy. Complete resection of the tumor, either at diagnosis or delayed until after chemotherapy, was the most significant predictor of event-free survival (EFS) in the German series of sacrococcygeal tumors (Fig. 63-14).[419] Second-look surgery was recommended for those with incomplete resection and had therapeutic benefit. Analysis of the data from the United States Pediatric Intergroup Trial (POG9049/CCG8882) also confirms that delayed resection did not have an adverse effect on prognosis.[416]

Most presacral lesions will be initially approached through a posterior transsacral incision. Superior

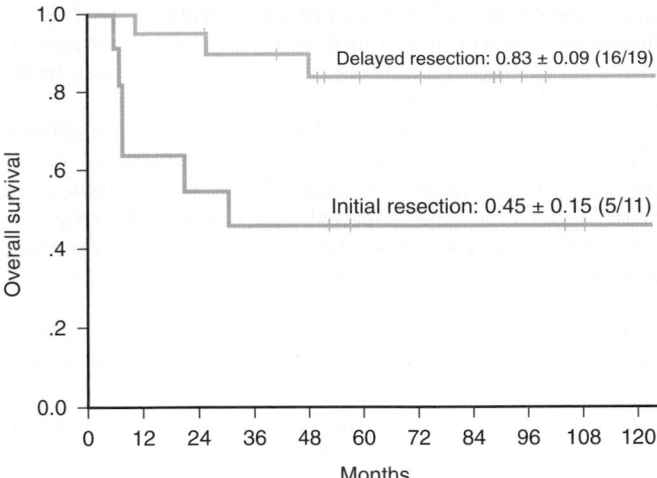

Figure 63-14 Five-year overall survival of 30 patients with locally advanced and metastatic malignant sacrococcygeal GCT (stage T2b M1) treated with initial resection versus delayed resection (P = .01, log-rank test). *(From Gobel U, Schneider DT, Calaminus G, et al: Multimodal treatment of malignant sacrococcygeal GCTs: a prospective analysis of 66 patients of the German cooperative protocols MAKEI 83/86 and 89. J Clin Oncol 19:1943–1950, 2001.)*

extension of the tumor into the pelvis often requires a laparotomy. If laparotomy is performed, retroperitoneal lymph nodes should be examined and biopsied if enlarged. In all cases, the coccyx must be completely removed en bloc with the primary tumor. The importance of the resection of the coccyx was first noted by Gross, who reported a recurrence rate of 38% of those who had not had coccygectomy and 0% of those who had had a coccygectomy.[430]

Surgical Approach to Testes Tumors

Risk of malignancy is age dependent with 38% to 74% of testicular tumors in the prepubertal age group having benign histology.[121,122] In prepubertal boys with localized tumors, those with normal tumor markers and imaging studies can be considered for testis sparing enucleation of the tumor. Because the most common sites of metastasis of a testicular GCT are the retroperitoneal lymph nodes, a pelvic/abdominal CT scan should be obtained preoperatively. If the CT scan is delayed until after surgical exploration of the inguinal region, reactive retroperitoneal lymphadenopathy may be noted on CT scans and may be difficult to differentiate from metastatic disease. Evaluating the lungs for pulmonary metastases with chest CT before surgery is advisable, because postoperative atelectasis can make evaluation for malignant disease more difficult. Tumor markers should also be obtained preoperatively, because these levels are important to confirm the initial diagnosis and to provide prognostic information. In addition, the rate of decline is important to be able to track postoperatively in patients, especially in patients with stage I disease who are being expectantly observed, reserving chemotherapy only for those patients who have demonstration of residual malignant disease.

The surgical approach for a scrotal tumor should be through an inguinal incision. Control of the testicular vessels and vas deferens is gained at the level of the inguinal ring. The testis is then mobilized from the scrotum. Occasionally, a large testicular mass cannot be mobilized out of the scrotum into the inguinal region, and in this situation the inguinal incision should be enlarged to the superior aspect of the scrotum in order to avoid tumor rupture during mobilization. A radical orchiectomy is then performed with high ligation of all cord structures at the level of the internal inguinal ring. In prepubertal boys who have a focal lesion with normal markers and metastatic imaging, tumor enucleation protecting the tumor capsule followed by frozen section should be considered. If the frozen section is consistent with teratoma, the testis can then be placed back in the scrotal position, because enucleation is adequate therapy for prepubertal testicular teratoma. In the postpubertal boy, however, even localized teratoma has malignant potential and orchiectomy ought to be undertaken.

Rate of adherence to surgical guidelines was evaluated among the 63 patients with stage I GCT of the testes who were treated with observation only on the last U.S. intergroup trial from 1990 through 1996.[431] Adherence to guidelines could be verified in only 69% of the patients. Likelihood of adherence was directly related to whether or not the surgeon thought the diagnosis was tumor preoperatively. In patients in whom the preoperative diagnosis was malignant tumor, the surgical guidelines were followed in 80% of patients, whereas among patients in whom another preoperative diagnosis was suspected (i.e., hydrocele, hernia, torsion), the guidelines were followed in only 17%. There was no difference in recurrence rate among those patients in whom the surgical guidelines were followed and among those for whom the guidelines were not followed, with the exception of patients who had had scrotal violations. Among the four patients with transscrotal violation, three had recurrence of disease.

Based on detailed review of the surgical procedures followed in the CCG-POG Intergroup Study (INT0098), the surgical guidelines in the case of scrotal violation were revised. In cases in which a scrotal orchiectomy has been performed without violation of the tumor capsule, the patient may still remain in stage I. If the cord structures show evidence of tumor spread, the patient should be upstaged to stage II. However, if a scrotal biopsy was performed as the initial procedure, the scrotum is considered to be contaminated and the patient should be treated as having stage II disease. Hemiscrotectomy, however, is no longer required. In addition, a "completion orchiectomy" with removal of all cord structures to the level of the internal ring should be performed.

Evaluation of Retroperitoneal Nodes in Pediatric Testicular Germ Cell Tumors

Lymphatic drainage of the testes is to the retroperitoneal nodes and to the nodes below the renal vessels. Right testicular tumors usually metastasize to the nodes between the aorta and the inferior vena cava (interaortocaval nodes). Left testicular tumors metastasize to the nodes lateral to the aorta (paraaortic).[432] Left supraclavicular nodes and pulmonary nodules have been observed in the absence of retroperitoneal adenopathy. In adults, it is estimated that up to 30% of patients have false negative CT scans; in the most recent U.S. intergroup study of stage I testicular cancer among boys younger than 10 years of age, 5% of patients had failure of normalization of tumor markers postoperatively (i.e., patients had occult disease that was not detected on initial CT scan (false-negative initial CT scan). In total, 22% of patients presumed to be in stage I at diagnosis eventually relapsed, but all were salvaged with chemotherapy with 100% survival.[399]

If the preoperative CT scan of the abdomen has identified enlarged (≥4 cm) retroperitoneal lymph nodes, biopsy is not necessary, and one may assume that this represents metastatic disease; the patient should be treated as having stage III disease. If retroperitoneal lymph nodes are between 2 and 4 cm, a biopsy should be performed. If the retroperitoneal nodes are smaller than 2 cm, a biopsy is not required; however, the tumor markers (AFP and β-HCG) should be observed and return to normal with appropriate decline according the half-life (see previous discussion of tumor markers). In adult males, 10% to 20% of nodes between the size of 1 and 2 cm contain metastatic disease.

If the decision is made to biopsy a suspected node of the prepubertal boy, the retroperitoneal procedure should simply be a lymph node excision, not a full retroperitoneal lymph node dissection. If no biopsy is performed and the nodes are enlarged (>2 cm), that patient should be treated as a patient with stage III disease. But in adolescents (as in adults), if a biopsy is being undertaken to evaluate nodal disease, then a nerve-sparing modified template retroperitoneal lymph node dissection (RPLND) should be employed, which some surgeons would expand to a full bilateral nerve-sparing RPLND if any of the initial nodes are positive on frozen section. RPLND is both diagnostic and potentially therapeutic. For further discussion of RPLND please see the section on treatment of adolescent boys with stage I testicular cancer.

Metachronous Testicular Cancer

In adults, 3% to 5% of men with testicular cancer have a metachronous tumor in the other testicle at diagnosis, and 2% of men subsequently develop a tumor in the contralateral testicle. These risks have not been quantified for pediatric patients and no formal evaluation of the contralateral testis is recommended besides that continued thorough physical examinations, although a patient should be advised of the likely need for continued surveillance of the contralateral testis. Patients who have developed a testicular tumor in a cryptorchid testis are at increased risk of malignancy in the normally descended contralateral testes.

Surgical Approach to Ovarian Tumors

The largest series of ovarian GCTs (66 cases) estimated rate of malignancy in an ovarian mass as 19% at ages 0 to 5 years, 14% at ages 6 to 10 years, and 33% at ages 11 to 15 years.[258] AFP and β-HCG should be determined preoperatively for ovarian tumors. If not done preoperatively, these markers should be sent from the operating room once the diagnosis is apparent. The goals of the initial exploration for a suspected ovarian tumor are to completely resect the tumor if it can be accomplished without sacrifice of adjacent organs and to completely evaluate the extent of disease.

Surgical guidelines for ovarian GCTs were originally based on the experience with ovarian epithelial carcinoma, in which aggressive surgical resection is associated with higher chance of survival. Application of those surgical guidelines to ovarian GCTs, which have a different pattern of spread and are also highly chemosensitive, is not warranted. It is clear from studies in adult women with GCTs that fertility-sparing surgery (i.e., performing an unilateral instead of bilateral salpingo-oophorectomy) had no adverse outcome on survival.[238] On the most recently completed U.S. Intergroup Trial for gonadal tumors (CCG8892/POG9048), surgeons adhered to the guidelines (derived from adult epithelial cancer) in only 2% of the patients,[418] but overall EFS and overall survival (OS) rates were nonetheless excellent.[433] Surgical omissions resulting in protocol noncompliance resulted from failure to biopsy bilateral nodes (97%), no omentectomy (36%), no peritoneal cytology (21%), and no contralateral ovary biopsy (59%). Among the patients in whom peritoneal cytology was examined, 25% of patients had malignant tumor found in what would otherwise been declared to be stage I disease. Biopsy of normal-appearing lymph nodes, omentum, and/or contralateral ovary very rarely, if ever, showed occult malignant disease.

Given the excellent overall survival, despite low adherence to the surgical guidelines on the Pediatric Intergroup Trial, the current surgical guidelines for pediatric ovarian GCT have been substantially revised. Given the high rate of positivity in the examination of peritoneal fluid, all patients with ascites present should have the fluid collected for cytology. In the absence of ascites, peritoneal washings should be conducted and sent for pathologic review. Any patient in whom cytology is not available should not be considered to be in stage I. The pelvic viscera should be examined, and pelvic and retroperitoneal lymph nodes should be palpated bilaterally. Only suspicious or enlarged lymph nodes should be biopsied. The omentum and peritoneal surfaces should also be palpated and visualized. If the omentum is adherent or has nodules or implants, partial or complete omentectomy that includes the lesions should be done. If the omentum does not appear grossly involved, an omentectomy does not need to be performed. Any nodules studding the peritoneal surfaces should be biopsied.

If only one ovary is involved, the tumor should be removed by unilateral oophorectomy. Attempts to preserve completely uninvolved fallopian tubes and the uterus should be made in all patients. Lesions adherent to the uterus may be managed by separation of the adherence if feasible or by biopsy only with planned second-look surgery after chemotherapy if necessary. The tumor capsule should not be aspirated. If the capsule is violated, either by the surgeon or because of rupture by the tumor or if there is microscopic capsule penetration seen by the pathologist in an apparently intact tumor, the patient should be upgraded to stage II (this is in contrast to adult staging guidelines in which a patient with capsular involvement is International Federation of Gynecology and Obstetrics [FIGO] stage IC). The ovary must be delivered intact and not removed in fragments. The contralateral ovary should only be biopsied if it appears involved with tumor; biopsy of a normal-appearing contralateral ovary is discouraged because of concern regarding possible adverse impact on future fertility. Bilateral ovarian lesions were present in only 6% of patients (n = 10) on the U.S. Pediatric Intergroup Study. Of these, four were benign teratomas and six were malignancies. If a patient has bilateral disease, preservation of as much normal ovarian parenchyma as possible should be the goal.

Surgical Approach to Mediastinal Germ Cell Tumors

The German MAKEI experience with mediastinal GCTs was analogous to the experience with sacrococcygeal tumors. Delayed resection increased the odds of complete resection of the primary tumor (10 of 11 patients at delayed resection vs. 6 out of 12 patients at primary resection) and complete resection was a strong predictor of more favorable outcome (EFS 0.94 ± 0.06 vs. 0.42 ± 0.33).[417] Therefore the surgeon must decide whether it is more prudent to attempt a primary resection or to obtain a biopsy and plan for delayed resection.

The resection may be through a lateral thoracotomy or median sternotomy, as determined by the site of the lesion. The margin of resection should include adherent nonvital structures such as the thymus and pericardium. Regional lymph nodes should be evaluated and biopsied when possible in all patients.

Surgical Approach to Extragonadal Tumors at Other Sites

YST (also referred to as *endodermal sinus tumor*) of the vagina is a rare tumor occurring exclusively in children younger than 3 years of age. The mass can be confused with sarcoma botryoides. Only small lesions that can be resected with vaginal preservation should be excised at initial presentation. In others, a careful vaginal examination and limited biopsy should be performed. After completion of chemotherapy, repeat evaluation and complete excision of residual disease should be considered, although oftentimes residual tissue is just scar tissue. A biopsy to guide the need for resection is a reasonable approach.

Malignant GCTs found at other locations should be completely excised if possible without sacrifice of adjacent organs. Biopsy only may be appropriate at the initial operation, with planned secondary procedures for delayed excision after chemotherapy. Any enlarged regional lymph nodes in the area should be sampled.

PROGNOSTIC FACTORS AT DIAGNOSIS OF PEDIATRIC GERM CELL TUMORS

Tumor markers have prognostic significance. In pediatric GCT, preoperative tumor markers have been evaluated, whereas in adult testicular cancer tumor markers evaluated at the time of initiation of chemotherapy are used as the benchmark, which is why it is important to obtain preoperative levels. In adult males with testicular cancer, the prognostic significance of tumor markers is well established. IGCCC pooled data on over 5000 men with testicular cancer; multivariate analysis identified prognostic factors that could divide patients into good, intermediate, and poor risk groups. Elevated tumor markers are one of the primary variables that determine risk group assignment in adults. Other adverse prognostic factors include mediastinal primary site and presence of nonpulmonary visceral metastases. LDH has been shown to be prognostic in adult males with testicular cancer but has not been shown to have prognostic significance in pediatric patients, although analyses to date have been underpowered to examine this issue.

Several retrospective studies in adult males with testicular cancer have shown that slower than expected decline in tumor markers after the initiation of treatment predicts both lower EFS and OS.[434-436] In an analysis of adult men with testicular cancer treated between 1986 and 1998 at Memorial Sloan Kettering, those with satisfactory decline in their tumor markers had an excellent 2-year survival rate (EFS 91%; OS 95%) compared with those who had unsatisfactory decline (EFS 69%, OS 72%).[436] A recent randomized trial among patients classified as having "IGCCC intermediate or poor risk" testicular cancer compared standard therapy, four cycles of BEP, to two cycles of BEP followed by 2 cycles of high-dose carboplatin, etoposide, and cyclophosphamide. Although the overall results of the trial did not show a difference in survival between the two arms, in the subgroup of 67 patients with unsatisfactory tumor marker decline, the 1 year durable complete response was 61% for the patients who received high-dose chemotherapy (HDCT) compared with 34% for those who received BEP alone.[437]

Evaluation of the prognostic significance of tumor markers in pediatrics has been limited by relatively small numbers enrolled on clinical trials. Nonetheless in data from the last U.S. pediatric intergroup trial, data from the United Kingdom's GC2 trial, and from the French TGM85 and TGM90 trials, an AFP of 10,000 IU/L or higher portends a worse prognosis for EFS.[418,438-441] In multivariate analysis of the U.K. data, AFP higher than 10,000 IU/L was a stronger predictor of relapse than site or stage; those with AFP greater than 10,000 IU/L had four times the risk of relapse. In two pediatric studies, AFP was not found to be prognostic, but both analyses were restricted only to patients with extragonadal primaries.[420,442] β-HCG and LDH was evaluated in the U.S. data and not shown to be of prognostic significance when using the cutpoints developed for adult men in the IGCCC data set.[418,438] Extragonadal tumor site was of prognostic significance in the United States, British, and French studies, although it was defined slightly differently in each study. Common to each study was the inclusion of mediastinal site, which is clearly associated with reduced EFS in all studies. Relative impact of other sites of extragonadal disease will require examination in a larger data set. The impact of satisfactory vs. unsatisfactory tumor marker decline has not been evaluated in pediatric patients with GCTs.

TREATMENT

Overview

Survival has improved markedly since the landmark publication by Einhorn in 1979 noting that widely metastatic testicular GCTs were curable with cisplatin-based regimens.[443] In 1981 Einhorn declared that "testicular cancer is the model of a curable neoplasm."[444] As it becomes more and more established, at least from long-term studies of adult men who have been successfully treated for testicular GCTs, that treatment is associated with significant long-term morbidities and even increased chance of mortality, oncologists need to concede that initial cure is not necessarily synonymous with normal life expectancy. Although highly curable, less toxic therapies need to be determined. Many patients require no treatment besides complete surgical resection; chemotherapy can be reserved to salvage only those patients who have recurrence. On the other end of the spectrum it is also apparent that for a subset of approximately 15% to 20% of patients, the standard cisplatin-based regimens are insufficient and more intensive chemotherapeutic strategies must be devised. A key part of future treatment strategies will be the ability to identify those patients at high risk of relapse at the time of their initial treatment and to design chemotherapeutic regimens that increase the odds of long-term survival both by optimal first-line therapies and salvage therapies for those who fail to respond.

Explanation of the Nomenclature

GCTs are generally divided into several categories when treatment is being discussed. The categories include: 1) teratoma, 2) immature teratoma, 3) seminoma/dysgerminoma, and 4) "other malignant" GCTs that include the histologies of YST (or endodermal sinus), embryonal carcinoma, and choriocarcinoma. GCTs can either present as a single histology, such as pure YST, or with a mixture of different histologies including histologies from all four categories (teratoma, immature teratoma, seminoma/dysgerminoma, and "other malignant"). The terminology is somewhat confusing in that a "malignant" GCT is shorthand for a GCT that contains at least one of the other malignant components, which means yolk sac, embryonal carcinoma, or choriocarcinoma. These histologies do have a more aggressive nature; however, both immature teratoma and seminoma/dysgerminoma are also malignant forms of GCTs. The general proviso is that the one must treat the most malignant form of the GCT. However, it is important to keep in mind what other histologies are present. For instance, if there is a significant portion of the original tumor that is mature or immature teratoma at diagnosis, this part of the tumor is not likely to respond to chemotherapy and it will likely be necessary to surgically excise the remaining teratoma at the end of the chemotherapeutic regimen.

Infantile Choriocarcinoma: A Rare but Rapidly Fatal Condition if Not Recognized

Infantile choriocarcinoma is an extremely rare entity that is a medical emergency and requires immediate institu-

tion of therapy. The disease is believed to be transplacentally acquired from a focus of choriocarcinoma that has arisen in the placenta as a variant of gestational trophoblastic disease. Choriocarcinoma is composed of cytotrophoblast, syncytiotrophoblast, and extravillous trophoblast, often mixed in random fashion surrounding areas of hemorrhage and necrosis.[69] Vascular invasion is a common feature of choriocarcinomas.

The median age at presentation was 1 month of age (range 0 days to 5 months).[11] Typical symptoms at diagnosis include severe anemia, failure to thrive, hepatomegaly, and seizures. Less commonly, infants can also have with hemoptysis and respiratory distress or signs of precocious puberty.[445,446] Marked elevations of β-HCG are typical (often $>1 \times 10^6$ IU/L).[12]

The disease is rapidly fatal if the syndrome is not recognized. Among 30 cases reviewed by Blohm and Gobel, two cases were diagnosed in stillborn children; in 19 cases, the diagnosis was made after death at postmortem examination.[445] Among those children who succumbed to the disease, the median time from initial symptoms to death was 21 days. Because of the rapid progression of this disease, treatment should not be delayed for histologic confirmation in an infant who shows a markedly elevated β-HCG and a clinical presentation consistent with infantile choriocarcinoma.

Single agent chemotherapy with methotrexate, which is usually sufficient as a single agent to treat gestational trophoblastic disease in the mother has never been curative in an infant with choriocarcinoma; multiagent chemotherapy is required.[447,448] In Blohm's series of 30 children, the five cases successfully treated received multiagent chemotherapy that included a platinum compound, either cisplatin or carboplatin, used in combination with etoposide. However, because of the rapid growth of these tumors, in several cases the platinum-etoposide combination was coupled with methotrexate administered either the week before or after the platinum regimen. Surgical resection of residual masses has been carried out in most patients at the end of the platinum-based therapy. Upfront surgical resection of tumor is definitely not advised in these patients because of the friability of the tumors, the chance of uncontrolled bleeding, and the delay that would be incurred in starting chemotherapy, as well as the usual fragile state of the infant at diagnosis.

If an infantile choriocarcinoma is diagnosed, the mother should also be screened for the disease. In the review by Blohm and Gobel, 60% of the mothers also had metastatic choriocarcinoma (17/30).[445] Since β-HCG is uniformly elevated in this disease, serial screening of the maternal β-HCG should be sufficient, although some physicians have advocated for radiologic examination of likely metastatic sites (lung, liver, brain) as well.

Seminoma and Dysgerminoma

The nomenclature of this subtype of pediatric GCT can be confusing. It is important to recognize that a tumor with the same histologic appearance has a different name depending on the site in which it arose. *Germinoma* typically refers to an intracranial lesion, usually in the pineal gland. *Dysgerminoma* describes a lesion in the ovary. *Seminoma* describes a lesion that arises in the testis.

Seminomas and dysgerminomas are much more common histologies in young and middle-aged adults than in adolescents. Diagnosis of a seminoma/dysgerminoma is exceedingly rare before the onset of puberty. However, in men overall seminomas account for approximately 50% of all testicular cancers, occurring most commonly in the fourth decade (Fig. 63-15).[261]

Because these tumors are exquisitely sensitive to radiotherapy, radiation was an important component of the treatment regimen. In patients with ovarian tumors, radiation resulted in sterilization of the remaining ovary; therefore since the 1980's chemotherapy with cisplatin-based therapy has replaced radiotherapy in the treatment of ovarian GCT. With longer follow-up observation of patients treated with radiotherapy, it became clear that there was reason for serious concerns about induction of secondary malignancies and cardiovascular disease in patients who received radiation therapy. In large prospective study, risk of cardiac events was 2.4 (95% CI, 1.04 to 5.5).[449] Risk of second malignant neoplasm is 2 (95% CI, 1.9 to 2.2).[450] An accepted standard now for stage I disease is surveillance with expected 15% to 20% relapse rate. With seminomas, relapses can occur quite late; 5% occur after 5 years, and there are anecdotal reports of relapses occurring after 10 years. Most pediatric radiotherapists would prefer not to use radiotherapy to treat a seminoma or dysgerminoma because of the risk of late effects; chemotherapy has replaced radiation as first-line therapy.

Treatment of these histologies has never been explicitly studied in pediatric clinical trials given their rarity, and hence treatment recommendations derive directly from the adult experience. The pediatric oncologist who is referred a patient with one of these diagnoses should consult with an adult oncologist and refer to an organization like National Cancer Care Network (NCCN) that maintains updated clinical practice guidelines for these tumors (http://www.nccn.org/).

TREATMENT OF STAGE I MALIGNANT NONSEMINOMATOUS GERM CELL TUMORS

Because much of the understanding about treatment options for pediatric stage I tumors derives from the adult experience, this work is reviewed in the following section.

Active Surveillance of Adult Men with Stage I Malignant Nonseminomatous Germ Cell Tumor Disease

The watch-and-wait strategy of active observation is based on a plethora of data from adult trials of men with stage I malignant GCT. Over 2000 adult patients have been enrolled on clinical trials of surveillance with a median follow-up range of at least 10 years.[451] Relapse rates range from 27% to 35%; 95% of relapses occur in the first 2 years after orchiectomy; almost all patients who relapse have "good risk" disease as defined by the IGCCC criteria; overall survival with chemotherapy is 98% to 99%.

An increasing concern is that patients who undergo surveillance are obligated to serial CT scans at regular intervals, which expose the patients to a dose of radiation that may subsequently be the cause of secondary malignancy. COG recommends scans every 3 months for the first year and every 6 months for the second year after diagnosis. However, a whole-trunk CT scan (chest/abdomen/pelvis) produces a radiation dose of 10 to 30 mSv.[452] It is recommended that exposure be limited to 100 mSv over 5 years.[453] Although it has been suggested that risk related to low doses of radiation may have been overestimated, a recent retrospective cohort study using data from 15 countries estimated that a cumulative exposure of 100 mSV would lead to a 9.7% increase in risk of all mortality from cancer, excluding leukemia, and a 19% increase in mortality because of leukemia.[454] Rustin et al. postulated that five total-body CT scans could therefore induce one second cancer in every 200 patients, which is the risk of death after stage I testicular cancer.[455] Therefore Rustin and colleagues designed a trial in adult men with stage I testicular cancer comparing a surveillance policy of two CT scans over the first year (at 3 and 12 months) with the standard surveillance policy of five CT scans over the first 2 years (3, 6, 9, 12, and 24 months).[455] Patients continued to have frequent clinical evaluations that included measurement of tumor markers and chest radiography (CXR; once per month in the first year, every 2 months in the second year, and every 3 months in the third year). There was no difference in overall relapse rate between the two surveillance groups, no increase in more advanced stage at relapse between the two groups, and no difference in overall survival. A major limitation of the study was that only 10% of the patients were at high risk for relapse on the basis of the presence of lymphovascular invasion (LVI), so it is not clear whether this schedule is vigilant enough for this group of patients. Given the increased radiosensitivity of children to the low-dose of ionizing radiation associated with CT scans, the schedule of surveillance in children with stage I GCTs deserves serious scrutiny.

Factors that Predict Relapse in Adult Stage I Nonseminomatous Germ Cell Tumor Patients on Surveillance Studies. Multiple studies have confirmed that the single most important prognostic factor is LVI, bifurcating risk into low risk (15% to 20%) and high risk (40% to 50%) for relapse. Although embryonal carcinoma is a significant prognostic variable in univariate analyses, its importance in multivariate models is subsumed by presence of LVI. No immunohistochemical markers, including MIB-1, p53, bcl-2, cathepsin D, or E-cadherin have added to the prognostic significance of LVI alone.[456-460]

Retroperitoneal Lymph Node Resection in Adult Men with Stage I Nonseminomatous Germ Cell Tumor

There is no doubt that surgical removal of retroperitoneal lymph nodes is known to comprise the "landing zones" for metastatic disease from the testes is the most accurate way to determine the stage of patient's cancer and is potentially therapeutic as well. Relapse in the surgical field is less than 1% after RPLND. The consensus of a

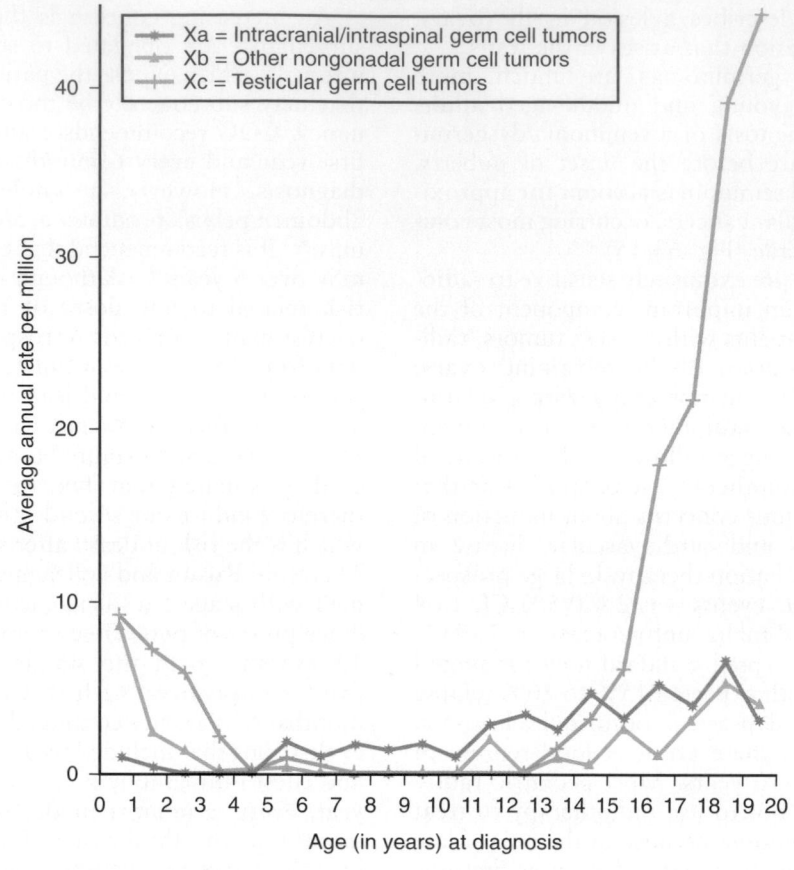

A

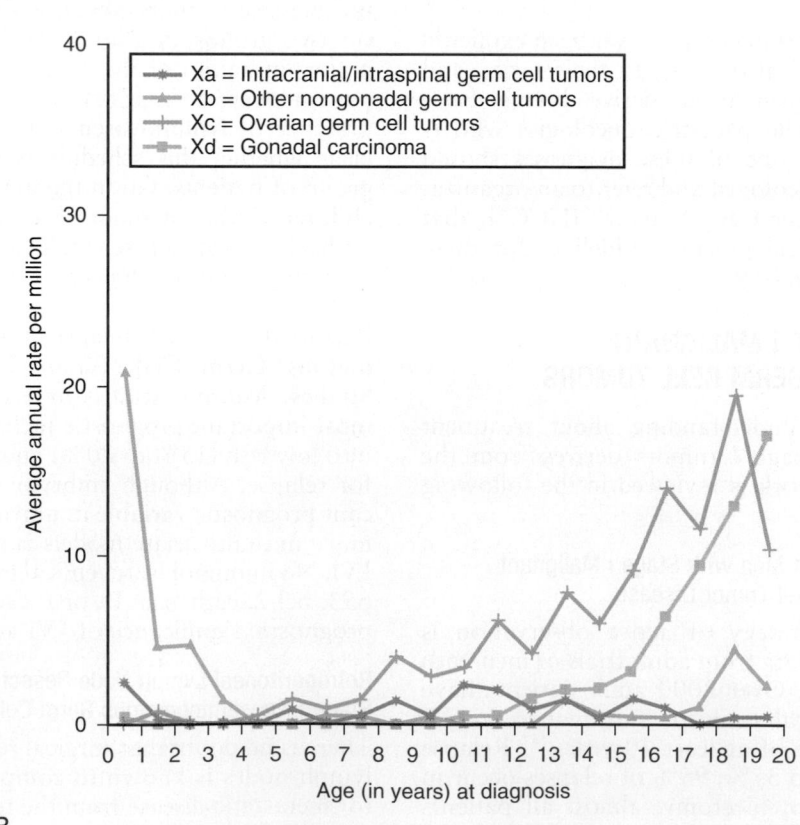

B

Figure 63-15 Incidence of germ cell tumors in the SEER program from 1973 to 1978 and 1994 to 1998. **A,** Males. **B,** Females. *(From McGlynn KA, Devesa SS, Sigurdson AJ, et al: Trends in the incidence of testicular GCTs in the United States. Cancer 97:63–70, 2003.)*

series of clinical trials has shown that between 30% and 50% of adult males with testicular stage I nonseminoma have occult metastases at RPLND that were not detected by radiologic scans. Surveillance for patients without an elevation of one of the tumor markers at diagnosis relies heavily on radiologic scans, and some patients prefer the certainty of RPLND in this particular situation.

A serious concern for any patient undergoing RPLND is nerve injury that interferes with the ability to ejaculate, causing retrograde ejaculation, or ejaculatory failure. Because of refinements in surgical technique and the development of so-called "nerve-sparing" approaches, it is estimated that preservation of ejaculatory function is as high as 90% to 95%, especially if the surgery is performed by an urologist who performs a high volume of these procedures per year (i.e., 10 to 20). The surgery can be the cause of uncommon but nonnegligible complications such as bowel complications, lymphocele, and chylous ascites. Referral of the adolescent male who chooses RPLND as primary therapy to a cancer center with a urologist who specializes in RPLND is warranted.

However, RPLND does not mean that chemotherapy will be avoided. Ten percent of patients with pathological stage 1 cancer experience relapse after RPLND (primarily in the lungs) and approximately one third of patients with stage II disease (or 10% to 15% of patients who undergo RPLND) have evidence of sufficiently extensive disease (multiple nodes, any node >2 cm, or any evidence of extranodal spread) that chemotherapy will be initiated immediately after RPLND. Usually at least 2 cycles of BEP is required. One argument in favor of primary (upfront) RPLND is that it may reduce the odds of having to perform RPLND after chemotherapy if there is residual disease. After chemotherapy, the operation is much more technically challenging because of the desmoplastic reaction to chemotherapy. Another advantage of primary RPLND is that it removes any concurrent teratoma, which is a chemoresistant form of GCT. Because a small percentage of teratomas can undergo malignant degeneration to non–germ cell malignancies that are much more difficult to treat, it is beneficial to resect these components of GCT early in course of treatment.

Adjuvant Chemotherapy for Stage I Testicular Nonseminomatous Germ Cell Tumors

Another option employed in men with clinical stage I nonseminomatous germ cell tumors (NSGCT) is adjuvant chemotherapy with one or two cycles of BEP. Although 11 studies have shown that the risk of relapse can be reduced to less than 2%, the concern remains that the majority of patients, conservatively at least 50%, have no further need for chemotherapy after the orchiectomy, and therefore treatment with BEP is overtreatment for a large percentage. Moreover, accumulating evidence of significant long-term side effects associated with three or four cycles of cisplatin-based therapy, including a marked increase in cardiovascular disease and risk of second malignancy (see "Late Effects") should invoke caution about the administration of even two cycles of the same therapy, because the relation between dose and late effect has not been quantified.

Active Observation of Pediatric Germ Cell Tumor Patients with Stage I Disease

On the U.S. Pediatric Intergroup Study (POG09048/CCG8891), boys younger than 11 years of age with stage I testicular malignant GCTs were observed after surgery (watch-and-wait strategy) and only given chemotherapy if tumor markers did not normalize as expected or if imaging revealed recurrent disease. Among the 63 patients enrolled on the protocol, 11 patients had progression of disease and received chemotherapy (four cycles of standard-dose PEB; see the following section on treatment); 80% of the recurrences occurred in the first year after surgery. The 6-year EFS of active observation was 78.5% ± 7%; however, all patients were salvaged with subsequent chemotherapy (6-year OS 100%).[431]

On the subsequent COG GCT study (AGCT0132), an initial strategy of surveillance after surgical resection was extended to girls with pediatric stage I malignant ovarian GCT (MOGCT) to determine whether overall survival could be preserved.[461] Between November 2003 and July 2011, 25 girls, ages 0 to 16 years (median age 12 years old) with stage I MOGCT were enrolled into the trial. Twenty-three patients had elevated AFP at diagnosis. Predominant histology was YST. Twelve patients had evidence of persistent or recurrent disease (EFS 52%; 95% CI, 31% to 69%). Median time to recurrence was 2 months. All patients had elevated AFP at recurrence; six had localized disease, two had metastatic disease, and four had tumor marker elevation only. Eleven of 12 patients with relapse were salvaged with chemotherapy (OS 96%; 95% CI, 74% to 99%) consisting of three cycles of "compressed PEB" (cisplatin 33 mg/m^2 and etoposide 167 mg/m^2 on days 1 through 3, bleomycin 15 U/m^2 on day 1; cycles repeated every 21 days). This trial demonstrated that 50% of stage I pediatric MOGCT can be spared with chemotherapy; a larger study is needed to ascertain whether prognostic factors exist for relapse of ovarian GCT, similar to LVI in adult male testicular cancer, and whether this strategy can be extended to older adolescents and young adults.

In the U.K. Germ Cell Tumor Study II that was conducted between 1989 and 1997, all gonadal (both testicular and ovarian) stage I tumors were observed without chemotherapy. Forty of 51 TGCT patients (78%) and 6 of 9 (66%) patients with ovarian stage I GCT were successfully treated with surgery alone. All patients who experienced recurrence after observation were cured with 4 to 6 cycles carboplatin, etoposide, bleomycin (JEB) chemotherapy. For details of JEB chemotherapy please see the section on treatment.

The Germans have used separate protocols for treating testicular tumors (MAHO protocols) and nontesticular, extracranial pediatric GCTs (MAKEI protocols). In the latest update of the MAHO protocols from 2002, the authors report on results from 1982 to 2001.[423] A watch-and-wait approach was taken for patients with stage I nonseminomatous testicular tumors, but only if the malignant histology was pure yolk sac, pure teratoma, pure immature teratoma, or pure seminoma. Boys with testicular tumors that included a malignant component other than yolk sac were treated with standard chemotherapy that consisted of platinum, vinblastine, and bleomycin (PVB). Of the 140 boys with stage I YST, 16 (13%) progressed and required standard chemotherapy 6 to 60 weeks after orchiectomy.[423] All but one of the 140 patients are alive and well. All boys with either mature teratoma (n = 40), immature teratoma (n = 19), or seminoma (n = 2) were cured with surgery alone.

On the MAKEI96 protocol, the observational strategy was extended to include stage I ovarian and extragonadal GCTs. Excluded from this surgery-only approach were extragonadal tumors that arose in the sacrococcygeal region. Children with primary sacrococcygeal tumors, regardless of stage, were treated with four cycles of cisplatin, etoposide, and ifosfamide (PEI), except for infants younger than 4 months of age, who were treated with four cycles of cisplatin and etoposide (PE; see "Treatment of Pediatric Germ Cell Tumors in Germany"). Results of this approach have not yet been published.

Chemotherapy for Pediatric Germ Cell Tumors (>Stage I)

Prechemotherapy Evaluation

Before initiating chemotherapy, studies should be done to establish a baseline for monitoring toxicity, and procedures should be undertaken to minimize risk of late effects. The postpubertal male patient should be encouraged to use a sperm bank, because a small percentage of male patients will be infertile after chemotherapy. Oocyte cryopreservation (egg freezing) should be considered in postpubertal females because of an ill-defined but apparently increased risk of infertility. In addition, patients who are to receive standard chemotherapy with PEB should have baseline measurements of their renal function by measuring the glomerular filtration rate (GFR), preferably with a chromium ethylenediaminetetraacetic acid (EDTA) clearance, pulmonary function tests (PFTs), including diffusing capacity of the lung for carbon monoxide (DLCO), and baseline audiometry that includes accurate measurements of the high-frequency region, because this is the region that is affected first by cisplatin-induced hearing loss.

History of Use of Chemotherapy Among Adult Men with Testicular Cancer

Treatment of pediatric GCTs derives in large part from knowledge gained in the treatment of adult men with testicular cancer. In 1979 Lawrence Einhorn, MD, reported in *Cancer Treatment Reports* that PVB (also referred to as the *Einhorn regimen*) cured a substantial portion of men with widely disseminated testicular cancer. A follow-up study showed that substitution of etoposide for vinblastine (PEB vs. PVB) was shown to be a superior regimen both in terms of increased efficacy in poor-risk patients and reduced neuromuscular toxicity,[462] and PEB became the standard of care. Finally, it was shown that three cycles of PEB was equivalent to four cycles of PEB among patients with good prognoses as defined by the IGCCC.[463] On this backbone of experience in the treatment of adult testicular cancer, the pediatric trials reviewed in the next section were developed.

Treatment of Pediatric Germ Cell Tumors in the United States

Before the use of chemotherapy, the outcome of children with GCTs was dismal; 3-year survival rates did not reach 20%.[212,464] In the mid 1970s, the first reports of effective chemotherapy regimens for pediatric GCTs were published.[465,466] These regimens were based on vincristine, dactinomycin, and cyclophosphamide (VAC) but also included radiation therapy as well. Although the survival for patients of average risk improved to approximately 60%, children with advanced-stage disease continued to have a very poor prognosis. After the Einhorn regimen of PVB was published in the late 1970s, showing that a high rate of cure was possible for men with metastatic testicular cancer,[443] cisplatin-based regimens were quickly adopted in pediatrics with marked improvement in outcome, even for patients with advanced stage disease. Ablin et al. initiated a regimen in the CCG (CCG861) that combined PVB with the drugs that had previously been shown to have activity: cyclophosphamide, actinomycin, and adriamycin.[453] At 18 weeks, patients in partial remission (PR) received radiation therapy and maintenance chemotherapy until 2 years after diagnosis. This protocol enrolled 93 patients with pediatric germ cell tumors, excluding patients with TGCTs and including patients with ovarian (n = 30), sacrococcygeal (n = 37), and mediastinal tumors (n = 17). Ovarian tumors had a 4-year OS rate and EFS rates of 67% and 63%, whereas extragonadal tumors had lower rates of survival (EFS, 48%; OS, 42%). Even though this protocol did include cisplatin, it was given at a low dose (60 mg/m^2) and dose intensity (every 9 weeks) so that its effectiveness was likely compromised.

Subsequently, the CCG and the POG initiated an intergroup study from 1990 to 1995. The intergroup study divided patients into two risk groups: the low-/intermediate-risk group included stage I/II gonadal MGCT patients (treated on POG9048/CCG8891),[467] and the high-risk group included stage III/IV gonadal MGCT and stages I through IV extragonadal MGCT (treated on POG9049/CCG8892).[433]

On the POG9048/CCG8891 protocol for treatment of low-stage gonadal tumors, only boys younger than 11 years of age were enrolled. Older boys were to be treated according to adult standards. Boys with stage I disease were treated with active observation (see "Treatment of Stage I Malignant Nonseminomatous Germ Cell Tumors"); boys with stage II testicular MGCT (including relapses of initially stage I testicular MGCT) and girls with stage I/II ovarian MGCT younger than 21 years of age received four cycles of standard-dose pediatric BEP (bleomycin 15 U/m^2 on day 1, etoposide 100 mg/m^2/day on days 1 through 5, and cisplatin 20 mg/m^2/day on days 1 through 5). On both the low-/intermediate-risk and high-risk arms of the intergroup study, bleomycin was reduced from a weekly dose used on adult protocols to once per cycle, or every 3 weeks, in order to reduce the incidence of pulmonary fibrosis. Of note, both the British and German investigators have similarly reduced the dose of bleomycin without apparent adverse results. It is important to realize, however, that this reduction in dosage has never been studied in a randomized trial that compares weekly dose, as bleomycin is administered in the adult trials, versus the once-every-3-week regimen introduced by pediatric oncologists. Patients were reevaluated with tumor markers and radiologic scans after four cycles. If either imaging or tumor markers suggested residual disease, patients underwent surgical exploration, and if viable tumor was found pathologically and/or if tumor markers did not normalize, the patient was given an additional two cycles of PEB.[467]

Patients with pure dysgerminoma/seminoma were excluded from the U.S. Pediatric Intergroup Trials. The treatment of pure immature teratoma on the U.S. Pediatric Intergroup Trial is discussed in "Mature and Immature Teratoma."

On the low-/intermediate-risk arm of the study, overall 6-year EFS was 94.5%, and 6-year OS was 95.7%.[467] Six-year EFS and OS by primary site were as follows: testicular stage II (100% and 100%), ovarian stage I (95% and 95%), and ovarian stage II (87% and 94%). Two patients underwent second-look surgery; one patient had evidence of residual malignant disease. Although 23% of patients had grade 3 to 4 hematologic toxicity, no delay in therapy was reported. No patient had grade 3 to 4 ototoxicity, renal toxicity or pulmonary toxicity. Two patients with primary ovarian tumors developed acute myelogenous leukemia (AML) at 5 and 32 months from start of therapy, but neither patient had the topoisomerase-induced 11q23 cytogenetic abnormality.[467]

To follow this trial the COG protocol AGCT0132, was opened in 2002 for low-risk (gonadal stage I patients, both ovarian and testicular) and intermediate-risk (stage II through IV gonadal tumors and stage I/II extragonadal tumors) patients. The aims of this trial were to evaluate a watch-and-wait strategy for low-risk patients, reserving chemotherapy for those who fail observation after surgery (see prior summary of results of the low risk trial). For patients who were judged to be of intermediate risk, the protocol evaluated the efficacy of three courses of PEB (rather than four courses, which had been used on the previous protocol) and whether the drugs can be given in a compressed manner over 3 days rather than over 5 days. Enrollment was completed in June 2012; analyses are ongoing.

The high-risk protocol of the previous Pediatric Intergroup Trial (POG9049/CCG8892) was a randomized clinical trial comparing standard-dose PEB (total cisplatin dose 100 mg/m^2) with high-dose PEB (HDPEB; total cisplatin dose 200 mg/m^2).[433] The results of the prior intergroup high-risk clinical trial for stage III/IV gonadal tumors and stage I to IV extragonadal MGCT did not show a significant difference in 6-year OS between HDPEB and PEB (92% vs. 86%); however, there was evidence of an increase in 6-year EFS among patients receiving HDPEB (89.6% ± 3.6% vs. 80.5 ± 4.8%; %, $P = 0.03$).[433] Overall 6-year EFS and OS by site and stage are as follows: testicular stage III (94% and 100%), testicular stage IV (88% and 91%), ovarian stage III (97% and 98%), ovarian stage IV (87% and 93%), extragonadal stage I and II (89% and 93%), extragonadal stage III (75% and 80%), and extragonadal stage IV (78% and 81%). The study was not powered to be able to examine response by site and stage, but in each subgroup there was a trend towards higher EFS and OS for patients treated with HDPEB. This difference was most pronounced in patients with extragonadal MGCT, in which it achieved borderline statistical significance. Patients with stage III/IV extragonadal tumors treated with HDPEB had a 2-year EFS of 84% compared with 74% for patients treated with standard-dose PEB ($P = 0.09$).

Toxicity was much greater on the HDPEB arm of the study. Fatal infections accounted for 7 deaths on the study, and 6 deaths occurred on the HDPEB arm. Hearing aids were needed in 67% of the patients treated with HDPEB. Three patients who initially had been diagnosed with a mediastinal MGCT developed hematologic malignancies posttreatment. Two patients developed AML; neither had the characteristic 11q23 abnormality usually associated with etoposide-induced leukemias. One patient developed erythrophagocytic syndrome.

Given the trend observed for better survival among patients with high-stage extragonadal GCTs on the HDPEB arm, a follow-up pilot study was designed incorporating amifostine (825mg/m^2/day) with the goal of reducing the observed toxicities of the higher dose of cisplatin, particularly the ototoxicity.[468] Among the 20 patients enrolled, 17 were females, median age was 1.6 years, and the primary site was sacrococcygeal in 15 patients. Although the EFS and OS were acceptable (83% and 85%), amifostine at this dose and schedule did not protect against ototoxicity; 75% of patients had significant hearing loss.

A second pilot study for patients with high-risk advanced stage extragonadal tumors has been completed by COG. In this trial, standard-dose PEB was combined with escalating doses of cyclophosphamide.[469] The three dose levels of cyclophosphamide were 1.2 gm/m^2, 1.8 g/m^2, and 2.4 gm/m^2. Nineteen patients were enrolled; 3 patients were nonevaluable for the assessment of dose limiting toxicity (DLT). Sixteen patients completed four cycles of induction, 11 had complete response, one had progressive disease, and four had a partial response. All four with partial response had a residual mass and underwent second look surgery and then completed two additional cycles of their assigned regimen. Only one patient, enrolled on the dosage of 1.8 g/m^2, experienced DLT during the first cycle of therapy manifested as grade 3 hyperglycemia. No other patient experienced DLT. The 4-year EFS and OS (± standard deviation) were 74% ± 7% and 89% ± 10%, respectively.[469] This observed EFS is not apparently different than what was observed with standard dose PEB in the prior intergroup study.

Treatment of Pediatric Germ Cell Tumors in the United Kingdom

From 1977 through 1988, patients in the United Kingdom were treated on United Kingdom Children's Cancer Study Group (UKCCG) Germ Cell Tumor Studies 1 (GC1).[470] This protocol compared five regimens that were used sequentially over the time interval: low-dose VAC, high-dose VAC, high-dose doxorubicin plus VAC (Adria-VAC),

PVB, and PEB. GC1 enrolled 52 patients who received chemotherapy until complete response was documented and then two more cycles after achieving complete remission (CR; CR +2). Outcome varied significantly by regimen; PEB was clearly the most effective.

In 1989 based on preliminary data showing efficacy of carboplatin in pediatric MGCT, the UKCCG initiated their second GCT study (GC2) in which cisplatin was replaced by carboplatin.[471] JEB consists of etoposide 120 mg/m^2/day for days 1 through 3 (total dose 360 mg/m^2); carboplatin on day 2 in at an area under the curve (AUC) of 7.9 (AUC formula: [6 × *uncorrected GFR*] + [15 × *surface area*]), equivalent to approximately 600 mg/m^2; and bleomycin 15 mg/ m^2 on day 3. Clinicians were urged to use the AUC formula to calculate the carboplatin dose rather than use a dose based on surface area, but 75% of the patients enrolled on the study were dosed according to the square-meter dose. It is important to note that this is a higher dose and dose-intensity of carboplatin than used in the French study of carboplatin in pediatric GCTs (TGM90), in which the results with carboplatin were inferior to those in a previous trial that had utilized cisplatin (TGM8589).[472,473] As was the practice with GC1, patients in GC2 received chemotherapy until a complete response was documented and then two further cycles.

The U.K. investigators have published an interim analysis of the patients treated between 1989 and 1997.[471] During this time, 184 patients younger than 16 years of age with either localized or metastatic extracranial GCTs were enrolled in GC2 and eligible for analysis. In total, JEB chemotherapy was administered to 137 patients. GC2 remained open to recruitment after analysis in 1997, and an additional 84 patients received JEB in this period, resulting in a total of 221 patients who eventually received chemotherapy. Patients with gonadal stage I tumors were observed without chemotherapy (watch-and-wait strategy). Forty of 51 patients with TGCTs (78%) and six of nine (66%) patients with ovarian stage I GCTs were successfully treated with surgery alone. All patients who experienced recurrence after observation were cured with JEB chemotherapy. The overall survival for all 137 JEB-treated patients at 5 years was 90.9% (95% CI, 83.8% to 95%) and EFS at 5 years was 87.8% (95% CI, 81.1% to 92.4%). Outcome by site, stage, histologic classification, and initial presurgical AFP level are summarized in Figure 63-6.[75] EFS according to site was 100% for testis, 90.7% for ovary, 86.5% for sacrococcygeal, and 75% for mediastinal. EFS according to stage was 100% for stage I, 93.8% for stage II, 84.8% for stage III, and 78% for stage IV. Toxicity was minimal with JEB. In the GC2 study, only one child had severe deafness (likely attributable to a middle-ear hemorrhage when the child had thrombocytopenia), and none had severe renal toxicity. However, carboplatin is more myelotoxic than cisplatin; 36% of the total number of courses were delayed more than 28 days. Second-look surgery was undertaken in 45 patients (33%) in GC2. Necrotic or fibrotic tissue was found in 24 patients (53%), mature or immature teratoma was found in 19 patients (42%), and only 2 patients were found to have viable tumor.

The United Kingdom Children's Cancer and Leukemia Group (UKCCLG) protocol (GC3) opened in May 2005. This protocol continues to use JEB chemotherapy as first line treatment. Patients with low-risk disease (stage 1 gonadal tumors) are treated surgically with close surveillance. Other patients receive four or six courses of JEB according to risk group stratification determined by site, stage, age, and AFP level. The study has closed; analyses are ongoing but not yet reported.

The results are similar to those reported by the U.S. POG/CCG Intergroup Study[433] and raise the question of whether it is necessary to continue treatment with cisplatin in pediatric patients, given the higher toxicity profile of cisplatin. The concern is that carboplatin has been shown to be inferior to cisplatin in five randomized clinical trials in adults with metastatic "good risk" testicular cancer.[474,475] However, the maximum dose used in the adult trials was 500 mg/m^2, and in two of the trials, the carboplatin was given every 28 days in a less dose-intense fashion.[476] Likewise in pediatric GCTs, the French showed that carboplatin was inferior to previous results of treating with cisplatin (TGM90 vs. TGM85); however both the dose (400 mg/m^2) and dose-intensity (once every 6 weeks) were low on the French trial.[472,473] Consideration of carboplatin as first-line therapy for low and intermediate risk pediatric germ cell patients is warranted.

Treatment of Pediatric Germ Cell Tumors in Germany

The German Society of Pediatric Oncology has used separate protocols for treating testicular tumors (MAHO protocols) and nontesticular, extracranial pediatric GCTs (MAKEI protocols). In the latest update of the MAHO protocols published in 2002, the authors report on results from 1982 through 2001.[477] A watch-and-wait approach was taken for patients with stage I testicular YSTs. All patients with stage I tumors who had a malignant component other than yolk sac, as well as patients with higher than stage I testicular tumors, were treated with "standard chemotherapy" that consisted of PVB (vinblastine 3.0 gm/m^2 on days 1 and 2, bleomycin 15 U/m^2 on days 1 through 3 as continuous infusion, and cisplatin 20 mg/m^2/day on days 4 through 8). Four cycles were given every 28 days. If there was not a complete response after 2 cycles, however, patients underwent exploratory laparotomy, and if viable disease was discovered, patients received four cycles of salvage therapy that consisted of PEI (etoposide 80mg/m^2/day on days 1 through 3, ifosfamide 1500 mg/m^2/day on days 1 through 4, and cisplatin 20 mg/m^2/day on days 2 through 5). If there was no evidence of disease at laparotomy, the patient received two more cycles of the standard PVB for a total of four courses. In toto, 59 patients received chemotherapy with an overall survival rate of 95%. Survival among patients with stage I and II disease was excellent; 41 of 42 patients survived. Among patients with stage III testicular cancer, 5 of 17 patients died despite the use of salvage chemotherapy.

The German MAKEI protocols (MAKEI83/86, MAKEI89, MAKEI96) specifically include only patients with either an ovarian or extragonadal primary tumor and exclude patients with a testicular primary tumor (treated on MAHO). In MAKEI83/86, patients were stratified into either low risk or high risk categories. The low-risk classification included only stage I ovarian tumors; these patients received four cycles of PVB. Patients in the high-risk group had stage II through IV ovarian and stage I through IIb extragonadal primary tumors. These patients received four cycles of PVB followed by four cycles of PEI. Because of concerns about the pulmonary toxicity associated with bleomycin and the neurotoxicity associated with vinblastine in the original Einhorn regimen, a modified Einhorn regimen was developed. Bleomycin was given before cisplatin, because cisplatin had been shown to reduce the clearance of bleomycin, as a continuous infusion over 3 days at 15 mg/m^2/day or 45 mg/m^2 per cycle. Cumulative dose of bleomycin was limited to 180 mg/m^2. This is substantially higher than the total dose of bleomycin patients receive on either U.S. or U.K. protocol, in which the per-cycle dose of bleomycin is only 15 units/m^2, and most patients receive between three and six cycles (or total cumulative dose of 45 to 90 U/m^2. The German dose of bleomycin is more analogous to the cumulative doses of bleomycin one would find on an adult protocol for treating GCTs, in which 30 units of bleomycin is administered weekly for 9 weeks for total cumulative dose on average of 270 units or 135 U/m^2 in a average adult with a body surface area (BSA) of 2 m^2. Vinblastine was administered at 50% the dose of the original Einhorn regimen to reduce the associated neurotoxicity.

In MAKEI89, changes were made to risk stratification, and the overall amount of chemotherapy administered was reduced. Risk level was stratified into three groups. The low-risk category remained stage I ovarian tumor; medium risk included ovarian stages II and III and extragonadal stage I and IIa tumors, and the high-risk group was comprised of extragonadal stage IIb, coccygeal stage I and IIb, and ovarian stage IV tumors. Therapy was reduced for these low- and intermediate-risk groups by 25% compared to MAKEI83/86. Patients in the low-risk group received three cycles of PEB, and patients at medium risk received three cycles of PEB followed by 3 cycles of PIV.

Outcome of the earlier MAKEI trials are as follows: on MAKEI83/86, the low-risk group achieved 94% EFS, whereas the high-risk group achieved 76% EFS. In MAKEI89, EFS on the low-risk arm was 91%, medium risk was 86%, and high risk was 83%. In terms of site, sacrococcygeal tumors had the lowest EFS without much significant change over time (74%, 80%, and 77% in MAKEI83, 86, and 89, respectively), whereas ovarian tumors had the best outcome with significant improvement over time (EFS 77%, 92%, and 90% on MAKEI83, 86, and 89, respectively).

In MAKEI96, several changes have been made to the risk stratification and recommended therapies. Chemotherapy is determined by site, stage, and degree of resection. Bleomycin was removed from all chemotherapy protocols. All patients with ovarian and extragonadal stage I tumors (except patients with stage I sacrococcygeal tumors) are initially treated with a watch-and-wait strategy. Children with sacrococcygeal primary tumors,

regardless of stage, are treated with four cycles of PEI (cisplatin 20 mg/m^2/day on days 1 though 5, etoposide 100 mg/m^2/day on days 1 through 3), and ifosfamide 1500 mg/m^2/day on days 1 through 5 as a continuous infusion). Infants younger than 4 months of age with sacrococcygeal primary tumors are treated with four cycles of PE, omitting the ifosfamide. Patients with primary ovarian tumors receive two cycles of either PE (completely resected) or PEI (incompletely resected), and patients with extragonadal primaries receive three cycles of either PE (completely resected) or PEI (incompletely resected). Patients with advanced stage ovarian and extragonadal primary tumors with poor prognosis are treated with four cycles of PEI. If the tumor was not completely excised at the onset of therapy, three cycles of PEI are given and then the patient undergoes resection. Postoperatively, an additional one to four cycles of PEI are administered depending on whether the tumor was completely or incompletely resected. In all MAKEI protocols diagnosis is based on imaging, tumor markers, and histology. In advanced/bulky disease, diagnosis could be based on markers and imaging, and a preoperative chemotherapy could be applied for downstaging.

The Dose of Bleomycin in Treatment of Pediatric Germ Cell Tumors

In adults, investigators have shown that bleomycin can be safely omitted in patients at "good risk" if the patient receives an additional (fourth) cycle of etoposide and cisplatin.[478] Concern about the possibility of bleomycin-induced pulmonary fibrosis has caused pediatric oncologists to evaluate the same issue. The British and American collaborative groups have reduced the dose of bleomycin from once a week to once per cycle (or once every 3 weeks).[433,471] This dose of bleomycin represents a 67% reduction in the total dose of bleomycin when compared to adult regimens. Since the institution of these changes (1989 in Britain and 1990 in the United States), there have been no reported cases of fatal pulmonary fibrosis in over 137 British cases of patients treated with JEB and 373 cases in the United States of patients treated with PEB. On MAKEI89, after two deaths occurred in children younger than age 2 years from pulmonary fibrosis, German investigators no longer treated children under 1 year of age with bleomycin (using instead etoposide and cisplatin [EP]), and children ages 1 to 2 years received half of the standard dose of bleomycin. However, the dose of bleomycin for older children on MAKEI83/86 and 89 was quite significant: 15 mg/m^2/day for 3 days with each cycle (total 45 mg/m^2/cycle). In MAKEI96, bleomycin was omitted entirely from the chemotherapeutic regimens for all patients. No decrement in survival has been observed since its deletion.

Other countries besides Germany have decided to delete bleomycin from use in pediatric patients. A Brazilian study has reported preliminary results using four cycles of EP with 5-year survival rates of 83% in patients at high risk.[479] The Italians also did not use bleomycin in the Italian cooperative study (TCG91), but their regimen, which alternated carboplatin and etoposide with vincristine, dactinomycin, and ifosfamide, produced suboptimal results, particularly in patients with higher stages of disease, compared with other pediatric germ cell trials.[480]

Mature and Immature Teratomas

Complete surgical excision is adequate therapy for pure mature teratomas. Mature teratomas are much more common than immature teratomas. It is estimated that mature teratomas of the ovary, also called *cystic teratoma* or *dermoid cyst,* account for 95% to 99% of all ovarian teratomas. Mature teratomas that contain an element of a malignant GCT (yolk sac, endodermal-sinus, choriocarcinoma, embryonal carcinoma) should be treated according to the guidelines for the treatment of malignant nonseminomatous GCTs discussed previously.

Immature teratomas are made up elements from the three germ layers and graded from 0 to 3 depending on the amount of immature neuroepithelium present in the tumor.[119] Grade has been shown to correlate with both stage and prognosis. Treatment for immature teratoma is more controversial and evolving.

A classic study by Norris et al reviewed 58 adult women with ovarian immature teratomas who had been treated with surgical resection alone and reported that 70% of women who had grade 3 tumors at diagnosis subsequently relapsed.[119] The recommendation was thus made that stage I grade 3 ovarian immature teratomas ought to be treated with chemotherapy.

Concern that the biology and behavior of immature teratoma might be different in childhood than adulthood led the U.S. pediatric oncology groups to investigate whether surgical resection was sufficient for immature teratoma, even among patients who had grade 3 tumors. Between 1990 and 1995, as part of the U.S. Intergroup Pediatric Study (POG9048/CCG8891), 73 patients with immature teratoma who had undergone a gross total resection were enrolled in the study.[168] Central review of grade showed 31.5% were grade 1; 38.4% were grade 2, and 30.1% were grade 3. Primary site of disease included ovarian (n = 44), testicular (n = 7), sacrococcygeal (n = 5), retroperitoneal (n = 7), and head/neck (n = 7). All pathology was centrally reviewed; 50 patients were confirmed to have pure immature teratoma, whereas 21 had microscopic foci of YST and two had microscopic foci of PNET. Because significant time had elapsed between the initial surgery and the central review of the pathology (typically at least 6 months), it was decided to continue to observe patients discovered to have a malignant focus at central pathology review. Tumor markers were elevated in 25 patients at diagnosis (AFP alone, 18; β-HCG alone, 5; both, 2). Overall, only one half of the patients with microscopic foci of YST had an elevated AFP at diagnosis (9 out of 20 patients). However, in ovarian tumors there is a tight correlation between an elevated AFP and presence of YST; 70% of patients shown to have microscopic foci of YST had an elevated AFP at diagnosis, whereas only 25% of patients with pure immature teratoma had an elevated AFP at diagnosis.[130] Elevation of AFP at diagnosis was also strongly correlated with stage and grade of the immature teratoma.[130]

With a median follow-up of 35 months, the overall 3-year EFS was 93%, with 3-year EFS of 97.8%, 100%, and 80% for ovarian, testicular, and extragonadal tumors respectively.[168] Five patients relapsed, all within 7 months of the original diagnosis; one had an ovarian primary tumor and 4 had extragonadal primary tumors. In retrospect at central pathology review, three of the five patients had YST present at diagnosis; one patient had PNET. The patient with PNET who had recurrence was resistant to platinum-based therapy. All of the other patients were successfully treated with PEB.

How to treat pure immature teratoma higher than stage I lacks clinical consensus and published data. There is generally a belief in the pediatric oncology community that the diagnosis of immature teratoma has different meaning and clinical significance in the newborn vs. the peripubertal period. In the newborn period, patients with incompletely resected immature teratomas are usually closely observed, reserving treatment (usually reoperation) for those who have recurrence. Immature teratoma in the peripubertal stage (older child and adult) is generally considered to be a malignant disease that warrants treatment with chemotherapy. Treatment with 3 to 4 cycles of standard-dose PEB is generally recommended for patients with higher than stage I pure immature teratoma in the United States, whereas in the United Kingdom all patients with immature teratoma, regardless of stage, site, and age are observed after surgical resection, even in the face of residual disease.[481]

In Germany, the German Society for Pediatric Oncology and Hematology (GPOH) has prospectively studied all extracranial testicular and nontesticular mature and immature teratomas since 1982 on successive MAHO and MAKEI protocols.[482] All pathology is centrally reviewed at a single institution, and grade of immaturity is classified according to Gonzalez-Crussi.[165] AFP and β-HCG are measured on all patients and by definition have to be within normal limits for age in order to establish the diagnosis of teratoma. Treatment of immature teratoma has varied over time. On MAKEI83/86, patients with incompletely resected immature teratoma grade 2 or 3 were treated with three cycles of VAC chemotherapy. On MAKEI89, chemotherapy (three cycles of PEB) was given to patients with incompletely resected immature teratomas of grade 3.

Overall, the completeness of the original tumor resection was the chief predictor of relapse. EFS after complete resection was 96%, whereas EFS was only 55% among those with incomplete resection at diagnosis. The Germans use a very strict definition of a complete resection. Complete resection of a coccygeal tumor was defined as resection of the tumor with its pseudocapsule and the coccygeal bone in one piece. Relapses occurred in 20% of patients with sacrococcygeal tumors, compared with 7% among patients with tumors at other extragonadal sites and only 2% of patients with ovarian primaries. Relapse rate was similar among patients treated with surgery alone vs. patients treated with chemotherapy on the basis of higher grade of immaturity. However, no malignant components were found at the time of relapse among the seven patients who relapsed after initial chemotherapy, whereas 15 of 29 patients who relapsed after surgery only as first treatment had a malignant component detectable in their recurrence.

Immature teratomas were more likely to relapse than mature teratomas; higher grade of immature teratoma was more likely to relapse than lower grade (grade 0 [mature], 10%; grade 1, 14%; grade 2, 21%; grade 3, 31%.).

On MAKEI96, patients with incompletely resected immature teratomas of grade 2 or 3 were stratified to either a watch-and-wait approach or to two courses of adjuvant chemotherapy. The therapy was switched from PEB to PEI, substituting ifosfamide 1500 mg/m²/day on days 1 through 5 for the bleomycin. However, because of low accrual, the randomization was stopped in the year 2000, and patients have been treated according to physician preference. 261 evaluable patients were enrolled.[482] Because the criteria for complete vs. incomplete resection were more highly scrutinized, the percentage of incompletely resected tumors rose from 10% to 34% on MAKEI96. However, this change was not associated with a reduced relapse rate in the patients whose tumors were completely resected (4.2%). However, the overall relapse rate decreased from 13.3% to 9.5% over that time. The authors are not certain whether this reflects better surgical procedures or a change in the distribution of the primary site of the tumor. The rates are similar to those reported in other studies.[425] It is easier to achieve a complete resection for a gonadal teratoma. Extragonadal teratomas are often adjacent to or infiltrating vital structures such as the sacral plexus in the case of the SCT or large vessels. Probability of relapse on MAKEI96 was not linked to the histologic grade of immaturity, as it had been on MAKEI 83/86/89. One-half of the relapses on MAKEI83/86/89 had a malignant component, whereas two thirds of the relapses on MAKEI96 had a malignant component, illustrating the malignant potential of the teratoma.

Growing Teratoma Syndrome

Growing teratoma syndrome describes the situation in which tumors are noted to enlarge either during chemotherapy or after chemotherapy in a patient with normalized tumor markers. Often mistaken as progression or recurrence, when these tumors are resected and examined pathologically, these tumors are comprised entirely of mature teratoma. The incidence of this phenomenon has been described in approximately 3% of men with testicular cancer[483] and in as high as 12% of women with ovarian GCT, particularly among women originally diagnosed with immature teratoma.[484] The hypothesized etiology is that the chemotherapy might induce differentiation of residual immature teratoma into a mature teratoma. Median interval between chemotherapy and first detection of growing teratoma syndrome was 9 months in a retrospective study of women with ovarian immature teratomas from the Institut Gustave-Roussy; however, the range extended from 1 month after treatment to 12 years after treatment.[484] The disease usually occurs at the site of prior disease; for instance, women known to have peritoneal deposits of tumor at diagnosis were noted to have peritoneal location for the growing teratoma syndrome. In most cases, the recurrence is treated with surgery only. In cases where total resection is not possible,

patients require continued surveillance. These patients can become quite ill if the tumor is not amenable to resection and impinges on organ function. A report in the *New England Journal of Medicine* described disease stabilization in three patients with nonresectable tumors who were treated with a CDK4/6 inhibitor; two patients had stable disease for 18 and 24 months at the time of publication.[362]

Extragonadal Tumors

Mediastinal Tumors

The Germans have reported on the outcome of pediatric mediastinal GCT as a separate entity.[417] Included in their report are all patients treated between 1983 and 1999 on German treatment protocols, including MAKEI83/86, 89, and 96. The authors examined the outcome of both mediastinal teratomas (both mature and immature; n = 21) and malignant GCTs of the mediastinum (n = 26). All the mediastinal GCTs diagnosed in the first year of life were teratomas (Fig. 63-16). The incidence of teratoma declined during infancy and adolescence; seminoma was not observed until after age 10.

Teratomas were surgically resected; no adjuvant chemotherapy or radiotherapy was given. Sixteen of the teratomas were mature; five were immature. All patients with teratoma underwent primary resection; surgery was microscopically complete in 17 of 21 patients. All patients with teratomas, regardless of the completeness of the tumor resection, were cured with surgery only.

Twelve of the 26 patients with MGCT had primary resection of the tumor that was complete in six of the 12. Four of the six patients with incomplete resections subsequently underwent second-look surgery, and all achieved a complete resection of the residual tumor. Eleven patients underwent delayed resection of the primary tumor after preoperative chemotherapy, and a complete resection was achieved in 10 of the 11 patients. Three patients did not undergo resection of the tumor;

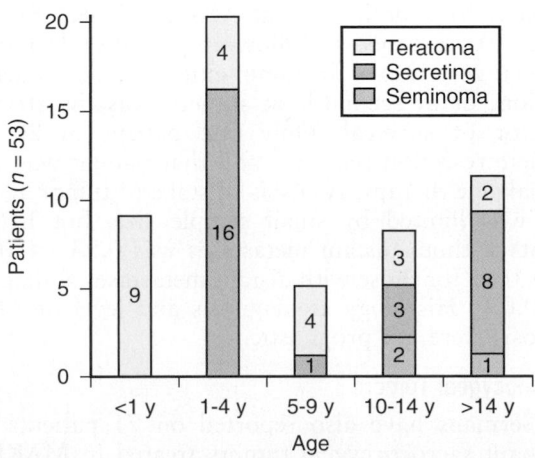

Figure 63-16 Age and histologic differentiation in all registered patients with mediastinal GCTs (*n* = 53; one patient with insufficient histopathology was excluded). *(From Schneider DT, Calaminus G, Reinhard H, et al: Primary mediastinal germ cell tumors in children and adolescents: results of the German cooperative protocols MAKEI 83/86, 89, and 96.* J Clin Oncol 18:832–839, 2000.)

TABLE 63-5   Summary of Treatment of Nonseminomatous Malignant Germ Cell Tumors in the United States, Germany, and the United Kingdom

	United States	Germany	United Kingdom
Testicular			
Stage I	W&W*	W&W for pure yolk sac Other: 2-3 cycles PVB	W&W
Stage II	3 cycles compressed PEB	2-3 cycles PVB	JEB[†]
Stage III-IV	3 cycles compressed PEB	2 cycles PVB, 4 cycles PEI	JEB
Ovarian			
Stage I ovarian	W&W	W&W	W&W
Stage II	3 cycles compressed PEB	2 cycles PE if completely resected 2 cycles PEI if incompletely resected	JEB
Stage III-IV	3 cycles PEB	4 cycles PEI	JEB
Extragonadal			
Stage I extragonadal	3 cycles compressed PEB	W&W except sacrococcygeal tumors; Stage I SCT: 4 cycles PE, PEI[‡]	W&W
Stage II	3 cycles compressed PEB	3 cycles PE if completely resected. 3 cycles PEI if incompletely resected	JEB
Stage III-IV	High risk protocol	4-5 cycles PEI Poor responder: 1 cycles PEI, 3 cycles HDPEI	JEB
Relapse	TIC +/− stem cell transplant	Local: 4 cycles local deep hyperthermia + PEI Disseminated: 1 cycles PEI, 3 cycles HDPEI	

HDPEI, High-dose cisplatin, etoposide, ifosfamide; *JEB,* carboplatin, etoposide, bleomycin; *PE,* cisplatin, etoposide; *PEB,* bleomycin, etoposide, cisplatin; *PEI,* cisplatin, etoposide, ifosfamide; *TIC,* taxol, ifosfamide, carboplatin; *W&W,* watch-and-wait strategy.
*Observation only after surgical excision of Stage I tumor with chemotherapy reserved for those who recur.
[†]4-6 Cycles; number of cycles determined by risk group stratification.
[‡]Depending on age: <4 months, PE; >4 months, PEI.

two patients had a CR to first-line therapy; and one patient had progressive disease on chemotherapy. Patients were treated with cisplatin-based regimens for a total of three to eight courses (details are shown in Table 63-5).[417] Excellent results on MAKEI83/86 encouraged the German investigators to reduce the maximum number of courses from eight to four or five cycles with no apparent detriment to overall survival. Overall 5-year EFS was 0.83 ± 0.05 at a median follow-up period of 41 months. Complete resection of the tumor either initially, at delayed resection, or at second-look surgery was the strongest predictor of survival. Only one patient of 20 with complete resection relapsed, and that patient was cured with salvage therapy. Analysis of stage of tumor at diagnosis was limited by small sample size, but EFS for patients without distant metastases was 0.93 ± 0.07 vs. 0.65 ± 0.17 for those with distant metastases at diagnosis (P = 0.09). Histology at diagnosis and level of AFP at diagnosis were not prognostic.

Sacrococcygeal Tumors

The Germans have also reported on 71 patients with malignant sacrococcygeal tumors treated in MAKEI83/86 and 89 from 1983 to 1995.[419] Of the 66 evaluable patients, there were 14 boys and 52 girls; median age was 17.4 months. Twelve patients had lymph node metastases, and 30 patients had distant metastases (lungs, 21; liver, 8; bones, 8). On histological examination, 45

patients had pure YST and 21 patients had mixed GCT. Treatment details of MAKEI83/86 and 89 are summarized in Table 63-5. Patients in MAKEI83/86 received a total of eight cycles of cisplatin-based therapy: four cycles of PVB followed by four cycles of PEI. Patients in MAKEI89 received a total of 6 cycles of cisplatin-based therapy: three cycles of PEB followed by three cycles of etoposide, ifosfamide, and cisplatin (VIP). EFS for the entire group was 0.76 ± 0.05, and OS was 0.81 ± 0.05. OS did not differ by protocol (MAKEI83/86 vs. 89) or by stage (T1 vs. T2). The most significant predictor of favorable outcome was the completeness of tumor resection. The completeness of this resection could either be established by tumor resection at initial diagnosis or at delayed resection after chemotherapy is given. Among patients with advanced and metastatic disease (T2b M1), those who had a delayed resection fared better than patients with an initial resection (5-year OS 0.83 ± 0.09 vs. 0.45 ± 0.15; P = 0.01). The presence of metastatic disease at diagnosis was only an adverse risk factor among those who had initial resection of their tumor at diagnosis. AFP levels at diagnosis were not prognostic, even when the analysis was restricted to children older than 1 year of age. The authors conclude that the therapeutic strategy of preoperative chemotherapy with delayed resection results in superior outcomes that abrogate prior reports that higher stage and higher pretherapy levels of AFP portend a worse prognosis.

An analysis of the prognostic factors among children with SCT treated on the U.S. intergroup study confirms the conclusions of the German report.[416] Seventy-four children with malignant SCT were randomized to receive either standard-dose PEB or HDPEB. Prognosis was excellent in this subgroup overall (4-year EFS 84% ± 6%; 4-year OS 90% ± 4%). Neither presence of metastatic disease nor delayed resection had an adverse effect on outcome. In this group of patients, AFP greater than 20,000 IU/L was associated with a higher than expected rate of failure.

Postchemotherapy Management

At the end of chemotherapy, full restaging should be undertaken, including radiologic imaging of the primary site and the most likely sites of nodal spread, chest CT, and measurements of tumor markers (AFP and β-HCG). If tumor markers are elevated and chest CT and pelvic/abdominal CT do not reveal the site of metastasis, a bone scan and brain MRI are indicated to look for other possible sites of metastatic disease. In the case in which tumor markers are elevated but no mass is detectable, a PET scan can sometimes be helpful in identifying occult disease. The recommended surveillance postchemotherapy is similar to that recommended for patients with stage I disease (see "Treatment of Stage I Malignant Non-seminomatous Germ Cell Tumors").

Postchemotherapy Retroperitoneal Lymph Node Dissection

If there is either a residual mass detected, surgery is recommended to remove the mass or to explore and biopsy any potentially involved residual lymph nodes. There is limited data on findings from second-look surgeries in children with GCTs. In the United Kingdom after completion of JEB chemotherapy, 15 out of 137 patients required surgery for residual mass seen on radiologic evaluation.[471] Half of the patients (53%) had necrosis or fibrosis; 42% were found to have immature or mature teratoma, and only two patients had viable tumors. The two patients who had viable tumors did not receive any further therapy after complete resection, and both remain in complete remission.

Postchemotherapy Retroperitoneal Lymph Node Dissection in Adult Men with Testicular Cancer

In a retrospective review from Memorial Sloan Kettering, 11% of men who underwent postchemotherapy RPLND had viable residual GCT; 49% had fibrosis, and 40% were found to have teratoma in the postchemotherapy surgical specimen.[437] In the subgroup of patients with teratomas, 85% had pure mature teratomas, 7% had immature teratomas, and 8% had teratomas with malignant transformation (to a non-GCT histology).[437] The median size of the node at postchemotherapy RPLND was 3.0 cm, but 18% of the patients discovered to have teratoma had a node smaller than 2 cm and 11% had a node smaller than 1 cm. The 5- and 10-year probabilities of relapse-free survival were 83% and 80%, respectively. There is debate in the adult testicular cancer community as to the optimal surgical approach: a modified RPLND template vs. bilateral infrahilar dissec-

tion. The complexity of these issues argue strongly for referral of the adolescent patient to a urologist well-versed in the data.[437,485]

Second-Look Surgery in Ovarian Malignancies

In adult women with epithelial ovarian carcinoma, second-look surgery postchemotherapy is performed on all patients to cytoreduce and has been found to improve prognosis. In adult women with malignant ovarian GCTs, however, it has been shown that the yield of second-look surgery, in the setting of a negative radiologic evaluation and normal tumors markers, has a very low probability of discovering occult residual malignant disease. A report by Gershenson et al. states that only 1 of 53 women with negative scans and tumor markers had viable tumor at second-look surgery.[164]

What should be chemotherapy if tumor is found? Standard of care if viable tumor is found at postchemotherapy lymph node resection has been two more cycles of the original chemotherapy. However, persistence of viable tumor after standard chemotherapy is increasingly viewed as evidence of resistant disease and anecdotally, most adult oncologists are now treating patient with salvage therapy in this setting.

Of note, in adults a higher-than-expected incidence of sarcoidosis has been noted in patients previously treated for GCTs.[434] Sarcoidosis should be considered in the differential diagnosis of any adolescent patient with pulmonary nodules or infiltrates or mediastinal adenopathy in the setting of negative tumor markers.

RELAPSE AND SALVAGE THERAPY

In the German experience, more than 90% of relapses occurred locally.[423] In an analysis of 22 patients with recurrent sacrococcygeal tumors previously treated on the German MAKEI protocols, the majority of patients (17 of 22) presented with local recurrence only. Two patients had only distant metastases, and three patients had combined local and distant recurrences.[346] Most relapses occurred within 6 months of completing primary therapy (median 5.5 months; range 0 to 21 months). Complete surgical resection of the relapse was associated with higher likelihood of continuous CR (5 of 7 patients in first relapse who had a microscopic CR of the relapsed tumor remained in CR). Only 1 of 5 patients who had distant metastases at relapse achieved a second continuous CR. Early vs. late relapse (<1 year vs. >1 year after diagnosis), AFP serum levels at relapse, and tumor size at relapse were not prognostic. These data contrast with those from adult men with TGCT in whom favorable prognostic factors at relapse include IGCCC "good risk" group at first diagnosis, testis as the primary site (vs. retroperitoneal or mediastinal), previous complete response to first line therapy, low tumor markers at relapse, and low-volume disease.

Salvage Therapy
Surgery

Unlike many other forms of cancer, surgical excision can be curative in chemorefractory GCTs in patients who have anatomically confined disease.[486] Most patients also require chemotherapy to achieve a second durable remission.

Chemotherapy

Several different regimens have been used in adult males with relapsed or refractory GCT. Vinblastine, ifosfamide, mesna, and cisplatin (VeIP; vinblastine 0.11mg/kg, cisplatin 25 mg/m^2 × 5, and ifosfamide 1.2 gm/m^2 × 5) results in a complete response in 50% of patients, but responses are durable in only 20% to 30% of cases.[460] More recently, investigators from Memorial Sloan Kettering have reported on a paclitaxel, ifosfamide, and cisplatin (TIP) regimen that substitutes paclitaxel for vinblastine (paclitaxel 250 mg/m^2, ifosfamide 1.2 gm/m^2 × 5, and cisplatin 20 mg/m^2 × 5), in which up to 70% of patients experience CR with durable CR rate of 63%.[487] Oxaliplatin and gemcitabine have both shown activity in phase II trials as single agents in men with relapsed testicular cancer.[488-490] Two recent single-institution reports of treatment of relapsed patients with high-dose chemotherapy (HDCT) have shown encouraging results. Kondagunla et al reported on the treatment of 48 patients with a poor response to standard BEP therapy who were treated with two cycles of paclitaxel and ifosfamide followed by three cycles of carboplatin and etoposide with peripheral blood stem cell (PBSC) support administered at 14-to 21-day intervals.[491] CR was obtained in 55% of patients, and 51% remain in remission at a median follow-up period of 40 months. Einhorn et al reported on the treatment of 184 patients with relapsed testicular cancer who were treated with two cycles of carboplatin and etoposide with PBSC support.[492] CR was obtained in 63% of patients with median follow-up time of 48 months; a high response rate was observed even among the subset of patients who had cisplatin-refractory disease, or had failed prior salvage regimens.

Limited data exist on optimal therapy for pediatric patients whose GCT has relapsed. A trial of paclitaxel, ifosfamide, and carboplatin (TIC; paclitaxel 135 mg/m^2, ifosfamide 1.8 gm/m^2 × 5, carboplatin 560 mg/m^2) is under investigation in the COG. The decision was made to use carboplatin rather than cisplatin for two reasons. First, children are more sensitive to the ototoxicity of cisplatin, and it is likely that many children would have serious hearing impairment if further courses of cisplatin were administered after PEB. Secondly, carboplatin has been shown to be potentially equally as efficacious as cisplatin in children with GCTs in the GC2 study conducted in the United Kingdom.[471] The study is evaluating response to two cycles of TIC. Additional therapy after two cycles of TIC (for instance, either to continue with TIC or to proceed to HDCT with stem cell transplant) is left to the physician's discretion.

Radiotherapy

Radiotherapy is not a standard part of salvage therapy in the United States and certainly not until standard second-line therapy has been attempted. However, in an analysis of outcome of patients with sacrococcygeal GCT tumors treated in Germany, Schneider et al report that 8 out of 22 patients received local irradiation after relapse, most in the situation of an incompletely resected tumor. None of the patients who received less than 45 Gy achieved a stable second CR, whereas 3 of 5 patients who received more than 45 Gy achieved a stable continuous remission.[346]

The Germans have also used regional deep hyperthermia successfully in the control of local recurrence, especially if it is applied early in the course of recurrence.[493] Cisplatin is a thermosensitizer, and thus this approach may be of use in overcoming cisplatin-resistant tumors.

Molecular Basis of Cisplatin Sensitivity and Resistance in Germ Cell Tumors

Compared to most other malignancies, GCTs are unusually responsive to chemotherapy, especially to cisplatin-based regimens (with the exception of teratomas, which are chemoresistant). The reasons for this exquisite sensitivity are not fully known, precluding a complete understanding of the mechanisms of cisplatin resistance, and hampering efforts to overcome chemoresistance in GCTs. Several features of GCTs are thought to contribute to their relative chemosensitivity.[494,495] In particular, GCTs may differ from other malignancies regarding uptake, efflux, and conjugation of cisplatin, as well as the cellular DNA repair and apoptotic response to cisplatin exposure. Uptake of cisplatin into GCTs may occur by passive or facilitated diffusion. Recent work has highlighted the role of copper transporter CTR1 in cisplatin uptake, and the significance of altered CTR1 expression in cisplatin-resistant solid tumors.[496-498] However, it is unclear whether CTR1 significantly affects cisplatin uptake into germ cells. Similarly, overexpression of proteins capable of exporting cisplatin, such as lung resistance protein (LRP) and multidrug resistance-related protein (MRP) 2 is not a consistent feature of cisplatin-resistant GCTs.[494,495,499,500] Conjugation of cisplatin to glutathione can limit its cytotoxicity and facilitate export; in germ cells this conjugation is mediated principally by the isoform of glutathione-S-transferase (GST) θ.[501-503] Strohmeyer et al reported an overall low level of GST enzyme activity in GCTs, and Mayer et al found consistent GST-θ expression in only 5 of 36 nonteratoma GCTs.[494,502] Thus low levels of GST activity may contribute to the activity of cisplatin in GCTs. However, in the Mayer et al study the differences between cisplatin-responsive and refractory tumors were not significant.

In the absence of compelling evidence that import or export mechanisms predominantly determine cisplatin's effect on GCTs, attention has focused on the role of DNA damage repair and apoptosis pathways in cisplatin-mediated cytotoxicity. Cisplatin causes bulky DNA adducts, which are removed via nucleotide excision repair (NER).[504] Most GCT cell lines exhibit low NER activity, which may be attributable to low expression levels of the NER proteins XPA, XPF, and ERCC1.[505-507] However, one study found no difference in XPA expression between cisplatin-sensitive and resistant tumors,[508] and restoring XPA expression to a testicular tumor cell line did not increase cellular resistance to cisplatin,[509] calling into question whether NER is an important factor in GCT response to cisplatin. Another DNA damage-repair pathway, mismatch repair (MMR), has also been investigated in relation to cisplatin treatment of GCTs. A hallmark of defects in the MMR pathway is the presence of microsatellite instability (MSI). Several studies have indicated a low level of MSI in GCTs, implying that the MMR system is generally intact in these tumors.[378,510,511] In the presence of DNA damage, the MMR pathway can trigger p53-dependent apoptosis,[512,513] and this response may explain the sensitivity of most GCTs to cisplatin. On the other hand, loss of MMR may confer chemoresistance. In one series, only 6% of unselected GCTs displayed MSI, whereas 45% of chemoresistant tumors exhibited MSI or low levels of MMR proteins.[378] In another study of GCTs, Velasco and co-workers found that low MMR expression and a high degree of MSI were associated with chemotherapy resistance, shorter time to recurrence, and poor survival.[514] Loss of MMR function is associated with genomic instability and the acquisition of secondary mutations that may enhance tumor survival or aggressiveness.[451,515,516] Thus the MMR system is an important determinant of cisplatin sensitivity in GCTs, and loss of MMR may signal a worse prognosis.

As mentioned, the MMR pathway not only functions to maintain genome integrity but is also one of the factors that triggers apoptosis in response to genotoxic damage such as that caused by cisplatin. Apoptosis, or programmed cell death, is a key determinant of the death or survival of cancer cells and the effectiveness of chemotherapy.[517-522] The tumor-suppressor protein p53 plays a central role in coordinating the apoptotic response to genotoxic damage,[523,524] and attention has focused on the role of the p53 pathway in chemotherapy of GCTs. Mutations in p53, which are commonly found in other tumor types, are rare in GCTs.[494,525] The presence of high levels of wildtype p53 protein in GCTs has been suggested to account for the unusual chemoresponsiveness of these tumors.[526,527] However, p53 deficiency per se does not prevent an apoptotic response to cisplatin in GCT cell lines,[528] and the presence or absence of wildtype p53 correlates poorly with clinical response to chemotherapy.[525] Thus the importance of wildtype p53 expression in determining the cisplatin response of GCTs is not clear. Also unclear is why GCTs treated with cisplatin predominantly exhibit apoptosis rather than undergoing cell-cycle arrest, senescence, or other p53-mediated responses. Despite the absence of p53 mutations, other mechanisms exist in GCTs to interfere with p53 function, including overexpression of the p53 inhibitor MDM2[529,530] and epigenetic silencing of p53 target genes.[531] Particularly interesting in this regard is the recent finding that the miR cluster miR-371-3 acts in GCTs to neutralize the p53 response to oncogenic stress.[295] In summary, there is suggestive evidence that specific features of GCTs, including their retention of a normal DNA damage repair, p53, and apoptosis pathways, may account for the unusual chemosensitivity of these cells. However, a simple loss of these mechanisms does not seem to account for the majority of cases of chemoresistance. Recently, CGH analysis has revealed genomic CNV of specific chromosomal regions associated with acquired cisplatin resistance,[532,533] and further exploration of the genes involved in these regions may shed light on the mechanisms underlying resistance.

Prospects for Targeted Therapy of Germ Cell Tumors

Cisplatin-based chemotherapy of GCTs has been highly effective and will continue to be a mainstay of treatment. However, the toxicity of these regimens, as well as the poor prognosis of cisplatin-resistant disease, points up the need for more specific, effective therapies. Such therapies will depend on advances in research focusing on the molecular mechanisms of germ cell tumorigenesis. To date, these mechanisms are only incompletely understood, but some case reports and small trials have raised intriguing prospects for targeted therapy of GCTs. The receptor tyrosine kinase c-kit oncogene is commonly overexpressed in seminomas, and activating mutations in c-kit have been described in seminomas,[199,243,372] suggesting that GCTs may be susceptible to treatment with the kinase inhibitor imatinib. Whereas case reports have documented efficacy of imatinib in seminoma[534] the majority of the described c-kit mutations in seminomas are insensitive to imatinib,[370] and a phase II trial of imatinib in six patients with c-kit–positive metastatic GCT failed to show significant antitumor activity.[490] Although c-kit remains a promising target in GCTs and other malignancies, it is clear that not all c-kit mutations will be susceptible to imatinib or other tyrosine kinase inhibitors (TKIs) currently in use.[535] Another potential TKI target, the epidermal growth factor receptor (EGFR) has also been investigated in relapsed or refractory GCTs. Several studies reported that EGFR is expressed in nonseminomas,[422,536,537] and a phase II study has been initiated to treat GCTs with erlotinib, a small-molecule EGFR inhibitor. Early reports that GCTs overexpress HER2/Neu and might be susceptible to trastuzumab (a chimeric anti-HER2/Neu antibody)[139] were not borne out by subsequent analyses.[538]

Differentiation therapy is another potential route to targeted therapy of GCTs. Based on the differentiating effect of retinoic acid on GCT cell lines in vitro, 16 patients with chemoresistant GCTs were treated with retinoic acid; no partial or complete responses occurred.[539]

Inhibition of tumor angiogenesis is a promising avenue under intense investigation for many tumor types. In GCTs, increased expression of the proangiogenic vascular endothelial growth factor (VEGF) correlates with tumor metastasis.[540,541] Trials are underway to evaluate the effect of inhibiting VEGF in patients with GCTs by using the small-molecule TKI sunitinib or the combination of oxaliplatin with the anti-VEGF antibody, bevacizumab.

It is important to note that most targeted therapy trials are based on preclinical models of adult GCTs; because the molecular pathogenesis of pediatric tumors likely differs from that of adults, targeted therapy developed for adult GCTs may not translate directly into clinical efficacy in children. More effort is required to define the "targets" for pediatric GCTs and to develop animal models that accurately model the human tumors. In both children and young adults, GCTs appear to arise from defects in early development.[1] Therefore particular attention should be given to examining developmental and stem-cell pathways such as the Wnt/β-catenin, BMP, notch, and hedgehog pathways. Intriguingly, a recent report describes activation of the Wnt/β-catenin pathway in immature teratomas and YSTs but not germinomas, embryonal carcinomas, or choriocarcinomas.[385] The emerging role of miRs in human cancer is another area with potentially great implications for understanding GCT pathogenesis.[390,542,543] Continued progress in molecular cytogenetics and pathway discovery in pediatric GCTs will be critical to the development of improved therapies.

LATE EFFECTS

There is limited data on both the short- and-long term side effects of treatment for GCTs among patients treated as children. GCTs are not included in the Childhood Cancer Survivor Study (CCSS), an invaluable source of information about late effects among children treated for other diagnoses. The only comprehensive survey of late effects of pediatric GCTs is a single-institution study from St. Jude's of 73 patients treated from 1962 through 1988; two thirds of patients had at least one major complication.[544] This study is limited for several reasons; first, the treatment of GCTs has changed radically since 1962 and even since 1988. In the era of the St. Jude study, the majority of patients received radiotherapy as part of their treatment; radiotherapy is seldom used today. The chemotherapy for GCTs during this era included VAC either alone or in combination with a cisplatin-based regimen. The inclusion of an alkylator, cyclophosphamide, in the older regimens radically changes the profile of expected toxicities. Cumulative doses of drugs were also much higher on the older regimens, because "maintenance" therapy often continued for a year, whereas total duration of current regimens is generally only 9 to 12 weeks. For these reasons, the toxicities described in the St. Jude report, such as the high prevalence of delayed pubertal development and ovarian failure, are related to either radiation or treatment with an alkylators, neither part of standard care today.

Other pediatric studies have focused primarily on short-term toxicity either occurring during the clinical trial or within the window of follow-up observation used to establish relapse rate. For instance, among 33 children treated with PEB in the GC1 study in the United Kingdom, 45% developed some degree of renal impairment and 10% developed auditory impairment (grades 1-3). One child developed AML while receiving PEB. There have been no deaths from bleomycin-induced pulmonary fibrosis after the dose of bleomycin was reduced to once per cycle every 3 weeks. There had been four deaths from pulmonary toxicity among children receiving weekly bleomycin. Of the 17 evaluable patients with SCT, four had neuropathic bladder and/or bowel and one child had shortening of one leg.[470,471] Among the 137 patients treated on GC2, which replaced carboplatin for cisplatin, only one patient had significant hearing loss, but this occurred after middle ear hemorrhages, and only patient died of pulmonary failure, and that patient had preexisting bronchopulmonary dysplasia.[470] All other renal and pulmonary toxicity noted on study was reversible. On the U.S. intergroup study, no patient died of pulmonary toxicity.

Late Effects Among Men Treated for Testicular Cancer

Physicians who care for long-term survivors of pediatric GCTs must be aware of and extrapolate from data emerging from follow-up studies of men treated for testicular cancer. Studies of adult men treated for testicular cancer are consistently demonstrating an increased risk of both cardiovascular disease and second malignant neoplasm. However, the limitations of this approach are twofold. One is that age at treatment likely has an important bearing on type and severity of toxicities. For instance, adults are much more likely to develop tinnitus or Reynaud phenomenon after cisplatin than children. Younger age at treatment, however, increases the risk of development of second malignant neoplasm. A concern about extrapolating from the data on men who have been treated with testicular cancer is that one must assume that the experience of men can be applied without revision to the experience of women, an assumption proven to be false in other clinical scenarios.

Cisplatin Levels Are Measurable for Years After Treatment

Cisplatin is a derived from platinum, a heavy metal like iron or lead. Recently it has become apparent that cisplatin is not completely excreted after treatment but is stored and slowly leaches back into the circulation over time. At autopsy, cisplatin can be measured in every tissue of the body,[545] and cisplatin levels are measurable for years after treatment.[546] In 45 patients, platinum plasma concentrations ranged between 1.42 and 2.99×10^{-3}ng/L.[547] Among adult testicular cancer survivors, the circulating level of cisplatin is highly correlated with the amount of persistent neuropathy reported after treatment.[548] The correlation of cisplatin levels with second malignant neoplasm (SMN) and cardiovascular disease has not been reported to date.

Risk of Cardiovascular Disease

In a nationwide cohort in the Netherlands of 2707 5-year survivors of testicular cancer, the standardized incidence ratio of myocardial infarction, angina pectoris, or congestive heart failure was 1.4.[549] In another study of long-term survivors, the relative risk (RR) of cardiovascular disease was estimated to be 2.59 for patients treated with chemotherapy compared with patients under surveillance (with median follow-up period of 10 years).[550] A partial explanation for this excessive morbidity and mortality is the higher prevalence of cardiovascular risk factors among survivors, including a 30% incidence of metabolic syndrome including hypertension, dyslipidemias, obesity, insulin resistance, and gonadal dysfunction[546,551] as compared with either patients treated with surgery and surveillance only or with normal population controls. However, the reason that patients treated with chemotherapy have higher prevalence of cardiovascular risk factors is not well understood. A possible factor contributing to cardiovascular morbidity may be the chemotherapy induces vasospastic disease, as evidenced by the high incidence (up to 50%) of Raynaud phenomenon postchemotherapy in adult survivors of testicular cancer.[552-555] Another explanation for premature onset of cardiovascular events may be direct damage to the endothelial cell. Evidence of endothelial cell damage is the high prevalence (22%) of microalbuminuria observed in long-term survivors.[556] Other authors report an increase in levels of von Willebrand factor in plasma and in the intimamedia thickness of the carotid artery after treatment as further evidence of endothelial cell toxicity.[557]

Risk of Second Malignant Neoplasm

Several studies of the risk of second malignancy among adult men treated for testicular cancer have been conducted.[450,558,559] In the first two studies published (n = 1025 and 1909) an increased risk of secondary malignancy, principally gastrointestinal cancers, was observed, but secondary cancers occurred only in patients who had received radiotherapy.[558,559] A subsequent study that utilized population-based cancer registries identified 40,576 survivors of testicular cancer who had developed a total of 2285 secondary solid cancers.[450,560] In this cohort, patients treated with chemotherapy alone exhibited a 1.8 fold excess risk of developing a second solid cancer, unlike prior studies in which risk appeared to be restricted to those who had been treated with radiotherapy. Treatment with radiotherapy did incur a higher risk (RR 2.0) than that observed with chemotherapy alone, and a synergistic effect between chemotherapy and radiation therapy was also observed (RR 2.9). This study was also the first to report an increased risk of supradiaphragmatic cancers (esophagus, pleura, and lung). Interestingly, cumulative risk at any given age increased with decreasing age at testicular cancer diagnosis. The authors estimated that a patient diagnosed with seminoma at age 20 would have a cumulative risk of solid cancer of 47% by age 75, compared with 36% for patient diagnosed at age 25 and 28% for a patient diagnosed at age 50. There was no plateau in the upward trend for risk throughout the 40 years of follow-up study, with serious implications for those diagnosed and treated at a young age.[450]

Risk of Secondary Leukemia

The development of secondary leukemia or myelodysplastic syndrome after treatment with epipodophyllotoxins is a well-described clinical syndrome usually involving a translocation of the *MLL* gene.[561] The risk of secondary leukemia among adult patients with testicular cancer has been estimated to be 0.6%.[562,563] An analysis of data that included children treated on the last U.S. intergroup national protocol for pediatric GCTs estimated the risk to be virtually identical (0.7%).[561] In a report of the German pediatric experience, 442 patients received chemotherapy, and 174 patients received chemotherapy and radiotherapy.[564] Six patients subsequently developed AML; four of the six had the classic cytogenetic abnormalities associated with topoisomerase II inhibitor-induced leukemias. Cumulative risk at 10 years for AML was 1% for children treated with chemotherapy alone

and 4.2% for children treated with both chemotherapy and radiotherapy.

Other Significant Late Effects

Bleomycin and Pulmonary Toxicity

Bleomycin is known to cause fatal pulmonary fibrosis in 1% to 2% of patients, but all patients experience some measurable decrement in pulmonary function while undergoing treatment. However, in adults, almost universally, pulmonary function tests recover to pretreatment values after completion of treatment.[565] Of more concern is the development of rapidly fatal adult respiratory distress syndrome (ARDS) in long-term survivors after general anesthesia. High concentrations of inspired oxygen have been implicated.[566,567] However, in a study reporting on the surgical management of patients that had been treated with bleomycin, the most significant predictor of postoperative oxygen saturation was the amount of blood transfused; intraoperative fractional oxygen was not significant in multivariate analysis.[568] These authors suggest that careful and conservative fluid management is at least as important as restriction of inspired oxygen during surgical procedures.

Most pediatric protocols have either deleted or significantly reduced the amount of bleomycin used so as to completely avoid the complication of fatal pulmonary fibrosis. It is not known how the reduction in dose will affect the development of ARDS during anesthesia posttreatment, and pediatric patients should be made aware of the risk.

Renal Toxicity

The glomerular filtration rate is decreased during treatment in almost all adult male patients, but most studies report restoration of renal function to approximately 85% of pretreatment value by 4 years off therapy.[475,565,569-571] Persistent salt-wasting (Ca, Mg, phosphate) has been reported in 20% of patients.[475,570] Men have also been reported to have elevated renin and aldosterone after therapy.[572]

Gonadal Function

Abnormal sperm counts and motility, and elevated follicle-stimulating hormone (FSH) indicative of impaired spermatogenesis have been documented in two thirds of men after orchiectomy and before any adjuvant treatment.[573,574] One study showed a similar clinical picture even before the initial orchiectomy.[571] Despite these abnormalities in spermatogenesis at diagnosis, a significant proportion of men recover both sperm number and function after treatment.[573,575,576] In one study, 50% of men who were azoospermic at baseline recovered sperm counts to at least 10×10^6 /mL, and 80% of patients who were oligospermic recovered normal sperm counts.[577] Elevated FSH (>2× upper limit of normal) was predictive of abnormal semen analysis both at baseline and also after treatment.[577] Semen recovery usually occurs in the first 2 years after completion of treatment, but improvement has been observed as late as 4 years after treatment.[571] Encouragingly, paternity rates posttreatment are quite high; most men (67% to 76%) who wished to father a child have succeeded.[578]

Persistent endocrine dysfunction has been documented in men after treatment for testicular cancer, particularly in the pituitary-gonadal axis.[553] Several authors note elevations of FSH (up to 75% of men), luteinizing hormone (LH; up to 50% of men),[208,553,569,579] and decreased testosterone (10% to 15%) in long-term survivors of testicular cancer.[553] One author noted that the volume of the remaining testis was reduced in those men who received chemotherapy compared with those who underwent surgery only.[580] Moderate testosterone deficiency, as documented in some long-term survivors, may have a broader systemic impact. For instance testosterone deficiency has been correlated with higher levels of serum cholesterol,[581] and lower testosterone levels are associated with lower levels of bone mineral density.[582] Site apparently was not related to endocrine dysfunction; patients with extragonadal primary tumors had the same profile of endocrine abnormalities.

CONCLUSIONS

Pediatric GCTs are a highly curable form of cancer. Several challenges remain. One objective of current research is to elucidate a better understanding of the underlying biologic etiology of these tumors. Work is also underway to improve upon the current ability to predict who is likely to fail first-line therapy. Better prognostication will allow a more refined approach to therapy, reducing the amount of therapy needed for those likely to be cured. Given the seriousness of the emerging late effects of therapy on rates of cardiovascular disease and SMN in men treated for testicular cancer, physicians must reweigh the risks of adjuvant chemotherapy versus either observation or primary RPLND. Conversely, the field is also challenged to find ways to intensify therapy for those for whom standard therapy is not sufficient. Finally, it is imperative that researchers and practitioners catalogue the late effects of treatment for children with GCTs so that they can adequately care for the majority of pediatric patients who will be cured.

References available online at ExpertConsult.

KEY REFERENCES

1. Oosterhuis JW, Looijenga LH: Testicular germ-cell tumours in a broader perspective. *Nat Rev Cancer* 5(3):210–222, 2005.
   This is a broad overview from leaders in the field that reexamines the biology of GCTs in the context of germ cell development.
2. Saitou M, Barton SC, Surani MA: A molecular programme for the specification of germ cell fate in mice. *Nature* 418(6895):293–300, 2002.
   This paper established the critical early events that lead to the emergence of the germline in developing embryos.
39. Runyan C, Schaible K, Molyneaux K, et al: Steel factor controls midline cell death of primordial germ cells and is essential for their normal proliferation and migration. *Development* 133(24):4861–4869, 2006.
   Using novel in vivo live imaging techniques, these authors established the Steel-kit pathway as a primary regulator of germ cell survival during PGC migration, a finding with implications for extragonadal GCTs.

48. Barton SC, Surani MA, Norris ML: Role of paternal and maternal genomes in mouse development. *Nature* 311(5984):374–376, 1984.
   A seminal paper that established the requirement of the maternal genome for proper embryonic development.
63. Ulbright TM: Germ cell tumors of the gonads: a selective review emphasizing problems in differential diagnosis, newly appreciated, and controversial issues. *Mod Pathol* 18(Suppl 2):S61–S79, 2005.
   A magisterial overview of GCT pathology with particular attention to the differing mechanisms of germ cell and somatic cell differentiation within GCTs.
168. Marina NM, Cushing B, Giller R, et al: Complete surgical excision is effective treatment for children with immature teratomas with or without malignant elements: a Pediatric Oncology Group/Children's Cancer Group Intergroup study. *J Clin Oncol* 17(7):2137–2143, 1999.
   A key study from the Children's Oncology Group that documents that surgery alone is sufficient for children with immature teratomas, including those with microscopic malignant elements. Patients who experienced recurrence were salvageable. Grade was not an important predictor of relapse or salvage.
260. Poynter JN, Amatruda JF, Ross JA: Trends in incidence and survival of pediatric and adolescent patients with germ cell tumors in the United States, 1975 to 2006. *Cancer* 116(20):4882–4891, 2010.
   The most current estimates of incidence and survival of pediatric GCTs.
291. Palmer RD, Barbosa-Morais NL, Gooding EL, et al: Pediatric malignant germ cell tumors show characteristic transcriptome profiles. *Cancer Res* 68(11):4239–4247, 2008.
   An in-depth analysis of gene expression in pediatric GCTs, demonstrating distinct transcriptional profiles that distinguish pediatric from adult GCTs.
293. Korkola JE, Houldsworth J, Feldman DR, et al: Identification and validation of a gene expression signature that predicts outcome in adult men with germ cell tumors. *J Clin Oncol* 27(19770384):5240–5247, 2009.
   This is an important contribution that used gene expression profiling to determine a signature associated with poor outcome in adult TGCTs.
295. Voorhoeve PM, le Sage C, Schrier M, et al: A genetic screen implicates miRNA-372 and miRNA-373 as oncogenes in testicular germ cell tumors. *Cell* 124(6):1169–1181, 2006.
   Among the very first demonstrations of a role for micro-RNAs in human cancer, this paper demonstrated the oncogenetic role of the miR37≈373 cluster in GCT pathogenesis.
296. Palmer RD, Murray MJ, Saini HK, et al: Malignant germ cell tumors display common microRNA profiles resulting in global changes in expression of messenger RNA targets. *Cancer Res* 70(7):2911–2923, 2010.
   Another important contribution from the Cambridge group describing the expression pattern of miRs in pediatric GCTs and the effect of altered miR expression on target mRNAs.
299. Murray MJ, Halsall DJ, Hook CE, et al: Identification of microRNAs from the miR-371~373 and miR-302 clusters as potential serum biomarkers of malignant germ cell tumors. *Am J Clin Pathol* 135(1):119–125, 2011.
   This paper describes the validation of specific miRs as novel serum tumor markers in GCTs.
363. Rapley EA, Turnbull C, Al Olama AA, et al: A genome-wide association study of testicular germ cell tumor. *Nat Genet* 41(7):807–810, 2009.
364. Turnbull C, Rapley EA, Seal S, et al: Variants near DMRT1, TERT and ATF7IP are associated with testicular germ cell cancer. *Nature Genet* 42:604–607, 2010.
   These two papers describe the UK and US Genome Wide Association Studies, which identified novel GCT susceptibility loci.
386. Neumann JC, Chandler GL, Damoulis VA, et al: Mutation in the type IB bone morphogenetic protein receptor Alk6b impairs germ-cell differentiation and causes germ-cell tumors in zebrafish. *Proc Natl Acad Sci U S A* 108(32):13153–13158, 2011.
   This paper describes a forward genetic screen for GCT susceptibility genes in zebrafish, resulting in the identification of the BMP pathway as a key regulator of differentiation in GCTs.

424. International Germ Cell Consensus Classification: A prognostic factor-based staging system for metastatic germ cell cancers. International Germ Cell Cancer Collaborative Group. *J Clin Oncol* 15(2):594–603, 1997.
    Landmark study of prognostic factors of outcome that has served as the basis for clinical trial design for adult men with testicular cancer since its publication.

431. Schlatter M, Rescorla F, Giller R, et al: Excellent outcome in patients with stage I germ cell tumors of the testes: a study of the Children's Cancer Group/Pediatric Oncology Group. *J Pediatr Surg* 38(3):319–324, 2003.
    A Children's Oncology Group study shows that boys with stage I testicular GCTs have ≈20% relapse rate but a 100% salvage rate.

433. Cushing B, Giller R, Cullen JW, et al: Randomized comparison of combination chemotherapy with etoposide, bleomycin, and either high-dose or standard-dose cisplatin in children and adolescents with high-risk malignant germ cell tumors: a pediatric intergroup study. Pediatric Oncology Group 9049 and Children's Cancer Group 8882. *J Clin Oncol* 22(13):2691–2700, 2004.
    A randomized study from the Children's Oncology Group that did not show overall advantage for high-dose cisplatinum, except perhaps in extragonadal GCTs, although this was a post-hoc analysis.

436. Mazumdar M, Bajorin DF, Bacik J, et al: Predicting outcome to chemotherapy in patients with germ cell tumors: the value of the rate of decline of human chorionic gonadotrophin and alpha-fetoprotein during therapy. *J Clin Oncol* 19(9):2534–2541, 2001.
    A seminal study that first demonstrated that a lack of adequate tumor-marker decline predicts adverse outcomes.

443. Einhorn LH: Combination chemotherapy with cis-dichlorodiammineplatinum (II) in disseminated testicular cancer. *Cancer Treat Rep* 63(9–10):1659-1662, 1979.
    This is the initial landmark study by Dr. Larry Einhorn that first demonstrated the activity of cisplatinum in testicular GCTs.

450. Travis LB, Fossa SD, Schonfeld SJ, et al: Second cancers among 40,576 testicular cancer patients: focus on long-term survivors. *J Natl Cancer Inst* 97(18):1354–1365, 2005.
    Definitive report of the two-fold rate of second malignant neoplasms (solid tumors) among patients treated with chemotherapy.

455. Rustin GJ, Mead GM, Stenning SP, et al: Randomized trial of two or five computed tomography scans in the surveillance of patients with stage I nonseminomatous germ cell tumors of the testis: Medical Research Council Trial TE08, ISRCTN56475197. The National Cancer Research Institute Testis Cancer Clinical Studies Group. *J Clin Oncol* 25(11):1310–1315, 2007.
    Study shows equal efficacy of a less frequent surveillance screening (2 scans in 2 years).

471. Mann JR, Raafat F, Robinson K, et al: The United Kingdom Children's Cancer Study Group's second germ cell tumor study: carboplatin, etoposide, and bleomycin are effective treatment for children with malignant extracranial germ cell tumors, with acceptable toxicity. *J Clin Oncol* 18(22):3809–3818, 2000.
    This study documents the excellent outcomes of pediatric germ cell patients treated on the British regimen of "JEB"-including carboplatin, etoposide, and bleomycin.

476. Shaikh F, Nathan PC, Hale J, et al: Is there a role for carboplatin in the treatment of malignant germ cell tumors? A systematic review of adult and pediatric trials. *Pediatr Blood Cancer* 60(4):587–592, 2013.
    A systematic meta-analysis of the adult data supporting the inferior efficacy of carboplatin in adult men with testicular cancer. The article points out that the pediatric trials have used higher doses of carboplatin and more frequent dosing and therefore the lack of efficacy in adult trials may be dose-related.

478. de Wit R, Roberts JT, Wilkinson PM, et al: Equivalence of three or four cycles of bleomycin, etoposide, and cisplatin chemotherapy and of a 3- or 5-day schedule in good-prognosis germ cell cancer: a randomized study of the European Organization for Research and Treatment of Cancer Genitourinary Tract Cancer Cooperative Group and the Medical Research Council. *J Clin Oncol* 19(6):1629–1640, 2001.
    This study serves as the basis for the current recommendation that three cycles of BEP (instead of the previous standard of four cycles) is sufficient therapy for patients with low-risk testicular cancer.

CHAPTER 64

Histiocytoses

Barbara A. Degar, Mark D. Fleming, Barrett J. Rollins, and Carlos Rodriguez-Galindo

CHAPTER OUTLINE

The histiocytoses constitute a collection of rare hematologic diseases that resist easy classification, at least in part because of the imprecise definition of "histiocyte." "Histiocyte" broadly refers both to cells of the macrophage lineage and to dendritic cells (DCs), only some types of which are derived from macrophages. The numerous descriptive and functional subsets of macrophages and DCs only add to the confusion. Nonetheless, their collective consideration is justified by a degree of uniformity in these childhood diseases that present with infiltration of bone, secondary lymphoid organs, or the liver, with or without concomitant involvement of other visceral organs. However, prognosis and treatment options are specific to the subtype, and thus an appreciation of the individual varieties of histiocytoses is mandatory.

This chapter is divided into two main sections that correspond to the two most common clinical histiocytic disorders, Langerhans cell histiocytosis (LCH) and hemophagocytic lymphohistiocytosis (HLH). Also included is a relatively brief discussion of non–Langerhans cell histiocytoses and Rosai-Dorfman disease. Each section will begin with a description of the normal counterpart(s) of the relevant histiocytes and their ontogeny to provide a context for describing how these cells are pathologically involved in the histiocytic disorders. Each section will also include a description of their clinical manifestations and current approaches to treatment.

TYPES OF DENDRITIC CELLS

The pathologic cells of LCH share some features with normal epidermal Langerhans cells (LCs), which are the primary antigen-presenting cells (APCs) of skin.[1] LCs are one type of the general class of APCs known as DCs because of the characteristic dendritelike structure they assume when activated. DCs are, in turn, just one of several types of APCs that are called "professional" because they can, by themselves, fully activate naive T lymphocytes by providing both the antigen/major histocompatibility complex ligand for T-cell receptor binding and the accessory signals required for full activation.[2,3]

Because DCs can also render T cells tolerant to specific antigens,[4] they have become a major focus of basic immunologic research. This research has revealed a surprising level of functional and phenotypic diversity among DCs, which will undoubtedly be relevant to the proliferative disorders affecting these cells. Several authors have provided helpful guides to thinking about and classifying DCs.[2,3,5,6] Overall, DCs can be divided into conventional and inflammatory types (Box 64-1). Conventional DCs are present in lymphoid and nonlymphoid organs in their basal state, and their primary function is to collect antigens for presentation to T cells in order to activate or tolerize them, depending on the antigen's source (i.e., nonself vs. self). Inflammatory DCs arise in response to

Box 64-1 Dendritic Cells

CONVENTIONAL DENDRITIC CELLS

MIGRATORY DENDRITIC CELLS

Migratory dendritic cells (DCs) gather antigen in peripheral tissues, then migrate to regional lymph nodes to present antigen to T lymphocytes
> *Examples: Langerhans cells, dermal DCs, interstitial DCs*

LYMPHOID TISSUE DENDRITIC CELLS

Lymphoid tissue DCs gather antigen within lymphoid tissue and present antigen to T lymphocytes within the same lymphoid tissue
> *Examples: thymic DCs, splenic DCs*

INFLAMMATORY DENDRITIC CELLS

Inflammatory DCs arise in response to inflammatory signals; they can gather antigen and present antigen to T lymphocytes and can secrete cytokines
> *Example: tumor necrosis factor and inducible nitric oxide synthase–producing DCs*

MUCOSAL DENDRITIC CELLS

Mucosal DCs are resident in mucosal surface tissues; they can gather antigen and present antigen to T lymphocytes and help direct responses toward activation or tolerance

PREDENDRITIC CELLS

Predendritic cells can develop DC function directly in response to inflammatory stimuli
> *Example: plasmacytoid DCs, monocytes*

Modified from Shortman K, Naik SH: Steady-state and inflammatory dendritic-cell development. Nat Rev Immunol 7:19–30, 2007.

specific inflammatory or infectious signals and are ordinarily not identifiable in the nonchallenged state. In addition to presenting antigen, these cells secrete cytokines and other mediators, including tumor necrosis factor (TNF), that enhance host defense.

Within the conventional DC category, one can distinguish between migratory DCs and DCs that reside in lymphoid tissue. Migratory DCs fulfill the sentinel role of this leukocyte class and include LCs, dermal DCs, and interstitial DCs of other organs. Migratory DCs shuttle between end organs that interface with the external world (e.g., skin or mucosa), in the case of LCs, and regional lymph nodes. This trafficking occurs at a low level in the basal state but can be greatly enhanced in the presence of foreign antigen or inflammatory challenges.[7-10] The migratory DC takes up antigen in the periphery and, once activated, travels to regional nodes either to present antigen itself or to transfer antigen to resident DCs in the node, which then perform the presentation function to T cells. Although the molecular signals that control this migratory behavior are not understood in detail, chemokines and their receptors play a large role.[11,12] In the case of LCs, resting cells express the chemokine receptor CCR6 whose ligand, CCL20, is secreted by cutaneous keratinocytes. Upon antigen uptake and activation, LCs downregulate CCR6 and in its place upregulate another chemokine receptor, CCR7, whose ligands, CCL19 and CCL21, are secreted by cells in regional lymph nodes. This receptor switch has the dual effect of neutralizing

the LC's anchor to the skin and attracting them to regional lymph nodes.

In contrast, DCs that reside in lymphoid tissue are nonmigratory. They make up most of the DCs populating the thymus and spleen and about half of the DCs in lymph nodes.[8,13] Unlike migratory DCs, which are mature when they appear in lymph nodes, resident DCs are immature, which allows them to take up, process, and present local antigens. Surface markers can distinguish several subsets of resident DCs, which are presumed to have specialized functions. In the mouse, these subsets include cluster of differentiation (CD)8+ and CD8– cells, and among the CD8– population are CD4+ and CD4– subpopulations.[14] Specific DC subsets also have characteristic gene expression profiles.[15]

LCs bear distinctive intracellular and extracellular markers that permit their distinction from DCs that reside in lymphoid tissue. The most characteristic surface marker is CD1a,[16] and the most characteristic ultrastructural feature is Birbeck granules, which are pentilaminar "tennis racket"–shaped cytoplasmic organelles that appear to be uniquely present in LCs.[17] Langerin, also known as CD207, is a cell surface marker for LCs that associates with Birbeck granules when internalized.[18] Langerin is a C-type lectin with specificity for sugars that contain mannose, suggesting that it may be involved in processing and trafficking of antigens that bear these sugars. Dectin-2 is another C-type lectin restricted to DCs,[19] and DEC-205 (CD205) is yet another lectin that is often used to identify LCs, although its expression is not as restricted to LCs as are the other lectins.[20] In the appropriate histologic context, from a diagnostic standpoint, CD1a and Langerin are the most reliable lineage-specific markers.[16]

Some authors also distinguish a group of so-called "predendritic cells" that do not ordinarily have DC functions or structure.[21,22] However, these cells can develop directly into DCs upon stimulation without the need for proliferation. One well-studied example is the plasmacytoid DC, which circulates as a nondescript mononuclear cell but acquires APC function and secretes large amounts of alpha interferon when activated.[23,24] Technically, using this definition, monocytes would also be predendritic cells. After exposure to interleukin (IL)-4 and granulocyte-macrophage colony-stimulating factor (CSF), monocytes become functional DCs, although their phenotype is closer to inflammatory DCs than conventional DCs.[25]

ORIGINS OF DENDRITIC CELLS

The availability of genetically modified mice that carry lineage-restricted markers has greatly expanded our understanding of the origins and development of DCs. Although mouse models have some limitations,[26] the major insight these animals provide is that a salient characteristic of DC ontogeny is flexibility. For example, although DCs generally have myeloid characteristics, all DC subtypes in the mouse can arise from either committed lymphoid or committed myeloid precursors.[27-29] Even though half of thymic DCs show evidence for immunoglobulin rearrangements, suggesting a lymphoid phenotype, they also transcribe the macrophage colony-stimulating factor (M-CSF) receptor gene, which is a myeloid characteristic.[30] Activation of fms-like tyrosine kinase–3 (FLT3), a growth factor receptor, is required for DC development, and it has been suggested that committed myeloid or lymphoid precursors expressing FLT3 can differentiate into DCs in the presence of FLT3 ligand.[31]

Splenic DCs have a relatively rapid turnover rate (every 3 days).[32] These cells are repopulated both by DC division and splenic precursors, as well as by bone marrow precursors. In contrast, LCs are very long-lived.[32] After their migration from the skin, the population is replenished from a pool of LC precursors in the skin, as well as by circulating monocytes.[33] The latter is dependent on the action of the chemokine CCL2 acting on its receptor CCR2.[34,35] Thus the ontogeny of LCs is distinct from that of splenic DCs. Immature DCs are more closely related to LCs but appear to be derived from noninflammatory monocytes that do not express CCR2.[36] Plasmacytoid DCs split off from conventional DCs early in development, consistent with their distinct functional characteristics.[37]

LANGERHANS CELL HISTIOCYTOSIS

The hallmark of LCH is the accumulation of LC-like DCs in one or more tissues or organs. The clinical manifestations of LCH are highly diverse. They result both from the direct, local effects of the growth and accumulation of pathologic LCs and the indirect, secondary effects these activated cells have on normal tissues, particularly cells of the immune system. Although the most commonly involved sites of disease are the bone and skin, virtually any organ or system may be involved. The pattern of involvement is not necessarily related to patterns of normal LC or DC migration.

Although the histiocytes in LCH share certain characteristics with LCs, such as expression of CD1a and the presence of Birbeck granules, recent reports suggest that mature LCs may not be the cell of origin for LCH histiocytes. In particular, a global analysis of gene expression suggested that LCH cells are more closely related to myeloid dendritic precursors than to LCs.[38] Whether this pattern of gene expression reflects a non-LC cell origin for LCH or is a consequence of LC transformation remains to be determined.

The fact that pathologic LCs are related to immunomodulatory cells and that they elicit inflammatory infiltrates suggests that LCH might be a reactive rather than a neoplastic disease. Indeed, ample precedent for this mechanism exists among the histiocytoses, including the secondary HLH syndromes that arise in the context of viral infection.[39] However, no reproducible reports exist of viral genomes recovered from LCH cells, and epidemiologic studies are not consistent with an infectious or environmental cause of LCH.[40,41,42,43] Rather, the preponderance of evidence indicates that LCH arises as a consequence of intrinsic genetic abnormalities. The most salient arguments that LCH is a neoplasm and not a reactive disease are as follows: (1) pathologic LCs are clonal,

as demonstrated by nonrandom X chromosome inactivation both in whole LCH tissue (in a proportion corresponding to the proportion of CD1a+ cells in the lesion)[42] and in sorted CD1a+ cells,[44] and (2) nearly 60% of LCH samples carry the oncogenic BRAF V600E variant.[45,46] Notably, the MAPK pathway, which would be activated constitutively in the presence of BRAF V600E, is uniformly activated in LCH cells regardless of the presence or absence of BRAF V600E, suggesting that alternative mechanisms of pathway activation are present in LCH samples that lack BRAF V600E. In some cases, other activating mutations of BRAF have been found.[46,47] Additional known mechanisms of BRAF activation, such as gene amplification or translocation, which occur in other diseases, have not been described in LCH.[45] Notably, although pulmonary LCH in adults is generally considered to be a polyclonal disease, more than 40% of pulmonary LCH cases contain BRAF V600E.[45] This finding suggests that a significant proportion of these cases are clonal[48] or that multiple independently developed clones of pulmonary LCH have BRAF V600E, giving the overall appearance of polyclonality.

Although BRAF mutations are among the most common molecular abnormalities found in all cancers, they are not present in other histiocytoses that affect children, such as juvenile xanthogranuloma (JXG) or Rosai-Dorfman disease.[45,49] However, BRAF V600E mutations are present in the histiocytes of about 50% of patients with Erdheim-Chester disease, a rare and aggressive non-LCH of adults.[49] Furthermore, treatment of patients who have BRAF V600E–positive Erdheim-Chester disease with a BRAF inhibitor led to dramatic clinical responses, indicating the pathogenetic importance of this mutation.[50] Interestingly, some of these patients had concomitant LCH that also responded to BRAF inhibition, suggesting that this therapeutic approach may be effective in patients who have BRAF V600E–positive LCH as well.

Activating mutations of BRAF are insufficient by themselves to produce neoplastic disease, and therefore additional molecular alterations are likely to be required for the development of LCH. One of the most common molecular abnormalities in LCH is overexpression of TP53,[51] suggesting that mutational inactivation of this pathway may contribute to pathogenesis. More such changes in other genes are likely to be discovered as advanced genomic analyses are applied to LCH samples.

Incidence

The incidence of LCH is difficult to determine precisely because of the rarity and marked clinical variability of the disorder. Estimates are in the range of 2.6 to 8.9 cases per million per year for children younger than 15 years,[52-55] corresponding to roughly one tenth the incidence of acute leukemia in childhood. LCH occurs in people of all races and all ages. Although the peak age at diagnosis is 2 years, LCH can present at any time from birth to old age. No evidence of seasonal variation has been noted in the time of presentation of LCH. Several studies have shown a slight male predominance.[56,57]

No known predisposing factors exist for the development of LCH in the majority of cases.[58] Studies have demonstrated concordance of the disorder in monozygotic twins, suggesting an inherited predisposition to LCH that might account for ~1% of cases.[59] However, a positive family history is lacking in most cases. Interestingly, isolated pulmonary LCH in adults is closely linked to cigarette smoking, and it often resolves with smoking cessation.[60] However, exposure to cigarette smoke has not been linked to pediatric LCH.[61] As previously noted, a significant proportion of pulmonary LCH cases also carry the activated BRAF V600E allele.

An intriguing (although incompletely understood) association exists between malignancy and LCH. Children with a history of cancer have an increased risk of LCH. Conversely, children with a history of LCH appear to have an increased risk of cancer. This finding suggests the possibility that underlying genetic abnormalities may place individual patients at increased risk for LCH.[62] Alternatively, the association between LCH and cancer may fall within the spectrum of secondary posttherapy effects, because irradiation and drugs such as etoposide are used to treat LCH and are known to induce tumor-promoting genotoxic injury. Several cases of LCH arising in the setting of T-cell acute lymphoblastic leukemia have been described, typically when the leukemia is in remission while the patient is receiving therapy or in the early posttherapy period.[63] A clonal link between the initial leukemia and pathologic LCs of LCH has been established in some cases, suggesting that the LCH represents a manifestation of the malignant clone rather than a distinct reactive or neoplastic process related to the leukemia or its therapy.[64,65] An intriguing link may exist to hairy cell leukemia, which also harbors BRAF V600E in the majority of cases.[66]

Clinical Features

The clinical manifestations of LCH are protean. Although patterns of clinical presentation have been described, the disease is appropriately viewed as a spectrum. LCH may involve a single site, multiple sites in a single organ system, or multiple organ systems. Many patients present with localized pain, soft tissue swelling, or skin rash. Less commonly, patients have symptoms of diabetes insipidus (DI), respiratory insufficiency, cytopenias, lymphadenopathy, liver dysfunction, or organomegaly.

In the past, three distinct clinical syndromes were described: eosinophilic granuloma, Hand-Schüller-Christian disease, and Letterer-Siwe disease.[67,68] "Eosinophilic granuloma," a term still commonly used by radiologists and orthopedists, refers to the presence of one or more lytic bone lesions. Hand-Schüller-Christian disease consists of the triad of bone defects, exophthalmos, and polyuria. Letterer-Siwe disease, a fulminant disorder of the reticuloendothelial system, is characterized by hepatosplenomegaly, lymphadenopathy, skin rash, bone lesions, anemia, and the tendency to bleed. This classification has important historic significance, but its applicability in the clinical setting is limited. Once it was recognized that the diverse manifestations of the disease share common histopathologic features, the three syndromes were unified under the term "histiocytosis X."[69] Categorizing patients based on the number and location of lesions and the presence or absence of organ involvement was shown to be useful in predicting prognosis and determining therapy.[70-74] Single-system LCH (SS-LCH) disease—which usually affects bone, less frequently affects skin, and rarely affects the lymph nodes, lung, or central nervous system—accounts for approximately two thirds of pediatric LCH cases. Involvement of two or more organ systems, referred to as multisystem LCH (MS-LCH), accounts for the remaining one third of cases. In about half of MS-LCH cases, "risk" organs (i.e., the liver, spleen, and hematopoietic system) are affected.[55,75] Thus far the presence of BRAF V600E does not correlate with disease extent or prognosis.

Pathology

A biopsy of lesional tissue is required to establish the diagnosis of LCH. The pathologic diagnosis is usually straightforward, but because the disease is rare, varied, and may mimic many other conditions, delay in diagnosis is common. LCH should be considered in any patient who presents with skeletal lesions, a persistent rash, chronically draining ears, central DI, unexplained lymphadenopathy, respiratory insufficiency with a reticulonodular pattern on a chest radiograph, hepatosplenomegaly, or cytopenias.

Once clinical suspicion is raised, the workup should proceed with a biopsy of the most accessible site of disease. Complete surgical excision of the lesion is generally unnecessary either for diagnosis or treatment. LCH lesions at all sites share common histopathologic features: accumulation of large neoplastic LCs with a moderate amount of dense pink cytoplasm and plump, distinctive "C-shaped," "coffee bean," or cleaved nuclei admixed with variable numbers of inflammatory cells, including T lymphocytes, macrophages, plasma cells, and eosinophils. The composition and architecture of the infiltrate characteristically differ according to the location. Osteolytic bone lesions often contain many nonneoplastic osteoclasts, as well as multinucleated tumor giant cells and large numbers of eosinophils, the latter speaking to the origin of the term "eosinophilic granuloma." Mature, "burned out" bone lesions may be difficult to distinguish from chronic osteomyelitis, which is often in the clinical and radiographic differential diagnosis. LCH infiltration of the skin typically involves the superficial dermis, with tumor cells infiltrating the epidermis (so-called "epidermotropism" or "exocytosis"), thus altering epidermal barrier function and leading to superinfection and the characteristic appearance of some LCH rashes. In all cases, the neoplastic LCs express the LC markers CD1a[16] and langerin,[76,77] as well as S100 protein[78] and fascin[79] (Fig. 64-1). Electron microscopy, which historically is used to demonstrate the presence of Birbeck granules indicative of the LC lineage, has little diagnostic utility at the present time. Cytogenetics or molecular studies are predominately needed to exclude other diseases with similar clinical presentations or histologies. Furthermore, no immunohistochemical or other laboratory methods are useful in

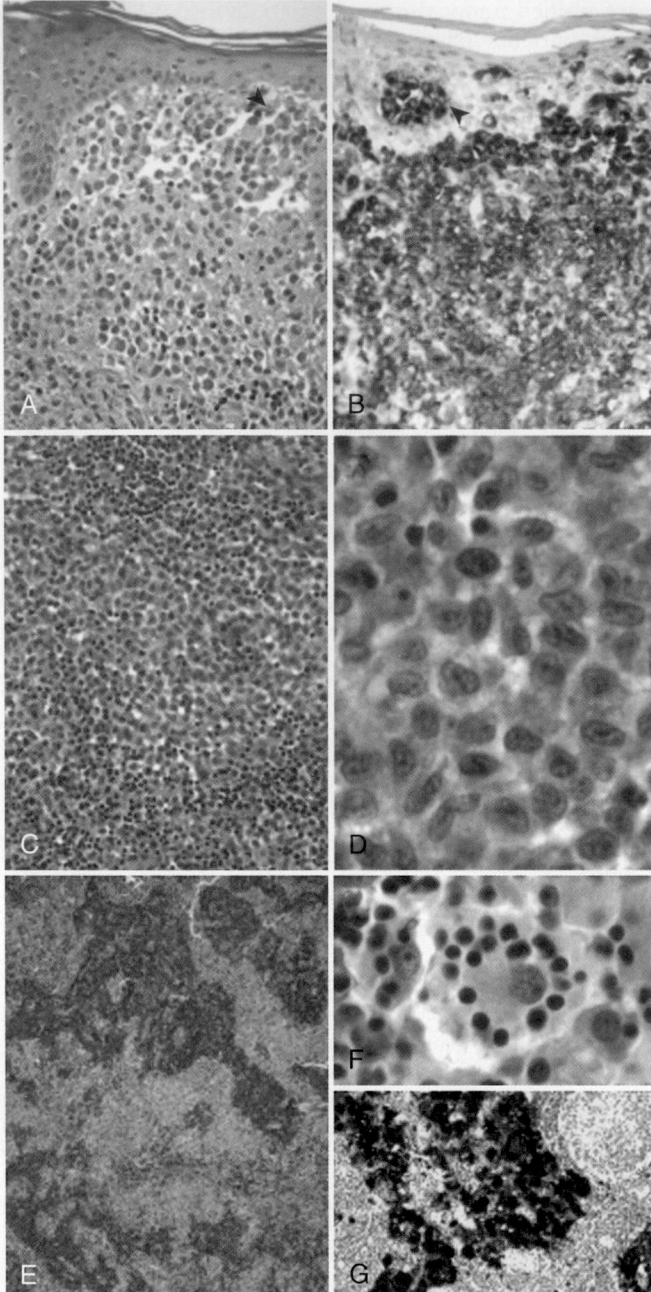

Figure 64-1 Histopathologic features of Langerhans cell histiocytosis (LCH) and sinus histiocytosis with massive lymphadenopathy (SHML). **A** and **B**, Hematoxylin and eosin (**A**) and CD1a immunostain (**B**) of LCH involving the skin. Lesional cells infiltrate the upper dermis and focally *(arrowheads)* involve the epidermis. **C** and **D**, Low-power (200× magnification, **C**) and high-power (1000× magnification, **D**) views of a hematoxylin and eosin–stained section of an LCH bone lesion. The low-power view (**C**) demonstrates tumor cells present in association with a mixed inflammatory infiltrate rich in eosinophils. The high-power view (**D**) illustrates the histologic features of the lesional Langerhans cells, including the characteristic "C-shaped" nuclei and abundant pink cytoplasm. **E, F,** and **G,** Low-power (40× magnification, **E**) and high-power (1000× magnification, **F**) views of a hematoxylin and eosin–stained section of SHML involving a lymph node. Pale areas in panel **E** represent dilated sinuses replaced by lesional histiocytes that are highlighted by an S100 immunostain in panel **G**. Panel **F** demonstrates a histiocyte that contains numerous lymphocytes, which is typical of the emperipolesis characteristic of SHML.

distinguishing clinically indolent from clinically aggressive forms of the disease.

Diagnostic Evaluation

In suspected LCH cases, evaluation for disease extent is indicated, starting with a history and physical examination.[80] A skeletal radiographic survey is recommended to comprehensively assess skeletal involvement. Abnormalities detected on plain radiographs may be followed by axial imaging to document the presence of a soft tissue mass.[81,82] Nuclear imaging (i.e., a bone scan or fluorodeoxyglucose positron emission tomography [FDG-PET]) complements the skeletal survey. Compared with plain radiographs, nuclear imaging tests detect active lesions on the basis of increased local metabolic activity. Active bone lesions usually show increased radiotracer uptake, whereas inactive lesions may be undetectable or appear "photopenic." FDG-PET appears to be the most sensitive imaging modality for the detection of lesions in persons with LCH, and it is particularly useful for following up on patients. Unlike a bone scan, PET is capable of detecting extraosseous lesions.[83-85]

Complete blood cell counts and liver function studies should be performed, and liver and spleen size should be assessed by physical examination. Abdominal ultrasound is indicated when laboratory studies are abnormal or if hepatosplenomegaly is present or suspected. The erythrocyte sedimentation rate may be elevated, but it is not a sensitive or specific disease indicator. Measurement of specific gravity of an early morning urine sample is an easy and inexpensive screening test for DI. A formal water deprivation test may be necessary to establish the diagnosis of DI. Magnetic resonance imaging (MRI) of the head should be performed in children with cranial bone lesions and when DI is suspected or confirmed. A chest radiograph should be performed in all cases, and a computed tomography (CT) scan of the chest should be performed if the radiograph findings are abnormal or if the patient has respiratory signs or symptoms. Additional evaluations such as upper/lower endoscopy and biopsies of bone marrow, skin, lymph nodes, and the liver should be considered in the appropriate clinical context.

Management

The approach to management of LCH must account for the variability in its clinical behavior. On one hand, LCH is an uncontrolled accumulation of a clonal population of cells, with the capacity to behave extremely aggressively and the potential to involve multiple sites and organ systems. The process may be driven, in part, by oncogenic variants of *BRAF*. In addition, it may be effectively treated with cytotoxic chemotherapy and radiotherapy and, based on preliminary reports, *BRAF* antagonists.[50] On the other hand, LCH is histologically benign, it sometimes resolves spontaneously, and it may respond to immunomodulatory or immunosuppressive agents. The historic uncertainty about the fundamental nature of LCH is reflected in the broad range of therapies that have been used to treat it.

Performing controlled clinical trials in persons with LCH has been challenging. As a consequence, the LCH literature is often descriptive, anecdotal, and retrospective. Since the 1980s, several collaborative groups have conducted prospective clinical trials that have led to standardization and improvements in treatment. An overall observation of these studies is that the treatment of LCH should match the clinical scenario. Patients with localized disease have an excellent prognosis with little or no intervention. For these children, the goal of therapy is to minimize symptoms and avoid long-term disability and potential late effects. In contrast, children with MS-LCH, especially those with involvement of the hematopoietic system or liver, are at significant risk for morbidity and mortality. For these children, aggressive treatment is justified.

Bone

Bone is the most commonly involved site, with bone involvement occurring in approximately 75% of children with LCH.[57] Although any bone(s) may be affected, the bones of the skull, pelvis, and vertebral bodies are most commonly affected[56] (Fig. 64-2). Bone pain (which is often worse at night), swelling, and a limp are typical presenting symptoms. Sometimes a history of local trauma precedes or coincides with the onset of symptoms. The typical plain radiographic appearance is of a smooth-edged, "punched-out" hole in the bone. Lesions of the long bones typically involve the diaphysis, but metaphyseal and epiphyseal lesions also occur. Involvement of a vertebral body may manifest as flattening or loss of height (vertebra plana) or as a wedge deformity. Axial imaging (CT and MRI) may show an associated soft tissue mass (Fig. 64-3). The radiographic differential diagnosis of osseous LCH lesions includes malignancy, especially Ewing sarcoma, leukemia or lymphoma, and osteomyelitis.

LCH of the bone may be unifocal (monostotic) or multifocal (polyostotic), and it may present in association with disease in other organ systems. Monostotic disease, which is the most common presentation of LCH (especially in older children), occurs in more than 50% of cases.[75,86] Children with LCH that is limited to a single bone have an excellent prognosis regardless of the treatment administered. Although various local and systemic therapies appear to be efficacious,[87] retrospective trials have failed to demonstrate a comparative advantage for any specific intervention or modality, including obser-

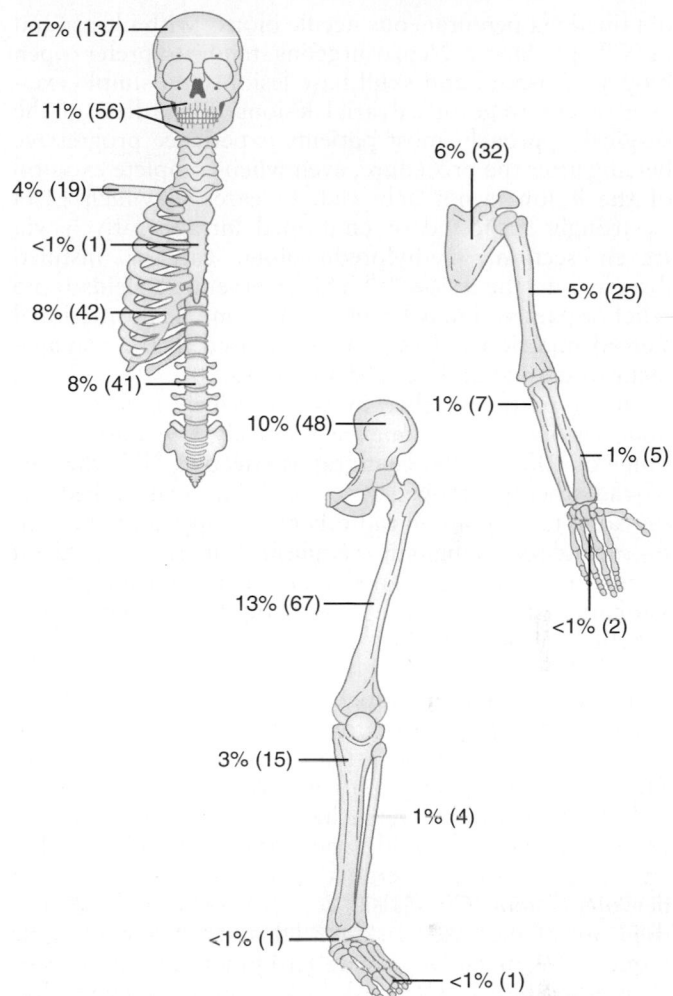

Figure 64-2 Anatomic distribution of 503 osseous lesions among 263 patients with Langerhans cell histiocytosis of bone. *(From Kilpatrick SE, Wenger DE, Gilchrist GS, et al: Langerhans' cell histiocytosis [histiocytosis X] of bone. A clinicopathologic analysis of 263 pediatric and adult cases. Cancer 76:2471–2484, 1995.)*

vation only, biopsy, curettage, simple excision, intralesional steroid instillation, local radiotherapy, or systemic therapy.[88,89]

Often the biopsy procedure performed to establish the diagnosis of LCH of the bone provides therapeutic benefit. In many cases, adequate tissue for diagnosis may be

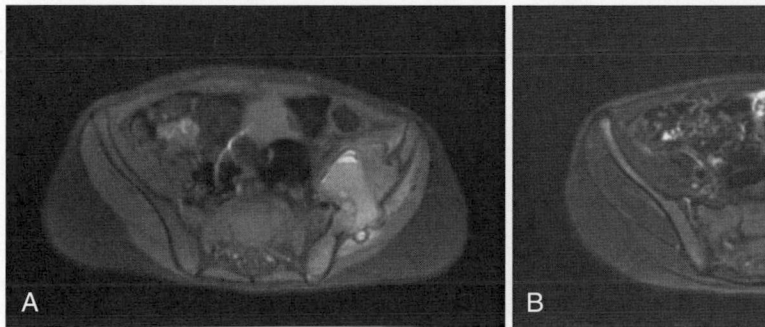

Figure 64-3 Magnetic resonance imaging scans of the pelvis of a 2-year-old boy with unifocal Langerhans cell histiocytosis of the left ilium. An expansile, destructive iliac lesion and large soft tissue mass (**A**) decreased dramatically in size within 3 months after an intralesional glucocorticoid injection (**B**).

obtained via percutaneous needle biopsy with ultrasound or CT guidance. Neurosurgeons tend to prefer open biopsy of orbital and skull base lesions and simple excision or curettage of calvarial lesions. Regardless of the surgical approach, most patients experience progressive healing after the procedure, even when complete excision of the lesion is not achieved. In cases in which LCH is strongly suspected or confirmed intraoperatively via frozen section, methylprednisolone can be instilled directly into the lesion.[90,91] This intervention yields rapid relief of pain and may hasten resolution.[92,93] Intralesional steroid injection is less commonly used in the management of cranial and vertebral lesions.

In the past, radiotherapy was routinely used to treat bone lesions. Even though a relatively low dose in the range of 600 to 1000 centigray is effective,[56,94,95] the role of radiotherapy in pediatric LCH has waned because the long-term risk of radiotherapy, especially the risk of secondary malignant neoplasms, is rarely justified in treatment of a benign disease. In the setting of disseminated disease, local radiotherapy contributes little benefit.[96]

Systemic therapy may be required for patients with monostotic LCH who experience unrelenting symptoms or are at significant risk for serious or permanent disability related to the location or extent of their lesion. This principle applies in patients with unifocal craniofacial bone involvement, including the orbit, temporal bone, mastoid, sphenoid, zygomatic, ethmoid, maxilla, paranasal sinuses, or cranial fossa (so-called "central nervous system [CNS]-risk" lesions), because these children are at increased risk for DI and other neurologic sequelae.[97] Currently it is standard practice to administer chemotherapy in "CNS-risk" cases, even though it has not been definitively established that treatment decreases the risk of neurologic complications.

Systemic therapy is also recommended for children with polyostotic (i.e., multifocal bone) LCH. In these patients, an important goal of treatment is to mitigate the risk of future reactivation,[71,75] because reactivation risk is approximately 40% for patients with multifocal bone disease versus 10% for patients with unifocal bone disease.[98] Children with SS-LCH of the bone who require systemic therapy—that is, those with CNS-risk lesions or multifocal bone involvement—are typically treated with the combination of vinblastine and prednisone (discussed later).

Skin

The skin is the second most commonly involved system in persons with LCH, with skin involvement occurring in about one third of patients.[54,55,71] Skin rashes may be extremely variable, and misdiagnosis is common. Cutaneous LCH may present as single or multiple nodules, vesicles, or scaly, seborrhea-like patches or plaques. Although the rash may be located anywhere on the body, it is typically most intense in the flexural areas, such as the neck, axillary, and inguinal folds. Involvement of the scalp, the ear canals, and the posterior auricular areas is also characteristic. Ear canal involvement may lead to chronic ear drainage that may be malodorous. Perineal and perianal rashes may be severe, persistent, and refractory to topical preparations.

Cutaneous involvement is more common in infants than in older children. Some infants with isolated cutaneous LCH prove to have a benign, self-healing disorder known as Hashimoto-Pritzker disease.[99,100] However, in infants who initially present with apparently isolated cutaneous LCH, MS-LCH may proceed to develop, and therefore self-healing cutaneous LCH is a diagnosis that can be made with accuracy only in retrospect.[101,102] The differential diagnosis of cutaneous LCH may include superficial candidiasis, seborrheic dermatitis ("cradle cap"), eczema, contact dermatitis, and viral exanthem. A skin biopsy is required to establish the diagnosis.

When treatment for cutaneous LCH is required, topical medications such as corticosteroid or nitrogen mustard may suffice.[103,104] Occasionally, systemic therapy is necessary to control extensive or severe skin involvement, especially when it is associated with pain, disfigurement, or infection. Alternatives such as psoralen ultraviolet A[105,106] or interferon[107] have been used with success in some patients who have resistant cutaneous involvement.

Central Nervous System

The brain and skull can be affected by LCH in a variety of ways, including extension of extraaxial bone-based lesions, hypothalamic-pituitary disease, intraparenchymal mass lesions, and later onset neurodegeneration.[108]

Hypothalamic-pituitary disease is the most common and best-characterized CNS manifestation of LCH. Infiltration of the pituitary stalk by lesional cells leads to deficiency of antidiuretic hormone and clinical DI.[109] Anterior pituitary deficiencies or panhypopituitarism may develop in some cases.[110] The diagnosis of DI may precede, coincide with, or occur years after the diagnosis of LCH. Estimates of the frequency of DI in persons with LCH vary considerably because of variability in study populations. One large retrospective review reported a 12% incidence of DI, with 6% having DI present at the time of LCH diagnosis. In this analysis, the risk of DI correlated significantly with the location and extent of LCH involvement. Children who have craniofacial lesions (CNS risk) or MS-LCH are at significantly higher risk for DI.[97]

Among children with a new presentation of DI, LCH is the cause in a significant proportion (approximately 15%) of cases.[111] Absence of posterior pituitary hyperintensity (the pituitary "bright spot") or thickening of the pituitary infundibulum[112] may be noted on brain imaging; however, these radiographic findings are neither sensitive nor specific for LCH. Their differential diagnosis includes brain tumors, especially germinoma, and inflammatory conditions such as hypophysitis. Investigation for other sites of LCH is worthwhile because detection and biopsy of extracranial lesions may allow histopathologic confirmation of the diagnosis without performing a pituitary stalk biopsy.[113]

Screening for DI in children who have LCH with use of a careful history is essential, and referral to an endocrinologist should be considered if symptoms of polyuria, polydipsia, nocturia, or dehydration are elicited. Urinary specific gravity greater than 1.015 weighs against a diagnosis of DI, and this reading can often be easily determined by analysis of a first-morning voided urine specimen. In cases in which the history or laboratory studies raise suspicion, a formal water deprivation test should be performed.

In general, DI is irreversible once it appears in patients with LCH. However, improvement has been reported in "early" DI cases when patients were treated promptly with chemotherapy.[114,115] At one time, emergent radiotherapy was recommended in patients with new onset DI. This recommendation has fallen out of practice because it is rarely, if ever, effective and is associated with potential long-term consequences.[116] Chemotherapy has no role in patients with established, long-standing DI who have no evidence of active LCH within or outside of the CNS.

Parenchymal CNS mass lesions in persons with LCH are composed of granulomas of CD1a+ cells admixed with other inflammatory cells. These lesions can occur in isolation or in association with disease in other organ systems. Depending on the extent and location, headaches, seizures, and focal neurologic symptoms may result. CNS mass lesions are managed with chemotherapy,[117] surgery, or radiotherapy.

Progressive neurodegeneration is an uncommon and poorly understood late event that arises years after LCH diagnosis.[118,119] Radiographically, it is characterized by signal abnormality confined to the brain stem and cerebellum on MRI.[120,121] Posterior fossa symptoms or neurocognitive dysfunction may be clinically apparent. Biopsy results show gliosis, neuronal cell loss, and lymphocytic infiltration without active CD1a+ cell infiltration.[109,122] The timing and course of this manifestation of LCH is quite variable, but it may be severe and progressive. No established treatment exists for neurodegeneration in patients with LCH. Retinoic acid[123] or low-intensity chemotherapy with or without immunoglobulin[38,124] may stabilize the disease or slow the rate of neurologic decline.

Other Sites

Lymph node involvement is occasionally present in the setting of MS-LCH, and sometimes it represents a single site of disease. The pathologic pattern of lymph node involvement is characteristically interfollicular and subtle.

The gastrointestinal tract is another uncommon site of disease in LCH, but its incidence may be underappreciated. When it does occur, it is usually in the context of multisystem involvement.[125] Clinical signs include diarrhea, bloody stools, failure to thrive, and hypoalbuminemia.[125-127] Gastrointestinal biopsies typically demonstrate a sparse infiltrate of LCs in the lamina propria.

Pulmonary involvement was historically thought to be an adverse prognostic feature, warranting its classification as a "risk" organ in early Histiocyte Society clinical trials. Involvement of the lung may be asymptomatic in up to half of affected children, with diffuse micronodular interstitial disease or cyst formation. Overt respiratory symptoms including tachypnea, chronic cough, dyspnea, and pneumothorax are seen in some patients. In children, pulmonary involvement occurs in the context of MS-LCH and is often accompanied by hematologic or hepatic dysfunction. Recent retrospective studies have shown that in the absence of other risk organ involvement, pulmonary involvement is not an independent negative prognostic indicator.[128-130] Interestingly, adults with LCH often present with disease limited to the lung, and their illness is closely linked to cigarette smoking. Cessation of smoking leads to resolution in the majority of patients.[60] Although traditionally described as a polyclonal disease, as many as 30% of cases may be clonal,[48] and a significant proportion harbor BRAF V600E.[45]

Risk Organs

Although the behavior of LCH is unpredictable, it is known that children with disease involving the hematopoietic system or liver are at highest risk for severe illness and death.[72,73] Conventionally, involvement of "risk" organs is defined by the presence of organ dysfunction, such as cytopenias, hyperbilirubinemia, and impaired hepatic synthetic function.[73] Risk organ involvement is typically a component of MS-LCH and is often associated with overt constitutional symptoms. Involvement of one or more risk organs occurs in approximately half of children with MS-LCH. Risk organ involvement is usually present at diagnosis, but it can develop later. It is clearly associated with young age, because more than half of children younger than 2 years manifest risk organ involvement. The association between young age and aggressive disease accounts for the perception that young age is an adverse prognostic feature.[53]

The presence of peripheral blood cytopenias in a patient with LCH is referred to as hematologic dysfunction and is taken to be synonymous with bone marrow involvement. Interestingly, however, evidence of bone marrow infiltration by morphologically apparent LCs is not typically seen. Most often the marrow contains a lymphohistiocytic infiltrate with hemophagocytosis that can be highly reminiscent of hemophagocytic syndromes (which will be discussed later), further illustrating that the neoplastic LCs retain some of the immunomodulatory function of their normal counterparts.[131-134] Splenomegaly is commonly seen in association with hematologic dysfunction as a consequence of organ infiltration, extramedullary hematopoiesis, and hemophagocytosis. Hypersplenism may contribute to cytopenias in these patients.

Hepatic dysfunction, like hematologic dysfunction, is associated with serious illness and a high risk of morbidity and mortality. Hepatic dysfunction is associated with any of the following findings: hepatomegaly, ascites, hyperbilirubinemia, increased serum concentrations of hepatic transaminases (especially γ-glutamyl transferase) and impaired hepatic synthetic function (hypoalbuminemia and hypoproteinemia). The pathogenesis of liver involvement is heterogeneous. In some cases hepatomegaly or transaminitis is a consequence of macrophage activation in a sinusoidal pattern in the liver and is associated with multisystem disease. In other cases, a cholestatic laboratory picture predominates, presumably resulting from the infiltration of hepatic bile ducts by CD1a+ LCs, even if these cells are not demonstrable upon a percutaneous liver biopsy.[135] In these patients, progressive hepatic dysfunction may lead over time to irreversible hepatic cirrhosis that requires liver transplantation, even after resolution of active LCH.[136]

Treatment of Multisystem LCH

Systemic therapy is indicated for all patients with MS-LCH and for some patients with SS- LCH, as previously described. The optimal therapy for this diverse group of patients is still not established. Over the years, a wide variety of immunosuppressive and cytotoxic drugs have demonstrated activity. Encouraging results were first published in the early 1960s using corticosteroids[137] and vinblastine.[138] Later, alkylating agents[139,140] and antimetabolites[141] were used. In the 1980s, the epipodophyllotoxin etoposide was shown to have particular cytotoxicity for cells of the monocyte/macrophage lineage. This agent showed promising results in children with refractory LCH and was subsequently studied in newly diagnosed patients.[142,143,144-146] More recently, the nucleoside analogs 2-chlorodeoxyadenosine (2-CdA)[147-150] and clofarabine[151,152] have shown promise in children with refractory LCH and in adults.[153] Regardless of the treatment regimen, survival among low-risk patients is excellent. However, a substantial proportion of high-risk patients still experience a progressive and fatal course despite therapy.[73,139,154,155]

The Deutsche Arbeitsgemeinschaft fur Leukamieforschung und Behandlung im Kindersalter (German Working Group for Research and Treatment of Leukemia in Childhood) performed two consecutive multicenter studies (known as DAL-HX 83 and DAL-HX 90) in which children with multifocal bone or MS-LCH were treated with a nonrandomized, risk-adapted, prospective, multidrug regimen. After initial therapy with prednisolone, vinblastine, and etoposide, children who had multisystem disease went on to receive 1 year of continuation therapy with prednisolone, vinblastine, etoposide, and mercaptopurine. In the DAL-HX 83 study, patients with organ dysfunction also received methotrexate. In these trials, approximately 67% of the patients who had organ dysfunction responded to therapy, with 42% of these patients experiencing subsequent disease reactivation. In contrast, the patients with multisystem disease who did not have organ dysfunction and the patients with multifocal bone disease had a roughly 90% response rate and a 20% reactivation rate.[71,156] Unfortunately, death due to refractory or progressive LCH occurred in about 20% of subjects in the DAL-HX studies. Mortality was restricted to children with disseminated disease, organ dysfunction, and an unfavorable response to initial therapy.

In 1991, The Histiocyte Society initiated LCH I, the first international, randomized clinical trial in persons with LCH. This study compared the efficacy of 6 months of vinblastine (arm A) versus etoposide (arm B) in children with multisystem disease.[142] The results showed that the two treatment arms, arms A and B, were equivalent in all respects, including response at week 6 (57% and 49%), toxicity (47% and 58%), probability of survival

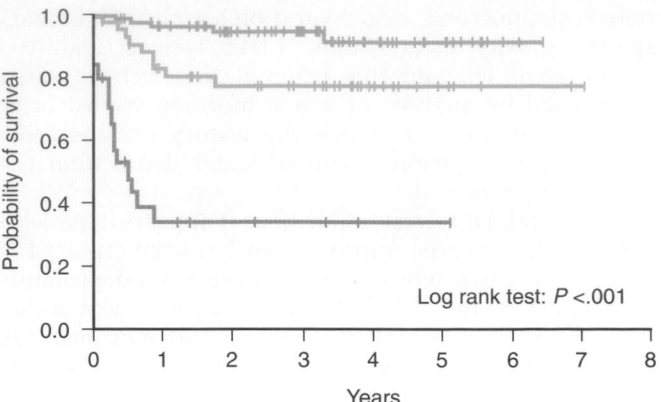

Figure 64-4 Results of the Langerhans cell histiocytosis (LCH) I clinical trial for the treatment of multisystem LCH in children. Survival related to response to treatment at week 6. The *solid line* represents responders ($n = 71/76$), the *dashed line* represents intermediate responders ($n = 32/41$), and the *dotted line* represents nonresponders ($n = 10/25$). *(From Gadner H, Grois N, Arico M, et al: A randomized trial of treatment for multisystem Langerhans' cell histiocytosis. J Pediatr 138:728–734, 2001.)*

(76% and 83%), probability of disease reactivation (61% and 55%), and probability of developing permanent sequelae (39% and 51%), including DI (22% and 23%). Of the 29 children in the study who died as a result of their disease, all had risk organ involvement. The probability of survival among the children older than 2 years who did not have risk organ involvement was 100%. Secondary acute myeloid leukemia developed in one patient in arm B. In light of the fact that etoposide was not superior to vinblastine in any measure, the study suggested that the added risk associated with it may not be justified.

Importantly, analysis of the LCH I study revealed that early response to therapy is an extremely powerful prognostic indicator in persons with MS-LCH. Children younger than 2 years who had MS-LCH and failed to respond to 6 weeks of initial therapy had a dismal 17% survival rate compared with an 88% survival rate in children who responded favorably (Fig. 64-4). The prognostic value of early response was confirmed in a retrospective analysis of the DAL-HX 83 and DAL-HX 90 studies.[157]

The Histiocyte Society's successor study, LCH II, intensified treatment for all patients and further explored the role of etoposide in persons with MS-LCH. All children received 6 weeks of initial therapy that consisted of continuous oral prednisone and weekly administration of vinblastine. Low-risk children who were risk organ negative received continuation therapy with pulse prednisone and vinblastine every 3 weeks for a total of 6 months. High-risk children who were risk organ positive also received mercaptopurine and were randomly assigned to either receive etoposide (arm B) or not receive etoposide (arm A) during both the initial and continuation phases. LCH II did not demonstrate a statistically significant benefit of the addition of etoposide in patients with MS-LCH; response at week 6 (63% vs. 71%), survival (74% vs. 79%), disease reactivation (46% in both arms) and permanent consequences (43% vs. 37%) were all similar in arms A and B, respectively. However, in comparison with the less-intensive therapy studied in the LCH I trial, the more intensive LCH II regimen did show a somewhat higher rapid response rate and lower mortality in children with risk organ involvement.[158]

LCH III opened for enrollment in 2001. For the highest risk group of subjects in this study—that is, the children with MS-LCH who had involvement of risk organs—methotrexate was added to the backbone of prednisone, vinblastine, and mercaptopurine in a randomized fashion. The total duration of therapy was lengthened to 12 months for all high-risk patients. Children without risk organ involvement were randomly assigned to receive vinblastine and prednisone for 6 versus 12 months. The study failed to demonstrate a benefit as a result of the addition of methotrexate to the standard backbone in multisystem high-risk patients. However, prolongation of therapy from 6 to 12 months in multisystem low-risk patients is associated with a significantly lower reactivation rate (a 3-year cumulative incidence of reactivation of 50% vs. 35%).[159]

Refractory Langerhans Cell Histiocytosis

Children with MS-LCH whose disease does not respond promptly to vinblastine and prednisone have an unfavorable prognosis, with survival rates in the range of 10% to 34%.[142,156] Unfortunately, LCH that is resistant to vinblastine and corticosteroid is often unresponsive to other conventional agents. 2-CdA, a nucleoside analog, has shown significant promise as salvage therapy in children with reactivated or refractory disease.[147,160,161] Dramatic responses to 2-CdA combined with cytarabine have been observed in children with refractory LCH who have hematologic dysfunction.[150] Also, the nucleoside analog clofarabine has demonstrated activity in a smaller number of reported cases of refractory MS-LCH.[151,152]

A small but growing number of children with refractory MS-LCH have been successfully treated with allogeneic hematopoietic cell transplantation (HCT).[162-166] Not surprisingly, toxicity is a significant obstacle in these very ill patients. Autologous transplantation has not resulted in durable responses.[167] Transplant regimens that incorporate reduced intensity conditioning are especially appealing in persons with refractory LCH and appear to be feasible, with lower transplant-related morbidity and mortality.[168,169]

Reactivation

Some children experience LCH reactivation after initial improvement or resolution of their disease. Most reactivations occur within 1 year of diagnosis, and almost all develop within 2 years.[75,170] Patients with MS-LCH are clearly at higher risk of reactivation than are patients with SS-LCH. Patients occasionally experience a chronic, relapsing, and remitting course with repeated reactivations. Aggressive radiographic surveillance for reactivation is generally discouraged, because the site of reactivation is unpredictable and the risk of imaging may outweigh the benefit of early diagnosis. However, monitoring physical examination and growth and development is advised, along with prompt evaluation of any new signs or symptoms. Elevation of the erythrocyte sedimentation rate and the platelet count can be a tip-off to disease reactivation.[171]

Bone is the most frequent site of LCH reactivation. Fortunately, reactivation in risk organs is distinctly uncommon in children who did not have risk organ involvement at presentation.[172] Localized reactivations, such as a single bony site or recurrent rash, may be effectively managed with local therapy alone (i.e., surgery or intralesional or topical administration of a corticosteroid). However, systemic therapy is often necessary in persons with reactivated disease to control symptoms, prevent permanent sequelae, and decrease the severity and frequency of subsequent reactivations. In contrast to recurrent malignancies in which acquired drug resistance limits the efficacy of cytotoxic drugs after previous exposure, in reactivated cases of LCH, medications used successfully in the setting of newly diagnosed disease often remain effective in the treatment of reactivation. When cytotoxic therapies such as corticosteroids, vinca alkaloids, antimetabolites, or nucleoside analogues fail to provide durable disease control or when adverse effects are limiting, more intensive and less conventional options are worth exploring. For these relatively rare cases, therapy must be individualized, keeping in mind the specific site(s), symptoms, and risk of the reactivation, as well as the specific adverse effects of therapy.

Alternatives to conventional therapy that have been used in bone reactivation include nonsteroidal antiinflammatory agents (e.g., indomethacin)[106] and bisphosphonates (e.g., pamidronate).[173,174] These agents may act to ameliorate pain but may not directly inhibit disease activity. Thalidomide has shown some efficacy in patients with low-risk LCH that is refractory to conventional therapy. The presumed mechanism of action is by inhibition of TNF or other cytokines.[175] Many children who undergo repeated reactivations experience permanent disabilities related to their LCH. Nonetheless, their overall likelihood of survival approaches 100%.[76]

Long-Term Consequences

Roughly half of survivors of LCH experience irreversible long-term consequences of their illness or, to a lesser extent, of the therapy they received. The incidence and pattern of sequelae strongly correlate with the initial extent and pattern of disease involvement; patients who experience multisystem disease and multiple reactivations are at highest risk.[170,176,177] A considerable fraction of irreversible complications observed in survivors of LCH were present at the time of diagnosis, and thus not all long-term complications are preventable.

Orthopedic complications are the most frequently observed permanent sequelae in survivors of SS-LCH. Examples include spinal deformity leading to scoliosis or kyphosis, dental loss due to involvement of the jaw, and facial asymmetry or proptosis due to involvement of orbital or facial bones. Although conductive hearing loss attributed to chronic inflammation of the middle and external ear is reversible, sensorineural hearing loss due to involvement of osseous structures is usually permanent when it occurs. Although permanent orthopedic and cosmetic consequences are relatively frequent, they do not necessarily adversely affect the quality of survival.[76]

DI is an irreversible condition in almost all cases in which it occurs, and a lifelong need for desmopressin is to be expected. Similarly, other endocrinopathies such as growth hormone deficiency and panhypopituitarism are not responsive to LCH-directed therapy but are managed with hormone supplementation. Awareness and close attention to growth and development are very important in the follow-up care of these patients.[97]

Rarely, survivors of LCH experience progressive end organ damage in the absence of demonstrable activity of LCs. Progressive hepatic cirrhosis with liver failure requiring liver transplantation is a rare but well-recognized late event.[136] A somewhat analogous process may occur in the lungs, leading to pulmonary fibrosis, cystic changes, or spontaneous pneumothorax. Adult survivors of pediatric LCH should be counseled to avoid exposure to cigarette smoke because of the potentially increased risk of developing pulmonary abnormalities.[178] Neurodegeneration, which was previously described, is the most dreaded late event in survivors of LCH.

Overview of Therapeutic Options

Approach to SS-LCH

Children with localized SS-LCH have an excellent prognosis. Most children with localized disease may be safely observed after a biopsy or resection is performed, without the need for additional intervention. Local therapy may be added to accelerate resolution of symptoms. In patients with craniofacial bone or multifocal bone disease or isolated CNS involvement, systemic therapy is indicated to control symptoms and to prevent reactivations and long-term (especially orthopedic and neuroendocrine) sequelae.

Approach to Low-Risk MS-LCH

Children with MS-LCH who do not have involvement of risk organs have an excellent prognosis. Because their course is generally favorable, maximizing response while minimizing short- and long-term toxicities is the primary objective. When possible, enrollment in a clinical trial is encouraged. The current standard of care in the United States is the combination of vinblastine and prednisone for a total duration of 12 months.

Approach to High-Risk MS-LCH

Thus far, up-front intensification of therapy has not been shown to improve outcome in children with MS-LCH who have involvement of risk organs. Children with high-risk features who respond favorably to standard chemotherapy have a good prognosis, but children who do not respond rapidly to standard treatment have a poor prognosis. For this group of patients, intensive chemotherapy, investigational agents, or HCT should be considered.

The role of *BRAF* inhibitors in patients whose LCH cells harbor oncogenic *BRAF* variants remains to be established. The increased risk of squamous cell carcinomas of the skin associated with the currently available inhibitors will likely restrict their use to patients with a poor prognosis in whom the benefits may outweigh the risks.

NON–LANGERHANS CELL HISTIOCYTOSES

In addition to LCH, a spectrum of other even rarer histiocytic lesions exists that affect both children and adults. In general they include a large number of clinically benign, not infrequently progressive dermatologic disorders that are pathologically characterized by proliferations of Langerhans-like cells, often with distinctive cytosolic features[179,180] (see Fig. 64-1). Other rare non-LCHs, most notably Erdheim-Chester disease and the "true" malignancies such as Langerhans cell sarcoma and histiocytic sarcoma,[181] have high mortality rates. With the exception of JXG and sinus histiocytosis with massive lymphadenopathy (SHML), these disorders will not be discussed further because of their rarity, and the reader is referred to several authoritative reviews on these diseases.[179,180]

Juvenile Xanthogranuloma

JXG is a generally benign tumoral proliferation of histiocytes with a CD1a–, S100–, Langerin–, CD68+, CD163+, fascin+ immunophenotype that, like LCH, is believed to be derived from dermal interstitial DCs. Lesions characteristically present as reddish to yellowish-brown cutaneous nodules in the head and neck region of children younger than 1 year of age; the median age of onset is 5 months, and tumors may be congenital. Multifocality is not uncommon, particularly in male infants.[180,182] An association exists with neurofibromatosis 1, Noonan syndrome, and juvenile myelomonocytic leukemia.[183] The natural history of most lesions is spontaneous regression, but they are often diagnosed by excisional biopsy, leaving little or no residual tumor. Extranodal involvement of the deep soft tissues, liver, spleen, conjunctivae, and the CNS—so-called systemic JXG—with or without cutaneous involvement occurs in nearly 5% of cases.[182,184] Although systemic lesions also typically regress, local disease, as in the eye and CNS, may lead to significant morbidity. Patients with systemic disease involving the CNS or liver have occasionally died of their disease.[182,184,185] In cases requiring treatment, single agents[186,187] or multiagent regimens similar to those used for persons with LCH have been employed with success.[188]

Sinus Histiocytosis with Massive Lymphadenopathy

SHML, also known by the eponym Rosai-Dorfman disease,[189] is an enigmatic histiocytic disorder associated with a proliferation of CD1a–, Langerin–, S100+, CD68+, CD163+, fascin+ histiocytes with abundant foamy cytoplasm.[180] Most characteristically, a subset of lesional histiocytes contains a large number of lymphocytes and other cells, but unlike in the hemophagocytic syndromes (discussed later), these cells are not contained within phagolysosomes. Rather, they are "just passing through" in invaginations of the cell membrane, in a process termed *emperipolesis*[190] (see Fig. 64-1). In lymph nodes, these histiocytes preferentially involve the nodal sinuses and secondarily the interfollicular areas, leading to remarkably huge lymphadenopathy, which gives the disease its name.

Because the SHML literature is largely retrospective, particularly since 1990 when a patient registry was last updated,[191] the reported patterns of clinical presentation and natural history of the disease are undoubtedly biased. Nevertheless, the prototypical clinical presentation is massive, painless cervical lymphadenopathy. In addition, up to 40% of patients present with extranodal disease, most commonly in the skin, upper respiratory tract, and bone.[191] The orbit and meninges are also not uncommon extranodal sites.[192,193] Although extensive nodal and extranodal (especially kidney, lower airway, and liver) disease and coexisting immunologic disorders tend to correlate with an adverse prognosis, it is apparent that many if not most cases remit spontaneously without therapy.[191,194,195] Constitutional symptoms including fever associated with neutrophilia, increased erythrocyte sedimentation rate, and polyclonal hypergammaglobulinemia that are often associated with SHML usually respond to systemic corticosteroids. In cases in which disease has compromised organ function, requiring therapy, no treatment modality is clearly preferred; surgical debulking and radiation therapy generally result in some amelioration, but the response to systemic chemotherapy—often a combination of alkylators, vinca alkaloids, and steroids—is inconsistent.[191,196]

MONOCYTES AND MACROPHAGES

Resident tissue macrophages play essential roles in host defense, especially when they populate tissues that face the external environment (e.g., alveolar macrophages in the lung). However, macrophages also contribute to tissue homeostasis through their repair and clearance activities. Functional and morphologic heterogeneity among macrophages has been long recognized, and identification of specific subsets has been aided by antibody-based identification of characteristic cell surface markers.[197] Some of these subsets may be involved in the histiocytoses of macrophage origin.

Among the macrophages active in host defense and inflammation, alveolar and gut macrophages are best understood. These cells express pattern recognition receptors and scavenger receptors that enhance recognition of microbial products,[198] are highly phagocytic, and are efficient antigen presenters. However, even within this category some degree of heterogeneity exists because gut macrophages tend to secrete lower amounts of proinflammatory cytokines. Kupffer cells are derived from macrophages and may also play a primarily defensive role in the host. In contrast, macrophages involved in homeostasis include osteoclasts and microglia.

Macrophages in secondary lymphoid organs show additional degrees of heterogeneity, with specific cell types occupying characteristic anatomic niches.[198,199] In the spleen, red pulp macrophages, which express high levels of the murine surface marker F4/80, are distinguishable from tingible body macrophages in the white pulp. Also present in the white pulp are metallophilic macrophages, which align adjacent to the marginal sinus.[200] Within the marginal zone itself are functionally distinct macrophages that express pattern recognition and scavenger receptors they may use to clear pathogens from the bloodstream.[201-203] These macrophages express much lower levels of the F4/80 marker than do red pulp macrophages. Similar subanatomic heterogeneity is observed in lymph nodes: macrophages in cortical regions express low levels of F4/80, whereas macrophages in the medullary sinuses, paracortex, and subcapsular sinuses express high levels of F4/80.[204]

In the absence of specific stimuli, tissue macrophages remain in a low-functioning, resting state. Activation induces functions that are characteristic of their host protection or homeostasis roles. Based on in vitro analyses, four distinct pathways of macrophage activation have been described.[205-207] "Classical" activation via interferon-γ or lipopolysaccharide induces microbicidal activities and upregulation of major histocompatibility complex class II expression. "Alternative" activation via IL-4 or IL-13 induces expression of genes that are involved in tissue repair or suppression of inflammation. "Innate" activation via toll-like receptor ligands also induces microbicidal activities. Finally, "deactivation" via IL-10 or transforming growth factor–β stimulation reduces class II expression and increases secretion of antiinflammatory cytokines. As clearly defined as these pathways are in vitro, little evidence exists as yet that they are relevant in vivo. However, secretion of cytokines by activated macrophage-derived cells may be a major pathophysiologic factor in histiocytoses.[208] The first and third mechanisms lead to the production of what are sometimes called "M1" macrophages, whereas the second and fourth mechanisms produce "M2" macrophages.[209]

Origins of Macrophages

For the most part, steady-state renewal of tissue macrophages appears to be accomplished by local proliferation of similar cell types. However, under conditions of rapid turnover such as inflammatory states, macrophages are replaced by bone marrow precursors—that is, circulating monocytes.[210] Recent findings have revealed substantial heterogeneity among circulating monocytes and the roles played by specific subsets in macrophage development.

Broadly defined, circulating monocytes can be separated into "classical" or inflammatory cells versus "resident" cells, which have a phenotype that closely resembles tissue macrophages.[197,211] Cell surface markers can distinguish these subsets: inflammatory monocytes are CD14hi CD16– in humans and Ly6C+ in mice; resident monocytes are CD14+ CD16+ in humans and Ly6C– in mice. Experiments in mice have tracked the fate of some of these cells.[212] For example, bone marrow–derived Ly6C+ cells, which express high levels of the chemokine receptor CCR2 and low levels of the chemokine receptor CX3CR1, enter the circulation. Ordinarily, these cells are very short-lived, but in inflammatory states, they are attracted to affected sites where they can differentiate into macrophages or DCs. Meanwhile, the precise process whereby circulating monocytes replenish resident macrophages (which are CCR2–, CX3CR1hi, Ly6C–) is unknown. Nonetheless, some of the signals that dictate tissue-specific macrophage differentiation are understood. For example, circulating mononuclear precursors that localize to bone will become osteoclasts under the influence of m-CSF and receptor activator of nuclear factor kappa-B ligand,[213] which may have pathophysiologic relevance in histiocytic disorders that attack bone.

HEMOPHAGOCYTIC LYMPHOHISTIOCYTOSIS

HLH is not a single disease entity but rather a syndrome consisting of clinical signs and laboratory abnormalities that result from the uncontrolled proliferation and activation of cells of the monocyte/macrophage lineage. Normally, monocytes and macrophages are responsible for phagocytosis of antigen and activation of other immune cells through the production of cytokines and chemokines. By way of their interactions with natural killer (NK) cells, macrophages are an important feature of the innate immune response. Additionally, they participate in adaptive immunity via their complex interactions with T cells. When pathogens, especially viral pathogens, are not rapidly eliminated by the innate immune response, the chemokines and cytokines produced by activated macrophages stimulate and perpetuate T-lymphocyte activation. Activated macrophages are themselves regulated by stimulatory and inhibitory factors that they and other immune cells produce. When this complex process escapes control, extremely potent and destructive inflammatory forces are unleashed. Uncontrolled macrophage activity is the hallmark of HLH. Although the pathogenetic mechanisms underlying the hyperinflammatory state in HLH are heterogeneous, the clinical consequences are shared.

The earliest published reports of hemophagocytic syndrome by Farquhar described four siblings who were afflicted in early infancy with fever, irritability, hepatosplenomegaly, and pancytopenia. Autopsy demonstrated histiocytic proliferation throughout the reticuloendothelial system with prominent hemophagocytosis.[214,215] The disorder was dubbed "familial haemophagocytic reticulosis" and was recognized as distinct from Letterer-Siwe disease (i.e., the disseminated form of LCH).[216] An autosomal-recessive pattern of inheritance was proposed. Subsequently, sporadic cases with similar clinical features were seen in association with viral infections,[217] bacterial infections,[218] and a host of other infections.[219] Concomitantly, it was observed that certain systemic illnesses, notably rheumatologic conditions and malignancies, occasionally led to the development of clinical features of hemophagocytic syndrome. In 1987, the Histiocyte Society adopted the unifying term *hemophagocytic lymphohistiocytosis* and defined a set of diagnostic criteria to assist clinicians and researchers. The criteria have subsequently been refined to account for advances in our understanding of the syndrome[220,221] (Box 64-2).

Incidence

HLH is broadly categorized into two forms: familial (FHL) and secondary (sHLH). Undoubtedly the delineation is an oversimplification, because significant clinical and perhaps even genetic overlap exists between the two forms. Importantly, FHL and sHLH may be indistinguishable at presentation.

In persons with FHL, an ordinary immune stimulus, such as a common viral exposure, triggers an unrestrained hyperinflammatory state as a result of the existence of an inherited, intrinsic defect in the patient's immunologic effector function. FHL is genetically heterogeneous, resulting from mutations that disturb the function of one or more of several proteins that participate in lymphocyte cytotoxicity. Approximately 1 in 50,000 live births are estimated to be affected by FHL.[222] A slight preponderance of males may be attributable to the occurrence of FHL in association with X-linked lymphoproliferative disorders.

In contrast, sHLH develops as a consequence of an intense immunologic stimulus in the form of an infection, malignancy, or inflammatory process in a person without an inherited immune defect. sHLH is more prevalent than

---

Box 64-2   Diagnostic Guidelines

DIAGNOSTIC GUIDELINES (1994)*

CLINICAL CRITERIA
- Fever
- Splenomegaly

LABORATORY CRITERIA
- Cytopenias (hemoglobin <9 g/L; platelets <100 × 109/L; neutrophils <1.0 × 109/L)
- Hypertriglyceridemia and/or hypofibrinogenemia (fasting triglycerides ≥3 SD, fibrinogen ≤3 SD of normal for age)

HISTOPATHOLOGIC CRITERIA
- Hemophagocytosis in marrow, spleen, or lymph nodes
- No evidence of malignancy

REVISED DIAGNOSTIC GUIDELINES (2004)

Molecular diagnosis consistent with hemophagocytic lymphohistiocytosis OR five of the following eight clinical, laboratory, and histopathologic criteria

CLINICAL CRITERIA
- Fever
- Splenomegaly

LABORATORY CRITERIA
- Cytopenias (hemoglobin <9 g/L; platelets <100 × 109/L; neutrophils <1.0 × 109/L)
- Hypertriglyceridemia or hypofibrinogenemia (fasting triglycerides ≥3 standard deviations, fibrinogen ≤3 standard deviations of normal for age)
- Hyperferritinemia (>500 μg/L)
- Elevated CD25 (≥2400 U/L)
- Low/absent natural killer function

HISTOPATHOLOGIC CRITERIA
- Hemophagocytosis in marrow, spleen, or lymph nodes with no evidence of malignancy

Data from Henter JI, Horne A, Arico M, et al: HLH-2004: diagnostic and therapeutic guidelines for hemophagocytic lymphohistiocytosis. Pediatr Blood Cancer *48:124–131, 2007; and Henter JI, Elinder G, Ost A: Diagnostic guidelines for hemophagocytic lymphohistiocytosis. The FHL Study Group of the Histiocyte Society.* Semin Oncol *18:29–33, 1991.*
*All criteria required. If hemophagocytic activity is not proven at presentation, further search is encouraged.

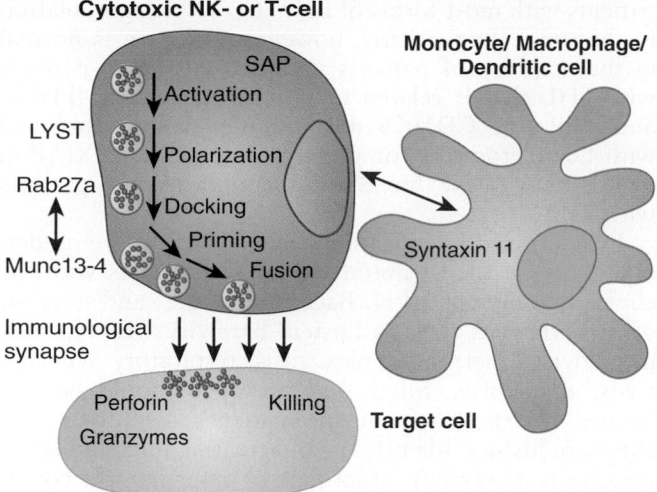

Figure 64-5 Mechanics of cytotoxic function revealed by hemophagocytic lymphohistiocytosis (HLH)-associated gene mutations. HLH-associated genetic abnormalities (in the indicated genes) may affect granule-dependent lymphocyte cytotoxicity by impairing trafficking, docking, priming for exocytosis, or membrane fusion of cytolytic granules. The function of this pathway may also be severely impaired by loss of functional perforin, the key delivery molecule for proapoptotic granzymes. Diverse mutations in this pathway all give rise to similar clinical phenotypes (albeit of variable severity). *LYST* (the gene affected in Chédiak-Higashi syndrome) is not portrayed because its function is not entirely clear, although it appears to play an important role in the maintenance of normally sized (and functional) cytolytic granules. *(From Jordan MB, Allen CE, Weitzman S, et al: How I treat hemophagocytic lymphohistiocytosis. Blood 118:4041–4052, 2011.)*

FHL,[223] but its true incidence in children and adults is not defined.

Clinical Features

The cardinal clinical features of HLH are persistent high fever, cytopenias, and splenomegaly, with or without hepatomegaly. Unquestionably, this constellation of signs and symptoms is not rare or specific. Furthermore, establishing the diagnosis is made more difficult by the fact that all clinical features of the disorder may not be initially or simultaneously present (Fig. 64-5).

Persistent and prolonged fever is essentially universal and is usually the first sign of illness. Signs of a routine childhood upper respiratory or gastrointestinal illness often accompany the fever. However, instead of resolving in the typical time course, constitutional symptoms generally progress in children who have HLH. At presentation, affected patients are usually acutely ill and require urgent evaluation and intervention.

Cytopenias that affect at least two cell lines are a key feature of HLH. Thrombocytopenia is almost always present. The platelet count may be normal or mildly depressed initially, but it often falls precipitously as the disease progresses. Normocytic anemia with reticulocytopenia is also common. In cytopenic patients, less than the expected increment may be seen in response to transfusions because of shortened survival of transfused blood cells. Leukopenia and neutropenia are more variably present.

Abdominal distention and hepatosplenomegaly are usually present and may be accompanied by jaundice and ascites. Biochemical evidence of liver dysfunction is typical, although it is not a universal feature of HLH. Hypertriglyceridemia,[224,225] increased transaminases, or hyperbilirubinemia may be present and may in a very young child raise the possibility of primary liver disease or a metabolic disorder. Impaired hepatic synthetic function and clotting factor consumption leads to hypofibrinogenemia and prolongation of the prothrombin and partial thromboplastin times. When coagulopathy is combined with thrombocytopenia, the risk of bleeding escalates.[226] Spontaneous hemorrhage, especially intracranially, may lead to acute decompensation and may raise an erroneous suspicion of child abuse.[227]

Typically, the serum ferritin level is markedly elevated in patients who have active HLH.[228,229] A serum ferritin level exceeding 10,000 µg/L is a highly sensitive and specific marker that supports the diagnosis.[230,231] However, although most patients with HLH have an increased ferritin level, not all patients demonstrate extreme hyperferritinemia. Furthermore, mild to moderate elevation in the serum ferritin level may be seen in disorders other than HLH, such as inflammatory conditions, infections, liver disease, hemochromatosis, and metabolic disorders. The precise mechanism of ferritin elevation in persons with HLH is unknown, but it is probably related both to increased synthesis of ferritin mediated by high levels of cytokines[232] and increased release of ferritin due to liver injury and red blood cell turnover.

In keeping with a state of generalized, uncontrolled inflammation, the levels of various cytokines are increased in patients with active HLH, including IL-2, IL-6, IL-8, IL-10, interferon, and TNF.[233-235] Cytokine levels are not routinely measured, but the soluble IL-2 receptor (also known as CD25) is available as a clinical laboratory test. CD25 elevation is a sensitive and reliable marker of HLH activity,[236] and it has been incorporated into the diagnostic criteria for HLH.[220] CD25 levels are also elevated in other disorders, especially lymphoid malignancies, but typically to a lesser degree.

The term *hemophagocytosis* describes the pathologic finding of activated, histologically benign macrophages engulfing erythrocytes, leukocytes, platelets, and their precursor cells (Fig. 64-6). This process is often assessed in the bone marrow, but it occurs throughout the reticuloendothelial system (i.e., in the liver, spleen, and lymph nodes) and sometimes in the CNS. Destruction of blood cells and their precursors leads to peripheral blood cytopenia(s), often in association with bone marrow hypercellularity. Analysis of the bone marrow is always recommended when a diagnosis of HLH is suspected, both to demonstrate hemophagocytosis and to rule out the presence of leukemia/lymphoma. Although the finding of hemophagocytosis in the bone marrow supports the diagnosis of HLH in the proper clinical context, it is not essential for the diagnosis or pathognomonic. In a series of 122 children with HLH from the Histiocyte Society's International Registry, only 75% had evidence of hemophagocytosis at diagnosis.[237] In some cases, repeated bone marrow analyses may be necessary to document hemophagocytosis. Neither the pathophysiologic basis for hemophagocytosis nor its precise mechanism is well

Clinical features

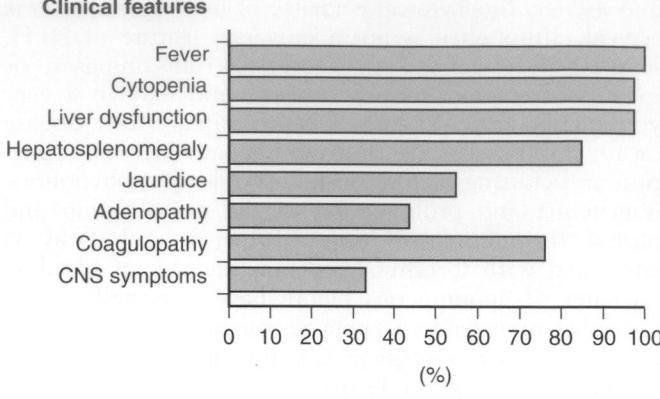

Laboratory findings

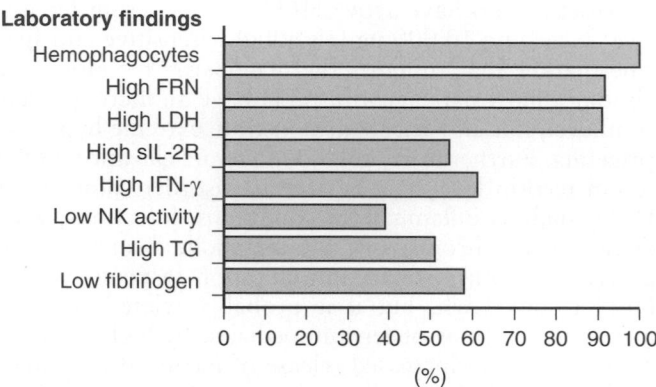

Figure 64-6 Incidence of clinical features and abnormal laboratory findings in 82 cases of hemophagocytic lymphohistiocytosis. *CNS,* Central nervous system; *FRN,* ferritin (normal range 8 to 78 μg/L); *IFN-γ,* interferon gamma; *LDH,* lactate dehydrogenase (normal range, 234 to 471 IU/L); *NK,* natural killer; *sIL-2R,* CD25 (normal range, <1090 U/mL); *TG,* triglycerides.[328]

understood. In HLH, hemophagocytosis is a reactive process that presumably results from the dysregulated immune response.

Despite the hyperactivity of the immune response in HLH and the presence of normal numbers of effector cells in many cases, targeted killing by these cells is depressed or absent. In the laboratory, impaired effector function may be demonstrated with use of a standard chromium release assay against K562 target cells. In the setting of active HLH of any variety, the functional activity of NK cells is usually impaired.[238] Manipulation of the conditions of the NK cell functional assay by the addition of mitogen or IL-2 or prolonged incubation times results in restoration of NK cell function in some patient samples.[239] It appears that the inability to reconstitute NK functional activity in vitro using modified assay conditions is associated with the familial form of the disease.[240] Some degree of correlation exists between the pattern of NK functional impairment and the molecular abnormality present in patients with FHL.[241,242]

Normally, when stimulated cytotoxic T cells and NK cells undergo exocytosis of lytic granules, expression of CD107a is induced on the cell surface, where it can be detected by flow cytometry. In a very high proportion of patients with most forms of FHL, CD107a degranulation is abnormal. Importantly, however, the assay is normal in the majority of patients with sHLH and in patients with FHL that is related to perforin deficiency (FHL2) and XLP. The CD107a degranulation assay, combined with flow cytometry for perforin and SAP and XIAP in males, may allow for rapid identification of patients with FHL.[243]

Evaluation for infectious agents should be undertaken as part of the initial workup in patients with the clinical features of HLH. Bacterial cultures and tests for other pathogens such as Epstein-Barr virus (EBV), cytomegalovirus, herpes simplex virus, respiratory syncytial virus, adenovirus, fungi, and protozoa should be performed on the basis of the patient's symptoms and exposure history. Identifying and treating infection when possible is a very important part of managing the condition of these critically ill patients. However, evidence of a bacterial, viral, or other infection in a patient with HLH does not discriminate between the familial and acquired forms of the disease. In fact, patients with FHL commonly present after an identifiable infectious trigger.[237] Conversely, a specific infectious trigger may not be identified in all patients who turn out to have infection-associated hemophagocytic syndrome. The possibility of a secondary infection must be assessed and managed conservatively in these patients, who are likely to be febrile and neutropenic and may be hemodynamically unstable.

A range of CNS symptoms including irritability, lethargy, seizures, and focal deficits may be seen. Analysis of the CSF may show pleocytosis (especially with activated monocytes present) or elevated CSF protein. Evidence of hemophagocytosis is present in a minority of cases. MRI of the brain may demonstrate a wide range of abnormalities.[244,245] CNS manifestations including neurologic symptoms, abnormal CSF, or both are reported in up to 63% of children at diagnosis,[246] and they develop in most if not all cases of advanced FHL.[247,248] Occasionally, neurologic symptoms represent the most conspicuous manifestation of illness, obscuring and delaying the correct diagnosis of HLH.[249] Pathologically, CNS involvement is variable, with meningeal inflammation at the mild end and multifocal brain infiltration with necrosis at the severe end of the clinical spectrum.[250] CNS involvement occurs in both FHL and sHLH.[251]

Familial Hemophagocytic Lymphohistiocytosis

FHL is predominantly a disease of early childhood. Although congenital cases do occur, most affected infants are born healthy and grow normally until the onset of symptoms in the first few months of life, often in association with an otherwise routine childhood infection. The peak age at diagnosis is 1 to 6 months, and it is estimated that approximately 70% are diagnosed within the first year of life. However, the age range at diagnosis is wide. FHL has been reported in patients beyond the fourth decade of life.[252-254]

As previously described, familial inheritance was recognized in the earliest descriptions of the clinical phenotype, and an autosomal-recessive pattern of inheritance

TABLE 64-1   Familial Hemophagocytic Lymphohistiocytosis Genes

Disease	Locus	Gene	Gene Symbol	Syndromic Associations
FHL1	9q22.1-23	Unknown	Unknown	None
FHL2	10q22	Perforin	PRF1	None
FHL3	17q25	Mammalian homologue of Caenorhabditis elegans (Unc13)	UNC13D	None
FHL4	6q24	Syntaxin-11	STX11	None
FHL5	19p13	Syntaxin binding protein 2	STXBP2	None
Griscelli syndrome type 2	15q21	RAS-associated protein (RAB27A)	RAB27A	Hypopigmentation, +/– neurodegeneration
Lysinuric protein intolerance	14q11.2	Solute carrier family 7, member 7	SLC7A7	Protein intolerance, malabsorption, failure to thrive
Chédiak-Higashi syndrome	1q42.1-42.2	Lysosomal trafficking regulator	LYST	Partial albinism, giant lysosomes/melanosomes, neutropenia, susceptibility to infection
XLP1	Xq25	Signaling lymphocyte activation molecule (SLAM)-associated protein (SAP)	SH2D1A	Sensitivity to Epstein-Barr virus infection, hypogammaglobulinemia, lymphoma
XLP2	Xq25	X-linked inhibitor of apoptosis	XIAP	Splenomegaly, hypogammaglobulinemia

was inferred for many cases.[255] It is evident that the familial forms of HLH can be subdivided into non-syndromic forms, in which the only or predominant clinical phenotype is a predisposition to hemophagocytic syndrome, and syndromic forms, in which hemophagocytosis is only one, often inconstant phenotype present in association with other systemic abnormalities, particularly pigmentation defects or immune deficiency (Table 64-1).

Early on, genetic linkage studies performed with large nonsyndromic FHL families indicated substantial genetic heterogeneity with potential linkage to several different loci, systematically named FHL1 to FHL5. FHL1, which was among the first to be mapped, continues to defy molecular characterization.[256] However, the genes responsible for FHL2, FHL3, FHL4, and FHL5 have been cloned and have led to remarkable insights into the pathogenesis of this group of disorders. Each encodes a component required for development or trafficking of a mature, fully capacitated cytotoxic lymphocyte or NK cell cytotoxic granule.

FHL2 is due to mutations in the gene that encodes perforin (PRF1).[257,258] Perforin is a component of T-lymphocyte and NK cell cytotoxic granules that is homologous to the pore-forming complement component C9, and like its homologue, it facilitates lysis of target cells by creating holes in cell membranes.[259] FHL2-associated mutations may lead to a complete lack of protein or a defect in protein maturation/transport, leading to varying degrees of perforin deficiency and lymphocyte-mediated cytotoxicity.[258,260]

Whereas FHL2 is attributed to primary defects in the effector function of cell-mediated toxicity itself, FHL3, FHL4, and FHL5 are attributed to mutations in protein components of the trafficking machinery required for exocytosis of cytotoxic granules. Prior to exocytosis, vesicles must associate or "dock" with the membrane, a process facilitated by soluble NSF-attachment proteins (SNAP) on the vesicular compartment surface and SNAP receptors (SNAREs) on the target membrane (Fig. 64-7). Mutations in the gene that encodes the putative vesicular SNAP, syntaxin-11 (STX11), are responsible for FHL4.[261] A mammalian homologue of the Caenorhabditis elegans protein UNC13, known as UNC13D (also known as MUNC13-4), is mutated in patients with FHL3.[262,263] UNC13 family members are thought to participate in preparing vesicles docked at the cell surface for fusion with the membrane—a process called "priming."[264,265] The binding of STX11 with STXBP2 regulates granule docking and initiation of SNARE complex formation. Mutations in STXBP2, also known as MUN18-2, are associated with FHL5, which is also often associated with colitis and hypogammaglobulinemia.[266-268] Thus it would appear that STX11, STXBP2, and UNC13D are necessary to deliver PRF1 extracellularly.[269] In toto, then, the deficiency of NK cell function in patients with FHL can be ascribed to a defect in the primary cytotoxicity effector pathway, leading to poor clearance of target cells and a

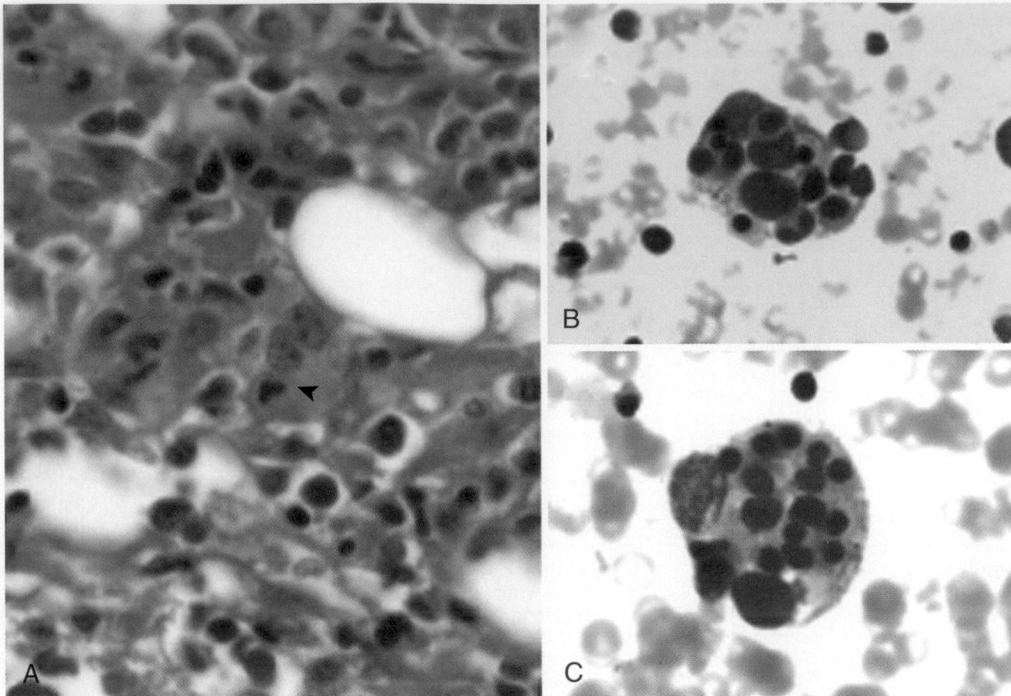

Figure 64-7 Histopathologic findings of hemophagocytic lymphohistiocytosis. **A,** A hematoxylin and eosin–stained bone marrow biopsy section (400× magnification) showing marrow infiltration by benign-appearing macrophages. A macrophage containing a phagocytosed neutrophil is indicated by the *arrowhead*. **B** and **C** show individual macrophages from a Wright-Giemsa–stained bone marrow aspirate smear (1000× magnification) that contain phagocytosed marrow elements, including mature eosinophils and erythroid precursors in **B** and numerous erythroid precursors and a band neutrophil in **C**.

continued state of immune activation, which is characteristic of the hemophagocytic syndromes.

Whereas the absolute frequency of disease-causing mutations in each of these genes varies greatly from publication to publication and population to population, it is evident that up to 80% of *molecularly defined* cases of FHL are attributable to mutations in *PRF1*, *UNC13D*, or *STXBP2*. *STX11* mutations are rare.[263,270-272] Despite the recent progress in the understanding of the genetic basis of FHL, a subset of presumptive FHL cases evade genetic characterization.

HLH Associated with Other Genetic Syndromes

HLH may occur in association with other inherited anomalies, including Chédiak-Higashi syndrome,[273] Griscelli syndrome type 2 (GS2),[274,275] lysinuric protein intolerance (LPI),[276] and X-linked lymphoproliferative syndrome (XLP1 and XLP2).[277,278] In these patients, hemophagocytosis is a variable feature, and it is not the sole manifestation of the disease. These disorders are diverse, with each disorder resulting from defects in distinct genes (Table 64-1).

Not coincidentally, the proteins encoded by the genes involved in several of these disorders each play a role in the process of cellular cytotoxicity. The GS2 protein labeled RAB27A, which is a small guanosine triphosphatase of the RAS-associated family, directly associates with the FHL3 protein labeled UNC13 and is similarly thought to regulate exocytosis.[279] Chédiak-Higashi syndrome, like GS2, gives rise to pigmentation defects and is also due to

mutations in a protein, LYST, that is involved in vesicular trafficking. Patients with XLP1 as a result of mutations in the Src homology 2 domain–containing gene 1A (*SH2D1A*), which functions as a lymphocyte signaling adapter, have a multifactorial humoral and cellular immune deficiency most saliently characterized by susceptibility to EBV infection, lymphoproliferative disorders, and dysgammaglobulinemia (see Chapter 24).[280] Defects in NK cell and T-cell development and function, including cytotoxicity, appear to predispose patients with XLP1 to HLH, particularly in the setting of primary EBV infection. How abnormalities in dibasic amino acid transport[281] should result in HLH is completely obscure; however, several persons with LPI have presented with HLH.[276]

Secondary Hemophagocytic Lymphohistiocytosis
Infection-Associated HLH

Virus-associated hemophagocytic syndrome was first described in a report of 19 adult patients, 14 of whom were immunocompromised.[217] Subsequently, it was shown that this disorder also may develop in immunocompetent persons. Although viruses, especially EBV and other members of the herpes virus group, are the most commonly identified infectious triggers, a host of other infectious agents have been implicated, including bacteria,[218] fungi, and protozoa (e.g., leishmania).[282] In a review of the 219 cases of infection-associated hemophagocytic syndrome reported in the medical literature between 1979 and 1995, 55% were attributed to EBV.[39] The clinical features of infection-associated HLH are identical to FHL, although the median age of onset is higher; about 50% of cases occurred in children younger than 3 years and 18% of cases occurred in children younger than 1 year. An interesting but as yet unexplained fact is that about half of reported cases are in people of Asian ancestry.

Malignancy-Associated HLH

HLH occurs rarely in association with a malignant neoplasm in children, and in these rare instances it is most frequently associated with T-cell malignancies. The association presents in two uncommon but somewhat distinct forms: during treatment for a known cancer in clinical remission (e.g., acute lymphoblastic leukemia)[283] or as a manifestation of an aggressive uncontrolled cancer that may be masked (e.g., T-cell or NK-cell leukemia/lymphoma). In the first case, the clinical features of HLH arise unexpectedly in a patient undergoing cancer chemotherapy, presumably as a result of iatrogenic immune dysregulation. An infectious trigger may or may not be identified.[284] In the latter case, which occurs more commonly in adults, the hemophagocytic syndrome is a feature of the hematologic malignancy itself.[285,286] It is proposed that the malignant clone potentiates a state of hypercytokinemia that results in the clinical signs and symptoms of HLH. Interestingly, some of these cancers are associated with EBV infection. The majority of the reported cases are in persons of Asian descent.

Macrophage Activation Syndrome

Macrophage activation syndrome (MAS) is a life-threatening complication of systemic inflammatory conditions that is characterized by all of the clinical symptoms and laboratory findings of HLH, leading to its classification as a form of sHLH. The syndrome was first described in 1985 in a report of seven children with systemic onset juvenile idiopathic arthritis (S-JIA).[287] Rheumatologic conditions other than JIA, such as systemic lupus erythematosus, may also be associated with the syndrome in both children and adults. Typically the syndrome develops years after the diagnosis, but it may occur early on or even concomitantly with the diagnosis of the rheumatologic disease.[288] With the onset of MAS, the chronically ill child may experience unremitting fever, a decrease in blood cell counts, and organomegaly. Interestingly, the erythrocyte sedimentation rate may decrease concomitant with the development of MAS. Flare-ups of the underlying disease, infection, and medication adverse effects not only mimic MAS but might also trigger the events.[289,290] Ravelli[290] proposed MAS diagnostic guidelines after examining clinical and laboratory characteristics of patients with active S-JIA compared with S-JIA–associated MAS. According to the guidelines, the diagnosis of MAS rests on the presence of two or more laboratory criteria (platelets $\leq 262 \times 10^9$/dL; aspartate aminotransferase >59 U/L; white blood cell count $\leq 4.0 \times 10^9$/dL; fibrinogen ≤ 2.5 g/L) or any two or more laboratory or clinical criteria (e.g., CNS dysfunction, hemor-

rhages, or hepatomegaly).[291] Distinguishing MAS from FHL and forms of sHLH can also be a challenge.[292]

It has been suggested that inherited defect(s) in one or more of the genes associated with FHL might confer predisposition to the development of MAS in the setting of rheumatologic disease or, moreover, to the development of the rheumatologic condition itself.[293] A review of 133 children with S-JIA and 384 matched unrelated control subjects failed to demonstrate an increased incidence of detectable abnormalities in the genes encoding perforin, MUNC13D, Granzyme B, or RAB27A.[294]

Recently, a form of sHLH has been observed in some children and adults treated with T-cell activating therapies using blinatumomab[295] and chimeric antigen receptor bearing T cells[296] for refractory leukemia. The cytokine release syndrome that occurs in this context may be successfully managed with corticosteroid and the IL-6 receptor antagonist tocilizumab. Remarkably, the development of cytokine release syndrome is associated with antileukemia efficacy in treated patients.

Management

The development of specific and effective therapy for HLH is hampered by the fact that affected patients demonstrate common clinical features despite variable underlying pathophysiologic conditions. Additionally, there may be little time to wait for diagnostic clarity in affected patients. Whether the patient has FHL or sHLH, the first objective of therapy is to cool down an overheated immune response. At the same time or later, the underlying basis of the patient's disease process must be determined and addressed.

Without therapy, FHL is rapidly and invariably fatal, usually within a month or two of presentation. A comprehensive literature review performed prior to the discovery of effective chemotherapy showed that only 12% of children survived 6 months and just 3 of 101 children survived long term.[297] sHLH is also a life-threatening condition, although the outcome is much more variable. It is estimated that without therapy, the mortality rate for EBV-associated HLH is approximately 50%.[39]

In 1980, Ambruso and colleagues[298] first reported the successful treatment of two infants who had presumed FHL with etoposide (VP-16). This report was an enormous step forward because no effective therapy for the disease had previously existed.[299] However, disease control proved to be transient in these and subsequent patients, with the CNS being a major site of treatment failure. To address the problem of CNS disease, cranial irradiation or intrathecal methotrexate was added to the combination of VP-16 and corticosteroid.[300] Systemic and CNS relapses remained a significant problem and few, if any, patients survived long term. In most of the reported cases, patients who received maintenance therapy with etoposide eventually died of refractory disease within 1 to 3 years.[300,301] Teniposide, also an epipodophyllotoxin, has been used in some patients who have HLH with roughly equivalent results.[302]

In 1986, the first successful matched sibling donor bone marrow transplant in a boy with FHL was described.[303] HCT was quickly recognized as the sole potentially curative modality for this group of patients who previously had no real possibility of cure. However, allogeneic transplantation, which is always a high-risk procedure, is particularly toxic in children with HLH. Control of the clinical signs of HLH prior to transplantation significantly improves the likelihood of a successful outcome.[304,305] Additionally, absence of CNS involvement and infection are favorable indicators.[237] These factors drive the preference for early transplantation, which should be performed as soon as possible after the achievement of disease control and prior to the onset of CNS manifestations or the acquisition of an opportunistic infection.

Initial Therapy

To standardize, improve, and study the treatment of this rare disease, the Histiocyte Society sponsored an international clinical trial that was named HLH-94.[306] This study and its successor, HLH-2004, defined a set of clear diagnostic criteria and laid out a nonrandomized treatment strategy that combined chemotherapy (etoposide, glucocorticoids, and intrathecal methotrexate in select cases), immunotherapy (cyclosporine A), and HCT (when possible in familial, refractory, or relapsing cases). The HLH-94 study enrolled 249 eligible children between 1994 and 2003. Because it is impossible to differentiate FHL from sHLH at onset in many cases, confirmation of familial disease was not required, and therefore both familial and secondary cases were included. Overall, 86% percent of the children responded to 8 weeks of initial therapy, approximately 60% of whom achieved nonactive disease. Factors associated with early death included marked hyperferritinemia, hyperbilirubinemia, and CSF pleocytosis at diagnosis and persistent fever, thrombocytopenia, and hyperferritinemia after 2 weeks of treatment.[307] Half of the patients taking HLH-94 underwent transplantation, with a median time between onset of therapy and HCT of 6 months. Overall survival at 5 years among the 124 patients who underwent HCT was 66% versus 54% for the entire study population. No patients with verified FHL survived without HCT.[307]

The combination of antithymocyte globulin (ATG), corticosteroid, and cyclosporine A (CSA) is an alternative to HLH-94 chemoimmunotherapy, although experience with it is more limited. Among 38 children with confirmed FHL who received one or two courses of rabbit ATG, complete resolution was achieved in 73% and partial improvement was noted in 24%. This finding includes responses seen among 10 children who had received prior immunosuppressive treatment (including steroids, CSA, or chemotherapy). All of the patients received maintenance therapy with CSA. Sixteen of 19 patients who proceeded to receive an allogeneic transplant after being treated with ATG as first-line therapy are long-term survivors. All patients who did not undergo transplantation died. The therapy was relatively well tolerated, although infusional and infectious complications were not trivial.[308,309]

Newer agents with inhibitory effects on T cells and cytokine production are being developed. These approaches are attractive because they may directly interfere with the hyperinflammation that is responsible for the clinical features of HLH without the adverse effects of cytotoxic chemotherapy. Alemtuzumab is a therapeutic monoclonal antibody that is directed against CD52, an antigen expressed on lymphocytes, NK cells, monocytes, and macrophages. Alemtuzumab seems to be effective as a bridge to transplant in patients with refractory HLH,[310] and it has been incorporated in reduced-intensity conditioning regimens in patients undergoing HCT for HLH.[310]

As stated previously, the CNS is not infrequently involved in children with HLH at diagnosis, and it is a major site of treatment failure in patients with advanced FHL. Prompt and aggressive initiation of systemic chemoimmunotherapy, followed by allogeneic stem cell transplant in familial, refractory, and relapsing cases, is the best strategy for minimizing the potential for CNS damage.[248] The role of CNS-directed therapy is not well established. Intrathecal methotrexate and cranial irradiation have been used in the context of systemic therapy. In the HLH-94 study, intrathecal methotrexate was reserved for patients in whom neurologic symptoms progressed or CSF abnormalities did not resolve after 2 weeks of systemic treatment. Interestingly, the same fraction of children (10 of 15) experienced normalization of neurologic symptoms by 2 months, whether or not they received intrathecal therapy. Intrathecal methotrexate does not appear to prevent the development of CNS manifestations in patients who do not undergo transplantation. Furthermore, intensive intrathecal methotrexate is not sufficient to reverse CNS manifestations in children with advanced FHL.[248] Cranial irradiation is now rarely used because of the lack of established efficacy and the potential long-term toxicities in these very young patients.

Management of Secondary HLH

HLH that is associated with EBV infection is the most common and best-studied type of infection-associated hemophagocytic syndrome, and it is the prototype of sHLH. Compared with children with infectious mononucleosis, children with EBV-HLH have higher EBV genome copy numbers as measured by quantitative polymerase chain reaction. The EBV copy number quickly decreases with the initiation of effective therapy and can be used as a marker of disease activity in these patients.[311] The role of antiviral agents (e.g., acyclovir) is not well established but is probably of limited benefit during the phase of active viral replication. Importantly, the need for immunosuppressive therapy is well established in these patients. The efficacy of HLH-94-based immunochemotherapy has been clearly demonstrated, yielding a survival rate of up to 90% in patients who are treated promptly.[312] Because of the potential short-term (myelosuppression) and long-term (secondary myelodysplastic syndrome/acute myelogenous leukemia) toxicities linked to etoposide,[313] its role has been specifically evaluated. Mortality was 14 times higher for patients with EBV-HLH who did not receive etoposide within the first 4 weeks after diagnosis.[314] The risk associated with a relatively short course of etoposide appears to be justified when weighed against the high risks of morbidity and mortality in these patients and the knowledge that delayed treatment yields inferior outcomes. In a series of 78 patients with EBV-HLH, most of whom were treated according to the HLH-94 study protocol, 75% remain disease free, with a median follow-up of 43 months. Reactivations occurred in approximately 20% of cases, and many of these patients were eventually cured by HCT.[315]

A complementary therapeutic strategy for EBV-HLH is the use of B-cell directed therapy, which reduces the burden of EBV-infected B cells. Two young men known to have XLP and who were diagnosed with acute infectious mononucleosis were treated with rituximab (anti-CD20 monoclonal antibody) in combination with corticosteroids and responded favorably.[316] Recently, a retrospective review of 42 patients with EBV-HLH, some of whom proved to have FHL, demonstrated that rituximab in combination with conventional HLH-directed therapy is well tolerated and leads to improvement in HLH disease manifestations and a reduction in the EBV viral load.[317]

When sHLH occurs in association with visceral leishmaniasis, a very uncommon infection in the United States, treatment of the underlying infection with amphotericin B is usually lifesaving.[282]

Treatment of HLH and MAS that is associated with malignancy must be individualized. When an active malignancy is responsible for the hemophagocytic syndrome, administration of tumor-directed cancer chemotherapy is the best treatment choice. The clinical features of HLH can be expected to resolve if the triggering cancer is controlled. For the very rare patients in whom HLH develops while they are receiving immunosuppressive therapy for a cancer that is in remission, the best strategy is not known.[318] Discontinuation of immunosuppressive therapy is beneficial in some cases but is not always possible. Treatment with corticosteroids and etoposide may be indicated. When standard therapy for HLH fails, HCT should be considered.

MAS and rheumatologic disease-associated HLH fall into a clinical spectrum within which there are no generally accepted distinctions or definitions. MAS is a term that arose in the rheumatology literature and has become more or less synonymous with reactive HLH. It is likely that many patients in this disease spectrum do not come to the attention of pediatric hematologists/oncologists because their cases are managed by pediatric or adult rheumatologists. Some differences in approach exist between the two groups of specialists. High-dose, parenteral, pulsed corticosteroids are usually used in the initial management of MAS. CSA may be effective when corticosteroids lack efficacy.[319] More recently, inhibitors of TNF—etanercept[320] and infliximab[321]—have been used successfully in patients with MAS that is refractory to steroids and cyclosporine.

In patients in whom HLH resolves completely and for whom a cause of the syndrome is not determined (i.e., they lack a positive family history or an identified genetic defect), HCT is not indicated. Very close monitoring in the period after cessation of therapy is warranted. Patients who remain well are presumed to have had sHLH. In the subset of patients who manifest signs of disease reactiva-

tion, chemoimmunotherapy should be promptly reinstituted to control the disease prior to HCT.

Supportive Care

Some of the improvement in prognosis observed in the past decades in persons with HLH is attributable to advances in supportive care. New onset and uncontrolled cases of HLH are typically characterized by the presence of multiple organ system dysfunction, including immunologic compromise, pancytopenia, hemorrhagic tendency, and hepatic and neurologic dysfunction. Hemodynamic instability, respiratory insufficiency, renal dysfunction, and electrolyte imbalance may be present. Immunosuppressive and myelosuppressive chemotherapy in these critically ill patients magnifies their risk for serious infection. A significant fraction of children with HLH succumb to opportunistic infection. Empiric antibiotics for febrile neutropenia and pneumocystis, along with fungal prophylaxis and intravenous immunoglobulin repletion, are suggested. These interventions—along with other supportive care measures, including aggressive blood product support—contribute substantially to the likelihood and quality of survival.

Hematopoietic Cell Transplantation

Multiple studies have demonstrated the necessity for an allogeneic transplant in the management of FHL. In the International Registry report of 122 children with HLH, HCT was performed in 29 children, for whom the 5-year survival after HCT was 66%. Most of the donors were fully matched or mismatched family donors, and only three children received transplants from unrelated donors. Among patients who did not undergo transplantation, the 5-year survival rate was only 10%, with just three children surviving long term.[237] Because only a minority of the patients received HCT, the 5-year event-free survival for the entire cohort of 122 patients was just 21%.

The fact that only approximately 20% of children in need of an allogeneic stem cell transplant have an available matched family donor accounts in part for the poor overall survival among patients in the International Registry. Aside from human leukocyte antigen compatibility, another limitation to the applicability of matched sibling donor transplantation in a genetic disorder such as HLH is the possibility that the sibling donor is at risk for developing the disease. These factors, combined with the knowledge that FHL is invariably fatal without transplantation, has led to the increased use of unrelated and alternative donors.[305,322,323] The 3-year overall survival rate was 44% among 16 children with HLH who underwent transplantation with marrow from unrelated donors. Among the 65 children on the HLH-94 protocol who underwent transplantation, approximately half of whom received marrow from an unrelated donor, the 3-year probability of survival was 62%. The impact of expanded access to HCT by increased use of alternative donors (among other factors) was borne out in the relatively high overall survival rate of 55% at 3 years in the HLH-94 study. Disease remission at the time of transplantation is associated with a superior outcome after HCT.[322] However, HCT should not be viewed as futile in a child

TABLE 64-2 Comparison of Langerhans Cell Histiocytosis and Hemophagocytic Lymphohistiocytosis

| | LANGERHANS CELL HISTIOCYTOSIS | | HEMOPHAGOCYTIC LYMPHOHISTIOCYTOSIS | |
	Single System	Multisystem	Primary	Secondary
Pathologic cell	Dendritic cell		Macrophage	
Histologic features	Clonal Langerhans cell proliferation (CD1a+, Langerin+) Mixed cellular infiltrate		Reactive macrophages (CD68+) hemophagocytosis	
Typical age at onset	Childhood	Infancy	Infancy	Childhood
Inheritance	Sporadic	Sporadic	Autosomal recessive	Sporadic
Clinical presentation	Bone pain/swelling Skin rash	Bone pain/swelling Skin rash, FTT, DI	Fever, hepatosplenomegaly, irritability, jaundice	
Laboratory/ radiographic features	Laboratory tests usually normal/lytic bone lesions	Cytopenia(s), liver dysfunction, bone lesion(s)	Cytopenias, ↑ferritin, ↓fibrinogen, ↑triglycerides, ↓NK function, ↑soluble CD25, abnormal CSF	
Treatment	Observation, vinblastine/steroids	Vinblastine/steroids	Etoposide/steroid/ CSA, HCT	Etoposide/steroid/CSA
Prognosis	Excellent	Variable Fatal in ≈25%	Fatal without HCT, Survival ≈50% with HCT	Variable Fatal in ≈20%

CD, Cluster of differentiation; *CSA,* cyclosporin A; *CSF,* cerebrospinal fluid; *DI,* diabetes insipidus; *FTT,* failure to thrive; *HCT,* hematopoietic cell transplantation; *NK,* natural killer.

with active disease, even involving the CNS, because many children with active disease at the time of HCT have done well.[324] Despite high early mortality rates, late reactivation of disease is very uncommon in patients who have undergone allogeneic HCT for FHL.[324]

The most commonly used myeloablative conditioning regimen for HCT in patients with HLH is the combination of busulfan, cyclophosphamide, etoposide, and ATG. Transplant-related mortality is very high with this approach; roughly one third of recipients of transplants die after myeloablative conditioning within the first few months as a result of infection, hepatopathy, pneumonitis, or uncontrolled disease.[325] Reduced-intensity conditioning is increasingly recommended in this setting because it is associated with a significantly higher likelihood of survival.[168,326] Establishment of stable, long-term donor chimerism is an issue, and donor lymphocyte infusion is indicated in many cases. For this reason, reduced-intensity conditioning is not suitable for patients for whom the only acceptable donor source is umbilical cord blood.

CONCLUSIONS

HLH is an acute, rapidly progressive, potentially life-threatening syndrome. The clinical features are the consequence of hyperinflammation and immune dysregulation, but the underlying mechanisms are diverse. Prompt recognition and initiation of therapy is warranted, even when diagnostic certainty is elusive. Initial therapy with etoposide and a corticosteroid with or without the addition of CSA is the standard of care in the United States. Analysis for defects in the genes known to be associated with the condition should be undertaken, although not

all familial cases will have a confirmatory genetic test. Assessment for triggers of secondary HLH should be pursued, but identification of an infectious trigger does not reliably differentiate FHL and sHLH. Children who have FHL based on a positive family history, the finding of a genetic abnormality, or a refractory or relapsing course should be referred for allogeneic hematopoietic stem cell transplant as soon as possible. Children not known to have FHL based on these criteria may be observed if they achieve disease resolution after 2 to 3 months of initial therapy. A comparison of some of the cardinal features of LCH and HLH is shown in Table 64-2.

References available online at ExpertConsult.

KEY REFERENCES

11. Dieu MC, Vanbervliet B, Vicari A, et al: Selective recruitment of immature and mature dendritic cells by distinct chemokines expressed in different anatomic sites. *J Exp Med* 188:373–386, 1998.
    This article, along with the article in reference 12, provide the first descriptions of sequential expression of CCR6 and CCR7 by DCs and their effects on patterns of dendritic cell migration.
12. Sallusto F, Schaerli P, Loetscher P, et al: Rapid and coordinated switch in chemokine receptor expression during dendritic cell maturation. *Eur J Immunol* 28:2760–2769, 1998.
    This article, along with the article in reference 11, provide the first descriptions of sequential expression of CCR6 and CCR7 by DCs and their effects on patterns of dendritic cell migration.
15. Hoeffel G, Wang Y, Greter M, et al: Adult Langerhans cells derive predominantly from embryonic fetal liver monocytes with a minor contribution of yolk sac-derived macrophages. *J Exp Med* 209:1167–1181, 2012.
    Demonstration of the yolk sac origin of LCs.
33. Ginhoux F, Tacke F, Angeli V, et al: Langerhans cells arise from monocytes in vivo. *Nat Immunol* 7:265–273, 2006.

The authors demonstrate a requirement for the CSF–1 receptor for the formation of LCs in mice and show that Gr-1(hi) circulating monocytes are precursors for LCs.

38. Allen CE, Li L, Peters TL, et al: Cell-specific gene expression in Langerhans cell histiocytosis lesions reveals a distinct profile compared with epidermal Langerhans cells. *J Immunol* 184:4557–4567, 2010.
   Use of gene expression profiles to demonstrate that LCH cells more closely resemble myeloid precursor cells than do mature LCs.

42. Willman CL, Busque L, Griffith BB, et al: Langerhans'-cell histiocytosis (histiocytosis X)—a clonal proliferative disease. *N Engl J Med* 331:154–160, 1994.
   Demonstration of clonality of nonpulmonary LCH cells.

45. Badalian-Very G, Vergilio JA, Degar BA, et al: Recurrent BRAF mutations in Langerhans cell histiocytosis. *Blood* 116:1919–1923, 2010.
   The first demonstration of a recurrent genomic abnormality in LCH and identification of a possible oncogenic driver.

50. Haroche J, Cohen-Aubart F, Emile JF, et al: Dramatic efficacy of vemurafenib in both multisystemic and refractory Erdheim-Chester disease and Langerhans cell histiocytosis harboring the BRAF V600E mutation. *Blood* 121:1495–1500, 2013.
   Demonstration of clinical responses to a BRAF inhibitor in patients with Erdheim-Chester disease with BRAF V600E mutations.

51. Weintraub M, Bhatia KG, Chandra RS, et al: p53 expression in Langerhans cell histiocytosis. *J Pediatr Hematol Oncol* 20:12–17, 1998.
   Demonstration of the high prevalence of p53 protein expression in LCH cells in the absence of detectable mutations.

69. Lichtenstein L: Histiocytosis X; integration of eosinophilic granuloma of bone, Letterer-Siwe disease, and Schuller-Christian disease as related manifestations of a single nosologic entity. *AMA Arch Pathol* 56:84–102, 1953.
   A proposal to unify eosinophilic granuloma of bone, Letterer-Siwe disease, and Schüller-Christian disease under the single category of histiocytosis X.

75. Titgemeyer C, Grois N, Minkov M, et al: Pattern and course of single-system disease in Langerhans cell histiocytosis data from the DAL-HX 83- and 90-study. *Med Pediatr Oncol* 37:108–114, 2001.
   Benign characterization of the course of disease in children with single-system LCH.

80. Haupt R, Minkov M, Astigarraga I, et al: Langerhans cell histiocytosis (LCH): guidelines for diagnosis, clinical work-up, and treatment for patients till the age of 18 years. *Pediatr Blood Cancer* 60:175–184, 2013.
   Consensus guideline for the diagnostic evaluation, treatment, and long-term follow-up of pediatric LCH.

108. Grois N, Fahrner B, Arceci RJ, et al: Central nervous system disease in Langerhans cell histiocytosis. *J Pediatr* 156:873–881, 881.e1, 2010.
   A comprehensive description of MRI changes, neuropathology, risk factors, clinical presentation, and behavior of central nervous system LCH.

119. Wnorowski M, Prosch H, Prayer D, et al: Pattern and course of neurodegeneration in Langerhans cell histiocytosis. *J Pediatr* 153:127–132, 2008.
   A description of the radiographic and clinical course of neurodegenerative LCH.

144. Gadner H, Grois N, Arico M, et al: A randomized trial of treatment for multisystem Langerhans' cell histiocytosis. *J Pediatr* 138:728–734, 2001.
   Results of LCH I demonstrating that vinblastine and etoposide are equally effective treatments for MS-LCH. Patients who do not respond within 6 weeks have an adverse prognosis.

152. Bernard F, Thomas C, Bertrand Y, et al: Multi-centre pilot study of 2-chlorodeoxyadenosine and cytosine arabinoside combined chemotherapy in refractory Langerhans cell histiocytosis with haematological dysfunction. *Eur J Cancer* 41:2682–2689, 2005.
   Demonstration of the efficacy and toxicity of cytarabine and cladribine combination chemotherapy in children with high-risk LCH that is refractory to standard therapy.

158. Minkov M, Grois N, Heitger A, et al: Treatment of multisystem Langerhans cell histiocytosis. Results of the DAL-HX 83 and DAL-HX 90 studies. DAL-HX Study Group. *Klin Padiatr* 212:139–144, 2000.
   Results of DAL-HX studies demonstrating superiority in comparison with LCH I (see reference 144) in children with MS-LCH treated with a more intensive and longer duration of therapy.

161. Gadner H, Minkov M, Grois N, et al: Therapy prolongation improves outcome in multisystem Langerhans cell histiocytosis. *Blood* 121:5006–5014, 2013.
   Results of the LCH III study demonstrating that longer treatment duration is associated with a decreased reactivation rate. The study also showed no benefit to the addition of methotrexate in risk organ–positive MS-LCH.

184. Janssen D, Harms D: Juvenile xanthogranuloma in childhood and adolescence: a clinicopathologic study of 129 patients from the Kiel pediatric tumor registry. *Am J Surg Pathol* 29:21–28, 2005.
   A very large case series detailing the typically benign clinical behavior of pediatric JXG.

191. Rosai J, Dorfman RF: Sinus histiocytosis with massive lymphadenopathy: a pseudolymphomatous benign disorder. Analysis of 34 cases. *Cancer* 30:1174–1188, 1972.
   The initial description of Rosai-Dorfman disease.

219. Risdall RJ, McKenna RW, Nesbit ME, et al: Virus-associated hemophagocytic syndrome: a benign histiocytic proliferation distinct from malignant histiocytosis. *Cancer* 44:993–1002, 1979.
   The first detailed description of virus-associated HLH and its relationship to familial HLH.

222. Henter JI, Horne A, Arico M, et al: HLH-2004: Diagnostic and therapeutic guidelines for hemophagocytic lymphohistiocytosis. *Pediatr Blood Cancer* 48:124–131, 2007.
   Careful characterization of HLH and recommendations for management.

232. Allen CE, Yu X, Kozinetz CA, et al: Highly elevated ferritin levels and the diagnosis of hemophagocytic lymphohistiocytosis. *Pediatr Blood Cancer* 50:1227–1235, 2008.
   Demonstrates the high sensitivity and specificity of extreme hyperferritinemia in the diagnosis of HLH.

245. Bryceson YT, Pende D, Maul-Pavicic A, et al: A prospective evaluation of degranulation assays in the rapid diagnosis of familial hemophagocytic syndromes. *Blood* 119:2754–2763, 2012.
   Details a diagnostic algorithm for familial HLH incorporating newer clinically available assays.

248. Horne A, Trottestam H, Arico M, et al: Frequency and spectrum of central nervous system involvement in 193 children with haemophagocytic lymphohistiocytosis. *Br J Haematol* 140:327–335, 2008.
   A description of the frequency and significance of central nervous system signs and symptoms in persons with HLH.

259. Stepp SE, Dufourcq-Lagelouse R, Le Deist F, et al: Perforin gene defects in familial hemophagocytic lymphohistiocytosis. *Science* 286:1957–1959, 1999.
   Identification of perforin deficiency in one of the genetic subsets of HLH. Identification of the molecular basis for other HLH subtypes followed (see references 263, 264, 268, 270, 279, and 280).

293. Ravelli A, Magni-Manzoni S, Pistorio A, et al: Preliminary diagnostic guidelines for macrophage activation syndrome complicating systemic juvenile idiopathic arthritis. *J Pediatr* 146:598–604, 2005.
   A proposed diagnostic guideline for MAS in children with underlying rheumatologic disease.

308. Henter JI, Samuelsson-Horne A, Arico M, et al: Treatment of hemophagocytic lymphohistiocytosis with HLH-94 immunochemotherapy and bone marrow transplantation. *Blood* 100:2367–2373, 2002.
   Results of the HLH-94 study, which demonstrated the efficacy of initial chemotherapy followed by stem cell transplantation in children with familial HLH.

311. Mahlaoui N, Ouachee-Chardin M, de Saint Basile G, et al: Immunotherapy of familial hemophagocytic lymphohistiocytosis with

antithymocyte globulins: a single-center retrospective report of 38 patients. *Pediatrics* 120:e622–e628, 2007.

A report on the efficacy of serotherapy in the initial management of familial HLH.

316. Imashuku S, Kuriyama K, Teramura T, et al: Requirement for etoposide in the treatment of Epstein-Barr virus-associated hemophagocytic lymphohistiocytosis. *J Clin Oncol* 19:2665–2673, 2001.

Establishes the indication for use of etoposide in the management of virus-associated HLH.

328. Marsh RA, Vaughn G, Kim MO, et al: Reduced-intensity conditioning significantly improves survival of patients with hemophagocytic lymphohistiocytosis undergoing allogeneic hematopoietic cell transplantation. *Blood* 116:5824–5831, 2010.

Demonstrates superior results using reduced intensity compared with conventional conditioning in patients with HLH undergoing allogeneic HCT.

CHAPTER 65

Rare Tumors of Childhood

John M. Goldberg, Alberto S. Pappo, and Michael Bishop

CHAPTER OUTLINE

This chapter covers the rare tumors of childhood. No attempt has been made to consider the rarest of the rare tumors, and the focus is on the more common of the rare pediatric tumors that do not fall into other categories covered in this text. The chapter is generally organized from top to bottom, with cancers of the head and neck at the beginning and cancers of the gastrointestinal tract discussed later in the chapter. The tumors discussed afflict mostly adults, and some are actually common cancers in older patients. Many are carcinomas and are more familiar to the oncologist who treats adults. These cancers tend to increase in incidence as children reach adolescence.

Evaluation of Surveillance, Epidemiology, and End Results (SEER) data has shown that 9.2% of all childhood cancers are carcinoma, and 75% of these cases are diagnosed in children between the ages of 15 and 19 years.[1] Of the cases in the study, 36% were thyroid carcinomas and 31% were melanomas. The next most common single carcinoma in children younger than age 19 years was nasopharyngeal carcinoma, which comprised 4.5% of these cases. Thus this chapter emphasizes discussion of melanoma, thyroid carcinoma, and nasopharyngeal carcinoma and reviews other rare tumors of childhood.

OROPHARYNGEAL CANCER

Oropharyngeal cancer of squamous cell histology in children remains uncommon.[2] Most of the children who develop epithelial cancer of the nose, ears, and throat are diagnosed with nasopharyngeal carcinoma, which is considered separately in this chapter. The use of smokeless tobacco, cigarette smoking, and alcohol consumption are well established risk factors for the development of squamous cell carcinoma in adults, and the continued use of these substances in Western children warrants monitoring for the development of adult types of squamous cell carcinoma of the oropharynx in children. Although such habits ultimately lead to increased risk for a variety of cancers and early death from heart disease, it remains a theoretical concern that the use of smokeless tobacco by children, particularly by male adolescents, could increase the incidence of these tumors during adolescence and young adulthood.

Duration of smoking increases risk for tobacco-related morbidity and mortality, including several cancers, and significant public health efforts have been aimed at reducing adolescent initiation of tobacco use.[3] Educational interventions have been shown to decrease the prevalence of cigarette and smokeless tobacco use in Massachusetts youth,[4] but restrictions on tobacco sales have a mixed record, because even a complete ban on sales of smokeless tobacco in Finland did not lead to a decrease in its use by adolescents.[5] Conversely, restrictions on smoking in public places have been demonstrated to decrease overall tobacco consumption (e.g., by up to 8% in Italy).[6] Overall trends of cigarette smoking among adolescents have decreased steadily since the mid-1990s. Rates of smoking for white, non-Hispanic twelfth grade students are significantly higher in comparison to Hispanic and African-American students.[3,7,8] Although smokeless tobacco use also declined during the late 1990s and early 2000s, recent data from Monitoring the Future and the National Youth Tobacco Survey have demonstrated increased use in recent years, with concurrent decreased reporting of perceived risk. These changes in trends are synchronous with aggressive marketing campaigns by tobacco companies of novel delivery forms of smokeless tobacco such as "snus" and dissolvable tobacco.[7,9]

The increasing prevalence of human papillomavirus (HPV) infection in adolescents and young adults has raised new concerns about the development of HPV-associated oral squamous-cell carcinoma in younger patients. HPV has recently been detected in approximately 26% of head and neck squamous-cell carcinomas; HPV16 was highly prevalent among these tumors.[10] Trends in adults show an increasing incidence in oral squamous-cell carcinomas despite declining use of tobacco in the United States because of the increasing prevalence of oral HPV infection.[11,12] A recent study showed 1.7% of 14- to 17-year-old adolescents and 5.6% of 18- to 24-year-old adults had oral HPV; male sex, number of sexual partners, tobacco use, open-mouth kissing, and oral sex have been associated with infection.[13,14] HPV is most often transmitted in adolescence and young adulthood; a quadrivalent vaccine for HPV that includes strains likely to cause oral cancers is now available and is recommended for both boys and girls.[15,16]

Few existing studies report outcomes of pediatric squamous-cell carcinomas. A population-based study of 54 pediatric patients with oral-cavity squamous-cell carcinoma had a 5-year disease-specific survival rate of 75%.[17] It is unlikely that many pediatric oncologists will be confronted by adult-type squamous-cell carcinoma of the head and neck, but it is likely that pediatric oncologists will be confronted with tobacco use in young adult and adolescent survivors of pediatric cancer. A St. Jude Children's Research Hospital study has found that 29% of surviving children treated on an acute myelogenous leukemia (AML) protocol were found to be cigarette smokers at follow-up examinations.[18] Although survivors of childhood cancer may not be seen often in the pediatric oncology clinic, tobacco use and prevention still merit mention during such visits.

Mucoepidermoid carcinoma of the salivary glands is still another type of head and neck carcinoma from which children suffer and is commonly associated with prior therapy for cancer, including radiation.[19] A study of childhood cancer survivors identified 23 cases of secondary head and neck malignancies; of the 14 secondary cancers that arose in the parotid gland, 10 were identified as mucoepidermoid carcinoma.[20] Most children are cured with surgery and sometimes surgery and radiation therapy. Any mass lesion or presenting complaint potentially related to a mass lesion in the salivary glands, particularly if found in a previous radiation field, should prompt a thorough evaluation with suspicion for this tumor.

NASOPHARYNGEAL CARCINOMA

Nasopharyngeal carcinoma is a cancer of the epithelial lining of the nasopharynx. It shows varying degrees of differentiation but is a type of squamous-cell carcinoma. Most cases have undifferentiated histology; the undifferentiated type is associated with Epstein-Barr virus (EBV) infection of the nasopharyngeal epithelium, and virus is found in the tumor cells.[21] It is the most common type of epithelial tumor of the head and neck in children, accounting for up to 50% of head and neck tumors in children. Incidence varies widely among populations and in relationship to exposure to EBV, environmental exposures such as preserved or salted fish, and geographic location. Rates in China are particularly high, and ethnic Chinese born in China who move to the West have a higher incidence of the disease than ethnic Chinese who are born in Western countries.[21] In the United States, this cancer is more common in the South and more prevalent in African-American children, who have incidence rates of the disease that approach those of the Chinese. These findings suggest interplay of genetic, viral, and environmental factors in the carcinogenesis of nasopharyngeal carcinoma.

Analysis of incidence and survival rates from SEER data has demonstrated improved survival for Asian-American patients compared to Caucasian and African-American patients. However, nasopharyngeal carcinoma-specific mortality is worse for adults than for children and adolescents, and survival rates in the adolescent and young-adult age ranges tend to be similar among races.[22-25]

Epidemiology

Nasopharyngeal carcinoma is more common in Asia and is strongly associated with Chinese ethnic origin within Asia, with some parts of China having incidence rates from 15 to 30 cases per 100,000 population.[21] There is also a higher incidence of the cancer in Turkey.[26,27] A bimodal age distribution has been suggested in nonendemic areas, with an early peak in adolescents age 15 to 19 years.[28] The actual cancer cells are infected by EBV, suggesting a possible role for immunosuppression in the pathogenesis of the tumor, or at least that immune augmentation could help prevent recurrence of nasopharyngeal carcinoma.[21] In Greenland and other regions with similar native populations, high rates of nasopharyngeal carcinoma have been found. Additionally, high rates for other cancers associated with EBV infection, such as various forms of uterine cancer, are more common in families with EBV and nasopharyngeal carcinoma.[29,30] Population-based screening based on EBV serology in endemic areas can help detect nasopharyngeal carcinoma early. However, this would be impractical in nonendemic areas.

Presentation

The typical presenting signs and symptoms of nasopharyngeal carcinoma include evidence of tumor mass in the nasopharynx such as epistaxis, nasal obstruction and discharge, Eustachian tube dysfunction, palsy of the fifth and sixth nerves relating to skull-based extension, and neck masses.[21] In children with epidemiologic factors making this disease more likely, clinicians must maintain a high index of suspicion for nasopharyngeal carcinoma and obtain imaging studies and consultation as necessary for these signs and symptoms. However, most children diagnosed with nasopharyngeal carcinoma in the United States are unlikely to have obvious epidemiologic associations for the cancer, and even in the United States EBV infection in childhood is common enough that screening based on evidence of EBV infection would be impractical.

Staging and Evaluation

Proper evaluation of patients suspected of having nasopharyngeal carcinoma includes computed tomography (CT) scan and/or magnetic resonance imaging (MRI) of the head and biopsy of appropriate tissue for diagnosis. A clinical examination is key to evaluate for any apparent lymph node spread. Although systemic evaluation, including laboratory testing, positron emission tomography (PET) scanning, whole-body anatomic scanning, and bone marrow biopsy can be considered, they have not been shown to improve staging accuracy in patients with nasopharyngeal carcinoma.[21]

All nasopharyngeal carcinoma cases are considered squamous-cell cancers, but the World Health Organization (WHO) classification of nasopharyngeal carcinoma defines type 1 histology as keratinizing squamous-cell carcinoma, a form of cancer more common in adults, versus the type 2 histology, which does not show keratinization on light microscopy but does show some differentiation. Type 3 histology is nonkeratinized and nondifferentiated and is associated with endemic nasopharyngeal carcinoma.[21] The majority of children with nasopharyngeal carcinoma have a presentation of undifferentiated or WHO type 2 or 3 histology.[23]

The American Joint Commission on Cancer (AJCC) tumor-nodes-metastasis (TNM) staging system (2010) is considered the most relevant for patients in the Western countries. The WHO staging system has fewer local (T) staging categories but seems to be adequate for patients in endemic areas.[21,31] The latest AJCC staging system is shown in Tables 65-1 and 65-2.

TABLE 65-1   Tumor-Nodes-Metastasis Definitions for Nasopharyngeal Carcinoma*

Primary Tumor (T)	Regional Lymph Nodes (N)	Distant Metastasis (M)
TX: Primary tumor cannot be assessed T0: No evidence of primary tumor Tis: Carcinoma in situ T1: Tumor confined to the nasopharynx, or tumor extends to oropharynx and/or nasal cavity without parapharyngeal extension[†] T2: Tumor with parapharyngeal extension[†] T3: Tumor involves bony structures of skull base and/or paranasal sinuses T4: Tumor with intracranial extension and/or involvement of cranial nerves, hypopharynx, orbit, or with extension to the infratemporal fossa/masticator space	NX: Regional lymph nodes cannot be assessed N0: No regional lymph node metastasis N1: Unilateral metastasis in cervical lymph node(s), ≤6 cm in greatest dimension; above the supraclavicular fossa and/or unilateral or bilateral; retropharyngeal nodes, ≤6cm in greatest dimension[‡] N2: Bilateral metastasis in cervical lymph node(s), ≤6 cm in greatest dimension; above the supraclavicular fossa[‡] N3: Metastasis in a lymph node(s)[‡] >6 cm and/or to supraclavicular fossa N3a: >6 cm in dimension N3b: Extension to the supraclavicular fossa[§]	M0: No distant metastasis M1: Distant metastasis

From Edge SB, Byrd DR, Compton CC et al, editors: AJCC: pharynx. In: AJCC cancer staging manual, ed 7, New York, 2010, Springer, p. 41–56.

*The distribution and prognostic impact of regional lymph-node spread from nasopharynx cancer, particularly of the undifferentiated type, are different from those of other head and neck mucosal cancers and justify the use of a different regional lymph-node classification scheme.
[†]Parapharyngeal extension denotes posterolateral infiltration of tumor.
[‡]Midline nodes are considered ipsilateral nodes.
[§]Supraclavicular zone or fossa is relevant to the staging of nasopharyngeal carcinoma and is the triangular region originally described by Ho. It is defined by three points: 1) the superior margin of the sternal end of the clavicle; 2) the superior margin of the lateral end of the clavicle; and 3) the point where the neck meets the shoulder. Note that this would include caudal portions of levels IV and VB. All cases with lymph nodes (whole or part) in the fossa are considered N3b.

TABLE 65-2   American Joint Committee on Cancer Stage Groupings for Nasopharyngeal Carcinoma*

Stage	Groupings
0	Tis, N0, M0
I	T1, N0, M0
II	T1, N1, M0
	T2, N0, M0
	T2, N1, M0
III	T1, N2, M0
	T2, N2, M0
	T3, N0, M0
	T3, N1, M0
	T3, N2, M0
IVA	T4, N0, M0
	T4, N1, M0
	T4, N2, M0
IVB	Any T, N3, M0
IVC	Any T, any N, M1

From Edge SB, Byrd DR, Compton CC et al, editors: AJCC: pharynx. In: AJCC cancer staging manual, ed 7, New York, 2010, Springer, p. 41–56.

*Results of radiation therapy for nasopharyngeal carcinoma (locoregional control and survival) are usually reported by T stage and N stage separately or by specific T and N subgroupings rather than by numerical stages I to IV. Outcome also depends on various biologic and technical factors related to treatment.

Treatment

Although nasopharyngeal carcinoma can be treated by radiation therapy only, it has been shown to be sensitive to chemotherapy in adults and children. Using chemotherapy may ultimately allow for curative radiotherapy at lower doses with less risk for late effects from head and neck radiotherapy.[21,24,26-27,32] A Pediatric Oncology Group (POG) study used four cycles of preirradiation chemotherapy with methotrexate with leucovorin, 5-fluorouracil (5-FU), and cisplatin to treat children with AJCC stage III or IV nasopharyngeal carcinoma. Children with stage I or II disease were treated with irradiation only. The 4-year event-free and overall survival rates were 77% ± 12% and 75% ± 12%, respectively.[24] Other agents used to treat nasopharyngeal carcinoma include bleomycin and doxorubicin.[27] More recently, the use of neoadjuvant chemotherapy with concomitant chemoradiation has demonstrated improved outcomes.[21,26-27] Xerostomia and dental problems are common adverse effects of treatment. Other long-term morbidities include sensorineural hearing loss, endocrinopathies, trismus, and recurrent infections.[33] Sensorineural hearing loss incidence has been noted to increase with the use of concomitant chemoradiotherapy.[34] Although both children and adults with nasopharyngeal carcinoma are at risk of developing secondary malignancies after treatment, the risk for children is 4.3 times the general population, compared with 1.4 for adults.[23] Current treatment strategies are investigating the use of intensity-modulated radiation therapy (IMRT) and amifostine to preserve salivary function[35,36] and to decrease acute and chronic sequelae of therapy.

THYROID CARCINOMA

This section summarizes the clinical-pathologic and therapeutic aspects of differentiated thyroid carcinoma in children and adolescents. Medullary thyroid carcinoma (MTC) and associated multiple endocrine neoplasia (MEN) syndromes are not discussed.

Epidemiology

The prevalence of palpable thyroid nodules in children is lower than that seen in adults (1.5% vs. 5%); despite this, thyroid nodules in children are five times more likely to be malignant than those in adults (25% vs. 5%).[37-39] Of the estimated 56,000 cases of thyroid cancer diagnosed in 2012, only 1.8% occur in patients under 20 years of age.[40] Furthermore, thyroid carcinoma accounts for 3% of all cancers in patients younger than 20 years, and 75% of these occur in patients between the ages of 15 and 19 years (Fig. 65-1).[41] Epidemiological studies suggest that the incidence of thyroid carcinoma has steadily increased over time and that it affects both low and high socioeconomic counties that were surveyed by the SEER registries.[42,43] In pediatrics, an increasing rate has been documented in the SEER registry for the years 1973 through 2007, with the rates being higher in whites, those aged between 15 and 19 years, girls, and in registries with predominantly white or Hispanic populations.[44]

Radioactive exposure to the neck is a well-established risk factor for the development of thyroid carcinoma.[45] Survivors of childhood cancer have up to a 14-fold excess risk of developing thyroid cancer if their thyroid gland received 20 to 25 Gy, and this malignancy accounts for 10% of all subsequent neoplasm in the survivor population.[46,47] A risk-prediction model for subsequent primary thyroid carcinoma in survivors of childhood cancer has been developed.[48] This model incorporates several variables including radiation and therapy information, age, sex, and a history of a thyroid nodule; the software to compute risk projections can be downloaded at http://dceg.cancer.gov/tools/riskassessment.[48]

Exposure to radioactive iodine and cesium isotopes after the Chernobyl accident resulted in a markedly increased rate of thyroid cancer in children; the estimated relative excess risk was estimated to be 5.6 per Gy of exposure in subjects with estimated doses of less than 1 Gy.[49-51] Other risk factors associated with the development of pediatric thyroid cancer include various genetic syndromes such as familial adenomatous polyposis (FAP), Cowden disease, Carney syndrome, and immune thyroid disorders such as Hashimoto thyroiditis.[37,52-54]

Pathology and Molecular Pathology

More than 90% of pediatric thyroid carcinomas have well-differentiated histology; papillary histology accounts for over 70% of cases, and follicular histology represents about 20% of cases. Medullary thyroid cancer is seen in fewer than 10% of pediatric cases of thyroid cancer and can be found in association with MEN syndrome types

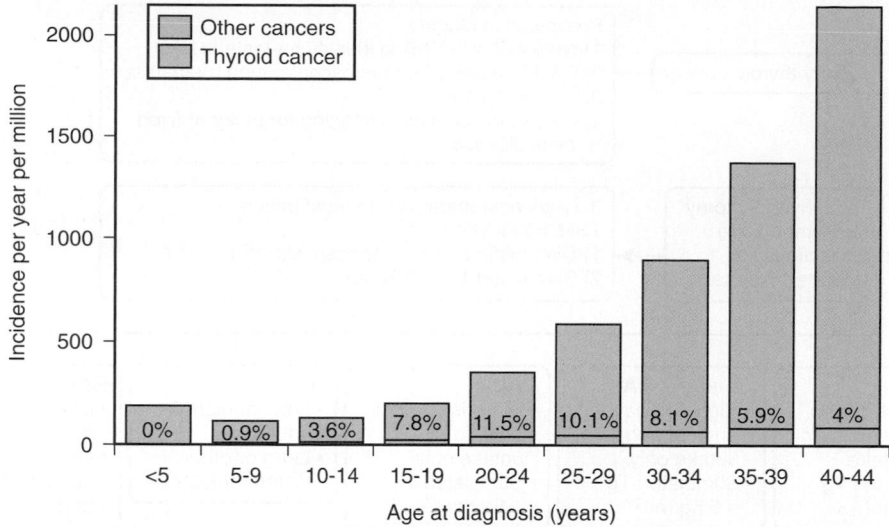

Figure 65-1 Incidence of thyroid carcinoma relative to all cancers, SEER 1975-2000. *(Data from Bleyer A, O'Leary M, Barr R, Ries LAG, editors: Cancer epidemiology in older adolescents and young adults 15 to 29 years of age, including SEER incidence and survival: 1975-2000 [NIH Publication No. 06-5767]. Bethesda, Md., 2006, National Cancer Institute.)*

2A and 2B.[55] The distribution of histologies varies slightly in cases with known radiation carcinogenesis; in a study of 740 children with thyroid cancer, of whom 92% were exposed to radiation at Chernobyl, 90% of cases were papillary, about 5% were follicular, and 0.4% were medullary.[56]

RET-PTC rearrangements have been documented in 50% to 60% of pediatric cases of papillary thyroid carcinoma and in up to 70% of radiation-induced pediatric papillary thyroid carcinoma.[54,57] *NTRK1* rearrangements and *AKAP9-BRAF* fusions have also been described in a small number of radiation-induced papillary tumors.[58-60] Unlike in adults, *BRAF* mutations are rarely seen in pediatric papillary tumors.[61-62] Follicular tumors are characterized by *RAS* mutations and peroxisome proliferator–activated receptor γ (PPARγ) rearrangements, whereas MEN-associated medullary thyroid carcinomas are characterized by germline-activating mutations of *RET.*[54,63]

Clinical Presentation and Staging

Most patients with thyroid carcinoma are older than 10 years and initially have an asymptomatic palpable thyroid nodule.[64] Younger age (<15 years), large fixed nodules, palpable adenopathy, history of radiation exposure, and diseases associated with an increased incidence of thyroid carcinoma such as FAP, Carney complex, Cowden syndrome, MEN types 2A or 2B, pheochromocytoma, and hyperparathyroidism should raise the suspicion for the presence of malignancy.

Children and adolescents with thyroid carcinoma are more likely to have nodal regional involvement, extrathyroid disease, and pulmonary metastases and are less likely to die from their disease than adults.[64] Ultrasound is a useful diagnostic technique, and most investigators prefer this method for evaluating thyroid nodules (Fig. 65-2).[37,64] Initial evaluation of a thyroid nodule should include measurements of serum thyroid-stimulating hormone (TSH), antithyroid peroxidase, antithyroid globulin antibodies,

and a neck ultrasound that evaluates the contralateral thyroid lobe and cervical nodes.[39] Screening for MTC using plasma calcitonin may not be cost-effective in children given its low prevalence in the pediatric population.[37,39,65] If the TSH level is low, raising the possibility of a hyperfunctional nodule, a thyroid technetium or iodine scan should be performed. Because of the higher likelihood of malignancy in children, it is recommended that all hyperfunctioning nodules be surgically removed in children, with further evaluation and treatment should the pathology be consistent with malignant disease.[65,66] Fine-needle aspiration biopsy is the most cost-effective and expeditious preoperative procedure to help distinguish benign from malignant thyroid nodules; a meta-analysis of 12 pediatric studies found that this procedure has a sensitivity of 94% and a specificity of 81% (see Fig. 65-2).[37,67] Preoperative staging should include a chest x-ray and a comprehensive neck ultrasound to evaluate the whole thyroid and lymph nodes.[64]

Prognostic Factors

Factors associated with an increased risk of progression include capsular invasion, soft-tissue invasion, positive margins of resection, age younger than 10 to 15 years, male sex, nonpapillary histology, distant metastases, and residual disease after surgery.[68,69,70] Survival for children with differentiated thyroid carcinoma approaches 100% (Fig. 65-3).

Treatment and Outcome

Surgery

Surgery is the mainstay of therapy for pediatric and adolescent thyroid carcinoma, and this procedure should be performed by a highly experienced thyroid surgeon.[64] Total thyroidectomy is the initial treatment of choice. especially in younger patients (<10 years) or those with a history of radiation exposure or a family history of

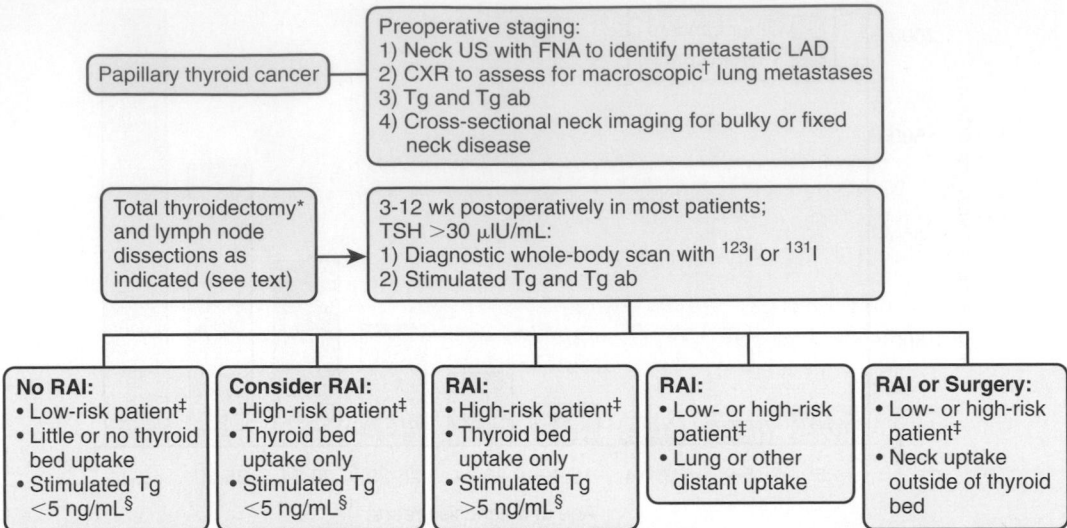

Figure 65-2 Initial evaluation and treatment of papillary thyroid cancer in children. *CXR*, Chest radiography; *FNA*, fine-needle aspiration; *LAD*, lymphadenopathy; *RAI*, radioactive iodine; *Tg*, thyroglobulin; *Tg ab*, thyroglobulin antibody; *TSH*, thyroid-stimulating hormone; *US*, ultrasound. *Rare cases where lobectomy may suffice. †Macroscopic lesions are considered to be larger than 1 cm. ‡Low-risk: primary tumor does not grossly invade the trachea, recurrent laryngeal nerve, esophagus, or other vital structures; nonbulky lymph node presentation; no evidence of distant metastatic disease. High risk: any of the previous features present. §Assumes negative Tg ab. ¶RAI if no macroscopic disease on US; surgery if macroscopic disease on US. (*From Waguespack SG: Initial management and follow-up of differentiated thyroid cancer in children.* J Natl Compr Canc Netw 8:1289–1300, 2010.)

thyroid cancer.[64] Many surgeons also advocate the upfront use of this procedure because pediatric thyroid carcinoma is associated with a high incidence of multifocal and metastatic disease, and follow-up screening with serum thyroglobulin is most useful after total thyroidectomy.[64,66] Lobectomy and isthmectomy can be considered in patients who have a low risk for recurrence such as adolescents with localized small (<1 cm) lesions.[64,71-73]

Lymph Node Dissection

Upfront nodal dissection has been shown to decrease the risk of surgical reintervention and nodal recurrence in children with thyroid carcinoma.[56,74] Current recommen-

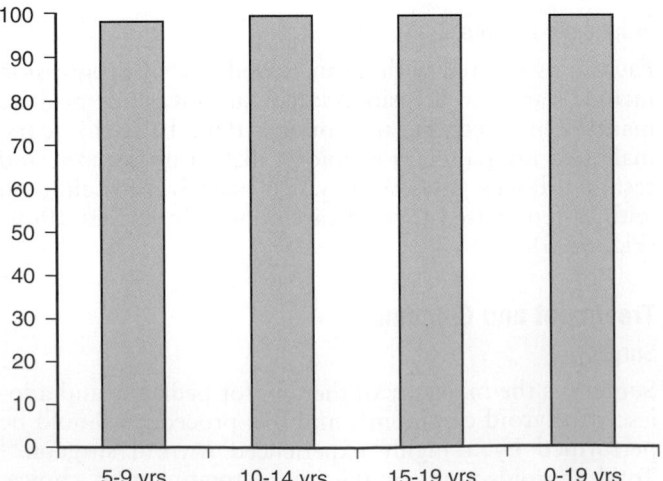

Figure 65-3 Five-year relative survival rates for thyroid carcinoma by age group, SEER 2002-2008.

dations favor the use of central compartment neck dissection, reserving less extensive surgeries for patients with small tumors and no evidence of nodal involvement by ultrasound (see Fig 65-2).[64]

Use of Radioactive Iodine

In adults, the use of radioactive iodine treatment to ablate residual thyroid or iodine-avid metastatic disease decreases the risk of distant metastases.[75] The goals for the use of this therapy in children includes ablation locoregional recurrence, elimination of residual sources of thyroglobulin production, and high remnant uptake that can obscure the presence of metastases and accurate detection of pulmonary metastatic disease.[76] The use of this therapy in children has been associated with a reduced recurrence risk in the thyroid and nodes independent of the surgical approach.[76] However, a recent study by Hay failed to show a significant difference in local and distant recurrence when this modality was used, and 73% of patients who died from a subsequent malignant neoplasm had received therapeutic irradiation postoperatively.[77] Radioactive iodine treatment should be reserved for children at high risk for disease recurrence, and a suggested measured approach for the postoperative use of this agent is shown in Figure 65-2.[64] When radioactive treatment is prescribed, TSH should be greater than 30 µIU/mL.[64] The dosing of this agent is not well established in children, and various centers follow the American Thyroid Association (ATA) guidelines for adults (*http://thyroidguidelines.net/revised/differentiated*). A posttherapy thyroid scan is usually obtained about 1 week after treatment, and this may identify additional sites of disease that were not apparent initially. Because of the risk of regrowth after TSH exposure, thyroid hormone suppression to achieve serum TSH levels between 0.1 and 0.5

µIU/mL is recommended in all pediatric patients with differentiated thyroid cancer.[64]

Targeted Therapies

A variety of "targeted" therapies have been developed for iodine-refractory differentiated thyroid carcinoma, and many of these agents have been approved for adult use.[78] Most of these therapies target RET and the vascular endothelial growth factor (VEGF) receptors but some also target platelet-derived growth factor β receptors (PDGFRβs), FGFR, MET, and endothelial growth factor (EGF) receptors.[78] Some of these agents include sorafenib, axitinib, motesanib, sunitinib, pazopanib, cabozantinib, and vandetanib.[78] In children sorafenib has been successfully used in a patient with refractory papillary thyroid carcinoma, and in a phase I/II study, vandetanib produced two partial responses in children with MEN2b-associated medullary thyroid carcinoma.[79,80]

Follow-Up Observation

Lifelong surveillance is recommended for children with thyroid carcinoma. A recent article recommends determination of suppressed thyroglobulin levels and antibodies every 3 to 6 months and a neck ultrasound every 6 to 12 months for the first 2 years of follow-up care.[64] If a patient was treated with radioactive iodine, a stimulated thyroglobulin test and whole body scan is recommended 1 year after initial treatment. About 25% of patients develop antibodies, and these interfere with the thyroglobulin assays. Declining antibody titers usually correlate with lower disease burden.[64]

BREAST TUMORS

Breast masses are rare in young children. During puberty, benign fibroadenomas are the most common cause of a palpable breast lump (Table 65-3).[81] The estrogen stimulation during adolescence may cause exaggerated growth of the stroma and epithelium in a localized breast lobule that characterizes a fibroadenoma. They have been found in as many as 20% of women between the ages of 15 and 25 years on autopsy studies.[82] Fibroadenoma occurring

TABLE 65-3   Breast Lesions in Adolescent Girls.

Abnormality	Incidence (%)
Fibroadenoma	68
Miscellaneous	27
Juvenile hypertrophy	2
Giant fibroadenoma	1
Phyllodes tumor	<1
Cancer	<1
Metastatic	38
Adenocarcinoma (lobular or ductal)	31
Lymphoma	13

Data from Neinstein LS: Breast disease in adolescents and young women. Pediatr Clin North Am 46:607–629, 1999.

in adolescence does not appear to be associated with concurrent or future breast carcinoma. Any dominant discrete breast mass in an adolescent should be reexamined at midcycle after one or two menstrual cycles. Persistent masses should be imaged by ultrasound (not mammography) and referred to a surgeon. Typically, malignant breast masses in children have similar imaging characteristics to malignant breast masses in adults, which can help guide the decision to perform more invasive evaluation.[83] Lesions typical for fibroadenoma are sometimes observed clinically; fine-needle aspiration or core biopsy can also be performed to confirm the diagnosis.[84] Most fibroadenomas in adolescents self-resolve or shrink.[85] Most boys with breast masses have gynecomastia that requires only reassurance and noninvasive supportive care. This is borne out by review of pathology specimens from teenage male patients who underwent resection of breast masses; nearly all such evaluations were negative.[86]

Phyllodes tumors are stromal tumors that present as rapidly growing but clinically benign masses. Although the median age of presentation is 45 years, they can occur in adolescence.[87] Benign phyllodes tumors of the breast are pathologically similar to a large fibroadenoma with more stromal cellularity. They are treated by resection with at least 1 cm margins.[88] Malignant phyllodes tumors are sarcomas with nuclear pleomorphism and mitotic activity; treatment requires a multimodality sarcoma approach. Five-year disease-free survival rates have been reported to be 96%, 74%, and 66% for benign, borderline, and malignant phyllodes tumors, respectively, in adults[89]; it is thought that adolescents have a more favorable outcome.[90]

Breast masses can also represent primary or metastatic sites of pediatric cancers such as rhabdomyosarcoma,[91] non-Hodgkin lymphoma, Hodgkin lymphoma, or neuroblastoma.[92]

Breast carcinoma in a patient under the age of 20 years is rare; five cases were seen at M.D. Anderson Cancer Center over 10 years, compared with 180 cases in patients between ages 20 and 30 years and 1347 in patients between ages 31 and 50 years.[93] The most common pathology is a juvenile secretory carcinoma that secretes mucin and mucopolysaccharide-containing material. It is treated by excision and lymph node biopsy. No studies have evaluated outcomes in patients younger that the age of 20 years with breast carcinoma, but multiple studies have shown that age younger than 30 or 35 years is an independent predictor of poor response.[93] The two younger age groups at particular risk of breast cancer are women who have received radiation to the breast, usually for lymphoma, and women who have a familial predisposition. These women should be taught breast self-examination and awareness at a young age.

PULMONARY TUMORS

Primary tumors of the lung are extremely rare in childhood, and metastatic pulmonary lesions far exceed the number of primary tumors.[94] Table 65-4 lists the most common pulmonary tumors in children.

TABLE 65-4   Pulmonary Tumors in Children

Malignant	Benign
Bronchial adenomas (40% to 60%)	Hamartomas
Carcinoid	Hemangiomas
Mucoepidermoid carcinoma	Lymphangioma
Adenoid cystic carcinoma	Leiomyomas
Pleuropulmonary blastoma (15%)	Myofibroblastic tumors
	Inflammatory myofibroblastic tumor
Bronchogenic carcinoma (10% to 15%)	Myofibromatosis
Adenocarcinoma	Congenital peribronchial myofibroblastic tumor
Small-cell carcinoma	Neurogenic tumors
Bronchoalveolar carcinoma	Mature teratoma
Squamous-cell carcinoma	
Undifferentiated carcinoma	
Fetal-lung adenocarcinoma	
Pulmonary mesothelioma	
Sarcomas (20% to 25%)	
Rhabdomyosarcoma	
Synovial sarcoma	
Hemangiopericytoma (solitary fibrous tumor)	
Leiomyosarcoma	
Angiosarcoma	
Bronchopulmonary fibrosarcoma	

Bronchial Adenomas

A large percentage of malignant pulmonary tumors in children are called bronchial adenomas, and although not benign, as the term implies, they are predominantly low grade in behavior. They include carcinoid tumor, mucoepidermoid carcinoma, and adenocystic carcinoma. Although pulmonary carcinoid tumors account for only 2% of all primary lung tumors in adults, between 40% and 85% of pediatric malignant lung lesions are carcinoids.[94-97] See "Carcinoid" for a more complete description of carcinoid and its management. Mucoepidermoid carcinomas (MECs)[98] and adenoid cystic carcinomas[99] are more often seen in the head and neck but can arise from mucous glands located in the respiratory submucosa.

Most bronchial adenomas are endobronchial; patients often have recurrent infections or obstructive pneumonitis before their diagnosis is determined (Fig. 65-4), and the most common presenting symptoms are cough, fever, or wheezing.[100-102] Although over 25% of adults with pulmonary carcinoid and MEC are asymptomatic, the figure is lower in children, who are less likely to have a radiographic study that would detect an incidental lesion.[103] Aggressive lesions can present with hemoptysis, chest pain, or pneumothorax in rare cases. It is extremely rare for patients with pulmonary carcinoid to show evidence of carcinoid syndrome in the absence of metastatic disease,[103] but a reported 2% to 4% of patients have Cushing syndrome.[101,104,105] A mass is usually detected by chest x-ray or chest CT, but endobronchial lesions may only be suspected by recurrent localized obstruction and volume loss (Fig. 65-5, A and B). Octreotide scans have a sensitivity of 80% to 90% for carcinoids and can be useful at diagnosis to assess for metastatic disease.[106]

More recently, PET CT imaging with the somatostatin analog ^{68}Ga-DOTATOC has shown sensitivity of 97% and specificity of 92% in identifying neuroendocrine tumors.[107] Diagnostic biopsy is usually obtained by flexible fiberoptic bronchoscopy (see Fig. 65-5, C). Lymph nodes can be involved, especially with higher grade tumors, but may also be enlarged as a reaction to obstructive pneumonitis rather than tumor.

The typical carcinoid tumor and low-grade MEC are pathologically bland and have a low rate of postresection recurrence or metastasis, even with local invasion.[95] The rarer atypical carcinoids and high-grade MEC have a higher mitotic rate and more necrosis and are more likely to behave aggressively.[97,108] The appropriate therapy is open resection of tumor and involved lymph node, the extent of which is determined by the centrality of the mass. Lobectomy or even pneumonectomy may be required for tumors of the main stem bronchus. Because adenoid cystic carcinomas can spread submucosally with circumferential bronchial involvement, the margin of resection should be determined intraoperatively by frozen sections of the bronchial margins.[94] Local recurrences of bronchial adenomas can occur, especially for MECs, but metastases are rare. Adenoid cystic carcinoma has a greater likelihood of distant metastases than MECs and a poorer overall survival rate.[94] Estimates for metastases from bronchial carcinoid range from 5% to 27%.[101,109,110]

When surgery is not curative, other therapies can be used but have shown limited success.[111] Octreotide, a somatostatin analogue used to treat the symptoms of carcinoid syndrome, has been known to stabilize carcinoid tumor growth but not result in regression; similarly, interferon has been used with a modest response. Radionuclide therapy with radiolabelled somatostatin analogs have also been investigated for carcinoids in adults and have demonstrated control of disease and symptom improvement in patients with metastatic disease.[112]

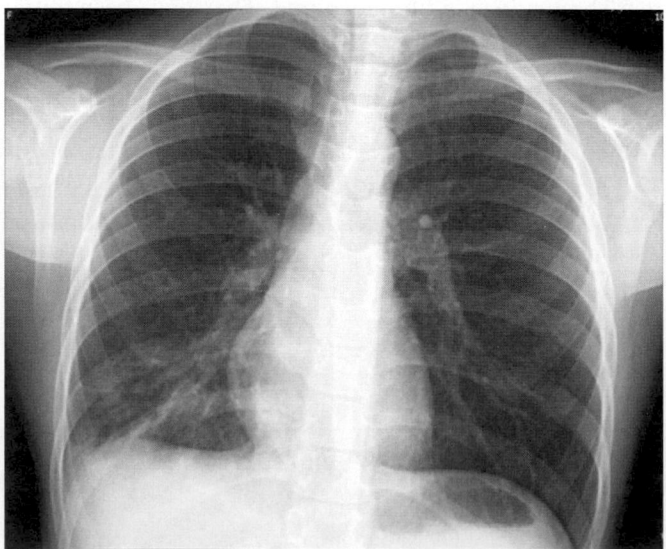

Figure 65-4 Plain radiograph of 9-year-old patient showing right lower-lobe infiltrate persistent over 1 month. Further workup revealed a right lower-lobe bronchus mucoepidermoid carcinoma.

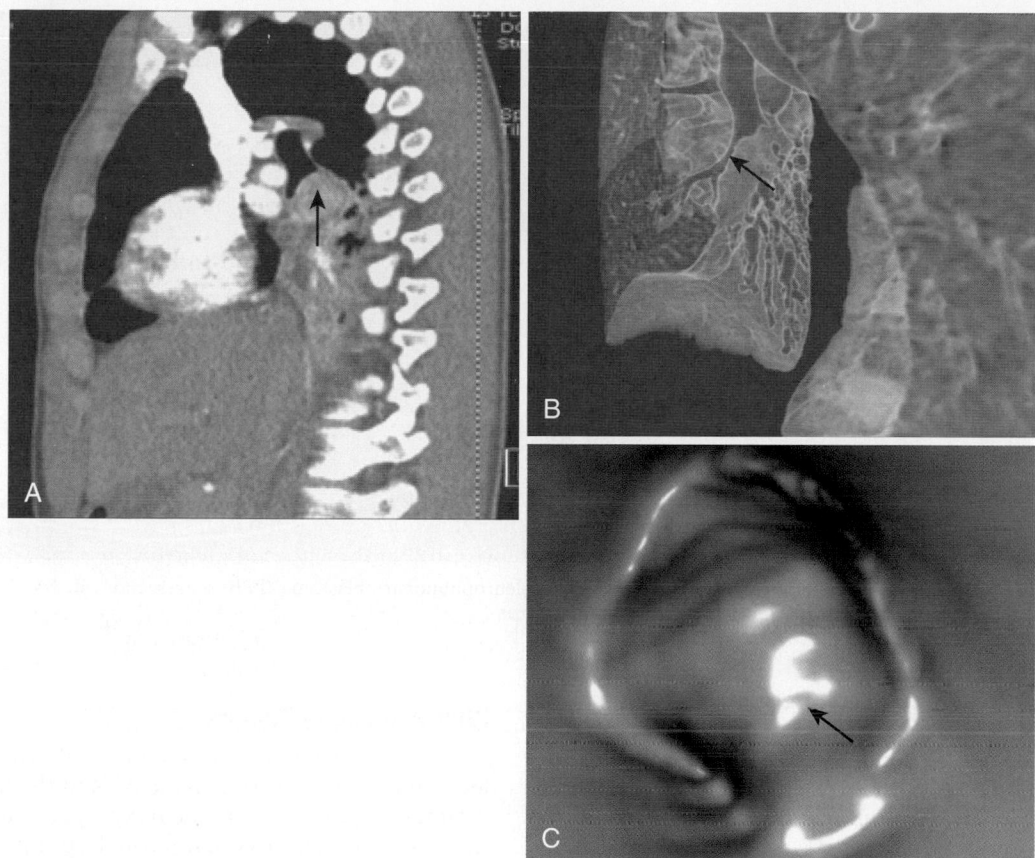

Figure 65-5 A, Carcinoid tumor *(arrow)* obstructing bronchus intermedius and causing peripheral consolidation of lung. **B,** Carcinoid tumor obstructing bronchus intermedius *(arrow)*. **C,** Carcinoid tumor *(arrow)* obstructing bronchus intermedius.

Cytotoxic chemotherapy for carcinoid and MECs has been used, but response rates, even with combination agents, are under 20%.[97,111] Novel molecular agents are being tested, including agents directed against VEGF, PDGFR, and mammalian target of rapamycin (mTor). Prognosis remains excellent for bronchial adenomas, even for locally invasive or high-grade tumors.

Pleuropulmonary Blastoma

Pleuropulmonary blastoma (PPB) in young children is distinct from pulmonary blastoma in adults; the pediatric tumor is composed of primitive blastema and neoplastic mesenchymal cells without epithelial malignant cells.[94,113] Since its initial description, there has appeared to be an increase in malformations and cancer in the afflicted child and family (Fig. 65-6).[114] Many pleuropulmonary blastomas are now known to be a part of a spectrum of dysplastic and neoplastic lesions that can arise from a constitutional mutation in *DICER1,* which is located on chromosome 14q and encodes a ribonuclease (RNase) endonuclease essential in the production of micro-ribonucleic acids (miRs). Other lesions that may arise as a result of germline *DICER1* mutations include ovarian sex-cord stromal tumors, cystic nephroma, embryonal rhabdomyosarcoma, ciliary body medulloepithelioma, nasal chondromesenchymal hamartoma, and multinodular goiter.[115-117] The tumor is located peripherally and can

be locally invasive. Most patients have symptoms of wheezing, respiratory distress, or pneumothorax. Pathologically there are three subtypes: type 1 PPB, which is exclusively cystic, without a macroscopically detectable solid component); type 2 PPB with solid and true cystic areas; and type 3 PPB, a true solid tumor.[113] PPBs (particularly type 1 cystic lesions) are often misdiagnosed as congenital pulmonary airway malformations (CPAMs) because of similar appearance on chest x-ray and CT imaging. Echocardiography may occasionally demonstrate extension into the thoracic great vessels and heart, and fatal embolic events have been reported in rare occurrences.[118]

Treatment involves resection. Adjuvant chemotherapy (doxorubicin, actinomycin, vincristine, and cyclophosphamide or ifosfamide), especially for types 2 and 3, may reduce the risk of recurrence[119] or can be used neoadjuvantly to improve the resectability of large lesions.[120] Radiation has been used adjuvantly or palliatively; its role is unclear. If left unresected, type 1 lesions may eventually progress to more aggressive subtypes with development of anaplasia. Prognosis correlates with subtype; type 1 PPB that is completely resected has a 5-year survival rate of 85% to 90%, whereas type 2 and 3 tumors have 45% to 60% survival rates.[121,122] Metastases can develop in up to 55% of patients with type 3 PPB; the most common sites are the brain and spinal cord and

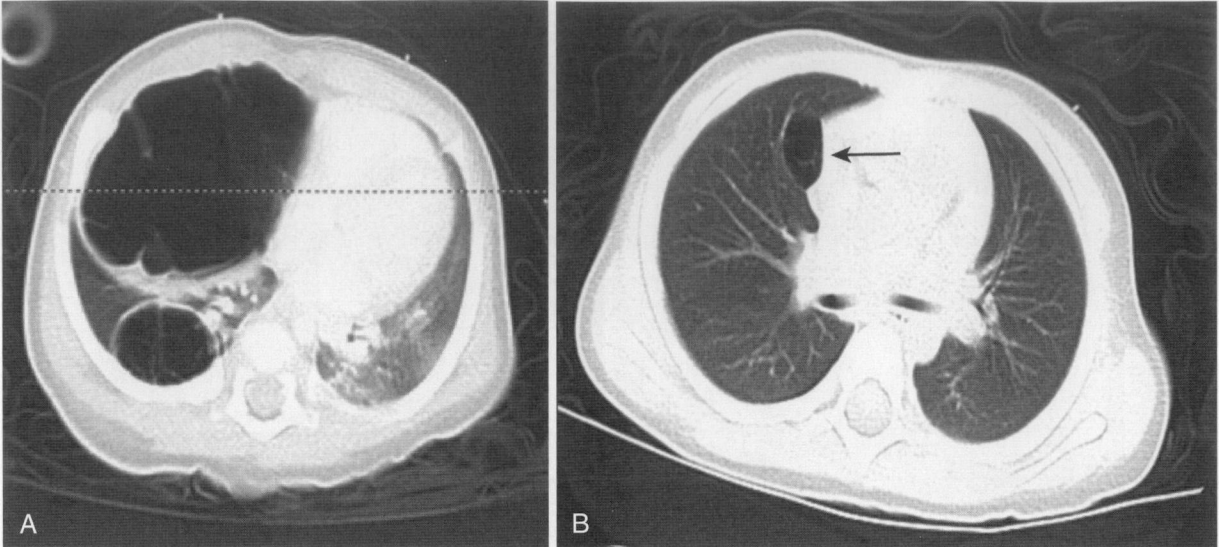

Figure 65-6 A, Two cystic lesions in 3-month-old infant found to be pleuropulmonary blastoma (PPB) on resection. **B,** Brother of patient with PPB in **A** with a benign cystic-adenomatoid carcinoma malformation *(arrow)*.

bone.[119,123] An international PPB registry has been established that collects clinical data on incident cases in an attempt to define the outcomes of patients with this rare disease. Families should be referred for genetic counseling to evaluate for the presence of a *DICER1* predisposition syndrome and risk of developing other related lesions.

Bronchogenic Carcinoma

Primary epithelial cancers of the lung are rarely seen in children; fewer than 100 cases have been reported in the literature. They are pathologically indistinguishable from the same tumors occurring in adults. Therapy should be planned after consultation with a medical oncologist experienced with lung cancers and in general should mimic the standard of care for adult tumors. When these histologies occur in children, they are often metastatic at diagnosis and have an aggressive course, high mortality, and average survival time of 7 months after diagnosis (Fig. 65-7).[94,97] Bronchioalveolar carcinoma (BAC) is a histology that accounts for less than 10% of lung malignancies in adults, with a mean age of presentation between the sixth and seventh decades. In children, mucinous BAC has been associated with CPAM type 1[94,124,125] and has also been reported as a second malignancy in osteosarcoma survivors.[126] Surgery is the primary treatment for BAC. Prognosis depends on nodal status and the resectability of the tumor; it appears to be slightly better for children than for adults with BAC or for children with other primary bronchogenic carcinomas.[127] Squamous cell carcinoma,[128] adenocarcinoma,[97] and small-cell lung cancer[129,130] are occasionally seen in children.[100] There is no clear causative pathway or association with environmental exposure, and most patients have no family history to suggest a genetic component. A rare form of adenocarcinoma in children is well-differentiated fetal adenocarcinoma (WDFA), which histologically resembles fetal lung and has an excellent prognosis.[97,131,132]

Other Pulmonary Tumors

Sarcomas arise from mesenchymal cells and therefore can develop from connective tissue cells in the lung. The most common types seen are hemangiopericytoma, synovial sarcoma, leiomyosarcoma, bronchopulmonary fibrosarcoma, and rhabdomyosarcoma.[94,100] Ewing sarcoma—peripheral primitive neuroectodermal tumor in the lung (Askin tumor)—is often pleural-based. Given its marked chemosensitivity, it should be treated with chemotherapy

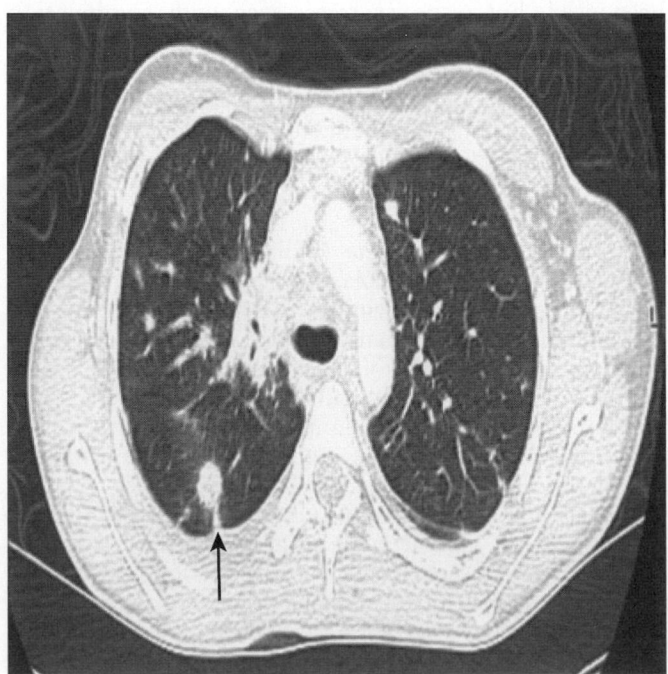

Figure 65-7 A 14-year-old patient with primary pulmonary poorly differentiated carcinoma *(arrow)* and lung, bone, lymphatic, hepatic, and adrenal metastases.

before surgical resection in contrast to almost all other lung tumors (see Chapter 61). Pleural mesothelioma is occasionally seen in children, with fewer than 100 cases in the literature and even fewer that have been confirmed by pathologic review.[133] Although there have been reports of assumed causation by asbestos exposure and chemotherapy and/or radiation for another malignancy, most cases appear in healthy children.[133,134] The tumor is similar to that in adult cases in its pathologic appearance and poor prognosis, with a median survival length of approximately 10 months.[135,136] Most cases are treated with a multimodality approach, but tumors are often diffuse and unresectable and are poorly responsive to chemotherapy and radiation. Current concepts in the therapeutic approach of adults with mesothelioma include the use of cisplatin and multitargeted antifolate chemotherapy[137] and aggressive surgery (extrapleural pneumonectomies).[138]

GASTROINTESTINAL STROMAL TUMORS

Epidemiology

Gastrointestinal stromal tumors (GISTs) are the most common mesenchymal neoplasm of the gastrointestinal tract in adults, with an incidence of 11 to 19.6 cases per million, which translates into 3300 to 6000 new cases per year.[139-141] GISTs are presumed to originate from the interstitial cells of Cajal, which regulate gastrointestinal motility.[142] Bardsley has characterized a putative interstitial cell of Cajal stem cell. This cell is capable of self-renewal and differentiation, has a KIT^low CD44+CD34+ phenotype, and is not dependent on KIT signaling for survival and proliferation.[143]

Gastrointestinal Stromal Tumors in Adults

The median age at diagnosis of GIST is approximately 60 years, and the disease has no sex predilection.[141,142] The most common presenting symptoms are abdominal pain, palpable mass, and gastrointestinal bleeding.[144] In adults, tumors range in size from 1 to 40 cm with a median size of 5 cm and most commonly arise in the stomach (60%) followed by the small intestine (30%) colon, rectum (5%), and esophagus (5%). About 95% of GISTs stain positive for CD117, and activating mutations of KIT (70% to 80%) and PDGFRα (~7%) are seen in nearly 90% of adult GISTs. About 12% to 15% of adult GISTs are wild-type for KIT and PDGFR, but mutations of other genes such as BRAF, SDHB, KRAS, and NRAS have been increasingly recognized (Table 65-5).[144]

Chemotherapy for unresectable or metastatic GISTs produces responses in fewer than 10% of patients, and the median survival for adults with metastatic disease is historically 20%.[145] The use of the tyrosine kinase inhibitor imatinib has revolutionized the treatment of GIST. Administration of this drug to adults with unresectable or metastatic GISTs produce responses in up to 85% of patients, and the median survival time for this group has increased to 58 months.[146] The likelihood of response to imatinib is correlated with the mutational genotype of the tumor; patients with KIT exon 11 mutations have significantly higher response rates to imatinib than patients

TABLE 65-5   Genetic Subtypes and Use of Imatinib in Selected Subsets of Adult Gastrointestinal Stromal Tumors

Genetic Type	Frequency of Total	Adjuvant Imatinib	Imatinib for Metastatic Disease
KIT mutated	80%		
Exon 11	67%	Yes, 400 mg/d	Yes, 400 mg/day
Exon 9	10%	Yes, 400 mg/day	Yes, 800 mg/day
Other	2%	Yes, 400 mg/day	Yes, 400 mg/day
PDGFR mutated			
Exon 12	5% to 8%		
Exon 14	1%	Yes, 400 mg/day	Yes, 400 mg/day
Exon 18	<1%	Yes, 400 mg/day	Yes, 400 mg/day
D842V	5%	No	No
Wild-type	12% to 15%		
BRAF V600	7% to 15%	?	?
SDH A,B,C,D	2%	?	?
HRAS/ NRAS	<1%	?	?
Other	2%	?	?

Modified from Corless CL, Barnett CM, Heinrich MC: Gastrointestinal stromal tumours: origin and molecular oncology. Nat Rev Cancer 11:865–878, doi:10.1038/nrc3143, 2011; and Blay JY, Le Cesne A, Cassier PA, Ray-Coquard IL: Gastrointestinal stromal tumors (GIST): a rare entity, a tumor model for personalized therapy, and yet ten different molecular subtypes. Discov Med 13:357–367, 2012.

with exon 9 mutations or no mutations.[147] A similar pattern has been documented for patients with PDGFR mutations; two thirds of patients with PDGFR lesions have the imatinib-resistant isoform D842V.[148] Suggested initial management of GISTs based on mutational status is shown in Table 65-5.

Pediatric Gastrointestinal Stromal Tumors and Succinate Dehydrogenase–Deficient Gastrointestinal Stromal Tumors

Epidemiology and Presenting Features

Pediatric GISTs account for 1% to 2% of all GISTs, but their true incidence in the United States is largely unknown.[149,150] Review of the SEER database from 2000 through 2009 revealed 23 cases of malignant GIST, and 14 were seen in patients between 15 and 19 years of age for an expected incidence of 0.06 per million among this age group. In children and adolescents these tumors present at a median age of 14 years and predominantly affect females. The most common presenting symptoms are gastrointestinal bleeding, abdominal pain, anemia, weight loss, vomiting and early satiety. About 20% of patients have metastatic disease at diagnosis, and approximately 10% have a history of Carney triad or Carney Stratakis syndrome (see below).[151,152,153] GISTs in younger patients more commonly arise in the stomach, tend to be multifocal and involve lymph nodes, more often contain epithelioid or mixed histology, and have a more indolent clinical course. Despite surgical resections, 30% to 80% of patients develop metastatic disease to lymph nodes, liver, or locoregional sites, but despite multiple recurrences, survival is close to 90%.[154]

Biology

In children and adolescents, GISTs can occur within the context of two genetic syndromes: Carney triad and Carney Stratakis syndrome.[155,156] Carney triad is characterized by pulmonary chondroma, GIST, and paraganglioma, whereas Carney Stratakis syndrome lacks the pulmonary chondromas. Furthermore, Carney triad is sporadic and its cause is not known, whereas Carney Stratakis syndrome is caused by germline inactivating mutations of succinate dehydrogenase (SDH) B, C, or D.[157] Unlike adult GIST in which KIT and PDGFR mutations are key for disease development, only about 15% of GIST tumors found in children have activating mutations of one of these two genes. Despite this their tumors still express KIT at comparable levels to those seen in adults.[151,158] In contrast to adult GISTs, pediatric tumors lack large-scale chromosomal or genomic aberrations and overexpress IGF1R, suggesting that this pathway should be investigated as a possible therapeutic target in these patients.[150,158-160]

About 10% of children with wild-type GIST and no history of paraganglioma have a heterozygous germline mutation of SDH B or C.[161] Additionally, wild-type GIST in patients under 20 years of age almost lack SDHB expression as determined by immunohistochemistry, and nearly 90% of SDHB-negative cases express IGF1R by immunohistochemistry.[162,163] SDHD germline mutations have been reported in cases of sporadic GIST and in association with familial paraganglioma.[157,164] Germline SDHA mutations have also been reported in sporadic GIST.[165] Interestingly, about 30% of SDHB-negative cases by immunohistochemistry also lack SDHA expression, and immunohistochemical loss is strongly associated with germline mutations of SDHA.[164] Given the markedly different biology of GIST in younger patients, some investigators prefer using the term SDH-deficient GIST to identify a preferentially younger population that has wild-type GIST and SDH-deficient driven tumors.

Treatment

GIST in younger patients has a more indolent course, and recurrences are common. For this reason, ultimate cure in this group of patients is unlikely and treatment options that combine the judicious use of surgery combined with selected medical therapies offer the best chance for disease control. Because of the rarity of this disease, it is recommended that children and adolescents with GIST be preferentially managed by a multidisciplinary team with expertise in sarcoma and gastrointestinal tumors.[166] Initial management of localized disease should include surgical resection with the goals of achieving a gross resection with an intact pseudocapsule and negative margins. Lymph-node sampling in younger patients should be considered. Gastrectomy and other extensive surgeries should be avoided, because recurrence is common; therefore wedge resections are preferred. The use of adjuvant imatinib in patients with wild-type high-risk tumors is not recommended. For patients with unresectable or metastatic disease who have a KIT or PDGFR mutation, treatment according to Table 65-5 or the National Comprehensive Cancer Network (NCCN) guidelines is recommended.[167] Wild-type or SDH-mutated GISTs do not usually respond to tyrosine kinase therapies used in adults, and in selected asymptomatic patients with active disease, careful observation and follow up care might offer the best approach. In patients who develop significant symptoms or progression, a trial of imatinib or sunitinib is warranted; in one series one partial response and five cases of disease stabilization were seen in children refractory to imatinib.[168] A trial using sunitinib in patients 6 to 21 years if age with wild-type GIST and a trial using the tyrosine kinase inhibitor directed against insulin-like growth factor 1 receptor (IGF1-R) OSI-906 in patients over 18 years with wild-type GIST are ongoing. Follow-up care should include imaging and examinations every 3 to 6 months for 5 years. The use of CT should be limited when possible, and use of MRI and plain chest radiographs encouraged.

CARCINOID TUMORS

Carcinoid tumors are tumors of neuroendocrine cells that derive from embryonic divisions of the gut. The most common locations for carcinoid tumors are in locations arising from the midgut: the appendix, small intestine, proximal colon, and rectum. Carcinoid tumor of the appendix is speculated to be the most common tumor of the gastrointestinal tract in children.[169] Tumors of the epithelial component of the bronchial mucosa arising from the foregut appear as carcinoid tumors of the lung and bronchus. Biologically, carcinoid tumor cells contain membrane-bound neurosecretory granules that contain hormones and biogenic amines. When serotonin, 5-hydroxyindole acetic acid (5-HIAA), and other metabolites of the granules are released, a syndrome of flushing, diarrhea, and abdominal cramps can occur. The syndrome rarely occurs in children, because it is associated with large tumor mass, hepatic metastases, or distant metastases.[170] Carcinoid tumors are one of the rarer tumors (less than 10%) seen in the autosomal dominant syndrome MEN type 1 (MEN1), which is caused by a mutation in the tumor suppressor gene MEN1 located at 11q13.[171,172] MEN1 may be involved in sporadic carcinoid tumors as well, as evidenced by loss of heterozygosity (LOH) on chromosome 11 or inactivated copies of the MEN1 gene.[173,174] Other possible contributors may be p53, K-ras-2, C-raf-1, and Bax/Bcl2.[172]

In a review of a 22-year period at St. Jude Children's Research Hospital, 0.08% of patients evaluated for malignancy had carcinoid tumors.[175] In that series, like others, the majority (approximately 60%) arose in the appendix. Pathologic examination of appendectomy specimens reveal carcinoid tumors in 0.23%, with the figure slightly lower in children than adults (Fig. 65-8).[170] Most patients with appendiceal carcinoid tumors have

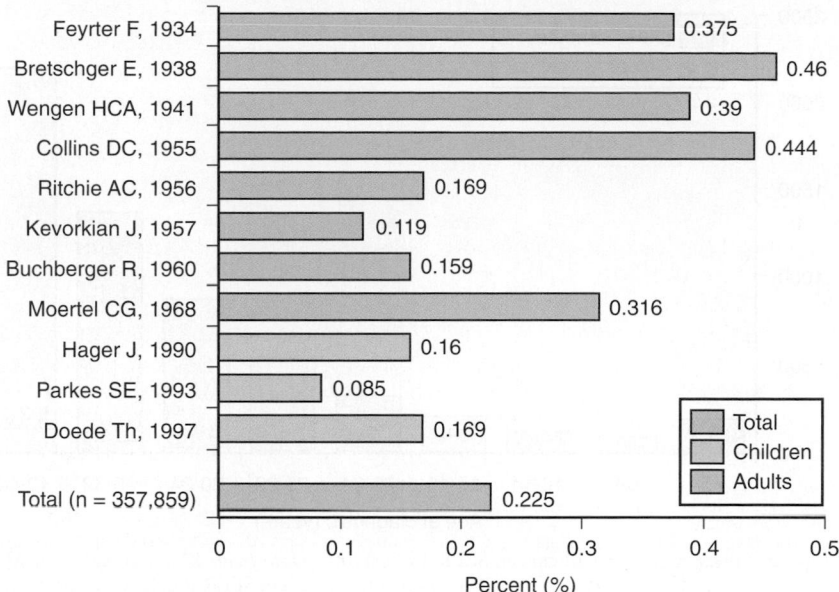

Figure 65-8 Percentage of appendectomy specimens found to have carcinoid tumors on pathologic examination. *(Modified from Doede T, Foss HD, Waldschmidt J: Carcinoid tumors of the appendix in children-epidemiology: clinical aspects and procedure.* Eur J Pediatr Surg 10:372–377, 2000.)

symptoms of acute appendicitis; others have chronic abdominal pain, or an incidental appendectomy is done during another surgical procedure. The diagnosis is rarely made preoperatively.

Appendiceal carcinoid tumors smaller than 1 cm rarely metastasize, and appendectomy alone is the appropriate therapy.[176] After a diagnosis of an appendiceal carcinoid tumor, it is reasonable to check levels of serum serotonin and chromogranin A and 24-hour urinary 5-HIAA, and abdominal imaging should be performed to look for metastases. Octreotide scans have a sensitivity of 80% to 90% for carcinoid tumors and can be useful at diagnosis to assess for metastases,[106,177] although there is a low incidence of distant disease in children. For appendiceal tumors larger than 2 cm, right hemicolectomy is advocated in adults[178]; there is controversy regarding its use for tumors between 1 and 2 cm and for children, for whom cecal or ileocecal resection may suffice.[179-181] Additionally, there are only rare cases of carcinoid tumors of the appendix with perforation described, but it is presumed that perforation in any carcinoid tumor would increase the risk for dissemination. The decision for hemicolectomy, particularly in those children with tumors having some high-risk features but size between 1 and 2 cm, must be made on a case-by-case basis.[182]

No deaths from pediatric appendiceal carcinoid have been reported in several large series with extended follow-up study.[169,180,181] In addition to increasing size, location at the base of the appendix and the presence of mucin-producing cells are thought to be poor prognostic indicators.[178] Given its rarity and benign behavior, recommended follow-up care is controversial. Several authors have recommended a schedule of monitoring serotonin metabolites, with or without abdominal ultrasonography, in patients whose tumor diameter was more

than 5 mm.[170,176] The findings that 14.6% of patients with appendiceal carcinoids in the SEER registry had synchronous or metachronous noncarcinoid malignant tumors,[183] that the risk of offspring carcinoid tumors (SIR 4.31) and secondary cancers (standardized incidence ratios [SIR] 2.15-3.31) was elevated in a Swedish registry study,[184] and several case reports of patients with secondary adenocarcinoma of the colon[175,185,186] have raised other questions of appropriate counseling and follow-up care for these patients. For the rare metastatic carcinoid tumor in childhood, treatment recommendations are based on experience in adult patients. Octreotide, a somatostatin analogue that has been used to treat the symptoms of carcinoid syndrome, has stabilized carcinoid tumor growth but not resulted in regression.[187] Similarly, interferon has been used with a modest response.[188] Recent efforts have demonstrated possible clinical activity of mTOR inhibitors and certain receptor tyrosine kinase inhibitors, but these initial findings await more follow-up investigation and larger studies.[189]

COLORECTAL CARCINOMA

In Western and developed countries, colorectal carcinoma is one of the most common malignant cancers and is responsible for significant morbidity and mortality. Conversely, colorectal carcinoma is rare in populations that do not have high rates of obesity and meat consumption. In the United States alone, approximately 153,000 patients per year are diagnosed with colorectal carcinoma, and approximately 52,000 deaths each year are attributed to it.[190] However, colorectal carcinoma is rare in children, with fewer than 100 cases per year in the United States as estimated by SEER data and approximately one case per million in those younger than age 20

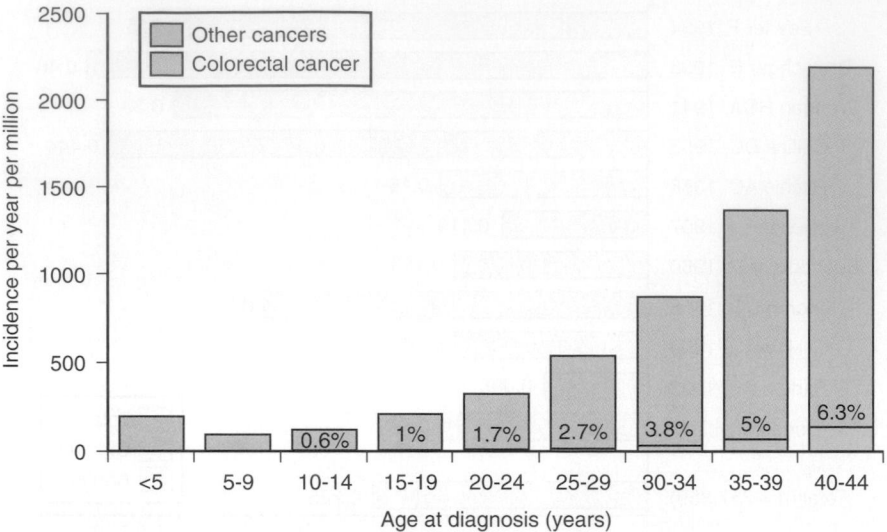

Figure 65-9 Incidence of colorectal cancer relative to all cancer, SEER 1975-2000. *(Data from Bleyer A, O'Leary M, Barr R, Ries LAG, editors: Cancer epidemiology in older adolescents and young adults 15 to 29 years of age, including SEER incidence and survival: 1975-2000 [NIH Publication No. 06-5767]. Bethesda, Md., 2006, National Cancer Institute.)*

years. The incidence of colorectal carcinoma relative to other cancers by age is shown in Figure 65-9, the 5-year survival rates of colorectal carcinoma by age are shown in Figure 65-10, and 5-year survival rates by age and stage are shown in Figure 65-11. Although case series offer suggestions about the biologic nature of this tumor in patients younger than 20 years, the rarity of this diagnosis in children means that comprehensive population-wide data are not available. Any case series from a large institution will be limited in number and by referral bias. Although many case series have suggested a higher stage at diagnosis for pediatric colorectal carcinoma and a prevalence of mucinous histology,[191,192] SEER data suggest that this disease in children more closely mirrors the adult

presentation and that referral bias could lead to the findings in the case series.

Most cases of colorectal carcinoma in adults occur sporadically and in association with lifestyle choices. Only approximately 10% of adults with colorectal carcinoma have an identified inherited or acquired predisposition to it. These include patients with the dominantly inherited FAP syndrome who have a mutation in the *FAP* tumor suppressor gene, patients with Lynch syndrome (also known as hereditary nonpolyposis colorectal cancer [HNPCC]) characterized by one of several defects in DNA mismatch repair genes, or patients with long-standing inflammatory bowel disease of more than 10 years' duration. It is not clear from the data whether

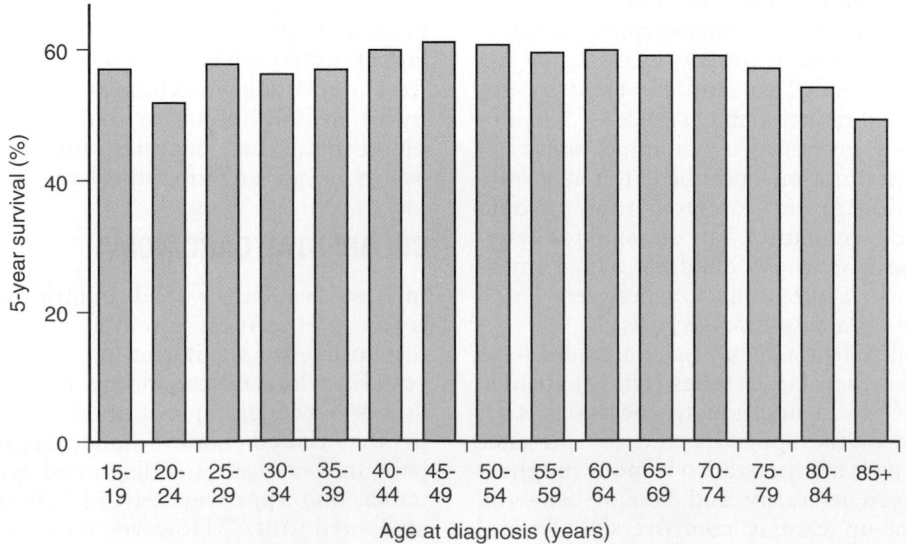

Figure 65-10 5-year survival rate for colorectal carcinoma, SEER 1975-1999. *(Data from Bleyer A, O'Leary M, Barr R, Ries LAG, editors: Cancer epidemiology in older adolescents and young adults 15 to 29 years of age, including SEER incidence and survival: 1975-2000 [NIH Publication No. 06-5767]. Bethesda, Md., 2006, National Cancer Institute.)*

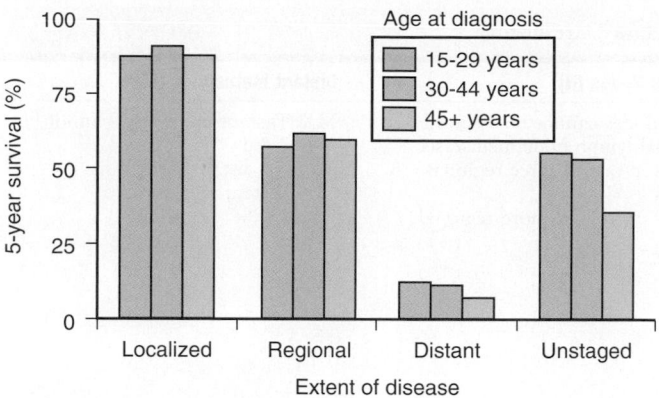

Figure 65-11 5-year survival rate for colorectal cancer by extent of disease, SEER 1975-2000. *(Data from Bleyer A, O'Leary M, Barr R, Ries LAG, editors: Cancer epidemiology in older adolescents and young adults 15 to 29 years of age, including SEER incidence and survival: 1975-2000 [NIH Publication No. 06-5767]. Bethesda, Md., 2006, National Cancer Institute.)*

children diagnosed with colorectal carcinoma are likely to have one of these common predispositions to the disease or if there is some other causative factor in these patients. Children with FAP, also known as Gardner syndrome, are commonly found to have myriad polyps on colonoscopy and many ultimately undergo prophylactic total colectomy before the age of 21 years because of symptoms (e.g., continued blood loss) or because of a strong family history of colon cancer. The vast majority of patients with FAP syndrome develop colorectal cancer by the age of 40 years. Many children who do undergo prophylactic colectomy are found to have dysplasia that was not apparent on routine screening colonoscopy.[193] Prophylactic colectomy is not clearly indicated in patients with Lynch syndrome, although in cases where there is lack of compliance with routine colonoscopy it may be appropriate.[194] Other syndromes associated with colorectal carcinoma include Bloom, Peutz-Jeghers, Turcot, Oldfield, and Rendu-Osler-Weber syndromes.[195-199]

Clinical Presentation

Colorectal carcinoma arises from the mucosal surface of the bowel, often growing from within a polyp. The tumor can cause intestinal obstruction through growth into the lumen of the bowel or can erode through the serosa and spread intraperitoneally. The early signs of colorectal carcinoma are difficult to separate from more common causes of abdominal complaints. Anemia, vague abdominal pain, bleeding, weight loss, and change in bowel habits have all been reported as the presenting complaint for children with colon cancer.[191] Many of these presenting complaints are common in pediatric care; it is possible that children who seek care with higher stages of colon cancer would have earlier diagnoses if they were adults, because an older adult with these complaints would likely be referred for colonoscopy. In two relatively large series reporting on this rare tumor in children, 0 of 20 and 3 of 30 patients had modified Dukes stage B tumors.[191-192] All other patients were stage C or D, and only 1 of 20 and 2 of 30 patients were alive without evidence of

disease when these reports were published. In these two series, 16 of 20 and 25 of 30 patients had tumors with mucinous histology, a higher rate than that reported for adults with colorectal carcinoma. Again, these dire statistics likely reflect referral patterns, although they demonstrate that children with colorectal carcinoma can have high-stage disease at diagnosis. Although vigilance for pediatric colorectal carcinoma remains important, in the absence of known risk factors for the disease, adult-oriented screening examinations such as colonoscopy, routine testing of stool for occult blood, and sigmoidoscopy are not indicated, because they would pick up many false-positives and would not be cost-effective.

Diagnosis and Staging

The diagnosis of colorectal carcinoma in children requires a high index of suspicion in patients with the typical presenting signs or symptoms and tissue acquisition. The exact procedure required to obtain tissue for diagnosis is best determined in consultation with surgical colleagues and depends on the patient's clinical situation. For some patients, complete resection before chemotherapy may be appropriate, but for others, particularly those known to have metastatic disease, chemotherapy or radiotherapy may make resection possible in previously unresectable cases, so a less invasive approach to diagnosis is warranted after careful consultation with a multidisciplinary team. Any patient undergoing resection should have up to 12 lymph nodes sampled in an attempt to determine whether the cancer has spread.[200] An expert panel convened by the American Society of Clinical Oncology has not recommended adjuvant chemotherapy for those adult patients with stage II colorectal carcinoma that can be fully surgically resected. Children tend to have more widespread disease at presentation; however in the absence of data to support a contrary approach, for children with disease that can be fully resected at initial diagnosis, surgical intervention and subsequent observation seem to be indicated.[201]

For pediatric patients discovered to have colorectal carcinoma, full staging should involve functional and anatomic imaging (see later) as would be carried out in adult patients. In adults, linked PET and CT scans are increasingly becoming the norm, because this modality helps link fluorodeoxyglucose (FDG)-avid lesions with actual sites of disease more efficaciously than separate PET and CT scans that cannot be linked because of bowel movement. Most large pediatric oncology centers now have access to linked PET and CT. Barium enema is sometimes used to help identify areas of concern before the diagnosis is made, and a bone scan can be used to identify bone metastases if there is concern that PET is not picking up lesions.[202] The AJCC staging for colorectal carcinoma is shown in Tables 65-6 and 65-7.

Treatment

Initial management of the patient is focused on the diagnostic and staging workup and on any surgical interventions that are urgently needed in the context of bowel-related emergencies such as perforation or obstruction. Consultation with medical oncologists experienced

TABLE 65-6   Tumor-Nodes-Metastasis Definitions for Colorectal Carcinoma

Primary Tumor (T)	Regional Lymph Nodes (N)[§]	Distant Metastasis (M)
TX: Primary tumor cannot be assessed T0: No evidence of primary tumor Tis: Carcinoma in situ: intraepithelial or invasion of the lamina propria* T1: Tumor invades submucosa T2: Tumor invades muscularis propria T3: Tumor invades through the muscularis propria into the subserosa or into nonperitonealized pericolic or perirectal tissues T4: Tumor directly invades other organs or structures and/or perforates visceral peritoneum[†,‡]	NX: Regional nodes cannot be assessed N0: No regional lymph node metastasis N1: Metastasis in one to three regional lymph nodes N2: Metastasis in four or more regional lymph nodes	MX: Distant metastasis cannot be assessed M0: No distant metastasis M1: Distant metastasis

From Colon and rectum. In Edge SB, Byrd DR, Compton CC, et al, editors: AJCC cancer staging manual, ed 7, New York, 2010, Springer, p. 143–164.

*Tis includes cancer cells confined within the glandular basement membrane (intraepithelial) or lamina propria (intramucosal) with no extension through the muscularis mucosae into the submucosa.

[†]Direct invasion in T4 includes invasion of other segments of the colorectum by way of the serosa; for example, invasion of the sigmoid colon by a carcinoma of the cecum.

[‡]Tumor that is adherent macroscopically to other organs or structures is classified T4. If no tumor is present in the adhesion microscopically, however, the classification should be pT3. The V and L substaging should be used to identify the presence or absence of vascular or lymphatic invasion.

[§]A tumor nodule in the pericolorectal adipose tissue of a primary carcinoma without histologic evidence of residual lymph node in the nodule is classified in the pN category as a regional lymph node metastasis if the nodule has the form and smooth contour of a lymph node. If the nodule has an irregular contour, it should be classified in the T category and also coded as V1 (microscopic venous invasion) or as V2 (if it was grossly evident), because there is a strong likelihood that it represents venous invasion.

in evaluating adult patients with colorectal carcinoma may help guide the workup.[203] Because of the potential for anemia from bleeding and liver involvement, as well as the potential for peritoneal seeding, complete blood counts, liver function tests, and kidney function tests with electrolyte levels should be obtained at diagnosis.[191] Carcinoembryonic antigen (CEA) should also be determined, although most series have found that children tend not to have heightened CEA at diagnosis,[191-192] and subsequently followed to survey for occult recurrence. Many chemotherapeutic agents can increase CEA, so care

should be taken when interpreting these values, especially when the patient is receiving oxaliplatin.[204] These patients should generally not have values checked until they have recovered from chemotherapy. If the patient did not have an elevated CEA level at diagnosis, the decision not to monitor subsequent levels to screen for occult relapse is reasonable but should be made in close consultation with medical oncology colleagues.

The treatment for children with colorectal carcinoma should be planned in conjunction with reports in the adult literature and with a medical oncologist experienced in treating gastrointestinal cancer in adults. Adult patients with stage II disease have not been shown to benefit from adjuvant chemotherapy if they have no evidence of disease after resection[201] and should undergo wide surgical resection with anastomosis if possible. It is reasonable to recommend careful observation after surgical treatment for children in this scenario in the absence of a clinical trial, because there is no standard of care therapy for these patients that has proven to reduce the risk for relapse. Although these patients should be considered for randomized controlled clinical trials, there are likely to be few trials available that include children younger than 18 years. If details of the case or of the surgical resection increase the concern that the patient could suffer a relapse, adjuvant therapy could be considered because the risk for recurrence could be from 51% to 73%.[205] The situation should include careful discussion between the oncologist and family. For patients with stage III or higher disease, chemotherapy has demonstrated a survival benefit for adults with colorectal carcinoma, and children should be treated in a similar fashion.[206] Patients with metastatic colorectal carcinoma should have their tumors tested for KRAS in codons

TABLE 65-7   American Joint Committee on Cancer Stage Groupings for Colorectal Carcinoma

Stage	Groupings
0	Tis, N0, M0
I	T1, N0, M0 T2, N0, M0
IIA	T3, N0, M0
IIB	T4, N0, M0
IIIA	T1, N1, M0 T2, N1, M0
IIIB	T3, N1, M0 T4, N1, M0
IIIC	Any T, N2, M0
IV	Any T, any N, M1

From Colon and rectum. In Edge SB, Byrd DR, Compton CC, et al, editors: AJCC cancer staging manual, ed 7, New York, 2010, Springer, p. 143–164.

12 or 13 in a Clinical Laboratory Improvement Amendment (CLIA)–certified laboratory. Those with tumors demonstrated to have *KRAS* mutations should not receive anti–epidermal growth factor receptor (EGFR) antibody therapy with chemotherapy, because it is not of benefit in these cases in adults.[207]

SEER data have suggested that the proportion of children with colorectal carcinoma who have high-stage disease at diagnosis mirrors that of adults with colorectal carcinoma. Thus at diagnosis many children have a higher stage disease that is fully resectable and that requires chemotherapy. These patients tend to have a poor prognosis. There are several regimens associated with prolonged survival for patients with metastatic colorectal carcinoma in adults based on the use of 5-fluorouracil (5-FU), oxaliplatin, and irinotecan in a variety of combinations. Bevacizumab (Avastin) is also being used in conjunction with these regimens, often as second-line therapy in adults, with the benefit of an improvement in survival.[208] Children with high-stage colorectal carcinoma have a poor prognosis, and any child successfully cured may have years of life added, so it may be reasonable for pediatric oncologists to add bevacizumab to the established regimens as frontline therapy. However, this depends somewhat on the clinical scenario. Bevacizumab has been tested in children with cancer in combination therapy, and a pediatric phase I trial of bevacizumab has been completed, so there is experience administering this agent to children.[209] New data also suggest that blocking VEGF with aflibercept has therapeutic benefit in colorectal carcinoma.[210] Further information on chemotherapy regimens for patients with colorectal carcinoma can be found at http://www.cancer.gov/cancertopics/pdq/treatment/colon/HealthProfessional/page4.

Screening and Preventive Therapy for At-Risk Children

Children with a family history of FAP syndrome should generally begin undergoing colonoscopy by the age of 10 or 12 years and should be observed closely by geneticists and pediatric gastroenterologists.[211,212] For such patients, prophylactic colectomy is essential to prevent death from colorectal carcinoma later in life. The decision to undergo total colectomy must be made in conjunction with the family history and timing of cancer onset in the pedigree, the clinical situation, and the child's wishes. Patients with HNPCC are unlikely to develop colorectal carcinoma before the age of 18 years, but the accepted standard for such patients is to begin regular colonoscopy at 20 years of age or at least 10 years earlier than the earliest onset of colorectal carcinoma in their pedigree.[213] For patients with inflammatory bowel disease, care should be based on standard practices for pediatric gastroenterology. Cyclooxygenase-2 (COX-2) inhibitors have been shown to reduce the risk for developing colorectal carcinoma in adults but are known to increase the risk for cardiovascular side effects, so they are not universally recommended for adults at risk of developing colorectal carcinoma.[214] These agents have been used in the pediatric oncology setting and may in the future be appropriate chemoprophylaxis for children at high risk for colorectal carcinoma.[215]

Follow-Up Observation

For the child with the sporadic occurrence of colorectal carcinoma who is cured by surgery or surgery and chemotherapy, careful observation must be recommended. However, there is little evidence available on the risk for such children to suffer recurrence or the risk for second malignancies later in life. Colorectal carcinoma is rare in children and often difficult to cure, so survivors are few. No large-scale randomized trials have documented the efficacy of a standard, postoperative monitoring program in adults to date. Therefore given the long latency period for relapse for young children, they should probably be screened with regular colonoscopy and radiologic evaluation of the lungs and perhaps PET scanning as well.[216,217] Because pediatric colorectal carcinoma is so rare, the child may suffer from a cancer predisposition syndrome and consideration should be given to such a diagnosis. The child may benefit from yearly colonoscopy and should be brought to medical attention with little delay for any blood in the stool or other symptoms of colon cancer. Screening for CEA at a reasonable interval could be considered but is associated with a high rate of false-positives in adults. It should probably only be used for children who had high levels at presentation and are healthy enough to undergo risky surgery if any liver or lung metastases are found early by screening.[216] Although the 5-year survival rate for low-stage colon cancer is excellent (approximately 90%), patients with metastatic disease have less than a 10% 5-year survival rate. For those who survive metastatic pediatric colorectal cancer, it is unclear for how long surveillance against relapse should be done, but follow-up care in a long-term survivor clinic is indicated.

URINARY BLADDER CARCINOMA

Rhabdomyosarcoma is a relatively common tumor affecting the urinary tract and is discussed elsewhere in this text (see Chapter 59). Malignant epithelial tumors of the bladder are extremely rare in children in the Western world; the incidence of bladder cancer in general is higher in Africa because of the inflammation caused by chronic parasitic infection with bilharzial and other organisms.[218] Boys are more likely than girls to be diagnosed with this.[219] The presenting signs and symptoms of transitional cell tumors of the bladder in children include gross painless hematuria, urinary tract infections, voiding difficulties, and even hematospermia.

If a child is suspected of having a bladder tumor, the differential diagnosis must include malignancies such as epithelial bladder cancer and rhabdomyosarcoma, as well as benign lesions such as inflammatory masses. In the absence of obvious clinical signs of a mass, these patients are usually seen first by the pediatric urologist. The initial workup should include urinalysis and culture, urine cytology, and imaging studies. CT or MRI can help define the lesion. Cystoscopy can help reveal the nature of the tumor and allow for biopsy of lesional tissue. Attempts at transurethral biopsy are a primary mode of obtaining a tissue diagnosis, with open procedures to be considered

Box 65-1	Ovarian Neoplasms

MALIGNANT TUMORS

1. Germ cell (65% to 70%)
2. Epithelial tumors (15%, including low malignant potential or borderline tumors)
   a. Adenocarcinoma
   b. Cystadenocarcinoma: mucinous, serous
   c. Endometrioid
   d. Clear-cell tumor
   e. Undifferentiated carcinoma
3. Stromal tumors (15%)
   a. Juvenile granulosa-cell tumors (JGCTs)
   b. Sertoli-Leydig cell tumors
   c. Sclerosing stromal tumors
   d. Gynandroblastoma
4. Miscellaneous (<5%)
   a. Burkitt lymphoma
   b. Carcinosarcoma (malignant mixed müllerian tumor)

BENIGN TUMORS

1. Germ cell
   a. Cystic teratoma (dermoid)
2. Epithelial
   a. Cystadenomas
   b. Mucinous
   c. Papillary and nonpapillary serous
3. Stromal tumors
   a. Granulosa cell
   b. Theca cell
   c. Fibromas

as a backup maneuver.[220] Because bladder cancer is uncommon in younger patients, delay in diagnosis is not uncommon for younger patients. However, the outcome for children and young adults with bladder carcinoma seems to be better than for adults, explained in part by more indolent clinical and biological features. Patient younger than 20 years of age at diagnosis, for instance, have a lower incidence of chromosome 9 abnormalities, *FGFR3* mutations, and few epigenetic alterations. Therefore treatment decisions must include careful consideration of late effects.[221]

OVARIAN TUMORS

Approximately 50% of tumors occurring in the ovary in children are nonneoplastic. Furthermore, the minority of neoplastic lesions are malignant, so that only 10% to 20% of ovarian masses in children are cancerous (Box 65-1).[222-224] In children and even in adolescents, surgical management plans should take into consideration the lower rate of malignancy than in adults and minimize the risk of compromising hormonal function and fertility.[225] Ovarian masses usually present with abdominal pain, bloating, distention, or dysmenorrhea. The most appropriate and widely used initial evaluation tool for an ovarian mass is ultrasonography, which can distinguish the size, origin, and cystic nature of the tumor.[226] If cystic, unilateral, and presumed benign, a laparoscopic procedure is appropriate. Otherwise, further workup with chest, abdomen, and/or pelvic CT and tumor markers such as β-human chorionic gonadotropin (β-hCG), α-fetoprotein (AFP), cancer antigen-125 (CA-125), and

CEA is required, and open laparotomy should be the surgical approach.[226] Ovarian tumors are staged by the International Federation of Gynecology and Obstetrics (FIGO) system (Table 65-8).

Of the neoplastic tumors, germ-cell tumors account for 65% to 70% (see Chapter 63). Epithelial carcinomas, the

TABLE 65-8   Carcinoma of the Ovary

Stage	Extent of Growth
I	Growth limited to the ovaries
IA	Growth limited to one ovary; no ascites present containing malignant cells; no tumor on the external surface; capsule intact
IB	Growth limited to both ovaries; no ascites present containing malignant cells; no tumor on the external surface; capsules intact
IC*	Tumor either stage IA or IB, but with tumor on surface of one or both ovaries or with capsule ruptured, ascites present containing malignant cells, or positive peritoneal washings
II	Growth involving one or both ovaries with pelvic extension
IIA	Extension and/or metastases to the uterus and/or tubes
IIB	Extension to other pelvic tissues
IIC†	Tumor either stage IIA or IIB, but with tumor on surface of one or both ovaries or with capsule(s) ruptured, ascites present containing malignant cells, or positive peritoneal washings
III	Tumor involving one or both ovaries, with histologically confirmed peritoneal implants outside the pelvis and/or positive retroperitoneal or inguinal nodes; superficial live metastases equals stage III; tumor limited to the true pelvis but with histologically proven malignant extension to small bowel or omentum
IIIA	Tumor grossly limited to the true pelvis, with negative nodes but with histologically confirmed microscopic seeding of abdominal peritoneal surfaces or histologically proven extension to small bowel or mesentery
IIIB	Tumor of one or both ovaries with histologically confirmed implants, peritoneal metastasis of abdominal peritoneal surface not exceeding 2 cm in diameter; nodes are negative
IIIC	Peritoneal metastasis beyond the pelvis >2 cm in diameter and/or positive retroperitoneal or inguinal nodes
IV	Growth involving one or both ovaries with distant metastases; if pleural effusion is present, there must be positive cytology to allot a case to stage IV; parenchymal liver metastasis equals stage IV

From Heintz AP, Odicino F, Maisonneuve P, et al: Carcinoma of the ovary: FIGO 6th Annual Report on the Results of Treatment in Gynecological Cancer. Int J Gynaecol Obstet 95(Suppl 1):S161–S192, 2006.

*International Federation of Gynecology and Obstetrics (FIGO) nomenclature, Rio de Janeiro, 1988.

†To evaluate the impact on prognosis of the different criteria for allotting cases to stage IC or IIC, it would be of value to know if rupture of the capsule was spontaneous or caused by the surgeon and if the source of malignant cells detected was peritoneal washings or ascites.

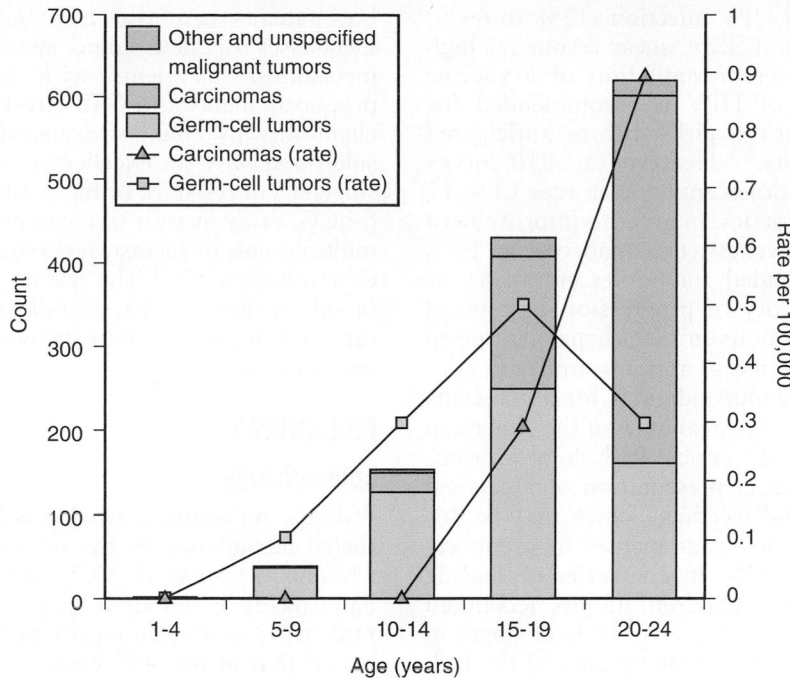

Figure 65-12 Incidence and rate per 100,000 cases of ovarian cancer in children and young adults, SEER-17 1998-2002.

most common ovarian tumor in adults, account for 15% to 20% of pediatric ovarian tumors, with most occurring after menarche when the rate increases markedly (Fig. 65-12). Unlike in adults, most pediatric epithelial ovarian tumors are localized, and pathologically most are of low malignant potential (borderline) or well differentiated.[224,227] Stage I tumors of potential low malignancy are appropriately treated by unilateral salpingo-oophorectomy alone, and have almost a 100% survival rate.[227] Surgery should include careful inspection of the peritoneum and contralateral ovary and lymph nodes.[228] For those rare children with invasive or advanced disease, platinum-based therapy developed for adult epithelial carcinomas has proven effective. Although a thorough family history should be obtained as a matter of course, studies suggest that breast cancer genes 1 and 2 (*BRCA1/2*), breast and ovarian cancer syndrome, and HNPCC syndrome account for few cases of epithelial cancer in women younger than age 30 years.[229-231]

Stromal Carcinomas

Tumors of the mesenchymal tissue of the ovary account for 15% of ovarian malignancies in pediatrics. Most present at an early stage and have a prognosis for survival higher than 85%.[232] Sertoli-Leydig tumors often cause overproduction of androgen precursors, producing virilizing symptoms of amenorrhea, masculinization, and hirsutism. Juvenile granulosa-cell tumors can overproduce estrogen and progesterone and present with precocious puberty. These tumors are sometimes classified with benign tumors, and many act in a benign fashion but have malignant potential and have been reported to metastasize and be fatal.[233] Nonlocalized tumors should be treated with adjuvant platinum-based chemotherapy with or without radiation.[234]

TUMORS OF THE CERVIX AND VAGINA

The most common nonovarian tumor of the female genital tract is rhabdomyosarcoma (82% in a registry series over 25 years in Great Britain), and the appearance of a protruding cluster-of-grapes vaginal mass in a young child is classic for sarcoma botryoides.[235,236] Cervical and vaginal carcinomas in children can be adenocarcinomas or squamous carcinomas; the ratio is skewed more toward adenocarcinoma in children than in adults. There is no known difference in causative factors, treatment, or prognosis between the two pathologies. Mesonephric adenocarcinoma is rare in adults but is a relatively more common subtype in children; it is thought to arise from mesonephric duct remnants and tends to arise deeply without reaching the endocervical surface.[237]

Cervicovaginal clear-cell adenocarcinomas are not associated with HPV infection. Rather, a peak of incidence in children and adolescent girls was a historic phenomenon caused by the maternal use of diethylstilbestrol (DES) therapy in pregnancy. Since its proscription, the tumor is again relatively uncommon in pediatrics. However, rates of non-DES cervical cancer in adolescents have been rising because of increasingly early sexual activity and higher rates of HPV infection.[238] HPV types 16 and 18 are the causative agents in more than 70% of cervical cancer. Around puberty the cervix has a particular biologic vulnerability to HPV infection, so that the sexually active adolescent has one of the highest risks of infection after exposure,[239] creating a risk for the development of squamous intraepithelial lesions that can progress over 10 to 15 years to invasive cervical cancer.[240] Recent data have shown that 27.8% of ninth-grade and 63.6% of twelfth-grade girls report having had sexual intercourse.[241] These sexually active female adolescents have high rates of genital HPV infection (13% to 64%) and abnormal Papanicolaou (Pap) smear results (as high as 38%).[239,240,242] The recent formulation of a vaccine against multiple strains of HPV is recommended for administration to 12-year-old girls—before anticipated initiation of sexual activity.[243] However, a 2010 survey found that only 32% of adolescent females ages 13 to 17 years complete the 3-dose series. In order to improve herd immunity and cost-effectiveness, the quadrivalent HPV vaccine is now recommended for adolescent males as well.[15-16] The natural history of progression of cervical abnormalities (from squamous intraepithelial lesions to cervical intraepithelial neoplasia) appears similar in adolescents and adults.[244] Recommendations for adolescents with abnormal Pap smears are available on the American Society for Colposcopy and Cervical Pathology website.

The most common clinical presentation of a cervical or vaginal tumor is vaginal bleeding, which may be difficult to distinguish from irregular menses in prepubescent and early pubescent girls. In one series evaluating causes of vaginal bleeding in children, tumors accounted for 11%.[245] These tumors often present at later stages in children and adolescents than adults because of the lack of screening Pap smears and hesitancy to perform pelvic examinations.[246]

Treatment includes surgical resection with lymph-node exploration and adjuvant radiation for residual disease or lymph nodes. This preference of surgery over radiation differs from therapy for adults because of the need to avoid radiation toxicity in younger, growing children. Novel uterus-sparing techniques (e.g., radical abdominal/vaginal trachelectomy) first adopted in adults to preserve fertility have been used successfully in children.[247,248] In a retrospective study of women younger than 25 years, localized cervical cancer had a 5-year survival rate of 91% and regional disease had a 5-year survival rate of 46%.[249] A series of 37 pediatric cases of vaginal and cervical adenocarcinoma from St. Jude Children's Research Hospital has found a 71% 3-year survival rate.[246] Other rare tumors reported in the cervix and vagina are alveolar soft parts sarcoma,[250,251] germ-cell tumors such as endodermal sinus (yolk sac) tumor and embryonal carcinoma,[236,252] and Wilms tumor.[253] These tumors are covered elsewhere in this text.

GESTATIONAL TROPHOBLASTIC TUMOR

Sexually active adolescents are at risk for these rare tumors, which arise as tumors of the products of conception. A hydatidiform mole, or molar pregnancy, is a uterine mass consisting only of placental-like tissue without an intact fetus. Pregnancies in those younger than 15 years have a sixfold risk of being molar.[254] Hydatidiform moles are treated by dilation and curettage with careful follow-up monitoring for resolution of elevated β-hCG levels.[255] Persistent or increasing β-hCG levels after a molar pregnancy, abortion, or term pregnancy indicate a malignant gestational trophoblastic tumor (GTT), the most aggressive of which is choriocarcinoma, a malignant tumor of the trophoblastic epithelium. The most common symptom is abnormal vaginal bleeding,

but patients can also have asymptomatic pulmonary metastases or neurologic symptoms caused by brain metastases.[256] Patients with nonmetastatic or good-prognosis metastatic GTT are treated with single-agent chemotherapy (methotrexate, dactinomycin, or etoposide), and have an excellent prognosis.[257,258] Those with single-agent resistant or high-risk metastatic disease (high β-hCG, delay in start of chemotherapy, brain metastases, multiple sites of metastases) require multiagent cytotoxic chemotherapy.[259-261] The use of platinum and etoposide-based regimens has significantly improved salvage rates for high risk patients who fail initial multiagent chemotherapy.[262]

MELANOMA

Epidemiology

Pediatric melanoma, which has been classified as an epithelial malignancy by the International Classification of Childhood Cancer (ICCC), accounts for 30% of epithelial cancers in children and adolescents.[41,55] Although rare, particularly among prepubertal patients, it is estimated that nearly 450 cases of pediatric melanoma are diagnosed each year in the United States in patients younger than age 20 years[31] and most cases affect 15- to 19-year-old adolescents, in whom this malignancy accounts for 7.1% of all cancers (Fig. 65-13).[41]

The incidence of melanoma in children younger than age 20 years increased by 2.9% per year from 1973 to 2001, with the highest rates of increase in adolescents.[263] Most melanomas in pediatric patients affect white females, and over 80% are localized. The female-to-male ratio increases with age, especially during adolescence, and there is a preponderance of nonwhite patients, nodular histology, and head and neck sites in patients younger than 10 years of age.[263]

Risk Factors

Melanoma can be transmitted transplacentally, but this is a very rare phenomenon that is associated with a dismal clinical outcome.[264] Other risk factors associated with the risk of melanoma in the pediatric population include the presence of a large congenital nevus, retinoblastoma, Werner syndrome, prior history of childhood cancer, xeroderma pigmentosum, neurocutaneous melanosis, immunosuppression, familial melanoma, and dysplastic nevi.[265-267]

Clinical Molecular and Pathologic Features

Pediatric melanoma resembles adult melanoma in its clinical presentation and can arise in a preexisting nevus or de novo. The classic ABCDEs of melanoma (asymmetry, border irregularity, color variegation, diameter larger than 6 mm, and an evolving lesion) are commonly reported in childhood and adolescent cases, but the presence of other lesions such as Spitz nevus or amelanotic lesions may make diagnosis difficult and delay the diagnosis. It is estimated that up to 60% of pediatric patients with melanomas are initially misdiagnosed.[266,268] The pathologic diagnosis of melanoma may be often difficult and challenging. Increasing evidence has suggested that

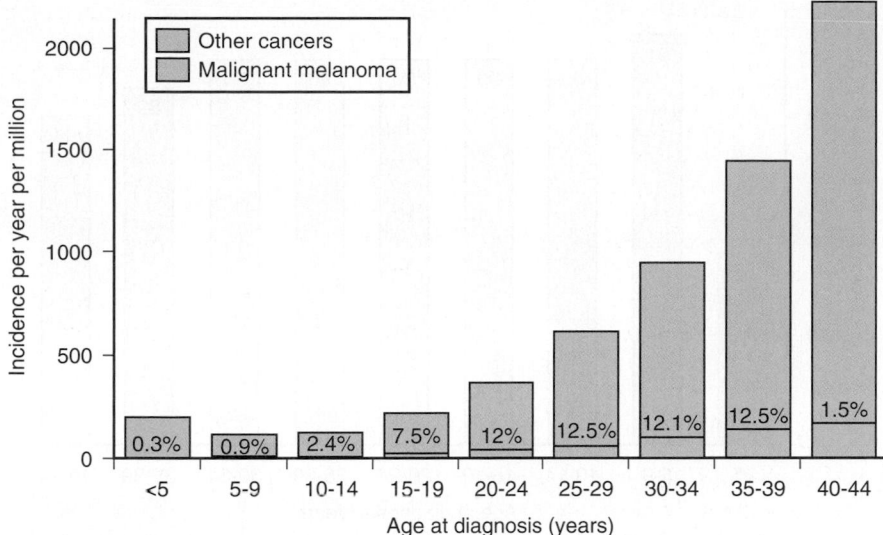

Figure 65-13 Incidence of malignant melanoma relative to all cancer, SEER 1975-2000.

pediatric melanoma may have a significant variability in its pathologic spectrum. The term *melanocytic lesion with unknown metastatic potential* has gained popularity in recent years, adding to the uncertainty and confusion of diagnosing pediatric melanoma.[269] The use of fluorescence in situ hybridization (FISH) probes sets that target 6 distinct chromosomal loci has identified 9p21 deletions and 6p25, 11q23 gains as markers of aggressive behavior.[270] About 50% of pediatric melanomas have a *BRAF V600* mutation that can be targeted with available therapies for adults.[271,272]

Diagnosis and Staging

Since there is no validated system for children, guidelines for diagnosing and staging children with melanoma have been extrapolated from adult studies. Adhering to the current AJCC guidelines for staging all pediatric patients with melanoma is recommended.[273] The use of routine imaging in children with melanoma has not been studied prospectively, but in one study 25% of patients with thicker lesions had evidence of distant disease on CT of the chest and abdomen. The routine use of PET imaging for staging pediatric melanoma has not been studied prospectively, but in adults it has not revealed a significant patient-relevant benefit.[274] Early detection and biopsy are imperative, and when melanoma is suspected the pathology report should include the type of melanoma, depth, mitotic count, and surgical margins. Nodal staging using sentinel node biopsy has become commonplace in pediatrics and should be performed in children with lesions greater than1 mm thick and may be considered in children with thinner lesions if they display one or more high risk features such as Clarks level of invasion IV or V, ulceration, and high mitotic rate (>0/mm²).[275]

Treatment and Outcome

Surgery is the treatment of choice for pediatric melanoma. For patients with lesions greater than 1 mm a wide

excision with a 1-cm margin is appropriate. For those that are 1 to 2 mm, a 1 to 2-cm margin is recommended, and for those thicker than 2 mm a 2-cm margin should be used.[276] After a positive sentinel node it is recommended that a patient be offered a complete lymph node dissection, because about 16% of these patients have occult nodal metastases; however, a survival advantage after this procedure has not been clearly demonstrated.[277,278] The administration of adjuvant high-dose interferon improves relapse-free survival in adult patients with high-risk melanoma, and this option should be offered to patients at high risk for recurrence.[279] Although single-institution studies suggest that high-dose interferon is well tolerated in children with melanoma, its use has not been studied prospectively in large numbers of patients.[280-282] Subcutaneous pegylated interferon for up to 5 years has been shown to prolong disease-free survival in adults with resected microscopic nodal disease and ulceration.[283] Its use in pediatrics has been limited, and results of clinical trials using this agent in children have not been yet published. Because *BRAF V600* mutations are seen in up to 50% of pediatric melanomas, the use of targeted therapies such as vemurafenib and dabrafenib should be explored further. There is a pediatric trial using vemurafenib for patients 12 to 17 years of age with measurable *BRAF V600* mutated melanoma. Ipilimumab, a monoclonal antibody directed against the inhibitory molecule cytotoxic T-lymphocyte antigen 4 (CTLA4), has improved survival in adults with metastatic melanoma, and a pediatric trial is being conducted.[284] In addition, other novel immunotherapies such as BMS-936558, a monoclonal antibody directed against programmed death receptor 1 (PD1), and BMS-936559, a monoclonal antibody directed against programmed cell death 1 ligand 1 (PDL1), has produced encouraging responses in adults with metastatic melanoma, but a pediatric trial is not available.[285,286] The overall survival of pediatric melanoma is stage-dependent and overall excellent, with

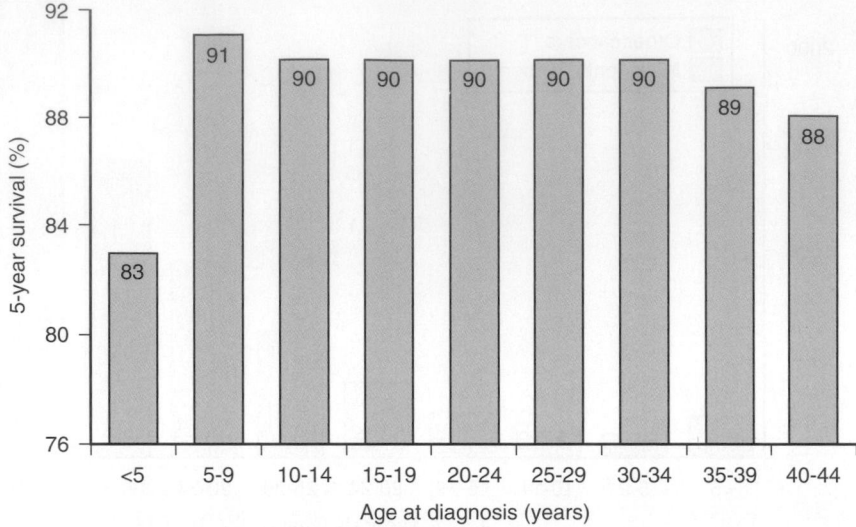

Figure 65-14 5-year survival rate for melanoma, SEER 1975-1999.

5-year survival rates in excess of 90% except in those who are younger than 10 years of age (Fig. 65-14).

References available online at ExpertConsult.

KEY REFERENCES

2. Weir HK, Thun MJ, Hankey BF, et al: Annual report to the nation on the status of cancer, 1975-2000, featuring the uses of surveillance data for cancer prevention and control. *J Natl Cancer Inst* 95(17):1276–1299, 2003.
   This work lays the foundation for the use of SEER data in this chapter.
10. Kreimer AR, Clifford GM, Boyle P, et al: Human papillomavirus types in head and neck squamous cell carcinomas worldwide: a systematic review. *Cancer Epidemiol Biomarkers Prev* 14(2):467–475, 2005.
    A systematic review of the role of HPV in head and neck cancer worldwide.
15. Advisory Committee on Immunization Practices (ACIP): Recommendations on the use of quadrivalent human papillomavirus vaccine in males, 2011. *MMWR Morb Mortal Wkly Rep* 60(50):1705–1708, 2011.
    Recommendations for the use of HPV vaccination in boys.
16. Committee on Infectious Diseases: HPV vaccine recommendations. *Pediatrics* 129(3):602–605, 2012.
    General recommendations for HPV vaccination in children.
24. Rodriguez-Galindo C, Wofford M, Castleberry RP, et al: Preradiation chemotherapy with methotrexate, cisplatin, 5-fluorouracil, and leucovorin for pediatric nasopharyngeal carcinoma. *Cancer* 103(4):850–857, 2005.
    Reports a cooperative group trial of chemotherapy for children with nasopharyngeal carcinoma.
41. Bleyer A, O'Leary M, Barr R: *Cancer epidemiology in older adolescents and young adults 15 to 29 years of age including SEER incidence and survival: 1975-2000*, Bethesda, Md, 2006, National Cancer Institute.
    A report based on the SEER database that demonstrated the unmet need for clinical trials in the adolescent and young adult age group.
69. Newman KD, Black T, Heller G, et al: Differentiated thyroid cancer: determinants of disease progression in patients <21 years of age at diagnosis: a report from the Surgical Discipline Committee of the Children's Cancer Group. *Ann Surg* 227(4):533–541, 1998.
    A report from a cooperative group on thyroid cancer in children.

83. Chung EM, Cube R, Hall GJ: From the archives of the AFIP: breast masses in children and adolescents; radiologic-pathologic correlation. *Radiographics* 29(3):907–931, 2009.
    Discusses the correlation between radiology and pathology in breast masses in young people.
93. Xiong Q, Valero V, Kau V, et al: Female patients with breast carcinoma age 30 years and younger have a poor prognosis: the MD Anderson Cancer Center experience. *Cancer* 92(10):2523–2528, 2001.
    Reports on the breast cancer experience in younger patients at MD Anderson Cancer Center over an extended time period.
94. Dishop MK, Kuruvilla S: Primary and metastatic lung tumors in the pediatric population: a review and 25-year experience at a large children's hospital. *Arch Pathol Lab Med* 132(7):1079–1103, 2008.
    A large series of children with lung tumors.
119. Priest JR, Hill DA, Williams GM, et al: Type I pleuropulmonary blastoma: a report from the International Pleuropulmonary Blastoma Registry. *J Clin Oncol* 24(27):4492–4498, 2006.
    A large series of pleuropulmonary blastoma cases.
131. Kantar M, Cetingul N, Veral A: Rare tumors of the lung in children. *Pediatr Hematol Oncol* 19(6):421–428, 2002.
    Reviews rare tumors of the lung in children.
137. Ellis P, Davies AM, Evans WK, et al: The use of chemotherapy in patients with advanced malignant pleural mesothelioma: a systematic review and practice guideline. *J Thorac Oncol* 1(6):591–601, 2006.
    A systematic review and guideline for therapy of mesothelioma.
139. Corless CL, Barnett CM, Heinrich MC: Gastrointestinal stromal tumours: origin and molecular oncology. *Nat Rev Cancer* 11(12):865–878, 2011.
    Background on GIST.
152. Pappo AS, Janeway KA: Pediatric gastrointestinal stromal tumors. *Hematol Oncol Clin North Am* 23(1):vii, 15–34, 2009.
    Background on pediatric GIST.
158. Janeway KA, Liegl B, Harlow A, et al: Pediatric KIT wild-type and platelet-derived growth factor receptor alpha-wild-type gastrointestinal stromal tumors share KIT activation but not mechanisms of genetic progression with adult gastrointestinal stromal tumors. *Cancer Res* 67(19):9084–9088, 2007.
    Begins to explain molecular differences between pediatric and adult GIST.
161. Janeway KA, Kim SY, Lodish M, et al: Defects in succinate dehydrogenase in gastrointestinal stromal tumors lacking KIT and PDGFRA mutations. *Proc Natl Acad Sci U S A* 108(1):314–318, 2011.
    Further explains the molecular underpinnings of pediatric GIST.

175. Spunt SL, Pratt CB, Rao BN, et al: Childhood carcinoid tumors: the St Jude Children's Research Hospital experience. *J Pediatr Surg* 35(9):1282–1286, 2000.

A large hospital series of children with carcinoid.

193. Vasudevan SA, Patel JC, Wesson DE: Severe dysplasia in children with familial adenomatous polyposis: rare or simply overlooked? *J Pediatr Surg* 41(4):658–661, 2006.

A review discussion of FAP in children.

194. Goodenberger M, Lindor NM: Lynch syndrome and MYH-associated polyposis: review and testing strategy. *J Clin Gastroenterol* 45(6):488–500, 2011.

A review with expert recommendations for patients with Lynch syndrome.

200. Compton C, Fenoglio-Preiser CM, Pettigrew N: American Joint Committee on Cancer Prognostic Factors Consensus Conference: Colorectal Working Group. *Cancer* 88(7):1739–1757, 2000.

Recommendations from a consensus conference for colorectal carcinoma.

207. Allegra CJ, Jessup JM, Somerfield MR, et al: American Society of Clinical Oncology provisional clinical opinion: testing for *KRAS* gene mutations in patients with metastatic colorectal carcinoma to predict response to anti-epidermal growth factor receptor monoclonal antibody therapy. *J Clin Oncol* 27(12):2091–2096, 2009.

A provisional opinion on the use of KRAS testing in colorectal carcinoma.

209. Glade Bender JL, Adamson PC, Reid JM, et al: Phase I trial and pharmacokinetic study of bevacizumab in pediatric patients with refractory solid tumors: a Children's Oncology Group Study. *J Clin Oncol* 26(3):399–405, 2008.

A report of the pediatric phase I study of bevacizumab.

215. Gibbon DG, Schaar D, Kamen B: A call to action: cancer in adolescents and young adults; an unrecognized healthcare disparity. *J Pediatr Hematol Oncol* 28(9):549–551, 2006.

A report describing the lack of progress in adolescents and young adults with cancer.

224. Hazard FK, Longacre TA: Ovarian surface epithelial neoplasms in the pediatric population: incidence, histologic subtype, and natural history. *Am J Surg Pathol* 37(4):548–553, 2013.

A review of pathology of ovarian tumors in children from one institution.

225. Cass DL, Hawkins E, Brandt ML, et al: Surgery for ovarian masses in infants, children, and adolescents: 102 consecutive patients treated in a 15-year period. *J Pediatr Surg* 36(5):693–699, 2001.

A review of treatment from a large number of children with ovarian masses.

263. Strouse JJ, Fears TR, Tucker MA, et al: Pediatric melanoma: risk factor and survival analysis of the surveillance, epidemiology and end results database. *J Clin Oncol* 23(21):4735–4741, 2005.

Uses SEER data to demonstrate the changing incidence of melanoma in the United States.

272. Chapman PB, Hauschild A, Robert C, et al: Improved survival with vemurafenib in melanoma with BRAF V600E mutation. *N Engl J Med* 364:2507–2516, 2011.

An initial report of vemurafenib, an agent approved specifically to treat BRAF mutant melanoma in adults.

280. Navid F, Furman WL, Fleming M, et al: The feasibility of adjuvant interferon alpha-2b in children with high-risk melanoma. *Cancer* 103:780–787, 2005.

Demonstrates the feasibility of administering adjuvant interferon alpha-2b to children with melanoma.

284. Hodi FS, O'Day SJ, McDermott DF, et al: Improved survival with ipilimumab in patients with metastatic melanoma. *N Engl J Med* 363(8):711–723, 2010.

Reported improved survival of adults with melanoma treated with ipilimumab, which is now approved for the treatment of adults with melanoma.

CHAPTER 66

Imaging in the Evaluation and Management of Childhood Cancer

Raja Shaikh, Sanjay P. Prabhu, and Stephan D. Voss

CHAPTER OUTLINE

The incidence of cancer in childhood is relatively rare when compared to the incidence in adults; approximately 6500 new cases are diagnosed in the United States each year. Nevertheless, cancer remains the second most common cause of death during childhood. Beginning in the mid-1960s treatment of childhood cancer has witnessed remarkable advances in chemotherapy, radiotherapy, and surgical intervention, with improvements in survival for the majority of pediatric malignancies. The imaging of children with malignancy has also evolved, with significant technical advances in both diagnostic and interventional radiology techniques. Faster magnetic reso-

nance (MR) and computed tomography (CT) scanners, three-dimensional (3D) acquisition and postprocessing techniques, and an increasing number of hybrid imaging technologies allow practitioners to image children more quickly, accurately, and safely, in addition to providing options for image-guided diagnostic and therapeutic procedures that historically required surgical intervention. This chapter provides an introductory overview of the various diagnostic imaging techniques available and a review of the imaging findings commonly seen in a broad spectrum of pediatric tumors. The chapter concludes with a discussion of diagnostic and therapeutic interventional

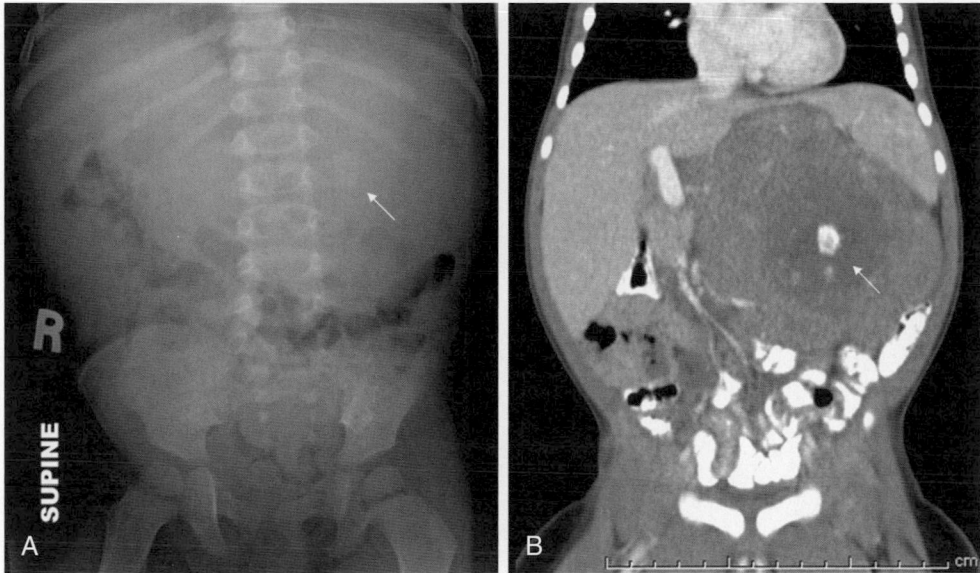

Figure 66-1 Neuroblastoma, detected incidentally. A 20-month-old infant fell, and caregivers felt a firm abdomen with no other symptoms. Abdominal radiograph (**A**) shows a calcified abdominal mass *(arrow)*, further characterized by CT (**B**) and found to be neuroblastoma.

radiologic techniques, surveillance imaging considerations, and finally a brief introduction to the evolving field of molecular imaging and novel imaging technologies.

TECHNICAL CONSIDERATIONS
Conventional Radiography

The decision to perform an imaging study on a child and the type of imaging that is selected very much depend on the patient's clinical history and physical examination findings. In young children with cancer, initial presenting symptoms and complaints are often nonspecific. An easily performed, relatively inexpensive imaging assessment like an x-ray is therefore appropriate as a first step in the evaluation. Conventional radiography is still commonly used as the first imaging examination undertaken both in children with suspected malignancy and in patients with nonspecific complaints that ultimately turn out to be related to neoplastic disease. These initial imaging studies provide valuable initial information that can help suggest a differential diagnosis and inform decision makers about subsequent imaging evaluations.

Although it is tempting to forego obtaining conventional radiographs in favor of cross-sectional imaging modalities such as ultrasound and CT, it is still appropriate in most instances to obtain conventional radiographs as a first step. Normal x-rays in certain settings may provide needed reassurance. Abnormal radiographs, on the other hand, provide a sensitive and accurate initial means of identifying pathology. For example, abdominal films allow assessment for bowel obstruction or perforation and may show solid mass lesions, abdominal calcifications, or areas of bone destruction (Fig. 66-1). Chest radiographs often reveal primary intrathoracic or mediastinal tumors and pulmonary metastases. Chest radiographs are also critical in suggesting impending airway compromise, pneumothorax, or pneumomediastinum and are rapidly obtained, easy to perform,

and fairly quickly interpreted. Oncologic emergencies are fortunately uncommon; however, cardiorespiratory emergencies in a child, such as pneumothorax or pneumomediastinum, airway compression secondary to a large mediastinal mass (Fig. 66-2), and malignant pericardial or pleural effusions can be effectively evaluated in the emergent setting by properly executed chest and abdominal radiographs. Indeed, a CT scan may be contraindicated if radiographs indicate the presence of significant airway compromise in the setting of a large mediastinal mass, because supine positioning with or without sedation may lead to further airway compression, impaired venous return, and acute cardiorespiratory collapse.[1]

Radiographs are essential for initial imaging of nonspecific orthopedic complaints such as pain and limp and may lead to the diagnosis of marrow infiltrative disorders such as leukemia and neuroblastoma (Fig. 66-3, *A*). Radiographs are also necessary for evaluation of primary bone tumors such as Ewing sarcoma and osteogenic sarcoma, where the presence of calcifications, periosteal reaction, bone destruction, and soft-tissue involvement are important in formulating an initial impression and plan. Conventional radiography also plays a role in specific conditions such as Langerhans cell histiocytosis, where skeletal surveys are still used to detect the lytic lesions characteristic of this disease (see Fig. 66-3, *B*). Whether whole body MRI or 18-fluorodeoxyglucose positron emission tomography (FDG-PET) scanning can be used to improve the sensitively and specificity of detecting these lesions has been the subject of several investigations.[2-5]

The role of fluoroscopy in the primary evaluation of pediatric oncology patients is limited and has been largely replaced by CT. CT provides the advantage of visualizing both endoluminal and surrounding mesenteric/intraperitoneal/retroperitoneal processes, for which traditional fluoroscopic evaluations are limited.

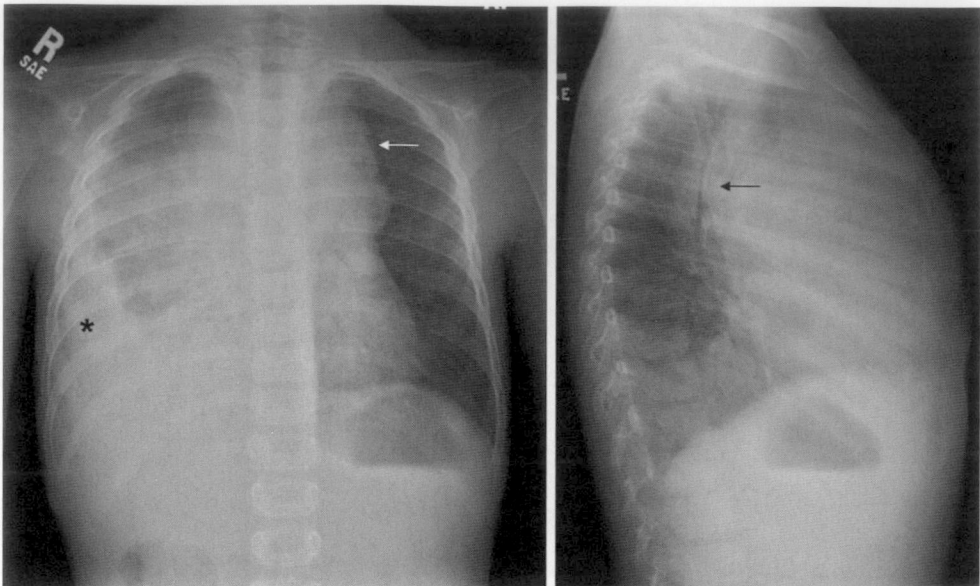

Figure 66-2 Incidentally discovered lymphoma. A 5-year-old boy, otherwise well, developed fever and cough and was treated for pneumonia. The chest x-ray, obtained for persistent symptoms, showed a large mediastinal mass *(white arrow)*. Note large pleural effusion *(asterisk)* and marked tracheal narrowing *(black arrow)*, placing this child at considerable risk for acute cardiorespiratory compromise. The biopsy showed T-cell lymphoblastic lymphoma.

Ultrasound

The use of ultrasound in pediatric radiology is ubiquitous. Ultrasonography is relatively inexpensive, can be done portably, involves no radiation, and in skilled hands can be used to accurately assess an anxious, moving child for whom sedation may pose additional risk. Technically ultrasound relies on the use of variable penetration and attenuation of sound waves by different tissue types. The routine ultrasound examination typically involves the combination of B-mode (brightness mode) scanning and either color or pulsed wave/duplex Doppler sonography to assess flow within vascular structures. As an initial screening modality, ultrasound is very sensitive at evaluating intraabdominal solid organ viscera and is the initial imaging modality of choice in the evaluation of Wilms tumor, neuroblastoma, and hepatoblastoma. Pelvic neoplasms, intraperitoneal free fluid, and musculoskeletal soft-tissue tumors can all be effectively evaluated by ultrasound.

Newer ultrasound imaging techniques rely on a large array of transducers, which afford high-resolution images independent of the size of the patient and depth of the lesion. Extended field-of-view image-processing algorithms offer the capability of visualizing large masses in their entirety along with their relationships to normal structures. Although not in routine clinical use, 3D ultrasound allows images to be displayed in multiple planes and may be useful in demonstrating relationships between solid-organ malignancies and adjacent normal structures.[6] Ultrasound contrast agents are in common use experimentally and have the potential to add to the diagnostic information obtained by conventional ultrasound, but they are not yet being used routinely in clinical practice.[7-9]

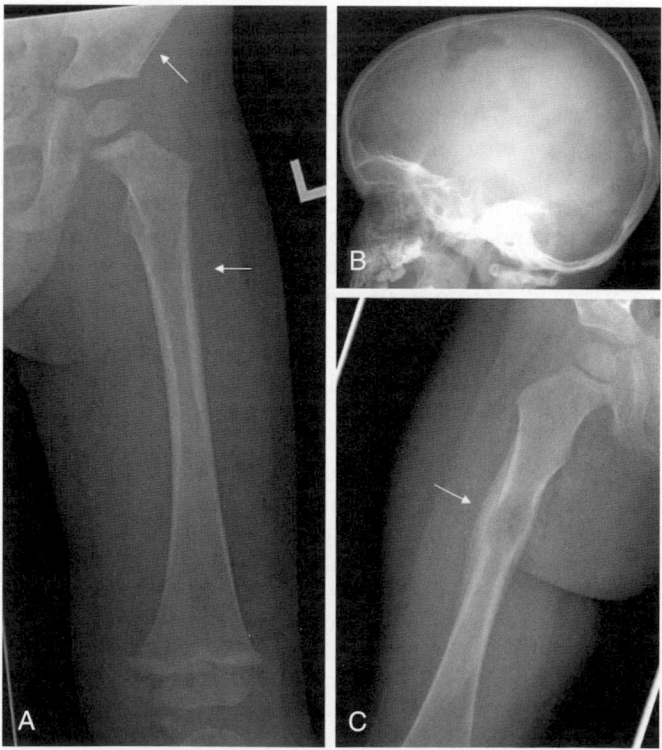

Figure 66-3 Two children with limp. **A,** 23-month-old child; hip and femur radiographs showed periosteal reaction involving femur and supraacetabular ilium *(arrows)*. The ultrasound revealed an abdominal mass, which on biopsy was neuroblastoma. **B** and **C,** 25 month-old-child with lytic skull lesion (**B**) that was revealed on a skeletal survey, which was obtained after extremity radiographs taken for limp identified a lytic femoral lesion with periosteal reaction (**C**). Biopsy showed Langerhans cell histiocytosis.

Ultrasound is also used intraoperatively to help identify lesions that are not visible, not palpable, or undetectable using other imaging techniques. Intraoperative ultrasound can also play an essential role in helping the surgeon identify a plane between tumor and adjacent normal tissue, which can be vital when tissue-sparing surgical techniques are desirable, such as nephron-sparing partial nephrectomy (see "Renal Masses") and partial hepatectomy.[10]

Computed Tomography

After ultrasound, CT scanning remains the primary imaging modality for evaluating most pediatric solid tumors. It is readily available in the majority of institutions, can be performed rapidly (often without sedation), and with newer generation scanners provides high spatial resolution and multiplanar viewing capabilities. CT scanning involves the use of a fan-shaped or cone-shaped x-ray beam generated by the x-ray tube rotating 360 degrees around the body part being examined. At the same time the x-ray tube rotation is occurring, the patient is moving longitudinally through the scanner, allowing the sequential and nearly simultaneous examination of multiple contiguous body parts. Once the x-rays pass through the patient, they strike an array of photodetectors that convert the x-ray energy into electrical signals, which are then used to reconstruct images from the region of the body through which the x-ray beam penetrated. The current generation of scanners are called *multidetector-row helical CT scanners* and rely on multiple detector rows (up to 256) to simultaneously acquire imaging information from larger segments of tissue.[11,12] This allows for more rapid scanning and also allows the reconstruction of imaging data in multiple planes with minimal artifact and image distortion. These multiplanar reconstructions also allow volumetric data to be evaluated, which may be important in assessing response to therapy.[13-14,15,16] In addition, the ability to view images in multiple planes with two-dimensional (2D) and 3D reconstructions and the ability to export images to robotic-assisted surgical devices is increasingly used by surgeons for both preoperative planning and intraoperative guidance in complicated cases.

For infants and anxious young children, it may be necessary for patients to be sedated in order to acquire high-quality imaging. In the majority of patients, sedation can be performed safely and effectively with skilled nursing staff and monitoring equipment.[17,18] In particular, sedation is usually necessary before infusion of intravenous contrast agents, because the contrast infusion may be startling to an otherwise calm child, and motion artifact severely compromises the image quality.

The use of intravenous contrast agents, particularly for the majority of pediatric solid tumors, is necessary to properly show relationships between primary neoplasms and adjacent structures. Although centers less experienced in the care of pediatric patients may consider performing scans without the use of intravenous contrast based on perceived increased risks of contrast reactions in children, a retrospective review of CT scanning results from over 12,000 contrast-enhanced studies performed over 5 years showed less than 0.5% incidence of contrast reactions (57 reported adverse events), with the vast majority being minor reactions. No severe contrast reactions occurred in infants or very young children.[19] Based on this and the results from other pediatric centers[20] there is little data to support the routine omission of intravenous contrast in the evaluation of children suspected of having malignancy. In particular, the use of nonionic low osmolar agents can be performed very safely in the majority of patients and are the contrast agents of choice in most large pediatric radiology departments. Enteric contrast is also recommended to opacify the bowel lumen, allowing better discrimination between normal viscera and potential sites of mesenteric or retroperitoneal lymph-node enlargement. Historically barium had been used, but this has been largely replaced by low-osmolar water-soluble contrast agents that can be mixed with water or juice, produce fewer streak artifacts, and do not affect other imaging studies such as PET and single-photon emission CT (SPECT) imaging.

Optimal imaging of the thorax for the purpose of evaluating the mediastinum and hilar structures requires the use intravenous contrast, whereas CT scanning of the chest to assess for pulmonary metastatic disease can generally be performed without the use of intravenous contrast. The use of multiplanar reconstructions and the ability to review slices in very thin sections improves detection of pulmonary nodules,[21,22] although the ability to discriminate benign from malignant pulmonary nodules based on CT is still limited.[23] In infants and small children who are either asleep or in whom quiet breathing can be encouraged, the speed with which current generation scanners can acquire images may allow noncontrast examinations of the chest to be performed without sedation. In older children for whom breath-holding is possible, image quality and sensitivity/specificity of pulmonary nodule detection is improved when images are obtained at the end of inspiration. If breath-holding is required for a child requiring sedation, anesthesia consultation should be obtained to determine the need for general anesthesia and endotracheal intubation versus using positive pressure laryngeal mask ventilation.[24]

The use of intravenous contrast agents also requires skill on the part of the radiologist in interpreting the examination, with awareness of potential causes of artifact. In particular, the spleen has a variable pattern of enhancement that is well appreciated but can be confused for splenic disease, particularly in the setting of lymphoma. Delayed scanning can usually help in discriminating artifact from disease.[25] In addition, acquisition of images at multiple phases after contrast infusion is often helpful in detecting subtle foci of disease that may only be seen at early arterial phases of enhancement, particularly in the liver (Fig. 66-4). Other lesions, in contrast, may only become evident after delayed enhancement, and knowledge of the typical patterns of enhancement for the particular disease that is being evaluated or suspected is important in determining the scanning technique.[26] It is still common to perform evaluations for hepatoblastoma in both hepatic arterial and portal venous phases in order to maximize sensitivity of lesion

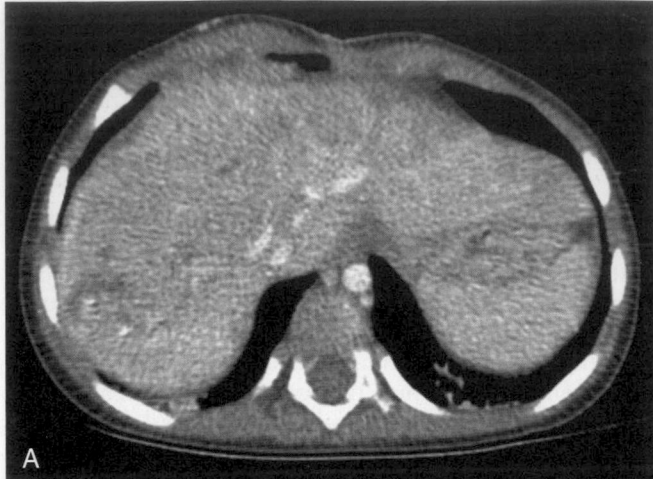

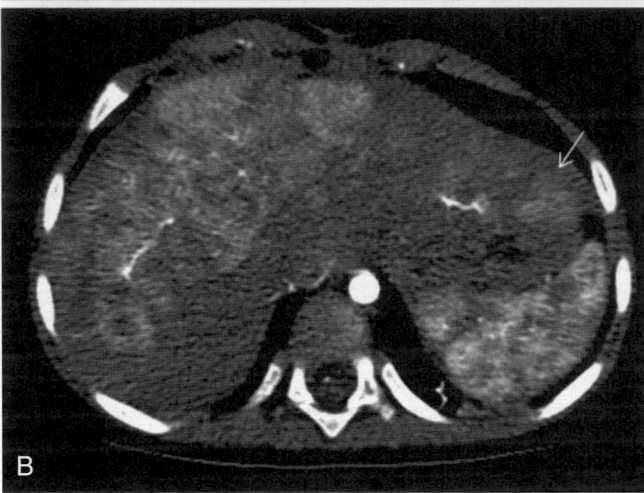

Figure 66-4 A 20-month-old child with unresectable hepatoblastoma, emphasizing the importance of multiphase scanning for optimal lesion detection. The presence of the left lateral segment lesion *(arrow)* was only seen on early arterial-phase scanning. Its identification determined surgical unresectability in this patient.

detection, delineate vascular anatomy, and provide optimal images to aid in surgical planning, although in many centers, improvements in abdominal MR image quality together with concerns about radiation related to repeated CT scanning have resulted in increasing use of MR imaging (MRI).[27]

Discussions of radiation dose in the setting of diagnostic CT scanning have become widespread in both the imaging and wider medical literature.[28-33] The data indicate measurable increases in incidence of malignancy attributable to radiation doses during diagnostic CT scanning, with cumulative increases in risk with increasing numbers of scans. Although these concerns are not to be underemphasized, particularly for otherwise well patients undergoing screening examinations, for patients with known malignancy or in whom malignancy is suspected, the relative benefit derived from the high-quality information achieved after diagnostic CT scanning almost always outweighs the modest incremental increase in risk associated with these techniques.[34] Nonetheless every effort should be made to limit the examination to involved

regions of the body and to minimize the frequency of scanning in these heavily evaluated patients, using the "as low as reasonably achievable" (ALARA) principle as guidance.[31,32,35-37]

Magnetic Resonance Imaging

The physical principles of MR image formation are beyond the scope of this chapter and can be reviewed in articles devoted to this subject.[38,39] MRI involves the use of an external magnetic field to orient protons (primarily contained in water molecules) within the body, after which radiofrequency pulses are applied with specific frequencies and orientations. These radiofrequency pulses force the protons aligned in the magnetic field to come out of alignment. After the radiofrequency energy is withdrawn, the protons gradually reassume their original alignment, or resonate, within the magnetic field. The process of relaxation is multidimensional, and the rate with which longitudinal and transverse relaxation (T1 and T2 relaxation times, respectively) occurs is dependent on the properties of the specific tissue. The energy released during this realignment process can be measured much in same way that a standard radio receiver acquires the signal (radiofrequency energy) from a radio station transmitter. This radiofrequency energy can be characterized both in terms of its spatial location and frequency, and this information in turn can be used to reconstruct images. The result is high resolution MR images obtained in multiple orientations and tissue planes with signal properties that reflect the tissue microenvironments within which the protons reside.

High field-strength and low field-strength magnets are in common clinical use. In general terms, with higher field strength there is a higher signal-to-noise ratio.[38,40] Despite this, the high field-strength magnets are susceptible to some image degradation and magnetic field artifact, and most imaging can be reliably performed at 1.5 and 3 Tesla. With lower field strengths, the signal-to-noise ratio is considerably diminished. There are a variety of radiofrequency coils that are utilized as receivers for the radiofrequency energy emitted during proton relaxation and reorientation. Newer coil designs allow for rapid scanning techniques and for high-resolution imaging of specific body parts to be performed.[38,41]

Multiple MR images of the same organ or tissue are typically generated; however, the imaging technique chosen results in different patterns of tissue contrast, allowing the unique features that characterize distinct components of an organ or tissue to be depicted. The tissue contrast that one observes is the result of the interplay between the externally applied magnetic field, the inherent properties of the tissue (i.e., freely mobile water protons or highly ordered soft-tissue protons), and the radiofrequency pulse-sequence parameters chosen to acquire the image. The tissue properties that have the greatest influence on image contrast are the proton density (PD) and the T1 and T2 proton relaxation times. Conventional MRI techniques are acquired with "T1- and T2- weighting," in which the tissue contrast is weighted to reflect differences in the T1 and T2 relaxation times among the different tissues. This is accomplished by varying the interval between which the radiofrequency pulses are applied (the pulse repetition time, or TR) and the time that is allowed before the emitted signal is received (the echo time, or TE). T1-weighted images typically have a short TR (300 to 600 msec) and short TE (10 to 20 msec) and emphasize T1 characteristics of tissues. On T1-weighted images, fat is typically bright, fluid has low signal intensity, and complex or proteinaceous fluid is of intermediate to high signal intensity. Conventional contrast agents used in MRI result in T1 shortening and therefore produce increased signal on T1-weighted images.

T2-weighted images have longer TR (greater than 2000 msec) and longer TE (greater than 80 msec). T2-weighted images obtained using standard techniques display simple fluid such as cerebrospinal fluid (CSF) or urine as bright in signal intensity, whereas fat is low in signal intensity. Muscle and solid organs, depending on their tissue make-up, have variable signal intensity on T2-weighted images. Beyond these simple T1- and T2-weighted images, specific pulses sequences can be created that eliminate fluid signal (fluid-attenuated inversion recovery, FLAIR) or provide fat suppression either using chemically selective fat suppression techniques or so-called *inversion recovery techniques*, in which the TE is selected to minimize signal from fat and maximize signal from non–fat-containing structures.

Diffusion-weighted MR imaging (DWI) has also emerged as an important technique for evaluation of malignancy.[42,43] DWI is sensitive to the molecular motion of water within the imaging volume and historically was developed for neuroradiologic applications, where it became routine for evaluation of CNS ischemia, identifying early areas of potentially reversible cellular damage by virtue of restricted water diffusion across ischemic cellular membranes. Tumors also commonly demonstrate restricted diffusion relative to surrounding tissue because of increased cellularity and reduced extracellular space. With improvements in gradient echo imaging techniques, DWI can help identify subtle sites of disease (Fig. 66-5) and in some instances distinguish benign from malignant disease.[44] DWI changes in response to therapy, with increasing free diffusion of water molecules in areas of cellular necrosis as opposed to the more restricted movement of water in cellular regions of a tumor, has also been shown to correlate with tumor necrosis induced by treatment, and is emerging as an important technique in assessing response to therapy.[45,46,47,48]

MRI angiography and MR spectroscopy are all standard imaging techniques in common practice in the evaluation of the central nervous system (CNS). MR angiography takes advantage of rapidly flowing blood moving in and out of the imaging slice. Alternatively, gadolinium (Gd)-enhanced MR angiography relies on the use of Gd-based contrast agents to display the vasculature. The use of dynamic enhanced MRI allows multiple acquisitions in a specific region such as a tumor to be obtained, and there is evidence to suggest that the relative rates of contrast uptake and perfusion in tumors may be a reflection of tumor cellularity and/or necrosis.[49,50]

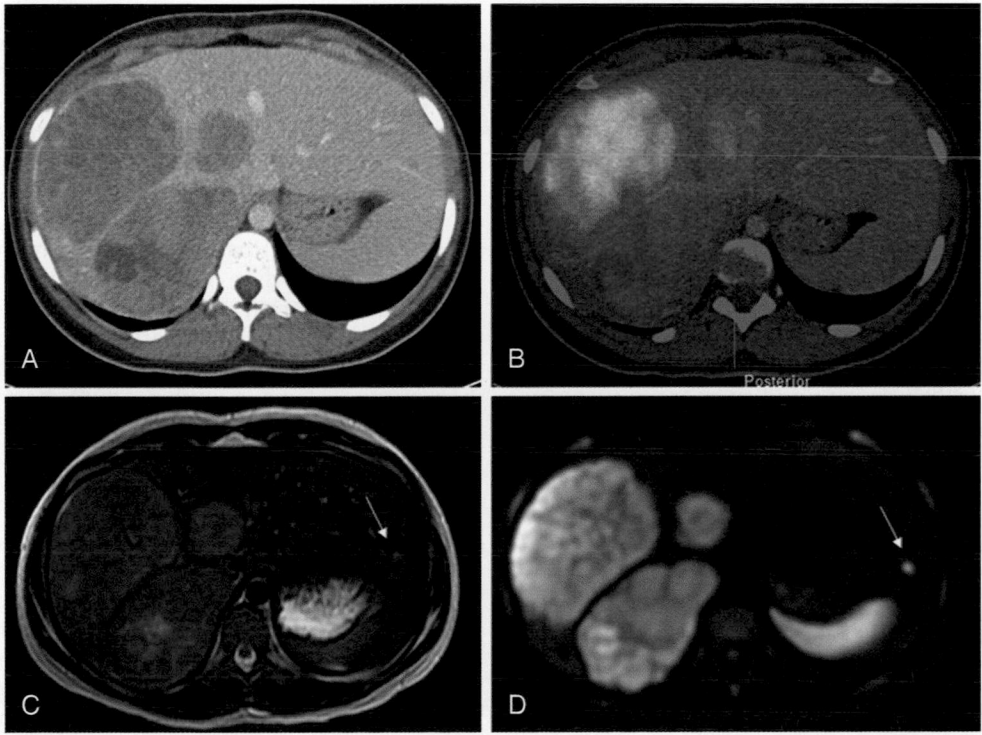

Figure 66-5 A 17-year-old adolescent with adrenocortical carcinoma primarily involving the right lobe. A small, metastatic deposit in the left lateral segment of the liver was not detectable by CT (**A**) or PET (**B**), is barely detectable on conventional T2-weighted MRI (**C**, *arrow*), but is easily seen on DWI (**D**, *arrow*).

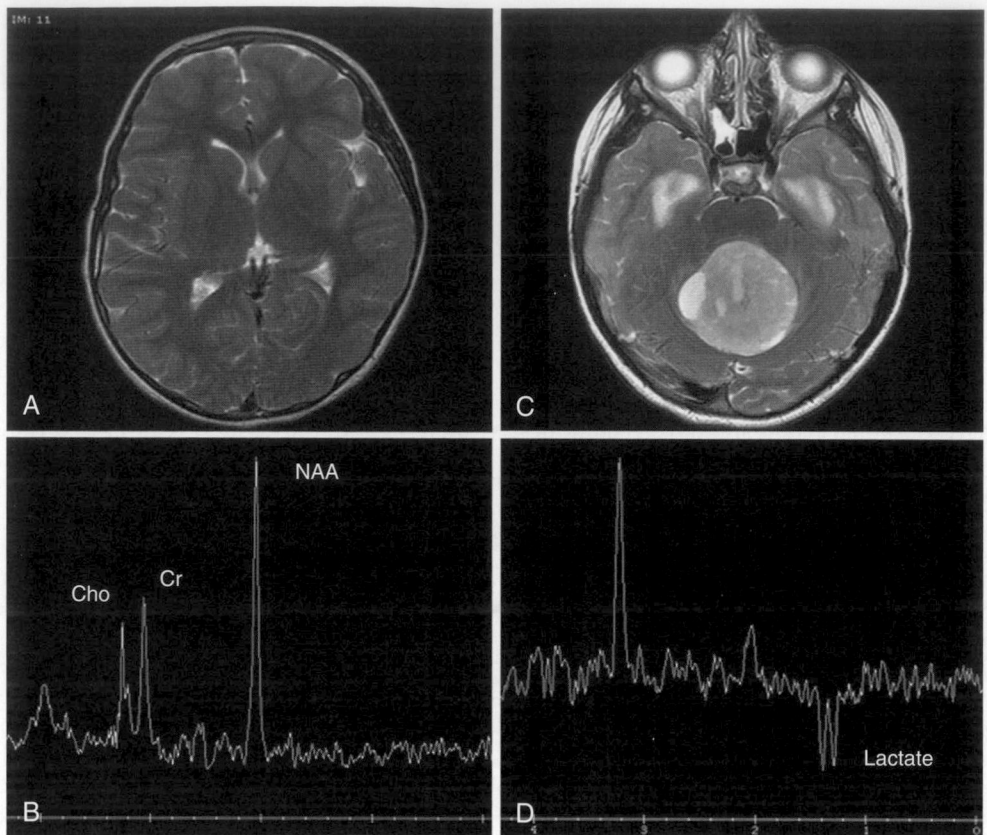

Figure 66-6 MRI and MR spectroscopy in a patient with medulloblastoma (**C** and **D**) compared with the normal MRI and spectrum on the left (**A** and **B**), demonstrating the increased Cho peak, decreased/absent NAA peak, and lactate peak characteristically seen in malignant lesions. *Cho,* Choline; *Cr,* creatine; *NAA,* N-acetylaspartate.

Contrast-enhanced angiography in particular may be useful as well for characterizing relationships of abdominal and mediastinal masses to critical adjacent vascular structures.

MR spectroscopy is used routinely in the evaluation of CNS tumors, where the metabolites N-acetylaspartate (NAA), creatine (Cr), and choline (Cho) have been defined and have specific and characteristic spectra. The use of spectroscopy, although not entirely diagnostic, adds additional information in evaluation of CNS tumors.[51,52] For example NAA is generally thought to correlate with neuronal density, whereas increases in Cho levels usually signify increases in cell density and membrane turnover, reflecting the relatively rapid metabolic rate and division of actively dividing tumors. NAA peaks are typically decreased or absent in pediatric brain tumors, and a decreased NAA/Cho ratio is a characteristic finding.[53,54] The presence of a prominent lactate peak, which is not usually present in the normal brain spectrum, signifies an increase in cellular hypoxia and necrosis (Fig. 66-6) and has been described in more malignant CNS neoplasms.[52] Because the obtainment of good spectral data relies on relatively static body parts, proton spectroscopy has not been used routinely outside the brain; however, investigations are underway to develop a better understanding of the spectra achieved in pediatric neoplasms outside the CNS.[55]

In addition to the use of spectroscopy and diffusion-weighted imaging for characterization of brain tumors, diffusion MR tractography based on diffusion tensor imaging (DTI) has rapidly become an important clinical tool that can delineate functionally important white matter tracts for surgical planning (Fig. 66-7). Tractography based on diffusion MR utilizes the correlation between water diffusion and brain structure to delineate the course of white matter pathways.[56] White matter tracts in the brain are highly organized into fasciculi comprised of densely packed axons. Axonal membranes, myelin, and other structures affect the pattern of Brownian motion of water within white matter. Tractography involves following the trajectory of the white matter tract from voxel to voxel in three dimensions by assuming that the direction of least restricted diffusion corresponds with the axon orientation.

While quantitative assessments of tissue microstructure are essential for many applications of diffusion MR, these measurements are not directly used for presurgical tractography.[57] Instead, the aim of presurgical tractography is to delineate the position of eloquent pathways such as the motor, sensory, visual, and language tracts. One of the goals of brain surgery is to avoid damage to eloquent cortex and subcortical white matter. DTI is the only noninvasive method available to segment the subcortical course of a white matter tract. Subcortical motor evoked

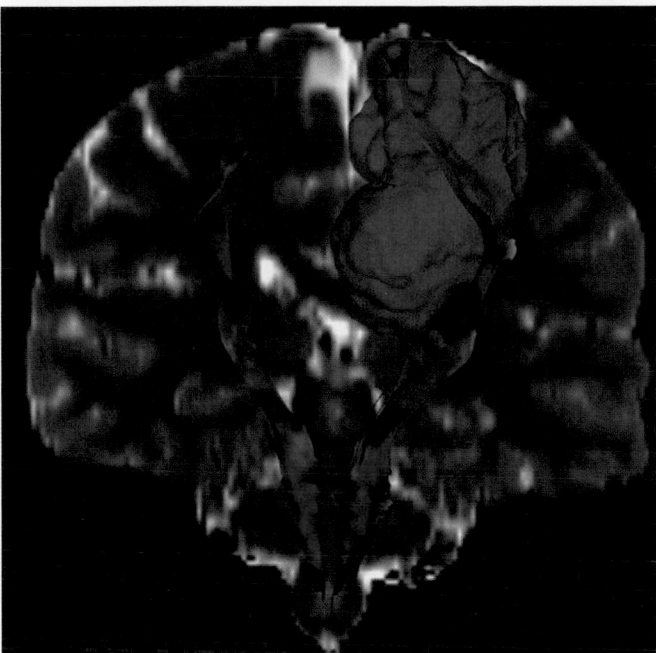

Figure 66-7 Diffusion MR tractography of the corticospinal tracts in a patient with a left-sided tumor showing displacement of the tracts by the tumor (*segmented and shown in red*).

potentials are often combined with tractography to preserve motor function.

Functional MRI (fMRI) using the blood oxygenation level–dependent (BOLD) method allows mapping out of the eloquent areas and is a noninvasive, repeatable, and flexible technique for studying brain function in the clinical setting (Fig. 66-8). It is often critical in surgical planning before resection of brain tumors and has become the standard of care for neurosurgical planning in centers where it is available. Although paradigms to measure eloquent cortices have not been standardized, simple tasks allow visualization of reliable maps for planning neurosurgical procedures. Current research indicates that patient-specific paradigm design can help refine the utility of fMRI for prognostication and recovery of function.[58] It should be noted that certain pathologic conditions and technical issues limit the interpretation of fMRI maps in clinical use and should be considered carefully.

Nuclear Medicine

PET has emerged as an important imaging tool in the evaluation of both adult and pediatric patients with malignancy. A number of textbooks and reviews have been dedicated to this topic and should be consulted for a more in depth discussion of this exciting technology.[59-68] The use of ^{18}F-fluorodeoxyglucose (^{18}F-FDG) has been routine in adult practice and is becoming increasingly commonplace in the evaluation of children with cancer.[69,70,72,128] FDG-PET scanning relies on the differential uptake of glucose by metabolically active tumor cells relative to surrounding tissues. The use of FDG-PET has been shown to be feasible in the majority of pediatric tumors[64,70] and is likely to play an important role in monitoring responses to therapy, particularly with agents

that do not produce immediate tumor shrinkage or cellular necrosis but do block specific metabolic pathways. Although flourine-18 (^{18}F) is the most common PET radionuclide used clinically, other agents are being developed and are in preclinical testing, including copper-64 (^{64}Cu)[73,74] and iodine-124 ([124]I)[75,76] and gallium-68 (^{68}Ga).[76] The use of biomarkers other than fluorodeoxyglucose is starting to emerge clinically, with compounds such as fluorinated thymidine (FLT) allowing deoxyribonucleic acid (DNA) synthesis and cellular proliferation to be directly imaged.[77]

Multiple studies have shown that the use of PET imaging alone, without the simultaneous review of anatomic imaging data acquired either by CT or MRI, results in high sensitivity of lesion detection but has an increased incidence of false positives and an overall decreased specificity. The use of correlative cross-sectional imaging improves the specificity of lesions detected by PET scanning and also increases the sensitivity with which lesions are detected by conventional imaging techniques.[78-80,81,82] As a result, integrated PET/CT scanners have rapidly replaced stand-alone PET imaging equipment in most centers, allowing the PET scan and CT scan to be obtained on the same instrument with the patient in the same position and orientation. This has revolutionized the use of PET scanning in evaluation of oncology patients, and in many institutions it is considered standard of care for PET scans and CT scans to be reviewed simultaneously by skilled radiologists and nuclear medicine physicians, who use the complementary information available from both imaging modalities to achieve greater confidence in rendering a diagnosis.[79,83] Current state-of-the

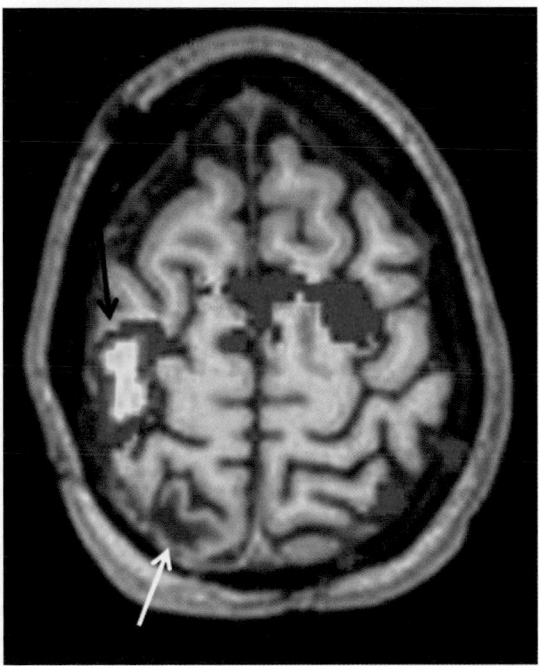

Figure 66-8 Functional MRI (fMRI) in an 18-year-old patient with a history of right posterior parietal oligoastrocytoma resection (*white arrow*), now showing epilepsy localized to around the surgical cavity. fMRI activation using left-finger tapping shows robust, right-lateralized activation of the primary motor cortex (*black arrow*) and subtle activation of midline supplementary motor cortex.

art equipment utilizes high-sensitivity multirow PET detectors and multidetector-row CT scanners, allowing imaging to be performed more rapidly, with greater sensitivity, and, depending on the equipment, can incorporate respiratory and cardiac gating functions to improve image quality. Postprocessing techniques, relying on newer software, also allow the functional data from PET scanners to be fused to MRI images acquired separately, much in the same way that the PET images are fused to their correlative CT data.

In 2011 the first integrated PET/MRI scanners were approved by the FDA for clinical use and have now been installed at a number of major academic centers in the United States, Europe, and Asia. As with PET/CT, the PET/MRI scanners allow the PET scan and MRI scan to be simultaneously acquired.[84-86] The advantages include lower radiation exposure, the ability to integrate quantitative MRI data with concurrently acquired functional PET data, and the increasing use of MRI for characterization of many pediatric malignancies. As additional PET tracers become available as well, PET/MRI is likely to have a significant impact on the imaging evaluation of pediatric oncology patients.[87]

In addition to PET scanning, conventional γ-emission planar and SPECT imaging is still an important element of pediatric oncology imaging.[88-90] In particular, ^{123}I-metaiodobenzylguanidine (MIBG) and technetium-99m (^{99m}Tc)-methylene diphosphonate (MDP) bone scintigraphy are routinely used in the evaluation of neuroblastoma patients.[91] Bone scintigraphy is also an important component of the sarcoma patient evaluation.[90] As with PET scanning, SPECT images can be fused to anatomic data acquired by either CT or MRI in order to provide correlative information and to confirm sites of abnormality and clarify areas of equivocal disease.[92] Integrated SPECT/CT systems are also available, which allows both SPECT and CT images to be acquired concurrently. Attenuation and scatter correction techniques can be used to further optimize SPECT image quality and potentially reduce tracer dose, as well as improve the accuracy of lesion colocalization.[93] In many instances performing the SPECT and CT simultaneously may also obviate the need for two sedations, further enhancing patient safety and the overall imaging experience.

STAGING CONSIDERATIONS

A detailed discussion of the different staging classifications used in pediatric oncology is beyond the scope of this chapter. Specific staging considerations are discussed in the disease-specific chapters elsewhere in this text. It is important to note, however, that there are unique staging systems in pediatric oncology, such as the International Neuroblastoma Staging System (INSS), the Wilms tumor staging system, the Hodgkin lymphoma staging system (Ann Arbor Staging), the non-Hodgkin lymphoma staging system (St. Jude Classification), and the Pretreatment Extent of Disease (PRETEXT) staging system for hepatoblastoma. Because these different staging systems do not simply rely on tumor size and nodal spread in determining disease stage (i.e., tumor-nodes-metastasis [TNM]

staging), the imaging evaluation must be tailored to reflect the type of malignancy being evaluated. The radiologist should work closely with the oncologist during the review of the initial imaging data in order to accurately determine the patient's disease stage and risk classification.

CENTRAL NERVOUS SYSTEM TUMORS

Primary CNS malignancies are the most common pediatric solid tumors, exceeded only by leukemia as a cause of pediatric cancer.[94,95] Although many of the pediatric CNS tumors are also seen in adults, there are several tumors that are unique to infancy and childhood and have characteristic imaging features and intracranial locations. The imaging evaluation should be directed at characterizing the location of the lesion (supratentorial or infratentorial) and determining whether the lesion is intraaxial or extraaxial. CT is usually the first imaging study performed to investigate children with suspected CNS tumors. Although the role of CT has been diminished by the increased use of MRI for imaging the brain, CT is still widely available and readily accessible in nearly all institutions. CT can effectively identify foci of hemorrhage or necrosis and can identify critical abnormalities such as brain edema or impending brain herniation. CT may also provide clues as to the histologic nature of the tumor, for example showing either a cystic or solid mass or the presence of subtle calcifications. Bone invasion into the adjacent skull is typically better depicted by CT, and particularly lesions at the base of the skull should include an evaluation by CT.

MRI of the brain, as with other parts of the body, provides enhanced spatial resolution and, with the variety of newly developed pulse sequences and imaging coils, can give highly specific functional and anatomic information about the lesion in question and the condition of the surrounding brain.[52,96] MR angiography can be performed during the same imaging evaluation and allows assessment of both arterial and venous systems. Obstruction to CSF flow can also be directly evaluated by MRI using specialized techniques aimed at monitoring CSF flow dynamics.

As described, advanced imaging techniques including MR spectroscopy, fMRI, and DTI[52] allow biochemical and metabolic characterization of focal lesions, assessment of functional activity in the brain, and direct evaluation of the structural integrity of CNS white-matter tracts, respectively. FDG-PET and PET scanning with newer radiotracers such as ^{18}F-thymidine may also be of additional value in delineating postsurgical margins from residual tumor and in predicting response to therapy.[97,98]

There are several classification systems for pediatric brain tumors. The most commonly used World Health Organization (WHO) classification of intracranial tumors is based on histopathologic characteristics and clinical course, with tumors further classified based on their intracranial location, specifically whether lesions are supratentorial or infratentorial. This classification system both allows a practical assignment of differential diagnoses to new CNS tumors based on their location and provides prognostic information related to histologic subtype and grade when this additional data becomes available.

Supratentorial Tumors

Astrocytomas

The most common supratentorial brain tumor is the astrocytoma, representing between 50% and 60% of all primary pediatric brain tumors.[99] Astrocytomas are seen in all age groups, and presenting symptoms are typically of intracranial pressure, with headache, nausea, and vomiting commonly seen. Astrocytomas can be reliably diagnosed by CT and MRI (Fig. 66-9). They range from benign to malignant in their histologic grade, with grade 1 lesions classified as benign, grade 2 as low-grade glioma, grade 3 as anaplastic glioma, and grade 4 as glioblastoma. The lesions are usually quite large with both solid and cystic components. Calcifications can occur but are unusual. Parietal, frontal, and temporal lobes are common sites of astrocytoma. On fluid-sensitive sequences, the cystic component of the lesion may show features of complex fluid, with decreased signal intensity relative to CSF on T2-weighted sequences. After contrast infusion, homogeneous enhancement of the solid component of the lesion is characteristic. Higher-grade, more malignant tumors often have less distinct margins, more heterogeneous enhancement, and increased peritumoral edema and mass effect.[100] Newer techniques including perfusion-weighted MRI and MR spectroscopy have been evaluated as noninvasive techniques to determine tumor angiogenesis and capillary permeability. For example, in higher-grade gliomas increased blood flow to the tumor lesion has been demonstrated using this technique.[101] Also, as the tumor grade increases to a more malignant variant, there is an increase in the Cho-to-NAA ratio, reflecting the increased metabolic activity present in higher grade lesions.[101,102] Complete surgical resection is often not possible because of involvement of adjacent major neural structures. The 5-year survival rate for low-grade astrocytomas is between 40% and 50%, with less than 5% survival for the higher-grade malignancies. Because of a propensity to spread to the spine via the CSF, the staging evaluation must also include imaging of the entire spine.

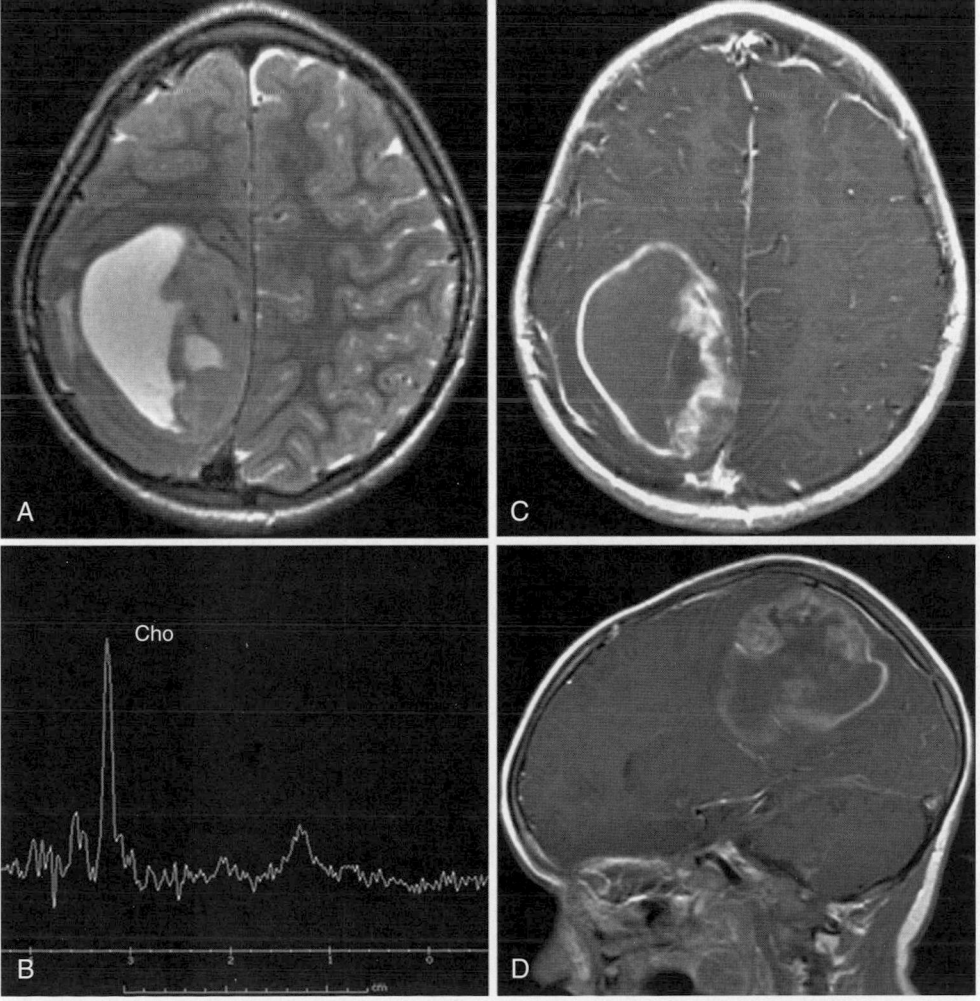

Figure 66-9 A 4-year-old patient with hemispheric astrocytoma. T2-weighted (A) and post-Gd T1-weighted images (C and D) show cystic and solid mass with peripheral enhancement located in the frontoparietal region. MRS from the solid component is notable for decreased N-acetylaspartate and elevated choline (Cho) and lipid peaks, typical of a highly cellular tumor (B).

The infratentorial/cerebellar form of astrocytoma, also known as *juvenile pilocytic astrocytoma,* is distinct from the diffuse supratentorial astrocytoma discussed here and is described in further detail below.

Oligodendrogliomas

Oligodendrogliomas, although common in adults, are relatively rare in children and adolescents.[103] The most common location is in the frontotemporal region, with less common involvement of the posterior fossa and spinal cord. Imaging evaluation shows a hypodense lesion on CT. Because the majority of these contain varying degrees of calcification, they are distinct as being the most common supratentorial tumor in childhood to calcify. The noncalcified solid component is typically isodense to the adjacent brain on CT. On MRI, the lesions are characterized by low signal intensity on T1-weighted images, hyperintensity on T2-weighted images, and minimal enhancement after infusion of gadolinium contrast (Fig. 66-10). Although these tend to be slow growing lesions, depending on their size there may be edema evident in the surrounding brain.

Gangliogliomas

Gangliogliomas and ganglioneuromas comprise about 5% of the pediatric brain tumors.[99] As with their counterparts in the peripheral nervous system, calcification is seen in up to 40% of the cases. The temporal lobes, frontoparietal lobes, and hypothalamic regions are the most common sites of involvement. The brainstem, posterior fossa, and spinal cord are less commonly involved. MRI demonstrates a low signal-intensity lesion on T1-weighted images with hyperintensity on T2-weighted

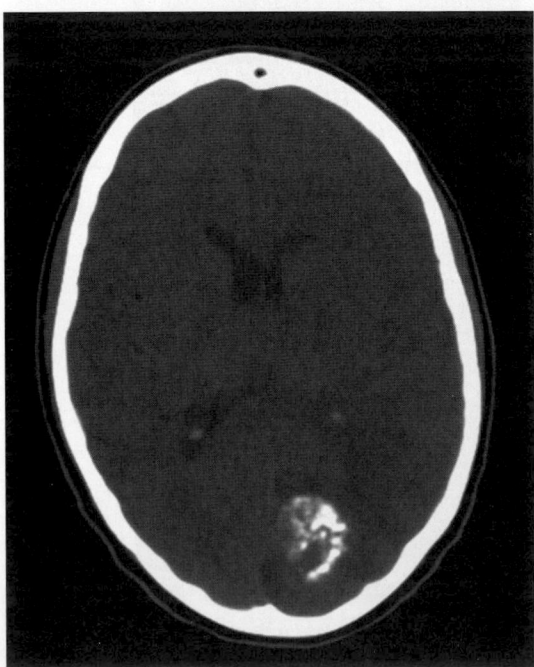

Figure 66-10 Oligodendroglioma. CT showing calcified low-attenuation lesion in the occipital cortex, with imaging features characteristic of oligodendroglioma.

images and hyperintense homogeneous enhancement after gadolinium infusion (Fig. 66-11).

Tumors of the midline deep gray matter, including the basal ganglia, thalamus, hypothalamus, and chiasmatic/optic pathway region tend to be astrocytomas.[95,104] As with the cerebral hemispheric astrocytomas, tumor grades range from benign to highly anaplastic. The imaging features are similar to the lesions located in the cerebral hemispheres with decreased signal intensity on T1-weighted images, hyperintensity on T2-weighted images, and variable contrast enhancement. Because of their location, behavioral changes, emotional and memory changes, movement disorders, visual abnormalities, and hydrocephalus are all common symptoms associated with these deep gray-matter tumors. Surgical resectability is often not possible, and the imaging evaluation is directed at identifying involvement of adjacent critical structures and monitoring posttherapy changes.[95]

Intraventricular tumors include choroid plexus papillomas, neurocytomas, and dermoid/epidermoid tumors. Choroid plexus papillomas/carcinomas are relatively common, making up between 10% and 20% of the intraventricular tumors identified in the first year of life and comprising approximately 5% of all CNS neoplasms.[103] The imaging features are characteristic and typically reveal large lobulated intraventricular lesions (Fig. 66-12). These tumors are highly vascular and are often associated with calcification and occasionally hemorrhage.[100,104] Depending on the size and location of the lesion, there may be obstructive hydrocephalus. MRI shows a low signal-intensity lesion on T1-weighted images with variable hyperintensity on T2-weighted images. Magnetic susceptibility is seen if hemorrhage is present, and after contrast infusion these lesions typically show marked contrast enhancement. The combination of a lobulated, intensely enhancing intraventricular lesion is nearly diagnostic of choroid plexus papilloma. Five percent to 10% of these lesions degenerate into choroid plexus carcinomas,[104] and this latter diagnosis is suggested by accompanying necrosis within the lesion and metastatic spread into the adjacent brain, either by direct extension into the adjacent brain or by CSF dissemination. Because of their intraventricular location, metastatic spread throughout the CNS via CSF dissemination is unfortunately common for choroid plexus carcinomas, resulting in a uniformly poor prognosis.[95]

Central Neurocytomas

Neurocytomas are rare in children and have imaging features that mimic oligodendroglioma, showing an intraventricular calcified mass with heterogeneous contrast enhancement. These tumors typically involve the lateral ventricle in the midline; however, surgical resection is necessary to distinguish this lesion from other intraventricular tumors such subependymal astrocytomas and ependymomas.

Midline Supratentorial Tumors

Tumors of the hypothalamic/suprasellar region include craniopharyngiomas, hypothalamic hamartomas, and pineal region tumors.

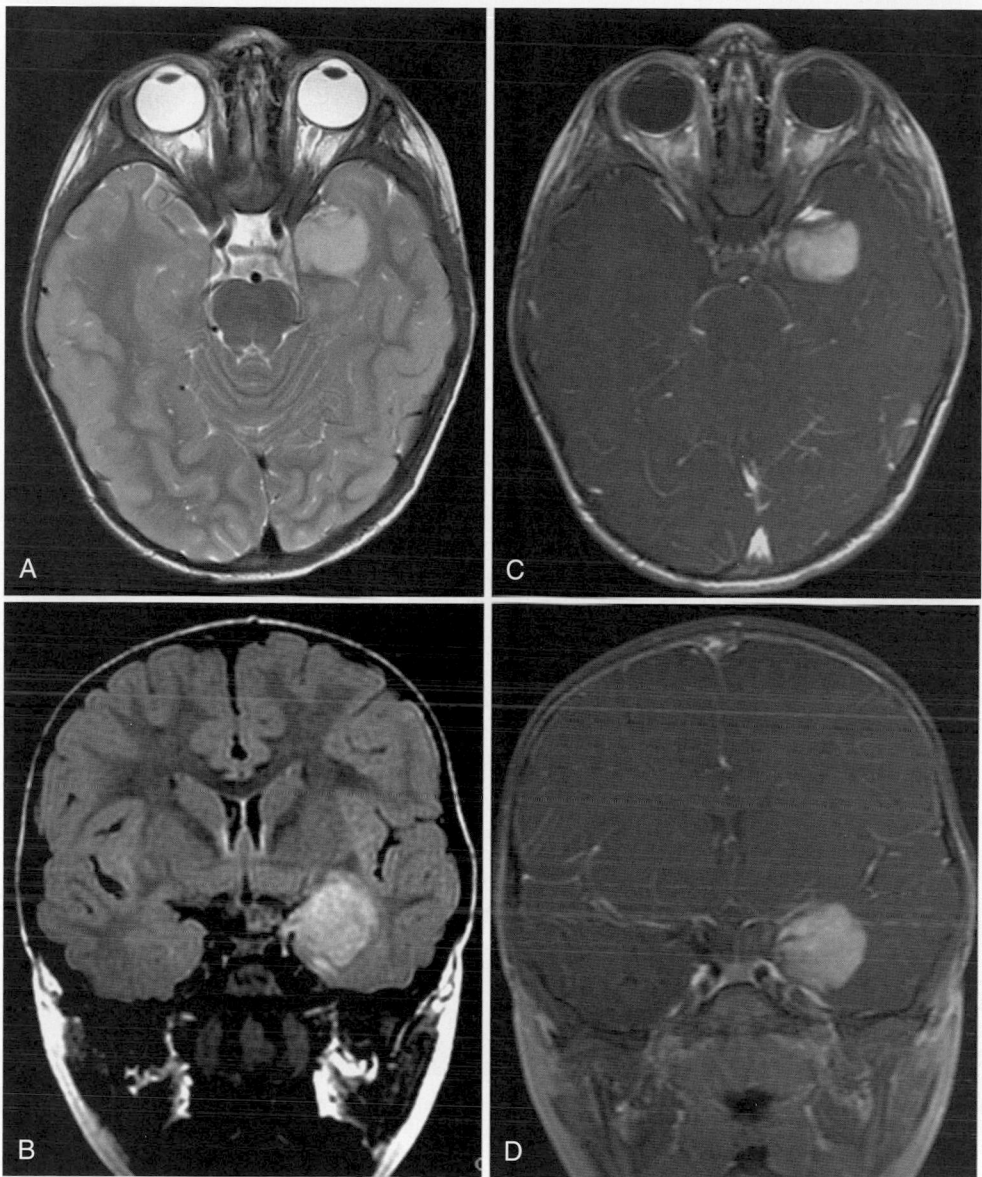

Figure 66-11 Ganglioglioma. A 4-year-old patient with left temporal-lobe ganglioma showing increased signal on T2-weighted images (**A**), and bright enhancement after gadolinium administration (**C** and **D**). Depending on their location, these lesions may be more conspicuous on fluid-attenuated FLAIR images (**B**).

Craniopharyngiomas

Craniopharyngioma is the most common suprasellar tumor.[100,104,105] It has fairly characteristic imaging features with lesions containing solid, cystic, and calcified elements. Symptoms usually result from increased intracranial pressure and local effects upon the hypothalamic pituitary region and optic chiasm. Because these are relatively slowly growing lesions, they may be quite large at diagnosis. The presence of a calcified suprasellar mass at CT scan is usually suggestive of the diagnosis; however, MRI is superior in evaluating the extent of involvement (Fig. 66-13). Depending on the type of material present in the cystic component of the mass, variable signal intensity on T1- and T2-weighted images may be seen.[106] It is common, for example, for the complex proteinaceous, cholesterol-laden fluid to be variably hyperintense on both T1- and T2-weighted images (see Fig. 66-13). After contrast infusion, the cyst wall commonly enhances. However, the solid components of the cyst often demonstrate inhomogeneous enhancement as well. Of note, craniopharyngiomas commonly cause T2 prolongation along the optic tracts. This is a nonspecific sign and has been reported in other tumors centered in this region. It is thought to signify optic tract edema caused by compression by the tumor.[107]

Pineal-Region Tumors

Pineal-region masses are characterized by their location in the quadrigeminal plate cistern. These tumors typically arise from primordial germ cells and include pineoblastomas, pineocytomas, and immature germ-cell tumors.[95,100,103,104] It is important to distinguish these

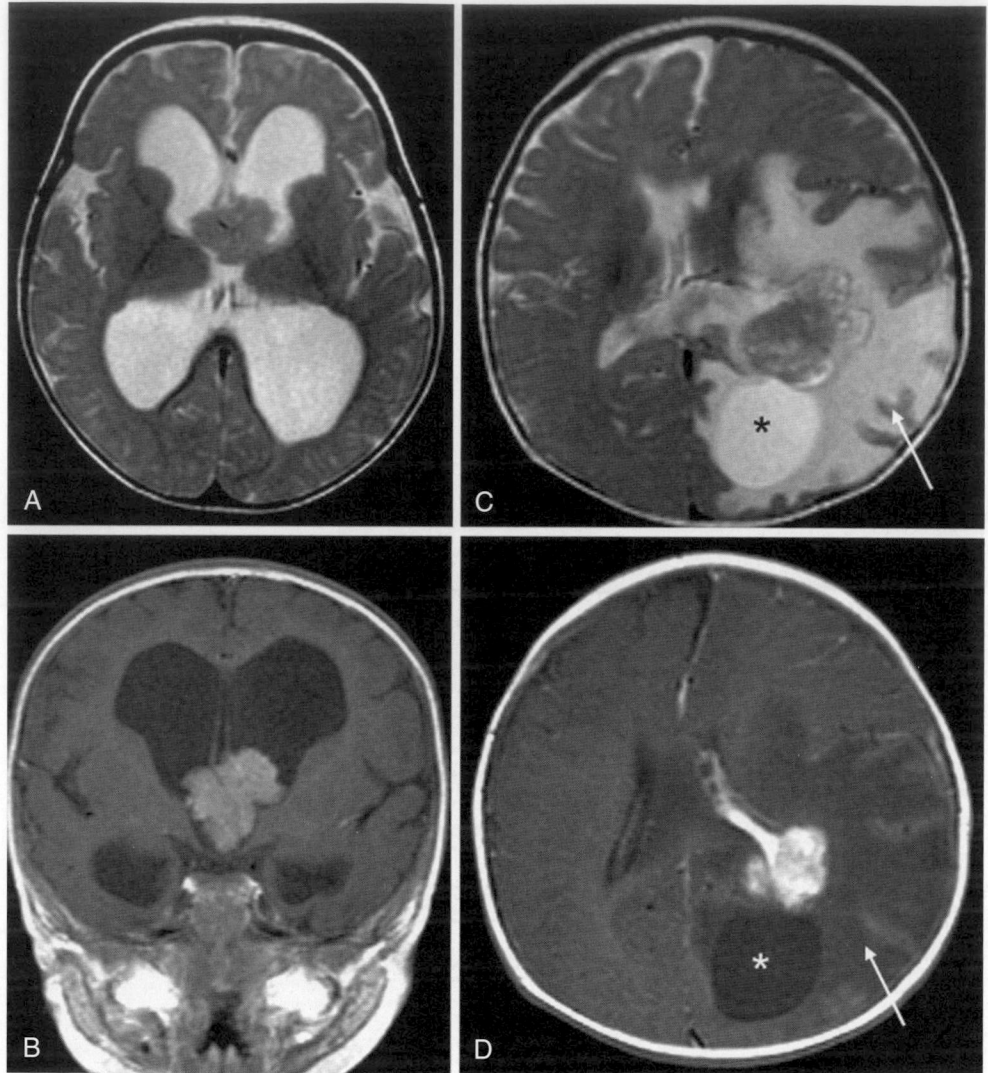

Figure 66-12 Choroid plexus papilloma. 8-month-old and 10-month-old infants, both with large lobulated lesions causing obstructive hydrocephalus. **A and B,** In one patient the tumor is centrally located, producing severe global hydrocephalus. **C and D,** In the other patient the peripheral location is accompanied by extensive vasogenic edema *(arrow)* and left occipital-horn hydrocephalus *(asterisk).*

neoplastic lesions from benign pineal cysts, which are commonly seen within the pineal gland. Pineal cysts have a characteristic appearance on both CT and MRI and do not distort or compress the adjacent ventricles. Simple pineal region cysts typically do not achieve sizes greater than 1 cm. Also of note is normal calcification within the pineal gland. Calcification is unusual before the age of 10 but is commonly seen in adolescents and older children.[108] Therefore the presence of calcification in the pineal region in an infant or young child should raise suspicion for a pineal region mass/germ-cell tumor and prompt further investigation.

Pineal-gland tumors, including pineocytomas and pineoblastomas, are relatively rare. Pineocytoma is benign and usually nonaggressive, whereas the pineoblastoma, representing an immature undifferentiated lesion, often metastasizes. Pinealoblastoma is also a component of the "trilateral retinoblastoma" and is seen with increased incidence in patients diagnosed with bilateral retinoblas-

toma. Pineocytomas are more often more calcified than pinealoblastomas. Pinealoblastomas are typically larger with low signal intensity on T1-weighted images, variable hyperintensity on T2-weighted images, and fairly homogeneous contrast enhancement (Fig. 66-14).[109] Very large pinealoblastomas frequently produce mass effect on the adjacent quadrigeminal cistern, and because of their large size often show areas of necrosis.

Germ-Cell Tumors

The pineal region is the most common location for intracranial germ-cell tumors.[110,111] Histopathologically these are most often germinomas and are usually associated with calcification. This is well demonstrated by CT. MRI is indicated to better delineate the extent of the noncalcified solid portion of the mass as well as heterogeneous cystic portions that may also be present. On T2-weighted images, the solid portion is typically hyperintense with bright enhancement after contrast infusion. Other tumors

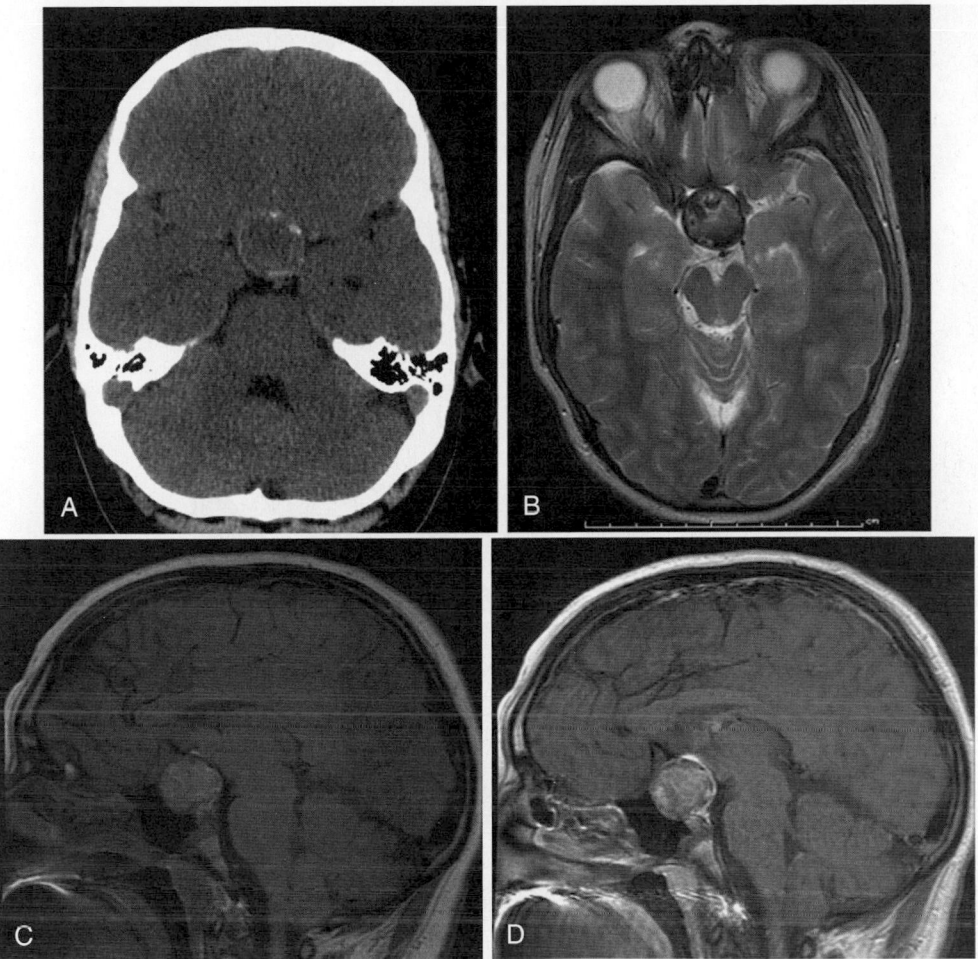

Figure 66-13 Craniopharyngioma. CT showing calcified suprasellar mass (**A**), with heterogeneous increased signal on both T2-weighted images (**B**) and T1-weighted images (**C**), with peripheral enhancement after gadolinium (**D**).

of germ-cell origin are also seen, with choriocarcinomas more commonly showing hemorrhagic components and displaying more aggressive features. Benign teratomas, in contrast, display imaging features more in keeping with their well-differentiated dermoid/epidermoid components, including low attenuation fluid on CT, hyperdense fluid on T1-weighted sequences, and heterogeneous contrast enhancement (Fig. 66-15).

Hypothalamic Hamartoma

This is a rare congenital lesion, usually identified in infants under the age of two. Seizure disorders are common, and these patients often have the presenting symptoms of intractable gelastic seizures. The presence of precocious puberty or diabetes insipidus may provide clinical clues to suggest this diagnosis.

On imaging, CT scanning shows an isodense mass in the region of the hypothalamus. There is little to no contrast enhancement either on CT or MRI.[112] On MRI, the lesion is usually isodense to the brain on T1-weighted images, minimally hyperintense on T2-weighted images, and interestingly may be hyperintense on FLAIR images (Fig. 66-16). Because of the location of these tumors,

surgical resection may be challenging, and MR- or CT-guided ablation techniques are now increasingly being used (Fig. 66-17).

Infratentorial Tumors

The most common lesions of the posterior fossa/cerebellum are juvenile pilocytic astrocytomas (JPAs) and medulloblastomas.[99]

Medulloblastomas

Medulloblastomas are slightly more common in incidence than cerebellar astrocytomas.[95] They typically occur in the first decade of life. Presenting symptoms usually relate to increased intracranial pressure secondary to obstructive hydrocephalus, most often related to mass effect upon the fourth ventricle. Medulloblastomas are highly malignant and have a propensity to disseminate and seed the CNS via the CSF route.[103] Hematogenous spread to other sites may also occur in medulloblastoma.

CT scanning is usually the first imaging study performed to evaluate new-onset nausea, vomiting, headache, or seizures. CT scanning usually demonstrates a hyperintense solid lesion within the cerebellum, often

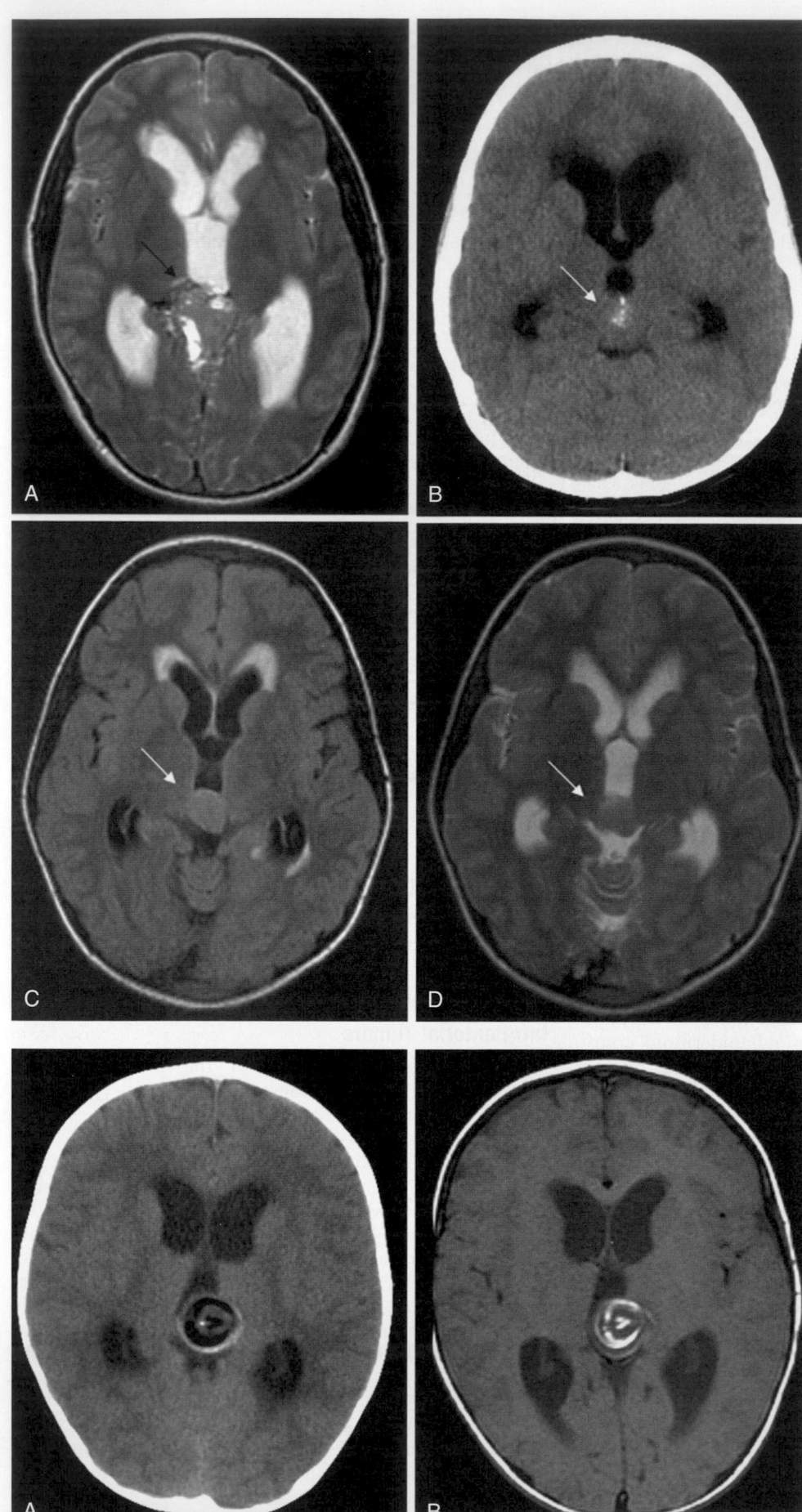

Figure 66-14 Pinealoblastoma. Two patients with pinealoblastoma. The larger cystic/solid mass seen in one patient causes obstruction and hydrocephalus at the level of the quadrigeminal plate cistern (**A**). In the accompanying case (**B**), even the smaller calcified mass causes hydrocephalus as a result of its central location abutting the ventricles. As noted in the text the lesions are often hyperintense on fluid-attenuated sequences (**C**, *FLAIR images*) and isointense to cortex on T2-weighted images (**D**).

Figure 66-15 Pineal germ-cell tumor. CT (**A**) and T1-weighted axial MRI (**B**) showing low attenuation fluid on CT and hyperintense fluid on T1-weighted sequences, typical of a well-differentiated pineal germ-cell tumor (teratoma).

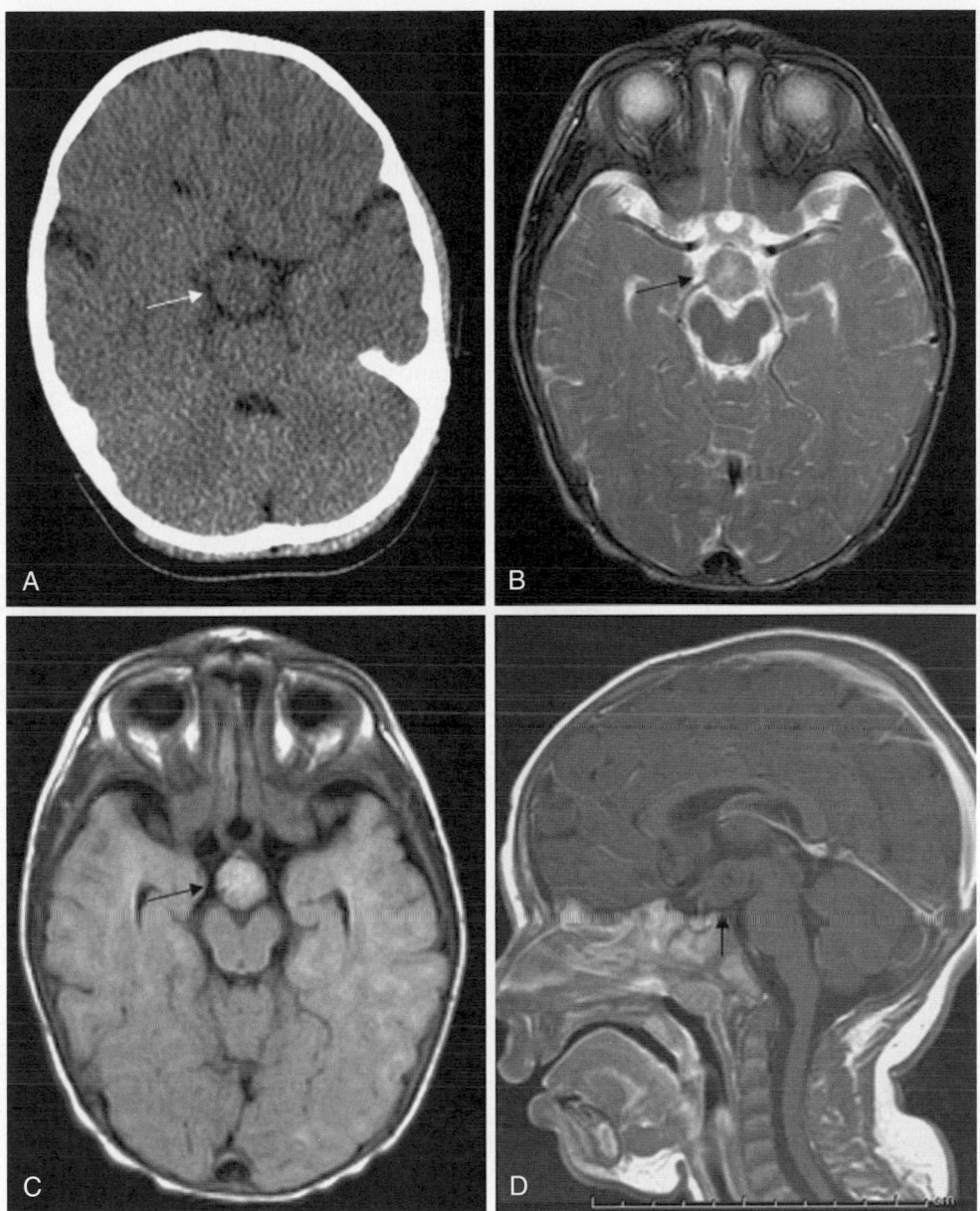

Figure 66-16 Hypothalamic hamartoma. **A,** CT shows a low density suprasellar/hypothalamic lesion. MRI shows the lesion to be isointense to brain on T2-weighted sequences (**B**), mildly hyperintense on FLAIR images (**C**), with no significant enhancement after gadolinium infusion (**D**).

near the midline (Fig. 66-18). MRI imaging is indicated to better characterize the lesions and to establish sites of local and metastatic spread. As with other highly cellular CNS tumors, on T1-weighted images medulloblastomas are usually hypointense relative to the adjacent cerebellum, with increased signal intensity on T2-weighted images (see Fig. 66-18) and homogeneous enhancement after gadolinium infusion.[100,104] Calcification and cystic areas are unusual in medulloblastoma. Because of the propensity to disseminate to other sites via the CNS, the staging evaluation must include a contrast-enhanced evaluation of the entire spine.

Cerebellar Astrocytomas

Astrocytomas are the next most common posterior fossa tumor.[95,99] As with their intracerebral counterpart, cere-

bellar astrocytomas range in histologic grade from benign to anaplastic. The characteristic juvenile pilocytic form makes up the majority of the cerebellar astrocytomas. Both cystic and solid components are normally present in this type of astrocytoma (Fig. 66-19). Calcification is unusual and occurs in 10% of tumors.[113] After resection, survival is excellent with a 10-year overall survival rate greater than 90%. As with medulloblastoma, CT scanning is usually the first imaging modality used to evaluate initial symptoms. CT shows a heterogeneous, predominantly cystic lesion in the posterior fossa, typically with a small mural nodule eccentrically along the margin of the tumor. These lesions are often midline, near the vermis, but may also be eccentric in location. MRI imaging is indicated to better characterize the extent of cerebellar involvement. Although the presence of a

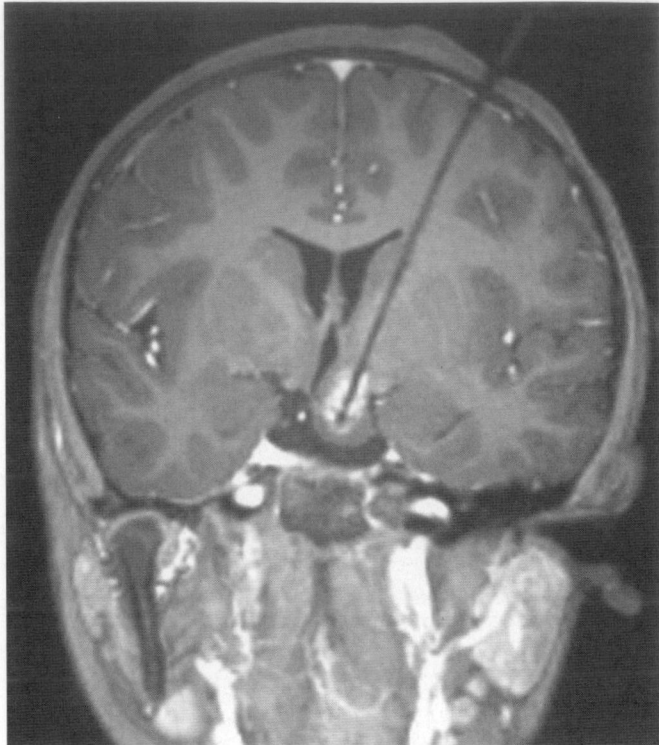

Figure 66-17 MRI-guided laser ablation of hypothalamic hamartoma in a 4-year-old female with medically intractable gelastic seizures. Coronal reformat of a magnetization-prepared rapid acquisition with gradient echo shows the needle tip within the lesion in the hypothalamus with enhancement around the tip indicating the areas that have been ablated by the procedure.

predominantly cystic component suggests a lower-grade neoplasm, foci of local/metastatic spread may be present and will be manifest as a focus of increased enhancement after contrast administration.[103] Therefore the imaging evaluation should include conventional T1- and T2-weighted imaging as well as postcontrast enhanced scanning in all three imaging planes. Because higher-grade neoplasms may also disseminate via the CSF, as with medulloblastoma, the initial staging evaluation should also include evaluation of the entire spine.

Brain-Stem Gliomas

Brain-stem gliomas make up the majority of the neoplasms involving the brain stem. These tumors are of astrocytoma origin and because of their location result in nearly uniformly poor survival.[95] These predominantly cellular solid lesions are best evaluated by MRI, and they typically appear as hypodense lesions on T1-weighted images, with increased signal intensity on T2-weighted images, and show heterogeneous enhancement.[100,103,104] Lower-grade lesions, or lesions with larger cystic components may only show very minimal contrast enhancement (Fig. 66-20). As with the other tumors in these locations, spread is most often via the CSF to other portions of the brain.

Ependymomas

After medulloblastomas and juvenile pilocytic astrocytomas, the next most common posterior fossa tumor is the ependymoma, constituting approximately 8% to 15% of intracranial neoplasms.[99] The majority of these tumors are benign and arise from the ependyma of the fourth ventricle. They typically present as a calcified intraventricular mass. Symptoms result from obstruction of CSF flow at the level of the fourth ventricle leading to obstructive hydrocephalus. There are two histologic types, with the

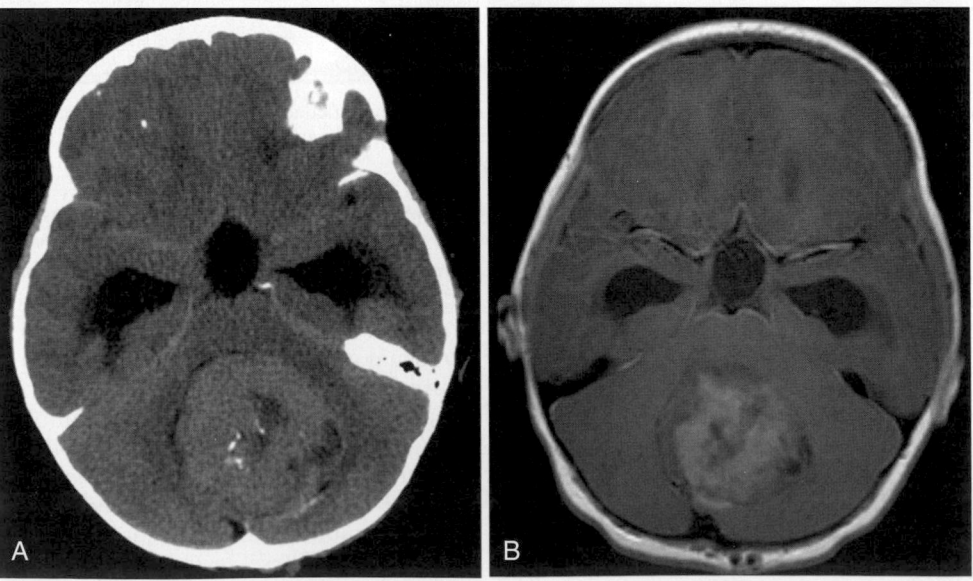

Figure 66-18 Medulloblastoma. **A,** Unenhanced CT shows hyperdense mass in the posterior fossa, compressing the fourth ventricle with resultant obstructive hydrocephalus. **B,** Gadolinium-enhanced T1-weighted MRI shows enhancement of the majority of the mass; these features are all consistent with a highly cellular medulloblastoma.

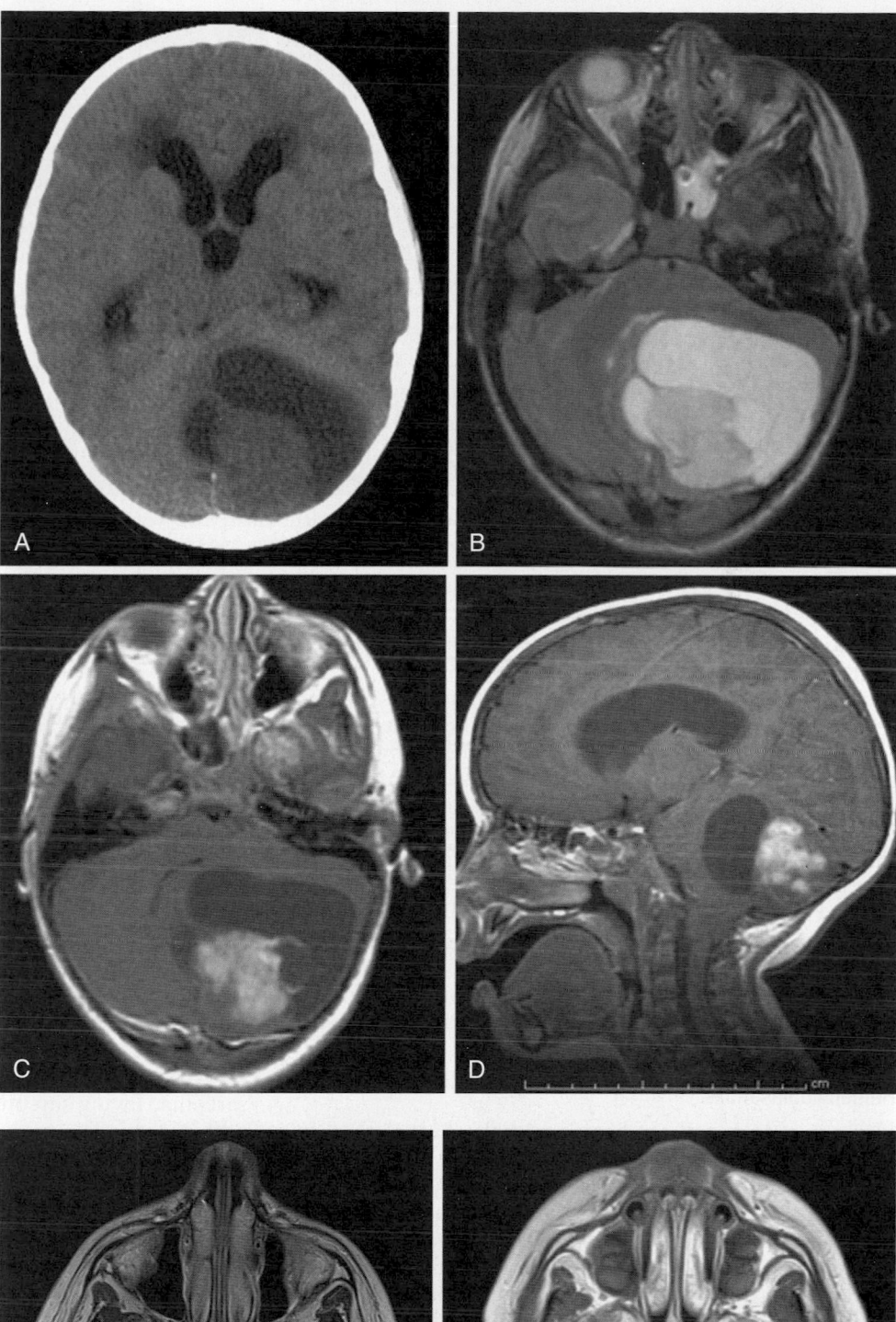

Figure 66-19 Cerebellar pilocytic astrocytoma. **A,** Unenhanced CT shows a large, predominantly cystic mass with a solid mural component in the posterior fossa with moderate hydrocephalus. **B,** T2-weighted MRI shows high signal-intensity cystic fluid and intermediate signal mural nodule. **C** and **D,** Only the mural nodule enhances after gadolinium infusion.

Figure 66-20 Low-grade pontine glioma. Axial T2 (**A**) and post-Gd T1-weighted (**B**) images show T2-bright lesion with faint enhancement of a small nodular component of the tumor along the lateral margin (*arrow*).

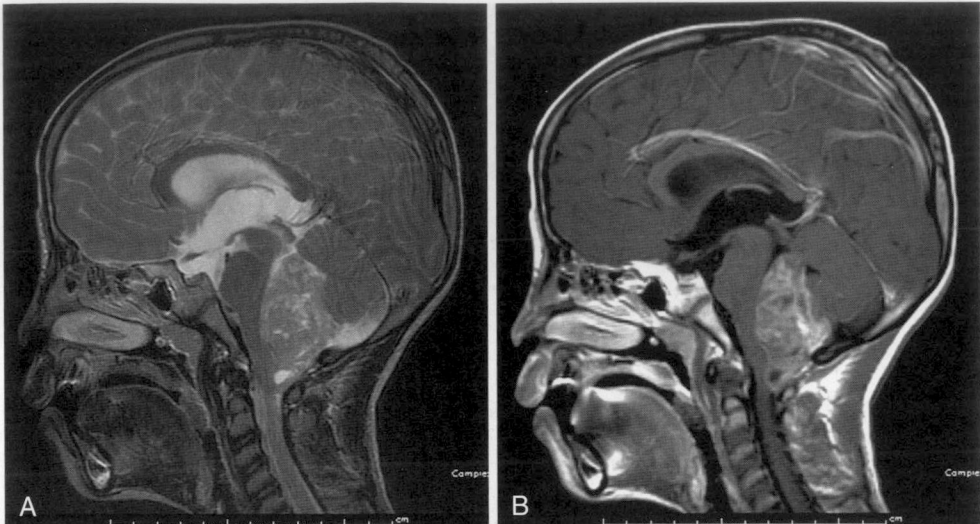

Figure 66-21 Ependymoma. A 7-year-old patient with the symptom of lethargy. T2-weighted (**A**) and gadolinium-enhanced (**B**) MRI show a large heterogeneously enhancing posterior fossa mass compressing the brain stem and beginning to extend out through the foramen magnum.

benign undifferentiated type more common, typically less invasive locally, and with a lower likelihood of CSF dissemination. Malignant anaplastic ependymomas, in contrast, tend to spread via the CSF early in the disease course to other sites within the CNS. Because of their propensity to insinuate through neural foramina, resulting in a lobulated appearance, ependymomas have a fairly characteristic appearance on imaging (Fig. 66-21). Depending on the degree of calcification, these lesions may be predominantly hypointense on T1- and T2-weighted images. In the absence of calcification, these are usually hyperintense lesions on T2-weighted images with heterogeneous intense enhancement after gadolinium infusion.[104] Because of their propensity to seed throughout the CSF and ventricular system, the imaging evaluation must include examination of both the brain and spinal canal.

Hemangioblastomas

Hemangioblastomas are benign vascular lesions that are more common in adults than children. However, the cerebellum is still the most common location in children, and multiple hemangioblastomas may be encountered in familial predisposition syndromes such as the von Hippel-Lindau disease.[114] The imaging features demonstrate a predominantly cystic lesion with an enhancing mural nodule that may be difficult to distinguish from JPAs. As with JPAs, these lesions show cystic characteristics on MRI with low signal intensity on T1-weighted images and T2 hyperintensity, with intense enhancement of the solid mural nodular component (Fig. 66-22). Depending on the size of the mural nodule, the degree of enhancement, and its location, these lesions may also be difficult to discriminate from a benign posterior fossa arachnoid cyst.

Metastatic Disease

Metastatic disease to the CNS may result from leptomeningeal seeding, hematogenous dissemination, or direct extension. Leptomeningeal seeding results from a number

of primary brain tumors, most notably medulloblastomas.[115] Leptomeningeal seeding can also result from non-CNS primary tumors and systemic malignancies.[116] The imaging appearance in this setting is similar to that of leptomeningeal dissemination occurring secondary to a primary CNS tumor.

Hematogenous metastases to calvarium or dura are most commonly seen in patients with neuroblastoma, leukemia, and lymphoma. These lesions present as lytic calvarial lesions or as nonspecific, enhancing dural masses. CNS involvement by leukemia is also common, although this is more often diagnosed by lumbar puncture and pathologic evaluation of the CSF rather than imaging.

Hematogenously disseminated metastases to the brain parenchyma are rare in childhood. When they do occur, primary tumors are sarcomas, particularly rhabdomyosarcoma, Ewing sarcoma,[117] and osteosarcoma. A tumor with a particular propensity to metastasize to the brain is the rhabdoid tumor of the kidney, and imaging of the CNS is essential in children with this diagnosis. Parenchymal metastases are usually multiple and located at the interface between the gray and white matter. They are associated with marked vasogenic edema and demonstrate avid enhancement secondary to loss of the blood-brain barrier.

Although the imaging features may be variable depending on the primary malignancy, the presence of any focal area of signal abnormality or enhancement with a known primary tumor should raise suspicion for metastatic spread of disease to the CNS.

Spinal Cord Tumors

In comparison to pediatric brain tumors, spinal cord tumors are relatively rare in children. The majority of the intramedullary spinal tumors in children are low-grade astrocytomas, with the remainder being ependymomas.[118,119] The imaging features of these lesions mimic

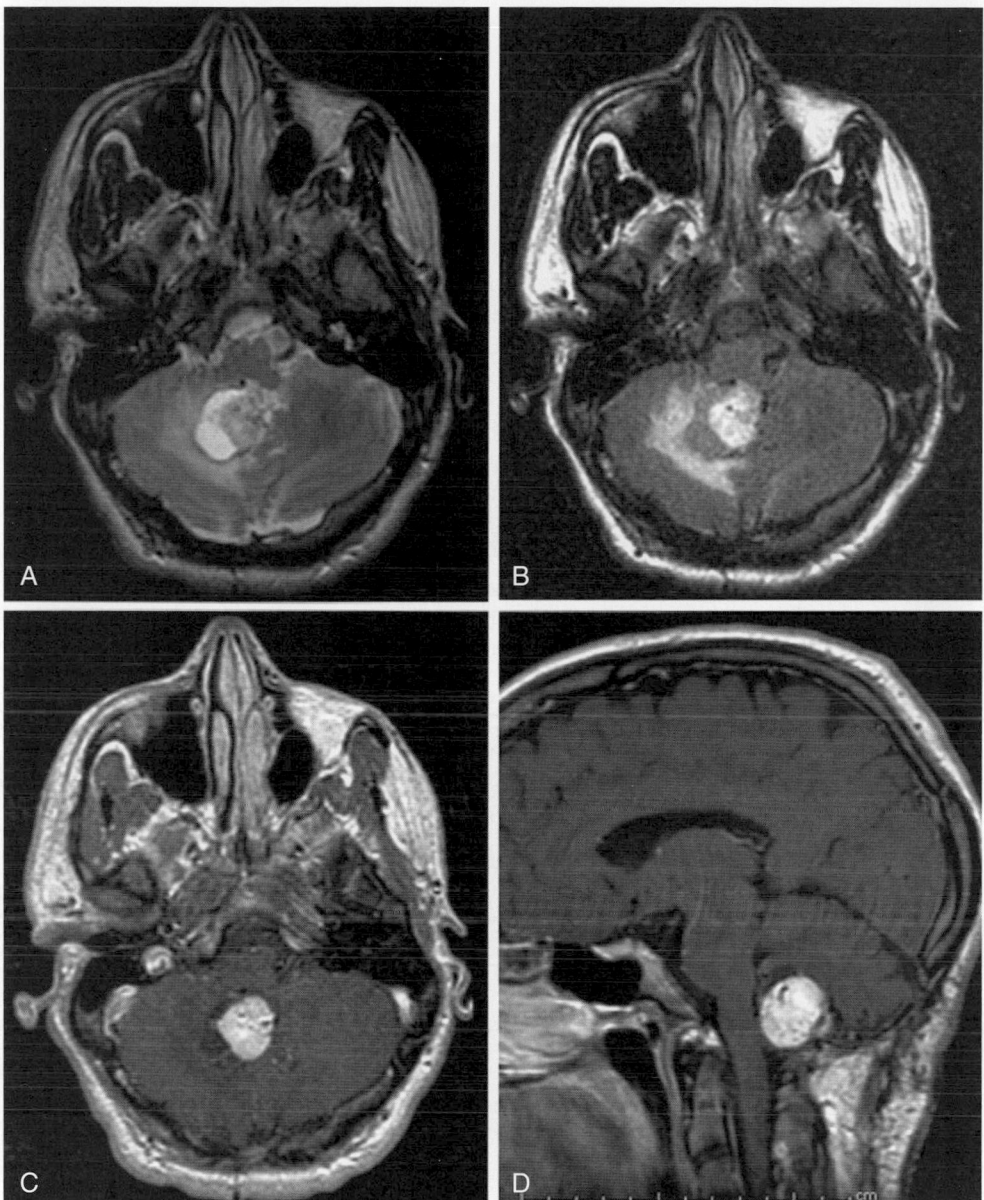

Figure 66-22 Hemangioblastoma. A 28-year-old patient with von Hippel-Lindau disease and cerebellar hemangioblastoma showing typical features on T2-weighted (**A**), fluid-attenuated FLAIR (**B**), and post-gadolinium enhanced images (**C** and **D**).

their intracranial counterparts. The imaging assessment is usually prompted by neurologic symptoms and should include multiplanar T1, T2, and post–gadolinium-enhanced imaging. Because it may be difficult to discriminate a primary intraspinal tumor from metastatic disease, imaging of the brain must also be performed.

As in the brain, the imaging examination should be directed at identifying the site of origin of the tumor. It should be possible to make a distinction between primary intramedullary tumors, extramedullary intradural tumors, and extradural/epidural lesions. This is important, because the majority of the spinal tumors in children are extramedullary. Intradural extramedullary lesions are, by definition, located within the subarachnoid space and are typically

the result of drop metastases, which as discussed earlier, spread via the CSF from primary brain tumors (Fig. 66-23). Their appearance on imaging mimics their counterparts in the brain. Extradural extramedullary tumors may arise from local extension of other primary neoplasms such as neuroblastoma, lymphoma, or Ewing sarcoma (Fig. 66-24). In evaluating these other primary pediatric neoplasms, when their location is adjacent to the vertebral column, it is essential that a thorough imaging evaluation be undertaken to evaluate the presence and extent of intraspinal involvement. In particular, with neuroblastoma, this will influence staging and surgical resectability. The presence of intraspinal extension may be suggested by CT, but will be typically better delineated by MRI (Fig. 66-25).

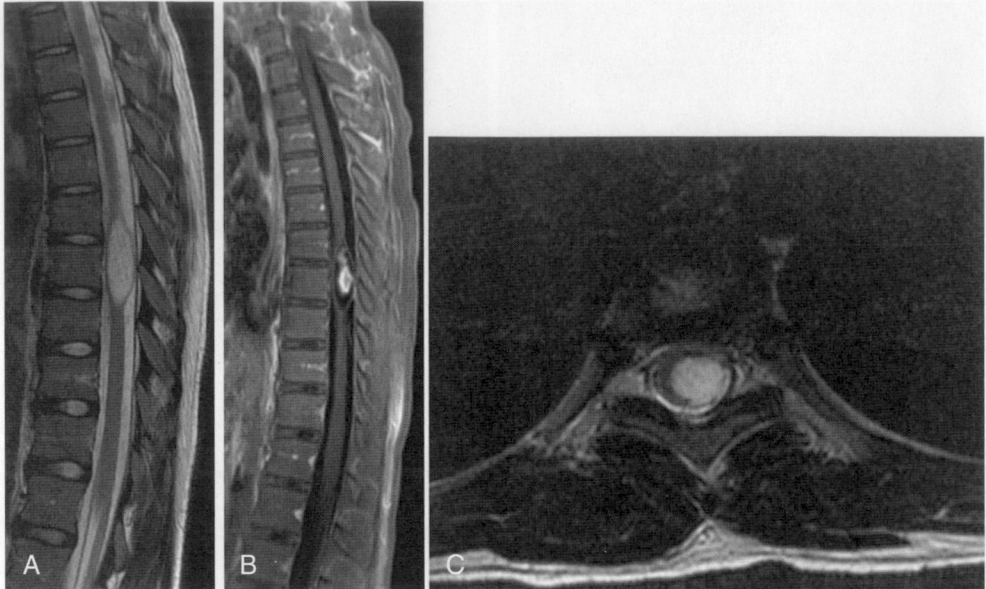

Figure 66-23 Spinal cord astrocytoma. Sagittal T2-weighted (**A**), sagittal post-Gd T1-weighted (**B**), and axial T2-weighted (**C**) images demonstrate a T2-hyperintense, ovoid lesion with enhancing central components consistent with a intramedullary thoracic spinal cord tumor. Pathology of resected specimen showed a low-grade astrocytoma.

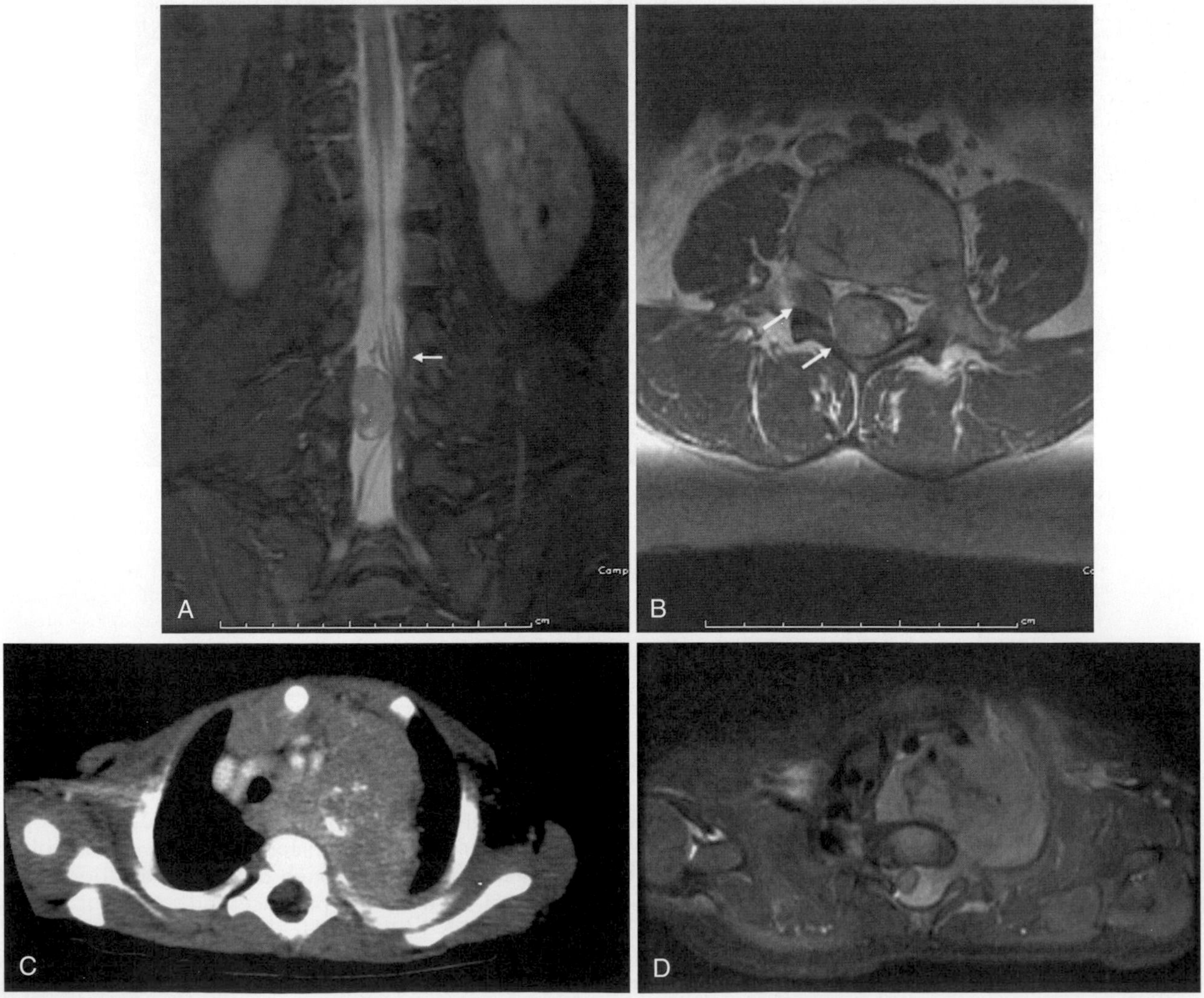

Figure 66-24 **A** and **B**, Coronal and axial MRI images show displacement of nerve roots and intension through the neural foramen in a patient with extramedullary intraspinal Ewing sarcoma. **C** and **D**, Patient with calcified left upper thoracic neuroblastoma initially detected on chest x-ray. MRI is superior in detecting the degree of intraspinal extension (**D**).

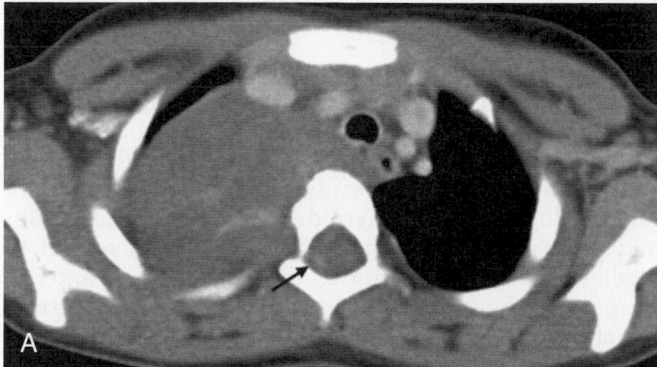

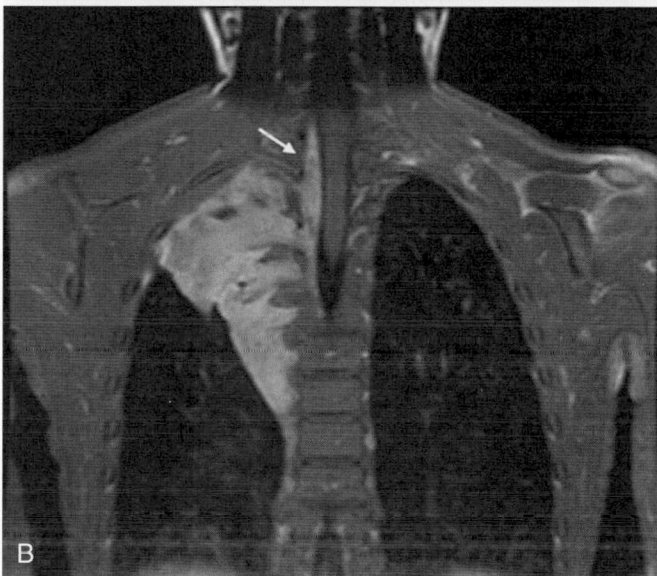

Figure 66-25 Upper thoracic paraspinal neuroblastoma. A 5-year-old patient with 2 weeks of upper-respiratory–infection symptoms. Chest x-ray revealed a right upper lobe opacity (not shown). This was found on CT to be a paraspinal mass. Intraspinal extension is evident on CT (**A**, *arrow*) but much better delineated by MRI (**B**, *arrow*).

PULMONARY AND INTRATHORACIC TUMORS

Thyroid and Parathyroid Tumors

Thyroid carcinoma in children is rare.[120] Three histologic subtypes are recognized in children, with the majority of patients (≈80%) having papillary carcinoma; follicular (≈15%) and medullary (≈5%) thyroid cancers occur less often. The risk is increased in patients with prior history or neck radiation or with predisposing familial syndromes (e.g., multiple endocrine neoplasia [MEN]).[120] Presentation is typically a painless mass in the thyroid gland. Ultrasound is the imaging modality of choice in evaluating the thyroid gland and is usually sufficient to characterize a palpable thyroid abnormality.[121] The goal of the ultrasound examination is to determine whether a cystic or solid mass is present (Fig. 66-26). The presence of increased flow and size of the mass is not reliable in distinguishing benign from malignant thyroid nodules. Malignant nodules are nearly always cold on ^{123}I-radioiodine scintigraphy relative to the surrounding thyroid gland.[121] Depending on the type of tumor, metastatic spread to adjacent lymph nodes and/or the lung may be present. In particular, papillary carcinoma of the thyroid often produces multiple small pulmonary nodules with a miliary distribution. These small pulmonary nodules may be challenging to detect by chest x-ray, and chest CT is indicated to provide increased sensitivity for lesion detection.[122] Bone metastases and thoracic lymph node involvement are common sites of extrapulmonary metastatic spread. [123]I or ^{131}I scintigraphy may also detect lesions not seen by conventional imaging (Fig. 66-27). The treatment of thyroid cancer in children includes total thyroidectomy and lymph-node dissection, followed by ^{131}I-radioiodine therapy for ablation of remnant thyroid tissue as well as to treat sites of micrometastatic disease not visualized by other imaging techniques or not amendable to surgical resection.[123] Diagnostic imaging is initially performed with ^{123}I-radioiodine to establish whether significant remnant tissue, iodine-avid lymph nodes, and metastatic disease are present in order to determine the appropriate therapeutic dose of ^{131}I-radioiodine. Higher doses are used for patients with extensive lymph-node involvement or

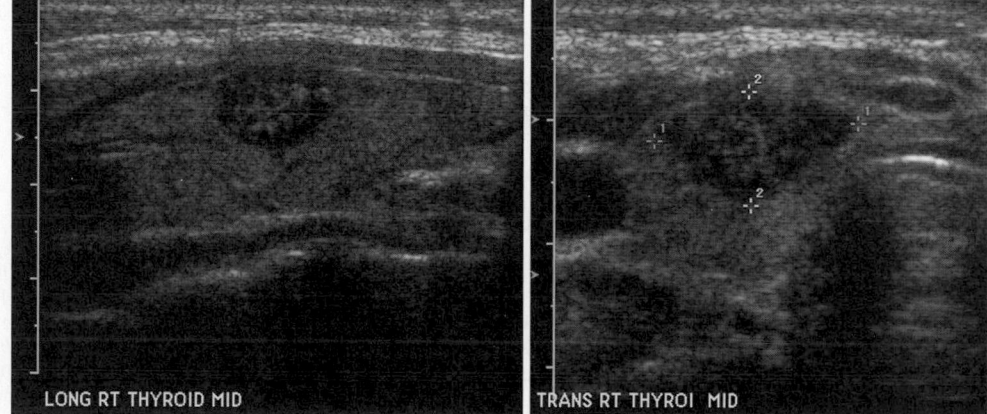

Figure 66-26 Follicular thyroid carcinoma. Palpable thyroid lesion with typical ultrasound imaging characteristics showing hypoechoic well-circumscribed mass. The mass is too small (≈1cm) to be accurately characterized by ^{123}I scintigraphy.

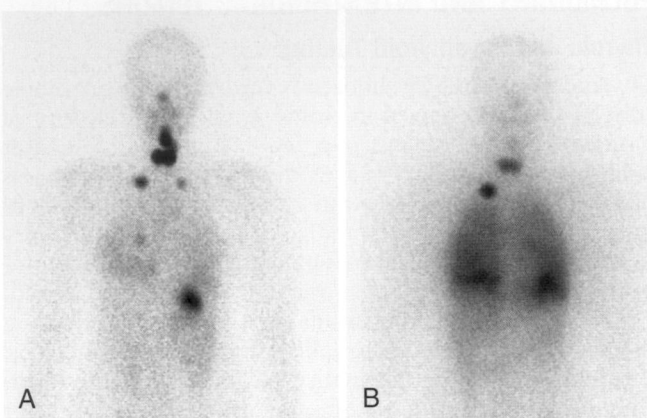

Figure 66-27 An 18-year-old patient with a history of stage-2 Hodgkin lymphoma treated with chemotherapy and radiation who developed a palpable thyroid nodule that was found to be papillary thyroid carcinoma. After thyroidectomy and lymph-node dissection, diagnostic imaging with ¹²³I radioiodine (**A**) shows intense uptake in the surgical bed, likely from remnant thyroid tissue, along with uptake in bilateral supraclavicular lymph nodes. Faint uptake is seen in the lungs. **B**, One week after therapy with ¹³¹I radioiodine, remnant tissue and nodal uptake is reduced; however; intense pulmonary uptake is present, compatible with widespread pulmonary micrometastatic disease.

metastatic spread, as opposed to those with only remnant thyroid tissue in the surgical bed. As shown in Figure 66-27, the higher doses of ¹³¹I used for therapy often allow sites of disease to be detected at the time of the post-therapy follow-up ¹³¹I scintigraphy examination that were not apparent on the initial diagnostic ¹²³I scan.

Abnormalities of the parathyroid gland usually come to clinical attention during evaluation of hypercalcemic states. Functional parathyroid hyperplasia and parathyroid adenomas have a similar imaging appearance and can be very well characterized by ultrasound. There is usually no need for additional imaging by CT. Because of the variable anatomic locations of the parathyroid glands, it may be difficult to identify all potential sites of abnormality by conventional anatomic imaging techniques. ⁹⁹ᵐTc-Methoxyisobutylisonitrile (MIBI) scintigraphy is very sensitive and specific at showing focal accumulation of radiotracer in sites of functional parathyroid activity and can be used to identify sites of otherwise occult disease (Fig. 66-28).

Mediastinal Masses

The mediastinum is located in the center of the thorax, between the two thoracic cavities, the diaphragm, and thoracic inlet. It is conventional to divide the mediastinum into anterior, middle, and posterior mediastinal compartments based on their location as seen on the lateral chest radiograph. Although there are no distinct tissue planes that delineate these compartments, this system of classification is useful in characterizing diseases based on their tissue of origin.[124] Classifying mediastinal masses within a single mediastinal compartment helps narrow the differential diagnosis, calls attention to the potential effect of the mediastinal mass upon adjacent compartmental structures, and therefore commonly guides clinical decision making.[125]

Anterior Mediastinal Masses

The anterior mediastinum is defined as the prevascular space situated between the sternum and the heart, pericardium, and great vessels. The anterior mediastinum extends superiorly from the thoracic inlet to the level of the diaphragm. Organs located in the anterior mediastinum include thymus, thyroid, and parathyroid glands and prevascular-space lymphoid tissue. With respect to mediastinal mass formation, the thymus and anterior mediastinal lymph nodes are the two most important structures to be considered.

In infants, it is important to distinguish normal thymus from a mediastinal mass. The normal thymus typically has an undulating contour and on chest radiographs can be accurately identified based on subtle deformity by the adjacent anterior ribs' costal cartilages (Fig. 66-29). The normal thymus can be quite large and may extend posteriorly between the superior vena cava and aorta in the middle mediastinum or superiorly into the lower neck, making the distinction from neoplasm difficult.[125,126] In the appropriate clinical setting thymic hyperplasia may also be seen and is characterized by a homogeneously enlarged thymus. The thymus also may rapidly involute in response to physiologic stress, and this can also provide an indirect means of confirming its identity as normal thymus.

Lymphoma. Lymphoma is the most common tumor arising in the mediastinum and most commonly arises in either the anterior mediastinum or middle mediastinum. Both Hodgkin and non-Hodgkin lymphomas can present as mediastinal masses. The imaging features of Hodgkin lymphoma characteristically reveal a bulky anterior mediastinal mass with a nodular appearance. In addition, Hodgkin lymphoma is characterized by contiguous lymph-node spread, which may aid in the distinction

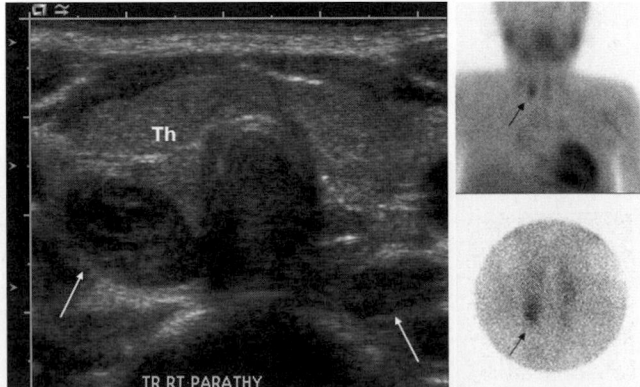

Figure 66-28 Parathyroid adenoma. Thyroid *(Th)* ultrasound showing a large hypoechoic mass on the right and a smaller lesion on the left *(arrows)* at the expected location of the parathyroid glands in an 11-year-old patient with end-stage renal disease and secondary hyperparathyroidism. The dominant mass on the *right* has corresponding increased uptake on ⁹⁹ᵐTc-MIBG scintigraphy, consistent with parathyroid adenoma. The lower levels of uptake in the smaller lesions are more in keeping with hyperplastic parathyroid tissue. ⁹⁹ᵐTc-MIBG is also effective at locating ectopically located parathyroid tissue (e.g., substernal) not visualized on thyroid ultrasound.

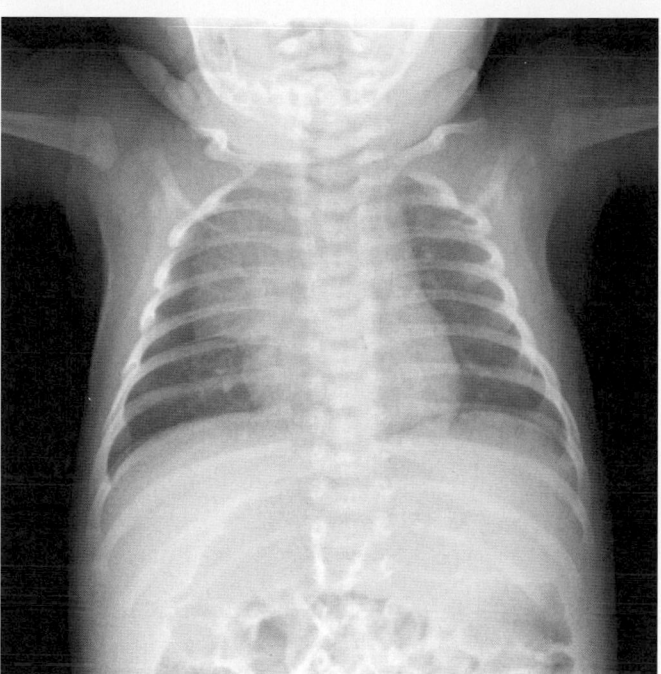

Figure 66-29 Anteroposterior chest radiograph of an infant shows prominent thymic shadow and undulating contour conforming to the adjacent ribs, findings all consistent with normal thymic tissue.

from other types of lymphoma. Approximately two thirds of pediatric patients with Hodgkin lymphoma show lymphadenopathy involving the mediastinum.[127] Non-Hodgkin lymphomas include lymphoblastic lymphoma and other subtypes.[127] Approximately one third of pediatric non-Hodgkin lymphomas have a mediastinal mass, and more than 50% of the lymphoblastic lymphomas have mediastinal involvement.[125] Although the distinction between some subtypes of non-Hodgkin and Hodgkin lymphoma may be difficult, acute T-lymphoblastic lymphomas often demonstrate a homogeneous infiltration and enlargement of the thymus gland with encasement/compression of the vessels (Fig. 66-30). All forms of lymphoma can result in significant tracheal compression/narrowing, vascular compression, and symptoms related to the superior mediastinal syndrome.[127,128] Pleural and pericardial effusions are seen in both non-Hodgkin and Hodgkin lymphomas of the mediastinum and are not a distinguishing feature. Bone-marrow involvement is seen in patients with either Hodgkin or non-Hodgkin lymphoma. Recent studies have shown that FDG-PET is a sensitive method for detecting bone-marrow involvement in children with Hodgkin lymphoma and can safely replace routine bone marrow biopsy for establishing the presence of marrow involvement.[129] Direct bone invasion by Hodgkin lymphoma is unusual; non-Hodgkin lymphomas often show more aggressive local involvement.

The imaging evaluation should always include a chest radiograph. In many instances this is the most important imaging study to guide the subsequent care of the patient. The presence of significant tracheal narrowing or tracheal displacement in the context of a large anterior mediastinal mass, particularly if accompanied by respiratory

symptoms (see Figs. 66-2 and 66-30), should raise immediate concern for impending respiratory/cardiopulmonary compromise and prompt intensive care unit (ICU)–level monitoring.[128] Pneumomediastinum and pneumothorax may also be identified on these initial imaging studies (see Fig. 66-30). The placement of the patient in a recumbent position for CT scanning may further exacerbate the patient's already tenuous respiratory status, impair central venous return, and result in an acute cardiorespiratory event. In this setting it may be necessary to delay CT imaging, and the staging evaluation will have to be postponed until stabilization of the patient's clinical status.

In a stable patient, staging of anterior mediastinal lymphomas must include imaging of the neck to evaluate the Waldeyer ring of lymphoid tissue and should also include the abdomen and pelvis. Intravenous contrast should be used to provide an accurate assessment of the mediastinal vascular structures. Oral contrast should be provided to opacify the bowel and aid in the distinction from mesenteric lymphadenopathy.

MRI, particularly with faster scanning techniques, may be effective in evaluating mediastinal masses and staging lymphoma[130,131] but currently does not have an established role in the more acute stages of the evaluation. Gallium scintigraphy previously and currently FDG-PET imaging are recognized as standard of care in identifying sites of metabolically active lymphoma and in identifying sites of disease otherwise undetected by conventional imaging techniques (Fig. 66-31). FDG-PET scanning, in particular, has also been shown to play an important role in the posttreatment evaluation, helping to stratify patients into early responder and nonresponder groups to allow appropriate modulation of therapy based on treatment response (Fig. 66-32).[90,132,133-135]

After treatment, particularly of Hodgkin disease, it is common for the mediastinal mass to slowly regress and for residual inflammatory tissue to persist even months after therapy.[136,137] In contrast, lymphoblastotic lymphomas often respond quite rapidly to therapy with very little residual soft-tissue abnormality remaining in the anterior mediastinum, even after a relatively short duration of treatment (Fig. 66-33).[138] The use of FDG-PET for early response assessment in Hodgkin lymphoma is now considered standard of care, with images being simultaneously acquired and coregistered as fused PET-CT images to distinguish persistent metabolically active disease from residual posttreatment inflammatory tissue.[139-141] There is a large body of literature from both pediatric and adult patients showing that the presence of residual metabolically active disease after two cycles of chemotherapy is prognostically significant, presumably reflecting chemosensitive versus chemoresistant disease.[133,142,143,144-146] Patients with residual CT abnormalities that are FDG-avid have a worse overall outcome as compared with patients whose scans are FDG-negative, which has led to a paradigm shift in Hodgkin lymphoma therapy such that patients in whom early response assessment shows no metabolically active disease would be eligible for reduced chemotherapy and radiation in an effort to reduce treatment-related complications.[144,147] Whether this approach will maintain the good outcomes (>90%

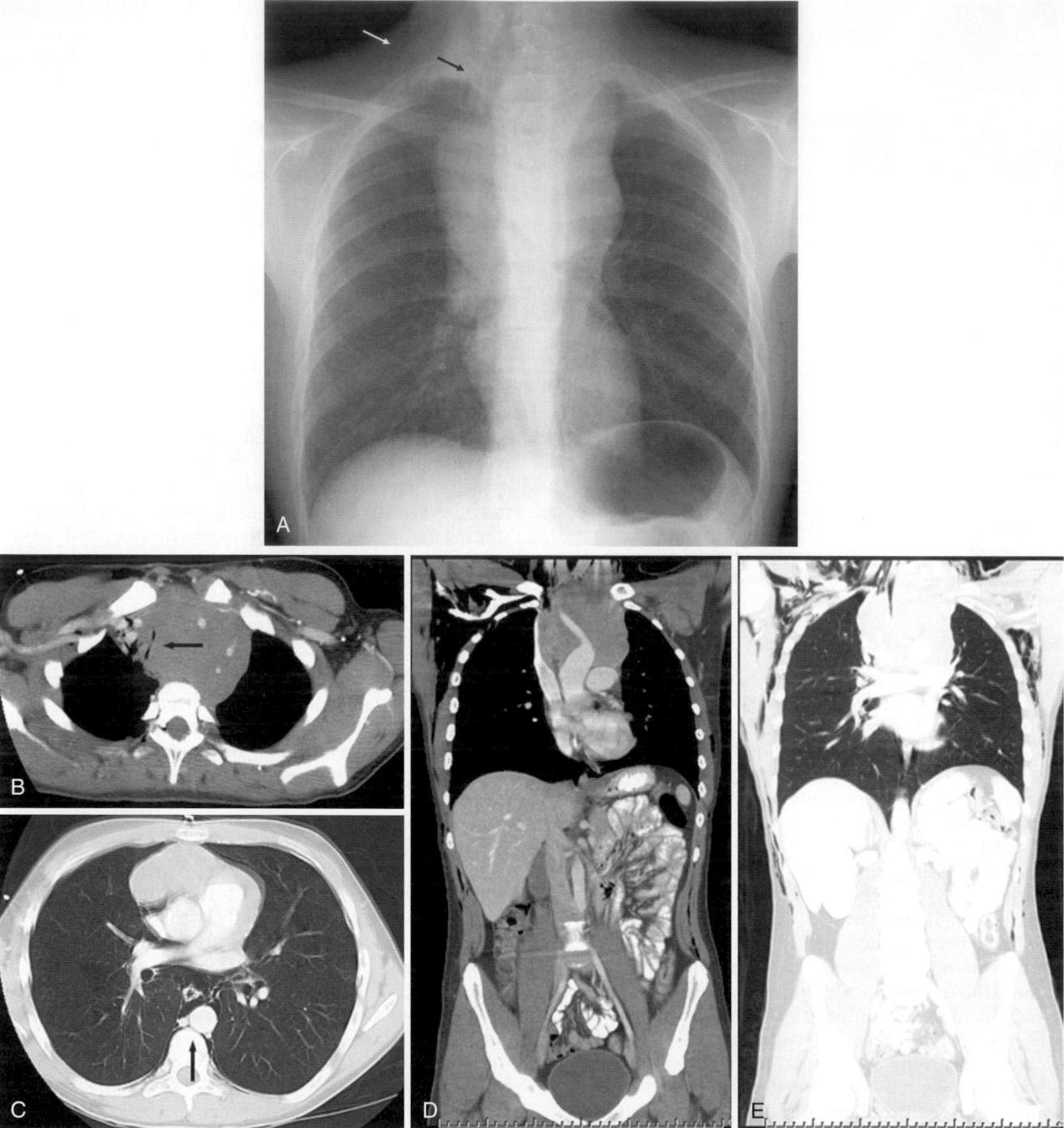

Figure 66-30 A, Chest x-ray showing marked tracheal deviation, pneumomediastinum, and subcutaneous emphysema along the right neck in a child with lymphoblastic lymphoma, emphasizing the severity of airway obstruction and potential for respiratory compromise *(arrows)*. B-E, CT shows large anterior mediastinal mass with mediastinal air around the heart, pulmonary vessels, aorta, and esophagus (C). The trachea is markedly narrowed *(arrow)*, likely the cause of the pneumomediastinum. Subcutaneous air is also evident in the anterior chest wall. Five days later the findings had progressed considerably (C and D).

overall survival) typically seen in Hodgkin lymphoma remains to be seen.[148,149] There is currently no convincing data showing the prognostic value of FDG-PET imaging in non-Hodgkin lymphoma.[150]

Germ-Cell Tumor. Mediastinal germ-cell tumors are primarily located in the anterior mediastinum near the

thymus gland and make up about 10% to 20% of all childhood mediastinal tumors. Germ-cell tumors are second only to lymphoma as the cause of a thymic/anterior mediastinal mass. When they present as predominately solid masses, they may be difficult to distinguish from lymphoma. Histologically, mature teratomas are the most common germ-cell tumor arising in the

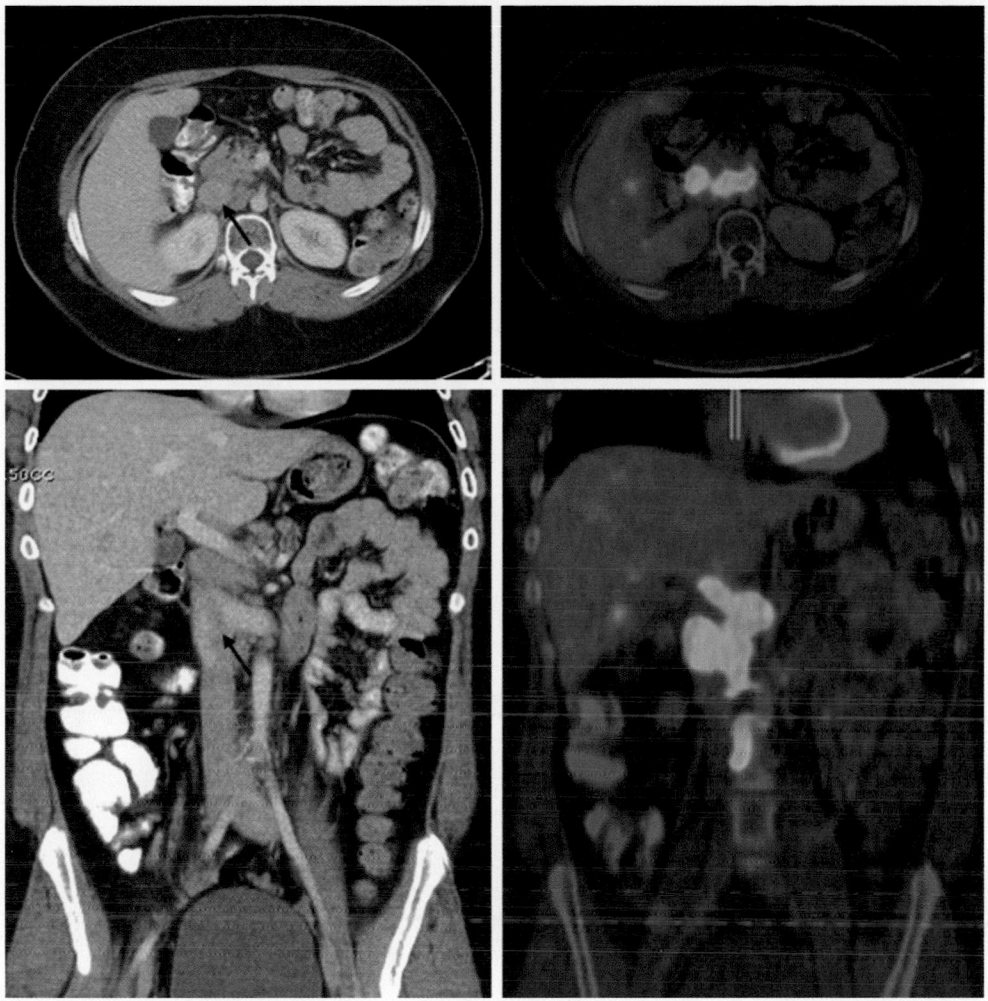

Figure 66-31 FDG-PET and image fusion delineate equivocal areas of abnormality on CT *(arrows)*, identifying foci of disease recurrence in a patient with Hodgkin lymphoma.

mediastinum.[151] At diagnosis, calcification of lymphoma is unusual, and the calcifications that are often present in teratoma may suggest the diagnosis. Germ-cell tumors are often asymptomatic and may be identified incidentally as mediastinal masses on chest radiographs obtained for other indications.[152] When symptoms are present, they are usually the result of compression of the tracheobronchial tree.

Either CT or MRI scanning are effective at further characterizing these masses. The presence of fluid attenuation, mixed attenuation fluids and gelatinous material, fat, and calcification all should suggest the diagnosis of mediastinal germ-cell tumor (Fig. 66-34). Ten percent to 20% of all mediastinal germ-cell tumors are malignant and present with signs of local invasion into the pleura or pericardium. Malignant tumors include seminomatous and nonseminomatous histologic subtypes. Seminomas tend to be noncalcified, bulky solid masses that either remain localized or spread to local lymph nodes, whereas other malignant germ-cell tumors display greater heterogeneity with cystic and solid elements and more aggressive, locally invasive features.[153] Germ-cell tumors may

rupture into the pleural or pericardial spaces, the lung parenchyma, or the tracheobronchial tree. Imaging evaluation should be directed at determining the extent of rupture and sites of tissue involvement. Chemical pneumonitis can result from parenchymal rupture, and expectoration of blood, hair, and sebaceous material can result from rupture into the airways.[154]

Thymic Masses

Thymoma. Thymoma is rare in children, accounting for less than 4% of pediatric mediastinal tumors.[125] As with adults, thymoma may present with symptoms related to associated autoimmune disorders, including myasthenia gravis, diabetes, and Hashimoto thyroiditis. Thymomas are typically solid, lobulated masses arising in or around the thymus (Fig. 66-35). The imaging evaluation should be directed at assessing for aggressive features such as invasion into adjacent pericardial or pleural structures. MRI and contrast-enhanced CT reveal a heterogeneously enhanced low-density mass that is isointense on T1-weighted images and mildly T2 hyperintense relative to muscle.[125] Both CT and MRI are excellent in

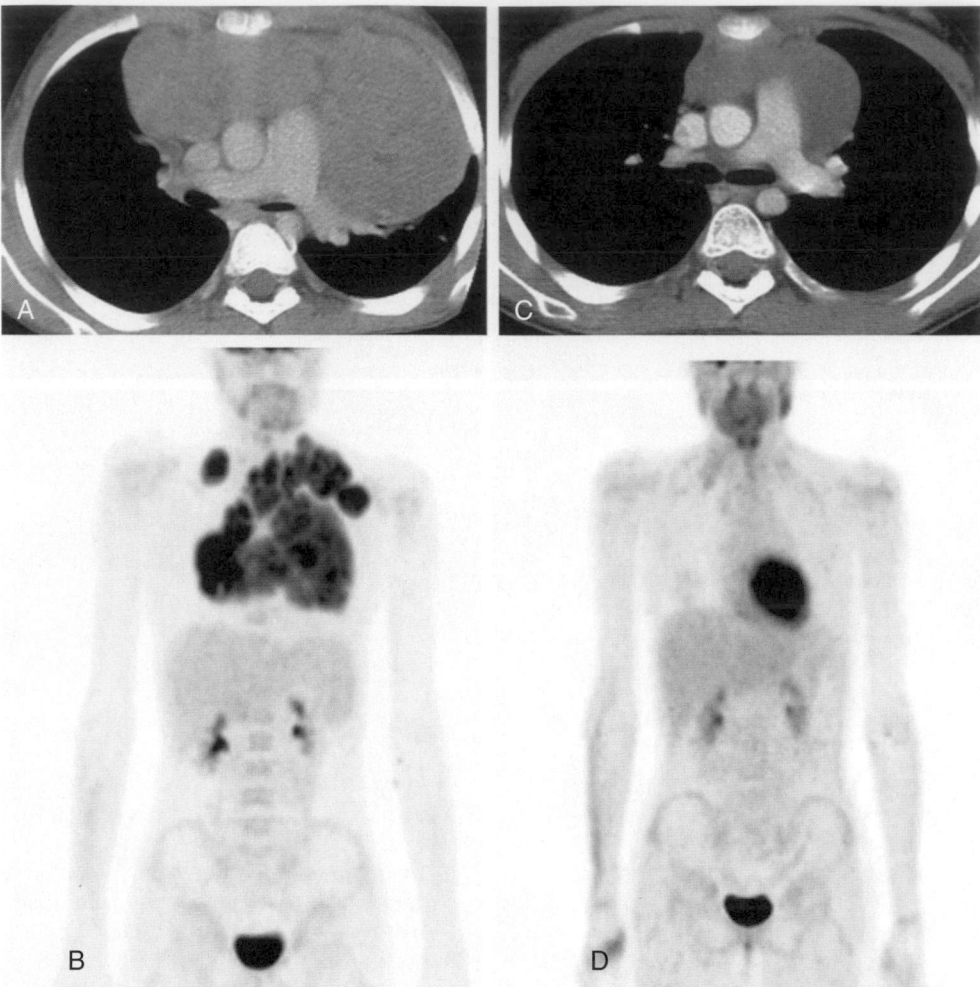

Figure 66-32 Hodgkin Lymphoma CT and FDG-PET obtained at diagnosis (**A** and **B**) and after 2 cycles of chemotherapy (**C** and **D**) show excellent functional and anatomic response to therapy. Residual mediastinal mass on CT with no residual FDG uptake emphasizes the potential importance of functional imaging in response assessment.

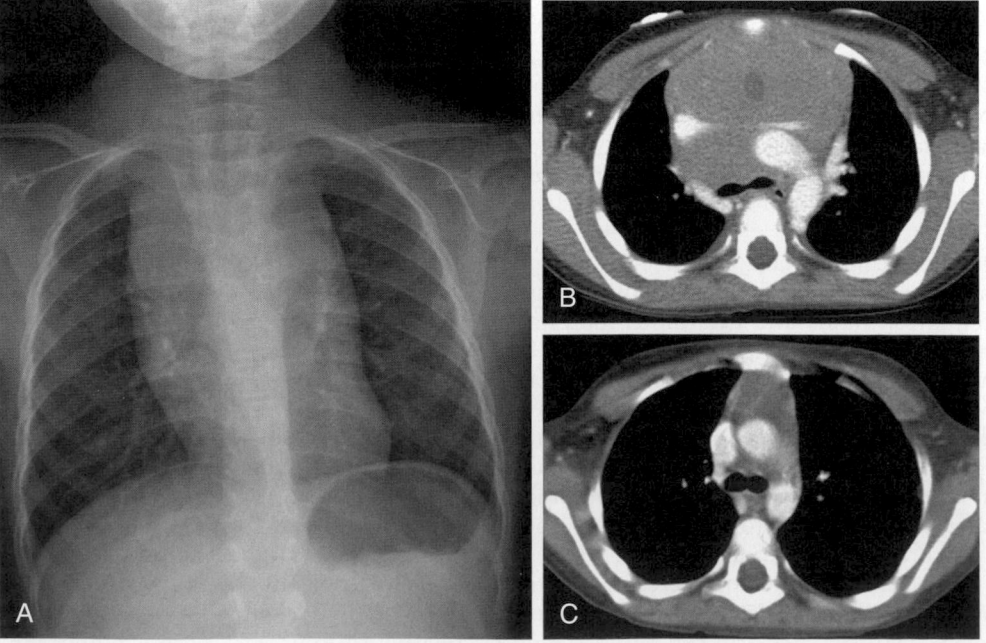

Figure 66-33 A 4-year-old child with T-cell ALL and a large mediastinal mass with airway and vascular compression seen by CXR (**A**) and CT (**B**), showing near complete resolution of the mass after just 2 weeks of therapy (**C**).

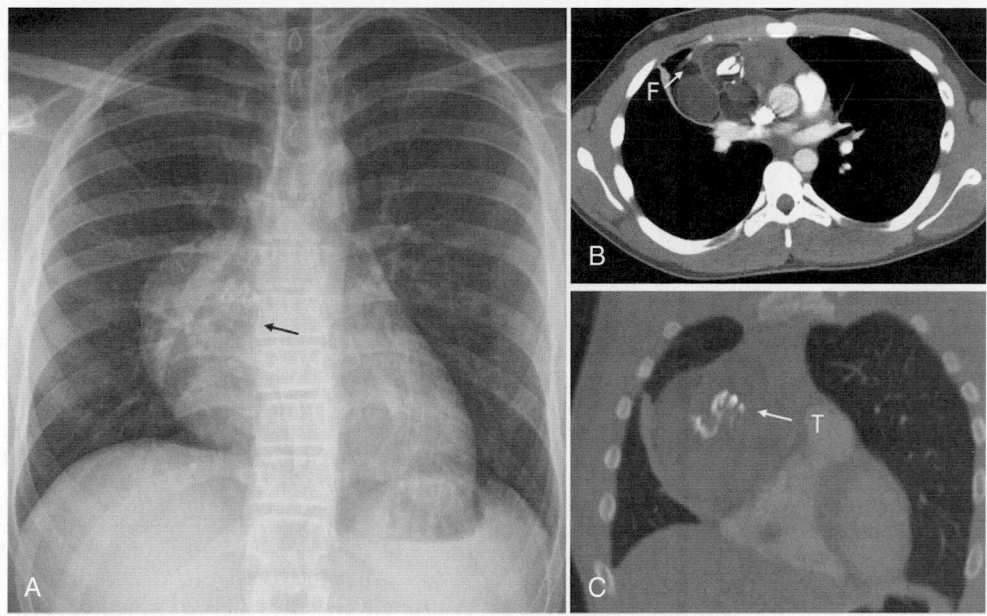

Figure 66-34 A 15-year-old boy with mediastinal mass seen incidentally on a chest x-ray obtained for pain after a football injury (**A**). Subsequent CT (**B** and **C**) shows fat *(F)* and adjacent solid elements in addition to calcification, in this case taking the form of tooth *(T)*, characteristic of germ cell tumor, in this case mature teratoma.

delineating the relationship of these masses to the adjacent vascular structures (see Fig. 66-35). Nodular pleural or pericardial thickening should raise concern for invasive thymoma. Because complete surgical resection is the most effective treatment for ensuring long-term survival for patients with thymoma, postsurgical radiation therapy may be considered when invasive features are present.[155]

Thymolipomas. Thymolipoma, in contrast to thymoma, is relatively more common, making up about 3% to 9% of pediatric thymic tumors.[156] These benign tumors are most often seen in older children, but they may present in infancy. These heterogeneous masses may contain calcification and cystic areas, making distinction from germ-cell tumors challenging. A predominantly fatty mass should, however, suggest the diagnosis of thymolipoma (Fig. 66-36). The fat characterization can be sensitively and specifically evaluated by MRI, showing a high signal-intensity mass on T1-weighted imaging with loss of signal on fat-suppressed images.[156] A low-attenuation mass with negative Hounsfield-unit density on either unenhanced or contrast-enhanced CT can also suggests the presence of a fat-containing mass (see Fig. 66-36).

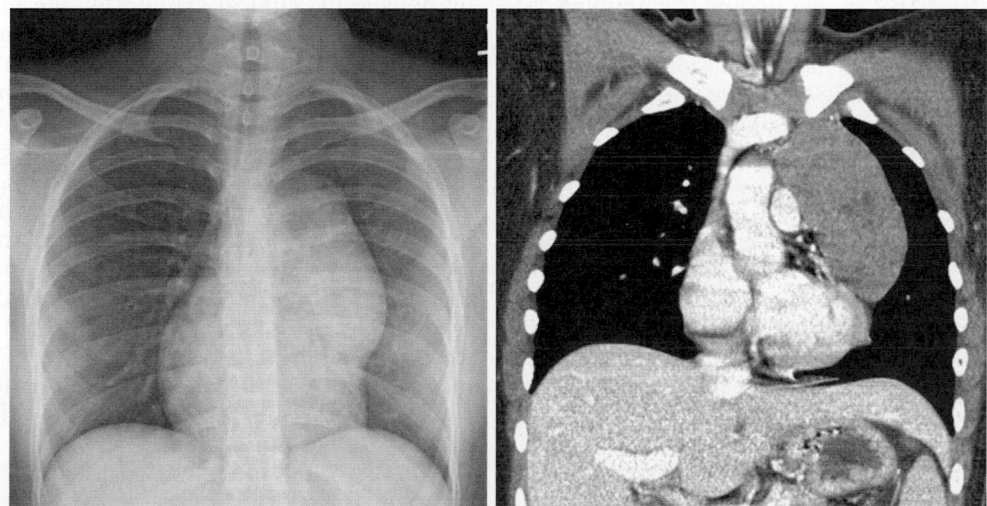

Figure 66-35 A 15-year-old girl with a 2-week history of chest pain. Chest x-ray and CT show a large, lobular, heterogeneous anterior mediastinal mass abutting the great vessels, with a poorly defined plane between the mass and normal mediastinal structures. Biopsy revealed thymoma, and the patient underwent complete resection.

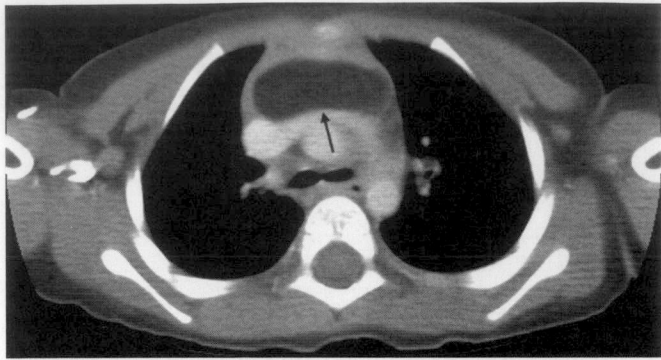

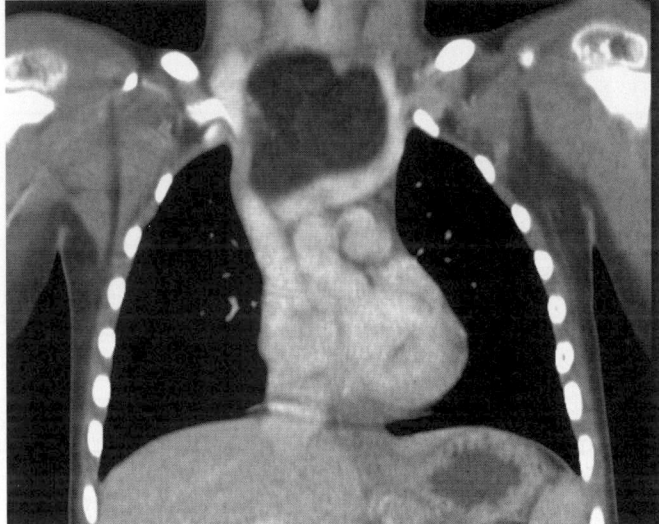

Figure 66-36 Thymolipoma in a child with an incidentally detected mediastinal mass on chest x-ray. Note the fat-density mass *(arrow)* located within the thymus.

Middle Mediastinum

Tracheobronchial Tree Masses. The middle mediastinum is defined as the vascular space including the pericardium/heart, the great vessels, and trachea/proximal bronchi and associated lymph nodes. Although the most common middle mediastinal mass is lymphoma, lymphoma is rarely isolated to the middle mediastinum and usually occurs in conjunction with a large anterior mediastinal mass. The most common masses isolated to the middle mediastinum are benign bronchopulmonary foregut malformations, including bronchopulmonary sequestration, congenital cystic adenomatoid malformation (C-CAM), and foregut/bronchogenic cysts.[124] These benign masses are not discussed further in this section except to emphasize that the distinction between cystic adenomatoid malformation and pleuropulmonary blastoma cannot be made on the basis of imaging alone (Fig. 66-37). Surgical resection and histopathologic evaluation is required to distinguish the benign C-CAM from its neoplastic counterpart.

Masses of the endobronchial tree are also exceedingly rare in children. The most common endobronchial neoplasm in children is the bronchial carcinoid tumor, making up about 50% of all bronchial neoplasms.[157] Although these tumors may secrete neuroendocrine peptides, the classic carcinoid syndrome is relatively unusual in children with bronchial carcinoids, and these patients are more likely to have presenting respiratory symptoms such as hemoptysis or lobar atelectasis/partial collapse caused by the obstructing endobronchial lesion (Fig. 66-38). These lesions are commonly hilar in location and may be very difficult to identify on chest radiographs. The presence of a persistent area of segmental or lobar collapse that does not resolve after appropriate therapy should prompt further investigation by CT scanning to directly assess the airways. Multidetector-row CT scans can provide exquisite 3D reformations of the airways and allow accurate detection of endobronchial abnormalities. Chest CT of patients with suspected endobronchial carcinoid tumor may be performed without intravenous contrast for the purpose of identifying the endobronchial lesion; however, contrast infusion typically shows prominent enhancement of these highly vascular lesions. There may be intraluminal, mural, and extraluminal components of these lesions, and the extraluminal extent of the lesion may exceed its intraluminal component.[158] Although the presence of calcification in an endobronchial mass should suggest the diagnosis of a carcinoid tumor, calcification is still relatively rare in childhood bronchial carcinoid tumors. Surgical resection is usually curative, and although the extent of local invasion around the primary lesion is variable, metastatic disease is relative rare (5% to 20%). Uptake of the neuroendocrine-specific radiotracer [111]I-octreotide provides highly specific scintigraphic imaging confirmation of the diagnosis (see Fig. 66-38, C and D) and may aid in identifying occult sites of metastatic disease. FDG-PET imaging of metabolically active carcinoid tumors has also been performed and, although not specific for neuroendocrine tumors, may prove to be a sensitive means of identifying occult metastases.

Mucoepidermoid carcinoma is the second most common primary bronchial neoplasm. These patients also have primarily respiratory presenting symptoms related to airway obstruction. Because primary airway neoplasia in children is rare and commonly characterized by nonspecific clinical symptoms, the diagnosis is often delayed and difficult to distinguish from infectious processes such as pneumonia. The most common finding on plain chest radiographs in patients with mucoepidermoid carcinoma is a central mass or nodule.[159,160] These tumors range from low to high grade, with high-grade neoplasms tending to invade the adjacent pulmonary parenchyma. As with carcinoid tumors, multidetector-row CT with multiplanar and 3D reformats can be used to accurately identify an airway abnormality.[160,161] However, in contrast to carcinoid tumors, mucoepidermoid carcinoma is relatively hypovascular and shows minimal enhancement. Recent studies have also suggested that FDG-PET imaging may be used to advantage in staging patients with mucoepidermoid carcinoma,[160] with intense FDG uptake visualized (Fig. 66-39).

Tumors of the heart and pericardium are very rare in children. The majority of these are rhabdomyomas arising from the neoplastic transformation of cardiac myocytes. There is a well-known association between cardiac rhabdomyoma and tuberous sclerosis (Fig. 66-40), with

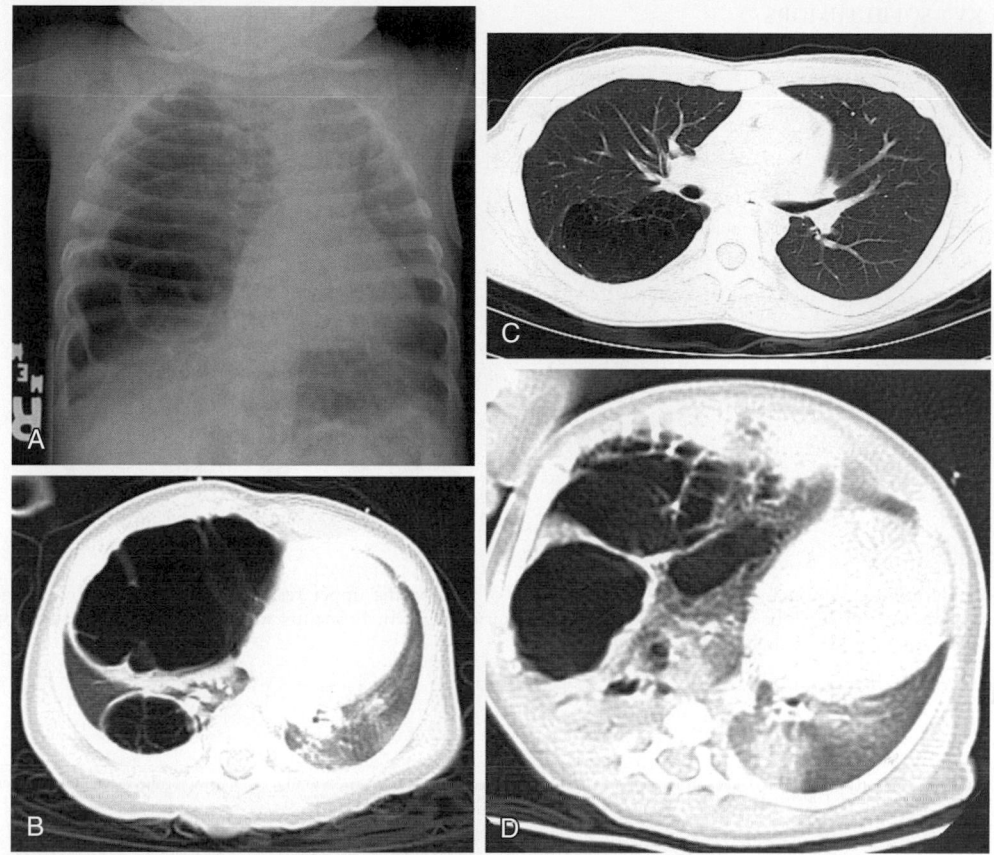

Figure 66-37 Pleuropulmonary blastoma (**A** and **B**). Note the difficulty in distinguishing this malignancy from C-CAM (**C** and **D**).

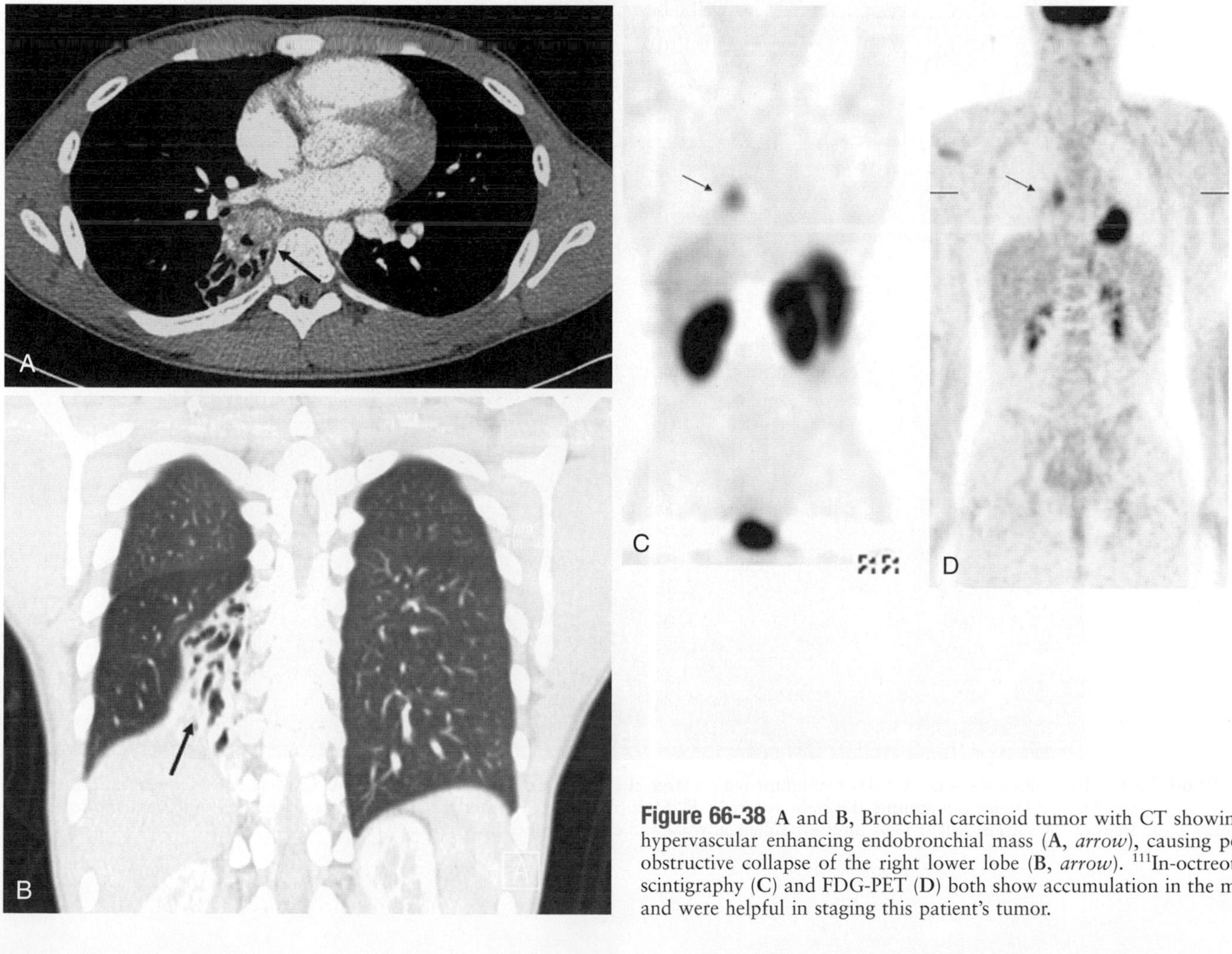

Figure 66-38 **A** and **B**, Bronchial carcinoid tumor with CT showing a hypervascular enhancing endobronchial mass (**A**, *arrow*), causing post-obstructive collapse of the right lower lobe (**B**, *arrow*). ^{111}In-octreotide scintigraphy (**C**) and FDG-PET (**D**) both show accumulation in the mass and were helpful in staging this patient's tumor.

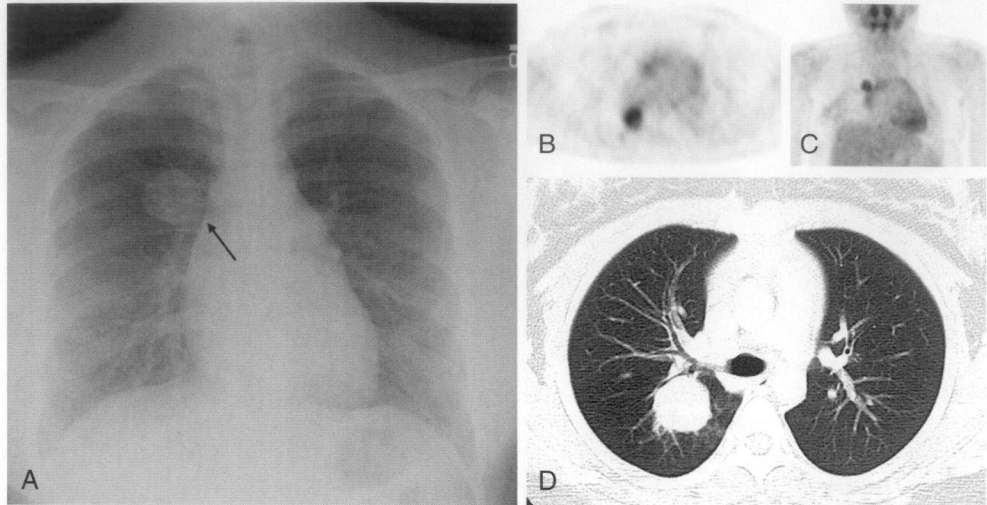

Figure 66-39 Mucoepidermoid carcinoma. Chest x-ray for symptoms of nonspecific upper respiratory infection showed right upper lobe mass (**A**). CT shows posterior segment upper lobe mass compressing the posterior segment bronchus with mild associated air-trapping (**D**). FDG-PET (**B** and **C**) showed intense uptake and was helpful for staging.

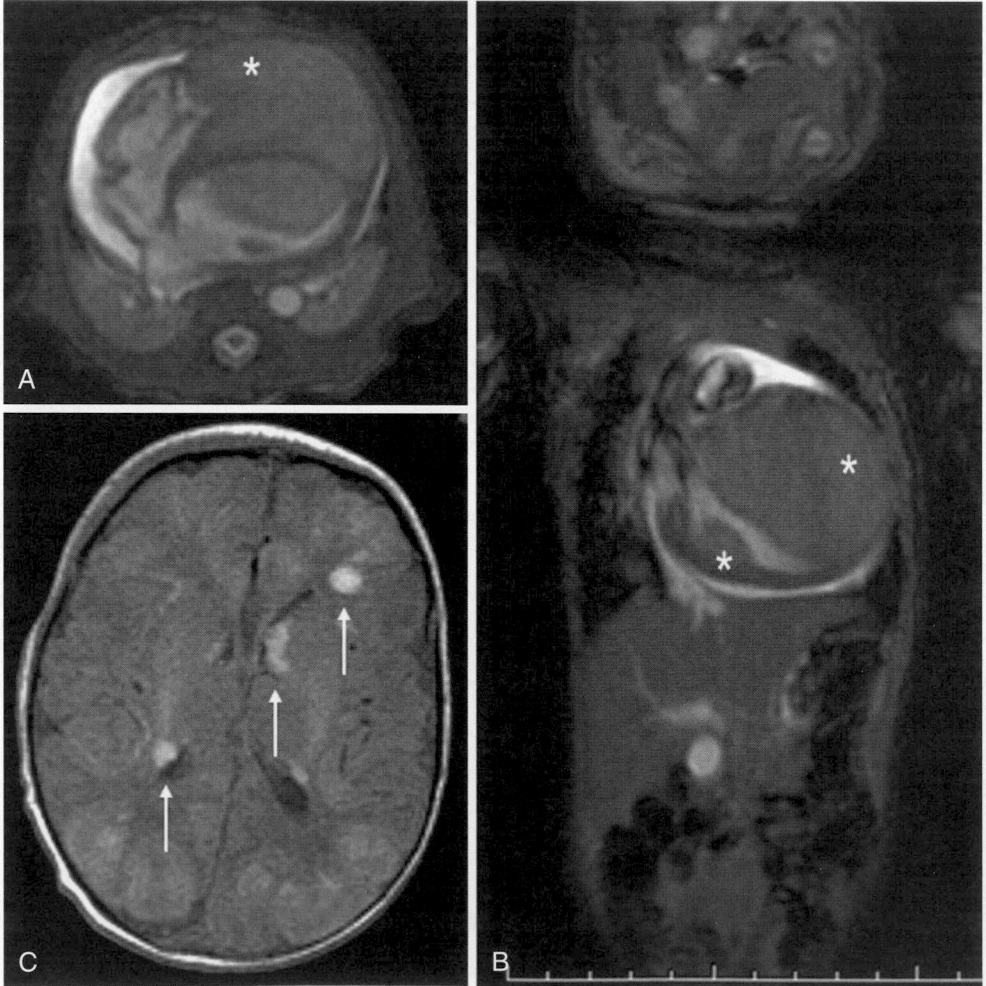

Figure 66-40 Cardiac rhabdomyoma. A 5-day-old infant with a large chest mass and tuberous sclerosis. **A,** Cardiac MRI showed multiple rhabdomyomas *(asterisks)*, the largest obliterating the right ventricle. **B,** Multiple smaller tumors are in the left ventricle, both adherent to the septum and along the free wall. **C,** Brain MRI shows multiple subependymal and cortical tubers *(arrows)*.

approximately half of the patients with this diagnosis having rhabdomyomas.[162] Indeed the presence of a rhabdomyoma should prompt further evaluation, because rhabdomyomas may be the initial presenting sign of tuberous sclerosis.

When symptoms are present, they are usually the result of tumor protruding into the cardiac lumen, resulting in outflow obstruction and congestive failure. Echocardiography is usually sufficient to suggest the diagnosis; however CT scanning and cardiac MRI are superior at defining the extent and attachments of these cardiac tumors and may be indicated for surgical planning. Cardiac fibromas and myxomas are much less common. Indeed it is more common to see secondary extension into the heart by other primary pediatric neoplasms such as neuroblastoma and Wilms tumor, both of which have a propensity to extend into the heart via the inferior vena cava (IVC); hepatoblastoma, which may show direct intracardiac extension (Fig. 66-41); and mediastinal lymphoma, which may result in chest wall/pericardial involvement. Contrast-enhanced CT scanning usually allows an accurate delineation of sites of local extension in the thorax. Either abdominal ultrasound, multiphase contrast-enhanced CT, or MRI can be used to demonstrate intravascular/intracardiac extension from primary abdominal malignancies.

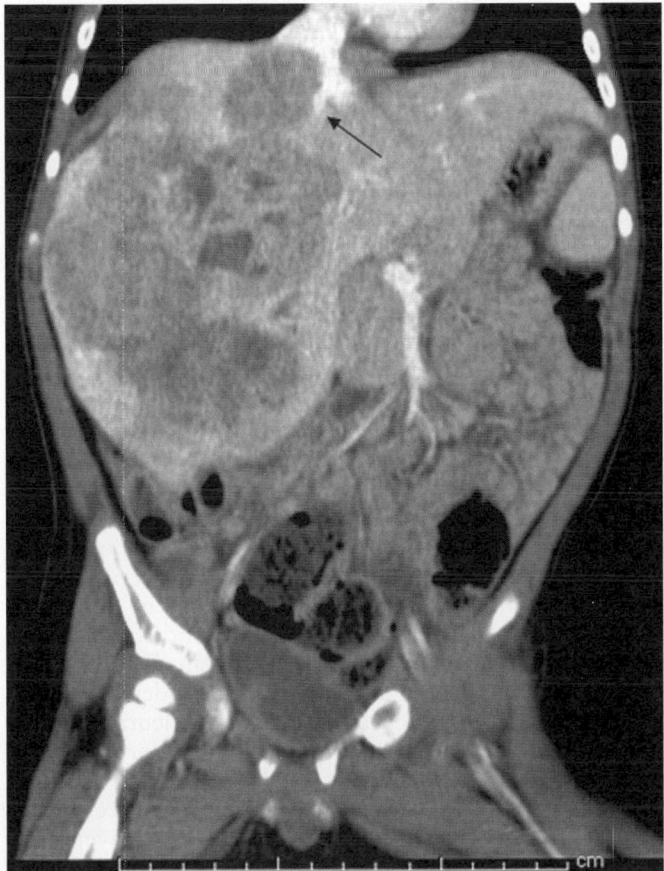

Figure 66-41 Coronal contrast-enhanced CT showing direct extension into the IVC in a 15-month-old patient with hepatoblastoma.

Posterior Mediastinal Masses

The posterior mediastinum is defined dorsally by the chest wall/vertebral column, ventrally by the pericardium and posterior wall of the great vessels, superiorly by the thoracic inlet, and inferiorly by the diaphragm. The primary components of the posterior mediastinum are the paravertebral sympathetic ganglia, azygos and hemiazygos veins, descending thoracic aorta, esophagus, and lymph nodes. The majority of the posterior mediastinal masses in children are neurogenic in origin[125,163] and include ganglion-cell tumors, nerve-sheath tumors, and other nervous-tissue neoplasms such as paragangliomas. Ganglion-cell tumors arise from sympathetic chain ganglia and range from well-differentiated and benign ganglioneuromas to malignant neuroblastomas. Ganglioneuroblastomas contain elements of both benign and malignant tissue types. The distinction between these different histologic subtypes cannot be made reliably based on imaging features, although age at presentation is important in narrowing the differential diagnosis. Neuroblastoma, the most common non-CNS solid tumor in children, typically occurs in young children with a median age at presentation of younger than 2 years and more than 95% of cases occurring by the age of 10 years. In contrast, the median age at presentation of ganglioneuroblastoma is approximately 5.5 years, whereas mature ganglioneuromas occur in later childhood/early adolescence, typically after the age of 10.[164] Whereas the majority of neuroblastomas occur in or around the adrenal gland, approximately 15% arise in the posterior mediastinum.[165]

It is important to emphasize that these lesions may be present in a child who is otherwise asymptomatic, and a thorough inspection of the chest radiograph using multiple windows and levels is necessary to identify small foci of disease. This is of particular importance, as shown in Figure 66-42, because a localized low-stage favorable histology neuroblastoma identified in a child under the age of 1 year may make the difference between being treated on low-risk protocols with higher likelihood of overall and disease-free survival versus more advanced stages of disease, when the patient's risk of relapse and treatment failure increases.[166] Primary intraabdominal neurogenic tumors may also have a significant posterior mediastinal extent and often have an associated posterior mediastinal/paravertebral component near the thoracic inlet (Virchow node). For this reason, it may be prudent to include imaging of the chest, in addition to the abdomen and pelvis, in the staging evaluation of patients with suspected neuroblastoma.

Radiographically, ganglion-cell tumors appear as paraspinal soft-tissue masses. Calcifications may be present. The presence of chest-wall invasion or destructive bony changes are more commonly seen with neuroblastoma, although benign ganglioneuromas can produce a considerable neural foraminal widening. As with primary adrenal neuroblastomas, staging should include ^{123}I-MIBG scintigraphy to assess for other sites of disease, including marrow involvement. ^{99m}Tc-MDP bone scintigraphy is also commonly performed to identify sites of

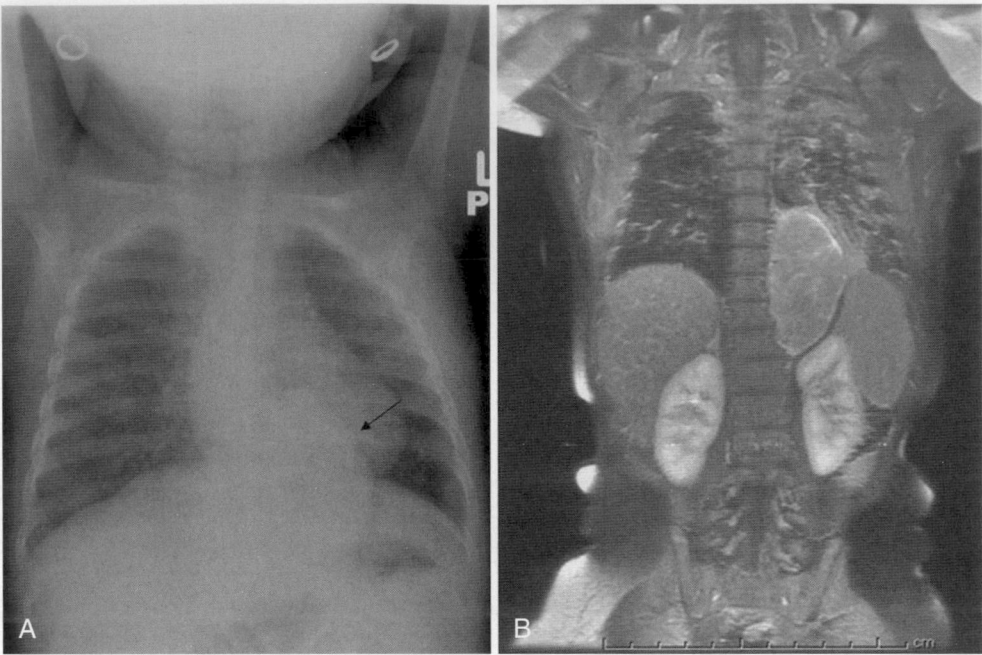

Figure 66-42 Posterior mediastinal neuroblastoma in a 5-month-old infant who showed symptoms of an upper respiratory infection. A posterior mediastinal mass was identified by chest x-ray (**A**) and MRI (**B**). Surgery revealed neuroblastoma. Subsequent staging confirmed low-stage disease.

cortical bone involvement,[91] although recent data suggests that bone scintigraphy rarely affects that clinical stage of the patient. The presence of a paraspinal mass can usually be adequately assessed by CT scanning, particularly with sagittal and coronal reconstructions. However, the extent of intraspinal extension is better depicted by MRI (Fig. 66-43).[125] MRI also provides a more accurate assessment of chest-wall involvement, nerve-root compression, and impingement upon the spinal cord. MRI of ganglion-cell tumors typically reveals a low signal-intensity lesion on T1-weighted images and intermediate to high signal intensity on T2-weighted and fast spin echo inversion recovery (FSEIR) images, with variable patterns of enhancement. Bone-marrow metastases are well demonstrated by MRI, with replacement of normal bone-marrow signal by areas of low signal intensity on T1-weighted images and high signal intensity on T2-weighted images. Indeed, several studies have suggested that MRI may be sufficient to identify sites of bone-marrow involvement in neuroblastoma, although is has not yet become common in clinical practice to rely on the MRI findings of bone-marrow involvement for staging of the patient.[167,168] The use of FDG-PET in neuroblastoma has received attention as an alternative to conventional imaging techniques.[91] However, a number of studies have shown variable patterns of FDG avidity in neuroblastoma, and FDG-PET has not yet been shown to offer a clear advantage over MIBG scintigraphy in either the staging or response assessment of patients with thoracic neuroblastoma.[169-171]

Nerve-sheath tumors, including schwannomas and neurofibromas may be similar in appearance to mature ganglion cell tumors, presenting as relatively sharply margined, lobulated paraspinal masses. The presence of rib erosions and neural foraminal widening is commonly seen with nerve-sheath tumors, although intraspinal extension is less common. Paraspinal paragangliomas are catecholamine-secreting tumors arising from extra-adrenal chromaffin cells present in sympathetic chain ganglia and occur much less often than either primary ganglion-cell or nerve-sheath neoplasms. Distinguishing between these tissue types is difficult on the basis of imaging, and surgical resection is the mainstay of therapy. Local recurrence can occur, however, and close imaging follow-up is necessary in these patients.

Chest-Wall/Pleural-Based Neoplasms

Most of these tumors are of mesenchymal origin and are primary neoplasms arising from the chest wall. They are relatively rare in infants and children, with a reported incidence of approximately 2% of all pediatric tumors.[172] The most common chest-wall neoplasms are the Ewing sarcoma family of tumors and primitive neuroectodermal tumors (PNETs), collectively known as Askin tumors. These tumors have a peak incidence between 10 and 15 years of age and are more common in males. Because of their origin within the chest wall and propensity to invade the adjacent bone, symptoms are commonly of a palpable mass or pain secondary to local extension. Chest radiography should be the first imaging study in the evaluation of these patients and is usually accurate at depicting sites of bone destruction, pleural effusion, and pleural thickening. CT and/or MRI are almost always performed to better delineate the extent of local disease. CT scanning of the chest is essential to assess for the presence of pulmonary metastatic disease (Fig. 66-44). For paravertebral and intercostal masses, MRI may also be necessary to identify and accurately delineate the extent of intraspinal involvement. FDG uptake is usually seen with these

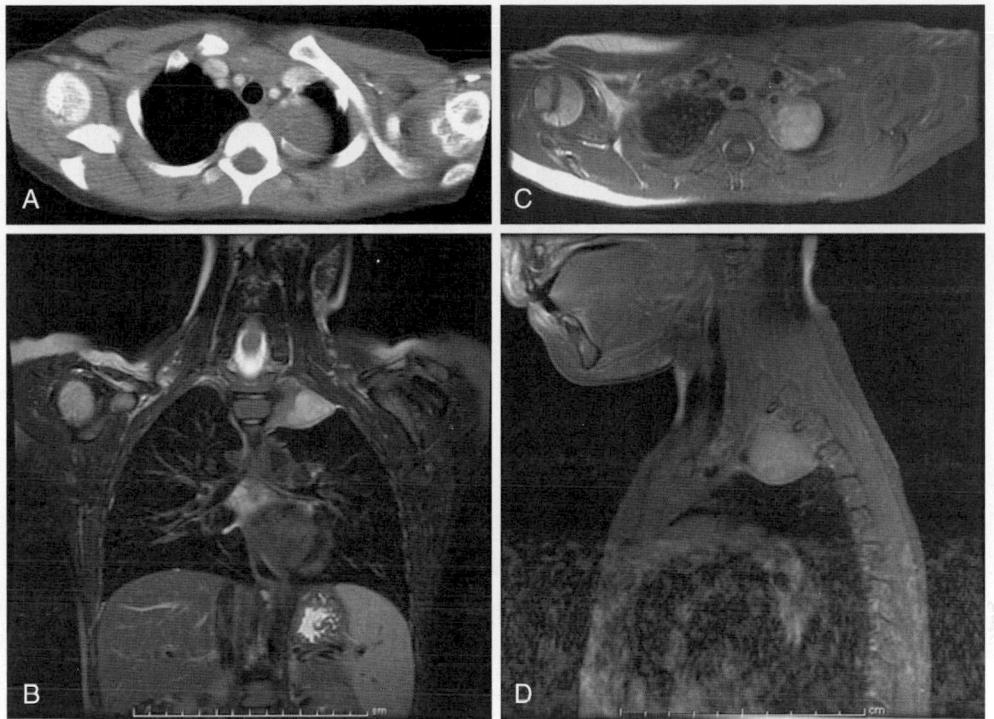

Figure 66-43 A 7-year-old child with a cough. Chest x-ray showed left upper lobe opacity. **A,** CT shows paraspinal mass. **B-D,** MRI shows the mass to much better advantage. Cor FSEIR and post–Gd-enhanced images (**C** and **D**) show the mass abutting the neural foramina and left subclavian vessels. MIBG scanning showed barely detectable uptake in the mature ganglioneuroma *(not shown).*

tumors,[173] and as with Ewing sarcomas of the appendicular skeleton, FDG-PET imaging should be considered both for identifying sites of occult disease that would otherwise go undetected and for monitoring responses to therapy when complete surgical resection cannot be achieved.[174-176]

Wide excision of the primary tumor is critical for local disease control, with variable response to radiation therapy and chemotherapy.[177,178] These chest-wall neoplasms are extremely malignant and can be quite destruc-tive, demonstrating extensive invasion into the airways, local vascular structures, and the lung parenchyma. There is a high rate of both metastatic spread and of local recurrence, and cure requires intensive therapy to control both distant and local disease. The presence of disseminated disease invariably results in a poor long-term outcome in patients with these aggressive poorly responsive tumors.[178]

Rhabdomyosarcoma is the most common soft-tissue sarcoma of childhood and is the second most common

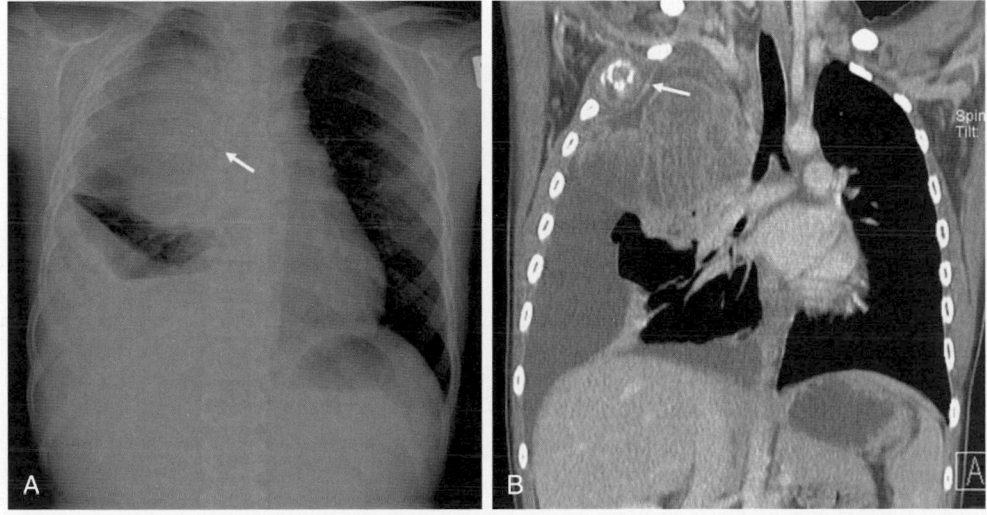

Figure 66-44 Ewing sarcoma of the chest wall in a 6-year-old patient with fever and a chest-wall mass detected by chest x-ray. **A,** Chest x-ray shows pleural effusion, central chest-wall mass *(arrow),* and partial lung collapse. **B,** Contrast enhanced CT shows a large, locally invasive chest wall mass with pleural involvement and rib destruction *(arrow).*

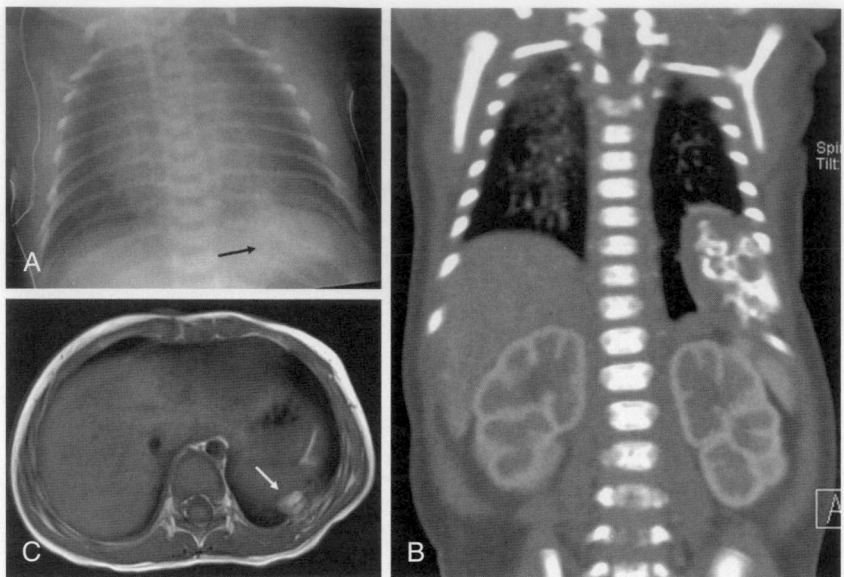

Figure 66-45 A 20-day-old infant with a prenatally diagnosed, calcified, left lower lung mass. Chest x-ray shows calcified mass (**A**, *arrow*) which on CT is seen to arise from posterolateral left ribs (**B**). T1-weighted MRI (**C**) shows presence of high signal intensity fat *(arrow)*, all consistent with the diagnosis of mesenchymal hamartoma.

malignancy of the chest wall in children.[177] Occurring in a younger population of children than thoracic Ewing sarcomas/PNETs, approximately 7% of pediatric rhabdomyosarcomas involve the chest wall and should be included in the differential diagnosis for a chest-wall mass occurring in children younger than the age of 10 years. Biopsy is necessary to make the diagnosis, and the imaging features are nonspecific, with considerable overlap between chest-wall Ewing sarcoma and rhabdomyosarcoma. Chest radiographs reveal a large unilateral chest mass, often with accompanying pleural thickening or effusion. As with Ewing sarcoma, there may be associated destructive rib changes. Cross-sectional imaging by either CT or MRI better delineates the extent of local disease spread. These tumors are heterogeneous in density on CT with variably increased signal on both T1- and T2-weighted MRI images. Contrast enhancement is heterogeneous, and these features likely reflect varying degrees of tumor necrosis. Tumor size, nodal status, and gross total tumor resection (upfront or delayed) have been shown to be significant predictors of event-free and overall survival. Tumors 5 cm or smaller were shown to be amenable to upfront surgical resection. Tumor size and the ability to achieve gross total resection were the strongest predictors of overall survival, with local recurrence after resection resulting in poor overall outcome.[179,180] As with other malignant sarcomas, FDG-PET has been used effectively in staging and response assessment in patients with rhabdomyosarcoma[181-184] and should be considered as an essential component of the imaging evaluation for these patients.

Mesenchymal Hamartomas

Mesenchymal hamartomas of the chest wall are rare, benign neoplasms occurring during infancy. The presence of a large chest-wall mass, often containing calcifications with associated rib destruction and chest-wall deformity should prompt this diagnosis. Because these lesions may contain a significant necrotic/cystic component, the distinction between Langerhans cell histiocytosis, lymphoma, and metastatic neuroblastoma may be difficult to make. These masses often become quite large, and the radiographic finding may be sufficient to suggest the diagnosis, showing a large calcified extrapleural mass with expansion/destruction of multiple ribs. CT or MRI allows more accurate measure of size, characterization of the soft-tissue component of the lesion, and mass effect on the lung and adjacent structures (Fig. 66-45).[185] In particular, the presence of hemorrhagic cystic components has been described as characteristic of these benign neoplasms.[185] There is some data to suggest that spontaneous resolution of these masses may also occur, although the extent of local invasion and tissue destruction may prompt surgical resection, which if complete, is usually curative. The importance of the imaging evaluation is to suggest this diagnosis in order to guide appropriate management of these benign lesions.

Pulmonary Metastases

Metastatic disease to the lung represents the most common pulmonary neoplasm encountered in childhood. The lung is a common site for metastatic disease spread but is an uncommon site in childhood for primary malignancy.

Extrathoracic pediatric tumors that are commonly associated with pulmonary metastases include Wilms tumor, rhabdomyosarcoma, hepatoblastoma, Ewing sarcoma, and osteosarcoma. Neuroblastoma does not typically result in hematogenously spread pulmonary metastases, although in its disseminated form, pulmonary metastases may be seen.

The imaging evaluation in a patient with a known primary malignancy with a propensity to metastasize to

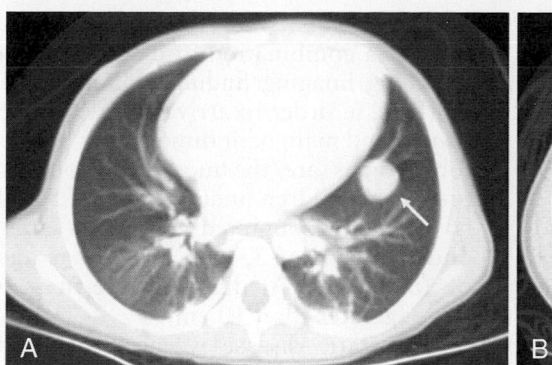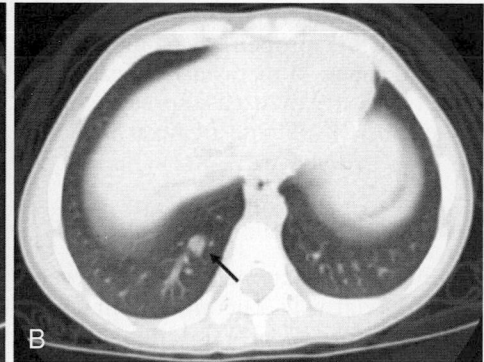

Figure 66-46 A 2½-year-old child with metastatic Wilms tumor. **A**, The nodule at the left lung base *(arrow)* was resected at diagnosis and found to be metastatic disease. **B**, The nodule at the right lung base discovered 1 year later was resected, and found to be a pulmonary hamartoma.

the lung should include chest CT. CT is more sensitive than conventional radiographs in detecting pulmonary metastatic disease, although the increased sensitivity of nodule detection has led to difficulty in distinguishing benign lesions from malignant pulmonary nodules (Fig. 66-46).[22,186] Once the staging evaluation has been completed and the absence of pulmonary metastatic disease and other sites of metastatic disease have been established, it may be reasonable to proceed with routine chest radiographs for subsequent follow-up care, reserving CT for patients with suspected relapse or at high risk for relapse. In particular, in osteosarcoma, which has a high frequency of developing pulmonary metastases and for whom resection of these metastases may be curative, routine follow up chest CT scanning is justifiable.

It is often difficult, particularly with small pulmonary nodules, to distinguish benign causes from malignancy.[22] Calcification within a pulmonary nodule is usually associated with benign causes (except in the case of osteosarcoma); however, there are no specific imaging findings that can be used to reliably make this distinction. Benign pulmonary nodules may result from postinflammatory change or represent small benign intrapulmonary lymph nodes. Short interval follow-up care and documentation of stability in areas of low suspicion is usually adequate to confirm the benign nature of these findings. For more suspicious or enlarging lesions, biopsy or surgical resection is necessary to arrive at a definitive diagnosis. The use of FDG-PET scanning has been advocated in an attempt to distinguish benign from malignant causes of pulmonary metastatic disease.[187] However, while CT can accurately identify lesions of only 1 to 2 mm in size, even the newest generation PET scanners have inherently lower limits of resolution, on the order of 5 mm, because of both the intrinsic spatial resolution of PET detectors and the distance traveled by positrons in the tissue before undergoing annihilation and emission of 511 keV coincident photons.

Controversy still exists as to the significance of pulmonary nodules detected by chest CT in patients with Wilms tumor.[188-190] There are conflicting data as to the importance of pulmonary nodules not visualized by chest radiography but detectable by chest CT in predicting relapse-free and overall survival in patients with Wilms

tumor, with the most recent data from the National Wilms Tumor Study Group (NWTSG) 4 and 5 showing that patients with lung lesions visible only on CT have improved event-free, but not overall, survival and do not appear to benefit from pulmonary radiation.[191] Nonetheless it has been shown that the sensitivity of malignant nodule detection is enhanced by CT,[188,189] and current treatment protocols routinely advocate the use of chest CT in staging these patients. In an effort to develop a better understanding of CT features that might distinguish benign from malignant pulmonary nodules,[188] current Children's Oncology Group (COG) Wilms tumor protocols call for surgical resection or biopsy of persistent, suspicious lung nodules detected by CT in patients with intermediate and high-risk disease.

CT scanning of the chest for the purposes of identifying pulmonary metastatic disease need not include intravenous contrast, and the presence of hyperdense contrast material in small pulmonary vessels may confound the interpretation of a subtle parenchymal nodules. In addition, multidetector-row CT scanners allow the acquisition imaging data to be reviewed in 1-mm thick increments or less, as well as in sagittal and coronal planes. This allows the radiologist to make an accurate judgment as to the presence or absence of a suspicious pulmonary nodule and distinguish it from branching vessels. There is no data to suggest that additional high-resolution CT (HRCT) imaging, which is performed using a different image acquisition technique, provides any additional benefit or higher resolution over the 1-mm thick slices obtained during the multidetector helical acquisition.[192] MRI for the detection of pulmonary nodules has been shown to be feasible,[193-195] but there are no studies showing that MRI can replace CT for the routine identification of pulmonary metastatic disease.[196] Similarly low-dose attenuation-correction CT images of the lungs obtained as part of combined PET/CT examinations are not sufficient to exclude small pulmonary nodules, and a diagnostic chest CT obtained during suspended inspiration is still recommended for evaluation of patients at risk and in whom pulmonary metastases will impact clinical management.[197,198]

Although the imaging features of small pulmonary nodules may be nonspecific and the difficulty in distinguishing benign from nonneoplastic etiologies is challenging, the presence and persistence of lung nodules in a child with a solid tumor that has a propensity to metastasize to the lung is usually indicative of metastatic disease. The use of CT in detecting these sites of disease spread remains an essential component of the staging of most pediatric solid tumors.

GASTROINTESTINAL TUMORS

Tumors of the gastrointestinal tract, including the visceral abdominal organs, are relatively uncommon in childhood. In neonates, the majority of intraabdominal masses are not malignant. Children commonly have nonspecific complaints such as abdominal pain, weight loss, or failure to thrive. The imaging evaluation should begin with abdominal radiographs. These often provide valuable initial information, such as the presence of calcifications, mass effect on adjacent visceral organs, and the presence of bowel obstruction or perforation. Abdominal ultrasound is often used to gain further information about a suspicious mass. Doppler assessment may help distinguish cystic from solid masses and delineate patterns of blood flow in and around a tumor. These initial imaging studies are usually sufficient to narrow the initial differential diagnosis and to guide the subsequent imaging evaluation by CT, MRI, and/or PET.

Liver

Although rare in infants and young children, tumors of the hepatobiliary tract are the most common of the gastrointestinal tract tumors seen in childhood.[199-201] Usually a combination of diagnostic studies is obtained, including imaging findings, clinical findings, and serum markers, in order to arrive at a definitive diagnosis. Both benign and malignant tumors may be encountered. Hepatoblastomas are the most common primary malignant tumors in children under the age of 5.[201] Hepatoblastoma is usually encountered in infants and young children under the age of 3, with an average age at presentation of 16 months. At diagnosis the mass is typically quite large (greater than 10 cm).

Metastatic disease is encountered in approximately 20% of the patients, with pulmonary metastases most common. The imaging evaluation should be directed at determining surgical resectability, establishing sites of metastatic disease, and monitoring response to chemotherapy. More than 90% of the children have elevated α-fetoprotein (AFP) levels at diagnosis; the presence of metastatic disease, high AFP levels, and a high PRETEXT stage of liver involvement by tumor are all associated with poor outcome.[202-204] Surgical resection alone is insufficient to achieve cure in most cases, and the combination of surgery and chemotherapy has resulted in 5-year overall survival rates of over 70%.[204]

Abdominal radiographs typically show an abdominal mass. Calcifications may be present, and pulmonary masses may be visible at the time of diagnosis at the lung bases (Fig. 66-47). Ultrasound should be the initial imaging test in a child with an abdominal mass and in hepatoblastoma reveals a large echogenic, intrahepatic

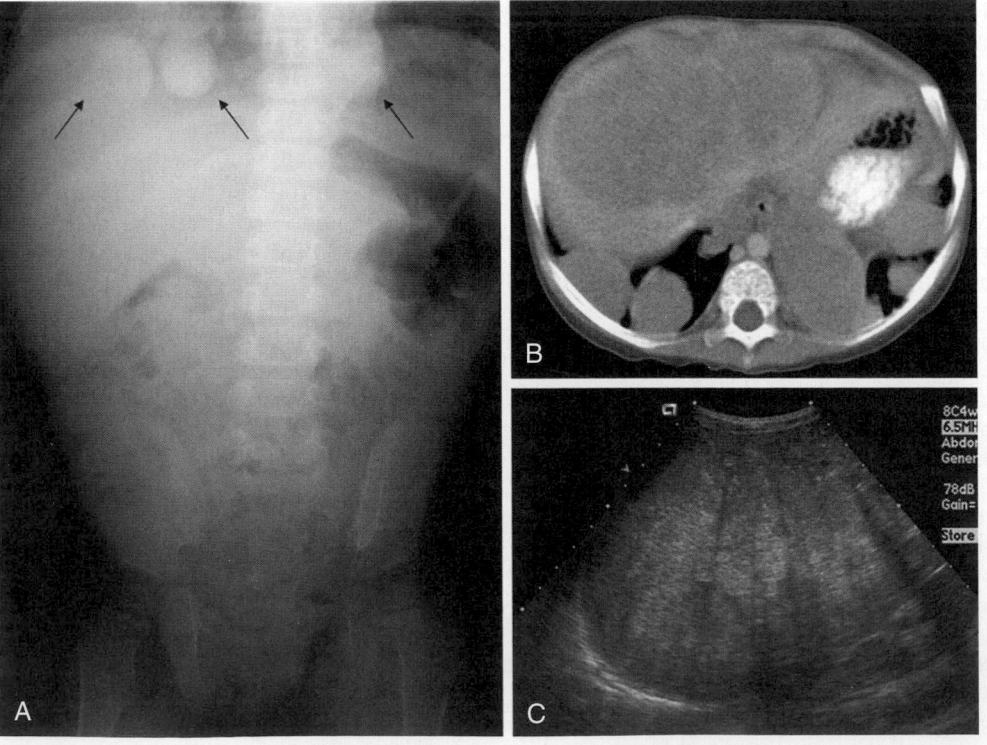

Figure 66-47 Hepatoblastoma. A 15-month-old patient with an abdominal mass found during the physical examination. **A,** Note lung metastases on the abdominal radiograph *(arrows);* **B,** extensive disease depicted on CT; and **C,** the difficulty discriminating the large echogenic mass from normal liver on ultrasound.

mass. It may be difficult with very large masses to define a margin between the hepatoblastoma and normal hepatic parenchyma (see Fig. 66-35). Hypoechoic areas may relate to necrosis or hemorrhage. Color Doppler imaging and pulsed-wave Doppler should be used routinely to assess for intravascular extension of tumor,[201,203] IVC invasion, and portal vein thrombosis, both of which may affect eligibility for liver transplantation.[205]

CT and or MRI are important to better define the relationship of the intra-hepatic mass to adjacent vascular structures, adjacent organs, and to determine the extent of hepatic involvement and surgical respectability.[203] This is best accomplished with biphasic CT or MR angiographic techniques and imaging should include scanning after early arterial and portal venous phases of contrast opacification, since small satellite lesions may only be visible on the early arterial phase imaging (see Fig. 66-2).[206] Typically, hepatoblastomas show a heterogeneous pattern of enhancement. Multiplanar reconstructions are also crucial, both in aiding surgical planning and in better delineating invasion into adjacent vascular structures (i.e., IVC invasion; portal venous thrombosis). MRI imaging typically shows heterogeneously T2-hyperintense lesions with variable patterns of enhancement after gadolinium contrast administration (Fig. 66-48). MRI may be of particular value in delineating subtle lesions that are inconspicuous on contrast enhanced CT scanning. The use of hepatobiliary contrast agents, which are taken up by normal functioning liver tissue but not by malignant liver lesions, as well as diffusion-weighted imaging, can further enhance lesion detection and characterization.[207] As shown in Fig. 66-49, the hepatobiliary agent gadoxetate (Eovist) identifies a poorly enhancing lesion on a background of normally enhancing hepatic parenchyma in a patent with unresectable hepatoblastoma.

The PRETEXT staging system was developed by the International Childhood Liver Tumors Strategy Group (SIOPEL) in an effort to develop a pretreatment imaging-based measurement of disease burden and surgical resectability as a basis for staging and risk stratification of children with hepatoblastoma.[203] In the PRETEXT system of staging the liver is divided into sections, based in part on Couinaud's system of segmental anatomy. PRETEXT staging is based on the number of adjacent liver sections involved with tumor (Table 66-1) and has been shown to be effective in predicting resectability and overall survival in patients who complete neoadjuvant chemotherapy.[208] Because the PRETEXT staging system relies almost entirely on the pretreatment imaging assessment, it is essential that MRI and/or CT scanning be performed using optimal scanning parameters (i.e., multiphasic technique, properly timed contrast bolus, sedation to minimize motion artifact) in order to provide and accurate assessment of the extent of liver involvement. The COG staging system, used widely throughout North America, historically had relied on intraoperative and postoperative assessment, with less dependence on preoperative imaging.[203] However, current protocols have adopted the SIOPEL recommendations for PRETEXT characterization to monitor response to neoadjuvant chemotherapy and determine surgical resectability.[209,210]

The presence of a rising AFP level in a patient previously free of detectable disease should prompt a thorough investigation to identify sites of recurrent disease. The detection of recurrent hepatoblastoma after chemotherapy and surgical resection may be challenging with conventional cross-sectional imaging techniques. Although there has been relatively little published experience using FDG-PET scanning to monitor early sites of disease recurrence, there are reports suggesting FDG-PET and/or CT can improve both the sensitivity and specificity of identifying early foci of disease recurrence.[72,211,212] Characterization by FDG-PET of unusual sites of disease relapse or equivocal abnormalities on CT and/or MRI

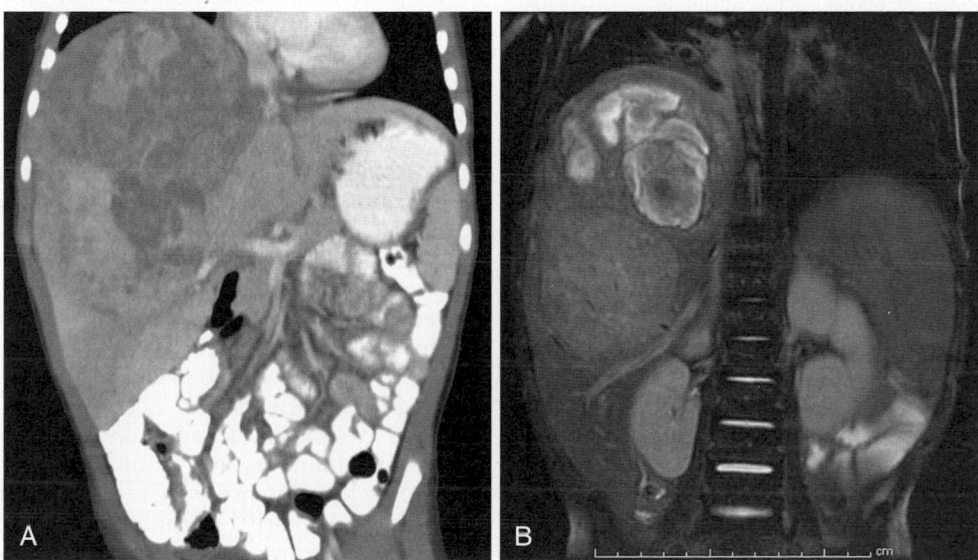

Figure 66-48 A 3-year-old patient with hepatoblastoma, showing superiority of MRI (**B**) in detecting the extent of liver involvement and the relationship to adjacent structures, as compared with CT (**A**).

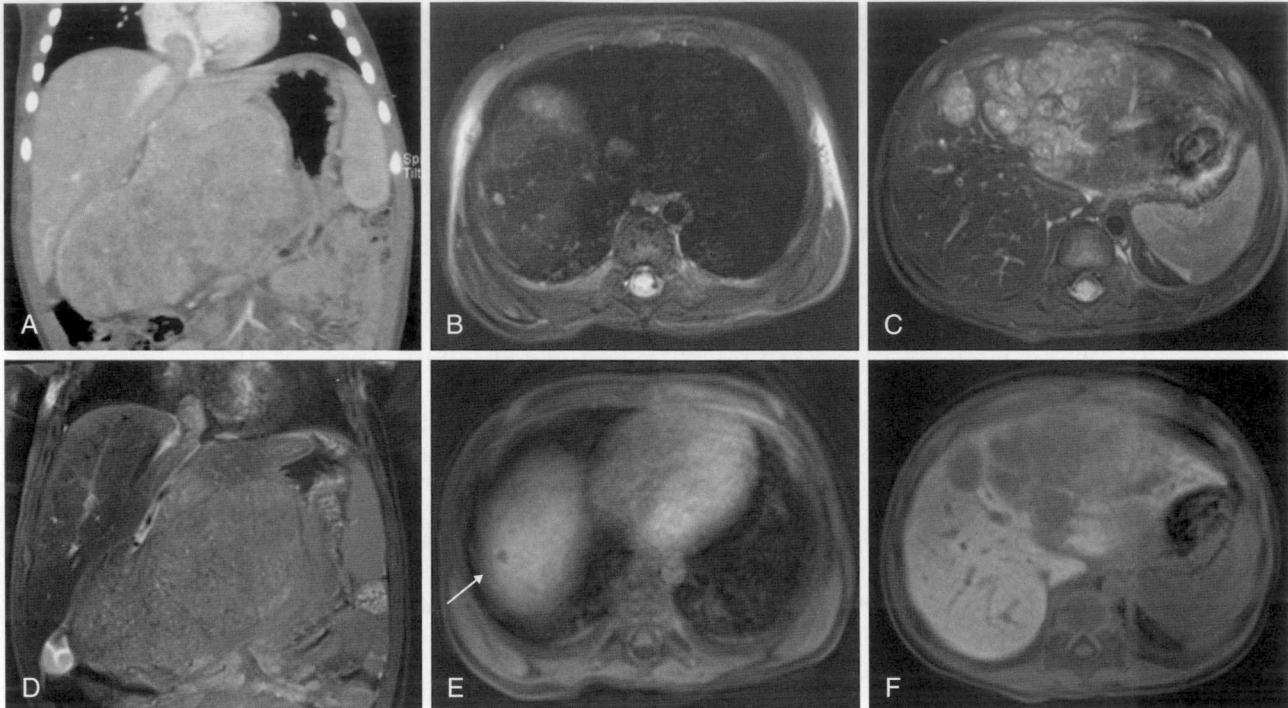

Figure 66-49 A 17-month-old infant with hepatoblastoma. CT angiogram (**A**), fat-suppressed T2-weighted (**B** and **C**) and contrast enhanced MRI (**D-F**) show a large exophytic liver mass with extension into the right atrium. Delayed postcontrast images after administration of the hepatocyte selective contrast agent gadoxetate (Eovist) identifies an additional tiny satellite lesion near the liver dome (**E,** *arrow*).

TABLE 66-1   Childhood Liver Cancer (Hepatoblastoma): PRETEXT Staging System[208]

Tumor Stage	Description
1	Tumor involves only one quadrant. Three adjoining liver quadrants are free of tumor.
2	Tumor involves two adjoining quadrants. Two adjoining quadrants are free of tumor.
3	Tumor involves three adjoining quadrants or two nonadjoining quadrants. One quadrant or two nonadjoining quadrants are free of tumor.
4	Tumor involves all four quadrants. There is no quadrant free of tumor.
Extrahepatic Considerations	
	V+: Involvement of the inferior vena cava and/or all three hepatic veins
	P+: Involvement of the main portal vein and/or both left and right branches
	E+: Extrahepatic disease in the abdomen
	M+: Distant metastases

PRETEXT, Pretreatment Extent of Disease.

may confirm the presence of metabolically active disease and guide subsequent treatment decisions (Fig. 66-50).

Hepatocellular Carcinomas

Hepatocellular carcinoma, although rare in childhood, is the second most common primary hepatic malignancy. It typically occurs in older children, with a mean age at diagnosis of approximately 12 years.[202] There is a slight male predominance and an association between development of hepatocellular carcinoma and preexisting liver disease, such as hepatitis B, biliary atresia, and Fanconi syndrome, as well as certain metabolic diseases such as hereditary tyrosinemia and glycogen storage disease.[202] The imaging features of hepatocellular carcinoma are not unique, and as for hepatoblastoma, ultrasound examination is often the first imaging study performed. Multiphase CT scanning with multiplanar reconstruction affords the greatest likelihood of detecting subtle lesions and in assessing relationships to adjacent structures and the vasculature,[200,206] although the use of diffusion-weighted MR imaging and hepatobiliary MR contrast agents has added to the appeal of MRI for evaluating these patients.[44,213] The CT appearance of hepatocellular carcinoma depends on tumor size and phase of contrast administration. Lesions are typically isointense or mildly hypointense relative to liver and show hyperattenuation on early arterial phase scanning, becoming isointense during later venous phases of imaging (Fig. 66-51). Early arterial phase, portal venous phase, and

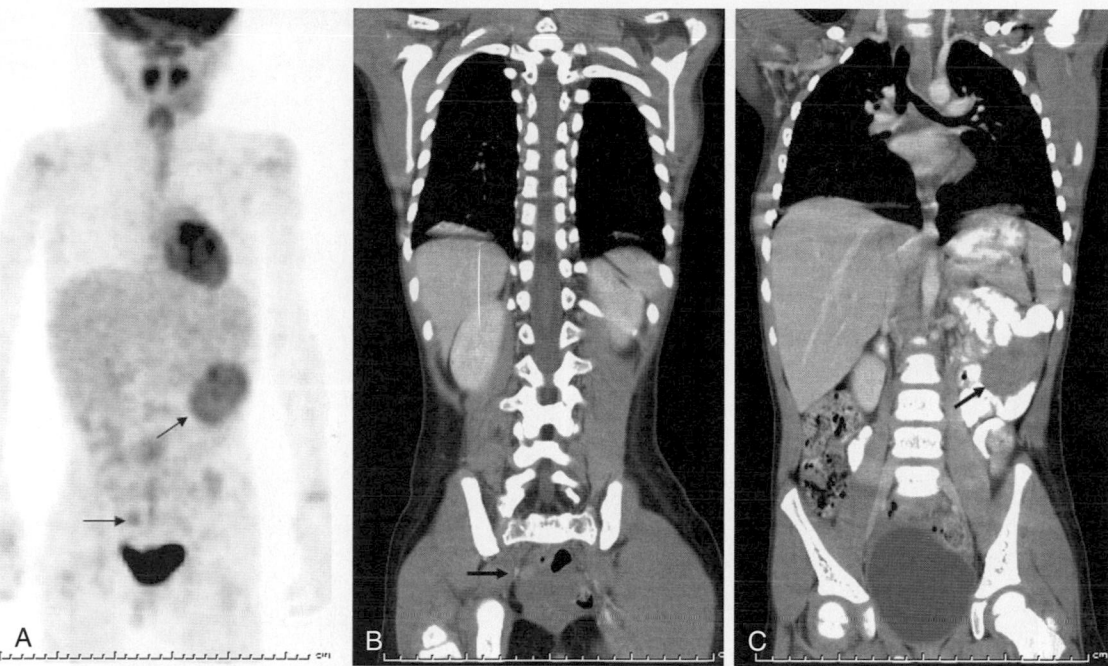

Figure 66-50 A 5-year-old girl with metastatic hepatoblastoma who had undergone resection of the primary mass. The patient was in remission with new rising AFP levels. FDG-PET (**A**) shows two foci of uptake *(arrows)*, corresponding to soft-tissue masses on CT in the mesentery (**B**) and deep pelvis (**C**, *arrows*). Surgery confirmed metastatic disease.

delayed equilibration venous phase images have all been shown to contribute to enhancing lesion conspicuity, providing the greatest sensitivity and specificity in lesion detection.[214] MR imaging, with opposed-phase imaging to detect microscopic fat and hepatobiliary agents to identify lesions with hepatocyte function can help in distinguishing hepatocellular carcinoma from benign liver lesions such as hepatic adenoma and focal nodular hyperplasia (FNH)[201]; however, biopsy may still be necessary to confirm the diagnosis (Fig. 66-52). Gadolinium-enhanced MRI, like CT, shows hyperenhancing lesions during early arterial phase imaging, with larger tumors showing variable signal intensity and patterns of enhancement[215] and absent enhancement on delayed hepatocyte phase imaging when hepatobiliary agents are used.

Superparamagnetic iron-oxide particles, which are taken up by Kupffer cells present in normal liver and in FNH, have been used to help differentiate hepatocellular carcinoma, which contains few if any Kupffer cells, from benign liver masses and to enhance lesion conspicuity relative to the surrounding liver tissue.[215]

The fibrolamellar form of hepatocellular carcinoma occurs in adolescents and has imaging features that are distinctive, showing a central scar and often associated with calcification (Fig. 66-53). Fibrolamellar hepatocellular carcinoma is not associated with elevated AFP, and overall survival is higher than in other forms of hepatocellular carcinoma, in part because of its presentation as a solitary localized mass amenable to complete surgical resection.[216] Ultrasound reveals a hypoechoic mass, often

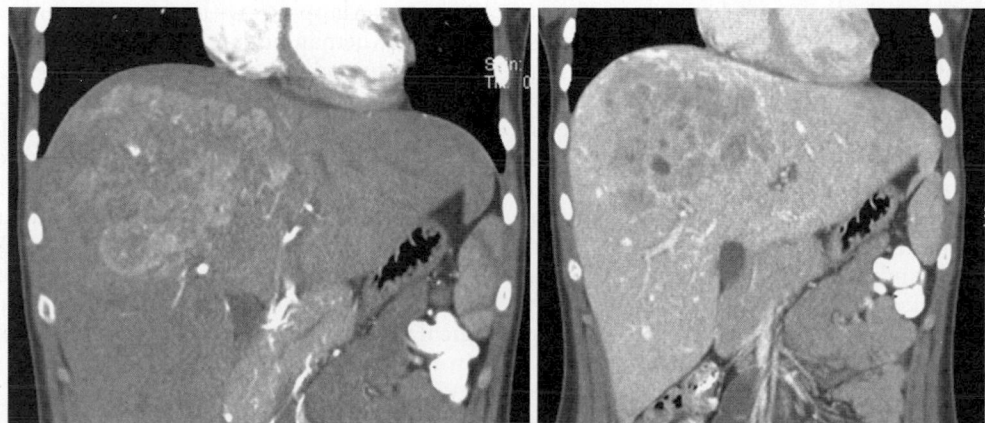

Figure 66-51 An 18-year-old female with fibrolamellar hepatocellular carcinoma. Biphasic contrast-enhanced CT demonstrates a large hyperenhancing lesion in the right lobe, which on delayed images becomes hypodense and less distinct from the background liver tissue.

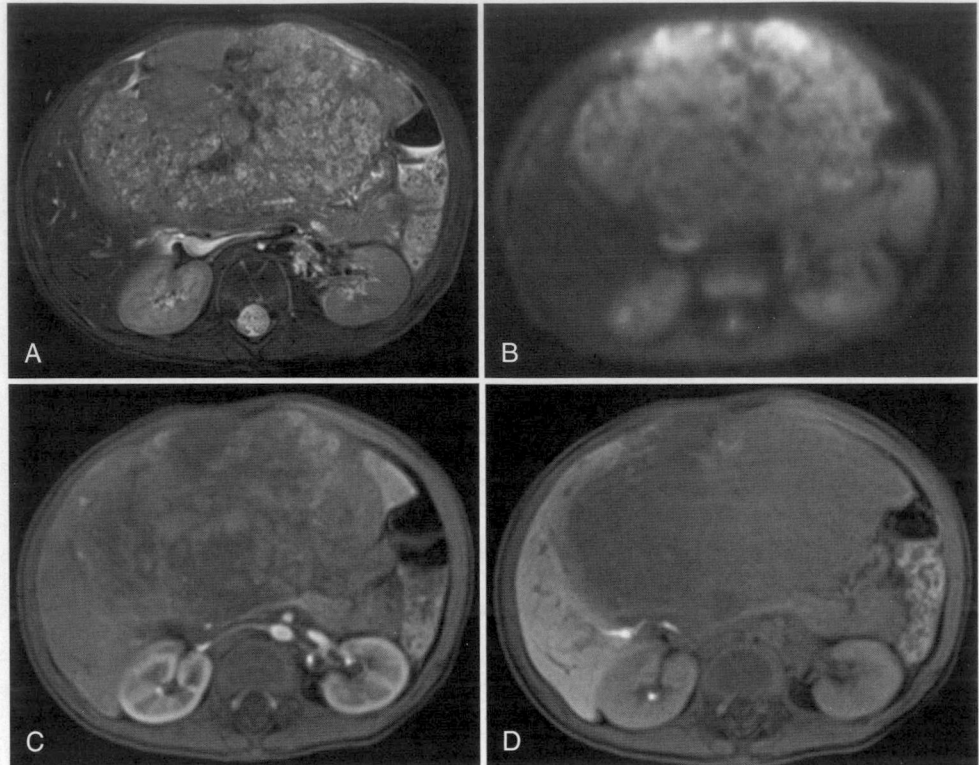

Figure 66-52 A 19-month-old child with hepatocellular carcinoma. T2-weighted (**A**) and DWI (**B**) images show a large heterogeneous mass in the left liver lobe with restricted diffusion. **C,** After Gd-contrast administration with gadoxetate (Eovist), early dynamic images shows heterogeneous enhancement. **D,** Delayed imaging shows absence of gadoxetate (Eovist) enhancement on the hepatocyte phase, in contrast to the enhancement of the adjacent normal liver.

with a focal central hyperechoic scar. After the initial characterization by ultrasound, CT or MRI is indicated for further staging. On CT, fibrolamellar hepatocellular carcinoma is usually relatively low attenuation, well-circumscribed mass with heterogeneous enhancement, initially becoming hyperintense relative to the surrounding liver parenchyma and ultimately becoming isointense to the liver during the equilibration phase of scanning. A nonenhancing central scar is seen in the majority of the cases (see Fig. 66-53).[217] On MRI, lesions are isointense to hypointense relative to the liver on T1-weighted images and isointense to hyperintense on T2-weighted sequences. The pattern on gadolinium enhancement is similar to that observed on CT, with lesions becoming hyperintense early after contrast infusion and ultimately isointense to liver on delayed scanning. The distinction between fibrolamellar hepatocellular carcinoma and FNH, both of which have similar imaging characteristics and patterns of early contrast enhancement, may be difficult to make (compare Figs. 66-53 and 66-54). However, as shown in Figure 66-54, the uptake and retention of a hepatobiliary contrast agent by the lesion on delayed hepatocyte phase imaging is nearly diagnostic of FNH.[213]

Embryonal Sarcomas (Hepatic Mesenchymomas)

Embryonal sarcomas of the liver are the fourth most common hepatic neoplasm in children after hepatoblastoma, hepatocellular carcinoma, and infantile hepatic

hemangioma. These tumors are highly malignant, usually present in later childhood (between the age of 6 and 10), and are typically accompanied by symptoms of abdominal pain and an abdominal mass. Embryonal sarcomas may be difficult to distinguish from mesenchymal hamartomas, although the latter tumors are more commonly diagnosed before the age of 2 years. At presentation embryonal sarcomas are often large and contain both cystic and solid areas with areas of necrosis. Ultrasound reveals a heterogeneous echogenic mass with many features overlapping with mesenchymal hamartoma and infantile hemangioma. Calcifications are rare. CT reveals a large hypodense mass, often with septations and areas of internal high attenuation; MRI shows a high signal-intensity lesion on T2-weighted images (Fig. 66-55), with predominantly low signal on T1-weighted images. After contrast enhancement, imaging by either CT or MRI demonstrates peripheral enhancement and central areas of heterogeneous signal intensity that likely reflect solid tumor elements, cystic spaces, necrosis, and foci of hemorrhage.[218] Despite being highly malignant, complete surgical resection and adjuvant chemotherapy can be curative in the majority of these patients.[202,219]

Mesenchymal Hamartomas

Mesenchymal hamartoma, in contrast to hepatoblastoma, is a predominantly cystic mass most often occurring in infants under the age of 2 years. It commonly

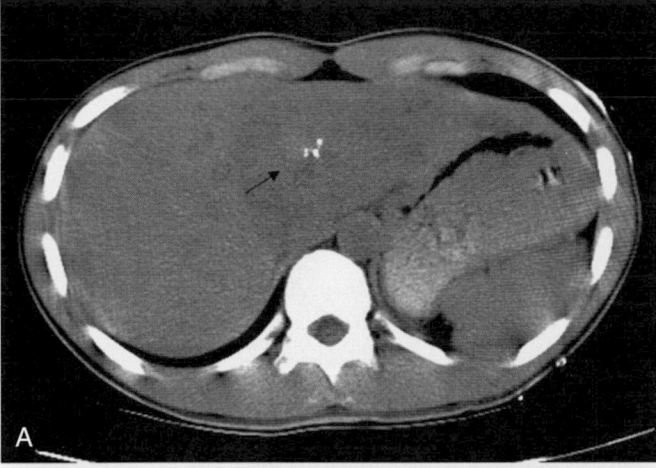

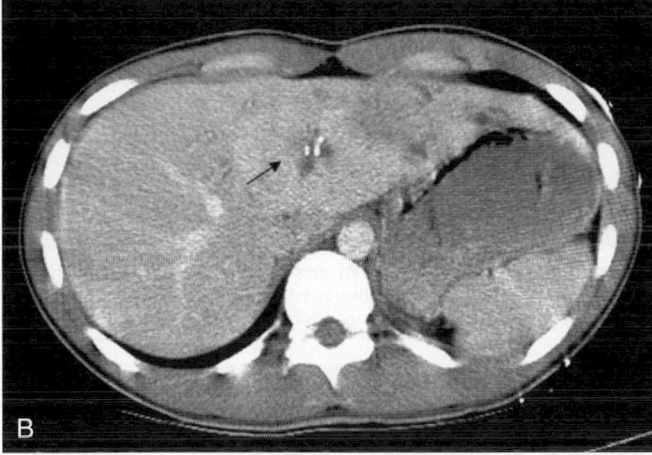

Figure 66-53 A 16-year-old patient with fibrolamellar hepatocellular carcinoma. Unenhanced (A) and contrast enhanced (B) CT show the calcifications and poorly enhancing central scar *(arrows)* typical of this form of hepatocellular carcinoma.

presents as a painless, palpable abdominal mass comprised of mesenchymal tissue, bile ducts, hepatocytes, and hematopoietic cells. In contrast to hepatoblastoma, which is the primary differential consideration in an infant, the AFP levels are normal. On imaging, radiographs reveal a large right upper quadrant mass. Calcifications, which are seen in hepatoblastoma, are unusual in mesenchymal hamartoma.[201] Ultrasound examination typically shows a complex, predominantly cystic mass. MRI and CT may be of value in further characterizing the lesion and typically show large multilocular cystic masses with septations. Only minimal enhancement is seen. Some of the masses may have a predominantly solid component yielding a so-called Swiss cheese appearance to the mass, and contributing to some difficulty in the differential diagnosis. MRI may also demonstrate the complex nature of the cystic fluid, with gelatinous, more complex fluids showing high signal on T1-weighted images instead of the more common T2 bright/ T1 dark serous fluid contained in the majority of the cysts (see Fig. 66-55). Treatment is surgical resection, and recurrence is uncommon.[202]

Infantile Hepatic Hemangiomas

Infantile hepatic hemangioma are proliferative endothelial cell neoplasms that may be solitary or may diffusely involve the liver. Infantile hepatic hemangiomas have characteristic phases of cellular proliferation followed by spontaneous involution. They are often referred to as *hepatic hemangioendothelioma*, creating some confusion in nomenclature and must be distinguished from epithelioid hemangioendothelioma.[220] The latter is a proliferative tumor with malignant potential that does not involute in contrast to the benign hepatic hemangioma. Infantile hepatic hemangiomas share the same growth characteristics as the more common cutaneous infantile hemangiomas. The majority present by 6 months of age, and about half are associated with cutaneous lesions. The majority of the infantile hepatic hemangiomas involute spontaneously, and adverse outcomes are only observed when there is massive hepatic involvement and arteriovenous (AV) shunting with accompanying high-output cardiac failure. The presence of extensive hepatic involvement and near complete replacement of the liver parenchyma occurs in the diffuse infantile hemangioma variant and is associated with profound hypothyroidism secondary to overproduction of type III iodothyronine deiodinase.[221]

Ultrasound is usually the first step in the evaluation and typically shows either focal or multiple hepatic masses with heterogeneous echotexture. It may be possible to identify a large draining varix or varices. Both arterial and venous waveforms are often detected, and calcifications may be present. More characteristic findings are seen on CT and MRI. MRI typically shows homogeneously hypointense lesions on T1-weighted imaging with heterogeneous hyperintense masses on T2-weighted images. After contrast enhancement, imaging by either CT or MRI reveals a typical pattern of peripheral contrast enhancement with gradual filling in centrally (centripetal enhancement) (Fig. 66-56, *A* and *B*).[222] Diffuse infantile hepatic hemangiomas may nearly completely occupy the entire liver parenchyma (see Fig. 66-56, *C* and *D*). The associated hypothyroidism is the result of the elaboration of deiodinase enzymes affecting thyroid hormone synthesis, which can in turn result in cardiac failure and neurologic impairment. These endocrinologic findings are important in securing the diagnosis, because the multiple hepatic masses may share overlapping imaging features with malignant hepatic lesions such as hepatoblastoma or metastatic neuroblastoma.

High-output cardiac failure associated with large varices and significant high-volume AV shunting can be effectively treated using interventional radiologic techniques, including coil and particle embolization. This may be essential in stabilizing the patient in order to initiate treatment to accelerate the involution of these benign proliferative lesions.[220]

Hepatic Adenoma

Other benign hepatic lesions include solitary hepatic adenomas. Hepatic adenomas are unusual in children in the absence of a predisposing condition, such as glycogen storage disease, galactosemia, or tyrosinemia. The

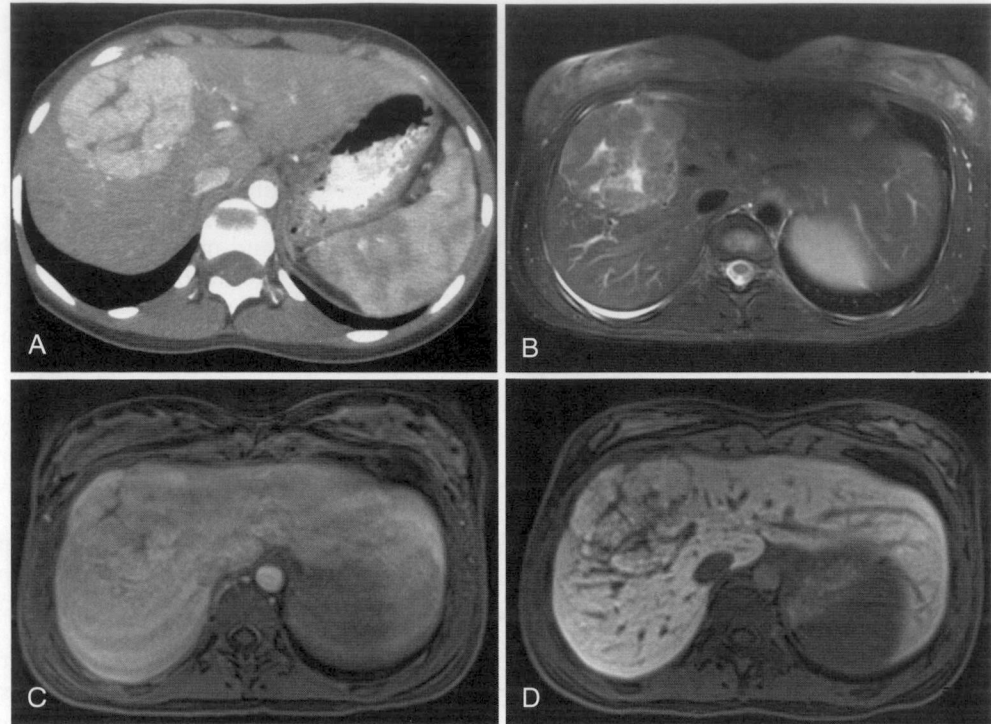

Figure 66-54 A 15-year-old patient with abdominal pain and a liver mass noted on outside CT (**A**). **B**, MRI performed with gadoxetate (Eovist) shows a mildly T2-hyperintense lesion that becomes isointense to liver shortly after contrast infusion (**C**), but that retains the contrast on delayed hepatocyte phase imaging (**D**). The features, together with the central nonenhancing scar, are characteristic of FNH.

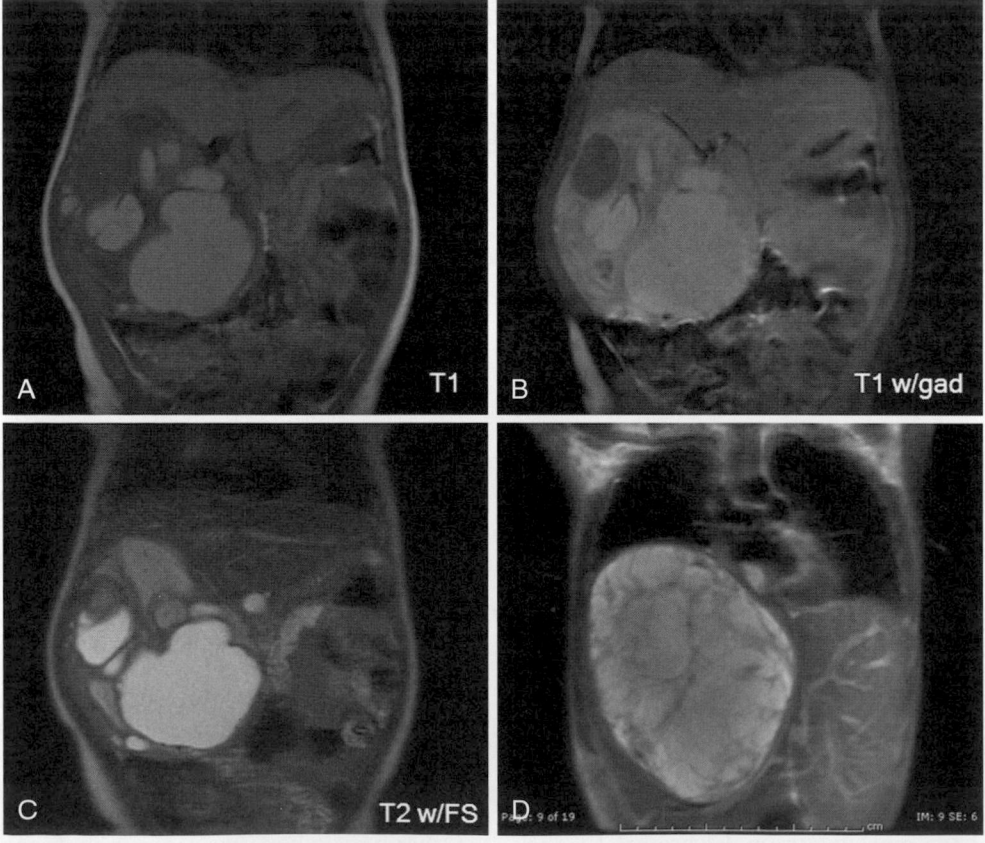

Figure 66-55 Mesenchymal hamartoma. MRI showing the complex nature of the multiple cysts in a 13-month-old infant with mesenchymal hamartoma. Note the importance of obtaining T1-weighted images before contrast administration (**A** and **B**), in addition to fluid-sensitive T2-weighted sequences (**C**), because areas of complex fluid may be T1 bright and should not be misinterpreted as enhancing solid components of the mass. Note the similarity to the large embryonal sarcoma shown in (**D**).

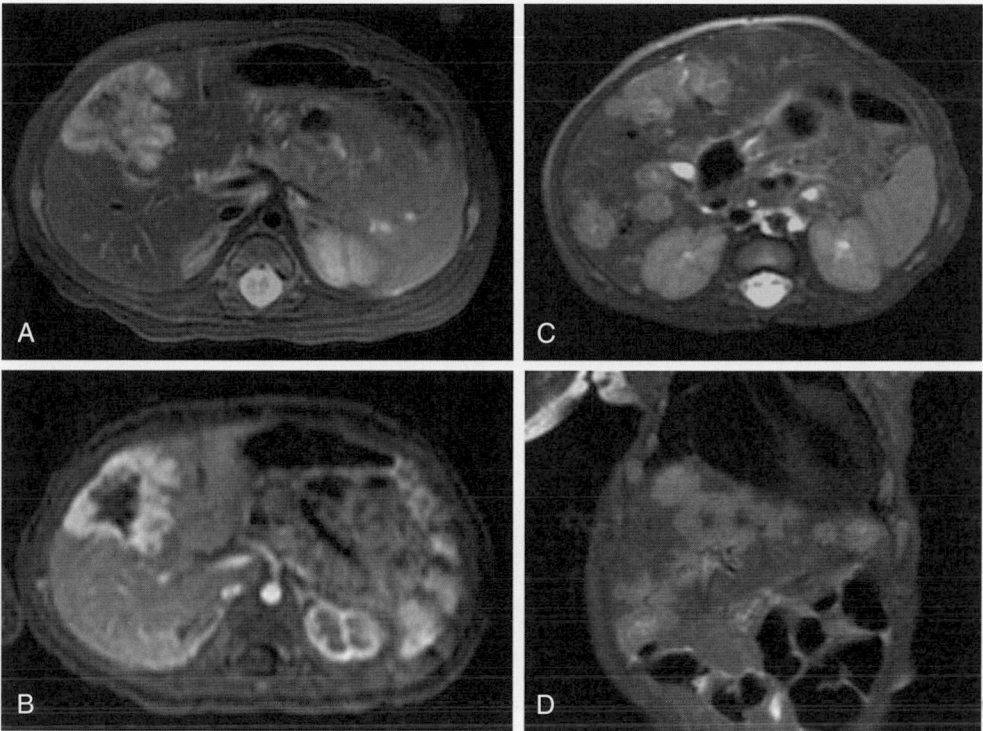

Figure 66-56 Involuting hepatic hemangioma and diffuse infantile hemangioma. Fat-suppressed T2-weighted (**A** and **C**) and post–gadolinium-enhanced (**B** and **D**) MRI showing large solitary peripherally enhancing lesion typical of involuting hepatic hemangioma (**A** and **B**) and the multifocal hepatic involvement in a patient with hypothyroidism and diffuse infantile hemangioma (**C** and **D**).

imaging features of hepatic adenomas are not specific, and imaging is usually directed at monitoring these lesions for increases in size and number. Rapid increase in size is generally considered to be an indication of degeneration of benign adenoma to hepatocellular carcinoma, particularly in patients with glycogen storage disease.[223] Regular surveillance, typically by ultrasound, is indicated in these patients. MRI should be considered to further aid in characterizing new or multiple lesions.

Focal Nodular Hyperplasia

FNH is rare in children, most commonly occurring in teenage and adolescent years.[224] It is usually found incidentally during imaging evaluation for other reasons. This benign lesion typically shows a central fibrous scar with surrounding hyperplastic hepatocytes and small bile ducts. As discussed, these imaging features are also seen in the fibrolamellar variant of hepatocellular carcinoma, and the distinction between FNH and fibrolamellar hepatocellular carcinoma may be difficult. CT and MRI scans usually show rapid homogeneous contrast enhancement during early arterial-phase imaging (see Figs. 66-53 and 66-54). Lesions then characteristically become isodense to the liver during later phases of enhancement, with the central scar remaining hypodense even during the delayed imaging period. With newer MRI imaging techniques performed either with iron-oxide particles that accumulate in reticuloendothelial cells (Kupffer cells) present in the hyperplastic FNH lesions or with hepatocyte selective gadolinium based agents such as gadoxetate (Eovist), the diagnosis of FNH[213,224] can generally be made with confidence. For equivocal cases, scintigraphy with ^{99m}Tc sulfur colloid can also be performed, although in practice this is rarely necessary. These masses may be monitored by ultrasound to ensure stability and do not typically require surgical resection unless they become symptomatic or undergo progressive enlargement. FNH has also been observed in patients who have completed therapy for nonhepatic primary tumors.[225-227] Whereas larger masses may be by detected by ultrasound or CT, it has been found that dynamic contrast-enhanced MRI is a highly sensitive technique for identifying these lesions. Occasionally these lesions can be characterized by ultrasound using high-resolution, high-frequency transducers; however, they are unequivocally shown by contrast-enhanced MRI (Figs. 66-57 and 66-58). These FNH lesions are also isointense to the liver on conventional imaging sequences and display rapid early arterial enhancement, after which they become nearly isointense to the liver and indistinguishable from the surrounding parenchyma. Hepatobiliary contrast agents are now used routinely to further characterize these lesions as benign FNH (see Fig. 66-53) and distinguish them from hepatic metastatic deposits. It is important recognize these characteristic patterns of enhancement so as to not mistake this benign entity for recurrent disease or a new site of disease relapse.

Other lesions occurring in the liver include sarcomatous tumors such as malignant angiosarcomas and rhabdomyosarcomas of the biliary tree, malignant vascular tumors, and metastatic disease. The most common metastatic lesions occurring in the liver include neuroblastomas, locally invasive and hematogenously-disseminated

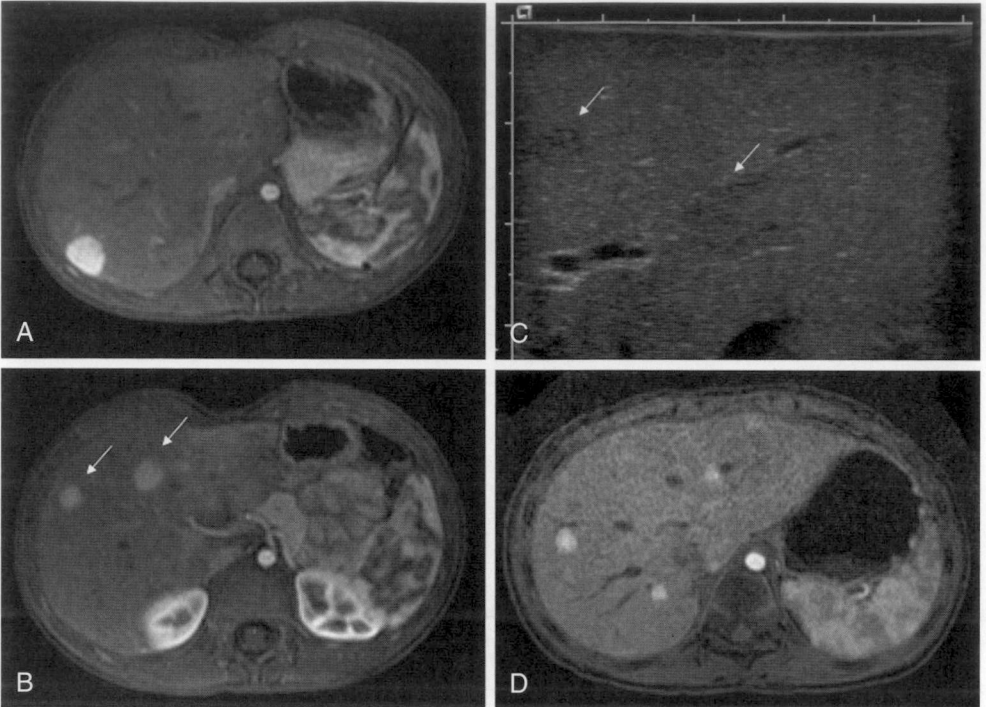

Figure 66-57 A 19-month-old boy with a history of treatment for stage 4 neuroblastoma. Follow-up MRI imaging using dynamic contrast enhancement shows multiple brightly enhancing lesions throughout the liver (**A** and **B**). These rapidly become isointense to liver during delayed scanning. They are not seen on any other sequences. The enhancement characteristics are typical of FNH. Intraoperative ultrasound localized lesions for biopsy (**C**) and confirmed them as FNH. Similar lesions in a 2-year-old patient treated in infancy for stage 4 neuroblastoma are shown in **D**.

Wilms tumors, rhabdomyosarcomas and Ewing sarcomas.[201] The imaging characteristics of these metastatic hepatic lesions are nonspecific with lesions characteristically hypoechoic on ultrasound relative to normal liver parenchyma, decreased attenuation on CT scan, low T1 and increased T2 signal intensity on T1- and T2-weighted MR images, respectively, and variable patterns of contrast enhancement with both CT and MRI.

Spleen

Primary tumors of the spleen are exceedingly rare.[228] Angiosarcomas have been reported but are not common in childhood. Involvement of the spleen by lymphoma and lymphoproliferative disease is the most common cause of malignant infiltration of the spleen.[229] Imaging evaluation by ultrasound often demonstrates multiple or

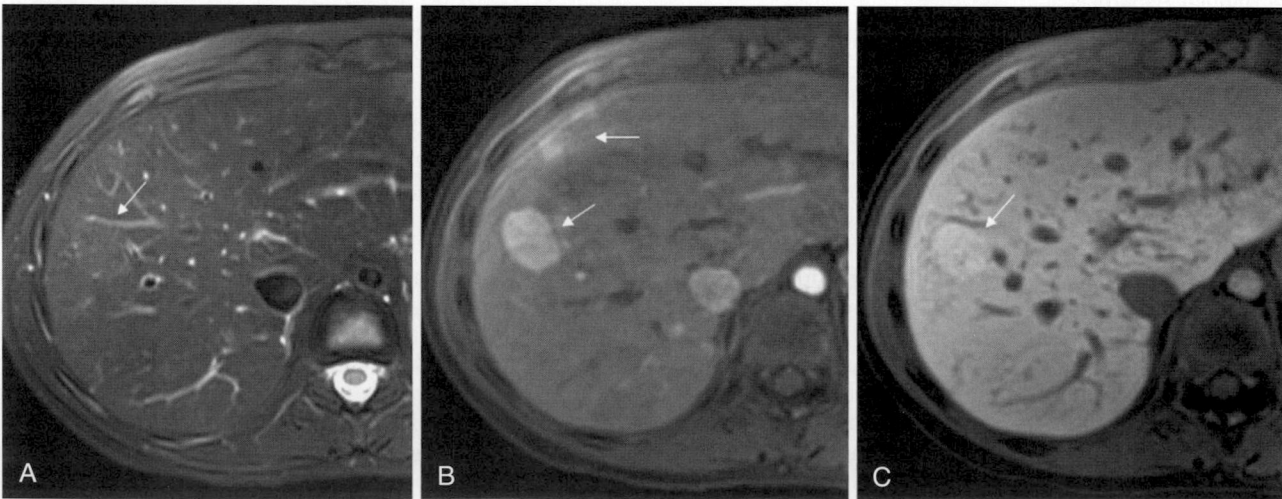

Figure 66-58 A 6-year-old patient treated for stage 4 neuroblastoma as an infant who developed multiple enhancing liver lesions proven to be FNH on biopsy. Subsequent MRI with gadoxetate (Eovist) shows representative lesions *(arrows)* to be isointense to liver on T2-weighted imaging (**A**), hyperenhancing on an early–arterial-phase image (**B**), and with persistent enhancement on the 20-minute delayed hepatocyte phase sequence (**C**). These features are characteristic of FNH.

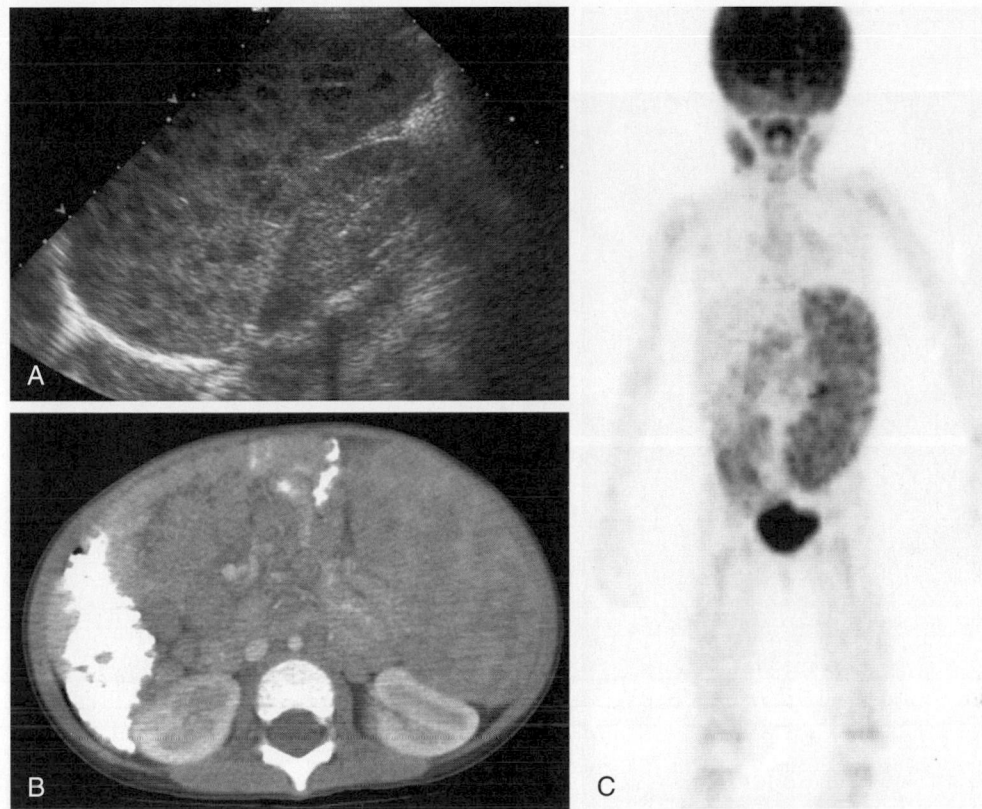

Figure 66-59 Lymphoproliferative disease. Ultrasound (**A**) and CT (**B**) demonstrate extensive splenic involvement and massive adenopathy in a patient with an unclassified lymphoproliferative disease. FDG-PET (**C**) shows multiple sites of disease and in particular confirms the extensive abnormalities in the spleen.

solitary hypoechoic masses (Fig. 66-59). CT scanning may be equivocal because of variable phases of splenic parenchymal enhancement. MRI, in contrast, can be very sensitive at detecting focal lesions that are occult by a CT and/or ultrasound. In the setting of lymphoma and lymphoproliferative disease, FDG-PET imaging has been shown to be an effective adjunctive imaging modality for detecting splenic involvement.[230,231] This is of importance both in determining the patient's stage of disease at diagnosis and in identifying sites of disease to be watched and assessed for response after treatment. In addition, the negative predictive value of PET/CT in discriminating between benign and malignant lesions has been emphasized both in patients with coexistent malignant disease and in patients without history of malignancy in whom a solid splenic mass is identified by other imaging techniques.[232]

Biliary Tract

Tumors of the gall bladder and bile ducts are rare in children, and include biliary rhabdomyosarcomas and cholangiocarcinomas, the latter of which occur in the setting of chronic ulcerative colitis. The initial imaging evaluation is usually by ultrasound, often for symptoms of biliary-tract obstruction such as pain, jaundice, and weight loss. Ultrasound may show evidence of bile-duct dilation and biliary-tract obstruction; however, identification of a focal mass usually requires additional evaluation by MRI/magnetic resonance cholangiopancreatography (MRCP), with diagnostic confirmation by endoscopic retrograde cholangiopancreatography (ERCP). Particularly in the setting of rhabdomyosarcoma, FDG-PET is of value in accurately determining the stage of disease.[184] Biliary rhabdomyosarcoma can arise from the intrahepatic or extrahepatic biliary bile ducts, gallbladder, cystic duct, or ampulla of Vater. At the time of presentation with obstructive jaundice and abdominal pain, these neoplasms are usually quite large, and as a result the distinction between biliary rhabdomyosarcoma, primary hepatic tumors arising in the hepatic hilum, pancreatic neoplasms, and renal/suprarenal masses may be challenging (Fig. 66-60).[233]

Pancreas

Primary tumors of the pancreas are rare in children, in contrast to adults. In addition, the types of tumors found in children differ from the adult tumors, in whom adenocarcinomas predominate. Pancreatic tumors can be classified into nonfunctional tumors of the exocrine pancreas and functional tumors of the endocrine pancreas, as well as secondary metastatic pancreatic neoplasia.[234]

Malignant epithelial neoplasms arising from the exocrine pancreas include pancreatoblastomas, and solid papillary epithelial neoplasms of the pancreas. Primary nonepithelial tumors of the pancreas are very rare and include lymphomas, rhabdomyosarcomas and primitive

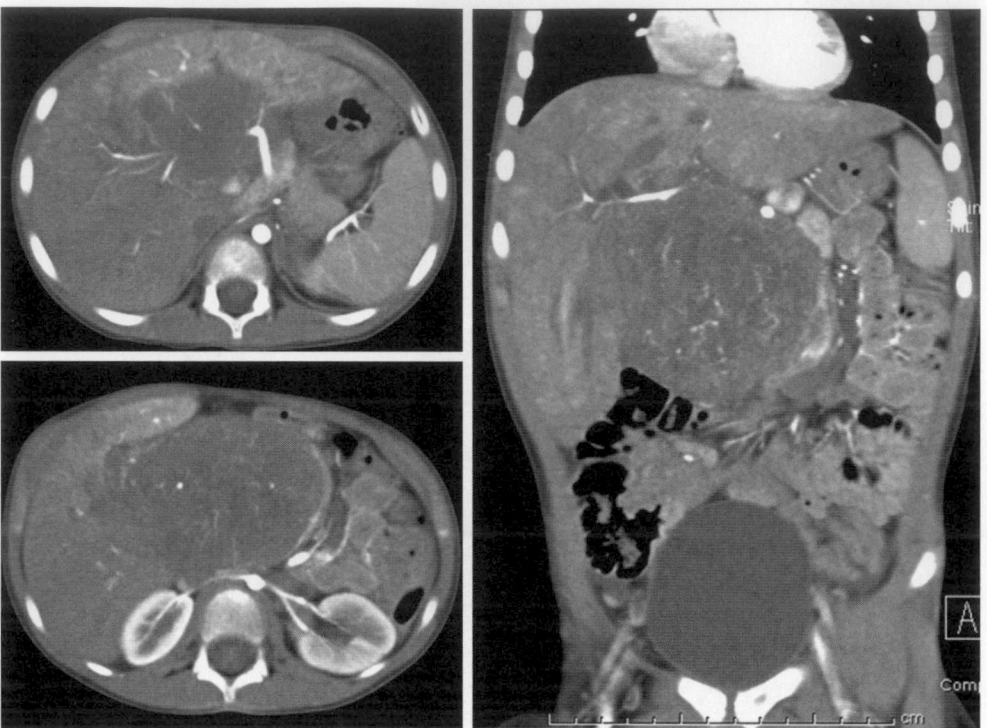

Figure 66-60 Biliary rhabdomyosarcoma. Dynamic contrast-enhanced CT reveals a large mass in the hepatic hilum, encasing the vessels and infiltrating adjacent structures. Note the lack of significant bile duct dilation, allowing the mass to become very large before producing symptoms of obstructive jaundice.

neuroectodermal tumors. Pancreatic endocrine neoplasms are rare in children, and they are usually associated with the multiple endocrine neoplasia syndrome. These include hormonally active tumors such as insulinomas, gastrinomas, VIPomas and glucagonomas.

Pancreatoblastomas

Pancreatoblastomas can occur at any age but are most common in children between the ages of 1 and 8 years. Pancreatoblastomas are reported as arising in or around the head of the pancreas in roughly half of the cases. Because they are nonfunctional, they are typically quite large at the time of diagnosis. Presenting symptoms include abdominal pain, nausea, and weight loss. Obstructive symptoms such as jaundice or pancreatitis are less common despite the large size of these masses, which has been attributed to the soft, gelatinous, and compliant consistency of these tumors.[235] These tumors are typically well encapsulated, have heterogeneous patterns of echogenicity on ultrasound, and show variable patterns of contrast enhancement on CT (Fig. 66-61). Calcifications are commonly seen and are probably the sequelae of hemorrhage and necrosis known to occur within these tumors. MRI shows a similar pattern of heterogeneous signal intensity and enhancement, with masses usually hypointense on T1-weighted images and variably hyperintense on T2-weighted and post–gadolinium-enhanced images. As with hepatoblastoma, pulmonary metastatic disease is often present, and the staging evaluation must include a CT of the chest. Because of their large size, the tissue of origin may be difficult to clearly delineate, and differential considerations includes exophytic hepatoblastoma, renal and suprarenal masses, and retroperitoneal neoplasms.[236]

Solid Pseudopapillary Neoplasms

Solid pseudopapillary neoplasms of the pancreas (also known as *solid* and *papillary epithelial neoplasms*)[237] are a rare primary pediatric pancreatic tumor. In contrast to other pancreatic tumors occurring in children, however, the prognosis after complete surgical resection is favorable.[238] Studies have reported up to a 90% survival rate after complete resection. In one small study, median age at presentation was 13 years, with abdominal pain, a palpable mass, dyspepsia, and pancreatitis the most common presenting symptoms.[238] On imaging, usually by ultrasound and/or CT, solid pseudopapillary tumors appear as solid, well-demarcated masses. On ultrasound there is heterogeneous echotexture, occasionally with fluid-filled cystic spaces (Fig. 66-62). CT shows a heterogeneous mass with peripheral contrast enhancement. Although these tumors are slow-growing tumors with low-grade malignant behavior, FDG uptake on PET imaging has been shown in solid papillary tumors of the pancreas.[239] FDG-PET scanning may therefore be of value in follow-up imaging to assess for recurrence. Despite

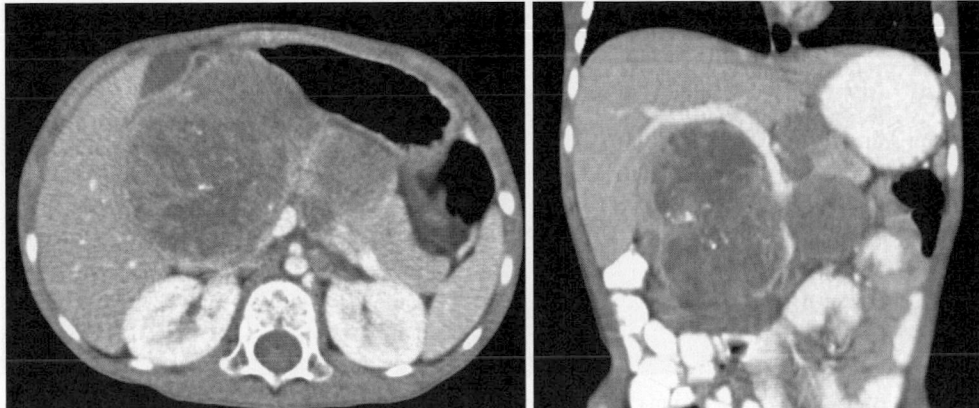

Figure 66-61 Pancreatoblastoma in a 4-year-old boy with a palpable abdominal mass. Contrast-enhanced CT shows a large, calcified retroperitoneal mass centered in the pancreas. Both adrenal glands were normal. Lung metastases were also present (not shown). The biopsy showed pancreatoblastoma.

high rates of overall 5-year survival, if metastases are present and not resectable, survival is poor with no clear, beneficial role reported for adjuvant chemotherapy or radiation therapy.[237]

Pancreatic Sarcomas

Mesenchymal tumors of the pancreas include rare synovial-cell sarcomas, myofibroblastic tumors, and metastatic rhabdomyosarcomas. Extremity rhabdomyosarcomas seem to have an unusual predilection for metastases to unusual cites such as the breast, ovary, testicle, and pancreas.[240] Two patients shown in Figure 66-63 had metastatic rhabdomyosarcoma to the pancreas. Local presentation may include pancreatitis and abdominal pain or may be incidental (see Fig. 66-48, *B*). A recent report from three major pediatric centers also noted an association of alveolar rhabdomyosarcoma with pancreatic metastasis,[241] emphasizing the importance of follow-up imaging in these patients and including an increasing role for routine FDG-PET/CT imaging to identify unusual sites of metastatic spread in patients with rhabdomyosarcoma.

Pancreatic Lymphomas

Burkitt lymphoma is well known to involve organs of the gastrointestinal tract, although isolated pancreatic involvement is unusual. Typically pancreatic involvement is accompanied by other sites of visceral and mesenteric disease. Diffuse pancreatic infiltration in the setting of Burkitt lymphoma is shown in Figure 66-64 in a child who had symptoms of pancreatitis. On ultrasound the pancreas was diffusely enlarged and heterogeneous in echogenicity. CT scan showed diffuse pancreatic enlargement, poor enhancement, and a homogeneous low attenuation. As is common for the rapidly dividing Burkitt lymphoma, a prompt response to chemotherapy was observed, with near complete resolution of pancreatic abnormalities 10 days after onset of chemotherapy.

Pancreatic Islet-Cell Tumors

Functioning islet-cell tumors of the pancreas are rare but important clinically because of symptomatic endocrine abnormalities that result from constitutive secretion of hormones normally tightly regulated by the endocrine

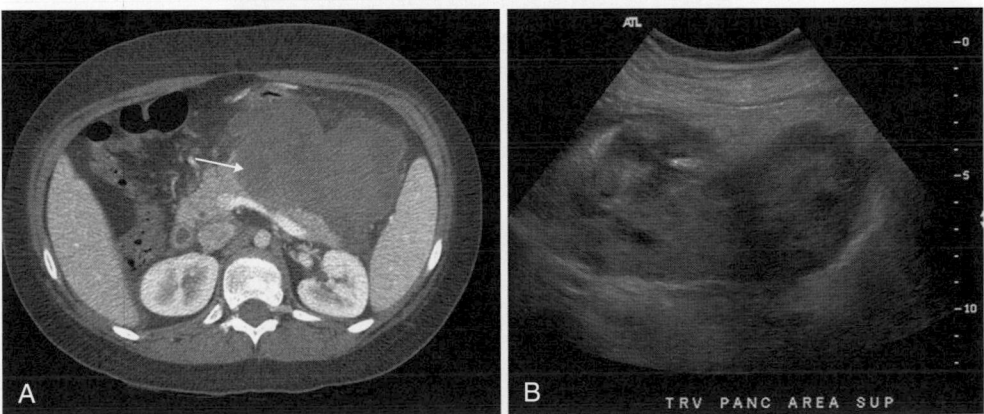

Figure 66-62 Pseudopapillary pancreatic tumor. This 9-year-old patient had hypertension and increased abdominal girth. **A,** CT shows a low attenuation, heterogeneously enhancing lobulated mass arising from the pancreatic body and tail *(arrow)*, which also abutted the greater curvature of the stomach (not shown). **B,** Ultrasound shows a lobulated solid mass that could not be distinguished from the pancreas.

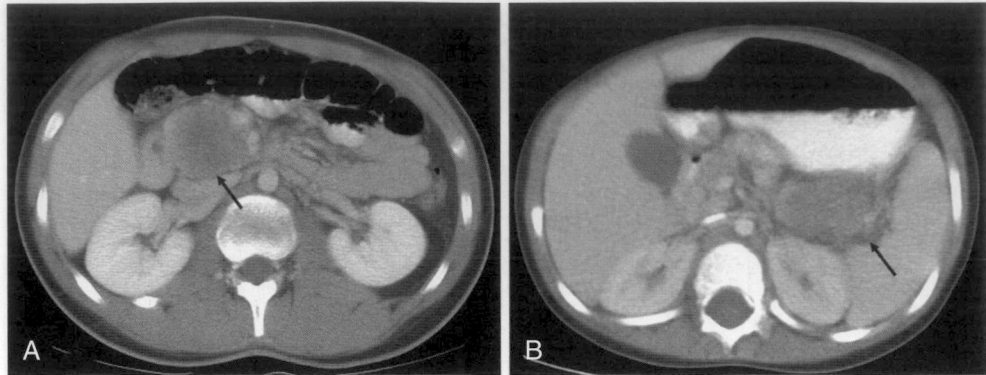

Figure 66-63 CT shows metastatic rhabdomyosarcoma to the pancreas in two patients with extremity rhabdomyosarcoma. **A,** The patient had symptoms of pain. **B,** The patient had no abdominal symptoms, and the lesion was detected by FDG-PET during routine surveillance.

pancreas. As shown in Figure 66-65, in which the patient had symptomatic hyperinsulinemic hypoglycemia, these tumors are often quite small and may be difficult to diagnose and characterize. As with other neuroendocrine neoplasms, optimal scanning techniques for detection of pancreatic islet-cell tumors include early arterial-phase scanning as part of a multiphase imaging technique. Thin sections (≈1 mm) are now routinely acquired by most multidetector-row CT scanners and the evaluation should include a careful review of sagittal and coronal reconstructed images. Although there are no controlled studies comparing CT and MRI in evaluating these tumors, a well-administered MRI examination with respiratory triggering/breath-holding, fast gradient-echo imaging, diffusion imaging, and dynamic-contrast administration is likely to yield comparable, if not superior results to CT. These small lesions are often difficult to see by conventional ultrasound; however, intraoperative ultrasound is invaluable for localizing small, nonpalpable lesions (see Fig. 66-65, *B*).

Alimentary Tract Tumors

Tumors of the gastrointestinal tract including the esophagus, stomach, and large and small bowel are rare in children. In the stomach, lymphomas, leiomyomas, lyomysarcomas, and adenocarcinomas are all rare as

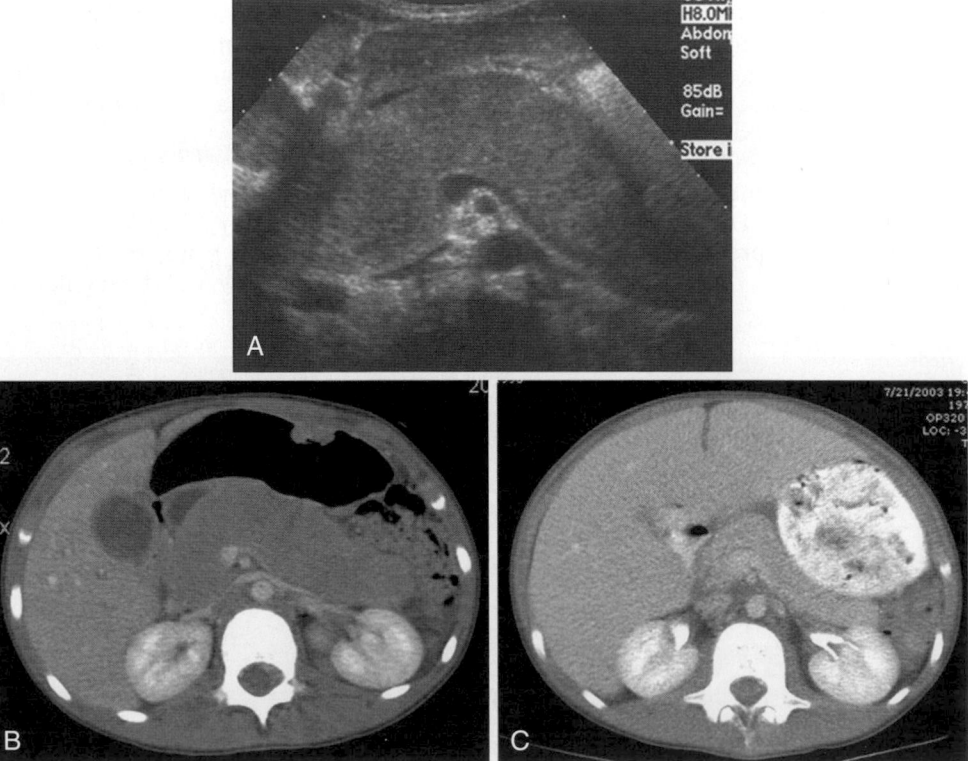

Figure 66-64 Burkitt lymphoma of the pancreas. An 8-year-old patient presented with pancreatitis. **A,** Ultrasound showed diffuse pancreatic infiltration, confirmed by CT (**B**), with disease limited to the pancreas. Ten days after initiating chemotherapy the pancreas appeared normal (**C**), typical of the rapid responses observed with Burkitt lymphoma.

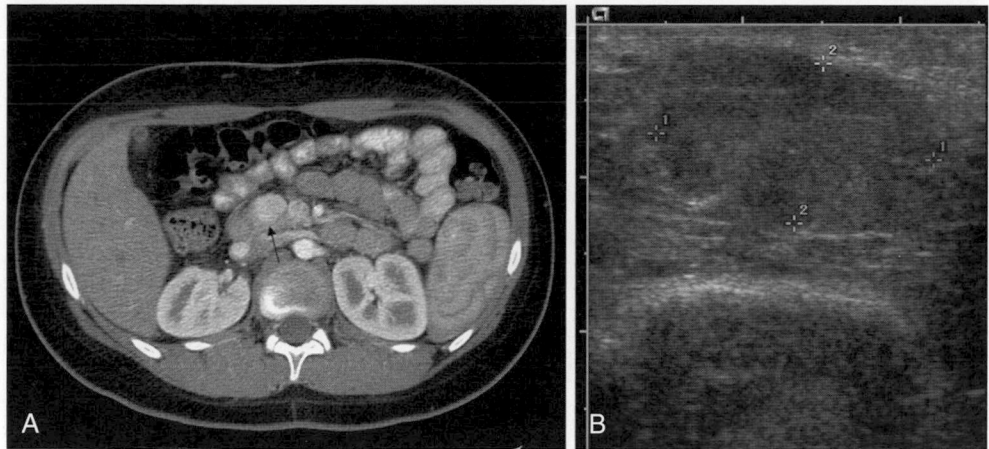

Figure 66-65 Pancreatic islet-cell tumor. This patient had profound hypoglycemia. **A,** CT shows a small enhancing lesion in the pancreatic head, adjacent to the superior mesenteric vein, detected only during the early arterial phase of scanning and consistent with insulinoma. **B,** Intraoperative ultrasound was essential to localize this small lesion before resection.

compared with adults. Gastrointestinal stromal tumors (GISTs) also have a low incidence in the pediatric population. Since early 2000, however, these tumors have attracted increased attention because of molecularly-targeted therapies (e.g., imatinib [Gleevec]) specifically inhibiting cell-surface receptors expressed on these cells. Although the majority of pediatric GISTs express a different cell-surface receptor mutation (*KIT* or *PDGFRA*)[242] and thus do not respond to imatinib like adult GISTs, the radiographic features are similar, with patients having a large mass closely apposed to the gastric wall. Depending on the size of the mass it may be difficult to distinguish between a pancreatic tumor invading the posterior gastric wall and a primary gastric tumor. On CT these tumors are often heterogeneous in attenuation with modest enhancement relative to the adjacent pancreatic tissue. For patients with localized disease, complete surgical resection is still the mainstay of treatment for this tumor, with targeted therapies being reserved for those patients with advanced or metastatic disease.[243] FDG-PET scanning has been shown to be important for staging and in follow-up evaluation, both as a measure of metabolic response to molecularly targeted therapy[243] and for early detection of small, local sites of relapse within the gastric wall that may be difficult to detect by conventional cross-sectional imaging techniques (Fig. 66-66).

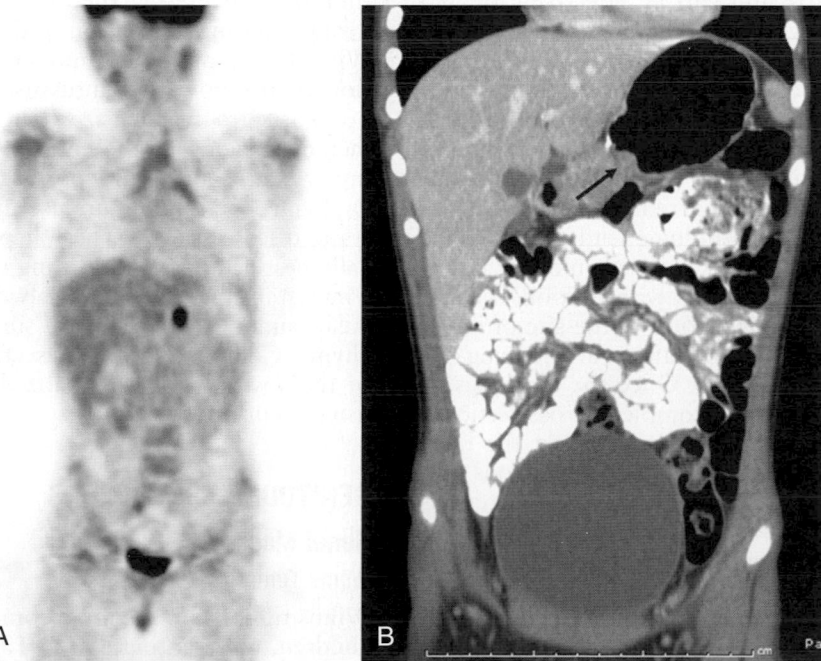

Figure 66-66 Images of a 9-year-old patient taken for routine follow-up examination after resection of a large GIST from the distal stomach. FDG-PET (**A**) shows intense focus of uptake in the upper abdomen, corresponding to a subtle nodular density seen by CT (**B**) along the greater curve of the stomach *(arrow)*. Endoscopic biopsy confirmed relapse at the resection margin.

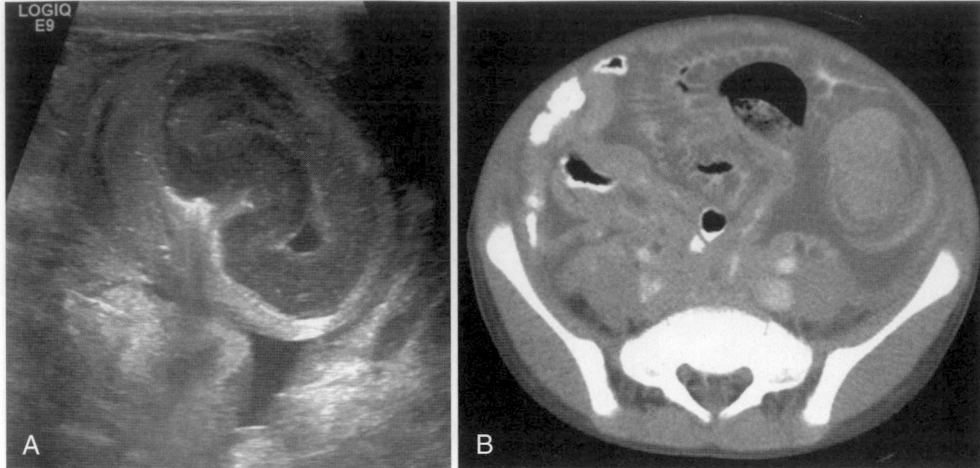

Figure 66-67 A 6-year-old patient with diffuse abdominal Burkitt lymphoma with symptoms of abdominal pain, diffuse bowel-wall thickening, adenopathy, ascites, and small-bowel intussusception, shown on both ultrasound (**A**) and CT (**B**).

The most common primary bowel malignancy in childhood is lymphoma. Small bowel is more often involved than large bowel, and this is most often non-Hodgkin lymphoma. Presentation is typically with abdominal pain, weight loss, anemia, gastrointestinal bleeding, or constipation. Intussusception or a palpable abdominal mass may bring the patient to attention sooner. In an older child (older than age 6 years) with intussusception, lymphoma should be the leading diagnostic consideration (Fig. 66-67). The majority of the small-bowel non-Hodgkin lymphomas are Burkitt lymphomas. These rapidly dividing tumors involve the bowel or small bowel/colonic mesentery and can become quite large and lead to intestinal obstruction. Burkitt lymphoma responds rapidly to chemotherapy and can be effectively treated with no residual imaging abnormalities seen.

The imaging evaluation may initially involve fluoroscopic/barium studies to assess nonspecific symptoms of abdominal pain. In the setting of suspected intussusception, conventional radiographs and ultrasound are usually sufficient to confirm the diagnosis. Attempts at hydrostatic or pneumatic enema reduction of intussusceptions occurring around pathologic lead points in the bowel because of lymphomatous infiltration of the bowel or mesentery should be undertaken with caution, because there is increased risk of perforation at the site of intussusception[244] and greater risk of failure at reducing the intussusception in these patients. Once the diagnosis of lymphoma has been made, a complete cross-sectional imaging (CT) staging examination, including the neck and chest, should be undertaken. Both intravenous and oral contrast are necessary for this evaluation. CT reveals bowel-wall thickening, mesenteric adenopathy, and often a large intraperitoneal/mesenteric mass. FDG-PET scanning has been shown to be effective in adult patients in staging and response assessment for non-Hodgkin lymphoma, and small case series have confirmed this finding in children, suggesting FDG-PET should probably be included in the diagnostic staging and posttreatment assessment of these patients.[245-248]

Adenocarcinomas of the colon and rectum are fortunately rare in children. As in adults, colonoscopy may provide the best early diagnosis for a suspected carcinomatous lesions. The staging evaluation for metastatic spread should involve imaging of the chest, abdomen, and pelvis, again with both intravenous and oral contrast. There is no clear role established for routine use of FDG-PET scanning in the staging of children with adenocarcinomas of the gastrointestinal tract.

Carcinoid tumors occurring in the gastrointestinal tract are rare and usually slow-growing but have malignant potential. The appendix is the most common location for carcinoid tumors. It is not uncommon for patients to show symptoms of acute appendicitis, with carcinoid tumors discovered at the time of appendectomy or incidentally during evaluation of the pathologic specimen.[249] When large, carcinoid tumors may also produce obstruction of the bowel or intussusception. Because of their propensity to metastasize to the liver, work-up should include imaging of the entire abdomen and pelvis with intravenous and oral contrast. Somatostatin receptor analogues (octreotide) are useful for occult sites of metastatic disease spread. These hepatic metastases are typically best demonstrated during the early arterial phase of contrast injection, which nicely delineates these hypervascular tumors relative to the surrounding hepatic parenchyma. Complete surgical resection remains the mainstay of therapy for disease localized to the appendix and is usually curative.[249]

GENITOURINARY TUMORS

Renal Masses

Wilms Tumors

Wilms tumors are the most common renal malignancy in children, representing 6% to 10% of all pediatric malignancies and making up greater than 80% of pediatric renal masses. The peak age of incidence is between 3 and 4 years, and bilateral disease is seen in between 5% and

TABLE 66-2 Childhood Wilms Tumor: National Wilms Tumor Study Group Staging[252]

Tumor Stage	Description
1	Tumor is limited to the kidney and is completely resected. The renal capsule is intact and tumor is not ruptured or biopsied before removal. No involvement of renal sinus vessels or evidence of the tumor at or beyond the margins of resection.
2	Tumor is completely resected, with no evidence of tumor at or beyond the margins of resection. Tumor extends beyond the kidney as evidenced by any one of the following: Regional extension of the tumor (i.e., penetration of the renal sinus capsule, or extensive invasion of the soft tissue of the renal sinus) Blood vessels within the nephrectomy specimen outside the renal parenchyma contain tumor.
3	Residual nonhematogenous intraabdominal tumor after surgery. Any one of the following may occur: Lymph nodes within the abdomen or pelvis are involved by tumor. Tumor implants are found on or penetrated through the peritoneal surface. Gross or microscopic tumor remains. Tumor is not completely resectable because of local infiltration. Tumor spillage occurs either before or during surgery, or tumor was biopsied before removal. Tumor is removed in more than one piece (e.g., tumor thrombus within the renal vein is removed separately from the nephrectomy specimen).
4	Hematogenous metastases (e.g., lung, liver, bone, brain) or lymph node metastases outside the abdominopelvic region are present.
5	Bilateral involvement by tumor is present at diagnosis.

10% of patients.[250,251] Wilms tumor is often associated with syndromes and nephroblastomatosis and typically presents as a painless, palpable abdominal mass. Occasionally, Wilms tumor is an incidental finding during a radiologic assessment for other indications such as trauma. Hypertension and hematuria only occur in about 25% of the cases.[250]

Tumor staging based on the NWTSG classification depends on surgical, pathological, and radiologic findings, and the imaging evaluation should be directed at determining spread to adjacent organs such as the pancreas, spleen, and liver and for intravascular extension into the renal vein, IVC, and right atrium (Table 66-2).[252] In addition, the imaging examination should assess for the presence of distant metastatic disease (lung and liver) and for the presence of contralateral kidney involvement.[251,253] Wilms tumor is a rapidly growing malignancy, and intraabdominal rupture at diagnosis, during chemotherapy, or at the time of surgical resection is a well-appreciated complication and a major risk factor for abdominal recurrence,[254] increasing the recurrence rate to as much as 20%.[255] Accurately identifying tumor rupture can be a challenge. In a recent review of 70 patients

treated through the COG, preoperative CT imaging was found to have moderate specificity (88%) but relatively low sensitivity (62%) in the detection of Wilms tumor rupture, although ascites seen outside of the cul-de-sac, irrespective of fluid density, was most predictive of rupture.[256] When tumor rupture is identified, these patients are upstaged and treated as having stage 3 disease.[251,253]

The initial examination is often a conventional abdominal x-ray obtained for symptoms of abdominal pain or a palpable mass. The typical findings include displacement of bowel and a masslike opacity in the abdomen. An ultrasound should serve as the initial evaluation and usually confirms the renal origin of the suspected mass. Sonographically Wilms tumors are often quite large with relatively homogeneous echogenicity. There may be focal areas of hypoechogenicity or cystic change. Calcifications are uncommon. Ultrasound is also accurate and sensitive at detecting intravascular invasion, and both color and Doppler imaging are effective at establishing vascular patency (Fig. 66-68). Intravascular extension occurs in 4% to 10% of patients with Wilms tumor but is rare in neuroblastoma, helping to differentiate between these two tumors.[253] In a recent study evaluating the diagnostic performance of CT versus Doppler ultrasound in identifying intravascular extension of Wilms tumor, investigators from the COG found CT to be superior to ultrasound for detection of intravascular and cavoatrial thrombus.[257] Nonetheless because ultrasound is often the initial examination performed in these patients, early identification of intravascular extension into the right atrium is essential and may increase the sedation/anesthesia risk for a child for whom subsequent CT or MRI is planned.

Once the diagnosis has been suggested by ultrasound, further imaging of suspected Wilms tumor requires either CT or MRI to accurately stage the disease. Multidetector-row CT scanning allows for rapid scanning and in some instances may allow sedation to be avoided. High-resolution imaging techniques with multiplanar reconstructions are essential in determining the extent of tumor spillage, local invasion, invasion into vascular structures, and presence of pulmonary metastatic disease. Early studies suggested that pulmonary metastases detected only by CT should not result in upstaging of the patient, relying on the chest x-ray to identify pulmonary metastases.[253] Subsequent work by European investigators in the International Society of Paediatric Oncology (SIOP) and in North America with the NWTSG identified a small cohort of patients with pulmonary lesions visualized only by CT scanning in whom disease stage would be advanced based on the CT results.[253] One study showed an increased risk of relapse in patients with positive CT findings.[258] Others, however, reported either no difference in prognosis between patients with positive or negative chest CT scans[189,259] or improvement in event-free survival rates, but with no impact on the overall survival rate and with no benefit from whole-lung radiation for patients with CT-only pulmonary nodules.[191] These studies are limited by their retrospective nature, and it remains controversial whether patients would have benefited from increased therapy.[251,253] Furthermore other investigators

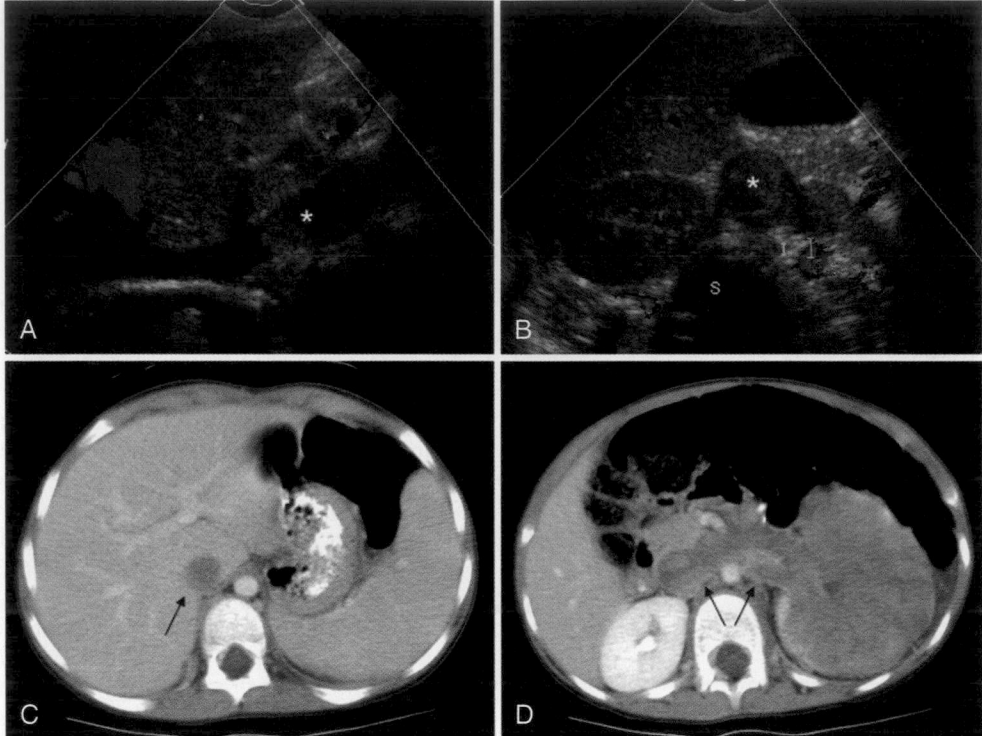

Figure 66-68 Wilms tumor. A 6-year-old child with a left renal Wilms tumor and left renal vein/IVC extension shown by ultrasound (**A** and **B**) and CT (**C** and **D**, *arrows*). Ultrasound confirms the complete absence of flow in the left renal vein and documents the level of intravascular invasion into the IVC *(asterisks)*. *s*, Spine.

have argued that CXR and CT data are concordant in the majority of cases,[190] and it as been shown that not all pulmonary lesions detected by CT represent metastases, even in the hands of experienced radiologists,[258] suggesting that surgical confirmation may be necessary to establish the malignant nature of suspicious lesions detected by CT in patients with Wilms tumor.[188] These considerations aside, it is current practice to obtain a chest CT for staging of all patients with Wilms tumor, with ongoing studies investigating the positive predictive value of this practice and its impact on overall clinical outcome.

Because of the need for chest CT in the staging evaluation, MRI is usually obtained for follow-up evaluation, either after resection or chemotherapy. In addition, MRI is the imaging modality of choice in monitoring nephrogenic rests that are seen in approximately 40% of patients with unilateral Wilms tumor and nearly all patients with bilateral Wilms tumors (Fig. 66-69).[260,261] Nephrogenic rests are remnants of primitive blastemal tissue that persist after birth and have the potential to transform into Wilms tumor. Nephroblastomatosis is the presence of multifocal or diffuse nephrogenic rests and is prevalent in patients with hemihypertrophy.[262] The distinction between nephrogenic rests and Wilms tumor may be difficult; however, there are certain distinguishing MRI features that may help discriminate between the two. On T1-weighted MRI images, Wilms tumors appear as well-defined heterogeneous masses with slightly lower signal intensity as compared with the adjacent renal cortex. On T2-weighted images Wilms tumors appear isointense to slightly hyperintense relative to the normal renal cortex.

After intravenous gadolinium-contrast administration, Wilms tumors typically enhance heterogeneously but less than the surrounding renal parenchyma. Nephrogenic rests also exhibit decreased signal intensity on T1-weighted images, but in contrast to Wilms tumors maintain low signal on T2-weighted images.[263-265] Furthermore, nephrogenic rests show minimal enhancement after contrast infusion relative to the normal renal parenchyma, whereas foci of Wilms tumors show heterogeneous enhancement.[263,264] A role for FDG-PET imaging in the routine management of patients with Wilms tumor has not been established. However, studies documenting increased FDG accumulation in metabolically active Wilms tumors[266,267] suggest there may be role for FDG-PET imaging in Wilms tumor staging, posttherapy response evaluation, and possibly in helping discriminate benign nephrogenic rests from foci of transformed malignant tumor.

As discussed in the next section, the major differential considerations in patients with suspected unilateral Wilms tumor are clear-cell sarcoma of the kidney and rhabdoid tumor of the kidney, although there are no characteristic imaging features to make this distinction.

Clear-Cell Sarcomas

Clear-cell sarcomas of the kidney (also know as *bone-metastasizing renal tumor of childhood*) were previously thought to be a histologically aggressive variant of Wilms tumors. They occur less often than Wilms tumor (4% to 5% of pediatric renal neoplasms), with an estimated 20 new cases diagnosed annually in the United States.[268]

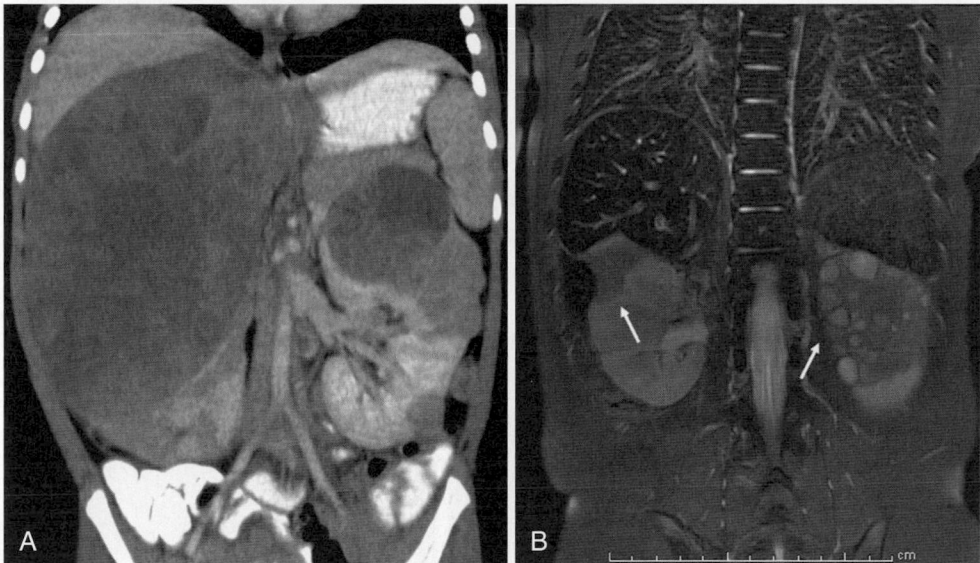

Figure 66-69 A 3-year-old patient with bilateral Wilms tumor, initially evaluated by CT (**A**). The patient underwent bilateral partial nephrectomies. **B,** MRI was used to monitor nephrogenic rests on both kidneys *(arrows)*, both for change in size and change in pattern of enhancement.

Although age at presentation ranges from infancy to the second decade, the peak incidence at about 2 to 3 years old closely parallels that of Wilms tumor, making differential diagnosis difficult. Bone metastases, which are unusual in Wilms tumor, occur commonly in patients with clear-cell sarcoma of the kidney and can have both osteolytic and osteoblastic activity.[250,262]

On imaging there are no specific features that allow distinction to be made from Wilms tumor.[269] Ultrasound confirms the renal origin of the mass, showing a heterogeneous mass with areas of hypoechogenicity and isoechogenicity reflecting cystic and solid elements within the mass. CT scanning is usually performed to more completely characterize the mass, assess for regional invasion, and check for metastatic disease. On CT, clear-cell sarcomas of the kidney are typically heterogeneous in attenuation with a variable pattern of contrast enhancement (Fig. 66-70). Vascular invasion is uncommon, and these tumors (in contrast to Wilms tumors) do not have a pseudocapsule and often infiltrate the adjacent renal parenchyma and perinephric spaces.[262] The most common site of metastatic spread is to locoregional lymph nodes, followed by metastases to the lung and bone.[270] Liver metastases also occur. As with Wilms tumor, the management of clear-cell carcinoma of the kidney involves a combination of nephrectomy and chemotherapy.[271] Clear-cell sarcomas are more aggressive than Wilms tumors with a higher relapse rate; the most common site of relapse is bone, and current recommendations include skeletal scintigraphy in follow-up screening examinations.

Rhabdoid Tumors of the Kidney

Rhabdoid tumors of the kidney are also extremely rare and are the most aggressive of the renal tumors in children. Previously thought to be a variant of Wilms tumor histology, they are now recognized as a discreet entity and

account for approximately 2% to 3% of pediatric renal tumors. Rhabdoid tumors tend to occur in young infants, with more than 80% occurring in patients under the age of 2 years (Fig. 66-71).[272]

CT, ultrasound, and MRI all show a large heterogeneous intrarenal mass that often involves the central renal hilum. There may be associated vascular invasion, and calcifications may be seen. Although there are no distinctive imaging features to reliably distinguish rhabdoid tumor of the kidney from Wilms tumor (see Fig. 66-66), the findings of calcification, subcapsular hematoma, and a lobular, centrally located heterogeneous renal mass have been reported as characteristic imaging findings in patients with rhabdoid tumors of the kidney.[273] In addition, the association between rhabdoid tumors of the kidney and the presence of primary brain tumors (posterior fossa tumors, including medulloblastomas, PNETs, astrocytomas, and medulloblastomas) and synchronous or metachronous brain metastases are considered a unique and distinctive feature of this tumor.[272,274] Once the diagnosis of rhabdoid tumor of the kidney is established, therefore, the subsequent staging and follow-up evaluations should always include imaging of the brain to assess for intracranial disease.

Renal-Cell Carcinomas

As children enter their teenage years, the incidence of Wilms tumor decreases and the incidence of renal-cell carcinoma rises. Although there have been rare reports of renal-cell carcinoma occurring in infancy, the vast majority occur in children in late adolescence.[250,262] Syndromes associated with renal-cell carcinoma include von Hippel-Landau syndrome, tuberous sclerosis, and Beckwith-Wiedemann syndrome. In contrast to adults, in whom hematuria is a common presenting complaint, children with renal-cell carcinoma more often have vague abdominal pain and an abdominal mass.

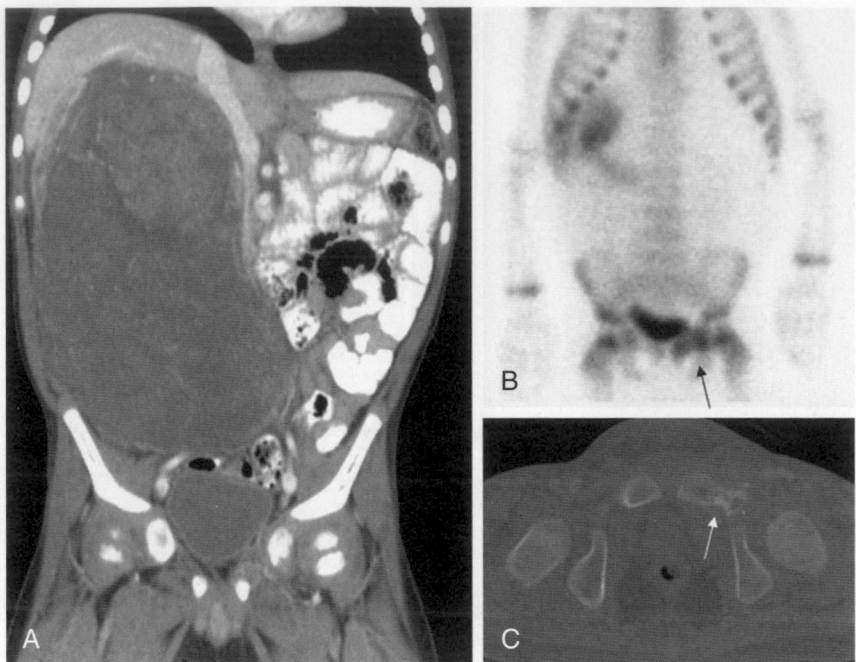

Figure 66-70 Clear-cell sarcoma of the kidney. A 2-year-old had symptoms of hip pain (x-rays were negative) and abdominal mass. Ultrasound (not shown) and CT (**A**) show heterogeneous masses with ill-defined margins, cystic and solid areas, and a variable pattern of contrast enhancement. Bone windows (**C**) revealed a destructive lesion in the left superior pubic ramus *(arrow)*, confirmed by bone scan (**B**), characteristic of the bone involvement seen with this renal neoplasm.

The imaging features of renal cell carcinoma and Wilms tumor overlap, although renal-cell carcinomas tend to show calcifications more often than Wilms tumors. Although renal cell carcinomas are more often bilateral and more commonly metastasize to bone than Wilms tumors, it is primarily the older age at presentation that favors renal-cell carcinoma over Wilms tumor. CT, MRI, and ultrasound all reveal a heterogeneous-appearing intrarenal mass. Multiple bilateral renal-cell carcinoma masses should suggest the diagnosis of von Hippel-Lindau syndrome.[272] Areas of cystic change may be seen, representing necrosis and hemorrhage, and calcifications are more common than in Wilms tumor (Fig.

66-72). After contrast infusion a heterogeneous pattern of contrast enhancement is seen on both CT and MRI. Local invasion into retroperitoneal lymph nodes and vascular invasion, particularly into the IVC, are common with renal-cell carcinoma and significantly influence the success of both primary surgical resection and overall prognosis. In some cases, when early-stage localized disease is established by CT and/or MRI, partial nephrectomy may be considered.[275,276] Intraoperative ultrasound can be valuable in guiding the surgeon and helping to define resection planes (Fig. 66-73). Because of increased incidence of bone metastases in renal-cell carcinoma, the staging evaluation should also include bone scintigraphy

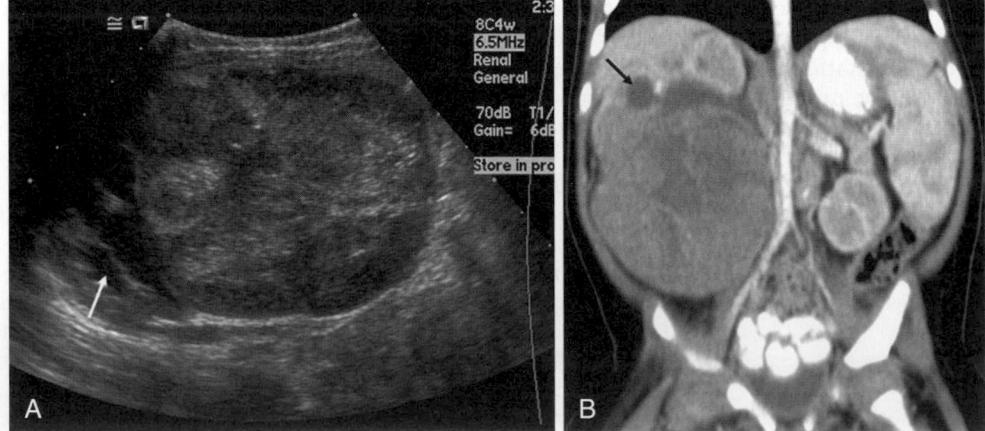

Figure 66-71 A 4-month-old patient with a palpable right renal mass. Ultrasound (**A**) and CT (**B**) show a centrally located lobulated mass causing obstruction of the right upper pole-collecting system *(arrows)*. On resection this was rhabdoid tumor. Note the difficulty in distinguishing this tumor from Wilms tumor (compare with Figs. 66-68 and 66-69).

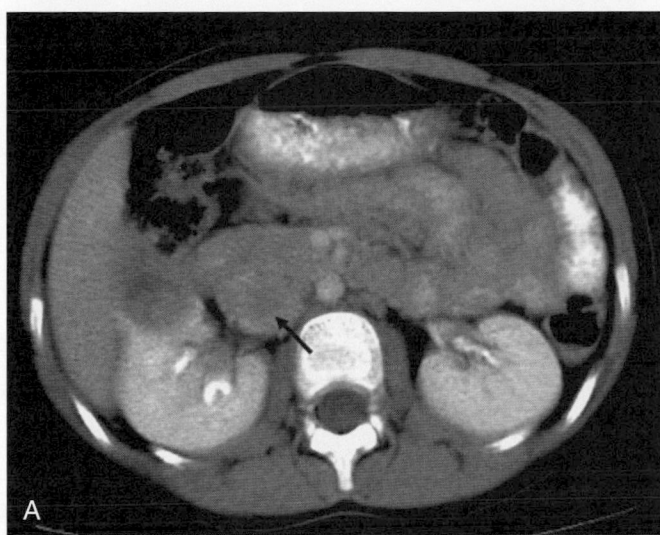

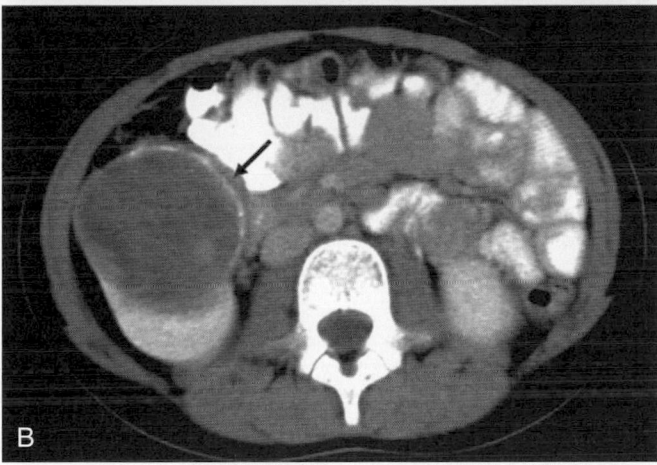

Figure 66-72 A 9-year-old child with a right renal mass that was found to be renal-cell carcinoma. Note the retroperitoneal lymph node spread (**A**, *arrow*), rim calcification (**B**, *arrow*), heterogeneous attenuation, and enhancement.

in addition to CT scanning of the chest, abdomen, and pelvis.

Congenital Mesoblastic Nephromas

Congenital mesoblastic nephromas, although not among the most common solid tumors in childhood, are the most common solid tumors of the neonatal period. They are benign tumor with almost three fourths of cases identified within the first year of life. With the advent of prenatal ultrasound screening, the incidence of early diagnosis is expected to increase. Infants typically have the presenting symptom of a large, palpable, abdominal mass. The imaging evaluation usually begins with ultrasound, showing a large, solid, renal mass that often involves the renal hilum (Fig. 66-74).[272] Although not a distinguishing feature, cystic elements are less commonly seen in mesoblastic nephroma than Wilms tumor. Congenital mesoblastic nephroma has been subdivided histologically into an aggressive high–cell-density variant and the classic variant, which has fewer active mitoses, less potential for local recurrence and metastasis, and overall better prognosis than the aggressive variant.[262,272] Hemorrhage, cysts, and necrosis, when present, are more often associated with the aggressive high–cell-density variant. Subsequent imaging by CT and/or MRI is usually performed to better characterize the intrarenal lesion and to assess for invasion into adjacent organs and structures (see Fig. 66-74). The imaging features alone do not allow distinction between mesoblastic nephroma and Wilms tumor,[270] and surgical resection is indicated. Because there may be poorly defined margins and the lack of a definable capsule, a surgical resection with wide margins is usually performed. The conventional benign histologic variant of this tumor is comprised primarily of benign connective tissue and mature mesenchymal cells, and prognosis is excellent if surgical resection is complete. Postoperative monitoring by ultrasound or MRI is still recommended, even with complete resection, for at least 1 year. With the aggressive cellular histologic variant, metastases and local spread of disease may require postoperative radiation and chemotherapy, and a more intensive follow-up imaging regimen should be directed at evaluating sites of local recurrence and typical metastatic spread (lungs, bone, and brain).[272]

Multilocular Cystic Nephromas

Multilocular cystic nephromas are benign renal tumors comprised almost entirely of coalescent cystic lesions with thin-walled septae.[277] Although the cystic appearance is distinctive, it is still not possible based on imaging features alone to discriminate between the cystic variant of Wilms tumor and the benign multilocular cystic nephroma. As with Wilms tumor, the typical age of presentation is between 2 and 5 years, with a smaller percentage occurring in young adults. Patients often have a large, painless, abdominal mass with no systemic symptoms.[272]

Radiographs may show a large abdominal mass displacing loops of bowel. The use of ultrasound is particularly important to demonstrate the cystic characteristics of these lesions, because CT scanning may simply show a large, low-attenuation mass with septations but not clearly demonstrate the hypoechoic cystic spaces revealed by ultrasound (Fig. 66-75). MRI shows characteristic fluid signal with low signal intensity on T1-weighted images and high signal intensity on T2-weighted images. After contrast enhancement, both by CT and MRI, enhancement of the thin-walled septae is seen, whereas the majority of the cystic mass remains unenhanced. Because the distinction between cystic Wilms tumor, clear-cell sarcoma, and multilocular cystic renal tumor cannot be made on the basis of imaging features, surgical resection is required for diagnosis.[270,271,277] Long-term prognosis is excellent; however, follow-up imaging is still necessary in the early stages postresection, because a low incidence of local recurrence is still possible.

Rare Renal Tumors

Two additional very rare tumors of infancy are the ossifying renal tumor of infancy and desmoplastic small round-cell tumors (Fig. 66-76). Both tumors characteristically calcify. Figure 66-76, *A* shows a renal hilar mass with

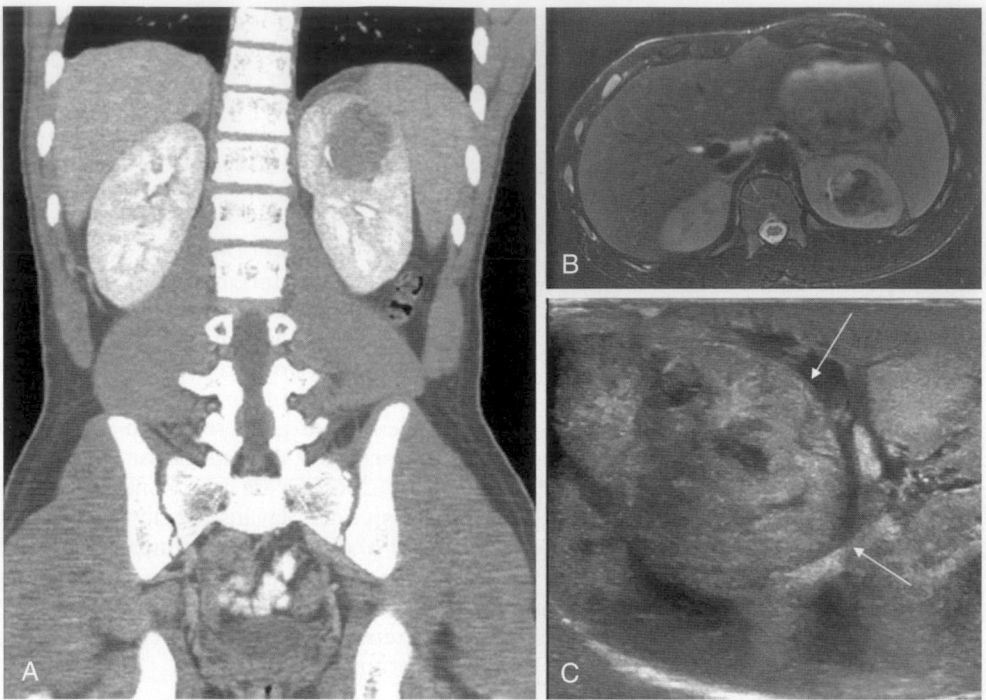

Figure 66-73 Renal-cell carcinoma in a 15-year-old patient with left flank pain and hematuria. Ultrasound showed left upper pole renal mass. CT (**A**) and MRI (**B**) show a low signal-intensity heterogeneously enhancing mass abutting the upper pole collecting system. Intraoperative ultrasound (**C**) defined a margin between the mass and renal parenchyma, vessels, and collecting system, allowing the patient to undergo partial nephrectomy of the upper pole.

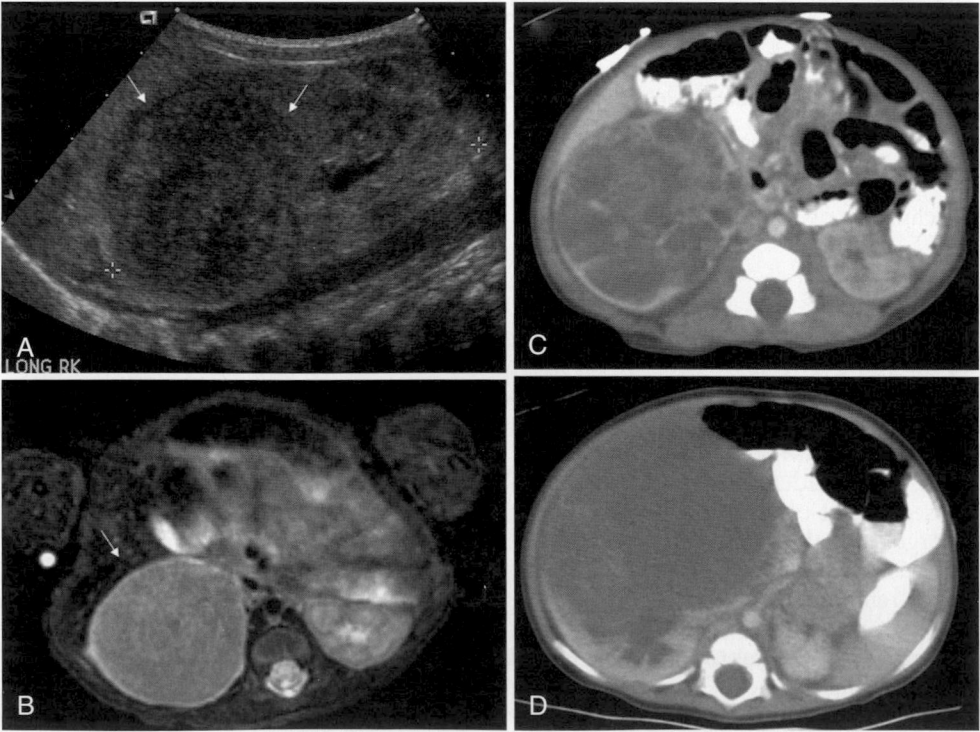

Figure 66-74 Congenital mesoblastic nephroma. **A** and **B** show a 7-day-old infant with a prenatally diagnosed solid right renal mass confirmed by ultrasound and MRI after birth. CTs from two other patients, newborn (**C**) and 5 months old (**D**), with large right renal masses showing both cystic and solid elements typical of congenital mesoblastic nephroma.

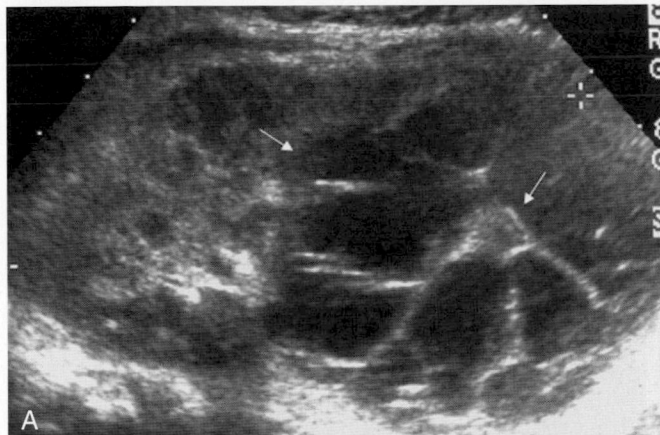

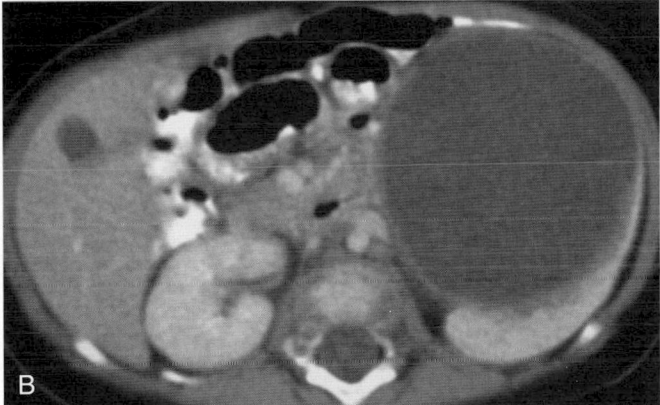

Figure 66-75 Multilocular cystic nephroma. Ultrasound shows a cystic left renal mass (A). Note how the cystic characteristics of these lesions and internal septations are not well demonstrated by CT (B), which simply shows a large low-attenuation mass, perhaps with thin internal septations.

extensive calcification that results from the ossifying renal tumors and is comprised of an osteoid core and osteoblastic tissue. Surgical resection is usually curative.[272] Desmoplastic small round-cell tumors are unusual as a primary renal neoplasm in children but have been reported.[278] As in other locations, these should be included in a differential for a calcified renal mass in a young child (see Fig. 66-76, B). Finally, metastatic disease to the

kidney is unusual except in the settings of leukemia and lymphoma.[262] Leukemic involvement of the kidney typically manifests as diffuse nephromegaly. Lymphomatous involvement more often presents with discrete foci of lymphomatous infiltration and occurs in both non-Hodgkin and Hodgkin lymphoma subtypes. Burkitt lymphoma and T-lymphoblastic lymphoma are the non-Hodgkin lymphoma types most commonly presenting with renal involvement. This is probably the result of hematogenous metastasis, and in the setting of Burkitt lymphoma is usually associated with extensive mesenteric and retroperitoneal lymphadenopathy.[272] In the case of leukemia, diffuse nephromegaly may also be accompanied by hepatosplenomegaly; however, generalized adenopathy is less common. Ultrasound is usually sufficient to identify renal involvement by leukemia and lymphoma. Additional imaging by either CT or MRI confirms the diagnosis, demonstrating low-density lesions with little enhancement relative to the surrounding renal parenchyma (Fig. 66-77).

Bladder Neoplasms

In children, tumors involving the urinary bladder are uncommon, with rhabdomyosarcoma being the most common malignancy encountered. Adult-type tumors such as transitional-cell carcinoma, fibroepithelial polyps, and adenomatous lesions are unusual.

Rhabdomyosarcomas

Pelvic rhabdomyosarcomas arise from the bladder wall, prostate, and vagina. Tumors arising in the bladder and prostate often result in obstruction of urinary flow, symptoms of dysuria and hematuria, and urinary retention. Vaginal rhabdomyosarcomas present as pelvic masses with vaginal bleeding and occasionally prolapse of tumor from the vaginal orifice onto the perineum.[279]

Imaging evaluation is initially by ultrasound with rhabdomyosarcomas of the bladder presenting either as diffuse bladder-wall thickening or as polypoid or "botryoid soft-tissue masses" protruding from the bladder wall into the bladder lumen. Color and Doppler flow demonstrate increased vascularity of these lesions. Cystourethrography may be helpful to assess the degree of functional impairment and usually demonstrates filling

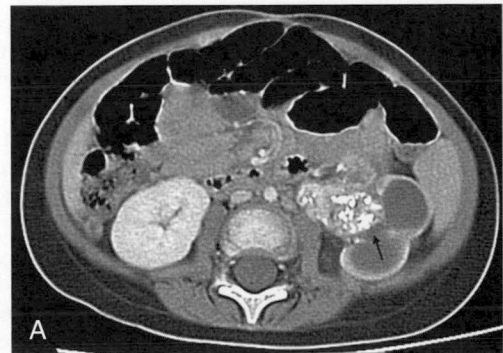
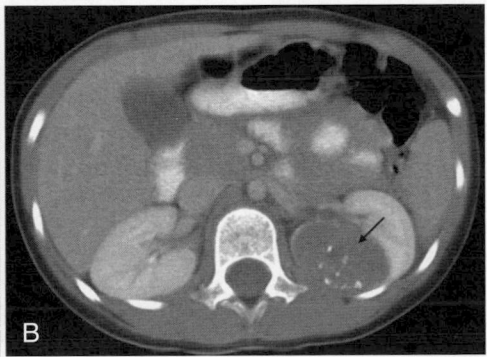

Figure 66-76 A, Ossifying renal tumor of infancy showing lobular renal hilar mass with extensive calcification *(arrow)* that results from the tumor being comprised of an osteoid core and osteoblastic tissue. B, Desmoplastic round-cell tumor of the kidney showing a well-circumscribed low-density mass in the left kidney with punctate calcifications *(arrow)* in a 6-year-old child who was being evaluated for hematuria.

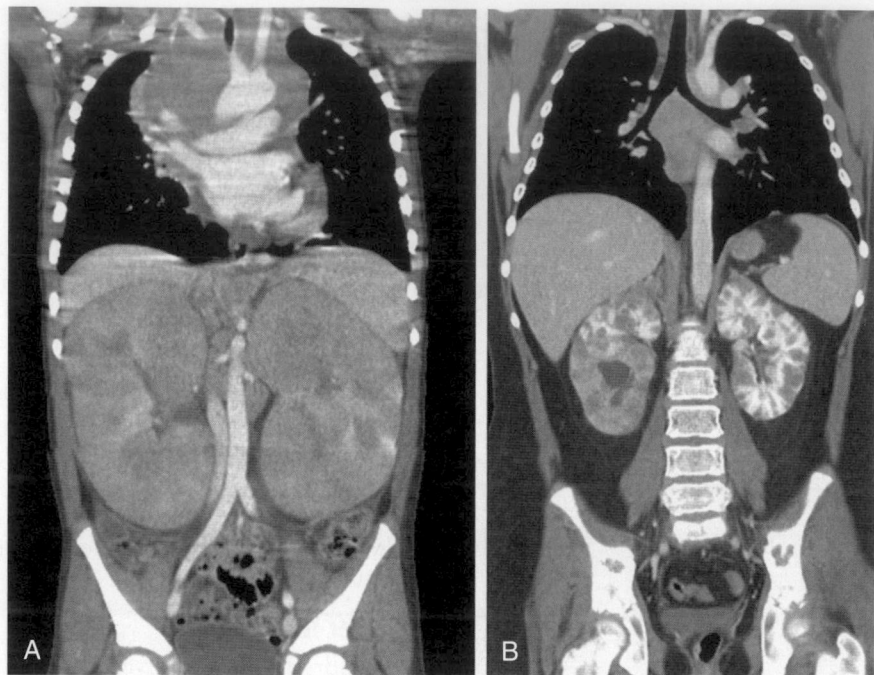

Figure 66-77 Renal involvement with leukemia and lymphoma. **A,** Diffuse renal enlargement and infiltration of the kidneys in a 6-year-old patient with T-cell lymphoblastic leukemia. This patient also had a large mediastinal mass at presentation. **B,** A 12-year-old patient with diffuse large B-cell lymphoma showing multifocal renal involvement as well as a mediastinal mass. Extensive bone involvement, seen under bone windows, is less evident here.

defects in the bladder, diminished bladder volume, and depending on the size and location of the lesion, obstruction to the flow of urine.

Contrast-enhanced CT scanning early after contrast infusion, after bladder filling, and after delayed bladder filling is helpful to assess the degree of local invasion. MRI, however, is preferable to characterize the lesion in multiple planes and to evaluate spread into adjacent pelvic organs and neurovascular structures.[280] Rhabdomyosarcomas typically show intermediate signal intensity on T1-weighted images with increased signal on T2-weighted images and heterogeneous or minimal enhancement on postcontrast images (Fig. 66-78). The imaging evaluation should be directed at assessing for local tumor extension into adjacent pelvic fat planes, adjacent lymph node enlargement, and involvement of the perivesical fat and adjacent musculature. Multiplanar fast-spin echo (FSE)–T2-weighted images with and without fat suppression are well-suited for detecting invasion of adjacent deep pelvic structures.

As with other rhabdomyosarcomas, metastases to the liver, bone, bone marrow, and lung occur, and the staging evaluation should include chest CT and bone scintigraphy. The role of FDG-PET in imaging rhabdomyosarcomas has not been the focus of any controlled prospective trials, but it has been observed[182,184,281] that rhabdomyosarcomas are usually FDG avid and that FDG-PET imaging can play in important role in identifying sites of occult disease, monitoring responses to therapy, and in evaluating equivocal foci of disease, either locally or at metastatic sites, that are identified by CT or MRI.[182]

ADRENAL/SUPRARENAL TUMORS

Neuroblastomas

Neuroblastomas are the most common non-CNS pediatric solid tumors and the third most common pediatric malignancy after leukemia and CNS tumors.[164,166] Greater than 90% of the cases occur in children younger than 5 years of age. Patients with neuroblastoma often have a painless abdominal mass. The most common site of origin is the retroperitoneum (adrenal gland), with other sites of origin in the posterior mediastinum, neck, and pelvis (at the level of the iliac bifurcation, the organ of Zuckerkandl).[164] Symptoms at presentation may also result from compression of adjacent organs, extension into the spinal canal, vascular compression/invasion, and bone involvement. Hypertension is seen in about 10% of patients and is caused by elevated catecholamine production. Paraneoplastic syndromes include the opsoclonus myoclonus syndrome and watery diarrhea. These symptoms commonly resolve after resection or chemotherapeutic treatment of the primary tumor.

The age and stage of disease remain the most important prognostic factors in neuroblastoma.[166] Infants (younger than 1 year of age) with localized disease have the highest rates of cure. Older patients with metastatic disease continue to be the most challenging population of patients to treat. The most widely-used staging system for neuroblastoma is the INSS (Table 66-3).[282,283] This involves a combination of radiographic, scintigraphic, surgical findings, and bone-marrow evaluation. Lower-stage disease is characterized by localized tumor involvement, whereas infiltration across the midline and/or

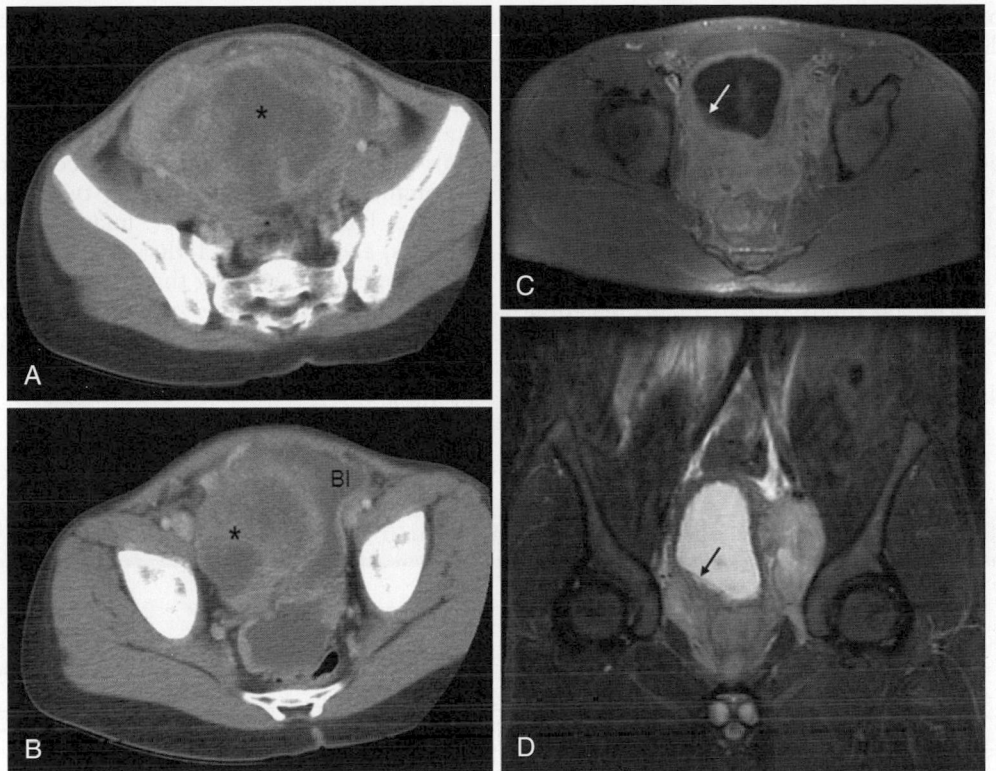

Figure 66-78 Rhabdomyosarcomas of the bladder and prostate. CT (**A** and **B**) shows large exophytic mass *(asterisk)* arising from the bladder wall and compressing the bladder lumen *(Bl)*. Contrast-enhanced (**C**) and FSEIR (**D**) MRI images show invasion of the bladder wall by prostatic rhabdomyosarcoma *(arrow)* showing the value of MRI over CT at demonstrating extent of invasion in the pelvis.

TABLE 66-3   Childhood Neuroblastoma: International Neuroblastoma Staging System[282,283]

Tumor Stage	Description
1	Localized tumor with complete gross excision with or without microscopic residual disease. Representative ipsilateral lymph nodes separate from the primary tumor are negative for tumor microscopically.
2A	Localized tumor with incomplete gross excision. Representative ipsilateral nonadherent lymph nodes are negative for tumor.
2B	Localized tumor with or without complete gross excision. Ipsilateral nonadherent lymph nodes are positive for tumor. Enlarged contralateral lymph nodes must be negative microscopically.
3	Unresectable unilateral tumor infiltrating across the midline, with or without regional lymph node involvement, or Localized unilateral tumor with contralateral regional lymph node involvement, or Midline tumor with bilateral extension by infiltration (unresectable) or by lymph node involvement. The midline is defined as the vertebral column.
4	Any primary tumor with dissemination to distant lymph nodes, bone, bone marrow, liver, skin, and/or other organs except as defined for stage 4S.

4S	Localized primary tumor as defined for stage 1, 2A, or 2B, and:
	    Dissemination limited to skin, liver, and/or bone marrow.
	    Limited to infants younger than 1 year.
	    Minimal marrow involvement (i.e., <10% of total nucleated cells in aspirate).
	        More extensive bone marrow involvement indicates stage 4 disease.
	    MIBG scan should be negative for disease in the bone marrow.

MIBG, Metaiodobenzylguanidine.

encasement of major blood vessels that results in surgical unresectability define stage 3 disease. Widespread disease with cortical bone, bone marrow, or visceral organ involvement is defined as stage 4 disease. A unique feature to the staging of patients with neuroblastoma is the category stage 4S (special), which is defined as localized primary tumor with dissemination limited to liver, skin, and less than 10% bone-marrow involvement.[166] Because current approaches to risk classification and treatment stratification for children with neuroblastoma vary greatly throughout the world the International Neuroblastoma Risk Group (INRG) classification system has recently been proposed to establish a consensus approach for pretreatment risk stratification. Disease stage, age, histo-logic category, grade of tumor differentiation, the status of the *MYCN* oncogene, chromosome 11q status, and DNA ploidy were identified the most significant factors impacting clinical outcome.[284,285] New guidelines for staging and imaging of neuroblastoma have also been proposed as a result of the INRG recommendations, with recommendations for reporting two stages of localized disease based on whether image-defined risk factors (IDRFs) are present.[286] IDRFs are imaging findings based on preoperative imaging that are likely to impact surgical management, including success of gross total resection and risk of postoperative complications. A summary of the INRG imaging recommendations and IDRFs is shown in Table 66-4.

TABLE 66-4   International Neuroblastoma Risk Group Classification and Image-Defined Risk Factors

Descriptions of New International Neuroblastoma Risk Group Tumor Stages[286]

Tumor Stage	Description*
L1	Localized tumor not involving vital structures as defined by the list of IDRFs and confined to one body compartment.
L2	Local-regional tumor with presence of one or more IDRFs.
M	Distant metastatic disease (except stage MS tumor).
MS	Metastatic disease in children younger than 18 months with metastases confined to skin, liver, and/or bone marrow.

Descriptions of IDRFs†[286]

Anatomic Region	Description
Multiple body compartments	Ipsilateral tumor extension within two body compartments (i.e., neck and chest, chest and abdomen, or abdomen and pelvis).
Neck	Tumor encasing carotid artery, vertebral artery, and/or internal jugular vein. Tumor extending to skull base. Tumor compressing trachea.
Cervicothoracic junction	Tumor encasing brachial plexus roots. Tumor encasing subclavian vessels, vertebral artery, and/or carotid artery. Tumor compressing trachea.
Thorax	Tumor encasing aorta and/or major branches. Tumor compressing trachea and/or principal bronchi. Lower mediastinal tumor infiltrating costovertebral junction between T9 and T12 vertebral levels.
Thoracoabdominal junction	Tumor encasing aorta and/or vena cava.
Abdomen and pelvis	Tumor infiltrating porta hepatis and/or hepatoduodenal ligament. Tumor encasing branches of superior mesenteric artery at mesenteric root. Tumor encasing origin of celiac axis and/or origin of superior mesenteric artery. Tumor invading one or both renal pedicles. Tumor encasing aorta and/or vena cava. Tumor encasing iliac vessels. Pelvic tumor crossing sciatic notch.
Intraspinal tumor extension	Intraspinal tumor extension (any location), provided that more than one third of spinal canal in axial plane is invaded, the perimedullary leptomeningeal spaces are not visible, or the spinal cord signal intensity is abnormal.
Infiltration of adjacent organs and structures	Pericardium, diaphragm, kidney, liver, duodenopancreatic block, and mesentery.

From References 285 and 286.
IDRF, Image-defined risk factors.
*Complete definitions of these stages are cited in the text.
†Conditions that should be recorded but are not considered IDRFs are multifocal primary tumors, pleural effusion with or without malignant cells, and ascites with or without malignant cells.

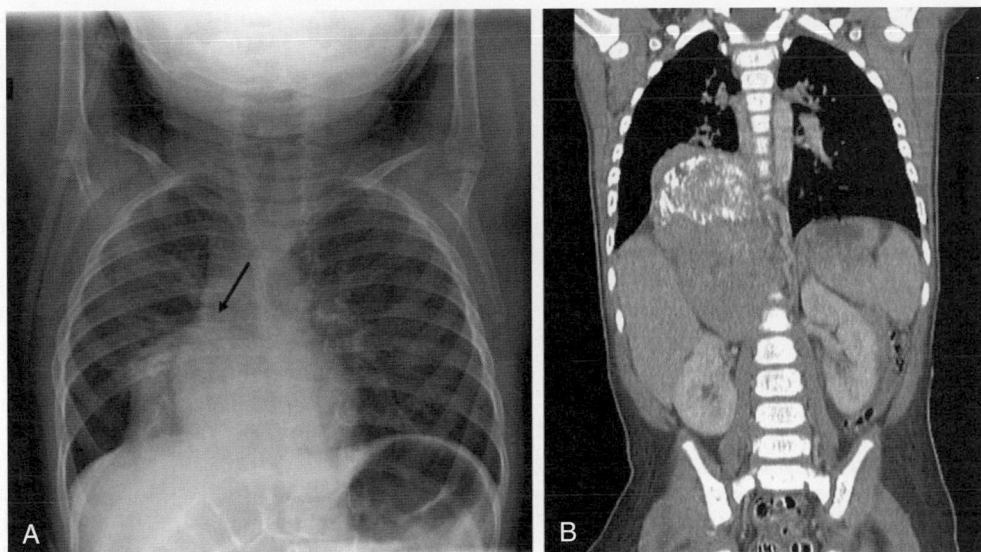

Figure 66-79 Neuroblastoma. **A,** Chest x-ray demonstrates calcified mass at the right lung base, seen on the lateral film to be posterior mediastinal (not shown). **B,** Coronal reconstructions from contrast-enhanced CT reveal a large, calcified right suprarenal mass with extension across the midline and into the thorax.

The initial imaging modalities used in evaluating patients with neuroblastoma are directed at the presenting symptoms. Abdominal films, chest radiographs, and skeletal films are usually obtained to assess abdominal distension, suspected pneumonia, or limp/extremity pain (see Figs 66-1 and 66-3; Fig. 66-79). Ultrasound is widely available and should be the first choice in evaluating a child with a suspected abdominal mass. Depending on the size of the mass, ultrasound can effectively demonstrate the presence of a retroperitoneal or suprarenal mass (Fig. 66-80) and is both sensitive and specific at evaluating for the presence of hepatic metastatic disease and localized vascular invasion. Calcifications are common in neuroblastoma and are seen sonographically as areas of acoustic shadowing. Depending on the age and size of the patient, intraspinal extension can also be detected.

CT scanning is widely used for defining the extent of primary tumor involvement and particularly with multiplanar reconstructions has become critical in the staging and surgical planning for patients with neuroblastoma (Fig. 66-81). The use of intravenous and oral contrast is essential in this evaluation, and scanning should include the chest, abdomen, and pelvis. The presence of intraspinal extension can often be detected by CT scanning; however, MRI is considered superior to CT in characterizing epidural extension or leptomeningeal spread of disease.[91] MRI, particularly with the advent of faster, whole-body scanning techniques together with diffusion weighted imaging, has also been advocated for use in determining extent of bone-marrow involvement.[167,287] In addition, MRI is effective in identifying unsuspected sites of bone and bone-marrow disease (Fig. 66-82), some of which may also be delineated by MIBG scintigraphy. MRI should also be considered for the monitoring of infants and children with low-risk disease, in whom treatment does not routinely involve radiotherapy and for

whom reduction in radiation exposure is desirable. Guidelines for incorporating CT and MRI findings into the new INRG specifications for IDRFs have been published (see Table 66-4).[286]

The staging and monitoring of patients with neuroblastoma also depends on the use of scintigraphic studies, including bone scanning and MIBG scintigraphy. ^{99m}Tc-MDP scintigraphy has historically been used to detect the presence of cortical bone metastases and has been shown to be superior to conventional radiography,[91] although with current multimodality imaging and staging protocols, it is not clear that bone-scan findings impact the clinical stage of the majority of patient over the age of 1 year (see Fig. 66-77, C). MIBG is a catecholamine analogue taken up by neuroblastoma cells. ^{123}I-MIBG has been used to localize neuroblastoma at primary sites (Fig. 66-83), as well as in bone, bone marrow, and lymph nodes, and is effective in identifying sites of disease in more than 90% of the patients.[91,288] In particular, sites of previously unsuspected disease in the bone marrow are effectively detected by MIBG. Normal uptake by the liver, however, does limit the use of MIBG in detecting small foci of hepatic disease, and uptake by normal adrenal tissue after contralateral adrenalectomy may make postoperative follow-up observation challenging. Nonetheless, the relative sensitivity and specificity of MIBG for detecting disease not evident by other techniques has led most investigators to routinely include MIBG scintigraphy in the diagnostic and posttreatment evaluation of neuroblastoma patients.[289,290]

Although large controlled studies are lacking, a number of smaller consortium studies have shown that MIBG scanning at the time of staging has prognostic significance and that early response to therapy as detected by MIBG scintigraphy correlates with overall response and event-free survival.[291-295,296] As a result, MIBG scoring systems have been proposed to allow enumeration of the number

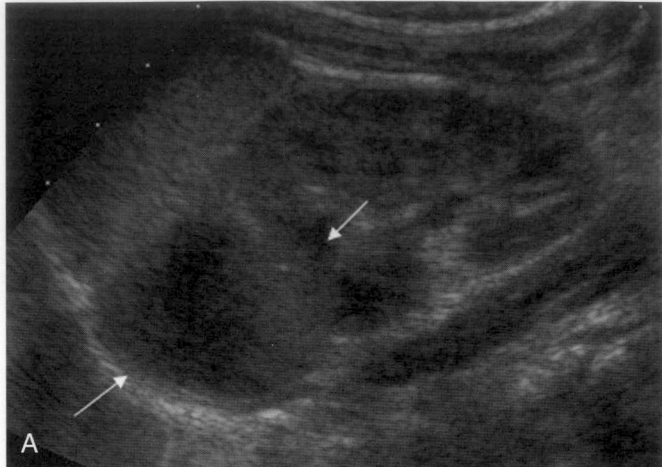

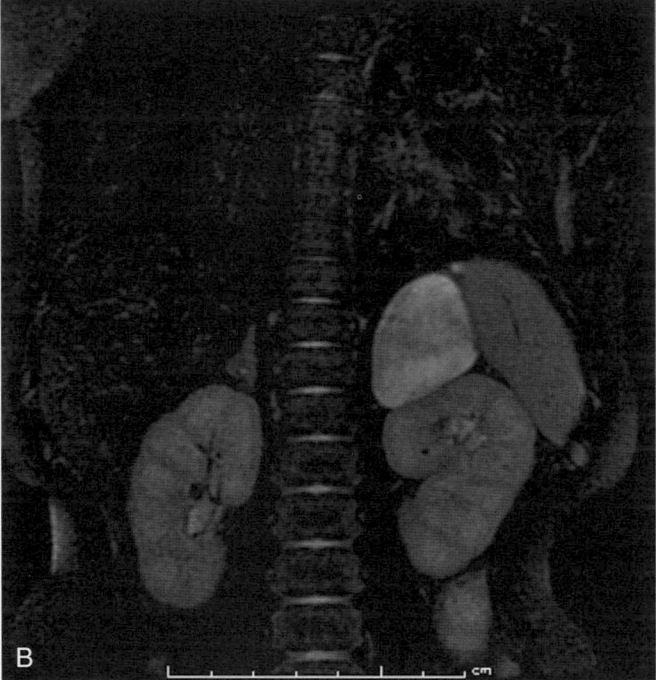

Figure 66-80 Neuroblastoma. Scans are of a 2-month-old infant being evaluated for vomiting. **A,** Ultrasound to assess for pyloric stenosis showed a well defined left suprarenal mass *(arrows)* confirmed by MRI **(B).**

of MIBG disease foci extent of MIBG avid disease, and have been used as a semi-quantitative means of monitoring responses to therapy, with good correlation with overall clinical response.[295,297,298]

FDG-PET imaging, although commonly used for many other tumor types, has not gained universal acceptance in the staging and follow-up evaluation of patients with neuroblastoma. PET scanning allows increased sensitivity and higher spatial resolution for disease detection.[70,299,300] However, discordant patterns of uptake,[169] combined with the general acceptance of MIBG scintigraphy and cross-sectional imaging for staging and response assessment, have resulted in the slow acceptance of FDG-PET in evaluation of patients with neuroblastoma.[91,169,301] Larger studies are needed to directly compare the sensitiv-

ity and specificity of FDG-PET with MIBG to determine the efficacy of FDG-PET imaging in the staging and post-treatment evaluation of patients with neuroblastoma.

Radiolabeled monoclonal antibodies, labeled with ^{131}I, ^{123}I, ^{99m}Tc, and ^{64}Cu, have all been used in both animal models and clinical models of neuroblastoma.[74,302,303] The antibodies upon which these imaging agents are based have mainly been directed against the disialoganglioside GD2, which has increased expression in neuroblastoma, and these same antibodies have been used clinically to treat patients with advanced stage disease.[304] However, the routine use of radioimmunodetection has still remained investigational in neuroblastoma patients.

Stage 4S neuroblastoma is unique among pediatric neoplasms. Identified in the early 1970s,[305] patients with this stage were identified as a "special" group with widespread neuroblastoma who had a favorable outcome. Criteria for defining these patients varied initially amongst cooperative groups. Currently, INSS stage 4S criteria include age younger than 1 year (increased to 18 months by the INRG) and localized primary tumor (not infiltrating across the midline and no contralateral lymph node involvement). Sites of metastatic involvement may include liver, skin, and bone marrow (less than 10% involvement). Patients with stage 4S disease comprise approximately 7% to 12% of all neuroblastoma cases, and despite extensive hepatic and primary site involvement, these tumors may completely resolve with observation alone and no additional chemotherapy (Fig. 66-84).

The importance of prenatal detection of neuroblastoma has also been emphasized recently in a study by Blackman, et al, in which a prenatal ultrasound and subsequent prenatal MRI delineated a large paraspinal mass.[306] In this case, the detection of spinal-cord compression by MRI combined with decreased fetal movement led to a rapid delivery, biopsy, further staging, and early initiation of treatment, which resulted in tumor response and preservation of lower-extremity neurologic function.

The opsoclonus myoclonus ataxia (OMA) syndrome is a paraneoplastic neurologic syndrome that has been associated with an occult neuroblastoma in up to 40% to 50% of patients.[307,308] Often the primary tumors associated with OMA syndrome are small, localized, and either paraspinal or extraabdominal. The identification of sites of disease is important, because symptoms may diminish or even resolve upon identification and treatment/resection of the neuroblastoma.[309,310] The imaging of patients with suspected OMA syndrome should include imaging of the chest, abdomen, and pelvis either by MRI or CT, as well as MIBG scintigraphy (Fig. 66-85).[91,311] MIBG scanning in particular has been shown to be both sensitive and specific for revealing occult neuroblastoma in patients with the OMA syndrome,[312] although with the availability of whole-body MRI, which affords a sensitive means of identifying sites of occult disease in a single examination, there is likely to be a shift in favor of whole-body MR screening for patients with OMA syndrome.

The distinction between neuroblastoma and its more differentiated counterparts ganglioneuroblastoma and ganglioneuroma cannot be made on the basis of imaging

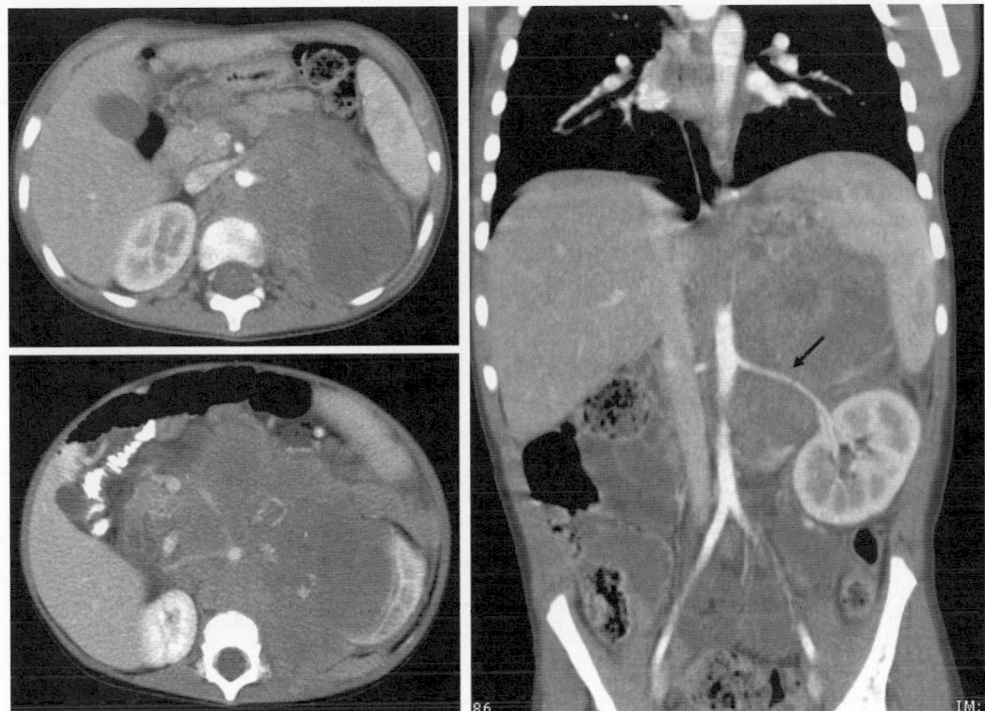

Figure 66-81 Neuroblastoma. Contrast-enhanced CT showing bulky retroperitoneal masses in two patients with encasement of vessels and extension across midline. Coronal reconstruction shows inferior displacement of the left kidney by the mass and demonstrate traction on the left renal artery *(arrow)*, which often leads to hypertension in such patients.

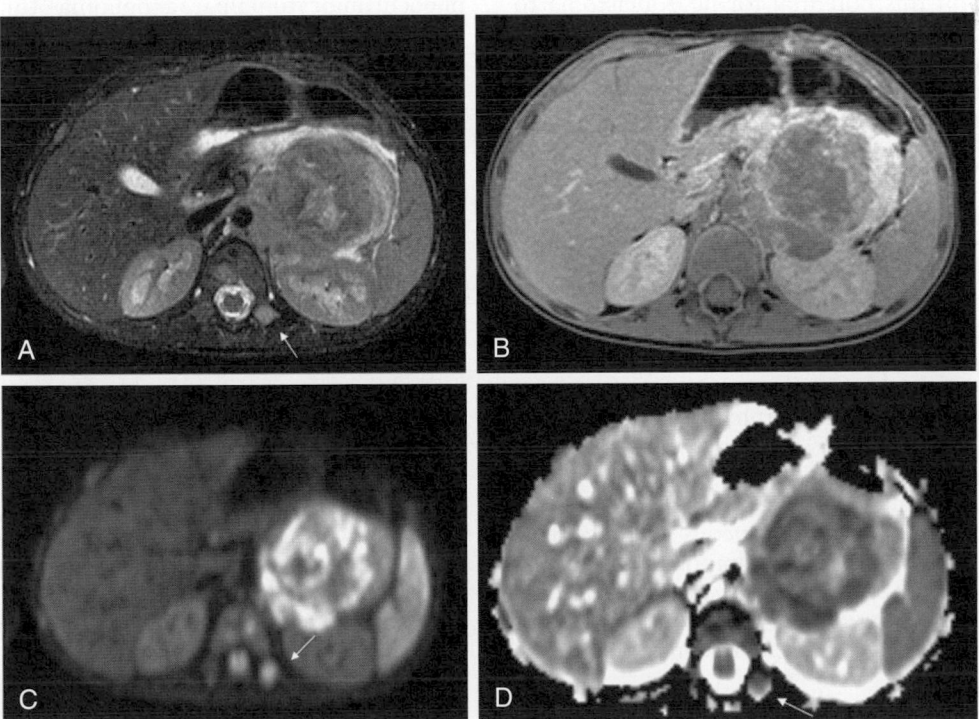

Figure 66-82 Stage 4 neuroblastoma. MRI shows left upper quadrant/retroperitoneal mass on T2-weighted (**A**) and post-Gd T1-weighted imaging (**B**). Diffusion-weighted imaging (**C**) and apparent diffusion coefficient (ADC) map (**D**) also reveal a focus of bone/bone-marrow involvement in the adjacent left vertebral pedicle *(arrow)* that is present but less conspicuous on the T2-weighted images and not seen on the post-Gd images.

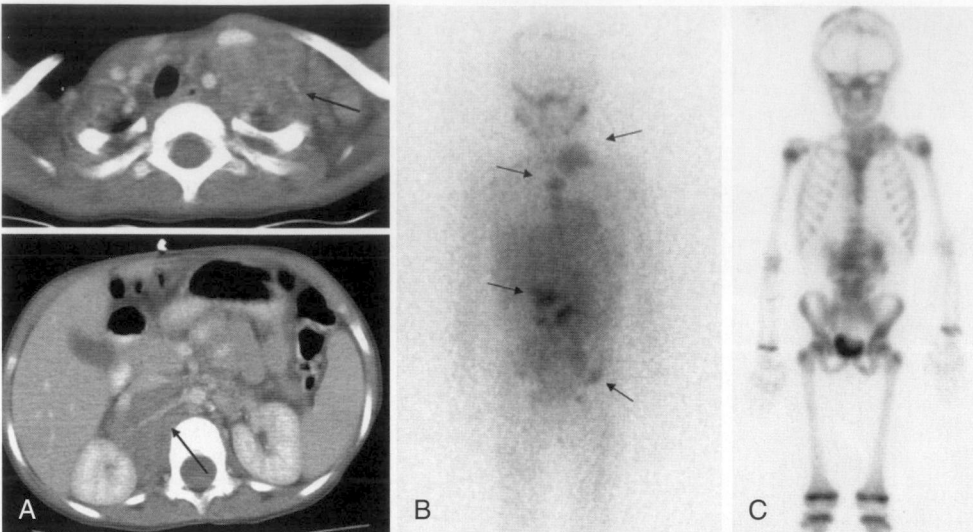

Figure 66-83 Neuroblastoma. Contrast enhanced CT (**A**) and MIBG (**B**) in a 5-year-old child showing intraabdominal, left supraclavicular, left acetabular, skull, and vertebral disease *(arrows)*. The thoracic vertebral disease is readily seen by MIBG but is not evident on CT. MDP bone scintigraphy (**C**) shows concordant uptake at most of these sites but does not reveal any additional sites of bone involvement; identifying additional sites would not have affected disease stage in this patient with stage 4 disease.

features alone.[164] Ganglioneuroma by definition shows completely differentiated stromal and cellular elements, with neuroblastoma containing less than 50% differentiated elements, and ganglioneuroblastoma intermediate between the two. Often patients who have responded to therapy will have residual lesions that remain MIBG avid and on biopsy are shown to be differentiated ganglioneuroma. In fact, novel treatment approaches are aimed at taking advantage of this potential for neuroblastoma to undergo differentiation, with cis-retinoic acid and its derivatives being used in an effort to accelerate the pathway toward differentiation.[313] Although biopsy/surgical resection is ultimately required to confirm the diagnosis, ganglioneuromas and ganglioneuroblastomas tend to be localized, with the most common sites of disease in the posterior mediastinum and retroperitoneum (Fig. 66-86). The age at presentation is also typically older than patients with neuroblastoma. Ganglioneuroma, like ganglioneuroblastoma and neuroblastoma, may accumulate MIBG, and MIBG uptake cannot be used to effectively discriminate between these distinct histopathologic entities.[314] Calcifications are often seen by CT and conventional radiography (see Fig. 66-86), and similar MRI appearances are seen with all three histopathologic types, with low signal intensity on T1-weighted images, intermediate to high signal intensity on T2-weighted images, and heterogeneous enhancement after gadolinium infusion. It is also important to recognize that sampling error can result after biopsy, and complete resection, if feasible, ensures a thorough sampling of the tumor specimen and a more confident diagnosis of ganglioneuroma.

Pheochromocytomas and Paragangliomas

Pheochromocytomas are rare pediatric tumors. They arise from chromaffin cells in the adrenal medulla or from cells of the extraadrenal sympathetic nervous system, where they are known as *paragangliomas*. In children these tumors are diagnosed from childhood to early adolescence, with a peak age range between 6 and 15 years. There is an increased incidence of pheochromocytoma in certain hereditary syndromes including the MEN syndromes IIA and IIB, von Hippel-Lindau disease, and neurofibromatosis type 1 (NF1). More recently pheochromocytoma/paraganglioma tumors have been associated with mutations in the succinate dehydrogenase gene family (*SDHB* and *SDHD*). The majority of these tumors (more than 80%) are located in the adrenal gland, with an increased likelihood of bilateral adrenal involvement in patients with MENII and von Hippel-Lindau disease.[315,316] Approximately 80% of patients have symptoms related to increased secretion of catecholamines, including sustained hypertension, headache, palpitations, anxiety, fatigue, and chest pain. Although these tumors are most often identified during the evaluation of clinical symptoms, they may also be discovered incidentally. The imaging features of pheochromocytoma are variable,[315] and while primary adrenal tumors are classically described on MRI as being hyperintense on T2-weighted images, low signal on T1 sequences, and showing a "salt and pepper" pattern of enhancement after contrast administration (Fig. 66-87),[315,317] these imaging characteristics are by no means specific for pheochromocytoma. ^{123}I-MIBG scintigraphy shows high specificity for pheochromocytoma and can be used to both identify lesions not seen by CT or MRI or to confirm the identity of abnormalities detected by cross-sectional imaging in patients with symptoms of catecholamine excess.[316,318] ^{18}F-dihydroxyphenylalanine (DOPA) PET and ^{18}F-fluorodopamine have both been shown to be superior to ^{123}I-MIBG, with greater sensitivity in detecting sites of metastatic disease,[319,320] although these agents are not in

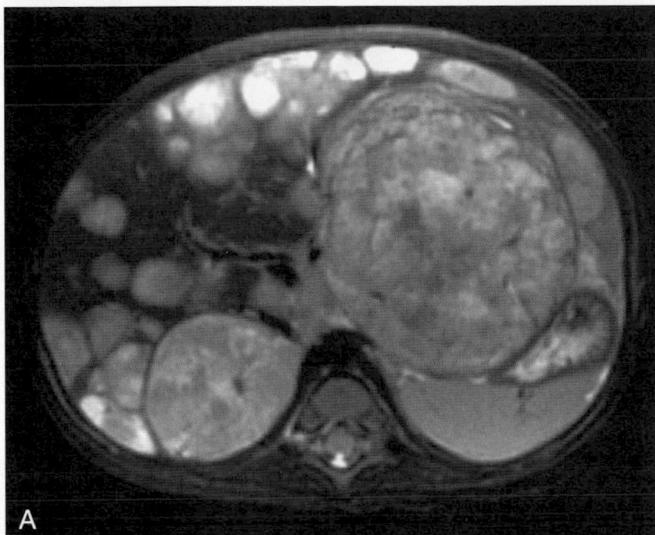

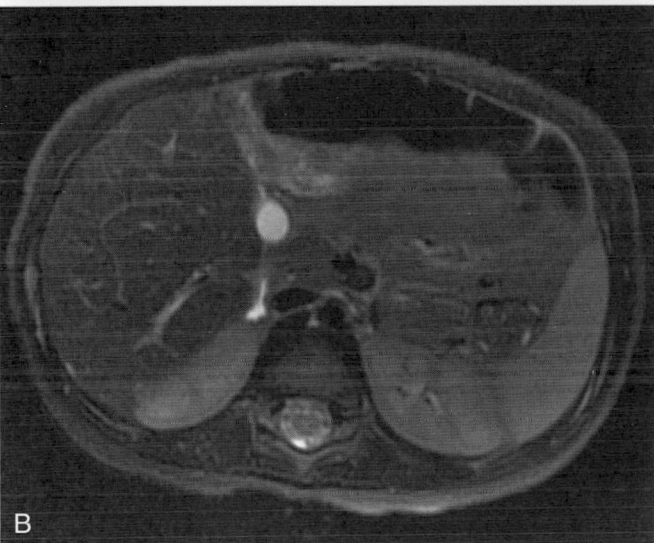

Figure 66-84 Stage 4S neuroblastoma. The patient is a 6-month-old baby with an abdominal mass. **A,** MRI shows extensive liver involvement. The infant was shown to have stage 4S disease. **B,** After 7 months of observation only and no chemotherapy, a repeat MRI shows near complete resolution of disease. This child continues with observation only.

routine use in the management of pediatric pheochromocytoma. Metastases are relatively uncommon in children (≈12%),[316] with the majority of patients having localized disease amenable to surgical resection. Higher rates of malignancy are seen in syndromic patients. Outcome is related to the presence and location of metastatic disease, with 5-year overall survival rates reported to be as high as 60% to 78% in patients with malignant metastatic tumors.[316]

GERM-CELL TUMORS

Gonadal and extragonadal germ-cell tumors are relatively rare in children, representing only about 1% of the tumors diagnosed in children under the age of 15 years.

The most common extragonadal sites of disease in older children are the mediastinum and brain, and these tumors are discussed separately in those respective sections. Sacrococcygeal germ teratomas are the most common germ-cell tumors occurring in infancy and account for approximately 40% of all teratomas identified in children.

Ovarian Germ-Cell Tumors

Ovarian germ-cell tumors include both benign and malignant neoplasms.[279] The majority of the ovarian tumors are benign, with the most common tumor being the mature cystic teratoma/dermoid cyst. Malignant ovarian tumors include neoplasms of both stromal- and germ-cell origin, the former including Sertoli-Leydig cell tumors, granulosa thecal-cell tumors, and undifferentiated stromal tumors. Malignant ovarian tumors of germ-cell origin include dysgerminomas, immature teratomas, endodermal sinus tumors, embryonal carcinomas, and choriocarcinomas.

The imaging evaluation of malignant ovarian germ-cell tumors should be directed at characterizing the primary lesion and identifying possible sites of metastatic spread of disease. Ultrasound is usually the first imaging study performed to identify and characterize a suspected primary ovarian and/or pelvic mass.[321] Ultrasound reliably distinguishes between cystic and solid lesions and is helpful to assess blood flow to the lesion. The presence of associated ascites may also aid in the differential diagnosis. Additional evaluation by MRI and/or CT is typically performed as needed to further characterize the primary lesion and to assess for locoregional and metastatic spread of disease.

Sonographically the benign/mature cystic teratoma may be a homogeneous echogenic mass or alternatively a predominantly fluid-filled mass with an echogenic mural nodule. The presence of fat, calcification, or fat-fluid levels are all common findings in mature cystic teratoma (Fig. 66-88).[279] Large masses may be better characterized by CT and MRI, with CT scanning showing low-density lesions of fat density and heterogeneous enhancement of the solid components. Calcifications, particularly microcalcifications, are effectively identified by CT.

The MRI findings are variable depending on the characteristics and tissue composition of the teratomatous elements.[321] Typically mature teratomas have areas of both high and low signal on both T1- and T2-weighted images, with suppression of signal on fat-suppressed T1-weighted sequences. As shown in Figure 66-88, the presence of calcification, teeth, or hair may be useful in confirming the diagnosis. Even in the presence of mature elements, surgical resection is indicated, because the imaging features cannot clearly discriminate between malignant components of mixed germ-cell tumors and the entirely benign mature counterparts. The presence of lymph node involvement, extension into contiguous organs/structures, hematogenous spread, and evidence of peritoneal/omental seeding all should suggest the presence of malignant disease.[279]

It is important to correlate the imaging findings with the age of the patient. Functional ovarian neoplasms such

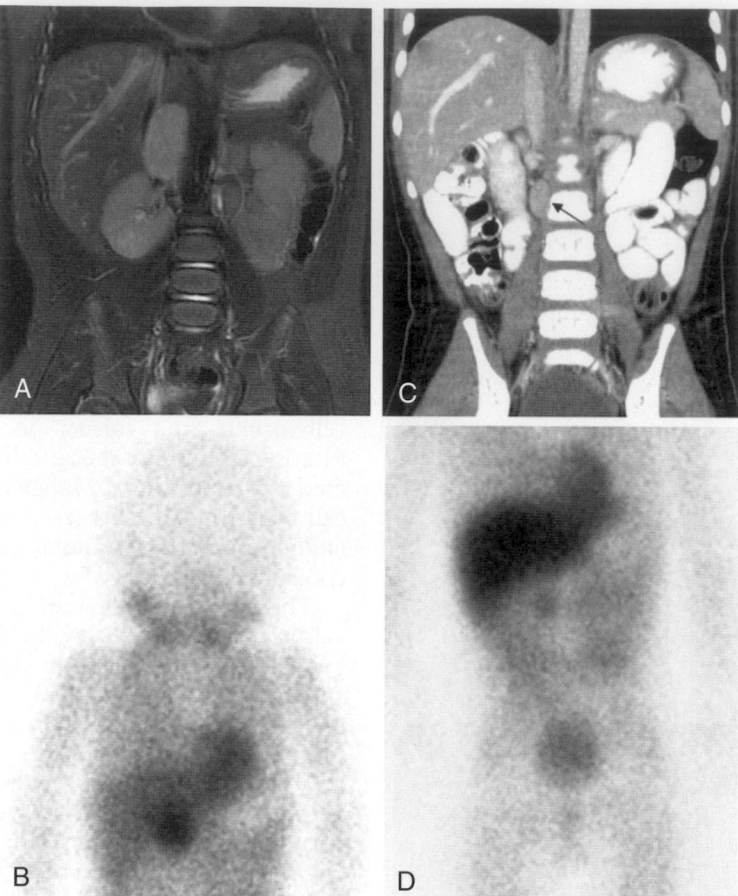

Figure 66-85 Two patients, ages 13 months (**A** and **B**) and 28 mo (**C** and **D**) with OMA syndrome secondary to occult neuroblastoma. MRI (**A**) and CT (**C**) show a right suprarenal mass (**A**) and subtle retroperitoneal lesion (**C**, *arrow*), both of which show focal MIBG uptake (**B** and **D**).

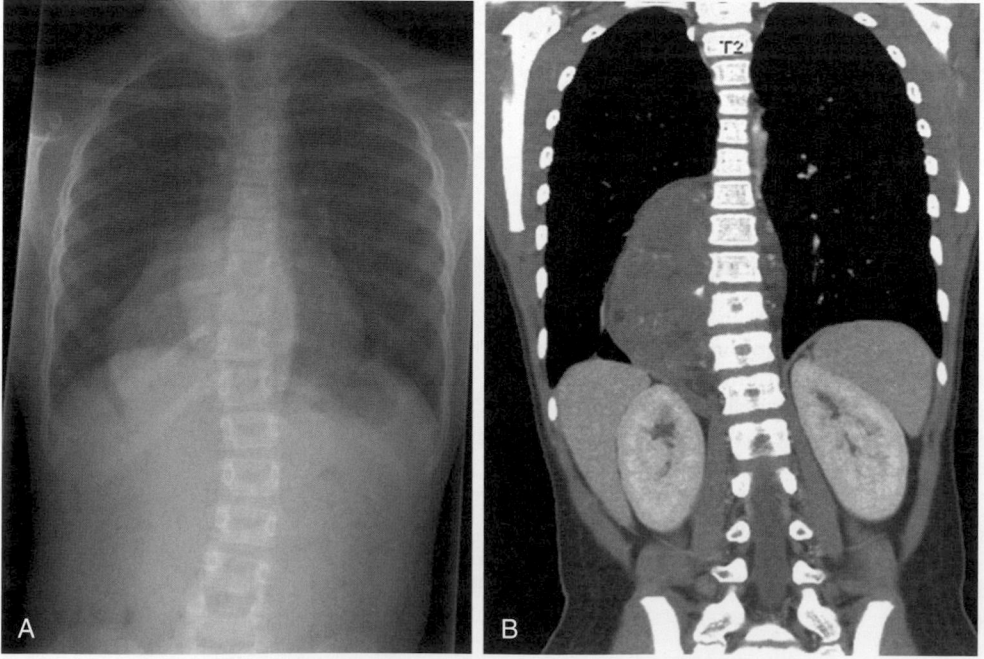

Figure 66-86 Ganglioneuroma in a 9-year-old child with back pain and scoliosis. Spine radiographs (**A**) and subsequent CT (**B**) showed a large paraspinal mass with calcifications also evident on CT. There was only faint MIBG uptake in the periphery of the mass (not shown), findings characteristic of mature ganglioneuroma.

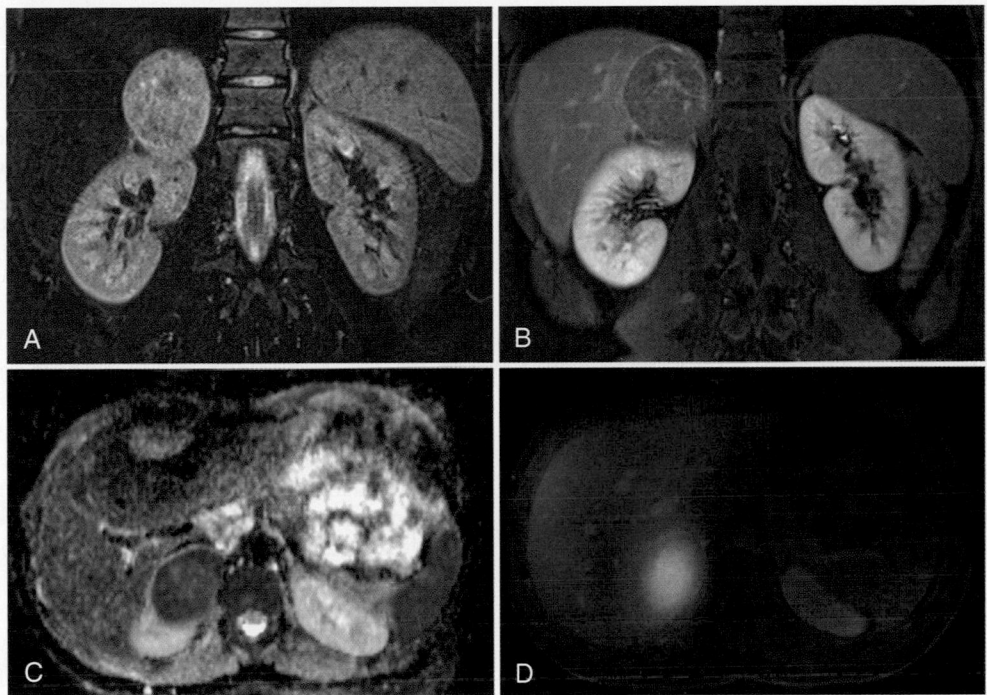

Figure 66-87 A 15-year-old patient with NF1 and an adrenal lesion detected on spine MRI. Coronal fat-suppressed T2-weighted (FSEIR) (**A**) and post-Gd fat-suppressed T1-weighted (**B**) images show a T2-bright lesion with a speckled ("salt & pepper") pattern of enhancement characteristic of pheochromocytoma. **C,** A DWI ADC map shows that the lesion has highly restricted diffusion. **D,** MIBG scintigraphy with SPECT images fused to the MRI show intense MIBG uptake in the lesion.

as granulosa thecal cell tumors may result in precocious puberty and sonographic findings that are discordant with the patient's age (Fig. 66-89). Correlation with serum hormone levels, AFP levels, and β human chorionic gonadotropin (HCG) levels is an important adjunct to the imaging evaluation.

The distinction between neoplastic masses of the ovary and nonneoplastic cysts, particularly hemorrhagic cysts, may be difficult. Nonneoplastic cysts are the most common etiologies for ovarian masses in infants and adolescent girls.[279,322] These hormonally responsive lesions arise as a result of follicular stimulation and corpus luteal maturation. Serial imaging by ultrasound is helpful in documenting stability and/or resolution of these benign processes and in making the distinction from their malignant neoplastic counterparts. Complex cysts and hemorrhagic cysts may be challenging to distinguish from solid neoplasms, and MRI with inclusion of fat suppression and magnetic susceptibility-weighted sequences can be helpful in discriminating fat-containing solid masses from complex hemorrhagic cysts.

Testicular Germ-Cell Tumors

Malignant testicular tumors are primarily of germ-cell origin, with the majority of these being malignant. The most common malignant testicular germ-cell tumor is the yolk sac, or endodermal sinus, tumor. Other malignant germ-cell tumors include embryonal carcinoma and teratocarcinoma. The benign teratomas seen more often in the ovary are less commonly encountered in the testes. Adult-type tumors such as seminomas and choriocarci-

nomas are less commonly encountered in infancy and begin to emerge around the time of puberty.[279]

Most testicular masses present with nontender scrotal swelling. Elevated serum AFP levels are common, and there is often spread to adjacent inguinal and retroperitoneal lymph nodes. The initial evaluation is usually by ultrasound to assess for the presence of a testicular mass and to distinguish between malignancy and nonneoplastic causes of scrotal swelling such as epididymorchitis, inguinal hernia or hydrocele, and testicular torsion. Sonographic features include an intratesticular mass with either increased or decreased echogenicity relative to the testicular parenchyma (Fig. 66-90). Color and Doppler assessments often reveal increased vascularity. The presence of an associated hydrocele, thickening of the spermatic cord, and extension of the mass through the tunica albuginea may indicate extratesticular spread of disease.[279] Once a mass has been confirmed, the staging evaluation should include imaging of the chest, abdomen, and pelvis to assess for regional lymph node spread and evidence of hematogenous disease spread, particularly to the liver and lungs.

FDG-PET imaging has been advocated in both the staging and follow-up evaluation of patients with malignant germ-cell tumors, with several studies showing the effectiveness of FDG-PET in identifying sites of disease that would otherwise have escaped detection on conventional cross-sectional imaging alone.[323-325] However, FDG-PET is unlikely to replace retroperitoneal lymph node sampling because of limitations in detecting small foci of disease.[326] In the only large prospective study

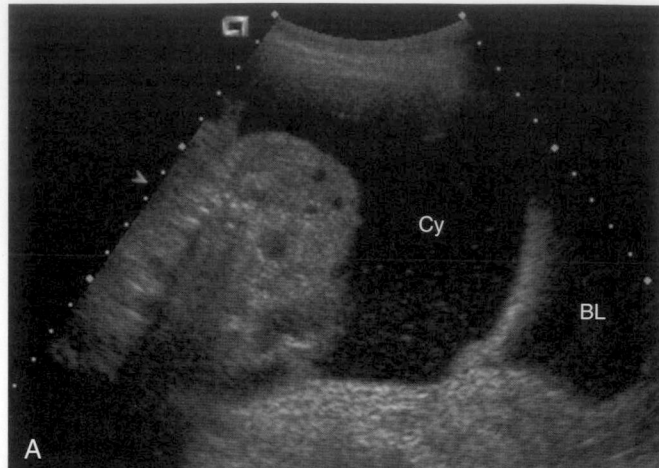

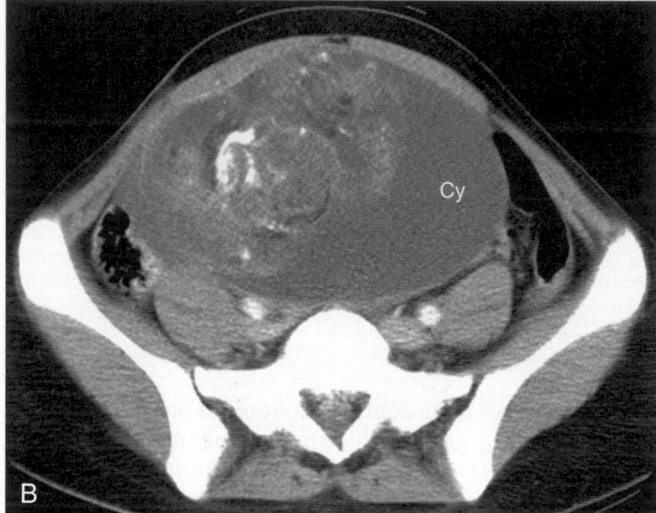

Figure 66-88 Mixed ovarian germ-cell tumor. Ultrasound shows a complex cystic and solid mass (**A**) that on CT showed areas of calcification within the solid mass (**B**), typical of germ-cell tumors.

available, posttherapy surveillance imaging with FDG-PET in patients with nonseminomatous germ-cell tumors did not confer a clinical benefit over CT and serum tumor markers for the prediction of tumor viability in residual masses.[327] Finally, there is a potential for false-negative findings on FDG-PET, particularly in the setting of mature, differentiated teratoma.[325]

Non–germ-cell tumors of the testes include Sertoli- and Leydig-cell tumors, both of stromal origin, as well as leukemia and lymphoma. Sertoli-cell tumors are more common in infancy, with Leydig-cell tumors occurring in early childhood and often accompanied by virilization or gynecomastia.

Sonographically, these testicular lesions are often heterogeneous and hypoechoic relative to the normal testicular parenchyma and usually demonstrate increased blood flow. MRI is not usually required to characterize the local site of disease; however, the MRI features of these testicular lesions include decreased signal intensity on T1-weighted images relative to the normal testicular parenchyma, increased T2 signal intensity, and heteroge-

neous enhancement. As with testicular germ-cell tumors, extension into the spermatic cord as well as inguinal and retroperitoneal lymph-node involvement, can be effectively demonstrated by MRI.

In children with cryptorchid testes, the presence of an undescended testicle is considered a predisposing factor leading to development of testicular tumors in childhood. Although the increased relative risk varies between published reports, there is little dispute that the risk of testicular cancer is increased in children and men with undescended testes.

Withdrawal of maternal estrogen at birth leads to a rise in testosterone and stimulation of testicular descent. Spontaneous descent of testes into the scrotum after 1 year of age is uncommon. The imaging evaluation of children with undescended testes should include a thorough ultrasound examination, with examination of the scrotum, inguinal canal regions, retroperitoneum, and kidneys. Often undescended testes can be located in the

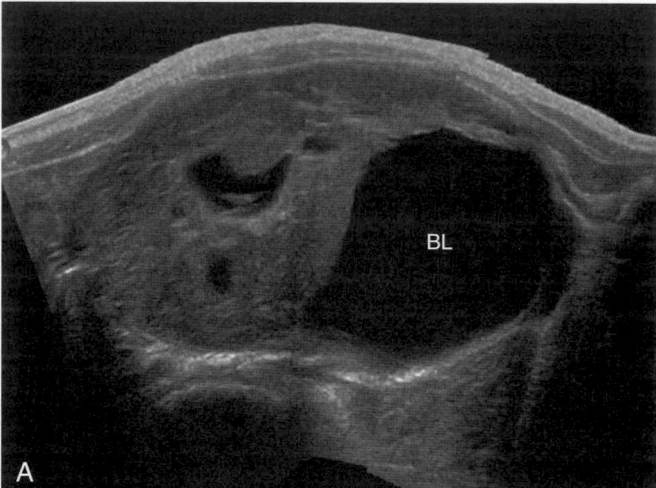

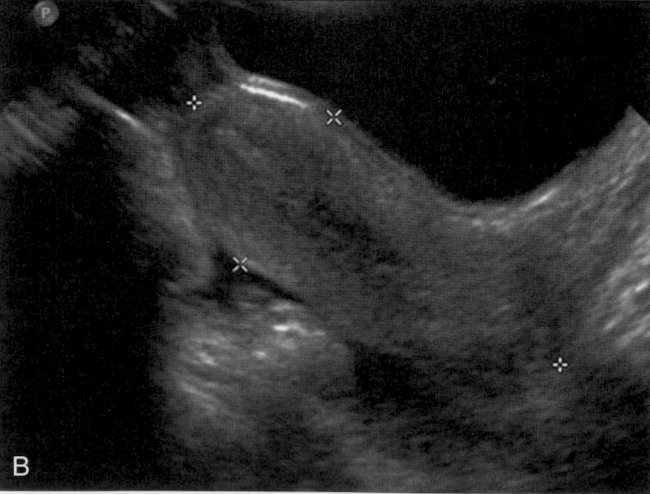

Figure 66-89 Granulosa-cell tumor. The images show a 5½-year-old child with the onset of menses. Luteinizing hormone/ follicle-stimulating hormone (LH/FSH): <0.1; estradiol: 144.5. Sagittal abdominal ultrasound image shows a mass adjacent to and above the bladder (*BL*) (**A**), likely arising from the left ovary. Note the post-pubertal appearance of the uterus (**B**), indicating a hormonally active mass.

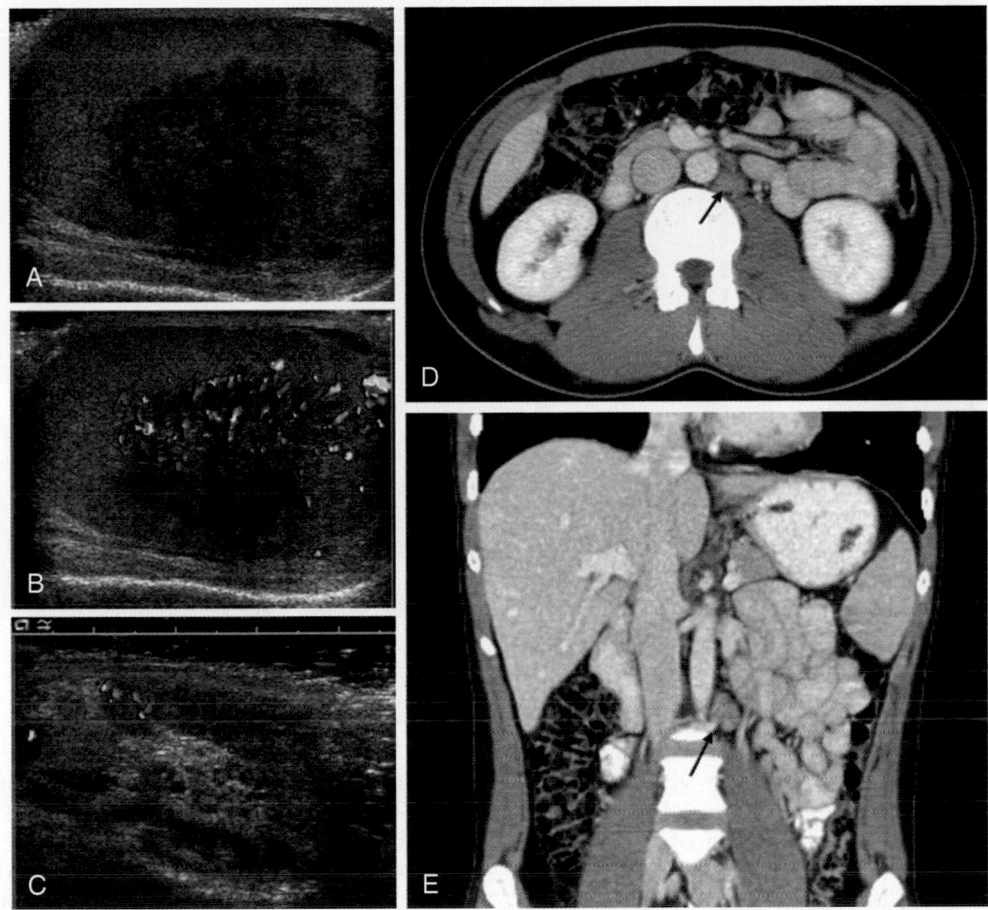

Figure 66-90 Testicular germ cell tumor (embryonal carcinoma). Images show an 18 year old patient with a palpable left testicular mass. Ultrasound shows hypoechoic mass (**A**) with increased vascularity and thickening of the epididymis and spermatic cord (**B** and **C**). A small hydrocele was also present. CT shows an enlarged left retroperitoneal lymph node that is suspicious for extratesticular spread of disease (**D** and **E**, *arrows*).

inguinal canal and effectively relocated in the scrotum by orchidopexy. The retroperitoneal location of the undescended testes, although less common, is associated with a higher risk of malignancy as compared with those located in the inguinal canal. MRI may also be helpful in identifying undescended testes not detectable by ultrasound, particularly in older children where the homogeneously T2-bright testes can often be located along the expected pathway of descent of the developing testes.

Sacrococcygeal Germ-Cell Tumors

Sacrococcygeal germ-cell tumors are the most common germ-cell tumors in children. These germ-cell neoplasms include mature and immature teratomas and endodermal sinus tumors. Both mature and immature teratomas are considered benign, whereas mixed malignant germ-cell tumors indicate the presence of both benign teratomatous elements and malignant yolk sac tumor elements. Most sacrococcygeal teratomas are detected in the newborn period, whereas yolk sac tumors may be discovered later in childhood.[328] With the advent of prenatal sonography and prenatal MRI, an extensive prebirth evaluation of the tumor is often performed, facilitating a prompt surgical resection.

Sacrococcygeal teratomas are commonly classified according to the system of Altman[329] as type I, predominantly external with a very small presacral component; type II, predominantly external with a significant intrapelvic component; type III, predominantly internal with both pelvic and intraabdominal components; and type IV, entirely presacral without significant intraabdominal or external extension. The incidence of malignant elements is closely linked to the type of tumor, with almost 40% of type IV tumors having malignant components.[279]

In addition to the prenatal imaging evaluation, both CT and MRI can be used to effectively stage sacrococcygeal teratomas.[328] MRI is preferable in determining the extent of adjacent muscular, neurovascular, and intraabdominal invasion. MRI findings also reflect the heterogeneous nature of these tumors, with variable signal intensity on T1-weighted images, increased signal intensity on T2-weighted images, and heterogeneous enhancement after contrast administration (Fig. 66-91).[280] The presence of calcification, bone, and other more mature tissue elements may be better seen on CT. Metastatic disease to the lung, liver, and draining retroperitoneal lymph nodes can occur, and CT scanning of the chest and abdomen is an important component of the staging evaluation.

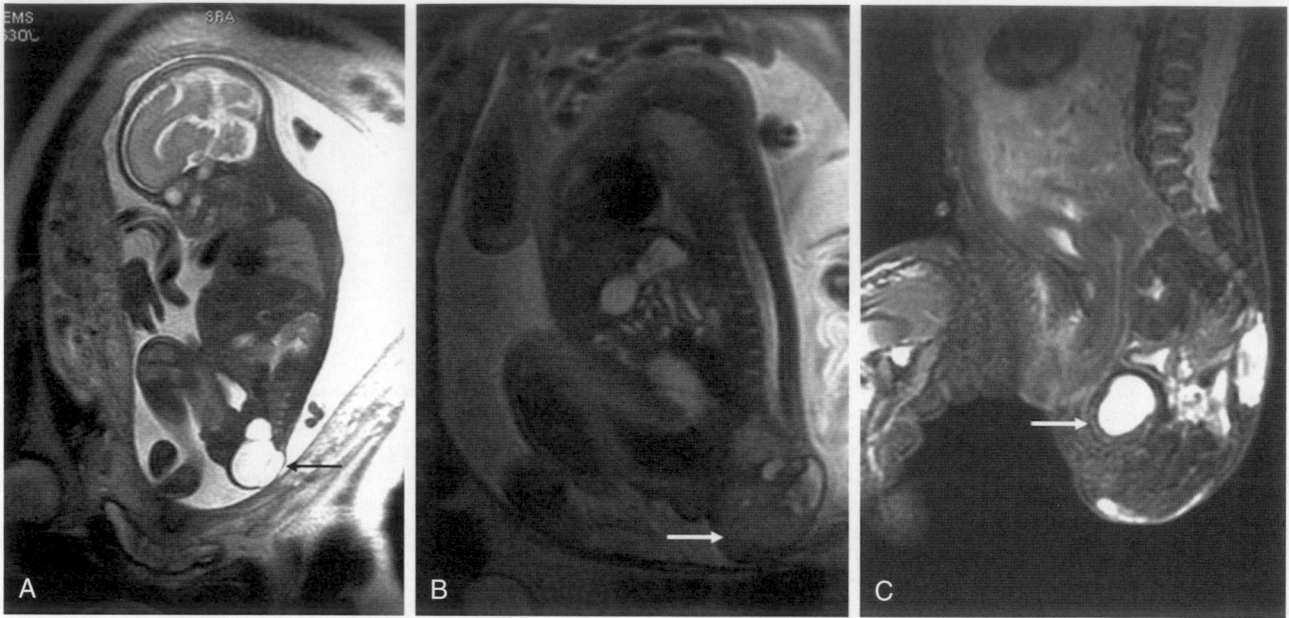

Figure 66-91 Sacrococcygeal germ-cell tumor. **A** and **B,** Prenatal MRI images show both cystic and solid elements within a large presacral mass. **C,** At birth the solid elements predominated, although large cystic spaces were still present.

Approximately 20% of these patients have pulmonary metastases at the time of diagnosis.[279]

These tumors arise from coccygeal tissue elements, and surgical resection must include resection of the coccyx. When complete resection can be accomplished, survival rates are greater than 95% with tumors that have benign mature teratomatous elements. The presence of malignant elements results in much lower rates of long-term survival.[279]

In addition to sacrococcygeal teratomas, other presacral solid masses must also be in the differential, including neuroblastoma and lymphoma. In particular, the distinction between presacral cystic neuroblastoma and a type IV germ-cell tumor may be difficult on the basis of imaging alone (Fig. 66-92). The presence of intraspinal extension, which is more commonly seen in neuroblastomas, is unusual in the setting of sacrococcygeal germ-cell tumors, aiding in the differential diagnosis. Predominantly cystic germ-cell tumors may also be difficult to distinguish from lumbosacral myelomeningoceles or the related fat-containing lipomyelomeningocele. Again the extent of intraspinal involvement, which is best demonstrated by MRI, may help in narrowing the differential diagnosis.

MUSCULOSKELETAL NEOPLASMS

Primary Bone Tumors

Pediatric bone tumors are relatively rare, comprising less than 5% of the new cancer diagnoses in children under the age of 9 years, and between 8% and 11% in children between the ages of 10 and 19 years. Osteosarcoma is the most common primary malignant bone tumor occurring in the first 2 decades of life. The remaining bone malignancies include the Ewing family of tumors (Ewing sarcoma) and primary lymphoma of the bone. Because

symptoms are frequently nonspecific, there is often a delay in diagnosis. The goal of the imaging evaluation is to establish a preliminary diagnosis,[330] because about half of the bone lesions detected in children are benign. Based on these preliminary assessments, a more detailed imaging evaluation can then be undertaken. It is beyond the scope of this review to discuss the nonmalignant lesions that may mimic malignancy; however, chronic osteomyelitis, osteoid osteoma, bone cysts, and stress-related injury are all included among the differential considerations for primary bone lesions.[331]

Conventional radiography is essential as a first step in the evaluation.[332] Radiographs afford high spatial resolution, can be readily obtained, are relatively inexpensive, and do not require sedation. Most importantly the radiographs are critical in guiding the next step in the evaluation based on the pattern of bone reaction/involvement and surrounding soft-tissue involvement. MRI is usually the imaging modality of choice to further characterize primary bone lesions.[330,331] MRI sequences should include at a minimum, T1- and T2-weighted imaging in at least two orthogonal planes as well as post–gadolinium-enhanced imaging. Fat suppression sequences are nearly always of value in distinguishing focal areas of enhancement from intramedullary fatty marrow or surrounding soft-tissue fat, whereas non–fat-suppressed T1-weighted sequences are invaluable for delineating the margins of marrow-space involvement. Fluid-sensitive sequences are highly sensitive but lack specificity: tumor, edema, hemorrhage, and focal fluid collections all may show increased signal on fluid-sensitive sequences. More importantly the fluid-sensitive sequences allow the examiner to closely assess the relationship of signal abnormalities in the bone and soft tissues to adjacent neurovascular structures. It remains controversial whether post–gadolinium-enhanced images, simple T1-weighted images, or fat-suppressed

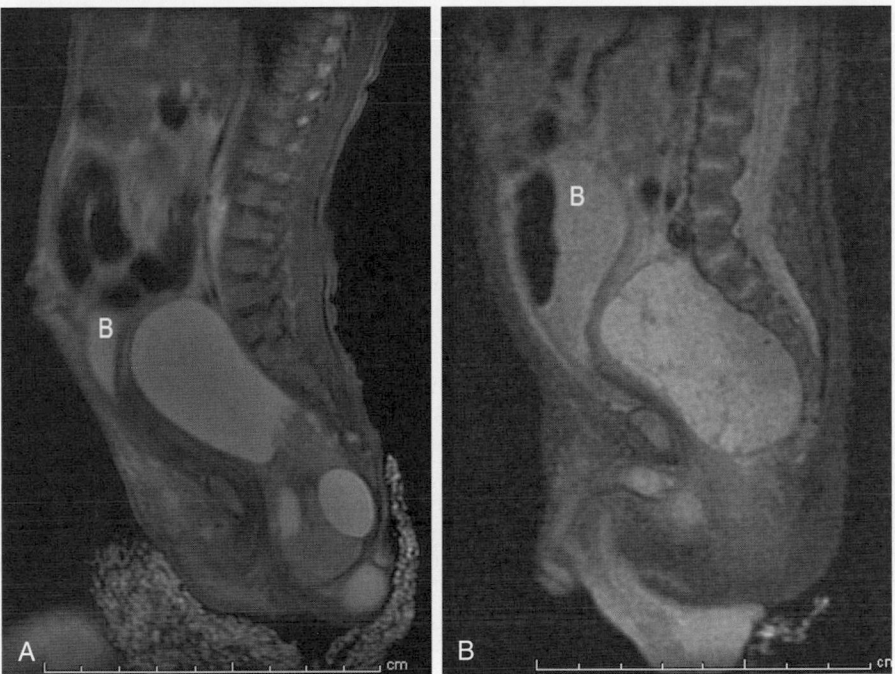

Figure 66-92 Sacrococcygeal germ-cell tumor (**A**) and cystic neuroblastoma (**B**). Two patients with prenatally diagnosed cystic presacral mass. Fluid-sensitive MRI showed similarly appearing complex cystic masses, both compressing the bladder *(B)*, with very similar imaging appearance, emphasizing the importance of including neuroblastoma in the differential for some sacrococcygeal teratomas.

T2-weighted images allow the best discrimination between the true intraosseous tumor margins and surrounding peritumoral edema and bone reaction. Dynamic contrast-enhanced MRI allows tumor vascularity and permeability to be measured directly, and in at one study of osteosarcoma patients, pretreatment patterns of intratumoral blood flow were identified as prognostic factors for event-free and overall survival, as well as being indicative of a histologic response to neoadjuvant therapy.[333] The technical challenges of performing these studies combined with complex postprocessing requirements has limited the more widespread acceptance of this technique.

CT has a relatively limited role in assessing the primary bone lesions, given the increased use of MRI. However, for focal bone lesions such as osteoid osteoma, CT is very helpful in characterizing the focal osseous abnormality. In addition, for primary bone tumors, particularly Ewing sarcoma involving the chest wall and ribs, CT may be preferable. The staging evaluation of primary bone tumors must also include a CT of the chest to assess for pulmonary metastatic disease. The use of bone scintigraphy, either using ^{99m}Tc or ^{18}F, is considered standard of care for assessing multifocal sites of disease.[90] FDG-PET imaging, although not in routine clinical practice, has been shown in several studies to be effective in detecting sites of lymph node spread and metastatic disease outside of the primary site and in helping determine the margin of metabolically active tumor involvement.[176,183,334-336] In addition FDG-PET has been effective at showing early responses to chemotherapy, and studies have shown that early responses to chemotherapy, manifest as decreased metabolic activity

and decreased FDG uptake, correlate with improved outcome and overall survival.[174,183,337-339]

Osteosarcomas

Osteosarcomas are the most common primary bone tumor occurring in children older than the age of 10 years (Ewing sarcoma being more common in younger children).[340-342] This may relate to the period of rapid bone growth occurring in early to mid adolescence, which corresponds to the peak incidence of osteosarcoma. The majority of osteosarcomas are of the classic high-grade histologic type with telangiectatic and surface osteosarcomas occurring less often (the latter two entities being divided into parosteal and periosteal subtypes). Osteosarcomas most commonly occur in the metaphysis of the rapidly growing ends of the long bones including the distal femur, proximal tibia, proximal femur, and proximal humerus. Involvement of the axial skeleton and flat bones is much less common, except where osteosarcoma has developed secondary to radiation treatment or chemotherapy. At diagnosis, approximately 20% of patients have pulmonary metastatic disease detectable by chest CT. Other sites of metastatic disease spread are unusual.

The radiographic appearance of osteosarcoma varies widely; however, the typical lesion is an aggressive, destructive lesion centered in the metaphysis (Fig. 66-93). Smaller lesions may show periosteal reaction, most commonly a sunburst-type reaction. The Codman triangle formation indicates periosteal new-bone formation with the free edge of the periosteal new bone disrupted by growth of the tumor mass (Fig. 66-94). A lamellated or onion skin–type periosteal reaction may also be seen in

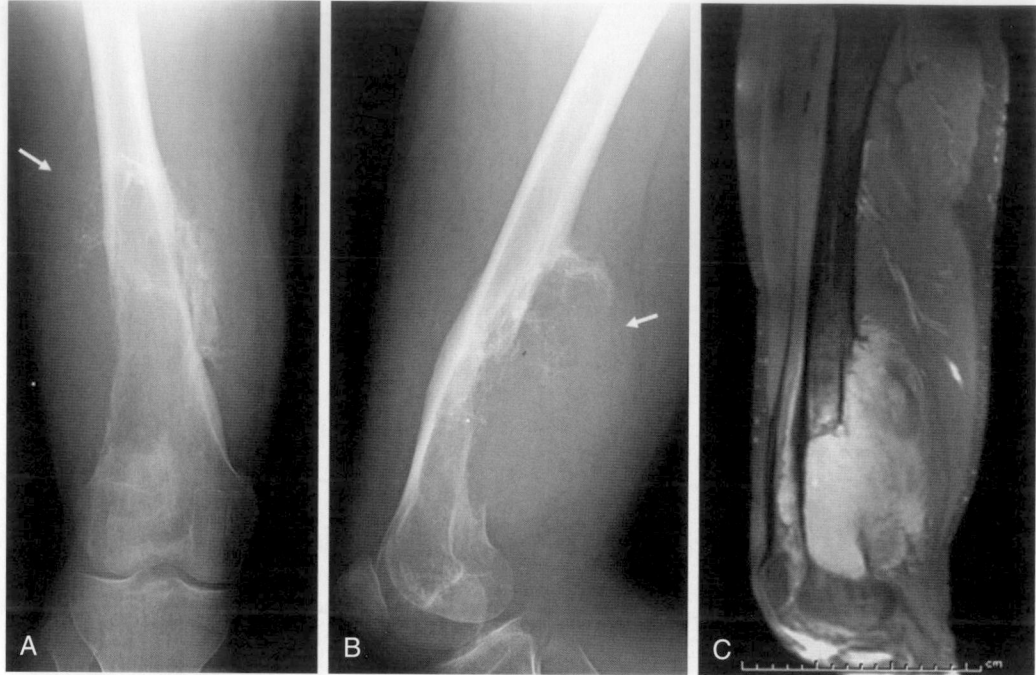

Figure 66-93 Osteosarcoma in a 19-year-old male with an enlarging right-leg mass. **A** and **B**, Radiographs show a large destructive lesion with extensive periosteal reaction. A large soft-tissue mass is also evident on the radiographs *(arrows)*. **C**, MRI shows better delineation of the associated soft-tissue mass and the extent of osseous involvement.

smaller lesions; however, this is more typically associated with Ewing sarcoma. Although the diagnosis of osteosarcomas is usually suggested by plain films, the films are relatively insensitive at determining the extent of disease. As noted, MRI is essential in determining the extent of long-bone involvement, the degree of soft-tissue involve-

ment, and the extent of invasion into adjacent neurovascular structures (see Fig. 66-94 and Fig. 66-95).[341,343] Although epiphyseal involvement and crossing of the growth plate by osteosarcoma is seen as unusual, reports have suggested that this may occur in as many as 80% of patients.

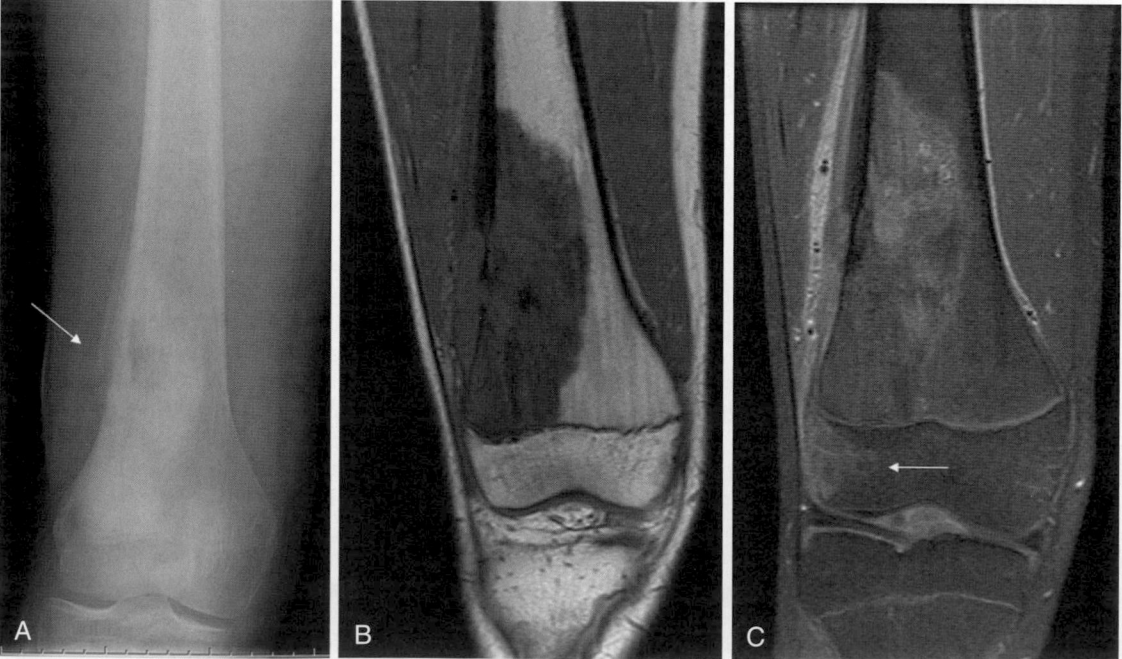

Figure 66-94 Osteosarcoma in a 16-year-old patient with leg swelling. **A**, Radiograph of the right femur shows a sclerotic lesion in the distal femoral metaphysis, with periosteal elevation and Codman's triangle *(arrow)*. **B** and **C**, T1-weighted MRI and post-Gd T1-weighted imaging show the extent of bone involvement and raise concern for epiphyseal extension of the tumor *(arrow)*.

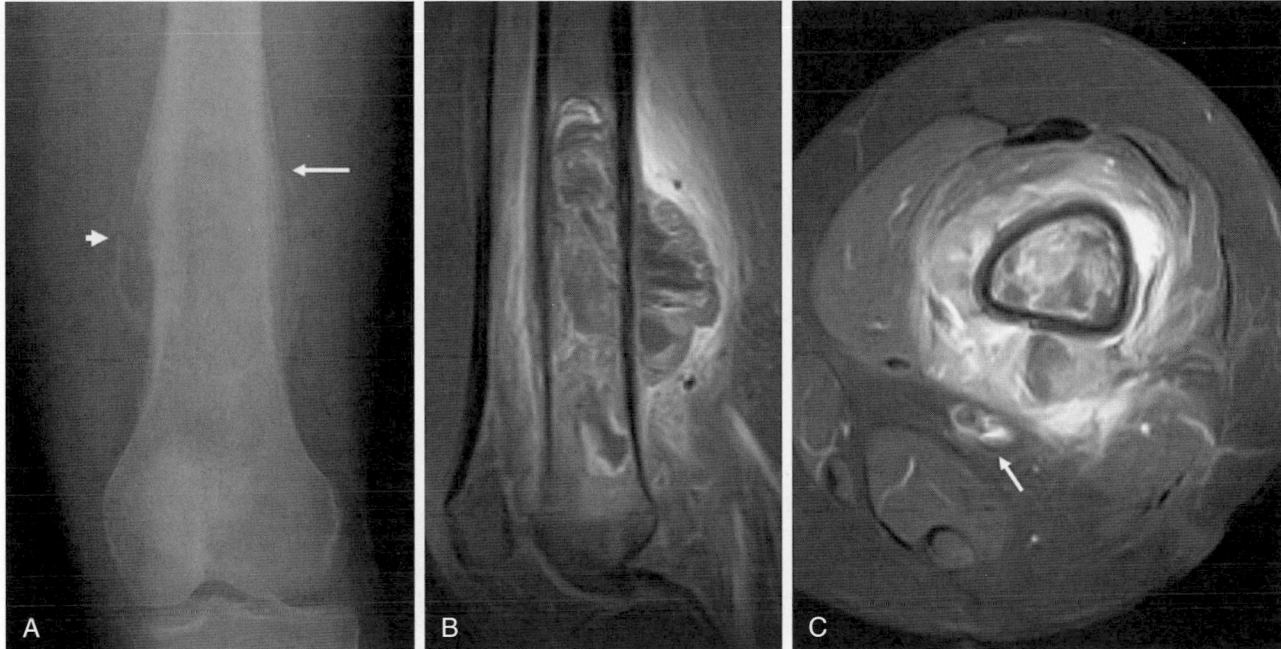

Figure 66-95 14-year-old girl with osteosarcoma. **A,** The radiograph shows a large, distal femoral destructive lesion with osteoblastic activity, lamellated periosteal reaction *(arrow),* and a Codman triangle *(arrowhead).* **B,** Contrast-enhanced MRI shows the associated soft-tissue mass to better advantage, as well as the extent of bone involvement. **C,** The axial MRI image shows the mass abutting the neurovascular bundle *(arrow)* but not encompassing it.

MRI is also helpful in characterizing the primary lesion. The presence of fluid-fluid levels, common to telangiectatic osteosarcoma, are best demonstrated by MRI (Fig. 66-96). The initial imaging evaluation should also assess for the presence of pathologic fracture and must include the joint proximal and distal to the primary lesion to aid in surgical planning and decision making. Skeletal scintigraphy and chest CT are necessary for the staging evaluation to assess for locoregional and distant metastatic disease.[341] Follow-up imaging is usually dictated by individual treatment protocols but typically includes imaging of the primary site of disease and chest

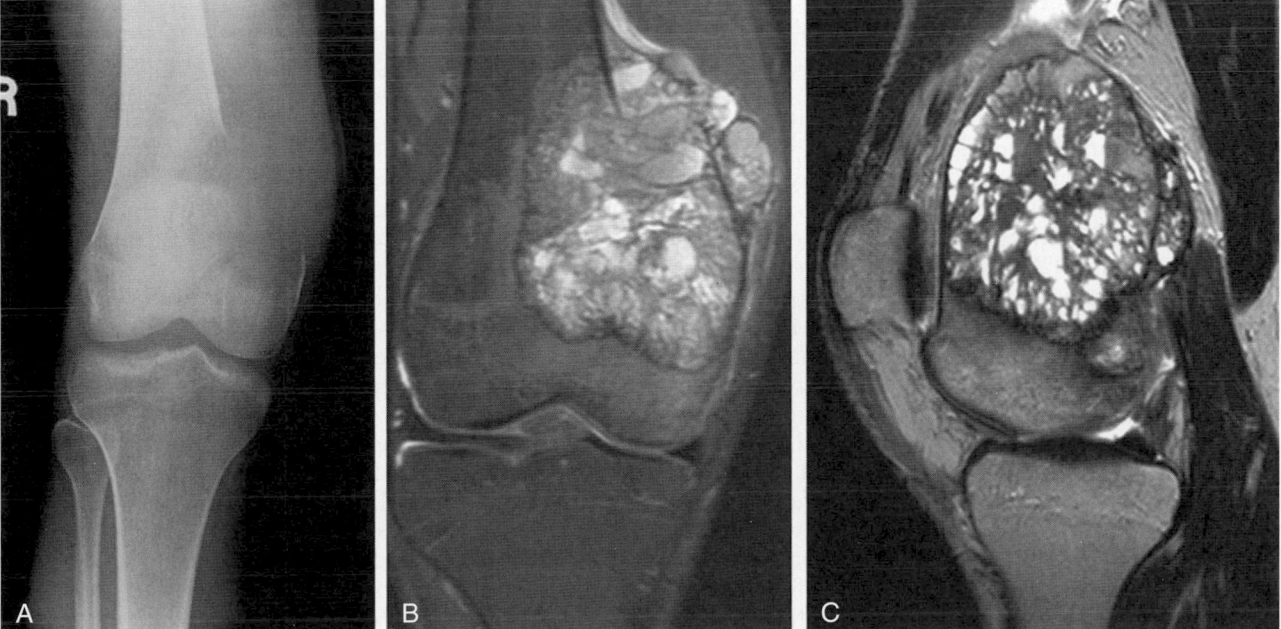

Figure 66-96 Osteosarcoma. This 18-year-old male experienced leg pain and swelling. **A,** Radiographs show a destructive lesion in the distal femur with an associated soft-tissue mass. Gadolinium contrast-enhanced **(B)** and fluid-sensitive FSEIR **(C)** MRI images demonstrate multiple fluids/fluid levels with heterogeneous contrast enhancement. The appearance is common in telangiectatic osteosarcoma, but in this patient with high-grade metastatic osteosarcoma the imaging features were the result of multiple solid and necrotic elements within the tumor.

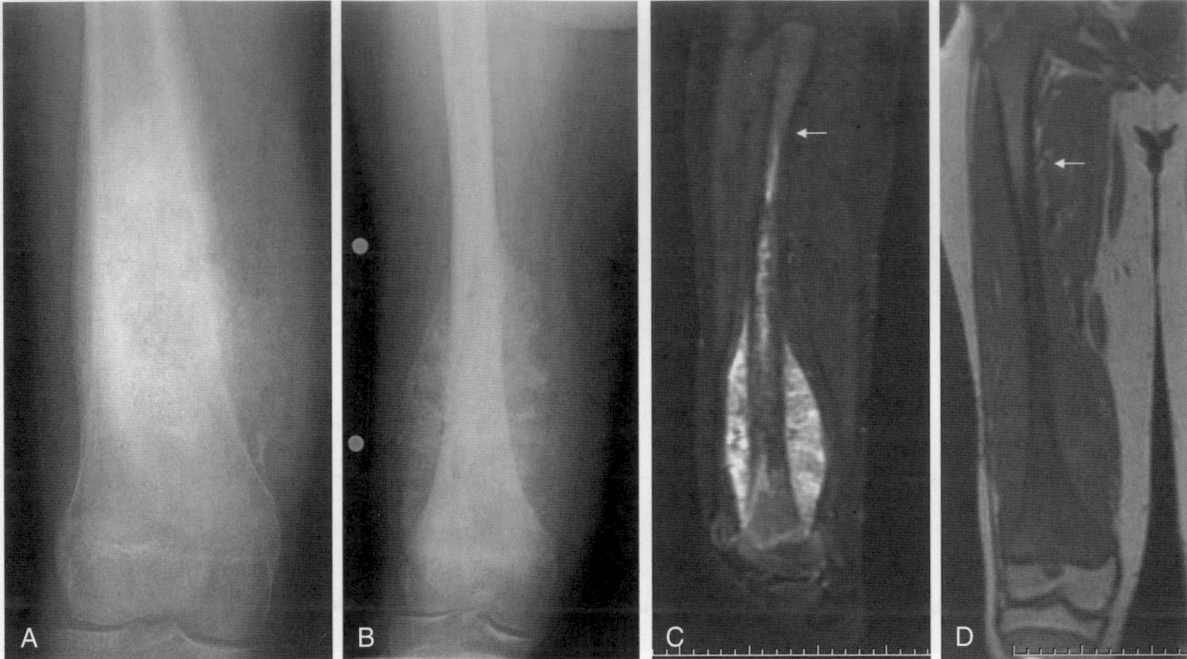

Figure 66-97 Ewing sarcoma. Radiographs from two patients with Ewing sarcoma show the "onion-skin" periosteal reaction characteristic of this tumor (**A**) and the sunburst periosteal reaction that is also commonly seen (**B**). FSEIR and T1-weighted MRI images from the patient demonstrate intramedullary high signal on the FSEIR images (**C**) and corresponding loss of normal intramedullary fat signal (**D**), indicating more widespread extension of tumor than was suggested by the radiographic findings and highlighting the importance of MRI in evaluating extent of disease in these patients.

CT. The presence of pulmonary nodules, both at diagnosis and as a site of relapse, is important prognostically,[344] and chest CT remains an essential part of the posttherapy evaluation in these patients. Unfortunately, there are no specific imaging features to distinguish benign from malignant pulmonary nodules,[22,186] and surgical resection remains essential for both definitive diagnosis and potential cure.[23]

Ewing Sarcomas

Ewing sarcomas are most often poorly differentiated tumors arising from the bone, although they may also arise from adjacent soft tissues. The primative neuroectodermal derivative of this tumor is known as the peripheral PNET (PPNET). Ewing sarcomas arising in a chest wall make up about 10% of the Ewing family of tumors. Clinically, pain and a palpable mass are the most common presenting complaints. As with osteosarcoma, the imaging evaluation should be initially directed at characterizing the primary site of abnormality. Anatomically, Ewing sarcomas occur with roughly equal distribution in the axial and appendicular skeleton, with about two thirds occurring in the pelvis and/or lower extremities. At the time of presentation, the size of the mass and extensive local invasion may make it difficult to determine whether the lesion has arisen primarily within the bone or within the surrounding soft tissue. Metastatic disease is also common at the time of diagnosis, with sites of metastatic disease reflecting hematogenous spread, including lung, bone, and bone marrow.

Radiographically, Ewing sarcoma of the bone is primarily a lytic lesion with a permeative destructive appearance.[345] The onion-skin or lamellated periosteal reaction is characteristically described with Ewing sarcoma, although it is not specific for this diagnosis. Other forms of periosteal reaction are also seen (Fig. 66-97), reflecting the variable degree of bone destruction and bone response to the tumor. There is usually a large accompanying soft-tissue mass. Particularly in the axial skeleton (pelvis and ribs), the soft-tissue component may predominate.

Plain radiographs should include imaging of the involved long bones, chest, and/or pelvis. MRI is indicated for further evaluating the appendicular skeleton and long bones, and as with osteosarcoma the entire length of the bone including the proximal and distal joints should be included. The choice of MRI pulse sequence is similar to that for osteosarcoma but should include at a minimum T1- and fat-suppressed T2-weighted images in orthogonal planes as well as post–gadolinium-enhanced images. The axial images, particularly T2-weighted, are useful for demonstrating the extent of subperiosteal and periosteal extension. Either sagittal or coronal images are effective at defining the margin of bone-marrow involvement and surrounding tissue edema.

Rib and chest wall lesions are best evaluated by CT. With multiplanar 3D image reconstruction capabilities on modern CT scanners, the extent of osseous involvement and adjacent lung/pleural involvement can usually be adequately demonstrated by CT (Fig. 66-98). For paraspinal lesions, MRI may be necessary to delineate intraspinal invasion. MRI is also useful in characterizing subtle abnormalities such as chest-wall muscle involvement and neurovascular involvement, particularly in the upper thorax and lung apices.

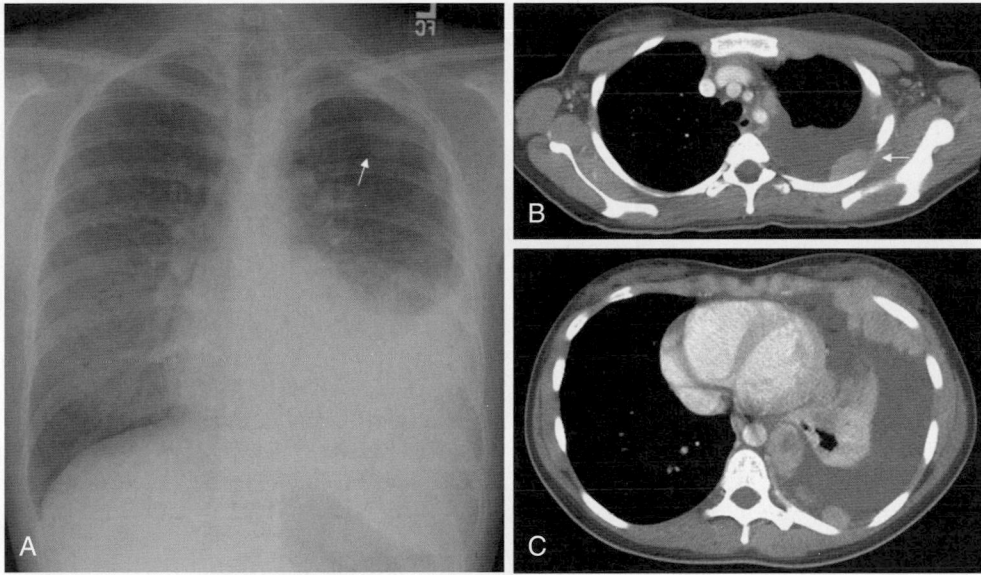

Figure 66-98 Ewing sarcoma of the chest wall. A 14-year-old girl with chest pain had a chest x-ray (**A**) that shows a large, left pleural effusion and multiple nodular densities *(arrow)* apparently arising from the chest wall/pleura. Contrast-enhanced CT (**B** and **C**) show extensive soft-tissue masses lining the chest cavity with large effusion and left lower lobe collapse. Biopsy showed Ewing sarcoma.

In contrast to osteogenic sarcoma, Ewing sarcoma does not typically show the presence of soft-tissue calcifications. Whole-body bone scintigraphy is effective at delineating sites of skeletal involvement; however, there is no clear evidence that skeletal scintigraphy is superior to MRI in characterizing local disease. FDG-PET imaging has been advocated in the staging evaluation of Ewing sarcoma, particularly with respect to identifying sites of occult bone-marrow metastatic disease. In addition, as with osteosarcoma, the use of FDG-PET has been advocated both for staging[336] and for monitoring response to therapy (Fig. 66-99).[80,174,335,337,339]

Other Bone Tumors

Primary lymphoma of the bone is a relatively unusual site of presentation in non-Hodgkin lymphoma but must be included in the differential diagnosis of a primary destructive lesion with intramedullary involvement. Radiographically the evaluation is similar to Ewing sarcoma, and biopsy is usually needed to confirm the diagnosis.

Although they are not primary bone neoplasms, leukemia and Langerhans-cell histiocytosis are both pediatric neoplastic conditions that may manifest with bone involvement (see Fig. 66-3). Leukemia, described below, often produces metaphyseal lucency and may result in an aggressive, permeative, moth-eaten appearance to the bone, occasionally accompanied by periosteal reaction. Pain is also common at this stage of bone reaction to the leukemic infiltration. Langerhans-cell histiocytosis can manifest either as localized disease or widespread osseous involvement. Typical osseous lesions are lytic on conventional radiographs. Because they are relatively slow growing and do not elicit a significant response from the surrounding bone, these lesions may go undetected by bone scintigraphy, and skeletal survey is still advocated to assess for the extent of osseous involvement in Langerhans-cell histiocytosis. Recent studies have also suggested that FDG-PET may be more sensitive both in determining sites of intraosseous involvement and in determining sites of soft-tissue involvement that would otherwise go undetected either by conventional scintigraphy or skeletal survey.[3]

Muscle/Soft-Tissue Tumors

The nonosseous musculoskeletal malignancies of childhood are typically sarcomas that arise from immature mesenchymal tissue. Rhabdomyosarcomas of skeletal-muscle origin comprise about half of the pediatric soft-tissue sarcomas.[342,346] The nonrhabdomyomatous soft-tissue sarcomas include fibrosarcomas, synovial sarcomas, alveolar soft-part sarcomas, malignant fibrous histiocytomas, and PPNETs. Ultimately the distinction between these different histologic subtypes is made pathologically. The imaging approach is directed at determining the size and extent of primary tumor involvement, the relationship to critical adjacent structures such as nerves and blood vessels, and local involvement of bone or regional lymph nodes. All of the soft-tissue sarcomas have a propensity to metastasize to the lung, and a CT of the chest should be performed at the time of diagnosis. Bone scintigraphy is also indicated to assess for additional sites of skeletal involvement, and FDG-PET is increasingly be used for staging and response assessment in pediatric soft-tissue sarcoma.

Rhabdomyosarcomas are the most common soft-tissue sarcomas of childhood, making up more than half of all soft-tissue sarcomas in children.[342] Although the head and neck and genitourinary tract are common sites of rhabdomyosarcoma presentation, about one fourth of these tumors are also located in the extremities. These are typically of the alveolar or undifferentiated histologic type.[347] The imaging characteristics are not specific, but feature a

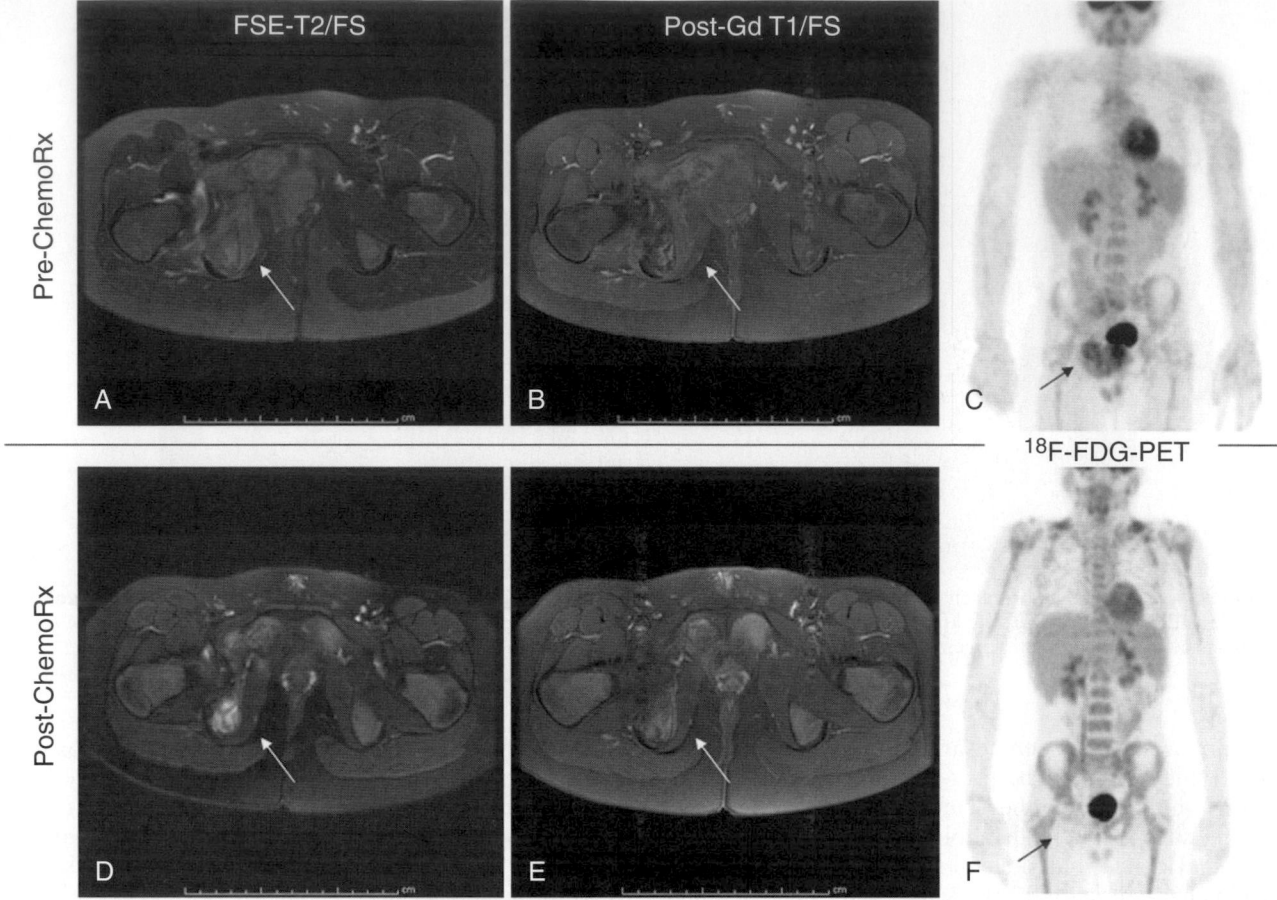

Figure 66-99 Ewing sarcoma response assessment. Images are of a 10-year-old child with nonmetastatic Ewing sarcoma of the right pelvis. T2-weighted (**A**) and contrast-enhanced T1-weighted (**B**) MRI images show an ill-defined enhancing mass centered in the right ischium with soft extension into the surrounding pelvis *(arrows)*. Pretreatment FDG-PET imaging (**C**) shows moderately intense uptake in the mass. After chemotherapy, MRI (**D** and **E**) shows persistent areas of increased T2 signal and enhancement *(arrows)*; FDG-PET shows no residual metabolic activity in the mass (**F**), demonstrating an excellent response to therapy and suggesting that the MRI findings may relate to a necrotic tumor and enhancing scar/granulation tissue rather than active disease.

T2-bright lesion localized in the deep soft tissues with extension along fascial planes (Fig. 66-100). After contrast infusion, these tend to be hypervascular tumors with bright enhancement. FDG-PET has been shown in several studies to yield intense FDG uptake and is likely to be of value in identifying sites of occult disease at the time of staging and in assessing response to therapy.[183,184,281]

Synovial Sarcoma

Synovial sarcomas typically occur in patients during their teenage years. Synovial sarcomas are the most common nonrhabdomyosarcomatous soft tissues in children,[346] and despite their name, they arise from undifferentiated mesenchymal cells that are typically located in a paraarticular location. They are more common in the lower extremities than in the upper extremities or axial skeleton and are often mistaken for other benign or incidental conditions.[348] Conventional radiographs are indicated for extremity lesions and show calcifications in about 30% of cases. MRI shows a lobulated lesion that is usually isointense to muscle on T1-weighted images and isointense to slightly hyperintense on T2-weighted images with a relatively homogeneous appearance.[349] After

contrast infusion, there is typically intense enhancement (Fig. 66-101). Although these findings are not specific for synovial sarcoma, the presence of a lobulated calcified lesion with the described MRI signal characteristics should suggest the diagnosis.

The clinical presentation is typically of a painless mass. Median duration of symptoms before presentation is approximately 14 months. The staging evaluation is important in predicting the overall survival of these patients. Patients with localized disease and/or with disease allowing gross total resection have an estimated 80% 5-year overall survival, as compared with patients who have metastatic disease at diagnosis and for whom the diagnosis is nearly always fatal.[350] Because these lesions most often occur in extremities, they may mimic benign disease such as synovial or ganglion cysts. The MRI examination must therefore include contrast enhancement in order to discriminate between a solid enhancing lesion and a predominantly fluid-containing cystic lesion (Fig. 66-102). Because of the importance of local control, imaging is also essential in determining resectability and in establishing the preoperative margins for surgical planning.

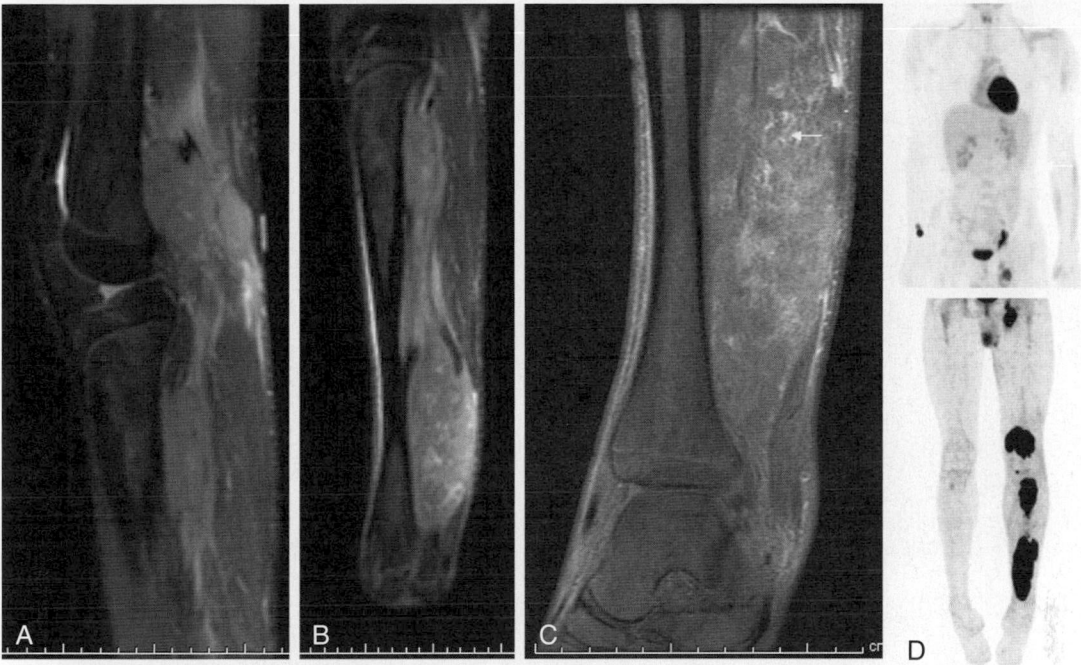

Figure 66-100 Rhabdomyosarcoma in a 16-year-old patient with a left leg mass. A and B, MRI findings show a T2 bright, enhancing (C) lesion localized in the deep soft tissues of the calf with extension proximally along fascial planes into the popliteal fossa. FDG-PET shows multiple sites of disease, including left inguinal lymph-node involvement that would not have been detected on the MRI. Biopsy showed alveolar rhabdomyosarcoma.

Tumor size has also been shown to be a key prognostic factor in synovial sarcoma, with lesions less than 5 cm resulting in a metastasis-free survival rate greater than 75%, in contrast to lesions greater than 5 cm in size. In patients with these lesions, the metastasis-free survival rate falls to less than 50%.[350] Synovial-cell sarcomas are typically FDG-avid tumors, and FDG-PET imaging should be considered at the time of staging to assess for locoregional lymph node spread and distant sites of metastatic disease that would adversely affect prognosis (see Fig. 66-102).

Malignant Peripheral Nerve-Sheath Tumor and Neurofibromatosis Type 1

Individuals with NF1 are at risk of developing benign and malignant tumors; the leading cause of mortality among these individuals is the development of malignant peripheral nerve-sheath tumors (MPNSTs). MPNSTs result from malignant degeneration of benign NF1 lesions, including plexiform neurofibromas (PNs).[351] In patients with extensive plexiform lesions, the diagnosis of malignant degeneration is challenging and classically relies on changes in lesion size and/or localized or unremitting pain, although these features are neither sensitive nor specific. Other than increase in size, no discriminating MRI features have been described to identify PNs potentially undergoing malignant degeneration into MPNSTs. A number of studies using FDG-PET in NF1 have demonstrated a significant difference in mean standardized uptake values (SUV) between benign and malignant lesions.[352-354] In a retrospective study of 19 children with NF1 who had cross-sectional imaging and correlative histopathologic data, Tsai et al. provided further data

supporting the hypothesis that benign and malignant lesions are distinguishable by FDG-PET imaging in children and that there is a correlation between SUV_{max} and tumor grade.[355] It is the authors' current practice to perform FDG-PET imaging on all patients who have NF1 with new clinical symptoms, change in lesion size, or identification of new lesions by CT or MRI. Lesions with an SUV_{max} greater than 4 are considered worrisome, warranting either more intensive monitoring or surgical resection (Fig. 66-103).

Infantile (Desmoid-Type) Fibromatosis

Infantile fibromatosis is a benign fibrous proliferation, although it can be locally aggressive and deforming.[356] Infantile desmoid-type fibromatosis must be distinguished from the congenital generalized fibromatosis, also known as *infantile myofibromatosis*.[357] This latter disorder is characterized by lesions consisting of both smooth muscle and fibroblastic spindle cells in contrast to the more differentiated fibroblastic cells seen in desmoid fibromatosis. The presence of deep soft-tissue involvement as well as visceral involvement of organs such as lung and liver has a worse prognosis than localized disease. The extent of involvement is optimally determined by MRI (Fig. 66-104), with lesions typically characterized by low signal on both T1- and T2-weighted sequences because of the relatively high collagen content in these tumors.[357]

It may be difficult based on imaging findings alone to distinguish between aggressive multifocal fibromatosis and congenital fibrosarcoma. The desmoid-type lesions, in contrast, tend to be localized and have a less aggressive appearance.

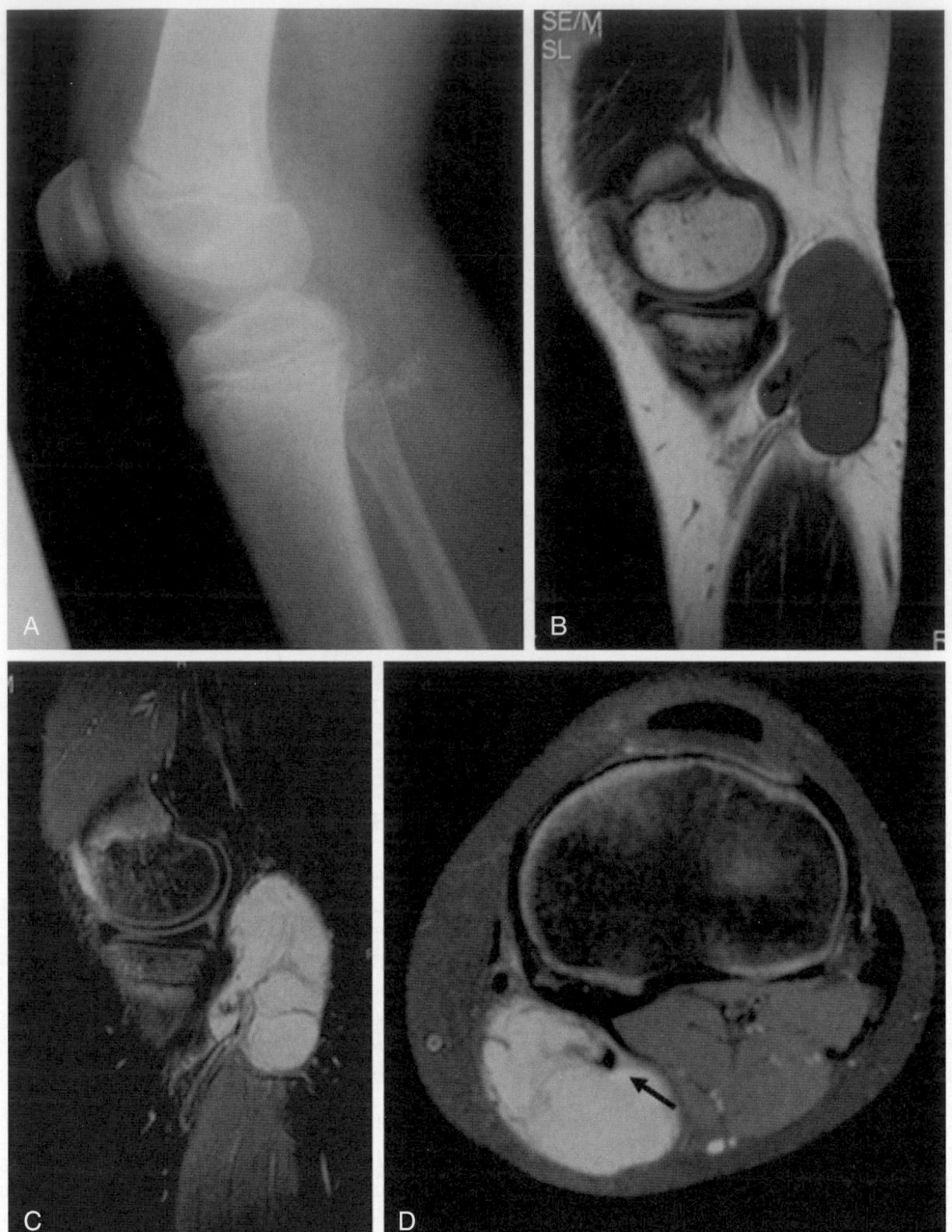

Figure 66-101 Synovial sarcoma. **A,** Radiograph of an 11-year-old child with a palpable leg mass showed a calcified mass behind the knee. MRI shows lobular mass in the medial compartment posterior to the knee, encasing the semi membranous tendon *(arrow)*, characterized by low signal on T1-weighted images (**B**), high signal on T2-weighted images (**C**) and intense contrast enhancement (**D**). These features are all characteristic findings in synovial sarcoma.

Other mesenchymal tumors, such as alveolar soft-part sarcomas, epithelioid sarcomas, and malignancy fibrous histiosarcomas are very rare in children and do not have distinctive imaging characteristics. As with the other mesenchymal tumors, lesions are typically isointense to slightly hyperintense on both T1- and T2-weighted images, with variable patterns of enhancement.

The distinction between liposarcoma and the benign lipoblastoma cannot be made on the basis of imaging alone, with both lesions showing high signal-intensity on T1-weighted images, decreased signal intensity on T2-weighted images, and minimal enhancement. As with the other malignant sarcomas, metastatic disease to the chest must be excluded, and the staging evaluation should include chest CT.

LYMPHOPROLIFERATIVE NEOPLASMS

Leukemias

Of the pediatric cancers approximately one third are leukemias, and together with brain tumors, leukemia accounts for over half of the childhood tumors.

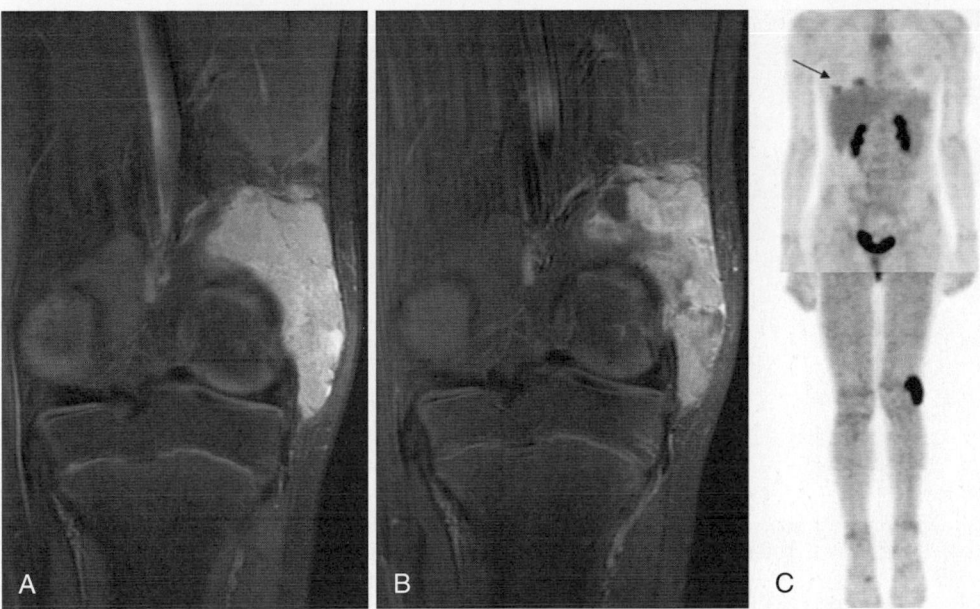

Figure 66-102 Synovial-cell sarcoma. Coronal fat-suppressed PD (**A**) and post-Gd T1-weighted MRI (**B**) shows a lobulated high signal-intensity enhancing lesion. The location and bright signal on fluid-sensitive sequences could be mistaken for a benign process; the pattern of contrast enhancement confirms a worrisome lesion. FDG-PET (**C**) shows intense uptake at the primary site and at least two focal pulmonary metastatic lesions *(arrow)*. This pattern of involvement and spread is common for synovial-cell sarcoma.

More than 75% of pediatric leukemia is acute lymphoblastic leukemia (ALL),[358] and the majority of the patients have B-lymphoblastic ALL, with 15% to 20% having T-cell ALL and 1% to 2% with mature B-cell ALL. Acute myelogenous leukemia (AML) makes up 15% to 20% of pediatric leukemia; the remainder are leukemic subtypes that are uncommon in children, such as chronic myelogenous leukemia and juvenile myelomonocytic leukemia.

The most common presenting symptoms and physical examination findings are nonspecific and include fever, bleeding, bone pain, lymphadenopathy, and splenomegaly. In addition to the fatigue, pallor, and anorexia, which

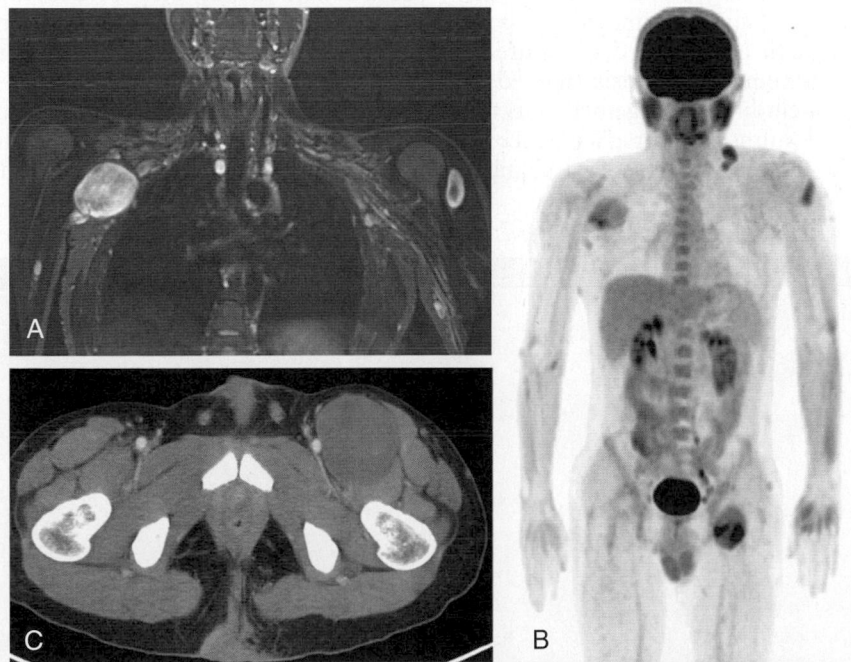

Figure 66-103 23-year-old patient with NF1 and multiple painful lesions. MRI shows T2-bright lesions in the right axilla and left deltoid (**A**), with corresponding FDG uptake (**B**). A CT scan of the pelvis shows low density left inguinal lesion (**C**) that has corresponding intense FDG uptake (**B**). SUV values and correlative histopathology of these lesions were: Left neck (not shown on MR) SUV: 4.97, atypical neurofibroma; right axilla SUV: 4.94, atypical neurofibroma; left deltoid SUV: 4.15:,atypical neurofibroma; left inguinal SUV: 9.33, low-grade malignant peripheral nerve sheath tumor.

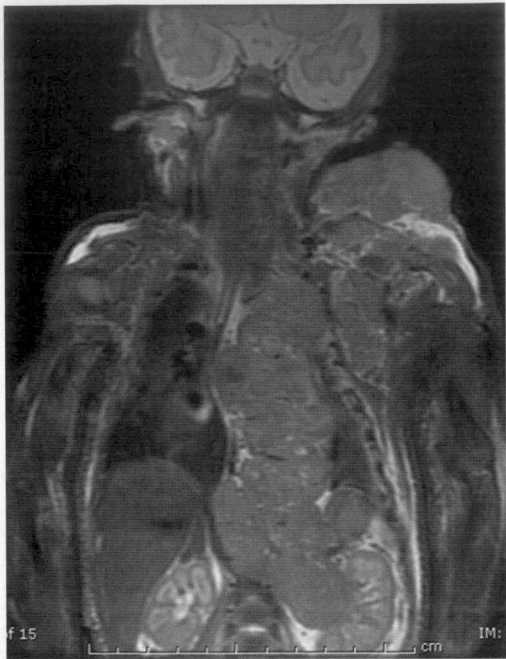

Figure 66-104 Infantile fibromatosis in a 4-week-old infant. The MRI shows extensive mediastinal, retroperitoneal, and intraabdominal disease. Biopsy showed infantile fibromatosis.

are seen in almost all patients with leukemia, hepatosplenomegaly and fever are seen in approximately two thirds of cases.[127]

Because of the nonspecific nature of presenting symptoms and physical examination findings, radiologic imaging may be useful in directing the next step in the evaluation. Common imaging findings include pulmonary edema secondary to high output cardiac failure in the setting of peripheral leukemic blast crisis (related to anemia); organomegaly including enlargement of the spleen, liver and heart; and pulmonary airspace opacities (related to leukostasis or infection).[359] Skeletal changes

can range from subtle metaphyseal lucent bands to frank bone destruction resulting from leukemic infiltration. CNS hemorrhage may be encountered as a result of leukostasis and thrombocytopenia in patients with high peripheral leukemic-cell counts.[360] Although such imaging finding alone do not make the diagnosis of leukemia, the initial imaging evaluation can be critical in assessing the overall physiologic burden of the patient's disease.

Imaging Findings

Peripheral skeletal lesions may be detected on conventional radiographs in approximately 25% of patients newly diagnosed with ALL.[127] In the patient with fatigue and poorly localized bone pain, metaphyseal lucent bands (leukemic lines) may be seen (Fig. 66-105). This finding was initially thought to represent leukemic infiltration in the submetaphyseal bone, although the discovery of elevated parathyroid hormone levels in patients with leukemia suggests paraneoplastic effects on bone resorption likely contribute to the observed radiographic changes.[361] Metaphyseal lucent lines are not unique to leukemia and may also be seen in other marrow-infiltrative malignancies such as neuroblastoma (see Fig. 66-3) and lymphoma and in response to physiologic stress such as infection, systemic inflammatory reactions, and radiation.

Metaphyseal lucent lines may be difficult to distinguish from the diffuse metaphyseal lucency, which represents a combination of direct leukemic infiltration of the bone and accompanying bone resorption. This pattern of infiltration typically results in a broad irregularity and more poorly demarcated pattern of metaphyseal lucency. It is also associated with pain and localized tenderness, and depending on the degree of bone destruction it may also be accompanied by focal lytic lesions. Leukemic infiltration of the bone can also yield a moth-eaten appearance with a marked pattern of periosteal reaction.

More advanced imaging techniques such as MRI may be helpful in demonstrating the extent of leukemic infiltration by showing both focal and diffuse replacement of

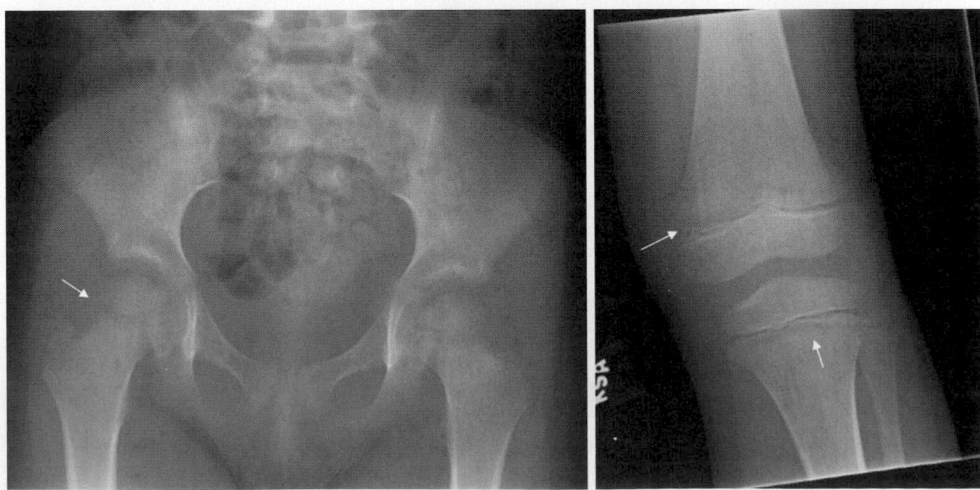

Figure 66-105 Leukemic lines. A 4½-year-old had child with limp and leg pain. Radiographs of the hips, pelvis, and knees show submetaphyseal lucency *(arrow)* and loss of the normal trabecular architecture, particularly in the femoral necks. Bone marrow aspiration confirmed leukemia.

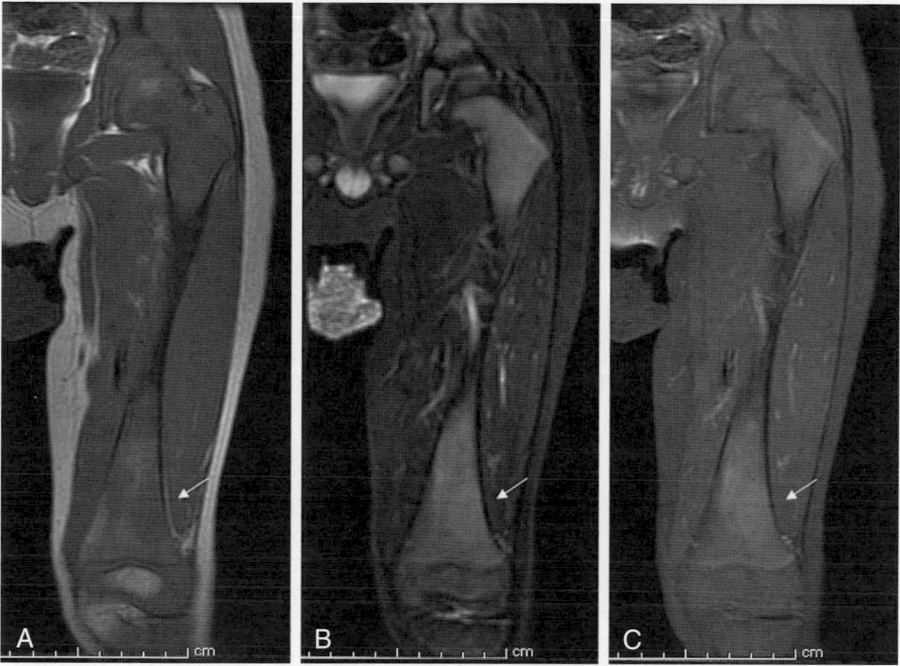

Figure 66-106 MRI of marrow infiltration in leukemia. A 3-year-old child experienced persistent limp and lower extremity pain. MRI showed patchy areas *(arrows)* of marrow replacement (A), heterogeneous increased signal (B), and enhancement (C) suggestive of diffuse marrow infiltration. Bone marrow aspiration confirmed B-cell ALL.

normal fatty marrow signal (Fig. 66-106).[127,362] However, heterogeneous patterns of marrow signal are a normal finding in children as hematopoietic marrow gradually converts to fatty marrow. Furthermore, therapeutic agents that stimulate bone-marrow recovery after ablative chemotherapy (e.g., granulocyte colony stimulating factor [G-CSF]) can mimic leukemic marrow replacement, and the extent of leukemic infiltration may be difficult to determine on the basis of MRI.[363,364]

In the setting of T-cell ALL, children and adolescents commonly experience wheezing as a result of accompanying large mediastinal masses (Fig. 66-107). The diffuse thymic infiltration seen in T-cell ALL (and T-cell lymphoblastic lymphoma) results in a bland, homogeneous-appearing mediastinal mass (Fig. 66-108). Pericardial and pleural effusions are common, as is leukemic infiltration of the kidneys. Despite the bulky disease that is often encountered at the time of presentation, T-ALL and lymphoblastic lymphomas respond rapidly to chemotherapy (see Fig. 66-33), and within a short time, radiographic studies typically return to normal, although the significance of incomplete response of the mediastinal mass to therapy with respect to overall outcome is uncertain.[365]

Childhood Acute Myelogenous Leukemia

AML represents a heterogeneous group of leukemias encompassing both the spectrum and extent of myeloid differentiation.[366] When patients with AML have high peripheral blast counts (leukocyte counts greater than 100,000/mm³), clinical leukostasis may result and is characterized by global CNS changes or respiratory distress caused by pulmonary vascular involvement. Imaging findings in the brain may suggest diffuse microvascular

thrombi (Fig. 66-109) without focal neurologic signs. CNS changes secondary to leukostasis may be difficult to detect by CT and standard MRI sequences, but they are readily demonstrated on paramagnetic susceptibility-sensitive gradient echo sequences because of the paramagnetic effects of hemoglobin breakdown products (i.e., hemosiderin) accumulating at sites of microvascular thrombus formation.

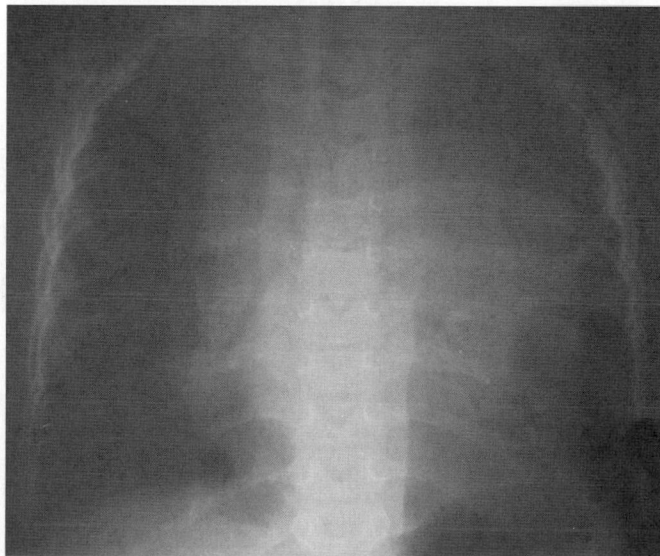

Figure 66-107 T-cell ALL in a 4-year-old child with first-time wheezing. Chest x-ray shows large mediastinal mass and narrowing of the proximal bronchi and air bronchograms, suggesting airway compression.

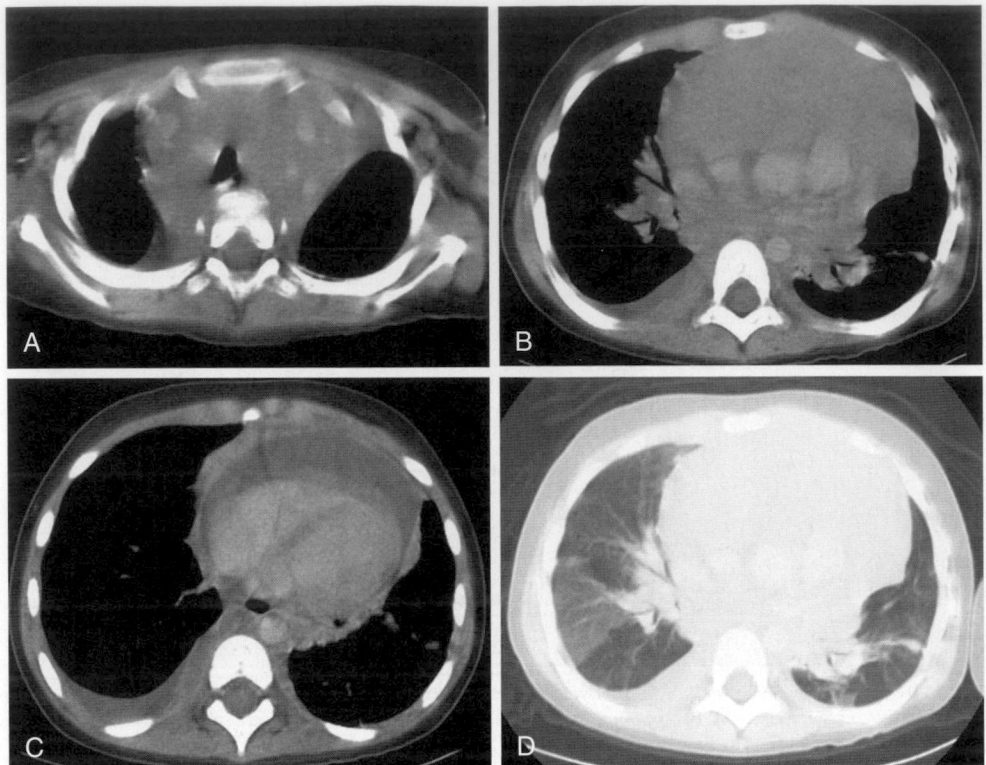

Figure 66-108 T-cell ALL. Shown are images of a 4-year-old child (see Fig. 66-107) with wheezing and mediastinal mass. Contrast-enhanced chest CT shows findings typical of T-cell lymphoblastic lymphoma, including mediastinal mass extending into the neck (**A**) with homogeneous density infiltrating the thymus (**A** and **B**). The mass causes marked airway compression and bronchial narrowing (**A** and **B**) and is associated with pericardial and pleural effusions (**C**) and mosaic lung attenuation (**D**) indicative of air-trapping and airway obstruction. Based on bone marrow involvement of greater than 50% marrow, the patient was diagnosed with T-cell lymphoblastic leukemia with a mediastinal mass.

Acute promyelocytic leukemia (APML) accounts for 5% to 10% of childhood AML and characteristically presents with a severe consumptive coagulopathy that is further exacerbated by cytotoxic chemotherapy because of cell lysis and release of procoagulant intracellular contents. The resulting coagulopathy can result in clinically significant bleeding, necessitating emergent imaging studies to assess for cerebral hemorrhage, which can be profound and rapidly progressive (see Fig. 66-109).

Extramedullary forms of AML, also called *chloromas* and *granulocytic sarcomas,* are seen in up to 10% of patients with AML and are also encountered in chronic myelocytic leukemia (CML) and myelodysplasia.[367] They are commonly asymptomatic; however, CNS involvement can result in mental status changes and lead to focal neurologic deficits. CNS chloromas are usually extraaxial and contiguous with the meninges. They may be virtually undetectable by CT, where they have similar to slightly increased attenuation relative to normal cortex. On MRI, these lesions are typically hypointense to isointense on T1-weighted imaging and heterogeneously isointense to hyperintense on T2-weighted imaging, with homogeneous contrast enhancement (Fig. 66-110).[367] Outside the CNS, chloromas may produce adjacent bone destruction and are often seen in the orbits, spine, paranasal sinuses, and the adjacent soft tissues,[367] as well as in the abdominal cavity (Fig. 66-111). Despite the uncommon presentation of this leukemic subset, extramedullary

disease in any form—including that presenting without evidence of bone-marrow disease—is still considered evidence of systemic disease and is usually treated as such, with a combination of local control (surgery, radiation) and systemic chemotherapy.[368]

Lymphomas

Pediatric lymphomas are classified as either Hodgkin or non-Hodgkin lymphomas.[369,370] Because there is considerable overlap in the imaging features, age at presentation and sites of involvement are useful in helping to distinguishing the types of disease.[127]

Hodgkin Lymphoma

In Hodgkin lymphoma, the bulky mediastinal mass characteristically seen radiographically (Fig. 66-112) is made up primarily of inflammatory cells with the malignant Reed-Sternberg cell, from which the histologic diagnosis of Hodgkin lymphoma is made, comprising only 10% or less of the cells in the bulky lymph-node mass.[127] Hodgkin lymphoma is typified by involvement of contiguous lymph-node groups[371,372] and is staged according to the extent of lymph-node involvement in distinct nodal sites.

Staging. The most commonly used staging system is the Ann Arbor system (Table 66-5),[372,373] which involves determining the extent and pattern of lymph-node

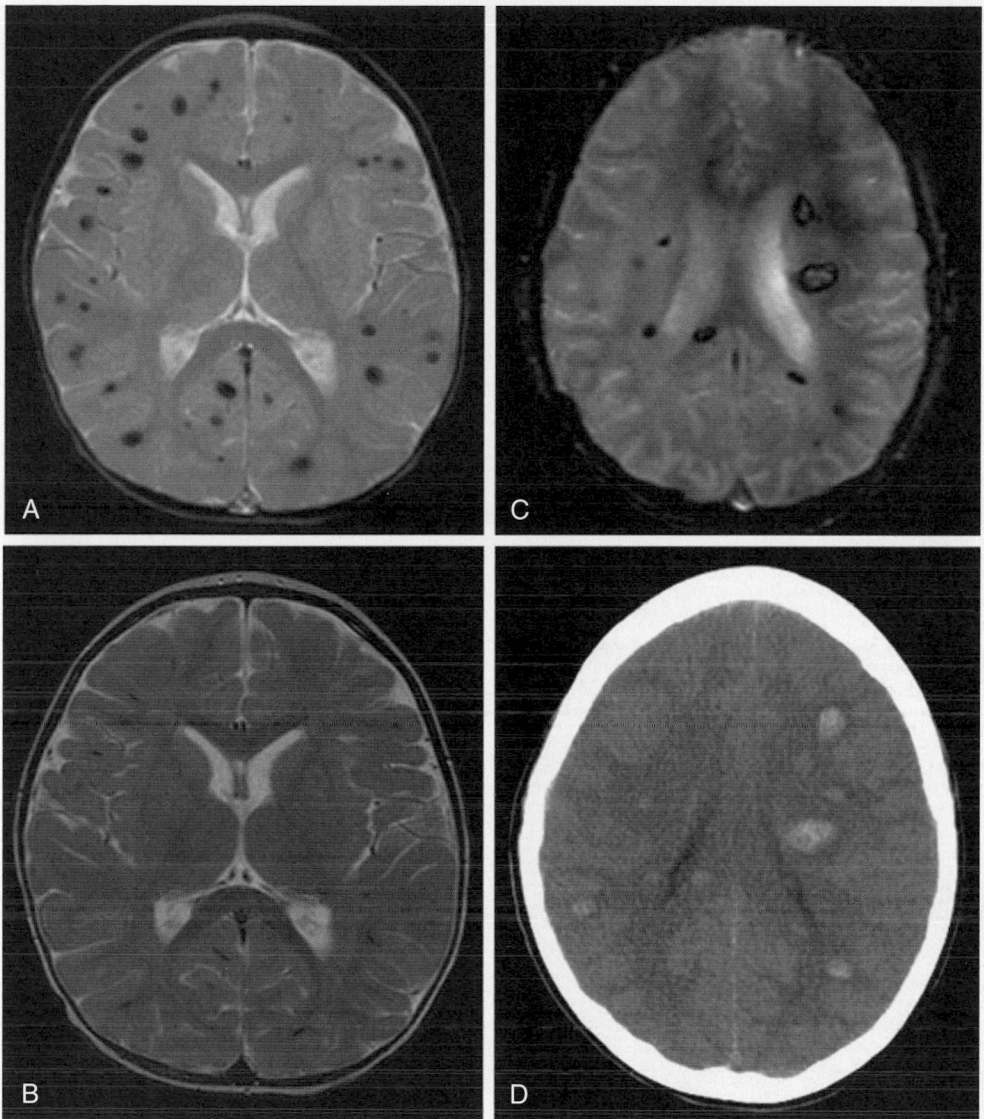

Figure 66-109 AML/APML. Gradient echo and FSE T2-weighted axial MRI images show the brain of a 17-month-old girl with AML who had a white blood cell count of greater than 300,000. Brain MRI obtained after the patient was stabilized showed multiple areas of paramagnetic susceptibility throughout the brain (**A**) with no corresponding T2 signal abnormality (**B**). Areas visualized were interpreted as foci of microthrombus formation secondary to leukostasis. A separate patient with APML had seizures, high white blood cell count, and a CT showing multiple foci of acute hemorrhage (**D**); the MRI showed multiple areas of paramagnetic susceptibility (**C**), likely caused by leukostasis with acute hemorrhage resulting from coagulopathy, reperfusion injury at sites of microthrombus formation, or both.

involvement. One unique feature of Hodgkin lymphoma relates to splenic involvement. For the purpose of disease staging, the spleen is consider localized lymphoid tissue, and lymphomatous infiltration of the spleen in Hodgkin lymphoma is not classified as stage 4 visceral metastatic disease, but rather as stage 3 disease.

The initial diagnosis is often prompted by chest x-ray evaluation for upper respiratory symptoms and vague constitutional symptoms such as fever and night sweats (see Fig. 66-112). At the time of diagnosis a mediastinal mass is encountered in more than two thirds of patients with Hodgkin lymphoma.[127,374] CT scanning is still the most commonly used cross-sectional modality for staging these patients. In addition to determining the extent of lymph-node involvement, pericardial and pleural effusions may be seen. Multiple sites of organ involvement may also be demonstrated, most commonly liver, spleen, and kidneys (Fig. 66-113). Children do not typically have symptoms referable to intraabdominal disease, so a thorough radiologic evaluation (intravenous and oral contrast-enhanced CT and FDG-PET) is essential to completely stage these patients. The staging evaluation for Hodgkin lymphoma should always include scanning of the neck to the level of the skull base in order to evaluate the nasopharyngeal and tonsillar lymphoid tissues (Waldeyer ring) for tumor involvement. Extensive involvement of the lymphoid tissue in Waldeyer ring may produce complete obliteration of the airway, requiring emergent intervention by a tracheostomy. As is true for all mediastinal lymphomas, the bulky anterior mediastinal mass

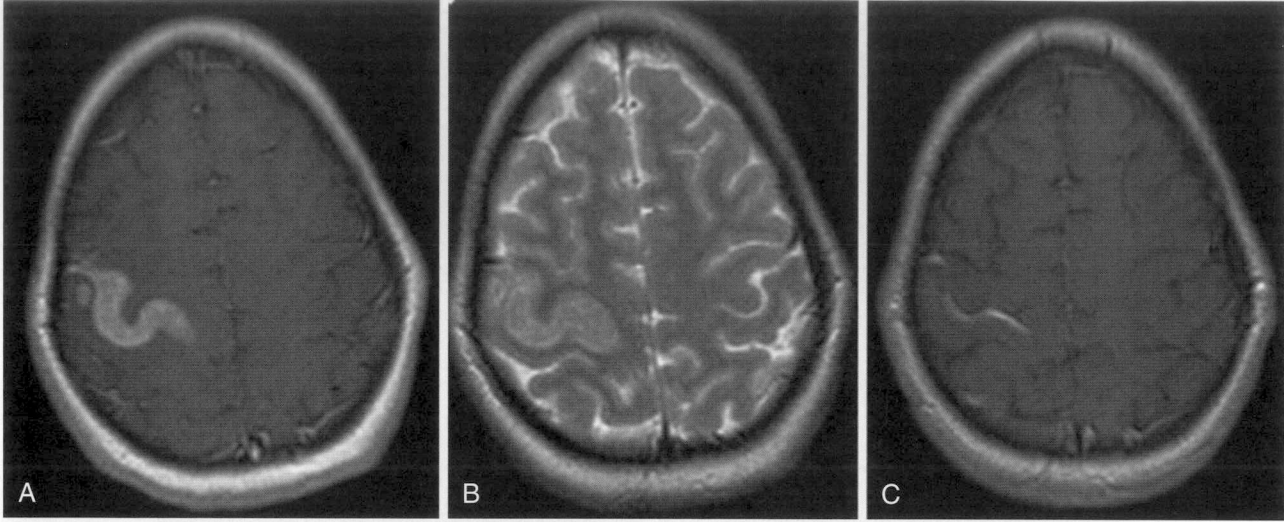

Figure 66-110 Chloroma in a 12-year-old patient with AML. Brain MRI shows typical findings of chloroma, including isointensity to cortex on T2-weighted images (**A**), homogeneous enhancement (**B**), and good response to radiation (**C**).

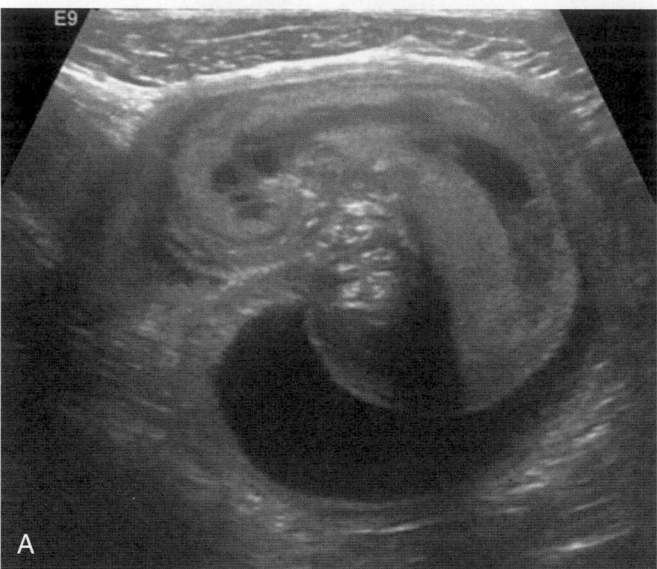

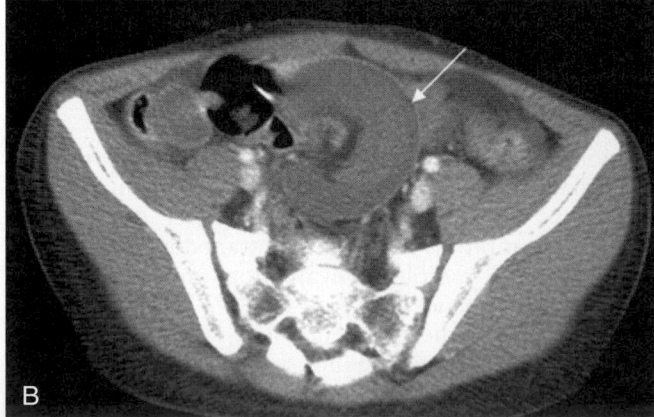

Figure 66-111 Extramedullary AML (chloroma). **A,** An 11-year-old boy with abdominal pain and vomiting had an ultrasound that revealed small-bowel intussusception. **B,** CT showed an abnormal mass involving the small bowel with apparent mural thickening *(arrow)*. At surgical resection this was found to be an isolated site of extramedullary AML (chloroma). The bone marrow biopsy was negative.

common in Hodgkin lymphoma may produce tracheal, bronchial, and central vascular compression (occasionally resulting in the superior vena cava [SVC] syndrome). Tracheal compression can result in acute airway compromise, particularly during procedures requiring general anesthesia and muscle relaxation. In addition, large anterior mediastinal masses can produce jugular vein thrombosis, venous sinus thrombosis, and CNS venous infarction (Fig. 66-114).

Pulmonary involvement in Hodgkin disease is unusual (seen in fewer than 5% of children under 10 years of age and fewer than 15% of adolescents),[374] but its identification often makes a difference in distinguishing stage 2 from stage 4 disease, resulting in dramatically different treatment regimens. Although pulmonary involvement can be quite extensive (Fig. 66-115), pulmonary nodules/masses that are associated with an ipsilateral hilar mass

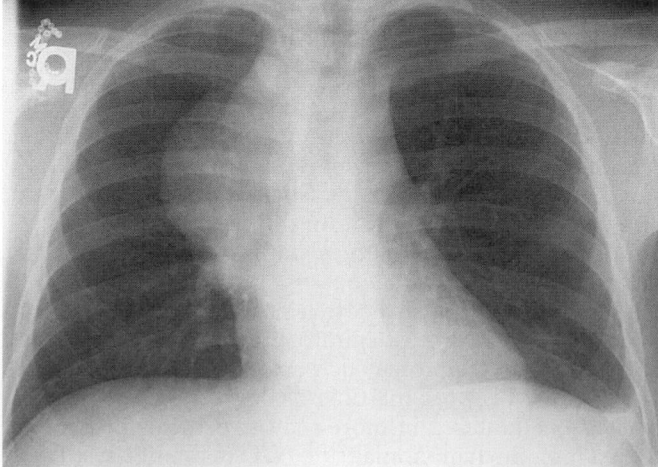

Figure 66-112 Hodgkin lymphoma. The chest x-ray of a patient with symptoms of a nonspecific upper respiratory infection shows an anterior mediastinal and paratracheal mass, as well as a small left effusion.

TABLE 66-5   Childhood Hodgkin Lymphoma: Ann Arbor Classification[372,373]

Tumor Stage	Description
1	Involvement of a single lymph node region, or Stage I(E): direct extension from that node to an adjacent extralymphatic region.
2	Involvement of two or more lymph node regions (number to be indicated) on the same side of the diaphragm, or Stage II(E): direct extension from any one of these lymph nodes to an adjacent extra-lymphatic organ.
3	Involvement of lymph node regions on both sides of the diaphragm. Stage III(E): may be accompanied by extension to an adjacent extralymphatic organ Stage III(S): may be accompanied by involvement of the spleen Stage III(E+S): involvement of both an adjacent extralymphatic organ and the spleen.
4	Noncontiguous involvement of one or more extralymphatic organs or tissues, with or without associated lymph-node involvement.

E, Extralymphatic spread of tumor into contiguous structures, to be distinguished from hematogenous spread; S, splenic involvement.

probably result in part from spread along peribronchial lymphatics,[371] although the distinction between local contiguous lymphatic spread and hematogenous dissemination can be challenging by CT.

As discussed in detail in the section on mediastinal masses, in addition to staging by CT, functional imaging with FDG PET is essential both for staging and monitoring response to therapy (see Figs. 66-31 and 66-32; Fig. 66-116). Historically, the time course to achieving gallium negativity was the initial functional imaging finding that correlated with event-free and overall survival.[375] However, with the ubiquitous use of FDG and modern day PET/CT scanners, gallium scintigraphy is rarely if ever performed for Hodgkin lymphoma.[135] FDG-PET imaging has been shown to impact staging and response assessment in a significant number of patients,* and its use in lymphoma has been incorporated into nearly all new clinical trials for Hodgkin lymphoma. As discussed earlier, there is growing evidence to suggest that early response to therapy, defined as rapid early resolution of previously FDG-avid sites of disease, even in the presence of residual disease by CT (see Fig. 66-32) or MRI, correlates with improved overall outcome.[144,149,378]

Using FDG-PET imaging to monitor changes in metabolic activity within the mediastinal mass provides an opportunity for making treatment decisions based on early response to therapy.[142,146] Based on studies in both adult and pediatric patients showing that patients with early metabolic responses to therapy have improved event-free and overall survival rates as compared with those who have residual PET abnormalities after the

initial two cycles of therapy,[144,379] response-based treatment paradigms have been implemented clinically to directly test whether FDG-PET imaging is a reliable prognostic indicator for predicting chemosensitivity of the tumor and ultimately clinical outcome. Early results evaluating both change in size of the mediastinal mass and change in the metabolic activity have suggested that outcomes will likely be best predicted by a combination of factors, including resolution of FDG uptake and significant change in size of the patient's sites of disease involvement as measured by CT and/or MRI.[380,381] There have been no large multicenter prospective trials in either adults or children testing whether relying solely on FDG-PET to determine if early response to therapy can be used to reduce chemotherapy and radiation therapy in those patients achieving a rapid early response (reserving intensified treatment regimens for those patients not achieving an early response),[149,379] although one study reported a higher rate of early relapses in patients for whom involved-field radiation was omitted based on early resolution of FDG-avid disease.[382]

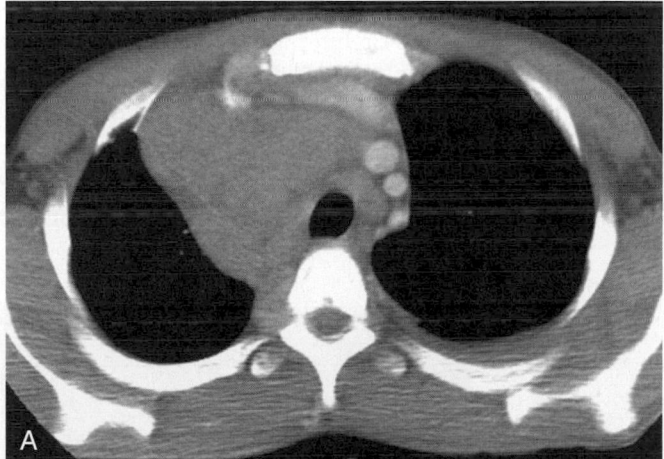

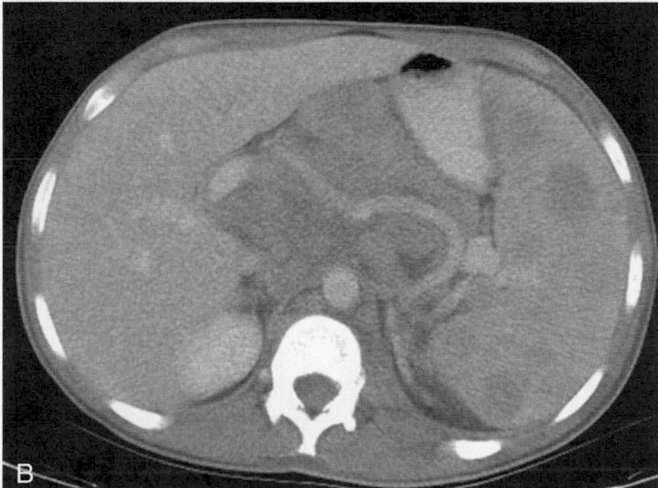

Figure 66-113 Hodgkin lymphoma. **A,** A contrast enhanced CT in patient whose chest x-ray is shown in Figure 66-112 shows the mediastinal mass and left pleural effusion. **B,** The images of the abdomen show extensive splenic, mesenteric, and retroperitoneal lymphadenopathy.

*133, 134, 139, 142-146, 245, 376, 377

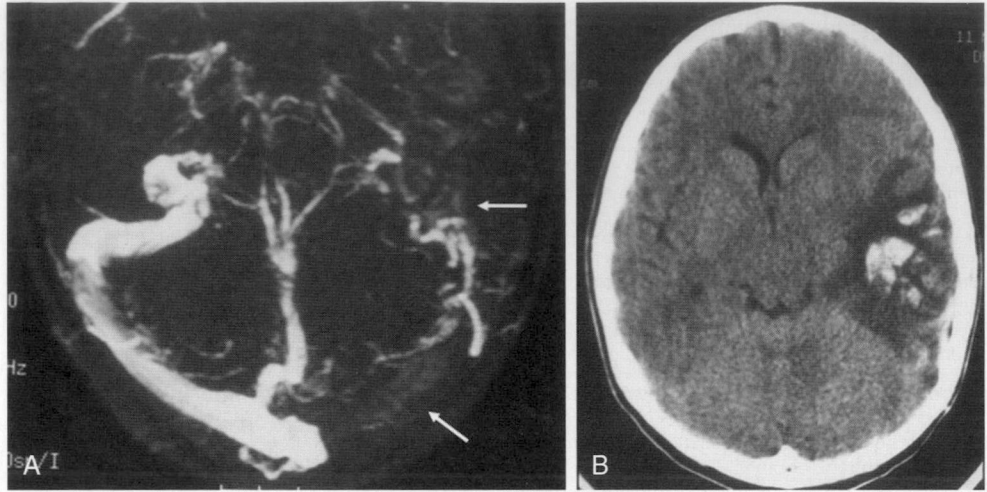

Figure 66-114 Hodgkin lymphoma. MR angiogram (**A**) and unenhanced head CT (**B**) in a patient with large mediastinal mass, brachiocephalic vein compression, and associated left jugular vein thrombosis show venous sinus thrombus involving the left transverse and sigmoid sinus *(arrows)* and associated hemorrhagic venous infarction. *(Images courtesy of Dr. Laureen Sena.)*

Given the importance of FDG-PET responses in dictating treatment decisions, an international team of experts reviewed the available data to arrive at the International Harmonization Project or International Working Group (IWG) consensus opinion regarding PET and CT criteria for determining disease and treatment response in lymphoma.[383,384] These are shown in Table 66-6, and are based on a revision of previous malignant lymphoma response criteria. Although the IWG criteria have not been validated in pediatric patients, the main challenge is

developing objective standards for assessing FDG-PET response. A number of proposals have been suggested for distinguishing residual low-level neoplastic FDG activity from background uptake.[142] The use of SUV measurements is still considered experimental and has not been universally accepted. The Deauville Criteria—receiving the greatest acceptance—are based on a five-point scale, with uptake greater than mediastinal blood pool but less than liver, considered to be background, with uptake greater than the liver considered suspicious for residual

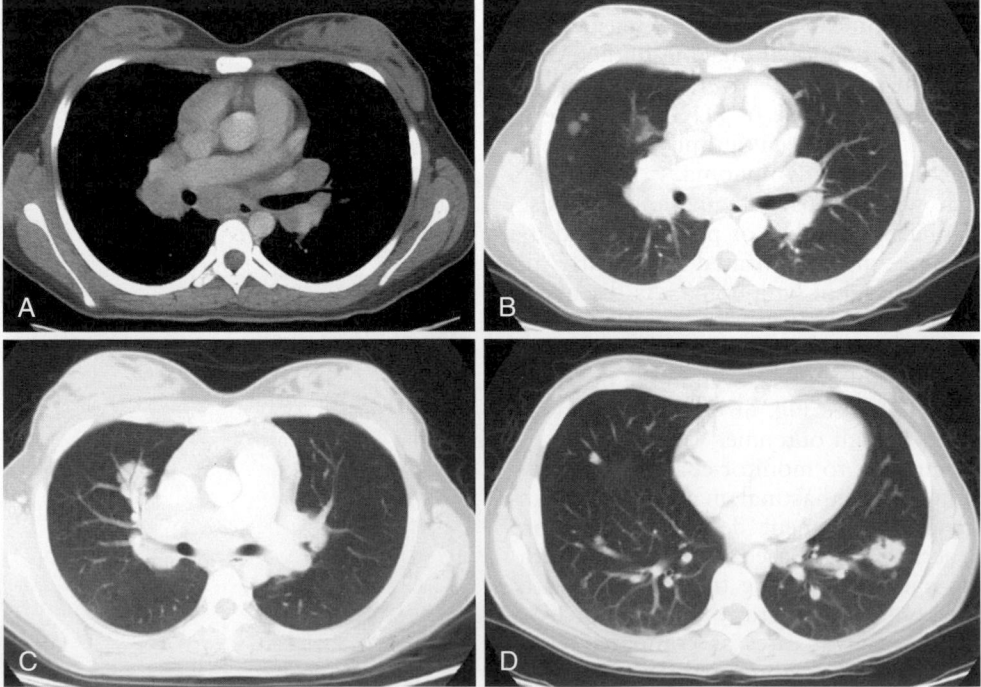

Figure 66-115 Hodgkin lymphoma and pulmonary involvement. This patient has extensive mediastinal and bilateral hilar nodal disease (**A**). The presence of discrete pulmonary nodules (**B** and **D**) may be the result of hematogenously spread disease, although contiguous spread along peribronchovascular lymphatics (**C** and **D**) is more common in Hodgkin lymphoma.

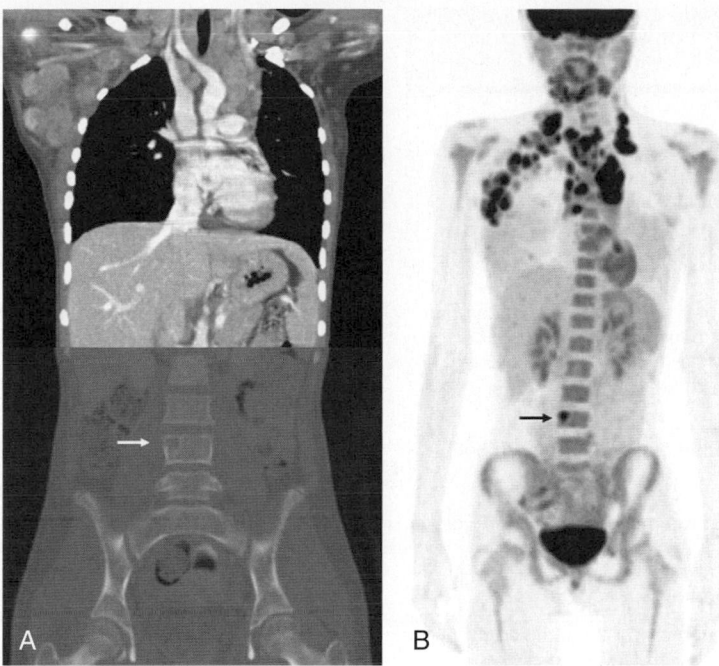

Figure 66-116 Hodgkin lymphoma and PET. Contrast-enhanced CT images of the chest, abdomen, and pelvis (**A**) show extensive mediastinal and axillary adenopathy, all of which is FDG avid. In addition, the PET scan (**B**) identifies a focus of FDG uptake at L4, corresponding to a subtle lytic lesion on CT, increasing the stage of this patient to stage 4. Note the background of low-level FDG uptake seen throughout the bone marrow, a common finding in Hodgkin lymphoma and reflective of a systemic inflammatory state associated with the disease rather an diffuse marrow infiltration.

TABLE 66-6 Summary of New International Working Group Criteria for PET and CT in Determining Response in Lymphoma[383]

Response	Criteria
CR*	FDG-PET completely negative. Residual lymph nodes/nodal masses allowed if FDG-negative. Bone marrow biopsy negative. Splenic/liver involvement must disappear. No new sites of disease.
PR	FDG positivity should be present in at least one previously involved site. Regression of measurable disease; no new sites of disease. ≥50% decrease in SPD of 6 dominant lymph nodes/nodal masses. ≥50% reduction in splenic/hepatic nodules, if present. Even if CR by other criteria, positive bone-marrow biopsy is considered PR.
SD	Failure to achieve PR, but not meeting PD criteria.
PD/Relapse	Any lesion increased in size by ≥50% from nadir. Any new lesion. PET should be positive in new/progressed lesions if ≥1.5 cm.

CR, Complete remission; *CT,* computed tomography; *FDG-PET,* 18-fluorodeoxyglucose positron emission tomography; *PD,* progressive disease; *PET,* positron emission tomography; *PR,* partial response; *SD,* stable disease; *SPD,* sum of the perpendicular diameters.
*New criteria include PET in definition of CR. PET considered positive if uptake is greater than mediastinal blood pool (lesions >2 cm) or above local background (lesions <2 cm).

metabolically active disease.[385] These criteria shown in Table 66-7 must be validated in larger treatment trials.

Non-Hodgkin Lymphomas

The non-Hodgkin lymphomas are a broad group of diseases.[127,370] Anaplastic large cell lymphoma often involves the soft tissues, skin, and bone, whereas Burkitt lymphoma most commonly presents with intraabdominal and mesenteric disease. Lymphoblastic lymphoma, particularly of the T-cell type, often presents with a mediastinal mass, although the appearance of the mass is characteristically distinct from the multilobulated bulky mass that is usually associated with Hodgkin disease. The distinction between T-cell lymphoblastic lymphoma and

TABLE 66-7 Five-Point Deauville Criteria for Determining FDG Response in Hodgkin Lymphoma[385]

Score	Semiquantitative Assessment of FDG Uptake
1	No uptake
2	Uptake less than mediastinal blood pool
3	Uptake greater than or equal to mediastinal blood pool but less than liver
4	Uptake greater than or equal to liver at any site
5	Markedly increased uptake at any site, including new sites of disease

FDG, Fluorodeoxyglucose.

TABLE 66-8   Childhood Non-Hodgkin Lymphoma: St. Jude (Murphy) Classification[386]

Tumor Stage	Description
1	A single tumor (extranodal) or nodal area is involved, excluding the abdomen and mediastinum.
2	Disease is limited to: A single tumor (extranodal) with regional node involvement, or Two or more tumors or nodal areas involved on one side of the diaphragm, or A primary gastrointestinal tract tumor (completely resected), with or without regional node involvement.
3	Tumors or involved lymph node areas occur on both sides of the diaphragm. Includes: Any primary intrathoracic (mediastinal, pleural, or thymic) disease Extensive primary intraabdominal disease Any paraspinal or epidural tumors
4	Tumors involve bone marrow (<25%) and/or central nervous system disease regardless of other sites of involvement.

its histologically-identical leukemic counterpart is made of the basis of bone-marrow aspirates; more than 25% marrow involvement results in a diagnosis of T-cell lymphoblastic leukemia.

Staging of non-Hodgkin lymphoma in most centers is according to the St. Jude Classification (Table 66-8).[386] Although there is considerable overlap in the imaging features of the lymphomas as shown in Figure 66-117, a localized anterior mediastinal mass that is not associated with other sites of significant contiguous lymph-node enlargement is more likely to be non-Hodgkin lymphoma. Non-Hodgkin lymphoma is also more likely to be disseminated at the time of diagnosis. Chest-wall and pericardial invasion is more common in the setting of non-Hodgkin lymphoma than in Hodgkin lymphoma (see Fig. 66-117).[370] The mediastinal mass in acute T-cell lymphoblastic lymphoma usually responds rapidly to chemotherapy, whereas other non-Hodgkin mediastinal lymphomas respond more slowly, with residual mediastinal abnormalities commonly seen even after multiple cycles of chemotherapy.

Non-Hodgkin lymphomas of the bone can present either primarily or in the setting of wide-spread metastatic disease. They often present with pathologic fracture and bone destruction[127] and may be difficult to distinguish from other processes.[387] MRI can be helpful in delineating the extent of marrow and adjacent soft-tissue involvement. Staging of non-Hodgkin lymphoma includes bone scintigraphy, which can be useful in distinguishing between localized osseous involvement and more widespread disease,[90] although it remains to be determined whether FDG-PET can replace bone scintigraphy in identifying sites of bone involvement in NHL.

Ileocecal involvement is common in non-Hodgkin lymphoma (Fig. 66-118). In the abdomen, intussusception in an older child should raise concern for a pathologic lead point caused by lymphoma. This is commonly seen in the setting of Burkitt lymphoma (see Figs. 66-67 and 66-118) but may also be seen in other forms of non-Hodgkin lymphoma.[127,370] The sporadic form of Burkitt lymphoma, which is more often encountered in Western and developed countries, is not etiologically linked to Epstein-Barr

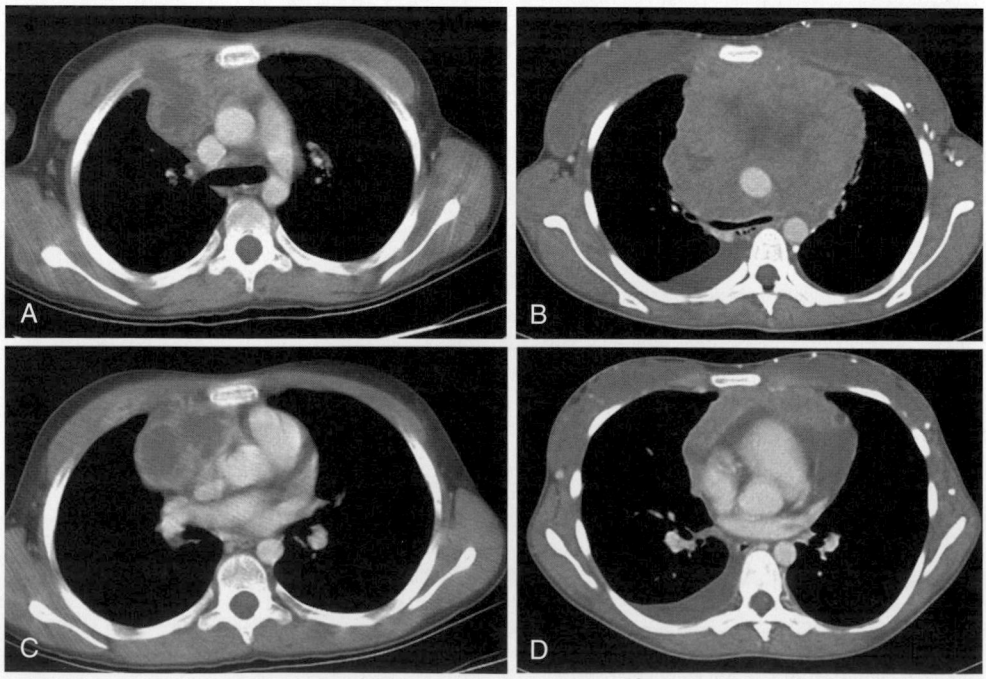

Figure 66-117 Non-Hodgkin lymphoma. Diffuse large B-cell (**A** and **B**) and B-cell–rich (**C** and **D**) non-Hodgkin lymphomas show chest wall and pericardial invasion that is more commonly seen in mediastinal non-Hodgkin lymphoma.

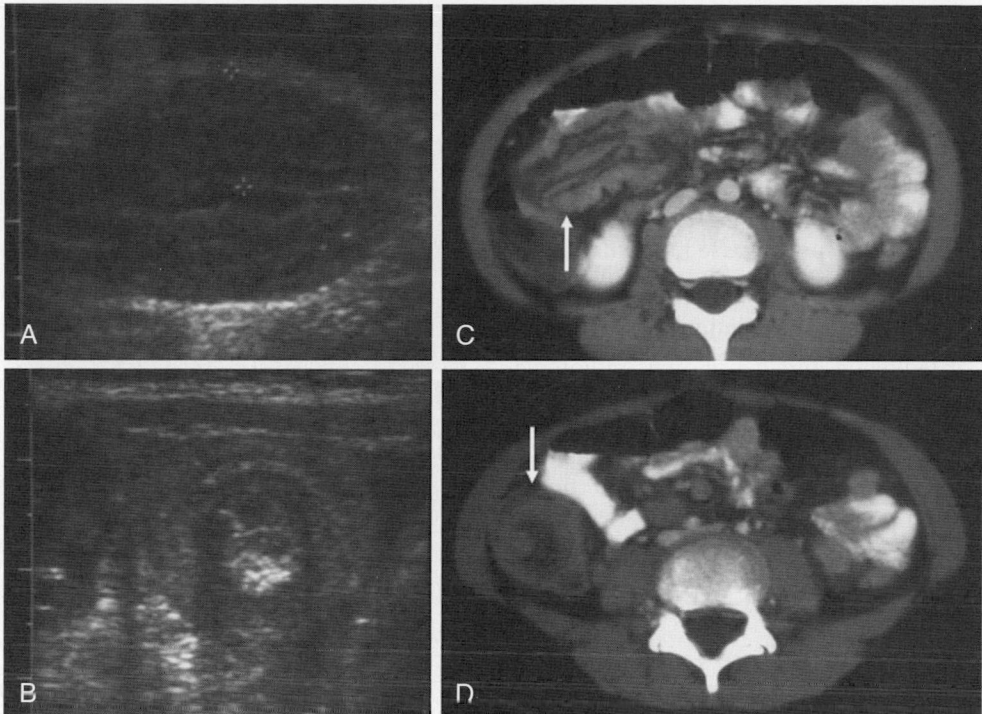

Figure 66-118 Non-Hodgkin lymphoma and intussusception. Ultrasound in a patient with Burkitt lymphoma (**A** and **B**) and CT in a patient with large-cell lymphoma (**C** and **D**) show typical features of intussusception, either small bowel/small bowel (**A** and **B**) or ileocolic (**C** and **D**).

virus (EBV) infection and has a pattern of bulky mesenteric and pelvic adenopathy, as well as involvement of multiple visceral organs including the liver, kidneys, and pancreas (see Fig. 66-64). Response of Burkitt lymphoma to chemotherapy is often quite rapid, with bulky disease responding within weeks. In contrast, the endemic form of Burkitt lymphoma, which is encountered in equatorial Africa, is usually associated with EBV infection (95%) and characteristically presents with jaw, orbit, paraspinal, and CNS involvement.[374]

Posttransplant lymphoproliferative disease (PTLD) is seen in the setting of both solid-organ and bone-marrow transplantation and results directly from the immunosuppression regimens used.[388] The lymphoproliferative disease, which is usually EBV-related, often responds to reduction in immunosuppression (Fig. 66-119). However, the lymphoproliferative disease may progress to an aggressive B-cell lymphoma, resulting in widespread malignant disease. PTLD can involve multiple organs and systems and responds variably to conventional lymphoma therapies. FDG-PET imaging is not routinely used in the management of PTLD, although some have advocated its use to improve early disease detection and staging.[389]

Just as with Hodgkin lymphoma, the role of FDG-PET imaging in non-Hodgkin lymphoma is currently being validated. Several studies of small cohorts of patients have indicated that FDG-PET is valuable both for staging and for predicting response to therapy in patients with

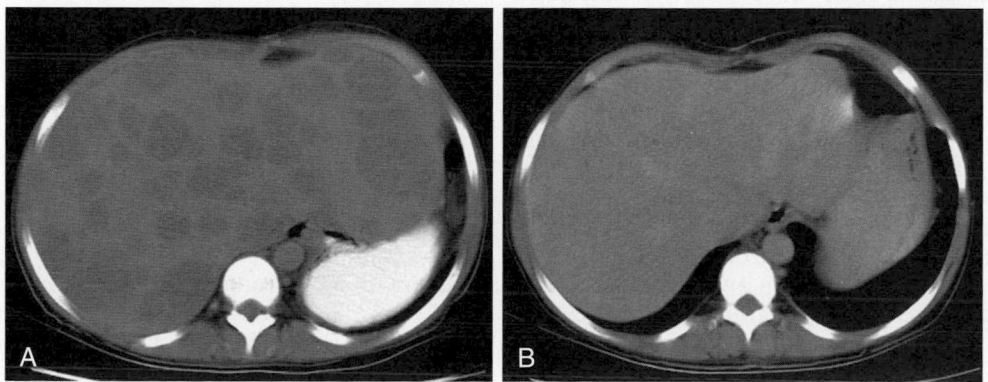

Figure 66-119 A 22-year-old patient with a renal transplant developed extensive PTLD involving the liver (**A**). **B**, Four months after reducing the immunosuppressive therapy, the PTLD had nearly completely resolved.

various forms of NHL.* As suggested by these studies, FDG-PET, particularly when combined with cross-sectional imaging either by CT or MRI, is extremely sensitive at detecting sites of disease that may not have otherwise been identified. It seems obvious that identifying the extent of disease should impact both staging and monitoring of treatment response; however; prospective trials are needed to determine whether FDG-PET response alone can by used to direct response-based modulation in therapy.

Sites of Relapse in Hematologic Malignancies

In the treatment of leukemia and lymphoma, radiologic evaluation plays an important role in monitoring for disease relapse. In addition to intramedullary (i.e., bone-marrow) relapse, common sites of extramedullary leukemic relapse include kidneys, spleen, CNS, and bone. Although less common, relapse to "sanctuary sites" such as the testicle can occur, both with diffuse organ infiltration and enlargement and with focal mass deposits (Fig. 66-120). Relapse to these sites may occur even in the setting of bone-marrow remission.

IMAGING TREATMENT COMPLICATIONS

Complications resulting from the treatment of pediatric malignancies are myriad. It is important to note that the radiographic manifestations of fungal and other infectious diseases may not be manifest during periods of profound neutropenia (Fig. 66-121). Often, abnormalities on imaging studies emerge only after peripheral neutrophil counts recover and infection-fighting white blood cells become available to mount an inflammatory response. Infectious complications commonly include localized as well as disseminated fungal infection. The extent of hepatic and splenic involvement may be better detected by MRI (Fig. 66-122).[394]

Cardiomyopathy results from cardiotoxic chemotherapy agents such as doxorubicin. Echocardiography has become the imaging modality of choice in monitoring patients with this complication. Pulmonary toxicity can range from subtle ground-glass opacity, which can be an early manifestation of bronchiolitis obliterans with organizing pneumonia (BOOP, or cryptogenic pneumonia) to frank interstitial pulmonary fibrosis.[395]

Children with cancer also have poorly understood hypercoagulable state. Pulmonary emboli and other sites of venous thrombosis occur at an increased incidence in these patients and may be detected either incidentally (Fig. 66-123) or in response to specific clinical symptoms.[396] Clinically the probability of thromboembolic disease may be difficult to assess. The presence of multiple known risks factors, including indwelling catheters, concurrent infection, immobility, dehydration, and chemotherapy all increase the risk of thromboembolic events in these patients,[397] and the clinician and radiologist must be vigilant in their respective examinations to enable

<hr />

*References 134, 136, 150, 246, 247, 390-393.

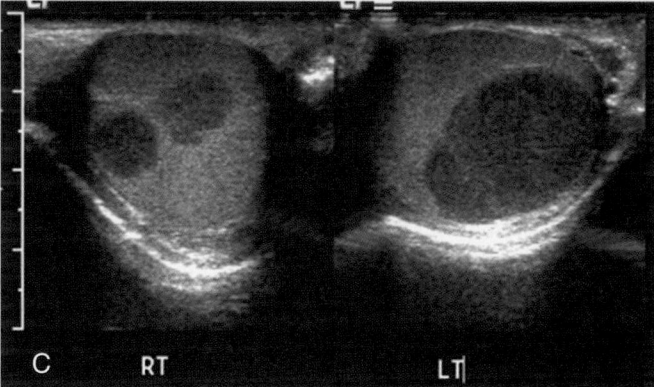

Figure 66-120 Scrotal relapse of leukemia. A 17-year-old patient with high risk ALL, s/p bone marrow transplant had painless scrotal swelling and palpable abnormalities on exam. Scrotal ultrasound shows multiple bilateral hypoechoic masses (**A** and **C**) (relative to testicular parenchyma) with increased blood flow to the masses (**B**), diagnostic of scrotal relapse.

early detection and treatment of these potentially live-threatening complications.

Gastrointestinal complications occur during periods of neutropenia and can range from typhlitis (with localized inflammation of the cecum) to extensive pancolitis and bowel necrosis (Fig. 66-124).[398,399] Asparaginase, which is included in many chemotherapy regimens for ALL and lymphoblastic lymphoma, results in pancreatitis in approximately 5% to 10% of patients. The severity of pancreatitis can range from a mild chemical pancreatitis to frank pancreatic necrosis and subsequent pseudocyst formation (Fig. 66-125). This is best evaluated initially by ultrasound, with CT reserved for persistent or worsening clinical pancreatitis or to assess for complications such as pseudocyst.[400]

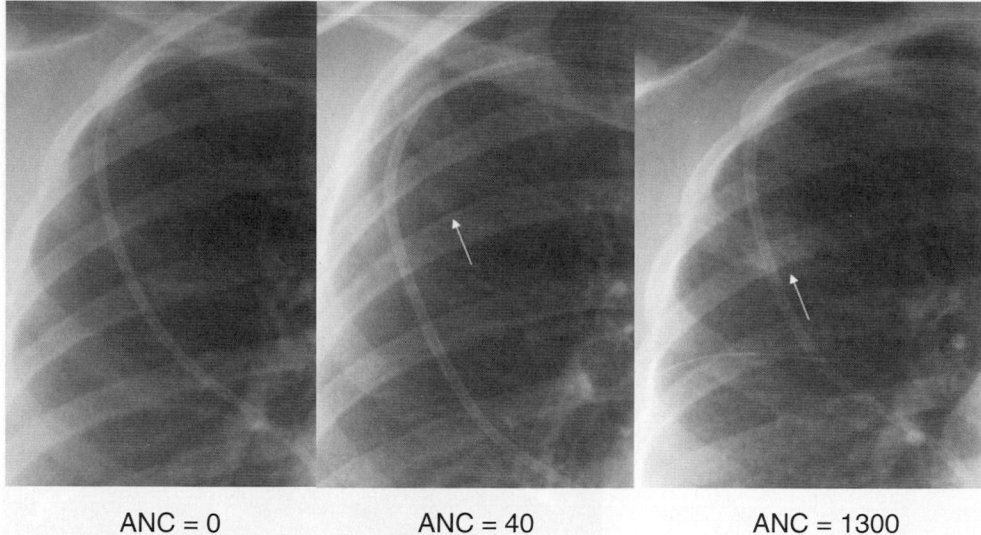

ANC = 0   ANC = 40   ANC = 1300

Figure 66-121 Imaging the patient with neutropenia. X-rays are of a 12-year-old patient with AML. Note the appearance of focal lung nodule *(Aspergillus)* as the patient's blood cell counts recover, suggesting that the appearance of infectious lesions in patients with neutropenia may be challenging to detect until the marrow has recovered after ablative chemotherapy.

Bony complications can arise after chronic treatment with corticosteroids and include osteopenia, fractures, bone-marrow infarcts, and osteonecrosis (Fig. 66-126), the latter of which is most typically seen in the hips and knees.[401] Second tumors, particularly musculoskeletal tumors, may be seen after radiation therapy. Osteochondromas involving the clavicles and sternoclavicular junction, for example, are common in patients with lymphoma who have received mantle radiation, particularly if radiation occurred at an early age. Malignant degeneration of these lesions is rare.

CNS changes can develop after radiation and chemotherapy. In one study, hemorrhagic events were seen in 4 of 120 children with ALL. All of these children had been disease-free for more than 2 years and had been treated with prior chemotherapy and cranial radiation.[402] These events are most commonly related to treatment-induced vasculopathy and may show diffuse or localized vasculopathy. Asparaginase may also produce venous sinus thrombosis, leading to profound neurologic deficits and areas of venous infarction (Fig. 66-127). Methotrexate, which is given both systemically as well as intrathecally for CNS prophylaxis in patients with high-risk ALL, may produce a leukoencephalopathy characterized by symmetric periventricular white-matter signal abnormalities. These changes may be transient or permanent. They are not specific to methotrexate and can be seen with other chemotherapeutic agents that penetrate the CNS.

Patients treated for cancer in childhood are also known to have an increased risk of developing second malignant neoplasms as a result of both cytotoxic chemotherapy and radiation therapy. In reports from the Childhood Cancer Survivor Study (CCSS), there was a 2.3-fold increase in second malignant neoplasms in children treated previously for cancer,[403] with patients who had Hodgkin lymphoma or Ewing sarcoma at greatest risk

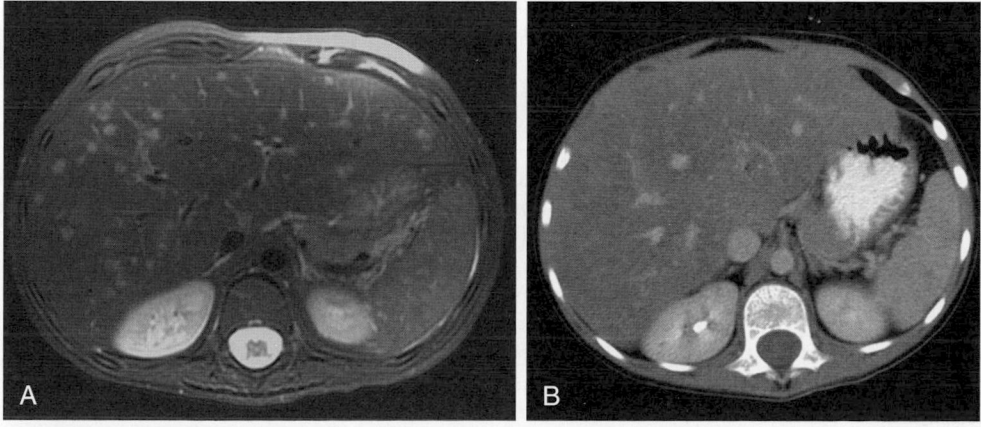

Figure 66-122 Imaging hepatosplenic fungal infection. MRI using fluid-sensitive FSEIR (or similar) sequences (**A**) is very sensitive for detecting lesions not seen with CT (**B**) or ultrasound.

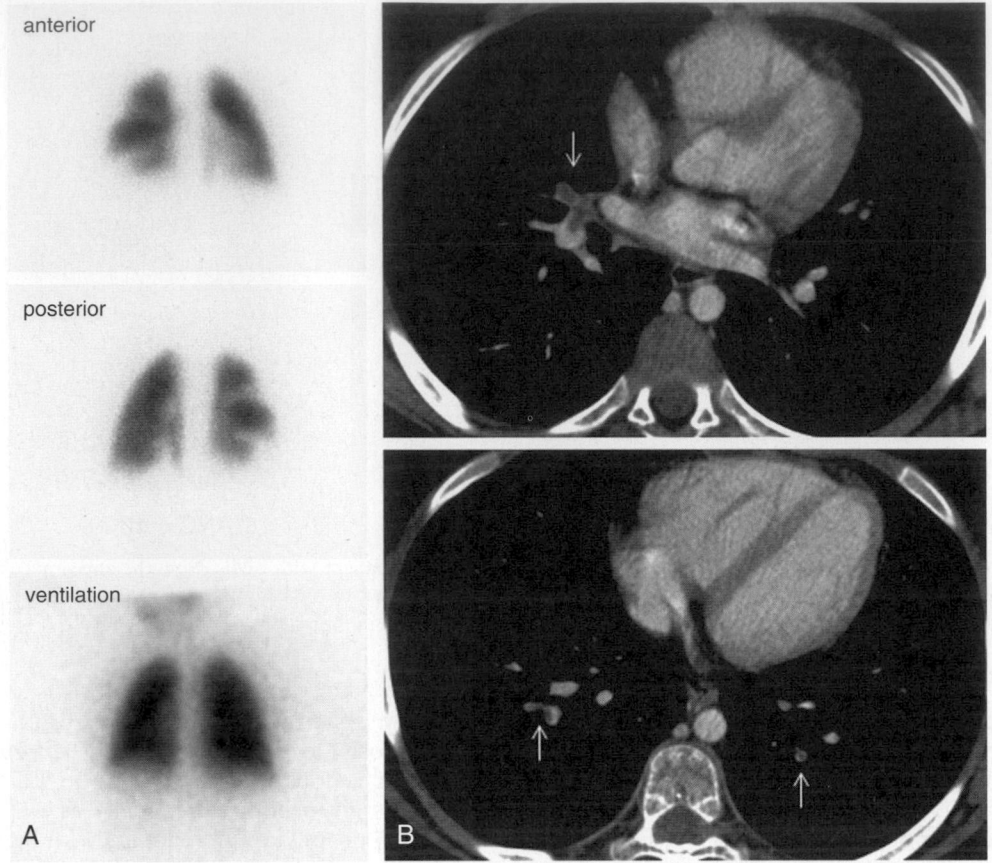

Figure 66-123 Pulmonary emboli. A 6-year-old boy with T-cell ALL had fever and neutropenia. CT scan of the chest identified multiple pulmonary emboli involving multiple lung segments (**B**). CT findings were confirmed by ventilation/perfusion scanning (**A**), which demonstrated multiple perfusion defects corresponding to involved segments identified by CT, but no corresponding ventilation defects.

(Fig. 66-128).[404] The most common second cancers include bone, breast, and thyroid cancer, as well as tumors of the CNS (meningioma and glioma) (Fig. 66-129).[405]

INTERVENTIONAL RADIOLOGY IN PEDIATRIC ONCOLOGY

Pediatric interventional oncology, also known as the "fourth pillar of cancer treatment" is an emerging specialty that offers an alternative resource when other options like surgery, chemotherapy, or radiation therapies have limited usefulness. This primarily involves use of minimally invasive techniques with image guidance for directly targeting tumors, both for diagnostic and for therapeutic reasons. When considering "tumors" broadly, to include nonneoplastic growths, pediatric interventional radiologists are involved in all aspects of management from diagnosis to treatment to offering palliative care. With regard to neoplastic disease, oncology-related pediatric interventional radiological procedures have traditionally been limited to diagnosis, management of complications, and procedures designed as auxiliaries to open surgery. Because of limitations such as the approval process for new devices, protocol-driven pediatric oncologic practice, and the inherent hesitation of trying new treatments in children, the development of

interventional oncology for children has been challenging.[406] Newer landmarks in pediatric therapeutic oncological interventions are under active development, but standards remain to be established. Although many broad principles in adult and pediatric interventions are the same, some specific aspects related to procedures in children deserve discussion, and are enumerated in the following list.

1) Informed consent: Because most pediatric patients younger than 18 years of age have parents or legal guardians, a detailed preprocedural discussion is necessary to educate them regarding possible complications, some of which may remain present throughout life. Many adolescent patients are able to participate actively in the decision-making process. This usually requires a detailed conversation that is simple, clear, and addressed in a way to make the parents and the child comfortable without inducing unwarranted fear of the procedural risks. It is appropriate to create a "child-friendly environment" to provide a sense of safety, security, and dedicated pediatric care.

2) Sedation and anesthesia: Almost all the procedures in children need general anesthesia or higher levels of sedation to minimize motion, help children tolerate pain better, and allow positioning during the

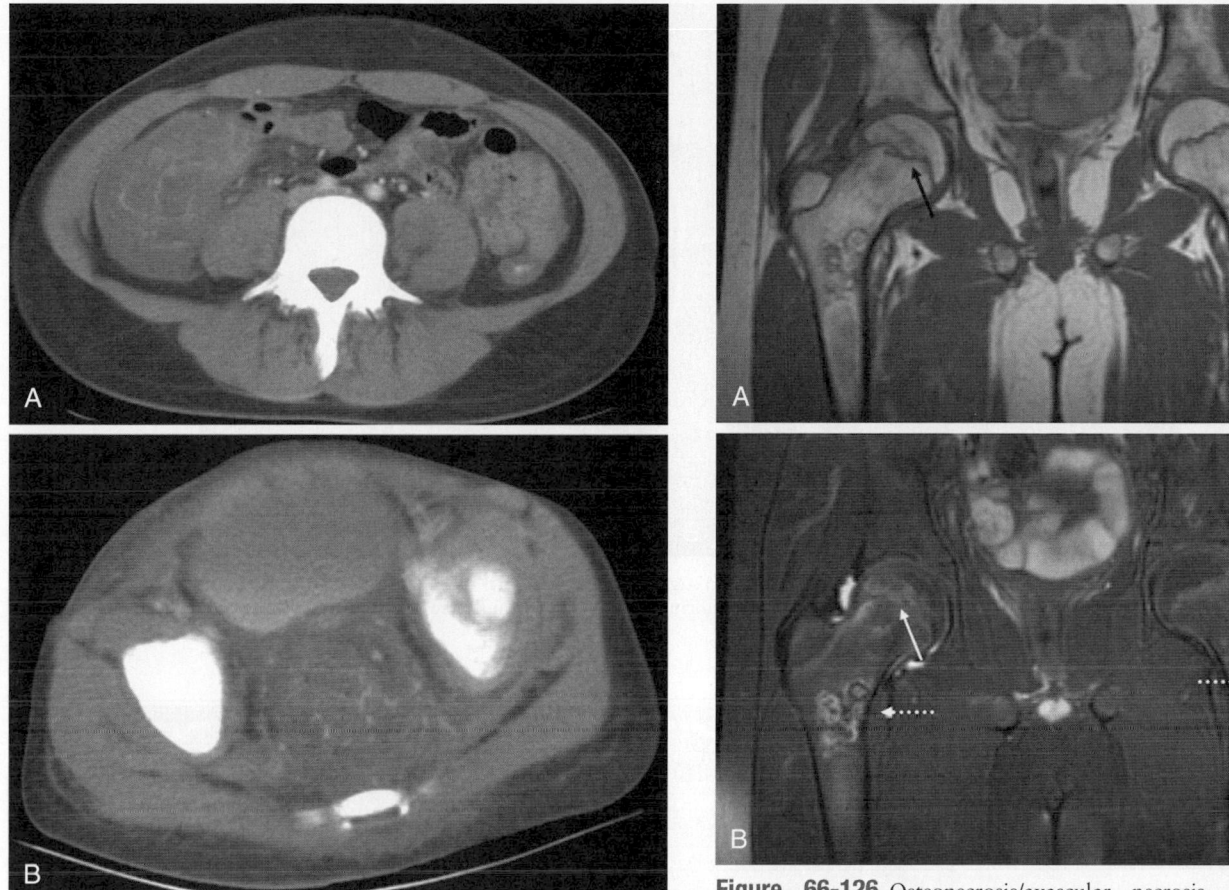

Figure 66-124 Contrast-enhanced CT in two patients with neutropenic colitis, showing disease primarily of the terminal ileum and cecum; i.e. typhlitis (**A**) and more extensive pancolonic disease with severe rectal necrosis that required diverting ileostomy (**B**).

Figure 66-126 Ostconccrosis/avascular necrosis. A 13-year-old patient with a history of high-risk ALL, receiving high dose steroids, experienced right hip pain. Unenhanced T1-weighted (**A**) and Gd-enhanced (**B**) MRI of the hips and pelvis show osteonecrosis of the right femoral head *(arrows)* and evidence of bone infarcts in both femoral necks *(dashed arrows)*.

procedure. Deep sedation or general anesthesia can provide some postprocedural amnesia, unlike adults who can tolerate most procedures under mild sedation and local anesthesia.

3) Equipment: Most available devices are designed for use in adults. Hence bench modifications of devices developed for adults are often performed to match the smaller body habitus of children.

4) Contrast and radiation: It is imperative that contrast doses be diligently monitored in children to minimize renal toxicity. Likewise, maximal efforts are directed to limit the radiation dose, because the cumulative effects of radiation are of major concern in children. Most interventional radiologists practicing in adult populations concern themselves largely with the deterministic effects of radiation

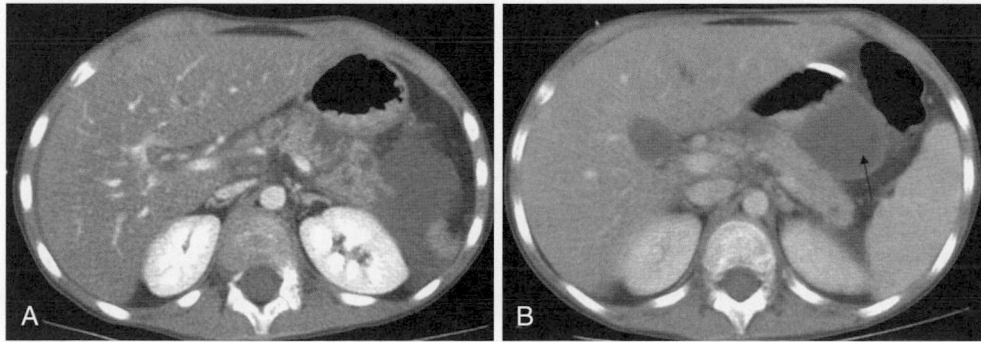

Figure 66-125 An 11-year-old with ALL receiving asparaginase developed severe pancreatitis (**A**) and subsequent pseudocyst formation *(arrow)*, with the pseudocyst closely adherent to the posterior wall of the stomach (**B**).

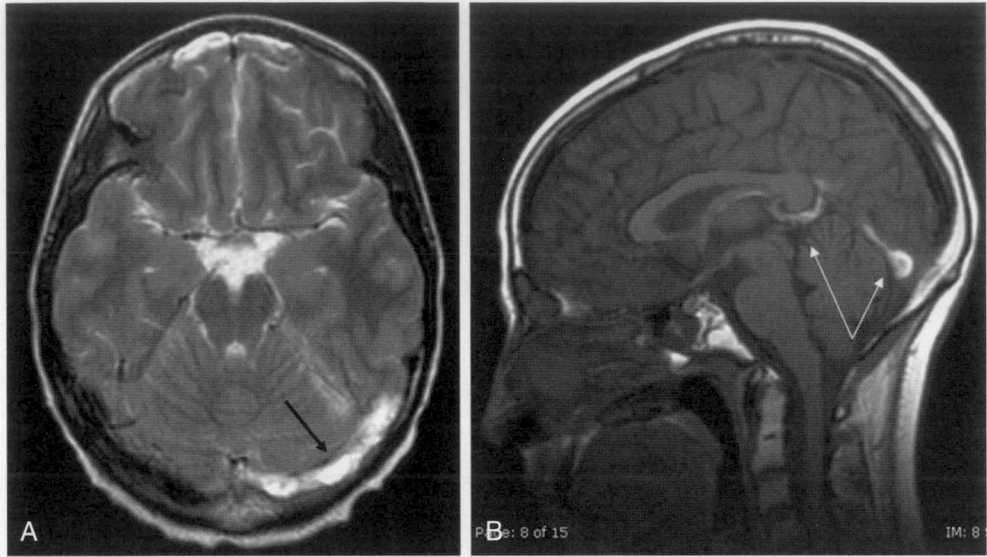

Figure 66-127 Cerebral sinus thrombosis. Axial T2-weighted (**A**) and sagittal T1-weighted (**B**) MRI in a 15-year-old patient with ALL, receiving asparaginase during induction therapy, shows high signal-intensity abnormality in the left transverse sinus, straight sinus, and deep cerebral veins *(arrows)*.

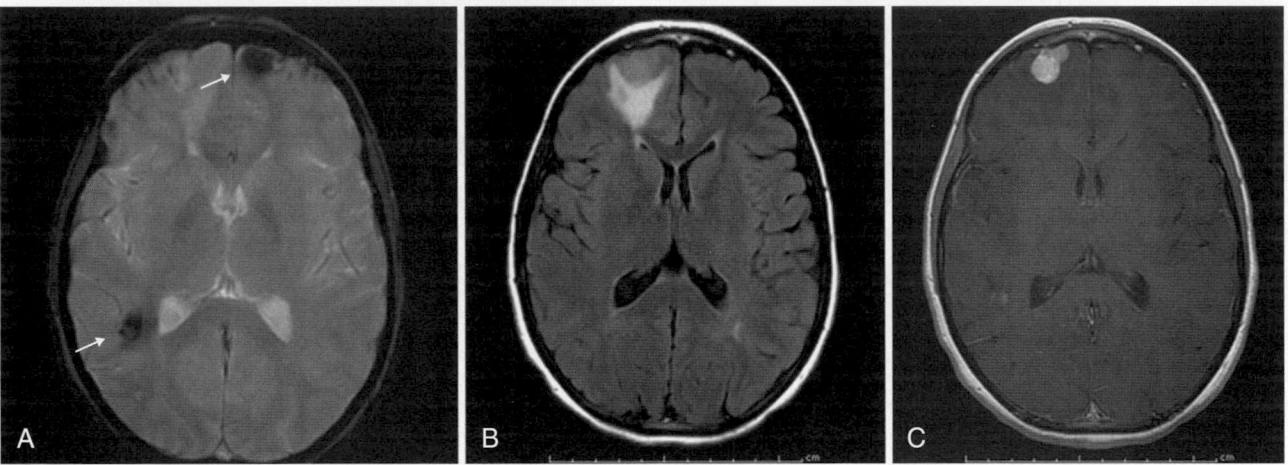

Figure 66-128 Radiation-related change and second malignancy. A 22-year-old patient was treated for ALL as a child with chemotherapy and craniospinal radiation therapy. Known cavernous angiomas (**A,** *arrows*) were being monitored routinely. She experienced seizures, and a new right frontal-lobe lesion seen on T2-FLAIR (**B**) and contrast-enhanced T1-weighted (**C**) MRI was found on resection to be high-grade sarcoma, presumably related to prior radiation.

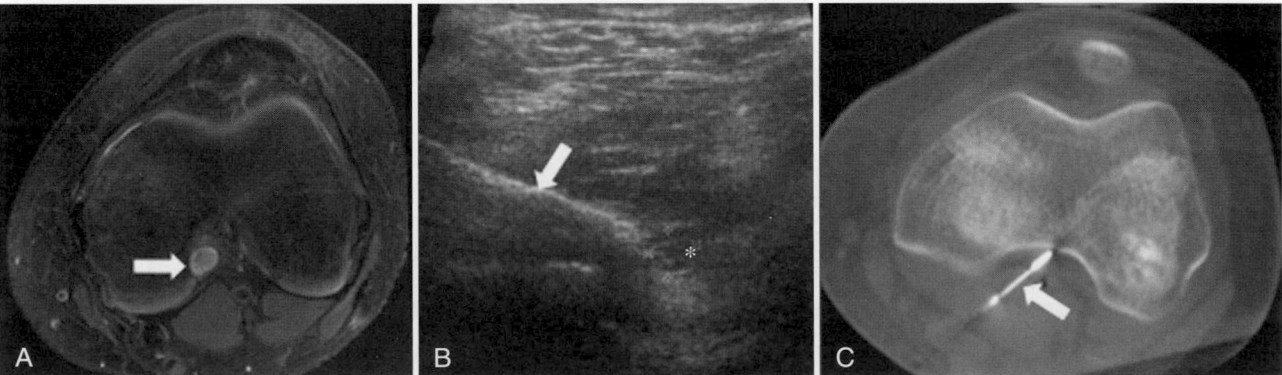

Figure 66-129 Percutaneous image-guided core needle biopsy. **A,** Axial T2-weighted fat inversion recovery MRI demonstrating a painful focal solid mass situated deep into the intercondylar notch of femur *(arrow)*. **B,** Ultrasound-guided access of the nodular lesion *(asterisk)* with a coaxial needle *(arrow)* **C,** Dyna CT images tumorstrating the biopsy needle deployed into the lesion *(arrow)* to obtain samples.

related to dose and time of exposure at the time of the procedure. These effects are usually manifest as damage to bone marrow, gastrointestinal mucosa, or skin. It is, however, the stochastic effects, those cumulative effects that are related to any exposure to ionizing radiation regardless of time or dose, that are far more concerning in the pediatric population than the adult.[407]

There is no minimum threshold radiation dose for stochastic effects to occur, and stochastic exposure (primarily related to DNA damage) may not manifest itself for decades. It is specifically in young children with many years of life ahead that these issues are of greatest concern. Additionally, many oncology patients are exposed to high-dose external-beam radiation as part of their treatment protocol, adding to the risk. The ALARA concept of radiation exposure is ubiquitous in radiology but is held to much higher standard in pediatric diagnostic imaging and pediatric interventional radiology, with risk of radiation exposure always weighed against the benefits of a given image-guided procedure, and every attempt is made to use the lowest possible radiation dose. Limiting the fluoroscopy time, low-dose pulse fluoroscopy, aggressive coning and filtering applied to the smallest possible region of interest, and maximal utilization of imaging modalities that are nonionizing are used to reduce radiation exposure.

5) Anatomic considerations: Children have a smaller body mass index, which can limit accessibility. In compact regions like the neck, continuous image guidance using ultrasound imaging or CT fluoroscopy is preferred during biopsies to avoid major blood vessels and nerves. In children these procedures are done with the use of general anesthesia, which may obscure immediate signs of nerve injury. Because of the smaller volume of subcutaneous fat and muscle bulk, the skin can be also vulnerable to injuries during ablation of tumors. These aspects of the procedure must be carefully considered during preprocedure planning.

6) Physiologic responses: Physiologic responses to intervention can be different in a child versus an adult. For example, vasospasm is commonly seen in children, making simple access or further intravascular manipulation more challenging. Children react to fluid imbalances and medications more quickly. Therefore close monitoring of fluid balance and drug dosages based on weight or body-surface area is mandatory; vigilant care on the part of specialized pediatric nurses and a pediatric anesthesia team is invaluable.

Role of Interventional Oncology

Generally, oncological interventions depend on the kind of care that is provided. This can be divided into the following areas: 1) diagnostic evaluation; 2) therapeutic care; and 3) supportive and palliative care.

Diagnostic Evaluation

Percutaneous Needle Biopsy

Core biopsy can provide tissue both for accurate histopathology, immunohistochemistry, and molecular pathology necessary for diagnosis and differentiation of childhood tumors. In some tumors like neuroblastomas, biopsy provides tissue not only for histologic classification but also for analysis of prognostic factors, such as *MYCN* and ploidy status.[408] Almost any mass can initially be biopsied using image-guided percutaneous needle biopsy. Ultrasound guidance is usually the imaging modality of choice given its real-time capability. Most biopsy needles are sonographically visible, and precise real-time targeting of most masses is possible, even in locations adjacent to vital structures (see Fig. 66-129). Other guidance modalities can be used for targeting, including CT and MR; these typically require general anesthesia. These authors often use Dyna CT with the I-guide technology to target areas situated in critical or compact zones (Fig. 66-130). Correlation with MRI or FDG-PET can guide the targeting to viable segments of tumor.

Evaluating tissues located in prior operative sites or within radiation fields can be challenging diagnostically

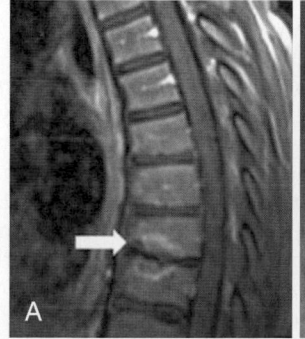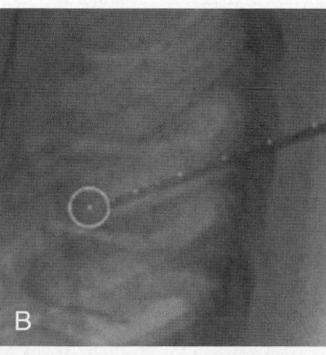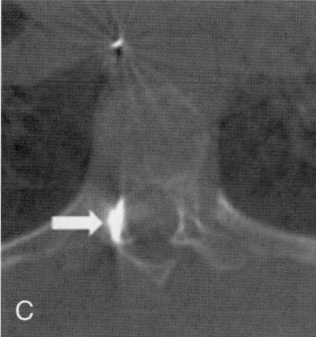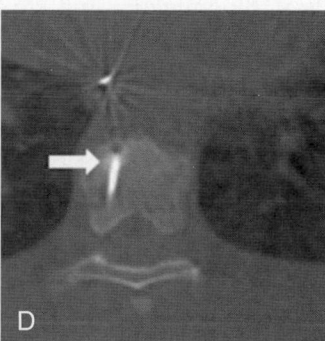

Figure 66-130 Percutaneous image-guided core needle biopsy. **A,** Sagital T1-weighted contrast enhanced MRI of the spine demonstrating an enhancing destructive lesion of contiguous vertebral endplates *(arrow)*. **B,** The more destructive of the endplates was targeted using the I-guide technology *(circle)* on Dyna CT. **C,** Transpedicular course *(arrow)* of the biopsy needle is seen on the Dyna CT image. **D,** The biopsy needle tip is safely positioned at the proposed biopsy site *(arrow)*.

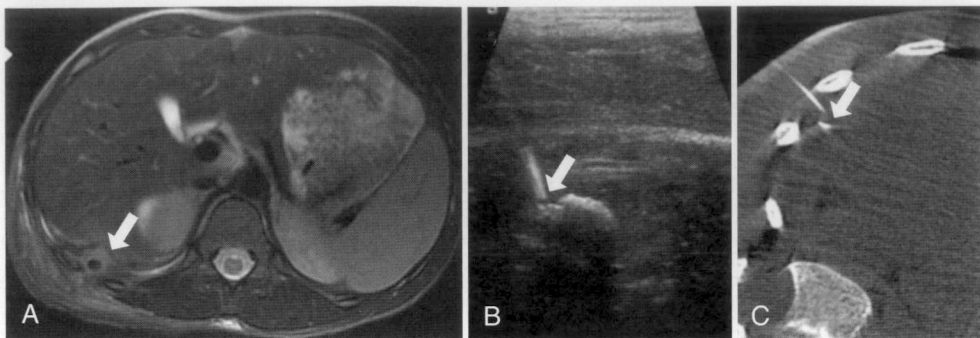

Figure 66-131 Needle localization. **A,** Axial T2 MRI of the abdomen demonstrating a hypointense, likely calcified, subhepatic nodule causing intense perilesional inflammation. An image-guided needle localization of this was requested before surgical exploration. **B,** Ultrasound-guided access toward the lesion *(arrow)* was performed. **C,** A hook was deployed *(arrow)* at the nodule to help localize the lesion at surgery as seen on Dyna CT image.

and can also be difficult to access, particularly when situated deep to vascular, neural, and bony structures. A multiple quadrant sampling or targeted sampling of FDG-avid areas should be planned, because intratumoral histologic heterogeneity could result in sampling artifacts that lead to incorrect prognostic histologic subgroup assignment,[408] which in turn may impact therapy. The most commonly biopsied structures include liver, renal and suprarenal tumors, mediastinal tumors, musculoskeletal tumors with associated soft tissue, and bony masses.

Obtaining a sample from the soft-tissue mass, bone mass and its interface is most helpful. Automated or semiautomated cutting needles in the range of sizes between 14-gauge and 20-gauge are available providing 1- to 2-cm throws. A coaxial core-needle biopsy technique is used, in which an initial puncture of the skin and the tumor capsule is made using a needle mounted on a coaxial outer cannula. A 16- or 18-gauge cutting needle (manual or spring-loaded) is then advanced via this outer cannula into the lesion, and several samples are obtained aiming at different tumor quadrants. This technique theoretically reduces the chance for tract seeding and also the possibility of bleeding and infection by limiting the number of punctures. Using the coaxial needle also allows the biopsy tract to be embolized if bleeding does not stop spontaneously or in patients with poor coagulation. For bone biopsies an 11- or 13-gauge needle permits the coaxial passage of a trephine Ackermann needle (Cook Medical, Bloomington, Ind.) to complete the bone biopsy. Smaller coaxial systems such as the Bonopty biopsy needle (Radi Medical Systems, Uppsala, Sweden) (12 and 14 gauge) are also available. Bony drills can be employed to obtain deeper access or access very hard bony lesions. Risks are smaller and rare and include bleeding, infection, and injury to the structures around the target.

Very tiny lesions or anatomically arduous areas can be subjected to fine-needle aspiration. Fine-needle aspiration can be obtained using a 20- to 22-gauge needle placed independently or coaxially via an 18- to 19-gauge needle. Whenever possible, the shortest and safest course to reach the lesion should be chosen. Accuracy, less invasiveness, low rate of complications, shorter recovery time, and ability to do targeted and multiquadrant sampling through minimal number of accesses are some of the

major benefits of image-guided percutaneous biopsies.[409-412] Available pooled data suggests that 95% of image-guided needle biopsies provide adequate sample for tissue diagnosis in childhood malignancies.[413] CT or sonography can be used preoperatively, using similar technique as for biopsy, to place Kopans localization hook wires (Cook Medical, Bloomington, Ind.) (Fig. 66-131) or coils or to inject a dye to help the surgeon easily find the lesion during operation.[414] The interventional radiologist also has the ability to place central venous lines or chemotherapy ports as part of the same interventional radiological procedure, precluding the need for a separate operating room visit and additional anesthesia.

Therapeutic Care

Therapies providing local control of tumors are widely used in adult interventional oncology practice. Indications for regional cancer treatments in children are still evolving and are based largely on experience extrapolated from the adult literature. These can be categorized broadly based on their principle of use: 1) transarterial embolization; 2) tumor ablation; 3) high intensity focused ultrasound; and 4) irreversible electroporation.

Embolization Therapy

This technique involves performing catheter angiography to determine the arterial perfusion to the tumor. After this, feeding vessels are selectively catheterized to deliver tumoricidal drugs or to create tumor ischemia by stopping the blood flow in these vessels.

Chemoembolization. This is also known as *transarterial chemoembolization (TACE)* in which chemotherapy is delivered by injecting a mixture of the chemotherapeutic agent with Ethiodol or particles, or as chemotherapeutic agent-impregnated beads, also known as *drug-eluting beads (DEBs)*. This technique concentrates the chemotherapy drug in the target tissues, with the embolization effectively prolonging the dwell time of the agent in the target with less systemic effect than intravenous or oral chemotherapy. In adults TACE has been widely used for hepatocellular carcinoma and hepatic colonic metastases. It has significantly prolonged 2-year survival rates up to 63% as compared to 27% with supportive care.[415]

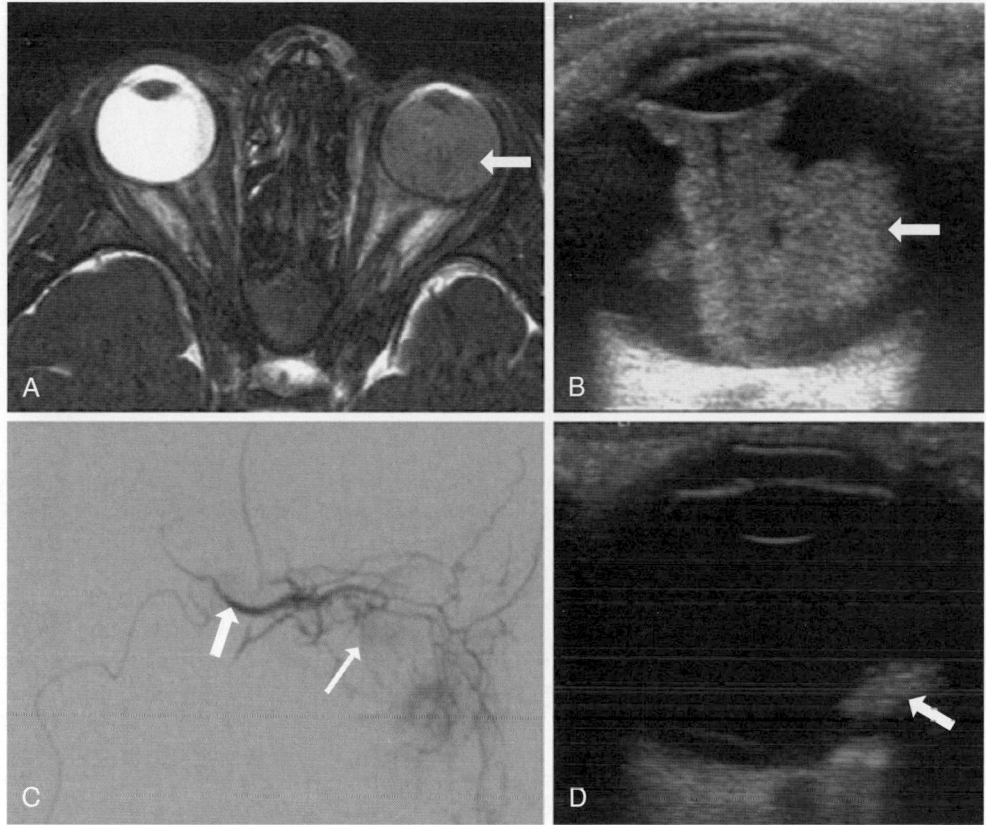

Figure 66-132 Intraarterial chemotherapy. **A**, Axial T2-weighted image of the orbits showing a hypointense retinoblastoma filling the entire left orbital cavity *(arrow)*. **B**, Ultrasound obtained during the first intraarterial chemotherapy demonstrating the hyperechoic intraorbital mass *(arrow)*. **C**, Selective left ophthalmic artery angiogram *(thick arrow)* before superselective chemotherapy demonstrating retinal blush *(thin arrow)*. **D**, Ultrasound obtained during the second intraarterial chemotherapy demonstrating the remarkable tumor shrinkage with a very small residual mass *(arrow)*.

Presurgical TACE for pediatric hepatoblastoma has been shown to decrease tumor volume without causing significant chemotoxicity, allowing for complete tumor removal.[416] In unresectable lung metastases having dual supply from pulmonary and bronchial arteries, TACE has been well tolerated as a palliative procedure.[417] TACE has also been used in osseous tumors[418] and in Wilms tumor, demonstrating prolonged time to tumor progression and increased survival compared with surgery alone.[419] Intraarterial chemotherapy for retinoblastoma has been widely accepted for pediatric tumors (Fig. 66-132).[420]

Radioembolization. In transarterial radioembolization (TARE) radioactive materials are used to embolize hepatocellular carcinomas with a technique similar to TACE. External radiation therapy in patients with diffuse hepatic malignancy does not improve overall survival,[421] in part because of the relatively low radiation tolerance of liver tissue when compared with the doses required for tumoricidal effect.[421,422] TARE is usually chosen for chemoinsensitive tumors or when chemotoxicity limit is reached. The technique also involves selective catheterization of the hepatic artery supplying the tumor and injecting yttrium-90 (^{90}Y) microspheres. This has been shown to have less toxicity, higher response rate with a longer time to disease progression, and a similar survival rate in patients with advanced hepatocellular carcinoma when compared with chemoembolization.[423] Potential complications include locoregional radiation effects, pulmonary irradiation, and gastric perforation. To reduce pulmonary or systemic irradiation a diagnostic study is initially performed by injecting ^{99m}Tc-labeled macroaggregated albumin (MAA) (the same tracer used for routine lung scans), allowing the hepatic-to-pulmonary artery shunt fraction to be estimated before embolization.[424] Preprocedure coil embolization of gastrointestinal collaterals prevents gastrointestinal irradiation.

Bland Embolization. This technique is mostly used palliatively in hypervascular tumors like hemangiomas[425] and angiosarcomas,[426] both to control symptoms and arrest tumor growth. It also used preoperatively to decrease the blood loss at surgical resection[427] or to reduce intractable blood loss in pediatric tumors.[428] It is occasionally used to arrest the growth of neuroblastoma metastases causing life-threatening hepatomegaly. The feeding arteries supplying the tumor are selectively catheterized and embolized with either polyvinyl alcohol (PVA) or Gelfoam particles, cutting off the blood supply to cause tumor shrinkage and necrosis (Fig. 66-133).

Ablation Therapy

Ablation results in local destruction of tumor using chemical or mechanical methods. Prior cross-sectional imaging

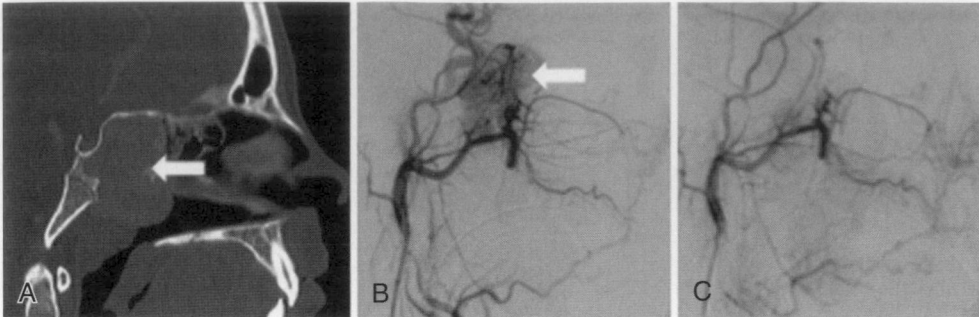

Figure 66-133 Juvenile nasopharyngeal angiofibroma. **A,** Sagittal-CT reconstructed image of the head demonstrates a large nasopharyngeal mass *(arrow)*. **B,** Selective internal maxillary artery injection demonstrating hypervascular nasopharyngeal mass *(arrow)*. **C,** After selective embolization with polyvinyl alcohol particles, there is near complete cessation of flow to the mass with preservation of the normal circulation.

is necessary in most patients to delineate the lesion and its relationship to critical structures like nerves, blood vessels, spinal cord, and hollow viscera, which are prone to injury during local ablation. This also helps plan the tract for probe placements and with assessment of the tumor volume to be treated. Local ablation techniques are most often used to treat hepatic tumors, desmoid tumors, and renal tumors and bony and pulmonary metastases.

Chemical Ablation. This is an established technique for treating hepatocellular carcinoma[429-433] and has been described for treating other solid tumors.[432] It is performed by percutaneously injecting and infiltrating the tumor with alcohol or acetic acid. The cytotoxic mechanism of action of ethanol is through cytoplasmic and membrane dehydration, denaturation of cellular proteins, and small-vessel thrombosis, resulting in coagulative necrosis. Acetic acid causes protein denaturation and dissolution of basement membrane and interstitial collagen, resulting in coagulative necrosis of tumor cells. Although these ablative techniques are technically simple, there is a small risk for nontarget tissue injury, including damage to adjacent blood vessels, nerves, organs, or overlying skin, especially if the tumor lacks a definite capsulation. Recently patients with desmoid tumors have been treated with acetic acid ablation.[434]

Thermal Ablation. These techniques provide cytolysis of the tumor cells either by thermal destruction or ionic agitation.

Radiofrequency Ablation. In this technique small probes are percutaneously directed into the tumor using

image guidance like CT or Dyna CT. A radiofrequency generator generates high-frequency (375-500 kHz) alternating current applied directly via these probes, producing ionic agitation and frictional heat, thereby causing coagulation necrosis in tumor target tissue. Because this involves an electric circuit, grounding pads applied to the patient are necessary to allow the exit of the current. Local tissue temperatures reach 60 to 100° C, adequate to produce the cytotoxic effect. Temperatures greater than 100° C are generally not beneficial, because this produces tissue vaporization and carbonization, impeding conductance of the thermal energy and limiting the size of the ablation zone.[435] The burn time varies between 6 and 12 minutes. Proper placement of the grounding pads in full contact with the skin without any air pockets is necessary to avoid burns.[436]

Different tissues conduct electrical currents to different degrees. Blood vessels and bile ducts disproportionately absorb current, creating heat sinks that can confound planned heating of target ablation zones. Strategies to limit the temperature drop include internal cooling of the probe with chilled water, diffusion of water along the electrode tines, or preembolizing the feeding arteries adjacent to the tumor.[435] In children, radiofrequency ablation is most commonly used to treat osteoid osteoma (Fig. 66-134), osteoblastomas, and chondroblastomas.[437] Radiofrequency ablation has been used for large hepatic adenomas,[438] Wilms tumor,[439,440] and desmoplastic round-cell tumors in children.[441] A phase I study to determine the toxicity of radiofrequency ablation for solid tumors in children concluded that toxicity is limited and that radiofrequency ablation may offer a local control alternative in carefully selected pediatric patients.[442]

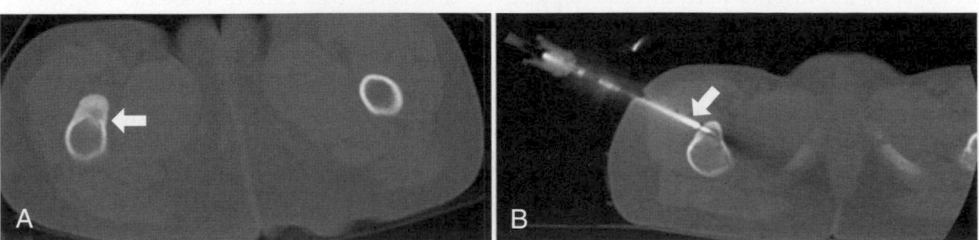

Figure 66-134 Radiofrequency ablation. **A,** Axial CT image of the hips demonstrates a painful sclerotic osteoid osteoma at the anterior cortex of the right femur *(arrow)*. **B,** The tumor was treated with radiofrequency ablation *(arrow)*, resulting in immediate resolution of pain and of the tumor at the follow-up examination.

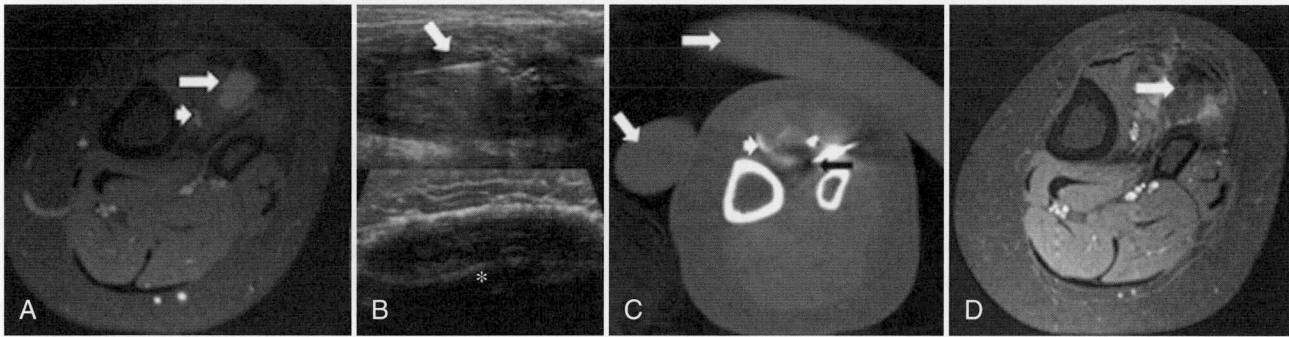

Figure 66-135 Cryoablation. **A,** Axial T1-weighted contrast-enhanced MRI of the left leg demonstrates a well-defined enhancing, recurrent desmoid tumor along the anterior aspect near the peroneus muscles *(arrow).* The tibial neurovascular bundle lies in the vicinity *(arrowhead).* **B,** The tumor was cryoablated using ultrasound guidance for probe placement *(arrow).* Posterior acoustic shadow from the ice ball formation seen at intraprocedural ultrasound *(asterisk).* **C,** Dyna CT monitoring during cryoablation. Contrast was used to create hydrodissection *(short arrow)* to protect the neurovascular bundle. A thermistor *(black arrow)* was positioned close to the neurovascular bundle to monitor temperature drop and prevent inadvertent nerve injury. Note the warm saline bags *(long arrows)* placed for skin protection during cryoablation. **D,** Follow-up postcontrast axial MRI of the leg demonstrates the loss of enhancement at the tumor ablation site *(arrow).*

Radiofrequency ablation has shown to be effective in pain palliation of painful bony metastases.[443,444]

Cryoablation. This is one of the oldest ablation techniques used and produces tissue destruction by applying nitrogen to surgically exposed tumors.[445] This technique has been surgically used (open or laparoscopic) to treat tumors. With newer imaging techniques that detect small cancers in early stages, together with the availability of smaller cryoprobes, these procedures are now being performed percutaneously using image guidance. The system involves a set of 11- to 17-gauge cryoprobes through which gases from pressurized cylinders are circulated to produce the desired effect of freezing and thawing. Argon gas is used to produce freezing (cooling), and helium gas is used to produce thawing (warming). The Joule-Thompson effect of rapid gas expansion is the basis for rapid cooling of the metallic cryoprobes when there is sudden release of highly pressurized argon gas from the probe. As low as −100° C is reached within a few seconds. On a similar principle, there is production of heat caused by rapid expansion of helium gas that causes local warming. These effects are used alternatingly in a cycle with two 10-minute freezes separated by a 5-minute passive thaw to optimize tumor destruction. There is irreversible tissue destruction that occurs at temperatures below −20 to −30° C. Mechanisms causing cell death are by direct freezing, denaturation of the cellular proteins, cell-membrane rupture, cell dehydration, and ischemic hypoxia.[435] There is formation of an ice ball at the tip of the cryoprobe, the size of which can be either fixed or varied (V-probe), depending on the type of probe used. The size of the ice ball with respect to the tumor volume coverage can be carefully monitored using CT[446] intermittently every 2 to 3 minutes.

Once adequate freezing of the tumor volume is achieved, cryoablation is stopped, thus preventing injury to the adjacent normal structures. Unlike radiofrequency ablation, there is very little or almost no pain after cryoablation. Additionally, larger tumors adjacent to critical structures can be treated more safely. Nerve injury, skin blistering, and bowel injury have been reported with this modality. However, these effects can be minimized by image-based planning, use of temperature monitoring probes to measure adjacent tissue temperatures, careful monitoring of ice ball formation, and use of tissue protection (Fig. 66-135) including hydro-dissection and warm saline bags over the skin. Cryoablation has been effectively used for treating desmoid tumors,[447] in palliation and local control of Ewing sarcoma,[448] and for painful bony metastases. Percutaneous cementoplasty has also been used as an adjuvant with radiofrequency ablation[449] and cryoablation in palliative pain management.

Microwave Ablation. This system consists of a microwave generator and a set of internally cooled antennas. Most microwave antennas are straight and needlelike with variations such as monopole, dipole, triaxial, choked, or slotted. These antenna shafts are as small as 17 gauge and are cooled by circulating chilled saline or by using compressed carbon-dioxide gas. This allows for delivery of higher powers for longer times to produce larger ablation zones. The generators emit 915 to 2450 MHz microwaves, creating high-speed microwaves that cause rapid vibration and rotation of the molecular dipoles within the ablation zone. This ionic agitation produces frictional heating and thermal coagulation of the tissue. Unlike radiofrequency ablation, the heating energy is deposited directly at the antenna rather than by creating a resistive heating circuit. This precludes the necessity of using grounding pads and chance of having skin burns. Additionally, there is less influence of tissue impedance factors like perfusion-mediated cooling. This system can create rapid heating of tumor tissue to greater than 100° C very quickly.[450] Multiple applicators can be safely placed in one session to optimize the ablation volume.[451,452] The use of microwave ablation has not been routine in children, but it is becoming more popular in adults for ablation of liver, lung,[453] and bone tumors.[454]

Laser Ablation. Although not widely used, laser ablation has also been used for treating tumors. An optical laser fiber transmits infrared light energy into the tumor to produce heat and coagulation necrosis.[435] The 17-gauge fibers are coaxially placed through 14-gauge guide needles, and the active tip is exposed. The size of induced zone of ablation depends on the laser wavelength, thermal and optical properties of the tissue, total duration of energy application, power used, diameter of the fiber, fiber tip, and number of fibers used sequentially or simultaneously for ablation.[455,456] An additional advantage of lasers is their MRI compatibility. Laser ablation has been used in the treatment of osteoid osteomas[457,458] and in lung metastases.[459]

High-Intensity Focused Ultrasound. Ultrasound waves generated by high frequency vibrations of up to 10 MHz are focused into a small discrete target region using a concave or parabolic arrangement.[460] When the local tissue absorbs this acoustic energy there is production of thermal energy, which creates coagulative tissue necrosis. Other changes, including tissue cavitation, microstreaming, and radiation forces generated during this process have been reported to contribute to the overall tumor lysis. Dose delivery to targeted tissues depends on the transducer array, the energy input, and the tissue attenuation that occurs between the transducer and the target.[461] This technique is entirely noninvasive and does not require incisions, general anesthesia, or blood transfusions, making it more appealing than the other modes of ablation. To minimize inadvertent injury to adjacent structures guidance and monitoring of acoustic therapy is critical. Sonography and MRI, especially in the obese,[462] can be used for image guidance and monitoring. Dynamic MRI temperature mapping to assess the ablative zone can also be performed.[463,464] Given the inherent behavior of ultrasound waves, this modality has limitations for lesions that are covered by bone or air-containing viscera, like bowel, which provide very high impedance to these waves. High-intensity focused ultrasound has been used in the treatment of desmoids,[465] bone,[466] and other solid tumors.[467]

Irreversible Electroporation. Irreversible electroporation (IRE) is novel technique in which high-voltage microsecond electrical pulses are applied through percutaneously placed probes into the tumor tissue. This technique causes tumor lysis by creating permanent pores in the cell membrane, which leads to apoptosis.[468] There is no generation of thermal energy; therefore critical structures like blood vessels, biliary ducts, and nerves are not adversely affected.[469,470] No grounding pads are necessary, thus avoiding possible skin burns. Most research on its application has been for pancreatic,[470] liver, pulmonary, and renal tumors.[471]

Supportive Care

Interventional radiologists play a major role in providing supportive care to cancer patients. These patients are usually referred after failed attempts at vascular accesses by other services or as an alternative to high-risk operations. By combining innovative approaches with image guidance and technical skill, these procedures provide a relatively safe and effective option in many difficult clinical situations for managing complex cancer patients.

Venous Access

Venous access in cancer patients is a major requirement for chemotherapy and nutritional support. It can also cause concern in small, underweight children with poor venous caliber. Maintenance of access can be problematic in patients with chronic venous stenosis resulting from long-standing line placement. Central line and peripherally-inserted central catheter (PICC) placements are commonly performed procedures in interventional radiology. These can be tunneled and partially buried underneath the skin at their exit points to provide a secure long-term intravascular access. Chemotherapy port placements can also be performed by interventional radiologists, a procedure ideally coordinated with the patient undergoing image-guided needle biopsy. This is shown to be safe and successful with a low rate of complications.[472,473] The initial vessel access is obtained using direct ultrasound guidance with a single anterior wall puncture, decreasing access time and complication rate and improving overall success of access.[474,475] Catheter position can be manipulated and confirmed simultaneously using fluoroscopy.

For central line placements or chemotherapy port placements, interventional radiologists prefer the internal jugular vein for access over the subclavian vein approach preferred by the surgeons (Fig. 66-136). This choice prevents the "pinch-off syndrome" caused by catheter kinking and is not associated with pneumothorax, hemothorax, and brachial plexus injury seen in the subclavian venous approach.[476] Chronic indwelling subclavian lines can also cause central venous stenosis. This has the disadvantage of precluding placement of dialysis fistulae in the upper extremity and making placement of peripherally inserted intravenous catheters more challenging.[477] Placement of these lines in interventional radiology is more accurate, less traumatic, and greatly reduces chances of inadvertent neurovascular injury. In patients with venous stenosis, venography can also be performed to assess for collateral patency and placement of venous lines using these pathways (Fig. 66-137). Paravertebral veins, internal thoracic veins, external jugular veins, although tenuous, can be safely accessed using sonographic guidance for placement of venous access in patients with inaccessible extremity veins.[478] Salvage procedures such as repositioning and removal of incorrectly positioned catheters (Fig. 66-138), fibrin stripping of occluded central venous catheters, and stenting of stenosed SVCs can also performed conveniently in interventional radiology.[476]

Ancillary Supportive Care

Interventional radiology also offers other supportive care in oncology patients, especially in palliative care. Enteric access for providing nutritional requirements becomes essential in cancer patients who feed poorly for a variety of reasons. Primary gastrostomy and transgastric jejunostomy tubes can be primarily placed with percutaneous nonendoscopic techniques using fluoroscopic guidance[479] and have the advantage of avoiding inadvertent bowel injury.[480] The transgastric tube may be inserted during the initial placement, avoiding the need for another tube

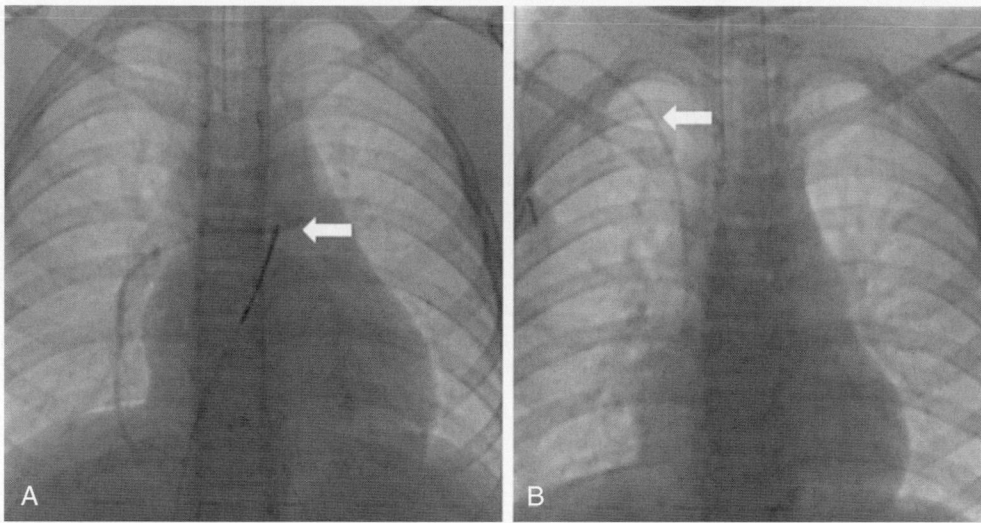

Figure 66-136 Port placement. **A,** Frontal chest radiograph demonstrates the migrated catheter of a chemotherapy port placed via the left subclavian vein. The proximal end of the catheter was floating in the main pulmonary artery with the distal end trapped in the lower branch of the right pulmonary artery. This was snared in the main pulmonary artery *(arrow)* and removed. **B,** A new chemotherapy port was then placed using a right internal jugular venous approach *(arrow)*.

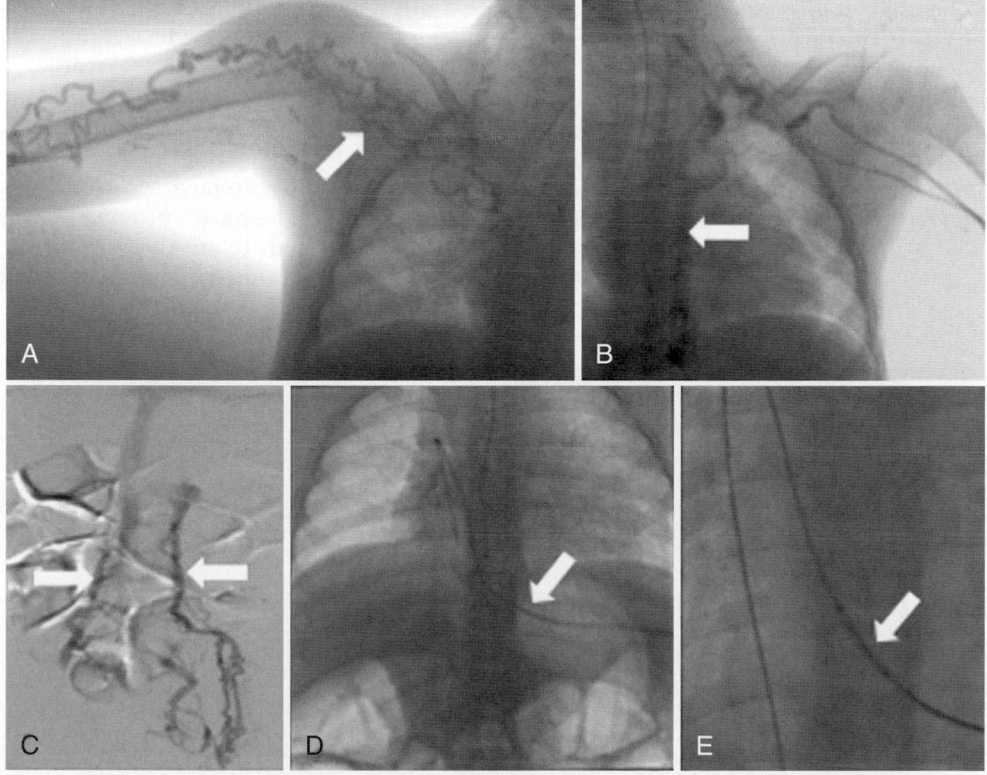

Figure 66-137 Difficult venous access. **A-C,** A patient with an imminent requirement for a central line had bilateral upper and lower extremity venograms demonstrating thrombosis of normal veins with extensive collateralization *(arrows)* diverting flow to the cava. **D,** Because of poor venous access, a posterior paravertebral vein was accessed, and a central line was inserted via the hemiazygos vein *(arrow)*. **E,** One year later there was line damage requiring an exchange. During the exchange there was extreme resistance at the access site with stenosis of the hemiazygos vein, which was angioplastied *(arrow)* to achieve successful exchange.

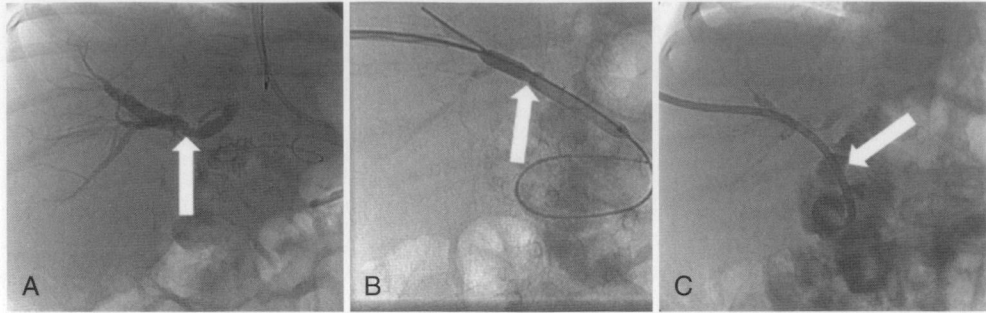

Figure 66-138 Hepatobiliary intervention. **A,** Percutaneous transhepatic cholangiogram in a liver transplant patient with elevated liver enzymes showing biliary strictures *(arrow).* **B** and **C,** The stricture at the confluence was dilated *(arrow* in **B)** and a biliary drain to the jejunum *(arrow* in **C)** was placed, relieving the patient's symptoms.

conversion, as is required for endoscopically placed tubes. The routine exchange of these tubes is performed in interventional radiology, providing a dedicated and consistent team for support in the maintenance of these tubes.

Certain complex procedures, including biliary interventions such as percutaneous cholangiograms (PTCs), percutaneous transhepatic biliary drain (PTBD) placements (see Fig. 66-138), percutaneous transhepatic intrabiliary biopsies, and cholecystostomies are occasionally performed in pediatric oncology patients but are more commonly encountered in adults. Interventional radiology procedures like PTBD placement and hepatic vein dilation are most often used after liver transplant in cancer patients. These include percutaneous and transjugular liver biopsies performed with ultrasonographic and fluoroscopic guidance for the diagnosis of graft disease; angioplasty and stent placement for treatment of vascular and biliary occlusion, stenosis, and stricture; and catheter placement for drainage of fluid collections.[481,482] In patients with portal hypertension a transjugular intrahepatic portosystemic shunt can be placed to decompress the liver as a bridge to transplantation.[483] In the genitourinary system, percutaneous nephrostomy catheter placements, nephroureteral catheters, ureteral stents, and suprapubic catheter placements for extrinsic abdominal or pelvic tumors causing urinary obstruction are all performed in interventional radiology (Fig. 66-139).[484]

Occasionally catheter-directed thrombolysis of the deep vein thrombosis in cancer patients[485] and placement of IVC filters to prevent pulmonary embolism are other supportive procedures performed by interventional radiologists. Patients with multivisceral transplants, including bowel transplant, may suffer recurrent chylous fluid accumulation. Intranodal lymphangiogram performed by accessing a groin node is a novel procedure that helps diagnose this condition and allows percutaneous embolization (Fig. 66-140) to treat this challenging posttreatment complication.

NEW IMAGING TECHNIQUES

Molecular Imaging

Historically the standard tools of radiology—CT, MRI, and ultrasound—have provided primarily anatomic information, with relatively little direct functional information being evident. Nuclear medicine imaging has

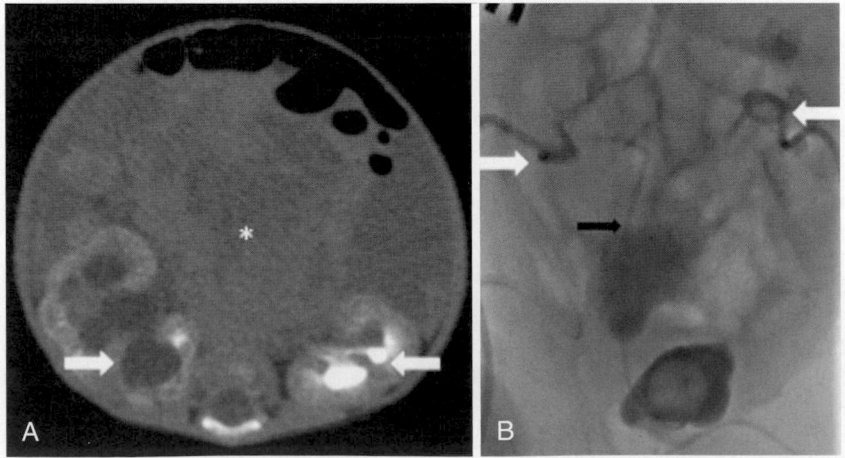

Figure 66-139 Genitourinary intervention. **A,** Axial CT image of the abdomen demonstrates a large rhabdoid tumor compressing the ureters and causing bilateral hydronephrosis. **B,** Bilateral percutaneous nephrostomy catheters *(white arrows)* and a right ureteric stent *(black arrow)* were placed to provide urinary diversion.

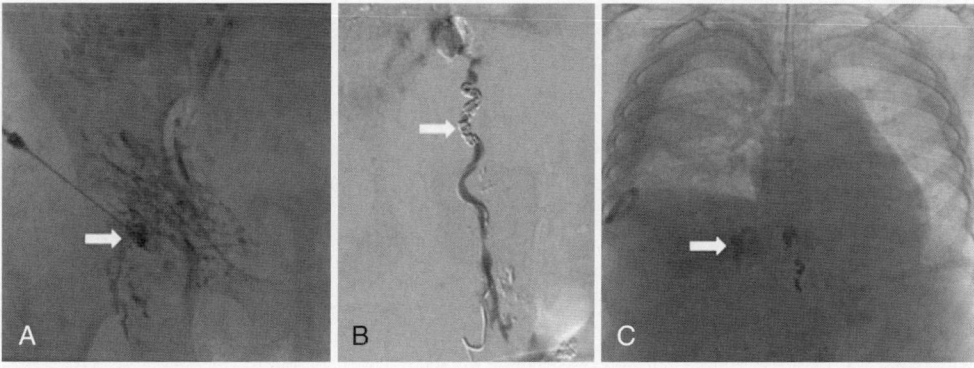

Figure 66-140 Intranodal lymphangiography and embolization. **A,** A child with recurrent chylous effusion after multivisceral transplant underwent intranodal lymphangiography *(arrow).* **B,** The cisternae chyli was percutaneously embolized with coils and glue *(arrow).* **C,** The persistent leak *(arrow)* that was causing recurrent pleural effusions stopped.

provided useful functional information but has been limited by the lack of accompanying anatomic detail available with conventional planar and SPECT techniques, although PET imaging has provided a considerable improvement in the anatomic resolution, particularly with the use of hybrid imaging approaches. Of the three major cross-sectional imaging technologies, MRI has come closest to providing direct information about cellular function, for example by employing diffusion-weighted imaging to assess regions of localized ischemia and using hydrogen (^1H) spectroscopy to derive metabolic information about specific regions being imaged. Functional MRI of the brain relies on relative changes in blood oxygen level in metabolically active tissues to yield exquisite information about cerebral activation in response to various stimuli. The relative success enjoyed by MRI in generating functional images derives mostly from the rich and varied information contained in the MR signal from different materials. Although most of the MR information being imaged routinely arises from the protons contained in hydrogen atoms from water molecules and lipids, a vast amount of metabolic information can also be derived from MR signals arising from molecules other than water.

The U.S. Food and Drug Administration (FDA), in its critical-path initiative, has emphasized the need to increase the speed, efficiency, and cost-effectiveness of drug development for cancer and other diseases.[486] Molecular imaging and functional imaging probes have great potential to identify and characterize disease-specific targets and to provide target- and treatment-specific imaging end points for therapy. In particular, as markers of biological response, imaging end points that characterize cellular vitality or apoptosis, receptor down-regulation, or functional inactivation, and treatment-specific changes to cellular metabolism will be critical in determining the success or failure of newer classes of molecular-based therapies. As has been learned with imatinib and gastrointestinal stromal tumors, noncytolytic therapies that slowly extinguish tumor metabolic activity do not immediately result in tumor shrinkage, and imaging techniques that directly measure tumor metabolism are necessary to directly reflect the response to

therapy.[487] In addition, for many molecularly targeted agents such as antibodies or receptor-targeted agents, it is unclear whether the agents ever localize in tumor in vivo. For these compounds, it is critical to develop surrogate end points of response. The ability to directly image the distribution and targeting of such agents in vivo would significantly benefit this assessment, particularly when there is a poor overall clinical response to therapy. Phase 1 trials of therapeutic agents in particular offer an opportunity to use imaging as means of establishing drug activity at a time when therapeutic efficacy may not be the primary or anticipated goal of therapy. As shown in Figure 66-141, in a phase I/II study of the insulinlike growth factor 1 receptor (IGF1R)–targeted agent cixutumumab[488] after just one 4-week cycle of therapy a child with metastatic fibrosarcoma showed a nearly complete metabolic response to therapy despite minimal change in tumor size. Conventional measures of response would have concluded there was no activity in this patient, highlighting the importance of molecular imaging techniques in assessing novel noncytolytic approaches to therapy.

Newer functional imaging approaches are also expected to impact treatment strategy and drug design with an emphasis on response-based treatment regimens. This allows patients with a high likelihood of response to be treated less aggressively, whereas those not responding to therapy are identified early and redirected into more aggressive therapeutic regimens.

Molecular imaging has been defined by the Commission on Molecular Imaging of the American College of Radiology as the "spatially localized and temporarily resolved sensing of molecular and other processes in vivo".[489] Although molecular imaging techniques, particularly in nuclear medicine, have been in use for many years, this terminology has recently been applied to the rapidly growing area of radiologic investigation aimed at developing tools to allow direct imaging of cellular and molecular events. Increasingly there has been recognition that the ability to perform multiparametric functional imaging is likely to provide the greatest insight into tumor or tissue biology and response to therapy by providing quantitative parameters (biomarkers) that derive from

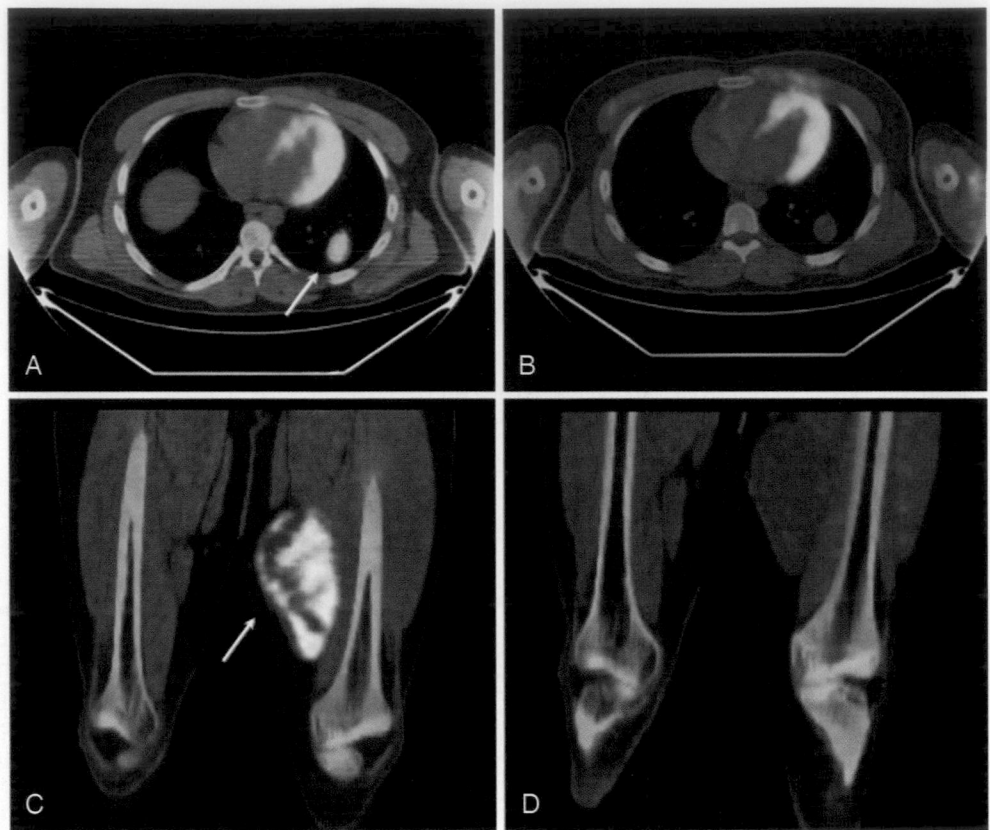

Figure 66-141 Reduction in FDG-PET activity with cixutumumab. Fused axial PET/CT of chest (**A** and **B**) and lower extremities (**C** and **D**) show increased uptake at baseline in metastatic left lower lobe lung nodule (**A**, *arrow*) and intense baseline uptake in a primary left midthigh mass at baseline (**C**, *arrow*) in a patient with metastatic fibrosarcoma. After 2 weeks of cixutumumab therapy, although the lung nodule had not changed in size, there was no significant residual FDG uptake remaining (**B**). Similarly, there was significant reduction in FDG uptake at the primary left thigh site with no apparent change in size of tumor (**D**) after 2 weeks of therapy. *(From Malempati, Weigel B, Ingle AM, et al: Phase I/II trial and pharmacokinetic study of cixutumumab in pediatric patients with refractory solid tumors and Ewing sarcoma: a report from the Children's Oncology Group.* J Clin Oncol *30:256–262, 2012.)*

merging the information obtained from different imaging techniques,[490] for example diffusion- and perfusion-weighted MRI results coupled with metabolic changes visible by PET imaging.[47]

Most of these investigations are still in the early stages of development[486,489,491,492] and include development of optical imaging probes, imaging gene expression, imaging marker genes, tracking cells in vivo, and developing targeted biomolecular conjugates to allow visualization of specific cellular and molecular events in vivo.[493,494] Perhaps the most fruitful area of research has been in the application of near-infrared fluorescent imaging to evaluation of malignant disease.[495-498] Fluorescence in the near-infrared range of the spectrum has been pursued, because these wavelengths penetrate biologic tissue further than visible or infrared light. Light in the visible spectrum is largely absorbed by abundant biomolecules such as hemoglobin that are present in most tissues, whereas light in the infrared range is almost completely absorbed by water.[499] The ability to image fluorescing tissues has long been in use in the laboratory setting but has not yet found clinical utility. The development of "smart" near-infrared fluorescent imaging probes has allowed tumor-specific enzymatic activity to be directly imaged by fluorescence. These probes are synthesized such that the near-infrared fluorophores are attached to a peptide scaffold that, by virtue of its amino acid sequence, can be selectively cleaved by tumor-specific proteases. Fluorescence of the near-infrared fluorophores is quenched because of their close proximity in the intact peptide scaffold. Upon enzymatic cleavage in the tumor, the fluorophores are released, and the resultant near-infrared fluorescent signal provides a specific signal, allowing tumor visualization. This technique has been used successfully to detect tumor-specific cathepsin activity in colon- and breast-cancer models[496] and more recently has been used for real-time hepatobiliary interventions.[493,500] Although the depth of penetration of near-infrared light still limits this technique to structures near the surface, near-infrared fluorescent imaging has been used with success intraoperatively for sentinel lymph node[501] identification and has great potential to provide guidance in determining tumor margins and sites of lymph node spread and in evaluating cavities and tissue linings such as the peritoneum, which are poorly imaged by other techniques.[502]

Magnetic Resonance Spectroscopy

Whole body MRI imaging uses the aggregate signal characteristics of a given tissue to generate high-resolution images that reveal information about both the anatomy and state of health of the tissue but give little direct information about the biochemical makeup of the tissue. In contrast, MR spectroscopy focuses on acquiring chemical information from small volumes of tissue, with the aim of characterizing the ongoing chemical processes that are unique to specific tissues. This is accomplished by separating the signal derived from specific tissue and cellular constituents into their different chemical forms. The protons contained within tissues experience a molecular environment that is unique to the tissue. These variations in molecular environment produce alterations or chemical shifts in the resonant frequency of the constituent protons. In theory, when the nuclear MR (NMR) signal is displayed as a function of resonant frequency, the different chemical forms in the tissue should yield a unique "spectroscopic fingerprint." In practice, large water and lipid peaks dominate the proton NMR spectra from biological tissues, with the less abundant elements giving lower signal. Because of the need to reduce heterogeneity of tissue within the voxel being interrogated, the small volumes of tissue evaluated by MR spectroscopy generally produce low signal, and prolonged imaging times are needed to acquire useful spectra. With prolonged imaging times, degradation of spectra from motion artifact occurs, and to date the majority of the routine spectroscopic examinations have focused on applications in the brain, where the tissues being examined remain relatively static.[52]

With higher field-strength magnets, faster scanning sequences, and advances in postprocessing techniques, ^{1}H-MR spectroscopy is increasingly being used for nonneurologic body applications. Some investigators have used ^{1}H-MR spectroscopy together with dynamic contrast-enhanced MRI to show that increases in vertebral marrow-fat content and accompanying decreases in marrow perfusion correlated with varying states of osteopenia and osteoporosis.[503] Others have evaluated the utility of ^{1}H-MR spectroscopy to characterize and monitor response to therapy in some pediatric solid tumors including neuroblastomas[504] and in adult prostate cancer.[505] Response of neuroblastoma to chemotherapy has been shown to correlate with decreases in cellular Cho peaks,[506] although this had not been validated against conventional imaging techniques in prospective clinical trials.

^{1}H-MR spectroscopy has also been used to characterize bone and soft-tissue tumors, with elevated Cho levels detected in lesions shown to have a malignant histology but not in the majority of benign lesions.[507] Quantitative spectroscopic measurement of trimethylamine concentration in MPNSTs has also been reported as having potential for the differentiation of benign and malignant lesions[508] and could be combined with FDG uptake for better characterization of these lesions. Several years ago, Preul et al. suggested that a pattern-recognition analysis of the biochemical information obtained from ^{1}H-MR spectroscopy of brain tumors could reliably distinguish benign, low grade, and high-grade tumors and suggested that specific tumor and nontumor "fingerprints" might ultimately provide an accurate noninvasive preoperative characterization of particular lesions.[509] Although considerable progress has been made, much work is still needed

to develop a similar "library" of characteristic spectra for other pediatric solid tumors.

Other nuclei that can be evaluated with MR scanners, particularly at higher field strengths, include ^{31}P-phosphorus, ^{13}C-carbon, and ^{23}Na-sodium. These nuclei all have lower gyromagnetic ratios than protons and resonate at lower frequencies than protons for a given field strength. The molecules and ions containing these nuclei are also much less abundant than water protons, so that the signal-to-noise ratios from these nuclei are low compared with those associated with proton MRI. As such, large voxels must be sampled from a given tissue in order to obtain a sufficient signal-to-noise ratio with a reasonable scan time. ^{31}P-MR spectroscopy enables the observation of energy metabolism and intracellular compartmentation through the signals of phosphomonoesters (PMEs), phosphodiesters (PDEs), inorganic phosphate (P_is), and nucleotide triphosphates, mainly adenosine triphosphate (ATP). Depending on the tissue being studied, a peak from phosphocreatine may also be seen (such as brain and muscle). When compared to ^{1}H-MR spectroscopy in the evaluation of bone and soft-tissue tumors, ^{31}P-MR spectroscopy was superior in identifying lesions shown to have a malignant histology.[507] Whether ^{31}P spectroscopic measurement of intratumoral changes in a phosphate metabolite profile will be feasible and valuable in response assessment remains to be validated.

SURVEILLANCE IMAGING

Surveillance imaging in pediatric oncology presents a unique challenge. Since the mid 1960s new treatment developments have continued to result in dramatic improvements in event-free and long-term overall survival rates for patients with many pediatric cancers.[510] For example, in Hodgkin lymphoma, long-term survival rates of greater than 90% can now be expected, with even higher rates of survival in lower-stage disease.[137,511] Along with these improvements in overall survival there has been a shift in the treatment paradigm. With efforts to develop criteria for upfront risk stratification coupled with response-based reduction in treatment intensity, current approaches are aimed at reducing late effects and improving overall treatment-related complications while preserving excellent long-term treatment outcome and survival. At the same time, advances in diagnostic imaging have led to a corresponding increase in number of imaging evaluations performed on these same patients.[512] Increases in use of conventional radiography, CT, MRI, and PET imaging, although providing important information about disease stage and response to therapy, are also costly and contribute to cumulative exposure to ionizing radiation, particularly from CT and nuclear medicine examinations.[512,513] Even though the doses of radiation from diagnostic imaging examinations are relatively low (particularly when compared with therapeutic doses) they are not without potential risk. With the improvements in patient outcome, a number of studies have begun to question the need for repeated high-intensity surveillance imaging and additional exposure to potentially harmful ionizing radiation for a population of patients who do very well once they have successfully completed therapy.[514-516] Patients with Hodgkin lymphoma often receive a large number of off-therapy imaging studies with no effect on overall patient outcome.[514] Similarly CT protocols that routinely include the pelvis in off-treatment surveillance of patients with Wilms tumor had no effect on disease detection and exposed gonadal tissue to potentially harmful additional radiation.[517] A recent study of patients with low-stage gonadal germ-cell tumors showed that tumor markers provided a sensitive and specific means of detecting patients with disease relapse; no relapses were identified in patients who were marker-negative.[518]

Taken together these studies underscore the need to reassess the frequency and type of surveillance imaging needed for the routine off-therapy monitoring of patients who have had successful treatment of their disease. Practitioners must be cognizant of the need to provide reassurance that disease relapse, if present, will be detected as early as possible while at the same time balancing these assurances against performing unnecessary, costly, and potentially harmful studies that have no impact on outcome.[519]

CONCLUSION

The approach to imaging pediatric oncology patients is rapidly evolving. The era when the radiologist played a peripheral role in the care of the child with cancer has been left behind. As outlined in this chapter, the imaging of children with cancer is complex and the role of radiology has changed. The development of new diagnostic imaging techniques and image-guided therapeutic interventions has lead to a new paradigm in which treatment designs are increasingly relying on imaging endpoints, with exciting opportunities and challenges to better detect, stage, and monitor malignant disease. The next decade of imaging will require close collaboration between the pediatric oncologist and the pediatric imaging specialist in order to determine which of these imaging techniques are best suited to these patients.

References available online at ExpertConsult.

KEY REFERENCES

12. Dalrymple NC, Prasad SR, Freckleton MW, et al: Informatics in radiology (infoRAD): introduction to the language of three-dimensional imaging with multidetector CT. *Radiographics* 25(5):1409–1428, 2005.
    Excellent overview of multidetector CT imaging.
15. Barnacle AM, McHugh K: Limitations with the Response Evaluation Criteria in Solid Tumors (RECIST): guidance in disseminated pediatric malignancy. *Pediatr Blood Cancer* 46(2):127–134, 2006.
    Systematic review of limitations with using Response Evaluation Criteria In Solid Tumors (RECIST) for evaluating common pediatric tumors.
16. Zhao B, Oxnard GR, Moskowitz CS, et al: A pilot study of volume measurement as a method of tumor response evaluation to aid biomarker development. *Clin Cancer Res* 16(18):4647–4653, 2010.
    Excellent pilot study on use of volumetric techniques for assessing tumor response.
19. Callahan MJ, Poznauskis L, Zurakowski D, et al: Nonionic iodinated intravenous contrast material-related reactions: incidence in large urban children's hospital—retrospective analysis of data in 12,494 patients. *Radiology* 250(3):674–681, 2009.
    Together with reference 20, required reading regarding incidence and severity of contrast reactions in children.
33. Brenner DJ: Slowing the increase in the population dose resulting from CT scans. *Radiation Res* 174(6):809–815, 2010.
    More recent review of current thinking regarding dose reduction in diagnostic imaging with emphasis on CT.
34. Nievelstein RA, Quarles van Ufford HM, Kwee TC, et al: Radiation exposure and mortality risk from CT and PET imaging of patients with malignant lymphoma. *Eur Radiol* 22(9):1946–1954, 2012.
    Excellent study with counterpoint position arguing for judicious use of CT where appropriate.
43. Padhani AR, Koh DM, Collins DJ: Whole-body diffusion-weighted MR imaging in cancer: current status and research directions. *Radiology* 261(3):700–718, 2011.
    Comprehensive review of DWI in oncologic imaging.
47. Padhani AR, Liu G, Koh DM, et al: Diffusion-weighted magnetic resonance imaging as a cancer biomarker: consensus and recommendations. *Neoplasia* 11(2):102–125, 2009.
    Excellent overview with recommendations for using MRI as an imaging biomarker; National Cancer Institute (NCI) consensus statement.
55. Margolis DJ, Hoffman JM, Herfkens RJ, et al: Molecular imaging techniques in body imaging. *Radiology* 245(2):333–356, 2007.
    Comprehensive summary of molecular imaging techniques; although somewhat dated, an excellent overview and introduction to molecular imaging.
58. Belyaev AS, Peck KK, Brennan NM, et al: Clinical applications of functional MR imaging. *Magn Reson Imaging Clin N Am* 21(2):269–278, 2013.
    Recent review of new applications and techniques for fMRI.
72. Franzius C: FDG-PET/CT in pediatric solid tumors. *Q J Nucl Med Mol Imaging* 54(4):401–410, 2010.
    Recent review of PET/CT in pediatric oncology.
81. Pfannenberg AC, Aschoff P, Brechtel K, et al: Value of contrast-enhanced multiphase CT in combined PET/CT protocols for oncological imaging. *Br J Radiol* 80(954):437–445, 2007.
    One of many articles showing the value of multimodality imaging in pediatric oncology.
86. Torigian DA, Zaidi H, Kwee TC, et al: PET/MR imaging: technical aspects and potential clinical applications. *Radiology* 267(1):26–44, 2013.
    Excellent and timely overview of an emerging new imaging technique.
87. Hirsch FW, Sattler B, Sorge I, et al: PET/MR in children: initial clinical experience in paediatric oncology using an integrated PET/MR scanner. *Pediatr Radiol* 43(7):860–875, 2013.
    Largest experience to date using integrated PET/MRI for pediatric oncology imaging.
101. Panigrahy A, Bluml S: Neuroimaging of pediatric brain tumors: from basic to advanced magnetic resonance imaging (MRI). *J Child Neurol* 24(11):1343–1365, 2009.
    Excellent overview of pediatric brain tumor imaging with emphasis on MRI.
120. Dinauer C, Francis GL: Thyroid cancer in children. *Endocrinol Metab Clin North Am* 36(3):779–806, vii, 2007.
    An important review of an uncommon pediatric tumor.
127. Guillerman RP, Voss SD, Parker BR: Leukemia and lymphoma. *Radiol Clin North Am* 49(4):767–797, vii, 2011.
    Comprehensive review of approaches to imaging the hematologic malignancies.
130. Kwee TC, Takahara T, Vermoolen MA, et al: Whole-body diffusion-weighted imaging for staging malignant lymphoma in children. *Pediatr Radiol* 40:1592–1602, 2010.
    Together with reference 131, important article investigating MRI for staging pediatric lymphoma.
133. Hutchings M, Loft A, Hansen M, et al: FDG-PET after two cycles of chemotherapy predicts treatment failure and progression-free survival in Hodgkin lymphoma. *Blood* 107(1):52–59, 2006.
    Together with reference 132, one of the early seminal articles showing predictive value of FDG-PET response on outcome in Hodgkin lymphoma.

142. Kluge R, Kurch L, Montravers F, et al: FDG PET/CT in children and adolescents with lymphoma. *Pediatric Radiol* 43(4):406–417, 2013.
    Excellent update on role of FDG-PET and CT in pediatric Hodgkin lymphoma.

144. Kostakoglu L, Cheson BD: State-of-the-art research on lymphomas: role of molecular imaging for staging, prognostic evaluation, and treatment response. *Front Oncol* 3:212, 2013.
    Recent update on role of FDG-PET and CT in assessing treatment response on Hodgkin lymphoma.

149. Hutchings M: FDG-PET response-adapted therapy: is 18F-fluorodeoxyglucose positron emission tomography a safe predictor for a change of therapy? *Hematol Oncol Clin North Am* 28(1):87–103, 2014.
    Together with reference 148, important articles challenging the notion that FDG-PET response will be the sole predictor of outcome in lymphoma therapy.

169. Sharp SE, Shulkin BL, Gelfand MJ, et al: ^{123}I-MIBG scintigraphy and 18F-FDG PET in neuroblastoma. *J Nucl Med* 50(8):1237–1243, 2009.
    Together with reference 170, important studies highlighting the limitations of FDG-PET in neuroblastoma.

174. Hawkins DS, Schuetze SM, Butrynski JE, et al: (18F)Fluorodeoxyglucose positron emission tomography predicts outcome for Ewing sarcoma family of tumors. *J Clin Oncol* 23(34):8828–8834, 2005.
    Important article showing improved outcome for patients with Ewing sarcoma who have good FDG-PET response to initial therapy. One of the few articles with outcome data.

191. Grundy PE, Green DM, Dirks AC, et al: Clinical significance of pulmonary nodules detected by CT and not CXR in patients treated for favorable histology Wilms tumor on national Wilms tumor studies-4 and -5: a report from the Children's Oncology Group. *Pediatr Blood Cancer* 59(4):631–635, 2012.
    Recent NWTSG update challenging the importance of CT-detected lung nodules on determining outcome in patients with metastatic Wilms tumor.

193. Chandarana H, Heacock L, Rakheja R, et al: Pulmonary nodules in patients with primary malignancy: comparison of hybrid PET/MR and PET/CT imaging. *Radiology* 268(3):874–881, 2013.
    Recent study comparing integrate PET/MRI and PET/CT for evaluating lung nodules.

213. Meyers AB, Towbin AJ, Serai S, et al: Characterization of pediatric liver lesions with gadoxetate disodium. *Pediatr Radiol* 41(9):1183–1197, 2011.
    Excellent study demonstrating the role of hepatocyte-selective MRI contrast agents in the majority of pediatric liver tumors.

221. Christison-Lagay ER, Burrows PE, Alomari A, et al: Hepatic hemangiomas: subtype classification and development of a clinical practice algorithm and registry. *J Pediatr Surg* 42(1):62–67, discussion 67–68, 2007.
    Important article presenting the currently accepted classification schema for pediatric hepatic hemangiomas.

250. Geller E, Kochan PS: Renal neoplasms of childhood. *Radiol Clin North Am* 49(4):689–709, vi, 2011.
    Excellent overview of pediatric renal tumors.

284. Cohn SL, Pearson AD, London WB, et al: The International Neuroblastoma Risk Group (INRG) classification system: an INRG Task Force report. *J Clin Oncol* 27(2):289–297, 2009.
    International task force report on new approach to risk classification in neuroblastoma.

285. Monclair T, Brodeur GM, Ambros PF, et al: The International Neuroblastoma Risk Group (INRG) staging system: an INRG Task Force report. *J Clin Oncol* 27(2):298–303, 2009.
    Important article on new approach to risk classification in neuroblastoma, with emphasis on imaging defined risk factors.

286. Brisse HJ, McCarville MB, Granata C, et al: Guidelines for imaging and staging of neuroblastic tumors: consensus report from the International Neuroblastoma Risk Group Project. *Radiology* 261(1):243–257, 2011.
    Important article with practical guidelines for incorporating imaging defined risk factors into risk classification in neuroblastoma.

295. Yanik GA, Parisi MT, Shulkin BL, et al: Semiquantitative mIBG scoring as a prognostic indicator in patients with stage 4 neuroblastoma: a report from the Children's Oncology Group. *J Nucl Med* 54(4):541–548, 2013.
    Role of MIBG response in determining outcome in advanced stage neuroblastoma, with emphasis on Curie scoring.

308. Brunklaus A, Pohl K, Zuberi SM, et al: Investigating neuroblastoma in childhood opsoclonus-myoclonus syndrome. *Arch Dis Child* 97(5):461–463, 2012.
    Imaging approach and diagnostic challenge in evaluating patients with OMS.

339. Hawkins DS, Conrad EU, 3rd, Butrynski JE, et al: (F-18)-fluorodeoxy-D-glucose-positron emission tomography response is associated with outcome for extremity osteosarcoma in children and young adults. *Cancer* 115(15):3519–3525, 2009.
    Outcome study showing improved survival in osteosarcoma patients with early FDG-PET response.

348. Bixby SD, Hettmer S, Taylor GA, et al: Synovial sarcoma in children: imaging features and common benign mimics. *AJR Am J Roentgenol* 195(4):1026–1032, 2010.
    Comprehensive review of important mimics of synovial-cell sarcoma.

355. Tsai LL, Drubach L, Fahey F, et al: (18F)-Fluorodeoxyglucose positron emission tomography in children with neurofibromatosis type 1 and plexiform neurofibromas: correlation with malignant transformation. *J Neurooncol* 108(3):469–475, 2012.
    One of several recent studies emphasizing the importance of FDG-PET and SUV measurements in predicting malignant degeneration of neurofibroma to MPNST.

373. Lister TA, Crowther D, Sutcliffe SB, et al: Report of a committee convened to discuss the evaluation and staging of patients with Hodgkin disease: Cotswolds meeting. *J Clin Oncol* 7(11):1630–1636, 1989.
    Classic paper establishing the current system of staging patients with Hodgkin lymphoma.

380. Kostakoglu L, Schoder H, Johnson JL, et al: Interim ((18)F)fluorodeoxyglucose positron emission tomography imaging in stage I-II non-bulky Hodgkin lymphoma: would using combined positron emission tomography and computed tomography criteria better predict response than each test alone? *Leuk Lymphoma* 53(11):2143–2150, 2012.
    Important study showing that both CT and FDG-PET contribute independently to predicting response to therapy.

383. Cheson BD, Pfistner B, Juweid ME, et al: Revised response criteria for malignant lymphoma. *J Clin Oncol* 25(5):579–586, 2007.
    Essential reading for response assessment criteria in the malignant lymphomas. This is the summary of the International Working Group.

384. Juweid ME, Stroobants S, Hoekstra OS, et al: Use of positron emission tomography for response assessment of lymphoma: consensus of the Imaging Subcommittee of International Harmonization Project in Lymphoma. *J Clin Oncol* 25(5):571–578, 2007.
    Together with reference 383, essential reading for response assessment criteria in the malignant lymphomas. This is the summary of the International Working Group's recommendations for use of PET in assessing response.

385. Meignan M, Gallamini A, Itti E, et al: Report on the Third International Workshop on Interim Positron Emission Tomography in Lymphoma held in Menton, France, 26–27 September 2011 and Menton 2011 consensus. *Leuk Lymphoma* 53(10):1876–1881, 2012.
    Important paper presenting recommendations on a semiquantitative 5-point scale for assessing residual FDG uptake during interim response assessment in Hodgkin lymphoma.

403. Meadows AT, Friedman DL, Neglia JP, et al: Second neoplasms in survivors of childhood cancer: findings from the Childhood Cancer Survivor Study cohort. *J Clin Oncol* 27(14):2356–2362, 2009.
    Summary of second malignant neoplasm incidence data from CCSS follow-up study of cancer survivors.

406. Becker GJ: Interventional oncology: perspectives on current scholarly productivity and potential for future growth. *Radiology* 257(2):309–312, 2010.
    Excellent review of emerging role of interventional radiology in the care of oncology patients.

424. Mahnken AH, Pereira PL, de Baere T: Interventional oncologic approaches to liver metastases. *Radiology* 266(2):407–430, 2013.

   Important recent report summarizing new interventional approaches to treating unresectable liver metastases.

444. Dupuy DE, Liu D, Hartfeil D, et al: Percutaneous radiofrequency ablation of painful osseous metastases: a multicenter American College of Radiology Imaging Network trial. *Cancer* 116(4):989–997, 2010.

   Important results from a large multicenter study of radiofrequency ablation in adult bone metastases.

476. Marcy PY: Central venous access: techniques and indications in oncology. *Eur Radiol* 18(10):2333–2344, 2008.

   Review of the role of interventional radiology in management of central venous access.

490. Padhani AR, Miles KA: Multiparametric imaging of tumor response to therapy. *Radiology* 256(2):348–364, 2010.

   Excellent overview of the emerging field of quantitative imaging and imaging biomarker development.

502. Vahrmeijer AL, Hutteman M, van der Vorst JR, et al: Image-guided cancer surgery using near-infrared fluorescence. *Nat Rev Clin Oncol* 10(9):507–518, 2013.

   Excellent up-to-date review of near-infrared fluorescent imaging and its emerging role in cancer diagnostics and image guided therapy.

510. Smith MA, Seibel NL, Altekruse SF, et al: Outcomes for children and adolescents with cancer: challenges for the twenty-first century. *J Clin Oncol* 28(15):2625–2634, 2010.

   Essential recent reference work from senior leaders in pediatric oncology, highlighting successes and challenges for the future of pediatric cancer care.

514. Voss SD, Chen L, Constine LS, et al: Surveillance computed tomography imaging and detection of relapse in intermediate- and advanced-stage pediatric Hodgkin lymphoma: a report from the Children's Oncology Group. *J Clin Oncol* 30(21):2635–2640, 2012.

   One of the first in a series of studies showing that routine surveillance imaging places little role in diagnosing relapse and improving patient outcome.

SUPPORTIVE CARE

CHAPTER 67

Infectious Disease in the Pediatric Cancer Patient

Lillian Sung, Brian T. Fisher, and Andrew Y. Koh

CHAPTER OUTLINE

INTRODUCTION

Infections are important issues faced by children with cancer. Invasive bacterial and fungal infections are problematic mainly in those receiving intensive treatment. Viruses may also be life-threatening in specific circumstances. Furthermore, non–life-threatening infections such as upper respiratory tract infection may still affect treatment and quality of life, particularly if febrile illnesses occur during neutropenia. In an effort to provide a comprehensive discussion of infection in pediatric cancer patients, this chapter focuses on general issues such as risk factors for infection, infection classification, and then approaches to intervention. Next, the chapter reviews major opportunistic pathogens, the risk factors and epidemiology of fever and neutropenia (FN), the therapeutic options for prophylaxis, infectious issues in pediatric cancer that are specific to low- and middle-income countries (LMIC), and recent directions involving preclinical research.

GENERAL ISSUES RELEVANT TO INFECTIONS

Risk Factors for Infection

Children with cancer are predisposed to infection for several reasons. The most common and important risk factor is neutropenia caused by myelosuppressive chemotherapy and cancer itself. Greater depth and duration of neutropenia are directly related to the risk of invasive bacterial and fungal infection and infectious mortality.[1,2] Corticosteroids are commonly used as anticancer therapy and as supportive care. The negative consequences of corticosteroids on the host immune system predispose to infections such as *Pneumocystis jiroveci*, other fungi, and bacteria and may be an independent risk factor for sepsis and infectious mortality.[3] Intensive chemotherapy also predisposes to infection through disruption of important protective anatomic barriers. The development of mucositis after chemotherapy administration provides a portal of entry for organisms colonizing the oral cavity and is a particularly important risk factor for viridans group streptococcal bacteremia.[4,5] Likewise, compromise of the gastrointestinal mucosa may clinically manifest as enteritis, typhlitis, and colitis and can facilitate translocation of enteric pathogens to the bloodstream. Beyond chemotherapy and corticosteroids, certain procedures performed in this patient population may predispose to infection. In many countries central venous lines (CVLs) are routinely used in patients with cancer, resulting in a risk for catheter-related bloodstream and local CVL site infections. Additionally, many children require surgery for various reasons, including tumor resection, and such procedures predispose to surgical site infection. Finally, children who receive allogeneic hematopoietic stem cell transplantation (HSCT) have a unique predisposition to infections related to graft-versus-host disease (GVHD) and therapies used to prevent and treat this complication of transplantation.[6]

Infection Classification

Infections can be classified by etiology as bacterial, fungal, viral, or protozoal, and these pathogens may infect sterile or nonsterile sites. The overall risk of infection varies depending on many factors, with intensity of chemotherapy being very important. Children who receive the most intensive chemotherapy include those with acute myeloid leukemia (AML). One study demonstrated that more than 60% of children with AML have at least one microbiologically documented infection during each phase of therapy, and the cumulative risk of infection-related mortality was 11 ± 2%.[7] In a subsequent pediatric AML analysis, more than 80% of children experienced at least one sterile site bacterial infection and 14% experienced at least one sterile site fungal infection throughout chemotherapy. The risk of sterile site bacterial infection was 30% to 60% per chemotherapy course.[8] In contrast, some children who receive non-myelosuppressive therapy such as those receiving maintenance therapy for acute lymphoblastic leukemia (ALL), have a very low risk of sterile site bacterial or fungal infections.[9]

Infections may also be classified by type of infection: microbiologically documented, clinically documented, or fever of unknown origin (FUO). In an analysis of children with cancer or recipients of HSCT presenting with FN, 80% of episodes were ultimately classified as FUO, 13% had a microbiologically confirmed etiology, 6% were clinically documented infection, and 2% were invasive mycosis.[9] The distribution of the etiology of FN will change depending on the presence of the aforementioned risk factors, especially the intensity of chemotherapy administered.

Intervention Approaches

The major approaches to reduction of infectious morbidity and mortality are prophylactic, empiric, and definitive treatment approaches. With prophylaxis, antimicrobials are administered before onset of fever or other clinical signs of infection. Empiric therapy consists of the administration of antimicrobial agents with early signs of infection, such as fever. Definitive treatment consists of administering specific antimicrobials once an infection has been documented.

MAJOR PATHOGENS

Bacteria

Bacteria are the most common cause of invasive infection in pediatric cancer patients. Over the last three decades, there has been a shift from gram-negative organisms being responsible for most infections in patients with cancer to gram-positive infections predominating.[10] The shift toward gram-positive agents has been attributed to the wide-spread use of CVLs, chemotherapy regimens associated with mucositis, and routine use of antibiotics with gram-negative activity.[11] The most common gram-positive infections are coagulase-negative staphylococci, viridans group streptococci, enterococci, and *Staphylococcus aureus*. The major types of gram-negative infections are *Escherichia coli, Klebsiella* species, and *Pseudomonas aeruginosa*.[9] Bacterial sterile site pathogens are most commonly tested for and isolated from blood culture, followed by urine and, less frequently, cerebrospinal fluid.

Fungi

Pediatric patients requiring intensive chemotherapy treatment for cancers such as AML, relapsed ALL, and allogeneic HSCT have the highest risk for invasive fungal infection (IFI) because of the resultant depth and duration of neutropenia. Additional IFI risk factors include mucositis, corticosteroid use, and antibiotic exposure.[12-20] The most common fungal infections in pediatric cancer are *Candida* spp. and *Aspergillus* spp.[21] Sterile site candidal infections typically occur in the blood and urine. In contrast, invasive aspergillosis typically involves the lungs, sinuses, gastrointestinal tract, and brain. Emerging fungal pathogens that are increasingly being encountered in pediatric oncology are Mucorales (formerly referred to as zygomycetes) and *Scedosporium* spp. These are particularly concerning because they tend to be fatal and are challenging to diagnose antemortem.[22,23]

P. jirovecii is a yeastlike fungal species that classically causes pneumonia in children with acute leukemia who do not receive *P. jirovecii* pneumonia (PCP) prophylaxis. In addition to chemotherapy exposure, corticosteroid use and age younger than 2 years are also risk factors for PCP.[24,25] PCP prophylaxis is considered standard care for many pediatric malignancies, including acute leukemia and HSCT recipients. Trimethoprim-sulfamethoxazole (TMP-SMX) is the prophylactic drug of choice. Although the optimal dosing regimen is not clear, administration regimens of 2 or 3 days per week are most common and have been shown to be reasonably effective.[26,27] Alternative regimens for allergy or other toxicities include oral dapsone, oral atovaquone, and inhaled pentamidine. Intravenous pentamidine is often used in children younger than 5 years who cannot tolerate the other options. However, clinicians should be aware that the effectiveness of intravenous pentamidine is questionable.[25]

Viral Infections

There are many viruses that can result in infections in pediatric cancer patients.[28] The list of potential agents continues to evolve with improved diagnostic abilities for previously unrecognized pathogens such as human metapneumovirus (HMPV). In one pediatric cancer series, respiratory syncytial virus (RSV) (31%) and rhinovirus (23%) were the most frequently detected respiratory viruses, followed by parainfluenza (12%) and influenza A (11%).[29] RSV usually does not cause life-threatening infections in children with cancer. However, in patients with AML and HSCT recipients who do acquire RSV, infection may progress to lower respiratory tract involvement. In this setting RSV infection is associated with a 14% case fatality rate in patients with AML and a 50% case fatality rate in pediatric HSCT recipients.[7,30] Adenovirus may also cause serious infection, particularly in HSCT recipients,[31] and is a frequent cause of death in this setting.[32-35] Other viral infections, including varicellazoster virus (VZV), influenza, and cytomegalovirus, are typically not life threatening in pediatric patients with cancer who are receiving less intense therapy, but they may cause severe infection and infectious mortality in the most intensively treated children. Conversely, some infections, such as severe acute respiratory syndrome (SARS), can cause fatal infection in immunocompetent patients but is rarely associated with severe illness in pediatric cancer.[36] It is hypothesized that an intact immune system is responsible for severity of illness and fatality in SARS, thus explaining this apparent paradox.

Protozoal Infections

In general, protozoal infections are not a common cause of fever in children with cancer in high-income countries, although these pathogens may be more prominent in some LMICs.[37]

FEVER AND NEUTROPENIA

FN is one of the most common complications of cancer therapy in pediatric patients. Episodes of FN are associated with considerable morbidity, reduction in quality of life (QoL), and high costs, and fatal outcomes still occur despite aggressive antimicrobial interventions.[2,38] Much research has been conducted in both adult and pediatric FN over the last several decades, which has allowed different therapeutic approaches to evolve while reducing mortality and improving other clinical endpoints.[39,40]

Initial Risk Stratification

Children with FN are not a homogenous group. Determining which children are at lower risk of complications can allow for a reduction in the intensity of therapy and monitoring. Conversely, identifying children at higher risk of complications can allow for escalation of therapy and closer observation.

In adults with FN, the risk stratification schema from the Multinational Association of Supportive Care in Cancer (MASCC) has been validated and is widely accepted as a standard approach. However, the MASCC score cannot be applied to children because age below 60 years and absence of chronic obstructive pulmonary disease are two items in the score and these are not applicable to pediatric patients.[41] At least 25 studies of risk prediction have been conducted in pediatric cancer.[42]

These studies have been highly variable using different pediatric cancer populations and different endpoints (e.g., bacteremia, "serious infection," death, and intensive care unit admission), making the results more difficult to interpret.

Although six of these low-risk stratification schemas have been validated in children (Table 67-1), identification of a single schema to be applied across all clinical scenarios has not been feasible, likely because of the divergence in clinical settings. Therefore clinicians should review the six validated low-risk stratification schemas, choose which schema matches their clinical setting, and determine whether the application of that schema is feasible for their center. For example, some rules use biomarkers such as C-reactive protein and would require expeditious analysis and return of results to be useful. Others require clinical judgment and thus require trained health care professionals to be readily available. There are no validated risk stratification schemas to identify the pediatric high-risk patient with FN.

Initial Investigations

At initial presentation, an evaluation for the cause of fever should be conducted. The evaluation begins with a careful history and physical examination, with the assessment focusing on potential sites of infection. Sites that merit particular attention are the mouth to search for herpes simplex virus stomatitis and dental abscess, the exit site and tunnel of CVLs, perianal region for cellulitis and perirectal abscess, and fingers and toes for paronychia.

The standard evaluation should include blood cultures, with further diagnostic testing dictated by clinical signs and symptoms. Blood cultures should be obtained from each lumen of the CVL if present. The utility of a peripheral blood culture at the initial evaluation of FN is controversial. There are seven studies that evaluated the contribution of peripheral blood cultures in addition to CVL cultures in adults and children with cancer or undergoing HSCT.[43-49] When these results were combined, 13% (95% confidence interval [CI] 8% to 18%) of all true bacteremias were identified only by the peripheral blood culture. This result is likely explained by false-negative CVL blood cultures when obtained culture volumes are small.[50] However, it is not known how failure to identify these episodes of bacteremia affect patient outcomes or whether this problem can be overcome by optimizing CVL blood culture volumes. Consequently, the role of peripheral blood culture remains uncertain.

Urinalysis and urine culture testing for the detection of urinary tract infections (UTIs) is also considered controversial in the setting of FN. In immunocompetent children, a UTI is often diagnosed when there is both evidence of pyuria on urinalysis and a positive culture. The state of neutropenia limits the ability to use pyuria as a diagnostic criterion,[51] and reliance on nitrite testing is not ideal because the test may be negative in younger children with UTI.[52] Therefore urinalysis testing has limited utility in the setting of FN. It may be reasonable to obtain a sterile urine culture and define the presence of a UTI on the culture results alone. However, sterile urine

TABLE 67-1   Validated Pediatric Risk Stratification Strategies for Low-Risk Patients

	Rackoff (1996)[132]	Alexander (2002)[133]	Rondinelli (2006)[134]	Santolaya (2001)[135]	Ammann (2003)[136]	Ammann (2010)[137]
Patient and disease-related factors	None	AML, Burkitt lymphoma, induction ALL, progressive disease, relapsed with marrow involvement	2 points for central venous catheter, 1 point for age ≤5 years	Relapsed leukemia, chemotherapy within 7 days of episode	Bone marrow involvement, central venous catheter, pre–B-cell leukemia	4 points for chemotherapy more intensive than ALL maintenance
Episode-specific factors	Absolute monocyte count	Hypotension, tachypnea/hypoxia <94%, new CXR changes, altered mental status, severe mucositis, vomiting or abdominal pain, focal infection, other clinical reason for in-patient treatment	4.5 points for clinical site of infection, 2.5 points for no URTI, 1 point each for fever >38.5°C, hemoglobin ≤70g/L	CRP ≥90 mg/L, hypotension, platelets ≤50 g/L	Absence of clinical signs of viral infection, CRP >50 mg/L, white blood cell count ≤500/μL, hemoglobin >100 g/L	5 points for hemoglobin ≥90 g/L, 3 points each for white blood cell count <300/μL, platelet <50 g/L
Rule formulation	Absolute monocyte count ≥ 100/μL = low risk of bacteremia HSCT = high risk	Absence of any risk factor = low risk of serious medical complication HSCT = high risk	Total score <6 = low risk of serious infectious complication HSCT = high risk	Zero risk factors or only low platelets or only <7 days from chemotherapy = low risk of invasive bacterial infection	Three or fewer risk factors = low risk of significant infection HSCT = high risk	Total score <9 = low risk of adverse FN outcome HSCT = high risk
Demonstrated to be valid*	USA Madsen 2002[138]	United Kingdom Dommett 2009[139]	Brazil Rondinelli 2006[134]	South America Santolaya 2002[140]	Europe Ammann 2010[137], Macher 2010[141]	Europe Miedema 2011[142]

Adapted from Lehrnbecher et al.[79]

ALL, Acute lymphoblastic leukemia; *AML*, acute myeloid leukemia; *CRP*, C-reactive protein; *CXR*, chest radiograph; *FN*, fever and neutropenia; *URTI*, upper respiratory tract infection; *USA*, United States of America.

*"Valid" refers to clinically adequate discrimination of a group at low risk of complications.

collection can be difficult in young children and infants and often requires urinary catheterization, a procedure that is seldom recommended for a neutropenic patient. Therefore where a clean-catch or midstream urine can be collected, the results of urinalysis and urine culture should be included in the initial FN investigations. It is important to remember that antibiotic administration should not be delayed to obtain a urine sample.

There are have been four studies,[53-56] including 540 episodes of FN, that investigated the impact of chest radiography (CXR) as a component of the initial FN evaluation. These studies indicate that pneumonia is detected in fewer than 5% of children without respiratory symptoms and that the omission of routine CXR does not lead to adverse outcomes.[53,57] Thus routine CXR should not be performed in asymptomatic children with FN.

Initial Antibiotic Therapy

In general, empiric antimicrobial therapy choices should provide good coverage for gram-negative organisms with some gram-positive coverage. In particular, for high-risk patients with FN, antibiotic therapy should include coverage for viridans group streptococci and *P. aeruginosa*. Various factors must be considered when determining an empiric antibiotic regimen, route of administration, and location of therapy. These factors include patient and family social factors, clinical presentation, ability of the hospital to support an ambulatory approach, availability and cost of drugs, and local hospital resistance patterns.

The role of combination antibiotic therapy versus monotherapy for FN has been debated. Monotherapy was supported by two metaanalyses that compared monotherapy versus an aminoglycoside-containing regimen in FN[58] and in immunocompromised patients with sepsis.[59] These analyses demonstrated that monotherapy is not inferior and is less toxic than combination therapy. The meta-analysis in FN observed fewer treatment failures with monotherapy (odds ratio [OR] 0.88, 95% CI 0.78 to 0.99) but included only four trials that enrolled patients younger than 14 years of age.[58] In the pediatric setting monotherapy was supported by a meta-analysis that found similar clinical outcomes when antipseudomonal penicillin monotherapy was compared to antipseudomonal penicillin plus an aminoglycoside.[60] Therefore monotherapy is suggested for FN in pediatric patients who are clinically stable and who are treated at centers with a low rate of resistant pathogens.

Monotherapy regimens that have been evaluated in children include antipseudomonal penicillins such as piperacillin-tazobactam and ticarcillin-clavulanic acid, antipseudomonal cephalosporins such as cefepime, and carbapenems such as meropenem or imipenem. In two pediatric-specific evaluations, treatment failure, mortality rates, and adverse effects were similar when antipseudomonal penicillins were compared with antipseudomonal cephalosporins or carbapenems.[61,62] There are potential downsides of carbapenems and cefepime. Carbapenems were associated with more pseudomembranous colitis compared with other beta-lactam antibiotics in a large meta-analysis.[62] Cefepime was associated with increased all-cause mortality in another large meta-analysis when compared to other beta-lactam treated patients.[62] However, these findings were not replicated in other studies.[53,63] Consequently, cefepime remains an option for empiric therapy. Ceftazidime monotherapy lacks adequate coverage against viridans group streptococci and resistant gram-negative organisms and thus should not be used if these organisms are of concern.[64]

Empiric glycopeptides (e.g., vancomycin) are not routinely recommended. A largely adult meta-analysis of 14 randomized controlled trials (RCTs) illustrated that inclusion of a glycopeptide did not lead to a difference in success (if addition of glycopeptide in the control arm was not considered failure) but was associated with more adverse effects.[65] Empiric glycopeptides should be reserved for patients who are clinically unstable or who have signs or symptoms suggestive of a gram-positive infection.

Considerations for Low-Risk Patients with Fever and Neutropenia

Patients with FN who are at lower risk of adverse outcomes may be appropriate for a reduction in therapy intensity. Two strategies commonly considered are outpatient management and oral antibiotic administration. These two strategies are commonly used together, and in adults with low-risk FN, outpatient management with oral antibiotics is recommended for selected patients.[20,41] Some experts have expressed concern that these recommendations may not be generalizable to children.[66] However, over the last several years data have emerged related to efficacy and safety, costs, QoL and preference considerations for different management strategies in pediatric FN.

Efficacy and Safety of Outpatient Management and Oral Antibiotic Administration

The advantages of outpatient management include better QoL for children[67] and a reduction in costs,[68] nosocomial infection,[69] and acquisition of resistant microorganisms.[70]

Outpatient management can be instituted at the onset of FN or after a brief period of hospitalization (step-down management). A meta-analysis synthesized the results of six RCTs, two of which were pediatric.[71] There was no difference in treatment failure with outpatient versus inpatient management (rate ratio [RR] 0.81, 95% CI 0.55 to 1.28) where the RR of less than 1 favored inpatient care. It is important to emphasize that failure was biased against outpatient care insofar as readmission was considered failure and this endpoint is applicable only to outpatients. No difference in mortality was demonstrated (RR 1.11, 95% CI 0.41 to 3.05). Results stratified by the two pediatric studies demonstrated similar findings as the overall analysis. The major concern with these data relates to the small number of children included; the two pediatric studies enrolled only 278 children. A subsequent systematic review combined all prospective randomized and nonrandomized pediatric trials that evaluated ambulatory or inpatient management within 24 hours of FN.[72] Among the 16 included studies, treatment failure was significantly less with outpatient management (15%) compared with inpatient management (27%, P = .04). There were no infection-related deaths among the 953 children treated as outpatients. Consequently, outpatient management appears to be a safe approach as long as appropriate patients can be selected and adequate follow-up monitoring is established. To institute outpatient management of FN, the institution must be able to identify low-risk patients and develop a program to monitor patients and expeditiously admit them in the case of deterioration. Social circumstances and travel considerations will dictate the feasibility of an ambulatory approach for a specific patient. The optimal frequency and nature of follow-up evaluations for children treated as outpatients for FN has not been determined, although daily clinic visits will rarely be feasible.

Oral antibiotic administration may be advantageous because it facilitates outpatient management, is usually less expensive, and does not require intravenous access. However, oral administration requires suspension formulation in younger children, and some children may refuse oral medication, particularly when they are unwell. There are two metaanalyses of RCTs that compared oral and parenteral antibiotic administration for FN; both did not restrict their review to low-risk patients. One included inpatient and outpatients (N = 2770),[73] whereas the other evaluated only outpatients (N = 1595).[71] Results were similar in both analyses, with no difference in treatment failure, mortality, or adverse effects of antibiotics by mode of administration. Results were similar when restricted to pediatric studies except for a trend toward lower risk of readmission for outpatient episodes treated with intravenous antibiotics compared with oral antibiotics (RR 0.52, 95% CI 0.24 to 1.09).[71] More data about the safety of oral administration were obtained from a meta-analysis of prospective pediatric trials, which instituted oral antibiotics within 24 hours of FN onset.[72] There was no difference in treatment failure among those who received oral versus intravenous antibiotics (20% versus 22%, P = .68). There was also no difference in the rate of antibiotic discontinuation resulting from adverse events (2% versus 1%, P = .73). No infection-related deaths were observed among the 676 children given oral antibiotics. To summarize, more readmissions were observed among children treated with oral antibiotics in the outpatient setting, although no difference in treatment failure or adverse events occurred and no child treated with oral antibiotics within 24 hours of FN onset died. Thus oral antibiotic administration may be appropriate if the health care team is confident that the child can tolerate this route reliably. Oral antibiotic regimens that have been used in pediatric FN include fluoroquinolone monotherapy, fluoroquinolone and amoxicillin-clavulanate, and cefixime.[72] One practical approach is to provide the first oral dose in the emergency or outpatient department to ensure that the child can tolerate oral administration of the planned empiric antibiotic. Discharge home would be contingent on successful administration. Even for children with low-risk FN who are managed as inpatients, oral administration may be advantageous because it is a more effective use of nursing resources and may facilitate early discharge depending on the reason for admission.

Costs

A pediatric cost-utility model demonstrated that outpatient management was the most cost-effective approach for children with low-risk FN.[68] Outpatient parenteral management was more cost-effective compared with outpatient oral management because of the higher rate of readmission among those who receive oral antibiotics. However, in sensitivity analyses, outpatient oral management may be more cost-effective depending on model assumptions. Inpatient management with intravenous antibiotic administration was the least cost-effective approach. These data suggest that outpatient management with intravenous or oral antibiotics is a better strategy for pediatric low-risk FN when probabilities, costs, and QoL are considered.

Preferences and Quality of Life

In implementing ambulatory and oral approaches for low-risk FN, consideration of patient and family preferences may facilitate program development. When asked which approach they preferred, approximately 50% of parents preferred inpatient intravenous management.[74,75] Both parents and children typically ranked inpatient intravenous management ahead of early discharge or ambulatory approaches.[75] A discrete choice experiment was used to assess preferences toward FN management.[76] Discrete choice experiment is an emerging method for the measurement of preferences in the face of multiple tradeoffs in health care. Parents were willing to tolerate only 2.1 (95% CI 1.1 to 3.2) clinic visits weekly to accept outpatient oral management. If a program were developed with clinic visits three times weekly and a 7.5% chance of readmission, the probability of parental acceptance of such an ambulatory program was 43% (95% CI 39 to 48%).[76]

Estimation of QoL is also important to conduct cost-utility analyses, as previously described. In one study in which parents and health care professionals compared inpatient intravenous and outpatient oral management,[74] respondents rated child QoL as higher at home compared with hospital. Compared with parents, health care professionals overestimated QoL for children at home and underestimated QoL for parents in hospital. In another study in which parents rated their children's QoL with different FN management options, early discharge and outpatient intravenous therapy were associated with the highest anticipated QoL.[75]

These data suggest that parents may have reservations about an ambulatory oral antibiotic approach. In a qualitative study the major themes identified when parents make decisions regarding site of care and route of drug administration were convenience and disruptiveness for the family, the child's physical and emotional health, and modifiers of parental decision making.[77] Reasons for preferring an inpatient approach include the inconvenience of clinic visits, apprehension regarding whether they can adequately monitor their child, and concerns related to oral antibiotic administration. In summary, although the child's QoL is anticipated to be better with outpatient management, many parents prefer inpatient management.

Modification of Empiric Antibacterial Therapy

After therapy for FN has been initiated, the initial empiric regimen should be adjusted to provide appropriate coverage for any positive microbiology results or identified clinical focus of infection. In patients in whom empiric glycopeptides or dual gram-negative coverage was initiated, reassessment at 24 to 72 hours should be conducted. In the absence of a specific microbiological reason to continue these agents, they should be discontinued. In the event of persistent fever, careful evaluation for an undetected source of infection is important. In this setting modification of antibiotics, including addition of empiric vancomycin, is not warranted in children who remain clinically stable.[78] Children who clinically deteriorate warrant broadening of empiric antibacterial therapy to include coverage for resistant gram-positive, gram-negative, and anaerobic organisms.

Empiric antibiotics should be discontinued if cultures are negative, the child is clinically well, fever has resolved, and there is evidence of neutrophil recovery.[79] One randomized trial of pediatric low-risk patients found that cessation of antibiotics on day 3 irrespective of count recovery versus continuation of antibiotics was associated with similar outcomes.[80] However, *Enterobacter* bacteremia occurred in one child in the early cessation study arm. Consequently, it is reasonable to discontinue antibiotics on day 3 in low-risk children with FN who have become afebrile with negative cultures as long as careful monitoring is in place. In high-risk patients the optimal duration of antibiotic therapy is unknown in the setting of persistent profound neutropenia. A small study of 33 high-risk patients suggested that cessation of empiric antibiotics on day 7 is associated with bacteremia and poor infection outcomes compared with continuation for 14 days.[81] Thus continuation of empiric antibiotics for at least 14 days for high-risk FN in the absence of evidence of neutrophil recovery is a reasonable strategy.

Evaluation for Invasive Fungal Infection and Empiric Antifungal Therapy

Children with FN and persistent or recurrent fever that persists 96 hours or more after initiation of broad-spectrum antibiotics and who are at higher risk of IFI should undergo an evaluation for fungal infection, including careful physical examination, blood and urine cultures, and computerized tomography (CT) of the chest.[82-85] The role of routine CT sinuses and imaging of the abdomen have not been defined in the standard investigation of IFI, although routine CT sinuses should not be conducted in children 2 years of age or younger because of insufficient pneumatization of the sinus cavities.[79] In children with demonstrated pulmonary lesions, investigations may include bronchoalveolar lavage and lung biopsy, although fatal bleeding may occur with biopsy of any angioinvasive mold lesion. Thus the decision to biopsy requires careful consideration.

Empiric antifungal therapy should consist of either caspofungin or liposomal amphotericin B (L-AmB) because these two therapies are similarly effective and L-AmB is slightly better and less nephrotoxic than amphotericin B deoxycholate.[86-88] Empiric antifungal therapy may be discontinued at resolution of severe neutropenia if the patient is clinically well without evidence of an IFI.

PROPHYLACTIC STRATEGIES

Antibacterial Prophylaxis

The approach to routine antibacterial prophylaxis is uncertain because the overall balance of benefit and harm is not clear.[20] Most of the interest has been focused on fluoroquinolones because of broad spectrum of activity, relative preservation of gastrointestinal tract anaerobic flora, high concentration in the feces, systemic bactericidal activity, tolerability, and lack of myelosuppression. A large meta-analysis of RCTs composed mostly of adult subjects found that antibiotic prophylaxis decreased the risk of death (RR 0.67, 95% CI 0.55 to 0.81), infection-related mortality (RR 0.58, 95% CI 0.55 to 0.81), and bacteremia (RR 0.052, 95% CI 0.46 to 0.59).[89] Some uncertainty remains regarding whether these benefits are applicable to contemporary patients given the changing spectrum of gram-positive and gram-negative bacteria over time.

The decision to use routine antibacterial prophylaxis must include consideration of the negative consequences of prophylaxis. These consequences appear to be important to clinicians because most North American and German centers do not routinely use antibacterial prophylaxis for children with AML.[90] Potentially harmful effects include predisposition to IFI, *Clostridium difficile* colitis, and potential contribution to evolving antibiotic resistance. Additionally, the physician must consider the toxicities of the specific antibiotic chosen. The previously cited meta-analysis of antibacterial prophylaxis also showed that prophylaxis was associated with more adverse events (RR 1.57, 95% CI 1.33 to 1.86).[89] Parents

also considered the frequency of administration, adverse effects, and costs in decision making related to antibacterial prophylaxis.[91]

Antifungal Prophylaxis

Because IFIs are relatively difficult to diagnose and effectively treat, there has been considerable interest in determining the effectiveness of a prophylactic approach, particularly in children undergoing allogeneic HSCT and children with AML, two populations at high risk for IFI.[92] Fluconazole prophylaxis was compared with placebo in two RCTs of allogeneic HSCT recipients.[93,94] Fluconazole decreased the occurrence of IFI because of a reduction in invasive candidiasis. Because children undergoing allogeneic HSCT are at risk for molds in addition to yeasts and because fluconazole does not provide any coverage against molds, there has been great interest in exploring the role of prophylactic antimold coverage. However, thus far agents with antimold activity, including micafungin, voriconazole, and amphotericin products, have not proved to have clinically significant advantages over fluconazole prophylaxis in the HSCT population.[95-97,98-100] Furthermore, some agents, such as itraconazole, showed a higher rate of toxicity leading to withdrawal[101] and agents such as amphotericin B led to infusion-related toxicities and renal toxicity.[102]

In pediatric AML a meta-analysis suggested that fluconazole significantly reduced the risk of IFI when the baseline rate was at least 15%.[103] The efficacy of itraconazole prophylaxis has also been explored. Although this agent has been shown to be effective compared with placebo or no therapy, no advantage over fluconazole or voriconazole has been demonstrated.[104-108] Posaconazole is an antifungal agent with broader antimold activity than voriconazole and thus represents a potentially better prophylactic option. In a randomized trial of patients with AML or myelodysplastic syndrome and prolonged neutropenia, posaconazole prophylaxis, when compared with fluconazole or itraconazole, reduced the rate of proven or probable IFI. Furthermore, overall survival rate was significantly better in posaconazole-treated patients.[109] However, only 16 adolescents between the ages of 13 and 18 years were included, and thus the generalizability of the results to children is limited. Furthermore, administration of posaconazole to children younger than 13 is challenging because of a lack of dosing information and the requirement to administer the drug orally with adequate food intake, which can be a challenge for children undergoing HSCT or those receiving chemotherapy for AML.

To better understand the contribution of mold-active prophylaxis, a systematic review of RCTs compared mold-active versus fluconazole prophylaxis in patients with cancer or those who underwent HSCT. Of 20 studies, children were included in four trials but only one trial was exclusively pediatric. Mold-active prophylaxis, when compared with fluconazole prophylaxis, significantly reduced the risk of IFI (RR 0.71, 95% CI 0.52 to 0.98), invasive aspergillosis (RR 0.53, 95% CI 0.37 to 0.75), and IFI-related mortality (RR 0.67, 95% CI 0.47 to 0.96). However, mold-active agents had significantly more associated adverse events leading to antifungal prophylaxis discontinuation or modification (RR 1.95, 95% CI 1.24 to 3.07). Mold-active prophylaxis did not influence overall mortality (RR 1, 95% CI 0.88 to 1.13).

Granulocyte and Granulocyte-Macrophage Colony Stimulating Factors

Granulocyte colony-stimulating factor (G-CSF) and granulocyte-macrophage colony-stimulating factor (GM-CSF) are hematopoietic colony-stimulating factors (CSFs) that reduce the duration and severity of neutropenia in chemotherapy recipients.[110,111] In a meta-analysis of 16 RCTs of prophylactic use of CSFs in pediatric patients with cancer, the mean rate of FN in the control arms was 57% (range 39 to 100%).[112] CSFs reduced the rate of FN (RR of 0.80, 95% CI 0.67 to 0.95), documented infection (RR 0.78, 95% CI 0.62 to 0.97), and amphotericin B use (RR 0.50, 95% CI 0.28 to 0.87). There was no difference infection-related mortality (RR 1.02, 95% CI 0.34 to 3.06).[112] A meta-analysis of prophylactic CSF administration in the HSCT setting found that CSFs reduced the risk of documented infections (RR 0.87, 95% CI 0.76 to 1) but did not significantly reduce infection-related mortality (RR 0.76, 95% CI 0.41 to 1.44). Finally, a meta-analysis of 148 trials that included any cancer or HSCT population found that CSFs did not reduce short-term all-cause mortality (RR 0.95, 95% CI 0.84 to 1.08). A reduction of infection-related mortality was shown, but this did not reach statistical significance (RR 0.82, 95% CI 0.66 to 1.02). CSFs reduced documented infections (RR 0.85, CI 0.79 to 0.92), microbiologically documented infections (RR 0.86, 95% CI 0.77 to 0.96), and FN (RR 0.71, 95% CI 0.63 to 0.80).[113] Consequently, CSFs reduce FN and infections but do not influence overall survival. Whether CSFs should be administered therefore should depend on preferences, QoL considerations, and costs.

Prevention of Central Line–Associated Bloodstream Infection

A central line–associated bloodstream infection (CLABSI) can be defined as a bloodstream infection occurring in the presence of a CVL (present during the 48-hour period before development of the infection) and not related to infection at another site.[114] The most common causes of CLABSI are coagulase-negative staphylococci, *S. aureus*, *Enterococcus* spp., and *Candida* spp.[115] An evidence-based guideline supported by multiple agencies, including the Centers for Disease Control and Prevention, has been developed.[116] Recommendations included providing education and training focused on insertion and maintenance of CVLs and in particular indications for their use and competencies around insertion technique. Other recommendations were to use maximum barrier precautions and greater than 0.5% chlorhexidine skin preparation before CVL insertion and to critically assess the need for a CVL on an ongoing basis. Finally, the guideline recommended consideration of chlorhexidine-impregnated sponges and antimicrobial- or antiseptic-impregnated short-term CVL if other strategies for CLABSI reduction are not successful.

INFECTIOUS ISSUES IN PEDIATRIC CANCER PATIENTS IN LOW- AND MIDDLE-INCOME COUNTRIES

Children who live in low- and middle-income countries (LMICs) make up the majority of pediatric patients with cancer worldwide. As a group, they have not benefited from the same improvements in cancer outcomes compared with children who live in high-income countries.[117] Excessive infection-related mortality has contributed to this survival gap. In one study from El Salvador, treatment-related mortality (TRM) was responsible for 50% of deaths in children with ALL and AML;[118] the 2-year cumulative incidence of TRM was 12.5 ± 1.7% for ALL and 35.1 ± 6.4% for AML. The most important cause of TRM was infections. In a second study of FN among all cancer types in El Salvador, 12.3% of episodes were noted to result in death.[119]

Given the excessive risk of infectious toxicity, the identification of modifiable risk factors becomes paramount in this setting. Among children with ALL (but not AML), low monthly income and low parental education were associated with significantly higher TRM.[118] A subsequent prospective observational study in El Salvador sought to determine the association between socioeconomic status and time to assessment and treatment of fever and with rates of sepsis and infectious mortality.[120] Among 269 febrile outpatient episodes, the major source of delay was time from fever onset to decision to seek care, with 75% of parents waiting 5 hours or more. Once the decision to seek care had been made, the median time to reach the hospital was 1.8 hours. Parents who were illiterate had a 12- to 16-hour delay in deciding to seek medical care compared with parents who were literate. Once the decision to seek medical care had been made, parental literacy did not influence time to reach hospital. Maternal illiteracy was an independent risk factor for sepsis (OR 3.2, 95% CI 1.2 to 8.1), and lower annual household income was associated with infectious death (OR 13.9, 95% CI 1.6 to 119.1). These findings suggest that poor socioeconomic status translates into a delay in deciding to seek care and receiving medical attention in febrile children with leukemia. Figure 67-1 summarizes the different factors that affect the rates of infections and infection outcomes for children receiving cancer care in high-income countries and LMICs. The factors in high-income countries are predominantly treatment-related issues, whereas the factors in LMICs also include social and economic issues. Therefore any intervention employed to reduce TRM in LMICs must be tailored to these socioeconomic factors.

RECENT DIRECTIONS INVOLVING PRECLINICAL RESEARCH

Continued laboratory and translational investigation are critical to ensuring new advances in infectious diseases supportive care for future pediatric oncology patients. The fields of synthetic biology, immunotherapy, and gut mucosal immunology hold particular promise for

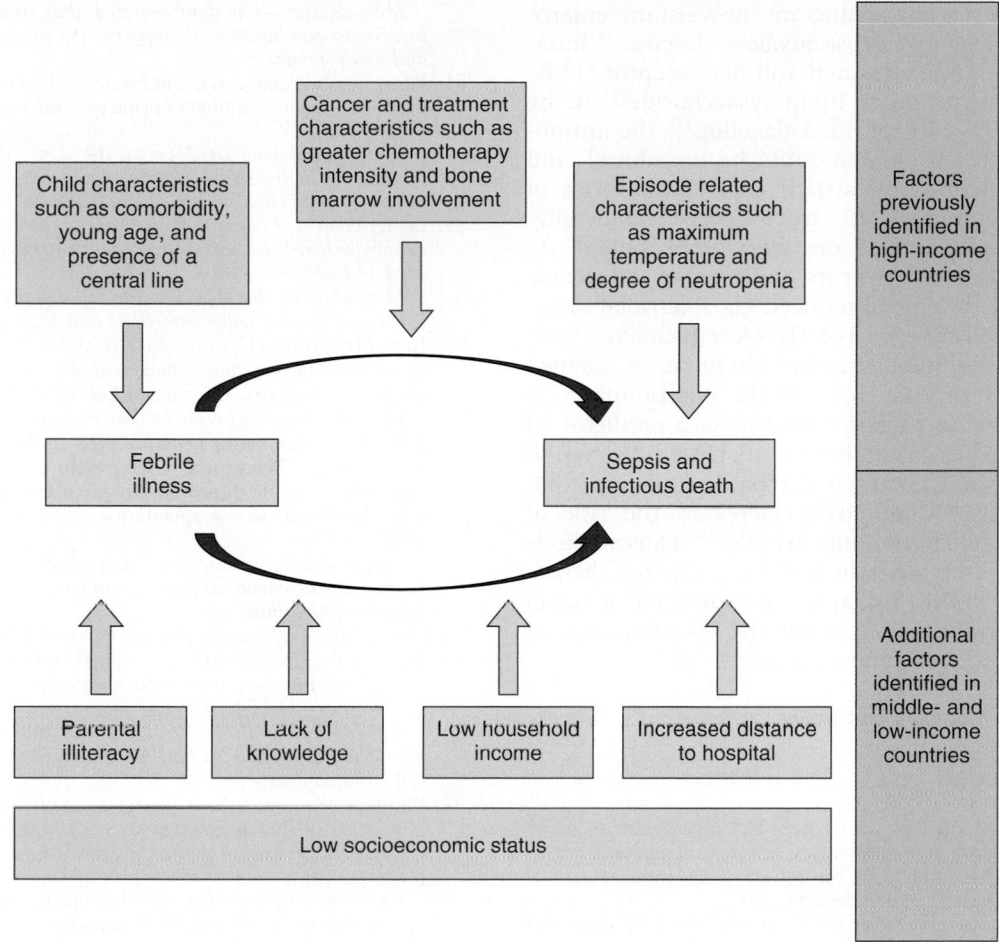

* Based on a systematic review in pediatric oncology. Factors listed are illustrative and not meant to be exhaustive.

Figure 67-1 Factors associated with sepsis and infectious deaths in pediatric acute leukemia in low- and middle-income countries. *(From Gavidia R et al: Low socioeconomic status is associated with prolonged times to assessment and treatment, sepsis and infectious death in pediatric Fever in el salvador.* PLoS One 7:e43639, 2012.)

novel methods of prevention and treatment of infectious diseases.

Synthetic biology is an emerging field focused on engineering biomolecular systems and cellular capabilities for a variety of applications, including the treatment of infections.[121] For example, bacteriophage (viruses that infect only specific bacteria) have been engineered to express a bacterial biofilm–degrading enzyme, dispersin B, that acts not only to rapidly degrade the biofilm matrix but also to kill 99.997% of the bacterial cells in the biofilm.[122] In another study synthetic adjuvants were designed by engineering bacteriophage to disrupt bacterial networks critical for antibiotic defense mechanisms, thereby resulting in significantly enhanced killing of bacterial strains by quinolones, beta-lactams, and aminoglycosides (in some cases a 5000-fold increase in killing).[123] Thus in the future bioengineered bacteriophages could help treat prosthetic device and CVL infections and also serve as adjuvants for treating antibiotic-resistant bacterial strains.

The use of immunotherapy in the prevention and treatment of infectious diseases is rapidly evolving. Adoptive transfer of antigen-specific T cells has proved to be an effective and powerful therapeutic tool in the prevention and treatment of viral infections (e.g., cytomegalovirus,[124] Epstein-Barr virus [EBV],[125] and adenovirus[126]) in immunocompromised hosts, but its use has been limited by the time needed to generate these cells. The technology has now advanced so that multivirus-specific (EBV, cytomegalovirus, adenovirus, BK, human herpes virus 6, RSV, and influenza) cytotoxic T lymphocytes (CTLs) can be generated within 10 days[127], and the possibility for using multivirus-specific CTLs for prophylaxis and treatment of viral infections, particularly in patients with leukemia and those undergoing HSCT, is encouraging.

The human microbiome, the aggregate of microorganisms that reside on and within the human host, has been shown to be critical for maintaining human immune function. Recent studies have shown that commensal microbes stimulate the gastrointestinal epithelium to produce antimicrobial proteins that act as a first line of defense against invading pathogenic bacteria.[128] When indigenous commensals are depleted after antibiotic administration, select pathogenic bacteria (e.g., vancomycin-resistant entero-cocci) can overgrow and cause invasive disease.[129] Interestingly, by stimulating intestinal Toll-like receptor (TLR) 4 by oral administration of lipopolysaccharide[129] or by stimulating TLR-5 with purified flagellin,[130] the antimicrobial protein RegIII gamma could be re-induced, and subsequently vancomycin-resistant enterococci levels in the murine gastrointestinal tract were significantly decreased and disseminated disease was prevented. As for human correlates, patients undergoing allogeneic HSCT uniformly developed reduced gut microbial diversity (as determined by deep 16S rRNA sequencing), with many patients exhibiting intestinal domination, defined as occupation of at least 30% of the microbiota by a single predominating bacterial taxon. As a predictor of outcomes, enterococcal domination increased the risk of vancomycin-resistant enterococcal bacteremia ninefold, and proteobacterial domination increased the risk of gram-negative bacilli bacteremia fivefold.[131] Thus methods for maintaining microbial homeostasis during chemotherapy and antibiotic therapies may provide a novel means for preventing colonization and dissemination of pathogenic microbes in cancer patients.

👆 *References available online at ExpertConsult.*

KEY REFERENCES

20. Freifeld AG, Bow EJ, Sepkowitz KA, et al: Clinical practice guideline for the use of antimicrobial agents in neutropenic patients with cancer: 2010 update by the Infectious Diseases Society of America. *Clin Infect Dis* 52:e56–e93, 2011.
    Clinical practice guideline for the management of fever and neutropenia developed by the Infectious Diseases Society of America.
42. Phillips RS, Lehrnbecher T, Alexander S, et al: Updated systematic review and meta-analysis of the performance of risk prediction rules in children and young people with febrile neutropenia. *PLoS ONE* 7:e38300, 2012.
    Systematic review of clinical prediction rules for fever and neutropenia risk factors among children with cancer.
58. Furno P, Bucaneve G, Del Favero A: Monotherapy or aminoglycoside-containing combinations for empirical antibiotic treatment of febrile neutropenic patients: a meta-analysis. *Lancet Infect Dis* 2:231–242, 2002.
    Meta-analysis that demonstrated that monotherapy was not inferior to combination therapy for the initial treatment of fever and neutropenia.
59. Paul M, Soares-Weiser K, Leibovici L: Beta lactam monotherapy versus beta lactam-aminoglycoside combination therapy for fever with neutropenia: systematic review and meta-analysis. *BMJ* 326:1111, 2003.
    Meta-analysis that demonstrated that monotherapy was not inferior to combination therapy for the initial treatment of fever and neutropenia.
81. Pizzo PA, Robichaud KJ, Gill FA, et al: Duration of empiric antibiotic therapy in granulocytopenic patients with cancer. *Am J Med* 67:194–200, 1979.
    Randomized trial of 7 versus 14 days of empiric antibiotic therapy for high-risk fever and neutropenia demonstrating that 7 days was associated with poor infection outcomes.
89. Gafter-Gvili A, Fraser A, Paul M, et al: Meta-analysis: antibiotic prophylaxis reduces mortality in neutropenic patients. *Ann Intern Med* 142:979–995, 2005.
    Meta-analysis that demonstrated that antibacterial prophylaxis is associated with fewer infections and improved survival.
91. Regier DA, Diorio C, Ethier MC, et al: Discrete choice experiment to evaluate factors that influence preferences for antibiotic prophylaxis in pediatric oncology. *PLoS ONE* 7:e47470, 2012.
    Discrete choice experiment that evaluated preferences for outpatient management of pediatric fever and neutropenia.
93. Goodman JL, Winston DJ, Greenfield RA, et al: A controlled trial of fluconazole to prevent fungal infections in patients undergoing bone marrow transplantation. *N Engl J Med* 326:845–851, 1992.
    Randomized controlled trial that illustrated the benefit of prophylactic fluconazole in patients undergoing hematopoietic stem cell transplantation.
94. Slavin MA, Osborne B, Adams R, et al: Efficacy and safety of fluconazole prophylaxis for fungal infections after marrow transplantation—a prospective, randomized, double-blind study. *J Infect Dis* 171:1545–1552, 1995.
    Randomized controlled trial that illustrated the benefit of prophylactic fluconazole in patients undergoing hematopoietic stem cell transplantation.
97. Wingard JR, Carter SL, Walsh TJ, et al: Randomized, double-blind trial of fluconazole versus voriconazole for prevention of invasive fungal infection after allogeneic hematopoietic cell transplantation. *Blood* 116:5111–5118, 2010.
    Randomized controlled trial that illustrated the lack of benefit of prophylactic voriconazole in patients undergoing hematopoietic stem cell transplantation.
109. Cornely OA, Maertens J, Winston DJ, et al: Posaconazole vs. fluconazole or itraconazole prophylaxis in patients with neutropenia. *N Engl J Med* 356:348–359, 2007.
    Randomized trial that illustrated that in patients with acute myeloid leukemia or myelodysplastic syndrome, prophylaxis with posaconazole, when compared with fluconazole or itraconazole, reduces the risk of invasive fungal infection and improves overall survival.
113. Sung L, Nathan PC, Alibhai SM, et al: Meta-analysis: effect of prophylactic hematopoietic colony-stimulating factors on mortality and outcomes of infection. *Ann Intern Med* 147:400–411, 2007.
    Systematic review illustrating that prophylactic colony-stimulating factors reduce infections but do not improve overall survival in patients with cancer who are undergoing hematopoietic stem cell transplantation.

CHAPTER 68

Oncologic Emergencies

Elizabeth A. Mullen and Eric Gratias

CHAPTER OUTLINE

Expert and timely management of emergent situations is crucial in the practice of pediatric oncology. Although many emergencies are common across the spectrum of pediatric patients, such as seizure, respiratory arrest, and electrolyte abnormalities, others stem from the underlying cancer or cancer-directed therapy and are unique to this population of patients. These types of emergencies require special consideration and specific management to minimize adverse outcomes. Emergencies related to space-occupying lesions, metabolic derangements caused by breakdown of tumor cells, and disruption of the hematopoietic system by invasion of cancer cells all in some way relate to disruption of the normal function of a cell or organ as a result of the abnormal presence of cancer cells. This disruption can be rapidly progressive and life-threatening, as when patients with T-cell lymphoblastic leukemia present with a mediastinal mass and respiratory compromise. The treatments directed toward cancer also carry significant toxicities and can result in uniquely emergent complications. Many chemotherapy agents result in a state of significant immune compromise and put patients at risk for unusual or opportunistic infections, as well as fulminant presentations of infection with more common organisms. All chemotherapy drugs carry

extensive profiles of possible adverse effects, and errors of administration or dosage can magnify toxicity; any available therapeutic interventions must be administered immediately. Appropriate management of an emergent pediatric oncologic situation requires a clear understanding of the specific underlying disease process and of the effects and consequences of cancer-directed therapies.

Symptoms in children who present with new diagnoses of cancer or are receiving cancer treatment are myriad. Therefore recognition of an emergency is not always straightforward, particularly in the young pediatric population, for whom obtaining an accurate history can be challenging. It is therefore imperative that the clinician maintain a high level of vigilance for the presentation of potentially life-threatening situations. A child with cough and mild respiratory distress is most likely to have a viral infection, but these symptoms also might be consistent with a child presenting with a marked mediastinal mass, developing leukostasis syndrome, or the onset of Pneumocystis pneumonia. A complaint of lower back pain in a child may relate to new physical activity or could represent developing spinal cord compression from a tumor. Pediatric oncologists need to be familiar with all pediatric oncologic emergent situations to evaluate and manage

2267

Box 68-1 Commonly Encountered Pediatric Oncologic Emergencies

DISEASE-RELATED

Anterior mediastinal mass
Increased intracranial pressure
Spinal cord compression
Leukocytosis and leukostasis
Tumor lysis syndrome
Disseminated intravascular coagulation

TREATMENT-RELATED

Fever and neutropenia, sepsis
Typhlitis
Pancreatitis
Vesicant infiltration
Methotrexate toxicity
All-*trans*-retinoic acid syndrome
Veno-occlusive disease
Intrathecal chemotherapy overdose
Central nervous system events such as seizure or CVA
Severe allergic reactions to chemotherapy agents or blood products

---

these high-risk patients appropriately. Rapid and appropriate triage of patient complaints is critical, because overlooked diagnoses, as well as inaction or inappropriate action, can have severe consequences.

Grouping of some emergent pediatric oncologic conditions into disease- and treatment-related events is presented in Box 68-1. Clear overlap exists among the conditions listed; for example, tumor lysis syndrome (TLS) can occur on presentation with a new diagnosis of leukemia or high-grade lymphoma, but it can be markedly worsened by initiation of chemotherapy. Similarly, superior vena cava syndrome (SVCS) can result from a new or recurrent presence of a mass lesion or as a complication of an indwelling catheter placed to deliver antineoplastic therapy. In this chapter our discussion will focus on several emergent situations unique to pediatric oncology patients, with a review of available data and overviews of current management strategies. The topics addressed in the chapter are anterior mediastinal mass, increased intracranial pressure, spinal cord compression, hyperleukocytosis and leukostasis, TLS, and selected chemotherapy toxicities. Several topics unique to the pediatric oncology patient are covered elsewhere in this text and will not be readdressed in this chapter (e.g., management of fever and neutropenia, typhlitis, veno-occlusive disease, all-*trans*-retinoic acid syndrome, transfusion medicine, and pain management). Situations that can occur in the pediatric oncology patient but that are not unique to this population, such as seizure, cerebral vascular injury, disseminated intravascular coagulation, and pancreatitis, will not be discussed here.

Although optimal management of many of these emergent situations has been difficult to study, given the relatively small number of patients presenting to each institution, a literature is evolving for many of these topics. Many institutions have established clinical practice guidelines to help manage the most common pediatric oncologic emergencies. Clinical practice guidelines provide uniform standards for management but must allow for adaptations for each specific clinical scenario. Uniform use of clinical guidelines with collection and analysis of outcomes has the potential to guide improvements in clinical practice.

ANTERIOR MEDIASTINAL MASSES

Definition

A commonly encountered oncologic emergency is the entity of anterior mediastinal mass. A clinician should always consider this entity in the differential diagnosis of a pediatric patient with new respiratory distress and must consider evaluation, even in asymptomatic patients presenting with any of the variety of cancers known to be associated with the occurrence of anterior mediastinal masses.

Space-occupying lesions occurring in the anterior mediastinum can impinge on vital structures, causing significant cardiac or airway compromise. The anterior mediastinum is defined as the anatomic compartment bounded by the sternum, thoracic inlet, and anterior border of the heart.[1] The presence of a mass in this region can cause SVCS, tracheobronchial compression, or compression of the heart or pulmonary vessels. The term *superior mediastinal syndrome* (SMS) has been used to denote the combination of great vessel and tracheobronchial tree compression. However, because these phenomena may be overlapping, particularly in the pediatric population, the terms SVCS and SMS are often used interchangeably.

Neoplasms that cause anterior mediastinal masses in the pediatric population and are associated with SVCS and/or tracheal compression include non-Hodgkin lymphoma (NHL), acute lymphoblastic leukemia (ALL), and Hodgkin lymphoma (HL),[2] as well as neuroblastoma, paraganglioma, germ cell tumors, sarcoma (including myeloid sarcoma), thymoma, desmoplastic round cell tumor, lymphangioma, inflammatory myofibroblastic tumor, and thyroid and parathyroid carcinaomas.[3-10] In a retrospective review of children with mediastinal masses treated at the Mayo Clinic, NHL and HL represented the majority of malignant causes of anterior mediastinal masses, although this review did not include patients with leukemia.[10] In a report on 3721 children with cancer treated at St. Jude Children's Research Hospital over a 15-year period, 24 children had superior vena cava (SVC) obstruction at initial presentation or with disease recurrence. Patients presenting with SVC obstruction at initial presentation included eight children with NHL, four with ALL, two with HL, one with neuroblastoma, and one with yolk sac tumor.[9] In contrast, in the adult population, small cell bronchogenic carcinoma is the most common underlying diagnosis associated with SVCS.[11]

SVCS was first described in a patient with a syphilitic aneurysm of the aorta in 1757.[12] The SVC is a thin-walled vessel with blood flowing under low pressure and is easily compressible by the enlargement of surrounding structures in the thorax. In persons with SVCS, compression and obstruction of the SVC cause restriction of blood return to the right atrium and impaired venous drainage from the upper extremities, head, and neck. Occlusion of

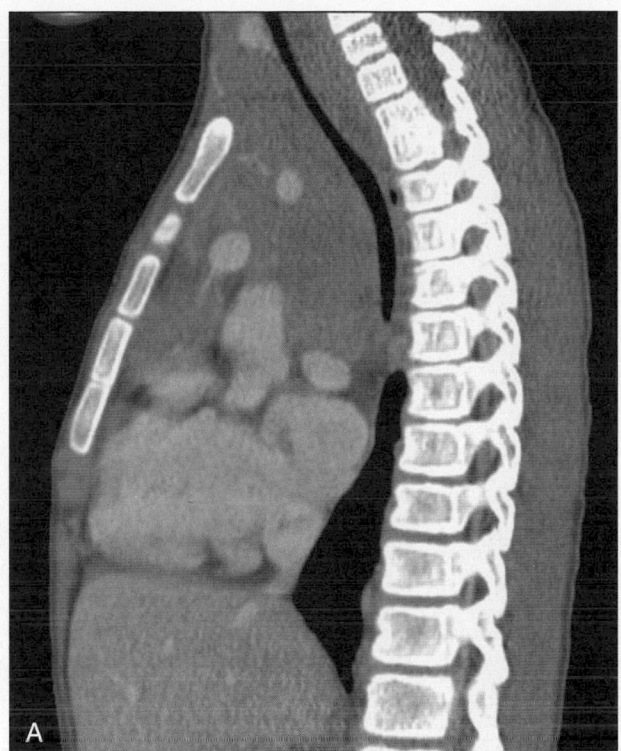

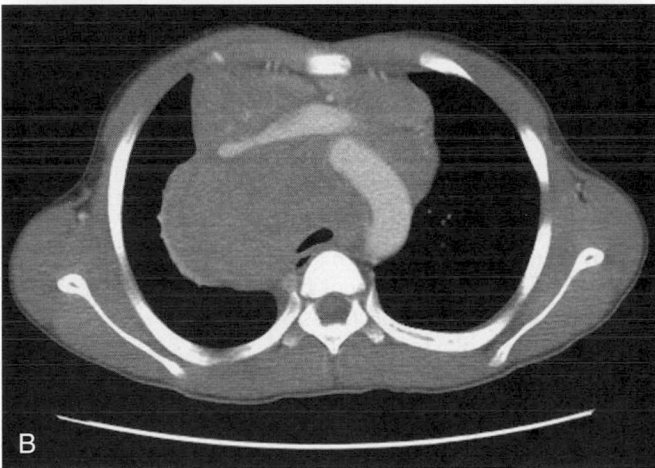

Figure 68-1 A chest computed tomography scan of a patient with Hodgkin disease. Sagittal (**A**) and axial (**B**) images show the significant effects of the mass on structures within the mediastinum, with marked narrowing of the trachea and superior vena cava. Remarkably, the patient was symptomatic only with exercise.

the SVC by thrombus—for example, as a complication of a central venous line—can also result in SVCS. Just as the SVC can be compressed by an anterior mediastinal mass, the trachea and main stem bronchi in children are relatively compressible and have smaller intraluminal diameters compared with these structures in adults, making the pediatric patient with an enlarging mass susceptible to respiratory compromise (Fig. 68-1).[10]

Clinical Presentation

Children with SMS can present with a constellation of signs and symptoms related to SVC and airway obstruc-

tion, including swelling, plethora, venous engorgement of the face, neck, and upper extremities, cough, hoarseness, orthopnea, cyanosis, anxiety, syncope, and altered mental status.[13,14] The child can present in extremis, with shock caused by cardiac compromise, or the child can present with respiratory failure, which more commonly occurs in malignancies with a higher growth fraction such as B- or T-lymphoblastic or mature B-cell lymphomas. Conversely, patients with more indolent tumors, such as HL, can present with impressively large masses and surprisingly little symptomatology (Fig. 68-2). Symptoms are often more profound with the patient in the supine position and may improve in the upright or prone position. In the supine position, thoracic volume is decreased because of decreased rib cage dimension and diaphragm position. In addition, blood flow to the mass itself can increase, causing further expansion of the mass.[1] Therefore pursuing testing such as computed tomography (CT) scanning in the supine position should be carefully considered, and patient tolerance of supine positioning should be evaluated before initiating cross-sectional imaging. Patients who are unable to tolerate supine positioning may require decubitus or prone positioning if CT evaluation is necessary during the initial workup, and some patients with extreme compression may not be able to tolerate any horizontal positioning prior to emergent cytoreductive therapy.

An anterior mediastinal mass may be suspected on the basis of medical history and physical examination and can be identified on a chest radiograph. Identifying patients at greatest risk for anesthetic complications is important in planning the diagnostic evaluation. Procedural sedation and anesthesia pose particular risks for

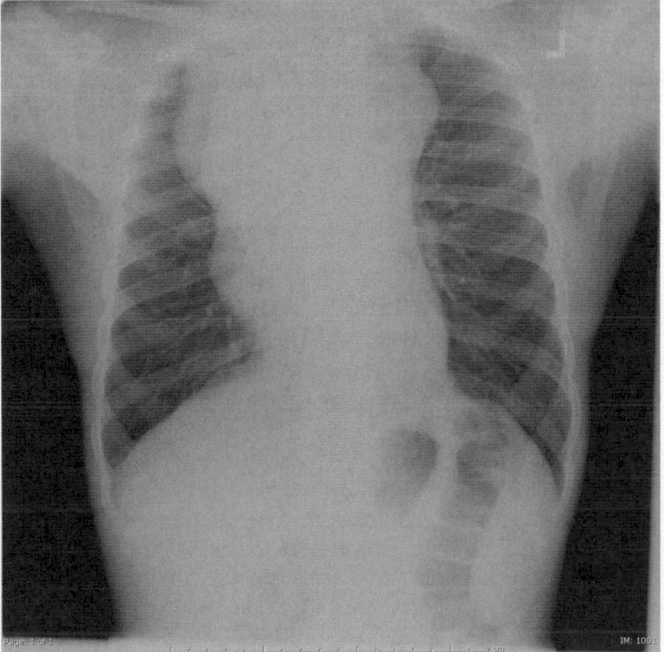

Figure 68-2 A chest radiograph of a patient with Hodgkin disease showing a markedly enlarged mediastinum. The patient had a several-month history of intermittent cough and had only mild respiratory symptoms at presentation.

patients with an anterior mediastinal mass, with the potential for cardiopulmonary collapse and death.[13-15] A patient whose respiratory status is stable while awake, with spontaneous respirations, may experience significant obstruction when anesthesia is induced. General anesthesia alters ventilatory mechanics, decreasing inspiratory muscle tone and functional residual capacity of the lung.[16] Chest wall tone is decreased by neuromuscular blockade. Airways are more compressible because of bronchial smooth muscle relaxation.[14] Positive pressure ventilation may further restrict an already narrowed airway.[17] In addition, general anesthetic agents can have negative inotropic effects and may contribute to decreasing cardiac output, precipitating hypoxemia, hypotension, or even cardiac arrest in patients with compression of the great vessels.[18]

Respiratory symptoms occur in 40% to 60% of children with anterior mediastinal masses, but correlation of symptoms with anesthetic risk can be challenging.[14,19] Orthopnea has been associated with increased anesthetic risk.[19,20] Posterior anterior and lateral chest radiographs can demonstrate tracheal compression but may not detect all cases.[19,21] CT can provide additional anatomic information, and patients with less than 50% of expected tracheal cross-sectional area on CT have been shown to be a high-risk group.[14,19] However, obstruction distal to the trachea may be more difficult to appreciate. Authors of a prospective study assessing tracheal area and pulmonary function testing have found that inducement of general anesthesia can be used safely in children who meet the minimum criteria of a tracheal area larger than 50% and predicted peak expiratory flow rate (PEFR) greater than 50%. Thirty-one children with mediastinal masses underwent pulmonary function testing in the sitting and supine positions along with CT prior to undergoing 34 surgical procedures. For children with less than 50% of predicted cross-sectional tracheal area (or with less than 50% of PEFR), only local rather than general anesthetic agents were used. Five patients had predicted tracheal areas larger than 50% but had a low PEFR and thus only local anesthetic agents were used. No intraoperative complications occurred in patients receiving anesthetic drugs when these criteria were used.[22]

Evaluation and Imaging

A definitive diagnosis is needed to initiate tumor-specific therapy, and the least invasive diagnostic methods possible should be pursued. If the peripheral blood smear is abnormal, a bone marrow aspiration or biopsy with use of a local anesthetic may prove sufficiently diagnostic. A biopsy of a peripheral lymph node, if present, may prove diagnostic. Serum α-fetoprotein or β-human chorionic gonadotropin may be positive in patients with mediastinal germ cell tumors, and these tests can be performed rapidly in many institutions. If a pleural effusion is present, pleural fluid aspiration may be possible with use of local anesthesia and may provide fluid for pathologic review and immunophenotypic and cytogenetic evaluation (Fig. 68-3).[23] Some patients whose only source of potential diagnostic tissue is the mediastinal mass will be

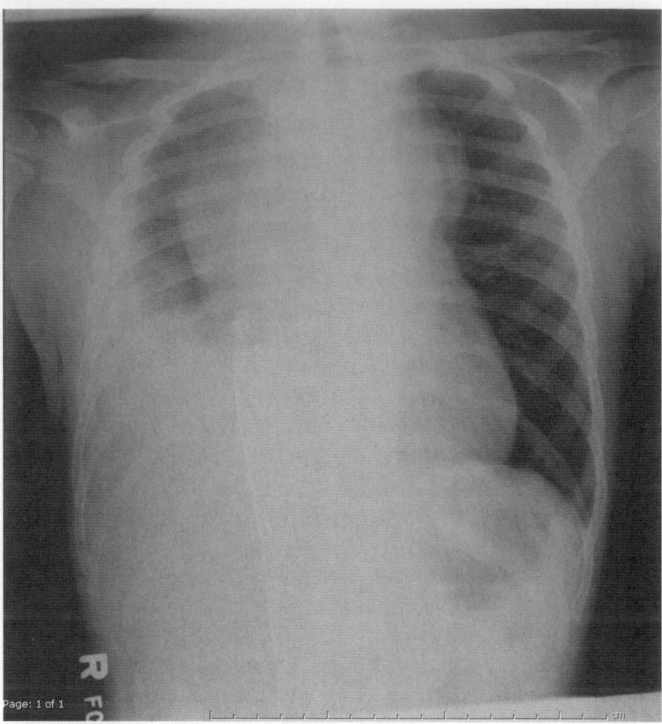

Figure 68-3 A chest radiograph of a patient who presented in near extremis, with facial swelling, plethora, and significant respiratory distress. The patient had a large anterior mediastinal mass and marked pleural effusion. T-cell lymphoblastic lymphoma was diagnosed from the pleural fluid.

able to tolerate percutaneous needle biopsy with use of a local anesthetic and anxiolytic-only sedation.

An accurate tissue diagnosis allows for initiation of the optimal specific treatment regimen. For many patients with anterior mediastinal masses, a general state of anesthesia will be able to be induced safely.[24] However, the cases of patients in extremis or those with rapidly evolving respiratory compromise who require sedation or inducement of general anesthesia are particularly challenging to manage. When proceeding with general anesthesia, some persons have advocated the preservation of spontaneous respiration when at all possible, avoidance of the use of muscle relaxants, being prepared to change the patient's position, and having an expert bronchoscopist and emergency cardiopulmonary bypass available.[15] Use of bilevel positive airway pressure for safe anesthesia in these settings has been reported recently.[25] Successful suprasedative dosing of dexmedetomidine has also been reported.[26] Use of extracorporeal membrane oxygenation in persons with anterior mediastinal masses who are experiencing cardiopulmonary failure has been reported.[27] Use of inhaled heliox, a helium-oxygen mixture, has been advocated in case reports to decrease resistance to airflow in obstructed airways, although its use in the setting of anterior mediastinal masses has not been studied.[28]

In recent years the surgical literature has included an increased focus on novel operative techniques to allow safe biopsy and/or resection in patients with large anterior mediastinal masses. Percutaneous biopsy has long been a standard approach in patients too unstable for inducement of general anesthesia, but advances in imaging technique allow for additional applications of this methodology, such as real-time ultrasound fusion with CT for biopsy guidance.[29] Additional modalities recently described as successful in a majority of patients include awake video-assisted thoracoscopic biopsy, the hemiclamshell approach, and the Chamberlain procedure (also known as anterior mediastinotomy).[30-32]

Treatment

In some clinical situations the risk of proceeding with diagnostic procedures is considered too great, and empiric therapy aimed at reducing the mass must be initiated. Emergent treatment modalities include radiation, intravenous steroids, and combination chemotherapy. Radiation has traditionally been used in emergency management of anterior mediastinal masses, because most lymphomas are radiosensitive. Daily radiation doses are based on those used for the presumed diagnosis that best fits the clinical data. Depending on the radioresponsiveness of the mass, prebiopsy radiation treatment will frequently obscure the tissue diagnosis, even with low-dose radiation therapy. Loeffler and colleagues[33] reported that in 8 of 10 patients younger than 30 years who underwent emergent prebiopsy radiation for a mediastinal mass, a tissue diagnosis could not be established because of uninterpretable pathologic specimens. Also of concern in the pediatric population is a risk of postradiation respiratory deterioration caused by swelling of the trachea after radiation. Concurrent administration of a steroid (e.g., dexamethasone at a dosage for airway edema, 0.5 to 2 mg/kg/day in divided doses every 6 hours) can be considered with the goal of preventing this complication but may also contribute to obscurity of the diagnosis because most untreated lymphomas are sensitive to steroids.

The emergent use of empiric chemotherapy includes the use of intravenous (IV) steroids or combination chemotherapy. Steroid therapy should be considered in the emergent management of proven or presumed ALL or lymphoblastic lymphoma. Careful attention must be directed to fluid management given concerns for TLS in the patient with the potential for cardiovascular compromise. Consideration of the use of rasburicase may be warranted. Steroid dosing based on ALL treatment protocols can be used (e.g., methylprednisolone, 32 to 48 mg/m²/day IV, divided every 8 to 12 hours). Steroid therapy may also be effective in the setting of other malignancies because of its potent antiinflammatory effect. Other chemotherapeutic agents for consideration in the emergent management of anterior mediastinal mass include cyclophosphamide, vincristine, and anthracyclines. Just as radiation may eliminate the ability to establish a definitive diagnosis, steroid therapy has also been reported to inhibit accurate diagnosis.[13] Without a definitive pathologic diagnosis, continued treatment of the patient for the presumed diagnosis that best fits the clinical data has been advocated. Masses that are not responsive to the previously described emergent therapies may require surgical intervention.

Conclusions

The evaluation of a child with a suspected anterior mediastinal mass or SVCS should be initiated rapidly once the diagnosis is considered to be a possibility. Great variability in the course of evaluation and treatment may be encountered, depending on the specifics of each clinical situation, including the clinical stability of the patient and the underlying diagnosis. A representative evaluation and treatment algorithm published in 2008 is outlined in Figure 68-4.[34] The clinician must adapt his or her care to the particular circumstances of the individual patient.

SPINAL CORD COMPRESSION

Spinal cord compression is overall a rare event in children, but several studies have shown an incidence of up to 5% in children with cancer.[35] The most frequent occurrence of spinal cord compression in children with cancer is during the initial presentation of the malignant process (67% of the time).[36] Although such a presentation often occurs with widely disseminated disease, spinal cord compression can also occur with a singular lesion as the initial presentation of a new diagnosis of cancer. In this scenario, along with preservation or restoration of lost neurologic functioning, proper diagnosis of the cancer through adequate tissue sampling is a management priority. Procurement of sufficient tissue for specialized testing and possible study enrollment is a lesser priority but still should be thoughtfully considered in the overall management plan. Spinal cord compression is also encountered in patients with relapsed and refractory disease, again as a single metastatic lesion or as widespread metastatic disease. In such situations, management strategies must take into account the likelihood of cure, the effect of interventions on the patient's quality of life, and the role of palliation.

The majority (71%) of tumors that cause spinal cord compression are extradural.[36] More than 50% of tumors causing spinal cord compression are found to be neuroblastoma, soft tissue sarcomas, Ewing sarcoma, or rhabdomyosarcoma. A wide variety of other tumors have been reported as causes of spinal cord compression and must be considered in the differential diagnosis. Tumors reported to date include osteosarcoma, Wilms tumor, metastatic central nervous system tumors, meningioma, pleuropulmonary blastoma, juvenile xanthogranuloma, adrenocortical carcinoma, acute myelogenous leukemia (AML), and lymphoma.[37-40]

Clinical Presentation

Back pain is the most common presenting sign of spinal cord compression and was present in 94% of 70 pediatric patients presenting with solid tumors and spinal cord compression.[36] Because recurrent back pain without known injury is a fairly uncommon complaint in children, spinal lesions and spinal cord compression should always be considered in the differential diagnosis of this complaint, even in the absence of neurologic findings. In pediatric patients known to have cancer, the index of suspicion must be particularly high. Any delay

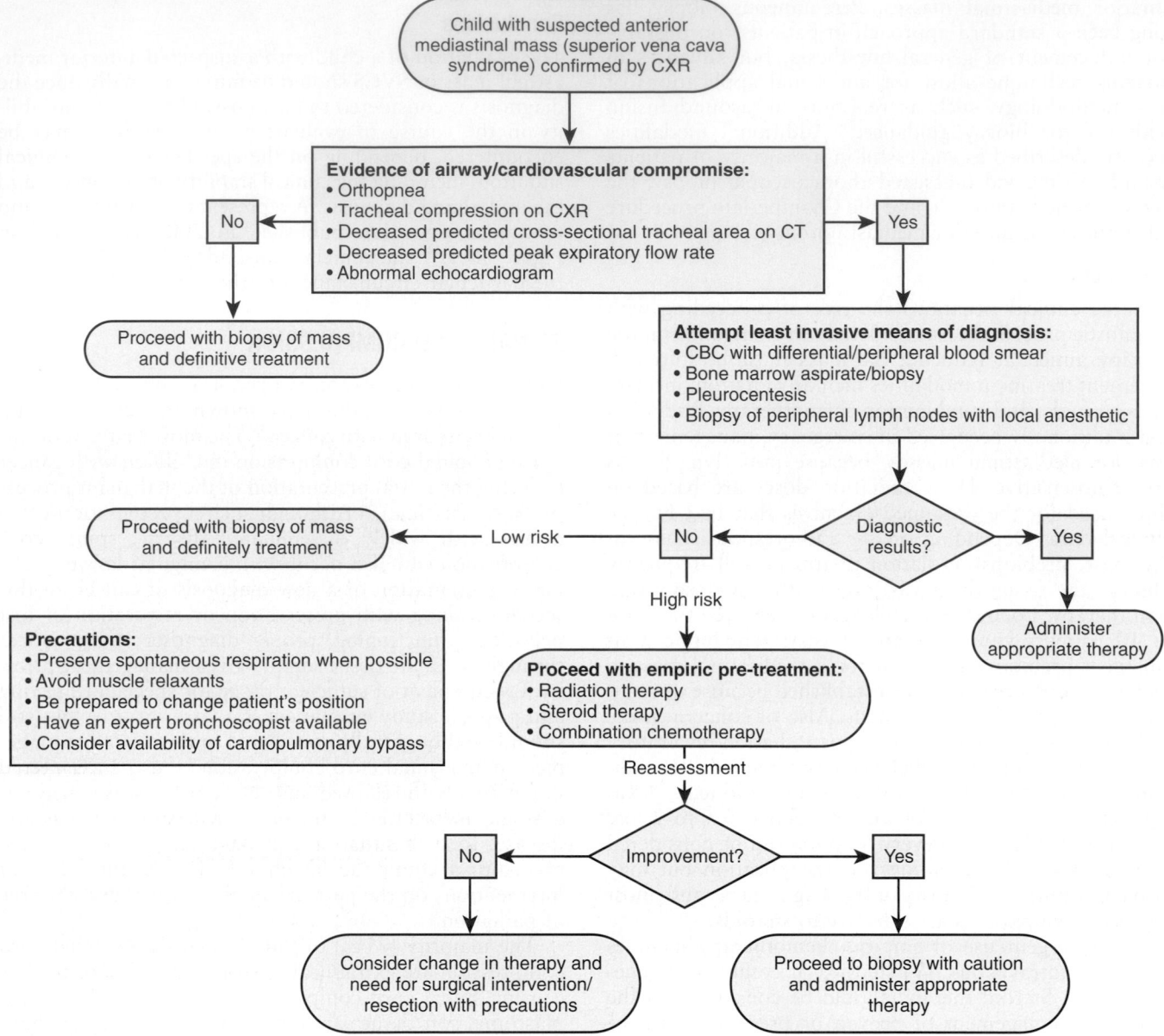

Figure 68-4 Algorithm for a patient with critical airways and an anterior mediastinal mass or superior vena cava syndrome.[34] *CBC,* Complete blood cell count; *CT,* computed tomography; *CXR,* chest x-ray.

in diagnosis of spinal cord compression may contribute significantly to morbidity. A thorough physical examination should accompany a complete history. The history should include characterization of pain, including onset and duration. Neurologic findings, if present, will vary, depending on the spinal level of the lesion and the degree of compression. In their series of children with systemic cancer and spinal cord disease, Lewis and coworkers[35] noted that localized spine tenderness is the most reliable clinical finding. A spectrum of ataxia, gait disturbance, and paraplegia can be observed. Sphincter dysfunction is most commonly seen as urinary retention or constipation. Localization of the level of epidural cord compression along the spine is suggested by the specific effects on strength, tendon reflexes, sensory level, Babinski

reflex, sphincter abnormalities, and rate of progression (Table 68-1).[35,41]

Evaluation and Imaging

When the possibility of spinal cord compression is considered, immediate evaluation should be undertaken. Spinal radiography is often the first-choice modality because it is quickly and easily undertaken. Plain films may be able to provide valuable clinical information rapidly, but one must be aware that they are positive in only approximately 30% of patients with spinal cord compression.[35] The presence of a compressive spinal lesion may be seen on a radiograph as a paraspinal soft tissue mass. In cases of neuroblastoma, calcifications are often present within the paraspinal mass. Classically,

TABLE 68-1 Epidural Cord Compression: Clinical Localization

	LOCATION		
Sign	**Spinal Cord**	**Conus Medullaris**	**Cauda Equina**
Weakness	Symmetrical; profound	Symmetrical; variable	Asymmetrical; may be mild
Tendon reflexes	Increased or absent	Increased knee; decreased ankle	Decreased; asymmetrical
Babinski	Extensor	Extensor	Plantar
Sensory	Symmetrical; sensory level	Symmetrical; saddle	Asymmetrical; radicular
Sphincter abnormality	Spared until late	Early involvement	May be spared
Progression	Rapid	Variable; may be rapid	Variable; may be slow

Modified from Lewis DW, Packer RJ, Raney B, et al: Incidence, presentation, and outcome of spinal cord disease in children with systemic cancer. Pediatrics 78:438–443, 1986.

neuroblastoma invading the spinal canal and intervertebral foramina may be visualized as a dumbbell-shaped lesion surrounding the spine. Other tumors can also have this appearance, emphasizing the importance of obtaining adequate tissue for diagnosis (Fig. 68-5). In many spinal lesions, lytic or sclerotic changes in adjacent bone are often observed on a radiograph. Diagnostic widening of interpeduncular distances and enlargement of the neural foramina can sometimes also be observed on radiographs.

Emergent magnetic resonance imaging (MRI) is essential when plain radiographs are negative and clinical suspicion still exists. MRI is also necessary for further delineation of lesions observed on plain radiographs. MRI has become widely accessible and thus it has replaced the previously used techniques of radionucleotide bone scanning, spinal CT with intrathecal contrast, and lumbar myelography. MRI offers the advantage of increased accuracy and a less invasive nature than previously used modalities. Careful comparison of axial, coronal, and sagittal images can help categorize spinal tumors as extradural, intradural-extramedullary, or intramedullary, thereby aiding in the differential diagnosis.[42] MRI sequences with and without use of gadolinium should be obtained for patients being evaluated for spinal cord compression. Contrast enhancement is less helpful for extradural tumors than for intradural-extramedullary or intramedullary lesions. Fat suppression techniques are most helpful for evaluating extradural lesions. It should also be remembered that it is important to image the entire spine to identify the possibility of involvement at several levels, even if the physical examination has localized the most likely area of compression.

MRI can also accurately detect compression and dislocation of the spinal cord. Coronal images can elucidate the degree of cranial and caudal extension on the intraspinal component of a mass lesion. Because of increased cellularity and high nuclear-to-cytoplasmic ratio, lesions are usually isodense to hypodense on T2-weighted images.[43] Cord edema can be seen as a hyperintense signal in T2-weighted images. Contrast enhancement is generally marked in the presence of intraspinal lesions. Diffusion tensor imaging has been recently described as a potentially beneficial additive sequence.[44]

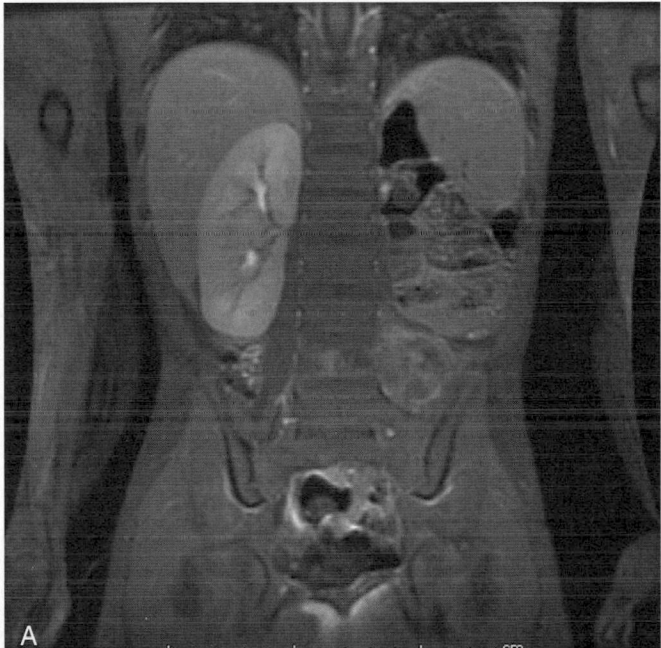

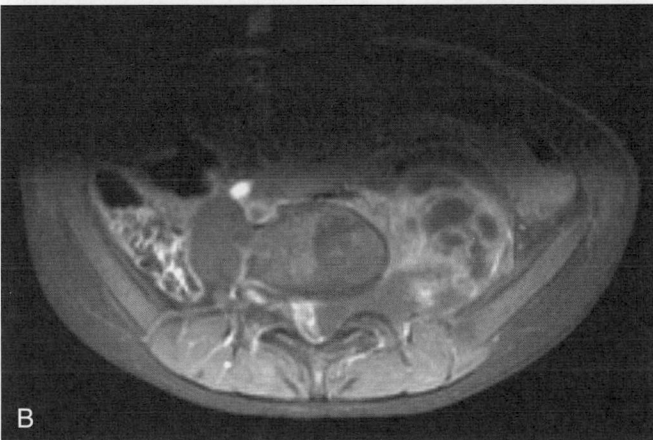

Figure 68-5 Magnetic resonance imaging after administration of gadolinium demonstrates a soft tissue retroperitoneal mass at the level of L4 with a dumbbell appearance on both coronal (**A**) and axial (**B**) views. The patient presented with a short history of leg pain and limp that progressed to the inability to ambulate, 2 years after the completion of therapy for Wilms tumor with a favorable histology.

If the clinical situation allows time for further radiologic evaluation, CT with bone windows can provide complementary information to MRI findings. Detailed information on bone architecture and cortical appearance is better obtained via CT.

Treatment

Treatment options for a patient presenting with spinal cord compression include surgery (laminectomy or laminotomy), chemotherapy, steroid therapy, and radiation therapy. The best choice of initial therapy will vary depending on the clinical situation. In many clinical situations use of more than one modality may be appropriate, and in some situations it is appropriate for more than one modality to be used simultaneously. The complexity of the choice of the best initial therapy stems largely from multiple competing therapeutic goals—the desire to act quickly to prevent further loss of neurologic function, the need to make an accurate diagnosis with sufficient biologic information for assignment of appropriate treatment, the hope of regaining any lost function existing at presentation, and the concern regarding the late effects of the available emergent treatment modalities. After providing a brief overview of the basic treatment options, we will present the conclusions of several clinical studies.

Surgery

Laminectomy is the most common surgical approach to relieve spinal cord compression caused by a solid tumor. Laminectomy involves removal of the bony arch, or lamina, of a vertebra. This procedure is often combined with biopsy and/or debulking of the tumor. The advantage of a laminectomy is the rapid decompression of the spinal cord. Laminectomy is generally accepted as the most likely modality to stabilize or improve lost neurologic function. Another significant advantage of laminectomy is the procurement of tumor tissue for proper histologic diagnosis and the option of obtaining tissue for relevant biology studies or possible protocol enrollment. The disadvantage of laminectomy is the high risk for late effects, with a significant percentage of patients experiencing kyphosis or scoliosis. Depending on the degree of spinal cord injury and how long symptoms have been present, laminectomy may not provide an advantage compared with treatment with chemotherapy only and may expose the child to risks of the surgical procedure and greater risks of long-term orthopedic sequelae.

The technique of osteoplastic laminotomy involves removal of part of the lamina above and below an affected nerve, with subsequent bracing for a period of 6 to 8 weeks. Although historically this technique is not commonly used, it may offer a decreased incidence of long-term sequelae and may be considered by the surgeon. Minimally invasive thoracoscopic approaches for decompression have been described.[45-48] Additionally, percutaneous approaches for decompression are increasing reported.[49,50]

Chemotherapy

Chemotherapy can be used successfully to reduce some neoplastic masses that cause spinal cord compression.

Use of chemotherapy has been most studied in cases of neuroblastoma or Ewing sarcoma that present with spinal cord compression, and chemotherapy has been used successfully to treat germ cell tumors as well.[51] In the rare cases of leukemic or lymphomatous infiltrates, chemotherapy is the clear standard initial therapy once the diagnosis has been established.

Advantages of upfront chemotherapy for lesions causing spinal cord compression are that chemotherapy is anatomically noninvasive and long-term surgical consequences may be avoided. In addition, patients may proceed with tumor-specific therapy without the need for delay from postoperative healing. However, the use of chemotherapy depends on first establishing an accurate pathologic diagnosis. In cases of metastatic tumor, it may be possible to make a diagnosis by biopsy of other primary or metastatic lesions. Identifying isolated paraspinal masses can be more diagnostically difficult. If surgery is avoided completely and chemotherapy is started presumptively, the possibility of an incorrect diagnosis will exist. Also, if no tissue is obtained, even though an isolated paraspinal mass may eventually be diagnosed as neuroblastoma on the basis of elevated urine catecholamine levels or positive metaiodobenzylguanidine activity, the opportunity to obtain valuable biologic information, such as histology, v-myc avian myelocytomatosis viral oncogene neuroblastoma derived homolog (MYCN) status, and other cytogenetic and molecular markers used to direct therapy could be lost.

In patients who experience spinal cord compression in the setting of relapsed disease, the choice of using chemotherapy rather than surgery or radiation therapy can become more complex, because the rate and overall likelihood of response can be substantially decreased in previously treated patients. Radiation therapy or surgeries may have been used previously and may limit these options in a relapse setting. Such clinical situations must be carefully weighed individually. The decision to initiate chemotherapy rather than to use surgery, radiation therapy, or comfort palliation must include consideration of the patient's overall chance of long-term cure, the history of treatment and response, and most importantly, the goals of treatment of the patient and family and the desired level of intensity of therapy.

In the patient with a new presentation of cancer, the choice of a chemotherapy regimen must be based on a clear identification of the malignant process. Once a diagnosis is known and a decision has been made to avoid surgery or radiation and commence with chemotherapy, standard frontline therapy for the malignancy that has been identified is accepted as the best initial chemotherapy in patients with spinal cord compression.

Dexamethasone

Dexamethasone is routinely recommended throughout the literature for the treatment of pediatric spinal cord compression. It is theorized that decreased swelling of the cord will help minimize neurologic damage through minimizing the effect of vasogenic edema and venous congestion. In a review of the adult literature compiled to create an evidence-based guideline for the emergency treatment of extradural spinal cord compression in adult patients, Loblaw and Laperriere[52] reviewed the available studies on the use of dexamethasone. They found strong evidence to support the use of high-dose dexamethasone with radiation therapy with improved outcome but significant associated toxicity.[53] They also reported evidence judged to be fair that dexamethasone does not need to be given to asymptomatic ambulatory patients with spinal cord compression receiving x-ray therapy.[54] Although no corresponding evidence is available to support the role of dexamethasone in improving outcome in spinal cord compression caused by solid tumors in pediatric patients, little substantial detrimental effect has been observed with the routine use of dexamethasone in the setting of acute spinal cord compression. Increased rates of infection and delayed wound healing are possible concerns. The use of gastric protectants is advised when administering dexamethasone in this setting and should include H2 blockers and/or proton pump inhibitors. Blood pressure and glucose levels should be monitored, and any increase above age norms should be treated appropriately.

In the case of a child presenting with a high index of suspicion of spinal cord compression caused by tumor and *any* neurologic compromise, rapid administration of dexamethasone at 1 to 2 mg/kg IV to be administered over 30 minutes is suggested. This dose should be administered prior to imaging. If no neurologic symptoms are present, lower oral dosing, 0.25 to 0.5 mg/kg every 6 hours, may be initiated while imaging is arranged. If the child is found to have a spinal lesion and radiation therapy is chosen as the modality for treatment of cord compression, use of moderate-dose dexamethasone is sometimes continued to decrease the effects of radiation-induced swelling and vasogenic edema.

Radiotherapy

Most tumors causing spinal cord compression in the pediatric population will respond to radiotherapy, and thus this modality can often be used emergently to relieve symptoms of spinal cord compression effectively. The benefits of its use include possible rapid response, reasonable tolerance, and avoidance of more invasive procedures. Potential drawbacks include interference with establishing a correct pathologic diagnosis, long-term effects on the spinal column (including stunted growth, cord damage, and scoliosis), thyroid dysfunction, and the risk of secondary malignancies. Additionally, young pediatric patients may require anesthesia for planning and delivery of radiotherapy fractions. For safety and accuracy, adequate imaging, usually through MRI, is required to define the length, depth, and width of the planned treatment field.

Several approaches can be used to deliver a therapeutic treatment dose.[55] Midline lesions, as well as lesions in the lumbar spine, may be treated through a parallel opposed anteroposterior-posteroanterior beam arrangement. A posterior field alone can be used for lesions in the thoracic spine. The cervical spine may be treated with opposed lateral fields in an effort to avoid the oral cavity. Conformal techniques can allow for more precise localization of the radiation therapy to the tumor volume. However, these methods require more elaborate planning and may delay the initiation of therapy. The potential benefit of a more conformal field must be weighed against the additional time and planning required.

Radiotherapy dose and schedule are determined by the pathologic diagnosis, extent of spinal involvement, possible coadministration of chemotherapy, and the patient's clinical situation (e.g., previously ambulatory or nonambulatory, overall life expectancy, likelihood of response to systemic therapy, and previous history of radiation therapy). A dosing range of 18 to 40 Gy can be used. Commonly used schedules include 30 Gy delivered in 10 fractions, 20 Gy given in 5 fractions, or up to 35 to 40 Gy spread over a more protracted course of 3 to 4 weeks. However, 8-Gy single fraction radiotherapy has been successfully used for palliation in patients with a grim prognosis and spinal cord compression, and a recent systematic review suggested that 30 Gy over 10 fractions was a preferred regimen for patients with a good prognosis.[56,57]

The concomitant use of dexamethasone with radiation therapy is often recommended. Dexamethasone is usually begun at a high dose prior to starting radiotherapy, continued at a lesser dose during the procedure, and tapered off after completion. The use of dexamethasone with a taper is thought to decrease some of the edema that can occur as a result of the radiotherapy. Although newer radiation modalities such as Gamma Knife radiosurgery and CyberKnife radiosurgery have been used in adult patients with spinal cord compression, pediatric use of these technologies for spinal cord compression has not been reported to date.[5,58]

Clinical Studies

Although much laudable investigation has been undertaken to address the best choice of initial therapy for children with spinal cord compression, no consensus has been reached to date. The available data are limited by relatively small sample sizes because of the overall rarity of spinal cord compression. Larger series tend to group multiple histologic diagnoses, which may respond differently to the interventions of chemotherapy, radiation, and surgery. Many of the studies also span long intervals and cannot necessarily take into account modernization of practice, improved imaging modalities, and improved therapeutic options.

Pollono and colleagues[36] have reported on a review of 70 pediatric patients with spinal cord compression treated at a single institution from 1984 to 2001; 71% were extradural tumors and 54% were soft tissue sarcomas or neuroblastoma. Figure 68-6 presents the algorithm by which these patients were diagnosed and treated. Patients with paraplegia of less than 96 hours' duration underwent laminectomy, as did patients with primary spinal cord tumor or isolated recurrence of main tumor, progression of symptoms after radiation or chemotherapy, or, if known, a radiation- and chemotherapy-resistant tumor. Surgery was avoided when the prognosis of the primary tumor was poor or risks were thought to outweigh benefits. Of patients with paraplegia, 57% became

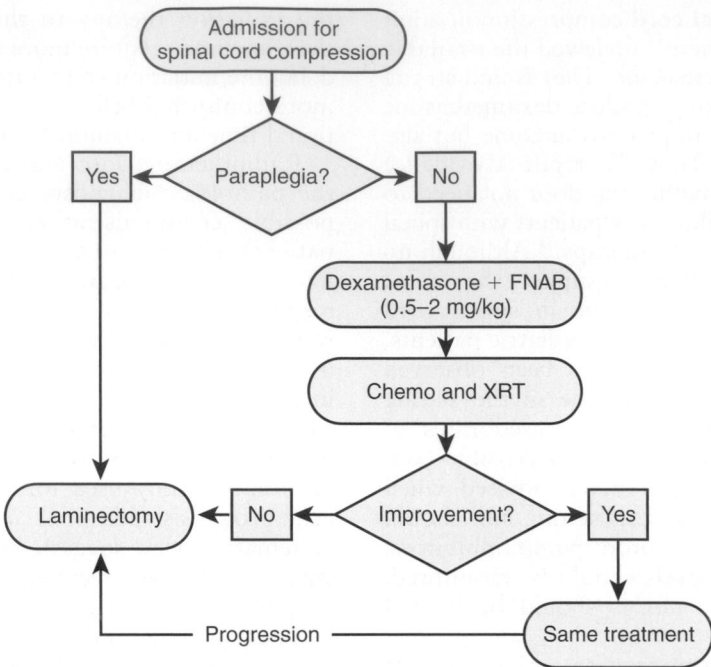

Figure 68-6 Algorithm for diagnosis and treatment of spinal cord compression. With tumor resection, paraplegia of less than 96-hour evolution in patients younger than 1 year and of less than 24 hours in older patients. *Chemo,* Chemotherapy; *FNAB,* fine-needle aspiration biopsy for diagnosis; *XRT,* x-ray therapy. *(Modified from Pollono D, Tomarchia S, Drut R, et al: Spinal cord compression: a review of 70 pediatric patients.* Pediatr Hematol Oncol *20:457–466, 2003.)*

ambulatory after undergoing a laminectomy, whereas only 14% improved after use of chemotherapy and radiation. In patients who presented without paraplegia and received medical treatment without surgery, 87% remained ambulatory. Overall survival was related to the original malignancy. These data suggest that patients with chemotherapy- and radiotherapy-sensitive tumors without evidence of progressive neurologic damage might be treated with chemotherapy and/or radiation therapy but that any indication of neurologic progression is a strong indication for laminectomy without delay.

The question of upfront chemotherapy versus surgery or radiation therapy for spinal cord compression has been most extensively studied in pediatric patients with neuroblastoma, because rapid improvement with initial chemotherapy has been demonstrated. The first reports on the use of chemotherapy as frontline therapy in children presenting with dumbbell neuroblastoma was published in 1984 by Hayes et al.[59] Eleven children with presenting neurologic symptoms were treated; 9 had complete recovery and 2 demonstrated sustained paraplegia. In 1989, Sanderson and coworkers[60] also reported encouraging results of two children with paraplegia and two with paraparesis who both demonstrated full neurologic recovery after treatment with vincristine, cisplatin, etoposide, and cyclophosphamide therapy. Since then, more investigations have been conducted on the use of frontline chemotherapy compared with neurosurgical intervention. Both prospective and retrospective studies have attempted to elucidate whether chemotherapy or surgery is the best initial choice of therapy, but the results yielded have conflicting conclusions. The variability in outcome likely reflects the difficulty of appropriately grouping patients based on initial presenting signs and extent of disease, as well as institutional practice variations and availability of resources.

A series of these studies has been well summarized by De Bernardi and colleagues.[43] Studies from several major international cooperative groups (Italy, Germany, Poland, United Kingdom, and United States) were reviewed. The Italian Cooperative Group for Neuroblastoma has reported a prospective study in which 26 patients with neuroblastoma and spinal cord compression were preferentially given chemotherapy rather than surgery or radiation therapy. Prior to this study, patients followed up between 1979 and 1998 by this group had been analyzed.[61] Retrospective analysis of the earlier patient group showed that radiotherapy, laminectomy, and chemotherapy have comparable ability to improve spinal cord compression. The prospective study also concluded that chemotherapy adequately relieves neurologic symptoms in most patients. Neurologic and orthopedic sequelae were seen in a large number of patients, including those who received chemotherapy only.

In another prospective study carried out by the French Society of Paediatric Oncology, 78 patients with intraspinal extension of neuroblastoma were treated, beginning in 1990.[62] Of these patients, 86% were initially treated with chemotherapy; 63% had a complete neurologic recovery and 21% had a partial neurologic recovery. Also, 13% failed to improve with chemotherapy, the disease of 1 patient progressed, 14% underwent primary surgery, 23% of initially symptomatic patients (10 of 43) had severe neurologic sequelae, 16% had mild sequelae, and 23% were reported to have severe orthopedic sequelae.

One of the largest series contained 83 patients registered for the Pediatric Oncology Group Neuroblastoma Biology Protocol 9047, in which 66 patients received upfront chemotherapy, 23 underwent primary laminectomy, 8 received initial radiotherapy, and 31 underwent initial surgical resection without laminectomy.[63] From this series of retrospectively collected data, it was concluded that patients with neurologic symptoms can be managed without laminectomy and that laminectomy should be reserved for patients who demonstrate progressive neurologic deterioration after initial chemotherapy. The likelihood of neurologic sequelae was found to be inversely related to the length of symptoms prior to initiation of treatment, and more severe sequelae were seen in patients presenting with more severe symptoms. Twenty-nine percent of patients had orthopedic sequelae, and the incidence was significantly lower in patients managed with chemotherapy compared with those who underwent laminectomy.

After a review of multiple studies, the primary conclusion of the neuroblastoma workshop was that a need exists for the creation of an international spinal cord compression registry.[43] The workshop group specified the need to standardize language and criteria to group patients with comparable degrees of neurologic compromise at presentation accurately and to characterize the late effects uniformly. A functional grading system proposed by Gilbert and colleagues[64] was used in some studies to aid in outcome analysis, but it has not been universally adopted (Table 68-2). This grading system notably does not take into account sphincter dysfunction, an important neurologic finding.

It was also concluded that chemotherapy is a reasonable initial approach, but laminectomy should be used for patients who demonstrate progressive neurologic symptoms after presentation or no restoration in the short term.[43] Patients with symptoms occurring within 96 hours of presentation may also be considered candidates for surgical intervention. It was also proposed that radiotherapy may be underused in spinal cord compression caused by neuroblastoma.

Because of the heterogeneity of pediatric malignancies, the findings of the neuroblastoma group cannot automatically be generalized for other types of cancer. Smaller series of outcomes of patients with Ewing sarcoma and intraspinal lesions have also described mixed use of upfront therapies, with variable outcomes. In a report of a series of seven patients with primary Ewing sarcoma of the spine, as well as a review of the literature, Sharafuddin and colleagues[65] noted the importance of the location (sacral or nonsacral) of the presenting lesion in the response to treatment. Differences in response in adult and pediatric patients were also noted. Figure 68-7 shows the algorithm that they proposed for the management of primary Ewing sarcoma of the spine. Initial chemotherapy or limited surgical decompression is recommended for all pediatric patients; surgical intervention is clearly indicated for patients who demonstrate progressive findings with medical treatment.

The rare cases of leukemia and lymphoma that present with spinal cord compression should be treated with initial chemotherapy. Radiotherapy can be considered for some special cases.

Late Effects

The long-term consequences of spinal cord compression and its management include neurologic compromise and orthopedic effects, and the choice of initial management heavily takes into account an attempt to minimize those late effects. A number of reports have supported the observation that neurologic sequelae are most related to the degree of presenting neurologic compromise; the more severe the neurologic compromise at presentation, the more likely long-term sequelae will be seen. Other studies have also shown that the duration of time between the development of neurologic symptoms and the initiation of therapy is inversely correlated with the degree of neurologic recovery.[49,63] Although laminectomy may be the most likely method to correct or prevent neurologic sequelae, it is clearly not necessary in all cases of spinal cord compression and carries the greatest risk of orthopedic sequelae. For patients with neuroblastoma in particular, the initial treatment for spinal cord compression did not demonstrate a clear impact on late effect frequency at a median follow-up of 8 years.[66] Orthopedic sequelae include scoliosis, growth impairment, and spinal instability. Orthopedic sequelae are related to the spinal level of the lesion and the age of the patient at treatment. The most severe sequelae are seen in patients with thoracic versus lumbar lesions and age younger than 12 months. Although a wide range of rates of sequelae has been reported, almost all studies have supported the observation of significantly greater orthopedic sequelae in patients who undergo surgery. In a study by Hoover and coworkers,[67] a scoliosis incidence of 67% was found in patients who underwent laminectomy compared with an incidence of 36% in patients who did not undergo laminectomy. Correlation between late effects, including differences in health-related quality of life and initial treatment, remain at the center of investigations into the optimal choice of initial therapy.

HYPERLEUKOCYTOSIS AND LEUKOSTASIS

Hyperleukocytosis is a clear, life-threatening pediatric oncologic emergency that requires immediate initiation of appropriate therapy. Marked metabolic abnormalities

---

TABLE 68-2　Functional Grading Scale of Spinal Cord Compression

Grade	Patient Function
1	Ambulatory, with or without weakness of lower extremities or ataxia
2	Not ambulatory, but able to lift legs against gravity when supine
3	Paraplegic and unable to move legs against gravity

Modified from Lewis DW, Packer RJ, Raney B, et al: Incidence, presentation, and outcome of spinal cord disease in children with systemic cancer. Pediatrics 78:438–443, 1986.

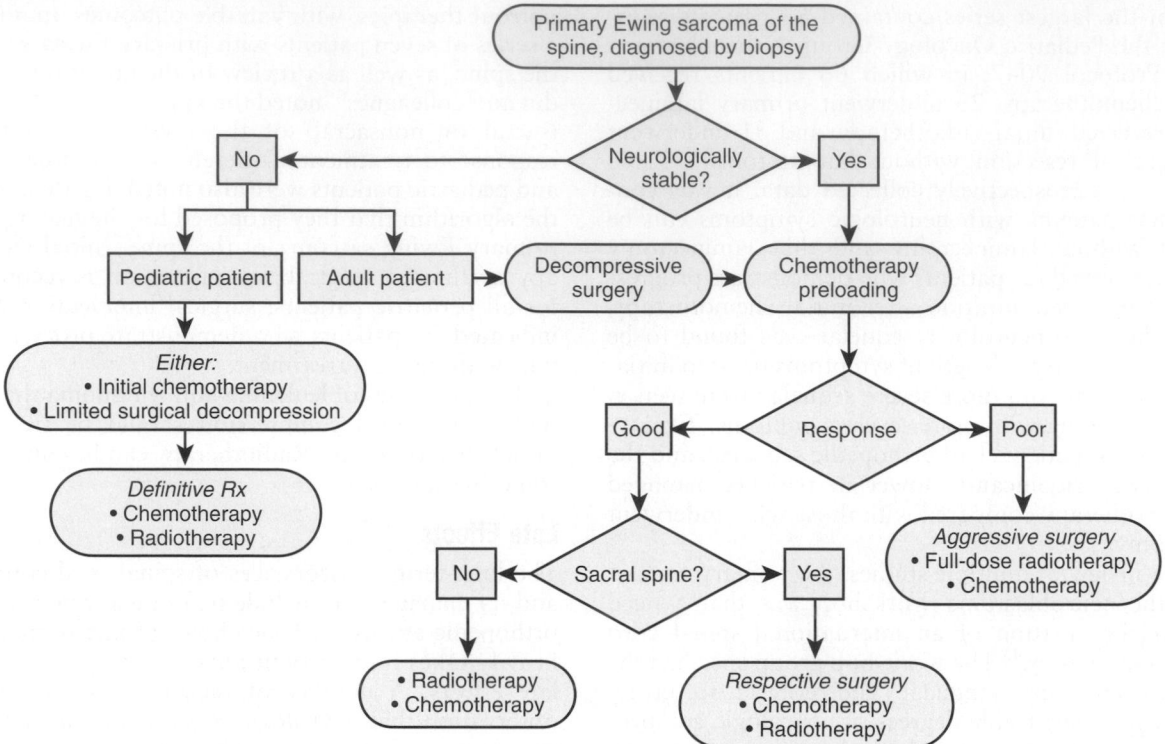

Figure 68-7 Proposed algorithm for the management of primary Ewing sarcoma of the spine. *Rx,* Therapy. *(Modified from Sharafuddin MJ, Haddad FS, Hitchon PW, et al: Treatment options in primary Ewing's sarcoma of the spine: report of seven cases and review of the literature. Neurosurgery 30:610–618, discussion 618–619, 1992.)*

and mild to severe pulmonary and neurologic symptoms can accompany the initial finding of hyperleukocytosis or can develop shortly after presentation. Stasis of leukemic cells within blood vessels and migration of blast cells into tissues can lead to the clinical entity of leukostasis, with mortality rates reported as high as 20% to 40%.[68-70] Despite the relative frequency of this true oncologic emergency and several varied therapeutic options, no data-driven management guidelines are available because of overall small numbers of patients, variability of clinical presentation, molecular differences in the underlying disease, and the difficulty of conducting randomized clinical trials with these constraints.

Definition

Hyperleukocytosis is generally accepted as a white blood cell (WBC) count higher than $100 \times 10^9/L$, although some studies have included patients with a WBC count higher than $50 \times 10^9/L$. It is estimated to occur in 5% to 20% of childhood leukemias and is seen most frequently in infant ALL and T-cell ALL. Hyperleukocytosis is more associated with certain subtypes of ALL and AML and is seen in almost all cases of childhood chronic myelogenous leukemia (Table 28-2). It has long been observed that the occurrence of leukostasis does not correlate directly with degree of hyperleukocytosis. Although hyperleukocytosis is seen more frequently in children with ALL, clinical leukostasis is seen more frequently in children with AML, particularly in M4 and M5 French-American-British subtypes. Clinical symptoms from

hyperleukocytosis generally occur at WBC counts higher than 200 to $300 \times 10^9/L$ in patients with AML and higher than 400 to $500 \times 10^9/L$ in patients with ALL.[71] However, symptoms of leukostasis have also been observed in patients with WBC counts lower than $100 \times 10^9/L$.[69,72,73]

Clinical Presentation

Clinical symptoms of leukostasis are dependent on the system affected. Any small vessels, and therefore any organs, can be at risk. Although pulmonary and neurologic symptoms are most often observed, involvement of many other systems has also been reported. Hyperleukocytosis has been reported to result in leukostasis, causing renal failure, papilledema, dactylitis, priapism or clitorism, acute myocardial infarction, and cardiac failure.[74-76] Histopathologic studies have demonstrated aggregates of blast cells and thrombi leading to occlusion of small vessels in multiple organs of patients with hyperleukocytosis.[77] Corresponding to observed clinical symptoms, postmortem examinations have shown profound infiltration of multiple organs, including brain (including retinal vessels), liver, spleen, adrenals, and pulmonary vasculature, and in the alveoli and connective tissue of the lungs. A striking image of leukemic infiltration of a coronary artery was obtained by Thornton and Levis[75] (Fig. 68-8, Table 68-3).

The observance of the clinical expression of leukostasis and the accompanying related comorbidities has evolved to a description of a leukostasis syndrome, which has been defined as a critical condition with severe metabolic

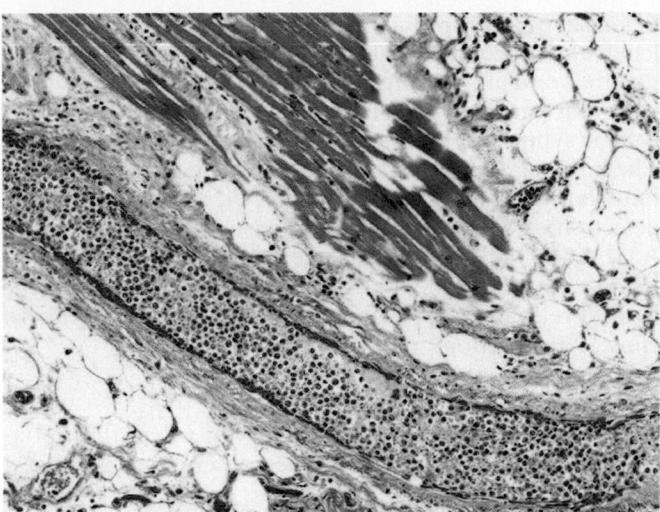

Figure 68-8 Small vessels throughout the body are at risk of occlusion in a patient with hyperleukocytosis. This image shows a coronary artery filled with fms-related tyrosine kinase 3–internal tandem duplication+ (FLT3-ITD+) acute myelogenous leukemia blasts. *(Modified from Thornton KA, Levis M: Images in clinical medicine: FLT3 mutation and acute myelogenous leukemia with leukostasis.* N Engl J Med 357:1639, 2007.)

abnormalities, tumor lysis syndrome, severe coagulopathy, and multiorgan failure that occurs in patients presenting with hyperleukocytic leukemia.[78,79]

Pathogenesis

The pathogenesis of leukostasis is under continued investigation as researchers have realized the importance and potential clinical relevance of understanding the pathophysiology involved. Increased blood viscosity is often postulated to contribute to the development of leukostasis. At high flow rates (in larger vessels), bulk viscosity of the blood is a function of the deformability of the blood cells and the fraction of blood represented by these cells.[72] The overall viscosity of the blood generally has been found not to increase, even with the marked increase in leukocytic cells, in part because of the corresponding decrease in erythrocrit with increasing leukocrit. In patients with associated moderate to severe anemia,

TABLE 68-3 Factors Associated With Occurrence of Hyperleukocytic Leukemias in Childhood

Acute Lymphoblastic Leukemia	Acute Myelogenous Leukemia
Age <1 year	Age <1 year
11q23	11q23
T cell with mediastinal mass	FAB M4 and M5
CNS involvement	FAB M3v
Hypodiploid	Inv 16
Philadelphia chromosome+	FLT3-ITD+*

CNS, Central nervous system; *FAB,* French-American-British; *FLT3-ITD,* fms-related tyrosine kinase 3–internal tandem duplication.
*FLT3 internal tandem duplication, shown in young adults.[74]

observed leukocrit levels greater than 20% to 25% are needed to demonstrate an objective increase in blood viscosity. Transfusion of red blood cells prior to reduction of the leukocyte count will increase the erythrocrit and can therefore result in hyperviscosity, which can be extremely deleterious to the patient, inducing clinical manifestations of hyperviscosity.

Blood viscosity in the microcirculation can increase because the viscosity is a function of the plasma viscosity and the deformability of the individual cells in the capillaries. Leukemic blasts are larger and less deformable than are erythrocytes or normal leukocytes. Flow in microvessels will slow if the diameter of the poorly deformable blast cell approaches that of the channel. Lymphoblasts range in size from 250 to 350 mm^3 and myeloblasts from 350 to 450 mm^3. It has been suggested that the larger size of myeloblasts compared with lymphoblasts helps account for the greater incidence of intracerebral hemorrhage that has been observed in patients who have AML compared with those who have ALL.[71] Histopathologic studies have revealed leukocyte thrombi and aggregates in the cerebral vasculature of patients with AML.

Appreciation of the role of adhesion molecules and the endothelial lining of the blood vessels is increasing. Laboratory observations have shown that expression of intracellular adhesion molecule–1, vascular cell adhesion molecule–1, and E-selectin can be induced in endothelial cells exposed to supernatants of blast cell cultures.[80] This effect was regulated by blast cell production of tumor necrosis factor-α and interleukin 1β. It is suggested that through this self-perpetuating interaction, leukemic blasts can promote their own adhesion to inactivated vascular endothelium. Alternate mechanisms of leukostasis have also been proposed and are being investigated, including molecular interactions directly between leukemic blast cells, leading to clumping and intravascular aggregates.

The molecular origin and subsequent cell phenotype is likely important to the role in developing leukostasis. The expression of CD56 neural cell adhesion molecule on leukemic blasts in a study of adult patients with AML was correlated with the development of severe clinical leukostatic syndrome.[78] In another study of adult patients with acute promyelocytic leukemia (APL, or level M3 AML), expression of CD13 (aminopeptidase N), a cell surface enzyme previously linked to tumor cell invasion, was highly associated with elevated leukocyte count and the development of all-*trans*-retinoic acid syndrome.[2] Further study in these intriguing areas of research is needed to confirm these findings and to test the applicability to pediatric patients. It is hoped that a better understanding of the underlying pathophysiology will lead to methods for early detection of patients at highest risk for severe leukostasis and eventually provide pharmacologic targets for disruption of the interaction of adhesion molecules, resulting in clinical improvements.

Clinical Presentation

Clinical manifestations of hyperleukocytosis and leukostasis can be myriad. Many patients with hyperleukocytosis are relatively asymptomatic. Clinical leukostasis can present subtly and evolve rapidly. Most commonly, pulmonary symptoms are observed. Tachypnea, oxygen desaturation, and dyspnea can occur and can progress rapidly to acute respiratory disease syndrome and respiratory failure. Neurologic symptoms can include headache, tinnitus, ataxia, behavioral changes, seizures, and stroke. Hemorrhagic stroke is a highly morbid complication of hyperleukocytosis and is seen most often in the microgranular variant of APL (level M3v AML). Often these patients have associated disseminated intravascular coagulation and thrombocytopenia, increasing their risk for hemorrhage.

Symptoms can rapidly worsen after initiation of therapy. It has been postulated that this phenomenon may be caused by release of intracellular components of blast cells after lysis, including enzymes that can lead to injury in surrounding tissue, such as alveolar damage and interstitial edema.[81] When using modern pediatric AML protocols for treatment and supportive care, early mortality in patients with AML who have hyperleukocytosis is very low, but hyperleukocytosis continues to be associated with inferior disease outcomes.[82,83] Additionally, Fong and coworkers[84] described unique anesthesia-related considerations for children with hyperleukocytosis and recommend close observation postoperatively for leukostasis-related pulmonary and neurologic events.

Authors of a number of studies have looked at the factors associated with more severe clinical events in patients with hyperleukocytic leukemias, with mixed conclusions. A clinical grading system has been proposed by Novotny and colleagues[79] (Table 68-4). The grading system groups patients into four categories: not present (0), possible (1), probable (2), and highly probable (3). The grading is based on the assumption that the severity

of presenting symptoms may indicate the probability of leukostasis, provided another cause for the symptoms is not found. This assumption is supported by the knowledge that patients with respiratory distress or severe neurologic symptoms have a much increased mortality rate.[85] The investigators used this clinical scoring system in conjunction with initial flow cytometry data to show that the detection of CD56 expression at baseline in patients with AML level M4 and M5 disease may identify patients at highest risk for fatal leukostasis. This approach has clear clinical relevance but requires further validation prior to clinical application.

Treatment

Definitive treatment for hyperleukocytosis is the initiation of appropriate induction chemotherapy as soon as a diagnosis is established. Previously, for many years the initiation of IV hydration, urinary alkalinization, and allopurinol was the clinical standard for the immediate initial treatment of hyperleukocytic acute leukemias. In 1995, Basade et al.[86] reported an 81.5% reduction in WBC count within a median of 36 hours in a cohort of pediatric patients who had ALL with the use of IV hydration, urinary alkalinization, and allopurinol. No treatment-related complications occurred in their patient cohort. Although studies have not yet been published, the availability of urate oxalate is likely to modify this practice, because many of these patients clearly meet criteria for high risk of TLS. Early therapy with urate oxalate has the potential to decrease the risk for TLS markedly in patients who have acute hyperleukocytic leukemias, which could decrease the number of patients in whom leukostasis syndrome develops, thereby positively affecting overall morbidity and mortality.

TABLE 68-4   Grading of Symptoms in Hyperleukocytic Leukemia*

Group	Probability of Leukostasis Syndrome	Severity of Symptoms	Pulmonary Symptoms	Neurologic Symptoms	Other Organ Systems
0	Not present	No limitations	No symptoms and no limitations in ordinary activities	No neurologic symptoms	No symptoms
1	Possible	Slight limitations	Mild symptoms and slight limitation during ordinary activity, comfortable at rest	Mild tinnitus, headache, dizziness	Moderate fatigue
2	Probable	Marked limitations	Marked limitation in activity because of symptoms, even during less than ordinary activity, comfortable only at rest	Slight visual disturbances, severe tinnitus, headache, dizziness	Severe fatigue
3	Highly probable	Severe limitations	Dyspnea at rest, oxygen or respirator required	Severe visual disturbances (acute inability to read), confusion, delirium, somnolence, intracranial hemorrhage	Myocardial infarction, priapism, ischemic necrosis

Modified from Novotny JR, Muller-Beissenhirtz H, Herget-Rosenthal S, et al: Grading of symptoms in hyperleukocytic leukaemia: a clinical model for the role of different blast types and promyelocytes in the development of leukostasis syndrome. Eur J Haematol 74:501–510, 2005.
*Probability of leukostasis deduced from the severity of symptoms attributable to leukostasis (no other obvious cause).

Additional measures to reduce the elevated WBC count and associated morbidities have been studied. Cranial radiation has been proposed to decrease the chance of intracerebral hemorrhage. Based on a study of adult patients with AML and a WBC count higher than $200 \times 10^9/L$, Wiernik and Serpick[87] have proposed the prophylactic use of 400 to 600 cGy of cranial radiotherapy to prevent intracranial hemorrhage. Several small series that used emergency cranial radiotherapy in pediatric patients with ALL and hyperleukocytosis were also reported, with a low incidence of intracranial hemorrhage.[88] However, subsequent experience has not consistently shown a beneficial effect of prophylactic cranial radiotherapy. Additionally, concerns exist about acute and chronic neuropsychiatric complications associated with cranial radiotherapy in pediatric patients, and thus it is rarely used for this indication in current practice.[89-91]

The use of low-dose prednisone as initial treatment for patients with ALL and hyperleukocytosis has been proposed, with the rationale of inducing a gradual blast cell lysis in an attempt to decrease the severity of metabolic derangements. Along with several other interventions, the use of low-dose prednisone was reviewed in a group of 124 patients with newly diagnosed ALL and a WBC count higher than $200 \times 10^9/L$ who were followed up by the Children's Cancer Study Group from 1981 to 1983.[91] All patients received IV hydration, urinary alkalinization, and allopurinol. Some patients received additional measures (e.g., low-dose prednisone, cranial radiation, exchange transfusion, and leukapheresis) in an attempt to decrease complications. It was concluded that pretreatment with low-dose prednisone does not correlate with fewer electrolyte abnormalities. However, many of the patients in this study received more than one additional treatment, complicating the analysis in this relatively small group of patients.

Leukapheresis and exchange transfusion have both been shown to be effective in reducing the total WBC and blast count. Patients weighing less than 12 kg usually are unable to undergo leukapheresis but may safely undergo exchange transfusion. Studies in pediatric patients have shown a mean reduction of 50% to 60% in WBC with exchange transfusion and leukapheresis.[90,92] However, the rate of WBC clearance with leukapheresis is inconsistent, and the overall benefit of this cytoreduction is unclear.[93]

In patients with ALL, the use of leukapheresis may decrease the risk of severe TLS. Patients with ALL and hyperleukocytosis in the Children's Cancer Study Group cohort who received leukapheresis or exchange transfusion appeared to show some benefit of the procedures, with a lower incidence of severe electrolyte abnormalities and renal dysfunction.[91] The same conclusion was reached by Bunin and Pui[71] in a series of 161 patients with ALL and hyperleukocytosis.

In the three largest studies in patients with AML that examined the role of leukapheresis, differing conclusions were reached. In a group of 22 patients with newly diagnosed AML (ages 12 to 74 years), it was found that decreasing the total WBC count through leukapheresis by at least 30% correlates with improved outcome in those patients.[94] In contrast, in a study by Porcu and col-

leagues,[85] 48 patients ages 8 to 79 years who had AML or chronic myelogenous leukemia and were in blast crisis underwent immediate cytoreduction with leukapheresis, and no correlation was found between the degree of cytoreduction and early mortality rate. In the largest study, Giles and coworkers[95] reviewed outcomes of 146 patients (ages 16 to 86 years) with AML, 71 of whom underwent leukapheresis. An association with decreased early mortality rate was found, but no improvement occurred in the overall survival rate.

The use of leukapheresis in patients with APL is greatly discouraged because increased rates of mortality have been observed in these patients, which are largely caused by the increased incidence of hemorrhage. Vahdat and colleagues[2] reported fatal or near-fatal hemorrhage in 9 of 11 patients with APL who underwent leukapheresis.

Hydroxyurea is known to be effective in reducing overall WBC and blast counts.[96] At the American Society of Hematology 2006 Annual Meeting, preliminary results of a randomized study on the use of hydroxyurea versus leukapheresis in patients with AML were presented, with equivalent outcome noted at 8 and 28 days and no difference in death rate.[97]

The possible benefits from a rapid reduction in WBC and blast count that can be achieved with leukapheresis or exchange transfusion need to be weighed against the risks of these procedures, which include obtaining adequate venous access and anticoagulation. The decision to initiate leukapheresis must also take into account the time to arrange these procedures, including mobilization of specialized blood bank personnel and possible transfer to tertiary centers where such specialized procedures are available. Institution of these procedures can be particularly deleterious if they delay initiation of definitive chemotherapy treatments. With increased use of urate oxalate, the benefit of leukapheresis in patients with ALL may need to be reassessed.

Conclusions

Acute leukemias presenting with hyperleukocytosis pose immediate clinical challenges to the treating pediatric oncologist and must be addressed rapidly and appropriately. Although many components of treatment of hyperleukocytosis are generally accepted, much ambiguity still exists about the appropriateness of many possible interventions. Although further study is appropriate, carrying out such studies poses many challenges. Box 68-2 groups treatment guidelines into those that have been shown to be clearly beneficial, those that have been shown to be harmful, and those of less certain benefit. It is hoped that translational research into the underlying pathophysiology of the leukostasis syndrome will lead to novel therapeutic modalities and pharmacologic interventions.

TUMOR LYSIS SYNDROME

TLS is the most commonly encountered pediatric oncologic emergency. Diagnosis and treatment strategies have evolved during the past decade with the development of new drug therapy. Morbidity and mortality have improved as the entity is now recognized and treated earlier in

Box 68-2   Clinical Guidelines for Patients With White Blood Cell Count Greater Than 50 × 10⁹ and Diagnosis of Acute Leukemia

RECOMMENDED FOR ALL PATIENTS WITH HYPERLEUKOCYTOSIS

- Institution of appropriate chemotherapy as soon as a diagnosis is made
- Careful clinical observation, neurologic examination, frequent laboratory evaluation per tumor lysis protocol, evaluation of renal function, chest radiograph, and oxygen saturation monitoring with supplemental oxygen as needed
- Treatment for TLS with IVF, alkalinization, and allopurinol OR rasburicase and no alkalinization; strong bias toward use of rasburicase if any parameters are met for high risk of TLS-increased uric acid, creatinine, LDH, potassium (see section on TLS)
- Correction of coagulopathy as appropriate with cryoprecipitate, FFP, vitamin K; special consideration of disseminated intravascular coagulation and risk of intracerebral hemorrhage in M4 or M5 level AML, and even greater risk in level M3v APL
- Platelet transfusion for platelet count <25 K or any clinical bleeding

RECOMMENDED IN SOME CLINICAL CIRCUMSTANCES

- Consider exchange transfusion or leukapheresis in patients with ALL and WBC >300-500 × 10⁹, or AML and WBC >100-200 × 10⁹, particularly if any pulmonary or neurologic symptoms exist
- Consider low-dose prednisone reduction phase prior to induction chemotherapy in patients with ALL and WBC >300-500 × 10⁹ (may decrease chance of TLS)

CONTRAINDICATED

- Avoid leukapheresis in patients with APL (substantially increases the risk of intracerebral hemorrhage)
- Avoid use of diuretics or transfusion of PRBC in patients with ALL and WBC >300-500 × 10⁹, or AML and WBC >100-200 × 10⁹ (confers increased risk of hyperviscosity and clinical leukostasis)

ALL, Acute lymphoblastic leukemia; *AML,* acute myelogenous leukemia; *APL,* acute promyelocytic leukemia; *DIC,* disseminated intravascular coagulation; *FFP,* fresh-frozen plasma; *IVF,* intravenous fluid; *LDH,* lactate dehydrogenase; *PRBC,* packed red blood cells; *TLS,* tumor lysis syndrome; *WBC,* white blood cell count.

presentation. New therapeutic interventions have become available and are more widely used.

Overview

After the incorporation of cytotoxic chemotherapy into the treatment of hematologic malignancies and solid tumors, recurrent observations were made of severe metabolic abnormalities associated with the onset of therapy.[98,99] The consistent occurrence of these metabolic and electrolyte imbalances, particularly in the setting of lymphoma and leukemia, eventually became recognized as TLS. TLS describes the metabolic derangements that occur as a result of spontaneous or treatment-related breakdown of tumor cells. The release of intracellular contents from the tumor cells into the bloodstream leads to the characteristic triad of hyperuricemia, hyperkalemia, and hyperphosphatemia. TLS is most commonly associated with initiation of therapy for cancers with massive tumor burden or high proliferative rates, such as ALL and Burkitt lymphoma. Predictors of TLS include the presence of bulky disease, adenopathy, hepatosplenomegaly, and a high leukocyte count. Additional risk factors for the development of severe TLS include

increased lactate dehydrogenase (LDH), uric acid, creatinine, and decreased urine output.[76,100,101] TLS can result in high morbidity and mortality, with possible rapid progression to multiorgan failure, and thus the prompt identification of patients at risk for this oncologic emergency and the institution of preventive measures are critical. Although the risk of developing TLS is highest at 12 to 72 hours after the initiation of chemotherapy, symptoms can also precede the initiation of therapy or occur as many as 7 days later. The main principles of TLS prevention and treatment include hydration and diuresis, careful monitoring of electrolyte abnormalities, and management of hyperuricemia. In this section, we will discuss the pathophysiology, incidence, and recent advances in the management of TLS.

Pathophysiology

Although TLS can occur spontaneously prior to the administration of chemotherapy, it is most commonly observed after the initiation of therapy. In tumors with a high proliferative rate, large tumor burden, and high chemosensitivity, the exposure of the tumor cells to cytotoxic chemotherapy leads to massive cell lysis, with the release of intracellular anions, cations, and breakdown products of nucleic acids and proteins into the bloodstream. This rapid efflux of intracellular contents can exceed the renal capacity for clearance and consequently can lead to the metabolic derangements and electrolyte imbalances observed in TLS. Hyperuricemia is the most common finding in TLS; it results from the release of intracellular nucleic acids and the subsequent catabolism of the purine nucleotides, adenosine and guanosine. Uric acid, the final product of both endogenous and dietary purine nucleotide catabolism, is normally generated in the liver by oxidation of xanthine to uric acid by xanthine oxidase (Fig. 68-9). Uric acid is a weak acid, with a pK_a of 5.4 to 5.7. At normal concentrations and at physiologic pH, 98% of uric acid is in the ionized form as urate, which is soluble in urine.[102] However, when uric acid is present in high concentrations in acidic urine, it can crystallize in the renal parenchyma, distal tubules, and collecting ducts, leading to intraluminal tubular obstruction and oliguria.

Hyperkalemia poses the greatest immediate threat of mortality because the rapid rise in serum potassium can result in severe arrhythmia and death. This life-threatening consequence of TLS is caused in part by the kidney's inability to excrete the massive quantities of intracellular potassium released from dying tumor cells. The kidney's inability to handle the excessive load of potassium can be amplified by renal dysfunction caused by precipitants such as uric acid. Hyperkalemia in the setting of TLS can be further exacerbated by concurrent metabolic acidosis or iatrogenic administration of potassium with IV fluids.

Hyperphosphatemia results from the rapid release of intracellular phosphorus from tumor cells, which can contain three to four times the amount of phosphorus in normal cells.[3,103] The development of hyperphosphatemia can also worsen in the setting of concurrent acute renal insufficiency as a result of uric acid precipitation. In TLS, the renal tubular capacity to reabsorb phosphorus can be

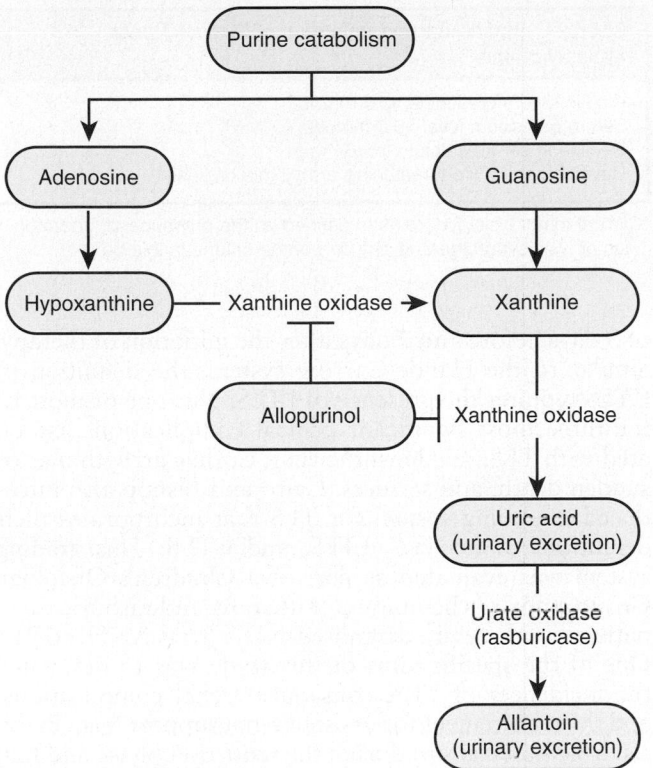

Figure 68-9 Pathophysiology of hyperuricemia in tumor lysis syndrome. Uric acid is a breakdown product of purine nucleotide catabolism. The current pharmacologic strategies for the management of hyperuricemia are allopurinol and rasburicase.

exceeded and lead to hyperphosphaturia. A cyclic process commences, in which the acute hyperphosphatemia and hyperphosphaturia can then lead to acute nephrocalcinosis and renal failure via precipitation of calcium phosphate crystals, further impairing the renal tubular reabsorption of phosphorus. The normal calcium × phosphorus product ranges between 30 and 55 mg^2/dL^2. When this product exceeds 70 mg^2/dL^2, the risk of calcium phosphate deposition in the kidney and other tissues is significant.[104] Metastatic calcification caused by calcium phosphate crystals in other soft tissues is rarely seen in TLS but has been described.[105] In addition, the precipitation of calcium phosphate can lead secondarily to asymptomatic or symptomatic hypocalcemia.

Incidence

The highest incidence of TLS occurs in ALL and high-grade NHL. A retrospective study of 102 patients with high-grade NHL found the incidence of TLS to be 42% based on laboratory evidence, although only 6% of the patients had clinically significant TLS.[106] Similarly, a pan-European retrospective chart review has reported TLS in 5.2% and 6.1% of patients with ALL and NHL, respectively.[107] This study also demonstrated a high incidence of mortality in patients with clinical TLS. Of the patients with TLS in this study, 17.5% died from TLS-related causes.

The incidence of TLS appears to be similar in the pediatric population. A retrospective study of 1192 pediatric patients with any form of NHL identified 63 patients (5.3%) with clinically significant TLS.[108] Among these 63 patients, two patients (3.2%) died within 48 hours of therapy because of electrolyte imbalances. However, another retrospective pediatric study has indicated that the incidence of TLS is significantly higher in patients with B-cell ALL or Burkitt lymphoma stage III or IV, with LDH greater than or equal to 500 units/L. Of the 218 patients who met these criteria initially (prior to the prophylactic use of urate oxidase), TLS developed in 35 (16.1%), and 20 (9.2%) became anuric.[109]

Other hematologic malignancies that have been less commonly associated with TLS include AML, chronic lymphocytic leukemia, and multiple myeloma. Only isolated case reports of TLS have been described in other hematologic malignancies, such as chronic myeloid leukemia in blast crisis, myeloproliferative disorders, and Hodgkin disease. TLS is also uncommon in solid tumors, which generally have a longer doubling time and a slow response to chemotherapy in comparison with lymphoproliferative malignancies. However, TLS can be seen in solid tumors that are highly chemosensitive or that have a high tumor burden, as in bulky, metastatic disease or in tumors that present with renal compromise. In the context of newly diagnosed solid tumors, renal compromise may occur from mass effect and compression. A literature review has identified 45 reported cases of TLS in solid tumors from 1977 to 2002.[110] Most of these cases occurred in tumors with a high response rate to cytotoxic therapy, such as small cell lung carcinoma, germ cell tumors, and breast carcinoma. Among the 45 reported cases, 16 patients (35.5%) died as a result of TLS. Risk factors for the development of TLS in persons with solid tumors were similar to those in persons with hematologic malignancies—increased LDH, hyperuricemia, and pretreatment renal impairment. However, the mortality rate caused by complications from TLS in these patients with solid tumors was higher than reported mortality rates in patients with hematologic malignancies. This finding may be the result of better implementation of prophylactic measures in patients with hematologic malignancies resulting from a greater awareness of TLS in this population.

Diagnosis

TLS should be anticipated in all new-onset oncology patients, with the highest concern for those presenting with a large tumor burden and concurrent laboratory abnormalities. Although many general criteria exist for TLS, a uniform, widely accepted definition for TLS is lacking. A standardized definition would enable a more exact determination of TLS incidence and would also improve the ability to evaluate and compare therapies for the prevention of TLS. Two classification systems for TLS have been developed and are variably followed, the Hande-Garrow system (Boxes 68-3 and 68-4) in 1993 and the Cairo-Bishop system in 2004. The Hande-Garrow classification system makes a distinction between laboratory and clinical TLS based on the observation that only a fraction of patients with TLS according to laboratory criteria experience clinically significant TLS.[106]

Box 68-3   **Hande-Garrow Definition of Laboratory Tumor Lysis Syndrome***

A 25% increase over pretreatment values in serum phosphate, potassium, uric acid, or urea nitrogen.
   or
A 25% decline in serum calcium.

*Any two of the metabolic changes must occur within 4 days of treatment.

Box 68-4   **Hande-Garrow Definition of Clinical Tumor Lysis Syndrome***

Rise in serum creatinine >2.5 mg/dL.
Serum potassium level >6.0 mmol/L.
Decline in serum calcium to <6 mg/dL.
Development of life-threatening arrhythmia or death.

*Clinical tumor lysis syndrome is defined as the presence of laboratory tumor lysis syndrome and any one of the criteria in this box.

Laboratory TLS (LTLS) designates patients who have laboratory evidence of metabolic changes as a result of tumor cell breakdown but who do not require any therapeutic intervention. Patients with any of the following metabolic changes occurring within the first 4 days of treatment are defined as having LTLS: (1) a 25% increase compared with pretreatment values in serum phosphate, potassium, uric acid, or urea nitrogen levels or (2) a 25% decline in the serum calcium level. Clinical TLS (CTLS) is designated in any patient with LTLS who also experiences one of the following: (1) a rise in the serum creatinine level greater than 2.5 mg/dL; (2) a serum potassium level greater than 6.0 mmol/L; (3) a decline in the serum calcium level to less than 6 mg/dL; (4) the development of a life-threatening arrhythmia; or sudden death. In practice, this classification system has several limitations. First, in requiring a 25% increase in the baseline laboratory value, the definition of LTLS does not account for patients who have preexisting abnormal laboratory values at presentation. In addition, the definition requires that the laboratory changes occur within 4 days of starting therapy, which excludes patients with clinical evidence of TLS at presentation or patients in whom TLS develops beyond 4 days of therapy. Additionally, any symptomatic hypocalcemia should alone constitute CTLS.[111]

The Cairo-Bishop classification system is a modified version of the Hande-Garrow system that aims to be more clinically relevant (Table 68-5).[112] For example, the definition of LTLS has been extended to include a window of 3 days before and 7 days after the initiation of therapy. Similar to the Hande-Garrow system, the definition of CTLS requires the presence of LTLS, plus one or more of the three most significant clinical complications associated with TLS: renal insufficiency, cardiac arrhythmias or sudden death, and seizures. Cairo and Bishop also introduced a grading system for TLS that incorporates their definitions of no TLS, LTLS, and CTLS. This grading system was evaluated as part of a Children's Oncology Group study of chemoimmunotherapy and rasburicase in patients with newly diagnosed NHL (trial ANHL01P1). One of the specific aims of this study was to determine the incidences of TLS, consequent renal complications, and the requirement for assisted renal support (e.g., dialysis or hemofiltration) during the reduction phase and first induction phase of therapy in children with newly diagnosed advanced-stage leukemia or lymphoma. It was found that the rasburicase was safe and well tolerated. Increased initial LDH was correlated with increased uric acid level, increased incidence of TLS, and lower glomerular filtration rate. Patients treated with rasburicase have only a 9% and 5% incidence of LTLS and CTLS, respectively. Importantly, a significant improvement in estimated glomerular filtration rate from day 0 to day 7 was found in patients after administration of rasburicase, and only 3% of patients required new-onset renal-assisted support after administration of rasburicase.[113]

Building on the Cairo-Bishop and Hande-Garrow definitions of LTLS and CTLS, an algorithm for the assessment

TABLE 68-5   Cairo-Bishop Grading Classification of Tumor Lysis Syndrome

Grade	LTLS	Creatinine Level	Cardiac Arrhythmia	Seizure
0	–	≤1.5 × ULN	None	None
I	+	1.5 × ULN	Intervention not indicated	None
II	+	>1.5-3.0 × ULN	Nonurgent medical intervention indicated	One brief generalized seizure, seizure(s) well controlled by anticonvulsants, infrequent focal motor seizures not interfering with ADLs
III	+	>3.0-6.0 × ULN	Symptomatic and incompletely controlled medically or controlled with device (e.g., defibrillator)	Seizure in which consciousness is altered, poorly controlled seizure disorder, breakthrough generalized seizures despite medical intervention
IV	+	>6.0 × ULN	Life-threatening (e.g., arrhythmia associated with CHF, hypotension, syncope, shock)	Seizures of any type that are prolonged, repetitive, or difficult to control (e.g., status epilepticus and intractable epilepsy)
V	+	Death	Death	Death

Modified from Cairo MS, Bishop M: Tumour lysis syndrome: new therapeutic strategies and classification. Br J Haematol 127:3–11, 2004.
ADLs, Activities of daily living; CHF, congestive heart failure; LTLS, laboratory tumor lysis syndrome; ULN, upper limit of normal.

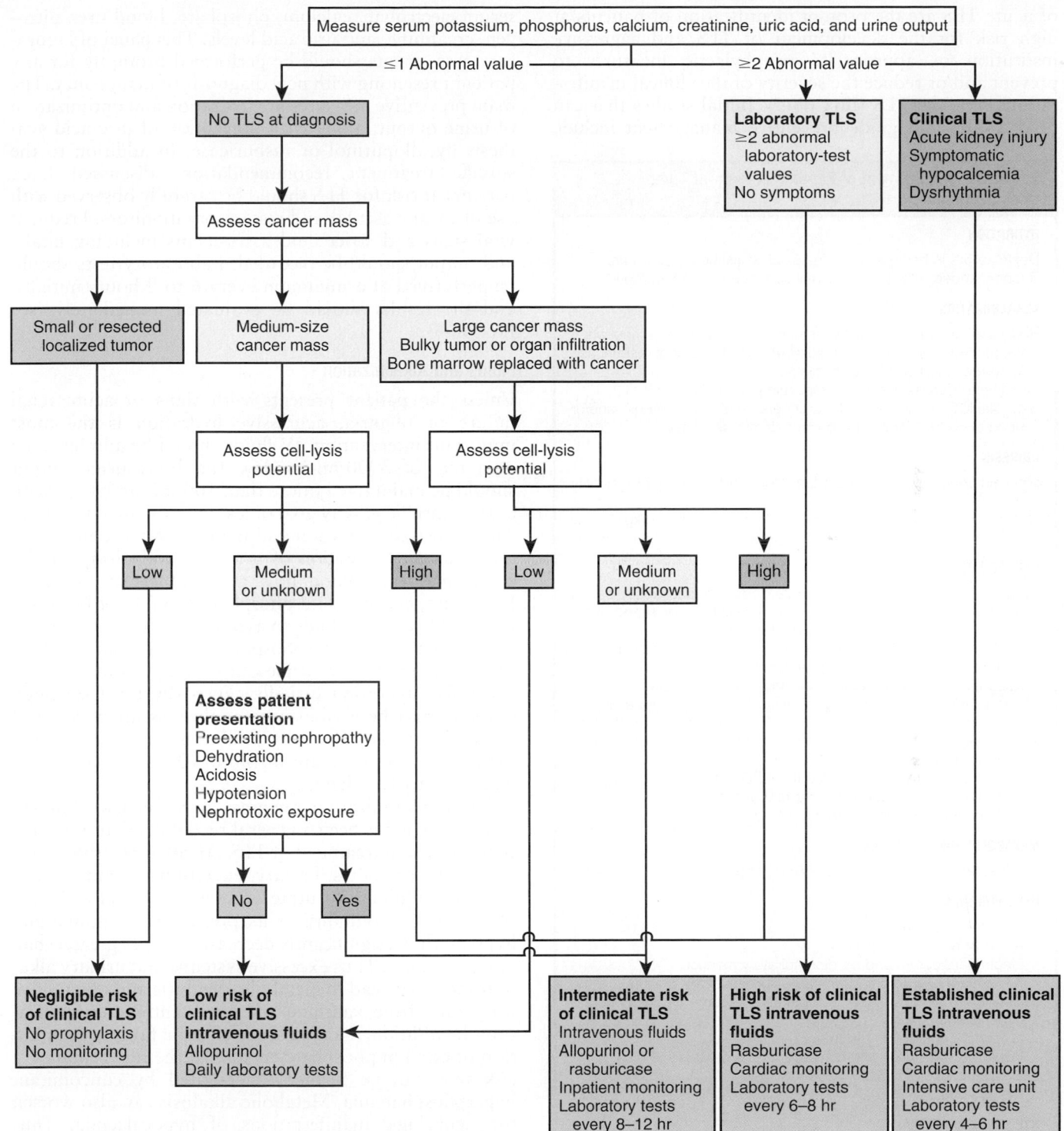

Figure 68-10 Proposed algorithm for assessment of tumor lysis syndrome *(TLS)*. *(Howard SC, Jones DP, Pui CH: The tumor lysis syndrome.* NEJM *364:1844–1854, 2011.)*

and initial management of TLS was proposed by Howard and colleagues (Fig. 68-10).[111] It is important to note that this guide is intended for a patient at the time of presentation, however; subsequent care and interventions should reflect the clinical course, expected or not, of the patient. When distinguishing the best classification group for a patient is difficult, it is always advisable to provide treatment as if the patient is in the higher risk group.

Clinical Manifestations and Treatment

Clinical manifestations of acute TLS include nausea, anorexia, cardiac arrhythmias, seizures, muscle cramps, tetany, oliguria or anuria, and alterations in consciousness. These symptoms primarily result from the electrolyte disturbances seen in TLS (described earlier). The most important objectives for the successful management of acute TLS are the prompt identification of patients at high risk for the development of TLS and aggressive institution of appropriate prophylactic measures to prevent and/or reduce the severity of the clinical manifestations of acute TLS (Box 68-5). Initial studies that can predict TLS and guide preventive management include

---

Box 68-5   Management of Patients at Risk for Tumor Lysis Syndrome

HYDRATION

Dextrose 5% in half-normal saline solution (without potassium)
Recommended rate: two times maintenance (125 mL/m^2/hour)

ALKALINIZATION

Routine alkalinization is not recommended; use with allopurinol when the primary concern is uric acid level and when use of rasburicase is contradicted or it is not available
Modify NaHCO$_3$ as needed to maintain urine pH at 7.0 to 8.0
Stop NaHCO$_3$ if the serum bicarbonate level is ≥30 mEq/L and/or urine pH is >8.0 or if hyperphosphatemia develops

DIURESIS

Maintain urine output at >100 mL/m^2/hour and urine specific gravity at <1.010
Consider furosemide (0.5 to 1.0 mg/kg) or mannitol (0.5 g/kg) for low urine output in the absence of hypovolemia

URIC ACID REDUCTION

Consider the role of allopurinol or urate oxidase (rasburicase), based on assessment of the potential of TLS, initial uric acid and phosphate level, drug availability, and G6PD status:
  Options: Allopurinol: by mouth, 100 mg/m^2 three times daily, or 10 mg/kg/day divided in three doses
  Rasburicase: IV, 0.2 mg/kg once daily for up to 5 days
    Indicated when serum creatinine is >1.5 times the upper limit or normal, or when uric acid is >7.0 mg/dL; consider at lower levels if the patient is assessed to be at high risk of TLS or if hyperphosphatemia exists
    Contraindicated in patients with G6PD deficiency
    Discontinue allopurinol if using rasburicase
    No bicarbonate necessary in IV fluid

METABOLIC ABNORMALITIES

Monitor serum electrolytes every 4 to 8 hours

HYPERKALEMIA

Moderate (≥6.0 mmol/L)
  Avoid IV and oral potassium
  Electrocardiogram and cardiorespiratory monitor
  Kayexalate (1 g/kg orally with 25% sorbitol every 6 hours)
Severe (>7.0 mmol/L and/or symptomatic)—same as for moderate hyperkalemia, plus:
  Albuterol nebulization treatment
  Insulin (0.1 units/kg) with concurrent 25% dextrose (2 mL/kg)
  Calcium gluconate (100 to 200 mg/kg)
  Dialysis

HYPERPHOSPHATEMIA

Moderate (≥5.0 mg/dL)—aluminum hydroxide 50-150 mg/kg/24 hours in divided doses every 4-6 hours
Severe (with symptomatic hypocalcemia)—dialysis, CVVH, and CVAH

HYPOCALCEMIA

Asymptomatic—no therapy
Symptomatic—calcium gluconate (50 to 100 mg/kg/dose)

CVAH, Continuous venoarterial hemofiltration; *CVVH*, continuous venovenous hemofiltration; *G6PD*, glucose-6-phosphate dehydrogenase; *IV*, intravenous; *NaHCO₃*, sodium bicarbonate; *TLS*, tumor lysis syndrome.

serum electrolyte, calcium, phosphate, blood urea nitrogen, creatinine, and uric acid levels. This panel of laboratory assessments should be performed promptly for any patient presenting with new diagnosis of malignancy. The main preventive measures are hydration and optimization of urine output, along with prevention of uric acid synthesis by allopurinol or rasburicase. In addition to the specific treatment recommendations discussed later, patients at risk for TLS should be carefully observed with use of cardiovascular and respiratory monitors. Frequent vital signs and strict fluid assessments including intake and output should be recorded. Laboratory tests should be performed at a minimum every 6 to 8 hours initially, and the results should be evaluated immediately (see Box 68-5).

Fluids and Alkalinization

Unless the patient presents with signs of acute renal failure or oliguria, aggressive hydration is the most important intervention. IV fluids should be administered at a rate of 3000 mL/m^2/day, and brisk urine output should be maintained (more than 100 mL/m^2/hour), with a urine specific gravity goal of less than or equal to 1.010. This increased hydration and increase in urine flow promotes urinary excretion of uric acid and phosphate by enhancing renal blood flow and glomerular filtration. Potassium, calcium, and phosphate should not be added to initial hydration fluids to avoid iatrogenic aggravation of hyperkalemia, hyperphosphatemia, or calcium phosphate precipitation. If urine output remains low despite aggressive hydration (usually caused by third spacing), diuretics may be used as long as there is no evidence of acute obstructive uropathy and/or hypovolemia. Commonly used diuretics are mannitol (0.5 g/kg) or furosemide (0.5 to 1.0 mg/kg).

Urine alkalinization remains controversial, although historically it has been a general recommendation for the prevention and treatment of TLS. An alkaline urine (urine pH ≥6.5) promotes urinary excretion of urate, with maximal solubility of urate occurring at a pH of 7.5.[114] However, the solubility of its precursors, xanthine and hypoxanthine, significantly decreases at a pH greater than or equal to 6.5. Thus excessive systemic and urinary alkalinization may lead to metabolic alkalosis and obstructive uropathies from xanthine and hypoxanthine crystallization. In addition, alkalinization of urine favors precipitation of calcium phosphate crystals in the renal tubules, a risk that can be further exacerbated by concomitant hyperphosphatemia. Metabolic alkalosis can also worsen the neurologic manifestations of hypocalcemia. Thus sodium bicarbonate should be used judiciously, with checks of urine pH with every void. If rasburicase is used, urine should not be alkalinized. If allopurinol is being used, alkalinization can be considered, but its use should be discontinued once serum uric acid normalizes, the dose should be decreased for urine pH greater than 8, and it must be discontinued if hyperphosphatemia develops.

Hyperkalemia

In the setting of TLS, hyperkalemia results from the massive efflux of intracellular potassium from dying tumor cells. Clinical manifestations include neuromuscular signs and symptoms such as muscle weakness, cramps, and paresthesias. Cardiac manifestations may include peaked T waves on an electrocardiogram, malignant arrhythmias, and conduction disturbances. Hyperkalemia is usually defined by a serum potassium level greater than or equal to 6.0 mmol/L. However, in the clinical setting of ongoing tumor lysis, a serum potassium level greater than 5.0 mmol/L and/or a trend of increasing values also merit intervention. Treatment of hyperkalemia is based on three approaches: driving extracellular potassium into cells, removing excess potassium from the body, and antagonizing the membrane effects of potassium. In asymptomatic patients, it is reasonable to begin simply with increased hydration with alkalinized fluids and diuresis with furosemide. The treatment of choice after alkalinization and optimization of urine output often is a potassium-binding cation exchange resin, such as sodium polystyrene sulfonate (1 g/kg/dose orally every 6 hours). This resin can also be given as a retention enema, but oral administration is more efficacious. Each gram of resin may bind as much as 1 mEq of potassium and release 1 to 2 mEq of sodium. For symptomatic patients, more rapid-acting treatments are required, such as insulin and β_2-adrenergic agonists, which drive potassium into cells by enhancing the activity of the Na+,K+ adenosine triphosphatase pump in skeletal muscle. Insulin is usually given as a bolus (0.1 unit/kg) with concurrent glucose infusion (25% dextrose, 2 mL/kg). Commonly used β_2-adrenergic agonists in the treatment of hyperkalemia are albuterol nebulizer treatments and IV epinephrine. Interventions commonly used in the fluid management of TLS, such as alkalinization and diuretics, can also help in the reduction of serum potassium. The increase in systemic pH with sodium bicarbonate results in hydrogen ion release from the cells as part of the buffering reaction; this change results in the movement of potassium into the cells to maintain electroneutrality. Loop and thiazide diuretics can lead to a transient lowering of serum potassium. Calcium directly antagonizes the inactivation of sodium channels and decreased membrane excitability caused by hyperkalemia. Thus calcium gluconate (100 to 200 mg/kg) can be given to stabilize myocardial conduction in cases of severe hyperkalemia or the presence of electrocardiographic abnormalities. Because concomitant hyperphosphatemia and alkalinization in the setting of TLS can increase the risk of calcium phosphate or calcium carbonate precipitation, calcium infusions should be given only when absolutely necessary. Finally, dialysis can be used if the conservative measures listed earlier are ineffective or if the hyperkalemia is severe.

Hyperphosphatemia

Clinical manifestations of severe hyperphosphatemia include nausea, vomiting, diarrhea, lethargy, and seizures. Physiologically, hyperphosphatemia increases the risk of tissue precipitation of calcium phosphate, which can subsequently lead to intrarenal calcification, acute obstructive uropathy, or symptomatic hypocalcemia. Hyperphosphatemia is usually defined by a phosphorus level greater than or equal to 5.0 mg/dL in children. Initial treatment for significant hyperphosphatemia consists of administration of oral forms of phosphate binders, such as aluminum hydroxide at a dosage of 50 to 150 mg/kg/day divided into equal doses every 6 hours. Acute severe hyperphosphatemia with symptomatic hypocalcemia can be life-threatening. However, given the real risk of worsening precipitation of calcium phosphate complexes, patients with hyperphosphatemia should not receive calcium infusions unless they have clinical symptoms of hypocalcemia. Patients with impaired renal function may require more aggressive therapy, such as peritoneal dialysis, hemodialysis, or continuous venovenous hemofiltration. Of these modalities, hemodialysis appears to be the most efficacious at clearing phosphorus.[115]

Hypocalcemia

During acute TLS, hypocalcemia commonly occurs because of precipitation of calcium phosphate, which in turn is a consequence of hyperphosphatemia. Many patients experience symptoms when their serum ionized calcium concentration is less than or equal to 0.7 mmol/L or their serum total calcium concentration is less than or equal to 7 mg/dL. Muscular manifestations of hypocalcemia include muscle cramps and spasms, paresthesias, and tetany. Cardiac abnormalities include ventricular arrhythmias, heart block, and hypotension. Neurologic complications include confusion, delirium, and seizures. Treatment of asymptomatic hypocalcemia is generally not recommended, particularly in the setting of hyperphosphatemia. In patients with severe hypocalcemia, IV calcium gluconate (50 to 100 mg/kg/dose) may be administered to correct marked or life-threatening clinical symptoms. However, this treatment may increase the risk of calcium phosphate deposition.

Hyperuricemia

Hyperuricemia is defined as serum uric acid greater than or equal to 8.0 mg/dL or a 25% increase from baseline 3 days before or 7 days after the initiation of chemotherapy. The major route of urate clearance is through the proximal renal tubule, and thus hyperuricemia develops when the excretory capacity of the renal tubule is exceeded. In combination with an acidic pH, hyperuricemia can lead to the formation of uric acid crystals in the renal tubule, resulting in intraluminal renal tubular obstruction and the development of acute renal dysfunction. The current pharmacologic strategies for the management of hyperuricemia are allopurinol and rasburicase.

Allopurinol was first approved for clinical use by the U.S. Food and Drug Administration in 1966 to treat patients with gout.[116] An isomer of hypoxanthine, allopurinol is rapidly converted in vivo to oxypurinol, which functions as a competitive inhibitor of xanthine oxidase. This irreversible inhibition of xanthine oxidase prevents the metabolism of xanthine and hypoxanthine to uric acid (see Fig. 68-9). In 1965, one of the first studies to examine the use of allopurinol in persons with TLS reported that 15 patients with leukemia or lymphoma had lowering of serum and urine uric acid levels after daily administration of allopurinol during the initiation of therapy.[117] A similar study was published in 1966, in which 33 patients with chronic leukemia, acute leukemia, or lymphoma had a dose-related reduction in uric acid after treatment with allopurinol.[118] This agent has since formed the backbone of both TLS prevention and treatment.

Allopurinol is available in two preparations, oral and IV, and they have similar efficacies. However, the IV formulation is considerably more costly and should be reserved for patients who are unable to take oral drugs. Allopurinol is administered at a dosage of 100 mg/m^2 every 8 hours by mouth (maximum, 800 mg/day) or 200 to 400 mg/m^2/day in one to three divided doses IV (maximum, 600 mg/day). A significant limitation of allopurinol is that it cannot reduce uric acid produced prior to its initiation. Patients with hyperuricemia at presentation will not have a reduction in uric acid levels for 2 to 3 days after the initiation of allopurinol because the removal of existing uric acid is dependent on renal clearance.[119] Another concern is that treatment with allopurinol can lead to increased levels of the uric acid precursors hypoxanthine and xanthine via inhibition of xanthine oxidase. Because xanthine is less soluble than uric acid, it is possible that high levels of xanthine may lead to xanthine nephropathy or xanthine renal stones. The clinical significance of this hypothesis is not clear because xanthine nephropathy has been rarely reported. In a study of 19 children with ALL who received allopurinol for tumor lysis syndrome, precipitated xanthine was significantly more likely to be found in the urine sediment of patients with high urine xanthine levels (>350 mg/dL). However, no difference was found in the incidence of precipitated xanthine in patients who did and did not experience acute renal failure.[114]

Urate oxidase provides an alternate approach for treating hyperuricemia by promoting the catabolism of uric acid to allantoin. Compared with uric acid, allantoin is five to ten times more water soluble and is easily excreted in urine.[120] Urate oxidase is an endogenous enzyme found in many mammalian species but not in humans. A nonrecombinant form of urate oxidase purified from the mold *Aspergillus flavus* has been demonstrated to reduce uric acid levels in patients at risk for TLS and has been available in Europe for more than 20 years. In the United States, a pediatric trial of this nonrecombinant urate oxidase was conducted in 126 children with newly diagnosed non–B-cell ALL. When compared with historic control subjects who were treated with allopurinol, patients treated with urate oxidase had significantly greater decreases in their blood uric acid levels (median maximal level during treatment, 2.3 vs. 3.9 mg/dL; $P <$ .001).[121] However, the nonrecombinant urate oxidase was also associated with significant acute hypersensitivity reactions, including anaphylaxis, in 4.5% of patients receiving the drug.

Subsequently, a recombinant form of urate oxidase (rasburicase) produced by a genetically modified *Saccharomyces cerevisiae* strain has become available and appears to have a lower incidence of hypersensitivity reactions. Rasburicase offers a potential advantage over allopurinol by affecting the direct breakdown of uric acid

and consequently leading to a more rapid lowering of serum uric acid levels. Faster normalization of uric acid levels also allows for earlier discontinuation of alkalinized fluids, which likely results in better excretion of other metabolites and avoids the increased risk of precipitation of calcium phosphate stones in the setting of overalkalinization. It should be noted that blood samples for uric acid measurement in patients receiving rasburicase therapy require special handling because of ex vivo degradation of uric acid by rasburicase at room temperature. To avoid falsely low uric acid levels, blood samples must be kept on ice and processed at 4°C within 4 hours of collection.

Pui and colleagues[122] initially administered rasburicase at a dose of 0.15 to 0.20 mg/kg IV for 5 to 7 days to 131 children with newly diagnosed leukemia or lymphoma. This study demonstrated a significant reduction of the median uric acid level by 4 hours after treatment, from 9.7 to 1 mg/dL in the 65 patients who presented with hyperuricemia and from 4.3 to 0.5 mg/dL in the remaining 66 patients. Rasburicase was very well tolerated in this study, with bronchospasm developing in 1 of 131 children. In addition, an open-label, multicenter, intent-to-treat, randomized, controlled trial was conducted to compare allopurinol with rasburicase in 52 pediatric patients with leukemia or lymphoma who were at high risk for TLS.[123] This study showed that patients randomized to rasburicase compared with allopurinol achieved an 86% versus 12% reduction of initial serum uric acid levels 4 hours after the first dose. In addition, no hypersensitivity reactions were observed in this study. Limitations of this study included its open-label design and the difficulty of generalizing these results to an adult population, although children up to age 17 years were included. Randomized controlled trials of allopurinol versus rasburicase have not been performed in the adult population.

Rasburicase is contraindicated in patients known to have glucose-6-phosphate dehydrogenase (G6PD) deficiency because the hydrogen peroxide generated in the breakdown of uric acid cannot be cleared by these patients.[120] The peroxide causes oxidative damage, resulting in hemolytic anemia and methemoglobinemia. The hemolytic anemia caused by rasburicase can be severe and can exacerbate renal damage in the setting of TLS. It is recommended that G6PD screening be performed before administration of rasburicase whenever possible.[124] Screening should be performed prior to transfusion with packed red blood cells to avoid false-negative results. If screening cannot be performed in a timely manner, the use of rasburicase should be avoided in patients who by ethnic background or family history have a significant risk of G6PD deficiency. Other adverse reactions associated with rasburicase include rare occurrences of hypersensitivity reactions, rash, increased liver enzyme levels, headache, vomiting, and nausea.[125] Because of the high incidence of hypersensitivity reactions associated with the nonrecombinant urate oxidase, several studies have measured antibody formation to rasburicase. In one study, no patients experienced hypersensitivity reactions and none of the 23 of 27 patient samples tested contained detectable levels of antibodies to rasburicase.[123] In another study, antibodies developed in 14% of patients, but none of these patients had hypersensitivity reactions.[123] It remains uncertain whether patients with detection of antibodies to rasburicase are at greater risk of hypersensitivity reactions with repeat courses. It has been suggested that patients with asthma and those with a high risk of hypersensitivity reactions based on allergy history should be monitored closely when receiving rasburicase.

Because of the high cost of rasburicase compared with allopurinol, it has been recommended that the use of rasburicase be reserved for patients with significant hyperuricemia at presentation or those at high risk of the development of severe TLS. The significant cost of rasburicase therapy has led several groups to evaluate the efficacy of single-dose therapy. Several published reports have demonstrated rapid reduction of uric acid levels with a single dose of rasburicase, with persistent effects for up to 7 days.[126,127] Thus single-dose therapy appears to be effective for both treatment and prophylaxis of hyperuricemia. However, when considering the use of rasburicase based on cost, it must be recognized that significant costs are also associated with complications of hyperuricemia and TLS, such as acute renal failure and dialysis. For example, a European study that examined the economic consequences of TLS management found that the main cost drivers in TLS are interventions requiring intensive care.[128] Thus studies aiming to analyze the cost difference between allopurinol and rasburicase should take into account the outcomes of acute renal failure and/or dialysis.

Uremia and Acute Renal Failure

Causes for renal dysfunction, azotemia, and rising creatinine levels can be multifactorial in persons with acute TLS. For example, any of the following conditions can result in renal injury: uric acid crystal obstructive uropathy, renal precipitation of calcium phosphate, renal tumor infiltration, xanthinuria, nephrotoxic drugs, or intravascular volume depletion. Despite appropriate medical management, some patients with increasing renal dysfunction and acute TLS require more aggressive measures, such as dialysis or hemofiltration. Indications for these therapies include metabolic derangements (e.g., hyperkalemia, hyperphosphatemia, hyperuricemia, hypocalcemia, and uremia) or volume overload that cannot be adequately controlled by medical management. Hemodialysis, peritoneal dialysis, and continuous hemofiltration (arteriovenous and venovenous) have been used in pediatric and adult populations for the treatment of TLS.[129-131] Peritoneal dialysis, although commonly used in many forms of acute renal failure, cannot be safely used in patients with intraabdominal tumors (e.g., Burkitt lymphoma) and is not recommended in the oncologic setting because of risk of infection in immunocompromised hosts.[115] The major advantage of hemodialysis compared with the other modalities is the rapidity with which electrolyte abnormalities can be corrected. However, hemodialysis can lead to large swings in plasma electrolyte levels and also can impose significant hemodynamic challenges. Continuous hemofiltration provides a more gradual method of correcting fluid and electrolyte disturbances and may serve as a safer alternative to hemodialysis in some cases. Unfortunately, little evidence relating to the comparison of the various dialysis modalities is available. Consultation with a nephrologist or an intensivist is recommended when weighing the options of hemofiltration and dialysis.

Conclusions

Tumor lysis syndrome is a constellation of metabolic derangements resulting from massive release of intracellular ions and nucleotides. Purine catabolism in the setting of TLS is particularly problematic for humans because of the lack of endogenous urate oxidase that can convert uric acid to the more soluble allantoin. The introduction of rasburicase has effectively reduced the incidence and severity of complications from hyperuricemia in patients at high risk for TLS. Although rasburicase appears to have great potential, many questions regarding its use remain unanswered.

COMPLICATIONS OF CHEMOTHERAPY

The use of chemotherapeutic agents carries risks for multiple acute and chronic toxicities and potential complications. Several oncologic emergencies related to the use of particular chemotherapeutic agents are summarized in this chapter. These emergencies must be recognized and managed effectively to prevent patient morbidity and mortality.

Vesicant Extravasation

Extravasation of vesicant chemotherapeutic agents can result in severe patient morbidity, with the development of extensive tissue damage. Vesicant agents include antitumor antibiotics (e.g., anthracyclines and dactinomycin), vinca alkaloids, epipodophyllotoxins, cisplatin, alkylating agents, and taxanes. Extravasation of anthracycline agents such as doxorubicin and daunorubicin can result in particularly severe and progressive tissue necrosis.[132] Importantly, the use of a central venous access device does not preclude the possibility of extravasation. Blood return or other evidence of patency, such as a dye study, is needed before a vesicant is administered in a central venous line. Once extravasation is suspected, usually because of swelling, redness, and pain at the injection site, administration of the agent should be stopped and assessment and treatment should be initiated.

Extravasation has traditionally been managed via the application of cold compresses, although this treatment is contraindicated with certain agents (such as vinca alkaloids and epipodophyllotoxins). Hyaluronidase may be used in certain situations to promote rapid dispersion of the infiltrate into surrounding tissue to lessen the severity of local tissue damage. Mechlorethamine extravasation can also result in tissue necrosis. The manufacturer recommends the local injection of sodium thiosulfate into the extravasation area, followed by topical application of ice. Vinca alkaloid extravasation management includes application of warm compresses and local injections of hyaluronidase.[133] Cooling the area has been recommended for taxane extravasation.[134]

Surgical debridement of affected areas may be required.[134] In 2007, the U.S. Food and Drug Administration approved dexrazoxane hydrochloride (Totect) for injection for the treatment of extravasation resulting from IV anthracycline chemotherapy.[135] In two studies, 57 evaluable patients underwent biopsy-proven extravasation of anthracycline from peripheral vein or central venous access sites. Totect was administered within 6 hours of extravasation for three doses, repeated 24 and 48 hours after the first dose. One patient required surgical intervention and the remaining patients had mild or no sequelae.[136] The use of Totect in the pediatric population has not been separately reported.

Methotrexate-Induced Renal Dysfunction

Because methotrexate is usually cleared exclusively by the kidneys, nephrotoxicity associated with high-dose methotrexate administration can be considered a true oncologic emergency. Although the strategies of hydration, alkalinization, and leucovorin rescue with close monitoring of methotrexate concentration and serum creatinine usually allow for safe administration of high-dose methotrexate, nephrotoxicity still occurs in some patients. Renal dysfunction was found to occur in approximately 1.8% of patients with osteosarcoma who were treated in clinical trials.[137] Renal dysfunction can result in persistently elevated methotrexate levels. Markedly delayed clearance of the drug amplifies methotrexate's other toxic effects, such as mucositis, hepatotoxicity, and myelosuppression.[138] In the patient with methotrexate-induced renal dysfunction, increasing leucovorin administration based on plasma methotrexate concentration remains a key intervention. Hemodialysis, hemoperfusion, therapeutic plasma exchange, and peritoneal dialysis have had limited success in this setting and may be useful in certain clinical situations.[137] Carboxypeptidase-G2 (known as CPDG2, glucarpidase, or Voraxaze), a recombinant bacterial enzyme, offers another emergency treatment option.[139,140] Glucarpidase provides hepatic elimination instead of renal clearance by metabolizing methotrexate to the inactive metabolite, 2,4-diamino-N10-methylpteroic acid.[141] Within minutes of administration, glucarpidase results in an average 97% reduction in plasma methotrexate concentration, allowing for continued management with leucovorin and supportive care. Glucarpidase is now commercially available and should be considered a standard component of treatment for patients with severe methotrexate-induced nephropathy.[142] Most cases of methotrexate-induced renal dysfunction resolve without long-term sequelae, and a single episode of nephrotoxicity does not automatically preclude future high-dose methotrexate use.[143]

Intrathecal Chemotherapy Overdose

Measures to prevent errors and overdose in the administration of intrathecal chemotherapeutic agents are key to avoiding this potentially devastating complication, and multistep safety systems have rendered these events rare in modern clinical practice. However, such errors continue to be reported, underscoring the importance of keeping plans for treatment and management in place in case such an adverse event occurs. Immediate response is crucial; case reports and small series highlight potential strategies.

Intrathecal overdose of methotrexate can result in seizures, coma, and death. Treatment options for intrathecal methotrexate overdose have traditionally included cerebrospinal fluid (CSF) drainage, ventriculolumbar CSF perfusion, systemic steroids, and systemic leucovorin.[137] Immediate removal of CSF has been advocated. The intrathecal use of leucovorin has not been advocated.[144] The intrathecal use of CPDG2 has also been reported.[145] In a 2004 report, Widemann et al.[137] presented results of a collaborative protocol assessing the intrathecal administration of CPDG2 in seven patients with cancer who had received accidental overdoses of intrathecal methotrexate, defined as a dose greater than 100 mg. These investigators found that methotrexate concentrations in the CSF declined by more than 98% in all patients and that all patients recovered completely from the overdose, except for two patients aged 61 and 77 years with memory impairment.[137] Four of the cases were pediatric cases, with ages ranging from 5 to 9 years. Three of these patients received a 600-mg dose of methotrexate, two underwent CSF exchange, and all were reported to have a complete recovery. It was concluded that CPDG2 should be considered for intrathecal methotrexate overdose.

One case report of an intrathecal overdose of cytarabine in a 4-year-old was managed with CSF exchange, and the patient survived.[146] At any dose, intrathecal vincristine is almost universally fatal and must be avoided at all costs.[147] As a result, the majority of active pediatric oncology practices have specific safety measures in place involving pharmacists, nurses, and physicians to prevent inadvertent administration of intrathecal vincristine. Clearly, preventive measures in prescribing, preparing, and delivering intrathecal chemotherapy remain essential.

References available online at ExpertConsult.

KEY REFERENCES

1. Robie DK, Gursoy MH, Pokorny WJ: Mediastinal tumors—airway obstruction and management. *Semin Ped Surg* 3:259–266, 1994.

    Comprehensive review of the concerns around large mediastinal massess causing compression of surrounding structures, and introduction of a treatment algorithm for managing patients with mediastinal masses.

2. Vahdat L, Maslak P, Miller WH, Jr, et al: Early mortality and the retinoic acid syndrome in acute promyelocytic leukemia: impact of leukocytosis, low-dose chemotherapy, PMN/RAR-alpha isoform, and CD13 expression in patients treated with all-trans retinoic acid. *Blood* 84:3843–3849, 1994.

    Review of patient developing retinoic acid syndrome during induction for APML, and report of outcomes for varied interventions for this syndrome.

3. Cohen LF, Balow JE, Magrath IT, et al: Acute tumor lysis syndrome. A review of 37 patients with Burkitt's lymphoma. *Am J Med* 68:486–491, 1980.

    Review of renal and metabolic complications during remission induction for patient with Burkitt lypoma, with the identification of the risk of hyperphosphatemia along with hyperkalemia and hyperuricemia.

19. Shamberger RC, Holzman RS, Griscom NT, et al: CT quantitation of tracheal cross-sectional area as a guide to the surgical and

anesthetic management of children with anterior mediastinal masses. *J Ped Surg* 26:138–142, 1991.

Frequently-sited work examining the correlation between tracheal cross-sectional area and anesthetic risk in children with anterior mediastinal mass.

34. Perger L, Lee EY, Shamberger RC: Management of children and adolescents with a critical airway due to compression by an anterior mediastinal mass. *J Ped Surg* 43:1990–1997, 2008.

A retrospective review of patients with critical airway due to compression by an anterior mediastinal mass, reviewing diagnostic workup with a focus on diagnostic biopsy. An algorithm for streamlining the choice of biopsy technique is suggested.

35. Lewis DW, Packer RJ, Raney B, et al: Incidence, presentation, and outcome of spinal cord disease in children with systemic cancer. *Pediatrics* 78:438–443, 1986.

36. Pollono D, Tomarchia S, Drut R, et al: Spinal cord compression: a review of 70 pediatric patients. *Ped Hematol Oncol* 20:457–466, 2003.

Both papers (References 35 and 36) present reviews of presentation of spinal cord compression in children with cancer and correlate outcomes with management approaches.

51. Grommes C, Bosl GJ, DeAngelis LM: Treatment of epidural spinal cord involvement from germ cell tumors with chemotherapy. *Cancer* 117:1911–1916, 2011.

Review of rare occurences of spinal cord involvement from germ cell tumors, and good response to chemotherapy only.

61. De Bernardi B, Pianca C, Pistamiglio P, et al: Neuroblastoma with symptomatic spinal cord compression at diagnosis: treatment and results with 76 cases. *J Clin Oncol* 19:183–190, 2001.

Review of patients with neuroblastoma with symptomatic spinal cord compression at diagnosis, showing comparable ability of radiotherapy, laminectomy, and chemotherapy to relieve or improve symptoms.

83. Inaba H, Fan Y, Pounds S, et al: Clinical and biologic features and treatment outcome of children with newly diagnosed acute myeloid leukemia and hyperleukocytosis. *Cancer* 113:522–529, 2008.

Review of 579 patients with newly diagnosed pediatric AML at a single center, correlating clinical and biologic features and treatment outcome. Early complications were highly associated with M4 and M5 FAB subytpes and patients with hyperleukocytosis and significantly lower post-remission 10 year event-free survival rate.

84. Sung L, Aplenc R, Alonzo TA, et al: Predictors and short-term outcomes of hyperleukocytosis in children with acute myeloid leukemia: a report from the Children's Oncology Group. *Haemat* 97:1770–1773, 2012.

Report of a Children's Oncology Group study, which included 1364 children with de novo AML, demonstrating an almost 20% occurrence of hyperleukocytosis at presentation, with correlation of poor outcome for this group in spite of currently available supportive care.

94. Chekol SS, Bhatnagar B, Gojo I, et al: Leukopheresis for profound hyperleukocytosis. *Transfus Apher Sci* 46:29–31, 2012.

Review of technical aspects of leukocytaphereis, justifying expectation of single 1-1.5 blood volume leukicytopheresis to reduce leukocyte count by 30% to 60%.

100. Zusman J, Brown DM, Nesbit ME: Hyperphosphatemia, hyperphosphaturia and hypocalcemia in acute lymphoblastic leukemia. *New Eng J Med* 289:1335–1340, 1973.

Early report of metabolic derangements noted during the presentation and treatment of acute lymphoblastic leukemia.

108. Annemans L, Moeremans K, Lamotte M, et al: Pan-European multicentre economic evaluation of recombinant urate oxidase (rasburicase) in prevention and treatment of hyperuricaemia and tumour lysis syndrome in haematological cancer patients. *Supp Care Cancer* 11:249–257, 2003.

Economic evaluation of the use of rasburicase demonstrating cost-saving and cost-effectiveness.

112. Howard SC, Jones DP, Pui CH: The tumor lysis syndrome. *New Eng J Med* 364:1844–1854, 2011.

Comprehenisve review of the current treatment of tumor lysis syndrome, with presentaion of strategies for risk assessment, prophylaxis, and therapy.

114. Galardy PJ, Hochberg J, Perkins SL, et al: Rasburicase in the prevention of laboratory/clinical tumour lysis syndrome in children with advanced mature B-NHL: a Children's Oncology Group Report. *Brit J Haematol* 163:365–372, 2013.

A report from a Children's Oncology Group study of patients on a therapeutic trial for advanced mature B-NHL, incorporating rasburicase prior to cytoreductive chemotherapy, demonstrating safety and efficacy in preventing new onset renal failure and association with significant improvement in GFR.

118. Krakoff IH, Meyer RL: Prevention of Hyperuricemia in Leukemia and Lymphoma: Use of Alopurinol, a Xanthine Oxidase Inhibitor. *JAMA* 193:1–6, 1965.

119. DeConti RC, Calabresi P: Use of allopurinol for prevention and control of hyperuricemia in patients with neoplastic disease. *New Eng J Med* 274:481–486, 1966.

Seminal papers (References 118 and 119) reporting the use of oral allopurinol in patients with neoplastic disease, describing successful decrease in serum uric acid with no significant toxicity.

136. Mouridsen HT, Langer SW, Buter J, et al: Treatment of anthracycline extravasation with Savene (dexrazoxane): results from two prospective clinical multicentre studies. *Annal Oncol* 18:546–550, 2007.

Descriptin of dexrazoxane as an effective and well-tolerated acute treatment for extravasation, mitigating the need for surgical resection in almost all cases.

137. Widemann BC, Balis FM, Shalabi A, et al: Treatment of accidental intrathecal methotrexate overdose with intrathecal carboxypeptidase G2. *J Natl Cancer Inst* 96:1557–1559, 2004.

Report of successful treatment of intrathecal methotrexate overdose with carboxypeptidase.

140. Widemann BC, Balis FM, Murphy RF, et al: Carboxypeptidase-G2, thymidine, and leucovorin rescue in cancer patients with methotrexate-induced renal dysfunction. *J Clin Oncol* 15:2125–2134, 1997.

Report of the efficacy of carboxypeptidase, along with leucovorin and thymidine, in instances of methotrexate-induced renal dysfunction.

CHAPTER 69

Nursing Care of Patients with Childhood Cancer

Patricia A. Branowicki, Kathleen E. Houlahan, Susanne B. Conley, and Nancy E. Kline

CHAPTER OUTLINE

HISTORY OF PEDIATRIC ONCOLOGY NURSING

Nursing is the largest health care occupation in the United States, representing 2.7 million jobs—a number that is expected to grow by 26% or more before 2020, faster than the national average of 14%.[1] Because its roots are embedded in daily life and the caretaking role women traditionally assumed throughout history, nursing was not recognized as a profession until the mid-1800s, when Florence Nightingale identified the need for specialized education and training and developed the underpinnings of modern-day nursing practice.[2]

The first nurses were considered generalists and cared for patients of all ages. Pediatric nursing emerged as a specialty in the early 20th century, when free-standing children's hospitals became more common.[2] During this time, pediatric oncology patients were often cared for by pediatric nurses (sometimes called tumor therapy nurses) who learned to care for oncology patients through experience and self-directed, on-the-job training.[3-5]

The subspecialty of pediatric oncology nursing first appeared in the late 1940s and early 1950s, when courses specific to cancer nursing were introduced by the American Cancer Society, the University of Washington, and the University of Minnesota School of Public Health.[1,4,6] It was formally recognized as a subspecialty practice in the mid-1970s, when more nursing schools began offering education specific to pediatric oncology, and a small cohort of nurses formed the Association of Pediatric Oncology Nurses (APON).[4,7,8] APON changed its name in 2006 to the Association of Pediatric Hematology/Oncology Nurses (APHON) and is considered the leading professional organization for registered nurses caring for children and adolescents with cancer and blood disorders.[9,10]

Over the years, the role of pediatric oncology nurses has evolved to match advances in cancer treatment. During the 1880s and early 1900s, the predominant treatment modality for cancer was surgery, and nursing care was focused primarily on relieving pain and meeting other postsurgical needs of patients.[6] Until the latter half of the 1900s, cancer was a metaphor for death and nurses had few resources available to care for the patients it affected. Children diagnosed with cancer commonly died, diagnostic techniques and treatment were often not available, and care was typically palliative.[4,5] The general attitude among health care professionals was that there was little to offer the person with cancer except a cheerful manner and a few comfort measures.[11]

After World War II, single-agent chemotherapy was introduced. This new therapy was administered only by physicians until the 1960s, when it was proposed that nurses assume this responsibility.[6] Today, chemotherapy is almost always administered by nurses, who as a discipline have been instrumental in developing standards for safe practice and education related to chemotherapy administration and symptom management.[7,12-14] Pediatric oncology nurses are also leaders in patient and family education, pain management, and palliative care. Over the past few decades, a number of advanced-practice nursing roles have gained prominence. The term *advanced practice nurse* applies to nurses in specialized roles, including clinical nurse specialists, nurse practitioners, certified nurse midwives, and nurse anesthetists, who have completed additional formal education and training. In pediatric oncology settings, it is the clinical nurse specialist and the pediatric nurse practitioner who are most commonly employed. Although their responsibilities vary among institutions, the clinical nurse specialist generally focuses on the education of the staff and of patients and families, whereas the pediatric nurse practitioner usually provides direct patient care in consultation with the patient's oncologist. As a primary oncology provider, the pediatric nurse practitioner follows patients and families over time and helps to formulate, implement, and evaluate the patient's plan of care. Depending on institutional, state, and federal regulations, a pediatric nurse practitioner may also prescribe medications and perform procedures, such as bone marrow biopsies and lumbar punctures. Standards and guidelines regarding professional behaviors and scope of practice developed by APHON and the American Nurses Association also guide the practice of advanced practice nurses.[15]

Each year, 10,000 children will receive a diagnosis of childhood cancer and 1.16 million children younger than the age of 15 years will be hospitalized with a cancer-related diagnosis.[16,17]Although the incidence of pediatric cancer has increased 29% during the past 20 years, advances in treatment have resulted in a long-term childhood survival rate of 79% for all childhood cancers.[18,19] Some selected childhood cancers have realized long-term

survival rates that now approach or exceed 95%.[16,18] Despite improving statistics where the 10-year survival rate is 75%, cancer is the second leading cause of death in children from birth to age 14 years.[20] Pediatric oncology nurses at all levels will continue to play critical roles in the care of children with cancer as new diagnostic and treatment techniques become available. Through persistence, vigilance, and dedication, nurses will shape the development and modification of practice standards that promote safe and effective pediatric cancer care.[7,21]

Nursing Education and Professional Certification

When nursing first emerged as a profession, nursing education was typically provided by hospital-based diploma programs.[22] Today, most diploma programs have closed and have been replaced by college- and university-based schools of nursing. Nurses specializing in pediatric oncology usually receive advanced training in all aspects of cancer and cancer treatment, including chemotherapy, management of complications related to therapy, pediatric oncology protocols, and the protection of human subjects.[23-25] In addition to this specialized training, APHON and most health care organizations recommend that pediatric oncology nurses obtain professional certification as another vehicle to confirm proficiency and demonstrate knowledge of pediatric oncology practice standards, although it is not a requirement for practice. Certification was first introduced in 1999, and since then more than 1700 registered nurses have become certified pediatric oncology nurses.[26,27-29]

OVERVIEW OF THE PEDIATRIC ONCOLOGY NURSE'S ROLE

The role of the nurse in the care of childhood cancer patients is well established.[30] Pediatric oncology nurses rely on their intellect, critical thinking abilities, expert communication skills, technical expertise, and up-to-date knowledge when caring for their patients.[25,31,32] These skills, when combined with intuition and caring, position pediatric oncology nurses to actively participate in and influence decisions concerning patient care and support, promote novel approaches to care, and optimize patient outcomes.[31-33]

When caring for patients, pediatric oncology nurses integrate information about the treatment modality with observations of how the patient and family are responding to treatment and whether additional education and support are needed. Much of a pediatric oncology nurse's practice is grounded in standards of care and professional performance defined by APHON. These standards apply to clinical settings across the continuum of care and serve as a guide for nurses practicing in all aspects of care, from prevention, early detection, ongoing physical and psychosocial care, and long-term survival. These standards of care also define activities associated with each step of the nursing process—a process that includes assessing the patient, identifying problems requiring nursing intervention, specifying expected outcomes, planning and implementing a nursing plan of care, and evaluating the child's progress (Table 69-1).[15] With the patient as the central

TABLE 69-1   The Nursing Process and Standards of Pediatric Oncology Nursing Care

Nursing Process	Standards of Care	Application: Case Study*
Assessment	The pediatric oncology nurse collects and documents data regarding the child and family.	• Obtained a patient history of severe chemotherapy-related nausea and vomiting during first treatment regimen.
Diagnosis	The nurse uses assessment data from nursing and other disciplines to identify problems and determine nursing diagnoses.	• Severe chemotherapy-related nausea despite antiemetics • New protocol regimen is highly emetogenic. • Assess the need for overnight hydration or next-day clinic infusion appointment for bolus to help with nausea control.
Outcomes Identification	The nurse identifies expected and desired outcomes specific to the patient and family and related to their physical and emotional health, education, growth and development, and effects of disease and treatment.	Expected outcomes: • Patient will experience little or no nausea during chemotherapy and postchemotherapy period. • Patient and family will communicate effectiveness of antiemetic and patient satisfaction with the regimen.
Planning	The nurse develops an individualized plan that prescribes interventions to attain expected outcomes.	• Resume previous antiemetics (ondansetron, corticosteroids, and scopolamine). Add new antiemetic, aprepitant. • Have patient maintain a diary describing nausea and individual drug effectiveness.
Implementation	The nurse implements the plan of care to achieve the expected outcomes for the child and family.	• Administer first antiemetic doses in clinic to monitor effectiveness, and review timing of doses.
Coordination of Care	The nurse coordinates the delivery of care to support transition across the continuum of care.	• College student describes past use of dronabinol and lorazepam to control nausea. Patient states that these agents made him feel "loopy" which impeded his ability to attend class and keep up with studies.
Health Teaching and Health Promotion	The nurse employs strategies to educate patient and family about maintaining health and providing a safe environment of care.	• Provided a detailed calendar outlining scheduled chemotherapy, predicted times of nausea, medication schedule, and escalation plan for unresolved nausea • Reviewed patient education materials associated with prescribed antiemetic agents. • Reviewed prn use of additional antiemetics
Evaluation	Working with other members of the care team, the nurse evaluates outcomes that have been achieved and follows the nursing process to adjust the plan of care as needed.	• Patient returned for cycle 2. Reviewed the drug diary with the patient to understand the duration of nausea and the patient's perspective on the effectiveness of the antiemetic regimen. • Patient reported no nausea, did not require supplemental antiemetics, and reported increased satisfaction with plan, noting that he had previously found the inability to control nausea extremely distressing.

From Association of Pediatric Oncology Nurses, American Nurses Association: Scope and standards of pediatric oncology nursing practice. *Silver Spring, Md., 2007, Nurses Books.*

*Applying the nursing process to the management of postchemotherapy nausea in a 19-year-old college student with relapsed Ewing sarcoma. Case study of a patient at Dana-Farber/Children's Hospital Cancer and Blood Disorders Center managed by primary nurse A. Carnes, BSN, RN, CPON.

focus, the ultimate goal is to reestablish a level of optimal wellness as defined by the patient and family.[34] The nursing process is dynamic and considers all dimensions of care; therefore, the plan of care is continually adjusted in response to changes in the patient's condition and treatment plan.[34]

As discussed in this chapter and highlighted in Box 69-1, pediatric oncology nurses are critical members of the oncology team, collaborating with colleagues and using an evidence-based approach to reduce the burden of cancer and meet the needs of patients and families.

The Nurse's Relationship with Patients, Families, and Other Providers

Meeting the varied needs of pediatric oncology patients and their families requires a broad range of professionals. For this reason, most pediatric cancer centers draw on an interdisciplinary team, replacing the physician-centered model that was more common in the early years of cancer care.[3] Today, members of the care team rely on one another's observations, knowledge, and skills, with physicians and nurses working as interdependent partners toward the care and cure of children with cancer.[5,35,36] Equally important is coordinated and ongoing interaction between the child, the family, and all members of the interdisciplinary team.

Patient- and Family-Centered Care

Partnering with patients and families is the cornerstone of patient- and family-centered care. A model of care delivery commonly practiced in pediatric oncology settings is based on the understanding that the family is the child's primary source of strength and support, that the perspectives and information provided by the family,

Box 69-1   The Role of the Pediatric Oncology Nurse in Reducing the Burden of Cancer: Ensuring Families' Needs Are Met

CARING PRACTICES

- Provides compassionate, developmentally appropriate care
- Considers cultural differences when developing and implementing a plan of care
- Minimizes pain and suffering
- Partners with patients and families to individualize approaches to care
- Develops and coordinates all aspects of patients' experiences across the continuum
- Collaborates with other disciplines to ensure optimal patient care
- Demonstrates caring practices toward all patients, families, and members of the health care system

COMMUNICATION AND COLLABORATION

- Serves as an advocate for the needs of the patients and families
- Exchanges ideas with other members of the clinical team to advance clinical practice and patient care
- Facilitates communication:
  - With the community
  - With the patients and families
  - Between the patients and physicians
  - Between the patients and other members of the health care team

EDUCATION AND LEARNING

- Teaches patients and families about the cancer diagnosis and its treatment
- Prepares patients and families to manage home care needs and transition back into the community
- Encourages techniques supporting compassionate clinical and emotional care
- Educates other members of the clinical team
- Creates educational materials for patients, families, and other health care providers
- Influences nursing practice at a local, national, and international level

CLINICAL INQUIRY AND SYSTEMS THINKING

- Uses clinical judgment and reasoning to care for patients effectively
- Guides pediatric oncology nursing practice by identifying key research areas
- Advances nursing science using the best available evidence as the basis for changes in practice
- Masters the skills and competencies necessary to maximize clinical outcomes
- Serves as a change agent
- Critically examines the environment, identifies opportunities for change, and introduces strategies to ensure safe care

Organizations are also urged to involve patients and families in defining and improving institutional policies and care delivery systems.[37]

Although patient- and family-centered care is now widely embraced by pediatric health care professionals, there was a time when parental visitation was permitted only on a limited basis, information related to a child's diagnosis was often withheld from the patient and the family for fear of increasing anxiety, and decisions surrounding care were made within a paternalistic framework.[21,40] Nurses were often caught in the middle when a patient did not know the diagnosis or the family was not involved in shared decision making.[6,21] The cultural shift to a family-centered focus, along with improvements in survival rates, have helped members of the health care team develop a keener understanding of the long-term effects of diagnosis and treatment as well as an appreciation for how physiologic and psychological sequelae impact the patient and their family members.[21] The patient- and family-centered approach has also helped parents to gain confidence in their ability to care for their child throughout the course of illness and has helped children and young adults to manage aspects of their own health care.[37] Nurses routinely partner with patients and families throughout the cancer patient's care, from diagnosis to end of life, involving patients and families in establishing short- and long-term goals. This is particularly important for children because it gives them a feeling of control and enhances their sense of autonomy.[41] Although the ability of the child to participate in goal setting and decision making depends in part on their maturity and cognitive capacities, approaches and techniques usually can be tailored to match their capabilities.

Meeting the Emotional and Developmental Needs of Patients and Families

Pediatric oncology nurses often spend long stretches of time with patients and families, particularly when patients are hospitalized or receiving outpatient chemotherapy.

Box 69-2   Patient- and Family-Centered Care: Guidelines for Providers

- **Respect and dignity.** Health care practitioners listen to and honor patient and family perspectives and choices. Patient and family knowledge, values, beliefs, and cultural backgrounds are incorporated into the planning and delivery of care.
- **Information sharing.** Health care practitioners communicate and share complete and unbiased information with patients and families in ways that are affirming and useful. Patients and families receive timely, complete, and accurate information to effectively participate in care and decision making.
- **Participation.** Patients and families are encouraged and supported in participating in care and decision making at the level they choose.
- **Collaboration.** Patients and families are also included on an institution-wide basis. Health care leaders collaborate with patients and families in policy and program development, implementation, and evaluation; in health care facility design; and in professional education, as well as in the delivery of care.

From the Institute for Patient- and Family-Centered Care: www.ipfcc.org.

the child, or the young adult are important to clinical decision making, and that the psychosocial and cultural needs of the family as well as the patient must be considered throughout the care process.[21,37,38,39] Guidelines developed by the Institute for Patient- and Family-Centered Care for clinicians interested in adopting a patient- and family-centered care model (Box 69-2) emphasize the importance of partnering with the patient and family throughout the course of treatment. Respecting the insights and perspectives of the parents regarding their child's needs, empowering the patient and family by providing them with information, and engaging the child in his or her own care are key aspects of the model.

Because of their frequent interactions with patients and families, nurses are often the first to recognize practical issues faced by families. Over time, many families view nurses as advocates; however, the nurses' role is not to provide all of the support families need but rather to nurture support systems and identify available resources that might be of help.

Developing trusting relationships with patients and families is essential to effective oncology nursing practice.[41] Nurses often gain this trust simply through the care provided, the hours spent at the patients' bedsides, and the efforts undertaken to meet the needs of patients and families while facilitating communication with other providers. Among children and adolescents, trust is often more readily gained when the actions of the nurse reflect an appreciation for developmental needs and when nurses are forthright, honest, and maintain developmentally appropriate boundaries regarding the behavior of the child or adolescent.[42-44]

In addition to the emotional needs of patients and families, children undergoing treatment for cancer are at risk for significant delays in growth and development, which are often functions of the length and type of treatment and the side effects that children experience.[45] Therefore, nurses caring for children with cancer incorporate developmentally supportive care into all phases of treatment. Such care requires knowledge of normal growth and development as well as an appreciation for the variations and abnormalities that may be encountered among children who are ill. A variety of approaches are used to support a patient's growth and development to help them reach their maximum personal potential. Providing age-appropriate care individualized to each patient, encouraging parental involvement, and fostering normalcy whenever possible by maintaining routines and usual activities are just a few of the strategies nurses use. Child-life specialists are routinely consulted to establish interventions for hospitalized children that are appropriate to developmental milestones.[46,47]

Educating Patients and Families

A hallmark of comprehensive pediatric oncology care is educating patients and families about the diagnosis and treatment, empowering them to make informed decisions and become active partners in the treatment process.[48,49-51] Because the care process typically spans multiple settings, patients and families are likely to receive information and instruction from a variety of clinicians and care providers. As a matter of course, teaching is a part of most patient encounters to help patients and families build skills and gain the self-confidence necessary to actively participate in ongoing care processes. When teaching patients and families, nurses adapt teaching methods to meet the educational needs of individual patients and families. Nurses supplement didactic instructions with written materials that augment topics covered in teaching sessions. Frequent opportunities to observe and practice the skills needed to manage care at home are typically offered. The use of technology for simulation and teaching is increasing as new educational formats become available.

Nurses have been instrumental on local, national, and international levels in developing educational materials for parents and age-appropriate materials for patients. In many hospitals and other care-delivery settings, nurses coordinate efforts to develop and evaluate educational materials on a wide range of topics, have the materials translated into various languages, and make them accessible to patients and families. A number of nursing organizations have also developed education resources. For example, APHON has developed a wide range of disease-specific pamphlets and education programs for patients and families that outline treatment options, side effects, and how to care for children at home.[52] The Children's Oncology Group also offers an informative website, a handbook, and numerous networking opportunities for parents.[53]

CARING FOR PATIENTS AND FAMILIES DURING THE DIAGNOSTIC PHASE

Receiving a diagnosis of childhood cancer is devastating and life altering.[54] For parents, the diagnostic phase is marked by extreme emotional, physical, and spiritual distress, with many describing the period of waiting and not knowing as one of the most difficult times in the journey.[55-57] It is during this waiting period that parents are often acutely aware that cancer is the probable diagnosis, but the type of cancer, the expected treatment, and the likely outcome have yet to be determined.[57] As a result, this is a time of uncertainty, with many fears stemming from the unknown and questions the clinical team may not yet be ready to answer. Some of the questions known to be plaguing the parents during this phase include the following: Will our child survive? What will the future hold? Will our child suffer? Will we be able to comfort and protect our child from pain?[51,56]

The nurse caring for a child suspected of having cancer is in a unique position to assess needs, identify cultural preferences, offer support and guidance, as well as ensure access to information needed to provide informed consent.[55,58] Because this period typically involves interactions with a variety of health care providers, the nurse supports coordination of this process to optimize communication between the patients and families and members of the health care team.[59] To do this, the nurse must possess a thorough understanding of the prediagnostic and diagnostic phases of pediatric malignancies that include, but are not limited to, the various tests and procedures commonly used for diagnosis.[55]

The Diagnostic Workup

Confirming a cancer diagnosis can be a long process because many of the initial symptoms imitate normal childhood illnesses.[55] The diagnostic workup includes obtaining a complete history of the current illness, the incidence and duration of symptoms, and the existence of any predisposing factors.[60] It is during this phase that the nurse completes a comprehensive assessment that includes a physical examination, developmental assessment, and measurement of vital signs, height, and weight. The height and weight are used to calculate the body surface area, a key measure if cancer is confirmed because it is used to determine chemotherapy doses in patients 1 year of age and older (weight in kilograms, rather than body surface area, is typically used to calculate doses for children younger than 1 year). Accurate measurement of body surface area is critical; therefore, it is common practice to have two nurses independently measure the initial height and weight and verify the calculations of body surface area.

Because the diagnostic phase involves numerous tests to determine the extent of disease, the nurse's role is focused on collecting specimens, coordinating the scheduling of the diagnostic workup, and partnering with the patient and family.[60] The nurse not only is responsible for ensuring that preparative regimens for specific tests are observed but also must facilitate the sequencing of various tests to ensure that procedures do not conflict with one another, that sufficient time is allotted for traveling from one department to another, and that tests are scheduled in a manner that permits judicious use of sedation.[60] Before each test, the nurse speaks with the patient and family explaining the test and how long it will take, discussing whether a contrast medium or sedation will be used, and answering any questions they may have about the procedure.

The diagnostic phase is emotionally and physically difficult, with diagnostic tests provoking anxiety and causing pain. Studies regarding the patient perception of pain suggest that the pain associated with invasive procedures and ultimate treatment for cancer is greater than the pain associated with the disease itself.[61,62] Fortunately, there are a wide array of pharmacologic and nonpharmacologic interventions available to minimize distress associated with pain and anxiety.

Informing Patients and Families of the Diagnosis

Once the diagnostic workup is complete and the type and extent of the cancer is known, news of the diagnosis is shared with the parents or guardian during a meeting with the physician and nurse. In some centers, this meeting is called the "Day One Talk." The purpose of this meeting is to review the extent of the disease, discuss the proposed treatment, consider whether alternatives to that treatment are available, and introduce and obtain informed consent in the patient's preferred language. If the proposed treatment is a research protocol, all issues related to the protocol, including the intent of the research, must be clearly explained to ensure informed decision making.[57] Studies regarding informed consent have found that parents of pediatric cancer patients often do not understand some of the issues related to participating in clinical trials, particularly that the purpose of research may be to benefit future patients rather than their own child.[63]

The Day One Talk typically represents the first step toward developing the patient-provider relationship forming the basis for future care. Determining who should be present during the meeting is not always simple, and parents often ask the physician or nurse for advice about whether the patient should be in attendance. Consideration should be given to including adolescents because they may assume that information later received is not completely true and that the diagnosis and treatment are worse than those stated in the information they have been given.[57] Including adolescents from the beginning may also help in later efforts to engage them in their own care. In cases involving younger children, a separate discussion tailored to the developmental level of the child is suggested, with the goal of informing the child about the treatment and clinical trial to obtain assent.[60]

Receiving the news that a child has cancer and hearing the complex treatment plan can be devastating for parents who may be overwhelmed with feelings of anger, fear, guilt, sadness, and self-blame. Because of this, parents may have difficulty retaining, processing, and understanding the information. The signed consent form detailing the aspects of treatment and chemotherapy information sheets may serve as useful references for parents after the meeting.[57]

If the patient is an adolescent, consideration must be given to the potential impact the treatment may have on fertility, as well as possible fertility-preservation options. It is generally recommended that this conversation take place as early as possible before beginning treatment. Some physicians choose to discuss fertility-related issues during the Day One Talk with a follow-up referral to reproductive specialists.[64]

Supporting Patients and Families after Diagnosis

After the Day One Talk, nurses provide ongoing support as patients and parents express fears and concerns. Once the diagnosis is made, patients and families are suddenly thrust into a complex plan of treatment that involves hospitals, ambulatory clinics, and home care agencies. Nurses help to arrange and coordinate appointments and other aspects of treatment, as well as facilitate collaboration and communication among care providers in various locations. During the weeks and months after the diagnosis, nurses carefully monitor patients and families for signs that suggest they may be having difficulty coping. If any signs of distress are observed, nurses work with colleagues on the health care team to formulate a plan to help patients, parents, and other family members manage their stress to enhance the family's chances for the best possible outcomes.[51] Many patients, parents, and family members benefit from working with psychosocial clinicians, attending family support groups, or having regularly scheduled family meetings, whereas others may require more intensive interventions.

NURSING IMPLICATIONS OF PEDIATRIC CANCER TREATMENT

The treatment of childhood cancer has evolved into an increasingly complex set of treatment modalities and methods. Although advances in treatment are responsible for marked improvements in survival rates, they have resulted in a broad range of side effects that require diligent monitoring and supportive therapy. Knowledgeable and well-trained pediatric oncology nurses are crucial to the safe and effective implementation of surgical, radiologic, and pharmacologic approaches to cancer treatment as well as to the management and oversight of clinical trials.

Nurses interact with patients during each treatment phase and in every care setting, making critical assessments and observations that guide decisions regarding the patients' care. Administering care specified by the treatment protocol, nurses continually monitor patients for complications and unexpected developments, offer emotional support to the patients and their families, and teach them what to expect during each treatment phase. Throughout the weeks, months, and years of care, nurses often develop a strong rapport with patients and families, becoming trusted sources of support and information.

Nursing Care Associated with Various Modes of Treatment

In this section, the specialized nursing care associated with the primary forms of pediatric oncology treatment—surgery, chemotherapy, radiation therapy, biotherapy, and hematopoietic stem cell transplant—are discussed. Complementary and integrative therapies and the nurse's role in clinical trials are also examined.

Surgery

Surgery is a major treatment approach for many pediatric solid tumors. Preoperative nursing care involves preparing patients and their families for the expected surgery and recovery by providing individualized teaching that is tailored to meet the unique needs of each patient and their family. In an effort to demystify the surgical experience, many hospitals offer programs that allow patients to visit the inpatient surgical unit, meet operating room nurses and other members of the staff, and see much of the equipment that will be used as part of the intraoperative care.[65]

During the postoperative period, nurses support the recovery process and promote healing. Close monitoring of vital signs and the overall clinical status, coughing and deep breathing, frequent position changes, and early ambulation are just a few of the nursing interventions introduced after surgery to prevent complications. Comprehensive postoperative care includes ongoing assessment of airway clearance, level of pain, signs and symptoms of fluid shifts, and infection. Fever is a common postoperative complication warranting careful monitoring and prompt treatment in pediatric oncology.[66]

Controlling postsurgical pain is a primary focus. Pain can have a profound effect on physical and emotional well-being, as well as discourage children from engaging in activities that promote recovery. Medications for pain control are typically initiated intraoperatively and are commonly continued for at least 72 hours after surgery or until the child is able to take medication by mouth.[67-70] During the postoperative period, nurses regularly assess for the presence of pain and the effectiveness of prescribed analgesics by observing the patient for signs of discomfort using age-appropriate pain-rating scales. Analgesics may be administered prior to activities such as walking or dressing changes to promote comfort and reduce the anxiety associated with procedures or activities that may cause pain.

Preparing patients and their families for discharge from the hospital after surgery typically begins before or at the time of admission. Discharge teaching involves a review of the care regimen, as well as coaching caregivers on how to perform aspects of physical care at home. Emphasis is placed on ensuring caregiver understanding of the signs and symptoms of potential complications, when they should contact a provider, and how to reach someone in the case of an emergency. Follow-up appointments with the surgical team and pediatric oncology providers are usually scheduled before discharge.

Chemotherapy

Chemotherapeutic agents are considered high-risk medications because of their narrow therapeutic index and the complexity of the treatment regimens in which they are used. If administered inappropriately, there is the potential for serious harm and even death.[71] Unlike other medications, administering chemotherapeutic agents to children introduces challenges because of the physiology of children, broad dosing ranges and schedules, widely differing protocols, weight-based dosing, and a high risk for toxicities.[13,14,72,73] Statistics revealing the incidence of medication errors have triggered widespread changes and standardization with all aspects of the medication process, from prescribing, dispensing and administration. The majority of medication errors occur at the time of administration (41%), followed by dispensing errors (38%) and prescribing errors (21%)[74] Because administering chemotherapy is the primary responsibility of pediatric oncology nurses, they are commonly viewed as the patient's last line of defense against medication errors.[75] Therefore, the provider may be viewed as the first line of defense with prescribers initiating the medication process. Because prescribing errors related to chemotherapy agents can have serious and even lethal effects, nurses in most institutions follow a special process to verify chemotherapy orders before the agent is administered. Each step of the verification process is designed to ensure chemotherapy is administered safely, the treatment protocol is observed, required pretreatment test results are within acceptable ranges, and the correct chemotherapy agent and dose are administered.[76] To minimize the risk for error, nurses complete specialized training and follow standards of practice for chemotherapy administration developed by APHON. In addition, they receive ongoing education relative to new agents and protocols before any new agents are introduced.[71]

Before administration of chemotherapy to a patient, the nurse reviews the patient's medical record and interviews the patient and family to determine past experience with chemotherapy, level of tolerance, and antiemetics used. During the interview, the nurse explains the current treatment plan, discusses each agent, reviews potential side effects, and completes a medication reconciliation process. The medication reconciliation process includes a review of chemotherapeutic agents, antiemetics, over-the-counter preparations, as well as herbal and nutritional supplements taken since the last visit. Querying the patient and family about medications reinforces an understanding of the treatment plan and medication doses providing an opportunity to evaluate compliance with the prescribed plan. The nurse also conducts an assessment to determine drug-specific side effects (e.g., constipation) to determine whether the chemotherapy can be administered as prescribed and if the symptom management plan should be adjusted.[73,77]

Because many chemotherapeutic agents are highly toxic, the National Institute of Occupational Safety and Health has developed standards to protect health care workers when handling or administering chemotherapy and caring for patients who have received chemotherapy.[78] The standards identify personal protective equipment such as gowns, gloves, and eye shields that must be worn by those handling chemotherapeutic agents. In addition, standards recommend the use of closed-system drug transfer devices to prevent accidental disconnection and exposure. Research has shown that complying with these standards limits long-term exposure.[79] Although some patients and families may be frightened when they first see nurses and other clinicians using protective equipment and procedures, most are quickly accepting once they understand the rationale for such measures. The safety concerns and precautions related to chemotherapy administration also apply to the patient's family, who must learn how to handle chemotherapeutic agents and the patient's body fluids. Body fluids can be a source of cytotoxic drugs and may pose a threat to the environment. As a result, special precautions for their disposal must be observed for 48 hours after chemotherapy administration, and family members should be given appropriate personal protective equipment and written instructions on how to handle the fluids safely. Family members of child-bearing age or who are pregnant should not prepare or administer cytotoxic drugs in the home. If they must handle the agent, they should minimize their risk by wearing appropriate protective equipment.[78]

During the time a patient is receiving a dose of chemotherapy, the nurse monitors parameters specific to the particular agent. In addition to monitoring temperature, blood pressure, and heart rate, the nurse observes the patient for signs of an allergic reaction and watches the access site for signs of possible extravasation or leakage of intravenous fluid into the tissues. Special precautions must be taken to prevent extravasation when administering a vesicant because these agents can cause blistering, severe tissue injury, or tissue necrosis if they extravasate.[80] If extravasation does occur, institutional polices and guidelines typically determine the appropriate actions to take.

After the chemotherapy has been administered, the nurse evaluates the effectiveness of the antiemetic regimen and monitors the patient for signs of toxicity and adverse effects. Detecting adverse effects early and taking quick action can minimize their severity. The nurse records the patient's response to treatment carefully because these observations are used by the care team to evaluate tolerance to treatment and determine whether changes need to be made in the overall plan of care.

For many families, the chemotherapy treatment phase is particularly difficult because they must cope with their own fears and anxieties while supporting the child or adolescent through treatment. Families often turn to the nurse for support and reassurance and find it comforting to work with a familiar and trusted team of nurses and providers. In some cases, families are asked to administer chemotherapy at home. Nurses work closely with these families to establish administration schedules, learn how to prepare and administer each medication safely, and understand which side effects to watch for and report (Box 69-3). They also teach the family about special considerations related to administering some agents. Most protocols and manufacturers now include specific instructions for these situations.

Radiation Therapy

Radiation therapy is a common form of treatment for pediatric malignancies. The advancement of new technologies such as proton beam therapy is promising. Evidence, however, is still emerging regarding the potential role these new technologies will have in maximizing disease control and achieving high-quality survivorship.[81] Often administered in an outpatient setting for a number of consecutive days and weeks, radiation therapy can have significant side effects in children. As part of the treatment planning process, most patients undergo radiation simulation to determine the radiation field. Simulation requires the use of markings, blocks, and immobilization devices to ensure that the radiation will be delivered consistently to the same location during each radiation session. Children younger than 4 years of age usually require sedation and central venous access for their simulation and radiation treatments.[82,83] Children between 4 and 6 years of age may be able to tolerate the sessions without sedation if distraction techniques and nursing support are made available. Children older than 7 years of age usually tolerate the treatments well and are able to cooperate during the sessions.[83]

Nursing care for a child undergoing radiation therapy includes discussing the treatment plan with the patient

Box 69-3   General Guidelines for Administering Chemotherapy by Family Members in the Home: What Families Need to Know

1. Treatment goals and plan, including the length of treatment, number of cycles and days of treatment
2. A schema or calendar that shows the general treatment plan
3. Names of all medications (brand and generic)
4. Indications for all medications
5. Doses of all medications, including the strengths
6. How to administer the medications
   a. Safe handling (e.g., disposal of waste products and management of chemotherapeutic exposure or spill)
   b. How to measure the medications, especially liquids
   c. What foods or drinks the medications can be mixed with or taken with
   d. What foods or drinks to avoid when taking the medications
7. How and when to take the medications (e.g., before or after meals, at bedtime)
8. The start and stop date or criteria for stopping
9. Expected and potential side effects and preventive measures for side effects
10. When to report side effects and whom to call

Data from references 71 and 77.

and family, describing what the simulation process involves, assessing the patient for side effects, and educating the patient and family how to prevent and manage side effects. Because the side effects of radiation therapy are related to the site that is irradiated, interventions to alleviate them vary accordingly. The mouth and skin are commonly affected, and all patients and families are taught proper mouth and skin care techniques before they begin treatment. Patients receiving radiation therapy in combination with chemotherapy or biotherapy are monitored closely because certain agents can produce an exacerbated effect known as radiation recall, a severe rash that requires special precautions and treatment.[82,83]

Biotherapy (Biologic Response Modifiers/Biologic Therapies/Targeted Therapy)

In recent years, biotherapy, also known as biologic response modifiers (BRMs), biologic therapies, and targeted therapy, has emerged as a treatment modality using immunologic mechanisms to eradicate tumor cells.[84] Biotherapy agents include a wide range of products such as vaccines, blood and blood components, allergenics, somatic cells, gene therapy, tissues, and recombinant therapeutic proteins.[76] For example, there are vaccines to help prevent cancers as well as those designed to treat cancer. Vaccines, such as the human papillomavirus vaccine, help protect against certain strains of viruses and ultimately may prevent some cancers. Alternatively, vaccines that treat cancers are intended to increase the patient's immune response with the goal of attacking cells with one or more specific antigens.[85]

Biologic therapies interact with the child's immune system to enhance the response to cancer and may cause toxicities influenced by the dose, route, and schedule of administration. The most common side effect of biotherapy is a flulike syndrome characterized by fever, chills, rigors, myalgias, headache, and fatigue.[86] The role of the nurse in caring for the patient receiving biotherapy includes obtaining baseline vital signs, administration of any prescribed medications, and close monitoring for side effects. During and after administration, the nurse observes the patient for tachycardia, hypotension, fever, chills, anaphylaxis, and signs of a local reaction. Nurses also teach the patient and family about potential side effects that might occur at home, when such side effects should be reported, and symptom management techniques.[86]

Hematopoietic Stem Cell Transplant

Hematopoietic stem cell transplant (HSCT) involves the intravenous infusion of autologous or allogeneic stem cells.[87] This modality is used to treat malignant and nonmalignant diseases, and more than 4000 HSCTs were performed in 2009-2010 in patients younger than the age of 20, revealing a 20% increase from 1993-1994.[87,88] Since its development in 1939 there have been advances in cell source; improved conditioning regimens; more exact human leukocyte antigen typing, thus improving donor and patient matches and increasing overall transplant survival; decreased incidence and severity of acute and chronic graft-versus-host disease; and improved rates of engraftment.[88,89]

In an effort to promote improvement in cellular therapy, regenerative medicine, and patient outcomes, more than 85% of all transplant facilities in the United States partner with the Foundation for the Accreditation of Cellular Therapy (FACT).[90] Founded in 1996, FACT has established standards for clinical and laboratory departments that apply to hematopoietic progenitor cells and other cells obtained from hematopoietic sources that include marrow, peripheral blood, and umbilical cord blood.[90] These standards are focused on processing the clinical use of cellular therapy products as well as ensuring that they are collected and processed using strict controls.[90] The primary role of the registered nurse is to participate in the coordination of the transplant and to ensure FACT standards related to nursing practice are understood and adhered to.

Preprocedure Phase. There are 75 pediatric FACT accredited HSCT centers in the United States.[90] As a result, many patients change providers and transfer care to one of these institutions for the duration of HSCT treatment. Nurses may help to facilitate patient transfer by coordinating aspects of the referral process, clinical evaluation, or preprocedure education in the patient and family's preferred language and counseling. The period before HSCT can be one of great anxiety for patients and families. Good communication between the referring institution and the transplant center helps to ensure a smooth transfer process and fosters trust between the families and the new provider. Preprocedure processes vary among institutions; however, most are focused on an exchange of information needed to appropriately plan for the transplant.

Inpatient Care. Although hospital mortality and complications after HSCT have decreased, hospital length of stay ranging between 2 weeks to several months requires an experienced, culturally competent multidisciplinary team.[91] Specially trained nurses familiar with the immune and hematopoietic systems, stem cell transplant concepts, and complex treatment protocols are key members of the team playing critical roles during each phase of the treatment process.[78] After admission, a core team of nurses is usually established to develop an individualized nursing plan of care and oversee the patient's nursing care throughout the hospitalization. By understanding the risk factors and potential complications associated with HSCT, the nursing team works closely with all members of the health care team to evaluate and revise the plan of care as needed. Throughout the patient's hospitalization nurses support the patient and family to ensure their understanding of the process, which includes careful monitoring, assessing the patient for side effects, and understanding adverse reactions associated with each type of transplant.[92]

Planning for discharge typically begins early in the hospitalization and becomes a higher priority as engraftment approaches. The nurse assists in the coordination of discharge, offering emotional support and providing education necessary to facilitate the transition of the patient and family back home. Discharge teaching should include instructions in the preferred language of the patient concerning medications that must be taken after discharge, the ambulatory treatment plan, the care that must be administered in the home, and arrangement of appropriate services. Careful discharge planning can reduce the anxiety many families experience as they transition home. In general, patients are required to remain in close proximity to the transplant center for the first 100 days after allogeneic transplant. Autologous transplant patients may be referred back to their primary physician once engraftment occurs and the risk for HSCT complications has decreased.[92]

Ambulatory Care and Acute Outpatient Follow-Up. After discharge from the hospital, outpatient care usually requires a combination of clinic and home care services. Some institutions provide housing close to the main hospital to allow for close supervision of the patient's status. Maintaining a consistent team of caregivers and good communication with the patient and family helps promote posttransplant recovery and minimizes toxicities and complications. HSCT patients continue to require treatment and close observation and may need to visit the oncology clinic as often as 5 days a week for the first few weeks. Outpatient nurses regularly assess the patient's physical status, administer prescribed treatment, and manage symptoms, particularly those associated with graft-versus-host disease and toxicities.

Clinical Trials

With approximately 60% of patients diagnosed with cancer younger than 29 years of age enrolling in clinical trials compared with less than 5% of adults with cancer, clinical trials are crucial to the treatment of children with cancer.[93] Most children receiving treatment today are either enrolled in a clinical trial or receiving therapy based on the findings of a previous clinical trial.

Permission to participate in a clinical trial must be obtained. If the patient is younger than the age of 18, permission must be granted by the patient's parent or guardian; however, many health care providers involved in treating young people believe that the child or adolescent should play a role in the decision to enter a research study, and they urge investigators to share information about the study with the child and obtain his or her assent or agreement to participate.[94,95] The National Commission for Protection of Human Subjects of Biomedical and Behavioral Research established age 7 as a reasonable minimum age for involving children in some kind of assent process.[94] After consenting to participate in a clinical trial, the child and family may have lingering questions about the study and turn to their nurse for clarification and more information. The nurse may arrange for them to meet again with the consenting physician to ensure that all questions have been addressed and that their decision to participate is truly informed.[95]

Once a patient has enrolled in a clinical trial, the research coordinator assigned to the trial, in partnership with the primary team, ensures that all required studies have been completed and that consent forms have been signed. Throughout the course of a trial, nurses help to oversee and maintain compliance with the study's protocol, provide ongoing staff education, and are primary collectors of the data used for dose adjustments and analyses. Nurses adhere to the principles of good clinical practices, including adequate human subject protection as a critical requirement to conducting research involving human subjects.[96] The role of the clinical research nurse includes, but is not limited to, administering investigational drugs; monitoring the patient's responses; assessing patient for adverse side effects in accordance with protocol criteria; collecting timed specimens according to the protocol schedule; and carefully documenting the start and stop times of drug administration.[97] Nurses also provide essential patient and family education and support, checking in with them frequently and bringing unresolved concerns to the attention of the team.[97,98]

Complementary and Alternative Medicine (Integrative Therapies)

It is not uncommon for a family whose child has been diagnosed with cancer to explore complementary and alternative medicine (CAM) at some point during the treatment process. CAM, also referred to as integrative therapies, includes practices and therapies that lie outside the realm of traditional medicine. They encompass a wide variety of approaches, including acupuncture, massage, imagery, energy healing, and prayer, as well as herbal, homeopathic, nutritional, and biologic therapies.[99] Although evidence that CAM improves immunity or promotes recovery is not well documented, the use of CAM among children and adolescents with cancer reportedly ranges between 46% and 85%.[100-102]

Even though CAM is not a replacement for standard pediatric oncology treatment, many patients and families view it as a form of adjunctive therapy that may be used to help relieve symptoms, cope with life-threatening illness, and improve well-being.[103] While working with a patient and family, pediatric oncology nurses and other providers should routinely assess whether the patient has used CAM. During all medication reviews, the patient and family should be asked to list any herbs and supplements the patient is taking. Although obtaining this information is an important part of the medication review process, many families report never having been asked about such practices.[103]

Patients often turn to nurses for information and insight about available therapies that might be useful to them. When trying to determine the best therapy for the patient, consideration should be given to the family's culture, spiritual beliefs, and practices and the patient's developmental level, education, and preferences.[99,104] Nurses' observations and documentation of a patient's response to CAM treatments are essential because they help providers gauge the impact of the treatments, as well as their potential interactions with individual therapies, and provide insight into the patient's coping strategies.

Symptom Management and Supportive Nursing Care

The advanced, complex treatment regimens designed to cure childhood cancer commonly produce multiple distressing side effects. Each treatment modality carries the potential for side effects that can occur during treatment or days, weeks, or even years after treatment. Side effects such as hair loss and low blood cell counts may be transient, whereas others, such as hearing loss and learning disabilities, can be permanent.[77,105] The most commonly reported side effects in children and adolescents with cancer include infection, bleeding, anemia, nutritional problems, nausea, vomiting, mucositis, fatigue, and pain.[61] Studies have found that children report nausea, fatigue, and pain as the most distressing.[106,107] Although many side effects can be effectively managed, some families believe suffering is to be expected among children with cancer. As a result, side effects may go unreported for a time and children may suffer unnecessary distress.[108,109]

Nurses help manage the side effects of cancer treatment by using strategies that have been tested and proven effective through research and evidence.[105] The nurse continually evaluates the effectiveness of symptom management strategies and, when necessary, collaborates with the interdisciplinary team to revise the plan so that it matches the needs and experiences of the individual patient. The following section summarizes specific nursing interventions associated with some of the most common and troubling side effects encountered in children with cancer.

Myelosuppression

Myelosuppression is a condition in which bone marrow activity is decreased, resulting in fewer red blood cells, white blood cells, and platelets.[110] It is the most common toxicity associated with radiation and many chemotherapeutic agents.[105] It can also occur with certain malignancies, such as leukemia, sarcoma, neuroblastoma, and lymphoma.[61] Patients receiving myelosuppressive agents commonly experience a nadir between 10 and 14 days after the end of treatment. With subsequent courses of myelosuppressive agents, the nadir and recovery from the nadir can be affected by the number and type of agents given and the timing of their administration.[105,111] Pediatric oncology nurses monitor a patient's response to treatment over time and anticipate complications of myelosuppression, such as infection, bleeding, and fatigue. Educating families to be aware of the signs and symptoms associated with complications related to myelosuppression, as well as when to report these symptoms, is an important part of the overall care of patients receiving cancer treatment.

Neutropenia

Neutropenia is characterized by an absolute neutrophil count of 1000 per mm^3 or less.[77] It is the most severe consequence of bone marrow suppression, increasing a patient's risk for potentially life-threatening infections, a risk that is higher when neutropenia is prolonged for more than 7 days. When neutropenia presents as fever, it must be treated as an emergency with broad-spectrum antibiotics administered as soon as possible.[112] The neutropenic patient often does not present with the routine signs of infection. In many cases, fever may be the only presenting symptom.[113,114]

Hand washing before and after contact with each patient minimizes the risk for microbial transmission and is the single most important method for preventing nosocomial infection.[115-117] BRMs can also help lower a patient's risk for infection by shortening the period of myelosuppression. These agents are usually given 24 hours after chemotherapy administration as a one-time subcutaneous injection or daily by the nurse, patient, or family member until the white blood cell count recovers.[118,119] Because many children associate subcutaneous injections with pain and fear, nurses use creative techniques and special devices to ameliorate the discomfort associated with these injections.

Major pathogens that cause infections in the neutropenic patients are bacteria, fungi, viruses, and protozoa, with gram-negative bacterial infections associated with higher mortality rates than all other causes of infection.[112] The administration of prophylactic antibiotics to prevent *Pneumocystis jiroveci* (formerly known as *Pneumocystis carinii*) pneumonia, a protozoal infection found in patients with prolonged neutropenia, is also a standard practice in many cancer treatment protocols.[120,121] These antibiotics are usually administered in an oral form and are commonly given throughout treatment. Getting children to take daily oral medications can be very distressing for parents of young children and adolescents. Teaching parents techniques that will help them to administer medications successfully and emphasizing the importance of the medications enhances the parents' ability to cope and has the potential to increase overall compliance with prescribed medication regimens.

Educating the patient and family about neutropenia is critically important. Elements of this education must include the meaning of blood cell counts, signs and symptoms of infection, an understanding that the time of greatest risk for infection occurs during nadir, and strategies to minimize the risk for infection (Box 69-4).[122,123] Because the family plays an important role in monitoring a patient for signs of infection, nurses also focus on teaching them when to contact the child's provider. Family members are taught how to take a temperature and that the presence of a fever may signal an emergency; they are instructed to call the provider whenever the child's temperature is higher than 38° C (100.4° F) on two occasions within 24 hours and to call immediately whenever it is higher than 38.5° C (101.3° F) (or per institutional guidelines). They are also taught to report any respiratory symptoms, shaking chills, and changes in the child's level of consciousness and are instructed not to administer acetaminophen unless directed to do so by the provider. In addition to reviewing these instructions regularly, nurses make sure family members have emergency contact information. Families must be taught the critical nature of fever and neutropenia and the importance of initiating antibiotics rapidly.

Early assessment and intervention are key to successfully managing a febrile neutropenic patient.[105] Whenever a fever is present, blood cultures are obtained from central venous access devices and peripheral sources. Broad-spectrum antibiotics are usually started within 60 minutes of the diagnosis of fever and neutropenia.[124] Treatment

---

Box 69-4 Neutropenic Precautions: Guidelines for Patients and Families

- Notify the physician if the child exhibits any of the following:
  - Oral or axillary temperature is ≥38.5°C (101.3°F) or is 38°(100.4°F)C two times within 24 hours
  - Oral lesions
  - Erythema at central venous access site
  - Open skin lesions
  - Perirectal laceration or irritation
  - Cough
  - Rhinorrhea
  - Tachypnea
  - Complaints of ear or throat pain
  - Diarrhea
  - Lethargy
- Perform meticulous hand washing.
- Do not take rectal temperatures or give suppositories.
- Avoid crowds and people who are sick.
- Do not share utensils with others.
- Do not let the child provide direct care to pets (e.g., the child should not change kitty litter).
- Do not keep reptiles or birds as pets.
- The child and siblings should not receive live-virus vaccines.
- Avoid exposure to mold (e.g., digging in soil).
- Practice good mouth care.

Data from references 122 and 123.

---

may be modified once the results of the culture and sensitivity are available and the specific organism has been identified. Antifungal therapy is often added if the patient's fever persists despite antibiotic treatment.

Most patients with fever and neutropenia are admitted to the hospital for treatment. During this time, nurses observe patients closely for signs and symptoms of septic shock by monitoring vital signs, peripheral perfusion, and intake and output. The patient's neurologic status is also monitored closely because lethargy, irritability, or a change in consciousness can indicate sepsis. Mouth care and perianal hygiene are performed on a routine basis. Rectal temperatures and suppositories are avoided in all neutropenic patients based on the risk for tearing the anal mucosa and introducing bacteria.

Anemia

Anemia can occur secondary to myelosuppression after chemotherapy or radiation therapy, most commonly appearing 7 to 10 days after treatment. It can also occur as a result of blood loss, metastasis to the bone marrow, or viral suppression.[105] Nurses routinely monitor all patients for symptoms of anemia, watching for pallor (particularly of the lips and conjunctiva), fatigue, tachycardia, gallop rhythm, headache, dizziness, dyspnea on exertion, and irritability.

Many children exhibit a high tolerance for low hemoglobin levels. Transfusions, however, are commonly necessary when the patient is symptomatic, hemoglobin is less than 7 g/dL, and the hematocrit is less than 21%. Recombinant human erythropoietin may be used to increase red cell recovery and decrease the need for transfusions, especially when the patient and family object to blood transfusions on the basis of religious beliefs. It takes erythropoietin 2 to 4 weeks to stimulate red cell precursors, whereas the effects of a transfusion are immediate.[118] Transfusion amounts are generally in the range of 10 to 20 mL/kg. Red blood cells should be leukoreduced to decrease alloimmunization and irradiated to inactivate T cells and reduce the risk for graft-versus-host reactions.[125]

Because the patient and family are often the first to note symptoms of anemia, the nurse focuses patient and family education on anemia, its symptoms, when it is most likely to occur, and how to manage symptoms at home, such as providing frequent rest periods. If a transfusion is ordered, nurses follow a standardized protocol to ensure that the blood product is administered safely and monitor the patient frequently for fever, chills, body aches, urticaria, pruritus, wheezing, respiratory distress, and other signs of reaction to transfusion.[105,126,127] Prior to the transfusion, a patient may require premedications to prevent transfusion reactions. Once the transfusion is complete, the nurse documents the patient's tolerance of the transfusion and whether premedications were administered. This information is important to guide future transfusions.

Thrombocytopenia

Thrombocytopenia, or a platelet count of less than 100,000/mm³, can be caused by myelosuppressive therapy, disease, or coagulopathy.[127] Thrombocytopenic patients are at risk for internal bleeding when the platelet count falls below 15,000 to 20,000/mm³.[127,128] Nurses instruct the patient and family in strategies for preventing injury, hence minimizing the chances that bleeding will occur (Box 69-5).[129] Nurses regularly assess a thrombocytopenic patient's risk for bleeding and communicate any

---

Box 69-5 Bleeding Precautions (Platelet Count <20,000/mm³): Guidelines for Patients and Families

- Notify the physician if the child exhibits any of the following:
  - Increased bruising
  - Evidence of bleeding
  - If a nosebleed occurs, pinch the nostrils together for at least 10 minutes. (Use gauze to pinch the nostrils, holding it between your thumb and forefinger.) Go to the emergency department if the bleeding persists after this time.
  - Change in level of consciousness
- Whenever the platelet level drops below 50,000/mm³, avoid skateboarding, trampolines, contact sports, and other activities that can cause bleeding.
- Always wear a helmet when riding a bicycle.
- Shave only with an electric razor.
- Clean teeth with a soft toothbrush or gauze. Do not use dental floss.
- Avoid sharp foods such as tortillas that can cause gum injury and bleeding.
- Avoid aspirin, aspirin products, and ibuprofen.
- To prevent straining, keep stools soft using prescribed laxatives and stool softeners.
- Avoid taking rectal temperature, enemas, and suppositories.
- Oral contraceptives may be prescribed to prevent excess bleeding during menses.
- Avoid sexual intercourse.

Modified from Elliott S: Thrombocytopenia. In Kline N, Brace-O'Neill J, Hooke M, et al, editors: Essentials of pediatric oncology nursing: a core curriculum, *2nd ed. Chicago, 2004, Association of Pediatric Oncology Nurses, p. 69–70.*

pertinent laboratory findings or symptoms to the clinical team. Platelets are commonly administered when patients are symptomatic, if below 50,000/mm³ and scheduled for a lumbar puncture, or in accordance with institutional or protocol guidelines. Patients receiving platelets are monitored carefully during and after the transfusion for signs of transfusion reaction.[125,127,128]

Fatigue

Fatigue is a major side effect of cancer treatment in children and adolescents.[130-132] Although defining fatigue in children undergoing cancer treatment has been challenging, children and adolescents can reliably describe the physical and mental symptoms associated with fatigue. Nurses routinely assess for fatigue throughout the course of treatment to determine possible factors that may contribute to fatigue, such as nutritional problems, pain, dehydration, and patterns of activity.[130,131] While caring for patients, nurses incorporate interventions designed to minimize fatigue. For example, with hospitalized children, incorporating adequate sleep time into the plan for the day and minimizing noise during sleep hours can sometimes be effective. In outpatient settings, nurses work with other members of the care team to avoid long waiting times to conserve and maximize energy, ensure adequate time for rest, and work with patients and families to optimize the patient's nutritional status. Other interventions and treatments that may decrease fatigue include pharmacologic assistance, physical activity, and distraction techniques. Integrative therapies that promote well-being and relaxation, such as massage and Reiki therapy, are increasingly employed in symptom management and show promise for relieving fatigue and promoting well-being.[99,103,104]

Nausea and Vomiting

Nausea and vomiting are common side effects of cancer treatment and described by patients as the second most distressing symptom after fatigue.[106] Uncontrolled vomiting can produce its own complications because it may quickly lead to dehydration and electrolyte imbalance. In some cases, nausea and vomiting can become dose-limiting side effects of chemotherapy if resolution requires a delay in treatment or a reduction in the chemotherapy dose.[76,105]

For a patient just beginning chemotherapy, the first cycle offers predictors of the chemotherapy's emetogenic potential. Antiemetics are typically ordered on the basis of symptoms observed during and after the cycle and adjusted according to the patient's response to subsequent cycles. The antiemetic regimen can also be adjusted to accommodate escalating doses of chemotherapy, as well as to manage breakthrough nausea and vomiting. Other interventions that may benefit some patients include antispasmodic therapy, relaxation techniques, acupuncture, and guided imagery.

Nurses routinely assess patients for nausea and vomiting during each chemotherapy cycle, obtaining information that helps in establishing and evaluating the effectiveness of the antiemetic regimen. They often encourage patients and families to maintain a diary describing the response to the antiemetic treatment and to list management strategies that the patient finds effective. Such information can help providers fine-tune the antiemetic regimen to the individual patient. When teaching patients and families about the regimen, nurses stress the importance of continuing antiemetics for the prescribed length of time.

Mucositis

Mucositis, or damage to the gastrointestinal cells and ulcerations of the mucosa, can develop as a result of chemotherapy or radiation therapy.[133] Ulcers that occur in the mouth are a dose-limiting toxicity that affects quality of life. Painful mouth ulcers make it difficult to eat and drink and can compromise a patient's nutritional status.[134,135]

Before treatment begins, patients are instructed to obtain dental care to ensure good oral hygiene and integrity. If applicable, they are usually asked to have their braces removed to decrease the potential for infection and gum irritation. Once treatment starts, nurses work closely with patients and families to ensure adequate oral hygiene and decrease the risk for mucositis. Upon meeting with patients and their families, nurses assess the patient's oral cavity and their baseline oral hygiene habits. The nurse instructs them in the techniques of good oral care, including rinsing the mouth frequently with water using a saline solution and a soft toothbrush or gauze to clean the teeth and gums three to four times a day.[105,136,137] Nurses also assess patients for mouth pain and discomfort and work with the care team to alleviate pain and promote adequate nutrition.

A wide variety of agents are marketed for the treatment and prevention of mucositis. Recent studies have shown that cold substances administered to the oral mucosa during chemotherapy administration (e.g., having patients suck on flavored ice popsicles) can help prevent mucosal cell damage.[133]

Pain

Pain is a common and distressing side effect of pediatric cancer and cancer treatment. Although techniques for managing pain effectively in children and adolescents are widely available, patients with cancer still experience unnecessary suffering. Inadequate pain assessment and poor communication between patients and providers are just two of the barriers to successful pain management. Other obstacles include lack of knowledge by health care providers about the manifestations of pain in pediatric patients and about how it is best managed. Taking the time to assess patients regularly to determine the type, cause, location, and intensity of pain will assist in developing an individualized management plan to relieve pain and optimize quality of life.

The use of a procedure room should be considered for hospitalized patients undergoing painful procedures in an effort to preserve the bed as a safe place. In addition, limiting the number of attempts by a single health care provider is one technique used to minimize discomfort. Whereas institution-specific procedures may define the process for managing multiple unsuccessful attempts by

---

Box 69-6   Common Myths and Barriers to Effective Pain Management in Children

ASSESSMENT

A child reports pain to the nurse or doctor.
If a child does not complain of pain, the child is not suffering.
It is always possible to determine whether a child is faking pain or truly suffering.
Active or sleeping children cannot be in pain.
Pain must have an evident stimulus; without one, a child cannot be feeling pain.
If a child is in pain, the parent would know it.

DIAGNOSIS

Infants have immature nervous systems and therefore feel less pain.
Children do not remember painful events.
Children become accustomed to pain and no longer feel it.
Children cannot communicate the location and intensity of pain.
Neurologically impaired children do not feel pain.
Adolescents are drug seekers.

PAIN MANAGEMENT

It is unsafe to administer opioids to children because of respiratory depression and addiction.
The best way to give an analgesic is intramuscularly.
It is unsafe to give narcotics through a central line.
Administering morphine means the patient is dying.

Modified from Jodarski K, Wilson K: Pain. In Kline NE, Brace-O'Neill J, Hooke MC, et al, editors. Essentials of pediatric oncology nursing: a core curriculum, 2nd ed. Glenview, IL, 2004, Association of Pediatric Oncology Nurses, p. 155.

one provider, if not otherwise specified it is recommended that a provider seek the assistance of another provider after three unsuccessful attempts.

Over the past decade, providers have become more aware of and concerned about pain in children, and efforts to understand and manage all aspects of pain have resulted in an overall improvement in pain management.[68,138] The creation of dedicated teams of clinicians who specialize in the treatment of pain has also contributed to the introduction of new drug combinations and techniques for the treatment and control of pain.[139]

Assessing Pain and Developing a Pain Management Plan. For pain to be effectively managed, dispelling the myths that exist regarding pain in children is important (Box 69-6) because believing any one of them can markedly compromise efforts to manage a patient's pain.[67,140] Although the most accurate and reliable indicator of pain remains the patient's report, many children cannot or do not consistently and independently report pain. Therefore health care providers must consider the physiologic and psychological components of pain and develop techniques for routine assessment.[67,68]

Finding the most effective pain management strategy begins with assessment. Nurses conduct routine pain assessments incorporating an understanding of the common types of pain and an appreciation of how pain is manifested by children at varying developmental stages. Because pain can affect patients differently, a comprehensive assessment typically includes the patient's pain threshold, fears related to particular drugs, cultural beliefs, anxiety level concerning pain control and, in adolescents and young adults, past use of alcohol or illicit drugs. A key component of the assessment also involves measuring the intensity of pain with an appropriate instrument. The most common scales use faces or numbers to gauge a patient's pain level. Scales that incorporate faces are particularly helpful in pediatrics because they can be understood by a variety of age groups and by patients who do not speak English.[141] Numerical scales, which generally ask the patient to rate pain on a scale of 1 to 10, are appropriate for children 5 years of age and older.[67,140,142]

Managing Pain and Stress during Invasive Procedures. Cancer treatment often involves numerous invasive procedures, such as bone marrow aspirations and lumbar punctures. Children with cancer perceive these procedures as extremely painful[143] and often report years later that the procedures were the most frightening and traumatic part of their cancer care.[134,144,145] Studies have demonstrated that children do not adapt to procedure-related pain; instead, the trauma and anxiety associated with procedures increases with repeated painful experiences.[61,143,146]

The pain and stress involved in procedures is commonly underestimated. Providers who believe that a procedure is brief and that sedation is time consuming may fail to manage procedural pain and anxiety with adequate attention. Offering support and preventing pain during procedures is the responsibility of nurses and physicians. A preprocedure assessment is usually conducted to determine the approach that is best suited to each particular patient.

Properly preparing a child to prevent trauma during the first procedure has been shown to have a direct impact on the ability of the child or adolescent to tolerate and cope with subsequent procedures.[134] A patient optimally managed through a combination of pain medication, careful timing, and parental support seems to be less anxious about and fearful of successive procedures.[142] A child who has had traumatic experiences during procedures in the past may demonstrate such symptoms as insomnia, anxiety, regression, and depression as the time for another procedure approaches.[61,140,145,146] If these symptoms do appear, providers should question whether past efforts to prevent or control pain have been adequate.

Researchers continue to build evidence for the best way to prepare a child for invasive procedures. Studies support general anesthesia as a safe and effective method of pain control and psychological support because procedural anesthesia does not require intubation and is accomplished quickly and effectively through the use of short-acting intravenous anesthetic agents.[143,147] If anesthesia services are not available, procedural sedation is recommended. Procedural sedation involves various pharmacologic combinations, most commonly an opioid analgesic such as fentanyl and a benzodiazepine such as midazolam, for anxiolysis and sedation.[142,144] Used in combination, these agents depress the level of consciousness while still allowing the child to maintain his or her airway independently and to respond to physical stimulation or verbal command. Carefully administering agents before and during the procedure can ensure a pain-free experience for children and adolescents.

A patient scheduled to receive general anesthesia or procedural sedation is ordered to have nothing to eat or drink for 6 to 8 hours before the scheduled procedure. An infant may have breast milk for up to 4 hours before and clear liquids until 2 hours before sedation. Ideally, the withholding of food and fluids begins at night and the procedure is performed early the following day to limit the child's distress. The nurse assisting with the procedure prepares the procedure room, ensuring that all necessary equipment such as oxygen saturation and cardiac monitor is available. For procedures performed with the patient under general anesthesia, the anesthesiologist ascertains that all the necessary anesthesia and emergency equipment is available, administers anesthetic agents, and monitors the patient. When procedural conscious sedation is used, the patient's physician or nurse practitioner usually determines the time of the procedure and prescribes the sedative agents to be used. The nurse assisting with the procedure initiates the time out, administers the prescribed sedative agents, and may also administer antiemetics if intrathecal chemotherapy is being given. During a procedure, the nurse carefully monitors vital signs and oxygenation. A pulse and oxygen saturation monitor is generally used throughout the procedure and for at least 30 minutes during the recovery period or until the patient's values return to baseline.[68,144]

For less invasive procedures, the application of a local anesthetic cream to the procedure site several hours before the procedure has been found to reduce pain. Applied in a thick layer (2 mm) and covered by an occlusive dressing that is left undisturbed for an hour, the anesthetic cream penetrates the skin and provides local anesthesia up to a depth of 5 mm for 2 to 3 hours. Anesthetic creams have been found to reduce the pain associated with a range of procedures, including venipuncture, lumbar puncture, injection, and accessing indwelling central venous lines.[148,149] In an ambulatory setting, a nurse may teach the parents to apply the cream before leaving home so it is at peak effectiveness on arrival at the hospital. The cream's effectiveness may be decreased by poor hydration and dark skin pigmentation and offers limited effectiveness in controlling the pain of bone marrow aspiration, which requires the addition of locally injected lidocaine and procedural sedation or anesthesia.

Stress Reduction Techniques. A child often benefits from having parents with them during a procedure. This is particularly true for toddlers and preschoolers for whom separation anxiety is a developmental issue. During the procedure, the parents should be positioned close to the child so they can offer reassurance and comfort and help the child use stress reduction and coping techniques. A parent who is uncomfortable staying with the child should be supported in that decision and given reassurance that the child will be well cared for and that a member of the team, such as a child life specialist or a member of the psychosocial staff, will be available to offer the child support.

A variety of behavioral techniques, such as music therapy, distraction, and relaxation methods, can be useful in reducing anxiety and managing the pain associated with cancer treatment and invasive procedures. Nurses routinely work with other members of the care team to identify techniques appropriate for the patient and to help the patient and family learn and use the techniques during treatment.[150] The appropriate stress-reduction techniques for a particular child are determined in part by the child's developmental age and individual preferences. An infant, for example, may benefit from sucking on a pacifier or sucrose nipple, whereas a toddler may be distracted by a book, a tactile toy, or music. Guided imagery often works well with a child of school age or older; an adolescent may prefer being distracted by a CD player with headphones or a video game. Medical play may also be used to help relieve a child's anxiety. Introduced before a procedure is performed, it allows the child to perform the procedure on a doll and to ask questions and examine equipment that will be used. Such play allows a child to gain insight into and understanding of the procedure and the sensations he or she will experience.[47,140]

Central Venous Catheters

Central venous catheters (CVCs) are one of the most important advances in the treatment and supportive care of children with cancer. The most commonly used CVCs are peripherally inserted central venous catheters, tunneled central venous lines, and implantable reservoirs inserted under the skin, also known as portacaths. Today, a CVC is considered integral to managing patient care; minimizing discomfort caused by placement of peripheral intravenous lines; and ensuring safe administration of blood products, parenteral nutrition, chemotherapy, antibiotics, and antifungal and other agents. CVCs can also be used to obtain blood samples and perform infusions in the patient's home.[149]

Complications associated with CVCs include local and systemic infections, central line–associated bloodstream infections (CLABSIs), septic thrombophlebitis, and endocarditis.[115] Other potential complications include bleeding, thrombus formation, and catheter damage or dislodgment. The complications can be significant, but the benefits of using CVCs generally outweigh the risks. To minimize and prevent complications, meticulous care of the CVC is required. Maintenance of a CVC requires special care to reduce the risk for infections. Extensive staff, patient, and family education must be conducted to ensure consistent and effective care of the CVC and the ability to identify the signs and symptoms of infection. To prevent the possibility of a nosocomial infection, caring for a patient with a CVC requires training in proper aseptic technique and good hand washing. In recent years, some institutions have found that a 15-second wipe of the cap prior to the entering line is the minimum necessary to remove bacteria. Guidelines developed by the manufacturer or institution-specific policies and procedures are designed to minimize the risk for infection and should be followed whenever a CVC is accessed.[117,121]

One of the most common complications in a CVC is a CLASBI. If a CLASBI is suspected, blood cultures are drawn immediately and antibiotic therapy is started. The administration of antibiotics for treatment of the infection should be alternated between the catheter's lumens, so that each lumen of a double- or triple-lumen catheter is used and the risk for colonizing an unused lumen is minimized. Depending on the institution's guidelines, the CVC may be removed, particularly if the patient has positive blood cultures 72 hours after antibiotics are initiated, evidence of tunnel infection, catheter-related septic shock, or occlusion of catheter that cannot be cleared by thrombolytic or chemical treatments.[124] If the CVC is not removed, parenteral antibiotic therapy usually continues for 7 to 10 days after a first negative blood culture is obtained in a patient who is not immunocompromised and for 10 to 14 days in an immunocompromised patient.[151,152]

Reduction of CLABSIs has become a national priority as well as an institutional one for many centers. CLABSIs are defined by the Centers for Disease Control and Prevention (CDC)/National Healthcare Safety Network (NHSN) and are a source of morbidity, mortality and increased medical costs.[153] The NHSN, established by the CDC, reported that in 2004 the mean among 54 pediatric intensive care units (PICUs) was 6.6 bloodstream infections per 1000 catheter-days, higher than many adult centers.[153] Recognizing the impact CLABSIs have on patients, families and institutions as well as in an effort to reduce infections, the National Association of Children's Hospitals and Related Institutions (NACHRI) partnered with clinical providers on a quality improvement initiative to examine bloodstream catheter infections in its (PICUs. Small tests of change were implemented and identified best practice, which included insertion and maintenance care bundles. Changes implemented resulted in a decrease of bloodstream infections from 5.40 per 1000 catheter-days to 3.10 per 1000 catheter-days. After 1 year the NACHRI PICU collaborative achieved a 43% reduction in catheter-associated bloodstream infection rates.[153] To date, pediatric oncology centers throughout the country are participating in a separate NACHRI collaborative specific to hematology, oncology, and stem cell transplant patients, with the goal of reducing bloodstream infections. Critical to prevention of CVC infections is focused education and training. Adherence to best practice and maintenance of the CVC, performance improvement plans, and nurse staffing are critical in prevention efforts to reduce bloodstream infections.[154]

Although a CVC is typically cared for by the nurse while a patient is in the hospital or clinic, the patient and family assume that responsibility at home. Patient and family education related to using and caring for the line at home is an important part of nursing care. Teaching begins before the line is inserted and covers a range of topics, such as proper technique for CVC dressing changes, how to flush the line with saline and heparin safely, and how to recognize the signs and symptoms of complications. Education of the patient and family consists of a series of demonstrations by the nurse of all procedures necessary to care for the CVC, followed by return-demonstrations by the parents. During the return-demonstration the nurse is able to evaluate technique and identify areas that need additional review. Other teaching materials, such as books and teaching dolls, may also be used. In addition to the management of the CVC, the patient and family are taught to identify the signs and symptoms of infection and to report untoward findings to the physician immediately. Family members are instructed to avoid giving antipyretics unless directed by the provider.

A patient with a CVC is also referred to a home care nursing service that provides nursing support and instruction in the child's home. The child's inpatient or clinic nurse works in collaboration with the home care agency to ensure that the supplies needed to care for the CVC and any prescribed medications are delivered to the patient's home.

Caring for Patients Across Multiple Treatment Locations

For many pediatric cancer patients, treatment spans months or years and takes place in multiple settings. Much of a patient's care is delivered through an ambulatory clinic, but many patients are hospitalized from time to time and also receive care from home care providers. Coordinating care across multiple sites and providers presents a complex challenge for the pediatric oncology care team as well as for the patient and family. Good communication, clear documentation, and careful planning are essential to safe and seamless care. Before a patient leaves a setting, the care team must develop a transition plan to ensure that the patient and family, as well as the team receiving the patient, are well informed about the patient's needs and treatment. In addition, nurses or social workers serving as case managers or care coordinators work with the primary care team to arrange for community services and obtain insurance approval for services and equipment the patient will need.[49,155]

Nursing agencies and other organizations in the community are often called on to help with a patient's care in the home. Some pediatric oncology patients may require home care nursing to assist with central line care, hyperalimentation, chemotherapy or antibiotic therapy, pain management, and psychological support. A home infusion company may also be involved to provide line care, infusion supplies, and pumps.

Although most patients receive the majority of their chemotherapy in an ambulatory clinic, some patients and families choose to administer chemotherapy at home, with the support of a home chemotherapy and infusion service. Research has shown that such home treatment programs are associated with lower total costs and yield no significant differences in patient outcomes.[156-158] Patients and families have noted that these programs not only help to decrease disruptions to their daily lives but also help reduce psychological distress.[159]

Whenever home care nurses or other community-based services are brought into a patient's home, the primary nurse from the inpatient or ambulatory setting should speak with the home care provider to provide a detailed patient history and outline specific home care needs. Written communication detailing specific flushing orders, cap changes, protocols, blood sampling, and when to call the doctor should also be provided. Once the patient is home, communication between the home care agency and the patient's providers must continue to ensure that the treatment plan is carried out appropriately and that the home care nurses know when and whom to call if they have questions or concerns.

PHARMACEUTICAL ADVANCES

Emerging Therapies

Advances in molecular biology and translational research will eventually allow selective targeting of tumor cells and radically change the way children with cancer are treated. Investigators who identify the underlying biology, potential obstacles to delivering the therapy, and the possible impact of new therapies on the practice of pediatric oncology will be preparing for the future of pediatric oncology. In recent years, treatment of genetically defined cancers—those cancers known to harbor specific genetic abnormalities—has moved away from general cytoxic chemotherapies toward agents that specifically target proteins and signaling pathways that cancer cells need for their growth. Called targeted therapies, these agents can induce dramatic clinical responses and offer significant therapeutic benefits in treating many previously hard-to-treat cancers, including certain melanomas, colorectal cancers, thyroid cancers, and advanced lung cancers.[160] As these therapies start to become available in clinical trials for children, pediatric oncology nurses will have to be educated regarding the agents, administration, adverse reactions, and side effects.

Patient Safety Considerations

Advances in the delivery of cancer therapies have reduced the risk for medication errors and improved patient safety. One of the most technologically advanced methods of reducing medication errors has been attributed to barcoding medication administration (BCMA). Until recently, general initiatives in place to reduce medication errors were limited to an institutional awareness of safety, examining the processes around medication administration to identify sources of error, and reviewing medication events. The advent of barcoding brought with it the ability of the nurse to verify the identification of the patient and prescribed medication via technology and thus not having to rely only on visually checking the medicine and patient to confirm that the "five rights" (right patient, drug, dose, route, and time) are correct. The literature has reported significant reductions in medication administration errors, from 50% to 90%, comparing retrospective data prior to BCMA with adverse event reporting after implementation and potential errors avoided.[75] One estimate is that BCMA may prevent more than 84,000 medication errors in the United States.[161]

SUPPORTING PATIENTS AND FAMILIES AT THE END OF TREATMENT

Usually, the patient and family eagerly await the completion of treatment. Its arrival, however, may be accompanied by uncertainty and fear. For some patients and families, ending treatment means a departure from the relative security of routine visits to the oncologist and signals a return to their pre-cancer world. This transition is typically accompanied by a whole host of worries about their child's future and the potential for recurrence. Some of the anxieties troubling a patient and family stem from the fear that once the cancer is no longer actively battled, the child will become more vulnerable to illness or disease. This anxiety is often heightened by the gradual loss of contact with the health care team as providers pay more attention to "sick families" and by the loss of the psychosocial support that the team has long provided.[21,162-164] Helping the patient and family transition from active treatment is an important part of comprehensive cancer care. The primary oncologist and nurse or nurse practitioner play key roles in this process because they provide much of the guidance and information that the patient and family need to transition from treatment successfully.[162,165]

The Emotional Impact of Transitioning from Treatment

For the patient and family, leaving the safety net provided by the health care team means they must adapt to living with the uncertainties of surviving cancer while reestablishing the life they had before cancer was diagnosed.[163-165] Often a patient finds it difficult to reassume the role of a well person and to integrate back into the contexts of family, school, and community.[163,164] Although the literature suggests that most childhood cancer survivors do relatively well from an emotional perspective, studies indicate that some survivors and their parents can exhibit trauma-related symptomatology and experience ongoing worry and alienation. For many survivors and families, the impact of the cancer experience stays with them long after treatment is over.[166-168]

The context of posttraumatic stress can help clinicians understand the long-term psychological reactions of the survivor and family.[168] The end of treatment may signal a return to normalcy from the providers' perspective, but it can hold a very different meaning for the patient and family. An individual's ability to reintegrate into the community and adjust to a "new normal" as a cancer survivor can be impacted by the psychological sequelae that result from prolonged uncertainty; the emotions, ranging from joy to unspeakable sadness; the restrictions the patient and family must still observe; and the extra work and overall loss associated with the cancer experience.[164,167]

Supporting the Transition

Patients' descriptions of their experiences after cancer treatment suggest that they and their families often need help in accepting and dealing with their new situations and circumstances.[162,163] Before providers can help patients and families, however, they must first understand the psychosocial impact of childhood cancer, as well as the heightened fears and the intense need for reassurance that families experience once treatment is over. These needs and fears may be especially evident when the child experiences common illnesses or during follow-up procedures and appointments.[21,165,166]

Nurses, physicians, and other providers can help to alleviate the fears of patients and families by validating the psychological distress that may surface at the end of treatment, by answering all questions, by providing honest feedback, and by helping them to begin to trust their ability to adjust to life after treatment.[41,164] Additional strategies include providing patients and families with ample opportunity to discuss concerns, acknowledging that fears of recurrence are normal, and preventing additional anxiety by ensuring that all posttreatment test results are reported to patients and families in as timely a manner as possible.[163]

The oncology team can also help to prepare patients and families for the challenges that lie ahead by teaching them about what to expect once treatment is over and by connecting them to programs that support the reintegration process. Support groups, programs that help with school reentry, camps that allow patients to socialize with other cancer survivors, and clinics that focus on cancer survival can all be instrumental in helping patients and families adjust to life after treatment.[163,169,170] Efforts to educate the patient and family and to support their transition from treatment can not only facilitate psychosocial adaptation but also improve the quality of life for cancer survivors.[165,171]

Because nurses are a primary source of support and information for patients and families, they play a critical role in ensuring a successful transition that is based on a unique understanding of the indicators of healthy transition: patient and family demonstration of an overall sense of well-being, observed mastery of skills required for home management, and well-being of the relationships among family members.[172] Nurses employ a variety of strategies to support transition after cancer treatment, which include, but are not limited to, an assessment of readiness, as well as the provision of materials and information about resources that patients can draw on once they leave the oncology setting. Information about programs and support groups for cancer survivors and written materials that outline follow-up care and potential side effects of treatment can be invaluable resources for patients and families as they leave the structure and security of the hospital and transition to other care settings.[162]

NURSING CARE OF CHILDHOOD CANCER SURVIVORS

The treatment of childhood cancer is one of the great medical success stories of the past 30 years. During this time, the cure rate for all childhood cancers has risen to 78%, resulting in a dramatic increase in the population of childhood cancer survivors.[173] Today, approximately 1 in 640 adults between the ages of 20 and 39 have a history of childhood cancer.[174] One unfortunate conse-

quence of this success is that late effects of childhood cancer treatment are now more commonly seen, effects that can occur during childhood or many years afterward, sometimes with devastating consequences. As many as two thirds of survivors experience late effects, and as many as a fourth experience an effect that is life-threatening.[174] Among the late effects that pose risks to cancer survivors are learning disabilities, infertility, heart problems, secondary tumors, and genetic issues.[162,169]

Although systematic and consistent follow-up of childhood cancer survivors is recommended, there is no consensus about where this care should be provided, who should provide it, or the detailed components that such care should entail.[174] The appropriate time to transfer care is also controversial and is dependent on the provider, although many suggest transitioning to long-term follow-up once a child has been off therapy for 2 years.

The primary pediatric oncology team, which typically has an intense investment in the childhood cancer survivor, may be reluctant to transition care to the primary provider; however, planning for the transition is essential and should begin well before follow-up care is needed. Developing a plan that includes detailed written information about the patient's specific cancer and treatment protocol ensures that the primary provider will have the necessary information to provide appropriate follow-up care. Other necessary information includes the medications the patient received (including dosages); the radiation therapy administered (including dosages); the surgical procedures performed; and any complications of therapy that the patient experienced. The oncology team should also equip the patient with documentation describing the cancer, its treatment, and possible long-term effects. Such a document in the form of a medical passport, notebook, or other transferable records is an important reference for the patient and for follow-up providers alike.

The patient and family should begin learning about late effects and follow-up care long before the end of treatment to ensure that they have a good understanding of the information presented and have a chance to ask questions and discuss concerns. Research on survivors of childhood cancer has shown that most survivors are unfamiliar with specific details of their diseases and treatments and are unaware of their risks for late effects.[170] One study found that only 30% of childhood and adolescent cancer survivors could provide adequate histories of their diseases and treatments.[175,176]

Providing a patient and family with information not only empowers them to advocate for adequate follow-up care but also prepares them to navigate the health care system and play an active role in monitoring and managing late effects once the cancer treatment ends.[177] Pediatric oncology nurses play a critical role in preparing the patient and family for the transition to follow-up care by teaching them about the disease, its treatment, and possible physical or psychological late effects. Although being careful not to overwhelm the patient and family with too much information, nurses should also address risks specific to that patient's treatment and offer guidance about how to self-monitor for late effects.[174,176] Information about organizations that offer resources for childhood cancer survivors, such as the Candlelighters Childhood Cancer Foundation and the National Children's Cancer Society, is also helpful, as are books and other written materials that provide additional practical information.[175,178]

Follow-Up Care and Care Settings

Over the past 10 years, many oncology centers have developed childhood cancer survivor clinics that monitor patients for late effects and provide treatment to improve survival rates and quality of life.[174] Centers that belong to the Children's Oncology Group are required to offer such a service. Care in these clinics is often provided by advanced practice nurses in collaboration with one or more pediatric oncologists. The nurses are trained in oncology and have extensive knowledge about survivorship issues and follow-up guidelines. During visits, nurses evaluate the patient's growth and development and conduct comprehensive screenings for late effects associated with the patient's particular cancer or treatment.[68] They also monitor the patient for systemic toxicities resulting from the cancer drugs and therapies they received. Some follow-up clinics are multidisciplinary in structure and offer the support of specialists, such as cardiologists, endocrinologists, fertility and genetic counselors, and social workers.

Although the number of specialized follow-up clinics is growing, most pediatric cancer survivors are followed by adult primary care providers. Childhood cancer survivors can also be encountered in a variety of other practice settings, such as primary pediatric settings and adult specialty clinics. Nurses and other providers in nononcology settings often have little experience working with survivors of childhood cancer and may not know about the possible consequences of cancer treatment or what to watch for. In addition, they often have little incentive to learn about the complex care required by childhood cancer survivors because many practices see very few such patients.[171]

Goals for the follow-up care of pediatric cancer survivors include identifying, preventing, treating, and curing late effects and bridging primary and special care services through education and outreach. To help support nononcology clinicians who are caring for pediatric oncology survivors, the Children's Oncology Group has developed a comprehensive set of guidelines for detecting and managing the late effects of childhood, adolescent, and young-adult cancers.[179] These guidelines were developed in a collaborative effort between the Nursing Discipline Committee of the Children's Oncology Group and the Late Effects Committee and are designed to enhance providers' awareness of potential late effects and to standardize the follow-up care of childhood cancer survivors.[177] The guidelines are risk based and exposure related and provide specific clinical recommendations for screening and managing late effects, beginning 2 years after cancer therapy has been completed. These guidelines can be obtained at no cost and, because they are on the Internet, they are readily accessible to primary care physicians, nurses, and the public.[179] Education materials developed by nursing experts are also available and can be used along with the guidelines to enhance the process of educating patients and empower patients to become proactive participants in their long-term follow-up care.[177,179]

The care of patients followed in nononcology settings can also be augmented by regular communication with the patients' pediatric oncology providers. Documentation of the cancers and the treatments given to patients (e.g., the medical notebook and other transferable records described earlier) is also an important reference for follow-up providers. Such communication, along with continuing education for community primary care providers, helps to ensure that survivors of childhood cancer receive comprehensive care and ongoing monitoring and treatment of late effects.[162] Nurses in nononcology settings may not be aware of the guidelines for follow-up care and may not be knowledgeable about the late effects of childhood cancer. Although the guidelines of the Children's Oncology Group are helpful, additional methods of training nurses about specific interventions required by the survivor population are needed.[180,181]

Follow-Up Nursing Care

Much of the care required by pediatric cancer survivors is the same as that required by other patients. For example, studies have indicated that survivors are at risk for establishing unhealthy lifestyle behaviors.[181] Because of this, nurses should use appropriate health promotion strategies and encourage survivors to exercise and maintain a healthy weight and balanced diet, avoid smoking, protect themselves from excessive sun exposure, and keep their consumption of alcohol to acceptable limits. Nurses working with adolescents, in particular, need to clarify the risks of unhealthy behaviors and encourage them to participate actively in decisions related to their health and follow-up care. Preventive screening techniques recommended for the general population (e.g., for colon, breast, and cervical cancer) should also be observed as minimum recommended follow-up.[174]

In addition to employing standard prevention and screening measures, nurses caring for pediatric cancer survivors must also help to monitor patients for late effects of cancer treatment. One of the most disturbing late effects for children and families is neurocognitive deficits. Childhood cancer survivors who received intrathecal chemotherapy or cranial irradiation or who were treated for tumors in the central nervous system are at particular risk for this late effect and should be routinely assessed for its symptoms. Patients with neurocognitive deficits may experience psychosocial problems and may have difficulties with school performance and academic achievement.[159] Memory loss and impaired intellectual or motor function can also occur and are more common in children, particularly girls, who received treatment when they were younger than 6 to 8 years of age.[182]

Survivors who have neurocognitive deficits are often placed in special education programs or programs for the learning-disabled and tend to have lower self-esteem than their siblings.[174] Families often describe the difficulties they encounter when dealing with learning issues, cognitive deficits, attention disorders, behavior disorders, and other problems associated with late effects relating to neurocognition. It is common for these families to need preparation for and assistance in working with school systems and help in obtaining referrals to and resources for neurocognitive testing. Nurses can play key roles in helping patients and families to obtain the support they need and should educate the survivors and families about three federal laws that ensure equal access to education. The Individuals with Disabilities Education Act requires states to provide free and appropriate education to all children between the ages of 3 and 21 years. The Americans with Disabilities Act prohibits discrimination against people with actual and perceived disabilities or histories of disability. The Rehabilitation Act prohibits schools that receive federal funding from discriminating against qualified students who have a history of cancer.[174] Nurses caring for pediatric cancer survivors should also become familiar with school reentry programs and advocate for continued identification of appropriate cognitive programs to promote the success of these children.

Nurses also play roles in identifying late effects related to hormones and fertility. The potential fertility issues and options for their treatment, including sperm or egg banking, should be discussed with patients and families at the time of diagnosis. Once patients enter long-term follow-up, nurses should routinely assess and document patients' sexual development, including their histories of menses, sexual function, and Tanner scale staging, and should provide education and support to patients pursuing fertility options.

SUPPORTING PATIENTS AND FAMILIES DURING RELAPSE AND RECURRENCE

Although the cure rate for pediatric cancers has improved significantly over the past few decades, recurrence of the disease is still possible and is a source of great anxiety for patients and families. Identifying and diagnosing recurrence at an early stage is among the goals of posttreatment surveillance programs because early detection may enhance the chances of successful treatment by means of a second-line protocol.[183]

Some patients and families liken the possibility of relapse to having the sword of Damocles hanging over their heads. Many begin to express fears of relapse and uncertainty as the end of cancer therapy draws near or soon after treatment is over. For patients and families who experience actual relapse, the news can be more devastating than receiving the initial diagnosis of cancer. Nurses, physicians, and other providers working with cancer patients and their families must be aware of the fear surrounding relapse and be prepared to help patients and families manage their anxiety and cope with relapse should it occur. In addition, it is important for the nurse to understand mechanisms and the guiding framework of resilience to effectively assist the patients and families in their adjustment to relapse. Examples of resilience pathways include positive coping, hope-derived meaning, and a spiritual perspective.[184]

Helping Patients and Families Cope with Fear of Relapse

With infants and very young children, the onus of fear related to relapse is generally carried by the parents. Once children reach school age, however, they, too, can experience fear of relapse and require the support of the oncology team. Some patients and families begin to raise the possibility of relapse during conversations with providers as they approach the end of treatment, whereas others do not address it until treatment is over. The fear may persist even after children or adolescents experience 5 cancer-free years, a time limit that is generally recognized as indicating recovery. In many cases the fear of relapse is brought on or is heightened by trigger events, such as the occurrence of minor illnesses or an increase in bruising.

Because outpatient nurses encounter patients and families frequently and are commonly primary sources of support, they may be the first to notice signs suggesting that patients or families are worried about relapse and they may be the first of the oncology team to whom the patients and families speak about their concerns. In addition to sharing their observations with other members of the team, nurses may recommend that patients and families meet with the oncology team's psychologist or social worker, who can help them identify ways of coping with fears and anxieties.

While encouraging patients and family members to verbalize their fears, nurses also emphasize the importance of maintaining a positive attitude because this benefits patients and families alike. Nurses also try to assess patients' siblings because they, too, can harbor fears of relapse and must be encouraged to verbalize these fears. In many centers, nurses or other providers have developed support groups for siblings that help them to express their feelings while engaging them in various activities, such as outings, discussion groups, or arts and crafts projects that allow them to spend time with others who have shared the same experience.

Recurrence

More upsetting than the fear of relapse is the experience of an actual relapse. The fear of recurrence can have a profound effect on patients and families, but experiencing actual relapse can be devastating. How families respond to the news of relapse has marked effects on the patients' responses to the illness and on the psychosocial environments in which they must continue to grow and develop.[56] Once parents are informed of a relapse, nurses and other members of the care team must help them manage their immediate emotional reactions so they can take necessary and curative actions on their children's behalf.[185] The behaviors of the nurses and the rest of the care team are critical in helping the patients and families cope and adapt as they endure what may be the greatest challenge of their lives.

Immediately after patients and families are told of recurrence, they are thrust once again into a state of waiting and not knowing.[56] During these difficult times, nurses support the patient and family by listening and providing them with opportunities to express their feelings. They may be confused about some of the information they have received and may feel angry, helpless, and overwhelmed as they contemplate decisions about additional treatment and realize they must once again take on the immense challenge of making decisions about their children's care. Collaborating with the health care team and coordinating the day-to-day care of siblings and work responsibilities may also add to parental distress. At this early stage, parents are especially dependent on physicians, nurses, and other health care professionals to communicate clearly and to share information about the illness and treatment that will help them plan and carry out their lives over the next weeks and months.[56]

At the time of recurrence, patients and families may express dissatisfaction with the initial treatment choice and may blame themselves for the treatment's ineffectiveness, calling themselves failures.[186] Parents often vacillate between hope for another remission and anticipatory grief while they struggle to determine whether they need to fight for cure or prepare for loss. These conflicting feelings are a part of coming to terms with the relapse, a process that involves limiting immediate emotional responses so they can take appropriate action.[185]

As treatment begins, patients and parents may become extremely vigilant about many of the details of therapy, such as the time a medication should be administered and the results of laboratory tests. Nurses and other providers must understand that such selective and watchful awareness is normal at this time and that it reflects the patients' and parents' need to gain control of the situation. During this time, parents often benefit from having predictable care routines and periods of time, however brief, in which they are free of any immediate worries. Such periods, parents say, help them to rest and recover from the burden of recurrence.[185] It is critical that the patient's needs for support not be overlooked or minimized in the mistaken belief that children are too young to understand the implications of recurrence. Research has shown that nurses who realize that school-aged children may be aware of the uncertainty associated with relapse support patients more appropriately than do nurses who believe the patients are unaware of the status of their disease.[187]

Studies show that parents who have experienced the relapse of their child's illness note the value of being kept apprised of treatment options and of how their children are responding to treatment.[185] Nurses address this need by speaking with family members during each encounter, reviewing what the families have been told, verifying information, answering questions, and helping them put new information into perspective.[56] Parents who have gone through the experience of the relapse of their child's illness also note the comfort they felt whenever providers demonstrated personal knowledge of or fondness for their children. Such actions, they said, told them that regardless of the treatment's outcome, their children would never be forgotten.[185]

NURSING CARE OF CHILDREN AT THE END OF LIFE

When efforts to treat the disease are unsuccessful, end-of-life care becomes critical.[188] As noted in a landmark report by the Institute of Medicine, the goal for children and families who face life-threatening diseases should be access to a health care system that provides "competent, consistent, and compassionate care that families can count on for support and solace as they experience a loved one's grave illness or death."[189] Unfortunately, many children who die of terminal illness in the United States do not receive aggressive supportive care at the end of life.[190] Historically, palliative care research in pediatrics has been difficult to conduct, owing to the sensitive nature of the topic and the reluctance of providers and parents to accept the inevitability of the situation at hand. Although this has been improving over time, additional efforts are needed to deliver more effective end-of-life care, educate professionals, and design supportive public services.[189] In spite of these challenges, many nurses and other health care providers have found that participating in end-of-life and bereavement care is a richly rewarding experience.

Nurses play critical roles in delivering end-of-life care because they provide most of the physical care while the patients are in the hospital and are key sources of support for patients and families while they are at home. The nurse has a unique appreciation of the patient's clinical condition, emotional needs, and family dynamics. Their observations and assessments are crucial to the efforts to keep the child comfortable and enhance quality of life. The family, or legal guardians, rely on the nurse as a give or vital information and support because they often have many questions and concerns.

End-of-Life and Palliative Care

Many of the challenges encountered when caring for patients and families at the end of life begin before the child enters the terminal phase of illness. Managing pain and other symptoms and coping with anxiety are issues for many patients with cancer. Palliative care, a specialized area of practice that focuses on preventing or relieving suffering and ensuring the best possible quality of life, is particularly important for patients at the end of life.[190,191]

Palliative care is both a philosophy of care and an organized, highly structured system of delivering care. Palliative care seeks to enhance patients' quality of life in the face of terminal illness. Palliative, or supportive, care should begin as soon as the child receives a diagnosis of a life-threatening condition and should continue throughout treatment until death, should it occur. The term *hospice care* refers to palliative care services (including therapeutic interventions and medical equipment) that are generally provided by a multidisciplinary group of physicians, nurses, chaplains, health aides, and bereavement counselors.[192]

An increasing number of hospitals and other health care organizations have organized teams of trained palliative care providers that consult with the patient's primary care team and provide guidance regarding the physical, emotional, developmental and spiritual needs of the child and family. These teams include physicians, nurses, social workers, and chaplains.

One of the most difficult decisions a family can face is deciding when to shift the focus from finding a cure to managing the end of a child's life. Historically, the conclusion that no curative options remain was arrived at solely by the treating physician. More recently, however, the parents or guardians have been routinely included in making end-of-life decisions, and the dying child may be included as well. In some cases, the family's decision about whether to shift the focus to end-of-life care may be complicated by an offer to participate in a clinical trial or to receive some form of innovative care. For the patient and the family these opportunities are usually unexpected, and deciding whether to participate in a trial or try a new treatment can be very difficult. Deciding what is right can also be difficult for health care providers who are also clinical investigators. They may experience discordance between their desire to advance science and improve the care of other children and their desire to protect the dying child by doing all that is in the child's best interest. This discordance may be lessened by the certainty that the dying child (when possible) and the family have been given all of the available information about the study and that they are making a well-informed decision.[193]

When discussing further treatment options or end-of-life care with a patient and family, clinicians must take the time to communicate clearly. How they approach the discussion should reflect appreciation of the child's developmental stage, how the child understands death, and awareness of the family's culture. The nurses who are caring for the child should be involved in the discussions because the family often calls on the nurse to interpret the information they have been given. A recent integrative review on parent perspectives on the care of their child at end of life found that recurring themes in the literature included poor communication with the health care team, inadequate emotional support, the parent's need to maintain their relationship with the child during end-of-life, availability of health care services impacting the child and family's quality of life, and the difficult decision to terminate life support.[194]

The nurse's primary goal when caring for a child or adolescent dying of cancer is to maximize the patient's quality of life. Nursing interventions are based on the patient's needs and on the patient's and family's style, values, spirituality, culture, and ways of relating to and interacting with others. To identify and support the unique needs of each patient and family, nurses assess the family's structure, dynamics, coping mechanisms, cognitive and emotional functioning, previous history with loss, family support system, and spiritual and religious beliefs on a continual basis, and the plan of care is developed and revised accordingly.

Nursing Care in the Inpatient Setting

Nurses focus on preventing illness, alleviating suffering, and protecting, promoting, and restoring health. However, when the restoration of health is no longer possible, the

care shifts to ensuring the highest possible quality of remaining life and a comfortable, dignified death. When a child is facing the death in the hospital, maintaining comfort and helping the patient and family cope are the major priorities. Often nurses provide all of the child's clinical and physical care so that parents and other family members are free to meet the emotional needs of the child.

During the hospital stay, a focus of care is to normalize the patient's daily activities. Depending on the child's age and developmental stage, this may mean encouraging parents to go for a walk with the child, read the child a story, or give the child a bath. Working with the other members of the care team, the nurse may introduce play therapy that helps the child to express and cope with fears and anxieties.[195] Throughout the child's hospitalization, the nurse should try to maintain consistent caregivers and routines, because this may decrease anxiety for the child and family.

Outpatient, Home, and Hospice Care

Many children with progressive cancer die at home. Helping a child or adolescent to die peacefully at home presents a multitude of challenges to the care team, but it is critically important because the support of providers can enhance the family's ability to cope with the child's death. In the United States, much of the palliative and hospice care outside the hospital is currently provided by specially trained community nursing agencies; however, palliative care is a rapidly growing specialty in medicine and nursing, and many new services are being developed by hospitals, skilled nursing facilities, and other groups and providers.

Nurses in hospital and clinic settings play central roles in helping to arrange for home-based services and to ensure good communication between home care providers and clinicians in the hospital and clinic. When a patient is hospitalized, an inpatient case manager (often a nurse or social worker) is usually charged with identifying and arranging the community resources. Once the patient is discharged, the outpatient pediatric oncology nurse usually coordinates communication between the clinic and the care providers in the community. If home care services are not available or are not covered by health insurance, outpatient nurses may play a more central role in coordinating care among the provider, patient, and family.[196]

Hospice is a philosophy of care that is rooted in the centuries-old idea of offering a place of shelter and rest, or "hospitality," to weary and sick travelers on long journeys. The term was first used in 1967 by Dame Cicely Saunders of St. Christopher's Hospice in London to describe specialized care for dying patients.[197] The hospice philosophy recognizes death as the final stage of life and seeks to enable patients to continue alert, pain-free lives and to manage other symptoms so that they may spend their last days with dignity and surrounded by their loved ones. Hospice affirms life and neither hastens nor postpones death. It treats the person rather than the disease and emphasizes the quality, rather than the length of, the person's life. Hospice care should be initiated when the patient can no longer benefit from curative treatment, and life expectancy is, at most, no longer than 6 months. If the patient's condition improves or the disease goes into remission, hospice discharge can be arranged and the patient can return to active treatment if they desire.

Hospice services provide family-centered care 24 hours a day, 7 days a week. Although it can be given in a hospital, nursing home, or private hospice facility, most hospice care in the United States is given in the patient's home, with a family member serving as the primary caregiver, and the hospice staff offering ongoing consultation, guidance, and support. Care is focused on relieving pain and other symptoms and providing social, emotional, and spiritual support. Many hospices also provide respite and bereavement care. Choosing a hospice service can be a difficult decision for patients and families, and nurses and other providers often help by assisting them in gathering information and helping them to choose a hospice service that will meet their needs. Because many providers are unfamiliar with the programs and hospice options that are available, The Joint Commission has created a list of questions that patients, families, and providers can use to guide their selection of a home care or hospice program.[198]

Unfortunately, pediatric hospice services are not as widely available as services for adults. Often the nursing agency that provides home care during treatment also provides palliative care at the end of life. Because round-the-clock, home-based pediatric nursing care is available only sporadically, most of the burden of care is placed on the parents. In some cases, enlisting the help of a surrogate caregiver to maintain daily routines and provide respite for the parents may be helpful.

Nurses are integral members of the hospice care team focusing on meeting the physical, emotional, and spiritual needs of patients and families. Hospice nurses work independently, providing care in settings that are removed from many of the resources available in hospitals. Although the limits, functions, and titles of nurses involved in hospice care may vary from state to state, all hospice nurses are guided by the same holistic hospice philosophy and by a position statement from the American Nurses Association regarding the care of the dying patient that reinforces the obligation to promote comfort and ensure aggressive efforts to relieve pain and suffering.

The primary role of hospice nurses is to coordinate the care of a patient at the end of life while maintaining a focus on comfort not cure. In the course of providing care within the patient's home, hospice nurses observe, assess, and record symptoms and work with the child's physician or nurse practitioner to develop and help the family implement a plan that ensures optimal end-of-life care. Family members caring for the patient rely on hospice nurses for guidance in identifying and treating symptoms and for instruction regarding who to call for assistance.

One of the major concerns at end of life is the fear of intractable pain that can lead to serious problems, such as sleeplessness, loss of morale, fatigue, irritability, restlessness, and withdrawal.[198] Because nurses often have the most frequent and continuous contact with patients, they play central roles in assessing and managing the patient's pain and other distressing symptoms at this critical time.

Bereavement Care

Grief and bereavement are highly individualized and are influenced by the family's culture, community, faith, and support system. For many grieving families, abruptly ending contact with health care providers can feel like abandonment.[188] There are organizations that developed bereavement care programs through which professionals, volunteers, other families, and community agencies work together to meet the needs of a family, should this be needed.

Nurses, physicians, and other care providers often experience grief when a patient dies. Some may identify with the family and feel sad about the death, whereas others may experience awkwardness and not know how to respond. Needs of health care providers working with dying children vary according to their personal and professional experiences. Contrary to popular belief, nurses and other clinicians do not become accustomed to working with dying children; however, caregivers who have developed coping skills over time are probably better equipped to deal with the care of a dying child.[186,196]

Nurses, and other providers, who cope effectively tend to recognize their own feelings, take advantage of support groups provided by the health care institution, have an established support network outside the hospital, understand their own limitations as health care providers, and feel their contributions to the patient's care have been positive. Those who detach themselves as the child's death approaches, or who become overly involved and focus on the dying child and the child's family to the exclusion of their own personal needs, tend to have a more difficult time coping with the child's death.[196]

Nursing Education about End-of-Life Care

The care of dying patients is enhanced when it is provided by nurses who are experienced in and knowledgeable about end-of-life care.[199] Among the barriers to providing optimal palliative care are lack of formal courses in palliative care, high reliance on trial-and-error learning, lack of strong role models, and limited access to services focusing on pain management and palliative care, although this has changed dramatically in the past 10 years.[200] Recognizing these barriers, many groups in the nursing community have made educating nurses regarding palliative and end-of-life care a priority.

In 1998, the American Association of Critical Care Nurses published a document specifying competencies that nursing students should acquire related to end-of-life care. Since then, APHON has developed a curriculum and standards related to end-of-life care for training nursing staff and the End-of-Life Nursing Education Consortium, which is composed of nationally recognized palliative care experts, has created a curriculum to train nurse educators in palliative and end-of-life care and prepare them for teaching nursing students and practicing nurses. To date, over 15,000 health care providers have been trained in the United States and 73 other countries.[199] Palliative care content has been included in licensing examinations for nurses and has been added to nursing textbooks.[200]

In addition to training staff nurses in end-of-life care, there is also a need for nurses who have advanced knowledge and skills in palliative care, and graduate nursing programs include palliative care tracks for nurse practitioner students.[200] Nurse practitioners and nurses at the bedside who have such expertise can play vital roles in caring for patients by leading organizations and programs that care for patients at the end-of-life.

ETHICAL NURSING PRACTICE

Complex patient care problems present themselves daily in pediatric oncology practices. Because of the interdisciplinary nature of pediatric oncology, many problems that involve ethical implications are foreseen, and anticipatory ethics is practiced.[201] Nurses dealing with ethical issues are guided by the Code of Ethics outlined by the American Nurses Association[202] (Box 69-7) and by the ethical standards for Pediatric Oncology Nursing Practice defined by APHON (Box 69-8).[15] These documents highlight fundamental principles of ethical practice, including respect for persons, beneficence, and justice that are considered basic to nursing and that underpin how nurses think when confronted by problems involving ethical tensions.[201,203]

Box 69-7   The American Nurses Association Code of Ethics for Nurses

1. The nurse, in all professional relationships, practices with compassion and respect for the inherent dignity, worth, and uniqueness of every individual, unrestricted by considerations of social or economic status, personal attributes, or the nature of health problems.
2. The nurse's primary commitment is to the patient, whether an individual, family group, or community.
3. The nurse promotes, advocates for, and strives to protect the health, safety, and rights of the patient.
4. The nurse is responsible and accountable for individual nursing practice and determines the appropriate delegation of tasks consistent with the nurse's obligation to provide optimum patient care.
5. The nurse owes the same duties to self as to others, including the responsibility to preserve integrity and safety, to maintain competence, and to continue personal and professional growth.
6. The nurse participates in establishing, maintaining, and improving health care environments and conditions of employment conducive to the provision of quality health care and consistent with the values of the profession through individual and collective action.
7. The nurse participates in the advancement of the profession through contributions to practice, education, administration, and knowledge development.
8. The nurse collaborates with other health professionals and the public in promoting community, national, and international efforts to meet health needs.
9. The profession of nursing, as represented by associations and their members, is responsible for articulating nursing values, for maintaining the integrity of the profession and its practice, and for shaping social policy.

From American Nurses Association: Code of ethics for nurses with interpretive statements, 2010. Accessed January 28, 2013 at http:// www.nursingworld.org/MainMenuCategories/EthicsStandards/ CodeofEthicsforNurses/Code-of-Ethics.pdf.

Box 69-8   Association of Pediatric Hematology and Oncology Nurses: Ethical Standards of Pediatric Oncology Nursing Practice

Standard: The pediatric oncology nurse respects the rights of all children and families and makes decisions and designs interventions that are in agreement with ethical principles.
Rationale: Advances in technology and genetics, along with scarce resources in health care, have created an environment in which ethical issues frequently arise. The pediatric oncology nurse should advocate for the rights of children with cancer as well as identify and help resolve ethical conflicts.
Measurement Criteria:
   The pediatric oncology nurse
- Understands and applies the basic ethical principles of autonomy (right to self-determination), beneficence (do what is in the best interest of the patient), nonmaleficence (do minimal harm), justice, and veracity (truth telling).
- Examines own beliefs relating to autonomy, rights of a minor, quality of life, death, suffering, truth telling, equality, and access to care.
- Identifies available resources, including the *Code of Ethics for Nurses with Interpretive Statements* (ANA, 2001) when formulating ethical decisions.
- Maintains confidentiality.
- Provides quality care to all children, regardless of race, culture, educational background, religious beliefs, socioeconomic status, or the ability to pay.
- Delivers care in a manner that preserves and protects patient autonomy, dignity, and rights.
- Acts as a patient advocate and assists children and families in developing skills so they can advocate for themselves.
- Identifies ethical conflicts and seeks to resolve them through multidisciplinary team discussions, including the child and family as appropriate.
- Addresses advance directives with young adults 18 years of age and older.
- Seeks to include minors in decision making as appropriate.
- Ensures that all children and families receive truthful information regarding diagnosis and treatment.
- Participates in the informed consent process by witnessing the signing of consent documents, obtaining ongoing education about research trials, answering the child and family's questions regarding their participation in research, and ensuring the child and family's continued desire to participate in the research trial.
- Reports illegal, incompetent, impaired, or unethical practices.
- Maintains therapeutic professional nurse-patient relationship with appropriate boundaries.

From Association of Pediatric Hematology/Oncology Nurses: Scope and standards of pediatric oncology nursing practice. Silver Spring, Md., 2007, Nurses Books.

Several factors must be present for high-quality, ethical nursing care to occur. Perhaps the most important factor is that the nurses themselves must be moral individuals, possessing integrity, courage, honesty, and a sense of justice.[195] Further, they must be willing to use these virtues to protect patients' rights to self-determination and to ensure that an individual's wishes, goals, and viewpoints are considered when managing care.[195,204,205] Nurses who frequently confront ethical issues benefit from forums that facilitate moral and ethical discussions, communication, and inquiry and that promote the exploration of options for patients. Guided sessions that focus on sorting through choices and their implications help nurses to gain a deeper understanding of nursing ethics and encourage them to embrace their role as patient advocate. The education provided by such forums not only helps nurses to develop skills needed to work through options when difficult situations arise but also helps them to cultivate the field of nursing ethics.[201]

The ways in which nurses approach ethical practice are somewhat different from the approaches used by other disciplines.[206] The differences may have their origins in the very core of each profession. Nursing and medicine, for example, often play complementary and virtually inseparable roles but have functionally different foci: nursing, a health-oriented profession, is focused predominantly on the care of patients and families while preserving and restoring health; medicine traditionally has been oriented toward the treatment, prevention, and cure of illness.[207] Because of these differences, the relationship that develops between patients and nurses can be very different from that which develops between patients and physicians.[208] Although both nurses and physicians serve as patients' advocates, the nurses' perspectives are informed by their proximity to the bedside, a proximity that allows nurses to develop unique relationships with patients and to witness directly the converging influences that surround care versus cure.[204,207,209]

During the course of pediatric oncology care, the varied and often complementary perspectives of each discipline have legitimate places in supporting the needs of patients and families. Nurses and physicians share responsibility for ensuring high-quality patient care and for achieving the best possible outcomes.[203] Further, because the uncertain nature of cancer renders the children and their families vulnerable, the practices of both disciplines must possess the moral virtues of honesty, courage, and justice and must reflect commitment to ethical principles.[195,209]

Ethical dilemmas related to care are often unavoidable. Nurses and physicians alike have the responsibility to manage with care the trust shown them by their patients. And when the right or good thing to do is not clear, they must have the moral courage to analyze critically and, if necessary, to challenge practices and health policies so as to ensure the best possible outcomes.[203,195,210,211]

FUTURE TRENDS IN ONCOLOGY NURSING

Change is intrinsic to the nursing profession and to pediatric oncology nursing, which remains a dynamic subspecialty that is subject to constant advances in technology and science and the introduction of new treatment regimens.[3,4,7] Faced with the potential for a nursing shortage, direct and deliberate strategies to integrate these changes into nursing education, practice, and research are required to ensure that pediatric oncology nurses are positioned to continue providing high-quality care.[7] In the coming years, as new treatments are introduced and more aspects of care shift to the outpatient setting and the home, it is expected that the role of the pediatric oncology nurse will continue to expand and assume greater importance. Remaining current with new developments in the field will make it possible for nurses to influence pediatric nursing practice effectively and to develop innovative strategies for managing the care of patients and families.[4,7,22]

No single discipline can accomplish all that is necessary for a patient; therefore collaboration is critical.[13] Research has shown that interdisciplinary collaboration is associated with improved outcomes, suggesting that intensifying nurse-physician partnerships based on mutual trust, respect, teamwork, and open communication is a priority.[21,22,35,212] Even though both nurses and physicians recognize the importance of collaboration, developing such partnerships may be a challenge.[213]

The primary focus of pediatric oncology nurses is healing rather than curing, but nurses will continue to play strategic roles in supporting the pursuit of a cure whenever possible.[22,32,214] As the consistent provider at the bedside, nurses have a distinct advantage to support translational research efforts. Leveraging this position by combining theory, research, science, and practice allows nurses to bring knowledge from the bench to the bedside and from the bedside to the bench.[215,216] The wide-ranging interests of pediatric oncology nurses and concerns include problems with care delivery systems, worries about meeting the needs of individual patients and families, and worries about national and global issues that impede clinicians' efforts to provide the best possible care to children with cancer.[216]

Moral and Sociopolitical Influences

The United States spends more on health care than most developed countries yet does not compare favorably with quality indicators of other high-performing health care systems.[217] The signing of the Patient Protection and Affordable Care Act in 2010 has been a catalyst of insurance reform and the introduction of cost reduction strategies within health care institutions. Viewed by some with skepticism and concern, the intent is to improve desired outcomes such as access, quality, equity, efficiency, and overall public health.[217] Although the aftereffects of health care reform on the health and well-being of children with cancer are not yet fully understood, in a setting of scarce resources understanding the multifaceted aspects of social and moral justification for health policy and the relationship to the various dimensions of well-being for children with cancer may be an initial signal of moral urgency for nurses who have a professional obligation to promote good health.[208]

With cancer identified as 1 of the 10 most expensive medical conditions, having generated an annual cost of $124.6 billion in 2010 alone, the National Cancer Institute predicts that costs associated with cancer care will reach $160 billion within the next 10 years as new targeted therapies are introduced.[218] Although much of the published data surrounding the rising costs of cancer care is associated with adult cancer treatment, the incidence of pediatric cancer has increased by 29% during the past 20 years. Long-term childhood survival rate of 79% for all childhood cancers and empirical reports also suggest there is increased complexity associated with childhood cancer treatment when compared with adult cancer.[17,18] The emergence of improved cure rates in pediatric cancer is now highlighting not only the cost of pediatric cancer care but also the long-term costs associated with survivorship. Nurses will need to fully use their unique knowledge, skill, and insight into the human experience developed by the interrelationships that occur with patient and families to facilitate an informed dialogue to influence health policy and reform at a local and national level through involvement in professional organizations such as the American Nurses Association and APHON.

Cancer Treatment and the Roles of Nurses

Current trends toward shorter hospital stays and more outpatient therapy demand that pediatric oncology providers change their focus and pay more attention to evaluating the burden of care that is placed on families and to supporting patients and families through the treatment process.[3,8,159,219] Helping patients and families to strengthen their personal support networks, learn about the disease, understand treatment options, and become knowledgeable about managing symptoms and side effects must continue to be a major focus for nursing and the entire health care team.[50,109,220]

Helping patients adjust to the diagnosis of cancer has become an increasingly important part of pediatric oncology nurses' roles. Research has shown that hope has a powerful influence on a patient's psychological and physiologic defenses.[221] These findings have significant implications for nurses, who work with patients and families to capitalize on their determination, courage, and optimism, helping them to develop a vision of hope, regardless of the child's age or the extent of disease.[221]

In the coming years, nursing's paradigm of professional practice will continue to shift toward a more holistic approach that requires knowledge of integrative therapies.[21,222] Therapies and interventions that strengthen the ability of the body and mind to influence healing are increasingly popular among pediatric oncology patients and families. As noted earlier, studies have found that as much as 85% of children and adolescents have used some form of integrative therapy.[101,102] These figures highlight the idea that developing an understanding of the risks and benefits of combining integrative therapies with traditional medicine is an important consideration for pediatric oncology nurses, now and in the future.[104,223] A committee formed by the Children's Oncology Group has highlighted the role of pediatric oncology nurses in CAM research and has noted that nurses are critical to the success of research in this area.[99]

Patient Safety

In 1979, NASA's Aerospace Human Factors Research Division linked inadequate communication, leadership, coordination, and decision-making skills, rather than pilot error, to most aviation accidents.[224] Since then, many health care organizations have translated this work into training courses designed to maximize teamwork among health care workers.[224] Clinicians participating in these courses have found that learning to communicate effectively and developing an understanding of one another's roles, responsibilities, and skills yields valuable insights and can positively influence the quality of patient care.[36] Such training programs will become increasingly important as organizations search for ways to minimize medical errors and improve the safety of the care environment.

Systems issues and other factors make many of the actions of nurses and physicians especially vulnerable to error. Nurses and physicians routinely make high-consequence decisions based on their knowledge and experience and an understanding of the relationship between patient-specific variables and environmental factors, such as work-flow patterns and the activities and norms of the patient care unit.[225] At times, these decisions are made in the context of factors such as conflicting goals, obstacles, unpredictability, poorly designed technology, constant change, hazards, and missing data that contribute to medical errors or near misses.[225] Maintaining vigilance in analyzing systems of care, identifying factors that contribute to errors or omissions, and introducing sustainable practice changes to promote safe patient care will continue to be a critical part of patient safety efforts.[226-228]

In many organizations, the growing focus on patient safety has impacted the culture of the work environment, shifting it from one that condones silence and blame to one that encourages open disclosure and promoting a team approach to problem solving.[229] Nurses in direct care roles confront patient safety directly and are important members of these problem-solving teams. They will continue to play critical roles in preventing medical errors and promoting safety in the health care environment.[229]

Self-Care

Nurses and physicians alike must find ways to preserve their interest in and passion for the work of caring for others. Although working to save, improve, or prolong the lives of others is rewarding, health care professionals often find that such work entails significant stress. This is particularly true in subspecialty practices like pediatric oncology, where patients are incredibly challenged by their diseases and often face uncertain futures. In addition to the emotional stress that stems from the focus on healing and helping, pediatric oncology providers often encounter workload and system constraints that contribute to chronic secondary stress and may lead to burnout or compassion fatigue.[230]

Understanding the concept of self-care and self-management is a pragmatic consideration for pediatric oncology nurses. Knowing how to renew oneself is critical to maximizing professional effectiveness and satisfaction.[21,22]

Nursing Research

The research training, methods, and rigor of nurse scientists are consistent with those of any other scientific disciplines. Through the lens of professional nurses, research questions spanning the continuum of the cancer trajectory guide oncology nursing care. Based on a holistic model (Fig. 69-1), the needs of the patient and family are addressed using evidence-based strategies that help them cope with the physical and emotional sequelae of the cancer experience.

Nurse scientists practicing in academic medical centers at the juncture of clinical practice and clinical or

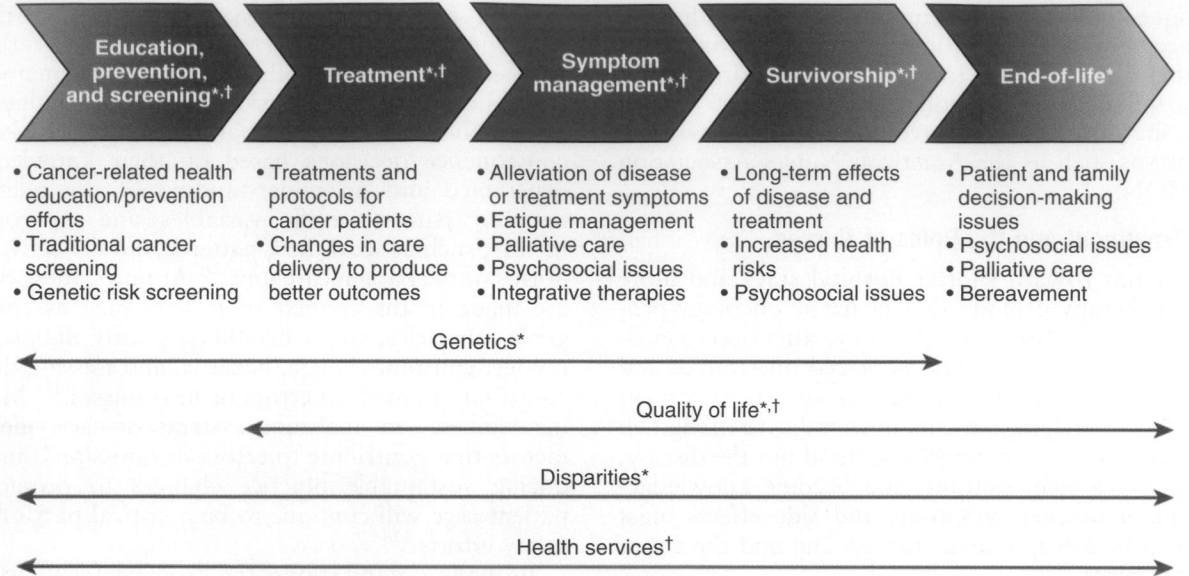

Figure 69-1 A continuum of oncology nursing research. *Research emphasis area of the National Institute of Nursing Research; †Priority area of the Oncology Nursing Society. *(From Bauer-Wu S, Epshtein A: Dana-Farber Cancer Institute, 2007.)*

patient-oriented research have made noteworthy strides in the past decade as nurses have sought to change clinical practice on the basis of existing evidence. This trend toward evidence-based practice is widespread in the nursing community. The past decade has also witnessed a trend toward clinically based nurse-scientists who can bridge the knowledge gap between academia and clinical practice. More doctorally prepared nurses contributing to science will help to support a shift in the research paradigm to one that is multidisciplinary in nature, with nurse-scientists contributing to large multisite studies. This shift means more nurse scientists will have to be trained as members of larger multidisciplinary research teams.

A review of studies conducted by nurse researchers and of surveys among oncology nurses suggests that future nursing research will continue to focus on understanding the full scope of the patient experience and on identifying nursing interventions that ease the hardship of disease for patients and families alike.[231-233] Some of the high-priority areas for future nursing research include the following:

- Understanding issues related to long-term survivorship
- Enhancing patients' quality of life, with a focus on the management of pain and symptoms
- Evaluating and improving care at the end of life
- Evaluating and promoting safe and effective nursing practice in all care settings, including the home
- Understanding families' perspectives to find ways to support patients and families
- Developing new ways to incorporate nursing research into practice and to promote and support interdisciplinary research

These priorities are consistent with the strategic plan and overall mission of the National Institute of Nursing Research (NINR) to advance the science of health by enhancing health promotion and disease prevention; improving quality of life by managing symptoms of acute and chronic illness; improving palliative and end-of-life care; enhancing innovation in science and practice; and developing the next generation of nurse-scientists.[234] They also reflect pediatric oncology nurses' appreciation for the ways in which cancer impacts patients and families and the toll it takes on their physical, psychological, and social well-being. The priorities also exhibit nursing's continued commitment to preventing illness; to alleviating suffering; to protecting, promoting, and restoring health; and to ensuring a comfortable and dignified death and the highest possible quality of life when the restoration of health is no longer possible.

The advances in pediatric oncology that have occurred over the past half century are responsible for a remarkable increase in the number of patients who are cured; however, many patients still face uncertain futures and require ongoing care and support by health care professionals. Although the benefits to patients and families of an interdisciplinary approach to care cannot be underestimated, it is widely acknowledged that pediatric oncology nurses play a vital role in the care of patients and families. The knowledge, skills, and caring practices demonstrated by expert pediatric oncology nurses not only enhance the abilities of patients and families to cope with diagnoses of cancer but also help to reduce the overall burden of the disease.

References available online at ExpertConsult.

KEY REFERENCES

8. Forte K: Pediatric oncology nursing: providing care through decades of change. *J Pediatr Oncol Nurs* 18:154–163, 2001.
    Pediatric oncology nursing practice has evolved over the years as new technology and trends in health care have necessitated change. Reflections of three pediatric oncology nursing leaders and a review of the literature demonstrate advances in treatment and supportive care.

15. Association of Pediatric Oncology Nurses, American Nurses Association: *Scope and standards of pediatric oncology nursing practice*, Silver Spring, MD, 2007, Nurses Books.

   Standards of practice and standards of professional performance are outlined for the pediatric oncology nurse and the pediatric oncology advanced practice registered nurse (APRN). The standards are critical for guiding pediatric oncology nurses in delivering high-quality nursing care.

27. Heiney S, Wiley F: Historical beginnings of a professional nursing organization dedicated to the care of children and adolescents with cancer and their families: the Association of Pediatric Oncology Nursing from 1974–1993. *J Pediatr Oncol Nurs* 13:196–203, 1996.

   In 1974, the Association of Pediatric Oncology Nurses (APON) was established based on the philosophy that pediatric oncology nursing is a specialty that requires specific knowledge and expertise in the care of children who have cancer. This distinction was formalized with the development of specialty certification in pediatric oncology nursing in 1993.

34. Curley M: *Synergy: The unique relationship between nurses and patients*, Indianapolis, IN, 2007, Sigma Theta Tau International.

   This model describes what nurses do based on levels of expertise and building of optimal nurse-patient relationships. Nurses from all roles and subspecialties can apply this framework to their practice.

38. Ponte PR, Conlin G, Conway J, et al: Making patient-centered care come alive. *J Nurs Admin* 33:82–90, 2003.

   The concept of patient-centered care is espoused in many health care organizations, yet implementing this framework has been challenging for many. This article describes how patient-centered care has been implemented within a major cancer center in the United States.

46. Hooke M: Psychosocial issues. In Kline N, Brace-O'Neill J, Hooke M, et al, editors: *Essentials of pediatric oncology nursing: a core curriculum*, ed 2, Chicago, 2004, Association of Pediatric Oncology Nurses, pp 196–227.

   Psychosocial issues including care of families, culturally sensitive care, spirituality, school reentry, and professional nurse-patient relationships are discussed with emphasis on pediatric and adolescent and young adult cancer patients.

49. Holm K, Patterson J, Gurney J: Parental involvement and family-centered care in the diagnostic treatment phases of childhood cancer: results from a qualitative study. *J Pediatr Oncol Nurs* 20:301–313, 2003.

   This qualitative study describes how parents of children with cancer participate in their child's medical care. Parents emphasized they advocated for their child during treatment, educated themselves about the disease and therapy, and worked with the medical team. Recommendations for practice included implementing a family-centered care approach and inclusion of parents regarding treatment decisions.

57. Mack J, Grier H: The day one talk. *J Clin Oncol* 22:563–566, 2004.

   This article describes the salient features of the discussion with parents at the time of their child's cancer diagnosis. Three main features of the talk are emphasized: the cancer diagnosis, treatment and causation.

59. Vaartio-Rajalin H, Leino-Kilpi H: Nurses as patient advocates in oncology care: activities based on literature. *Clin J Oncol Nurs* 15:526–532, 2011.

   This literature review found that oncology nurses assessed their patients both physically and psychologically and developed plans of care, starting with the diagnosis. The literature emphasizes the importance of patient education regarding cancer treatment and the informed consent process.

75. Cescon D, Etchells E: Barcoded medication administration: a last line of defense. *JAMA* 299:2200–2202, 2008.

   The two processes from which preventable accidental disconnection and exposure most commonly arise are medication prescribing and administration. Barcoded medication administration (BCMA) systems are a last line of defense against medication errors and warrant greater advocacy and implementation.

78. Conley S: Safe handling of chemotherapy and biotherapy agents. In Kline N, Hesselgrave J, O'Hanlon-Curry J, editors: *The pediatric chemotherapy and biotherapy curriculum*, ed 3, Chicago, 2011, Association of Pediatric Oncology Nurses, pp 65–69.

   Occupational exposure risks and exposure prevention guidelines including personal protective equipment, preparation and administration guidelines, disposal of chemotherapy, body fluid guidelines, exposure guidelines, spill management, and safe handling in the home are discussed.

108. Fochtman D: The concept of suffering in children and adolescents with cancer. *J Pediatr Oncol Nurs* 23:92–102, 2006.

   Individual suffering needs to be defined and measured by self-report (as opposed to parent or staff report) to gain an accurate, complete holistic picture of the nature and scope of the child's and adolescent's suffering. Knowledge of how children and adolescents experience suffering would enable practitioners to design interventions to prevent or ameliorate this suffering.

111. Hockenberry M: Symptom management research in children with cancer. *J Pediatr Oncol Nurs* 21:132–136, 2004.

   A review of the literature revealed that children with cancer continue to experience distressing physical symptoms caused by the disease and treatment. The purpose of this article is to provide a concise overview of the most common symptoms experienced by children with cancer including pain, nausea and vomiting, nutritional concerns, mucositis, and fatigue.

121. Kline N: Prevention and treatment of infection. In Baggott C, Kelly K, Fochtman D, et al, editors: *Nursing care of children and adolescents with cancer*, ed 4, Philadelphia, 2011, WB Saunders.

   As immunity wanes during cancer treatment children and adolescents become susceptible to infections. A comprehensive review of bacterial, viral, and fungal infections is presented along with prevention and treatment guidelines.

153. Margolis P, Muething S, Brilli J, et al: Quality transformation efforts: decreasing PICU catheter-association bloodstream infections: NACHRI's. *Pediatrics* 125:206, 2010.

   The purpose of this multiinstitutional study was to develop and evaluate effective catheter-care practices to reduce pediatric catheter-associated bloodstream infections (CA-BSI). Results suggested that the main reasons for additional reductions in pediatric CA-BSI rates are issues that surround daily maintenance care for central lines, and additional research is needed to define the optimal maintenance bundle to reduce CA-BSIs in children.

154. Secola R, Lewis M, Pike N, et al: "Targeting to zero" in pediatric oncology: a review of central venous catheter–related bloodstream infections. *J Pediatr Oncol Nurs* 29:14–27, 2012.

   The purpose of this review of the literature is to summarize existing adult and pediatric data on central venous catheter–related bloodstream infections and explore nursing models of central venous catheter care that may improve pediatric oncology patient outcomes.

193. Hinds P, Kelly P: Helping parents make and survive end of life decisions for their seriously ill child. *Nurs Clin North Am* 3:465–474, 2010.

   American parents of chronically ill children prefer to be involved in decision making about their ill child's end-of-life care. Parents report that having access to understandable information about their child's health status influences their ability to participate in end-of-life decisions.

196. Fochtman D: Palliative care. In Baggott C, Fochtman D, Foley G, et al, editors: *Nursing care of children and adolescents with cancer and blood disorders*, Chicago, 2011, Association of Pediatric Oncology Nurses, pp 468–501.

   The focus of pediatric palliative care is to enhance the quality of life for the terminally ill child by preventing and alleviating suffering using the skills and knowledge of a specialized care team. Pediatric palliative care focuses on pain and symptom management, information sharing and advance care planning, practical, psychosocial and spiritual support, and coordination of care.

199. American Association of Colleges of Nursing: The End-of-Life Nursing Education Consortium (ELNEC), 2013. Accessed March 1, 2013 at <http://www.aacn.nche.edu/elnec/about/fact-sheet>.

   The ELNEC program is a national initiative to provide nurses with training in palliative care. More than 17,500 nurses and other health care providers from all 50 states and 77 additional countries have received ELNEC training.

202. American Nurses Association: Code of Ethics for Nurses with Interpretive Statements, 2010. Accessed January 28, 2013 at <http://www.nursingworld.org/MainMenuCategories/Ethics Standards/CodeofEthicsforNurses/Code-of-Ethics.pdf>.

The code of ethics for nurses outlines the nonnegotiable ethical obligations and duties of individuals entering nursing practice and is an expression of nursing's understanding of its commitment to society.

224. Oriol M: Crew research management. *J Nurs Admin* 36:402–406, 2006.

Lessons from the aviation industry, which long ago acknowledged that most errors were the result of poor communication and coordination rather than individual mistakes, are applied to the health care setting. Examples are given of how health care organizations have successfully adopted aviation's curriculum called "Crew Resource Management," which promotes and reinforces the conscious, learned team behaviors of cooperation, coordination, and sharing.

234. National Institute of Nursing Research: Bringing Science to Life: NINR Strategic Plan, 2011. Accessed February 24, 2013 at <https://www.ninr.nih.gov/sites/www.ninr.nih.gov/files/ninr-strategic-plan-2011.pdf>.

Released in 2011, the NINR strategic plan identifies 25 years of accomplishments in nursing science, specifically those that have the greatest potential to improve the health of the nation. The plan is based on the idea that individuals would benefit from being actively involved in maintaining their own health from prevention of disease and self-management of illness.

CHAPTER 70

Palliative Care in Pediatric Oncology

Jennifer W. Mack, Elana Evan, Janet Duncan, and Joanne Wolfe

CHAPTER OUTLINE

More than 2000 children die each year in the United States of cancer-related causes, and many more are living with advanced cancer.[1] In children with cancer, it is not always possible to determine whether the disease will be responsive to cancer-directed therapy, nor is it possible to determine which type of path the dying process will take. Some children may die suddenly and unexpectedly, such as a child undergoing bone marrow transplant who experiences a treatment-related complication. Others may experience a steady and fairly predictable decline, such

as the child with a progressive brainstem glioma after radiation therapy. Most children with progressive cancer will experience varying periods of chronic illness punctuated by crises, one of which may prove fatal. An example of this type of path may involve a child with relapsed metastatic neuroblastoma who may be palliated long term before experiencing a life-ending event.

Although intensive, interdisciplinary supportive care, that is, palliative care, is essential for all children with cancer, it is especially critical for children living with

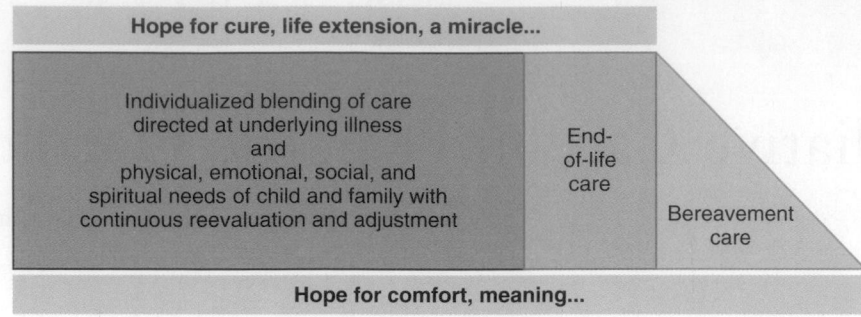

Figure 70-1 Pediatric palliative care includes individualized integration of palliative care principles to ensure combined hopes of varying degrees related to life extension and comfort, both of which can last throughout the child's life. End-of-life care is an important component of palliative care when the focus of care is almost entirely on comfort, although hope for a miracle can persist. Bereavement care needs can be intense and long lasting, gradually lessening over time.

more advanced stages of cancer. Involvement of palliative care services has been shown to improve symptom detection and identification of communication needs among children with advanced cancer,[2] but as of 2008, only 58% of Children's Oncology Group institutions had dedicated palliative care services available, suggesting that there is still room for improvement.[3] Nonetheless in recent years there has been greater awareness and integration of palliative care and, with this, care more consistent with its principles.[4]

Palliative care, as defined by the World Health Organization,[5] is an approach to care that improves the quality of life of patients with life-threatening illness and their families, through the prevention and relief of suffering by means of early identification, assessment, and treatment of pain and other problems, whether physical, psychosocial, or spiritual. The organization's definition of palliative care appropriate for children and their families is as follows:

- Palliative care for children is the active total care of the child's body, mind, and spirit and also involves giving support to the family.
- Palliative care begins when illness is diagnosed and continues regardless of whether a child receives disease-directed treatment.
- Health care providers must evaluate and alleviate a child's physical, psychological, and social distress.
- Effective palliative care requires a broad multidisciplinary approach that includes the family and makes use of available community resources; it can be successfully implemented even if resources are limited.
- Palliative care may be provided in tertiary care facilities, community health centers, and the home.

Hospice and Palliative Medicine (HPM) became a formal physician subspecialty in 2006, and, currently, to become board eligible, a physician needs to complete a 1-year accredited fellowship program. However not all children with cancer require care by a HPM subspecialist or pediatric palliative care (PPC) team. Basic palliative care knowledge, skills, and behaviors should be known to all clinicians who care for children with life-threatening illnesses and conditions. The role of the HPM subspecialist and team is to provide clinical consultation for more complex situations, to provide education and training,

and to improve palliative care outcomes for all children and families through quality improvement and research.

In fact both data[6,7] and clinical experience favor a blended approach to care that includes disease-directed treatments together with palliative or comfort care. This approach is most often favored by parents, who commonly hope for life prolongation while also desiring maximal comfort and minimal pain and suffering for their child (Fig. 70-1). Pediatric palliative care should not be a choice between life-prolonging treatments (e.g., chemotherapy for cancer) and palliative care. Rather pediatric palliative care should be integrated into an overall care plan that is individualized and adaptable over changing circumstances.

INTEGRATING PALLIATIVE CARE FROM THE TIME OF DIAGNOSIS

Although palliative care and end-of-life care are often considered to be a single entity, it is important to note that palliative care can be initiated at any time, not just in the end-of-life period. Rather than being restricted to the last phase of life, palliation includes attention to symptoms from the time of diagnosis. Palliative care also allows for discussion of goals and preferences for care long before death occurs.

In addition rather than precluding intensive life-prolonging care, palliative care can be complementary to therapy with curative intent. With the inclusion of palliative care early in the disease course, children can benefit from attention to symptoms and quality of life concurrent with efforts to control disease. Parents often have many goals of care beyond cure or life prolongation. Parents of children who died of cancer, for example, recall holding simultaneous goals of extending life and minimizing suffering during their child's treatment course.[7,8] Concurrent disease-directed care and attention to the physical, psychosocial, and spiritual needs of the child and family may be the optimal approach to meeting these seemingly conflicting goals.

Among some pediatric cancer patients, such as children with pontine gliomas, the pattern of progression is relatively predictable, making planning for the end of life a logical part of care from diagnosis. Patients with other cancers, however, may have long periods of disease control and relative clinical stability. Although ultimately the child may be expected to die of the disease, which relapse or acute decompensation will result in death can be very difficult to predict. Early relapses may be responsive to intensive treatment, and the timing of death may be difficult to predict.

For a child with relapsed neuroblastoma, for instance, many years may elapse between the first recurrence and death. At any moment in time, the use of intensive chemotherapy may seem reasonable and may offer significant hope of life prolongation and remediation of symptoms. However repeated intensive therapies including chemotherapy-related toxicity may not coincide with the family's wishes for the end of the child's life and may be associated with unnecessary suffering for the child. Even when families choose life-extending measures, they should have the opportunity to do so in the context of an understanding of the expected path of illness.

Advantages of Early Integration of Palliative Care

Before the patient is clearly in the last phase of life, physicians may find it difficult to initiate conversations about a poor prognosis.[9] But the majority of parents of children with cancer say they want prognostic information, even when the news is upsetting.[10] Patients and families who are poorly prepared for death tend to choose more intensive disease-directed care at the end of life.[8,11] Without realistic information, they may not have the opportunity to make choices for care that are consistent with their values.

Just as physicians sometimes prefer not to discuss prognosis, pediatricians sometimes consider palliative care to be equivalent to hospice care. As a result they may integrate palliative care concepts such as advanced care planning and anticipatory guidance only once curative options have been exhausted.[12] Yet families may find earlier integration of palliative care to be helpful. A study of bereaved family members of adult cancer patients, for example, found that half believed that palliative care was provided too late in the disease course, whereas less than 5% believed palliative care referrals occurred too early.[13] Physician communication was found to be an important contributing factor; families who believed that the physician had communicated effectively about the patient's prognosis and end-of-life care were less likely to believe that palliative care was introduced too late.

Early initiation of palliative care facilitates attention to symptoms and quality of life. Involvement of palliative care services improves symptom detection and identification of communication needs among children with advanced cancer.[2] Similarly adults with advanced cancer tend to experience improvement in symptoms, including pain, anorexia, nausea, vomiting, sleeplessness, and constipation, after referral to palliative care services. In addition patients who receive palliative care frequently experience improvements in overall quality of life and well-being.[14]

It is also possible that early discussions about palliative care can help parents to cope with the death. Mothers who experience the sudden death of a child tend to have more intense grief than mothers whose children die after a chronic condition.[15] These findings raise the possibility that emotional and psychological adjustment before a child's death can help parents to cope with the loss of the child over time.

Perhaps most importantly parents value preparation for the end-of-life period. In a study of bereaved parents of children with cancer, physician communication about what to expect in the end-of-life care period was a component of high-quality care.[16] Parents who felt prepared for the circumstances surrounding the child's death were also more likely to consider care to be of high quality overall. Communication with parents in advance of the child's death may allow them to process and be prepared for the death before it happens and to make choices about end-of-life care that are right for them and their child.

Box 70-1 gives some general guidance for discussion about end-of-life preferences.[17,18] Even if the patient's outcome is uncertain, death can be discussed as a possibility so that the patient has opportunities to express goals for care.

Enhancing Integration of Palliative Care When Cure is No Longer Possible

Although integration of palliative care from the time of diagnosis is often ideal, sometimes a clinical event such as relapse or a severe complication makes it necessary to discuss a poor prognosis for the first time. A transition from care intended to cure the child can be experienced as a terrible loss for families. However as with discussions about care at the time of diagnosis, honest communication about the child's prognosis can help the family make reasonable decisions about care, based on their values.[19]

Delays in parental understanding of a poor prognosis can affect the care they choose for their children. In a study of parents of children who died of cancer, parents recalled understanding that the child was likely to die about 3 and one half months after the physician realized this. Earlier parental realization of the low likelihood of cure was associated with increased hospice use and decreased cancer-directed therapy in the end-of-life care period.[8] Although parents sometimes have difficulty accepting a poor prognosis, the difficulty physicians have in communicating a poor prognosis also contributes to parents' overly optimistic expectations about cure.[20]

MAKING THE TRANSITION TO PALLIATIVE CARE

Discussing a Change in Prognosis

A statement that physicians can use when introducing this discussion with parents is, "Although I had hoped that your child's disease would be cured and your child could live a long life, I am now worried that this is no longer possible."[18] Acknowledging the sadness of the situation, responding to the parent's emotions, and allowing for silence can also be helpful. Parents may ask about treatment options, but such discussion should not obscure the fact that the child's disease is unlikely to be cured.

Box 70-1 Communicating with Children and Families About Integrating Palliative Care

BEGINNING THE CONVERSATION

"What is your understanding of what is ahead for your child?"

"Would it be helpful to talk about how his or her disease may affect him or her in the months and years ahead?"

"As you think about what is ahead for your child, what would you like to talk about with me? What information can I give you that would be helpful to you?"

INTRODUCING THE POSSIBILITY OF DEATH

"I am hoping that we will be able to control the disease, but I am worried that this time we may not be successful."

"Although we do not know for certain what will happen for your child, I do not expect that your child will live a long and healthy life; most children with this disease eventually die because of the disease."

"I have been noticing that your child seems to be sick more and more often. I have been hoping that we would be able to make him or her better, but I am worried that his or her illness has become more difficult to control and that soon we will not be able to help him or her to get over these illnesses. If that is the case, he or she could die of his or her disease."

ELICITING GOALS OF CARE

"As you think about your child's illness, what are your hopes?"

"As you think about your child's illness, what are your worries?"

"As you think about your child's illness, what is most important to you right now?"

"You mentioned that what is most important to you is that your child be cured of his or her disease. I am hoping for that, too. But I would also like to know more about your hopes and goals for your child's care if the time comes when a cure isn't possible."

INTRODUCING PALLIATION

"Although I hope that we can control your child's disease as long as possible, at the same time I am hoping that he or she feels as good as possible each day."

"Although it is unlikely that this treatment will cure your child's disease, it may help him or her to feel better and possibly to live longer."

TALKING ABOUT WHAT TO EXPECT

"Would it be helpful to talk about what to expect as your child's illness gets worse?"

"Although we cannot predict exactly what will happen to your child, most children with this disease eventually have [difficulty breathing]. If that happens to your child, our goal will be to help him or her feel as comfortable as possible. We can use medications to help control his or her discomfort."

TALKING TO CHILDREN

"What are you looking forward to most of all?"

"Is there anything that is worrying you or making you feel afraid?"

"Is there anything about how you are feeling that is making you feel worried or afraid?"

From Mack JW, Wolfe J: Early integration of pediatric palliative care: for some children, palliative care starts at diagnosis. Curr Opin Pediatr *18:10–14, 2006.*

The physician might respond to such requests by saying, for instance, "It is possible that treatment might help your child to feel better and possibly live longer; the hope would be for the treatment to control the cancer for as long as possible." Although these conversations are difficult for families and for medical providers, such honesty can help parents to make the best possible decisions for their child. In addition although honest provision of information is important, physicians may be able to clarify the goals of care without needing to have parents necessarily openly acknowledge that cure is not likely; this approach may be preferable to some parents.

Discussing Goals of Care

An important aspect of providing care for children with cancer is an understanding of the goals of care. Often these goals are identified by the parents, but adolescents and even younger children are often able to define priorities for their care as well.[21] Understanding goals of care allows the medical team to make recommendations for care that fit with patient and family values. In addition goals of care, and conversations about these goals, provide another window into parents' perceptions of what is ahead.

A discussion about goals of care can be started by asking parents what is most important to them as they think about what is ahead for the child.[18] Specific questions about hopes for the future and worries about what is ahead can also be useful. Often parents will verbalize general goals, such as maintaining a good quality of life for as long as possible, minimizing suffering, prolonging life, or curing the child's cancer. Parents often hold more than one goal and may have separate goals for cancer-directed and symptom-directed therapy; for example, goals of cancer-directed therapy may be to cure or to prolong life, whereas goals of symptom-directed therapy may be to lessen suffering and maximize quality of life.[8,7] Although such goals may appear to be conflicting, holding more than one goal of care is normal, and physicians can make plans for care with both sets of goals in mind.

Acceptance of the parents' goals is an important aspect of acknowledging the parents' values, even when the goals are not in concert with the physicians' goals. At times, however, parents will continue to articulate a goal of cure, when the medical team believes that such an outcome is not possible. Understanding what the parent would want if the child cannot be cured can help the medical team to make plans for care. Back and colleagues[22] have recommended that the physician ask what the family would want if cure is not possible, a strategy described as hoping for the best but preparing for the worst. This strategy allows the medical team to have a conversation about what the family would want in such a situation.

Even when parents hold goals of cure, physicians need to have clear discussions about the goals of treatment, especially cancer-directed treatment. Depending on the circumstances, the oncologist may want to express goals of controlling the disease for as long as possible, for example. When the purpose of treatment is to help cancer research, with little hope of direct benefit to the child, that goal also should be stated.

In addition to the specific nature of goals of care, parents also consider a number of other values while they make these difficult decisions. For example parents sometimes think about what it means to be a good parent to their child as one compass for decision making.[23] Parents may believe, for instance, that a good parent would focus on preserving the child's life, would make unselfish decisions in the child's best interest, or show the child that he or she is loved. In addition to helping parents clarify their own wishes, having conversations about the meaning of the good parent role can help clinicians to reinforce that role as the child's illness progresses.

Similarly parents may use phrases to sum up the things that are most important to them: "I want the best for my child;" "I have to fight;" "I want my child to have quality of life."[24] By listening for and probing these phrases, clinicians partner with parents in clarifying their goals and making decisions. Ultimately these conversations about parents' values allow clinicians and the parents themselves to recognize their values, enact them in the child's care, and work together during these very difficult times.

Eliciting Children's Goals

Children and adolescents may express goals in general terms, like their parents, or they may have very specific wishes, such as staying at home, spending time with siblings, or minimizing invasive procedures.[21,25,26,27] Knowing about these goals, which can be elicited by asking children for their hopes and worries, and what is most important to them when they think about what is ahead, can allow the medical team to work toward meeting any specific hopes or needs.

Creating a Plan for Care Based on Goals

Once goals of care have been elicited, then a plan of care can be made. It is important to acknowledge that this plan is flexible and may change frequently. Importantly each family is unique, and even with similar goals there may be very different plans of care. As previously mentioned, pediatric palliative care should be integrated while a family is seeking a life-prolonging or potentially curative therapy. Therefore a plan of care may include preventative therapies, looking for life-prolonging or curative therapies, rehabilitation, and intensive quality of life and symptom management.[28] Having parents consider these questions may help them with decision making.

- How will this treatment affect my child's quality of life?
- What is likely to happen without this treatment?
- How will the treatment change my child's prognosis?
- What will it be like for my child (and family) to go through this treatment?
- Are there other options we should consider that might have the same outcome but with a different approach?

Particularly as cure becomes less likely, helping parents to think deeply about what brings a child joy or which experiences provide quality of life may help their decision making. Ideally the child will be included in these decisions and plan of care. In one study, children aged 8 to 17 years wanted to be told if they were dying and adolescents in particular wanted to participate in palliative care decisions.[29]

Appointing a Health Care Proxy

For patients older than 18 years, the decision of whom to appoint as a health care proxy may provide an opportunity for discussion of care preferences. This document, often completed on admission to the hospital, allows the patient to designate someone to make medical decisions if the patient is unable to do so. The proxy ideally makes decisions based on knowledge of what the patient would want in various situations and not on what the proxy would want or believe to be appropriate. Most hospitals have standard forms that are completed by the patient and an admissions staff person. This could be an opportunity to explore the true wishes of the young adult patient and lead to rich discussion and meaningful decision making.

Resuscitation Status and Other Aspects of Advance Care Planning

Advance care planning may include (1) designation of a decision maker or, for those older than 18 years old, choosing a health care proxy; (2) discussion of the illness and prognosis; (3) establishment of goals of care; (4) discussion of preferences for resuscitation, artificial nutrition and hydration, and palliative sedation; (5) primary location of care and death; and (6) discussion about organ or tissue donation, including autopsy, and preferences for funeral arrangements.[30] Advanced care planning is a process that requires time and often occurs through multiple conversations and at different phases of the child's illness.

Of note many clinicians believe that these conversations happen later than they should.[31] Clinicians cite multiple barriers to discussions about advance care planning, especially unrealistic parent expectations about the child's illness, differences between clinicians' and parents' understanding of prognosis, and a lack of parent readiness to have these conversations. Clinician perceptions about parent understanding or readiness, however, should not preclude having these conversations. Physicians also report that they often do not know what to say.[31]

Fortunately several resources are available to assist in these discussions. *Five Wishes* (for those >18 years) (available at www.agingwithdignity.org) is a legal document in 37 states. This document presents information and questions in a way that enhances communication about these difficult subjects, and it addresses what kinds of nonmedical interventions would be wanted, such as music, prayer, presence of family, and so on. *My Wishes* (for those <18 years) (also available at www.agingwithdignity.org) is not a legal document, but through simple questions and the opportunity to write and draw it affords the child or adolescent the opportunity to communicate his or her wishes. In addition *Voicing My Choices* has been recently developed for adolescents and young adults aged 16 to 28, using materials from *Five Wishes* and modified after interviews with adolescent and young adult patients with cancer or who are infected with human immunodeficiency virus.[26] This work involves four priority areas, which can serve as a model for younger patients as well: the ability to express and document preferences for (1) the medical treatment they want and the treatment they do not want; (2) how they would like to be cared for; (3) information they want family and friends to know; and (4) how they want to be remembered.

Other techniques may be helpful, such as asking an adolescent to name his or her wishes, realistic or not. The provider may also ask a question such as, "What is your understanding of your illness now?" Another technique is to suggest that the adolescent write, with a trusted person, such as a child life specialist, psychosocial clinician, or parent, what questions he or she would like to ask of the health care team. Ideally advance care planning among adolescents is family centered, with the family and adolescent both taking part in shaping wishes for care, in an effort to develop a plan for care that all can support.[32] Doing so can allow families to understand their adolescent's wishes and ultimately carry out these wishes.

Making Recommendations

Even when curative therapies are no longer sought, families report wanting recommendations regarding available interventions. Most do not want the burden of making decisions completely on their own. Providers may believe that, especially when there are treatments with uncertain or marginal benefit, plans for care should be the parents' choice. However parents can often be best supported by providers who clearly discuss the positives and negatives of each treatment or therapy and then recommend a treatment in the context of the family's goals and values. This can apply to a wide spectrum of situations such as participating in a phase I or II clinical treatment trial, putting in a chest tube for pleural effusions, using intravenous antibiotics to treat an infection, or instituting a do not resuscitate (DNR) order. Clinicians who make recommendations can alleviate this burden from the parents and help to minimize the parents' sense of regret and responsibility for choices that ultimately allow death to occur.

COMMUNICATING PLANS FOR CARE

A plan of care must then be communicated to all involved in the child's care. Consistency and honesty are among what bereaved parents tell us is most important.[33] Written documentation of team meetings, family meetings, and the care plan is essential. Documentation can also help to communicate plans of care with other providers, such as the home care team or those providing emergency services. Along with a home DNR or comfort care form, for instance, a letter that documents the child's situation and plans for care can be carried by the parents to help ensure that any care providers they encounter know their goals for care. By partnering with the child and family, the health care team in the hospital or home has the opportunity to enhance quality of life while the child is living and affect the grieving and bereavement that will follow for the family.

Talking with Children about Advanced Illness

To tell or not to tell? This is the question that typically arises when parents and health care providers of children with life-threatening illnesses face the issue of discussing prognosis with children. Health care providers have reported a wide range (10% to 80%, with a median 45% prevalence) of open discussions among parents and children regarding the child's impending death.[34] Of a sample of 429 parents in Sweden, 34% discussed death with their child, and none of those parents regretted having this discussion. When children were given the information that their illness was terminal, most (63%) received it from the parent and physician together.[35] In addition, several studies have shown that children as young as 6 to 10 years old are willing to participate in end-of-life decision making.[21,36] Parents' and health care providers' distress in navigating these communication processes (especially regarding death) may prevent children and families from accessing appropriate and timely pediatric palliative care.[37]

Parents may be reluctant to discuss death with their child because of the understandable worry that such a conversation may be very upsetting to the child. However children may have some understanding that death is likely but, because they sense the parents' distress, may feel unable to discuss this topic with a parent. This choice often stems from concern for the parent's well-being. Providing the child with an opportunity to talk, however, can be therapeutic for the child. We therefore often encourage parents to allow for such an opportunity. For parents to initiate discussion, they need to be supported for their efforts in broaching and carrying out these difficult conversations with their child.[38] When parents were asked how they best could be supported during end-of-life care of their child, they responded by saying that respect for the family's role, comfort, spiritual care, access to care and resources, communication, support for parental decision making, and caring/humanism were central.[39]

By describing to parents a nonthreatening mode of communication when carrying out discussions with their child, centered on exploring what the child knows and what the child may be worrying about and hoping for in the time ahead, we can often reassure parents that this conversation will be sensitive and guided by the needs of the child.

The needs and wishes of the individual child should guide how communication takes place and its content. A child's age and level of cognitive development as well as the changing comprehension of death by age can help shape the appropriate conversations regarding the prognosis, treatment choices, and end-of-life decisions; however, all this information cannot necessarily predict what a child understands about death.[40] Furthermore depending on the disease (e.g., brain tumor), the act of communication may be functionally difficult on the part of the child.[41] Thus careful assessment of a child's physical abilities, maturity, level of comprehension, and coping abilities rests on the family and health care team. Himelstein[30] explains appropriate communication interventions (i.e., language, details, expression, participation) based on age (Table 70-1). Chesler and colleagues found that the age at which the child was diagnosed with cancer was strongly and significantly related to the amount of information the parents provided about the illness: the older the child, the more information was given.[42]

TABLE 70-1   Development of Death Concepts and Spirituality in Children

Age Range	Characteristics	Predominant Concepts of Death	Spiritual Development	Interventions
0-2 yr	Has sensory and motor relationship with environment. Has limited language skills. Achieves object permanence. May sense that something is wrong.	None	Faith reflects trust and hope in others. Need for sense of self-worth and love.	Provide maximal physical comfort, familiar persons, transitional objects (favorite toys), and consistency. Use simple physical communication.
>2-6 yr	Uses magical and animistic thinking. Is egocentric. Has thinking that is irreversible. Engages in symbolic play. Is developing language skills.	Believes death is temporary and reversible, like sleep. Does not personalize death. Believes death can be caused by thoughts.	Faith is magical and imaginative. Participation in ritual becomes important. The need for courage is important.	Minimize separation from parents. Correct perceptions of illness as punishment. Evaluate for sense of guilt and assuage if present. Use precise language (dying, dead).
>6-12 yr	Has concrete thoughts.	Develops adult concepts of death. Understands that death can be personal. Is interested in physiology and details of death.	Faith concerns right and wrong. Eternal interpretations may be accepted as the truth. Ritual is connected with personal identity.	Evaluate child's fears of abandonment. Be truthful. Provide concrete details if requested. Support child's efforts to achieve control and mastery. Maintain access to peers. Allow child to participate in decision making.
>12-18 yr	Has generality of thinking. Sees reality as objective. Is capable of self-reflection. Sees body image and self-esteem as paramount.	Explores nonphysical explanations of death.	Internal interpretations start to be accepted as the truth. Relationship with God or higher power evolves. Meaning, purpose, hope, and the value of life are sought.	Reinforce child's self-esteem. Allow child privacy. Promote child's independence. Promote access to peers. Be truthful. Allow child to participate in decision making.

From Himmelstein BP, Hilden JM, Boldt AM, et al: Pediatric palliative care. N Engl J Med 350:1752–1762, 2004.

However, in another study that retrospectively collected information regarding psychosocial variables on 45 pediatric oncology patients who died, it was found that children between the ages of 3 to 6 years had more information about their own death from their parents than older children between the ages of 7 to 11 years. The investigators concluded that perhaps children in the younger age group had a "magical concept" of death, thus making it easier for caregivers to discuss end of life with these younger children.[43] Hurwitz and colleagues provide questions and statements children raise about dying at various ages, thoughts that guide the behavior, their underlying developmental understanding of death, and strategies and responses that can help children in these situations (Table 70-2).

Assessing the child's level of autonomy, perception of threat and safety, and individual coping style can help the clinician determine how to communicate with the child regarding palliative care. Independence and individuation will vary. For example, some adolescents, especially those who have close relationships with their parents, may not make a lot of the day-to-day decisions on their own and depend on their parents' authority and life experience for critical decision making. Other adolescents may be accustomed to "heading" the household and making many of the daily decisions for a family.[44]

Understanding the child's family history with regard to illness and experience with death are important components to consider when broaching sensitive issues within palliative care. A child who has previously witnessed a relative die or suffer from a serious illness and observed his or her family's grief may have unique needs related to this experience. Children who are accustomed to making decisions along with their siblings may request to have siblings present during important decision-making events.

Understanding whether the child has a current and/or premorbid history of anxiety and/or depression is also critical in how information is delivered during advanced care planning discussions.[45]

TABLE 70-2 Statements About Dying at Various Stages of Development

Examples of Questions and Statements About Dying	Things That Guide Behavior	Developmental Understanding of Dying	Strategies and Responses to Questions and Statements About Dying
1-3 Years			
"Mommy, after I die, how long will it be before I'm alive again?" "Daddy, will you still tickle me while I'm dead?"	Understanding of accidental events, of future and past time, and of the difference between living and not living is limited.	Death is often viewed as continuous with life. Life and death are often considered alternate states, like being awake and being asleep, or coming and going.	Maximize physical comfort, familiar persons, and favorite toys. Be consistent. Use simple physical contact and communication to satisfy the child's need for sense of self-worth and love. "I will always love you." "You are my wonderful child, and I will always find a way to tickle you."
3-5 Years			
"I have been a bad boy, so I have to die." "I hope the food is good in heaven."	Concepts are crude and irreversible. The child may not distinguish between reality and fantasy. Perceptions dominate judgment.	The child sees death as temporary and reversible and not necessarily universal (only old people die). Because of their egocentricity, the child often believes that he or she has somehow caused the death or views it as a punishment. Death is like an external force that can get you and may be personified (e.g., the bogeyman).	Correct the child's perception of illness as punishment. Maximize the child's time with his or her parents. A child of this age may be concerned about how the family will function without him or her. Help parents accept and appreciate the openness of these discussions. Reassure the child and help parents lessen guilt that the child may feel about leaving by using honest and precise language. "When you die, we will always miss you, but we will know that you are with us and that you are in a safe, wonderful place" (perhaps with another loved one who has died).
5-10 Years			
"How will I die? Will it hurt? Is dying scary?"	The child begins to demonstrate organized, logical thought. Thinking becomes less egocentric. The child begins to problem-solve concretely, reason logically, and organize thoughts coherently. However he or she has limited abstract reasoning.	The child begins to understand death as real and permanent. Death means that your heart stops, your blood does not circulate, and you do not breathe. It may be viewed as a violent event. The child may not accept that death could happen to himself or herself or to anyone he or she knows but starts to realize that people he or she knows will die.	Be honest and provide specific details if they are requested. Help and support the child's need for control. Permit and encourage the child's participation in decision making: "We will work together to help you feel comfortable. It is very important that you let us know how you are feeling and what you need. We will always be with you, so you do not need to feel afraid."
10-13 Years			
"I'm afraid if I die my mom will just break down. I'm worried that when I die, I'll miss my family or forget them or something."	Thinking becomes more abstract, incorporating the principles of formal logic. The ability to generate abstract propositions, multiple hypotheses, and their possible outcomes becomes apparent.	The child begins to understand death as real, final, and universal. It could happen to him or her or family members. The biologic aspects of illness and death and details of the funeral may begin to interest the child. The child may see death as a punishment for poor behavior. The child may worry about who will care for him or her if a parent or caregiver dies. He or she needs reassurance that he or she will continue to be cared for and loved.	Help reinforce the adolescent's self-esteem, sense of worth, and self-respect. Allow and respect the adolescent's need for privacy, but maintain his or her access to friends and peers. Tolerate the teenager's need to express strong emotions and feelings. Support the need for independence, and permit and encourage participation in decision making. Although I will miss you, you will always be with me and I will rely on your presence in me to give me strength."

TABLE 70-2   Statements About Dying at Various Stages of Development (Continued)

Examples of Questions and Statements About Dying	Things That Guide Behavior	Developmental Understanding of Dying	Strategies and Responses to Questions and Statements About Dying
14-18 Years			
"This is so unfair!" "I cannot believe how awful this cancer has made me look." "I just need to be alone!" "I can't believe I'm dying. ... What did I do wrong?"	Thinking becomes more abstract. Adolescence is marked by risk-taking behavior that seems to deny the teenager's own mortality. At this stage, the teenager needs someone to use as a sounding board for his or her emotions.	A more mature and adult understanding of death develops. Death may be viewed as an enemy that can be fought against. Thus dying may be viewed by the teenager as a failure, as giving up.	"I can't imagine how you must be feeling. You need to know that despite it all, you are doing an incredible job of handling all of this. I'd like to hear more about what you are hoping for and what you are worrying about."

From Hurwitz CA, Duncan J, Wolfe J: Caring for the child with cancer at the close of life: "there are people who make it, and I'm hoping I'm one of them." JAMA 292:2141–2149, 2004.

Within the framework of the American culture is the diversity of the various ethnic and religious cultural subgroups that utilize a range of guiding principles with regard to illness and truth-telling. It is critical to assess the family's identification with their particular culture and inquire what their beliefs are with regard to communication with children about issues pertaining to advanced care,[46] because this may vary from the protective approach (shielding young patients and siblings from full knowledge of the disease) to a more open approach.[42,47] Although every family's style of disclosing sensitive information may be different for a variety of reasons, health care providers should consider how parents may feel if they do not prepare their child for impending death, because this has been shown to have long-term implications for parental grief.[48]

Techniques for Communication

In many instances communicating with children regarding palliative care issues is best received when healthcare professionals are aware of the child's level of desired information and concurrently reinforce the primary role of parents.[49] Children between the ages of 8 and 17 years who were interviewed about disclosure regarding their diagnosis and prognosis reported a range of views about the form of disclosure they preferred: a few believed it was better to hear the news at the same time as their parents, some thought it was more appropriate for their parents to be told first, and others reported no strong feelings either way.[50] Patients reported the roles their parents performed in facilitating communication with their health care team: asking questions for them, being the source of information, and reframing the information from the health care team so they could understand it better. Some children reported feeling "protected" by the parent's executive role in screening the communication with doctors and "marginalized" by the nonparticipant status.[49] Parents of cancer survivors indicated that the shielding of

information that took place (i.e., preference regarding whether to provide information to their child about prognosis and treatment options) depended on their child's age and emotionality.[51]

The range of views reported by pediatric patients exemplifies the necessity for tailoring one's approach of communication to the individual child. The most beneficial method for determining the most appropriate way to communicate with a particular child is by spending time with him or her. A provider who knows the child well may be best suited for this conversation whenever possible. Prior to the delivery of information, it is helpful to uncover what the child already knows. This can be done through direct conversation or through nonverbal communication (e.g., drawing and symbolic play). Storytelling, such as using the experience of another family with a child or a loved one facing death, may be another modality that can be used by parents and health care providers to broach sensitive topics related to death.[52] Ensuring privacy, confidentiality, and support can facilitate the trust that is needed for the child to disclose what it is that he or she already knows. The next step is finding out what the child wants to know. Then the clinician can give information in small amounts, responding to the child's reactions and feelings; and can remind the child that there will be additional opportunities to discuss the issues of concern.[40]

Listening

Listening to a child cannot be underrated nor underutilized. Because a child confronting a life-threatening illness is at his or her most vulnerable, listening to the child can be a very powerful tool in placing some of the control back in the hands of the child.[53] Allowing moments for silence in the discussion only reinforces this acknowledgement that the clinician is listening.[53] Providing a child with a tape recorder can be another method for empowering the child. This allows the child to record his or her questions for the upcoming appointment with the clinician, and also allows them to record the clinician's answers so they can be reviewed if necessary.[54] Asking about and listening to the child's priorities and providing choices, when possible, may allow the child to participate in "life-enhancing experiences even at the close of life."[55(p 746)] Listening to the voice of the parent(s) goes hand-in-hand with listening to the child to provide comprehensive family-centered care; it can provide helpful information about the child and make the health care provider a better listener for the child. Listening to the parent without the presence of the child can also be a valuable tool in certain instances when the child's presence may restrict communication.[56]

SPIRITUALITY

Spirituality can be regarded as a multidimensional (mind, body, spirit), unique expression that brings individuals hope, meaning, and purpose.[57] Spirituality is related to, but different from, religion, such that "spirituality is a dynamic state of being in which the individual seeks connectedness, whereas, religion represents the beliefs, values, practices, and rituals that are an observable aspect of a person's spirituality."[58(p 56)] Spirituality is often "inexpressible" whereas religion is marked by greater structure.[57] A child can have a "highly developed awareness of spiritual concepts without ever having been part of a formal religious group."[59(p 271)]

Spirituality in Children

Similar to the development of cognitive abilities, children display a developing awareness of spiritual needs, meaning, or purpose within their lives at various ages. During infancy, children find meaning in their daily life through unconditional love and trust. Toddlers desire self-assertion, worthiness, and success when performing new skills. Preschoolers and school-aged children tend to derive their satisfaction from learning concepts of right/wrong, impulse control, and the benefits of peer socialization. Adolescents find purpose in their developing independence, individuality, and a deeper relationship with a higher being.[59] For a child with a life-threatening illness, spiritual concerns often include a need for unconditional love, forgiveness, hope, safety and security, and development of a legacy. Children also often experience loneliness and loss of wholeness.[60] It can be helpful for children of all ages to be assured that they bring meaning to their families lives and that when they are no longer alive they will be remembered by their family.[57,61]

Children, in general, more than adults, tend to attribute an illness to "internal" (personal) factors, as opposed to "external" (environmental) factors. Children younger than the age of 7 years, who have yet to develop the ability to think abstractly, often see illness as a form of punishment for something they have done wrong (immanent justice belief).[58] Although some older children may attribute the illness to internal causes to maintain control, others are able to attribute the illness to external causes but also seek out the meaning and purpose of their illness—a task that is very often spiritual.[58]

The Spiritual Assessment

Because children tend to reflect the religious and spiritual values of their parents and family, a family-centered assessment of spirituality is often helpful. Providing spiritual care for parents can prepare them for the questions children ask, such as, "Why is God doing this?" or "What is heaven like"? Parents need assurance that there is no specific "right answer."[62]

One method for conducting a spiritual assessment is through the use of the B-E-L-I-E-F questions:[63]

Belief system (e.g., Does your family take part in religious events/rituals? Have you discussed the idea of afterlife with your child? Do you believe in a higher power that influences your life?)

Ethics or values (e.g., What are the values you believe are most central to your family?)

Lifestyle (e.g., Are there rituals or dietary practices that you/your family follow?)

Involvement in a spiritual community (e.g., Are you involved with a spiritual community?)

Education (e.g., Do you/your family receive or have received religious education?)

Future events (In the near future, are there any religious rites of passage set to occur for you or your family members? What role would you like the members of your faith community to play in the spiritual care of your child?).

However most spiritual counselors and chaplains discourage the use of a "checklist format" in assessing spirituality. Instead questions could be posed to the family and/or to the child in a conversation format depending on the situation.[59] Clinically effective pediatric spiritual assessments are conducted in narrative form and may use words, pictures, music, and play, thus inviting a child to explain his or her sources of strength and areas of fear. Discussions with children and their families regarding spirituality early on in the disease course can help bring meaning to what the family is enduring and can provide hope and comfort at end of life.[60] Assessing children's developmental understanding of faith using Fowler's stages of faith[64] can be helpful in knowing how to lead these spiritual conversations with children directly and how to guide parents in doing so:

Stage 1: Intuitive Projective Faith (2-7 years) is when children's thinking is filled with fantasy and notions of faith are based on stories usually told by parents and other caretakers.

Stage 2: Mythic-Literal Faith (7-12 years) incorporates children's knowledge of cause-and-effect relationships into separating fact from fantasy when constructing an understanding of faith and their religious expression.

Stage 3: Synthetic-Conventional Faith (12-21 years) is when adolescents are able to use abstract reasoning skills to develop their own spiritual identity by separating out what has been told to them and creating new connections between faith-based stories and their own beliefs.

Facing obstacles, challenges, and adversity in life often engenders spiritual thoughts and prompts adults and children alike to ask questions of a higher power, such as, "why me?" "why my child?" It is natural that spirituality is a significant issue for families of children with cancer.[57,65] Pastoral care providers at children's hospitals estimate that more than half of child patients can benefit from spiritual care for fear, anxiety, coping with pain, and familial difficulties.[66] Providers in this study identified three major barriers to providing spiritual care: "inadequate training of health care providers to detect patients' spiritual needs, inadequate staffing of the pastoral care office, and being called to visit with patients and families too late to provide all the spiritual care which could have been provided."[67(p e70)] When the focus of clinical care is on "the cure" for children, treatment discussions focus on medical facts and issues centered on resolving the "problem" with medications or therapies; spirituality, in palliative care, by contrast, is more about a journey of meaning, where there may be no clear solution.[57] Providing spiritual care to dying children and families requires the professional to face his or her own issues with spirituality, something not all individuals have done or are ready to do.[57] Children's spirituality tends to be overlooked and, as a result, children may be more likely to feel unheard, invalidated, and alone in the end-of-life period.[68] A focus on spiritual beliefs during the end-of-life period is not only critical to the dying patient but also can have implications for bereavement outcomes, such that people who profess stronger spiritual beliefs may experience a more rapid and complete sense of closure after the death of a loved one.[69]

SCHOOL

Going to school provides multiple benefits for the school-aged child with cancer. It is the child's peer group; it is the child's chance for discovery, mastery, and socialization.[70] Most children want to continue with their class unless they have not been well supported or they feel unable to participate. With the family and child's permission, creative solutions for participation can allow the child to remain in school often until just days before death. Preparation of school staff and classmates is important, as is a willingness on the family's part to allow for candid information about the child's illness and treatment course.

Ideally this information is shared soon after a child is diagnosed. Often hospital or clinic staff will travel to the child's school and provide information through a "back to school" program. The question frequently arises during these sessions as to whether the child/friend/peer will survive. Most school-aged children have known an adult with cancer, some who have survived and some who have not. Addressing this question in a hopeful way while acknowledging the uncertainty is essential. In all instances if the child dies, it is important for schools and communities to have a plan about ways to communicate this information and support classmates' questions, fears, and feelings.

One possible disturbing aspect of school attendance by the ill child may be the change in the child's physical condition. Reassuring classmates of the child's unchanging personhood may be necessary. Explaining absences, altered appearance, and altered ability to participate in regular class activities may also be helpful.

For the ill child to attend school, school staff and medical providers may need to be creative. Perhaps the child is allowed to attend for half days or just for lunch or on special activity days. Even limited time can be meaningful for the child and his or her peers. An individualized education plan (IEP) tailored to the needs of the child can also allow resources to be mobilized. An ill child should be able to receive home or hospital schooling, and some may be able to complete computer courses or stay in touch with the classroom via teleconferencing.

Advance Care Planning and the School System

As a child's disease progresses, the family and medical team may decide together that a DNR order should be in effect. This can present challenges as to how to honor this within a child's community. Many states are in the process of adopting medical orders for life-sustaining treatment[71] to provide consistent communication regarding advanced care decisions for loved ones no matter what the location of care. However most school districts do not have guidelines or policies to deal with this kind of situation, and those that do have policies typically prohibit school staff from honoring an order that would limit attempts on resuscitation.[72] Nonetheless ethical principles of beneficence, nonmaleficence, and autonomy have been offered as justification for honoring limits on attempts at resuscitation for the student.[72,73] At this point each child, family, and school will need to come to some clear agreement of whether abiding by medical orders for life-sustaining treatment would be observed if the child was at school during a life-ending event.[74-76]

Grief and Bereavement in the School

Finally anticipatory grief and bereavement needs of classmates and school staff must be considered. Resources are available (e.g., www.dougy.org); however affording the training and opportunities for staff to integrate this into their knowledge and experiential repertoire may be challenging. It may be helpful for the oncology clinicians who helped treat the child as well as palliative care staff to do an in-service or advise school personnel.[77] Because children with life-threatening illness are living longer, however, acceptance of their goals to enhance their quality of life must be honored whenever possible.

INTERDISCIPLINARY CARE

The interdisciplinary team is an essential aspect of palliative care for children.[28] How else could we possibly address the physical, social, emotional, and spiritual needs of the child with a life-threatening illness and the family as well?[78] Ideally the team is providing care from the time of diagnosis through death and bereavement.[18,28,79,80] Because care may occur in the hospital, home, or community, most often the child has a primary team (pediatrician or oncologist) whose members take the lead in day-to-day management. Most often the team consists of a physician, nurse practitioner or nurse, and social worker. Other core team members include a psychologist, chaplain, child life specialist, and case manager. The needs of the child and family require an entire team to provide the holistic care that is synonymous with palliative care.

Interdisciplinary care occurs with the child and family as partners. Priorities of the family are elicited, with their values, beliefs, and culture taken into account as recommendations are made that inform the necessary decision making. Family meetings, especially those used to address goals of care, include the parents, the child if appropriate, and interdisciplinary team members, so that information, emotional cues, and nonverbal language may be appreciated from different perspectives. This format also allows for a response that may address the issues holistically. In addition to those already mentioned, at times an interpreter, physical therapist, teacher, respiratory therapist, nutritionist, or pharmacist is present for the family meeting. Importantly, research has shown that when the physician is working with a psychosocial clinician there is closer agreement between the physician and parents in the understanding of the child's prognosis.[8]

Interdisciplinary care is essential so that not only the child's and parents' needs can be addressed but also those of the extended family, community groups, and the hospital, clinic, and home care staff. Particularly when doing a home visit, it is helpful to have several team members present so that physical and emotional needs of the patient, parents, and siblings may receive attention. Each team member carries the responsibility to inform, teach, and reach out to colleagues. Depending on one's clinical setting, there inevitably will be times that different team members are called on to take the lead.

Pediatric palliative care is particularly challenging. As providers, we have "an obligation to nurture relationships that can hold within their embrace both vulnerability and suffering: that which is experienced by our child patients and their families, and that which we experience within ourselves."[81] The depth and meaning of this care touches us at our core. We need the expertise, support, and companionship that interdisciplinary care provides.

COORDINATION OF CARE

The coordination of care for a child with a life-threatening illness who moves between hospital, home, clinic, and perhaps a rehabilitation facility is daunting. Despite the efforts of many providers, parents often report feeling overwhelmed with the responsibility of care and coordination of services, particularly in the home. There are many barriers to coordination of pediatric palliative care services, including lack of available staff to provide home-based services; limited training of staff in pediatric palliative and hospice care; few resources for services; limited agencies with comprehensive services; and insufficient systems to support communication and coordination between sites of care.[30] Ideally each hospital, clinic, community, or home care agency has designated personnel to perform coordination tasks for the child and family and has protocols specifying a standard of practice.[28]

Thankfully, in the United States a growing number of home care agencies have developed palliative care programs that serve as a bridge to hospice services for children not yet meeting hospice eligibility criteria (<6 months to live) or for those seeking intensive disease-directed therapies. Previously the reimbursement structure and use of medical technology (e.g., intravenous nutrition, assistive respiratory support), experimental therapies, and/or need for block hours of nursing care had precluded enrollment of children on the hospice benefit.

Importantly section 2302 of the recent Patient Protection and Affordable Care Act, termed the "Concurrent Care for Children Requirement" (CCCR) has eliminated the requirement that Medicaid patients younger than 21 years forgo curative or life-prolonging therapies to be eligible for hospice. Therefore Medicaid programs in every state are now required to provide concurrent curative/life-prolonging treatment and hospice services for hospice-eligible children. The development of systems to make such concurrent care a reality has been slow and, in the meantime, a number of state-based pediatric palliative care coalitions have formed to jumpstart access to home-based pediatric hospice/palliative care services, using strategies such as Medicaid waivers or state plan amendments to increase coverage for hospice services. For example Massachusetts implemented a statewide pediatric palliative care program in 2006.[82]

LOCATION OF DEATH

At the end of life, children and families often benefit from intensive support. It is generally assumed that children would prefer to be at home to die, although approximately half of children with progressive cancer die in the hospital,[83] as do the majority of infants and children who die in the United States.[84] In a study from the United Kingdom, research showed that of children dying in the hospital, 85.7% died in the intensive care unit, with the trend having increased over the years from 1997 to 2004.[85] Families and children need to feel safe and well cared for and given permission, if possible, to choose location of care, be that at home, in the hospital, or a hospice house. Asking children where they would most like to be even if they are very sick and what is most important to them is often very instructive.

Although seemingly contradictory, the philosophy of palliative care can be successfully integrated into a hospital setting, including the intensive care unit, when the focus of care also includes the prevention or amelioration of suffering and improving comfort and quality of life. All interventions that affect the child and family need to be assessed in relationship to these goals. This proactive approach focuses on what "we can do" not what we cannot do. We might ask what can we offer that will improve the symptoms and quality of this child's life (e.g., radiation therapy, a trip to the garden, a special visit from a pet) and provide the most meaning and control for their family instead of asking what interventions are not going to be offered. Staff needs education, support, and guidance because pediatric palliative care, like other types of intensive care, is an area of specialty.

Preparation for Home Care

Preparing parents for events that may occur at home is essential. Even if they may not want to talk about this, written materials can be offered. Anticipating likely symptoms, ways to manage the symptoms, what resources will best match needs, and who will be available on call 24/7 to the family is key to making the transition to home successful. The child's primary inpatient or clinic providers must work closely with the case managers and social workers who know the intricacies of insurance benefits, home care nurses, and durable medical equipment vendors and who can determine what each can and will provide. It is also important to reach out to the primary care provider, who may have important insights to the home environment and resources in the community.

Even the most experienced families still need maximum physical and emotional supports in the home to care for a child who is facing the end of life. The goal is to have enough support in place so that parents can simply be "parents" and so that family interactions and events may become meaningful experiences.

Hospice Services

For those families and children who know they want to be at home, hospice services can be invaluable. Many hospice agencies now have palliative care programs, which offer greater flexibility and broaden the scope of care. There are many barriers, however, to provision of hospice services to children even with the new legislation section 2302 of the Patient Protection and Affordable Care Act.[78] Many fewer children than adults die, and so maintaining a staff that is willing and able to provide care to children can be challenging. Families and practitioners often see hospice as "giving up," and it remains difficult to change this assumption. There is a prognostic requirement of life expectancy of less than 6 months, and this can be a significant emotional barrier for families and clinicians. Financially provision of hospice may also be a struggle, because hospice is mandated to provide all the personnel, medications, equipment, and supplies that the child needs and this is capped at a per diem rate.[86] The financial concerns may be mitigated with successful implementation of the Affordable Care Act, which should be reassessed over time.

The first free-standing pediatric palliative care center in the United States, the George Mark House, opened in 2004, and other pediatric hospice houses have followed. Some adult hospice houses are now willing and equipped to accept a child, with the hospice staff often appreciating the support of a previously involved pediatric palliative care team. In addition to hospice care there is a monumental unmet need for many families who are in desperate need of respite care for their child, who may have a prolonged palliative care path ahead of them.

Despite these barriers, palliative care, respite care, and hospice care for all children with life-threatening conditions is the recommendation of the Committee on Bioethics and Committee on Hospital Care.[80] Importantly when experienced in caring for children, hospice teams are ideally suited to provide comprehensive home-based services to the child, siblings, parents, and extended family. Hospice programs often have physicians, nurses, social workers, chaplains, and bereavement staff, art therapists, music therapists, pet therapists, and volunteers who can provide integrative therapies such as massage and Reiki.[87]

CANCER-DIRECTED THERAPY

Parents often wish to continue some form of cancer-directed therapy in the end-of-life care period and are more likely to favor using cancer treatment at the end of life than clinicians.[88] The choice of cancer-directed therapy should be considered in the context of goals of care. For example if a parent's primary goal is to minimize the child's suffering, then an option that causes few distressing side effects and that necessitates few interventions may be a reasonable choice, if parents wish to continue to provide cancer-directed therapy.

Some regimens with limited toxicity have established efficacy in relapsed or refractory tumors. For example, daily oral etoposide has been used in children with refractory solid tumors, with limited resulting toxicity and with the possibility of tumor response.[89-93] Oral temozolomide has had similar results in children with neuroblastoma.[94] In refractory acute lymphoblastic leukemia, maintenance-type regimens of 6-mercaptopurine, low dose methotrexate, vincristine, and prednisone may be effective without causing significant side effects. Antibody therapies, such as rituximab for children with B-cell malignancies, and molecular agents, such as imatinib in potentially responsive cancers, may also offer palliation with limited toxicity. Other examples of therapies with limited toxicity can be found in the literature.

Other parents may wish to continue more intensive regimens of chemotherapy. Recent work has found that, when prescribing chemotherapy for children with no realistic chance for cure, oncologists consider the potential toxicity of the chemotherapy, family preferences, and the potential that therapy will decrease cancer-related symptoms.[95] However, nearly half of oncologists studied had prescribed chemotherapy to meet parental wishes, and many oncologists' recent experiences with end-of-life chemotherapy did not meet their goals of prescribing. Thus physicians should ensure that such regimens offer reasonable hope of meeting the parents' and child's goals of care.

Parents may also wish to pursue experimental options such as those provided on phase I clinical trials. In general the likelihood of significant benefit from agents offered on phase I trials is limited, typically under 8%, even in children.[96] Misconceptions about the purpose of phase I trials are common; as with other clinical trials, many subjects believe that the purpose of such a trial is to benefit them personally rather than to benefit future patients.[97] When clinical trials are offered, clarity about the purpose of the trial is important so that parents and children can make informed decisions about whether such therapy will help to meet their goals. In addition such therapies do not preclude concurrent attention to symptoms and quality of life. In fact attention to life prolongation and symptoms simultaneously may best meet the needs of children with advanced cancer and their families.[98,99]

Other cancer-directed options to be considered include local irradiation or surgery. If a single lesion is causing significant pain or other symptoms, then localized radiation therapy may offer palliation with few systemic side effects. Radiation therapy directed at an isolated painful bony metastasis is one such example. Surgery can be similarly beneficial, but a frank team discussion with the surgeon about the possibility of recovery and the likelihood of recurrence can help in consideration of the likelihood that the child will benefit from the surgery. Debulking of a rapidly growing abdominal tumor, for example, may provide little benefit, in contrast to control of a single painful metastasis by radiation or surgery. A consistent recommendation between the oncologist and surgeon or radiation oncologist should be provided to the family.

Physicians sometimes feel an obligation to describe cancer-directed therapy as either "curative" or "palliative." Such a distinction may be difficult, however, because at times cancer-directed therapy may offer some chance of cure, even if this chance is low, as well as some possibility of symptom palliation and life extension. In addition this distinction may be difficult for families, who may hold more than one goal for care. We recommend rather than using a label of curative or palliative, that cancer-directed therapy be discussed in terms of the goals for care. For example we may be able to tell parents that the goals of a particular therapy are to control the disease for as long as possible, with a very small possibility of cure, and with a higher likelihood of decreasing symptoms for a period of time. If cure is clearly not a goal of therapy, then that also should be stated.

Families who have been accustomed to using cancer-directed therapy at every recurrence may continue to pursue such options even when the medical team believes that the likelihood of benefit is extremely low. Unfortunately previous work suggests that parents may regret decisions made about end-of-life cancer treatment in retrospect,[100,101] especially if treatment involved suffering.[100] Thus clinicians should do everything possible to ensure thoughtful decision-making prospectively. In addition when such situations arise, the team should reach consistent recommendations about cancer-directed therapy and should not offer therapies with no chance of benefit and a high risk for harm. However patients and families will have different preferences for end-of-life care; and for some families, continuing to "battle cancer" until the time of death may hold personal meaning. The team should therefore follow the same standards for communication that we have described earlier: assess the family's understanding of prognosis, allow for further communication about the prognosis if needed, elicit goals of care, come to a team consensus about plans for care that fit with goals, and make recommendations for care based on family and patient goals and the team's consensus. Intensive interventions may be chosen by families who have overly optimistic perceptions of prognosis[8,11]; ongoing communication about the child's prognosis may allow families to readjust goals and to choose interventions that offer realistic chances of benefit. The team should never be obligated to provide care that is considered to be inappropriately harmful and in such cases should work with hospital ethics teams to define appropriate responses to family requests. But beyond the reaches of harm, families who make thoughtful decisions about care for their children should be allowed to do so, even when plans for care do not match the ideals of staff members.

SYMPTOM-DIRECTED THERAPY

Managing symptoms for the child with a life-threatening condition is of utmost importance. Parents and children are partners in care and the experts regarding the symptoms and treatments that make the most sense based on their goals and values. Managing symptoms can be complicated and difficult. In research by Wolfe and colleagues, parents reported that 89% of children who died of cancer suffered a lot or a great deal from at least one symptom in the last month of life.[6] In a nationwide study in Sweden, parents of children who died of malignancies reported that pain in particular had a profound impact on their children.[102] Not surprisingly parents are quite distressed by these symptoms, especially changes in behavior and appearance, pain, weakness, fatigue, and dyspnea.[103]

Importantly there is also evidence of progress. A more recent study by Wolfe and associates documented less suffering from pain and dyspnea near death for children who died in the years after their initial study.[4] Thus a culture of awareness and attention to symptoms as well as intensive efforts at management may be able to mitigate the suffering children experience at the end of life.

Many of the symptoms we describe are addressed in detail in Chapter 71, "Symptom Management in the Child with Cancer." We have therefore limited our discussion to management of common symptoms in the setting of more advanced illness. Medications used in managing common symptoms are listed in Table 70-3.

Pain

Pain should be considered a medical emergency; over 80% of children with advanced cancer experience pain.[6,104] Pain affects not only the physical being but also the emotional and spiritual being. Often pain is accompanied by anxiety and emotional or spiritual distress. It is important to address each coexisting or contributing factor to pain. Parents often express extreme helplessness and distress when the child is suffering in pain.

The child's report of pain is an essential aspect of assessment.[105] Reliable scales that are consistent in the hospital and home are available, but assessment can be challenging, particularly with the nonverbal child. A knowledge of the child's usual behaviors and previous experience with pain management and with children with similar diagnoses can be helpful.[106] Tailored assessment tools can allow parents to equate behaviors with comfort or pain on an individualized rating scale.[107,108]

Treatment of pain should be followed by assessment for effective relief. The current WHO pain guidelines

TABLE 70-3   Medication Guidelines for Symptom Management

Symptom	Medication	Dosage	Comment
Anorexia	Megestrol acetate	100 mg PO bid; if no effect in 2 wk, double dose to 200 mg bid	Use only in children >10 yr
	Dronabinol	2.5-5 mg/m²/dose q4h	Use only in children >6 yr; contraindicated in depression
	Dexamethasone	0.3 mg/kg/day PO/IV	Use only in children >2 yr
	Cyproheptadine	0.25 mg/kg/day divided twice daily; age-dependent maximum daily dose: ≤6 yr: 12 mg/day; 7-14 yr: 16 mg/day; ≥15 yr: 32 mg/day	
Agitation	Haloperidol	0.01 mg/kg PO tid prn; for acute onset: 0.025-.05 mg/kg PO; may repeat 0.025 mg/kg in 1 hour prn	
Anxiety	Fluvoxamine	25 mg/day; may increase by 25 mg every 4-7 days up to 200 mg/day	Rarely can worsen depression or cause suicidality
Constipation	Glycerin suppository	One suppository PR qd	
	Lactulose	5-10 mL q2h until stools	
	Polyethylene glycol (MiraLax)	0.8 g/kg/day PO; maximum dose 17 g/day PO	Always dissolve dose in 4-8 oz of liquid
	Children's Senokot liquid	2-6 yr: 2.5-3.75 mL qd 6-12 yr: 5-7.5 mL qd	
	Pediatric Fleets enema	One PR qd prn	
	Methylnaltrexone	0.15 mg/kg SQ every other day prn	
Depression	Fluvoxamine	25 mg/day; may increase by 25 mg every 4-7 days up to 200 mg/day	Rarely can worsen depression or cause suicidality
	Methylphenidate	5 mg orally in the morning and at noon	Not recommended for children <6 yr
Dyspnea	Morphine sulfate immediate release	0.1 mg/kg PO q1-4h	Starting dose, no ceiling
	Lorazepam	Starting dose 0.025-0.1 mg/kg PO/IV q4h Maximum dose: 0.5 mg/kg	
Fatigue	Methylphenidate	5 mg orally in the morning and at noon	Not recommended for children <6 yr
Fever	Acetaminophen	15 mg/kg PO q4h	
	Ibuprofen	10 mg/kg PO q6-8h	
Insomnia	Melatonin	3 to 5 mg given 3 to 4 hours before an imposed sleep period	
	Trazodone	0.75-1 mg/kg PO at bedtime	Not recommended in children <10 years of age
	Nortriptyline	0.1 mg/kg PO at bedtime	
Nausea and vomiting Mild-moderate	Diphenhydramine	1 mg/kg PO q6-8h prn	
	Metoclopramide	0.25 mg/kg PO q8h prn	
Severe	Ondansetron	0.15 mg/kg PO q8h prn	
	Dexamethasone	0.3 mg/kg/day PO/IV	Maximum dose 10 mg/kg/day PO/IV
	Lorazepam	0.025-0.1 mg/kg q8h prn	Maximum 3 mg/day
Pruritus	Diphenhydramine	1 mg/kg PO/IV q4h prn	
	Hydroxyzine	0.5 mg/kg PO q8h prn	
	Hydrocortisone 1% cream	q6-8h	

Continued on following page

TABLE 70-3   Medication Guidelines for Symptom Management (Continued)

Symptom	Medication	Dosage	Comment
Pain			
Mild pain	Acetaminophen	15 mg/kg PO q4h prn or around the clock	Available in 160 mg/5 mL suspension or 80 mg/mL
Moderate to severe pain	Morphine sulfate immediate release	*<6 mo:* 0.1 mg/kg PO q3-4h *>6 mo to 50 kg:* 0.3 mg/kg PO q3-4h for opioid-naïve patient Titrate by 50%-100%/dose Prescribe breakthrough dose of 0.15 mg/kg PO q15-30 min.	
	Time-released morphine (MS Contin, Oramorph, Kadian)	Total daily dose divided by 2 determines q12h dose (approximately 1 mg/kg PO q8 or 12h). Breakthrough dose approximately 10% of the 24 hour total given q1-2h	
	Oxycodone	0.1 mg/kg q3-4h PO	
	Hydromorphone	0.03-0.08 mg/kg q4h PO	
	Fentanyl patch	*2-12 yr:* Do not exceed 15 µg/kg every 72 hours.	
	Methadone	0.1 mg/kg PO/IV bid or tid	No dose adjustments for 72 hours due to long half-life of drug; available in liquid
Adjuvant analgesics			
Bony metastases	Ibuprofen	10 mg/kg PO q6h	
	Choline magnesium trisalicylate	25 mg/kg PO tid	
Neuropathic pain	Nortriptyline	0.5mg/kg at bedtime	Maximum dose: 150 mg/ day
	Gabapentin	*Initial dose:* 10-15 mg/kg/day divided q8h. Titrate if needed to 50 mg/kg/day; not to exceed 2400 mg/day	
Severe visceral distention or bony disease	Prednisone	*Oral solution:* 1 mg/kg/day or bid with food	
Secretions	Scopolamine	1.5-mg patch, apply topically, every 72 hours	
	Glycopyrrolate	0.04-0.1 mg/kg PO q4-8h	
	Hyoscyamine sulfate	*<2 yr:* 4 gtts PO q4h prn (0.125 mg/mL solution) *2-12 yr:* 8 gtts PO q4h prn (0.125 mg/mL solution)	Maximum: 24 gtts/day
Seizures	Lorazepam	0.1 mg/kg PO/SL/PR, may repeat q 15 min × 3 doses 4 mg single dose	Parents should be advised to contact physician if used
	Diazepam rectal gel (Diastat)	*2–5 yr:* 0.2 mg/kg q 15 min × 3 doses *6-11 yr:* 0.3 mg/kg q 15 min × 3 doses *>11 yr:* 0.2 mg/kg q 15 min × 3 doses	Parents should be advised to contact physician if used

recommend the first step for mild pain and the second step for moderate to severe pain.[109,110] This approach suggests moving from weak analgesics, such as acetaminophen, to stronger analgesics such as opioids, although, depending on the presenting pain, strong analgesics may be initiated at the outset. Codeine should no longer be used in children. Although it was previously recommended, prescribing codeine should generally be avoided because of its side effect profile and lack of superiority over nonopioid analgesics. Furthermore, relatively common genetic polymorphisms in the *CYP2D6* gene lead to wide variation in codeine metabolism. Specifically, 10% to 40% of individuals carry polymorphisms causing them to be "poor metabolizers" who cannot convert codeine to its active form, morphine, and therefore are at risk for inadequate pain control; others are "ultrametabolizers" who may even experience respiratory depression from rapid generation of morphine from codeine. It is therefore preferable to use a known amount of the active agent, morphine.[111]

Plans for treatment should be based on the child's report of pain, the type of pain, the history of pain medicine use, and the parent's understanding of the pain and possible treatment options.

The child and parents should be educated about the basic principles of self-report, around-the-clock dosing, and the need for frequent reevaluation. Particularly when a family is facing the end of the child's life, the meaning of a recommendation for a medicine such as morphine sulfate cannot be underestimated.[112-115] Often myths of opioid use need to be explored and education, reassurance, and rationale provided. Using opioids also necessitates the prophylactic treatment of common side effects.

In addition to analgesic agents, there are a variety of adjuvant therapies that may be used to alleviate pain (see Chapter 71, "Symptom Management in Children with Cancer"). Increasingly families are also being encouraged to use nonpharmacologic strategies such as distraction, heat, cold, positioning, and touch. Children may also benefit from acupuncture, hypnosis, Reiki, and guided imagery, particularly if it has been used during the earlier days of treatment.[116-121]

Occasionally a child suffers from severe pain due to malignancy and needs massive opioid infusions. Collins and colleagues found that 6% of children with terminal malignancy were in this category of needing more than 3 mg/kg of morphine dose equivalent per hour. Eight of 12 required epidural or subarachnoid infusion and/or sedation.[122] Children may also experience rapidly escalating symptoms of pain, dyspnea, and or agitation. For these situations it has been beneficial to have templated orders, created by an interdisciplinary group of clinicians, so that sound principles and standard management can be executed at the bedside.[123]

Transitioning a child from the hospital to home with adequate symptom management may pose challenges to the home care system. Strategies such as using concentrated elixir that can be administered buccally, by mouth, or by gastrostomy tube or using transdermal medications such as a fentanyl patch[124,125] may be of benefit. Long-acting agents such as methadone and transdermal fentanyl may be given in conjunction with shorter-acting agents administered intravenously, subcutaneously, or orally. Compounding pharmacies can assist with multiple drug combinations for ease of administration in a variety of preparations. Many home care agencies, including hospice, are able to provide intravenous patient-controlled analgesia in the home setting as well. Finally exploring the potential use of midazolam or propofol infusions with the home care or hospice agency[126] may help determine what can realistically be provided for the child in extreme circumstances at home.

Dyspnea

Similar to pain dyspnea is subjective and can be caused by a multitude of factors. Having the child report the degree of distress associated with dyspnea, using a scale similar to a visual analogue scale for pain, may be helpful.[127] Recommended interventions should be congruent with the child's and family's goals, whether for extending life, relieving suffering, being in the hospital, or remaining at home. For instance if pneumonia is diagnosed, some families may choose parenteral antibiotics, others enteral antibiotics, or others strictly symptom relieving measures, such as treating fever and dyspnea. Diuretics may be given for situations involving fluid overload, and thoracentesis can be considered for pleural effusions, although such interventions may not provide effective palliation in patients with extensive parenchymal disease.[128] Transfusion can be considered if the level of red blood cells is low with the hope of increasing oxygenation potential.

Oxygen is often considered for dyspnea.[129] In a study in adult patients with advanced cancer, Philip and colleagues found that patients reported relief with either room air or oxygen by nasal prongs.[130] Interestingly they also found poor correlation between dyspnea complaints and measured oxygen saturation levels. In the hospital it may be easy to provide oxygen, whereas at home opening a window or providing a fan, to provide facial cooling in the areas subserved by the second and third branches of the trigeminal nerve, in addition to positioning and relaxation techniques, may be useful.

Finally opioid medications intravenously, subcutaneously, or orally can provide relief[131,132] and can be used without hastening death or suppressing respirations. Dyspnea can often be relieved with a lower opioid dose than that used for pain; a starting dose that is 25% to 30% of the opioid dose used for pain is often effective, although the dose should then be titrated to symptom relief. Nebulized opioids have been used, although studies have not confirmed efficacy of this route.[133] Emerging data among adults also suggest that low-dose long-acting opioids may improve symptom relief in chronic dyspnea.[134] In addition anxiety often precedes or follows episodes of dyspnea and may be relieved by benzodiazepines,[135,136] hypnosis, or other relaxation techniques.

Airway Obstruction

Airway obstruction and the resulting "noisy breathing" from excessive secretions and relaxation of oropharyngeal muscles can be very distressing to families. Usually deep suctioning is not helpful and may cause discomfort. Rather explaining that this is a natural result of the physiologic decline and that it is not distressing to the child may be reassuring. Anticholinergics may be used to decrease secretions[137,138] as well as decreasing parenteral or enteral fluids, if they are being given. However overly thickened secretions can lead to airway obstruction and greater distress; thus careful titration of interventions is warranted.

A somewhat different situation occurs when tumor progression causes airway obstruction. In our experience, the respiratory distress that occurs in this situation can be quite difficult to control, even with massive opioid doses. If the child appears to be gasping and uncomfortable despite opioid therapy, then palliative sedation may be warranted. In this case extensive discussions with the family and providers must occur so consensus is reached and it is clear that the goal is to sedate the child and relieve his or her symptoms and not to hasten death.

Gastrointestinal Symptoms

Nausea and Vomiting

Just over half of parents of children who have died of cancer report that nausea and vomiting were present at the end of life, often with significant associated suffering.[6,139,140] Such symptoms sometimes go unrecognized and untreated by physicians,[6,140,141] and even when treatment is offered, efficacy may be limited. Physicians should therefore assess for nausea and vomiting carefully, attend to symptoms promptly, and pay close attention to the efficacy of treatment.

Vomiting is stimulated by the gastrointestinal tract, after local receptor stimulation by obstruction, stasis, or toxins; by the pharynx, due to mucous or mucosal breakdown; by the medullary vomiting center, in response to cortical, gastrointestinal, or chemoreceptor trigger zone stimulation; or by the cortex, in response to elevated intracranial pressure or emotional and sensory stimuli. Chapter 71, "Symptom Management in Children with Cancer," provides further detail on causes of nausea and vomiting in cancer patients. Because the cause may define the most effective therapy, the most likely cause should be considered in evaluation and treatment of the patient.[142]

At end of life chemoreceptor trigger zone stimulation by toxins such as medications (chemotherapeutic agents, antibiotics, and opioids) and metabolic byproducts of uremia or hepatic failure in the blood and cerebrospinal fluid is a particularly common cause of nausea. In addition to effects on the chemoreceptor trigger zone, opioids induce nausea by decreasing gut motility and thereby causing gastroparesis and constipation. Patients may particularly experience nausea and vomiting after dose escalation, but this typically resolves after 3 to 4 days at a stable dose.[136] Opioid-induced nausea and vomiting are usually responsive to antiemetic therapy, especially with 5-hydroxytryptamine antagonists.[136,143,144]

Another important cause of nausea and vomiting in the end-of-life period is bowel obstruction, which deserves particular consideration in patients with abdominal tumors. Management of obstruction is discussed later in this chapter.

Refractory nausea and vomiting in the end-of-life setting have been effectively treated with antipsychotics such as olanzapine[145] and haloperidol. Also of note dexamethasone may have limited efficacy against nausea and vomiting in the end-of-life setting,[146] in contrast to its efficacy with chemotherapy-induced nausea, unless specific corticosteroid-responsive causes such as increased intracranial pressure or bowel obstruction are present. Finally because sights, smells, and the child's emotional state can contribute to nausea, management of distress and any environmental triggers should be considered. Nonpharmacologic therapies such as hypnosis and acupuncture may also be effective.

Constipation

Constipation is a common cause of pain and distress at the end of life,[6,139,140] particularly owing to opioid use for pain. Opioids cause constipation by decreasing colonic motility and secretions and by increasing fluid absorption in the colon. Preventive measures should always be considered at the time of initiation of opioids, with an osmotic and motility agent typically prescribed at initiation. Although many opioid-related side effects tend to decrease over time, constipation tends to remain a problem throughout the period of opioid use.[136]

Other important causes of constipation in the end-of-life care period are decreased patient mobility and decreased oral fluid and nutritional intake.[147] In addition cord compression and bowel obstruction due to intraabdominal tumor should be considered as possible causes.

Unless evaluation reveals an underlying cause such as bowel obstruction[148] or cord compression, therapy should be similar to that used for any child with cancer, regardless of phase of life. Because fluid intake is often limited at the end of life, however, fiber supplementation is not generally useful and can sometimes increase constipation. Similarly stool softeners alone are often inadequate and should instead be replaced by or combined with osmotic agents or stimulants.

For opioid-induced constipation, subcutaneous methylnaltrexone can also be used to relieve constipation. About half of patients will experience laxation after the first dose,[149] and subsequent doses can be given every other day as needed. Despite properties as a mu opioid receptor antagonist, methylnaltrexone has not been found to precipitate pain or withdrawal.[149]

Bowel Obstruction

Intestinal obstruction, such as from an abdominal tumor, is an important cause of refractory nausea and vomiting in the end-of-life care period.[142] Goals of care and the patient's quality of life may guide the choice of treatment. Therapeutic surgical options include bypass of the intestinal obstruction or placement of a venting gastrostomy tube. However nonsurgical alternatives exist for patients who wish to avoid surgery or who have limited ability to tolerate invasive measures.[150] Options for medical management include corticosteroids, which can be useful in relieving obstruction,[151] and octreotide, which can markedly decrease nausea and vomiting by reducing gastrointestinal secretions.[152] Octreotide can be administered subcutaneously and can be used in the outpatient setting if desired. The combination of morphine, scopolamine, and haloperidol has also been used to relieve cramping and nausea and vomiting.

Anorexia and Cachexia

Cachexia is a common finding in patients with advanced cancer. Poor nutritional intake and increased metabolic demands related to cancer appear to be its primary underlying causes. Mechanisms for increased catabolism, including lipolysis and proteolysis, are complex and likely mediated in part by cytokines.[153-155]

Anorexia compounds the problem. This too is mediated by a number of factors, including gastrointestinal (nausea, constipation, mucositis, dysphagia), other physical (pain), medication-related (impaired taste, decreased hunger), and psychological (depression) factors. Often multiple factors contribute to anorexia in any patient, and treatment should be directed at the individual causes when such causes can be discerned.[154,155]

Plans for care should include assessment of the meaning of this syndrome to individual patients and families. Some children and families will not be significantly bothered by anorexia and cachexia, but other children and families will find wasting to be extremely distressing, conjuring up the concern that the child is starving to death. Although severe cancer-related wasting is associated with poor outcomes in adult cancer patients,[156] increased nutrition is not enough to reverse this process.[157,158] Physicians may be able to address concerns about starvation by explaining that the cancer itself may be responsible for this condition and that increased nutritional intake often cannot halt this process. Goals for management should instead focus on symptoms, such as nausea or constipation, associated with this process. Another important goal is the maintenance of the child's level of function.[159]

Treatment of any underlying causes including associated psychological and spiritual issues should be a first step in management. Additional options such as enteral or parenteral[160] nutrition can be considered in light of overall goals of care and the efficacy of treatment for underlying causes. If the family wishes to institute artificial nutrition, it can be helpful to discuss the fact that, as the child's cancer progresses, there may be some point at which supplemental nutrition is no longer providing significant benefits relative to its actual or potential harms. The family and physician may wish over time to reassess the degree to which supplemental nutrition is meeting the goals of care, with the thought that, at some point, discontinuation of supplemental nutrition may make the most sense for the child. Discussion of this issue with families at the time of institution of supplemental nutrition may make reconsideration of this intervention less distressing for families as the child's illness progresses.

Pharmacologic therapeutic options include corticosteroids, which can increase appetite and nutritional intake. Their effect tends to wane after 4 weeks. Cyproheptadine is a safe and effective way to promote weight gain in children with cancer.[161] Cannabinoids such as dronabinol can also increase appetite, as can megestrol acetate.[162] Because megestrol acetate is associated with severe adrenal suppression in children with cancer,[163] it should be used with caution; some have recommended routine corticosteroid replacement for children on megestrol.[163]

Nutrition and Hydration

Near the end of life, fluid and nutritional needs diminish. Because parents often identify provision of nutrition as one of their important roles, physicians should prepare parents for the expected decrease in fluid and nutritional needs as the end of life approaches. Preparation for decreased urine output, as a manifestation of waning perfusion rather than of dehydration, can also be helpful.

Most studies suggest that nutrition and hydration can be withheld or limited in the end of life period without causing suffering.[164-166] In fact continued feeding via gastrostomy or nasogastric tube may be associated with abdominal discomfort or nausea when the child is in the last stages of life. In a study of bereaved parents who had made decisions to forgo artificial nutrition and hydration for their children, parents perceived deaths to be peaceful and comfortable.[167] Many of these parents chose to forgo artificial nutrition and hydration when the child developed feeding intolerance, suggesting that continued artificial nutrition may have increased discomfort.

One study of terminally ill adult cancer patients, however, suggests that some degree of parenteral hydration may improve symptoms associated with dehydration.[168] Even in this study, limited volumes of parenteral fluid were sufficient to improve symptoms. Parenteral hydration also has the potential to affect other choices about care, such as the location in which families feel most comfortable receiving care, the need for medical services at the end of life, and the need for intravenous or subcutaneous access.

When the choice is made not to provide supplemental hydration or nutrition at the end of life, it is helpful to pay close attention to symptoms of dehydration, hunger, or thirst, with the goal of treating any symptoms that arise. Often noninvasive measures such as moistening the lips or providing small tastes of food or fluid are enough to provide comfort.

Fatigue

Fatigue shapes the types of activities that children with life-limiting illnesses choose to participate in and has the potential to significantly diminish a child's quality of life.[169] Parents consider fatigue to be the most common symptom in the last month of life and the course of greatest distress for dying children.[6,170] Unfortunately this symptom is also the least likely to be treated.[6]

In general fatigue is a multidimensional symptom with both physical elements (muscle weakness, decreased energy) and cognitive or affective elements (difficulty concentrating, maintaining attention, lack of motivation and interest).[171] In a retrospective study of children who died of cancer, parents reported that 96% of children experienced fatigue in the last month of life. Nausea and vomiting, anorexia, and fear were other symptoms independently associated with fatigue.[172]

Younger children and adolescents with cancer define fatigue differently; younger children emphasize the physical aspects of the symptom, whereas adolescents describe multiple dimensions and distinguish between mental and physical fatigue.[173] Parents of children with cancer note that physical and emotional dimensions of fatigue create significant disruptions for the entire family.[174] Parents describe mood changes in the child and also report delays around the household and family activities because of the need to accommodate the fatigued child.[174] Fatigue also tends to limit children who wish to attend school until the very end of the illness, rather than receive private tutoring from a teacher in the hospital.[169] For children who remain in the hospital, fatigue also impacts cognitive function and mood due to interrupted sleep patterns that are mostly a result of frequent awakenings throughout the night and daytime hours.[175]

Opioid analgesics contribute to diminished levels of energy as well as a decreased ability to concentrate in children with advanced disease.[169] Coexisting or contributing factors include anemia, infection, pain, depression, and anxiety.[171,176] Assessment instruments commonly utilized to assess fatigue in cancer patients measure severity, onset, course, duration, and distress and concurrently assess other correlated symptoms, yet these assessment tools are not widely used. Furthermore the development of more sensitive instrumentation could assist practitioners in conducting a more comprehensive assessment of fatigue and, thus, provide more effective treatment of this symptom.[177]

Fatigue can seriously affect pediatric quality of life.[169] Multimodal approaches to treatment may be most effective; treatment of anxiety, depression, and sleep disturbance can also mitigate fatigue. Psychostimulants such as methylphenidate can be used to increase wakefulness, particularly when patients have opioid-related somnolence,[178] although they have not been formally evaluated in children. Because methylphenidate has a short duration of action, patients can control the timing of doses to coincide with important events during the day, such as time with family and friends. Blood transfusions, exercise programs (including physiotherapy),[179] psychosocial interventions, acupuncture, rest and relaxation (including playing/socializing), and nutrition and hydration counseling can also help alleviate fatigue.[171,174,180] A qualitative study conducted by Hinds and colleagues[173] reported differing views regarding successful fatigue interventions among patients, parents, and staff: whereas parents and staff considered themselves the primary responders to the child's fatigue and source of alleviation, patients stated rest and distraction as their first choice for alleviating symptoms of fatigue.

Psychological Symptoms

Psychological symptoms (including worrying, sadness, nervousness, and irritability) are among the most common symptoms experienced by children with cancer.[181,182] Some authors have reported that children with cancer as young as 7 years "can report clinically relevant and consistent information about their symptom experience" including psychological symptoms.[181(p 14)] Through interviews with children with life-threatening illness, Woodgate and colleagues[183] have identified a symptom experience described by children as: "I am hurting ... My heart is sad." Children may have difficulty distinguishing between such symptoms, instead experiencing them as more of an "overall state," such as "experiences that cause ... mental distress or suffering ... from feeling sick to being scared."[183(p 811)] In adult studies of cancer patients, the notion of neuropsychological symptom clusters (including depressive symptoms, cognitive disturbance, fatigue, sleep disturbance, and pain) may help shed light on the mechanisms behind these symptoms. It is hypothesized that proinflammatory cytokines may underlie the first stage of development of these symptoms; however, more research is needed to fully understand the role of these cytokines and how this information can be used to effectively treat this cluster of symptoms.[184] This phenomenon of a "cluster" of symptoms is also noted in quantitative studies in which children reported high levels of symptom distress, suggesting an "interplay between psychological and physical symptoms," especially between psychological symptoms and the physical symptom of pain.[182] Additionally when disease advances, it may be challenging for children to discuss with their loved ones and with the health care team some of the emotional issues that arise.

Depression

Children with life-threatening illness have been reported to experience symptoms of depression and may also meet diagnostic criteria for clinical depression. Gothelf found that 16 of 63 adolescents with cancer (25.4%) met the *Diagnostic and Statistical Manual of Mental Disorders*, fourth edition (DSM-IV) criteria for major depressive disorder.[185] Children older than 12 years, with a diagnosis of acute lymphocytic leukemia, receiving opiate analgesics, or undergoing radiation therapy were all significantly more likely to receive antidepressant medication.[186] Adolescents with higher levels of self-reported depression and lower levels of self-esteem had higher rates of nonadherence to medication; these same teens had lower rates of survival at a 6-year follow up.[187] Collins and colleagues found that roughly 36% of 159 children with cancer between the ages of 10 and 18 reported "feeling sad"; of this group, 17.5% rated its frequency as "a lot to almost always," 59.6% rated its intensity as "moderate to very severe," and 39.5% rated the distress it caused as "quite a bit to very much."[182]

In a younger cohort of children (ages 7 to 12) with cancer, Collins and colleagues[181] determined that 10.1% of the children surveyed reported feeling sad. Of this group, 53% reported feeling sad "a medium amount to almost all the time" on a scale of frequency, 60% reported feeling sad "a medium amount to a lot" on a scale of intensity, and 50% reported their sadness causing "a medium amount to very much" distress.[181] A slightly different story unfolds when Dejong and colleagues conducted a review of studies on depression in pediatric cancer published between 1980 and 2004. The majority of studies reviewed was cross-sectional and conducted, at the most, 5 years after diagnosis. In almost all the studies either no significant differences between depression rates in children with cancer and normal control subjects or significantly lower depression scores among the cancer group were found.[188]

There is mixed evidence that rates of sadness in children with cancer increase as disease advances. Parents have reported that a significant portion (up to 65%) of their children experience sadness during the terminal phase[139,189] and that sadness was the psychological symptom their child experienced most during the child's physical decline.[189] The well-being of children who died between the ages of 9 and 15 years was moderately or severely affected by depression, although similar results were not found among children who died before the age of 4 years.[139]

Risk factors for depression in children with cancer include parental depression and perceived stress and social support; age and illness severity are not consistently associated with depression.[188] However variation in findings across studies may be attributed to factors such as having multiple informants about the child's symptoms. Another confound in conducting accurate assessments of depression relate to the presence of other cancer symptoms or to the medications being taken to alleviate these symptoms, which may exacerbate or mask the symptoms of depression.[190]

Anxiety

Anxiety appears to be quite common in children with life-threatening illnesses.[181,182] In a sample of 149 children between the ages of 7 and 12, 20.1% reported feeling "worry."[181] Of those children, 43% experienced it a "medium amount to a lot" (intensity), 43% experienced it "a medium amount to almost all the time" (frequency), and 30% reported that it caused them "a medium amount to very much" distress. Among 160 older children with cancer,[182] 35.4% reported feeling "worry." Of these children, 66.1% reported that worry was "moderate to very severe," 28.6% reported a frequency between "a lot and almost always," and 27.2% reported the worry caused "quite a bit to very much" distress.

In children with advanced disease, levels of anxiety have been described by parents and health care providers. Researchers studied the medical records of 28 children who died of cancer to understand their end-of-life experiences; 53.6% of the children were documented as experiencing anxiety.[140] In a separate study of 164 symptom assessments collected in the last month of life, 50.0% of children reported "no problem" with anxiety/depression, 27.4% reported a "minor problem," and 17.7% reported a "major problem."[190] Anxiety was found to significantly influence the prevalence of pain.[191] Additionally exposure to physical pain early in life and/or a history of frequent painful medical procedures is associated with fear and anxiety during successive medical procedures, and, in turn, may have implications for future medical nonadherence and other related problems.[192] In the documentation of the symptom experiences of 30 children who died of cancer, worrying and nervousness were two of three symptoms "for which the proportion of children suffering a high level of distress ('quite a bit' to 'very much') was more than 50%."[170(pp 597–598)]

Parents of children who died of cancer were surveyed about their child's symptom experiences during the last month of life and reported, that among other symptoms, their child's sense of well-being was moderately or severely affected by anxiety.[139] Children older than 9 years were reported to be more troubled by anxiety than younger children.[139]

Qualitatively, children have described anxiety and fear together: "I am scared ... I don't know what is going to happen to me."[193(p 811)]; often children and families experienced a fear so strong that they could "not focus their thoughts on anything but the cancer and [it paralyzed] children and families from participating in life."[193(p 811)] In children undergoing cancer treatment, anxiety has been commonly linked to the experience of nausea, vomiting, insomnia, nightmares, and rashes. Younger children may act out behaviorally (kicking, fighting).[194] In children with advanced disease, children who identified themselves as feeling "scared" explained that the feeling was often the result of "painful treatments or procedures, experiencing unexpected and new symptoms, and experiencing feelings that there was a greater chance for relapse or death ... sometimes the fear experienced by children would be so great this led them to not to talk about the symptom(s) or event(s) that caused them to experience such intense fear and anxiety."[193(p 811)] Parents have described how they handled the fear that their children with cancer experience and note that they dealt with their child's fear by providing a sense of reassurance and security for their child up until the point when they needed to reprioritize their energies on their child's physical health rather than assuage their fears.[195]

Treatment of Depression and Anxiety

Pain, anxiety, distress, and suffering in children with advanced disease are interrelated; thus, providing relief for each of these symptoms is important. Given this reality, depression and anxiety, especially as they relate to other symptoms such as pain, should be treated simultaneously. Depression and anxiety screening programs[196,197] have been documented as operating successfully in oncology outpatient settings and should be adopted as standard practice to the continuum of pediatric care in all ages.

When treating depression and/or depressive symptoms of children in palliative care, a combination of medication and psychosocial therapies is optimal. Fluvoxamine and other types of serotonin reuptake inhibitors may be effective for those children with cancer who also exhibit symptoms of depression and anxiety. In one study of adolescents receiving chemotherapy for advanced cancer, 25.4% of those given fluvoxamine experienced a significant decrease in the somatic and nonsomatic symptoms of major depressive disorder with few side effects.[185] Methylphenidate also has antidepressant properties and may have a more rapid onset of antidepressant effects than other agents.[198] Other antidepressants may also be effective, as may counseling or psychotherapy or, ideally, a combination of medications and psychotherapy when indicated.

In contrast benzodiazepines in isolation are believed to be overused for chronic anxiety. Although medications can be effective in palliative care, therapeutic interventions that address a child's anxiety must be tailored to his or her condition, age, and temperament.[199] In children undergoing cancer treatment as well as at the terminal phases of the disease, supportive therapies such as hypnosis appear to be beneficial.[200,201] Pretend play has been suggested for younger children undergoing cancer treatment,[121] whereas telehealth[202] and virtual reality[203] technologies are on the cutting edge of providing effective forums to provide cost-efficient and convenient methods of support for diverse age groups of pediatric patients and their families.

Sleep Disturbance

Sleep disturbance in children who are critically ill typically takes the form of insomnia-type symptoms (involving difficulties in falling asleep, trouble staying asleep, early-morning awakening, complaints of nonrestorative sleep) and/or periods of too much sleep. When Goldman and colleagues[191] surveyed the records of children with terminal cancer, the prevalence of children who reported that too much sleep was a problem almost doubled between the point of entry into the study ("palliative phase") to the last month of life.

Data on the quality of sleep of children with critical illness found that children infected with human immunodeficiency virus slept approximately 1 hour less than healthy children, had more nightmares, and had more general sleep problems.[204] Children with serious illness[205] also slept significantly less on nights when they were experiencing pain, compared with nights that were pain free, and "reported poor sleep on an average of 43% percent of days with pain and 3% of days without pain."[206]

Predictors of sleep disturbance among cancer patients include pain, breathing difficulty, headaches, hot flashes, limb movements, frequent urination, nausea, and vomiting.[207] Patients who received greater amounts of radiation had poorer sleep.[208] In a study of adolescents with chronic pain, the investigators found a correlation between more frequent pain and daytime sleepiness and longer-lasting pain and later bedtimes; furthermore, sleep/wake problems (irregular sleep habits, hard time falling asleep or waking up) were associated with reduced social/emotional well-being.[211]

Psychological consequences of impaired sleep include feelings of fatigue, impaired daytime functioning, mood disturbances,[210] as well as an negative impact on quality of life, ability to cope, and perception of illness severity.[207] Cancer patients with sleep disturbances also reported high correlations between difficulty falling asleep and fatigue, early awakening and fatigue, and difficulty falling asleep and anxiety. Study results also support the idea that depression, anxiety, and sleep disturbances are related as are cancer-related pain, fatigue, and sleep disturbances.[211,212]

Treatments for problems with sleep include pharmacologic and nonpharmacologic modalities. Pharmacologic treatments include melatonin,[213] the tetracyclic antidepressant trazodone and the tricyclic antidepressants,[210] and antipsychotics (especially for cancer patients with delirium).[207] Psychological and behavioral interventions for sleep disturbance include stimulus control, sleep restriction, sleep education, relaxation training, and combinations of the aforementioned therapies.[210] In cases in which sleep problems are linked to symptoms or correlated with a disorder, treatment of the underlying condition may improve the sleep problems.

Anemia and Bleeding

Decisions about treatment of anemia should center on the child's quality of life and the expectations of the family and providers. For a child whose major complaint is fatigue, significant dizziness, tachycardia or dyspnea, a red blood cell transfusion may add to quality of life.[214] For some children and families, however, the need to travel to a center and spend half a day for associated medical care may make transfusions less desirable.

Fear of profuse bleeding in the setting of thrombocytopenia at the end of life is worrisome for providers and family members. As with red cells, platelet transfusions are not possible in the home setting; therefore careful planning and consideration are necessary so as not to disrupt the child's last days. Families may tolerate only treating symptomatic bleeding or may choose prophylactic scheduling of transfusions at a clinic or nearby hospital.[215] When children are at high risk for bleeding at home, parents and providers may want to develop a plan that minimizes distress to the child if this should occur. For example, ways to apply pressure for a nosebleed or having dark-colored linens on hand may be recommended in this situation.

Mucosal bleeding can sometimes be controlled with less invasive measures.[216] For example, aminocaproic acid can be used orally or intravenously to inhibit fibrinolysis.[217] Nausea is a common side effect, and aminocaproic acid should be avoided in patients who have hematuria. Topical options include fibrin sealants.[217] The tannins present in black teas can also help to stop bleeding. At home, patients can wet a tea bag with cool water and press it onto bleeding gums.

Fever and Infection

Parents of children with cancer are well aware of the consequences of fever and neutropenia during the child's treatment course. At the end of life, it may be appropriate to think about the role of antibiotics in a different way. Fevers may be due to infection; however, they may be due to the underlying disease. If a fever and associated symptoms can be ameliorated with acetaminophen and other simple measures, this may be most beneficial to the child. Other families may feel more comfortable with a course of oral or parenteral antibiotics, whether the child is an inpatient or outpatient. If this is the case, it may be helpful to plan for a time-limited course, after which antibiotics may be discontinued if no infection has been detected. Over time, parents who prefer antibiotic therapy may become more comfortable with only antipyretic treatment if they see that their child can tolerate this management strategy. Meeting with parents and the child to determine what investigative measures and treatment fit with their family goals will help to determine provider recommendations.[218]

Central Nervous System Symptoms
Seizures

Although seizures tend to be associated with limited suffering for the patient, parents often find seizures to be highly distressing at the end of life. Seizures may occur near the end of life as a result of central nervous system disease, electrolyte abnormalities, fever, or hypoxia. For any patient at home and deemed to be at risk for seizures, rectal diazepam should be available. At times seizure prophylaxis with an antiepileptic agent or benzodiazepine may also be desirable, especially if a patient is at high risk.

Increased Intracranial Pressure

Children with intracranial tumors are at risk for experiencing symptoms of increased intracranial pressure as the disease progresses. Common signs and symptoms include headache, vomiting, and somnolence. Although invasive therapies, such as surgical debulking or ventricular shunting, can be considered, the efficacy of such treatments may not be enduring in the end-of-life setting; tumor growth can quickly block a shunt or lead to recurrence of elevated pressure. Administration of dexamethasone can be effective in alleviating symptoms, and the dosing can be titrated as new symptoms arise or if initial symptoms wane. Dexamethasone-associated side effects, including mood changes, cushingoid appearance, and hunger with subsequent weight gain can be a source of distress to patients, and such side effects should therefore be part of ongoing discussion about dose titration. Radiation therapy may also be considered to decrease tumor size and thereby decrease symptoms at least temporarily.

Spinal Cord Compression

Spinal cord compression is relatively uncommon in the end-of-life setting for children with cancer, but it has the potential to severely impact quality of life at the end of life. Early diagnosis and management maximizes the chances of preservation of function.[219] Presenting symptoms include sensory and motor changes as well as bowel and bladder function abnormalities. Prompt imaging, typically with magnetic resonance imaging, can confirm the diagnosis. Dexamethasone can be used to decrease edema at the site of compression, thereby reducing symptoms and preserving neurologic function.[220] A local intervention such as neurosurgical intervention or radiation therapy is the mainstay of treatment, because decompression surgery plus radiation therapy increases the chances of recovery to ambulation.[221] However the specific intervention recommended should take the patient's overall functional status and goals of care into consideration.

Swallowing Impairment

Patients with brainstem involvement of a central nervous system tumor may develop swallowing impairment as one manifestation of disease progression. Such impairment has important implications for nutrition and hydration and may place patients at risk for aspiration pneumonia. Symptoms of coughing or choking when eating or drinking should be regarded as signs of aspiration and evaluated carefully. A swallowing study can establish which consistencies of liquids and solids the patient can tolerate without aspirating. If thin liquids cannot be tolerated, then additives can be used to thicken liquids until they are of tolerable consistency.

Some patients are unable to tolerate adequate nutrition and hydration without a significant risk for aspiration. A trial of a nasogastric tube may be a short-term option, or gastrostomy tube placement can allow long-term sustenance while minimizing food-related aspiration risks. This choice may be most appropriate in patients who are expected to live and to have a reasonable quality of life for some time. Even with a gastrostomy tube, patients remain at risk for aspiration of oropharyngeal secretions. Pharmacologic drying of secretions can offer some help, but most patients remain at risk for aspiration pneumo-nia. Chemical pneumonitis is also a risk in patients with reflux, and so acid control may also be beneficial.

For some families, placement and use of a gastrostomy tube may not be consistent with a goal of minimizing procedures or risks as opposed to allowing a more natural end of life to unfold. Such families may choose to either limit nutrition and hydration or to continue to provide oral nutrition and hydration despite the inherent risks. When eating provides significant pleasure to the patient, choosing to maintain oral feeding or even continuing to offer "tastes" may positively impact quality of life. For ease some families may choose to use a gastrostomy tube for nutrition and medication administration. Such decisions should be made with sensitivity to the role of parents in providing sustenance for their children and the social interaction inherent in meal time.

WHEN DEATH IS IMMINENT

Escalating Symptoms

For children with chronic conditions and progressive disease, escalating symptoms may occur over days, hours, or minutes. Ideally family goals are known and interventions can be recommended that are consistent.[79] A palliative care team often can assist the primary providers by anticipating what interventions are likely to be the most helpful and to cause the least suffering and in strategizing about how to carry out plans for care. It may be helpful to have an emergency symptom management plan (including pharmacologic and nonpharmacologic interventions) in place to initiate during an inpatient admission or at home. This process facilitates efforts of all involved to anticipate and proactively manage physical and emotional symptoms.

Families need to be reassured that there is no "right" place to be as the child nears end of life. Instead, families should choose what best meets the needs of the child and whole family. Homecare services vary widely between regions and countries.[87,222,223] Hospitals may have the advantage of multiple providers, quicker access to therapies, and even a special room such as a "comfort corner," but it is never "home."

For a patient experiencing extreme distress in the hospital, one strategy is to have algorithms or template orders in place for intravenous administration of medications with starting doses and resources to be accessed. Such an escalating situation for a child at our institution prompted nurses, physicians and pharmacists to develop a set of orders for management of escalating pain, dyspnea or agitation, using morphine, fentanyl, or hydromorphone, to improve care in these relatively rare but highly demanding cases.[123] Some general recommendations for rapid escalation include the following:[123]

- Bedside titration when symptoms arise, with intravenous bolus dosing every 10 to 15 minutes until pain is relieved
- Initial bolus dose of 10% of the 24-hour intravenous morphine dose for patients already on opioids
- Increase of intravenous bolus dose by 30% to 50% every third dose for unrelieved pain

- Initiation of continuous infusion once pain is relieved, with additional dosing, approximately equivalent to hourly rate, for breakthrough pain
- Increase of hourly intravenous rate and bolus by 30% to 50% when pain is unrelieved by existing regimen

At some institutions, a 24-hour on-call palliative care service or pain treatment service is available for assistance. Often allowing children who are facing the end of life to be directly admitted to their usual inpatient unit, with staff members who know them, will lessen the anxiety of the family and child and allow for faster, individualized care.

Palliative Sedation

Palliative sedation may be considered in rare circumstances. Sedation for refractory symptoms requires pain and palliative care expertise and a trusting relationship with the child and parents of the dying child. It must be clear that it is not the same as euthanasia and is not intended to hasten death, although parents who are desperate to see their child at peace may ask for that. When a child's refractory or unendurable symptoms cannot be managed by the "best standard" with opioids, benzodiazepines, and all other adjuncts, then palliative sedation may be warranted.[224,225]

Palliative sedation has the expressed outcome of relieving patient suffering and is considered only when physical and/or psychological symptoms are refractory to all other reasonable medical and complementary therapies.[226,227] Medications are most commonly started by a continuous infusion and titrated to the effect that the patient and/or parents and medical team have agreed upon. The most common agents used are anxiolytic sedatives, sedating antipsychotics, barbiturates, or general anesthetics.[126,226,228,229] Suggested dosing may be found in *Fast Facts*[230] available at www.eperc.mcw.edu or the *National Hospice and Palliative Care Compendium*.[231]

Before beginning palliative sedation, a frank discussion needs to be held with the family as well as the health care team so that any questions, concerns, or misgivings may be addressed.[232] Staff and/or family members may express ethical concerns that may be addressed by the pain or palliative care team, chaplaincy, or ethics consultation service. Ethical principles, including the "principle of double effect" and "principle of proportionality," justify the use of such measures when the benefits outweigh possible unintended but foreseeable consequences. Allowing for a full discussion of any ethical concerns, as well as the consistent intent to relieve suffering,[232] may be helpful. The patient and/or family and staff need to agree on the symptoms, amount of distress, and reasonable outcomes of interventions. Being certain that the patient and family have had the opportunity to express any final thoughts or feelings while the loved one is awake and conversant may be important to reduce the subsequent potential for regret.

Talking with Parents About What to Expect

Parents usually want to know and often ask what to expect as their child nears death.[16] In particular parents often want to know how to achieve comfort for their child, both with medications and with nonpharmacologic interventions. Once it is clear that there is very little likelihood of the child's clinical situation being stable or improving, families want to know when their child will die. Using parameters of prognosis such as "hours to days," "days to weeks," or "weeks to months" can be helpful because so often more specific prognostication is wrong.

Families want to know what death will look like and what to look for, so that they may be ready and be present at the moment of death. Some may wish to keep cardiac and respiratory monitors turned on to help them be prepared and know when it might be "safe" to leave the bedside, if only momentarily. It may be helpful to describe likely physical changes such as decreased mobility, weakness, loss of interest in eating or drinking, and decreased interest in interacting.[83] Being frank about decreased urine output, cool and mottled extremities, vital sign and breathing changes, respiratory congestion, and decreased level of consciousness in the final days can allow the parents to recognize the situation when it occurs.

At this time, it is important to help families focus on being with their child in whatever way is helpful to the child and family. Highlighting what family members can do for their loved one, for example, a simple hand or foot massage, retelling favorite family stories, playing music, praying, reading poems, and simply being present are examples.

Despite our best efforts, not every death is peaceful. Although assuring families that we will do everything possible to alleviate suffering and allow for a peaceful death, we cannot make promises. Some families interpret this as their child "fighting to the end." Making sure staff is present, listening, and responding to anyone's distress. During such times, it is important to reaffirm the positive role of the parents, siblings, and grandparents throughout the child's life.

Talking about Autopsy

The discussion about autopsy is often dreaded by staff, and sometimes it is avoided altogether, although ideally it is discussed by a trusted caregiver before the death. Some families ask about organ/tissue donation, and autopsy may be discussed similarly. Some families may believe that the child has "been through enough"; however some believe that this is a way to advance science and help other children who may suffer from the same condition. Autopsy may answer some of the questions about disease, cause of death, or side effects of treatments. Tissue or organ donation, including donation to science through autopsy, may be a part of a child's legacy. Studies have shown adults and children are altruistic even when facing death,[233] and so autopsy may be offered as a kind of "gift" to future affected children, to medical science, and to the training of physicians who are seeking cures to diseases. In addition to inviting the family to meet for a bereavement visit, inviting them to review the autopsy results with trusted providers and a pathologist may allow lingering questions or concerns that may be causing parental distress to be explored.[234]

Care of the Child's Body after Death

After death, whether at home or in the hospital, families often value the opportunity to have time for memory-making activities, family rituals, sharing of stories, and having staff come to pay respect. They may also want to participate in washing or dressing the body. In the hospital, one of the most difficult moments comes when the family leaves the hospital without their child. Having one staff member stay with the body while another accompanies the family to the lobby may be comforting. At home sometimes a parent chooses to carry the body to the hearse rather than have staff remove the body. Again having home care/hospice staff be present through this time may assist the family by bearing witness and holding the sacred space in an unspoken way. Finally, reassuring the family of bereavement follow-up allows them to know that continued contact will occur and is available.

AFTER DEATH

Bereavement Care for Families

Bereavement is a term used to describe the overall experience of family members and friends in the periods before, during, and after the death of a loved one.[235] It includes the unique grief (the emotional/internal process experienced as a result of the loss) that family members and loved ones feel as well as the mourning process (the more external process related to changing one's environment as a result of the loss) for the loss of a child.[236]

Bereavement begins upon the diagnosis of any pediatric life-limiting condition, because the diagnosis, in itself, signifies a loss of normal life and the beginning of significant emotional and physical adaptations on the part of the family. Health care providers can begin to support the family before the death of the child by helping the family to stay connected with the child, communicate effectively with the child, process the concept of the "appropriate death," and develop memories. In addition, health care providers may help the family to negotiate the medical system, obtain respite care, and assist with the "prethinking" of the funeral.[237] Having this type of system in place before the death of the child can help the family begin to adapt to life without their child.[238]

The grieving process for families who have just lost a child is typically fraught with the ache of coming to the realization that they will no longer see or be with their child. This process is often layered with a sense of guilt as well—guilt that stems from questioning their treatment decisions, thoughts that they caused the illness, as well as guilt from perhaps giving more attention to the ill child than other siblings.[237] The two-track model of bereavement, described by Rubin,[239,240] can guide interventions in dealing with the grief of family member by first (track one) assessing the individual's functioning (for example his or her feelings of anxiety, depression, guilt, return to work) and then (track two) assessing the relationship of the individual to the deceased person, even as it continues to evolve and change in meaning over the course of the surviving relative's life span. Similarly via review of recent literature on parent grief, Davies rejects certain notions that bonds with the deceased individual must be broken for grief to be resolved or to obtain closure. Instead she concludes that "exploring the significance of their children's lives, as well as the continuing influence they have through continuing bonds, may be regarded as a positive means [of] dealing with bereavement."[241(p 510)] Others emphasize attempting to understand patterns of individual differences in grieving families and how continuing the bond with the deceased while relinquishing certain ties can be adaptive to the family functioning on a long-term basis.[242]

Spinetta and colleagues measured the after-death (up to 3 years after the death) adaptation of parents whose child had died from cancer. Of 23 sets of parents interviewed, most had "adequately mastered" a return to normal activities, become active and zestful again, become able to confront physical reminders of their child, and had no regret of the past. Other tasks, such as resolving remaining questions and healing relationships with siblings, were found to be more difficult for the bereaved parents.

Four to 6 years after the death of a child due to cancer, bereaved parents were more likely to report depression, low to moderate psychological well-being, and anxiety compared with nonbereaved parents. Overall self-reports of continued grief were associated with more anxiety and depression. The risk for depression and anxiety for bereaved parents resembled that of nonbereaved parents 7 to 9 years after the death of the child; however parents were at an increased risk if their child was 9 years or older at the time of death.[243,244]

Immediate supportive bereavement interventions can take place during end-of-life care. In-depth qualitative interviews with 10 mothers of children who died of a variety of life-limiting illnesses revealed four main needs of the mothers during the end of their children's lives: time with their dying child, space and privacy to be with their dying child, time to be with their child's body after death, and space and privacy to be with their child's body after death. Mothers who did not have time, quiet space, and dignity expressed distress and anguish over the unavailability of these things.[245] In a study of 156 bereaved parents, Lichtenthal and colleagues[246] explored how parents brought meaning to the loss of their child. Through qualitative analysis of these parent interviews, *meaning making* was broken down into two themes: (1) sense-making (the use of spirituality and religious beliefs in finding meaning) and (2) benefit-finding (the increased need to offer help and compassion for others' suffering). The support of *meaning making* for bereaved parents can be a valuable tool for balancing the act of maintaining ties with their deceased child while also facilitating the relinquishing of some ties that may complicate grief.

Shortly after their child's death, many parents cited that the attendance of members of health care team at their child's memorial or funeral service tended to be helpful in coping with their loss. Parents also found that formal support groups where they could speak with other parents who had similar experiences, follow-up contact with the health care team to discuss results of the autopsy, contact with the health care team on significant days (e.g., anniversaries of the death, Mother's or Father's Day), and guidance in how to help siblings cope with the loss of a brother or sister proved to be beneficial while they mourned their loss.[247] Other, more long-term, types of supportive care for bereaved families included individual grief counseling for one or both parents, couples counseling, family counseling, and social support groups,[237] including Internet support groups.[248]

Care of Siblings

Siblings of children with cancer are deeply affected by their experiences of the sibling's illness and its effects within the family.[249] Siblings experience profound life changes as a result of the illness and experience intense positive and negative feelings.[250] Bereaved siblings are at increased risk for low self-esteem, have lower levels of personal maturity, and experience more difficulties falling asleep than nonbereaved siblings.[251] In addition the family dynamic and their role within the family are often altered by the illness.[250]

The experiences of bereaved siblings are particularly intense. Their bereavement is often marked by feelings of anger, guilt, jealousy, and sadness.[252] A particular area of distress reported by siblings is a lack of involvement in the dying process.[252] Parents in particular may choose not to involve the sibling closely in the end-of-life period so as to protect them.[253] However it is possible that limited involvement is even more problematic for some siblings than being closely involved in the end-of-life period. Care providers should encourage open communication and allow involvement in care to the extent that siblings wish. Helping parents to understand that such involvement can be healing may be useful.

Care of Staff

Providing care to children with life-limiting illnesses and their families can be one of the most worthwhile acts a health care professional can offer. At the same time providing pediatric palliative care services can place both uniquely physical and emotional demands on the health care team. Pediatric oncologists need to be aware of the impact of these stressors on themselves and colleagues and take the appropriate steps in maintaining both a healthy physical and emotional well-being. Zambrano and associates[254] investigated how general practitioners processed the death of their adult patients. The general practitioners who participated in the study used the metaphor of a "death journey" that involved five different moments that depicted their experience with dying patients: private acknowledgment, communication of prognosis, continuity of care, the moment of death, and looking after the family. A model of self-awareness for grief in caregiving as described here is a positive step in acknowledging the very normal emotions that practitioners experience when caring for sick patients and thus opens the door for self-care and prevention of burnout at each stage of the caregiving process.

Stressors identified by hospice nurses and physicians have included care of patients with intractable symptoms, difficult communication issues, administrative concerns and paperwork, too many patients dying at the same time, the expectation (among family members, other staff, or self-imposed) that all the patient's problems can be fixed, as well as becoming overinvolved in the care of their patients.[255-257] When pediatric residents were asked to rate their personal experiences regarding death, similar emotional stressors such as guilt and feelings of responsibility over the child's death were prevalent.[258]

Self-care can take the form of staff support sessions, educational seminars, as well as mechanisms created within the medical system to relieve professionals of patient service time to restore physical and emotional well-being. Methods for staff support can include regular, confidential debriefing sessions consisting of time for reflection with opportunities for staff to share challenges as well as effective ways for coping with these challenges.[259] These debriefing sessions can either have a specific focus (e.g., processing the death of an individual child) or can have a more general focus that might take into account the day-to-day issues that arise from providing pediatric oncology and palliative care services.[260] Other types of staff support sessions can take the form of annual or semi-annual memorial services to give health care teams a designated day to remember those children they cared for throughout the year.[255,261]

Often a combination approach of providing educational seminars regarding palliative care topics as well as time set aside to discuss and process emotions can be quite effective in gathering a larger crowd of professionals who may not necessarily attend one type or another. For example a combination approach could include a 1-day[262] or several-day death and bereavement retreat for residents to help them achieve the following goals: gain experience in talking about child death with parent; practice being in emotional situations; provide knowledge about autopsy, organ donation, and ministry; provide resources for supporting the family; gain insight into the impact of death on themselves and prevent burnout from stress; and provide resources to better understand the parents' perspective.[263-265]

Sumner suggests opportunities for professional growth for the seasoned professional as well as new providers of pediatric oncology and palliative care services through mentorship programs. This type of program would encourage, for example, a new physician or pediatric oncology provider be partnered with an "expert colleague."[255] The mentor, in turn, may develop the sense of satisfaction of self-efficacy in training a new member of the team in providing pediatric palliative care.

ONGOING CHALLENGES

High-quality palliative care is now an expected standard,[28,80] and Hospice and Palliative Medicine has been recognized as a formal medical subspecialty.[266] The American Academy of Pediatrics set the following as a minimum standard for pediatric palliative care: "Excellence in pediatric palliative care is essential for hospitals and other facilities caring for children. Program development in pediatric palliative care, along with community outreach and public education, must be a priority of tertiary care centers serving children."[80]

Although the principles of pediatric palliative care have been defined and refined over recent decades, notable challenges remain in all domains of care, including communication, symptom management, coordination of care, and bereavement. The field of pediatric palliative care is still in need of rigorous research efforts, and these efforts should be integrated into curricula across disciplines and at all levels. Further advocacy aimed at creating greater opportunity for children to receive palliative care across care settings is essential.[28]

References available online at ExpertConsult.

KEY REFERENCES

2. Zhukovsky DS, Herzog CE, Kaur G, et al: The impact of palliative care consultation on symptom assessment, communication needs, and palliative interventions in pediatric patients with cancer. *J Palliat Med* 12:343–349, 2009.
   A study demonstrating that palliative care consultation can identify symptom control and communication needs.
3. Johnston DL, Nagel K, Friedman DL, et al: Availability and use of palliative care and end-of-life services for pediatric oncology patients. *J Clin Oncol* 26:4646–4650, 2008.
   This study evaluated the availability of palliative care services in Children's Oncology Group institutions; only 58% of these institutions had such services available.
4. Wolfe J, Hammel JF, Edwards KE, et al: Easing of suffering in children with cancer at the end of life: is care changing? *J Clin Oncol* 26:1717–1723, 2008.
   A follow-up study looking at changes in care after the institution of palliative care services.
6. Wolfe J, Grier HE, Klar N, et al: Symptoms and suffering at the end of life in children with cancer. *N Engl J Med* 342:326–333, 2000.
   This study evaluated the prevalence of symptoms and suffering at the end of life among children with cancer. Many children received aggressive treatment and experienced significant suffering.
7. Bluebond-Langner M, Belasco JB, Goldman A, et al: Understanding parents' approaches to care and treatment of children with cancer when standard therapy has failed. *J Clin Oncol* 25:2414–2419, 2007.
   This ethnographic study evaluated parents' decisions about care for their children with relapsed disease and a poor prognosis. Most parents wished to continue cancer therapy even after standard therapy had failed.
8. Wolfe J, Klar N, Grier HE, et al: Understanding of prognosis among parents of children who died of cancer: impact on treatment goals and integration of palliative care. *JAMA* 284:2469–2475, 2000.
   This study identified delayed parental recognition of a child's poor prognosis relative to physician recognition. Earlier parental recognition of a poor prognosis was associated with a greater use of palliative measures.
9. Murray SA, Kendall M, Boyd K, et al: Illness trajectories and palliative care. *BMJ* 330:1007–1011, 2005.
   This article describes different illness trajectories and the ways that trajectory of illness impacts the use of palliative care.
10. Mack JW, Wolfe J, Grier HE, et al: Communication about prognosis between parents and physicians of children with cancer: parent preferences and the impact of prognostic information. *J Clin Oncol* 24:5265–5270, 2006.
    This study evaluated parent preferences for prognostic information and found that most parents want prognostic information even if they also find it upsetting.
12. Thompson LA, Knapp C, Madden V, et al: Pediatricians' perceptions of and preferred timing for pediatric palliative care. *Pediatrics* 123:e777–e782, 2009.
    This study evaluated pediatricians' beliefs about the optimal timing of palliative care. Most equated palliative care with hospice and referred patients only when there was no possibility of cure.
15. Seecharan GA, Andresen EM, Norris K, et al: Parents' assessment of quality of care and grief following a child's death. *Arch Pediatr Adolesc Med* 158:515–520, 2004.
    This study evaluated the relationship between perceived care quality and experiences with grief after a child's death. Satisfaction with care was generally high despite grief.
16. Mack JW, Hilden JM, Watterson J, et al: Parent and physician perspectives on quality of care at the end of life in children with cancer. *J Clin Oncol* 23:9155–9161, 2005.
    This study evaluated factors associated with parent ratings of the quality of care their child received near death. Physician communication was a primary determinant of quality of care ratings.
17. Hurwitz CA, Duncan J, Wolfe J: Caring for the child with cancer at the close of life: "there are people who make it, and I'm hoping I'm one of them." *JAMA* 292:2141–2149, 2004.
    This article provides guidance for conversations with children and parents near the end of life, including identifying and supporting goals of care.
21. Hinds P, Drew D, Oakes LL, et al: End-of-life care preferences of pediatric patients with cancer. *J Clin Oncol* 23:9055–9057, 2005.
    Adolescent patients were interviewed after making end-of-life decisions about care; many of their decisions focused on the needs of their loved ones.
23. Hinds PS, Oakes LL, Hicks J, et al: "Trying to be a good parent" as defined by interviews with parents who made phase I, terminal care, and resuscitation decisions for their children. *J Clin Oncol* 27:5979–5985, 2009.
    The researchers evaluated parents' perspectives on end-of-life decision-making for their children and found that many were guided by their feelings about what it means to be a good parent.
24. Renjilian CB, Womer JW, Carroll KW, et al: Parental explicit heuristics in decision-making for children with life-threatening illnesses. *Pediatrics* 131:e566–e572, 2013.
    This study evaluated heuristics used by parents of children with life-threatening illness as they made decisions about care.
26. Wiener L, Zadeh S, Battles H, et al: Allowing adolescents and young adults to plan their end-of-life care. *Pediatrics* 130:897–905, 2012.
    This study describes the development of the Voicing My Choices planning guide for young people with life-threatening illness.
28. Field MJ, Behrman RE; Institute of Medicine (U.S.) Committee on Palliative and End-of-Life Care for Children and Their Families: *When children die: improving palliative and end-of-life care for children and their families*, Washington, DC, 2003, National Academy Press.
    This Institute of Medicine report describes the state of palliative care for children.
30. Himelstein BP, Hilden JM, Boldt AM, et al: Pediatric palliative care. *N Engl J Med* 350:1752–1762, 2004.
    This review describes central issues in pediatric palliative care.
31. Durall A, Zurakowski D, Wolfe J: Barriers to conducting advance care discussions for children with life-threatening conditions. *Pediatrics* 129:e975–e982, 2012.
    This study evaluated clinician perspectives on barriers to advance care planning discussions. Lack of parent understanding of prognosis was perceived as a major barrier.
32. Lyon ME, Jacobs S, Briggs L, et al: Family-centered advance care planning for teens with cancer. *JAMA Pediatr* 167:460–467, 2013.
    These authors offered advance care planning interventions for adolescents with cancer and found that interventions were associated with decisions to limit treatments.
35. Kreicbergs U, Valdimarsdottir U, Onelov E, et al: Talking about death with children who have severe malignant disease. *N Engl J Med* 351:1175–1186, 2004.
    This study found that parents who choose not to talk with their children about the child's imminent death may regret not having done so.

61. Hexem KR, Mollen CJ, Carroll K, et al: How parents of children receiving pediatric palliative care use religion, spirituality, or life philosophy in tough times. *J Palliat Med* 14:39–44, 2011.
This study found that many parents draw on religion, spirituality, or life philosophy when caring for a child with advanced illness.

71. Bomba PA, Vermilyea D: Integrating POLST into palliative care guidelines: a paradigm shift in advance care planning in oncology. *J Natl Compr Canc Netw* 4:819–829, 2006.
This article describes the use of POLST (Physician Orders for Life-Sustaining Treatment) in the oncology setting.

88. Tomlinson D, Bartels U, Gammon J, et al: Chemotherapy versus supportive care alone in pediatric palliative care for cancer: comparing the preferences of parents and health care professionals. *Can Med Assoc J* 183:E1252–E1258, 2011.
This study found that parents are more likely than clinicians to desire aggressive treatment for their children at the end of life.

95. Kang TI, Hexem K, Localio R, et al: The use of palliative chemotherapy in pediatric oncology patients: a national survey of pediatric oncologists. *Pediatr Blood Cancer* 60:88–94, 2013.
This study describes oncologists' experiences prescribing palliative chemotherapy; 40% of oncologists described prescribing chemotherapy in order to respect parental wishes.

100. Mack JW, Joffe S, Hilden JM, et al: Parents' views of cancer-directed therapy for children with no realistic chance for cure. *J Clin Oncol* 26:4759–4764, 2008.
This study found that, although many parents chose chemotherapy at the end of life for their own children, not all would recommend it to others, especially if they believed their child had suffered as a result of chemotherapy.

109. Persisting pain in children package: WHO guidelines on the pharmacological treatment of persisting pain in children with medical illnesses. 2012. Accessed August 13, 2013 at <http://whqlibdoc.who.int/publications/2012/9789241548120_Guidelines.pdf>.
These guidelines offer information about pain treatment for children.

167. Rapoport A, Shaheed J, Newman C, et al: Parental perceptions of forgoing artificial nutrition and hydration during end-of-life care. *Pediatrics* 131:861–869, 2013.
This qualitative study evaluated parental experiences of forgoing artificial nutrition and hydration at the end of their child's life.

196. Kersun LS, Rourke MT, Mickley M, et al: Screening for depression and anxiety in adolescent cancer patients. *J Pediatr Hematol Oncol* 31:835–839, 2009.
This study found that adolescents report relatively low levels of anxiety and depression, especially compared with physicians' reports about adolescents.

244. Rosenberg AR, Baker KS, Syrjala K, et al: Systematic review of psychosocial morbidities among bereaved parents of children with cancer. *Pediatr Blood Cancer* 58:503–512, 2012.
This systematic review summarized findings about psychosocial outcomes among bereaved parents of children with cancer. Parents had increased risks for anxiety, depression, prolonged grief, and poor quality of life.

CHAPTER 71

Symptom Management in Children with Cancer

Christina K. Ullrich, Amy Louise Billett, and Charles B. Berde

CHAPTER OUTLINE

Progress in understanding the causes of pediatric cancer, as well as advances in cancer-directed therapies, hold great promise for curing and extending the lives of many children diagnosed with cancer. However, as advances in medicine and technology improve the survival of children with life-threatening illnesses, attention to health-related quality of life and progress in symptom management have not kept pace with advances in disease-directed therapies. As a result a population of children exists who are living with cancer and have suboptimally controlled symptoms.

Amelioration of symptoms experienced by a child with cancer does far more than reduce the suffering caused by the troublesome symptoms. Control of physical symptoms may allow attention to be focused on other issues faced by family members who are living with a child's cancer, such as psychosocial concerns or existential distress, and it may allow them to participate in activities and interactions that are important for maximizing quality of life. In fact, symptom burden is highly associated with quality of life in children with cancer[1] and is one of the most significant determinants of quality of life in adolescents and young adults with cancer.[2] In some instances, improved control of symptoms may enhance the delivery of optimal cancer-directed therapy as well. Finally, optimal symptom control throughout the illness trajectory may also shape the child's and family's long-lasting impressions of their experience with cancer.

In many instances, relief from distressing symptoms is possible with a myriad of modalities available today. Pediatric oncologists play a key role in managing symptoms in their patients. Symptom management requires actively partnering with families to assess not only the presence of symptoms but also the impact of uncontrolled symptoms on their daily lives, as well as to implement appropriate symptom-directed interventions. Ideally such attention to symptoms occurs in the context of attention to the child's overall condition so that the impact of symptoms on the child's overall quality of life is appreciated.

The vast majority of children who have cancer experience multiple symptoms that could be ameliorated but are not addressed.[3,4,5,6,7] For example, Collins and colleagues[3] asked 10- to 18-year-old children about the symptoms they experienced during the past week. Symptoms included lack of energy (49%), pain (49%), nausea (45%), lack of appetite (40%), and itching (33%).[3] The prevalence of uncontrolled symptoms in children with cancer is likely to stem from a variety of systemwide causes, including inadequate formal training dedicated to symptom management, a focus on cancer-directed treatment, and time constraints.

In addition, a lack of systematic research in the pediatric population, particularly with regard to non–pain-related symptoms, leads to a lack of evidence or standards on which to base interventions. Many symptom-directed interventions for children at this time are based on extrapolation from adult studies or even individual or anecdotal experiences. Some guidelines exist that are strongly evidence based, such as the National Comprehensive Care Network (NCCN) Guidelines for Pediatric Cancer Pain, which is encouraging.[8] As advances in pediatric oncology extend into the realm of symptom management, additional guidelines for non–pain-related symptoms will become available to help pediatric oncologists attend to their patients' symptoms.

The promising survival rates that have resulted from discoveries in pediatric oncology have led to increasing attention to health-related quality of life and the human costs of cancer care.[9] With such a shift, efforts to understand and ameliorate the myriad of symptoms experienced by children with cancer are likely to be increasingly supported in the coming years.

PAIN

Pain is defined as "an unpleasant sensory and emotional experience associated with actual or potential tissue damage or described in terms of such damage."[10] This symptom is the most studied and best understood of all cancer symptoms in adults and children alike. However, despite such attention, pain is often suboptimally controlled.

Families and children confronting cancer often worry about potential pain due to the disease and its treatment. In fact, pain is the most feared problem for children with cancer.[11] To some extent, their concern is justified. For example, Collins and colleagues[3] demonstrated that children with cancer experience multiple symptoms, including pain. Among 160 children ages 10 to 18 years with cancer, pain was the second most common symptom, with a prevalence of 49.1%. In addition, 61.6% reported pain that was moderate to very severe in the 48 hours prior to completing the questionnaire, and 40.9% reported pain that occurred "a lot" to "almost always." Moreover, the pain experienced by children was distressing—"quite a bit" to "very much" in 39.1% of respondents.

Pain control provides a variety of benefits beyond the amelioration of suffering. Prompt pain relief is needed to prevent central sensitization, a centrally mediated hyperexcitability response that may result in escalating pain. Uncontrolled pain also leads to a physiologic stress response with a variety of effects such as altered metabolism and immune function. Control of pain with appropriate analgesia in the perioperative period can reduce some of these effects and prevent complications.[12]

Epidemiology

In general, pain experienced by children with cancer may be caused by a variety of entities, including the disease itself (e.g., tumor invasion of bone, viscera, or the peripheral or central nervous system [CNS] or compression of the spinal cord), treatment (e.g., mucositis, radiation-induced dermatitis, and drug-induced neuropathy) or procedures (e.g., venipuncture, lumbar puncture, and bone marrow aspiration or biopsy, as well as postoperative pain). Authors who performed a cross-sectional analysis of pain in inpatient children with cancer found that the most frequent cause of pain was adverse effects of antitumor therapy.[13] Evidence also indicates that children who have solid tumors outside of the CNS have more pain and higher opioid requirements.[14]

Because the majority of pediatric cancers respond at least initially to treatment, most of the pain that children experience early in the disease trajectory is related to procedures and treatment. Later, if the cancer progresses, pain is more likely to be due to tumor extension. In a series of structured interview surveys conducted by Ljungman and colleagues,[15] 49% of children with cancer experienced pain at diagnosis. Procedure- and treatment-related pain were the most significant types of pain at the start, and although procedure-related pain improved, treatment-related pain did not improve. In addition, measurement of pain intensity was rarely performed.[15]

A significant barrier to pain management in children stems from the fact that research and development of evidence-based practice guidelines in pediatrics lag behind that in adults. The NCCN and World Health Organization (WHO) have developed comprehensive guidelines for managing pain in children with cancer,[16] but in many instances, pain management in children relies on extrapolation from adult data, anecdotal reports, and personal experience.

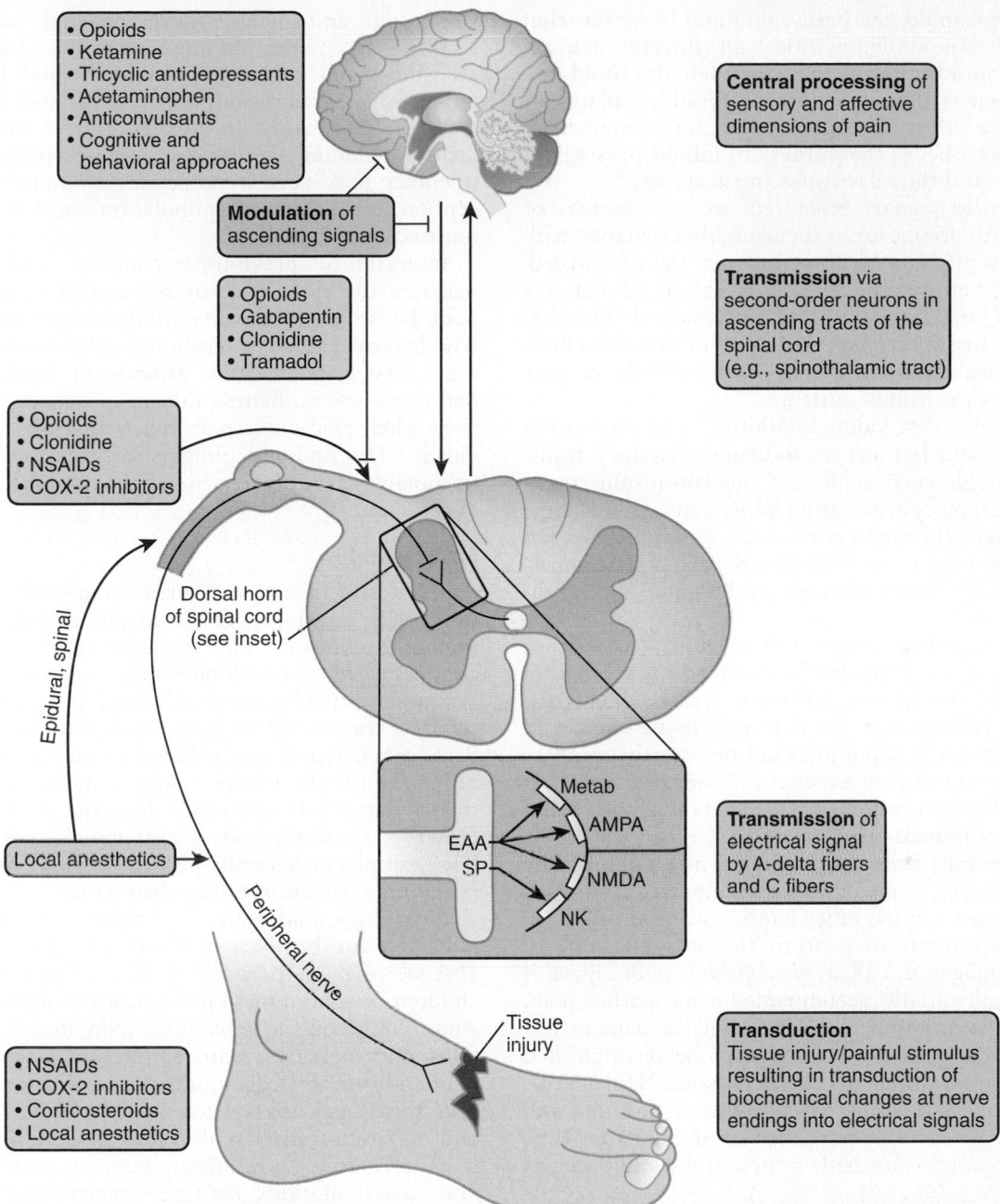

Figure 71-1 Anatomic illustration of a nociceptive pathway and corresponding analgesic action sites. Major elements of nociception are indicated in *blue boxes*. Analgesics are indicated in *green boxes*. *Inset*, Neurotransmission and neuromodulation in the dorsal horn of the spinal cord. Analgesics: *COX-2*, Cyclooxygenase-2; *NSAIDs*, nonsteroidal antiinflammatory drugs. Neurotransmitters: *EAA*, Excitatory amino acids; *SP*, substance P. Receptors: *AMPA*, Alpha-amino-3-hydroxy-5-methyl-4-isoxazolepropionic; *Metab*, metabotropic; *NK*, neurokinin; *NMDA*, N-methyl-d-aspartate.

Children may also experience incidental, non–cancer-related pain. Other pain-inducing disorders such as migraines, recurrent abdominal pain, or injuries seen in the general pediatric population can also occur in children with cancer. These causes of pain unrelated to the cancer diagnosis should always be included in the differential diagnosis of pain in children who have cancer.

Pathophysiology

Nociception is a complex process whereby actual (or potential) tissue damage is perceived as pain by an individual. In many instances pain is a protective mechanism that alerts a person to tissue injury. Nociception may be thought to occur on three levels: peripheral, spinal, and supraspinal (Fig. 71-1). Through transduction, the primary afferent nociceptors, which are thinly myelinated A-delta and unmyelinated C fibers, transmit biochemical changes at the sensory nerve endings that are generated by painful (chemical, thermal, or mechanical) stimuli into electrical signals. Stimulation of such nerve endings in the periphery may be increased or decreased by molecules such as prostaglandins, leukotrienes, bradykinin, and histamine. For example, the bradykinin and histamine that accompany tissue inflammation can directly activate nociceptors, in addition to reducing their threshold and increasing their response to suprathreshold stimulation.[17] The analgesic effect of nonsteroidal antiinflammatory drugs (NSAIDs) lies in their ability to inhibit prostaglandin synthesis and thus desensitize nociceptors.[18]

The electrical signals generated are propagated, or transmitted, to second-order neurons that synapse with sensory nociceptors in the dorsal horn of the spinal cord. Second-order neurons convey signals via ascending tracts in the spinal cord, including the anterolateral spinothalamic tracts, to supraspinal sites that include the brainstem, thalamus, and cortical areas involved in the sensory and affective dimensions of pain.

For example, descending inhibitory pathways from the thalamus and brainstem modulate excitatory transmission through such inhibitory neurotransmitters as serotonin, norepinephrine, and endogenous opioids. Several pharmacologic interventions such as opioids and tricyclic antidepressants (TCAs) exert their analgesic effects through such inhibitory processes at the spinal and supraspinal levels.

Pain is a complex sensory and emotional experience that involves nociception but is modified by a range of contextual and psychological factors. Because the experience of pain is subjective, the degree of tissue injury and therefore nociceptive input does not necessarily correlate with the intensity of pain experienced. Interventions that may reduce the perception of pain include hypnosis and relaxation techniques.

Pain that results from stimulation of intact neurons by impulses reflecting tissue injury or inflammation is called *nociceptive pain*. On the other hand, pain resulting from abnormal excitability of neurons (for example, due to neuronal damage) is called *neuropathic pain*. Even if tissue damage initially accompanied neuropathic pain, neuropathic pain may persist long after the damage has resolved. Nociceptive pain often may be distinguished from neuropathic pain by its characteristics. Neuropathic pain frequently is described as burning or shooting and is often associated with paresthesias or allodynia (i.e., elicitation of pain by normally nonpainful stimuli such as light touch).

Factors Influencing a Child's Experience of Pain

As a subjective experience, many factors have an impact on a child's experience of pain. Recognizing such factors can facilitate an understanding of the pain as it is experienced by the child and facilitate development of an effective pain treatment plan. The experience of pain shapes learning in infancy and throughout life. The neurobiologic mechanisms underlying nociception develop during the third trimester. Specific cortical responses to noxious stimuli can be demonstrated in 32-week preterm infants using evoked potentials or near-infrared spectroscopy. The nature of pain as a conscious experience in young infants remains a subject of speculation and controversy.[19]

Factors influencing the perception and meaning of pain that occurs after infancy are both individual and contextual and include developmental and cognitive factors (e.g., understanding, control, expectation, and relevance) and behavioral and emotional factors (e.g., anxiety, fear, frustration, anger, guilt, and isolation), as well as familial and cultural factors.[20-22] A variety of other factors including age, gender, pain acceptance, and pain tolerance have been hypothesized to influence pain perception in the pediatric population and have been summarized elsewhere.[23]

Importantly, previous encounters with pain may heighten the experience of subsequent encounters with pain. For example, children newly diagnosed with cancer who had inadequate procedural analgesia when undergoing a first bone marrow aspirate or lumbar puncture had more severe distress during subsequent procedures, even when efficacious pain relief was subsequently provided.[24] This finding highlights the need to provide effective analgesia to prevent both present and future painful experiences.

Assessment

Pain assessment and measurement provide the foundation for addressing pain effectively. Regular assessment of pain may improve pain management[25,26] and should be conducted in a developmentally appropriate manner. When permitted by the child's developmental status, self-report is considered the gold standard in pain assessment. Because self-report can include bias and error, behavioral observations, physiologic changes, and clinician/parental report may be incorporated into the pain assessment. However, these methods also have inherent limitations. For example, tachycardia may reflect fever or intravascular volume depletion rather than pain.

Physiologic and behavioral signs and symptoms can indicate pain, but lack of these signs does not indicate absence of pain, particularly in chronically or very ill children, in whom these indicators are unreliable. In one study comparing a behavioral pain measure with two self-report measures, many children who reported severe pain showed few behavioral pain indicators.[27] In addition, these signs are not necessarily specific for pain itself and may reflect distress that may or may not be related to pain. Parental and clinician estimates of the child's pain also have limitations, because clinicians and parents frequently underestimate pain.[28,29]

Examples of symptom assessment tools for children of various ages and developmental capacities are demonstrated in Figure 71-2. These tools may be helpful in assessing symptoms and measuring severity before and after interventions. However, they are not all validated specifically for the population of children with cancer.[30] A given tool should be used consistently with a given child. When the assessment reveals the presence of pain, further inquiry regarding the nature of the pain (e.g., the character of the pain and aggravating and alleviating factors) and the meaning that the pain holds for the child and the family is in order.

Self-Report Instruments

Many children 3 years of age or older are able self-report their symptoms. Because some young children,

FLACC Behavioral Scale: Recommended for Children <3 Years of Age

Categories*	Scoring*		
	0	**1**	**2**
Face	No particular expression or smile	Occasional grimace or frown, withdrawn, disinterested	Frequent to constant quivering chin, clenched jaw
Legs	Normal position or relaxed	Uneasy, restless, tense	Kicking, or legs drawn up
Activity	Lying quietly, normal position, moves easily	Squirming, shifting back and forth, tense	Arched, rigid, or jerking
Cry	No cry (awake or asleep)	Moans or whimpers; occasional complaint	Crying steadily, screams or sobs, frequent complaints
Consolability	Content, relaxed	Reassured by occasional touching, hugging, or being talked to, distractable	Difficulty to console or comfort

A

Wong-Baker FACES Pain Rating Scale: Recommended for Children ≥3 Years of Age

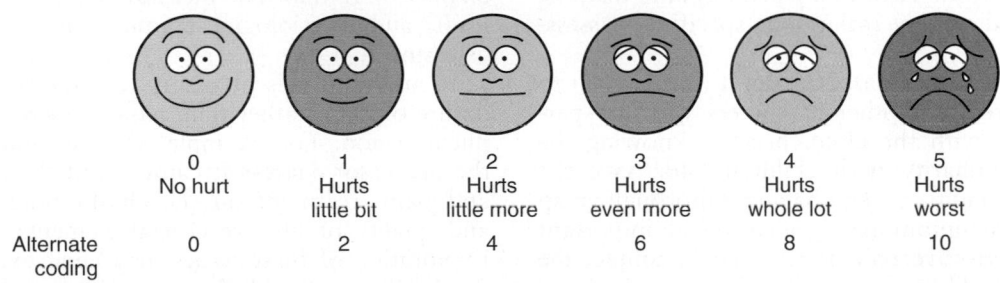

	0 No hurt	1 Hurts little bit	2 Hurts little more	3 Hurts even more	4 Hurts whole lot	5 Hurts worst
Alternate coding	0	2	4	6	8	10

Brief word instructions: Point to each face using the words to describe the pain intensity. Ask the child
B to choose face that best describes own pain and record the appropriate number.

Numerical Rating Scale: Recommended for Children ≥8 Years of Age

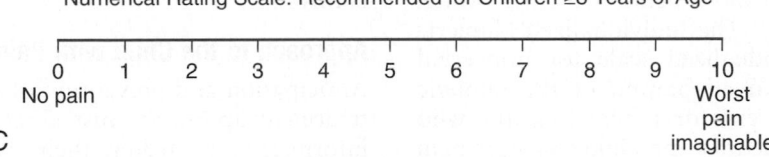

C

Figure 71-2 Pain assessment instruments. **A,** The Face, Legs, Activity, Cry, Consolability *(FLACC)* Scale, recommended for use in children younger than 3 years. Each of the five categories is scored from 0 to 2, which results in a total score between 0 and 10. **B,** The Wong-Baker FACES Pain Rating Scale, recommended for children 3 years of age and older. Brief word instructions: Point to each face, using the words to describe the pain intensity. Ask the child to choose the face that best describes his or her own pain and record the appropriate number. **C,** The Numerical Pain Rating Scale, recommended for children 8 years and older. *(A, From Merkel SI, Voepel-Lewis T, Shayevitz JR, et al: The FLACC: A behavioral scale for scoring postoperative pain in young children.* Pediatr Nurs *23:293–297, 1997; **B** and **C,** Modified from Hockenberry MJ, Wilson D, Winkelstein ML:* Wong's essentials of pediatric nursing, *ed 7, St. Louis, 2005, Mosby, p. 1259.)*

particularly those who are chronically ill, may be more mature than their chronologic age, the responses even of young children should be heeded. Self-report scales for children include faces scales, color analogue scales, visual analogue scales,[31] the Poker Chip Tool,[32] and numeric rating scales. With the faces scales, such as the Wong-Baker Faces Scale[33] and the Bieri Faces Pain Scale,[34] the child is asked to match how he or she feels with one of the faces. Color analogue scales and faces scales can be used by most children ages 4 years and older. Faces scales differ psychometrically; an example is the use of a smiling face for the "no pain" anchor in the Wong-Baker Faces

Scale versus a neutral face for the "no pain anchor" in the Bieri Faces Pain Scale. Although children often report that they like using the Wong-Baker Scale, some researchers regard the use of a neutral face for the "no pain anchor," as in the Bieri Faces Pain Scale, to be psychometrically more specific. With the visual analogue scale, a child selects a point on a line that represents the intensity of his or her pain. These scales have been extensively studied and are appropriate for children 8 years and older.

Numeric rating scales do not require any equipment, are simple to use, and are already used frequently with adults. These scales require numeracy and the ability to think and express oneself in quantitative terms and thus are most appropriate for use in children who are at least 8 years of age.[35] Children younger than 8 years may provide an unreliable numeric response because, although they can count, they have do not have an understanding of the quantitative meaning of numbers.[35] All quantitative scales are based on the concept of counting, which is a universal concept for children who have this developmental capacity. It is therefore possible to develop quantitative tools for pain measurement that are appropriate for children of virtually all cultures.[36]

Behavioral Observation Scales

Behavioral and physiologic cues are particularly useful in preverbal children and in children who are not able to verbalize their symptoms because of cognitive impairment, developmental capacity, or sedation. Such scales may rely on facial expressions,[37] motor or verbal responses, or combinations of behavioral and autonomic responses.[38] Behavioral scales may actually rate distress, including fear and anxiety, rather than specifically assessing pain per se.

When using behavior to assess pain, it is important to partner with parents or other caretakers who are particularly familiar with the child, because knowing the child, having familiarity with children who have the same or similar conditions, and having a thorough grasp of the science of symptom management are all important components of effective pain relief.[39] For example, the Paediatric Pain Profile was created to be a usable document for parents to assess and record their child's pain behavior. It is a well-validated instrument that uses behavioral cues, including changes in facial expression, vocal sounds, posture and movements, sleeping, eating, and mood, to assess pain.[40] The Individualized Numeric Rating Scale is an individualized scale for nonverbal children.[41] This scale is an adaptation of the numeric rating scale; it allows parents or other clinicians who know the child well to identify the child's typical pain behavior and rank that behavior on a standard scale from 0 to 10.

The Face, Legs, Activity, Cry, Consolability (FLACC) tool was originally designed to score postoperative pain in children ages 2 to 7 years[42] but has also been validated for postoperative use in children with cognitive impairment.[43] Use of this instrument may be advantageous because it employs a variety of types of measures such as activity and facial expression. Further work in the area of pain assessment in children with developmental or cognitive impairment is needed because children in these vulnerable populations are less likely to be assessed for pain, in addition to receiving less analgesic medication.[44]

The previously discussed assessment scales largely reduce pain assessment to the measurement of pain intensity. Although such pain assessment is an oversimplification, the scales permit rapid evaluation of pain and rapid institution of interventions aimed at ameliorating pain. Such scales are also key outcome measures in evaluations of pain-relieving interventions. Findings from a recent study, however, highlight the fact that such a simple screening for pain intensity fails to identify many persons who have significant functional interference from pain or pain significant enough to trigger a physician visit.[45] Regardless of the scale used, if clinical pain indicators are unclear, a trial of measures to ameliorate pain may clarify the cause of distress or pain.

Beyond Assessment Instruments

Beyond use of formal assessment tools, key elements in the history include alleviating/exacerbating factors; the quality, location, onset, and severity of pain; and the degree of impact on the child's function and well-being. Understanding the child's previous experiences with pain and strategies that have been used successfully in the past to address pain are also key components of the history and may inform the treatment plan. To this end a multidimensional indicator of pain can help the clinician understand the existence, intensity, and location of pain that a child is experiencing. Use of techniques that employ more than one measure (e.g., self-report, behavioral, and physiologic) permit a more accurate pain assessment.

In addition, it is necessary to understand the holistic nature of pain, rather than pain as merely a physiologic phenomenon. For example, the meaning of the pain, the degree of distress it causes, and the impact of pain and pain treatment on the child's functional capacity and quality of life are crucial elements of the history. Exploration of these issues may elicit exacerbating and potentially modifiable factors related to the pain experience. Finally, it is important to gain a clear understanding of the beliefs that the child and family have about pain, as well as their treatment goals in terms of pain control.

Approach to the Child with Pain

Anticipation and prevention of pain is the most effective treatment approach. Just as children and parents need information regarding their cancer treatment so they know what to expect, informing them in a sensitive manner about the symptoms they may expect and strategies available for reducing their symptoms can reduce anxiety about the unknown. In many cases, without open conversations in which expectations can be addressed, the imagined reality that is substituted is far worse than the true reality. By helping children understand what will happen and how the treatment or procedure will work, their fear and anxiety may be allayed, thereby reducing the symptoms they may actually experience.

When a child reports pain, careful assessment with use of history and physical examination is imperative to generate a complete differential diagnosis. Determination of the underlying cause of pain may inform consideration of which modalities are likely to be most effective in alleviating it. Both pharmacologic and nonpharmacologic (e.g., cognitive, behavioral, physical, and supportive) approaches should be considered, including addressing factors that are likely to affect the child's experience of pain. Once a pain treatment plan is implemented, pain should be regularly reassessed. The goal of pain management should be to achieve the degree of comfort that the child finds satisfactory.

To provide optimal pain control and prevent breakthrough pain, analgesics should in most cases be administered "By the ladder, by the clock, by the appropriate route, by the child" (WHO), and behavioral, physical, and cognitive supports should be provided throughout treatment. Pain of a moderate to severe rating should be treated with analgesics that are administered around the clock, with rescue doses of the same or an alternative analgesic available. Families often find it helpful to understand that preemptive analgesia is far more effective than catch-up analgesia administered for established pain.

Finally, the dosing interval as determined by the pharmacokinetics of the agents considered and the feasibility of their administration by caregivers should also be considered.

WHO Guidelines

The WHO guidelines previously provided a three-step approach to cancer-related pain in children and adults. For mild pain in a child who is not taking any analgesics, an NSAID or acetaminophen was suggested. For moderate pain, a short-acting weak opioid (e.g., codeine) was recommended, and for severe pain, a strong opioid was recommended (e.g., morphine).

The three-step WHO guidelines, which were widely publicized for cancer-related pain, provided an effective approach to pain control for many adults, with published success rates of 69% to 100%.[46-48] However, the three-step ladder consisting of nonopioids, weak opioids, and strong opioids may not be appropriate for some patients with cancer, particularly those with advanced disease. In fact, studies have shown that a two-step ladder in which treatment passes directly from step I (nonopioids) to step III (strong opioids) for mild to moderate pain provides superior pain relief.[49,50] Some medications historically used in step II (e.g., codeine and tramadol) are unlikely to provide better control of moderate pain compared with continuation of acetaminophen and NSAIDs (unless contraindicated) along with titrated doses of a strong opioid. Furthermore, codeine presents safety and efficacy concerns (discussed later), and few data exist to guide the administration of tramadol or other intermediate-potency analgesic agents in children. For these reasons, the most recent WHO guidelines for the management of pain in children with cancer (or other medical illness) are now based on a two-step approach.[51]

The WHO guidelines, which provide an effective, systematic approach to pain that includes strong opioids, have facilitated other WHO initiatives, such as increasing worldwide access to essential medicines for children with painful conditions. The WHO approach, however, may not adequately emphasize a multidisciplinary approach from the start, and thus opportunities to use adjuvant medications (e.g., steroids and local anesthetics) and cognitive or behavioral interventions to reduce pain and pathologic responses to pain may be missed.

Analgesic Medications and Interventions
Nonopioid Analgesics

Nonopioid analgesics are appropriate for mild pain in a child who is not already receiving analgesics. Nonopioid analgesics include acetaminophen, NSAIDs, salicylates, and selective cyclooxygenase (COX-2) inhibitors.

Nonopioid analgesics are frequently used as monotherapy for mild pain and are used together with opioids for more severe pain. Unlike opioids, they do not cause sedation, tolerance, and respiratory depression. When given as an adjuvant to opioids, they enhance analgesia.[52,53] To this end they may be opioid-sparing (i.e., decreasing the amount of opioid required for adequate analgesia),[54,55] thereby also limiting opioid-associated adverse effects. A recent randomized double-blind study of infants who underwent noncardiac surgery demonstrated that children randomly assigned to receive intermittent intravenous (IV) paracetamol with morphine as needed for rescue required only about one third as much rescue morphine as children randomly assigned to receive an IV placebo.[56] Combinations of nonopioids and opioids are available, although dosing of such a combination is often limited by the maximum dose of the nonopioid.

Salicylates and NSAIDs

Salicylates and NSAIDs nonspecifically inhibit cyclooxygenase enzymes, thereby blocking production of a variety of prostaglandins that mediate pain, inflammation, fever, and platelet function, protect gastric mucosa, and maintain a physiologic distribution of blood flow in the liver and kidneys. The permanent effects of aspirin on platelet function via permanent acetylation of cyclooxygenase are of particular concern in patients who have thrombocytopenia because the antiplatelet effect lasts even after the drug has been metabolized. Choline magnesium salicylate (Trilisate) is a salicylate that provides many of the same benefits as those provided by other salicylates or NSAIDs without known antiplatelet activity. Salicylates, however, have been associated with Reye syndrome in children younger than 2 years.

No particular NSAID or route of administration has been found to be superior over another. Even ketorolac, the only parenteral NSAID widely used in the United States, is no more effective than orally administered NSAIDs, especially if doses are compared in an equitoxic range. A single NSAID dose is roughly equivalent to 5 to 10 mg of intramuscular morphine in adults and has fewer adverse effects.[57] NSAIDs are commonly regarded as having a ceiling effect with no added benefit at supramaximal doses, although the doses commonly recommended (based on safety concerns) remain well below the ceiling in most cases. NSAIDs can cause nephropathy, gastritis, and bleeding from reversible platelet dysfunction, a characteristic that may limit their use in patients with cancer who are thrombocytopenic. COX-2 inhibitors (e.g., celecoxib) selectively block production of prostaglandins that mediate inflammation and pain without impairing platelet function and with fewer effects on gastric mucosal integrity compared with traditional NSAIDs, particularly with short-term use.[58,59] Concerns have been raised regarding effects of COX-2 inhibitors on the risk of cardiovascular events in adults. Evidence does not currently indicate that these concerns extend to children with neoplasms, including the small subgroup of children with tumors or vascular anomalies who have an increased risk of thrombotic events.

Acetaminophen

Acetaminophen is a nonopioid analgesic that reduces pain and fever. It may act in part by inhibiting prostaglandin synthesis in the CNS. Unlike salicylates and NSAIDs, which inhibit peripheral cyclooxygenases, it does not have peripheral antiinflammatory properties. Acetaminophen is available in a variety of oral formulations, as an IV formulation (approved in the United States for children ≥2 years), and as a rectal suppository, although rectal administration should be avoided in neutropenic patients. When not contraindicated, rectal administration is helpful for children unwilling or unable to take oral medications, although its absorption is slow and variable, peaking at 70 minutes.[60] Because rectal absorption is less efficient, single doses of 30 to 40 mg/kg can be administered.[60] Subsequent doses should be smaller (20 mg/kg), and the interval between doses should be increased to 6 to 8 hours.[60,61] Dosing of oral or IV acetaminophen is limited to 75 mg/kg/day or a maximum of 4 g/day (whichever is smaller) because of the risk of hepatic toxicity.

Opioid Analgesics

General Considerations. Guidelines for initial opioid dosages are presented in Table 71-1 and are discussed in

TABLE 71-1　Guidelines for Initial Dosages for Opioid Analgesics*

Drug	EQUIANALGESIC DOSES		USUAL STARTING IV OR SUBCUTANEOUS DOSES AND INTERVALS		Ratio of Parenteral to Oral Dose	USUAL STARTING ORAL DOSES AND INTERVALS	
	Parenteral	Oral	Child <50 kg	Child ≥50 kg		Child <50 kg	Child ≥50 kg
Morphine	10 mg	30 mg (long term) 60 mg (single dose)	Bolus: 0.1 mg/kg every 2-4 h Infusion: 0.03 mg/kg/h	Bolus: 5-8 mg every 2-4 h Infusion: 1.5 mg/h	1:3 (long term) 1:6 (single dose)	Immediate release: 0.3 mg/kg every 3-4 h Sustained release: 20-35 kg: 10-15 mg every 8-12 h 35-50 kg: 15-30 mg every 8-12 h	Immediate release: 5-20 mg every 3-4 h Sustained release: 30-45 mg every 8-12 h
Oxycodone	NA	15-20 mg	NA	NA	NA	0.1-0.2 mg/kg every 3-4 h	5-10 mg every 3-4 h
Methadone[†]	10 mg	10-20 mg	0.1 mg/kg every 4-8 h	5-8 mg every 4-8 h	1:2	0.1-0.2 mg/kg every 4-8 h	5-10 mg every 4-8 h
Fentanyl	100 μg (0.1 mg)	NA	Bolus: 0.5-1.0 μg/kg every 1-2 h Infusion: 0.5-2.0 mg/kg/h	Bolus: 25-50 μg every 1-2 h Infusion: 25-100 μg/h	NA	NA	NA
Hydromorphone	1.5-2 mg	6-8 mg	Bolus: 0.02 mg/kg every 2-4 h Infusion: 0.006 mg/kg/h	Bolus: 1 mg every 2-4 h Infusion: 0.03 mg/h	1:4	0.04-0.08 mg/kg every 3-4 h	2-4 mg every 3-4 h
Meperidine (pethidine)[‡]	75-100 mg	300 mg	Bolus: 0.8-1.0 mg/kg every 2-3 h	Bolus: 50-75 mg every 2-3 h	1:4	2-3 mg/kg every 3-4 h	100-150 mg every 3-4 h

Modified from Berde CB, Sethna N: Analgesics for the treatment of pain in children. N Engl J Med 347:1094–1103, 2002. All doses are approximate and should be adjusted according to clinical circumstances. Recommendations are modified from previous summary tables, including those of a consensus statement from the World Health Organization and the International Association for the Study of Pain. IV, Intravenous; NA, not applicable.

*Doses are for patients older than 6 months of age. In infants younger than 6 months, initial per-kilogram doses should begin at roughly 25% of the per-kilogram doses recommended here. Higher doses are often required for patients receiving mechanical ventilation.

[†]Use of methadone requires additional vigilance because it can accumulate and produce delayed sedation. If sedation occurs, doses should be withheld until sedation resolves. Thereafter, doses should be substantially reduced; the interval between doses should be extended to 8 to 12 hours, or both.

[‡]Use of meperidine, especially long-term use, should generally be avoided if other opioids are available, because its metabolites can cause seizures.

greater detail in this section. Ultimately, the correct dose of opioid is the dose that provides the desired analgesia with acceptable adverse effects. In general, intolerable adverse effects are usually the dose-limiting factor, as opposed to opioids having a ceiling effect. This situation should be explained to parents, as well the fact that, with rare exceptions, *children with cancer who receive opioids for pain control do not become addicted to opioids.* Addiction is an aberrant psychiatric condition in which the person exhibits maladapted, drug-seeking behavior. True addiction is comparatively rare in patients with cancer-related pain. Children who exhibit exaggerated pain behaviors (e.g., demanding pain medication and engaging in manipulative behaviors) are far more likely to be demonstrating pseudoaddiction, in which case their behavior is a reflection of poorly controlled pain.

Addiction should be distinguished from dependence, that is, a physiologic response to opioids in which abrupt removal leads the patient to experience symptoms of withdrawal. It may be helpful to draw a parallel to blood pressure medication, the abrupt cessation of which causes an undesired rebound hypertensive effect because the body has adjusted to the presence of the antihypertensive drug. Addiction should also be distinguished from tolerance, which is another physiologic response of the body to the presence of opioids that requires increasing doses to achieve the same analgesic effect. *The need to adjust dosing to account for tolerance is not an indication of addiction.* Other processes that can resemble tolerance, including opioid-induced hyperalgesia, are discussed later in this chapter.

Opioids do not need to be saved for cases of extreme pain, because increasing pain can often be managed by increasing the opioid dose. In addition, when escalating doses provide marginal benefit, rotating to an alternative opioid may provide better analgesia. It may be helpful to explain to parents that good pain control from the start may improve pain control overall and actually minimize the amount of opioid that is ultimately needed because when good pain control is achieved, the need to use large doses required to catch up to uncontrolled pain can be avoided.

Some children who have cancer, particularly advanced cancer, require extremely high doses of opioids. For example, in a sample of children with advanced cancer, Collins and colleagues[62] found that in some patients the opioid infusions ranged more than 100-fold from 3.8 to 518 mg per hour of morphine equivalent.

Some studies conducted in vitro and in animal models have demonstrated that opioids may promote cancer cell growth by affecting processes such as tumor cell proliferation and migration. For example, opioids at physiologically relevant concentrations promote tumor angiogenesis.[63,64] In addition, the opioid receptor antagonist naloxone and the COX-2 inhibitor celecoxib inhibit angiogenesis, tumor growth, and metastasis in rodents.[64,65] However, other studies demonstrate growth-inhibiting effects of opioids and have been reviewed elsewhere.[66] No evidence to date demonstrates opioid-associated promotion of tumor growth in humans. These preliminary findings should not, by themselves, lead to the conclusion that use of opioids to relieve cancer-related pain should be avoided. The data accumulated to date regarding the potential risks of opioids and the benefits of adequate analgesia are insufficient to recommend limiting opioid use for analgesia.

Developmental Pharmacology. Elements of renal clearance such as glomerular filtration and tubular secretion increase in the first few weeks of life, such that renal clearance commensurate with adult clearance is achieved by 8 months. When compared with children and adults, neonates and infants have reduced hepatic clearance as a result of hepatic enzyme immaturity. In addition, children 2 to 6 years of age have higher clearance than do adults because of a larger liver mass to body weight ratio.[67] As a result, drugs may need to be administered more frequently in children than they are in adults. Other age-related differences, such as changes in body composition and plasma concentrations of drug-binding proteins, can also influence pharmacokinetics.

Choice of Opioid. The usual starting opioid is morphine because of its low cost, wide availability, multiple routes of administration, and familiarity to clinicians. Because of its long history of use in children, it should be considered the first-line opioid in this population unless specific reasons exist to consider alternatives. Alternative opioids including oxycodone, hydromorphone, and semisynthetic and synthetic compounds such as fentanyl and methadone can be used in children. Use of alternative opioids may be predicated on availability, route of administration, presence of organ impairment, and the patient's prior experience with particular opioids.

Renal Failure. Metabolites of morphine, oxycodone, and hydromorphone (discussed later) may accumulate during renal failure. Some metabolites have analgesic activity, which may lead to delayed opioid toxicity (opioid neurotoxicity will be discussed later). For this reason, dosing intervals may need to be increased in patients with renal dysfunction. The pharmacokinetics of alternative opioids such as fentanyl and methadone are not changed with renal impairment, making these opioids better choices in this setting.

Hepatic Failure. Because glucuronidation is relatively well preserved in persons with liver failure, opioids metabolized by glucuronidation (i.e., morphine, hydromorphone, and buprenorphine) are generally better choices than those metabolized by oxidation via liver cytochromes (e.g., oxycodone, fentanyl, and methadone) in this setting.[68] However, because of shunting in persons with liver cirrhosis, the bioavailability of glucuronidated opioids may be increased. For this reason, initial opioid doses should be lower in persons with hepatic impairment.

Weak Opioids. Tramadol is an atypical analgesic with some direct noradrenergic and serotonergic agonist action and with an active metabolite that is a weak opioid. Tramadol has numerous drug-to-drug interactions that should be considered. For example, it can produce seizures by itself, but this risk is greatly increased when tramadol is administered in combination with several classes of antidepressants. It is available in oral immediate and extended-release preparations and in combination formulations with acetaminophen.

Although codeine has historically been recommended as a weak opioid for mild to moderate pain, it has several limitations. The variable expression of the CYP2D6 enzyme that biotransforms codeine leads to unpredictable levels of the active metabolite, morphine. In the fetus, CYP2D6 activity is absent, and in children younger than 5 years, CYP2D6 activity is less than 25% that of adult activity.[51] Furthermore, certain genotypes are associated with reduced enzyme activity, regardless of age. In a study of 96 children randomly assigned to receive either morphine and diclofenac or codeine and diclofenac after an adenotonsillectomy, it was found that 47% of children had genotypes associated with reduced enzyme activity and that neither morphine nor its metabolites were detected in 36% of children with reduced CYP2D6 activity genotypes who received codeine, although the study did not account for other factors influencing catalytic rate, such as gene copy number.[69] Such "poor metabolizers" of codeine were more likely to have uncontrolled pain and to require rescue medication.

On the other hand, persons who are "ultrarapid metabolizers" may possess multiple copies of the CYP2D6 gene responsible for codeine metabolism or have genotypes associated with rapid metabolism and may therefore be at risk for adverse effects such as respiratory depression from rapid generation of morphine from codeine. Several pediatric deaths from codeine administered after a tonsillectomy and/or an adenoidectomy have resulted from such ultrarapid metabolism. It is for this reason that the U.S. Food and Drug Administration (FDA) has issued a "boxed warning" and deemed codeine contraindicated in this setting.

In a variety of painful conditions in children, provision of codeine provides no benefit greater than that of NSAIDs. When codeine, ibuprofen, and acetaminophen monotherapy were compared in children with musculoskeletal trauma who presented to an emergency department, ibuprofen provided superior analgesia.[70] In the posttonsillectomy setting, codeine in combination with acetaminophen caused more nausea with no difference in pain or postoperative bleeding.[71] A meta-analysis also found that weak opioids (i.e., codeine) in combination with NSAIDs fail to provide superior analgesia to that provided by NSAIDs alone[57] but do have significantly more adverse effects. Based on these findings, in our view, very few instances exist in which codeine is a preferred choice among opioids.

Some opioids exhibit partial mu receptor agonist activity (e.g., buprenorphine), kappa agonist activity (e.g., nalbuphine), or mixed agonist activity (e.g., butorphanol and pentazocine). Although these opioids have predominantly agonist activity, some have significant antagonist activity as well, and thus they may reduce the effect of pure mu agonists given concurrently. In general they do not provide superior analgesia, although they may have fewer gastrointestinal (GI) or respiratory adverse effects and may be considered for individual patients who have limiting adverse effects with other opioids. Currently the greatest use of buprenorphine in the United States is for substance abuse treatment. It has been used by multiple routes for treatment of cancer-related pain in children, particularly in countries with greater impediments to the prescribing of morphine, methadone, or other opioids. Authors of a recent small prospective case series reported reasonable effectiveness and tolerability of transdermal buprenorphine for children with cancer.[72]

Strong Opioids. Meperidine is a strong opioid that should be avoided in most cases because of its adverse effect profile and lack of superiority to the strong opioids described in the next sections. For example, repeated doses of meperidine lead to accumulation of its metabolite, normeperidine, which in turn causes neuroexcitatory symptoms including agitation, tremors, myoclonus, and seizures.[73] In a double-blind trial comparing morphine with meperidine administered via patient-controlled analgesia (PCA), it was found that morphine resulted in better analgesia and had no more adverse effects than did meperidine.[74] In low doses, meperidine reduces postoperative shivering or rigors associated with amphotericin infusion.

Morphine. Morphine is the most frequently prescribed opioid in children and is the best studied opioid in this population. It offers flexibility in terms of routes of administration. It is also available in a controlled-release formulation, and multiple randomized controlled trials have shown that this formulation can effectively control cancer-related pain when administered every 12 hours.[75] Morphine is extensively metabolized by glucuronidation in the liver to morphine 3-glucuronide (M3G) and morphine 6-glucuronide (M6G). M3G does not bind mu receptors and has no analgesic activity but may contribute to some of the neuroexcitatory adverse effects of morphine.[76] On the other hand, M6G does bind mu receptors and is a potent analgesic.[77,78]

Oxycodone. Oxycodone is a semisynthetic derivative of morphine. Although it is frequently categorized as a weak opioid appropriate for mild to moderate pain (and is frequently administered in combination with acetaminophen), this categorization is a reflection of its use at low doses. In fact, a meta-analysis showed that oxycodone is as efficacious an analgesic as morphine or hydromorphone.[79] This meta-analysis also showed no difference between oxycodone and morphine in terms of adverse effects such as dry mouth, sedation, or nausea.[79] Oxycodone itself has no ceiling effect or dose limit, although dosing may be limited when it is administered in combination with nonopioid agents such as acetaminophen. Although it is available in parenteral formulations in other countries, in the United States it is only available in an oral formulation. The oral formulation is available in an extended-release preparation.

Oxycodone is predominantly metabolized by CYP3A4 to inactive products. A secondary pathway involving CYP2D6 may lead to generation of the active opioid oxymorphone in patients with ultrarapid metabolizing variants. Although cases of apnea and death associated with excessive conversion from oxycodone to oxymorphone have been published, the prevailing impression is that pharmacogenomic variation overall leads to less variance in effect for oxycodone compared with codeine. Oxycodone pharmacokinetics have been studied in children,[80] but there is a need for additional pediatric pharmacokinetic/pharmacodynamic studies that include oxymorphone assay, pharmacodynamic end points, and contemporary genotyping.

Hydromorphone. Hydromorphone may be administered orally, intravenously, or subcutaneously. Although it was previously thought that hydromorphone has less neurotoxicity, hydromorphone metabolites have recently been shown to convey neuroexcitatory adverse effects. One advantage of hydromorphone compared with morphine is that its higher potency allows for smaller subcutaneous volumes to be delivered when this route of administration is utilized.

Fentanyl. Fentanyl may be given intravenously with rapid onset of action and short duration of action (20 to 30 minutes). For this reason fentanyl is frequently used as an analgesic for brief, painful procedures. Rapid administration of fentanyl may cause chest wall rigidity that requires reversal with naloxone or even neuromuscular blockade and positive pressure ventilation.[81] In occasional patients, fentanyl may be better tolerated than other opioids, in part because it is associated with less histamine release[82] and creates no metabolites that may produce neurotoxicity.

Fentanyl transdermal patches last 72 hours and are a convenient parenteral mode of drug delivery that is preferred by many adults.[83,84] These patches have also been used successfully in children who have chronic pain.[85] Although wide within-individual variability in fentanyl absorption exists, intraindividual absorption is reported to be stable.[86,87] In addition, hyperhidrosis, hypertrichosis, and the localization of patches on the skin do not appear to affect fentanyl absorption.[86] Because the onset of action is at least 12 hours, and because some fentanyl remains in the system for 72 hours after patch removal, transdermal fentanyl lacks flexibility for close titration for rapidly changing pain severity. The smallest patch size (12 µg/h) may be too large a dose for some children. For children as young as 2 years who had previously taken opioids and had developed some degree of tolerance, transdermal fentanyl was found to be a safe and well-tolerated alternative to oral opioid treatment.[85] The reservoir design of the patch prevents the patch from being cut to adjust the dose delivered. Transdermal fentanyl should be avoided in patients who have not previously taken opioids because it may result in respiratory depression.

In addition to rapid onset of action and transdermal application, fentanyl provides several other benefits. When renal function is impaired, fentanyl does not accumulate to the same extent as morphine.[88] Some studies have demonstrated that transdermal fentanyl appears to cause less constipation than does oral morphine, but it is unknown whether this observation is related to the route or the drug.[89-91]

In adults or children already receiving 60 mg/day of morphine, oral transmucosal fentanyl citrate (OTFC, or Actiq) provides extremely rapid control of incident pain, with an onset of action of 5 to 10 minutes. This rapid onset of action is due to its lipophilic nature, as well as because this route bypasses first-pass hepatic metabolism. Because of the rapidity of its onset of action, OTFC has been used to provide analgesia for brief, painful procedures without the requirement for IV access.[92] OTFC is also quite useful for patients who have breakthrough pain. In a double-blind, double-dummy, randomized, crossover study of adult patients with cancer who had incident (breakthrough) pain, it was found that OTFC reduced pain intensity more effectively than did immediate-release oral morphine, and OTFC was favored over immediate-release morphine sulfate by more patients after the study.[93] No conversion ratio is available for OTFC, and careful titration is needed to determine the correct dose. No correlation exists between the effective OTFC dose and the around-the-clock dose of an opioid.[94] For this reason the lowest strength (200 µg) should be tried first. If inadequate pain relief is achieved in 20 minutes, this dose may be repeated.

The fentanyl buccal tablet is another preparation of fentanyl that is rapidly absorbed through effervescent action through the oral mucosa. Patients should be taking at least 60 mg/day of oral morphine so they have opioid tolerance to safely receive a fixed dose of fentanyl with such rapid onset of action through the oral mucosa. The need for this degree of tolerance is highlighted by recent experiences with buccal/sublingual fentanyl tablets, which, when (inappropriately) administered to opioid-naive patients, may result in life-threatening respiratory depression.

Methadone. Methadone may be given orally (it is available as a tablet or liquid) or intravenously. One advantage to methadone in the pediatric population is that it is the only long-acting opioid widely available in liquid formulation. In addition, it is relatively inexpensive to manufacture, costing 90% less than extended-release morphine.[95] Methadone also exhibits unique receptor-binding properties in that the l-isomer binds mu opioid receptors and the d-isomer binds the N-methyl-d-aspartate (NMDA) receptor. Because the NMDA receptor is involved in opioid tolerance, opioid hyperalgesia, and neuropathic pain, it may be a useful opioid in these clinical situations, which are discussed later. For these reasons, administration of methadone for analgesic purposes has become more popular in recent years.

The variable pharmacologic half-life of methadone, which ranges from 12 to 150 hours, may result in delayed toxicity (e.g., sedation and hypoventilation) that can occur many days after initiation of the drug.[96] The analgesic half-life of methadone is commonly cited as 4 to 6 hours,[97] although some patients can require minimal rescue analgesia with dosing at 8- or 12-hour intervals. In addition, equianalgesic dose conversion from other opioids is variable and depends in part on the dose of the previous opioid. Its potency relative to morphine is highly dependent on the previous morphine dose.[98,99] A very convenient website, www.globalrph.com/narcoticonv.htm, can be used to assist in dose conversions. It should be emphasized that even with these calculations, enormous individual variability exists, and close follow-up is required to avoid delayed oversedation.

Methadone is metabolized through several cytochromes and therefore interacts with a variety of other medications. Individual variation in cytochrome expression may account in part for significant blood concentration variability in patients.[100,101] Methadone, in conjunction with other medications, may prolong the QTc interval.[102] It is unclear whether this phenomenon explains the otherwise unexplained increased incidence of sudden cardiac arrest in adults receiving methadone therapy.[103] Until the potential for methadone to pose cardiotoxicity is better understood, it should be used cautiously in children who have underlying cardiac conditions or those at risk for prolonged QTc. Although methadone has several advantages, it also has some unique features that require familiarity with this agent for safe and effective use. The majority of pediatric oncologists rarely, if ever, prescribe methadone.[104] Lack of familiarity with methadone pharmacodynamics, effectiveness, and dosing equivalence are the most common reasons cited for prescribing other opioids rather than methadone.

Oxymorphone. Oxymorphone is the active metabolite of oxycodone and is available as a rectal suppository. An extended-release oral formulation has also recently been approved.

Opioid Starting Doses. For the opioid-naive patient, recommended starting doses are listed in Table 71-1. For infants younger than 6 months, the starting dose should be roughly one fourth the weight-scaled dose suggested in the table and titrated to effect. Opioids should be administered with caution in patients who have disordered control of respiration, altered mental status, or altered drug metabolism. This is not to say, however, that opioids should be withheld from these patients. In fact, opioids can be safely delivered and adequate analgesia achieved with careful titration to effect.

Routes and Methods of Administration. Medication should be given by the simplest, most effective, and least distressing route. Other considerations that should guide the choice of route include the severity and type of pain, the ability of the child to tolerate a given route due to developmental or personal factors, and the ability of the caregivers to administer medication via certain routes.

Oral. When possible, the oral route of administration should be attempted first. In general, the time for opioids to reach peak effect is about 60 minutes with the oral route. Most extended-release preparations are available in tablets or capsules. For children who cannot swallow tablets or capsules but who would benefit from an extended-action preparation or agent, liquid methadone can be used. If the child has a gastrostomy tube, ultra–extended-release morphine (given every 24 hours) may be suspended (*but not crushed*) and administered via a gastrostomy tube. Ultra–extended-release morphine allows once-daily oral dosing, but unintended chewing or crushing may lead to overdose from immediate release of the morphine.[105,106] Opening the capsules and sprinkling the drug onto applesauce may be an appropriate administration technique for adults[105] but should be avoided in young children. Ultra–extended-release morphine may be

considered for adolescents, but in younger children who may be at risk for accidentally chewing the capsules, these preparations should generally be avoided.

For intermittent dosing, oral opioids prepared as concentrated drops may provide analgesia without the requirement of swallowing larger volumes of liquid. Concentrated morphine may be helpful for children who are unable to reliably take oral opioids because of their neurodevelopmental capacity or nausea and vomiting.

Rectal. Suppositories containing hydromorphone and morphine may be administered rectally. In addition, controlled-release morphine tablets may be given rectally.[107] Although the published potency of rectal opioids approximates that of oral opioids,[108] the pharmacokinetic properties of morphine, that is, first-pass metabolism to the active metabolite M6G by the portal circulation, should be considered when considering rectal administration. For example, Wilkinson and colleagues[107] determined that the area under concentration-time curves for morphine metabolites were approximately twice those achieved after rectal administration. The maximal concentration of morphine and its metabolites was lower and the time to achieve peak levels was longer for rectal administration. In this study, the variation in morphine kinetics did not correspond with altered pain ratings.[107] Although it is reasonable to start with 1:1 (oral to rectal) equianalgesic dosing of morphine, adjustments in the dose or dosing interval should be anticipated.

Transdermal. Fentanyl and buprenorphine are the only opioids manufactured in transdermal formulations. The transdermal route for delivery of fentanyl or buprenorphine provides some advantages. Other opioids such as morphine may be compounded as transdermal formulations, but absorption of these other opioids via this route is unreliable, and alternative means of opioid administration are almost invariably available.

Intravenous. Use of the IV route, when appropriate, may provide rapid and reliable administration. In general, the time for morphine to reach its peak effect is about 15 minutes via this route. The IV route is frequently used for patients who have severe pain or for children who are unable to take oral medications, such as children who are in the final stages of life.[14]

Subcutaneous. All IV opioids may be administered subcutaneously, although methadone may cause local irritation if infused continuously.[109] Delivery of opioids by this route dose adds approximately 30 minutes to the time of peak effect obtained by IV administration. This route is simple to use and requires only a portable syringe driver to administer the medication through a butterfly needle. In addition, it confers consistent delivery and easy titration without the requirement for IV access. Needles are changed every week or more often if skin irritation occurs, and this task can often be performed by a family member. In our experience, children can absorb 2 mL per hour, whereas adults can absorb 3 to 5 mL per hour. Higher doses of opioids may exceed these volume limits. In such cases, switching to a more potent opioid, such as hydromorphone, may be necessary.

Patient-Controlled Analgesia. PCA can provide a continuous IV or subcutaneous infusion of opioid to provide basal control of pain, as well as a bolus, which provides relief from breakthrough pain. The PCA delivery system allows patients to manage their pain themselves, and no lag time exists between the request and delivery of a bolus dose for uncontrolled pain, increasing their sense of control over their pain. In one study comparing continuous infusion morphine with PCA, it was found that patients who used PCA required less total opioid while receiving equivalent control of the pain of mucositis associated with bone marrow transplantation.[110]

Because opioid-induced sedation generally occurs before respiratory depression, it is rare for a patient to administer boluses to himself or herself to the point of respiratory depression. PCA delivery has been used in the pediatric population with safety and efficacy. PCA does not increase the incidence of opioid-related complications, including sedation.[111] Clinical protocols for calculating the PCA commencement opioid dose and subsequent opioid-dose escalation can facilitate the safe and efficacious implementation of PCA.[112] Thorough assessment of PCA use includes the total daily dose, ratio between continuous and bolus opioid, amount of baseline and breakthrough pain, and response to the bolus dose. A common recommendation is to adjust the continuous (basal) rate to supply roughly two thirds of the patient's daily opioid requirement. Although this starting point is reasonable for most oncology patients with persistent disease-related pain, individual circumstances exist in which the parameters should be modified. For example, in the setting of brief, severe, episodic pain, it may be reasonable to use a lower basal rate and give more generous boluses. In postoperative care, considerable variation exists in the use of basal infusions. Our practice is to use them for operations expected to result in more severe pain and/or in patients who are likely to underdose themselves. Conversely, we tend to avoid basal infusions or use very low basal rates for patients who have less painful surgery, for patients who have received other nonopioid methods of analgesia (e.g., peripheral nerve blocks or plexus blocks), or for patients who have factors that increase respiratory risks.

PCA has been used successfully in children as young as 4 years of age.[113] PCA may also be administered by surrogates, commonly as nurse-controlled analgesia or parent-controlled analgesia, or collectively as PCA-by-proxy. In theory the safety of PCA is maximized when the patient self-administers the medication, because when the patient falls asleep, he or she stops pushing the button. Because the proxy assesses the child's pain and provides the bolus dose, the safety feature inherent in a PCA to prevent respiratory depression is overridden, but when it is used appropriately it is associated with only rare respiratory or neurologic complications.[114] Overall, the safety of nurse-controlled analgesia is well established and is widely used for both opioid-tolerant and opioid-naive infants and children. Greater controversy persists with parent-controlled PCA, although experience with this arrangement is mounting.[115] Our general practice is to greatly limit its use for routine care of opioid-naive postoperative infants and children but to use it widely for opioid-tolerant infants and children in palliative care, especially at home. Guidelines to increase the safety of PCA by proxy have been proposed.

Intrathecal. Opioids may be administered intrathecally and are considered later in the "Invasive Approaches to Pain Management" section.

Regardless of the route utilized, if the patient has continuous pain, a regimen providing continuous pain control should be implemented. To establish a patient's true analgesic needs, short-acting opioids, which can be easily titrated, may be administered for the first 24 to 48 hours. Based on the amount of opioid required during the initial interval, a longer acting opioid may then be substituted, with provision of an as-needed short-acting opioid available for incident or breakthrough pain.

Whatever the regimen, ensuring proper follow-up assessment is critical to ensure appropriate analgesia and to evaluate for potential opioid-associated adverse effects. Because constipation is a predicted and preventable adverse effect of opioids, a bowel regimen to prevent this adverse effect should always be instituted and adjusted as necessary whenever opioids are started or escalated.

Breakthrough Pain. Breakthrough pain is a transitory exacerbation of pain that occurs when pain is otherwise relatively controlled or stable at baseline. Patients with chronic cancer-related pain and superimposed breakthrough pain have worse overall pain, more impaired functioning, and higher psychological distress than do patients with chronic cancer-related pain alone.[116] Breakthrough pain may occur as a result of incident pain (i.e., pain due to a stimulus, such as movement or coughing) or end-of-dose failure, or it may be spontaneous in nature (such as lancinating pain attacks in persons with postherpetic neuralgia).

In a prospective study of pediatric inpatients with cancer it was found that 57% experienced one or more episodes of breakthrough pain during the preceding 24 hours, with each episode lasting seconds to minutes and most commonly characterized by the children as "sharp" and "shooting."[117]

Breakthrough pain may be challenging in that its onset may be unpredictable and rapid, and it may be more severe than pain typically experienced at baseline. For these reasons, use of a pain diary may be particularly important in detecting patterns and factors associated with breakthrough pain. If end-of-dose breakthrough pain occurs, the total daily around-the-clock dose may be increased by 25%, although this increase may lead to intolerable adverse effects. Alternatively, the dosing interval may be shortened.

Breakthrough pain should be approached as other types of pain are approached, with (1) consideration of the underlying triggers and interventions aimed at the underlying problem, (2) optimization of the scheduled analgesic regimen, and (3) use of adequate analgesics for episodic pain, that is, rescue medication. The rescue dose to treat such breakthrough pain should be the equivalent to the dose used every 4 hours, or 5% to 10% of the total daily opioid dose. For predictable incident pain, a short-acting opioid given just prior to the activity may be helpful. When the breakthrough pain has neuropathic features, consideration should be given to adjunctive use of analgesics with specificity for these types of pain, that is, anticonvulsants or antidepressants, as will be discussed later.

OTFC may safely provide very rapid pain relief in patients receiving the equivalent of 60 mg/day of oral morphine, as was previously discussed. It may be especially useful when breakthrough pain is unpredictable and short-lived. Other hydrophilic agents such as morphine are often administered sublingually for breakthrough pain but have a longer onset of action. A recent small study indicates that the rapid onset of action of methadone may make it a useful agent for treatment of breakthrough pain.[118]

Dose Escalation. When a patient who is already receiving oral or IV opioids has severe pain that persists despite a dose of breakthrough opioid medication, the dose should be increased by 50% to 100% and repeated. Once adequate analgesia is reached, the total amount given over 4 hours to determine the "effective dose" for every 4 hours should be calculated.[8] If more than two rescue doses are used in a 24-hour period, the total standing dose should be increased.

For patients receiving continuous IV opioids, a rescue dose for breakthrough pain should be provided that consists of 50% to 200% of the hourly infusion every 15 minutes as needed. For the sake of simplicity, use of multiple different short-acting opioids is discouraged.

Opioid Tolerance. The response to acquired tolerance to an opioid is usually to increase the opioid dose. When this approach is not feasible because of opioid adverse effects such as neuroexcitability, rotating to a different opioid may be an option. Because the NMDA receptor plays a role in opioid tolerance, methadone, with its attendant NMDA antagonist properties, may control pain that is otherwise refractory to opioids.[119] The addition of adjuvant NMDA receptor antagonists such as ketamine may also reverse opioid tolerance. In animals, as well as in some patients, chronic administration of opioids can generate a condition of generalized hyperalgesia, meaning that new painful stimuli produce a greater intensity of pain than would have occurred with the same stimulus for that subject in an opioid-naive state. Opioid-induced hyperalgesia is discussed in greater detail later.

Opioid Rotation. Opioid rotation, or switching, may also be indicated as a result of intolerable adverse effects or route of administration. Equianalgesic tables are useful for conversion from one opioid to another and are widely available. Although no evidence exists to demonstrate the superiority of one opioid over another in such a switch, the strategy of changing opioids may be successful in alleviating dose-limiting adverse effects or opioid tolerance in children. For example, Drake and colleagues[120] found that opioid rotation resolved adverse effects in 90% of children without loss of analgesia or the need to increase morphine equivalents. In fact, because of the phenomenon of incomplete tolerance, the equianalgesic dose of the second opioid should be decreased by 20% when a patient is transitioned from one opioid to another. The phenomenon of incomplete tolerance is particularly pronounced when converting to methadone,[98,99] likely because of the ability of the d-isomer of methadone to act as an NMDA receptor antagonist.[121]

Opioid Withdrawal and Opioid Tapering. Opioid withdrawal is a physiologic response. Sudden discontinuation of opioids in a patient who has been taking long-standing opioids may prompt a withdrawal syndrome characterized by irritability, restlessness, dysphoria, anxiety, muscle aches, sweating, piloerection, diarrhea, nausea, vomiting, yawning, and sneezing. Withdrawal may be prevented by tapering opioids. Opioid doses may be safely cut in half without precipitating withdrawal. Continued tapering may be achieved by halving the dose every 3 days. An alternative strategy is to reduce the total daily dose by 10% per day. Maintaining the rescue dose at its original dose during the tapering process allows for effective treatment of breakthrough pain that may occur as the dose is tapered.

Opioid Adverse Effects. Nonrespiratory adverse effects from opioids include constipation, nausea, pruritus, somnolence/sedation, and, particularly at high doses, neurotoxicity. A prospective study of pediatric oncology patients found that in children receiving morphine, postoperatively, 38% had vomiting, 32% had nausea, and 24% had constipation.[122] The high incidence of nausea and vomiting in this population is likely confounded by postoperative nausea and vomiting.

Opioid-associated sedation typically self-resolves within a few days of the institution of opioids. In some cases the sedation observed when instituting opioids is not an adverse effect of opioids per se but rather a result of an exhausted patient finally able to sleep once pain is controlled. Nausea experienced by some patients upon starting opioids similarly self-resolves within a few days and is often relieved with use of an antiemetic. Switching to a different opioid due to nausea within the first 3 days of opioid therapy may be premature. Opioid-associated urinary retention is an uncomfortable symptom that may respond to a switch to an alternative opioid. Anecdotally, urinary retention in some patients may respond to selective alpha-1A antagonists such as tamsulosin, which are commonly prescribed for adults with lower urinary tract outflow obstruction. Urinary retention, frequency, or urgency should prompt a focused consideration of a range of oncologic and neurologic causes, as well as effects of other medications in addition to opioids, such as anticholinergics and antihistamines. Management of opioid-associated sedation/fatigue, constipation, pruritus, and nausea are further discussed in the sections of this chapter dedicated to these specific symptoms.

If adverse effects persist despite appropriate interventions, rotation to a different opioid may be helpful. Overall, at this point no clear evidence exists that one particular opioid has a different adverse effect profile than another opioid. Patients may exhibit different sensitivities to different opioids because of individual variability in opioid receptors, pharmacokinetics, and metabolism. Inroads have recently been made in understanding which genetic variants may influence a particular person's response to opioids. For example, certain variants of the multidrug resistance 1 gene (formerly *MDR1*, now called *ABCB1*) or the gene encoding catechol-O-methyltransferase *(COMT)* are associated with CNS adverse effects, such as drowsiness or confusion.[123] A very promising recent approach to reducing opioid adverse effects involves identifying opioid agonists with "ligand biasing" of actions on opioid receptors that preferentially act via G proteins rather than via beta-arrestin signaling.[124]

Opioid-associated adverse effects may be also improved with a reduction in opioid dose, which may be achieved without loss of analgesic effect if a coanalgesic medication is added. For example, when gabapentin and morphine are combined they provide better analgesia from neuropathic pain at lower doses of each drug than either does as a single agent.[125]

Opioid-Induced Neurotoxicity. Opioid-induced neurotoxicity is typically encountered when opioid doses are rapidly increased, when high doses of an opioid are used, or in the setting of renal failure. The patient may describe increased sensitivity to pain (hyperalgesia), pain in response to nonpainful stimuli (allodynia), worsening pain despite increasing doses of opioids, or pain that appears to spread. Other findings of neurologic hyperexcitability such as myoclonus, delirium, or seizures may also be present. Opioid-induced hyperalgesia is likely due to accumulation of neurotoxic opioid metabolites such as M3G or hydromorphone-3-glucuronide. Such metabolites activate presynaptic calcium channels that release glutamate, which in turn activates NMDA receptors and depolarized postsynaptic neurons in the CNS.[126]

If signs or symptoms of opioid neurotoxicity develop, the opioid should be decreased or changed to one with potentially less neurotoxic effects, such as fentanyl or methadone. The addition of a nonopioid analgesic may lessen the amount of opioid required. An alternative mode of analgesia such as intrathecal, regional, or local analgesia may be used in place of systemic opioids. If needed, parenteral ketamine, an NMDA receptor antagonist, may also be initiated to reduce NMDA receptor-mediated neurotoxicity.[127]

Myoclonus is frequently relieved by a benzodiazepine such as diazepam. Opioids may also play a role in the development of delirium; the reader is referred to the section in this chapter dedicated to mental status changes.

Management of Opioid Overdose. Respiratory depression occurs as a result of opioid receptor blockade of CO_2 chemoreceptors in the medulla. The risk of respiratory depression from opioids is indeed small when opioids are dosed and titrated judiciously. Scenarios in which opioids may cause respiratory depression are the development of renal failure or a sudden decrease in pain, such as after a neurolytic block if opioid doses are not adjusted.

Respiratory depression characterized by hypopnea alone is not in and of itself an indication for opioid reversal with naloxone. In fact, administration of oxygen and reduction of the subsequent dose may be the only actions needed. For a true respiratory emergency, naloxone should be administered by (1) diluting the 0.4 mg/mL ampule in 10 mL saline solution and (2) administering 1 mL IV or subcutaneously every 3 minutes until respiratory depression improves. If the patient is taking long-acting opioids, repeated doses of naloxone or a naloxone infusion may be required, with the hourly dose being the dose initially required to overcome respiratory depression. Overadministration of naloxone will block opioid receptors, resulting in withdrawal that may be characterized by severe pain and sympathetic instability.

Adjuvant Treatments

Radiotherapy

Radiotherapy is commonly used to relieve pain such as localized bone metastases. In a review of 13 randomized trials in adults with painful bone metastases who received either radiotherapy or radioisotope injection for pain, it was found that 27% achieved total pain relief and 42% attained a 50% level of pain relief. The largest trial found that the median duration of complete pain relief was 12 weeks. A variety of fractionation schedules were used, and no clear difference between schedules was found.[128]

Antidepressants

TCAs and serotonin and norepinephrine reuptake inhibitors (e.g., duloxetine) may relieve neuropathic pain and are discussed in more detail later.

Steroids

Pain attributable to swelling, such as headache from increased intracranial pressure, bone pain, nerve pain from compression by a tumor, and hepatic capsular pain, may be responsive to steroids. A common starting dose is 10 mg followed by 4 mg four times a day in larger patients. Dosages of 10 mg/m² followed by 4 mg/m² four times a day can be used in smaller patients. If the response is favorable, the steroid dose should gradually be reduced to the lowest effective dose. A medication to provide concurrent gastric protection should also be prescribed.

Anticonvulsant Agents

Anticonvulsant agents control neuropathic pain by preventing peripheral nerve excitation. Carbamazepine has been widely studied for neuropathic pain such as trigeminal neuralgia. However, carbamazepine interacts with many other drugs and may suppress bone marrow function, limiting its usefulness in patients with cancer. Oxcarbazepine is a carbamazepine derivative that acts via use-dependent blockade of sodium channels. Overall, compared with carbamazepine, oxcarbazepine appears to result in fewer risks for hematologic, dermatologic, and hepatic complications. Hyponatremia can occur, and electrolytes should be monitored in the first weeks of therapy or with dose escalation. Gabapentin and pregabalin are newer anticonvulsants that lack such interactions and bone marrow toxicity. These agents target both excitatory and inhibitory neurotransmitters through inhibition of sodium and voltage-gated calcium channels.

Gabapentin may be sedating, requiring gradual initiation (i.e., a 5 to 7 mg/kg/dose by mouth three times a day, with a gradual increase every 3 days) and titration to effect. Reports of pediatric uses of gabapentin and pregabalin for treatment of chronic neuropathic pain are limited to case series. For any of the anticonvulsants, effects on mood, sedation, and mental clarity are quite variable.

Clonidine

Clonidine is an alpha-agonist drug that historically has been used to treat hypertension or opioid withdrawal. It may also be used for neuropathic pain or to enhance analgesia from opioids. Clonidine may be administered orally or transdermally, which is an additional benefit in the pediatric population. Clonidine has also been used in children for hyperactivity or steroid-associated psychiatric symptoms. Sedation is common.

Ketamine

Ketamine is an effective adjuvant analgesic that is useful for its opioid-sparing and opioid-sensitizing capabilities, particularly in persons experiencing difficult pain syndromes such as neuropathic pain.[129] Although the evidence is scant, reports exist of its usefulness in relieving refractory pain in children with cancer.[130] Ketamine may on occasion cause hallucinations and depersonalization/derealization. Such effects are more common in adults and may be prevented or treated with a benzodiazepine.

Invasive Approaches to Pain Management

In a small subgroup of patients, aggressive titration of analgesics and adjuvants still results in a circumstance of inadequate analgesia and/or intolerable adverse effects, including intolerable sedation. In some situations consideration of regional anesthetic approaches may be appropriate; the most common approaches are infusions of analgesics and local anesthetics via indwelling intrathecal, epidural, or plexus catheters. A number of considerations influence the choice of these methods, including the wishes of the patient and his or her surrogate in terms of balancing analgesia, alertness, and the risks and inconveniences of a technologic approach; availability of expert personnel for both catheter placement and ongoing management; and consideration of the nature of the pain, the expected course of the disease, and disease-related symptoms. Because a number of technical and management issues cannot be readily extrapolated from similar infusions in adults or from perioperative infusions in children, consultation with clinicians who have experience in these techniques is encouraged. In adults, a track record exists of using implantable programmable pumps that can be refilled at a frequency ranging from weekly to every several months. One study indicated benefits of these systems with regard to pain, quality of life scores, and even longevity.[131]

In children with cancer, it is generally necessary to combine small amounts of a local anesthetic along with opioids in the spinal infusion. Because of the relatively low potency and low solubility of existing local anesthetics, this requirement makes it impractical to use the programmable pumps commonly used in adults. Therefore in a majority of these cases, our preference has been to use implanted intrathecal ports rather than implanted pumps. The procedure to place these ports is performed in the operating room with use of general anesthesia while the patient is in the lateral position. The intrathecal catheters are advanced cephalad from spinal entry near L3-L4 under fluoroscopic guidance to position the tips near the spinal dorsal horn levels (rather than the exiting nerve root levels) relevant to the sites of greatest pain. The reader is referred to Figure 564 in the atlas by Clemente[132] for illustration of the spinal dorsal horn levels.

As an example, for refractory pain due to pelvic or lower extremity tumors predominantly involving lumbosacral dermatomes, we advance the catheter tips to a level around T11. Catheters are tunneled subcutaneously and connected to a port that is positioned over the lower ribs near the anterior axillary line.

In the setting of refractory pain due to advanced cancer, our view is that coagulopathy in most cases should not be regarded as a major contraindication to this procedure. If necessary, platelets and/or fresh-frozen plasma are infused immediately before and during the procedure as guided by coagulation parameters.

Use of indwelling ports is preferable for the sake of sterility and skin care. Ports are accessed with Huber needles similar to those used for IV ports. Dilute local anesthetics are generally required for adequate analgesia (particularly with movement), and they can generally be titrated in a manner that preserves reasonable lower body motor functioning. Depending on the adverse-effect profile seen with opioids and local anesthetics, other spinal analgesics may be included in the mixture, including clonidine and ketamine.

Although the epidural route can be used, our experience is that the intrathecal route is more reliable over a longer time frame because of several factors, including the development of adhesions or fibrosis in the epidural space over periods of months with use of high-concentration infusions and because of the phenomenon of tolerance to local anesthetics, which can be overcome very readily with intrathecal dosing but with much greater difficulty with prolonged epidural dosing. Clinicians' estimates of prognosis and longevity are often imprecise. Our general recommendation is that, if invasive approaches are being considered in the first place, the most versatile system available should be chosen to be implanted—that is, one most likely to work successfully for the short term (i.e., a few weeks) as well as longer term (i.e., months to a year) and least likely to require a repeat procedure. One potential early complication of this procedure is cerebrospinal fluid leak, leading to headache in the days after placement. In two cases we have returned to the operating room several days later to resolve this problem with a fluoroscopically guided epidural blood patch. The introduction of spinal analgesic medication and the corresponding adjustment of systemic analgesics require careful attention because of the potential for oversedation and even respiratory depression. Because the intensity of afferent nociceptive transmission is diminished by the spinal medications, the stimulating effect of this nociceptive activity on alertness and respiratory drive is also diminished.

Occasionally in patients who have a tumor that involves a single peripheral nerve or nerve plexus, indwelling tunneled catheters can be placed percutaneously along the nerve or in the plexus sheath. Our preference is to use a combination of ultrasound and nerve stimulation guidance. These peripheral and plexus catheters can be extremely helpful if the pain remains highly localized. In a majority of cases, however, the tumor spreads beyond these more limited distributions, and we have therefore generally favored intraspinal infusions because of greater versatility in covering pain arising from a broader area. For similar reasons, our general preference is to choose intraspinal drug infusions rather than neurolytic nerve blocks except in very restricted circumstances, such as the use of a neurolytic celiac plexus blockade for a tumor that is almost entirely restricted to the upper abdominal solid viscera. Celiac plexus blockade has a good track record for treatment of refractory pain due to pancreatic cancer in adults. It affects visceral innervation only and produces no somatic sensory or motor deficits. Adverse effects such as diarrhea or orthostatic hypotension tend to be relatively short-lived and tolerable. For children and adolescents, our preference is to perform this procedure with use of general anesthesia with the patient in the prone position, using alcohol as the neurolytic agent. We use a posterior approach with computed tomography (CT) guidance, in collaboration with an interventional radiologist. Interventional approaches for pain in children were recently reviewed.[133]

Psychological and Nonpharmacologic Approaches to Pain

Because of the multifactorial nature of the experience of pain, a multidisciplinary approach is often helpful in optimizing pain management. With use of psychosocial assessment it may be possible to identify and address factors that contribute to pain that analgesic interventions alone cannot address.

Depending on the developmental capacity of the child, interventions such as preparatory play, distraction, imagery, relaxation, deep breathing, hypnosis, and behavioral management can reduce anxiety and fear associated with pain. A child life specialist, psychologist, complementary medicine practitioner, or other specialist may be able to provide some of these interventions.

A variety of cognitive and behavioral approaches to pain and invasive procedures may be helpful to reduce pain and distress experienced by the child. In a study of 56 children aged 3 to 13 years, delivery of a cognitive-behavioral intervention was compared with preprocedure administration of diazepam or cartoon watching prior to bone marrow aspiration.[134] The cognitive-behavioral intervention consisted of breathing exercises, positive reinforcement, and imagery or distraction to provide the child with imaginative and cognitive tools to cope with procedural stress. Overall, children who received the cognitive-behavioral intervention had lower

pulse rates and distress and pain scores when compared with children who either received diazepam or watched cartoons. However, during the actual aspiration procedure, no difference was found between groups, suggesting that it did not ameliorate distress associated with the intense experience of the actual procedure.[135] Cognitive behavioral therapy (CBT) does provide children with mechanisms for coping with distressing procedures and may explain why children who receive CBT display less distress after the procedure compared with children who receive an anesthestic via a mask but do not receive CBT.[136]

Hypnotherapy can be performed in children as young as 4 years.[137] Hypnosis can reduce procedural pain (e.g., from a bone marrow aspirate) and postoperative pain in children, as well as anticipatory nausea and dyspnea. In a randomized controlled trial of 30 children (ages 5 to 15 years) with cancer who were undergoing bone marrow aspiration, children who received either hypnosis or CBT reported less pain and anxiety compared with their baseline symptoms or control subjects who did not receive either intervention. Children who underwent hypnosis also demonstrated less procedure-related distress than did those in the other two groups.[138]

Music, art, and play therapy may also be helpful in reducing anxiety associated with procedures. For example, soft lullaby music reduces heart rates in children undergoing the application or removal of a cast.[139] Even when specific nonpharmacologic techniques are not employed, some behavioral strategies should always be used, including appropriately preparing the child, giving the child choices when possible, providing developmentally appropriate and honest explanations, and providing positive reinforcement. Patient education is also an important component of addressing pain.

Many patients find integrative therapies (i.e., therapies complementary to traditional medical approaches) to be of benefit in coping with stress, reducing the effects of treatment and illness, providing a sense of control, and enhancing quality of life.[140] In a survey of adults participating in cancer clinical trials, 63% used at least one type of integrative therapy, with an average use of two therapies per patient.[140] Few clinicians are aware of these practices and thus should routinely inquire about them.

Although many practices such as acupuncture, massage, and healing touch seem promising in reducing cancer-related pain, the evidence base supporting these therapies is weak. Barriers to the publication of such trials include issues of study quality and design such as small study size, high attrition rates, and lack of a comparison arm, particularly in fields where the placebo effect may be high.[141] Studies with adequate power and duration and sham controls are needed to evaluate the efficacy of these interventions for cancer-related pain.

Pediatric Cancer Pain Syndromes

Although pain should be approached with a systematic approach and the use of analgesics, including opioids and adjuvants, certain cancer-related pain syndromes may respond to particular treatments.

Tumor-Mediated Pain

GI obstruction may cause pain. Management of GI obstruction is discussed in the section entitled "Other Gastrointestinal Symptoms." Visceromegaly or invasion of organs, which often presents as a poorly localized, dull pain, is best treated with opioids, radiation, nerve blockade, or epidural/intrathecal techniques. Involvement of nerve or bone may result in neuropathic or bone pain, which is discussed later. Liver capsular pain may be alleviated by steroids.[142] Elevated intracranial pressure may present as headache and vomiting and may respond to steroids or surgical decompression. In situations in which inflammation is thought to contribute to pain, the pain may respond to steroids or NSAIDs.

Pain Related to Administration of Antineoplastic Therapy

Antineoplastic therapy may produce a variety of pain syndromes. Injection of chemotherapy into a peripheral vein may cause local transient pain or phlebitis. Extravasation of a vesicant such as vincristine or anthracycline may cause local pain, burning, swelling, and/or redness, as well as tissue necrosis. These symptoms are most likely to occur when the agent is injected peripherally. Preclinical data showed that dexrazoxane, a reversible topoisomerase II catalytic inhibitor, reduced the number, severity, and duration of wounds that developed in a dose-dependent manner after extravasation.[143] In a single-arm, open-label study of 53 humans with anthracycline extravasation, dexrazoxane was well tolerated. In this uncontrolled trial, one patient required surgical resection (1.8%).[144]

Intrathecal chemotherapy may cause arachnoiditis, which is associated with fever, headache, nuchal rigidity, nausea, and vomiting. A new liposomal formulation of cytarabine appears to have an increased risk of arachnoiditis in children, which can be mitigated with systemic dexamethasone.[145]

Prolonged steroid administration may result in avascular necrosis, which occurs most often in the hip.[146] NSAIDs may help provide relief for this painful condition, although if the pain is severe, opioid therapy may be indicated. Pamidronate is a bisphosphonate that holds promise in reducing symptoms and increasing function in children who have painful osteonecrosis due to steroid therapy for acute lymphoblastic leukemia (ALL).[147,148]

Bone Pain

Infiltration of bone is often experienced as a constant aching, which may be relieved by steroids, NSAIDs, or opioid analgesics. Isolated bone metastases may be treated with local treatments such as external beam radiation or surgical techniques such as vertebral body or long bone stabilization or other more invasive treatments for pain (see "Invasive Approaches to Pain Management"). Bisphosphonates, which reduce osteoclastic bone resorption, may be helpful when analgesics or radiotherapy are inadequate for the management of painful bone metastases.[149] Diffuse bone metastases may also be treated with radioisotopes, but radioisotopes may cause myelosuppression.

Bone pain may also be caused by filgrastim or pegfilgrastim.[150] Although the mechanism underlying such pain has not been clearly established, it is frequently attributed to filgrastim-stimulated marrow expansion. In a study of 100 adults receiving care in a community oncology practice, 79% experienced either moderate or severe bone pain due to use of pegfilgrastim. Pain was either diffuse or located in the lower extremities/hips or back. For persons with the most severe pain, the mean duration of pain was 2.8 days after the injection. NSAIDs provided relief for 74% of persons with moderate pain. Some persons with severe pain received opioids, but opioids provided relief in only 45% of patients. Interestingly, patients with lymphoma who were receiving concurrent steroids as lymphoma-directed therapy did not have significantly less bone pain.

Filgrastim-induced bone pain has not been well studied in children, although anecdotally it appears to occur less frequently in children than in adults. In a relatively small study of 28 children with cancer who received pegfilgrastim (100 μg/kg with a maximum dose of 6 mg for a total of 126 doses) after myelosuppressive chemotherapy, four children reported bone pain.

Although use of antihistamines to treat filgrastim-associated bone pain has been reported,[151] no clinical trials have been performed to evaluate this practice. Until evidence indicates that antihistamines reduce this type of bone pain, antihistamines should not be used at the exclusion of established analgesic practices.

Mucositis

Mucositis is a common problem for children after chemotherapy, radiation, or bone marrow transplantation. It is particularly problematic in children undergoing high-dose chemotherapy or head and neck radiotherapy. Mucositis is associated with increased risk of infection and may impair intake of adequate nutrition. It usually self-resolves within 14 days or upon recovery of the bone marrow. The WHO has developed a mucositis rating scale that ranges from 0 (no visible evidence of mucositis, no pain, able to eat solids, and able to drink) to 4 (erythema, ulceration present, significant pain, and inability to eat or drink). Prophylactic antiviral or antifungal therapy does not decrease the incidence of mucositis. However, superinfection should be considered and cultures should be obtained when mucositis appears to be more severe or prolonged than anticipated.

Historically the mainstay of pain control for mucositis has been parenteral opioid therapy, usually via PCA. This mechanism of analgesia delivery is both safe and effective for this purpose.[112] An adjuvant mouthwash containing diphenhydramine, 2% viscous lidocaine, and liquid antacid (e.g., Maalox) in a 1 : 1 : 1 formulation may be used in children older than 2 years who can spit out the medication rather than swallowing it. Topical application of straight viscous lidocaine carries the risk of systemic absorption if the mucositis is widespread. Although the true risk of aspiration due to local anesthesia of glottic structures is unclear, some centers avoid using this strategy because of this concern. A supersaturated calcium phosphate mouth rinse moistens and lubricates the oral cavity. Although results of studies of this agent have been mixed, the majority of studies support its use to reduce the severity/duration of mucositis and the pain associated with it. The Children's Oncology Group is currently conducting a study of this rinse in preventing mucositis in children who are undergoing hematopoietic stem cell transplantation.

Other measures to alleviate mucositis include regular administration of oral sucralfate during chemotherapy, low-dose laser therapy, and gum chewing.[152-154] Results of studies evaluating the efficacy of the free radical scavenger amifostine in reducing mucositis have been inconsistent.[155] Severe mucositis can also cause abdominal pain, which is best treated with opioids. Perineal pain due to mucositis may also be addressed with a topical barrier cream to soothe and protect the area.

Recent advances in the understanding of the pathogenesis of mucositis have led to the development of targeted therapies. For example, palifermin is a keratinocyte growth factor that mediates epithelial cell growth and reduces epithelial cell apoptosis, factors that both appear to be important processes in the evolution of mucositis. Palifermin reduces mucosal injury as manifested by decreased mucositis duration and severity and a reduced need for analgesics and parenteral nutrition in adults undergoing high-dose chemotherapy and radiotherapy requiring peripheral blood stem cell rescue. In one study of adults undergoing high-dose therapy with autologous stem cell rescue, the incidence of WHO grade 4 mucositis was reduced from 62% to 20% ($P < .001$).[156]

The role of L-glutamine in mucositis has also been recently investigated. Depletion of L-glutamine is associated with epithelial damage, and increased levels are associated with healing. The role of uptake-enhanced L-glutamine suspension (AES-14) in reducing mucositis has recently been studied. In a placebo-controlled crossover study of 326 women undergoing chemotherapy for breast cancer, AES-14 reduced mucositis incidence and severity.[157] In addition, AES-14 demonstrated a carryover effect, with patients receiving AES-14 before placebo having a lower risk of mucositis.

Neuropathic Pain

Neuropathic pain may occur from infiltration or compression of nerves, nerve damage from surgery, herpes zoster, or adverse effects from antineoplastic therapies such as vinca alkaloids, cisplatin, oxaliplatin, or bortezomib. Children often describe it as burning or shooting pain, and it may be accompanied by dysesthesia or hyperalgesia.

Neuropathic pain may be related to chronic pain states whereby chronic afferent input into the dorsal horn of the spinal cord leads to a hyperactive state. Mediators of this condition are excitatory amino acids, such as glutamate, which bind to the NMDA receptor. The NMDA/glutamate receptor is a calcium channel involved in opioid-resistant pain, neuropathic pain, allodynia, and hyperalgesia. NMDA receptor binding may lead to lasting increases in neuronal excitability, leading to persistence of neuronal hyperactivity. The end result of such a phenomenon is hyperalgesia, allodynia, spontaneous pain,

and phantom limb pain, even after the painful stimulus has resolved. Methadone, with its NMDA receptor antagonist properties, may be the most appropriate opioid for neuropathic pain. However, no clear evidence from studies in humans shows that methadone is superior to other opioids in treating neuropathic pain.[158] In addition, other approaches such as nerve blocks or adjuvant NMDA receptor antagonists may disrupt ongoing nociceptive input and neuronal hyperexcitability.

Most therapies for neuropathic pain have been evaluated in non–cancer-related neuropathic pain syndromes such as diabetic neuropathy. Medications for neuropathic pain include TCAs and the newer atypical antidepressants venlafaxine and duloxetine. TCAs often relieve neuropathic pain more quickly and at lower doses than are required to treat depression. TCAs reduce neuropathic pain by inhibiting serotonin and norepinephrine uptake, which increases transmission of inhibitory signals in the spinal cord. For children experiencing disturbed sleep, amitriptyline, a TCA that leads to greater sedation, may be a good choice. However, amitriptyline also has more anticholinergic effects such as xerostomia and constipation, in which case nortriptyline is an alternative TCA.

Duloxetine is the first antidepressant to be approved by the U.S. FDA for treatment of neuropathic pain, and in a recent multicenter randomized placebo-controlled crossover trial, it was demonstrated to reduce chemotherapy-induced painful peripheral neuropathy.[159] Anticonvulsants such as topiramate, pregabalin, or gabapentin may also be effective.[125,160,161] In the cancer population, gabapentin effectively reduced tumor-related neuropathic pain in a randomized controlled study of adults already receiving opioids, with lower average pain intensity scores and less dysesthesia in the gabapentin group.[162] In some instances when tumors incite pain because of spinal cord compression, dexamethasone may reduce pain.[163] Other interventions such as topical lidocaine or capsaicin, transcutaneous electrical nerve stimulation, surgical decompression, or nerve blocks may also relieve neuropathic pain.

Phantom Limb Pain

Phantom limb pain is a common phenomenon in children who undergo amputation of an extremity.[164] It may be experienced as either stump pain or the type of pain experienced preoperatively, and it appears to improve over time.[164,165] Phantom limb pain appears to be associated with preoperative limb pain.[164] For this reason it is best approached with preemptive regional anesthesia. In our practice, regional anesthesia is used widely for anesthetic and analgesic management of amputations in children. The widespread use of ultrasound guidance has increased the reliability of continuous peripheral nerve blockade via indwelling catheters.

Additional measures to treat phantom limb pain include anticonvulsants, TCAs, and topical agents such as Lidoderm. Some small series have reported success with gabapentin[166] and topiramate for phantom limb pain.[167] A preliminary observational study found that use of a prosthesis to support limb use was associated with reduced phantom limb pain when compared with cosmetic prosthesis use.[168] A few studies suggest that therapy with mirrors may relieve phantom limb pain, although the limitations of these studies, including small sample size, preclude definitive conclusions.[169,170]

Pain Related to Graft-Versus-Host Disease

Graft-versus-host disease (GVHD) may cause a variety of pain syndromes. It is a common cause of abdominal pain in children undergoing bone marrow transplantation.[171] Along with diarrhea, nausea/vomiting, weight loss, dysphagia, and early satiety, abdominal pain/cramping may occur in gut GVHD.[172] Antimuscarinic/anticholinergic agents such as scopolamine may reduce colic from smooth muscle spasms. However, gut GVHD may be so severe that opioids are required for analgesia.[113]

Oral GVHD usually does not cause pain. Development of oral pain is associated with ulceration or involvement of the soft palate.[173,174] When evaluating pain in the setting of oral GVHD, one should also consider a concomitant infection such as herpes simplex virus or candidiasis. Oral GVHD pain is usually reduced with GVHD-directed treatment such as topical steroids or topical FK506 rinses. Pain associated with vulvovaginal GVHD may also respond to topical steroids or topical cyclosporine.[175,176] Other types of GVHD, such as myositis or fasciitis, may require systemic analgesia.

Postoperative Pain

A broader discussion of treatment of postoperative pain in children and adolescents than that presented here can be found elsewhere.[177,178]

Cancer surgery is often distressing and anxiety provoking for children and their parents. Unless specifically contraindicated, anxiolytic premedication with benzodiazepines should be considered routine, using oral or IV routes as appropriate. For patients who were treated with opioids on a regular basis before surgery, it is necessary to increase postoperative analgesic dosing accordingly. It is a common mistake to select routine parameters for opioid infusions or PCA for these patients, which invariably results in underdosing and inadequate analgesia.

For major tumor resections in the lower extremities, pelvis, abdomen, and thorax, we make extensive use of epidural infusions for postoperative analgesia. Epidural analgesia in children requires specific training regarding the technical aspects, as well as pediatric-specific management protocols and a level of acute pain service coverage that permits optimal dose adjustment. For patients receiving epidural infusions who were opioid tolerant before surgery, it may be necessary to provide a systemic opioid along with an epidural opioid postoperatively (despite a widespread "taboo" against this combination); alternately, larger than usual dosing of epidural opioids, the addition of epidural clonidine, or other approaches may be necessary to account for the patient's preexisting opioid tolerance, which may be accompanied by hyperalgesia. Peripheral nerve and plexus catheters placed via ultrasound guidance are increasingly being used for surgery on the limbs. For thoracotomies, ultrasound-guided continuous paravertebral catheters are a promising alternative to thoracic epidural catheters.

Procedure-Related Pain

Brief procedures involving the use of needles, including venipunctures, IV cannulation, lumbar punctures, and bone marrow biopsies and aspirates, are a major component of cancer care and a major source of distress for patients. Approaches to management of these interventions should be individualized, based on consideration of the child's age, temperament, coping style, and past pain experiences, as well as the intensity of the procedure (e.g., bone marrow biopsy is more painful than a simple venipuncture).

Explanations provided prior to procedures should be tailored according to the child's age, developmental status, and coping style. The presence of the parents can be helpful, especially when the parents have been coached to help facilitate positive coping. Parents should be present to provide support, not to hold the child or assist the clinicians.

A variety of products are available to provide needle-free skin analgesia. These products include local anesthetic creams such as eutectic mixture of local anesthetics (EMLA), ELA-Max, tetracaine gel (Ametop), patches such as Synera, needleless injection systems such as Zingo, and lidocaine iontophoresis. These products differ in their onset time, propensity for vasodilation or vasoconstriction, cost, and availability in different countries. In a busy clinic, use of these topical anesthetic techniques is facilitated by standing order policies so they can be applied at an appropriate time before the planned procedure.

Several cognitive-behavioral approaches have been shown to be effective in reducing a child's procedure-related distress, including hypnosis, guided imagery, and related approaches to achieving a relaxed or dissociated state. These approaches have the virtue of safety and generalizability. A patient who learns these techniques for one setting can apply them to other situations.

Conscious sedation, deep sedation, or brief general anesthesia can be very effective in alleviating the pain and distress of lumbar punctures and bone marrow biopsies and aspirates. The approach chosen will depend in part on the individual patient, the intensity of pain involved in the procedure, the degree of immobility required (e.g., for radiation therapy or magnetic resonance imaging), and available resources.

Considerable variation exists in the choices of drugs, the depth of sedation, and the personnel involved in different aspects of sedation. In some hospitals a two-tiered approach is taken, with lower risk patients receiving sedation administered by oncologists and nurses and higher risk patients cared for by pediatric anesthesiologists.

Other hospitals use a different two-tiered approach, with sedation for low- to intermediate-risk patients being administered by nurses and pediatric subspecialists from a sedation service who have specific expertise (e.g., pediatric intensivists or pediatric emergency physicians) and utilization of pediatric anesthesiologists to care for higher risk patients, those having more extensive procedures, or those requiring higher degrees of immobility. For example, for a cooperative, relatively healthy 12-year-old undergoing a lumbar puncture, a regimen that involves conscious sedation with midazolam and fentanyl and topical local anesthesia followed by local anesthetic infiltration is likely to be safe and effective. Conversely, a 2-year-old with a history of a very difficult to manage airway and cardiomyopathy who is undergoing bone marrow aspiration, biopsy, and a lumbar puncture would be at higher risk and therefore might be referred for management by a pediatric anesthesiologist.

In our view, regardless of local decisions about which specific specialists are involved in which procedures, pediatric oncologists need to advocate for sufficient institutional resources to ensure that effective and safe approaches to conscious sedation and general anesthesia are available for all children with cancer. Some general recommendations for sedation programs are listed in Box 71-1.

More detailed discussions of individual drugs and outcomes of pediatric sedation may be found elsewhere.[179,180]

Reassessing Interventions for Pain

Careful reassessment to determine response to therapy is a key component in effectively addressing pain. In addition to reducing pain, interventions seek to reduce distress and functional impairment and enhance quality of life. Pain relief measures do not necessarily achieve all of these goals. For example, in one survey of adults with non–cancer-related pain, even when the degree of pain was controlled for, persons receiving opioid therapy did not have improved quality of life or improved function.[181] Therefore in addition to evaluation of whether pain relief is attained, determination of whether increased functional capacity and increased quality of life is achieved is crucial in symptom management.

Barriers to Effective Pain Management

Increasing interest in pain and pain treatment in recent years has resulted in a better understanding of pathophysiologic mechanisms of pain, better treatment options, and greater availability of treatment for pain. However, these advances have not necessarily resulted in a reduced prevalence of pain in patients with cancer.[182]

This paradox is due in part to the multitude of barriers to effective pain management. Clinician-related barriers include a focus on cure at the exclusion of attention to symptoms, lack of familiarity with pain management, fear of either regulatory repercussions for prescribing opioids or diversion of the medications to persons for whom the opioid is not prescribed, and underappreciation of the multifactorial nature of the experience of pain. Patient-related factors may include fear of addiction; fear of adverse effects, including respiratory depression; fear that treating pain with opioids is equivalent to "giving up"; and the misperception that opioids should be "saved" for severe pain.

Educational strategies for clinicians and families alike are likely to surmount many of these barriers to pain management. In addition, partnership with the child and family may enhance attention to this important issue and provide added opportunities for addressing barriers to treating pain adequately. For example, a randomized clinical trial tested the effectiveness of the PRO-SELF Pain Control Program, which actively involves adult patients and families in the pain management plan; findings included decreased pain intensity scores, an increased number of appropriate analgesic prescriptions, and increased analgesic intake in oncology outpatients who had pain from bone metastasis when compared with standard care.[183] Such an approach is endorsed by the American Pain Society and is likely to contribute greatly to overcoming barriers to successful pain management.

NAUSEA AND VOMITING

Pathophysiology

Vomiting may be caused by a wide variety of triggers, including motion, insult to the GI tract, hormonal changes, medications, and emotions. Vomiting is a complex process that involves both the central and peripheral nervous systems, with both biologic and psychological mechanisms playing a role.

During the past three decades strides have been made in understanding the pathophysiologic components of

---

Box 71-1 Recommendations for Pediatric Oncology Sedation Programs

1. A standardized preprocedure history and physical should be performed to identify factors that might modify risk (e.g., airway anomalies, respiratory difficulties, and cardiac compromise).
2. Use of procedure checklists should be encouraged.
3. Nothing by mouth guidelines should be consistent with those recommended for children undergoing general anesthesia.
4. Clinicians who are performing the procedure should have undivided attention during the procedure (e.g., their beeper and phone should be carried by someone else), and they should ensure that all necessary supplies (including kits, sterile supplies, chemotherapy, and tubes) are already in the room before bringing the child into the room or initiating sedation.
5. Children receiving sedation should receive continuous monitoring, including a dedicated observer, continuous use of pulse oximetry, and regular recording of vital signs.
6. All procedure locations should have at least the following supplies, equipment, or systems at hand:
   a. Wall or tank oxygen supplies
   b. Wall or portable suction devices
   c. Monitoring equipment
   d. Airway equipment, including bags and suitably sized masks, laryngoscopes, endotracheal tubes, oral airways, and laryngeal mask airways
   e. An emergency cart, such as a code cart
   f. Communication protocols (often assisted by a code button or phone system)
7. After the procedure, children require observation until they meet standardized recovery criteria, and often for a period of time thereafter. During recovery, and especially when they no longer appear sedated, children remain at significant risk for injuries caused by falling, hitting their head on bed rails, and so forth.
8. Observation and administration of medications should be performed by a clinician with no additional responsibilities—that is, not by the clinician performing the procedure. These clinicians should have training and competency in pediatric acute care and pediatric airway management.
9. Clinics and hospitals performing pediatric sedation should track outcomes related to efficacy (from a child-centered viewpoint) and safety to facilitate system-based improvements in quality of care.

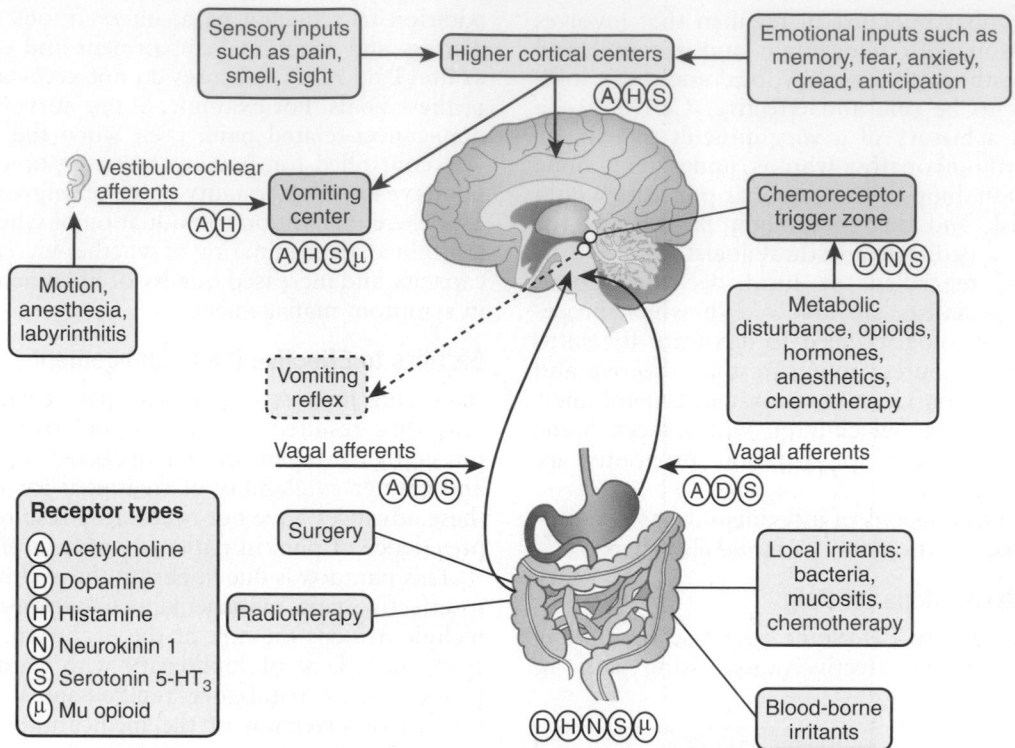

Figure 71-3 The pathogenesis of chemotherapy-induced nausea and vomiting.

nausea and vomiting and in the development of agents aimed at them. Investigations have focused primarily on chemotherapy-induced nausea and vomiting (CINV). Prior to the 1990s, dopamine was the major neurotransmitter recognized as being important in mediating CINV, and dopamine blockade was the mainstay of therapy for CINV.

Vomiting is mediated by the vomiting center in the medullary lateral reticular formation. This center is not a discrete entity but instead is a group of loosely organized neurons in the medulla that are activated in a sequential manner during emetogenesis.[184,185] Sources of afferent input to the nucleus tractus solitarius in the vomiting center include the chemoreceptor trigger zone (CTZ), the viscera (via vagal and sympathetic afferents), the midbrain, the vestibular system, and the cerebral cortex (Fig. 71-3). Vomiting occurs when the vomiting center emits coordinated efferent impulses to several targets including the diaphragm, abdominal wall musculature, esophagus, and stomach.

Chemotherapy-Induced Nausea and Vomiting

Chemotherapy can lead to nausea and vomiting through several mechanisms. One mechanism is by stimulation of the CTZ, which lies in the area postrema, in the floor of the fourth ventricle. Although the CTZ is part of the CNS, it contains chemoreceptors outside the blood-brain barrier that can detect emetogenic agents present in the circulation, as well as in the spinal fluid. However, evidence suggests that chemotherapy stimulates the CTZ indirectly because (1) it is unlikely that the CTZ has specific receptors that are activated by each type of chemotherapy agent; (2) the latency time to the onset of emesis is not compatible with direct action of the drugs on the CTZ; and (3) vagotomy and sympathectomy prevent cisplatin-induced emesis in the ferret, indicating that these inputs are needed for chemotherapy-induced vomiting to occur.[186,187]

Chemotherapy can also stimulate the vomiting center directly.[184] In addition, chemotherapeutic agents can stimulate the gut, leading to release of serotonin. This release in turn stimulates the vagus nerve, which activates the vomiting center, either directly or via impulses to the CTZ.[188] The central cortex may also be involved in CINV by mediating emotions such as anxiety that play a role in the genesis of nausea.

Several neurotransmitter pathways are known to play a role in nausea and vomiting. Whereas histamine and muscarinic receptors are prominent in vomiting associated with motion sickness,[189] serotonin, dopamine, and substance P appear to be particularly important in CINV.[190] Central blockade of the D2 subtype of dopamine receptors in the area postrema and vomiting center is the mechanism of action of antidopaminergic antiemetics such as metoclopramide. It was later found that in addition to dopamine receptor antagonism, metoclopramide was an antagonist of the 5-hydroxytryptamine 3 (5-HT3) receptor,[191,192] prompting interest in the role of this receptor in nausea and vomiting.[184]

Serotonin is produced by enterochromaffin cells in the gut and is also found in multiple locations in the CNS. Several observations in both animals and humans confirmed that serotonin plays a major role in acute CINV. Cisplatin and cyclophosphamide-induced vomiting in the ferret was drastically reduced with the administration of intravenous, intraperitoneal, or intracerebral injection of serotonin S3 receptor antagonists.[193] Serotonin receptor blockers and serotonin receptor blockade inhibited chemotherapy-induced vomiting in ferrets[186,194-197] and in other animal systems.[198,199] Depletion of serotonin stores was shown to also prevent cisplatin-induced vomiting.[200]

In humans, studies by Cubeddu et al.[201] demonstrated that strongly emetogenic regimens containing cisplatin or dacarbazine resulted in a marked increase in serotonin metabolites in plasma and urine with a time course similar to CINV symptoms in patients. In addition, treatment with a serotonin synthesis inhibitor inhibited both cisplatin-induced vomiting and increases in serotonin metabolites.[201] The relationship between other chemotherapeutic agents and markers of serotonin metabolism has been further explored, with more emetogenic regimens resulting in higher serotonin metabolite levels.[201] Chemotherapeutic agents appear to be toxic to the enterochromaffin cells lining the upper small intestine, resulting in generation of free radicals and release of serotonin.[187]

5-HT3 receptors are present in the GI tract as well as vagal afferents. They are also found throughout the human brainstem, including a high concentration in the CTZ.[202] Serotonin antagonists injected into the area postrema inhibit cisplatin-induced emesis in the ferret,[193] but it appears that 5-HT3 receptor antagonists also exert their antiemetic effect at the level of the peripheral nervous system via serotonin blockade in the vagal nerve.[203,204]

Substance P, which binds to the tachykinin neurokinin NK1 receptor, has more recently been implicated in mediating vomiting. Substance P is a neuropeptide found in both the CNS and in the GI tract. Because of its localization pattern and its ability to induce vomiting when administered intravenously, substance P was suspected to play a role in the genesis of vomiting.[205] NK1 receptor antagonists appeared promising in that they inhibited vomiting induced by a range of agents known to produce vomiting by both central and peripheral mechanisms in the ferret.[206,207] The site of antiemetic action of NK1 receptor antagonists has not yet been clearly defined. It may occur peripherally, at the level of vagal motor neurons that control relaxation of the gastric fundus.[185] Investigation of the time course of the antiemetic effects of a 5-HT3 antagonist and the NK1 receptor antagonist aprepitant indicates that serotonin may mediate the early vomiting process (within the first 8 to 12 hours of cisplatin administration), whereas later vomiting may be mediated by the binding of substance P to NK1 receptors.[203]

Classification of CINV

Acute and Delayed CINV. Acute CINV, also known as posttreatment CINV, is traditionally defined as nausea and vomiting that occurs within the first 24 hours after administration of chemotherapy. Delayed CINV occurs 24 hours after chemotherapy and may last up to 5 days. Delayed CINV is typically associated with certain chemotherapeutic agents such as cisplatin and peaks 48 to 72 hours after administration of chemotherapy.[208] The incidence of delayed CINV is as high as 89% in patients who receive cisplatin-based chemotherapy without antiemetic prophylaxis.[209] The incidence of delayed CINV in patients who do receive antiemetic prophylaxis is as high as 73%.[210]

Because not all acute CINV antiemetics are effective for delayed CINV and specific treatment for delayed symptoms may not be prescribed, delayed CINV may be more severe than acute CINV. The recent introduction of the NK1 receptor antagonist aprepitant has provided new options for controlling delayed CINV. However, it remains clear that the single best predictor of delayed CINV is acute CINV and that *control of acute CINV is a key factor in preventing delayed CINV*.[208,211,212] For example, in a cohort of 705 patients receiving chemotherapy for the first time, when acute CINV was completely controlled with ondansetron plus dexamethasone, 92% had complete control of delayed CINV. However, of the patients who did have acute CINV, only 41% had complete control of delayed CINV.[212]

Although some pharmacologic agents to control delayed CINV have been developed, lack of recognition of this problem remains a major barrier to its effective management. Grunberg et al.[213] demonstrated that in a cohort of patients receiving moderately emetogenic chemotherapy for the first time, clinicians overestimated control of CINV, and this discrepancy was particularly notable for delayed CINV, in which case control of symptoms was overestimated by 21% to 28%. More than 75% of clinicians underestimated the incidence of delayed CINV.[213] This misperception may in part explain the observation that fewer than half of persons who experience delayed CINV receive adequate prophylaxis that conforms to established guidelines.[214] Given the extent to which delayed CINV negatively affects the lives of persons undergoing chemotherapy,[215] improved practice, in conjunction with pharmacologic advances, is needed to reduce suffering from delayed CINV.

Relatively little information has been published regarding delayed vomiting in children. Pinkerton and colleagues[216] found that of 27 children who received cisplatin, cyclophosphamide, or carboplatin and ondansetron, 9 (33%) experienced delayed emesis. In a larger prospective study of pediatric patients who did not receive antiemetics during the delayed phase after chemotherapy, two of six children (33%) who received highly emetogenic antineoplastics (cyclophosphamide, cisplatin, or carboplatin) and 12 of 110 children (11%) who received other chemotherapeutic agents experienced delayed vomiting, although the accuracy of the incidence of delayed vomiting in the "high risk" group is limited by the small number of children in that group.[217] As has been appreciated in adult patients, children who vomited in the acute phase were significantly more likely to have delayed vomiting (45%) compared with children who did not experience significant acute vomiting (13%). In addition, chemotherapy lasting 2 or more consecutive days was associated with a significantly higher rate of delayed vomiting (39%) compared with chemotherapy administered on a single day (13%). In our experience, many children experience delayed CINV.

Anticipatory Nausea

Anticipatory nausea and vomiting is a conditioned response that occurs in anticipation of planned chemotherapy when vomiting has been poorly controlled in previous cycles. In adults, anticipatory nausea and vomiting occurs in one quarter of adults receiving chemotherapy[218] and is associated with higher anxiety, a history of severe acute CINV, and a history of delayed CINV.[218-221]

A similar pattern is seen in the pediatric population, with the severity of distress from nausea/vomiting, greater expectation for severe nausea/vomiting, and the severity of the nausea/vomiting that is actually sustained all corresponding with a higher likelihood of anticipatory CINV.[222-224] Anticipatory nausea/vomiting is most likely to develop within the first 4 months of therapy, usually occurs hours before treatment, and is most severe at the actual time that chemotherapy is administered.[222] Anticipatory nausea and vomiting in children appears to have features consistent with a conditioned response. These features suggest that this type of nausea and vomiting is a learned response, which explains why it is refractory to typical antiemetics.

Measurement and Assessment

Measurement. Although nausea and vomiting are often lumped together, as in the term "CINV," they may be regarded as two distinct phenomena. Nausea may be accompanied by physiologic changes such as pallor, sweating, or feeling hot or cold, but it is essentially a subjective experience that is measured by patient report. For this reason nausea cannot be studied in models other than humans. On the other hand, vomiting can be objectively measured. For this reason it is invariably used as the outcome of choice when evaluating interventions for nausea and vomiting. Complete control of CINV is a frequently used outcome and is defined as the absence of any vomiting for a defined period after administration of chemotherapy. That being said, vomiting does not always accompany nausea, and changes in vomiting do not necessarily reflect a concomitant change in nausea.

Although they can occur together, nausea occurs more frequently than does vomiting.[210,213,225] Much attention has been focused on the prevention of vomiting, which is an important goal because previous uncontrolled vomiting may stimulate anticipatory vomiting in subsequent cycles of chemotherapy. However, nausea is also an important symptom to assess and control because it too impairs functioning and quality of life, even in the absence of vomiting.[215,226-229] Finally, although advances such as the 5-HT3 receptor antagonists may have improved chemotherapy-associated vomiting, related posttreatment nausea has not improved.[230] For all these reasons, attention to both nausea and vomiting is needed. Research that reports only vomiting as an outcome is a limited endeavor,

and interpretations of assessments that rely solely on vomiting should be made with care.

Instruments have been developed to measure the subjective phenomenon of nausea in adults.[231,232] Instruments to assess nausea in children, including children who are preverbal, have been described but are not in widespread use.[233,234] One strategy for assessing nausea in children is to have them use a simple analogue or numeric scale to rate the severity of their nausea. It is known that children 5 years and older can reliably use a color analogue scale to report the severity of their pain[235] and that children 7 years and older can report pain with a visual analogue scale[31] or a numeric scale, and thus it is likely that they can report their nausea with similar reliability. A nausea scale of 0 to 10 with six faces (the Baxter Retching Faces BARF scale) for use in children ages 7 to 18 years who have nausea for a number of reasons has recently been demonstrated to have convergent and discriminant validity, as well as responsiveness.[236]

Hinds et al.[237] have shown that a symptom distress instrument that includes nausea assessment, which was designed for adults, is reliable and valid in adolescents with cancer. Other symptom distress scales that include nausea assessment, most notably the Memorial Symptom Assessment Scale, are also reliable and valid in children.[3,4]

Within the pediatric population, parental report is also an important source of information when assessing nausea and vomiting. In one small study of CINV, parent-child dyads were found to have a moderate to strong association when reporting symptoms of nausea and vomiting.[238] Studies by Zeltzer et al.[239,240] have also showed a high degree of correlation between parental and child reports of nausea, although Tyc et al.[241] have found that parents tend to underestimate their child's nausea.

Assessment. When nausea and vomiting in patients with cancer are considered, attention is often focused on CINV. When evaluating a patient with nausea/vomiting, however, it is imperative that other causes be considered in the differential diagnosis.

A full assessment of a patient with nausea and vomiting that extends beyond quantification of the severity of the symptom permits the generation of a complete differential diagnosis. Only in this way can all possible mechanisms and therefore all potentially efficacious interventions be entertained.

Features such as whether the nausea and vomiting is acute or chronic and intermittent or constant, along with whether it is associated with any particular factors, are important to consider. Other elements of the history, such as whether vomiting is projectile, bowel patterns, current medications, and prior history of nausea and vomiting, can also be helpful in delineating the cause and therefore finding potentially effective interventions. For example, obtaining a history that suggests constipation as the cause of nausea and vomiting will lead to a workup and treatment plan that is entirely different than if the cause is suspected to be chemotherapy or labyrinthitis.

Another important component of the history is an assessment of the impact of the symptom on the patient's

---

Box 71-2 Patient-Related Risk Factors for Developing Chemotherapy-Induced Nausea and Vomiting

- History of previous chemotherapy and prior chemotherapy-induced nausea and vomiting
- Prechemotherapy nausea
- Prechemotherapy anxiety
- Female sex
- History of motion sickness
- Low performance status
- Low social functioning

---

daily functioning and quality of life. Specific instruments to address these aspects have been developed, such as the Morrow Assessment of Nausea and Emesis, which is a self-report form that allows adults to assess their experience with acute, delayed, and anticipatory CINV.[242]

Predictors of Nausea and Vomiting

The likelihood of CINV development and CINV severity is determined by both treatment-related and patient-related factors (Box 71-2). The particular agent used is the primary treatment-related risk factor for CINV, but higher dosages of the agent, shorter infusion rates, combinations with other agents, and repeated cycles of chemotherapy can also increase the risk of CINV.[204,243,244] When combination chemotherapy is given, antiemetics should be prescribed based on the most emetogenic chemotherapy drug and with the consideration that some combinations may potentially act synergistically in creating CINV.

Patient-related factors, as determined in the adult population, also appear to affect the risk for developing CINV (Box 71-2).[226,245,246] In one multivariate analysis, low social functioning, prechemotherapy nausea, and female sex were found to be predictive of more severe CINV.[226] Patients with a history of vomiting in a previous cycle are at greater risk of vomiting with the subsequent cycle[247] in part, perhaps, because of anticipatory vomiting. Use of patient-reported outcomes from previous chemotherapy cycles is critical when prescribing antiemetics. An assessment of the intended treatment, as well as the patient's individual risk factors, may help determine which patients are more at risk for the development of CINV and therefore in need of more intensive prophylaxis or rescue therapy.

Principles of Pharmacologic Therapy

Prevention of acute CINV is a key element in reducing delayed CINV. Because (1) the development of anticipatory CINV is based on prior experience, (2) severity of acute CINV predicts delayed CINV severity, and (3) rescue therapy is inadequate once nausea and vomiting have developed, the best approach to CINV and other situations in which nausea and vomiting may develop (e.g., in the postoperative period) is to prevent these symptoms from occurring in the first place. Although it is best to take a targeted approach based on the inciting cause and the suspected underlying pathophysiology and/or evidence demonstrating superiority of certain agents

TABLE 71-2 Schematic Approach to Chemotherapy-Induced Nausea and Vomiting*

Type of CINV	Prophylaxis	Breakthrough[†]
Acute CINV		
High risk	5-HT3 receptor antagonist Dexamethasone Aprepitant[‡] Lorazepam ± scopolamine patch, metoclopramide, or cannabinoid if needed	Same as prophylaxis, initially as needed, then scheduled
Moderate or low risk	5-HT3 receptor antagonist Dexamethasone ± lorazepam, scopolamine patch, metoclopramide, or cannabinoid if needed	
Delayed CINV	Ondansetron Aprepitant Dexamethasone ± metoclopramide, cannabinoid, as needed	Same as prophylaxis, initially as needed, then scheduled
Anticipatory CINV	Prevention of CINV Lorazepam Nonpharmacologic approaches	Lorazepam

CINV, Chemotherapy-induced nausea and vomiting; *5-HT3*, 5-hydroxytryptamine 3.
*Points to consider:
- Choose appropriate prophylactic antiemetics based on emesis risk, determined by patient-related risk factors and the emetogenicity of the chemotherapeutic agent(s) being used.
- Assess the effect of the antiemetic regimen regularly.
[†]If breakthrough CINV occurs, strategies may be to (1) add a new agent, (2) change the dose or schedule of antiemetics in use but not already maximized, or (3) change administration of existing "as-needed" antiemetics to scheduled administration. In addition, the prophylaxis regimen for subsequent chemotherapy cycles should be augmented.
[‡]If ≥12 years of age.

or classes in different situations, it is not always possible to know which agent to choose first. Guidelines for the initial choice of antiemetics, as well as dosing, are provided in Tables 71-2 and 71-3. In this situation, use of one (or two) agents with titration of the dose and the addition of other agents if necessary might be the best strategy. For CINV, which is thought to be mediated through several pathways, a combination of antiemetics is usually warranted. This approach is particularly necessary with use of highly emetogenic chemotherapy, in which case monotherapy is almost always insufficient.

Drugs used to manage CINV include true antiemetics and adjuvants. Adjuvant medications may be used to allay anxiety, induce amnesia, or induce sleep. Although many of these agents have been investigated in adults, evidence regarding their use in children, including optimal dosing and potential adverse effects, is frequently much more limited. When evidence regarding dosing in the pediatric population is available, it is presented in this chapter. However, in many circumstances we must rely on evidence from adult studies and extrapolate appropriate dosing. Furthermore, guidelines and standard practices in

TABLE 71-3   Classes of Antiemetics, Dosing, and Routes of Administration

Class	Dose and Route	Indication	Notes
5-HT3 Receptor Antagonists			
Ondansetron	0.15 mg/kg dose PO every 8 h or 0.45 mg/kg/dose PO every 24 h, not to exceed 24 mg 0.15 mg/kg (not to exceed 8 mg/dose) IV every 8 h; no single dose should exceed 16 mg due to risk of QT prolongation	First-line therapy for prophylaxis of high-, moderate-, or low-risk CINV or breakthrough CINV	May cause constipation and/or headache; available as an oral disintegrating tablet (that contains phenylalanine) or may be extemporaneously prepared For patients with electrolyte abnormalities, congestive heart failure, bradyarrhythmias, or patients taking other medications with the potential to cause QT prolongation, consider ECG monitoring
Granisetron	<50 kg: 20 µg/kg IV/PO daily; maximum dose 1 mg ≥50 kg: 1 mg IV/PO daily	First-line prophylaxis for high-, moderate-, or low-risk CINV or breakthrough CINV	Available as an oral solution For patients with electrolyte abnormalities, congestive heart failure, bradyarrhythmias, or patients taking other medications with the potential to cause QT prolongation, consider ECG monitoring
Dolasetron	≥2 yr: 1.8 mg/kg IV or PO as a single dose; maximum single dose 100 mg		May be extemporaneously prepared For patients with electrolyte abnormalities, congestive heart failure, bradyarrhythmias, or patients taking other medications with the potential to cause QT prolongation, consider ECG monitoring
Dopamine Antagonist			
Metoclopramide	0.5 mg/kg IV or PO daily (for prophylaxis) 0.5 mg/kg IV or PO every 6 h (for breakthrough CINV) 1 mg/kg IV or PO every 6 h (for severe breakthrough CINV or if lower dose is ineffective)	High-risk prophylaxis; breakthrough CINV	High-dose metoclopramide: Prescribe with diphenhydramine and continue diphenhydramine for 24 h after the last dose to prevent EPS; if the metoclopramide dose is ≤1 mg/kg and the patient weighs >40 kg, scopolamine may be considered Treat EPS with diphenhydramine or benztropine
Corticosteroid			
Dexamethasone	≤BSA 1 m²: 10 mg/m² IV or PO daily BSA >1 m²: 10-12 mg IV or PO daily; may use 20 mg as a single dose on day 1	High-risk prophylaxis for acute or delayed CINV; breakthrough CINV	Contraindicated in patients receiving pulmonary radiation therapy Consider lower dose if given with an NK-1 receptor antagonist
NK1 Antagonist			
Aprepitant	≥45kg: 125 mg PO ×1 on day 1, then 80 mg PO daily on days 2 and 3	Prophylaxis of acute or delayed CINV	Limited data in pediatrics CYP3A4 substrate and inhibitor of metabolism of drugs that are CYP3A4 substrates including chemotherapeutic drugs (such as vincristine, irinotecan, imatinib, among others) and nonchemotherapeutic drugs (e.g., corticosteroids)
Anticholinergic			
Scopolamine	1.5-mg patch applied transdermally; change every 72 h	High-risk prophylaxis; breakthrough CINV	Use only if >40 kg (the patch cannot be cut); may cause dry mouth and/or blurred vision
Cannabinoid			
Dronabinol	2.5-5 mg/m²/dose PO every 6 h (10 mg/dose maximum)	High-risk prophylaxis; breakthrough CINV	Do not use in children <6 yr; use with caution if 6-12 yr; may cause confusion, ataxia, hallucinations; no IV form
Anxiolytic			
Lorazepam	<20 kg: 0.025 mg/kg IV or PO every 6 h 20-40 kg: 0.0125 mg/kg IV or PO every 6 h >40 kg: 0.5-2 mg IV or PO every 6 h	High-risk prophylaxis; breakthrough; anticipatory CINV	May cause confusion, sedation, hallucinations, or memory impairment; avoid use of dose greater than 0.5 mg unless proven tolerance of 0.5 mg

BSA, Body surface area; *CINV,* chemotherapy-induced nausea and vomiting; *ECG,* electrocardiogram; *EPS,* extrapyramidal side effects; *IV,* intravenous; *NK1,* neurokinin 1; *PO,* by mouth.

adults may involve formulations of medications that cannot be adjusted for pediatric patients (e.g., capsules or patches). Use of medications in children that are only available in tablet or capsule form also may not be feasible for developmental or psychological reasons.

Dopamine Receptor Antagonists

Dopamine receptor antagonists include the butyrophenones (e.g., droperidol), phenothiazines (e.g., prochlorperazine), and substituted benzamides (e.g., metoclopramide; refer to the "Metoclopramide" section later in this chapter). Until the advent of 5-HT3 receptor antagonists and other antiemetics in the 1990s, dopamine-blocking agents were widely used. Use and efficacy of these agents are limited by their adverse effects, which include sedation and extrapyramidal symptoms (EPS). Children may be at higher risk for EPS, although EPS can often be prevented by concomitant administration of an anticholinergic agent such as diphenhydramine. Scopolamine, an antiemetic in its own right, is sometimes also used for this purpose. We have experience using scopolamine for EPS prophylaxis when the metoclopramide dose is less than or equal to 1 mg/kg/day and the patient weighs 40 kg or more.

Metopimazine, a phenothiazine derivative, is used as an adjunct to 5-HT3 antagonists to treat CINV. Although it is not marketed in North America, metopimazine is used for children in Europe, and a recent small study demonstrated improved emetic control when it was combined with ondansetron compared with ondansetron monotherapy. Olanzapine, an atypical antipsychotic agent, has fewer extrapyramidal effects than do older agents. In small studies in which it is combined with other antiemetics for CINV prophylaxis, olanzapine showed promise in preventing or treating CINV.[248] Chlorpromazine and droperidol both may cause prolongation of the QT interval, and droperidol has been associated with serious cardiac adverse events. Extreme caution, including electrocardiogram monitoring, should be exercised if these agents are used, particularly in patients at risk for arrhythmias. Today use of droperidol is usually limited to the operative period in patients who do not respond to other agents.

5-HT3 Receptor Antagonists

5-HT3 receptor antagonists became the mainstay of therapy in the prevention and treatment of acute CINV since their introduction in the 1990s, when they were shown to be superior to the majority of preexisting antiemetics such as prochlorperazine[249] and metoclopramide,[250-255] even when highly emetogenic chemotherapy such as cisplatin is administered.[251-253]

Compared with other agents, the superiority of 5-HT3 receptor antagonists in preventing acute CINV in children has also been confirmed.[256-260] The efficacy of these agents appears to be further enhanced by the addition of a corticosteroid.[261-263] In one study of 33 children, ondansetron plus dexamethasone provided a complete response in 61% of patients, whereas ondansetron alone provided a complete response in only 21% of patients.[262] Ondansetron has also been shown to reduce acute CINV

compared with placebo when chemotherapy is delivered intrathecally.[264]

First-generation agents in this class include ondansetron, dolasetron, and granisetron. Taken together, the data on these agents indicate that these agents are equally effective when given at equivalent doses.[265-271,272] These agents also appear to be equivalent in children, including in situations involving high-dose therapy such as preparative regimens for hematopoietic stem cell transplant.[273-275] In one small study it was found that, compared with tropisetron, ondansetron better controlled acute CINV resulting from use of moderately emetogenic agents. However, no difference was found between the two agents with regard to controlling acute CINV resulting from use of highly emetogenic agents.

5-HT3 antagonists are quite well tolerated by children,[263] with the most common adverse effects reported being mild headache and constipation.[264] 5-HT3 inhibitors, in conjunction with a corticosteroid, are now recommended as first-line therapy for children who receive moderately to highly emetogenic chemotherapy.[246,276]

Efficacy and tolerability of daily administration of high-dose ondansetron (24 mg or 32 mg by mouth daily) has been compared with a smaller dose (8 mg by mouth) given twice daily in adults. A large dose given daily is well tolerated in adults.[277] In a large multicenter, randomized trial, the 24-mg daily dose provided the highest complete control of nausea and vomiting.[278] The superiority of more intensive dosing has been confirmed by other investigators.[279-282] The efficacy of 32 mg compared with 24 mg has also been confirmed by Tsavaris.[283] However, because of the risk for QT interval prolongation in the IV formulation, the 32-mg IV dose is no longer available, and single (daily) doses exceeding 24 mg are not recommended.

Oral and IV routes of administration have been shown to be equally effective in both adults and children.[284-287] Ondansetron, dolasetron, and granisetron are all available in IV formulations and as an oral tablet. Ondansetron is available as an oral dissolving tablet and as an oral liquid; these two preparations are especially attractive in the pediatric population. Granisetron may be extemporaneously compounded by an apothecary. Successful administration of 16 mg of ondansetron daily as a suppository has been described in adults[288] but not in children.

A second-generation 5-HT3 receptor antagonist, palonosetron, differs from its predecessors in its stronger affinity for the 5-HT3 receptor and its prolonged plasma half-life (four times that of the other 5-HT3 antagonists), qualities that may enhance its duration of action.[289,290] In randomized trials in adults, single doses of palonosetron appear to be at least as good in the prevention of acute CINV as single doses of first-generation antagonists delivered 30 minutes before administration of moderately emetogenic chemotherapy. Furthermore, the single dose of long-lasting palonosetron provides better protection from delayed CINV.[291-293] Because of these findings, palonosetron is recommended rather than first-generation 5-HT3 receptor antagonists for adults receiving highly or moderately emetogenic chemotherapy.[294] In pediatric patients palonosetron may prove to be a useful agent in the prevention of acute CINV during multiple-day therapy (in which acute CINV is repeatedly induced) and for the prevention of delayed CINV. Although administration of palonosetron for the prevention of CINV in children has been described,[295,296] further study of dosing, safety, and efficacy is needed before palonosetron can be recommended for children.

Corticosteroids

Corticosteroids are frequently used as antiemetics, although their mechanism of action is unclear. Dexamethasone is the best-studied corticosteroid and the primary one in use today, although success with methylprednisolone has been described. The typical dexamethasone dose used for adults is 10 to 20 mg per day. Our starting dose for children is 10 mg/m^2, to a maximum of 10 mg/day. For persistent vomiting, this dose may be doubled to a maximum of 10 mg given twice a day. If administered with an NK1 receptor antagonist, the corticosteroid dose should be halved.

Dexamethasone provides moderate protection from CINV, including delayed CINV, when used alone.[297-299] Dexamethasone has been shown to be as effective as metoclopramide for acute CINV in adults receiving moderately and highly emetogenic chemotherapy without the extrapyramidal effects of metoclopramide.[300,301]

Dexamethasone is especially useful in preventing delayed CINV from cisplatin, cyclophosphamide, and doxorubicin[302-307] and may be even more effective for this purpose when combined with metoclopramide.[209] Dexamethasone is also very effective in potentiating the action of other antiemetics, including 5-HT3 inhibitors[308] and metoclopramide.[304,306,307,309-312]

In the pediatric population, dexamethasone combined with ondansetron provided significantly more protection from acute CINV that occurred as a result of highly emetogenic agents than did ondansetron monotherapy; 77% of children receiving ondansetron monotherapy had at least one episode of vomiting, compared with 39% who received ondansetron with dexamethasone.[262]

The benefit of improved protection from CINV must be weighed against the risks of corticosteroids. Adverse effects of corticosteroids include metabolic effects, gastritis, insomnia, hypertension, immune dysregulation, impaired wound healing, and adverse psychiatric effects such as emotional lability and, more rarely, psychosis. In general, short courses of corticosteroids do not usually produce significant adverse effects and are often very well accepted and tolerated by patients.[297] Potential beneficial effects of corticosteroids are preservation of appetite and promotion of energy.

Other potential risks include a decrease in action of a biologic response modifier or induction of radiation pneumonitis when a steroid is withdrawn from patients who have undergone lung radiation.[313,314] Caution is advised if corticosteroids are used as antiemetics in conjunction with a treatment regimen that is associated with a high risk of infection or GI toxicity such as induction regimens for acute myelogenous leukemia. Concomitantly administered corticosteroids may further increase these risks. Concerns about the impact of steroids on the blood-brain barrier have led to a desire to avoid the use of steroids as an antiemetic in patients with brain tumors, although chemotherapy-specific data are lacking.[315] The use of steroids may be prohibited when they are already part of a patient's chemotherapeutic regimen.

Metoclopramide

Metoclopramide, a procainamide derivative, exerts antiemetic effects via both a central mechanism (dopamine receptor blockade in the CTZ) and a peripheral mechanism (promotion of gastric emptying).[316] It has been recognized as an effective antiemetic for adults for the past two decades[317] as monotherapy or in conjunction with dexamethasone,[318] lorazepam,[319] or both.[320] Low-dose metoclopramide (i.e., 0.1 mg/kg/dose) is effective in treating postoperative nausea and in promoting gastric emptying.

At high doses, metoclopramide also serves as a serotonin receptor antagonist[191,192] and provides better protection from CINV.[247] For these reasons, metoclopramide is usually given at high doses for CINV. At such higher doses, however, patients—and, in particular, children—are at a greater risk for extrapyramidal adverse effects such as dystonia and akathisia. In a dose-related toxicity study in children, significant extrapyramidal toxicity was observed at doses of 2 mg/kg or higher,[321] and for this reason, high-dose metoclopramide is given with diphenhydramine to decrease the risk of extrapyramidal adverse effects.[247] Extrapyramidal adverse effects can occur up to 24 hours later in patients who receive multiple daily doses of metoclopramide, and thus diphenhydramine administration should continue until 24 hours after the last dose of metoclopramide. We have also had personal experience using transdermal scopolamine as an anticholinergic agent in patients receiving no more than 1 mg/kg/day of metoclopramide. Because of the association of tardive dyskinesia with high-dose or long-term administration of metoclopramide, the FDA issued a boxed warning about this risk in 2009.

Cannabinoids

Delta-9-tetrahydrocannabinol (THC) is the active ingredient in cannabis, or marijuana. THC was approved by the FDA in 1985 for the treatment of emesis. Synthetic THC, called dronabinol (Marinol), has since become available. It is formulated in sesame oil and is available as 2.5- or 5-mg gelatin capsules. A homologue of THC, nabilone, is also now available in the United States.

THC binds to the CB1 receptor found in the central and peripheral nervous systems, as well as the CB2 receptor, which is found in nonneural tissues. THC exerts its antiemetic effect as a receptor agonist, in contrast to other antiemetics, which typically serve as receptor antagonists. THC also interacts with dopaminergic, serotonin, monoaminergic, noradrenergic, and opioid systems, which are pathways that mediate both emesis and pain.

Sallan and colleagues[321a] demonstrated that in patients who have CINV that is not controlled by standard antiemetic therapy, THC provided better complete protection from CINV (in 36 of 79 subjects) than did prochlorperazine (in 16 of 78 subjects). Interestingly, patients younger than 20 years had a higher proportion of complete responses than did older patients. Persons in the THC group also had significantly higher food intake. Adverse effects from cannabinoid administration include sedation, mood alterations (such as euphoria and dysphoria), dizziness, hallucinations, and arterial hypotension. Because of these potential adverse effects, cannabinoids are not typically considered first-line agents for CINV prophylaxis but are added to a regimen if first-line agents are not adequate for prophylaxis or breakthrough CINV.

An advantage of cannabinoids is their utility in treating pain. They are known to bind to kappa and delta receptors and act synergistically with opioids, a feature that may be useful when treating children with both nausea and pain.[322] In addition, they are frequently used to stimulate appetite in patients who are not experiencing nausea or vomiting per se.

NK1 Receptor Antagonists

Aprepitant and its prodrug, fosaprepitant, are the only approved NK1 receptor antagonists. NK1 receptor antagonists are particularly effective in preventing delayed CINV, a historically difficult symptom to prevent. A study was performed to compae cisplatin-naive patients who received granisetron plus dexamethasone on day 1 and either (1) aprepitant (then called L-754,030) on day 1 or (2) aprepitant on days 1 through 5 or (3) placebo on days 1 through 5. In the aprepitant arms, 93% and 94% of subjects had no acute vomiting, compared with 67% in the placebo arm who had no vomiting. Subjects in the aprepitant arms also experienced significantly better complete protection from delayed vomiting (82% and 78%) compared with subjects who received a placebo (33%). In addition, minimal or no nausea was noted in 49% and 48% of subjects in the aprepitant arms and in 25% of subjects who received a placebo.[323]

Other studies have replicated these impressive findings in terms of control of delayed CINV, but thcy have not demonstrated the improved protection from acute CINV seen in the aforementioned study.[324,325] For example, in a double-blind multicenter trial of 351 patients, aprepitant with dexamethasone provided no benefit in preventing acute emesis when compared with the combination of granisetron and dexamethasone; however, the addition of aprepitant to granisetron and dexamethasone more than doubled the efficacy of this regimen in preventing delayed vomiting.[324]

Aprepitant is generally vcry well tolerated by adults and adolescents and is easily administered by mouth daily. In addition, it appears to decrease delayed cisplatin-induced CINV that has been established to be refractory to the combination of 5-HT3 antagonists and dexamethasone.[326] The efficacy of aprepitant appears to be sustained over multiple cycles of chemotherapy.[326,327]

Aprepitant is usually administered for 3 consecutive days, because administration on additional days has not been shown to provide better protection from CINV. A pilot study comparing 1-day versus 3-day administration of aprepitant in the prevention of acute and delayed CINV in patients who were receiving highly emetogenic chemotherapy demonstrated no significant difference between the regimens.[328] Additional studies are needed to confirm the noninferiority of the single-day aprepitant regimen.

Studies of the efficacy and safety of aprepitant in children are rare and quite limited methodologically. Use of aprepitant in children as young as 11 years using adult dosing (125 mg on day 1 and 80 mg daily on days 2 and 4) has been reported.[329-331] In the only published prospective trial of aprepitant in children, 46 children aged 11 to 19 years who received emetogenic chemotherapy along with ondansetron and dexamethasone for 4 days were randomly assigned to also receive aprepitant or placebo for 3 days. In this study, which was designed to evaluate pharmacokinetics and tolerability, it was found that aprepitant was well tolerated but that febrile neutropenia occurred more often in children who received aprepitant, although the overall infection rate was higher in the placebo group. The limited sample size may have contributed to these findings and prevented statistical significance in the assessment of efficacy. The study demonstrated that pharmacokinetics in adolescents is similar to that of adults, and it is therefore reasonable to administer the adult dose to this age group.[331] Administration of a lower dose (80 mg/day for 3 days) to smaller children (<20 kg) has been described, but the efficacy of this rcgimcn in preventing CINV was not reported.[330]

Fosaprcpitant is an IV prodrug of aprepitant that is approved for administration in adults as a one-time dose prior to the administration of chemotherapy. Administration of this one-time dose given with ondansetron and dexamethasone provides protection from acute and delayed CINV that is equivalent to a regimen of aprepitant, ondansetron, and dexamethasone.[332] Fosaprepitant dosing in children is currently bcing studied.

Aprepitant is a CYP3A4 enzyme pathway substrate and inhibitor and therefore may alter levels of drugs metabolized via this pathway. Concomitant administration with aprepitant may raise the level of drugs such as dexamethasone, methylprednisolone, fentanyl, cyclophosphamide, thiotepa, vincristine, or etoposide.[333,334] For this reason aprepitant should be prescribed with care to avoid potential interactions, and the patient should be monitored closely for such interactions. It has been suggested that when aprepitant is coadministered with dexamethasone for CINV prophylaxis, the dexamethasone dose should be decreased by 50%.[335] Aprepitant does not appear to alter the pharmacokinetics of ondansetron or granisetron.[336] Aprepitant should be used with caution in patients who take warfarin.[337]

Other Agents

Lorazepam is often used as an adjuvant to true antiemetics because of its anxiolytic and amnestic properties. Early studies evaluating the addition of lorazepam found that patients reported less anxiety and preferred regimens that contained this additional agent, although it did cause more sedation.[338-340] The acute antiemetic effect of several agents is enhanced when lorazepam is given concomitantly.[341-343] Interestingly, the addition of lorazepam to regimens that contained dexamethasone as prophylaxis against delayed CINV from cisplatin appears to decrease delayed CINV as well.[303,341]

Scopolamine is a muscarinic antagonist that is known to reduce motion sickness. It is inadequate as monotherapy for CINV,[344] but in conjunction with other antiemetics such as metoclopramide and dexamethasone, it reduces cisplatin-induced CINV.[345] Scopolamine is administered as a 1.5-mg transdermal patch applied behind the ear that releases 0.5 mg/day and must be changed every 3 days. Because the patch is only available in the 1.5-mg size and cannot be cut, we normally reserve it for children who weigh 40 kg or more. Adverse effects from scopolamine include dry mouth, blurry vision, and mydriasis from systemic effects. Mydriasis on the side ipsilateral to the patch from unintentional touching of the patch followed by rubbing of the eyes can also occur.[346]

Antihistamines such as dimenhydramine, hydroxyzine, and diphenhydramine are effective in reducing the nausea associated with vertigo and motion sickness. For CINV management, diphenhydramine is often given in regimens containing high-dose metoclopramide to prevent extrapyramidal effects. Diphenhydramine does not, however, enhance the antiemetic effect of metoclopramide,[347,348] and apart from preventing extrapyramidal effects, it should not be used for CINV management.

Olanzapine is an atypical antipsychotic agent that binds to several receptors, including dopamine, serotonin, and to a lesser extent histamine and muscarinic receptors. Because of its action at multiple receptor sites implicated in CINV, it may hold promise as a therapy for CINV. In a small study of 10 adult patients receiving moderately to highly emetogenic chemotherapy with olanzapine, palonosetron, and dexamethasone as antiemetic prophylaxis, 100% had complete protection from nausea and vomiting in the first 24 hours after chemotherapy, with 50% and 75% of patients protected from nausea and vomiting, respectively, on days 2 to 5.[349] Olanzapine is consequently included in some guidelines for adults with CINV. No studies evaluating olanzapine for children with CINV have been published.

Gabapentin has also been evaluated for CINV in adults.[350] One study showed a decrease in peak nausea scores for both acute and delayed CINV, indicating that this agent may also hold promise as a therapy for CINV.

Special Cases

Delayed Vomiting. Until very recent years, steroids and metoclopramide were the primary agents used to control delayed vomiting,[209,305,320] with modest protection from delayed CINV in 48% to 57% of adult patients. Some studies have demonstrated efficacy of 5-HT3 antagonists in preventing delayed CINV[351,352] and providing better protection when compared with existing drugs such as prochlorperazine.[353] However, the majority of studies have demonstrated that the addition of a 5-HT3 receptor antagonist to the standard therapy, dexamethasone, does not confer greater protection from delayed CINV.[211,212,354-357] In a meta-analysis of the efficacy of 5-HT3 antagonists, these antagonists did not confer protection from delayed CINV significantly beyond that provided by dexamethasone monotherapy. When

ondansetron plus dexamethasone was compared with metoclopramide plus dexamethasone in randomized controlled trials, 5-HT3 was equivocal at best.[358-360]

In one pediatric study evaluating ondansetron for acute and delayed CINV after treatment with carboplatin, cisplatin, Adriamycin with cyclophosphamide, or ifosfamide, ondansetron prevented acute CINV in 87% of children. Its efficacy in preventing delayed CINV was not nearly as high; it prevented only 20% of children from experiencing nausea and 50% of children from vomiting after administration of cisplatin or ifosfamide. A reasonable approach would be to start with dexamethasone and metoclopramide. In children who do not tolerate or who do not respond to metoclopramide, a 5-HT3 antagonist such as ondansetron may then be tried as an alternative.

In adults, some of the best protection from delayed CINV is conferred by the combination of a single dose of palonosetron with three doses of aprepitant and concurrent dexamethasone. In one study, this regimen provided a complete response (no emesis and no rescue medication) for 88% of patients in the acute period and 78% during the delayed period.[361] Evidence for the efficacy of palonosetron in preventing delayed CINV is limited to single-day administration regimens. Interest in consecutive daily dosing of palonosetron to cover multiday chemotherapy has been expressed. Multiple dosing of palonosetron has recently been approved for adults.

Numerous studies in adults have demonstrated the effectiveness of aprepitant for delayed CINV, as previously described. Because most studies of aprepitant have been in the setting of single-day emetogenic treatment, it can be difficult to know how best to utilize this drug in the setting of the multiday regimens common in pediatrics. It is our practice to give the drug for up to 5 days, which may or may not continue beyond the end of the emetogenic treatment.

Anticipatory Nausea. Because anticipatory CINV it is a learned response, typical antiemetics are generally ineffective. The best strategy for preventing CINV is the prevention of CINV in previous courses of chemotherapy.[213] Because anxiety plays a key role in anticipatory nausea, use of an anxiolytic such as lorazepam may be effective.

Breakthrough Emesis. Breakthrough emesis is defined as vomiting that occurs in spite of optimal preventive therapy. Although no studies of breakthrough emesis have been performed and no widely accepted standards are available, a reasonable approach is (1) ensuring that the patient is receiving maximal doses of current antiemetics and (2) adding a rescue agent from a category different from those the patient is already receiving. Although breakthrough agents may be started on an as-needed basis, scheduled administration may be needed during the current or future cycles.

Radiation-Induced Nausea and Vomiting

Radiation-induced nausea and vomiting occurs acutely in more than 90% of adult patients who receive total body

TABLE 71-4   Emetogenicity of Chemotherapeutic Agents and Radiotherapy Fields Commonly Used in Pediatrics

Modality	RISK OF EMESIS			
	High (>90%)	Moderate (30%-90%)	Low (10%-30%)	Minimal (<10%)
Chemotherapy	Carmustine (BCNU)	Arsenic trioxide	Cyclophosphamide	2-Chloroxydeadenosine
	Cisplatin	Carboplatin	($\leq$750 mg/m^2)	(cladribine)
	Cyclophosphamide	Clofarabine	Cytarabine (<1000 mg/m^2)	Asparaginase
	(>1500 mg/m^2)	Cyclophosphamide	Etoposide (VP-16)	Bortezomib
	Dacarbazine (DTIC)	(750-1500 mg/m^2)	5-Fluorouracil	Bleomycin
	Dactinomycin	Cytarabine (>1000 mg/m^2)	Gemcitabine	Busulfan
	Ifosfamide ($\geq$500 mg/m^2)	Cytarabine (intrathecal)	Imatinib	Decitabine
	Lomustine (CCNU)	Daunorubicin	Methotrexate (50-	Fludarabine
	Mechlorethamine	Doxorubicin	1000 mg/m^2)	Hydroxyurea
	(nitrogen mustard)	Epirubicin	Mitomycin	Mercaptopurine
	Procarbazine	Idarubicin	Mitoxantrone	Methotrexate (<50 mg/m^2)
	Thiotepa ($\geq$300 mg/m^2)	Ifosfamide (<500 mg/m^2)	Topotecan	Monoclonal antibodies
		Irinotecan	Vinblastine	(e.g., rituximab)
		Melphalan (>50 mg/m^2)	Vorinostat	Thioguanine
		Methotrexate		Vincristine
		(>1000 mg/m^2)		Vinorelbine
Radiotherapy	Total-body irradiation	Abdominal-pelvic	Cranium	Other (e.g., extremity)
	Upper abdomen	Craniospinal	Lower thorax	
	(moderate to high risk)	Hemibody irradiation	Mantle	

irradiation for bone marrow transplantation and within 30 to 60 minutes in 80% of adults who receive single high-dose/large-field hemibody irradiation. Radiation-induced nausea and vomiting may also occur within 2 to 3 weeks in about 50% of adults who receive fractionated radiotherapy to the abdomen.[362] The incidence and severity of radiotherapy-induced nausea and vomiting is largely related to the location of the radiation field, as indicated in Table 71-4. In a prospective study of adults undergoing radiotherapy, the two radiotherapy-related risk factors for nausea and vomiting were the site of irradiation and the field size, with significantly more vomiting in persons who received radiation to the upper abdomen and in those with a radiation field size greater than 400 cm^2.[363] The only patient-related factor was previous experience with cancer chemotherapy. Because radiation to the upper/mid hemibody results in an increase in circulating serotonin metabolites and because of the efficacy of 5HT-3 receptor antagonists in this setting, it has been proposed that serotonin mediates radiation-induced emesis.[364]

In patients receiving single-dose radiation to the upper abdomen, ondansetron has been demonstrated to be superior to metoclopramide in reducing vomiting and nausea.[365] In a randomized controlled trial comparing ondansetron with prochlorperazine in adults receiving fractionated radiotherapy to the abdomen, 43 (61%) of patients in the ondansetron arm and 23 (35%) of patients in the prochlorperazine arm had a complete response, that is, complete protection from emesis throughout their entire treatment course (P = .002). However, no difference was found in the incidence or severity of nausea in the two groups.[366] Although no controlled trials have been performed in the pediatric population, studies have demonstrated its efficacy and tolerability during radiotherapy.[367] Dolasetron has also been used successfully to prevent nausea

after a single high-dose fraction of radiotherapy to the upper abdomen.[368]

The addition of dexamethasone to ondansetron appears to confer a slight benefit to ondansetron, even for multiply fractionated radiation to the upper abdomen.[369] Current adult guidelines recommend prophylaxis with a 5-HT3 receptor antagonist before each fraction and for 24 hours after the last fraction for patients at high or moderate risk of radiation-induced vomiting (i.e., total body irradiation and radiation directed at the upper abdomen); prophylaxis or rescue with a 5-HT3 receptor antagonist in the low-risk group (i.e., those with radiation directed at the lower thorax, pelvis, or cranium); and rescue with a dopamine or 5-HT3 antagonist in the minimal risk group (i.e., patients with radiation directed at the head and neck, extremities, and breast).[370] One study evaluating ondansetron in children undergoing radiotherapy has been performed.[367] In this study it was found that ondansetron provided 60% protection in children undergoing radiation therapy for a brain tumor, although no control subjects were used for comparison.

Postoperative Vomiting

Postoperative nausea and vomiting (PONV) is a common problem in all pediatric patients. Recent studies have demonstrated that dexamethasone is effective in preventing acute and late PONV.[371-373] Droperidol is also an effective agent, but given the high level of sedation, risk of EPS, and the recent concern of cardiotoxicity, this agent is no longer considered first-line prophylaxis.[374] A significant number of studies have evaluated the efficacy of ondansetron in preventing PONV in children, and this agent is considered the drug of choice for this situation.[374,375] Pooled analyses, however, show that the efficacy lies primarily in an antiemetic effect rather than an antinausea effect.[375]

A recent controlled study of adults undergoing surgery also showed that scopolamine may be a promising agent in preventing PONV in adults, although it caused the symptom of dry mouth to a considerable degree.[376] Two large adult studies have recently shown that one dose of aprepitant is superior to ondansetron in preventing postoperative vomiting; however, only one study found a significant reduction in postoperative nausea.[377,378]

Vomiting from Other Causes

Opioid-Induced Nausea and Vomiting

Although reactions to opioids are frequently, and incorrectly, labeled as an allergy, they can cause nausea and vomiting. Such effects are mediated through (1) direct effects of opioids on the CTZ, (2) effects on the vestibular apparatus, and (3) signals from the gut as a result of constipation. Except when it is due to constipation, opioid-related nausea and vomiting tends to improve with repeated dosing of the opioid. Therefore a reasonable strategy is to provide an antiemetic with the first few doses of the opioid, particularly if the patient is at risk for nausea and vomiting. This strategy prevents the problem of the patient being labeled as "allergic" to the opioid.

Although no evidence is available to indicate that one opioid is more emetogenic than another, it is commonly believed that morphine and codeine are the most likely opioids to cause nausea and vomiting. If nausea and vomiting in response to an opioid persist despite use of antiemetics, it may be reasonable to consider changing the opioid or route of administration. Because tolerance to the emetogenic effect of the initial opioid usually develops in a few days, however, it may be difficult to know whether it was tolerance or the change in opioid that improved symptoms.

Data comparing antiemetics for opioid-induced nausea and vomiting are limited. One study compared 24 mg of daily ondansetron with either metoclopramide, 10 mg by mouth three times a day, or placebo. No differences were detected in the three arms, although the study was terminated prematurely as a result of accrual difficulties.[379] In another study of adults receiving opioids for postsurgical pain, single doses of either 8 or 16 mg of ondansetron provided better emetic control than did a single 10-mg dose of metoclopramide. One report also indicates that ondansetron may be effective in preventing nausea and vomiting from morphine administered via the spine.[380] Recent publications have also demonstrated that the addition of a low-dose naloxone infusion may reduce opioid-related adverse effects, including nausea, without affecting analgesia in both adults and children.[381-383]

Disease-Related Vomiting

Outside of direct treatment-related nausea and vomiting, disease processes themselves may cause nausea and vomiting through a variety of mechanisms, including increased intracranial pressure, GI obstruction, altered gut motility, organ capsule distension, or GVHD. For example, altered gut motility appears to contribute to nausea and vomiting in patients recovering from bone marrow transplantation.[384-386] Interestingly, recent reports

have indicated that mirtazapine, a new serotonin-norepinephrine reuptake inhibitor, improves nausea and vomiting in patients with gastroparesis from a variety of causes, but mirtazapine has not been studied for this purpose in patients undergoing bone marrow transplantation or in children.[387-390]

In addition, other processes that may or may not be related to the disease process or its treatment, such as GI infection, may be present. The mnemonic V.O.M.I.T. may be used to review the possible underlying causes of nausea and vomiting so that a targeted approach to the situation may be undertaken.[391] This mnemonic indicates that nausea and vomiting may be due to vestibular problems, obstruction of the bowel (including constipation), gut dysmotility, infection and inflammation, and toxins. Remarkably little is known about the effectiveness of antiemetics for these causes, and treatment of the underlying problem may be the best strategy. Ondansetron has a modest effect in controlling vomiting that occurs as a result of acute gastroenteritis.[392]

Nonpharmacologic Interventions

Acupuncture and behavioral therapies are some of the best-studied nonpharmacologic interventions for CINV. Electroacupuncture reduced vomiting but not nausea in women undergoing myeloablative chemotherapy when compared with control subjects.[393] In children, P6 acupoint injections are as effective as droperidol in preventing postoperative nausea and vomiting.[394]

Acupressure and acustimulation have also been studied as interventions to mitigate CINV. In one relatively large study of 739 patients who were randomly assigned to use an acupressure band, an acustimulation band, or no band, persons who received acupressure bands had less nausea on the day of treatment, but no differences in delayed nausea were found.[395] In pooled analyses of trials evaluating acupuncture-point stimulation, these interventions reduced the proportion of acute vomiting but not the severity of nausea. When broken down by modality, stimulation with needles and electroacupuncture reduced vomiting but not nausea. Acupressure reduced nausea but not vomiting, but these studies were not controlled.[396]

In children receiving chemotherapy, behavioral interventions such as hypnosis and cognitive distraction reduce nausea, vomiting, and the extent to which these symptoms bothered the children, and these effects were maintained even after the interventions were discontinued and chemotherapy was continued.[239] Behavioral interventions such as hypnosis and systemic desensitization also appear to be useful in treating anticipatory nausea, a phenomenon with a strong learned component.[397,398] Progressive muscle relaxation has been shown to reduce the duration of CINV in women with breast cancer but not the intensity or frequency of nausea or vomiting episodes.[399]

Role of the Patient and Family

Because patients who anticipate CINV may be more likely to actually experience it, discussing the role of interventions to prevent or mitigate CINV may enhance the efficacy of these interventions. Patients and families should also be encouraged to record their symptoms in a diary and to notify their medical team of uncontrolled symptoms when they occur, particularly because uncontrolled acute nausea is associated with increased incidence of both delayed nausea and anticipatory nausea with future chemotherapy. The phenomenon of delayed nausea should specifically be addressed, because children and their parents are usually at home and unable to be observed at the time the child may experience these symptoms.

Strategies to enhance patients' sense of control over their treatment may also improve their experience. In one small study of adults with CINV that was controlled with IV antiemetics via a pump, the patients who were able to control the pump themselves used less antiemetic.[400] More recent studies in both adults and children indicate that a continuous infusion, patient-controlled pump is well tolerated, safe, and effective in controlling CINV.[401,402] Patients should be encouraged to explore strategies for nonpharmacologic management if these options are of interest, because they appear to have little downside and can also add to the patient's sense of control over his or her experience.

Future Directions

Significant advances have been made in the past few decades with regard to managing nausea and vomiting, particularly CINV; however, more remains to be done to improve the management of these symptoms in children. More knowledge is needed regarding assessment of the symptom of nausea, looking beyond the quantification of vomiting, along with the determination of a child's risk for the development of nausea to begin with.

Pharmacogenomics may play a role in finding candidate genes that may predict emetic sensitivity and responsiveness to antiemetic therapy, which may help clinicians identify patients who are unlikely to respond to conventional therapies. Optimal regimens for multiple-day and high-dose chemotherapy or bone marrow transplantation, as well as new strategies for control of delayed and refractory symptoms, are also needed. Exploration of drugs, such as the new atypical antipsychotic medications or new small molecules, may contribute to this area.

For children in particular, more evidence of efficacy and adverse effects are needed, as are evidence-based guidelines for CINV management to address the wide variations in practice that exist. Finally, knowledge of nausea and vomiting in children historically has been based on CINV or postoperative situations. Much remains to be learned regarding non–chemotherapy-related nausea and vomiting.

OTHER GASTROINTESTINAL SYMPTOMS

Constipation

Constipation is the passage of hard feces that typically occurs with difficulty and decreased frequency. Most children who experience constipation have no history of bowel dysfunction prior to their cancer diagnosis. Children who have cancer are predisposed to the development of constipation when compared with healthy children because of their decreased fluid intake, variable diet, and decreased mobility, in addition to specific cancer- and treatment-related causes. Constipation may be caused by direct effects of the cancer such as a tumor that obstructs the intestinal lumen, infiltrates enteric nerves and muscles, or causes spinal cord compression or cauda equina syndrome. Cancer-directed therapy, particularly neurotoxic agents such as vinca alkaloids, may also cause constipation. In addition, use of opioids may be one of the most important causes of constipation in this population.

Constipation may lead to painful bowel movements, which some children respond to by withholding stool, further exacerbating the problem. Constipation may lead to significant distress, discomfort (e.g., pain, nausea, and bloating), and embarrassment for some children. Medical complications may include GI obstruction, urinary obstruction, or infection.

Constipation is usually due to altered GI motility and/or altered fluid handling. Intestinal motility is controlled by neuronal, endocrine, and luminal factors. Acetylcholine is the chief neurotransmitter that mediates peristalsis. Serotonin also plays an important role in mediating the gut's response to luminal contents. Opioids lead to constipation by reducing intestinal motility and secretions and increasing fluid absorption and blood flow,[403] as well as by decreasing sensitivity to luminal contents. The effects of opioids on the gut do not appear to be strongly related to the dose.

Evaluation of the patient with constipation includes a thorough history and physical examination. If not contraindicated by a condition such as neutropenia or mucositis, a rectal examination may facilitate the distinction of lower (rectosigmoid) constipation from "colonic inertia" or high obstruction and may also allow assessment of anal sphincter tone and examination for fissures or hemorrhoids. When the diagnosis of constipation is unclear, a radiograph of the kidneys, ureters, and bladder may facilitate the diagnosis.

In addition to medical interventions, the treatment of constipation includes strategies such as provision of a comfortable, easily accessible toilet or commode and addressing issues such as lack of privacy and the need for care providers to help the patient with toileting. Although physical activity is associated with colonic peristalsis, increasing exercise does not necessarily reduce constipation.[404] In addition, the child's medications should be reviewed and dosing of constipating medications such as opioids, TCAs, antihistamines, and 5-HT3 receptor antagonists such as ondansetron and neuroleptics should be altered, if possible. For example, transdermal fentanyl may be less constipating than oral morphine.[405] Patients taking methadone have less of a laxative requirement than do patients taking morphine or hydromorphone, perhaps because methadone provides analgesia by binding to both opioid and NMDA receptors.[406]

Medical management of constipation relies on stool softeners, osmotic agents, and irritant stimulants that increase bowel motility. Softeners, by acting as detergents, soften the stool. Osmotic agents include lactulose, polyethylene glycol, and magnesium salts and increase secretion of water into the lumen. Osmotic agents that increase stool volume actually also facilitate contraction of the bowel wall musculature, thereby increasing bowel motility. Polyethylene glycol is a tasteless agent that may be mixed with a beverage of the child's choice, making it an attractive option for children. In addition, because it is a large polymer that is not degraded by bacteria, it causes less bloating and flatulence than other osmotic agents.[407]

Irritant stimulants such as senna and bisacodyl stimulate contraction and increase secretion. Both of these agents act quickly and are most appropriately used in single doses for temporary constipation. When a hard, leading edge of stool is detected in the rectal vault on examination, it may need to be addressed with use of rectal laxatives (i.e., stimulant suppositories or enemas) if these are acceptable to the child and are not contraindicated because of neutropenia. In the neutropenic child requiring rectal laxatives, administration of antibiotics may prevent bacterial translocation during these maneuvers. As a last resort, manual disimpaction may be required for impacted, hard stool in the rectal vault. Manual disimpaction is a very uncomfortable and distressing procedure for many children and should be avoided if possible.

Although increased fiber intake may be a useful strategy for reducing constipation in healthy persons, patients with cancer may be unable to consume enough fiber to prevent constipation. Inadequate fluid intake directly contributes to constipation but also reduces the efficacy of fiber and increases the risk of obstruction due to a gelatinous mass from inadequately hydrated fiber.[403]

The most effective approach to predictable constipation due to opioids or vinca alkaloids is prevention. Because constipation is one adverse effect of opioids to which patients do not develop tolerance, opioids should always be prescribed with a bowel regimen including a stool softener and stimulant. Despite wide recognition of the constipating effects of opioids, as many as 26% of health care providers who prescribe opioids fail to provide bowel prophylaxis.[408] Other barriers to effective prevention of constipation include (1) difficulty in convincing patients to take a medication to *prevent* another symptom, (2) multiple daily dosing for softeners and laxatives, and (3) adverse effects from these agents such as abdominal pain, cramping, and loose stools.[403]

Methylnaltrexone, a novel agent that may be given orally, intravenously, or subcutaneously to treat opioid-induced constipation, has recently been evaluated in adults.[409,410] This opioid receptor antagonist binds to peripheral mu opioid receptors and does not cross the blood-brain barrier. As such it does not reverse analgesia or induce withdrawal but reliably results in a prompt bowel movement, often within minutes of parenteral administration. It may provide added benefits of treating other peripheral opioid adverse effects such as nausea, pruritus, and urinary retention. It provides the added benefit of relieving opioid-induced constipation without the addition of an enteral medication. Methylnaltrexone is contraindicated in the setting of mechanical GI obstruction or an acute surgical abdomen. Although a pediatric study is required to determine the optimal pediatric methylnaltrexone dose, in one retrospective study it was found that after administration of methylnaltrexone at a mean dose of 0.15 mg/kg/dose, 10 of 19 patients (53%) had a bowel movement within 30 minutes and an additional 4 patients (for a total of 14/19, or 74%) did so within 4 hours of administration.[383]

Bowel Obstruction

Bowel obstruction may result from tumor (malignant bowel obstruction) or other entities such as strictures or postradiation fibrosis obstructing the intestinal lumen. Factors that reduce bowel propulsion such as electrolyte imbalance, opioids, and vinca alkaloids may also contribute to bowel obstruction. Bowel obstruction may occur anywhere from the gastroduodenal junction distally and typically causes abdominal pain, colic, distension, and nausea and vomiting.

Management options for obstruction depend on the site and the underlying cause of the obstruction, the patient's functional status and prognosis, and the goals of care of the patient and family. Treatment modalities for obstruction include surgery, endoscopic procedures, radiation, and medical interventions. For these reasons, decisions regarding management of obstruction may likely involve an interdisciplinary discussion with the family.

Surgery, either by laparoscopy or laparotomy, is often the primary treatment for a mechanical bowel obstruction. Such techniques may allow for resection or bypass of the obstruction and perhaps placement of a venting gastrostomy or a stoma distally. Obstructions may also sometimes be stented endoscopically. Consultation with a surgeon to determine the likelihood of success of the procedure and the potential for obstruction to recur in light of the patient's medical condition may be helpful. Even if obstruction is likely to recur, for some patients it may be reasonable to consider surgery if it is likely to restore bowel function or reduce symptoms for a period. For example, a relatively minor surgery such as gastrostomy placement may allow for venting of an upper obstruction, reducing nausea and vomiting and allowing the patient to eat for comfort.

For some patients, such as those with advanced disease and poor functional status, medical management may be more appropriate than surgery. A variety of medical interventions may break the cycle of obstruction, distension, and secretion. These interventions are aimed at relieving symptoms and potentially reducing the obstruction to allow some degree of enteral nutrition.

Antimuscarinic/anticholinergic agents such as scopolamine reduce colic from smooth muscle spasm and reduce GI secretions. Scopolamine may be administered intravenously, subcutaneously, or transdermally. Because it crosses the blood-brain barrier, it may cause CNS effects such as delirium; glycopyrrolate, which does not cross the blood-brain barrier, is sometimes used as an alternative.

Octreotide is a somatostatin analogue that is a potent antisecretogogue. By inhibiting several hormones, as well as neurotransmission, in the GI tract, it reduces splanchnic blood flow and peristalsis, reduces gastric and intestinal secretions, and increases the absorption of water and salts from the intestine. Octreotide may be given subcutaneously or intravenously, and a long-acting injection formulation is available for once-monthly dosing for patients taking a stable dose.

In a randomized trial of 68 adults with an inoperable malignant bowel obstruction who were receiving an anticholinergic agent, antiemetics, and an opioid, those who also received octreotide had significantly reduced nausea, vomiting, anorexia, and fatigue, although no difference in pain was appreciated.[411] In an uncontrolled study of 27 adults who had an inoperable malignant bowel obstruction, a combination of octreotide, dexamethasone, metoclopramide, opioids, and other agents produced a 90% recovery rate.[412] This regimen reduced vomiting, restored intestinal motility, and allowed for oral feedings.

Other medications that may be helpful include prokinetic drugs such as metoclopramide, which reverses peristalsis from obstruction and decreases nausea and need not be reserved only for partial obstruction. Other pharmacologic interventions include corticosteroids, which decrease inflammation and edema and reduce nausea. For some patients, a venting gastrostomy tube may reduce symptoms. IV hydration may reduce nausea and sedation.[413] Both surgical approaches and medical hydration/nutrition, however, are supportive measures that should be considered in light of the patient's prognosis and the goals of the patient and family.

Diarrhea

Diarrhea is defined as the frequent occurrence of loose stools, often with urgency. Patients' definitions of diarrhea may vary, and when it is a presenting complaint, it must be accurately characterized, particularly with regard to how the patient's bowel habits have changed compared with his or her baseline. In addition to potentially causing significant medical complications, diarrhea may be debilitating for patients. It may cause life-threatening dehydration and electrolyte imbalance in addition to malnutrition and immune impairment. Attendant mucosal injury may also predispose patients to sepsis. Diarrhea may cause physical discomfort with cramping and painful perianal skin breakdown and emotional distress for children and caregivers.

Diarrhea may occur as a direct effect of a malignancy (e.g., a carcinoid, a GI stromal tumor, or medullary cancer of the thyroid), although this occurrence is relatively rare in pediatric cancers. Secretory diarrhea can occur in rare cases of neuroblastoma with associated vasoactive intestinal polypeptide secretion. Diarrhea may also result from chemotherapy, as will be discussed later. Radiation to the abdomen or pelvis may cause mucosal damage, prostaglandin release, and bile salt malabsorption, which in turn increase peristalsis and cause diarrhea. Radiation-induced enteritis frequently occurs during the third week of fractionated therapy.[414] Another form of treatment-related diarrhea is gut GVHD after bone marrow transplant. In gut GVHD, inflammatory infiltrates of activated lymphocytes, plasma cells, and eosinophils cause intestinal mucosal damage, in turn leading to diarrhea and sometimes bleeding.[415] Mucosal damage from cancer treatment may increase the risk of superinfection, which can further exacerbate diarrhea and other GI symptoms.

Other causes of diarrhea in patients with cancer include bacterial overgrowth, which may occur with changes in anatomy after surgery, as well as bona fide infection. In particular, patients with cancer are prone to *Clostridium difficile* infections largely as a result of the frequent administration of antibiotics. Infection leads to diarrhea through mucosal injury and impaired absorption, although malabsorption may occur for other reasons, such as a surgically shortened gut or fistula that reduces absorptive capacity.

Diarrhea may also be caused by medications, including antibiotics and magnesium (in electrolyte supplements or antacids). Furthermore, diarrhea may be seen in association with constipation, either as a result of impaction constipation with overflow or leakage or laxatives used to treat constipation.

In general, treatment of diarrhea depends on the underlying cause. If needed, rehydration should be undertaken with correction of electrolyte imbalance. Patients should be advised that food intake is secondary to maintenance of hydration during an episode of diarrhea. Dairy products should be avoided because of secondary lactase deficiency. In addition, a topical skin barrier such as Desitin may be applied to protect the skin from irritation. Symptomatic management with opioids, and in the case of severe diarrhea, octreotide, is discussed later in the context of chemotherapy-induced diarrhea (CID), but it is applicable to diarrhea from a wide variety of causes.

Chemotherapy-Induced Diarrhea

CID is seen with increasing frequency as an adverse effect of new chemotherapeutic agents. It is a common adverse effect of agents such as 5-fluorouracil, irinotecan, capecitabine, and docetaxel. Irinotecan may cause acute diarrhea immediately after administration of the drug through cholinergic mechanisms; the diarrhea may be treated with an anticholinergic agent such as atropine. Irinotecan commonly causes delayed diarrhea, usually at least 24 hours after administration. Irinotecan is conjugated by the liver to form SN-38, which is then deconjugated back to the active agent in the intestinal lumen by bacteria. The irinotecan is then able to directly exert toxic effects on colonic epithelium, resulting in diarrhea.[416,417] The late onset secretory diarrhea is best prevented by antibiotics, and if necessary, it is treated with loperamide.

Loperamide is the opioid of choice for diarrhea because it acts locally in the gut and is only very minimally absorbed. By slowing peristalsis and promoting water reabsorption, it reduces stool frequency and volume, as well as urgency. If systemic absorption is less of a concern, other opioids such as morphine may be used as well. Loperamide may be discontinued after the patient has been free of diarrhea for 12 hours, but in the case of radiation-induced diarrhea, loperamide should be continued for the duration of radiation treatment.[414] In cases in which CID is severe or complicated (i.e., with moderate to severe cramping, decreased performance status, fever, neutropenia, and bleeding or dehydration), administration of octreotide should be considered.[414] Octreotide is also effective in cases of diarrhea refractory to loperamide,[418] and it has been shown to be effective in reducing diarrhea associated with GVHD.[419] In a small study of pediatric patients receiving irinotecan, it was found that activated charcoal taken three times a day during irinotecan administration reduced the severity and frequency of diarrhea and improved chemotherapy tolerability and continuation rates.[420]

DYSPNEA

Dyspnea is defined as the uncomfortable or abnormal awareness of breathing. Patients may describe dyspnea in a variety of ways, including chest tightness, air hunger, choking, or heavy breathing. Dyspnea is clearly an important source of suffering in children and adults alike, triggering feelings of fear, anxiety, and loss of control and impairing quality of life.[421] In addition, family members are distressed by witnessing a loved one with this symptom.[422]

Dyspnea may occur in patients with malignant involvement of the respiratory tract. Direct effects of malignancy such as airway obstruction by tumor or a malignant pleural effusion are possible. Treatment-related complications such as pulmonary fibrosis, pneumonitis, or GVHD after hematopoietic stem cell transplantation may cause dyspnea. Other respiratory processes that result in dyspnea include pulmonary edema, pulmonary embolus, pneumonitis, or a restrictive physiology due to tumor, ascites, or organomegaly. Patients with cardiac pathologic conditions such as anthracycline-induced congestive

heart failure or pericardial effusion may also experience dyspnea. Despite the multitude of potential causes of dyspnea, it may also occur in patients who have no respiratory or cardiac involvement at all. For example, in the National Hospice Study it was found that 24% of terminally ill adults with cancer who reported dyspnea had no known cardiac or pulmonary disease.[423] In cases in which no known underlying respiratory or cardiac disease exists, dyspnea may stem from multiple causes, including muscle weakness from deconditioning or poor nutritional status, anemia, metabolic derangements, fluid shifts, or anxiety.

Dyspnea may occur at any point during the clinical course but is most notably observed at the end of life. In the National Hospice Study it was found that 70% of 1754 terminally ill adults experienced dyspnea in the last 6 weeks of life.[423] Dyspnea, particularly dyspnea at the severe end of the spectrum, is associated with shorter survival. For example, as a symptom by itself or in association with other parameters, it is a prognostic indicator of more rapid mortality in adults with advanced cancer.[424]

Pathophysiology

The respiratory center that processes input from the respiratory system and coordinates respiratory activity is located in the medulla and pons. Afferent input arises from peripheral mechanoreceptors in respiratory muscles, the chest wall, the lungs, and the upper airway, as well as central and peripheral chemoreceptors and pulmonary vagal afferents (Fig. 71-4). Chemoreceptors detect low Po_2 and high Pco_2 in the blood and send this input to

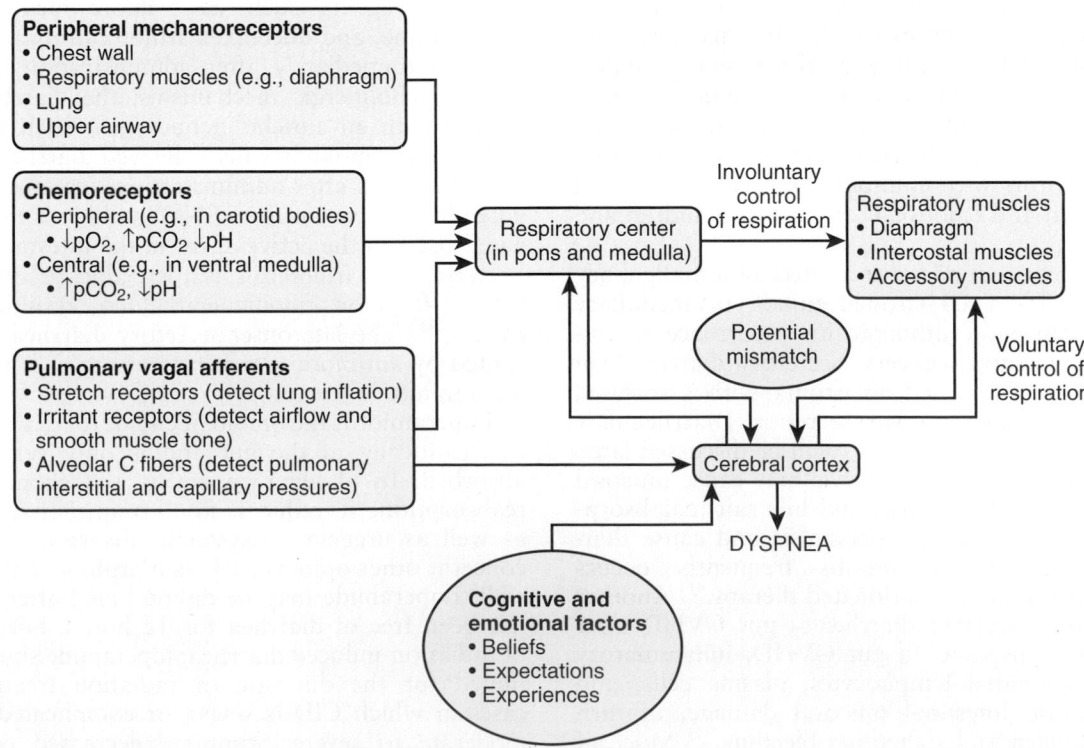

Figure 71-4 The pathophysiology of dyspnea.

the respiratory center. Pulmonary vagal afferents are activated by input from stretch receptors and irritant receptors, and they also trigger activity in tracts that project to the cerebral cortex. Based on this sensory input, the respiratory center coordinates the respiratory apparatus consisting of the diaphragm, intercostal muscles, and accessory muscles. The cerebral cortex integrates sensory input, motor output, and cognitive and emotional input to create the sensation of breathing.[425]

The phenomenon of dyspnea occurs when the afferent sensory input to the brain—for example, input from mechanoreceptors in the chest wall—fails to match the outgoing motor signal emanating from the brain.[426] Situations in which such mismatch may occur include (1) increased work of breathing such as when breathing against increased resistance or with weakened muscles; (2) chemical changes such as hypercapnia and hypoxemia; and (3) neuromechanical dissociation such as when sensory input from a given inspiratory effort does not match the input anticipated by the brain.[425] The interpretation of this mismatch, or perceived dyspnea, by the cerebral cortex is affected by the individual's expectations, experiences, and beliefs, making the sensation of dyspnea highly subjective and individual.

Diagnosis and Assessment

Neither clinical signs such as respiratory rate or oxygen saturation nor laboratory data such as arterial blood gases and hemoglobin concentration are reliable predictors of dyspnea. Because objective data correlates poorly with dyspnea, the gold standard for measuring and assessing dyspnea is the patient's self-report. The visual analogue scale[427] and Borg scale[428] are among the most widely used in adults. The Borg scale is a 10-point scale with descriptive anchors at the ends. A numeric rating scale has also been evaluated in adult oncology patients, with a 0/1 out of 10 score having a 98% sensitivity and a 54% specificity. A score greater than 1 is predictive of dyspnea that may impair daily function and is recommended as a threshold score requiring further evaluation.[429] The Dalhousie dyspnea scale was developed to meet the need for a pediatric dyspnea assessment instrument.[430] This pictorial instrument actually contains three scales depicting three subconstructs of dyspnea including throat closing, chest tightness, and effort. This instrument was tested in children with asthma or cystic fibrosis and in healthy children. Children 8 years or older used the instrument reliably. Our review of the literature did not yield any instruments that have been specifically developed for the measurement of dyspnea in the younger pediatric population.

Further assessment of dyspnea necessitates a history that should include triggers or exacerbating factors, alleviating factors, severity, and description of degree of functional impairment. Indications of complications such as infection, GVHD, and cardiac compromise should be sought, as should potential treatment-related causes such as chemotherapy and radiotherapy. Potential causes of dyspnea unrelated to malignancy such as asthma should also be considered. Finally, contributing psychosocial factors such as anxiety should be explored because emo-

tional and cognitive factors may influence how the individual interprets dyspnea as a symptom.

Evaluation beyond a thorough physical examination depends upon the suspected cause of dyspnea. Studies that may provide useful information include a complete blood cell count, noninvasive measures including pulse oximetry and capnometry, selective assessment of venous or arterial blood gases, and a chest radiograph. Additional tests that may also be considered include pulmonary function testing, an axial chest CT scan, an echocardiogram, an electrocardiogram, and a spiral CT or ventilation-perfusion scan to assess for a pulmonary embolus.

Management

Targeted approaches to treat dyspnea depend upon the underlying cause and may include medical therapies such as chemotherapy, antibiotics, or diuretics. Procedural interventions may include pleurocentesis and stenting of the airways to relieve the obstruction or surgical removal of the obstruction. Consideration of such interventions should weigh the likely benefits and burdens for the child in light of his or her medical condition.

Rapid and effective strategies for symptomatic management of dyspnea are available and applicable both for patients who are candidates for targeted approaches and for those in whom such interventions are not appropriate. The mainstays of symptomatic management include opioids and oxygen. Other agents such as anxiolytics, steroids, and bronchodilators may also be of benefit, particularly if an inflammatory or bronchospastic component is suspected.

Opioids

Several studies in adult patients with cancer support the use of opioids as an effective intervention for dyspnea.[431-434] Brucra et al.[431] and Mazzocato et al.[433] conducted randomized placebo-controlled crossover studies demonstrating that opioids relieved dyspnea and furthermore did not cause clinically important respiratory depression. No studies demonstrating the efficacy of opioids for dyspnea in children have been published, although based on clinical experience, they appear to be as effective and safe in children as in adults.

The mechanism(s) by which opioids relieve dyspnea has/have not yet been clearly elucidated. Opioid receptors present in both the peripheral nervous system and the CNS may play a role relieving dyspnea when they are bound. Opioids may alleviate dyspnea by blunting the effect of hypercapnia or hypoxia on ventilation, relieving anxiety, or modifying the sensation of dyspnea, akin to their ability to modify the sensation of pain.

The dose required to relieve dyspnea is often relatively small, even when a patient is not opioid-naive. For example, Allard and colleagues[434] showed that a 25% increase in the baseline dose controlled breakthrough dyspnea for up to 4 hours. Our standard practice for opioid-naive patients is to start by administering 0.025 mg/kg of morphine intravenously (i.e., 25% of 0.1 mg/kg, the typical starting dose for pain) and titrating as indicated. In addition to short-acting preparations, long-acting preparations such as sustained-relief morphine are effective treatments for dyspnea.[435]

Because opioid receptors are present in the lower respiratory tract, it was postulated that nebulized opioids might alleviate dyspnea. Case reports of inhaled morphine and fentanyl in adolescents with cystic fibrosis[436,437] and a small uncontrolled study in patients with cancer who used inhaled morphine fentanyl to reduce dyspnea held promise in this regard.[438] A crossover study conducted by Bruera and colleagues[439] comparing subcutaneous and nebulized morphine suggested that both routes of administration may reduce dyspnea, but perhaps because of a small sample size or placebo effect, a difference between the two routes could not be excluded. In addition, several other studies have not demonstrated efficacy of nebulized opioids. Until larger studies are conducted that use standardized doses of opioid and consistent delivery methods, evidence is insufficient to support this method of delivery for dyspnea.[440]

Oxygen

When hypoxemia is suspected to be the cause of dyspnea, administration of oxygen to reverse hypoxemia may relieve this symptom. However, it is likely that most patients who have dyspnea either are not hypoxemic or do not have dyspnea as a result of hypoxemia alone. For example, in a study of adults with advanced cancer and dyspnea, only 40% were hypoxic.[441]

Studies evaluating oxygen compared with air for relief of dyspnea in both hypoxemic and nonhypoxemic adults show no clear superiority of oxygen compared with air.[442-445] An explanation for the comparability of flowing oxygen and air in relieving dyspnea is based on the ability of both to stimulate mechanoreceptors in the trigeminal nerve. Receptors in the distribution of the trigeminal nerve appear to influence induced dyspnea in healthy subjects.[446] In addition, administration of cold air appears to improve dyspnea in patients with chronic obstructive pulmonary disease.[447] Therefore provision of flowing air or oxygen could potentially reduce dyspnea through this mechanism. Trigeminal nerve stimulation may explain why experiencing cool, moving air provided by a fan or open window also seems to reduce dyspnea.

Anxiolytics

Although anxiety may worsen perceived dyspnea and dyspnea may induce anxiety, evidence to date does not support the routine use of anxiolytics to treat dyspnea, particularly not as a first-line agent. Dyspnea is a common symptom in persons who have panic attacks or anxiety disorder. However, anxiety may contribute less to coexisting dyspnea than has been traditionally thought. Recent work reveals that in adults with advanced cancer, anxiety explained only 10% of the variance in dyspnea. Use of an anxiolytic agent to alleviate anxiety may be appropriate when anxious symptoms are particularly prominent and are thought to have a significant influence on a patient's interpretation of the sensation of dyspnea. Anxiolytics may also be indicated for sedation to manage escalating dyspnea at the end of life, as discussed in Chapter 69, which covers palliative care.

Nonpharmacologic Interventions

To the extent that the cerebral cortex mediates the sensation of dyspnea, interventions that modify cognitive and emotional factors such as breathing/relaxation training that influence the interpretation of dyspnea may be helpful. In healthy adults undergoing induced dyspnea, distraction of subjects did not change dyspnea severity ratings but did decrease the perceived unpleasantness of the dyspnea.[448] Increased support, such as is provided in the nurse-run dyspnea clinic studied by Bredin and the one described by Booth, may reduce dyspnea by providing education, cognitive and behavioral training, and psychosocial support.[449]

Escalating Dyspnea

The symptom of dyspnea may escalate at the end of life. Respiratory changes and the development of secretions are discussed in Chapter 69, which covers palliative care. Refractory, distressing dyspnea such as may occur at the end of life is an indication for consideration of palliative sedation, as described in Chapter 70.

Future Directions

Much remains to be learned regarding the physiologic features and mechanisms of dyspnea. Once these features and mechanisms are better understood, targeted interventions may be developed to ameliorate this challenging symptom for which we currently have relatively few treatment options. Within the pediatric realm, a better understanding of how children sense and interpret this highly subjective symptom is needed. This understanding in turn may enable development of methods to measure and assess this symptom, allowing the care team to better understand how it affects children and evaluate dyspnea-directed interventions.

COUGH

Cough can be a distressing symptom and may lead to dyspnea, vomiting, sleep disruption, and chest or throat pain. Topical antitussives act on receptors in the respiratory tree to reduce cough. Nebulized lidocaine has been described to ease an intractable cough at the end of life.[450] Symptomatic treatment for a significant cough usually entails administration of an opioid to suppress the cough reflex in the medulla. Dextromethorphan and codeine are most commonly used, although all opioids have antitussive activity.

FATIGUE

Cancer-related fatigue has been defined by the NCCN as a "distressing persistent, subjective sense of tiredness or exhaustion related to cancer or cancer treatment that is not proportional to recent activity and interferes with usual functioning."[451] Fatigue is a complex symptom that may have physical, cognitive, and emotional components. In addition, fatigue is subjective and highly individual, and thus patients may experience and interpret fatigue differently. Patients may describe fatigue in a wide variety of ways (Box 73-3). Nevertheless, adults with cancer-related fatigue almost universally report that (1) it is unresponsive to rest, (2) it is not proportional to activity, and (3) it pervades multiple areas of their life. Clearly, this type of fatigue is not the fatigue of everyday life. Recent work in adult cancer survivors reveals that fatigue may be long-lived, lasting for months to years after cancer-directed treatment has been completed.[452,453] In pediatric cancer survivors, fatigue is the only factor associated with both poor physical and psychosocial health-related quality of life.[454]

Impact

It is well established that fatigue is the most common symptom in patients with cancer.[455,456] One survey of published studies on cancer-related fatigue in adults found that fatigue was present in 50% to 75% of patients at diagnosis, with the prevalence increasing to 80% to 96% in patients undergoing chemotherapy and to 60% to 93% in patients receiving radiotherapy.[457] In children, fatigue is less well studied but has been shown to be the most common symptom.[5] For example, Wolfe and colleagues[5] found that fatigue was the most common symptom in children with advanced cancer, with 96% of children experiencing fatigue. Collins also found that in a cross-sectional study of children aged 10 to 18 years who had current or previous cancer, lack of energy was the most common symptom, affecting 49.7%.

According to adult patients with cancer, fatigue is the most distressing of all the symptoms they experience, creating profound physical, psychological, and financial burdens that can impair quality of life and diminish hope.[458] It not only leads to a decrement in physical ability but also to a sense of loss of control, loneliness, and isolation. In the Fatigue II study of 379 adults undergoing treatment for cancer, 60% ranked fatigue as the symptom affecting their life the most.[458] According to the parents in the study by Wolfe et al.,[5] fatigue caused "a great deal" or "a lot" of suffering in 57% of children approaching the end of life. In another study, Jalmsell et al.[6] reported that of 449 parents of children who had died from cancer, 86% reported that fatigue significantly affected their child's well-being. Adolescents who have cancer also report that fatigue significantly affects their physical, social, and psychological well-being.[459] Higher self-reported fatigue in adolescents is also negatively associated with quality of life.[460]

In addition to causing suffering, concerns regarding fatigue as an adverse effect of disease-directed or symptom-directed treatment may limit therapy. Fatigue is documented to be the most common adverse effect of chemotherapy and radiotherapy in adults.[457,461] In adults, treatment-related fatigue can be severe enough to prevent maximal treatment and disease control,[451,462] although in children, fatigue is rarely cited as a reason to reduce therapy. In terms of symptom-related treatment, pain may be inadequately relieved when concerns regarding opioid-related fatigue or sedation inhibit optimal opioid administration.[463,464] When fatigue is not controlled, patients are forced to choose between adequate analgesia

with somnolence and mental clouding and less sedation at the price of increased pain.

Approach

Despite its prevalence and impact, fatigue frequently is not addressed by clinicians and patients alike. In a large multicenter study of 1317 adults with cancer, only 52% of those with fatigue reported it to their physician.[465] One significant barrier to addressing fatigue is the perception on the part of the care team that fatigue, although undesirable, does not have a significant adverse affect on patients. In the Fatigue I study it was found that although oncologists believe that pain adversely affects their patients to a greater degree than fatigue (61% vs. 37%), patients with cancer believed that fatigue adversely affected their daily lives more than pain (61% vs. 19%).[456] This disparity may be due in part to clinicians' personal understanding of day-to-day fatigue that leads them to believe they understand the reality of cancer-related fatigue. Other barriers to addressing fatigue may include (1) a belief that fatigue is "normal" or "to be expected" in a patient with cancer; (2) a paucity of descriptors for patients to adequately convey the various manifestations of fatigue; (3) the clinician's lack of familiarity with options to ameliorate fatigue; (4) a disease-directed focus to the exclusion of attention to symptoms; and (5) system-related problems such as time pressures or reimbursement difficulties.

Measurement and Assessment of Fatigue in Children

The NCCN provides guidelines for fatigue management in adults and children that calls for screening for fatigue at every visit using a 1 to 10 scale.[451] Although use of such a scale has not been validated in children, this type of scale may generally be used reliably in children 7 years and older.

Once screening identifies fatigue, it should be further assessed, although universally accepted means for assessing fatigue in either adults or children do not exist. Several unidimensional and multidimensional scales for assessment in adults and a few pediatric instruments are available. One, developed by Hockenberry and colleagues[466] is for children with cancer. Although it is part of a series of instruments that evaluate fatigue in pediatric oncology patients from the perspective of the child, parent, and staff,[466] it was derived from interviews with only 13 children and has not yet been prospectively evaluated. Another instrument, the PedsQL Multidimensional Fatigue Scale,[467] measures child and parent perceptions of fatigue in pediatric patients. This instrument has been studied in healthy children and in children with cancer.[467]

Even when a formal assessment instrument is not used to assess fatigue, clinicians should explore a variety of possible manifestations of fatigue that the child/adolescent and the adult caregiver may identify (Box 71-3). Exacerbating and alleviating factors, the pattern of fatigue, and the degree to which the symptom is affecting the child's life can then be explored. In assessing fatigue it may be helpful to bear in mind that children tend to conceptualize fatigue as a physical sensation, whereas adolescents alternate or merge the physical concept with mental

Box 71-3   **Manifestations of Fatigue**

PHYSICAL

- Weakness
- Physical tiring
- Heaviness

COGNITIVE

- Mental clouding
- Poor concentration
- Impaired memory

EMOTIONAL

- Depression
- Apathy
- Irritability
- Decreased motivation

ENERGY

- Tiredness
- Lethargy
- Low energy
- Decreased endurance

SLEEP

- Insomnia
- Hypersomnia
- Somnolence
- Nonrestorative sleep

From Ullrich C, Mayer O: Assessment and management of fatigue and dyspnea in pediatric palliative care. Pediatr Clin North Am 54:735–756, 2007.

tiredness.[468] On the other hand, parents and staff conceptualize fatigue as a symptom that interferes with the child's ability to participate in a variety of activities and may be manifested by physical, emotional, and mental changes. Investing the time to fully assess a report of fatigue may frequently yield important clues regarding the cause of the fatigue; these clues are valuable because few diagnostics tests exist to determine the cause of fatigue.

Associated Factors

Fatigue may stem from concomitant, interrelated causes including physical factors, psychological factors, and disrupted sleep (Fig. 71-5). Investigations aiming to uncover the cause of fatigue exist only in adults and consist of retrospective and prospective analyses of factors associated with fatigue. No studies have been published that evaluate objective factors associated with fatigue in children with cancer.

For simplicity, factors considered to be associated with fatigue may be categorized into physical and psychosocial factors, with the realization that many patients experience fatigue as a result of a combination of factors. For example, in adults undergoing chemotherapy or radiotherapy, fatigue correlates with both physical factors (symptom distress) and psychological factors (e.g., depression, anxiety, anger, or confusion).[469] Another study of adult patients with cancer similarly determined that both physical factors (severity of pain and dyspnea) and psychological symptoms (anxiety and depression) were associated with the experience of fatigue.[455]

In adults, certain sociodemographic factors are also associated with fatigue. For example, the demographic factors of being employed or living alone were significantly associated with the symptom of fatigue.[470] Although children are unlikely to experience fatigue related to these exact sociodemographic considerations, the stress induced by these financial or caregiver concerns can affect children and the fatigue that they experience.

Physical Factors

Physical factors contributing to fatigue include direct effects of the underlying disease and adverse effects of treatment of the underlying illness. Unrelieved symptoms are also likely to contribute to a patient's fatigue. In adults, overall symptom distress is associated with the report of fatigue.[471] Conversely, treatment for symptoms such as pain or dyspnea may also contribute to fatigue.

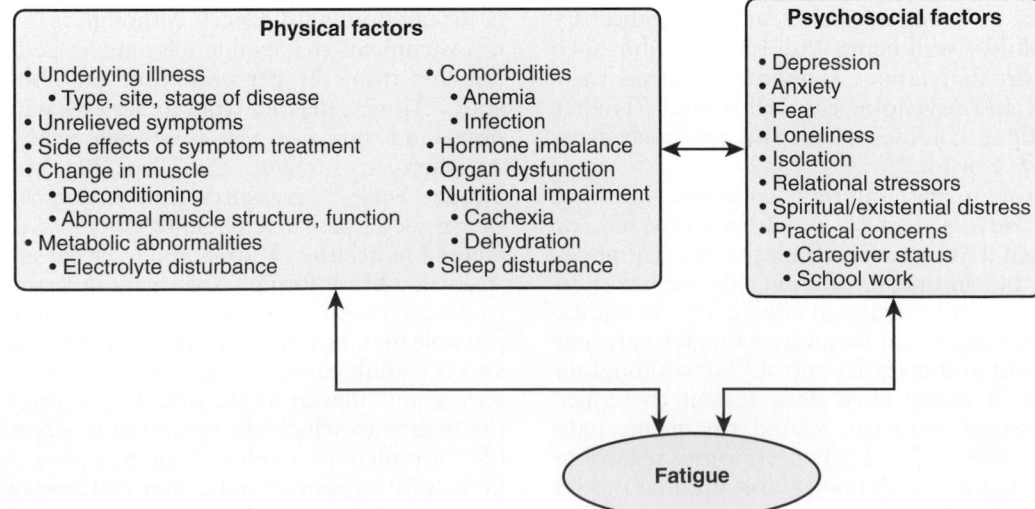

Figure 71-5 A conceptual model of fatigue.

Because a variety of medications including benzodiazepines, opioids, and antihistamines may cause fatigue, thoroughly reviewing the patient's medications may reveal medications that cause fatigue. Finally, a variety of comorbidities such as organ dysfunction (e.g., renal, hepatic, cardiac, pulmonary, or endocrine dysfunction), electrolyte imbalance, poor nutritional status, and infection may contribute to fatigue.

Anemia is a well-established cause of fatigue in a variety of patient populations. In adults with cancer, it has been demonstrated to be associated with fatigue and impaired quality of life. In some adults with advanced cancer, anemia is not significantly related to fatigue.[472,473] Thus anemia may not fully account for the fatigue experienced by some patients, suggesting that correction of anemia may or may not decrease fatigue.

Like anemia, hypothyroidism is associated with fatigue in patients with and without cancer. Other endocrine abnormalities that are associated with the experience of fatigue include hypothalamic-pituitary axis alterations[474] and hypogonadism, which is also associated with negative mood and cachexia.[475-477]

Deconditioning from decreased activity may lead to fatigue, which in turn lessens activity and may further exacerbate fatigue. A variety of muscle abnormalities that have been described in patients with cancer may be associated with fatigue.[478] Finally, muscle wasting (cachexia) is associated with fatigue, perhaps because of the cytokines proposed to mediate cachexia such as tumor necrosis factor, which are also thought to contribute to the sensation of fatigue.[474]

Psychosocial Factors

Psychosocial factors such as depression and anxiety, existential or spiritual suffering, and stress from practical concerns may all be related to fatigue. When psychological factors such as fatigue and depression coexist, depressed mood may be a contributor or a consequence of fatigue. For example, when characterized by withdrawal and decreased participation in activities in an adolescent, fatigue may be a manifestation of depression. On the other hand, the experience of fatigue may lead to isolation, decreased engagement in activities, and impaired quality of life, all of which may contribute to depression.

Sleep Disturbance

Sleep disturbance, manifested as decreased quantity or quality of sleep, results from factors including unrelieved physical or psychological symptoms or environmental factors, such as distortion of sleep architecture by medications or sleep disruptions that occur in the hospital.[479,480] Impaired sleep may in turn worsen the physical or psychological distress experienced by patients. Although a decrement in the quantity or quality of sleep may contribute to fatigue, cancer-related fatigue may occur independent of changes in sleep.[481]

Interventions

An algorithm for approaching the symptom of fatigue is presented in Figure 71-6. Although fatigue is frequently multifactorial, targeting underlying factors that are suspected to contribute to fatigue can improve this symptom. Even when no particular contributing factor is identified, nonspecific interventions may ameliorate fatigue. For example, exercise and stimulants are effective interventions that reduce fatigue. Educating the patient and his or her family about fatigue is important in helping them understand fatigue and its impact, as well as the available options for addressing it. Strategies to optimize function and facilitate adaptation to fatigue such as realistic goal setting, modifying activities, and conserving energy should also be reviewed.

Exercise

Curtailing activity is a natural reaction to fatigue, and oncologists report recommending activity in response to the complaint of fatigue.[456] Several randomized controlled trials in adults have demonstrated that exercise actually reduces fatigue, and in some instances it also ameliorates psychological symptoms such as depression and anxiety. For example, a 6-week walking program for women undergoing radiotherapy for breast cancer improved fatigue as well as anxiety, depression, and sleep disturbance.[482] Finally, exercise can also provide a variety of physical benefits, including improved strength and function.

Psychosocial Interventions

Strategies to address psychological factors include both pharmacologic and nonpharmacologic approaches. Psychological interventions such as psychotherapy and support group participation may reduce fatigue,[483] as can increased support from clinicians such as intensive nursing support.[484] If depression or anxiety are suspected to contribute to fatigue, a trial of a pharmacologic agent such as an antidepressant or anxiolytic may be of benefit, recognizing that some drugs in each of these classes may exacerbate sedation and fatigue. If other stressors are uncovered, such as spiritual suffering or concerns about practical matters, professionals such as a chaplain, resource specialist, or staff at school should be approached for assistance.

Sleep

If sleep disturbance is suspected, reducing factors that impair sleep and strategizing with patients to improve sleep hygiene are a necessary first step. If indicated by persistent or severe sleep impairment, pharmacologic interventions such as benzodiazepines, benzodiazepine receptor agonists, and antidepressants with sedating qualities (e.g., TCAs, trazodone, and mirtazapine) may be tried. It is important to keep in mind, however, that benzodiazepines and antihistamines in particular may have paradoxic effects in children and that the benzodiazepine receptor agonists have not yet been well studied in young children.

Pharmacologic Interventions

Correction of Anemia. Correcting anemia associated with cancer or chemotherapy with erythropoietin is a strategy often used in adult oncology. Some studies support this practice in adults, demonstrating that

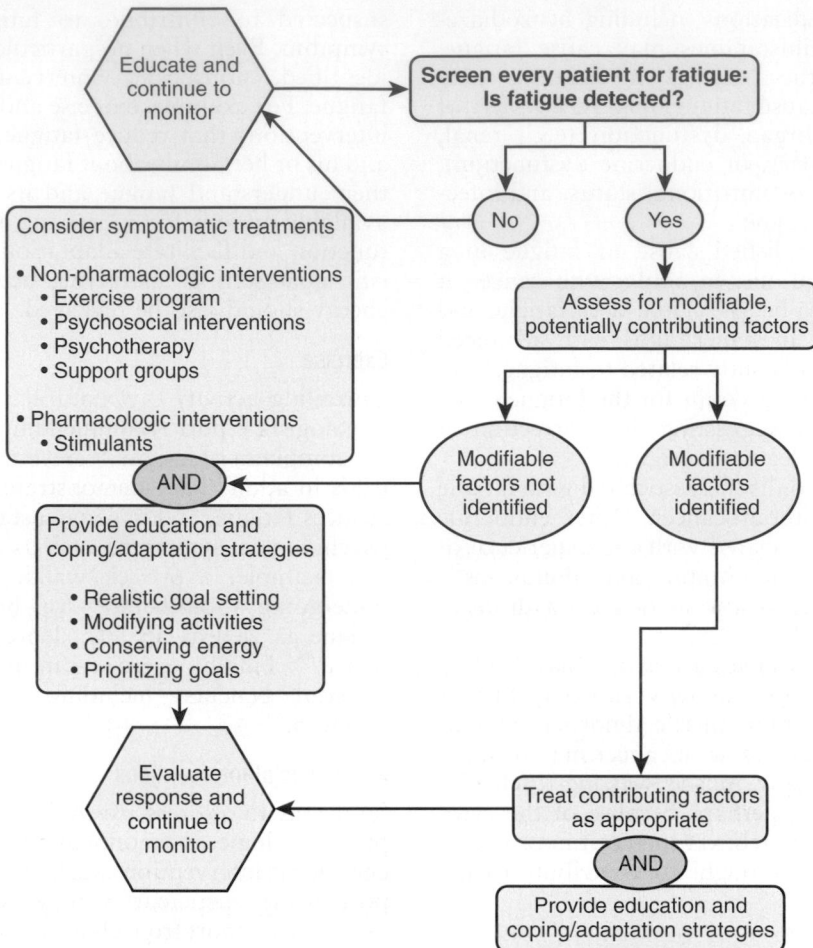

Figure 71-6 An algorithm for fatigue management.

improving anemia may also improve fatigue-related quality of life.[485] However, correction of anemia with erythropoietin has not been as widely pursued in pediatric oncology practice, in part because no evidence exists that treatment of anemia with erythropoietin improves quality of life. The one published study examining this question in children failed to show that health-related quality of life improved with correction of anemia.[486] The authors provide several possible explanations for this finding, but the lack of association between correction of anemia and quality of life and fatigue suggests that focusing on anemia at the exclusion of other suspected causes of fatigue and decreased quality of life may lead to inadequate treatment of fatigue. If erythropoietin is used, recent concerns that it is associated with more rapid tumor progression, thrombosis, and increased mortality in adults[487-489] should be kept in mind. If anemia is suspected as a cause of fatigue, transfusion support is an alternative to erythropoietin therapy.

Stimulants. The stimulant with the best-established efficacy in ameliorating fatigue in adults who have serious illness is methylphenidate. This agent reduces fatigue in adults with cancer and human immunodeficiency virus, regardless of the underlying cause.[490,491] In one study of adults with cancer-related fatigue, patients had significantly less fatigue after they started taking methylphenidate.[492] However, studies have not consistently demonstrated the efficacy of methylphenidate in reducing fatigue. These discrepancies are likely due to the variation in dosing and titration procedures, as well as heterogeneity in fatigue assessment instruments and the study populations evaluated. Methylphenidate is advantageous in that it improves cognition and exerts direct analgesic and antidepressant actions,[490,492,493] and one study reports success in improving cognition in children who have survived cancer.[494] A case series documenting successful treatment with methylphenidate of opioid-related sedation in children who have cancer has been published,[495] but currently no randomized controlled trials have been published that evaluate its efficacy or tolerability in children with cancer-related fatigue.

Methylphenidate has a history of extensive use in children with attention deficit hyperactivity disorder[496] and has a well-established track record in terms of being safe and well tolerated by children. The most prevalent adverse effect of methylphenidate is decreased appetite, which we attempt to mitigate by giving the first dose after breakfast. Despite concerns that methylphenidate should be used with caution in children at risk for seizure, open-label and controlled trials in adults and children with attention deficit hyperactivity disorder and epilepsy do not support this concern (reviewed by Baptista-Neto et al.[497] in 2008). For example, a recent study in children with epilepsy found no increase in seizure frequency and in fact observed beneficial electroencephalogram changes with methylphenidate.[498] Modafinil may be considered as an alternative to methylphenidate, although significantly less pediatric experience exists with this agent. Modafinil has been used with success to treat children with narcolepsy[499] and excessive daytime sleepiness associated with Prader-Willi syndrome[500] and to treat adults with fatigue associated with multiple sclerosis or sedation due to opioids.[501,502] However, no studies evaluating its use in children to treat cancer-related fatigue have been published.

Integrative Therapies

Adult patients with fatigue are more likely to use dietary and herbal supplements,[503] which may be related to patients' perceptions that conventional medicine offers no effective interventions for fatigue. Patients reporting fatigue should be questioned regarding potential use of dietary and herbal supplements. A randomized controlled study evaluating ginseng in adults found that subjects who received 1000 mg per day for 8 weeks had significantly improved fatigue scores when compared with subjects who received a placebo.[504]

Future Directions

Despite its prevalence and impact, fatigue is frequently underrecognized and underappreciated, particularly in comparison with other symptoms. Particular areas of need in the management of fatigue include a better developed assessment method, increased understanding of causes of fatigue, and interventions targeted at specific causes of fatigue.

PRURITUS

Pruritus, also referred to as itching, may occur in children who have cancer for a variety of reasons. As a paraneoplastic symptom it may be associated with malignancy, such as Hodgkin lymphoma or other types of lymphoma. Other disorders such as mastocytosis, iron deficiency, and polycythemia vera may cause pruritus. Pruritus may also occur with organ dysfunction such as hypothyroidism, hyperparathyroidism, liver dysfunction (i.e., cholestasis) or renal dysfunction (uremia),[505] as well as infection of the skin. Pruritus may also be iatrogenic and occur as a result of cancer-directed therapy, as in the pruritic rash caused by growth factor receptor inhibitors[506]—for example, in skin GVHD after hematopoietic stem cell transplantation. Pruritus may also result from a variety of other medications, as well as blood products. Rarely, pruritus may be a manifestation of an underlying psychiatric or neurologic disorder. In general, pruritus associated with a systemic disease is generalized, more gradual in onset, and accompanied by normal appearing skin.[505]

Although pain and pruritus are distinct sensations, they are mediated by the same neural pathways. Stimulation of unmyelinated C fibers that are situated in the dermal-epidermal junction (which are more superficial than those responsible for detecting pain) creates impulses that travel to the dorsal root ganglia and cross to the contralateral spinothalamic tract and ultimately to the somatosensory cortex. Neurotransmitters thought to mediate the sensation of pruritus include the amines, histamine and serotonin, opioids, eicosanoids, neuropeptides, and cytokines. Histamine, which is released primarily in the skin from mast cells, mediates pruritus via H1 and H2 receptors. The superficial C fibers are especially sensitive to histamine release. By binding to 5-HT3 receptors on C fibers, serotonin also plays a role in inducing pruritus. Finally, endogenous opioids also appear to affect itching, potentially through both central and peripheral mechanisms.

Pruritus triggers the urge to scratch through a spinal reflex, and scratching transiently relieves pruritus. However, persistent scratching can worsen pruritus and lead to more serious consequences, such as skin breakdown and infection. Pruritus is likely worsened by a variety of factors including dry skin, pain, boredom, or anxiety. Conversely, distraction and competing stimulation of the skin such as by painful stimuli may reduce this symptom.

Opioid-induced pruritus is a common problem in patients treated with systemic opioids. For example, Maxwell and colleagues[382] found that as many as 77% of children who received IV morphine by PCA experienced pruritus. The incidence of pruritus with use of opioids administered via the spine is also high, occurring in 20% to 90% of patients, particularly in the postoperative setting. The incidence of itching with spinal opioids appears lower in opioid-tolerant patients who have advanced cancer.[507] Whereas the itching associated with systemic opioids is usually widespread, the itching observed with spinal opioids tends to be more segmental.[505]

Although opioids do cause histamine release from mast cells, this phenomenon does not seem to account for most of the pruritus attributed to opioids, for several reasons. First, fentanyl does not cause histamine release, but it may still cause pruritus.[507] Second, opioids administered via the spine (e.g., morphine in doses up to fiftyfold lower than those used systemically) can produce intense and prolonged itching despite evoking negligible peripheral histamine release. Third, as will be detailed later, antihistamines are much less effective for opioid-induced itching compared with interventions that influence opioid-receptor coupling to G-protein–mediated intracellular actions. Possible explanations for opioid-induced pruritus include central activation of itch centers, activation of serotonergic pathways, and opioid-receptor–mediated activation of G-stimulatory proteins.

Interventions

Effective control of pruritus is important to provide comfort, improve quality of life, and prevent potential worsening of any underlying dermatologic condition or complications, such as infection. Treatment should be targeted to the suspected underlying cause, if possible. For example, the most effective treatment for pruritus resulting from Hodgkin lymphoma is cancer-directed therapy. Similarly, stenting of the bile duct, if clinically appropriate, is the most effective treatment for cholestatic pruritus. Depending on the degree and extent of involvement, pruritic GVHD may be treated with systemic immunosuppression, topical steroids, or topical tacrolimus.[508] Pruritus from histamine-mediated reactions (e.g., allergic reactions) often responds to antihistamines such as diphenhydramine. These agents should not be used indiscriminately or without regard for the underlying cause because they may contribute to mental status changes such as sedation, confusion, and delirium.

Antihistamines are typically ineffective in persons with cholestatic or uremic pruritus. Cholestyramine is effective in reducing pruritus associated with cholestasis, presumably by binding bile salts or other accumulated pruritogens. Randomized placebo-controlled trials have shown that cholestatic pruritus is relieved by naloxone or its oral equivalent, naltrexone, perhaps through opioid receptors thought be activated in this clinical condition.[509-511] Ondansetron may also reduce itch from cholestasis.[512-514] Cholestatic pruritus has also been reported to respond to midazolam in the absence of sedation, with the effect purportedly achieved through increased γ-aminobutyric activity.[515] For uremic pruritus, studies have yielded conflicting results for both the efficacy of ondansetron[516,517] and naltrexone.[518,519] Uremic and postburn pruritus, both considered forms of neuropathic itch, are relieved with use of either gabapentin or pregabalin.[520,521]

Biologic cancer treatments, such as epidermal growth factor receptor inhibitors, commonly cause pruritus. A single published study supports the use of aprepitant (125 mg on day 1 and 80 mg daily on days 2 and 3) for pruritus associated with erlotinib.[2] It is hypothesized that neuropeptide substance P activates mast cells in the lesional skin of persons who are treated with erlotinib, and because it is an NK-1 receptor antagonist, aprepitant may ameliorate itch.[522]

Interventions for Opioid-Associated Pruritus

Despite the widespread use of antihistamines for treatment of opioid-induced pruritus, data on their effectiveness in this setting are remarkably sparse, and some randomized controlled trials indicate lack of effectiveness.[523] One study found that hydroxyzine was superior to placebo in a postoperative setting, but most other trials have shown no differences between antihistamines and placebo.[523] Similarly, we have been unable to identify any trials showing effectiveness of the less-sedating antihistamines, such as cetirizine, fexofenadine, or loratadine, for opioid-induced itching.

Several studies, including a prospective, randomized controlled trial in children and adolescents receiving postoperative analgesia with a morphine PCA, have shown that low-dose naloxone infusions (0.25 µg/kg/h) reduce opioid-induced pruritus, and to a lesser extent nausea, without increasing opioid requirements or pain scores.[381,382,524] More recently, a prospective dose-finding study found a higher naloxone dose (1 µg/kg/h) to be more consistently effective in preventing opioid-induced adverse effects.[383] When low-dose naloxone infusions and

nalbuphine are used to treat itching in patients who are quite opioid-tolerant, some uncertainty exists regarding whether to begin with lower or higher infusion rates or doses, but the 1 µg/kg/h rate appears to be appropriate for this population as well.

Systemic opioid-induced pruritus may be addressed by opioid rotation.[525] In one study of 90 children receiving morphine, hydromorphone, or fentanyl for postoperative pain, it was found that pruritus was more severe in the morphine group.[526] To our knowledge, however, no other studies have demonstrated superiority of one opioid over another in terms of pruritus.

Low-dose systemic infusions of opioid antagonists are widely used for patients receiving opioids administered via epidural and spinal routes. Nalbuphine is a mixed-agonist antagonist that is widely used to treat itching (as well as nausea and other adverse effects) from systemic and neuraxial opioids. A common dosing schedule is 0.01 to 0.02 mg/kg IV every 6 hours, to a maximum total dose of 1.5 mg. Note that these doses are fivefold to tenfold lower than the starting doses recommended when nalbuphine is administered as an analgesic.

Ondansetron has been shown to reduce systemic opioid-associated scratching, although the reduction in opioid-induced itching was not statistically significant.[527] Ondansetron reduces pruritus from intrathecal morphine,[528-530] although the mixed opioid agonist nalbuphine may be superior to ondansetron for this purpose.[531]

Our clinical impression, unconfirmed by data, is that pruritus is a more significant problem in the initial weeks of opioid use and that for many patients with advanced cancer who are receiving escalating doses of opioids, pruritus becomes less problematic as opioid tolerance progresses.

Topical Approaches

Any potential skin irritants such as perfumed skin products and harsh detergents should be avoided. When dry skin is thought to compound itching, application of a moisturizer may be helpful. Medicated baths containing oatmeal or baking soda, as well as the application of ice or cold compresses, may quell the itching sensation. Topical agents such as capsaicin (0.025% cream) or Sarna lotion containing camphor and menthol may also soothe skin. Successful use of topical naltrexone to relieve pruritus in persons with atopic dermatitis has recently been reported, suggesting that opioid receptors are involved in a variety of pruritic conditions, although this strategy remains experimental at this point.[532]

Other Potential Therapies for Pruritus

Several antidepressants have been used to treat pruritus. In adult dermatology practice, TCAs, especially doxepin, are widely used. TCAs appear to reduce itch and pain due to postherpetic neuralgia. Paroxetine has been implicated in providing relief from pruritus in a variety of situations, including paraneoplastic itch, opioid-induced itch, and pruritus associated with polycythemia vera. In a small randomized controlled trial of 26 patients with pruritus from a variety of nondermatologic causes, Zylicz[532a] found that one third of patients experienced a modest improvement in pruritus with paroxetine, although it was not reported which patients benefited. In addition, some patients received concurrent cisapride, a 5-HT3 receptor antagonist, which could have accounted for the improvement in pruritus through serotonergic mechanisms.[533] The antidepressant mirtazapine, which has 5-HT2, 5-HT3, H1 antagonist, and noradrenergic activity, was reported to ameliorate pruritus in a case series of four patients with either cholestatic, uremic, or paraneoplastic pruritus. It is unclear whether it is serotonergic blockage at the peripheral or central level that reduces pruritus or whether sedation per se contributed to its efficacy. Other medications used for neuropathic pain, such as anticonvulsants and systemic local anesthetics, have also occasionally been used for patients with refractory pruritus.

MOOD DISORDERS AND MENTAL STATUS CHANGES

Depression

Children with cancer may experience depression that predates their cancer diagnosis or develops after their cancer diagnosis. The reported prevalence of depression in children with cancer varies, likely because of differences in assessment techniques and the populations studied. In general, it does not appear that children with cancer have more psychological symptoms, including depression, than do other children.[534-536] For example, Noll and colleagues[535] found no significant differences in measures of depression, anxiety, or loneliness between children with cancer and their classroom peers. Psychologists have proposed that the similarity in depression diagnosis rates is due to use of avoidant or repressive styles of coping with the cancer experience.[537,538]

Physical symptoms stemming from cancer or its treatment can also occur in people with depression and in fact may be diagnostic criteria for depression. Adults diagnosed with major depression have been shown to have higher rates of such nonspecific symptoms, including fatigue, decreased appetite, and sleep disturbance.[539] Standardized screening measures for healthy children have not been validated in the pediatric oncology population. Clinicians may find it helpful to rely on psychological symptoms such as guilt, hopelessness, worthlessness, or anhedonia to make the diagnosis of depression. However, clinicians have been demonstrated to underestimate psychosocial symptoms such as depression and anxiety in children with cancer.[540]

Risk factors for the development of depression in children with cancer include perceived stress, lack of social support, not receiving open information about their diagnosis and prognosis at the initial stage of the disease, and parental anxiety.[537,541,542] Cancer survivors are also at risk for depression.[543,544] For example, adolescents who had cancer as children are 1.5 times more likely to have depression or anxiety[544] and are at higher risk for suicidal ideation than are their siblings.[545] Depression in this case may be due to impaired social functioning as a result of cancer or its treatment.[543]

Oncologists play a crucial role in screening patients for psychological disorders and for implementing first-line treatments for depression and anxiety (described later). Involvement of a psychosocial team is crucial. Most oncologists prescribe selective serotonin reuptake inhibitors (SSRIs), although some only do so in conjunction with a mental health consultation for the child.[546] Options for medical interventions for depression include TCAs, SSRIs, and newer selective serotonin norepinephrine reuptake inhibitors. TCAs are rarely used for depression because of their anticholinergic adverse effects and the lack of efficacy data in children. SSRIs appear to be the most commonly prescribed class of antidepressants in children with cancer.[547,548]

No particular antidepressant has been demonstrated to be superior to another in the pediatric cancer population. Instead, the choice of antidepressant should be determined by the characteristics, including adverse effect profiles, of different agents. For example, mirtazapine may be an optimal agent for a child with anorexia or difficulty sleeping. Likewise, a TCA may be the treatment of choice for a child with concomitant neuropathic pain. A modest increase in suicidal ideation has been noted in studies evaluating children treated with SSRIs compared with placebo.[549] The FDA now requires labeling of all antidepressants to warn clinicians of such a risk.[550] Although the meaning of the increased risk is unclear, initiation of an antidepressant warrants discussion of the risks and benefits with families and close monitoring of children for worsening depression or signs of suicidality. Some medications such as tramadol, triptans, and linezolid interact with SSRIs, increasing the risk of serotonin syndrome. Children with depression who do not respond to these measures, and children with suicidal ideation or complex psychological symptoms, should be referred for formal psychiatric evaluation.

Evaluation of screening for depression, longitudinal studies of mood disorders and their predictors, and prospective evaluation of interventions for children with cancer and depressive symptoms are clearly needed to better understand and ameliorate depression in children with cancer.

Anxiety

Children with cancer may experience anxiety that is situation-dependent (e.g., related to treatment). Such anxiety may respond to anxiolytic medications administered prior to treatment, as well as cognitive or behavioral interventions. Such nonpharmacologic interventions are described in more detail in the section on pain. Other types of anxiety in children should be approached with an exploration of potentially contributing factors (e.g., stress related to family or school) and referral for increased psychosocial support. A child with anxiety who meets the criteria for a psychiatric anxiety disorder (e.g., generalized anxiety disorder and panic disorder) or a child whose anxiety significantly impairs his or her function should be referred for psychiatric evaluation.

Delirium

Delirium is a state of disturbed consciousness or level of arousal characterized by an inability to focus or to maintain or divert attention. Delirium has a rapid onset and results in significant confusion for the patient. Delirious patients may have mumbling speech, perceptual disturbances with delusion or hallucinations, or alterations in their sleep/wake cycle. Patients may exhibit hyperalert-hyperactive delirium with anxiety, agitation, or even aggression. Alternatively, patients may have hypoalert-hypoactive delirium, characterized by slowed reactions and difficulty focusing. Delirium is a disturbing symptom for patients and may be extremely distressing for caregivers.[551]

Delirium may be caused by metabolic disturbances (e.g., hypoglycemia or electrolyte abnormalities), CNS pathology, liver or kidney dysfunction, infection, constipation, or urinary obstruction. The most common cause of delirium is a drug effect. The most common offending medications are anticholinergics, corticosteroids, benzodiazepines, and opioids. For this reason, delirium should never be treated with escalation of opioid therapy unless uncontrolled pain is suspected. Instead, the opioid dose should be decreased if possible or converted to an alternative opioid. In addition, psychoactive medications should be discontinued, if possible, and a neuroleptic such as haloperidol should be inititated. In fact, a randomized controlled trial of haloperidol versus chlorpromazine or lorazepam for adults with human immunodeficiency virus and delirium was halted early because of adverse effects in the lorazepam arm. Haloperidol should be initiated by dose escalation similar to the process used for treating pain.

Atypical antipsychotic medications have also been used successfully in adults with delirium, although no trials comparing them with haloperidol have been performed.[552] For delirium with significant agitation, benzodiazepines may be considered, but they may cause paradoxic exacerbation of symptoms. Regardless of the pharmacologic agent used, concomitant nonpharmacologic interventions should always be used as well. Measures to reduce stimulation in the environment or to orient the patient, such as a familiar person remaining with the patient and frequent orientation to time and place, may be helpful.

Corticosteroid-Induced Mood and Behavior Disturbance

Psychiatric abnormalities including depression, mania, hypomania, and psychosis, as well as cognitive changes due to corticosteroid therapy, are well described. Among children with ALL, both dexamethasone and prednisone are associated with neurobehavioral adverse effects, and preschool-aged children appear to be at greater risk for these effects.[553] Such alterations are reversible with dose reduction or discontinuation of treatment. However, dose reduction or discontinuation of corticosteroids administered for antineoplastic purposes, as in therapy for ALL, may not be possible. Reports of successful use of olanzapine or promethazine for steroid-associated psychosis or mood disturbance have been published. Risperidone also appears to be an effective short-term pharmacologic agent for corticosteroid-related mood disturbance or psychosis related to corticosteroid treatment for ALL.[554]

References available online at ExpertConsult.

KEY REFERENCES

3. Collins JJ, Byrnes ME, Dunkel IJ, et al: The measurement of symptoms in children with cancer. *J Pain Symptom Manage* 19(5):363–377, 2000.
   This article describes the development and psychometric testing of the Memorial Symptom Assessment Scale, a widely used symptom assessment scale for children 10 to 18 years of age who have cancer.

5. Wolfe J, Grier HE, Klar N, et al: Symptoms and suffering at the end of life in children with cancer. *N Engl J Med* 342(5):326–333, 2000.
   This seminal article describes the symptoms and suffering experienced by children with advanced cancer from the perspective of a large cohort of bereaved parents.

7. Goldman A, Hewitt M, Collins GS, et al: Symptoms in children/young people with progressive malignant disease: United Kingdom Children's Cancer Study Group/Paediatric Oncology Nurses Forum Survey. *Pediatrics* 117(6):e1179–e1186, 2006.
   Using self-report data from 164 children and adolescents with progressive cancer, the investigators report symptoms experienced by children and adolescents with cancer. Symptoms included some that are often unrecognized, including anorexia, weight loss, and weakness. The prevalence and nature of symptoms experienced varied between cancer types.

9. National Institutes of Health: State-of-the-science statement on symptom management in cancer: pain, depression, and fatigue. *NIH Consens State Sci Statements* 19(4):1–29, 2002.
   This statement by a multidisciplinary panel summarizes available evidence regarding the symptoms of cancer-related pain, depression, and fatigue.

12. Anand KJ, Hickey PR: Pain and its effects in the human neonate and fetus. *N Engl J Med* 317(21):1321–1329, 1987.
    This article presents evidence that nociceptive activity is present in the neonate and fetus, a relatively novel opinion at the time, and calls for humane considerations to be factored into the decisions regarding analgesic and anesthetic techniques even in young, nonverbal patients.

16. World Health Organization: *WHO guidelines on the pharmacological treatment of persisting pain in children with medical illnesses,* Geneva, Switzerland, 2012, World Health Organization.
    These guidelines present an approach to the pharmacologic treatment of pain in children with medical illness, including the recently revised analgesic ladder (which now has two rather than three steps).

22. Franck LS, Greenberg CS, Stevens B: Pain assessment in infants and children. *Pediatr Clin North Am* 47(3):487–512, 2000.
    This review presents the wide-ranging considerations to be included in the assessment of pain in infants and children.

41. Solodiuk J, Curley MA: Pain assessment in nonverbal children with severe cognitive impairments: the Individualized Numeric Rating Scale (INRS). *J Pediatr Nurs* 18(4):295–299, 2003.
    This article presents a novel pain assessment tool for nonverbal children, which could also be used in assessment of pain in children with cancer who are preverbal or nonverbal with cognitive impairment.

51. Smith AW, Bellizzi KM, Keegan TH, et al: Health-related quality of life of adolescent and young adult patients with cancer in the United States: The Adolescent and Young Adult Health Outcomes and Patient Experience Study. *J Clin Oncol* 31(17):2136–2145, 2013.
    This article presents findings from the Adolescent and Young Adult Health Outcomes and Patient Experience (AYA HOPE) study, involving a cohort of 523 AYA patients with cancer. AYAs had significant decrements in physical and mental health–related quality of life domains and experienced higher levels of fatigue.

55. Michelet D, Andreu-Gallien J, Bensalah T, et al: A meta-analysis of the use of nonsteroidal antiinflammatory drugs for pediatric postoperative pain. *Anesth Analg* 114(2):393–406, 2012.
    This meta-analysis provides definitive evidence that perioperative nonsteroidal antiinflammatory drugs reduce opioid consumption and result in less postoperative nausea and vomiting. Although

the study is based in the postoperative setting, clinicians in other scenarios in which nonsteroidal antiinflammatory drugs are a viable option should consider their use, given their opioid-sparing effect.

56. Ceelie I, de Wildt SN, van Dijk M, et al: Effect of intravenous paracetamol on postoperative morphine requirements in neonates and infants undergoing major noncardiac surgery: a randomized controlled trial. *JAMA* 309(2):149–154, 2013.

This randomized controlled trial demonstrated that infants undergoing major surgery who received intermittent intravenous paracetamol required less morphine for analgesia than did those in the placebo group, providing evidence that paracetamol may also be opioid-sparing.

62. Collins JJ, Grier HE, Kinney HC, et al: Control of severe pain in children with terminal malignancy. *J Pediatr* 126(4):653–657, 1995.

In this retrospective medical record review it was found that standard dosing of opioids controls cancer-related pain in most children, although a group requiring massive opioid infusions exists and is associated with solid tumors metastatic to the spine and major nerves.

69. Williams DG, Patel A, Howard RF: Pharmacogenetics of codeine metabolism in an urban population of children and its implications for analgesic reliability. *Br J Anaesth* 89(6):839–845, 2002.

This United Kingdom–based study demonstrated that reduced ability to metabolize codeine to morphine (due to genetic variation in the cytochrome P450 enzyme CYP2D6) is relatively common. This finding suggests that codeine may provide unreliable analgesia for a significant number of children.

70. Clark E, Plint AC, Correll R, et al: A randomized, controlled trial of acetaminophen, ibuprofen, and codeine for acute pain relief in children with musculoskeletal trauma. *Pediatrics* 119(3):460–467, 2007.

In this randomized, controlled trial comparing acetaminophen, ibuprofen, and codeine for relief of pain in children with musculoskeletal injury, ibuprofen provided a significant decrease in pain score, and neither codeine nor acetaminophen provided adequate analgesia.

111. Berde CB, Lehn BM, Yee JD, et al: patient-controlled analgesia in children and adolescents: a randomized, prospective comparison with intramuscular administration of morphine for postoperative analgesia. *J Pediatr* 118(3):460–466, 1991.

This randomized prospective comparison of morphine patient-controlled analgesia (PCA) and PCA with continuous morphine infusion found that PCA is a safe and effective method of postoperative pain relief in children and adolescents.

114. Anghelescu DL, Faughnan LG, Oakes LL, et al: Parent-controlled PCA for pain management in pediatric oncology: is it safe? *J Pediatr Hematol Oncol* 34(6):416–420, 2012.

This retrospective review of self-administered patient-controlled analgesia (PCA), nurse-controlled PCA, and parent-controlled PCA found that parent-controlled PCA by authorized parents was as safe as the other methods of PCA administration.

149. Wong R, Wiffen PJ: Bisphosphonates for the relief of pain secondary to bone metastases. *Cochrane Database Syst Rev* (2):CD002068, 2002.

This Cochrane review of 30 randomized controlled studies found evidence supporting the use of bisphosphonates for relief of pain from bone metastases and recommended that bisphosphonates be considered, particularly when analgesics or radiotherapy provide inadequate pain control.

159. Smith EM, Pang H, Cirrincione C, et al: Effect of duloxetine on pain, function, and quality of life among patients with chemotherapy-induced painful peripheral neuropathy: a randomized clinical trial. *JAMA* 309(13):1359–1367, 2013.

In this multicenter, randomized, double-blind, placebo-controlled crossover trial it was found that duloxetine therapy resulted in decreased pain in adults who had chemotherapy-induced peripheral neuropathy.

177. Greco C, Berde C: Pain management for the hospitalized pediatric patient. *Pediatr Clin North Am* 52:995–1027, 2005.

This article provides a comprehensive review of pain assessment and treatment in hospitalized children.

215. Bloechl-Daum B, Deuson RR, Mavros P, et al: Delayed nausea and vomiting continue to reduce patients' quality of life after highly and moderately emetogenic chemotherapy despite antiemetic treatment. *J Clin Oncol* 24(27):4472–4478, 2006.

In this study, a multicenter prospective evaluation of adults receiving highly or moderately emetogenic chemotherapy, it was found that even with modern antiemetic therapy, more than half of patients experienced delayed nausea, and that of the adults who did not experience nausea and vomiting during the first 24 hours, 23% experienced delayed nausea and vomiting that affected daily life. Nausea had a stronger negative impact on patients than did vomiting.

224. Tyc VL, Mulhern RK, Barclay DR, et al: Variables associated with anticipatory nausea and vomiting in pediatric cancer patients receiving ondansetron antiemetic therapy. *J Pediatr Psychol* 22(1):45–58, 1997.

This study is one of the few studies to examine anticipatory nausea and vomiting in children with cancer. Children expecting severe postchemotherapy vomiting and those more distressed by nausea and vomiting were more likely to experience anticipatory nausea and vomiting.

248. Mizukami N, Yamauchi M, Koike K, et al: Olanzapine for the prevention of chemotherapy-induced nausea and vomiting in patients receiving highly or moderately emetogenic chemotherapy: a randomized, double-blind, placebo-controlled study. *J Pain Symptom Manage* 47(3):542–550, 2014.

This randomized, double-blind, placebo-controlled trial of adults receiving highly or moderately emetogenic chemotherapy and antiemetic therapy with a 5-hydroxytryptamine 3 receptor antagonist, steroid, and neurokinin-1 receptor antagonist compared patients who also received 5 mg/day olanzapine with patients who received placebo. The olanzapine group reported a higher rate of total control of vomiting, less nausea, and higher quality of life.

294. Basch E, Prestrud AA, Hesketh PJ, et al: Antiemetics: American Society of Clinical Oncology clinical practice guideline update. *J Clin Oncol* 29(31):4189–4198, 2011.

This update to the American Society of Clinical Oncology clinical practice guidelines, although not specific to the pediatric population, addresses equivalency of the neurokinin-1 receptor antagonists fosaprepitant and aprepitant and includes recommendations regarding selection of 5-hydroxytryptamine 3 receptor antagonists and management of patients undergoing radiation therapy with a high risk of emesis.

324. McCrea JB, Majumdar AK, Goldberg MR, et al: Effects of the neurokinin1 receptor antagonist aprepitant on the pharmacokinetics of dexamethasone and methylprednisolone. *Clin Pharmacol Ther* 74(1):17–24, 2003.

This study evaluated the effect of coadministration of aprepitant with dexamethasone or methylprednisolone and determined that aprepitant resulted in increased plasma concentrations of both corticosteroids, suggesting that in the setting of coadministration with aprepitant, the corticosteroid dose should be decreased.

327. de Wit R, Herrstedt J, Rapoport B, et al: Addition of the oral NK1 antagonist aprepitant to standard antiemetics provides protection against nausea and vomiting during multiple cycles of cisplatin-based chemotherapy. *J Clin Oncol* 21(22):4105–4111, 2003.

Given the concern that patients receiving cisplatin-based chemotherapy are at risk for a decreased response rate after repeated cycles of chemotherapy, this study evaluated patients who received aprepitant in addition to a standard antiemetic regimen. Study results indicate that patients who received aprepitant had better and more sustained protection against chemotherapy-induced nausea and vomiting over the course of multiple cycles.

410. Yuan CS, Foss JF, O'Connor M, et al: Methylnaltrexone for reversal of constipation due to chronic methadone use: a randomized controlled trial. *JAMA* 283(3):367–372, 2000.

This randomized controlled trial was one of the first to demonstrate that methylnaltrexone can reverse opioid-associated constipation. Administration of intravenous methylnaltrexone induced laxation and reversed the slowing of oral cecal–transit time by opioids.

456. Vogelzang NJ, Breitbart W, Cella D, et al: Patient, caregiver, and oncologist perceptions of cancer-related fatigue: results of a tripart assessment survey. The Fatigue Coalition. *Semin Hematol* 34(3 Suppl 2):4–12, 1997.

This survey-based study demonstrates the need for increased oncologist awareness and appreciation of the impact of cancer-related fatigue on patients. Despite its impact, patients often do not discuss fatigue with their oncologist and believe it is a symptom to be endured. This study highlights the multiple opportunities that may exist for improving care for patients with cancer-related fatigue.

458. Curt GA, Breitbart W, Cella D, et al: Impact of cancer-related fatigue on the lives of patients: new findings from the Fatigue Coalition. *Oncologist* 5(5):353–360, 2000.

This study describes the prevalence and impact of fatigue on adults, including its emotional, social, physical, and economic impact on patients with cancer and their caregivers.

495. Yee JD, Berde CB: Dextroamphetamine or methylphenidate as adjuvants to opioid analgesia for adolescents with cancer. *J Pain Symptom Manage* 9(2):122–125, 1994.

This case series describes the use of psychostimulants to counteract opioid-associated analgesia in children with cancer. The findings were encouraging, and future prospective controlled studies are needed to assess the efficacy and safety of stimulants for this indication.

547. Pao M, Ballard ED, Rosenstein DL, et al: Psychotropic medication use in pediatric patients with cancer. *Arch Pediatr Adolesc Med* 160(8):818–822, 2006.

In this retrospective review of children receiving cancer care it was found that psychotropic medications are commonly prescribed. The review calls attention to the need for trials to evaluate the safety and efficacy of these agents in children with complex medical illness who are experiencing mood disturbance and anxiety.

CHAPTER 72

Childhood Cancer Survivorship

Lynda Vrooman, Lisa Diller, and Lisa B. Kenney

CHAPTER OUTLINE

HISTORY AND OVERVIEW	Renal System
Recognition of Late Effects	Genitourinary System
Early Mortality	Gastrointestinal System
Identifying Risk Factors for Late Effects	**OTHER LATE EFFECTS**
Interpreting Late Effects Research	Infections
General Principles of Late Effects	Dental Problems
SECOND CANCERS	Psychosocial Function
Secondary Solid Tumors	**SPECIAL CONSIDERATIONS FOR THE**
Hematologic Malignancies	**HEMATOPOIETIC STEM CELL TRANSPLANT**
ORGAN SYSTEM LATE EFFECTS	**SURVIVOR**
Cardiovascular System	**FOLLOW-UP CARE OF CHILDHOOD CANCER**
Pulmonary System	**SURVIVORS**
Endocrine System	Models of Survivorship Care
Central Nervous System	Comprehensive Clinical Evaluation
Reproductive System	**FUTURE DIRECTIONS**

With ongoing advances in the diagnosis and treatment of childhood cancers, increasing numbers of children and adolescents diagnosed with cancer are becoming long-term survivors. However, even as higher cure rates are achieved, there is increasing recognition that the diagnosis and treatment of cancer during childhood and adolescence can have lifelong implications for health and well-being. Cancer therapy administered during critical periods of growth and development render childhood cancer survivors vulnerable to a variety of physical and emotional disorders often referred to as "late effects." Some late effects can be diagnosed soon after completion of cancer-directed therapy, and others may not manifest until decades later. The severity of late effects ranges from minor disabilities to chronic conditions and even life-threatening morbidities, including second cancers, cardiac disease, and pulmonary dysfunction. Severe late effects can reduce a survivor's life expectancy.

Although remarkable progress has been made in advancing our understanding of the adverse health outcomes associated with treatment of childhood cancer, survivors continue to experience significant long-term morbidity related to late effects. Increasingly it is recognized that the care of the child or adolescent diagnosed with cancer does not end with the completion of therapy but continues on the path into adulthood. Clinical focus during survivorship care shifts from treatment of the primary cancer and screening for its recurrence to the prevention, detection, and management of adverse consequences of prior therapy. Ultimately, ongoing research may result in the reduction or even elimination of late effects and in improved quality of life for childhood cancer survivors.

HISTORY AND OVERVIEW

Prior to 1950, children and adolescents who developed cancer rarely survived. The first generation of survivors primarily consisted of children with Hodgkin lymphoma, sarcoma, and Wilms tumor who were successfully treated with surgery and high-dose, large-field radiation therapy.[1-4] The widespread use of multiagent chemotherapy, beginning in the 1970s, resulted in dramatic increases in survival for the most common childhood cancer, acute

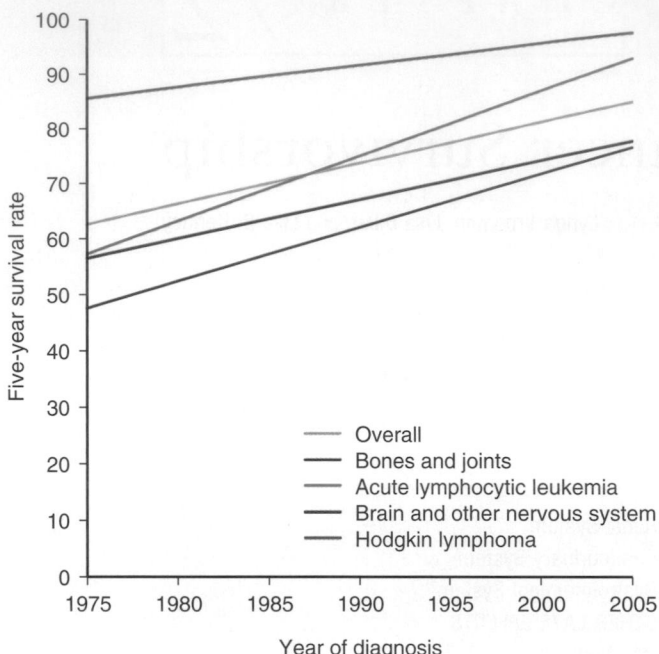

Five-year survival rate

— Overall
— Bones and joints
— Acute lymphocytic leukemia
— Brain and other nervous system
— Hodgkin lymphoma

Year of diagnosis

Note: Data represent linear trendline.
Surveillance, Epidemiology, and End Results (SEER) Program (www.seer.cancer.gov)

Figure 72-1 Trends in 5-year cancer survival by selected diagnosis, age younger than 20 years, 1975 to 2005. *(Data from Howlader N, Noone AM, Krapcho M, et al, editors: SEER cancer statistics review, 1975-2010. Bethesda, Maryland, National Cancer Institute. Accessed at http://seer.cancer.gov/csr/1975_2010/. Modified from November 2012 SEER data submission, posted to the SEER website, April 2013.)*

leukemia, and continued improvement in survival for other pediatric cancers as well.[5] By the mid-1970s, many forms of childhood cancer became treatable, and potentially curable. Continuing advances in treatment options for childhood cancer have continued to improved survival. Children with cancer have also benefited from improvements in diagnostic testing, resulting in earlier and more precise diagnosis and more timely delivery of necessary treatment. Enhanced supportive care including advances in intensive care, blood banking, and management of infectious disease and acute toxicities of therapy also contributed to successful outcomes. Currently, the overall 5-year survival for childhood cancer exceeds 80%, and for some cancer diagnoses 5-year survival is above 95% (Fig. 72-1).[6] There are estimated to be more than 300,000 adult survivors of childhood cancer in the U.S. population, and this number continues to grow by approximately 10,000 survivors each year.[7]

Recognition of Late Effects

Along with these remarkable advances in survival there is a growing recognition that treatment for childhood cancer is associated with long-term complications or "late effects." Late effects can be defined as adverse health outcomes experienced by childhood cancer survivors associated with previous cancer–directed therapy;

these outcomes reduce survival or affect the "quality" of survival. Some late effects can be life threatening and contribute to the increased risk for early mortality observed in adults who are long-term survivors of childhood cancer. Other late effects, such as neurocognitive impairment, physical deformity, and infertility, can limit survivors' social or economic opportunities and impair their overall quality of life. In contrast, some late effects may be "positive" effects, such as increase in psychological resiliency and decrease in smoking rates and the rates of other high-risk behaviors compared with those in the rest of the population.[8,9]

Second cancers, cardiopulmonary disease, and infertility were among the first treatment-associated late effects recognized in childhood cancer survivors. These first descriptions were based on clinical observations in small numbers of the earliest survivors of childhood cancer treated primarily with surgery and irradiation in the 1960s.[10-12] Early clinical observations created awareness about late effects and identified the need for further research defining treatment-related health outcomes in the growing numbers of survivors of childhood cancer.

Early Mortality

Follow-up studies of the earliest cohorts led to the observation that childhood cancer survivors are at risk for early mortality. These studies showed that late recurrence of the primary cancer and treatment-associated complications resulted in decreased long-term survival, 80% at 20 years after diagnosis compared with 97% expected survival in the age-matched general population.[13,14] The majority of premature deaths observed in survivors in these early studies were attributed to late relapse, whereas treatment-associated second cancers and major organ toxicity accounted for 30% of deaths.[13-16] It was also recognized that the risk for dying of a treatment-related cause increased with increasing intensity of therapy.[15,16] Although late recurrence accounts for the majority of premature deaths observed in childhood cancer survivors, the risk for relapse diminishes over time while the risk for therapy-related mortality persists beyond 25 years of follow-up.[17-21] Figure 72-2 depicts all-cause mortality in 5-year survivors of childhood cancer, and Figure 72-3 demonstrates all-cause mortality by underlying cancer diagnosis.[21] It remains to be determined if current treatment protocols that are specifically designed to reduce late effects will continue to improve very long-term survival by reducing the risk for therapy-related mortality.

Identifying Risk Factors for Late Effects

After the early descriptive studies, registry-based investigations of larger groups of childhood cancer survivors were undertaken with the aim of identifying specific risk factors for late effects. These included the National Cancer Institute's "Five Center Study," a registry-based cohort that enrolled 2490 adult 5-year survivors diagnosed with cancer between 1945 and 1975 at age younger than 20 years who were followed prospectively for reproductive outcomes, second cancers, and mortality[22]; the "Late Effects Study Group," a multiinstitutional cohort that analyzed the occurrence of second cancers in 9170

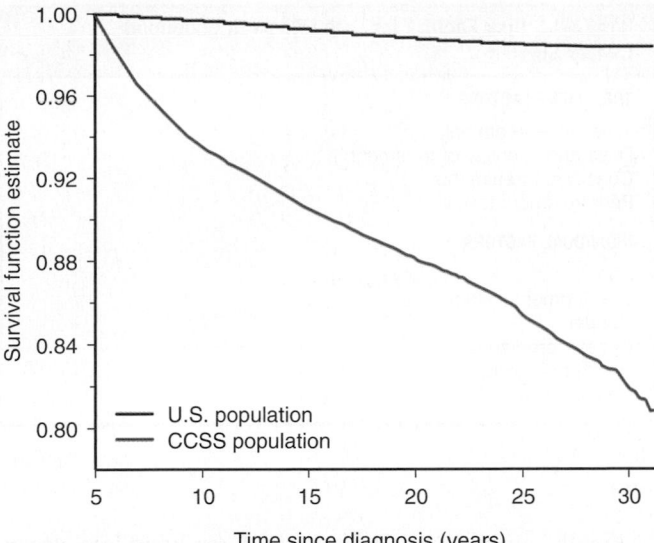

Figure 72-2 All-cause mortality in 5-year survivors of childhood cancer diagnosed from 1970 to 1986, age younger than 21 years. *(From Armstrong GT, Liu Q, Yasui Y, et al: Late mortality among 5-year survivors of childhood cancer: a summary from the Childhood Cancer Survivor Study.* J Clin Oncol 27:2328–2338, 2009).

two-year survivors of childhood cancer diagnosed between 1936 and 1979[23]; and cancer registry–based studies in the United Kingdom,[24] the Netherlands,[25] and the Nordic countries (Denmark, Finland, Iceland, Norway, Sweden)[26] from the same early treatment era and beyond. These epidemiologic studies analyzed the association between specific treatments and adverse health outcomes of interest. Relative risks were calculated to compare rates of outcomes under study in cancer survivors with rates in a control population. Collectively these investigations made significant contributions to the understanding of late effects. Limitations of such studies of late-occurring outcomes included that recruitment was often not complete, resulting in a possible overrepresentation of childhood cancer survivors who were experiencing health conditions related to their prior therapy. In addition, some of the late effects observed in these cohorts were associated with historic treatments that have been replaced by more modern modalities. However, despite such limitations, these studies identified the relationships, now well accepted, between cancer therapy and early mortality, radiation therapy and secondary cancers, and alkylating agents and gonadal dysfunction.[16,22,27,28]

To address the limitations of prior studies, the development of "survivor" cohorts to be followed prospectively was undertaken by investigators in North America and Europe. In North America, a multiinstitutional follow-up study of a cohort of over 14,000 childhood cancer survivors (the Childhood Cancer Survivor Study [CCSS]) was created, evaluating late effects in survivors diagnosed from 1970 to1986, at age younger than 21 years, and surviving at least 5 years from diagnosis.[29] A recent expansion of the CCSS to include survivors treated between 1986 and 1999 will yield important analyses of the effects of more "modern" therapies, as well as reflect

a more ethnically and racially diverse population in North America.[30] The CCSS uses self-reported questionnaires to obtain health outcomes and analyzes the association between outcome and treatment variables documented in abstracted medical records. The primary end points investigated by the CCSS included second cancers, mortality, and heart disease. Large registry-based cohort studies of childhood cancer survivors treated in Great Britain, France, the Netherlands, and the Nordic countries are ongoing and continue to contribute to our understanding of survivorship.[20,31-33] Within these cohort studies, the prevalence of and the risk factors for the development of late effects after childhood cancer have been better elucidated.

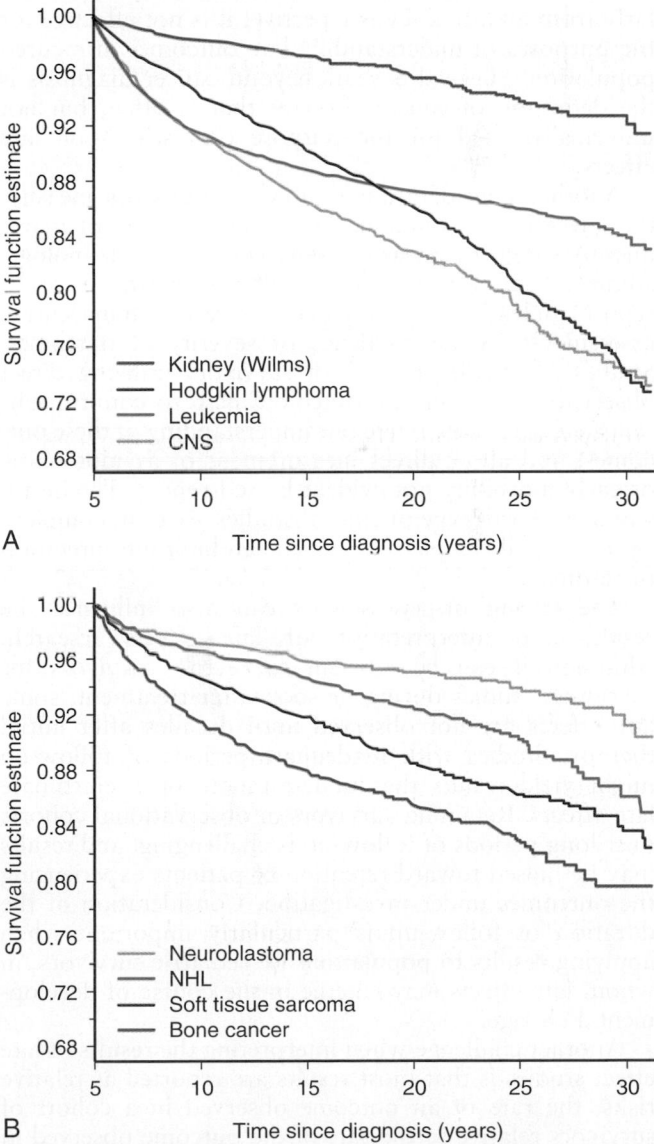

Figure 72-3 A and B, All causes of mortality, 5-year survivors of childhood cancer diagnosed 1970 to 1986, age younger than 21 years, by original cancer diagnosis. *CNS*, Central nervous system; *NHL*, non-Hodgkin lymphoma. *(From Armstrong GT, Liu Q, Yasui Y, et al: Late mortality among 5-year survivors of childhood cancer: a summary from the Childhood Cancer Survivor Study.* J Clin Oncol 27:2328–2338, 2009.)

Interpreting Late Effects Research

Advances continue to be made in recognizing and categorizing adverse health outcomes in childhood cancer survivors. However, the study of late effects in cancer survivors has inherent challenges that must be considered when interpreting research findings. First, there is not universal implementation of a definition for "cancer survivor." The definition chosen for a particular investigation determines eligibility for studies and dictates how results can be interpreted and generalized to specific populations of survivors. The Office of Cancer Survivorship at the U.S. National Cancer Institute considers an individual a cancer survivor from the moment of cancer diagnosis through the balance of his or her life regardless of degree of cancer control.[34] Although this definition is meaningful, particularly from an advocacy perspective, it is not effective for the purposes of understanding late outcomes in a cured population. Survival 5 years beyond cancer diagnosis is the definition of cancer survivor that is often, but not universally, used for the purpose of research on late effects.

Another consideration is how investigators measure the late effect or outcome of interest. Self-report is frequently used to measure outcomes in epidemiologic studies of late effects. Although it is cost-effective, self-report can lead to reporting bias that results in inaccurate assessments of the incidence or severity of outcomes. Studies of smaller groups of survivors utilizing direct observation to delineate outcomes help to confirm self-reported outcomes, refine our understanding of these outcomes, and allow direct measurement of asymptomatic or early morbidity not evident by self-report. The disadvantages of this type of clinical studies are cost, complexity, and small sample size, which can limit interpretation of results.

The timing of assessments can also influence the results and interpretation of late effects research. Although it can be efficient to recruit survivors for follow-up studies during or soon after treatment, some late effects are not observed until decades after initial therapy. Studies with inadequate periods of follow-up might yield results that underestimate or overestimate late effects. Retaining survivors in observational cohorts over long periods of follow-up is challenging, and results may be biased toward retention of patients experiencing the outcomes under investigation. Consideration of the duration of follow-up is particularly important when applying results to populations of pediatric survivors, in whom late effects may emerge in the course of developmental change.

Another challenge when interpreting the results of late effect studies is that most results are reported as relative risks, the rate of an outcome observed in a cohort of survivors relative to the rate of the outcome observed in a control population. Elevated relative risks must be interpreted and communicated with caution, because even the smallest increase in an otherwise very rare outcome results in a very large relative risk; however, even a small or statistically insignificant increase in relative risk might have important clinical implications.

> **Box 72-1   Risk Factors for Late Effects in Childhood Cancer Survivors**
>
> **TREATMENT FACTORS**
>
> Time since treatment
> Dose and intensity of treatment
> Concurrent treatments
> Prior treatment toxicities
>
> **INDIVIDUAL FACTORS**
>
> Age
> Developmental stage
> Gender
> Genetic predisposition
> Health behaviors
> Comorbidities

Finally, an inherent difficulty with studying late effects is that treatments for cancer continue to evolve; therefore the health outcomes of interest in follow-up studies are often reflective of historic or outdated treatments. Methodology does not exist to address this issue, so treatment era must be taken into consideration when interpreting the results of these investigations. Duration of follow-up, treatment era, cohort eligibility, and outcome measures are all aspects of study design that merit careful consideration when interpreting results of late effects research studies.

General Principles of Late Effects

Epidemiologic studies investigating the association between treatment and risk for adverse health outcomes have led to general principles that contribute to our thinking about an individual survivor's potential for developing late effects (Box 72-1). A childhood cancer survivor's risk for developing late effects depends on the nature of prior treatment as well as individual characteristics, such as age at exposure, gender, or time since exposure.

First, the dose and intensity of the treatment is frequently correlated with risk for late effects. In general, survivors exposed to larger doses of therapy have worse outcomes. For example, risk for male infertility after treatment with gonadotoxic chemotherapy is directly related to dose; males exposed to the highest cumulative doses have the greatest risk for future infertility.[35] In addition, a survivor's likelihood for late effects is increased if there is exposure to more than one modality with related toxicities. For example, survivors treated concurrently with mediastinal radiation and cardiotoxic chemotherapy are at greater risk for cardiac late effects than those treated with either of those modalities alone.[36]

Organ toxicity associated with a single treatment exposure can manifest clinically as different late effects depending on the timing of the clinical assessment. For example, consider a postmenarchal female adolescent treated with gonadotoxic chemotherapy. During treatment she might experience acute reversible amenorrhea. Years later, after resolution of acute menorrhea, the woman might experience infertility secondary to premature menopause.

Over time, the same woman might have osteoporosis as a secondary late effect of chronic estrogen deficiency. Neurocognitive impairment after central nervous system (CNS) therapy provides another example of how the timing of assessment influences detection of late effects. Children treated with CNS therapy might not manifest treatment-related neurocognitive deficits until they reach a time when school work, employment responsibilities, or social interactions require more complex cognitive function. The clinical manifestations of a single treatment exposure can change over time and are influenced by the physical, emotional, and social needs of the individual survivor.

Duration of follow-up also influences the potential for late effects. Some irradiation-associated late effects, especially secondary malignancies, have long latency periods, with increases in cumulative incidence over time. In contrast, other treatment-related toxicities can be acute and resolve (bone marrow suppression) or occur late and be progressive (pulmonary fibrosis). The leukemogenic potentials of specific forms of chemotherapy appear to be associated with fairly discrete time frames after exposures: topoisomerase inhibiters are associated with occurrence of secondary leukemias within months of exposure and rarely beyond 5 years, whereas alkylating agents are associated with a later onset and a later, but still predictable plateau in cumulative incidence at 10 years after exposure.[37] In addition, acute chemotherapy organ toxicity can predict late toxicity. For example, chemotherapy-associated renal toxicity diagnosed during therapy can persist as a chronic condition or resolve and be diagnosed again as chronic renal disease decades after treatment. Although treatment exposures are the largest determinants of future late effects, a survivor's age or developmental stage during cancer treatment and his or her sex, family history, existing comorbidities, and health behaviors can all modulate risk for the development of late effects. In general, younger age at treatment is associated with a higher risk and/or greater severity for late effects. Children treated with cranial irradiation during the critical period of rapid brain development (<2 years old) are at greater risk for neurocognitive late effects than children treated when they are older.[38] In addition, female survivors are at greater risk than males for some late effects, including chemotherapy-associated cardiomyopathy, neurocognitive impairment, and second cancers, although the explanation for this gender difference is not clear.[39-42]

Underlying genetic predisposition for cancer (contributing etiologically to the primary cancer occurrence) will influence the risk for secondary cancers, as has been observed in hereditary retinoblastoma and nevoid basal cell carcinoma syndrome. In some patients, the only marker of this predisposition will be family history or a feature of the primary tumor itself (young age at occurrence, occurrence in paired organs). Predisposition to late effects based on genetic background is an area of great interest in survivorship research. Those survivors with a genetic predisposition to chronic medical conditions, such as heart disease, may be at greater risk for treatment-associated chronic conditions, such as radiation-associated

coronary artery disease.[43] Recent genome-wide association studies have identified risk-specific polymorphisms that may become clinically relevant for predicting the risk for late effects and allow for potential tailoring of primary cancer therapy or follow-up. Most associations that have been described—for example, for ototoxicity after cisplatin exposure[44] or second cancer after irradiation[45]—await further validation. In addition, common medical comorbidities associated with aging, such as hypertension or hypercholesterolemia, may contribute to a survivor's risk for a variety of medical late effects, including chronic renal disease, heart disease, and cerebrovascular disease. Modifiable health behaviors such as diet, exercise, smoking, and sun exposure may also modulate a survivor's risk for late effects.

High rates of chronic health conditions have been described in adult survivors of childhood cancer.[46,47] In the CCSS cohort, the relative risk for a severe or life-threatening chronic condition in survivors when compared with siblings was 8.2 (95% confidence interval [CI], 6.9 to 9.7).[46] In the St. Jude Lifetime Cohort Study, the cumulative prevalence of a chronic condition was 95.5% (9%% CI, 94.8% to 98.6%) by age 45 years and 80.5% (95% CI, 73.0% to 86.6) for a severe or life-threatening or disabling condition.[47] The following section provides an overview of late effects experienced by survivors of childhood cancer. A summary of selected treatment-associated late effects is presented in Table 72-1.

SECOND CANCERS

Second cancers are the leading cause of treatment-related mortality in 5-year survivors. In the CCSS cohort, second cancers accounted for 13% of deaths overall and for 60% of deaths defined as treatment related.[17] Most often, a new cancer diagnosed in a survivor can be associated with a prior treatment exposure, such as radiation therapy or alkylating agent chemotherapy. Genetic cancer predisposition may also contribute to a survivor's risk for subsequent cancers. In addition, survivors, like all aging individuals, develop cancers that are not related to prior treatment or known genetic predisposition and these cancers will become more prevalent as the childhood cancer survivor population ages. To date, there are no data that address the comparative morbidity and mortality from these adult-onset cancers and whether survivors will be compromised in their ability to receive or respond to known effective therapies.

Overall, the likelihood of a childhood cancer survivor being diagnosed with a second primary cancer is three to six times greater than the risk in the aged-matched general population.[33,48-51] At 20 years after diagnosis, the cumulative incidence of second cancers in childhood cancer survivors is estimated at 3.2% to 4.2%.[48-50] In the British Survivorship Cohort, 5% of survivors had developed a secondary cancer by 38 years of age; this cumulative incidence of cancer would be expected at age 54 in a comparable, nonsurvivor population.[33] Clinical and demographic factors that increase the risk for second cancers include primary diagnosis, exposure to radiation, attained age, and chemotherapy with alkylating

TABLE 72-1   Selected Late Effects by Treatment Exposure

Treatment	Late Effect	Comments	Reference
Alkylating agents (busulfan, carmustine, lomustine, mechlorethamine, procarbazine, cyclophosphamide, ifosfamide, dacarbazine, melphalan)	Secondary leukemia/ myelodysplasia	Melphalan and mechlorethamine more leukemogenic than cyclophosphamide Median latency 4-6 years Dose-response relationship	23-25, 143-145
	Premature menopause	Risk factors: increasing cumulative total dose, concurrent pelvic radiation, increasing age, older age at treatment Myeloablative doses are associated with ovarian failure. Cryopreservation of oocytes or embryos are interventions to preserve fertility.	341, 343, 344
	Male infertility	Risk of azoospermia increases with increasing cumulative dose; spermatogenesis may recover over time. Highest dose is associated with impaired testosterone production. Pretreatment semen cryopreservation and testicular sperm extraction are interventions to preserve fertility.	35, 349, 351, 352
Anthracyclines (daunorubicin, doxorubicin, mitoxantrone, idarubicin)	Clinical heart failure	Risk factors: female gender, age <5 yr, cumulative doxorubicin equivalent dose >250-300 mg/m^2, concurrent radiation	152, 155, 156, 158, 175-177
Bleomycin, carmustine, busulfan (pulmonary toxic chemotherapies)	Pulmonary fibrosis	No plateau in incidence observed Radiation exposure an additional risk factor	215, 219
Platinum compounds (cisplatin, carboplatin)	High-frequency hearing loss	Cumulative dose cisplatin >450 mg/m^2 Risk factors: dose, age <5 yr Carboplatin ototoxic at myeloablative dose	326-329
	Speech frequency hearing loss	Cumulative dose cisplatin >720 mg/m^2 Rarely observed cumulative dose cisplatin <360 mg/m^2 Risk factors: dose, age <5 yr Carboplatin ototoxic at myeloablative dose	326-329
Topoisomerase II inhibitors (epipodophyllotoxins and anthracyclines)	Secondary leukemia	Median latency 1-3 yr Frequent administration increases risk (weekly/twice weekly).	24, 146-148, 149, 150
Any irradiation	Secondary sarcoma	Risk factors: increasing radiation dose, concurrent alkylating agent or anthracycline chemotherapy, young age at diagnosis, primary diagnosis of sarcoma or retinoblastoma, family history of sarcoma	66, 110-115
	Nonmelanomatous skin cancer	Fifty percent of survivors will have multiple lesions. Basal cell carcinoma—linear dose-response	118-120
	Melanoma	Risk factors: radiation dose >15 Gy, prior history melanoma, retinoblastoma, familial melanoma	115, 116
Cranial and head/neck irradiation (including TBI)	Growth hormone deficiency	High prevalence (85%-100%) with median dose 45-55 Gy Observed at 18-24 Gy, with lower prevalence and longer latency	223, 229-231
	Obesity	Risk factors: ≥20 Gy cranial radiation, female gender	282, 283, 285
	Hypothyroidism	Primary—direct neck radiation ≥10 Gy Central hypothyroidism—cranial dose >35 Gy Dose-response relationship with no plateau in incidence observed after neck radiation	93, 223, 226
	Thyroid cancer	Risk factors: radiation dose 15-30 Gy, young age at treatment, female gender	93-103
	Brain tumors	The most common pathologic processes are meningioma and glioma. Risk increases with increasing dose.	41, 122, 126
	Head and neck carcinoma	Parotid gland carcinoma most common; secondary head and neck carcinoma Risk of salivary gland carcinoma increases linearly with dose.	51, 67, 68, 138
	Stroke	Mean cranial radiation dose ≥30 Gy increased risk for both leukemia and brain tumor survivors. Highest risk after cranial dose ≥50 Gy	210, 212
	Dental abnormalities	Risk factors: age at diagnosis <5 yr, higher-dose radiation	416-419

TABLE 72-1   Selected Late Effects by Treatment Exposure (Continued)

Treatment	Late Effect	Comments	Reference
Chest irradiation (chest, mantle, lung, mediastinal, TBI)	Coronary artery disease	Increased risk with high-dose exposure	32, 36, 188, 192
	Cardiac valve disease	Increased risk with high-dose exposure	36, 43, 198
	Breast cancer	Risk factors: increasing radiation dose, age 10-30 years at diagnosis Latency: 10-15 years Ovarian failure reduces risk.	61, 82-85
	Lung fibrosis	Pulmonary—toxic chemotherapy an additional risk factor	216-219
	Lung cancer	Greatest risk in Hodgkin lymphoma survivors Increased risk in smokers	51, 65, 67, 85
	Thyroid cancer	Risk factors: radiation dose 15-30 Gy, young age at treatment, female gender	93-103
	Hypothyroidism	Risk factors: increasing radiation dose, older age at diagnosis, female gender No plateau in incidence observed over time	93, 223
Abdominal irradiation (abdominal, periaortic, flank)	Gastrointestinal cancer	Risk factors: dose >30 Gy; concurrent treatment with alkylating agents; increasing radiation dose and increasing radiation volume	72, 73, 130
Pelvic irradiation (pelvic, inverted "Y," TBI)	Genitourinary cancer	Modestly increased risk overall; greatest risk for cancers of the female genital tract, bladder cancer, and renal cell carcinoma Risk factors: renal cell carcinoma renal irradiation, platinum-based chemotherapy, primary diagnosis of neuroblastoma	51, 67, 131
	Premature menopause	Risk factors: dose (≥ 1 to ≤ 20 Gy) and concurrent alkylating agent chemotherapy Pelvic radiation >10 Gy associated with ovarian failure Cryopreservation of oocytes or embryos is intervention to preserve fertility.	341-344
	Male hypogonadism	Risk of irreversible azoospermia >2 Gy Higher dose associated with impaired testosterone production, >20 Gy Pretreatment semen cryopreservation and testicular sperm extraction are interventions to preserve fertility.	264, 339, 349

TBI, Total-body irradiation.

agents or epipodophyllotoxins.[33] Diagnoses that confer the greatest risk for subsequent cancers include Hodgkin lymphoma (standardized incidence ratio [SIR], 8.7),[51] Ewing sarcoma (SIR, 8.5),[51] and retinoblastoma (relative rate [RR], 15).[49]

Genetic predisposition for second cancers results from an inherited or spontaneous germline mutation in a known or presumed cancer susceptibility gene. Characteristic findings in family cancer predisposition syndromes are younger age at cancer diagnosis, cancer in two or more generations, two or more cancers in an individual, and rare forms of cancer in combination.[52,53] An example of a rare cancer predisposition syndrome that is associated with pediatric malignancies is Li-Fraumeni syndrome, which is associated with germline mutations in the tumor suppressor gene *TP53*. It is inherited as an autosomal dominant trait and has a high penetrance with cancer risk of 50% by age 40 years.[52] The cancers most commonly observed in Li-Fraumeni syndrome are soft tissue sarcomas, breast cancer, leukemia, osteosarcoma, adrenocortical cancer, and brain tumors.

Survivors with an underlying genetic predisposition for cancer are more susceptible to treatment-associated secondary malignancies. This is demonstrated in survivors of retinoblastoma who carry a mutation in the *RB1* gene. Those with hereditary retinoblastoma treated with irradiation for their primary cancer have a cumulative risk for second cancers of 58% at 50 years, compared with 26% if not treated with irradiation.[54] There are other rare genetic syndromes that are associated with an increased susceptibility to pediatric cancers and subsequent adult-onset secondary cancers, and increasing evidence suggests that a substantial percentage of children with cancer may have an underlying cancer predisposition syndrome that might inform risk for subsequent cancers.[55] Genome-wide association studies of patients with and without secondary cancers may reveal polymorphisms associated with increased risk; for example, a study of Hodgkin lymphoma survivors who received irradiation identified two variants at genetic locus 6q21 that are associated with increased risk for a subsequent cancer.[45] Further work in this field may determine which survivors should undergo more intensive surveillance or prophylaxis for secondary cancer. All survivors of childhood cancer should be assessed for risk for secondary cancer based on a possible cancer predisposition, with attention to the family history as it evolves, development of benign disorders (e.g., polyps or hamartomatous lesions), as well as assessment of the pediatric history, including the primary diagnosis and age at diagnosis. Referral for genetic counseling for survivors of childhood cancer is increasingly important, because recent studies suggest that early genetic diagnosis and subsequent tumor surveillance may result in early diagnosis of secondary cancers in patients with known cancer predisposition syndromes (Box 72-2).[56,57]

Secondary Solid Tumors

Cancer that develops in a prior radiation field is the most common type of second cancer observed in survivors.[33,51] Risk estimates for second cancers have been reported from populations of survivors treated with irradiation during historic treatment eras when the modes of radiation therapy routinely used in clinical practice were different than current practices. In current oncology practice, orthovoltage radiation has been eliminated, thus reducing radiation doses to nontumor tissues such as skin, bones, and soft tissue. Large-dose extended-field radiation therapy is increasingly being replaced by involved-field lower-dose radiation therapy or conformal radiation therapy, often in combination with chemotherapy. It is assumed that this change in clinical practice aimed at reducing exposure to radiation will result in a lower incidence of radiogenic cancer; however, no "safe" dose of therapeutic radiation has been established and irradiation-associated cancers have been observed at what would be considered the lowest treatment doses.[58,59] In general, risk factors for irradiation-associated second cancers include treatment with radiation doses greater than 30 Gy, radiation in combination with alkylating agent chemotherapy, young age at exposure, more than 10 years beyond treatment, and the presence of a cancer predisposition syndrome.[25,27,60] Of particular concern is the observation that the cumulative incidence of irradiation-associated cancers does not plateau in groups of survivors followed for up to 50 years after their therapy for childhood cancer.[27,61-64] Second cancer risk is modulated by lifestyle choices; for example, adult survivors of Hodgkin lymphoma who smoke after exposure to chest irradiation have a 20-fold greater risk for secondary lung cancer compared with survivors who are nonsmokers.[65]

Box 72-2   Indications for Cancer Genetic Counseling in Childhood Cancer Survivors

FAMILY HISTORY

- Cancer in first-degree relatives
- Relatives with cancer at early age
- Cancer in two or more generations
- Individual with two or more cancers
- Rare cancers in combination
- Cancer in paired organs

PRIMARY CHILDHOOD CANCER DIAGNOSIS

- Adrenal cortical carcinoma
- Choroid plexus carcinoma
- Melanoma
- Pleuropulmonary blastoma
- Renal cell carcinoma
- Retinoblastoma
- Rhabdoid tumor
- Sarcoma

MEDICAL HISTORY

IMMUNODEFICIENCY SYNDROME

- X-linked lymphoproliferative syndrome
- Wiskott-Aldrich syndrome

GENETIC SYNDROME

- Beckwith-Weidemann syndrome
- WAGR/Denys-Drash syndrome
- Hereditary leiomyomatosis and renal cell carcinoma
- Familial adenomatous polyposis
- Juvenile polyposis syndrome
- Peutz-Jeghers syndrome
- Cowden syndrome
- Bannayan-Riley-Ruvalcaba syndrome
- Von Hippel-Lindau disease
- Hereditary paraganglioma–pheochromocytoma

- Nevoid basal cell carcinoma
- Noonan syndrome
- Blooms syndrome
- Diamond-Blackfan anemia
- Fanconi anemia
- Ataxia-telangiectasia
- Neurofibromatosis
- Tuberous sclerosis
- Carney complex
- Xeroderma pigmentosum
- Turcot syndrome
- Rubenstein-Taybi syndrome
- Simpson-Golabi-Behmel syndrome
- Costello syndrome

KNOWN CARRIER OF CANCER PREDISPOSITION GENE MUTATION

- *ATM*
- *TP53*
- *APC*
- *RB1*
- *WT1*
- *PTCH*
- *MLH1, MLH2*
- *BRCA1, BRCA2*
- *NF1, NF2*
- *MEN1, MEN2*
- *DICER-1*
- *PTEN*
- *VHL*

PHYSICAL FINDINGS

- Dysmorphic features
- Skin lesions
- Hemihypertrophy

Data from Genetics Home Reference: Your guide to understanding genetic conditions. Accessed at http://ghr.nlm.nih.gov; and Schneider K: Counseling about cancer: strategies for genetic counseling. *New York, 2011, John Wiley & Sons.*

All tissues and organs are vulnerable to cancer induction by exposure to radiation. However, some tissues, such as thyroid and breast tissue, have greater sensitivity to radiation. Excluding low-grade nonmelanomatous skin cancer and (benign) meningiomas, the most frequently reported irradiation-associated second cancers in 5-year survivors of childhood cancer followed in the CCSS are, in order, breast cancer, thyroid cancer, CNS cancers, soft tissue sarcomas, and bone sarcomas.[48,66] Additional irradiation-associated second cancers reported in survivors, especially with longer follow-up intervals, include carcinomas of the head and neck (primarily parotid gland), colon cancer and other gastrointestinal cancers, lung cancer, and carcinomas of the genitourinary tract.[33,51,67,68-72,73] The most common second cancers observed in childhood cancer survivors are described next.

Breast Cancer

Breast cancer is one of the most frequently diagnosed irradiation-associated second cancers in childhood cancer survivors. Women treated with mantle, mediastinal, chest, spinal, whole-lung, and total-body irradiation during childhood or adolescents are at risk for secondary breast cancer.[27,61,62,68,74,75,76-81] Large cohort studies of childhood Hodgkin lymphoma survivors report a fifteen- to thirty-fold increased risk for irradiation-associated secondary breast cancer compared with the age-matched general population. Risk estimates vary by characteristics of the cohort, including radiation dose, age at therapy, and duration of follow-up. The cumulative incidence of secondary breast cancer is as high as 12% to 35% at 20 years after therapy for Hodgkin lymphoma, and the incidence does not plateau with longer duration of follow-up.[27,61,62,68,74-79]

Female survivors at greatest risk for secondary breast cancer are those treated between the age of 10 and 30 years with chest radiation doses greater than 20 Gy.[76,82]

Studies have demonstrated a linear dose-response relationship between radiation dose and risk for secondary breast cancer.[76,83,84] The typical latency of irradiation-associated breast cancer is 10 to 15 years after therapy; however, secondary breast cancer has been reported in women as young as 20 years of age and as soon as 4 years after primary diagnosis.[61,85] Secondary breast cancer is most often associated with chest irradiation for Hodgkin lymphoma; however, it is important to recognize that women treated with chest irradiation for any childhood cancer diagnosis have increased risk for subsequent breast cancer, as illustrated in Figure 72-4.[61] Survivors of primary sarcomas not treated with chest irradiation also have an increased risk for secondary breast cancer (RR, 7).[61] Interestingly, survivors with therapy-induced ovarian dysfunction have a relative decreased risk for irradiation-associated breast cancers compared with survivors with normal ovarian function.[61,76,83] Although very rare, sporadic cases of male breast cancer have been reported in men treated with whole-lung irradiation as children.[10]

The most common type of breast cancer diagnosed in survivors is invasive ductal carcinoma; adverse biologic features (e.g., hormone-receptor negativity) may be more common in these childhood cancer survivors than in the general population.[61,74,86-88] Similar to findings in the general population, secondary breast cancer is detectable by radiographic imaging and has an excellent prognosis when treated in the earliest stages.[86] Breast cancer treatment options for survivors, however, can be limited by the therapy received for their childhood cancer. Specifically, prior anthracycline exposure and concern for potential cardiotoxicity may limit the use of adjuvant systemic chemotherapy with doxorubicin and the concern for tissue necrosis with repeated exposure to chest irradiation limits the option of breast-conserving surgery for some women.[86]

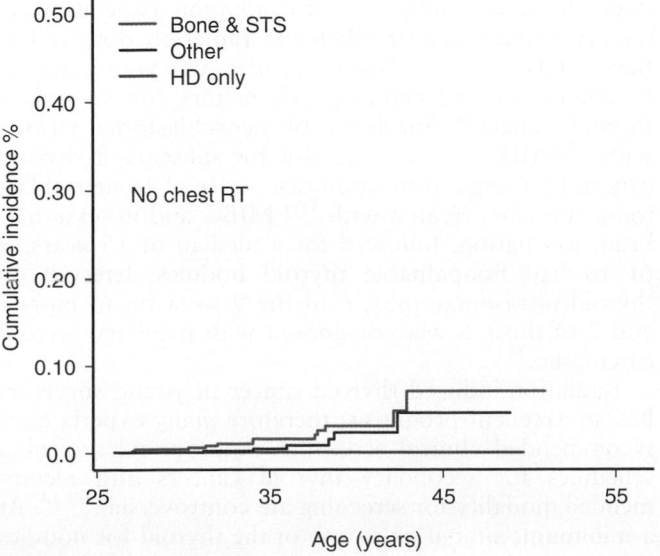
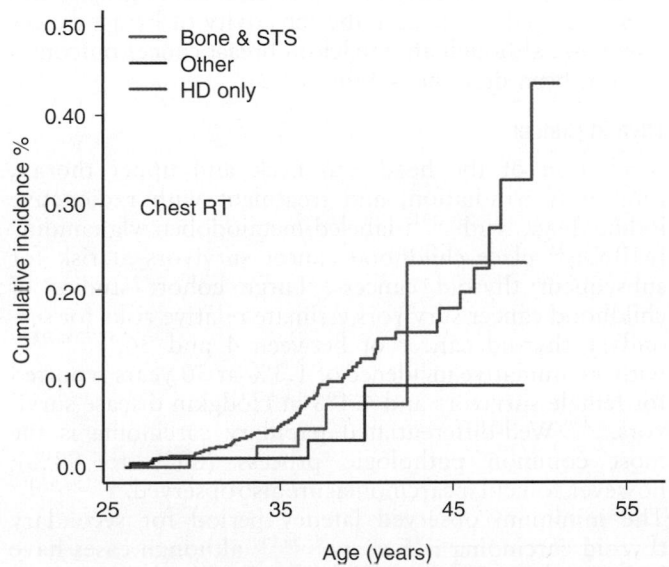

Figure 72-4 Cumulative incidence of breast cancer in survivors of Hodgkin lymphoma, sarcomas, and other diagnosis exposed and not exposed to chest radiation therapy *(RT)*, as a function of attained age. *STS*, Soft tissue sarcoma. *(From Kenney LB, Yasui Y, Inskip PD, et al: Breast cancer after childhood cancer: a report from the Childhood Cancer Survivor Study.* Ann Intern Med *141:590–597, 2004.)*

TABLE 72-2   Evaluation of Childhood Cancer Survivors for Irradiation-Associated Second Cancers

	Treatment Risk Factors	Clinical Evaluation	Special Considerations
Breast Cancer	Any chest irradiation Spinal irradiation TBI	Monthly breast self-examination Biannual clinical breast examination Breast MRI Mammogram	Current recommendations are to begin annual radiologic screening 8 years after irradiation or age 25 years, whichever occurs last.
CNS Tumor	Cranial irradiation Head /neck irradiation TBI	Annual neurologic examination Head MRI	Imaging studies are indicated for new or persistent neurologic symptoms.
Colorectal Cancer	Any abdominal irradiation Pelvic irradiation Spinal irradiation TBI	Colonoscopy Computed tomographic colonoscopy (CTC)	Current recommendations are to begin colonoscopy 10 years after radiation or age 35, whichever occurs last. CTC is not universally recommended as an alternative to colonoscopy in high-risk populations.
Thyroid Cancer	Neck irradiation Chest irradiation TBI MIBG	Annual clinical thyroid examination Thyroid ultrasound evaluation	Routine ultrasound screening is not currently recommended but should be considered for survivors with difficult clinical examination.
Skin Cancer	Any irradiation	Annual skin cancer screening Monthly skin self-examination	Practicing skin cancer prevention has potential to reduce risk.

Data from www.cancer.org/healthy/findcancerearly/cancerscreeningguidelines; www.uspreventiveservicestaskforce.org/recommendations.htm; *and* www.survivorshipguidelines.org.
TBI, Total-body irradiation.

Current screening recommendations for childhood cancer survivors treated with chest radiation published by the Children's Oncology Group include monthly self-breast examination, annual clinical breast examination, and annual breast magnetic resonance imaging (MRI) and mammography starting 8 years after treatment or age 25 whichever comes last.[89] Guidelines published by the American Cancer Society also advocate mammography and annual breast MRI, but suggest MRI only for women treated with chest irradiation between the ages of 10 and 30 years.[90] The addition of MRI to mammography has been reported to increase the sensitivity of breast cancer screening, although an impact on breast cancer outcomes has not been described (Table 72-2).[91]

Thyroid Cancer

Irradiation of the head and neck and upper thorax, total-body irradiation, and treatment with radioactive iodine (e.g., with ^{131}I-labeled-metaiodobenzylguanidine [MIBG])[92] place childhood cancer survivors at risk for subsequent thyroid cancers. Large cohort studies of childhood cancer survivors estimate relative risks for secondary thyroid cancer of between 4 and 36,[51,77,85,93-98] with a cumulative incidence of 1.3% at 30 years reported for female survivors and 4.4% in Hodgkin disease survivors.[85,99] Well-differentiated papillary carcinoma is the most common pathologic process (63% to 80%); however, follicular carcinomas are also observed.[68,85,96,97,100] The minimum observed latency period for secondary thyroid carcinoma is 5 years,[85,96,100] although cases have been reported closer to the time of original diagnosis.[85] At 20 years of follow-up, the relative risk for thyroid carcinoma remains increased[85,101] and a plateau in

incidence has not been observed beyond 40 years of follow-up.[102] The risk for thyroid cancer is related to radiation dose; but unlike most other radiation-induced second cancers, the risk for thyroid cancer is greatest at lower doses of 15 to 30 Gy and beyond 30 Gy there is a decline in risk.[95,96,103] This finding demonstrates that thyroid tissue has enhanced sensitivity to radiation toxicity and supports the "cell kill" hypothesis that suggests higher doses of radiation cause cell death, which reduces the initiation of carcinogenesis observed at lower doses.[95] Although there is conflicting evidence, chemotherapy does appear to modify risk for irradiation-associated secondary thyroid cancer when the radiation dose is less than 20 Gy.[95,97,99,103] Female gender and young age at treatment are independent risk factors for secondary thyroid cancer.[85] Survivors of neuroblastoma treated with ^{131}I-MIBG are also at risk for subsequent thyroid cancer. In a single-institution case series of 16 neuroblastoma survivors treated with ^{131}I-MIBG and no external-beam irradiation, followed for a median of 15 years, 9 of 16 had nonpalpable thyroid nodules detected on thyroid ultrasonography, 6 of the 9 went on to biopsy, and 2 of those 6 were diagnosed with papillary thyroid carcinoma.[92]

Radiation-induced thyroid cancer in young survivors has an excellent prognosis; therefore many experts have recommended clinical screening. Appropriate screening schedules for secondary thyroid cancers and recommended modality for screening are controversial.[104-107] At a minimum, annual palpation of the thyroid for nodules by an experienced examiner is recommended.[89] Routine screening to detect subclinical thyroid nodules with high-resolution ultrasonography has been recommended by some investigators but remains controversial.[105,106] Ultrasound screening has the benefit of detecting smaller non-palpable nodules but has the consequence of false-positive findings and potential for unnecessary biopsies.[106,107] Thyroid nodules do have ultrasound characteristics that are of concern for malignancy (hypoechogenicity, irregular margins, microcalcification). However, these findings are not diagnostic[108] and fine-needle aspiration of nodules larger than 1.0 cm or with suspicious features is usually necessary to evaluate for malignancy. Serial ultrasonography is then recommended to monitor thyroid nodules that are small or benign on biopsy.[108] Although clinical practice is moving toward using ultrasound to screen asymptomatic high-risk survivors for thyroid cancer, screening should be considered only after a discussion of the potential risks and benefits (see Table 72-2).

In general, irradiation-associated thyroid cancer is treated the same as other thyroid cancers and has an excellent prognosis. Thyroid surgery is indicated for nodules that are enlarging, are of indeterminate pathology on fine-needle aspiration, or are positive on fine-needle aspiration for malignancy.[108] Total thyroidectomy is often recommended to survivors because irradiation-associated thyroid cancers can be multicentric and because benign nodules can accompany clinically undetectable malignant lesions.[108] Finally, there is indirect evidence to support that exogenous thyroid hormone use reduces the risk for secondary thyroid cancer by suppressing thyroid stimulating hormone (TSH)-induced proliferation of thyroid nodules. Although not proven to reduce risk for thyroid cancer, the use of exogenous thyroid hormone to suppress thyroid proliferation is supported by data that show a decrease in incidence of new thyroid nodules in patients treated with exogenous thyroid hormone after partial thyroidectomy (34% vs. 14%).[109]

Sarcomas

Survivors treated with radiation are at increased risk for secondary cancer of the bone and soft tissue in the radiation field. Although secondary sarcomas are most often associated with irradiation, survivors of primary sarcoma and hereditary retinoblastoma who have not had prior radiation therapy also have an increased risk, suggesting a genetic predisposition.[54,110,111] Risk estimates for secondary sarcoma vary by type of sarcoma and composition of the study cohort.[60,63,110,112,113] The CCSS cohort, which did not include survivors of retinoblastoma, reports an overall ninefold increased risk for secondary sarcomas and an absolute excess risk of 32.5 per 100,000 person-years.[110] Secondary sarcomas occurring after childhood cancer include multiple histologic subtypes such as osteosarcoma, nonrhabdomyosarcoma soft tissue sarcomas, primitive neuroectodermal tumors (Ewing sarcoma), and malignant peripheral nerve sheath tumors, as well as rarer sarcoma subtypes.[110] The median latency for secondary sarcomas is 11 years, with increased risk persisting beyond 20 years.[63,110] Reported risk factors for subsequent sarcomas include higher doses of radiation, primary diagnosis of sarcoma or hereditary retinoblastoma, younger age at diagnosis, alkylating agent exposure, anthracycline exposure, and family history of sarcoma.[63,110,112-114] A nested case-control study of secondary sarcomas in the CCSS cohort identified a dose-response relationship between radiation dose and risk for secondary sarcomas, with elevations in risk ratios with higher radiation doses: 10 to 29.9 Gy (odds ratio [OR], 15.6; 95% CI, 4.5 to 53.9), 30 to 49.9 Gy (OR, 16.0; 95% CI, 3.8 to 67.8), and more than 50 Gy (OR, 114.1; 95% CI, 13.5 to 964.8).[66] Risk factors other than irradiation associated with increases in risk for secondary sarcoma in this study included primary cancer diagnosis of sarcoma or Hodgkin lymphoma and anthracycline exposure.[66]

For survivors of hereditary retinoblastoma treated with irradiation, the risk for subsequent bone sarcomas is as high as 400-fold with a cumulative incidence at 20 years of 14.1% and the relative risk for soft tissue sarcomas is 140 with 50-year cumulative incidence of 13%.[60,63,111] Radiation exposure and underlying genetic predisposition both contribute to risk for secondary sarcomas in retinoblastoma survivors.[60,63,111]

Routine radiographic screening for secondary sarcomas is currently not recommended. Survivors at risk for secondary sarcomas should be counseled to report new pain, lesions, or masses in the radiation field and should be promptly evaluated for any signs or symptoms suggestive of a secondary sarcoma. As survivors enter follow-up care, providers should consider obtaining baseline imaging of any previously irradiated site, so these studies are then available for comparison should symptoms suggestive of a new malignancy develop. There is no established role for secondary sarcoma surveillance for survivors of hereditary sarcoma predisposition syndromes (Li-Fraumeni syndrome, hereditary retinoblastoma), although the role of whole-body MRI is currently under investigation.

Skin Cancer

Melanoma and nonmelanomatous skin cancers are reported with increased incidence in survivors. The relative risk for melanoma is 2.5 to 9.0 in childhood cancer survivors, with a median latency of 15 to 18 years.[48,51,115,116] Survivors of hereditary retinoblastoma, familial melanoma syndromes, and those with a prior history of melanoma all have an increased risk for subsequent melanoma independent of irradiation.[49,55,111,117] Although the association between therapeutic radiation and melanoma is not firmly established,[116] a case-control study of 16 survivors with secondary melanoma in a European cohort of 4000 childhood cancer survivors found an association between secondary melanoma and exposure to more than 15 Gy of radiation.[115] In contrast, basal cell carcinomas and squamous cell carcinomas are known to be more common in radiation-exposed survivors (RR, 6.3), with 90% of all nonmelanomatous skin cancers diagnosed in previously irradiated fields.[118,119] A linear dose-response relationship is described for basal cell carcinomas, with an excess odds ratio of 1.09 per Gy of radiation.[120] Also of note, these low-grade skin cancers can be recurrent, and almost half of survivors diagnosed will have multiple lesions.[119] The prognosis for secondary skin cancers is excellent with early diagnosis; therefore routine screening

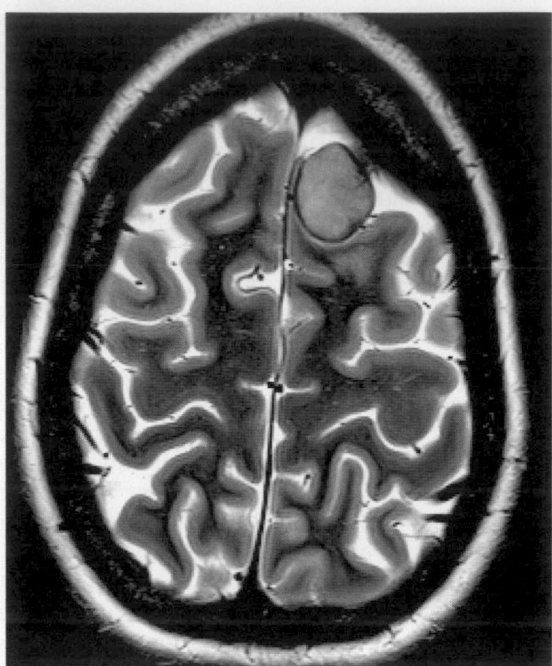

Figure 72-5 MR image of meningioma in a 20-year-old with a history of relapsed acute lymphoblastic leukemia, with therapy including total-body irradiation, presenting with headache. Note frontal mass. Pathology was consistent with meningioma.

with skin examinations is recommended.[121] Because ultraviolet radiation from the sun is known to contribute to skin cancer risk; patients should be routinely educated about preventive strategies such as aggressive sun exposure protection (see Table 72-2).

Central Nervous System Tumors

Past exposure to cranial irradiation is considered the most important risk factor for the development of subsequent CNS tumors in survivors of childhood cancer.[41,122] The most common pathologic processes include meningioma (Fig. 72-5) and glioma; however, other tumors such as primitive neuroectodermal tumor or medulloblastoma have been reported.[41,49,123-125] In a report from the British Childhood Cancer Survivor Study, the standardized incidence ratio for development of a subsequent glioma was 10.8 (95% CI, 8.5 to 13.6),[126] and in the CCSS cohort it was 8.7 (95% CI, 6.2 to 11.6).[41] Higher standardized incidence ratios have been reported for meningioma,[122] and meningioma is the most common subsequent CNS tumor 10 years or more after a childhood cancer diagnosis.[41,124] There is an established dose-response relationship between cranial radiation dose and incidence of secondary CNS tumors. In the CCSS cohort, Neglia and colleagues reported an excess relative risk of 1.06 per Gy of cranial irradiation for meningiomas and 0.3 per Gy for gliomas.[41] In the British Childhood Cancer Survivor Study cohort, Taylor and colleagues reported that the risk for glioma and for meningioma each increased linearly with increasing radiation dose.[126] Several studies have suggested that the increased risk for development of meningioma does not appear to plateau.[118,123,127] In a

report from the CCSS, among survivors with no previous diagnosis of meningioma at 25 years after a primary CNS tumor, the cumulative incidence of meningioma at 30 years was 3.5% (95% CI, 0.9% to 6.1%).[123] The contribution of chemotherapy to the risk for CNS malignancies is controversial. Laboratory investigations have suggested an association between radiation-induced brain tumors and thiopurine-based chemotherapy related to a deficiency in the enzyme thiopurine methyltransferase (TPMT).[128] In the British Childhood Cancer Survivor Study cohort, a higher cumulative dose of intrathecal methotrexate was associated with the development of meningioma.[126] In the CCSS cohort, after adjusting for radiation dose, chemotherapy exposure did not alter the survivor's secondary brain tumor risk.[41]

The role of routine surveillance for secondary CNS tumors with neuroimaging in asymptomatic childhood cancer survivors requires further investigation. Single-institution series of neuroimaging screening have reported high rates of meningioma.[127,129] For example, in a prospective study of 76 survivors of acute lymphoblastic leukemia that was treated with cranial irradiation and who were screened with MRI every 3 to 6 years for 20 years, Goshen and colleagues detected 16 meningiomas (15 asymptomatic) and one glioma.[127] Cumulative incidence in this screened population was 14.8% at 20 years.[127] Surgical resection of these secondary CNS tumors was recommended for 12 of the 16 survivors, with one surgical complication reported.[127] Whether early detection of meningiomas in asymptomatic survivors might reduce morbidity and minimize neurologic complications by facilitating surgical intervention remains to be determined. Survivors with a prior history of cranial irradiation should be educated about the potential for late-occurring CNS tumors and instructed to report new or persistent neurologic signs or symptoms (see Table 72-2).

Other Cancers

Secondary carcinomas of the gastrointestinal tract, genitourinary organs, lung, and head and neck region are observed in survivors of childhood cancer and are associated with radiation exposure and longer follow-up times. In general, irradiation-associated carcinomas (like colon cancers) occur at an earlier age than is seen in the general population, thereby supporting recommendations for early initiation of cancer screening and aggressive evaluation of symptoms suggestive of possible secondary malignancy.

Large cohorts of childhood cancer survivors report relative risks for gastrointestinal cancers between 4.6 and 7.0.[33,49,67,68,72,73] A European cooperative cohort study found the risk for secondary gastrointestinal malignancies greatest after abdominal radiation dose greater than 30 Gy (SIR, 9.7); however, lower-dose radiation was also associated with increased risk (10 to 29 Gy, SIR 5.2).[72] Alkylating agent chemotherapy is consistently found to be independently associated with an increased risk for gastrointestinal cancer.[72,73,130] The most common irradiation-associated secondary gastrointestinal malignancy is colorectal cancer, with a standardized incidence ratio of 3.6 to 13 and as high as 63.4 (95%

CI, 15.7 to 71.8) reported in a cohort of Hodgkin lymphoma survivors.[68,72,73,130] In a British cohort of 18,000 childhood cancer survivors, the 50-year cumulative incidence of colorectal cancer for those treated with direct abdominal radiation was 1.4% (95% CI, 0.7 to 2.6).[33] The St. Jude Children's Research Hospital cohort of over 13,000 childhood cancer survivors found a 40-year cumulative incidence of secondary colorectal cancer of 1.4% ± 0.53%).[130] In this study, the risk for colorectal cancer increased by 70% with each 10-Gy increase in radiation dose and increasing radiation volume also significantly increased risk. Current recommendations for screening of survivors treated with abdominal radiation therapy are to begin colon cancer screening earlier than what is recommended for the general population (10 years after completing radiation therapy or age 35 years, whichever comes last), although the benefit of early surveillance has not been established in this high-risk population (see Table 72-2).[89]

Of note, gastric cancers and esophageal cancers are also observed in greater numbers than expected for age in survivors of pediatric Hodgkin lymphoma.[68,85] Common symptoms such as dysphagia and dyspepsia should be evaluated aggressively, with a low threshold for utilizing endoscopy or imaging to rule out malignant or premalignant conditions in exposed survivors.

Overall, the relative risk for genitourinary cancer is modestly elevated (SIR, 1.9; 95% CI, 1.6 to 2.4),[33] with elevated relative risks for secondary malignancies of the female genital tract (SIR, 2.1; 95% CI, 1.4 to 3.2),[51] secondary renal cell carcinoma (SIR, 8.0; 95% CI, 5.2 to 11.7),[131] and secondary bladder cancer (SIR, 5.1; 95% CI, 2.1 to 12.4).[67] Data from the CCSS show the risks for secondary renal carcinoma are primary diagnosis of neuroblastoma (SIR, 85.8; 95% CI, 38.4% to 175.2%), renal-directed radiation therapy of 5 Gy or greater (RR, 3.8; 95% CI, 1.6 to 9.3), and platinum-based chemotherapy (RR, 3.5; 95% CI, 1.0 to 11.2).[131] Secondary urinary bladder cancer is associated with both radiation therapy and cyclophosphamide chemotherapy, with the risk dependent on dose and duration of therapy.[67,132-135] An adult series of more than 6000 non-Hodgkin lymphoma survivors treated with cyclophosphamide reported 31 cases of bladder cancer (RR, 4), and no significantly increased risk was observed at doses less than 20 g/m^2.[133] In a British cohort of 18,000 childhood cancer survivors, 17 were diagnosed with bladder cancer (RR, 4); risk factors were diagnosis of hereditary retinoblastoma, treatment with chemotherapy, male gender, and longer follow-up.[135] In another series of adults treated with prolonged cyclophosphamide for nonmalignant disease, 5% developed secondary bladder cancer at a median of 8.5 years and all diagnoses were preceded by symptoms of microscopic hematuria.[136] Although the absolute excess risk for bladder cancer in childhood cancer survivors is low, routine monitoring with urinalysis of survivors exposed to pelvic radiation, large cumulative dose of cyclophosphamide, and those with hereditary retinoblastoma should be considered.

Cancer of lung and bronchus is diagnosed more commonly in childhood cancer survivors than the general population (SIR, 3.4; 95% CI, 1.9 to 6.1),[51] with greater risk observed in cohorts of pediatric Hodgkin lymphoma survivors (SIR, 5.1 to 27.2).[67,85] In a meta-analysis of secondary lung cancer in Hodgkin lymphoma survivors, the largest risk for secondary lung cancer was observed among patients diagnosed age 15 to 24 years (RR, 8.76; 95% CI, 4.55 to 16.89).[137] Treatment with alkylating agents and irradiation are both associated with increased lung cancer risk.[67] In addition, studies of adult survivors of Hodgkin lymphoma have shown that smoking increased lung cancer risk more than twentyfold. Aggressive smoking cessation interventions and routine surveillance with radiographic imaging have been suggested for this high-risk population of survivors, although the use of spiral computed tomography has not been studied in the survivors who had chest irradiation.

Survivors are also at increased risk for secondary head and neck carcinomas (SIR, 10.8 to 14.1), with mucoepidermoid carcinoma of the parotid gland the most frequently observed diagnosis.[51,67,68] In a CCSS analysis of secondary salivary gland carcinomas, the incidence was thirty-ninefold higher in survivors compared with the general population (95% CI, 25.4 to 57.8).[138] The analysis also demonstrated that risk increased linearly with radiation dose (excess RR, 0.36/Gy; 95% CI, 0.06 to 2.5).[138] Interestingly, modifiable health behaviors including cigarette smoking and alcohol intake were not associated with increased risk for head and neck cancers in childhood cancer survivors.[138]

Hematologic Malignancies

Childhood cancer survivors are at an increased risk for developing subsequent hematologic malignancies, particularly secondary acute myelogenous leukemia. Overall, the relative risk for secondary acute leukemia in childhood cancer survivors is reported from 7 to 20.[23,24,48,49,68,77,139,140] An increased risk for secondary leukemia is described after treatment of a primary solid tumor[139] and after treatment of acute lymphoblastic leukemia, particularly with exposure to a topoisomerase II inhibitor.[141] In an analysis of survivors of cancer diagnosed when younger than 20 years of age, utilizing the Surveillance, Epidemiology, and End Results (SEER)-9 database, the cumulative incidence of secondary hematologic malignancy at 5 years was 0.2% (± 0.03%) and at 10 years it was 0.4% (± 0.04).[142] In contrast to irradiation-associated malignancies, the latency for leukemogenesis associated with chemotherapy is within the first 10 years after treatment, with the greatest risk observed in the first 5 years off therapy. In a study of 4202 survivors of childhood solid tumors, the relative risk of leukemia was 20 at 3 to 5 years and then decreased to 2.2 by 10 years off therapy.[139] Of interest, in this same study a second peak in secondary leukemia was observed at 20 years or more of follow-up (RR, 14.8); this finding has not been observed in studies with shorter follow-up periods.[24,48,62]

Acute leukemias and myelodysplasia are associated with exposure to high cumulative doses of alkylating agents and topoisomerase II inhibitors, including epipodophyllotoxins and anthracyclines. The alkylating agents presenting the greatest concern for secondary leukemia risk are melphalan and mechlorethamine, when compared with cyclophosphamide and ifosfamide.[23,25,143] Secondary leukemias induced by exposure to high-dose alkylating agents are classically considered to be preceded by myelodysplasia, have a median latency of 4 to 6 years, are more often diagnosed in older children, and are often associated with losses or deletions of chromosome 5 or 7.[37] Higher cumulative dose of alkylating agents is associated with a greater risk for the development of secondary acute myelogenous leukemia.[144] Interestingly, more recent pediatric studies demonstrated lower overall rates of leukemia after alkylating agent exposure[139,145] than earlier studies,[23,24] likely reflecting the trend of treatment with lower cumulative doses of less leukemogenic alkylating agents in more modern cohorts.

Topoisomerase II–induced leukemias, on the other hand, typically do not have an indolent course, have a relatively short latency (median, 1 to 3 years), are diagnosed in younger children, and are associated with a balanced chromosomal translocation 11q23 and, less frequently, 21q22.[24,37,146,147] Some have reported an increased risk for secondary acute myelogenous leukemia with higher cumulative epipodophyllotoxin dose. For example, in a case-control study of 61 cases of secondary leukemia in childhood survivors, Le Deley and colleagues reported a greater than twentyfold increased risk for leukemia after exposure to greater than 6 g/m² of epipodophyllotoxins and a sevenfold increased risk after exposure to either 1.2 to 6 g/m² epipodophyllotoxins or greater than 170 mg/m² of anthracyclines compared with lower doses of these agents.[145] However, other investigators have not demonstrated a relationship between higher cumulative epipodophyllotoxin dose and the development of secondary acute myelogenous leukemia.[148,149] Schedule of administration of epipodophyllotoxins may contribute to the risk for secondary leukemia, because prolonged infusions (twice weekly, weekly) have been found to be an independent risk factor for development of leukemia.[148,150]

The contributory role of therapeutic doses of radiation in the development of secondary leukemia is debated. Although some studies find no association between leukemia and exposure to radiation therapy,[49,139,148] others studies have documented subsequent leukemia in survivors after exposure to radiation in the absence of chemotherapy.[24,37,139] In addition, specific host factors, such as polymorphisms of DNA repair genes, may contribute to susceptibility to secondary acute myelogenous leukemia.[144]

The prognosis of secondary acute myelogenous leukemia is generally considered to be poor.[37,146] In the SEER-9 analysis cited earlier, the 5-year overall survival for patients with secondary hematologic malignancies was 31% ± 4.7%.[142] In a report of 24 children with secondary myelodysplastic syndrome or acute myelogenous leukemia, those with secondary myelodysplastic syndrome or acute myelogenous leukemia had lower rates of remission with induction therapy and poorer overall and event-free survival when compared with patients with de novo acute myelogenous leukemia.[151] Further investigation is needed to determine the optimum strategies for preventing and treating secondary leukemia.

ORGAN SYSTEM LATE EFFECTS

Cardiovascular System

Cardiac disease is the leading cause of treatment-related morbidity and noncancer mortality observed in childhood cancer survivors.[152] In an analysis of late mortality among 5-year survivors of childhood cancer from the CCSS cohort, childhood cancer survivors were seven times more likely to die of cardiac-related events compared with expected population-based rates of cardiac-related deaths.[21] Indeed, childhood cancer survivors have been reported to be at significantly increased risk, compared with a sibling cohort, for the development of congestive heart failure (RR, 15.1; 95% CI, 4.8 to 47.9,), coronary artery disease (RR, 10.4; 95% CI, 4.1 to 25.9), and cerebrovascular accidents (RR, 9.3; 95% CI, 4.1 to 21.2).[46] The treatments most often associated with cardiac morbidity and mortality are anthracycline chemotherapy and cardiac irradiation.[21] A recent cohort study assessing the long-term risk for clinically validated, symptomatic cardiac events in 5-year survivors of childhood cancer demonstrated that higher cumulative anthracycline dose or higher cumulative radiation dose was associated with higher risk ratio for cardiac events. Survivors with both anthracycline and cardiac irradiation exposures had the highest cumulative incidence of cardiac events, with nearly one in eight survivors treated with both exposures developing a serious cardiac event.[36] Risk factors for late onset anthracycline cardiotoxicity (occurring 1 year beyond completion of therapy) have been assessed in multiple studies and include higher cumulative anthracycline dose, history of acute cardiac toxicity, combined exposure with other cardiotoxic therapy, female sex, younger age at exposure (<5 years old), and longer duration of follow-up.[42,153-158] Irradiation of the heart as a consequence of irradiation to the chest for treatment of childhood cancer can cause both functional and anatomic cardiac disease. Mantle field, whole-lung fields, left- or whole-abdominal irradiation, spinal irradiation, and total-body irradiation all put a survivor at risk for cardiac late effects.[155,159-162] Irradiation-associated cardiac late effects include constrictive pericarditis,[163] myocardial fibrosis,[164] cardiomyopathy, coronary artery disease, valvular abnormalities, conduction disturbances, and vascular disease.[43,155,159] Similar to other irradiation-associated late effects, cardiac toxicity is observed more frequently in those survivors treated at the youngest age, receiving higher radiation dose volumes to the heart, and followed the longest.[159,160]

Nonanthracycline chemotherapeutic agents, including cyclophosphamide, cytarabine, cisplatin, and ifosfamide, have also been associated with cardiotoxicity.[152] In addition, children and adolescents are increasingly being treated with newer agents with unclear cardiac risks. For example, tyrosine kinase inhibitors (imatinib mesylate, sorafenib, and sunitinib) have been associated with cardiac toxicity with exposure in adulthood.[165,166] Cardiac risks with prolonged exposures to newer agents in large cohorts of pediatric patients are yet to be defined.

The spectrum and nature of cardiac late effects experienced by childhood cancer survivors suggest a need for regular screening with one or more cardiac imaging modalities. Risk-based screening recommendations for childhood cancer survivors exposed to cardiotoxic therapies have been published by the Children's Oncology Group as part of the "Late Effect Guidelines" as well as by other groups.[89,167,168] However, these guidelines have not been tested for efficacy in terms of reduction of cardiac mortality or morbidity. Survivors exposed to cardiotoxic therapy should be informed about their risk for cardiac disease and should also be made aware of activities that present potential stressors to already impaired cardiac function, including smoking, pregnancy, and anesthesia.

Cardiomyopathy

Cardiomyopathies diagnosed in childhood cancer survivors after completion of therapy are associated with both anthracycline chemotherapy and cardiac irradiation. Survivors are at risk for both systolic and diastolic left ventricular dysfunction, which can lead to clinical heart failure.[169-171] Anthracycline-associated cardiotoxicity can be classified as acute, early onset (<1 year after anthracycline exposure), or late onset (>1 year after anthracycline exposure),[158] although it is not clear to what extent these categories reflect differences in underlying pathophysiology.[172] Anthracyclines are considered to be directly toxic to cardiac myocytes, with exposure resulting in reduced myocyte mass and impaired function of cardiac muscle. Subclinical anthracycline cardiotoxicity is measured as diminished left ventricular contractility and a thinning of the left ventricular wall. Thinning of ventricular walls causes elevated wall stress, which increases afterload, and ultimately can progress to symptomatic left ventricular failure. In children, loss of cardiac myocytes at a young age can result in impaired cardiac growth and function relative to somatic growth, which contributes to the observed decrease in left ventricular systolic function.[42,173] Anthracycline-associated late cardiac toxicity can manifest as asymptomatic cardiac dysfunction detected by echocardiogram or other modalities or symptomatic dysfunction and the classic signs of heart failure.[155,156] Longitudinal and long-term follow-up data support that cardiac abnormalities diagnosed in childhood cancer survivors treated with anthracyclines are persistent and progressive.[174,175] In a Dutch cohort of more than 800 anthracycline-exposed childhood survivors, the cumulative incidence of anthracycline-induced clinical heart failure increased with the duration of follow-up; there was a cumulative incidence of 2.6% at 10 years and 5.5% at 20 years, with no evidence of plateau in incidence with longer duration of follow-up.[157] Of further concern, the incidence of asymptomatic left ventricular dysfunction detected by cardiac screening is reported to be as high as 50% to 60%.[153,176] However, the long-term clinical implications of subtle echocardiographic abnormalities in asymptomatic individuals are not fully determined.

Many risk factors for anthracycline-associated cardiomyopathy have been identified. The major risk factor for anthracycline cardiomyopathy is cumulative dose ("doxorubicin equivalent"). Equivalent dose takes into consid-

TABLE 72-3 Calculation of Anthracycline (Doxorubicin) Isotoxic Dose Equivalents*

Anthracycline	Conversion Factor
Doxorubicin	Total dose (mg/m²) × 1
Daunorubicin	Total dose (mg/m²) × 1
Mitoxantrone	Total dose (mg/m²) × 4
Idarubicin	Total dose (mg/m²) × 5
Epirubicin	Total dose (mg/m²) × 0.67

From the Children's Oncology Group long-term follow-up guidelines for survivors of childhood, adolescent, and young adult cancers, *Version 4.0. Accessed at www.survivorshipguidelines.org, October 2013.*
*Estimation of anthracycline isotoxic dose equivalents for use in calculation of total cumulative anthracycline dose.

eration exposure to different anthracyclines and can be calculated using conversion factors (Table 72-3). Survivors exposed to cumulative doses of doxorubicin equivalents greater than 250 to 300 mg/m² appear to be at greatest risk for cardiomyopathy.[19,42,157,175,177,178] The dose-dependent relationship between anthracyclines and subsequent congestive heart failure was demonstrated in the Dutch cohort, where the greatest risk for congestive heart failure was at a dose greater than 300 mg/m² (RR, 8), and no congestive heart failure was observed at doses less than 150 mg/m².[157] However, others have shown that survivors treated with low cumulative dose (45 mg/m²) also have asymptomatic cardiac abnormalities detectable on an echocardiogram,[174] suggesting that exposure to anthracycline at any dose poses potential risk for late cardiotoxicity.

Additional reported risk factors for the development of anthracycline-associated cardiomyopathy include history of acute cardiac toxicity during treatment, combined exposure with other cardiotoxic therapy, female sex, younger age at exposure (<5 years of age), and longer duration of follow-up.[42,153-157] Cardiotoxicity diagnosed during or within 1 year of completion of therapy is considered a risk factor for late cardiotoxicity.[152] Furthermore, survivors exposed to anthracycline therapy and concurrent mediastinal radiation are considered to be at risk for cardiomyopathy at lower total anthracycline dose.[160] Increasingly, genetic variants that may predispose to anthracycline cardiotoxicity are being explored.[177,179] A recent evaluation from the Children's Oncology Group demonstrated that patients with *CBR3* V244M homozygous G genotype with low- to moderate-dose anthracycline exposure were at an increased risk for cardiomyopathy.[177]

Interventions aimed at preventing or reducing long-term anthracycline-associated cardiotoxicity in childhood cancer survivors include limiting anthracycline doses in most therapeutic regimens to less than 300 mg/m², adding cardioprotectants such as dexrazoxane to anthracycline-based regimens, and prescribing afterload-reducing agents to prevent progression of asymptomatic dysfunction to overt heart failure. Data from clinical trials in childhood ALL show that the addition of cardio-protectants did not adversely affect survival.[180] Although an early analysis of a Pediatric Oncology Group clinical trial for Hodgkin lymphoma, which randomized the use of dexrazoxane as a cardioprotectant, demonstrated a possible increase in second cancers with dexrazoxane exposure,[181] a larger cohort of survivors of childhood acute lymphoblastic leukemia treated with dexrazoxane did not demonstrate an increased risk for second cancers.[182] Childhood cancer survivors diagnosed with anthracycline-associated left ventricular dysfunction have been treated with angiotension-converting enzyme inhibitors with the aim of reducing afterload and preventing the progression of left ventricular dysfunction to heart failure. In a longitudinal study of 18 survivors with left ventricular dysfunction, treated with enalapril and followed for a median of 10 years, all initially showed improvement in left ventricular function. The effects, however, were transient, lasting 6 to 10 years, followed by deterioration of left ventricular function over time.[183] However, given results from large studies of medical interventions for patients with asymptomatic left ventricular dysfunction (who have not received anthracyclines), as well as data from adult cancer patients,[184,185] many cardiologists who evaluate and treat adults with anthracycline-induced cardiomyopathy will intervene with angiotensin-converting enzyme inhibitors. Future investigations should be directed at testing interventions to prevent cardiac injury during therapy and to prevent progression of asymptomatic left ventricular dysfunction to overt cardiac disease in survivors.

Irradiation-associated cardiomyopathy is most often restrictive, with impaired diastolic function, although systolic dysfunction may also be observed.[163,164] Radiation is believed to induce injury to the myocardial microvasculature, which in turn causes myocardial ischemia, and ultimately myocardial fibrosis, resulting in diastolic dysfunction.[37] Studies have demonstrated a significant incidence of diastolic dysfunction in asymptomatic patients who undergo radiation therapy.[159,186,187] In a small cohort of Hodgkin lymphoma survivors treated with a median mediastinal dose of 35 Gy, evaluated at a mean of 9 years after therapy, 20% had evidence of diastolic dysfunction on cardiac imaging.[186] The extent to which these changes are progressive, and whether subclinical dysfunction will result in clinical heart failure over time, is unknown. As noted earlier, there is a significantly increased risk for cardiotoxicity with combined exposure to both anthracyclines and irradiation.[36,159,188]

Screening for cardiomyopathy with serial echocardiograms is currently recommended for survivors treated with anthracyclines and/or thoracic radiation therapy, with the frequency of echocardiogram screening depending on the individual survivor's risk for cardiomyopathy as determined by age at exposure, cumulative treatment dose, and concurrent treatment with thoracic irradiation.[89] The use of newer modalities for screening, such as cardiac MRI, is an area of active investigation.[189] The extent to which screening will result in a reduction in cardiac morbidity and mortality in survivors remains unknown.

Coronary Artery Disease

Survivors treated with thoracic irradiation are at increased risk for the development of radiation-associated coronary artery disease (CAD), which is an established cause of early mortality.[109,190] Radiation injury to the coronary arteries is considered to be caused by acute endothelial damage followed by subsequent initiation or acceleration of atherosclerosis.[152,160] Irradiation-associated coronary artery stenosis is most common in the proximal coronary arteries, which are not necessarily shielded during cardiac blocking.[191] In a historic cohort, childhood Hodgkin lymphoma survivors treated with more than 40 Gy of mediastinal radiation had a fortyfold excess risk for fatal myocardial infarction compared with an age-matched general population.[192] A report on 314 Hodgkin lymphoma survivors treated at age younger than 20 years found a fivefold increased risk for myocardial infarction at a median of 19 years after treatment,[188] and a British cohort that included 2158 Hodgkin lymphoma survivors treated at age younger than 25 years found a nineteenfold increased risk for death from myocardial infarction.[32] A recent study assessing the long-term risk for clinically validated, symptomatic cardiac events in 5-year survivors of childhood cancer demonstrated a significantly increased 30-year cause-specific cumulative incidence of cardiac ischemia for survivors treated with cardiac irradiation compared with survivors treated without cardiac irradiation (2.2% [95% CI, 0% to 4.7%] vs. 0.3% [95% CI, 0% to 0.8%], $P = .01$)].[36] Modern irradiation techniques are designed to reduce radiation to the coronary arteries, although reduction in irradiation-associated CAD has not yet been proven.

The risk for asymptomatic CAD in survivors is described in many studies; however, optimal screening and interventions to detect and treat irradiation-associated cardiovascular disease have not been determined. Survivors at risk for irradiation-associated CAD are advised to adopt preventive measures commonly used to reduce the risk for atherosclerotic CAD in the general population (aggressive treatment of hypertension, diabetes, obesity, dyslipidemias). Although the efficacy of such measures is not proven in this population, at least one cardiac risk factor was present in all survivors who developed CAD in a single-institution study of 415 Hodgkin lymphoma survivors[43]; these data suggest that standard cardiovascular risk–reducing strategies might be beneficial to survivors.

Stress echocardiograms can be used as a noninvasive method to detect asymptomatic ischemic heart disease by observing stress-induced wall motion abnormalities. Noninvasive nuclear scintigraphy has also been considered to screen survivors for asymptomatic CAD. A report of screening 294 asymptomatic Hodgkin lymphoma survivors treated at a median age of 25 years with more than 35 Gy found 20% had electrocardiographic findings consistent with prior ischemia and 14% had abnormal stress echocardiograms or stress-induced perfusion defects by nuclear scintigraphy.[193] The survivors with abnormal nuclear perfusion studies who went on to cardiac catheterization were diagnosed with irradiation-induced microvascular damage in the myocardium that was not amendable to surgical intervention.[193] This study showed that the increased sensitivity of adding perfusion scanning in addition to stress echocardiography was at the expense of decreased specificity, with false-positive detection of disease not amendable to intervention. This calls into question the benefit of adding nuclear studies to routine screening of asymptomatic survivors for CAD. The roles of modalities such as CT angiography, MR angiography, and coronary artery calcium scores in the childhood cancer survivor population are yet to be established.[152,194]

Surgical treatment of CAD in survivors with prior radiation exposure can be complicated by mediastinal fibrosis, myocardial fibrosis, and the coexistence of other irradiation-associated morbidities, including valvular disease, conduction abnormalities, and pulmonary dysfunction.[195] In a recent report from Wu and colleagues, adults with irradiation-associated heart disease undergoing cardiothoracic surgery had significantly higher mortality compared with a matched control population undergoing similar procedures.[196] The high surgical risk in patients with irradiation-associated heart disease should be carefully considered when planning surgical interventions.

Arrhythmias

A full spectrum of cardiac arrhythmias and conduction disturbances have been reported in childhood cancer survivors treated with both irradiation and anthracyclines. These include atrioventricular nodal bradycardia, sick-sinus syndrome, complete and incomplete heart block, prolonged QT interval, and serious ectopy (ventricular tachycardia).[197] In a series of 48 survivors of pediatric Hodgkin lymphoma treated with mediastinal irradiation (median dose, 40 Gy), 75% were found to have conduction abnormalities.[198] The most frequent conduction disturbance was right anterior bundle branch block, the most anterior structure in the conduction system.[198] These arrhythmias are rarely symptomatic; however, the clinical concern is that conduction abnormalities may be progressive.[197,198] Because conduction abnormalities typically are asymptomatic, they usually are detected in association with other irradiation-induced cardiac abnormalities.[197,198]

Valvular Disease

The mitral, aortic, and tricuspid valves can all be affected by irradiation-associated fibrous endocardial thickening.[199] Valvular insufficiency is more common than valvular stenosis, but stenosis tends to be more severe, requiring intervention.[43,199,200] The frequency of left-sided valvular regurgitation is reported to be 16% to 24% in chest-irradiated survivors of Hodgkin lymphoma screened by echocardiography at a median of 10 years, and valvular dysfunction was not observed at a radiation dose less than 30 Gy.[200,201] In a cohort of 48 long-term survivors of pediatric Hodgkin lymphoma (median age at diagnosis, 16 years; median dose, 40 Gy), left-sided regurgitation was noted in 36% and valvular defects were detected in 42%.[198] In a recent report, the 30-year cause specific

cumulative incidence of symptomatic valvular disease in survivors treated with cardiac irradiation was 2.5% (95% CI, 0% to 5.0%), compared with 0.1% (95% CI, 0% to 0.3%) for those treated without cardiac irradiation.[36] Valvular defects can be progressive, which is of particular concern for young survivors.[199] In a single-institution series of 415 survivors of Hodgkin lymphoma who received mediastinal irradiation, clinically significant valvular dysfunction developed in 6.2% at a median of 22 years.[43] In this cohort, aortic stenosis was the most common clinically significant valve lesion and when results were compared with those of an age-matched general population the relative risk for needing valve surgery was eightfold higher in survivors. The only treatment risk identified for significant valvular disease in this cohort was irradiation technique that resulted in a higher total dose to the heart.[43] Symptoms of valvular heart disease are the same in survivors as the general population, and valve function can be monitored by routine echocardiographic screening.

Pericarditis

The incidence of late-occurring irradiation-associated pericarditis has been significantly reduced by modern irradiation techniques.[202,203] In historic cohorts of children treated with orthovoltage mediastinal irradiation, 7% to 15% developed symptomatic constrictive pericarditis,[203,204] compared with 0% to 2.5% of children treated with megavoltage therapy.[203,205,206] Although the incidence of pericarditis has been significantly reduced in recent cohorts, older childhood cancer survivors continue to be at risk for pericarditis. Presenting signs and symptoms include pleuritic chest pain, shortness of breath, a friction rub, and electrocardiographic changes. A survivor presenting with symptomatic pericarditis is at risk for progressing to cardiac tamponade.[198] Management includes pericardiocentesis and pericardiectomy,[203] which are high-risk procedures in this patient population with known risks for other irradiation-associated cardiac morbidities.

Cerebrovascular Disease

Survivors treated with irradiation to the head and neck are at risk for the development of clinically significant premature cerebrovascular disease. Irradiation-induced cerebrovascular disease can encompass numerous abnormalities, such as moyamoya disease, vascular malformations including venous-based cavernous malformations (cavernomas) or intracranial aneurysms, and extracranial internal carotid stenosis.[207] Abnormalities such as cavernous malformations may be asymptomatic and noted incidentally on follow-up imaging or may present as neurologic symptoms such seizures, headache, or with hemorrhage, potentially necessitating surgical interventions.[208] Intracranial aneurysms can be life threatening.[209] There are limited long-term data on the risk for late-occurring cerebrovascular disease in survivors of childhood cancer. Data from the CCSS, based on self-report, demonstrated an increased risk for stroke in survivors of brain tumors (RR, 29) and of leukemia (RR, 6.4) when compared with sibling controls, and risk for stroke was associated with a mean cranial irradiation dose greater than or equal to 30 Gy. In addition, among leukemia and brain tumor survivors who did not receive cranial radiation therapy, the risk for stroke remained significantly increased when compared with siblings.[210] CCSS data also demonstrate an increased risk for stroke among survivors of Hodgkin lymphoma (RR, 4.32), with mantle irradiation strongly associated with subsequent stroke.[211] Importantly, in the CCSS cohort, smoking was associated with a threefold excess risk for stroke in survivors of Hodgkin lymphoma. In a study investigating cerebrovascular mortality in a French/United Kingdom cohort of 4227 five-year survivors of childhood cancer, at a median follow-up 29 years after radiation to the brain, the risk for death from cerebrovascular disease increased linearly with local radiation dose to the prepontine cistern. Survivors who received greater than 50 Gy to the prepontine cistern had a notably increased risk for death from cerebrovascular disease (RR, 17.8).[212]

Risk-based surveillance for cerebrovascular disease currently includes careful assessment by history and physical examination for neurologic and neurocognitive signs and symptoms. Neuroimaging is indicated for diagnostic assessment in symptomatic patients. The Children's Oncology Group Guidelines recommend consideration of baseline Doppler ultrasonography of carotid vessels 10 years after radiation therapy to the neck in those with radiation exposure of more than 40 Gy.[89] In a report on 30 childhood cancer survivors who received neck irradiation, Meeske and colleagues noted an increase in carotid disease on carotid ultrasound assessment compared with healthy control subjects, including in those treated with lower doses of radiation (18 to 30 Gy).[213] Further investigations are needed to better define risks and to inform screening recommendations. Abstinence from smoking should be emphasized. Aggressive medical management of other risk factors associated with cerebrovascular disease in the general population should also be advised.

Modifiable Cardiovascular Risk Factors

As noted earlier, attention to modifiable cardiovascular risk factors, such as obesity, hypertension, diabetes mellitus, dyslipidemia, and smoking, may be particularly important in the care of survivors of childhood cancer. A recent assessment from the CCSS found that two or more cardiovascular risk factors were reported by 10.3% of survivors. In this report, acquisition of modifiable cardiovascular risk factors, particularly hypertension, increased the risk for severe, life-threatening, and fatal cardiac events.[214] These results reinforce the importance of early diagnosis and careful management of modifiable cardiovascular risk factors in survivors.

Pulmonary System

Pulmonary toxicities as a consequence of cancer-directed therapy can range in severity from asymptomatic abnormalities on pulmonary function testing to life-threatening disease. Childhood cancer survivors are at increased risk for death from pulmonary complications. In an analysis of late mortality among 5-year survivors from the CCSS cohort, childhood cancer survivors were 8.8 times more likely to die of a pulmonary event compared with the U.S. population (age-, calendar year-, and sex-matched).[21] Therapeutic exposures, including radiation therapy, certain chemotherapeutic agents (bleomycin, carmustine, lomustine, busulfan, and cyclophosphamide), thoracic surgery, and hematopoietic stem cell transplantation, are associated with late pulmonary complications.[215] Recognition of these toxicities informed changes in upfront cancer-directed therapies, such as the reduction or elimination of radiation therapy and bleomycin in the treatment of Hodgkin lymphoma.

The late effects of radiation therapy on the respiratory system include reduced lung volumes, pulmonary fibrosis, and decreased chest wall growth. Risk factors for radiation-induced pulmonary late effects include concurrent pulmonary toxic chemotherapy, lung radiation dose greater than 15 Gy, spinal irradiation, and total-body irradiation.[216-218] Data from the CCSS cohort showed an increased risk for pulmonary fibrosis (RR, 4.3), emphysema (RR, 2.0), abnormal chest wall development (RR, 5), and chronic pneumonia (RR, 2.2) in those survivors who had chest irradiation. At 20 years after diagnosis, chest irradiation was associated with a cumulative incidence of pulmonary fibrosis of 3.5%.[219]

Treatment with chemotherapy including bleomycin, busulfan, cyclophosphamide, and nitrosoureas is also associated with the development of pulmonary fibrosis.[215,220,221] In the CCSS cohort, an increased risk for pulmonary fibrosis was seen in those exposed to bleomycin (RR, 1.4), carmustine (RR, 1.6), and busulfan (RR, 2.1).[219] A plateau in cumulative incidence of pulmonary fibrosis was not observed up to 15 years after diagnosis in survivors treated with chemotherapy alone or in combination with radiation therapy.[219]

Current long-term follow-up guidelines include obtaining a baseline chest radiograph and pulmonary function testing, including spirometry and diffusing capacity, in survivors with significant risk factors for late pulmonary toxicity.[89] Attention to smoking abstinence and cessation is also recommended. Reports of worsening bleomycin-associated pulmonary fibrosis after exposure to 100% oxygen suggest that survivors receive a pulmonary evaluation before undergoing anesthesia and avoid situations with increased oxygen concentrations such as scuba diving.[222]

Endocrine System
Hypothalamic-Pituitary Dysfunction

Hypothalamic pituitary dysfunction is a potential late effect in childhood cancer survivors who undergo radiation therapy for CNS, orbital, facial, or nasopharyngeal cancers. CNS tumors of the optic pathway, hypothalamus, or suprasellar region can also cause long-term hypothalamic-pituitary dysfunction as a result of hypothalamic injury from tumor growth or surgical resection. The incidence of pituitary hormone deficiencies after cranial irradiation varies by radiation dose and other treatment factors, such as age at therapy and duration of follow-up.[223] The reported range in prevalence of anterior pituitary deficiencies after a median dose of 45 to 55 Gy cranial radiation is as follows: growth hormone (GH), 85% to 100%; TSH, 3% to 60%; luteinizing hormone/follicle-stimulating hormone (LH/FSH), 5% to 40%, and adrenocorticotropic hormone, 4% to 30%.[223] This variability is a result of differences in cohort composition as well as different measures used to define hormone deficiencies. The GH pathway is the most sensitive to radiation and, therefore, GH deficiency is the most likely manifestation of hypothalamic hypopituitarism in survivors treated with cranial irradiation. The pituitary-thyroid, gonadal, and adrenal axes are less sensitive to late onset radiation toxicity, and, as such, centrally mediated deficiencies of these hormones are usually not observed in survivors treated with cranial irradiation below the range of 35 Gy.[186,224-228]

Growth Hormone Deficiency. The severity and latency of GH deficiency diagnosed in survivors is related to cranial irradiation dose. GH deficiency can be observed after doses as low as 18 to 24 Gy with late onset typically more than 10 years after therapy, whereas a cranial dose of more than 30 Gy can result in GH deficiency within 5 years after treatment.[229] This suggests that after a dose threshold of 18 to 25 Gy the incidence of GH deficiency increases with increased period of follow-up.[230,231] Clinical features of GH deficiency in survivors who have cranial irradiation can include poor growth, increased fat mass, reduction in lean body mass, decreased strength and exercise tolerance, adverse lipid profile, and decreased bone mineral density (BMD). These clinical features can be improved by GH replacement.[232] However, the use of GH replacement in GH-deficient survivors after they obtain final height is controversial, with more to be determined regarding the long-term benefits, safety, and risks for GH replacement in GH-deficient survivors in adulthood.[230,233]

The safety of GH replacement in childhood cancer survivors with regard to the risk for cancer recurrence or the development of a second primary cancer is controversial. Several studies report a lack of association between history of treatment with GH and primary cancer recurrence.[234-237] In a report from the CCSS, there was no documented increased risk for primary cancer recurrence in GH-treated survivors. However, exposure to GH was associated with an increased risk for second neoplasms (RR, 3.21; 95% CI, 1.88 to 5.46). An updated report from the CCSS continued to demonstrate this association (RR, 2.15; 95% CI, 1.33 to 3.47).[235,238] The association between development of second cancers and GH treatment is based on relatively few events and could be confounded by ascertainment bias (GH-treated patients could have had increased surveillance) and suggests the need for further study. The frequency and duration of screening for GH deficiency in childhood cancer survivors, the long-term effects and safety of GH replacement therapy, and the utility of long-term replacement therapy beyond attainment of final height require further investigation.

Skeletal Toxicities

Skeletal toxicities, including low BMD and osteonecrosis are increasingly recognized potential complications of therapy for childhood cancer. In children and adolescents undergoing treatment for cancer, acquisition of peak bone mass may be compromised. Cancer-directed treatment exposures, nutritional deficiencies, or physical inactivity can all contribute to decreased BMD in the setting of treatment of childhood cancer.[239] Risk factors for low BMD identified in cohorts of childhood cancer survivors include prior treatment with corticosteroids, methotrexate, cranial irradiation, and total-body irradiation. Survivors with hypogonadism, nutritional deficiencies, and prolonged immobilization or physical inactivity are also at risk for low BMD.[240-243] In the general population, osteoporosis-associated fractures result in significant morbidity and mortality; however, the association between low BMD and fracture risk has not been established for childhood cancer survivors. A report from the CCSS did not note an increased prevalence of fracture in adult survivors of childhood cancer compared with siblings[244]; however, the risks for long-term skeletal morbidity with advancing age remain to be defined.

Baseline bone density evaluation has been advised upon entry into survivorship care for those with treatment exposures associated with low BMD.[89] Dual-energy x-ray absorptiometry (DXA) is a commonly used modality that provides quantitative measurement of bone mineral content and indirect calculation of BMD. DXA has well-established normative pediatric values. However, as a two-dimensional technique, DXA has limitations and cannot provide direct volumetric measurements of BMD and is confounded by bone size.[245] Use of other modalities such as quantitative computed tomography (QCT) has been largely investigational.[246] Nutritional counseling to ensure sufficient intake of calcium and vitamin D in the diet, and supplementation in the setting of inadequate intake, has been recommended.[239] Management of conditions associated with decreased BMD, such as GH deficiency and hypogonadism, could potentially enhance bone health; however, the overall potential risks and benefits of such interventions with limited available data on long-term bone health outcomes must be considered.

Childhood cancer survivors are at increased risk for the development of osteonecrosis (also referred to as avascular necrosis). Osteonecrosis typically effects weight-bearing joints and can result in pain, loss of function, and joint collapse requiring surgical intervention including joint replacement. Cancer treatment exposures associated with the development of osteonecrosis include glucocorticoid therapy and irradiation,[247-249] with several studies indicating that exposure to dexamethasone is associated with a greater risk for osteonecrosis than exposure to prednisone.[249,250] Treatment as an adolescent has consistently been identified as a risk factor for the development of osteonecrosis.[249,250] Osteonecrosis has been identified as an acute toxicity of cancer therapy, with potential long-term impact on the quality of life of survivors. In the CCSS cohort, the 20-year cumulative incidence of osteonecrosis was 0.43%, with survivors 5.6 times more likely to have reported osteonecrosis compared with siblings. The risk for osteonecrosis was greatest among survivors of allogeneic stem cell transplant for underlying diagnoses of leukemia and in survivors of acute lymphoblastic leukemia, acute myelogenous leukemia, and bone sarcoma.[249] In this study, the cumulative incidence of osteonecrosis increased with time after treatment. Whether this reflects the worsening of previously asymptomatic bony lesions or a continued risk for the development of new lesions over time is unclear. Indeed, data are limited on the longitudinal outcomes of those diagnosed with osteonecrosis and more remains to be determined about the risk for late-occurring osteonecrosis.

In addition, bone and soft tissue in treatment fields are vulnerable to irradiation-induced hypoplasia and fibrosis, resulting in reduced or uneven skeletal growth. Survivors treated with irradiation that included the spine (>12 Gy) and long bones are at risk for scoliosis, shortened trunk height, and growth asymmetry.[251,252]

Disorders of Glucose Metabolism

Survivors of childhood cancer appear to be at increased risk for the development of insulin resistance and diabetes mellitus (DM). In a cross-sectional evaluation of survivors of childhood acute lymphoblastic leukemia, Oeffinger and colleagues noted that survivors of this type of leukemia treated with and without cranial irradiation had an increased prevalence of insulin resistance when compared with a cohort composed of older individuals from the same community.[253] In a report from the CCSS, the prevalence of DM was almost twice as high in childhood cancer survivors compared with siblings, with an increased risk for DM associated with total-body irradiation (OR, 7.2; 95% CI, 3.4 to 15; $P <.001$), abdominal irradiation (OR, 2.7; 95% CI, 1.9 to 3.8; $P <.001$), and younger age at diagnosis.[254] This increased risk for DM with abdominal radiation exposure in this cohort appeared to be independent of body mass index (BMI). Survivors of acute lymphoblastic leukemia who had cranial irradiation were 1.6 times as likely as siblings to report DM (after adjustment for BMI). [254] Survivors treated with total-body irradiation or with abdominal irradiation have been reported to have an increased risk for DM in several recent reports.[254-257] A report of 2520 survivors from France and the United Kingdom demonstrated a dose-response relationship between irradiation to the tail of the pancreas, where beta cells are concentrated, and risk for DM (RR of DM, 11.5% [95% CI 3.9 to 34] with 10 Gy or more to the tail of the pancreas).[257] Irradiation to other part of the pancreas was not associated with an increased risk for DM in this study. Further investigation of the mechanisms of development of DM and the interplay between treatment-related and modifiable risk factors in survivors is needed. Screening for DM should be considered in survivors, with implementation of aggressive risk-reduction strategies as clinically indicated.

Thyroid Disorders

The thyroid gland is extremely sensitive to radiation toxicity; subsequently, thyroid abnormalities are among the most common irradiation-induced morbidities after childhood cancer therapy. Childhood cancer survivors exposed to thyroid radiation as a consequence of direct neck irradiation for Hodgkin lymphoma, sarcomas, nasopharyngeal or oropharyngeal carcinomas, and other tumors are at risk for thyroid abnormalities. The clinical manifestations of thyroid irradiation injury include hypothyroidism, hyperthyroidism, thyroid nodules, and thyroid cancer. Because even low doses and scatter radiation can damage thyroid tissue, survivors who received seemingly distant irradiation such as whole-lung irradiation, craniospinal irradiation, and total-body irradiation for bone marrow transplant are also at risk for thyroid abnormalities. In addition, neuroblastoma survivors treated with ^{131}I-MIBG are at risk for hypothyroidism.[92,258] Although coadministration of potassium iodide is considered protective, a single-institution follow-up study of 16 survivors, a median 15 years after treatment, found 8 of 16 with clinical hypothyroidism. Primary hypothyroidism (low thyroxine [T4] level with elevated TSH or compensated normal T_4 with elevated TSH) is the most common thyroid abnormality observed after thyroid irradiation.[93] Survivors in the CCSS cohort had a seventeenfold increased risk for hypothyroidism, compared with siblings.[93] The incidence of hypothyroidism increases with increasing radiation dose to the thyroid; at 20 years after treatment with 35 to 44.99 Gy the cumulative incidence is 35%, and with 45 Gy or more the cumulative incidence is 50%.[93] Risk factors identified for hypothyroidism are larger dose of radiation, older age at diagnosis, and female gender.[93] Although the greatest risk for hypothyroidism occurs the first 5 years after treatment, no plateau for thyroid disease has been observed and cumulative incidence continues to rise beyond 20 years of follow-up.[93] Central hypothyroidism (low TSH, low T_4) can be observed as a late toxicity of cranial irradiation to the hypothalamic pituitary axis, although centrally mediated deficiencies are usually not observed in survivors treated with cranial irradiation below 35 Gy.[224,226,229] Hyperthyroidism is an uncommon late effect and is sometimes observed after high-dose thyroid irradiation greater than 35 Gy.[93] Irradiation-induced thyroid nodules are commonly detected in survivors treated with head and neck irradiation. A recent cohort study of over 3000 survivors reported the cumulative incidence of irradiation-associated thyroid adenomas as 5.5% (95% CI, 4.2 to 7.2) at 40 years of follow-up.[259] A small cohort study of Hodgkin lymphoma survivors reported the median latency of thyroid nodules as 10 years (range, 1 to 25 years) after therapy, and in this study only 10% of nodules detected by physical examination or screening ultrasonography were malignant.[107]

Recommended screening for survivors at risk for irradiation-associated thyroid disease include annual palpation of the thyroid by a skilled examiner and annual measurements of serum thyroid hormones beginning 1 year after completion of therapy.[89,93] Thyroid replacement therapy is successful in treating irradiation-associated hypothyroidism. Treatment with thyroxine to suppress elevated TSH may reduce the frequency of benign nodules.[260] Routine ultrasound screening of asymptomatic survivors is controversial, because the majority of thyroid nodules detected in survivors have an indolent course and a minority of the nodules are malignant.[107] Survivors with palpable thyroid nodules are advised to undergo high-resolution thyroid ultrasonography with fine-needle aspiration of any large or suspicious nodules. Nodules with benign pathology can be followed by serial ultrasonography and resampled if there is interval change, and patients whose nodules that have indeterminate or malignant pathology are referred for thyroidectomy. Total thyroidectomy is often recommended to survivors because irradiation-associated thyroid cancers can be multicentric, the remaining thyroid is at risk for malignancy, and occult malignancy has been detected in nodules believed preoperatively to be benign.[108]

Parathyroid Disorders

Neck irradiation is associated with an increased incidence of hyperparathyroidism. Studies of adults treated with head and neck irradiation for nonmalignant conditions during childhood show a 2.5-fold increased risk for hyperparathyroidism, with a prolonged latency of 25 to 50 years.[223,261-263] Hyperparathyroidism was diagnosed in 10% (5/53) of childhood cancer survivors treated with head and neck irradiation who underwent surgery for thyroid disease at a single institution, with a latency of 15 to 34 years.[264] Survivors treated with neck irradiation as children should have monitoring of their serum calcium concentration as they approach older adulthood, especially if they have thyroid disease.

Short Stature

Many factors can contribute to growth disturbances in childhood cancer survivors, and it may be challenging to isolate a specific cause for diminished height in an individual child. Final height in survivors can be directly affected by cancer therapy and indirectly affected by treatment-related hormonal deficiencies and poor nutrition. Identified independent risk factors for diminished final height in childhood cancer survivors include treatment with cranial irradiation (related to GH deficiency), treatment with total-body irradiation, treatment with spinal irradiation, and young age at diagnosis (<age 13 years, with children <age 4 years at greatest risk).[265-269] Survivors of pediatric brain tumors and of leukemia who undergo cranial or craniospinal irradiation are at particular risk for short stature. In a report from the CCSS, among survivors of acute lymphoblastic leukemia significant risk factors for short stature included diagnosis before puberty, female sex, higher-dose cranial radiation therapy (≥20 Gy), and irradiation of the spine.[270] In a CCSS report assessing 921 brain tumor survivors, nearly 40% of survivors were below the 10th percentile for height. Risk factors included earlier age at diagnosis and higher doses of radiation therapy to the hypothalamic-pituitary axis.[267]

Irradiation-associated bone hypoplasia and fibrosis can directly impede skeletal growth, such that radiation fields that include the spine or lower extremities can result in diminished adult final height.[267,271,272] Irradiation-associated spinal deformities (kyphosis or scoliosis) can also impact final adult height.[251,252,271,272] Prolonged use of corticosteroids can impair longitudinal growth and reduce final adult height. Proposed mechanisms of corticosteroid-induced growth suppression include suppression of pituitary growth hormone secretion, reduction of insulin-like growth factor type 1 production by the liver, and possibly impaired action of insulin-like growth factor type 1 on bone, all of which contribute to diminished growth.[241,271,273] Antimetabolite chemotherapy is associated with decreased bone growth and diminished final height in some clinical studies.[241] This finding is supported by animal and in vitro models, which demonstrate that antimetabolite chemotherapy damages growth plate chondrocytes and impairs growth.[274]

Loss of height velocity during a prolonged course of treatment without subsequent catch-up growth can also result in diminished final attained height. Interruption of growth during the active treatment period can be related to the malignant process itself, poor nutrition, or growth suppression by therapy.[266,275] In a single-institution study of final height in survivors of childhood acute lymphoblastic leukemia, decrease in height growth scores in children undergoing active treatment was noted as soon as 6 months after beginning therapy.[266]

Treatment-induced deficiencies of GH, thyroid hormone, testosterone, and estrogen can all contribute to reduced final height in survivors. The effect of hormone deficiencies on final height can be minimized by early recognition and use of hormone replacement therapy.[276,277] Precocious puberty, a late effect observed after cranial irradiation, can also indirectly result in diminished final height because early onset of puberty reduces the time interval of prepubertal growth.[278] Cranial irradiation for CNS leukemia prophylaxis (18 to 24 Gy) is associated with relatively early and precocious puberty in girls, and higher doses of cranial irradiation often used to treat brain tumors can precipitate early puberty in both males and females.[278]

All childhood cancer survivors, and especially survivors exposed to therapies particularly associated with growth impairment such as total-body irradiation and cranial irradiation, should be monitored for appropriate growth during and after therapy.

Obesity

Obesity has been reported as a potential late complication in survivors of childhood cancer. Obesity is frequently defined as a BMI greater than the 95th percentile for age, or greater than or equal to 30 after age 21 years.[279] Irradiation-induced hypothalamic damage has been implicated in the pathogenesis of obesity in childhood cancer survivors, resulting in impaired growth, low metabolic rate, altered body composition, and dysregulation of eating behaviors.[265,280,281] Indeed, cranial irradiation has been identified as a risk factor for obesity in adult survivors of acute lymphoblastic leukemia.[282,283] A study of 1765 young adult acute lymphoblastic leukemia survivors enrolled in the CCSS identified female gender (RR, females 2.6, males 1.9), younger age at diagnosis in females (<4 years of age), and treatment with a radiation dose greater than 20 Gy during cranial irradiation as risk factors for obesity.[282] Treatment with lower-dose radiation therapy or chemotherapy only was not associated with an increased risk for obesity in this study. In a follow-up longitudinal analysis of changes in obesity and BMI among adult survivors of acute lymphoblastic leukemia from the CCSS, survivors treated with cranial radiation therapy had a significantly greater increase in BMI when compared with the sibling cohort. The rate of increase was not significantly increased for survivors treated with chemotherapy alone.[283] In contrast, a prospective study measuring BMI of 422 children with acute lymphoblastic leukemia and non-Hodgkin lymphoma before, during, and after completion of therapy found no difference in the rate of BMI increase between irradiated and nonirradiated children and concluded that high BMI at diagnosis was the best predictor of adult obesity in survivors of these malignancies.[284]

Physical inactivity as a consequence of treatment-associated morbidities, including cardiopulmonary disease that limits exercise tolerance, neurocognitive disabilities that limit coordination and participation, chronic pain, genetic factors, and social factors, all likely contribute to the obesity observed in survivors. Green and colleagues assessed risk factors for obesity among 9284 adult CCSS participants. In a multivariable analysis, impaired physical function, hypothalamic/pituitary irradiation, use of paroxetine, and younger age at cancer diagnosis were each independent predictors of obesity, whereas meeting the Centers for Disease Control and Prevention guidelines for physical activity and a reported moderate amount of anxiety were associated with a reduced risk for obesity. This study, including the findings of an association of a specific antidepressant and of poor physical functioning with obesity, highlights the importance of further investigation of the interplay between obesity, pharmacologic exposures, physical activity, and other modifiable risk factors.[285] Survivor care should include education regarding the long-term health consequences of obesity and the reduction of modifiable risk factors for this late effect.

Metabolic Syndrome

An increased risk for metabolic syndrome and/or its component parts has been observed in survivors of childhood cancer.[286-288] Metabolic syndrome is a grouping of component physiologic disturbances that is associated with an increased risk for developing cardiovascular disease and diabetes mellitus. Although there are various definitions of metabolic syndrome in the literature, definitions generally include measures of obesity, insulin resistance, dyslipidemia, and hypertension.[289] Identified treatment-related risk factors associated with metabolic syndrome in childhood cancer survivors include cranial irradiation and total-body irradiation.[287,288] Older attained age and a sedentary lifestyle have also been implicated.[290] Because metabolic syndrome is an established risk factor for cardiovascular disease and diabetes mellitus in the general population, aggressive management of modifiable cardiovascular risk factors in survivors is warranted.

Central Nervous System

Therapy for childhood cancer can result in long-term adverse sequelae on function of the CNS and sensory organs. Surgery, radiation therapy, and chemotherapy used to treat brain tumors and solid tumors in the head and neck region and cranial irradiation and chemotherapy used as CNS prophylaxis for leukemia and lymphoma can all contribute to neurologic, cognitive, and sensory deficits observed in survivors.

Neurocognitive Impairment

There is a broad spectrum of neurocognitive impairments observed in childhood cancer survivors. These include deficits in executive functioning (planning and organization), sustained attention, memory (visual sequencing and temporal memory), processing speed, visuomotor integration, and diminished intelligence. As a result of these deficits, survivors may experience learning difficulties, academic failure, and behavioral changes.[38,291-297] Neurocognitive impairment is observed in survivors treated with cranial radiation. Methotrexate, administered intrathecally as CNS prophylaxis or at high doses systemically (single dose >1000 mg/m^2), is also associated with neurocognitive late effects.[291,298] Indeed, neurocognitive impairment has been noted in adult survivors of acute lymphoblastic leukemia treated with chemotherapy alone (without cranial irradiation).[299] Brain tumor survivors treated with surgery alone are at risk for neurocognitive impairment attributable to direct brain injury from tumor growth, surgical resection, hydrocephalus, and seizures.[300]

Risk factors for neurocognitive impairment in childhood cancer survivors treated with radiation include higher dose, young age at exposure (<3 years), female gender, and personal or family history of learning disabilities.[38,293-295,301,302] Additional risk factors include total-body irradiation exposure and concurrent treatment with dexamethasone, methotrexate, or cytarabine.[293] Lower-dose cranial irradiation as CNS prophylaxis for leukemia/lymphoma (18 to 24 Gy) is more commonly associated with information processing or learning disabilities,[38] whereas higher-dose cranial irradiation necessary to treat brain tumors is more often associated with global cognitive impairments and diminished intelligence.[294] Neurocognitive deficits are persistent,[299] and new deficits may emerge over time or become evident during periods of increasing cognitive demands.[293] Armstrong and colleagues reported that adult survivors of childhood acute lymphoblastic leukemia who received 24 Gy of cranial irradiation had increased immediate and delayed memory impairment. In addition, survivors who received 24 Gy of cranial irradiation were found to function at a level one to two decades older than their chronologic age on delayed memory assessments, raising concern for early onset of cognitive impairment.[303]

Formal neurocognitive testing is used to diagnose cognitive impairments. A full battery of tests administered by specially trained psychologists is indicated to evaluate the full spectrum of potential deficits. Survivors diagnosed with neurocognitive impairments should be referred to specialized services at the treating center or in the community to facilitate access to educational, rehabilitation, social, and vocational resources. Cognitive remediation, educational interventions with individualized learning programs, and family support that address survivor specific needs are all necessary for survivors to meet full educational potential.[293,304]

Neurologic Deficits

Surgery for brain tumors and head and neck cancers can result in permanent neurologic deficits that are specific to the location of the primary cancer. For example, postoperative cerebellar mutism may persist years beyond the surgical resection of a posterior fossa tumor.[305] In addition, postoperative hydrocephalus, infections, and seizures can evolve into chronic neurologic conditions that result in neurologic deficits that can be stable or progressive over time.[40]

Peripheral sensory and motor neuropathy presenting as weakness, paresthesias, or pain and episodic vasospasm of the digits (Raynaud phenomenon) are potentially late effects associated with vincristine and vinblastine therapy.[306-308] Treatment-induced neuropathy might restrict survivors from physical activity; however, impaired motor performance, measured in a cohort of 128 childhood cancer survivors, was not associated with cumulative vincristine dose,[309] nor was prolonged vincristine exposure associated with physical inactivity observed in acute lymphoblastic leukemia survivors in the CCSS cohort.[310] Management of these late effects is primarily symptomatic, and a trial of agent used to treat neuropathic pain or prevent peripheral vascular spasm can be considered.[89,306]

Irradiation-induced cerebrovascular disease, such moyamoya disease, vasculitis, and vascular malformations (venous-based cavernous malformations or intracranial aneurysms) have been reported.[207,311-313] Late onset of seizures was reported in 6.5% of brain tumor survivors in the CCSS cohort and cortical irradiation of greater than 30 Gy was associated with a twofold risk for this complication.[40] Also in the CCSS cohort, an increased risk for late-occurring stroke was reported among survivors of brain tumor (RR, 29), leukemia (RR, 6.4), and Hodgkin lymphoma (RR, 4.32).[210,211] Rare neurologic late effects of radiation therapy associated with higher doses of radiation (>50 Gy) include focal brain necrosis and spinal cord myelitis.

Leukoencephalopathy, presenting as spasticity, ataxia, dysarthria, dysphagia, hemiparesis, or seizures, is a rare complication of treatment of childhood cancer and has been associated with cranial irradiation with doses of radiation greater than 18 Gy as well as chemotherapy with methotrexate and dexamethasone. Signs and symptoms of leukoencephalopathy may present without imaging abnormalities (brain MRI, MR angiography, CT); conversely, findings on neuroimaging (white matter changes, cerebral atrophy, dystrophic calcifications, mineralizing microangiopathy) do not necessarily correlate with clinical severity.[314-316] Leukoencephalopathy has also been described as a late manifestation of childhood histiocytic syndromes with no known treatment association.[317]

Late-onset neurologic complications can present as a variety of nonspecific neurologic symptoms, including headache, seizure, hemiparesis, or other focal findings. Neuroimaging is indicated for diagnostic assessment.

Neurovascular abnormalities or irradiation-associated abnormalities of the brain parenchyma can also be incidental findings on neuroimaging obtained for other indications. The role of screening with neuroimaging in asymptomatic survivors is not yet defined, with no current data to support that screening asymptomatic survivors reduces morbidity or mortality from neurologic complications. However, cancer survivors who have received cranial irradiation and have nonspecific neurologic symptoms might benefit from early evaluation by a neurologist and/or early neuroimaging.

Vision

Childhood cancer survivors' vision may be impaired by surgery, localized irradiation, total-body irradiation, or chemotherapy with corticosteroids. Visual late effects are both anatomic and functional, including cataracts, orbital hypoplasia, lacrimal gland atrophy, conjunctival corneal damage, retinopathy, glaucoma, and optic nerve damage.[40,318-320] Cataracts are a visual late effect frequently diagnosed in bone marrow transplant survivors and survivors treated with cranial irradiation. Bone marrow transplant conditioning regimens that include total-body irradiation are associated with significant risk for cataract development that can require surgical intervention.[321,322] Chemotherapy-based conditioning regimens are not as likely to induce cataracts, and those that develop are usually less severe and do not requiring intervention.[321,322] Survivors with visual symptoms, those with a history of an ocular tumor, those who received total-body irradiation, or those treated with cranial, orbital, or ocular irradiation are at highest risk for late-onset ocular complications and should receive ongoing follow-up by an ophthalmologist.[40,89,320,321]

Hearing

Hearing loss is a late effect experienced by childhood cancer survivors exposed to head and neck radiation and/or platinum-based chemotherapy. Radiation fields that include the temporal bone and adjacent soft tissues can cause impaired auditory function.[40] Low-dose cranial irradiation alone (as was administered to leukemia patients) is unlikely to cause hearing loss; however, sensorineural hearing loss can occur at cranial doses greater than 50 Gy and at lower doses (40 to 50 Gy) when combined with ototoxic chemotherapy, especially when the treatment sequence is chemotherapy administered after irradiation.[40,323,324] In a series of 157 children with brain tumors treated by radiation therapy only with a median dose of 54 Gy, the cumulative incidence of hearing loss in the speech frequency range was 27% at 5 years after therapy.[325] The cumulative incidence of hearing loss steadily increased over the 9-year follow-up period, and no plateau was observed.[325]

The effect of platinum-based chemotherapy exposure on hearing is dose and age dependent. Children treated at a younger age (<5 years) are more vulnerable to cisplatin ototoxicity at any dose level.[326,327] The incidence of high-frequency hearing loss (4000 to 8000 Hz) is up to 50% in children treated with more than 450 mg/m^2 cumulative dose of cisplatin.[326] Hearing loss in the speech range (500 to 3000 Hz) is rarely reported at cumulative cisplatin doses less than 360 mg/m²; however, it has been reported at cumulative doses as low as 360 mg/m², and the incidence is as high as 22% to 25% at cumulative dosages greater than 720 mg/m².[323,326] Cisplatin ototoxicity is typically bilateral and irreversible, and children with normal hearing at the completion of platinum therapy, who have not undergone cranial irradiation, are unlikely to have subsequent loss of hearing.[326] Survivors treated with carboplatin in nonmyeloablative doses do not appear to be at risk for hearing loss, but carboplatin-containing conditioning regimens used in stem cell transplant can contribute to hearing impairment.[328,329] Genetic polymorphisms associated with an increased risk for cisplatin-induced hearing loss in children have been identified.[44] Such findings await further validation but reflect a potential for tailoring treatment and/or follow-up based on the genetic risk for chemotherapy-associated ototoxicity.

The role of otoprotectants, such as amifostine, administered before or during cancer therapy, has not been established, and studies are ongoing in this area.[330] To minimize risk, clinicians should minimize exposure to other ototoxins, including aminoglycoside antibiotics and furosemide. In assessing a survivor, prior and current exposure to all ototoxic agents should be considered in the assessment of auditory function. The contribution of environmental factors (e.g., use of headphones, occupational exposures) to hearing loss in the young survivor population has not been documented.[329] Survivors with treatment exposures that put them at risk for hearing loss or those with symptoms of hearing impairment should have serial auditory evaluations, and those diagnosed with hearing impairments should be prescribed hearing aids and classroom or workplace accommodations as indicated. Early intervention for auditory problems is particular important in the survivor population because hearing loss has the potential to compound already existing social, developmental, and cognitive impairments.

Reproductive System

Reproductive function depends on the complex interaction of hormonal, anatomic, and psychosocial factors. Treatment of childhood cancer directed at the brain, spinal cord, pelvis, genitourinary organs, and gonads can all impair future reproductive potential. Therapy that is directly toxic to the ovaries and testes predisposes survivors to primary hypogonadism resulting in both diminished sex hormone production (testosterone, estrogen) and damage to oocytes and spermatocytes. Secondary hypogonadism, impaired secretion of gonadotropins (LH, FSH), can be the result of radiation and surgery to the hypothalamic-pituitary axis. Alternation of the neurovascular or structural anatomy of the reproductive organs or reduction in the volume of gonadal tissue by radiation and surgery can also impair reproductive function. As with most late effects, chemotherapy-associated gonadotoxicity is directly related to the individual agent and cumulative dose. Specifically, the alkylating agents cyclophosphamide and procarbazine pose a greater risk for gonadal dysfunction than cisplatin and dacarbazine.[35,331-333] In general, the ovary is less vulnerable to chemotherapy-induced damage than the testis. As with other late effects, irradiation-associated toxicity to the ovaries and testes is dependent on the radiation dose and field. The availability of established fertility preservation strategies for patients newly diagnosed with cancer (semen cryopreservation, oophoropexy, oocyte cryopreservation) may improve long-term fertility outcomes for survivors treated with gonadotoxic therapy.[334-337]

Females

Ovarian dysfunction can be a result of acute ovarian toxicity that persists or premature ovarian failure. The majority of prepubertal and adolescent girls receiving standard-dose chemotherapy will retain or recover ovarian function; however, those receiving high-dose alkylating agents, conditioning for bone marrow transplant, or those exposed to pelvic irradiation are at risk for irreversible ovarian toxicity, which manifests as both estrogen deficiency and infertility.[338-341] Of note, irradiation to the pelvis, abdomen, or spine may include the ovaries in the field. Ovarian doses greater than 10 Gy can result in complete ovarian failure, requiring hormone replacement therapy.[342,343] Survivors treated with both radiation therapy and gonadal-toxic chemotherapy have a worse prognosis for ovarian function.[344,345] Cranial irradiation that has a radiation dose greater than 22 Gy to the hypothalamic-pituitary access is associated with reduced fertility, and use of more than 30 Gy is associated with ovarian failure as a result of impaired secretion of gonadotropins (LH, FSH).[346] Survivors diagnosed with ovarian failure should be offered treatment with hormone replacement therapy in consultation with an endocrinologist.

Survivors who retain or recover ovarian function after completing therapy are at risk for premature menopause (defined as cessation of menses prior to age 45 years). Risk factors for premature menopause include increasing age, older age at treatment, increasing radiation dose to the ovaries, and increasing cumulative dose of alkylating agents.[344,345] The pathophysiology of therapy-induced premature menopause is reduction in number of ovarian follicles, which supports the finding that prepubertal girls with the greatest reserve of follicles are less vulnerable to premature ovarian failure than older survivors. In the historic Five-Center Study, which included 1067 female survivors, the risk for reaching early menopause (age <25 years) for those treated between the ages of 13 and 19 years was four times greater than sibling controls.[347] Increased risk for premature menopause was observed in survivors treated with irradiation below the diaphragm (RR, 3.7), alkylating agents (RR, 9.2), or both (RR, 27). In this historical cohort, 42% of women treated with irradiation below the diaphragm and alkylating agents had reached menopause by age 31 years.[347] The overall relative risk for premature menopause in survivors in the CCSS cohort was thirteenfold higher than sibling controls, with a cumulative incidence of 8% by age 40.[345] In this study, the cumulative incidence of menopause for survivors exposed to alkylating agents only was 5% at age 35 years and increased to 15% by age 40 years, and survivors exposed to both radiation therapy and alkylating agents had a cumulative incidence of menopause of 15% at age 30 years that increased to 30% by age 40 years.[345] Of note, the threshold dose of cumulative alkylating agent exposure below which ovarian function is preserved has not been determined, and in pelvic irradiation even the lowest radiation doses (1 to 99 cGy) are associated with premature menopause.[345]

Survivors who retain ovarian function but are at risk for premature menopause should be educated about their potentially reduced window of fertility and offered referral to fertility specialists for counseling and intervention. Clinical tests to predict the precise timing of menopause are not available; however, the serum antimüllerian hormone level is promising as a predictor of ovarian reserve and is likely to be recommended for routine monitoring of cancer survivors at risk for premature menopause in the near future.[341] Hormonal interventions to potentially prolong ovarian function have not been clinically effective.[341] Cryopreservation of embryos (which require a partner or sperm donor) is an option for a survivor who anticipates early menopause. Recent successes in the techniques of cryopreservation of eggs during the period of ovarian function create new options for survivors at risk for premature menopause.[341,348]

Males

Males treated with alkylating agents as children and adolescents are at risk for infertility secondary to impaired testicular germ cell function and low testosterone resulting from Leydig cell insufficiency.[349] Alkylating agent gonadal toxicity is dose dependent, and pubertal status or age at exposure is not protective.[35,225,350] Of note, the majority of male survivors with alkylating agent–induced infertility will have normal testosterone production, with normal sexual function and secondary sexual characteristics. Abnormal semen analyses have been observed with cumulative cyclophosphamide doses greater than 5.0 to 7.5 g/m². However, Leydig cell insufficiency (elevated serum LH, normal testosterone) or Leydig cell failure (elevated LH, low testosterone) is associated with higher total cyclophosphamide doses (>20 g/m²).[35,351,352] Survivors treated with unilateral orchiectomy and not exposed to additional gonadal toxic therapy usually maintain adequate testicular function.[353]

A survivor's risk for irradiation-induced testicular dysfunction depends on radiation dose and age at exposure. Testicular germ cells are very sensitive to radiation damage. Changes in spermatogenesis can be observed after doses as low as 0.1 Gy, and irreversible azoospermia usually occurs after doses greater than 2 Gy.[339] In contrast, testosterone production is usually preserved with testicular doses up to 20 Gy. Irreversible damage to testicular germ cell and endocrine function usually occurs after exposure to more than 20 Gy of radiation, requiring androgen replacement therapy. However, survivors who are beyond puberty at the time of diagnosis can usually tolerate higher doses of radiation before loss of testicular endocrine function.[265]

Although reduced testicular volume on physical examination, elevated serum gonadotropins (e.g., FSH), and low serum inhibin B suggest infertility, the only definitive measures of a survivor's potential fertility is by semen analysis or paternity. Of note, male survivors with ejaculatory azoospermia diagnosed by semen analysis soon after completion of therapy have the potential to recover spermatogenesis many years later.[352,354] Thus a sexually active survivor who is not contemplating paternity must be counseled about birth control, even if he has had an abnormal semen analysis in the past. Furthermore, survivors with ejaculatory azoospermia who desire biologic paternity may be candidates for the surgical procedure of testicular biopsy with sperm extraction.[355] These men should be referred to a urologist with this expertise for consultation.

Survivors with delayed onset of puberty or symptoms of hypoandrogenism should be screened with morning serum testosterone, LH, and FSH evaluation. If results are abnormal, testosterone replacement therapy should be guided by the appropriate subspecialist. Of note, serum testosterone levels normally decline with advancing age, so survivors at risk for treatment-associated hypoandrogenism should have serum testosterone levels reevaluated as they reach older adulthood.

Sexual Function

Surgery or irradiation of the pelvis or lumbar spine, treatment-associated hormonal insufficiencies, medical comorbidities, and the social and emotional changes associated with a cancer experience may predispose childhood cancer survivors to sexual dysfunction. An emerging literature on the prevalence and risk factors for sexual dysfunction in young adult survivors of childhood cancer shows a higher than expected prevalence of both males (20% to 32%) and females (37% to 52%) reporting a problem in one or more areas of sexual function.[356-359] Normal sexual function is dependent on the complex interplay of both physical and social and emotional factors. Physical factors that can cause sexual dysfunction include disruption of normal pelvic anatomy from pelvic or spinal surgery or irradiation, hormonal deficiency, increasing age, and emotional distress.[349] Survivors at the greatest risk for psychosexual dysfunction include those diagnosed during adolescence, those with a brain tumor, and those with poor health status; these factors may be related to social isolation and delayed psychosexual development.[356,358,359] Because sexual function is an important aspect of quality of life and all survivors are at risk for psychosexual dysfunction related to their cancer experience, it is recommended that all adolescent and young adult survivors have an assessment of their sexual function as part of follow-up care.[360] The assessment for sexual dysfunction in the childhood cancer survivor includes a thorough psychosexual history, sexual history, medical history, and physical examination, including Tanner staging. Sexual history should include detailed questions about social relationships; body image; sexual experiences; libido; for women, lubrication genital sensation, orgasm, dyspareunia, and postcoital bleeding; and for men, nocturnal emissions, spontaneous erections, orgasm, and quality of ejaculate. If sexual dysfunction is a concern, consultation with gynecologist, urologist, or psychotherapist is indicated.

Pregnancy

Women who undergo abdominal or pelvic irradiation who are able to conceive children are at risk for complications of their pregnancy and delivery. Irradiation-induced damage to uterine muscle and blood flow adversely affects survivors' prognosis for a healthy full-term pregnancy.[361] Pelvic and abdominal radiation fields that include the uterus are associated with pregnancy complications, including spontaneous abortions, preterm labor, low-birth-weight infants, infants who are small for gestational age (SGA), neonatal death, and postpartum hemorrhage.[343,362,363,364-369] A report on more than 4000 pregnancies from the CCSS showed that the only risk factor for adverse pregnancy outcomes was pelvic irradiation, which was associated with low-birth-weight infants (RR, 1.84). No other treatment factor was a risk for any adverse pregnancy outcome in this large cohort.[362,363] When the analysis was restricted to 2201 liveborn children of 1264 survivors in the CCSS cohort, maternal uterine irradiation (>5 Gy) was associated with prematurity (OR, 3.5), low birth weight (OR, 6.8), and SGA infants (OR, 4.0).[364] Estrogen therapy does increase uterine size and stimulate blood flow but is not shown to improve uterine muscular function.[370]

Survivors with therapy-associated cardiac toxicity (either subclinical or overt) are at risk for pregnancy-associated congestive heart failure and should be monitored before pregnancy, during pregnancy, and after delivery by obstetricians aware of potential complications.[157,371] Peripartum acute congestive heart failure has been described in survivors treated with anthracyclines and chest irradiation; however, the incidence has not been determined.[157,371] One study of 37 anthracycline-exposed pregnant women showed that prepregnancy left ventricular dysfunction was a risk factor for acute congestive heart failure during pregnancy, supporting the need to closely monitor at-risk survivors.[371] Survivors with risks for other organ toxicities such as endocrinopathies, pulmonary fibrosis, and renal insufficiency should also be meticulously evaluated and monitored before pregnancy, during pregnancy, and after delivery.

Offspring

Many studies have investigated the possible association between exposure to cancer therapy during childhood and a mutagenic or teratogenic effect on future offspring. Fortunately, no study to date has found in increased risk for either congenital anomalies or cancer in the offspring of adult survivors of nonhereditary childhood cancer treated before conception.[35,372-381] This is true for both male and female survivors of childhood cancer and survivors treated with both chemotherapy and radiation therapy. Of note, survivors of childhood cancers that are associated with genetic syndromes and hereditary cancer predisposition (e.g., Cowden syndrome, Li-Fraumeni syndrome, retinoblastoma) are at increased risk for their offspring being diagnosed with cancer. These survivors should be referred for genetic counseling and genetic testing as desired and appropriate (see Box 72-2). Preimplantation genetic testing may be available to survivors with a known mutation in a cancer predisposition gene who are contemplating pregnancy.[382,383]

Renal System

Chronic renal disease is a late effect associated with irradiation to the kidneys as part of an abdominal field or total-body irradiation; chemotherapy with ifosfamide and high-dose cisplatin; nephrectomy, especially in combination with other nephrotoxic therapy; and treatment with other nephrotoxic agents, including antibiotics and immunosuppressants. The pathophysiology of irradiation injury to the kidney is progressive arteriolonephrosclerosis, resulting from irradiation injury of the renal microvasculature with subsequent secondary damage to the glomeruli and tubules. Irradiation-associated renal injury is dose related, and the threshold dose is approximately 15 Gy; however, nephrectomy and exposure to other nephrotoxic agents lower that threshold.[384,385] In a cohort of bone marrow transplant survivors treated with fractionated total-body irradiation, 12 to 14 Gy over 3 to 4 days, late renal dysfunction was reported in 35% of acute lymphoblastic leukemia survivors and 71% of neuroblastoma survivors.[385] Modern conditioning regimens with altered fractionation should reduce the incidence of renal insufficiency in transplant survivors.

Chemotherapy with cisplatin at doses greater than 200 mg/m^2 can cause nephropathy secondary to glomerular or tubular injury. This injury is usually acute and reversible; however, it can be stable or progressive.[386] Carboplatin does not appear to be associated with long-term nephrotoxicity.[387] Ifosfamide nephrotoxicity is also a result of glomerular or tubular injury and presents most often as renal tubular acidosis.[388] The greatest risk for ifosfamide nephrotoxicity is at total dose greater than 45 g/m^2, and age younger than 3 years.[388] Combination nephrotoxic chemotherapy, nephrectomy, and therapy with nephrotoxic antibiotics all contribute to survivors' risk for long-term renal damage.[389-392]

The risk for chronic renal disease in survivors treated with unilateral nephrectomy alone appears to be minimal.[393] However, data suggest that patients treated with unilateral nephrectomy do manifest subclinical evidence of early reversible renal injury detectable by elevated urine levels of microalbumin.[394,395] A study linking Wilms tumor survivors in the National Wilms Tumor Study group to the U.S. End-Stage Renal Disease registry followed for a median of 11 years showed a low risk for end-stage chronic renal failure in nonsyndromic Wilms tumor survivors (cumulative incidence, 0.6% at 20 years).[393] These data suggest that Wilms tumor survivors with clinically detectable renal dysfunction will not routinely progress to end-stage renal disease.[393] Of note, this cohort has not reached an age when survivors might be at the greatest risk for chronic renal failure.[393] Survivors of Wilms tumor with the highest cumulative incidence of chronic renal failure at 20 years are survivors with predisposition syndromes such as Denys-Drash syndrome (74%), WAGR syndrome (36%), genitourinary abnormalities (7%), and survivors with bilateral disease

(12%).[396-398] Survivors of Wilms tumor with progressive tumor in the contralateral kidney or nephrogenic rests and survivors who have undergone irradiation have also been identified as having an increased risk for renal dysfunction.[396-398]

Survivors treated with nephrotoxic therapy should be routinely monitored for early clinical signs of renal dysfunction, including hypertension, proteinuria, and elevated serum creatinine concentration. Survivors with the earliest signs of renal injury might benefit from therapeutic interventions with angiotensin-converting enzyme inhibitors to reverse or halt progression of renal injury. Survivors with a single kidney should be counseled to adopt health behaviors to maintain kidney health, including hydration, avoidance of prolonged use of nonsteroidal antiinflammatory drugs, prompt treatment of urinary tract infections, and meticulous control of coexisting diabetes and hypertension.

Genitourinary System

In addition to the renal late effects discussed previously, survivors of childhood cancer are also at risk for toxicity to the genitourinary system from surgery, treatment with pelvic and whole-abdominal irradiation, and alkylating agent chemotherapy. Genitourinary surgery can result in long-term functional impairments, including urinary incontinence and sexual dysfunction. The primary late effects associated with irradiation include fibrosis or hypoplasia of the anatomic components of the male and female genitourinary systems, including urinary bladder, ureter, urethra, prostate, vagina, and uterus, resulting in chronic pain or dysfunction. Survivors experiencing anatomic or functional genitourinary late effects, including sexual dysfunction, should be referred to a gynecologist or urologist as indicated for evaluation and management of their symptoms.

Chemotherapy with cyclophosphamide and ifosfamide has been associated with protracted hemorrhagic cystitis and bladder fibrosis, although this late effect has been reduced by concurrent therapy with mesna.[399,400] Hemorrhagic cystitis that develops beyond the time of therapy more often has a viral etiology or is associated with chronic graft-versus-host disease (GVHD) in transplant survivors.[401] Although the risk for bladder pathology in childhood cancer survivors is low, routine monitoring with urinalysis of survivors exposed to cyclophosphamide and ifosfamide is clinically indicated.

Gastrointestinal System

Potential late effects of cancer therapy on the gastrointestinal system are late onset surgical complications such as adhesions, small bowel obstruction, and fecal incontinence[402]; irradiation-induced functional impairment; and secondary neoplasms of the gastrointestinal tract and hepatobiliary system.[67] Hepatic fibrosis is a rare late complication of antimetabolite chemotherapy (methotrexate, mercaptopurine, thioguanine), and the fibrosis typically follows acute hepatic toxicity such as venoocclusive disease.[403-405] As with other organ systems, irradiation can result in functional impairment and second cancers of the gastrointestinal organs consequently exposed to radiation as a result of location in a treatment field. The clinical spectrum of irradiation-induced gastrointestinal toxicity that has been reported includes salivary gland dysfunction, esophageal stricture, Barrett esophagus, hepatic fibrosis and cirrhosis, focal nodular hyperplasia, cholelithiasis, and chronic enterocolitis.[405,406] In the CCSS, survivors had nearly twice the risk for gastrointestinal disease than that observed in the sibling cohort. Survivors were more likely to require colostomy/ileostomy (RR, 5.6 [95% CI, 2.4 to 13.1]), undergo liver biopsy (RR, 23.1 [95% CI, 7.5 to 77.8]), or self-report cirrhosis (RR, 8.9 [95% CI 2.0 to 40.0]).[407] Risk factors for gastrointestinal toxicity in long-term survivors included older age at diagnosis (>10 years), high-dose alkylating agent and/or anthracycline exposure, abdominal irradiation, and abdominal surgery.[407] Of note, survivors were more likely to have more than one gastrointestinal condition than their siblings and more frequently reported common conditions such as diarrhea, ulcers, polyps, and heartburn.[407]

Common gastrointestinal symptoms reported by a childhood cancer survivor, such as abdominal pain and heartburn, should be evaluated in the context of his or her treatment history. A survivor's risk for a serious gastrointestinal pathologic process should be considered when planning a diagnostic workup and therapy for common symptoms. Children requiring abdominal surgery as part of their cancer therapy are at risk for late onset small bowel obstruction and should be educated about his late effect.[408] Because survivors exposed to abdominal irradiation are considered to be at higher risk for colon cancer, and self-report polyps at greater frequency,[407] they are advised to begin colon cancer screening earlier than what is recommended for the general population (10 years after completing radiation therapy or age 35 years, whichever comes last).[67,89]

OTHER LATE EFFECTS

Infections

Late-occurring infectious complications can result from surgery, transfusions, immunosuppression, and radiation therapy. Childhood cancer survivors who had a surgical splenectomy as part of their staging for Hodgkin lymphoma are at lifelong risk for potentially fatal bacterial sepsis with encapsulated organisms. Survivors who received more than 40 Gy of abdominal or left flank irradiation are considered functionally asplenic and have a similar risk for sepsis.[409] These survivors must be continually reminded of their risk and educated to receive immediate medical evaluation and prophylactic antibiotic therapy for fever or other signs of sepsis. Immunizations against *Streptococcus pneumoniae, Haemophilus influenzae,* and *Neisseria meningitidis* are also recommended for this high-risk group.[410] Hematopoietic stem cell transplant survivors receiving immunosuppression for chronic GVHD are also at risk for ongoing infectious complication and should be considered for prophylactic antibiotics.[411] Older survivors treated in the United States are at risk for transfusion-acquired chronic hepatitis B if they received blood products prior to 1972; for hepatitis C if they received blood products prior to 1993; and for human immunodeficiency virus if they received blood products between 1977 and 1985.[412] Irradiation to the sinuses for a primary sarcoma or CNS tumor at doses greater than 30 Gy is associated with chronic bacterial sinusitis.[413] Survivors who received therapy that is associated with a risk for pulmonary disease such as lung irradiation or total-body irradiation and those with cardiac disease should receive annual influenza vaccine. Survivors with known irradiation-associated valve disease should receive appropriate antibiotic prophylaxis for subacute bacterial endocarditis.[414] Survivors at risk for infectious complications should be educated about their risks and informed of the necessity for preventive strategies.

Dental Problems

Childhood cancer survivors are at risk for dental late effects. Survivors treated with head and neck irradiation are at risk for root shunting, microdontia, hypodontia, and craniofacial abnormalities resulting in severe cosmetic or functional impairment necessitating surgical or orthodontic intervention.[415-417] The risk for dental facial abnormalities is greatest in survivors treated at the youngest age and with higher doses of radiation. Survivors treated with chemotherapy prior to the complete eruption of their permanent teeth are at risk for tooth agenesis, root thinning or shortening, and enamel dysplasia.[417,418] Neuroblastoma survivors and leukemia survivors treated with cranial irradiation have a particularly high incidence of dental abnormalities (71% and 94%, respectively) most likely associated with young age at treatment.[416,417] In a report from the CCSS, when compared with the sibling cohort, survivors were more likely to report microdontia, hypodontia, root abnormalities, abnormal enamel, teeth loss (six or more), severe gingivitis, and xerostomia. Radiation exposure of 20 Gy or more to dentition was associated with an increased risk for one or more dental abnormalities. Children diagnosed at age younger than 5 years treated with alkylating agents also had increased risk for one or more dental abnormalities.[419] All childhood cancer survivors should be advised to have regular dental care, including cleanings, fluoride applications, and appropriate imaging to evaluate tooth development.[89]

Psychosocial Function

The experience of having childhood cancer and its associated treatment can have long-term effects on a survivor's emotional and social functioning. Common disorders of emotional function, such as depression, anxiety, and posttraumatic stress disorders are reported more frequently in populations of childhood cancer survivors than in both their siblings and the general population.[420,421] Serious emotional distress, such as suicidal symptoms, is also reported more commonly in survivors. In a report from the CCSS, adult survivors of childhood cancer were at increased risk for suicidal ideation compared with the sibling control cohort (7.8% of survivors reported suicidal ideation compared with 4.6% of controls [OR, 1.79; 95% CI, 1.4 to 2.4]). In survivors, suicidal ideation was associated with a primary diagnosis of CNS malignancy, depression, and poor current physical health.[422] There is no known increased incidence of psychiatric disorders such as schizophrenia or other psychoses in childhood cancer survivors, with the exception of survivors of brain tumors. A Dutch study of over 3700 childhood cancer survivors found that brain tumor survivors had an excess risk for psychiatric hospitalizations for diagnoses that included psychoses of somatic and cerebral causes, psychiatric disorders in somatic disease, and schizophrenia.[423]

Challenges to normal social functioning such as educational remediation, employment discrimination, insurance discrimination, marital dissatisfaction, social isolation, and poor health-related quality of life have all been reported more frequently in survivors of childhood cancer.[424-433] The majority of childhood cancer survivors will not experience significant psychosocial dysfunction as a result of their cancer experience or cancer therapy; however, survivors of childhood CNS malignancies and those treated with cranial irradiation are more vulnerable to psychosocial morbidity. These survivors, in particular, should be routinely monitored for emotional distress and social disability.

SPECIAL CONSIDERATIONS FOR THE HEMATOPOIETIC STEM CELL TRANSPLANT SURVIVOR

The comprehensive clinical evaluation of the hematopoietic stem cell transplant (HSCT) survivor requires that the clinician consider all aspects of the survivor's pretransplant history, transplant course, posttransplant immune function, and disease status. In assessing the risk for late effects in a survivor of HSCT, both the treatments associated with the condition that led to the transplant and the therapies associated with the transplant must be considered. The modality, dose, and intensity of the conditioning regimens for HSCT are major factors that determine the survivor's risk for late effects. Total-body irradiation used as conditioning for HSCT may contribute to the organ-specific toxicity of prior chemotherapy, such as cardiotoxicity from anthracyclines,[188] ototoxicity from platinum agents,[324] and gonadotoxicity of alkylating agents.[344] The transplant history should be reviewed for complications that occurred during the course of transplant, such as acute pneumonitis or renal failure, which might add to the survivor's risk for late onset organ toxicity.[221,385] Survivors who received an allogeneic HSCT are at risk for chronic GVHD that can be associated with severe chronic illness. Long-term consequences of chronic GVHD can include joint contractures, polymyositis, vaginal stenosis, alopecia, vitiligo, scleroderma, lichenoid skin lesions, xerostomia, lichenoid or atrophic oral lesions, xerophthalmia, keratoconjunctivitis, esophageal strictures, malabsorption, cholestasis, bronchiolitis obliterans, and obstructive airway disease. Survivors with chronic GVHD and those on chronic immunosuppressive regimens have an increased risk for infection.[411] Comprehensive assessment of the HSCT must also include posttransplant immunization history to ensure revaccination was accomplished at appropriate intervals after transplant.

FOLLOW-UP CARE OF CHILDHOOD CANCER SURVIVORS

The need for specialized follow-up care for childhood cancer survivors is evident, given the numerous morbidities associated with childhood cancer treatment and the potential for survivors to develop complications decades after treatment. The prevalence of chronic health conditions observed in young adult survivors of childhood cancer is 62% in the CCSS cohort and 58% in a single-institution cohort of survivors from the United Kingdom.[46,434] In the CCSS, almost a third of patients had a severe or life-threatening health condition, and the cumulative incidence of a severe or disabling health condition approached 50% at 30 years after the diagnosis of childhood cancer.[46] A survivor's self-reported health status, including self-assessment of functional health, general health, mental health, and pain, has been described in several cohorts of young adult survivors of childhood cancer. Impaired health status is reported in more than 75% of adult survivors surveyed in Canada, 58% of adult survivors in a British cohort, and 48% of adult survivors in the CCSS.[434-436]

Although childhood cancer survivors are at risk for a variety of treatment-related health conditions as they age, they are not necessarily knowledgeable about the specifics of their cancer diagnosis and treatment, nor are they proactive about their future health or adherent to follow-up recommendations. Of the young adult survivors surveyed in the CCSS cohort, only 72% could accurately report their diagnosis; and although the majority were knowledgeable about the general type of therapy they received (e.g., chemotherapy, surgery, irradiation), only 70% of those receiving radiation therapy could report the site.[437] Furthermore, an analysis of cancer screening practices of the young adults in the CCSS cohort showed that adherence was not optimal[438] and in a separate analysis it was shown that the proportion of survivors who remain in long-term follow-up decreases with increasing years since completion of therapy.[439] The high prevalence of chronic health conditions, poor health status, knowledge deficits, and suboptimal adherence to follow-up recommendations all support the need for comprehensive specialized follow-up care of childhood cancer survivors, including both provision of health care services and risk education.

Models of Survivorship Care

Comprehensive survivor programs have been developed at pediatric cancer centers to provide long-term, specialized, risk-based, follow-up care to childhood cancer survivors. A survey of Children's Oncology Group institutions found 87% provide survivorship care and 59% have specialized late effects programs.[440] The ideal components of follow-up care systems include review of disease treatment and history, screening for and diagnosing late effects, a plan for long-term surveillance, coordination of subspecialists, provision of psychosocial support, counseling on education and occupation, coordination of transition to adult care, education and outreach to survivors in the community, education of professionals (primary care providers, educators), and research. The optimal patterns and models of care for childhood cancer survivors have not been well studied. A model endorsed by leaders of existing pediatric long-term follow-up clinics contains the following elements: clinic services under the direction by a pediatric oncologist with expertise in survivorship care; staffing by advanced degree nurses to provide and coordinate patient care; and access to social workers, psychologists, a referral network of medical and surgical specialists with survivorship expertise, and ongoing care provided in the community with periodic center-based follow-up.[441] This model assumes frequent bidirectional communication between survivors, primary care providers, and oncologists with clear delineation of responsibilities for ongoing care. In general, these comprehensive, center-based programs have the proven advantage of providing multidisciplinary expertise and survivor education and have the facility for research in cancer survivorship. Common challenges these programs face are limited financial and personnel resources; inadequate capacity to meet the needs of growing numbers of survivors; and limited access because of geography, insurance, or lack of awareness on the part of the primary care providers or the individual survivor.[441,442] These and other alternative models for extending and improving care delivered to childhood cancer survivors have been proposed but have not been formally evaluated in terms of feasibility and efficacy.

Current efforts to retain survivors in long-term follow-up have focused on introducing and reinforcing the concept of life-long follow-up at critical transition points on the cancer care continuum (Fig. 72-6). Two specific points that have become the focus of educational interventions are the time periods around completion of planned cancer treatment and again when a survivor is an emerging adult. Transition programs for those who recently completed therapy are designed to educate survivors regarding treatment-related risks and to introduce issues related to survivorship early after cancer treatment. The goal of these programs is to bridge the period between active therapy and survivorship follow-up care and subsequently reduce the knowledge deficit and loss to follow-up seen in prior cohorts of long-term survivors.[443] Similarly, transition programs for survivors who have reached the age of adolescence or young adulthood are designed to support adolescent or young adult survivors as they transfer care to adult-oriented health care services. Ideally, these transition programs address the transfer of knowledge about disease, treatment, and future health risks from parents to adolescent or young adult survivor; enhance the survivor's cognitive competence/self-efficacy; and help with access to and confidence in adult providers.[444] Research is needed to test the efficacy of these transition specific programs to improve the participation of childhood survivors in lifelong term follow-up care.

Comprehensive Clinical Evaluation

Independent of the setting in which it occurs, the clinical evaluation of the childhood cancer survivor should include a comprehensive treatment summary, thorough

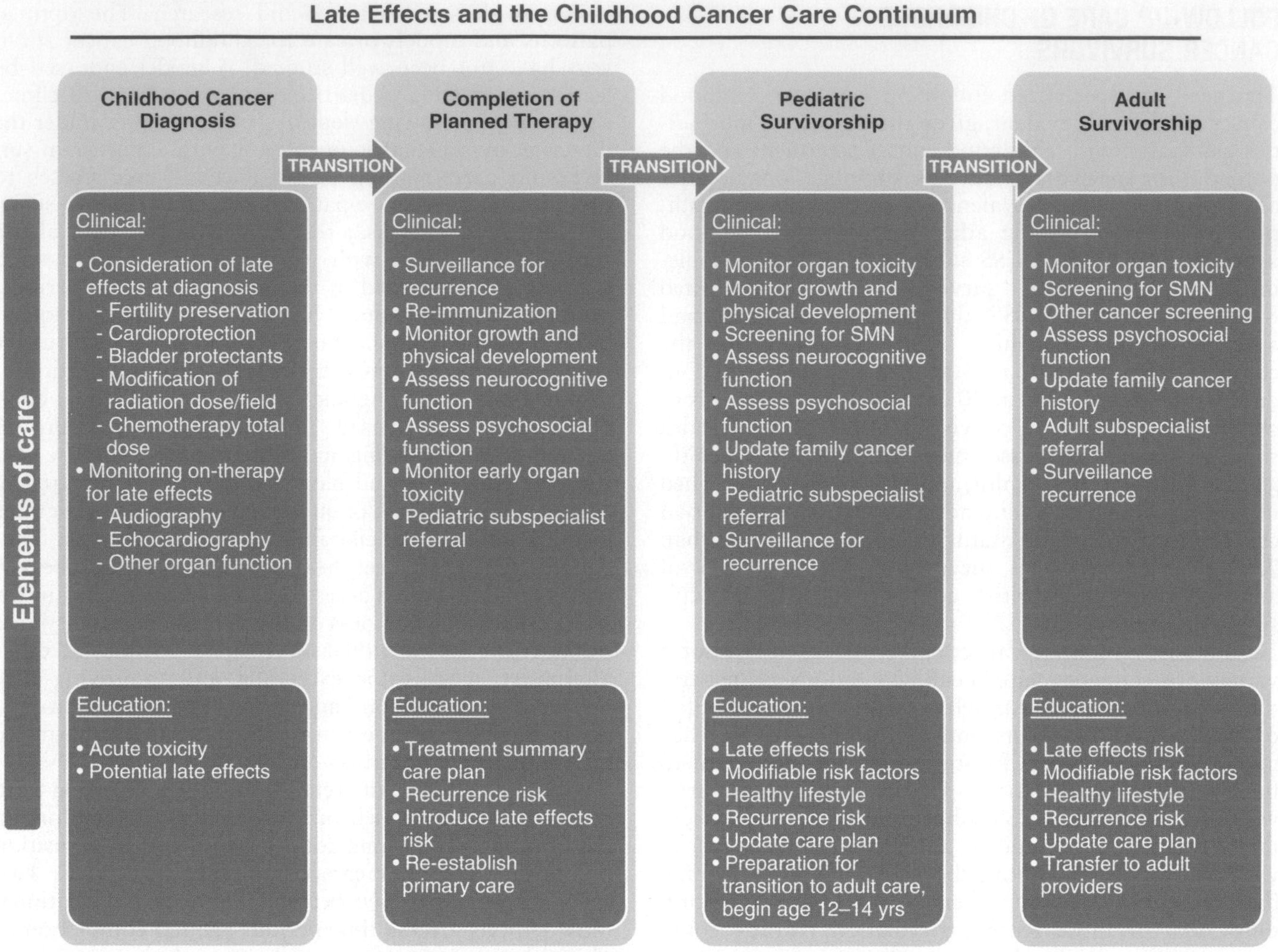

Late Effects and the Childhood Cancer Care Continuum

Figure 72-6 Late effects and the childhood cancer care continuum.

physical examination, and a care plan that includes recommendations for diagnostic or screening tests as indicated. The results of the evaluation should be summarized, documented, and communicated to the survivor and all health care providers participating in the survivor's care.

Treatment Summary

Information about prior diagnosis and treatment exposures is necessary for a health care provider to begin a comprehensive childhood cancer survivor's evaluation. This critical information is likely contained in a pediatric oncology "treatment summary." Details about diagnosis that are necessary for the survivor follow-up evaluation include age at diagnosis, presenting symptoms, results of diagnostic and staging evaluation, and pathology. Specifics of radiation therapy (field and dose); chemotherapy (specific agents and cumulative doses); surgeries (splenectomy, organ resections, and biopsies); and blood transfusions are all important component of a survivor's treatment history that contribute to the assessment of future health risks. Information about any required modifications in treatment, major acute complications of therapy, and ongoing treatment-related issues, such as

chronic GVHD, should be available at the time of evaluation. For a provider not familiar with a survivor's prior therapy, a treatment summary can usually be obtained from the treating institution. A sample treatment summary template is provided in Figure 72-7. A summary of late effects associated with curative treatments for the most common childhood cancer diagnoses is presented in Table 72-4.

Medical History and Physical Examination

As in all medical assessments, obtaining and documenting a history of current and past medical problems is important to the childhood cancer survivor evaluation. Past medical history, including birth history, surgeries, and medical conditions that preceded the cancer diagnosis, may be pertinent. For older survivors, menstrual history, reproductive history, and obstetric history all contribute important information to the follow-up evaluation. Information about current medications and chronic medical conditions should also be obtained. Survivors should specifically be asked about any late effects diagnosed or treated to date, including subsequent cancers.

Treatment Summary

Current Name:	Medical Record Number:
Name at Diagnosis:	Date of Birth:

Diagnosis:	Site(s):
Presenting Symptoms:	
Date of Diagnosis:	Protocol:
Date of Recurrence:	Site(s):
Relapse Protocol:	Date of Treatment Completion:
Complications During Treatment	

Chemotherapy

Agent:	Total Dose:
Agent:	Total Dose:
Agent:	Total Dose:
Agent:	Total Dose:
Agent:	Total Dose:

Radiotherapy

Date:	Site:	Dose:

Bone Marrow Transplant

Date:	Allo/Auto	Allo Donor / HLA Matching
Chemotherapy Conditioning (include doses):		

TBI / Other Radiotherapy	Site:	Dose:	Fractions:
Acute GvHD (Grade, site)	Chronic GvHD (Grade, site)	Treatment	

Surgery

Site:	Date:

Medical History

Complications After Treatment Completion:

Family History:

Recent Studies

Test:	Date:	Results:

Figure 72-7 Example of childhood cancer survivor treatment summary template. *(Modified from Skinner R, Wallace WHB, Levitt GA, editors: Therapy-based long-term follow-up practice statement, 2nd ed. United Kingdom, 2005, Children's Cancer Study Group. Accessed at http://www.ukccsg.org.uk/public/followup/PracticeStatement/APPENDICES-g.pdf.)*

TABLE 72-4   Potential Late Effects Associated With Curative Therapies for Common Childhood Cancers

Primary Cancer	Categories of Treatment-Associated Late Effects					
	Secondary Malignancy (Associated Therapy)	Cardiovascular/Pulmonary (Associated Therapy)	Musculoskeletal (Associated Therapy)	Neurologic/Developmental (Associated Therapy)	Endocrine/Reproductive (Associated Therapy)	Other (Associated Therapy)
Leukemia	MDS/leukemia (*Alkylating agents, topoisomerase inhibitors*) Skin cancer Meningiomas CNS tumors (*Cranial irradiation*)	Cardiomyopathy Arrhythmias (*Anthracyclines*)	Decreased bone mineral density (*Corticosteroids, MTX*) Osteonecrosis (*Corticosteroids*) Short stature (*Corticosteroids, Cranial irradiation*) Dental abnormalities (*Cranial irradiation*)	Learning disabilities (*Cranial irradiation, intrathecal therapy*) Vasculopathy (*Cranial irradiation*) Cataracts (*Corticosteroids, cranial irradiation*) Peripheral neuropathy Raynaud phenomenon (*Vincristine*)	GH deficiency Obesity (*Cranial irradiation*) Hypogonadism Azoospermia (*Testicular irradiation*) Infertility Hypogonadism (*Alkylating agents*)	Alopecia (*Cranial irradiation*)
Brain tumor	CNS tumors Meningiomas Skin cancer (*Cranial/spinal irradiation*) MDS/leukemia (*Alkylating agents, topoisomerase inhibitors*)	Cardiac dysfunction (*Spinal irradiation*)	Scoliosis Short stature (*Cranial/spinal irradiation*) Dental abnormalities (*Cranial irradiation*)	Learning disabilities (*Cranial irradiation/ neurosurgery*) Cataracts Neurosensory deficits Vasculopathy (*Cranial irradiation*) Seizures Hydrocephalus (*Neurosurgery*) Hearing loss (*Platinum compounds, cranial irradiation*) Peripheral neuropathy Raynaud phenomenon (*Vincristine*)	Hypothalamic-hypopituitarism GH deficiency Obesity (*Cranial irradiation*) Infertility Hypogonadism (*Alkylating agents*)	Renal insufficiency (*Platinum compounds, ifosfamide*) Alopecia (*Cranial irradiation*)
Hodgkin lymphoma	Thyroid cancer Breast cancer Lung cancer Upper GI cancer Sarcomas Skin cancer (*Mantle irradiation*) Colon cancer GU cancers Skin cancer (*Abdominal, pelvic irradiation*) MDS/leukemia (*Alkylating agents, topoisomerase inhibitors*)	Carotid artery stenosis Coronary artery disease Valvular heart disease Cardiomyopathy Pericardial fibrosis Arrhythmia (*Mantle irradiation*) Cardiomyopathy Arrhythmias (*Anthracycline*)	Scoliosis Short stature (*Thoracic irradiation*) Osteopenia Osteoporosis (*Corticosteroids*)		Thyroid disease (*Mantle irradiation*) Infertility Hypogonadism (*Pelvic irradiation/ alkylating agents*)	High-risk pregnancy (*Irradiation, anthracyclines*) Life-threatening bacterial sepsis (*Splenectomy*) GI strictures (*Mantle irradiation*) Pulmonary fibrosis (*Mantle irradiation, bleomycin*)

Neuroblastoma	Skin cancer Sarcomas (*Any irradiation*) Breast cancer Thyroid cancer (*Thoracic irradiation*) MDS/leukemia (*Alkylating agents, topoisomerase inhibitors*)	Cardiomyopathy Arrhythmias (*Anthracycline*)	Scoliosis Short stature (*Thoracic irradiation, TBI*)	Hearing loss (*Platinum compounds*)	Thyroid disease (*Thoracic irradiation*) Infertility Hypogonadism (*Alkylating agents*)	Renal insufficiency (*Platinum compounds, ifosfamide, abdominal irradiation*) Pulmonary fibrosis (*Thoracic irradiation*) Small bowel obstruction (*Abdominal surgery*) Horner syndrome Scoliosis (*Thoracic surgery*)
Wilms tumor	Colon cancer Skin cancer Sarcoma (*Abdominal irradiation*) Skin cancer Breast cancer Lung cancer (*Lung irradiation*)	Cardiomyopathy Arrhythmias (*Anthracycline*)	Scoliosis Short stature (*Abdominal irradiation*)	Peripheral neuropathy Raynaud phenomenon (*Vincristine*)	Infertility Hypogonadism (*Alkylating agents*)	Small bowel obstruction (*Abdominal surgery*) Renal insufficiency (*Nephrectomy, abdominal irradiation*) Pulmonary fibrosis (*Lung irradiation*) High-risk pregnancy (*Irradiation, anthracyclines*)
Sarcoma	MDS/leukemia (*Alkylating agents, topoisomerase inhibitors*) Cancer of the skin/bone/soft tissue/organs in the treatment field (*Irradiation*)	Cardiomyopathy Arrhythmias (*Anthracycline*)	Hypoplasia of the bone/soft tissue in irradiation field (*Irradiation*) Deformity of bone/soft tissue (*Surgery*) Dental abnormalities (*Irradiation*)	Hearing loss (*Platinum compounds*) Peripheral neuropathy Raynaud phenomenon (*Vincristine*)	Infertility Hypogonadism (*Alkylating agents*)	Renal insufficiency (*Platinum compounds, ifosfamide*) High-risk pregnancy (*Irradiation, anthracyclines*) Dysfunction of the organs in the treatment field (*Irradiation*)

CNS, Central nervous system; *GH*, Growth hormone; *GI*, gastrointestinal; *GU*, genitourinary; *MDS*, myelodysplastic syndrome; *MTX*, methotrexate; *TBI*, total-body irradiation.

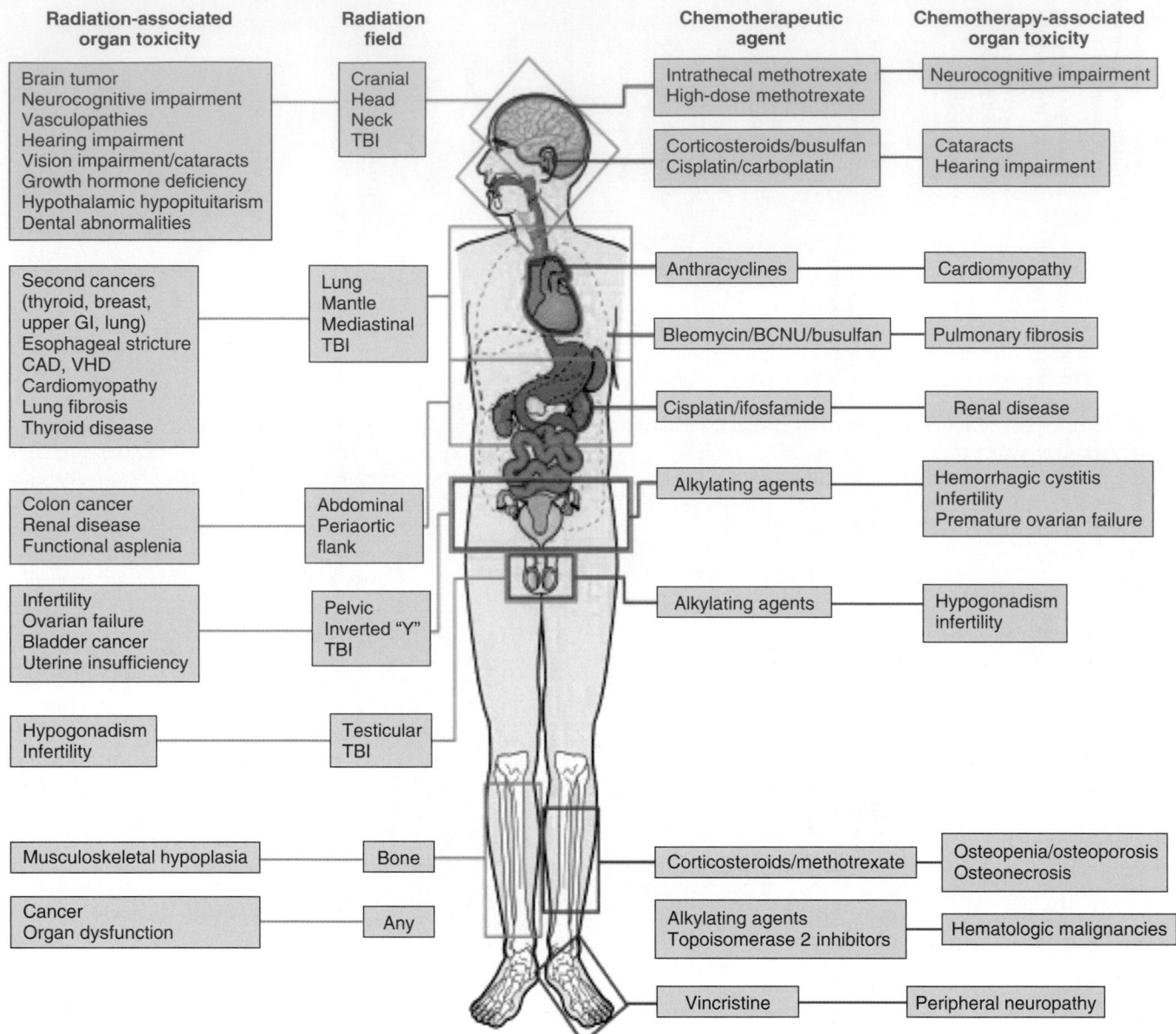

Figure 72-8 Late effects associated with common treatments for childhood cancer by organ systems. *CAD,* Coronary artery disease; *GI,* gastrointestinal; *TBI,* total-body irradiation; *VHD,* valvular heart disease.

Family history of chronic diseases, mental illness, and family cancer history are also an important part of the comprehensive survivor evaluation. Cancer diagnosed in first-degree relatives (parents, offspring, siblings) in a pattern suggestive of a hereditary cancer predisposition syndrome should be noted and appropriate referrals to cancer geneticists considered (see Box 72-2). A family history that includes other children with cancer raises particular concerns about hereditary cancer syndromes, as does a family history of genetic syndromes associated with cancer predisposition. A survivor's family history of common chronic diseases should be noted, with special attention to conditions for which the survivor may have treatment-related risk factors, such as heart disease, osteoporosis, or depression. Family history should be updated and reassessed at each subsequent evaluation.

All survivors should be asked about educational attainment and special education services or needs. For older survivors, employment history and insurance status are also critical to determining health care needs. Health behaviors including exercise, diet, sleep, tobacco use, alcohol use, and nonprescription drug use are also important aspects of the follow-up assessment. To further evaluate a survivor's emotional and physical needs not addressed in a medical history, survivors should be asked about their relationships with family and peers, sexual activity, and current living arrangements.

A comprehensive childhood cancer survivor's evaluation also includes a review of current and recent symptoms. This review of symptoms should include special consideration of symptoms known to be associated with specific late effects. Symptoms should be evaluated in light of the increased prior probability of significant morbidity compared with similar-aged patients. For example, a complaint of chronic headaches or sinus problems in a patient with a history of head and neck irradiation should be evaluated in light of the risk for radiogenic tumors; a young patient with dyspnea or chest pain might undergo a cardiac evaluation with a lower threshold than a patient who was not exposed to cardiotoxic therapies as a child.

A thorough physical examination including a skin examination and neurologic examination are also part of a childhood cancer survivor's routine evaluation. Radiation fields in particular should be examined carefully for any skin changes, masses, or lesions. A careful thyroid examination is indicated, in particular for patients who received radiation to the head, neck, chest or upper spine. Head, trunk, and limbs should be examined for growth disturbances related to surgery or irradiation, such as limb-length discrepancies, spinal deformity, and facial bone deformity. Major organ toxicity associated with specific chemotherapy agents and radiation fields commonly used to treat pediatric cancers is illustrated in Figure 72-8. Transplant survivors should be examined for signs of chronic GVHD.

Diagnostic and Screening Tests

The health care provider evaluating the childhood cancer survivor should arrange for diagnostic or screening tests and subspecialty consultations based on the survivor's treatment risks, symptoms, or other findings. The provider should recommend surveillance studies assessing primary disease recurrence if indicated; studies to assess organ function in any organs potentially affected by cancer therapy; and specialist consultation to evaluate findings or potential health risks. Depending on exposures, age, and gender, screening studies to assess for second cancers such as mammography or colonoscopy should be considered. Clinical guidelines developed by the Children's Oncology Group are available to help direct clinicians in the evaluation of survivors of childhood, adolescent, and young adult cancer.[89] These risk-based, treatment-related guidelines are intended to provide screening recommendations for late effects commonly observed in survivors.

Assessment and Follow-Up Plan

A childhood cancer survivor's risk for each late effect should be interpreted in light of his or her treatment history, past medical history, family history, symptoms, and physical examination. All findings and test results from the comprehensive survivor evaluation should be summarized in a survivorship care plan, and recommendations and plans for follow-up should be documented and communicated to the patient and all providers involved in the patient's care. Acknowledging the potential complexity of the survivorship care plan, the provider should prioritize the follow-up recommendations for the survivor and family and emphasize that this advice is limited by our current knowledge of late effects and based on future probabilities.

In summary, the successful follow-up care for the childhood cancer survivor depends on thorough evaluation with attention to possible late effects and effective communication with patient, family, and other providers involved in ongoing care.

FUTURE DIRECTIONS

Advances in the treatment of childhood cancer have resulted in growing numbers of survivors. Epidemiologic studies show that survivors of childhood cancer are likely to experience adverse health-related consequences of their treatment, and the potential to develop late effects appears to be lifelong. Although remarkable progress has been made in describing the late effects experienced by childhood cancer survivors and their associated risk factors, future research is needed to continue to decrease incidence and morbidity and to improve the quality of life for current and future survivors. In response, survivorship research is focused on three main areas: changes in primary cancer therapy that are focused on decreasing incidence of late toxicity; improvements in care to decrease the incidence or severity of particular late effects; and changes in the health care systems to ensure that all survivors have access to best practices to detect and manage late effects.

Current treatment protocols for childhood cancer are designed to minimize late effects without compromising survival. The strategies that have been investigated or are under investigation include eliminating or reducing exposures to specific chemotherapies with known late toxicities, such as anthracyclines and alkylating agents, developing chemoprotectant agents, reducing radiation dose and field, and delaying radiation therapy for very young children.[445-451] Studies to quantify the efficacy of these strategies to obviate late effects while maintaining survival are forthcoming. Current strategies for primary treatment of standard-risk acute lymphoblastic leukemia, localized Hodgkin lymphoma, Wilms tumor, and neuroblastoma designed to reduce late effects have resulted in excellent outcomes, with low incidence of both recurrence and treatment-related late effects, to date.[180,448,451,452]

Another strategy to reduce late morbidity in childhood cancer survivors is the identification of individuals with heightened susceptibility for specific treatment-associated late effects. One potential method of identification is genetic polymorphism testing, which identifies individuals with a genotype that is known to increase susceptibility to treatment-associated toxicity, such as second cancers, obesity, and cardiac disease.[128,453-455] Testing could be done before cancer treatment and the results used to modify treatment plans to account for an individual's genetic susceptibility for late effects. For example, lower-dose radiation therapy might be indicated for an individual identified by genetic polymorphism testing as having a genotype associated with irradiation-induced second cancers. Similarly, genetic polymorphism testing could be done decades after therapy to identify survivors at risk for late effects, which would inform screening recommendations and eligibility for preventive interventions.

Health services research focused on understanding cancer survivor care and studying improvements in care is ongoing. As the current population of childhood cancer survivors ages, health care delivery to this group will become more complex and will include integration of treatment-related risks and adult-onset morbidity. Optimal and innovative methods of patient (and health care provider) education that achieve this integration will need to be elucidated and disseminated to ensure the best possible quality of life for survivors of childhood cancer.

The care of the child diagnosed with cancer does not end with the completion of therapy. Consequently, pediatric oncology providers need to have a working knowledge of the potential late effects of curative therapy for childhood cancer and are responsible to communicate information about late effects to survivors, their families, and other health care providers involved in the care of childhood cancer survivor. Pediatric survivorship research has made significant contributions to advance our understanding of long-term treatment–associated morbidities, and current therapeutic protocols are designed with the intention of minimizing known late effects. However, despite progress, childhood cancer survivors remain vulnerable to many long-term treatment related morbidities. Ongoing efforts in research and clinical care for childhood cancer survivors must be directed toward improving and extending follow-up care, at developing interventions for individuals identified as being at risk for specific late effects, and at optimizing management of late effects with the ultimate aim of improving quality of life for all current and future childhood cancer survivors.

> ▶ *References available online at ExpertConsult.*

KEY REFERENCES

10. Li FP, Cassady JR, Jaffe N: Risk of second tumors in survivors of childhood cancer. *Cancer* 35:1230–1235, 1975.

   This study is one of the first descriptions of the association between treatment of childhood cancer and the development of second primary malignancies decades after treatment. In this single-institution study researchers reported the 20-year cumulative probability of a second cancer (12% SE 4%). They describe the association between therapeutic radiation and second cancers as well as suggest that host susceptibility may be an etiologic factor.

21. Armstrong GT, Liu Q, Yasui Y, et al: Late mortality among 5-year survivors of childhood cancer: a summary from the Childhood Cancer Survivor Study. *J Clin Oncol* 27:2328–2338, 2009.

   This is a comprehensive summary of the CCSS mortality data based on a cohort of 20,483 childhood cancer survivors, representing 337,334 person-years of observation, linked to the National Death Index and death certificates. Overall cumulative mortality, patterns of late death over time, cause-specific mortality, and specific treatment-related risk factors for late mortality are described.

29. Robison LL, Mertens AC, Boice JD, et al: Study design and cohort characteristics of the Childhood Cancer Survivor Study: a multi-institutional collaborative project. *Med Pediatr Oncol* 38:229–239, 2002.

   The CCSS is a consortium of 25 North American institutions representing one of the largest and most extensively characterized cohorts of childhood and adolescent cancer survivors (diagnosed prior to age 21 years with selected cancer diagnoses, diagnoses between 1970-1986, and survival for at least 5 years). This reference is a description of the methodology used to develop the CCSS, which serves as a resource for addressing risk for second malignancies, endocrine and reproductive outcomes, cardiopulmonary complications, and psychosocial implications among childhood cancer survivors.

33. Reulen RC, Frobisher C, Winter DL, et al: Long-term risks of subsequent primary neoplasms among survivors of childhood cancer. *JAMA* 305:2311–2319, 2011.

   The British Childhood Cancer Survivor Study is a population-based cohort of 17,981 5-year survivors of childhood cancer diagnosed with cancer when younger than 15 years between 1940 and 1991 in Great Britain, followed up through December 2006. In this study the cohort is used to investigate the long-term risks of subsequent primary neoplasms in survivors of childhood cancer, to identify the cancer types that contribute most to long-term excess risk, and to identify subgroups of survivors at substantially increased risk for particular subsequent primary neoplasms.

36. van der Pal HJ, van Dalen EC, van Delden E, et al: High risk of symptomatic cardiac events in childhood cancer survivors. *J Clin Oncol* 30:1429–1437, 2012.

   This cohort study assessing the long-term risk for clinically validated, symptomatic cardiac events in 5-year survivors of childhood cancer demonstrated that higher cumulative anthracycline dose or higher cumulative radiation dose was associated with higher risk ratio for cardiac events. Survivors with both anthracycline and cardiac irradiation exposures had the highest cumulative incidence of cardiac events, with nearly one in eight survivors treated with both exposures developing a serious cardiac event.

46. Oeffinger KC, Mertens AC, Sklar CA, et al: Chronic health conditions in adult survivors of childhood cancer. *N Engl J Med* 355:1572–1582, 2006.

   This report from the Childhood Cancer Survivor Study details chronic health conditions in adult survivors of childhood cancer. The relative risk for a severe or life-threatening chronic condition in survivors when compared with siblings was 8.2 (95% CI, 6.9-9.7).

47. Hudson MM, Ness KK, Gurney JG, et al: Clinical ascertainment of health outcomes among adults treated for childhood cancer. *JAMA* 309:2371–2381, 2013.

   This report of clinically ascertained health outcomes among adult survivors of childhood cancer from the St. Jude Lifetime Cohort Study presents the prevalence and adverse health outcomes of 1713 adult survivors of childhood cancer. Survivors underwent comprehensive, risk-based clinical assessment. The cumulative prevalence of a chronic condition was estimated as 95.5% (95% CI, 94.8%-98.6%) and the cumulative prevalence of a severe or life-threatening/disabling condition was estimated as 80.5% (95% CI, 73.0%-86.6%) by age 45 years.

51. Friedman DL, Whitton J, Leisenring W, et al: Subsequent neoplasms in 5-year survivors of childhood cancer: the Childhood Cancer Survivor Study. *J Natl Cancer Inst* 102:1083–1095, 2010.

   In this study, the CCSS cohort was used to update the incidence of and risk for subsequent neoplasms occurring 5 years or more after the childhood cancer diagnosis from 14,359 5-year survivors in the CCSS who were at a median age of 30 years (range, 5 to 56 years) at follow-up. Cumulative incidence of subsequent neoplasm at 30 years, standardized incidence ratios, excess absolute risks for invasive second malignant neoplasms, and relative risks for subsequent neoplasms are presented. The study confirms that as childhood cancer survivors progress through adulthood, risk for subsequent neoplasms increases and there is no evidence of risk reduction with increasing duration of follow-up.

55. Garber JE, Offit K: Hereditary cancer predisposition syndromes. *J Clin Oncol* 23:276–292, 2005.

   This review highlights the most common hereditary cancer syndromes and a number of rare syndromes in which particular progress has been made. The prevalence, penetrance, tumor spectrum, and underlying genetic defects are discussed and then summarized in a table in which a comprehensive listing of known hereditary cancer syndromes is provided.

61. Kenney LB, Yasui Y, Inskip PD, et al: Breast cancer after childhood cancer: a report from the Childhood Cancer Survivor Study. *Ann Intern Med* 141:590–597, 2004.

This study identifies risk factors for secondary breast cancer beyond chest radiation therapy among female survivors of childhood cancer. In the CCSS cohort, breast cancer risk for female survivors was independently associated with prior chest radiation therapy, primary diagnosis of bone and soft tissue sarcoma, family history of breast cancer, and history of thyroid disease. In addition, prior pelvic radiation was found to reduce breast cancer risk.

67. Bassal M, Mertens AC, Taylor L, et al: Risk of selected subsequent carcinomas in survivors of childhood cancer: a report from the Childhood Cancer Survivor Study. *J Clin Oncol* 24:476–483, 2006.

    This study describes childhood cancer survivors' risk for subsequent carcinomas other than the three most common (breast, thyroid, and skin) using standardized incidence ratios calculated from the CCSS cohort and Surveillance, Epidemiology, and End Results program data. Young survivors of childhood cancers were found to be at increased risk for developing subsequent carcinomas typically associated with older adulthood, including those of the genitourinary system, head and neck area, and gastrointestinal tract.

73. Henderson TO, Oeffinger KC, Whitton J, et al: Secondary gastrointestinal cancer in childhood cancer survivors: a cohort study. *Ann Intern Med* 156:757–766, 2012.

    This analysis from the CCSS characterizes risk factors for childhood cancer survivors to develop secondary gastrointestinal cancer. Results show the greatest risk for subsequent gastrointestinal cancer is prior abdominal radiation; however, high-dose procarbazine and platinum chemotherapy were also found to independently increase the risk.

75. Travis LB, Hill DA, Dores GM, et al: Breast cancer following radiotherapy and chemotherapy among young women with Hodgkin disease. *JAMA* 290:465–475, 2003.

    This matched case-control study of 3817 female Hodgkin lymphoma survivors provides a detailed analysis of the relative risk for secondary breast cancer associated with both radiation dose delivered to site of breast cancer or to ovaries and with the cumulative dose of alkylating agent chemotherapy. Results of this study support the importance of hormonal stimulation for the development of radiation-induced breast cancer, as evidenced by the reduced risk associated with ovarian damage from alkylating agents or ovarian radiation.

89. Children's Oncology Group: *Long-Term follow-up guidelines for survivors of childhood, adolescent and young adult cancers, version 3.0,* Arcadia, CA, 2008, Children's Oncology Group. Accessed at: http://www.survivorshipguidelines.org/.

    These Children's Oncology Group Long-Term Follow-Up Guidelines for Survivors of Childhood, Adolescent, and Young Adult Cancer (COG-LTFU Guidelines) are evidence-based recommendations for screening and management of late effects of therapeutic exposures. They are updated by a multidisciplinary panel based on current literature review and expert consensus.

93. Sklar CA, Whitton J, Mertens A, et al: Abnormalities of the thyroid in survivors of Hodgkin's disease: data from the Childhood Cancer Survivor Study. *J Clin Endocrinol Metab* 85:3227–3232, 2000.

    Treatment of childhood cancer is associated with a variety of thyroid abnormalities. This early analysis from the CCSS comparing Hodgkin lymphoma survivors to sibling controls describes relative risks for hypothyroidism, hyperthyroidism, thyroid nodules, and thyroid cancer. It also characterizes the interaction between various patient and treatment variables. Female sex, radiation dose, and younger age at diagnosis were found to be independent risk factors for thyroid cancer.

110. Henderson TO, Whitton J, Stovall M, et al: Secondary sarcomas in childhood cancer survivors: a report from the Childhood Cancer Survivor Study. *J Natl Cancer Inst* 99:300–308, 2007.

    Childhood cancer survivors are at increased risk for secondary sarcomas. This analysis from the CCSS determined the incidence of secondary sarcomas and examined factors associated with the risk for developing secondary sarcomas. In a multivariable model, increased risk for secondary sarcoma was associated with radiation therapy, with a primary diagnosis of sarcoma, and with treatment with anthracyclines.

126. Taylor AJ, Little MP, Winter DL, et al: Population-based risks of CNS tumors in survivors of childhood cancer: the British Childhood Cancer Survivor Study. *J Clin Oncol* 28:5287–5293, 2010.

    A large cohort study of CNS tumors in survivors of childhood cancer from the British Cancer Survivor Study linked to national population–based cancer registries investigated treatment-related risk factors. Investigators found that the risk of secondary meningioma increases linearly and independently with increased dose of radiation to meningeal tissue and also with increased dose of intrathecal methotrexate. The risk for secondary glioma/primitive neuroectodermal tumors also increased linearly with dose of therapeutic radiation.

130. Nottage K, McFarlane J, Krasin MJ, et al: Secondary colorectal carcinoma after childhood cancer. *J Clin Oncol* 30:2552–2558, 2012.

    In this nested case-control study of 13,048 childhood cancer survivors from St Jude Children's Research Hospital, the long-term risk for secondary adenocarcinoma of the colon or rectum is reported to be 10-fold greater in survivors compared with the age-matched general population. Matched-pairs analyses found that radiation and alkylator exposure are associated with increased risk for secondary colorectal carcinoma and that the risk is proportional to dose and volume of radiation received. These data support the recommendation for early colon cancer screening for survivors receiving high-risk exposures.

152. Lipshultz SE, Adams MJ, Colan SD, et al: Long-term cardiovascular toxicity in children, adolescents, and young adults who receive cancer therapy: pathophysiology, course, monitoring, management, prevention, and research directions: a scientific statement from the American Heart Association. *Circulation* 128:1927–1995, 2013.

    This detailed report provides a comprehensive review of long-term cardiovascular toxicity associated with treatment of malignancy in childhood, adolescence, and young adulthood.

210. Bowers DC, Liu Y, Leisenring W, et al: Late-occurring stroke among long-term survivors of childhood leukemia and brain tumors: a report from the Childhood Cancer Survivor Study. *J Clin Oncol* 24:5277–5282, 2006.

    This report assesses the incidence of and risk factors for late-occurring stroke among survivors of childhood leukemia and brain tumors. The relative risk for stroke for leukemia survivors was 6.4 (95% CI, 3.0-13.8) and for brain tumor survivors it was 29.0 (95% CI, 13.8-60.6) compared with a sibling comparison group.

214. Armstrong GT, Oeffinger KC, Chen Y, et al: Modifiable risk factors and major cardiac events among adult survivors of childhood cancer. *J Clin Oncol* 31:3673–3680, 2013.

    In this assessment of adult survivors of childhood cancer from the CCSS, two or more cardiovascular risk factors were reported by 10.3% of survivors. In this report, acquisition of modifiable cardiovascular risk factors, particularly hypertension, increased the risk for a severe, life-threatening, and fatal cardiac event, reinforcing the importance of early diagnosis and careful management of modifiable cardiovascular risk factors in survivors.

219. Mertens AC, Yasui Y, Liu Y, et al: Pulmonary complications in survivors of childhood and adolescent cancer: a report from the Childhood Cancer Survivor Study. *Cancer* 95:2431–2441, 2002.

    In this report from the CCSS, survivors of childhood cancer were found to have a significantly increased risk for pulmonary complications compared with siblings, including an increased risk of lung fibrosis, recurrent pneumonia, and use of supplemental oxygen.

223. Cohen LE: Endocrine late effects of cancer treatment. *Endocrinol Metab Clin North Am* 34:769–789, xi, 2005.

    This review article describes the endocrinopathies that are associated with the treatment of childhood cancers, specifically hypothalamic-pituitary, thyroid, and gonadal dysfunction, as well as osteopenia-osteoporosis and obesity. The article also addresses the risk factors for endocrine complications, including the underlying disease, treatment with cytotoxic agents, and radiation therapy.

249. Kadan-Lottick NS, Dinu I, Wasilewski-Masker K, et al: Osteonecrosis in adult survivors of childhood cancer: a report from the Childhood Cancer Survivor Study. *J Clin Oncol* 26:3038–3045, 2008.

In the CCSS cohort, the 20-year cumulative incidence of osteonecrosis was 0.43%, with survivors 5.6 times more likely to have reported osteonecrosis compared with siblings. The risk for osteonecrosis was greatest among survivors of allogeneic stem cell transplant for underlying diagnoses of leukemia in survivors of acute lymphoblastic leukemia, acute myelogenous leukemia, and bone sarcoma.

299. Krull KR, Brinkman TM, Li C, et al: Neurocognitive outcomes decades after treatment for childhood acute lymphoblastic leukemia: a report from the St. Jude Lifetime Cohort Study. *J Clin Oncol* 31:4407–4415, 2013.

     In this report, adult survivors of childhood acute lymphoblastic leukemia were found to have significant and pervasive neurocognitive impairment.

341. Metzger ML, Meacham LR, Patterson B, et al: Female reproductive health after childhood, adolescent, and young adult cancers: guidelines for the assessment and management of female reproductive complications. *J Clin Oncol* 31:1239–1247, 2013.

     This is a comprehensive review of the literature that informed the COG-LTFU guidelines task force recommendations for the assessment and management of female reproductive complications after treatment of childhood, adolescent, and young adult cancers. Topics include all aspects of female reproductive and sexual health, including hypogonadism, precocious puberty, and reduced fertility. Also reviewed is current knowledge in other areas relevant to the reproductive health of female survivors of childhood cancer, including investigational fertility preservation, interventions for infertility, and sexual function.

349. Kenney LB, Cohen LE, Shnorhavorian M, et al: Male reproductive health after childhood, adolescent, and young adult cancers: a report from the Children's Oncology Group. *J Clin Oncol* 30:3408–3416, 2012.

     This is a comprehensive review of the literature that informed the COG-LTFU guidelines task force recommendations for the assessment and management of male reproductive complications after treatment of childhood, adolescent, and young adult cancers. This review presents an overview of male reproductive complications, including hypoandrogenism, precocious puberty, reduced fertility, and sexual dysfunction. Risk factors, clinical assessment, and interventions for each of the treatment-associated complications, as put forth in the guidelines, are discussed.

363. Green DM, Whitton JA, Stovall M, et al: Pregnancy outcome of female survivors of childhood cancer: a report from the Childhood Cancer Survivor Study. *Am J Obstet Gynecol* 187:1070–1080, 2002.

     This study reviews self-reported pregnancy outcome among female participants in the Childhood Cancer Survivor Study to determine the effect of prior treatment with radiation therapy or chemotherapy for cancer diagnosed during childhood or adolescence on pregnancy loss, live births, and birth weight. This large study did not identify adverse pregnancy outcomes for female survivors treated with most chemotherapeutic agents; however, the offspring of women who received pelvic irradiation are at risk for low-birth-weight infants.

407. Goldsby R, Chen Y, Raber S, et al: Survivors of childhood cancer have increased risk of gastrointestinal complications later in life. *Gastroenterology* 140:1464–1471, 2011.

     This study from the Childhood Cancer Survivor Study cohort evaluates the incidence of long-term gastrointestinal disease for childhood cancer survivors and identifies treatment-related risk factors. Compared with siblings, survivors had increased risk for late onset complications of the upper gastrointestinal tract, liver, and lower gastrointestinal tract. Older age at diagnosis, intensified therapy, abdominal radiation, and abdominal surgery increased the risk for certain gastrointestinal complications.

419. Kaste SC, Goodman P, Leisenring W, et al: Impact of radiation and chemotherapy on risk of dental abnormalities: a report from the Childhood Cancer Survivor Study. *Cancer* 115:5817–5827, 2009.

     In this report from the CCSS, survivors when compared with siblings, were more likely to report microdontia, hypodontia, root abnormalities, abnormal enamel, teeth loss, severe gingivitis, and xerostomia.

422. Recklitis CJ, Diller LR, Li X, et al: Suicide ideation in adult survivors of childhood cancer: a report from the Childhood Cancer Survivor Study. *J Clin Oncol* 28:655–661, 2010.

     In this report from the CCSS, adult survivors of childhood cancer were at increased risk for suicidal ideation compared with the sibling control cohort. In survivors, suicidal ideation was associated with a primary diagnosis of central nervous system malignancy, depression, and poor current physical health.

CHAPTER 73

Psychosocial Care of the Child and Family

Cori Liptak, Lonnie M. Zeltzer, and Christopher J. Recklitis

CHAPTER OUTLINE

The diagnosis and treatment of cancer represents a major challenge for the family and the individual child. For most families, coping with a child's cancer will be the most stressful and difficult experience they will face. Although the majority of families will make an adequate adjustment,[1-4] coping with the diagnosis and the subsequent challenges of treatment is a difficult and demanding process.[5-9] In this chapter we will address the emotional and psychosocial needs of children and their families while the child receives a diagnosis of cancer and undergoes therapy, and describe some resources and interventions that may be useful. This chapter is intended primarily for oncologists, nurse practitioners, and other medical professionals who are seeking to understand and attend to the psychosocial needs of children with cancer. In each section we highlight the issues facing the child and family and suggest supportive strategies or interventions that may be helpful. A description of the psychosocial clinician's role is included in certain sections so that oncology providers can better understand and collaborate with psychosocial clinicians, but readers looking for a detailed description of psychosocial assessment and treatment

techniques will need to look beyond this chapter to more comprehensive treatments of the subject.[4,10,11,12,13] Given the great variability in oncology diagnoses and treatments, as well as individual differences in children and families, we will focus on the issues that are most common in this population. Beginning with the crisis of diagnosis and proceeding chronologically through the treatment period to the end of therapy, we will address the issues that are expected to arise for most families.

CONCEPTUAL MODELS GUIDING THE PSYCHOSOCIAL CARE OF CHILDREN AND FAMILIES

In approaching the topic of psychosocial care for the child and family, we have adopted a conceptual model developed by Anne Kazak[14] that illustrates the different levels of need seen in families of children with cancer (Fig. 73-1). In this model, adapted from the preventative mental health model,[14] Kazak represents the distribution of families along the continuum of needs in the form of a pyramid, with the least acute needs at the bottom and

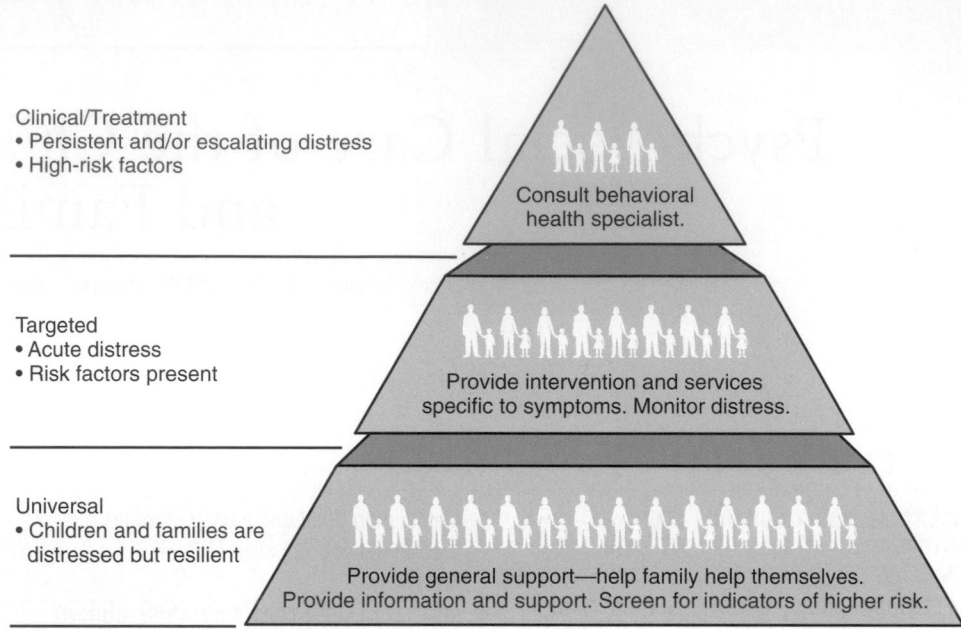

Figure 73-1 Pediatric psychosocial preventative health model. *(From Kazak AE: Pediatric psychosocial preventative health model [PPPHM]: research, practice, and collaboration in pediatric family systems medicine. Fam Syst Health 24:381–395, 2006.)*

the most acute needs at the top. The largest section of the pyramid at the bottom represents the majority of patients and families who have expected levels of distress but generally have adequate resources and may benefit from information and psychosocial support. Moving up the pyramid, the second largest group of families represented have more significant needs according to Kazak, either because of existing risk factors or the presence of more acute distress. Finally, at the top of the pyramid is the smallest group of families, whose level of distress is in the clinical range and for whom some significant behavioral or psychiatric intervention is required. This chapter focuses on describing the needs of the largest group of families with "universal" or expected needs and discussing the support strategies and interventions that can be helpful for them. In addition we address some of the special issues that are likely to be seen in the "targeted" group of families such as noncompliance or marital conflicts that are not typical but that the treatment team should be aware of and be prepared to address. In the less common situations in which patients or parents require significant mental health interventions, referrals to specialists are necessary; these situations will be discussed briefly at the end of this chapter.

The ecological and developmental perspectives are also essential for understanding the experience of the child and family going through cancer therapy. Urie Bronfenbrenner (1917-2005) created the modern concept of the ecology of human development.[15] In his model no one factor operates in isolation, and the biopsychosocial model is considered within a developmental context. At the core of the model, the child has genetic and environmental influences on emotions, cognition, and behavior. In addition the child's own responses to the environment

not only influence his or her emotions, thoughts, and behaviors but in turn influence the microenvironment.[16,17] For example a child who responds to new situations with aggression or fear will elicit different responses from medical providers than will a child who responds with curiosity, and in that way the child shapes the environment to which he or she was initially reacting. At the next level of the model, the family system is a powerful factor that directly affects the child and shapes many of the child's interactions with the environment. Family factors including family composition, parental emotional states, socioeconomic status, and other family stressors will influence the child's experience of illness.[18-22] For example parental depression might reduce the extent of nurturing and support provided to a child with cancer. Recommendations for family-centered care as the primary model of care delivery for children are supported by this aspect of the model (Fig. 73-2).[20]

Finally, at the broadest level, racial, ethnic, community, and cultural factors can have an impact on the entire family/child system (Fig. 73-3).[23]

From a developmental perspective, children go through five recognizable stages of development from the newborn period until adulthood. These stages typically are thought of as infant, toddler, preschool, school age, and adolescence. Different developmental tasks are associated with each stage, and the needs for information, support, and care will vary in relation to the developmental stage of the child. A review of how to communicate with sick children during different developmental stages is provided by Rushforth.[24] Pediatric health care providers are accustomed to tailoring their general approach to patients and families according to the child's developmental stage and will draw on these skills and experience

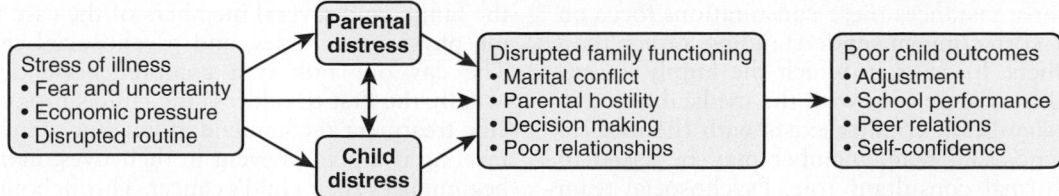

Figure 73-2 Family stress model. *(Modified from Conger KJ, Rueter MA, Conger RD: The role of economic pressure in the lives of parents and their adolescents: the family stress model. In Crockett LJ, Silbereisen RJ, editors:* Negotiating adolescence in times of social change. *Cambridge, England, 2000, Cambridge University Press, p. 201–233.)*

when working with children who have cancer. For example infants generally need a significant degree of parental soothing and physical contact, as do toddlers, yet toddlers need room for explanation and consistency in the environment. Preschool-aged children can understand simple information that can help reduce fears of the unknown. School-aged children need to have opportunities for peer interaction, as well as clear communication. Adolescents have a need for the development of autonomy and identity formation. When little room for individual choice is perceived by the adolescent, the drive for independence can lead to maladaptive coping, such as nonadherence to medications or refusals to come to the clinic or undergo medical procedures. Adolescents with cancer by necessity become more dependent upon their parents for physical and emotional needs and may have self-image issues related to weight loss or baldness, because during this developmental period perceptions of peer acceptance are important and sexuality develops as well.[25,26] The specific needs of the adolescent patient are discussed in a separate section.

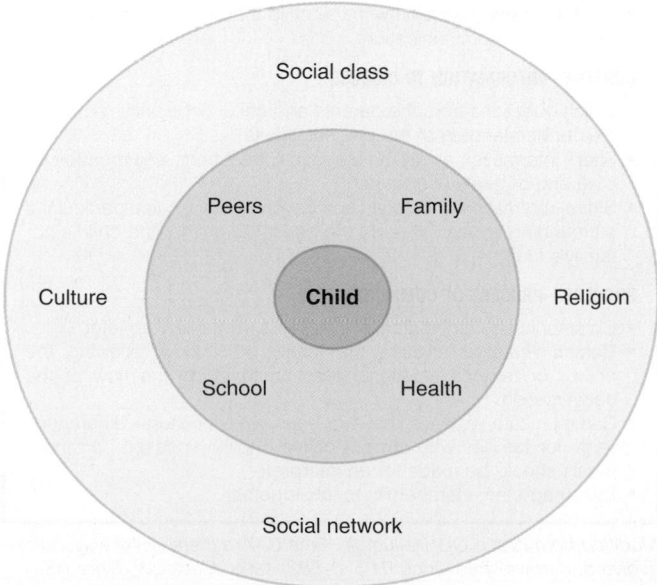

Figure 73-3 Child health from an ecological perspective. *(Modified from Kazak AE: Pediatric psychosocial preventative health model [PPPHM]: research, practice, and collaboration in pediatric family systems medicine.* Fam Syst Health *24:381–395, 2006.)*

PROFESSIONAL ROLES AND A TEAM APPROACH TO PSYCHOSOCIAL CARE

No single individual is able to provide for all the psychosocial needs of the child and family undergoing cancer therapy. In many pediatric oncology settings a team approach[27-30] is used, with the team composed of both medical and psychosocial care providers. The composition of the medical members of the team vary from setting to setting, but the team generally includes an attending oncologist, a surgeon, and a radiation oncologist (if these treatment modalities are indicated), as well as other oncology care providers such as an oncology fellow, a nurse practitioner or physician's assistant, and an oncology nurse. Psychosocial members of the team may include a resource specialist, social worker, psychologist, child life specialist, or psychiatrist. Variation in the professions included in the psychosocial support team in a particular treatment setting generally has more to do with local culture and tradition than with the specific training or skills of a particular profession. Although each psychosocial discipline has its particular focus or specialized skill set[31-38] (e.g., prescriptive authority or psychological testing) in working with children who have cancer and their families, considerable overlap between their roles is likely.

Psychosocial professionals have several important roles on the care team. The primary role may be as a consultant to other members of the team, including the patient and the family.[39-42] Because all team members will be interacting and providing some level of information and support, they will need to attend to psychosocial concerns, and developing a consistent approach to support of the family is essential.[43] As a consultant, the psychosocial team members should conduct a preliminary assessment of the child and family to understand their history, preferred ways of coping, important supports, and potential sources of vulnerability. Using this knowledge of the family, the psychosocial care provider may be able to help the other team members understand the family's individual needs and consider best approaches for supporting them. Similarly when the patient or family has questions and concerns that are not resolved in the course of routine care, the psychosocial care provider may help them work on solving the issue and think about how to help them raise their concerns with the medical team. The emphasis of these consultations is on improving communication between the family and the medical team, and in most instances these consultations focus on clarifying and correcting misunderstanding rather than resolving conflicts. In cases in which the family is very reluctant to address a concern with the medical team, or when a more significant conflict exists with the medical team, the psychosocial team member may be asked to play a more formal consultant role. Psychosocial team members also fulfill the role of direct service providers to patients and families, providing individual or family meetings to offer support to the parents, patient, or family, as well as education and preparation for surgery and other medical procedures. Support groups run by psychosocial and/or nursing staff in the inpatient or outpatient setting may be very helpful for meeting families' educational and emotional needs.[44-47] Finally, the psychosocial provider's role often includes consultation and liaison with outside agencies and community resources.[48-51] This aspect may include assisting families in accessing financial and insurance resources, contacting schools, tutors, and other child care agencies, and helping identify additional support services in the community, including referrals for psychotherapy when appropriate.

CRISIS OF A CANCER DIAGNOSIS

The cancer diagnosis and the events leading up to it are typically frightening, complex, and unfamiliar.[7,8,52] The diagnosis period, which can be thought of as beginning when the child first comes to medical attention until a clear diagnosis and treatment plan are made, is foremost a period of uncertainty. At some point in this period, parents are told cancer is possible or even likely, but it may take time before a definitive diagnosis is made. During this period their child's symptoms may persist and the child often must face painful diagnostic tests and procedures.

Until their child is diagnosed, most families have never thought about childhood cancer and don't know anyone who has had to face it. Whereas families facing common stressful life events can be guided by their prior experiences and the experience of their friends and family, the cancer diagnosis pushes them beyond the realm of ordinary experience. Not surprisingly parents are typically overwhelmed emotionally and cognitively while they try to understand their child's illness. In addition parents may describe feelings of unreality, "like this is not really real." Children's immediate reactions to illness depend largely on their age, their symptoms, and the medical procedures they have had to undergo. Except in cases of older adolescents, it is most often the parents who are most anxious to learn the diagnosis and are the first ones to be informed of the diagnosis of cancer.

Presenting the Diagnosis and Plan for Treatment: Day One Talk

The diagnostic period comes to a close when the treatment team has made a clear diagnosis of the child's cancer and communicates this diagnosis and related treatment plan to the patient and family. Often referred to as the "day one talk," this conversation with the family usually takes place in the form of a treatment conference between the family and several members of the care team, including physicians, nurses, and psychosocial care providers. The day one talk is a comprehensive discussion and usually the first to address the child's prognosis and specific treatment recommendations. For many families this meeting is a pivotal event in their lives, marking the real beginning of their child's cancer. Throughout the diagnostic phase most families maintain hope that the child does not in fact have cancer, so the day one talk is similar to other situations in which a physician must communicate bad news to the family. The literature on communicating bad news about a child's health[53-57] may be relevant, and recommendations from these noncancer settings may be instructive. Box 73-1 provides a summary of essential points for communicating the diagnosis.

Although the medical details discussed will vary from one family to the next, challenges in communicating diagnostic, prognostic, and treatment information are consistent across families and can be considered and planned for.[58-61] Planning is essential for a successful meeting with the family, and although there may be pressure from family or medical staff to have the conversation as soon as possible, some minimal amount of scheduling and organization will be required. A written protocol for communicating the diagnosis has been recommended,[60] with the expectation that this protocol will

---

Box 73-1   Summary of Essential Points: Principles for Communicating the Diagnosis

STRUCTURE—ORGANIZATION

- Establish an initial plan for communication.
- Communicate in a private and comfortable space where interruptions will be minimized.
- Communicate with the parents, child, and other family members, if desired. Nursing staff and psychosocial workers should also be included whenever possible.
- Hold a separate session with the child if he or she is not present for the initial communication.

CONTENT—INFORMATION TO DISCUSS

- Solicit questions from the parents and child, especially regarding their understanding of the present illness.
- Share information about the diagnosis, treatment, and the plan for cure and/or goals of treatment.
- Share information on lifestyle and psychosocial issues, particularly surrounding causation (e.g., the cancer is neither the child's nor family's fault).

PROCESS—PROCESS OF COMMUNICATION

- Communicate immediately at diagnosis and follow-up later.
- Communicate at a pace the family can follow, allowing the child's or family's emotional reaction to guide the flow of the conversation.
- Communicate in ways that are sensitive to cultural differences (e.g., for families who are not native English speakers, arrangements should be made for an interpreter).
- Encourage the entire family to talk together.

Modified from Krahn GL, Hallum A, Kime C: Are there good ways to give bad news? Pediatrics 91:578–582, 1993; Mack JW, Grier HE: The day one talk. J Clin Oncol 22:563–566, 2004; and Masera G, Chesler MA, Jankovic M, et al: SIOP Working Committee on Psychosocial Issues in Pediatric Oncology: guidelines for communication of the diagnosis. Med Pediatr Oncol 28:382–385, 1997.

be tailored to meet the needs of the patient and family. Conducting the meeting in a private space while all participants are free from interruptions is very important, as is scheduling the meeting so that the important members of the family and care team can attend. Because families typically find the day one talk overwhelming[58,62-64] and may not remember many of the details discussed, some practitioners recommend providing written material or making a tape recording of the meeting for the parents to review subsequently.[63,65-68] Reassuring families that they are not expected to remember all of the details discussed can reduce their sense of information overload, as will making explicit the critical pieces of information they are being asked to focus on.

In addition to the oncologists directly caring for the patient, the day one talk should include nurses and psychosocial caregivers whenever possible.[69,70] The organization and roles of the medical center staff are often confusing to families, and taking time to introduce the different members of the team and describe their roles is essential. Both parents should attend, and they should be offered the opportunity to include other family members involved in the care of the child. Whether to include the child in all or part of this session or to arrange for a separate session for the child will depend largely on the age of the child and the parents' preference. Although a subsequent meeting with a smaller group consisting of parents and one or two medical professionals may be more appropriate for younger children,[71-73] including adolescents in the day one talk can help them develop trust in the medical team and invest in their own care.[58,74]

The principal goal of the meeting is to provide the family with an overview of the child's diagnosis, the treatment recommendations, and the prognosis. It is important to directly elicit questions the patient or family may have and to provide sufficient time to discuss their concerns. Mack and Grier[58] emphasize the opportunity to address the family's questions about what may have caused the child's cancer and particularly to correct misconceptions that may lead to a sense of blame or responsibility for the cancer. Communicating prognostic information to the family is critical because it is likely to have an impact on their understanding of the treatment recommendations,[75,76] but delivering this information can be difficult, especially when the prognosis is guarded or poor. How much to rely on a numeric presentation of this information is a question that frequently arises, and some evidence indicates that patients may misunderstand the information[77-79] if it is not carefully explained. Numeric information about risk, such as 5-year survival rates, should not be avoided altogether because many families want this information,[80] but care should be taken to ensure that parents receive the information in the way they find most useful and that they understand the information that is provided. Recommendations for treatment should be presented, beginning with a general overview of the modalities used and the timing and setting for treatments. The introduction of consent forms and discussion of known and likely adverse effects (short term and long term) should follow after the family understands the general outline of the treatment.

If a separate session for the child is held, the same general information about diagnosis, prognosis, and treatment plan should be covered. The information will need to be tailored to the developmental level and the particular concerns of the patient, such as the ability to return home and to school, to see friends, and to participate in sports or other activities.[74] Children should be told about specific expectable adverse effects such as hair loss, with an emphasis on concrete ways in which their appearance or activities may be affected. Older children and adolescents may be able to engage directly with the medical providers, but younger children may be more comfortable talking with their parents, who can elicit their questions and reinforce what medical providers communicate to the child directly. Most professionals will emphasize the importance of the children knowing the name of their disease and that it is cancer. Parents may initially shy away from this direct approach and particular words like "cancer," and they may need some preparation for how to talk with their child and what words to use. Understandably many parents feel protective toward their children and may wish to avoid using the words "cancer" or "leukemia." It is important to help parents understand that honesty, even about potentially frightening information, can decrease anxiety and be supportive for children in the long term because they can grow to trust that adults are not withholding information and that they need not fear unpleasant surprises. Similarly it is important to explain that the word "cancer" is commonly used with pediatric patients and that it is important for children not to feel that their condition is so frightening it cannot be named or spoken about. It can be helpful to share with parents that the climate of open communication with young patients comes from lessons learned in past treatment eras when communication was not open, which contributed to children's anxiety and fear about their disease. With this sort of preparation, most parents can begin to feel comfortable with open communication with the child. Parents from different cultural backgrounds,[73,81,82] or those who are unused to open discussions of illness, may not easily accept this openness and naming of the disease, and some careful negotiation and compromise may be required to reach an agreement of what words to use and topics to discuss with the patient. Over time families may become more comfortable being open with the patient themselves, while they meet other families and children whom they see are comfortable with this type of open discussion. In an elegant description of the day one talk in pediatric oncology, Mack and Grier[58] highlight the importance of forming an alliance between the family and the medical provider and the ways in which this alliance can affect adjustment to the diagnosis. In particular they emphasize the importance of listening closely, making an emotional connection with the family, and acknowledging the overwhelming impact of the diagnosis on every aspect of the family's life. Although they provide some very specific guidelines for the information that should be discussed, they conclude, "...listening and the openness of silence may be more important than the words themselves."[58]

Parents' Reactions to a Child's Diagnosis

Many factors can contribute to the overwhelming nature of the cancer diagnosis. The word "cancer" continues to have a significant social stigma,[83-88] as well as personal connotations. For many parents, their personal experiences with cancer may be limited to relatives who were diagnosed later in life and may not have survived long after diagnosis. Although it can be helpful to learn about these personal associations with cancer, it is very important to clearly correct parents' explicit or implicit assumptions as they apply to their child's illness. Families who have lost family members to cancer may need very explicit explanations that a parent's or grandparent's experience with prostate or lung cancer may have little in common with a child's diagnosis of cancer.

In the context of a new diagnosis, most parents will experience many intense emotional reactions and may even report psychiatric symptoms of acute stress.[5,89] They are typically frightened and anxious about their child's prognosis and distraught at the thought of their child's physical suffering. If many days or weeks elapse between the child's initial symptoms and the diagnosis, parents may feel angry at medical providers, whom they believe "missed the diagnosis" or did not listen to them or to their child. Parents' belief that there was a delay in diagnosis may also contribute to feeling angry at themselves. Parents are ordinarily active agents in shaping every aspect of their child's care and well-being and may feel quite dismayed at how helpless they feel to protect their ill child. This sense of responsibility may lead many parents to feel responsible for their child's situation, perhaps blaming themselves for not bringing the child to medical attention earlier or for not understanding the significance of a child's initial symptoms.[2,7,8,90,91] In some cases this sense of responsibility and the need to understand the cause of the child's illness may make parents (or other family members) wonder if they themselves are responsible for the cancer. Examples of these thoughts, many of which are not entirely rational, might be wondering if allowing their child to use certain electrical devices, or bringing some kind of contamination into the home from a work site, may have contributed to the cancer.[2,7,8,91] For families coping with neurofibromatosis, Li-Fraumeni syndrome, or other genetic predispositions, a child's diagnosis of cancer may weigh more heavily on parents and leave them more vulnerable to psychosocial distress. The psychosocial care provider can play a crucial role in helping families reframe these difficulties, which will allow them to cope more effectively. In addition encouraging families to pursue a consultation with a genetics counselor can be an important intervention in helping families gain increased knowledge about the genetic predisposition to cancer and develop strategies to decrease stigma and fear and increase appropriate management of risk. Listening to the family in crisis and providing reassurance can be the most useful responses for all members of the care team. Normalizing parents' reactions by letting them know that parents almost universally feel overwhelmed and that intense emotional reactions are normal responses to their child's illness can

help reassure them that they are not "going crazy" and they won't be judged for their reactions by the care team.[2,3,7,44,92,93] One reason parents feel overwhelmed is their awareness that they are facing a more complicated, frightening, and demanding challenge than they may have ever faced before. Although it is helpful to acknowledge the feeling of facing this seemingly overwhelming challenge, it is also useful to let parents know that families do cope well, and with some assistance and support, there is every reason to believe their family will cope successfully, even though that may be difficult to imagine at the beginning of treatment.[52,94-97]

During the crisis of diagnosis, many families will benefit from concrete structuring from the care team. Parents often need to be encouraged to focus on their own self-care and may need encouragement to mobilize their social supports to meet their acute needs, such as arranging extended time off from work or asking friends and extended family to help with other tasks. Many parents can benefit from some active problem solving,[52,92,98-100] with staff helping them to identify needs, generate possible solutions, and then select and implement a potential solution. Social workers and resource specialists on the care team may be helpful in identifying sources of practical support (e.g., transportation, meals, and lodging), sorting through insurance issues, and helping solve problems with regard to meeting the needs of the patient and family.

Occasionally some parents experience such a strong need to act in the face of their child's illness that they make decisions that can be premature or even impulsive. For example some parents have quit their jobs, mortgaged their homes, or moved their residence even before knowing the details of their child's treatment and taking time to consider these major life decisions. Although parents need to decide for themselves how their family will adjust and cope with the demands of the child's illness and treatment, it is appropriate for members of the care team to caution against making impulsive decisions and support them in making short-term plans for managing the health crisis that can be revised as circumstances change or new information becomes available.

During the crisis period parents can experience a wide range of intense emotional reactions. In most cases parents' reactions can be managed with education and support from the care team. Specialized services from a psychosocial care provider, usually a psychologist or social worker, can be particularly useful in helping parents identify and begin to cope with their emotional reactions.[92,101-103] Many of these reactions will be of short duration because parents often report feeling less overwhelmed after they have heard a definitive diagnosis and can focus on the demands of a treatment plan. Research has demonstrated that the initial psychological distress experienced by mothers at the time of diagnosis tends to steadily improve as long as 6 months after the diagnosis.[104] In rare cases parents may have emotional reactions that are more enduring or problematic,[2,12,105,106] which may require more targeted intervention during the crisis period. Situations involving confusion about the child's diagnosis or requiring a prolonged diagnostic evaluation

TABLE 73-1   Factors Associated with Increased Psychosocial Distress

Family Factors	Disease Factors	Environment/Resource Factors
Single-parent families	Unclear diagnosis(es)	Financial problems (e.g., job loss or debts)
Preexisting chronic or mental health	Poor prognosis	Isolation (e.g., lack of family and/or problems with peer support)
Concurrent illness or injury in family (e.g., parent or sibling illness)	Prolonged or intense treatment(s) (e.g., bone marrow transplant)	Language differences (e.g., foreign national or immigrant)
Marital problems (e.g., separation and/or divorce)	Disfiguring disease or treatment(s) (e.g., amputation)	Transportation (e.g., no car to get to the hospital)
Family problems (e.g., emotional or learning difficulties)	Disease status (e.g., relapse or recurrence)	Minimal or no health insurance
Recent stressful life events (e.g., job and/or school problems, a move, or relocation)		

Modified from Hersh SP, Wiener LS: Psychosocial support for the family of the child with cancer. In Pizzo PA, Poplack DG, editors: Principles and practice of pediatric oncology. Philadelphia, 1989, J.B. Lippincott Company, p. 897–891; Kazak AE, Cant MC, Jensen MM, et al: Identifying psychosocial risk indicative of subsequent resource use in families of newly diagnosed pediatric oncology patients. J Clin Oncol 21:3220–3225, 2003; and Lansky SB, List MA, Ritter-Sterr C: Psychiatric and psychological support of the child and adolescent with cancer. In Pizzo PA, Poplack DG, editors: Principles and practice of pediatric oncology. Philadelphia, 1989, J.B. Lippincott Company, p. 885–896.

period are more stressful for parents and may be more likely to cause significant distress. Similarly parents who are managing other significant stressors such as having a parent or other family member with medical needs and parents with preexisting psychological problems will be more likely to have symptoms that interfere with their ability to function (Table 73-1).[2,12] Examples of these problematic reactions might include manifesting signs of clinical depression or anxiety, not being able to care for themselves adequately (i.e., not sleeping or eating), or being so frustrated and angry that they cannot consistently collaborate with medical providers. In these situations in which parents' reactions will have a negative impact on the child and have the potential to interfere with the treatment process, it is important to address the situation directly with the parents and make appropriate referrals for intervention.

Interventions for parents experiencing these problematic reactions may require more intensive services from some members of the care team, as well as consultation with and referral to other individuals. The underlying problems may predate the child's cancer, but the focus of intervention during the crisis of diagnosis may appropriately be alleviation of symptoms. Parents showing signs of severe distress should be evaluated by an appropriate psychosocial team member or be referred to a mental health provider who can assess their psychological status and refer them for any urgent intervention they may need. In addition to supportive therapy and the problem-solving approaches previously described, psychopharmacologic intervention may be particularly helpful for parents who have severe anxiety or depressive reactions, severe sleep disturbance,[107,108] or a preexisting psychopathologic diagnosis. Pastoral counseling may be useful for parents whose faith is an important source of support and for those experiencing a "crisis of faith" as they struggle to make meaning of their child's illness.[109-111]

Children's Reactions to Diagnosis

Children will react to their diagnosis and initial treatment on the basis of their developmental level, their own individual temperament and past experiences, and to a large degree on how their parents cope with the new diagnosis and treatment.[112,113] Typically the infant, toddler, and especially the preschooler will be more concerned about changes in routine and the normal home environment, separation from family, especially the primary caregiver, and bodily intrusion through physical examinations and medical procedures for diagnostic or treatment purposes. Strange environments will disrupt normal awake/sleep patterns, and sleep deprivation can reduce the child's normal self-regulation effectiveness. For example infants who had been able to sleep through the night at home might have constant awakenings. Separation from the primary caregiver(s) then becomes an even larger issue if the parent is not present during the night or during bodily intrusion episodes to help comfort the child. Clearly this need for the parents suggests that, when possible, it is better for parents to create "shifts" to be with the child as much as possible, day and night. Such parental support also means that the issue of support for parents, both emotionally and in practical ways, needs to be addressed.[114] Stressed parents who cope poorly will not be able to help their child self-soothe well.[15,115]

One issue that the medical team can address is the manner in which examinations and procedures are carried out. For example Chen and colleagues[116,117] found that children had memories of stressful and painful procedures that affected their experience and behaviors during subsequent procedures. Asking the parent to leave the room while a team of doctors and nurses in white coats enter the child's room to carry out examinations is more likely to help create an uncooperative child who will become conditioned to be anxious around anyone with a white coat. Having one member of the team develop a relationship with the child, from toddlerhood through adolescence, will be helpful in establishing the child's trust of the nonfamily "team." Establishing a system for families in the hospital that sets clear guidelines for providers as they enter a child's room can prevent significant distress. For example psychosocial providers or child life specialists can create a sign for the door that reminds providers to introduce themselves when they enter the room, let the child know up front what is going to be required of them, and hold medical discussion outside the room when appropriate. Respecting such requests fosters rapport, reiterates the message that the child and family are part of the team, and promotes the sense of being "heard" by the medical team.

For the very young child, procedures that can be performed competently and quickly while distracters are present (e.g., iPad apps, bubbles, party blowers, cartoons, and stories) can reduce fear of future procedures and help the child develop a sense of control and cooperation. The use of positive reinforcement is helpful in an effort to pair "scary" novel and intrusive experiences with positive, pleasurable experiences. The use of behavioral strategies (e.g., breathing, relaxation, imagery, and behavioral charts) can provide parents with ways to support their child in these novel and intrusive situations and help the child develop a sense of security and mastery, and they give parents the opportunity to feel successful in the context of challenging medical demands. Additionally it may be useful to encourage the family to bring in a "transitional object" for their child (e.g., a favorite blanket or stuffed animal) to bring the familiarity of "home" into the hospital.

School-aged children will be interested in concrete answers to their questions about hospitalization, expectations with regard to medical examinations, and specifics about what to expect in unfamiliar situations. Encouraging parents to answer questions directly, even when the topics may be uncomfortable, will foster open communication and minimize the chance that the child will create "answers" based on faulty assumptions that can be anxiety provoking.[118-120] Parents should be reminded that this is not a one-time discussion and that providing their child with information, even upsetting information, can decrease uncertainty about the illness and potentially improve psychological functioning.[121]

While children develop an increased understanding of their illness, they may ask, "Am I going to die?" Psychosocial providers can help guide parents in providing answers to this question based on a child's age and diagnosis. It is important for parents to acknowledge the severity of the disease while highlighting the fact that the medical team has a treatment for the illness. Answers to this question will vary based on a child's medical condition, particularly in the case of relapse. Exploring a child's thoughts and fears around illness and death can be helpful; however, providing reassurance that he or she will be well taken care of and not left alone and that his or her symptoms will be treated is critical.[119]

Adolescents are likely to want to know more information about their illness and treatment. Simple responses to questions often will not satisfy them, and parents will need to understand that adolescents may potentially turn to alternative sources beyond their parents for important information. A child or adolescent who has formed a relationship with a member of the treating team can ask questions of that team member that might seem difficult to ask parents.[122,123] Some adolescents feel a need to "protect" their parents from more stress by not acknowledging to their parents their own fears, anger, and worries. Encouraging adolescents to talk about what they have learned from their medical providers, the Internet, and their peers will help eliminate misinformation and confusion while empowering adolescents to seek information in their own way. Developing a sense of mastery over the medical information can lead to a feeling of control and confidence that can be helpful for teenagers.

Finally, children of all ages often regress when they are scared, and parents need to know that changes in the child's behavior are not unusual.[124] Psychosocial providers can normalize behavioral reactions for parents and subsequently minimize the distress associated with particular behaviors. For instance a preschooler who has just been toilet trained may begin having accidents, and it is imperative that parents recognize that this behavior is a normal response to a stressor and that they should not focus too heavily on that behavior during a time of crisis. The following guidelines are related to children's reactions to diagnosis and treatment:[125]

- Many parents need help talking with their child, who is often scared and needs some explanation and education along with his or her parents.
- A variety of disciplines, such as child life, nursing, social work, and psychology, can all be helpful to parents, siblings, and pediatric patients. Interventions relating to preparation for medical procedures, supportive work with parents and other family members, and psychoeducation are important. Connections with other children and families who are having similar experiences can be helpful.
- Keys to getting through diagnostic procedures are good preparation and good pharmacologic and psychological pain and anxiety management.

Education and Information about Treatment

Most treatment regimens put an enormous information burden on the family. Children are often treated with several modalities (such as surgery, radiation, and/or chemotherapy) and may receive a large number of medications, as well as a variety of blood tests and other diagnostic procedures. Although adolescents may be active in their own care to some extent, parents are responsible for understanding and managing their child's treatment, especially during outpatient phases of treatment when parents will need to work with home care agencies, administer treatments themselves, and monitor their child's health. To meet these demands, parents require detailed information about their child's treatment regimen and reactions that can be expected.[101,102,126,127] Most of this detailed information will be provided by nursing and medical care providers. Patients and families are generally quite resilient and successfully accommodate even the most demanding treatment regimens, but initial apprehension about being able to understand and implement these regimens is common. Staff may need to present information several times and reinforce verbal exchanges with written materials. While remaining optimistic and encouraging families to develop competence, it is also important for providers to recognize the complexity of what they are asking of families and the burden it imposes. Normalizing the common feelings of anxiety and "information overload" while focusing on problem solving in the face of new demands is an important role for the psychosocial clinician. Talking with other families who are undergoing similar treatment can be particularly helpful,[102,103,126,128,129] and many centers offer education and support groups for new patients and families. In addition a wide variety of books useful to parents[130-135] and helpful for patients and siblings[136-146] may be available from hospitals, libraries, and booksellers.

Among older children and adolescents, interest in or openness to learning more about their illness and treatment can be highly variable. Because they have more developed cognitive and language abilities than younger children, older children can ask more questions and understand more about their treatment, and like parents, they may receive educational information from nursing staff as previously described. To the extent of their capabilities, adolescents should be encouraged to participate in their own treatment by learning about their medications and schedule, helping with simple self-care activities such as routine care for a central venous line (CVL), and learning the best ways for them to cope with adverse effects or medical procedures. In some cases adolescents may not be interested in some of this information or may feel disinclined to assume even basic self-care responsibilities. It is not uncommon for adolescents to feel overwhelmed by information about their disease, particularly given the typical developmental milestones they are attempting to navigate.[147] Feelings of distress associated with a loss of autonomy may lead adolescent patients to become more withdrawn. It can be helpful to empathize with adolescents' plight of feeling "pushed around" while actively working with them to develop adaptive coping strategies that may lessen their feelings of helplessness. It is often important to point out that although many aspects of the situation cannot be changed (i.e., you have cancer, you need treatment, and the treatment will cause you to miss school), some aspects can be changed (e.g., you can maintain ties with friends through texting, social media, or visits, you can keep up with school work, and you can plan a party or an outing to celebrate an upcoming treatment milestone). It can be overwhelming for parents to include adolescents in difficult conversations about their illness and treatment, but adopting a model of shared decision making with adolescent patients in the early stages of treatment can empower patients, improve comprehension and understanding of the treatment plan and toxicities, and enhance communication among parents, patients, and providers.[148,149]

The Internet

In addition to obtaining medical information from medical teams, outside consultations, and family and friends, parents also gather information from the Internet. The ability to access information quickly and conveniently is appealing to parents who can feel overwhelmed during medical discussions. Given that it is common for patients and parents to use the Internet to gain knowledge about their disease and treatment, it is crucial that medical providers help families identify appropriate websites where they can access accurate information. In particular providers should consider providing parents with a list of recommended websites. These websites may include local resources affiliated with the treating institution, disease-specific resources, and general pediatric cancer sites facilitated by reputable organizations such as the Children's Oncology Group, Pediatric Cancer Research Foundation, National Cancer Institute, and the American Childhood Cancer Organization (e.g., www.curesearch.org, www.pcrf-kids.org, www.cancer.gov, and www.acco.org). The National Cancer Institute website offers educational materials in both English and Spanish. Ensuring accuracy of information is important not only for the parents' understanding but also for that of adolescent patients who frequently access the Internet.[150,151] Using a search engine to research a cancer diagnosis and treatment does not always lead to relevant content.[152] In addition the readability of websites is highly variable,[152] and the information provided on some websites may be difficult for some parents and patients to understand, potentially leading to additional confusion at an already challenging time. Potential exposure to difficult material (e.g., prognosis, individual narratives, and grief) without the immediate support of the medical team can be a particular concern. Having a discussion with families about the dangers of exploring too broadly on the Internet early in the diagnosis and treatment period is important so they can avoid exposure to potentially upsetting information.

Despite the potential challenges associated with gathering information via the Internet, this avenue provides some clear advantages for parents and patients, and research is burgeoning in this area to best meet the needs of the families.[153] Open patient-physician communication with regard to gathering information, asking questions, and researching treatment options and plans can help minimize confusion or distress based on misinformation obtained via the Internet. This approach represents a movement away from the more paternalistic approach, and medical providers can encourage families to conduct their own research and come back with questions or concerns.

ADJUSTING TO TREATMENT

While the child and family come to understand the diagnosis and treatment plan, their focus begins to shift from managing uncertainty to coping with the demands of treatment. Although parents in particular will continue to worry about their child's prognosis for years to come, the day-to-day demands of treatment along with the other demands of work and family life become increasingly salient. Families often experience a subjective sense of relief associated with a reduction in uncertainty, but they may also have an increased sense of burden. During the crisis of a new diagnosis, parents usually take time off from work and temporarily set aside many practical concerns. With the initiation of treatment, parents and children typically need to return to their regular roles and responsibilities while also taking on the new responsibilities associated with treatment. During this period of adjusting to treatment, families often benefit from continued psychosocial assessment, education, and support. In actual practice, encounters with the patient and family will blend these three objectives, especially at the initiation of treatment, but they are presented separately here for clarity of presentation.

Psychosocial Assessment of the Patient and Family

Experienced psychosocial care providers generally have a way of conducting an assessment that is comfortable for them and generates the relevant information. For illustrative purposes, a general approach to the assessment interview will be outlined here and in Box 73-2. The process of the interview should include time for the family members to speak about their concerns, but the provider will need to actively direct the conversation to ensure that the necessary topics are covered. In an interview with both parents if possible, the provider may begin by asking about the general family history and then focus on the patient's premorbid functioning, a developmental history, and the relevant history of any other children. Details of the patient's functioning at school and relationships with peers and siblings should be solicited, as well as prior experience with stressful situations and any behavioral, developmental, or emotional concerns prior to the cancer diagnosis. In learning more about the parents, it is useful to know the basic outline of their families of origin, their current work or family roles, and any religious and cultural traditions that may affect their ability to cope with the illness. It is important to know if the family has had to cope with significant stressors in the past and if any other significant problems exist in the family at present. If the parents are divorced or not married, understanding this history, as well as the practical and legal aspects of any custody arrangements, is critical. Understanding the family's practical and social resources is also an important component of the assessment.

The assessment of the pediatric patient will vary significantly depending on the child's age and medical status. With an infant or toddler, the child will be seen along with the parent, and the goals may be to observe the parent-child interaction, appreciate the child's temperament and reaction to the medical setting, and establish the psychosocial provider as a friendly and nonthreatening presence. With older children the goals will also include directly assessing their reaction to their illness as they are able to express it verbally or in play. Because children typically have met many health care providers in the hospital or clinic, it is important for the provider to begin by introducing himself or herself, describing the purpose of the meeting, and reassuring the child that there will be no medical examination or use of needles during the meeting. With most children, even into adolescence, the assessment can be greatly facilitated by including action, such as unstructured play, a walk in the hospital, a craft, or a game.

With preschool and school-aged children, familiar activities such as drawing or symbolic play with dolls or puppets can serve the dual purpose of engaging them and

---

Box 73-2 Psychosocial Assessment Interview of the Patient and Family

STRUCTURE OF INTERVIEW

- One to three intake meetings with patients and parents, conducted by a mental health professional.
- Meetings held in a relaxed, nonthreatening setting.
- Written summary of assessment to be shared with the treatment team.

ASSESSMENT CONTENT

ILLNESS CONTEXT

- Initial presentation of the illness.
- Diagnosis, prognosis, and anticipated treatment.
- Previous child and family experiences with physical health problems and behavioral problems.
- Family's coping, especially cohesiveness, communication style, and ways of resolving conflicts.

CHILD PATIENT

- History
  - Developmental—milestones, temperament, delays.
  - Medical—previous diagnoses and responses to medical care.
  - Behavioral—energy level, moods, and sleeping/eating habits before and after the illness.
  - School and Social—relationships with parents, siblings, and peers, educational history, and functioning in school.
- Response to diagnosis and coping style.

PARENT AND FAMILY

- Background and History.
  - Basic structure and involvement of extended family.
  - Sources of social support.
  - Relationships, sources of conflicts, and cohesion.
  - Physical and mental health.
  - Sibling relationships.
  - Parent education and employment.
  - Religious beliefs and cultural traditions.
  - Parenting styles.
- Initial Response to the Diagnosis
  - Knowledge and understanding of diagnosis.
  - Level of distress—emotional and physical symptoms.
  - Strength and vulnerabilities during the crisis.
  - Coping styles and experienced need for support.
  - Expectations and sources of stress and anxiety.

RESOURCES

- Housing.
- Names and ages of family members living at home (e.g., siblings and grandparents).
- Available support for work, neighborhood, and school.
- Financial status.
- Health insurance.
- Involvement within the community and social supports.
- Travel time and transportation to treatment center.
- Resources available during the child's ongoing medical treatment.

Modified from Hersh SP, Weiner LS, Figueroa V, et al: Psychiatric and psychosocial support for the child and family. In Pizzo PA, Poplack DG, editors: Principles and practice of pediatric oncology, ed 3, Philadelphia, 1997, Lippincott-Raven, p. 1241–1266.

---

providing an expressive medium through which they can relate their concerns. When children are engaged in this type of play, the provider can assess them by observing or participating in the play, as well as by asking them questions about their illness, their medical care, and how they are coping (e.g., "What has been the hardest part about being a patient?"). For older children, questions about life before cancer including friends, hobbies, and school activities can be a good starting place before asking about their illness and how they are coping with their medical care. It is important to ask older children directly about any worries, anxiety, and symptoms of depression or hopelessness, as well as how the adults involved in their care can best help and support them.

Adolescents may have very personal concerns about how their illness will affect them, such as by causing them to miss an upcoming social event or interfering with a particular friendship or a dating or romantic interest; such concerns may not be immediately apparent to the parents or the medical team. Asking explicitly about what they anticipate will be difficult about their treatment plan is an important part of the assessment, as is inquiring about ways they believe they will deal with the challenges of treatment. Family systems often shift in response to a child's illness, and it can be important to understand the changes adolescents may have experienced and how those changes may be affecting them, especially because adolescents in treatment may become more dependent on their parents and spend more time with them than they normally would. Because adolescents often believe that the patient role limits their privacy, agreeing ahead of time with parents and adolescents about what information from the adolescent interview will need to be discussed with parents and what information everyone agrees can be kept confidential will be important.

After concluding the interview with the patient, it is important to give feedback to the parents about what was discussed, the child's main concerns, and generally how the patient is coping with the illness and the demands of treatment. If the psychosocial care provider has specific recommendations for further assessment or intervention, they should be explained to the parent and patient. For illustrative purposes this description has emphasized the information that should be gathered in the assessment, but the process of the interview should accommodate both the goal of assessment and the goals of education and support.

Support for Parents and Families during Treatment

Families may require very different levels of psychosocial support during treatment, and even within a single family, needs will vary over time. Ideally psychosocial support can be offered to patients and families in a flexible way that can be tailored to their individual needs. This flexible approach requires some ongoing assessment and communication with families about their coping and adjustment, as well as the ability to quickly adjust the level of services offered to each family. Families typically require more intensive involvement from the psychosocial care provider during the diagnostic period and the beginning of treatment,[104,154] as previously described. Some families may continue to have high levels of emotional distress or ongoing problems adjusting to treatment (Table 73-1) and will require continued regular meetings with a psychosocial provider, but many families will not have this need. For families who are adjusting adequately to the routine of treatment, their need for psychosocial care often decreases. For these families the psychosocial care

provider may briefly check in with patients and parents in the context of their regular medical care. These brief visits may be useful for assessing their adjustment and reinforcing previously offered suggestions and interventions. The psychosocial team may also offer information about educational and support groups, which can be particularly helpful for parents adjusting to treatment.

With any decrease in intensity of direct psychosocial involvement, care should be taken to ensure that patients and families do not feel abandoned by the psychosocial care provider. In most clinical settings a team model is used in which medical providers and psychosocial clinicians are in frequent communication so parents can be assured that when important medical changes occur that have potential psychological implications, psychosocial care providers will be informed and will intervene as appropriate. It is important to review with parents the expected challenges that may arise during the course of treatment (described in the next section) and encourage them to contact the psychosocial care provider if they need assistance with these or other issues that arise.

If some adjustment problems arise during the course of treatment, such as problems at school or difficulties with discipline, the psychosocial care provider should offer symptom-focused interventions such as educational support, behavioral intervention, or other counseling. Typically this intervention may involve a small number of sessions delivered as part of the patient's regular medical visits or a referral for short-term therapy within the treating institution or in the community. While the presenting issue is resolved, children and families will typically return to their previous level of adjustment, and the intervention can be tapered off and discontinued.

Some families will experience brief periods of intense emotional distress related to the stress of cancer treatment. These episodes may occur when they are facing painful or unpleasant therapies or when treatment complications arise. Intervention for moderate to severe distress could include an increase in the intensity of routine psychosocial support services, consultation with additional mental health providers to provide crisis intervention, psychiatric assessment, and use of psychopharmacology for patients or other family members. In the outpatient setting, referral to outpatient providers in the community will also be important.

Some children and families will require a more intensive level of psychosocial care consistently throughout treatment. In most cases these families have high emotional distress, multiple stressors, or limited resources, which can often be recognized during the psychosocial assessment (see the previous section). For most of these children and families, regular ongoing psychosocial services will need to be provided for much or all of the treatment period. In these cases the psychosocial care provider should consider several types of intervention, such as play therapy, cognitive-behavioral treatment, and parent guidance. Referral to other specialists, either within the treating medical center or in the community, is useful when specialized services are needed (e.g., psychopharmacology) or the child or family needs more intensive treatment than can be accommodated within the oncology clinic. Referral for outside services such as psychopharmacology or individual or family therapy is particularly useful in cases of some preexisting mental illness, family conflicts, or multiple major stressors.

Few families will present with psychological distress or behavioral problems that cannot be successfully managed with routine psychosocial care along with some provision for brief intensive interventions.[14] Usually families that cannot be managed in this way are those with many other stressors occurring at the same time or families that include an individual with a preexisting psychiatric disorder, such as major mental illness, substance abuse, or severe personality disorder. When families have multiple stressful events occurring simultaneously, such as a second illness in the family, a major loss, or economic instability, they may require more psychosocial support at the cancer center, as well as referral to additional outside agencies. Preexisting psychiatric disorders should be evaluated as part of the psychosocial assessment. Vulnerable persons at high risk for worsening of symptoms or relapse should be referred for mental health treatment or counseled about the need to access treatment quickly if symptoms recur. Communication between the psychosocial providers on the oncology team and outside mental health providers can be helpful to share a common understanding of the child's cancer treatment status and updates about the mental health status of the family member in treatment, but this communication needs to be undertaken in a limited manner that preserves privacy.

Families with consistently active psychosocial needs can present a challenge to the care team because of their emotional distress and the demands they may make on staff time. By providing consultation to the nursing and oncology staff, the psychosocial care provider can help the treatment team formulate an understanding of the family's needs and coordinate an appropriate and consistent response.

School

Shortly after diagnosis, questions often arise regarding the child's academic needs and how these needs will be met. Will the child be able to attend school, or will a tutor be provided until the child is able to return to the classroom? How is the treatment course likely to interfere with the child's ability to succeed academically? Will the child meet the academic requirements to be promoted to the next grade, or is it likely that the child will need to repeat a grade? These types of questions will need to be addressed by the family, school, and medical team.

School represents an important locus for the child's cognitive, social, and emotional development, and maintaining participation in or reconnecting with school should be a priority when planning the child's treatment and care.[155,156] For the child resuming school responsibilities can feel overwhelming given the demands of treatment. Adverse effects of treatment can have a negative impact on motivation, concentration, and processing speed, making the transition back to school challenging. Despite the issues resuming academic work promptly will minimize the disruption to academic progress and maximize the child's ability to reengage in school-related tasks. Because many children will be unable to attend school during at least part of their treatment, home- or hospital-based tutoring along with a structured schedule that provides the child with the exact time and duration of school-related work often promotes compliance.

Parents and caregivers must commit themselves to providing the necessary structure and support to promote the child's academic progress, even when juggling numerous other responsibilities. Parents should be encouraged to let the tutors be responsible for assisting children with their academic work and avoid the urge to "help" children with their homework. Extended absences from school can lead to increased anxiety at the time of reentry and potential avoidance behavior. Psychosocial providers can work closely with patients, parents, and school personnel to help ease a child back into school while addressing anxiety issues.

The medical team is often called upon to provide the school with relevant information about the child's ability to attend to academic responsibilities or any vulnerability the child may have as a result of treatment (e.g., risk of infection, susceptibility to illness, and potential cognitive and/or physical deficits). School personnel may be especially anxious when the child initially returns to school, resulting in multiple calls to the treating physician. Parents will play a critical role in educating the school about their child's situation and advocating for the child's needs. Many parents benefit from consultation with psychosocial providers about how best to negotiate the return to school and often find written guides for parents[131,135] to be helpful. Some clinics have established "school reentry" programs in which staff members (e.g., child life, nursing, and mental health professionals) visit schools to present information to teachers and classmates about the child's diagnosis and treatment.[157-159] This proactive approach can be effective in providing medical information to the school nurse and other staff, as well as helping to answer questions that teachers and classmates may have about the returning child's condition and needs. In most cases, these efforts will result in a plan for school reentry that is appropriate and comfortable for the child and parents.

If a child will need specialized instruction because of his or her illness or consequences of treatment, an individualized education plan (IEP) will be required. Federal laws, as well as the laws in several states, require that children with disabilities be accommodated in their schools,[160-162] and parents who suspect their child will need some accommodation should speak with the school's special education director and refer to their state's Department of Education website for information about the special education procedures in their location. In most cases, parents will need to begin the process by making a written request for an evaluation. This evaluation is conducted by the school, often with significant input from medical and psychosocial providers involved in the child's cancer treatment. If as a result of the evaluation the child is found to be eligible for special education services, an IEP will be developed and implemented by the school. If the child does not qualify for specialized education services, he or she may still qualify for accommodations under the Federal Rehabilitation Act, often referred to as a "504 plan."[163] A 504 plan may ensure appropriate accommodation for problems in physical mobility, fatigue, attendance, or other needs of the child that affect school performance but do not require specialized instruction. The IEP determination process can be time consuming and frustrating for parents who have already had to negotiate complex health and insurance systems for their child. Parents should educate themselves about their state's education laws and the federal laws that govern accommodation of children with medical conditions and disabilities[161,162,164] and consult with psychosocial providers who understand the system and academic needs. If significant issues are encountered in securing appropriate accommodations, parents may want to consider enlisting the services of educational advocates[165] to assist them in negotiating with their school.

Peer Relationships

Relationships with peers at any developmental level provide a child or adolescent with crucial components for successful adaptation, including a sense of connection, friendship, and support. This role of peer relationships is as true for children diagnosed with cancer as it is for their healthy peers. Several research studies have focused on the role of peer relationships in the coping and adjustment of children and adolescents with cancer.[166-170] Although parents have been identified as a primary source of nurturance, support, and information for children with cancer,[168] research findings suggest that relationships either with healthy peers or with peers diagnosed with cancer are also extremely important. For example adolescents diagnosed with cancer who report close friendships have been noted to experience increased social support,[148,167] increased feelings of hope,[171] and an ease in communicating about their cancer experience.[168] Additional research suggests that adolescents with cancer view peer relationships as vital to the continued development of their independence and identity, which are areas that can easily be derailed by illness.[169,172]

Studies examining other aspects of peer interactions reveal somewhat mixed results. Some findings have suggested that both children and adolescents who are diagnosed with cancer have fewer friends than their same-aged peers[168,173] and that this trend may continue after treatment has been completed.[174,175] Other findings have indicated that children diagnosed with cancer may be socially isolated and withdrawn,[176] despite the fact that their popularity and number of friendships are comparable with those of their peers.[177] Whether these results reflect a change in the nature or quality of peer interactions because of illness-related factors (e.g., prolonged hospitalizations, significant school absences, or the inability to engage in recreational activities) is difficult to determine.

Given the importance of peer relationships in the course of normal development and the potential for disruption to these relationships during diagnosis and treatment, members of the medical team must support connections with peers whenever possible.[178] This support may include encouraging parents to facilitate peer interactions at home and at the hospital and to work with educators to establish opportunities for the child to visit school for lunch or a single class so that peer connections can continue when the child is not well enough to attend school regularly. When appropriate, medical staff can also support an adolescent patient who wishes to share the clinic experience with a friend and invite the friend to attend an outpatient appointment. These opportunities, although often limited by the impact of treatment, help children with cancer and their peers maintain crucial relationships that will improve posttreatment adjustment. Encouraging parents to allow children and adolescents to have contact with peers who are also diagnosed with cancer can be extremely important. The Internet and social media sites can be very helpful when treatment prevents school attendance. Although parents will want to ensure that the sites that children are using are appropriate, technology that provides ways for children to share pictures, play video games with friends online, video chat, or text can be important ways for them to maintain contact with peers. Participation in summer camps or activities offered through the clinic or hospital provide opportunities for children and adolescents to enjoy activities with peers who have a shared medical experience and can improve self-concept.[179]

EXPECTABLE CHALLENGES DURING TREATMENT

Although psychosocial needs vary considerably between families, certain challenges commonly arise while children progress through their cancer treatment. Some of these challenges are directly related to coping with the demands of treatment, and others have to do with managing the ongoing demands of work, school, and family life while also managing the added stressors of cancer and its treatment. Understanding these challenges can help families anticipate when and how they may need to mobilize their resources. Psychosocial care providers can provide anticipatory guidance with regard to these concerns and facilitate access to appropriate intervention as needed.

Coping with Treatment and Adverse Effects

About 25 years ago, adolescents with cancer reported that their treatment and its adverse effects were the worst things about having cancer.[180] The nausea and vomiting accompanying chemotherapy and the pain associated with procedures such as lumbar punctures and bone marrow aspirations were particularly distressing.[181-184] Treatment of these adverse effects has significantly improved since then. Fairly effective antiemetic drugs are available, and for most patients, procedures are carried out after induction of light or deep sedation or general anesthesia. Despite these advances, children still find chemotherapy, radiation therapy, and various procedures to be very unpleasant and a source of significant apprehension and distress.[185-190] A variety of studies have documented the effects of hypnotherapy, memory evaluation, and other behavioral therapies in reducing adverse effects in this population.[116,191-198] Reducing procedure-related pain, anxiety, and nausea and vomiting associated with chemotherapy and radiation therapy is critically important for reduction of risk factors for posttraumatic stress disorder, long-term pain, and psychological distress in survivors.[1,105,199-210] The topics of pain and symptom management are treated more extensively in Chapter 71.

Maintaining Child and Family Routines
Basic Needs

In the aftermath of a pediatric cancer diagnosis, family members must find ways to attend to basic needs and responsibilities. Although this process can be difficult, family members must eventually shift their focus from the diagnosed child and the isolation of the hospital room to life outside of the hospital. For many families, this process may include working to understand their insurance coverage and medical costs or negotiating with employers regarding the use of vacation or sick leave to care for their child. Grocery shopping, cleaning the house, paying bills, and keeping up with the laundry are additional activities that constitute a typical week for the average family—activities that were likely ignored or attended to by others during the early stages of diagnosis and treatment.

Transitioning from managing a medical crisis to managing the more mundane tasks of everyday life can be challenging but can also reintroduce a sense of normalcy. The reality of financial pressures can necessitate the transition back to work and create additional stress on the family system. Even with excellent insurance coverage, the costs associated with treatment can be significant, particularly for parents or caregivers who have been away from work since the child's diagnosis.

After the initial phase of treatment, parents and caregivers typically attempt to piece together a plan that will allow the family to function effectively and attend to basic needs. This plan will likely take into account the child's medical appointments (both scheduled and unscheduled), the child's school reentry and ongoing attendance, parent or caregiver work responsibilities, attention to the academic and social needs of the child and the child's siblings, and other family commitments and responsibilities. The ability of the family to successfully develop and implement this plan is dependent upon a number of factors, including characteristics of individual family members (e.g., coping style, organizational skills, and cognitive abilities), the functioning of the family as a whole (e.g., cohesion, adaptability, and flexibility), and the response of community members (e.g., a supportive network of friends, the flexibility of employers, and the commitment of school personal).

Understandably attending to basic needs and securing resources is crucial to the successful treatment of the child and the overall functioning of the family, and thus it is essential that members of the medical team support the family in their efforts to meet basic needs whenever possible. This support might include the timely completion of medical forms that will facilitate the implementation of educational services, helping eligible families secure appropriate financial resources, helping families access specialized nursing services in the home, allowing for flexibility in the scheduling of appointments to accommodate a long commute to the clinic, or simply being willing to listen empathically when parents discuss the challenges they face.

Discipline

The diagnosis and treatment of cancer in a child can disrupt every facet of family functioning, including expectations that parents have about their child's behavior and their ability to effectively set limits and exercise appropriate discipline. Understandably many parents and caregivers are unable or unwilling to discipline their children given the difficult medical circumstances in which the family finds itself. A child's behavioral outbursts that may include hitting, kicking, and screaming are seen as a natural consequence of a very difficult and unnatural situation. Disruptions to daily routines, invasive medical procedures, medication adverse effects, and the child's "just feeling lousy" can provide more than sufficient rationale to let the child's behavior remain unchecked. In addition parents and caregivers may be wrestling with their own feelings of guilt, sadness, anxiety, or exhaustion that can make it increasingly difficult to impose behavioral expectations, even for parents who previously demonstrated consistent and appropriate behavior management techniques with their children.

For children whose parents or caretakers are unable to provide effective discipline during treatment, the short- and long-term consequences can be disastrous. For example a child who does not experience appropriate limit setting may feel out of control and unsafe, leading to further behavioral disruption. Behavioral outbursts and noncompliance can interfere with medical care and have an impact on effective working relationships with staff. Inappropriate behavior can spread quickly to siblings who learn through observation that parental authority has been eroded, increasing the overall chaos within the family system. By the time the child's treatment ends months or years later, it can be extremely difficult, if not impossible, to reestablish expectations for appropriate behavior.

To avoid these short- and long-term consequences, parents and caregivers need to provide clear and consistent expectations for their child's behavior as quickly as possible after diagnosis. It is essential to acknowledge to the child that the pain and disruption associated with diagnosis and treatment often causes frustration, sadness, anger and despair and that this is expected. However it is equally essential to convey to the child that expressing emotions through appropriate means is imperative.

Members of the medical team should work with parents to reestablish appropriate discipline practices. During the initial phase of treatment, the team's assessment of the family should include questions about the parents' approach to discipline and strategies that are both effective and ineffective in managing their child's behavior. Understanding parenting styles[211] and the child's prior experiences with discipline can be extremely helpful in predicting possible reactions in both the child and parent. Encouraging parents to utilize an authoritative approach—that is, clear, firm limit setting coupled with appropriate encouragement of independence—will help children be more successful at negotiating the difficulties associated with diagnosis and treatment. A more punitive and authoritarian style will likely increase the anxiety and fear the child is already experiencing, whereas an indulgent or permissive style can foster noncompliance and increased disrespect of others.

A number of behavioral techniques can be used to increase a child's compliance and to minimize disruptive behavior. First, taking the parent aside, acknowledging the challenges of disciplining a sick child, and offering suggestions will be more effective than openly criticizing the parent's poor behavior management in front of the child. When the child's behavior interferes with medical care, staff should encourage and support authoritative parenting. Such encouragement might include staff modeling of behavior management techniques such as giving the child clear instructions ("You need to sit on the table, and you can hold dad's hand"), praise ("I really appreciate how you answered my questions; you've done a great job"), and attention ("Because you were so cooperative and we finished your dressing change so quickly, I have a few minutes to look at your baseball cards, if you'd like to show them to me"). Praise and attention are examples of positive reinforcement, approaches that increase the likelihood that the child will behave the same way in the future.

Behavioral techniques such as "sticker charts" can be implemented with the help of mental health practitioners or child life specialists. Developing a sticker chart includes identifying a behavior the team needs the child to perform (e.g., taking medication), as well as a reward that increases the child's willingness to engage in the behavior. Each time the child behaves appropriately, a sticker is applied to the chart, and after a specified number of stickers have been achieved, a predetermined reward is given. The reward must be given frequently enough that the child experiences the benefits of his or her efforts. When available these techniques should be used in conjunction with psychosocial services from mental health practitioners familiar with the treatment of medically compromised children. Parent education and guidance, as well as counseling or psychotherapy, can be helpful in supporting parents and caregivers in maintaining discipline while providing children with appropriate outlets for their feelings. Many parents will benefit from referral to parenting support groups and books about effective discipline.[212,213]

Siblings

The siblings of children diagnosed with cancer have a unique and often difficult road from the moment a brother or sister is diagnosed with cancer. The uncertainty experienced in the context of a cancer diagnosis and the impact it has on a family system has significant implications for siblings. Siblings spend a significant amount of time with caregivers other than parents, and despite the best parental intentions, they can get shuffled around from place to place while the ill sibling is in the hospital. Although parents may work diligently to attend to the needs of all their children, the parents are often overwhelmed and overburdened, and as a result the siblings of the diagnosed child often feel ignored and excluded, contributing to feelings of jealousy, guilt, anxiety, and sadness.[214,215] The type of challenges that are faced and how a sibling responds are greatly dependent on developmental level. For example preschoolers may experience significant anxiety related to prolonged separation from caregivers who remain at the hospital with the patient, whereas adolescents may be more concerned about details of their sibling's treatment and prognosis.

Siblings of children with cancer have been the subjects of numerous studies designed to investigate their adjustment and adaptation after the diagnosis of their brother or sister.[214,216-223] Findings suggest that most siblings experience some level of stress associated with the treatment of the ill child, especially in the first few months,[154,224] and that this stress may lead to deterioration in normal functioning. Siblings may demonstrate a range of externalizing and internalizing problems, including withdrawal from friends and activities, disturbances in eating and sleeping, temper tantrums, depressed mood, and anxiety.[219,220,225-229] A few studies have documented positive effects, particularly in older siblings, who may exhibit higher levels of empathy and maturity.[216,222,230-232]

Despite years of research highlighting the challenges encountered by siblings of children with cancer, relatively few targeted interventions have been developed for this group. A systematic review of the literature identified studies using individual intervention, camp, and group support to evaluate the impact on sibling psychological adjustment. Findings indicated that participation in interventions improved siblings' depressive symptoms, medical knowledge, and health-related quality of life.[233] Ideally interventions should address sibling adjustment throughout the treatment process rather than at specific phases (e.g., diagnosis or at the time of a bone marrow transplant).[234] General guidelines for improving sibling adjustment include involving the sibling in developmentally appropriate discussions as early as possible, educating the sibling about the illness and treatment course, encouraging the sibling to visit the hospital, and providing opportunities for supportive interactions (e.g., sibling support groups, individual counseling, and summer camp experiences).[215,235] Programs such as SuperSibs, a nonprofit organization for siblings of pediatric cancer patients,[236] provide opportunities for siblings to feel valued and heard through activities and services. Feelings of frustration, anger, jealousy, or guilt need to be acknowledged and normalized, and younger siblings may need to be reassured that the illness of their brother or sister was in no way attributable to anything they may have said or done. Having siblings maintain a routine by attending school or day care, socializing with friends, or engaging in various extracurricular activities provides structure and a sense of normalcy during a very challenging time for the family and increase the opportunities for social support when parents and caregivers are busy attending to the ill child. For siblings who demonstrate ongoing emotional distress or significant difficulties in returning to their regular school, family, and social routines, a consultation with a psychosocial provider should be recommended. Depending on the sibling's needs and available resources, they may be able to provide some short-term supportive therapy or make a referral to community or school-based resources.

Transitions and Changes in Care

While families transition from one phase of cancer care to another, they often experience the change as a loss. In each phase of treatment, children and families adapt, even unwittingly, to difficult circumstances of treatment, and when these circumstances change, they experience disruption in their new routines and habits. Parents may be particularly susceptible and often appreciate the irony of having spent days or week feeling "trapped" in the hospital, only to find themselves later terrified to leave it. Children may miss the special care they received in certain settings, the reassurance and attention they received from nursing staff, relationships they developed with other children, and the relaxed expectations that may apply when they are undergoing intensive treatment. Many kinds of transitions in care can be challenging to families, but discharges from the hospital and the transition from active treatment to going "off therapy" may be among the most stressful,[237-241] especially for parents. During these transitions it is especially important for providers to be sensitive to the likelihood that families will feel anxious and unsure, even while the treatment is "progressing." Providers may naturally tend to emphasize only the positive aspects of a transition, but this approach is likely to increase feelings of anxiety and isolation. Providers should normalize families' feelings by asking about their uncertainty or ambivalence with regard to moving to a new phase of treatment and should reassure them that these reactions are common. Asking, "How does it feel now that you are getting ready to go home?" is much more useful to the family than a well-intentioned statement of "Oh, you must be so happy to be going home." Acknowledging that a transition may require the patient and family to adapt to new routines and providers or manage aspects of the medical care more independently is important, as is reassuring the family that there will be continued support for them during the transition period.

For families beginning a new phase of treatment, such as outpatient radiation or chemotherapy, a tour of the new treatment area, introductions to new providers, and opportunities to meet other children and families can be very helpful. Child life specialists can be particularly helpful to children acclimating to new treatment settings and modalities. Families transitioning from active therapy to off-treatment care can experience significant uncertainty and emotional distress, especially when treatment has lasted for a year or longer. Although some families find the end of therapy a great relief, many families are surprised to find themselves experiencing anxiety, uncertainty, and feelings of helplessness reminiscent of feelings they had during the crisis period of diagnosis.[238] For these families it is helpful to normalize their reactions, helping them to understand that during active therapy their anxiety was kept at bay by the demands of treatment, the frequent contact with providers, and the rituals of medical care. While the demands of treatment decrease, they may find themselves looking back and reflecting on all they have been through since diagnosis. In addition the cessation of treatment raises concerns about the possibility of relapse, and less frequent visits to the oncologist may make parents in particular worry about how their child's health will be monitored. Because the off-therapy transitions can be a time of increased stress and uncertainty for many families, it is helpful to anticipate these needs by offering additional psychosocial support either in individual meetings with families or through parent support groups. In addition to providing increased emotional support, programs providing tailored medical information for families ending treatment, such as a summary of the child's treatment and their schedule for off-treatment and follow-up care, can be effective for reducing anxiety and uncertainty.[238]

Home Care

Children's cancer treatment will often require that some specialized care be provided in the home. Depending on the specifics of the child's treatment, specialized care may include taking oral medications or nutritional supplements, caring for a CVL, or receiving injections or intravenous medications. Care in the home setting is critical to allowing children and families to leave the medical setting and return home to normal routines, but it also represents a significant new responsibility for parents and children.[242,243] Over time, providing care in the home can give both parents and patients a way to feel active and competent in managing their own care, but at least initially it can be a source of burden and anxiety. Parents may feel overwhelmed both by the technical aspects of home care they must learn to provide, such as flushing a CVL or giving an injection, as well as by the sense of responsibility for monitoring their child's health. Children can feel confused about why their home setting is being "invaded" by the medical world they had hoped to leave behind in the hospital, and some resistance to treatment may emerge. Receiving care from the parent rather than a medical provider can be a relief for some children but may raise problems for other children. Parents' discomfort or unfamiliarity can be unsettling for children, and the parent as medical provider can be an awkward change of roles in the family. Young children may experience difficulty in having parents shift from an emotionally supportive role to being the hands-on person providing their care, and thus they may become resistant to certain aspects of their care, such as taking oral medications. Older children and adolescents may want to assert their independence and be directly involved in their care but may not know how to do so. They may also be ambivalent, with some adolescents alternately striving for independence and exhibiting dependence and passivity.

Practical education from nursing staff is vital for parents and children assuming responsibility for home care.[242,244] The availability of home care nurses to provide some of this care, monitoring, and education is also critical. Nursing and psychosocial professionals can also offer important emotional support by normalizing feelings of uncertainty and responsibility and by promoting the development of a sense of competence by patients and families. For children of all ages it is useful for parents and providers to consider how the child can be involved in his or her care in a way that will help the child feel some mastery and sense of control. If problems with a child's compliance are anticipated or develop at home, the psychosocial care provider should work with the family to develop a behavioral plan to address the problems. Supporting the parents in their role, helping them to set clear and consistent expectations, implementing a reward system with tokens, and helping the child find a way to be appropriately active in his or her care can all be useful interventions. With older children and adolescents, a token reward system such as a sticker chart is less likely to be effective, and some negotiation of roles and responsibilities will often be more helpful. Family members may need to be encouraged to be more flexible and try involving different family members or different schedules to manage their home care. In these cases the psychosocial care provider may want to involve other members of the treatment team such as nurses, nutritionists, or pharmacists in considering how the home care plan can be adapted for the needs of a particular family. Peer support from other families and patients may also be helpful.

SPECIAL ISSUES THAT MAY ARISE DURING TREATMENT

Marital Adjustment

A pediatric cancer diagnosis has immediate and significant consequences for those connected to the ill child, most notably the parents. Although the level of care a child will require through the treatment process will depend on several factors, including the severity of illness and the child's developmental level, most children undergoing cancer treatment will require significant support from at least one parent or caregiver. Many families find that managing the child's hospitalizations, clinic visits, daily medications, adverse effects of treatment, and other illness-related factors is a full-time job, often leaving the responsible adult feeling overwhelmed. With one parent now dedicated to caring for the ill child, the other parent is often left to support the family financially, attend to other children, and ensure that the household continues to function effectively. Not surprisingly these circumstances can present significant challenges to all aspects of family functioning and can test the marital relationship. Understanding how these circumstances affect the child and family is complex and necessitates the consideration of several factors, such as parental coping, family cohesion and organization, emotional expression, and marital satisfaction.[245]

Given the challenges that parents must face after their child has been diagnosed, one might predict that marital relationships would suffer as a result. Research has suggested that although parents of children with cancer were no more likely to divorce than other parents and that marriages generally remain stable,[246-248] marital dissatisfaction and distress do increase.[249-251] Specifically Hoekstra-Weebers and colleagues[249] noted that marital dissatisfaction was associated with higher levels of psychological distress 6 and 12 months after diagnosis, but not at the time of diagnosis. Schuler and colleagues[250] found that parents, especially mothers, experienced distress with regard to adjusting to new demands. Similarly Dahlquist and colleagues[94,251] reported that marital distress was predicted by general emotional distress and a discrepancy between the couple's perceived anxiety levels. Although pediatric cancer may strain marital relationships and accentuate differences in parental coping styles, these results suggest that couples are committed to remaining in their marriages, perhaps to minimize any additional disruption to the family and to the diagnosed child. Given that marital distress appears to increase over the course of the child's treatment and may not be evident at diagnosis when clinical assessments are initiated, it may be helpful for medical staff to monitor parental functioning over time and to seek consultation from mental health colleagues when marital tension is evident and could potentially affect the adjustment of the child and family.

Nonadherence

The ability to adhere to treatment regimens is an important clinical issue that has ramifications for overall disease outcome and clinical trial data.[252] In pediatric oncology, nonadherence can be used to refer to failure to attend medical appointments, undergo chemotherapy or take other medications as directed, and comply with clinical research requirements.[253] Nonadherence can have significant implications such as inaccurate conclusions regarding medication efficacy, skewed research findings for experimental protocols, and even a decreased chance for survival.[254] In one study nonadherence with oral cancer treatment was found in nearly 60% of adolescents and 33% of children younger than 13 years.[255]

The adherence literature has consistently demonstrated that adolescents are at greater risk for nonadherence compared with younger or older patients.[254,256-258] The nonadherence rates for adolescents receiving cancer treatment are consistent with findings of nonadherence in other chronic diseases such as cystic fibrosis[259] and diabetes.[260] The nonadherence demonstrated in the literature is likely related to the developmental tasks associated with adolescence. On a practical level, because adolescents spend more time away from their parents, the parents (especially those who are working or caring for other children) may naturally expect the adolescent to remember when to take medications and to take them more independently. Psychologically adolescents naturally develop an increased sense of autonomy and move away from being dependent on parents, which may make it more complicated to negotiate how their medication use will be monitored.[147] Although most parents and adolescents may fully intend to adhere to medication schedules, the combination of the adolescent's need to exert some level of independent functioning, the need to fully integrate adolescents into school and social settings where parents may have less opportunity for oversight, and multiple demands on parents can increase noncompliance and create opportunities for miscommunication and conflict with regard to who is responsible for ensuring adherence to treatment.[252]

Despite the belief of adolescents that they can take care of themselves, they face a number of challenges in adhering to a complicated oral treatment regimen. Their neurocognitive abilities may not be appropriately developed, and executive functioning challenges may interfere with their capacity to organize medication schedules. In addition many adolescents may not adhere to treatment recommendations if the treatment schedule or medication adverse effects interfere with pleasurable activities. Psychosocial care providers can be helpful in terms of potentially preventing adherence issues by encouraging parents and providers to include adolescents, when developmentally appropriate, more fully in their medical care. Simply raising the issue can be valuable, because letting families know that trouble with ongoing adherence to medication is not unusual can help many parents and patients acknowledge the issue and talk more openly about it. Research has demonstrated that including adolescents in the treatment decision-making process increases their sense of autonomy and improves treatment adherence.[257] In addition, working with the medical providers to factor in flexibility, when appropriate, to accommodate the social needs of adolescent patients may help increase adherence.

A number of individual, family, and treatment characteristics have been linked to treatment adherence. Die-Trill and Stuber[255] found that characteristics of the child such as behavioral problems, poor self-image, poor insight regarding prognosis, and poor coping mechanisms were positively correlated with nonadherence. Family predictors of nonadherence included parental depression and an increase in the number of siblings. Treatment intensity and the number of medications needed for effective treatment also increase nonadherence. Die-Trill and Stuber[255] identified additional factors that promote treatment adherence, including increased anxiety in female patients and increased obsessive-compulsive behaviors in parents of male patients.

Recent research on adherence has begun to utilize advances in technology to move beyond self-report and pill counting to incorporate electronic monitoring devices on pill bottles and blood work. In one such study Bhatia and colleagues[254] identified nonadherence in 44% of children with acute lymphoblastic leukemia and found that 59% of the relapses were related to nonadherence to medication regimens. In addition ethnic differences in adherence were reported, with Hispanic patients having significantly higher rates of nonadherence when compared with other ethnic groups. Patients from single-parent homes were also at greater risk for nonadherence. It is likely that in such households, adolescents are more likely to be responsible for medications, and given the issues previously raised, they have difficulty adhering to the recommended medical treatment.

Although a significant amount of literature has been devoted to nonadherence in adolescent patients, issues associated with adherence can also be a result of parent error. Protocols that involve oral regimens have increased, subsequently requiring parents to be responsible for appropriate dosing and administration. A multisite study of medication errors in the home revealed that one in two patients were exposed to at least one, if not more than one, medication error when medications were administered in the home. These errors mostly entailed inaccurate dosing or missed doses.[261] It is important that the medical team consistently monitor patients and parents regarding the use of oral medications, and if nonadherence or errors are suspected, education and training should be provided to support families in adhering to what can often be complicated treatment regimens.

Given that adherence is essential for the safe and successful treatment of pediatric cancer, a number of interventions can be incorporated to increase adherence, such as educating parents and patients about the prescribed medical treatment and the medical ramifications of not taking medications as recommended. It is also important to understand the neurocognitive capabilities of patients and families and factor that knowledge into helpful strategies that can be used to aid organizational and memory issues, thus helping parents to develop supportive relationships with their children that will allow the use of appropriate behavioral techniques.

Depression and Anxiety

Given the many challenges that children and adolescents face during the course of cancer treatment, many investigators have hypothesized that children with cancer are at risk for higher levels of depression and anxiety. Research findings to date are mixed, with some studies suggesting emotional and behavioral maladjustment, including depression and anxiety, in children with cancer[262-264] and other studies showing less behavioral or emotional disruption in these children.[265,266] Social support and effective parenting throughout treatment appear to provide protection from the adversity encountered by the child with cancer[266] and may be important buffers against serious psychological distress in patients.

Given the stress associated with the diagnosis and treatment of pediatric cancer, some level of heightened anxiety and depression is to be expected, although these symptoms may not be of sufficient intensity to reach clinical significance and may not be consistent with a psychiatric diagnosis. The inability to attend school, participate in extracurricular activities, and socialize with friends, coupled with invasive procedures, nausea, and hair loss, would leave even the most well-adjusted child or adolescent struggling to maintain appropriate functioning. Given the likelihood that most patients will experience at least some transient symptoms of anxiety and depression, the tasks for providers and parents is to identify these symptoms, assess their level of intensity and functional significance, and plan for appropriate interventions to address them.

The medical team, with the assistance of parents or caregivers, should consistently assess the child's mood and behavior for signs of emotional difficulty, comparing current functioning with functioning prior to diagnosis. The team may ask why a child is no longer playing his or her favorite video games, being disrespectful toward nursing staff, refusing physical therapy, or ignoring visitors. Anhedonia, sleep disturbance, irritability, and social isolation are some of the signs and symptoms of depression that are commonly seen in children and adolescents coping with cancer treatment. For most patients these symptoms will be mild to moderate in severity and can be thought of as reflecting expectable reactions to the illness and demands of treatment. Supportive care provided by nurses, parents, and child life specialists to minimize physical discomfort, empathize with the frustrations and disappointments of being a patient, and promote opportunities to find some pleasurable activities can be useful for most of these individuals. Similarly nightmares, heightened reactivity, and worry about future health problems or medical procedures are indicators of anxiety commonly encountered in children with cancer. Parents and providers can often help patients with these symptoms by providing reassurance, offering information about the medical course, providing the opportunity to express their worry openly, and teaching some relaxation and distraction techniques.

When symptoms of depression or anxiety do not respond to routine supportive care, cause significant distress, or otherwise interfere with the child's ability to engage in essential daily activities or comply with medical care, a specialized mental health evaluation should be sought. This evaluation drawing on information from the patient, family, and medical team, should be focused on determining the extent and severity of behavioral and psychological symptoms, the relevant psychiatric disorders, if any, as well as deficits in knowledge or coping skills that may need to be addressed. Based on this information, the mental health specialist should be able to recommend which of a variety of types of interventions such as cognitive-behavioral therapy, expressive therapy, play therapy, psychopharmacology, or family therapy would be most appropriate. Psychological assessment can be complicated by questions of whether a pediatric patient's physical symptoms are secondary to the physical cancer or are evidence of psychological disturbance.[267-269] The physical effects of treatment and adverse effects of medications may mimic symptoms of depression or anxiety and interfere with an accurate diagnosis. While working to understand how medical factors can contribute to the presentation of psychological symptoms, it is important not to dismiss these symptoms too quickly as manifestations of physical illness. Hedstrom and colleagues[270] found that medical and nursing staff underestimate the level of depression and anxiety in adolescents with cancer, underscoring the need to carefully consider depression and anxiety as problems in this group.

Relapse and Recurrence

Patients and families who experience a relapse or recurrence of cancer can be expected to enter a second crisis period. Similar to the initial crisis of diagnosis, families experience a cognitive and emotional overload; they often are overwhelmed with fear and anxiety at the same time they are trying to understand the medical implications of the return of the cancer. Families typically feel shocked by news of a relapse. For many families, faith in their medical care, trust in the world, and hope for future treatment are severely challenged.

The initial approach to this new crisis should draw on the elements of psychosocial support described in the section on the crisis of diagnosis, including provision of psychosocial support and participation in a new treatment conference or "day one talk." In the context of a relapse, emotional distress and disbelief are to be expected, and parents, older patients, and siblings may be distraught. Presenting information about prognosis after relapse can be even more difficult, because the prognosis is typically less favorable, and patients and families who previously may have been reassured may now need to be told that cure is less likely or even not to be expected. Families need to have accurate medical information presented to them in a way they can understand, but perhaps just as important, they need to feel that the physicians and other providers are committed to continuing to care for them. For some patients and families a recurrence may be experienced as a personal failure, and the team should be careful to readdress this issue of blame and causality in the context of relapse or recurrence. In cases in which a new treatment plan means transferring care to a new clinical service (e.g., as in the case of a bone marrow transplant) or referral to a new care team or hospital, great care should be taken to ensure that patients and families do not feel abandoned.

The psychosocial challenges facing the patient and family after relapse depend to a large extent on the subsequent treatment that is planned and the extent to which cure remains the goal of treatment. When potentially curative treatment is planned, patients face the challenge of reengaging in a new and potentially more intensive therapy regimen. Patients and families already burdened by an initial treatment may have more trouble adjusting to new demands along with increased anxiety and the psychological experience of "starting over" with a new treatment. Psychosocial care providers should be prepared to reassess the patient and family in this new context and offer emotional support and crisis intervention. Psychosocial providers should also anticipate new issues that could emerge such as financial stress, parent depression, patient behavioral problems, or emotional distress and be prepared to help the family address these issues.

For some patients the likelihood of cure after relapse or recurrence is remote. For these patients, treatment options may include palliative care or experimental therapies. Learning that a cure for the cancer is unlikely and that the patient may be expected to die of his or her disease is devastating for the family. Parents and patients are likely to be terrified and overwhelmed, and care providers may feel unsure about how to help these families. Communication between the physicians and other members of the team is especially important at this juncture,[80] and care should be taken to communicate directly to patients as well as parents and to provide honest information in a sensitive manner. Psychosocial providers should participate in team meetings with the family, assess the needs of the patient, parents, and other family members, and offer crisis intervention and emotional support. They should anticipate that symptoms of depression, hopelessness, and anxiety may become significant in one or more family members and be prepared to offer clinical care and/or referrals to other specialists or community agencies. A more comprehensive discussion of care for the dying child is included in Chapter 70.

SPECIAL POPULATIONS

Adolescents

Adolescence is traditionally seen as a time of transition and growing independence. The diagnosis of cancer during this developmental stage has the potential to disrupt normal functioning and limit the attainment of specific goals that move the adolescent from childhood into adulthood. Research has considered several important areas related to the psychosocial adjustment of adolescents with cancer, including family factors, psychological factors, and socialization factors.[26,209]

Mental health professionals have noted that children and adolescents often function as well or as poorly as their parents during stressful life events. The psychological adjustment of adolescents with cancer was noted to be better when maternal distress was low[271] and maternal adjustment was high.[272] In addition adolescents benefited from the ability of family members to introduce a sense of normalcy and felt more supported during treatment when family members demonstrated flexibility.[148] Some adolescents noted that stressful family relationships impeded successful adjustment to the illness.[273] These data taken together suggest that the adolescent's family is crucial to the adolescent's successful coping and illness management. The medical team should encourage open communication between family members that will promote positive interactions and allow for the ongoing assessment of individual functioning. Psychosocial support should extend beyond the adolescent patient to all family members to ensure the healthy functioning of the entire family system. When problems in an adolescent's behavior or coping are identified, providers should be mindful that some family-focused assessment and intervention may be indicated.

Psychologically adolescents typically possess cognitive abilities that allow for a more sophisticated understanding of their illness and treatment than would be found with younger children. Adolescents often seek information[102,126] and feel empowered by their understanding, which may in turn facilitate their active participation in treatment decisions, thereby increasing their use of effective coping strategies and their overall sense of control.[25] However the ability to understand illness-related information does not guarantee increased psychological adjustment. In fact some adolescents may feel overwhelmed by extensive medical information and corresponding treatment decisions, increasing the level of stress and potential psychological maladjustment. To ensure that the adolescent is appropriately informed, a careful assessment must be conducted to evaluate how information is processed and understood by the adolescent and what amount and type of information will be most helpful. Because adolescents may feel that opportunities to achieve increased independence (e.g., attaining a driver's license) are limited as a result of their illness,

including the adolescent in treatment discussions, facilitating effective coping strategies, and encouraging participation in the decision-making process may promote an increased sense of autonomy.[274]

Socially the adolescent's ability to engage with peers, participate in extracurricular activities, or attend school while undergoing treatment is often very limited. Immediately after diagnosis, extensive support is often available to the adolescent and the adolescent's family. However, as treatment progresses and the initial shock associated with the diagnosis decreases, support from friends, teachers, and others in the community may be less consistent. With time friends may return their focus to school and other activities, leaving the diagnosed adolescent feeling isolated and left out.[126,175,209,275] Evan and Zeltzer[25] suggest that developmental level plays a significant role in the type of support that an adolescent both provides and seeks. Encouraging flexibility and support with regard to an adolescent's participation in his or her usual activities, such as attending school, attending social events, and spending time with friends, can help adolescents feel "normal" and may increase adherence to treatment.[253] Encouraging the adolescent patient to bring a friend to a clinic appointment can also be helpful to bridge the divide between peers and the medical setting for some adolescents. Research findings suggest that adolescents with cancer seek social support from same-aged peers encountering similar developmental issues[276] and from parents and other adults who have a wider range of life experiences that may be relevant to overcoming their illness.[275]

Studies have considered several factors related to the development of successful adolescent social relationships, including the importance of self-esteem and sexual identity.[26,277-282] For example, findings suggest that adolescents who are absent from school may begin to experience academic difficulties that have a negative impact on their self-confidence and self-esteem. This decrease in self-confidence and self-esteem undermines the adolescent's attempt to form and sustain social relationships. Other findings highlight sexual identity and the significant role that sexual identity plays in adolescent relationships and developing self-esteem.[26] The adolescent diagnosed with cancer may have a negative body image as a result of treatment-related adverse effects (e.g., hair loss, procedural/surgical scars, and weight gain or loss)[283-286] and more limited opportunities for both formal and informal sex education, impeding healthy sexual development and positive self-esteem.[287] Evan and colleagues[26] suggest assessing the adolescent's cognitive, social, developmental, and family functioning, both to determine the most appropriate ways to enhance sexual health and self-esteem and to recommend opportunities to assume personal control and interact with other adolescents who may be encountering similar experiences.

Social support and social relationships are essential to successful adjustment during the treatment course and beyond. Although parents and other family members typically provide the primary, day-to-day support needed by the adolescent patient to successfully complete treatment, peer relationships are equally valuable, because they allow adolescents to remain connected to other key aspects of their life that exist outside of their treatment. Members of the medical staff can also provide important interpersonal connections that can greatly improve the adolescent's social functioning. The medical team should work to understand how cancer is adversely affecting the adolescent's peer relationships and encourage peer interactions by supporting the adolescent's return to school and participation in peer-related activities when feasible. For adolescents who have been dating, cancer often interferes with their ability to develop these relationships or to maintain contact with a boyfriend or girlfriend. For the sexually active adolescent, the illness may also raise questions about whether they need to limit their sexual activities because of treatments or risks for infection. Counseling and information on contraception and prevention of sexually transmitted diseases should be provided to sexually active adolescents in keeping with recommended practices for this age group.[288,289] Because parents may not be privy to all of their adolescent child's romantic or sexual activities, it is important that providers discuss these issues with adolescents in private and provide appropriate support and information.

Neurooncology

The literature has indicated that, in general, children and adolescents treated for cancer will have a positive adjustment to treatment and that once the acute crisis of diagnosis has passed, they tend to adapt positively.[290,291] The diagnosis of a pediatric brain tumor is often more complicated given the location of the tumor, the toxicities of treatment, the possibility of long-term medical late effects, and the poor prognosis associated with many pediatric brain tumors.[292,293] Research has often indicated that patients diagnosed with central nervous system (CNS) tumors are at greater risk for psychological difficulties, neurocognitive deficits, poor functional outcomes, and decreased quality of life when compared with children treated for other cancers.[174,290,294-298] In addition disease-related fear, uncertainty, loss of control, and depression have been found to be heightened among parents of children treated for a CNS tumor when compared with parents of children who have acute lymphoblastic leukemia or acute myeloid leukemia.[294] Issues associated with diagnosis, the impact of treatment on immediate and long-term functioning, and the morbidity associated with CNS tumors are factors contributing to the increased risk for psychological distress among parents.

The terms "benign" and "malignant" are often the nomenclature by which we understand the gravity of a particular diagnosis. However in pediatric neurooncology, very little is benign. Children and adolescents die of both benign and malignant tumors. Regardless of the label, persons with both benign and malignant tumors require treatment (e.g., surgery, chemotherapy, radiation, or autologous stem-cell transplant) that comes with significant demands that can be challenging for patients and families. Parents are often in the position of consenting to a treatment that will cause significant late effects and will have a negative impact on quality of life for their child, all in the hope for a cure. The stress associated with

making this decision in the context of trying to integrate new diagnostic information, the input of family and friends, and the abundance of material on the Internet can be extremely overwhelming for parents. Many families opt to seek second opinions at other institutions, which can be helpful but also can make treatment decisions more complex. Psychosocial care providers can help parents process information, encourage additional conversations with medical providers, and facilitate coping styles that most effectively support decision making.

Given that the cancer is located in the brain, all treatment interventions come with a number of risks. An insult to the brain can have an impact on motor skills, cognition, vision, speech/language, and emotional regulation. Although some of the postoperative complications can improve, it is also possible that a patient may not return to his or her presurgical level of functioning,[299] which has significant implications for self-esteem and self-identity. Psychosocial providers working with children with brain tumors need to recognize the impact of loss, grieving related to permanent changes in functioning, despair pertaining to the need for extensive rehabilitation, and uncertainty about the future. These issues are prevalent not just for the patient but for the family as a whole. Providing the space in which a patient and family can grieve, while dealing with ongoing medical stressors, is important for future psychological adjustment. Patients may believe that they are unable to engage with peers because of their limitations; however, guidance about how to encourage participation in activities is crucial. For patients who may not be able to engage in athletics, ongoing participation on the sports team through a team manager position or scorekeeper can be instrumental in keeping patients connected to peers, bolstering self-confidence, and fostering the attainment of developmental milestones.

Although significant improvements have occurred in the survival rate for some pediatric brain tumors, some diagnoses are still associated with a very poor prognosis. The medical team is often faced with the difficult task of telling a family that their child is not likely to survive, while preserving some hope through the form of treatment options. Psychosocial care providers can serve as an important support during the meeting, provide guidance with regard to having additional family members at the meeting, and validate the challenges of making treatment decisions. Because of advancements in treatment, parents are often faced with the challenge of deciding between clinical trials, none of which has data regarding efficacy. Parents are often overwhelmed at this time while they process the news of the diagnosis, the prognosis, and the treatment options. It is crucial that psychosocial clinicians assess the parents' psychological history and current functioning to identify interventions that are required immediately to help facilitate decision making and treatments that will provide symptom relief on a long-term basis.

Hematopoietic Stem Cell Transplant

Similar to patients with CNS tumors, patients and families for whom stem-cell transplant is the recommended treatment are at increased risk for psychosocial complications during and after treatment in terms of their overall psychological adjustment.[300,301] Increased vulnerability to psychological distress and the posttraumatic symptoms described in the literature that are associated with the stem-cell transplant experience can be attributed to factors associated with treatment risks, morbidity, the stress associated with simply trying to get to the point of transplantation, restrictions and isolation, and the late effects associated with treatment.

The process of getting disease in remission or eliminating any residual disease can be an anxiety-provoking start to the challenges of transplantation. Patients and families often experience anticipatory anxiety as they await news from screening tests that will clear the patient to move forward with the transplant process. At the same time, significant stress is associated with finding an appropriate donor. Many patients have siblings who are eligible to be the donor, and although they are certainly fortunate in terms of having a good match, this process becomes complicated and plays into multiple layers of family dynamics. Sibling donors have been shown to be at risk for posttraumatic stress disorder, anxiety, and low self-esteem.[302-304] Psychosocial care providers play an important role by conducting donor evaluations that provide the medical information donors need to ensure that they understand the process. Psychosocial care providers also provide the psychological support and care required to ensure that the donor is not being coerced into the procedure and understands the possibility of both a positive and negative outcome and that neither outcome is associated with the donor process. Parents now have to worry about the emotional and medical functioning of both the sibling and the patient, leading to increased vulnerability for distress.[305]

Parents with a child who requires a bone marrow transplant are in the position of choosing a treatment that will irrevocably change the course of their child's life because of the toxicities of treatment. The adverse effects of transplantation can include hearing loss, infertility, renal failure, cardiac dysfunction, growth and gonadal failure, secondary malignancies, neurocognitive delay, and possible death. Discussion of the potential risk of death is part of the consenting process and indicates the intensity of the treatment and the potential psychological trauma that can result for both patients and parents. Indeed retrospective studies have indicated that parental distress tends to be at its highest before the actual transplant procedure.[306,307] This information is crucial in terms of determining points of intervention, given that the literature has shown that fewer maternal depression symptoms are associated with improved patient outcomes after the transplant procedure.[308] Ensuring that patients and families have been provided with appropriate medical information up front and ample opportunity to ask questions of the medical team is one way that psychosocial care providers can help empower families before the transplant procedure.[309] A thorough assessment that includes identification of significant parental psychological distress well before the start of transplant process is important to ensure that potential psychotropic

interventions have ample opportunity to take effect before the patient enters the hospital.

Given the intensity of the treatment, the extended period of hospitalization, and the potential for significant medical complications, families should be followed closely by their psychosocial care provider throughout the transplant process. Use of cognitive-behavioral interventions such as relaxation strategies and guided imagery can be helpful for both patients and caregivers. Implementation of behavioral plans that provide positive reinforcement to the patient with regard to the significant demands of treatment can be very helpful. Given the significant stress associated with transplant procedure, as well as the isolation that can occur for caregivers, parent support groups can be extremely helpful in connecting parents with others going through similar experiences, allowing for parental self-care, and providing a forum for discussion of worries and challenges. Many medical institutions also incorporate family-centered rounds or regularly scheduled family meetings to keep lines of communication open, provide an opportunity for parents to ask questions of the team, and address any logistical or systemic issues that may be negatively affecting the family's adjustment to the transplant. Keeping in close contact with medical, nursing, and child life care providers is critical to providing the best care for these families who are at significant psychosocial risk.

Once patients have completed the transplant and are discharged from the hospital, they must participate in an intensive outpatient plan that can include multiple trips to the hospital or clinic per week, use of multiple medications, and restriction in terms of social contact. Given the immunocompromised status of patients after transplantation, they are not allowed to attend school or be in an enclosed space with a lot of people. This restriction can be extremely difficult for children and adolescents who can be essentially cut off from their peers. This period is also anxiety provoking because parents are concerned about the possibility of complications, infections, and the potential for disease relapse. Parents are often on high alert with increased vigilance regarding oral intake, participation in physical/occupational/speech therapies, and/or hygiene. Adolescent patients in particular may have significant difficulty in managing a hypervigilant parent in the context of their limited control. Power struggles between patients and parents are not uncommon, and anticipatory guidance with regard to these potential challenges early in the process with a focus on prevention can be an important role for the psychosocial clinician.

With the significant limitations placed on daily functioning as a result of the intensive treatment and the very real possibility of disease relapse despite the transplant, it is understandable that patients who have undergone bone marrow transplant are at increased risk for psychological distress, both acutely and long term.[301] Clinicians should be aware that subsets of patients are more likely to experience psychological difficulties, specifically patients who are dealing with debilitating adverse effects such as graft-versus-host disease (GVHD) and its treatment. Results from the Bone Marrow Transplant Survivor Study indicated that active chronic GVHD was associated with somatic and global psychological distress.[310] In addition, the use of corticosteroids in the management of GVHD is another factor associated with depression and diminished quality of life.[311]

Despite the risks, some reports in the literature demonstrate that many survivors of bone marrow transplant have a good health-related quality of life within 12 months after the transplant procedure, particularly if they are not affected by severe adverse effects of treatment.[300,312] Parents and children may have very different perspectives on the child's progress and adaptation after transplant, making it important to include both patient and parent perspectives whenever possible.[301,313,314] Parents may experience elevations in distress during the acute phase of the transplant process, but the distress typically resolves approximately 4 to 6 months after the transplant for most parents. Nonetheless subgroups of parents exhibit distress after the transplant that is significant enough to meet the criteria for posttraumatic stress disorder or to be classified as having posttraumatic stress symptoms; families with lower socioeconomic backgrounds have been noted to be at particular risk.[315] With this in mind, clinicians should incorporate assessment of social and psychological functioning of the patient and the family into the routine follow-up of patients undergoing a transplant. Informing patients and families that ongoing psychological or social problems are not uncommon after transplant may help families be forthcoming about their functioning and help those who have significant difficulties to accept a referral for more specialized assessment and treatment.

References available online at ExpertConsult.

KEY REFERENCES

4. Patenaude AF, Kupst MJ: Psychosocial functioning in pediatric cancer. *J Pediatr Psychol* 30:9–27, 2005.
   This article describes the development of the pediatric psychooncology field and summarizes the outcomes and challenges faced during childhood cancer and survivorship. The article identifies avenues for future psychosocial research and longitudinal studies focusing on the increasing number of pediatric cancer survivors.
10. Brown RT: *Comprehensive handbook of childhood cancer and sickle cell disease: A biopsychosocial approach,* New York, 2006, Oxford University Press.
    This extensive handbook for practitioners addresses the psychosocial factors involved in caring for pediatric patients who have cancer or sickle cell disease.
13. Kazak AE, Rourke MT, Alderfer MA, et al: Evidence-based assessment, intervention and psychosocial care in pediatric oncology: a blueprint for comprehensive services across treatment. *J Pediatr Psychol* 32:1099–1110, 2007.
    This article describes the research and clinical experience at one institution (Children's Hospital of Philadelphia) and describes the institutional framework for providing psychosocial care to children and families during pediatric cancer. The experience-based combination of two models (the Pediatric Psychosocial Preventative Health Model and the Traumatic Stress Model) is used to address and support families at all levels of psychosocial need.
14. Kazak AE: Pediatric Psychosocial Preventative Health Model (PPPHM): research, practice, and collaboration in pediatric family systems medicine. *Fam Syst Health* 24:381–395, 2006.
    This article provides a three-tiered pyramidal model (universal, targeted, clinical) for categorizing families of acutely and chronically ill children at varying levels of psychosocial risk. The

Pediatric Psychosocial Preventative Health Model, in combination with evidence-based assessment tools, aims to screen for families at highest risk of psychosocial distress and guide supportive services to match their level of need in the pediatric health care system.
25. Evan EE, Zeltzer LK: Psychosocial dimensions of cancer in adolescents and young adults. *Cancer* 107:1663–1671, 2006.
    This article reviews the evidence-based literature available with regard to caring for adolescents and young adults with cancer. Factors pertinent to the psychological adjustment of adolescent and young adult patients and the clinical implications of late effects are discussed. Practical examples of empirical interventions to address psychosocial challenges for adolescent and young adult patients are presented.
43. Masera G, Spinetta JJ, Jankovic M, et al: Guidelines for a therapeutic alliance between families and staff: a report of the SIOP Working Committee on Psychosocial Issues in Pediatric Oncology. *Med Pediatr Oncol* 30:183–186, 1998.
    This document was developed by the International Society of Paediatric Oncology Working Committee on Psychosocial Issues in Pediatric Oncology. It addresses the therapeutic alliance between families and staff and the overarching goal of curing cancer while minimizing medical and psychological toxicities.
58. Mack JW, Grier HE: The day one talk. *J Clin Oncol* 22:563–566, 2004.
    This article outlines a thoughtful and sensitive approach for physicians who need to inform the family of a child's cancer diagnosis. The article provides concrete suggestions for the content and structure of the "day one" talk, emphasizing an approach that is empathic and supportive to patients and families.
64. Levi RB, Marsick R, Drotar D, et al: Diagnosis, disclosure, and informed consent: learning from parents of children with cancer. *J Pediatr Hematol Oncol* 22:3–12, 2000.
    The authors report on a retrospective study of parental perception surrounding their child's cancer diagnosis and the process of informed consent. Focus groups were conducted and themes associated with receiving the diagnosis, how to improve the informed consent process, and lack of control were discussed. Limitations were identified in parental understanding of the distinction between the treatment, research participation, and other aspects of the cancer experience.
80. Mack JW, Wolfe J, Grier HE, et al: Communication about prognosis between parents and physicians of children with cancer: parent preferences and the impact of prognostic information. *J Clin Oncol* 24:5265–5270, 2006.
    The authors of this study examined parents' preferences for prognostic information in regard to their child's cancer diagnosis. Parents were surveyed and findings indicated that the majority of parents wanted as much prognostic information as possible and wanted that information to be in numbers. Although some parents found the information distressing, they were no less likely to want the information.
104. Dolgin MJ, Phipps S, Fairclough DL, et al: Trajectories of adjustment in mothers of children with newly diagnosed cancer: a natural history investigation. *J Pediatr Psychol* 32:771–782, 2007.
     This study assessed posttraumatic stress symptoms (PTSS) in mothers of children who were diagnosed with cancer, the relationships between sociodemographic and psychosocial distress over time, and whether particular subgroups of mothers could be identified based on trajectory of adjustment. Mothers completed standardized measures at the time of diagnosis, 3 months, and 6 months. Findings indicated mildly elevated negative affectivity and PTSS at the time of diagnosis, but improvement over time. The study was able to identify subgroups of mothers who were likely to have particularly trajectories of adjustment.
105. Kazak AE, Boeving CA, Alderfer MA, et al: Posttraumatic stress symptoms during treatment in parents of children with cancer. *J Clin Oncol* 23:7405–7410, 2005.
     This study examined posttraumatic stress symptoms (PTSS) in mothers and fathers of children receiving treatment for cancer and in relation to treatment variables. Parents completed questionnaires and data were obtained from oncologists regarding treatment intensity. With the exception of one parent, all participants reported PTSS. In families in which both parents participated in the study, 80% had at least one parent report moderate to severe

PTSS. *Treatment-related variables were minimally associated with PTSS.*

117. Chen E, Craske MG, Katz ER, et al: Pain-sensitive temperament: does it predict procedural distress and response to psychological treatment among children with cancer? *J Pediatr Psychol* 25:269–278, 2000.

    This intervention study examined pain sensitivity and distress in children undergoing lumbar punctures (LPs). Baseline data were gathered on pain sensitivity, and then children were randomized into the psychological intervention arm or control group. Findings demonstrated that children who reported high pain sensitivity had higher levels of anxiety and pain prior to and during the LP. Children who had higher pain sensitivity and who received the intervention had significant decreases in distress with time, whereas children with high pain sensitivity who did not receive the intervention reported elevated LP distress with time.

130. Sourkes BM: *Armfuls of time: the psychological experience of the child with a life-threatening illness,* Pittsburgh, 1995, University of Pittsburgh Press.

    This seminal work on the emotional experience of the ill child provides clinical material that highlights the value and importance of a multidisciplinary approach. Using play therapy vignettes and stories from patients and their families, a rich description is provided of the challenges faced when experiencing a life-threatening disease and the interventions that can provide support around the issues of diagnosis, treatment, and loss.

154. Houtzager BA, Oort FJ, Hoekstra-Weebers JE, et al: Coping and family functioning predict longitudinal psychological adaptation of siblings of childhood cancer patients. *J Pediatr Psychol* 29:591–605, 2004.

    This study examined the relationships between coping and family functioning in siblings of children with cancer. Assessments were conducted at four time points across 2 years since the cancer diagnosis. Findings indicated that at initial assessment (1 month after the diagnosis), psychological adjustment was impaired, but that it normalized over time. Optimism and having the sibling involved were noted as protective factors. Sibling age, gender, and coping style were noted to help identify at-risk siblings.

172. Zebrack B, Bleyer A, Albritton K, et al: Assessing the health care needs of adolescent and young adult cancer patients and survivors. *Cancer* 107:2915–2923, 2006.

    In response to the literature demonstrating that adolescent and young adult (AYA) patients have not had improvement in cancer outcomes compared with other populations, this study sought to identify the health and supportive care needs of AYA patients and survivors. Findings from surveys of medical providers and young adults survivors indicated agreement in a number of areas of importance across health care professionals and AYA survivors. However the importance of meeting same-aged peers with cancer was rated significantly higher for AYA survivors. This study identified areas in which resources could be useful in potentially changing the gap in cancer outcomes between the population as a whole and AYA patients.

174. Vannatta K, Gartstein MA, Short A, et al: A controlled study of peer relationships of children surviving brain tumors: teacher, peer, and self ratings. *J Pediatr Psychol* 23:279–287, 1998.

    This original research evaluated the behavioral reputation and acceptance of pediatric brain tumor survivors. Children (ages 8 to 18 years) were compared with nonchronically ill peers and data were gathered from peers, teachers, and patients. In comparison with same-aged classmates, children diagnosed with brain tumors were reported to be more socially isolated and received fewer friendship nominations. Issues associated with fatigue and school absence were reported. This article represents the initial work that highlighted the significant social struggles experienced by pediatric brain tumor survivors.

198. Zeltzer LK, Dolgin MJ, LeBaron S, et al: A randomized, controlled study of behavioral intervention for chemotherapy distress in children with cancer. *Pediatrics* 88:34–42, 1991.

    This article reports on a prospective trial comparing hypnotherapy for reduction of chemotherapy-related distress with distraction/relaxation therapy and an attention control condition. Hypnotherapy was found to be superior to other conditions, with the results discussed in the context of complex interactions between biologic and psychological factors contributing to nausea and related adverse effects of chemotherapy.

210. Zebrack BJ, Gurney JG, Oeffinger K, et al: Psychological outcomes in long-term survivors of childhood brain cancer: a report from the childhood cancer survivor study. *J Clin Oncol* 22:999–1006, 2004.

    This study evaluated the psychological outcomes of the pediatric neurooncology participants in the Childhood Cancer Survivor Study. Data for survivors and siblings were utilized and levels of psychological distress were consistent with reports in the general population. Survivors reported high levels of distress and depressive symptoms compared with siblings. Higher distress was associated with female gender, low household income, lower educational attainment, unemployment, poor health, and not being married. This study indicates that although treatment for pediatric brain tumors may not be associated with higher distress than the general population, the social difficulties experienced by survivors may be what puts them at greater risk for psychological challenges.

215. Spinetta JJ, Jankovic M, Eden T, et al: Guidelines for assistance to siblings of children with cancer: report of the SIOP Working Committee on Psychosocial Issues in Pediatric Oncology. *Med Pediatr Oncol* 33:395–398, 1999.

    This document establishes a framework for the psychosocial care of siblings in pediatric oncology as developed by the International Society of Paediatric Oncology Working Committee on Psychosocial Issues in Pediatric Oncology, instituted in 1991. It outlines the general principles for helping siblings throughout various phases of treatment, including relapse, palliation, and death.

216. Sloper P: Predictors of distress in parents of children with cancer: a prospective study. *J Pediatr Psychol* 25:79–91, 2000.

    This study investigated parental psychological distress in both mothers and fathers of children with cancer at 6 and 18 months after diagnosis. Relationships between illness, illness appraisal, resources, and coping were examined. Findings demonstrated elevated levels of distress for both mothers and fathers that were consistent with time. Internal factors such as appraisal and coping were associated with maternal distress, whereas external factors such as employment issues and the number of hospital admissions were associated with paternal distress. This article highlights the importance of identifying at-risk parents so appropriate supports can be put into place early during the treatment process.

253. Butow P, Palmer S, Pai A, et al: Review of adherence-related issues in adolescents and young adults with cancer. *J Clin Oncol* 28:4800–4809, 2010.

    This review article examines studies that investigated medication adherence in the adolescent and young adult (AYA) oncology population between the years 1980–2008. Lack of adherence has been associated with higher risk of relapse, more adverse effects, and poor outcomes. The review highlighted the methodologic issues found in the AYA adherence literature, including a lack of clarity around defining the AYA age range and a lack of representation of oncologic diagnoses beyond leukemia and lymphoma. Reported rates of nonadherence range are broad, from 27% to 60%. Consistent predictors of adherence include openness of family relationships and support.

254. Bhatia S, Landier W, Shangguan M, et al: Nonadherence to oral mercaptopurine and risk of relapse in Hispanic and non-Hispanic white children with acute lymphoblastic leukemia: a report from the Children's Oncology Group. *J Clin Oncol* 30:2094–2101, 2012.

    This original research report describes a prospective study of the prevalence and impact of nonadherence with oral mercaptopurine in a cohort of 327 patients treated for acute lymphoblastic leukemia. Using a medication event-monitoring system, findings show that nonadherence is associated with relapse of disease, ethnicity, and patient age.

283. Pendley JS, Dahlquist LM, Dreyer Z: Body image and psychosocial adjustment in adolescent cancer survivors. *J Pediatr Psychol* 22:29–43, 1997.

    This study evaluated body image and social adjustment in adolescent cancer survivors and healthy peers. Participants completed questionnaires and a videotaped interview. Raters who were blind to medical history rated the attractiveness of the participants.

Survivors reported being less involved in social activities compared with the comparison group. Survivors who had been off treatment for a longer period reported lower self-worth, higher social anxiety, and more negative body image. Despite the self-report around these difficulties, these long-term survivors were not rated as less attractive by observers. This article provides evidence that psychological adjustment issues and body image difficulties may not fully emerge until well after treatment completion.

290. Zeltzer LK, Recklitis C, Buchbinder D, et al: Psychological status in childhood cancer survivors: a report from the Childhood Cancer Survivor Study. *J Clin Oncol* 27:2396–2404, 2009.

     This article reviews findings from the Childhood Cancer Survivor Study regarding psychosocial adjustment, health-related quality of life (HRQOL), and life satisfaction. Comparisons are made between siblings and survivors and to normative data when available. Overall most survivors are psychologically healthy and report satisfaction with their lives; a significant proportion of survivors report more symptoms of psychological distress and poorer physical HRQOL. Risk factors for psychological distress and poor HRQOL are brain tumor diagnosis, female sex, lower educational attainment, unmarried status, presence of a major medical condition, and treatment with cranial radiation and/or surgery. Psychological distress also predicted poor health behaviors, including smoking, alcohol use, fatigue, and altered sleep.

310. Sun CL, Francisco L, Baker KS, et al: Adverse psychological outcomes in long-term survivors of hematopoietic cell transplantation: a report from the Bone Marrow Transplant Survivor Study (BMTSS). *Blood* 118:4723–4731, 2011.

     The authors report on a large cohort study of survivors of hematopoietic cell transplantation. Psychological outcomes were assessed in bone marrow transplant (BMT) survivors and sibling control subjects. Survivors of BMT reported significantly higher levels of psychological distress than did their siblings, with those who had been exposed to prednisone reporting global distress across somatization, anxiety, and depression scales. High levels of somatization were reported, particularly for patients with graft-versus-host disease.

312. Parsons SK, Phipps S, Sung L, et al: NCI, NHLBI/PBMTC First International Conference on Late Effects after Pediatric Hematopoietic Cell Transplantation: health-related quality of life, functional, and neurocognitive outcomes. *Biol Blood Marrow Transplant* 18:162–171, 2012.

     The authors of this article review the late effects in survivors of pediatric hematopoietic stem cell transplantation in the domains of health-related quality of life, physical function, and neurocognitive function.

314. Jobe-Shields L, Alderfer MA, Barrera M, et al: Parental depression and family environment predict distress in children before stem cell transplantation. *J Dev Behav Pediatr* 30:140–146, 2009.

     This study examined the factors of parental and family environment variables in relation to the severity of distress in children slated to receive a stem cell/bone marrow transplant. Parental depression, family cohesion, and expressiveness were found to predict child distress, and parental depression, when high, was associated with elevated child distress regardless of family environment. This study provides evidence that parental psychological functioning prior to transplant is a predictor of child psychological adjustment.

CHAPTER 74

Ethical Considerations in Pediatric Oncology Clinical Trials

Raymond Barfield, Philip M. Rosoff, and Eric Kodish

CHAPTER OUTLINE

HISTORIC PERSPECTIVE

WHAT IS "CONSENT" IN PEDIATRICS?

ASSENT IN CHILDHOOD CANCER TRIALS

PEDIATRIC CLINICAL TRIALS

Minimal Risk

Phase I and II Trials in Pediatric Oncology

Phase III Trials and Clinical Equipoise

SPECIAL CONSIDERATIONS FOR CANCER TRIALS
USING ALLOGENEIC HEMATOPOIETIC STEM
CELL TRANSPLANTATION

MODELS AND TOOLS FOR ETHICAL DECISION
MAKING IN PEDIATRIC CLINICAL TRIALS

FURTHER CHALLENGES IN PEDIATRIC CLINICAL
ONCOLOGY TRIALS

Bioinformatics and Genomics

Globalization

CONCLUSION

Ethical decision making is a fundamental goal common to both clinical medicine and clinical research trials of all types. Broad attempts have long been made to thoroughly explicate the elements of ethical decision making that are common to both settings. However this goal has been pursued with increased vigor since the exposure of human moral abuses in the United States Public Health Service–sponsored Tuskegee Syphilis Study and by the Nuremberg trials and President Clinton's Advisory Committee on Human Radiation Experiments. The practical yield has been the production of highly influential documents such as the Belmont Report, the Declaration of Helsinki and its several versions, guidelines produced for the International Arena by the Council for International Organizations of Medical Sciences, and most recently, the adoption of the Universal Declaration of Bioethics and Human Rights in October 2005 by the United Nations Educational, Scientific, and Cultural Organization. Common to these efforts are principles such as respect for persons, beneficence, and justice. Table 74-1 lists selected guidelines for research ethics. But how do general principles translate into practical action that is ethically sound for the practitioner faced with a particular clinical situation, for the clinical research physician considering whether to offer a phase I trial to a patient, and for the investigator whose nontherapeutic trials pose some risks?

The issues become considerably more complex when the patient or research participant is a child and the decision maker is not the person facing the possibility of risk or benefit. This issue poses special challenges in both pediatric clinical medicine and pediatric clinical research. The challenges are made more acute by the fact that they are not static. The considerations change as a child grows in age and experience and as we move from standard-of-care therapy to clinical trials, which, as recently argued, involve the standard of care for future children, the results of which have been a remarkable success story.[1,2,3] Indeed it may be that survival percentages for adolescents and young adults with "pediatric" cancers have lagged behind those of younger patients in part because of their lower rates of participation in clinical trials.[4] Further the issues do not remain static across all types of clinical trials.[5] A child enrolled in a phase III clinical trial for newly diagnosed, standard-risk leukemia faces a situation very different from that of a child who has had multiple relapses of leukemia and whose family must choose between a phase I trial and a Make-A-Wish trip to the Grand Canyon.

This chapter begins with a brief historic review of the unique issues in pediatric medicine and pediatric clinical trials. It then moves to issues of parental permission and assent—issues that draw on, but are not fully informed by, the many studies of informed consent in adults. The differences in language and approach required as patients progress from phase III trials to phase I trials and palliative care are examined. After these more general issues, we will consider more specific questions, such as those raised by autopsy, stem cell transplantation, advances in

TABLE 74-1   Selected Guidelines on Ethics of Biomedical Research with Human Subjects

Guideline	Source	Year and Revisions
Nuremberg Code	Fundamental; Nuremberg Military Tribunal decision in *United States v Brandt*	1947
Declaration of Helsinki	World Medical Association	1964, 1975, 1983, 1989, 1996
Belmont Report	National Commission for the Protection of Human Subjects of Biomedical and Behavioral Research	1979
International Ethical Guidelines for Biomedical Research Involving Human Subjects	Council for International Organizations of Medical Sciences in collaboration with World Health Organization	Proposed in 1982; revised, 1993
45 CFR 46, Common Rule	Other: U.S. DHHS and other federal agencies	DHHS guidelines in 1981; Common Rule, 1991
Guidelines for Good Clinical Practice Trials on Pharmaceutical Products	World Health Organization	1995
Good Clinical Practice: Consolidated Guidance	International Conference on Harmonisation of Technical Requirements for Registration of Pharmaceuticals for Human Use	1996
Convention of Human Rights and Biomedicine	Council of Europe	1997
Guidelines and Recommendations for European Ethics Committees	European Forum for Good Clinical Practice	1997
Medical Research Council Guidelines for Good Clinical Practice in Clinical Trials	Medical Research Council, United Kingdom	1998
Guidelines for the Conduct of Health Research Involving Human Subjects in Uganda	Uganda National Council for Science and Technology	1998
Ethical Conduct for Research Involving Humans	Tri-Council Working Group, Canada	1998
National Statement on Ethical Conduct in Research Involving Humans	National Health and Medical Research Council, Australia	1999

From Emanuel EJ, Wendler D, Grady C. What makes clinical research ethical? JAMA 283:2701–2711, 2000.
CFR, Code of Federal Regulations; DHHS, Department of Health and Human Services.

technology, conflict of interest, insurance, ethics consultation, and international bioethics.

HISTORIC PERSPECTIVE

For hundreds of years, medical research has involved children as subjects.[6] Edward Jenner first used an experimental smallpox vaccine on his own 1-year-old son at the end of the eighteenth century. At the end of the nineteenth century, a 9-year-old child was the first human recipient of Louis Pasteur's rabies vaccine.[7] However it was not until the first half of the twentieth century that regulations governing such experimental therapy began to be established and the importance of consent and parental permission became clearer.

The informed consent of human research subjects was first officially advocated in the Nuremberg Code, a code of ethics that grew out of the trial of German physicians who conducted egregious human experiments in Nazi concentration camps during World War II. However because this important code emphasized the absolute requirement of informed consent, it implicitly excluded children—who cannot give informed consent—from participating in research on human subjects.[8]

The issue was more explicitly addressed in 1964, when the World Medical Association adopted a set of research ethics principles now known as the Declaration of Helsinki.[9,10] This set of principles established the priority of the human subjects' interests over those of science and society, and it sanctioned the participation of children in research if permission was given by the child's responsible guardian.

Interestingly experiments were performed on children after the publication of the Nuremberg Code, which implicitly excluded children from research, and before the Declaration of Helsinki, which explicitly allowed such research under specific conditions. One of the most important of these experiments was a series of radiation exposure experiments. Among participating institutions was the Fernald School in Framingham, Massachusetts and the Massachusetts Institute of Technology with funding from the Quaker Oats Company, in which children deemed mentally retarded were fed radioactive iron and calcium in their cereal.[11] President Clinton's Advisory

Committee on Human Radiation Experiments revealed the ethical consequences of inadequate parental permission in these experiments.[12]

Another important set of experiments on children at that time occurred at the Willowbrook institution (located on New York's Staten Island) and was designed to follow the natural history of hepatitis in children deemed mentally retarded.[13,14] Newly arrived children were infected with hepatitis virus by housing them with others already known to be infected. Participating children were kept in a special unit with better conditions and nutrition, and children whose parents agreed to participation were admitted more rapidly. The lead investigator did require a thorough consent process that included a 2-week waiting period for full deliberation. However because Willowbrook was so crowded, critics subsequently argued that the expedited admission and special treatment amounted to coercion. These two cases underscored the need for ethical review and oversight of human subjects research involving children, even when parental permission is obtained.

The United States Congress became increasingly concerned about research ethics during the early 1970s, in part because of the syphilis study involving poor black men conducted by the U.S. Public Health Service at the Tuskegee Institute. As a result the National Commission for the Protection of Research Subjects of Biomedical and Behavioral Research was formed, and it published the Belmont Report in 1979.[15] This report embraced three principles that are now familiar and accepted as crucial for research involving human subjects: respect for persons, beneficence, and justice. The principle of beneficence acknowledges the Hippocratic maxim "do no harm" and extends it to include maximizing the possible benefits and minimizing the possible harms to research subjects (minimizing harms is often formulated separately as a fourth principle, nonmaleficence).[16] The principle of beneficence is operative in any discussion weighing the risks and benefits of research on human subjects, especially when the subject is a minor. The principle of justice concerns the right and fair distribution of the benefits of research, as well as the burdens, an issue that has a particular urgency when clinical treatment and research are considered globally. The concept of respect for persons includes two principles: that individuals be treated as autonomous agents and that those with less autonomy are entitled to protection. The latter principle is especially relevant in pediatrics and is somewhat fluid in its definition because of the growing autonomy of pediatric patients as they approach adulthood.

Given the past abuse of research subjects who were harmed in studies that they did not understand and for which they had not given meaningful permission, it is understandable that "informed consent" has become the dominant concept in discussion about ethical research on human subjects. However recent arguments have been put forth that informed consent is not always necessary for ethical clinical research, nor is it sufficient to qualify research as ethical. A recent review of major codes and declarations relating to research with human subjects led to the proposal that there be seven requirements for ethical clinical research.[17-20] The research must lead to enhancement of health or knowledge. It must be methodologically rigorous. Selection of study sites and of individual subjects should be determined by scientific objectives and the potential for and distribution of risks and benefits. Given standard clinical practice and the research protocol, risks should be minimized, the potential for benefits should be enhanced, and risks must be outweighed by potential benefits to individuals and knowledge for society. Individuals should be informed about the research and provide voluntary consent. Research subjects should have their privacy protected, have the opportunity to withdraw, and have their well-being monitored. These requirements are thorough and persuasive, but they still must be adapted to the conditions under which the research is conducted. Factors of health, economy, culture, religion, and technology will affect how these requirements are translated into concrete, ethical action. For this reason, the specific context in which the research is conducted will affect ethical deliberation.

Ethical decision making in therapeutic and research efforts for children comprises all of the previously discussed considerations, plus the profoundly salient fact that the recipient of the risk or benefit is not the person who makes the decisions. The minor may not be capable of assimilating sufficient information to meaningfully participate in an "informed choice." One need not enter the arena of international bioethics to find challenges to the role of "autonomy" in ethical decision making: such challenges are the daily fare in pediatric medicine and research, because children's "autonomy" is an issue that changes from day to day.

WHAT IS "CONSENT" IN PEDIATRICS?

The Nuremberg Code provides one starting point for understanding the meaning and importance of informed consent. The statement in this code that "the voluntary consent of human subjects is absolutely essential" has been interpreted as legal capacity, a power of free choice based on knowledge and comprehension.[21] Consent, which was once seen as a single event, has come to be understood to be more of a process.[22] It is not surprising, with the development of guidelines and goals for consent, that the process has become more intentional and more highly scrutinized.

The dominant theoretical framework for morally valid informed consent requires that four criteria be met: disclosure, understanding, voluntariness, and competence. Briefly, the core set of information that must be *disclosed* includes (1) facts (such as risks, benefits and alternatives) that patients (subjects) and providers believe are relevant to the decision, (2) the recommendation of the professional, and (3) the purpose, nature, and limitations of consent. *Understanding* goes beyond disclosure because, although the elements disclosed can be objectively stated, true understanding involves many variables and is more difficult to assess. Establishing and documenting understanding remains a great challenge, because information that has been disclosed but not understood contributes little to the ideal paradigm of informed consent.

Voluntariness—another complex notion susceptible to interpretation—means at least that a decision is made without constraints of coercion or manipulation. Finally, *competence*, which is conventionally understood as the ability to perform a task, has also become a complex concept the definitions of which derive from law, psychiatry, and philosophy. At base a person's competence (or perhaps more accurately expressed as cognitive capacity) to make a particular decision relates to the person's ability to understand and think rationally about available choices, to weigh the benefits and burdens and risks within the context of his or her life and values, and then to use that understanding and logic to make a rational decision.

In the context of complex pediatric medical therapy or research, the process of consent is influenced by the fact that parents are making high-stakes decisions on behalf of their own child. The Children's Cancer Group (CCG) conducted studies that showed that a sense of pressure is perceived by parents when making the consent decision for intervention in the context of childhood cancer.[23] However a more recent study indicated that despite significant dissatisfaction with the consent process among CCG clinician-investigators, most parents were satisfied with it.[24] The same study indicated that the parents' satisfaction did not constitute adequate informed consent.

Even among clinicians assessment of the process of informed consent varies. The experience of the clinician is relevant in this assessment. Simon et al.[25] found that clinicians with 10 or fewer years of experience were more likely to say that the most important goal of informed consent is to explain the disease and treatment and were more likely to suggest to parents that other children might benefit from the research. The same study found that in the end, when reports from clinicians and parents are compared, clinicians are dissatisfied with aspects of consent that parents seem far more satisfied with. For example, clinicians expressed concern about information overload and about the fact that the consent discussion often occurs while the parents are still in a state of shock about the diagnosis.

Further insights into this difference have been gained from a number of studies addressing the perspectives of parents of children with cancer. One such study used three focus groups of parents of children with cancer to retrospectively examine their perceptions of the informed consent process.[26] High levels of stress were consistently reported, which were attributed to efforts to cope with multiple demands, including assimilating their child's diagnosis, nurturing and supporting the child, understanding the information given to them about the diagnosis and treatment, getting to know an entirely new group of people involved in the child's care, and participating in the child's treatment. Another important point was that the parents did not consistently distinguish research from their child's medical treatment. This finding underscores the importance of clearly explaining that research is optional during the process of "informing." If no distinction is made between research and treatment, the goal of informing has not been met. Physician-investigators often experience tension between their role

as the patient's physician and their role as a researcher offering participation in a clinical trial designed to contribute to generalizable knowledge. This tension suggests that someone besides the physician-investigator should conduct the consent process. The study also suggested that the nature of clinical research, as well as the difference between research and proven current therapy, might be difficult for parents to grasp.

These conclusions were supported by a second study in which parents of children with newly diagnosed cancer were interviewed.[27] All of the participants recalled the diagnosis, and most (80%) recalled survival statistics. However only slightly more than half knew that the treatment protocol involved research and understood the concept of randomization. This finding is striking when coupled with the fact that three fourths of the parents thought that alternatives to enrollment in a randomized protocol had been insufficiently discussed. Because randomization is such an important tool for answering certain clinical questions, this finding suggests that greater emphasis be placed on explaining unfamiliar concepts during the process of "informing." Again, in this study, the majority of participants were satisfied with the consent process.

A study by Kodish and colleagues[28] confirmed the difficulty of effectively conveying the meaning of randomization during the consent process in pediatric leukemia trials. In this multisite study, informed consent conferences were observed and audiotaped and were then compared with information acquired in interviews with parents shortly after the conference. The investigators found that although randomization was explained in 83% of cases, 50% of the parents did not understand it. Further, parents who did not understand randomization were more likely to consent to the randomized study than did those who did understand it, although this difference was not statistically significant ($P = .07$). These findings led to several recommendations for improving understanding, including a clear explanation of the differences between the randomized trial and off-study therapy, assessment of parental understanding of randomization, and further explanation when the idea was not yet grasped.

Other efforts have been made to improve the process of informed consent in pediatrics, especially in the case of complex clinical trials. For example, a study by the Children's Oncology Group (COG) assessed the possibility of staged consent; investigators had the option of obtaining consent over a 28-day period using a staged approach.[29] This option allowed parents and patients more time to discuss and absorb facts about the disease, the purpose of the trial, the design of the study, and the potential risks. Several measures in this study suggested benefit from the staged approach. There was greater understanding of treatment choices and of the distinction between a randomized controlled trial and standard therapy with the staged approach (80% understanding) than in the other studies (62.5%, $P = .05$).

Contemporary medicine will require the introduction of new methods of informing patients and parents to meet the ethical imperative of informed consent in pediatric trials. Informed consent documents for cancer

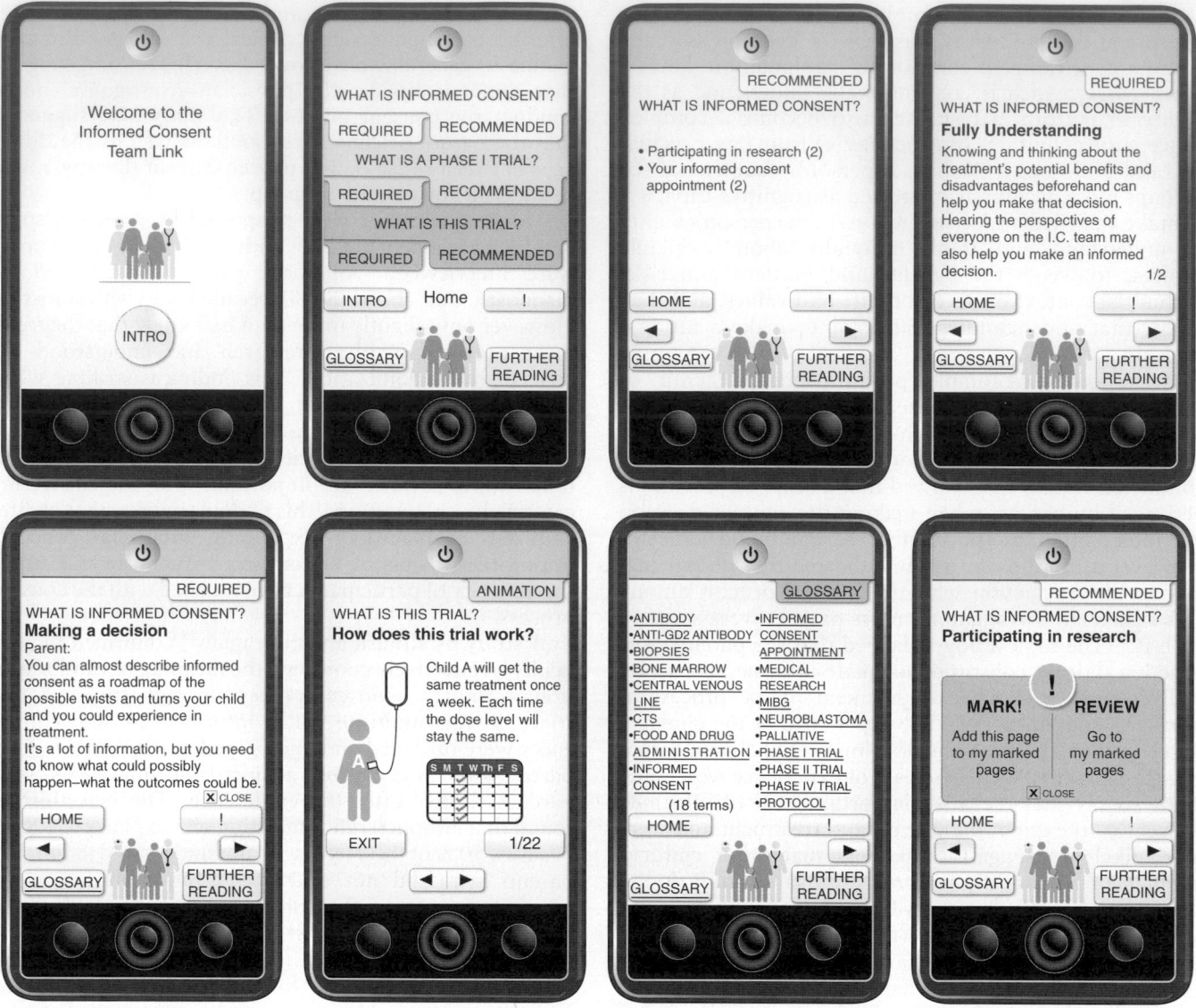

Figure 74-1 The Informed Consent Team Link, a prototype device to augment the process of informed consent in phase I trials. This device was developed through multidisciplinary user-centered research and design. The aim of such efforts is to use technological and educational advances to address the widening gap between the average capacity to understand concepts and the advances in medical technology and research.

clinical trials are sometimes long and difficult to understand, with language that serves less to protect human subjects than to decrease institutional liability.[30] Therefore some advances may take the form of technologic and educational methods to explain ever more complex medicine and research to people not formally trained in a medical discipline. One such example is a device known as the Informed Consent Team Link (Fig. 74-1). This device was designed to help families understand phase I trials, which present daunting challenges to fully informed consent. The design was based on information from focus groups of parents, physicians, nonphysician health care workers, and teenaged patients. Among the elements considered important were (1) the need for a "big picture" overview that would create a context for details, (2) delivery of information in small chunks, (3) use of multiple modes of information delivery, and (4) prioritization of information. Such basic observations provided a basis

for the design of a device that uses interactive technology, voice, animation, and health education principles to deliver information about phase I trials. Because of children's apparently natural affinity for interactive electronic devices, this approach may be helpful in addressing assent as well.

Concepts about the nature of consent in pediatrics are evolving with changes in contemporary medicine. For example some persons argue that informed consent may be too restrictive a concept and that "valid consent" should be substituted.[31] The three aspects of valid consent are personal competence (Does the patient have the capacity to make the decision?), procedural competence (Is the consent given correctly?), and material competence (Is the procedure consented to appropriate for valid consent?). The concept of valid consent has been explored in the pediatric context by the Society for Industrial and Organizational Psychology Working Committee on

Psychosocial Issues in Pediatric Oncology.[32] The value of this notion, they suggest, is that it emphasizes the patients' or parents' understanding of what is being consented to and recognizes that there are both rational and nonrational aspects to the decision-making process that must be understood. The underlying concern is that informed consent has come to mean legally signed documentation rather than real understanding, insofar as that is possible. Because parents come from different backgrounds and because children of different ages differ in their ability to grasp complex concepts, the level of understanding that is attainable may vary from situation to situation. The notion of valid consent acknowledges this fact and counters the idea that a signed document is equivalent to informed consent.

The four elements of informed consent previously mentioned—disclosure, understanding, voluntariness, and competence—are useful for informed consent in adults, but informed consent in pediatrics is complicated by the fact that three parties are involved (parent, child, and clinician/investigator) and that the research subject is the child. In pediatrics, it is not autonomy (the basis of the four components of consent) that takes precedence but rather the best interest of the child.[33] The best-interests notion is clearer in a purely clinical setting than in a research setting, in which interventions are designed to contribute to general knowledge. Despite the difficulty of approximating truly informed consent in the setting of pediatrics, and especially pediatric research, the obligation to advance pediatric medicine lends urgency to continued efforts to offer the closest possible approximation to informed consent.

One important aspect of the difference between informed consent in adult and pediatric medicine and research is the fact that in pediatrics, informed consent is better thought of as a combination of parental permission and (as appropriate) the more complex concept of the assent of the child.

ASSENT IN CHILDHOOD CANCER TRIALS

The ethics of assent is one of the most difficult issues faced in pediatric clinical trials. Many adolescents, and even some younger children, possess the elements of competence or health care decision-making capacity (setting aside for the moment the legal definitions, which hinge on age rather than capacity). This is especially true, perhaps, of children who are exposed to long-term clinical trials and to the environment of a children's hospital for long periods. Certainly younger children are not developmentally capable of comprehending complex protocols, but they do have some level of understanding that increases with age and experience.[34] How should assent be understood and when should it be required? But first, what do we actually mean by "assent" and how can it be distinguished from consent?

Consent refers to an active affirmative agreement to something by an autonomous agent (i.e., a person). It is capable of being given by anyone who meets the minimal criteria of being in the state of mind and body to be an autonomous agent; generally, most adults would qualify

as long as they were not placed in a situation in which their decisions might be suspected to be the result of some form of coercion. The ability to give consent is also context and subject dependent in the sense that most people are generally not competent in all spheres of their lives: for instance, many persons who are perfectly capable to make health care decisions or even agree to participate in research may not be competent to make (informed) decisions about automobile repair. For the purposes of this discussion, the relevant area in which cognitive capacity is important is in the domain of health care (and associated human subjects research). In the United States the legal age of consent is 18 years for most realms (nearly all jurisdictions, however, permit older adolescents who have not yet reached the age of 18 years to make some types of health care decisions [i.e., give consent], usually in regard to reproductive medical issues).[35] Assent is a more complex concept; in general it describes a less active form of agreement to a proposed procedure or action, rather than the more active and involved consent. It is used in an attempt to engage children and adolescents in the process of consent that must be given by parents or other authorized surrogate decision makers.[36,37] However what may qualify as acceptable assent (a grudging or sullen nod of the head or a more energetic and participatory form of positive interaction) remains an area of reasonable concern.

Far less is known about assent than about consent. Much remains to be learned about the practices of institutional review boards (IRBs), the perceptions of parents, clinicians, and children about consent, and the methods that might be most effective in the process of assent. Several studies have looked into these issues and documented the need for further work to address variability in IRB practices and the implementation of assent. One study found that half of IRBs have a method they require investigators to follow when determining which children are capable of assent, whereas half have no such method, and the majority of IRBs rely on investigators' judgment.[38] IRBs need guidance on the implementation of requirements regarding assent. Authors of a second study compared standards for assent, as well as consent forms approved by 55 local IRBs, when reviewing three standardized multicenter research protocols.[39] Standards varied widely; 35 had separate forms and simplified language for assent, and 31 specified lower age ranges for obtaining assent in three studies. For a hypertension study, the age at which assent was required ranged from 6 to 15 years;, for a pain study, the age range was 6 to 12 years; and for a respiratory failure study, the range was 7 to 12 years. It is not clear why some IRBs consider a child of 6 years to be capable of assent while others do not require assent until a child is 15 years old.

Do the regulations help us understand assent? Most research on children is governed by subpart D of 45 Code of Federal Regulations (CFR) 46, which provides additional protections for children (as vulnerable subjects) beyond those specified in subpart A of 45 CFR 46. Subpart D, added in 1983, outlines three categories of research that a local IRB can approve: research not

TABLE 74-2   Categories of Pediatric Research and Requirements for Institutional Review Board Approval

Level of Risk	PROSPECT OF DIRECT BENEFIT	
	No	**Yes**
Minimal risk	Approval by IRB permitted (46.404), conditioned on: • Permission from one parent or guardian • Assent of child, unless waived on capacity grounds	
Greater than minimal risk	Approval by IRB permitted (46.406), conditioned on: • Minor increase over minimal risk • Research involves experiences commensurate with those inherent in children's actual or expected medical, dental, psychological, social, or educational circumstances • Intervention or procedure is likely to yield generalizable knowledge about the subject's disorder or condition that is of vital importance for understanding or ameliorating that condition or disorder • Permission from both parents, if reasonably available • Assent of child, unless waived on capacity grounds	Approval by IRB permitted (46.405), conditioned on: • Risks are justified by anticipated benefit to subjects • Relation of anticipated benefit to risk is at least as favorable as that presented by available alternatives • Permission from one parent or guardian • Assent of child, unless waived on capacity grounds or grounds of prospect of direct benefit that "is available only in the context of the research"
Not otherwise approvable, but presents the opportunity to understand, prevent, or alleviate a serious problem affecting the health or welfare of children	Approval requires U.S. Department of Health and Human Services approval after consultation with an expert panel and opportunity for public review and comments (46.407), conditioned on: • Research presents reasonable opportunity to further understanding, prevention, or alleviation of a serious problem affecting health or welfare of children • Permission from both parents, if reasonably available • Assent of child, unless waived on capacity grounds	

From Joffe S, Fernandez CV, Pentz RD, et al: Involving children with cancer in decision-making about research participation. J Pediatr 149:862–868, 2006.

involving greater than minimal risk to participants (45 CFR 46.404), research involving greater than minimal risk but with the prospect of direct benefit to individual participants (45 CFR 46.405), and research involving no greater than a minor increase over minimal risk (with no prospect of direct benefit) but likely to provide generalizable knowledge of the subject's condition or disorder that is vital to understanding or ameliorating it (45 CFR 46.406; Table 74-2).[40] Local IRBs cannot approve research that does not fall into one of these categories, and performance of the research is possible only if two conditions are met: (1) the local IRB finds that the research provides a reasonable opportunity to further the understanding, prevention, or alleviation of a serious problem affecting the health and welfare of children, and (2) the protocol is approved by the Secretary of Health and Human Services, after soliciting the opinions of an expert panel and providing for a period of public comment (45 CFR 46.407). According to these regulations governing research on children, assent means "a child's voluntary affirmative agreement to participate in research. Mere failure to object should not, absent affirmative agreement, be construed as assent" (45 CFR 46.402). If the IRB determines that the participants in certain categories of age and maturity are capable of providing assent, investigators must obtain it to proceed. When assent is required, a child's refusal is generally binding.

Can an IRB waive the requirement for assent? Yes, but only if (1) the intervention or procedure offers the possibility of direct benefit that is important to the health or well-being of the child and this intervention or procedure is only available in the research context (45 CFR 46.408[a]) or (2) the IRB determines that children below a certain age in a certain situation or with a certain condition have such a limited capacity to participate in the decision that they cannot reasonably be consulted.

The requirements are difficult to apply, especially in the context of clinical trials for childhood cancer. Most of the children are enrolled in research studies in which the therapy is prolonged and carried out in the context of profound physical, spiritual, and psychological stress. The Bioethics Committee of the COG convened an international multidisciplinary task force to address assent in 2003. This group identified a number of problems with the regulatory framework.[41] In brief the regulations do not take adequate account of the dynamic moral and cognitive development of children and thus allow a child either to have no formal role in decision making or to have the power of veto. Nor do the guidelines make clear what constitutes meaningful assent, and so they leave IRBs and investigators with uncertainty about when they have or have not hit the mark (although other groups have provided guidance in this area).[42,43] The regulations do not take into account the fact that some clinical research is more complex than other research, and thus some research may be more accessible to the understanding of children than other research. The regulations say that permission from the guardians and assent from the child are distinct decisions, and they do not take into account the manner in which parents and children make decisions together. Finally, cultures in which autonomy is less emphasized are not accommodated by a regulation

Box 74-1 **Principles Governing Children's Participation in Research Decisions**

1. Investigators should always respect children as persons. In particular, investigators together with parents should honor children's developing autonomy in decisions about research.
2. Investigators should respect parents' roles in guiding their children's moral development and assessing their best interests. For example, parents should have discretion to determine the degree to which children should be encouraged to participate in activities that benefit others.
3. Policies regarding assent, as well as decisions of Institutional Review Boards with respect to particular protocols, should be sufficiently flexible to accommodate the wide range of medical, psychological, and contextual circumstances seen in pediatric oncology.

From Joffe S, Fernandez CV, Pentz RD, et al: Involving children with cancer in decision making about research participation. J Pediatr *149:862–868, 2006.*

that potentially sets parental prerogatives against a child's veto power.[44]

Taking into account these factors, the COG Task Force offered three principles governing children's participation in research decisions (Box 74-1). A number of specific recommendations followed from these principles. The Task Force acknowledged that in some settings the principles offered will sometimes conflict. Therefore the recommendations emphasize the importance of establishing procedures for the resolution of conflict rather than attempting to define universal rules. In that way the absence of universal rules governing decisions in families with, perhaps, different cultural backgrounds and assumptions does not end conversation and negotiation. This approach is especially valuable in an increasingly pluralistic society and a global culture of information sharing. Much work remains to be done to understand the processes of communication and learning and the interactions that comprise the permission-assent process.

The flexibility of the approach using conflict resolution acknowledges that the obligation to obtain assent may change, depending on the time and situation, even for the same child. For example assent considerations may differ between a 9-year-old child with standard-risk leukemia who may obtain considerable benefit from enrollment in a phase III leukemia trial and a 9-year-old child who has leukemia that has relapsed multiple times and for whom a phase I trial is being considered. Similarly, a child at the beginning of a 2 and one half-year course of therapy for leukemia will be different in age, maturity, vocabulary, experience, and capacity to understand by the end of that course of therapy (Fig. 74-2). Developmentally appropriate approaches to help the child understand the experience do not have the restrictions and limitations that accompany the binding aspects of assent.

For older adolescents assent should be approached in the same way as adult informed consent, even though parental permission may be required.[45,46] Some adolescents may have the capacity for consent but may choose to have their parents make decisions about their participation in research.[47] Several studies have recently assessed assent in adolescents.[48,49] Our understanding of the

differences between parents' and adolescents' perceptions of research is growing as we learn more about the assessment of risk (i.e., concern for physical safety) versus aversion (psychological discomfort).[50] More than 3000 adolescents in the United States alone die of chronic illness and cancer each year. In such situations when adolescents meet the criteria for functional competence, the broad ethical consensus is that decisional authority should be granted to them regardless of their legal decisional status.[51] However this is an area in which a wide divergence exists between what ethics may demand but the law allows. Most states and jurisdictions do not permit minors to be sole participants in medical decision making, including consenting to participate in research, unless they have been emancipated according to the laws of the state in which they reside. This restriction does not imply that adolescents should not fully participate in the decision-making process, and there certainly is no legal proscription against their doing so; it simply underlines the difference between good ethical clinical (and research) practice and the legal framework. It might perhaps be better stated that in these situations, if the adolescent is going to be a research subject, assent is necessary but not sufficient.

PEDIATRIC CLINICAL TRIALS

The majority of children with cancer are enrolled in clinical trials.[52] This systematic evaluation of interventions is largely responsible for the dramatic improvement in survival during the past 40 years. A number of important ethical concepts influence the design and execution of these trials. Permission and assent have already been discussed. Other important issues include the distinction between therapeutic and nontherapeutic research, the various concepts of minimal risk and clinical equipoise, and the considerations that distinguish phase I and II trials from phase III trials.

As previously described and in Table 74-2, reports published by the National Commission for Subjects of Biomedical and Behavioral Research formed the basis of current regulations governing research with human subjects, including children. One of the most important

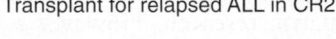

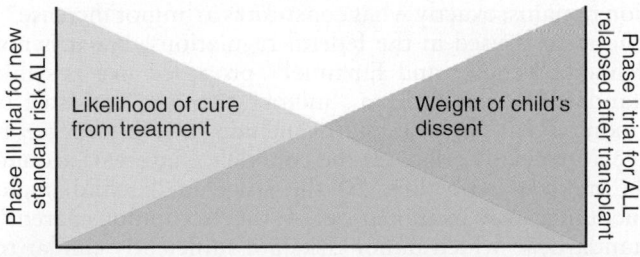

Figure 74-2 The weight of childhood dissent changes as the likelihood for direct benefit (in the form of cure or extension of life) diminishes, as with a patient who goes through a phase III trial for standard risk leukemia, relapses, undergoes transplantation in second remission, relapses, and goes on to consider phase I trials. *ALL,* Acute lymphoblastic leukemia; *CR2,* second complete remission.

distinctions made was between research that does, versus does not, offer the prospect of direct benefit to the child. Some elements of a clinical trial may offer the prospect of direct benefit (for example, chemotherapy for acute lymphoblastic leukemia), whereas other elements may not (e.g., biologic and pharmacokinetic studies designed to improve future trials). What are the general criteria used to determine whether the latter sorts of research are permissible?

Minimal Risk

The central ethical concept that guides discussion of pediatric research that has no prospect of direct benefit is "minimal risk." The Belmont Report defines minimal risk as "the probability and magnitude of physical or psychological harm that is normally encountered in the daily lives, or in the routine medical or psychological examination, of healthy children." The question that immediately arises is which children's lives should be the basis for deciding what is "normally encountered in daily life." These risks can vary widely, not only from country to country but within subgroups in a single country. Even if the notion of "harms or discomforts that average, healthy, normal children may encounter" (as clarified by the National Bioethics Advisory Commission) can be roughly agreed upon as a standard, the question remains whether it is ever acceptable for a parent to give permission for any risk greater than minimal risk in the absence of direct benefit to the child.

Because of concern that the "minimal risk" standard would exclude some pediatric research that is important and appropriate, the National Commission allowed parental discretion in giving permission for research that exposes children to a "minor increase" over minimal risk, given the fact that parents routinely permit their children to participate in activities, such as contact sports, that present more than a minimal risk, and given the potential benefits of such research to others. Therefore a "minor increase" over minimal risk is permissible if the proposed research involves only procedures that such children might normally experience because of their medical condition and if the proposed research has the potential to yield vitally important knowledge for understanding or ameliorating the child's particular condition.

The permissibility of a "minor increase" over minimal risk provides a conceptual way to avoid barriers to important pediatric research. However a difficult question remains: exactly what constitutes a "minor increase"? The term is used in the federal regulations, but it is not defined. Wendler and Emanuel[53] proposed five possible standards for defining a "minor" increase consistently among IRBs. These standards include (1) a fixed percentage above daily risks, (2) the confidence intervals around the risks of daily life, (3) the risks an ill child might encounter in an examination, (4) the "scrupulous parent" standard, in which minor risks are sufficiently similar to the child's past experiences in daily life, and (5) the "socially acceptable" risk standard.

Wendler and Emanuel[53] argue that the fifth standard is the most reasonable. The "socially acceptable" risk standard takes as its starting point the fact that some children encounter greater risks in daily life than others. The socially acceptable risk standard allows risks that are greater than those faced every day by healthy children, but it limits the risks to those that are socially acceptable. The socially acceptable risks greater than those experienced by the average healthy child may be more closely defined through research. In any case this standard tethers the concept of "minor increase over minimal risk" to an evaluation that is nonarbitrary, that does not impede important beneficial research, and that does not justify greater risks for ill children simply because their daily lives are filled with more risk (due to their disease and its treatment).[54] An alternative to the approach taken by Wendler and Emanuel has been suggested by Nelson and Ross.[55] They argue that the "scrupulous parent" standard is ethically justifiable and that such an approach incorporates both minimal risk and a minor increase over minimal risk within a uniform standard that should be applicable to all children.[55]

Phase I and II Trials in Pediatric Oncology

Phase I studies have the unique primary objective of assessing the maximum tolerated dose and estimating toxic effects in human subjects, in contrast to phase II and phase III studies, which explicitly assess the efficacy and relative safety of interventions. Phase I studies in children are important because the pharmacokinetics and toxic effects of drugs differ between children and adults. Therefore if drugs were used in the general pediatric population without phase I testing in children, the incidence of adverse effects would be unpredictable. Additionally some diseases are unique, or nearly unique, to the pediatric population, including a number of pediatric cancers.[56] Prohibition of phase I studies in children would limit the ability of the research community to develop new drugs that target uniquely pediatric diseases.

Phase I studies are typically dose-escalation trials in which some children receive a dose unlikely to be of any benefit while others receive a dose that is toxic. Therefore phase I studies do not fit the category of minimal risk nor, many would argue, of a "minor increase" over minimal risk. Much of the controversy about phase I studies in children, therefore, centers on whether they offer sufficient direct benefit to justify the risks, both from a purely ethical point of view and from the regulatory point of view.

What is the likelihood of harms and benefits in phase I oncology trials? A recent review of abstracts and reports of the results of phase I cancer trials submitted to the American Society of Clinical Oncology (ASCO) from 1991 to 2002 found that the death rate from toxicity was 0.54%, with an overall objective response rate of 3.8%, and that risks decreased over time.[57] A National Cancer Institute–sponsored study of adult phase I oncology trials run between 1991 and 2002 found an overall response rate of 10.6%. The response rates in "classic" single-agent phase I trials were lower (4.4%), whereas those that included at least one Food and Drug Administration (FDA)–approved anticancer agent had a response rate of 17.8%.[58] In pediatric oncology phase I trials, the response rate (both partial and complete responses) has been reported to be between 4% and 9.6%.[59,60] However the (causal) relationship or correlation between dose and response is rarely reported, and the small number of subjects at any dose level would preclude any sort of definitive conclusion from being drawn. The overall rate of death due to toxicity was 0.49%. That said, in any single phase I trial centered around a single drug, considerable variability in outcomes can exist among the research subjects recruited. Hence it is reasonable to conclude that few children entered in phase I trials die from study-drug–related toxicity and a very small percentage may derive some therapeutic benefit. Unfortunately no feasible mechanism exists to abstract what might be called the "pain and suffering" effects of trial participation or whether—as has been reported for adults enrolled in similar studies—there may be an avoidance of engaging in appropriate end-of-life discussions and planning.[61] Finally, at least one study has suggested that parents may feel compelled by their child's physician to enroll in phase I trials.[62] These observations suggest the idea of "collusion" between doctors and patients to temper the discussion of bad news with the hope that may be imparted by treatment.[63]

Can phase I trials be viewed as offering a prospect of direct benefit in the context of pediatric oncology? The pediatric medical and bioethics communities are divided on this question. The fact is that most people who enroll in phase I trials hope for personal benefit, although they know that the trial is designed to test toxicity.[64-66] The concern exists that such a "therapeutic misconception" may encourage false hope for cure and lead parents to make decisions that do not take into account all of the elements that make up "the child's best interest."[67,68] This phrase refers to the mistaken belief by clinical trial subjects (especially those participating in early-phase studies, such as phase I) that the principal purpose or goal of the trial is therapeutic, rather than data generation.[69,70,71,72,73] Clearly the primary scientific goal is not therapeutic, and the fundamental purpose of these trials is to gather data on toxicity, physiologic tolerability, and dosage. However it is very difficult to communicate such bare facts to families. Much of the confusion is derived from the emotional tension of the situation, the hopes and fears of parents (and patients), the fact that treating physicians often are involved in discussing the clinical options available for terminally ill patients, and the mixed messages that are both transmitted and received by families during these conversations.[74-76] The simple fact of the matter is that parents may not wish to hear "the truth" and their physicians may not wish to transmit it. Although many persons consider this problem to be almost insuperable, some attempts have been made to combat it with mixed success.[77] Nevertheless it remains a significant complicating factor that contributes to the ethical complexity of performing pediatric phase I trials.

On the other hand because only patients for whom known therapies have failed are usually eligible for phase I trials, these trials may be viewed as offering a relative prospect of direct benefit, although the chance of controlling the disease is small.[78] Such a view would bring phase I research under CFR 46.405 of the federal regulations,

but it has been criticized because such a classification (in which risk is justified by potential benefit) fails to take into account the researcher's focus on safety rather than efficacy. From the latter point of view, phase I research would be approvable only under CFR 46.407, in which the research is reviewed and approved by a panel appointed by the Secretary of the Department of Health and Human Services—a time-consuming effort that requires both national and local IRB review.

One critic of the "direct benefit" argument also questions the approval of phase I trials under CFR 46.407 because the required review process delays providing benefit to children and adds little to the meaningful protection of children. This author has suggested that a new category of research offering the potential for "secondary direct benefit" be added to the regulations.[79] Such a category would require (1) that the risks be justified by the likelihood that the research will yield generalizable knowledge, (2) that the research be commensurate with the lived experience of those with the disease or condition, (3) that the research offer a potential secondary benefit that is otherwise not available (a potential therapeutic benefit even though the trial lacks therapeutic intent), and (4) that consent requirements be met. Work that addresses gaps in the understanding of phase I trials and the federal regulations governing them should take high priority in pediatric medical ethics research. A recent essay supports phase I trials in children using an interesting and somewhat novel argument.[80] Morris[80] suggests that most children who would be eligible for the types of phase I trials that may involve more than minimal risk (independent of how it may be defined) would of course be afflicted with the disease or condition for which the agent under study is under investigation (for future possible therapeutic use). Furthermore it is likely that the experience of this disease would have acquainted both the child and his or her parents with many of the tests and procedures used as part of the trial (such as phlebotomy). Because they would also have an inherent interest in the outcome of such studies (both for the present and the future), they (and local, institutional IRBs) should be extended some moral flexibility in interpreting what should be interpreted as "minimal risk."

Phase II trials play an important role in all areas of cancer therapy. They provide the initial assessment of treatment efficacy and identify agents for further investigation in phase III studies.[81] These studies, although experimental, are clearly therapeutic in intent and thus the therapeutic misconception is not as germane. Phase II studies are likely to increase in number as high-throughput screening of compounds identifies more candidate anticancer drugs and more molecularly targeted agents and biologic agents become available. This fact will raise many important ethical questions in pediatric clinical trials, because phase II studies specifically evaluate drug efficacy before benefit is clearly demonstrated. Therefore it is vital that families and patients be fully informed about alternatives.

We should mention the attraction for incorporating nonrandomized phase II trials into therapeutic phase III studies, the so-called "phase II window." This approach was quite popular for some time because of the belief that previously untreated, "chemotherapy-naive" patients would constitute a population that would better represent the efficacy of a given agent compared with heavily pretreated patients whose response rates might be diminished both because of cross-resistance to other drugs and decreased performance status. This technique has come under significant ethical and statistical criticism, and in 2010, a consensus statement from the National Institute Clinical Trial Design Task Force was issued that called for the elimination of single-arm studies of this type and their replacement with better designed trials (although the Task Force did express the caveat that unique situations may exist in which nonrandomized, window designs might be appropriate).[82,83] Many stand-alone phase II COG studies have had this design, and it is rarely used in phase III studies (only one as of this writing). Therefore although phase II windows and single-arm studies still exist, the future of this form of design is questionable.

Finally, a word should be said about the use of drugs that are still under investigation in an "off-label" capacity. FDA-approved agents have been demonstrated to be safe and effective by FDA standards and thus receive approval for one or more indications. Many of these approved agents that have not yet been shown to have similar efficacy or a justifiable safety profile in children are nonetheless used in a phase II–like practice, but without the protections of an IRB-approved clinical trial (including rigorous and supervised informed consent and an adverse event reporting framework). Data about the frequency of this practice in children have not yet been published, but Peppercorn and colleagues[84] have reported this practice among adult oncologists, even when a clinical study incorporating the same drug(s) and for which the patient is eligible is available. Although it may be imagined that many studies use drugs that are only available via the trial, this situation is not actually the fact in adult oncology. In pediatrics this observation would be even more germane because it is rare for an agent to be available for children (especially for phase II and III trials) without first being tested and approved in adults.[85] The widespread use of this practice is worrisome for several reasons: First, it tends to undermine the clinical trial enterprise if physicians are willing to prescribe (off-label) investigational drugs in the same clinical setting in which they are being investigated. Such use also can lead to the failure to notice uncommon toxicities that may be more easily detected within the stricture of a formal clinical trial. Second, it is argued that such use results in the conduct of research without the significant human subjects oversight. Third, this practice exposes children to more than minimal risk, but the (relative) safety of patients cannot be ensured as it would be in a clinical trial with formal tracking of adverse events.[86] Finally, this practice represents a missed opportunity for more phase II trials to be conducted with sufficient statistical power to enable substantive conclusions about their significance to be drawn.[87,88] Thus this practice exposes patients (subjects) to potential risk without even the compensatory benefit of contributing valuable scientific knowledge to the general community.

Phase III Trials and Clinical Equipoise

If the concept of minimal risk demarcates the upper limit of nontherapeutic research, the notion of clinical equipoise is central (although not unproblematic) to ethical thought about randomization in clinical research. Clinical equipoise requires that if patients are to be randomly assigned to one of two interventions in a clinical trial, real doubt must exist—in the medical community as a whole, if not in the mind of the investigator—about which of the two interventions is superior. This requirement is said to provide one answer to the possible conflict of interest that clinical investigators can experience in the dual role of researcher and physician.[89]

At least two sources of confusion are presented by all forms of clinical trials, especially in pediatrics. First, sick children are first and foremost patients, which creates a special and unique fiduciary relationship between the patient and his or her doctor. This relationship also establishes a duty on the part of the doctor toward the patient that confers certain responsibilities to act in the patient's best interest.[90,91] This relationship should be distinguished from that of an investigator to a research subject, which is defined within the parameters of federal regulations (previously described).[92] In pediatric hematology-oncology, physicians often occupy both roles simultaneously, which can present significant conflicts (although not necessarily straightforward conflicts of interest). For example if the treating physician is also in some way involved in the design or implementation of the clinical trial under discussion with a patient and his family, she (the doctor) may have a conflict. Enrolling in the trial may not necessarily be to the best advantage or well-being of the patient as defined by him (and his surrogates) and his physician, but participating in the trial as a subject could be beneficial to the investigator (the doctor). In these situations it may be advisable for the treating physician to avoid caring for patients with diagnoses that may make them eligible for the trial for which he or she is responsible. For physicians whose relationship to the study is peripheral, in a manner that could perhaps be described as administrative (as is often the case for many, if not most, treating physicians with COG clinical trials), the conflict is minimal. However in a number of institutions, participation in "therapeutic" (i.e., phase II and III) trials may be remunerative, if not to the doctor, to the local group that employs the physician, by way of financial reimbursements to (partially) cover the cost of performing clinical trials. Although these rewards are hardly profitable, they do raise the specter of a conflict and may need to be addressed. A commitment to transparency may be sufficient in these cases. Second—and we admit that this may be more of a theoretical concern—years of experience have demonstrated the enormous benefit bestowed by the cooperative group clinical trial enterprise in pediatric oncology. Of course this progress would only have been possible with the recruitment (by physicians) and participation (by patients/subjects) in many clinical trials during the past four decades. The ongoing dedication of families, patients, and pediatric oncologists to this endeavor has been crucial to its success. Hence it could be perceived that there is a not-so-subtle pressure to enroll as many (eligible) patients as possible in group clinical studies (both therapeutic and nontherapeutic); indeed, failure to enroll sufficient numbers may result in institutional sanctions, up to and including suspension from the Group and thus an inability to access study protocols and documents (see the COG website for details). However, the recognition that this cooperative endeavor has been both productive and protective of patient (and subject) welfare is well understood and accepted. Nevertheless, the conflicts and the potential for their intensification and complexity remains and actually could increase as more pharmaceutical industry clinical trials are incorporated into the cooperative clinical trial group apparatus.

Does the physician's "therapeutic obligation" require the provision of the best possible care or simply of competent care?[93] The concept of clinical equipoise has been challenged from a number of perspectives. Some critics argue that therapeutic medicine and clinical research are distinct types of activity that require distinct ethical frameworks and that the concept of "clinical equipoise" cannot provide a unifying ethical framework.[94,95] Clinical equipoise has also been criticized as especially problematic in developing countries, where the lack of resources may not support trials that test new treatments against established therapies or placebo. The requirement for clinical equipoise could make it difficult to justify the search for interventions that, although they provide significant benefit for less money, are known not to be the most effective interventions.[96,97]

Several other considerations are important in evaluating the concept of clinical equipoise. First, the conditions for establishing true equipoise are not objective, based as they are on unverified judgments that are open to bias.[98,99] Second, if clinical equipoise is not always a reliable foundation for randomized studies, how do we resolve the conflicts that can be posed by clinical investigators' dual roles? Finally, although adults may be able to negotiate the ambiguities of clinical equipoise in a clinical trial, children cannot do so. In light of the previous discussion regarding the best interest of the child (or the attempt to avoid harm to the child), no phase III randomized pediatric trial should be conducted unless genuine doubt exists about which of two or more alternatives is better.

Recently a new approach to bringing together research and clinical care has begun to emerge. The Institute of Medicine has called for the transformation of health systems into "learning health care systems" that are able to study and continuously improve their practices. Learning health care systems pursue a wide range of investigations, including those aimed at quality improvement and better clinical effectiveness. An active question is whether the data collection and monitoring central to learning health care systems should be construed as research, and if so, what type of ethical oversight it should have.[100]

Finally, a great deal of discussion has ensued about the responsibility of investigators to communicate the results of clinical trials to patients and their families, irrespective of the outcome of the studies. Surveys have suggested that patients who have enrolled in trials (or who have been enrolled by their parents) retain an interest in the outcome.[102-105] Thus there is good reason to believe that a continuation of the respect we pay to patients, and the diligence and responsibility owed to study participants/subjects, would warrant the formal reporting of the results of trials to them, even taking into consideration the time lag that is intrinsic to the completion of a large study, the maturing of the data, and the challenges associated with communicating complex information of this type. Furthermore, the variety of data that can be collected from the trial—including intricate genetic and other biologic marker data—will require careful consideration to decide what information would be most important to communicate. The issue of conveying genetic or genomic information has proven to be particularly problematic, and to date the challenge has resisted consensus solutions.[106-108]

SPECIAL CONSIDERATIONS FOR CANCER TRIALS USING ALLOGENEIC HEMATOPOIETIC STEM CELL TRANSPLANTATION

Many patients with high-risk cancers (especially leukemias) that are resistant to standard chemotherapy may be cured with hematopoietic stem cell transplantation (HSCT). As in other areas of pediatric oncology, most such patients are treated according to research protocols or treatment plans recently derived from research protocols. Because of the continuing, rapid changes in the field of HSCT, ethical considerations, such as the specifics of the risk/benefit analysis, are rapidly changing as well.

The issues that apply to pediatric oncology trials in general are also relevant to those that include HSCT. However HSCT raises additional questions. Unlike most phase III trials, transplantation for cancer is usually a second-line medical procedure aimed at cure after a patient has been treated with other therapies. Common indications for transplantation in patients with malignant disease include lack of response to conventional chemotherapy and a known high risk of relapse despite conventional therapy. In both cases patients have been treated prior to transplantation, and the education received in this experience will be relevant to the consent process (the same, of course, can be said for phase I trials). Patients' and parents' familiarity with the language of pediatric oncology makes the discussion about transplantation easier in some ways than the discussion about a phase III trial in the context of a newly diagnosed childhood malignancy. However these considerations are primarily cognitive. What about other issues?

No studies have examined noncognitive considerations in consent for pediatric HSCT, but one study addressed the relative value of receiving full information in decision making among adult patients.[109] The findings provide interesting information that might in part guide future assessments of the unique characteristics of consent and assent in pediatric HSCT. The study had an unusual hypothesis: in the context of a potentially life-saving procedure, when there are no treatment alternatives that have a reasonable chance of cure, factors other than the effort to fully inform have the greatest influence on the patient's decision-making process. The notion of "voluntary" action is complex in such cases, because the patients' life-threatening illness has "forced" them to consider HSCT as an option. Four factors were considered by patients, according to this study: (1) a full understanding of the treatment, (2) trust in the physician, (3) trust in the treatment team, and (4) the best chance for a good outcome. The most important factor was "best chance for a good outcome," and the least important factor was "a full understanding of the treatment."

This finding is relevant to any high-risk, complex intervention (such as transplantation) in which the patient's life is at stake. The lack of alternative therapies that offer the real possibility of cure limits the voluntariness of the decision, and trust in the physician and the health care team may become more significant than understanding of the treatment. Given the vulnerability of these patients, this fact underscores the importance of careful attention to the therapeutic rationale of treatment, as well as the relationship of the patient and family to the health care team, especially when the intervention has not been established as the standard of care.

Another significant difference between cancer chemotherapy trials and those using allogeneic HSCT is the fact that HSCT involves two patients—the recipient and the donor. Different issues arise depending on whether the donor is a matched unrelated, matched related, cord blood, or haploidentical donor. These differences are, in part, based on the fact that the matched unrelated donor is a stranger, the matched related donor is a brother or sister, and the haploidentical donor is usually a parent. The patient's course and outcome affect the donor in various ways, depending on the relationship of the donor to the patient, and this effect is relevant to the ethical issues involved in HSCT cancer clinical trials.

More than 7 million people are registered as potential bone marrow or peripheral blood stem cell donors for the 70% of candidates for HSCT who do not have a matched sibling donor.[110] The risks of bone marrow donation are small; life-threatening complications occur in approximately 0.1% of healthy donors.[111] Ninety-five percent of peripheral blood stem cell (PBSC) donors do well with only minor complaints.[112] In matched unrelated–donor transplantation, one must consider the donor's rights as well as the patient's rights. These issues were outlined in a review by the World Marrow Donor Association.[113] First, donor autonomy must always be honored. At a minimum, this means that the consequences of each act in the process (as they bear on both the donor and the patient) must be explained to the donor. The informed consent process and document must stipulate the donor's right to withdraw at any time (even during the pretransplant conditioning) and must state the possible consequences of withdrawal. The donor registry cannot pressure or coerce donors, although the center/registry has the right to exclude a donor.

No one is obligated to join a donor registry, but a donor who does join a registry with clear knowledge of the expectations voluntarily incurs some moral obliga-

tion. This obligation grows as the process continues: a donor at the point of donation for a patient who is being conditioned has a greater obligation than does a person who is only at the stage of registering, because the patient has undergone a treatment that creates considerable vulnerability and has done so because of the expectation that the donor will follow through. Therefore donor centers are obligated to communicate clearly with donors to avoid disrupting the recipient's treatment plan if possible.

Limits exist to a donor's obligation. Sometimes a clinical situation is such that optimal care of a patient would require additional cell products from the donor, such as T cells or additional stem cells. The donor does not have a legal obligation to continue donating cells or bone marrow after the original donation.

Donor unavailability remains a problem that bears upon decision making because the treatment plan is dependent upon such variables. When donor unavailability rates over 1 year were examined by the National Marrow Donor Program, the worldwide registry of volunteer unrelated stem cell donors, some interesting facts were discovered.[114] Initially when a donor search is started, a request is made for confirmatory typing. Approximately 20% of all donors were permanently deferred at the time of confirmatory testing, and another 12% were temporarily unavailable (because of such things as pregnancy, high-risk exposure, job change, and location change). Donation centers differed considerably. The self-identified racial or ethnic group of the donor affected the likelihood that the donor would be available when requested. These findings suggest important areas in which practical improvement might be achieved: better medical screening, better collection of contact information, better education about the details of the commitment, and movement toward a pressure-free environment. Other important issues that bear upon ethical decision making, such as cultural sensitivity and route of contact, must be studied further. The overall goal is to structure the donor registry in such a way that donor availability is maximized through better recruitment, retention, and contact.

A second important source of hematopoietic stem cells in pediatric oncology transplant trials are sibling donors, many of whom are minors. Although the process of donation has been designed to minimize the coercion of unrelated donors, sibling donors may experience a variety of pressures. The ethical question centers on the coercion of a younger child who is dependent on the parents to provide permission for the donation. One central related ethical question concerns what, if anything, constitutes a benefit to the donor. The sibling donor can experience psychological, spiritual, and physical stress like that experienced by the HSCT recipient. The pain and anxiety among adult sibling donors of bone marrow or PBSC has been described.[115-118] Further, refusal to donate can be perceived as resulting in the loss of a sibling, even though the loss is actually due to the underlying disease. Because the variable of developmental age is added in pediatrics, the issue is more complex. Whether or not the transplant actually occurs, if the sibling dies, the complexity is compounded.[119] In many areas of family life, parents are allowed to give more weight to the interest of one child than to those of another or of the family in general; therefore some persons advocate leaving the decision of whether a minor child should donate bone marrow to a sibling in the hands of the parents.[120] Regardless of how such issues are ultimately resolved, the sibling donors clearly deserve all developmentally appropriate information at the beginning of the process and full psychological support throughout and after the procedure.

Sibling donor interviews provide helpful information. Irrespective of transplant outcome, pediatric sibling donors report a perception of having "no choice" about becoming a donor, whether the sense of constraint is derived from outside pressure (indicated by participants' use of the words "guilt," "propaganda," "privileged," and "conned") or from the donor's own beliefs.[121] Hesitancy may arise not from a lack of concern for the sibling's health but rather from fear of the procedure and of pain. Donors whose recipient sibling died offered a unique perspective. Anger, guilt, and blame were common emotions expressed and seemed to be most difficult to deal with in cases in which the death was directly related to graft failure or graft-versus-host disease. These issues have not been studied enough to draw substantial conclusions, but enough is known to raise questions about competence to consent, the weight accorded to a child's refusal to donate, the limits of the parents' decision-making power, and the worrisome specter of what may constitute battery in the face of a child's refusal. One might override the refusal of a 5-year-old, but what about that of a 10-year-old, a 13-year-old, or a 17-year-old?

Another important issue in the case of sibling donors for pediatric HSCT is the fact that siblings who are not chosen as donors are susceptible to ambivalent feelings of relief, disappointment, and guilt.[122] If siblings are involved in the screening process, issues of psychological well-being and respect for persons meet. In one study that compared sibling donors with sibling nondonors, nondonors had more school-related problems than did donors, and a third of siblings in both groups reported moderate to severe posttraumatic stress.[123-125] Medical encounters with a nondonor sibling may well show suffering that would not have occurred apart from the process of being screened for stem cell donation. Caregivers owe this person as much respect as they owe any patient.

Both case and common law have reasonably established that potential donors who have achieved legal majority (age 18 years or emancipation by a court) may not necessarily or generally be compelled to donate bone marrow (or other organs) irrespective of who the prospective beneficiary may be and the relationship between the two (although the legal history of this situation is complex).[126] The state of affairs for minors who are possible donors is considerably more involved. In 2010 the Committee on Bioethics of the American Academy of Pediatrics (AAP) endorsed the view that minors could serve as donors provided that five conditions were met: (1) "there [should] be no medically equivalent histocompatible adult relative who is willing and able to donate; (2) there [must] be a strong personal and positive relationship between the donor and recipient ... this is important, in part, to increase the likelihood that the donor will experience some psychological benefit; (3) there [should] be some likelihood that the recipient will benefit from transplantation; (4) the clinical, emotional, and psychosocial risks to the donor be minimized and be reasonable in relation to the benefits expected to accrue to the donor and the recipient; and (5) parental permission and donor assent be obtained."[127] The AAP also suggested that a "donor advocate" be appointed to help the donor "... (and parents) understand the process and procedures and to protect and promote the interests and well-being of the donor. As such the donor advocate ... should not be involved in direct patient care of the potential transplant recipient." The statement did not describe any further the identity of this advocate. Although presumably he/she could be a guardian ad litem appointed by a court, we suspect most institutions would wish to avoid the potential cumbersome process of applying to a court unless necessary. Not surprisingly this position has generated some controversy, including the opposition of the parent (whose child had severe aplastic anemia and who received a sibling marrow transplant) and other objections to the donor advocate requirement.[128,129] The AAP (and others) defended this requirement, and at present their position stands.[130,131]

However a recent case from Alabama in which a 6-year-old girl was required to "donate" split-thickness skin for grafting onto her severely burned identical twin sister suggests that the legal landscape for these cases may still be in a state of some flux.[132] Does this case (and others like it) suggest that under certain conditions involving desperately ill children who may possibly benefit from an allogeneic stem cell transplant, a minor sibling can be compelled to be a donor? Although the image of a child being forced to undergo a painful procedure, protesting all the way, is disconcerting, one can certainly imagine forms of parental pressure that are brought to bear to persuade a reluctant child to proceed with donation. Indeed the opposition to the possibly interdictive role of the "advocate" is the source of at least some of the objections to the AAP position. However most of the cases under discussion (or dispute) concern potential donors who are quite young. For those who may be in the mid to late teenage years, the answer is quite a bit more complicated. As children mature, they become more able to participate in health care decision making, as previously noted. However this increasing cognitive capacity does not accord with the laws in most states that do not extend legal decision-making authority to so-called "mature minors." Nevertheless the legal facts may conflict not only with our moral intuitions but with more mundane biology: it may be physically very difficult (if not completely improper) to force a 15- or 16-year-old to submit to bone marrow or PBSC harvesting if he or she does not agree to be a donor. Indeed the role of the advocate under these circumstances would be superfluous. Unfortunately this fact implies that the objections of a (small) 6-year-old count for far less than those of an adult-sized teenager, even though legally they are similarly inconsequential in the overwhelming majority of states.

A third, increasingly prominent source of stem cells is cord blood. Initial concerns about early clamping of the umbilical cord to obtain the maximum number of cells have been allayed, but other ethical questions remain.[133] Should the cord blood be linked to the identity of the donor so that unsafe units can be identified if the donor is later disqualified (e.g., by genetic testing)? The controversy centers on concerns about loss of privacy for donors. Because the cord blood deoxyribonucleic acid holds genetic information (the social implications of which are not clear at this time), the donor is potentially vulnerable to inappropriate disclosure.[134] A related issue concerns what the limits for cord blood testing ought to be and what one should do with the results. Clearly, some testing is needed to avoid unnecessary risk to the recipient. However in 1994, the Institute of Medicine recommended that children should not be tested for abnormal genes unless the disease has an effective curative or preventative treatment that must be initiated early in life.[135] This view was also endorsed more recently in a comprehensive report from the President's Commission on Bioethics.[136] Thus it may be that samples should be tested broadly to protect the recipient but that the testing should be performed in a blinded way to protect the donor. The details of this issue will require further thought and debate as more is learned about the human genome and prediction of disease. However this approach does not address the use of these samples for general genetic research, which is a related but altogether different question (discussed later).

The fourth source of stem cells used in pediatric clinical oncology trials is the haploidentical donor, usually a parent. The advantage of this sort of transplant is the ready availability of a partially matched donor. No research has been performed on the impact of this sort of transplant on parents and families, but it would not be surprising if the issues seen with sibling donation were compounded when the parent is the donor, including feelings of guilt when the child has severe graft-versus-host disease or graft failure. Another important question is whether there is a limit to acceptable parental sacrifice, and if so, what it is. For example one would not allow a parent to donate his or her heart, but intermediate scenarios include those in which a parent donates a portion of a lung, kidney, or liver in the face of posttransplant complications.

Finally, autologous stem cell reconstitution after myeloablation, mostly for solid tumors (frequently inaccurately referred to as "transplants"), is worth mentioning. Although these procedures do not raise the types of ethical challenges associated with allogeneic transplants of various sorts, they do often take the form of phase II single-arm trials for which little evidentiary support may exist and that are statistically underpowered, as explained earlier in this chapter. The classic example of this situation was the story of stem cell treatment for advanced breast cancer, but similar cases have occurred with childhood tumors as well, including Ewing sarcoma and rhabdomyosarcoma in which apparently excellent outcomes are compared with historic control subjects.[137-140] This observation does not imply that there are not clinical situations in which this therapy may provide significant benefits (as in stage IV, poor-risk neuroblastoma or relapsed Hodgkin disease).[141-143] Although this issue would appear to be straightforward and its resolution similarly so, it has proven to be surprisingly resilient over the years. The significant point is that this intervention can, and should, be used in a manner that is designed to address an important clinical question in a manner that could provide a reliable (and presumably reproducible) answer.

MODELS AND TOOLS FOR ETHICAL DECISION MAKING IN PEDIATRIC CLINICAL TRIALS

As important as the individual issues (such as consent, assent, and clinical equipoise) are, they make the most sense in both the clinical and research settings when they are considered within a larger framework for ethical decision making. Such a framework takes into account fundamental moral principles such as respect for persons, individual and cultural variation, the importance of full information, and the relevance of an individual's experience of illness to the concrete process of decision making. Although it is essential to have a sound foundational understanding of ethical principles as they apply to both the clinical and research settings, it is equally important to emphasize the vital role that facts play. "Good ethics begins with good facts" is an epigram often cited but not trivialized by its pithiness. Comprehensive knowledge about the facts of a case and possession of much information as possible about the patient and his or her family situation can be critical to the pediatric oncologist's role as caregiver and advisor. Incorporated in this approach is also an understanding of the prognosis, along with an appreciation (which should be communicated to the patient and family) of the limits and inherent uncertainty of the prognosis and what this signifies.

The Individualized Care Planning and Coordination (ICPC) model for ethical decision making developed by Baker and colleagues[144] combines the various elements of decision making in such a way that they are intentionally and systematically addressed (to ensure nothing is missed) and revisited using the care model (so that changes over time are acknowledged and responded to). The model begins by establishing a foundation based on the principles of competence, empathy, compassion, communication, and quality (Fig. 74-3). The aims of this model are to attend to quality of life, healing, and suffering from the start of a life-threatening illness. The ICPC model has three steps, each of which has three components (Fig. 74-4, Table 74-3).

The first step, relationship, is made up of three interrelated components: understanding the illness experience, sharing relevant information, and needs assessment. Without comprehending the illness experience of the child and the family, the clinician will be unable to proceed to seeking the best interest of the child and the decision-making process. This may be especially true at the extreme of consideration of phase I clinical trials toward the end of the child's life. Similarly, no decision

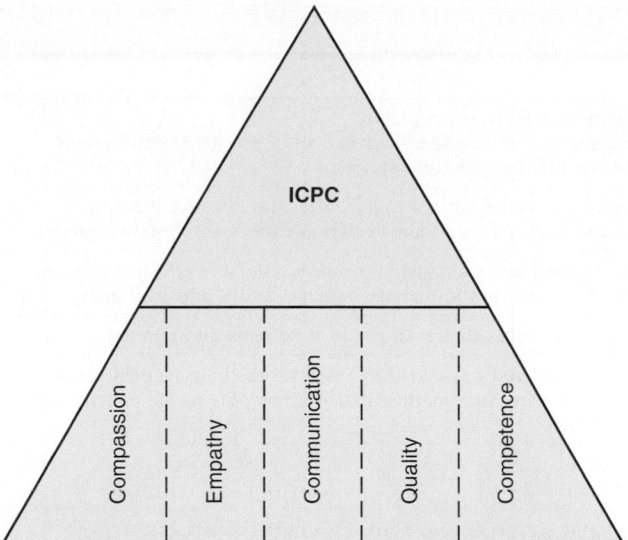

Figure 74-3 Foundation of the Individualized Care Planning and Coordination *(ICPC)* model. *(Modified from Baker JN, Barfield RC, Hinds PS, et al: A model to facilitate decision making in pediatric stem cell transplantation: the individualized care planning and coordination model. Biol Blood Marrow Transplant 13:245–254, 2007.)*

can realistically address the best interest of the child unless all persons involved in the decision-making process have the needed information. This issue can be difficult when the relevant information is bad news; several studies have shown that the bearer of bad news can elicit strong negative reactions from family members that, in turn, make the clinician reluctant to deliver bad news (an effect known as the "MUM effect").[145-147] Communication of sufficient information for ethical decision making can also be truncated in approximately 10% of cases by lack of training and communication of the pediatric oncologist.[148] A comprehensive needs assessment—not just an assessment of medical needs—is also vital to the process of ethical decision making in both clinical medicine and clinical oncology trials (see Table 74-3). Such comprehensive assessments can inform the decision-making processes by incorporating relevant changes in a patient's needs.

The second step in the ICPC model is negotiation in which goals, prognoses, and treatment options are considered. Although the prognosis for cure can be dynamic because of advances in the science of pediatric oncology, prognostic information is helpful to patients and families as they make decisions.[149,150] Another relevant consideration is that more than one relevant prognosis exists—more, that is, than the prognosis for cure—such as the prognosis for life prolongation and the prognosis for relief of suffering. These two prognoses are relevant, relate intimately to the goals of care, and are profoundly important aspects of ethical decision making in pediatric oncology.

After the range of prognostic elements has been considered, it is possible to move on to a discussion of what the goals are to be—goals that may change as the prognosis changes (Fig. 74-5).[151] In a phase III clinical trial, cure may be the dominant goal. However for a child who

has had multiple relapses and whose family is considering a phase I trial, ethical decision making will involve a reassessment of goals in light of the best interest of the child, including a reassessment of the child's expressed values. Assessment and prioritization of the values of the child—especially, perhaps, in the context of a low probability of cure—is an area in which much research remains to be done. Among novel projects being assessed is the use of interactive technologies (tapping into the "video-game" culture) to augment the expressive ability of younger children (Fig. 74-6).

Each potential goal with its associated prognosis is related in turn to a treatment option aimed at achieving the goal to the extent possible (i.e., as limited by scientific progress). If families see that supportive care is available to help them achieve their goals, they are less likely to feel abandoned and to fear discontinuation of therapies with curative intent.[152] Ethical decision making takes into account prognoses, goals, and treatment options and

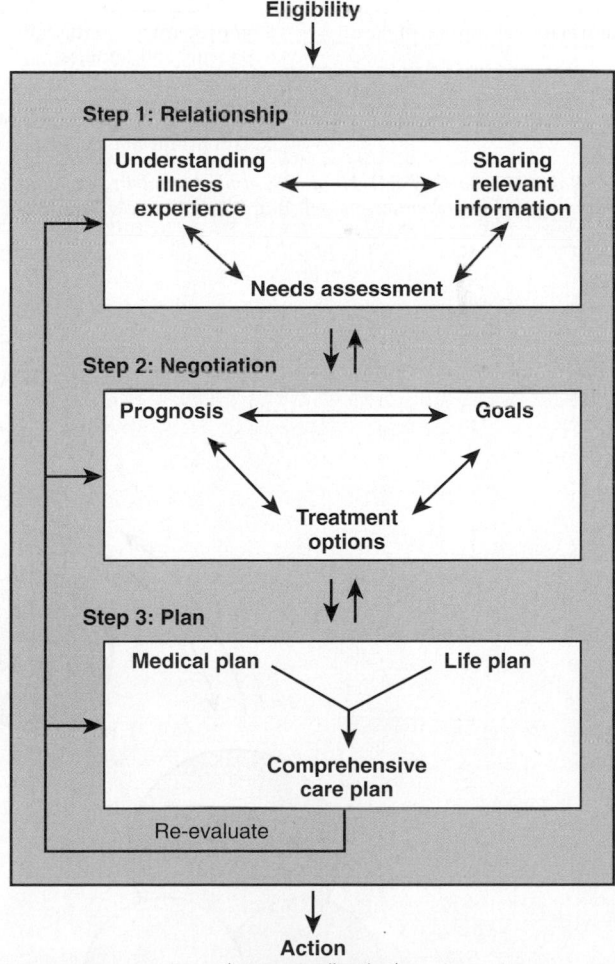

Figure 74-4 The three-step individualized care planning and coordination model. *(Modified from Baker JN, Barfield RC, Hinds PS, et al: A model to facilitate decision making in pediatric stem cell transplantation: the individualized care planning and coordination model. Biol Blood Marrow Transplant 13:245–254, 2007.)*

TABLE 74-3   Domains of Interdisciplinary Needs Assessment

Assessment Domain	Examples
Structure and process of care	Specialty-level trained symptom management experts are available. The setting of care should meet the preferences, needs, and circumstances of the patient and family. The care plan is based on a comprehensive interdisciplinary assessment.
Physical aspects of care	Symptoms and adverse effects are assessed and managed in a timely, safe, and effective manner. Symptoms and side effects are assessed and managed in a manner that is patient and family centered.
Psychological and psychiatric aspects of care	Psychological and psychiatric needs are assessed and managed in a timely, safe, and effective manner. Grief and bereavement program is available to assess and manage patient, family, and staff grief.
Social aspects of care	Comprehensive interdisciplinary assessment identifies the social needs of patients and families.
Spiritual, religious, and existential aspects of care	Spiritual and existential dimensions are assessed and responded to based on the best available evidence. Spiritual and existential dimensions are approached in a manner that is acceptable to the patient and family as they pertain to the patient's illness.
Cultural aspects of care	Needs are assessed in a culturally sensitive manner. Specific patient and family cultural needs are assessed.
Care of the imminently dying	During this stage of the illness trajectory, the comprehensive needs assessment continues. Signs and symptoms of impending death are assessed, recognized, communicated, and treated as needed.
Ethical and legal aspects of care	Health care professionals assess and attempt to incorporate the values, goals, and preferences of each patient and family. The need for ethics consultation should be assessed based on the comprehensive needs assessment and discordant steps in the process (i.e., cure as a primary goal in end-stage cancer).
Informational aspects of care	Comprehensive interdisciplinary assessment identifies the informational and educational needs of patients and families. Specific patient and family information is provided in a timely manner.
Relational aspects of care	As a part of the generation of a life plan, the relational needs of the patient and family are assessed. Relationships are assessed and augmented throughout the illness trajectory.

From Baker JN, Barfield RC, Hinds PS, et al: A model to facilitate decision making in pediatric stem cell transplantation: the individualized care planning and coordination model. Biol Blood Marrow Transplant 13:245–254, 2007.

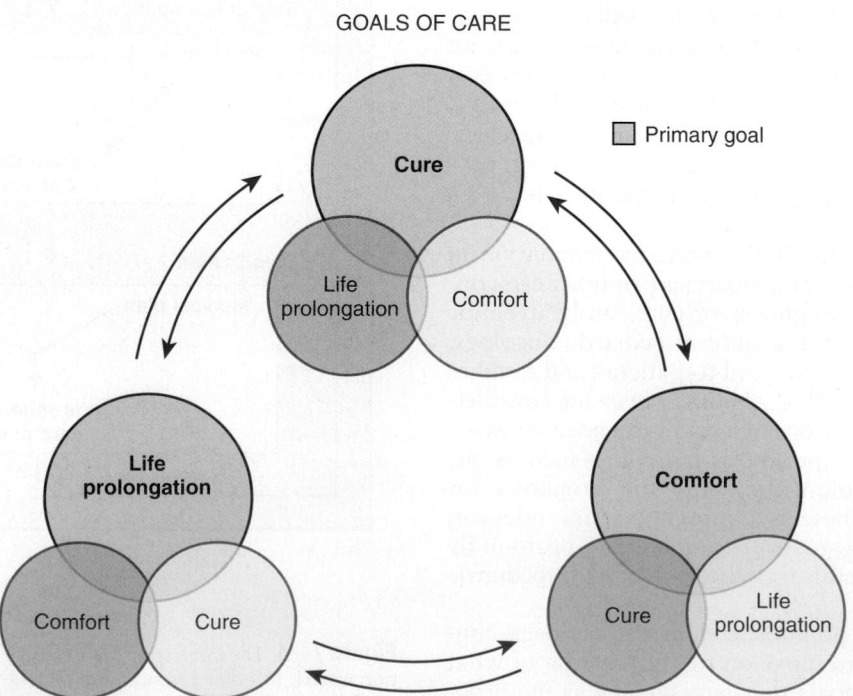

Figure 74-5 Goals of care. *(Modified from Baker JN, Barfield RC, Hinds PS, et al: A model to facilitate decision making in pediatric stem cell transplantation: the individualized care planning and coordination model. Biol Blood Marrow Transplant 13:245–254, 2007.)*

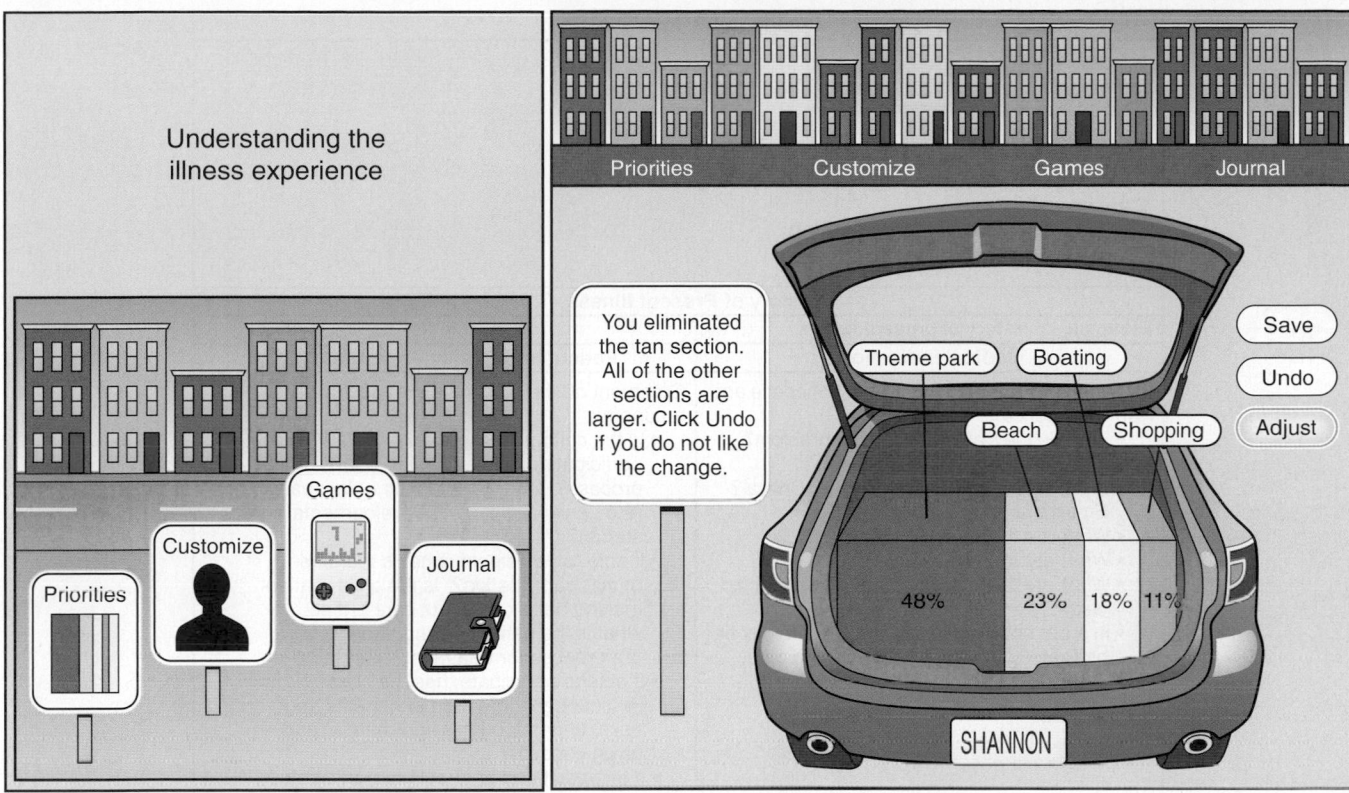

Figure 74-6 "The Treasure Box" prototype uses children's attraction to electronic games to help them express their priorities and values in the context of ethical decision making regarding phase I trials.

involves shared decision making by the family, the patient, and the clinicians. This process leads to the third step of the ICPC, the comprehensive care plan.

The ethical decision-making process that yields a comprehensive plan takes into account consent, assent, full disclosure of information, and attention to the variety of ways that families and individuals prioritize values. The comprehensive care plan includes both a medical plan (decisions about medical treatment and symptom management) and a life plan (addressing personal goals and family needs). The former might carry more weight when the goals emphasize cure, and the latter might carry more weight for a patient with incurable disease.[153]

The value of such an approach is that it can clarify complex ethical decision making in settings such as the intensive care unit (with the extraordinary advances in sustaining biologic life) and can clarify the goals of care. A useful tool that complements the ICPC is the "four box" method developed by Jonsen and colleagues,[154] which offers specific questions that can add content to the information categories relevant to comprehensive ethical decision making (Fig. 74-7). This more detailed set of questions in the categories of medical information, family preferences, contextual details, and quality of life expands those put forward by the President's Commission in 1983 and by the publication *Deciding to Forgo Life-Extending Treatment*.[155] The five considerations offered by the Commission for determining the best interest of the child in such situations are the amount of suffering and potential for relief, the severity of dysfunction

or the potential for restoration of function, expected duration of life, potential for personal satisfaction and enjoyment of life, and the potential to develop a capacity for self-determination.

These issues are very complex, and it is beyond the scope of this chapter to discuss them in depth. However both the moral and spiritual outlook of families (and the emerging and solidifying views of patients) and physicians can become entangled in an elaborate mixture of feelings and facts that may have a profound influence on the types of decisions that emerge during discussions at or near the end of life.[156,157,158,159,160,161] The often-heard directive to "do everything" may be interpreted in a variety of ways, including offering further therapies both in and out of the context of sanctioned clinical trials. Complicating these clinically challenging situations is the influence of both radical uncertainty about prognosis and the underrecognized influence of anecdotal experience.[162-164] When to transition to comfort care only in the dying pediatric cancer patient—or, for that matter, when to concede that a patient is actually dying—remains a dilemma, but one that should be managed in an individualized manner for each patient and his or her family.

FURTHER CHALLENGES IN PEDIATRIC CLINICAL ONCOLOGY TRIALS

Bioinformatics and Genomics

In the past two decades we have seen an unprecedented increase in the international sharing of information and

Demographic Information
Name: Date: Length of visit: Physician of record: Prepared by (name of scribe): Present (all participants with titles for future reference): Care coordinator: ____ First decision--making meeting ____ Update

History of Present Illness
Summary of history of present illness.

Medical Indications	Patient and Family Preferences
Comment on the principles of beneficence and nonmaleficence: • What is the patient's medical problem? History? Diagnosis? Prognosis? • Is the problem acute? Chronic? Critical? Emergent or reversible? • What are the goals of treatment? • What are the probabilities of success? • What are the plans in case of therapeutic failure? • In sum, how can this patient and family be benefited by medical and nursing care, and how can harm be avoided?	Comment on the principle of respect for autonomy: • Is the child-patient capable of participating in the decision--making process? Is there evidence of incapacity (e.g., age, cognitive or developmental status)? • If able to participate, what is the extent of that participation? Is the child--patient making decisions about care? If so, what is the patient stating about preferences for treatment? • If able to participate, has the child--patient been informed of benefits and risks, understood this information, and given consent? • If incapacitated or unable to participate, who is making decisions on his or her behalf? Is the parent or surrogate using appropriate standards for decision-making? • Has the patient, parent, or surrogate expressed prior preferences (e.g., Advance Directives)? • Is the patient, parent, or surrogate unwilling or unable to cooperate with medical treatment? If so, why? • In sum, are the patient and family's rights to choose being respected to the extent possible in ethics and law? Do they know they have a choice?

Quality of Life	Contextual Features
Comment on the principles of beneficence, nonmaleficence, and respect for autonomy: • What are the prospects, with or without treatment, for a return to normal life? • What physical, mental, and social deficits is the patient likely to experience if treatment succeeds? What is the impact on the family? • Are there biases that might prejudice the provider's evaluation of the patient's quality of life? • Is the patient's present or future condition such that his or her continued life might be judged undesirable? • Is there any plan and rationale to forego treatment? • Are there plans for comfort and palliative care?	Comment on the principles of loyalty and fairness: • What are the rights of the child relative to the rights of the family? • Are there family issues that might influence treatment decisions? • Are there provider issues that might influence treatment decisions? • Are there financial and economic factors? • Are there religious or cultural factors? • Are there limits on confidentiality? • Are there problems of allocation of resources? • How does the law affect treatment decisions? • Is clinical research or teaching involved? • Is there any conflict of interest on the part of the providers of the institution?

Discussion
Summary of key discussion points.

Plan
Summary of action plan.

Figure 74-7 Decision-making communication tool. *(From Jonsen AR, Siegler M, Winslade WJ: Clinical ethics: a practical approach to ethical decisions in clinical medicine, ed 6, New York, 2006, McGraw-Hill.)*

ideas. This fact has allowed more rapid dissemination of useful information and has also increasingly uncovered disparities in access to technology, availability of resources, and ethical values, all of which bear on the ethics of pediatric clinical oncology trials when considered from a global perspective.

Technological advances that are revolutionizing the diagnosis and treatment of childhood cancer (and other childhood disorders) bring with them new ethical issues.[165] These complex ethical questions challenge us to develop a coherent approach that accommodates the diversity of political, religious, cultural, philosophical, and vocational backgrounds that bear upon the discussion.

Bioinformatics is one area demonstrating rapid advances. Bioinformatics attempts large-scale organization of information, including genomic data, protein expression data, and molecular interactions.[166] Genomics is revolutionizing the diagnosis and treatment of cancer.[167] High-throughput microarrays can profile the expression patterns of tens of thousands of genes simultaneously.[168] This technology offers much promise. Similarly, it raises a number of important ethical questions. If a disease gene or disease susceptibility gene profile is discovered, should a subject be notified? Should the subject's family also be notified, or is this a breech of confidentiality?[169]

ASCO has recommended that genetic testing for cancer predisposition be offered when (1) the individual has a personal history, family history, or features suggestive of genetic cancer susceptibility, (2) the test can be adequately interpreted, and (3) the result will aid in a diagnosis or in the medical or surgical management of a patient or family member who has a hereditary risk for cancer.[170] ASCO has also recommended that the regulatory oversight of laboratories providing such tests be strengthened and that federal laws be established to prohibit discrimination by health care providers, employers, and insurance agencies on the basis of such information. Although some persons maintain that genetic discrimination will not affect insurance coverage, several surveys have shown that the public fears this possibility.[171,172,173] One important legislative step that has been taken to address these concerns is the Genetic Nondiscrimination Act of 2008 (Box 74-2).[174]

In pediatric oncology, the ethical issue is even more complex because surrogate decision makers make decisions that may affect the research subjects' future employability, insurability, and privacy. Further, as technology grows more complex, the gap between technology and meaningful understanding on the part of the family/patient widens (a growing challenge to "informed consent"). Can the surrogate decision makers understand fully the implications of their decision? How much can be expected of a parent without special training?

Pharmacogenomics is the subcategory of genomics research that has perhaps the most immediate potential impact in pediatric clinical oncology trials. This area, too, has enormous potential to benefit children but also creates the potential for social and economic discrimination and abuse of information in genomic databases. Pharmacogenomics combines human genomics with pharmacogenetics to study the role of the individual's genetic makeup in

the individual's response to a drug.[175] The promise of this approach is that patients can receive individually tailored medical therapy and dosing. This technology advances the important concept of risk stratification, which historically has led to better protection of children with lower risk cancers from excess toxicity while ensuring that children with higher risk disease are not undertreated.

Pharmacogenomics raises several ethical questions. For example an economic question exists: Might pharmacogenomic criteria eventually become regulatory requirements for the development and testing of medicines?[176] Because the pharmaceutical industry functions on a business model, it is unlikely to develop medicines that will benefit only a small, narrowly defined group of patients. This dilemma is familiar to investigators in pediatric oncology. Orphan drugs might therefore become more common. How should economic risk be weighed against the potential clinical benefit for a small group of patients? Second, if pharmacogenomics information suggests only that a child is more or less likely to benefit from a drug, what likelihood threshold would exclude the child from the use of a drug? Ten percent? Thirty percent? If a child is less likely to respond to a drug, is an insurance company obligated to pay for the drug?[177] If genetic variance peculiar to an ethnic group is found, what are the political, social, and economic implications? Might these be used to decide whether to develop certain medicines for certain populations?[178]

Globalization

Such questions about the impact of technology present a contrast to the ethical issues involved in pediatric oncology trials in low-income countries.[179] The cure rates of many diseases in children differ substantially between high-income and low-income countries.[180] The interventions that have the greatest impact in such countries are often not therapies per se but are rather aimed at reducing the substantial relapse rate caused by, for example, abandonment of treatment—the main cause of treatment failure in low-income countries. Remedial interventions

---

> **Box 74-2 Genetic Information as Defined by the Genetic Information Nondiscrimination Act of 2008**
>
> - An individual's genetic tests (including genetic tests done as part of a research study).
> - Genetic tests of the individual's family members (defined as dependents and up to and including fourth-degree relatives).
> - Genetic tests of any fetus of an individual or family member who is a pregnant woman, and genetic tests of any embryo legally held by an individual or family member utilizing assisted reproductive technology.
> - The manifestation of a disease or disorder in family members (family history).
> - Any request for, or receipt of, genetic services or participation in clinical research that includes genetic services (genetic testing, counseling, or education) by an individual or family member.
> - Genetic information does not include information about the sex or age of any individual.

From Office for Human Research Protections, Department of Health and Human Resources: Genetic Information Nondiscrimination Act of 2008. Accessed June 10, 2014 at www.hhs.gov/ohrp/policy/gina.pdf.

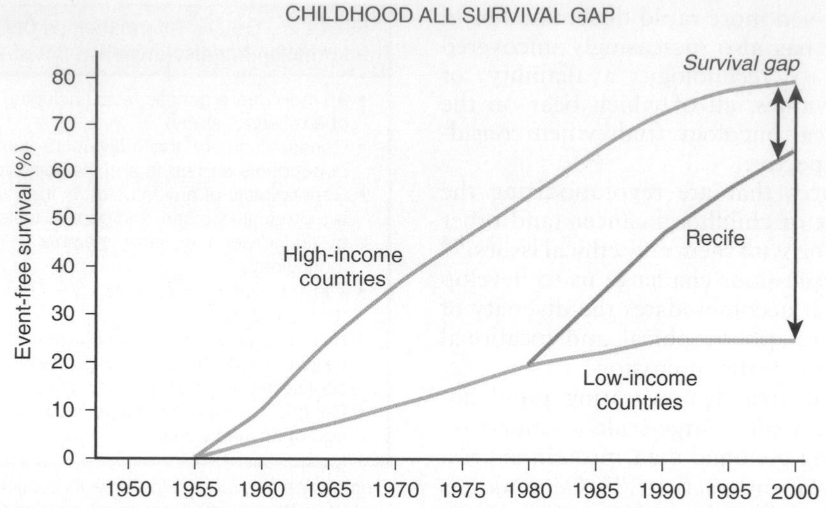

CHILDHOOD ALL SURVIVAL GAP

Figure 74-8 Five-year event-free survival of children with acute lymphoblastic leukemia in high-income countries versus low-income countries. Interventions to reduce the loss of patients to follow-up (e.g., making work available near the hospital so the parents are able to make sufficient income to feed other children) increased the survival rate in Recife, Brazil. *(Modified from Howard SC: Delivering global oncology care. Accessed June 10, 2014 at* http://www.cure4kids.org/public/873.*)*

can have a significant impact.[181] St. Jude Children's Research Hospital collaborated with a pediatric cancer center in Recife, Brazil, to reduce abandonment of therapy by providing family support such as housing, work, and food, and the 5-year event-free survival rate of children with acute lymphoblastic leukemia rose from 32% in the 1980s to 63% in 2000 (Fig. 74-8). Similarly, in El Salvador, the 4-year survival rate for children with acute lymphoblastic leukemia increased from 5% to 46% for high-risk cases and 69% for standard-risk cases.[182] Such success has underscored the promise of international collaborative clinical care and research for children with cancer. Many challenges remain, however.

One important challenge is that of ethical oversight of international research in pediatric oncology. Researchers in low-income countries often have little or no access to a functional research ethics committee. However institutions in high-income countries require (in part under the guidance of federal regulations) that adequate ethical oversight be in place as a prerequisite for cooperative clinical research. Collaborative research that uses the strategy of "twinning" institutions in high-income countries with those in low-income countries can produce important advances, as previously described, but the lack of ethical oversight can preclude these collaborations. Researchers cannot report such work in high-profile journals. The International Committee of Medical Journal Editors requires that reports of research involving human subjects document established mechanisms of human subject protection.

The Council for International Organizations of Medical Sciences guidelines state that researchers and institutions in high-income countries sponsoring research in low-income countries have an ethical obligation to improve the capacity for human participant protection in these countries. However in a survey of 203 clinical researchers in low-income countries, 44% reported that their studies were not reviewed by the country's ministry

or department of health, and 25% reported that their studies underwent no ethical review by a research ethics committee, IRB, or ministry or department of health.[183]

Federal regulations require that clinical trials conducted in low-income countries in collaboration with U.S. institutions must meet the ethical standards for trials based in the United States. However within the framework of these ethical standards, the research procedures can be adapted to local needs, conditions, and culture.[184] Advancing the development of research ethics in developing countries will open future possibilities for international collaboration that can increase the survival of children with cancer worldwide. Such trials do not necessarily require advanced technology to address the root causes of the disparate survival rates of children in low-income versus high-income countries. Addressing this disparity is itself an ethical imperative.

Although performing clinical trials in impoverished countries in an ethically justifiable manner is laudable, it fails to address the issue of whether the results of such studies will be able to be used to practically benefit future patients. For example within the confines of a trial in a developing country, the sponsor may provide the drugs free of charge to the subjects. However once the trial was complete and, say, the experimental arm was proven to be a significant improvement over the control arm of a phase III study for leukemia, would the expensive agents required to bestow the benefits of the therapy be available for future patients to receive and hence gain the advantages of such treatment? It is unlikely that multiple pharmaceutical companies would continue to make their products available without cost in perpetuity. Another approach that has been suggested is to perform trials with truncated versions of the "first world" model in an attempt to discern if less expensive and perhaps simpler options exist to obtain similar therapeutic outcomes. Of course this would be adjusting treatment to acknowledge the reality of the clinical situations in poor countries and hoping to transmit some (rather than no) benefit, but it also preserves an altered standard of care for people (patients) who already endure the excessive burdens associated with poverty.[185,186] In addition the enactment of the (U.S.) Pediatric Exclusivity Provision, which provides a financial incentive to drug companies to study agents in children that have heretofore only been approved in adults, has generated a large amount of international research, but it is unclear whether the subjects and future children for whom the drugs are appropriate but who live outside the home countries of these pharmaceutical companies will continue to benefit.[187,188] How this situation will ultimately settle out and what the landscape will look like remain to be resolved.[189,190]

CONCLUSION

Pediatric clinical trials present some of the most challenging ethical issues in modern medicine. Children are inherently vulnerable, and yet they are in need of the best, most effective, and least toxic therapies. Much is at stake in childhood cancer. New therapies are developed through research, and yet in pediatric trials, the person who is experiencing the risk is not the same person who is deciding whether the child participates. Many questions will require further thought and discussion and empiric research for the questions amenable to such approaches. Children do not have legal status as decision makers, and yet persons who care for children in pediatric clinical trials know how mature a child's perception can be, even that of a young child. What weight should be given to their opinions? More globally, how should we respond to the disparity of wealth in prioritizing pediatric research goals, even within the boundaries of a developed nation? How should we navigate cultural and political differences that influence the ethical considerations in international clinical trials?

Advancing excellent care of children around the world who have catastrophic diseases such as cancer depends upon clinical trials. Good clinical trials require ethical decision making at every level. Two questions regarding advances in therapy for childhood cancer must always be asked at the same time: "What *can* be done next?" and "What *should* be done next?" The means for answering the first question is scientific. The means for answering the second question is often more philosophical, drawing on many sources of wisdom and insight that are not intrinsically scientific in their approach. History has taught us that scientific advances without ethical considerations can become horrific. Similarly, wisdom without scientific advances cannot further the effort to cure sick children. Medical science committed to ethical research offers the best possibility for continuing to advance the care of children with cancer.

References available online at ExpertConsult.

KEY REFERENCES

2. Smith MA, Seibel NL, Altekruse SF, et al: Outcomes for children and adolescents with cancer: challenges for the twenty-first century. *J Clin Oncol* 28:2625–2634, 2010.

Incidence, survival, and mortality data for childhood cancers were analyzed in this article to provide an overview of current statistics to examine the impact of past research discoveries as a means to direct future research.

25. Simon C, Eder M, Raiz P, et al: Informed consent for pediatric leukemia research: clinician perspectives. *Cancer* 92:691–700, 2001.

Clinicians from five major medical centers were interviewed to learn their perspectives on the informed consent process for a pediatric leukemia trial. Clinicians' race, gender, and experience practicing were correlated with several items. Clinicians provided their view of the informed consent process and provided suggestions for improvement.

27. Kupst MJ, Patenaude AF, Walco GA, et al: Clinical trials in pediatric cancer: parental perspectives on informed consent. *J Pediatr Hematol Oncol* 25:787–790, 2003.

Parents of children newly diagnosed with cancer were interviewed to learn their perspective on the informed consent process for a clinical trial. Recollection for items such as diagnosis, treatment, and general statistics were high, but understanding of certain aspects of clinical trials was low.

28. Kodish E, Eder M, Noll RB, et al: Communication of randomization in childhood leukemia trials. *JAMA* 291:470–475, 2004.

This report analyzed physicians' explanations of and parents' understanding of randomizations in randomized clinical trials for childhood leukemia. Physicians explained randomization in most cases, but half of the parents did not understand the concept. The presence of a nurse and discussing specific aspects of the clinical trial were shown to increase the understanding of randomization, and parents who did not understand randomization were likely to be of the racial minority and lower socioeconomic status.

39. Kimberly MB, Hoehn KS, Feudtner C, et al: Variation in standards of research compensation and child assent practices: a comparison of 69 institutional review board-approved informed permission and assent forms for 3 multicenter pediatric clinical trials. *Pediatrics* 117(5):1706–1711, 2006.

This study was carried out to review child participant assent and compensation by looking at informed permission, assent, and consent forms. These forms were found to offer compensation in three instances: reimbursement for travel and food expenses, for inconveniencing the participant, and for the participant's time. Compensation varied between $0 and $1400. Most of the forms included assent documentation, and a little over half included a separate form written for children and specified at which age to provide assent.

50. Brody JL, Scherer DG, Annett RD, et al: Voluntary assent in biomedical research with adolescents: a comparison of parent and adolescent views. *Ethics Behav* 13:79–95, 2003.

Parent and adolescent perspectives on an asthma research vignette, including a final decision of whether or not to participate, were compared; 74% of the time parents and their children agreed on research participation, with both claiming to be the responsible party for the decision.

53. Wendler D, Emanuel EJ: What is a "minor" increase over minimal risk? *J Pediatr* 147(5):575–578, 2005.

The additional protections for children involved in research require the interpretation and application of three different levels of risk: minimal risk, minor increase over minimal risk, and more than a minor increase over minimal risk. Wide variability exists in the categorization of various research procedures according to these levels of risk. Noting that the federal regulations do not define a minor increase over minimal risk, the authors propose that this level of risk be interpreted as socially acceptable risks that are nevertheless greater than the risks ordinarily encountered by healthy children (i.e., minimal risk).

55. Nelson RM, Ross LF: In defense of a single standard of research risk for all children. *J Pediatr* 147:565–566, 2005.

In response to the article on minor risk by Wendler and Emanuel[53] (2005), this article argues that the ethical justification for this standard appears tautological, endorsing those risks that are "acceptable" to society and rejecting those that are "unacceptable" to society without explaining why certain risks would or would not be considered socially acceptable. As an alternative, the authors believe that the "scrupulous parent" standard is ethically justifiable and incorporates both minimal risk and a minor increase over minimal risk within a uniform standard that should be applicable to all children.

59. Kim A, Fox E, Warren K, et al: Characteristics and outcome of pediatric patients enrolled in phase I oncology trials. *Oncologist* 13:679–689, 2008.

    Analyses presented in this article aimed to define characteristics, toxicity risk, and outcomes of pediatric phase I trial participants. A higher risk for a dose-limiting toxicity was associated with drug dose and prior radiation, and the median survival rate was 5 months from the time of subject enrollment.

62. Maurer SH, Hinds PS, Spunt SL, et al: Decision making by parents of children with incurable cancer who opt for enrollment on a phase I trial compared with choosing a do not resuscitate/terminal care option. *J Clin Oncol* 20:3292–3298, 2010.

    Decision making for parents who just enrolled their child on a phase I trial and those who had chosen a do not resuscitate order or terminal care were compared. They were asked for the rationale of their decision, how they define a good parent, and what clinician behaviors supported this definition. Both groups desired clinician support and believed a good parent was supportive, present, and sacrificed for the child. Participants who chose a clinical trial indicated that they felt compelled to continue with care, whereas the other group expressed quality of life concerns.

66. Tomlinson D, Bartels U, Hendershot E, et al: Factors affecting treatment choices in paediatric palliative care: comparing parents and health professionals. *Eur J Cancer* 47:2182–2187, 2011.

    Factors influencing parents' and health care professionals' decision making for chemotherapy or supportive care in pediatric palliative care were compared. Parents rated hope, increased survival time, and the child's quality of life as most important to their decision, which were significantly higher than the physicians' ratings. Physicians placed a higher importance on the family's financial considerations.

71. Miller FG, Brody H: A critique of clinical equipoise. Therapeutic misconception in the ethics of clinical trials. *Hastings Cent Rep* 33:19–28, 2003.

    A predominant ethical view holds that physician-investigators should conduct their research with therapeutic intent. Because a physician offering a therapy would not prescribe second-rate treatments, the experimental intervention and the best proven therapy should appear equally effective. "Clinical equipoise" is necessary. The authors argue that this perspective is flawed, that the ethics of research and of therapy are fundamentally different, and that clinical equipoise should be abandoned.

76. Cousino MK, Zyzanski SJ, Yamokoski AD, et al: Communicating and understanding the purpose of pediatric phase I cancer trials. *J Clin Oncol* 30:4367–4372, 2012.

    Parents of children enrolled in a phase I clinical trial were interviewed and their responses were analyzed for understanding of three core components of a phase I trial: dose escalation, dose limiting toxicity, and safety. Physician disclosure was also measured. The child was present in 83 of the 85 conferences analyzed. Only a third of parents exhibited understanding of the scientific goals, and another third exhibited no understanding. Parents of a higher socioeconomic status and racial majority status were more likely to understand. Physician explanation of goals were associated with parent understanding but were not explained in all cases.

77. Marshall PA, Magtanong RV, Leek AC, et al: Negotiating decisions during informed consent for pediatric phase I oncology trials. *J Empir Res Hum Res Ethics* 7:51–59, 2012.

    Sixteen informed consent conferences for a pediatric phase I trial were examined to identify communication steps and what influences the negotiation. It was found that families and patients attempt to gain control and autonomous decision making by negotiating microdecisions in drug logic and logistics and administration and/or scheduling, which unfold in a four-step process.

108. Kollek R, Petersen I: Disclosure of individual research results in clinico-genomic trials: challenges, classification and criteria for decision-making. *J Med Ethics* 37:271–275, 2011.

    Although an ethical obligation to report findings of clinical research to trial participants is increasingly recognized, it is unclear how such a process should be organized. The authors present a classification of different actors, processes, and data involved in the feedback of research results pertaining to an individual. They go on to discuss the types of difficulties that must be faced when returning individual research results to trial participants and present a stepwise model to trigger the individual feedback process.

121. MacLeod KD, Whitsett SF, Mash EJ, et al: Pediatric sibling donors of successful and unsuccessful hematopoietic stem cell transplants (HSCT): a qualitative study of their psychosocial experience. *J Pediatr Psychol* 28:223–230, 2003.

    This study was a qualitative review of the psychosocial experience of pediatric sibling donors' successful and unsuccessful hematopoietic stem cell transplants. Siblings who were in the unsuccessful transplant group had a higher negative impact, reported feelings of guilt, and were less likely to experience positive effects. According to both groups, psychological aspects were of greater importance than physical aspects.

126. Coleman DL, Rosoff PM: The authority of "mature minors" to consent to general medical treatment. *Pediatrics* 131:786–793, 2013.

    The law has developed a broad "mature minor exception" to the general requirement of parental consent in abortion cases and has additionally carved out numerous specific status-based and condition-based exceptions to that requirement. Because of this, it is not always easy for medical professionals who treat adolescents to ascertain the applicable law. In this article, the authors discuss the underlying differences between medical ethics and law that have caused some of the confusion in this area, and they set out the most current legal rules governing adolescent decision-making authority in general medical settings.

134. Sugarman J, Kaalund V, Kodish E, et al: Ethical issues in umbilical cord blood banking. Working Group on Ethical Issues in Umbilical Cord Blood Banking. *JAMA* 278:938–943, 1997.

    Umbilical cord blood (UCB) technology is increasingly important. In this article the authors argue for several important conclusions regarding UCB. UCB banking for autologous use is associated with even greater uncertainty than is banking for allogeneic use. Marketing practices for UCB banking in the private sector require close attention. There must be continued work to ensure that recruitment for banking and use of UCB are equitable. The process of obtaining informed consent for collection of UCB should begin before labor and delivery.

144. Baker JN, Barfield RC, Hinds PS, et al: A model to facilitate decision making in pediatric stem cell transplantation: the individualized care planning and coordination model. *Biol Blood Marrow Transplant* 13:245–254, 2007.

    The authors introduce the individualized care planning and coordination (ICPC) model as a practical approach to facilitate ethical and effective decision making in pediatric stem cell transplantation settings. The ICPC is a three-step model comprising (1) relationship—understanding the illness experience from the perspective of the patient and family, sharing relevant information, and assessing ongoing needs; (2) negotiation—prognosticating, establishing goals of care, and discussing treatment options; and (3) plan—generating a comprehensive plan of care that includes life and medical plans. Based on a foundation of a care of competence, empathy, compassion, communication, and quality, the ICPC model aims to diminish contentious family-staff interactions that can lead to mistrust and help guide treatment decision making.

148. Hilden JM, Emanuel EJ, Fairclough DL, et al: Attitudes and practices among pediatric oncologists regarding end-of-life care: results of the 1998 American Society of Clinical Oncology survey. *J Clin Oncol* 19:205–212, 2001.

    Members of the American Society of Clinical Oncology were surveyed to gain an understanding of the attitudes, practices, and challenges its members experience when caring for end-of-life care patients. Clinicians reported a lack of formal education in pediatric palliative care and a need for strong mentors. The absence of a palliative care team was reported as impeding quality care for patients and reducing the effectiveness of communication between clinicians and patients.

153. Whitney SN, Ethier AM, Fruge E, et al: Decision making in pediatric oncology: who should take the lead? The decisional priority in pediatric oncology model. *J Clin Oncol* 24:160–165, 2006.

    The authors propose a new model of decision making in pediatric oncology to reconcile the discrepancies that exist between how ethicists and clinicians view the decision-making process for patients. Emphasis is placed on distinguishing decisional priority from decisional authority and on having clinicians encourage parents to assume decisional priority for their child.

156. Curlin FA, Chin MH, Sellergren SA, et al: The association of physicians' religious characteristics with their attitudes and self-reported behaviors regarding religion and spirituality in the clinical encounter. *Med Care* 44:446–453, 2006.

The relationship between physicians' religious beliefs and their self-reported behaviors on religion and spirituality in the clinical setting was examined. Clinicians indicated that it was appropriate to discuss these topics when the patient initiates the discussion and that they often are encouraging of the patients' own beliefs and practices. Clinicians who indicate they are more religious are more likely to address religion and spirituality in the clinical setting.

158. Ecklund EH, Cadge W, Gage EA, et al: The religious and spiritual beliefs and practices of academic pediatric oncologists in the United States. *J Pediatr Hematol Oncol* 29:736–742, 2007.

The religious and spiritual beliefs of pediatric oncologists were compared with those of the general public, because it is recognized that religion and spirituality are important to the care of seriously ill patients. Many oncologists described themselves as spiritual, while also reporting that they did not have a religious identity.

160. Seale C: The role of doctors' religious faith and ethnicity in taking ethically controversial decisions during end-of-life care. *J Med Ethics* 36:677–682, 2010.

In this study the author compares ethnicity and religious faith in the medical and general United Kingdom populations and reports on their associations with ethically controversial decisions taken when providing care to dying patients. Based on the study's findings, the author advocates for greater acknowledgement of the relationship of doctors' values with clinical decision making.

164. Fagerlin A, Wang C, Ubel PA: Reducing the influence of anecdotal reasoning on people's health care decisions: is a picture worth a thousand statistics? *Med Decis Making* 25:398–405, 2005.

This study was designed to assess participants' decision making when given a quiz or pictograph versus anecdotal information and how heavily each was relied upon. The use and influence of anecdotal information decreased when participants were presented with statistical information in a pictograph.

165. Feigin RD: Prospects for the future of child health through research. *JAMA* 294:1373–1379, 2005.

Advances made possible through genomics, proteomics, and the application of nanosystem technology, coupled with a greater understanding of the influence of the environment on human genes, will enhance our ability to prevent, modify, or cure numerous childhood disorders. This article reviews some of the more pressing and important causes of morbidity and mortality in children, discusses the manner in which some of the newer technologies may be applied to investigations of these disorders, and offers predictions concerning the effect that new discoveries may have in ameliorating the morbid consequences of childhood diseases.

The author highlights the need to design and implement prospective long-term studies to determine the most effective ways to reduce the burden of preventable problems, which are rooted in societal issues.

172. Nowlan W: Human genetics. A rational view of insurance and genetic discrimination. *Science* 297:195–196, 2002.

The Human Genome Project has committed a portion of its annual budget to the study of the ethical, legal, and social implications (ELSI) of genetics research. The assertion that discrimination in health insurance is a real problem pervades the ELSI literature, despite compelling evidence that at worst the threat is theoretical. The author reviews this evidence and also argues that genetic discrimination in the area of life insurance is unlikely to become a significant social problem.

182. Howard SC, Pedrosa M, Lins M, et al: Establishment of a pediatric oncology program and outcomes of childhood acute lymphoblastic leukemia in a resource-poor area. *JAMA* 291:2471–2475, 2004.

The cure rate for childhood acute lymphoblastic leukemia (ALL) differs markedly between developed and developing countries. The authors assess the effect of a multidisciplinary team approach and protocol-based therapy on the event-free survival of children with ALL in an area with limited resources over 22 years. The 5-year event-free survival improved steadily with implementation of a range of changes over time. The authors conclude that the treatment of childhood ALL in a dedicated pediatric oncology unit using a comprehensive multidisciplinary team approach, protocol-based therapy, and local support and funding is associated with improved outcomes in a resource-poor area.

185. Glickman SW, McHutchison JG, Peterson ED, et al: Ethical and scientific implications of the globalization of clinical research. *N Engl J Med* 360:816–823, 2009.

Economic globalization is an important development of the past half century. The authors address several important questions related to this development. Who benefits from the globalization of clinical trials? What is the potential for exploitation of research subjects? Are trial results accurate and valid, and can they be extrapolated to other settings? In this article, they discuss recent trends in and underlying reasons for the globalization of clinical research, highlight important scientific and ethical concerns, and propose steps for the harmonization of international clinical research.

188. Pasquali SK, Burstein DS, Benjamin DK, et al: Globalization of pediatric research: analysis of clinical trials completed for pediatric exclusivity. *Pediatrics* 126:e687–e692, 2010.

This study was conducted to assess the setting in which pediatric research is conducted and its influence in the globalization of pediatric research. Studies under the U.S. Pediatric Exclusivity Provision were included that reported trial data between 1998 and 2007. Fifty-four countries were represented in conducting pediatric research, and the majority of published research was conducted at locations outside the United States.

Reference Values in Infancy and Childhood

Carlo Brugnara

APPENDIX 1   Hematologic Values* in Normal Fetuses at Different Gestational Ages

Week of Gestation	Hemoglobin (g/dL)	RBCs (×10⁶/mL)	Hematocrit (%)	Mean Corpuscular Volume (fL)	Total WBCs (×10⁶/µL)	Corrected WBCs (×10⁶/µL)	Platelets (×10⁶/µL)
18-21 (N = 760)	11.69 ± 1.27	2.85 ± 0.36	37.3 ± 4.32	131.1 ± 11.0	4.68 ± 2.96	2.57 ± 0.42	234 ± 57
22-25 (N = 1200)	12.2 ± 1.6	3.09 ± 0.34	38.59 ± 3.94	125.1 ± 7.8	4.72 ± 2.82	3.73 ± 2.17	247 ± 59
26-29 (N = 460)	12.91 ± 1.38	3.46 ± 0.41	40.88 ± 4.4	118.5 ± 8.0	5.16 ± 2.53	4.08 ± 0.84	242 ± 69
>30 (N = 440)	13.64 ± 2.21	3.82 ± 0.64	43.55 ± 7.2	114.4 ± 9.3	7.71 ± 4.99	6.4 ± 2.99	232 ± 87

Modified from Forestier F, Daffos F, Catherine N, et al: Developmental hematopoiesis in normal human fetal blood. Blood 77:2360, 1991.
RBCs, Red blood cells; WBCs, white blood cells.
*Hematologic data obtained with a Coulter S plus II instrument. Total WBC count included nucleated red blood cells. Corrected WBC count included only WBCs, after subtracting the nucleated red cell component, based on a 100-cell manual differential.

APPENDIX 2   WBC Manual Differential Counts in Normal Fetuses at Different Gestational Ages

Week of Gestation	Lymphocytes (%)	Neutrophils (%)	Eosinophils (%)	Basophils (%)	Monocytes (%)	Nucleated RBCs (% of WBCs)
18-21 (N = 186)	88 ± 7	6 ± 4	2 ± 3	0.5 ± 1	3.5 ± 2	45 ± 86
22-25 (N = 230)	87 ± 6	6.5 ± 3.5	3 ± 3	0.5 ± 1	3.5 ± 2.5	21 ± 23
26-29 (N = 144)	85 ± 6	8.5 ± 4	4 ± 3	0.5 ± 1	3.5 ± 2.5	21 ± 67
>30 (N = 172)	68.5 ± 15	23 ± 15	5 ± 3	0.5 ± 1	3.5 ± 2	17 ± 40

From Forestier F, Daffos F, Catherine N, et al: Developmental hematopoiesis in normal human fetal blood. Blood 77:2360, 1991.
RBCs, Red blood cells; WBCs, white blood cells.

APPENDIX 3   Hematologic Values for Cord Blood (Vaginal Delivery and Cesarean Section*)

Characteristic	Study Sample (N = 167)		Vaginal Delivery (N = 63)		Cesarean Section (N = 104)		P-value[2]
	Median	Range	Median	Range	Median	Range	
WBC (×10^9 per l)	15.1	5.54-39.7	18.4	12.0-34.1	13.6	8.54-39.7	<0.0001
RBC (×10^{12} per l)	4.7	3.46-6.62	4.78	3.89-6.30	4.62	3.46-6.62	NS
Hb (g l^{-1})	174	130-234	176	140-230	171	130-234	NS
Hct (%)	53.6	40.1-73.1	54.7	41.9-73.1	52.6	40.1-72.2	NS
MCV (fl)	112	97.7-127	114	105-127	112	97.7-125	NS
MCH (pg)	36.5	31.4-41	36.5	31.4-41	36.6	32-39.9	NS
MCHC (g l^{-1})	324	303-359	323	308-359	324	303-344	NS
RDW (%)	17.4	14.2-23.6	17.4	14.9-23.6	17.4	14.2-23.3	NS
PLT (×10^9 per l)	270	161-607	297	169-607	254	161-424	0.0053
MPV (fl)	8.7	7.5-11.5	8.7	7.7-11.4	8.8	7.5-11.5	NS
Plateletcrit (%)	0.24	0.15-0.48	0.26	0.15-0.48	0.23	0.15-0.36	0.0056
CD34+ cells (×10^6 per l)	43.9	7.14-253	47.7	15.9-253	39.9	7.14-120	0.007

From Eskola M, Juutistenaho S, Aranko K, et al: J Perinatol 2011; 258–262. Data obtained with Sysmex K-1000 analyzer (Sysmex, Kobe Japan).

Hb, Hemoglobin; Hct, hematocrit; MCH, mean corpuscular hemoglobin; MCHC, mean corpuscular hemoglobin concentration; MCV, mean corpuscular volume; MPV, mean platelet volume; NS, not significant; plateletcrit, MPV × PLT; PLT, platelet; RBC, red blood cell; RDW, red blood cell distribution width; WBC, white blood cell.

*aP-values of the differences between vaginal delivery and cesarean section. The concentrations were standardized to exclude the varying effect of the anticoagulant.

APPENDIX 4   Hematologic Values* for Normal Cord Blood

	Mean ± SD		Mean ± SD
Red Blood Cells		% HYPER (MCHC >41 g/dL)	0.6 ± 0.3
Hb (g/dL)	15.3 + 1.3	% MICRO (MCV <61 fL)	0.8 ± 0.3
Hct (%)	49 ± 5	% MACRO (MCV >120 fL)	31.8 ± 9.7
RBC (×10^6/μL)	4.3 ± 0.4	**Reticulocytes**	
MCV (fL)	112 ± 6	%	3.63 ± 1.11
MCH (pg)	36.2 ± 2.2	Absolute reticulocytes (×10^9/L)	156.1 ± 47.7
MCHC (g/dL)	30.9 ± 1.3	MCVr (fL)	125.8 ± 7.3
CHCM (g/dL)	30.4 ± 1.2	CHCMr (g/dL)	25.6 ± 1.2
% HYPO (MCHC <28 g/dL)	17.3 ± 11.9	CHr (pg)	31.3 ± 1.4

Modified from Diagne I, Archambeaud MP, Diallo D, et al: Parametres erythrocytaires et reservés en fer dans le sang du cordon. Arch Fr Pediatr 2:208, 1995; and from G Tchernia, personal communication. Data obtained in 142 specimens with H*2 Technicon analyzer.

CHCM, Cell hemoglobin concentration mean; CHCMr, reticulocyte cell hemoglobin concentration mean; CHr, reticulocyte hemoglobin content; Hb, hemoglobin; Hct, hematocrit; % HYPER, % hyperchromic red cells; % HYPO, % hypochromic red cells; % MACRO, % macrocytic red cells; MCH, mean corpuscular hemoglobin; MCHC, mean corpuscular hemoglobin concentration; MCV, mean corpuscular volume; MCVr, reticulocyte mean corpuscular volume; % MICRO, microcytic red cells; RBC, red blood cell; SD, standard deviation.

*Values obtained with Technicon H*2 and H*3 Hematology analyzers (Bayer Diagnostics) in neonates delivered at term with weight ≥2500 g.

APPENDIX 5   Red Cell and Reticulocyte Indices, Serum Iron Status Markers in Cord Blood

Parameter	Mean	SD	Reference Range*
Blood Count and Cellular Indices			
Hb, g/L	159	15	146-189
HCT, L/L	0.49	0.05	0.44-0.58
MCV, fL	109	4	102-118
MCVr, fL	124	6	115-136
MCH, pg	35	1	33-38
MCHC, g/L	325	10	306-342
%Retic, %	4.0	0.8	2.6-5.4
IRF-H, %	24.1	7.8	10.2-40.0
CHm, pg	34.9	1.3	32.5-37.2
CHr, pg	35.6	1.3	33.1-38.6
%HYPOm, %	3.0	3.0	0.4-9.9
%HYPOr, %	42.0	15.6	18.3-76.8
Serum Measurements			
TfR, mg/L	2.0	0.7	1.2-4.0
Ferritin, μg/L	198	137	45-636
TfR-F index	0.95	0.43	0.49-2.1
Iron, μmol/L	27.4	7.7	12.2-42.1
Transferrin, g/L	2.0	0.4	1.2-2.9
TfSat, %	55	19	21-111

From Ervasti M, Kotisaari S, Sankilampi U, et al: The relationship between red blood cell and reticulocyte indices and serum markers of iron status in the cord blood of newborns. Clin Chem Lab Med 45:1000–1003, 2007. Hematologic data obtained in 199 full-term newborn infants with a ADVIA 120 analyzer (Siemens Diagnostic Solutions, Terrytown, NY).

CHm, Cellular hemoglobin in red blood cells; CHr, cellular hemoglobin in reticulocytes; Hb, hemoglobin; HCT, hematocrit; %HYPOm, percentage of hypochromic red blood cells; %HYPOr, percentage of hypochromic reticulocytes; IRF-H, high immature reticulocyte fraction; MCH, mean cell hemoglobin; MCHC, mean cell hemoglobin concentration; MCV, mean cell volume of red blood cells; MCVr, mean cell volume of reticulocytes; %Retic, proportion of reticulocytes; TfR, transferrin receptor; TfR-F index, transferrin receptor/log (ferritin); TfSat, transferrin saturation.

*For reference range calculations, only samples in which Hb was greater than 146 g/L were included.

APPENDIX 6   Erythroblast and Leukocyte Counts in Umbilical Cord Blood*

Type of Delivery	Erythroblast Count (×10⁹/L)	Leukocyte Count (×10⁹/L)
Spontaneous, vaginal (N = 55)	0.75 (0.0-5.3)	13.8 (7.25-48.0)
Elective cesarean section (N = 39)	0.30 (0.0-0.49)	10.6 (6.2-17.7)
Emergency cesarean section (N = 55)	1.10 (0.0-15.9)	13.5 (4.2-40.3)

From Thilaganthan B, Athansasiou S, Ozmen S, et al: Umbilical cord blood erythroblast count as an index of intrauterine hypoxia. Arch Dis Child 70:F192, 1994.

*Values are expressed as mean (range). Erythroblast counts were significantly higher in the spontaneous vaginal and emergency cesarean section groups compared with the elective cesarean group.

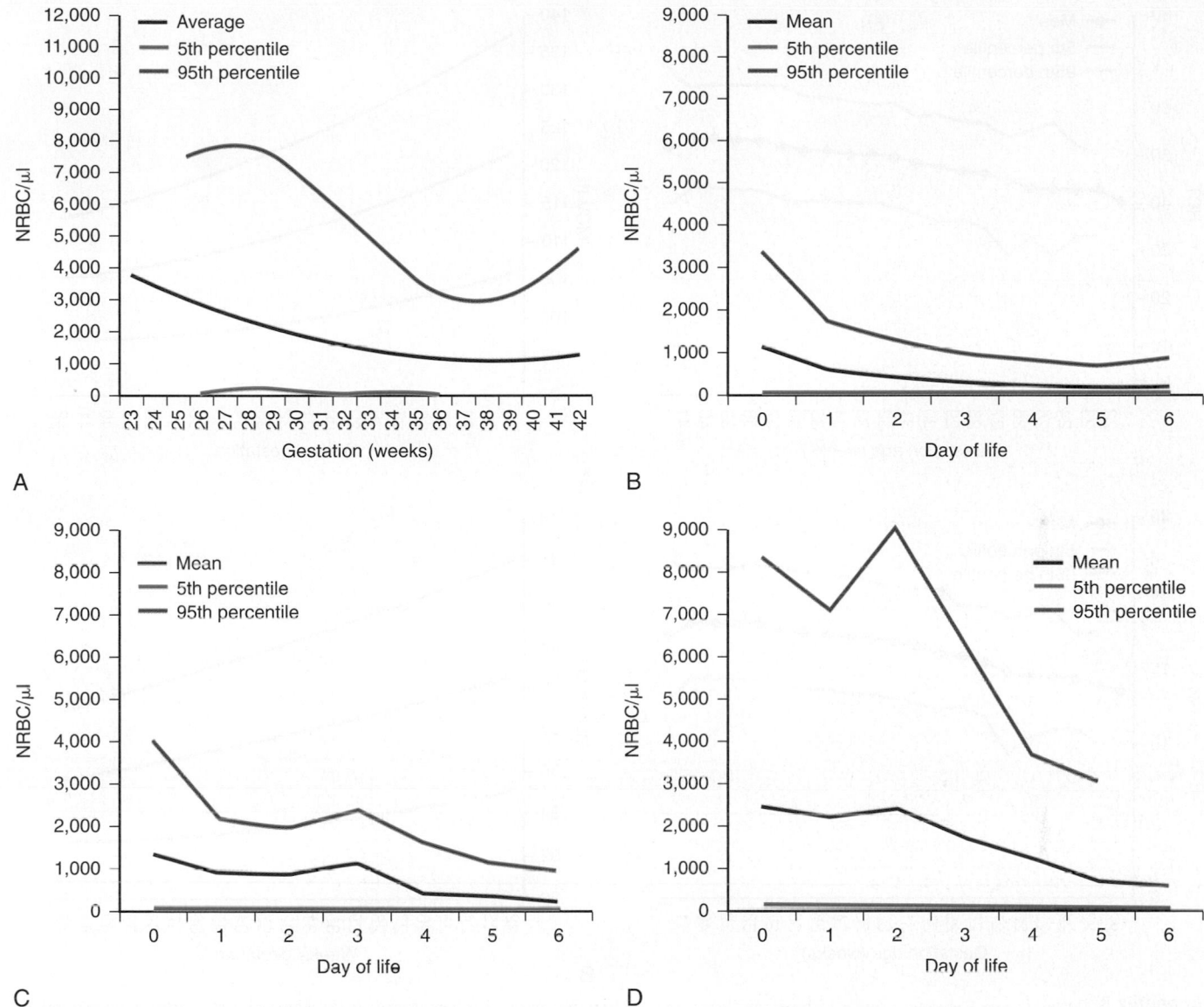

Appendix 7 A, Reference ranges for blood concentrations of NRBC on the day of birth are displayed according to gestational age. The lower and upper lines represent the 5% and 95% limits, and the middle line represents the mean value. B-D, Reference ranges for blood concentrations of NRBC during the first 7 days following birth are shown. The lower and upper lines represent the 5% and 95% limits, and the middle line represents the mean value. B, Reference range for neonates 1 to 36 weeks' gestation at birth. C, Range for neonates 30 to 35 weeks' gestation at birth. D, Range for neonates 1 to 30 weeks' gestation at birth. *(From Christensen RD, Henry E, Andres RL et al. Reference ranges for blood concentrations of nucleated red blood cells in neonates. Neonatol 99:289–294, 2011.)*

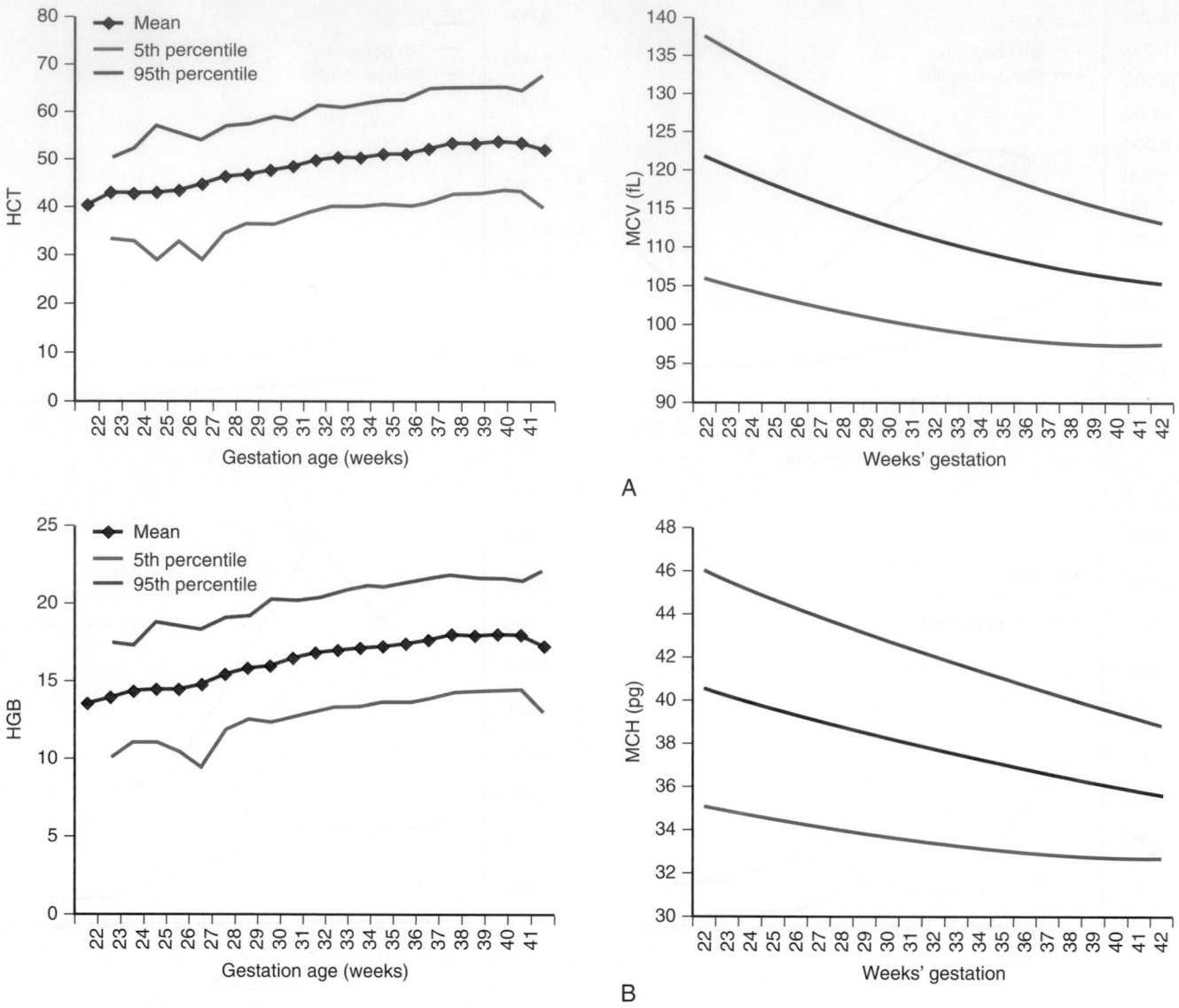

Appendix 8 *Left Column*, Reference ranges (5th percentile, mean, and 95th percentile) for hematocrits *(top)*, Hemoglobin *(bottom)*, both obtained during the first 6 hours after birth among patients 22 to 42 weeks gestation. *Right Column (top and bottom)*, Expected range of values for mean corpuscular volume (MCV, *a*) and mean corpuscular hemoglobin (MCH, *b*) for neonates on the first day after birth. The upper and lower boundaries incorporate 95% of the measured values. *(Left column, From Christensen RD, Henry E, Jopling J, et al: The CBC: reference ranges for neonates. Semin Perinatol 33:3–11, 2009; Right column, From Christensen RD, Jopling J Henry E et al. The erythrocyte indices of neonates, defined using data from over 12000 patients in a multihospital health care system. J Perinatol 28:24–28, 2008.)*

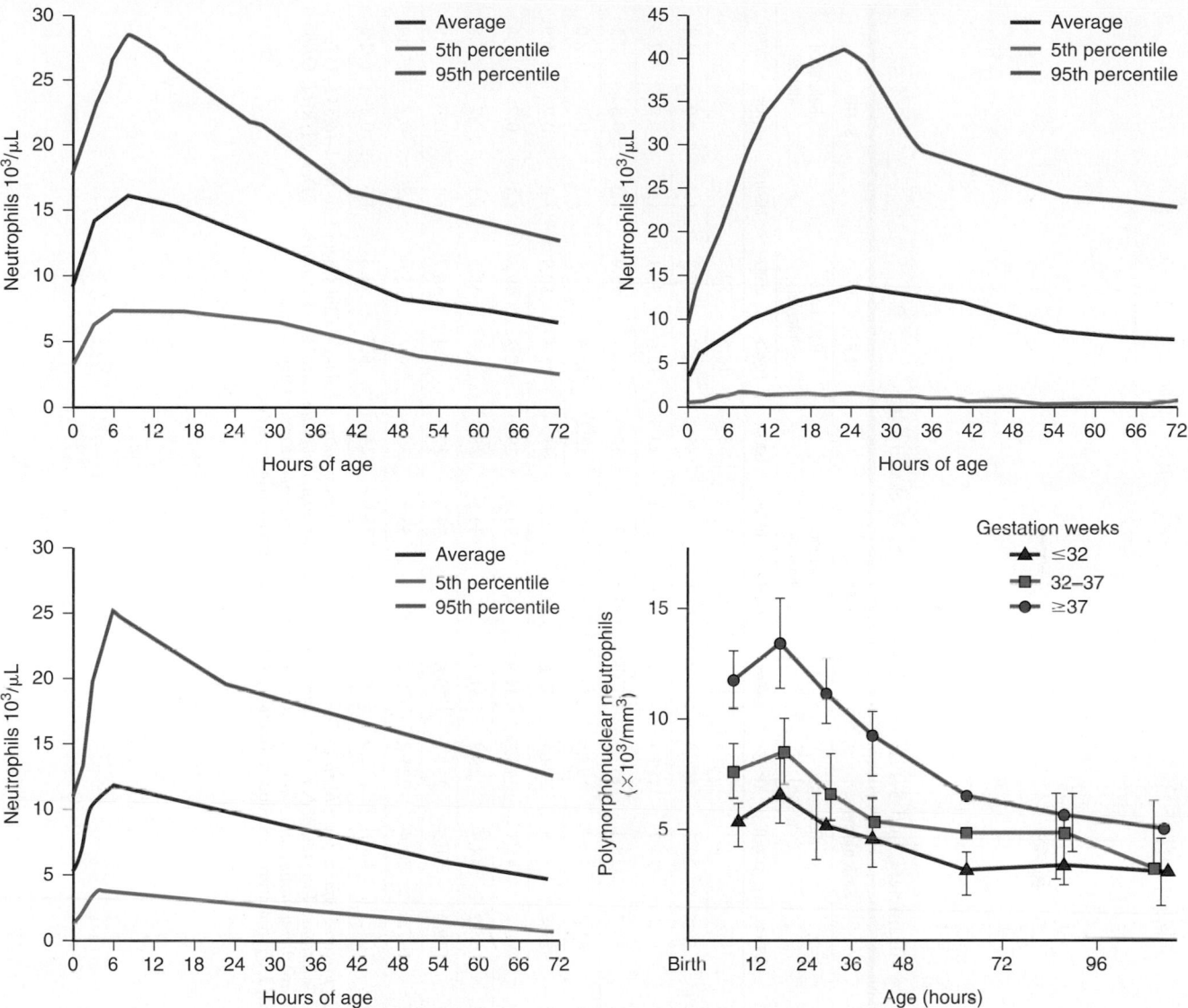

Appendix 9 *Top Left,* Reference ranges for blood neutrophil concentrations during the first 72 hours after the birth of term and near-term (36 weeks' gestation) neonates. A total of 12149 values were obtained for the analysis. The 5th percentile, the mean, and the 95th percentile values are shown. *Bottom Left,* Reference ranges for blood neutrophil concentration during the first 72 hours after the birth of 28 to 36 weeks' gestation preterm neonates. A total of 8896 values were obtained for the analysis. The 5th percentile, the mean, and the 95th percentile values are shown. *Top Right,* Reference ranges for blood neutrophil concentration during the first 72 hours after the birth of 28 weeks' gestation preterm neonates. A total of 852 values were obtained for the analysis. The 5th percentile, the mean, and the 95th percentile values are shown. *Bottom right,* Changes in polymorphonuclear neutrophils after birth in three groups with different gestational ages. Total white blood cell (WBC) counts were obtained with a Coulter S analyzer; manual differential counts were performed on 200 nucleated cells. *(Top and Bottom Left and Top Right, From Christensen RD, Henry E, Jopling J, et al: The CBC: reference ranges for neonates. Semin Perinatol 33:3–11, 2009; Bottom Right, Modified from Coulombel L, Dehan M, Tchernia G, et al: The number of polymorphonuclear leukocytes in relation to gestational age in the newborn. Acta Paediatr Scand 68:709, 1979.)*

APPENDIX 10   Reference Ranges for Hb, HCt, Reticulocyte Parameters, and S-TfR During the First 15 Weeks of Life

Age, Week	Hb			Hct			Reticulocyte			CHr			IRF			S-TfR		
	MEAN	Reference Interval LOWER	UPPER	MEAN	Reference Interval LOWER	UPPER	MEAN	Reference Interval LOWER	UPPER	MEAN	Reference Interval LOWER	UPPER	MEAN	Reference Interval LOWER	UPPER	MEAN	Reference Interval LOWER	UPPER
0.5	150.5	101.8	222.4	0.45	0.30	0.65				35.7	31.5	39.9	36.6	13.5	59.7			
1.5	138.7	97.9	196.3	0.41	0.29	0.58	59.5	20.2	175.6	35.0	31.1	38.9	35.5	13.7	57.2	1.4	0.9	2.4
2.5	128.8	94.0	176.5	0.38	0.28	0.52	66.8	24.7	181.1	34.3	30.6	38.1	34.3	13.6	55.1	1.3	0.8	2.3
3.5	120.6	90.0	161.5	0.36	0.27	0.47	74.1	29.2	187.9	33.7	30.1	37.4	33.3	13.1	53.4	1.3	0.8	2.1
4.5	113.8	86.2	150.3	0.34	0.26	0.44	81.2	33.7	195.8	33.1	29.5	36.7	32.2	12.4	52.1	1.2	0.7	2.0
5.5	108.3	82.5	142.1	0.32	0.25	0.42	87.9	37.8	204.3	32.6	29.0	36.2	31.3	11.6	50.9	1.2	0.7	1.9
7.0	101.9	77.8	133.7	0.30	0.23	0.39	96.7	43.1	216.7	31.9	28.3	35.5	29.9	10.3	49.6	1.1	0.7	1.8
9.0	96.9	73.5	127.7	0.29	0.22	0.38	105.2	48.4	228.8	31.2	27.5	34.8	28.4	8.6	48.1	1.1	0.7	1.8
11.0	94.9	71.7	125.7	0.28	0.21	0.37	109.0	51.3	231.9	30.6	26.9	34.3	27.0	7.4	46.7	1.1	0.7	1.9
13.0	96.1	72.6	127.3	0.28	0.21	0.37	107.6	51.4	225.2	30.2	26.5	33.9	25.9	6.7	45.0	1.2	0.7	2.0
15.0	100.5	75.9	133.1	0.30	0.22	0.39	101.2	48.1	212.9	30.0	26.4	33.6	24.9	6.7	43.3	1.3	0.8	2.2

From Mäkela E, Takal TI, Suomine P, et al: Hematological parameters in preterm infants from birth to 16 weeks of age with reference to iron balance. Clin Chem Lab Med 46:551–557, 2008. Hematologic data obtained with ADVIA 120, Siemens Medical Solutions, Tarrytown, NY. S-TfR measured with an automated immunoturbidimetric methos (IDeA sTfR-IT, Orion Diagnostica), Espoo, Finland. Ferritin assayed with Elecsys ferritin electrochemiluminescence immunoassay on a Modular E analyzer (Roche Diagnostics).
CHr, Reticulocyte hemoglobin content; Hb, hemoglobin; Hct, hematocrit; IRF, immature reticulocyte fraction; S-Tfr, soluble transferrin receptor.

APPENDIX 11   Reference Ranges for Ferritin During the First 15 Weeks of Life

| Age, Week | Ferritin* | | | Ferritin, No Transfusions* | | |
| | MEAN | Reference Interval | | MEAN | Reference Interval | |
		LOWER	UPPER		LOWER	UPPER
1.5	221.4	77.0	636.8	215.5	73.5	631.6
2.5	199.9	65.6	609.2	178.5	56.9	559.8
3.5	180.4	52.8	616.5	149.2	43.9	507.2
4.5	162.8	41.4	640.2	125.9	34.1	465.4
5.5	147.0	32.3	668.4	107.2	26.8	429.7
7.0	126.0	22.6	702.3	85.7	19.2	382.1
9.0	102.6	14.9	708.7	65.7	13.3	324.6
11.0	83.5	10.6	659.1	52.3	10.1	271.7
13.0	68.0	8.2	563.0	43.2	8.3	224.0
15.0	55.3	6.9	444.8	37.0	7.5	182.9

From Mäkela E, Takal TI, Suomine P, et al: Hematologic parameters in preterm infants from birth to 16 weeks of age with reference to iron balance. Clin Chem Lab Med 46:551–557, 2008. Ferritin assayed with Elecsys ferritin electrochemiluminescence immunoassay on a Modular E analyzer (Roche Diagnostics).

*The information under the column "Ferritin" shows values calculated for the neonates who had not been transfused during the preceding 2 weeks of measurements. The information under the column "Ferritin, no transfusions" shows the values calculated for those neonates who had not been transfused at all (indicating ferritin level development in the most stable preterm neonates).

APPENDIX 12   Reference Ranges for CBC, Reticulocytes, Ferritin, and S-TfR During the First Year of Life in Preterm and Full-Term Infants

Age, Weeks	Hb, g/L		Hct		RBC count, ×10¹²/L		MCV, fL		MCH, pg		Retic, ×10⁹/L	
	Mean	95% RI	Mean	95% RI	Mean	95% RI	Mean	95% RI	Mean	95% RI	Mean	95% RI
Preterm												
20	112.2	92.0-136.8	0.327	0.271-0.395	4.03	3.15-4.92	81.6	73.2-90.0	28.1	25.2-31.0	77.4	39.0-153.5
25	116.8	98.7-138.1	0.340	0.287-0.401	4.27	3.48-5.07	80.1	72.3-88.0	27.7	24.8-30.5	69.7	36.7-132.5
30	120.8	103.6-140.9	0.351	0.300-0.411	4.47	3.70-5.25	79.0	71.2-86.7	27.3	24.4-30.3	64.1	34.3-119.6
35	124.3	106.7-144.7	0.360	0.309-0.421	4.64	3.83-5.44	78.1	70.1-86.0	27.1	24.0-30.2	60.1	32.4-111.8
40	127.0	108.5-148.6	0.368	0.315-0.431	4.76	3.92-5.60	77.5	69.3-85.7	26.9	23.7-30.1	57.6	30.9-107.2
45	129.0	109.6-151.8	0.374	0.319-0.438	4.85	3.98-5.71	77.3	68.9-85.6	26.8	23.5-30.0	56.3	30.1-105.1
50	130.2	110.3-153.6	0.378	0.323-0.442	4.89	4.03-5.75	77.3	69.0-85.6	26.7	23.6-29.9	56.1	30.0-105.2
55	130.6	111.1-153.6	0.380	0.326-0.442	4.90	4.07-5.73	77.6	69.6-85.7	26.8	23.7-29.8	57.2	30.3-107.7
60	130.2	112.0-151.3	0.379	0.329-0.437	4.87	4.11-5.62	78.2	70.7-85.8	26.9	24.0-29.7	59.4	31.1-113.5
Full-Term												
20	120.0	102.2-140.9	0.345	0.293-0.407	4.32	3.76-4.87	80.3	74.2-86.4	27.9	25.6-30.2	45.5	25.3-82.2
25	118.9	101.9-138.8	0.345	0.296-0.402	4.38	3.84-4.92	79.0	73.1-84.9	27.3	24.9-29.6	45.2	25.1-81.5
30	118.3	101.5-137.7	0.345	0.298-0.400	4.44	3.90-4.98	78.1	72.3-83.9	26.8	24.3-29.2	45.4	26.1-78.9
35	118.0	101.5-137.3	0.346	0.300-0.400	4.48	3.93-5.03	77.6	71.8-83.4	26.5	23.9-29.0	46.0	27.6-76.6
40	118.2	102.0-137.1	0.348	0.303-0.400	4.51	3.96-5.06	77.4	71.6-83.2	26.3	23.7-28.9	47.1	28.8-76.8
45	118.9	102.9-137.3	0.351	0.307-0.401	4.54	3.99-5.08	77.6	71.7-83.5	26.3	23.6-29.0	48.7	28.7-82.5
50	120.0	104.2-138.1	0.354	0.313-0.402	4.55	4.01-5.08	78.2	72.2-84.1	26.5	23.8-29.2	50.9	26.9-96.3
55	121.5	105.4-140.0	0.359	0.319-0.403	4.55	4.04-5.06	79.1	73.1-85.1	26.9	24.2-29.6	53.7	23.9-121.0

Age, Weeks	Ferritin, µg/L		S-TfR, mg/L		CHr, pg		WBC count, × 10⁹/L		Platelet count, × 10⁹/L	
	Mean	95% RI	Mean	95% RI	Mean	95% RI	Mean	95% RI	Mean	95% RI
Preterm										
20	37.8	7.37-193.9	1.52	1.07-2.16	29.8	26.6-33.1	9.48	5.63-16.0	478	294-777
25	30.1	7.48-120.8	1.54	1.10-2.15	29.6	26.4-32.8	9.60	5.73-16.1	465	290-744
30	24.7	7.06-86.6	1.56	1.12-2.16	29.4	26.2-32.7	9.71	5.82-16.2	452	286-714
35	21.1	6.41-69.5	1.57	1.14-2.17	29.3	26.0-32.6	9.83	5.92-16.3	439	280-687
40	18.6	5.80-59.9	1.59	1.16-2.19	29.2	25.9-32.6	9.94	6.01-16.5	427	274-663
45	17.1	5.41-53.8	1.61	1.17-2.21	29.2	25.8-32.6	10.1	6.09-16.6	415	268-642
50	16.2	5.25-49.8	1.63	1.18-2.25	29.3	25.8-32.7	10.2	6.17-16.8	403	260-623
55	15.9	5.31-47.5	1.65	1.18-2.30	29.4	25.8-32.9	10.3	6.24-17.0	391	252-607
60	16.2	5.44-47.9	1.67	1.18-2.36	29.5	25.9-33.2	10.4	6.31-17.2	380	244-593
Full-Term										
20	71.7	21.5-239.7	1.49	1.06-2.08	29.8	27.4-32.1	9.36	5.84-15.0	426	282-646
25	51.1	16.1-162.2	1.52	1.08-2.12	29.2	25.7-32.6	9.19	5.73-14.7	415	269-640
30	38.5	11.5-128.7	1.54	1.09-2.19	28.8	24.7-32.9	9.02	5.57-14.6	404	258-634
35	30.6	8.76-107.0	1.57	1.09-2.27	28.7	24.5-32.9	8.85	5.37-14.6	394	247-628
40	25.8	7.46-89.1	1.60	1.08-2.37	28.9	25.1-32.6	8.68	5.14-14.7	383	237-621
45	22.9	7.01-75.0	1.63	1.07-2.48	29.2	26.4-32.1	8.52	4.88-14.9	373	227-614
50	21.6	6.78-68.6	1.66	1.05-2.62	29.9	27.6-32.2	8.36	4.61-15.2	363	218-607
55	21.5	5.90-78.0	1.69	1.04-2.76	30.8	27.0-34.5	8.21	4.33-15.5	354	209-599

From Takale TI, Mäkelä E, Suomine P, et al: Blood Cell and iron status analytes of preterm and full-term infants from 20 weeks onward during the first year of life. Clin Chem Lab Med 48:1295–1301, 2010. Hematologic data obtained with ADVIA 120, Siemens Medical Solutions, Tarrytown, NY. S-TfR measured with an automated immunoturbidimetric methos (IDeA sTfR-IT, Orion Diagnostica), Espoo, Finland. Ferritin assayed with Elecsys ferritin electrochemiluminescence immunoassay on a Modular E analyzer (Roche Diagnostics).
CBC, Complete blood count; CHr, reticulocyte hemoglobin content; Hb, hemoglobin; Hct, hematocrit; MCH, mean corpuscular hemoglobin; MCV, mean corpuscular volume; RBC, red blood cell; Retic, reticulocyte; RI, reference interval; S-Tfr, soluble transferrin receptor; WBC, white blood cell.

Hematocrit (%)

Age Range	AA 2.5 M	2.5 F	50 M	50 F	95 M	95 F	97.5 M	97.5 F	MW 2.5 M	2.5 F	50 M	50 F	95 M	95 F	97.5 M	97.5 F
1	31.0		36.0		39.0		39.5		32.0		37.0		40.0		41.0	
2-3	32.0		36.0		39.0		39.5		33.0		37.0		40.5		41.0	
4-6	33.0		37.0		41.0		42.0		34.0		38.0		42.0		42.5	
7-10	34.0		38.0		42.0		42.0		35.0		39.5		43.5		45.0	
11-14	35.0	33.0	40.0	38.0	45.0	43.0	46.0	43.5	36.5		42.0	40.0	47.5	44.0	48.0	45.0
15-18	38.0	32.0	44.0	38.0	49.0	42.0	51.0	43.5	40.0	34.0	46.0	40.0	50.0	43.5	51.5	44.5

Hemoglobin (g/dL)

Age Range	AA 2.5 M	2.5 F	50 M	50 F	95 M	95 F	97.5 M	97.5 F	MW 2.5 M	2.5 F	50 M	50 F	95 M	95 F	97.5 M	97.5 F
1	10.4		12.0		13.1		13.2		10.5		12.5		13.7		13.9	
2-3	10.8		12.0		13.4		13.5		11.0		12.6		13.9		13.9	
4-6	11.0		12.5		14.0		14.1		11.7		12.9		14.2		14.2	
7-10	11.2		12.7		14.1		14.4		12.0		13.5		14.7		15.0	
11-14	11.8	10.6	13.6	12.9	15.2	14.4	15.4	14.7	12.6	12.3	14.3	13.7	16.0	14.9	16.1	15.0
15-18	12.9	10.7	14.9	12.8	16.5	14.2	16.7	14.6	13.7	11.5	15.4	13.7	17.0	14.9	17.2	15.0

Red blood cell count ($10^6/mm^3$)

Age Range	AA 2.5 M	2.5 F	50 M	50 F	95 M	95 F	97.5 M	97.5 F	MW 2.5 M	2.5 F	50 M	50 F	95 M	95 F	97.5 M	97.5 F
1	4.10		4.65		5.25		5.40		4.10		4.60		5.20		5.50	
2-3	4.00		4.50		5.30		5.50		4.00		4.50		5.05		5.10	
4-6	3.90		4.50		5.30		5.40		4.00		4.50		5.05		5.20	
7-10	4.00		4.50		5.25		5.45		4.05		4.60		5.20		5.30	
11-14	4.10	3.70	4.70	4.40	5.50	5.00	5.80	5.20	4.30	4.00	4.85	4.60	5.50	5.10	5.60	5.25
15-18	4.10	3.60	5.00	4.40	5.80	5.00	5.90	5.30	4.45	3.80	5.15	4.50	5.65	4.95	5.75	5.05

Mean cell volume (fL)

Age Range	AA 2.5 M	2.5 F	50 M	50 F	95 M	95 F	97.5 M	97.5 F	MW 2.5 M	2.5 F	50 M	50 F	95 M	95 F	97.5 M	97.5 F
1	63.0		77.0		87.0		88.0		71.0		79.5		84.0		85.5	
2-3	64.0		80.0		88.0		88.5		74.0		81.5		88.5		89.0	
4-6	67.0		82.5		89.0		90.5		77.0		84.0		90.0		90.5	
7-10	72.0		84.0		91.5		92.5		78.0		85.0		90.0		90.5	
11-14	73.0	71.0	85.5		93.5		95.0		80.0		87.0		92.5		93.5	
15-18	75.0	71.0	87.0		94.5		95.5		81.0		89.0		95.0		95.5	

Mean cell hemoglobin concentration (g/dL)

Age Range	AA 2.5 M	2.5 F	50 M	50 F	95 M	95 F	97.5 M	97.5 F	MW 2.5 M	2.5 F	50 M	50 F	95 M	95 F	97.5 M	97.5 F
1	32.3		33.4		34.8		35.0		32.4		34.0		35.0		35.1	
2-3	31.7		33.6		34.9		35.0		32.6		34.1		35.4		35.7	
4-6	31.8		33.8		35.2		35.4		32.9		34.2		35.5		35.7	
7-10	31.4		33.8		35.0		35.2		32.6		34.1		35.4		35.7	
11-14	31.7		33.7		34.8		34.8		32.6		34.0		35.1		35.1	
15-18	32.0		33.4		34.8		34.8		32.5		33.9		35.1		35.2	

Mean cell hemoglobin (pg)

Age Range	AA 2.5 M	2.5 F	50 M	50 F	95 M	95 F	97.5 M	97.5 F	MW 2.5 M	2.5 F	50 M	50 F	95 M	95 F	97.5 M	97.5 F
1	20.2		25.8		29.4		29.5		23.5		27.0		29.0		29.3	
2-3	21.0		26.7		29.9		30.8		24.5		28.0		30.0		30.3	
4-6	22.0		27.7		30.7		30.8		26.0		28.8		30.0		31.0	
7-10	23.3		28.3		31.2		31.6		26.3		29.0		31.0		31.2	
11-14	24.0	22.8	29.0		31.0	32.0	32.2		26.6		29.5		31.5		31.9	
15-18	24.2	22.9	29.3		32.0		32.8		27.0		30.2		32.5		32.8	

Red cell distribution width ($10^9/L$)

Age Range	AA 2.5 M	2.5 F	50 M	50 F	95 M	95 F	97.5 M	97.5 F	MW 2.5 M	2.5 F	50 M	50 F	95 M	95 F	97.5 M	97.5 F
1	11.5		13.4		15.6		15.9		11.8		13.1		15.5		17.0	
2-3	11.6		12.7		14.8		15.2		11.4		12.4		14.1		14.6	
4-6	11.4		12.4		13.7		15.1		11.4		12.2		13.2		13.5	
7-10	11.3		12.5		13.7		14.1		11.4		12.2		13.2		13.4	
11-14	11.4		12.4		14.0	14.5	16.0		11.3		12.2		13.4		13.6	
15-18	11.2		12.5		13.5	15.9	16.8	18.3	11.4		12.2		13.2	13.8	13.6	14.4

White blood cell count ($10^3/mm^3$)

Age Range	AA 2.5 M	2.5 F	50 M	50 F	95 M	95 F	97.5 M	97.5 F	MW 2.5 M	2.5 F	50 M	50 F	95 M	95 F	97.5 M	97.5 F
1	5.0		8.0		11.5		13.2		6.0		9.5		16.5		17.5	
2-3	4.0		6.8		10.0		11.0		5.5		8.0		12.0		13.0	
4-6	4.0		6.5		9.2		10.0		5.0		7.5		11.5		12.5	
7-10	3.3		6.0		9.3		11.4		4.5		7.3		11.0		11.5	
11-14	3.3		6.0		9.0		10.0		4.5		7.0		11.0		11.5	
15-18	3.0	4.0	5.5	6.3	9.0		9.7		5.1		7.0		11.0		12.0	

Neutrophil count ($10^3/mm^3$)

Age Range	AA 2.5 M	2.5 F	50 M	50 F	95 M	95 F	97.5 M	97.5 F	MW 2.5 M	2.5 F	50 M	50 F	95 M	95 F	97.5 M	97.5 F
1	1.0		2.6		4.6		4.6		1.5		3.1		6.2		7.4	
2-3	1.0		2.8		4.8		7.5		1.5		3.3		6.3		7.7	
4-6	1.0		2.8		5.2		5.8		1.7		3.5		6.7		7.9	
7-10	1.1		2.5		5.7		6.8		1.8		3.6		6.7		7.2	
11-14	1.2		2.8		5.7	5.6	7.0		1.9		3.4	4.1	6.7	7.5	7.4	8.2
15-18	1.1	1.6	2.7	3.2	5.7		6.8	5.9	2.3		3.5	4.6	7.0	7.9	7.9	8.3

Lymphocyte count ($10^3/mm^3$)

Age Range	AA 2.5 M	2.5 F	50 M	50 F	95 M	95 F	97.5 M	97.5 F	MW 2.5 M	2.5 F	50 M	50 F	95 M	95 F	97.5 M	97.5 F
1	1.8		4.1		6.0		6.7		2.5		5.0		8.5		9.5	
2-3	1.1		3.4		5.0		5.4		5.0		3.6		6.0		6.3	
4-6	1.1		2.7		4.6		5.1		1.5		3.0		4.8		4.7	
7-10	1.3		2.3		3.7		4.0		1.5		2.7		4.0		4.5	
11-14	1.3		2.3		3.4		3.8		1.3		2.4		3.6		3.8	
15-18	1.4		2.1		3.2		3.3		1.2		2.0		3.6		3.5	

Monocyte count ($10^3/mm^3$)

Age Range	AA 2.5 M	2.5 F	50 M	50 F	95 M	95 F	97.5 M	97.5 F	MW 2.5 M	2.5 F	50 M	50 F	95 M	95 F	97.5 M	97.5 F
1	0.40		0.60		1.38		1.66		0.45		0.80		1.40		1.50	
2-3	0.30		0.60		0.92		1.03		0.35		0.60		0.95		0.95	
4-6	0.30		0.50		0.90		0.90		0.35		0.60		0.95		1.10	
7-10	0.20		0.50		0.90		1.00		0.30		0.60		0.90		0.90	
11-14	0.25		0.50		0.80		0.85		0.30		0.55		0.90		0.97	
15-18	0.30		0.50		0.88		0.95		0.35		0.50		0.87		0.90	

Eosinophil ($10^3/mm^3$)

Age Range	AA 2.5 M	2.5 F	50 M	50 F	95 M	95 F	97.5 M	97.5 F	MW 2.5 M	2.5 F	50 M	50 F	95 M	95 F	97.5 M	97.5 F
1	0.10		0.30		1.00		1.10		0.10		0.20		0.70		0.80	
2-3	0.00		0.20		0.70		0.90		0.10		0.20		0.75		0.90	
4-6	0.05		0.30		0.80		0.95		0.05		0.25		0.75		0.80	
7-10	0.10		0.20		0.90		1.00		0.10		0.20		0.75		1.00	
11-14	0.00		0.20		0.55		0.60		0.05		0.15		0.70	0.80		0.70
15-18	0.00		0.15		0.45		0.55		0.05		0.15		0.55	0.40	0.50	

Platelet count ($10^3/mm^3$)

Age Range	AA 2.5 M	2.5 F	50 M	50 F	95 M	95 F	97.5 M	97.5 F	MW 2.5 M	2.5 F	50 M	50 F	95 M	95 F	97.5 M	97.5 F
1	225		330		475		480		235		375		510		555	
2-3	220		335		480		490		225		335		470		530	
4-6	220		315		440		470		225		325		440		460	
7-10	210		310		420		435		200		295		410		435	
11-14	180		275		380	410	410	430	190		280		495		420	
15-18	165	185	245	265	340	375	360	400	180		270		345	400	360	420

Mean platelet volume (fL)

Age Range	AA 2.5 M	2.5 F	50 M	50 F	95 M	95 F	97.5 M	97.5 F	MW 2.5 M	2.5 F	50 M	50 F	95 M	95 F	97.5 M	97.5 F
1	6.3		7.6		8.8		9.0		6.3		7.2		8.0		8.4	
2-3	6.5		7.5		8.7		8.8		6.2		7.3		8.6		8.8	
4-6	6.4		7.7		9.2		9.6		6.5		7.5		8.6		8.9	
7-10	6.7		8.1		9.1		9.4		6.6		7.8		9.2		9.6	
11-14	6.8		8.2		9.7		10.3		6.7		8.1		9.5		9.7	
15-18	7.0		8.2		10.1		10.8		6.9		8.2		9.9		10.2	

Appendix 13 *From Cembrowski GS, Chan J, Cheng C, Bamforth FJ. NHANES 1999-2000 Data used to create comprehensive health-associated race-, sex-, and age-stratified pediatric reference intervals for the Coulter MAXM. Lab Hematol 10:245–246, 2004. Presented at the annual meeting of the International Society for Laboratory Hematology, Barcelona, Spain, May 2004. Numerical summary kindly provided by GS Cembrowski, MS Cembrowski, KA Versluys, 2013. Original Graphs at http://www.mylaboratoryquality.com/hematologyri1x.htm.*

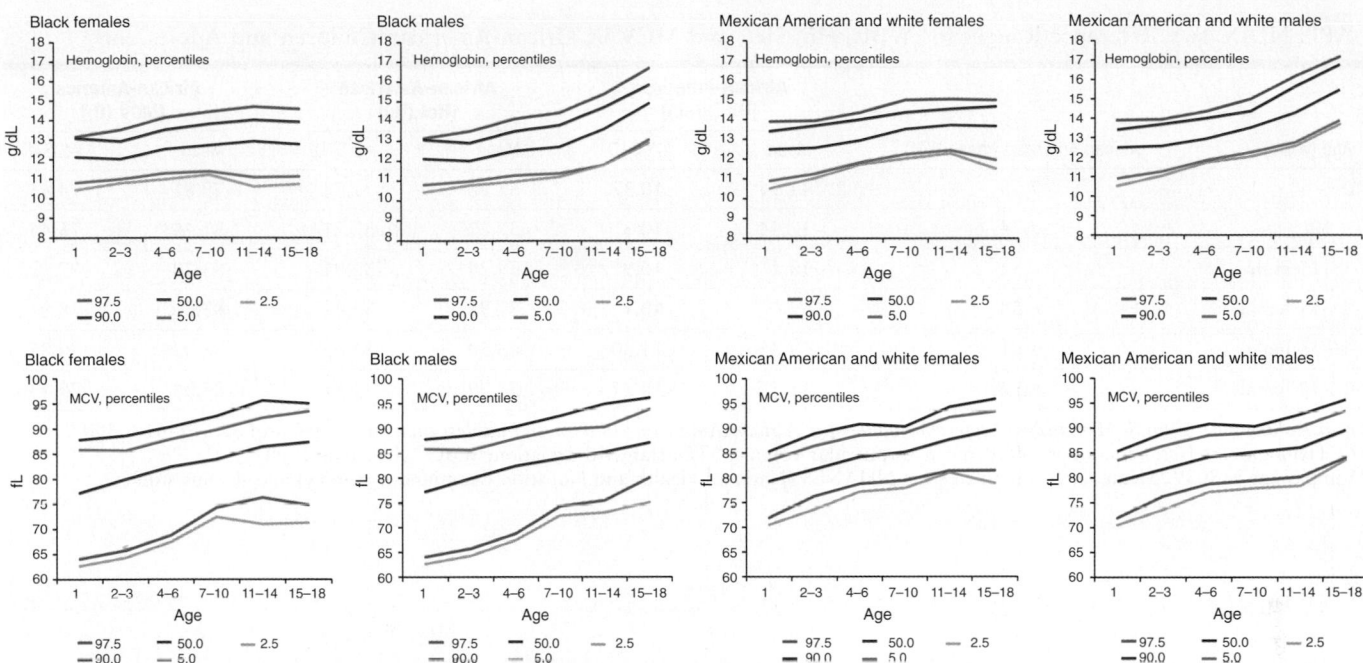

Appendix 14 Hb and MCV percentile curves for African American and Mexican American/Caucasian girls and boys. *Top row,* Hb percentile curves for African American girls and boys and for Mexican American and Caucasian girls and boys. *Bottom row,* MCV percentile curves for African American girls and boys and for Mexican American and Caucasian girls and boys. *(From Cembrowski GS, Chan J, Cheng C, Bamforth FJ: NHANES 1999-2000 Data used to create comprehensive health-associated race-, sex-, and age-stratified pediatric reference intervals for the Coulter MAXM. Lab Hematol 10:245–246, 2004. Presented at the annual meeting of the International Society for Laboratory Hematology, Barcelona, Spain, May 2004. Numerical summary kindly provided by GS Cembrowski, MS Cembrowski, KA Versluys, 2013. Original Graphs at http://www.mylaboratoryquality.com/hematologyri1x.htm.)*

Ferritin (ng/mL)

| | African-American | | | | | | | | Mexican American & Caucasian | | | | | | | |
| | 2.5 Percentile | | 50.0 Percentile | | 95.0 Percentile | | 97.5 Percentile | | 2.5 Percentile | | 50.0 Percentile | | 95.0 Percentile | | 97.5 Percentile | |
Age Range	M	F	M	F	M	F	M	F	M	F	M	F	M	F	M	F
1	8		20		45		50		5		20		60		65	
2-3	8		26		63		70		5		20		55		65	
4-6	11		35		72		77		7		25		60		70	
7-10	17		42		86		100		7		28		62		75	
11-14	11	8	35		95	81	100	88	7		28		60		80	70
15-18	15	3	50	25	160	82	204	100	15	5	52	25	125	70	140	85

Iron (µg/dL)

| | African-American | | | | | | | | Mexican American & Caucasian | | | | | | | |
| | 2.5 Percentile | | 50.0 Percentile | | 95.0 Percentile | | 97.5 Percentile | | 2.5 Percentile | | 50.0 Percentile | | 95.0 Percentile | | 97.5 Percentile | |
Age Range	M	F	M	F	M	F	M	F	M	F	M	F	M	F	M	F
1	25		60		130		140		18		60		120		125	
2-3	25		70		110		120		18		75		130		135	
4-6	30		80		130		140		20		75		140		155	
7-10	20		75		125		130		25		75		140		150	
11-14	30	20	80	70	135		145		30		85		165	150	170	160
15-18	30	20	105	85	140		150		45	25	105	85	185	150	210	150

Appendix 15 *From Cembrowski GS, Chan J, Cheng C, Bamforth FJ. NHANES 1999-2000 Data used to create comprehensive health-associated race-, sex-, and age-stratified pediatric reference intervals for the Coulter MAXM. Lab Hematol 10:245–246, 2004. Presented at the annual meeting of the International Society for Laboratory Hematology, Barcelona, Spain, May 2004. Numerical summary kindly provided by GS Cembrowski, MS Cembrowski, KA Versluys, 2013. Original Graphs at http://www.mylaboratoryquality.com/hematologyri1x.htm.*

APPENDIX 16   Reference Ranges for WBC, Hb, Hct, and MCV in African-American Children and Adolescents*

Age (years)	African American (mean WBC)	African-American [Hb (g/dL)]		African-American [Hct (%)]		African-American [MCV (fl)]	
		Mean	−2 STD	Mean	−2 STD	Mean	−2 STD
2-5	7.33	11.94	10.37	35.98	31.54	79.81	74.65
6-10	6.74	12.44	10.3	37.27	32.71	81.44	76.45
11-15 male	6.32	13.2	10.97	39.29	32.91	83.20	77.99
11-15 female	6.58	12.67	10.1	37.95	33.41	83.60	78.01
16-18 male	5.91	14.35	11.30	43.50	37.62	86.02	80.85
16-18 female	6.92	12.55	10.27	37.39	31.87	85.26	79.43

From Robins EB, Blum S: Hematologic reference values for African American children and adolescents. Am J Hematol 82:611–614, 2007.
Hb, Hemoglobin; Hct, hematocrit; MCV, mean corpuscular volume; STD, standard deviation; WBC, white blood cell.
*Sample size is 5039. Mean values obtained from NHANES (National Health and Nutrition Examination Survey) and Robins studies.

APPENDIX 17   WBC and ANC Mean Values and Reference Intervals*

	12-18 Years: WBC		>18 Years: WBC		12-18 Years: ANC		>18 Years: ANC	
	N		N		N		N	
NHBM	401	3.2-9.3 (5.6)	547	3.1-9.9 (6.1)	401	1.0-6.2 (2.9)	547	1.3-6.6 (3.1)
MAM	493	4.1-11.4 (6.9)	776	4.1-11.4 (7.1)	492	1.8-8.2 (4.1)	776	2.1-7.9 (4.2)
NHWM	342	4.1-11.4 (6.8)	1473	4.1-11.8 (7.0)	342	1.8-7.2 (3.8)	1471	2.1-8.0 (4.3)
MAM, NHWM	835	4.1-11.4 (6.8)	2249	4.1-11.6 (7.1)	834	†	2247	2.1-8.0 (4.3)
NHBF	329	3.7-10.1 (6.2)	344	3.4-11 (6.3)	329	1.2-6.6 (3.1)	344	1.4-7.5 (3.4)
MAF	401	4.1-12.0 (7.6)	552	4.5-11.8 (7.5)	401	1.9-8.4 (5.3)	550	2.2-8.0 (4.9)
NHWF	322	4.1-11.3 (7.2)	1222	3.9-11.6 (7.0)	322	1.9-7.7 (4.0)	1221	2.0-7.9 (4.7)
MAF, NHWF	723	†	1774	†	723	†	1771	2.0-7.9 (4.8)

From Lim EM, Cembrowski G, Cembrowski M, et al: Race-specific WBC and neutrophil count reference intervals. J Lab Clin Hematol 32:590–597, 2010.
ANC, Absolute neutrophil count; MAF, female Mexican American; MAM, male Mexican American; NHBF, female non-Hispanic black; NHBM, male non-Hispanic black; NHWF, female non-Hispanic white; NHWM, male non-Hispanic white; WBC, white blood cell.
*Data are presented as reference intervals (2.5-97.5 percentile limits) and mean values (in parentheses).
†Could not be pooled because of variation within and between populations.

APPENDIX 18   Activities of RBC Enzymes

Enzyme	Activity at 37° C (mean ± SD)
Acetylcholinesterase	36.93 ± 3.83
Adenosine deaminase	1.11 ± 0.23
Adenylate kinase	258 ± 29.3
Aldolase	3.19 ± 0.86
Bisphosphoglyceromutase (2,3- diphosphoglyceromutase)	4.78 ± 0.65
Catalase	$15.3 ± 2.4 × 10^4$
Enolase	5.39 ± 0.83
Epimerase	0.23 ± 0.06
Galactokinase	0.029 ± 0.004
Galactose-1 phosphate uridyltransferase	28.4 ± 6.94
Glucose phosphate isomerase	60.8 ± 11.0
Glucose-6-phosphate dehydrogenase	8.34 ± 1.59
WHO method	12.1 ± 2.09
Glutamic oxaloacetic transaminase without PLP	3.02 ± 0.67
Glutamic oxaloacetic transaminase with PLP	5.04 ± 0.90
γ-Glutamylcysteine synthetase	0.43 ± 0.04
Glutathione peroxidase	30.82 ± 4.65
Glutathione reductase without FAD	7.18 ± 1.09
Glutathione reductase with FAD	10.4 ± 1.50
Glutathione S-transferase	6.66 ± 1.81
Glyceraldehyde phosphate dehydrogenase	226 ± 41.9
Hexokinase	1.78 ± 0.38
Hypoxanthine phosphoribosyltransferase	1.72 ± 0.30
Lactate dehydrogenase	200 ± 26.5
Methemoglobin reductase	2.60 ± 0.71
Monophosphoglyceromutase	37.71 ± 5.56
NADH-methemoglobin reductase	19.2 ± 3.85 (30°)
NADPH diaphorase	2.26 ± 0.16
Phosphofructokinase	11.01 ± 2.33
Phosphoglucomutase	5.50 ± 0.62
Phosphoglycerate kinase	320 ± 36.1
Phosphoglycolate phosphatase	1.23 ± 0.10
Pyrimidine 5' nucleotidase	0.11 ± 0.03
Pyruvate kinase	15.0 ± 1.99
6-Phosphogluconate dehydrogenase	8.78 ± 0.78
Triose phosphate isomerase	2111 ± 397

From Beutler E, Blum KG: In Altman PL, Dittmer DS, editors: Human health and disease. *Bethesda, Md., Federation of American Societies for Experimental Biology, 1977, p. 156; and Beutler E:* Red cell metabolism: a manual of biochemical methods, *3rd ed, Orlando, Fla., Grune & Stratton, 1984.*

FAD, Flavin adenine dinucleotide; *NADH,* reduced nicotinamide adenine dinucleotide; *NADPH,* reduced nicotinamide adenine dinucleotide phosphate; *PLP,* pyridoxal 5-phosphate; *SD,* standard deviation; *WHO,* World Health Organization.

APPENDIX 19 Levels of Intermediate Metabolites in Normal Adult Erythrocytes

Metabolite	Abbreviation	CONCENTRATION (mean ± 1 SD)		
		nmol/g Hb	nmol/mL Red Cells	μmol/L in Whole Blood
Adenosine-5′-diphosphate	ADP	6635 ± 105	216 ± 36	—
Adenosine-5-monophosphate	AMP	62 ± 10	21.1 ± 3.4	—
Adenosine-5-triphosphate	ATP	4230 ± 290 (whites) 3530 ± 301 (blacks)	1438 ± 99 1200 ± 102	—
2,3-Diphosphoglycerate	2,3-DPG	1227 ± 1870	4171 ± 636	—
Glutathione	GSH	6570 ± 1040	2234 ± 354	—
Glutathione (oxidized)	GSSG	12.3 ± 4.5	4.2 ± 1.53	—
Glucose-6-phosphate	G6P	82 ± 22	27.8 ± 7.5	—
Fructose-6-phosphate	F6P	27 ± 5.8	9.3 ± 2.0	—
Fructose-6-diphosphate	FDP	5.6 ± 1.8	1.9 ± 0.6	—
Dihydroxyacetone phosphate	DHAP	27.6 ± 8.2	9.4 ± 2.8	—
3-Phosphoglyceric acid	3-PGA	132 ± 15.0	44.9 ± 5.1	—
2-Phosphoglyceric acid	2-PGA	21.5 ± 7.35	7.3 ± 2.5	—
Phosphoenolpyruvate	PEP	35.9 ± 6.47	12.2 ± 2.2	—
Creatine		1310 ± 310 (male) 1500 ± 250 (female)	445 ± 105 510 ± 85	—
Lactate		—	—	932 ± 211
Pyruvate		—	—	53.3 ± 21.5

From Beutler E: Red cell metabolism: a manual of biochemical methods, 3rd ed. Orlando, Fla., 1984, Grune & Stratton.
SD, Standard deviation.

APPENDIX 20 Red Cell Enzyme Activity in Premature and Term Neonates, Adults, and Adult Reticulocytes

	Premature Infants (N = 11)	Term Infants (N = 10)	Normal Adults (N = 50)	95% Adult* Reticulocytes
Hexokinase (HK)	3.6 ± 0.6[a]	2.7 ± 0.3[a]	1.15 ± 0.35	9.9[a]
Glucosephosphate isomerase (PGI)	94.5 ± 15.2[a]	88 ± 16[a]	67.7 ± 12.0	95.7[c]
Phosphofructokinase (PFK)	8.0 ± 1.3[d]	7.1 ± 1.5[c]	8.4 ± 3.4	14.1[d]
Aldolase (ALD)	4.3 ± 0.8[c]	5.3 ± 1.7[b]	3.55 ± 1.07	9.5[a]
Triosephosphate isomerase (TIM)	2961 ± 1378[d]	1787 ± 380[d]	2700 ± 700	3220[d]
Glyceraldehyde-3-phosphate dehydrogenase (GAPDH)	131 ± 76[d]	164 ± 45[d]	134 ± 93	240[d]
Phosphoglycerate mutase (PGK)	591 ± 114[b]	436 ± 119[b]	312 ± 86	438[d]
Diphosphoglycerate mutase (DPGM)	8.3 ± 3.6[c]	6.7 ± 1.9[c]	5.3 ± 2.5	7.3[d]
Enolase (ENO)	15.1 ± 3.4[a]	14.6 ± 2.1[a]	7.8 ± 2.2	8.1[d]
Pyruvate kinase (PK)	19.4 ± 3.5[a]	17.3 ± 2.5[a]	11.4 ± 2.8	54.2[a]
Glucose-6-phosphate dehydrogenase (G6PD)	21.3 ± 3.8[a]	19.1 ± 4.3[a]	10.9 ± 3.8	30.6[a]
6-Phosphogluconate dehydrogenase (6PGD)	9.1 ± 2.1[d]	9.9 ± 1.6[c]	8.4 ± 1.0	14.4[a]
Glutathion reductase (GR)	9.5 ± 1.7[a]	11.0 ± 2.6[a]	7.2 ± 2.2	11.3[c]
Acetyl choline esterase (ACE)	17.5 ± 3.5[a]	18.5 ± 4.1[a]	36.9 ± 3.8	44.4[c]

From Jansen G, Koenderman L, Rijksen G, et al: Characteristics of hexokinase, pyruvate kinase, and glucose-6-phosphate dehydrogenase during adult and neonatal reticulocyte maturation. Am J Hematol 20:203–215, 1985.
*Obtained after Percoll density gradient centrifugation of red cells from a patient with a hemolytic syndrome. Statistical interpretation versus normal adult group: [a]P <.001; [b]P <.01; [c]P <.1; [d]not significant.

APPENDIX 21   Red Cell Glycolytic Intermediate Metabolites in Normal Adults, Term Infants, and Premature Infants*

Metabolite	Normal Adults (10)	Term Infants (10)	Premature Infants (11)	Normals (5)
Glucose-6-phosphate	24.8 ± 9.8	45.2 ± 8.7	66.8 ± 34.8	27 ± 2.4
Fructose-6-phosphate	5.4 ± 1.0	9.9 ± 2.3	20.5 ± 8.9	11 ± 2.5
Fructose, 1,6-diphosphate	4.6 ± 1.0	3.8 ± 0.7	3.6 ± 0.8	5 ± 0.9
Dihydroxyacetone phosphate	4.9 ± 3.5	11.9 ± 5.0	18.6 ± 10.7	12 ± 3.7
Glyceraldehyde-3-phosphate	2.6 ± 0.7	1.9 ±1.6	6.5 ± 3.2	4 ± 1.5
3-Phosphoglycerate	61.6 ± 12.4	58.2 ± 14.4	47.5 ± 14.2	48 ± 16.1
2-Phosphoglycerate	4.3 ± 1.8	4.9 ± 1.6	4.4 ± 2.5	7 ± 1.7
Phosphoenolpyruvate	8.8 ± 2.6	7.6 ± 2.9	7.4 ± 3.0	12 ± 0.9
Pyruvate	73.5 ± 33.1	70.4 ± 32.3	78.4 ± 4.15	71 ± 17.7
2,3-Diphosphoglycerate	4423 ± 1907	3609 ± 800	3152 ± 2133	4000

From Oski FA: Red cell metabolism in the newborn infant: V. Glycolytic intermediates and glycolytic enzymes. Pediatrics 44:87, 1969.
*Infant samples were obtained from newborns weighing more than 2800 g whose gestational age was 39 weeks or greater. Blood was drawn within 24 hours of birth. All the newborns were clinically healthy. Adult samples were obtained from healthy normal volunteers.

APPENDIX 22   RBC Enzyme Activity* in ELBWI Infants and Premature and Normal Adults (Whole Blood and Reticulocyte Rich)

	Normal Adult (N = 28) Mean ± SD	ELBWI (N = 28) Mean ± SD	Reticulocyte Rich (N = 20) Mean ± SD	ELBWI Versus Reticulocyte Rich	ELBWI Versus Normal Adults
Hexokinase (HK)	1.05 ± 0.11	3.28 ± 0.47	3.45 ± 1.78	NS	High (P <.0001)
Glucosephosphate isomerase (GPI)	58.4 ± 5.0	83.4 ± 6.2	65.2 ± 8.5	High (P <.0001)	High (P <.0001)
Phosphofructokinase (PFK)	13.3 ± 1.7	10.1 ± 1.6	15.8 ± 2.4	Low (P <.0001)	Low (P <.0001)
Aldolase (ALD)	3.09 ± 0.53	4.73 ± 5.13	5.12 ± 0.94	NS	High (P <.0001)
Triosephosphate isomerase (TPI)	1760 ± 253	2215 ± 339	2077 ± 375	NS	High (P <.0001)
Glyceraldehyde-3-phosphate dehydrogenase (GA3PD)	191 ± 34	252 ± 39	232 ± 51	NS	High (P <.0001)
Phosphoglycerate kinase (PGK)	288 ± 31	469 ± 67	355 ± 43	High (P <.0001)	High (P <.0001)
Monophosphoglycerate mutase (MPGM)	23.5 ± 2.8	33.8 ± 6.9	29.9 ± 5.3	High (P = .0412)	High (P <.0001)
Enolase (ENL)	6.9 ± 1.0	23.9 ± 3.0	9.3 ± 1.7	High (P <.0001)	High (P <.0001)
Pyruvate kinase (PK)	16.3 ± 2.1	29.7 ± 4.0	27.6 ± 8.1	NS	High (P <.0001)
Lactate dehydrogenase (LDH)	195 ± 17	248 ± 28	264 ± 34	NS	High (P <.0001)
Glucose-6-phosphate dehydrogenase (G6PD)	7.6 ± 0.8	18.1 ± 2.2	12.8 ± 2.0	High (P <.0001)	High (P <.0001)
6-Phosphogluconate dehydrogenase (6PGD)	8.1 ± 1.0	8.2 ± 1.5	13.2 ± 1.8	Low (P <.0001)	NS
Glutathione reductase (GR)	7.1 ± 1.2	9.2 ± 1.8	7.8 ± 1.8	High (P = .0090)	High (P <.0001)
GR + flavin adenine dinucleotide (FAD)	9.9 ± 1.6[b]	10.9 ± 1.7[b]	10.4 ± 1.7	NS	NS
Glutathione peroxidase (GSH-Px)	31.8 ± 5.7	22.5 ± 4.0	41.3 ± 7.4	Low (P <.0001)	Low (P <.0001)
Adenylate kinase (AK)	252 ± 35	132 ± 18	253 ± 26	Low (P <.0001)	Low (P <.0001)
Adenosine deaminase (ADA)	1.25 ± 0.33	0.96 ± 0.30	1.60 ± 0.60	Low (P <.0001)	Low (P = .0010)
Acetylcholinesterase (AchE)	31.7 ± 4.7	16.7 ± 3.3	37.6 ± 10.1	Low (P <.0001)	Low (P <.0001)
Pyrimidine 5'-nucleotidase	9.1 ± 1.4	17.0 ± 4.0	19.1 ± 4.5	ns	High (P <.0001)
NADH methemoglobin reductase (MetHbR)	14.9 ± 1.8[b]	11.5 ± 2.1[a]	14.1 ± 2.3[a]	Low (P = .0087)	Low (P <.0001)
Catalase (CAT)	13.6 ± 2.1[b]	11.8 ± 2.7[a]	15.6 ± 3.2[a]	Low (P = .0048)	Low (P = .0459)
Reduced glutathione (GSH) (mg/dL RBC)	67.8 ± 9.3	76.9 ± 13.8	69.4 ± 12.0	NS	High (P = .0059)

From Miyazono Y, Hirono A, Miyamoto Y, et al: Erythrocyte enzyme activities in cord blood of extremely low-birth-weight infants. Am J Hematol 62:88–92, 1999.
ELBWI, Extremely low-birth-weight infants (birth weight <1000 g); Hb, hemoglobin; NS, not significant; RBC, red blood cell; SD, standard deviation.
*All enzyme activities are represented as units/g Hb, except for CAT (10^4 units/g Hb) and P5N (μmol Pi liberated/hr/g Hb). [a]N = 12; [b]N = 20.

APPENDIX 23   G6PD Reference Values for G6PD-Normal and –Deficient Males and Females with Probable Genotypes

Category (U/g Hb)	No.	Median Value	IQR	Min-Max	G6PD Phenotype	Probable Genotype*†
Male (N = 1502)						
<7.0	243 (16.2%)	0.28	0.21-0.39	0.01-6.20	Deficient	Deficient hemizygote
≥9.0	1256 (83.8%)	18.76	17.27-21.68	9.00-34.66	Normal	Normal hemizygote
Female (N = 1298)						
<7.0	81 (6.2%)	4.84	0.45-6.16	0.06-6.96	Deficient	Deficient homozygote
7.0-9.4	64 (4.9%)	8.61	7.67-9.00	7.04-9.46	Intermediate	Heterozygote
≥9.5	1153 (88.8%)	18.36	16.21-20.63	9.54-35.50	Normal	Normal homozygote

*In females, because of nonrandom X chromosome inactivation among heterozygotes, accurate genotype categories may be difficult to determine based on phenotype. The term "probable" genotype is therefore used.

†Male genotype based on phenotype may be assumed with reasonable accuracy.

APPENDIX 24   Hemoglobin A Content in Male and Female Newborns According to Birth Weight

Birth Weight (g)	Males Hb A (%)	Females Hb A (%)
<1501	7.1 ± 1.3 (9)	13.2 ± 11.3 (14)
1501-2000	12.2 ± 8.2 (36)	13.1 ± 10.4 (44)
2001-2500	12.6 ± 5.2 (139)	14.9 ± 6.5 (206)*
2501-3000	15.8 ± 6.4 (635)	17.8 ± 6.2 (776)*
3001-3500	18.2 ± 6.5 (1289)	19.9 ± 6.8 (1204)*
3501-4000	20.0 ± 6.6 (803)	20.9 ± 7.2 (590)*
4001-4500	19.7 ± 6.3 (200)	22.6 ± 8.6 (94)*
>4500	21.7 ± 7.0 (45)	20.9 ± 7.2 (20)

From Galacteros F, Guilloud-Bataille M, Feingold J: Sex, gestational age, and weight dependency of adult hemoglobin concentration in normal newborns. Blood 78:1121, 1991.

HbA, Hemoglobin A.

*P <.05 between male and female newborns.

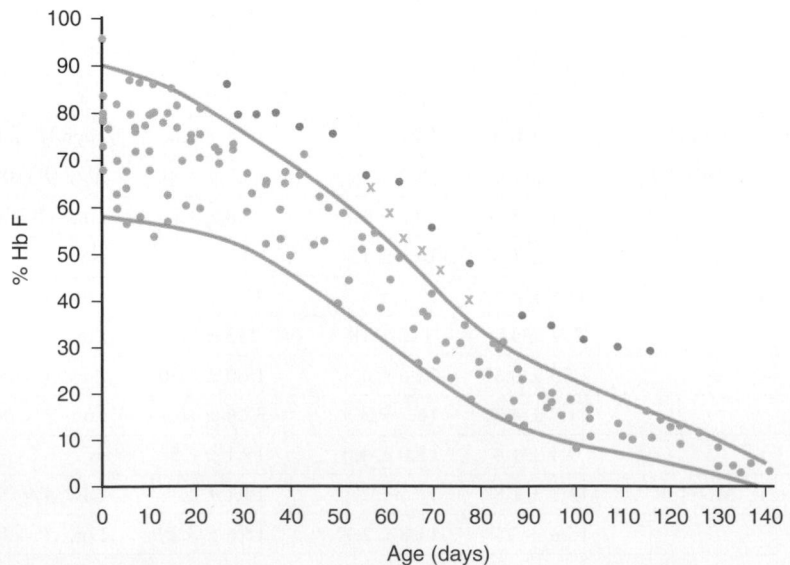

Appendix 25 Relative concentration of hemoglobin F in infants and its variation with age. The region between the curved lines contains 120 observations in 17 normal children. (From Garby L, Sjolin S. Development of erythropoiesis. Acta Paediatr 51:245, 1962.)

APPENDIX 26   Percentage of Hemoglobins F and A2 in the Newborn and Adult*

	% Hb F (Gα:Aα ratio)	% Hb A2
Newborn	60-90 (3:1)	<1.0
Adult	<1.0 (2:3)	1.6-3.5

From Altman PL, Dittmer DS, editors: Human health and disease. Bethesda, MD, 1977, Federation of American Societies for Experimental Biology, p. 159.
Hb, Hemoglobin.
*The α chains of fetal hemoglobin contain either a glycyl residue or an alanyl residue at position 136. The Gα:Aα ratio in the newborn undergoes a considerable change between the third and fourth months of life, at which time it approximates that of the Hb F of adults.

APPENDIX 27   Methemoglobin Levels in Normal Children*

	METHEMOGLOBIN (g/dL)					METHEMOGLOBIN AS PERCENTAGE OF TOTAL HEMOGLOBIN				
	No. Cases	No. Det.	Mean	Range	Standard Dev.	No. Cases	No. Det.	Mean	Range	Standard Dev.
Prematures (birth-7 days)	29	34	0.43	(0.02-0.83)	±0.07	24	28	2.3	(0.08-4.4)	±1.26
Prematures (7-72 days)	21	29	0.31	(0.02-0.78)	±0.19	18	23	2.2	(0.02-4.7)	±1.07
Prematures (total)	50	63	0.38	(0.02-0.83)	±0.10	42	51	2.2	(0.08-4.7)	±1.10
Cook County Hospital, prematures (1-14 days)	8	8	0.52	(0.18-0.83)	±0.08	—	—	—	—	—
Newborns (1-10 days)	39	39	0.22	(0.00-0.58)	±0.17	25	30	1.5	(0.00-2.8)	±0.81
Infants (1 month-1 year)	8	8	0.14	(0.02-0.29)	±0.09	8	8	1.2	(0.17-2.4)	+0.78
Children (1-14 years)	35	35	0.11	(0.00-0.33)	±0.09	35	35	0.79	(0.00 2.4)	±0.62
Adults (14-78 years)	30	30	0.11	(0.00-0.28)	±0.09	27	27	0.82	(0.00-1.9)	±0.63

From Kravitz H, Elegant LD, Kaiser E, et al: Methemoglobin values in premature and mature infants and children. Am J Dis Child 91:2, 1956.
*The premature and full-term infants were free of known disease. None had respiratory distress or cyanosis. Analysis of milk and water ingested by these infants revealed a nitrate level less than 0.027 ppm. The premature infants routinely received vitamin C orally each day from the seventh day of life.

APPENDIX 28   Hemoglobin, Serum Transferrin Saturation, Serum Ferritin*, and Red Cell Indices in Adolescents (15-16 Years of Age)†

		PERCENTILE				
	Mean ± SD	10th	25th	50th	75th	90th
Boys						
Hb (g/dL)	14.7 ± 0.831	135	14.2	14.7	15.2	15.7
Transferrin saturation (%)	32.7 ± 10.25	21.2	25.7	31.7	38.6	46.3
Serum ferritin (μg/L)	26.4 ± 17.71	13.2	22	29	40.8	52
MCV (fL)	88.4 ± 3.87	83.5	85.5	88.1	90.9	93.2
RDW (%)	13.0 ± 0.95	12.3	12.5	12.9	13.2	13.5
MCH (pg)	29.4 ± 1.43	27.7	28.6	29.2	30.2	31.0
Girls						
Hb (g/dL)	13.4 ± 0.763	12.3	12.9	13.4	13.9	14.3
Transferrin saturation (%)	29.9 ± 10.7	17.2	22.8	29	35.2	43.4
Serum ferritin (μg/L)	18.2 ± 1.98	7.5	12	18.2	28.5	41.5
MCV (fL)	90.1 ± 3.86	84.8	87.6	90.3	92.8	94.8
RDW (%)	12.8 ± 0.71	12.1	12.4	12.7	13.2	13.6
MCH (pg)	29.6 ± 1.43	27.8	28.8	29.5	30.6	31.3

From Hallberg L, Hulten L, Lindstedt G, et al: Prevalence of iron deficiency in Swedish adolescents. Pediatr Res 34:680–687, 1993.
Hb, Hemoglobin; MCH, mean corpuscular hemoglobin; MCV, mean corpuscular volume; RDW, red blood cell volume distribution width; SD, standard deviation.
*Data for serum ferritin are presented as geometric means ± antilog of logarithmic values.
†Data collected in 197 to 207 boys and 215 to 220 girls, from ages 15 to 16.

APPENDIX 29   Hemoglobin and Iron Status Indicators According to Age

	2 m			6 m			9 m		
	Mean ± SD	5-95 Percentiles	N	Mean ± SD	5-95 Percentiles	N	Mean ± SD	5-95 Percentiles	N
Hemoglobin (g/L) (mmol/L)	115 ± 8 7.1 ± 0.5	101-130 6.3-8.1	68	116 ± 9 7.2 ± 0.6	105-130 6.5-8.1	57	117 ± 7 7.3 ± 0.5	103-129 6.4-8	94
Serum ferritin* (μg/L)	301	134-675	63	59	23-140	54	37	17-78	84
Erythrocyte protoporphyrin (nmol/l erythrocytes)	679 ± 185[†]	479-1148	65	475 ± 109	304-659	48	556 ± 133[†]	369-763	83
Serum transferrin (μmol/L)	26 ± 4[†]	20-33	65	31 ± 4	24-38	57	35 ± 7[†]	26-47	90
Serum iron (μmol/L)	13.1 ± 3.5[†]	7.5-19.1	59	9.9 ± 3.1	6.3-17.3	46	8.8 ± 3.4	3.9-14.9	80
Transferrin saturation (%)	26 ± 8[†]	15-40	59	16 ± 6	10-29	46	13 ± 6	5-25	77
Mean red cell volume (fl)	86 ± 5[†]	78-94	64	76 ± 4	69-82	49	76 ± 6	68-85	89

From Michaelsen KF, Milman N, Samuelson G: A longitudinal-study of iron status in healthy Danish infants—effects of early iron status, growth velocity and dietary factors. Acta Paediatr 84:1035–44, 1995.
m, Months; SD, standard deviation.
*Geometric mean values.
[†]Significantly different (P <.001) from values at 6 months (Student's paired t-test).

APPENDIX 30   Serum Ferritin, Iron, Total Iron-Binding Capacity, and Transferrin Saturation in Children and Adolescents

Age	Male Subjects		Female Subjects	
Ferritin	ng/mL	μg/L	ng/mL	μg/L
1-30 d*	6-400	6-400	6-515	6-515
1-6 m*	6-410	6-410	6-340	6-340
7-12 m*	6-80	6-80	6-45	6-45
1-5 y[†‡]	6-24	6-24	6-24	6-24
6-9 y[†‡]	10-55	10-55	10-55	10-55
10-14 y[‡]	23-70	23-70	6-40	6-40
14-19 y[‡]	23-70	23-70	6-40	6-40
Iron	μg/dL	μmol/L	μg/dL	μmol/L
1-5 y[†‡]	22-136	4-25	22-136	4-25
6-9 y[†‡]	39-136	7-25	39-136	7-25
10-14 y[‡]	28-134	5-24	45-145	8-26
14-19 y[‡]	34-162	6-29	28-184	5-33
Iron-Binding Capacity				
1-5 y[†‡]	268-441	48-79	268-441	48-79
6-9 y[†‡]	240-508	43-91	240-508	43-91
10-14 y[‡]	302-508	54-91	318-575	57-103
14-19 y[‡]	290-570	52-102	302-564	52-101

APPENDIX 30 Serum Ferritin, Iron, Total Iron-Binding Capacity, and Transferrin Saturation in Children and Adolescents (Continued)

Age	Male Subjects	Female Subjects
Transferrin Saturation		
1-5 y[††‡]	0.07-0.44	0.07-0.44
6-9 y[††‡]	0.17-0.42	0.17-0.42
10-14 y[‡]	0.11-0.36	0.02-0.40
14-19 y[‡]	0.06-0.33	0.06-0.33
Transferrin	**U/L (Males and Females)**	
0-5 d[§]	1.43-4.46	
1-3 y[§]	2.18-3.47	
4-6 y[§]	2.08-3.78	
7-9 y[§]	2.25-3.61	
10-13 y[§]	2.24-4.42	
14-19 y[§]	2.33-4.44	

d, Days; *m*, months; *y*, years.

[*] Soldin SJ, Morales A, Albalos F, et al: Pediatric reference ranges on the Abbott IMx for FSH, LH, prolactin, TSH, T_4, T_3, free T3, T-uptake, IgE, and ferritin. *Clin Biochem* 28:603, 1995. Study based on hospitalized patients; values represent 2.5th and 97.5th percentiles.

[†] No significant differences between males and females; range derived from combined data.

[‡] Lockitch, G; Halstead, AC; Wadsworth, et al: Age- and sex-specific pediatric reference intervals and correlations for zinc, copper, selenium, iron, vitamins A and E, and related proteins. *Clin Chem* 34:1625, 1988. Study based on healthy children; values represent the 0.025 and 0.975 fractiles. Transferrin saturation calculated from iron (μmol/L)/total iron binding capacity. Note that the lower reference limits for serum iron and transferrin saturation in this study are below the limits used to define acceptable levels for these two analytes (O'Neal RM, Johnson OC, Schaefer AE: Guidelines for classification and interpretation of group blood and urine data collected as part of the National Nutrition Survey. *Pediatr Res* 4:103, 1970.)

[§] Lockitch, G; Halstead, AC; Quigley G, et al: Age- and sex-specific pediatric reference intervals: study design and methods illustrated by measurement of serum proteins with the Behring LN nephelometer. *Clin Chem* 34:1618, 1988. Results are 2.5th and 97.5 percentiles.

APPENDIX 31 Reference Ranges for Erythrocyte Zinc Protoporphyrin in Children and Adolescents

Age Groups	Blood ZPP Reference Ranges 2.5th–97.5th Percentiles (μg/dL)*		Blood ZPP Reference Ranges 2.5th–97.5th Percentiles (μmol/mol heme)		N	
	Males	Females	Males	Females	Males	Females
0-12 months	8.5-34.5	9-40	15.6-63.5	16.6-73.6	145	203
13-24 months	10-34	11-32	18.4-62.6	20.2-58.9	605	725
2-5 years	5-35	10-31	9.2-64.4	18.4-57.0	1926	1822
6-9 years	6-31	9-30	11.0-57.0	16.6-55.2	522	408
10-17 years	5.5-31.5	5-33.5	10.1-58.0	9.2-61.6	61	61
Total					3259	3219

From Soldin OP, Miller M, Soldin SJ: Pediatric reference ranges for zinc protoporphyrin. Clin Biochem 36:21–25, 2003.

ZPP, Zinc protoporphyrin.

*Multiply μg/dL by 1.83 to convert to μmol/mol heme.

APPENDIX 32 Reference Ranges for Serum Transferrin Receptor in Children and Adolescents*

Age Groups	2.5% Reference Limit mg/L	97.5% Reference Limit mg/L
6 months to 4 years	1.5 (1.4-1.5)	3.3 (3.1-3.4)
4 to 10 years	1.3 (1.3-1.4)	3.0 (2.9-3.2)
10 to 16 years	1.2 (1.1-1.2)	2.7 (2.7-2.8)
>16 years	0.9 (0.9-1.0)	2.3 (2.2-2.4)

From Suominen, P, Virtanen A, Lehtonen-Veronmaa M, et al: Regression-based reference limits for serum transferrin receptor in children 6 months to 16 years of age. Clin Chem 47:935–937, 2001.
*The 95% confidence interval for each limit is given in parentheses.

APPENDIX 33 Percentile Distributions for Plasma Folate, RBC folate, Vitamins B_6 and B_{12}, Holotranscobalamin, and Total Homocysteine of Healthy European Adolescents 12.5 to 17.49 Years of Age

		PF(nmol/L)	RBC Folate nmol/L	PLP (nmol/L)	Cbl (pmol/L)	Holo-TC (pmol/L)	tHcy (μmol/L)
	N	1049	1040	974	1051	1017	1050
	Mean	18.7	784.2	63.2	349.4	63.4	7.4
	SD	10.5	340.9	51.9	143.5	33.7	3.8
Percentile	2.5	6.4	315.5	16.6	154.4	27.4	3.7
	5	7.6	378.8	20.0	170.8	30.9	3.9
	10	9.1	428.9	25.0	193.0	35.2	4.4
	25	11.8	553.0	34.7	240.0	44.4	5.4
	50	16.0	721.9	49.1	319.0	57.8	6.7
	75	22.1	942.3	75.7	434.9	73.0	8.4
	90	31.7	1214.0	113.9	557.0	91.7	10.5
	95	39.0	1389.3	149.7	638.0	107.1	12.3
	97.5	46.4	1582.6	187.3	696.0	127.1	15.7

Cbl, Cobalamin; *Holo-TC*, holotranscobalamin; *PF*, plasma folate; *PLP*, pyridoxal 5-phosphate; *RBC*, red blood cell; *SD*, standard deviation.

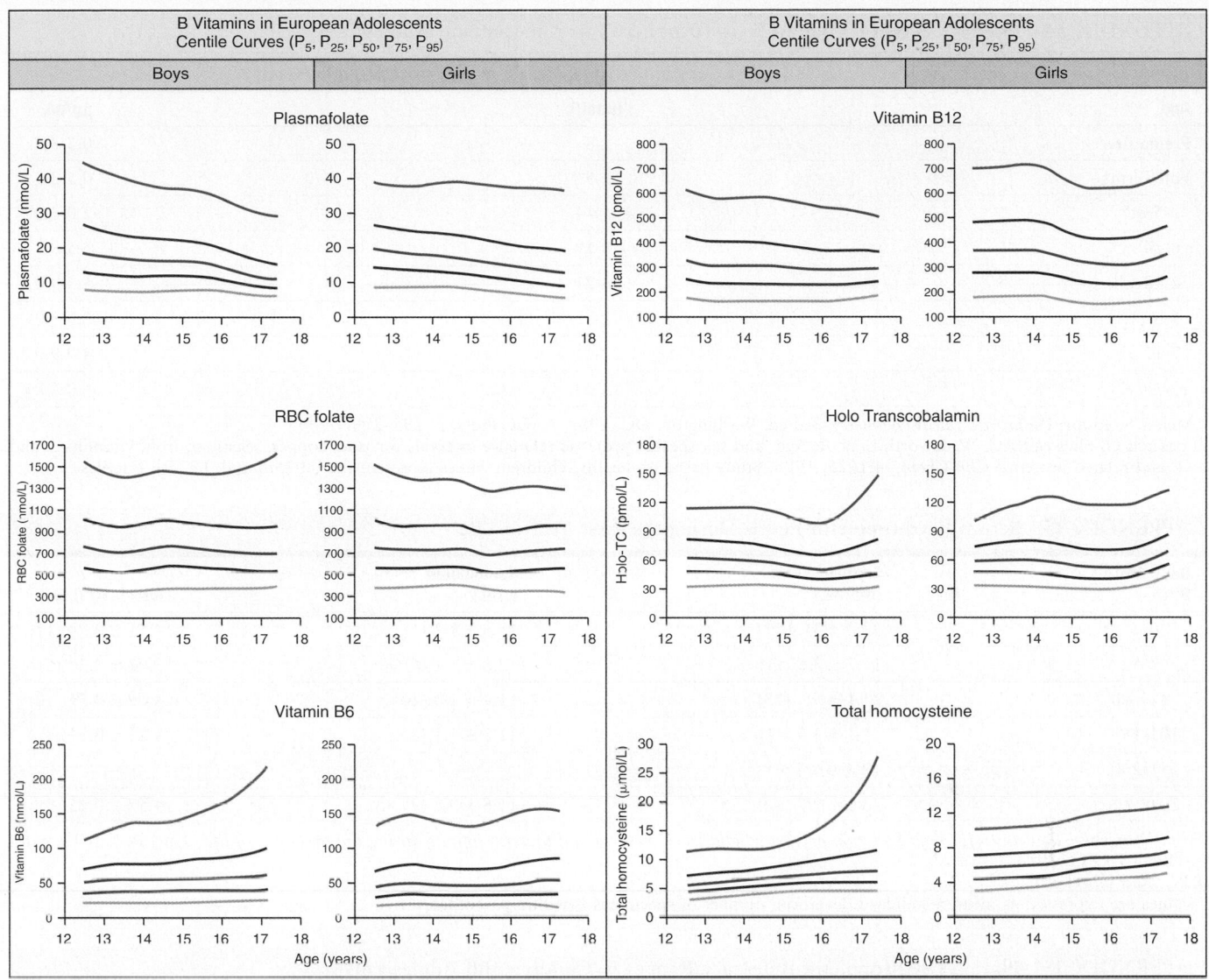

Smoothed (LMS method) centile curves (*from the bottom to the top*: P5, P25, P50, P75, P95) of plasma folate (nmol/L), red blood cell folate (nmol/L), vitamin B₆ (pmol/L), vitamin B₁₂ (pmol/L), holo-transcobalamin (pmol/L), and total homocysteine (μmol/L) concentrations in males and females. *Cbl,* Cobalamin; *Holo-TC,* holo-transcobalamin; *PF,* plasma folate; *PLP,* pyridoxal phosphate or Vitamin B₆; *RBC folate,* red blood cell folate; *tHcy,* total homocysteine. *(From Gonzalez-Gross M, Benser J, Breidenassel C, et al: Gender and age influence blood folate, vitamin B12, vitamin B6, and homocysteine levels in European adolescents: the Helena Study. Nutr Res 32:817–826, 2012.)*

APPENDIX 34 Plasma Levels of Vitamin E (α-Tocopherol) in Children and Adolescents

Age	MALES AND FEMALES	
	μmol/L	μg/mL
Premature*	1-8	0.5-3.5
Full Term	2-8	0.5-3.5
2-5 m*	5-14	2.0-6.0
6-24 m*	8-19	3.5-80
2-12 y*	13-21	5.5-9.0
1-6 y†	7-21	3.0-9.0
7-12 y†	10-21	4.0-9.0
13-19 y†	13-24	6.0-10.1

*Meites S, editor: *Pediatric clinical chamistry,* 3rd ed. Washington, DC, 1989, AACC Press, p. 295–296.
†Lockitch G, Halstead AC, Wadsworth L, et al: Age- and sex-specific pediatric reference intervals for zinc, copper, selenium, iron, vitamins A and E and related proteins. *Clin Chem* 34:1625, 1988. Study based on healthy children; values represent the 0.025th and 0.975th fractiles.

APPENDIX 35 Serum Erythropoietin Levels During the First Year of Life*

Days After Birth	Erythropoietin (mU/mL)	Hemoglobin (g/dL)	RBC (×10⁶/μL)
0-6	33.0 ± 31.4 (11)	15.6 ± 2.2 (11)	4.51 ± 0.74 (11)
7-50	11.7 ± 3.6 (7)	12.8 ± 1.1 (5)	3.92 ± 0.35 (5)
51-100	21.1 ± 5.5 (13)	11.4 ± 1.0 (10)	4.09 ± 0.51 (10)
101-150	15.1 ± 3.9 (5)	11.2 ± 1.1 (3)	4.21 ± 0.31 (3)
151-200	17.8 ± 6.3 (6)	—	—
>201	23.1 ± 9.7 (10)	11.8 ± 0.8 (9)	4.57 ± 0.25 (9)

From Yamashita H, Kukita J, Ohga S: Serum erythropoietin levels in term and preterm infants during the first year of life. Am J Pediatr Hematol Oncol 16:213, 1994.
RBC, Red blood cell.
*Values are expressed as mean ± standard deviation; number of specimens is within parentheses.

APPENDIX 36 Plasma Erythropoietin Reference Ranges in Children and Adolescents*

Age (y)	MALE SUBJECTS		FEMALE SUBJECTS	
	2.5%	97.5%	2.5%	97.5%)
1-3	1.7	17.9	2.1	15.9
4-6	3.5	21.9	2.9	8.5
7-9	1.0	13.5	2.1	8.2
10-12	1.0	14.0	1.1	9.1
13-15	2.2	14.4	3.8	20.5
16-18	1.5	15.2	2.0	14.2

From Krafte-Jacobs B, Williams J,. Soldin SJ, Plasma erythropoietin reference ranges in children. J Pediatr 126:601, 1995.
y, Years.
*Data obtained from a total of 1122 hospitalized and outpatient children ages 1 to 18 years. Levels found in anemic patients cannot be compared with normal values. In fact, as long as the erythropoietin-generating apparatus in the kidney is efficient, serum levels increase exponentially as the hematocrit concentration decreases. Serum erythropoietin must therefore be evaluated in relation to the degree of anemia, and every single laboratory should determine the exponential regression of serum erythropoietin versus hematocrit (or hemoglobin) in a home-made reference population of anemic subjects and define the 95% confidence limits. The patients gathered to calculate a reference regression equation should have an anemia with a single simple mechanism and no evidence of either renal failure or excessive cytokine production (i.e., normal values for C-reactive protein and α_2-globulins). Patients with chronic iron-deficiency anemia caused by nonneoplastic and noninflammatory chronic blood loss have the advantages of being easily found, unequivocably defined, and homogeneous. They could become the universal reference population, although patients with hemolytic anemia or thalassemia intermedia also may be studied as reference subjects. Serum erythropoietin levels are also much higher for hemoglobin concentration in hypoplastic than in hyperplastic states. Thus for the same hemoglobin concentration, serum erythropoietin levels are lower in thalassemia intermedia than in Diamond-Blackfan anemia.

APPENDIX 37 Membrane Lipid Composition of Fetal Erythrocytes

	G1 20-25 wk (N = 8)	G2 28-35 wk (N = 7)	G3 38-41 wk (N = 7)	G4 Adults (N = 10)
Cholesterol (μg/μg prot.)	0.22 ± 0.01	0.23 ± 0.01	0.22 ± 0.01	0.23 ± 0.01
Phospholipids (μg/μg prot.)	0.70 ± 0.14	0.81 ± 0.07	0.89 ± 0.16	0.93 ± 0.11
CH/PL	0.36 ± 0.05	0.30 ± 0.03	0.26 ± 0.02	0.27 ± 0.02
Phospholipids				
Sphingomyelin (%)	30.11 ± 0.91	30.64 ± 0.65	31.97 ± 2.62	30.83 ± 0.3
Phosphatidylcholine (%)	30.30 ± 0.48	30.17 ± 1.0	26.78 ± 0.30*	26.88 ± 0.4*
Phosphatidylinositol (%)	3.76 ± 0.29	3.70 ± 0.24	3.39 ± 0.2	3.38 ± 0.21
Phosphatidylserine (%)	11.75 ± 1.24	11.87 ± 0.8	12.73 ± 0.31	12.02 ± 0.81
Phosphatidic acid (%)	2.98 ± 0.11	2.99 ± 0.22	2.79 ± 0.12	2.81 ± 0.18
Phosphatidylethanolamine (%)	20.93 ± 0.6	20.68 ± 1.33	22.25 ± 0.63	21.82 ± 0.43
Fatty Acids				
16:0 (%)	22.51 ± 0.92	25.31 ± 0.78*	22.95 ± 0.73	23.02 ± 0.79
18:0 (%)	17.74 ± 0.92	17.52 ± 0.51	18.18 ± 0.33	17.92 ± 0.46
18:1w9 (%)	13.03 ± 0.21	11.74 ± 0.38*	10.70 ± 0.30	10.57 ± 0.33
18:1 bw7 (%)	1.75 ± 0.12	1.57 ± 0.07	1.73 ± 0.08	1.59 ± 0.07
18:2w6 (%)	4.81 ± 0.36	4.85 ± 0.42	4.38 ± 0.31	4.18 ± 0.32
20:3w6 (%)	2.40 ± 0.14	2.79 ± 0.1 1	3.42 ± 0.11*†	3.59 ± 0.11*
20:4w6 (%)	21.95 ± 0.5	23.13 ± 0.4	22.36 ± 0.46	22.47 ± 0.48
22:4w6 (%)	3.76 ± 0.34	4.28 ± 0.19	4.98 ± 0.23*	5.31 ± 0.40*
22.5w3 (%)	1.29 ± 0.19	1.45 ± 0.04	1.76 ± 0.17	1.63 ± 0.15
22:6w3 (%)	9.41 ± 0.71	8.79 ± 0.26	9.49 ± 0.46	9.48 ± 0.52
Fatty Acids of Phosphatidylcholine				
16:0 (%)	40.40 ± 2.10	40.78 ± 1.74	35.75 ± 2.76	32.12 ± 2.58
18:0 (%)	9.36 ± 0.48	9.32 ± 0.53	12.27 ± 0.57*	13.07 ± 0.51*
18:1w9 (%)	20.10 ± 0.82	15.96 ± 0.65*	14.63 ± 0.56*	12.23 ± 0.88*
18:1 bw7 (%)	3.51 ± 0.15	3.05 ± 0.15	3.62 ± 0.21	3.45 ± 0.18
18:2w6 (%)	6.37 ± 0.47	6.94 ± 0.5	8.71 ± 0.78	10.42 ± 0.9*
20:3w6 (%)	1.97 ± 0.15	2.92 ± 0.20*	4.89 ± 0.28	6.05 ± 0.21*
20:4w6 (%)	16.23 ± 0.98	17.18 ± 14.2	14.21 ± 1.17	14.12 ± 1.74
22:4w6 (%)	0.54 ± 0.06	0.57 ± 0.07	0.73 ± 0.09	0.73 ± 0.08
22.5w3 (%)	0	0.35 ± 0.07	0.42 ± 0.03	0.22 ± 0.03
22:6w3 (%)	1.93 ± 0.16	2.6 ± 0.47	3.73 ± 0.43*	4.37 ± 0.49*
Fatty Acids of Phosphatidylethanolamine				
16:0 (%)	29.83 ± 0.83	30.19 ± 1.71	30.20 ± 1.44	28.55 ± 1.23
18:0 (%)	11.62 ± 0.68	10.36 ± 0.64	9.16 ± 0.57*	7.63 ± 0.58*
18:1w9 (%)	17.25 ± 1.20	16.44 ± 0.22	17.36 ± 0.33	16.17 ± 0.62
18:1 bw7 (%)	1.63 ± 0.08	1.22 ± 0.05	1.59 ± 0.15	1.28 ± 0.13
18:2w6 (%)	3.01 ± 0.2	2.71 ± 0.15	3.11 ± 0.20	4.52 ± 0.26*
20:3w6 (%)	1.61 ± 0.11	1.82 ± 0.16	2.16 ± 0.14*	2.4 ± 0.12*
20:4w6 (%)	22.85 ± 0.68	24.22 ± 1.4	21.60 ± 0.98	23.6 ± 1.5
22:4w6 (%)	3.95 ± 0.29	4.92 ± 0.52	5.14 ± 0.27*	5.5 ± 0.43*
22.5w3 (%)	1.52 ± 0.16	1.37 ± 0.09	1.65 ± 0.17	1.72 ± 0.12
22:6w3 (%)	7.81 ± 0.30	7.27 ± 0.45	8.01 ± 0.42	9.00 ± 0.88

From Colin FC, Gallois Y, Rapin D, et al: Impaired fetal erythrocytes' filterability: relationship with cell size, membrane fluidity, and membrane lipid composition. Blood 79:2148, 1992.

CH, Cholesterol; PL, phospholipids; SEM, standard error of the mean; wk, weeks.

Results are expressed at mean ± SEM, P <.05 versus G1(*) or G2(†).

APPENDIX 38 Geometric Data* for Unfractionated, Top, and Bottom Neonatal and Adult Erythrocytes

	Neonatal	Adult
Volume (fL)		
Unfractionated	107.3 ± 5.6[†‡]	90.5 ± 4.4[‡]
Top	130.8 ± 13.1[†‡]	99.2 ± 6.3[‡]
Bottom	89.4 ± 5.9[†]	80.3 ± 4.0
Surface Area (μm²)		
Unfractionated	153.5 ± 7.0[†‡]	137.1 ± 6.7[‡]
Top	186.1 ± 10.6[†‡]	150.6 ± 8.4[‡]
Bottom	108.5 ± 8.2[†]	118.6 ± 6.2
Surface Area/Volume		
Unfractionated	1.43 ± 0.04[†‡]	1.51 ± 0.04
Top	1.43 ± 0.05[†]	1.51 ± 0.03
Bottom	1.21 ± 0.05[†]	1.51 ± 0.04
Diameter (μm)		
Unfractionated	8.8 ± 0.4[‡]	7.9 ± 0.4
Top	9.8 ± 0.4[†‡]	8.6 ± 0.5[‡]
Bottom	6.9 ± 0.5	7.5 ± 0.4
Mean Thickness (μm)		
Unfractionated	1.76 ± 0.10[‡]	1.84 ± 0.13
Top	1.70 ± 0.11	1.71 ± 0.11[‡]
Bottom	2.39 ± 0.13[†]	1.83 ± 0.14
Surface Area Index		
Unfractionated	1.40 ± 0.05[‡]	1.41 ± 0.04[‡]
Top	1.49 ± 0.07[‡]	1.46 ± 0.05[‡]
Bottom	1.12 ± 0.04[†]	1.33 ± 0.04

From Linderkamp O, Friederichs E, Meiselman HJ: Mechanical and geometrical properties of density-separated neonatal and adult erythrocytes. Pediatr Res 34:688–693, 1993.

*Data are presented as mean ±SD for 10 nenonatal and 10 adult samples.

[†]Significant difference (P <.05 unpaired † test) between adult and neonatal erythrocytes.

[‡]Significant difference (P <.05 paired † test) between top or bottom fraction and unfractionated erythrocytes.

Age Group	No of Studies	Estimated Mean Circulating Blood Volume, mL/kg (95% CI)	Test of Homogeneity*	
			Q Statistic	p
All subjects	21	80.0 (77.4–82.5)	46.53	0.16
Premature newborns 0–30 d	3	91.5 (77.3–105.7)	0.18	0.91
Full-term newborns 0–24 h	16	87.7 (83.2–92.3)	11.69	0.70
Full-term newborns 1–7 d	6	91.7 (84.0–99.4)	2.40	0.79
Full-term newborns 7–30 d	2	86.0 (75.6–96.4)	0.09	0.76
Children 1–6 mo	6	84.0 (77.2–90.7)	2.68	0.75
Children 6–24 mo	9	75.4 (68.5–82.3)	8.74	0.36
Children 2–5 yr	6	75.7 (70.7–80.7)	7.26	0.20
Children 5–12 yr	4	74.9 (67.3–82.6)	2.98	0.39
Children 12–18 yr	4	71.4 (66.2–76.5)	1.90	0.59

This compilation was obtained using study-level data from all studies.
*p >.05 indicates that results of the included studies are homogeneous and can be combined.

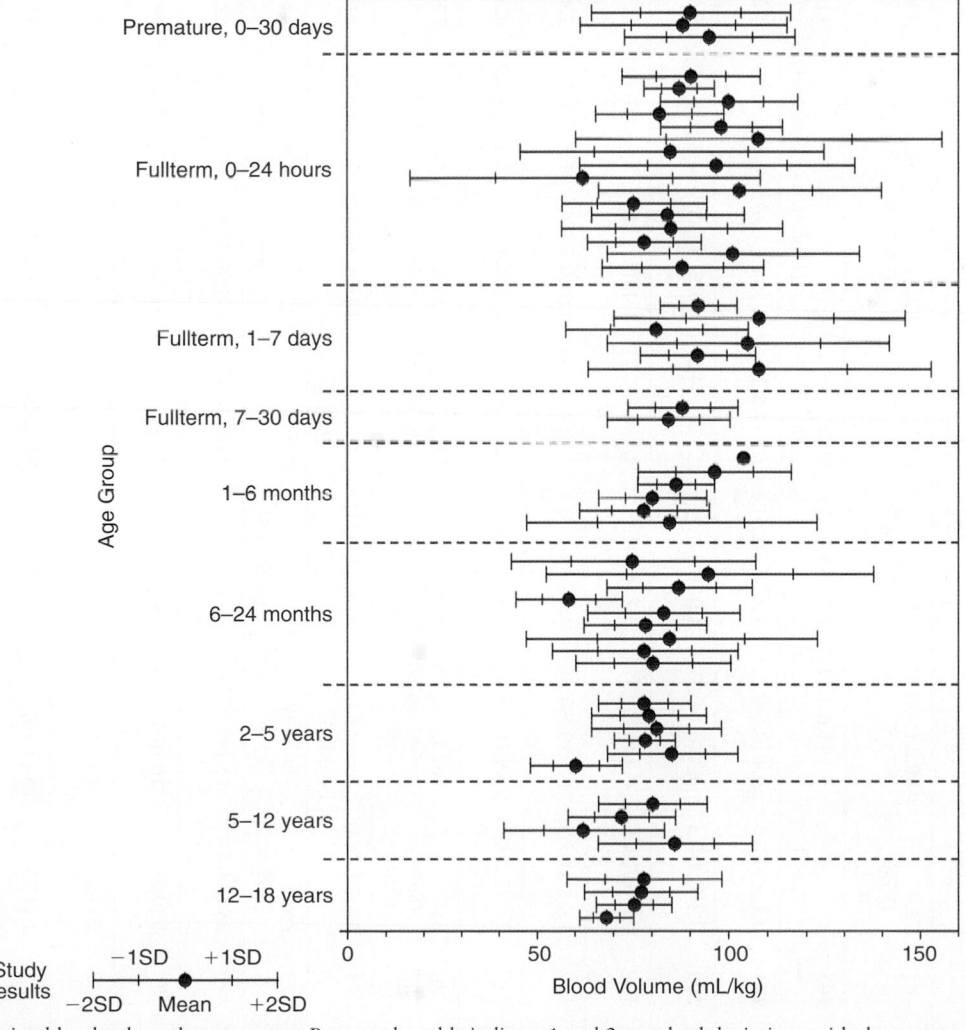

Appendix 39 Circulating blood volume by age group. Bars on the table indicate 1 and 2 standard deviations with the center point indicating study mean blood volume. *(From Riley AA, Arakawa Y, Worley S, et al. Circulating blood volumes: a review of measurement techniques and a meta-analysis in children. ASAIO 56:260–264, 2010.)*

APPENDIX 40   Percentages and Absolute Counts for Total B cells and B-Cell Subsets*

	Number	Cord Blood	0-6 Months	6-12 Months	1-2 Years	2-3 Years	3-4 Years	4-6 Years	6-9 Years	9-12 Years	12-15 Years	15-18 Years
Total B cells	90	11.5 (7.6-15.5)	31.3 (20.5-40.9)	26.1 (11.1-45.4)	21.1 (16.3-26.8)	25.7 (17.3-30.3)	20.0 (14.4-25.1)	17.9 (7.9-22.5)	16.5 (8.5-20.2)	13.1 (4.3-18.2)	12.3 (7.8-23.7)	11.5 (7.8-15.1)
RBE B cells	83	15.5 (5.6-30.7)	27.6 (17.1-32.2)	15.4 (9.3-26.7)	14.8 (9.7-17.9)	10.2 (3.6-21.4)	9.1 (6.4-13.9)	9.3 (6.8-11.5)	5.8 (3.4-9.0)	6.4 (2.9-23.8)	4.8 (1.5-7.3)	5.2 (1.5-19.1)
Naive B cells	83	75.9 (55.6-81.3)	60.2 (55.2-73.9)	73.7 (57.5-84.7)	65.7 (61.5-68.7)	68.7 (50.4-78.5)	66.5 (49.7-77.1)	59.1 (52.3-72.1)	52.6 (47.8-69.8)	57.2 (51.5-73.3)	70.6 (64.6-80.1)	64.7 (59.0-81.1)
CD27+IgM+IgD+memory B cells	145	4.6 (1.3-11.5)	4.5 (1.6-10.1)	5.9 (3.4-14.0)	10.2 (4.6-15.0)	7.6 (5.1-12.3)	8.3 (4.8-16.1)	11.4 (6.7-18.1)	10.4 (6.3-22.0)	10.3 (6.5-22.2)	9.0 (4.7-15.5)	7.6 (4.6-16.8)
CD27+IgM+IgD−memory B cells	145	0.1 (0.0-0.3)	0.4 (0.1-0.7)	1.1 (0.4-2.6)	1.9 (1.6-2.6)	2.3 (1.6-6.6)	4.5 (0.9-9.3)	4.3 (2.0-9.5)	6.9 (2.0-11.8)	2.9 (1.8-13.3)	2.8 (1.6-11.3)	3.8 (0.9-9.1)
CD27+IgG+memory B cells	100	0.2 (0.1-0.5)	0.3 (0.1-0.4)	1.0 (0.4-1.7)	2.3 (1.5-4.2)	3.3 (0.8-6.3)	4.3 (1.8-6.2)	5.6 (0.8-10.3)	6.1 (2.7-14.0)	4.7 (1.5-8.8)	5.4 (2.1-9.4)	4.7 (0.8-11.7)
CD27+IgA+memory B cells	100	0.2 (0.1-0.6)	0.4 (0.2-0.5)	0.7 (0.3-1.0)	1.3 (0.8-1.7)	1.4 (0.7-2.9)	1.8 (1.0-3.5)	2.6 (1.0-3.9)	3.5 (1.1-6.1)	2.4 (1.3-6.1)	2.6 (1.2-3.8)	2.6 (0.2-4.6)
CD27−IgG+memory B cells	100	1.4 (1.1-2.3)	0.7 (0.5-0.8)	1.2 (0.4-2.9)	2.1 (0.7-2.6)	1.7 (0.5-3.4)	1.5 (1.1-3.9)	2.4 (0.7-6.8)	4.1 (1.8-6.5)	2.6 (0.7-4.4)	3.1 (1.1-8.0)	2.6 (0.6-28.4)
CD27−IgA+memory B cells	100	2.5 (2.2-4.7)	1.8 (1.4-2.4)	2.4 (1.4-4.4)	2.5 (1.0-4.3)	2.1 (1.3-5.8)	2.5 (1.3-4.9)	3.3 (1.6-4.9)	4.1 (1.1-5.7)	2.6 (1.2-10.3)	3.1 (1.1-5.3)	4.0 (0.8-5.6)
Total B cells	90	858 (559-1054)	1623 (961-3679)	1717 (571-3680)	1115 (871-1553)	1157 (686-1732)	709 (359-1552)	593 (278-1022)	418 (296-784)	338 (116-555)	284 (119-578)	210 (114-436)
RBE B cells	73	89 (72-164)	459 (164-1184)	214 (70-821)	143 (109-278)	143 (41-248)	72 (23-95)	41 (24-98)	33 (13-63)	24 (12-35)	14 (2-41)	10 (6-41)
Naive B cells	73	698 (439-800)	988 (627-2136)	1378 (420-2181)	738 (586-955)	757 (346-1356)	470 (244-724)	344 (149-618)	263 (154-413)	233 (60-300)	193 (83-398)	153 (72-257)
CD27+IgM+IgD+memory B cells	90	25 (24-34)	61 (49-179)	71 (30-396)	116 (40-177)	87 (50-148)	62 (27-210)	62 (32-164)	48 (24-135)	35 (9-109)	21 (10-74)	20 (10-39)
CD27+IgM+IgD−memory B cells	90	0 (0-2)	10 (6-19)	16 (2-42)	21 (16-34)	33 (19-53)	27 (6-113)	24 (7-98)	32 (7-65)	9 (3-34)	7 (3-39)	10 (2-40)
CD27+IgG+memory B cells	90	2 (1-3)	4 (1-15)	13 (9-44)	28 (13-55)	38 (6-57)	29 (13-95)	32 (4-73)	26 (13-74)	16 (4-49)	11 (7-32)	8 (2-51)
CD27+IgA+memory B cells	90	1 (1-1)	5 (3-10)	69 (21-106)	16 (8-20)	17 (8-26)	10 (6-54)	13 (4-26)	13 (5-35)	9 (3-26)	7 (4-13)	4 (1-20)
CD27−IgG+memory B cells	90	12 (12-16)	12 (5-20)	22 (8-48)	22 (8-35)	20 (4-51)	18 (4-27)	15 (4-28)	17 (8-35)	7 (4-20)	8 (3-22)	5 (1-49)
CD27−IgA+memory B cells	90	21 (14-24)	30 (17-50)	51 (15-85)	26 (11-48)	31 (10-70)	18 (5-75)	17 (6-42)	18 (5-34)	10 (7-35)	10 (1-17)	10 (2-17)

IG, Immunoglobulin; RBE, recent bone marrow emigrants.

*Total B cells (defined as CD19+ lymphocytes) as percentage of total lymphocytes. B-cell subsets as percentage of total B cells. Values are presented as medians (value range). Recent bone marrow emigrants were defined as CD19+IgD+CD10+ B cells, which brightly express CD38 and are CD27− and IgM+.

APPENDIX 41   Lymphocyte Subsets in Term and Premature Neonates in the First Week of Life*

		Term (N = 21)	Premature (N = 104)	Healthy Premature (N = 36)	Sick Premature (N = 68)
Total leukocytes	—	15.44 ± 1.42	13.63 ± 0.94	13.81 ± 1.12	13.54 ± 1.32
Lymphocytes	—	3.51 ± 0.38	5.47 ± 0.23	6.04 ± 0.36	5.18 ± 0.28
CD2	%	67 ± 4	72 ± 1.5	77 ± 3	70 ± 2
	A	2.65 ± 0.34	3.97 ± 0.20	4.61 ± 0.33	3.63 ± 0.24
CD4	%	45 ± 2	47 ± 1.5	52 ± 2	45 ± 2
	A	1.56 ± 0.20	2.58 ± 0.14	3.16 ± 0.14	2.29 ± 0.17
CD8	%	13 ± 1	12 ± 0.5	12.6 ± 0.7	12 ± 0.6
	A	0.57 ± 0.13	0.67 ± 0.04	0.73 ± 0.07	0.64 ± 0.05
CD20	%	5.3 ± 0.4	6.4 ± 0.4	5.6 ± 0.4	6.8 ± 0.6
	A	0.18 ± 0.03	0.34 ± 0.03	0.34 ± 0.04	0.34 ± 0.03
CD21	%	9.1 ± 0.6	8.6 ± 0.5	6.8 ± 0.6	9.5 ± 0.7
	A	0.33 ± 0.06	0.44 ± 0.03	0.39 ± 0.04	0.47 ± 0.05

From Series IM, Pichette J, Carrie C, et al: *Quantitative analysis of T and B cell subsets in healthy and sick premature infants.* Early Hum Dev 26:143, 1991.
A, Absolute cell count; *SEM*, standard error of the mean.
*Values are expressed as mean ± SEM; %, relative %; A, Absolute cell count × 10^9/L.

APPENDIX 42 Absolute Counts for Total T Cells, T-Cell Subsets, sjTRECs, and T-Cell Ratios in Children and Adolescents

	No.	Cord Blood	0-6 Months	6-12 Months	1-2 Years	2-3 Years	3-4 Years	4-6 Years	6-9 Years	9-12 Years	12-15 Years	15-18 Years
Leukocytes ($\times10^9$/l)	98	nd	10.8 (4.7-14.8)	12.1 (6.6-13.6)	8.7 (7.4-14.3)	9.5 (6.6-12.9)	8.5 (5.0-11.2)	8.4 (6.7-11.9)	7.0 (4.0-12.5)	6.0 (5.3-11.2)	5.9 (4.1-8.3)	5.9 (4.8-7.4)
Lymphocytes ($\times10^9$/l)	98	nd	5.2 (3.2-9.8)	6.4 (3.8-9.3)	5.6 (4.6-6.0)	4.4 (2.8-6.4)	3.7 (2.2-5.9)	3.4 (2.8-4.8)	3.0 (1.8-5.0)	2.7 (2.1-4.0)	2.4 (1.5-2.8)	2.1 (1.5-2.7)
Total CD4$^+$ T cells	98	nd	1985 (1294-4012)	2721 (1327-4455)	2073 (1902-2977)	1469 (925-2477)	1044 (646-2331)	1186 (1000-1931)	992 (641-1453)	970 (695-1473)	904 (608-1217)	809 (560-1067)
CD25$^+$CD127$^-$CD4$^+$ T cells (regulatory)	73	nd	208 (64-282)	136 (74-280)	107 (79-162)	63 (42-69)	78 (30-126)	58 (41-86)	47 (18-86)	36 (23-89)	41 (25-64)	26 (19-41)
CD27$^+$ CD45RO$^-$ (naive)	73	nd	175 (55-251)	123 (60-237)	100 (57-147)	41 (27-49)	58 (16-93)	33 (21-58)	28 (10-61)	25 (9-52)	20 (10-40)	16 (7-23)
CD45RO$^+$ (memory or effector)	73	nd	21 (9-36)	25 (11-43)	18 (9-26)	20 (13-27)	20 (10-38)	26 (11-31)	20 (8-30)	20 (10-36)	19 (12-32)	11 (8-23)
CD27$^+$CD45RO$^-$CD4$^+$ T cells (naive)	98	nd	1856 (1164-3712)	2512 (1134-4204)	1797 (1565-2794)	1153 (685-2055)	882 (430-1871)	894 (630-1414)	661 (375-1096)	596 (441-1109)	523 (311-781)	469 (335-725)
CD31$^+$	73	nd	1684 (781-2695)	1920 (788-2564)	1188 (961-1597)	824 (438-1037)	908 (296-1446)	644 (493-1054)	460 (244-894)	442 (313-785)	304 (239-477)	325 (207-585)
CD27$^+$CD45RO$^+$CD4$^+$ T cells (memory)	98	nd	130 (110-299)	230 (119-355)	241 (112-314)	293 (210-442)	236 (155-476)	357 (222-502)	266 (195- 27)	262 (215-489)	328 (232-373)	242 (201-419)
CD27$^-$CD45RO$^+$CD4$^+$ T cells (memory effector)	98	nd	6 (1-17)	9 (5-67)	12 (4-18)	16 (10-34)	16 (5-51)	39 (11-50)	28 (14-97)	45 (26-75)	29 (19-59)	25 (15-78)
CD27$^-$CD45RO$^-$CD4$^+$ T cells (effector)	98	nd	7 (1-14)	4 (3-37)	8 (3-11)	3 (1-12)	4 (2-10)	3 (1-7)	3 (1-10)	10 (0-28)	2 (1-101)	2 (1-21)
CD45RO$^+$CD4$^+$	98	nd	139 (111-315)	240 (126-378)	245 (121-329)	311 (224-456)	251 (167-499)	399 (234-534)	304 (216-497)	322 (246-564)	357 (252-417)	273 (216-490)
Total CD8$^+$ T cells	98	nd	747 (394-1865)	850 (593-1517)	892 (667-1473)	733 (394-1197)	868 (365-1255)	852 (602-1203)	628 (249-1440)	652 (426-991)	447 (228-577)	399 (216-499)
CD27$^+$CD45RO$^-$CD8$^+$ T cells (naive)	98	nd	669 (345-1635)	789 (499-1423)	834 (637-1113)	526 (336-927)	673 (248-999)	573 (442-733)	426 (203-961)	448 (267-683)	325 (165-424)	257 (118-312)
CD27$^+$CD45RO$^+$CD8$^+$ T cells (memory)	98	nd	28 (14-260)	40 (26-127)	34 (8-127)	66 (38-239)	105 (32-228)	156 (62-402)	103 (35-256)	100 (72-262)	82 (32-153)	96 (30-166)
CD27$^-$CD45RO$^+$CD8$^+$ T cells (memory effector)	98	nd	1 (0-18)	1 (0-67)	1 (0-47)	5 (2-77)	18 (2-106)	36 (3-67)	16 (2-109)	18 (3-51)	5 (3-26)	10 (1-26)
CD27$^-$CD45RO$^-$CD8$^+$ T cells (effector)	98	nd	5 (0-50)	3 (1-123)	5 (1-193)	15 (5-174)	25 (7-218)	40 (5-310)	20 (3-198)	50 (8-155)	5 (3-59)	20 (3-65)
CD45RO$^+$CD8$^+$ T cells	98	nd	29 (14-268)	41 (26-177)	35 (8-174)	74 (41-314)	151 (36-246)	196 (79-425)	134 (38-296)	123 (77-303)	89 (35-163)	111 (33-189)

Parameter	No.										
CD4+ T-cell sjTREC content (per cell)	78	0.098 (0.080-0.173)	0.180 (0.083-0.343)	0.225 (0.047-0.251)	0.130 (0.018-0.377)	0.093 (0.016-0.299)	0.057 (0.023-0.342)	0.032 (0.014-0.190)	0.030 (0.013-0.102)	0.045 (0.007-0.108)	0.037 (0.017-0.058)
CD8+ T-cell sjTREC content (per cell)	77	0.112 (0.096-0.172)	0.145 (0.060-0.222)	0.151 (0.043-0.206)	0.078 (0.022-0.285)	0.085 (0.021-0.239)	0.036 (0.015-0.289)	0.032 (0.011-0.152)	0.034 (0.016-0.104)	0.047 (0.009-0.120)	0.031 (0.012-0.055)
CD4+ T-cell sjTREC number	71	nd	484 (188-1206)	436 (105-626)	142 (25-585)	102 (36-625)	71 (24-433)	33 (13-289)	22 (19-118)	36 (5-94)	24 (14-56)
CD8+ T-cell sjTREC number	70	nd	131 (41-345)	113 (39-145)	65 (12-267)	54 (19-293)	32 (13-181)	17 (5-219)	18 (8-85)	10 (3-68)	13 (4-26)
Total CD4+/CD8+ T-cell ratio	109	2.8 (2.2-4.3)	2.6 (1.9-5.5)	2.7 (1.4-3.7)	2.4 (1.3-3.0)	1.6 (0.9-2.7)	1.6 (0.9-2.3)	1.6 (1.0-3.0)	1.6 (0.9-2.5)	2.2 (1.5-3.7)	2.2 (1.4-4.0)
Naive CD4+/CD8+ T-cell ratio	109	2.9 (2.2-4.3)	2.8 (1.9-5.5)	2.7 (1.5-3.5)	2.2 (1.4-2.8)	1.7 (0.9-2.5)	1.7 (1.0-2.3)	1.5 (0.9-2.6)	1.6 (0.8-2.1)	1.7 (1.1-3.1)	1.7 (1.3-4.6)
Naive/memory CD4+ T-cell ratio	109	18.4 (11.8-61.9)	13.2 (9.0-18.6)	7.1 (4.8-22.8)	3.8 (2.6-5.4)	3.1 (1.9-5.4)	2.8 (1.4-4.3)	1.9 (1.3-3.2)	1.9 (1.2-3.1)	1.5 (1.0-2.7)	1.7 (1.0-2.7)
Naive/memory CD8+ T-cell ratio	109	22.2 (11.5-71.8)	25.0 (5.1-36.3)	23.4 (8.4-116.1)	7.6 (2.3-14.4)	4.6 (2.0-15.9)	3.1 (1.4-9.2)	3.8 (2.0-6.5)	3.7 (1.5-6.4)	3.6 (2.3-7.8)	2.4 (1.1-8.6)
Naive/(memory or effector) Treg ratio	80	5.7 (3.4-18.1)	6.9 (4.9-8.8)	5.3 (4.2-9.2)	4.2 (2.5-13.2)	2.4 (1.1-5.0)	1.9 (1.5-3.0)	1.5 (1.0-2.5)	1.2 (0.6-2.4)	1.1 (0.6-2.0)	1.2 (0.6-2.4)

From van Gent R, van Tilburg CM, Nibbelke EE, et al: Refined characterization and reference values of the pediatric T- and B-cell compartments. Clin Immunol 133:95–107, 2009.
Absolute counts $\times 10^6$ per liter blood, unless stated differently. Values are presented as medians (value range). Counts of T-cell subsets in boldface, whereas counts of specific cell populations within these T-cell subsets in italics. No., Number of individuals; *nd*, not determined.
sjTREC numbers $\times 10^6$ per liter blood. Values are presented as medians (value range). Naive = CD27+CD45RO−; memory = CD27+CD45RO+; effector = CD27−CD45RO+; Treg indicates regulatory T cells, which are defined as CD25+CD127−CD4+ T cells.

APPENDIX 43 Absolute Numbers of T Lymphocytes

Population	N	Cord Blood	N	1 w-2 m	N	2-5 m	N	5-9 m	N	0-15 m	N	15-24 m	N	2-5 y	N	5-10 y	N	10-16 y	N	>16 y*	N
Lymphocytes (total)	136	5.4 (3.1-9.4)	18	5.7 (2.9-11.4)	11	6.5 (3.4-12.2)	12	5.8 (1.8-18.7)	13	6.3 (3.2-12.3)	10	4.1 (1.4-12.1)	10	2.7 (1.4-5.5)	11	2.4 (1.2-4.7)	15	2.4 (1.4-4.2)	15	2.3 (1.2-4.1)	21
B lymphocytes	136	0.54 (0.14-2.0)	18	0.81 (0.18-3.5)	11	1.1 (0.52-2.3)	12	0.90 (0.13-6.3)	13	0.94 (0.11-7.7)	10	0.76 (0.16-3.7)	10	0.49 (0.18-1.3)	11	0.29 (0.10-0.80)	15	0.30 (0.12-0.74)	15	0.23 (0.064-0.82)	21
NK cells	136	1.2 (0.5-3.1)	18	0.51 (0.14-1.9)	11	0.44 (0.097-1.99)	12	0.52 (0.068-3.9)	13	0.50 (0.071-3.5)	10	0.47 (0.055-4.0)	10	0.18 (0.061-0.51)	11	0.20 (0.070-0.59)	15	0.33 (0.092-1.2)	15	0.34 (0.10-1.2)	21
T lymphocytes	136	3.1 (1.4-6.8)	18	4.0 (1.9-8.4)	11	4.5 (2.2-9.2)	12	4.0 (1.4-11.5)	13	4.4 (2.4-8.3)	10	2.5 (0.7-8.8)	10	1.9 (0.85-4.3)	11	1.8 (0.77-4.0)	15	1.6 (0.85-3.2)	15	1.5 (0.78-3.0)	21
Helper T lymphocytes	136	2.2 (1.0-4.8)	18	3.0 (1.5-6.0)	11	3.3 (1.6-6.5)	12	2.7 (1.0-7.2)	13	3.0 (1.3-7.1)	10	1.6 (0.4-7.2)	10	1.1 (0.5-2.7)	11	1.0 (0.4-2.1)	15	0.9 (0.4-2.1)	15	1.0 (0.5-2.0)	21
Cytotoxic T lymphocytes	136	0.8 (0.2-2.7)	18	0.9 (0.3-2.7)	11	1.0 (0.3-3.4)	12	1.1 (0.2-5.4)	13	1.2 (0.4-4.1)	10	0.7 (0.2-2.8)	10	0.6 (0.2-1.8)	11	0.6 (0.2-1.7)	15	0.6 (0.3-1.3)	15	0.5 (0.2-1.2)	21
Naive helper T cells	125	1.8 (0.9-3.9)	18	2.7 (1.3-5.7)	10	3.1 (1.6-6.0)	11	2.5 (0.8-7.6)	11	2.7 (1.1-6.4)	10	1.3 (0.2-7.5)	10	0.8 (0.3-2.3)	11	0.7 (0.2-2.5)	13	0.6 (0.2-1.7)	15	0.5 (0.1-2.3)	15
Terminally differentiated helper T cells	125	0.00079 (0.00021-0.003)b	18	0.0005 (0.00017-0.0015)	10	0.0011 (0.00024-0.0053)	11	0.0027 (0.0000047-0.4)b	11	0.0021 (0.000081-0.077)b	10	0.0015 (0.0001-0.033)b	10	0.0017 (0.000025-0.016)b	11	0.0011 (0.000025-0.025)b	13	0.0016 (0.00004-0.051)b	15	0.0037 (0.000098-0.068)b	15
Effector memory helper T cells	125	0.00067 (0.00017-0.0026)	18	0.0017 (0.00011-0.026)	10	0.0064 (0.002-0.021)	11	0.0093 (0.0012-0.072)	11	0.013 (0.00043-0.12)b	10	0.011 (0.00085-0.15)	10	0.018 (0.0035-0.089)	11	0.023 (0.003-0.17)	13	0.033 (0.0051-0.21)	15	0.053 (0.013-0.22)	15
Central memory helper T cells	125	0.39 (0.075-2.0)	18	0.39 (0.09-1.7)	10	0.35 (0.053-2.2)	11	0.32 (0.083-1.3)	11	0.39 (0.19-0.8)	10	0.17 (0.001-0.65)b	10	0.33 (0.16-0.66)	11	0.18 (0.0037-0.51)b	13	0.3 (0.12-0.74)	15	0.43 (0.18-1.1)	15
Naive cytotoxic T cells	125	0.36 (0.023-1.3)b	18	0.55 (0.14-2.2)	10	0.69 (0.29-1.65)	11	0.7 (0.15-3.2)	11	0.58 (0.14-2.46)	10	0.31 (0.03-3.1)	10	0.24 (0.053-1.1)	11	0.24 (0.042-1.3)	13	0.22 (0.078-0.64)	15	0.13 (0.016-1.0)	15
Terminally differentiated cytotoxic T- cells	125	0.095 (0.012-0.75)	18	0.086 (0.015-0.48)	10	0.1 (0.013-0.82)	11	0.22 (0.017-2.8)	11	0.22 (0.029-1.7)	10	0.16 (0.055-0.46)	10	0.14 (0.025-0.53)	11	0.14 (0.057-0.34)	13	0.12 (0.035-0.42)	15	0.084 (0.025-0.28)	15
Effector memory cytotoxic T cells	125	0.044 (0.0074-0.26)	18	0.042 (0.0094-0.19)	10	0.056 (0.0024-0.4)b	11	0.1 (0.0076-1.4)	11	0.13 (0.0076-2.1)	10	0.1 (0.016-0.63)	10	0.12 (0.024-0.59)	11	0.14 (0.045-0.41)	13	0.11 (0.016-0.81)	15	0.16 (0.04-0.64)	15
Central memory cytotoxic T cells	125	0.04 (0.0011-0.16)b	18	0.071 (0.013-0.38)	10	0.059 (0.0006-0.19)b	11	0.037 (0.0018-0.15)b	11	0.034 (0.012-0.092)	10	0.022 (0.0048-0.11)	10	0.017 (0.0043-0.064)	11	0.016 (0.0061-0.043)	13	0.014 (0.0023-0.086)	15	0.024 (0.0047-0.12)	15
CD197-/- cytotoxic T cells	125	0.56 (0.13-2.4)	18	0.65 (0.18-2.3)	10	0.81 (0.31-2.1)	11	0.96 (0.18-5.0)	11	0.86 (0.25-3.0)	10	0.5 (0.1-2.4)	10	0.37 (0.12-1.2)	11	0.38 (0.1-1.5)	13	0.36 (0.16-0.8)	15	0.23 (0.06-0.83)	15
Recent thymic emigrants	126	1.7 (0.71-4.2)	18	2.2 (1.0-4.9)	10	2.7 (1.4-5.2)	11	2.2 (0.8-6.2)	11	2.3 (0.9-5.8)	10	1.1 (0.17-7.4)	10	0.71 (0.19-2.6)	11	0.59 (0.2-1.7)	14	0.48 (0.15-1.5)	15	0.34 (0.05-2.4)	15
NK-T cells	136	0.034 (0.0056-0.21)	18	0.025 (0.0069-0.091)	11	0.035 (0.013-0.09)	12	0.047 (0.0044-0.51)	13	0.049 (0.0075-0.33)	10	0.038 (0.0065-0.23)	10	0.06 (0.015-0.25)	11	0.064 (0.012-0.34)	15	0.075 (0.016-0.35)	15	0.096 (0.023-0.41)	15

Cell type	n; value (range)	n; value (range)	n; value (range)	n; value (range)	n; value (range)	n; value (range)	n; value (range)	n; value (range)	n; value (range)	n; value (range)
CXCR5+ memory helper T cells	102; 0.0019 (0.00052-0.0066)	14; 0.0063 (0.00067-0.06)	11; 0.024 (0.0062-0.089)	11; 0.041 (0.015-0.11)	10; 0.048 (0.011-0.2)	10; 0.045 (0.015-0.14)	10; 0.048 (0.013-0.17)	9; 0.047 (0.013-0.16)	8; 0.047 (0.014-0.16)	10; 0.067 (0.024-0.19)
Regulatory T cells	124; 0.144 (0.065-0.319)	18; 0.23 (0.083-0.64)	10; 0.25 (0.12-0.53)	11; 0.21 (0.06-0.74)	11; 0.21 (0.063-0.69)	10; 0.12 (0.02-0.77)	11; 0.076 (0.039-0.15)	11; 0.073 (0.02-0.27)	12; 0.078 (0.033-0.19)	16; 0.067 (0.025-0.18)
TCR-αβ	127; 2.8 (1.1-6.9)	18; 3.7 (1.6-8.6)	10; 4.3 (2.2-8.3)	11; 3.8 (1.2-12.0)	11; 4.0 (2.0-8.0)	10; 2.2 (0.6-8.5)	11; 1.5 (0.6-4.3)	11; 1.5 (0.6-3.7)	15; 1.4 (0.7-2.8)	16; 1.4 (0.6-3.3)
Double negative T cells	123; 0.028 (0.01-0.079)	18; 0.022 (0.0055-0.086)	10; 0.034 (0.0082-0.14)	11; 0.046 (0.016-0.14)	11; 0.04 (0.012-0.14)	10; 0.033 (0.011-0.1)	10; 0.047 (0.016-0.14)	11; 0.032 (0.01-0.1)	14; 0.027 (0.009-0.078)	13; 0.023 (0.0069-0.074)
Helper T cells	123; 1.9 (0.8-4.7)	18; 2.8 (1.2-6.2)	10; 3.1 (1.6-6.0)	11; 2.5 (0.83-7.8)	11; 2.7 (1.0-7.0)	10; 1.4 (0.3-7.0)	10; 1.0 (0.4-2.8)	11; 0.91 (0.36-2.8)	15; 0.85 (0.34-2.1)	13; 0.85 (0.3-2.4)
Cytotoxic T cells	123; 0.73 (0.23-2.4)	18; 0.85 (0.23-3.1)	10; 1.1 (0.4-2.8)	11; 1.2 (0.27-5.2)	11; 1.2 (0.36-3.8)	10; 0.65 (0.17-2.5)	10; 0.54 (0.17-1.7)	11; 0.57 (0.21-1.5)	14; 0.54 (0.21-1.5)	13; 0.45 (0.12-1.7)
Double positive T cells	123; 0.039 (0.0073-0.21)	18; 0.049 (0.015-0.17)	10; 0.059 (0.014-0.24)	11; 0.035 (0.0063-0.19)	11; 0.027 (0.0066-0.11)	10; 0.014 (0.0023-0.088)	10; 0.012 (0.0033-0.043)	11; 0.0081 (0.0036-0.018)	14; 0.0091 (0.0032-0.026)	13; 0.012 (0.0023-0.06)
TCR-γδ	127; 0.087 (0.03-0.25)	18; 0.12 (0.013-1.0)	10; 0.17 (0.056-0.51)	11; 0.18 (0.038-0.89)	11; 0.21 (0.07-0.63)	10; 0.16 (0.041-0.64)	10; 0.16 (0.027-0.96)	11; 0.16 (0.027-0.96)	15; 0.15 (0.039-0.54)	16; 0.071 (0.025-0.2)
Double negative T cells	123; 0.059 (0.02-0.17)	18; 0.075 (0.0077-0.73)	10; 0.094 (0.026-0.34)	11; 0.12 (0.032-0.43)	11; 0.14 (0.047-0.43)	10; 0.12 (0.027-0.5)	10; 0.13 (0.021-0.85)	11; 0.13 (0.033-0.54)	15; 0.13 (0.039-0.44)	13; 0.056 (0.019-0.17)
Helper T cells	123; 0.014 (0.0034-0.061)	18; 0.02 (0.0039-0.1)	10; 0.03 (0.01-0.086)	11; 0.017 (0.0056-0.051)	11; 0.013 (0.00092-0.17)	10; 0.008 (0.00087-0.073)	10; 0.0047 (0.001-0.021)	11; 0.0028 (0.00051-0.015)	14; 0.0022 (0.000041-0.012)	13; 0.001 (0.000012-0.0076)
Cytotoxic T cells	123; 0.011 (0.0027-0.046)	18; 0.012 (0.00025-0.14)b	10; 0.04 (0.012-0.13)	11; 0.043 (0.004-0.45)	11; 0.046 (0.004-0.45)	10; 0.03 (0.005-0.19)	10; 0.019 (0.0019-0.2)	11; 0.019 (0.0051-0.069)	14; 0.02 (0.0021-0.19)	13; 0.013 (0.0018-0.094)
Double positive T cells	123; 0.0005 (0.000098-0.0026)	18; 0.00082 (0.000012-0.0057)	10; 0.0021 (0.00029-0.015)	11; 0.0011 (0.000097-0.012)	11; 0.0058 (0.000067-0.005)	10; 0.00041 (0.000038-0.0045)	10; 0.0003 (0.000038-0.0045)	11; 0.0002 (0.000034-0.0011)	14; 0.0002 (0.00002-0.0021)	13; 0.0002 (0.000035-0.0011)

From Schatorjé EJH, Gemen EFA, Driessen GJA, et al: Paediatric reference values for the peripheral T cell compartment. Scand J Immunol 75:436–444, 2012.

m, Months; *w*, weeks; *TCR*, T-cell receptor; *y*, years.

*The right limit of this tolerance interval was based on the original values (see Methods).

APPENDIX 44   Reference Ranges for Dendritic Cell Subpopulations in Peripheral Blood for Different Age Groups*

Dendritic Cell Subpopulations	AGE GROUPS			
	0-<2 (N = 16)	2-<5 (N = 19)	5-<10 (N = 27)	10-<18 (N = 38)
mDC/µl PB	16 (7-30)	15 (6-28)	13 (6-24)	10 (5-19)
mDC (%)	0.16% (0.08-0.24)	0.19% (0.09-0.30)	0.19% (0.09-0.34)	0.16% (0.08-0.33)
pDC/ µl PB	17 (8-38)	16 (7-34)	15 (6-29)	13 (5-23)
pDC (%)	0.19% (0.09-0.38)	0.19% (0.09-0.38)	0.20% (0.08-0.39)	0.20% (0.08-0.40)

From Heinze A, Elze MC, Kloess S, et al. Age-matched Dendritic cell subpopulations reference values in Childhood. Scand J Immunol 77:213–220, 2013
%, Relative count per peripheral leukocytes; mDC, myeloid dendritic cell; PB, peripheral blood; pDc, plasmacytoid dendritic cell.
*Absolute counts (cells/µL), percentage of dentritic cells within the leucocytes population in PB: median and percentiles (5th to 95th percentile). Age expressed in years.

APPENDIX 45   Tibial Bone Marrow Cell Populations of Normal Infants from Birth to 18 Months of Age*

Cell Type	MONTH										
	0 (N = 57)[†]	1 (N = 71)	2 (N = 48)	3 (N = 24)	4 (N = 19)	5 (N = 22)	6 (N = 22)	9 (N = 16)	12 (N = 18)	15 (N = 12)	18 (N = 19)
Small lymphocytes	14.42 ± 5.54	47.05 ± 9.24	42.68 ± 7.90	43.63 ± 11.83	47.06 ± 8.77	47.19 ± 9.93	47.55 ± 7.88	48.76 ± 8.11	47.11 ± 11.32	42.77 ± 8.94	43.55 ± 8.56
Transitional cells	1.18 ± 1.13	1.95 ± 0.94	2.38 ± 1.35	2.17 ± 1.64	1.64 ± 1.01	1.83 ± 0.89	2.31 ± 1.16	1.92 ± 1.39	2.32 ± 1.90	1.70 ± 0.82	1.99 ± 1.00
Proerythroblasts	0.02 ± 0.06	0.10 ± 0.14	0.13 ± 0.19	0.10 ± 0.13	0.05 ± 0.10	0.07 ± 0.10	0.09 ± 0.12	0.07 ± 0.09	0.02 ± 0.04	0.07 ± 0.12	0.08 ± 0.13
Basophilic erythroblasts	0.24 ± 0.25	0.34 ± 0.33	0.57 ± 0.41	0.40 ± 0.33	0.24 ± 0.24	0.47 ± 0.33	0.32 ± 0.24	0.31 ± 0.24	0.30 ± 0.25	0.38 ± 0.37	0.50 ± 0.34
Early erythroblasts	0.27 ± 0.26	0.44 ± 0.42	0.71 ± 0.51	0.50 ± 0.38	0.28 ± 0.30	0.55 ± 0.36	0.41 ± 0.30	0.39 ± 0.28	0.39 ± 0.27	0.46 ± 0.36	0.59 ± 0.34
Polychromatic erythroblasts	13.06 ± 6.78	6.90 ± 4.45	13.06 ± 3.48	10.51 ± 3.39	6.84 ± 2.58	7.55 ± 2.35	7.30 ± 3.60	7.73 ± 3.39	6.83 ± 3.75	6.04 ± 1.56	6.97 ± 3.56
Orthochromatic erythroblasts	0.69 ± 0.73	0.54 ± 1.88	0.66 ± 0.82	0.70 ± 0.87	0.34 ± 0.30	0.46 ± 0.51	0.38 ± 0.56	0.39 ± 0.48	0.37 ± 0.51	0.50 ± 0.65	0.44 ± 0.49
Extruded nuclei	0.47 ± 0.46	0.16 ± 0.17	0.26 ± 0.22	0.19 ± 0.12	0.16 ± 0.17	0.14 ± 0.11	0.16 ± 0.22	0.22 ± 0.25	0.23 ± 0.25	0.17 ± 0.12	0.21 ± 0.19
Late erythroblasts	14.22 ± 7.14	7.60 ± 4.84	13.99 ± 3.82	11.40 ± 3.43	7.34 ± 2.54	8.16 ± 2.58	7.85 ± 4.11	8.34 ± 3.31	7.42 ± 4.11	6.72 ± 1.80	7.62 ± 3.63
Early/late erythroblasts ratio[‡]	1:50	1:15	1:18	1:22	1:23	1:15	1:17	1:19	1:17	1:15	1:10
Fetal erythroblasts	14.48 ± 7.24	8.04 ± 5.00	14.70 ± 3.86	11.90 ± 3.52	7.62 ± 2.56	8.70 ± 2.69	8.25 ± 4.31	8.72 ± 3.34	7.81 ± 4.26	7.18 ± 1.95	8.21 ± 0.19
Blood reticulocytes	4.18 ± 1.46	1.06 ± 1.13	3.39 ± 1.22	2.90 ± 0.91	1.65 ± 0.73	1.38 ± 0.65	1.74 ± 0.80	1.67 ± 0.52	1.79 ± 0.79	2.10 ± 0.91	1.84 ± 0.46

Continued on following page

APPENDIX 45 Tibial Bone Marrow Cell Populations of Normal Infants from Birth to 18 Months of Age (Continued)

| Cell Type | MONTH | | | | | | | | | | |
	0 (N = 57)[†]	1 (N = 71)	2 (N = 48)	3 (N = 24)	4 (N = 19)	5 (N = 22)	6 (N = 22)	9 (N = 16)	12 (N = 18)	15 (N = 12)	18 (N = 19)
Neutrophils											
Promyelocytes	0.79 ± 0.91	0.76 ± 0.65	0.78 ± 0.68	0.76 ± 0.80	0.59 ± 0.51	0.87 ± 0.80	0.67 ± 0.66	0.41 ± 0.34	0.69 ± 0.71	0.67 ± 0.58	0.64 ± 0.59
Myelocytes	3.95 ± 2.93	2.50 ± 1.48	2.03 ± 1.14	2.24 ± 1.70	2.32 ± 1.59	2.73 ± 1.82	2.22 ± 1.25	2.07 ± 1.20	2.32 ± 1.14	2.48 ± 0.94	2.49 ± 1.39
Early neutrophils	4.74 ± 3.43	3.27 ± 1.94	2.81 ± 1.62	3.00 ± 2.18	2.91 ± 2.01	3.60 ± 2.50	2.89 ± 1.71	2.48 ± 1.46	3.02 ± 1.52	3.16 ± 1.19	3.14 ± 1.75
Metamyelocytes	19.37 ± 4.84	11.34 ± 3.59	11.27 ± 3.38	11.93 ± 13.09	6.04 ± 3.63	11.89 ± 3.24	11.02 ± 3.12	11.80 ± 3.90	11.10 ± 3.82	12.48 ± 7.45	12.42 ± 4.15
Bands	28.89 ± 7.56	14.10 ± 4.63	13.15 ± 4.71	14.60 ± 7.54	13.93 ± 6.13	14.07 ± 5.48	14.00 ± 4.58	14.08 ± 4.53	14.02 ± 4.88	15.17 ± 4.20	14.20 ± 5.23
Mature neutrophils	7.37 ± 4.64	3.64 ± 2.97	3.07 ± 2.45	3.48 ± 1.62	4.27 ± 2.69	3.77 ± 2.44	4.85 ± 2.69	3.97 ± 2.29	5.65 ± 3.92	6.94 ± 3.88	6.31 ± 3.91
Late neutrophils	55.63 ± 7.98	29.08 ± 6.79	27.50 ± 6.88	31.00 ± 11.17	31.30 ± 7.80	29.73 ± 7.19	29.84 ± 6.74	29.86 ± 7.36	30.77 ± 8.69	34.60 ± 7.35	32.93 ± 7.01
Early/late neutrophil ratio	1:12	1:9	1:9	1:9	1:11	1:8	1:10	1:12	1:10	1:10	1:10
Total neutrophils	60.37 ± 8.66	32.35 ± 7.68	30.31 ± 7.27	34.01 ± 11.95	34.21 ± 8.61	33.12 + 8.34	32.75 ± 7.03	32.33 ± 7.75	33.79 ± 8.76	37.76 ± 7.32	36.06 ± 7.40
Total eosinophils	2.70 ± 1.27	2.61 ± 1.40	2.50 ± 1.22	2.54 ± 1.46	2.37 ± 4.13	1.98 ± 0.86	2.08 ± 1.16	1.74 ± 1.08	1.92 ± 1.09	3.39 ± 1.93	2.70 ± 2.16
Total basophils	0.12 ± 0.20	0.07 ± 0.16	0.08 ± 0.10	0.09 + 0.09	0.11 ± 0.14	0.09 ± 0.13	0.10 ± 0.13	0.11 ± 0.13	0.13 ± 0.15	0.27 ± 0.37	0.10 ± 0.12
Total myeloid cells	63.19 ± 9.10	35.03 ± 8.09	32.90 ± 7.85	36.64 ± 2.26	36.69 ± 8.91	35.40 ± 8.54	34.93 ± 7.52	34.18 ± 8.13	35.83 ± 8.84	41.42 ± 7.43	38.86 ± 7.92
Monocytes	0.88 ± 0.85	1.01 ± 0.89	0.91 ± 0.83	0.68 ± 0.56	0.75 ± 0.75	1.29 ± 1.06	1.21 ± 1.01	1.17 ± 0.97	1.46 ± 1.52	1.68 ± 1.09	2.12 ± 1.59
Miscellaneous											
Megakaryocytes	0.06 ± 0.15	0.05 + 0.09	0.10 ± 0.13	0.06 ± 0.09	0.06 ± 0.06	0.08 ± 0.09	0.04 ± 0.07	0.09 ± 0.12	0.05 ± 0.08	0.00 ± 0.00	0.07 ± 0.12
Plasma cells	0.00 ⊥ 0.02	0.02 ± 0.06	0.02 ± 0.05	0.00 ± 0.02	0.01 ± 0.03	0.05 ± 0.11	0.03 ± 0.07	0.01 + 0.03	0.03 + 0.07	0.07 ± 0.12	0.06 ± 0.08
Unknown blasts	0.31 ± 0.31	0.62 ± 0.50	0.58 + 0.50	0.63 ± 0.60	0.56 ± 0.53	0.50 ± 0.37	0.56 ± 0.48	0.42 ± 0.50	0.37 ± 0.33	0.46 ± 0.32	0.43 ± 0.45
Unknown cells	0.22 ± 0.34	0.21 ± 0.25	0.16 ± 0.24	0.19 ± 0.21	0.23 ± 0.25	0.17 ± 0.22	0.10 ± 0.15	0.14 ± 0.17	0.11 ± 0.14	0.13 ± 0.18	0.20 ± 0.23
Damaged cells	5.79 ± 2.78	5.50 ± 2.46	5.09 ± 1.78	4.75 ± 2.30	4.80 ± 2.29	4.86 ± 1.25	5.04 ± 1.08	4.89 ± 1.60	5.34 ± 2.19	4.99 ± 1.96	5.05 ± 2.15
Total	6.38 ± 2.84	6.39 ± 2.63	5.94 ± 1.94	5.63 ± 2.36	5.66 ± 2.30	5.66 ± 1.41	5.78 ± 1.16	5.55 ± 1.74	5.90 ± 2.03	5.65 ± 2.02	5.81 ± 2.16

From Rosse C, Kraemer MJ, Dillon TL, et al: Bone marrow cell populations of normal infants; the predominance of lymphocytes. J Lab Clin Med 89:1228, 1997.

*Percentages of cell types (mean ± standard deviation) is tibial bone marrow of infants from birth to 18 months of age. Data were obtained from normal American infants of black, white, and Asian racial origin. The changes in the marrow during the first 18 months of postnatal life are based on different counts of 1000 cells classified on stained smears on each of 10 serial marrow samples aspirated from the same population of infants. Criteria for including bone marrow data in this study consisted of absence of any clinical evidence of disease, normal rate of growth, and normal serum protein and transerffin saturations.

[†]N = number of infants studied at each stage.

[‡]Expressed in round figures for facilitating comparison. Means ± standard deviation were calculated from values obtained in individual infants, and statistical comparisons were performed.

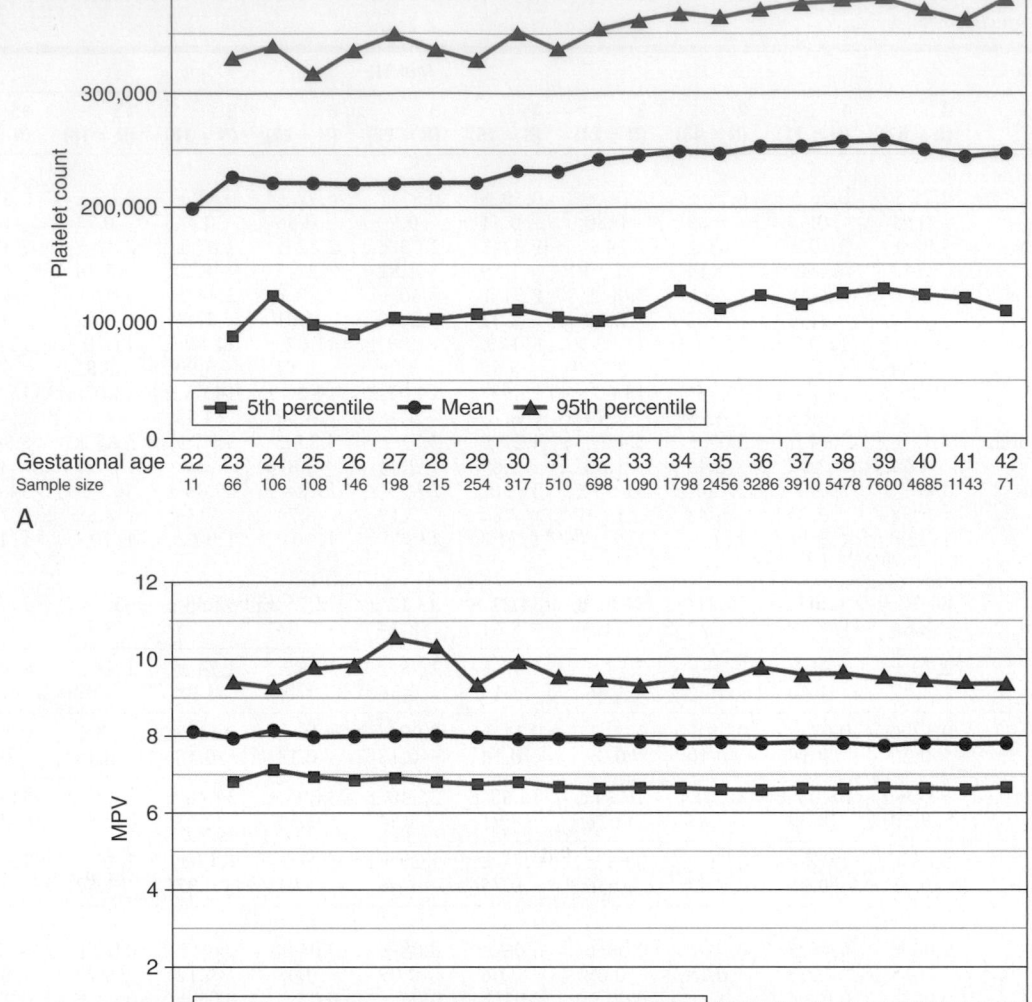

A

B

Appendix 46 The first recorded platelet counts (A) and MPV determinations (B) obtained in the first three days after birth, are shown for neonates of 22 to 42 weeks gestation. Mean values are given by the red line and the 5th and 95th percentiles are given by the green and blue lines. **A,** Initial platelet counts. (b) Initial MPV measurement. Platelet values were measured using automated Beckman Coulter Hematology Analyzers (Beckman Coulter Inc., Fla., USA). *(From Wiedmeier SE, Henry E, Sola-Visner MC, et al: Platelet reference ranges for neonates, defined using data from over 47 000 patients in a multihospital healthcare system.* J Perinatol *29:130–136, 2009.)*

APPENDIX 47   Circulating Platelet Counts and Serum TPO Levels at Different Ages*

Age Categories	Platelet Count (10⁹/L)	Serum TPO (fmol/L)
Core blood	288 ± 53	3.73 ± 1.48 (1.44-6.74)
2 days	303 ± 48	5.92 ± 1.4 (4.33-9.18)
5 days	338 ± 59	4.32 ± 0.94 (2.38-5.76)
1 month	343 ± 72	3.77 ± 1.45 (2.25-7.60)
2-11 months	365 ± 49	2.10 ± 0.69 (1.04-4.24)
1-2 years	314 ± 78	2.23 ± 0.89 (0.43-4.54)
3-4 years	304 ± 66	1.97 ± 0.67 (0.98-3.73)
5-6 years	303 ± 65	1.67 ± 0.66 (0.58-3.14)
7-10 years	295 ± 58	1.39 ± 0.63 (0.53-2.94)
11-15 years	251 ± 40	1.24 ± 0.40 (0.49-1.99)
Adult	234 ± 48	0.83 ± 0.36 (0.25-1.72)

From Ishiguro A, Nakahata T, Matsubara K, et al: Age-related changes in thrombopoietin in children: reference interval for serum thrombopoietin levels. Br J Haematol 106(4):884–888, 1999.
TPO, Thrombopoietin.
*All values for children are significantly different (P <.001, Mann-Whitney U test) from values for adults. Data are expressed as mean ± standard deviation. The range of values for TPO is reported in parentheses.

APPENDIX 48   Comparison of Selected Coagulation Factor Values in Newborns*

Age	Fibrinogen (mg/dL)	F II (U/mL)	F VIII (U/mL)	F IX (U/mL)	F XII (U/mL)	Antithrombin (U/mL)	Protein C (U/mL)
Term							
Hathaway and Bonnar (1987) and Manco-Johnson et al. (1988)†	240 (150)	0.52 (0.25)	1.5 (0.55)	0.35 (0.15)	0.44 (0.16)	0.56 (0.32)	0.32 (0.16)
Andrew et al. (1987, 1988)‡	283 (177)	0.48 (0.26)	1.0 (0.50)	0.53 (0.25)	0.53 (0.20)	0.63 (0.25)	0.35 (0.17)
Corrigan (1992)§	246 (150)	0.45 (0.22)	1.68 (0.50)	0.40 (0.20)	0.44 (0.16)	0.52 (0.20)	0.31 (0.17)
Preterm							
Hathaway and Bonnar (1987) and Manco-Johnson et al. (1988)†	300 (120)	0.45 (0.26)	0.93 (0.54)	0.41 (0.20)	0.33 (0.23)	0.40 (0.25)	0.24 (0.18)
Andrew et al. (1987, 1988)‡	243 (150)	0.45 (0.20)	1.1 (0.50)	0.35 (0.19)	0.38 (0.10)	0.38 (0.14)	0.28 (0.12)
Corrigan (1992)§	240 (150)	0.35 (0.21)	1.36 (0.21)	0.35 (0.10)	0.22 (0.09)	0.35 (0.10)	0.28 (0.12)

From Hathaway W, Corrigan J: Report of scientific and standardization subcommittee on neonatal hemostasis. Thromb Haemost 65:323, 1991.
*Data are expressed as mean and lower limits of normal. Preterm = 30- to 36-weeks' gestational age.
†Hathaway W, Bonnar J: Hemostatic disorders of the pregnant woman and newborn infant. New York, 1987, Elsevier; Manco-Johnson M, Marlar R, et al: Severe protein C deficiency in newborn infants. J Pediatr 113:359, 1988.
‡Andrew M, Paes B, Milner R, et al: Development of the human coagulation system in the full-term infant. Blood 70:165, 1987; Andrew M, Paes B, Milner R, et al: Development of the human coagulation system in the healthy premature infant. Blood 72:1651, 1988.
§Corrigan JJ Jr: Normal hemostasis in fetus and newborn. coagulation. In Polin RA, Fox WW, editors: Fetal and neonatal physiology. Philadelphia, 1992, Saunders, p. 1368–1371.

APPENDIX 49   Reference Ranges for Coagulation Parameters*, Inhibitors, and Fibrinolysis in Preterm Newborns

	Premature SGA Newborns (N = 68) (Mean ± SD and 2.5th to 97.5th Percentile)	Premature SGA Newborns (N = 71) (Mean ± SD and 2.5th to 97.5th Percentile)	S
[1]INR	1.35 ± 0.22 (1.02-2.09)	1.32 ± 0.20 (1.02-1.85)	NS
[1]PT(sec)	16.6 ± 2.1 (13.2-23.1)	16.4 ± 1.98 (13.3-21.4)	NS
[2]APTT(sec)	51 ± 11 (35.4-97.6)	51 ± 12 (34.2-102.9)	NS
[1]Fibrinogen (mg/dL)	158 ± 46 (65-243)	183 ± 80 (64-478)	0.029
[1]IIc (%)	37.6 ± 6.5 (23.4-53)	37.2 ± 9 (20.5-58)	NS
[1]Vc (%)	61 ± 22 (23-128)	62 ± 20.4 (22.6-120)	NS
[1]VIIc (%)	61.2 ± 20.5 (17.9-116.5)	68.8 ± 23.7 (27.8-124.2)	NS
[1]VIIIc (%)	142 ± 80 (26-389)	116 ± 57 (28-276)	0.041
[2]IXc (%)	32 ± 22 (11.8-107.5)	28 ± 11 (11.6-60.5)	NS
[1]Xc (%)	41.2 ± 9.7 (18.2-65.5)	41.5 ± 10 (27.0-68.7)	NS
[1]XIc (%)	33.5 ± 14.2 (11.3-76.9)	30.5 ± 11.0 (13.2-60.4)	NS
[1]XIIc (%)	50 ± 22 (16-110.7)	47 ± 24 (12.7-119.6)	NS
[1]AT Act (%)	37.2 ± 11.0 (19.5-67.8)	39.0 ± 13.7 (16.7-80.3)	NS
[2]PC Act (%)	24 ± 8 (11.0-50.3)	24 ± 9 (10.4-52)	NS
[1]Free PS Act (%)	31.5 ± 9.0 (17-57)	31.1 ± 5.9 (20-47.6)	NS
[2]APCR	2.3 ± 0.30 (1.32-3.13)	2.2 ± 0.34 (1.43-3.16)	0.017
[2]tPA (ng/ml)	13.8 ± 8.2 (4.5-44.1)	11.4 ± 7.0 (3.2-34.6)	0.021
[2]PAI-1 (ng/ml)	55.3 ± 24.4 (14.9-102.6)	46 ± 24 (16.5-122)	0.019
[1]VWF Ag (%)	202 ± 64 (105-355)	193 ± 59 (95-339)	NS

From Mitsiako G, Giougi E, Chatziioannidis I, et al: Haemostatic profile of healthy premature small for gestational age neonates. Thromb Res 126:103–106, 2010.
1, T test; 2, Mann-Whitney U test; Act, activity; Ag, antigenic value; c, coagulant activity; D, difference; NS, not significant; S, significance.
*All parameters were determined utilizing a STA Compact Analyzer and reagents from Diagnostica Stago (Asnières sur Seine, France).

APPENDIX 50   Reference Ranges for Coagulation Tests in Healthy, Full-Term Newborns Compared with Normal Adults*

Test	Newborns	Adults	P<
PT (sec)	13.1 ± 0.9	11.9 ± 0.6	.0001
aPTT (sec)	35 ± 4.5	28.8 ± 2.7	.0001
Platelets (×10⁹/L)	214 ± 55	258 ± 66	.0001
Fibrinogen (mg/dL)	251 ± 51	262 ± 44	NS
Factor II (%)	73 ± 7	100 ± 15	.0001
Factor V (%)	93 ± 13	98 ± 19	NS
Factor VII (%)	88 ± 12	95 ± 18	.005
Factor VIII (%)	113 ± 38	92 ± 21	.0001
Factor IX (%)	86 ± 18	94 ± 16	.003
Factor X (%)	72 ± 10	97 ± 15	.0001
Hematocrit (%)	59 ± 3.0	44 ± 2.5	.0001

From Cerneca F, de Vonderweid U, Simeone R, et al: The importance of hematocrit in the interpretation of coagulation tests in the full-term newborn infant. Hematologica 79:25, 1994.
*Data were obtained in 71 newborns and 100 adults and expressed as mean ± standard deviation. Samples were collected with a constant anticoagulant-to-blood ration, based on a previous determination of hematocrit level.

APPENDIX 51   Template Bleeding Time in Neonate According to Gestational Age and in Children and Adolescents*

| | ≤28 Weeks | | | 29-32 Weeks | | | 33-37 Weeks | | | ≥ 38 Weeks | | |
DOL	BT	PL	MPV	BT	PL	MPV	BT	PL	MPV	BT	PL	MPV
1	204 ± 80	255.5 ± 69.4	8.9 ± 1.2	207 ± 105	286.6 ± 81.1	10.8 ± 1.0	157 ± 68	307.0 ± 106.1	10.6 ± 0.8	107 ± 38	315.9 ± 80.9	10.5 ± 1.4
10	152 ± 59	286.0 ± 81.1	9.7 ± 1.3	146 ± 79	300.9 ± 124.3	10.4 ± 1.4	163 ± 92	347.6 ± 93.9	10.7 ± 1.1	88 ± 31	344.2 ± 99.4	10.5 ± 1.6
30	104 ± 45	277.5 ± 99.8	9.9 ± 1.4	173 ± 86	306.1 ± 125.0	10.5 ± 1.4	146 ± 92	314.1 ± 120.9	10.3 ± 1.3	82 ± 39	352.3 ± 139.3	11.3 ± 1.2

From Del Vecchio A, Latini G, Henry E, et al: *Template bleeding times of 240 neonates born at 24 to 41 weeks gestation.* J Perinatol 28:427–431, 2008.

BT, Bleeding time; DOL, day of life; MPV, mean platelet volume; PL, platelets.

*Patients were tested on either day of life 1 (N 1/420 in each gestational age group), day of life 10 (N 1/420 per group), or day of life 30 (N 1/420 per group).

Bleeding Time in Children*

Age (y)	Number of Subjects	Bleeding Time (s)
0-2	33	180 ± 30
2-4	33	240 ± 60
4-9	75	300 ± 60
9-18	66	300 ± 70
0-18	201	270 ± 60
Adults	90	320 ± 90

From Aversa LA, Vázquez A, Peñalver JA, et al: *Bleeding time in normal children.* J Pediatr Hematol Oncol 17:25, 1995.

s, Seconds; y, years.

*Values are expressed as mean ± standard deviation, using a disposable Simplate method.

APPENDIX 52   Reference Ranges for Global Coagulation Assays in Children and Adolescents

Assay	Method	1-6 Months N = 29[†] (14M/15F)	7-12 Months N = 25[‡] (19M/6F)	1-5 Years N = 57 (35M/22F)	6-10 Years N = 56 (29M/27F)	11-18 Years N = 50[§] (24M/26F)	> 19 Years N = 52 (27F/25M)
PT (sec)	Thromborel S	12.5/12.8*[‖]	12.2/12.4*[‖]	12.1/12.2*[‖]	12.6/12.6*[‖]	12.8/12.6*[‖]	11.7/11.8*
	BCS	11.2-15.5	11.4-13.5	11.2-13.4	11.5-14.0	11.4-13.8	10.7-12.9
	Innovin	10.7/10.7 *	10.6/10.6*	10.6/10.6 *	10.9/10.9*[‖]	10.8/10.9*[‖]	10.5/10.6*
	CA-1500	10.0-12.7	9.5-12.8	10.0-11.4	10.2-11.6	10.1-11.9	9.7-11.4
PT (%)	Thromborel S	92/89*[‖]	95/93*[‖]	97/96*[‖]	91/91*[‖]	89/91*[‖]	101/101*
	BCS	64-108	81-105	81-108	76-104	78-105	88-116
	Innovin	103/104*	106/106*	106/106*	100/100*[‖]	101/100*	108/108*
	CA-1500	72-122	71-128	89-121	86-116	81-118	89-129
APTT (sec)	Pathromtin SL	41/42*[‖]	39/39*[‖]	36/37*[‖]	37/37*[‖]	35/36*[‖]	34/34*
	BCS	33-56	32-49	31-44	31-44	30-43	27-40
	Actin FS	29/29*[‖]	28/28*[‖]	27/27*[‖]	28/28*[‖]	27/27*[‖]	25/25*
	CA-1500	21-33	24-33	24-30	25-32	25-30	22-28
TT (sec)	Thromboclotin	19.2/20.0[‖]	18.0/18.0	17.0/17.2	17.5/17.4	17.4/17.8	17.4/17.5
	CA-1500	16.2-24.9	15.4-21.1	15.3-19.7	14.5-19.9	15.2-24.0	15.5-20.5
BT (sec)	Batroxobin	21.0/21.4[‖]	20.2/20.5	20.2/20.3	20.2/20.2	19.8/19.9	20.1/20.1
	Reagent CA-1500	19.7-25.0	19.1-24.0	18.8-22.7	19.1-21.5	18.8-21.5	18.7-22.4

Grimminck B, Geerts J, et al: *Age dependency of coagulation parameters during childhood and puberty.* J Thromb Haemost 10:2254–2263, 2012.

APTT, Activated partial thromboplastin time; BCS, Behring Coagulation System; BT, batroxobin time; CA-1500, Sysmex CA-1500 Analyzer; F, female; M, male; PT, prothrombin time; sec, seconds; TT, thrombin time.

*Indicates statistically significant difference between devices for the student's t-test.

[†]n = 28 for APTT with the BCS.

[‡]n = 24 for PT, TT, and BT with the CA-1500.

[§]n = 49 for batroxobin time (one sample was excluded because of an extremely outlying result of 13.3 seconds). Data are presented as median/ mean with t-test results of between methods and age comparisons in the first row, whereas the second row shows the boundaries including 90% of the central population.

[‖]Indicates statistically significant difference between child groups and adults for the student's t-test.

APPENDIX 53   Reference Ranges for Single Coagulation Factors in Children and Adolescents

Assay	Method	1-6 Months N = 29[†] (14M/15F)	7-12 Months N = 25[‡] 19M/6F	1-5 Years N = 57[§] 35M/22F	6-10 Years N = 56[¶] 29M/27F	11-18 Years N = 50[‖] 24M/26F	> 19 Years N = 52[†] 27F/25M
Fbg (g/L)	Multifibren U	2.2/2.3[#]	2.3/2.6[#]	2.5/2.7*	2.3/2.6[#]	2.3/2.5[#]	2.9/3.0
	BCS	1.5-3.8	1.8-4.8	1.9-3.9	2.0-3.9	1.9-3.7	2.1-4.2
	Dade Thrombin	1.9/2.0[#]	2.2/2.3[#]	2.4/2.5[#]	2.3/2.4[#]	2.3/2.4[#]	2.7/2.8
	CA-1500	1.3-3.3	1.6-4.0	1.7-3.5	1.8-3.6	1.8-3.3	2.0-3.9
FII (%)	Thromborel S	93/91[#]	98/99[#]	104/105[#]	99/99[#]	96/99[#]	117/119
	BCS	66-112	83-132	85-126	78-121	78-132	96-147
	Innovin	86/86[#]	95/97[#]	102/103[#]	97/98[#]	92/94[#]	114/116
	CA-1500	60-109	77-134	81-126	77-116	70-120	93-151
FV (%)	Thromborel S	114/114	114/117*	108/111	97/99[#]*	95/99[#]*	112/113*
	BCS	82-145	97-148	85-153	80-123	76-132	84-149
	Innovin	118/110[#]	102/102[#]*	102/104[#]	93/92*	87/87*	89/91*
	CA-1500	56-148	66-141	68-143	62-127	55-119	57-128
FVII (%)	Thromborel S	98/97[#]	96/98[#]	99/99[#]*	96/98[#]*	100/101[#]*	105/108
	BCS	54-126	74-131	81-117	79-119	75-130	86-142
	Innovin	93/91[#]	89/88	84/85[#]*	86/87[#]*	86/86[#]*	101/101
	CA-1500	38-129	41-148	61-111	61-127	55-115	67-146
FVIII (%)	Pathromtin SL	90/96[#]	95/100[#]	109/109[#]*	100/101[#]*	109/108[#]*	123/123*
	BCS	58-144	59- >152	76-143	68-137	70-148	87- >152
	Actin FS	108/107[#]	116/119[#]	124/125[#]*	118/119[#]*	118/122[#]*	133/140*
	CA-1500	67-141	70-213	83-170	75-163	80-166	96-216
FIX (%)	Pathromtin SL	53/57[#]	64/68[#]	77/78[#]	78/80[#]	84/85[#]	102/104*
	BCS	41-87	42-109	58-99	57-106	60-117	78-139
	Actin FS	57/57[#]	71/72[#]	78/78[#]	77/80[#]	87/89[#]	110/116*
	CA-1500	44-78	46-114	63-97	60-108	72-116	87-174
FX (%)	Thromborel S	90/90[#]	100/99[#]	104/104[#]	95/95[#]	88/94[#]*	112/115
	BCS	66-132	74-124	84-129	74-120	73-128	90-149
	Innovin	88/87[#]	97/99[#]	101/100[#]	92/92[#]	84/86[#]*	110/114
	CA-1500	55-120	67-146	75-124	69-118	66-117	78-159
FXI (%)	Pathromtin SL	83/80[#]	86/88[#]	100/100	95/96[#]	88/91[#]	104/104*
	BCS	54-101	65-125	72-134	75-127	72-122	77-130
	Actin FS	85/82[#]	88/91[#]	104/104[#]	99/100[#]	93/95[#]	115/113*
	CA-1500	57-105	64-129	74-134	78-131	78-122	83-158
FXII (%)	Pathromtin SL	75/72[#]	88/81[#]	95/92[#]	96/90[#]	96/89[#]	102/101
	BCS	29-112	35-113	44-127	41-122	44-116	52-140
	Actin FS	76/74[#]	82/82[#]	88/87[#]	92/88[#]	92/88[#]	106/108
	CA-1500	28-116	31-126	36-122	37-123	43-122	53-165
FXIII (%)	Berichrom FXIII	96/99[#]	97/97[#]	99/100[#]	104/103[#]	99/97[#]	116/115
	BCS	63-152	42-128	71-139	76-133	64-133	68- >156

Appel IM, Grimminck B, Geerts J, et al: Age dependency of coagulation parameters during childhood and puberty. J Thromb Haemost 10:2254–2263, 2012.

BCS, Behring Coagulation System; CA-1500, Sysmex CA-1500 Analyzer; F, female; Fbg, fibrinogen; M, male; PT, prothrombin time; sec, seconds.

*Indicates statistically significant difference between devices for the student's t-test.

[†]n = 28 for FVII, FVIII, FIX, FX with the BCS and n = 27 for FXIII.

[‡]n = 24 for Fbg, FII, FV, FVII, FX, and FIX with the CA-1500, n = 23 for FXI with the BCS and n = 18 for FXIII.

[§]n = 53 for FXI with the BCS and n = 50 for FXIII.

[‖]n = 48 for FXI with BCS and FXIII; n = 51 for FXI with BCS, and n = 49 for FXIII. Data are presented as median/mean with t-test results of between methods and age comparisons in the first row, whereas the second row shows the boundaries including 90% of the central population.

[¶]n = 55 for FII with the CA-1500, n = 53 for FXI with BCS, and n = 51 for FXIII.

[#]Indicates statistically significant difference between child groups and adults for the student's t-test.

APPENDIX 54   Reference Values for the Inhibitors of Coagulation in Healthy Children Aged 1 to 16 Years Compared with Adults*

| Coagulation Inhibitors | AGE | | | |
| | 1 to 5 y | 6 to 10 y | 11 to 16 y | Adult |
	Mean (Boundary)	Mean (Boundary)	Mean (Boundary)	Mean (Boundary)
ATIII (U/mL)	1.11 (0.82-1.39)	1.11 (0.90-1.31)	1.05 (0.77-1.32)	1.0 (0.74-1.26)
α_2M (U/mL)	1.69 (1.14-2.23)[†]	1.69 (1.28-2.09)[†]	1.56 (0.98-2.12)[†]	0.86 (0.52-1.20)
C_1-Inh (U/mL)	1.35 (0.85-1.83)[†]	1.14 (0.88-1.54)	1.03 (0.68-1.50)	1.0 (0.71-1.31)
α_1AT (U/mL)	0.93 (0.39-1.47)	1.00 (0.69-1.30)	1.01 (0.65-1.37)	0.93 (0.55-1.30)
HCII (U/mL)	0.88 (0.48-1.28)[†]	0.86 (0.40-1.32)[†]	0.91 (0.53-1.29)[†]	1.08 (0.66-1.26)
Protein C (U/mL)	0.66 (0.40-0.92)[†]	0.69 (0.45-0.93)[†]	0.83 (0.55-1.11)[†]	0.96 (0.64-1.28)
Protein S				
Total (U/mL)	0.86 (0.54-1.18)	0.78 (0.41-1.14)	0.72 (0.52-0.92)	0.81 (0.60-1.13)
Free (U/mL)	0.45 (0.21-0.69)	0.42 (0.22-0.62)	0.38 (0.26-0.55)	0.45 (0.27-0.61)

From Andrew M, Vegh P, Johnston M, et al: Maturation of the hemostatic system during childhood. Blood 80:1998, 1992.
y, Years.
*All values are expressed in units per milliliter, where for all factors pooled plasma contains 1.0 U/mL, with the exception of free protein S, which contains a mean of 0.4 U/mL. All values are given as a mean, followed by the lower and upper boundary encompassing 95% of the population. Between 20 and 30 samples were assayed for each value for each age group. Some measurements were skewed because of a disproportionate number of high values. The lower limits, which exclude the lower 2.5% of the population, are given.
[†]Values that are significantly different from those of adults.

APPENDIX 55   Reference Ranges for Coagulation Inhibitors in Children and Adolescents[||]

Assay	Method	1-6 Months N = 29[†] 14M/15F	7-12 Months N = 25[‡] 19M/6F	1-5 Years N = 57 35M/22F	6-10 Years N = 56 29M/27F	11-18 Years N = 50 24M/26F	>19 Years N = 52 27F/25M
AT (%)	INNOVANCE AT, BCS	105/104[§] 81-126	110/109[§] 90-132	110/109[§] 93-128	108/107[§] 92-122	104/104[§] 90-119	116/115 97-133
	Berichrom AT CA-1500	106/103[§] 78-129	110/108[§] 88-132	113/113* 97-129	110/109[§] 97-122	105/106[§] 93-122	113/114 98-131
PS (%)	Protein S Ac BCS	78/19[§] 60-103	81/80[§] 61-95	85/83[§] 65-99	84/84*[§] 63-97	82/86[§] 69-119	101/105* 83- >130
	Protein S Ac CA-1500	84/83[§] 59-99	85/82[§] 59-110	85/87[§] 60-115	87/89*[§] 63-116	90/90[§] 62-126	116/114* 86- >130
PC (%)	Protein C Reagent, BCS Berichrom	70/71[§] 41-115	83/85[§] 60-117	97/97[§] 63-133	98/97[§] 62-134	100/103[§] 71-144	120/118 78-148
	Protein C CA-1500	66/67[§] 43-102	76/78[§] 59-103	88/92[§] 71-125	90/92[§] 75-120	93/96[§] 70-131	114/115 83-153

Appel IM, Grimminck B, Geerts J, et al: Age dependency of coagulation parameters during childhood and puberty. J Thromb Haemost 10:2254–2263, 2012.
AT, Antithrombin; BCS, Behring Coagulation System; CA-1500, Sysmex CA-1500 Analyzer; F, female; M, male; PT, prothrombin time; sec, seconds.
*Indicates statistically significant difference between devices for the student's t-test.
[†]N = 28 for PS with CA-1500 and N = 27 for PC with BCS.
[‡]N = 24 for AT with CA-1500.
[§]Indicates statistically significant difference between child groups and adults for the student's t-test.
[||]Data are presented as median/mean with t-test results of between methods and age comparisons in the first row, whereas the second row shows the boundaries including 90% of the central population.

APPENDIX 56 Reference Ranges for D-dimer, α_2-Antiplasmin, and Plasminogen in Children and Adolescents

Assay	Method	1-6 Months N = 29[†] 14M/15F	7-12 Months N = 25[†] 19M/6F	1-5 Years N = 57 35M/22F	6-10 Years N = 56 29M-27F	11-18 Years N = 50 24M/26F	>19 Years N = 52 27F/25M
D-dimer (mg/L FEU)	INNOVANCE D-dimer, BCS	0.28/0.50* <0.17-2.81	0.25/0.46* <0.17-3.32	0.19/0.25 <0.17-0.64	0.19-0.24 <0.17-0.49	<0.17/0.28 <0.17-0.99	<0.17/0.21 <0.17-0.44
	INNOVANCE D-dimer, CA-1500	0.33/0.39* <0.19-3.49	0.27/0.34* <0.19-10.9	0.20/0.27 <0.19-0.65	0.20/0.26 <0.19-0.52	<0.19/0.27 <0.19-0.75	<0.19/0.23 <0.19-0.48
α_2-antiplasmin (%)	Berichrom α_2- antiplasmin, CA-1500	122/121 103-139	123/125* 100-151	128/128* 107-145	119/121 103-140	114/113* 97-126	118/119 103-133
Plasminogen (%)	Berichrom Plasminogen, CA-1500	81/79* 56-102	93/94* 66-115	104/106* 84-130	99/99* 75-126	95/99* 83-128	112/117 92-150

Appel IM, Grimmick B, Geerts J, et al: Age dependency of coagulation parameters during childhood and puberty. J Thromb Haemost 2254–2263, 2012.

BCS, Behring Coagulation System; *CA-1500*, Sysmex CA-1500 Analyzer; *F*, female; *FEU*, fibrinogen equivalent units; *M*, male; *PT*, prothrombin time; *sec*, seconds.

Data are presented as median/mean with t-test results of between methods and age comparisons in the first row, whereas the second row shows the boundaries including 90% of the central population.

*Indicates statistically significant difference between child groups and adults for the student's t-test. Differences between devices for D-dimer were statistically not significant for student's t-test.

[†]N = 28 for D-dimer with CA-1500; N = 24 for α_2-antiplasmin and plasminogen.

APPENDIX 57 Reference Intervals for FVIII: C, VWF: Ag, and VWF: RCo and Relation to ABO (H) Blood Group*

Coagulation Factors (%)			AGE GROUP			
	1-3 Months	4-6 Months	7-12 Months	13 Months-4 Years	5-9 Years	10-18 Years
FVIII: C						
All	96 (68-179) N = 40 26M/14F	93 (71-147) N = 47 20M/27F	117 (67-178) N = 45 30M/15F	113 (78-177) N = 242 188M/54F	110 (78-182) N = 127 89M/38F	119 (79-185) N = 71 39M/32F
Blood group A/B/AB	95 (67-176) N = 22	97 (78-144) N = 29	117 (78-178) N = 26	122[†] (85-182) N = 127	120[†] (81-189) N = 62	134[†] (84-202) N = 32
Blood group O	93 (70-181) N = 16	88 (65-181) N = 18	119 (59-187) N = 19	104 (70-153) N = 108	99 (78-166) N = 64	102 (68-161) N = 39
VWF: Ag						
All	143 (81-191) N = 38 25M/13F	110 (66-190) N = 47 20M/27F	105 (60-154) N = 45 30M/15F	89 (54-149) N = 240 187M/53F	90 (59-151) N = 126 89M/37F	99 (55-170) N = 71 39M/32F
Blood group A/B/AB	122 (88-186) N = 20	113 (77-166) N = 29	108 (66-146) N = 26	99[†] (65-150) N = 126	106[†] (60-174) N = 62	124[†] (85-193) N = 32
Blood group O	163 (78-191) N = 16	100 (60-245) N = 18	95 (51-183) N = 19	80 (53-125) N = 107	76 (58-126) N = 63	80 (51-150) N = 39
VWF: RCo						
All	136 (72-196) N = 40 26M/14F	105 (54-206) N = 47 20M/27F	96 (54-151) N = 45 30M/15F	87 (51-145) N = 242 188M/54F	87 (47-159) N = 127 89M/38F	89 (45-163) N = 70 38M/32F
Blood group A/B/AB	135 (83-186) N = 22	120 (57-206) N = 29	111 (60-153) N = 26	93[†] (55-153) N = 127	97[†] (51-181) N = 62	113[†] (50-181) N = 32
Blood group O	139 (67-205) N = 16	91 (52-288) N = 18	85 (35-151) N = 19	78 (40-126) N = 108	72 (40-133) N = 64	73 (43-135) N = 38

Klarmann D, Eggert C, Geisen C, et al: Association of ABO(H) and I blood group system development with von Willebrand factor and Factor VIII plasma levels in children and adolescents. Transfusion 50:1571–1580, 2010.

*For each assay the first two rows show the median and the central 90% reference intervals. The second two rows show the number (N) of individual samples and the ratio of males (M) to females (F) for each group.

[†]Blood group A/b/AB values are significantly different from blood group O values (P <.01 Mann-Whitney test).

APPENDIX 58   Reference Values for the Fibrinolytic System in Healthy Children Aged 1 to 16 Years Compared with Adults

	AGE			
	1 to 5 y	**6 to 10 y**	**11 to 16 y**	**Adult**
	Mean (Boundary)	*Mean (Boundary)*	*Mean (Boundary)*	*Mean (Boundary)*
Plasminogen (U/mL)	0.98 (0.78-1.18)	0.92 (0.75-1.08)	0.86 (0.68-1.03)	0.99 (0.77-1.22)
Tissue plasminogen activator (TPA) (ng/mL)	2.15 (1-4.5)*	2.42 (1.0-5)*	2.16 (1-4)*	4.90 (1.4-8.4)
α₂-antiplasm (α-AP) (U/mL)	1.05 (0.93-1.17)	0.99 (0.89-1.10)	0.98 (0.78-1.18)	1.02 (0.68-1.36)
Plasminogen activator inhibitor (PAI) (U/mL)	5.42 (1-10)	6.79 (2-12)*	6.07 (2-10)	3.60 (0-11)

From Andrew M, Vegh P, Johnston M, et al: Maturation of the hemostatic system during childhood. Blood 89:1998, 1992.
For α2-AP, values are expressed as units per millimeter, where pooled plasma contains 1 U/mL. Values for TPA are given as nanograms per millimeter. Values for PAI are given as U/mL, where 1 U of PAI activity is defined as the amount of PAI that inhibits 1 IU of human-single chain TPA. All values are given as the mean, followed by the lower and upper boundary encompassing 95% of the population (boundary).
*Values that are significantly different from those of adults.

APPENDIX 59   Endogenous Plasma Concentrations of Thrombin-Antithrombin Complexes (TATs) and Prothrombin Fragment 1.2 (F1.2) in Children and Adults*

	1-5 Years	**6-10 Years**	**11-16 Years**	**20-45 Years**
TAT (µg/L)	2.3 ± 0.08	2.38 ± 0.13	2.8 ± 0.18	2.15 ± 0.09
F1.2 (nm/L)	1.04 ± 0.06	0.87 ± 0.07	0.82 ± 0.06	0.83 ± 0.06

From Andrew M, Mitchell L, Vegh P, et al: Thrombin regulation in children differs from adults in the absence and presence of heparin. Thromb Haemost 72:836, 1994.
*Data are expressed as mean ± standard error of the mean.

APPENDIX 60   Coagulation Screening Tests and Factor Levels in Fetuses and Full-Term Newborns

	FETUSES (WEEKS' GESTATION)				
Parameter	**19-23 (N = 20)**	**24-29 (N = 22)**	**30-38 (N = 22)**	**Newborns (N = 60)**	**Adults (N = 40)**
PT (s)	32.5 (19-45)	32.3 (19-44)†	22.6 (16-30)*	16.7 (12.0-23.5)*	13.5 (11.4-14.0)
PT (INR)	6.4 (1.7-11.1)	6.2 (2.1-10.6)†	3.0 (1.5-5.0)*	1.7 (0.9-2.7)*	1.1 (0.8-1.2)
APTT (s)	168.6 (83-250)	154.0 (87-210)†	104.8 (76-128)†	44.3 (35-52)*	33.0 (25-39)
TCT (s)	34.2 (24-44)*	26.2 (24-28)*	21.4 (17.0-23.3)	20.4 (15.2-25.0)†	14.0 (12-16)
Factor					
I (g/L Von Clauss)	0.85 (0.57-1.50)	1.12 (0.65-1.65)	1.35 (1.25-1.65)	1.68 (0.95-2.45)†	3.0 (12-16)
I Ag (g/L)	1.08 (0.75-1.50)	1.93 (1.56-2.40)	1.94 (1.30-2.40)	2.65 (1.68-3.60)†	3.5 (2.50-5.20)
IIc(%)	16.9 (10-24)	19.9 (11-30)*	27.9 (15-50)†	43.5 (27-64)†	98.7 (70-125)
VIIc (%)	27.4 (17-37)	33.8 (18-48)*	45.9 (31-62)	52.5 (28-78)†	101.3 (68-130)
IXc (%)	10.1 (6-14)	9.9 (5-15)	12.3 (5-24)†	31.8 (15-50)†	104.8 (70-142)
Xc (%)	20.5 (14-29)	24.9 (16-35)	28.0 (16-36)†	39.6 (21-65)†	99.2 (75-125)
Vc (%)	32.1 (21-44)	36.8 (25-50)	48.9 (23-70)†	89.9 (50-140)	99.8 (65-140)
VIIIc (%)	34.5 (18-50)	35.5 (20-52)	50.1 (27-78)†	94.3 (38-150)	101.8 (55-170)
XIc (%)	13.2 (8-19)	12.1 (6-22)	14.8 (6-26)†	37.2 (13-62)*	100.2 (70-135)
XIIc (%)	14.9 (6-25)	22.7 (6-40)	25.8 (11-50)†	69.8 (25-105)†	101.4 (65-144)
PK (%)	12.8 (8-19)	15.4 (8-26)	18.1 (8-28)†	35.4 (21-53)†	99.8 (65-135)
HMWK (%)	15.4 (10-22)	19.3 (10-26)	23.6 (12-34)†	38.9 (28-53)†	98.8 (68-135)

From Reverdiau Moalic P, Delahouse B, Body G, et al: Evaluation of blood coagulation activators and inhibitors in the healthy human fetus. Blood 88:900, 1996.
Ag, Antigenic value; c, coagulant activity.
Values are the mean, followed in parentheses by the lower and upper boundaries including 95% of the population.
*P <.05
†P <.01

APPENDIX 61   Coagulation Inhibitors in Fetuses and Full-Term Newborns

| Parameter | FETUSES (WEEKS' GESTATION) | | | Newborns (N = 60) | Adults (N = 40) |
	19-23 (N = 20)	24-29 (N= 22)	30-38 (N = 22)		
AT (%)	20.0 (12-31)*	30.0 (20-39)	37.1 (24-55)†	59.4 (42-80)†	99.8 (65-130)
HCII (%)	10.3 (6-16)	12.9 (5.5-20)	21.2 (11-33)†	52.1 (19-99)†	101.4 (70-128)
TFPI (ng/ML)	21.0 (16.0-29.2)	20.6 (13.4-33.2)	20.7 (10.4-31.5)†	38.1 (22.7-55.8)†	73.0 (50.9-90.1)
PC Ag (%)	9.5 (6-14)	12.1 (8-16)	15.9 (8-30)†	32.5 (21-47)†	100.8 (68-125)
PC Act (%)	9.6 (7-13)	10.4 (8-13)	14.1 (8-18)*	28.2 (14-42)†	98.8 (68-129)
Total PS (%)	15.1 (11-21)	17.4 (14-25)	21.0 (15-30)†	38.5 (22-55)†	99.6 (72-118)
Free PS (%)	21.7 (13-32)	27.9 (19-40)	27.1 (18-40)†	49.3 (33-67)†	98.7 (72-128)
Ratio of free PS to total PS	0.82 (0.75-0.92)	0.83 (0.76-0.95)	0.79 (0.70-0.89)†	0.64 (0.59-0.98)†	0.41 (0.38-0.43)
C4b-BP (%)	1.8 (0.6)	6.1 (1-12.5)	9.3 (5-14)	18.6 (3-40)†	100.3 (70-124)

From Reverdiau Moalic P, Delahouse B, Body G, et al: Evaluation of blood coagulation activators and inhibitors in the healthy human fetus. Blood 1996;88:900, 1996.
Values are the mean, followed in parentheses by the lower and upper boundaries including 95% of the population.
Ag, Antigenic value; AT, antithrombin; c, coagulant activity; HCII, heparin cofactor II; TFPI, tissue factor pathway inhibitor; PC, protein C; PS, Protein S; C4b-BP, C4b binding protein.
*P <.05
†P <.01

APPENDIX 62   Age-Specific and Sex-Specific Pediatric Reference Intervals for C3, C4, and high sensitivity C-reactive Protein

| | | CHEMISTRY | | | | | | | | | |
| | | FEMALE REFERENCE INTERVAL | | | | | MALE REFERENCE INTERVAL | | | | |
Analyte	Age	Lower Limit	Upper Limit	No. of Samples	Lower Limit Confidence Interval	Upper Limit Confidence Interval	Lower Limit	Upper Limit	No. of Samples	Lower Limit Confidence Interval	Upper Limit Confidence Interval
C3, mg/dL	0-14 days	50	121	155	42-57	118-130	50	121	155	42-57	118-130
	15 days to < 1 year	51	160	151	31-55	150-165	51	160	151	31-55	150-165
	1 to <19 years	83	152	877	82-87	151-157	83	152	877	82-87	151-157
C4, mg/dL	0 to <1 year	7	30	353	5-8	28-32	7	30	353	5-8	28-32
	1 to <19 years	13	37	864	12-13	36-38	13	37	864	12-13	36-38
Hs-CRP, mg/L	0 to 14 days	0.3	6.1	139	0.2-0.4	5.4-6.3	0.3	6.1	139	0.2-0.4	5.4-6.3
	15 days to <15 years	0.1	1.0	653	0.1-0.1	0.9-1.1	0.1	1.0	653	0.1-0.1	0.9-1.1
	15 to <19 years	0.1	1.7	196	0.1-0.1	1.6-1.9	0.1	1.7	196	0.1-0.1	1.6-1.9

From Colantino DA, Kyriakopoulou, Chan MK, et al: Closing the gaps in pediatric laboratory reference intervals: a CALIPER Database of 40 biochemical markers in a healthy and multiethnic population of children. Clin Chem 58:854–868, 2012.

APPENDIX 63   Serum Acid Glycoprotein (AGP), α_1-Antitrypsin (α_1-AT), and Haptoglobin Levels Reference Ranges at Different Ages

Age (Years)	Acid Glycoprotein (g/L)			α_1-Antitrypsin (g/L)			Haptoglobin (g/L)		
	2.5th	50th	97.5th	2.5th	50th	97.5th	2.5th	50th	97.5th
Males									
1	0.52	0.88	1.47	0.87	1.40	1.91	0.07	1.11	3.1
4	0.50	0.84	1.42	0.89	1.44	1.96	0.05	0.83	2.31
7	0.49	0.83	1.39	0.90	1.45	1.98	0.04	0.74	2.05
10	0.47	0.80	1.34	0.91	1.46	1.99	0.04	0.68	1.90
14	0.44	0.74	1.25	0.86	1.38	1.88	0.27	0.81	1.63
18	0.46	0.78	1.31	0.83	1.34	1.83	0.31	0.93	1.87
20	0.47	0.80	1.34	0.83	1.33	1.82	0.32	0.98	1.97
30	0.51	0.87	1.46	0.82	1.31	1.79	0.38	1.15	2.31
Females									
1	0.63	1.07	1.80	0.92	1.48	2.02	0.08	1.38	3.84
4	0.54	0.92	1.55	0.90	1.44	1.97	0.06	0.95	2.63
7	0.51	0.86	1.45	0.89	1.43	1.95	0.05	0.81	2.26
10	0.49	0.83	1.40	0.88	1.42	1.94	0.04	0.74	2.05
14	0.48	0.80	1.35	0.88	1.41	1.93	0.31	0.95	1.90
18	0.46	0.78	1.31	0.92	1.48	2.02	0.35	1.07	2.14
20	0.46	0.77	1.31	0.92	1.49	2.03	0.37	1.11	2.23
30	0.50	0.83	1.40	0.90	1.45	1.98	0.40	1.22	2.45

From Ritchie, RF, Palomaki GE, Neveux LM, et al:Reference distributions for the positive acute phase proteins, alpha1-acid glycoprotein (orosomucoid), alpha-antitrypsin, and haptaglobin: a comparison of a large cohort to the world's literature. J Clin Lab Anal 14(6):265–270, 2000; see also Ritchie, RF, Palomaki GE, Neveux LM, et al: Reference distributions for the positive acute phase serum proteins, alpha1-acid glycoprotein (orosomucoid), alpha1-antitrypsin, and haptoglobin: a practical, simple and clinically relevant approach in a large cohort. J Clin Lab Anal 14(6):284–292, 2000.

APPENDIX 64   Plasma Levels of Immunoglobulin A in Males and Females

Age	g/L	mg/dL
Lockitch et al (1988)*		
0-12 m	0.00-1.00	0-100
1-3 y	0.24-1.21	24-121
4-6 y	0.33-2.35	33-235
7-9 y	0.41-3.68	41-368
10-11 y	0.64-2.46	64-246
12-13 y	0.70-4.32	70-432
14-15 y	0.57-3.00	57-300
16-19 y	0.74-4.19	74-419
Children's Hospital†		
Newborn	0.00-0.11	0-11
1-3 m	0.06-0.05	6-50
4-6 m	0.08-0.90	8-90
7-12 m	0.16-1.00	16-100
1-3 y	0.20-2.30	20-230
3-6 y	0.50-1.50	50-150
Adult	0.50-2.00	50-200

m, Month; *y,* year.

*Lockitch G, Halstead AC, Quigley G, et al: Age- and sex-specific pediatric reference intervals: study design and methods illustrated by measurement of serum proteins with the Behring LN nephelometer. *Clin Chem* 34:1618, 1988. Results are expressed as 2.5th and 97.5th percentiles.

†Children's Hospital, Boston, Massachusetts, by laser nephelometry (Dade-Behring BN2).

APPENDIX 65   Serum Levels of Immunoglobulin D in Males and Females

Age	mg/L
Cord blood*	0.04-1.02
Adult†	2.0-173

*Ownby DR, Johnson CC, Peterson EL: Maternal smoking does not influence cord serum IgE or IgD concentrations. *J Allergy Clin Immunol* 88:555, 1991. Values constitute 95% of the measured samples.

†Tozawa T, Nakata N, Adachi K: Serum IgD concentrations in normal individuals 20-39 years of age. *Rinsho Byori Jpn J Clin Pathol* 42:656, 1994.

APPENDIX 66 Serum Levels of Immunoglobulin E in Males and Females

Age	IU/mL
Cord blood*	0.02-2.08
<1 y†	0-6.6
1-2 y†	0-20.0
2-3 y†	0.1-15.8
3-4 y†	0-29.2
4-5 y†	0.3-25.0
5-6 y†	0.2-17.6
6-7 y†	0.2-13.1
7-8 y†	0.3-46.1
8-9 y†	1.8-60.1
9-10 y†	3.6-81.0
10-11 y†	8.0-95.0
11-12 y†	1.5-99.7
12-13 y†	3.9-83.5
13-16 y†	3.3-188.0
<3 y‡	<30
<10 y‡	<200
10-14 y‡	<500
Adult‡	<120

	Females (KIU/L)	Males (KIU/L)
0-12 m§	0-20	2-24
1-3 y§	2-55	2-149
4-10 y§	8-279	4-249
11-15 y§	5-295	7-280
16-18 y§	7-698	5-268

KIU/L, Kilo international units/L; m, months; y, years.
*Ownby DR, Johnson CC, Peterson EL: Maternal smoking does not influence cord serum IgE or IgD concentration. J Allergy Clin Immunol 88:555, 1991. Values constitute 95% of the measured samples.
†Lindenberg RE, Arroyave C: Levels of IgE in serum from normal children and allergic children as measured by an enzyme immunoassay. J Allergy Clin Immunol 78:614, 1986.
‡Children's Hospital, Boston, Massachusetts.
§Soldin SJ, Morales A, Albalos F, et al: Pediatric reference ranges on the Abbott IMx for FSH, LH, prolactin, TSH, T4, T3, free T3, T-uptake, IgE, and ferritin. Clin Biochem 28:603, 1995. Study based on hospitalized patience; values represent 2.5th and 95.7th percentiles.

APPENDIX 67 Plasma Levels of Immunoglobulin M in Males and Females

Age	g/L	mg/dL
Lockitch et al. (1988)*		
0-12 m	0.0-2.16	0-216
1-3 y	0.28-2.18	28-218
4-6 y	0.36-3.14	36-314
7-9 y	0.47-3.11	47-311
10-11 y	0.46-2.68	46-268
12-13 y	0.52-3.57	52-357
14-15 y	0.23-2.81	23-281
16-19 y	0.35-3.87	35-387
Children's Hospital†		
Newborn	0.05-0.30	5-30
1-3 m	0.15-0.70	15-70
4-6 m	0.10-0.90	10-90
7-12 m	0.25-1.15	25-115
1-3 y	0.30-1.20	30-120
3-6 y	0.22-1.0	22-100
Adult	0.50-2.0	50-200

m, Months; y, years.
*Lockitch G, Halstead AC, Quigley G, et al: Age- and sex-specific pediatric reference intervals: study design and methods illustrated by measurement of serum proteins with the Behring LN nephelometer. Clin Chem 34:1618, 1988. Results are expressed as 2.5th and 97.5th percentiles.
†Childen's Hospital, Boston, Massachusetts, by laser nephelometry (Dade-Behring BN2).

APPENDIX 68 Plasma Levels of Immunoglobulin G in Males and Females

Age	g/L	mg/dL
Lockitch et al. (1988)*		
0-12 m	2.73-16.60	273-1660
1-3 y	5.33-10.78	533-1078
4-6 y	5.93-17.23	593-1723
7-9 y	6.73-17.34	673-1734
10-11 y	8.21-18.35	821-1835
12-13 y	8.93-18.23	893-1823
14-15 y	8.42-20.13	842-2013
16-19 y	6.46-18.64	646-1864
Children's Hospital†		
Newborn	7.0-1.30	700-1300
1-3 m	2.80-7.50	280-750
4-6 m	2.0-12.0	200-1200
7-12 m	3.0-15.0	300-1500
1-3 y	4.0-13.0	400-1300
3-6 y	6.0-15.0	600-1500
Adult	6.0-13.4	600-1344

m, Months; y, years.
*Lockich G, Halstead AC, Quigley G, et al: Age- and sex-specific pediatric reference intervals: study design and methods illustrated by measurement of serum proteins with the Behring LN nephelometer. Clin Chem 34:1618, 1988. Results are expressed as 2.5th and 97.5th percentiles.
†Childen's Hospital, Boston, Massachusetts, by laser nephelometry (Dade-Behring BN2).

APPENDIX 69   Reference Intervals for IgG Subclasses on Dade Behring Nephelometer by Age Groups

Age Group (months)	Patients (N)	Median (g/L)	2.5th Percentile (g/L)	97.5th Percentile (g/L)
1 to 6 m				
IgG	12	4.3	2.3	9.5
IgG1	12	3.0	1.5	7.9
IgG2	12	0.84	0.36	1.40
IgG3	12	0.22	0.09	0.86
IgG4	12	0.048	0.006	0.460
6 to 12 m				
IgG	17	4.1	2.3	7.3
IgG1	15	3.2	1.7	5.8
IgG2	15	0.51	0.26	1.30
IgG3	17	0.25	0.10	0.92
IgG4	15	0.022	0.004	0.370
12 to 18 m				
IgG	16	6.8	4.1	12.1
IgG1	16	5.3	3.2	9.2
IgG2	16	0.76	0.26	1.50
IgG3	16	0.31	0.12	0.88
IgG4	14	0.060	0.007	0.370
18 m to 2 y				
IgG	21	6.2	2.8	9.9
IgG1	21	5.0	2.6	7.8
IgG2	21	0.77	0.42	2.20
IgG3	21	0.22	0.11	0.97
IgG4	20	0.063	0.017	0.750
2 to 3 y				
IgG	47	7.0	3.7	11.7
IgG1	47	5.6	2.7	9.4
IgG2	46	0.99	0.44	1.90
IgG3	47	0.22	0.09	0.63
IgG4	46	0.101	0.023	0.590
3 to 4 y				
IgG	37	8.6	3.8	17.9
IgG1	37	6.3	2.8	13.7
IgG2	37	1.15	0.44	3.00
IgG3	37	0.29	0.13	0.84
IgG4	37	0.129	0.005	1.140
4 to 6 y				
IgG	76	9.4	5.6	15.4
IgG1	76	6.8	3.8	11.7
IgG2	76	1.43	0.73	2.90
IgG3	76	0.37	0.13	0.75
IgG4	73	0.282	0.013	1.570
6 to 9 y				
IgG	62	9.4	6.0	14.6
IgG1	62	6.3	4.2	9.9

Continued on following page

Age Group (months)	Patients (N)	Median (g/L)	2.5th Percentile (g/L)	97.5th Percentile (g/L)
IgG2	62	1.72	0.63	3.50
IgG3	62	0.38	0.17	0.88
IgG4	61	0.288	0.010	1.210
9 to 12 y				
IgG	43	9.4	5.5	15.2
IgG1	43	6.7	3.6	11.2
IgG2	43	1.92	0.89	3.60
IgG3	43	0.43	0.23	0.83
IgG4	43	0.381	0.052	1.560
12 to 18 y				
IgG	86	10.7	6.5	14.6
IgG1	86	6.9	3.9	10.0
IgG2	86	2.47	1.02	4.50
IgG3	86	0.42	0.14	1.02
IgG4	84	0.412	0.061	1.860

From Lepage N, Huang SH, Nieuwenhuys, et al: Pediatric reference intervals for immunoglobulin G and its subclasses with Siemens immunonephelometric assays. Clin Biochem 43:694–696, 2010.

APPENDIX 70   Serum Levels of Immunoglobulin Light Chains in Males and Females

Age	Kappa g/L	Lamba g/L
Newborn	7.7-8.7	1.7-1.9
Premature	3.1-4.9	1.6-1.9
1 m	3.6-4.8	1.6-2.0
2 m	2.4-2.7	1.6-1.7
3 m	1.7-2.5	1.0-1.3
4 m	1.9-2.4	0.8-1.0
5 m	2.0-3.2	1.0-1.1
1 y	3.0-5.3	0.9-1.2
2 y	3.6-6.4	1.3-1.5
3 y	4.1-5.4	1.1-1.4
4 y	4.8-8.3	1.2-1.7
5 y	5.4-7.1	1.3-1.7
6 y	6.0-8.5	1.6-1.7
7 y	4.6-7.5	1.4-1.8
8 y	7.3-9.1	1.4-1.7
9 y	7.1-9.6	1.5-1.8
10 y	8.2-9.6	1.3-1.9
11 y	6.0-8.3	1.4-1.8
12 y	8.2-9.6	1.7-2.0
13 y	8.2-10.5	1.4-1.7
14 y	8.0-10.8	1.9-2.2
15 y	7.2-11.0	1.7-2.3
16 y	7.0-11.2	1.5-2.2

From Herkner KR, Salzer H, Bock A, et al: Pediatric and perinatal reference intervals for immunoglobulin light chains kappa and lambda. Clin Chem 38:548, 1992.
m, Months; y, years. Results expressed as 10th and 90th percentiles.

APPENDIX 71 Selected Biochemical Parameters in Cord Blood

	Cord Blood (Term)	Cord Blood (Preterm)	Adult or Maternal Blood
Erythrocytes			
Magnesium (mmol/L)*	1.76 ± 0.15 (44)	—	—
Copper (μmol/L)*	12.9 ± 3.0 (39)	—	—
Zinc (μmol/L)*	40.4 ± 13.6 (44)	—	—
Ferritin (ag/cell)[†]	265 (47)	92.7 (47)	
Serum/Plasma			
Ferritin (μg/L)[†]	56.8 (47)	17.7 (47)	—
Free riboflavin (nM)[†]	20.2 (31)[‖]	25.0[‖]	4.7 (31)
Flavocoenzymes (nM)[‡]	55.8 (31)[‖]	71.8[‖]	90.7 (31)
Vitamin B2 (nM) [‡]	77.2 (31)[‖]	92.6[‖]	94.9 (31)
Flavocoenzymes uptake(nmol/min per kg)[‡]	0.4	1.5[¶]	—
Free riboflavin release (nmol/min per kg)[†]	0.2	0.4[¶]	—
Selenium (μmolL)[§]	1.04 ± 0.21[‖]	0.89 ± 0.27[‖]	1.56 ± 0.27
Retinol (μmol/L)[§]	0.66 ± 0.22[‖]	0.52 ± 0.12[‖]	1.26 ± 0.45
Alpha-Tocopherol (μmol/L)[§]	7.10 ± 2.1[‖]	8.81 ± 2.8[‖]	32.4 ± 9.2
Glutathione peroxidase (U/L)[§]	456 ± 108[‖]	305 ± 89[‖]	873 ± 176

*Speich M, Micat A, Acget JC, et al: Magnesium total calcium, phosphorus, copper and zinc in plasma and erythrocytes of venous cord blood from infants of diabetic mothers: comparison with a reference group by logist discriminant analysis. *Clin Chem* 38:2002, 1992. Values expressed as mean ± SD; number of samples in parentheses.

[†]Carpani G, Marini F, Ghisoni C, et al: Red cell and plasma ferritin in a group of normal fetuses at different ages of gestation. *Eur J Haematol* 49:260, 1992.

[‡]Zempleni J, Link G, Bitsch I: Intrauterine vitamin B2 uptake of preterm and full-term infants. *Pediatr Res* 38:585, 1995. Concentrations measured in the umbilical vein are reported in this table; values for umbilical artery are reported in the chapter text as well.

[§]Dison PJ, Lockitch G, Halstead AC, et al: Influence of maternal factors on cord and neonatal plasma micronutrient levels. *Am J Perinatol* 10:30, 1993. Data obtained in 107 term, 23 preterm (<32 weeks) and 58 maternal samples.

[‖]P<.05 compared with full term.

[¶]P<.05 compared with adult/maternal.

APPENDIX 72   Reference Ranges for Serum Ferritin, Folate, and Cobalamin in Children and Adolescents*

Analyte	Age	MALE RIs						FEMALE RIs					
		No. of Samples	Geometric Mean	Lower Limit	Upper Limit	Lower Limit CI	Upper Limit CI	No. of Samples	Geometric Mean	Lower Limit	Upper Limit	Lower Limit CI	Upper Limit CI
Ferritin, ng/mL	4 to <15 days	127	288.4	99.6	717.0	63.1 to 122.9	648.7 to 741.2	127	288.4	99.6	717.0	63.1 to 122.9	648.7 to 741.2
	15 days to <6 months	172	109.2	14.0	647.2	9.8 to 22.1	521.5 to 734.2	172	109.2	14.0	647.2	9.8 to 22.1	521.5 to 734.2
	6 months to <1 year	140	41.7	8.4	181.9	4.6 to 8.9	167.1 to 250.4	140	41.7	8.4	181.9	4.6 to 8.9	167.1 to 250.4
	1 to <5 years	126	25.1	5.3	99.9	4.0 to 9.6	80.9 to 167.0	126	25.1	5.3	99.9	4.0 to 9.6	80.9 to 167.0
	5 to <14 years	497	34.3	13.7	78.8	12.9 to 15.4	73.0 to 86.6	497	34.3	13.7	78.8	12.9 to 15.4	73.0 to 86.6
	14 to <16 years	**65**	**39.3**	**12.7**	**82.8**	**10.0 to 15.7**	**74.5 to 87.9**						
	16 to <19 years	88	55.6	11.1	171.9	7.6 to 17.3	149.7 to 188.4						
	14 to <19 years							151	25.7	5.5	67.4	4.4 to 5.9	61.4 to 78.8
Folate (serum), ng/mL	5 days to <1 year	235	NA	10.6	NA	8 to 11.7	NA	235	NA	10.6	NA	8 to 11.7	NA
	1 to <3 years	50	NA	3.9	NA	0 to 6.4	NA	50	NA	3.9	NA	0 to 6.4	NA
	3 to <6 years	90	NA	11.9	NA	11.1 to 12.8	NA	90	NA	11.9	NA	11.1 to 12.8	NA
	6 to <8 years	70	NA	13.1	NA	10.2 to 14.4	NA	70	NA	13.1	NA	10.2 to 14.4	NA
	8 to <12 years	284	NA	11.4	NA	11.2 to 12.6	NA	284	NA	11.4	NA	11.2 to 12.6	NA
	12 to <14 years	144	NA	11.9	NA	10.8 to 12.3	NA	144	NA	11.9	NA	10.8 to 12.3	NA
	14 to <18 years	342	NA	7.9	NA	6.6 to 8.7	NA	342	NA	7.9	NA	6.6 to 8.7	NA
Cobalamin, pg/mL	5 days to <1 year	257	652	259	1576	181 to 274	1509 to 1620	257	652	259	1576	181 to 274	1509 to 1620
	1 to <9 years	267	744	283	1613	229 to 340	1420 to 1769	267	744	283	1613	229 to 340	1420 to 1769
	9 to <14 years	374	596	252	1125	234 to 291	1078 to 1207	374	596	252	1125	234 to 291	1079 to 1208
	14 to <17 years	217	493	244	887	214 to 261	848 to 925	217	493	244	888	214 to 262	848 to 926
	17 to <19 years	127	428	203	811	192 to 224	783 to 885	127	428	203	812	192 to 225	783 to 885

From Bailey D, Colantonio D, Kyriakopoulou L, et al: Marked biological variance in endocrine and biochemical markers in childhood: establishment of pediatric reference intervals using healthy community children from the Canadian Laboratory Initiative for Pediatric Reference Intervals Cohort Clinical Chemistry Clin Chem 59:1393–405, 2013.

CI, Confidence interval; NA, not applicable.

Bold and underlined values indicate sex-specific differences within age partitions.

APPENDIX 73   Reference Ranges for Selected Biochemical Markers in Children and Adolescents*

Analyte	Age	FEMALE REFERENCE INTERVAL					MALE REFERENCE INTERVAL				
		Lower Limit	Upper Limit	No. of Samples	Lower Limit Confidence Interval	Upper Limit Confidence Interval	Lower Limit	Upper Limit	No. of Samples	Lower Limit Confidence Interval	Upper Limit Confidence Interval
Bilirubin (direct), mg/dL	0 to 14 days	0.33	0.71	171	0.29-0.36	0.67-0.73	0.33	0.71	171	0.29-0.36	0.67-0.73
	15 days to <1 year	0.05	0.30	108	0.04-0.06	0.27-0.33	0.05	0.30	108	0.04-0.06	0.27-0.33
	1 to <9 years	0.05	0.20	281	0.05-0.05	0.18-0.20	0.05	0.20	281	0.05-0.05	0.18-0.20
	9 to <13 years	0.05	0.29	181	0.05-0.10	0.28-0.33	0.05	0.29	181	0.05-0.10	0.28-0.33
	13 to <19 years	**0.10**	**0.39**	**177**	**0.05-0.11**	**0.34-0.46**	**0.11**	**0.42**	**170**	**0.10-0.12**	**0.40-0.43**
Bilirubin (total), mg/dL	0 to 14 days	0.19	16.60	166	0.10-0.29	15.04-17.88	0.19	16.60	166	0.10-0.29	15.04-17.88
	15 days to <1 year	0.05	0.68	245	0.05-0.10	0.63-0.73	0.05	0.68	245	0.05-0.10	0.63-0.73
	1 to <9 years	0.05	0.40	270	0.05-0.05	0.36-0.42	0.05	0.40	270	0.05-0.05	0.36-0.42
	9 to <12 years	0.05	0.55	135	0.05-0.10	0.50-0.61	0.05	0.55	135	0.05-0.10	0.50-0.61
	12 to <15 years	0.10	0.70	161	0.05-0.10	0.64-0.81	0.10	0.70	161	0.05-0.10	0.64-0.81
	15 to <19 years	0.10	0.84	219	0.05-0.11	0.81-0.89	0.10	0.84	219	0.05-0.11	0.81-0.89
Iron, µg/dL	0 to <14 years	16	128	588	15-21	123-138	16	128	588	15-21	123-138
	14 to <19 years	**20**	**162**	**143**	**13-31**	**138-185**	**31**	**168**	**138**	**11-42**	**153-184**
Magnesium, mg/dL	0 to 14 days	1.99	3.94	133	1.80-2.19	3.77-4.11	1.99	3.94	183	1.80-2.19	3.77-4.11
	15 days to <1 year	1.97	3.09	145	1.85-2.11	3.01-3.21	1.97	3.09	145	1.85-2.11	3.01-3.21
	1 to <19 years	2.09	2.84	897	2.09-2.11	2.82-2.87	2.09	2.84	897	2.09-2.11	2.82-2.87
	15 to <19 years	130	250	227	124-142	239-257	130	250	227	124-142	239-257
LDH, U/L	0 to 14 days	309	1222	197	267-360	1116-1257	309	1222	197	267-360	1116-1257
	15 days to <1 year	163	452	145	94-173	428-483	163	452	145	94-173	428-483
	1 to <10 years	192	321	370	189-199	314-333	192	321	370	189-199	314-333
	10 to <15 years	**157**	**272**	**141**	**130-162**	**258-308**	**170**	**283**	**125**	**138-175**	**277-286**
	15 to <19 years	130	250	227	124-142	239-257	130	250	227	124-142	239-257

From Colantonio DA, Kyriakopoulou, Chan MK, et al: Closing the gaps in pediatric laboratory reference intervals: a CALIPER database of 40 biochemical markers in a healthy and multiethnic population of children. Clin Chem 58:854-868, 2012.

LDH, Lactate dehydrogenase.

*Bold and underlined values indicate sex-specific differences within age partitions.

APPENDIX 74 Reference Ranges for Selected Biochemical Markers in Children and Adolescents*

Analyte	Age	Lower Limit	Upper Limit	No. of Samples	Lower Limit Confidence Interval	Upper Limit Confidence Interval	Lower Limit	Upper Limit	No. of Samples	Lower Limit Confidence Interval	Upper Limit Confidence Interval
Albumin G, g/dL	0 to 14 days	3.3	4.5	191	3.2-3.3	4.4-4.6	3.3	4.5	191	3.2-3.3	4.4-4.6
	15 days to <1 year	2.8	4.7	156	2.6-3.0	4.5-5.3	2.8	4.7	156	2.6-3.0	4.5-5.3
	1 to <8 years	3.8	4.7	298	3.8-3.9	4.6-4.7	3.8	4.7	298	3.8-3.9	4.6-4.7
	8 to <15 years	4.1	4.8	388	4.1-4.1	4.8-4.9	4.1	4.8	388	4.1-4.1	4.8-4.9
	15 to <19 years	**4.0**	**4.9**	**119**	**3.9-4.1**	**4.8-4.9**	**4.1**	**5.1**	**123**	**4.1-4.2**	**5.0-5.2**
Albumin P, g/dL	0 to 14 days	2.8	4.1	182	2.6-2.9	4.0-4.2	2.8	4.1	182	2.6-2.9	4.0-4.2
	15 days to <1 year	2.5	4.6	153	2.1-2.7	4.4-4.7	2.5	4.6	153	2.1-2.7	4.4-4.7
	1 to <8 years	3.5	4.5	298	3.5-3.6	4.5-4.6	3.5	4.5	298	3.5-3.6	4.5-4.6
	8 to <15 years	3.7	4.7	390	3.7-3.8	4.6-4.7	3.7	4.7	390	3.7-3.8	4.6-4.7
	15 to <19 years	**3.5**	**4.9**	**119**	**3.5-3.6**	**4.8-4.9**	**3.8**	**5.0**	**123**	**3.7-3.9**	**4.8-5.0**
Prealbumin, mg/dL	0 to 14 days	2	12	127	2-2	10-12	2	12	127	2-2	10-12
	15 days to <1 year	5	24	137	4-7	22-25	5	24	137	4-7	22-25
	1 to <5 years	12	23	148	12-13	22-23	12	23	148	12-13	22-23
	5 to <13 years	14	26	359	13-14	25-27	14	26	359	13-14	25-27
	13 to <16 years	18	31	187	15-18	30-33	18	31	187	15-18	30-33
	16 to <19 years	**17**	**33**	**96**	**0-17**	**32-34**	**20**	**35**	**95**	**0-20**	**34-36**
Total protein, g/dL	0 to 14 days	5.3	8.3	158	5.0-5.4	8.0-8.5	5.3	8.3	158	5.0-5.4	8.0-8.5
	15 days to <1 year	4.4	7.1	152	4.2-4.6	6.9-7.4	4.4	7.1	152	4.2-4.6	6.9-7.4
	1 to <6 years	6.1	7.5	209	5.8-6.2	7.5-7.6	6.1	7.5	209	5.8-6.2	7.5-7.6
	6 to <9 years	6.4	7.7	118	6.3-6.5	7.6-7.8	6.4	7.7	118	6.3-6.5	7.6-7.8
	9 to <19 years	6.5	8.1	588	6.5-6.6	8.0-8.2	6.5	8.1	588	6.5-6.6	8.0-8.2
Haptoglobin, mg/dL	0 to 14 days	0	10	64	0-0	9-10	0	10	64	0-0	9-10
	15 days to <1 year	7	221	129	7-7	203-234	7	221	129	7-7	203-234
	1 to <12 years	7	163	444	7-7	150-168	7	163	444	7-7	150-168
	12 to <19 years	7	179	418	7-12	172-191	7	179	418	7-12	172-191
Transferrin, mg/dL	0 to <9 weeks	104	224	188	99-111	217-233	104	224	188	99-111	217-233
	9 weeks to <1 year	107	324	104	93-118	310-337	107	324	104	93-118	310-337
	1 to <19 years	220	337	878	216-223	333-342	220	337	878	216-223	333-342

From Colantonio DA, Kyriakopoulou, Chan MK, et al: Closing the Gaps in Pediatric Laboratory Reference Intervals: A CALIPER Database of 40 Biochemical Markers in a Healthy and Multiethnic Population of Children. Clin Chem 58:854-868, 2012.
Albumin G, Albumin assay with bromcresol green; Albumin P, albumin assay with bromcresol purple.
Bold and underlined values indicate sex-specific differences within age partitions.

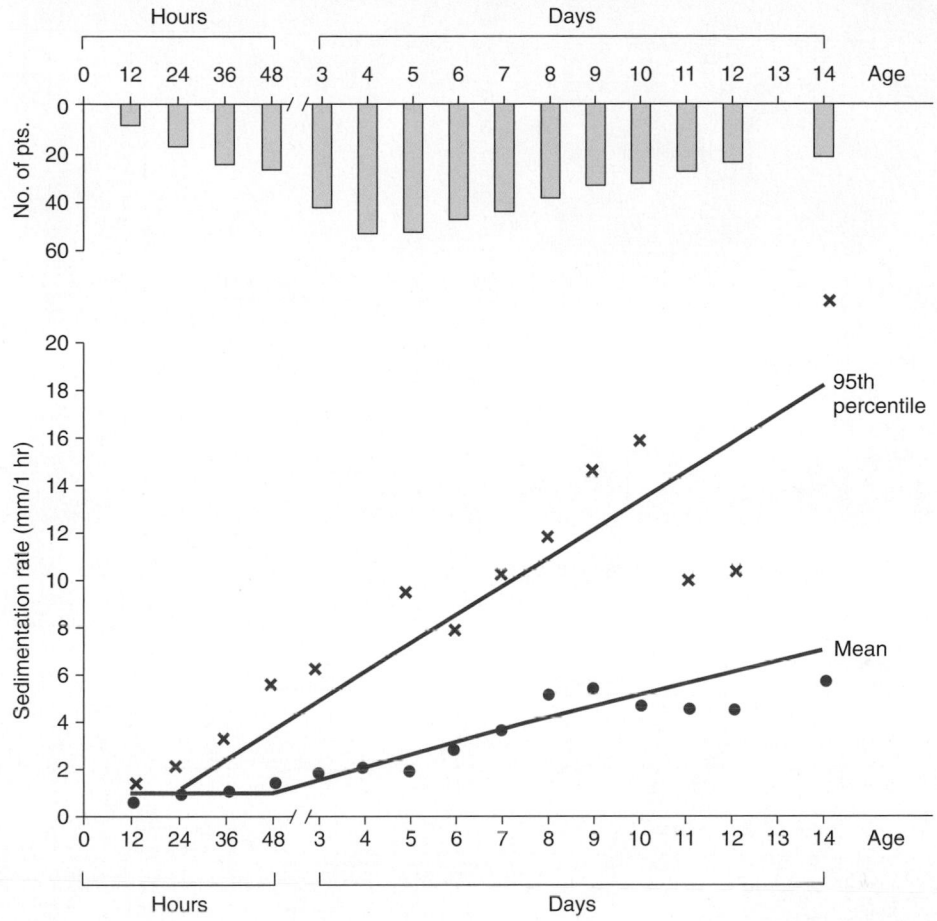

Appendix 75 Sedimentation rate in the newborn period. The erythrocyte sedimentation rate was measured in capillary blood in healthy full-term and low-birth-weight newborns. Normal values ranged from 1 mm/h at 12 hours of age to 17mm/h at 14 days of age. All values of neonates with hematocrit values less than 40% were corrected to 40%. *(From Adler SM, Denton RL: The erythrocyte sedimentation rate in the newborn period.* J Pediatr *86:942, 1975.)*

INDEX

Page numbers followed by "f" indicate figures, "t" indicate tables, and "b" indicate boxes.

Infants *(Continued)*
neuroblastoma, scans/ultrasound, 2208f
ossifying renal tumor, lobular renal hilar mass, 2203f
peripheral blood smear, hemolysis (presence), 73
pineoblastoma, 1867-1868
reticulocyte values, 71f
Rh disease, late anemia, 69
Rh erythroblastosis fetalis, neonatal blood sample, 83f
Rh/Kell alloimmunization, 69
testicular teratoma, 2061-2062
testicular yolk sac tumor, 2063
thalassemia, birth rate (decrease), 767f
thymic shadow, anteroposterior chest radiograph, 2169f
Infant tumors, 1864-1869
clinical presentation, 1865
management, 1865-1866
issues, 1866-1869
Infection
bacterial infections, 1173-1174
childhood ALL, 1246-1248
classification, 2258
developing world, 1182
early child care/preschool experiences, 1247
hematologic aspects, 1173-1182
hematologic signs, 1170-1173
index pregnancy, 1246
antibiotic use/immunizations, 1246-1247
infection-associated HLH, 2116-2117
invasive fungal infection, evaluation, 2263
issues, 2257-2258
pathogens, 2258-2259
prophylaxis/treatment, 263-265
protozoal infections, 2259
risk factors, 2257-2258
viral infections, 1175-1181, 2258-2259
Infectious diseases, 1170-1182
Infectious mononucleosis, 1175-1179
acute lymphoblastic leukemia, relationship, 1538
atypical lymphocytes (Downey cells), 1178f
clinical manifestations, 1175-1176
complications, 1176-1178, 1176t
epidemiology, 1175
laboratory diagnosis, 1178-1179
laboratory features, 1177t
treatment, 1179
Infectious suppression, 68
Inflammasomes, 789
Inflammation, anemia (iron abnormalities), 370
Inflammatory cells, fascicles, 1968f
Inflammatory disease/transplantation (treatment), monoclonal antibodies/fusion proteins (impact), 877t
Inflammatory myofibroblastic tumor (IMT), 1371, 1963
composition, 1362f
spindled/plump myofibroblasts, 1963f
Inflammatory response
humoral mediators, 783-785
pathologic consequences, 799-800
Informatics, 1268
clustering/classification, 1268
sample size, 1268
validation, 1268

Informed consent, 2238
Informed Consent Team Link, prototype device, 2464f
Infratentorial tumors, 2159-2165
Infusion-related toxicities, 1151
Ingestion
cellular disorders, 828-829
disorders, 828-829
Inheritance
dyskeratosis congenita (DC), 209-210
Fanconi anemia, 194
preshortened telomeres, 218f
Inherited bleeding disorders, pregnancy (relationship), 1198
Inherited bone marrow failure syndromes (IBMFSs), 182
clinical studies, 45-47
isolated cytopenias, association, 229-251
pancytopenia, association, 187-229
types, 183t-186t
Inherited connective tissue disorders, 1170
Inherited disorders, SCN (association), 245t
Inherited hypercoagulable states, pregnancy (relationship), 1198-1199
Inherited platelet disorders
integrins, presence, 1015
platelet membrane/receptors, 999-1002
qualitative disorders, 999
Inherited thrombocytopenias, 247-250
syndromes, 248t-249t
Inherited thrombotic disorders, patient management, 1071-1074
Inhibitory antibodies, presence, 1036-1038
Inhomogenous fields, Bragg peaks (presence), 1481f
Initial antibiotic therapy, 2260-2261
Initially metastatic osteosarcoma, 2049-2050
Initial risk stratification, 2259
Innate immune system, recognition (activation), 1453
Innate immunity, acquired immunity (contrast), 852t
Inpatient setting, nursing care, 2313
In situ hybridization (ISH)
chromogenic in situ hybridization (CISH), 1355f
flexibility, substrate options, 1348
fluorescence-activated cell-sorting (FACS), usage, 1347-1351
resolution, 1348
Institutional Review Board approval, pediatric research/requirements categories, 2466t
Insulin-like growth factors
osteosarcoma, 2038-2039
receptor signaling, pediatric solid tumors (relationship), 1330-1331
role, 1900
Integral membrane proteins, 462-479
glycophorin A (GPA), 473
glycophorin C/D (GPC/GPD), interactions, 487-488
Integrins
activation, 960f
presence, 1015
Intensity-modulated proton therapy (IMPT), 1480-1481
Intensity-modulated radiation therapy (IMRT), 1802
Intensity-modulated radiotherapy (IMRT), 1478-1479
Intentional biomodulation, 1442

Intercalary resection, usage, 1518f
Intercellular adhesion molecules (ICAMs), 787f
Intercellular iron transport, 348-349
Intercytoplasmic bridging (malaria), 1211f
Interdisciplinary needs assessment, domains, 2476t
Interfant 99 trial, 1619f
Interferon alfa, usage, 1086
Interferons, 16, 1455
Interferon-stimulated response element (ISRE), 31
Intergroup Rhabdomyosarcoma Study, Surgical-Pathologic Grouping System, 1953t
Interleukin 1 (IL-1), 19-20
gene family, 16
impact, 19-20
Interleukin 2, 1456
Interleukin 2 receptor (IL-2R), usage, 8
Interleukin 3 (IL-3), 17-18
Interleukin 5 (IL-5), 16-17
Interleukin 6 (IL-6), 19-20
IL-6 gp130
complex ligands, 23
signal-transducing system, usage, 20
impact, 20
Interleukin 7 (IL-7), 1456-1457
Interleukin 11 (IL-11), 19-20
receptor complex, IL-6 gp130 signal-transducing system (usage), 20
Interleukin 13 (IL-13), separation, 23
Interleukin 14 (IL-14), separation, 23
Interleukin 15 (IL-15), 1457
Interleukins, 17-18
Interlocus IG/RCR gene rearrangements/translocations, 1383-1385
Intermediate metabolites, levels, 2498t
Intermediate tumors, soft tissue tumor World Health Organization classification, 1947t-1948t
Intermittent red cell transfusion (childhood), 1129b
International Bone Marrow Transplant Registry Severity Index (aGVHD), 268t
International Classification for Intraocular Retinoblastoma, 1758b, 1758f
International neuroblastoma pathology classification, 1691t
International neuroblastoma risk group pretreatment classification, 1697t
International neuroblastoma risk group staging system, 1696t
International neuroblastoma staging system, 1695t
International Neuroblastoma Staging System (childhood neuroblastoma), 2205t
International Retinoblastoma Staging System, 1759b
International Society of Paediatric Oncology (SIOP), 1499-1500
histologic risk classification schema, COG schema (comparison), 1718t
postchemotherapy histologic classification system, 1717-1718
studies, findings, 1732t
Intestinal Cajal cells, SCF dependence, 18
Intestinal lumen, acquired malabsorptive disorders, 331
Intestinal ulceration, 61
Intestine, bilirubin conjugates (presence), 107
Intraarterial chemotherapy, 2243f